BRAUNWALD'S

HEART DISEASE

A TEXTBOOK OF CARDIOVASCULAR MEDICINE

Edited by

Douglas P. Zipes, MD, MACC
Distinguished Professor of Medicine, Pharmacology, and Toxicology
Director, Division of Cardiology and the Krannert Institute of Cardiology
Indiana University School of Medicine
Indianapolis, Indiana

Peter Libby, MD
Mallinckrodt Professor of Medicine
Harvard Medical School
Chief, Cardiovascular Division
Brigham and Women's Hospital
Boston, Massachusetts

Robert O. Bonow, MD
Goldberg Distinguished Professor of Cardiology
Northwestern University Feinberg School of Medicine
Chief, Division of Cardiology
Northwestern Memorial Hospital
Chicago, Illinois

Eugene Braunwald, MD, MD (Hon), ScD (Hon), FRCP
Distinguished Hersey Professor of Medicine
Harvard Medical School
Chairman, TIMI Study Group
Brigham and Women's Hospital
Boston, Massachusetts

VOLUME 1

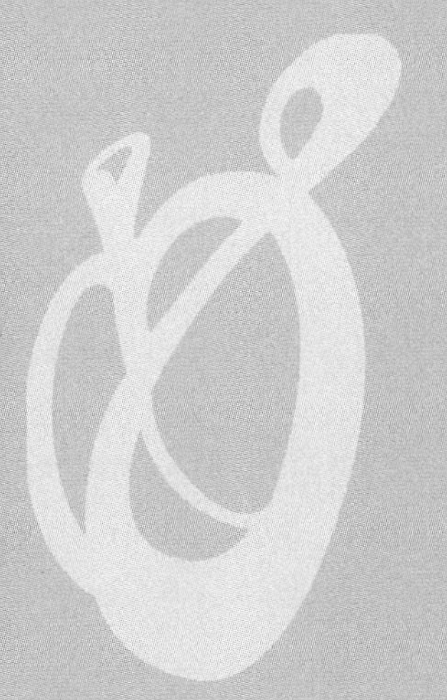

BRAUNWALD'S HEART DISEASE

A TEXTBOOK OF CARDIOVASCULAR MEDICINE

7th Edition

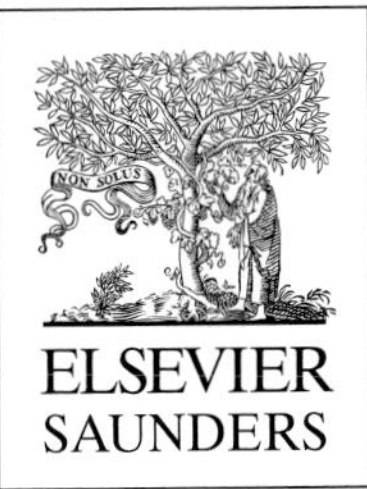

ELSEVIER
SAUNDERS

The Curtis Center
170 S Independence Mall W 300E
Philadelphia, Pennsylvania 19106

BRAUNWALD'S HEART DISEASE: A Textbook of Cardiovascular Medicine, Seventh Edition

Two-volume set	0-7216-0509-5
Single volume	0-7216-0479-X
Two-volume e-dition	1-4160-00038-0
Single volume e-dition	1-4160-00014-3
International edition	0-8089-2305-6
Indian edition	0-8089-2334-X

NOTICE

Medicine is an ever-changing field. Standard safety precautions must be followed, but as new research and clinical experience broaden our knowledge, changes in treatment and drug therapy may become necessary or appropriate. Readers are advised to check the most current product information provided by the manufacturer of each drug to be administered to verify the recommended dose, the method and duration of administration, and contraindications. It is the responsibility of the licensed prescriber, relying on experience and knowledge of the patient, to determine dosages and the best treatment for each individual patient. Neither the publisher nor the authors assume any liability for any injury and/or damage to persons or property arising from this publication.

Library of Congress Cataloging-in-Publication Data

Braunwald's heart disease : a textbook of cardiovascular medicine / [edited by] Douglas P. Zipes . . . [et al.].—7th ed.
p. ; cm.
Rev. ed. of: Heart disease / edited by Eugene Braunwald, Douglas P. Zipes, Peter Libby. 6th ed. 2001.
Includes bibliographical references and index.
ISBN 0-7216-0509-5 (2 vol. set)—ISBN 0-7216-0479-X (Single vol.)—ISBN 0-8089-2305-6 (International ed.)
1. Heart—Diseases. 2. Cardiology. I. Title: Heart disease. II. Zipes, Douglas P. III. Braunwald, Eugene—Heart disease.
[DNLM: 1. Heart Diseases. 2. Cardiovascular Diseases. WG 210 B825 2005]
RC681.H36 2005
616.1′2—dc22 2004050808

Publishing Director: Anne Lenehan
Managing Editor, Developmental Editorial: Deborah Thorp
Publishing Services Manager: Frank Polizzano
Senior Project Manager: Robin E. Davis
Design Manager: Steven Stave

Printed in the United States of America.

Last digit is the print number: 9 8 7 6 5 4 3 2 1

To:

Joan, Debra, Jeffrey, and David

Beryl, Oliver, and Brigitte

Pat, Rob, and Sam

Elaine, Karen, Allison, and Jill

CONTRIBUTORS

Stephan Achenbach, MD
Assistant Professor of Medicine and Cardiology, Friedrich-Alexander University School of Medicine; Staff Cardiologist, Division of Cardiology, Department of Medicine, University Hospital Erlangen, Erlangen, Germany
Computed Tomography of the Heart

David H. Adams, MD
Marie-Josée and Henry R. Kravis Professor and Chair, Department of Cardiothoracic Surgery, Mount Sinai Medical Center, New York, New York
Medical Management of the Patient Undergoing Cardiac Surgery

Elliott M. Antman, MD
Professor of Medicine, Harvard Medical School; Director, Samuel A. Levine Cardiac Unit, Brigham and Women's Hospital, Boston, Massachusetts
ST-Elevation Myocardial Infarction: Pathology, Pathophysiology, and Clinical Features; ST-Elevation Myocardial Infarction: Management; Medical Management of the Patient Undergoing Cardiac Surgery

Karen Antman, MD
Deputy Director for Translational and Clinical Sciences, National Cancer Institute, National Institutes of Health, Bethesda, Maryland
The Patient with Cardiovascular Disease and Cancer

Piero Anversa, MD
Professor, Department of Medicine, Cardiovascular Research Institute, New York Medical College, Valhalla, New York
Myocardial Regeneration

William F. Armstrong, MD
Professor of Medicine, University of Michigan; Associate Clinical Chief, Division of Cardiology, Associate Chair, Department of Internal Medicine, University of Michigan Health System, Ann Arbor, Michigan
Echocardiography

Donald S. Baim, MD
Professor of Medicine, Harvard Medical School; Director, Center for Integration of Medicine and Innovative Technology, Partners Healthcare System and Brigham and Women's Hospital, Boston, Massachusetts
Percutaneous Coronary and Valvular Intervention

Leora B. Balsam, MD
Resident in Surgery, Department of Surgery, Stanford University School of Medicine, Stanford, California
Heart Transplantation

Arthur J. Barsky, MD
Professor of Psychiatry, Harvard Medical School; Director, Psychiatric Research, Brigham and Women's Hospital, Boston, Massachusetts
Psychiatric and Behavioral Aspects of Cardiovascular Disease

Kenneth Lee Baughman, MD
Professor of Medicine, Harvard Medical School; Director, Advanced Heart Disease Section, Brigham and Women's Hospital, Boston, Massachusetts
Myocarditis

Joshua A. Beckman, MS, MD
Assistant Professor of Medicine, Harvard Medical School; Associate Physician, Cardiovascular Division, Brigham and Women's Hospital, Boston, Massachusetts
Diabetes Mellitus, the Metabolic Syndrome, and Atherosclerotic Vascular Disease

George A. Beller, MD
Ruth C. Heede Professor of Cardiology and Professor of Medicine, University of Virginia School of Medicine; Department of Internal Medicine, Cardiovascular Division, University of Virginia Health System, Charlottesville, Virginia
Relative Merits of Cardiac Diagnostic Techniques

Michael A. Bettman, MD
Professor of Radiology, Dartmouth Medical School, Hanover, New Hampshire
The Chest Radiograph in Cardiovascular Disease

Robert O. Bonow, MD
Goldberg Distinguished Professor of Cardiology, Northwestern University Feinberg School of Medicine; Chief, Division of Cardiology, Northwestern Memorial Hospital, Chicago, Illinois
Care of Patients with End-Stage Heart Disease; Nuclear Cardiology; Cardiac Catheterization; Valvular Heart Disease

Eugene Braunwald, MD, MD (Hon), ScD (Hon), FRCP
Distinguished Hersey Professor of Medicine, Harvard Medical School; Chairman, TIMI Study Group, Brigham and Women's Hospital, Boston, Massachusetts
The History; Physical Examination of the Heart and Circulation; Pathophysiology of Heart Failure; Clinical Aspects of Heart Failure; Pulmonary Edema, High-Output Failure; ST-Elevation Myocardial Infarction: Pathology, Pathophysiology, and Clinical Features; Unstable Angina and Non–ST Elevation Myocardial Infarction; Chronic Coronary Artery Disease; Valvular Heart Disease; The Cardiomyopathies

Michael R. Bristow, MD, PhD
Professor of Medicine and Head, Division of Cardiology, University of Colorado Health Sciences Center, Denver, Colorado
Drugs in the Treatment of Heart Failure; Management of Heart Failure

Hugh Calkins, MD, FACC, FAHA
Professor of Medicine, Johns Hopkins University School of Medicine; Director, Arrhythmia Service and Clinical Electrophysiology Laboratory, Johns Hopkins Hospital, Baltimore, Maryland
Hypotension and Syncope

Christopher P. Cannon, MD
Associate Professor of Medicine, Harvard Medical School; Senior Investigator, TIMI Study Group, Cardiovascular Division, Brigham and Women's Hospital, Boston, Massachusetts
Approach to the Patient with Chest Pain; Unstable Angina and Non–ST Elevation Myocardial Infarction

John D. Carroll, MD
Professor of Medicine, Division of Cardiology, University of Colorado Health Sciences Center; Director, Cardiac and Vascular Center and Director, Interventional Cardiology, University of Colorado Hospital, Denver, Colorado
Assessment of Normal and Abnormal Cardiac Function

Agustin Castellanos, MD
Professor of Medicine, University of Miami School of Medicine; Director, Clinical Electrophysiology, University of Miami/Jackson Memorial Medical Center, Miami, Florida
Cardiac Arrest and Sudden Cardiac Death

Bernard R. Chaitman, MD
Professor of Medicine and Director, Cardiovascular Research, St. Louis University School of Medicine, St. Louis, Missouri
Exercise Stress Testing

Jonathan M. Chen, MD
Assistant Professor of Surgery, Columbia University College of Physicians and Surgeons; Attending Surgeon, New York Presbyterian Hospital, New York, New York
Assisted Circulation in the Treatment of Heart Failure

Wilson S. Colucci, MD, FACC
Thomas J. Ryan Professor of Medicine; Professor of Physiology; Director, Myocardial Biology Unit, Boston University School of Medicine; Chief, Cardiovascular Medicine, Boston Medical Center, Boston, Massachusetts
Pathophysiology of Heart Failure; Clinical Aspects of Heart Failure; Pulmonary Edema, High-Output Failure; Primary Tumors of the Heart

Mark A. Creager, MD
Professor of Medicine, Harvard Medical School; Director, Vascular Center; Simon C. Fireman Scholar in Cardiovascular Medicine, Brigham and Women's Hospital, Boston, Massachusetts
Diabetes Mellitus, the Metabolic Syndrome, and Atherosclerotic Vascular Disease; Peripheral Arterial Diseases

Adnan S. Dajani, MD
Professor Emeritus of Pediatrics, Wayne State University School of Medicine; Director Emeritus, Division of Infectious Diseases, Children's Hospital of Michigan, Detroit, Michigan
Rheumatic Fever

Werner G. Daniel, MD
Professor of Medicine and Cardiology, Friedrich-Alexander School of Medicine; Division of Cardiology, Department of Medicine, University Hospital Erlangen, Erlangen, Germany
Computed Tomography of the Heart

Charles J. Davidson, MD
Professor of Medicine, Northwestern University Feinberg School of Medicine; Chief, Cardiac Catheterization Laboratories, Northwestern Memorial Hospital, Chicago, Illinois
Cardiac Catheterization

Vasken Dilsizian, MD
Professor of Medicine and Radiology, University of Maryland School of Medicine; Director of Cardiovascular Nuclear Medicine and Cardiac Positron Emission Tomography, University of Maryland Medical Center, Baltimore, Maryland
Nuclear Cardiology

Pamela S. Douglas, MD
Ursula Geller Professor of Medicine, Chief, Cardiovascular Medicine, Duke University Medical Center, Durham, North Carolina
Cardiovascular Disease in Women

Kim A. Eagle, MD
Albion Walter Hewlett Professor of Internal Medicine; Chief, Clinical Cardiology; Clinical Director, Cardiovascular Center, University of Michigan Health System, Ann Arbor, Michigan
Anesthesia and Noncardiac Surgery in Patients with Heart Disease

Andrew C. Eisenhauer, MD
Assistant Professor of Medicine and Radiology, Harvard Medical School; Director, Interventional Cardiovascular Medicine Service, Brigham and Women's Hospital, Boston, Massachusetts
Endovascular Treatment of Noncoronary Obstructive Vascular Disease

Uri Elkayam, MD
Professor of Medicine, University of Southern California Keck School of Medicine, Los Angeles, California
Pregnancy and Cardiovascular Disease

Linda L. Emanuel, MD, PhD
Buehler Professor of Geriatric Medicine and Director, Buehler Center of Aging, Northwestern University Feinberg School of Medicine, Chicago, Illinois
Care of Patients with End-Stage Heart Disease

Anthony L. Estrera, MD
Assistant Professor of Cardiothoracic and Vascular Surgery, University of Texas Health Science Center, Houston, Texas
Traumatic Heart Disease

Farzan Filsoufi, MD
Assistant Professor of Cardiothoracic Surgery, Mount Sinai School of Medicine, New York, New York
Medical Management of the Patient Undergoing Cardiac Surgery

Stacy D. Fisher, MD
Department of Cardiology, Sinai Hospital of Baltimore, Johns Hopkins University; Mid-Atlantic Cardiovascular Associates, Baltimore, Maryland
Cardiovascular Abnormalities in HIV-Infected Individuals

Lee A. Fleisher, MD, FACC
Professor of Anesthesia and Medicine, University of Pennsylvania School of Medicine; Chair, Department of Anesthesia, University of Pennsylvania Health System, Philadelphia, Pennsylvania
Anesthesia and Noncardiac Surgery in Patients with Heart Disease

J. Michael Gaziano, MD, MPH
Associate Professor of Medicine, Harvard Medical School; Chief, Division of Aging, Brigham and Women's Hospital; Director, Massachusetts Veterans Epidemiology and Research Information Center (MAVERIC), Boston VA Healthcare Systems, Boston, Massachusetts
Global Burden of Cardiovascular Disease; Primary and Secondary Prevention of Coronary Heart Disease

Jacques Genest, MD
Professor of Medicine, McGill University; Chief, Cardiology, McGill University Medical Center, Montréal, Québec, Canada
Lipoprotein Disorders and Cardiovascular Disease

Bernard J. Gersh, MD, DPhil, FRCP
Professor of Medicine, Mayo College of Medicine; Consultant, Division of Cardiovascular Diseases, Mayo Clinic, Rochester, Minnesota
Chronic Coronary Artery Disease

Michael M. Givertz, MD
Assistant Professor of Medicine, Harvard Medical School; Co-Director, Cardiomyopathy and Heart Failure Program, Brigham and Women's Hospital, Boston, Massachusetts
Clinical Aspects of Heart Failure; Pulmonary Edema, High-Output Failure

Ary L. Goldberger, MD
Associate Professor of Medicine, Harvard Medical School; Director, Margret and H. A. Rey Laboratory for Nonlinear Dynamics in Physiology and Medicine, Beth Israel Deaconess Medical Center, Boston, Massachusetts
Electrocardiography

Samuel Z. Goldhaber, MD
Associate Professor of Medicine, Harvard Medical School; Staff Cardiologist and Director, Venous Thromboembolism Research Group; Director, Anticoagulation Service, Brigham and Women's Hospital, Boston, Massachusetts
Pulmonary Embolism

Antonio M. Gotto, Jr., MD, DPhil
Stephen and Suzanne Weiss Dean, Provost for Medical Affairs, Professor of Medicine, Weill Medical College of Cornell University, New York, New York
Lipoprotein Disorders and Cardiovascular Disease

William J. Groh, MD, MPH
Associate Professor of Medicine, Indiana University School of Medicine, Indianapolis, Indiana
Neurological Disorders and Cardiovascular Disease

David L. Hayes, MD
Professor of Medicine, Mayo Medical School, Mayo Clinic College of Medicine; Chair, Division of Cardiovascular Diseases and Internal Medicine, Mayo Clinic, Rochester, Minnesota
Cardiac Pacemakers and Cardioverter-Defibrillators

Otto M. Hess, MD
Professor of Cardiology, Swiss Cardiovascular Center, University Hospital, Bern, Switzerland
Assessment of Normal and Abnormal Cardiac Function

L. David Hillis, MD
Professor and Vice Chair, Department of Medicine; James M. Wooten Chair in Cardiology, University of Texas Southwestern Medical Center, Dallas, Texas
Toxins and the Heart

Mark A. Hlatky, MD
Professor of Health Research and Policy and Professor of Cardiovascular Medicine, Stanford University School of Medicine; Attending Physician, Stanford University Medical Center, Stanford, California
Economics and Cardiovascular Disease

Gary S. Hoffman, MS, MD
Professor of Medicine, Cleveland Clinic Lerner College of Medicine of Case Western Reserve University; Professor of Medicine and Harold C. Schott Chair of Rheumatic and Immunologic Diseases; Director, Center for Vasculitis Care and Research, Cleveland Clinic, Cleveland, Ohio
Rheumatic Diseases and the Cardiovascular System

David R. Holmes, Jr., MD
Professor of Medicine, Mayo Clinic College of Medicine; Consultant, Mayo Clinic Saint Marys Hospital, Rochester, Minnesota
Primary Percutaneous Coronary Intervention in the Management of Acute Myocardial Infarction

Sharon A. Hunt, MD
Professor of Cardiovascular Medicine, Stanford University Medical Center, Stanford, California
Heart Transplantation

Eric M. Isselbacher, MD
Assistant Professor of Medicine, Harvard Medical School; Co-Director, Thoracic Aortic Center, Director, Cardiac Unit Associates, Massachusetts General Hospital, Boston, Massachusetts
Diseases of the Aorta

Samer Kabbani, MD
Assistant Professor of Medicine, University of Vermont College of Medicine; Attending Cardiologist, Fletcher Allen Health Care, Burlington, Vermont
Pericardial Diseases

Norman M. Kaplan, MD
Clinical Professor of Internal Medicine, University of Texas Southwestern Medical Center, Dallas, Texas
Systemic Hypertension: Mechanisms and Diagnosis; Systemic Hypertension: Therapy

Adolf W. Karchmer, MD
Professor of Medicine, Harvard Medical School; Chief, Division of Infectious Diseases, Beth Israel Deaconess Medical Center, Boston, Massachusetts
Infective Endocarditis

Morton J. Kern, MD
Professor of Medicine, Saint Louis University School of Medicine; Director, Cardiac Catheterization Laboratory, Saint Louis University Hospital, St. Louis, Missouri
Coronary Blood Flow and Myocardial Ischemia

Irwin Klein, MD
Professor of Medicine, New York University School of Medicine, New York, New York; Chief, Division of Endocrinology, North Shore University Hospital, Mannasset, New York
Endocrine Disorders and Cardiovascular Disease

Barbara A. Konkle, MD
Associate Professor of Medicine and of Pathology and Laboratory Medicine; Director, Penn Comprehensive Hemophilia and Thrombosis Program, University of Pennsylvania School of Medicine and Health System, Philadelphia, Pennsylvania
Hemostasis, Thrombosis, Fibrinolysis, and Cardiovascular Disease

Peter C. Kouretas, MD, PhD
Cardiothoracic Transplantation Fellow, Department of Cardiothoracic Surgery, Stanford University School of Medicine; Staff Physician and Clinical Instructor, Stanford University Hospital, Stanford, California
Heart Transplantation

Ronald M. Krauss, MD
Adjunct Professor, Department of Nutritional Sciences, University of California, Berkeley, Berkeley, California; Senior Scientist and Director, Atherosclerosis Research, Children's Hospital Oakland Research Institute, Oakland, California
Nutrition and Cardiovascular Disease

Meir H. Kryger, MD, FRCPC
Professor of Medicine, University of Manitoba Department of Medicine; Director, Sleep Disorders Centre, St. Boniface Hospital Research Centre, Winnipeg, Manitoba, Canada
Sleep Disorders and Cardiovascular Disease

Richard E. Kuntz, MD
Associate Professor of Medicine and Chief, Division of Clinical Biometrics, Harvard Medical School, Boston, Massachusetts
Percutaneous Coronary and Valvular Intervention

Gary E. Lane, MD
Assistant Professor, Mayo Medical School; Director, Cardiac Catheterization Laboratory, Mayo Clinic St. Luke's Hospital, Jacksonville, Florida
Primary Percutaneous Coronary Intervention in the Management of Acute Myocardial Infarction

Richard A. Lange, MD
Professor of Medicine and E. Cowles Andrus Professor of Cardiology, Johns Hopkins University School of Medicine, Baltimore, Maryland
Toxins and the Heart

Thomas H. Lee, MSc, MD
Professor of Medicine, Harvard Medical School; Network President, Partners Healthcare System, Boston, Massachusetts
Measurement and Improvement of Quality of Cardiovascular Care; Guidelines: Electrocardiography; Guidelines: Exercise Stress Testing; Guidelines: Use of Echocardiography; Guidelines: Nuclear Cardiology; Guidelines: Management of Heart Failure; Guidelines: Ambulatory Electrocardiography and Electrophysiological Testing; Guidelines: Cardiac Pacemakers and Cardioverter-Defibrillators; Guidelines: Treatment of Hypertension; Approach to the Patient with Chest Pain; Guidelines: Primary Percutaneous Coronary Intervention in Acute Myocardial Infarction; Guidelines: Unstable Angina; Guidelines: Chronic Stable Angina; Guidelines: Percutaneous Coronary and Valvular Intervention; Guidelines: Management of Valvular Heart Disease; Guidelines: Infective Endocarditis; Guidelines: Pregnancy; Guidelines: Reducing Cardiac Risk with Noncardiac Surgery

Annarosa Leri, MD
Associate Professor, Department of Medicine, Cardiovascular Research Institute, New York Medical College, Valhalla, New York
Myocardial Regeneration

Martin M. LeWinter, MD
Professor of Medicine and of Molecular Physiology and Biophysics, University of Vermont College of Medicine; Director, Heart Failure Program, Fletcher Allen Health Care, Burlington, Vermont
Pericardial Diseases

Peter Libby, MD
Mallinckrodt Professor of Medicine, Harvard Medical School; Chief, Cardiovascular Division, Brigham and Women's Hospital, Boston, Massachusetts
The Vascular Biology of Atherosclerosis; Risk Factors for Atherothrombotic Disease; Lipoprotein Disorders and Cardiovascular Disease; Diabetes Mellitus, the Metabolic Syndrome, and Atherosclerotic Vascular Disease; Peripheral Arterial Diseases

Stuart Linas, MD
Professor of Medicine, University of Colorado Health Sciences Center; Chief, Nephrology, Denver Health, Denver, Colorado
Drugs in the Treatment of Heart Failure

Steven E. Lipshultz, MD
Professor and Chair, Department of Pediatrics; Professor of Medicine and of Epidemiology and Public Health, University of Miami School of Medicine; Chief of Staff, Holtz Children's Hospital of the University of Miami–Jackson Memorial Medical Center, Miami, Florida
Cardiovascular Abnormalities in HIV-Infected Individuals

Brian D. Lowes, MD
Associate Professor of Medicine, University of Colorado Health Sciences Center; Director, Heart Failure Program, University Hospital, Denver, Colorado
Management of Heart Failure

Brian F. Mandell, MD, PhD
Professor of Medicine, Cleveland Clinic Lerner College of Medicine of Case Western Reserve University; Vice Chair of Medicine for Education, Cleveland Clinic, Cleveland, Ohio
Rheumatic Diseases and the Cardiovascular System

JoAnn E. Manson, MD, DrPH
Professor of Medicine and Elizabeth F. Brigham Professor of Women's Health, Harvard Medical School; Chief, Division of Preventive Medicine, Co-Director, Connors Center for Women's Health and Gender Biology, Brigham and Women's Hospital, Boston, Massachusetts
Primary and Secondary Prevention of Coronary Heart Disease

Daniel B. Mark, MD, MPH
Professor of Medicine, Duke University Medical Center; Director, Outcomes Research, Duke Clinical Research Institute, Durham, North Carolina
Economics and Cardiovascular Disease

Andrew R. Marks, MD
Professor and Chair, Department of Physiology and Cellular Biophysics; Professor of Medicine; Clyde and Helen Wu Professor of Molecular Cardiology, Columbia University College of Physicians and Surgeons
The Patient with Cardiovascular Disease and Cancer

Barry J. Maron, MD
Director, Hypertrophic Cardiomyopathy Center, Minneapolis Heart Institute Foundation, Minneapolis, Minnesota; Adjunct Professor of Medicine, Tufts University School of Medicine, Boston, Massachusetts
Cardiovascular Disease in Athletes

Kenneth L. Mattox, MD
Professor and Vice Chair, Michael E. DeBakey Department of Surgery, Baylor College of Medicine; Chief of Surgery Service and Chief of Staff, Ben Taub General Hospital, Houston, Texas
Traumatic Heart Disease

Peter A. McCullough, MD, MPH
Consultant Cardiologist and Chief, Division of Nutrition and Preventive Medicine, William Beaumont Hospital, Royal Oak, Michigan
Interface Between Renal Disease and Cardiovascular Illness

Vallerie V. McLaughlin, MD
Associate Professor of Medicine and Director, Pulmonary Hypertension Program, University of Michigan Health System, Ann Arbor, Michigan
Pulmonary Hypertension

John M. Miller, MD
Professor of Medicine, Indiana University School of Medicine; Director, Clinical Cardiac Electrophysiology, Clarian Health System, Indianapolis, Indiana
Diagnosis of Cardiac Arrhythmias; Therapy for Cardiac Arrhythmias

David M. Mirvis, MD
Professor and Director, Center for Health Services Research, University of Tennessee, Memphis, Tennessee
Electrocardiography

David A. Morrow, MD, MPH
Assistant Professor of Medicine, Harvard Medical School; Associate Physician, Brigham and Women's Hospital, Boston, Massachusetts
Chronic Coronary Artery Disease

Robert J. Myerburg, MD
Professor of Medicine and Physiology, University of Miami School of Medicine; Director, Division of Cardiology, University of Miami–Jackson Memorial Hospital, Miami, Florida
Cardiac Arrest and Sudden Cardiac Death

Elizabeth G. Nabel, MD
Scientific Director, National Heart, Lung, and Blood Institute, National Institutes of Health, Bethesda, Maryland
Principles of Cardiovascular Molecular Biology and Genetics

Yoshifumi Naka, MD, PhD
Herbert Irving Assistant Professor of Surgery, Division of Cardiothoracic Surgery, Columbia University College of Physicians and Surgeons; Adjunct Assistant Professor of Cardiothoracic Surgery, Cornell University Weill Medical College; Director, Cardiac Transplantation and Mechanical Circulatory Support Program, Division of Cardiothoracic Surgery, New York Presbyterian Hospital, New York, New York
Assisted Circulation in the Treatment of Heart Failure

Carlo Napolitano, MD, PhD
Senior Scientist, Molecular Cardiology Laboratories, IRCCS Fondazione S. Maugeri, Pavia, Italy
Genetics of Cardiac Arrhythmias

Richard W. Nesto, MD
Associate Professor of Medicine, Harvard Medical School, Boston; Chair, Department of Cardiovascular Medicine, Lahey Clinic Medical Center, Burlington, Massachusetts
Diabetes and Heart Disease

Jeffrey E. Olgin, MD
Associate Professor in Residence and Chief, Cardiac Electrophysiology, University of California, San Francisco, School of Medicine, San Francisco, California
Specific Arrhythmias: Diagnosis and Treatment

Lionel H. Opie, MD, DPhil, DSc, MD (Hon)
Director, Hatter Institute and Cape Heart Center, Faculty of Health Sciences, University of Cape Town; Senior Physician, Department of Medicine, Groote Schuur Hospital, Cape Town, South Africa
Mechanisms of Cardiac Contraction and Relaxation

Richard C. Pasternak, MD
Associate Professor of Medicine, Harvard Medical School; Director, Preventive Cardiology and Cardiac Rehabilitation, Massachusetts General Hospital, Boston, Massachusetts
Comprehensive Rehabilitation of Patients with Cardiovascular Disease

Dudley Pennell, MD, FRCP, FACC, FESC
Professor of Cardiology, Imperial College; Director, Cardiovascular Magnetic Resonance Unit, Royal Brompton Hospital, London, United Kingdom
Cardiovascular Magnetic Resonance

Joseph K. Perloff, MD
Streisand/American Heart Association Professor of Medicine and Pediatrics, Emeritus, Founding Director, Ahmanson/UCLA Adult Congenital Heart Disease Center, David Geffen School of Medicine at UCLA; Los Angeles, California
Physical Examination of the Heart and Circulation

Jeffrey J. Popma, MD
Associate Professor of Medicine, Harvard Medical School; Director, Interventional Cardiology, Brigham and Women's Hospital, Boston, Massachusetts
Coronary Angiography and Intravascular Ultrasound Imaging; Percutaneous Coronary and Valvular Intervention

J. David Port, PhD
Associate Professor of Medicine and Pharmacology, University of Colorado Health Sciences Center, Denver, Colorado
Drugs in the Treatment of Heart Failure

Silvia G. Priori, MD, PhD
Associate Professor, University of Pavia School of Cardiology; Director of Molecular Cardiology, IRCCS Fondazione S. Maugeri, Pavia, Italy
Genetics of Cardiac Arrhythmias

Reed E. Pyeritz, MD, PhD
Professor of Medicine and Genetics, Chief, Division of Medical Genetics, University of Pennsylvania School of Medicine, Philadelphia, Pennsylvania
Genetics and Cardiovascular Disease

Andrew N. Redington, MD, MBBS, MRCP(UK), FRCP(UK), FRCPC
University of Toronto; Head, Division of Cardiology, Hospital for Sick Children, Toronto, Ontario, Canada
Congenital Heart Disease

Stuart Rich, MD
Professor of Medicine and Director, Center for Pulmonary Heart Disease, Rush Medical College, Chicago, Illinois
Pulmonary Hypertension

Paul M. Ridker, MD, MPH
Eugene Braunwald Professor of Medicine, Harvard Medical School; Director, Center for Cardiovascular Disease Prevention, Brigham and Women's Hospital, Boston, Massachusetts
Risk Factors for Atherothrombotic Disease; Primary and Secondary Prevention of Coronary Heart Disease

Robert C. Robbins, MD
Associate Professor, Department of Cardiothoracic Surgery, Stanford University School of Medicine and Stanford Hospital, Stanford, California
Heart Transplantation

David Robertson, MD
Elton Yates Professor of Medicine, Pharmacology, and Neurology; Director, General Clinical Research Center, Vanderbilt University School of Medicine, Nashville, Tennessee
Cardiovascular Manifestations of Autonomic Disorders

Rose Marie Robertson, MD
Professor of Medicine, Vanderbilt University School of Medicine; Chief Science Officer, American Heart Association, Nashville, Tennessee
Cardiovascular Manifestations of Autonomic Disorders

Dan M. Roden, MD
Professor of Medicine and Pharmacology and Director, Division of Clinical Pharmacology, Vanderbilt University School of Medicine, Nashville, Tennessee
The Principles of Drug Therapy

Eric A. Rose, MD
Morris and Rose Milstein/Johnson & Johnson Professor and Chair, Department of Surgery; Surgeon-in-Chief, Columbia University College of Physicians and Surgeons; Director, Surgical Service, New York Presbyterian Hospital, New York, New York
Assisted Circulation in the Treatment of Heart Failure

Kenneth Rosenfield, MD
Lecturer on Medicine, Harvard Medical School; Director, Cardiac and Vascular Invasive Services, Massachusetts General Hospital, Boston, Massachusetts
Endovascular Treatment of Noncoronary Obstructive Vascular Disease

Michael Rubart, MD
Assistant Scientist, Indiana University School of Medicine, Indianapolis, Indiana
Genesis of Cardiac Arrhythmias: Electrophysiological Considerations

Marc S. Sabatine, MD, MPH
Instructor in Medicine, Harvard Medical School; Associate Physician, Cardiovascular Division, Brigham and Women's Hospital, Boston, Massachusetts
Primary Tumors of the Heart

Andrew I. Schafer, MD
Frank Wister Thomas Professor and Chair, Department of Medicine, University of Pennsylvania School of Medicine and Health System, Philadelphia, Pennsylvania
Hemostasis, Thrombosis, Fibrinolysis, and Cardiovascular Disease

Frederick J. Schoen, MD, PhD
Professor of Pathology and Health Sciences and Technology, Harvard Medical School; Executive Vice Chair, Department of Pathology, Brigham and Women's Hospital, Boston Massachusetts
Primary Tumors of the Heart

J. Sanford Schwartz, MD
Professor of Medicine and Health Management and Economics, University of Pennsylvania School of Medicine and The Wharton School, Philadelphia, Pennsylvania
Clinical Decision-Making in Cardiology

Janice B. Schwartz, MD
Clinical Professor of Medicine, Divisions of Cardiology and Clinical Pharmacology, University of California, San Francisco, School of Medicine; Director, Research, Jewish Home of San Francisco, San Francisco, California
Cardiovascular Disease in the Elderly

Peter J. Schwartz, MD
Professor of Cardiology, University of Pavia, Pavia, Italy
Genetics of Cardiac Arrhythmias

Jeffrey F. Smallhorn, MBBS, FRACP, FRCPC
University of Toronto; Hospital for Sick Children, Toronto, Ontario, Canada
Congenital Heart Disease

Nancy K. Sweitzer, MD, PhD
Assistant Professor of Medicine, University of Wisconsin Medical School; Director, Heart Failure Program, University of Wisconsin Hospital and Clinics, Madison, Wisconsin
Cardiovascular Disease in Women

Judith Therrien, MD, FRCPC
McGill University, Department of Medicine; Sir Mortimer B. Davis Jewish General Hospital, Montréal, Québec, Canada
Congenital Heart Disease

James E. Udelson, MD
Associate Professor of Medicine and Radiology, Tufts University School of Medicine; Associate Chief, Division of Cardiology; Director, Nuclear Cardiology; Co-Director, Heart Failure Center, Tufts–New England Medical Center, Boston, Massachusetts
Nuclear Cardiology

Matthew J. Wall, Jr., MD
Professor, Michael E. DeBakey Department of Surgery, Baylor College of Medicine; Deputy Chief of Surgery, Chief of Cardiothoracic Surgery, Ben Taub General Hospital, Houston, Texas
Traumatic Heart Disease

Gary D. Webb, MD, FRCPC
Bitove Family Professor of Adult Congenital Heart Disease and Professor of Medicine, University of Toronto; Director, Toronto Congenital Cardiac Centre for Adults, Toronto General Hospital, Toronto, Ontario, Canada
Congenital Heart Disease

Joshua Wynne, MD, MBA, MPH
Professor of Medicine, Wayne State University; Attending Physician, Detroit Medical Center, Detroit, Michigan
The Cardiomyopathies; Myocarditis

Clyde W. Yancy, MD
Professor of Medicine (Cardiology) and Medical Director, Heart Failure and Heart Transplantation, University of Texas Southwestern Medical Center; Associate Dean of Clinical Affairs, St. Paul University Hospital, Dallas, Texas
Heart Disease in Varied Populations

Douglas P. Zipes, MD, MACC
Distinguished Professor of Medicine, Pharmacology, and Toxicology, Director, Division of Cardiology and the Krannert Institute of Cardiology, Indiana University School of Medicine, Indianapolis, Indiana
Genesis of Cardiac Arrhythmias: Electrophysiological Considerations; Diagnosis of Cardiac Arrhythmias; Therapy for Cardiac Arrhythmias; Cardiac Pacemakers and Cardioverter-Defibrillators; Specific Arrhythmias: Diagnosis and Treatment; Hypotension and Syncope; Cardiovascular Disease in the Elderly; Neurological Disorders and Cardiovascular Disease

PREFACE

The preface to the previous (sixth) edition of *Heart Disease* began, "The accelerating advances in cardiology since the publication of the fifth edition of *Heart Disease* have required the most extensive changes yet made in any revision." That statement applies with even greater emphasis to this edition. The exponential growth curve of new knowledge has never been steeper, and the seventh edition of *Braunwald's Heart Disease* has been created to meet that challenge.

The appearance of the book has been changed radically: the cover shows a holographic MRI of a heart, alternating between systole and diastole, and the pages within are in full color, both to enhance reader appeal and to make figures and images more realistic and understandable. We now have an e-dition that provides electronic access to the entire book and enables the reader to download any figures or tables to his or her own computer and to use them in a PowerPoint format for lectures. The book contains 569 tables and 1503 figures, and the accompanying CD contains additional images and video clips. Finding a particular fact can be done with a flip of a finger in the e-dition, as a reader can electronically scan pages, facts, figures, and references. We recognize that books published on a four-year cycle cannot hope to keep current with the incredible pace of new observations. Therefore, by scanning and summarizing the important articles in the literature, and posting those commentaries on the e-dition site, we will update the e-dition *weekly*. Updates will be keyed to related book content. Finally, having recognized the important issues of professionalism and ethics, for the first time we have included an index listing of potential conflict of interest associations for all contributors.

The contents of this edition have also been comprehensively upgraded. As expected, all of the 51 chapters in the sixth edition that have been retained for the current edition have been thoroughly revised and updated. In addition, 36 new chapters have been included, whose topics range from clinical decision-making to cardiovascular manifestations of autonomic disorders. Fifty-seven new authors have made contributions. Thus, the state-of-the-art information serving as the foundation of the text's intellectual vitality has been retained and strengthened in this edition. Bibliographic citations have been generally limited to sources published in 1998 or later, to avoid the accretion of references that can consume valuable pages without offering the utility of fresh content. Earlier references can be obtained from the reviews cited and from previous editions. We continue to present an understanding of basic mechanisms underlying disease states, but we also emphasize the practical evaluation and treatment of patients with these problems, as well as provide a compendium of current guidelines for the reader's convenience.

Part I includes the general considerations of cardiovascular disease, with chapters on the global burden, economics, *clinical decision making,* assessment of quality of cardiac care, principles of drug therapy*, and *care of patients with end-stage heart disease*.

Part II continues the tradition of the previous edition, emphasizing history and physical examination, electrocardiography, exercise stress testing, and echocardiography. However, recognizing the increasing importance of new imaging techniques, we include new chapters on *radiology of the heart and great vessels, nuclear cardiology, magnetic resonance imaging, computed tomography*, cardiac catheterization, and coronary angiography and intravascular ultrasonography, as well as a chapter that places the various imaging modalities into perspective.

Heart failure has emerged as one of the most important problems in cardiology, as is reflected in **Part III**. It comprises a chapter on understanding mechanisms of cardiac contraction, *assessment of cardiac function*, pathophysiology of heart failure and its clinical aspects, two chapters on pharmacological treatment, and chapters on *assisted circulation* and *transplantation*.

Almost a quarter of all deaths in the U.S. are due to sudden death, most commonly from a rhythm disturbance, and **Part IV** deals with that issue, beginning with the genesis of arrhythmias. We have a new chapter addressing the growing importance of *genetics and arrhythmias*, and then continue with diagnosis, treatment, pacemakers and defibrillators, specific arrhythmias, cardiac arrest, and syncope.

Preventive cardiology is a mainstay of the cardiologist's role, and we devote multiple chapters to this important initiative in **Part V**, including the biology of atherogenesis, risk factors, hypertension (two chapters), lipoprotein disorders, *diabetes, nutrition*, prevention of coronary heart disease, and *rehabilitation*. In view of the growing importance of diabetes in the practice of cardiology, the current edition now includes a new chapter devoted to the vascular complications of this common condition.

Part VI includes the section on coronary disease, which accounts for the vast majority of heart disease in developed countries. The chapters include *understanding coronary blood flow and ischemia, approach to the patient with chest pain*, pathophysiology, clinical features, and management of ST-segment elevation myocardial infarction (MI), *percutaneous coronary intervention in MI*, unstable angina and non–ST-elevation MI, *chronic coronary artery disease, diabetes and heart disease*, percutaneous coronary and valvular intervention, aortic diseases, peripheral vascular diseases, and *endovascular treatment of noncoronary obstructive vascular disease*.

The rest of the book addresses somewhat less common, but still very important, problems. **Part VII** includes chapters on *congenital heart disease*, valvular heart disease, infective endocarditis, cardiomyopathies, *myocarditis*, HIV and the heart, *toxins*, primary cardiac tumors, *pericardial diseases*, traumatic heart disease, pulmonary embolism and pulmonary hypertension, and *sleep disorders*. **Part VIII** focuses on aspects of molecular biology and genetics. The chapters include *general principles of molecular biology needed by physicians*, genetics, and *myocardial regeneration*.

Part IX focuses on special populations of patients with cardiovascular disease, including *elderly patients, women*, pregnant patients, athletes, patients undergoing cardiac and *noncardiac surgery*, and patients belonging to *varied populations*. **Part X** fills remaining gaps by including cardiovascular disease and disorders of other organs, such as *endocrine disorders*, hematologic issues, rheumatic fever and rheumatic diseases, *oncologic disorders*, behavioral issues, neurological disorders, *renal disorders*, and *autonomic dysfunction*.

Companion volumes continue to supplement the information in *Braunwald's Heart Disease*, and they now include

*New chapters indicated in italics.

Heart Disease Review and Assessment, sixth edition (Lilly), Cardiovascular Therapeutics, second edition (Antman), Molecular Basis of Cardiovascular Disease, second edition (Chien), Clinical Trials in Heart Disease, second edition (Manson), Heart Failure (Mann), Marcus' Cardiac Imaging, second edition (Skorton), Acute Coronary Syndromes (Theroux), and Clinical Cardiovascular Imaging (St. John Sutton and Rutherford). Companion volumes in other areas of cardiology are planned for the near future. The seventh edition of *Braunwald's Heart Disease* continues to serve as the anchor for this collection of books, all of which help the busy scientist and clinician keep up with contemporary issues in cardiovascular diseases.

As always, the goal of this textbook is to educate, stimulate, and serve as a resource for all professionals caring for patients with cardiovascular disease. We are certain that the e-dition will add significant value to accomplishing that end. We could not have accomplished this goal without the help of our editorial associates, Janet Hutcheson, Karen Williams, Cynthia Escobedo, and Kathryn Saxon. The staff at Elsevier has been extremely supportive, and has tolerated our frequent requests for changes to make the book even better. To our editor, Anne Lenehan, developmental editor, Deborah Thorp, and project manager, Robin Davis, we give our thanks.

On the cover is a holographic magnetic resonance image of a cross section of the heart of Dr. Saptarsi Haldar in end-systole and end-diastole courtesy of Dr. Raymond Kwong, both of Brigham and Women's Hospital, reproduced with both of their permissions.

Finally, we thank you, the reader, from medical student to skilled clinician, for showing support for this textbook over the years. You, and our patients, are the driving forces to make this the kind of effort that contributes meaningfully to the education of cardiovascular specialists.

Douglas P. Zipes

Peter Libby

Robert O. Bonow

Eugene Braunwald

2004

PREFACE *Adapted from the First Edition*

Cardiovascular disease is the greatest scourge affecting the industrialized nations. As with previous scourges—bubonic plague, yellow fever, and smallpox—cardiovascular disease not only strikes down a significant fraction of the population without warning but also causes prolonged suffering and disability in an even larger number. In the United States alone, despite recent encouraging declines, cardiovascular disease is still responsible for almost 1 million fatalities each year and more than half of all deaths; almost 5 million persons afflicted with cardiovascular disease are hospitalized each year. The cost of these diseases in terms of human suffering and of material resources is almost incalculable. Fortunately, research focusing on the causes, diagnosis, treatment, and prevention of heart disease is moving ahead rapidly.

In order to provide a comprehensive, authoritative text in a field that has become as broad and deep as cardiovascular medicine, I chose to enlist the aid of a number of able colleagues. However, I hoped that my personal involvement in the writing of about half of the book would make it possible to minimize the fragmentation, gaps, inconsistencies, organizational difficulties, and impersonal tone that sometimes plague multiauthored texts.

Since the early part of the 20th century, clinical cardiology has had a particularly strong foundation in the basic sciences of physiology and pharmacology. More recently, the disciplines of molecular biology, genetics, developmental biology, biophysics, biochemistry, experimental pathology, and bioengineering have also begun to provide critically important information about cardiac function and malfunction. Although *Heart Disease: A Textbook of Cardiovascular Medicine* is primarily a clinical treatise and not a textbook of fundamental cardiovascular science, an effort has been made to explain, in some detail, the scientific bases of cardiovascular diseases.

Eugene Braunwald, 1980

CONTENTS

PART III ▪ Heart Failure 457

PART IV ▪ Arrhythmias, Sudden Death, and Syncope 653

PART V ▪ Preventive Cardiology 921

Look for these other titles in the Braunwald's HEART DISEASE family!

Antman: *Cardiovascular Therapeutics, 2nd Edition: A Companion to Braunwald's Heart Disease*

Chien: *Molecular Basis of Cardiovascular Disease, 2nd Edition: A Companion to Braunwald's Heart Disease*

Lilly: *Heart Disease Review and Assessment to Accompany Heart Disease, Sixth Edition*

Mann: *Heart Failure: A Companion to Braunwald's Heart Disease*

Manson, Buring, Ridker and Gaziano: *Clinical Trials in Heart Disease, 2nd Edition: A Companion to Braunwald's Heart Disease*

St. John Sutton and Rutherford: *Clinical Cardiovascular Imaging: A Companion to Braunwald's Heart Disease*

Theroux: *Acute Coronary Syndromes: A Companion to Braunwald's Heart Disease*

PART I 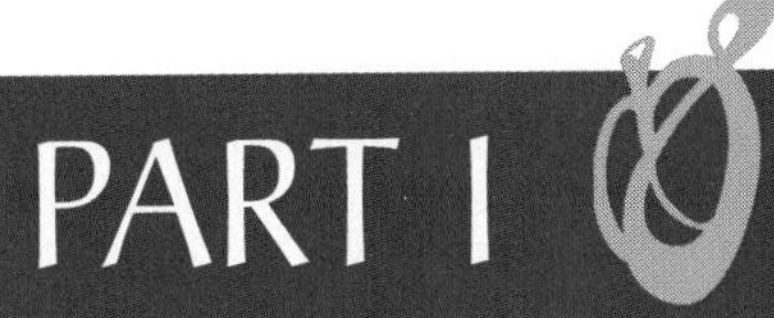

General Considerations of Cardiovascular Disease

CHAPTER 1

Global Burden of Cardiovascular Disease

J. Michael Gaziano

Over the past two centuries, the Industrial and Technological Revolutions and their associated economic and social transformations have resulted in dramatic shifts in the diseases responsible for illness and death. Cardiovascular disease (CVD) has emerged as the dominant chronic disease in many parts of the world, and early in the 21st century it is predicted to become the main cause of disability and death worldwide. In this chapter, trends in global patterns of disease and the increasing burden of CVD are summarized. The chapter begins with an explanation of the concept of the epidemiological transition, followed by a synopsis of this transition in the United States. This is followed by reviews of the current burden of cardiovascular and other chronic diseases in various regions of the world and global trends in the rates of CVD as well as rates of risk behaviors and factors. The chapter ends with a discussion of the diverse challenges that the increasing burden of CVD poses for the various regions of the world and potential solutions to this global problem.

The Epidemiological Transitions

At the beginning of the 20th century, CVD accounted for less than 10 percent of all deaths worldwide. At the beginning of the 21st century, CVD accounts for nearly half of all deaths in the developed world and 25 percent in the developing world.[1,2] By 2020, it is predicted that CVD will claim 25 million lives annually and that coronary heart disease (CHD) will surpass infectious disease as the world's number one cause of death and disability.

This global rise in CVD is the result of a dramatic shift in the health status of individuals around the world during the course of the 20th century. Equally important, there has been an unprecedented transformation in the dominant disease profile, or the distribution of diseases responsible for the majority of cases of death and debility. Before 1900, infectious diseases and malnutrition were the most common causes of death. These have been gradually supplanted in some (mostly developed) countries by chronic diseases such as CVD and cancer, thanks largely to improved nutrition and public health measures. As this trend spreads to and continues in developing countries, CVD will dominate as the major cause of death by 2020, accounting for at least one in every three deaths (Fig. 1–1).[2]

This shift in the diseases that account for the lion's share of mortality and morbidity is known as the *epidemiological transition*.[3,4] Never occurring in isolation, the epidemiological transition is tightly intertwined with changes in personal and collective wealth (economic transition), social structure (social transition), and demographics (demographic transition). Because the epidemiological transition is linked to the evolution of social and economic forces, it takes place at different rates around the world.

At the beginning of the third millennium, national health and disease profiles

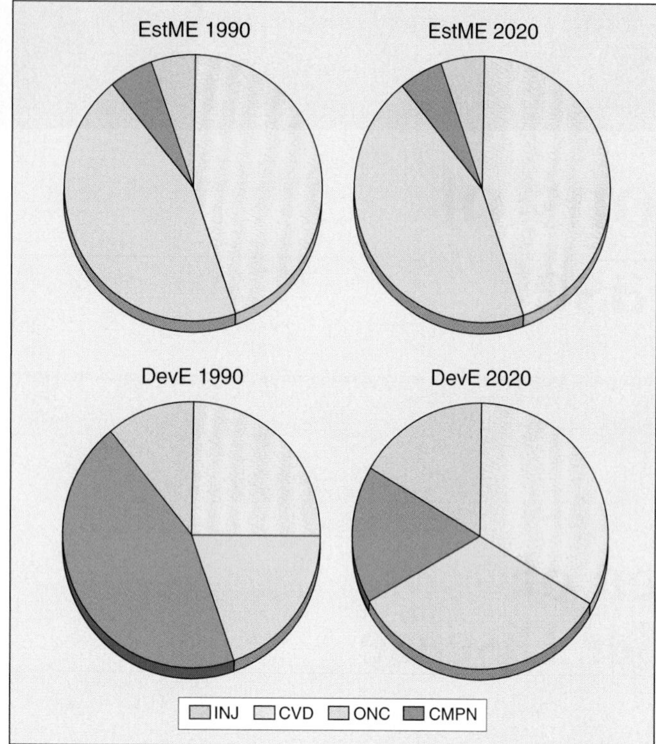

FIGURE 1–1 Changing pattern of mortality, 1990 to 2020. EstMe, Established market economies; DevE, developing economies; INJ, injury; CVD, cardiovascular disease; ONC, other noncommunicable diseases; CMPN, communicable, maternal, perinatal, and nutritional diseases. (From Murray CJL, Lopez AD: The Global Burden of Disease. Cambridge, MA, Harvard School of Public Health, 1996.)

vary widely by country and by region. For example, life expectancy in Japan (81.4 years) is more than twice that in Sierra Leone (34.2 years).[1] In a similar vein, communicable, infectious, maternal, perinatal, and nutritional diseases—the group I diseases defined by Murray and Lopez in their comprehensive analysis of the global burden of disease[2]—account for just 6 percent of deaths in so-called developed countries, compared with 33 percent in India.[2] The vast differences in burden of disease are readily apparent across three broad economic and geographical sectors of the world (Table 1–1). These include the established market economies (EstME) of Western Europe, North America, Australia, New Zealand, and Japan; the emerging market economies (EmgME) of the former socialist states of Eastern Europe; and the developing economies (DevE), which can further be subdivided into six geographical regions: China, India, other Asian countries and islands, sub-Saharan Africa, the Middle Eastern Crescent, and Latin America and the Caribbean. Currently, CVD is responsible for 45 percent of all deaths in EstME, 55 percent of all deaths in EmgME, and only 23 percent of the deaths in DevE.

An excellent model of the epidemiological transition has been developed by Omran.[3] He divides the transition into three basic ages: pestilence and famine, receding pandemics, and degenerative and man-made diseases (Table 1–2). Olshansky and Ault added a fourth stage, delayed degenerative diseases.[4] It is possible that a fifth stage (discussed later) may be emerging in some countries. Although any specific country or region enters these ages at different times, the progression from one to another tends to proceed in a predictable manner.

The Age of Pestilence and Famine

From the epidemiological standpoint, humans evolved under conditions of pestilence and famine and have lived with them for most of recorded history. This age is characterized by the predominance of malnutrition and infectious disease and by the infrequency of CVD as a cause of death. High fertility rates are offset by high infant and child mortality, resulting in a mean life expectancy on the order of approximately 30 years. In the countries that eventually became today's established market economies, the transition through the age of pestilence and famine was relatively slow, beginning in the late 1700s and developing throughout the 1800s. Competing influences prolonged the transition—improvements in the food supply early in the Industrial Revolution that by themselves would have reduced mortality were offset by concentration of the population in urban centers, which led to increases in mortality due to communicable diseases such as tuberculosis, cholera, dysentery, and influenza.

Although the transition through the age of pestilence and famine occurred much later in the emerging market economies and the developing economies, it has also taken place more rapidly, driven largely by the transfer of low-cost agricultural products and technologies and well-established, lower-cost public health technologies. Much of the developing world has emerged from the age of pestilence and famine. In sub-Saharan Africa and parts of India, however, malnutrition and infectious disease remain leading causes of death.

The Age of Receding Pandemics

Rising wealth and the resultant increase in the availability of food help usher in the second phase of the epidemiological transition. Improved nutrition decreases early deaths due to

TABLE 1–1 Burden of Disease for the Three Economic Regions of the World

Sector	Population (Millions) (Percentage of Total World Population)		Cardiovascular Disease (%)		Other Noncommunicable Diseases* (%)		Communicable, Maternal, Perinatal, and Nutritional Conditions (%)		Injuries (%)	
	1990	*2010*	*1990*	*2010*	*1990*	*2010*	*1990*	*2010*	*1990*	*2010*
EstME†	798 (15.2)	874 (12.4)	44.6	43.1	42.8	45.1	6.4	6.2	6.2	5.5
EmgME‡	346 (6.6)	363 (5.2)	54.6	55.0	29.5	32.2	5.6	3.5	10.3	8.8
DevE§	4124 (78.3)	5764 (82.3)	23.0	31.0	17.0	31.2	41.9	24.7	10.7	12.0

*Includes cancer, diabetes, neuropsychiatric conditions, congenital anomalies, and respiratory, digestive, genitourinary, and musculoskeletal diseases.
†EstME = established market economies: United States, Canada, Western Europe, Japan, Australia, and New Zealand.
‡EmgME = emerging market economies: former socialist states of Russian Federation.
§DevE = developing market economies: China, India, other Asian countries and islands, sub-Saharan Africa, Middle Eastern Crescent, and Latin America and the Caribbean.
Adapted from Murray CJL, Lopez AD: The Global Burden of Disease. Cambridge, MA, Harvard School of Public Health, 1996.

TABLE 1–2 Four Typical Stages of the Epidemiological Transition

Stage	Description	Typical Proportion of Deaths due to Cardiovascular Disease (%)	Predominant Types of Cardiovascular Disease
Pestilence and famine	Predominance of malnutrition and infectious diseases as causes of death; high rates of infant and child mortality; low mean life expectancy	<10	Rheumatic heart disease, cardiomyopathies due to infection and malnutrition
Receding pandemics	Improvements in nutrition and public health lead to decrease in rates of deaths due to malnutrition and infection; precipitous decline in infant and child mortality rates	10-35	Rheumatic valvular disease, hypertension, CHD, stroke
Degenerative and man-made diseases	Increased fat and caloric intake and decreased physical activity lead to emergence of hypertension and atherosclerosis; with increased life expectancy, mortality from chronic, noncommunicable diseases exceeds mortality from malnutrition and infectious diseases	35-65	CHD, stroke
Delayed degenerative diseases	Cardiovascular diseases and cancer are the major causes of morbidity and mortality; better treatment and prevention efforts help avoid deaths among those with disease and delay primary events. Age-adjusted CVD mortality declines; CVD affecting older and older individuals	40-50	CHD, stroke, congestive heart failure

CHD = coronary heart disease; CVD = cardiovascular disease.
Adapted from Omran AR: The epidemiologic transition: A theory of the epidemiology of population change. Milbank Mem Fund Q 49:509, 1971; and Olshansky SJ, Ault AB: The fourth stage of the epidemiologic transition: The age of delayed degenerative diseases. Milbank Q 64:355, 1986.

malnutrition and may also reduce susceptibility to infectious diseases. Increased personal and public wealth is associated with public health measures that contribute still further to declines in infectious diseases. These advances, in turn, increase the productivity of the average worker, further improving the economic situation. The change most characteristic of this phase is a precipitous decline in infant and child mortality accompanied by a substantial increase in life expectancy. Examples of countries in this phase of the epidemiological transition are the United States early in the 20th century and China today, where approximately 29 percent of deaths are due to CVD and only 16 percent are due to communicable disease.[2] Changes in nutrition and other aspects of life style that cause lower rates of communicable, maternal, perinatal, and nutritional diseases eventually lead to a greater incidence of CVD.

The Age of Degenerative and Man-Made Diseases

Continued improvements in economic circumstances, combined with urbanization and radical changes in the nature of work-related activities, lead to dramatic life-style changes in diet, activity levels, and behaviors such as smoking. During the age of pestilence and famine, most of the population is deficient in total caloric intake relative to daily caloric expenditure. Easier access to less expensive foods and increased fat content increase total caloric intake, whereas mechanization results in lower daily caloric expenditure. This disparity leads to a higher mean body mass index, blood pressure, and levels of plasma lipids and blood sugar. These changes set the stage for the emergence of hypertensive diseases and atherosclerosis. Cancer rates also rise rapidly during the age of degenerative and man-made diseases. As the average life expectancy increases beyond 50 years, mortality from largely chronic noncommunicable diseases—dominated by CVD—exceeds mortality from malnutrition and infectious diseases.[5,6] Countries currently in this phase of the epidemiological transition are the emerging market economies of the former Soviet socialist states.

The Age of Delayed Degenerative Diseases

In the fourth phase of the epidemiological transition, CVD and cancer remain the major causes of morbidity and mortality. In the industrialized nations, however, major technological advances such as coronary care units, bypass surgery, percutaneous coronary interventions, and thrombolytic therapy are available to manage the acute manifestations of CVD, and preventive strategies such as smoking cessation and blood pressure management are widely implemented. As a result of better treatment and widespread primary and secondary prevention efforts, deaths are prevented among people with disease and primary events are delayed. Life expectancy continues to creep upward as age-adjusted CVD mortality tends to decline, with the average age of people affected by CVD getting increasingly older.

Is There a Fifth Phase of the Epidemiological Transition?

Troubling trends in certain risk behaviors and risk factors may be foreshadowing a new phase of the epidemiological transition. In many parts of the industrialized world, physical activity continues to decline while total caloric intake increases at alarming rates, with the combination resulting in an epidemic of obesity. As a result, rates of type 2 diabetes, hypertension, and lipid abnormalities associated with obesity are increasing. These trends are particularly evident in children. These changes are occurring at a time when measurable improvements in other risk behaviors and risk factors such as smoking have slowed. If these risk factor trends continue, age-adjusted CVD mortality rates, which have declined over the past several decades in developed countries, could increase in the coming years. Evidence that we are approaching an inflection point in the CVD mortality curves is provided by the slowing of the rate of decline in the past few years. This is especially true for age-adjusted stroke death rates.

Changes in Cardiovascular Disease through the Epidemiological Transitions

During the transition from the age of pestilence and famine to the age of delayed degenerative diseases, changes occur in both the character of CVD and total rates of CVD.[6] During the age of pestilence and famine, CVD accounts for only 5 to 10 percent of mortality, with the major forms of CVD related to infection and malnutrition, largely rheumatic heart disease and the infectious and nutritional cardiomyopathies. Given the potentially long latent period of these diseases, they are apparent well into the age of receding pandemics, when they persist as major causes of death along with emerging hypertensive heart disease and stroke. During the age of receding pandemics, CVD accounts for 10 to 35 percent of deaths. CHD rates tend to be low relative to stroke rates. In addition, risk behaviors and risk factors that will foreshadow the next phase become more widespread. During the age of degenerative and man-made diseases, increased caloric intake (particularly from saturated animal fats and processed vegetable fats), reduced daily activity, increased smoking rates, and related changes in the prevalence of hypertension, diabetes, and hyperlipidemia result in further increases in hypertensive diseases and rapid increases in CHD and peripheral vascular disease. During this phase, 35 to 65 percent of all deaths are due to CVD. Typically, the rate of CHD deaths greatly exceeds that of stroke by a ratio of 2:1 to 3:1.

In the fourth phase of the epidemiological transition, the age of delayed degenerative diseases, age-adjusted death rates from CVD begin to fall, leveling off somewhere below 50 percent of total mortality. The decline in stroke rates tends to precede the decline for CHD; thus, the ratio of CHD to stroke deaths increases, typically to between 2:1 and 5:1 (Fig. 1–2).

The decline in CVD rates is the result of two factors: better access to health technology and adoption of healthier life styles. Improvements in health technology and better access to it decrease the likelihood of death among patients presenting with acute manifestations of atherosclerotic disease, although better survival means more and more individuals living longer with conditions such as angina pectoris, congestive heart failure, and cardiac arrhythmias.

Reductions in risk behaviors and factors may make even greater contributions to the decline in age-adjusted rates of death. In many cases, these are the result of concerted efforts by public health and health care communities. In other cases, secular trends also play a role. For example, the widespread availability of fresh fruits and vegetables all year long in developed countries, and thus increased consumption, may have contributed to declining mean cholesterol levels before effective drug therapy was widely available. In general, however, even though age-adjusted rates of CVD continue to decline during the final phase of the epidemiological transition, the prevalence of CVD increases as the population ages.

ECONOMIC, SOCIAL, AND DEMOGRAPHIC TRANSITIONS

As mentioned earlier, several parallel transformations accompany the epidemiological transition. These include economic, demographic, and social transitions that pave the way for major shifts in a population's health and the nature of the diseases that account for most of the mortality and morbidity.

ECONOMIC TRANSITION. The economic transition is characterized by rising levels of personal wealth. This is usually reflected in increasing per capita income, per capita gross domestic product (GDP), or gross national product (GNP).

SOCIAL TRANSITION. The social transition is driven by industrialization and the changes that accompany it, including urbanization, the development of a public health infrastructure, wider access to health care, and increasing application of health technologies. Industrialization tends to spark a large number of social changes. It is typically accompanied by urbanization, a major social force that has a significant impact on the epidemiological transition. Urbanization affects living standards and life style and affords the opportunity to develop organized health care systems.

In virtually every region of the world, there has been a shift from rural to urban life. For example, in the United States, 60 percent of the population lived in rural settings at the beginning of the 20th century compared with only 20 percent at the beginning of the 21st century. In Asia, Africa, and Latin America, a similar shift has occurred over the second half of the 20th century (Fig. 1-3).

DEMOGRAPHIC TRANSITION. *Demographic transition* refers to shifts in the age structure of a population due to declining fertility and increased survival. During the age of pestilence and famine, individuals 20 years of age and younger may account for 40 to 50 percent of the

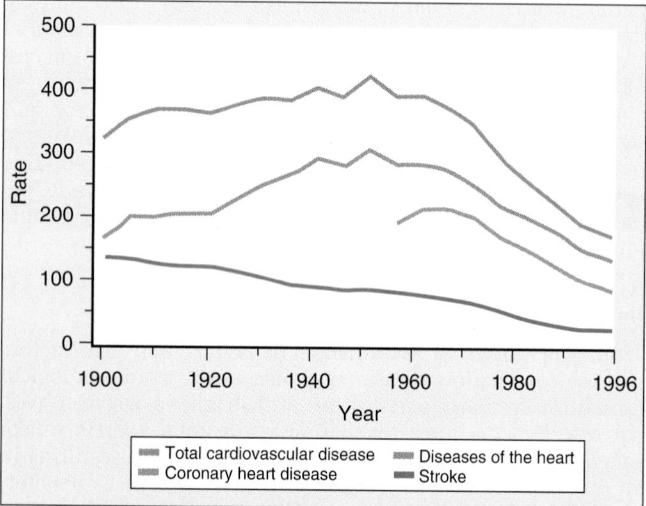

FIGURE 1–2 Increase and decline in heart disease rates through the epidemiological transition in the United States, 1900 to 1996. Rate is per 100,000 population, standardized to the 1940 U.S. population. Diseases are classified according to International Classification of Diseases (ICD) codes in use when the deaths were reported. ICD classification revisions occurred in 1910, 1921, 1930, 1939, 1949, 1958, 1968, and 1979. Death rates before 1933 do not include all states. Comparability ratios were applied to rates for 1970 and 1975. (From Achievements in public health, 1900-1999: Decline in deaths from heart disease and stroke—United States, 1900-1999. MMWR Morbid Mortal Wkly Rep 48:649, 1999.)

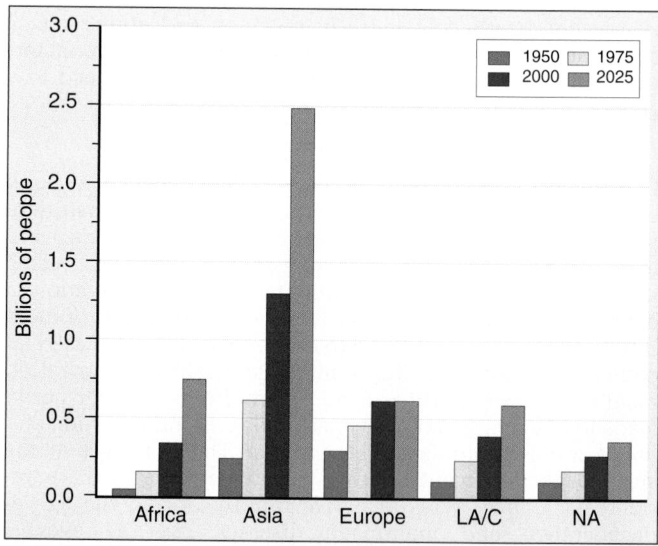

FIGURE 1–3 Number of people living in urban areas, 1950, 1975, 2000, and 2025. LA/C, Latin America and Caribbean; NA, North America. (From Population Division, Department of Economic and Social Affairs: World Urbanization Prospects: The 2001 Revision. New York, United Nations Secretariat, 2002. Number ESA/P/WP.173.)

population. As child and infant mortality rates are reduced in the age of receding pandemics, rapid gains are seen in life expectancy, and the proportion of individuals 20 years of age and younger decreases. Declines in mortality rates are generally followed by declining fertility rates, further flattening the shape of the population distribution curve. As population growth rates fall, the mean age of the population continues to rise slowly as individuals live longer.

The life-style changes associated with the economic and social transitions cause shifts in the profile of risk behaviors and risk factors for disease. These include decreased physical activity, increased smoking, and dramatic changes in diet.

RATE OF CHANGE OF THE EPIDEMIOLOGICAL TRANSITION

Several factors influence how early or how quickly the epidemiological transition occurs in a given country or region. (1) The rate of economic growth relative to population growth affects the rate of adoption of life styles characteristic of established market economies. (2) Regional economic influences can cause great disparities in the rates of transition within a region. (3) The development of low-cost public health technologies, as well as falling costs of unhealthy aspects of the Western life style such as cigarette smoking and consumption of highly processed food, permits currently developing countries to make transitions more rapidly.

SOCIOECONOMIC CLASS. Even within a given country, segments of the population may undergo the transition at varying rates. These factors are related to economic, social, or cultural factors. In fact, epidemiological transitions occur at different rates across economic groups, generally beginning among those with higher socioeconomic status and eventually spreading to those with lower socioeconomic status. The decline in rates of malnutrition and communicable diseases as well as the rise in coronary risk factors and behaviors occur first in the privileged classes; increases in rates of stroke and CHD soon follow. Later, as the middle class grows, the epidemiological transition spreads to a broad enough sector of the population to have a measurable impact on population rates. As more and more of the burgeoning middle class passes through the second and third phases of the transition, CVD and cancer rates become the population's dominant causes of death and disability. People in the lower socioeconomic strata tend to acquire the risk factors and behaviors last, in part because of their economic situation and in part because they tend to engage in more physical activity at work. Compared with people in the upper and middle socioeconomic strata, those in the lowest stratum are less likely to have access to advanced treatments and to acquire and apply information on modification of risk factors and behaviors. Thus, CVD mortality rates decline later among those with lower socioeconomic status. In a developed country such as Canada, for example, CVD mortality rates are highest among the poorest individuals (Fig. 1-4).[7]

The Epidemiological Transition in the United States

Like other established market economies, the United States has proceeded through four stages of the epidemiological transition. Recent trends, however, suggest that the rates of decline of some chronic and degenerative diseases have slowed, suggesting the possibility that the United States is entering a fifth phase characterized by the epidemic of obesity. Given the large amount of economic, social, demographic, and health data available (Table 1–3), the United States is used as a reference point for later comparisons.

THE AGE OF PESTILENCE AND FAMINE

The United States, like virtually all other countries and regions, was born into pestilence and famine. Infectious diseases killed many of the earliest immigrants to the New World. About half of the Pilgrims arriving in the New World in November of 1620 died of infection and malnutrition by the following spring. In addition, the infectious diseases the immigrants brought with them from Europe had a devastating impact on Native American populations.

At the end of the 1800s, the U.S. economy was still largely agrarian, with more than 60 percent of the population living in rural settings. However, industrialization and urbanization were well under way. Per capita income was increasing, and the food supply was improving. Modest gains in life expectancy were apparent throughout the 19th century. By 1900, life expectancy had increased to 47.8 years for men and 50.7 years for women.[8] Infectious diseases—largely tuberculosis, pneumonia, and diarrheal diseases—accounted for more deaths than any other cause.[9] CVD accounted for less than 10 percent of all deaths. Tobacco products were out of the economic reach of a large segment of the population.

THE AGE OF RECEDING PANDEMICS

Early in the 20th century, the pace of industrialization accelerated. The shift from a rural, agriculture-based economy to an urban, industry-based economy had a number of consequences on cardiovascular risk behaviors and factors. Food supplies had become abundant, but urbanization required a dramatic shift in dietary staples. The railway network in place at the turn of the century was capable of moving foodstuffs from the farm to the city. But because the trains were not refrigerated, perishable foodstuffs such as fresh fruits and vegetables could not readily be transported, whereas cereal grains and livestock could. Large slaughter houses and meat-packing plants were established in or near urban areas. As a result, consumption of fresh fruits and vegetables declined and consumption of meat and grains increased, resulting in diets that were higher in fat and processed carbohydrates.[10] In addition, the manufacture of factory-rolled cigarettes made them more portable and more affordable for the mass population.[11]

RAPID SOCIAL CHANGES. The population of urban areas outnumbered that of rural areas for the first time by 1920. By 1930, 56 percent of the population was living in or near urban centers. Infectious disease mortality rates had fallen dramatically, from a crude death rate of approximately 800 per 100,000 population in 1900 to approximately 340 per 100,000 people.[9] Largely as a result of rapidly declining infant, childhood, and adolescent mortality from malnutrition and infectious diseases, life expectancy increased by 10 years between 1900 and 1930, to 57.8 years for men and 61.1 years for women. At the same time, cigarette smoking was on the rise. Age-adjusted CVD mortality rates, at approximately 390 per 100,000 people, were in the midst of their steady climb up from slightly more than 300 per 100,000 people in 1900. This increase was largely driven by rapidly rising CHD rates.

EMERGENCE OF A PUBLIC HEALTH INFRASTRUCTURE. By 1900, a public health infrastructure had emerged: 40 states had health departments and many larger towns had major public works efforts to improve water supply and sewage systems.[9] Municipal use of chlorine to disinfect water was becoming widespread, and improvements in food handling such as pasteurization were introduced.[12] The health care system was growing but still largely comprised general practitioners providing care in the office or home; hospitals were largely for the indigent. The Flexner Report of 1910, which took a careful look at the quality of medical education in the United States and Canada,[13] was the first step toward organized quality improvement in health care personnel that, along with other public health changes, was responsible for dramatic declines in infectious disease mortality rates throughout the century (Fig. 1-5).

THE AGE OF DEGENERATIVE AND MAN-MADE DISEASES

By the middle of the 20th century, the United States was predominantly an urban, industrial economy, with 64 percent of the population living

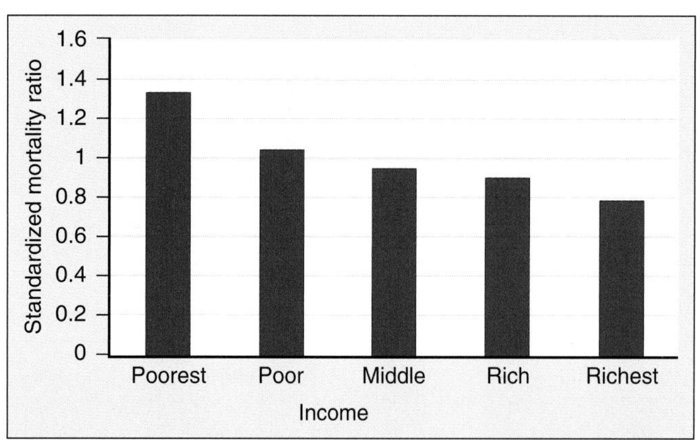

FIGURE 1–4 Cardiovascular disease standardized mortality ratios by neighborhood income for Canadians of European ancestry, ages 35 to 74, in 1986 and 1991. (From Sheth T, Nair C, Nargundjar M, et al: Cardiovascular and cancer mortality among Canadians of European, south Asian, and Chinese origin from 1979 to 1993: An analysis of 1.2 million deaths. Can Med Assoc J 161:132, 1999.)

TABLE 1–3 Trends in the United States During the 20th Century

	1900	1930	1970	2000
Population (millions)	76	123	203	281
Median income (real dollars)	NA	$15,050 (1947)	$26,333	$29,058
Age-adjusted cardiovascular disease mortality (n/100,000)	325	390	699	341
Age-adjusted coronary heart disease mortality (n/100,000)	NA	NA	448	186
Age-adjusted stroke mortality (n/100,000)	140	100	148	57
Urbanization (%)	39	56	74	76
Life expectancy (yr)	49.2	59.3	70.8	76.9
Smoking				
Cigarettes per capita (n)	54	1185	3969	1977
Smokers (%)	NA	NA	37.4	23.3
Total caloric intake (kcal)	3500	3300	3200	3800
Fat intake (% of total calories)	31.6	37.3	41.2	33
Cholesterol level (mg/dl)	NA	NA	216	204
Overweight or obese (%)	NA	NA	47.7	64.5

NA = not available.

Sources: *Population*: US Census Bureau. *Per capita income*: U.S. Bureau of the Census: Current Population Reports, P60-203, Measuring 50 Years of Economic Change Using the March Current Population Survey. Washington, DC, U.S. Government Printing Office, 1998; and U.S. Bureau of the Census: Money Income in the United States, 2000, P60-213. Washington, DC, U.S. Government Printing Office, 2001. *Cardiovascular disease, coronary heart disease, stroke mortality*: Morbidity & Mortality: 2002 Chart Book on Cardiovascular, Lung, and Blood Diseases. Betuesda, MD, National Heart, Lung, and Blood Institute, 2002. *Urbanization*: Measuring America: The Decennial Censuses, 1790 to 2000: U.S. Bureau of the Census, 2002. *Life expectancy*: Arias E: United States life tables, 2000. *In* National Vital Statistics Report vol 51, no 3. Atlanta, GA, National Center for Health Statistics, Centers for Disease Control and Prevention, 2002. *Smoking*: Federal Trade Commission: Cigarette report for 2001. (http://www.ftc.gov/os/2003/06/2001cigreport.pdf) Accessed on 1 July 2003. *Total caloric intake and fat intake*: Nutrient content of the US food supply, 1909-1994: a summary. Washington, DC, US Department of Agriculture, 1998; and Kennedy ET, Bowman SA, Powell R: Dietary-fat intake in the US population. J Am Coll Nutr 18:207, 1999. *Cholesterol level and obesity*: National Center for Health Statistics: Health, United States, 2002. (http://www.cdc.gov/nchs/data/hus/hus02.pdf) Accessed on 15 July 2003.

in urban and suburban settings. With continued mechanization and urbanization, activity levels declined considerably. The rise of suburbs meant that more and more people were driving to work or to shopping rather than walking or bicycling. Prevalence of smoking, one of the major contributors to premature mortality and chronic disease, hit its zenith among adult men at 57 percent in 1955 and among women 10 years later at 34 percent.[14] Annual per capita consumption of cigarettes peaked in 1963 at 4345, or more than half a pack per day for every American.[11]

By 1965, per capita income had risen to approximately $10,000 (in 1997 adjusted dollars).[15] Deaths from infectious diseases had fallen to fewer than 50 per 100,000 population per year, and life expectancy was up to almost 70 years. However, almost 52 percent of men and 34 percent of women were smokers, and fat consumption represented 41 percent of total calories. Age-adjusted CHD mortality rates were at their peak, at approximately 225 per 100,000 people. Stroke rates were also high, at 75 per 100,000.

GROWTH OF THE HEALTH CARE INDUSTRY

One of the most remarkable changes in the years after World War II was the growth of the health care industry. Only some of this growth was stimulated by rises in per capita GDP. In the private sector, the growth of labor unions propelled a major expansion in private health care insurance. In fact, by the late 1950s, more than two thirds of the working U.S. population had some form of private insurance.[16] The federal government also played an important role. Increases in federal funding (the Hill Burton Act of 1948) led to the construction of more hospitals to deal with the acute manifestations of chronic illnesses. These new hospitals drew on the great successes of the military hospitals.[17] In 1966, two key federal insurance programs, Medicare and Medicaid, provided access to medical care for the medically indigent and the elderly. The Health Professions Education Assistance Act of 1966, which provided capitation grants to medical schools, doubled medical school enrollment over the next two decades through expanded class size and estab-

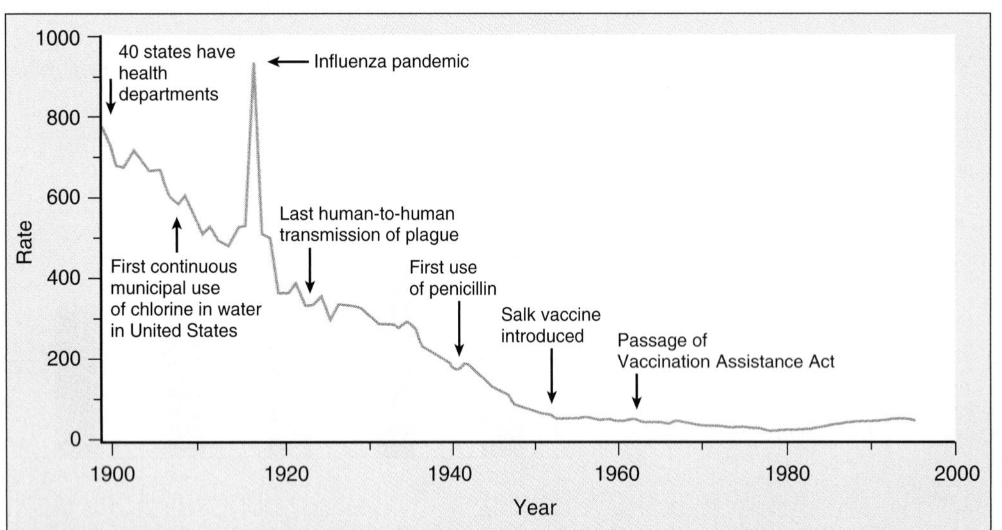

FIGURE 1–5 Decline in mortality due to infectious diseases in the United States, 1900 to 1996. Rate is per 100,000 population per year. (Data on chlorine use from American Water Works Association: Water chlorination principles and practices: AWWA manual M20. Denver, American Water Works Association, 1973. From Achievements in public health 1900-1999: Control of infectious diseases. MMWR Morbid Mortal Wkly Rep 48:621, 1999. Adapted from Armstrong GL, Conn LA, Pinner RW: Trends in infectious disease mortality in the United States during the 20th century. JAMA 281:61, 1999.)

TABLE 1–4 Cardiovascular Disease, United States, 2000

Type	Prevalence* (Millions)	Crude Mortality (Thousands)†	Percentage of Total Deaths†	Rate per 100,000 Population†
Cardiovascular disease	61.8	936.9	38.9	340.4
Hypertension	50	44.6	1.8	16.2
Ischemic heart disease	12.9	515.2	21.4	187.2
Stroke	4.7	167.6	7.0	60.9
Arrhythmia	3.9	37.6	1.6	13.6
Congestive heart failure	4.9	51.5	2.1	18.7
Rheumatic heart disease	NA	3.5	0.2	1.3
Valvular disease (nonrheumatic)	NA	19.7	0.8	7.2

Type	Annual Events* (Thousands)
Myocardial infarction	1100
New	650
Recurrent	450
Stroke	700
New	500
Recurrent	200
CABG	519
PTCA	561
Valve surgery	87
Total costs	$351.8 billion
Direct	$204.3 billion
Indirect	$142.5 billion

*Data from American Heart Association: 2003 Heart and Stroke Statistical Update. Dallas, TX, American Heart Association, 2003.

†From Miniño AM, Arias E, Kochanek KD, et al: Deaths: Final Data for 2000. National Vital statistics reports, vol 50, no 15. Hyattsville, MD, 2002, National Center for Health Statistics.

CABG = coronary artery bypass grafting; CDC, Centers for Disease Control and Prevention; NA = not available; PTCA = percutaneous transluminal coronary angioplasty.

lishment of new medical schools. The establishment of the National Institutes of Health, spurred largely by scientific achievements in medicine made during World War II, not only promoted health-related research but also transformed medical education by providing financial support for the establishment of full-time medical school faculty.

The Age of Declining Degenerative Diseases

A decline in age-adjusted CVD mortality rates began in the mid-1960s, and there have been substantial reductions in rates of mortality from both stroke and CHD since then.[18] These reductions have occurred among both whites and blacks, among men and women, and in all age groups. Age-adjusted CHD mortality rates have fallen approximately 2 percent per year, and stroke rates have fallen 3 percent per year (see Fig. 1–2). Table 1–4 gives a snapshot of CVD in 2000, the last year for which complete statistics are available.

DECLINE IN CARDIOVASCULAR DISEASE MORTALITY. Two main factors have been attributed to the decline in CVD mortality rates: therapeutic advances and prevention measures targeted at people with CVD and those potentially at risk for it.[19-21] Treatments once considered advanced, including the establishment of emergency medical systems, coronary care units, and the widespread use of new diagnostic and therapeutic technologies such as echocardiography, cardiac catheterization, angioplasty, bypass surgery, and implantation of pacemakers and defibrillators are now considered the standard of care. Advances in the pharmaceutical industry have also had a major impact on both primary and secondary prevention. Efforts to improve the acute management of myocardial infarction led to the development of life-saving drugs such as beta blockers, percutaneous coronary intervention thrombolytics, angiotensin-converting enzyme inhibitors, and others (see Chaps. 46 and 47).[22] The widespread use of an "old" drug, aspirin, has also reduced the risk of dying of acute or secondary coronary events. Low-cost pharmacological treatment for hypertension (see Chap. 38) and the development of highly effective cholesterol-lowering drugs such as statins have also made major contributions to reducing deaths from CVD in both primary and secondary prevention (see Chaps. 39 and 42). Such shifts are reflected in the burgeoning cost of medical care. In 1965, Americans spent approximately 5.9 percent of the GDP ($42 billion in unadjusted dollars) on health care.[23] In 2001, the last year for which complete statistics are available, we spent 14.1 percent of the GDP ($1.4 trillion in unadjusted dollars), or $5035 per capita.[24]

In concert with these advances, public health campaigns have also hammered home the message that certain behaviors increase the risk of CVD and that life-style modifications are particularly effective ways to reduce risk. One such success is with smoking cessation. In 1955, 57 percent of men smoked cigarettes,[14] whereas today 26 percent of men smoke. Among women, the prevalence of smoking has fallen from a high of 34 percent in 1965 to 21 percent today. Campaigns beginning in the 1970s resulted in dramatic improvements in the detection and treatment of hypertension.[18] This likely had a profound and immediate effect on stroke rates and a more subtle effect on CHD rates. Similar public health messages concerning saturated fat and cholesterol are largely responsible for the decline in overall fat consumption as a percentage of total calories from approximately 45 percent in 1965 to 34 percent in 1995[25] and the decline in population mean cholesterol levels from 220 mg/dl in the early 1960s to 203 mg/dl in the early 1990s.[18]

A main characteristic of the age of declining degenerative diseases is the steadily rising age at which a first CVD event occurs or at which people die of CVD (Fig. 1–6). Despite declines in age-adjusted mortality, the aging of the population will cause CVD to remain the predominant cause of morbidity and mortality. This, in turn, leads to ever-increasing numbers of individuals with CVD as well as ever-increasing health expenditures related to its treatment. In 2000, for example, CVD was the first-listed diagnosis for 6.3 million inpatients.[26] Hospital discharges included 781,000 for acute myocardial infarction; 716,000 for cardiac dysrhythmias; 999,000 for congestive heart failure; 1,221,000 for cardiac catheterizations; 519,000 for bypass surgery; 1,025,000 for percutaneous coronary interventions; and 327,000 for insertions or revision of a pacemaker or defibrillator. In addition, there were 981,000 hospital discharges for stroke.[27]

At the beginning of the 21st century, the nation is fully industrialized, with only 2 percent of the population involved in farming and a per capita GDP of approximately $36,300. Life expectancy at birth is 74.1 years for men and 79.5 years for women, and at age 65 is 16.3 years for men and 19.2 for women.[28] CVD continues to be the predominant cause of morbidity and mortality, but it afflicts an older

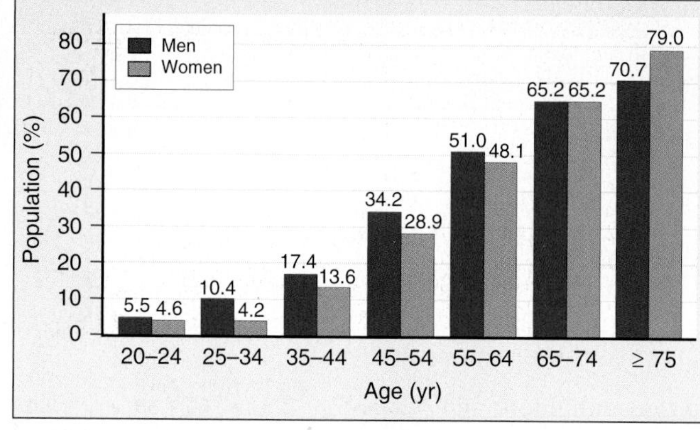

FIGURE 1–6 Estimated prevalence of cardiovascular disease in Americans 20 years of age and older. (From American Heart Association: 2003 Heart and Stroke Statistical Update. Dallas, American Heart Association, 2003.)

population than it did in the middle of the century. Although age-adjusted CVD rates continue to fall, the rate of decline began slowing in the 1990s, with virtually no change in stroke rates for the last 5-year period for which data are available. CHD rates may also be leveling off, owing in part to a slowing in the rate of decline in risk factors such as smoking and increases in other risk factors such as obesity and physical inactivity.

Is the United States Entering a New Phase of the Epidemiological Transition?

Although rates of CHD and stroke death fell 2 to 3 percent per year through the 1970s and 1980s, the rate of decline has slowed.[21] Overweight and obesity are increasing at an alarming pace, and only a minority of the population meets minimal physical activity recommendations. This has resulted in increases in diabetes and hypertension. Rates of detection and treatment of hypertension are stagnant.[29] The decline in smoking rates has leveled off, with approximately 26 percent of men and 21 percent of women classified as current smokers.[14] Even more troubling are increases in childhood obesity and physical inactivity, leading to large increases in diabetes and hypertension among younger individuals.[30,31] These troubling changes in CVD risk behaviors and factors may slow the rate of decline and could even contribute to increases in age-adjusted rates of CVD in the coming years.

Current Worldwide Variations in the Global Burden of Cardiovascular Disease

An epidemiological transition much like the one that occurred in the United States is occurring throughout the world. As in the United States, worldwide CVD rates have risen steadily throughout the 1900s. At the close of the 20th century, 28 percent of all deaths worldwide were due to CVD, whereas communicable diseases accounted for 34 percent of the total.[2] With the ongoing global transition, dominated by the transition in the developing world, CVD is predicted to be the number one cause of death by 2020, accounting for 36 percent of all deaths, whereas communicable diseases will account for barely half that, at 15 percent.[2]

Looking behind the global transition reveals vast discrepancies in regional rates of change. These wide variations began to appear early in the 20th century. Although most of the world remained in the phase of pestilence and famine, economic circumstances in several relatively confined regions changed rapidly, accelerating the pace of their epidemiological transitions. Thus, the global burden of CVD is best understood by examining the differential rates of change in each economic region. In addition to variability in the rate of the transition, there are unique regional features that have modified aspects of the U.S.-style transition in various parts of the world.

In terms of economic development, the world can be divided into two broad sectors, as described in Table 1–1: (1) the developed world, which can be further subdivided into the established market economies (EstME) and the emerging market economies (EmgME); and (2) the developing economies (DevE). Given the diversity within the DevE, it is useful to further subdivide it into six distinct economic/geographic regions: China, India, other Asian countries and Pacific islands, sub-Saharan Africa, the Middle Eastern Crescent, and Latin America and the Caribbean. Currently, four of every five people live in countries with developing economies, and it is these countries that are driving the rates of change in the global burden of CVD.

Like the United States, the rest of the EstME are largely in the fourth phase of the epidemiological transition, with CVD accounting for 45 percent of all deaths in 1990 and communicable diseases accounting for well under 10 percent (see Table 1–1). The EmgME are generally in the third phase of the transition, with CVD accounting for 54 percent of deaths. In the DevE overall, 23 percent of deaths are due to CVD, whereas communicable diseases account for 42 percent of deaths. Across the six subgroups of the DevE, however, there remains a high degree of heterogeneity with respect to the phase of the epidemiological transition, as illustrated by the dominant disease rates in each region (Table 1–5). In sub-Saharan Africa, communicable disease rates still far exceed those of chronic diseases, placing it in the first phase (pestilence and famine). Within regions, there is a great deal of heterogeneity. Some regions of India, for example, appear to be in the first phase, characterized by high rates of infectious and communicable disease, whereas others are in the second or even the third phase. The Middle East appears to be in the third phase of the epidemiological transition. This section briefly describes the difficulties in assessing and comparing disease rates around the world and discusses the regional rates, as well as highlights within-region variations.

Established Market Economies

At the beginning of the 21st century, approximately 840 million people (13.6 percent of the world's population) live in the established market economies of the United States, Canada, Australia, New Zealand, Western Europe, and Japan. In these countries, CHD rates tend to be twofold to fivefold higher than stroke rates. Table 1–6 demonstrates this tendency in selected European countries. There are two notable exceptions. In Portugal, stroke rates for both men and women are higher than CHD rates. The same is true for Japan, where stroke is responsible for far more fatalities than CHD.

Rapid declines in CHD and stroke rates since the early 1970s signal that the EstME countries are in the fourth phase of the epidemiological transition, the age of delayed degenerative diseases. In general, stroke rates have fallen faster than CHD rates, increasing the CHD-to-stroke ratio. In the United States, for example, stroke rates over the past three decades have fallen an average of 3 percent per year, whereas CHD rates have fallen approximately 2 percent per year.

The rates of CVD in Western Europe tend to be similar to those in the United States. However, the absolute rates vary threefold among the countries of Western Europe with a clear north/south gradient, with higher CHD and stroke rates in the

TABLE 1–5 Mortality and Disability-Adjusted Life Years Lost by Disease Category in the Developing World

	Region						
	China	*India*	*Other Asia*	*SSA*	*MEC*	*LatAm*	*Total*
Deaths (%)							
CMPN	15.8	51.0	39.6	64.8	42.7	31.3	41.9
Injury	11.5	8.6	10.1	12.5	9.9	12.9	10.7
Non-CVD, non-CMPN	43.8	16.1	25.9	12.8	19.0	29.5	24.3
All CVD	28.9	24.2	24.4	9.9	28.4	26.2	23.0
Ischemic heart disease	8.6	12.5	8.3	2.5	13.4	11.6	9.0
Stroke	14.3	4.8	7.0	4.7	4.7	8.3	7.5
Rheumatic heart disease	1.8	0.7	0.2	0.2	0.5	0.3	0.7
Other CVD	3.4	5.2	7.3	1.7	8.3	5.3	4.7
Disability-adjusted life-years (%)							
CMPN	24.2	56.4	44.7	65.9	47.7	35.3	48.7
Injury	17.6	14.6	14.4	15.4	11.1	16.4	15.2
Non-CVD, non-CMPN	47.2	20.9	30.8	14.9	28.2	40.3	27.9
All CVD	11.0	8.1	10.1	3.9	11.1	7.9	8.2
Ischemic heart disease	2.9	3.5	2.2	0.8	3.5	3.0	2.5
Stroke	5.2	1.5	2.5	1.6	1.6	2.5	2.4
Rheumatic heart disease	1.1	0.5	0.1	0.2	0.5	0.2	0.5

CMPN = communicable, maternal, perinatal, and nutritional diseases; CVD = cardiovascular disease; LatAm = Latin America; MEC = Middle Eastern Crescent; SSA = sub-Saharan Africa.
Adapted from Murray CJL, Lopez AD: The Global Burden of Disease. Cambridge, MA, Harvard School of Public Health, 1996.

TABLE 1–6 Age-Adjusted, All-Cause and Cardiovascular Mortality in European Countries, 1990-1992*

Country	All Causes	CVD	CHD	Stroke
Established market economies				
Spain				
Men	1323	399	181	93
Women	578	180	52	57
France				
Men	1361	330	142	67
Women	552	122	36	35
Portugal				
Men	1673	593	207	267
Women	805	305	73	158
Finland				
Men	1691	834	631	110
Women	1718	837	587	132
Scotland				
Men	1846	886	655	139
Women	1103	441	273	107
Economies in transition				
Russian Federation				
Men	2881	1343	767	409
Women	1223	657	288	178
Ukraine				
Men	2940	1490	749	606
Women	1379	830	342	408

CHD = coronary heart disease; CVD = cardiovascular disease.
*Per 100,000 men and women aged 45-75 years. From World Heart Federation: Impending Global Pandemic of Cardiovascular Diseases. Barcelona, Prous Science, 1999.

north. The highest CVD rates in the European established market economies (two to three times higher than the median rates) are in Finland, Northern Ireland, and Scotland, where CVD-related mortality exceeds 800 deaths per 100,000 for men and 500 deaths per 100,000 for women.[32] The lowest CVD rates are in the Mediterranean countries of Spain and France, where annual CVD rates are less than 400 and 200 per 100,000 for men and women, respectively. Although both stroke and CHD rates are higher in northern Europe, the disparity in CHD rates is much greater. For example, male CHD rates are 362 percent higher in Finland than in Spain, whereas stroke rates are only 49 percent higher.[32] CVD rates in Canada, New Zealand, and Australia are similar to rates in the United States.

JAPAN. This country is unique among the EstME. As its rates of communicable disease fell in the early part of the 20th century, stroke rates increased dramatically; and by the middle of the century they were the highest in the world. CHD rates, however, did not rise as sharply as they did in other industrialized nations and have remained lower than in any other industrialized country. Overall CVD rates have fallen 60 percent since the 1960s, largely due to a decrease in age-adjusted stroke rates. Japanese men and women currently have the highest life expectancies in the world: 84.7 years for women and 77.9 years for men.[1] The difference between Japan and other industrialized countries may stem in part from genetic factors, but it is more likely that the average plant-based, low-fat diet and resultant low cholesterol levels have played a more important role. As is true for so many countries, Japanese dietary habits are undergoing substantial changes. In the last half of the 20th century, there was an estimated 9.3-fold increase in annual per capita consumption of meat, a 5.2-fold increase in egg consumption, a 7.4-fold increase in milk and dairy consumption, and a 5.3-fold increase in consumption of fats and oils.[33] These changes may explain possible recent increases in CHD.

CH 1

As a group, the EmgME countries have the highest rates of CVD mortality in the world. However, there is substantial variability, with some countries experiencing increasing CVD mortality and others experiencing a decline. Overall rates are similar to those seen in the United States in the 1960s, when CVD was at its peak. Although CHD is generally more common than stroke, the CHD-to-stroke ratio is relatively low, approximating 1 : 1 in several countries. This suggests that the EmgME are largely in the third phase of the epidemiological transition.

Within the EmgME, CVD mortality rates vary widely. The highest CVD mortality rates are in Ukraine (1490 for men and 830 for women per 100,000 population) and Russia (1343 and 657 per 100,000), and the lowest rates are in Slovenia (692 and 313 per 100,000).[32] CVD rates for women are particularly high compared with rates in EstME countries. In the former Soviet and Eastern Bloc countries, CVD predominates as the leading cause of death, accounting for approximately 54 percent of deaths, whereas communicable diseases account for only 6 percent. As expected in this phase of the transition, the average age of people who develop and die of CVD is lower than that in the established market economies.

One major difference between the EstME and the EmgME countries is that CVD mortality rates are not falling in many of the latter countries. On the contrary, since the dissolution of the Soviet Union, there has been a surprising increase in CVD rates in some of these countries. In the former socialist countries of the Russian Federation, Belarus, Ukraine, Estonia, Latvia, and Lithuania, there has been a remarkable increase in CVD rates since 1990. In Russia, life expectancy for men has dropped precipitously since 1986, from 71.6 to 59 years today, but has declined only slightly for women, standing now at 72.2 years. The causes of this decline in life expectancy are not entirely clear. Rapid increases in per capita alcohol consumption may represent one possible cause for the increasing CVD rates that underlie this decline. Inadequate health care infrastructure and lack of institution of preventive public health measures also may contribute to worsening CVD mortality rates.

CVD rates have been stable in Bulgaria, Romania, Hungary, and Poland. The only two emerging market economies in which age-adjusted CVD rates have been declining are the Czech Republic and Slovenia. Even so, CVD rates remain generally higher than in Western European countries (Fig. 1–7).

Developing Economies

Approximately 80 percent of the world's inhabitants live in developing economies (DevE). In general, communicable diseases are nearly twice as likely to cause death than CVD in the DevE. Overall, CVD mortality rates are approximately 23 percent, although this represents only 8.2 percent of total lost disability-adjusted life years (DALYs) because cardiovascular diseases tend to affect an older segment of the population than communicable diseases. An infant death due to malnutrition, for example, results in more lost DALYs than a CHD death in the sixth decade of life. There are vast differences within and between the regions and countries that make up the DevE—some are still in the age of pestilence and famine, whereas others are in the second or even third phase of the epidemiological transition (see Table 1–5).

The character of CVD varies greatly by region. Reporting of CVD event rates is often based on sampling rather than on true national data collection efforts. In China, stroke rates far exceed CHD rates, whereas in India the reverse is true. Rheumatic heart disease remains a major problem in India, China, and sub-Saharan Africa but is less of a problem in other Asian countries and Latin America (Table 1–7).

Many factors contribute to the heterogeneity between and within regions of the DevE. First, the distinct regions are at various stages of the economic and social transitions. Second, vast differences in life style and behavioral risk factors exist. For example, per capita consumption of dairy products (and thus consumption of saturated fat) is much higher in India than it is in China. Third, racial and ethnic differences may lead to altered susceptibilities to various forms of CVD. Finally, social, cultural, political, and economic considerations result in vast disparities in the health care structure in each region.

CHINA. The People's Republic of China accounts for one fifth of the world's population; 69 percent of its inhabitants live outside urban centers. Since the 1950s, life expectancy in China has doubled from 35 years to 70 years. Over the same period, the rate of mortality from CVD increased threefold as a percentage of total deaths, from 12 to 36 percent.[34] As in Japan, stroke is by far the leading cause of cardiovascular death. Hemorrhagic stroke predominates over ischemic stroke, and stroke rates are higher among women than men. These lower rates of CHD and high rates of stroke may be due to genetic factors; however, it has also been hypothesized that overall low serum cholesterol levels may contribute to high rates of hemorrhagic stroke.[35]

There appears to be a north/south gradient, with higher CVD rates in northern China than in southern

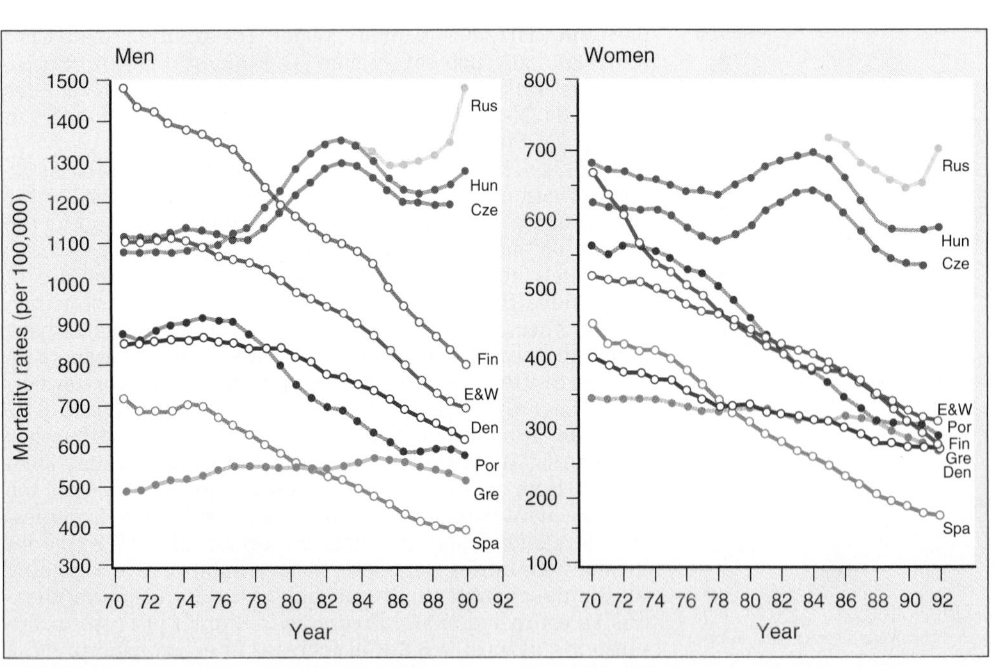

FIGURE 1–7 Time trends in mortality from cardiovascular disease in selected European countries, 1970 to 1992, among men and women aged 45 to 74. Fin = Finland; Hun = Hungary; Rus = Russia; Cze = Czechoslovakia; Por = Portugal; Spa = Spain; Gre = Greece; Den = Denmark; E&W = England and Wales. (From Sans S, Kesteloot H, Kromhout D: The burden of cardiovascular diseases mortality in Europe: Time trends in mortality from CVD in selected European countries. Eur Heart J 18:1231, 1997.)

TABLE 1–7 Rheumatic Heart Disease, Mortality Estimates for 2000

Sector	Number of Deaths (Thousands)	CVD Mortality (%)	DALYs (Thousands)	CVD DALYs (%)
EstME	21	0.6	15	0.8
EmgME	26	1.0	38	2.3
DevE	338	2.8	5697	4.8
India	80,000	2.7	1569	5.5
China	192,000	5.8	2384	8.7
Other Asia	13,000	0.7	159	0.8
Sub-Saharan Africa	19,000	1.8	62	4.7
Middle Eastern Crescent	25,000	1.4	76	3.8
Latin America, Caribbean	9,000	0.8	18	1.9

CVD = cardiovascular disease; DALYs = disability-adjusted life-years; DevE = developing economies; EmgME = emerging market economies; EstME = established market economies.
Adapted from Murray CJL, Lopez AD: The Global Burden of Disease. Cambridge, MA, Harvard School of Public Health, 1996.

China. As is the case in most DevE, there is also an urban/rural gradient for CHD, stroke, and hypertension, with higher rates in urban centers. Regional differences exist in CVD rates, although they are not as great as those seen in India and sub-Saharan Africa. This is likely due to the system of resource distribution that results in less regional difference in the standard of living compared with Africa or India. In general, China appears to be in the third stage of a Japanese-style epidemiological transition, with CVD rates higher than 35 percent, although dominated by stroke and not CHD as they are in the EstME and EmgME. Major features of the transition in China are the rapidly rising rates of cigarette smoking and hypertension, much of which remains untreated.

INDIA. One sixth of the world's population lives in India; approximately three quarters of the more than 1 billion people reside in rural settings. Accurate country-wide data on cause-specific mortality are not available, as death certificate completion is not uniform and the country does not have a centralized registry for CVD deaths. CVD accounts for 24 percent of total deaths.[2] As expected, CVD mortality rates tend to be higher in urban than in rural areas, and CVD is much more prevalent among the upper and middle classes.[36,37]

In contrast to China and much of the rest of Asia, CHD appears to be the dominant form of CVD in India. In 1960, CHD represented 4 percent of all CVD deaths, whereas in 1990 the proportion was greater than 50 percent.[38] CHD death rates are currently about three times higher than stroke rates. This statistic is somewhat unexpected, because stroke tends to be a more dominant factor early in the epidemiological transition. This finding may reflect inaccuracies in cause-specific mortality estimates. However, it may suggest metabolic differences in response to the Western life style of higher-fat diets and lower levels of activity. Based on migration studies, it has been suggested that Indians have an exaggerated insulin insensitivity in response to this life-style pattern that may differentially increase rates of CHD and stroke. Furthermore, the proportion of calories derived from fat, much of which comes from dairy products, is significantly higher in India than in other parts of the developing world.

Although rates of communicable disease remain high, accounting for 51 percent of all deaths and 56 percent of all lost DALYs,[2] the rates are falling rapidly. Thus, India appears to be early in the second phase of the transition, with the urban upper classes in the third phase. As in China, rheumatic heart disease continues to be a major cause of morbidity and mortality (see Table 1-7). Certain remote areas, however, are still in the age of pestilence and famine, with CVD accounting for less than 10 percent of total deaths.[39]

SOUTHEAST ASIA. The diversity of economic circumstances in the countries of Southeast Asia is reflected in the status and character of the epidemiological transition across the region. In South Korea, for example, 57 percent of the population resides in urban centers and the mean annual per capita GNP is $9700, whereas in Cambodia only 19 percent of the population lives in urban centers and the per capita GNP is $240. Average life expectancy in South Korea is 72 years, compared with 53 years in Cambodia.

The rapid economic expansion occurring in several Southeast Asian countries has been accompanied by the expected shift to urbanization and associated life-style changes. In the most industrialized countries, such as Singapore, CVD rates mirror those in the EstME and EmgME, with CVD predominating as a major cause of death and CHD mortality rates twice as high as stroke mortality rates. In other less developed parts of Asia, such as Indonesia and Sri Lanka, the character of disease is similar to that of China. In still others, such as Vietnam and Cambodia, pestilence and famine still predominate.

SUB-SAHARAN AFRICA. In spite of large regional variations, sub-Saharan Africa remains largely in the first phase of the epidemiological transition, with more than 40 percent of all deaths due to infectious and parasitic diseases (see Table 1–5). Life expectancies, as a result, are the lowest in the world.[1] As is the case in India, accurate country-wide data are not generally available, and most data come from urban centers and sampling in rural areas. Overall, CVD is responsible for approximately 10 percent of all deaths in sub-Saharan Africa, with stroke representing the dominant form, in keeping with patterns characteristic of the earlier phases of the epidemiological transition. Even in urban centers, CHD was rare in the middle part of the 20th century.[40] With increasing urbanization, average daily physical activity among urban dwellers is falling and smoking rates are increasing. Hypertension has emerged as a major public health concern, and hypertensive heart disease accounts for the dominance of stroke.[39] Rheumatic heart disease and cardiomyopathies, the latter due mostly to malnutrition, various viral illnesses, and parasitic organisms, are also important causes of CVD mortality and morbidity.

Almost 75 percent of the 40 million adults and children living with HIV/AIDS reside in sub-Saharan Africa.[41] This devastating epidemic is having significant effects on virtually all aspects of health and health care in the region and will definitely influence the natural history of cardiovascular disease. Cardiac involvement is a common sequela of infection with human immunodeficiency virus (HIV) (see Chap. 61). In an autopsy study of adults who died of acquired immunodeficiency syndrome (AIDS), 19 percent had cardiac abnormalities related to HIV infection.[42] Cardiac manifestations can become apparent even earlier in the course of HIV infection. In a prospective study of 952 asymptomatic HIV-infected adults, 8 percent had significant left ventricular dysfunction over 60 months of follow-up.[43] Other cardiovascular-related manifestations of HIV/AIDS include pericardial effusion, infective endocarditis, malignancies such as myocardial Kaposi sarcoma, and myocardial B-cell immunoblastic lymphoma, arrhythmias, and right ventricular and pulmonary disease.[44]

Children with HIV/AIDS are also prone to infection-related cardiovascular disease. These include fetal and congenital cardiovascular malformations, left ventricular dysfunction, myocarditis, vascular disease, dysrhythmias, pericardial disease, cardiovascular tumors, and pulmonary hypertension.[45] In a retrospective study of 68 children with AIDS, predictors of serious cardiac events included recurrent bacterial infections, AIDS-related wasting, encephalopathy, and male gender.[46]

Although much of this research has been conducted in developed countries, reports from Africa describe similar cardiac manifestations of HIV infection.[47,48] At present, few countries in sub-Saharan Africa have the resources to cope adequately with the AIDS epidemic, and few patients receive medications proven to slow the progression of the disease. Thus, opportunistic infections will continue to overshadow cardiac manifestations of AIDS. With the development of public health infrastructures capable of dealing with this disease, cardiac abnormalities should be expected with greater frequency in clinical practice. Use of highly active antiretroviral therapy may further increase the cardiovascular complications of HIV infection.[49,50]

LATIN AMERICA AND THE CARIBBEAN. As a whole, Latin America appears to be in the third phase of the epidemiological transition, although there are vast regional differences. Today, approximately 31 percent of all deaths are attributable to CVD, a figure that is expected to increase to 38 percent by 2020.[2] Although CHD rates are higher than stroke rates (although not to the degree seen in EstME), the combination of these two accounts for more than 75 percent of CVD in this region. CVD rates are beginning to decline in some countries in Latin America and the Caribbean. However, those countries with the lowest CVD rates are facing the steepest increases in CVD mortality rates.[51] Rheumatic heart disease appears to be declining in most countries in this region. Chagas disease remains a major problem in Argentina, Bolivia, Brazil, Chile, Colombia, Costa Rica, Ecuador, El Salvador, Guatemala, Honduras, Mexico, Nicaragua, Paraguay, Peru, Uruguay, and Venezuela, where as much as 30 percent of the population may be infected with the parasite responsible for this disease.

MIDDLE EASTERN CRESCENT. In this region, increasing economic wealth has been characteristically accompanied by urbanization but uncharacteristically accompanied by increasing fertility rates as infant and childhood mortality rates declined. This has resulted in rapid population growth and a young mean age of the population (i.e., 44 percent younger than 15 years of age). The rate of mortality from CVD is increasing rapidly, and CVD is now the leading cause of death, accounting for 25 to 45 percent of total deaths. The adoption of a Western diet has occurred at a rapid rate. As in the established market economies, CHD is the predominant cause of CVD, with about three CHD deaths for every stroke death. Rheumatic heart disease remains a major cause of morbidity and mortality, but the number of hospitalizations for rheumatic heart disease is rapidly declining. This region is entering the third phase of the transition.

Global Trends in Cardiovascular Disease

Estimating global trends in the burden of disease, particularly CVD, is aided by examining regional trends. Because 80 percent or more of the world's population lives in the DevE, global rates of CVD are largely driven by rates in these countries. The acceleration of worldwide CVD rates, for example, is occurring as most DevE countries are entering the second and third phases of the epidemic transition. This section summarizes global and regional estimates for 1990 and 2020 provided by Murray and Lopez.[2]

In 1990, the world population stood at 5.3 billion. CVD accounted for more than 14.3 million deaths, or 28.4 percent of the world's 50 million deaths (Table 1–8). Of these, 6.3 million deaths were due to CHD (44 percent of CVD deaths) and 4.4 million were due to stroke (31 percent of CVD deaths). An estimated 133 million lost DALYs, or 9.7 percent of the total DALYs, were due to CVD.

Expectations for 2020

THE ESTABLISHED MARKET ECONOMIES. By 2020, it is estimated that the world's population will reach 7.8 billion, with much of the growth occurring in the DevE countries (see Table 1–8). In the EstME, population growth (up 13 percent from 1990 to 905 million people) will be fueled by emigration from the DevE. Even this substantial growth, however, represents a gradually shrinking proportion of the world's population, from 15.1 percent in 1990 to 11.5 percent in 2020. In the EmgME, growth will be more modest (up only 5 percent to 365 million people) and also represents a falling world share, from 6.5 percent in 1990 to 4.6 percent in 2020.

TABLE 1–8 Contribution of Various Categories of Disease to Global Mortality

	Population (Millions)	Total Deaths (Millions)	Total Deaths (%)							
			CMPN	*Injury*	*Non-CMPN, Non-CVD*	*All CVD*	*IHD*	*Stroke*	*RHD*	*Other CVD*
1990										
World	5267	50.4	34.2	10.1	27.4	28.4	12.4	8.7	0.7	6.7
EstME	798	7.12	6.4	6.2	42.8	44.6	23.4	11.1	0.3	12.0
EmgME	346	3.8	5.6	10.3	29.5	54.6	27.1	16.9	0.7	10.0
DevE	4124	39.5	41.9	10.7	24.3	23.0	9.0	7.5	0.7	5.7
2020										
World	7844	68.3	15.1	12.3	36.4	36.3	16.3	11.3	0.7	8.1
EstME	905	8.6	6.2	5.2	46.3	42.3	22.5	10.6	0.2	9.1
EmgME	365	4.8	2.9	8.6	34.8	53.7	27.0	16.3	0.5	9.9
DevE	6573	54.8	17.6	13.7	34.9	33.8	14.3	10.9	0.8	12.1

CMPN = communicable, maternal, perinatal, and nutritional diseases; CVD = cardiovascular disease; DevE = developing economies; EmgME = emerging market economies; EstME = established market economies; IHD = ischemic heart disease; RHD = rheumatic heart disease.

Adapted from Murray CJL, Lopez AD: The Global Burden of Disease. Cambridge, MA, Harvard School of Public Health, 1996.

Continued rapid growth in the DevE will increase their population by more than 60 percent, from 4.1 billion people in 1990 to 6.6 billion in 2020, or 84 percent of the world's people. By 2020, CVD will be responsible for an estimated 25 million deaths annually (36.3 percent of all deaths), more than twice the number of deaths caused by the combination of communicable, maternal, perinatal, and nutritional conditions. As deaths from these conditions fall from 34.2 percent of the total to 15.1 percent, CVD takes on greater significance. In terms of lost DALYs, those due to CVD are expected to double between 1990 and 2020, from less than 10 percent to greater than 20 percent.

In the EstME, the modest decline in CVD death rates begun in the latter third of the 20th century will continue, with the proportion of total deaths falling from 44.6 to 42.3 percent. The rate of decline, however, appears to be slowing. The absolute number of deaths as well as the prevalence of CVD will continue to increase as the population continues to age. In terms of lost DALYs, the proportion due to CVD will remain stable at about 19 percent.

THE EMERGING MARKET ECONOMIES. In the EmgME, there will be little change in the overall proportion of deaths due to CVD (54.6 percent in 1990 and 53.7 percent in 2020). As a reflection of the anticipated decreases in DALYs lost due to communicable, maternal, perinatal, and nutritional diseases, lost DALYs due to CVD will increase as a proportion of the total (23.2 percent in 1990 to 26 percent in 2020). The average age of those persons afflicted with CVD will increase.

THE DEVELOPING MARKET ECONOMIES. In the DevE, an estimated 9 million persons died of CVD in 1990. By 2020, that figure will more than double to more than 18 million persons annually, accounting for approximately three fourths of all CVD deaths worldwide. What will drive this overall rapid rise in CVD mortality rates in the DevE? One major factor is the projected 60 percent increase in population between 1990 and 2020. Another is that most of the countries that make up the DevE will have entered the third phase of the epidemiological transition by 2020. Substantial declines in communicable disease rates, from 41.2 percent in 1990 to 17.6 percent in 2020, will increase the proportion of DALYs lost due to CVD by more than 50 percent (8.2 percent in 1990 to 13.8 percent in 2020). Because CVD will afflict a younger population in the DevE than in the more developed economies, more than 100 of the 133 million DALYs lost to CVD (75 percent) will occur in this region.

Only in China and sub-Saharan Africa will stroke rates far exceed CHD rates and remain the predominant form of CVD, accounting for about half of all CVD deaths. In the other Asian countries and Latin America, CHD rates will be only slightly greater than stroke rates, whereas the CHD-to-stroke ratio will exceed 2 in India and the Middle Eastern Crescent.

Regional Trends in Risk Factors

As indicated earlier, the global variation in CVD rates is related to temporal and regional variations in known risk behaviors and factors. Discussions of the strength of the associations of the various factors with CVD are found elsewhere in this text (see Chap. 36). Ecological analyses of major CVD risk factors and mortality demonstrate high correlations between expected and observed mortality rates for the three main risk factors—smoking, serum cholesterol, and hypertension[52,53]—and suggest that many of the regional variations are based on differences in conventional risk factors. This section focuses on regional differences in these risk factors that help explain regional variations in the rate and character of the epidemiological transition. Today, the adoption of risky behaviors such as smoking and eating a Western-type diet has preceded the development of advanced health care delivery systems due to economic realities in the DevE.

Tobacco

Smoking represents an important and rapidly growing avoidable global cause of CVD and total death. Worldwide, more than 1.3 billion people smoke cigarettes or other tobacco products.[54] Tobacco currently causes an estimated 4.9 million deaths annually (8.8 percent of all deaths). This represents 1 million more tobacco-related deaths than in 1990, with the increase being most marked in developing countries.[1] If current smoking patterns continue, by 2020 the global burden of disease attributable to tobacco will reach 9 million deaths annually, with 7 million of these in developing countries.[55]

Regionally, the highest per capita cigarette consumption rates are in Europe at 2080 per year, followed closely by the countries of the Western Pacific with 1945 per day and the Americas with 1530; they are the lowest in Africa, where annual per capita consumption is 480 cigarettes (Fig. 1–8).[56]

In the market economies, smoking rates are declining, with the most substantial changes in the EstME. In the United States, for example, 42 percent of adults smoked in 1965, whereas only 23 percent currently smoke.[14] Over the same period, per capita consumption declined from 4200 cigarettes per year to well under 2000.[57] Among young men and women, smoking rates increased through the 1990s but now appear to be declining.[58,59] In the EmgME countries, smoking rates are extremely high—59 percent of men and 26 percent of women smoked in 1995—but are stable or falling.[60]

In the DevE, tobacco represents an important cash crop and source of employment, two things that are often in short supply. On average, about 48 percent of adult men smoke, and smoking rates are increasing about 3.4 percent per year.[56] In some countries included in the DevE, smoking rates among men are staggeringly high, reaching 73 percent in Vietnam[61] and even higher in parts of Nepal.[62] Throughout the developing world, women have traditionally represented only a small proportion of the number of smokers. That is certain to change. In terms of sheer numbers, the number of women living in the DevE will rise from 2.6 billion in 1990 to 3.9 billion by 2020. As women's spending power increases, tobacco companies are targeting them as customers even as woman-specific health education and quitting programs are rare.[63]

A unique feature of the DevE is easy access to smoking during the early stages of the epidemiological transition due

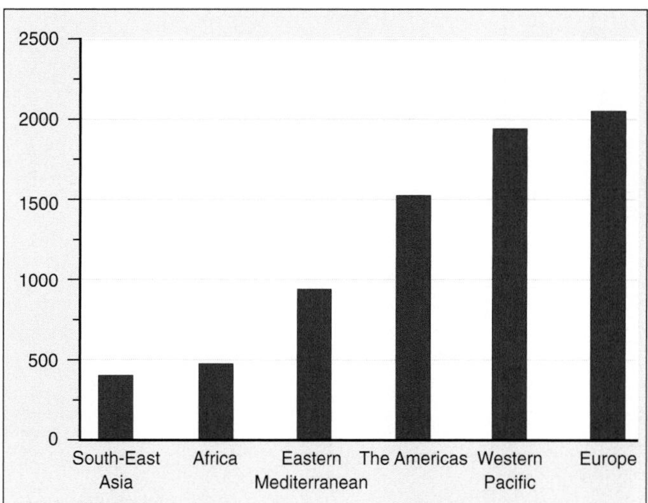

FIGURE 1–8 Annual per capita cigarette consumption in major regions of the world, 2000 estimates. (From World Health Report 1999: Making a Difference. Geneva, World Health Organization, 1999.)

to the availability of relatively inexpensive tobacco products. In the established market economies, cigarette smoking peaked late in the third phase of the transition. In many DevE that are in the first or second stages, however, male smoking rates already exceed the peak rates of the EstME, and rates are expected to continue rising among both men and women. The impact of more widespread smoking earlier in the epidemiological transition means a more rapid increase in CVD rates as the DevE enter the third phase of the transition. In China, which is in the early stages of the epidemiological transition, the 1996 National Prevalence Survey determined that 63 percent of men (but only 3.8 percent of women) were current smokers.[64] A massive retrospective study of 1 million deaths estimated that tobacco was responsible for 13 percent (600,000 deaths) of total mortality in China in 1990 and will account for 3 million deaths a year by 2025.[65]

Diet (see Chap. 41)

With regard to cardiovascular disease, a key element of dietary change is an increase in intake of saturated animal fats and hydrogenated vegetable fats, which contain atherogenic trans fatty acids, along with a decrease in intake of plant-based foods. Although dietary habits clearly vary from country to country, intake of dietary fat tends to be low in many DevE and high in many EstME and generally increases with annual per capita income (Fig. 1–9). Fat contributes less than 20 percent of calories in rural China and India,[66] less than 30 percent in Japan,[67] and well above 30 percent in the United States. Caloric contributions from fat appear to be falling in the EstME. In the United States, for example, the percent of calories from fat has steadily declined over the past 30 years, from 45 percent of calories in 1965 to 34 percent in 1994, although the total amount of fat in the diet has increased slightly since 1989.[68]

Even in the DevE, which are broadly characterized by low fat intake, fat intake varies greatly and tends to increase with industrialization and urbanization. For example, although dietary fat accounts for less than 20 percent of total calories in rural China, in urban areas it contributes more than 30 percent of calories.[69]

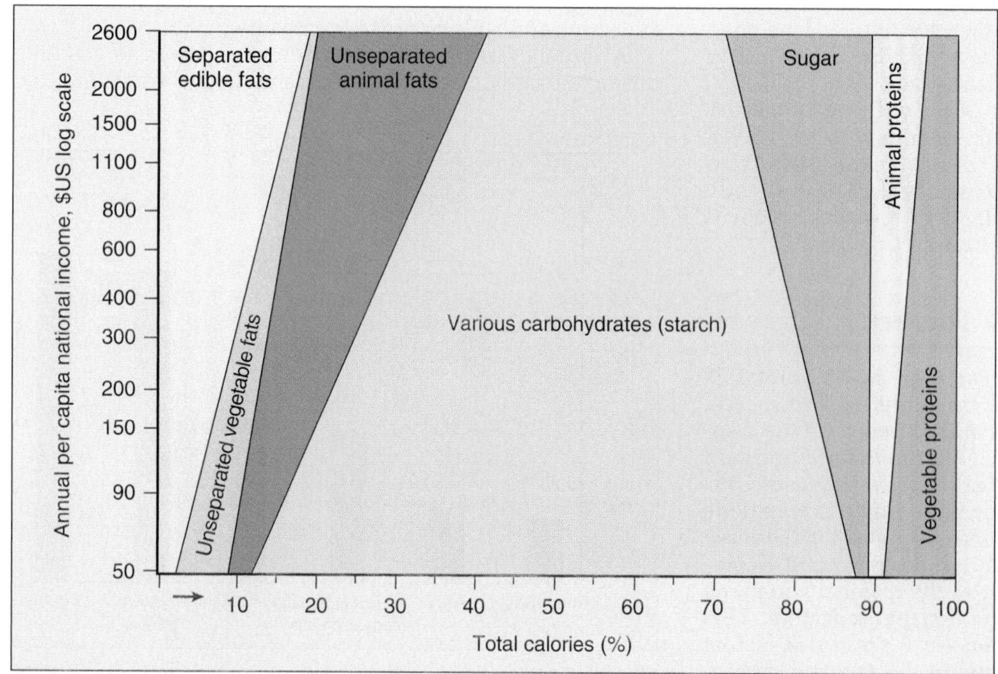

FIGURE 1–9 Association between income and dietary intake, based on country-level sources of energy. (From Drwenowski A, Popkin BM: The nutrition transition: New trends in the global diet. Nutr Rev 55:31, 1997.)

Physical Inactivity

One byproduct of the increased mechanization that accompanies the economic transition is decreased physical activity. In the market economies, the widespread prevalence of physical inactivity produces a high population-attributable risk of cardiovascular consequences. In the United States, approximately 25 percent of the population does not participate in any leisure-time physical activity and only 22 percent report engaging in sustained physical activity for at least 30 minutes on 5 or more days a week (the current recommendation).[70,71] The shift from physically demanding, agriculture-based work to largely sedentary industry- and office-based work is occurring throughout the developing world. This is also accompanied by a switch from physically demanding transportation to mechanized transportation.

Obesity (see Chap. 41)

Obesity is clearly associated with increased risk of CHD. However, much of this risk may be mediated by other CVD risk factors, including hypertension, diabetes mellitus, and lipid profile imbalances. Whereas rates of smoking and hypertension tend to increase early in the epidemiological transition, obesity tends to increase later. Worldwide, obesity accounts for approximately 58 percent of diabetes cases, 21 percent of ischemic heart disease cases, 8 to 42 percent of certain cancers, and more than 10 percent of deaths.[1]

In the mid-1980s, the World Health Organization's MONICA Project sampled 48 populations for cardiovascular risk factors. In all but one male population (China), and in most of the female populations, between 50 percent and 75 percent of adults aged 35 to 64 years were overweight or obese.[72] A later follow-up study showed that the prevalence of obesity has continued to increase.[73]

In many EstME, mean body mass index is rising at an alarming rate even as mean plasma cholesterol levels are falling and age-adjusted hypertension levels remain fairly stable during the fourth phase (the age of delayed degenerative diseases).[74] In the United States, this is occurring among all sectors of the population; however, rates are increasing faster among minorities and women.[75] Overweight and obesity are not limited to market economies. In many of the DevE countries, obesity appears to coexist with undernutrition and malnutrition. Although the prevalence of obesity in DevE countries is certainly less than among the market economies, it is on the rise there as well.[74] A study in Mauritius, for example, documented rapid increases in obesity between 1987 and 1992,[76] whereas another study estimated that 44 percent of African women living in the Cape Peninsula were obese.[77]

Excess weight early in life not only increases the likelihood of adult obesity, but it also increases the prevalence of weight-related disorders, including CVD. Further increases in the prevalence of overweight and obesity are to be expected if data on childhood and adolescent obesity are any indication. In Great Britain, for example, waist size and body mass index among youths aged 11 to 16 years increased significantly between 1977 and 1997.[78]

Lipid Levels

The causal association between plasma cholesterol levels and risk of CVD is indisputable. Low levels of high-density lipoproteins and elevated triglycerides are also clearly associated with excess risk of CVD, and this association holds across racial and ethnic divisions. The lipid profile appears to have a greater impact on CHD than on stroke. Worldwide, high cholesterol levels are estimated to cause 56 percent of global ischemic heart disease and 18 percent of strokes, amounting to 4.4 millions deaths annually.[1]

As countries move through the epidemiological transition, mean population plasma cholesterol levels tend to rise. Social and individual changes that accompany urbanization clearly play a role, because plasma cholesterol levels tend be higher among urban residents than among rural residents. This shift is largely driven by greater consumption of dietary fats—primarily from animal products and processed vegetable oils—and decreased physical activity. Cross-cultural differences in mean cholesterol levels reflect this pattern. In rural Nigeria, which is early in the epidemiological transition, mean cholesterol levels are 120 mg/dl (3.1 mmol/l),[79] whereas in the heavily industrialized United States and northern Europe, which are in the fourth phase, mean cholesterol levels are 200 mg/dl (5.2 mmol/l) and 240 mg/dl (6.2 mmol/l),[80] respectively. In the established market economies, mean population cholesterol levels are generally falling. Japan is something of an exception to this pattern, with only relatively recent increases in average serum cholesterol levels.[81,82] This may help explain why CHD rates did not increase in the third phase of Japan's epidemiological transition. If plasma cholesterol levels continue to rise, however, CHD rates may follow in the coming years. In the emerging market economies, mean population cholesterol levels also tend to be high, but levels are stable or rising.

In the DevE, there is wide variation in mean population cholesterol levels. In Asia, cholesterol levels rose steadily in the last decades of the 20th century, generally faster in urban areas than in rural areas.[83] Once as low as 115 mg/dl (3 mmol/l), mean total cholesterol levels now tend to be at or above 190 mg/dl (5 mmol/l). In Singapore, mean population levels reached 250 mg/dl (6.5 mmol/l) in the mid-1980s, but have since fallen. In many countries in Latin America and the Caribbean, cholesterol levels approach those of northern Europe. A population survey in Bogotá, Colombia, for example, found that 46 percent of men had serum cholesterol levels greater than 250 mg/dl (6.5 mmol/l).[84] In sub-Saharan Africa, mean cholesterol levels in rural areas are similar to the low levels seen in China, whereas levels are considerably higher in urban centers.[85] Given the high level of global capacity to produce Western-style food products at low cost, developing countries can now afford to adopt a Western dietary life style earlier in the economic transition than was possible in the past.

As is true for hypertension, rates of hypercholesterolemia are increasing far faster than the resources needed for widespread detection and treatment. Thus, the impact of both of these on atherosclerosis may be far greater than they have been in developed economies.

Hypertension

Hypertension is clearly a risk factor for CHD and stroke (see Chaps. 36 and 37). Elevated blood pressure is an early hallmark of the epidemiological transition. Rising mean population blood pressure is apparent as countries industrialize; emigration from less developed to more developed countries, as well as emigration from rural to urban settings, results in increasing blood pressure levels among emigrants. Among urban-dwelling men and women in India, for example, the prevalence of hypertension is 25.5 percent and 29.0 percent, respectively, whereas it is just 14.0 percent and 10.8 percent, respectively, among those living in rural communities.[86] Although the relative increase in mortality associated with a given increase in blood pressure is similar in various regions of the world, the absolute risk at the same blood pressure level varies greatly.[87] In addition, the overall impact of hypertension may vary depending on the proportion of individuals in a country who have untreated hypertension.

Worldwide, approximately 62 percent of strokes and 49 percent of cases of ischemic heart disease are attributable to suboptimal (<115 mm Hg systolic) blood pressure, and it is thought to account for more than 7 millions deaths annually.[1]

In the EstME, hypertension remains a major cause of CVD morbidity and mortality despite high rates of detection and treatment. Given the relationship of increasing blood pressure with advancing age, the prevalence of hypertension is increasing in most (aging) established market economies. In most of the EstME, the proportion of the population with untreated hypertension is declining, although in the United States there has been a slight reversal of this trend.[29] In the EmgME, the prevalence of hypertension is at least as high as it is in the EstME, whereas rates of treatment are much lower. This may explain, at least in part, the higher stroke rates in these countries in relation to CHD rates.

Across the DevE countries, hypertension rates are quite variable. One major concern in these countries is the high rate of undetected, and therefore untreated, hypertension. In northern Asian countries such as China and South Korea, hypertension is rapidly increasing,[88] with higher rates in urban areas than rural areas. The high rates of hypertension, especially undiagnosed hypertension, throughout Asia likely contribute to the high prevalence of hemorrhagic stroke. An analysis of several large cohort studies from mainland China, Hong Kong, Japan, Singapore, South Korea, Taiwan, Australia, and New Zealand with more than 3 million person-years of follow-up demonstrated continuous log-linear associations between systolic blood pressure and risks of stroke, ischemic heart disease, and total cardiovascular death down to at least 115 mm Hg.[89]

In contrast, rates of hypertension remain relatively low in sub-Saharan Africa. However, the attributable risk of hypertension in urban centers is exceedingly high in most countries of this region owing to lack of available treatment. Data on mean blood pressure levels in the population are limited. High rates of hypertension are apparent only in urban centers, where there are a significant number of hospitalizations for hypertension, largely owing to the very low rates of detection and treatment.[39,90]

In Latin America and the Caribbean, as well as in the Middle Eastern Crescent, hypertension rates are also quite variable. A review of Latin American hypertension studies published between 1995 and 2000, for example, showed overall prevalence of hypertension ranging from 11.1 percent in Chile to 43.0 percent in Cuba, and hypertension control ranging from 22 percent in Chile to 58 percent in Mexico.[91] In these regions, as in others, hypertension rates tend to be highest in more affluent countries and urban centers. However, even in rural areas hypertension can be prevalent. In a screening program in a rural district of Ecuador, 36 percent of the 4284 individuals screened had hypertension; only 4 of these cases were well controlled by treatment.[92] During 2.5 years of follow-up, hypertension-related cardiovascular disease was the main cause of death.

Diabetes Mellitus (see Chap. 40)

Diabetes and impaired glucose tolerance represent strong risk factors for vascular disease, including CHD, cerebrovascular disorders, and peripheral vascular disease. As a consequence of, or in addition to, increasing body mass index and decreasing levels of physical activity, worldwide rates of diabetes—predominantly type 2 diabetes, or non-insulin-dependent diabetes mellitus—are on the rise. According to World Health Organization models, the number of persons with diabetes will swell from 135 million people in 1995 to 300 million in 2025, a 35 percent increase in worldwide prevalence (from 4.0 to 5.4 percent).[93] The largest increases in prevalence of diabetes will be in China (up 68 percent between 1995 and 2025) and India (up 59 percent), followed by Latin America and the Caribbean (41 percent), other Asian countries and the Pacific Islands (41 percent), and the Middle Eastern Crescent (30 percent). The market economies will experience increases between 26 percent and 28 percent.

The prevalence of diabetes varies greatly by geographic region, race, and ethnic composition. There appear to be clear genetic susceptibilities of various racial and ethnic groups. For example, Pima Indians living in the southwestern United States are eight times more likely to develop diabetes than the general U.S. population.[94] Hispanic Americans also tend to have higher rates than white Americans.[95] Migration studies suggest that South Asians and Indians also tend to be at higher risk than those of European extraction.

Diabetes mellitus is associated with a number of other CVD risk factors, including high triglyceride levels, low high-density lipoprotein levels, central obesity, and hypertension. In relative terms, the attributable risk of diabetes is higher in women than in men.

Future Challenges

Although the concept of the epidemiological transition offers tremendous insight into how and why CVD is emerging as the predominant global cause of morbidity and mortality, it does not mandate that this must be so. As has been seen from the experience of established market economies, CVD rates rise in a predictable fashion with increasing rates of risk factors and behaviors. It is equally true that population-based and individual interventions can have an impact on both the rates and the consequences of CVD. This raises the possibility of altering the epidemiological transition to blunt the increase in regional CVD rates or to hasten their decline. The transfer of lower-cost health and food technologies from the EstME to the DevE has produced great gains in the fight against communicable diseases and clearly helped hasten the transition out of the age of pestilence and famine. It is possible that similar interventions could alter the course of later stages.

Given the multifactorial nature of CVD, no single solution will be generally applicable to all geographic and economic regions of the world. In this section are outlined the major challenges facing each economic region, and the various strategies to address these problems are discussed. Appropriate regional strategies depend on a number of factors, including a country or region's stage in the epidemiological transition, the rate of change of the epidemiological transition, individual and collective resources, and cultural and political factors.

Three complementary strategies can be used to reduce morbidity and mortality from CVD (Table 1–9). First, the overall burden of CVD risk factors in the entire population can be lowered through population-wide public health measures. These include detection and surveillance strategies, public education campaigns, and the institution of low-cost, population-wide preventive interventions. National campaigns against cigarette smoking are an example of the public health approach. The second approach involves identifying and targeting higher risk subgroups of the population who stand to benefit the most from moderate, cost-effective prevention interventions. This involves screening and targeting preventive interventions such as treatment of hypertension and cholesterol. Third, resources can be allocated to acute and chronic higher-cost treatments as well as secondary prevention interventions for those with clinically manifest disease. Typically, resources are allocated simultaneously to all three strategies; however, this three-pronged approach has been implemented mostly in EstME with abundant financial resources for health care. In the following sections are outlined the major challenges and possible solutions for each region.

TABLE 1–9 Complementary Strategies to Reduce Morbidity and Mortality due to Cardiovascular Disease

Lower overall burden of risk factors in the entire population through population-wide public health measures such as detection and surveillance strategies, public education campaigns, and the institution of low-cost, population-wide preventive interventions.
Identify and target higher-risk subgroups of the population who stand to benefit the most from moderate, cost-effective prevention interventions through screening and targeting preventive interventions such as treatment of hypertension and cholesterol.
Allocate resources to acute and chronic higher-cost treatments and secondary prevention interventions for those with clinically manifest disease.

Established Market Economies

Although CVD mortality rates have fallen in most EstME, several important challenges remain. First, socioeconomic and racial disparities in CVD rates continue to linger. In the United States, for example, although rates of CVD mortality have fallen across the population, there are still wide disparities between racial and ethnic groups. Thus, a major goal will be to accelerate the widespread application of preventive and therapeutic technologies to all racial, ethnic, and socioeconomic groups.

Second, the rate of declining CVD mortality appears to be stagnating. Over the past 5 years in the United States, age-adjusted stroke mortality rates have not changed and the decline in CHD rates has slowed. These may be the result of troubling trends in a number of coronary risk factors: although older men and women continue to stop smoking, young adults and teenagers, particularly young women, are smoking at increasing rates; the rates of those appropriately treated for hypertension has decreased slightly in the past 5 years; obesity and diabetes rates are accelerating rapidly. Perhaps most troubling are observations of increasing rates of obesity and decreasing rates of physical activity in children. Taken together, these trends may explain the flattening of mortality curves and may also explain why mortality rates have fallen faster than CVD incidence rates.

In the absence of efforts to reverse these trends in risk factors, we may once again see increasing rates of CVD. More public health dollars need to be directed at anti-smoking efforts that target high-risk groups such as teenage girls and at broader application of guidelines for detecting and managing hypertension and hyperlipidemia. Effective strategies to increase activity and reverse trends in obesity and diabetes must be developed and implemented.

Third, the prevalence of CVD will continue to increase with the increasing mean age of a population even if that population's age-adjusted mortality rates continue to decline. In addition, incremental advances in therapeutic health technology and secondary prevention have led to increasing numbers of people surviving with CVD, which consumes increasing amounts of resources. With the institution of many life-saving strategies among those who present with acute manifestations of atherosclerotic disease, more and more individuals are surviving acute events such as myocardial infarction. For example, approximately one third of those who presented to hospitals with acute myocardial infarction in the 1950s died. Today, in-hospital mortality is less than half that, despite the fact that sicker and older patients are presenting to the hospital. Furthermore, CHD is being diagnosed in increasing numbers of individuals before cardiovascular events. Thousands of pacemakers and defibrillators are implanted each year. As more and more individuals survive longer with CVD, the prevalence of congestive heart failure increases, even as mortality from congestive heart failure is declining.[96,97] Thus, the management of congestive heart failure will consume more and more health care resources.[98] A major challenge for most established market economies will be the increasing financial burden of the management of CVD. More efficient and cost-effective strategies for treating CVD will have to be developed.

Emerging Market Economies

The EmgME region is largely in the third phase of the epidemiological transition. However, the resources available are considerably less than those available in the EstME. Annual per capita GNP in the EmgME ranges from about $1000 to $5000, less than the United States spends per capita on health care alone. This mandates making careful choices in terms of allocating health care dollars to each of the three strategies outlined earlier (see Table 1–9).

In the EmgME, the two overarching goals are to manage the increasing number of people with CVD and to hasten the transition from the third to the fourth phase of the epidemiological transition. This will likely enhance overall productivity in the region, because during the third phase of the epidemiological transition, CVD, and particularly CHD, often afflicts individuals at the age of highest productivity. In terms of challenges facing the former socialist countries, the region can be divided into two categories: those countries with stable or declining rates and those countries with increasing CVD rates. For countries with stable or declining rates, the three-pronged approach used in the EstME should serve as a model. For those countries experiencing rapid rises in CVD rates, an important first step will be implementing more centralized efforts at compiling data on rates of disease and risk factors and then determining the major country-specific contributors to the rise. All countries in this economic sector need more careful tracking and assessment of risk factors in terms of population-attributable risk. Better tracking of CVD rates and risk factors will allow for more careful allocation of scarce preventive resources.

National guidelines that have been developed in the EstME need to be adapted for the EmgME. However, Western guidelines should be modified, taking into account public health and healthcare infrastructure and economic realities. Governments should initiate major public health initiatives aimed at life-style factors, including lowering rates of smoking and drinking, modifying diet, and increasing physical activity. Major public health priorities should include smoking cessation and the detection and control of hypertension, both of which are highly cost effective. The targeting of higher-risk individuals for higher-cost preventive strategies such as pharmacological lowering of cholesterol and blood pressure will initially need to be confined to areas such as urban centers, where the burden is high and the necessary laboratory-based health care infrastructure is available.

Throughout this economic sector, improvements in health care delivery systems will be needed to manage the already high rates of CVD prevalent in these countries. Careful attention must be paid to the transfer of lower-cost health technology, keeping in mind the considerably lower annual health care expenditures in the EmgME countries compared with those in the EstME. An intervention such as the more widespread and appropriate use of aspirin and beta blockers during acute myocardial infarction is an example of an extremely cost-effective life-saving therapy that should be implemented universally before extensive resources are directed at higher-cost interventions such as angioplasty. Personnel issues must also be addressed, given the general shortage of health care professionals in the EmgME.

Developing Economies

The problems facing the DevE may be the most challenging. These countries have rapidly increasing burdens of CVD early in their economic transitions. They often do not have the per capita resources needed to create the three-pronged type of public health and health care infrastructure currently available in the EstME. In many DevE, per capita health care expenditures are less than $50 per year. In addition, there are a number of competing national priorities, including the stimulation of economic growth, social and political change, and the devastation wrought by communicable diseases.

Rising CVD rates will eventually exert a drag on economic growth. Early in the epidemiological transition, CVD deaths occur among younger individuals as opposed to later in the transition. Thus, the economic impact on both the family and national productivity is greater in developing economies than in established market economies. The loss of the head of a household from CVD (or any other disease) has a devastating impact on the health and well-being of the entire family. In Bangladesh, for example, when there is an adult death, a child who depends on that adult has a 12-fold higher probability of death.[99] At present, the data on the economic consequences of CVD in the DevE are limited. Much more work is needed to refine estimates that would permit more thoughtful allocation of health care resources.

As mentioned earlier, the epidemiological transition has been accelerated at least in part by an efficient translation of risk behaviors and the rise in risk factors from the EstME to the DevE early in the economic transition. The rapid spread of cigarette smoking is a prime example of this. A major challenge for developing countries is to attempt to change the natural history of the epidemiological transition. That such alterations are possible is evident from the experience of Japan, in which CHD rates were kept relatively low during a fairly rapid economic transition to an industrial-based economy. Although imbedded cultural practice such as diet likely played a large role, the Japanese experience illustrates that the nature of the transition is variable.

As is true for the EmgME, a critical first step in developing a comprehensive plan for many of the DevE is better assessment of cause-specific mortality and morbidity as well as the prevalence of the major preventable risk factors for CVD. In many areas of the DevE, reliable estimates of the prevalence and incidence of CVD as well as risk behaviors and factors are not available. Improved estimates would enable better allocation of resources based on country-wide burdens of disease. Beginning first in the urban centers and then moving out to rural areas, government agencies will need to make careful assessments of, and create longitudinal surveillance of, rates of disease and risk factors for which low-cost strategies are available. High priorities include smoking and hypertension, for which the population-attributable risks are likely to be high and the cost efficacy favorable. The strategy for the detection and management of high cholesterol must be carefully tailored for each region due to higher costs. Public health approaches aimed at educating the general population about diet and exercise may be useful, but precise estimates of cost efficacy are not available on these even for EstME countries. Drug therapy for cholesterol lowering is likely less cost effective than short-term smoking cessation programs or managing hypertension with low-cost medications.

Once these initial assessments have been made, resources should be carefully allocated to each prong of the overall strategy (see Table 1–9), with most resources dedicated to the first two—national programs for population-wide prevention and guidelines for screening and targeted interventions. Such programs must be based on the population-attributable risk and the available resources. These guidelines must be implemented with low-cost campaigns. Such prevention-directed efforts could blunt the rise in disease rates already apparent in many developed countries. Given the extreme limitations in per capita health care resources in many DevE, the allocation of resources to higher-cost strategies for treating CVD may divert resources from the potentially more effective population-wide efforts. Thus, efforts targeted at interventions and high-technology therapeutics may have to be parsimoniously implemented only in those urban areas where risk is highest. Assistance in the transfer of health care and preventive technologies from countries with developed economies will greatly enhance regional efforts in countries with developing economies.

Summary and Conclusions

We are now halfway through a two-century transition in which CVD will dominate as the major cause of death and disease. Although CVD rates are declining in the EstME, they are increasing in virtually every other region of the world. From a worldwide perspective, the rate of change in the global burden of CVD is accelerating, reflecting the change in the developing economies, which represent more than 80 percent of the world's population, as they move rapidly through the second and third phases of the epidemiological transition. The consequences of this epidemic will be substantial on many levels—individual mortality and morbidity, family suffering, and staggering economic costs, both the direct costs of diagnosis and treatment and the indirect costs of lost productivity.

Each region of the world faces major challenges presented by the epidemic of CVD. There is no single global solution to the rising burden of CVD, given the vast differences in social, cultural, and economic circumstances. The EstME must minimize disparities to reverse unfavorable trends in CVD risk factors and behaviors and deal with the increasing prevalence of CVD in an aging population. To hasten the transition from the third to the fourth phase of the epidemiological transition, the EmgME must find ways to efficiently care for increasing numbers of individuals with CVD as well as to deploy lower-cost prevention strategies. The most complex challenges are those facing the DevE. They must dedicate often minuscule resources to better assessment of rates of death, disease, and CVD risk factors. The allocation of resources to lower-cost preventive strategies will likely be more cost effective than dedicating resources to high-cost management of CVD.

The EstME must continue to bear the burden of research and development into every aspect of prevention and treatment. Through further expansion of the knowledge base, particularly regarding the economic consequences of various treatment and prevention strategies, it is possible that the efficient transfer of low-cost preventive and therapeutic strategies may alter the natural course of the epidemiological transition in every part of the world and thus reduce the excess global burden of preventable CVD.

REFERENCES

Epidemiological Transitions

1. World Health Report 2002: Reducing risks, promoting healthy life. Geneva, World Health Organization, 2002.
2. Murray CJL, Lopez AD: The Global Burden of Disease. Cambridge, MA, Harvard School of Public Health, 1996.
3. Omran AR: The epidemiologic transition: A theory of the epidemiology of population change. Milbank Mem Fund Q 49:509, 1971.
4. Olshansky SJ, Ault AB: The fourth stage of the epidemiologic transition: The age of delayed degenerative diseases. Milbank Q 64:355, 1986.
5. Pearson TA, Jamison DT, Trijo-Gutierrez H: Cardiovascular disease. *In* Jamison DT (ed): Disease Control Priorities in Developing Countries. New York, Oxford University Press, 1993, pp 577-599.
6. Pearson TA: Global perspectives on cardiovascular disease. Evidence Based Cardiovasc Med 1:4, 1997.
7. Sheth T, Nair C, Nargundkar M, et al: Cardiovascular and cancer mortality among Canadians of European, south Asian and Chinese origin from 1979 to 1993: An analysis of 1.2 million deaths. CMAJ 161:132, 1999.
8. National Center for Health Statistics: US Decennial Life Tables for 1989-91, Some Trends and Comparisons of United States Life Table Data, 1900-91. Hyattsville, MD, 1999. DHHS-99-1150-3.
9. Control of infectious diseases. MMWR Morb Mortal Wkly Rep 48:621, 1999.
10. Center for Nutrition Policy: Nutrient content of the US food supply, 1909-1994: A summary. Washington, DC, U.S. Department of Agriculture, 1998.
11. Office on Smoking and Health: Reducing the health consequences of smoking: 25 years of progress. A report of the Surgeon General. Rockville, Maryland, US Department of Health and Human Services, Public Health Service, Centers for Disease Control, 1989. DHHS Publication No. (CDC) 89-8411.
12. Safer and healthier foods. MMWR Morb Mortal Wkly Rep 48:905, 1999.
13. Flexner A: Medical education in the United States and Canada: A report to the Carnegie Foundation for the Advancement of Teaching. Boston, Merrymount Press, 1910.
14. Office on Smoking and Health: Smoking prevalence among U.S. adults. Centers for Disease Control and Prevention, 2002. (*http://www.cdc.gov/tobacco/research_data/adults_prev/prevali.htm*)
15. U.S. Bureau of the Census: Measuring 50 years of economic change using the March Current Population Survey. Washington, DC, U.S. Government Printing Office, 1998, pp P60-203.
16. Starr P: The social transformation of American medicine. New York, Basic Books, 1982.
17. Feldstein PJ: Health care economics. Albany, NY, Delmar Publishers, 1998.
18. Decline in deaths from heart disease and stroke—United States, 1900-1999. MMWR Morb Mortal Wkly Rep 48:649, 1999.
19. Goldman L, Cook EF: The decline in ischemic heart disease mortality rates: An analysis of the comparative effects of medical interventions and changes in lifestyle. Ann Intern Med 101:825, 1984.
20. Hunink MG, Goldman L, Tosteson AN, et al: The recent decline in mortality from coronary heart disease, 1980-1990. The effect of secular trends in risk factors and treatment. JAMA 277:535, 1997.
21. Cooper R, Cutler J, Desvigne-Nickens P, et al: Trends and disparities in coronary heart disease, stroke, and other cardiovascular diseases in the United States: Findings of the national conference on cardiovascular disease prevention. Circulation 102:3137, 2000.
22. Hennekens CH, Albert CM, Godfried SL, et al: Adjunctive drug therapy of acute myocardial infarction—evidence from clinical trials. N Engl J Med 335:1660, 1996.
23. Levit KR, Cowan CA, Lazenby HC, et al: National health spending trends, 1960-1993. Health Aff (Millwood) 13:14, 1994.
24. Levit K, Smith C, Cowan C, et al: Trends in U.S. health care spending, 2001. Health Aff (Millwood) 22:154, 2003.
25. Anand RS, Basiotis PP: Is total fat consumption really decreasing? Washington, DC, US Department of Agriculture, Center for Nutrition Policy and Promotion, 1998. *http://www.usda.gov/agency/cnpp/insght5a.PDF.*
26. American Heart Association: 2003 Heart and Stroke Statistical Update. Dallas, American Heart Association, 2003.
27. Kozak LJ, Hall MJ, Owings MF: National Hospital Discharge Survey: 2000. Hyattsville, MD, National Center for Health Statistics, Centers for Disease Control and Prevention, 2002. Vital Health Statistics, Series 13, No. 153.
28. Arias E: United States life tables, 2000. Hyattsville, MD, National Center for Health Statistics, Centers for Disease Control and Prevention, 2002. National Vital Statistics Report vol 51, no 3.
29. Chobanian AV, Bakris GL, Black HR, et al: The Seventh Report of the Joint National Committee on Prevention, Detection, Evaluation, and Treatment of High Blood Pressure: The JNC 7 Report. JAMA 289:2560, 2003.
30. Fagot-Campagna A, Pettitt DJ, Engelgau MM, et al: Type 2 diabetes among North American children and adolescents: An epidemiologic review and a public health perspective. J Pediatr 136:664, 2000.
31. American Diabetes Association: Type 2 diabetes in children and adolescents. Diabetes Care 23:381, 2000.

Worldwide Variations

32. Sans S, Kesteloot H, Kromhout D: The burden of cardiovascular diseases mortality in Europe. Task Force of the European Society of Cardiology on Cardiovascular Mortality and Morbidity Statistics in Europe. Eur Heart J 18:1231, 1997.

33. Drewnowski A, Popkin BM: The nutrition transition: New trends in the global diet. Nutr Rev 55:31, 1997.
34. Yao C, Wu Z, Wu Y: The changing pattern of cardiovascular diseases in China. World Health Stat Q 46:113, 1993.
35. Okumura K, Iseki K, Wakugami K, et al: Low serum cholesterol as a risk factor for hemorrhagic stroke in men: A community-based mass screening in Okinawa, Japan. Jpn Circ J 63:53, 1999.
36. Singh RB, Niaz MA, Thakur AS, et al: Social class and coronary artery disease in a urban population of North India in the Indian Lifestyle and Heart Study. Int J Cardiol 64:195, 1998.
37. Singh RB, Sharma JP, Rastogi V, et al: Social class and coronary disease in rural population of north India. The Indian Social Class and Heart Survey. Eur Heart J 18:588, 1997.
38. Reddy KS: Cardiovascular diseases in India. World Health Stat Q 46:101, 1993.
39. Bertrand E: Cardiovascular disease in developing countries. *In* Dalla Volta S (ed): Cardiology. New York, McGraw-Hill, 1999, pp 825-834.
40. Muna WF: Cardiovascular disorders in Africa. World Health Stat Q 46:125, 1993.
41. Report on the global HIV/AIDS epidemic. Geneva, United Nations Programme on HIV/AIDS, 2002.
42. Barbaro G, Di Lorenzo G, Grisorio B, Barbarini G: Cardiac involvement in the acquired immunodeficiency syndrome: A multicenter clinical-pathological study. Gruppo Italiano per lo Studio Cardiologico dei Pazienti Affetti da AIDS. AIDS Res Hum Retroviruses 14:1071, 1998.
43. Barbaro G, Di Lorenzo G, Grisorio B, Barbarini G: Incidence of dilated cardiomyopathy and detection of HIV in myocardial cells of HIV-positive patients. Gruppo Italiano per lo Studio Cardiologico dei Pazienti Affetti da AIDS. N Engl J Med 339:1093, 1998.
44. Fisher SD, Lipshultz SE: Epidemiology of cardiovascular involvement in HIV disease and AIDS. Ann N Y Acad Sci 946:13, 2001.
45. Starc TJ, Lipshultz SE, Easley KA, et al: Incidence of cardiac abnormalities in children with human immunodeficiency virus infection: The prospective P2C2 HIV study. J Pediatr 141:327, 2002.
46. Al-Attar I, Orav EJ, Exil V, et al: Predictors of cardiac morbidity and related mortality in children with acquired immunodeficiency syndrome. J Am Coll Cardiol 41:1598, 2003.
47. Danbauchi SS, Okpapi JU: Cardiovascular involvement in HIV/AIDS: Report of 3 cases. West Afr J Med 20:261, 2001.
48. Nzuobontane D, Blackett KN, Kuaban C: Cardiac involvement in HIV infected people in Yaounde, Cameroon. Postgrad Med J 78:678, 2002.
49. Barbaro G: Cardiovascular manifestations of HIV infection. Circulation 106:1420, 2002.
50. Currier JS: Cardiovascular risk associated with HIV therapy. J Acquir Immune Defic Syndr 31 Suppl 1:S16; discussion S24, 2002.
51. Nicholls ES, Peruga A, Restrepo HE: Cardiovascular disease mortality in the Americas. World Health Stat Q 46:134, 1993.

Regional Trends in Risk Factors

52. Kuulasmaa K, Tunstall-Pedoe H, Dobson A, et al: Estimation of contribution of changes in classic risk factors to trends in coronary-event rates across the WHO MONICA Project populations. Lancet 355:675, 2000.
53. The World Health Organization MONICA Project: Ecological analysis of the association between mortality and major risk factors of cardiovascular disease. Int J Epidemiol 23:505, 1994.
54. Shafey O, Dolwick S, Guindon EG: Tobacco Control: Country Profiles. 2nd ed. Atlanta, American Cancer Society, World Health Organization, and International Union Against Cancer, 2003.
55. Peto R, Lopez A: Future worldwide health effects of current smoking patterns. *In* Koop CE, Pearson CE, Schwarz MR (eds): Critical Issues in Global Health. San Francisco, Jossey-Bass, 2001.
56. World Health Report 1999: Making a Difference. Geneva, World Health Organization, 1999.
57. Cigarette report for 2001. Federal Trade Commission, 2003. (*http://www.ftc.gov/os/2003/06/2001cigreport.pdf*)
58. Trends in cigarette smoking among high school students—United States, 1991-2001. MMWR Morb Mortal Wkly Rep 51:409, 2002.
59. Wechsler H, Rigotti NA, Gledhill-Hoyt J, Lee H: Increased levels of cigarette use among college students: A cause for national concern. JAMA 280:1673, 1998.
60. Jha P, Chaloupka FJ: Curbing the epidemic: Governments and the economics of tobacco control. Washington, DC, The World Bank, 1999.
61. Jenkins CN, Dai PX, Ngoc DH, et al: Tobacco use in Vietnam: Prevalence, predictors, and the role of the transnational tobacco corporations. JAMA 277:1726, 1997.
62. Pandey MR, Neupane RP, Gautam A: Epidemiological study of tobacco smoking behaviour among adults in a rural community of the hill region of Nepal with special reference to attitude and beliefs. Int J Epidemiol 17:535, 1988.
63. Mackay J: Women and tobacco: International issues. J Am Med Womens Assoc 51:48, 1996.
64. Yang G, Fan L, Tan J, et al: Smoking in China: Findings of the 1996 National Prevalence Survey. JAMA 282:1247, 1999.
65. Liu BQ, Peto R, Chen ZM, et al: Emerging tobacco hazards in China: 1. Retrospective proportional mortality study of one million deaths. BMJ 317:1411, 1998.
66. Janus ED, Postiglione A, Singh RB, Lewis B: The modernization of Asia: Implications for coronary heart disease. Council on Arteriosclerosis of the International Society and Federation of Cardiology. Circulation 94:2671, 1996.
67. Research Committee on Serum Lipid Level Survey 1990 in Japan: Current state of and recent trends in serum lipid levels in the general Japanese population. J Atheroscler Thromb 2:122, 1996.
68. Kennedy ET, Bowman SA, Powell R: Dietary fat intake in the US population. J Am Coll Nutr 18:207, 1999.
69. Du S, Lu B, Zhai F, Popkin BM: A new stage of the nutrition transition in China. Public Health Nutr 5:169, 2002.
70. U.S. Department of Health and Human Services: Healthy People 2010: Understanding and Improving Health. Washington, DC, U.S. Government Printing Office, 2000.
71. Physical activity trends—United States, 1990-1998. MMWR Morb Mortal Wkly Rep 50:166, 2001.
72. Keil U, Kuulasmaa K: WHO MONICA Project: Risk factors. Int J Epidemiol 18:S46, 1989.
73. Dobson AJ, Evans A, Ferrario M, et al: Changes in estimated coronary risk in the 1980s: Data from 38 populations in the WHO MONICA Project. World Health Organization. Monitoring trends and determinants in cardiovascular diseases. Ann Med 30:199, 1998.
74. Obesity: Preventing and managing the global epidemic. Geneva,World Health Organization, 2000. Technical Report Series, No 894.
75. Mokdad AH, Ford ES, Bowman BA, et al: Prevalence of obesity, diabetes, and obesity-related health risk factors, 2001. JAMA 289:76, 2003.
76. Hodge AM, Dowse GK, Gareeboo H, et al: Incidence, increasing prevalence, and predictors of change in obesity and fat distribution over 5 years in the rapidly developing population of Mauritius. Int J Obes Relat Metab Disord 20:137, 1996.
77. Steyn K, Jooste PL, Bourne L, et al: Risk factors for coronary heart disease in the black population of the Cape Peninsula. The BRISK study. S Afr Med J 79:480, 1991.
78. McCarthy HD, Ellis SM, Cole TJ: Central overweight and obesity in British youth aged 11-16 years: Cross sectional surveys of waist circumference. BMJ 326:624, 2003.
79. Erasmus RT, Uyot C, Pakeye T: Plasma cholesterol distribution in a rural Nigerian population—relationship to age, sex and body mass. Cent Afr J Med 40:299, 1994.
80. Verschuren WM, Jacobs DR, Bloemberg BP, et al: Serum total cholesterol and long-term coronary heart disease mortality in different cultures: Twenty-five-year follow-up of the seven countries study. JAMA 274:131, 1995.
81. Kuzuya M, Ando F, Iguchi A, Shimokata H: Changes in serum lipid levels during a 10 year period in a large Japanese population: A cross-sectional and longitudinal study. Atherosclerosis 163:313, 2002.
82. Yamada M, Wong FL, Kodama K, et al: Longitudinal trends in total serum cholesterol levels in a Japanese cohort, 1958-1986. J Clin Epidemiol 50:425, 1997.
83. Khoo KL, Tan H, Liew YM, et al: Lipids and coronary heart disease in Asia. Atherosclerosis 169:1, 2003.
84. INCLEN Multicentre Collaborative Group: Risk factors for cardiovascular disease in the developing world. A multicentre collaborative study in the International Clinical Epidemiology Network (INCLEN). J Clin Epidemiol 45:841, 1992.
85. Walker AR, Sareli P: Coronary heart disease: Outlook for Africa. J R Soc Med 90:23, 1997.
86. Singh RB, Sharma JP, Rastogi V, et al: Prevalence of coronary artery disease and coronary risk factors in rural and urban populations of north India. Eur Heart J 18:1728, 1997.
87. van den Hoogen PC, Feskens EJ, Nagelkerke NJ, et al: The relation between blood pressure and mortality due to coronary heart disease among men in different parts of the world. Seven Countries Study Research Group. N Engl J Med 342:1, 2000.
88. Gu D, Reynolds K, Wu X, et al: Prevalence, awareness, treatment, and control of hypertension in China. Hypertension 40:920, 2002.
89. Lawes CM, Rodgers A, Bennett DA, et al: Blood pressure and cardiovascular disease in the Asia Pacific region. J Hypertens 21:707, 2003.
90. Seedat YK: Hypertension in developing nations in sub-Saharan Africa. J Hum Hypertens 14:739, 2000.
91. Ordunez P, Silva LC, Rodriguez MP, Robles S: Prevalence estimates for hypertension in Latin America and the Caribbean: Are they useful for surveillance? Rev Panam Salud Publica 10:226, 2001.
92. Anselmi M, Avanzini F, Moreira JM, et al: Treatment and control of arterial hypertension in a rural community in Ecuador. Lancet 361:1186, 2003.
93. King H, Aubert RE, Herman WH: Global burden of diabetes, 1995-2025: Prevalence, numerical estimates, and projections. Diabetes Care 21:1414, 1998.
94. Knowler WC, Pettitt DJ, Saad MF, Bennett PH: Diabetes mellitus in the Pima Indians: Incidence, risk factors and pathogenesis. Diabetes Metab Rev 6:1, 1990.
95. Harris MI, Flegal KM, Cowie CC, et al: Prevalence of diabetes, impaired fasting glucose, and impaired glucose tolerance in U.S. adults. The Third National Health and Nutrition Examination Survey, 1988-1994. Diabetes Care 21:518, 1998.

Future Challenges

96. Haldeman GA, Croft JB, Giles WH, Rashidee A: Hospitalization of patients with heart failure: National Hospital Discharge Survey, 1985 to 1995. Am Heart J 137:352, 1999.
97. Changes in mortality from heart failure—United States, 1980-1995. MMWR Morb Mortal Wkly Rep 47:633, 1998.
98. Malek M: Health economics of heart failure. Heart 82 Suppl 4:IV11, 1999.
99. Howson CP, Reddy KS, Ryan TJ, Bale JR (eds): Control of cardiovascular disease in developing countries. Washington, DC, National Academy Press, 1998.

CHAPTER 2

Economics and Cardiovascular Disease

Mark A. Hlatky • Daniel B. Mark

The United States leads the world in spending on health care, whether measured as a percentage of gross domestic product or as dollars per capita. The decisions made by physicians control the bulk of these expenditures, and society has increasingly called for greater stewardship of the vast resources that doctors command. This chapter discusses some of the key economic principles that underlie clinical and health policy decision-making and reviews important economic studies evaluating management of cardiovascular disorders.

Key Economic Principles

Alternative Uses

A key principle of economics is that all resources have alternative uses, so devoting resources to any particular activity makes them unavailable for different, and perhaps better, uses. Society's application of resources to medical care diminishes the resources available for alternative programs, such as public safety, assistance to the elderly or the poor, or environmental protection. This same principle applies to the resources earmarked to health care: the resources devoted to implantable defibrillators within a health care system might be used to meet alternative health needs, such as treatment of heart failure, prenatal care programs, or provision of vaccinations. Thus, the goal of health economics is to define the most efficient use of the resources available to provide health care to a population of patients.

Societal Perspective

Economic analyses most often employ the societal perspective: how will society as a whole benefit from the new clinical program and what will society have to pay for it? In contrast, clinicians are focused on individual patients. Their traditional role is to be the patient's advocate, to do what is possible for the patient before them, regardless of the value provided to society. Thus, economic analysis is a policy tool for informing spending about populations, not a tool for assisting with bedside decision-making.

Law of Diminishing Returns

An economic principle of special relevance to medicine is the so-called "law of diminishing returns," indicated schematically in Figure 2–1. As resources are initially applied to a particular end, the returns are large, but as further resources are applied, the returns become progressively smaller to the point that there is no further gain, and perhaps even a loss, with application of additional resources. This type of response is familiar to clinicians caring for patients; in the case of acute myocardial infarction (MI), for example, access to defibrillation and hospital monitoring provides great benefits, and the addition of reperfusion therapy further improves patient outcomes. The provision of yet more care may improve outcomes a bit further, but eventually maximum benefit is obtained—this point has been termed the "flat of the curve." A key economic insight is that it is not optimal for society to have medical care operate on the flat of the curve, but rather have it operate on the upsloping portion of the curve (see Fig. 2–1) because the resources that would be spent in moving along the flat of the curve have better alternative uses. A major goal of economic analysis of cardiovascular care is to find the optimal level of resources for a given clinical problem.

As exemplified in Figure 2-1, a key economic measure of value is the cost of adding another unit of medical benefit, or the slope of the curve.[1-3] In economic analysis, the costs and effects of an intervention are always compared with an explicitly defined alternative. Thus, cost-effectiveness analysis assesses the marginal (or incremental) costs required to improve outcomes by one unit. The cost-effectiveness ratio is defined as follows:

$$\frac{\text{Cost}_{\text{new}} - \text{Cost}_{\text{old}}}{\text{Effect}_{\text{new}} - \text{Effect}_{\text{old}}}$$

where $Cost_{new}$ is the total cost of the new program, $Cost_{old}$ is the total cost of the old program, and $Effect_{new}$ and $Effect_{old}$ indicate the medical effectiveness of the new and old programs, respectively. The cost of a program should include all relevant costs: the intervention itself (e.g., streptokinase for an acute MI); the cost of complications induced (e.g., bleeding, stroke) and averted (e.g., heart failure) by therapy; and the costs of concomitant treatments (e.g., mechanical coronary revascularization). The effectiveness of a medical intervention should be assessed using outcomes directly relevant to patients, such as survival and quality of life. Economic analysis commonly measures effectiveness in "quality-adjusted life-years" (QALYs) to assess on a common scale both of these dimensions of improved clinical outcome. Laboratory-based outcome measures (e.g., ejection fraction, serum cholesterol level) are intermediate, surrogate markers of ultimate patient benefit and therefore are not used in economic analysis.

Economies of Scale

A final economic principle of relevance to medical care is that the production of goods and services is often more efficient in larger quantities due to "economies of scale." Costs per patient are lower when the high fixed costs of specialized equipment (e.g., an angiography suite) are spread over more

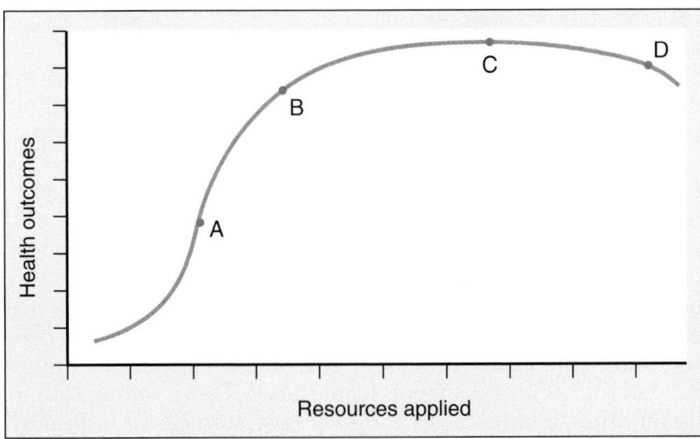

FIGURE 2–1 General relationship between application of health care resources (horizontal axis) and health outcomes (vertical axis). At Point A, outcomes are improving rapidly with increased resources, and treatment is cost-effective. At Point B, outcomes are still improving with increased resources, but at a rate that is less cost-effective. At Point C, increased resources are no longer improving outcome (i.e., "flat at the curve"), and at Point D increased resources actually lead to worse outcomes, through iatrogenic complications and overtreatment.

patients. Also, large-volume facilities can negotiate price discounts from suppliers and achieve more flexible use of personnel with their larger staff. In medical care, there is also evidence that higher patient volumes are associated with greater technical proficiency and better clinical outcomes.[4,5] Of course, beyond a certain scale, the clinical and cost advantages of higher patient volumes will be diminished and the disadvantages may increase (e.g., poorer communication, an impersonal approach to patient care). Nevertheless, there is strong empirical evidence of the value of maintaining a minimum level of clinical volume in procedures such as coronary angioplasty and coronary bypass surgery and in the care of critically ill patients such as those with acute MI.

Medical Costs

Provision of medical care requires resources: the time and energy of physicians, nurses, and other health care professionals; specialized facilities such as intensive care units, angiography suites, and operating rooms; and costly drugs and supplies. Use of these resources has a cost, even if medical care is provided "for free." In principle, the best measure of this cost is what economists term the *opportunity cost*, or what has been lost by not applying resources to their next best use. As a practical matter, cost is measured by the prices paid in a competitive market. The overall cost of a medical program can then be measured as $\Sigma_i P_i Q_i$, where P_i is the price for resource i, Q_i is the quantity of resource i that is used, and the summation is over all i resources used in care of the patient. Modern hospital cost accounting systems facilitate such "microcosting" of medical care services. When microcosting is not feasible, an alternative measure of hospital cost has been found by multiplying the charge for the service by a correction factor (the ratio of costs to charges) from the hospital's annual financial report to the Centers for Medicare and Medicaid Services.

In medical economic studies, the cost of an intervention includes all relevant costs, regardless of who pays for them. The cost of an angioplasty might be borne in part by the insurance company, in part by the patient (e.g., prescription drugs after discharge), and in part by the hospital (e.g., costs over the contracted insurance payment amount). An expensive new therapy in the angioplasty laboratory may reduce total costs in the year after the procedure and therefore be quite economically attractive. Nevertheless, a hospital may resist using the new therapy because its costs are increased. Even programs that save total medical costs can create economic winners and losers, whose incentives and disincentives can distort optimal resource allocation from a societal perspective.

Medical costs and benefits are typically spread over long time intervals, which leads to two related issues regarding measurement. Inflation changes the units of cost measurement, such that a dollar in the year 2003 does not have the same value as a dollar in 2008: it is therefore necessary to standardize all costs to a single metric, such as 2008 dollars. A separate issue is that even if there were no cost inflation, it is still preferable to be paid today than to be paid in 5 years, and, conversely, it is preferable to repay a debt sometime in the future than to repay it immediately. To adjust for these time preferences, medical economic studies typically discount future costs and medical benefits by 3% per year.[2]

Analysis of Specific Interventions

Economic analysis has been applied to treatment of acute illness (e.g., acute MI), procedures (e.g., coronary bypass surgery), treatment of chronic illness (e.g., heart failure), prevention of disease (e.g., reduction of high cholesterol levels), or the use of diagnostic tests (e.g., coronary angiography). In the remainder of this chapter, we illustrate the principles of economic analysis by discussing cardiovascular management strategies drawn from each of these areas. Detailed review of the economics of all cardiovascular therapies is beyond the scope of this chapter.

Application of economic analysis to medical care can be illustrated by the use of thrombolytic therapy for acute MI. Timely reperfusion of the occluded coronary artery improves survival of the patient with an acute MI, and this survival benefit is maintained over long-term follow-up.[6] The added cost of treating an acute MI patient with reperfusion therapy needs to be weighed against the long-term benefit to assess the value provided by this treatment strategy.

The value of streptokinase administration for acute MI compared with no reperfusion therapy can be analyzed using cost-effectiveness analysis. For the purpose of this example, we assume that streptokinase costs \$270 per treatment, and that costs of medical care are otherwise equal in treated and untreated MI patients. We further assume that hospital survival is improved from 88% to 92% by streptokinase treatment, and that the life-expectancy of MI survivors is 15 years, regardless of whether they were treated with streptokinase. Based on these assumptions, the incremental cost-effectiveness of streptokinase for the treatment of acute MI can be calculated as follows:

$$\frac{\Delta\text{Cost}}{\Delta\text{Life expectancy}} = \frac{\$270 - 0}{(0.92)(15\text{ yr}) - (0.88)(15\text{ yr})}$$
$$= \frac{\$270}{0.6\text{ yr}} = \$450/\text{life-year added}$$

Thus, the expenditure of \$450 on average adds a year to the life of a patient with an acute MI. To judge whether streptokinase therapy for acute MI represents a good value for the money spent (i.e., is "economically attractive") requires a standard of comparison. Renal dialysis currently costs about \$50,000 per patient per year in the United States. The cost of dialysis is covered by the publicly funded Medicare program and provides a good benchmark of how much society is willing to spend to add a life-year. Programs that cost up to \$50,000 per year of life added are generally considered economically attractive, whereas programs with cost-effectiveness ratios greater than \$100,000 per year of life added are generally considered to be economically unattractive. Based on these benchmarks, streptokinase therapy for acute MI is a very economically attractive intervention.

Acute Coronary Syndromes (see Chap. 49)

Thrombolytic Agents

Treatment of acute coronary syndromes (MI, unstable angina) with reperfusion, antithrombotic, and anticoagulant regimens has been extensively investigated. While clinically diverse, these therapies share common features from the perspective of economic evaluation. The therapies for acute coronary syndromes are typically short-term in duration and expensive, and they provide benefit to patients mainly by reducing the short-term risk of hospital death and/or MI.

Tissue plasminogen activator (t-PA) has been extensively studied for the treatment of acute MI. t-PA is much more expensive than streptokinase, the first thrombolytic agent shown to be effective for MI. The cost-effectiveness of t-PA was assessed in the randomized GUSTO-1 trial.[7] In GUSTO-1, the cost of therapy was assessed by assigning standardized costs to each resource consumed (e.g., hospital days, cardiac angiography) and summing the costs over all resources used. Apart from the cost of the thrombolytic agents themselves, hospital and follow-up costs were quite similar in t-PA-treated and streptokinase-treated patients, and the added cost of t-PA ($2200 vs. $270) was not offset by cost savings in other aspects of the patient's care. The 30-day survival rate of t-PA-treated patients was improved by 1%, and the life expectancy of survivors was projected to be 15.4 years. Using these data, the cost-effectiveness of t-PA relative to streptokinase was $27,100 per year of life saved, which was economically attractive by the previously described benchmarks.[7]

The use of streptokinase and t-PA for acute MI provides a striking example of the economic principle of diminishing returns. The greatest gain in clinical outcome comes from using the cheapest effective thrombolytic agent (streptokinase) for acute MI, which improves survival by 4% or more in absolute terms at a net cost of about $270 per patient. t-PA improves survival by a further 1% in absolute terms, but at an added cost of more than $1900 per patient. Thus, the cost-effectiveness of streptokinase relative to placebo ($450 per life-year added) is more favorable than the cost-effectiveness of t-PA relative to streptokinase ($27,100 per life-year added). Simple and cheap therapies usually provide most of the potential improvement in outcomes for a given clinical condition, with smaller and smaller marginal improvements coming at greater and greater cost. This example also illustrates the comparative nature of economic evaluations—the value of a treatment can be assessed only in light of the therapeutic alternatives.

Angioplasty (see Chap. 52)

Primary angioplasty for acute MI has been compared with thrombolytic therapy in several clinical trials, some of which also included an economic evaluation. A quantitative overview of randomized trials showed the survival of patients with acute MI treated with angioplasty is better than patients treated with thrombolysis.[8] The results of economic analysis have been less consistent, with primary angioplasty being less expensive in some studies but more expensive in others.[9-11] The net economic effect of primary angioplasty depends on the patterns of coronary angiography and revascularization in patients treated with thrombolysis. Primary percutaneous coronary intervention (PCI) strategy is relatively less expensive when angiography is routinely performed after thrombolysis, since many patients would have received PCI in the same admission anyway. The primary PCI strategy is more expensive when angiography is infrequent after thrombolysis, however, since primary PCI leads to expensive revascularization procedures that would not otherwise have been performed. A formal cost-effectiveness analysis of primary PCI relative to thrombolysis showed it to be cost-effective when performed in hospitals with existing cardiac angiography laboratories and minimal delay to therapy.[12] This analysis also suggested that it would not be economically justified to build new catheterization laboratories solely to provide primary PCI.[12]

Newer developments in primary coronary intervention for acute MI include the use of stents and adjunctive glycoprotein IIb/IIIa inhibitor therapy, each of which adds to the cost of the procedure. Formal economic evaluations have not yet been reported.

Anticoagulation and Antiplatelet Regimens (see Chap. 80)

Anticoagulant and antiplatelet regimens in the treatment of patients with unstable angina and acute MI have been investigated intensively in clinical trials. Since the newer agents of these classes tend to be more expensive than the standard alternatives (heparin, aspirin), economic evaluation is important. Economic evaluations are difficult to perform in these settings, however, because some or all of the benefit of these therapies comes from reducing nonfatal MI, not hospital mortality. The economic analysis must therefore assess the long-term value of preventing a nonfatal MI.

In one study, low-molecular-weight heparin (enoxaparin) improved clinical outcomes and lowered overall hospital costs relative to unfractionated heparin, largely because the $75 greater cost of enoxaparin was more than recouped by reducing the need for costly revascularization procedures in patients with recurrent ischemia.[13] The combination of better clinical outcomes and lower cost, termed a "dominant" strategy because no tradeoffs between cost and outcome are involved, is clearly economically attractive. Use of eptifibatide, a glycoprotein IIb/IIIa inhibitor, in patients with acute coronary syndrome improved clinical outcomes, primarily nonfatal MI, at a net cost of $1014 per patient. The cost-effectiveness ratio for this drug appears economically attractive ($16,500 per life-year added) based on the assumption that prevention of a nonfatal MI increases life expectancy by approximately 2 years.[14]

Cardiac Procedures and Devices

CORONARY BYPASS GRAFTING (see Chap. 50). In 2001, there were 305,000 coronary bypass surgeries in the United States, as well as 1,051,000 coronary angioplasty procedures.[15] With a total cost of roughly 20 billion dollars a year, the use of coronary revascularization procedures has spurred extensive economic evaluation.

Coronary artery bypass graft surgery (CABG) is an effective treatment for angina in symptomatic patients and extends life expectancy in patients with extensive coronary disease. An overview of randomized clinical trials of surgery versus medical therapy[16] suggests that patients with left main disease may live more than 0.6 years longer after CABG, patients with three-vessel disease may live more than 0.5 years longer, and patients with one- or two-vessel disease may live more than 0.16 years longer (life extension was estimated only over the first 10 years of follow-up). These data suggest that CABG is more economically attractive in patients with more extensive coronary disease at higher risk of death, since the absolute improvement in survival is greatest in these patients whereas the cost of the surgery is roughly the same. An early classic study[17] found that the cost-effectiveness of CABG versus medical therapy for left main disease was $3800 per year of life added, a highly favorable ratio. More recent analyses[18] confirm that the cost-effectiveness of CABG is most favorable in patients with higher clinical risk (more extensive coronary disease, reduced left ventricular function), and greater degrees of angina.

PERCUTANEOUS CORONARY INTERVENTION (see Chap. 52). Despite the extensive use of coronary angioplasty, few randomized trials have compared it with medical therapy. The RITA-2 trial[19] found better angina relief but more cardiac events in patients with stable angina treated by angioplasty compared with medical therapy. Economic data from RITA-2[20] documented that the higher initial cost among the angioplasty patients (2793 British pounds) was undiminished after 3 years of follow-up. A formal cost-effectiveness evaluation of angioplasty compared with medical therapy has not yet been reported.

Coronary angioplasty and bypass surgery have been directly compared in several randomized trials conducted in patients with multivessel disease. The clinical results of these studies have been quite consistent in showing significantly less angina and slightly lower mortality in surgery patients.[21] Economic analysis in the RITA,[22] EAST,[23] ERACI,[24]

BARI,[25] and ARTS[26] trials all documented significantly lower initial costs with coronary angioplasty, roughly one half to two thirds the cost of bypass surgery. The initial cost advantage of angioplasty was almost completely lost over the subsequent follow-up as a result of the frequent need for repeat coronary revascularization procedures among angioplasty-treated patients. At 5 to 8 years of follow-up, the total medical costs averaged 4% to 6% lower in balloon angioplasty patients than in surgery patients.[27,28] The introduction of coronary stents may alter the relative costs of angioplasty and bypass surgery.[26] While long-term follow-up has not yet been reported in the ARTS and SOS trials, which used stents extensively, 1-year follow-up of ARTS shows a $3000 cost advantage for the stent-assigned patients. Economic analysis suggests that bypass surgery is more cost-effective than angioplasty in patients with more extensive coronary disease (i.e., three-vessel disease), whereas angioplasty has a significant cost advantage in patients with less extensive disease, albeit with somewhat less angina relief.[25]

Coronary stents have now become a standard part of percutaneous revascularization. Stents reduce the need for emergency bypass surgery after initial angioplasty and significantly reduce the likelihood of restenosis and repeat revascularization.[29] Use of stents substantially increases the cost of the revascularization procedure, but the higher cost of the stent is only partially offset by the lower incidence of repeat revascularization.[30,31] Consequently, the total cost of patients treated with coronary stents remains 7% to 12% higher than that of patients treated with balloon angioplasty at 1 year of follow-up, with an equivalent incidence of death and nonfatal MI. Drug-coated stents have further reduced the rate of repeat revascularization procedures,[32] but the economic implications of these devices are uncertain. Preliminary data from the SIRIUS trial suggest that the $2880 higher initial cost of patients assigned to a sirolimus-coated stent was narrowed over 1 year of follow-up to only $309 by reduced costs of repeat revascularization procedures.[33] The clinical and economic effects of drug-coated stents in various patient groups are currently undefined and are the subject of ongoing investigation.

IMPLANTABLE CARDIOVERTER DEFIBRILLATOR (see Chap. 31). The implantable cardioverter defibrillator (ICD) has reduced total mortality by 26% among patients at high risk for sudden cardiac death.[34] Because implantation of a defibrillator costs $30,000 or more, many investigators have questioned whether the ICD is worth its high cost.

Several randomized trials have reported data on economic as well as clinical outcomes, including MADIT-1,[35] AVID,[36] and CIDS.[37] In each study, the early costs among ICD patients were considerably higher than those of conventionally treated patients (Table 2–1). Over the next 3 to 5 years, the ICD patients had lower costs, but these savings were only a fraction of the initial ICD cost. With randomized trials showing that ICD-treated patients have higher costs and reduced mortality, cost-effectiveness was performed based on primary data from the trials. The cost-effectiveness of the ICD was most favorable in MADIT-1 (US$27,000 per life-year added) and least favorable in CIDS (C$214,000 per life-year added), primarily because of the degrees of mortality reduction found in the two trials (54% versus 20%). A limitation of the cost-effectiveness analysis within randomized clinical trials is that some clinical benefits and costs occur only after longer follow-up and are not included in the analysis. Lifetime costs and survival were projected for patients with life-threatening ventricular arrhythmias by Owens and coworkers,[38] who found that a 26% relative risk reduction by the ICD translates to a cost-effectiveness ratio of $40,000 per year of life added, a ratio that is in the range generally acceptable in the United States. A current dilemma in health policy is whether prophylactic ICD placement is justified and is worth the expenditure of more than 1 billion dollars per year.

TABLE 2–1 Costs in Implantable Cardiac Defibrillator (ICD) Treated and Conventionally Treated Patients

Study	Costs		
	ICD	*Conventional*	*Difference*
MADIT-1[35] (US$)			
Initial therapy	44,565	18,880	25,685
4-year follow-up	52,995	57,100	–4,105
Total	97,560	75,980	21,580
AVID[36] (US$)			
Initial therapy	66,629	34,059	32,570
Follow-up	9,604	14,594	–4,990
Total	76,233	48,653	27,580
CIDS[37] (C$)			
Initial therapy	48,874	7,927	40,948
Follow-up	38,840	30,673	8,167
Total	87,715	38,600	49,115

These studies illustrate several general points about the economic evaluation of procedures and devices. The initial cost of procedures and devices is often quite high, but long-term follow-up is needed to assess the total net cost of the procedure relative to alternative therapies. An expensive procedure may have some or all of its incremental costs recouped through prevention of costly adverse events, such as in the case of bypass surgery relative to balloon angioplasty. The higher cost may be only partially offset by later savings (e.g, coronary stents) or barely recovered at all (e.g., implantable defibrillators). Nevertheless, high initial costs of procedures and devices may be justified if survival is sufficiently improved or quality of life enhanced. These considerations emphasize the importance of a long-term perspective in the economic evaluation of devices and procedures, so that their full costs and benefits can be assessed.

Chronic Disease: Heart Failure (see Chaps. 23, 24)

Economically efficient management of a chronic disease such as heart failure is very different from that of an acute illness or a surgical procedure. In cases of chronic diseases, the cost of care is spread over many years instead of being concentrated at the outset of treatment. Similarly, the benefits of treatment accrue only over a period of prolonged follow-up. Most medical care for chronic disease is delivered in an ambulatory, outpatient setting, and patient adherence to prescribed regimens has a substantial impact on the efficacy of therapy. Improvements in clinical and economic outcomes may come either from better therapies or from better ways to deliver established therapies, or both.

Angiotensin-converting enzyme inhibitors have significantly improved survival of patients with heart failure in randomized trials.[39] An economic appraisal of enalapril therapy based on the SOLVD trial results[40] suggested that the added cost of enalapril was completely offset by the cost savings from fewer hospitalizations for heart failure. Projections of lifetime costs and life expectancy performed using a model suggested that the net lifetime cost per patient was only $25 and that life expectancy was increased by 0.30 life years,[40] yielding an extremely favorable cost-effectiveness ratio of $83 per life-year added. An economic analysis based on the SAVE trial in patients with an ejection fraction less than 40% after an acute MI suggested that captopril therapy was economically attractive for this indication, with more favorable cost-effectiveness ratios in older patients than in younger patients.[41] An overview of economic analyses of heart failure treatment[42] suggests that the use of angiotensin-converting enzyme inhibitors is generally economically attractive.

An overview of randomized trials shows that beta blockade reduces mortality by 35% among patients with congestive heart failure,[43] with hospital admissions for heart failure reduced by a similar degree. A cost-effectiveness model based on published data from clinical trials found that beta blockers for heart failure have a cost-effectiveness ratio between $2500 and $6700 per life-year added,[44] which is certainly acceptable when judged against common benchmarks.

Most hospital admissions for heart failure result from lack of patient adherence to drug or dietary regimens,[45] suggesting that disease management programs could improve clinical outcomes and economic outcomes. An overview of 11 randomized trials[46] found that hospitalizations were reduced by 13% and overall costs were generally lowered by various disease management programs.

Disease Prevention (see Chap. 42)

Disease prevention is very important from a clinical perspective. Some preventive measures are very effective and inexpensive, as exemplified by vaccination programs for common infectious diseases that cut risk by more than 90% at the cost of only a few dollars. Most preventive measures are less effective in reducing the risk of disease and far more costly to implement. Vaccines are relatively inexpensive because they are given only two or three times, whereas drugs to lower serum cholesterol or high blood pressure are given daily for decades. Thus, the cost-effectiveness of preventive programs varies considerably according to the intervention, its effectiveness, and its cost.[47]

Hypercholesterolemia has long been established as a strong, consistent risk factor for coronary atherosclerosis, and HMG-CoA-reductase inhibitors ("statins") clearly reduce the risk of death and nonfatal cardiovascular events.[48] The cost-effectiveness of this class of drugs has been controversial, largely because of the heterogeneity of patients considered for lipid-lowering therapy. Secondary prevention trials have consistently shown substantial reductions in the absolute rate of cardiac events in patients treated with statins. The efficacy of cholesterol lowering in primary prevention (i.e., subjects at high risk of heart disease but without evidence of clinical disease) has been demonstrated in several large randomized trials.

The cost-effectiveness of HMG-CoA reductase therapy to prevent coronary heart disease varies from extremely favorable values in secondary prevention settings to quite unfavorable in some primary prevention settings.[49] The reason for this wide variation is that higher risk patients have a greater absolute benefit from treatment than lower risk patients. The 4S trial[50] of secondary prevention found that lipid-lowering treatment reduced mortality by 32 deaths per 1000 patients treated (Table 2–2). In contrast, the WOSCOPS study[51] of primary prevention found an absolute mortality difference of 5 per 1000 patients treated. The greater clinical efficacy of secondary prevention over primary prevention implies that lipid-lowering therapy is more economically attractive in the secondary prevention setting. Furthermore, the prevention of nonfatal myocardial infarction and revascularization offsets more of the cost of drug therapy in the secondary prevention setting, enhancing its economic attractiveness. Even within the primary prevention setting, treatment of higher risk patients (i.e., those with multiple risk factors, higher cholesterol levels) provides greater absolute risk reduction and hence is more cost-effective than is the treatment of lower risk patients. Formal cost-effectiveness studies suggest that primary prevention with HMG-CoA reductase therapy in low-risk patients is economically unattractive, whereas treatment of higher risk patients is quite cost-effective.[49,52] Clinical guidelines stress the importance of tailoring therapy to the patient's risk profile[53] to achieve optimal results.

Cigarette smoking clearly increases the risk of coronary heart disease events, with evidence of risk reduction after quitting in numerous nonrandomized studies. Although the effectiveness of a physician's advice to stop smoking is low, it does induce some smokers to quit, and because such advice has such a low cost, it has a favorable cost-effectiveness ratio of less than $1000 per year of life added.[54] Use of nicotine replacement strategies as part of a smoking cessation program adds to the number of patients who quit smoking and has a favorable cost-effectiveness ratio.[55] Hospital-based smoking cessation programs have also been shown to be cost-effective.[56] Smoking cessation is a particularly attractive preventive measure, since the interventions are generally short-term and of relatively low cost, and smoking cessation has highly beneficial effects on both cardiac and noncardiac diseases (e.g., various cancers, emphysema) and thus adds considerably to life expectancy.

Diagnostic Testing

Proper selection of diagnostic tests to evaluate various clinical problems has become more challenging as a result of the collision between the forces of technologic innovation, which develop many new tests to examine different facets of a particular disease, and the forces of economic restraint, which insist on their cost-effective use. Economic evaluation of diagnostic tests starts from the premise that the information provided by a test has value only if physicians use the information to change therapy and the change in therapy then improves clinical outcomes. Thus, the effectiveness of a test is gauged not solely by its information content but by its ultimate, indirect effects on patient outcomes.

Tests that provide clinical value do so by adding to what is already known about the patient. In practical terms, the test needs to add independent information to what is available from the clinical history, physical examination, and simpler, cheaper tests. The information value of myocardial perfusion scans in the diagnosis of coronary artery disease, for example, must be judged by how much unique diagnostic and prognostic information they add to the clinical examination and the simpler stress electrocardiogram. The evaluation of diagnostic tests by measuring the incremental value of information they provide is analogous to the way that therapies are evaluated by documenting what they add compared with the best available alternative (e.g., how much better is t-PA than streptokinase for treatment of acute MI). But the additional requirement placed on diagnostic tests is that they add enough information to modify decision-making. A test that is statistically more accurate does not provide value from an economic perspective unless the additional accuracy leads to improved clinical decisions. Demonstrations of a statistical improvement in diagnostic accuracy with new tests are common, but evaluations of the effects of this extra accuracy on clinical management are rare.

The evaluation of chest pain is a critical diagnostic problem that has been carefully analyzed in many studies. Early studies focused on the incremental information provided by noninvasive testing, most commonly the exercise electrocardiogram. These studies, by application of Bayes' rule, showed that the difference between pretest and posttest probability of disease was greatest among patients with an intermediate pretest probability of disease (i.e., between 15% and 85%). More recent

TABLE 2–2 Clinical and Economic Outcomes of Randomized Trials of Lipid-Lowering

	Reductions Per 1000 Patients (n)			Cost per Patient ($)		
Study	*Deaths*	*Myocardial Infarction*	*Revascularization*	*Drug Treatment*	*Complications Prevented*	*Net*
Primary prevention						
WOSCOPS	5	19	8	3700	100	3600
AFCAPS	4	26	31	4654	524	4130
Secondary prevention						
4S	32	47	59	4650	3900	780
CARE	11	18	47	5550	1660	3890

cost-effectiveness analysis extended the earlier studies by considering the health outcomes resulting from detecting (or failing to detect) underlying coronary disease amenable to coronary revascularization.[57-59] These analyses suggest that immediate coronary angiography is reasonable in patients with a very high pretest likelihood of coronary disease, such as an older man with typical exertional angina. In patients with an intermediate probability of coronary disease, noninvasive testing is generally economically attractive in comparison with no testing (cost-effectiveness ratios roughly $30,000 per QALY added), whereas coronary angiography without prior noninvasive testing is not (cost-effectiveness ratio >$65,000 per QALY added, depending on patient characteristics). Alternative noninvasive tests (exercise electrocardiography, exercise single photon emission computed tomography perfusion imaging, stress echocardiography) are close enough in cost-effectiveness that the determining factors in choosing among them are the likelihood of an indeterminate test result and the degree of local expertise with each alternative. The cost-effectiveness of all diagnostic strategies for chest pain are more favorable when stringent, outcome-based guidelines for coronary revascularization are followed.

The use of routine coronary angiography in survivors of acute MI has been controversial, in large part due to conflicting evidence on the efficacy of routine versus selective angiography practices.[60-63] The VANQWISH trial found that routine angiography initially cost $4500 more than a conservative, ischemia-guided strategy, and that this cost difference narrowed to $2200 after 1 years.[64] TIMI-18 found a similar pattern of costs, with the invasive strategy costing $1667 more initially, narrowing to $670 at 6 months' follow-up.[65] FRISC-II also found the invasive approach to be more costly over 1 year.[66] Thus, these clinical trials consistently found the invasive strategy to be more costly than a conservative ischemia-guided approach. The cost-effectiveness of the invasive strategy depended on the clinical results of the trial more than the economic outcomes. Studies that found better clinical results from the invasive strategy (TIMI-18 and FRISC-II) judged it cost-effective, whereas the trial that found poorer clinical outcomes in the invasive strategy (VANQWISH) judged it to be not economically attractive. A synthesis of the clinical and economic evaluations has not yet been performed, but these disparate findings underscore that economic assessment must be closely tied to clinical evaluation. While costs can be readily measured, determination of value requires weighing the added costs against the improvement in outcomes.

Developments in Economic Analysis

Cost-effectiveness analysis has been applied to clinical medicine for just over 20 years. The initial studies were based largely on decision models and related analytical methods and were of more interest to researchers than to clinicians. After considerable experience, consensus on some aspects of the methodology of economic analysis has been reached, although several areas of controversy remain.[1-3] The most important recent development in cost-effectiveness analysis has been the inclusion of economic endpoints as part of randomized trials, providing rigorous evaluation of the efficacy of therapies. As in all arenas of clinical research, the methods of economic evaluation in clinical trials have become more sophisticated, with application of economic models to extend clinical trial findings.[67] Future developments in cost-effectiveness analysis include wider application of economic evaluations in international settings, improved cost-identification methods, and continued development of statistical methods appropriate to cost and outcome data from clinical trials.[68]

REFERENCES

Law of Diminishing Returns

1. Russell LB, Gold MR, Siegel JE, et al: The role of cost-effectiveness analysis in health and medicine. Panel on Cost-Effectiveness in Health and Medicine. JAMA 276:1172, 1996.
2. Weinstein MC, Siegel JE, Gold MR, et al: Recommendations of the Panel on Cost-Effectiveness in Health and Medicine. JAMA 276:1253, 1996.
3. Siegel JE, Weinstein MC, Russell LB, et al: Recommendations for reporting cost-effectiveness analyses. Panel on Cost-Effectiveness in Health and Medicine. JAMA 276:1339, 1996.

Economies of Scale

4. McGrath PD, Wennberg DE, Dickens JD, et al: Relation between operator and hospital volume and outcomes following percutaneous coronary interventions in the era of the coronary stent. JAMA 284:3139, 2000.
5. Tu JV, Austin PC, Chan BTB: Relationship between annual volume of patients treated by admitting physician and mortality after acute myocardial infarction. JAMA 285:3116, 2001.

Analysis of Specific Interventions

6. Franzosi MG, Santoro E, De Vita C, et al: Ten-year follow-up of the first megatrial testing thrombolytic therapy in patients with acute myocardial infarction. Results of the Gruppo Italiano per lo Studio della Sopravivenza nell'Infarto-1 Study. Circulation 98:2659, 1998.

Acute Coronary Syndromes

7. Mark DB, Hlatky MA, Califf RM, et al: Cost effectiveness of thrombolytic therapy with tissue plasminogen activator as compared with streptokinase for acute myocardial infarction. N Engl J Med 332:1418, 1995.
8. Keeley EC, Boura JA, Grines CL: Primary angioplasty versus intravenous thrombolytic therapy for acute myocardial infarction: A quantitative review of 24 randomised trials. Lancet 361:13, 2003.
9. Gibbons RJ, Holmes DR, Reeder GS, et al: Immediate angioplasty compared with the administration of a thrombolytic agent followed by conservative treatment for myocardial infarction. N Engl J Med 328:685, 1993.
10. Stone GW, Grines CL, Rothbaum D, et al: Analysis of the relative costs and effectiveness of primary angioplasty versus tissue-type plasminogen activator: The primary angioplasty in myocardial infarction (PAMI) trial. J Am Coll Cardiol 29:901, 1997.
11. Every NR, Parsons LS, Hlatky M, et al: A comparison of thrombolytic therapy with primary coronary angioplasty for acute myocardial infarction. Myocardial Infarction Triage and Intervention investigators. N Engl J Med 335:1253, 1996.
12. Lieu TA, Gurley RJ, Lundstrom RJ, et al: Projected cost-effectiveness of primary angioplasty for acute myocardial infarction. J Am Coll Cardiol 30:1741, 1997.
13. Mark DB, Cowper PA, Berkowitz SD, et al: Economic assessment of low-molecular-weight heparin (enoxaparin) versus unfractionated heparin in acute coronary syndrome patients. Results from the ESSENCE randomized trial. Circulation 97:1702, 1998.
14. Mark DB, Harrington RA, Lincoff AM, et al: Cost effectiveness of platelet glycoprotein IIb/IIIa inhibition with eptifibatide in patients with non-ST elevation acute coronary syndromes. Circulation 101:366, 2000.

Coronary Procedures and Devices

15. Hall MJ, DeFrances CJ: 2001 National Hospital Discharge Survey. Advance data from vital and health statistics; no. 332. Hyattsville, MD, National Center for Health Statistics, 2003.
16. Yusuf S, Zucker D, Peduzzi P, et al: Effect of coronary artery bypass graft surgery on survival: Overview of 10-year results from randomised trials by the Coronary Artery Bypass Graft Surgery Trialists Collaboration. Lancet 344:563, 1994.
17. Weinstein MC, Stason WB: Cost-effectiveness of coronary artery bypass surgery. Circulation 66:III-56, 1982.
18. Wong JB, Sonnenberg FA, Salem DN, et al: Myocardial revascularization for chronic stable angina: Analysis of the role of percutaneous transluminal coronary angioplasty based on data available in 1989. Ann Intern Med 113:852, 1990.
19. RITA-2 Trial Participants: Coronary angioplasty versus medical therapy for angina: The second Randomised Intervention Treatment of Angina (RITA-2). Lancet 350:461, 1997.
20. Sculpher M, Smith D, Clayton T, et al: Coronary angioplasty versus medical therapy for angina: Health service costs based on the second Randomized Intervention Treatment of Angina (RITA-2) trial. Eur Heart J 23:1291, 2002.
21. Hoffman SN, TenBrook JA, Wolf MP, et al: A meta-analysis of randomized controlled trials comparing coronary artery bypass graft with percutaneous transluminal coronary angioplasty: One- to eight-year outcomes. J Am Coll Cardiol 41:1293, 2003.
22. Henderson RA, Pocock SJ, Sharp SJ, et al: Long-term results of RITA-1 trial: Clinical and cost comparisons of coronary angioplasty and coronary-artery bypass grafting. Lancet 352:1419, 1998.
23. Weintraub WS, Mauldin PD, Becker E, et al: A comparison of the costs of and quality of life after coronary angioplasty or coronary surgery for multivessel coronary artery disease: Results from the Emory Angioplasty Versus Surgery Trial (EAST). Circulation 92:2831, 1995.
24. Rodriguez A, Mele E, Peyregne E, et al: Three-year follow-up of the Argentine randomized trial of percutaneous transluminal coronary angioplasty versus coronary artery bypass surgery in multivessel disease (ERACI). J Am Coll Cardiol 27:1178, 1996.
25. Hlatky MA, Rogers WJ, Johnstone I, et al: Medical care costs and quality of life after randomization to coronary angioplasty or coronary bypass surgery. N Engl J Med 336:92, 1997.
26. Serruys PW, Unger F, Sousa JE, et al: Comparison of coronary-artery bypass surgery and stenting for the treatment of multivessel disease. N Engl J Med 344:1117, 2001.
27. Weintraub WS, Becker ER, Mauldin PD, et al: Costs of revascularization over eight years in the randomized and eligible patients in the Emory Angioplasty Versus Surgery Trial (EAST). Am J Cardiol 86:747, 2000.
28. Hlatky MA, Boothroyd DB, Johnstone IM: Economic evaluation in long-term clinical trials. Statist Med 21:2879, 2002.
29. Brophy JM, Belisle P, Joseph L: Evidence for use of coronary stents: A hierarchical Bayesian meta-analysis. Ann Intern Med 138:777, 2003.
30. Cohen DJ, Krumholz HM, Sukin CA, et al: In-hospital and one-year economic outcomes after coronary stenting or balloon angioplasty. Circulation 92:2480, 1995.

31. Serruys PW, van Hout B, Bonnier H, et al: Randomised comparison of implantation of heparin-coated stents with balloon angioplasty in selected patients with coronary artery disease (Benestent II). Lancet 352:673, 1998.
32. Morice M, Serruys PW, Sousa JE, et al: A randomized comparison of a sirolimus-eluting stent with a standard stent for coronary revascularization. N Engl J Med 346:1773, 2002.
33. Sorelle R: Cardiovascular news. Circulation 107:9024e, 2003.
34. Ezekowitz JA, Armstrong PW, McAlister FA: Implantable cardioverter defibrillators in primary and secondary prevention: A systematic review of randomized, controlled trials. Ann Intern Med 138:445, 2003.
35. Mushlin AI, Hall WJ, Zwanziger J, et al: The cost-effectiveness of automatic implantable cardiac defibrillators: Results from MADIT. Circulation 97:2129, 1998.
36. Larsen G, Hallstrom A, McAnulty J, et al: Cost-effectiveness of the implantable cardioverter-defibrillator versus antiarrhythmic drugs in survivors of serious ventricular tachyarrhythmias. Results of the Antiarrhythmics Versus Implantable Defibrillators (AVID) Economic Analysis Substudy. Circulation 105:2049, 2002.
37. O'Brien BJ, Connolly SJ, Goeree R, et al: Cost-effectiveness of the implantable cardioverter defibrillator: Results from the Canadian Implantable Defibrillator Study (CIDS). Circulation 103:1416, 2001.
38. Owens DK, Sanders GD, Harris RA, et al: Cost-effectiveness of implantable cardioverter defibrillators relative to amiodarone for prevention of sudden cardiac death. Ann Intern Med 126:1, 1997.

Chronic Disease: Heart Failure

39. Flather MD, Yusuf S, Køber L, et al: Long-term ACE-inhibitor therapy in patients with heart failure or left-ventricular dysfunction: A systematic overview of data from individual patients. Lancet 355:1575, 2000.
40. Glick H, Cook J, Kinosian B, et al: Costs and effects of enalapril therapy in patients with symptomatic heart failure: An economic analysis of the studies of left ventricular dysfunction (SOLVD) treatment trial. J Cardiac Fail 1:371, 1995.
41. Tsevat J, Duke D, Goldman L, et al: Cost-effectiveness of captopril therapy after myocardial infarction. J Am Coll Cardiol 26:914, 1995.
42. Weintraub WS, Cole J, Tooley JF: Cost and cost-effectiveness studies in heart failure research. Am Heart J 143:565, 2002.
43. Brophy JM, Joseph L, Rouleau JL: β-blockers in congestive heart failure: A Bayesian meta-analysis. Ann Intern Med 134:550, 2001.
44. Gregory D, Udelson JE, Konstam MA: Economic impact of beta blockade in heart failure. Am J Med 110:74S, 2001.
45. Chin MH, Goldman L: Factors contributing to the hospitalization of patients with congestive heart failure. Am J Public Health 87:643, 1997.
46. McAlister FA, Lawson FME, Teo KK, et al: A systematic review of randomized trials of disease management programs in heart failure. Am J Med 110:378, 2001.

Disease Prevention

47. Krumholz HM, Weintraub WS, Bradford WD, et al: Task Force #2—The cost of prevention: Can we afford it? Can we afford not to do it? J Am Coll Cardiol 40:603, 2002.
48. Ross SD, Allen IE, Connelly JE, et al: Clinical outcomes in statin treatment trials: A meta-analysis. Arch Intern Med 159:1793, 1999.
49. Prosser LA, Stinnett AA, Goldman PA, et al: Cost-effectiveness of cholesterol-lowering therapies according to selected patient characteristics. Ann Intern Med 132:769, 2000.
50. Scandinavian Simvastatin Survival Study Group: Randomised trial of cholesterol lowering in 4444 patients with coronary heart disease: The Scandinavian Simvastatin Survival Study (4S). Lancet 344:1383, 1994.
51. Shepherd J, Cobbe SM, Ford I, et al: Prevention of coronary heart disease with pravastatin in men with hypercholesterolemia. N Engl J Med 333:1301, 1995.
52. Brown AD, Garber AM: Cost effectiveness of coronary heart disease prevention strategies in adults. Pharmacoeconomics 14:27, 1998.
53. Third Report of the National Cholesterol Education Program (NCEP) Expert Panel on Detection, Evaluation, and Treatment of High Blood Cholesterol in Adults (Adult Treatment Panel III): Final report. Circulation 106:3143, 2002.
54. Cummings SR, Rubin SM, Oster G: The cost-effectiveness of counseling smokers to quit. JAMA 261:75, 1989.
55. Song F, Raftery J, Aveyard P, et al: Cost-effectiveness of pharmacological interventions for smoking cessation: A literature review and a decision analytic analysis. Med Decis Making 22(Suppl):S26-S37, 2002.
56. Meenan RT, Stevens VJ, Hornbrook MC, et al: Cost-effectiveness of a hospital-based smoking cessation intervention. Med Care 36:670, 1998.

Diagnostic Testing

57. Shaw LJ, Hachamovitch R, Berman DS, et al: The economic consequences of available diagnostic and prognostic strategies for the evaluation of stable angina patients: An observational assessment to the value of precatheterization ischemia. J Am Coll Cardiol 33:661, 1999.
58. Kuntz KM, Fleischmann KE, Hunink MG, et al: Cost-effectiveness of diagnostic strategies for patients with chest pain. Ann Intern Med 130:709, 1999.
59. Garber AM, Solomon NA: Cost-effectiveness of alternative test strategies for the diagnosis of coronary artery disease. Ann Intern Med 130:719, 1999.
60. Boden WE, O'Rourke RA, Crawford MH, et al: Outcomes in patients with acute non-Q-wave myocardial infarction randomly assigned to an invasive as compared with a conservative management strategy. N Engl J Med 338:1785, 1998.
61. FRagmin and Fast Revascularisation during InStability in Coronary artery disease (FRISC II) Investigators: Invasive compared with non-invasive treatment in unstable coronary-artery disease: FRISC II prospective randomised multicentre study. Lancet 354:708, 1999.
62. Cannon CP, Weintraub WS, Demopoulos LA, et al: Comparison of early invasive and conservative strategies in patients with unstable coronary syndromes treated with the glycoprotein IIb/IIIa inhibitor tirofiban. N Engl J Med 344:1879, 2001.
63. Fox KAA, Poole-Wilson PA, Henderson RA, et al: Interventional versus conservative treatment for patients with unstable angina or non-ST-elevation myocardial infarction: The British Heart Foundation RITA 3 randomised trial. Lancet 360:743, 2002.
64. Barnett PG, Chen S, Boden WE, et al: Cost-effectiveness of a conservative, ischemia-guided management strategy after non-Q-wave myocardial infarction: Results of a randomized trial. Circulation 105:680, 2002.
65. Mahoney EM, Jurkovitz CT, Chu H, et al: Cost and cost-effectiveness of an early invasive vs conservative strategy for the treatment of unstable angina and non-ST-segment elevation myocardial infarction. JAMA 288:1851, 2002.
66. Janzon M, Levin LA, Swahn E, et al: Cost-effectiveness of an invasive strategy in unstable coronary artery disease: Results from the FRISC II invasive trial. Eur Heart J 23:31, 2002.

Developments in Economic Analysis

67. Hlatky MA: Role of economic models in randomized clinical trials. Am Heart J 137:S41, 1999.
68. Diehr P, Yanez D, Ash A, et al: Methods for analyzing health care utilization and costs. Annu Rev Public Health 20:125, 1999.

CHAPTER 3

Clinical Decision-Making in Cardiology

J. Sanford Schwartz

Despite continuing significant advances in medical knowledge and technology, skilled clinical decision-making remains the cornerstone of medical practice. The goal of medical decision-making is to optimize patients' health and health care. This optimization requires integration and application of cognitive skills, medical knowledge, and judgment with social, cultural, and interpersonal sensitivity. Medical decision-making is a multistep process, involving problem identification, selection and assessment of diagnostic information, and choice of interventions.

Medical decision-making is challenging. Medical decisions involve high stakes and are characterized by imperfect information and complex problems that vary in presentation and response to treatment. Medical information is voluminous, widely dispersed, rapidly changing, often conflicting, and of uncertain validity and reliability. Important information is often not available.

All clinical information has diagnostic value, albeit imperfect and subject to error, with imperfect validity and reliability. Thus, all medical decisions are subject to some degree of uncertainty. Paradoxically, the tremendous progress of medical science, while enhancing our ability to diagnose and manage disease and disability, has made medical decision-making ever more complex and difficult.

Medical decision-making is further complicated by *variation* in disease among biological systems and in preferences and values across individuals; *uncertainty* of medical information; and *scarcity* of resources, with resulting need to allocate resources and address trade-offs among benefits, risks, and costs. The decision-making task is made more complex by social, organizational, economic, and environmental factors, including the need to incorporate the perspectives, preferences, values, and needs of patients, families, and providers; highly fragmented financing and delivery systems; inadequate clinical information systems; and misaligned incentives.

The goal of this chapter is to provide a basic framework for approaching, evaluating, and organizing medical information. The chapter discusses cognitive psychological, behavioral, and environmental aspects of decision-making; assessment and use of diagnostic tests; and evaluation and selection of medical practices and interventions. Decision-making related to resource constraints and cost-effectiveness, an increasingly important component of medical decision-making, is discussed in Chapter 2.

Cognitive, Behavioral, and Environmental Influences on Decision-Making

Decision-Making Models

Medical judgment is an inferential process applied to incomplete and inherently uncertain information, requiring integration of observational and diagnostic data with current understanding of disease processes and responses to interventions. Medical reasoning is complex and incompletely understood, involving a combination of heuristic, probabilistic, causal, and deterministic processes.

The first step in medical decision-making involves problem identification and definition through observation, clinical examination, and diagnostic testing. Generation and evaluation of diagnostic hypotheses provide a framework for collection and interpretation of diagnostic information. Medical reasoning and problem solving are iterative, involving modification, refinement, elimination, and addition of diagnostic alternatives. Hypotheses are verified for coherence, adequacy, and parsimony until a limited set of working hypotheses are produced.

Probabilistic reasoning explicitly considers the relationships and associations between clinical variables and is used to reduce the uncertainty inherent in medical decisions. Probabilistic reasoning consists of (1) estimation of prevalence (prior, preexisting, or pretest probability); (2) assessment of conditional probability (frequency of associations between variables and candidate diagnoses and normal individuals); and (3) mathematical calculation of revised probabilities.

Causal reasoning is fundamental to modern medical practice. Causal thinking provides a coherent conceptual framework for explaining clinical observations and outcomes by simulating the natural history of disease and determining the consistency among findings, scientific knowledge, and models of physiology and pathophysiology. Causal models are commonly used when abnormal findings or events are not congruent or compatible with normal physiology. The validity of causal models is a function of the strength, correlation, congruity, and contiguity in time between findings and events.

Deterministic (categorical) reasoning involves use of unambiguous rules derived from medical knowledge to simplify practice and reduce cognitive burden (e.g., ordered, simple structured algorithms to facilitate performance of specific clinical tasks). Frequently used for common, relatively straightforward problems, deterministic thinking is not well suited to complex problems, high levels of uncertainty, multiple complaints, and situations in which underlying logic cannot be precisely defined. Advances in information technology will enhance the utility and practical application of deterministic reasoning.

Heuristic Reasoning

Heuristics are shortcuts used to help cope with cognitive and psychological limitations and reduce information complexity to a manageable level. As expertise increases, data collection, interpretation, and action become more selective and more automatic. Although generally helpful, they may lead to predictable decision-making errors.

Information is interpreted in light of past experience and the context in which it occurs; perceptions are selective and strongly influenced by beliefs, experiences, and expectations. Knowledge and experience may accentuate the impact of preconceived notions on observations (e.g., the same heart sounds may be interpreted somewhat differently depending on what the physician expects to hear). Problem formulation and interpretation are influenced by how information is *framed* (e.g., information ordering or formatting, use of value-laden phrases, presenting events as gains or losses). For example, framing an alternative as trying to "help the patient" versus "doing nothing" biases the decision in favor of intervention.

Decision-making is influenced by inherent human psychological and cognitive factors and constraints. Short-term memory capacity is limited (the average person can consider only up to seven alternatives simultaneously). Memory is context dependent and fallible. Rather than representing accurate recall of past experiences or events, memories are reconstructed from separately stored pieces of information, with missing details filled in by logical inference, resulting in a new blended memory. Medical decisions can be distorted by "cognitive dissonance," aligning beliefs with behavior (either before or after the fact) to reduce or eliminate psychological inconsistencies and contradictions. Thus, before engaging in important medical decisions, physicians should consider how they are motivated by prior belief or expectation to interpret data and how the same findings might be otherwise interpreted in the absence of such motives and expectations.

Physicians often attempt to classify patients' conditions on the basis of their similarity to other patients' conditions (*representativeness).* Although often useful in formulating diagnoses or estimating response to therapy, the representativeness heuristic may, by inappropriately focusing on misleading or noninformative components of clinical presentation, lead to misestimated probabilities (e.g., the frequent underestimation of the probability of acute ischemia in women presenting with chest discomfort), failure to consider the prevalence of alternative possibilities, insensitivity to sample size (giving equal weight to large and small trials although observations based on larger samples should engender greater confidence than those derived from smaller samples), misconceptions of chance (e.g., assuming that if a rare adverse event occurs it will not occur again in the near future), regression to the mean (e.g., failing to recognize that patients tend to present when symptoms worsen and thus misattributing therapeutic benefit to normal waxing and waning of symptoms), and undercorrection for correlation (e.g., overestimating the value of diagnostic tests that measure highly correlated information).

Similarly, there is a tendency to estimate an event's likelihood by the ease with which its occurrence can be recalled (*availability)*, resulting in overestimating the probability of events that are familiar, salient, easily imaginable, or recent (e.g., the tendency to assess the likelihood that a patient will respond to a specific antihypertensive drug on the basis of one's experience the last several times the drug was prescribed rather than data from large, rigorous clinical trials) or attempting to predict events that are inherently not predictable (illusory correlation).

Diagnostic information is obtained in a temporal sequence, with initial probability estimates revised as new information becomes available. However, earlier probability estimates (even when based on incomplete information) are typically insufficiently adjusted for subsequent information (*adjustment and anchoring*). For example, initial information suggesting nonischemic chest pain (premenopausal woman) followed by information more suggestive of coronary artery disease (exertional substernal chest discomfort) may result in a lower estimate of the probability of coronary ischemia than if the order of information presentation was reversed. The tendency to view events that already happened as relatively inevitable and obvious (*hindsight bias)* also distorts probability estimates by assigning a higher pre-event probability after the fact than was estimated before the event.

Reduction of Psychological and Heuristic Errors

Cognitive errors occur in all stages of diagnostic reasoning—hypothesis generation, information gathering and processing, data diagnosis, and treatment. The best way to avoid or minimize such errors is to be aware of their existence and undertake conscious actions to override them. Thus, physicians should address the tendency to develop inappropriately narrow search sets by consciously considering alternative perspectives and expanding consideration of the range of potential diagnostic and therapeutic alternatives; reduce uncertainty of predictions by increasing confidence intervals, maintaining alternative hypotheses longer, replacing rejected hypotheses with new hypotheses (instead of just narrowing options as additional information is collected), and seeking and recognizing correlated information; vigilantly seek evidence that either supports competing diagnoses or does not support the working hypothesis, especially for rare but catastrophic conditions; keep accurate records; and explicitly consider why or how results might have turned out differently. Decision-making errors can also be reduced by recognizing common statistical errors, including the narrower confidence intervals associated with larger studies and greater experience, using regression to the mean, and distinguishing between association and causality and statistical versus clinical significance (as may occur in very large studies, where small differences may be statistically significant but not clinically important).

Behavioral and Environmental Influences

Medical decision-making is often presented as a rational, logical sequence, driven by dispassionate evaluation of scientific knowledge. However, medical decisions are influenced by a variety of behavioral, social, organizational, and environmental factors.

People are inherently social organisms; we take behavioral cues from and are concerned with how we are viewed by others (especially our patients and our colleagues). Increasingly, medical decisions are made in conjunction with other people. However, group judgment and decision-making are prone to biases, including insufficient consideration of challenging or disconfirming information, resulting in overconfidence and self-reinforcing judgments and behavior (group attribution error) and polarization of opinion. *Typically, groups perform better than the average member but not as well as the best member.* Errors attributable to group judgment and decision-making can be reduced by brainstorming independently rather than in a group and, within groups, encouraging dissent and criticism, refraining from stating personal preferences at the outset, and appointing a "devil's advocate." For particularly important decisions, decision-making may be improved by creating independent groups to consider the same question and inviting qualified outside experts and colleagues to challenge the group consensus.

*Physicians' characteristics (*age, knowledge, training, attitudes, experience, practice setting and organization, geographical location, social integration, personality traits, and general decision style such as attitude toward risk) influence decisions, as does *how information is communicated* (characteristics of the message, messenger, and the medium and setting in which it is communicated). Although medical information is communicated through a variety of channels (journals and textbooks, continuing medical education, professional societies, advertising, public media), opinion leaders are most influential. Characteristics of the information itself (e.g., cost, risk, ability to apply, ease of reversibility) also affect decisions.

Education (including clinical practice guidelines) has a major influence on decision-making. However, acceptance and credibility of education are a function of the sponsor, format and context, and previous education and training. Educational efforts can also be distorted or undermined if they conflict with other incentives, practice style, regulations, or professional and local norms and values.

The environment in which medicine is practiced also strongly influences medical decision-making. Administrative structure, process, and regulation can influence physicians' decision-making through construction or elimination of barriers and timely provision of cues, reminders, feedback, and support. However, unless particularly potent or cumbersome, such factors are often easily bypassed and rapidly extinguished. Feedback of credible, relevant data, especially by respected sources and provided on a timely basis (e.g., expert-generated computer reminders at the time of service), may strongly influence medical decisions. Monetary incentives are powerful influencers of decision-making and practice but are difficult to calibrate and must be aligned and consistent with professional, social, cultural, and organizational knowledge, values, and norms. Thus, a wide range of factors exert powerful influence on medical decisions, especially when aligned in combination with one another and reinforced over time.

Diagnostic Decision-Making

Diagnostic tests are used to define medical problems with sufficient precision to guide management of patients. Diagnostic tests are useful to the degree that they provide new information that beneficially affects subsequent diagnostic work-up, clinical management, and health outcome. New information alone is of little value if it does not alter patients' care or health.

Interpretation and use of a diagnostic test are driven by the clinical objective, the test's ability to discriminate between the presence or absence of disease, and the safety, efficacy, effectiveness, and cost-effectiveness of testing and therapy (Fig. 3–1).

For every clinical condition, there is a probability of disease above which intervention is indicated, the "test-treatment threshold," and a probability below which the disease can be excluded with sufficient confidence and other diagnostic possibilities considered, the "test–no treatment threshold." When the probability of disease is between these

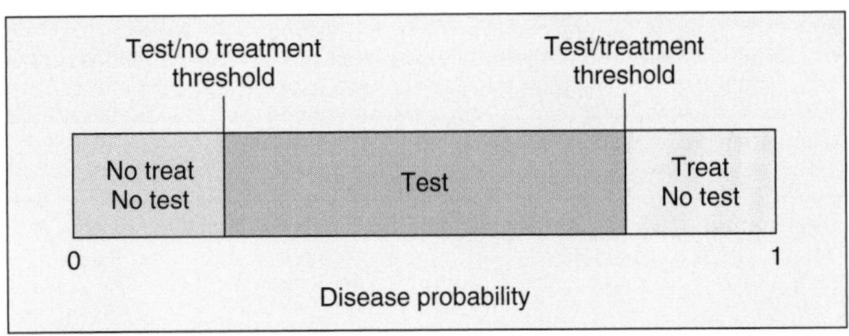

FIGURE 3–1 Schematic diagram of threshold theory of decision-making. (Adapted from Pauker SAG, Kassirer JP: The threshold approach to clinical decision making. N Engl J Med 302:1109, 1980.)

two thresholds, diagnostic tests, singly or in combination, are useful to the degree that they move the probability of disease either above the test-treatment threshold or below the test–no treatment threshold.

Treatment and testing thresholds are determined by diagnostic test performance characteristics (sensitivity and specificity) and the risks, costs, and benefits (mortality, morbidity, and quality of life) of treatment options. Less effective, riskier, or more costly therapy raises both the test-treatment threshold and the test–no treatment threshold (i.e., greater diagnostic certainty is required to institute treatment but less certainty is needed to exclude the disease). Conversely, less diagnostic certainty is required before instituting therapy or testing (lower test-treatment threshold and lower test–no treatment threshold) the more effective, safer, and less costly the treatment. Reduced test risk and cost and improved test performance widen the probability range in which testing is appropriate (higher test-treatment threshold and lower test–no treatment threshold), whereas increased test cost and risk and reduced sensitivity and specificity narrow the range for testing (lower test-treatment threshold and higher test–no treatment threshold). The more serious the disease (i.e., the greater its morbidity and mortality), the lower the test and treatment thresholds.

Diagnostic Test Performance

Although diagnostic tests must be both precise and reliable (yield a consistent result) and valid and accurate (yield a correct result), the primary measure of diagnostic test performance is the ability to distinguish between the presence and absence of a disease. An ideal diagnostic test perfectly discriminates those with disease (true positives [TPs]) and without disease (true negatives [TNs]). However, diagnostic tests detect markers imperfectly correlated with the presence or absence of disease. Thus, in their simplest dichotomous form (interpreted as either positive or negative), two types of misclassification errors occur: people free of a disease incorrectly classified as diseased (false-positives [FPs]) and people with a disease incorrectly classified as nondiseased (false-negatives [FNs]).

Before ordering a diagnostic test, the physician needs to consider the probability of the test's correctly identifying people with and without the disease. *Sensitivity* refers to the proportion of people with disease correctly identified by a diagnostic test, *specificity* the proportion of those without the disease correctly identified by the diagnostic test as nondiseased. When a test has been obtained, however, the physician needs to know the probability that a positive test correctly indicates the presence of disease *(predictive value positive [PV+])* and a negative test correctly identifies those without disease *(predictive value negative [PV–])* (Table 3–1).

For example, exercise stress test performance for detecting coronary ischemia among 1465 men with exercise-induced chest pain, with 1.0 mm of horizontal or downward-sloping

TABLE 3–1 Test Performance Characteristics

	Disease Present	Disease Absent	
Test positive	True-positive (TP)	False-positive (FP)	TP + FP
Test negative	False-negative (FN)	True-negative (TN)	FN + TN
	TP + FN	FP + TN	

Sensitivity = true positives/all patients with disease = TP/TP + FN.
Specificity = true negatives/all patients without disease = TN/TN + FP.
PV+ = true positives/all patients with positve tests = TP/TP + FP.
PV− = true negatives/all patients with negative tests = TN/TN + FN.

TABLE 3–2 Exercise Stress Test Performance Characteristics for Ischemic Congestive Heart Disease in Men Undergoing Cardiac Catheterization

	CHD Present			CHD Absent	
EST positive	815	TP	FP	115	**930**
EST negative	208	FN	TN	327	**535**
	1023			**442**	

Sensitivity = TP/TP + FN = TP/CHD+ = 815/1023 = 0.80.
Specificity = TN/TN + FP = TN/CHD− = 327/442 = 0.74.
PV+ = TP/TP + FP = TP/EST+ = 815/930 = 0.88.
PV− = TN/TN + FN = TN/EST− = 327/442 = 0.61.
CHD = congestive heart disease; EST = exercise stress test; FN = false-negative; FP = false-positive; PV = predictive value; TN = true-negative; TP = true-positive.
Adapted from Weiner DA, Ryan TJ, McCabe CH, et al: Exercise stress testing: Correlation among history of angina, ST-segment response and prevalence of coronary artery disease in the Coronary Artery Surgery Study (CASS). N Engl J Med 301:230, 1979.

ST segment depression, was compared with the resting baseline electrocardiogram (ECG) for at least 0.08 second (considered a positive test) and using the presence of 70 percent narrowing of one or more major coronary arteries on cardiac catheterization as the reference standard against which the exercise stress test was judged (Table 3–2).

Test sensitivity and specificity are not affected by disease prevalence or the pretest probability of disease. In contrast, PV+ increases and PV− decreases as the pretest probability of disease increases. Thus, the higher the prevalence or pretest probability of disease, the more likely a positive test result is to represent a true positive and the less likely a negative test result correctly identifies those without disease. If the pretest probability of disease is very high, even a negative test does not exclude the disease. Conversely, if the pretest probability of disease is very low, a positive test probably represents a false-positive result (Table 3–3).

Biases in Assessing Diagnostic Test Performance

Diagnostic test evaluation is frequently confounded by biases that tend to overstate the diagnostic test performance. The greater the discrepancy between study conditions and the setting in which the test is used, the less applicable the study results are to clinical practice.

REFERENCE ("GOLD") STANDARD PROBLEMS. Test performance should be assessed in relation to an independent reference ("gold") standard that establishes the presence or absence of a disease. However, true disease status is often hard to determine because of safety, cost, ethical, and scientific constraints. Imperfect reference standards result in misclassification errors, distorting estimates of test sensitivity

TABLE 3–3 Relationship Between Predictive Value of Positive Test and Disease Pretest Probability or Prevalence for Hypothetical Tests with Varying Test Sensitivity and Specificity

Pretest Probability	Sensitivity 0.90 Specificity 0.90	Sensitivity 0.95 Specificity 0.95	Sensitivity 0.99 Specificity 0.99
0.001	0.009	0.019	0.09
0.01	0.08	0.16	0.50
0.02	0.15	0.28	0.67
0.05	0.32	0.50	0.84
0.50	0.90	0.95	0.99

From Mulley AG: The selection and interpretation of diagnostic tests. *In* Goroll AH, May L, Mulley AG (eds): Primary Care Medicine. Philadelphia, Lippincott, 1987, p 7.

and specificity. For example, although coronary angiography is an appropriate reference standard for establishing a diagnosis of coronary vessel occlusion, it does not detect patients at increased risk for a cardiac event with nonocclusive coronary lesions (e.g., chemically unstable, thin-walled coronary plaque).

SPECTRUM BIAS. Diagnostic tests should be evaluated on a spectrum of diseased and nondiseased subjects sufficient to estimate test performance in clinically relevant subgroups, including healthy subjects with no disease as well as patients without the disease but with common comorbid conditions, recent onset of asymptomatic disease, established asymptomatic disease, established symptomatic disease, advanced disease, end-stage disease, and other diseases affecting the same anatomical organs. Evaluation of diagnostic tests on an unrepresentative sample results in overestimation of test sensitivity and specificity. For example, exercise stress test sensitivity varies with disease severity (highest in three-vessel disease; intermediate in other multivessel disease; lowest in non–left main single-vessel disease), lesion location (highest for left main lesions and progressively declining for left anterior descending, right coronary, and left circumflex lesions, respectively), and symptom presentation (highest in patients with classical exertional substernal discomfort)[1,2] (see Chap. 10).

REFERRAL, VERIFICATION, AND WORK-UP BIAS. Referral bias occurs when the outcome of the test being evaluated is used to determine which subjects are further evaluated by the reference standard (e.g., the more risky, expensive, or uncomfortable the reference standard, the greater this bias). The specificity of exercise radionuclide angiography was lower in practice than in initial published studies, as physicians used the test to select patients for further, more invasive evaluation by cardiac catheterization.[3] Because people with positive results on the test being evaluated are more likely to receive the reference test, work-up bias often overstates the sensitivity but underestimates the specificity of the test being evaluated.[4]

BLINDED INTERPRETATION. Results of the test being evaluated should be interpreted without knowledge of the reference standard test result or the true diagnosis. When such blinded, independent test interpretation does not occur, test sensitivity and specificity may be overestimated.

UNINTERPRETABLE RESULTS. Uninterpretable or nondiagnostic test results are common. A patient may not be able to exercise to the level of exertion required for a stress test; technicians vary in their ability to obtain high-quality echocardiograms of obese patients or to avoid attenuation of the inferior wall on single-photon emission computed tomography. Such uninterpretable test reports commonly are not included in calculation of diagnostic test performance, resulting in overestimation of test sensitivity, and are especially important when comparing alternative diagnostic tests when the frequency of uninterpretable test results differs among tests.

TEST-INTERPRETER UNIT. A diagnostic test's performance depends on both the test characteristics and the expertise of the person performing the test. This dependence is particularly important for many cardiac tests for which specifics of imaging agents, protocols, and technician and interpreter experience and skill affect test performance. The more important such factors, the more difficult it is to compare or generalize diagnostic performance across tests, interpreters, and sites.

Selection and Use of Diagnostic Tests

True-positive results allow selection of appropriate management, reduce patients' morbidity and mortality, and improve patients' function. True-negative results provide reassurance and avoid unnecessary risk, inconvenience, and cost. In contrast, false-positive results lead to unnecessary testing and treatment and can increase anxiety, and false-negative results lead to delayed or missed diagnosis and treatment, with associated adverse outcomes, unnecessary testing, and increased uncertainty and anxiety.

Tests with high sensitivity are preferred when the costs of missing a diagnosis are high; treatment is effective, safe, and inexpensive; false-positive results do not result in serious harm; and the goal is to minimize false-negative results (as in screening or when attempting to exclude a disease). Tests with high specificity are desired when the goal is to minimize false-positive results: the lower the effectiveness and the greater the risk and expense of therapy (e.g., surgery), the more false-positive results cause serious harm.

Selection of diagnostic tests varies according to the diagnostic process stage (Table 3–4). For example, although a history of chest discomfort has modest sensitivity for clinically significant acute ischemic coronary heart disease, it is not specific (i.e., has a high false-positive rate). Thus, physicians commonly evaluate such patients with an imaging test (e.g., exercise stress test, stress echocardiography, nuclear stress test) that, although more expensive and difficult to perform, has higher sensitivity. However, tests with very high specificity (e.g., coronary angiography) are required before initiating expensive or risky interventions.

The clinician can optimize sensitivity and specificity either by carefully selecting among alternative tests with different test performance characteristics or by altering the cutoff point of a test to emphasize *either* sensitivity *or* specificity (but not both simultaneously).

TABLE 3–4 Test Performance Characteristics Desired at Different Stages of Diagnosis

Objective	Desire	Avoid	Risk	Cost
Screening, case finding	High sensitivity	FN	Minimal	Low
Disease exclusion, R/O disease	High sensitivity	FN	Minimal-moderate	Low-moderate
Disease confirmation, R/in disease	High specificity	FP	Minimal-high	Low-high

FN = false-negative; FP = false-positive; R/in = rule in; R/O = rule out.

Screening

Diagnostic tests are commonly used for screening (detection of disease or elevated risk of disease in apparently well patients prior to the onset of symptoms). Because of the low prevalence of disease among screened populations, tests used for screening purposes always produce a high false-positive rate (low PV+). Unless screening is confined to a population at very high risk (50 percent), even the best screening tests yield more false-positive than true-positive results. Furthermore, the large majority of people being screened do not benefit. Thus, screening is best confined to serious diseases for which safe and effective treatment exists and early detection and treatment significantly improve patients' outcomes. A screening test itself must have high sensitivity (to minimize false-negative results) and specificity and be safe, inexpensive, convenient, and acceptable to the targeted screening population. In addition, because performance of the screening test will result in many false-positive results, appropriate follow-up tests with sufficiently high diagnostic performance and safety and reasonable cost must be available to identify and exclude those without the disease and to confirm the presence of disease in those affected. For this reason, generally even the best screening tests are best confined to populations and patients at increased risk for disease as determined by known risk factors.

The effectiveness and benefits of screening tests and screening testing programs are often overestimated. In deciding whether to screen for a disease, one must determine whether early diagnosis improves outcome. A common pitfall in the evaluation of screening programs is to measure the time between disease detection and death. *Lead time*, the interval between disease detection by screening and the time of usual symptomatic diagnosis, is a function of the rate of biological progression of a disease and screening test sensitivity. Screening effectiveness is often overestimated as a result of artifactual survival prolongation resulting from earlier disease detection in the absence of increased effectiveness of earlier intervention (*lead time bias*); enhanced participation by people more likely to adhere to recommended therapy (*adherence* or *compliance bias*); and unrepresentative impact of detection of prevalent cases in early screening cycles, which have a disproportionate number of slowly progressive cases relative to a larger proportion of more rapidly progressive incident cases in subsequent screening cycles (*prevalence bias*). Therefore, it is essential that promising screening tests and programs be rigorously evaluated by randomized clinical trials over multiple screening cycles before being widely adopted.

Information Content

A diagnostic test's value is a function of the amount of new additional information provided. Even the best diagnostic test does not contribute new diagnostic information when one is certain that the disease either is present or absent. Conversely, diagnostic tests provide the greatest diagnostic information the more uncertain one is prior to testing (intermediate prevalence or pretest probability).

Diagnostic tests are commonly interpreted dichotomously as either positive or negative. The information content of a diagnostic test is greater when one also considers the degree of positivity, as a slightly abnormal test is more likely to be a false-positive result than a markedly abnormal test, which is more likely to be a true-positive. For example, an exercise stress test with 3 mm of ST segment depression at an early stage of exercise is more likely to be a true-positive than an exercise stress test with 1 mm of ST depression at high levels of extended exertion. Similarly, a strongly negative test result is more likely to represent a true-negative than a slightly negative test result, which is more likely to be a false-negative. Borderline test results are commonly of limited diagnostic value. Thus, considering the extent of exercise stress test positivity provides approximately one-third more diagnostic information than interpreting the test as either positive or negative.[5,6]

Use of Likelihood Ratios in Clinical Practice

Sensitivity and specificity are difficult to use clinically because of the computational complexity of revising probabilities. Odds ratios (and likelihood ratios, which express test performance in terms of odds) are interchangeable with probabilities (Table 3–5), can be multiplied by each other, and thus are easier to use to revise disease probability at the bedside.

The likelihood ratio of a positive test (LR+) represents the TP/FP ratio for an interval test result and is obtained by calculating the probability of the positive test result among diseased subjects divided by the probability of the same positive test result among nondiseased subjects.

$$LR+ = \frac{\text{probability (result x)/patients with disease}}{\text{probability (result x)/patients without disease}}$$

TABLE 3–5 Conversion Between Probability and Odds

Odds	Probability
9 : 1	0.90
4 : 1	0.80
3 : 1	0.75
2 : 1	0.67
1 : 1	0.50
1 : 2	0.33
1 : 3	0.25
1 : 4	0.20
1 : 9	0.10

$$\text{Odds} = \frac{\text{probability}}{1-\text{probability}}$$

Pretest odds × likelihood ratio = posttest odds

where

$$\text{Pretest odds} = \frac{\text{pretest probability disease}}{1-\text{pretest probability disease}}$$

$$\text{Posttest odds} = \frac{\text{posttest probability disease}}{1-\text{pretest probability disease}}$$

or

$$LR+ = \frac{\text{sensitivity}}{1-\text{specificity}}$$

$$= \frac{\text{probability of T+/patients with disease}}{\text{probability of T+/patients without disease}}$$

An LR+ greater than 1 indicates that the posttest probability of disease is greater than the pretest probability of disease, whereas an LR+ less than 1 indicates that the test result lowered the probability of disease (i.e., the posttest probability of disease is lower than the pretest probability of disease). The higher a test's likelihood ratio, the more likely the test result is to occur in a person with the disease as opposed to a person who is free of the disease, the more likely it is to be a true-positive, and the higher the posttest probability of disease. By providing information for ranges of test results, likelihood ratios maximize the information provided by diagnostic tests. A simple nomogram can be used to convert subjective estimated pretest probability of disease to posttest disease probability for a given LR+, facilitating its clinical use. A literature-based pooled estimate of the diagnostic performance of exercise stress test for congestive heart disease in patients with chest pain syndromes was developed by Diamond and colleagues[7] for various magnitudes of exercise-induced horizontal or downward-sloping ST segment depression, using 50 percent diameter narrowing of at least one coronary artery as the reference standard. Using a dichotomous result criterion of 1.0 ST segment depression as a positive test, exercise stress test sensitivity 0.65 and specificity 0.89. Considering the *degree* of test positivity improves discrimination between those with and without disease (Table 3–6 and Fig. 3–2).

Receiver Operating Characteristic Curves

Diagnostic test sensitivity and specificity depend on the cutoff point chosen between a normal and an abnormal test result. Selection of a cutoff point such that no disease-free people are incorrectly categorized as having disease (specificity = 1.0) results in many false-negative results and low test sensitivity. Conversely, a cutoff point that results in correct identification of all people with disease (sensitivity = 1.0) misclassifies disease-free people as having disease (increased FP), resulting in low test specificity.

A receiver operating characteristic curve is a plot of test sensitivity versus 1 – specificity as the definition of positive test is varied across the full range of clinically relevant values.[8] Table 3–7 illustrates the trade-offs among test sensitivity (true-positive rate), specificity (true-negative rate), and 1 – specificity (false-positive rate) for alternative ST segment positivity criteria for the exercise stress test.

TABLE 3–6 Interval Exercise Stress Test Likelihood Ratios

EST Positivity Criteria (mm ST Segment Depression)	Sensitivity (TP Rate)	1 – Specificity (FP Rate)	Likelihood Ratio (Sensitivity/1 – Specificity)
$0.0 \le ST < 0.5$	0.143	0.625	0.23
$0.5 \le ST < 1.0$	0.208	0.227	0.92
$1.0 \le ST < 1.5$	0.233	0.110	2.12
$1.5 \le ST < 2.0$	0.088	0.021	4.19
$2.0 \le ST < 2.5$	0.133	0.012	11.08
$2.5 \le ST$	0.195	0.005	39.0

EST = exercise stress test; FP = false-positive; TP = true-positive.
Adapted from Diamond GA, Forrester JS: Analysis of probability as an aid in the clinical diagnosis of coronary-artery disease. N Engl J Med 300:1350, 1979.

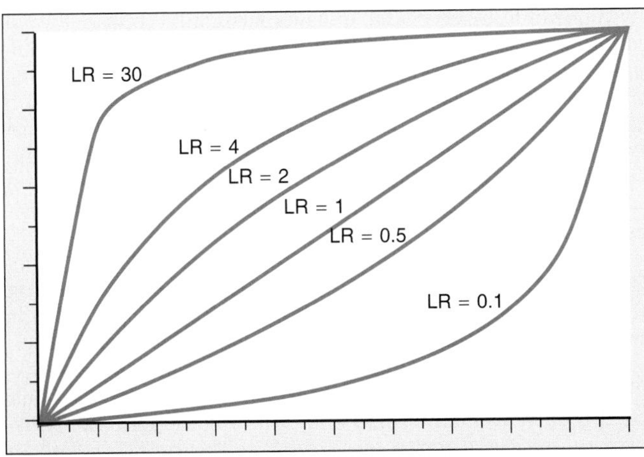

FIGURE 3–2 Relationship of alternative diagnostic test likelihood ratios for a positive test result to pretest and posttest disease probability.

TABLE 3–7 Relationship Between ST Segment Depression Criterion and Exercise Stress Test Sensitivity and Specificity

ST Segment (mm)	Sensitivity	Specificity	1 – Specificity
≥0.5	0.86	0.77	0.23
≥1.0	0.65	0.89	0.11
≥1.5	0.42	0.98	0.02
≥2.0	0.33	0.99	0.01
≥2.5	0.20	0.995	0.005

From Diamond GA, Forrester JS: Analysis of probability as an aid in the clinical diagnosis of coronary artery disease. N Engl J Med 300:1350, 1979.

Given the inherent trade-off between sensitivity and specificity as a test's positivity criterion is varied over a range of cutoff points,[9,10] it is not appropriate or informative to discuss either test sensitivity or specificity without consideration of the other, as test sensitivity can always be increased by adopting a more lenient positivity criterion but only at the expense of decreased specificity and vice versa.

The optimal diagnostic test cutoff point is a function of disease prevalence and estimated pretest probability of disease; test sensitivity and specificity; and the risks, costs, and benefits of correct and incorrect diagnoses (themselves a function of disease severity and the safety, effectiveness, and cost of therapeutic interventions).

$$\frac{\text{sensitivity}}{1-\text{specificity}} = \frac{\text{net cost TN} - \text{net cost FP}}{\text{net cost TN} - \text{net cost FN}} \times \frac{\text{posttest probability no disease}}{\text{posttest probability disease}}$$

Published diagnostic test cutoff points are generally more subjectively determined and thus may not be the most appropriate clinical values to use.

COMPARISON OF PERFORMANCE OF ALTERNATIVE DIAGNOSTIC TEST SYSTEMS. The performance of competing diagnostic tests must be compared over a range of cutoff points, which requires a receiver operating characteristic curve. When using receiver operating characteristic curves to compare the performance of competing diagnostic tests, the superior diagnostic technology is higher and farther to the left in the receiver operating characteristic curve (i.e., sensitivity is greater for any given level of specificity and vice versa), and the greater the area under the receiver operating characteristic curve (or the greater the ROC curve area within a clinically relevant range of test cutoff points), the better the diagnostic test.[7]

TABLE 3–8 Combination Testing: Exercise Stress Test and Radionuclide Angiocardiography

Test Combination Positivity Criterion	Sensitivity	Specificity
EST	0.88	0.46
RNA	0.92	0.34
EST or RNA	0.96	0.29
EST and RNA	0.65	0.68

EST = exercise stress test; RNA = radionuclide angiocardiography.
Campos CT, Chu HW, D'Agostino HJ Jr, Jones RH: Comparison of rest and exercise radionuclide angiocardiography and exercise treadmill testing for diagnosis of anatomically extensive coronary artery disease. Circulation 67:1204, 1983.

Using Tests in Combination

For most problems, multiple diagnostic tests are used in combination to provide the diagnostic information required to guide patients' management. Multiple testing offers the advantages of increased information, improved diagnosis, speed of diagnosis, convenience, and, in some circumstances, reduced cost. However, multiple tests expose patients to increased risks and costs and, at times, diagnostic and therapeutic delay. In addition, as the number of diagnostic tests performed increases, the opportunity for discrepancies among test results increases substantially, increasing the complexity of test interpretation.

When multiple tests are performed, one must adopt criteria for interpreting discrepant test combinations. A test combination may be interpreted as positive if *all* tests are positive (conjunctive positivity criterion). Conversely, a test combination may be interpreted as positive if *any* of the tests performed are positive (disjunctive positivity criteria). Disjunctive criteria for interpreting test combinations increase sensitivity and decrease specificity relative to the individual tests, whereas conjunctive criteria decrease sensitivity but increase specificity relative to the individual tests (Table 3–8).

Thus, conjunctive criteria are preferred when false-positive results are undesirable and specificity is to be maximized. Disjunctive testing is used when false-negative results are undesirable and sensitivity is to be maximized.

TEST CORRELATION AND CONDITIONAL DEPENDENCE. Tests used in combination are often partially correlated with each other. The greater correlation among tests, the less additional information gained from using tests in combination. Tests that measure different aspects of a suspected pathological condition or use different methods of diagnosis (e.g., serological tests and imaging tests) are more likely to provide independent information than test combinations using similar methods.

SEQUENTIAL VERSUS CONCURRENT TESTING. When tests are used in combination, they can be performed either concurrently or sequentially, with performance of subsequent tests based on the results of previous tests. Concurrent test strategies result in faster diagnosis but involve performance of more tests than sequential testing. Thus, sequential testing is generally more appropriate when problem evolution is slow and when costs of slower diagnosis are lower (e.g., outpatients), test risk is high, and the costs of delayed therapy are low. Concurrent testing is preferred when problem evolution is rapid and costs of delay are high (e.g., hospitalized patients), test risk is low, and costs of delayed treatment are high.

Therapeutic Decision-Making

The goal of therapy is to improve the patient's outcome and health. Medical interventions are assessed in terms of *safety* (acceptable side effects), *efficacy* (net benefit under ideal conditions), *effectiveness* (net benefit under routine conditions), and *cost-effectiveness* (incremental benefits relative to incremental costs). Because all interventions in practice have some benefit and risk, the challenge is to determine the trade-offs between benefit and risk in specific patients (i.e., how much net benefit, in which patients, under what conditions).

Therapeutic decision-making requires (1) identifying and defining the potential courses of action, (2) estimating the various potential resulting outcomes and their likelihood of occurrence, (3) assessing the value of each outcome on the basis of the trade-offs between risk and benefit (especially difficult when selecting among alternative competing options), and (4) assessing how patients value alternative outcome states. Although most clinical decisions are made subjectively using a combination of approaches and principles previously discussed, quantitative decision support methods can assist the physician with this complex and challenging task.

Predictive models use various forms of statistical and mathematical regression and related techniques (e.g., neural networks) to identify a parsimonious set of clinical variables that predict a disease state or outcome of therapy. For example, the Jones criteria provide a predictive model for rheumatic fever (see Chap. 82), Framingham risk equations estimate risk of developing congestive heart disease (see Chaps. 21 and 22), and models have been developed to predict the risk of coronary artery bypass graft surgery and coronary angioplasty (see Chap. 52). Predictive models are merely mathematical diagnostic tests, and their interpretation and use are thus subject to the principles described previously for diagnostic tests.

Decision support models are used for a wide range of clinical decisions, ranging from complex problems characterized by high uncertainty, risk, or cost to standardization of management for common, routine problems. Decision models (of which decision analysis is currently the most common and familiar) are prescriptive decision aids (i.e., they seek to improve medical decision-making by proposing how decisions should be made rather than describing how decisions actually are made). In addition to help in guiding clinical decisions, such models are particularly useful for informing clinical decision-making: organizing the salient issues for traditional clinical decision-making, identifying (through single-variable or multivariable sensitivity analysis, where the point estimates of model parameters are varied across a range of plausible values) the critical elements that drive decisions and therefore need to be most precisely defined, and explicitly clarifying trade-offs among safety, effectiveness, and cost.

Decision support models structure clinical decisions, precisely defining the question to be addressed; identifying relevant exhaustive, mutually exclusive alternative actions that may be undertaken and their potential outcomes; and estimating the probability that events will occur and their associated costs and values (i.e., "utilities"). Parameter values are estimated and integrated from the best available experimental (randomized trials), quasiexperimental (observational cohort and case-control studies), and nonexperimental (meta-analysis, models, expert opinion) studies. The expected value of each decision path is calculated and aggregated at each decision node, with the decision providing the highest expected utility the preferred management option. Sensitivity analyses identify the impact of alternative estimates on outcome and decisions and provide an estimate of the robustness of findings.

The primary advantage of decision modeling is its structured, explicit nature, which forces systematic examination of the problem and assignment of explicit values, avoids information processing errors, and focuses attention on parameters that drive clinical decisions. The primary disadvantages are their complexity to develop and explain and the difficulty in maintaining and updating the models. Thus, even when not directly applicable at the point of care of patients, such models are extremely useful for informing general clinical approaches and for guiding development of clinical guidelines.

In theory, in making decisions the physician should act as the patient's agent, choosing the management option the patient would prefer if the patient possessed the same medical information as the physician. For many medical problems there is more than one reasonable management alternative, and the choice is frequently driven by the patient's values and preferences for alternative beneficial outcomes and tolerance for potential adverse events and effects of disease sequelae. Because the physicians' knowledge of the patients' preferences and values is generally incomplete, patients' values and preferences in terms of risk and various potential benefits need to be identified and incorporated into clinical decisions.

Decision support interventions and systems are increasingly attractive methods to supplement physicians' knowledge, providing physicians with reminders and cues by providing timely feedback. However, decision support systems are complex to develop, keep current, and implement, although timely support is facilitated by increasing computerization and especially by the advent of computerized medical record systems.[9-11]

REFERENCES

1. Pauker SG, Kassirer JP: Decision analysis. N Engl J Med 316:250, 1987.
2. Black ER, Panzer RJ, Mayewski RJ, Griner PF: Characteristics of diagnostic tests and principles for their use in quantitative decision making. *In* Black ER, Bordley DR, Tape TG, Panzer RJ (eds): Diagnostic Strategies for Common Medical Conditions. Philadelphia, American College of Physicians, 1999, p 7.
3. Mulley AG: The selection and interpretation of diagnostic tests. *In* Goroll AH, May L, Mulley AG (eds): Primary Care Medicine. Philadelphia, Lippincott, 1987, p 7.
4. Froelicher VF, Myers J: Exercise and the Heart. 3rd ed. Philadelphia, WB Saunders, 1999.
5. Choi BC: Sensitivity and specificity of a single diagnostic test in the presence of work-up bias. J Clin Epidemiol 45:581, 1992.
6. Begg CB, Greenes RA, Iglewicz B: The influence of uninterpretability on the assessment of diagnostic tests. J Chron Dis 39:575, 1986.
7. Diamond GA, Forrester JS: Analysis of probability as an aid in the clinical diagnosis of coronary-artery disease. N Engl J Med 300:1350, 1979.
8. Diamond GA, Hirsch M, Forrester JS, et al: Application of information theory to clinical diagnostic testing. The electrocardiographic stress test. Circulation 63:915, 1981.
9. Hershey JC, Cebul RD, Williams SV: Clinical guidelines for using two dichotomous tests. Med Decis Making 6:68, 1986
10. Schwartz JS, Kinosian B, Pierskalla W, Lee H: Strategies for screening blood for HIV virus antibody: Use of a decision support system. JAMA 264:1704, 1990.
11. Schwartz JS, Dans PE, Kinosian BP: Human immunodeficiency virus test evaluation, performance, and use: Proposals to make good tests better. JAMA 259:2574, 1988.

CHAPTER 4

Measurement and Improvement of Quality of Cardiovascular Care

Thomas H. Lee

Measurement of Quality

In recent years, the measurement and improvement of quality of cardiovascular care have grown in importance due to several factors, including methodological advances in measurement of quality and changes in the health care environment. This trend has been made possible by clinical research that has helped define "evidence-based medicine" for cardiovascular disease—that is, knowledge of which interventions improve patient outcomes. Insight into which interventions should be delivered has naturally led to interest in the reliability with which high-quality care is delivered. At first, health services researchers were the main users of data on quality of cardiovascular care, but today their methods are widely used in quality improvement programs and in publicly available "report cards" for insurance plans, hospitals, and individual physicians.

Interest in such report cards has been intensified by public concerns about quality in the United States and other countries. In 1999, the U.S. Institute of Medicine issued a report that showed serious problems stemming from medical errors leading to harm to patients.[1] In 2001, a follow-up report entitled "Crossing the Quality Chasm" identified major system problems as the source of many errors.[2] During this period, organizations in several countries began disseminating information on quality of care by health care providers to the public to encourage the development of a consumer-based marketplace in which patients use data to improve the quality of their care.[3]

A third report from the Institute of Medicine, released in 2002,[4] recommended that "purchasing strategies should provide rewards to providers who achieve higher levels of quality." Particularly in the United States and England, the health care marketplace began witnessing the introduction of a variety of incentive programs that reward physicians and hospitals whose performance data suggest superior care.

In fact, measurement of quality of cardiovascular care had been building momentum throughout the 1990s, and numerous agencies in the United States are actively involved in the development of measures and dissemination of data (Table 4–1).[5] Statewide report cards on cardiac surgery and percutaneous coronary interventions for hospitals and individual physicians have been introduced in some states.[6-8] The National Committee for Quality Assurance (NCQA) developed measures of quality for managed care organizations known as HEDIS (Healthplan Employers Data and Information Set).[9,10] Most recently, measures for cardiovascular quality of care delivered by hospitals have been introduced by the Joint Commission on Accreditation of Healthcare Organizations (JCAHO),[11] and data on volume of cardiovascular procedures have been disseminated via organizations such as Leapfrog.[12] This phenomenon has not been limited to the United States; detailed data on cardiovascular and other outcomes are available via the Internet for hospitals in the United Kingdom[13] and other countries.

GUIDELINES AND PERFORMANCE MEASURES. Amid calls for caution and expression of concern, health care professionals have responded with a variety of initiatives aimed at improving care. The most prominent of these responses in cardiovascular medicine has been the development of guidelines, particularly those from the American College of Cardiology (ACC) and the American Heart Association (AHA).[14,15] These guidelines often provide the basis for measures of quality (also known as performance measures), but serve a different purpose. Guidelines are written to describe a consensus on the diagnostic or therapeutic interventions appropriate for most patients in most circumstances. Guidelines are written with the expectation that individual physicians will use discretion in the treatment of individual patients, and *not* follow the guidelines in certain cases. Key guidelines are summarized in this text.

In contrast, performance measures build upon the consensus expressed in guidelines to define "rules" or standards of care. As summarized by an AHA/ACC working group, "Performance measures should be explicit actions, performed for carefully specified, easily identified (using clear administrative and/or easily documented clinical criteria) patients for whom adherence should be advocated in all but the most unusual circumstances".[16] When these standards are not met, the implication is that an error has occurred (e.g., failure to recommend aspirin for patients with acute myocardial infarction).

Therefore, performance measures tend to be written to define the minimum standards of adequate care, as opposed to the targets that might define excellent care. For example, NCQA uses a HEDIS measure for cholesterol management in patients who have had acute myocardial infarction, coronary artery bypass graft surgery, or percutaneous coronary interventions. Guidelines from the National Heart, Lung, and Blood Institute encouraged physicians to pursue a target low-density lipoprotein (LDL) cholesterol level below 100 mg/dl for this population,[17] but, as of 2003, the HEDIS measure required managed care organizations to report the percent-age of such patients who achieved an LDL level below 130 mg/dL. The NCQA rationale was that although experts agreed that a level below 100 mg/dl reflects excellent care, the strength of evidence is such that physicians should be faulted only if they allowed patients with coronary disease to have a level above 130 mg/dl.[18]

The practical implication of this relationship between performance measures and guidelines in cardiovascular medicine is that quality measures are usually closely linked to class I indications from the ACC/AHA guidelines—that is, conditions for which there is evidence or general agreement that a given procedure or treatment is useful and effective. Failure to perform

TABLE 4–1 Key Organizations Involved in Measurement of Quality of Cardiovascular Care

Organization	Major Activity	Focus	Web Site
American College of Cardiology (ACC)	Guidelines Applied in Practice (GAP) ACC/AHA Task Force on Performance Measures	Health care providers	www.acc.org
American Heart Association (AHA)	Get with the Guidelines ACC/AHA Task Force on Performance Measures	Health care providers	www.americanheart.org
American Medical Association (AMA)	Physician Consortium for Quality Improvement	Physicians	www.ama-assn.org
Centers for Medicare & Medicaid Services (CMS) (Formerly the Health Care Financing Administration, or HCFA)	National Heart Care Project	Physicians and hospitals	www.cms.gov
Joint Commission on the Accreditation of Healthcare Organizations (JCAHO)	ORYX Initiatives	Accreditation of hospitals	www.jcaho.org
Leapfrog	Publication of volume data for cardiac procedures at hospitals	Hospitals	www.leapfroggroup.org
National Committee for Quality Assurance (NCQA)	Healthplan Employers Data and Information Set (HEDIS) Heart Stroke Provider Recognition Program	Accreditation of health plans; physician provider recognition programs	www.ncqa.org
National Quality Forum	Hospital Performance Measures Project	Hospitals	www.qualityforum.org

Adapted from Sperttus JA, Radford MJ, Every NR, et al: Challenges and opportunities in quantifying the quality of care for acute myocardial infarction: Summary from the Acute Myocardial Infarction Working Group of the American Heart Association/American College of Cardiology First Scientific Forum on Quality of Care and Outcomes Research in Cardiovascular Disease and Stroke. Circulation 107:1681, 2003.

interventions that are less strongly supported by evidence is too often a matter of judgment to use as a quality measure.

METHODOLOGICAL ISSUES. Many of the methodological issues that affect clinical research influence the measurement of cardiovascular quality, with two major additional themes. First, the performance data for individual physicians and hospitals may be made public in some cases; as a general rule, the more widely data are disseminated, the greater the demand for methodological rigor. Second, the collection and analysis of data for quality measurement is rarely funded as well as in clinical trials. Thus, the desire for methodological rigor must be weighed against the cost of collecting and analyzing the data.

Claims Data. The least expensive type of information used for quality measurement is claims data, which are collected for the purposes of mediating payment, not promoting quality of care; thus, there is little or no quality control for claims data regarding issues such as the accuracy of diagnoses. These data have the advantage of being readily available for large populations, but error rates in diagnoses are high, and information that is not required for payment is unavailable (e.g., whether heart failure is due to systolic or diastolic dysfunction, or whether blood pressure levels were controlled).

Retrospective Chart Review. This method can be used to collect more accurate clinical data, but such reviews are expensive and are complicated by the existence of multiple medical records for most patients. Patients generally have separate records at each hospital to which they have been admitted as well as at the office of their primary care physicians and the specialists from whom they have received care; none of these records is complete unless all of these health care providers are part of an integrated delivery system with a single electronic medical record. Even when all records are available for review, data collection from paper records is limited by the completeness, accuracy, and legibility of record-keeping.

Prospective Data Collection. Key data collection for quality measurement is becoming an increasingly common and important tactic for quality improvement. Standard dataforms for patients undergoing cardiac surgery or percutaneous coronary intervention (PCI) are now used at many medical centers. At some institutions, the data collected via these protocols are used for institutional databases or for inter-institutional collaborations, such as the Northern New England Cardiovascular Disease Study Group.[19] Many hospitals now report data on specific cardiovascular patient populations to national databases such as the Society of Thoracic Surgery or the American College of Cardiology's National Catheterization Data Registry. Participation in such databases allows comparison of institutional performance to regional and national benchmarks.

Collection of Patient Outcome Data. Collection of patient outcome data (e.g., 1-year mortality or functional status) is expensive and difficult. Administrative sources such as the National Death Index can provide information on whether individual patients have died within the United States; analogous resources are available in many other countries. However, obtaining information on the cause of death or on the status of patients who have not died requires interviews or surveys. Even when such data are available, the results should be adjusted for clinical and socioeconomic factors that are likely to influence the results. Therefore, many quality measures focus on processes such as the use of medications (e.g., beta blockers after acute myocardial infarction) or tests (e.g., measurement of LDL cholesterol) that are expected to lead to better outcomes.

DEFINITION OF QUALITY. A variety of definitions of quality have been proposed, reflecting the complexity of the health care system and its heterogeneous stakeholders. One of the most widely cited is that of the Institute of Medicine: "The degree to which health services for individual and populations increase the likelihood of desired health outcomes and are consistent with current professional knowledge."[20]

Error Reduction

An increasingly popular operational definition of quality is based on error reduction and the recognition that there are three major types of errors in health care: errors of underuse, overuse, and misuse (Table 4–2).[2,21] *Underuse* is the failure to provide a medical intervention when it is likely to produce a favorable outcome for a patient, such as the failure to prescribe an angiotensin-converting enzyme inhibitor for a patient with left ventricular dysfunction. *Overuse* occurs when an intervention becomes common practice even though its benefits do not justify the potential harm or costs, such as performance of exercise testing in asymptomatic patients with a low risk for cardiovascular disease. *Misuse* occurs when a preventable complication eliminates the benefit of an intervention. An example is continued administration of a statin to a patient with muscle tenderness and weakness, suggesting possible myopathy.

The relationship between guidelines and these three types of errors is close and complex. In ACC/AHA guidelines, class I indications sometimes define "rules" that, if not applied for an appropriate patient, would suggest an error of underuse. Class III indications define potential errors of overuse. The ACC/AHA guidelines tend to focus on two aspects of quality:

- Complying with evidence-based medicine (i.e., doing the right thing for the patient)
- Procedural quality (i.e., performing interventions correctly)

Failure to comply with evidence-based medicine may constitute an error of underuse (e.g., failure to use a beta blocker after acute myocardial infarction) or an error of overuse (e.g., performance of coronary angiography in a patient without clinical evidence of coronary artery disease). Failure to perform an intervention correctly can constitute an error of misuse (e.g., continued administration of a statin in a patient with symptoms of myopathy).

Structure, Process, Outcome. For deeper analysis of quality of health care, Donabedian and others recommend organization of evaluation into three categories—structure, process, and outcome (see Table 4–2).[22] *Structure* describes the components of the local health care system; relevant characteristics include the nurse-to-patient ratios, board certification status of physicians, and availability of computerized physician order entry systems and electronic medical records. *Process* elements of care describe the reliability with which key functions are performed (e.g., smoking cessation counseling for patients with coronary artery disease, administration of angiotensin-converting enzyme inhibitors to patients with left ventricular dysfunction). *Outcome* measures describe clinical outcomes such as mortality and morbidity or efficiency outcomes such as length of stay and overall costs.

TABLE 4–2 Key Frameworks for Measurement and Improvement of Quality

Framework	Components
Error reduction	Errors of overuse Errors of underuse Errors of misuse
Donabedian[22]	Structure Process Outcome
Institute of Medicine[2]	Safe Effective Patient-centered Timely Efficient Equitable

A third framework that is increasingly used by organizations to assess their quality of care is that of the Institute of Medicine (see Table 4–2), which describes six dimensions that should serve as aims for improvement. In this structure, measures should be developed to reflect the goal of making health care safe, effective, patient-centered, timely, efficient, and equitable.[2]

- Safe—avoiding injuries to patients from the care that is intended to help them.
- Effective—providing services based on scientific knowledge to all who could benefit and refraining from providing services to those not likely to benefit (avoiding underuse and overuse, respectively).
- Patient-centered—providing care that is respectful of and responsive to individual patient preferences, needs, and values and ensuring that patient values guide all clinical decisions.
- Timely—reducing waits and sometimes harmful delays for both those who receive and those who give care.
- Efficient—avoiding waste, including waste of equipment, supplies, ideas, and energy.
- Equitable—providing care that does not vary in quality because of personal characteristics such as gender, ethnicity, geographic location, and socioeconomic status.

Many organizations are developing an array of measures, with one or two measures in each of these areas.

The ACC and AHA have articulated their own basic principles for selecting performance measures (Table 4–3).[16] Using these principles, AHA/ACC workgroups have reviewed specific domains for measurement of quality for patients with acute myocardial infarction and heart failure (Tables 4–4 and 4–5).[23] Their review notes that no major structural measures of quality fulfill all five of the principles described in Table 4–3. It comments that the evidence and infrastructure to support process measures are more fully developed for acute myocardial infarction than any other medical condition, but these measures are influenced by patient-specific factors such as the long list of relative contraindications to the use of beta blockers. The use of patient outcomes is plagued by expense and the difficulty of performing adequate risk adjustment. The workgroups supported internal use of such performance measures but expressed concern about public dissemination due to methodological limitations.

VOLUME AS A MARKER FOR QUALITY OF CARE. A surrogate marker for quality that is used by the public and by professional organizations is procedure volume. The relationship between volume and patient outcomes has been demonstrated in numerous studies focusing on hospitals and on physicians.[24-31] These relationships are complex; for some procedures, outcomes are associated with the volume for the hospital, whereas for other procedures, outcomes are associated with the volume for the individual physician.[25] The relationship between hospital volume and mortality for major cardiac surgical procedures from one major study is shown in Table 4–6 and Figure 4–1.[26] These findings were based on Medicare claims data from 1994 to 1999, and the study was the largest of its kind to date. Based on such research, organizations in the United States and abroad are publishing volume data for major procedures on their Internet sites to help patients choose their hospital for surgery.[12,13]

The ACC/AHA guidelines acknowledge research on the relationship between volume and outcome in guidelines, such as those for the use of PCI for patients with acute myocardial infarction.[32] These guidelines recommend that PCI should be performed by experienced operators at high-volume facilities (see Table 48G–1).[32] For patients without acute myocardial infarction, these guidelines recommend performance of PCI by higher volume operators

TABLE 4–3 Basic Principles for Selection of Performance Measures

Principle	Comment
1. The performance measure must be meaningful.	Any potential performance measure must either be a meaningful outcome to patients and society or be closely linked to such an outcome.
2. The measure must be valid and reliable.	To serve as a useful marker of health care quality, it must be possible to measure the structure, process, or outcome of interest.
3. The measure can be adjusted for patient variability.	Interpretation of quality assessments necessitates that the observed outcomes/rates of process adherence be adjusted so that the observed differences between health care systems are due to the performance of those systems and not patient characteristics.
4. The measure can be modified by improvements in the processes of care.	To be a useful measure of quality, there must be an opportunity for motivated providers to improve their performance. This requires that the measures have variability after risk adjustment among providers. In addition, evidence should be available that suggests that alterations in the process of care can favorably influence this measure.
5. It is feasible to measure the performance of health care providers.	Although certain performance measures, such as health status, may fulfill all other criteria, the expense of collecting baseline and follow-up health status may be too great for a health care system to perform on a routine basis. Sensitivity to the fiscal implications of assessing certain performance measures may require limited sampling or avoidance altogether of certain potential measures of health care quality.

Adapted from Quality of Care and Outcomes Research in CVD and Stroke Working Groups: Measuring and improving quality of care: A report from the American Heart Association/American College of Cardiology first scientific forum on the assessment of healthcare quality in cardiovascular disease and stroke. Circulation 101:1483, 2000.

TABLE 4–4 Measures of Quality for Acute Myocardial Infarction

Type	Measures
Structure	Prehospital evaluation, triage, and treatment. Access to invasive and noninvasive cardiac tests and procedures, including transfer protocols to appropriate facilities when the necessary equipment or personnel is not available. Appropriately trained staff with access to cardiovascular specialists for management of patients with complications. Protocols or other management programs that ensure timely delivery of required therapies. Systems to ensure patient education, rehabilitation, and follow-up. Quality-improvement programs that provide for collection and review of data on care that can also be used to identify areas for improvement.
Process	Use of beta blockers at discharge and during admission. Use of aspirin at discharge and during admission. Timely and appropriate acute reperfusion (fibrinolysis or primary angioplasty) The use of angiotensin-converting enzyme inhibitors for patients with depressed left ventricular systolic function. Risk factor assessment and life-style counseling. Cholesterol status assessment and management.
Outcome	Death Readmission Physiological endpoints (e.g., achievement of blood pressure or cholesterol targets) Patient health status Patient satisfaction

TABLE 4–5 Measures of Quality for Heart Failure

Type	Measures
Structure	Availability of clear, evidence-based guidelines. Mechanism to systematically monitor patient care and outcomes. Organizational structure to move patients to appropriate level of care (e.g., access to an advanced heart failure facility). Availability of programs to address end-of-life needs.
Process	Clear documentation of left ventricular function. Use of angiotensin-converting enzyme inhibitors for patients with left ventricular systolic dysfunction. Use of digoxin for patients hospitalized with heart failure and left ventricular systolic dysfunction. Use of beta blockers for patients with NYHA Class II and III heart failure, left ventricular dysfunction, and no contraindication to beta blockers.
Outcome	Mortality Readmission Resource consumption Health status Satisfaction with care

TABLE 4–6 Annual Volume Categories for Hospitals Performing Cardiac Surgery

	Coronary Artery Bypass Graft Surgery (n)	Aortic and Mitral Valve Replacement (n)
Very low	<230	<43
Low	230-348	43-74
Medium	349-549	75-119
High	550-849	120-199
Very high	>849	>199

From Birkmeyer JD, Siewers AE, Finlayon EVA, et al: Hospital volume and surgical mortality in the United States. N Engl J Med 346:1128, 2002.

(>75 cases/year) with advanced technical skills (e.g., subspecialty certification) at high-volume centers (>400 cases/year), associated with on-site cardiovascular surgical programs, except in underserved areas that are geographically far removed from major centers (see Table 52G–1).

Current Quality of Cardiovascular Care

Some of the most comprehensive data on the quality of cardiovascular care have come from the Community Quality Index (CQI) study,[33] which draws upon medical records and self-reported information from random samples of patients

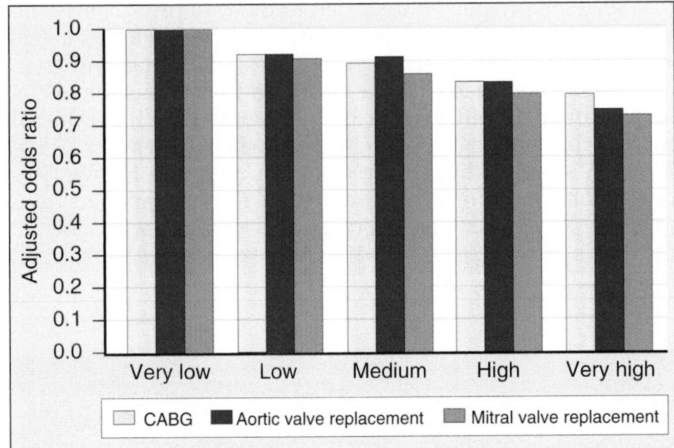

FIGURE 4–1 Relationship of hospital volume and adjusted odds ratio for mortality. Data from reference 26. See Table 4–6 for definition of volume categories. (Data from Birkmeyer JD, Siewers AE, Finlayson EVA, et al: Hospital volume and surgical mortality in the United States. N Engl J Med 346:1128, 2002.)

from 12 U.S. metropolitan areas (Boston, MA; Cleveland, OH; Greenville, SC; Indianapolis, IN; Lansing, MI; Little Rock, AR; Miami, FL; Newark, NJ; Orange County, CA; Phoenix, AZ; Seattle, WA; and Syracuse, NY). For this study, investigators selected acute and chronic conditions that represented the leading causes of death and disability and developed indicators to assess potential problems with overuse and underuse of key processes. A sampling of the indicators for cardiovascular conditions and the total number of indicators used are summarized in Table 4–7, along with the percentage of recommendations that had been followed for the 6712 study participants. The full list of measures is available at *http://www.rand.org/health/mcglynn_appa.pdf.*

Rates of compliance with recommendations ranged from 68% for care of coronary disease to 25% for atrial fibrillation. For example, only 45% of patients presenting with a myocardial infarction received beta blockers, and only 61% of participants with a myocardial infarction who were appropriate candidates for aspirin therapy received this drug. It was concluded that patients received about half of the interventions supported by evidence from clinical trials.

HOSPITALS. For hospitals in the United States, measures of cardiovascular care mandated by the JCAHO have recently become important foci for quality improvement. These measures are part of a program called the ORYX Initiative, which integrates outcomes and other performance measurement data into the accreditation process for hospitals. Two of the core foci of the ORYX initiative are acute myocardial infarction and heart failure. It is anticipated that these data will be made public within a few years.

Health services researchers, the JCAHO, and other organizations have converged on several measures of quality of hospital care for acute myocardial infarction and for heart failure (Table 4–8). Review of medical records for Medicare

TABLE 4–7 Selected Cardiovascular Quality of Care Indicators and Classifications Used in the Community Quality Index Study

Condition	Examples of Selected Indicators	Percentage of Recommended Care Received (95% Confidence Interval)
Atrial fibrillation (10 indicators)	Patients with atrial fibrillation >48 hours' duration or of unknown duration who are undergoing elective electrical or chemical cardioversion should receive anticoagulation for at least 3 weeks prior to cardioversion unless they have had a transesophageal echocardiogram within 24 hours of cardioversion that indicates no clot. Patients with atrial fibrillation started on warfarin should have an INR checked within 1 week of the first dose. Patients with atrial fibrillation >48 hours' duration or of unknown duration who do not have contraindications to warfarin should receive warfarin if they are younger than 65 years, with one or more other risk factors for stroke.	25 (18-31)
Congestive heart failure (36 indicators)	Ejection fraction assessed before medical therapy Angiotensin-converting enzyme inhibitors for patients with congestive heart failure and an ejection fraction <40%	64 (55-72)
Coronary artery disease (37 indicators)	Counseling on smoking cessation Avoidance of nifedipine for patients with an acute myocardial infarction	68 (64-72)
Diabetes (13 indicators)	Diet and exercise counseling Angiotensin-converting enzyme inhibitors for patients with proteinuria	45 (43-48)
Hyperlipidemia (7 indicators)	Treatment of high low-density cholesterol levels in patients with coronary artery disease	49 (44-53)
Hypertension (27 indicators)	Life-style modification for patients with mild hypertension Pharmacotherapy for uncontrolled mild hypertension Change in treatment when blood pressure is persistently uncontrolled	65 (53-67)

For full list, see http://www.rand.org/health/mcglynn_appa.pdf.
Data from McGlynn EA, Asch SM, Adams J, et al: The quality of health care delivered to adults in the United States. N Engl J Med 348:2635, 2003.

patients hospitalized from 1998 to 2001 suggests that improvement appears to be taking place for most of these measures.[34] Data for this study were collected by Medicare Quality Improvement Organizations in each state, based on chart reviews of up to 750 inpatients with acute myocardial infarction and up to 800 patients with congestive heart failure per state. However, these data also show marked regional variability. For example, in 2000-2001, use of beta blockers in appropriate patients after acute myocardial infarction varied from 57% in Arkansas to 95% in Rhode Island. Use of an angiotensin-converting enzyme inhibitor for patients with heart failure and an ejection fraction below 0.40 ranged from 43% in Arkansas to 82% in Wyoming and 81% in Vermont.

PHYSICIANS. Cardiovascular surgeons and cardiologists who perform PCI are evaluated on their actual outcomes data via public report cards in some states. In these reports, analyses attempt to adjust for the risk of complications and for emergency procedures, allowing calculation of a risk-adjusted mortality rate for individual physicians and hospitals. Thus far, limited data suggest that the public does not use such data extensively,[35,36] although the public disclosure of performance data is believed to be a powerful driver for individual institutions to improve their care.[8]

Nonprocedural care by physicians is often assessed by HEDIS measures developed by NCQA (Table 4–9).[10] These measures were developed for evaluation of health maintenance organizations, and therefore most rely on analyses of medical and pharmacy claims data. In recent years, however, there has been a shift toward measures that are less focused on measuring processes and are more closely tied to patient outcome. Therefore, measures have been introduced that require review of medical records for some data (e.g., blood pressure and LDL cholesterol levels).

A program called the Heart/Stroke Recognition Program was introduced in 2003 by NCQA in collaboration with the American Heart Association and the American Stroke Association. This program is designed to identify physicians who are providing excellent care to patients who have cardiovascular disease or a history of stroke. It is a voluntary program in which physicians seeking "recognition" must audit a sample of their office records and report on their rates of success in meeting specific performance measures (Table 4–10). A similar physician recognition program for diabetes care has been administered by NCQA for several years, and some employers now pay a bonus to physicians who meet its standards for each of their patients with diabetes. This same

TABLE 4–8 Quality Indicators for Inpatient Care for Medicare Patients

Topic	Indicator	Median State Rates* 1998-1999	Median State Rates* 2000-2001
Acute myocardial infarction	Administration of aspirin within 24 hours of admission	84	85
	Aspirin prescribed at discharge	85	86
	Administration of beta blocker within 24 hours of admission	64	69
	Beta blocker prescribed at discharge	72	79
	Angiotensin-converting enzyme inhibitor prescribed at discharge for patients with left ventricular ejection fraction <0.40	71	74
	Smoking cessation counseling given during hospitalization	40	43
	Time to angioplasty (minutes)	41	45
	Time to thrombolytic therapy (minutes)	120	107
Heart failure	Evaluation of ejection fraction	65	70
	Angiotensin-converting enzyme inhibitor prescribed at discharge for patients with left ventricular ejection fraction <0.40	69	68

*In this study, rates of performance of each measure were calculated from chart reviews in each state. The figures in these columns represent the median performance among the 50 U.S. states.

Data from Jencks SF, Haft ED, Cuerdon T: Change in the quality of care delivered to Medicare beneficiaries, 1998-1999 to 2000-2001. JAMA 289:305, 2003.

TABLE 4–9 Cardiovascular HEDIS Measures

Measure	Description	Mean Performance* (%)
Beta blocker treatment after a heart attack	The percentage of patients ≥35 yrs who were hospitalized and discharged alive during the measurement year with a diagnosis of acute myocardial infarction and who received an ambulatory prescription for beta blockers upon discharge.	92.5
Controlling high blood pressure	The percentage of patients 45-85 yrs who had a diagnosis of hypertension and whose blood pressure was adequately controlled (≤140/90) during the measurement year.	55.4
Cholesterol screening	The percentage of patients 18-75 yrs who had evidence of an acute cardiovascular event (hospitalization for acute myocardial infarction, coronary artery bypass graft, or percutaneous transluminal coronary angioplasty) and whose low-density lipoprotein cholesterol was screened in the year following the event.	77.1
Cholesterol management	The percentage of patients with an acute cardiovascular event whose low-density lipoprotein cholesterol was screened and controlled to less than 130 mg/dl in the year following the event.	59.3

*Data are for commercial population for 2001. Data from http://www.ncqa.org/sohc2002/

TABLE 4–10 Measures of the Heart/Stoke Provider Recognition Program of the National Committee for Quality Assurance
Blood pressure testing
Proportion of patients with blood pressure <130/85 mm Hg
Lipid testing
Proportion of patients with low-density lipoprotein cholesterol <100 mg/dl
Use of aspirin or other antithrombotics
Smoking status and cessation advice

bonus framework may be extended to the Heart/Stroke Recognition Program.

Improvement Strategies

The American College of Cardiology and a wide range of other organizations are attempting to develop and disseminate tools for improvement in the reliability of delivery of evidence-based cardiovascular care. The ACC's Guidelines Applied in Practice Initiative used tactics known as continuous quality improvement (CQI) to help physicians and hospitals improve compliance with guidelines.[37] These CQI tools are based on principles adapted from industrial manufacturers and seek to improve quality and efficiency through repetitive cycles of process and outcomes measurement, design and implementation of interventions to improve the processes of care, followed by remeasurement to assess the impact of interventions.[38]

Research that has evaluated the impact of CQI programs on quality of cardiovascular care have yielded encouraging results. One report demonstrated a positive impact from interventions to improve care for acute myocardial infarction led by local opinion leaders in 37 centers,[39] and collaboratives in which surgeons share data and best practices have been associated with improved outcomes in cardiac surgery.[19] Other studies, however, have been unable to demonstrate significant effects from well-designed CQI programs.[40]

In a large recent study of CQI for improvement of cardiac surgery,[41] the investigators randomly assigned 359 hospitals that performed coronary artery bypass grafting on 267,917 patients between January 2000 and July 2002 and that participated in the Society of Thoracic Surgeons National Cardiac Database. The hospitals were randomly assigned to a control arm or to one of two groups that used CQI interventions aimed at improving preoperative use of beta blockade in all patients and internal mammary artery graft utilization in elderly patients. The intervention groups received measure-specific information, including a call to action to a physician leader, educational products, and periodic longitudinal data with benchmark information. This intervention led to a significant increase in the use of beta blockade at intervention sites (by 7.3% vs 3.6%) and a trend toward an increase in use of internal mammary grafts. Both interventions were associated with statistically significant increases in these practices at lower volume coronary artery bypass grafting sites.

The simplest application of CQI principles is utilization of critical pathways, which are standardized protocols that define the key steps and their timing for procedures or for care of common syndromes such as acute chest pain.[42,43] Whether critical pathways actually improve efficiency and quality is unclear, as some data suggest that improvement associated with them may result simply from focusing physicians' and nurses' attention on the patient population, not from the protocols themselves.[44]

Several studies have demonstrated that outcomes of patients with acute myocardial infarction and other serious cardiovascular conditions are improved if they receive their acute and post-hospitalization care from a cardiologist as opposed to generalist physician.[45-47] Other data demonstrate that team-based care and longitudinal programs known as disease management can improve care for patients with acute myocardial infarction and heart failure.[48,49]

REFERENCES

1. Kohn LT, Corrigan JM, Donaldson MS, et al: To Err is Human: Building a Safer Health System. Washington, DC, National Academy Press, 1999.
2. Committee on Quality of Health Care in America: Crossing the Quality Chasm. Washington, DC, National Academy Press, 2001.
3. Galvin R, Milstein A: Large employers' new strategies in health care. N Engl J Med 347:939, 2002.
4. Leadership by Example, Coordinating Government Roles in Improving Health Care Quality. Washington, DC, National Academy Press, 2002.
5. Bodenheimer T: The American health care system: The movement for improved quality in health care. N Engl J Med 340:488, 1999.
6. Hannan EL, Kilburn H, Racz M, et al: Improving the outcomes of coronary artery bypass surgery in New York State. JAMA 271:761, 1994.
7. Ghali WA, Ash AS, Hall RE, Moskowitz MA: Statewide quality improvement initiatives and mortality after cardiac surgery. JAMA 277:379, 1997.
8. Chassin MR: Achieving and sustaining improved quality: Lessons from New York State and cardiac surgery. Health Aff (Millwood) 21:40, 2002.
9. Iglehart JK: The National Committee for Quality Assurance. N Engl J Med 335:995, 1996.
10. National Committee for Quality Assurance (NCQA): Measuring the Quality of America's Health Care: The Health Plan Employer Data and Information Set (HEDIS). Vol. 2003. Washington, DC; NCQA 2003.
11. Joint Commission on Accreditation of Healthcare Organizations. (http://www.jcaho.org/)
12. Leapfrog Group. (http://www.leapfroggroup.org/)
13. (http://www.drfoster.co.uk/)
14. Gibbons RJ, Smith S, Antman E: American College of Cardiology/American Heart Association clinical practice guidelines: Part I: Where do they come from? Circulation 107:2979, 2003.
15. Gibbons RJ, Smith S, Antman E: American College of Cardiology/American Heart Association clinical practice guidelines: Part II: Evolutionary changes in a continuous quality improvement project. Circulation 107:3101, 2003.
16. Quality of Care and Outcomes Research in CVD and Stroke Working Groups: Measuring and improving quality of care: A report from the American Heart Association/American College of Cardiology first scientific forum on the assessment of healthcare quality in cardiovascular disease and stroke. Circulation 101:1483, 2000.
17. National Cholesterol Education Program: Detection and Treatment of High Blood Cholesterol in Adults (Adult Treatment Panel III) NIH Publication No. 02-5215. 2002.
18. Lee TH, Cleeman JI, Brundy SM, et al: Clinical goals and performance measures for cholesterol management for secondary prevention of coronary heart disease. JAMA 283:94, 2000.
19. O'Connor GT, Plume SK, Olmstead EM, et al, for the Northern New England Cardiovascular Disease Study Group: A regional intervention to improve the hospital mortality associated with coronary artery bypass graft surgery. JAMA 275:841, 1996.
20. Chassin MR, Galvin RW: The urgent need to improve health care quality. JAMA 280:1000, 1998.
21. Lee TH: A broader concept of medical errors. N Engl J Med 347:1965, 2002.
22. Donabedian AL: The quality of care: How can it be assessed? JAMA 260:1743, 1988.
23. Sperttus JA, Radford MJ, Every NR, et al: Challenges and opportunities in quantifying the quality of care for acute myocardial infarction: Summary from the Acute Myocardial Infarction Working Group of the American Heart Association/American College of Cardiology First Scientific Forum on Quality of Care and Outcomes Research in Cardiovascular Disease and Stroke. Circulation 107:1681, 2003.
24. Epstein AE: Volume and outcome—it is time to move ahead. N Engl J Med 346:1161, 2002.
25. Halm EA, Lee C, Chassin MR: Is volume related to quality in health care? A systematic review and methodologic critique of the medical literature. Ann Intern Med 137:511, 2002.
26. Birkmeyer JD, Siewers AE, Finlayson EVA, et al: Hospital volume and surgical mortality in the United States. N Engl J Med 346:1128, 2002.
27. Malenka DJ, McGrath PD, Wennberg DE, et al: The relationship between operator volume and outcomes after percutaneous coronary interventions in high volume hospitals in 1994-1996: The northern New England experience. Northern New England Cardiovascular Disease Study Group. J Am Coll Cardiol 34:1471, 1999.
28. Jollis JG, Peterson ED, DeLong ER, et al: The relation between the volume of coronary angioplasty procedures at hospitals treating Medicare beneficiaries and short-term mortality. N Engl J Med 331:1625, 1994.
29. Magid DJ, Calonge BN, Rumsfeld JS, et al: Relation between hospital primary angioplasty volume and mortality for patients with acute MI treated with primary angioplasty vs thrombolytic therapy. JAMA 284:3131, 2000.
30. Canto JG, Every NR, Magid DJ, et al: The volume of primary angioplasty procedures and survival after acute myocardial infarction: National Registry of Myocardial Infarction 2 Investigators. N Engl J Med 342:1573, 2000.

31. Maynard C, Every NR, Chapko MK, et al: Outcomes of coronary angioplasty procedures performed in rural hospitals. Am J Med 108:710, 2000.
32. Smith SC Jr, Dove JT, Jacobs AK, et al: ACC/AHA guidelines for percutaneous coronary intervention: A report of the American College of Cardiology/American Heart Association Task Force on Practice Guidelines (Committee to Revise the 1993 Guidelines for Percutaneous Transluminal Coronary Angioplasty). J Am Coll Cardiol 37:2239, i-lxvi, 2001.
33. McGlynn EA, Asch SM, Adams J, et al: The quality of health care delivered to adults in the United States. N Engl J Med 348:2635, 2003.
34. Jencks SF, Huff ED, Cuerdon T: Change in the quality of care delivered to Medicare beneficiaries, 1998-1999 to 2000-2001. JAMA 289:305, 2003.
35. Schneider EC, Epstein AM: Use of public performance reports: A survey of patients undergoing cardiac surgery. JAMA 27:1638, 1998.
36. Schneider EC, Epstein AM: Influence of cardiac-surgery performance reports on referral practices and access to care: A survey of cardiovascular specialists. N Engl J Med 335:251, 1996.
37. Mehta RH, Montoye CK, Gallogly M, et al: Improving quality of care for acute myocardial infarction: The Guidelines Applied in Practice (GAP) Initiative. JAMA 287:1269, 2002.
38. Berwick DM: Continuous improvement as an ideal in health care. N Engl J Med 320:53, 1989.
39. Soumerai SB, McLaughlin TJ, Gurwith JH, et al: Effect of local medical opinion leaders on quality of care for acute myocardial infarction. JAMA 279:1358, 1998.
40. Krumholz H, Amatruda J, Smith GL, et al: Randomized trial of an education and support intervention to prevent readmission of patients with heart failure. J Am Coll Cardiol 39:83, 2002.
41. Ferguson TB, Peterson ED, Coombs LP, et al: Use of continuous quality improvement to increase use of process measures in patients undergoing coronary artery bypass graft surgery. A randomized controlled trial. JAMA 290:49, 2003.
42. Pearson SD, Goulart-Fisher D, Lee TH: Critical pathways as a strategy for improving care: problems and potential. Ann Intern Med 123:941, 1995.
43. Nichol G, Walls R, Goldman L, et al: A critical pathway for management of patients with acute chest pain who are at low risk for myocardial ischemia: recommendations and potential impact. Ann Intern Med 127:996, 1997.
44. Pearson SD, Kleefield SF, Roukop JR, et al: Critical pathways intervention to reduce length of hospital stay. Am J Med 110:175, 2001.
45. Jollis JG, DeLong ER, Peterson ED, et al: Outcome of acute myocardial infarction according to the specialty of the admitting physician. N Engl J Med 335:1880, 1996.
46. Ayanian JZ, Hauptman PJ, Guadagnoli E, et al: Knowledge and practices of generalist and specialist physicians regarding drug therapy for acute myocardial infarction. N Engl J Med 331:1136, 1994.
47. Chen J, Radford MJ, Wang Y, et al: Care and outcomes of elderly patients with acute myocardial infarction by physician specialty: The effects of comorbidity and functional limitations. Am J Med 108:460, 2000.
48. DeBusk RF, Miller NH, Superko HR, et al: A case-management system for coronary risk factor modification after acute myocardial infarction. Ann Intern Med 120:721, 1994.
49. Rich MW, Beckham V, Wittenberg C, et al: A multidisciplinary intervention to prevent the readmission of elderly patients with congestive heart failure. N Engl J Med 333:1190, 1995.

CHAPTER 5

The Principles of Drug Therapy

Dan M. Roden

Importance of Correct Drug Use

In 2001, Americans spent $191 billion on pharmaceuticals.[1] Adverse drug reactions are estimated to be the fourth to sixth most common cause of death in the United States, to cost $19 to 27 billion annually, and to account directly for 2% to 3% of all hospital admissions. The prevalence of heart disease and the increasing utilization of not only acute interventional therapies but also long-term preventive therapies translate into a dominant role of cardiovascular drugs in these costs: 19% of all drug costs ($36 billion) in 2001.[1] Moreover, with increasing success not only in heart disease but also in other therapeutic arenas, cardiovascular physicians are increasingly encountering patients receiving multiple medications with which they may not have complete comfort and familiarity. The goal of this chapter is to outline principles of drug action and interaction that allow the safest and most effective therapy in an individual patient.

The Key Decision in Drug Therapy: Risk versus Benefit

The fundamental assumption underlying administration of any drug is that the real or expected benefit exceeds the anticipated risk. The benefits of drug therapy are initially defined in small clinical trials, perhaps involving several thousand patients, prior to a drug's marketing and approval. Ultimately, the efficacy and safety profile of any drug is determined after the compound has been marketed and used widely in hundreds of thousands of patients.

When a drug is administered for the acute correction of a life-threatening condition, the benefits are often self-evident; insulin for diabetic ketoacidosis, nitroprusside for hypertensive encephalopathy, or lidocaine for ventricular tachycardia are examples. Extrapolation of such immediately obvious benefits to other clinical situations may not be warranted, however. The efficacy of lidocaine to terminate ventricular tachycardia led to its widespread use as a prophylactic agent in cases of acute myocardial infarction, until it was recognized that, in this setting, the drug does not alter mortality. The outcome of the Cardiac Arrhythmia Suppression Trial (CAST) highlights the difficulties in extrapolating from an incomplete understanding of physiology to chronic drug therapy. CAST tested the hypothesis that suppression of ventricular ectopic activity (a recognized risk factor for sudden death for myocardial infarction) would reduce mortality; this notion was highly ingrained in cardiovascular practice in the 1970s and 1980s. In CAST, sodium channel–blocking antiarrhythmics did suppress ventricular ectopics, but also unexpectedly increased the rate of mortality threefold. In this instance, the use of arrhythmia suppression as a "surrogate" marker for a desired drug action, reduction in mortality, was inappropriate because the underlying pathophysiology was incompletely understood. Similarly, reduced contractility in cases of heart failure has led to development of a series of drugs with positive inotropic activity, but these also show an increase in mortality, likely due to drug-induced arrhythmias.[2] Nevertheless, clinical trials with these agents do suggest symptom relief. Thus, the prescriber and the patient may elect therapy with positive inotropic drugs, because of this benefit, and recognizing the risk. These examples illustrate the continuing personal relationship between the prescriber and the patient and emphasize the needs for a clear understanding of the expected benefit of therapy, and a clear understanding of disease pathophysiology and its response to drug therapy, in the drug development and prescribing processes.

The risks of drug therapy may be a direct extension of the pharmacological actions for which the drug is actually being prescribed. Excessive hypotension in a patient taking an antihypertensive agent or bleeding in a patient taking a platelet IIb/IIIa receptor antagonist are examples. In other cases, adverse effects develop as a consequence of pharmacological actions that were not appreciated during a drug's initial development and use in patients. Rhabdomyolysis with HMG-CoA reductase inhibitors, angioedema during angiotensin-converting enzyme (ACE) inhibitor therapy, or torsades de pointes during treatment with "noncardiovascular" drugs such as thioridazine or pentamidine are examples. However, these rarer but very serious events may become evident only after a drug has been marketed and extensively used. Even rare adverse effects can alter the overall perception of risk versus benefit and can prompt removal of the drug from the market, particularly if alternate, safer therapies are available; for example, withdrawal of the first insulin-sensitizer, troglitazone, after recognition of hepatotoxicity was further spurred by availability of other new drugs in this class. Further, investigation of the pathophysiology underlying these unusual events has defined new mechanisms underlying variable responses to drug therapy.

Variability in Drug Action

Drugs interact with specific molecular targets to effect changes in whole organ and whole body function. The targets with which drugs interact to produce beneficial effects may or may not be the same as those with which drugs interact to produce adverse effects. Drug targets may be in the circulation, at the cell surface, or within cells. Many newer drugs have been developed to specifically interact with a desired drug target; examples of such targets are HMG-CoA reductase, angiotensin-converting enzyme, G-protein coupled receptors (α, β, AT1, histamine, and many others), and platelet IIb/IIIa receptors. On the other hand, many drugs widely used in cardiovascular therapeutics were developed at a time when the technology to identify specific molecular targets simply was not available; digoxin, amiodarone, and aspirin are examples. In some cases, such agents turn out to have rather specific molecular targets: digoxin's major effect is by inhibition of Na-K-ATPase, whereas aspirin permanently acetylates a specific serine residue on the cyclooxygenase enzyme. However, with the cloning of multiple isoforms of cyclooxygenase has come the recognition that aspirin is in fact targeting multiple molecules; more specific inhibitors have therefore been developed, and their effects are being evaluated in patients with cardiovascular and other types of disease.

MECHANISMS UNDERLYING VARIABILITY IN DRUG ACTION. Two major processes determine how the interaction between a drug and its target molecule can generate variable drug actions in the patient (Fig. 5–1). The first, *pharmacokinetics*, describes drug delivery to and removal from the target molecule and includes the processes of absorption, distribution, metabolism, and excretion. These are collectively termed "drug disposition." Robust techniques—applicable across drugs and drug classes—to analyze drug disposition have been developed and result in a series of principles that can be used to adjust drug dosages to enhance the likelihood of a beneficial effect and to minimize toxicity.

The second process, *pharmacodynamics*, describes how the interaction between a drug and its target generates downstream molecular, cellular, whole organ, and whole body effects. Pharmacodynamic sources of variability in drug action arise from the specifics of the target molecule and the biological context in which the drug-target interaction occurs; thus, methods for analysis of pharmacodynamics tend to be drug class specific. In practice, pharmacodynamic variability often arises as a consequence of disease, especially the disease for which the drug is being prescribed.

One source of pharmacodynamic variability is variability in the target molecule itself; this can arise because of genetic factors, discussed subsequently, or because disease alters the number of target molecules or their state (e.g., changes in extent of phosphorylation). A second source of pharmacodynamic variability arises from our increasing understanding of the molecular pathophysiology of disease: the interaction between drugs and their target molecules occurs in a complex biologic context, so variability in this biology (often a consequence of disease) can affect the extent to which a drug produces desired or undesired effects. Examples include high dietary salt that can inhibit the antihypertensive action of beta blockers, or hypokalemia that increases the risk for drug-induced QT prolongation. The latter clinical observation led to experiments at the basic level to define the underlying mechanism, and these results in turn highlight the value of aggressive potassium supplementation in patients with both congenital and acquired long QT syndromes.

PHARMACOGENETICS AND PHARMACOGENOMICS. This contemporary view of drug actions identifies a series of molecules that mediate drug actions in patients: drug metabolizing enzymes, drug transport molecules, drug targets, and molecules modulating the biology in which the drug-target interaction occurs. The vast majority of these molecules are proteins, so variations in the genes that encode them may therefore contribute to variability in drug actions. Isolated examples of familial aggregation of unusual responses to drug therapy have been recognized for decades and defined the field of *pharmacogenetics*. Such rare aberrant responses recognized in families generally arise as a result of mutations, usually defined as rare DNA variants that are associated with a disease phenotype. With the sequencing of the human genome has come the recognition that DNA variants are extremely common, occurring on average in 1 of 300 base pairs; such variants—termed *polymorphisms*—may or may not alter gene expression or function. The nascent field of *pharmacogenomics* is attempting to define common polymorphisms, or sets of polymorphisms, that underlie variability in drug action.[3] Ultimately, it may be possible to genotype individuals prior to prescribing medications to ensure that benefit is maximized and risk minimized: the concept of "pre-prescription genotyping."

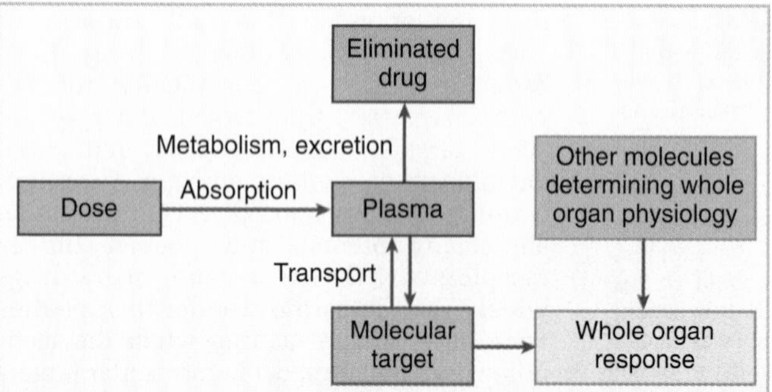

FIGURE 5–1 A model for understanding variability in drug action. When a dose of a drug is administered, the processes of absorption, metabolism, excretion, and transport determine its access to specific molecular targets that mediate beneficial and toxic effects. The interaction between a drug and its molecular target then produces changes in molecular, cellular, whole organ, and ultimately whole patient physiology. This molecular interaction occurs in a complex biologic milieu modulated by multiple factors (some of which are disturbed to cause disease). DNA variants in the genes responsible for the processes of drug disposition (green), the molecular target (blue) or the molecules determining the biological context in which the drug-target interaction occurs (tan) all can contribute to variability in drug action.

Pharmacokinetics

Administration of an intravenous drug bolus results in maximal drug concentrations at the end of the bolus and then a decline in plasma drug concentrations over time (Fig. 5–2A). The simplest case is one in which this decline occurs monoexponentially over time. A useful parameter to describe this decline is the *half-life* (t1/2), the time in which 50% of the drug elimination occurs; after two half-lives, 75% of the drug has been eliminated, after three half-lives 87.5%, and so on.

In some cases, the decline of drug concentrations following administration of an intravenous bolus dose is multiexponential. The most common explanation is that drug is not only eliminated (represented by the terminal portion of the time-concentration plot) but also undergoes more rapid *distribution* to peripheral tissues. Just as elimination may be usefully described by a half-life, distribution half-lives can also be derived from curves such as those shown in Figure 5–2B.

The plasma concentration measured immediately after a bolus dose can be used to derive a volume into which the drug is distributed. When the decline of plasma concentrations is multiexponential, multiple distribution compartments can be defined; these *volumes of distribution* can be useful in considering dose adjustments in cases of disease, but rarely correspond exactly to any physical volume such as plasma or total body water. Indeed, with drugs that are highly tissue bound (such as some antidepressants), volume of distribution can exceed total body volume by orders of magnitude.

Drugs are often administered by nonintravenous routes, such as oral, sublingual, transcutaneous, or intramuscular. With such routes of administration, two differences arise from the intravenous route (see Fig. 5–2A). First, concentrations in plasma demonstrate a distinct rising phase as drug slowly enters plasma. Second, the total amount of drug that actually enters the systemic circulation may be less than that achieved by the intravenous route. The relative amount of drug entering by any route, compared to the same dose administered intravenously, is termed *bioavailability*. Bioavailability may be reduced because drug undergoes metabolism prior to entering the circulation or because drug is simply not absorbed from its site of administration.

Clearance is the most useful way of quantifying drug elimination. Clearance can be viewed as a volume that is "cleared" of drug in any given period of time. Clearance may be organ specific (e.g., renal clearance, hepatic clearance) or whole body clearance.

With repeated doses, drug levels accumulate to a *steady state*, the condition under which the rate of drug administration is equal to the rate of drug elimination in any given period of time. As illustrated in Figure 5–3, the elimination half-life describes not only the disappearance of a drug but also the time course by which a drug accumulates to steady state. It is important to distinguish between steady-state plasma concentrations, achieved in four to five elimination half-lives, and steady-state drug effects, which may take longer to achieve. For some drugs, clinical effects develop immediately upon access to the molecular target: nitrates for angina, nitroprusside to lower blood pressure, and sympathomimetics to treat shock are examples. In other situations, drug effects follow plasma concentrations, but with a lag. An active metabolite may need to be generated to achieve drug effects. Time may be required for translation of the drug effect at the molecular site to a physiologic end point. Inhibition of synthesis of vitamin K–dependent clotting factors by warfarin ultimately leads to a desired elevation of INR, but the development of this desired effect occurs only as levels of clotting factors fall. Penetration of a drug into intracellular or other tissue sites of action may be required prior to development of drug effect; this is widely cited to explain the lag time between administration of amiodarone dosages and development of its effects, although the exact mechanism underlying this phenomenon remains elusive.

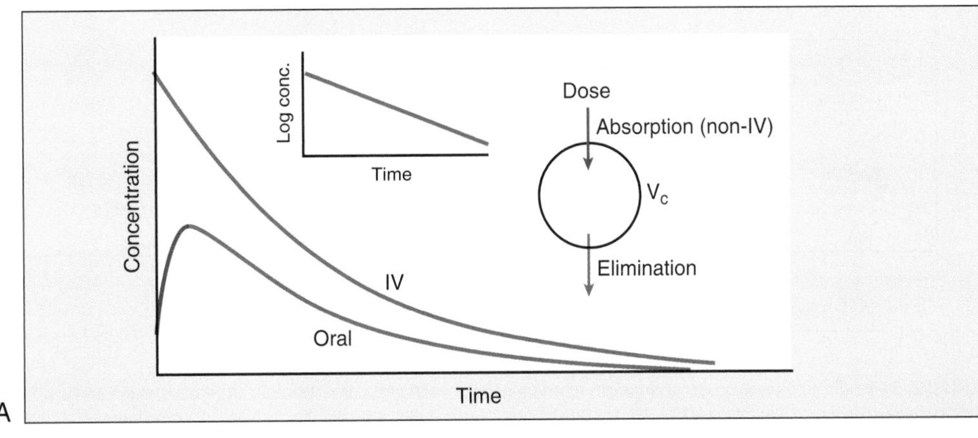

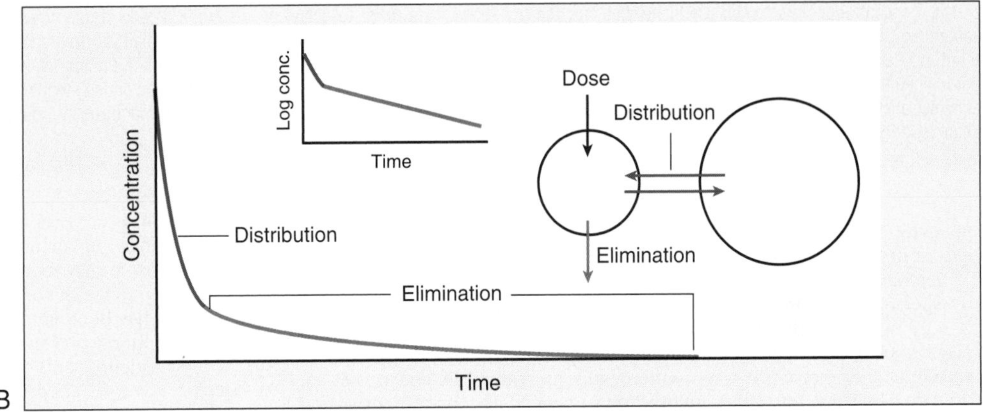

FIGURE 5–2 Models of plasma concentrations as a function of time after a single dose of a drug. **A.** The simplest situation is one in which a drug is administered as a very rapid intravenous bolus into a volume (V_c) into which it is instantaneously and uniformly distributed. Elimination then takes place from this volume. In this case, drug elimination is monoexponential; that is, a plot of the logarithm of concentration versus time is linear, as shown in the inset. When the same dose of drug is administered orally, a distinct absorption phase is required prior to drug entry into V_c. Most absorption (shown here in red) is completed prior to elimination (shown in green), although the processes overlap. In this example, the amount of drug delivered by the oral route is less than that delivered by the intravenous route, assessed by the total areas under the two curves, indicating reduced bioavailability. **B.** In this example, drug is delivered to the central volume, from which it is not only eliminated but also undergoes distribution to the peripheral sites. This distribution process is more rapid than elimination, resulting in a distinct biexponential disappearance curve.

Pharmacokinetic Principles in Managing Drug Therapy

BIOAVAILABILITY AND DOSE ADJUSTMENT. Some drugs undergo such extensive presystemic metabolism that the amount of drug required to achieve a therapeutic effect is much greater (and often much more variable) than that required for the same drug administered intravenously. Thus, small doses of propranolol (5 mg) may achieve heart rate slowing equivalent to that observed with much larger oral doses (80-120 mg). Propranolol is actually well absorbed but undergoes extensive metabolism in the intestine and the liver prior to entering the systemic circulation. Another example is amiodarone, the physicochemical characteristics of which make it only 30% to 50% bioavailable when it is administered orally (the drug is highly lipophilic and thus has limited water solubility). Thus, an intravenous infusion 0.5 mg/min (720 mg/day) is equivalent to 1.5 to 2 gm/day orally.

DISTRIBUTION. Rapid distribution can alter the way in which drug therapy should be initiated. When lidocaine is administered intravenously, it displays a prominent and rapid distribution phase (t1/2 = 8 min) prior to slower elimination (t1/2 = 120 min). As a consequence, an antiarrhythmic effect of lidocaine may be transiently achieved but very rapidly lost following a single bolus, due not to elimination but to rapid distribution. Administration of higher bolus doses to circumvent this problem results in dose-related toxicity, often seizures. Hence, administration of a lidocaine loading dose of 3 to 4 mg/kg should occur over 10 to 20 minutes, as a series of intravenous boluses (e.g., 50-100 mg every 5-10 min) or an intravenous infusion (e.g., 20 mg/min over 10-20 min).

CLEARANCE MECHANISMS. The mechanisms underlying drug elimination from the body are metabolism and excretion. Drug metabolism most often occurs in the liver, although extrahepatic metabolism (in the circulation, the intestine, the lungs, and the kidneys) is increasingly well defined. "Phase I" drug metabolism generally involves oxidation of the drug by specific drug-oxidizing enzymes, a process that renders the drug more water-soluble (and hence more likely to undergo renal excretion). Additionally, drugs or their metabolites often undergo conjugation with specific chemical groups ("phase II") to enhance water solubility; these conjugation reactions are also catalyzed by specific transferases.

The most common enzyme systems mediating drug metabolism are those of the P450 superfamily, termed CYPs. Multiple CYPs are expressed in human liver and other tissues. A major source of variability in drug action is variability in CYP activity, due to variability in CYP expression and/or genetic variants that alter CYP activity. The most abundant CYP in human liver and intestine is CYP3A4 and a closely related isoform, CYP3A5. These CYPs metabolize up to 50% of clinically used drugs. CYP3A activity varies widely among individuals, for reasons that are not entirely clear. One mechanism underlying this variability is the presence of a polymorphism in this CYP3A5 gene that reduces its activity.[4] Table 5–1 lists CYPs and other drug-metabolizing enzymes and emphasizes that genetic variants that alter function are well recognized with some CYPs (2D6, 2C9, 2C19), and a number of phase II enzymes.[5] Table 5–1 also points out that the frequencies of polymorphisms in these genes may vary among ethnic groups and is one explanation for interethnic variability in drug response; another is variability in the frequency of polymorphisms in the genes whose function determines pharmacodynamics, discussed further later.

Reduction in clearance, by disease, drug interactions, or genetic factors, will increase drug concentrations and hence drug effects. An exception is drugs whose effects are mediated by generation of active metabolites. In this case, inhibition of drug metabolism may lead to accumulation of the parent drug but loss of therapeutic efficacy. The anticonvulsant phenytoin is an inhibitor of CYP2C9; when phenytoin is started in a patient receiving the angiotensin receptor blocker losartan, blood pressure control may be lost because of failure of biotransformation of losartan to its active metabolite.[6] This is in contrast to phenytoin effects on CYP3A substrates. In this case, phenytoin acts as a potent inducing agent, increasing gene transcription. Thus, administration of

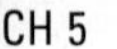

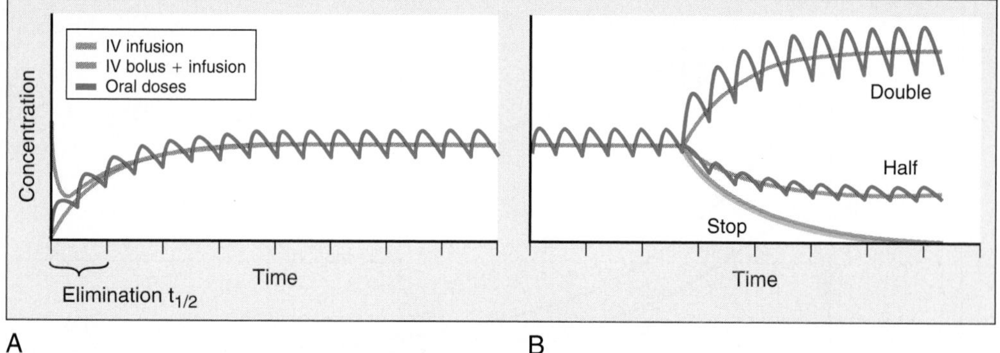

FIGURE 5–3 Time course of drug concentrations when treatment is started or dose is changed. **A.** The hash lines on the abscissa indicate one elimination half-life (t1/2). With a constant rate intravenous infusion (gold), plasma concentrations accumulate to steady state in four to five elimination half-lives. When a loading bolus is administered with the maintenance infusion (blue), plasma concentrations are transiently higher but may dip, as shown here, prior to achieving the same steady state. When the same drug is administered by the oral route, the time course of drug accumulation is identical; in this case, the drug was administered at intervals of 50% of a t1/2 (magenta). Steady-state plasma concentrations during oral therapy fluctuate around the mean determined by intravenous therapy. **B.** This plot shows that dosages are doubled or halved, or the drug is stopped during steady-state administration, and the time required to achieve the new steady state is four or five half-lives and is independent of the route of administration.

phenytoin actually increases CYP3A activity and hence leads to altered effects of CYP3A substrates through this mechanism.

Excretion of drugs, generally into the urine or bile, is accomplished by specific drug-transport molecules, whose level of expression and genetic variation are only now being explored. In fact, drug transporters play a role not only in drug elimination, but also in drug uptake into many cells, including hepatocytes and enterocytes. As with CYPs and other drug-metabolizing enzymes, multiple genes encoding multiple drug uptake and efflux transporters are being identified. The most widely recognized of these is P-glycoprotein, the product of expression of the *MDR1* gene. Originally identified as a factor mediating multiple drug resistance in patients with cancer, *MDR1* expression is now well recognized in normal enterocytes, hepatocytes, renal tubular cells, the endothelium of the capillaries forming the blood-brain barrier, and the testes. In each of these sites, P-glycoprotein expression is restricted to the apical aspect of polarized cells, where it acts to enhance drug efflux. In intestine, P-glycoprotein pumps substrates back into the lumen, thereby limiting bioavailability. In the liver and kidney, it promotes drug excretion into bile or urine. In the central nervous system capillary endothelium, P-glycoprotein-mediated efflux is an important mechanism limiting drug access to the brain.[7]

Clinical Relevance of Polymorphic Drug Metabolism: The Concept of High-Risk Pharmacokinetics

The absence of a specific pathway for drug metabolism, due to genetic factors or to the administration of other drugs, has variable clinical consequences. When a drug uses multiple pathways for its elimination, absence of one of these is unlikely to have major clinical consequences because elimination can be accomplished by alternate pathways. On the other hand, a drug eliminated by only a single pathway carries with it the liability that absence of activity of that pathway will lead to marked accumulation of drug in plasma, failure to form downstream metabolites, and thus a risk of unusual drug responses.

One example was the antihistamine terfenadine, which is eliminated almost exclusively by CYP3A metabolism in the intestine and the liver. Terfenadine itself is a highly potent QT-prolonging agent and is biotransformed to a noncardioactive metabolite (fexofenadine) that mediates the compound's antihistamine actions. Coadministration of terfenadine with CYP3A inhibitors such as ketaconazole or erythromycin led to inhibition of presystemic metabolism, striking elevations of plasma terfenadine concentrations, marked QT prolongation, and torsades de pointes. As a consequence, the drug was withdrawn from the market, and fexofenadine is now marketed as a widely used antihistamine (Allegra).

Similarly, CYP3A inhibition appears to increase the risk of rhabdomyolysis with some but not all HMG-CoA reductase inhibitors, through mechanisms that are not completely understood[8]; fibrates also increase this risk, though the mechanisms are uncertain.

Administration of CYP2D6-metabolized beta blockers to patients with defective enzyme activity (on a genetic basis or due to coadministration of inhibitors) produces exaggerated heart rate slowing. Similarly, the weak beta-blocking actions of the antiarrhythmic propafenone are increased in this setting. The widely used analgesic codeine undergoes CYP2D6-mediated bioactivation to an active metabolite, morphine, and patients with defective CYP2D6 activity display reduced analgesia.[9] A small group of individuals with multiple functional copies of CYP2D6, and hence *increased* enzymatic activity, has been identified; in this group codeine may produce nausea and euphoria, presumably due to rapid morphine generation. Similarly, some antidepressants are CYP2D6 substrates; for these drugs, cardiovascular adverse effects are more common in CYP2D6 poor metabolizers, whereas therapeutic efficacy is more difficult to achieve in ultra-rapid metabolizers.

The concept of high-risk pharmacokinetics extends from drug metabolism to transporter-mediated drug elimination. The most widely recognized example is digoxin, which is eliminated primarily by P-glycoprotein-mediated efflux into bile and urine. Administration of wide range of structurally and mechanistically unrelated drugs has been empirically recognized to increase digoxin concentrations, and the common mechanism appears to be inhibition of P-glycoprotein-mediated elimination (see Table 5–1).[7]

Pharmacodynamics and the Genetics of Drug Responses

Drugs can exert variable effects, even in the absence of pharmacokinetic variability. As indicated in Figure 5–1, this variability can arise as a function of variability in the molecular targets with which drugs interact to achieve their (beneficial and adverse) effects, as well as variability in the broader biologic context within which the drug-target interaction takes place. Simple examples illustrate the point that this is a common mechanism for variability in drug action: the effect of lytic therapy in a patient with no clot is manifestly different from that in a patient with acute coronary thrombosis; the arrhythmogenic effects of digitalis depend on serum potassium; the vasodilating effects of nitrates, beneficial in patients with coronary disease with angina, can be catastrophic in patients with aortic stenosis.

DNA variants in key genes controlling this biological context (as well as genes encoding drug targets themselves) are increasingly recognized as contributors to variability in drug action. Many examples of associations between DNA polymorphisms and disease severity are now reported; there are fewer reports of polymorphisms modulating responses to cardiovascular drugs, and examples are listed in Table 5–2. It is important to recognize that genomic science is in its

TABLE 5–1 Proteins Important in Drug Metabolism and Elimination

Protein	Substrates	Interacting drugs	Genetics
CYP3A4, CYP3A5	Erythromycin, clarithromycin Quinidine, mexiletine Many benzodiazepines Cyclosporine, tacrolimus Many antivirals HMG CoA reductase inhibitors (atorvastatin, simvastatin, lovastatin; not pravastatin) Many calcium channel blockers	*Inhibitors:* Antivirals: ritonavir and others Amiodarone Erythromycin, clarithromycin (not azithromycin) Ketaconazole, itraconazole Many calcium channel blockers *Inducers:* Rifampin Efavirenz, nevirapine St. John's wort Phenytoin Pioglitazone	Highly variable activity in vivo Common coding region polymorphism in CYP3A5 may contribute; more common in blacks than whites No common coding region polymorphisms in CYP3A4
CYP2D6	Some beta-blockers: propranolol, timolol, metoprolol, carvedilol Propafenone Desipramine and other tricyclics Codeine Debrisoquine Dextromethorphan	*Inhibitors:* Amiodarone Fluoxetine Quinidine Paroxetine *Inducers:* Rifampin	Multiple loss of function alleles described. Common (25%) in white and black populations; homozygotes (7%) display the PM phenotype. Reduction of function alleles described in Asian populations but PMs rare. Ultra-rapid metabolizers due to multiple functional copies of CYP2D6 described especially in northern Africa.
CYP2C9	Warfarin Phenytoin Tolbutamide Glyburide Losartan, irbesartan	*Inhibitors:* Amiodarone Zafirlukast *Inducers:* Rifampin Barbiturates	Heterozygotes for common (>50% in some populations) loss of function alleles display reduced enzymatic activity and may have lower warfarin dose requirements. Very low warfarin dose requirements in homozygotes.
CYP2C19	Omeprazole Mephenytoin Nelfinavir		PMs common (~20%) in Asian populations.
P-glycoprotein	Digoxin Fexofenadine Cyclosporine, tacrolimus Many anticancer agents Many antivirals	*Inhibitors:* Amiodarone Quinidine Ketoconazole Erythromycin Itraconazole Verapamil Cyclosporine	DNA polymorphisms common; clinical significance uncertain
N-acetyl transferase	Procainamide Hydralazine Isoniazid		Whites and blacks: 50% fast acetylators, 50% slow acetylators, no non-acetylators Asians: mostly fast acetylators Slow acetylators: increased risk of the lupus syndrome Slow acetylators; increased risk of hepatotoxicity
Thiopurine methyl-transferase	6-mercaptopurine Azathioprine		Homozygotes for loss of function mutations (1/300): increased risk for bone marrow aplasia at usual doses Rapid metabolizers: suboptimal therapeutic response
Pseudo cholinesterase	Succinylcholine		Rare homozygote null individuals: prolonged apnea
UDP-glucuronosyl-transferase	Irinotecan		Polymorphisms cause Gilbert syndrome Enhanced toxicity of some anticancer drugs

More detailed CYP listing available at http://medicine.iupui.edu/flockhart/
PM = Poor metabolizer.

infancy; therefore, reported associations such as these require independent confirmation and assessment of clinical importance and cost-effectiveness before they can or should enter clinical practice.

Polymorphisms in the β_1 and β_2 receptor genes have been associated with variability in heart rate slowing and blood pressure effects with beta blockers and beta agonists.[10-12] An example of tumor genotype determining response to therapy is the anticancer drug herceptin, which is effective only in cancers that do not express the herceptin receptor; since the drug also potentiates anthracycline-related cardiotoxicity, toxic therapy can be avoided in patients who are receptor-negative.[13]

The ACE gene includes a common polymorphism (termed insertion/deletion, or I/D) that determines ACE activity. DD individuals, homozygous for the D allele, have higher plasma ACE activity and thus higher concentrations of the pressor peptide angiotensin than do II individuals. DD patients with heart failure have a worse prognosis than do II or ID subjects and yet have a better response to beta blockers.[14] Almost certainly, this action does not reflect a direct interaction between beta blockers and the ACE protein; rather, the ACE polymorphism likely alters the milieu in which the beta blocker interacts with beta receptors to ameliorate the prognosis in patients with heart failure. Similarly, the effect of hormone replacement therapy on high-density lipoprotein cholesterol has been linked to a polymorphism in the estrogen receptor,[15] and susceptibility to stroke in patients receiving diuretics to a polymorphism in the adducin gene that plays a role in renal tubular sodium transport.[16] Torsades de pointes during QT-prolonging antiarrhythmic therapy has been linked to polymorphisms in ion channel genes; in addition, this adverse effect sometimes arises in patients with clinically latent congenital long QT syndrome, emphasizing the interrelationship among disease, genetic background, and drug therapy.[17,18]

Principles of Dosage Optimization

The goals of drug therapy should be defined prior to initiation of drug treatment. These may include acute correction of serious pathophysiology, acute or chronic symptom relief, or changes in "surrogate" endpoints (such as blood pressure or serum cholesterol or INR) that have been linked to beneficial outcomes in target patient populations. The lessons of CAST and of positive inotropic drugs should make prescribers skeptical about such surrogate-guided therapy in the absence of controlled clinical trials.

When the goal of drug therapy is to acutely correct a disturbance in physiology, the drug should be administered intravenously, in doses designed to rapidly achieve a therapeutic effect. This approach is best justified when benefits clearly outweigh risks. As discussed earlier with lidocaine, large intravenous drug boluses carry with them a risk of enhancing drug-related toxicity, so even with the most urgent of medical indications, this approach is rarely appropriate. An exception is adenosine, which must be administered as a rapid bolus because it undergoes extensive and rapid elimination from plasma by uptake into virtually all cells; as a consequence, a slow bolus or infusion rarely achieves sufficiently high concentrations at the desired site of action (the coronary artery perfusing the atrioventricular node) to terminate arrhythmias.

The time required to achieve steady-state plasma concentrations is determined by elimination half-life, as discussed earlier. The administration of a loading dose may abbreviate this time, but only if the kinetics of distribution and elimination are known *a priori* in an individual subject and the correct loading regimen is chosen; otherwise, overshoot or undershoot during the loading phase may occur. Thus, the initiation of drug therapy by a loading strategy should be used only when the indication is acute.

Two dose-response curves describe the relationship between drug dose and the expected cumulative incidence of a beneficial effect or an adverse effect (Fig. 5–4). The distance along the X axis describing the difference between these

TABLE 5–2 DNA Polymorphisms Implicated in Variable Pharmacodynamics in Cardiovascular Medicine*

Drug	Gene	Reported Association
QT-prolonging drugs	KCNH2/KCNE2 (HERG/MiRP1)†	Increased torsades de pointes risk in patients with KCNE2 T8A[18]
QT-prolonging drugs	KCNQ1 (KvLKQT1)† MinK (KCNE1)[1] SCN5A†	Increased torsades de pointes risk in patients with KCNE1 D85N, SCN5A S1102Y[22,23]
Beta-blockers	β_1- and β_2-adrenergic receptor	Altered extent of heart rate slowing or blood pressure lowering[10-12]
ACE inhibitors	ACE	Decreased response in DD subjects[24]
β-blockers	ACE	Increased response in DD subjects[19]
Fluvastatin	ABCA1 transporter LDL receptor Paraoxonase	Variable low-density lipoprotein lowering[25-27]
Pravastatin	Cholesteryl ester transfer protein	Variable regression of atherosclerosis[28]
Estrogen	Estrogen receptor	Variable high-density lipoprotein elevation[15]
Lipid-lowering therapy	Hepatic lipase	Variable lipid lowering[29]
Antiplatelet drugs	Platelet glycoprotein IIIa	Variable antiplatelet effects ex vivo[30]
Amiloride	Epithelial sodium channel	Antihypertensive effect in black subjects[31]
Antihypertensive drugs	β_3 G-Protein subunit	Variable blood pressure lowering[32]
Diuretics	α-adducin	Variable myocardial infarction or stroke incidence during antihypertensive therapy[16] Variable blood pressure response (especially with ACE I/D)[33]
ACE inhibitor	Bradykinin B2 receptor	ACE-inhibitor cough[34]

ACE = angiotensin-converting enzyme.
*DNA variants that modulate pharmacokinetics are listed in Table 5–1.
†Mutations in these genes, causing the long QT syndrome, may be clinically silent until challenge with QT prolonging drugs

curves, often termed the *therapeutic ratio* (or index or window), provides an index of the likelihood that a chronic dosing regimen that provides benefits without adverse effects can be identified. Drugs with especially wide therapeutic indices can often be administered at infrequent intervals, even if they are rapidly eliminated (left panels, Fig. 5–4).

When expected adverse effects are serious, the most appropriate treatment strategy is to start at very low doses and re-evaluate the necessity for increasing drug dosages once steady-state drug effects have been achieved. This approach has the advantage of minimizing the risk of dose-related adverse effects but carries with it a need to titrate doses to efficacy. Only when stable drug effects are achieved should increasing drug dosage to achieve the desired therapeutic effect be considered.

The risk of sotalol-related torsades de pointes increases with drug dosage, and so the starting dose should be low. In other cases, anticipated toxicity is relatively mild and manageable. Here, it may be acceptable to start at dosages greater than the minimum required to achieve a therapeutic effect, accepting a greater than minimal risk of adverse effects; some antihypertensives can be administered in this fashion. However, the principle of using the lowest dose possible to minimize toxicity, particularly toxicity that is unpredictable and unrelated to recognized pharmacologic actions, should be the rule.

Occasionally, dose escalation into the high therapeutic range results in no beneficial drug effect and no side effects. In this circumstance, the prescriber should be alert to the possibility of drug interactions, at the pharmacokinetic or pharmacodynamic level. Depending on the nature of the anticipated toxicity, dose escalation beyond the usual therapeutic range may occasionally be acceptable, but only if anticipated toxicity is not serious and is readily manageable.

PLASMA CONCENTRATION MONITORING. For some drugs, curves such as those shown in Figures 5–4A and B relating drug concentration to cumulative incidence of beneficial and adverse effects can be generated. With such drugs, monitoring plasma drug concentrations to ensure that they remain within a desired therapeutic range (i.e., above a minimum required for efficacy and below a maximum likely to produce adverse effects) may be a very useful adjunct to therapy. Monitoring drug concentrations may also be useful to ensure compliance and to detect pharmacokinetically based drug interactions that underlie unanticipated efficacy and/or toxicity at usual dosages. Samples for measurement of plasma concentrations should generally be obtained just prior to the next dose, at steady state. These "trough" concentrations provide an index of the minimum plasma concentration expected during a dosing interval.

On the other hand, patient monitoring, whether by plasma concentration or other physiologic indices, to detect incipient toxicity is best accomplished at the time of anticipated peak drug concentrations. Thus, patient surveillance for QT prolongation during sotalol therapy is best accomplished 1 to 2 hours after administration of a dose of drug at steady state.

There may be a lag between the time courses of drug in plasma and of drug effects, as described earlier. In addition, monitoring plasma drug concentrations relies on the assumption that the concentration measured is in equilibrium with that at the target molecular site. Importantly, it is only the fraction of drug that is not bound to plasma proteins that is available to achieve such equilibration. Variability in the extent of protein binding can therefore affect the free fraction and the anticipated drug effect, even in the face of apparently therapeutic total plasma drug concentrations. Basic drugs such as lidocaine and quinidine not only are bound to albumin but also bind extensively to α_1-acid glycoprotein, an acute phase reactant whose concentrations are increased in a variety of "stress" situations, including acute myocardial infarction. Because of this increased protein binding, drug effects may be blunted despite "therapeutic" drug concentrations in these situations.

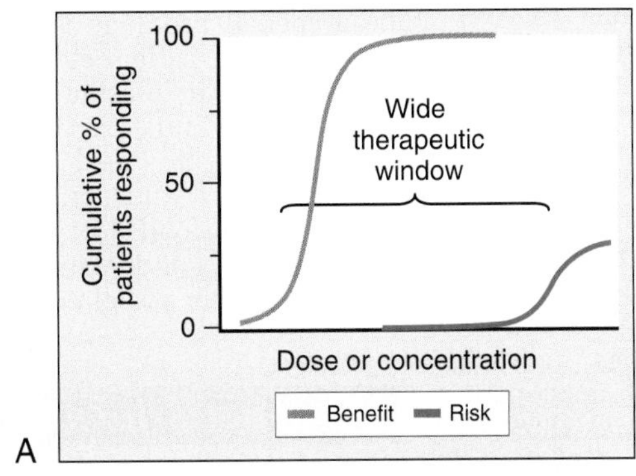

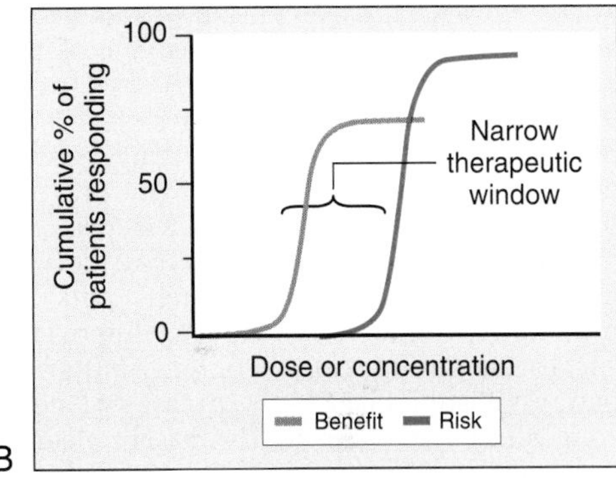

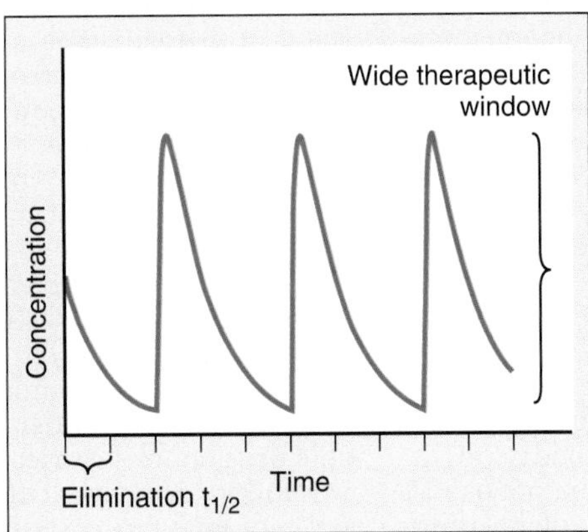

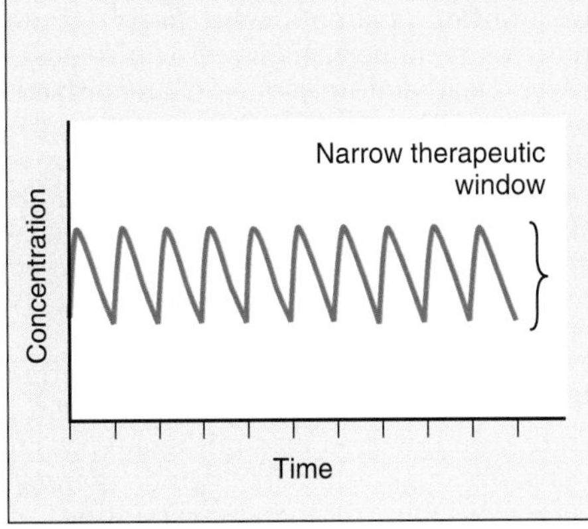

FIGURE 5–4 The concept of a therapeutic ratio. **A** and **B,** Dose- (or concentration) response curves: the solid line in each panel describes the relationship between dose and cumulative incidence of beneficial effects and the dotted line the relationship between dose and dose-related adverse effects (risk). A drug with a wide therapeutic ratio displays separation between the two curves, a high degree of efficacy, and a low degree of dose-related toxicity **(A).** Also, the toxicity would be expected to be mild and readily reversible. Under these conditions, a wide therapeutic ratio can be defined. In part **B,** on the other hand, the curves describing cumulative efficacy and cumulative incidence of adverse effects are positioned near each other, the incidence of adverse effects is higher, and the expected beneficial response is lower; these characteristics define a narrow therapeutic ratio. **C** and **D,** Steady-state plasma concentrations with oral drug administration as a function of time with wide (left) and narrow (right) therapeutic ratios. The hash marks on the abscissae indicate one elimination half-life. When the therapeutic window is wide **(C),** drug administration every three elimination half-lives can produce plasma concentrations that are maintained above the minimum for efficacy and below the maximum beyond which toxicity is anticipated. Panel **D** shows the opposite situation. To maintain plasma concentrations within the narrow therapeutic range, the drug must be administered more frequently.

It is unusual for a healthy patient to receive chronic drug therapy with a single agent. Rather, the rule is polypharmacy in patients with varying degrees of specific organ dysfunction. Although treatment with an individual agent may be justified, the practitioner should also recognize the risk of unanticipated drug effects, particularly drug toxicity, in these settings.

The presence of advanced renal disease mandates that the dosages of drugs eliminated primarily by renal excretion be reduced. Digoxin, dofetilide, and sotalol are examples. A requirement for dose adjustment in cases of less severe renal dysfunction is dictated by available clinical data, and the likelihood of serious toxicity if drug accumulates in plasma due to impaired elimination. Renal failure reduces the protein binding of some drugs (e.g., phenytoin); in this instance, a total drug concentration value in the therapeutic range may actually represent a toxic value of unbound drug.

Very advanced liver disease is characterized by decreased hepatic drug metabolism and portocaval shunts that decrease clearance (and particularly first-pass clearance). Moreover, such patients frequently have other profound disturbances of homeostasis, such as coagulopathy, severe ascites, and altered mental status. These pathophysiologic features of advanced liver disease can profoundly affect not only the dose of a drug required to achieve a potentially therapeutic effect but also the perception of risks and benefits, thereby altering the prescriber's assessment of the actual need for therapy.

Heart disease similarly carries with it a number of disturbances of drug elimination and drug sensitivity that may alter either the therapeutic doses or the practitioner's perception of the desirability of therapy, based on evaluation of risks and benefits. Patients with left ventricular hypertrophy often have baseline QT prolongation, and thus risks of QT-prolonging antiarrhythmias may increase; most guidelines suggest avoiding QT-prolonging antiarrhythmics in such patients (see Table 72–3). In cases of heart failure, hepatic congestion can lead to decreased clearance and thus an increased risk for toxicity with usual doses of certain drugs. Some sedatives, lidocaine, and beta blockers are examples. In addition, patients with heart failure may demonstrate reduced renal perfusion and require dose adjustments on this basis. Heart failure is also characterized by a redistribution of regional blood flow. This can lead to reduced volume of distribution and enhanced risk for drug toxicity. Lidocaine is probably the best-studied example: loading doses of lidocaine should be reduced in patients with heart failure because of altered distribution, whereas maintenance doses should be reduced in cases both of heart failure and of liver disease because of altered clearance.

Age is also a major factor in determining drug doses as well as sensitivity to drug effects. Doses in children are generally administered on a milligram per kilogram body weight basis, although firm data to guide therapy are often not available. Variable postnatal maturation of drug disposition systems may present a special problem in the neonate. Elderly persons often have reduced creatinine clearance, even in the face of a normal serum creatinine level, and dosages of renally excreted drugs should be adjusted accordingly. Systolic dysfunction with hepatic congestion is more common in the elderly. Vascular disease and dementia are common in the elderly and can lead to increased postural hypotension and risk of falling. Thus, therapies such as sedatives, tricyclic antidepressants, or anticoagulants should be initiated only when the practitioner is convinced that the benefits of such therapies outweigh this increased risk.

Drug Interactions

Multiple mechanisms, and examples, of interactions on a pharmacokinetic or pharmacodynamic basis have been presented in this chapter. Table 5–3 summarizes these and other mechanisms that may underlie important drug interactions. Drug interactions may be based on altered pharmacokinetics (absorption, distribution, metabolism, and excretion). In addition, drugs can interact at the pharmacodynamic level. A trivial example is coadministration of two antihypertensive drugs leading to excessive hypotension. Similarly, coadministration of aspirin and warfarin leads to an increased risk for bleeding, although benefits of the combination can also be demonstrated.

The most important principle in approaching a patient receiving polypharmacy is to recognize this potential. A complete medication history should be obtained from each patient at regular intervals; patients will often omit topical medications such as eye drops, "health food" supplements, and medications prescribed by other practitioners unless specifically prompted. Each of these, however, carries a risk of important systemic drug actions and interactions. Beta blocker eye drops can produce systemic beta blockade, particularly with CYP2D6 substrates in patients with defective CYP2D6 activity. St. John's wort induces CYP3A and P-glycoprotein activity and thus can markedly lower plasma concentrations of drugs such as cyclosporine and oral contraceptives.[19,20] As with many other interactions, this may not be a special problem as long as both drugs are continued. However, if a patient stabilized on cyclosporine stops taking St. John's wort, plasma concentrations of the drug can rise dramatically and toxicity ensue. Similarly, initiation of St. John's wort may lead to markedly lowered cyclosporine concentrations and a risk of organ rejection. A number of other "health foods" have been associated with very serious drug toxicity and withdrawal from the market; phenylpropanolamine-associated stroke is one recent example.[21]

Prospects for the Future

The last 20 years have seen dramatic advances in the treatment of heart disease, due in no small part to the development of highly effective and well tolerated drug therapies, such as HMG-CoA reductase inhibitors, ACE inhibitors, and beta blockers. These developments, along with improved nonpharmacological approaches, have led to dramatically enhanced survival of patients with advanced heart disease. Thus, polypharmacy in an aging and chronically ill population is becoming increasing common. In this milieu, drug effects become increasingly variable, reflecting interactions among drugs, underlying disease and disease mechanisms, and genetic backgrounds.

An increasing understanding of the genetic basis of variable drug actions carries with it the promise of reducing such variability. However, the logistics of implementing such a strategy and the costs of individualizing therapy based on genetics are major outstanding issues. An alternate view is that effective therapies are available and have not been adequately delivered to populations that would benefit. The two views are not mutually exclusive. In the face of such increasing complexity, the relationship between the individual prescriber and the individual patient remains the centerpiece of modern therapeutics. Each initiation of drug therapy represents a new clinical experiment, and prescribers must be continually vigilant regarding the possibility of unusual drug effects that may provide initial clues to unanticipated and important mechanisms of beneficial and adverse drug effects.

TABLE 5–3 Drug Interactions: Mechanisms and Examples

Mechanism	Drug	Interacting Drug	Effect
Decreased bioavailability	Digoxin	Antacids	Decreased digoxin effect due to decreased absorption
Increased bioavailability	Digoxin	Antibiotics	By eliminating gut flora that metabolize digoxin, some antibiotics may increase digoxin bioavailability. Note: some antibiotics also interfere with P-glycoprotein (expressed in the intestine and elsewhere), another effect that can elevate digoxin concentration.
Induction of hepatic metabolism	*CYP3A substrates:* Quinidine Mexiletine Verapamil Cyclosporine	Phenytoin Rifampin Barbiturates St. John's wort	Loss of drug effect due to increased metabolism Similar effects with the CYP2C9 substrate warfarin, except with phenytoin
Inhibition of hepatic metabolism	*CYP2C9:* Warfarin Losartan	Amiodarone Phenytoin	Decreased warfarin requirement Diminished conversion of losartan to its active metabolite, with decreased antihypertensive control
	CYP3A substrates: Quinidine Cyclosporine HMG-CoA reductase inhibitors: lovastatin, simvastatin, atorvastatin; not pravastatin Cisapride, terfenadine, astemizole*	Ketoconazole Itraconazole Erythromycin Clarithromycin Some calcium blockers Some HIV protease inhibitors (especially ritanovir)	Increased risk for drug toxicity
	CYP2D6 substrates: Beta blockers (see Table 5–1) Propafenone Desipramine Codeine	Quinidine (even ultra-low dose) Fluoxetine	Increased beta-blockade Increased beta-blockade Increased adverse effects Decreased analgesia (due to failure of biotransformation to the active metabolite morphine)
Inhibition of drug transport	*P-glycoprotein substrates:* Digoxin	Amiodarone Quinidine Verapamil Cyclosporine Itraconazole Erythromycin	Digoxin toxicity
	Renal tubular transport: Dofetilide	Verapamil Cimetidine	Slightly increased plasma concentration and QT effect
	Monoamine transporter substrates: Guandrel	Tricyclic antidepressants	Blunted antihypertensive effects
Pharmacodynamic interactions	Aspirin + warfarin		Increased therapeutic anti-thrombotic effect; increased risk of bleeding
	Nonsteroidal anti-inflammatory drugs	Warfarin	Increased risk of gastrointestinal bleeding
	Antihypertensive drugs	Nonsteroidal anti-inflammatory drugs	Loss of blood pressure lowering
	QT-prolonging antiarrhythmics	Diuretics	Increased torsades de pointes risk due to diuretic-induced hypokalemia
	Supplemental potassium	Angiotensin-converting enzyme inhibitors	Hyperkalemia
	Sildenafil	Nitrates	Increased and persistent vasodilation; risk of myocardial ischemia

*These drugs have been withdrawn or their availability highly restricted because they can produce torsades de pointes, particularly when their metabolism is inhibited.

REFERENCES

Importance of Correct Drug Use

1. (http://cms.hhs.gov/statistics/nhe/historical/t2.asp; http://www.americanheart.org/downloadable/heart/ 10461207852142003HDSStatsBook.pdf)
2. Cohn JN, Goldstein SO, Greenberg BH, et al: A dose-dependent increase in mortality with vesnarinone among patients with severe heart failure. Vesnarinone Trial Investigators. N Engl J Med 339:1810, 1998.

Variability in Drug Action

3. Roden DM, George AL Jr: The genetic basis of variability in drug responses. Nat Rev Drug Discovery 1:37, 2002.
4. Kuehl P, Zhang J, Lin Y, et al: Sequence diversity in CYP3A promoters and characterization of the genetic basis of polymorphic CYP3A5 expression. Nat Genet 27:383, 2001.
5. Meyer UA: Pharmacogenetics and adverse drug reactions. Lancet 356:1667, 2000.
6. Fischer TL, Pieper JA, Graff DW, et al: Evaluation of potential losartan-phenytoin drug interactions in healthy volunteers. Clin Pharmacol Ther 72:238, 2002.
7. Fromm MF, Kim RB, Stein CM, et al: Inhibition of P-glycoprotein-mediated drug transport: A unifying mechanism to explain the interaction between digoxin and quinidine. Circulation 99:552, 1999.

Clinical Relevance of Polymorphic Drug Metabolism

8. Thompson PD, Clarkson P, Karas RH: Statin-associated myopathy. JAMA 289:1681, 2003.
9. Caraco Y, Sheller J, Wood AJ: Impact of ethnic origin and quinidine coadministration on codeine's disposition and pharmacodynamic effects. J Pharmacol Exp Ther 290:413, 1999.

Pharmacodynamics

10. Sofowora GG, Dishy V, Muszkat M, et al: A common beta1-adrenergic receptor polymorphism (Arg389Gly) affects blood pressure response to beta-blockade. Clin Pharmacol Ther 73:366, 2003.
11. Dishy V, Sofowora GG, Xie HG, et al: The effect of common polymorphisms of the beta2-adrenergic receptor on agonist-mediated vascular desensitization. N Engl J Med 345: 1030, 2001.
12. Johnson JA, Terra SG: β-Adrenergic receptor polymorphisms: Cardiovascular disease associations and pharmacogenetics. Pharm Res 19:1779, 2002.
13. Chien KR: Myocyte survival pathways and cardiomyopathy: Implications for trastuzumab cardiotoxicity. Semin Oncol 27:9, 2000.
14. McNamara DM, Holubkkov R, Janosko K, et al: Pharmacogenetic interactions between β-blocker therapy and the angiotensin-converting enzyme deletion polymorphism in patients with congestive heart failure. Circulation 103:1644, 2001.
15. Al Khatib SM, Granger CB, Huang Y, et al: Sustained ventricular arrhythmias among patients with acute coronary syndromes with no ST-segment elevation: Incidence, predictors, and outcomes. Circulation 106:309, 2002.
16. Psaty BM, Smith NL, Heckbert SR, et al: Diuretic therapy, the alpha-adducin gene variant, and the risk of myocardial infarction or stroke in persons with treated hypertension. JAMA 287:1680, 2002.
17. Yang P, Kanki H, Drolet B, et al: Allelic variants in long QT disease genes in patients with drug-associated torsades de pointes. Circulation 105:1943, 2002.
18. Sesti F, Abbott GW, Wei J, et al: A common polymorphism associated with antibiotic-induced cardiac arrhythmia. PNAS 97:10613, 2000.

Drug Interactions

19. Dresser GK, Schwarz UI, Wilkinson GR, et al: Coordinate induction of both cytochrome P4503A and MDR1 by St John's wort in healthy subjects. Clin Pharmacol Ther 73:41, 2003.
20. Zhou S, Gao Y, Jiang W, et al: Interactions of herbs with cytochrome P450. Drug Metab Rev 35:35, 2003.
21. Kernan WN, Viscoli CM, Brass LM, et al: Phenylpropanolamine and the risk of hemorrhagic stroke. N Engl J Med 343:1826, 2000.
22. Splawski I, Timothy KW, Tateyama M, et al: Variant of SCN5A sodium channel implicated in risk of cardiac arrhythmia. Science 297:1333, 2002.
23. Wei J, Yang IC, Tapper AR, et al: *KCNE1* polymorphism confers risk of drug-induced long QT syndrome by altering kinetic properties of IKs potassium channels. Circulation 100:I-495, 1999.
24. Kuznetsova T, Staessen JA, Wang JG, et al: Antihypertensive treatment modulates the association between the D/I ACE gene polymorphism and left ventricular hypertrophy: A meta-analysis. J Hum Hypertens 14:447, 2000.
25. Turban S, Fuentes F, Ferlic L, et al: A prospective study of paraoxonase gene Q/R192 polymorphism and severity, progression and regression of coronary atherosclerosis, plasma lipid levels, clinical events and response to fluvastatin. Atherosclerosis 154:633, 2001.
26. Salazar LA, Hirata MH, Quintao EC, et al: Lipid-lowering response of the HMG-CoA reductase inhibitor fluvastatin is influenced by polymorphisms in the low-density lipoprotein receptor gene in Brazilian patients with primary hypercholesterolemia. J Clin Lab Anal 14:125, 2000.
27. Lutucuta S, Ballantyne CM, Elghannam H, et al: Novel polymorphisms in promoter region of ATP binding cassette transporter gene and plasma lipids, severity, progression, and regression of coronary atherosclerosis and response to therapy. Circ Res 88:969, 2001.
28. Kuivenhoven JA, Jukema JW, Zwinderman AH, et al: The role of a common variant of the cholesteryl ester transfer protein gene in the progression of coronary atherosclerosis. The Regression Growth Evaluation Statin Study Group. N Engl J Med 338:86, 1998.
29. Zambon A, Deeb SS, Brown BG, et al: Common hepatic lipase gene promoter variant determines clinical response to intensive lipid-lowering treatment. Circulation 103:792, 2001.
30. Szczeklik A, Sanak M, Undas A, et al: Platelet glycoprotein IIIa P1A polymorphism and effects of aspirin on thrombin generation response. Circulation 103:33e, 2001.
31. Baker EH, Duggal A, Dong Y, et al: Amiloride, a specific drug for hypertension in black people with T594M variant? Hypertension 40:13, 2002.
32. Siffert W: Cardiovascular pharmacogenetics: On the way toward individually tailored drug therapy. Kidney Int Suppl 84:S168, 2003.
33. Sciarrone MT, Stella P, Barlassina C, et al: ACE and alpha-adducin polymorphism as markers of individual response to diuretic therapy. Hypertension 41:398, 2003.
34. Mukae S, Aoki S, Itoh S, et al: Bradykinin B2 receptor gene polymorphism is associated with angiotensin-converting enzyme inhibitor-related cough. Hypertension 36:127, 2000.

CHAPTER 6

Care of Patients with End-Stage Heart Disease

Linda L. Emanuel • Robert O. Bonow

Care for the incurable patient has been a defining part of medicine from its earliest origins, as reflected in the emphasis on comfort in the writings of 5th century BC Greek physician Hippocrates.[1] In recent decades, advances in cardiopulmonary resuscitation, cardiovascular surgery, and implantable devices have stimulated medical ethics discussions of who should receive resuscitation and when life really ends. End-of-life and palliative care more generally remain a defining part of the practice of cardiology. For instance, the primary indication for coronary artery bypass, stents (see Chap. 50), and other procedures is symptom control and quality of life; in this sense, a significant amount of care provided by cardiologists is quality palliative care. At the same time, consideration of the types of care sought by those who are facing death and dying needs more attention.[2-4] For instance, one study found that of the 15 guidelines on congestive heart failure (see Chap. 24), none had significant mention of palliative care and only six had moderate mention.[5] By explicitly integrating palliative care considerations into the new patient assessment, treatment decision-making, continuity of care planning, and systems of care delivery, cardiovascular medicine can further advance the quality of care it provides.[6]

Epidemiology (see Chap. 1)

The characteristic cardiovascular death is sudden (see Chap. 33). However, cardiovascular conditions are also chronic and can afflict children and young adults as well as the elderly. In 2000, about 65 million Americans had chronic cardiovascular conditions, and between 1976 and 1980, approximately 1 million children and young adults were living with congenital heart defects.

The site of death has also evolved. Nearly 60% of Americans died as inpatients in hospitals in 1980; by 2000, about 40% died in the hospital. Although this trend corresponds with patient and family preferences, patients with cardiovascular disease are least represented among those receiving home care and hospice care. In 2000, approximately 20% of all decedents received hospice care, with cancer patients accounting for more than 70% of hospice users. Among patients with nine cancer diagnoses, 15% to 34% of decedents used hospice, whereas among patients with myocardial infarction and congestive heart failure diagnoses, 7% and 8% of decedents, respectively, used hospice.[7] Patients in need of palliative care can be ambulatory, in long-term care, or in the hospital. Consequently, palliative care is needed in a full range of settings.

Palliative Care

Because terminally ill patients have a wide variety of advanced diseases, often with multiple symptoms demanding relief and requiring a noninvasive therapeutic regimen to be delivered in a commodious care setting, their care requires some of the most complex and demanding cognitive skills for assessments and interventions. Fundamental to ensuring quality palliative and end-of-life care is a focus on four broad domains of the illness experience: (1) physical symptoms; (2) mental or psychological symptoms; (3) social needs, including relationships, practical issues, and economic issues; and (4) existential or spiritual needs. Palliative care also includes support for the family, including for their bereavement. Recent empirical studies have confirmed that these domains coincide with the experiences and preferences for care of patients with advanced illness and for their families. A whole-person assessment screens for and evaluates needs in each of these four domains. Goals for care are discerned and decided on in discussion with the patient and/or family based on the assessment in each of these domains. Although physicians are responsible for certain, especially technical, interventions and for coordinating the interventions, they depend on an interdisciplinary team and the family to provide all of them. Importantly, failing to address any one of the domains is likely to preclude a good death, and therefore a well coordinated, effectively communicating interdisciplinary team takes on special importance in end-of-life care.

Assessment, Goals, and Care Planning

WHOLE-PERSON ASSESSMENT. The assessment of physical and mental symptoms should follow a modified version of the traditional history and physical examination that emphasizes symptoms. Questions should discern sources of suffering and how much these symptoms interfere with the patient's life. Standardized assessment questions are available from clinically relevant scales such as the Memorial Symptom Assessment Scale; these have the advantage of ensuring that the assessment is comprehensive. For a patient with late end-stage disease for whom the care goal is quality of being, tests and aspects of the physical examination that are uncomfortable should be carefully evaluated for their benefit-to-burden ratio for the patient. Since a focused physical examination may be all that is reasonable, these skills need to be well developed.

In the area of social needs, health care providers should screen for financial needs, the status of important relationships, care giving needs, and access to medical care. Relevant questions may include the following: *How often is there someone to feel close to? How much help do you need with things like getting meals or getting around? How much trouble do you have getting the medical care you need?* In the area of existential needs, providers should assess distress and the patient's sense of being emotionally and existentially settled and of finding purpose or meaning.[8] Helpful assessment questions can include the following: *How much are you able to find meaning since your illness began?* It is helpful to ask about the patient's perception of his or her care, as follows: *How much do you feel your doctors and nurses respect you? How clear is the information from us about what to expect regarding your illness? How much do you feel that the medical care you are getting fits with your goals?* If concern is detected in any areas, deeper evaluation questions are warranted.[9]

COMMUNICATION. Communication is arguably as powerful an intervention in medicine as any invasive procedure. Poor communication has significant adverse consequences, and quality communication allows for navigating difficult situations in the best available fashion. Communication requires both effective "signal output" and effective reception, so the clinician must assist the patient and family with their ability to receive difficult information as well as offer the information in an accessible way.

A seven-step guide for communicating important information has been developed by Buckman: (1) Prepare, mentally and physically by (2) setting up a quiet environment with room for face-to-face discussion and accommodating items such as a chair, a box of tissues, a pen and paper to write down information, and perhaps a beverage. (3) Begin by asking what the patient and/or family know and/or understand and then (4) ask how they prefer to receive new information and how much they want who to know. (5) Give the new information according to their preferences. (6) Allow for emotional responses and (7) plan for the next steps in care, including identification of the next concrete steps.[10] See Table 6–1 for suggested wording and the rationale behind each step.

PROGNOSIS. Among patients with an equally poor prognosis, 75% of cancer patients reported that they knew they would likely die, whereas only 54% of non-cancer patients, many of whom had cardiac diagnoses, reported the same.[11,12]

TABLE 6–1 Elements of Communicating Bad News: The P-SPIKES Approach

Acronym	Steps	Aim of the Interaction	Preparations, Questions, or Phrases
P	Preparation	Mentally prepare for the interaction with the patient and/or family.	Review what information needs to be communicated. Plan how you will provide emotional support. Rehearse key steps and phrases in the interaction.
S	Setting of the interaction	Ensure the appropriate setting for a serious and emotionally charged discussion.	Ensure that patient, family, and appropriate social supports are present. Devote sufficient time—do not squeeze in a discussion. Ensure privacy and prevent interruptions by people or beeper. Bring a box of tissues.
P	Patient's perception and preparation	Begin the discussion by establishing the baseline and whether the patient and family can grasp the information. Ease tension by having the patient and family contribute.	Start with open-ended questions to encourage participation. Possible phrases to use: *What do you understand about your illness?* *When you first had symptom X, what did you think it might be?* *What did Dr. X tell you when he sent you here?* *What do you think is going to happen?*
I	Invitation and information needs	Discover what information needs the patient and/or family have and what limits they want regarding the bad information.	Possible phrases to use: *If this condition turns out to be something serious, do you want to know?* *Would you like me to tell you the full details of your condition? If not, then who would you like me to talk to?*
K	Knowledge of the condition	Provide the bad news or other information to the patient and/or family sensitively.	Do not just dump the information on the patient and family. Interrupt and check that the patient and family are understanding. Possible phrases to use: *I feel badly to have to tell you this, but. . . .* *Unfortunately, the tests showed. . . .* *I'm afraid the news is not good. . . .*
E	Empathy and exploration	Identify the cause of the emotions—e.g. poor prognosis. Empathize with the patient and/or family's feelings. Explore by asking open-ended questions.	Strong feelings in reaction to bad news are normal. Acknowledge what the patient and family are feeling. Remind them that such feelings are normal even if frightening. Give them time to respond. Remind patient and family you won't abandon them. Possible phrases to use: *I imagine this is very hard for you.* *You must be upset. Tell me how you are feeling.* *I wish the news were different.* *I'll do whatever I can to help you.*
S	Summarizing and strategic planning	Delineate for the patient and the family the next steps, including additional tests or interventions.	It is the unknown and uncertain that increase anxiety. Recommend a schedule with goals and landmarks. Provide your rationale for the patient and/or family to accept or reject. If the patient and/or family are not ready to discuss the next steps, schedule a follow-up visit.

Adapted from Buchman R: How to Break Bad News: A Guide for Health Care Professionals. Baltimore, Johns Hopkins University Press, 1992.

The established gap between prognosis in late-stage cardiovascular conditions and the patients' expectation of death, the continuous stream of life-prolonging cardiovascular therapies and devices, the difficulty in establishing accurate prognoses in individual cases, and the need to sustain hope may be only four of multiple factors that conspire to keep poor prognosis from triggering appropriate forms of palliative care.

Clinicians should provide population-based statistics regarding prognosis to patients and families and allow these statistics rather than individual predictions to trigger the kinds of whole-patient assessments and continuous goal assessment conversations that follow palliative care guidelines. This in turn will allow patients and families not only to follow plans for care that are appropriate but also to achieve the kinds of psychological, social, and existential engagements that people tend to seek when going through the last stages of life.[13-15] Generally, clinicians should share population-based prognosis at the time of diagnosis and then introduce a palliative care framework of whole-patient assessment and continuous goal adjustment from the time when clinical indicators suggest a prognosis of 6 months or less. When sharing prognostic information, use language such as, *"Of all the people with your condition in America, about half will go on to live for more than 3 years and about half will die within 3 years."* Continue by saying something like this: *"We will hope for the best but also plan for the worst so that we are not caught unprepared and you can live your life with a positive attitude."* The conversation can go further if the clinician then says something such as, *"Many people have special things they want to accomplish in this phase of their life, such as a project, a trip, or coming to terms in a personal relationship. I encourage you to think about what that might be for you so that I can do my best to tailor our medical care to your goals."* For patients with cardiovascular illnesses, it is often helpful to point out that, *"The good news is that we can expect you to feel well and function pretty normally. Often people with cardiac disease avoid the long phases of disability and suffering that other illnesses can cause. The counterpart is that people sometimes do not engage in the growth that often comes at the end of life or they become overly fearful of dying suddenly. Preparation of the kind we just mentioned can bring the best of both worlds. So let's keep an open discussion about your goals for care."*

CONTINUOUS GOAL ASSESSMENT. Goals for care are numerous. They range from cure of a specific condition, to delaying the course of an incurable disease, to adapting to progressive disability without disrupting the family, to finding peace of mind or personal meaning, to dying in a manner that leaves loved ones with a positive "departure memory." Discernment of goals for care can be approached through a seven-step protocol: (1) Ensure that information is as complete as is reasonably possible and is understood by all relevant parties (see sections on Whole-Patient Assessment and on Communication). (2) Explore what the patient and family are hoping for. (3) Share all the options with the patient and family. Delineate some relevant goals that are also realistic. (4) Respond empathetically to the patient and family as they adjust to declining realistic expectations. (5) Make a plan, emphasizing what can be done toward the realistic goals. (6) Follow through with the plan. (7) Review and revise this plan periodically, considering at every encounter whether the goals of care should be reviewed with the patient and/or family. If a patient or family member has difficulty letting go of an unrealistic goal, suggest that while hoping for the best, it is still prudent to have a plan for other outcomes as well.

ADVANCE CARE PLANNING. Advance care planning is a process of planning for future medical care in case the patient becomes incapable of making medical decisions. Ideally, it starts before a health care crisis or the terminal phase of an illness. However, although 80% of Americans endorse advance care planning, only 20% have actually made advance care plans. A similarly small proportion of health care providers have completed their own advance care planning. A good first step is for health care providers to start with themselves. Personal planning makes the providers aware of the critical and charged choices in the process and allows them to truthfully tell their patients that they have done this themselves. With experience, advance care planning discussions need not take long.

Steps in effective advance care planning involve the following: (1) introducing the topic, (2) structuring a discussion, (3) reviewing plans that have been discussed by the patient and family, (4) documenting the plans, (5) updating them periodically, and (6) implementing the advance care directive (Table 6–2). Raising the topic can be done efficiently as a routine matter, analogous to insurance or estate planning, and is recommended for all patients. Structuring a focused discussion (step 2) is the central skill. Identify the health care proxy and recommend his or her involvement in the discussion. Select a worksheet, preferably one that has been evaluated and demonstrated to produce reliable and valid expressions of patient preferences, and orient the patient and proxy to it. Discuss with the patient and proxy one scenario as an example to demonstrate how to think about the issues. It is often helpful to begin with a scenario in which the patient is likely to have settled preferences, such as being in a persistent vegetative state. Ask the patient and proxy to discuss and complete the worksheet for the other scenarios. If appropriate, suggest that they involve family members in the discussion. On a return visit, go over the patient's preferences, checking and resolving any medical or logical inconsistencies. After having the patient and proxy sign the document, place it in the medical chart and be sure that copies are provided to relevant family members and care sites. Since patients' preferences can change, review these documents periodically or after an illness episode or personal experience.

Types of Documents. Two broad types of advance care planning documents exist. The first includes living wills or instructional directives; these advisory documents describe the types of decisions that should direct care. Some are specific, delineating scenarios and interventions. Among these, some are for general use and others are for a specific type of disease, such as cancer or human immunodeficiency virus; some are available in multiple languages.[16] Less specific directives can be general statements or can describe the values that should guide decisions. Health care proxy forms appoint an individual to make decisions. A combined directive that both directs care and designates a proxy is generally recommended, and the directive should clearly indicate whether the patient's preferences or the proxy's choice should take precedence if they conflict.

The U.S. Supreme Court has established that patients have a constitutional right to refuse or terminate life-sustaining interventions, and that mentally incompetent patients may do so by having previously provided "clear and convincing evidence" of their advance preferences.[17,18] As of 2003, all states and the District of Columbia also have living will or health care proxy legislation. State variations exist but are less important than they could be, since the Constitution has been interpreted to require states to honor any clear advance care directive. A potentially misleading distinction relates to statutory as opposed to advisory documents. Statutory documents are drafted to fit relevant state statutes. They tend to be written with the goal of protecting clinicians from legal action if they follow the patient's stated wishes. Advisory documents are drafted to reflect the patient's wishes. Both are legal, the first under State and the second under common or

TABLE 6–2 Steps in Advance Care Planning

Step	Goals to be Achieved and Measures to Cover	Useful Phrases or Points to Make
Introducing advance care planning	Ask the patient what he or she knows about advance care planning and if he or she has already completed an advance care directive. Indicate that you as a physician have completed advance care planning. Indicate that you try to perform advance care planning with all patients regardless of prognosis. Explain the goals of the process as empowering the patient and ensuring that you and the proxy understand the patient's preferences. Provide the patient with relevant literature, including the advance care directive that you prefer to use. Recommend that the patient identify a proxy decision-marker who should attend the next meeting.	"I'd like to talk with you about something I try to discuss with all my patients. It's called advance care planning. In fact, I feel that this is such an important topic that I have done this myself. Are you familiar with advance care planning or living wills?" "Have you thought about the type of care you would want if you ever became too sick to speak for yourself? That is the purpose of advance care planning." "There is no change in health that we have not discussed. I am bringing this up now because it is sensible for everyone, no matter how well or ill, old or young." Have many copies of advance care directives available, including in the waiting room, for patients and families.
Structured discussion of scenarios and patient preferences	Affirm that the goal of the process is to follow the patient's wishes if the patient loses decision-making capacity. Elicit the patient's overall goals related to health care. Elicit the patient's preferences for specific interventions in a few salient and common scenarios. Help the patient define the threshold for withdrawing and withholding interventions. Define the patient's preference for the role of the proxy.	Use a structured worksheet with typical scenarios. Begin the discussion with persistent vegetative state and consider other scenarios, such recovery from an acute event with serious disability, asking the patient about his or her preferences regarding specific interventions, such as ventilators, nasogastric feedings, and CPR proceeding to less invasive interventions, such as blood transfusions and antibiotics.
Review the patient's preferences	After the patient has made choices of interventions, review them to ensure that they are consistent and that the proxy is aware of them.	
Document the patient's preferences	Formally complete the advance care directive and have witness sign it. Provide a copy for the patient and the proxy. Insert a copy into the patient's medical record.	
Update the directive	Periodically, and with major changes in health status, review with the patient the existing choice made and make any modifications.	
Apply the directive	The directive goes into effect only when the patient becomes unable to make medical decisions for him- or herself. Re-read the directive to be sure about its content. Discuss your proposed actions based on the directive with the proxy.	

constitutional law. However, it is simpler to honor a statement that complies with all laws, so if a patient is not using a statutory form, then it is appropriate to attach a statutory form to the advance care directive being used.

Interventions

PHYSICAL SYMPTOMS AND THEIR MANAGEMENT. The most common physical and psychological symptoms among all terminally ill patients include pain, fatigue, insomnia, anorexia, dyspnea, depression, anxiety, and nausea and vomiting (Table 6–3). In the last days of life, terminal delirium is also common. Patients with advanced cancer experience an average of 11.5 symptoms. Statistics on symptoms for late-stage cardiovascular patients are not available. However, almost one third of cardiovascular deaths involve additional causes, so the cardiologist managing patients in end-stage disease should be able to manage symptoms from noncardiac conditions as well. Symptom management skills are well described elsewhere.[19]

SOCIAL NEEDS AND THEIR MANAGEMENT.

Financial Burdens. Dying can impose substantial economic strains on patients and families (see Chap. 2). In the United States, about 20% of terminally ill patients and their families have to spend more than 10% of family income on health care costs over and above health insurance premiums. Between 10% and 30% of families have sold assets, used savings, or taken out a mortgage to pay for the patient's health care costs. Nearly 40% of terminally ill patients report that the cost of their illness was a moderate or great economic hardship for their family.

One source of economic burden is related to medical costs. The second, more universal source of economic burden is a decline in the patient's income. In 20% of cases, a family member stopped working to provide care. Economic burden is associated with poor physical functioning and needs for housekeeping, nursing, and personal care. That is, more

TABLE 6–3 Managing Changes in the Patient's Condition during the Final Days and Hours

Change in the Patient's Condition	Potential Complication	Family's Possible Reaction and Concern	Advice and Intervention
Profound fatigue	Bedbound with development of pressure ulcers that are prone to infection, malodor, and pain, as well as joint pain.	Patient is lazy and giving up.	Reassure family and caregivers that terminal fatigue will not respond to interventions and should not be resisted. Use an air mattress if necessary.
Anorexia	None	Patient is giving up. Patient will suffer from hunger and will starve to death.	Reassure family and caregivers that the patient is not eating because he or she is dying; not eating at the end of life does not cause suffering or death. Forced feeding, whether oral, parenteral, or enteral, does not reduce symptoms or prolong life.
Dehydration	Dry mucosal membranes (see below).	Patient will suffer from thirst and die of dehydration.	Reassure family and caregivers that terminal dehydration does not cause suffering because patients lose consciousness before any symptom distress. Intravenous hydration can worsen symptoms of dyspnea by pulmonary or peripheral edema as well as prolong dying process.
Dysphagia	Inability to swallow oral medications needed for palliative care.		Do not force oral intake. Discontinue unnecessary medications that may have been continued including antibiotics, diuretics, antidepressants, and laxatives. If swallowing pills is difficult for patient, convert essential medications (analgesics, antiemetics, anxiolytics, and psychotropics) to oral solutions, buccal, sublingual, or rectal administration.
"Death rattle"—noisy breathing		Patient is choking and suffocating.	Reassure the family and caregivers that this is caused by secretions in the oropharynx and the patient is not choking. Reduce secretions with scopolamine (0.2-0.4 mg Sc every 4 hours or 1-3 patches every 3 days) Reposition patient to permit drainage of secretions. Do not suction. Suction can cause patient and family discomfort and is usually ineffective.
Apnea, Cheyne-Stokes respirations, dyspnea		Patient is suffocating.	Reassure family and caregivers that unconscious patients do not experience suffocation or air hunger. Apneic episodes are frequently a premorbid change. Opioids or anxiolytics may be used for dyspnea. Oxygen is unlikely to relieve dyspneic symptoms and may prolong the dying process.
Urinary or fecal incontinence	Skin breakdown if days until death. Potential transmission of infectious agents to caregivers.	Patient is dirty, malodorous, and physically repellent.	Remind family and caregivers to use universal precautions. Frequent changes of bedclothes and bedding. Use diapers, urinary catheter, or rectal tube if diarrhea or high urine flow occur.
Agitation or delirium	Day/night reversal. Hurt to self or caregivers.	Patient is in horrible pain and going to have a horrible death.	Reassure family and caregivers that agitation and delirium do not necessarily connote physical pain. Depending on the prognosis and goals of treatment, consider evaluating for causes of delirium and modify medications. Manage symptoms with haloperidol, chlorpromazine, diazepam, or midazolam.
Dry mucosal membranes	Cracked lips, mouth sores, and candidiasis can also cause pain. Malodor.	Patient may be malodorous, physically repellent.	Use baking soda mouthwash or saliva preparation every 15-30 minutes. Use topical nystatin for candidiasis. Coat lips and nasal mucosa with petroleum jelly every 60-90 minutes. Use ophthalmic lubricants every 4 hours or artificial tears every 30 minutes.

debilitated and less well-off patients experience greater economic burdens. Economic burdens tend to increase the psychological distress of families and patients. Assistance from a social worker, early on if possible, to ensure access to available benefits may be helpful. Many people are unaware of options, including insurance benefits, the Family Medical Leave Act, and other sources of assistance.

Relationships. Closing the narrative of lived relationships is a nearly universal need. When asked if sudden death or death after an illness is preferable, respondents often initially select the former but soon change to the latter as they reflect on the importance of saying goodbye. Bereaved family members who have not had the chance to say goodbye often have a difficult grief process. Since many of the deaths in cardiology are sudden (see Chaps. 32 and 33), this issue is of particular importance. Patients and their families should be encouraged to settle what they would like to, even though it is more difficult to anticipate the time of death.

Care of seriously ill patients requires efforts to facilitate the types of encounters and time spent with family and friends that are necessary to meet these needs. Family and close friends may need to be accommodated with unrestricted visiting hours for inpatients, including, in some cases, sleeping near the patient even in institutional settings. Assistance for patients and family members who are unsure about how to create or help preserve memories, whether by providing materials such as a scrap book or memory box or by offering suggestions and informational resources, can be deeply appreciated. Taking photographs and creating videos or audiotapes can be especially helpful to patients with life-shortening illness who have younger children.

Family Caregivers. Caring for seriously ill patients places a heavy burden on families. Families are required to provide transportation, homemaking, and other services. Typically, paid professionals, such as home health nurses and hospice, supplement family care giving; only about one quarter of all caregiving is exclusively paid professional assistance. The trend toward more out-of-hospital deaths will increase reliance on families for end-of-life care. About three quarters of the caregivers of terminally ill patients are female—wives, daughters, and even sisters. Consequently, women tend to be able to rely less on family for caregiving assistance and may need more paid assistance. About 20% of terminally ill patients report substantial unmet needs for nursing and personal care.

This makes it imperative to inquire about unmet needs and facilitate family or paid professional services. Assistance from religious or community groups can often be mobilized by phone calls from the medical team to someone the patient or family identifies.

Existential Needs and Their Management. Dying is one of the ultimate existential challenges. Religion and spirituality are important to dying patients. Approximately 70% of patients report becoming more religious or spiritual when they became terminally ill, and many find comfort in practices such as prayer. Some studies suggest that women and older patients are more likely to experience greater interest in religion and spirituality. On the other hand, about 20% of terminally ill patients become less religious, frequently feeling alienated by becoming terminally ill. For other patients, the need is for existential meaning and purpose that is distinct from, and maybe even an antireligious form of, spirituality. Among patients with cardiovascular conditions, clinical experience suggests that fear of sudden death is common. Further, the well-recognized accomplishment of personal growth and relationship resolution characteristic among patients who foresee death in the near future is less apparent among patients with cardiovascular illnesses.[20] This may reflect the rarer recognition of mortality among heart patients as compared with cancer patients.

Health care providers are often hesitant about involving themselves in the religious, spiritual, and existential experiences of their patients, because it may seem private, related to alternative lifestyles, or "soft." But physicians and other members of the interdisciplinary team should be able to at least detect spiritual need. Screening questions have been developed for a physician's spiritual history taking. Spiritual distress can amplify other types of suffering and even masquerade as, for instance, intractable physical pain or anxiety. The screening questions in the whole-person assessment are usually sufficient. Deeper evaluation and intervention is rarely appropriate for the physician unless no other member of the team is available or suitable. Pastors may be helpful, whether from the medical institution or from the patient's community.

Precisely how religious practices, spirituality, and existential explorations can be facilitated and improve end-of-life care is not well established. In at least one study, only 36% of respondents indicated that a clergy member would be comforting. Nevertheless, this increase in religious and spiritual interest among a substantial proportion of dying patients underscores the importance of inquiring how this need can be addressed in individual patients.

Managing the Last Stages of Life

WITHDRAWING AND WITHHOLDING LIFE-SUSTAINING TREATMENT. For centuries, it has been deemed ethical to withhold or withdraw life-sustaining interventions. For patients who are incompetent and terminally ill but have not completed an advance care directive, next-of-kin can exercise this right, although this may be restricted in some states depending on how clear and convincing the evidence is of the patient's preferences. In theory, a patient's right to refuse medical therapy can be limited by four countervailing interests: (1) preservation of life; (2) prevention of suicide; (3) protection of third parties such as children; and (4) preserving the integrity of the medical profession. In practice, these interests almost never override the right of competent patients or incompetent patients who have left explicit advance care directives to decline unwanted intervention.

Physicians' Orders Regarding Cardiopulmonary Resuscitation and Other Life-Sustaining Treatments. Whenever a patient is a suitable candidate for a Do Not Resuscitate (DNR) order, he or she deserves to have had a comprehensive discussion about goals of care, a plan of care, and possibly also advance care planning. Use of predesigned forms such as the Physicians Orders for Life-Sustaining Treatments (POLST) in place of limited DNR orders can encourage these more comprehensive and coherent approaches to creating plans of care. In general, an isolated DNR order with no reference to other life-sustaining treatment preferences can be considered a red flag that should prompt a physician to include or return to a whole-patient assessment and a comprehensive plan for care with goal-tailored treatment choices.

Mechanical Ventilation. Perhaps the most challenging intervention to withdraw is mechanical ventilation. There are two approaches: "terminal extubation," which is the removal of the endotracheal tube, and "terminal wean," which is the gradual reduction of the FIO_2 or ventilator rate. Some physicians recommend the terminal wean because patients do not develop upper airway obstruction and the distress caused by secretions or stridor with this approach; however, it is reported that terminal weaning can prolong the dying process. To ensure comfort for conscious or semiconscious patients, a common practice is to inject a bolus of midazolam (2-4 mg) prior to withdrawal followed by 5 to 10 mg of morphine and a continuous infusion of morphine (50% of the bolus dose per hour). (Higher doses are needed for patients already receiving anxiolytics and opioids.) Remove any neuromuscular blocking agents so that patients can show any discomfort, which in turn can allow medication titration or additional boluses of morphine or midazolam. Families need to be warned that up to 10% of patients unexpectedly survive for 1 day or more after mechanical ventilation is stopped.

FUTILE CARE. Beginning in the late 1980s, some commentators argued that physicians could terminate futile treatments demanded by families of terminally ill patients. There is no objective definition or standard of futility. The term conceals subjective value judgments about when a treatment is not beneficial. A more practical approach acknowledges that in many cases in which futility concerns are raised, there are underlying communication gaps or unresolved personal issues that are best dealt with in team or family meetings. Occasionally, true value differences exist; these may be best handled with assistance from an ethics committee.

EUTHANASIA AND PHYSICIAN-ASSISTED SUICIDE. Terminating life-sustaining intervention and providing opioids to manage symptoms are not to be confused with euthanasia or physician-assisted suicide. Both the former, unlike the latter, have long been considered ethical by the medical profession and legal by courts.

A growing body of data indicates that depression, hopelessness, and worries about loss of dignity or autonomy are the primary factors motivating a desire for euthanasia or physician-assisted suicide. While any of these can occur in patients with cardiovascular conditions, there appear to be fewer requests in this population than among patients with cancer or acquired immunodeficiency syndrome. Perhaps the characteristic sudden death among cardiac patients helps to avoid some of the fears of indignity and dependence associated with a slow, highly symptomatic decline. Nonetheless, multiple symptoms and chronic disability do occur in patients with end-stage heart disease, and requests for physician-assisted suicide or euthanasia also occur. Cardiologists should know how to respond to such requests.

After receiving a request for euthanasia or physician-assisted suicide, the physician should probe with empathetic, open-ended questions to help elucidate the underlying cause for the request such as: *"What makes you want to consider this option?"* Endorsing either moral opposition or moral support for the act tends to be counterproductive, lending an impression either of being judgmental or of endorsing the worthlessness of the patient's life. Health care providers must reassure the patient of continued care and commitment. Simultaneously, the patient should be educated about (1) alternative, less controversial options, such as symptom management and withdrawing any unwanted treatments; (2) the reality of euthanasia and/or physician-assisted suicide, since the patient is likely to have misconceptions about its effectiveness; and (3) the legal implications of the choice. As indicated, depression, hopelessness, and other symptoms of psychological distress, as well as physical suffering and economic burdens, are likely factors motivating the request. Health care providers should identify the factors motivating the request and aggressively treat those factors. After these interventions and clarification of options, most patients proceed with a less controversial approach of declining life-sustaining interventions, possibly including refusal of nutrition and hydration.

CARE DURING THE LAST HOURS. Most lay people have limited experiences with the actual dying process and death. They frequently do not know what to expect of the final hours, and afterwards. There is no rehearsal and no second chance. Therefore, the family must be prepared, especially if the plan is for the patient to die at home.

For patients with heart failure, there may be several last days of life with characteristic pathophysiologic changes such as increased orthopnea and nocturnal dyspnea. Patients experience extreme weakness and fatigue and become bed bound. This can lead to bedsores. If death is imminent and the sores are causing less distress than the dressing changes and frequent turning do, it is reasonable to cease these usual types of care. Dry mucosal membranes should be cared for with frequent oral swabbing, lip lubricants, and artificial tears. These activities can provide the family with a form of care to substitute for those that no longer help, such as feeding. With loss of the gag reflex and dysphagia, patients can also accumulate airway and pharyngeal secretions, producing noises during respiration sometimes called "the death rattle." Scopolamine can reduce this condition. Dying patients also have changes in respiration with periods of apnea or Cheyne-Stokes breathing. Decreased intravascular volume and cardiac output cause tachycardia, hypotension, peripheral coolness, and livedo reticularis (skin mottling). Patients can also have urinary and fecal incontinence at death as the sphincters lose their tone. Most importantly, changes occur in consciousness and neurological function, leading to two very different paths to death (Fig. 6–1). Patients with hallucinations and seizures may need a palliative care specialist's attention.

Each of these terminal changes can cause distress to patients and families. Informing families of what to expect, even by providing an information sheet, can help relieve this distress. For instance, it can be calming to know that patients stop eating because they are dying, not dying because they have stopped eating, or that the "death rattle" is not a sign of suffocation, or that mottling tends to mean that death is near.

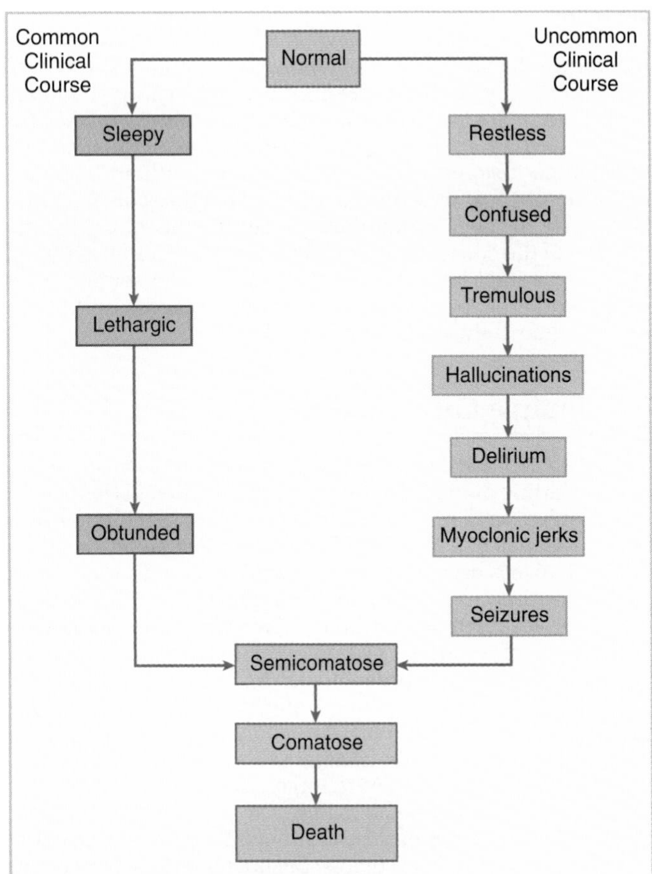

FIGURE 6–1 Common and uncommon clinical courses of the last days of terminally ill patients . (Adapted from Advance Planning. Module 4: Palliative Care. *In* Ferris FD, Flannery JS, McNeal HB, et al (eds): A Comprehensive Guide for the Care of Persons with HIV Disease. Mount Sinai and Casey Hospice, Toronto, Ontario, 1995. Available at http://www.cpsonline.info/content/resources/hivmodule4.html.)

It is claimed that hearing and touch are the last senses to stop functioning. Families should be encouraged to communicate with and touch the patient, even if he or she is unconscious.

When the plan is for the patient to die at home, the family needs to know how to determine when death has occurred, including the cardinal signs of cessation of cardiac function and respiration, fixed pupils, coolness, changes in skin color and texture, and incontinence. Remind the family that the eyes may remain open. It helps to have a plan of who the family and caregivers will contact when the patient is dying or has died. Without a plan, they may panic and call 911, unleashing a cascade of unwanted events from arrival of emergency personnel and resuscitation to hospital admission. Family and caregivers should be instructed to contact hospice, the covering physician, or the on-call member of the palliative care team. There is no reason to contact the coroner, unless the state requires it for all deaths. Similarly, unless foul play is suspected, the health care team need not contact the coroner either.

Just after the patient dies, even the best prepared family may experience shock and bereavement and be distraught. They need time to assimilate the event and be comforted. Health care providers should write a bereavement card or letter to the family. It can be appropriate, although it is not obligatory, to attend the funerals of patients to lend support to the grieving family and to find an opportunity for closure for the physician.

Death is a strong predictor of poor health and even mortality for the surviving spouse. It may be important to alert the spouse's physician about the death so that he or she can be aware of symptoms that might require professional attention.

SUDDEN DEATH. Sudden death may "short-change" patients of the growth that often happens in the last phase of life and that may make it easier for bereaved family members to accommodate to the death. Even adult children of patients who have died suddenly may be excessively influenced by the sudden disappearance of their parent, without a chance to say goodbye, and by the fear of suffering the same fate. Preparedness through discussion, planning, and engaging the benefits of the consciously trodden last paths in life can help, as can extended bereavement counseling. The services of a social worker or other professional with expertise in the area should almost always be considered.

Palliative Care Services

HOW AND WHERE. For nearly two decades, hospice has been a leading model of palliative care services. Patients who use hospice tend to appreciate the care, and their families tend to adjust better than others in similar situations.[21] In 1983, Medicare began paying for hospice services under Part A, the hospital insurance part of reimbursement. To be eligible, a patient must be certified by two physicians as having a prognosis of 6 months or less if the disease runs its usual course. Prognoses are probabilistic by their nature; patients are not required to die within 6 months but rather to have a condition from which half the people with it would be deceased within 6 months. Patients sign a hospice enrollment form that states their intent to forgo curative services related to their terminal illness, but they can still receive medical services for other comorbid conditions. Patients can also disenroll and re-enroll later; that is, the hospice Medicare benefit can be reinvoked later in order to secure traditional Medicare benefits in the interim. Payments to hospice are per diem rather than fee-for-service and are intended to cover comprehensive care, including physician services for the medical direction of the interdisciplinary team, regular home care visits by registered nurses and licensed practical nurses, home health aide and homemaker services, dietary counseling, chaplain services, social work services, and bereavement counseling as well as medical equipment, supplies, and medications. Additional clinical care, including care by the primary physician, is covered by Medicare Part B, even while the hospice Medicare benefit is in place. By 1996, the mean length of enrollment in hospice was 65 days, with the median being less than 24 days. Since then, the length of enrollment has declined. Physicians should initiate earlier referrals to hospice to allow more time for patients to receive palliative care.

Until relatively recently, hospice had been the main way of securing palliative services for terminally ill patients. Efforts are now directed at ensuring continuity of palliative care across settings and through time. Increasingly, these same types of palliative care services are available as consultative services in hospitals, in day care and other outpatient settings, and in nursing homes. For instance, in the United States, although the vast majority of hospice care is provided in residential homes, just over 10% now occurs in nursing homes. In addition, palliative care consultations for non-hospice patients can be billed as for other consultations under Medicare Part B, the physician reimbursement part. Many supporters believe that palliative care should be offered to patients regardless of their prognosis. A patient and his or her family should not have to make an "either curative care or palliative care" choice, in large part because it can be psychologically stressful to embrace mortality. Although provision of palliative care, as needed, from the onset of illness onward is ideal, discontinuities in care can make this challenging. Documentation of goals, orders for life-sustaining treatment that are comprehensive and standardized,[22] advance care planning, and the date of the most recent update can help coordinate care across care sites, among members of the care team, and along the illness trajectory of changing goals for care.

OUTCOME MEASURES. Care near the end of life cannot be measured by most of the traditional validated outcome measures, since palliative care does not consider death a bad outcome. Similarly, family and patients may seek different elements of quality of life that are not included in standard measures when their active engagement is with dying well. Symptom control, enhanced family relationships, and quality of bereavement are difficult to measure and are rarely the primary focus of carefully developed or widely used outcome measures. Nevertheless, outcomes are as important in end-of-life care as in any other field of medical care. Specific end-of-life care instruments are being developed both for assessment and for outcome measures, such as The Brief Hospice Inventory, NEST, and the Palliative Care Outcomes Scale. The field of end-of-life care is ready to enter an era of evidence-based practice and continuous improvement within established institutions.

Acknowledgment

Portions of this chapter are derived from previous writings by Ezekiel and Linda Emanuel.

RESOURCES

The Education in Palliative and End-of-Life Care (EPEC) Project: www.epec.net.
The End of Life/Palliative Education Resource Center (EPERC): www.eperc.mcw.edu.
The National Comprehensive Cancer Network (NCCN) palliative care guidelines, 2002: www.nccn.org.

REFERENCES

1. Asimov I: Asimov's Biographical Encyclopedia of Science and Technology. 2nd ed. Garden City, NY, Doubleday, 1982.

2. Hanratty B, Hibbert D, Mair F, et al: Doctor's perceptions of palliative care for heart failure: Focus group study. Br Med J 325:581, 2002.
3. Easson AM, Crosby JA, Librach SL: Discussion of death and dying in surgical textbooks. Am J Surg 182:34, 2001.
4. Rabow MW, McPhee SJ: Deficiencies in end-of-life care content in medical textbooks. J Am Geriatr Soc 50:397, 2002.
5. Personal communication from R. Arnold.
6. Emanuel L, Alexander C, Arnold R, et al: Palliative care in disease management guidelines. Copies available from American Hospice Foundation, 2004, Washington, DC.
7. Iwashyna T, Zhang JX, Christakis NA: Disease-specific patterns of hospice and related healthcare use in an incidence cohort of seriously ill elderly patients. J Pall Med 5:531, 2002.

Assessment Goals and Care Planning

8. Lo B, et al: Discussing religious and spiritual issues at the end of life: A practical guide for physicians. JAMA 287:749, 2002.
9. Emanuel LL, Alpert H, Emanuel EJ: Concise screening questions for clinical assessments of terminal care: The needs near the end of life care screening tool (NEST). J Palliat Med 4:465, 2001.
10. Buckman R: How to break bad news: A guide for health care professionals. Baltimore, The Johns Hopkins University Press, 1992, pp 65-97.
11. Lamont EB, Christakis NA: Complexities in prognostication in advanced cancer: JAMA 290:98, 2003.
12. Foley K: *In* Seale & Cartwright, 1994.
13. Emanuel EJ, Emanuel LL: The promise of a good death. Lancet 351(Suppl 2):SII21, 1998.
14. Singer PA, et al: Quality end-of-life care: Patients' perspectives. JAMA 281:163, 1999.
15. Webb M: The Good Death: The New American Search to Reshape the End of Life. New York, Bantam Books, 1997.
16. Emanuel LL: The Health Care Directive: Learning how to draft advance care documents. J Am Geriatrics Soc 39:1221, 1991. (www.medicaldirective.org)
17. President's Commission for the Study of Ethical Issues in Medicine and Biomedical and Behavioral Research: Deciding to Forego Life-Sustaining Treatment. Washington, DC, US Government Printing Office, 1983.
18. *Vacco v Quill*, 95-1858; and *State of Washington v Glucksberg*, 96-110.

Interventions

19. An ASCO Curriculum: Optimizing Cancer Care—The importance of symptom management. Vols I & II. Dubuque, IA, Kendal/Hunt Publishing Company, 2001, p 52002.
20. Byock I: Dying Well: The Prospect for Growth at the End of Life, New York, Putnam/Riverhead, 1998.
21. Christakis NA, Iwashyna TJ: The health impact of health care on families: A matched cohort study of hospice use by decedents and mortality outcomes in surviving, widowed spouses. Soc Sci Med 57:465, 2003.
22. Center for Ethics in Health Care: Physician Orders for Life-Sustaining Treatment (POLST) forms. Portland, OR, Oregon Health Sciences University, 1997.

PART II

Examination of the Patient

CHAPTER 7

The History

Eugene Braunwald

Importance of the History

Specialized examinations of the cardiovascular system, presented in Chapters 9 through 18, provide a large portion of the database required to establish a specific anatomical diagnosis of cardiac disease and to determine the extent of functional impairment of the heart. The development and application of these methods are a triumph of modern medicine. However, their appropriate use is to supplement but not to supplant a careful clinical examination. The clinical examination, consisting of the history and physical examination (see Chap. 8), remains the cornerstone of the assessment of the patient with known or suspected cardiovascular disease. For example, the initial clinical evaluation is at least as accurate in predicting coronary anatomy and survival as the exercise stress test.[1] There is a temptation in cardiology, as in many other areas of medicine, to carry out expensive, and occasionally uncomfortable or even hazardous, procedures to establish a diagnosis when a detailed and thoughtful history and a thorough physical examination are sufficient. Obviously, it is undesirable to subject patients to the unnecessary risks, discomfort, and expenses inherent in many specialized tests when a diagnosis can be made on the basis of the clinical examination or when management will not be altered significantly as a result of these tests.

With the increasing emphasis on the cost of medical care, it is likely that there will be a resurgence of interest in the relatively inexpensive clinical examination. On the other hand, it must be appreciated that there may be little correlation between the intensity of symptoms and the severity of heart disease; asymptomatic persons may have a life-threatening condition, whereas persons with many symptoms referable to the cardiovascular system may have no or mild heart disease.

THE ROLE OF THE HISTORY. The overreliance on laboratory tests has increased as physicians attempt to use their time more efficiently by delegating responsibility for taking the history to an assistant or nurse or even by limiting the history to a questionnaire. I consider this to be an undesirable trend for the patient with known or suspected heart disease. First, it must be appreciated that the history remains the richest source of information concerning the patient's illness,[2] and any practice that might diminish the quality or quantity of information provided by the history is likely ultimately to impair the quality of care. Second, the physician's attentive and thoughtful taking of a history establishes a bond with the patient. This bond is frequently valuable in securing the patient's compliance in following a complex treatment plan, undergoing hospitalization for an intensive diagnostic workup or a hazardous operation, and, in some instances, accepting that heart disease is not present at all.

A careful history allows the physician to evaluate the impact of the disease, or the fear of disease, on the various aspects of the patient's life and to assess the patient's personality, affect, and emotional stability; often it provides a glimpse of the patient's responsibilities, fears, aspirations, and threshold for discomfort as well as the likelihood of compliance with one or another therapeutic regimen. Whenever possible, the physician should question not only the patient but also relatives or close friends to obtain a clearer understanding of the extent of the patient's disability and the impact of the disease on both the patient and the family. For example, the patient's spouse is much more likely than the patient to provide a history of Cheyne-Stokes (periodic) respiration.

The combination of the widespread fear of cardiovascular disorders and the deep-seated emotional, symbolic, and sometimes even religious connotations surrounding the heart may, on the one hand, lower the threshold for the development of symptoms that mimic those of organic heart disease in persons with normal cardiovascular systems. On the other hand, they may cause so much dread that serious symptoms are denied by patients with established heart disease. Patients with established heart disease are often frightened, anxious, and/or depressed; these symptoms may be as troubling as those resulting from the pathophysiology of their disorder. These and other psychological symptoms can be identified only by a careful history.[2]

TECHNIQUE. Several approaches can be employed in obtaining the medical history. I believe that patients should first be given the opportunity to relate their experiences and complaints in their own way. Although time consuming and likely to include much seemingly irrelevant information, this technique provides considerable insight into the patient's intelligence, emotional make-up, and attitude toward his or her symptoms and gives the patient the satisfaction that he or she has been "heard" by the physician. After the patient has given an account of the illness, the physician should direct the discussion and obtain information concerning the onset and chronology of symptoms; their location, quality, and intensity; the precipitating, aggravating, and alleviating factors; the setting in which the symptoms occur and any associated symptoms; and the response to therapy.

Of course, a detailed general medical history, including the personal past history, occupational history, nutritional history, and review of systems, must be obtained. Of particular interest is a history of thyroid disease, recent dental extractions or manipulations, or catheterization of the bladder as well as a report of earlier examinations that showed abnormalities of the cardiovascular system as reflected in restriction from physical activity at school and in rejection for life insurance, employment, or military service. Personal habits such as exercise, cigarette smoking, alcohol intake, and parenteral use of drugs—illicit and otherwise—should be ascertained. The medications taken and the reasons given to the patient should be obtained.

Adults should be routinely questioned about the presence of or history of the major risk factors for coronary artery disease (see Chap. 36): cigarette smoking, hypertension, hypercholesterolemia, diabetes mellitus, and a family history of premature coronary artery disease. The exact nature of the patient's work, including physical and emotional stresses, should be assessed. The increasing appreciation of the importance of genetic influences in many forms of heart disease (see Chap. 70) underscores the importance of the family history.

Myocardial and coronary function that may be adequate at rest are often inadequate during exertion; therefore, specific attention should be directed to the influence of activity on the patient's symptoms. Thus, a history of chest discomfort and/or undue shortness of breath that appears only during activity is characteristic of heart disease, whereas the opposite pattern (i.e., the appearance of symptoms at rest and their remission during exertion) is almost never observed in patients with heart disease but is more characteristic of functional disorders.

It is important also to assess the "tempo" of the progression of symptoms. A decline in the threshold for severe anginal discomfort across a 2-week period is much more likely to signify a high risk of an adverse outcome, such as cardiac death or myocardial infarction, than a similar decline occurring over 2 years. Similarly, the history of a "breakthrough" of symptoms despite maintenance of a previously successful regimen should be noted, because it, too, may be a harbinger of a poor outcome and may dictate a change in therapeutic strategy.

As the patient relates the history, important nonverbal clues are often provided. The physician should observe the patient's attitude, reactions, and gestures while being questioned, as well as the choice of words or emphasis. Tumulty has aptly likened obtaining a meaningful clinical history to playing a game of chess[3]: "The patient makes a statement and based upon its content, and mode of expression, the physician asks a counter-question. One answer stimulates yet another question until the clinician is convinced that he understands precisely all of the circumstances of the patient's illness."

Cardinal Symptoms of Heart Disease

Dyspnea (see Chap. 22)

Dyspnea is defined as an abnormally uncomfortable awareness of breathing[4]; it is one of the principal symptoms of cardiac and pulmonary disease and ranges from an increased awareness of breathing to intense respiratory distress.[5,6] Dyspnea occurs after strenuous exertion in normal, healthy, well-conditioned subjects and after only moderate exertion in those who are healthy but unaccustomed to exercise (dyspnea of deconditioning). It should therefore be regarded as abnormal only when it occurs at rest or at a level of physical activity not expected to cause this symptom.

Dyspnea is associated with a wide variety of diseases of the heart and lungs, chest wall, and respiratory muscles as well as with anxiety.[7] Among patients with cardiac dyspnea, this symptom is most commonly associated with and caused by pulmonary congestion, as occurs in cases of left ventricular failure or mitral stenosis. The interstitial and alveolar edema stiffens the lungs and stimulates respiration by activating "J" receptors in the lung. Less frequently, cardiac dyspnea occurs secondary to a reduced cardiac output, without pulmonary engorgement, as in cases of tetralogy of Fallot. Table 7–1 provides a list of the various syndromes that may cause dyspnea and the primary pathophysiological mechanisms that are responsible. Both Borg and Noble[8] and the American Thoracic Society (Table 7–2)[9] have developed scales that are useful in quantitating the severity of dyspnea.

The sudden development of dyspnea suggests pulmonary embolism, pneumothorax, acute pulmonary edema, pneumonia, or airway obstruction. In contrast, in most forms of chronic heart failure, dyspnea progresses slowly over weeks or months. Such a protracted course may also occur in patients with a variety of unrelated conditions, including obesity, pregnancy, and bilateral pleural effusion. Inspiratory dyspnea suggests obstruction of the upper airways, whereas expiratory dyspnea characterizes obstruction of the lower airways. Exertional dyspnea suggests the presence of organic diseases, such as left ventricular failure (see Chap. 22) or chronic obstructive lung disease (see Chap. 67), whereas dyspnea developing at rest may occur in patients with pneumothorax, pulmonary embolism, pulmonary edema, or anxiety neurosis.

Dyspnea that occurs only at rest and is absent on exertion is almost always functional. A functional origin is also suggested when dyspnea, or simply a heightened awareness of breathing, is accompanied by brief stabbing pain in the region of the cardiac apex or by prolonged (more than 2 hours) dull chest pain. It is often associated with difficulty in getting enough air into the lungs, claustrophobia, and sighing respirations that are relieved by exertion, by taking a few deep breaths, or by sedation. Dyspnea in patients with panic attacks is usually accompanied by hyperventilation. A history of relief of dyspnea by bronchodilators suggests asthma as the cause, whereas relief of dyspnea by rest and diuretics suggests left ventricular failure. Dyspnea accompanied by wheezing may be secondary to left ventricular failure (cardiac asthma) or primary bronchial constriction (bronchial asthma).

In patients with chronic heart failure, dyspnea is a clinical expression of pulmonary venous and capillary hypertension (see Chap. 22). It occurs either during exertion or in resting patients in the recumbent position, in whom it is relieved promptly by sitting upright or standing (orthopnea). Patients with left ventricular failure soon learn to sleep on two or more pillows to avoid this symptom. In patients with heart failure, dyspnea is often accompanied by edema of the lower extremities, upper abdominal pain (due to congestive hepatomegaly), and nocturia.

TABLE 7–1 Disorders Causing Dyspnea and Limiting Exercise Performance, Pathophysiology, and Discriminating Measurements

Disorders	Pathophysiology	Measurements that Deviate from Normal
Pulmonary		
Air flow limitation	Mechanical limitation to ventilation, mismatching of $\dot{V}A/\dot{Q}$, hypoxic stimulation to breathing	$\dot{V}E$ max/MVV, expiratory flow pattern, VD, VT; $\dot{V}O_2$ max, $\dot{V}E/\dot{V}O_2$, $\dot{V}E$ response to hyperoxia, (A – a) PO_2
Restrictive	Mismatching $\dot{V}A/\dot{Q}$, hypoxic stimulation to breathing	
Chest wall	Mechanical limitation to ventilation	$\dot{V}E$ max/MVV, $PACO_2$, $\dot{V}O_2$ max
Pulmonary circulation	Rise in physiological dead space as fraction of VT, exercise hypoxemia	VD/VT, work-rate-related hypoxemia, $\dot{V}O_2$ max, $\dot{V}E/\dot{V}O_2$, (a – ET)PCO_2, O_2-pulse
Cardiac		
Coronary	Coronary insufficiency	ECG, $\dot{V}O_2$ max, anaerobic threshold $\dot{V}O_2$, $\dot{V}E/\dot{V}O_2$, O_2-pulse, BP (systolic, diastolic, pulse)
Valvular	Cardiac output limitation (decreased effective stroke volume)	
Myocardial	Cardiac output limitation (decreased ejection fraction and stroke volume)	
Anemia	Reduced O_2-carrying capacity	O_2-pulse, anaerobic threshold $\dot{V}O_2$, $\dot{V}O_2$ max, $\dot{V}E/\dot{V}O_2$
Peripheral circulation	Inadequate O_2 flow to metabolically active muscle	Anaerobic threshold $\dot{V}O_2$, $\dot{V}O_2$ max
Obesity	Increased work to move body; if severe, respiratory restriction and pulmonary insufficiency	$\dot{V}O_2$-work-rate relationship, PAO_2, $PACO_2$, $\dot{V}O_2$ max
Psychogenic	Hyperventilation with precisely regular respiratory rate	Breathing pattern, PCO_2
Malingering	Hyperventilation and hypoventilation with irregular respiratory rate	Breathing pattern, PCO_2
Deconditioning	Inactivity or prolonged bed rest; loss of capability for effective redistribution of systemic blood flow	O_2-pulse, anaerobic threshold $\dot{V}O_2$, $\dot{V}O_2$ max

$\dot{V}A$ = alveolar ventilation; $\dot{Q}$ = pulmonary blood flow; $\dot{V}E$ = minute ventilation; MVV = maximum voluntary ventilation; VD/VT = physiological dead space/tidal volume ratio; O_2 = oxygen; $\dot{V}O_2$ = O_2 consumption; (A – a)PO_2 = alveolar-arterial PO_2 difference; (a – ET)PCO_2 = arterial-end tidal PCO_2 difference.
Modified from Wasserman D: Dyspnea on exertion: Is it the heart or the lungs? JAMA 248:2042, 1982, Copyright 1982, the American Medical Association.

TABLE 7–2 American Thoracic Society Scale of Dyspnea

Descriptions	Grade	Degree
Not troubled by shortness of breath when hurrying on the level or walking up a slight hill	0	None
Trouble by shortness of breath when hurrying on the level or walking up a slight hill	1	Mild
Walks more slowly than people of the same age on the level because of breathlessness or has to stop for breath when walking at own pace on the level	2	Moderate
Stops for breath after walking about 100 yards or after a few minutes on the level	3	Severe
Too breathless to leave the house; breathless on dressing or undressing	4	Very severe

From Fishman AP: Approach to the patient with respiratory symptoms. *In* Fishman's Pulmonary Diseases and Disorders. 3rd ed. New York, McGraw-Hill, 1998, pp 361-393.

Paroxysmal nocturnal dyspnea is caused by interstitial pulmonary edema and sometimes intraalveolar edema, most commonly as a consequence of left ventricular failure (see Chap. 22). This condition, usually beginning 2 to 4 hours after the onset of sleep and often accompanied by cough, wheezing, and sweating, may be quite frightening. Paroxysmal nocturnal dyspnea is often ameliorated by the patient's sitting on the side of the bed or getting out of bed; relief is not instantaneous but usually requires 15 to 30 minutes. Although paroxysmal nocturnal dyspnea secondary to left ventricular failure is usually accompanied by coughing, a careful history often discloses that the dyspnea precedes the cough, not vice versa. Nocturnal dyspnea associated with pulmonary disease is usually relieved after the patient rids himself or herself of secretions rather than specifically by sitting up.

Patients with pulmonary embolism usually experience sudden dyspnea that may be associated with apprehension, palpitation, hemoptysis, or pleuritic chest pain (see Chap. 66). The development or intensification of dyspnea, sometimes associated with a feeling of faintness, may be the only symptom of the patient with pulmonary emboli. Pneumothorax and mediastinal emphysema also cause acute dyspnea, accompanied by sharp chest pain. Dyspnea is a common "anginal equivalent" (see Chap. 50), that is, a symptom secondary to myocardial ischemia that occurs in place of typical anginal discomfort. This form of dyspnea may or may not be associated with a sensation of tightness in the chest, is present on exertion or emotional stress, is relieved by rest (more often in the sitting than in the recumbent position), is similar to angina in duration (i.e., 2 to 10 minutes), and is usually responsive to or prevented by nitroglycerin.

APPROACH TO THE PATIENT. The approach to the patient is shown in Figure 7–1. Measurement of Brain Natriuretic Peptide (BNP) has been shown to be a valuable laboratory test in the evaluation of dyspnea, especially in patients presenting to the Emergency Department[11] (see Chaps. 21 and 22).

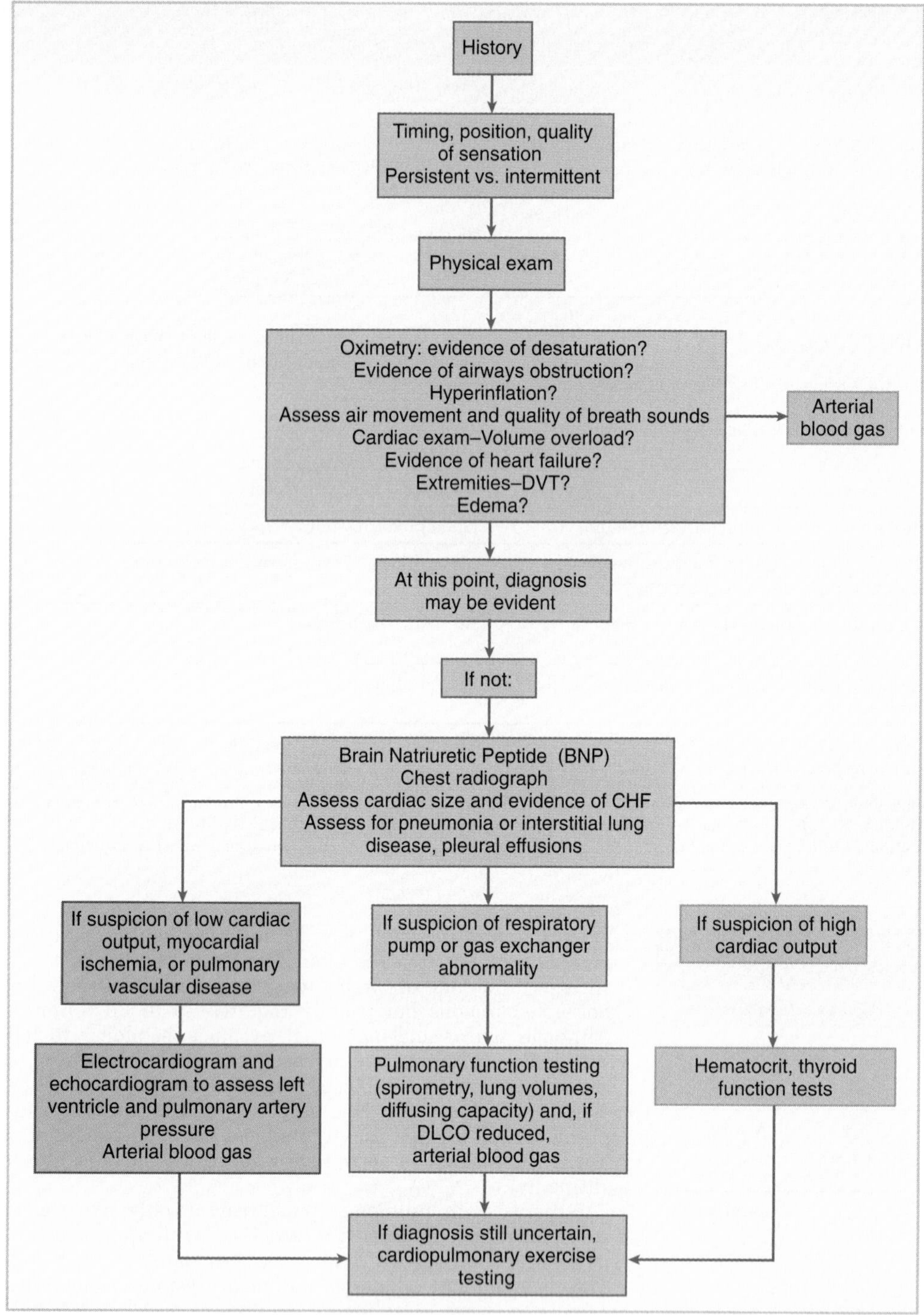

FIGURE 7–1. Algorithm for the evaluation of the patient with dyspnea. The pace and completeness with which one approaches this framework depend on the intensity and acuity of the patient's symptoms. In the patient with severe, acute dyspnea, for example, an arterial blood gas measurement may be one of the first laboratory evaluations, whereas it might not be obtained until much later in the work-up in a patient with chronic breathlessness of unclear cause. A therapeutic trial of a medication, for example, a bronchodilator, may be instituted at any point if one is fairly confident of the diagnosis based on the data available at that time. DVT = deep venous thrombosis; CHF = congestive heart failure; DLCO = diffusing capacity of the lung for carbon monoxide. (From Schwartzstein RM, Feller-Kopman, D.: Approach to the patient with dyspnea. *In* Braunwald E, Goldman L [eds]: Primary Cardiology. 2nd ed. Philadelphia, WB Saunders, 2003, pp 101-116.)

Chest Pain or Discomfort

(see Chaps. 45, 46, and 49)

Although chest pain or discomfort is one of the cardinal manifestations of heart disease, such pain may originate not only in the heart but also (1) in a variety of noncardiac intrathoracic structures, such as the aorta, pulmonary artery, bronchopulmonary tree, pleura, mediastinum, esophagus, and diaphragm; (2) in the tissues of the neck or thoracic wall, including the skin, thoracic muscles, cervicodorsal spine, costochondral junctions, breasts, sensory nerves, and spinal cord; and (3) in subdiaphragmatic organs such as the stomach, duodenum, pancreas, and gallbladder (Table 7–3). Pain of functional origin or factitious pain may also occur in the chest.

In obtaining the history of a patient with chest pain, it is helpful to have a mental checklist and to ask the patient to describe the location, radiation, and character of the discomfort; what causes and relieves it, especially the extent and timing of relief by sublingual nitroglycerin; the duration, frequency, and pattern of recurrence of the discomfort; the setting in which it occurs; and associated symptoms. It is also particularly useful to observe the patient's gestures. The patient's clenching of the fist in front of the sternum while describing the sensation (Levine sign) is a strong indication of an ischemic origin of the pain.

QUALITY OF DISCOMFORT. Angina pectoris may be defined as a discomfort in the chest and/or adjacent area associated with myocardial ischemia but without myocardial necrosis.[12-15] *Angina* means tightening, not pain. Thus, the discomfort of angina often is described not as pain at all but rather as an unpleasant sensation; "pressing," "squeezing," "strangling," "constricting," "bursting," and "burning" are some of the adjectives commonly used to describe this sensation. "A band across the chest," "a weight in the center of the chest," and "a vise tightening around the chest" are other frequent descriptors.

It is characteristic of angina pectoris that the intensity of effort required to incite it may vary from day to day and throughout the day in the same patient, but often a careful history will uncover explanations for this, such as meals ingested, weather, emotions, and the like. The anginal threshold is lower in the morning than at other times of the day. When the threshold for angina is quite variable, defies any pattern, and is prominent at rest, the possibility that myocardial ischemia is caused by coronary

TABLE 7–3 Cardiovascular Causes of Chest Pain

Condition	Location	Quality	Duration	Aggravating or Relieving Factors	Associated Symptoms or Signs
Angina	Retrosternal region: radiates to or occasionally isolated to neck, jaw, epigastrium, shoulder, or arms—left common	Pressure, burning, squeezing, heaviness, indigestion	<2-10 min	Precipitated by exercise, cold weather, or emotional stress; relieved by rest or nitroglycerin; atypical (Prinzmetal) angina may be unrelated to activity, often early morning	S_4, or murmur of papillary muscle dysfunction during pain
Rest or unstable angina	Same as angina	Same as angina but may be more severe	Usually <20 min	Same as angina, with decreasing tolerance for exertion or at rest	Similar to stable angina, but can be pronounced. Transient cardiac failure can occur
Myocardial infarction	Substernal and can radiate like angina	Heaviness, pressure, burning, constriction	Sudden onset, 30 min or longer, but variable	Unrelieved by rest or nitroglycerin	Shortness of breath, sweating, weakness, nausea, vomiting
Pericarditis	Usually begins over sternum or toward cardiac apex and can radiate to neck or left shoulder; often more localized than the pain of myocardial ischemia	Sharp, stabbing, knifelike	Lasts many hours to days; may wax and wane	Aggravated by deep breathing, rotating chest, or supine position; relieved by sitting up and leaning forward	Pericardial friction rub
Aortic dissection	Anterior chest; can radiate to back	Excruciating, tearing, knifelike	Sudden onset, unrelenting	Usually occurs in setting of hypertension or predisposition such as Marfan syndrome	Murmur of aortic insufficiency, pulse or blood pressure asymmetry; neurological deficit
Pulmonary embolism (chest pain often not present)	Substernal or over region of pulmonary infarction	Pleuritic (with pulmonary infarction) or angina-like	Sudden onset; minutes to <1 hr	Can be aggravated by breathing	Dyspnea, tachypnea, tachycardia; hypotension, signs of acute right-sided heart failure, and pulmonary hypertension with large emboli; rales, pleural rub, hemoptysis with pulmonary infarction
Pulmonary hypertension	Substernal	Pressure; oppressive		Aggravated by effort	Pain usually associated with dyspnea; signs of pulmonary hypertension

From Andreoli TE, Bennett JC, Carpenter CCJ, Plum F: Evaluation of the patient with cardiovascular disease. *In* Cecil Essentials of Medicine, 4th ed. Philadelphia, WB Saunders, 1997, p 11.

spasm should be considered.[15] A history of prolonged, severe anginal chest discomfort accompanied by profound fatigue often signifies acute myocardial infarction. Thus, a careful history not only may indicate the cause of the pain (i.e., myocardial ischemia) but also can provide a clue to the mechanism.

When dyspnea is an "anginal equivalent," the patient may describe the mid-chest as the site of the shortness of breath, whereas true dyspnea is usually not well localized. Other anginal equivalents are discomfort limited to areas that are ordinarily sites of secondary radiation, such as the ulnar aspect of the left arm, lower jaw, teeth, neck, or shoulders, and the development of gas and belching, nausea, "indigestion," dizziness, and diaphoresis. When angina radiates to the arms, it is often described as a "painful heaviness." Anginal equivalents above the mandible or below the umbilicus are quite uncommon.

LOCATION. Embryologically, the heart is a midline viscus; thus, cardiac ischemia produces symptoms that are characteristically felt substernally or across both sides of the chest (Fig. 7–2). Some patients complain of discomfort only to the left or less commonly only to the right of the midline. If the pain or discomfort can be localized to the skin or superficial structures and can be reproduced by localized pressure, it usually arises from the chest wall and is not caused by myocardial ischemia. If the patient can point directly to

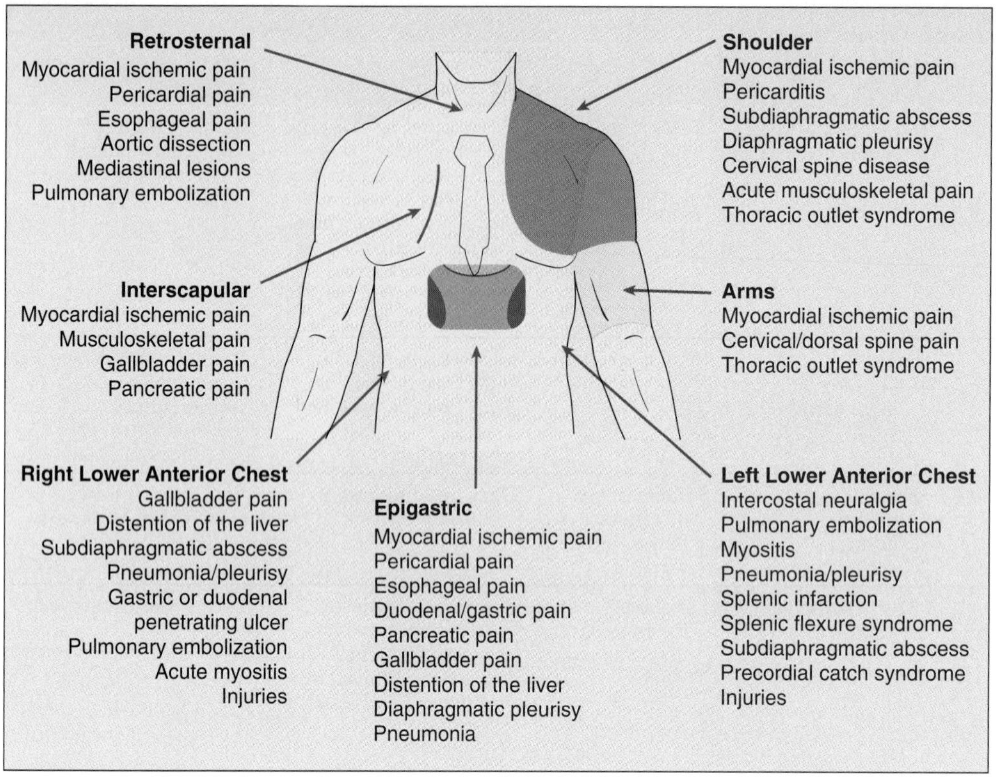

Retrosternal
Myocardial ischemic pain
Pericardial pain
Esophageal pain
Aortic dissection
Mediastinal lesions
Pulmonary embolization

Interscapular
Myocardial ischemic pain
Musculoskeletal pain
Gallbladder pain
Pancreatic pain

Right Lower Anterior Chest
Gallbladder pain
Distention of the liver
Subdiaphragmatic abscess
Pneumonia/pleurisy
Gastric or duodenal penetrating ulcer
Pulmonary embolization
Acute myositis
Injuries

Epigastric
Myocardial ischemic pain
Pericardial pain
Esophageal pain
Duodenal/gastric pain
Pancreatic pain
Gallbladder pain
Distention of the liver
Diaphragmatic pleurisy
Pneumonia

Shoulder
Myocardial ischemic pain
Pericarditis
Subdiaphragmatic abscess
Diaphragmatic pleurisy
Cervical spine disease
Acute musculoskeletal pain
Thoracic outlet syndrome

Arms
Myocardial ischemic pain
Cervical/dorsal spine pain
Thoracic outlet syndrome

Left Lower Anterior Chest
Intercostal neuralgia
Pulmonary embolization
Myositis
Pneumonia/pleurisy
Splenic infarction
Splenic flexure syndrome
Subdiaphragmatic abscess
Precordial catch syndrome
Injuries

FIGURE 7–2. Differential diagnosis of chest pain according to location where pain starts. Serious intrathoracic or subdiaphragmatic diseases are usually associated with pains that begin in the left anterior chest, left shoulder, or upper arm, the interscapular region, or the epigastrium. The scheme is not all inclusive (e.g., intercostal neuralgia occurs in locations other than the left, lower anterior chest area). (From Miller AJ: Diagnosis of Chest Pain. New York, Raven Press, 1988, p 175.)

pectoris. Angina may also be precipitated by strong emotion or fright, by a nightmare, by working with the arms over the head, by hurrying, by cold exposure, or by smoking a cigarette. Prinzmetal (variant) angina characteristically occurs at rest and may or may not be affected by exertion[15]; however, classic angina, although most often precipitated by effort, may progress to unstable angina, which is characterized by ischemic discomfort at rest (see Chap. 49).

DIFFERENTIAL DIAGNOSIS. Chest pain that occurs after protracted vomiting can be due to the Mallory-Weiss syndrome (i.e., a tear in the lower portion of the esophagus). Pain that occurs while the patient is bending over is often radicular and can be associated with osteoarthritis of the cervical or upper thoracic spine. Chest pain occurring on moving the neck can be due to a herniated intervertebral disc.

the site of discomfort with the tip of a finger, and if that site is quite small (<3 cm in diameter), it is usually not angina pectoris.

Pain that is localized to the region of or under the left nipple or that radiates to the right lower chest is usually noncardiac in origin and may be functional or due to costochondritis, gaseous distention of the stomach, or the splenic flexure syndrome.[16] Like other symptoms arising in deeper structures, angina tends to be diffuse and eludes precise localization. Although pain due to myocardial ischemia often radiates to the arm, especially the ulnar aspect of the left arm, wrist, epigastrium, or left shoulder, such radiation may also occur in patients with pericarditis and disorders of the cervical spine. Radiation of pain from the chest to the neck and jaws is typical of myocardial infarction.

DURATION. The duration of the pain is important in determining its origin. Angina pectoris is relatively brief, usually lasting from 2 to 10 minutes. However, if the pain is very brief (i.e., a momentary, lancinating, sharp pain, or other discomfort that lasts less than 15 seconds), angina can usually be excluded; such a short duration points instead to musculoskeletal pain, pain due to a hiatal hernia, or functional pain. Chest pain that is otherwise typical of angina but that lasts for more than 10 minutes or occurs at rest is typical of unstable angina.[12] Chest pain lasting for hours can be seen with acute myocardial infarction, pericarditis, aortic dissection, musculoskeletal disease, herpes zoster, anxiety, and cocaine abuse.[13]

PRECIPITATING AND AGGRAVATING FACTORS. Angina pectoris occurs characteristically on exertion, particularly when the patient is hurrying or walking up an incline. Thus, the development of chest discomfort or pain during walking, typically in the cold and up an incline or against a wind, especially after a heavy meal, is typical of angina

ESOPHAGEAL AND OTHER GASTROINTESTINAL PAIN

Substernal and epigastric discomfort after swallowing can be caused by esophageal spasm or esophagitis, often with acid reflux, with or without a hiatal hernia.[17-19] These conditions can also be associated with substernal or epigastric burning pain that is brought on by eating or by lying down after meals and that can be relieved by antacids. Pain due to esophageal spasm has many of the features of and may be difficult to differentiate from angina pectoris. A history of acid reflux into the mouth (water brash) and/or dysphagia can be a useful diagnostic clue pointing to esophageal disease. The chest discomfort secondary to esophageal reflux is most common after meals, occurs in the supine position or on bending, and can be relieved by nitroglycerin.

The discomfort produced by peptic ulcer disease is characteristically located in the mid-epigastrium. It can also resemble angina pectoris, but its characteristic relationship to food ingestion and its relief by antacids are important differentiating features. The pain of acute pancreatitis, like that of acute myocardial infarction, may be predominantly in the epigastrium. However, unlike the pain of myocardial infarction, pancreatic pain is usually transmitted to the back, is position sensitive, and can be relieved in part by leaning forward.[16]

OTHER CAUSES

The chest discomfort of unstable angina[12] and acute myocardial infarction (see Chaps. 46 and 49) is similar in quality, location, and character to that of chronic stable angina pectoris; however, it usually radiates more widely than does chronic stable angina, is more severe, and therefore is generally referred to by the patient as true pain rather than discomfort. The development of pain in patients with these conditions is usually unrelated to unusual effort or emotional stress, often with the patient at rest or even sleeping. Characteristically, nitroglycerin does not provide complete or lasting relief. The chest discomfort of pulmonary hypertension (see Chap. 67) may be identical to that of typical angina[20]; it is caused by right ventricular ischemia or dilation of the pulmonary arteries.

Acute pericarditis (see Chap. 64) is frequently preceded by a history of a viral upper respiratory infection. The inflammation causes pain that is sharper than anginal discomfort, is more left sided than central, and is often referred to the neck, upper shoulders, and back. The pain of pericarditis lasts for hours and is little affected by effort but is often aggravated by breathing, turning in bed, swallowing, or twisting the body; unlike the discomfort produced by ischemia, the pain of acute pericarditis may lessen when the patient sits up and leans forward.

Aortic dissection (see Chap. 53) is suggested by the sudden development of persistent, very severe pain with radiation to the back and into the lumbar region, often in a patient with a history of hypertension. An expanding thoracic aortic aneurysm may erode the vertebral bodies and cause localized, severe, boring pain that may be worse at night.

Chest-wall pain due to costochondritis or myositis is common in patients who present with fear of heart disease.[21] It is associated with local costochondral and muscle tenderness, which can be aggravated by moving or coughing. Chest-wall pain can also accompany chest injury. In patients with the Tietze syndrome, the discomfort is localized to swollen costochondral and costosternal joints, which are painful on palpation. When herpes zoster affects the left chest, it can mimic myocardial infarction. However, its persistence, its localization to a dermatome, the extreme sensitivity of the skin to touch, and the appearance of the characteristic vesicles allow recognition of this condition. The preeruptive stage of herpes zoster can mimic myocardial ischemia as a tight localized band across the chest.

The pain of pulmonary embolism (see Chap. 66) usually commences suddenly and in patients who are at rest, and it is accompanied by shortness of breath. It is typically described as tightness in the chest and is accompanied or followed by pleuritic chest pain (i.e., sharp pain in the side of the chest that is intensified by respiration or cough). Functional or psychogenic chest pain (see Chap. 84) can be one feature of an anxiety state called *Da Costa syndrome* or *neurocirculatory asthenia*.[22-24] It differs from angina pectoris in that it is usually localized to the cardiac apex and consists of a dull, persistent ache that lasts for hours and is often accentuated by or alternates with attacks of sharp, lancinating stabs of inframammary pain of 1 or 2 seconds' duration. The condition may occur with emotional strain and fatigue, bears little relation to exertion, and may be accompanied by precordial tenderness. Attacks can be associated with palpitation, hyperventilation, numbness and tingling in the extremities, sighing, dizziness, dyspnea, generalized weakness, faintness, severe fatigability, and a history of panic attacks and other signs of emotional instability or depression. The pain may not be completely relieved by any medication other than analgesics, but it is often attenuated by many types of interventions, including rest, exertion, tranquilizers, and placebos. Patients with Da Costa syndrome usually are young (<40 years), are female, and have high scores on depression and anxiety scales.[24]

RELIEF OF PAIN

Rest and sublingual nitroglycerin characteristically relieve the discomfort of chronic stable angina in 1 to 5 minutes. If more than 10 minutes transpire before relief, the diagnosis of chronic stable angina becomes questionable and instead unstable angina, acute myocardial infarction, or pain not caused by myocardial ischemia at all is the cause. Although nitroglycerin commonly relieves the pain of angina pectoris, response to this drug is nonspecific, since the discomfort caused by esophageal spasm and esophagitis can also be relieved. Angina pectoris is alleviated by quiet standing or sitting; sometimes resting in the recumbent position does not relieve angina. Chest pain secondary to acute pericarditis is characteristically relieved by leaning forward, whereas pain that is relieved by food or antacids may be due to peptic ulcer disease or esophagitis. Pain that is alleviated by holding the breath in deep expiration is commonly due to pleuritic inflammation. Some patients with upper gastrointestinal disease or anxiety report relief of symptoms after belching.

CHEST PAIN IN WOMEN (see Chap. 73). Chest discomfort that is atypical for angina pectoris is more common in women than in men, perhaps because of the higher prevalence of vasospastic and of microvascular angina and nonischemic causes of chest pain in women.[25-27] Women with epicardial coronary artery disease more often report chest discomfort at rest, during sleep, or during mental stress than do men.

ACCOMPANYING SYMPTOMS. The physician should always be concerned about the patient with the combination of severe chest discomfort and profuse sweating. This combination frequently signals a serious disorder, such as acute myocardial infarction but also acute pulmonary embolism or aortic dissection. Severe chest pain accompanied by nausea and vomiting is also often due to myocardial infarction. The latter diagnosis, as well as pneumothorax, pulmonary embolism, or mediastinal emphysema, is suggested by pain associated with shortness of breath. Chest pain accompanied by palpitation may be due to the acute myocardial ischemia precipitated by a tachyarrhythmia-induced increase in myocardial oxygen consumption in the presence of coronary artery disease. Chest pain accompanied by hemoptysis suggests pulmonary embolism with infarction or lung tumor, whereas pain accompanied by fever occurs in patients with pneumonia, pleurisy, and pericarditis. Functional pain is commonly accompanied by frequent sighing, anxiety, or depression.

APPROACH TO THE PATIENT (see Chap. 45). This is summarized in the algorithm shown in Figure 7-3 (see also Fig. 45-3). After administration of emergency treatment, if necessary, a focused history and physical examination should allow determination of a cardiac or possible cardiac cause. The 12-lead electrocardiogram and cardiac markers of necrosis (CK-MB and troponin) are then helpful in guiding therapy.[28,29]

Cyanosis

Cyanosis, both a symptom and a physical sign, is a bluish discoloration of the skin and mucous membranes resulting from an increased quantity of reduced hemoglobin or of abnormal hemoglobin pigments in the blood perfusing these areas.[30,31] It may go unnoticed by the patient and is more commonly described by a family member. There are two principal forms of cyanosis: (1) central cyanosis, characterized by decreased arterial oxygen saturation due to right-to-left shunting of blood or impaired pulmonary function, and (2) peripheral cyanosis, most commonly secondary to cutaneous vasoconstriction due to low cardiac output or exposure to cold air or water; if peripheral cyanosis is confined to a single extremity, localized arterial or venous obstruction should be suspected. A history of cyanosis localized to the hands suggests Raynaud's phenomenon. Patients with central cyanosis due to congenital heart disease or pulmonary disease characteristically report that it worsens during exertion, whereas the resting peripheral cyanosis of congestive heart failure may be accentuated only slightly, if at all, during exertion.

Central cyanosis usually becomes apparent at a mean capillary concentration of 4 gm/dl reduced hemoglobin (or 0.5 gm/dl methemoglobin). In general, a history of cyanosis in light-skinned people is rarely elicited unless arterial saturation is 85 percent or less; in people with darker skin, arterial saturation has to drop far lower before cyanosis is perceptible.

Although a history of cyanosis beginning in infancy suggests a congenital cardiac malformation with a right-to-left shunt, hereditary methemoglobinemia is another, albeit rare, cause of congenital cyanosis; the diagnosis of this condition is supported by a family history of cyanosis in the absence of heart disease.

A history of cyanosis limited to the neonatal period suggests the diagnosis of atrial septal defect with transient right-to-left shunting or, more commonly, pulmonary parenchymal disease or central nervous system depression. Cyanosis beginning at the age of 1 to 3 months may be reported when spontaneous closure of a patent ductus arteriosus causes a reduction of pulmonary blood flow in the presence of right-sided obstructive cardiac anomalies, most commonly tetralogy of Fallot. If cyanosis appears at the age of 6 months or later in childhood, it may be due to the development or progression of obstruction to right ventricular outflow in patients with ventricular septal defect. A history of the development of cyanosis in a patient with congenital heart disease between 5 and 20 years of age suggests Eisenmenger syndrome with right-to-left shunting as a consequence of a progressive increase in pulmonary vascular resistance (see Chap. 56). Cyanosis secondary to a pulmonary arteriovenous fistula also usually appears first in childhood.

Syncope (see Chap. 34)

Loss of consciousness results most commonly from reduced perfusion of the brain. The history is extremely valuable in

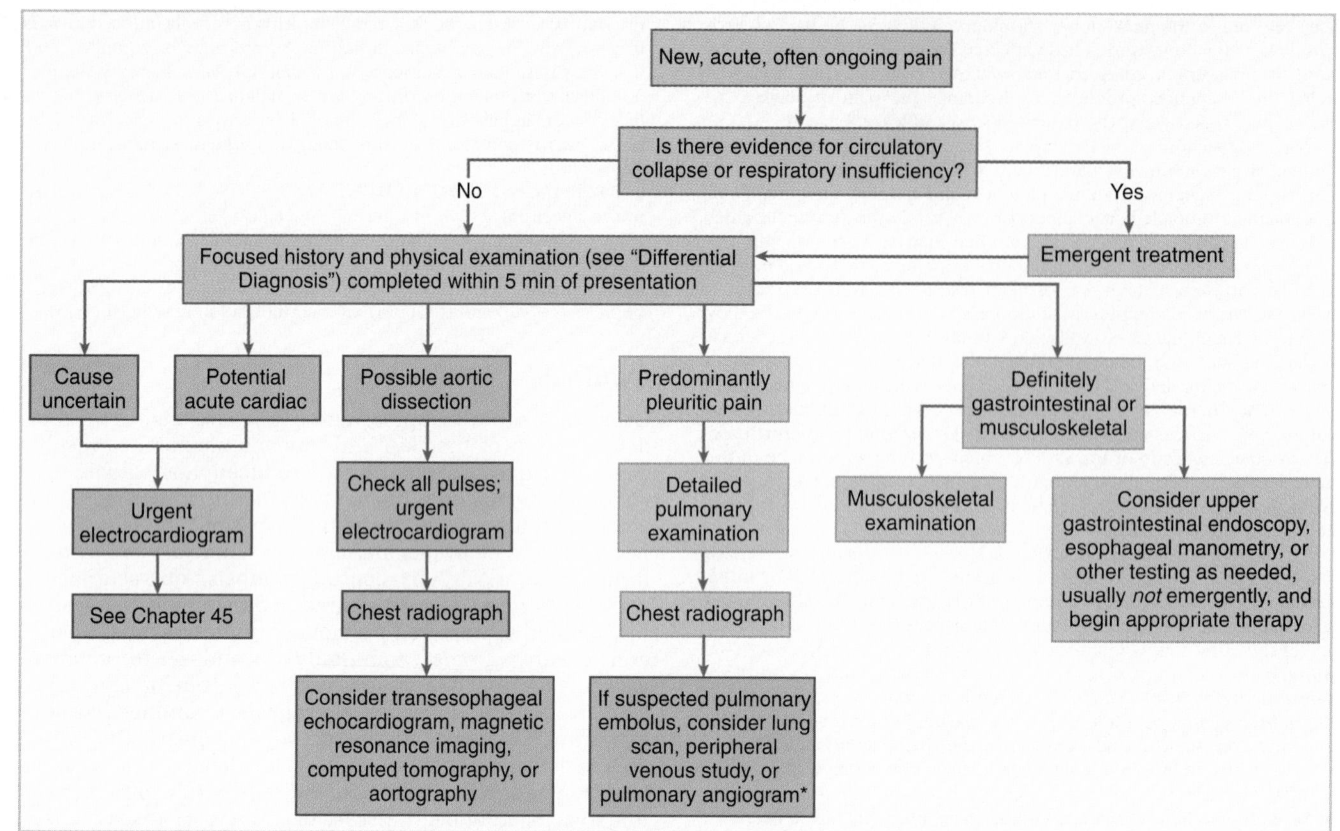

FIGURE 7–3. Diagnostic approach to the patient with new, acute, often ongoing chest pain. *Spiral computed tomographic scan should also be considered. (From Goldman L: Approach to the patient with chest pain. *In* Braunwald E, Goldman L [eds]: Primary Cardiology. 2nd ed. Philadelphia, WB Saunders, 2003, pp 83-100, Adapted from Goldman L: Chest discomfort and palpitation. *In* Fauci A, Braunwald E, et al [eds]: Harrison's Principles of Internal Medicine. 14th ed. New York, McGraw-Hill, 1998, p 61.)

the differential diagnosis of syncope. Several daily attacks of loss of consciousness suggest (1) Stokes-Adams attacks (i.e., transient asystole or ventricular fibrillation in the presence of atrioventricular block); (2) other cardiac arrhythmias; or (3) a seizure disorder (i.e., petit mal epilepsy). These diagnoses are suggested when the loss of consciousness is abrupt and occurs over 1 or 2 seconds; a more gradual onset suggests vasodepressor syncope (i.e., the common faint) or syncope due to hyperventilation or, much less commonly, hypoglycemia.

CARDIAC SYNCOPE. This condition is usually of rapid onset without aura and is usually not associated with convulsive movements, urinary incontinence, or a postictal confusional state. Syncope in aortic stenosis[32-34] is usually precipitated by effort. Patients with syncope secondary to a convulsive disorder often have a prodromal aura preceding the seizure. Injury from falling is common, as are urinary incontinence and a postictal confusional state, associated with headache and drowsiness. Unconsciousness developing gradually and lasting for a few seconds suggests vasodepressor (neurocardiogenic) syncope or syncope secondary to postural hypotension[35,36] (see Chap. 87), whereas a longer period of unconsciousness suggests aortic stenosis or hyperventilation. Hysterical fainting is usually not accompanied by any untoward display of anxiety or change in pulse, blood pressure, or skin color, and there may be a question whether any true loss of consciousness occurred. It is often associated with paresthesias of the hands or face, hyperventilation, dyspnea, chest pain, and feelings of acute anxiety.

REGAINING CONSCIOUSNESS. Consciousness is usually regained quite promptly in patients with syncope of cardiovascular origin but more slowly in patients with convulsive disorders. When consciousness is regained after vasodepressor syncope, the patient is often pale and diaphoretic with a slow heart rate, whereas after a Stokes-Adams attack, the patient's face is often flushed and there may be cardiac acceleration.

DIFFERENTIAL DIAGNOSIS. A family history of syncope or near-syncope can often be elicited in patients with hypertrophic cardiomyopathy (see Chap. 59) or ventricular tachyarrhythmias associated with QT prolongation (see Chap. 29). A history of syncope during childhood suggests the possibility of obstruction to left ventricular outflow—valvular, supravalvular, or subvalvular aortic stenosis. In patients with hypertrophic cardiomyopathy, syncope may be posttussive and occurs characteristically in the erect position, when arising suddenly, after standing erect for long periods, and during or immediately after cessation of exertion. Patients with syncope secondary to orthostatic hypotension may have a history of drug therapy for hypertension or of abnormalities of autonomic function, such as impotence, disturbances of sphincter function, peripheral neuropathy, and anhidrosis.[36]

Calkins and coworkers demonstrated the value of the clinical history in differentiating between serious arrhythmias (ventricular tachycardia or atrioventricular block) and neurocardiogenic syncope. Features predictive of the former were male gender, age older than 54 years, two or fewer episodes of syncope, and duration of warning of 5 seconds or less. On the other hand, features of syncope due to neurocardiogenic syncope included palpitations, blurred vision, nausea, diaphoresis, or lightheadedness before syncope, and nausea, warmth, diaphoresis, or fatigue after syncope.[37]

Palpitation (see Chap. 29)

Palpitation is a common symptom defined as an unpleasant awareness of the forceful or rapid beating of the heart. Patients describe it as pounding, jumping, racing, or irregularity of the heart beat, a "flip flopping" or "rapid fluttering" in the chest, or pounding in the neck.[38-40] It can be brought about by a variety of disorders involving changes in cardiac rhythm or rate, including all forms of tachycardia, ectopic beats, compensatory pauses, augmented stroke volume due to valvular regurgitation, hyperkinetic (high cardiac output) states, and the sudden onset of bradycardia. In the case of premature contractions, the patient is more commonly aware of the post-extrasystolic beat than of the premature beat itself.

DIFFERENTIAL DIAGNOSIS. Palpitation characterized by a slow heart rate may be due to atrioventricular block or sinus node disease. When palpitation begins and ends abruptly, it is often due to a paroxysmal arrhythmia such as paroxysmal atrial or junctional tachycardia, atrial flutter, or atrial fibrillation, whereas a gradual onset and cessation of the attack suggest sinus tachycardia and/or an anxiety state. A history of chaotic, rapid heart action suggests the diagnosis of atrial fibrillation; fleeting and repetitive palpitation suggests multiple ectopic beats. A history of dizziness, presyncope, or syncope with palpitations may be due to ventricular tachycardia and may be an ominous prognostic sign.

Some patients have taken their pulse during palpitation or have asked a companion to do so. A regular rate between 100 and 140 beats per minute suggests sinus tachycardia, a regular rate of approximately 150 beats per minute suggests atrial flutter, and a regular rate exceeding 160 beats per minute suggests paroxysmal supraventricular tachycardia.

A history of palpitation during strenuous physical activity is normal, whereas palpitation during mild exertion suggests either that the individual is severely deconditioned or the presence of heart failure, atrial fibrillation, anemia, or thyrotoxicosis. When palpitation can be relieved suddenly by stooping, breath-holding, or induced gagging or vomiting (i.e., by vagal maneuvers), the diagnosis of paroxysmal supraventricular tachycardia is suggested. Palpitation followed by angina suggests that myocardial ischemia has been precipitated by increased oxygen demands induced by the rapid heart rate. Palpitations are frequently accompanied by, and are often caused by, anxiety, panic reactions, or emotionally startling experiences.[40]

A directed history is useful in elucidating the cause of palpitation (Table 7–4). Is there a history of cocaine or amphetamine abuse? Thyrotoxicosis? Anemia? Do the palpitations occur after heavy cigarette smoking or caffeine ingestion? Is there a family history of syncope, arrhythmia, or sudden death?

DIAGNOSTIC APPROACH TO THE PATIENT. The diagnostic approach is shown in Figure 7–4. The key decision points are the determination of whether structural heart disease is present and whether the patient complains of severe symptoms, including syncope and presyncope.

Edema

LOCALIZATION. Localization is helpful in elucidating the cause of edema.[41,42] Unilateral leg edema is most commonly due to deep venous thrombosis or cellulitis. A history of edema of the legs that is most pronounced in the evening is characteristic of heart failure or bilateral chronic venous insufficiency. Inability to fit the feet into shoes is a common early symptom. In most patients, any visible edema of both lower extremities is preceded by a weight gain of at least 3 to 5 kg. Cardiac edema is generally symmetrical. As it progresses, it usually ascends to involve the legs, thighs, genitalia, and abdominal wall. In patients with heart failure who are largely confined to bed, the edematous fluid localizes in the sacral area. Edema may be generalized (anasarca) in patients with the nephrotic syndrome, severe heart failure, and hepatic cirrhosis. These three conditions can be distinguished by consideration of the history, physical examination, and simple laboratory tests (Table 7–5).

A history of edema around the eyes and face is characteristic of the nephrotic syndrome, acute glomerulonephritis, angioneurotic edema, hypoproteinemia, and myxedema. A history of edema limited to the face, neck, and upper arms may be associated with obstruction of the superior vena cava, most commonly by carcinoma of the lung, lymphoma, or aneurysm of the aortic arch. A history of edema restricted to one extremity is usually due to venous thrombosis or lymphatic blockage of that extremity.

ACCOMPANYING SYMPTOMS. A history of dyspnea associated with edema is most frequently due to heart failure, but it may also be observed in patients with large bilateral pleural effusions, elevation of the diaphragm due to ascites, angioneurotic edema with laryngeal involvement, and pulmonary embolism. When dyspnea precedes edema, the underlying disorder is usually left ventricular dysfunction, mitral stenosis, or chronic lung disease with cor pulmonale. A history of jaundice suggests that edema may be of hepatic origin, whereas edema associated with a history of ulceration and pigmentation of the skin of the legs is most commonly due to chronic venous insufficiency or postphlebitic syndrome. When cardiac edema is not associated with

TABLE 7–4 Items to be Covered in History of Patient with Palpitation

Does the Palpitation Occur:	If So, Suspect:
As isolated "jumps" or "skips"?	Extrasystoles
In attacks known to be of abrupt beginning, with a heart rate of 120 beats/min or over, with regular or irregular rhythm?	Paroxysmal rapid heart action
Independent of exercise or excitement adequate to account for the symptom?	Atrial fibrillation, atrial flutter, thyrotoxicosis, anemia, febrile states, hypoglycemia, anxiety state
In attacks developing rapidly though not absolutely abruptly, unrelated to exertion or excitement?	Hemorrhage, hypoglycemia, tumor of the adrenal medulla
In conjunction with the taking of drugs?	Tobacco, coffee, tea, alcohol, epinephrine, ephedrine, aminophylline, atropine, thyroid extract, monoamine oxidase inhibitors
On standing?	Postural hypotension
In middle-aged women, in conjunction with flushes and sweats?	Menopausal syndrome
When the rate is known to be normal and the rhythm regular?	Anxiety state

From Goldman L, Braunwald E: Chest discomfort and palpitation. *In* Isselbacher KJ, Braunwald E, et al (eds). Harrison's Principles of Internal Medicine, 13th ed. New York, McGraw-Hill, 1994.

CH 7

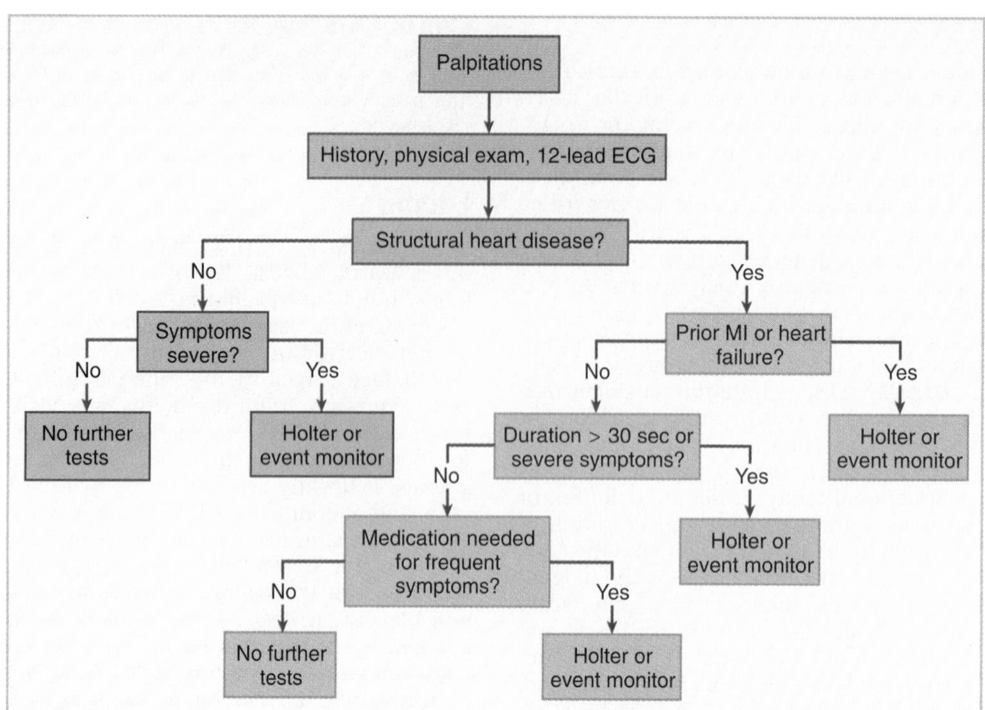

FIGURE 7–4. Diagnostic approach to the patient with palpitations. (From Hlatky MA: Approach to the patient with palpitations. *In* Braunwald E, Goldman L [eds]: Primary Cardiology, 2nd ed. Philadelphia, WB Saunders, 2003, pp 129-136.)

TABLE 7–5 Principal Causes of Generalized Edema: History, Physical Examination, and Laboratory Findings

Organ System	History	Physical Examination	Laboratory Findings
Cardiac	Dyspnea with exertion prominent—often associated with orthopnea—or paroxysmal nocturnal dyspnea	Elevated jugular venous pressure, ventricular (S_3) gallop; occasionally with displaced or dyskinetic apical pulse; peripheral cyanosis, cool extremities, small pulse pressure when severe	Elevated urea nitrogen-to-creatinine ratio common; elevated uric acid; serum sodium often diminished; liver enzymes occasionally elevated with hepatic congestion
Hepatic	Dyspnea infrequent, except if associated with a significant degree of ascites; most often a history of ethanol abuse	Frequently associated with ascites; jugular venous pressure usually normal or low; blood pressure typically lower than in patients with renal or cardiac disease; one or more additional signs of chronic liver disease (jaundice, palmar erythema, Dupuytren contracture, spider angiomas, male gynecomastia or testicular atrophy, caput medusae); asterixis and other signs of encephalopathy may be present	If severe, reductions in serum albumin, cholesterol, other hepatic proteins (transferrin, fibrinogen); liver enzymes may or may not be elevated, depending on the cause and acuity of the liver injury; tendency toward hypokalemia, respiratory alkalosis; magnesium and phosphorus levels often markedly reduced if associated with ongoing ethanol intake; uric acid typically low; macrocytosis from folate deficiency
Renal	Usually chronic; associated with uremic signs and symptoms, including decreased appetite, altered (metallic or fishy) taste, altered sleep pattern, difficulty concentrating, restless legs or myoclonus; dyspnea can be present, but is generally less prominent than in patients with heart failure	Blood pressure often high; hypertensive or diabetic retinopathy in selected cases; nitrogenous fetor; periorbital edema may predominate; pericardial friction rub in advanced cases with uremia	Elevation of serum creatinine and urea nitrogen most prominent; also frequent hyperkalemia, metabolic acidosis, hyperphosphatemia, hypocalcemia, anemia (usually normocytic)

S_3, third heart sound.

From Chertow GM: Approach to the patient with edema. *In* Braunwald E, Goldman L (eds): Primary Cardiology. 2nd ed. Philadelphia, WB Saunders, 2003, pp 117-127.

orthopnea, it may be due to interference with filling of the right side of the heart, such as tricuspid valve disease or constrictive pericarditis. A history of leg edema after prolonged sitting (particularly in the elderly) may be due to simple venous stasis and not be associated with disease at all.

COUGH

Cough, one of the most frequent of all cardiorespiratory symptoms, may be defined as an explosive expiration that provides a means of clearing the tracheobronchial tree of secretions and foreign bodies.[43,44] It can be caused by a variety of infectious, neoplastic, or allergic disorders of the lungs and tracheobronchial tree. Cardiovascular disorders most frequently responsible for cough include those that lead to pulmonary venous hypertension, interstitial and alveolar pulmonary edema, pulmonary infarction, and compression of the tracheobronchial tree (aortic aneurysm).

Cough due to pulmonary venous hypertension secondary to left ventricular failure or mitral stenosis tends to be dry, irritating, spasmodic, and nocturnal. When cough accompanies exertional dyspnea, it suggests either chronic obstructive lung disease or heart failure, whereas in a patient with a history of allergy and/or wheezing, cough is often concomitant with bronchial asthma. A history of a combination of cough with hoarseness without upper respiratory disease may be due to pressure of a greatly enlarged left atrium on an enlarged pulmonary artery compressing the recurrent laryngeal nerve.

The character of the sputum may be helpful in the differential diagnosis. Thus, a cough producing frothy, pink-tinged sputum occurs in cases of pulmonary edema, whereas blood-streaked sputum suggests tuberculosis, bronchiectasis, carcinoma of the lung, or pulmonary infarction.

HEMOPTYSIS

The expectoration of blood or of sputum, either streaked or grossly contaminated with blood, may be due to (1) escape of red blood cells into the alveoli from congested vessels in the lungs (acute pulmonary edema); (2) rupture of dilated endobronchial vessels that form collateral channels between the pulmonary and bronchial venous systems (mitral stenosis); (3) necrosis and hemorrhage into the alveoli (pulmonary infarction); (4) ulceration of the bronchial mucosa or the slough of a caseous lesion (tuberculosis); (5) minor damage to the tracheobronchial mucosa, produced by excessive coughing of any cause, which can result in mild hemoptysis; (6) vascular invasion (carcinoma of the lung); or (6) necrosis of the mucosa with rupture of pulmonary-bronchial venous connections (bronchiectasis).

The history is often decisive in pinpointing the cause of hemoptysis.[43,45] Recurrent episodes of minor bleeding are observed in patients with chronic bronchitis, bronchiectasis, tuberculosis, and mitral stenosis. Rarely, these conditions result in the expectoration of large quantities of blood (i.e., more than one-half cup). Massive hemoptysis can also be due to rupture of a pulmonary arteriovenous fistula; exsanguinating hemoptysis may occur with rupture of an aortic aneurysm into the bronchopulmonary tree.

Hemoptysis associated with shortness of breath suggests mitral stenosis (see Chap. 57); in this condition, the hemoptysis is often precipitated by sudden elevations in left atrial pressure with effort, especially during pregnancy, and is attributable to rupture of small pulmonary or bronchopulmonary anastomosing veins. Blood-tinged sputum in patients with mitral stenosis may also be due to transient pulmonary edema; in these circumstances, it is usually associated with severe dyspnea. A history of hemoptysis associated with acute pleuritic chest pain suggests pulmonary embolism with infarction. Hemoptysis associated with congenital heart disease and cyanosis suggests Eisenmenger syndrome.

FATIGUE

Fatigue is among the most common symptoms in patients with impaired cardiovascular function. However, it is also one of the most nonspecific of all symptoms. In patients with impaired systemic circulation as a consequence of a depressed cardiac output, fatigue may be associated with muscular weakness. In other patients with heart disease, fatigue may be caused by drugs, such as beta-adrenoceptor blocking agents. It may be the result of excessive blood pressure reduction in patients treated too vigorously for hypertension or heart failure. In patients with heart failure, fatigue may also be caused by excessive diuresis and by diuretic-induced hypokalemia. Extreme fatigue sometimes precedes or accompanies acute myocardial infarction.

OTHER SYMPTOMS

Nocturia is a common early complaint in patients with congestive heart failure. Anorexia, abdominal fullness, right upper quadrant discomfort, weight loss, and cachexia are symptoms of advanced heart failure (see Chap. 22). Anorexia, nausea, vomiting, and visual changes are important signs of digitalis intoxication (see Chap. 23). Nausea and vomiting occur frequently in patients with acute myocardial infarction. Hoarseness may be caused by compression of the recurrent laryngeal nerve by an aortic aneurysm, a dilated pulmonary artery, or a greatly enlarged left atrium. A history of fever and chills is common in patients with infective endocarditis (see Chap. 58).

The History in Specific Forms of Heart Disease

Just as the history is of central importance in determining whether a specific symptom is caused by heart disease, it is equally valuable in elucidating its cause. A few examples are given here, whereas considerably greater detail is provided in chapters that deal with each specific disease entity.

HEART DISEASE IN INFANCY AND CHILDHOOD (see Chap. 56)

The history is particularly helpful in establishing the diagnosis of congenital heart disease. In view of the familial incidence of certain congenital malformations (see Chap. 70), a history of congenital heart disease, cyanosis, or heart murmur in the family should be ascertained. Rubella in the first 2 months of pregnancy is associated with a number of congenital cardiac malformations (patent ductus arteriosus, atrial and ventricular septal defect, tetralogy of Fallot, and supravalvular aortic stenosis). A maternal viral illness in the last trimester of pregnancy may be responsible for neonatal myocarditis. Exertional syncope in a child with congenital heart disease suggests a lesion in which the cardiac output is fixed, such as aortic or pulmonic stenosis. Exertional angina in a child suggests severe aortic stenosis, pulmonary stenosis, primary pulmonary hypertension, or anomalous origin of the left coronary artery. A history of syncope or faintness with straining and associated with cyanosis suggests tetralogy of Fallot.

In infants or children with cardiac murmurs, it is important to ascertain by history as precisely as possible when the murmur was first detected. Murmurs due to either aortic or pulmonic stenosis are usually audible within the first 48 hours of life, whereas those produced by a ventricular septal defect are usually apparent a few days or weeks later. On the other hand, the murmur produced by an atrial septal defect often is not heard until age 2 to 3 months.

Frequent episodes of pneumonia early in infancy suggest a large left-to-right shunt, and a history of excessive diaphoresis occurs in patients with left ventricular failure, most commonly due to ventricular septal defect in this age group. A history of squatting is most frequently associated with tetralogy of Fallot or tricuspid atresia. Dysphagia in early infancy suggests the presence of an aortic arch anomaly such as double aortic arch or an anomalous origin of the right subclavian artery passing behind the esophagus. A history of headaches, weakness of the legs, and intermittent claudication is compatible with the diagnosis of coarctation of the aorta. Weakness or lack of coordination in a child with heart disease suggests cardiomyopathy associated with Friedreich ataxia or muscular dystrophy (see Chap. 85). A cerebrovascular accident in a cyanotic patient may be due to cerebral thrombosis or abscess or paradoxical embolization.

MYOCARDITIS AND CARDIOMYOPATHY. Rheumatic fever (see Chap. 81) is suggested by a history of sore throat followed by rash and chorea (St. Vitus dance). Chorea is characterized by twitching or clumsiness for a few months in childhood, as well as by frequent episodes of epistaxis and growing pains (i.e., nocturnal pains in the legs). A history of dyspnea following an influenza-like illness with myalgia suggests acute myocarditis. Carcinoid heart disease (see Chap. 59) is associated with a history of diarrhea, bronchospasm, and flushing of the upper chest and head. A history of diabetes, particularly if resistant to insulin and associated with bronzing of the skin, suggests hemochromatosis, which can be associated with heart failure due to cardiac infiltration.

Amyloid heart disease (see Chap. 59) is often associated with a history of postural hypotension and peripheral neuropathy. Hypertrophic cardiomyopathy (see Chap. 59) is often associated with a family history of this condition and sometimes with a family history of sudden death. The characteristic symptoms are angina, dyspnea, and syncope, which occur during or immediately after exercise.

HIGH-OUTPUT HEART FAILURE. Patients with symptoms of heart failure (breathlessness and excess fluid accumulation) with warm extremities often have high-output heart failure (see Chap. 22). They should be questioned about a history of anemia and of its common causes and accompaniments, such as menorrhagia, melena, peptic ulcer, hemorrhoids, sickle cell disease, and the neurological manifestations of vitamin B_{12} deficiency. Also, in such patients an attempt should be made to elicit a history of thyrotoxicosis (weight loss, polyphagia, diarrhea, diaphoresis, heat intolerance, nervousness, breathlessness, muscle weakness, and goiter [see Chap. 79]). Patients with beriberi heart disease responsible for high-output heart failure often have a history characteristic of peripheral neuritis, alcoholism, poor eating habits, fad diets, or upper gastrointestinal surgery.

COR PULMONALE. Patients with chronic cor pulmonale (see Chap. 67) frequently present with a history of smoking, chronic cough and sputum production, dyspnea, and wheezing relieved by bronchodilators. Alternatively, they have a history of pulmonary emboli, phlebitis, and the sudden development of dyspnea at rest, with palpitations, pleuritic chest pain, and, in the case of massive infarction, syncope.

PERICARDITIS. In patients in whom pericarditis or cardiac tamponade is suspected (see Chap. 64), an attempt should be made to elicit a history of chest trauma, a recent viral infection, recent cardiac surgery, neoplastic disease of the chest with or without radiation therapy, myxedema, scleroderma, tuberculosis, or contact with tuberculous patients. In patients with chronic constrictive pericarditis, ascites often precedes edema, which in turn usually precedes exertional dyspnea.

INFECTIVE ENDOCARDITIS. The diagnosis of infective endocarditis is suggested by a history of fever, severe night sweats, anorexia, and weight loss and embolic phenomena expressed as hematuria, back pain, petechiae, tender finger pads, and a cerebrovascular accident (see Chap. 58).

Drug-Induced Heart Disease

Because a wide variety of cardiac abnormalities can be induced by drugs, a meticulous history of drug intake is of great importance. Table 7–6 summarizes the major drugs responsible for various cardiovascular manifestations.

TABLE 7–6 Cardiovascular Manifestations of Adverse Reactions to Drugs

Acute Chest Pain (Nonischemic)	**Cardiomyopathy**	**Hypertension**
Bleomycin	Adriamycin	Clonidine withdrawal
	Daunorubicin	Corticotropin
Angina Exacerbation	Emetine	Cyclosporine
Alpha blockers	Lithium	Erythropoietin
Beta-blocker withdrawal	Phenothiazines	Glucocorticoids
Ergotamine	Sulfonamides	Monoamine oxidase inhibitors with sympathomimetics
Excessive thyroxine	Sympathomimetics	Nonsteroidal anti-inflammatory drugs
Hydralazine		Oral contraceptives
Methysergide	**Fluid Retention/Congestive Heart Failure/Edema**	Sympathomimetics
Minoxidil	Beta-blockers	Tricyclic antidepressants with sympathomimetics
Nifedipine	Calcium blockers	
Oxytocin	Carbenoxolone	**Pericardial Effusion**
Vasopressin	Diazoxide	Minoxidil
	Estrogens	Oral contraceptives
Arrhythmias	Mannitol	Thromboembolism
Adenosine	Minoxidil	
Adriamycin	NSAIDs	**Prolonged QT Interval/Torsades de Pointes**
Anticholinesterases	Phenylbutazone	Amiodarone
Atropine	Steroids	Amitriptyline
Beta blockers	Verapamil	Chlorpromazine
Daunorubicin		Diphenylhydramine
Digitalis	**Pericarditis**	Disopyramide
Emetine	Emetine	Haloperidol
Erythromycin	Hydralazine	Ibutilide
Guanethidine	Methysergide	Pentamidine
Lithium	Procainamide	Procainamide
Papaverine		Sotalol
Pentamidine	**Hypotension (see also Arrhythmias)**	Terfenadine
Phenothiazines, particularly thioridazine	Amiodarone	Trimethoprim-sulfamethoxazole
Sympathomimetics	Calcium channel blockers, e.g., nifedipine	
Terfenadine		
Theophylline	**Diuresis**	
Thyroid hormone	Interleukin-2	
Tricyclic antidepressants	Levodopa	
Verapamil	Morphine	
	Nitroglycerin	
Atrioventricular Block	Phenothiazines	
Clonidine	Protamine	
Methyldopa	Quinidine	
Verapamil	Sildenafil	

Modified from Wood AJ: Adverse reactions to drugs. *In* Braunwald E, Fauci A, Kasper D, et al (eds): Harrison's Principles of Internal Medicine. 15th ed. New York, McGraw-Hill, 2001. Copyright © by McGraw-Hill, Inc. Used by permission of McGraw-Hill Book Company.

Catecholamines, whether administered exogenously or secreted by a pheochromocytoma (see Chap. 79), may produce myocarditis and arrhythmias. Digitalis glycosides can be responsible for a variety of tachyarrhythmias and bradyarrhythmias as well as gastrointestinal, visual, and central nervous system disturbances (see Chap. 23). Paradoxically, the administration of antiarrhythmic drugs is one of the major causes of serious cardiac arrhythmias (see Chap. 29). For example, quinidine may cause QT prolongation, ventricular tachycardia of the torsades de pointes variety, syncope, and sudden death, presumably due to ventricular fibrillation.

Disopyramide, beta-adrenoceptor blockers, and the calcium channel antagonists diltiazem and verapamil may depress ventricular performance, and, in patients with ventricular dysfunction, these drugs may precipitate heart failure. Alcohol is also a potent myocardial depressant and may be responsible for the development of cardiomyopathy (see Chap. 59), arrhythmias, and sudden death. Tricyclic antidepressants may cause orthostatic hypotension and arrhythmias. Lithium, also used in the treatment of psychiatric disorders, can aggravate preexisting cardiac arrhythmias, particularly in patients with heart failure in whom the renal clearance of this ion is impaired. Cocaine can cause coronary spasm with resultant myocardial ischemia, myocardial infarction, and sudden death (see Chap 62).[13,46]

The anthracycline compounds doxorubicin (Adriamycin) and daunorubicin, which are widely used because of their broad spectrum of activity against various tumors, may cause or intensify left ventricular failure, arrhythmias, myocarditis, and pericarditis (see Chap. 83). Cyclophosphamide, an antineoplastic alkylating agent, may also cause left ventricular dysfunction, whereas 5-fluorouracil and its derivatives may be responsible for angina secondary to coronary spasm. Radiation therapy to the chest may cause acute and chronic pericarditis (see Chap. 64), pancarditis, or coronary artery disease; furthermore, it may enhance the aforementioned cardiotoxic effects of the anthracyclines.

Assessing Cardiovascular Disability
(Table 7–7)

One of the greatest values of the history is in categorizing the degree of cardiovascular disability, so that a patient's status can be followed over time, the effects of a therapeutic intervention assessed, and patients compared with one another. The Criteria Committee of the New York Heart Association has provided a widely used classification that relates functional activity to the ability to carry out "ordinary" activity.[47] The term *ordinary* is, of course, subject to widely varying interpretation, as are terms such as *undue fatigue* that are used in this classification, and this has limited its accuracy and reproducibility. More recently, the New York Heart Association changed its evaluation from functional activity to a broader one, called *cardiac status*, which takes account

TABLE 7–7 A Comparison of Three Methods of Assessing Cardiovascular Disability

Class	New York Heart Association Functional Classification	Canadian Cardiovascular Society Functional Classification	Specific Activity Scale
I	Patients with cardiac disease but without resulting limitations of physical activity. Ordinary physical activity does not cause undue fatigure, palpitation, dyspnea, or anginal pain.	Ordinary physical activity, such as walking and climbing stairs, does not cause angina. Angina with strenuous or rapid or prolonged exertion at work or recreation.	Patients can perform to completion any activity requiring ≤7 metabolic equivalents (e.g., can carry 24 lb up eight steps; carry objects that weigh 80 lb; do outdoor work [shovel snow, spade soil]; do recreational activities [skiing, basketball, squash, handball, jog/walk 5 mph])
II	Patients with cardiac disease resulting in slight limitation of physical activity. They are comfortable at rest. Ordinary physical activity results in fatigue, palpitation, dyspnea, or anginal pain.	Slight limitation of ordinary activity. Walking or climbing stairs rapidly, walking uphill, walking or stair climbing after meals, in cold, in wind, or when under emotional stress, or only during the few hours after awakening. Walking more than two blocks on the level and climbing more than one flight of ordinary stairs at a normal pace and in normal conditions.	Patients can perform to completion any activity requiring ≤5 metabokic equivalents (e.g., have sexual intercourse without stopping, garden, rake, weed, roller skate, dance fox trot, walk at 4 mph on level ground) but cannot and do not perform to completion activities requiring ≥7 metabolic equivalents.
III	Patients with cardiac disease resulting in marked limitation of physical activity. They are comfortable at rest. Less than ordinary physical activity causes fatigue, palpitation, dyspnea, or anginal pain.	Marked limitation of ordinary physical activity. Walking one to two blocks on the level and climbing more than one flight in normal conditions.	Patients can perform to completion any activity requiring ≤2 metabolic equivalents (e.g., shower without stopping, strip and make bed, clean windows, walk 2.5 mph, bowl, play golf, dress without stopping) but cannot and do not perform to completion any activities requiring ≥5 metabolic equivalents.
IV	Patient with cardiac disease resulting in inability to carry on any physical activity without discomfort. Symptoms of cardiac insufficiency or of the anginal syndrome may be present even at rest. If any physical activity is undertaken, discomfort is increased.	Inability to carry on any physical activity without discomfort—anginal syndrome *may be* present at rest.	Patients cannot or do not perform to completion activities requiring ≥2 metabolic equivalents. *Cannot* carry out activities listed above (Specific Activity Scale, Class III).

From Goldman L, Hashimoto B, Cook EF, Loscalzo A: Comparative reproducibility and validity of systems for assessing cardiovascular functional class: Advantages of a new specific activity scale. Circulation 64:1227, 1981. Copyright 1981, American Heart Association.

of symptoms and other data gathered from the patient.[47] Cardiac status is classified as (1) uncompromised, (2) slightly compromised, (3) moderately compromised, and (4) severely compromised.

Somewhat more detailed and specific criteria were provided by the Canadian Cardiovascular Society,[48] but this classification is limited to patients with angina pectoris. Goldman and coworkers[49] developed a specific activity scale in which classification is based on the estimated metabolic cost of various activities. This scale appears to be more reproducible and to be a better predictor of exercise tolerance than either the New York Heart Association classification or the Canadian Cardiovascular Society criteria.

A key element of the history is to determine whether the patient's disability is stable or progressive. A useful way to accomplish this is to inquire whether a specific task that now causes symptoms (e.g., dyspnea after climbing two flights of stairs) did so 3, 6, and 12 months previously. Precise questioning on this point is important because a gradual reduction of ordinary activity as heart disease progresses may lead to an underestimation of the apparent degree of disability.[50]

REFERENCES

1. Sandler G: The importance of the history in the medical clinic and the cost of unnecessary tests. Am Heart J 100:928, 1980.
2. Sapira JD: The history. *In* The Art and Science of Bedside Diagnosis. Baltimore, Urban & Schwartzenberg, 1990, pp 9-45.
3. Tumulty PA: Obtaining the history. *In* The Effective Clinician. Philadelphia, WB Saunders, 1973, pp 17-28.
4. Scano G, Ambrosino N: Pathophysiology of dyspnea. Lung 180:131, 2002.
5. Schwartzstein RM, Feller-Kopman D: Approach to the patient with dyspnea. *In* Braunwald E, Goldman L (eds): Primary Cardiology, 2nd ed. Philadelphia, WB Saunders, 2003, pp 101-116.
6. Mahler DA, Fierro-Carrion G, Baird JC: Evaluation of dyspnea in the elderly. Clin Geriatr Med 19:19, 2003.
7. Michaelson E, Hollrah S: Evaluation of the patient with shortness of breath: An evidence based approach. Emerg Med Clin North Am 17:221, 1999.
8. Borg G, Noble B: Perceived exertion. *In* Wilmore JH (ed): Exercise and Sports. Science Reviews. New York, Academic Press, 1974, pp 131-153.
9. American Thoracic Society: Dyspnea: Mechanisms, assessment, and management. A consensus statement. Am J Respir Crit Care Med 159:321, 1999.
10. Logeart D, Saudubray C, Beyne P, et al: Comparative value of Doppler echocardiography and B-type natriuretic peptide assay in the etiologic diagnosis of acute dyspnea. J Am Coll Cardiol 40:1794, 2002.
11. Collins SP, Ronan-Bentle S, Storrow AB: Diagnostic and prognostic usefulness of natriuretic peptides in emergency department patients with dyspnea. Ann Emerg Med 41:532, 2003.
12. Yeghiazarians Y, Braunstein JB, Askari A, et al: Unstable angina pectoris. N Engl J Med 342:101, 2000.
13. Weber JE, Shofer FS, Larkin GL, et al: Validation of a brief observation period for patients with cocaine-associated chest pain. N Engl J Med 348:510, 2003.
14. Crea F, Gaspardone A: Mechanisms and significance of anginal pain. Cardiologia 44:233, 1999.
15. Mayer S, Hillis LD: Prinzmetal's angina. Clin Cardiol 21:243, 1998.
16. Horwitz LD, Groves BM (eds): Signs and Symptoms in Cardiology. Philadelphia, JB Lippincott, 1985.
17. Boivin M, Peterson WG: Management of complicated gastroesophageal reflux disease: Atypical chest pain. Can J Gastroenterol 11:91B, 1997.
18. Lemire S: Assessment of clinical severity and investigation of uncomplicated gastroesophageal reflux disease and noncardiac angina-like chest pain. Can J Gastroenterol 11:37B, 1997.
19. Chauhan A, Mullins PA, Taylor G, et al: Cardioesophageal reflex: A mechanism for "linked angina" in patients with angiographically proven coronary artery disease. J Am Coll Cardiol 27:1621, 1996.
20. Zimmerman D, Parker BM: The pain of pulmonary hypertension: Fact or fancy? JAMA 246:2345, 1981.
21. Spalding L Reay E, Kelly C: Cause and outcome of atypical chest pain in patients admitted to hospital. J R Soc Med 96:122, 2003.
22. Carter CS, Servan-Schreiber D, Perlstein WM: Anxiety disorders and the syndrome of chest pain with normal coronary arteries: Prevalence and pathophysiology. J Clin Psychiatry 58:70, 1997.
23. Mayou R: Chest pain, palpitations, and panic. J Psychosom Res 44:53, 1998.
24. Serlie AW, Erdman RA, Passchier J, et al: Psychological aspects of non-cardiac chest pain. Psychother Psychosom 64:62, 1995.
25. Douglas PS, Ginsberg GS: The evaluation of chest pain in women. N Engl J Med 334:1311, 1996.
26. Marroquin OC, Holubkov R, Edmindowicz D, et al: Heterogeneity of microvascular dysfunction in women with chest pain not attributable to coronary artery disease: Implications for clinical practice. Am Heart J 145:628, 2003
27. D'Antono B, Dupuis G, Fleet R, et al: Sex differences in chest pain and prediction of exercise-induced ischemia. Can J Cardiol 19:515, 2003.
28. Goldman L: Approach to the patient with chest pain. *In* Braunwald E, Goldman L (eds): Primary Cardiology, 2nd ed. Philadelphia, WB Saunders, 2003, pp 83-101.
29. Rao SV, Ohman EM, Granger CB, et al: Prognostic value of isolated troponin elevation across the spectrum of chest pain syndromes. Am J Cardiol 91:936, 2003.
30. Braunwald E: Hypoxia and cyanosis. *In* Kasper DL, et al (eds): Harrison's Principles of Internal Medicine. 16th ed. New York, McGraw-Hill, 2005.
31. Fishman AP: Cyanosis and clubbing. *In* Fishman A, et al (eds): Fishman's Pulmonary Diseases and Disorders. 3rd ed. New York, McGraw-Hill, 1998, pp 382-383.
32. Linzer M, Yang EH, Estes NA III, et al: Diagnosing syncope: I. Value of history, physical examination, and electrocardiography. Clinical Efficacy Assessment Project of the American College of Physicians. Ann Intern Med 126:989, 1997.
33. Linzer M, Yang EH, Estes NA III, et al: Diagnosing syncope: II. Unexplained syncope. Clinical Efficacy Assessment Project of the American College of Physicians. Ann Intern Med 127:76, 1997.
34. Kochar MS: Management of postural hypotension. Curr Hypertens Rep 2:457, 2000.
35. Cadman CS: Medical therapy of neurocardiogenic syncope. Cardiol Clin 19:203, 2001.
36. Mathias CJ, Kimber JR: Postural hypotension: Causes, clinical features, investigation and management. Annu Rev Med 50:317, 1999.
37. Calkins H, Shyr Y, Frumin H, et al: The value of the clinical history in the differentiation of syncope due to ventricular tachycardia, atrioventricular block, and neurocardiogenic syncope. Am J Med 98:365, 1995.
38. Zimetbaum P, Josephson ME: Evaluation of patients with palpitations. N Engl J Med 338:1369, 1998.
39. Hlatky MA: Approach to the patient with palpitations. *In* Braunwald E, Goldman L (eds): Primary Cardiology. 2nd ed. Philadelphia, WB Saunders, 2003, pp 129-136.
40. Barsky AJ: Palpitations, arrhythmias, and awareness of cardiac activity. Ann Intern Med 134:832, 2001.
41. Braunwald E: Edema. *In* Kasper DL, et al (eds): Harrison's Principles of Internal Medicine. 16th ed. New York, McGraw-Hill, 2005.
42. Chertow GM: Approach to the patient with edema. *In* Braunwald E, Goldman L (eds): Primary Cardiology. 2nd ed. Philadelphia, WB Saunders, 2003, pp. 117-128.
43. Weinberger S: Cough and hemoptysis. *In* Kasper DL, et al (eds): Harrison's Principles of Internal Medicine. 16th ed. New York: McGraw-Hill, 2005.
44. Patrick H, Patrick F: Chronic cough. Med Clin North Am 79:361, 1995.
45. Corder R: Hemoptysis. Emerg Med Clin North Am 21:421, 2003.
46. Isner JM, Chokshi SK: Cocaine and vasospasm. N Engl J Med 321:1604, 1989.
47. The Criteria Committee of the New York Heart Association: Nomenclature and Criteria for Diagnosis. 9th ed. Boston, Little, Brown, 1994.
48. Campeau L: Grading of angina pectoris. Circulation 54:522, 1975.
49. Goldman L, Hashimoto B, Cook EF, Loscalzo A: Comparative reproducibility and validity of systems for assessing cardiovascular functional class: Advantages of a new specific activity scale. Circulation 64:1227, 1981.
50. Goldman L, Cook EF, Mitchell N, et al: Pitfalls in the serial assessment of cardiac functional status: How a reduction in "ordinary" activity may reduce the apparent degree of cardiac compromise and give a misleading impression of improvement. J Chronic Dis 35:763, 1982.

CHAPTER 8

Physical Examination of the Heart and Circulation

Eugene Braunwald • Joseph K. Perloff

Importance of the Physical Examination

A common pitfall in cardiovascular medicine is the failure by the cardiologist to recognize that a patient's heart disease is part of a systemic illness. Equally important is the failure by the noncardiologist to recognize the presence of a cardiac disorder that is a component of a systemic illness whose major effect may be on other organ systems. To avoid these two pitfalls, patients known to have or suspected of having heart disease require not only a detailed examination of the cardiovascular system but also a careful general physical examination. For example, the presence of coronary artery disease should prompt a careful search for frequent noncardiac concomitant conditions such as atherosclerosis of the carotid arteries and of the arteries of the lower extremities and aorta. Conversely, the very high incidence (approximately 50 percent) of coronary artery disease in patients with cerebrovascular disorders must be considered in dealing with patients with these conditions.

As stated by Mangione and coworkers,[1] "There are still many reasons to promote the teaching of bedside diagnostic skills such as cardiac auscultation. Among these are cost-effectiveness, the possibility of making inexpensive serial observations, the early detection of critical findings, the intelligent and well-guided selection of costly diagnostic technology, and the therapeutic value of the physical contact between physician and patient."

Shaver and Tavel have pointed out that in this era of cost containment in the practice of medicine, and the great expense of many "high-tech" diagnostic procedures, the physical examination remains a relatively inexpensive, useful "test."[2,3] An additional benefit is that the actual physical contact, that is, the "laying on of hands" by the physician creates a valued closer bond with the patient at a time when the patient's encounter with the medical care system is often so impersonal.

The General Physical Examination

General Appearance

An assessment of the patient's general appearance is usually begun with a detailed inspection at the time that the history is being obtained.[4-7] The general build and appearance of the patient, the skin color, and the presence of pallor or cyanosis should be noted, as well as the presence of shortness of breath, orthopnea, periodic (Cheyne-Stokes) respiration (see Chap. 22), and distention of the neck veins. If the patient is in pain, is he or she sitting quietly (typical of angina pectoris); moving about, trying to find a more comfortable position (characteristic of acute myocardial infarction); or most comfortable sitting upright (heart failure) or leaning forward (pericarditis)? Simple inspection also reveals whether the patient's whole body shakes with each heartbeat and whether Corrigan pulses (bounding arterial pulsations, as occur with the large stroke volume of severe aortic regurgitation, arteriovenous fistula, or complete atrioventricular [AV] block) are present in the head, neck, and upper extremities. Malnutrition and cachexia, which occur in severe chronic heart failure (see Chap. 22), may also be readily evident. The distinctive general appearance of the Marfan syndrome (see Chap. 70) is often apparent: long extremities with an arm span that exceeds the height; a longer lower segment (pubis to foot) than upper segment (head to pubis); and arachnodactyly (spider fingers).

HEAD AND FACE

Examination of the face often aids in the recognition of many disorders that can affect the cardiovascular system. For example, myxedema (see Chap. 79) is characterized by a dull, expressionless face, periorbital puffiness, loss of the lateral eyebrows, a large tongue, and dry, sparse hair. An earlobe crease occurs more frequently in patients with coronary artery disease than in those without this condition.[8] Bobbing of the head coincident with each heartbeat (de Musset sign) is characteristic of severe aortic regurgitation. Facial edema may be present in patients with tricuspid valve disease or constrictive pericarditis.

EYES

External ophthalmoplegia and ptosis due to muscular dystrophy of the extraocular muscles occur in patients with the Kearns-Sayre syndrome, which may be associated with complete heart block. Exophthalmos and stare occur in patients with hyperthyroidism, an important cause of high-output cardiac failure (see Chaps. 22 and 79). Blue sclerae can be seen in patients with osteogenesis imperfecta, a disorder that may be associated with aortic dilatation, regurgitation, and dissection and with prolapse of the mitral valve (see Chap. 70).

FUNDI

Examination of the fundi allows classification of arteriolar disease in patients with hypertension and may also be helpful in the recognition of arteriosclerosis. Beading of the retinal artery may be present in patients with hypercholesterolemia. Hemorrhages near the discs with white spots in the center (Roth spots) occur in patients with infective endocarditis. Embolic retinal occlusions can occur in patients with rheumatic heart disease, left atrial myxoma, and atherosclerosis of the aorta or arch vessels. Papilledema can be present not only in patients with malignant hypertension (see Chap. 37) but also in those with cor pulmonale with severe hypoxia (see Chap. 67).

SKIN AND MUCOUS MEMBRANES

Central cyanosis (due to intracardiac or intrapulmonary right-to-left shunting) involves the entire body, including warm, well-perfused sites such as the conjunctivae and the mucous membranes of the oral cavity. Peripheral cyanosis (due to reduction of peripheral blood flow, such as occurs in patients with heart failure and peripheral vascular disease) is characteristically most prominent in cool, exposed areas that may not be well perfused, such as the extremities, particularly the nail beds and nose. Polycythemia can often be suspected from inspection of the conjunctivae, lips, and tongue, which are darkly congested in cases of polycythemia and pale in cases of anemia.

Bronze pigmentation of the skin and loss of axillary and pubic hair occur in patients with hemochromatosis (which may result in cardiomyopathy owing to iron deposits in the heart). Jaundice may be observed in patients after pulmonary infarction as well as in patients with congestive hepatomegaly or cardiac cirrhosis. Lentigines, which are small brown macular lesions on the neck and trunk that begin at about age 6 and do not increase in number with sunlight, are observed in patients with pulmonic stenosis and hypertrophic cardiomyopathy.[9]

Several types of xanthomas (cholesterol-filled nodules) are found either subcutaneously or over tendons in patients with hyperlipoproteinemia (see Chap. 39). Premature atherosclerosis frequently develops in these individuals. Tuberoeruptive xanthomas, present subcutaneously or on the extensor surfaces of the extremities (Fig. 8–1), and xanthoma striatum palmare, which produce yellowish, orange, or pink discoloration of the palmar and digital creases, occur most commonly in patients with type III hyperlipoproteinemia. Patients with xanthoma tendinosum (i.e., nodular swellings of the tendons, especially of the elbows, extensor surfaces of the hands, and Achilles tendons) usually have type II hyperlipoproteinemia. Eruptive xanthomas are tiny yellowish nodules, 1 to 2 mm in diameter on an erythematous base, that may occur anywhere on the body and are associated with hyperchylomicronemia and are therefore often found in patients with type I and type V hyperlipoproteinemia.

Hereditary telangiectases are multiple capillary hemangiomas occurring in the skin, lips (Fig. 8–2), nasal mucosa, and upper respiratory and gastrointestinal tracts and resemble the spider nevi seen in patients with liver disease. When present in the lung, they are associated with pulmonary arteriovenous fistulas and cause central cyanosis.

EXTREMITIES

A variety of congenital and acquired cardiac malformations are associated with characteristic changes in the extremities. Among the congenital lesions, short stature, cubitus valgus, and medial deviation of the extended forearm are characteristic of Turner syndrome (see Chap. 56). Patients with the Holt-Oram syndrome[10] (atrial septal defect with skeletal deformities) often have a thumb with an extra phalanx, a so-called fingerized thumb, which lies in the same plane as the fingers, making it difficult to appose the thumb and fingers. In addition, they may exhibit deformities of the radius and ulna, causing difficulty in supination and pronation.

Arachnodactyly is characteristic of Marfan syndrome (see Chap. 70). Normally, when a fist is made over a clenched thumb, the thumb does not extend beyond the ulnar side of the hand, but it usually does so in patients with Marfan syndrome.

Systolic flushing of the nail beds, which can be readily detected by pressing a flashlight against the terminal digits (Quincke sign), is a sign of aortic regurgitation and of other conditions characterized by a greatly widened pulse pressure. Differential cyanosis, in which the hands and fingers (especially on the right side) are pink and the feet and toes are cyanotic, is indicative of patent ductus arteriosus with reversed shunt due to pulmonary hypertension (see Chap. 67); this finding can often be brought out by exercise. On the other hand, reversed differential cyanosis, in which cyanosis of the fingers exceeds that of the toes, suggests Taussig-Bing anomaly with pulmonary vascular disease and reversed flow through a patent ductus arteriosus. Alternatively, it may occur with transposition of the great arteries, pulmonary hypertension, preductal narrowing of the aorta, and reversed flow through a patent ductus arteriosus.[11]

CLUBBING OF THE FINGERS AND TOES

Clubbing of the digits is characteristic of central cyanosis (cyanotic congenital heart disease or pulmonary disease with hypoxia) (Fig. 8–3). It may also appear within a few weeks of the development of infective endocarditis. The earliest forms of clubbing are characterized by increased glossiness and cyanosis of the skin at the root of the nail.[12] After obliteration of the normal angle between the base of the nail and the skin, the soft tissue of the pulp becomes hypertrophied, the nail root floats freely, and its loose proximal end can be palpated. In the more severe forms of clubbing, bony changes occur (i.e., hypertrophic

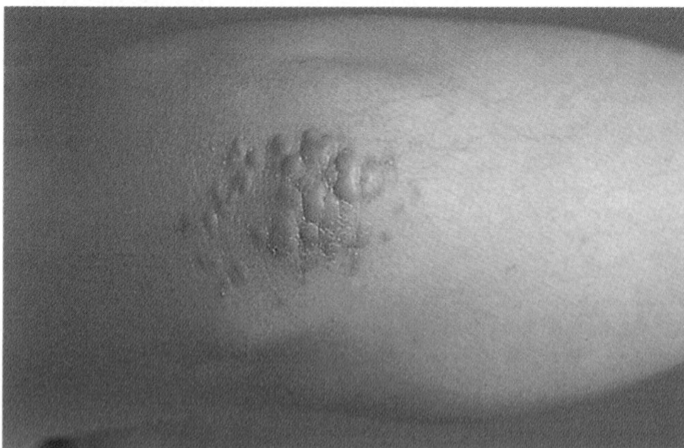

FIGURE 8–1 Eruptive xanthomas on the elbow. Lipid deposition in the skin (xanthoma tuberosum) can be seen in young patients with homozygous familial hypercholesterolemia. It affects the buttocks and palms. There is also joint involvement. (From Zatouroff M: Physical Signs in General Medicine. 2nd ed. London, Mosby-Wolff, 1996, p 99.)

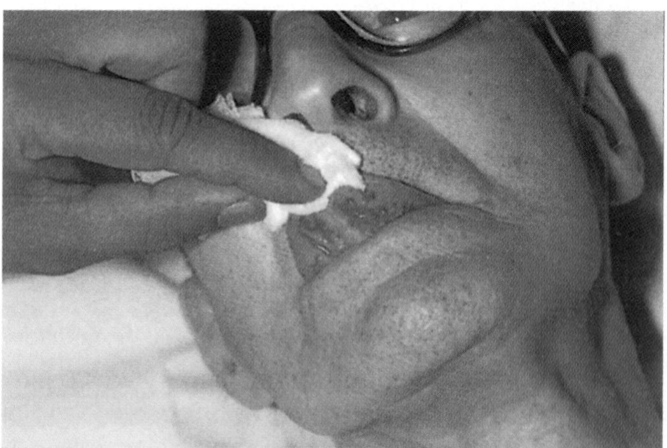

FIGURE 8–2 Telangiectasia of the mouth and cheek (Osler-Weber-Rendu disease). (From Zatouroff M: Physical Signs in General Medicine. 2nd ed. London, Mosby-Wolff, 1996, p 168.)

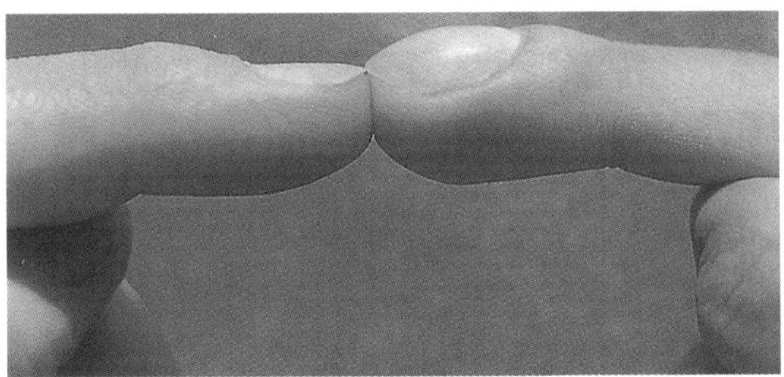

FIGURE 8–3 Nail clubbing (right) and a normal nail (left). (From Zatouroff M: Physical Signs in General Medicine. 2d ed. London, Mosby-Wolff, 1996, p 239.)

osteoarthropathy); these changes involve the terminal digits and in rare instances even the wrists, ankles, elbows, and knees. Unilateral clubbing of the fingers is rare but can occur when an aortic aneurysm interferes with the arterial supply to one arm.

Osler nodes are small, tender, purplish erythematous skin lesions caused by infected microemboli and occurring most frequently in the pads of the fingers or toes and in the palms of the hands or soles of the feet,[13] whereas Janeway lesions are slightly raised, nontender hemorrhagic lesions in the palms of the hands and soles of the feet; both of these lesions as well as petechiae occur in patients with infective endocarditis (see Chap. 58). When petechiae occur under the nail beds, they are termed *splinter hemorrhages.*

EDEMA. The presence of edema of the lower extremities is a common finding in patients with congestive heart failure (see Chap. 22)[14]; however, if it is present in only one leg, it is more likely due to obstructive venous or lymphatic disease than to heart failure. Firm pressure on the pretibial region for 10 to 20 seconds may be necessary for the detection of edema. In patients confined to bed, edema appears first in the sacral region. Edema may involve the face in children with heart failure of any cause and in adults with heart failure associated with marked elevation of systemic venous pressure (e.g., constrictive pericarditis and tricuspid valve disease).

Chest and Abdomen

Examination of the thorax should begin with observations of the rate, effort, and regularity of respiration. The shape of the chest is important as well; thus, a barrel-shaped chest with low diaphragm suggests emphysema, bronchitis, and cor pulmonale. Inspection of the chest is an integral part of the cardiac examination. It may reveal a bulging to the right of the upper sternum caused by an aortic aneurysm. The latter can also produce a venous collateral pattern caused by obstruction of the superior vena cava. *Kyphoscoliosis* of any cause can cause cor pulmonale; this skeletal abnormality, as well as pectus excavatum (funnel chest)[15,16] and pectus carinatum (pigeon breast), is often present in patients with Marfan syndrome.

Left ventricular failure and other causes of elevation of pulmonary venous pressure can cause pulmonary rales; wheezing is sometimes audible in patients with pulmonary edema (cardiac asthma).

Painful enlargement of the liver may be due to venous congestion; the tenderness disappears in cases of long-standing heart failure. Hepatic systolic expansile pulsations occur in patients with severe tricuspid regurgitation, and presystolic pulsations can be felt in patients with tricuspid stenosis and sinus rhythm. Patients with constrictive pericarditis also often have pulsatile hepatomegaly, the contour of the pulsations resembling those of the jugular venous pulse in this condition. When firm pressure over the abdomen causes cervical venous distention (that is, when there is abdominojugular reflux, right-sided heart failure[17]) constrictive pericarditis (see later), or tricuspid valve disease is usually present. Ascites is also characteristic of heart failure, but it is especially characteristic of tricuspid valve disease and chronic constrictive pericarditis.

Splenomegaly can occur in the presence of severe congestive hepatomegaly, most frequently in patients with constrictive pericarditis or tricuspid valve disease. The spleen may be enlarged and painful in patients with infective endocarditis as well as after splenic embolization. Splenic infarction is frequently accompanied by an audible friction rub.

Both kidneys may be palpably enlarged in patients with hypertension secondary to polycystic disease. Auscultation of the abdomen should be carried out in all patients with hypertension; a systolic bruit secondary to renal artery stenosis may be audible near the umbilicus or in the flank.

Atherosclerotic aneurysms of the abdominal aorta are usually readily detected on palpation of the abdomen below the umbilicus (see Chap. 53), except in markedly obese patients. In patients with coarctation of the aorta, no abdominal pulsations are palpable despite the presence of prominent arterial pulses in the neck and upper extremities; arterial pulses in the lower extremities are reduced or absent.

Jugular Venous Pulse

Important information concerning the dynamics of the right side of the heart can be obtained by observation of the jugular venous pulse.[5,18-21] The internal jugular vein is ordinarily examined; the venous pulse can usually be analyzed more readily on the right than on the left side of the neck, because the right innominate and jugular veins extend in an almost straight line cephalad to the superior vena cava, thus favoring transmission of hemodynamic changes from the right atrium, whereas the left innominate vein is not in a straight line and may be kinked or compressed by a variety of normal structures, by a dilated aorta, or by an aneurysm.

During the examination, the patient should be lying comfortably. Although the head should rest on a pillow, it must not be at a sharp angle from the trunk. One can examine the jugular venous pulse effectively by shining a light tangentially across the neck. Most patients with heart disease are examined most effectively in the 45-degree position, but in patients in whom venous pressure is high, a greater inclination (60 or even 90 degrees) is required to obtain visible pulsations, whereas in those in whom jugular venous pressure is low, a lesser incline (30 degrees) is desirable.

The internal jugular vein is located deep within the neck, where it is covered by the sternocleidomastoid muscle and is therefore not usually visible as a discrete structure except in the presence of venous hypertension. However, its pulsations are transmitted to the skin of the neck, where they are usually easily visible. Sometimes examiners experience difficulty in differentiating between the carotid and jugular venous pulses in the neck, particularly when the latter exhibits prominent v waves, as occurs in patients with tricuspid regurgitation, in whom the valves in the internal jugular veins may be incompetent. There are several helpful clues to avoid this difficulty, however:

1. The arterial pulse is a sharply localized rapid movement that may not be readily visible but that strikes the palpating fingers with considerable force; in contrast, the venous pulse, although more readily visible, often disappears when the palpating finger is placed lightly on or below the pulsating area.
2. The arterial pulse usually exhibits a single upstroke, whereas (in patients in sinus rhythm) the venous pulse has two peaks and two troughs per cardiac cycle.
3. The arterial pulsations do not change when the patient is in the upright position or during respiration, whereas venous pulsations usually disappear or diminish greatly in the upright position and during inspiration, unless the venous pressure is greatly elevated.
4. Compression of the root of the neck does not affect the arterial pulse but usually abolishes venous pulsations, except in the presence of extreme venous hypertension.

Two principal observations can usually be made from examination of the neck veins: the level of venous pressure and the type of venous wave pattern. To estimate jugular venous pressure, the height of the oscillating top of the distended proximal portion of the internal jugular vein, which reflects right atrial pressure, should be determined. The upper limit of normal is 4 cm above the sternal angle, which corresponds to a central venous pressure of approximately 9 cm H_2O, since the right atrium is approximately 5 cm below the sternal angle. When the veins in the neck collapse in a subject breathing normally in the horizontal position, it is likely that the central venous pressure is subnormal. When obstruction of veins in the lower extremities is responsible for edema, pressure in the neck veins is not elevated and the abdominal-jugular reflux is negative.

ABDOMINAL-JUGULAR REFLUX. With the patient positioned to make the jugular vein easily visible, steady, firm pressure is supplied to the periumbilical region for 10 to 30 seconds with the patient breathing quietly[17-20]; increased respiratory excursions, straining, and the Valsalva maneuver should be avoided. In normal subjects, jugular venous pressure rises less than 3 cm H_2O and only transiently while abdominal pressure is continued, whereas in patients with right or left ventricular failure and/or tricuspid regurgitation, the jugular venous pressure remains elevated for more than 15 seconds. A positive abdominal-jugular reflux suggests right ventricular systolic and/or diastolic dysfunction, tricuspid valve disease, constrictive pericarditis, or central venous pressure.

PATTERN OF THE VENOUS PULSE. The events of the cardiac cycle, shown in Figure 19–19 provide an explanation for the details of the jugular venous waveform (Fig. 8–4). The A wave in the venous pulse results from venous distention due to right atrial systole, whereas the X descent is due to atrial relaxation and descent of the floor of the right atrium during right ventricular systole. The C wave, which occurs simultaneously with the carotid arterial pulse, is an inconstant wave in the jugular venous pulse and/or interruption of the X descent after the peak of the A wave. The continuation of the X descent after the C wave is referred to as the X′ descent. The V wave results from the rise in right atrial pressure when blood flows into this chamber during ventricular systole when the tricuspid valve is shut, and the Y descent (i.e., the downslope of the V wave) is related to the decline in right atrial pressure when the tricuspid valve reopens. After the bottom of the Y descent (the Y trough) and beginning of the A wave is a period of relatively slow filling of the atrium or ventricle, the diastasis period, a wave termed the H wave.

ALTERATIONS IN DISEASE. Elevation of jugular venous pressure reflects an increase in right atrial pressure and occurs in cases of heart failure, reduced compliance of the right ventricle, pericardial disease, hypervolemia, obstruction of the tricuspid orifice, and obstruction of the superior vena cava. During inspiration, the jugular venous pressure normally declines but the amplitude of the pulsations increases. Kussmaul sign[19,20] is a paradoxical rise in the height of the jugular venous pressure during inspiration, which typically occurs in patients with chronic constrictive pericarditis and sometimes in patients with congestive heart failure and tricuspid stenosis.

The A wave is particularly prominent in patients with conditions in which the resistance to right atrial contraction is increased, such as right ventricular hypertrophy, pulmonary hypertension, and tricuspid stenosis (see Fig. 8–4A). The A wave can also be tall in cases of left ventricular hypertrophy when the thickened ventricular septum interferes with right ventricular filling. Tall A waves are present in patients with sinus rhythm and tricuspid stenosis or atresia, right atrial myxoma, or reduced compliance and/or marked hypertrophy of the right ventricle. Cannon (amplified) A waves are noted in patients with AV dissociation when the right atrium contracts against a closed tricuspid valve. In cases of atrial fibrillation, the A wave and X descent disappear and the V wave and Y descent become more prominent. In cases of right ventricular failure and sinus rhythm, there may be increases in

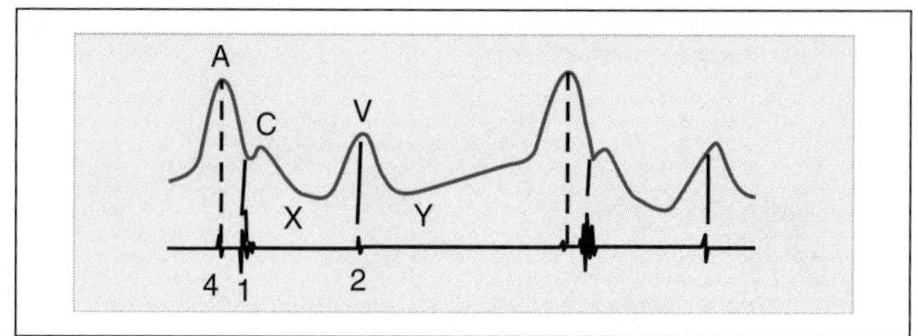

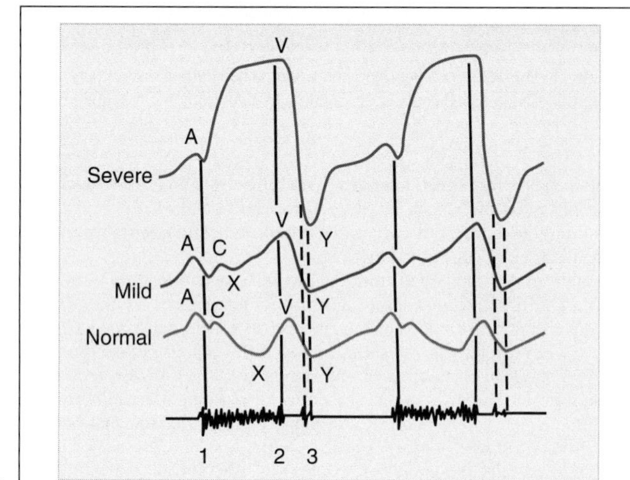

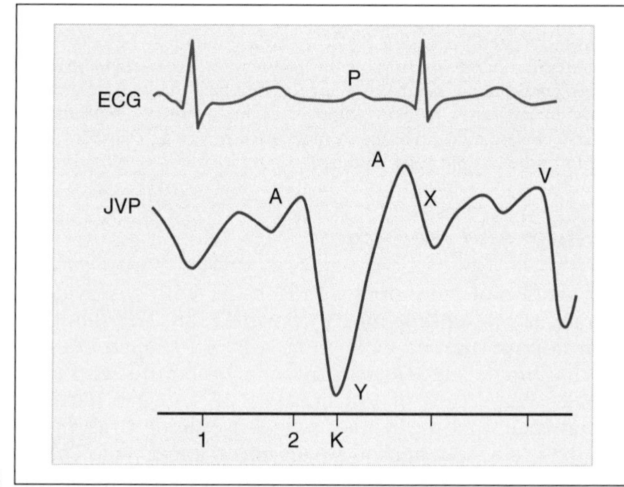

FIGURE 8–4 Common abnormalities of the venous pulse. **A,** Large A waves associated with elevated right ventricular end-diastolic pressure or decreased right ventricular compliance. Increased A wave size or giant A waves are seen when there is severe right ventricular hypertrophy, usually associated with right ventricular systolic hypertension. A right ventricular S4 is often present in such cases. **B,** Augmented V wave in tricuspid regurgitation. As reflux across the tricuspid valve increases in severity, the systolic V valve becomes higher as well as broader. The X descent disappears and the Y descent is progressively accentuated with increasing severity of tricuspid regurgitation. With severe tricuspid regurgitation, the systolic wave may be so dominant as to mimic the carotid arterial pulsations; the entire lower neck will swell with each right ventricular systole. **C,** Constrictive pericarditis. In this condition, right ventricular diastolic pressure is greatly elevated. This elevation results in a prominent Y descent following tricuspid valve opening. The abrupt rise in venous pressure during right ventricular filling is due to the noncompliant right ventricular chamber encased in an unyielding pericardial shell. The venous pulse contour in constrictive pericarditis often takes on an M or W configuration. A pericardial knock (K), a high-frequency early diastolic filling sound, typically is present. (From Abrams J: Synopsis of Cardiac Physical Diagnosis. 2nd ed. Boston, Butterworth Heinemann, 2001, pp 23-35.)

prominence of both A and V waves. A steeply rising H wave is observed (or recorded) in patients with restrictive cardiomyopathy, constrictive pericarditis, and right ventricular infarction. The X descent may be prominent in patients with large A waves, as well as in patients with right ventricular volume overload (atrial septal defect).

Constrictive pericarditis (see Fig. 8–4C) is characterized by a rapid and deep Y descent followed by a rapid rise to a diastolic plateau (H wave) without a prominent A wave; occasionally, the X descent is prominent in patients with this condition as well, causing a W-shaped jugular venous pulse. However, it is in patients with cardiac tamponade that the X descent is most prominent. A prominent V wave or a C-V wave (i.e., fusion of the C and V waves in the absence or attenuation of an X descent) occurs in patients with tricuspid regurgitation, sometimes causing a systolic movement of the earlobe (see Fig. 8–4B, *center*) and a right-to-left head movement with each ventricular systole. Equal A and V waves are seen in patients with atrial septal defect; the Y descent is gradual when right atrial emptying is impeded, as in tricuspid stenosis, and rapid when it is unimpeded, as in tricuspid regurgitation. A steep Y descent is seen in patients with any condition in which there is myocardial dysfunction, ventricular dilatation, and an elevated central venous pressure.

Sphygmomanometric Measurement of Arterial Pressure

One can estimate systolic arterial pressure without a sphygmomanometer by gradually compressing the brachial artery while palpating the radial artery; the force required to obliterate the radial pulse represents the systolic blood pressure, and, with practice, one can often estimate this level within 15 mm Hg. Ordinarily, however, a sphygmomanometer is used to obtain an indirect measurement of arterial pressure. The cuff should fit snugly around the arm, with its lower edge at least 1 inch above the antecubital space, and the diaphragm of the stethoscope should be placed close to or under the edge of the sphygmomanometer cuff. The width of the cuff selected should be at least 40 percent of the circumference of the limb to be used.

The standard size, with a 5-inch-wide cuff, is designed for adults with an arm of average size. When this cuff is applied to a large upper arm or a normal adult thigh, arterial pressure is overestimated, leading to spurious hypertension in the obese patient (arm circumference >35 cm)[22]; when it is applied to a small arm, the pressure is underestimated. The cuff width should be approximately 1.5 inches in infants and small children, 3 inches in young children (2 to 5 years), and 8 inches in obese adults. The rubber bag should be long enough to extend at least halfway around the limb (10 inches in adults). In patients with rigid, sclerotic arteries, the systolic pressure may also be overestimated, by as much as 30 mm Hg. Mercury manometers are, in general, more accurate and reliable than the aneroid type; the latter should be calibrated at least once yearly.

BLOOD PRESSURE IN THE UPPER EXTREMITIES. To measure arterial pressure in an upper extremity,[23,24] the patient should be seated or lying comfortably and relaxed, the arm should be slightly flexed and at heart level, and the arm muscles should be relaxed. The cuff should be inflated rapidly to approximately 30 mm Hg above the anticipated systolic pressure. The cuff is then deflated slowly, no faster than 3 mm Hg/sec; the pressure at which the brachial pulse can be palpated is close to the systolic pressure.

The cuff should be deflated rapidly after the diastolic pressure is noted and a full minute allowed to elapse before pressure is remeasured in the same limb. Although excessive pressure on the stethoscope head does not affect systolic pressure, it does erroneously lower diastolic readings.

BLOOD PRESSURE IN THE LOWER EXTREMITIES. With the patient lying on the abdomen, an 8-inch-wide cuff should be applied with the compression bag over the posterior aspect of the mid-thigh and should be rolled diagonally around the thigh to keep the edges snug against the skin. Auscultation should be carried out in the popliteal fossa. To measure pressure in the lower leg, an arm cuff is placed over the calf and auscultation is carried out over the posterior tibial artery. Regardless of where the cuff is applied, care must be taken to avoid letting the rubber part of the balloon of the cuff extend beyond its covering and to avoid placing the cuff on so loosely that central ballooning occurs.

KOROTKOFF SOUNDS. There are five phases of Korotkoff sounds (i.e., sounds produced by the flow of blood as the constricting blood pressure cuff is gradually released). The first appearance of a clear, tapping sound (phase I) represents the systolic pressure. These sounds are replaced by soft murmurs during phase II and by louder murmurs during phase III, as the volume of blood flowing through the constricted artery increases. The sounds suddenly become muffled in phase IV, when constriction of the brachial artery diminishes as arterial diastolic pressure is approached. Korotkoff sounds disappear in phase V, which is usually within 10 mm Hg of phase IV.

Diastolic pressure measured directly through an intraarterial needle and external manometer corresponds closely to phase V. In cases of severe aortic regurgitation, however, when the disappearance point is extremely low, sometimes 0 mm Hg, the sound of muffling (phase IV) is much closer to the intraarterial diastolic pressure than is the disappearance point (phase V). When the difference between phases IV and V of the Korotkoff sounds exceeds 10 mm Hg, both pressures should be recorded (e.g., 142/54/10 mm Hg).

Korotkoff sounds may be difficult to hear and arterial pressure difficult to measure when arterial pressure rises at a slow rate (as in cases of severe aortic stenosis), when the arteries are markedly constricted (as in cases of shock), and when the stroke volume is reduced (as in cases of severe heart failure). Very soft or inaudible Korotkoff sounds can often be accentuated by having the patient dilate the blood vessels simply by opening and closing the fist repeatedly. Sometimes in states of shock, the indirect method of measuring blood pressure is unreliable and arterial pressure should be measured through an intraarterial needle.

The Auscultatory Gap. The auscultatory gap is a silence that sometimes separates the first appearance of the Korotkoff sounds from their second appearance at a lower pressure. The phenomenon tends to occur when there is venous distention or reduced velocity of arterial flow into the arm. If the first muffling of sounds is considered to be the diastolic pressure, it will be overestimated. If the second appearance is taken as the systolic pressure, it will be underestimated. On the other hand, sounds transmitted through the arterial tree from prosthetic aortic valves may be responsible for falsely high readings.

BLOOD PRESSURE IN THE BASAL CONDITION. To determine arterial pressure in the basal condition, the patient should have rested in a quiet room for 5 to 10 minutes. It is desirable to record the arterial pressure in both arms at the time of the initial examination; differences in systolic pressure between the two arms that exceed 10 mm Hg when measurements are made simultaneously or in rapid sequence[24] suggest obstructive lesions involving the aorta or the origin of the innominate and subclavian arteries or supravalvular aortic stenosis (in which pressure in the right arm exceeds that in the left). In patients with vertebral-basal artery insufficiency, a difference in pressure between the arms may signify that a subclavian "steal" is responsible for the cerebrovascular symptoms.

To be certain from physical examination that the systolic pressure is different in the two arms or in the upper and lower extremities, two examiners should measure the pressures simultaneously and then switch extremities and measure the pressures again.

ORTHOSTATIC HYPOTENSION. To determine whether orthostatic hypotension is present, arterial pressure should be determined with the patient in both the supine and the erect positions. Regardless of the patient's posture, however, the brachial artery should be at the level of the heart to avoid superimposition of the effects of gravity on the recorded pressure.

Normally, the systolic pressure in the legs is up to 20 mm Hg higher than in the arms, but the diastolic pressures are usually virtually identical. The recording of a higher diastolic pressure in the legs than in the arms suggests that the thigh cuff is too small. When systolic pressure in the popliteal artery exceeds that in the brachial artery by more than 20 mm Hg (Hill sign), aortic regurgitation is usually present.[25] Blood pressure should be measured in the lower extremities in patients with hypertension to detect coarctation of the aorta or when obstructive disease of the aorta or its immediate branches is suspected.

Arterial Pulse

The volume and contour of the arterial pulse are determined by a combination of factors, including the left ventricular stroke volume, the ejection velocity, the relative compliance and capacity of the arterial system, and the pressure waves that result from the antegrade flow of blood and reflections of the arterial pressure pulse returning from the peripheral circulation (Table 8–1).[25,26] Bilateral palpation of the carotid, radial, brachial, femoral, popliteal, dorsalis pedis, and posterior tibial pulses should be part of the examination of all cardiac patients (Fig. 8–5). The frequency, regularity, and shape of the pulse wave and the character of the arterial wall should be determined.

The carotid pulse provides the most accurate representation of the central aortic pulse.[26,27] The brachial artery is the vessel ordinarily most suitable for appreciating the rate of rise of the pulse and the contour, volume, and consistency of the peripheral vessels. This artery is located at the medial aspect of the elbow, and it may be helpful to flex the patient's arm to improve palpation; palpation of the artery should be carried out with the thumb exerting pressure on the artery until its maximal movement is detected. A normal rate of rise of the arterial pulse suggests that there is no obstruction to left ventricular outflow, whereas a pulse wave of small amplitude with normal configuration suggests a reduced stroke volume.

THE NORMAL PULSE. The pulse in the ascending aorta normally rises rapidly to a rounded dome (Fig. 8–6); this initial rise reflects the peak velocity of blood ejected from the left ventricle. A slight anacrotic notch or pause is frequently recorded, but only occasionally felt, on the ascending limb of the pulse. The descending limb of the central aortic pulse is less steep than is the ascending limb, and it is interrupted by the incisura, a sharp downward deflection related to closure of the aortic valve. Immediately thereafter, the pulse wave

TABLE 8–1 Classification of Abnormal Pulses

Name	Meaning	Comments
General Abnormalities		
Hypokinetic	Related to a decreased rate of LV pressure development, a decreased LV stroke volume, and/or obstruction of LV outflow	Low amplitude, may or may not have a slow rate of rise
Hyperkinetic	Related to an increased rate of LV pressure development and/or to a large LV stroke volume with decreased peripheral resistance	Prominent fluctuation in the diameter of an artery Pulse pressure can be: Increased (aortic regurgitation, patent ductus arteriosus, arteriovenous fistulas, fever, anemia, exercise) Normal (HOCM, MR)
Specific Abnormalities		
Pulsus parvus et tardus	Pulse with slow rate of pressure increase, small pulse pressure, late	AS
Bisferiens pulse	A pulse with two palpable beats during systole	Occurs in HOCM and in mixed AS/AR. Can also occur in cases of rapid ejection of an increased stroke volume (e.g., exercise, fever, patent ductus arteriosus) Best appreciated in the carotid artery
Dicrotic pulse	A twice-beating or double pulse produced by a combination of the systolic wave followed by an exaggerated dicrotic (diastolic) wave	Low-volume pulse, with shortened ejection period. Observed both in central and peripheral arteries. Observed in cases of cardiac tamponade, hypovolemic shock, severe cardiac failure
Pulsus alternans	Beats occur at constant intervals but with a regular alternation of the peak of the pressure pulse and/or the rate of rise of the ascending limb.	Strong and weak pulses occur in consecutive beats. Pulses alternate in systolic pressure by ≥20 mm Hg Caused by alternating strength of cardiac contraction with consecutive beats, signifies severely depressed cardiac function Best palpated in radial or femoral artery
Bigeminal pulse	Regular coupling of two beats with the interval between a pair of beats greater than between the coupled beats themselves.	Observed with premature ectopic beats coupled to a sinus beat, 3 : 2 Wenckebach atrioventricular block and nonconducted atrial premature systole following every second sinus beat
Pulsus paradoxus	Abnormal exaggeration (>10 mm Hg) of the normal decrease in systolic blood pressure during inspiration	Observed in cases of cardiac tamponade, constrictive pericarditis, restrictive cardiomyopathy, hypotensive shock, severe obstructive pulmonary disease, large pulmonary embolism

AR = aortic regurgitation; AS = aortic stenosis; HOCM = hypertrophic obstructive cardiomyopathy; LV = left ventricular; MR = mitral regurgitation.
Modified from Vlachopoulos C, O'Rourke M: Genesis of the normal and abnormal pulse. Curr Prob Cardiol 25:297, 2000.

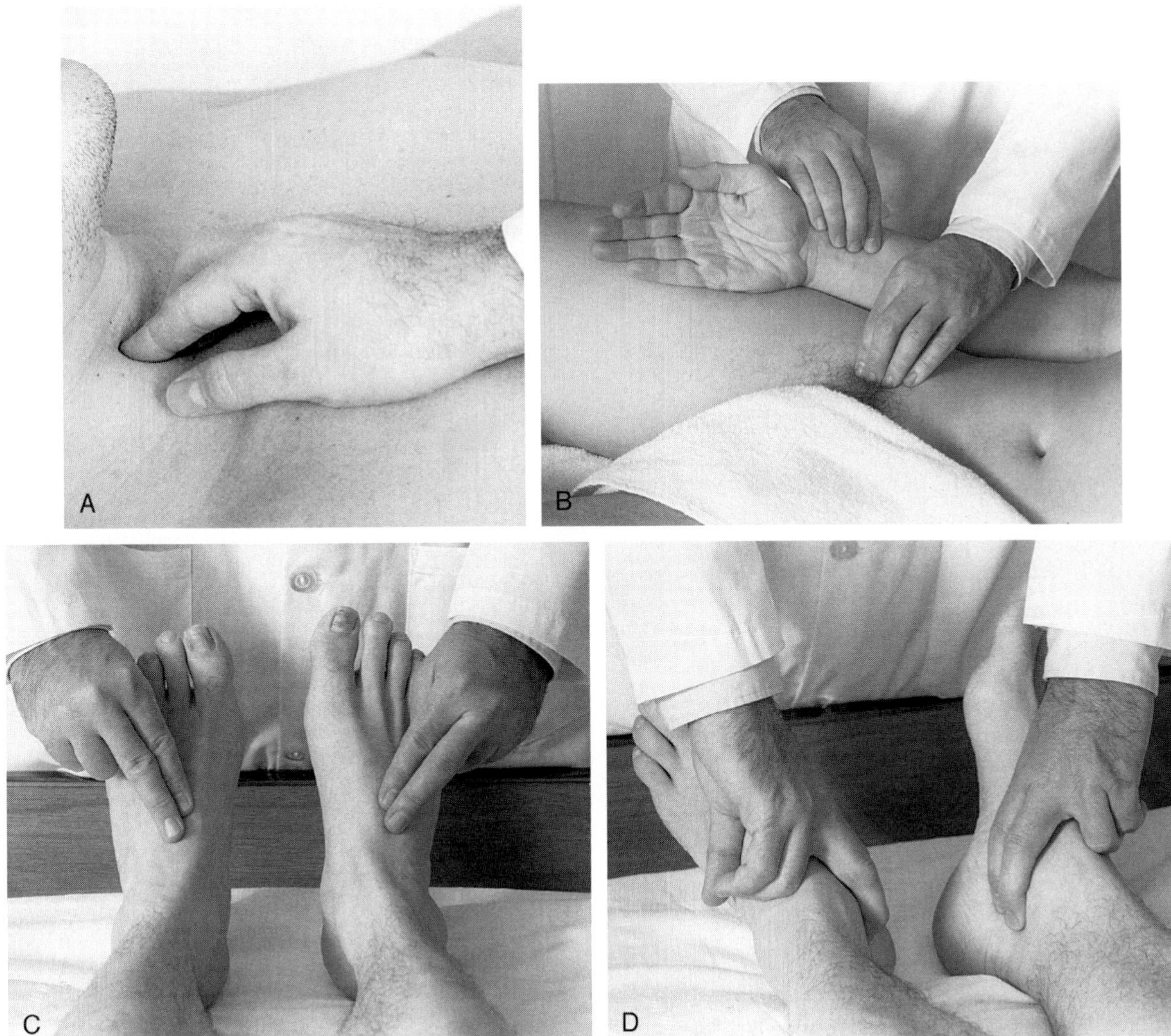

FIGURE 8–5 **A,** Technique for evaluating the carotid artery pulsations. **B,** Technique for timing pulses in the femoral and radial arteries. **C,** Technique for palpation of the dorsalis pedis arteries. **D,** Technique for palpation of the posterior tibial arteries. (From Swartz MH [ed]: Textbook of Physical Diagnosis: History and Examination. 3rd ed. Philadelphia, WB Saunders, 1998, pp 300, 329, and 330.)

rises slightly and then declines gradually throughout diastole. As the pulse wave is transmitted to the periphery, its upstroke becomes steeper, the systolic peak becomes higher, the anacrotic shoulder disappears, and the sharp incisura is replaced by a smoother, later dicrotic notch followed by a dicrotic wave.[26-28] Normally, the height of this dicrotic wave diminishes with age, hypertension, and arteriosclerosis. In the central arterial pulse (central aorta and innominate and carotid arteries), the rapidly transmitted impact of left ventricular ejection results in a peak in early systole, referred to as the *percussion wave;* a second, smaller peak, the *tidal wave,* presumed to represent a reflected wave from the periphery, can often be recorded but is not normally palpable. In older subjects, however, particularly those with increased peripheral resistance, as well as in patients with arteriosclerosis and diabetes, the tidal wave may be somewhat higher than the percussion wave; that is, the pulse reaches a peak in late systole. In peripheral arteries, the pulse wave normally has a single sharp peak.

ABNORMAL PULSES. When peripheral vascular resistance and arterial stiffness are increased, as in patients with hypertension or with the increased arterial stiffness that accompanies normal aging, there is an elevation in pulse wave velocity and the pulse contour has a more rapid upstroke and greater amplitude.[29] Reduced or unequal carotid arterial pulsations occur in patients with carotid atherosclerosis and with diseases of the aortic arch, including aortic dissection, aneurysm, and Takayasu disease (see Chap. 53). The pulses of the upper extremities may be reduced or unequal in a variety of conditions, including supravalvular aortic stenosis, arterial embolus or thrombosis, anomalous origin or aberrant path of the major vessels, and cervical rib or scalenus anticus syndrome. Asymmetry of right and left popliteal pulses is characteristic of iliofemoral obstruction. Weakness or absence of radial, posterior tibial, or dorsalis pedis pulses on one side suggests arterial insufficiency. In cases of coarctation of the aorta, the carotid and brachial pulses are bounding, rise rapidly, and have large volumes, whereas in the lower extremities, the systolic and pulse pressures are reduced, their rate of rise is slow, and there is a late peak. This delay in the femoral arterial pulses can usually be readily detected by simultaneous palpation of the femoral and brachial arterial pulses (see Fig. 8–5B).

In patients with fixed obstruction to left ventricular outflow (valvular aortic stenosis and congenital fibrous subaortic stenosis), the carotid pulse rises slowly (pulsus tardus) (see Fig. 8–6B); the upstroke is frequently characterized by a thrill (the carotid shudder); and the peak is reduced, occurs late in systole, and is sustained. There is a notch on the upstroke of the carotid pulse (anacrotic notch) that is so

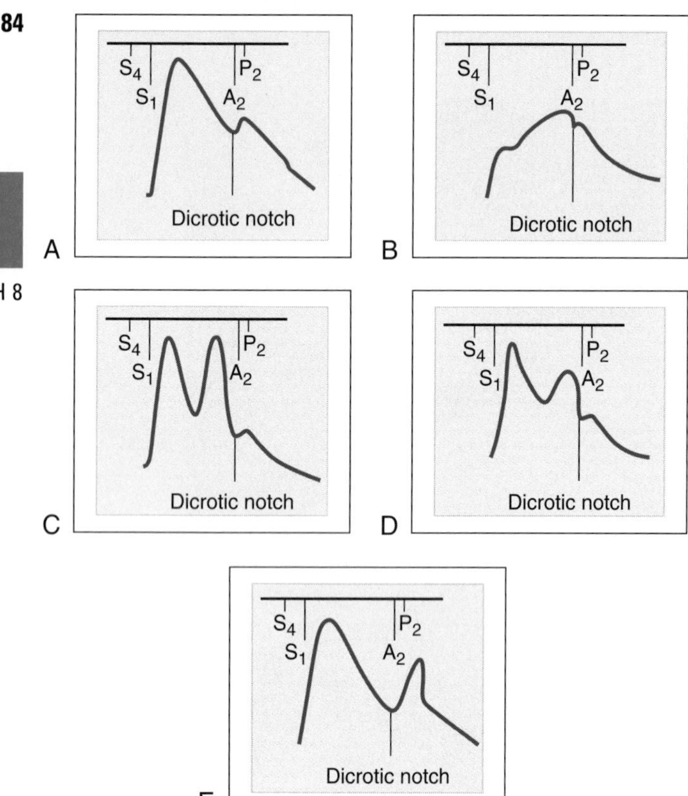

FIGURE 8–6 Schematic diagrams of the configurational changes in carotid pulse and their differential diagnoses. Heart sounds are also illustrated. **A,** Normal. **B,** Anacrotic pulse with a slow initial upstroke. The peak is close to S_2. These features suggest fixed left ventricular outflow obstruction, such as occurs with valvular aortic stenosis. **C,** Pulsus bisferiens with both percussion and tidal waves occurring during systole. This type of carotid pulse contour is most frequently observed in patients with hemodynamically significant aortic regurgitation or combined aortic stenosis and regurgitation with dominant regurgitation. It is rarely observed in patients with mitral valve prolapse or in normal individuals. **D,** Pulsus bisferiens in hypertrophic obstructive cardiomyopathy. It is rarely appreciated at the bedside by palpation. **E,** A dicrotic pulse results from an accentuated dicrotic wave and tends to occur in patients with sepsis, severe heart failure, hypovolemic shock, cardiac tamponade, and aortic valve replacement. A_2 = aortic component of the second heart sound; P_2 = pulmonic component of the second heart sound; S_1 = first heart sound; S_4 = atrial sound. (From Chatterjee K: Bedside evaluation of the heart: The physical examination. *In* Chatterjee K, Parmley W [eds]: Cardiology: An Illustrated Text/Reference. Philadelphia, JB Lippincott, 1991, pp 3.11-3.51; and Braunwald E: The clinical examination. *In* Braunwald E, Goldman L [eds]: Primary Cardiology. 2nd ed. Philadelphia, Elsevier, 2003, pp 36.)

distinct that two separate waves can be palpated in what is termed an *anacrotic pulse. Pulsus parvus* is a pulse of small amplitude, usually because of a reduction of stroke volume. *Pulsus parvus et tardus* refers to a small pulse with a delayed systolic peak, which is characteristic of severe aortic stenosis. This type of pulse is more readily appreciated by palpating the carotid rather than a more peripheral artery. Patients with severe aortic stenosis and heart failure usually exhibit simply a reduced pulse amplitude (i.e., pulsus parvus), and the delay in the upstroke is not readily apparent. However, this delay is readily recorded. In elderly patients with inelastic peripheral arteries, the pulse may rise normally despite the presence of aortic stenosis.

The carotid arterial pulse may be prominent or exaggerated in a patient with any condition in which pulse pressure is increased, including anxiety, the hyperkinetic heart syndrome, anemia, fever, pregnancy, or other high cardiac output states (see Chap. 22), as well as in patients with bradycardia and peripheral arteriosclerosis with reduction in arterial distensibility. In patients with mitral regurgitation or ventricular septal defect, the forward stroke volume (from the left ventricle into the aorta) is usually normal but the fraction ejected during early systole is greater than normal; hence, the arterial pulse is of normal volume (the pulse pressure is normal) but the pulse may rise abnormally rapidly.[30] Exaggerated or bounding arterial pulses may be observed in patients with an elevated stroke volume, with sympathetic hyperactivity, and in patients with a rigid, sclerotic aorta. In patients with aortic regurgitation, there is a very brisk rate of rise with an increased pulse pressure.

AORTIC REGURGITATION. The *Corrigan* or *water-hammer pulse* of aortic regurgitation consists of an abrupt upstroke (percussion wave) followed by rapid collapse later in systole but no dicrotic notch. Corrigan pulse reflects a low resistance in the reservoir into which the left ventricle rapidly discharges an abnormally elevated stroke volume, and it can be exaggerated by raising the patient's arm. In cases of acute aortic regurgitation, the left ventricle may not be significantly dilated, and premature closure of the mitral valve may occur and limit the volume of aortic reflux; therefore, the aortic diastolic pressure may not be very low, the arterial pulse not bounding, and the pulse pressure not widened despite a serious abnormality of valve function (see Chap. 57).

Signs characteristic of severe chronic aortic regurgitation include "pistol shot" sounds heard over the femoral artery when the stethoscope is placed on it (Traube sign); a systolic murmur heard over the femoral artery when the artery is gradually compressed proximally; a diastolic murmur when the artery is compressed distally (Duroziez sign[25]), and Quincke sign (phasic blanching of the nail bed). Of these, Duroziez sign is the most predictive of severe aortic regurgitation. Bounding arterial pulses are also present in patients with patent ductus arteriosus or large arteriovenous fistulas; those in hyperkinetic states such as thyrotoxicosis, pregnancy, fever, and anemia; those in severe bradycardia; and in arteries proximal to coarctation of the aorta. In patients with the Hill sign[25] of aortic regurgitation (or any condition leading to an increased stroke volume or the hyperkinetic circulatory state), the indirectly recorded systolic pressures in the lower extremities exceed that in the arms by more than 20 mm Hg. Other signs of increased pulse pressure include Becker sign (visible pulsations of the retinal arterioles) and Mueller sign (pulsating uvula).

BISFERIENS PULSE. A bisferiens pulse (see Fig. 8–6C) is characterized by two systolic peaks, the percussion and tidal waves, separated by a distinct midsystolic dip; the peaks may be equal, or either one may be larger. This type of pulse is detected most readily by palpation of the carotid and, less commonly, of the brachial arteries. It occurs in conditions in which a large stroke volume is ejected rapidly[31] and is observed most commonly in patients with pure aortic regurgitation or with a combination of aortic regurgitation and stenosis; it may disappear as heart failure supervenes (see Fig 8–6D).[26,31]

A bisferiens pulse also occurs in patients with hypertrophic obstructive cardiomyopathy, but the bifid nature may only be recorded, not palpated; on palpation, there may merely be a rapid upstroke. In these patients, the initial prominent percussion wave is associated with rapid ejection of blood into the aorta during early systole, followed by a rapid decline as obstruction becomes manifest in midsystole and by a tidal (reflected) wave. In some patients with hypertrophic cardiomyopathy with no or little obstruction to left ventricular outflow, the arterial pulse is normal or simply hyperkinetic in the basal state, but obstruction and a bisferiens pulse can be elicited by means of the Valsalva maneuver or inhalation of amyl nitrite. Occasionally, a bisferiens pulse is observed in patients in hyperkinetic circulatory states, and very rarely it occurs in normal individuals.

DICROTIC PULSE. Not to be confused with a bisferiens pulse, in which both peaks occur in systole, is a dicrotic pulse, in which the second peak is in diastole immediately after S_2 (see Fig. 8–6E).[27-29,31-33] The normally small wave that follows aortic valve closure (i.e., the dicrotic notch) is exaggerated and measures more than 50 percent of the pulse pressure on direct pressure recordings and in which the dicrotic notch is low (i.e., near the diastolic pressure). A dicrotic wave may be present in normal hypotensive subjects with reduced peripheral resistance, as occurs in fever, and it may be elicited or exaggerated by inhalation alone or the inhalation of amyl nitrite. Rarely, a dicrotic pulse is noted in healthy adolescents or young adults, but it usually occurs in conditions such as cardiac tamponade,[29] severe heart failure, and hypovolemic shock, in which a low stroke volume is ejected into a soft elastic aorta. In patients with these conditions, the dicrotic pulse is due to a reduction of the systolic wave with preservation of the incisura.

PULSUS ALTERNANS (ALTERNATING STRONG AND WEAK PULSES). Mechanical alternans is a sign of depression of left ventricular function (see Chap. 22).[34,35] Although more readily recognized on sphygmomanometry, when the systolic pressure alternates by more than 20 mm Hg, pulsus alternans can be detected by palpation of a peripheral (femoral or brachial) pulse more frequently than by a more central pulse. Palpation should be carried out with light pressure and with the patient's breath held in mid-expiration to avoid the superimposition of respiratory variation on the amplitude of the pulse. Pulsus alternans is generally accompanied by alternation in the intensity of the Korotkoff sounds and occasionally by alternation in intensity of the heart sounds. Rarely, pulsus alternans is so marked that the weak beat is not perceived at all.[36] Aortic regurgitation, systemic hypertension, and reducing venous return by administration of nitroglycerin or by tilting the patient into the upright position all exaggerate pulsus alternans and assist in its detection. Pulsus alternans, which is frequently precipitated by a premature ventricular contraction, is characterized by a regular rhythm and must be distinguished from pulsus bigeminus, which is usually irregular.

PULSUS BIGEMINUS. A bigeminal rhythm is caused by the occurrence of premature contractions, usually ventricular, after every other beat and results in alternation of the strength of the pulse, which can be confused with pulsus alternans. However, in contrast to the pulsus alternans, in which the rhythm is regular, in pulsus bigeminus the weak beat always follows the shorter interval. In normal persons or in patients with fixed obstruction to left ventricular outflow, the compensatory pause after a premature beat is followed by a stronger-than-normal pulse. In patients with hypertrophic obstructive cardiomyopathy, however, the post-premature ventricular contraction beat is weaker than normal because of increased obstruction to left ventricular outflow (see Chap. 59).[37]

PULSUS PARADOXUS. Pulsus paradoxus is an exaggerated reduction in the strength of the arterial pulse during normal inspiration due to an exaggerated inspiratory fall in systolic pressure (more than 10 mm Hg during quiet breathing) (see Chap. 64). When marked (i.e., an inspiratory reduction of pressure greater than 20 mm Hg), the paradoxical pulse can be detected by simple palpation of the brachial arterial pulse[38]; in severe cases, there is inspiratory disappearance of the pulse. Milder degrees of a paradoxical pulse can be readily detected on sphygmomanometry: the cuff is inflated to suprasystolic levels and is deflated slowly at a rate of about 2 mm Hg per heartbeat; the peak systolic pressure during exhalation is noted.[39,40] The cuff is then deflated even more slowly, and the pressure is again noted when Korotkoff sounds become audible throughout the respiratory cycle. Normally, the difference between the two pressures should not exceed 10 mm Hg during quiet respiration. (Pulsus alternans can also be detected by this maneuver by noting whether peak systolic pressure or the intensity of the Korotkoff sounds alternates when the breath is held.)

Pulsus paradoxus represents an exaggeration of the normal decline in systolic arterial pressure with inspiration. It results from the reduced left ventricular stroke volume and the transmission of negative intrathoracic pressure to the aorta. It is a frequent, indeed characteristic, finding in patients with cardiac tamponade,[41,42] occurs less frequently (in about half) in patients with chronic constrictive pericarditis,[19] and is also observed in patients with emphysema and bronchial asthma (who have wide respiratory swings of intrapleural pressure),[39] as well as in patients with hypovolemic shock, pulmonary embolus, pregnancy, and extreme obesity. Aortic regurgitation tends to prevent the development of pulsus paradoxus despite the presence of cardiac tamponade. Reversed pulsus paradoxus (an inspiratory rise in arterial pressure) may occur in hypertrophic obstructive cardiomyopathy.

THE ARTERIAL PULSE IN VASCULAR DISEASE (see Chap. 54). Examination of the arterial pulses is of critical importance in the diagnosis of extracardiac obstructive arterial disease. Systematic bilateral palpation of the common carotid, brachial, radial, femoral, popliteal, dorsalis pedis,[42] and posterior tibial vessels (see Fig. 8–5C and D), as well as palpation of the abdominal aorta (both above and below the umbilicus), should be part of every examination in patients suspected of having ischemic heart disease.[43] A normal aorta is often palpable above the umbilicus, but a palpable aorta below the umbilicus suggests the presence of an aneurysm of the abdominal aorta. To diminish cold-induced vasoconstriction, peripheral pulses should be palpated after the patient has been in a warm room for at least 20 minutes. Absent or weak peripheral pulses usually signify obstruction. However, the dorsalis pedis and posterior tibial arteries may be absent in approximately 2 percent of normal persons because they pursue an aberrant course.

Arterial bruits should be sought at specific anatomical sites. When the lumen diameter is reduced by approximately 50 percent, a soft short systolic bruit is heard; as the obstruction becomes more severe, the bruit becomes high pitched, louder, and longer. With approximately 80 percent diameter reduction, the murmur spills into early diastole, but it disappears with more severe stenosis or complete occlusion. Arterial bruits are augmented by elevation of the cardiac output (e.g., as occurs in patients with anemia), by poor development of collaterals, and by increased arterial outflow (as occurs with regional exercise).

The Cardiac Examination

Inspection

The cardiac examination proper should commence with inspection of the chest, which can usually best be accomplished with the examiner standing at the side or foot of the bed or examining table.[4] Respirations—their frequency, regularity, and depth—as well as the relative effort required during inspiration and exhalation, should be noted. Simultaneously, one should search for cutaneous abnormalities, such as spider nevi (seen in patients with hepatic cirrhosis and Osler-Weber-Rendu disease). Dilation of veins on the anterior chest wall with caudal flow suggests obstruction of the superior vena cava, whereas cranial flow occurs in patients with obstruction of the inferior vena cava. Precordial prominence is most striking if cardiac enlargement developed before puberty, but it may also be present, although to a lesser extent, in patients in whom cardiomegaly developed in adult life, after the period of thoracic growth.

A heavy muscular thorax, contrasting to less developed lower extremities, can occur in patients with coarctation of the aorta, in which collateral arteries may be visible in the axillae and along the lateral chest wall. The upper portion of the thorax exhibits symmetrical bulging in children with stiff lungs in whom the inspiratory effort is increased. A "shield chest" is a broad chest in which the angle between the manubrium and the body of the sternum is greater than normal, and it is associated with widely separated nipples; shield chest is frequently observed in patients with Turner and Noonan syndromes (see Chap. 56). Careful note should be made of other deformities of the thoracic cage, such as kyphoscoliosis, which may be responsible for cor pulmonale (see Chap. 67); and ankylosing spondylitis, sometimes associated with aortic regurgitation (see Chap. 82).

Pectus excavatum,[15,16] a condition in which the sternum is displaced posteriorly, is commonly observed in patients with Marfan syndrome, homocystinuria, Ehlers-Danlos syndrome, and Hunter-Hurler syndrome and in a small fraction of patients with mitral valve prolapse. This thoracic deformity rarely compresses the heart or elevates the systemic and pulmonary venous pressures, and the signs of heart disease are more often apparent rather than real.[44] Displacement of the heart into the left thorax, prominence of the pulmonary artery, and a parasternal midsystolic murmur, all key features of this deformity, may falsely suggest the presence of organic heart disease. Lack of normal thoracic kyphosis (i.e., the straight back syndrome) is often associated with expiratory splitting of S_2, a parasternal midsystolic murmur, and prominence of the pulmonary artery on radiography.

CARDIOVASCULAR PULSATIONS. Cardiovascular pulsations should be looked for on the entire chest but specifically in the regions of the cardiac apex, the left parasternal region, and the third left and second

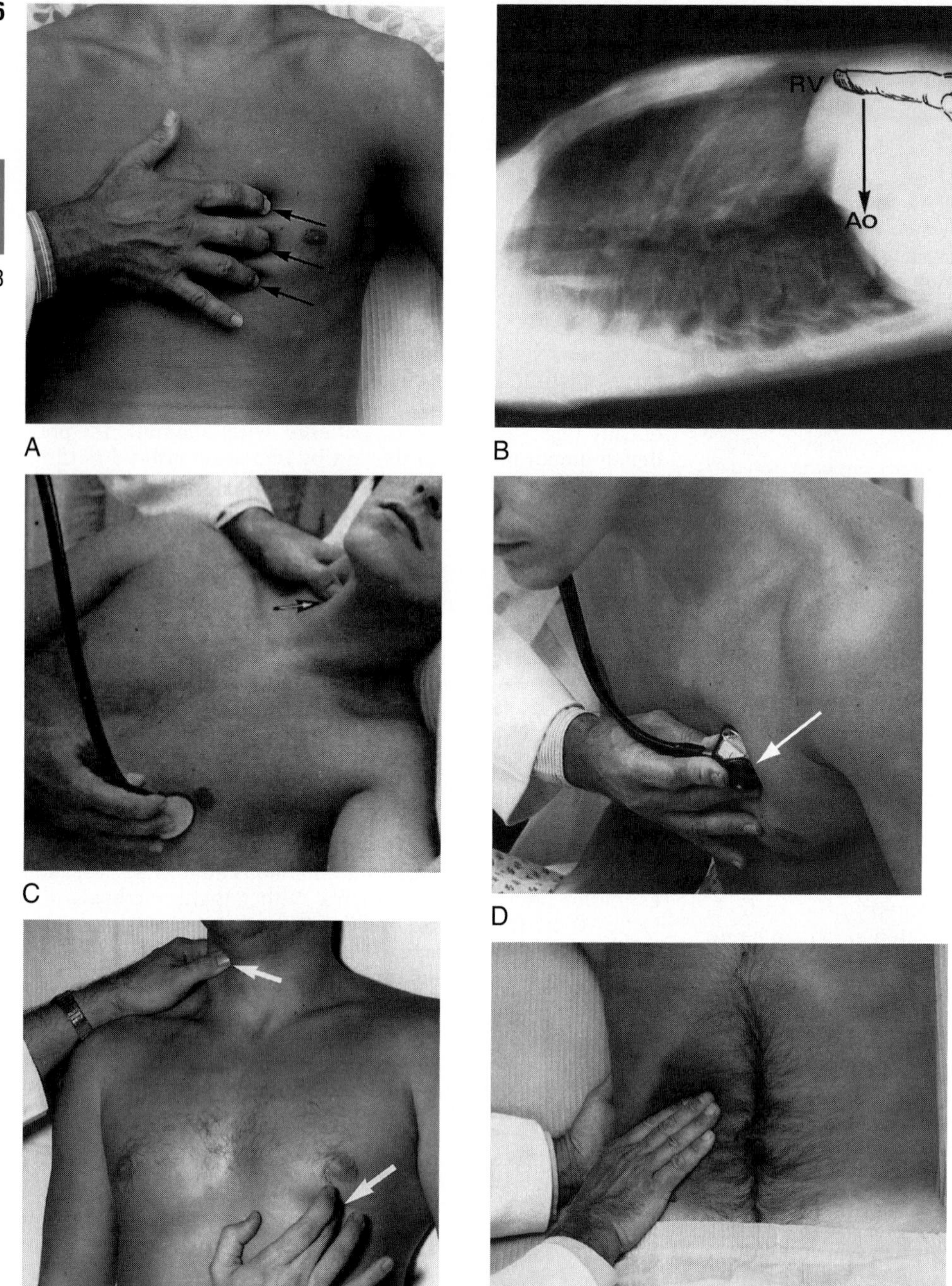

FIGURE 8–7 **A,** Palpation of the anterior wall of the right ventricle by applying the tips of three fingers in the third, fourth, and fifth interspaces, and left sternal edge (arrows), during full held exhalation. Patient is supine with the trunk elevated 30 degrees. **B,** Subxiphoid palpation of the inferior wall of the right ventricle (RV) with the relative position of the abdominal aorta (Ao) shown by the arrow. **C,** The bell of the stethoscope is applied to the cardiac apex while the patient lies in a partial left lateral decubitus position. The thumb of the examiner's free left hand is used to palpate the carotid artery for timing purposes. **D,** The soft, high-frequency early diastolic murmur of aortic regurgitation or pulmonary hypertensive regurgitation is best elicited by applying the stethoscopic diaphragm very firmly to the mid-left sternal edge. The patient leans forward with breath held in full exhalation. **E,** Palpation of the left ventricular impulse with a fingertip (arrow). The patient's trunk is 30 degrees above the horizontal. The examiner's right thumb palpates the carotid pulse for timing purposes. **F,** Palpation of the liver. The patient is supine with knees flexed to relax the abdomen. The flat of the examiner's right hand is placed on the right upper quadrant just below the expected inferior margin of the liver; the left hand is applied diametrically opposite. (From Perloff JK: Physical Examination of the Heart and Circulation. 3rd ed. Philadelphia, WB Saunders, 2000.)

right intercostal spaces. Prominent pulsations in these areas suggest enlargement of the left ventricle, right ventricle, pulmonary artery, and aorta, respectively. A thrusting apex exceeding 2 cm in diameter suggests left ventricular enlargement; systolic retraction of the apex may be visible in cases of constrictive pericarditis. Normally, cardiac pulsations are not visible lateral to the midclavicular line; when present there, they signify cardiac enlargement unless there is thoracic deformity or congenital absence of the pericardium. Shaking of the entire precordium with each heartbeat can occur in patients with severe valvular regurgitation, large left-to-right shunts, especially patent ductus arteriosus, complete AV block, hypertrophic obstructive cardiomyopathy, and various hyperkinetic states. Aortic aneurysms may produce visible pulsations of one of the sternoclavicular joints of the right anterior thoracic wall.

Palpation

Pulsations of the heart and great arteries that are transmitted to the chest wall are best appreciated when the examiner is positioned on the right side of a supine patient. To palpate the movements of the heart and great arteries, the examiner should use the fingertips or the area just proximal thereto. Precordial movements should be timed with the simultaneously palpated carotid pulse or auscultated heart sounds.[45] The examination should be carried out with the chest completely exposed and elevated to 30 degrees, with the patient both supine and in the partial left lateral decubitus positions (Fig. 8–7).[2] Rotating the patient into the left lateral decubitus position with the left arm elevated over the head causes the heart to move laterally and increases the palpability of both normal and pathological thrusts of the left ventricle. The subxiphoid region, which allows palpation of the right ventricle, should be examined with the tip of the index finger during held inspiration. Obese, muscular, emphysematous, and elderly persons may have weak or undetectable cardiac pulsations in the absence of cardiac abnormality, and thoracic deformities (e.g., kyphoscoliosis, pectus excavatum) can alter the pulsations transmitted to the chest wall. In the course of cardiac palpation, precordial tenderness may be detected; this finding can result from costochondritis (Tietze syndrome) and can be an important indication that chest pain is not due to myocardial ischemia.

LEFT VENTRICLE. The left ventricular impulse, also referred to as the cardiac impulse, the apex beat, and the apical thrust, is normally produced by left ventricular contraction and is the lowest and most lateral point on the chest at which the cardiac impulse can be appreciated and is normally above the anatomical apex. Normally, the left ventricular impulse is medial and superior to the intersection of the left midclavicular line and the fifth intercostal space and is palpable as a single, brief outward motion. Although it may not be palpable in the supine position in as many as half of all normal subjects older than 50 years of age, the left ventricular impulse can usually be felt in the left lateral decubitus position. Displacement of the apex beat lateral to the midclavicular line or more than 10 cm lateral to the midsternal line is a sensitive but not specific indicator of left ventricular enlargement. However, when the patient is in the left lateral decubitus position, a palpable apical impulse that has a diameter of more than 3 cm is an accurate sign of left ventricular enlargement.[46] Thoracic deformities—particularly scoliosis, straight back, and pectus excavatum—can result in the lateral displacement of a normal-sized heart.

APEX CARDIOGRAM. This recording reflects the movement of the chest wall and represents the pulsation of the entire left ventricle. Its contour differs from what is perceived on palpation of the apex.

SYSTOLIC MOTION

During isovolumetric contraction, the heart normally rotates counterclockwise (as one faces the patient), and the lower anterior portion of the left ventricle strikes the anterior chest wall, causing a brief outward motion followed by medial retraction of the adjacent chest wall during ejection. The peak outward motion of the left ventricular impulse occurs simultaneously with, or just after, aortic valve opening; then the left ventricular apex moves inward. In asthenic persons, in patients with mild left ventricular enlargement, and in subjects with a normal left ventricle but an augmented stroke volume, as occurs in anxiety and other hyperkinetic states, and in cases of mitral or aortic regurgitation, the cardiac impulse may be overactive but with a normal contour; that is, the outward thrust during systole is exaggerated in amplitude but is not sustained during ejection.

HYPERTROPHY AND DILATATION. With moderate or severe left ventricular concentric hypertrophy, the outward systolic thrust persists throughout ejection, often lasting up to the second heart sound,[47] and this motion is accompanied by retraction of the left parasternal region. The left ventricular heave or lift, which is more prominent in patients with concentric hypertrophy than in those with left ventricular dilatation without volume overload, is characterized by a sustained outward movement of an area that is larger than the normal apex; that is, it is more than 2 to 3 cm in diameter. In patients with left ventricular enlargement, the systolic impulse is displaced laterally and downward into the sixth or seventh interspaces. In patients with volume overload and/or sympathetic stimulation, the left ventricular impulse is hyperkinetic; that is, it is brisker and larger than normal.

OTHER CONDITIONS. Left ventricular aneurysm produces a larger-than-normal area of pulsation of the left ventricular apex. Alternatively, it may produce a sustained systolic bulge several centimeters superior to the left ventricular impulse, sometimes termed an *ectopic impulse*.

A double systolic outward thrust of the left ventricle is characteristic of patients with hypertrophic obstructive cardiomyopathy (see Chap. 54), who may also often exhibit a typical presystolic cardiac expansion, thus resulting in three separate outward movements of the chest wall during each cardiac cycle.[48] Constrictive pericarditis is characterized by systolic retraction of the chest, particularly of the ribs in the left axilla (Broadbent sign).

DIASTOLIC MOTION

The outward motion of the apex characteristic of rapid left ventricular diastolic filling is most readily palpated with the patient in the left lateral decubitus position and in full exhalation. The outward motion is accentuated when the inflow of blood into the left ventricle is accelerated. This occurs in cases of mitral regurgitation, when the volume of the left ventricle is increased or when its function is impaired.[4] This motion is the mechanical equivalent of and occurs simultaneously with a third heart sound (S_3).

PRESYSTOLIC EXPANSION. When the atrial contribution to ventricular filling is augmented, as occurs in patients with reduced left ventricular compliance associated with concentric left ventricular hypertrophy, myocardial ischemia, and myocardial fibrosis, a presystolic pulsation (usually accompanying a fourth heart sound [S_4]) is palpable, resulting in a double outward movement of the left ventricular impulse. This presystolic expansion is most readily discernible during exhalation, when the patient is in the left lateral decubitus position, and it can be confirmed by detecting the motion of the stethoscope placed over the left ventricular impulse or by observing the motion of an X mark over the left ventricular impulse. Presystolic expansion of the left ventricle can be enhanced by sustained handgrip. In patients with ischemic heart disease, presystolic pulsation is usually associated with a reduction in left ventricular compliance.

RIGHT VENTRICLE

Except in the first few months of life, the right ventricle normally is not palpable. A palpable anterior systolic movement (replacing systolic retraction) in the left parasternal region, best felt by the proximal palm or fingertips and with the patient supine, usually represents right ventricular enlargement or hypertrophy.[4] In patients with pulmonary emphysema, even an enlarged right ventricle is not readily palpable at the left sternal edge but is better appreciated in the subxiphoid region. Exaggerated motion of the entire parasternal area (i.e., a hyperdynamic impulse with normal contour) usually reflects increased right ventricular stroke volume, as occurs in patients with atrial septal defect or tricuspid regurgitation.

PULMONARY ARTERY

Pulmonary hypertension and increased pulmonary blood flow frequently produce a prominent systolic pulsation of the pulmonary trunk in the second intercostal space just to the left of the sternum. This pulsation is often associated with a prominent left parasternal impulse, reflecting right ventricular enlargement, or with hypertrophy and a palpable shock synchronous with the second heart sound, reflecting forceful closure of the pulmonic valve.

LEFT ATRIUM

An enlarged left atrium or a large posterior left ventricular aneurysm can make right ventricular pulsations more prominent by displacing the right ventricle anteriorly against the left parasternal area; in patients with severe mitral regurgitation, an expanding left atrium may be responsible for marked left parasternal movement, even in the absence of right ventricular hypertrophy. Movement imparted by the systolic expansion of the left atrium can be appreciated by placing the index finger of one hand at the left ventricular apex and the index finger of the other in the left parasternal region in the third intercostal space.

AORTA. Enlargement or aneurysm of the ascending aorta or aortic arch may cause visible or palpable systolic pulsations of the right or left sternoclavicular joint and may also cause a systolic impulse in the suprasternal notch or the first or second right intercostal space.[4]

THRILLS

The flat of the hand or the fingertips usually best appreciate thrills, which are vibratory sensations that are palpable manifestations of loud, harsh murmurs having low- to medium-frequency components. Because the vibrations must be quite intense before they are felt, far more information can be obtained from the auscultatory than from the palpatory features of heart murmurs. High-pitched murmurs such as those produced by valvular regurgitation, even when loud, are not usually associated with thrills.

PERCUSSION

Palpation is far more helpful than is percussion in determining cardiac size. However, in the absence of an apical beat, as occurs in patients with pericardial effusion or in some patients with dilated cardiomyopathy, heart failure, and marked displacement of a hypokinetic apical beat, the left border of the heart can be approximately outlined by means of percussion. Also, percussion of dullness in the right lower parasternal area may, in some instances, aid in the detection of a greatly enlarged right atrium. Percussion aids materially in determining visceral situs, that is, in ascertaining the side on which the heart, stomach, and liver are located.

Cardiac Auscultation

Principles and Technique

The modern binaural stethoscope is a well-crafted, airtight instrument with earpieces selected for comfort, with metal tubing joined to single flexible 12-inch-long, thick-walled rubber tubing (internal diameter of 1/8 inch), and with dual chest pieces—diaphragm for high frequencies, bell for low or lower frequencies—designed so that the examiner can readily switch from one chest piece to the other.[49,50] When the bell is applied with just enough pressure to form a skin seal, low frequencies are accentuated; when the bell is pressed firmly, the stretched skin becomes a diaphragm, damping low frequencies. Variable pressure with the bell provides a range of frequencies from low to medium.

Cardiac auscultation is best accomplished in a quiet room with the patient comfortable and the chest fully exposed. The topographical areas for auscultation (Fig. 8–8) are best designated by descriptive terms: cardiac apex, left and right sternal borders interspace by interspace, and subxiphoid. Auscultation should begin at the cardiac apex (best identified in the left lateral decubitus) and contiguous lower left sternal edge (inflow), proceeding interspace by interspace up the left sternal border to the left base and then to the right base (outflow). In addition, the stethoscope should be applied regularly to the axillae, the back, the anterior chest on the opposite side, and above the clavicles. In patients with increased anteroposterior chest dimensions (emphysema), auscultation is often best achieved by applying the stethoscope in the epigastrium (subxiphoid).

During auscultation, the examiner is generally on the patient's right; three positions are routinely employed: left lateral decubitus (assuming left thoracic heart), supine, and sitting. One should begin auscultation by applying the stethoscope to the cardiac apex with the patient in the left lateral decubitus position (see Fig. 8-7C). Identification of S_1 can usually be established by simultaneous palpation of the carotid artery with the thumb of the free left hand. Once the S_1 is identified, analysis then proceeds by systematic, methodical, sequential attention to early, middle, and late systole; S_2; then early, middle, and late diastole (presystole); and returning to S_1. When auscultation at the apex has been completed, the patient is turned into the supine position. Each topographical area—lower to upper left sternal edge interspace by interspace and then the right base—is interrogated using the same systematic sequence of analysis (see Fig. 8-7D).

Assessment of pitch or frequency ranging from low to moderately high can be achieved by variable pressure of the stethoscopic bell, whereas for high frequencies the diaphragm should be employed. It is practical to begin by using the stethoscopic bell with varying pressure at the apex and lower left sternal edge, changing to the diaphragm when the base is reached. Low frequencies are best heard by applying the bell just lightly enough to achieve a skin seal. High-frequency events are best elicited with firm pressure of the diaphragm, often with the patient sitting, leaning forward in full, held exhalation.

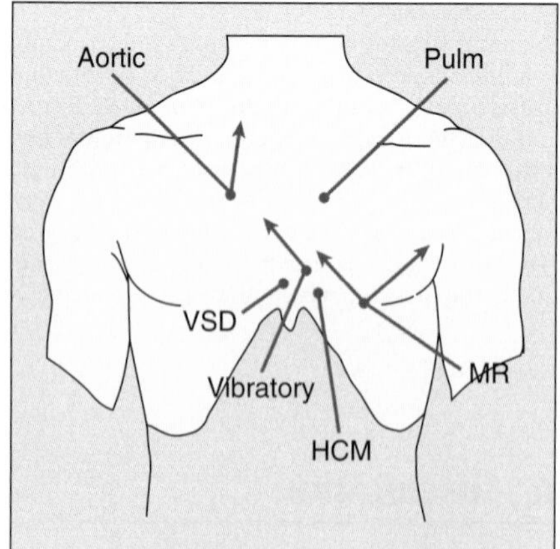

FIGURE 8–8 Maximal intensity and radiation of six isolated systolic murmurs. HCM = hypertrophic cardiomyopathy; MR = mitral regurgitation; Pulm = pulmonary; VSD = ventricular septal defect. (From Barlow JB: Perspectives on the Mitral Valve. Philadelphia, FA Davis, 1987, p 140.)

Heart Sounds

Heart sounds are relatively brief, discrete auditory vibrations that can be characterized by intensity (loudness), frequency (pitch), and quality (timbre). S_1 identifies the onset of ventricular systole, and S_2 identifies the onset of diastole. These two auscultatory events establish a framework within which other heart sounds and murmurs can be placed and timed.[4,48,50]

The basic heart sounds are the S_1, S_2, S_3, and S_4 (Fig. 8–9). Each of these events can be normal or abnormal. Other heart sounds are, with few exceptions, abnormal or iatrogenic (e.g., prosthetic valve sounds, pacemaker sounds). Heart sounds within the framework established by S_1 and S_2 are designated as "early systolic, midsystolic, late systolic," and "early diastolic, mid-diastolic, late diastolic (presystolic)."[2]

For example, an early systolic sound might be an ejection sound (aortic or pulmonary) or an aortic prosthetic sound. Midsystolic and late systolic sounds are typified by the click or clicks of mitral valve prolapse but occasionally are "remnants" of pericardial rubs. Early diastolic sounds are represented by opening snaps (usually mitral), an early S_3 (constrictive pericarditis, less commonly mitral regurgitation), the opening of a mechanical inflow prosthesis, or the abrupt seating of a pedunculated mobile atrial myxoma ("tumor plop"). Mid-diastolic sounds are generally S_3 or summation

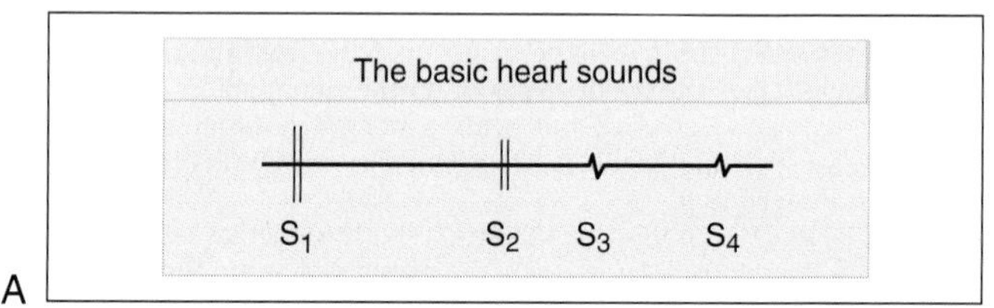

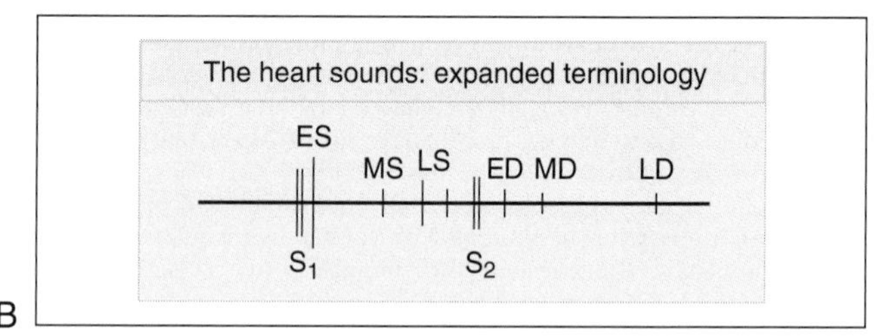

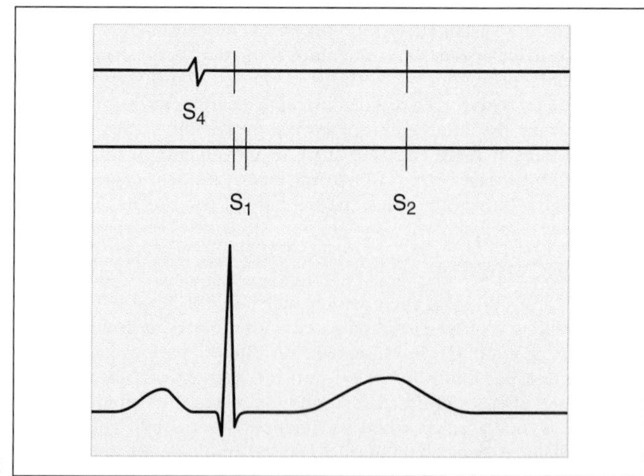

FIGURE 8–9 **A,** The basic heart sounds consist of the first heart sound (S_1), the second heart sound (S_2), the third heart sound (S_3), and the fourth heart sound (S_4). **B,** Heart sounds within the auscultatory framework established by S_1 and S_2. The additional heart sounds are designated as early systolic (ES), midsystolic (MS), late systolic (LS), early diastolic (ED), mid-diastolic (MD), and late diastolic (LD) or presystolic. **C,** Upper tracing illustrates a low-frequency S_4, and the lower tracing illustrates a split S_1, the two components of which are of the same quality.

TABLE 8–2 Factors Affecting the Intensity of S_1
Loud S_1
Short PR interval (<160 msec)
Tachycardia or hyperkinetic states
"Stiff" left ventricle
Mitral stenosis
Left atrial myxoma
Holosystolic mitral valve prolapse
Soft S_1
Long PR interval (>200 msec)
Depressed left ventricular contractility
Premature closure of mitral valve (e.g., acute aortic regurgiation)
Left bundle branch block
Extracardiac factors (e.g., obesity, muscular chest, chronic obstructive pulmonary disease, large breasts)
Flail mitral leaflet

From Abrams J: Synopsis of Cardiac Physical Diagnosis. 2nd ed. Boston, Butterworth Heinemann, 2001, p 60.

sounds (synchronous occurrence of S_3 and S_4). Late diastolic or presystolic sounds are almost always S_4 sounds, rarely pacemaker sounds.

First Heart Sound

S_1 consists of two components (see Fig. 8–9C). The initial component is most prominent at the cardiac apex when the apex is occupied by the left ventricle. The second component, if present, is normally confined to the lower left sternal edge, is less commonly heard at the apex, and is seldom heard at the base. The first major component is associated with closure of the mitral valve and coincides with abrupt arrest of leaflet motion when the cusps, especially the larger and more mobile anterior mitral cusp, reach their fully closed positions. The origin of the second component of S_1 has been debated but is generally assigned to closure of the tricuspid valve based on an analogous line of reasoning.[4,48-51]

Opening of the semilunar valves with ejection of blood into the aortic root or pulmonary trunk usually produces no audible sound in the normal heart. In cases of complete right bundle branch block, S_1 is widely split as a result of delay of the tricuspid component.[52] In cases of complete left bundle branch block, S_1 is single as a result of delay of the mitral component.[53]

When S_1 is split, its first component is normally louder. The softer second component is confined to the lower left sternal edge but may also be heard at the apex. Only the louder first component is heard at the base. The intensity of the S_1, particularly its first major audible component, depends chiefly on the position of the bellies of the mitral leaflets, especially the anterior leaflet, at the time the left ventricle begins to contract. S_1 is therefore loudest when the onset of left ventricular systole finds the mitral leaflets maximally recessed into the left ventricular cavity, as in the presence of a rapid heart rate, a short PR interval (Table 8-2),[54] short cycle lengths in atrial fibrillation, or mitral stenosis with a mobile anterior leaflet. When this mobility is lost, the intensity of S_1 decreases.

Early Systolic Sounds

Aortic or pulmonary ejection sounds are the most common early systolic sounds (Table 8–3).[55] *Ejection sound* is preferred to the term *ejection click*, with the latter designation best reserved for the midsystolic to late systolic clicks of mitral valve prolapse (see Chap. 57). Ejection sounds coincide with the fully opened position of the relevant semilunar valve, as in congenital aortic valve stenosis (Fig. 8–10), bicuspid aortic valve in the left side of the heart, or pulmonary valve stenosis in the right side of the heart.[4,48,50] Ejection sounds are relatively high frequency events and, depending on intensity, have a pitch similar to that of S_1. An ejection

TABLE 8–3 Conditions Associated with Ejection Sound or Click
Aortic
Congenital valvular aortic stenosis
Bicuspid aortic valve
Aortic regurgitation
Aortic aneurysm
Aortic root dilatation
Systemic hypertension
Severe tetralogy of Fallot
Pulmonic
Pulmonary valve stenosis
Idiopathic dilatation of the pulmonary artery
Atrial septal defect
Chronic pulmonary hypertension
Tetralogy of Fallot (with pulmonic valve stenosis)
Pseudo-ejection sound
Prominent splitting of S_1
Increased T_1 (Ebstein's anomaly; atrial septal defect)
Hypertrophic cardiomyopathy
Early nonejection click of holosystolic mitral valve prolapse
High-pitched S_4 (S_1 confused for ejection sound)

From Abrams J: Synopsis of Cardiac Physical Diagnosis. 2nd ed. Boston, Butterworth Heinemann, 2001, p 100.

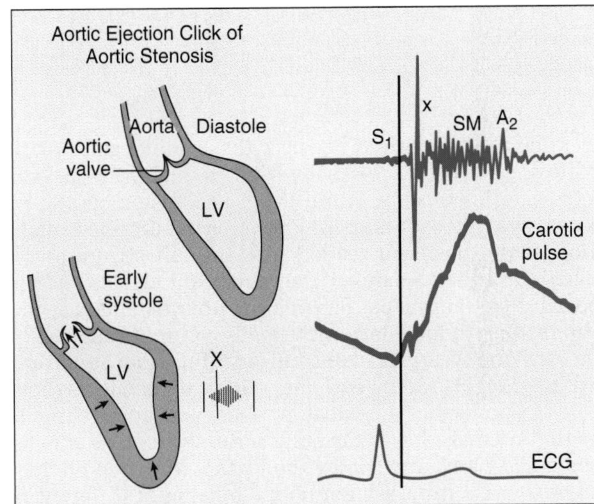

FIGURE 8–10 Ejection click associated with aortic stenosis due to a congenitally bicuspid valve. Note the high-frequency, high-amplitude sound that follows S_1 and is coincident with the onset of ejection into the aorta. The aortic ejection sound is formed by sudden cessation of the opening motion of the abnormal valve leaflets (doming). Note also the delayed carotid upstroke and long systolic murmur. (From Abrams J: Synopsis of Cardiac Physical Diagnosis. 2nd ed. Boston, Butterworth Heinemann, 2001, p 135.)

sound originating in the aortic valve (congenital aortic stenosis or bicuspid aortic valve) or in the pulmonary valve (congenital pulmonary valve stenosis) indicates that the valve is mobile because the ejection sound is caused by abrupt cephalad doming.[56] Less certain is the origin of an ejection sound within a dilated arterial trunk distal to a normal semilunar valve (Fig. 8–11A). Origin of the sound is assigned either to opening movement of the leaflets that resonate in the arterial trunk or to the wall of the dilated great artery. Aortic ejection sounds do not vary with respiration.

Midsystolic to Late Systolic Sounds

The most common midsystolic to late systolic sounds are associated with mitral valve prolapse (see Chap. 57).[4,57] The

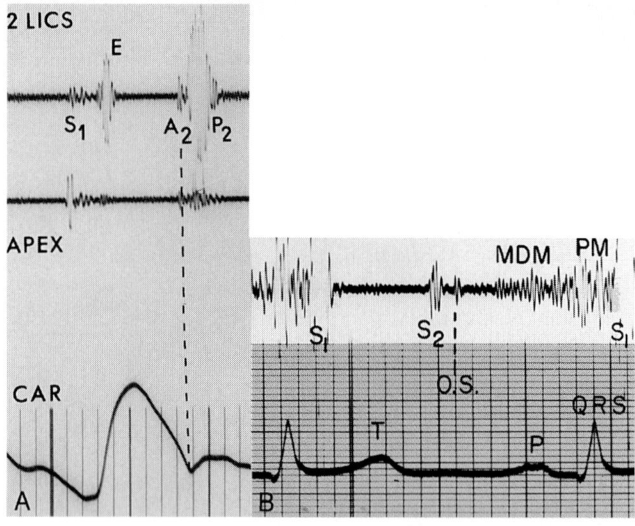

FIGURE 8–11 **A,** Tracings from a 32-year-old woman with an ostium secundum atrial septal defect, pulmonary hypertension, and a small right-to-left shunt. In the second left intercostal space (2 LICS), the first heart sound is followed by a prominent pulmonary ejection sound (E). The second sound remains split. The pulmonic component (P_2) is very loud and is transmitted to the apex. CAR = carotid pulse. **B,** Phonocardiogram recorded in the left lateral decubitus position over the left ventricular impulse in a patient with pure rheumatic mitral stenosis. The first heart sound (S_1) is loud. The second heart sound (S_2) is followed by an opening snap (OS). There is a mid-diastolic murmur (MDM). The prominent presystolic murmur (PM) goes up to the subsequent loud S_1.

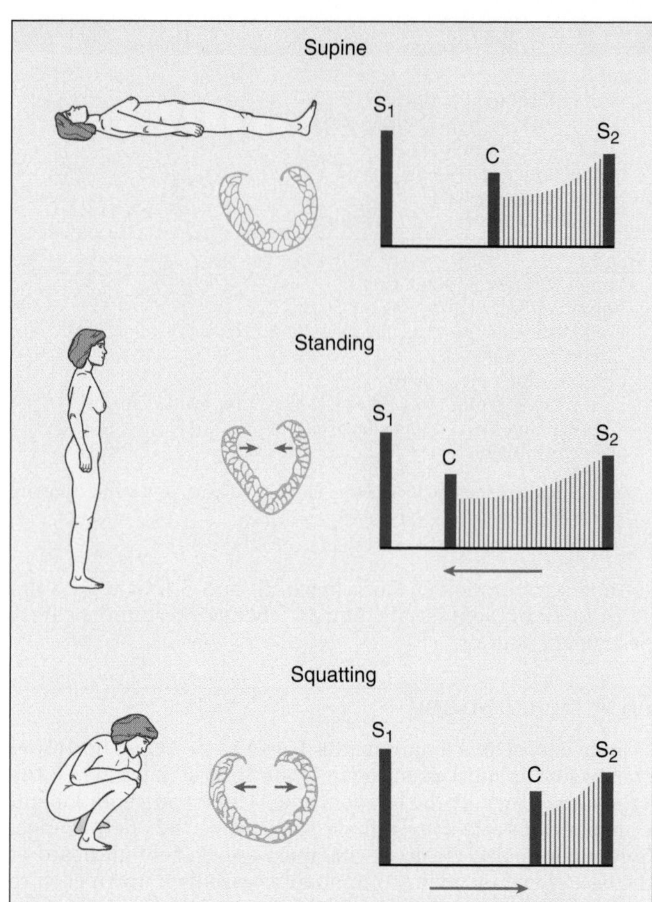

FIGURE 8–12 A midsystolic nonejection sound (C) occurs during mitral valve prolapse and is followed by a late systolic murmur that crescendos to the second heart sound (S_2). Standing decreases venous return; the heart becomes smaller; C moves closer to the first heart sound (S_1) and the mitral regurgitant murmur has an earlier onset. With prompt squatting, venous return increases; the heart becomes larger; C moves toward S_2 and the duration of the murmur shortens. (From Shaver JA, Leonard JJ, Leon DF: Examination of the Heart. Part IV: Auscultation of the Heart. Dallas, American Heart Association, 1990, p 13. Copyright 1990, American Heart Association.)

term *click* is appropriate because these midsystolic to late systolic sounds are of relatively high frequency. Midsystolic to late systolic clicks of mitral valve prolapse coincide with maximal systolic excursion of a prolapsed anterior leaflet (or scallop of the posterior leaflet) into the left atrium and are ascribed to sudden tensing of the redundant leaflets and elongated chordae tendineae. Physical or pharmacological interventions that reduce left ventricular volume, such as the Valsalva maneuver, or a change in position from squatting to standing (Fig. 8–12) causes the clicks to occur earlier in systole.[57] Conversely, physical or pharmacological interventions that increase left ventricular volume, such as squatting or sustained hand grip, delay the clicks. Multiple clicks are thought to arise from asynchronous tensing of different portions of redundant mitral leaflets, especially the triscalloped posterior leaflet.

Second Heart Sound (Table 8–4)

S_2, like S_1, has two components. The first component of the second heart sound is designated "aortic" (A_2) and the second "pulmonic" (P_2) (Fig. 8–13).[58,59] Each component coincides with the incisura of its great arterial pressure pulse. Inspiratory splitting of S_2 is due chiefly to a delay in P_2, less to earlier timing of A_2.[60] During inspiration, the pulmonary arterial incisura moves away from the descending limb of the right ventricular pressure pulse because of an inspiratory increase in capacitance of the pulmonary vascular bed, delaying P_2.[61] Exhalation has the opposite effect. The earlier inspiratory timing of A_2 is attributed to a transient reduction in left ventricular volume coupled with unchanged impedance (capacitance) in the systemic vascular bed. Normal respiratory variations in the timing of S_2 are therefore ascribed principally to the variations in impedance characteristics (capacitance) of the pulmonary vascular bed and secondarily to an inspiratory increase in right ventricular volume as originally proposed. When an increase in capacitance of the pulmonary bed is lost because of a rise in pulmonary vascular resistance, inspiratory splitting of S_2 narrows and, if present at all, reflects an increase in right ventricular ejection time and/or earlier timing of A_2.

The frequency compositions of the aortic and pulmonary components of S_2 are similar, but their normal amplitudes differ appreciably, the aortic component being the louder, reflecting the differences in systemic (aortic) and pulmonary arterial closing pressures. Splitting of S_2 is most readily identified in the second left intercostal space, because the softer P_2 is normally confined to that site, whereas the louder A_2 is heard at the base, sternal edge, and apex.[4,58]

ABNORMAL SPLITTING OF THE SECOND HEART SOUND (Fig. 8–14). Three general categories of abnormal splitting are recognized: (1) persistently single, (2) persistently split (fixed or nonfixed), and (3) paradoxically split (reversed). When S_2 remains single throughout the respiratory cycle, one component is absent or the two components are persistently synchronous. The most common cause of a single S_2 is inaudibility of the P_2 in older adults with increased anteroposterior chest dimensions. In the setting of congenital heart disease, a single S_2 due to absence of the pulmonary component is a feature of pulmonary atresia, severe pulmonary valve stenosis, dysplastic pulmonary valve, or complete transposition of the great arteries. Conversely, a single S_2 due to inaudibility of the A_2 occurs when the aortic

TABLE 8–4 Causes of Splitting of the Second Heart Sound

Normal Splitting	Reversed Splitting
Delayed pulmonic closure	**Delayed aortic closure**
Delayed electrical activation of the right ventricle	Delayed electrical activation of the left ventricle
Complete right bundle branch block (proximal type)	Complete left bundle branch block (proximal type)
Left ventricular paced beats	Right ventricular paced beats
Left ventricular ectopic beats	Right ventricular ectopic beats
Prolonged right ventricular mechanical systole	Prolonged left ventricular mechanical systole
Acute massive pulmonary embolus	Complete left bundle branch block (peripheral type)
Pulmonary hypertension with right-sideed heart failure	Left ventricular outflow tract obstruction
Pulmonic stenosis with intact septum (moderate to severe)	Hypertensive cardiovascular disease
Decreased impedance of the pulmonary vascular bed (increased hangout)	Arteriosclerotic heart disease
Normotensive atrial septal defect	Chronic ischemic heart disease
Idiopathic dilatation of the pulmonary artery	Angina pectoris
Pulmonic stenosis (mild)	Decreased impedance of the systemic vascular bed (increased hangout)
Atrial septal defect, postoperative (70%)	Poststenotic dilatation of the aorta secondary to aortic stenosis or insufficiency
Early aortic closure	Patent ductus arteriosus
Shortened left ventricular mechanical systole (left ventriculer ejection time)	**Early pulmonic closure**
Mitral regurgitation	Early electrical activation of the right ventricle
Ventricular septal defect	Wolff-Parkinson-White syndrome, type B

Modified from Shaver JA, O'Toole JD: The second heart sound: Newer concepts. Parts 1 and 2. Mod Concepts Cardiovasc Dis 46:7 and 13, 1977.

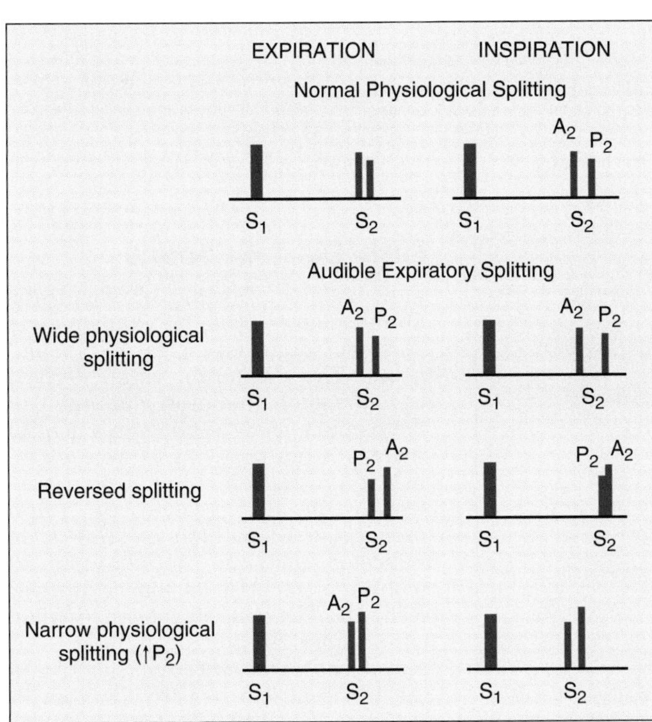

FIGURE 8–13 **Top,** Normal physiological splitting. During expiration (left), the aortic (A_2) and pulmonic (P_2) components of the second heart sound are separated by less than 30 milliseconds and are appreciated as a single sound. During inspiration (right), the splitting interval widens, and A_2 and P_2 are clearly separated into two distinct sounds. **Bottom,** Audible expiratory splitting. In contrast to normal physiological splitting, two distinct sounds are easily heard during expiration. Wide physiological splitting is caused by a delay in P_2. Reversed splitting is caused by a delay in A_2, resulting in paradoxical movement; that is, with inspiration P_2 moves toward A_2, and the splitting interval narrows. Narrow physiological splitting occurs in patients with pulmonary hypertension, and both A_2 and P_2 are heard during expiration at a narrow splitting interval because of the increased intensity and high-frequency composition of P_2. (From Shaver JA, Leonard JJ, Leon DF: Examination of the Heart, Part IV, Auscultation of the Heart. Dallas, American Heart Association, 1990, p 17. Copyright 1990, American Heart Association.)

valve is immobile (severe calcific aortic stenosis) or atretic (aortic atresia).

Persistent Splitting of S_2. This term applies when the two components remain audible (or recordable) during both inspiration and exhalation (see Fig. 8–14). Persistent splitting may be due to a delay in P_2, as in cases of simple complete right bundle branch block,[58] or to early timing of the A_2, as occasionally occurs in cases of mitral regurgitation. Normal directional changes in the interval of the split (greater with inspiration, lesser with exhalation) in the presence of persistent audibility of both components defines the split as *persistent* but not *fixed*.

Fixed Splitting of S_2. This term applies when the interval between the A_2 and P_2 is not only wide and persistent but also remains unchanged during the respiratory cycle.[50] Fixed splitting is an auscultatory hallmark of uncomplicated ostium secundum atrial septal defect (Fig. 8–15; see Chap. 56). A_2 and P_2 are widely separated during exhalation and exhibit little or no change in the degree of splitting during inspiration or with the Valsalva maneuver. The wide splitting is caused by a delay in the P_2 because a marked increase in pulmonary vascular capacitance prolongs the interval between the descending limbs of the pulmonary arterial and right ventricular pressure pulses ("hangout"), and therefore delays the pulmonary incisura and the P_2. The capacitance (impedance) of the pulmonary bed is appreciably increased, and the right ventricular stroke volume is not influenced by respiration, so there is little or no additional increase during inspiration and little or no inspiratory delay in the P_2. Phasic changes in systemic venous return during respiration in patients with atrial septal defect are associated with reciprocal changes in the volume of the left-to-right shunt, minimizing respiratory variations in right ventricular filling. The net effect is the characteristic wide, fixed splitting of the two components of the S_2.[55]

Paradoxical (Reversed) Splitting of S_2. This term refers to a reversed sequence of semilunar valve closure, the P_2 preceding the A_2. Common causes of paradoxical splitting are complete left bundle branch block[62] or a right ventricular pacemaker, both of which are associated with initial activation of the right side of the ventricular septum, and delayed activation of the left ventricle owing to transseptal (right-to-left) depolarization.[63] When the S_2 splits paradoxically, its

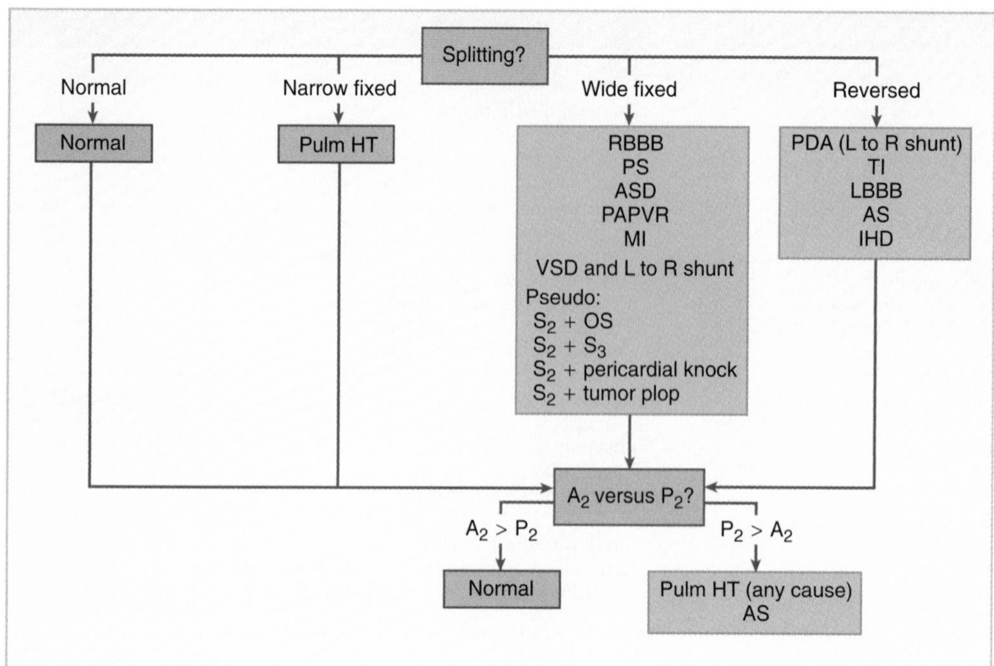

FIGURE 8–14 Decision tree for splitting of the second heart sound (S_2). A_2 = aortic valve closure; AS = aortic stenosis; ASD = atrial septal defect; IHD = ischemic heart disease; L to R shunt = left-to-right shunt; LBBB = left bundle branch block; MI = mitral insufficiency; OS = opening snap; P_2 = pulmonic valve closure; PAPVR = partial anomalous pulmonary venous return; PDA = patent ductus arteriosus; PS = pulmonic stenosis; Pulm HT = pulmonary hypertension; RBBB = right bundle branch block; S_3 = third heart sound; TI = tricuspid insufficiency; VSD = ventricular septal defect. (From Braunwald E: The clinical examination. *In* Braunwald E, Goldman L [eds]: Primary Cardiology. 2nd ed. Philadelphia, Elsevier, 2003; and Sapira JD: The Art and Science of Bedside Diagnosis. Baltimore, Urban and Schwartzenberg, 1990.)

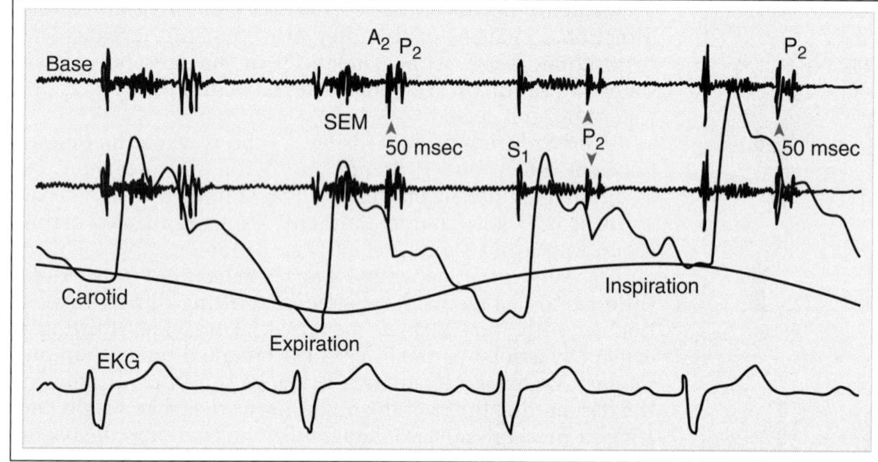

FIGURE 8–15 Simultaneous base and apex phonocardiograms recorded with the carotid pulse during quiet respiration in a young woman with a large atrial septal defect. Wide fixed splitting of the second heart sound (S_2) is present, and the pulmonic component (P_2) is easily recorded at the apex. A prominent systolic ejection murmur (SEM) is recorded at the base and is attributable to the large stroke volume across the right ventricular outflow tract. The tricuspid component of S_1 is prominent at the apex. EKG = electrocardiogram. (From Shaver JA: Innocent murmurs. Hosp Med 14:8, 1978. Copyright 1999, Quadrant Healthcom, Inc.)

two components separate during exhalation and become single (synchronous) during inspiration (see Fig. 8–13). Inspiratory synchrony is achieved as the two components fuse because of a delay in the P_2, less to earlier timing of the aortic component.

ABNORMAL LOUDNESS (INTENSITY) OF THE TWO COMPONENTS OF S_2

Assessment of intensity requires that both components be compared when heard simultaneously at the same site. The relative softness of the normal P_2 is responsible for its localization in the second left intercostal space, whereas the relative loudness of the normal A_2 accounts for its audibility at all precordial sites (see earlier). An increase in intensity of the A_2 occurs with systemic hypertension. The intensity of A_2 also increases when the aorta is closer to the anterior chest wall, owing to root dilatation or transposition of the great arteries or when an anterior pulmonary trunk is small or absent, as in pulmonary atresia.[55]

A loud P_2 is a feature of pulmonary hypertension, and the loudness is enhanced by dilatation of a hypertensive pulmonary trunk. An accentuated P_2 can be transmitted to the middle or lower left sternal edge and, when very loud, throughout the precordium to the apex and right base. A moderate increase in loudness of the P_2 sometimes occurs in the absence of pulmonary hypertension when the pulmonary trunk is dilated, as in cases of ostium secundum atrial septal defect or when there is a decrease in anteroposterior chest dimensions (loss of thoracic kyphosis) that places the pulmonary trunk closer to the chest wall.[64]

Early Diastolic Sounds

The opening "snap" of rheumatic mitral stenosis is the best known early diastolic sound (see Figs. 8–11B and 8–26). The diagnostic value derived from the pitch, loudness, and timing of the opening snap in the assessment of rheumatic mitral stenosis was established by Wood in his classic monograph, *An Appreciation of Mitral Stenosis*.[65] An audible opening snap indicates that the mitral valve is mobile, or at least its longer anterior leaflet is. The snap is generated when superior systolic bowing of the anterior mitral leaflet is rapidly reversed toward the left ventricle in early diastole in response to high left atrial pressure. The mechanism of the opening snap is therefore a corollary to the loud S_1, which is generated by abrupt superior systolic displacement of a mobile anterior mitral leaflet that was recessed into the left ventricle during diastole by high left atrial pressure until the onset of left ventricular isovolumetric contraction (see earlier). The designation "snap" is appropriate because of the relatively high frequency of the sound.

The timing of the opening snap relative to the A_2 has important physiological meaning.[4] A short A_2/opening snap interval generally reflects the high left atrial pressure of severe mitral stenosis. In older subjects with systolic hypertension, however, mitral stenosis of appreciable severity can occur without a short A_2/opening snap interval because the elevated left ventricular systolic pressure takes longer to fall below the left atrial pressure. In the presence of atrial fibrillation, the A_2/opening snap interval varies inversely with cycle length, because (all else being equal) the higher the left atrial pressure (short cycle length), the earlier the stenotic valve opens and vice versa.

Early diastolic sounds are not confined to the opening snap of rheumatic mitral stenosis but include the pericardial "knock" of chronic constrictive pericarditis.[66] The term "knock" has also been applied to an early diastolic sound in patients with pure severe mitral regurgitation with reduced left ventricular compliance. Both the pericardial knock and the knock of mitral regurgitation are rapid filling sounds that are early and loud because a high-pressure atrium rapidly decompresses across an unobstructed mitral valve into a recipient ventricle whose compliance is impaired.

Early diastolic sounds are sometimes caused by atrial myxomas (see Chap. 63).[67] The generation of such a sound, called a tumor "plop," requires a mobile myxoma attached to the atrial septum by a long stalk. The "plop" is believed to result from abrupt diastolic seating of the tumor within the right or left AV orifice.[67]

An early diastolic sound can also be generated by the opening movement of a mechanical prosthesis in the mitral position. This opening sound is especially prominent with a ball-in-cage prosthesis (Starr-Edwards) and less prominent with a tilting disc prosthesis (Bjork-Shiley).

Mid-diastolic and Late Diastolic (Presystolic) Sounds (Fig. 8–16)

Mid-diastolic sounds are, for all practical purposes, either normal or abnormal S_3 sounds, and most, if not all, late diastolic or presystolic sounds are S_4 sounds. Each sound coincides with its relevant diastolic filling phase.[68] In sinus rhythm, the ventricles receive blood during two filling phases. The first phase occurs when ventricular pressure drops sufficiently to allow the AV valve to open; blood then flows from atrium into ventricle. This flow is designated the "rapid filling phase," accounting for about 80 percent of normal ventricular filling. The rapid filling phase is not a passive event in which the recipient ventricle merely expands in response to augmented inflow volume. Rather, ventricular relaxation is an active, complex, energy-dependent process (see Chaps. 19 and 20).

S_3 is generated during the rapid filling phase.[69] The second filling phase—diastasis—is variable in duration, usually accounting for less than 5 percent of ventricular filling. The third phase of diastolic filling is in response to atrial contraction, which accounts for about 15 percent of normal ventricular filling. S_4 is generated during the atrial filling phase. Both S_3 and S_4 occur within the recipient ventricle as that chamber receives blood. The addition of either an S_3 or an S_4 to the cardiac cycle produces a triple rhythm. If both S_3 and S_4 are present, a quadruple rhythm is produced. When diastole is short or the PR interval is long, S_3 and S_4 occur simultaneously to form a summation sound.[4]

Children and young adults often have a normal (physiological) S_3 but do not have a normal S_4. A normal S_3 sometimes persists beyond the age of 40 years, especially in women. After that age, however, especially in men, S_3 is likely to be abnormal. An S_4 is sometimes heard in healthy older adults without clinical evidence of heart disease, particularly after exercise.[4] Such observations have led to the conclusion, still debated, that such an S_4 may be normal in the elderly.

ATRIAL CONTRIBUTION TO FILLING. Because an S_4 requires active atrial contribution to ventricular filling, the sound disappears when coordinated atrial contraction ceases, as in atrial fibrillation. When the atria and ventricles contract independently as in complete heart block, an S_4 or summation sound occurs randomly in diastole because the relationship between the P wave and the QRS of the electrocardiogram is random. S_3 and S_4 are events caused by rapid ventricular filling, so obstruction of an AV valve, by impeding ventricular inflow, removes one of the prime preconditions for the generation of these filling sounds. Accordingly, the presence of an S_3 or S_4 implies an unobstructed (or relatively unobstructed) AV orifice on the side of the heart in which the sound originates. An S_3 or S_4 originating from the right ventricle often responds selectively and distinctively to respiration, becoming more prominent during inspiration.[4] The inspiratory increase in right atrial flow is converted into an inspiratory augmentation of both mid-diastolic and presystolic filling.

S_3 and S_4, either normal or abnormal, are relatively low frequency events that vary considerably in intensity (loudness), that originate in

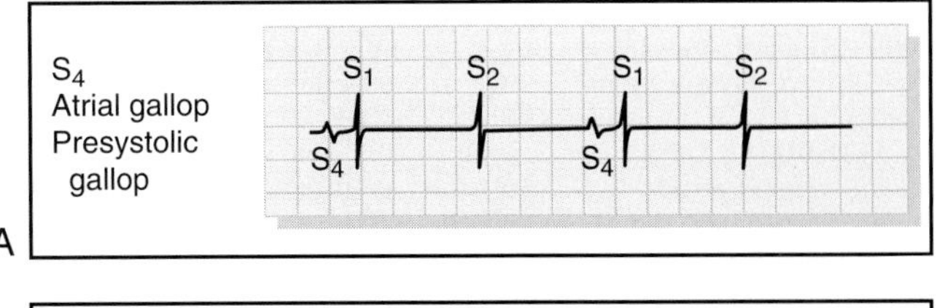

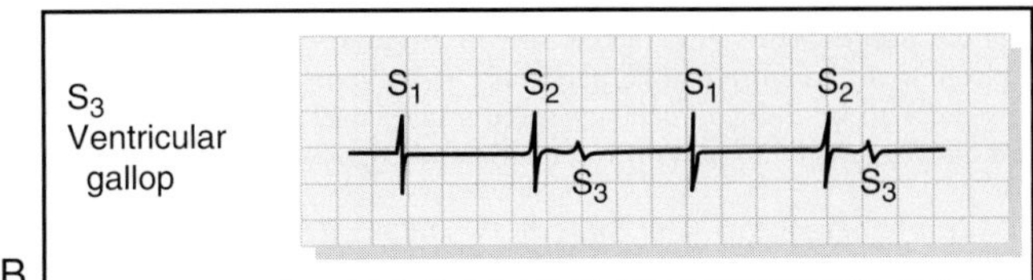

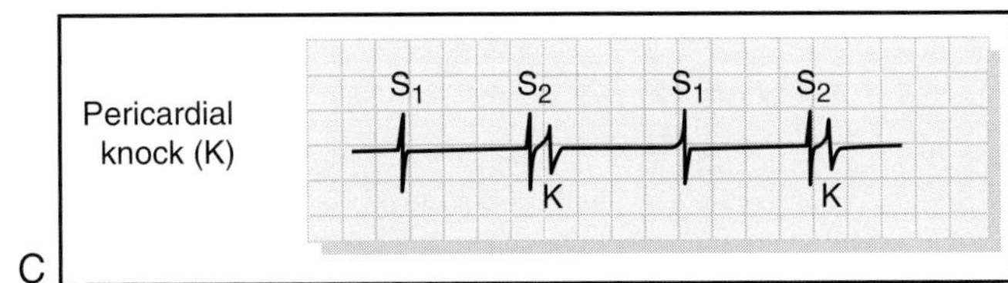

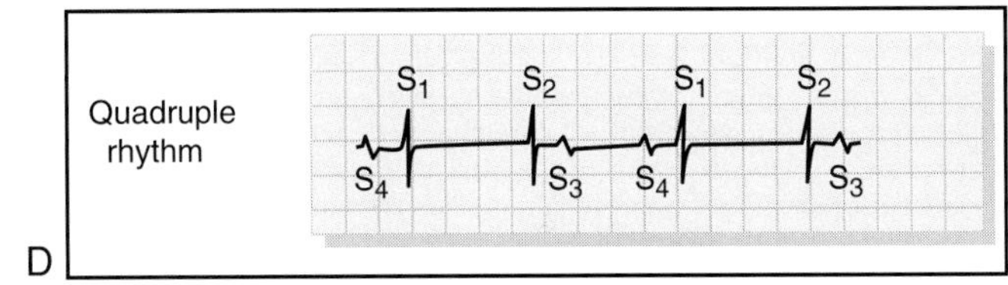

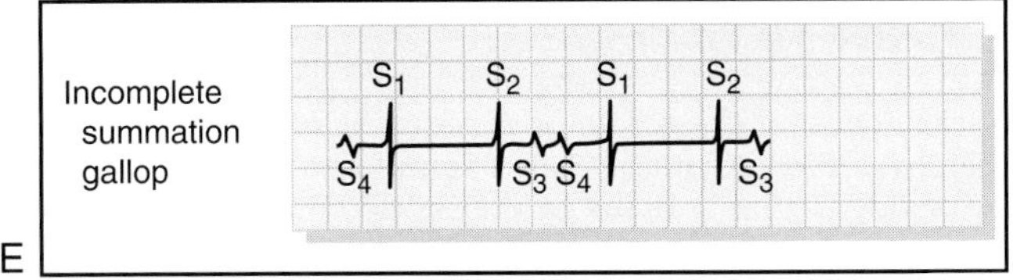

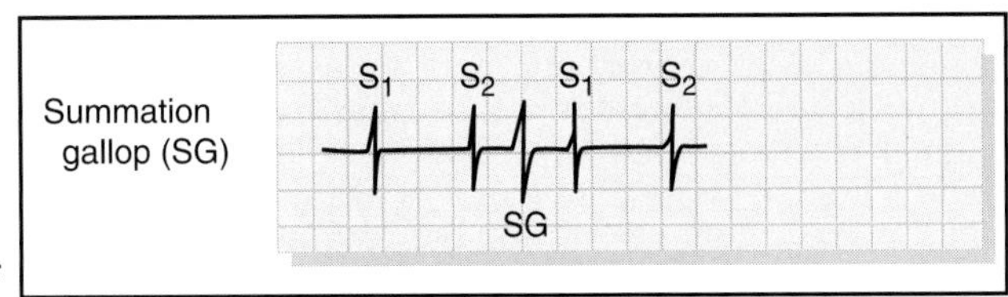

FIGURE 8–16 Diastolic filling sounds. **A,** the fourth heart sound (S_4) occurs in presystole and is frequently called an *atrial* or *presystolic gallop.* **B,** The third heart sound (S_3) occurs during the rapid phase of ventricular filling. It is a normal finding that is commonly heard in children and young adults but disappears with increasing age. When it is heard in a patient with cardiac disease, it is called a pathologic S_3 or ventricular gallop and usually indicates ventricular dysfunction or atrioventricular valvular incompetence. **C,** In constrictive pericarditis, a sound in early diastole, the pericardial knock (K) is heard earlier and is louder and higher pitched than the usual pathologic S_3. **D,** A quadruple rhythm results if both S_4 and S_3 are present. **E,** At faster heart rates, S_3 and S_4 occur in rapid succession and may give the illusion of a mid-diastolic rumble. **F,** When the heart rate is sufficiently rapid, the two rapid phases of ventricular filling reinforce each other, and a loud summation gallop (SG) may appear; this sound may be louder than either S_3 or S_4 alone. S_1 = first heart sound; S_2 = second heart sound. (From Braunwald E: The clinical examination. *In* Braunwald E, Goldman L [eds]: Primary Cardiology. 2nd ed. Philadelphia, Elsevier, 2003, pp 29-46; and Shaver JA: Examination of the Heart. Part 4: Auscultation. Dallas, American Heart Association, 1990.)

either the left or right ventricle, and that are best elicited when the bell of the stethoscope is applied with just enough pressure to provide a skin seal. An S_3 or S_4 originating from the left ventricle should be sought over the left ventricular impulse identified with the patient in the left lateral decubitus position. An S_3 or S_4 originating from the right ventricle should be sought over the right ventricular impulse (lower left sternal edge, occasionally subxiphoid) with the patient supine. An understanding of these simple principles sets the stage for bedside detection. The same principles can be used to advantage to distinguish an S_4 preceding a single S_1 from splitting of the two components of the S_1 (see Fig. 8-9C). The two components of S_1 are similar in frequency (pitch) although not in intensity (loudness) but differ in pitch from a preceding S_4. Selective pressure with the bell of the stethoscope enhances these distinctions.

AUDIBILITY OF S_3. This is improved by isotonic exercise that augments venous return and mid-diastolic AV flow. A few sit-ups usually suffice to produce the desired increase in venous return and acceleration in heart rate that increase the rate and volume of AV flow. Venous return can be increased by simple passive raising of both legs with the patient supine. The heart rate is also transiently increased by vigorous coughing. Left ventricular S_4, especially in patients with ischemic heart disease, can be induced or augmented when resistance to left ventricular discharge is increased by sustained hand-grip (isometric exercise; see later).

In the presence of sinus tachycardia, atrial contraction may coincide with the rapid filling phase, making it impossible to determine whether a given filling sound is an S_3, an S_4, or a summation sound. Carotid sinus massage transiently slows the heart rate, so the diastolic sound or sounds can be assigned their proper timing in the cardiac cycle.[4]

CAUSES OF S_3 AND S_4. The normal S_3 is believed to be caused by sudden limitation of longitudinal expansion of the left ventricular wall during brisk early diastolic filling.[70-73] The majority of abnormal S_3 sounds are generated by altered physical properties of the recipient ventricle and/or an increase in the rate and volume of AV flow during the rapid filling phase of the ventricle. An abnormal S_4 occurs when augmented atrial contraction generates presystolic ventricular distention (an increase in end-diastolic segment length) so that the recipient chamber can contract with greater force.[74-76] Typical substrates are the left ventricular hypertrophy of aortic stenosis or systemic hypertension or the right ventricular hypertrophy of pulmonary stenosis or pulmonary hypertension in the right side of the heart.[74] S_4 sounds are also common in ischemic heart disease and are almost universal during angina pectoris or acute myocardial infarction.

Heart Murmurs

A cardiovascular murmur is a series of auditory vibrations that are more prolonged than a sound and are characterized according to timing in the cardiac cycle, intensity (loudness), frequency (pitch), configuration (shape), quality, duration, and direction of radiation.[4,50,77] When these features are established, the stage is set for diagnostic conclusions.[2,76,78] The principal causes of heart murmurs are listed in Table 8–5.

Intensity or loudness is graded from 1 to 6, based on the original recommendations of Samuel A. Levine in 1933. A grade 1 murmur is so faint that it is heard only with special effort. A grade 2 murmur is soft but readily detected; a grade 3 murmur is prominent but not loud; a grade 4 murmur is loud (and usually accompanied by a thrill); a grade 5 murmur is very loud. A grade 6 murmur is loud enough to be heard with the stethoscope just removed from contact with the chest wall. The factors affecting the loudness of heart murmurs are listed in Table 8–6. Frequency or pitch varies from high to low. The configuration or shape of a murmur is best characterized as crescendo, decrescendo, crescendo-decrescendo (diamond-shaped), plateau (even), or variable (uneven). The duration of a murmur varies from short to long, with all gradations in between. A loud murmur radiates from its site of maximal intensity, and the direction of radiation is sometimes diagnostically useful.

There are three broad categories of murmurs: systolic, diastolic, and continuous. A systolic murmur begins with or after S_1 and ends at or before S_2 on its side of origin. A

TABLE 8–5 Principal Causes of Heart Murmurs

A. Organic Systolic Murmurs
- 1. Midsystolic (ejection)
  - a. Aortic
    - (1) Obstructive
      - (a) Supravalvular—supraaortic stenosis, coarction of the aorta
      - (b) Valvular—aortic stenosis and sclerosis
      - (c) Infravalvular—HOCM
    - (2) Increased flow, hyperkinetic states, aortic regurgitation, complete heart block
    - (3) Dilatation of ascending aorta, atheroma, aortitis, aneurysm of aorta
  - b. Pulmonary
    - (1) Obstructive
      - (a) Supravalvular—pulmonary arterial stenosis
      - (b) Valvular—pulmonic valve stenosis
      - (c) Infravalvular—infundibular stenosis
    - (2) Increase flow, hyperkinetic states, left-to-right shunt (e.g., ASD, VSD)
    - (3) Dilatation of pulmonary artery
- 2. Pansystolic (regurgitant)
  - a. Atrioventricular valve regurgitation (MR, TR)
  - b. Left-to-right shunt to ventricular level

B. Early Diastolic Murmurs
- 1. Aortic regurgitation
  - a. Valvular: rheumatic deformity; perforation postendocarditis, posttraumatic, postvalvulotomy
  - b. Dilatation of valve ring: aorta dissection, annuloectasia, cystic medial necrosis, hypertension
  - c. Widening of commissures: syphilis
  - d. Congenital: biscuspid valve, with VSD
- 2. Pulmonic regurgitation
  - a. Valvular: postvalvulotomy, endocarditis, rheumatic fever, carcinoid
  - b. Dilatation of valve ring: pulmonary hypertension; Marfan syndrome
  - c. Congenital: isolated or associated with tetralogy of Fallot, VSD, pulmonic stenosis

C. Mid-Diastolic Murmurs
1. Mitral stenosis
2. Carey-Coombs murmur (mid-diastolic apical murmur in acute rheumatic fever)
3. Increased flow across nonstenotic mitral valve (e.g., MR, VSD, PDA, high-output states, and complete heart block)
4. Tricuspid stenosis
5. Increased flow across nonstenotic tricuspid valve (e.g., TR, ASD, and anomalous pulmonary venous return)
6. Left and right atrial tumors

D. Continuous Murmurs
1. PDA
2. Coronary arteriovenous fistula
3. Ruptured aneurysm of sinus of Valsalva
4. Aortic septal defect
5. Cervical venous hum
6. Anomalous left coronary artery
7. Proximal coronary artery stenosis
8. Mammary souffle
9. Pulmonary artery branch stenosis
10. Bronchial collateral circulation
11. Small (restrictive) ASD with mitral stenosis
12. Intercostal arteriovenous fistula

A and *C*, Modified from Oram S (ed): Clinical Heart Disease. London, Heinemann, 1981. *D*, Modified from Fowler NO (ed): Cardiac Diagnosis and Treatment. Hagerstown, MD, Harper & Row, 1980.

ASD = atrial septal defect; HOCM = hypertrophic obstructive cardiomyopathy; MR = mitral regurgitation; PDA = patent ductus arteriosus; TR = tricuspid regurgitation; VSD = ventricular septal defect.

From Norton PJ, O'Rourke RA: Approach to the patient with a heart murmur. *In* Braunwald E, Goldman L, (eds): Primary Cardiology. 2nd ed. Philadelphia, Elsevier, 2003, pp 151–168.

TABLE 8–6 Factors Affecting the Loudness of Heart Murmurs

Increased intensity
High cardiac output (hyperdynamic) states
Thin chest wall
Narrow thoracic diameter; for example, "straight back," pectus excavatum
Anemia (decreased blood viscosity)
Tortuous aorta (close to chest wall)
Decreased intensity
Obesity
Muscular or thick chest wall
Obstructive lung disease
Barrel chest (increased anteroposterior diameter)
Pericardial thickening or fluid
Decreased cardiac output (congestive heart failure, low ejection fraction)

From Abrams J: Synopsis of Cardiac Physical Diagnosis. 2nd ed. Boston, Butterworth Heinemann, 2001, p 115.

diastolic murmur begins with or after S_2 and ends before the subsequent S_1. A continuous murmur begins in systole and continues without interruption through the S_2 into all or part of diastole. The following classification of murmurs is based on their timing relative to S_1 and S_2.

Systolic Murmurs

Systolic murmurs are classified according to their time of onset and termination as midsystolic, holosystolic, early systolic, or late systolic (Fig. 8–17).[77,79,80] A midsystolic murmur begins after S_1 and ends perceptibly before S_2. The termination of a systolic murmur must be related to the relevant component of S_2. Accordingly, midsystolic murmurs originating in the left side of the heart end before A_2; midsystolic murmurs originating in the right side of the heart end before P_2. A holosystolic murmur begins with S_1, occupies all of systole, and ends with the S_2 on its side of origin. Holosystolic murmurs originating in the left side of the heart end with A_2, and holosystolic murmurs originating in the right side of the heart end with P_2.

The term *regurgitant systolic murmur*, originally applied to murmurs that occupied all of systole, has fallen out of use because "regurgitation" can be accompanied by holosystolic, midsystolic, early systolic, or late systolic murmurs.[2] Similarly, the term *ejection systolic murmur*, originally applied to midsystolic murmurs, should be discarded, because midsystolic murmurs are not necessarily due to "ejection."[4]

MIDSYSTOLIC MURMURS. Midsystolic murmurs occur in five settings: (1) obstruction to ventricular outflow, (2) dilatation of the aortic root or pulmonary trunk, (3) accelerated systolic flow into the aorta or pulmonary trunk, (4) innocent (normal) midsystolic murmurs,[55] and (5) some forms of mitral regurgitation. The physiological mechanism of outflow midsystolic murmurs reflects the pattern of phasic flow across the left or right ventricular outflow tract as originally described by Leatham (Fig. 8–18).[58] Isovolumetric contraction generates S_1. Ventricular pressure rises, the semilunar valve opens, flow commences, and the murmur begins. As flow proceeds, the murmur increases in crescendo; as flow decreases, the murmur decreases in decrescendo. The murmur ends before ventricular pressure drops below the pressure in the central great artery, at which time the aortic and pulmonary valves close, generating A_2 and P_2.

AORTIC VALVE STENOSIS (see Chap. 57)**.** This is associated with a midsystolic murmur, which may have an early systolic peak and a short duration, a relatively late peak and a prolonged duration, or all gradations in between. Whether long or short, however, the murmur retains a symmetrical diamond shape beginning after S_1 (or with an aortic ejection sound), rising in crescendo to a systolic peak, and declining in decrescendo to end before A_2. The high-velocity jet within the aortic root results in radiation of the murmur upward, to the right (second right intercostal space), and into the neck. An important variation occurs in older adults with previously normal trileaflet aortic valves rendered sclerotic or stenotic by fibrocalcific changes. The accompanying murmur in the second right intercostal space is harsh, noisy, and impure (see Fig.

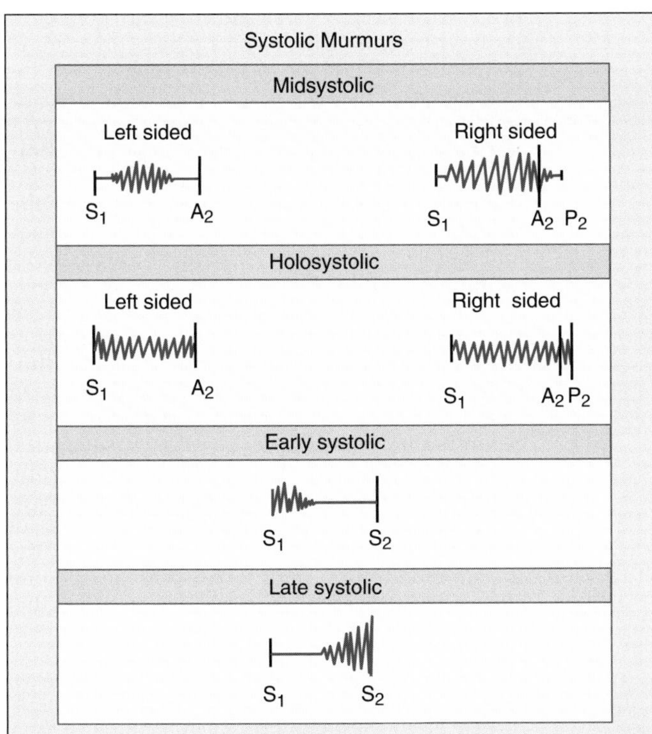

FIGURE 8–17 Systolic murmurs as illustrated here are descriptively classified according to their time of onset and termination as midsystolic, holosystolic, early systolic, and late systolic. The termination of the murmur must be related to the component of the second heart sound on its side of origin, that is, the aortic component (A_2) for systolic murmurs originating in the left side of the heart and the pulmonic component (P_2) for systolic murmurs originating in the right side of the heart.

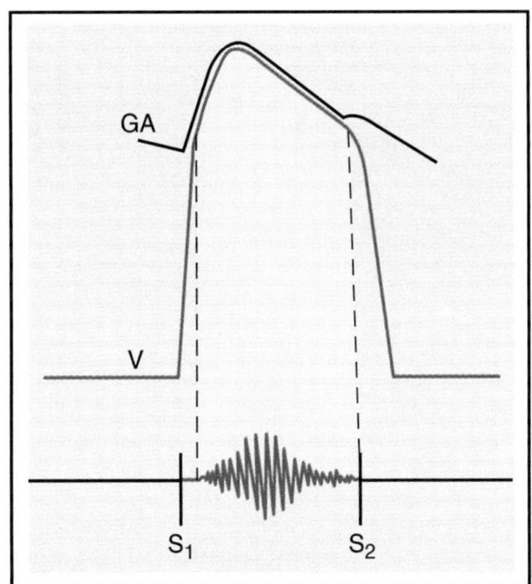

FIGURE 8–18 Illustration of the physiological mechanism of a midsystolic murmur generated by phasic flow into aortic root or pulmonary trunk. Ventricular (V) and great arterial (GA) pressure pulses are shown with phonocardiogram. The midsystolic murmur begins after the first heart sound (S_1), rises in crescendo to a peak as flow proceeds, then declines in decrescendo as flow diminishes, ending just before the second heart sound (S_2) as ventricular pressure falls below the pressure in the great artery.

8-10), whereas the murmur over the left ventricular impulse is pure and often musical.

The high-frequency apical midsystolic murmur of aortic sclerosis or stenosis should be distinguished from the high-frequency apical murmur of mitral regurgitation, a distinction that may be difficult or impossible, especially if A_2 is soft or absent. However, when premature ventricular contractions are followed by pauses longer than the dominant cycle length, the apical midsystolic murmur of aortic stenosis or sclerosis increases in intensity in the beat after the premature contraction, whereas the intensity of the murmur of mitral regurgitation (whether midsystolic or holosystolic) remains relatively unchanged. The same patterns hold after longer cycle lengths in atrial fibrillation.

PULMONARY VALVE STENOSIS (see Chap. 56). This is prototypical of a midsystolic murmur originating in the right side of the heart.[55] The murmur begins after S_1 or with a pulmonary ejection sound, rises in crescendo to a peak, then decreases in a slower decrescendo to end before a delayed or soft P_2. The length and configuration of the murmur are useful signs of the severity of obstruction.[55] When the ventricular septum is intact (Fig. 8-19, *left*), as obstruction becomes more severe, the murmur lengthens and envelops A_2, and P_2 becomes softer. When obstruction to right ventricular outflow is accompanied by a ventricular septal defect (tetralogy of Fallot), the midsystolic murmur becomes shorter with increased severity of obstruction (see Fig. 8-19, *right*).

ACCELERATED FLOW. Short, soft midsystolic murmurs originate within a dilated aortic root or dilated pulmonary trunk. Midsystolic murmurs are also generated by rapid ejection into a normal aortic root or pulmonary trunk, as during pregnancy, fever, thyrotoxicosis, or anemia. The pulmonary midsystolic murmur of ostium secundum atrial septal defect results from rapid ejection into a dilated pulmonary trunk (see Fig. 8-17).

INNOCENT (NORMAL) MURMURS. These are, except for the systolic mammary souffle, all midsystolic.[53] The normal vibratory midsystolic murmur (Still murmur) is short, buzzing, pure, and medium in frequency (Fig. 8-20) and is believed to be generated by low-frequency periodic vibrations of normal pulmonary leaflets at their attachments or periodic vibrations of a left ventricular false tendon.[81,82] A second type of innocent midsystolic murmur occurs in children, adolescents, and young adults and represents an exaggeration of normal ejection vibrations within the pulmonary trunk. This normal pulmonary midsystolic murmur is relatively impure and is best heard in the second left intercostal space, in contrast to the vibratory midsystolic murmur of Still, which is typically heard between the lower left sternal edge and apex. Normal pulmonary midsystolic murmurs are also heard in patients with diminished anteroposterior chest dimensions (e.g., loss of thoracic kyphosis).

The most common form of "innocent" midsystolic murmur in older adults has been designated the "aortic sclerotic" murmur (see earlier). The cause of this functionally benign murmur is fibrous or fibrocalcific thickening of the bases of otherwise normal aortic cusps as they insert into the sinuses of Valsalva.[55] As long as the fibrous or fibrocalcific thickening is confined to the base of the leaflets, the free edges remain mobile. No commissural fusion and no obstruction occur. The Gallavardin dissociation phenomenon associated with such an aortic valve was described earlier.

MIDSYSTOLIC MURMUR OF MITRAL REGURGITATION. The clinical setting is usually ischemic heart disease associated with left ventricular regional wall motion abnormalities. The physiological mechanism responsible for the midsystolic murmur of mitral regurgitation in this setting reflects impaired integrity of the muscular component of the mitral apparatus, with early systolic competence of the valve, and midsystolic incompetence, followed by a late systolic decline in regurgitant flow. These midsystolic murmurs are unrelated to "ejection."

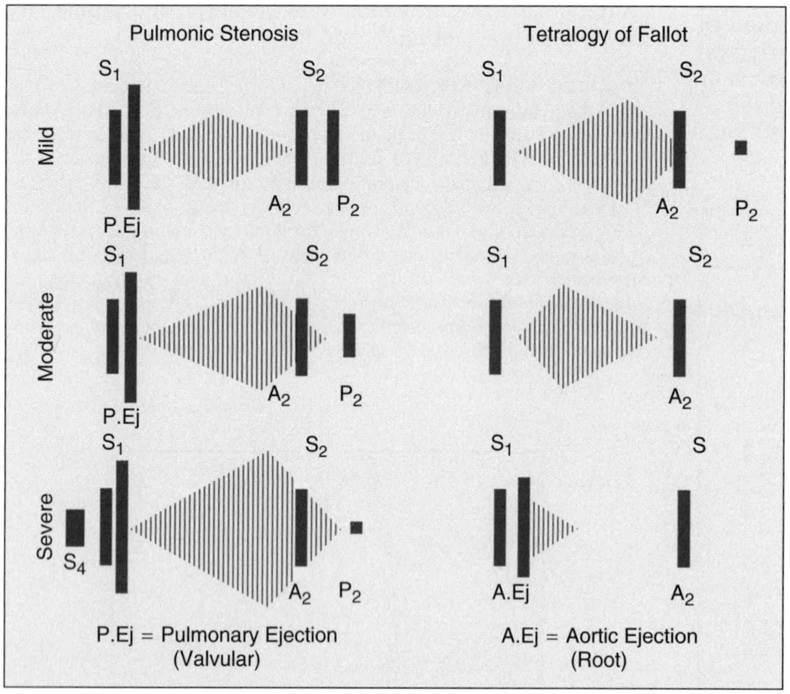

FIGURE 8–19 **Left,** In cases of valvular pulmonic stenosis with intact ventricular septum, right ventricular systolic ejection becomes progressively longer, with increasing obstruction to flow. As a result, the murmur becomes louder and longer, enveloping the aortic component of the second heart sound (A_2). The pulmonic component (P_2) occurs later, and splitting becomes wider but more difficult to hear because A_2 is lost in the murmur and P_2 becomes progressively fainter and lower pitched. As pulmonic diastolic pressure progressively decreases, isometric contraction shortens until the pulmonary valvular ejection sound fuses with the first heart sound (S_1). In cases of severe pulmonic stenosis with concentric hypertrophy and decreasing right ventricular compliance, a fourth heart sound appears. **Right,** In cases of tetralogy of Fallot with increasing obstruction at the pulmonic infundibular area, an increasing amount of right ventricular blood is shunted across the silent ventricular septal defect, and flow across the obstructed outflow tract decreases. Therefore, with increasing obstruction the murmur becomes shorter, earlier, and fainter. P_2 is absent in patients with severe tetralogy of Fallot. A large aortic root receives almost all cardiac output from both ventricular chambers, and the aorta dilates and is accompanied by a root ejection sound that does not vary with respiration. (From Shaver JA, Leonard JJ, Leon DF: Examination of the Heart. Part IV: Auscultation of the Heart. Dallas, American Heart Association, 1990, p 45. Copyright 1990, American Heart Association.)

HOLOSYSTOLIC MURMURS. Just as the term *midsystolic* is preferable to *ejection systolic*, the term *holosystolic* is preferable to *regurgitant* because holosystolic murmurs are not necessarily due to regurgitant flow. A holosystolic murmur begins with S_1 and occupies all of systole up to the S_2 on its side of origin (see Figs. 8–17 and 8–21).[4,50] Such murmurs are generated by flow from a vascular bed whose pressure or resistance throughout systole is higher than the pressure or resistance in the vascular bed receiving the flow. Holosystolic murmurs occur in the left side of the heart with mitral regurgitation, in the right side of the heart with high-pressure tricuspid regurgitation, between the ventricles through a restrictive ventricular septal defect, and between the great arteries through aortopulmonary connections.

The timing of holosystolic murmurs reflects the physiological and anatomical mechanisms responsible for their genesis. Figure 8–21 illustrates the mechanism of the holosystolic murmur of mitral regurgitation or high-pressure tricuspid regurgitation. Ventricular pressure exceeds atrial pressure at the very onset of systole (isovolumetric contraction), so regurgitant flow begins with the S_1. The murmur persists up to or slightly beyond the relevant component of the S_2, provided that ventricular pressure at end systole exceeds atrial pressure and provided that the AV valve remains incompetent.

Direction of radiation of the intraatrial jet of mitral regurgitation determines the chest wall distribution of the murmur.[83] When the direction of the intraatrial jet is forward and medial against the atrial septum near the origin of the aorta, the murmur radiates to the left sternal edge, to the base, and even into the neck. When the flow generating the murmur of mitral regurgitation is directed posterolaterally within the left atrial cavity, the murmur radiates to the axilla, to the angle of the left

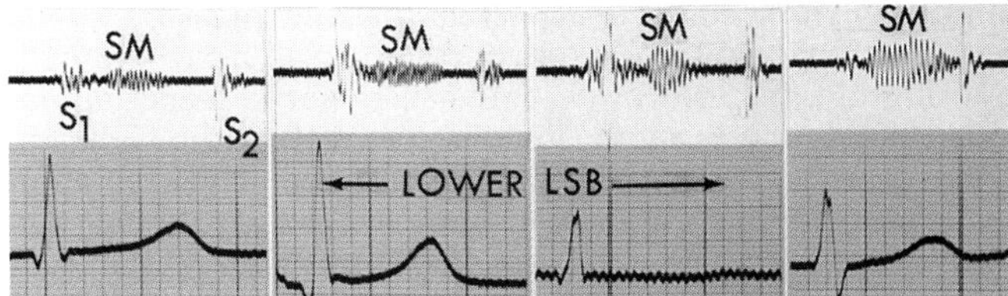

FIGURE 8–20 Four vibratory midsystolic murmurs (SM) from healthy children. These murmurs, designated *Still murmur*, are pure, medium frequency, relatively brief in duration, and maximal along the lower left sternal border (LSB). The last of the four murmurs was from a 5-year-old girl who was febrile. After defervescence, the murmur decreased in loudness and duration.

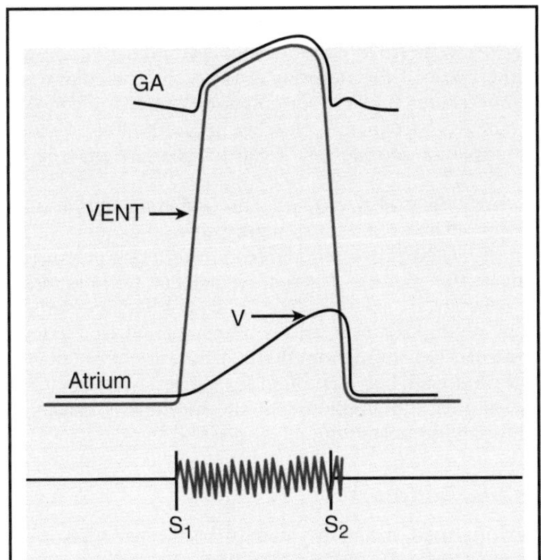

FIGURE 8–21 Illustration of great arterial (GA), ventricular (VENT), and atrial pressure pulses with phonocardiogram showing the physiological mechanism of a holosystolic murmur in some forms of mitral regurgitation and in high-pressure tricuspid regurgitation. Ventricular pressure exceeds atrial pressure at the very onset of systole, so regurgitant flow and murmur commence with the first heart sound (S_1). The murmur persists up to or slightly beyond the second heart sound (S_2) because regurgitation persists to the end of systole (ventricular pressure still exceeds atrial pressure). V = atrial v wave.

scapula, and occasionally to the vertebral column, with bone conduction from the cervical to the lumbar spine.

The *murmur of tricuspid regurgitation* is holosystolic when there is a substantial elevation of right ventricular systolic pressure, as schematically illustrated in Figure 8–21. A distinctive and diagnostically important feature of the tricuspid murmur is its selective inspiratory increase in loudness—Carvallo sign. The tricuspid murmur is occasionally audible only during inspiration. The increase in intensity occurs because the inspiratory augmentation in right ventricular volume is converted into an increase in stroke volume and in the velocity of regurgitant flow. When the right ventricle fails, this capacity is lost; thus, Carvallo sign vanishes.

The murmur of an uncomplicated restrictive ventricular septal defect (see Chap. 56) is holosystolic because left ventricular systolic pressure and systemic resistance exceed right ventricular systolic pressure and pulmonary resistance from the onset to the end of systole. Holosystolic murmurs are perceived as such in patients with large aortopulmonary connections (aortopulmonary window, patent ductus arteriosus) when a rise in pulmonary vascular resistance abolishes the diastolic portion of the continuous murmur, leaving a murmur that is holosystolic or nearly so.[55]

EARLY SYSTOLIC MURMURS. Murmurs confined to early systole begin with S_1, diminish in decrescendo, and end well before S_2, generally at or before midsystole (see Fig.

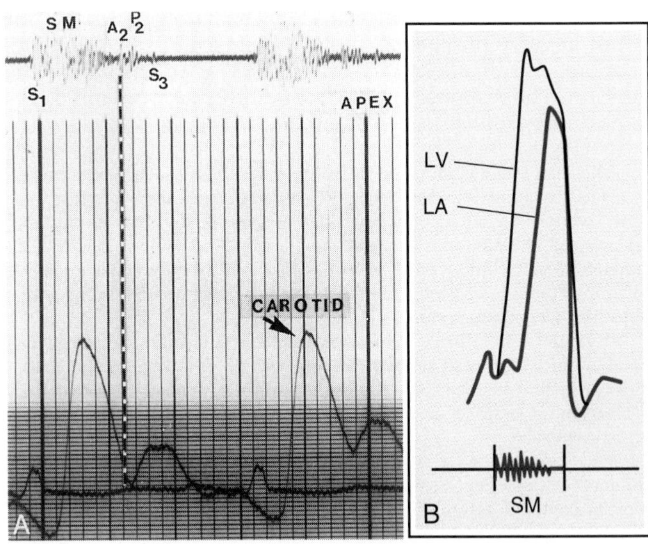

FIGURE 8–22 **A,** Phonocardiogram recorded from the cardiac apex of a patient with acute severe mitral regurgitation due to ruptured chordae tendineae. There is an early systolic decrescendo murmur (SM) diminishing if not ending before the aortic component (A_2) of the second heart sound. **B,** Left ventricular (LV) and left atrial (LA) pressure pulses with schematic illustration of the phonocardiogram showing the relationship between the decrescendo configuration of the early systolic murmur and late systolic approximation of the tall left atrial v wave and left ventricular end-systolic pressure. Regurgitant flow diminishes or ceases. The murmur therefore is early systolic and decrescendo, paralleling the hemodynamic pattern of regurgitation. P_2 = pulmonic component of the second heart sound; S_1 = first heart sound; S_3 = third heart sound.

8–17). Certain types of mitral regurgitation, tricuspid regurgitation, or ventricular septal defects are the substrates.

Acute severe mitral regurgitation is accompanied by an early systolic murmur or a holosystolic murmur that is decrescendo, diminishing if not ending before S_2 (Fig. 8–22A).[84] The physiological mechanism responsible for this early systolic decrescendo murmur is acute severe regurgitation into a relatively normal-sized left atrium with limited distensibility. A steep rise in left atrial V wave approaches the left ventricular pressure at end systole; a late systolic decline in left ventricular pressure favors this tendency (see Fig. 8–22B). The stage is set for regurgitant flow that is maximal in early systole and minimal in late systole. The systolic murmur parallels this pattern, declining or vanishing before S_2.

An early systolic murmur is a feature of tricuspid regurgitation with normal right ventricular systolic pressure.[85] An example is tricuspid regurgitation caused by infective endocarditis in drug abusers. The mechanisms responsible for the timing and configuration of the early systolic murmur of low-pressure tricuspid regurgitation are analogous to those just described for mitral regurgitation. The crest of the right atrial V wave reaches the level of normal right ventricular pressure in later systole; the regurgitation and murmur are therefore chiefly, if not exclusively, early systolic. These murmurs are of medium frequency because normal right ventricular systolic pressure generates comparatively low velocity regurgitant flow, in contrast to elevated right ventricular systolic pressure, which generates a high-frequency holosystolic murmur (see earlier).

Early systolic murmurs also occur through ventricular septal defects, but under two widely divergent anatomical and physiological circumstances. A soft, pure, high-frequency, early systolic murmur localized to the middle or lower left sternal edge is typical of a very small ventricular septal defect in which the shunt is confined to early systole.[55] A murmur of similar timing and configuration occurs through a nonrestrictive ventricular septal defect when an elevation in pulmonary vascular resistance decreases or abolishes late systolic shunting.

LATE SYSTOLIC MURMURS. The term *late systolic* applies when a murmur begins in middle to late systole and proceeds up to the S_2 (see Fig. 8–17). The late systolic murmur of mitral valve prolapse is prototypical (see Fig. 8–12).[86] One or more middle to late systolic clicks often introduce the murmur. The responses of the late systolic murmur and clicks to postural maneuvers are illustrated in Figure 8–12.

The late systolic murmur of mitral valve prolapse is occasionally replaced by an intermittent, striking, and sometimes disconcerting systolic "whoop" or "honk," either spontaneously or in response to physical maneuvers. The whoop is of high frequency, musical, widely transmitted, and occasionally loud enough to be disturbing to the patient. The musical whoop is thought to arise from mitral leaflets and chordae tendineae set into high-frequency periodic vibration.

SYSTOLIC ARTERIAL MURMURS. Systolic murmurs can originate in anatomically normal arteries in the presence of normal or increased flow or in abnormal arteries because of tortuosity or luminal narrowing. Detection of systolic arterial murmurs requires auscultation at non-precordial sites.

The supraclavicular systolic murmur, often heard in children and adolescents, is believed to originate at the aortic origins of normal major brachiocephalic arteries.[55] The configuration of these murmurs is crescendo-decrescendo, the onset is abrupt, the duration is brief, and the intensity at times is surprisingly loud, with radiation below the clavicles. Normal supraclavicular systolic murmurs decrease or vanish in response to hyperextension of the shoulders, which is achieved by bringing the elbows back until the shoulder girdle muscles are drawn taut.

In older adults, the most common cause of a systolic arterial murmur is atherosclerotic narrowing of a carotid, subclavian, or iliofemoral artery. A variation on this theme is the "compression artifact" that can be induced in the femoral artery in the presence of free aortic regurgitation. When the femoral artery is moderately compressed by the examiner's stethoscopic bell, a systolic arterial murmur is generated. Further compression causes the systolic murmur to continue into diastole, a sign described in 1861 by Duroziez.[55] The eponym is still in use.

A systolic "mammary souffle" is sometimes heard over the breasts because of increased flow through normal arteries during late pregnancy or more especially in the postpartum period in lactating women.[55] The murmur begins well after S_1 because of the interval between left ventricular ejection and the arrival of flow at the artery of origin.

A systolic arterial murmur is present in the interscapular region over the site of coarctation of the aortic isthmus.[55] Transient systolic arterial murmurs originating in the pulmonary artery and its branches are occasionally heard in normal neonates because the angulation and disparity in size between the pulmonary trunk and its branches set the stage for turbulent systolic flow. These normal or innocent pulmonary arterial systolic murmurs disappear with maturation of the pulmonary bed, generally within the first few weeks or months of life.[55] Similar if not identical pulmonary arterial systolic murmurs are generated at sites of congenital stenosis of the pulmonary artery and its branches. Rarely, a pulmonary arterial systolic murmur is caused by luminal narrowing after a pulmonary embolus.[74]

Diastolic Murmurs

Diastolic murmurs, like systolic murmurs, are classified according to their time of onset as early diastolic, mid-diastolic, or late diastolic (presystolic) (Fig. 8–23). An early diastolic murmur begins with A_2 or P_2, depending on its side of origin. A mid-diastolic murmur begins at a clear interval after S_2. A late diastolic or presystolic murmur begins immediately before S_1.

Early Diastolic Murmurs

CHRONIC AORTIC REGURGITATION. An early diastolic murmur originating in the left side of the heart occurs in cases of aortic regurgitation (see Chap. 57). This murmur is heard best with the diaphragm of the stethoscope, with the patient leaning forward and during a held, deep exhalation (see Fig. 8–7D). The murmur begins with the aortic component of S_2 (Fig. 8–24A), that is, as soon as left ventricular pressure falls below the aortic incisura. The configuration of the murmur tends to reflect the volume and rate of regurgitant flow. In cases of chronic aortic regurgitation of moderate severity, the aortic diastolic pressure consistently and appreciably exceeds left ventricular diastolic pressure, so the decrescendo is subtle and the murmur is well heard throughout diastole. In cases of chronic severe aortic regurgitation, the decrescendo is more obvious, paralleling the dramatic decline in aortic root diastolic pressure. Selective radiation of the murmur of aortic regurgitation to the right sternal edge implies aortic root dilatation, as in patients with Marfan syndrome. When an inverted cusp is set into high-frequency periodic vibration by aortic regurgitation, the accompanying murmur is musical, early diastolic, and decrescendo (see Fig. 8–24B).

ACUTE AORTIC REGURGITATION. The diastolic murmur of acute severe aortic regurgitation differs importantly from the murmur of chronic severe aortic regurgitation as just described (Fig. 8-25). When regurgitant flow is both sudden *and* severe (as may occur in cases of infective endocarditis or aortic dissection), the diastolic murmur is relatively short because the aortic diastolic pressure rapidly equilibrates with the steeply rising diastolic pressure in the unprepared, nondilated left ventricle; the pitch of the murmur is likely to be medium and it may be quite soft (grade 2). These auscultatory features are in contrast to the long, pure, high-frequency, blowing and often loud (grade 4) early diastolic murmur of chronic severe aortic regurgitation (see Figs. 8-24 and 8-25).

Pulmonary Regurgitation. The Graham Steell murmur of pulmonary hypertensive pulmonary regurgitation begins with a loud P_2 because the elevated pressure exerted on the incompetent pulmonary valve begins at the moment that right ventricular pressure drops below the pulmonary arterial incisura. The high diastolic pressure generates high-velocity regurgitant flow and results in a high-frequency blowing murmur that may last throughout diastole. Because of the persistent and appreciable difference between pulmonary arterial and right ventricular diastolic pressures, the amplitude of the murmur is usually relatively uniform throughout most, if not all, of diastole.

Mid-Diastolic Murmurs

By definition, mid-diastolic murmurs begin at a clear interval after S_2 (Figs. 8–23 and 8–26). The majority of mid-diastolic murmurs originate across mitral or tricuspid valves during the rapid filling phase of the cardiac cycle (AV valve obstruction or abnormal patterns of AV flow) or across an incompetent pulmonary valve in the absence of pulmonary hypertension.

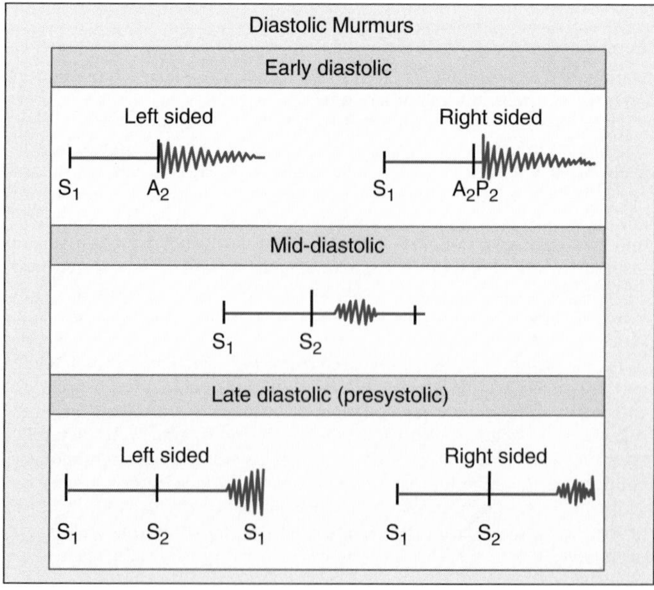

FIGURE 8–23 Diastolic murmurs are descriptively classified according to their time of onset as early diastolic, mid-diastolic, or late diastolic (presystolic). Diastolic murmurs originate in either the left or the right side of the heart.

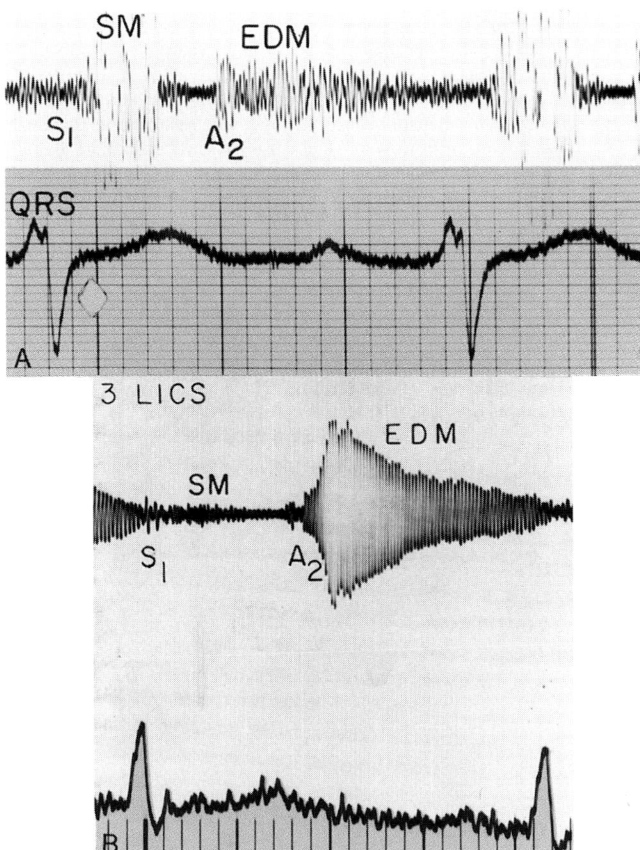

FIGURE 8–24 **A,** Phonocardiogram recorded from the mid-left sternal edge of a patient with chronic pure severe aortic regurgitation. An early diastolic murmur (EDM) proceeds immediately from the aortic component of the second heart sound (A_2). The murmur has an early crescendo followed by a late long decrescendo. There is a prominent midsystolic flow murmur (SM) across an unobstructed aortic valve. **B,** Phonocardiogram in the third left intercostal space (3 LICS) records a high-frequency, musical, early diastolic decrescendo murmur (EDM) caused by eversion of an aortic cusp. S_1 = first heart sound; SM = midsystolic murmur.

The mid-diastolic murmur of rheumatic mitral stenosis is a prime example.[87] The murmur characteristically follows the mitral opening snap (see Fig. 8–11B). Because the murmur originates within the left ventricular cavity, transmission to the chest wall is maximal over the left ventricular impulse. Care must be taken to place the bell of the stethoscope lightly against the skin precisely over the left ventricular impulse with the patient turned into the left lateral decubitus position (see Fig. 8–7C). Soft mid-diastolic murmurs are reinforced when the heart rate and mitral valve flow are transiently increased by vigorous voluntary coughs or a few sit-ups. In patients with atrial fibrillation, the duration of the mid-diastolic murmur is a useful sign of the degree of obstruction at the mitral orifice. A murmur that lasts up to S_1 even after long cycle lengths indicates that the stenosis is severe enough to generate a persistent gradient even at the end of long diastoles.

The mid-diastolic murmur of tricuspid stenosis occurs in the presence of atrial fibrillation. The tricuspid mid-diastolic murmur differs from the mitral mid-diastolic murmur in two important respects: (1) the loudness of the tricuspid murmur increases with inspiration, and (2) the tricuspid murmur is confined to a relatively localized area along the left lower sternal edge. The inspiratory increase in loudness occurs because inspiration is accompanied by an augmentation in right ventricular volume, by a fall in right ventricular diastolic pressure, and by an increase in gradient and flow rate across the stenotic tricuspid valve.[4] The murmur is localized to the lower left sternal edge because it originates within the inflow portion of the right ventricle and is transmitted to the overlying chest wall.

Mid-diastolic murmurs across unobstructed AV valves occur in the presence of augmented volume and velocity of flow. Examples in the left side of the heart are the mid-diastolic flow murmur of pure mitral regurgitation and the mid-diastolic mitral flow murmur that accompanies a large left-to-right shunt through a ventricular septal defect (Fig. 8-27A). Mid-diastolic murmurs due to augmented flow across unobstructed tricuspid valves are generated by severe tricuspid regurgitation or by a large left-to-right shunt through an atrial septal defect (see Fig. 8-27B). These mid-diastolic murmurs indicate appreciable AV valve incompetence or large left-to-right shunts and are often preceded by an S_3, especially in the presence of mitral or tricuspid regurgitation.

Short, mid-diastolic AV flow murmurs occur intermittently in patients with complete heart block when atrial contraction coincides with the phase of rapid diastolic filling. These murmurs are believed to result from antegrade flow across AV valves that are closing rapidly during filling of the recipient ventricle. A similar mechanism is believed to be responsible for the Austin Flint murmur (see Fig. 8-25).[88,89]

A mid-diastolic murmur is a feature of pulmonary valve regurgitation, provided that the pulmonary arterial pressure is not elevated. The diastolic murmur typically begins at a perceptible interval after P_2 is crescendo-decrescendo, and ends well before the subsequent S_1.[55] The diastolic pressure exerted on the incompetent pulmonary valve is negligible at the inception of P_2, so regurgitant flow is minimal. Regurgitation accelerates as right ventricular pressure dips below the diastolic pressure in the pulmonary trunk; at that point, the murmur reaches its maximum intensity. Late diastolic equilibration of pulmonary arterial and right ventricular pressures eliminates regurgitant flow and abolishes the murmur before the next S_1.

Late Diastolic or Presystolic Murmurs

A late diastolic murmur occurs immediately before S_1, that is, in presystole (see Fig. 8–23). With few exceptions, the late

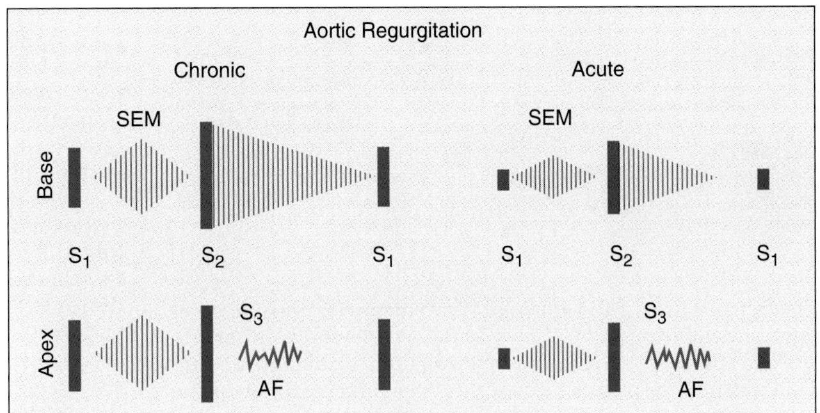

FIGURE 8–25 Contrast between the auscultatory findings in patients with chronic and acute aortic regurgitation. In a patient with chronic aortic regurgitation, a prominent systolic ejection murmur resulting from the large forward stroke volume is heard at the base and the apex and ends well before the second heart sound (S_2). The aortic diastolic regurgitant murmur begins with S_2 and continues in a decrescendo fashion, terminating before the first heart sound (S_1). At the apex, the early diastolic component of Austin Flint murmur (AF) is introduced by a prominent third heart sound (S_3). A presystolic component of the AF is also heard. In cases of acute aortic regurgitation, there is a significant decrease in the intensity of the systolic ejection murmur compared with that of chronic aortic regurgitation because of the decreased forward stroke volume. The S_1 is markedly decreased in intensity because of preclosure of the mitral valve, and at the apex the presystolic component of the AF murmur is absent. The early diastolic murmur at the base ends well before S_1 because of equilibration of the left ventricle and aortic end-diastolic pressures. Significant tachycardia is usually present. (From Shaver JA: Diastolic murmurs. Heart Dis Stroke 2:100, 1994.)

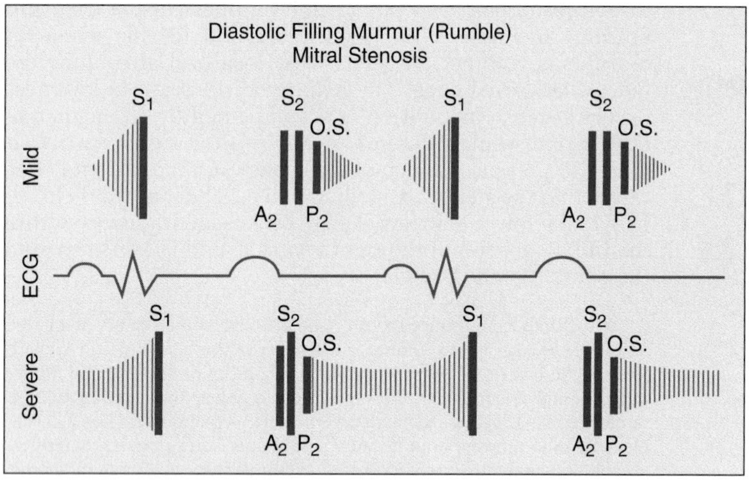

FIGURE 8–26 Diastolic filling murmur (rumble) in mitral stenosis. In cases of mild mitral stenosis, the diastolic gradient across the valve is limited to the two phases of rapid ventricular filling in early diastole and presystole. The rumble may occur during either period or during both periods. As the stenotic process becomes severe, a large pressure gradient exists across the valve during the entire diastolic filling period, and the rumble persists throughout diastole. As the left atrial pressure becomes greater, the interval between aortic component of the second heart sound (A_2) and the opening snap (O.S.) shortens. In cases of severe mitral stenosis, secondary pulmonary hypertension develops and results in a loud pulmonic component of the second heart sound (P_2) and the splitting interval usually narrows. S_1 = first heart sound; S_2 = second heart sound; ECG = electrocardiogram. (From Shaver JA, Leonard JJ, Leon DF: Examination of the Heart. Part IV: Auscultation of the Heart. Dallas, American Heart Association, 1990, p 55. Copyright 1990, American Heart Association.)

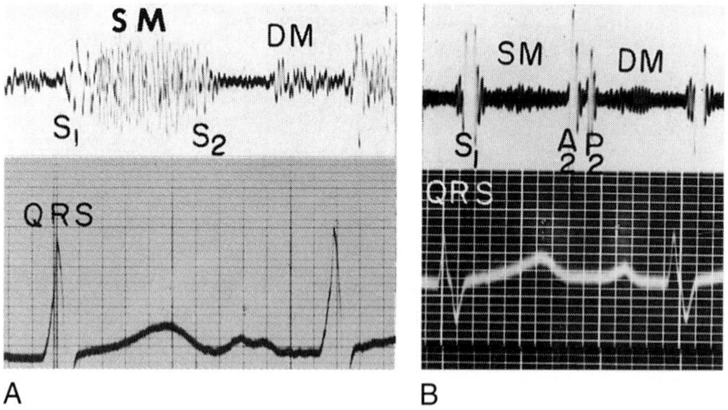

FIGURE 8–27 **A,** Phonocardiogram recorded at the apex of a patient with a moderately restrictive ventricular septal defect and increased pulmonary arterial blood flow. The mid-diastolic murmur (DM) results from augmented flow across the mitral valve. **B,** Phonocardiogram at the lower left sternal edge of a patient with an ostium secundum atrial septal defect and increased pulmonary arterial blood flow. A mid-diastolic murmur resulted from augmented flow across the tricuspid valve. SM = holosystolic murmur; S_1 = first heart sound; S_2 = second heart sound; A_2 and P_2 = aortic and pulmonic components of a conspicuously split S_2.

diastolic timing of the murmur coincides with the phase of ventricular filling that follows atrial systole and implies the presence of sinus rhythm and coordinated atrial contraction. Late diastolic or presystolic murmurs usually originate at the mitral or tricuspid orifice because of obstruction, but occasionally because of abnormal patterns of presystolic AV flow.

The best known presystolic murmur accompanies rheumatic mitral stenosis in sinus rhythm as AV flow is augmented in response to an increase in the force of left atrial contraction (Figs. 8–11B and 8–28A).[65] Presystolic accentuation of a mid-diastolic murmur is occasionally heard in patients with mitral stenosis with atrial fibrillation, especially during short cycle lengths; however, the timing is actually early systolic, and the mechanism differs from the true presystolic murmur as described earlier and as shown in Figure 8–28A.

TRICUSPID STENOSIS. In patients with tricuspic stenosis who are in sinus rhythm, a late diastolic or presystolic murmur typically occurs in the absence of a perceptible mid-diastolic murmur (see Fig. 8–28B). This is so because the timing of tricuspid diastolic murmurs reflects the maximal acceleration of flow and gradient, which is usually negligible until a powerful right atrial contraction occurs.[4] The presystolic murmur of tricuspid stenosis is crescendo-decrescendo and relatively discrete, fading before S_1 (see Fig. 8–28B). This is in contrast to the presystolic murmur of mitral stenosis, which tends to rise in a crescendo up to S_1 (see Fig. 8–28A). The most valuable auscultatory sign of tricuspid stenosis in sinus rhythm is the effect of respiration on the intensity of the presystolic murmur. Inspiration increases right atrial volume, provoking an increase in right atrial contractile force that coincides with a fall in right ventricular end-diastolic pressure. The result is an increase in the tricuspid gradient, in the velocity of tricuspid flow, and in the intensity of the tricuspid stenotic presystolic murmur (Fig. 8–29).

THE AUSTIN FLINT MURMUR (see Fig. 8–25). In 1862, Austin Flint described a presystolic murmur in patients with aortic regurgitation and proposed a mechanism that was astonishingly perceptive[88-91]: "Now in cases of considerable aortic insufficiency, the left ventricle is rapidly filled with blood flowing back from the aorta as well as from the auricle, before the auricular contraction takes place. The distention of the ventricle is such that the mitral curtains are brought into coaptation; and when the auricular contraction takes place, the mitral direct current passing between the curtains throws them into vibration and gives rise to the characteristic blubbering murmur."[88]

Continuous Murmurs

The term *continuous* appropriately applies to murmurs that begin in systole and continue without interruption through S_2 into all or part of diastole (Fig. 8–30). The presence of murmurs throughout both phases of the cardiac cycle (holosystolic followed by holodiastolic) is not the criterion for the designation "continuous." Conversely, a murmur that fades completely before the subsequent S_1 may be continuous, provided that the systolic portion of the murmur proceeds without interruption through S_2.

Continuous murmurs are generated by uninterrupted flow from a vascular bed of higher pressure or resistance into a vascular bed of lower pressure or resistance without phasic interruption between systole and diastole. Such murmurs are due chiefly to (1) aortopulmonary connections, (2) arteriovenous connections, (3) disturbances of flow patterns in arteries, and (4) disturbances of flow patterns in veins (Table 8–7).

The best known continuous murmur is associated with the aortopulmonary connection of patent ductus arteriosus (see Chap 56; Fig. 8–31). The murmur characteristically peaks just before and after S_2, which it envelops, decreases in late diastole (often appreciably), and may be soft or even absent before the subsequent first heart sound.[55] George Gibson's description in 1900 was even more precise.[92] "It persists through S_2 and dies away gradually during the long pause. The murmur is rough and thrilling. It begins softly and increases in intensity so as to reach its acme just about, or immediately after, the incidence of the second sound, and from that point gradually wanes until its termination."

ARTERIOVENOUS CONTINUOUS MURMURS. These can be congenital or acquired and are represented in part by arteriovenous fistulas, coronary arterial fistulas, anomalous origin of the left coronary artery from the pulmonary trunk, and communications between the sinus of Valsalva and the right side of the heart.[55] The configuration, location, and intensity of arteriovenous continuous murmurs vary considerably among these different lesions. Acquired systemic arteriovenous fistulas are created surgically by forearm shunts for hemodialysis. Congenital arteriovenous continuous murmurs occur when a coronary arterial fistula enters the pulmonary trunk, right atrium, or right ventricle. At the right ventricle, the continuous murmur can be either softer or louder in systole, depending on the degree of compression exerted on the fistulous coronary artery by right ventricular contraction.[55] Rupture of a congenital aortic sinus aneurysm into the right side of the heart results in a continuous murmur that tends to be louder in either systole or diastole, sometimes creating a to-and-fro impression.[55]

ARTERIAL CONTINUOUS MURMURS. These originate in either constricted or nonconstricted arteries. A common example of a continuous murmur arising in a constricted artery is carotid or femoral arterial atherosclerotic obstruction. Not surprisingly, these murmurs are characteristically louder in systole and more often than not are purely systolic.

Disturbances of flow patterns in normal, nonconstricted arteries sometimes produce continuous murmurs. The "mammary souffle" described earlier,[4] an innocent murmur heard during late pregnancy and the puerperium, is an arterial murmur that, when continuous, is typically louder in systole and maximal over either lactating breast.

Continuous murmurs in nonconstricted arteries originate in the large systemic-to-pulmonary arterial collaterals in certain types of cyanotic congenital heart disease, typically tetralogy of Fallot with pulmonary atresia. These continuous murmurs are randomly located throughout the thorax because of the random location of the aortopulmonary collaterals.[55] They are also heard in coarctation of the aorta (see Chap. 56).

CONTINUOUS VENOUS MURMURS. These are well represented by the innocent cervical venous "hum" (Fig. 8-32). The hum is by far the most common type of normal continuous murmur, universal in healthy children, and frequently present in healthy young adults, especially during pregnancy. Thyrotoxicosis and anemia, by augmenting cervical venous flow, initiate or reinforce the venous hum. The term *hum* does not necessarily characterize the quality of these cervical venous murmurs, which may be rough and noisy and are occasionally accompanied by a high-pitched whine.[55] The hum is truly continuous, although

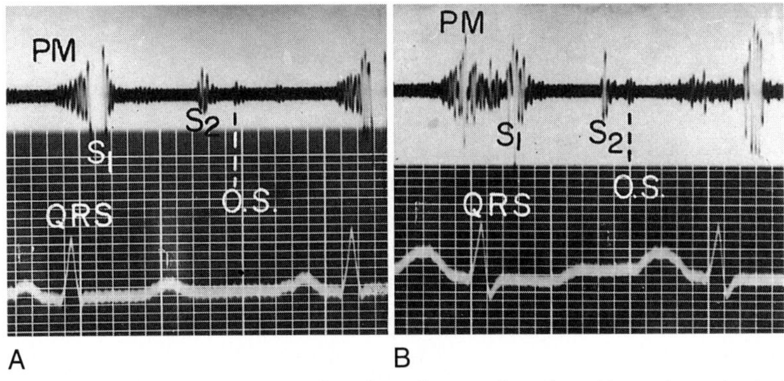

FIGURE 8–28 **A,** Phonocardiogram from the cardiac apex of a patient with pure rheumatic mitral stenosis. A presystolic murmur (PM) rises in a crescendo that is interrupted by a loud first heart sound (S_1). **B,** Phonocardiogram from the lower left sternal edge of a patient with rheumatic tricuspid stenosis. The first cycle is during inspiration and is accompanied by a prominent presystolic murmur (PM) that is crescendo-decrescendo, decreasing before the S_1. During exhalation (second cycle), the presystolic murmur all but vanishes. S_2 = second heart sound; OS = mitral opening snap.

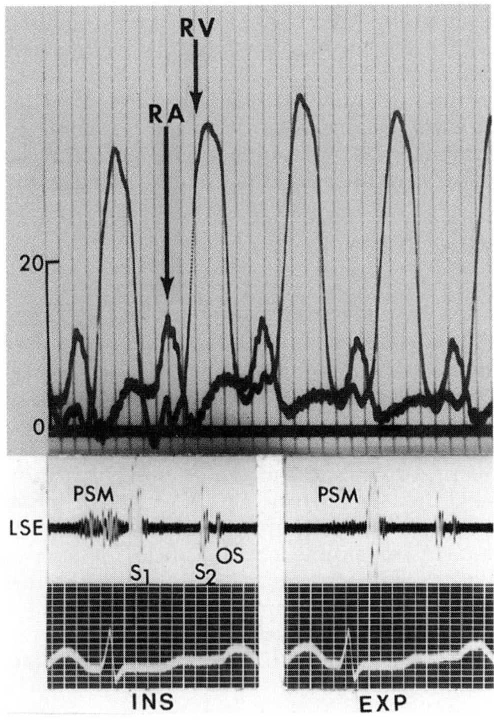

FIGURE 8–29 Pressure pulses and phonocardiogram illustrating the physiological mechanism of the respiratory variation in the presystolic murmur of tricuspid stenosis. During inhalation, a fall in intrathoracic pressure and an increase in systemic venous return result in an increase in the right atrial (RA) A wave and a decline in right ventricular (RV) end-diastolic pressure, so the presystolic murmur (PSM) increases in loudness. During exhalation, the right atrial A wave declines, the RV diastolic pressure increases, the tricuspid gradient is at its minimum, and the PSM all but vanishes. LSE = left sternal edge; S_1 = first heart sound; S_2 = second heart sound; INS = inspiration; EXP = expiration.

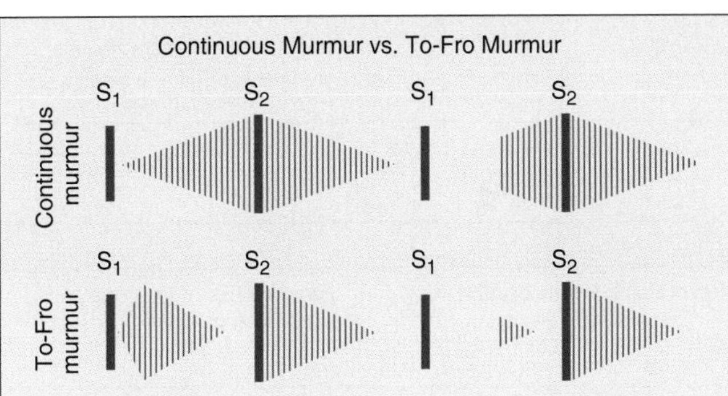

FIGURE 8–30 Comparison of continuous murmurs and to-fro murmurs. During abnormal communication between high-pressure and low-pressure systems, a large pressure gradient exists through the cardiac cycle, producing a continuous murmur. A classic example is patent ductus arteriosus. At times, this type of murmur is confused with a to-fro murmur, which is a combination of systolic ejection murmur and a murmur of semilunar valve incompetence. A classic example of a to-fro murmur is aortic stenosis and regurgitation. A continuous murmur crescendos to around the second heart sound (S_2), whereas a to-fro murmur has two components. The midsystolic ejection component decrescendos and disappears as it approaches S_2. S_1 = first heart sound. (From Shaver JA, Leonard JJ, Leon DF: Examination of the Heart. Part IV: Auscultation of the Heart. Dallas, American Heart Association, 1990, p 55. Copyright 1990, American Heart Association.)

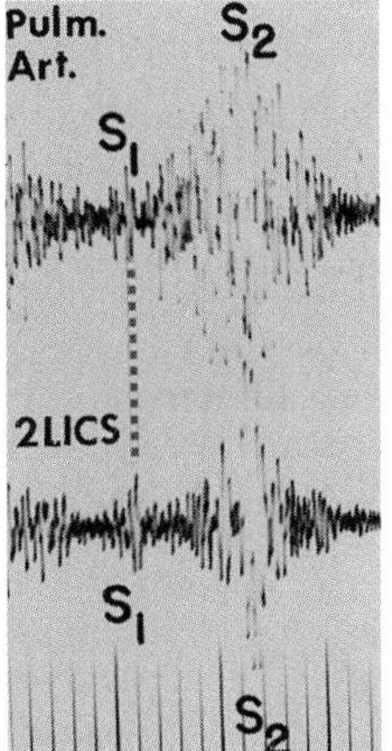

FIGURE 8–31 The classic continuous murmur of patent ductus arteriosus recorded from within the main pulmonary artery (upper tracing) and simultaneously on the chest wall at the second left intercostal space (2LICS). The murmur "begins softly and increases in intensity so as to reach its acme just about, or immediately after, the incidence of the second sound, and from that point gradually wanes until its termination," as originally described by Gibson in 1900.[92] Pulm. Art. = pulmonary artery; S_1 = first heart sound; S_2 = second heart sound.

TABLE 8–7 Differential Diagnosis of Continuous Thoracic Murmurs (in Order of Frequency)

Diagnosis	Key Findings
Cervical venous hum	Disappears on compression of the jugular vein
Hepatic venous hum	Often disappears with epigastric pressure
Mammary souffle	Disappears on pressing hard with stethoscope
Patent ductus arteriosus	Loudest at second left intercostal space
Coronary arteriovenous fistula	Loudest at lower sternal borders
Ruptured aneurysm of sinus of Valsalva	Loudest at upper right sternal border, sudden onset
Bronchial collaterals	Associated signs of congenital heart disease High-grade coarctation Brachial pedal arterial pressure gradient
Anomalous left coronary artery arising from pulmonary artery	Electrocardiographic changes of myocardial infarction
Truncus arteriosus	
Pulmonary artery branch stenosis	Heard outside the area of cardiac dullness
Pulmonary arteriovenous fistula	Same as above
Atrial septal defect with mitral stenosis or atresia	Altered by the Valsalva maneuver
Aortic-atrial fistulas	

Adapted from Sapira JD: The Art and Science of Bedside Diagnosis. Baltimore, Urban & Schwartzenberg, 1990.

typically louder in diastole. The mechanism of the venous hum is unsettled. Silent laminar flow in the internal jugular vein may be disturbed by deformation of the vessel at the level of the transverse process of the atlas during head rotation designed to elicit the hum.[93]

Approach to the Patient with a Heart Murmur

Although a careful physical examination with emphasis on detailed auscultation is useful in establishing a cardiac diagnosis or excluding serious cardiac disease in a patient with a heart murmur, echocardiography is decisive in confirming the diagnosis and determining the severity of the condition (Fig. 8–33). As delineated by O'Rourke,[77] the approach to the patient with a heart murmur depends on its intensity, timing, location, response to maneuvers, and the presence of other cardiac and noncardiac symptoms and signs. Patients with diastolic murmurs, or continuous murmurs that are not cervical venous hums, or mammary souffles of pregnancy, should ordinarily go to two-dimensional and Doppler echocardiography, and subsequent work-up, including cardiac consultation, is guided by the echocardiographic findings. In general, echocardiography is also advised for patients with systolic murmurs having the following characteristics: (1) loud murmur (i.e., grade 3 or higher); (2) holosystolic or late systolic murmur, especially at the left sternal edge or apex; (3) systolic murmurs that become louder or longer during the strain of the Valsalva maneuver (suggesting the diagnosis of hypertrophic obstructive cardiomyopathy or

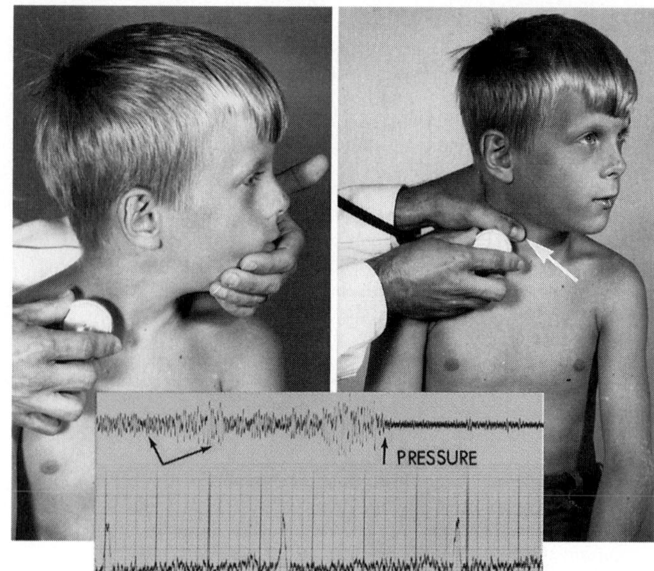

FIGURE 8–32 The phonocardiogram shows the continuous murmur of a normal venous hum. The diastolic component is louder (paired arrows). Digital pressure over the right internal jugular vein (vertical arrow) abolishes the murmur. The photographs show maneuvers used to elicit or abolish the venous hum. **Left,** The bell of the stethoscope is applied to the medial aspect of the right supraclavicular fossa as the examiner's left hand grasps the patient's chin from behind and pulls it tautly to the left and upward, stretching the neck. **Right,** The patient's head has returned to a more neutral position, and digital compression of the right internal jugular vein (arrow) abolishes the hum.

mitral valve prolapse respectively); (4) other systolic murmurs in patients with clinical findings suggesting infective endocarditis (see Chap. 58), thromboembolism, or syncope; (5) a systolic murmur accompanied by an abnormal electrocardiogram.

According to this schema, a large majority of patients with heart murmurs (i.e., patients with grade 1 or grade 2 midsystolic murmurs) without any other clinical manifestations of cardiac disease ordinarily do not require extensive work-up.

Pericardial Rubs (see Chap. 64)

In sinus rhythm, the typical pericardial "rub" is triple phased, that is, midsystolic, mid-diastolic, and presystolic. Recognition is simplest when all three phases are present and when the characteristic superficial scratchy, leathery quality is evident. Pericardial rubs may be more readily detected when the patient is on elbows and knees (Fig. 8–34), a physical maneuver designed to increase the contact of visceral and parietal pericardium (see earlier). The term *rub* is appropriate because the auscultatory sign is generated by abnormal visceral and parietal pericardial surfaces "rubbing" against each other. In the supine position, firm pressure with the stethoscopic diaphragm during full held exhalation reinforces visceral and parietal pericardial contact and accentuates the rub. Apposition of visceral and parietal pericardium can be even better achieved by examination while the patient rests on elbows and knees.

Of the three phases of the pericardial rub, the systolic phase is the most consistent,[94] followed by the presystolic phase. In atrial fibrillation, the presystolic component necessarily disappears. The diagnosis of a pericardial rub is least secure when only one phase remains, which is typically the midsystolic. The most common clinical setting in which pericardial rubs are heard is immediately after open heart surgery. However, auscultation often detects instead a "crunch" synchronous with the heartbeat, especially in the left lateral decubitus position. This is not a pericardial rub but is Hamman sign caused by air in the mediastinum.[95] Pericardial rubs are frequently audible in patients with acute pericarditis. They may become softer or even disappear in the presence of a large pericardial effusion.

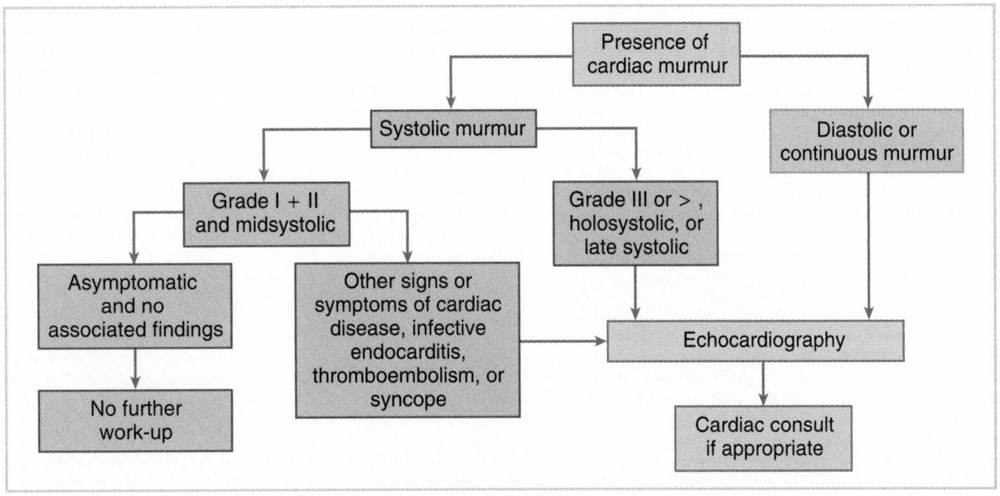

Presence of cardiac murmur
Systolic murmur
Diastolic or continuous murmur
Grade I + II and midsystolic
Grade III or >, holosystolic, or late systolic
Asymptomatic and no associated findings
Other signs or symptoms of cardiac disease, infective endocarditis, thromboembolism, or syncope
Echocardiography
No further work-up
Cardiac consult if appropriate

FIGURE 8–33 A schematic approach to the work-up of a patient with a cardiac murmur according to whether the murmur is probably innocent or secondary to cardiac pathology. This algorithm is particularly relevant to children and adults younger than 40 years, and echocardiography is recommended before cardiac consultation. (From Norton PJ, O'Rourke RA: Approach to the patients with a heart murmur. *In* Braunwald E, Goldman L [eds]: Primary Cardiology. 2nd ed. Philadelphia, Elsevier, 2003.)

Dynamic Auscultation

Dynamic auscultation refers to the technique of altering circulatory dynamics by a variety of physiological and pharmacological maneuvers and determining the effects of these maneuvers on heart sounds and murmurs.[96,97] The conditions and interventions most commonly employed in dynamic auscultation include respiration, postural changes, the Valsalva maneuver, premature ventricular contractions, isometric exercise, and one of the vasoactive agents—amyl nitrite, methoxamine, or phenylephrine.

Respiration

SECOND HEART SOUND. The splitting of S_2 is most audible along the left sternal border and can usually be appreciated when A_2 and P_2 are separated by more than 0.02 second. The effects of respiration on the splitting of the second heart sound were discussed earlier (see Second Heart Sound).

DIASTOLIC SOUNDS AND EJECTION SOUNDS. When S_3 and S_4 originate from the right ventricle, they are characteristically augmented during inspiration and diminished during exhalation, whereas they exhibit the opposite response when they originate from the left side of the heart. Like other left-sided events, the opening snap of the mitral valve may become softer during inspiration and louder during exhalation, owing to respiratory alterations in venous return, whereas the opening snap of the tricuspid valve behaves in the opposite fashion. Inspiration also diminishes the intensity of ejection sounds in pulmonary valve stenosis because the elevation of right ventricular diastolic pressure causes partial presystolic opening of the pulmonary valve and therefore less upward motion of the valve during systole. On the other hand, respiration does not affect the intensity of aortic ejection sounds, except in cases of tetralogy of Fallot with pulmonary atresia.

MURMURS. Respiration exerts more pronounced and consistent alterations on murmurs originating from the right than from the left side of the heart. During inspiration, the diastolic murmurs of tricuspid stenosis (see Fig. 8–29) and low-pressure pulmonary regurgitation, the systolic murmurs of tricuspid regurgitation (Carvallo sign),[98] and the presystolic murmur of Ebstein anomaly may all be accentuated. The inspiratory reduction in left ventricular size in patients with mitral valve prolapse increases the redundancy of the mitral valve and therefore the degree of valvular prolapse; consequently, the midsystolic click and the systolic murmurs occur earlier during systole and may become accentuated.[99]

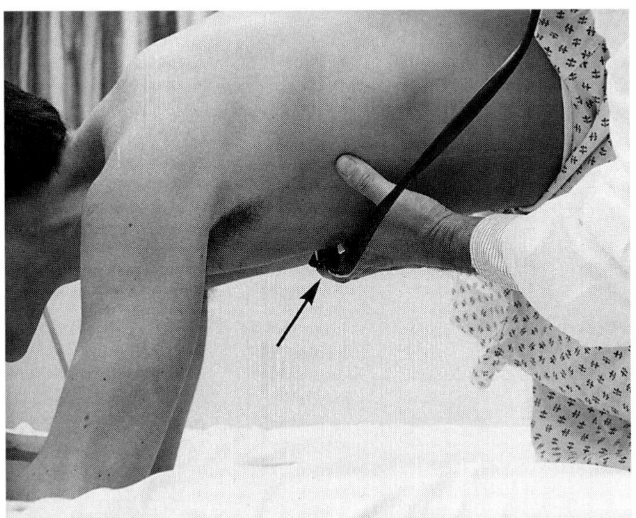

FIGURE 8–34 A technique for eliciting a pericardial rub. The diaphragm of the stethoscope is firmly applied to the precordium (arrow) while the patient rests on elbows and knees.

THE VALSALVA MANEUVER. This maneuver consists of a relatively deep inspiration followed by forced exhalation against a closed glottis for 10 to 20 seconds. The patient should first be instructed on how to perform the maneuver. Simulation by the examiner is a simple means of doing so. The examiner then places the flat of the hand on the abdomen to provide the patient with a force against which to strain and to permit assessment of the degree and duration of the straining effort.[100,101]

The normal response to the Valsalva maneuver consists of four phases. Phase I is associated with a transient rise in systemic arterial pressure as straining commences. Phase II is accompanied by a perceptible decrease in systemic venous return, systolic pressure, and pulse pressure (small pulse) and by reflex tachycardia. Phase III begins promptly with cessation of straining and is associated with an abrupt, transient decrease in arterial pressure. Phase IV is characterized by an overshoot of systemic arterial pressure and reflex bradycardia. During phase II, S_3 and S_4 are attenuated and the A_2-P_2 interval narrows or is abolished. As stroke volume and systemic arterial pressure fall, the systolic murmurs of aortic and pulmonary stenosis and of mitral and tricuspid regurgitation diminish and the diastolic murmurs of aortic and pulmonary regurgitation and of tricuspid and mitral stenosis soften. As left ventricular volume is reduced, the systolic murmur of hypertrophic obstructive cardiomyopathy amplifies and the click and late systolic murmur of mitral valve prolapse begin earlier. In phase III, the sudden increase in systemic venous return is accompanied by wide splitting of the S_2 and by augmentation of murmurs and filling sounds in the right side of the heart. Murmurs and filling sounds in the left side of the heart return to control levels and may transiently increase during the overshoot of phase IV.

In patients with atrial septal defect, mitral stenosis, or heart failure, the Valsalva maneuver provokes a "square wave" response, negating the four phases and their auscultatory equivalents. The Valsalva maneuver should not be performed in patients with ischemic heart disease because of the accompanying fall in coronary blood flow.

THE MULLER MANEUVER. This maneuver is the converse of the Valsalva maneuver but is less frequently employed because it is not as useful. In this maneuver, the patient forcibly inspires while the nose is held closed and the mouth is firmly sealed for about 10 seconds. The Muller maneuver exaggerates the inspiratory effort, widens the split S_2, and augments murmurs and filling sounds originating in the right side of the heart.

POSTURAL CHANGES AND EXERCISE (Fig. 8-35)

Sudden assumption of the lying position from the standing or sitting position or sudden passive elevation of both legs results in an increase in venous return, which augments first right ventricular and, several cardiac cycles later, left ventricular stroke volume. The principal auscultatory changes include widening of the splitting of S_2 in all phases of respiration and augmentations of right-sided S_3 and S_4 and, several cardiac cycles later, left-sided S_3 and S_4. The systolic murmurs of pulmonic valve stenosis and aortic stenosis, the systolic murmurs of mitral and tricuspid regurgitation and ventricular septal defect, and most functional systolic murmurs are augmented. On the other hand, because left ventricular end-diastolic volume is increased, the systolic murmur of hypertrophic obstructive cardiomyopathy is diminished and the midsystolic click and late systolic murmur associated with mitral valve prolapse are delayed and sometimes attenuated (see Fig. 8-12).

Rapid standing or sitting up from a lying position or rapid standing from a squatting posture has the opposite effect; in patients in whom there is relatively wide splitting of S_2 during exhalation—a finding that may be confused with fixed splitting—the width of the splitting is reduced, so that a normal pattern emerges during the respiratory cycle. No change in splitting occurs in patients with true fixed splitting. The decrease in venous return reduces stroke volume and innocent pulmonary flow murmurs as well as the murmurs of semilunar valve stenosis and of AV valve regurgitation. The auscultatory changes in hypertrophic cardiomyopathy and mitral valve prolapse are opposite to those on assumption of the lying posture just described.

SQUATTING. A sudden change from standing to squatting increases venous return and systemic resistance simultaneously. Stroke volume and arterial pressure rise, and the latter may induce a transient reflex bradycardia. The auscultatory features include augmentation of S_3 and S_4 (from both ventricles) and as a consequence of an increase in stroke volume, the systolic murmurs of pulmonary and aortic stenosis and the diastolic murmurs of tricuspid and mitral stenosis become louder, with right-sided events preceding left-sided events. Squatting may make audible a previously inaudible murmur of aortic regurgitation.

The elevation of arterial pressure increases blood flow through the right ventricular outflow tract of patients with tetralogy of Fallot and increases the volume of mitral regurgitation and of the left-to-right shunt through a ventricular septal defect, thereby increasing the intensity of the systolic murmur in these conditions. Also, the diastolic murmur of aortic regurgitation is augmented consequent to an increase in aortic reflux. The combination of elevated arterial pressure and increased venous return increases left ventricular size, which reduces the obstruction to outflow and thus the intensity of the systolic murmur of hypertrophic obstructive cardiomyopathy; the midsystolic click and the late systolic murmur of mitral valve prolapse are delayed.

OTHER POSITIONAL CHANGES. Assumption of the left lateral recumbent position accentuates the intensity of S_1, S_3, and S_4 originating from the left side of the heart; the opening snap and the murmurs associated with mitral stenosis and regurgitation; the midsystolic click and late systolic murmur of mitral valve prolapse; and the Austin Flint murmur associated with aortic regurgitation. Sitting up and leaning forward (see Fig. 8-10D) make the diastolic murmurs of aortic and pulmonary regurgitation more readily audible.

Stretching the neck to elicit a venous hum is illustrated in Figure 8-32. Passive elevation of the legs with the patient supine transiently increases venous return and augments S_3.

ISOMETRIC EXERCISE. This can be carried out simply and reproducibly using a calibrated handgrip device or hand ball. (It is useful to carry out isometric exercise bilaterally simultaneously.) Isometric exercise should be avoided in patients with ventricular arrhythmias and myocardial ischemia, both of which can be intensified by this activity. Handgrip should be sustained for 20 to 30 seconds, but a Valsalva maneuver during the handgrip must be avoided. Isometric exercise results in transient but significant increases in systemic vascular resistance, arterial pressure, heart rate, cardiac output, left ventricular filling pressure, and heart size.

As a consequence, (1) S_3 and S_4 originating from the left side of the heart become accentuated; (2) the systolic murmur of aortic stenosis is diminished as a result of reduction of the pressure gradient across the aortic valve[102]; (3) the diastolic murmur of aortic regurgitation and the systolic murmurs of rheumatic mitral regurgitation and ventricular septal defect increase in intensity; (4) the diastolic murmur of mitral stenosis becomes louder consequent to the increase in cardiac output; and (5) the systolic murmur of hypertrophic obstructive cardiomyopathy diminishes and the systolic click and late systolic murmur of mitral valve prolapse are delayed because of the increased left ventricular volume.

PHARMACOLOGICAL AGENTS (see Fig. 8-35)

AMYL NITRITE. Inhalation of amyl nitrite is carried out by placing an ampule in gauze near the supine patient's nose and then crushing the ampule. The patient is asked to take three or four deep breaths over 10 to 15 seconds, after which the amyl nitrite is removed. The drug produces marked vasodilatation, resulting in the first 30 seconds in a reduction of systemic arterial pressure and 30 to 60 seconds later in a

Diagnosis	Systolic Murmur	Second Sound	Effect of Posture: Erect	Effect of Posture: Squatting	Amyl Nitrite	Phenyl-ephrine
			Changes in intensity of systolic murmur			
1. Hypertrophic obstructive cardiomyopathy		Variable ie - reversed partially reversed narrow or normal	↑	↓	↑	↓
2. Mitral regurgitation a. Pure severe		widely split	↓	↑	↓	↑
b. Papillary muscle dysfunction		normal or partially reversed	↑↓	↑	↓	↑
c. Billowing posterior leaflet		normal	↑↓	↑	↓	↑
d. Rheumatic of moderate degree		slightly wide	↓	↑	↓	↑
3. Valvular aortic stenosis: mild to mod		narrow or partially reversed	↓	↑	↑	—
3. Valvular aortic stenosis: marked		reversed	↓	↑	↑	—
4. Ventricular septal defect		slightly wide	– ↓	↑	↓	↑
5. Innocent vibratory systolic murmur		normal	↓	—	↑	↓

— No change from control ↑ ↑ Degree of increase ↓ ↓ Degree of decrease

FIGURE 8–35 Diagrammatic representation of the character of the systolic murmur and of the second heart sound in five conditions. The effects of posture, amyl nitrite inhalation, and phenylephrine injection on the intensity of the murmur are shown. (Modified from Barlow JB: Perspectives on the Mitral Valve. Philadelphia, FA Davis, 1987, p 138.)

reflex tachycardia, followed in turn by a reflex increase in cardiac output, velocity of blood flow, and heart rate.[4,97,101,103] The major auscultatory changes occur in the first 30 seconds after inhalation. S_1 is augmented, and A_2 is diminished. The opening snaps of the mitral and tricuspid valves become louder, and as arterial pressure falls, the A_2/opening snap interval shortens. An S_3 originating in either ventricle is augmented, owing to greater rapidity of ventricular filling; but because mitral regurgitation is reduced, the S_3 associated with this lesion is diminished. The systolic murmurs of aortic valve stenosis, pulmonary stenosis, hypertrophic obstructive cardiomyopathy, tricuspid regurgitation, and functional systolic murmurs are all accentuated.

The response to amyl nitrite is useful in distinguishing (1) the systolic murmur of aortic stenosis (which is augmented) from that of mitral regurgitation (which is diminished)[103]; (2) the systolic murmur of tricuspid regurgitation (augmented) from that of mitral regurgitation (diminished); (3) the systolic murmur of isolated pulmonary stenosis (augmented) from that of tetralogy of Fallot (diminished); (4) the diastolic rumbling murmur of mitral stenosis (augmented) from the Austin Flint murmur of aortic regurgitation (diminished); and (5) the early blowing diastolic murmur of pulmonary regurgitation (augmented) from that of aortic regurgitation (diminished).

In patients with tetralogy of Fallot, the reduction of arterial pressure increases the right-to-left shunt and decreases the blood flow from the right ventricle to the pulmonary artery and diminishes the midsystolic murmur. The increase in cardiac output augments the diastolic murmurs of mitral and tricuspid stenosis and of pulmonary regurgitation and the systolic murmur of tricuspid regurgitation. However, as a result of the fall in systemic arterial pressure, the systolic murmurs of mitral regurgitation and ventricular septal defect, the diastolic murmurs of aortic regurgitation, and the Austin Flint murmur as well as the continuous murmurs of patent ductus arteriosus and of systemic arteriovenous fistula are all diminished. The reduction of cardiac size results in an earlier appearance of the midsystolic click and late systolic murmur of mitral valve prolapse; the intensity of the systolic murmur exhibits a variable response.

METHOXAMINE AND PHENYLEPHRINE. These agents increase systemic arterial pressure and exert an effect opposite to that of amyl nitrite. Phenylephrine is preferred because of its shorter duration of action; when administered intravenously it elevates systolic pressure by approximately 30 mm Hg for only 3 to 5 minutes. Both drugs cause reflex bradycardia and decreased contractility and cardiac output. They should not be used in the presence of congestive heart failure and systemic hypertension.

After administration, the intensity of S_1 is usually reduced, and the A_2/mitral opening snap interval becomes prolonged. The responses of S_3 and S_4 are variable. As a result of the increased arterial pressure, the diastolic murmur of aortic regurgitation, the systolic murmurs of mitral regurgitation, ventricular septal defect, and tetralogy of Fallot, and the continuous murmurs of patent ductus arteriosus and systemic arteriovenous fistula all become louder. On the other hand, as a consequence of the increase in left ventricular size, the systolic murmur of hypertrophic obstructive cardiomyopathy becomes softer and the click and late systolic murmur of mitral valve prolapse are delayed. The reduction in cardiac output diminishes the systolic murmur of aortic valve stenosis, functional systolic murmurs, and the diastolic murmur of mitral stenosis. The rumbling diastolic murmurs of mitral regurgitation and the Austin Flint murmur also diminish.

REFERENCES

The General Physical Examination

1. Mangione S, Nieman LZ, Gracely E, et al: The teaching and practice of cardiac auscultation during internal medicine and cardiology training: A nationwide survey. Ann Intern Med 119:47, 1993.
2. Shaver JA: Cardiac auscultation: A cost-effective diagnostic skill. Curr Probl Cardiol 20:441, 1995.
3. Tavel M: Cardiac auscultation: A glorious past—but does it have a future? Circulation 93:1250, 1996.
4. Perloff JK: Physical Examination of the Heart and Circulation. 3rd ed. Philadelphia, WB Saunders, 2000.
5. Roldan CA, Abrams J (eds): Evaluation of the Patient with Heart Disease: Integrating the Physical Exam and Echocardiography. Philadelphia: Lippincott Williams & Wilkins, 2002, pp 383.
6. Swartz MH (ed): Textbook of Physical Diagnosis: History and Examination. 3rd ed. Philadelphia, WB Saunders, 1998.
7. O'Rourke RA, Braunwald E: Physical Examination of the Cardiovascular System. *In* Kasper DL et al (eds): Harrison's Principles of Internal Medicine. 16th ed. New York: McGraw-Hill, 2005.
8. Kirkham N, Murrels T, Melcher SH, Morrison EA: Diagonal ear lobe creases and fatal cardiovascular disease: A necropsy study. Br Heart J 61:361, 1989.
9. Woywodt A, Welzel J, Haase H, et al: Cardiomyopathic lentiginosis/LEOPARD syndrome presenting as sudden cardiac arrest. Chest 113:1415, 1998.
10. Basson CT, Cowley GS, Solomon SD, et al: The clinical and genetic spectrum of the Holt-Oram syndrome (heart-hand syndrome). N Engl J Med 330:885, 1994.
11. Buckley MJ, Mason DT, Ross J Jr, Braunwald E: Reversed differential cyanosis with equal desaturation of the upper limbs: Syndrome of complete transposition of the great vessels with complete interruption of the aortic arch. Am J Cardiol 15:111, 1965.
12. Fishman AP: Approach to the patient with respiratory symptoms. *In* Fishman AP (ed): Pulmonary Diseases and Disorders. New York, McGraw-Hill, 1998, pp. 361-394.
13. Yee J, McAllister CK: The utility of Osler's nodes in the diagnosis of infective endocarditis. Chest 92:751, 1987.
14. Braunwald E: Edema. *In* Kasper DL, et al (eds): Harrison's Principles of Internal Medicine. 16th ed. New York, McGraw-Hill, 2005.
15. Willekes CL, Backer CL, Mavroudis C: A 26-year review of pectus deformity repairs, including simultaneous intracardiac repair. Ann Thorac Surg 67:511, 1999.
16. Fonkalsrud EW, Bustorff-Silva J: Repair of pectus excavatum and carinatum in adults. Am J Surg 177:121, 1999.
17. Wiese J: The abdominojugular reflux sign. Am J Med 109:59, 2000.
18. Butman SM, Ewy GA, Standen JR, et al: Bedside cardiovascular examination in patients with severe chronic heart failure: Importance of rest or inducible jugular venous distension. J Am Coll Cardiol 22:968, 1993.
19. Perloff JK: The jugular venous pulse and third heart sound in patients with heart failure. N Engl J Med 345:612, 2001.
20. Bilchick KC, Wise RA: Paradoxical physical findings described by Kussmaul: Pulsus paradoxus and Kussmaul's sign. Lancet 359:1940, 2002.
21. Drazner MH, Rame JE, Stevenson LW, Dries DL: Prognostic importance of elevated jugular venous pressure and a third heart sound in patients with heart failure. N Engl J Med 345:574, 2001.
22. Linfors EW, Feussner JR, Blessing CL, et al: Spurious hypertension in the obese patient: Effect of sphygmomanometer cuff size on prevalence of hypertension. Arch Intern Med 144:1482, 1984.
23. Nelson WP, Egbert AM: How to measure blood pressure accurately. Prim Cardiol 10:14, 1984.
24. Gould BA, Hornung RS, Kieso HA, et al: Is the blood pressure the same in both arms? Clin Cardiol 8:423, 1985.
25. Sapira JD: Quincke, de Musset, Duroziez, and Hill: Some aortic regurgitations. South Med J 74:459, 1981.
26. Vlachopoulos C, O'Rourke M: Genesis of the normal and abnormal pulse. Curr Prob Cardiol 25:297, 2000.
27. Perloff JK: The physiologic mechanisms of cardiac and vascular physical signs. J Am Coll Cardiol 1:184, 1983.
28. Brown DV: Dicrotic pulse in pericardial tamponade. J Cardiothorac Vasc Anesth 16:742, 2002.
29. Safar ME, Levy BI, Struijker-Boudier H: Current perspectives on arterial stiffness and pulse pressure in hypertension and cardiovascular diseases. Circulation 107:2864, 2003.
30. Elkins RC, Morrow AG, Vasko JS, Braunwald E: The effects of mitral regurgitation on the pattern of instantaneous aortic blood flow: Clinical and experimental observations. Circulation 36:45, 1967.
31. Talley JD: Recognition, etiology, and clinical implications of pulsus bisferiens. Heart Dis Stroke 3:309, 1994.
32. Smith D, Craige E: Mechanisms of the dicrotic pulse. Br Heart J 56:531, 1986.
33. Talley JD: Dicrotism: Examples and review of the dicrotic pulse. J Ark Med Soc 92:507, 1996.
34. Morpurgo M, Boutarin J: Right-sided pulsus alternans: A neglected phenomenon. Cardiologia 40:803, 1995.
35. Lab MJ, Seed WA: Pulsus alternans. Cardiovasc Res 27:1407, 1993.
36. Rosenthal E: Extreme pulsus alternans presenting as 2:1 electromechanical dissociation. Br Heart J 74:695, 1995.
37. Brockenbrough EC, Braunwald E, Morrow AG: A hemodynamic technic for the detection of hypertrophic subaortic stenosis. Circulation 23:189, 1961.
38. Fowler NO: Pulsus paradoxus. Heart Dis Stroke 3:68, 1994.
39. Pearson MG, Spence DP, Ryland I, Harrison BD: Value of pulsus paradoxus in assessing acute severe asthma. BMJ 307:659, 1993.
40. Jay GD, Onuma K, Davis R, et al: Analysis of physician ability in the measurement of pulsus paradoxus by sphygmomanometry. Chest 118:348, 2000.
41. Swami A, Spodick DH: Pulsus paradoxus in cardiac tamponade: A pathophysiologic continuum. Clin Cardiol 26:215, 2003.
42. Mowlavi A, Whiteman J, Wilhelmi BJ, et al: Dorsalis pedis arterial pulse: Palpation using a bony landmark. Postgrad Med J 78:746, 2002.
43. Hirsch AT: Recognition and management of peripheral arterial disease. *In* Braunwald E, Goldman L (eds): Primary Cardiology. 2nd ed. Philadelphia: Elsevier, 2003.
44. Beiser GD, Epstein SE, Stampfer M, et al: Impairment of cardiac function in patients with pectus excavatum. N Engl J Med 287:267, 1972.

The Cardiac Examination

45. Abrams J: Precordial palpation. *In* Horwitz LD, Groves BM (eds): Signs and Symptoms in Cardiology. Philadelphia, JB Lippincott, 1985, pp. 156-177.
46. Ellen SD, Crawford MH, O'Rourke RA: Accuracy of precordial palpation for detecting increased left ventricular volume. Ann Intern Med 99:628, 1983.
47. Ellen SD, et al: Accuracy of precordial palpation for detecting increased left ventricular volume. Ann Intern Med 99:628, 1983.
48. Ranganathan N, Juma Z, Sivaciyan V: The apical impulse in coronary heart disease. Clin Cardiol 8:20, 1985.

49. Adolph RJ: In defense of the stethoscope. Chest 114:1235, 1998.
50. Abrams J: Synopsis of cardiac physical diagnosis. 2nd ed. Boston: Butterworth Heinemann, 2001.

Heart Sounds

51. O'Toole JD, Reddy PS, Curtiss EL, et al: The contribution of tricuspid valve closure to the first heart sound: An intracardiac micromanometer study. Circulation 53:752, 1976.
52. Brooks N, Leech G, Leatham A: Complete right bundle branch block: Echophonocardiographic study of the first heart sound and right ventricular contraction times. Br Heart J 41:637, 1979.
53. Burggraf GW: The first heart sound in left bundle branch block: An echophonocardiographic study. Circulation 63:429, 1981.
54. Leech G, Brooks N, Green-Wilkinson A, Leatham A: Mechanism of influence of PR interval on loudness of first heart sound. Br Heart J 43:138, 1980.
55. Perloff JK: The Clinical Recognition of Congenital Heart Disease. 5th ed. Philadelphia, WB Saunders, 2003.
56. Mills PG, Brodie B, McLaurin L, et al: Echocardiographic and hemodynamic relationships of ejection sounds. Circulation 56:430, 1977.
57. Lembo NJ, Dell'Italia JL, Crawford MH, O'Rourke RA: Bedside diagnosis of systolic murmurs. N Engl J Med 318:1572, 1988.
58. Leatham A: Splitting of the first and second heart sounds. Lancet 2:607, 1954.
59. Kupari M: Aortic valve closure and cardiac vibrations in the genesis of the second heart sound. Am J Cardiol 52:152, 1983.
60. Curtiss EI, Matthews DG, Shaver JA: Mechanism of normal splitting of the second heart sound. Circulation 51:157, 1975.
61. Shaver JA, Nadolny RA, O'Toole JD, et al: Sound-pressure correlates of the second heart sound. Circulation 49:316, 1974.
62. Xiao HB, Faiek AH, Gibson DG: Re-evaluation of normal splitting of the second heart sound in patients with classical left bundle branch block. Int J Cardiol 45:163, 1994.
63. Hultgren HN, Craige E, Nakamura T, Bilisoly J: Left bundle branch block and mechanical events of the cardiac cycle. Am J Cardiol 52:755, 1985.
64. Tokushima T, Utsunomiya T, Ogawa T, et al: Contrast-enhanced radiographic computed tomographic findings in patients with straight back syndrome. Am J Card Imaging 10:228, 1996.
65. Wood P: An appreciation of mitral stenosis: I. Clinical features. BMJ 1:1051, 1954; II. Investigations and results. BMJ 1:1113, 1954.
66. Tyberg TI, Goodyer AVN, Langou RA: Genesis of the pericardial knock in constrictive pericarditis. Am J Cardiol 46:570, 1980.
67. Bass NM, Sharatt GJP: Left atrial myxoma diagnosed by echocardiography with observations on tumor movement. Br Heart J 35:1332, 1973.
68. Van de Werf F, Minten J, Carmeliet P, et al: Genesis of the third and fourth heart sounds. J Clin Invest 73:1400, 1984.
69. Van de Werf F, Boel A, Geboers J, et al: Diastolic properties of the left ventricle in normal adults and in patients with third heart sounds. Circulation 69:1070, 1984.
70. Drzewiecki GM, Wasicko MJ, Li JK: Diastolic mechanics and the origin of the third heart sound. Ann Biomed Eng 19:651, 1991.
71. Glower DD, Murrah RL, Olsen CO, et al: Mechanical correlates of the third heart sound. J Am Coll Cardiol 19:450, 1992.
72. Downes TR, Dunson W, Stewart K, et al: Mechanism of physiologic and pathologic S_3 gallop sounds. Am Soc Echocardiol 5:211, 1992.
73. Tribouilloy CM, Enriquez-Sarano M, Mohty D, et al: Pathophysiologic determinants of third heart sounds: A prospective clinical and Doppler echocardiographic study. Am J Med 111:96, 2001.
74. Adolph RJ: The fourth heart sound. Chest 115:1480, 1999.
75. Baracca E, Scorzoni D, Brunazzi MC, et al: Genesis and acoustic quality of the physiological fourth heart sound. Acta Cardiol 50:23, 1995.
76. Ishikawa M, Sakata K, Maki A, et al: Prognostic significance of a clearly audible fourth heart sound detected a month after an acute myocardial infarction. Am J Cardiol 80:619, 1997.

Heart Murmurs

77. O'Rourke R: Approach to the patient with a heart murmur. *In* Braunwald E, Goldman L (eds): Primary Cardiology. 2nd ed. Philadelphia: Elsevier, 2003, pp 155-173.
78. Grewe K, et al: Differentiation of cardiac murmurs by auscultation. Curr Probl Cardiol 13:699, 1988.
79. Lembo NJ, et al: Bedside diagnosis of systolic murmurs. N Engl J Med 318:1572, 1988.
80. Ecchells E, et al: Does this patient have an abnormal systolic murmur? JAMA 277:564, 1997.
81. Joffe HS: Genesis of Still's innocent systolic murmur. Br Heart J 67:206, 1992
82. Donnerstein RL, Thomsen VS: Hemodynamic and anatomic factors affecting the frequency content of Still's innocent murmur. Am J Cardiol 74:508, 1994.
83. Perloff JK, Roberts WC: The mitral apparatus: Functional anatomy of mitral regurgitation. Circulation 46:227, 1972.
84. Ronan JA, Steelman RB, DeLeon AC, et al: The clinical diagnosis of acute severe mitral insufficiency. Am J Cardiol 27:284, 1971.
85. Rios JC, Massumi RA, Breesman WT, Sarin RK: Auscultatory features of acute tricuspid regurgitation. Am J Cardiol 23:4, 1969.
86. Fontana ME: Mitral valve prolapse and floppy mitral valve: Physical examination. *In* Mitral Valve: Floppy Mitral Valve, Mitral Valve Prolapse, Mitral Valvular Regurgitation. 2nd ed. Armouk, NY, Futura, 2000, pp 283-304.
87. Fortuin NJ, Craige E: Echocardiographic studies of genesis of mitral diastolic murmurs. Br Heart J 35:75, 1973.
88. Flint A: On cardiac murmurs. Am J Med Sci 44:23, 1862.
89. Landzberg JS, Tflugfelder PW, Cassidy MM, et al: Etiology of the Austin Flint murmur. J Am Coll Cardiol 20:408, 1992.
90. Reddy PS, Curtiss EL, Salerni R: Sound-pressure correlates of the Austin Flint murmur: An intracardiac sound study. Circulation 53:210, 1976.
91. Berman P: Austin Flint—America's Laennec revisited. Arch Intern Med 148:2053, 1988.
92. Gibson GA: Persistence of the arterial duct and its diagnosis. Edinb Med J 8:1, 1900.
93. Cutforth R, Wideman J, Sutherland RD: The genesis of the cervical venous hum. Am Heart J 80:488, 1970.
94. Spodick DH: Auscultatory phenomena in pericardial disease. *In* Spodick DH: The Pericardium: A Comprehensive Textbook. New York, Marcel Dekker, 1997, pp 27-39.
95. Hamman L: Mediastinal emphysema. JAMA 128:1, 1945.

Dynamic Auscultation

96. Grewe K, Crawford MH, O'Rourke RA: Differentiation of cardiac murmurs by dynamic auscultation. Curr Probl Cardiol 13:671, 1988.
97. Lembro NJ, Dell'Italia LJ, Crawford MH, O'Rourke RA: Bedside diagnosis of systolic murmurs. N Engl J Med 318:1572, 1988.
98. Cha SD, Gooch AS: Diagnosis of tricuspid regurgitation. Arch Intern Med 143:1763, 1983.
99. Barlow JB: Perspectives on the Mitral Valve. Philadelphia, FA Davis, 1987.
100. Vrewe K, Crawford MH, O'Rourke RA: Differentiation of cardiac murmurs by dynamic auscultation. Curr Probl Cardiol 13:671, 1988.
101. Nishimura RA, Tajik AJ: The Valsalva maneuver and response revisited. Mayo Clin Proc 61:211, 1986.
102. McCraw DB, Siegel W, Stonecipher HK, et al: Response of the heart murmur intensity to isometric (handgrip) exercise. Br Heart J 34:605, 1972.
103. Barlow J, Shillingford J: The use of amyl nitrite in differentiating mitral and aortic systolic murmurs. Br Heart J 20:162, 1958.

CHAPTER 9

Electrocardiography

David M. Mirvis • Ary L. Goldberger

The electrocardiogram (ECG), as used today, is the product of a series of technological and physiological advances pioneered over the past two centuries.[1] Early demonstrations of the heart's electrical activity reported during the last half of the 19th century, for example, by Marchand and others, were closely followed by direct recordings of cardiac potentials by Waller in 1887. Invention of the string galvanometer by Willem Einthoven in 1901 provided a reliable and direct method for registering electrical activity of the heart. By 1910, use of the string galvanometer had emerged from the research laboratory into the clinic.

Subsequent achievements built on the very solid foundation supplied by the early electrocardiographers. The result has become a widely used and invaluable clinical tool for the detection and diagnosis of a broad range of cardiac conditions, as well as a technique that has contributed to the understanding and treatment of virtually every type of heart disease. Electrocardiography remains the most direct method for assessing abnormalities of cardiac rhythm. Furthermore, the ECG is essential in the management of major metabolic abnormalities such as hyperkalemia and certain other electrolyte disorders, as well as in assessing drug effects and toxicities such as those caused by digitalis, antiarrhythmic agents, and tricyclic antidepressants. More than 7 million ECGs are performed in the United States each year, making ECG the most commonly performed as well as the oldest cardiovascular laboratory procedure.

Fundamental Principles

Use of the ECG for any of these clinically important purposes is the final outcome of a complex series of physiological and technological processes. This sequence is depicted in Figure 9-1. First, an extracellular cardiac electrical field is generated by ion fluxes across cell membranes and between adjacent cells. These ion currents are synchronized by cardiac activation and recovery sequences to generate a cardiac electrical field in and around the heart that varies with time during the cardiac cycle. This electrical field passes through numerous other structures, including the lungs, blood, and skeletal muscle before reaching the body surface. These elements, known as *transmission factors,* differ in their electrical properties and perturb the cardiac electrical field as it passes through them.

The potentials reaching the skin are then detected by electrodes placed in specific locations on the extremities and torso and configured to produce leads. The outputs of these leads are amplified, filtered, and displayed by a variety of electronic devices to construct an ECG recording. Finally, diagnostic criteria are applied to these recordings to produce an interpretation. The criteria have statistical characteristics that determine the clinical utility of the findings. Each of these steps influences the final product—the clinical ECG—and are considered in detail in this chapter to provide a foundation for considering the common abnormalities found in clinical practice and as a basis for further learning.

GENESIS OF THE CARDIAC ELECTRICAL FIELD

CARDIAC ELECTRICAL FIELD GENERATION DURING ACTIVATION. Transmembrane ionic currents are ultimately responsible for the cardiac potentials that are recorded as an ECG. Current may be analyzed as though carried by positively charged or negatively charged ions. Through a purely arbitrary choice, electrophysiological currents are considered to be the movement of positive charge. A positive current moving in one direction is equivalent to a negative current of equal strength moving in the opposite direction.

The process of generating the cardiac electrical field during activation can be illustrated by considering the events in a single cardiac fiber, 20 mm in length, that is activated by a stimulus applied to its left-most margin (Fig. 9-2A). Transmembrane potentials (V_m) are recorded as the difference between intracellular and extracellular potentials (ϕ_e and ϕ_i, respectively). Figure 9-2B plots V_m along the length of the fiber at the instant during the propagation (t_o) at which activation has reached the point designated as X_0. As each site is activated, the polarity of the transmembrane potential is converted from negative to positive. Thus, sites to the left of the point X_0, which have already undergone excitation, have positive transmembrane potentials (that is, the inside of the cell is positive relative to the outside of the cell), whereas those to the right of X_0 (which remain in a resting state) have negative transmembrane potentials. Near the site undergoing activation (site X_0), the potentials reverse polarity over a short distance.

Figure 9-2C displays the direction and magnitude of transmembrane currents (I_m) along the fiber at the instant (t_o) at which excitation has reached site X_0. Current flow is inwardly directed in fiber regions that have undergone activation (that is, to the left of point X_0) and outwardly directed in neighboring zones still at rest (that is, to the right of X_0). Sites of outward current flow are *current sources* and those with inward current flow are *current sinks.* As depicted in the figure, current flow is most intense in each direction near the site of activation X_0. Because the border between inwardly and outwardly directed currents is relatively sharp, we can visualize these currents as though they were limited to the sites of maximal current flow, as depicted in Figure 9-2D, and separated by distance d that is usually 1.0 mm or less. As activation proceeds along the fiber, the source-sink pair moves to the right at the speed of propagation for the particular type of fiber.

Two point sources of equal strength but of opposite polarity located very near each other, such

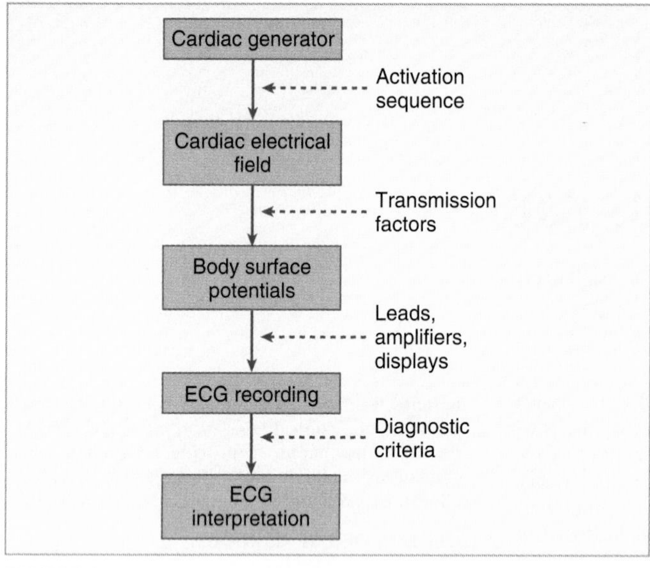

FIGURE 9–1 Schematic representation of the factors resulting in recording the electrocardiogram (ECG). The major paths leading to the ECG are marked by solid arrows and factors influencing or perturbing this path are shown with dashed arrows.

as the current source and the current sink depicted in Figure 9-2D, can be represented as a *current dipole*. Thus, activation of a fiber can be modeled as a current dipole that moves in the direction of propagation of activation. Such a dipole is fully characterized by three parameters: strength or dipole moment, location, and orientation. In this case, the location of the dipole is the site undergoing activation (point X_0), and its orientation is in the direction of activation (that is, from left to right along the fiber). Dipole moment is proportional to the rate of change of intracellular potential with respect to distance along the fiber, that is, action potential shape.

A current dipole produces a characteristic potential field with positive potentials projected ahead of it and negative potentials projected behind it. The actual potential recorded at any site within this field is directly proportional to the dipole moment, inversely proportional to the square of the distance from the dipole to the recording site, and directly proportional to the cosine of the angle between the axis of the dipole and a line drawn from the dipole to the recording site.

This example from one cardiac fiber can be generalized to the more realistic case in which multiple adjacent fibers are activated in synchrony to produce an activation front. Activation of each fiber creates a dipole oriented in the direction of activation. The net effect of all the dipoles in this wave front is a single dipole equal to the (vector) sum of the effects of all the simultaneously active component dipoles. Thus, an activation front propagating through the heart can be represented by a single dipole that projects positive potentials ahead of it and negative potentials behind it.

This relationship between activation direction, orientation of the current dipole, and polarity of potentials is a critical one in electrocardiography. It describes a fundamental relationship between the polarity of potentials sensed by an electrode and the direction of movement of an activation front: an electrode senses positive potentials when an activation front is moving toward it and negative potentials when the activation front is moving away from it.

The dipole model, though useful in describing cardiac fields and understanding clinical electrocardiography, has significant theoretical limitations. These limits derive primarily from the inability of a single dipole to accurately represent more than one wave front that is propagating through the heart at any one instant. As will be discussed, during much of the time of ventricular excitation, more than one wave front is present.

Solid Angle Theorem. One important and commonly used method of estimating the potentials projected to some point away from an activation front is an application of the *solid angle theorem*. A *solid angle* is a geometric measure of the size of a region when viewed from a distant site. It equals the area on the surface of a sphere of unit radius constructed around an electrode that is cut by lines drawn from the recording electrode to all points around the boundary of the region of interest.

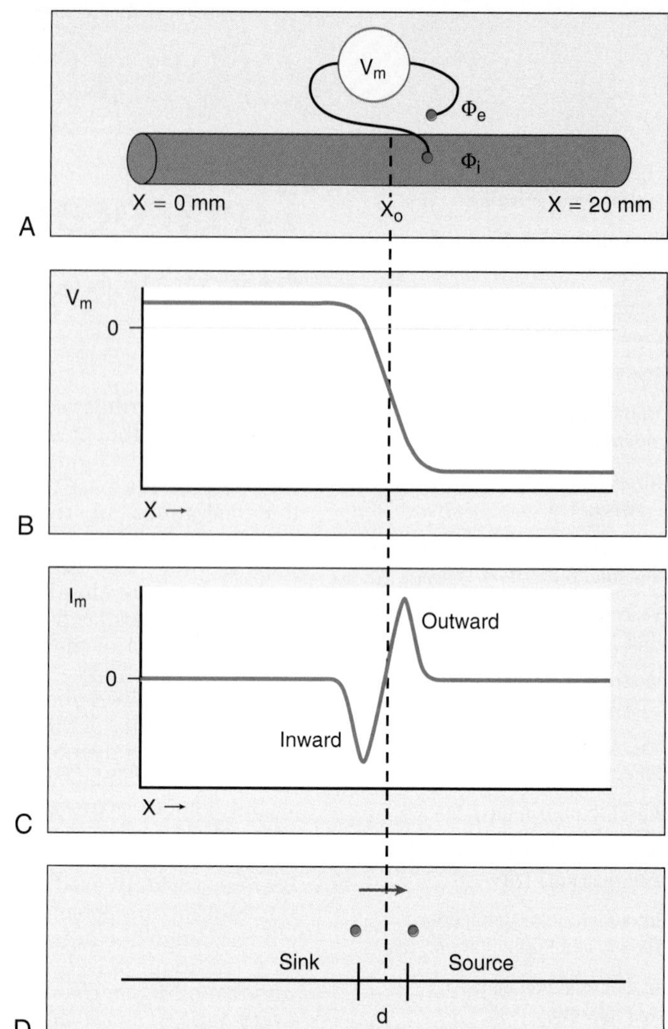

FIGURE 9–2 Example of potentials and currents generated by the activation of a single (e.g., ventricular) cardiac fiber. **A,** Intracellular (ϕ_i) and extracellular (ϕ_e) potentials are recorded with a voltmeter (Vm) from a fiber 20 mm in length. The fiber is stimulated at site X = 0 mm, and propagation proceeds from left to right. **B,** Plot of transmembrane potential (Vm) at the instant in time at which activation reaches point X_0 as a function of the length of the fiber. Positive potentials are recorded from activated tissue to the left of site X_0, and negative ones are registered from not yet excited areas to the right of site X_0. **C,** Membrane current (I_m) flows along the length of the fiber at time t_0. The outward current is the depolarizing current that propagates ahead of activation site X_0, while an inward one flows behind site X_0. **D,** Representation of the sites of peak inward and outward current flow as two point sources, a sink (at the site of peak inward current flow) and a source (at the site of peak outward current flow) separated by distance d. The dipole produced by the source-sink pair is represented by the arrow. (Modified from Barr RC: Genesis of the electrocardiogram. *In* MacFarlane PW, Lawrie TDV [eds]: Comprehensive Electrocardiography. New York, Pergamon, 1989.)

This region may be a wave front, a zone of infarction, or any other region in the heart.

The solid angle theorem states that the potential recorded by a remote electrode (Φ) is defined by the following equation:

$$\Phi = (\Omega/4\pi)(V_{m2} - V_{m1})K$$

where Ω is the solid angle, $V_{m2} - V_{m1}$ is the potential difference across the boundary under study, and K is a constant reflecting differences in intracellular conductivity. This equation indicates that the recorded potential equals the product of two factors. First, the solid angle reflects spatial parameters, such as the size of the boundary of the region under study and the distance from the electrode to that boundary. The potential will rise as the boundary size increases and as the distance to the electrode shrinks. A second set of parameters includes nonspatial factors, such as the potential difference across the surface and intracellular and extracellular conductivity. Nonspatial effects include, as one example, myocardial ischemia, which changes transmembrane action potential shapes and alters conductivity.

CARDIAC ELECTRICAL FIELD GENERATION DURING VENTRICULAR RECOVERY. The cardiac electrical field during recovery (phases 1 through 3 of the action potential) differs in fundamental ways from that described for activation. First, intercellular potential differences and hence the directions of current flow during recovery are the opposite of those described for activation. As a cell undergoes recovery, its intracellular potential becomes progressively more negative. Hence, for two adjacent cells, the intracellular potential of the cell whose recovery has progressed further is more negative than that of an adjacent, less recovered cell. Intracellular currents then flow from the less toward the more recovered cell. An equivalent dipole can then be constructed for recovery, just as for activation. Its orientation, however, points from less to more recovered cells. Thus, the recovery dipole is oriented away from the direction of propagation of the activation front, that is, in the direction opposite that of the activation dipole.

The moment, or strength, of the recovery dipole also differs from that of the activation dipole. As described previously, the strength of the activation dipole is proportional to the rate of change in transmembrane potential. Rates of change in potential during the recovery phases of the action potential are considerably slower than during activation, so that the dipole moment at any one instant during recovery is less than during activation.

A third difference between activation and recovery is the rate of movement of the activation and recovery dipoles. Activation is rapid (as fast as 1 msec in duration) and occurs over only a small distance along the fiber. Recovery, in contrast, lasts 100 msec or longer and occurs simultaneously over extensive portions of the fiber.

These features result in characteristic ECG differences between activation and recovery patterns. All other factors being equal (an assumption that is often not true, as described later), ECG waveforms generated during recovery of a linear fiber with uniform recovery properties may be expected to be of opposite polarity, lower amplitude, and longer duration than those due to activation. As will be described, these features are explicitly demonstrated in the clinical ECG.

THE ROLE OF TRANSMISSION FACTORS. These activation and recovery forces exist within a complex three-dimensional physical environment (the *volume conductor*). The structures within the volume conductor modify the cardiac electrical field in significant ways. They are called *transmission factors* to emphasize their effects on transmission of the cardiac electrical field throughout the body and can be grouped into four broad categories: cellular factors, cardiac factors, extracardiac factors, and physical factors.

Cellular factors determine the intensity of current fluxes that result from local transmembrane potential gradients and include intracellular and extracellular resistance and the concentration of relevant ions, especially the sodium ion. Lower ion concentrations reduce the intensity of current flow and lower extracellular potentials.

Cardiac factors affect the relationship of one cardiac cell to another. Two major factors are (1) *anisotropy*, that is, the property of cardiac tissue that results in greater current flow and more rapid propagation along the length of a fiber than transversely, and (2) the presence of connective tissue between cardiac fibers that disrupts effective electrical coupling between adjacent fibers. These factors alter the paths of extracellular currents and produce changes in the amplitude and configuration of recorded electrograms. Recording electrodes oriented along the long axis of a cardiac fiber register larger potentials than do electrodes oriented perpendicular to the long axis, and waveforms recorded from fibers with little or no intervening connective tissue are narrow in width and smooth in contour, whereas those recorded from tissues with abnormal fibrosis are prolonged and heavily fractionated.

Extracardiac factors encompass all the tissues and structures that lie between the activation region and the body surface, including the ventricular walls, intracardiac and intrathoracic blood volume, the pericardium, and the lungs, as well as skeletal muscle, subcutaneous fat, and skin. These tissues alter the cardiac field because of differences in the electrical resistivity of adjacent tissues, that is, the presence of electrical inhomogeneities within the torso. For example, intracardiac blood has much lower resistivity (162 Ω-cm) than do the lungs (2150 Ω-cm). When the cardiac field encounters the boundary between two tissues with differing resistivity, the field is altered.

Other transmission factors reflect basic laws of physics. First, changes in the distance between the heart and the recording electrode reduce potential magnitudes in accord with the inverse square law; that is, amplitude decreases in proportion to the square of the distance. A related factor is the effect of eccentricity. The heart is located eccentrically within the chest; it lies closer to the anterior than to the posterior of the torso, so that the right ventricle and the anteroseptal aspect of the left ventricle are located closer to the anterior chest wall than are other parts of the left ventricle and the atria. Therefore, ECG potentials will be higher anteriorly than posteriorly, and waveforms projected from the anterior of the left ventricle to the chest wall will be greater than those generated by posterior ventricular regions.

As a result of all of these factors, body surface potentials have an amplitude of only 1 percent of the amplitude of transmembrane potentials and are smoothed in detail so that surface potentials have only a general spatial relationship to the underlying cardiac events. The modifying effect of these physical structures is a biophysical one dependent on the physical properties of the structures and the related laws of physics, in contrast to the biological cardiac generators, whose output is dependent on cellular structure and physiological and biochemical processes. Thus, ECG potentials on the body surface are dependent on both biological and biophysical properties.[2] Although changes in torso inhomogeneities within physiological ranges appear to have little impact on ECG potentials,[3] pathological changes such as those produced by anasarca do have an impact on the ECG recording.[4]

Recording Electrodes and Leads

Potentials generated by the cardiac electrical generator and modified by transmission factors are processed by a series of electrical and electronic devices to yield a clinical ECG (Fig. 9–3). They are first sensed by electrodes placed on the torso that are configured to form various types of leads.

ELECTRODE CHARACTERISTICS. Electrodes used to sense the cardiac electrical field are not passive devices that merely detect the field. Rather, they are intricate systems that are affected by the properties of the dermal and epidermal layers of the skin, the electrolytic paste applied to the skin, the electrode itself, and the mechanical contact between the electrode and skin. The net effect is a complex electrical circuit that includes resistances, capacitances, and voltages produced by these different components and the interfaces between them. Each of these factors modifies the cardiac potentials registered by the electrodes before they are displayed as an ECG.

The ECG leads can be subdivided into two general types, *bipolar leads* and *unipolar leads*. A bipolar lead consists of two electrodes placed at two different sites. These leads register the difference in potential between these two sites. The actual potential at either electrode is not known, and only the difference between them is recorded. One electrode is designated as the positive input; the potential at the other, or negative, electrode is subtracted from the potential at the positive electrode to yield the bipolar potential.

Unipolar leads, in contrast, measure the absolute electrical potential at one site. To do so requires a *reference site*—that is, a site at which the potential is deemed to be zero. The reference site may be a location far away from the active electrode (as in an experimental preparation) or, as in clinical electrocardiography, a specially designed electrode configuration (described later). The unipolar recording is then the potential sensed by a single electrode at one site—the *recording* or *active* or *exploring electrode*—in relation to the designated zero or reference potential.

Clinical Electrocardiographic Lead Systems

The standard clinical ECG includes recordings from 12 leads. These 12 leads include three *bipolar* (leads I, II, and III), six *unipolar precordial leads* (leads V_1 through V_6), and three *modified unipolar limb leads* (the augmented limb leads aV_r, aV_l, and aV_f). Definitions of the positive and negative inputs for each lead are listed in Table 9–1.

BIPOLAR LIMB LEADS. Bipolar limb leads record the potential differences between two limbs, as detailed in Table 9–1 and illustrated in Figure 9–4. As bipolar leads, the output is the potential difference between two limbs. Lead I

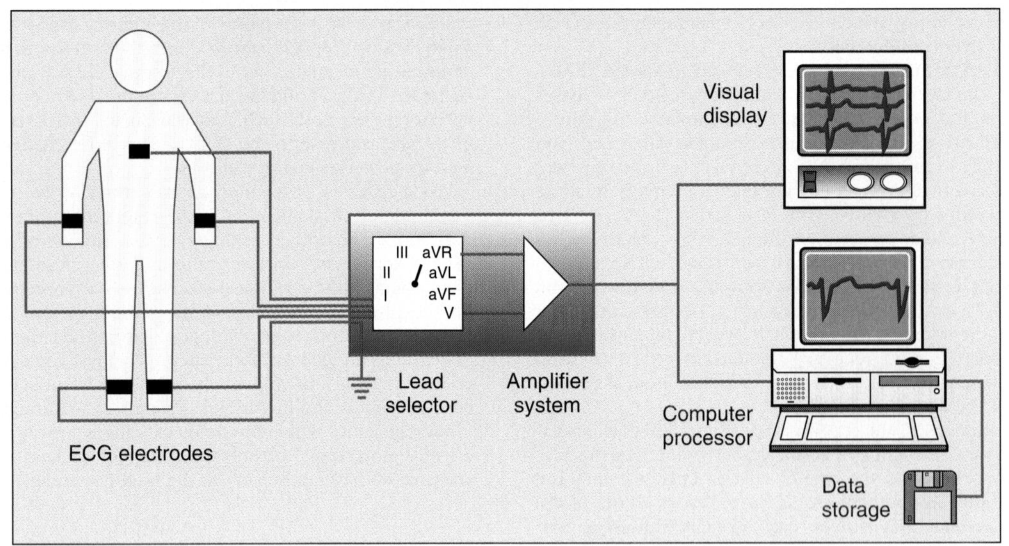

FIGURE 9–3 Components used in the recording and processing of an electrocardiogram. (From Mirvis DM: Electrocardiography: A Physiologic Approach. St Louis, Mosby-Year Book, 1993.)

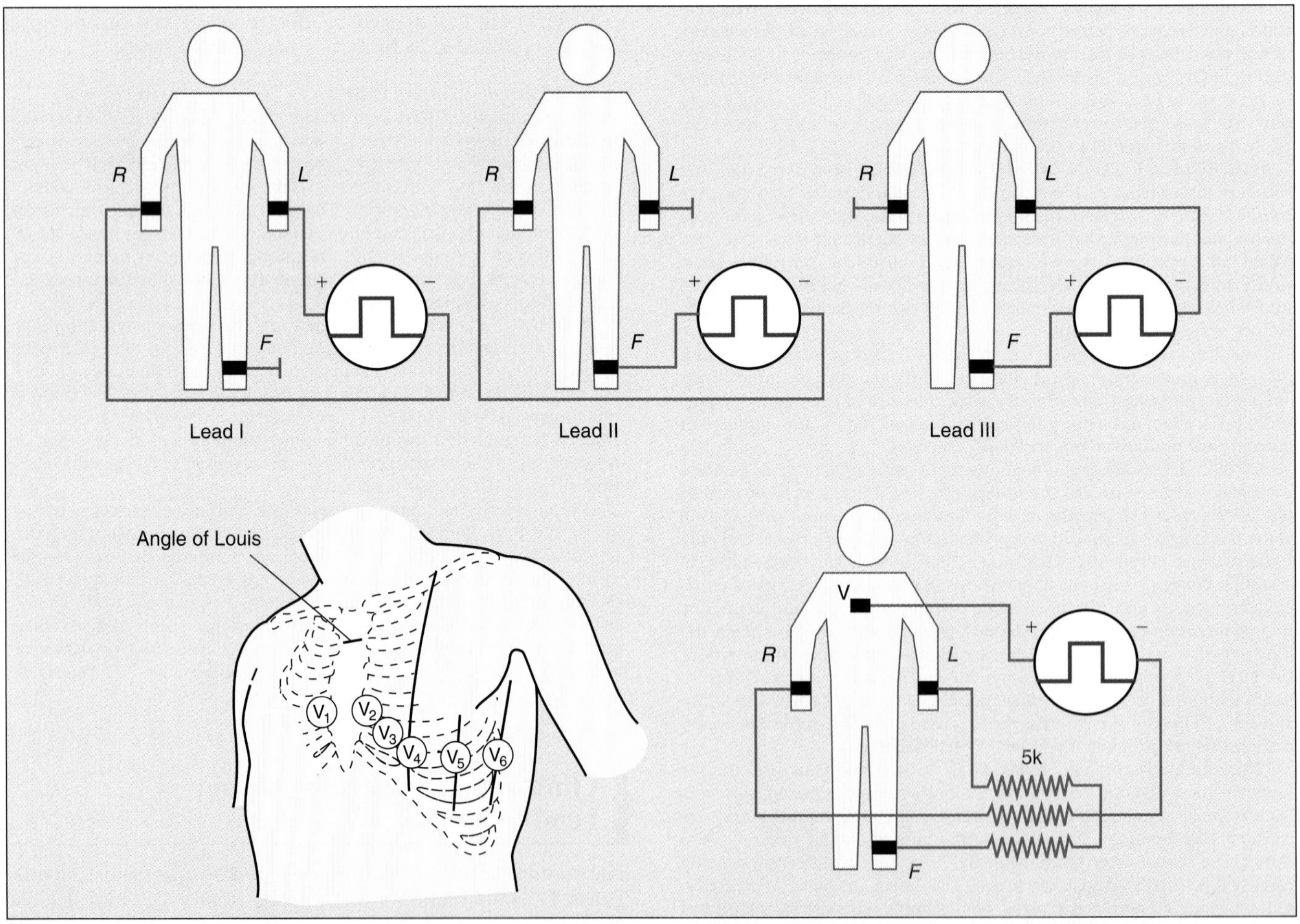

FIGURE 9–4 **Top,** Electrode connections for recording the three bipolar limb leads I, II, and III. R, L, and F indicate locations of electrodes on the right arm, the left arm, and the left foot, respectively. **Bottom,** Electrode locations and electrical connections for recording a unipolar precordial lead. Left, The positions of the exploring electrode (V) for the six precordial leads. Right, Connections to form the Wilson central terminal for recording a precordial (V) lead. (From Goldberger AL: Clinical Electrocardiography: A Simplified Approach. 6th ed. St Louis, CV Mosby, 1999.)

TABLE 9–1	Location of Electrodes and Lead Connections for the Standard 12-Lead Electrocardiogram and Additional Leads	
Lead Type	**Positive Input**	**Negative Input**
Bipolar limb leads		
Lead I	Left arm	Right arm
Lead II	Left leg	Right arm
Lead III	Left leg	Left arm
Augmented Unipolar Limb Leads		
aV_r	Right arm	Left arm plus left leg
aV_l	Left arm	Right arm plus left leg
aV_f	Left leg	Left arm plus left arm
Precordial Leads*		
V_1	Right sternal margin, 4th intercostal space	Wilson central terminal
V_2	Left sternal margin, 4th intercostal space	Wilson central terminal
V_3	Midway between V_2 and V_4	Wilson central terminal
V_4	Left midclavicular line, 5th intercostal space	Wilson central terminal
V_5	Left anterior axillary line†	Wilson central terminal
V_6	Left midaxillary line†	Wilson central terminal
V_7	Posterior axillary line†	Wilson central terminal
V_8	Posterior scapular line†	Wilson central terminal
V_9	Left border of spine†	Wilson central terminal

*The right-sided precordial leads V_3R to V_6R are taken in mirror image positions on the right side of the chest.
†Leads V_5 to V_9 are taken in the same horizontal plane as V_4.

represents the potential difference between the left arm (positive electrode) and the right arm (negative electrode), lead II displays the potential difference between the left foot (positive electrode) and the right arm (negative electrode), and lead III represents the potential difference between the left foot (positive electrode) and the left arm (negative electrode). The electrode on the right foot serves as a ground and is not included in these leads.

The electrical connections for these leads are such that the potential in lead II equals the sum of potentials sensed in leads I and III. That is,

$$I + III = II$$

This relationship is known as *Einthoven's law* or Einthoven's equation.

UNIPOLAR PRECORDIAL LEADS AND THE WILSON CENTRAL TERMINAL. The unipolar precordial leads register the potential at each of the six designated torso sites (see Fig. 9–4, bottom, left panel) in relation to a theoretical zero reference potential. To do so, an exploring electrode is placed on each precordial site and connected to the positive input of the recording system (see Fig. 9–4, bottom, right panel).

The negative, or reference, input is composed of a compound electrode (that is, a configuration of more than one electrode connected electrically) known as the *Wilson central terminal.* This terminal is formed by combining the output of the left arm, right arm, and left leg electrodes through 5000-Ω resistances (see Fig. 9–4, bottom, right panel). The result is that each precordial lead registers the potential at a precordial site with reference to the average potential on three limbs. The potential recorded by the Wilson central terminal remains relatively constant during the cardiac cycle, so the output of a precordial lead is determined predominantly by time-dependent changes in the potential at the precordial site.

AUGMENTED UNIPOLAR LIMB LEADS. The three augmented limb leads aV_r, aV_l, and aV_f are modified or augmented unipolar leads. The exploring electrode (Fig. 9–5) is the right arm electrode for lead aV_r, the left arm electrode for lead aV_l, and the left foot electrode for aV_f. It is the reference electrode that is modified. Instead of consisting of a full Wilson central terminal composed of the output from three limb electrodes, the reference potential for the augmented unipolar limb lead is the mean of the potentials sensed by only two of the three limb electrodes; the electrode used for the exploring electrode is excluded from the reference electrode. For lead aV_l, for example, the exploring electrode is on the left arm and the reference electrode is the mean output of the electrodes on the right arm and the left foot. Similarly, for lead aV_f, the reference potential is the mean of the output of the two arm electrodes.

This modified reference system was designed to increase the amplitude of the output. The output of the limb leads without augmentation tended to be small, in part because the same electrode potential was included in both the exploring

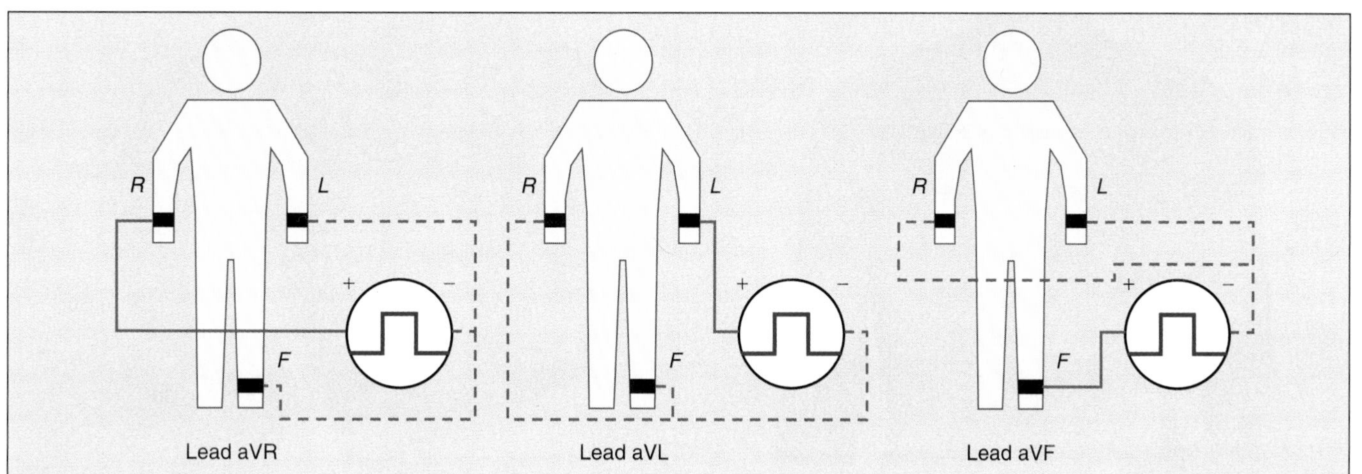

FIGURE 9–5 Electrode locations and electrical connections for recording the three augmented unipolar leads aV_r, aV_l, and aV_f. Dotted lines indicate connections to generate the reference electrode potential.

and the reference potential input. Eliminating this duplication results in a theoretical increase in amplitude of 50 percent.

OTHER LEAD SYSTEMS. Other lead systems can be used for specific purposes. For example, additional unipolar right precordial leads can be used to assess right ventricular lesions, and locations posterior to V_6 can be used to help detect acute posterior-lateral infarctions[5] (see Table 9-1). Such posterior locations include lead V_7 with the exploring electrode at the left posterior axillary line at the vertical level of V_6, lead V_8 with the exploring electrode on the left midscapular line, lead V_4R with the exploring electrode on the right midclavicular line in the 4th intercostal space, and so forth. A vertical parasternal bipolar pair can facilitate detection of P waves for diagnosing arrhythmias.

Precordial and anterior-posterior thoracic electrode arrays of up to 150 (or more) electrodes can be used to display the spatial distribution of body surface potentials as body surface isopotential maps.[6] Other arrays have sought to reduce rather than expand the number of electrodes and reconstruct the full 12-lead ECG from as few as three bipolar leads.[7] Modified lead systems are also used in ambulatory ECG recording and exercise stress testing, as described elsewhere, and for bedside cardiac monitoring.

Other lead systems that have had clinical utility include those designed to record a vectorcardiogram (VCG). The VCG depicts the orientation and strength of a single cardiac dipole or vector at each instant during the cardiac cycle. Lead systems for recording the VCG are referred to as *orthogonal systems* because they record the three orthogonal or mutually perpendicular components of the dipole moment: the horizontal (x axis), frontal (y axis), and sagittal or anteroposterior (z axis) axes. An example of a normal VCG is shown in Figure 9-6. Clinical use of the VCG has waned in recent years, but the VCG can be useful in certain situations, and, as described below, vectorial principles remain essential to understanding the physiology and pathology of ECG waveform genesis.[8]

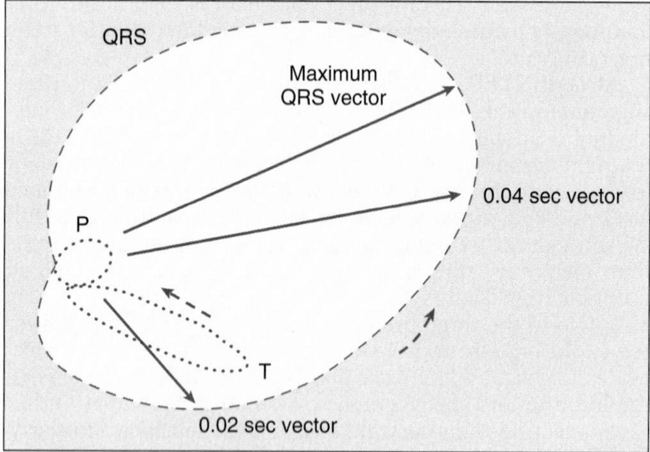

FIGURE 9–6 Example of a frontal plane vectorcardiogram. The three loops (QRS, T, and P) mark the ends of instantaneous vectors during the P wave, the QRS complex, and the T wave. Long arrows correspond to heart vectors 0.02 and 0.04 second into the QRS complex, at the instant of maximal vector strength during the QRS complex. Short arrows identify the direction in which the QRS and T loops are inscribed.

LEAD VECTORS AND HEART VECTORS

A lead can be represented as a vector (the *lead vector*). For simple bipolar leads, such as leads I, II, and III, the lead vectors are directed from the negative electrode toward the positive one (Fig. 9-7). For unipolar leads such as the augmented limb and precordial leads, the origin of the lead vectors lies at the midpoint of the axis connecting the electrodes that make up the compound electrode. That is, for lead aV_L, the vector points from the midpoint of the axis connecting the right arm and left leg electrodes toward the left arm (see Fig. 9-7, left). For the precordial leads, the lead vector points from the center of the torso to the precordial electrode site (see Fig. 9-7, right).

Instantaneous cardiac activity can also be approximated as a single dipole representing the vector sum of the various active wave fronts (the *heart vector*). Its location, orientation, and intensity vary from instant to instant because of the changing pattern of cardiac activation.

The amplitude and polarity of the potentials sensed in a lead equal the length of the projection of the heart vector on the lead vector multiplied by the length of the lead vector:

$$V_L = (H)(\cos \theta)\ (L)$$

where L and H are the length of the lead and heart vectors, respectively, and θ is the angle between the two vectors, as illustrated in Figure 9-8.

If the projection of the heart vector on the lead vector points toward the positive pole of the lead axis, the lead will record a positive potential. If the projection is directed away from the positive pole of the lead axis, the potential will be negative.

The lead axes of the six frontal plane leads can be overlaid to produce the hexaxial reference system. As depicted in Figure 9-9, the six lead axes divide the frontal plane into 12 segments, each subtending 30 degrees.

The Electrical Axis

The concepts of the heart vector and the lead vector allow calculation of the mean electrical axis of the heart. The mean force during activation is represented by the area under the QRS waveform measured as millivolt-milliseconds. Areas above the baseline are assigned a positive polarity and those

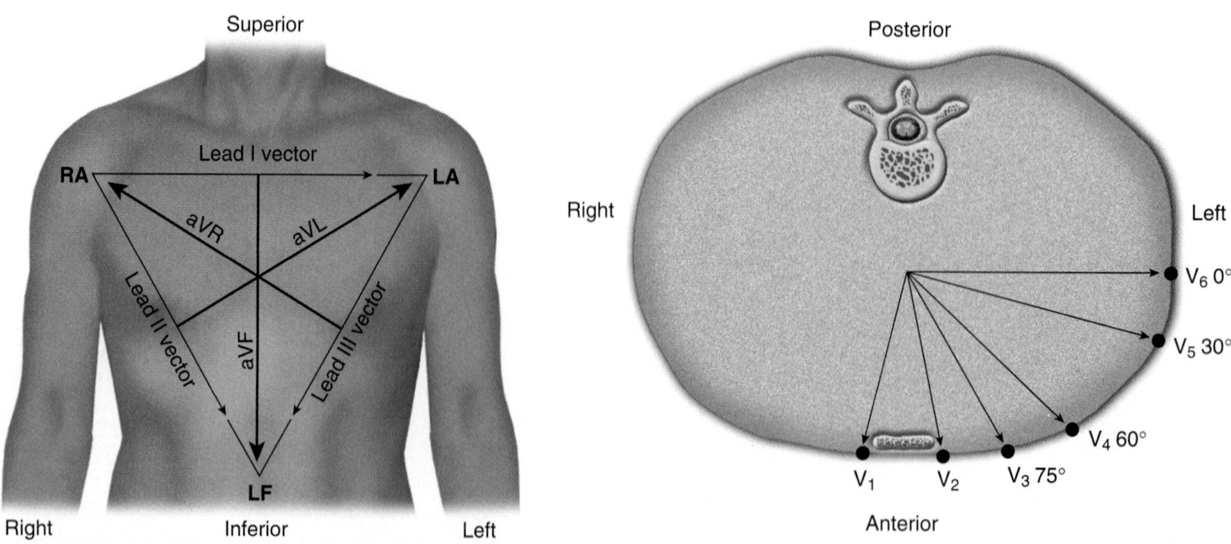

FIGURE 9–7 Lead vectors for the three bipolar limb leads, the three augmented unipolar limb leads **(left)**, and the six unipolar precordial leads **(right)**.

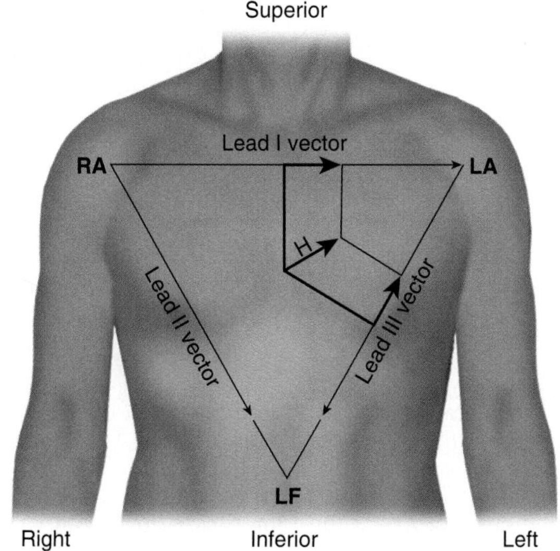

FIGURE 9–8 The heart vector H and its projections on the lead axes of leads I and III. Voltages recorded in lead I will be positive and potentials in lead III will be negative.

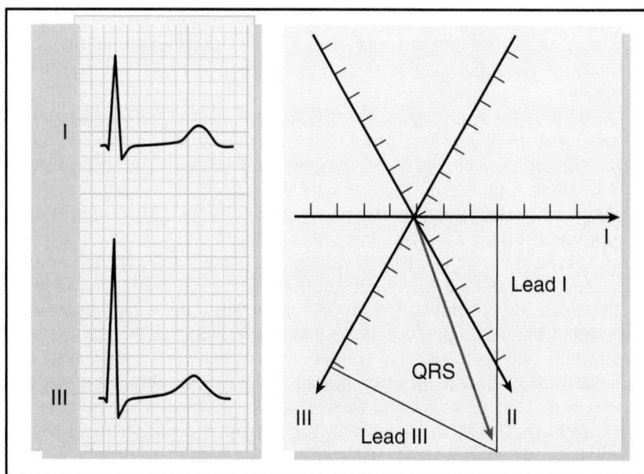

FIGURE 9–10 Calculation of the mean electrical axis during the QRS complex from the areas under the QRS complex in leads I and III. Magnitudes of the areas of the two leads are plotted as vectors on the appropriate lead axes, and the mean QRS axis is the sum of these two vectors. (From Mirvis DM: Electrocardiography: A Physiologic Approach. St Louis, Mosby-Year Book, 1993.)

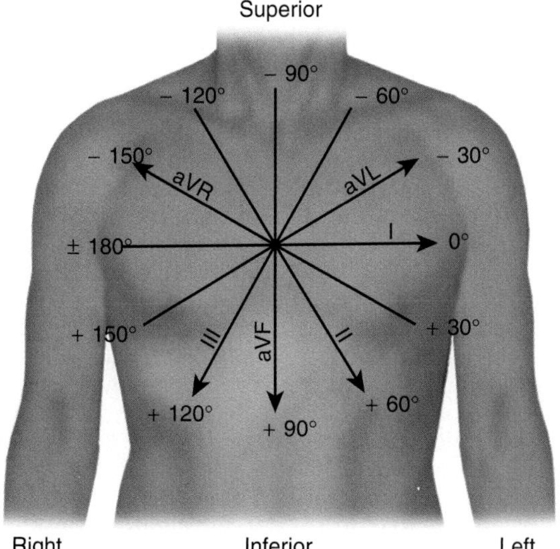

FIGURE 9–9 The hexaxial reference system composed of the lead axes of the six frontal plane leads. The lead axes of the six frontal plane leads have been rearranged so that their centers overlay one another. These axes divide the plane into 12 segments, each subtending 30 degrees. Positive ends of each axis are labeled with the name of the lead.

below the baseline have a negative polarity. The overall area equals the sum of the positive and the negative areas.

The process for computing the axis of the mean force during activation is illustrated in Figure 9–10. It is the reverse of that used to compute potential magnitudes in the leads from the orientation and moment of the heart vector. The area in each lead (typically two are chosen) is represented as a vector oriented along the appropriate lead axis in the hexaxial reference system (see Fig. 9–9), and the mean electrical axis equals the resultant or the sum of the two vectors. An axis directed toward the positive end of the lead axis of lead I, that is, oriented directly away from the right arm and toward the left arm, is designated as an axis of 0 degrees. Axes oriented in a clockwise direction from this zero level are assigned positive values and those oriented in a counterclockwise direction are assigned negative values.

The mean electrical axis in the horizontal plane can be computed in an analogous manner by using the areas and the lead axes of the six precordial leads (see Fig. 9–7, right). A horizontal plane axis located along the lead axis of lead V_6 is assigned a value of 0 degrees, and those directed more anteriorly have positive values.

This process can be applied to compute the mean electrical axis for other phases of cardiac activity. Thus, the mean force during atrial activation will be represented by the areas under the P wave, and the mean force during ventricular recovery will be represented by the areas under the ST-T wave. In addition, the instantaneous electrical axis can be computed at each instant during ventricular activation by using voltages at a specific instant rather than using areas to calculate the axis.

The orientation of the mean electrical axis represents the direction of the activation front in an "average" cardiac fiber. The direction of the front, in turn, is determined by the interaction of three factors: the anatomical position of the heart in the chest, the properties of the cardiac conduction system, and the activation properties of the myocardium. Differences in the anatomical position of the heart within the chest would be expected to change the relationship between cardiac regions and the lead axes and would thus change recorded voltages. Similarly, changes in conduction patterns, even of minor degree, can significantly alter relationships between activation (or recovery) of various cardiac areas and, hence, the direction of instantaneous as well as mean electrical force. In practice, differences in anatomy contribute relatively little to shifts in axis; the major influences on the mean electrical axis are the properties of the conduction system and cardiac muscle.

Electrocardiographic Display Systems

Another group of factors that determines ECG waveforms includes the characteristics of the electronic systems used to amplify, filter, and digitize the sensed signals. ECG amplifiers are differential amplifiers; that is, they amplify the difference between two inputs. For bipolar leads, the differential output is the difference between the two active leads; for unipolar leads, the difference is between the exploring electrode and the reference electrode. This differential configuration significantly reduces the electrical noise that is sensed by both inputs and hence is canceled. The standard amplifier gain for routine electrocardiography is 1000 but can vary from 500 (*half-standard*) to 2000 (*double standard*).

Amplifiers respond differently to the range of signal frequencies included in an electrophysiological signal. The *bandwidth* of an amplifier defines the frequency range over which the amplifier accurately amplifies the input signals. Waveform components with frequencies above or below the bandwidth can be artifactually reduced or increased in amplitude. In addition, recording devices include high- and low-pass filters that intentionally reduce the amplitude of specific frequency ranges of the signal. Such reduction in amplitude may be done, for example, to reduce the effect of body motion or line voltage frequencies, that is, 60 Hz interference. For routine electrocardiography, the standards of the American Heart Association require a bandwidth of 0.05 to 100 Hz.

Amplifiers for routine electrocardiography include a capacitor stage between the input and the output terminals; they are *capacitor coupled.* This configuration blocks direct-current (DC) voltage while permitting flow of alternating-current (AC) signals. Because the ECG waveform can be viewed as an AC signal (which accounts for the waveform shape) that is superimposed on a DC baseline (which determines the actual voltage levels of the recording), this coupling has significant effects on the recording process. First, unwanted DC potentials, such as those produced by the electrode interfaces, are eliminated. Second, elimination of the DC potential from the final product means that ECG potentials are not calibrated against an external reference level. ECG potentials must be measured in relation to an internal standard. Thus, amplitudes of waves are measured in millivolts or microvolts relative to another portion of the waveform. The TP segment, which begins at the end of the T wave of one cardiac cycle and ends with onset of the P wave of the next cycle, is usually the most appropriate internal ECG baseline.

An additional issue is the digitizing or sampling rate for computerized systems. Too low a sampling rate will miss brief signals such as notches in QRS complexes or brief bipolar spikes and reduce the precision and accuracy of waveform morphologies. Too fast a sampling rate may introduce artifacts, including high-frequency noise, and requires excessive digital storage capacity. In general, the sampling rate should be at least twice the frequency of the highest frequencies of interest in the signal being recorded. Standard electrocardiography is most commonly performed with a sampling rate of 500 Hz, with each sample representing a 2 msec period.

Cardiac potentials can be processed for display in numerous formats. The most common of these formats is the classic scalar ECG. Scalar recordings depict the potentials recorded from one lead as a function of time. For standard electrocardiography, amplitude is displayed on a scale of 1 mV to 10 mm vertical displacement and time as 400 msec/cm on the horizontal scale. Other display formats are used for ambulatory electrocardiography and for bedside ECG monitoring.

The Normal Electrocardiogram

The heart is activated with each cardiac cycle in a very characteristic manner determined by the anatomy and physiology of working cardiac muscle and the specialized cardiac conduction systems. The waveforms and intervals that make up the standard ECG are displayed in the diagram in Figure 9–11, and a normal 12-lead ECG is shown in Figure 9–12. The

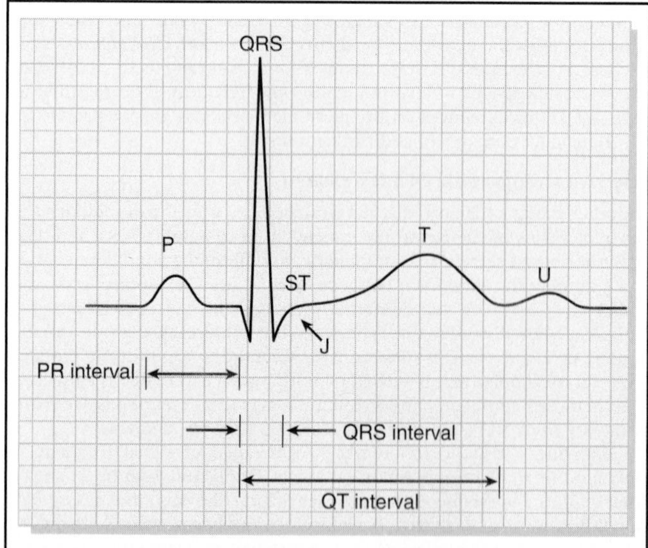

FIGURE 9–11 The waves and intervals of a normal electrocardiogram. (From Goldberger AL: Clinical Electrocardiography: A Simplified Approach. 6th ed. St Louis, CV Mosby, 1999.)

TABLE 9–2 Normal Values for Durations of Electrocardiographic Waves and Intervals in Adults

Wave/Interval	Duration (msec)
P wave duration	<120
PR interval	<120
QRS duration	<110-120*
QT interval (corrected)	≥440-460*

*See text for further discussion.

P wave is generated by activation of the atria, the *PR segment* represents the duration of atrioventricular (AV) conduction, the *QRS complex* is produced by activation of both ventricles, and the *ST-T wave* reflects ventricular recovery. Table 9–2 includes normal values for the various intervals and waveforms of the ECG.

Atrial Activation and the P Wave

Atrial activation[9,10] under normal conditions begins with impulse generation in the atrial pacemaker complex in or near the sinoatrial (SA) node. The rate of discharge of the SA node, and hence the heart rate, is determined by parasympathetic and sympathetic tone, the intrinsic properties of the SA node, extrinsic factors such as mechanical stretch, and various pharmacological effects (see Chap. 27).

HEART RATE VARIABILITY. Increasing attention is being directed to the beat-to-beat changes in heart rate, termed *heart rate variability,* to gain insight into neuroautonomic control mechanisms and their perturbations with aging, disease, and drug effects.[11] For example, high-frequency (0.15-0.5 Hz) fluctuations mediated by the vagus nerve occur phasically, with heart rate increasing during inspiration and decreasing during expiration. Attenuation of this respiratory sinus arrhythmia, and related short-term heart rate variability, is a consistent marker of physiological aging and also occurs with diabetes mellitus, congestive heart failure, and a wide range of other cardiac and noncardiac conditions that alter autonomic tone.[12] Lower frequency (0.05-0.15 Hz) physiological oscillations in heart rate are associated with baroreflex activation and appear to be jointly regulated by sympathetic and parasympathetic interactions. A variety of complementary signal processing techniques are being developed to analyze heart rate variability, including the very low-frequency (<0.05 Hz) components and circadian rhythms. These methods include time-domain statistics, frequency-domain techniques based on spectral (Fourier) methods, and tools derived from nonlinear dynamics. For further discussion, see Chapter 29.

Once the impulse leaves this pacemaker site within the SA node, atrial activation spreads in several directions. First, propagation is rapid along the crista terminalis and moves anteriorly toward the lower portion of the right atrium. It also spreads across the anterior and posterior surfaces of the atria toward the left atrium. The last area to be activated is over the inferolateral aspect of the left atrium, which is activated by convergence of these anterior and posterior wave fronts moving from right to left. Although right atrial activation begins before activation of the left atrium, activation occurs simultaneously in both atria during much of the overall atrial activation time. At the same time, activation spreads through the interatrial septum, beginning high on the right side and moving around the fossa ovalis to reach the top of the interventricular septum. These patterns are largely determined by the complex anatomical and functional properties of the atrial musculature.

The pattern of atrial activation noted above produces the normal P wave. Activation beginning high in the right atrium

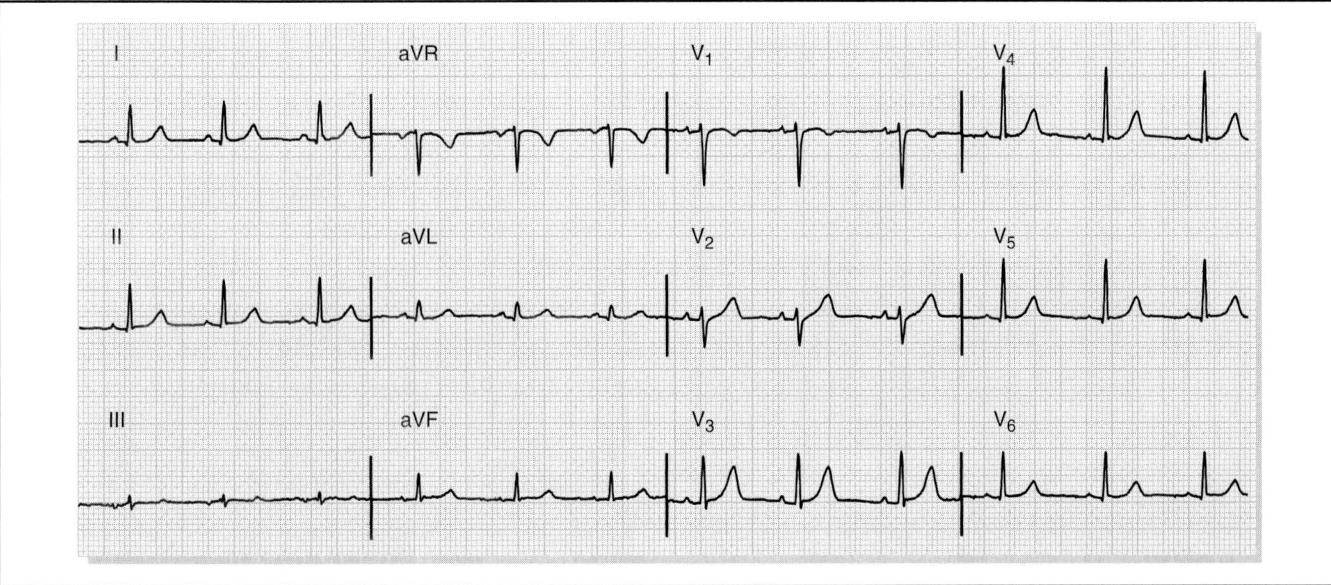

FIGURE 9–12 Normal electrocardiogram recorded from a 48-year-old woman. The vertical lines of the grid represent time, with lines spaced at 40 msec intervals. Horizontal lines represent voltage amplitude, with lines spaced at 0.1 mV intervals. Every fifth line in each direction is typically darkened. The heart rate is approximately 72 beats/min; the PR interval, QRS, and QT_c durations measure about 140, 84, and 400 msec, respectively; and the mean QRS axis is approximately +35 degrees.

and proceeding simultaneously leftward toward the left atrium and inferiorly toward the AV node corresponds to a mean frontal plane P wave axis of approximately 60 degrees. Based on this orientation of the heart vector, normal atrial activation projects positive or upright P waves in leads I, II, aV_l, and aV_f. The pattern in lead III may be either upright or downward, depending on the exact orientation of the mean axis, that is, upright if the mean axis is more positive than +30 degrees and downward otherwise.

P wave patterns in the precordial leads correspond to the direction of atrial activation wavefronts in the horizontal plane. Atrial activation early in the P wave is over the right atrium and is oriented primarily anteriorly; later it shifts posteriorly as activation proceeds over the left atrium. Thus, the P wave in the right precordial leads (V_1 and, occasionally, V_2) is commonly biphasic, with an initial positive deflection followed by a later negative one. In the more lateral leads, the P wave is upright and reflects right-to-left spread of the activation fronts.

P wave duration is normally less than 120 msec and is usually measured in the lead with the widest P wave. The amplitude in the limb leads is normally less than 0.25 mV and the terminal negative deflection in the right precordial leads is normally less than 0.1 mV in depth.

Atrial depolarization is followed by atrial repolarization. The potentials generated by atrial repolarization are not usually seen on the surface ECG because of their low amplitude (usually less than 100 μV) and because they are superimposed on the much higher amplitude QRS complex. They may be observed as a low-amplitude wave with a polarity opposite that of the P wave (the T_a wave) during heart block and may have special significance in influencing ECG patterns during exercise testing. Deviation of the PR segment (corresponding to the atrial ST segment) is, as described later, also an important marker of acute pericarditis and, more rarely, atrial infarction.

Atrioventricular Node Conduction and the PR Segment

The PR segment is the isoelectric region beginning with the end of the P wave and ending with the onset of the QRS complex. It forms part of the PR interval, which extends from the onset of the P wave to the onset of the QRS complex. The PR interval is usually best measured in the leads with the shortest PR intervals (to avoid missing various preexcitation syndromes). The normal PR interval measures 120 to 200 msec in duration.

The PR segment is the temporal bridge between atrial activation and ventricular activation. It is during this period that activation of the AV node, the bundle of His, the bundle branches, and the intraventricular specialized conduction system occurs. As noted earlier, atrial repolarization also occurs during this period. Most of the conduction delay during this segment is due to slow conduction within the AV node.

Upon exiting the AV node, the impulse traverses the bundle of His to enter the bundle branches and then travels through the specialized intraventricular conduction paths to finally activate ventricular myocardium. The PR segment appears isoelectric because the potentials generated by these structures are too small to produce detectable voltages on the body surface at the normal amplifier gains used in clinical electrocardiography. The standard ECG detects only activation and recovery of working myocardium, not the specialized conduction system. Signals from elements of the conduction system have been recorded from the body surface by using very high gains (over 25,000) and signal-averaging techniques or, in clinical settings, from intracardiac recording electrodes placed against the base of the interventricular septum near the bundle of His, as described in Chapter 29.

Ventricular Activation and the QRS Complex

Ventricular excitation is the product of two temporally overlapping functions, endocardial activation and transmural activation. Endocardial activation is guided by the anatomical distribution and physiology of the His-Purkinje system. The broadly dispersed ramifications of this tree-like (fractal) system[13] and the rapid conduction within it result in depolarization of most of the endocardial surfaces of both ventricles within several milliseconds and the simultaneous activation of multiple endocardial sites.

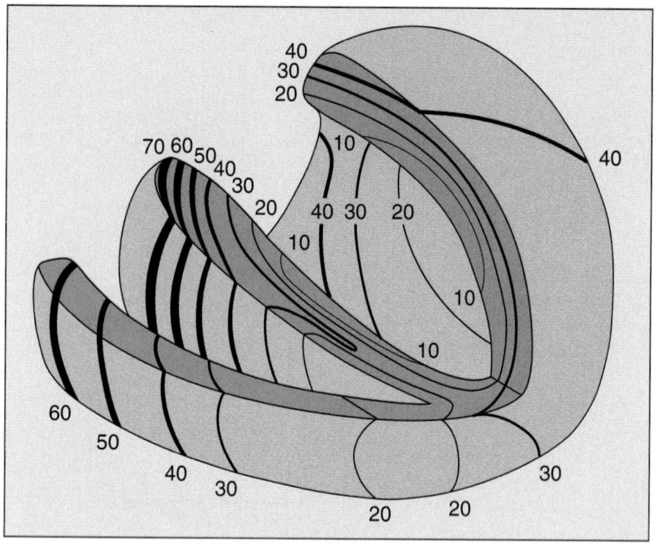

FIGURE 9–13 Activation sequence of the normal right and left ventricles. A portion of the left and right ventricles has been removed so that the endocardial surfaces of the ventricles and the interventricular septum can be seen. Isochrone lines connect sites that are activated at equal instants after the earliest evidence of ventricular activation. (From Durrer D: Electrical aspects of human cardiac activity: A clinical-physiological approach to excitation and stimulation. Cardiovasc Res 2:1, 1968.)

The sequence of ventricular endocardial activation is depicted in Figure 9–13. Earliest activity begins in three sites: (1) the anterior paraseptal wall of the left ventricle, (2) the posterior paraseptal wall of the left ventricle, and (3) the center of the left side of the septum. These loci generally correspond to the sites of insertion of the three branches of the left bundle branch. Wavefronts spread from these sites in anterior and superior directions to activate the anterior and lateral walls of the left ventricle. The posterobasal areas of the left ventricle are the last to be activated. Septal activation begins in the middle third of the left side and spreads across the septum from left to right and from apex to base.

Excitation of the right ventricle begins near the insertion point of the right bundle branch close to the base of the anterior papillary muscle and spreads to the free wall. The final areas to be involved are the pulmonary conus and the posterobasal areas. Thus, in both ventricles, the overall endocardial excitation pattern begins on septal surfaces and sweeps down and around the anterior free walls to the posterior and basal regions in an apex-to-base direction.

The activation fronts then move from endocardium to epicardium. Excitation of the endocardium begins at sites of Purkinje-ventricular muscle junctions and proceeds by muscle cell-to-muscle cell conduction in an oblique direction toward the epicardium.

LIMB LEADS. The sequence of endocardial and transmural activation results in the characteristic waveforms of the QRS complex. QRS patterns are described by the sequence of waves constituting the complex. An initial negative deflection is called the *Q wave;* the first positive wave is the *R wave;* and the first negative wave after a positive wave is the *S wave.* A second upright wave following an S wave is an *R′ wave.* Tall waves are denoted by capital letters and smaller ones by lowercase letters. A monophasic negative complex is referred to as a *QS complex.* Thus, for example, the overall QRS complex may be described as qRS if it consists of an initial small negative wave (the q wave) followed by a tall upright one (the R wave) and a deep negative one (an S wave). In an RSr′ complex, initial R and S waves are followed by a small positive wave (the r′ wave). In each case, the deflection must cross the baseline to be designated a discrete wave.

Septal Q Waves. The complex pattern of activation described can be simplified into two vectors representing septal and left ventricular free wall activation (Fig. 9–14). Initial activation of the interventricular septum corresponds to a vector oriented from left to right in the frontal plane and anteriorly in the horizontal plane, as determined by the anatomical position of the septum within the chest. This arrangement produces an initial positive wave in leads with axes directed to the right (lead aVr) or anteriorly (lead V_1). Leads with axes directed to the left (leads I, aV_l, V_5, and V_6) will register initial negative waves (septal q waves). These initial forces are normally of low amplitude and are brief (less than 30–40 msec).

Absence of these septal q waves is often a normal variant and not associated with any cardiac disease. However, absence or, particularly, loss of septal q waves may be a sign of septal infarction, various forms of conduction defects, or fibrosis, and commonly correlates with other ECG evidence of myocardial infarction and left ventricular mechanical dysfunction.[14-16]

Subsequent parts of the QRS complex reflect activation of the free walls of the left and right ventricles. Because right ventricular muscle mass is considerably smaller than that of the left ventricle, it contributes little to normal QRS complexes recorded in the standard ECG. Thus, the second phase of the normal QRS can be considered to represent only left ventricular activity with relatively little oversimplification.

Axis Positions. The forms of the QRS complex frontal plane leads are variable and reflect differences in the mean QRS electrical axis. The normal mean QRS axis in adults lies between −30 degrees and +90 degrees. Mean QRS axes more positive than +90 degrees represent *right axis deviation,* and those more negative than −30 degrees represent *left axis deviation.* Mean axes lying between −90 and −180 degrees (or equivalently between +180 and +270 degrees) are referred to as *extreme axis deviations.* The designation *indeterminate axis* is applied when all six extremity leads show biphasic (QR or RS) patterns; this finding can occur as a normal variant or may be seen in a variety of pathological conditions.

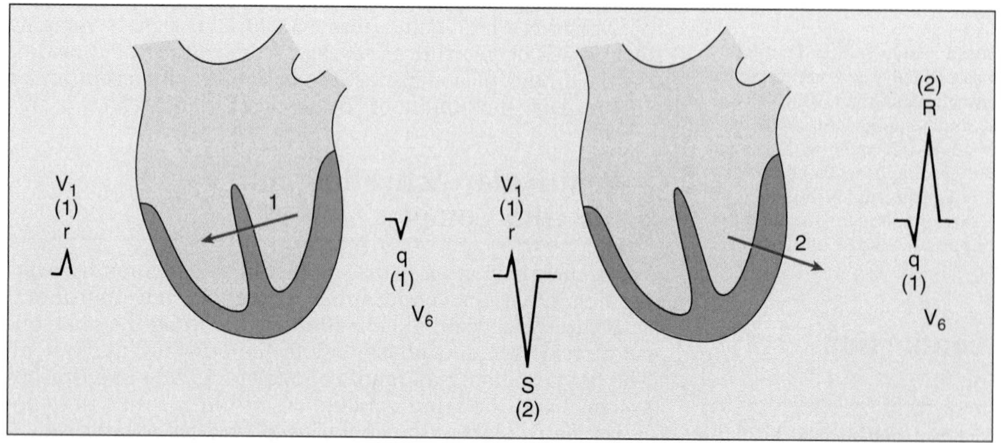

FIGURE 9–14 Schematic representation of ventricular depolarization as two sequential vectors representing septal **(left)** and left ventricular free wall **(right)** activation. QRS waveforms generated by each stage of activation in leads V_1 and V_6 are shown.

The wide span of the normal axis results in a range of QRS patterns, especially in the inferior leads. This characteristic can be understood by referring to the hexaxial reference system in Figure 9–9. If the mean axis is near 90 degrees, the QRS complex in leads II, III, and aV_f will be predominantly upright with qR complexes; lead I will record an isoelectric RS pattern because the heart vector lies perpendicular to the lead axis. This configuration is commonly referred to as a *vertical heart* position, although it is not necessarily related to the anatomical position of the heart within the chest. If the mean axis is nearer 0 degrees, the patterns will be reversed; lead I (and aV_l) will register a predominantly upright qR pattern, and leads II, III, and aV_f will show rS or RS patterns, a configuration often referred to as a *horizontal heart* pattern.

PRECORDIAL LEADS. In the precordial leads V_1 and V_2, free wall activation generates S waves following the initial r waves generated by septal activation. These S waves are produced by the spread of activation in the free wall to the left and posteriorly, with generation of a heart vector directed away from the axes of these leads. Thus, these leads are characterized by rS patterns.

Patterns in the midprecordial leads V_3 and V_4 are more variable. Potentials sensed in these leads reflect, as in the case of the right precordial leads, the activation front in the ventricular free wall approaching the exploring electrode, followed by its moving leftward and posteriorly to more remote regions of the left ventricle. This front generates an R or r wave and later an S wave to produce rS or RS complexes in these leads. As the exploring electrode moves laterally to the left, however, the R wave becomes more dominant and the S wave becomes smaller because of the greater time period during which the activation front moves toward the positive end of the electrode.

Thus, in the precordial leads, the QRS complex is usually characterized by consistent progression from an rS complex in the right precordial leads to a qR pattern in the left precordial leads. The point during this transition at which the pattern changes from an rS to an Rs configuration, that is, the lead in which an isoelectric RS pattern is present, is known as the *transition zone* and normally occurs in leads V_3 or V_4. An example of a normal precordial QRS pattern is shown in Figure 9–12. Transition zones shifted to the right, to lead V_2, are referred to as *early transitions,* and those shifted leftward to V_5 or V_6 are *delayed transitions.* These variations in the horizontal plane axis are sometimes described as *counterclockwise* and *clockwise rotations*, respectively, of the heart, although these descriptors do not necessarily correlate with cardiac anatomical findings.[17]

QRS DURATION. The upper normal value for QRS duration is traditionally given as less than 120 msec (and often as <110 msec) measured in the lead with the widest QRS duration. In a survey of 1224 healthy men with normal QRS morphology and frontal plane axis, the 98 percent upper boundary of QRS duration measured by a multilead, automated computer algorithm was 116 msec. Women, on average, have somewhat smaller QRS durations than men (by about 5 to 8 msec).

INTRINSICOID DEFLECTION. An additional feature of the QRS complex is the intrinsicoid deflection. An electrode overlying the ventricular free wall will record a rising R wave as transmural activation of the underlying ventricular free wall proceeds. Once the activation front reaches the epicardium, the full thickness of the wall under the electrode will be in an active state, with no propagating electrical activity. At that moment, the electrode will register negative potentials from remote cardiac areas still undergoing activation. The sudden reversal of potential with a sharp downslope is the intrinsicoid deflection and marks the timing of activation of the epicardium under the electrode.

Ventricular Recovery and the ST-T Wave

The normal ST-T wave begins as a low-amplitude, slowly changing wave (the *ST segment*) that gradually leads to a larger wave, the *T wave.* Onset of the ST-T wave is the junction, or *J point*, and is normally at or near the isoelectric baseline of the ECG (see Figs. 9–11 and 9–12).

The polarity of the ST-T wave is generally the same as the net polarity of the preceding QRS complex. Thus, T waves are usually upright in leads I, II, aV_l, aV_f, and the lateral precordial leads. They are negative in lead aVr and variable in leads III and V_1 through V_3.

Recovery, like activation, occurs in a characteristic geometrical pattern. Differences in recovery timing occur both across the ventricular wall and between regions of the left ventricle. Transmural differences in recovery times are the net result of two effects—differences in action potential duration across the ventricular wall and the relatively slow spread of activation across the wall. As activation moves from endocardium to epicardium, sites further away from the endocardium are activated later and later in sequence. However, action potential durations are longest near the endocardium and shortest near the epicardium, which produces a transmural gradient in recovery periods. Differences in action potential duration are greater than differences in activation times, so recovery is completed near the epicardium before it is completed near the endocardium. For example, one endocardial site may be excited 10 msec earlier than the overlying epicardium (that is, transmural activation may require 10 msec), and the action potential duration at the endocardium may be 22 msec longer than on the epicardium. As a result, recovery will be completed 12 msec earlier in the epicardium than in the endocardium.

The resulting recovery dipole will then be directed from sites of less recovery (the endocardium) toward sites of greater recovery (near the epicardium). The orientation of this dipole is in the same direction as transmural activation dipoles. This orientation is opposite to the expected direction as described earlier in this chapter; this difference is due to the presence of nonuniform recovery properties across the wall. If recovery times were uniform across the wall (or if differences in recovery times were less than differences in transmural activation times), the recovery dipole would have been directed toward the endocardium, that is, in the direction opposite the activation dipole. The result, in normal persons, is concordant QRS and ST-T wave patterns.

Regional differences in recovery properties likewise exist. Under normal conditions, it is the transmural gradients that predominantly determine ST patterns. However, as will be described, these regional differences account for the discordant ST-T patterns observed with intraventricular conduction defects.

THE QRST ANGLE. This concordance between orientation of the QRS complex and ST-T wave can also be expressed vectorially. An angle can be visualized between the vector representing the mean QRS force and that representing the mean ST-T force—the *QRST angle.* This angle in the frontal plane is normally less than 60 degrees and usually less than 30 degrees. Abnormalities of the QRST angle reflect abnormal relationships between the properties of activation and recovery.

THE VENTRICULAR GRADIENT. If the two vectors representing mean activation and mean recovery forces are added, a third vector known as the *ventricular gradient* is created. This third vector represents the net area under the QRST complex. The concept of the ventricular gradient was originally developed to assess differences in the properties of ventricular activation and recovery. According to this concept, the more variability that exists in regional repolarization properties, the greater the difference between the QRS and ST-T areas will be. In other words, the ventricular gradient correlates with the magnitude of regional differences in recovery properties. In addition, because changes in activation patterns produced, for example, by bundle branch block cause corresponding changes in recovery patterns (see later), no change in the ventricular gradient typically results. The ventricular gradient should thus allow a measure of regional recovery properties that is independent of the activation pattern. This measurement has possible relevance to the genesis of reentrant arrhythmias that are due, in part, to abnormal regional variations in refractory periods.

THE U WAVE. The T wave may be followed by an additional low-amplitude wave known as the *U wave.* This late repolarization wave, usually less than 0.1 mV in amplitude, normally has the same polarity as the preceding T wave and is largest in the midprecordial leads and at slow heart rates. Its basis in cardiac electrophysiology is uncertain; it may be caused by repolarization of the Purkinje fibers, by the long action potential of midmyocardial cells (M cells), or by delayed repolarization in areas of the ventricle that undergo late mechanical relaxation.[18,19]

THE QT INTERVAL. A final interval of the ECG waveform is the QT interval, which is measured from the beginning of the QRS complex to the end of the T wave in the lead with the longest interval and without prominent U waves.[20] It includes the total duration of ventricular activation and recovery and, in a general sense, corresponds to the duration of the ventricular action potential.

The normal QT interval is defined by its duration, measured in milliseconds. Like the ventricular action potential duration, the duration of the QT interval decreases as heart rate increases. Thus, the normal range for the QT interval is rate dependent. One formula for relating QT interval duration to heart rate was developed by Bazett in 1920. The result

is computation of a corrected QT interval, or QT_c, by using the following equation:

$$QT_c = QT/(R - R)^{1/2}$$

where the QT and RR intervals are measured in seconds. The normal QT_c is generally accepted to be less than or equal to 440 msec. Some studies suggest that it may be 20 msec longer,[20a] and it is slightly longer, on average, in women (see Chap. 32). When the T wave overlaps with the beginning of a U wave, the QT interval is sometimes referred to as the *QT(U) interval*; this designation is particularly appropriate when considering the ECG effects of certain metabolic abnormalities that alter the duration of repolarization and the amplitude of the U wave (see later).

The Bazett formula, while widely used to adjust the QT interval duration for the effects of heart rate, has limited accuracy in predicting the effects of heart rate on the QT interval.[20,20b] Many other formulas and methods for correcting the QT interval for the effects of heart rate, including logarithmic, hyperbolic, and exponential functions, have been developed and tested, but they also have limitations. These limitations result from both physiological and computational problems. The substantial variation in the relationship between QT interval duration and heart rate among different patient groups reduces the accuracy of any single correction formula. In addition, these formulas do not account for the effects of autonomic tone on the QT interval independent of the effects on rate. They also do not account for the relatively slow adaptation of repolarization to changes in rate; for example, several minutes may be required for the QT interval to reach a new steady state after an abrupt change in heart rate. The normal corrected QT interval can vary by more than 75 msec during a 24-hour period.[20b]

A second property of the QT interval is that its duration is lead dependent; that is, the duration of the QT interval varies from lead to lead. In normal persons, the QT interval varies between leads by up to 50 msec and is longest in the midprecordial leads V_2 and V_3. This range of intervals, referred to as *QT interval dispersion*, may be related to electrical instability and the risk of ventricular arrhythmogenesis, as described further below.[21]

NORMAL VARIANTS. These descriptions of the waveforms of the normal ECG represent patterns most often observed in normal adults. Understanding the limitations of assigning and interpreting the normal ranges of ECG measurements is important. Values for many of the intervals and amplitudes to be described vary widely within the population as a function of age, race, gender, body habitus, and the geometric position of the heart within the torso. Variation may also occur within an individual over time as a function of autonomic tone and activity level. Thus, what is normal in one condition may be abnormal in another. Some variations have already been described in this chapter, including, for example, variations in rate, QRS axis, and QT intervals.

Common variations occur in patterns of the ST segment and the T wave. These variations are important to recognize because they may be mistaken for significant abnormalities; for example, as many as 40% of Olympic athletes have "abnormal" electrocardiograms, whereas fewer than 5% of these athletes have structural cardiac disease.[22] ST-T patterns are affected by maneuvers that change autonomic tone. For example, changing body position, hyperventilating, drinking cold water, and performing the Valsalva maneuver can produce modest ST segment depression and slight T wave inversion in as many as one third of subjects.

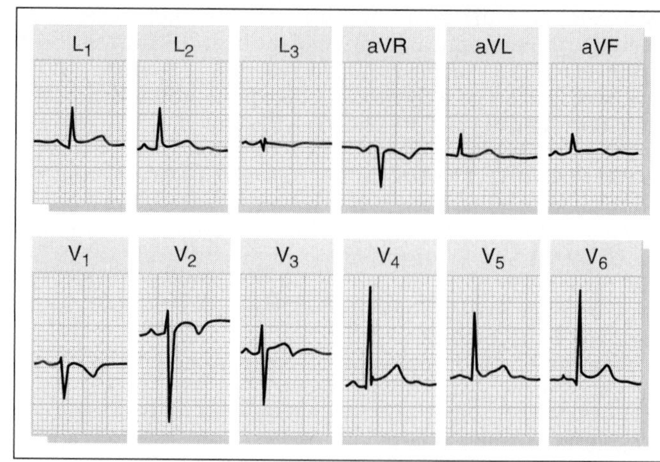

FIGURE 9–15 Normal tracing with a juvenile T wave inversion pattern in leads V_1, V_2, and V_3, as well as early repolarization pattern manifested by ST segment elevation in leads I, II, aV_f, V_4, V_5, and V_6. (Courtesy of C. Fisch, M.D.)

T waves can be inverted in the right precordial leads (Fig. 9–15). In adults, this inversion reflects the uncommon, but not necessarily abnormal, persistence of patterns commonly seen in infants and children. T waves can be inverted in all precordial leads at birth and usually become more limited to the right side of the chest as time passes; by the age of 10 years, T wave inversion is generally limited to leads V_1 and V_2. A persistent juvenile pattern is more common in women than in men and among the black population than among other racial or ethnic groups.

Second, the ST segment can be elevated, especially in the midprecordial leads (Fig. 9–16). The elevation begins from an elevated J point, is usually concave in form, is commonly associated with notching of the downstroke of the QRS complex, and can reach 0.3 mV in amplitude.[23,24] This pattern is more common at slow than at rapid heart rates and is most prevalent in young adults, especially among black men. Although this physiological ST segment elevation pattern is commonly referred to as *early repolarization*, clinical studies have failed to demonstrate an earlier than normal onset of ventricular recovery. This physiologic variant may be related to relative enhancement of vagal tone in healthy subjects and is also prevalent in those with high (T5 or above) spinal cord injuries where sympathetic outflow is interrupted.[25]

The Abnormal Electrocardiogram

Atrial Abnormalities

Various pathological and physiological events alter the normal sequence of atrial activation and produce abnormal P wave patterns in the ECG. Three general categories of P wave changes are described here, including those reflecting abnormal sites or patterns of activation, those caused by left atrial abnormalities, and those resulting from right atrial abnormalities.

Abnormal Sites of Atrial Activation

Shifts in the site of initial activation away from the SA node to other, ectopic sites can lead to major changes in the pattern of atrial activation and, hence, in the morphology of P waves.[26] These shifts can occur either as escape rhythms if the normal SA nodal pacemaker fails or as accelerated ectopic rhythms if the automaticity of an ectopic site is enhanced (see AV dissociation, Chapter 32). The resulting ECG abnormalities most commonly include recording negative P waves in the leads in which P waves are normally upright (leads I, II, aV_f, and V_4 through V_6), with or without shortening of the PR interval.

P wave patterns can suggest the site of impulse formation based on simple vectorial principles. For example, a negative P wave in lead I can predict a left atrial rhythm. Inverted P waves in the inferior leads normally correspond to a posterior atrial site. However, because of the uncertainties with this localization, these ECG patterns can, as a group, be referred to as *ectopic atrial rhythms*. Apparent left atrial rhythms can arise in the pulmonary veins and play a role in precipitating atrial fibrillation (see Chap. 32).

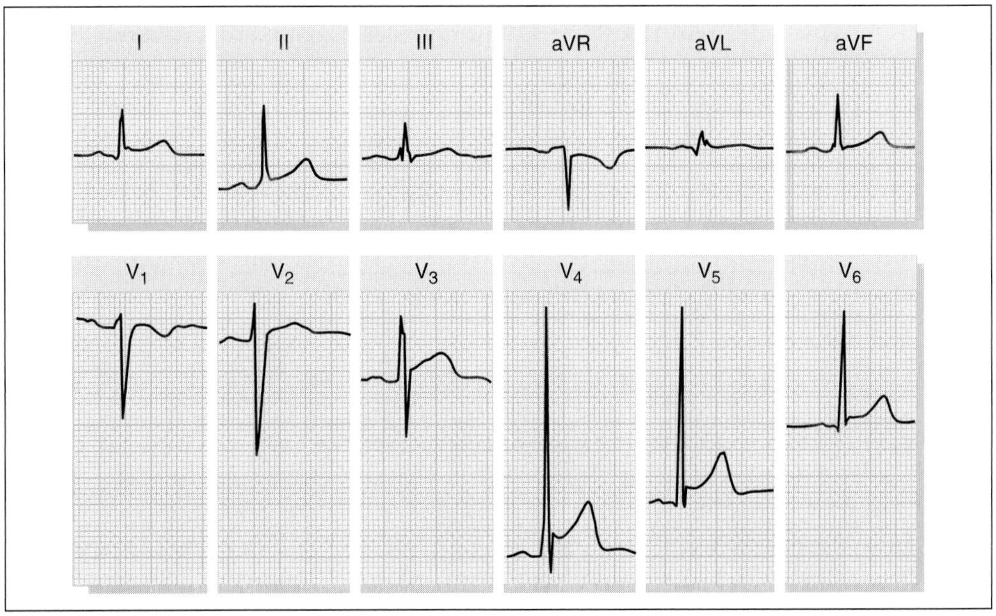

FIGURE 9–16 Normal variant pattern with functional ST elevations ("early repolarization" variant). These benign ST segment elevations are usually most marked in the midprecordial leads (V_4 here). Note the absence of reciprocal ST depression (except in lead aV_r), as well as the absence of PR segment deviation, which may be helpful in the differential diagnosis of ischemia and pericarditis, respectively. Note also that lead II has a baseline recording shift. (From Goldberger AL: Myocardial Infarction: Electrocardiographic Differential Diagnosis. 4th ed. St Louis, Mosby-Year Book, 1991.)

Left Atrial Abnormality

ECG ABNORMALITIES. Anatomical or functional abnormalities of the left atrium alter the morphology, duration, and amplitude of the P waves in the clinical ECG. Specific abnormalities include increases in the amplitude and duration of the P wave in the limb leads, as well as an increase in the amplitude of the terminal negative portion of the P wave in lead V_1. These features are illustrated in Figures 9–17 and 9–18.

DIAGNOSTIC CRITERIA. Commonly used criteria for diagnosing left atrial abnormality are listed in Table 9–3.

MECHANISMS FOR ECG ABNORMALITIES. Abnormal ECG patterns can reflect increases in left atrial mass or chamber size or conduction delays within the atria. Increasing mass causes increased P wave amplitudes. Because the left atrium is activated (in general) late during P wave inscription, the increased electrical force accounts for the prolonged P wave duration and the augmented P terminal force in the right precordial leads.

These patterns also correlate with a delay in interatrial conduction. This delay prolongs P wave duration and shortens the PR segment. It also reduces the overlap between right and left atrial activation, so the ECG patterns generated by each atrium may be separated as two humps in lead II (*P mitrale*).

DIAGNOSTIC ACCURACY. The diagnostic accuracy of these criteria is limited. Comparison of the various ECG abnormalities to echocardiographic criteria for left atrial enlargement demonstrates limited sensitivity but high specificity for standard ECG criteria. For example, recent studies have demonstrated that the presence of classic P mitrale patterns has a sensitivity of only 20 percent but a specificity of 98 percent for detecting echocardiographically enlarged left atria.[27] Other studies have reported better correlations of these ECG abnormalities with ventricular dysfunction (e.g., with reduced ventricular compliance) than with atrial morphology. Because of the correlation of these ECG features with high atrial pressure, intraatrial conduction defects, and ventricular dysfunction, as well as increased atrial size, these ECG abnormalities are preferably referred to as criteria for left atrial abnormality rather than left atrial enlargement.

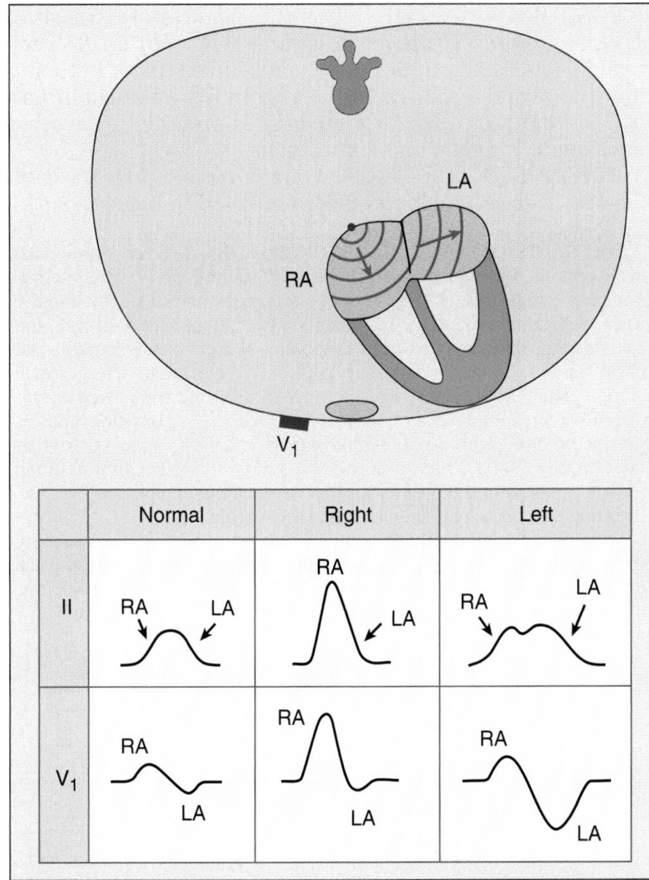

FIGURE 9–17 Schematic representation of atrial depolarization **(diagram)** and P wave patterns associated with normal atrial activation **(left panel)** and with right **(middle panel)** and left **(right panel)** atrial abnormalities. (Modified from Park MK, Guntheroth WG: How to Read Pediatric ECGs. 3rd ed. St Louis, Mosby-Year Book, 1993.)

TABLE 9–3 Common Diagnostic Criteria for Left and Right Atrial Abnormalities*

Left Atrial Abnormality	Right Atrial Abnormality
Prolonged P wave duration of >120 msec in lead II	Peaked P waves with amplitudes greater than 0.25 mV in lead II (P pulmonale)
Prominent notching of the P wave, usually most obvious in lead II, with an interval between the notches of >40 msec (P mitrale)	Rightward shift of the mean P wave axis to above 75 degrees
Ratio between the duration of the P wave in lead II and the duration of the PR segment of >1.6	Increased area under the initial positive portion of the P wave in lead V_1 to >0.06 mm-sec
Increased duration and depth of the terminal negative portion of the P wave in lead V_1 (the P terminal force) so that the area subtended by it exceeds 0.04 mm-sec	
Leftward shift of the mean P wave axis to between −30 and +45 degrees	

*In addition to criteria based on P wave morphologies, right atrial abnormalities are suggested by QRS changes, including (1) Q waves (especially qR patterns) in the right precordial leads without evidence of myocardial infarction and (2) low amplitude (under 600 μV) QRS complexes in lead V_1 with a threefold or greater increase in lead V_2.

CLINICAL SIGNIFICANCE. The ECG findings of left atrial abnormality are associated with more severe left ventricular dysfunction in patients with ischemic heart disease and with more severe valve damage in patients with mitral or aortic valve disease. Patients with left atrial changes also have a higher than normal incidence of paroxysmal atrial tachyarrhythmias.

Right Atrial Abnormality

ECG ABNORMALITIES. The ECG features of right atrial abnormality are illustrated in Figures 9–17 and 9–18. They include abnormally high P wave amplitudes in the limb and right precordial leads. As in the case of left atrial abnormality, the term *right atrial abnormality* is preferred over other terms such as *right atrial enlargement.*

DIAGNOSTIC CRITERIA. Criteria commonly used to diagnose right atrial abnormality are listed in Table 9–3.

MECHANISMS FOR ECG ABNORMALITIES. Greater right atrial mass generates greater electrical force early during overall atrial activation, with production of taller P waves and augmentation of the initial P wave deflection in lead V_1. In patients with chronic lung disease, the abnormal P pattern may reflect a more vertical heart position within the chest caused by pulmonary hyperinflation rather than true cardiac damage. The QRS changes commonly associated with right atrial abnormalities correspond to the underlying pathologic condition that is producing the right atrial hemodynamic changes—right ventricular hypertrophy (RVH), which produces tall R waves in the right precordial leads, and a shift of the position of the heart within the chest by obstructive lung disease, which produces initial Q waves.

DIAGNOSTIC ACCURACY. The finding of right atrial abnormality has limited sensitivity but high specificity. Echocardiographic correlations have shown, for example, that P pulmonale has very low sensitivity but very high specificity for detecting right atrial enlargement.

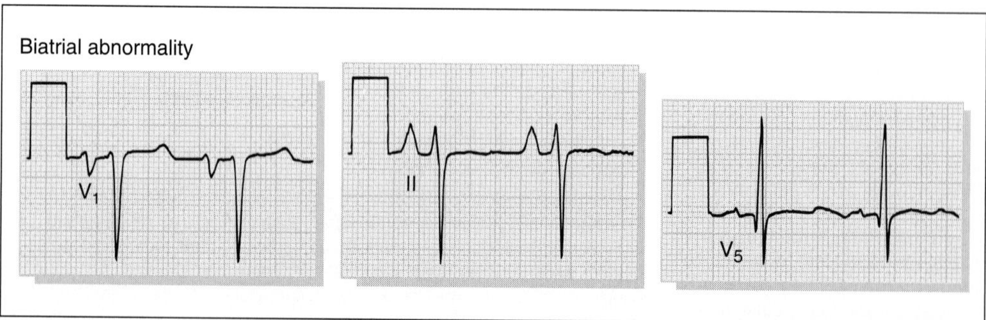

FIGURE 9–18 Biatrial abnormality, with tall P waves in lead II (right atrial abnormality) and an abnormally large terminal negative component of the P wave in lead V_1 (left atrial abnormality). The P wave is also notched in lead V_5.

CLINICAL SIGNIFICANCE. Patients with chronic obstructive pulmonary disease and this ECG pattern have more severe pulmonary dysfunction, as well as significantly reduced survival.[28] However, comparison of ECG and hemodynamic parameters has not demonstrated a close correlation of P wave patterns and right atrial hypertension.

Other Atrial Abnormalities

Patients with abnormalities in both atria—that is, *biatrial abnormality*—can have ECG patterns reflecting each defect. Suggestive findings include large biphasic P waves in lead V_1 and tall and broad P waves in leads II, III, and aV_f (see Fig. 9–18).

P wave and PR segment changes can also be seen in patients with atrial infarction or pericarditis. The changes caused by these conditions are described later in this chapter.

Ventricular Hypertrophy and Enlargement

Left Ventricular Hypertrophy and Enlargement

ECG ABNORMALITIES. Left ventricular hypertrophy (LVH) or enlargement produces changes in the QRS complex, the ST segment, and the T wave. The most characteristic finding is increased amplitude of the QRS complex. R waves in leads facing the left ventricle (that is, leads I, aV_l, V_5, and V_6) are taller than normal, whereas S waves in leads overlying the right ventricle (that is, V_1 and V_2) are deeper than normal. These changes are illustrated schematically in Figure 9–19.

ST-T wave patterns vary widely in patients with left ventricular enlargement and hypertrophy. ST segment and T wave amplitudes can be normal or increased in leads with tall R waves. In many patients, however, the ST segment is depressed and followed by an inverted T wave (Fig. 9–20). Most often, the ST segment slopes downward from a depressed J point and the T wave is asymmetrically inverted. These repolarization changes usually occur in patients with QRS changes but can appear alone. Particularly prominent inverted T waves, or so-called *giant negative T waves*, are characteristic of hypertrophic cardiomyopathy with predominant apical thickening, especially in patients from the Pacific Rim (*Yamaguchi syndrome*) (see Fig. 9–49).

Other ECG changes seen in cases of LVH include widening and notching of the QRS complex. An increase in QRS duration beyond 110 msec and a delay in the intrinsicoid deflection may reflect the longer duration of activation in a thickened ventricular wall or damage to the ventricular conduction system. Notching of the QRS complex may also be observed.

These ECG features are most typical of LVH induced by pressure or "systolic overload" of the left ventricle. Volume overload or "diastolic overload" can produce a somewhat different ECG pattern, including tall, upright T waves and sometimes narrow (less than 25 msec) but deep (0.2 mV or greater) Q waves in leads facing the left side of the septum (Fig. 9–20). The diagnostic value of these changes in predicting the underlying hemodynamics is, however, very limited.

MECHANISMS FOR ECG ABNORMALITIES. High voltages can be produced by any of several mechanisms. They can be due directly to an increase in left ventricular mass. This increase in mass is due to an enlargement in cell size, with an increase in surface area increasing transmembrane current flow and an increase in the number of intercalated disks enhancing intercellular current flow. This effect is augmented by an increase in the size of activation fronts moving across the thickened wall; these larger wavefronts subtend larger solid angles and result in higher body surface voltage.

The high voltage as well as QRS prolongation can also be due to conduction system delays. The delay in intrinsicoid deflection is a result of the prolonged transmural activation time required to activate the thickened wall, as well as delayed endocardial activation. Notching of the QRS complex can be produced by the fractionation of activation wavefronts by intramural scarring associated with wall thickening and damage.

In addition, changes in transmission factors can contribute to ECG abnormalities. Left ventricular enlargement can shift the position of the heart so that the lateral free wall lies closer than normal to the chest wall, which, as described earlier, would increase body surface potentials in accordance with the inverse square law.

Also, ventricular dilatation increases the size of the highly conductive intraventricular blood pool. This enhanced blood volume results in an increase in potentials produced by transmural activation fronts, a phenomenon referred to as the *Brody effect.*

Repolarization abnormalities can reflect a primary disorder of repolarization that accompanies the cellular processes of hypertrophy. Alternatively, they can reflect subendocardial ischemia. Patients with coronary artery disease have a higher prevalence of ST-T abnormalities with LVH than do those without coronary artery disease. Ischemia can be induced in the absence of coronary artery disease by the combination of high oxygen demand caused by high wall tension and limited blood flow to the subendocardium of the thickened wall.

DIAGNOSTIC CRITERIA. Many sets of diagnostic criteria for LVH have been developed on the basis of these ECG abnormalities (Fig. 9–21). Details of widely used criteria are presented in Table 9–4. Most commonly used methods assess the presence or absence of LVH as a binary function based on an empirically determined

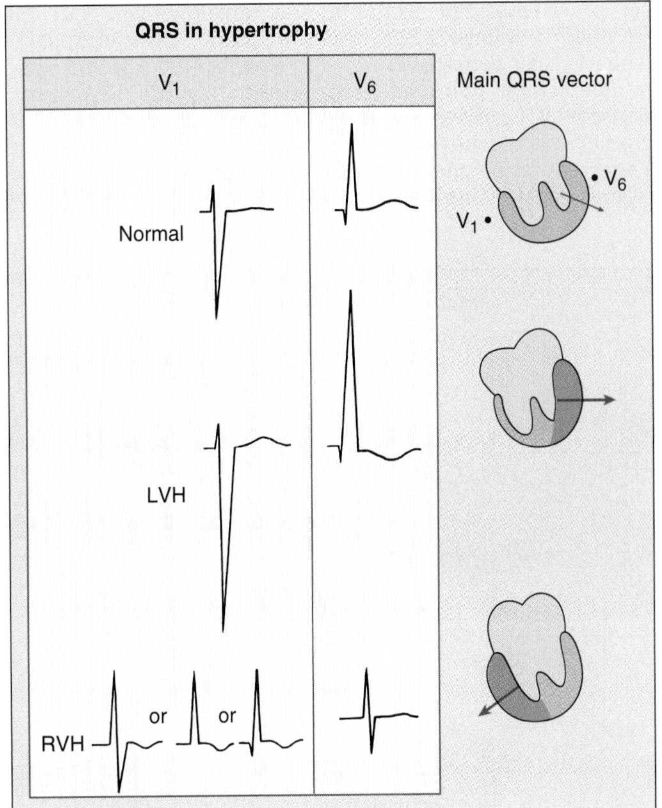

FIGURE 9–19 Left ventricular hypertrophy (LVH) increases the amplitude of electrical forces directed to the left and posteriorly. In addition, repolarization abnormalities can cause ST segment depression and T wave inversion in leads with a prominent R wave (formerly referred to as a "strain" pattern). Right ventricular hypertrophy (RVH) can shift the QRS vector to the right; this effect is usually associated with an R, RS, or qR complex in lead V_1, especially when due to severe pressure overload. T wave inversions may be present in the right precordial leads. (From Goldberger AL: Clinical Electrocardiography: A Simplified Approach. 6th ed. St Louis, CV Mosby, 1999.)

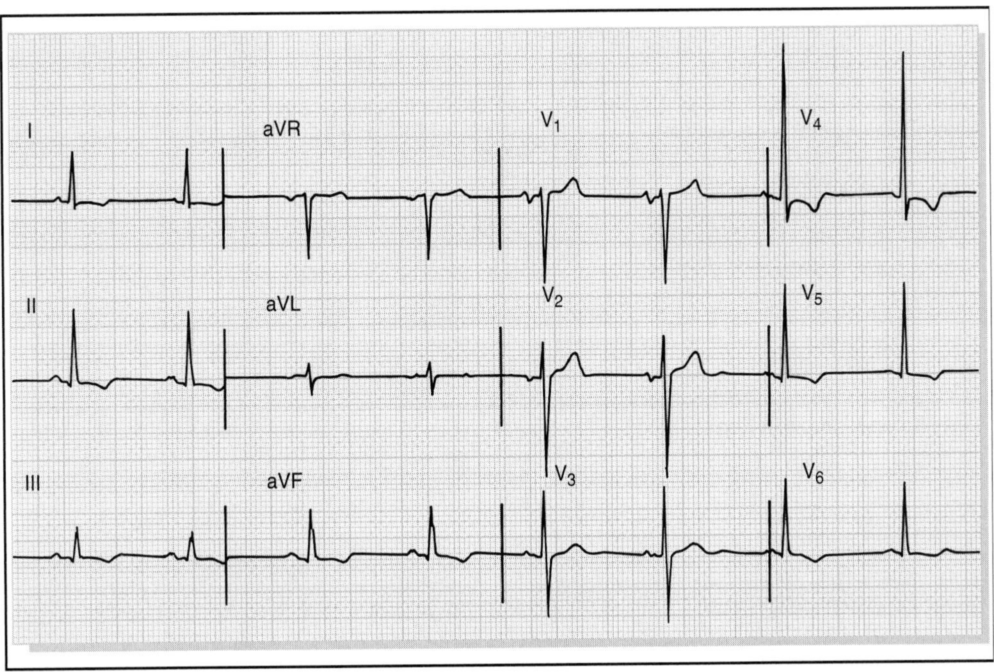

FIGURE 9–20 Marked left ventricular hypertrophy (LVH) pattern with prominent precordial lead QRS voltages. ST depression and T wave inversion can be seen with severe LVH in leads with a predominant R wave (compare with Fig. 9–21). Left atrial abnormality is also present.

set of criteria. For example, the Sokolow-Lyon and the Cornell[29,30] voltage criteria require that voltages in specific leads exceed certain values. The Romhilt-Estes point score system assigns point values to amplitude and other criteria; definite LVH is diagnosed if 5 points are computed, and probable LVH is diagnosed if 4 points are computed. The Cornell voltage-duration method includes measurement of QRS duration as well as amplitudes.

Other methods seek to quantify left ventricular mass as a continuum. Diagnosis of LVH can then be based on a computed mass that exceeds an independently determined threshold. Two recently developed sets of criteria applying this approach are the Cornell regression equation and the Novacode system.

Diagnostic Accuracy. The relative diagnostic accuracy of these methods has been tested by radiographic, echocardiographic, and autopsy measurements of left ventricular size as standards. In general, these studies have reported low sensitivity and high specificity. Sensitivities are lowest (approximately 10 to 30 percent) for the Sokolow-Lyon and Romhilt-Estes criteria and higher for the Cornell voltage and voltage-duration criteria and for the Cornell and Novacode regression methods (35 to 50 percent). In contrast, specificities for all measures vary from 85 percent to 95 percent. Thus, all methods are limited as screening tests in which high sensitivities (few false-negatives) are critical but have good reliability as diagnostic tests when few false-positives are desired.

Repolarization abnormalities associated with ECG findings increase the correlation with anatomical LVH. ST and T wave abnormalities

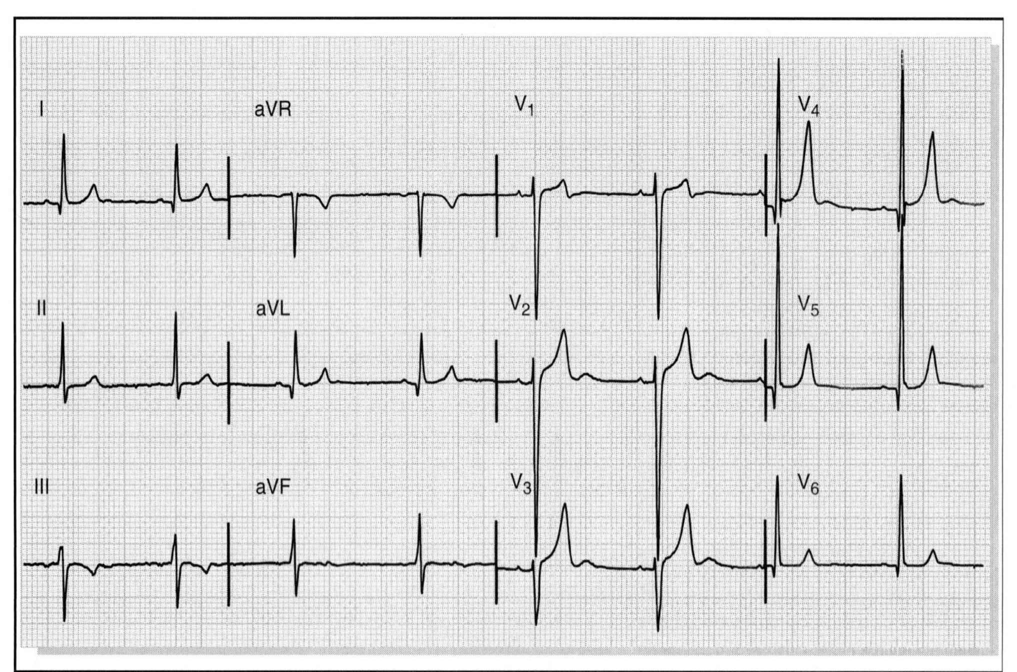

FIGURE 9–21 Left ventricular hypertrophy with prominent positive anterior T waves from a patient with severe aortic regurgitation. This pattern has been described with "diastolic overload" syndrome but has limited sensitivity and specificity. Serum potassium level was normal.

TABLE 9–4 Common Diagnostic Criteria for Left Ventricular Hypertrophy

Measurement	Criteria	
Sokolow-Lyon index	$S_{V1} + (R_{V5}$ or $R_{V6}) > 3.5$ mV $R_{aVl} > 1.1_{l}$ mV	
Romhilt-Estes point score system*	Any limb lead R wave or S wave ≥2.0 mV *or* S_{V1} or $S_{V2} \geq 3.0$ mV *or* R_{V5} to $R_{V6} \geq 3.0$ mV ST-T wave abnormality (no digitalis therapy) ST-T wave abnormality (digitalis therapy) Left atrial abnormality Left axis deviation (≥30 degrees) QRS duration ≥90 msec Intrinsicoid deflection in V_5 or V_6 ≥50 msec	3 points 3 points 3 points 3 points 1 point 3 points 2 points 1 point 1 point
Cornell voltage criteria	$S_{V3} + S_{aVl} \geq 2.8$ mV (for men) $S_{V3} + S_{aVl} \geq 2.0$ mV (for women)	
Cornell regression equation	Risk of LVH = $1/(1 + e^{-exp})$, where exp = 4.558 – 0.092 ($R_{aVl} + S_{V3}$) – 0.306 T_{V1} – 0.212 QRS – 0.278 PTF_{V1} – 0.859 (sex), voltages are in mV, QRS is QRS duration in msec, PTF is the area under the P terminal force in lead V_1 (in mm-sec), and sex = 1 for men and 2 for women; LVH is present if exp < –1.55.	
Cornell voltage-duration measurement[55]	QRS duration X Cornell Voltage <2436 QRS duration X sum of voltages in all leads >17,472	
Novacode criterion (for men)	LVMI (gm/m²) = –36.4 + 0.010 R_{V5} + 0.20 S_{V1} + 0.28 $S^{\dagger}_{III}$ + 0.182 $T_{(neg)}V_6$ – 0.148 $T_{(pos)}$aVr + 1.049 $QRS_{duration}$ where neg and pos refer to amplitudes of the negative and positive portions of the T waves, respectively; $S^{\dagger}_{III}$ indicates the amplitude of the S, Q, and QS wave, whichever is larger	

LVH = left ventricular hypertrophy; LVMI = left ventricular mass index.
*Probable left ventricular hypertrophy is diagnosed if 4 points are present and definite left ventricular hypertrophy is diagnosed if 5 or more points are present.

are associated with a three-fold greater prevalence of anatomical LVH in patients without coronary artery disease and a fivefold greater risk among patients with coronary disease.[31] The prevalence of anatomical LVH increases with the magnitude of the ST-segment depression.[32]

Which diagnostic criteria are met may have pathophysiological and clinical implications. Most patients with ECG criteria for LVH meet criteria for one set of criteria but not others.[30] Those meeting Cornell criteria have different patterns of left ventricular geometry than do those meeting Sokolow-Lyon criteria.[33]

Accuracy of the diagnostic criteria vary with demographic and related features of the populations studied. For example, precordial voltages are often higher among African Americans than among white persons, which leads to a higher prevalence of false-positive ECG diagnoses of left ventricular hypertrophy among African Americans with hypertension.[34]

Several reasons can be suggested for the limited accuracy of these criteria. Many of the clinical studies that were used to define the criteria included a disproportionate number of white men, thus limiting applicability of the tests to other populations. In addition, the criteria for dichotomous tests such as the Sokolow-Lyon and Cornell voltage criteria are based on quantitative differences in normally occurring measures, that is, QRS voltage, between normal and abnormal cohorts. These tests by their nature are limited to detecting only the extreme end of the spectrum of LVH, because milder degrees overlap with findings in normal populations. Finally, these voltage measurements are subject to the influence of many noncardiac factors, such as body habitus, which blurs the distinction between normal and abnormal.[35]

CLINICAL SIGNIFICANCE. The presence of ECG criteria for LVH identifies a subset of the general population with a significantly increased risk for cardiovascular morbidity and mortality.[36] This increased risk is particularly apparent in women and in people in whom ST-T wave abnormalities are present; the relative risk of cardiovascular events for patients with LVH voltage criteria alone is approximately 2.8, whereas the relative risk increases to more than 5.0 if ST segment depression is also present.[37] Interestingly, positive diagnoses of LVH by Sokolow-Lyon criteria and by Cornell criteria have independent prognostic value.[38]

In patients with cardiac disease, the ECG finding of LVH correlates with more severe disease, including higher blood pressure in hypertensive patients and greater ventricular dysfunction in patients with hypertension or coronary artery disease. In contrast, effective treatment of hypertension reduces ECG evidence of LVH and decreases the associated risk of cardiovascular mortality (see Chap. 38).

Patients with repolarization abnormalities have, on average, more severe degrees of LVH and more commonly have symptoms of left ventricular dysfunction, in addition to a greater risk of cardiovascular events.

Right Ventricular Hypertrophy and Enlargement

ECG ABNORMALITIES. The right ventricle is considerably smaller than the left ventricle and produces electrical forces that are largely concealed by those generated by the larger left ventricle. Thus, for RVH to be manifested on the ECG, it must be severe enough to overcome the concealing effects of the larger left ventricular forces. In addition, increasing dominance of the right ventricle changes the ECG in fundamental ways, whereas an enlarged left ventricle produces predominantly quantitative changes in underlying normal waveforms.

The ECG changes associated with moderate to severe concentric hypertrophy of the right ventricle include abnormally tall R waves in anteriorly and rightward directed leads (leads aV_r, V_1, and V_2) and deep S waves and abnormally small r waves in leftward directed leads (I, aV_l, and lateral precordial leads) (Fig. 9–22). These changes result in a reversal of normal R wave progression in the precordial leads, a shift in the frontal plane QRS axis to the right, and sometimes the presence of S waves in leads I, II, and III (so-called *$S_1S_2S_3$ pattern*).

Several other ECG patterns of RVH also exist. Less severe hypertrophy, especially when limited to the outflow tract of the right ventricle that is activated late during the QRS complex, produces less marked changes. ECG abnormalities may be limited to an rSr′ pattern in V_1 and persistence of s (or S) waves in the left precordial leads. This pattern is typical of right ventricular volume overload as produced by an atrial septal defect.

Chronic Obstructive Pulmonary Disease. Chronic obstructive pulmonary disease can induce ECG changes by producing RVH, changes in the position of the heart within the chest, and hyperinflation of the lungs (Fig. 9–23). QRS changes caused by the insulating and positional changes produced by hyperinflation of the lungs include reduced amplitude of the QRS complex, right axis deviation in the

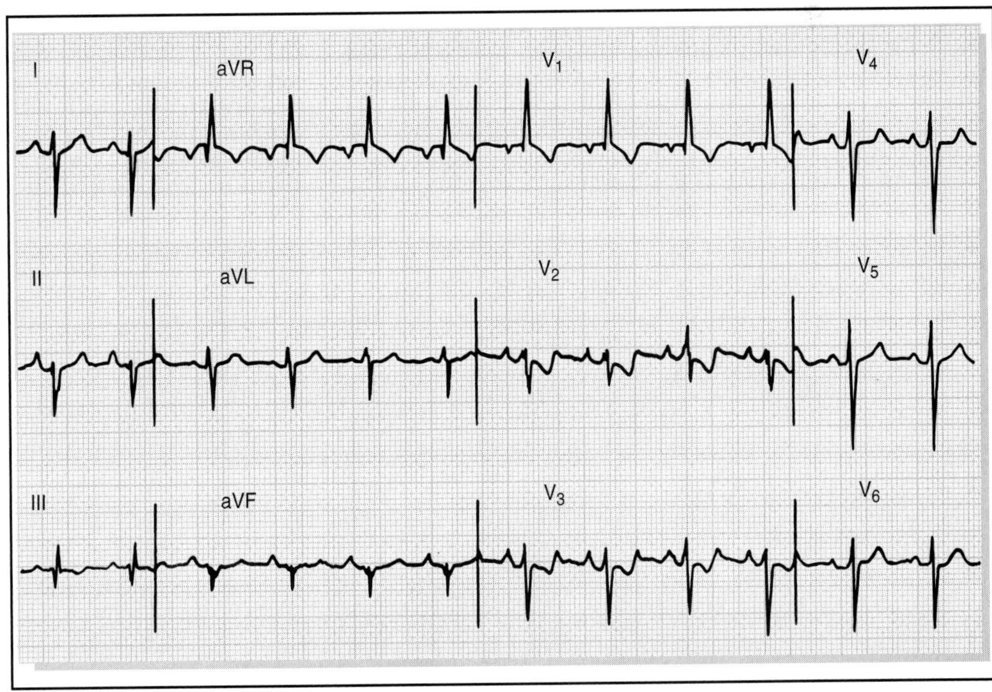

FIGURE 9–22 Right ventricular hypertrophy pattern most consistent with severe pressure overload. Note the combination of findings, including (1) a tall R wave in V_1 (as part of the qR complex), (2) right axis deviation, (3) T wave inversion in V_1 through V_3, (4) delayed precordial transition zone (rS in V_6), and (5) right atrial abnormality. An S_1Q_3 pattern is also present and can occur with acute or chronic right ventricular overload syndromes.

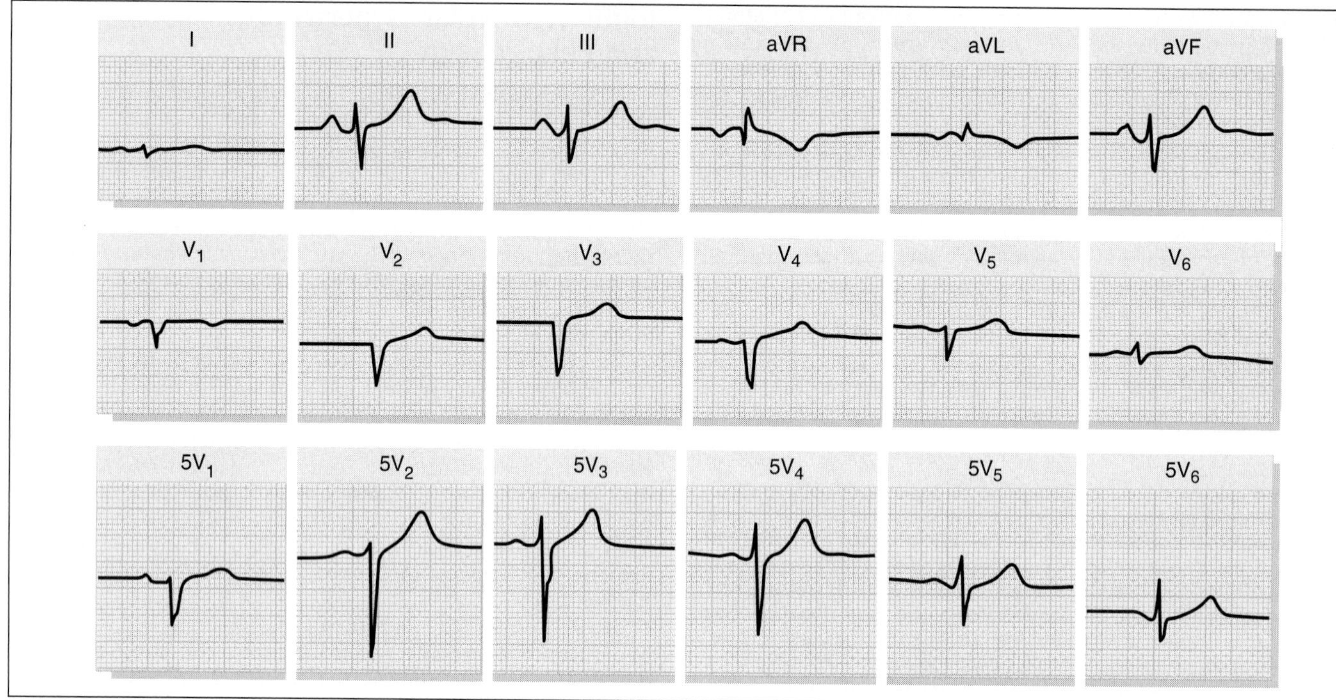

FIGURE 9–23 Pulmonary emphysema simulating anterior infarction in a 58-year-old man with no clinical evidence of coronary disease. Note the relative normalization of R wave progression with placement of the chest leads an interspace below their usual position ($5V_1$, $5V_2$, and so forth). (From Chou TC: Pseudo-infarction (noninfarction Q waves). *In* Fisch C [ed]: Complex Electrocardiography. Vol 1. Philadelphia, FA Davis, 1973.)

frontal plane, and delayed transition in the precordial leads (probably reflecting a vertical and caudal shift in heart position because of hyperinflation and a flattened diaphragm). Evidence of true RVH includes (1) marked right axis deviation (more positive than 110 degrees), (2) deep S waves in the lateral precordial leads, and (3) an $S_1Q_3T_3$ pattern, with an S wave in lead I (as an RS or rS complex), an abnormal Q wave in lead III, and an inverted T wave in the inferior leads.

Pulmonary Embolism. Finally, acute right ventricular pressure overload such as produced by pulmonary embolism can produce a characteristic ECG pattern (Fig. 9–24), including (1) a QR or qR pattern in the right ventricular leads; (2) an $S_1Q_3T_3$ pattern with an S wave in lead I and new or increased Q waves in lead III and sometimes aV_f, with T wave inversions in those leads; (3) ST segment deviation and T wave inversions in leads V_1 to V_3; and (4) incomplete or complete right bundle branch block (RBBB). Sinus tachycardia is usually present. Arrhythmias such as atrial fibrillation can also occur. However, even with major pulmonary artery obstruction, the ECG is notoriously deceptive and may show little more than minor or nonspecific waveform changes, or it may even be normal. The classic $S_1Q_3T_3$ pattern occurs in only about 10 percent of cases of acute pulmonary embolism (see Chaps. 66 and 67). Furthermore, the specificity of this finding is limited, because it can occur acutely with other causes of pulmonary hypertension.

DIAGNOSTIC CRITERIA. These ECG abnormalities form the basis for the diagnostic criteria for RVH. The most commonly relied on criteria for the ECG diagnosis of RVH are listed in Table 9–5.

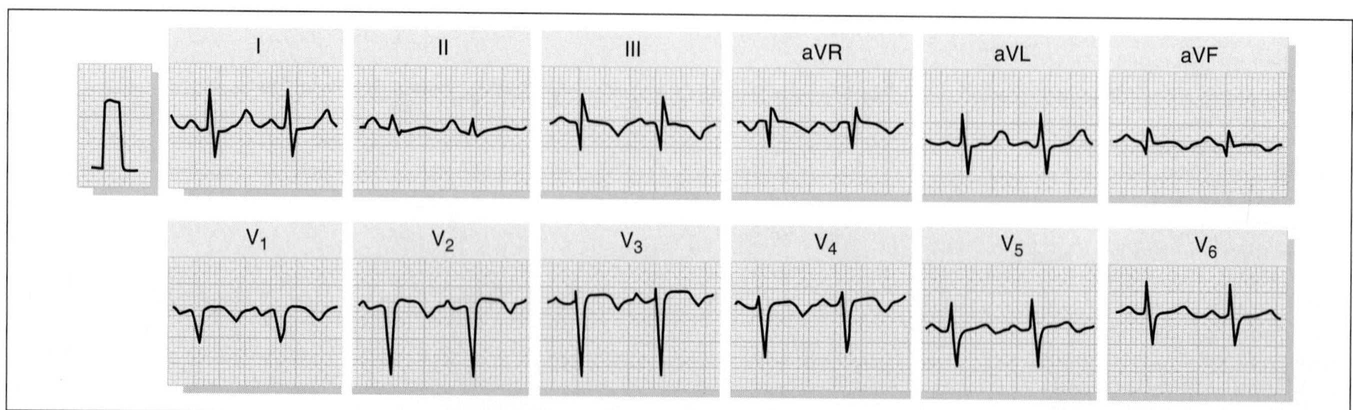

FIGURE 9–24 Acute cor pulmonale secondary to pulmonary embolism simulating inferior and anterior infarction. This tracing exemplifies the classic pseudoinfarct patterns sometimes seen: an $S_1Q_3T_3$, a QR in V_1 with poor R wave progression in the right precordial leads ("clockwise rotation"), and right precordial to midprecordial T wave inversion (V_1 to V_4). Sinus tachycardia is also present. The S_1Q_3 pattern is usually associated with a QR or QS complex, but not an rS, in aV_f. Furthermore, acute cor pulmonale per se does not cause prominent Q waves in II (only in III and aV_f). (From Goldberger AL: Myocardial Infarction: Electrocardiographic Differential Diagnosis. 4th ed. St Louis, Mosby-Year Book, 1991.)

TABLE 9–5 Common Diagnostic Criteria for Right Ventricular Hypertrophy

Criterion	Sensitivity (%)	Specificity (%)
R in $V_1 \geq 0.7$ mV	<10	—
QR in V_1	<10	—
R/S in $V_1 > 1$ with R > 0.5 mV	<25	89
R/S in V_5 or $V_6 < 1$	<10	—
S in V_5 or $V_6 \geq 0.7$ mV	<17	93
R in V_5 or $V_6 \geq 0.4$ mV with S in $V_1 \geq 0.2$ mV	<10	—
Right axis deviation (≥+90 degrees)	<14	99
S_1Q_3 pattern	<11	93
$S_1S_2S_3$ pattern	<10	—
P pulmonale	<11	97

From Murphy ML, Thenabadu PN, de Soyza N, et al: Reevaluation of electrocardiographic criteria for left, right and combined cardiac ventricular hypertrophy. Am J Cardiol 53:1140, 1984

MECHANISMS FOR ECG ABNORMALITIES. These ECG patterns result from three effects of RVH. First, current fluxes between hypertrophied cells are stronger than normal and produce higher than normal voltage on the body surface. Second, activation fronts moving through the enlarged right ventricle are larger than normal and produce higher surface potentials, as predicted by the solid angle theorem. Third, the activation time of the right ventricle is prolonged. This last effect is particularly important in producing ECG changes; right ventricular activation now ends after the completion of left ventricular activation, so its effects are no longer canceled by the more powerful forces of the left ventricle and may merge in the ECG. Because the right ventricle is located anteriorly as well as to the right of the left ventricle, the effects produce increased potentials in leads directed anteriorly and to the right, especially late during the QRS complex. As noted, changes in cardiac position in patients with obstructive lung disease can produce ECG changes without intrinsic cardiac electrophysiological derangements.

Diagnostic Accuracy. The sensitivity and specificity of the individual ECG criteria are also shown in Table 9–5. As in the case of ECG criteria for other abnormalities, the sensitivities of individual criteria are low and specificities are high. If any one feature is present, the sensitivity rises to more than 50 percent with a specificity of more than 90 percent; requiring any two features to make a diagnosis markedly reduces the sensitivity and raises the specificity to very high levels. These low sensitivities may reflect the marked degree of hypertrophy required to produce ECG abnormalities.

CLINICAL SIGNIFICANCE. The ECG evidence of RVH has limited value in assessing the severity of pulmonary hypertension or lung disease. QRS changes do not generally appear until ventilatory function is significantly depressed, with the earliest change commonly being a rightward shift in the mean QRS axis, and correlation with either ventilatory function or hemodynamics is poor. The presence of right atrial abnormality, an $S_1S_2S_3$ pattern, or both is associated with reduced survival, especially if an increased arterial-alveolar oxygen gradient is also present. ECG findings of acute right ventricular overload in patients with pulmonary embolism correspond to obstruction of more than 50 percent of the pulmonary arterial bed and significant pulmonary hypertension.

Biventricular Enlargement

Enlargement or hypertrophy of both ventricles produces complex ECG patterns.[39] In contrast to biatrial enlargement, the result is not the simple sum of the two sets of abnormalities. The effects of enlargement of one chamber may cancel the effects of enlargement of the other; for example, anterior forces produced by RVH may be canceled by enhanced posterior forces generated by LVH. In addition, the greater left ventricular forces generated in LVH increase the degree of RVH needed to overcome the dominance of the left ventricle.

Because of these factors, specific ECG criteria for either RVH or LVH are seldom observed with biventricular enlargement. Rather, ECG patterns are usually a modification of the features of LVH and include (1) tall R waves in both the right and left precordial leads, (2) vertical heart position or right axis deviation in the presence of criteria for LVH, (3) deep S waves in the left precordial leads in the presence of ECG criteria for LVH, or (4) a shift in the precordial transition zone to the left in the presence of LVH. The presence of prominent left atrial abnormality or atrial fibrillation with evidence of right ventricular or biventricular enlargement (especially LVH with a vertical or rightward QRS axis) should suggest chronic rheumatic valvular disease (Fig. 9–25) (see Chap. 57).

Intraventricular Conduction Delays and Preexcitation

The ECG patterns described in this section reflect abnormalities in the conduction system (see Chap. 29).

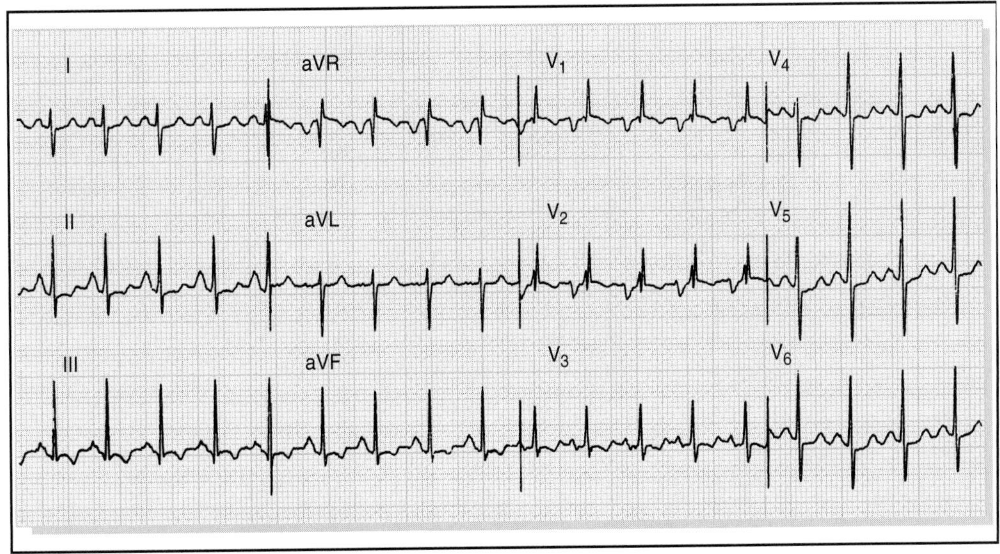

FIGURE 9–25 This electrocardiogram from a 45-year-old woman with severe mitral stenosis shows multiple abnormalities. The rhythm is sinus tachycardia. Right axis deviation and a tall R wave in lead V_1 are consistent with right ventricular hypertrophy. The very prominent biphasic P wave in lead V_1 indicates left atrial abnormality/enlargement. The tall P waves in lead II suggest concomitant right abnormality. Nonspecific ST-T changes and incomplete right bundle branch block are also present. The combination of right ventricular hypertrophy and marked left or biatrial abnormality is highly suggestive of mitral stenosis. (From Goldberger AL: Clinical Electrocardiography: A Simplified Approach. 6th ed. St Louis, CV Mosby, 1999.)

Fascicular Blocks

Under normal conditions, activation of the left ventricle begins simultaneously at the insertion sites of the fascicles. Delayed conduction in a fascicle—*fascicular block*—results in activation of these sites sequentially rather than simultaneously. This produces an abnormal sequence of early left ventricular activation that, in turn, leads to characteristic ECG patterns. Even modest delays in conduction through the affected structure may be enough to alter ventricular activation patterns sufficiently to produce characteristic ECG patterns; complete block of conduction is not required.

LEFT ANTERIOR FASCICULAR BLOCK. Damage to the left anterior fascicle is a very common occurrence because of the delicate nature of the structure. The ECG features of left anterior fascicular block (LAFB) are listed in Table 9–6 and illustrated in Figure 9–26. The most characteristic finding is marked left axis deviation. However, LAFB is not synonymous with left axis deviation. Axis shifts to between −30 and −45 degrees commonly reflect other conditions, such as LVH, without conduction system damage and are best referred to as *left axis deviation* rather than LAFB.

TABLE 9–6 Common Diagnostic Criteria for Unifascicular Blocks

Left anterior fascicular block
Frontal plane mean QRS axis of −45 to −90 degrees with rS patterns in leads II, III, and aV_f and a qR pattern in lead aV_l
QRS duration less than 120 msec
Left posterior fascicular block
Frontal plane mean QRS axis of ±120 degrees
RS pattern in leads I and aV_l with qR patterns in inferior leads
QRS duration of less than 120 msec
Exclusion of other factors causing right axis deviation (e.g., right ventricular overload patterns, lateral infarction)

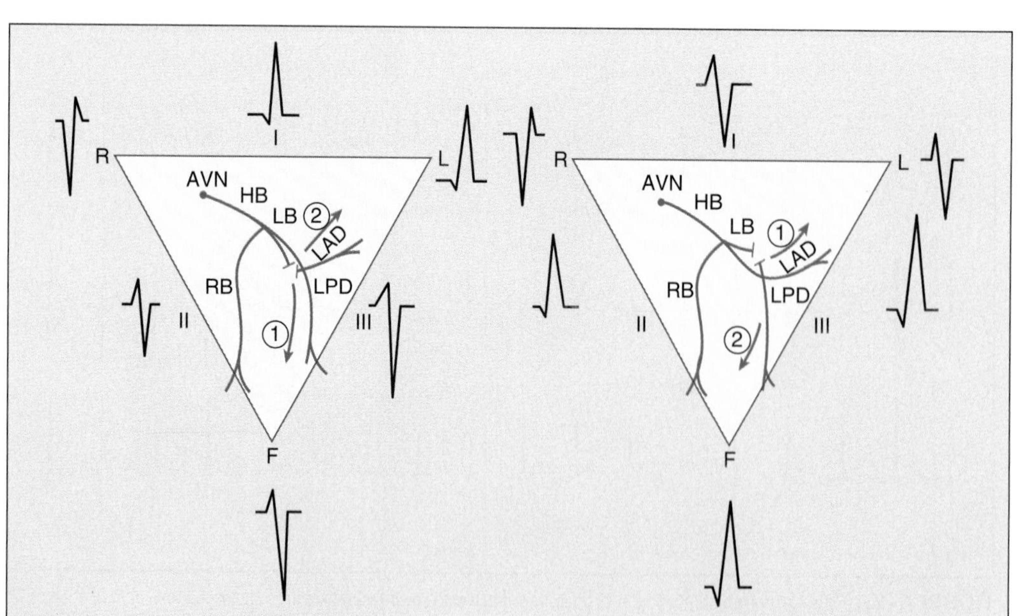

FIGURE 9–26 Diagrammatic representation of fascicular blocks in the left ventricle. Interruption of the left anterior fascicle (LAF) **(left)** results in an initial inferior (1) followed by a dominant superior (2) direction of activation. Interruption of the left posterior fascicle (LPF) **(right)** results in an initial superior (1) followed by a dominant inferior (2) direction of activation. AVN = atrioventricular node; HB = His bundle; LB = left bundle; RB = right bundle. (Courtesy of C. Fisch, M.D.)

Left axis shift is a result of delayed activation of the anterosuperior left ventricular wall. Delayed activation causes unbalanced inferior and posterior forces early during ventricular activation and unopposed anterosuperior forces later during the QRS complex. The abnormal pattern results in initial r waves followed by deep S waves in the inferior leads (left axis deviation with rS patterns) and a qR pattern in left-looking leads (leads aV_l and usually V_5 and V_6). Initial q waves in these leads reflect the normal left-to-right activation of the septum. LAFB can also produce prominent changes in the precordial leads; V_4 through V_6 commonly show deep S waves related to superiorly directed late QRS forces. The overall QRS duration is not prolonged; fascicular block alters only the sequence of left ventricular activation but does not by itself prolong the overall duration of ventricular excitation or the QRS complex.

Left anterior fascicular block is common in persons without overt cardiac disease, as well as in persons with a wide range of diseases. It has minimal or no independent prognostic significance. Commonly associated cardiac and systemic conditions include myocardial infarction, especially occlusion of the left anterior descending coronary artery, LVH, hypertrophic and dilated cardiomyopathy, and degenerative diseases. The development of LAFB with rS complexes in II, III, and aV_f can mask the Q waves of a prior inferior myocardial infarction.

LEFT POSTERIOR FASCICULAR BLOCK. Conduction delay in the left posterior fascicle is considerably less common than delay in the anterior fascicle because of its thicker structure and more protected location near the left ventricular inflow tract. Conduction delay results in sequential activation of the anterosuperior left ventricular free wall, followed by activation of the inferoposterior aspect of the left ventricle, that is, the reverse of the pattern observed with LAFB.

The ECG features of left posterior fascicular block (LPFB), listed in Table 9–6 and illustrated in Figure 9–26, reflect this altered activation pattern. Right axis deviation with rS patterns in leads I and aV_l, as well as qR complexes in the inferior leads, is the result of early unopposed activation forces from the anterosuperior aspect of the left ventricle (producing the initial q and r waves) and late unopposed forces from the inferoposterior free wall (generating the late S and R waves). As in the case of LAFB, the overall activation time of the ventricles is not prolonged and the QRS duration remains normal.

Left posterior fascicular block, like LAFB, can occur in patients with almost any cardiac disease but is unusual in otherwise healthy persons. Other conditions that enhance electrical forces from the right ventricle, such as right ventricular enlargement and extensive lateral infarction, can produce similar ECG patterns and must be excluded before a diagnosis of LPFB is made.

OTHER FORMS OF FASCICULAR BLOCK. The ECG evidence of left septal fascicular block has also been described. These patterns are adduced to reflect conduction delay in the third fascicle of the left bundle branch system—the septal fascicle—that inserts high on the left side of the interventricular septum. Among the ECG changes that are attributed to this form of block is the absence of septal q waves reflecting an abnormal sequence of septal activation.[16]

Left Bundle Branch Block

Left bundle branch block (LBBB) results from conduction delay or block in any of several sites in the intraventricular conduction system, including the main left bundle branch, in each of the two fascicles, or, less commonly, within the fibers of the bundle of His that become the main left bundle branch. The result is extensive reorganization of the activation pattern of the left ventricle.

ECG ABNORMALITIES. LBBB produces a prolonged QRS duration, abnormal QRS complexes, and ST-T wave abnormalities (Fig. 9–27). Commonly accepted diagnostic criteria for LBBB are listed in Table 9–7. Basic requirements include a prolonged QRS duration to 120 msec or beyond; broad, sometimes notched R waves in leads I and aV_l and the left precordial leads; narrow r waves followed by deep S waves in the right precordial leads; and absent septal q waves. R waves are typically tall and S waves are deep. The mean QRS axis with LBBB is highly variable; it can be normal, deviated to the left or, less often, deviated to the right.[40] Left axis deviation is associated with more severe conduction system disease that includes the fascicles as well as the main left bundle,[41] whereas right axis deviation suggests dilated cardiomyopathy with biventricular enlargement.[40] In addition to these features, some electrocardiographers require a delayed intrinsicoid deflection (60 msec or greater) to diagnose LBBB.

ST-T wave changes are also prominent with LBBB. In most cases, the ST wave and the T wave are discordant with the QRS complex; that is, the ST segment is depressed and the T wave is inverted in leads with positive QRS waves (leads I, aV_l, V_5, and V_6), while the ST segment is elevated and the T wave is upright in leads with negative QRS complexes (leads V_1 and V_2).

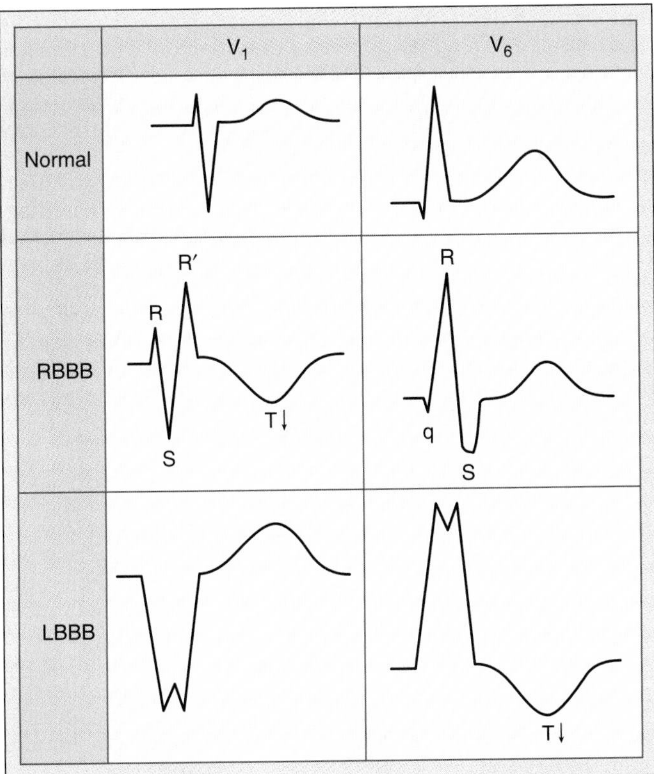

FIGURE 9–27 Comparison of typical QRS-T patterns in right bundle branch block (RBBB) and left bundle branch block (LBBB) with the normal pattern in leads V_1 and V_6. Note the secondary T wave inversions (arrows) in leads with an rSR′ complex with RBBB and in leads with a wide R wave with LBBB. (From Goldberger AL: Clinical Electrocardiography: A Simplified Approach. 6th ed. St Louis, CV Mosby, 1999.)

TABLE 9–7 Common Diagnostic Criteria for Bundle Branch Blocks

Complete left bundle branch block
QRS duration ≥120 msec
Broad, notched R waves in lateral precordial leads (V_5 and V_6) and usually leads I and aV_l
Small or absent initial r waves in right precordial leads (V_1 and V_2) followed by deep S waves
Absent septal q waves in left-sided leads
Prolonged intrinsicoid deflection (>60 msec) in V_5 and V_6*
Complete right bundle branch block
QRS duration ≥120 msec
Broad, notched R waves (rsr′, rsR′, or rSR′ patterns) in right precordial leads (V_1 and V_2)
Wide and deep S waves in left precordial leads (V_5 and V_6)

*Criterion required by some authors.

An incomplete form of LBBB may result from lesser degrees of conduction delay in the left bundle branch system. Left ventricular activation begins, as in complete LBBB, on the right side of the septum, but much of left ventricular activation occurs through the normal specialized conduction system. ECG features include (1) loss of septal q waves (reflecting reversal of the normal pattern of septal activation), (2) slurring and notching of the upstroke of R waves (because of the presence of competing activation fronts), and (3) modest prolongation of the QRS complex (between 100 and 120 msec).

MECHANISMS FOR ECG ABNORMALITIES. The ECG abnormalities of LBBB result from an almost completely reorganized pattern of left ventricular activation. Initial septal activation occurs on the right (rather than on the left) septal surface, resulting in the absence of normal septal q waves in the ECG.

The excitation wave then spreads slowly, by conduction from muscle cell to muscle cell, to the left side of the septum; the earliest left ventricular activation begins as late as 30 to 50 msec into the QRS complex. Endocardial activation of the left ventricle may then require an additional 40 to more than 180 msec, depending largely on the functional status of the distal left bundle and Purkinje systems.[42] Thus, the overall QRS complex is prolonged and can be very wide in patients with, for example, diffuse ventricular scarring from prior myocardial infarction.

Once left ventricular activation begins, it proceeds in a relatively simple and direct manner around the free wall and, finally, to the base of the heart. This is in contrast to the multicentric, overlapping patterns of activation seen under normal conditions. Direct progression of activation across the left ventricle projects continuous positive forces to left-sided leads and continuous negative ones to right-sided leads. Spread predominantly through working muscle fibers rather than the specialized conduction system results in notching and slurring as a consequence of discontinuous anisotropy, as described earlier.

The discordant ST-T wave pattern is a result of the transventricular recovery gradients referred to earlier. With LBBB, the right ventricle is activated and recovers earlier than the left, so recovery vectors or dipoles are directed toward the right and away from the left. Hence, positive ST-T waves will be registered over the right ventricle and negatives ones over the left ventricle. These transventricular gradients play only a minor role in normal conduction because the simultaneous activation of multiple regions cancels the forces that they produce; with bundle branch block, activation is sequential, so cancellation is reduced. Because the ST-T wave changes with LBBB are generated by abnormalities in conduction, they are called *secondary T wave abnormalities*; as will be discussed later, ST-T wave changes produced by direct abnormalities of the recovery process are referred to as *primary T wave abnormalities.*

CLINICAL SIGNIFICANCE. LBBB usually appears in patients with underlying heart disease. It is associated with significantly reduced long-term survival and with 10-year survival rates as low as 50 percent, probably reflecting the severity of the underlying cardiac disease. Among patients with coronary artery disease, the presence of LBBB correlates with more extensive disease, more severe left ventricular dysfunction, and reduced survival rates. The duration of the QRS complex in LBBB correlates inversely with left ventricular ejection fraction.[43] Patients with associated left or right axis deviation have more severe clinical manifestations.

In addition to the hemodynamic abnormalities produced by these underlying conditions, the abnormal ventricular activation pattern of LBBB itself induces hemodynamic perturbations, including abnormal systolic function with dysfunctional contraction patterns, reduced ejection fraction and lower stroke volumes, and abnormal diastolic function; reversed splitting of the second heart sound and functional mitral regurgitation are common. In addition, functional abnormalities in phasic coronary blood flow and reduced coronary flow reserve caused by delayed diastolic relaxation[44] often result in septal or anteroseptal defects on exercise perfusion scintigraphy in the absence of coronary artery disease. Pharmacological vasodilator stress testing with dipyridamole or adenosine, or stress echocardiography (exercise or dobutamine), appear more specific than standard exercise scintigraphy in diagnosing left anterior descending coronary stenosis in the presence of LBBB.[45,46]

A major impact of LBBB lies in obscuring or simulating other ECG patterns. The diagnosis of LVH is complicated by the increased QRS amplitude and axis shifts intrinsic to LBBB; in addition, the very high prevalence of anatomical LVH in combination with LBBB makes defining criteria with high specificity difficult. The diagnosis of infarction may be obscured; as will be described, the emergence of abnormal Q waves with infarction is dependent on a normal initial sequence of ventricular activation, which is absent with LBBB. In addition, ECG patterns of LBBB, including low R wave amplitude in the midprecordial leads and ST-T wave changes, can simulate anterior infarct patterns.

Right Bundle Branch Block

Right bundle branch block is a result of conduction delay in any portion of the right-sided intraventricular conduction system. The delay can occur in the main right bundle branch itself, in the bundle of His, or in the distal right ventricular conduction system. The latter is the common cause of RBBB after right ventriculotomy performed, for example, to correct the tetralogy of Fallot. The high prevalence of RBBB corresponds to the relative fragility of the right bundle branch, as suggested by the development of RBBB after minor trauma produced by right ventricular catheterization.

ECG ABNORMALITIES. Major features of RBBB are illustrated in Figure 9–27, and commonly used diagnostic criteria are listed in Table 9–7. As with LBBB, the QRS complex duration exceeds 120 msec. The right precordial leads show prominent and notched R waves with rsr′, rsR′, or rSR′ patterns, while leads I, aV$_l$, and the left precordial leads demonstrate wide S waves that are longer in duration than the preceding R wave. Septal q waves are preserved because the initial ventricular activation remains unchanged. The ST-T waves are, as in LBBB, discordant with the QRS complex, so T waves are inverted in the right precordial leads (and other leads with a terminal R′ wave) and upright in the left precordial leads and in leads I and AV$_l$.

The mean QRS axis is not altered by RBBB. Axis shifts can occur, however, as a result of the simultaneous occurrence of fascicular block along with RBBB. This concurrence of RBBB with either LAFB (producing left axis deviation) or LPFB (producing right axis deviation) is termed *bifascicular block*.

Features indicative of incomplete RBBB, produced by lesser delays in conduction in the right bundle branch system, are commonly seen. This finding is most frequently characterized by an rSr′ pattern in lead V$_1$ with a QRS duration between 100 and 120 msec.

MECHANISMS FOR ECG ABNORMALITIES. With delay or block in the proximal right bundle branch system, activation of the right side of the septum is initiated after slow transseptal spread of activation from the left septal surface. The right ventricular free wall is then excited slowly, with variable participation of the specialized conduction system. The result is delayed and slowed activation of the right ventricle with much or all of the right ventricle undergoing activation after depolarization of the left ventricle has been completed.

Because left ventricular activation remains relatively intact, the early portions of the QRS complex are normal. Delayed activation of the right ventricle causes prolongation of the QRS duration and a reduction in the cancellation of RV activation forces by the more powerful left ventricular activation forces. The late and unopposed emergence of right ventricular forces produces increased anterior and rightward voltage in the ECG. Discordant ST-T wave patterns are generated by the same mechanisms as for LBBB; with RBBB, recovery forces are directed toward the earlier-activated left ventricle and away from the right. Although these ECG changes of incomplete RBBB are commonly attributed to conduction defects, they can reflect RVH without intrinsic dysfunction of the conduction system.

CLINICAL SIGNIFICANCE. RBBB is a common finding in the general population, and many persons with RBBB have no clinical evidence of structural heart disease. In the group without overt heart disease, the ECG finding has no prognostic significance. However, the new onset of RBBB does predict a higher rate of coronary artery disease, congestive heart failure, and cardiovascular mortality. When cardiac disease is present, the coexistence of RBBB suggests advanced disease with, for example, more extensive multivessel disease and reduced long-term survival in patients with ischemic heart disease. An entity known as the *Brugada syndrome* has been described in which a RBBB-like pattern with persistent ST segment elevation in the right precordial leads is associated with susceptibility to ventricular tachyarrhythmias and sudden cardiac death[47] (see Chap. 32).

Right bundle branch block interferes with other ECG diagnoses, although to a lesser extent than does LBBB. The diagnosis of RVH is more difficult to make with RBBB because of the accentuated positive potentials in lead V$_1$. RVH is suggested, although with limited accuracy, by the presence of an R wave in lead V$_1$ that exceeds 1.5 mV and a rightward shift of the mean QRS axis. The usual criteria for LVH can be applied but have lower sensitivities than with normal conduction. The combination of left atrial abnormality or left axis deviation with RBBB also suggests underlying LVH.

Multifascicular Blocks

The term *multifascicular block* refers to conduction delay in more than one of the structural components of the specialized conduction system—that is, the left bundle branch, the left anterior and posterior fascicles of the left bundle branch, and the right bundle branch. Conduction delay in any two fascicles is called *bifascicular block,* and delay in all three fascicles is called *trifascicular block.* The term *bilateral bundle branch block* is sometimes used to refer to concomitant conduction abnormalities in the left and right bundle branch systems.

Bifascicular block can have several forms. These include (1) RBBB with LAFB, which is characterized by the ECG pattern of RBBB plus left axis deviation beyond −45 degrees (Fig. 9–28), (2) RBBB with LPFB, with an ECG pattern of RBBB and a mean QRS axis deviation to the right of +120 degrees (Fig. 9–29), or (3) LBBB that may be caused by delay in both the anterior and posterior fascicles. This form of LBBB represents one of the inadequacies of current ECG terminology and the simplification inherent in the trifascicular schema of the conduction system. The electrophysiological consequences of these abnormalities are discussed in Chapters 29, 30, and 31.

Trifascicular block involves conduction delay in the right bundle branch plus delay in either the main left bundle branch or both the left anterior and the left posterior fascicles. The resulting ECG pattern is dependent on (1) the relative degree of delay in the affected structures, and (2) the shortest conduction time from the atria to the ventricles through any one fascicle. Ventricular activation begins at the site of insertion of the branch with the fastest conduction time and spreads from there to the remainder of the ventricles. For example, if delay in the right bundle branch is less than the delay in the left main bundle branch, activation will begin in the right ventricle and the QRS pattern will resemble that of LBBB. If the delay were greater in the right bundle branch than in the left bundle branch, the ECG pattern would be that of RBBB. The fascicle with the greatest delay can vary with, for example, the heart rate and lead to changing or alternating conduction patterns, as illustrated in Figure 9–30.

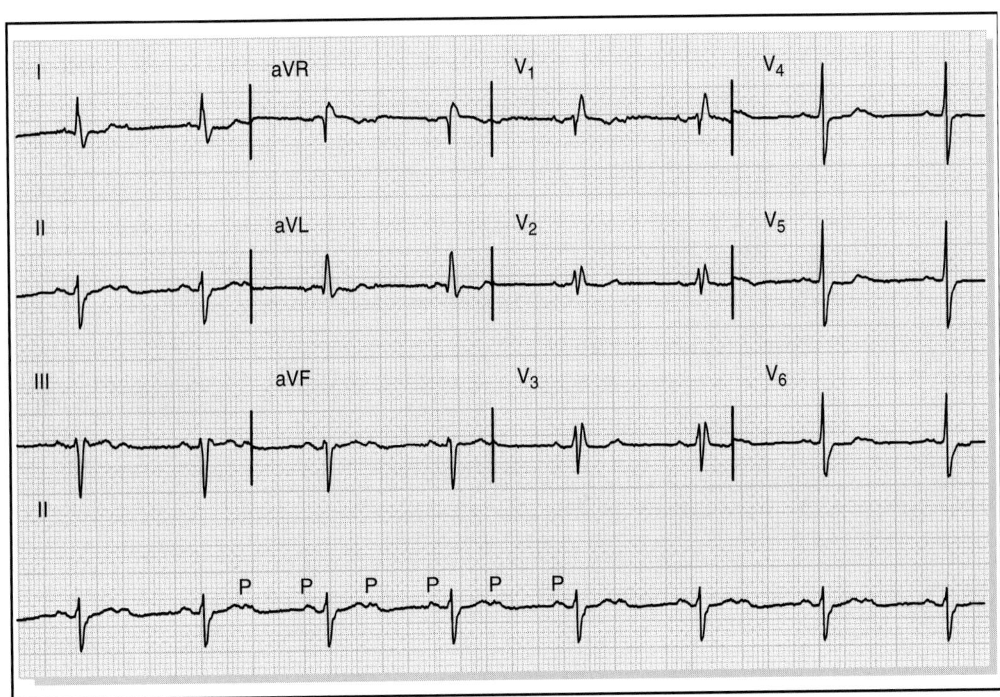

FIGURE 9–28 Sinus rhythm at 95 beats/min with 2:1 atrioventricular block. Conducted ventricular beats show a pattern consistent with bifascicular block with delay or block in the right bundle and left anterior fascicle. The patient underwent pacemaker implantation for presumed infra-Hisian block.

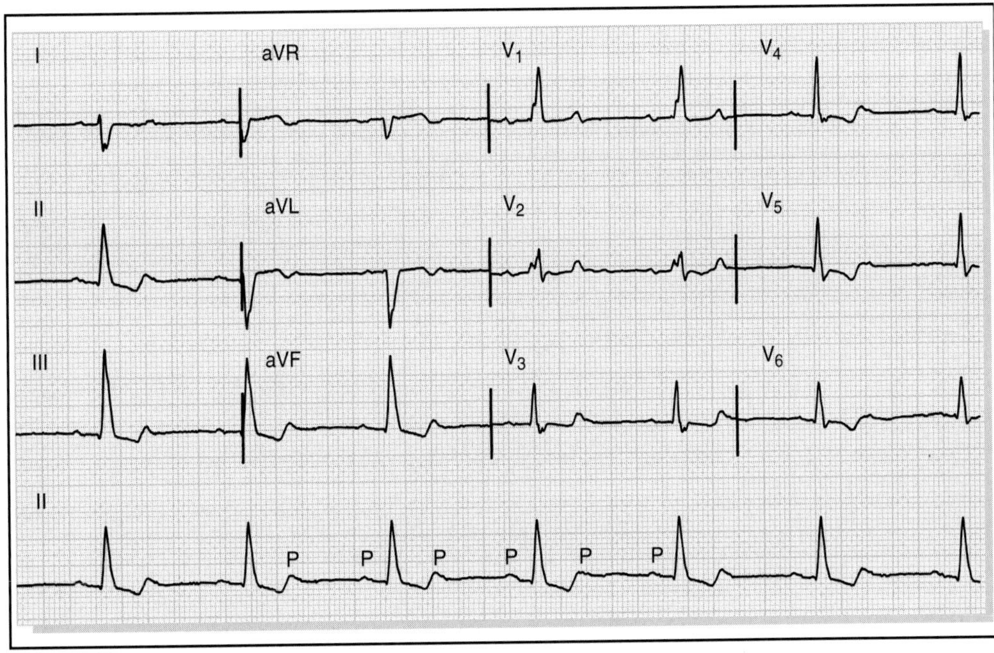

FIGURE 9–29 Sinus rhythm with a 2:1 atrioventricular block. QRS morphology in the conducted leads is consistent with bifascicular block with delay or block in the right bundle and left posterior fascicle. Subsequently, complete heart block was also noted. The patient underwent pacemaker implantation for presumed infra-Hisian block.

What distinguishes ECG patterns of trifascicular block from those of bifascicular block is an increased overall AV conduction interval that results specifically from prolongation of the His-ventricular time. In bifascicular block, conduction time through the unaffected fascicle (and hence, overall AV conduction time) is normal. In trifascicular block, however, the delay in conduction through even the least affected fascicle is abnormal and results in relative prolongation of the overall AV conduction interval. (Note that only delay, not block, of conduction is required. If block were present in all fascicles, conduction would fail and complete heart block would result. This situation is perhaps best illustrated by cases of alternating bundle branch block [see Fig. 9-30]; if the block were total in one bundle branch, development of block in the other would produce complete AV block rather than a change in bundle branch block patterns.) Thus, a diagnosis of trifascicular block requires an ECG pattern of bifascicular block *plus* evidence of prolonged AV conduction.

Detecting AV conduction delay is best accomplished by intracardiac recordings as a prolongation of the His-ventricular interval. On the surface ECG, AV conduction delay may be manifested as a prolonged PR interval. However, the PR interval includes conduction time in the AV node as well as in the intraventricular conduction system. Prolonged intraventricular conduction may be insufficient to extend the PR interval beyond normal limits, whereas a prolonged PR interval can reflect delay in the AV node rather than in all three intraventricular fascicles. Thus, the finding of a prolonged PR interval in the presence of an ECG pattern of bifascicular block is not diagnostic of trifascicular block, whereas the presence of a normal PR interval does not exclude this finding (see Chap. 29).

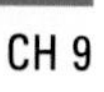

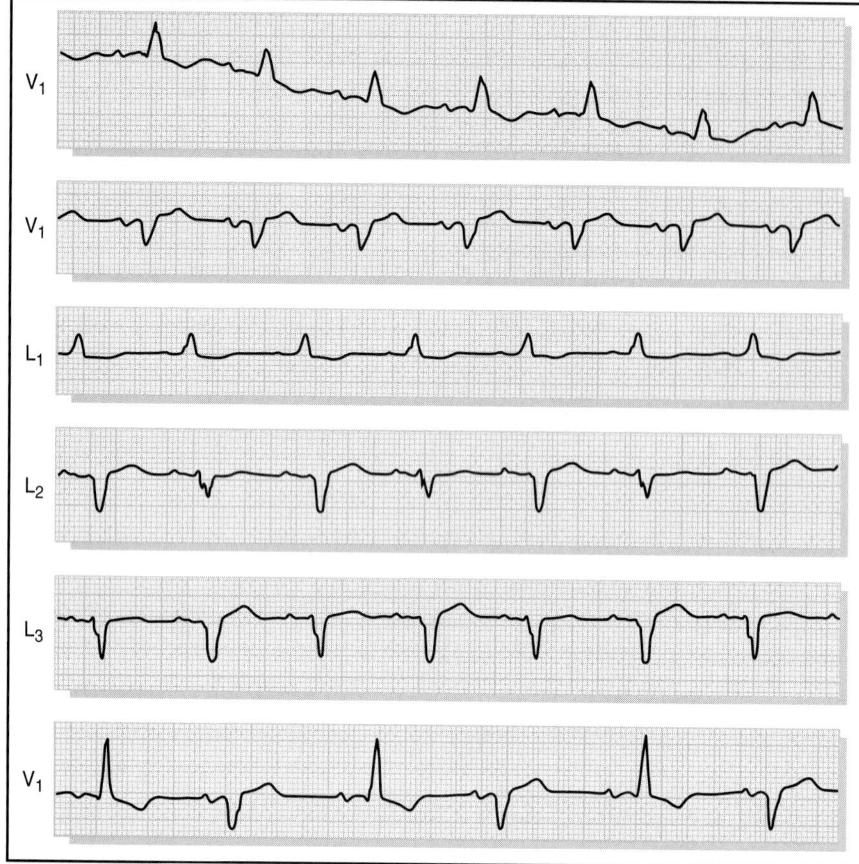

FIGURE 9–30 Multifascicular block manifested by alternating bundle branch blocks and PR intervals. **Top panel,** V_1 right bundle branch block (RBBB) with a PR interval of 280 msec. **Middle panel,** V_1 left bundle branch block (LBBB) with a PR interval of 180 msec. **Lower panel,** RBBB alternating with LBBB, along with alternation of the PR interval. The electrocardiographic records shown in leads I, II, and III (L1 to L3) exhibit left anterior fascicular block. An alternating bundle branch block of this type is consistent with trifascicular conduction delay. (From Fisch C: Electrocardiography of Arrhythmias. Philadelphia, Lea & Febiger, 1990, p 433.)

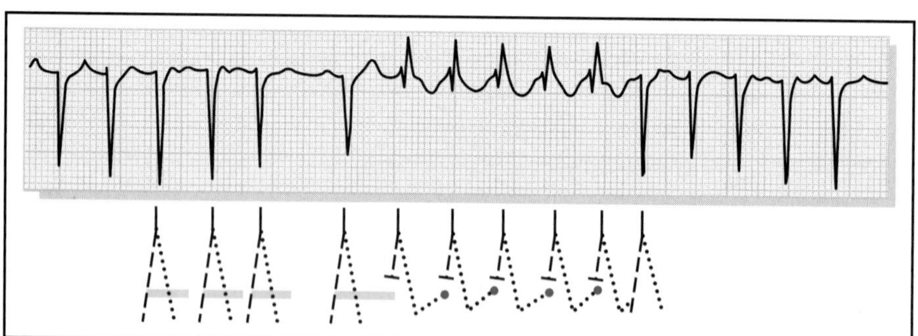

FIGURE 9–31 Atrial tachycardia with a Wenckebach (type I) second-degree atrioventricular (AV) block, ventricular aberration resulting from the Ashman phenomenon, and probably concealed transseptal conduction. The long pause of the atrial tachycardia is followed by five QRS complexes with right bundle branch block (RBBB) morphology. The RBBB of the first QRS reflects the Ashman phenomenon. The aberration is perpetuated by concealed transseptal activation from the left bundle (LB) into the right bundle (RB) with block of anterograde conduction of the subsequent sinus impulse in the RB. Foreshortening of the R-R cycle, a manifestation of the Wenckebach structure, disturbs the relationship between transseptal and anterograde sinus conduction, and RB conduction is normalized. In the ladder diagram below the tracing, the solid lines represent the His bundle, the dashes represent the RB, the dots represent the LB, and the solid horizontal bars denote the refractory period. P waves and the AV node are not identified in the diagram. (Courtesy of C. Fisch, M.D.)

The major clinical implication of a multifascicular block is its relation to advanced conduction system disease. It may be a marker for advanced myocardial disease and may identify patients at risk for heart block (see Figs. 9–28 and 9–29), as discussed in Chapters 30 and 31.

Rate-Dependent Conduction Block (Aberration)

Intraventricular conduction delays can result from the effects of changes in the heart rate, as well as from fixed pathological lesions in the conduction system. Rate-dependent block or aberration can occur at either high or low heart rates. In acceleration (tachycardia)-dependent block, conduction delay occurs when the heart rate exceeds a critical value. At the cellular level, this aberration is the result of encroachment of the impulse on the relative refractory period (usually in phase 3 of the action potential) of the preceding impulse, which results in slower conduction. This form of block is relatively common and can have the ECG pattern of RBBB or LBBB (Figs. 9–31 and 9–32).

In deceleration (bradycardia)-dependent block, conduction delay occurs when the heart rate falls below a critical level. Although the mechanism is not clearly established, it may reflect abnormal phase 4 depolarization of cells so that activation occurs at lower resting potentials. Deceleration-dependent block is less common than acceleration-dependent block and is usually seen only in patients with significant conduction system disease (Fig. 9–33).

Other mechanisms of ventricular aberration include concealed conduction (anterograde or retrograde) in the bundle branches (see Figs. 9-31 and 9-32), premature excitation, depressed myocardial conduction as a result of drug effects or hyperkalemia (see Fig. 9-52, top), and the effect of changing cycle length on refractoriness (the Ashman phenomenon) (see Chaps. 29 and 32). The duration of the refractory period is a function of the immediately preceding cycle length: the longer the preceding cycle, the longer the subsequent refractory period. Therefore, abrupt prolongation of the immediately preceding cycle can result in aberration as part of a long cycle–short cycle sequence. These so-called Ashman beats usually have a RBBB morphology (see Fig. 9-31).

WOLFF-PARKINSON-WHITE PREEXCITATION. This abnormality is discussed in Chapter 32.

Myocardial Ischemia and Infarction

The ECG remains a key test in the diagnosis of acute and chronic coronary syndromes.[48] The findings vary considerably, depending importantly on four major factors: (1) the duration of the ischemic process (acute vs. evolving/chronic), (2) its extent (transmural vs. nontransmural), (3) its topography (anterior vs. inferior-posterior and right ventricular), and (4) the presence of other underlying abnormalities (e.g., LBBB, Wolff-Parkinson-White

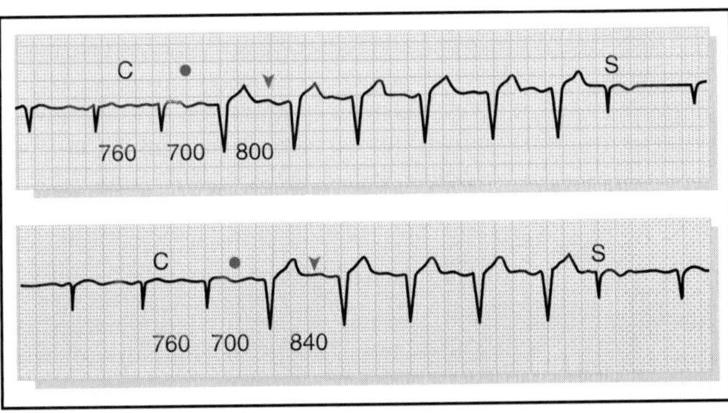

FIGURE 9–32 Acceleration-dependent QRS aberration with the paradox of persistence at a longer cycle and normalization at a shorter cycle than what initiated the aberration. The duration of the basic cycle (C) is 760 msec. Left bundle branch block (LBBB) appears at a cycle length of 700 msec (dot) and is perpetuated at cycle lengths of 800 (arrowhead) and 840 (arrowhead) msec; conduction normalizes after a cycle length of 600 msec. Perpetuation of LBBB at a cycle length of 800 and 840 msec is probably due to transseptal concealment, similar to that described in Figure 9–31. Unexpected normalization of the QRS (S) following the atrial premature contraction is probably due to equalization of conduction in the two bundles; however, supernormal conduction in the left bundle cannot be excluded. (From Fisch C, Zipes DP, McHenry PL: Rate dependent aberrancy. Circulation 48:714, 1973.)

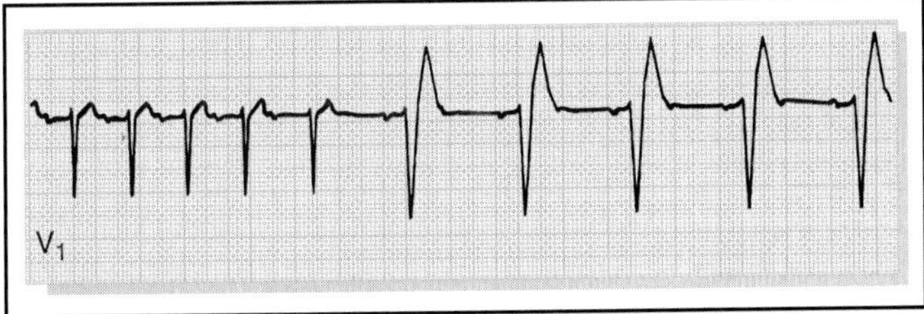

FIGURE 9–33 Deceleration-dependent aberration. The basic rhythm is sinus with a Wenckebach (type I) atrioventricular (AV) block. With 1 : 1 AV conduction, the QRS complexes are normal in duration; with a 2 : 1 AV block or after the longer pause of a Wenckebach sequence, left bundle branch block (LBBB) appears. Slow diastolic depolarization (phase 4) of the transmembrane action potential during the prolonged cycle is implicated as the cause of the LBBB. (Courtesy of C. Fisch, M.D.)

syndrome, or pacemaker patterns) that can mask or alter the classic patterns.

Repolarization (ST-T Wave) Abnormalities

The earliest and most consistent ECG finding during acute ischemia is deviation of the ST segment as a result of a current-of-injury mechanism. Under normal conditions, the ST segment is usually nearly isoelectric because virtually all healthy myocardial cells attain approximately the same potential during early repolarization, that is, during the plateau phase of the ventricular action potential.

Ischemia, however, has complex time-dependent effects on the electrical properties of myocardial cells. Severe, acute ischemia can reduce the resting membrane potential, shorten the duration of the action potential in the ischemic area, and decrease the rate of rise and amplitude of phase 0 (Fig. 9–34). These changes cause a voltage gradient between normal and ischemic zones that leads to current flow between these regions. These currents of injury are represented on the surface ECG by deviation of the ST segment.

Both *diastolic* and *systolic injury currents* have been proposed to explain ischemic ST elevations (Fig. 9-35). According to the diastolic-current-of-injury hypothesis, ischemic ST elevation is attributable to negative (downward) displacement of the electrical "diastolic" baseline (the TQ segment of the ECG). At least partly because of transmembrane

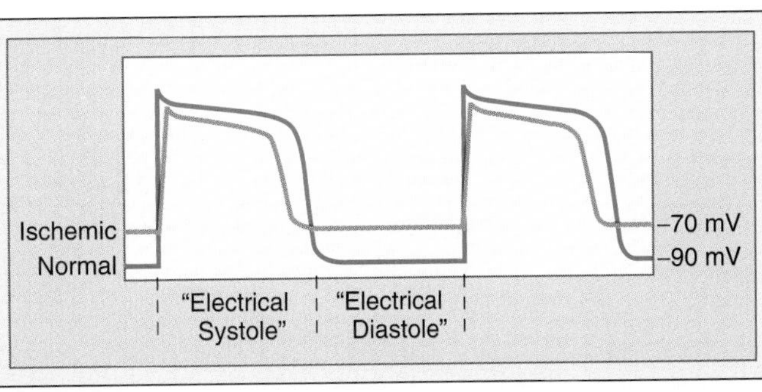

FIGURE 9–34 Acute ischemia may alter ventricular action potentials by inducing lower resting membrane potential, decreased amplitude and velocity of phase 0, and an abbreviated action potential duration (pathological early repolarization). These electrophysiological effects create a voltage gradient between ischemic and normal cells during different phases of the cardiac electrical cycle. The resulting currents of injury are reflected on the surface electrocardiogram by deviation of the ST segment (see Figure 9–35).

leakage of intracellular potassium ions, ischemic cells may remain relatively depolarized during phase 4 of the ventricular action potential (i.e., lower membrane resting potential) (see Fig. 9-34).[49] Depolarized muscle carries a negative extracellular charge relative to repolarized muscle. Therefore, during electrical diastole, current (the diastolic current of injury) will flow between the partly or completely depolarized ischemic myocardium and the neighboring normally repolarized uninjured myocardium. The injury current vector will be directed away from the more negative ischemic zone toward the more positive normal myocardium. As a result, leads overlying the ischemic zone will record a negative deflection during electrical diastole and produce depression of the TQ segment.

TQ segment depression, in turn, appears as ST segment elevation because the ECG recorders in clinical practice use AC-coupled amplifiers that automatically "compensate" for any negative shift in the TQ segment. As a result of this electronic compensation, the ST segment will be proportionately elevated. Therefore, according to the diastolic-current-of-injury theory, ST segment elevation represents an apparent shift. The true shift, observable only with DC-coupled ECG amplifiers, is the negative displacement of the TQ baseline.

Current evidence suggests that ischemic ST elevations (and hyperacute T waves) are also related to systolic injury currents. Three factors may make acutely ischemic myocardial cells relatively positive in comparison to normal cells with respect to their extracellular charge during electrical systole (QT interval). These are (1) pathological early repolarization (shortened action potential duration), (2) decreased action potential upstroke velocity, and (3) decreased action potential amplitude (see Fig. 9-34). The presence of one or more of these effects will establish a voltage gradient between normal and ischemic zones during the QT interval such that the current-of-injury vector will be directed toward the ischemic region. This systolic-current-of-injury mechanism will result in primary ST elevation, sometimes with tall positive (hyperacute) T waves.

When acute ischemia is transmural (whether caused by diastolic or systolic injury currents or both), the overall ST vector is usually shifted in the direction of the outer (epicardial) layers, and ST elevation and sometimes tall positive (hyperacute) T waves are produced over the ischemic zone (Fig. 9–36). Reciprocal ST depressions can appear in leads reflecting the contralateral surface of the heart. Occasionally, the reciprocal changes can be more apparent than the primary ST elevations. When ischemia is confined primarily to the subendocardium, the overall ST vector typically shifts toward the inner ventricular layer and the ventricular cavity such that the overlying (e.g., anterior precordial) leads show ST segment depression with ST elevation in lead aV_r (see Fig. 9–36). This subendocardial ischemic pattern is the typical finding during spontaneous episodes of angina pectoris or during symptomatic or asymptomatic ("silent") ischemia induced by exercise or pharmacological stress tests (see Chaps. 10 and 46).

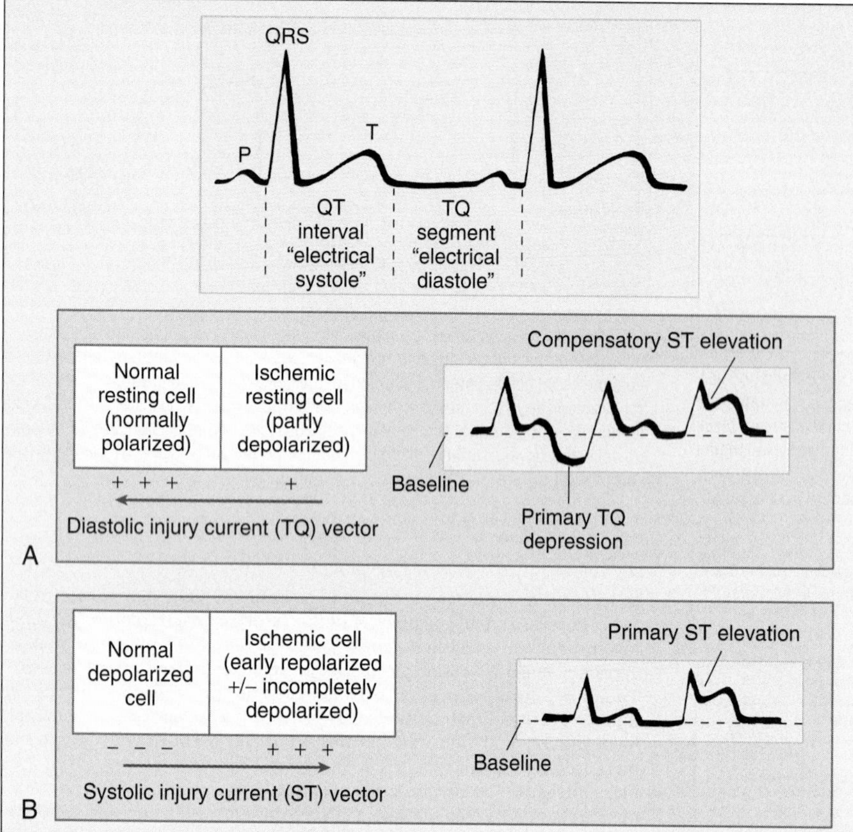

FIGURE 9–35 Pathophysiology of ischemic ST elevation. Two basic mechanisms have been advanced to explain the elevation seen with acute myocardial injury. **A,** Diastolic current of injury. In this case (first QRS-T complex), the ST vector will be directed away from the relatively negative, partly depolarized, ischemic region during electrical diastole (TQ interval), and the result will be primary TQ depression. Conventional alternating-current electrocardiograms compensate for the baseline shift, and an apparent ST elevation (second QRS-T complex) results. **B,** Systolic current of injury. In this case, the ischemic zone will be relatively positive during electrical systole because the cells are repolarized early and the amplitude and upstroke velocity of their action potentials may be decreased. This injury current vector will be oriented toward the electropositive zone, and the result will be primary ST elevation. (Modified from Goldberger AL: Myocardial Infarction: Electrocardiographic Differential Diagnosis. 4th ed. St Louis, Mosby-Year Book, 1991.)

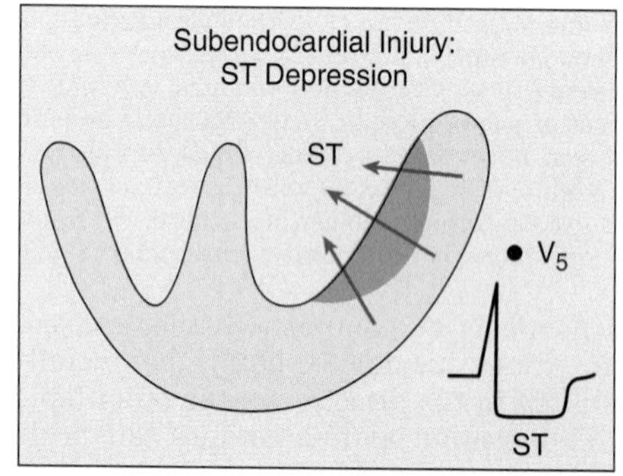

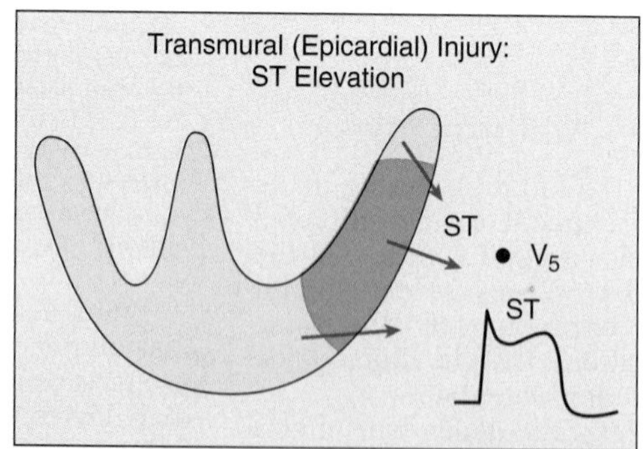

FIGURE 9–36 Current-of-injury patterns with acute ischemia. With predominant subendocardial ischemia **(A)**, the resultant ST vector is directed toward the inner layer of the affected ventricle and the ventricular cavity. Overlying leads therefore record ST depression. With ischemia involving the outer ventricular layer **(B)** (transmural or epicardial injury), the ST vector is directed outward. Overlying leads record ST elevation. Reciprocal ST depression can appear in contralateral leads.

Multiple factors can affect the amplitude of acute ischemic ST deviations. Profound ST elevation or depression in multiple leads usually indicates very severe ischemia. Conversely, prompt resolution of ST elevation following thrombolytic therapy[50] or primary angioplasty[51] is a specific marker of successful reperfusion. These relationships are not universal, however, since severe ischemia or even infarction can occur with slight or even absent ST-T changes. Furthermore, a relative increase in T wave amplitude (hyperacute T waves) can accompany or precede the ST elevations as part of the injury current pattern attributable to ischemia with or without infarction (Fig. 9–37).

QRS Changes

With actual infarction, depolarization (QRS) changes often accompany repolarization (ST-T) abnormalities (Fig. 9–38). Necrosis of sufficient myocardial tissue can lead to decreased R wave amplitude or Q waves in the anterior, lateral, or inferior leads as a result of loss of electromotive forces in the infarcted area. Local conduction delays caused by acute ischemia can also contribute to Q wave pathogenesis in selected cases. Abnormal Q waves were once considered markers of transmural myocardial infarction, while subendocardial (nontransmural) infarcts were thought to not produce Q waves. However, careful experimental and clinical ECG-pathological correlative studies have indicated that transmural infarcts can occur without Q waves and that subendocardial infarcts can sometimes be associated with Q waves.[52] Accordingly, infarcts are better classified electrocardiographically as "Q wave" or "non-Q-wave" rather than transmural or nontransmural, based on the ECG. The findings may be somewhat different with posterior or lateral infarction (Fig. 9–39). Loss of depolarization forces in these regions can reciprocally *increase* R wave amplitude in lead V_1 and sometimes V_2, rarely without causing diagnostic Q waves in any of the conventional leads.

The differential diagnosis of prominent right precordial R waves is given in Table 9–8.

Evolution of Electrocardiographic Changes

Ischemic ST elevation and hyperacute T wave changes occur as the earliest sign of acute infarction and are typically followed within a period ranging from hours to days by evolving T wave inversion and sometimes Q waves in the same lead distribution (see Fig. 9–38). T wave inversion from evolving or chronic ischemia correlates with increased ventricular action potential duration, and these ischemic changes are often associated with QT prolongation. The T wave inversion can resolve after days or weeks or persist indefinitely. The extent of the infarct may be an important determinant of T wave evolution.[53] In one series, T waves that were persistently negative for more than 1 year in leads with Q waves were associated with a

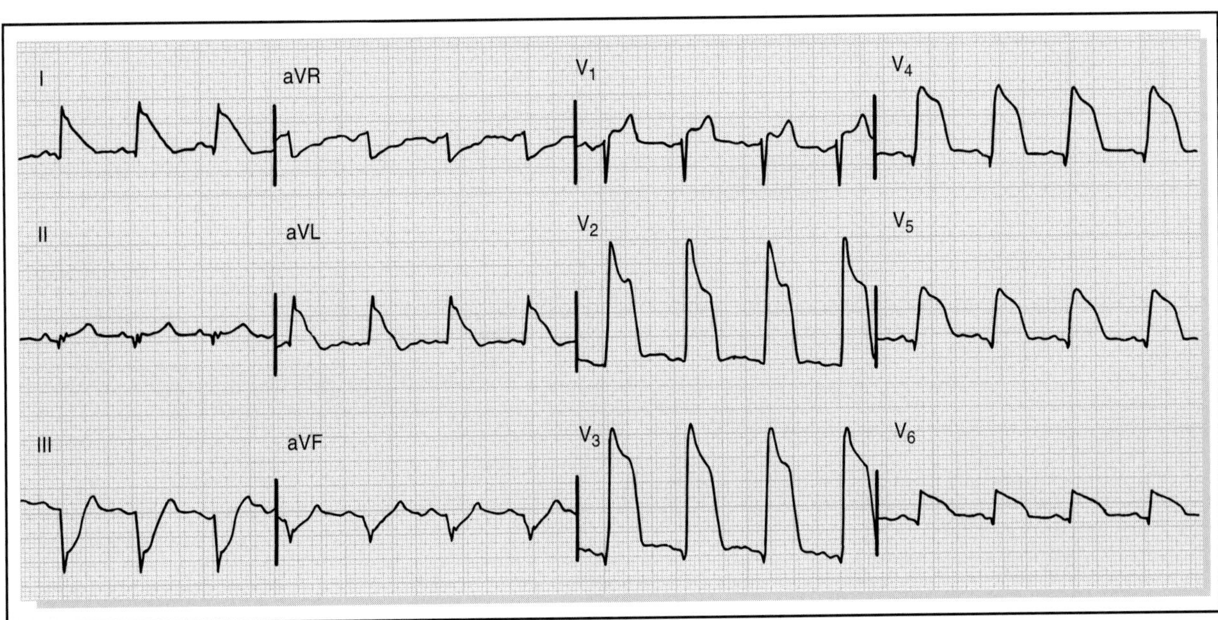

FIGURE 9–37 Hyperacute phase of extensive anterior-lateral myocardial infarction. Marked ST elevation melding with prominent T waves is present across the precordium, as well as in leads I and aV_l. ST depression, consistent with a reciprocal change, is seen in leads III and aV_f. Q waves are present in leads V_3 through V_6. Marked ST elevations with tall T waves caused by severe ischemia are sometimes referred to as a *monophasic current-of-injury* pattern. A paradoxical increase in R wave amplitude (V_2 and V_3) may accompany this pattern. This tracing also shows left axis deviation with small or absent inferior R waves, which raises the possibility of a prior inferior infarct.

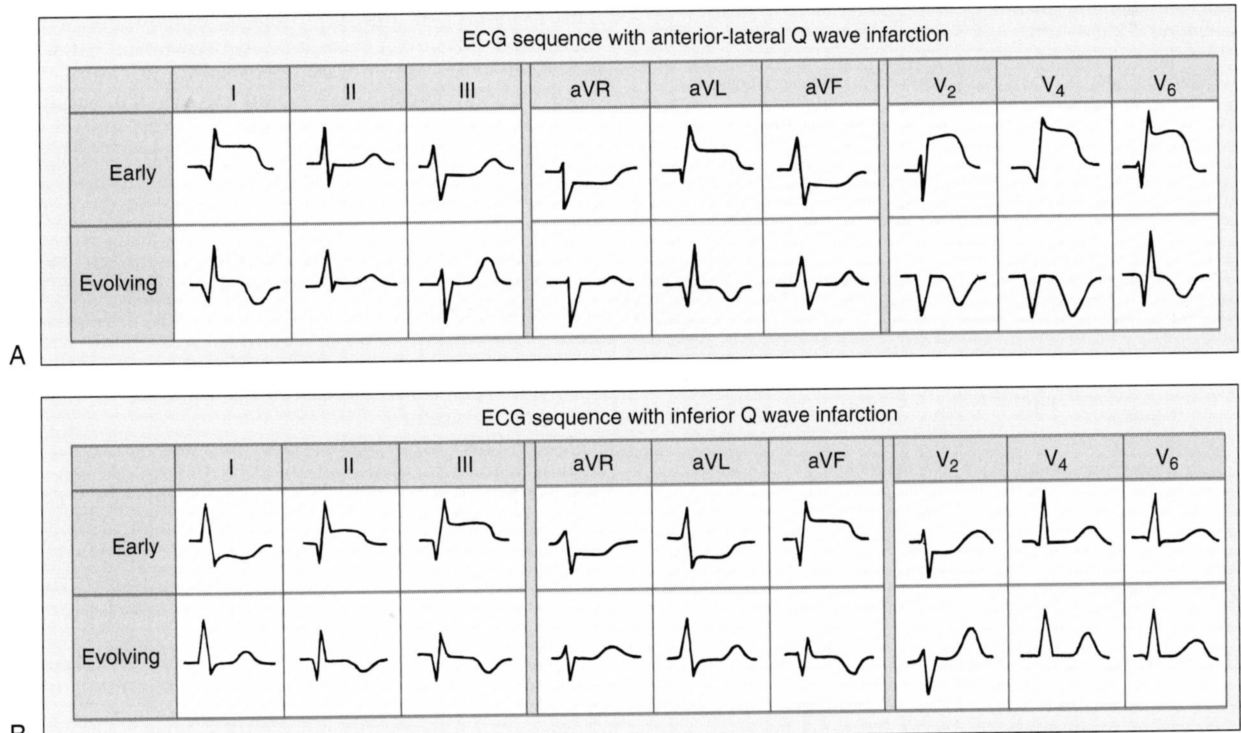

FIGURE 9–38 Sequence of depolarization and repolarization changes with **(A)** acute anterior-lateral and **(B)** acute inferior wall Q wave infarctions. With anterior-lateral infarcts, ST elevation in leads I, aV_l, and the precordial leads can be accompanied by reciprocal ST depression in leads II, III, and aV_f. Conversely, acute inferior (or posterior) infarcts can be associated with reciprocal ST depression in leads V_1 to V_3. (Modified from Goldberger AL: Clinical Electrocardiography: A Simplified Approach. 6th ed. St Louis, CV Mosby, 1999.)

transmural infarction with fibrosis of the entire wall; in contrast, T waves that were positive in leads with Q waves correlated with nontransmural infarction with viable myocardium within the wall.

In the days to weeks or longer following infarction, the QRS changes can persist or begin to resolve. Complete normalization of the ECG following Q wave infarction is uncommon but can occur, particularly with smaller infarcts and when the left ventricular ejection fraction and regional wall motion improve. This is usually associated with spontaneous recanalization or good collateral circulation[54] and is a good prognostic sign. In contrast, persistent Q waves and ST elevation several weeks or more after an infarct correlate strongly with a severe underlying wall motion disorder (akinetic or dyskinetic zone), although not necessarily a frank ventricular aneurysm. The presence of an rSR′ or similar

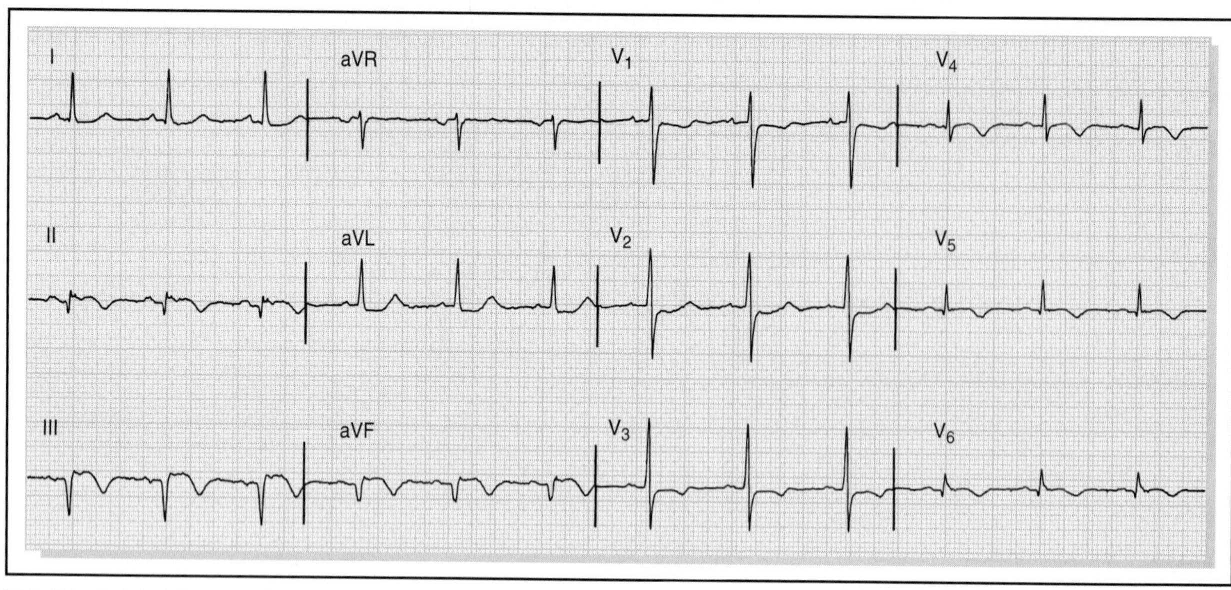

FIGURE 9–39 Evolving inferoposterolateral infarction. Note the prominent Q waves in II, III, and aV_f, along with ST elevation and T wave inversion in these leads, as well as V_3 through V_6. ST depression in I, aV_l, V_1, and V_2 is consistent with a reciprocal change. Relatively tall R waves are also present in V_1 and V_2.

TABLE 9–8 Differential Diagnosis of Tall R Waves in V_1/V_2

Physiological/positional factors
Misplacement of chest leads
Normal variants
Displacement of heart toward right side of chest (dextroversion): congenital or acquired
Myocardial injury
Posterior (and/or lateral) myocardial infarction (see Fig. 9–39)
Duchenne muscular dystrophy (see Chap. 71)
Ventricular enlargement
Right ventricular hypertrophy (usually with right axis deviation)
Hypertrophic cardiomyopathy
Altered ventricular depolarization
Right ventricular conduction abnormalities
Wolff-Parkinson-White patterns (caused by posterior or lateral wall preexcitation)

Modified from Goldberger AL: Clinical Electrocardiography: A Simplified Approach. 6th ed. St Louis, CV Mosby, 1999.

complex in the mid-left chest leads or lead I is another reported marker of ventricular aneurysm.

Other Ischemic ST-T Patterns

Reversible transmural ischemia caused, for example, by coronary vasospasm may cause transient ST segment elevation (Fig. 9–40). This pattern is the ECG marker of Prinzmetal variant angina (see Chap. 49). Depending on the severity and duration of such noninfarction ischemia, the ST elevation can either resolve completely within minutes or be followed by T wave inversion that can persist for hours or even days. Some patients with ischemic chest pain have deep coronary T wave inversion in multiple precordial leads (e.g., V_1 through V_4), with or without cardiac enzyme elevations. This finding is typically caused by severe ischemia associated with a high-grade stenosis in the proximal left anterior descending coronary artery system (LAD-T wave pattern). The T wave inversion can actually be preceded by a transient ST elevation that resolves by the time the patient arrives at the hospital. These T wave inversions, in the setting of unstable angina, can correlate with segmental hypokinesis of the anterior wall and suggest a "myocardial stunning" syndrome. The natural history of this syndrome is unfavorable, with a high incidence of recurrent angina and myocardial infarction. On the other hand, patients whose baseline ECG already shows abnormal T wave inversion can experience paradoxical T wave normalization (pseudonormalization) during episodes of acute transmural ischemia (Fig. 9–41). The four major classes of acute ECG-coronary artery syndromes in which myocardial ischemia leads to different ECG findings are summarized in Figure 9–42.

ISCHEMIC U WAVE CHANGES. Alterations in U wave amplitude or polarity have been reported with acute ischemia or infarction. For example, exercise-induced transient inversion of precordial U waves has been correlated with severe stenosis of the left anterior descending coronary artery.[55] Rarely, U wave inversion can be the earliest ECG sign of acute coronary syndromes.

QT INTERVAL DISPERSION. Increasing interest has been shown in the effects of acute myocardial ischemia and infarction on the disparity among QT intervals in various ECG leads, referred to as *QT dispersion*.[56] The greater the difference between maximum and minimum QT intervals, that is, increased QT dispersion, the greater the variability in myocardial repolarization. An increased index has been proposed as a marker of arrhythmia risk after myocardial infarction and as a marker of acute ischemia with atrial pacing.[56] The practical utility of QT dispersion measurements, in patients with coronary syndromes and certain other cardiac pathologies, is a focus of ongoing investigation and debate[57] (see Chap. 27).

Localization of Ischemia or Infarction

The ECG leads are more helpful in localizing regions of transmural than subendocardial ischemia. As examples, ST elevation and/or hyperacute T waves are seen in (1) one or more of the precordial leads (V_1 through V_6) and in leads I and aV_l with acute transmural anterior or anterolateral wall ischemia; (2) leads V_1 to V_3 with anteroseptal or apical[58] ischemia; (3) leads V_4 to V_6 with apical or lateral ischemia; (4) leads II, III, and aV_f with inferior wall ischemia; and (5) right-sided precordial leads with right ventricular ischemia. Posterior wall infarction, which induces ST elevation in leads placed over

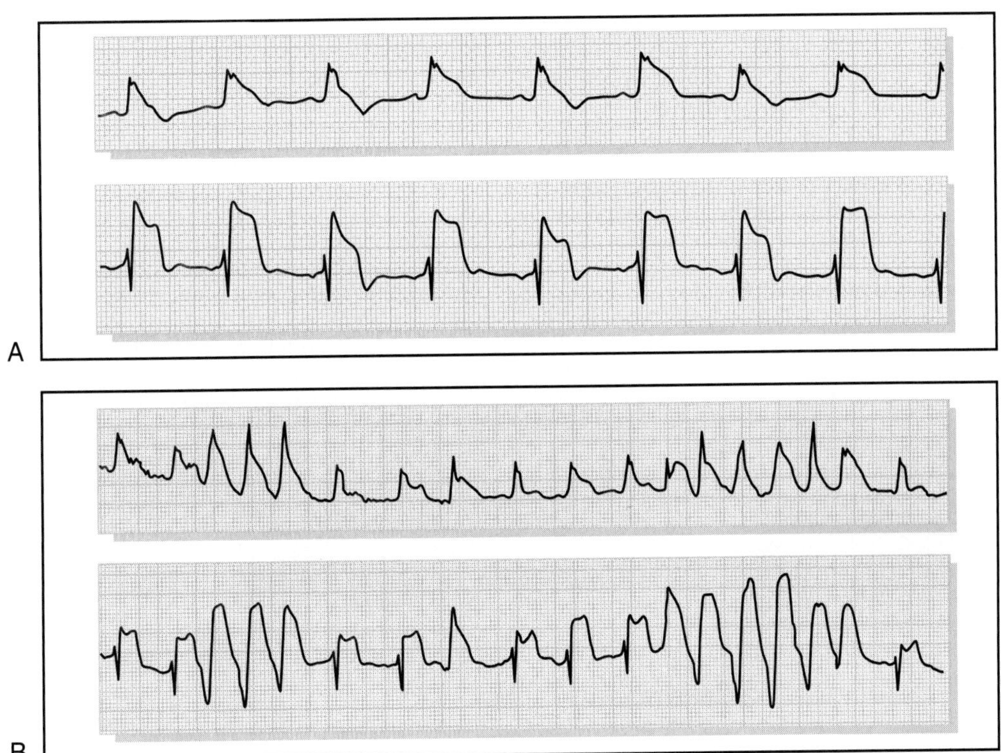

FIGURE 9–40 **A,** Prinzmetal angina with ST segment and T wave alternans. **B,** ST segment and T wave alternans associated with nonsustained ventricular tachycardia. (Courtesy of C. Fisch, M.D.)

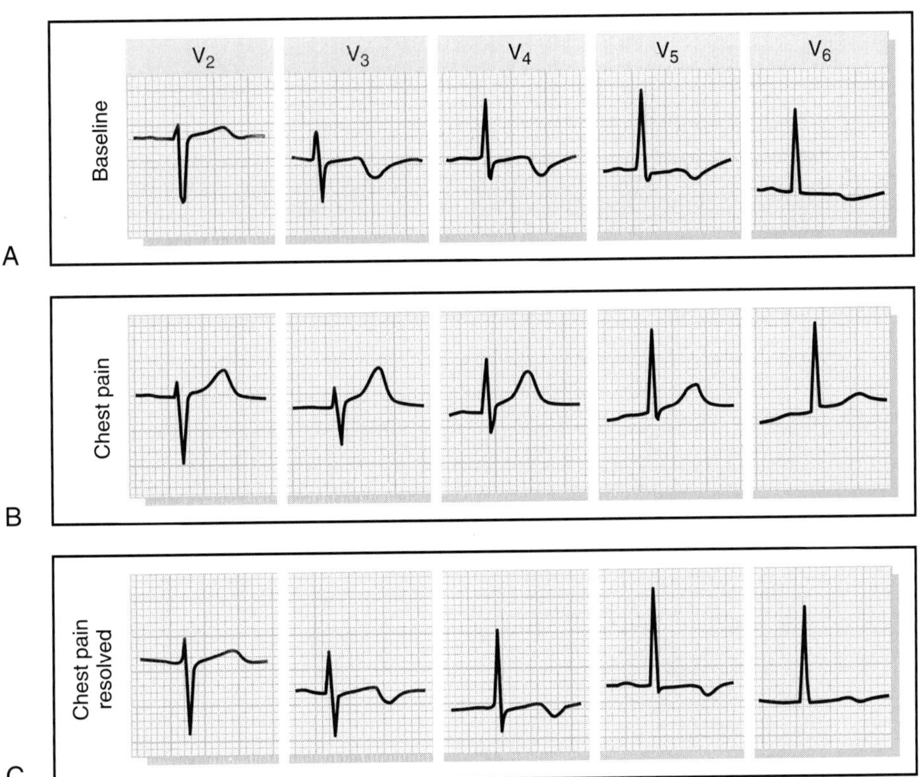

FIGURE 9–41 Pseudo (paradoxical) T wave normalization. **A,** The baseline electrocardiogram of a patient with coronary artery disease shows ischemic T wave inversion. **B,** T wave "normalization" during an episode of ischemic chest pain. **C,** Following resolution of the chest pain, the T waves have reverted to their baseline appearance. (From Goldberger AL: Myocardial Infarction: Electrocardiographic Differential Diagnosis. 4th ed. St Louis, Mosby-Year Book, 1991.)

the back of the heart, such as leads V_7 to V_9,[5,59] can be induced by lesions in the right coronary artery or left circumflex artery. These lesions can produce both inferior and posterior-lateral injury, which may be indirectly recognized by reciprocal ST depression in leads V_1 to V_3.[60] Similar ST changes can also be the primary ECG manifestation of anterior subendocardial ischemia. Posterior inferior wall infarction with reciprocal changes can be differentiated from primary anterior wall ischemia by the presence of ST segment elevations in posterior leads.

The ECG can also provide more specific information about the location of the occlusion within the coronary system *(the culprit lesion)*.[48] In patients with an inferior wall myocardial infarction, the presence of ST segment elevation in lead III exceeding that in lead II, particularly when combined with ST elevation in V_1, is a useful predictor of occlusion in the proximal to midportion of the right coronary artery (Fig. 9–43). In contrast, the presence of ST segment elevation in lead II equal to or exceeding that in lead III, especially in concert with ST depression in leads V_1 to V_3 or ST elevation in leads I and aV_1, strongly suggests occlusion of the left circumflex coronary artery or a distal occlusion of a dominant right coronary artery. Right-sided ST elevation is indicative of acute right ventricular injury[61,62] and usually indicates occlusion of the proximal right coronary artery. Of note is the finding that acute right ventricular infarction can project an injury current pattern in leads V_1 through V_3 or even V_4, thereby simulating anterior infarction. In other cases, simultaneous ST elevation in V_1 (V_2R) and ST depression in V_2 (V_1R) can occur (Fig. 9–43). These and many other criteria proposed for localization of the site of coronary occlusion based on the initial ECG[48,63-67] require additional validation in test populations.

In some cases, ischemia can affect more than one region of the myocardium (e.g., inferolateral) (see Fig. 9–38). Not uncommonly, the ECG will show the characteristic findings of involvement in each region. Sometimes, however, partial normalization can result from cancellation of opposing vectorial forces. Inferior lead ST segment elevation accompanying acute anterior wall infarction suggests either occlusion of a left anterior descending artery that extends onto the inferior wall of the left ventricle

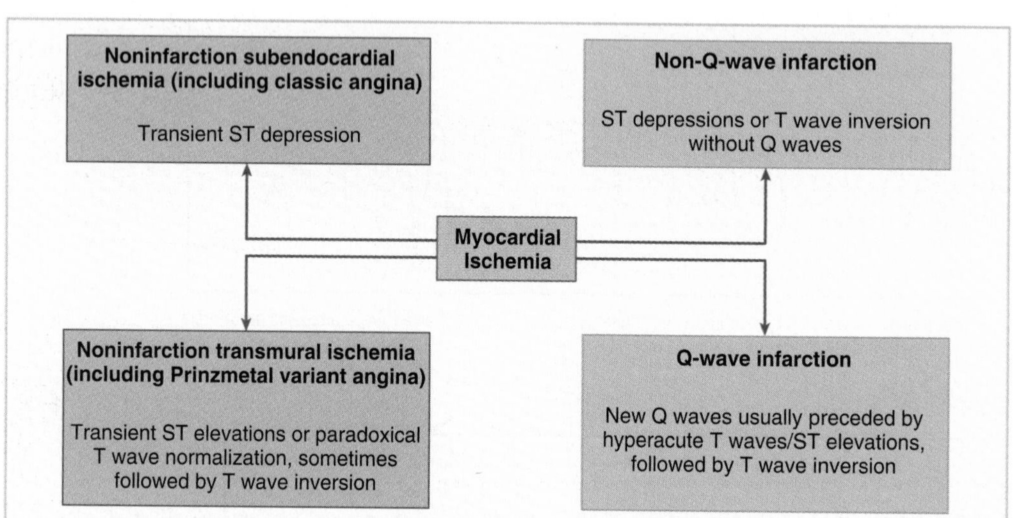

FIGURE 9–42 Variability of electrocardiogram (ECG) patterns with acute myocardial ischemia. The ECG may also be normal or nonspecifically abnormal. Furthermore, these categorizations are not mutually exclusive. For example, a non-Q-wave infarct can evolve into a Q wave infarct, ST elevation can be followed by a non-Q-wave infarct, or ST depression and T wave inversion can be followed by a Q wave infarct. (Modified from Goldberger AL: Myocardial Infarction: Electrocardiographic Differential Diagnosis. 4th ed. St Louis, Mosby-Year Book, 1991.)

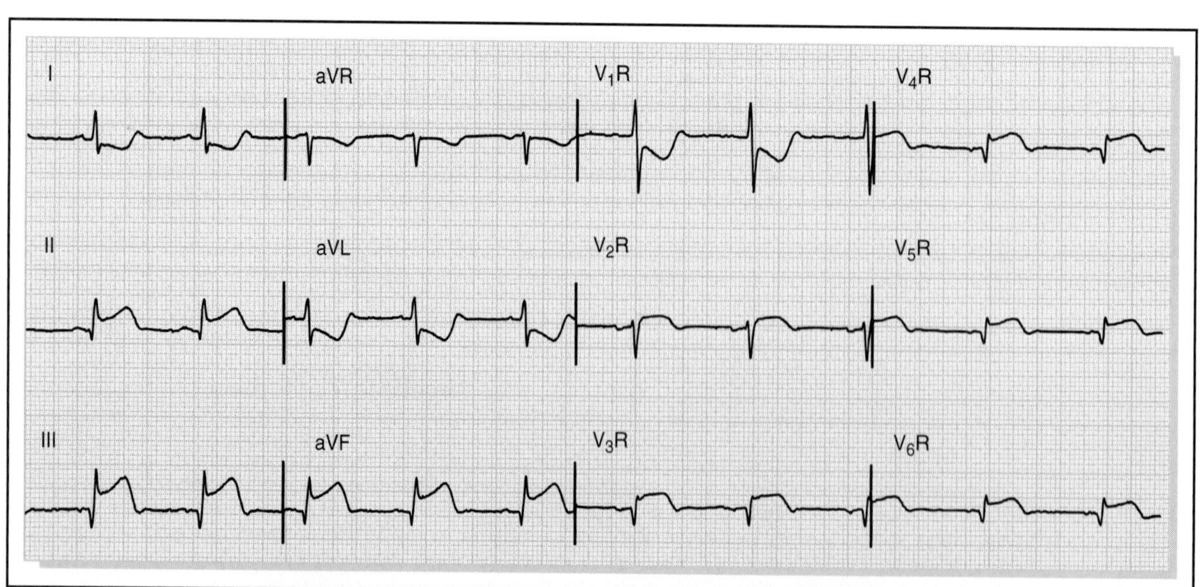

FIGURE 9–43 Acute right ventricular infarction with acute inferior wall infarction. Note the ST elevation in the right precordial leads, as well as in leads II, III, and aV_f, with reciprocal change in I and aV_l. ST elevation in lead III greater than in lead II and right precordial ST elevation are consistent with proximal to middle occlusion of the right coronary artery. The combination of ST elevation in conventional lead V_1 (V_2R here) and ST depression in lead V_2 (lead V_1R here) has also been reported with acute right ventricular ischemia/infarction.

(the "wrap around" vessel) or multivessel disease with jeopardized collaterals.[68]

Electrocardiographic Diagnosis of Bundle Branch Blocks and Myocardial Infarction

The diagnosis of myocardial infarction is often more difficult in cases in which the baseline ECG shows a bundle branch block pattern, or a bundle branch block develops as a complication of the infarct. The diagnosis of Q wave infarction is not usually impeded by the presence of RBBB, which affects primarily the terminal phase of ventricular depolarization. The net effect is that the criteria for the diagnosis of a Q wave infarct in a patient with RBBB are the same as in patients with normal conduction (Fig. 9–44). The diagnosis of infarction in the presence of LBBB is considerably more complicated and confusing, because LBBB alters both the early and the late phases of ventricular depolarization and produces secondary ST-T changes. These changes may both mask and mimic the findings of myocardial infarction. As a result, considerable attention has been directed to the problem of diagnosing acute and chronic myocardial infarction in patients with LBBB[69,70] (Fig. 9–45).

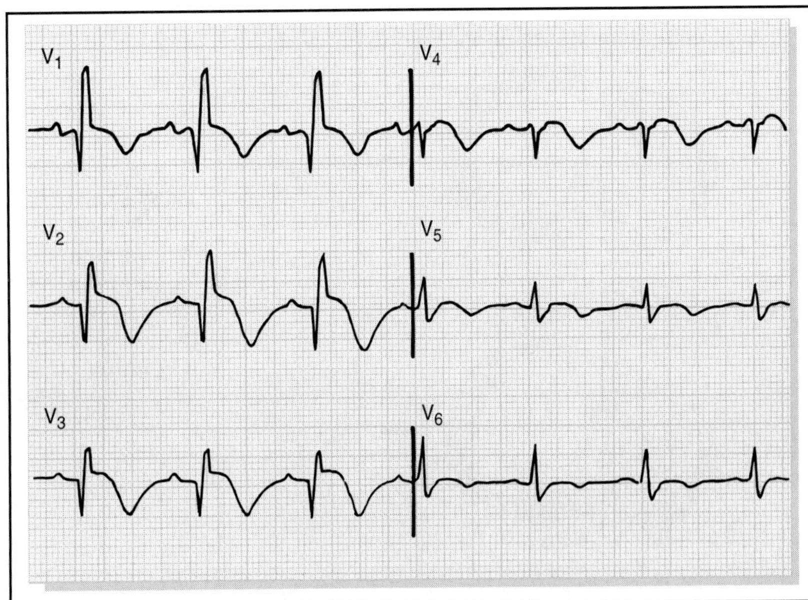

FIGURE 9–44 Right bundle branch block with acute anterior infarction. Loss of anterior depolarization forces results in QR-type complexes in the right precordial to midprecordial leads, with ST elevations and evolving T wave inversions (V_1 through V_6).

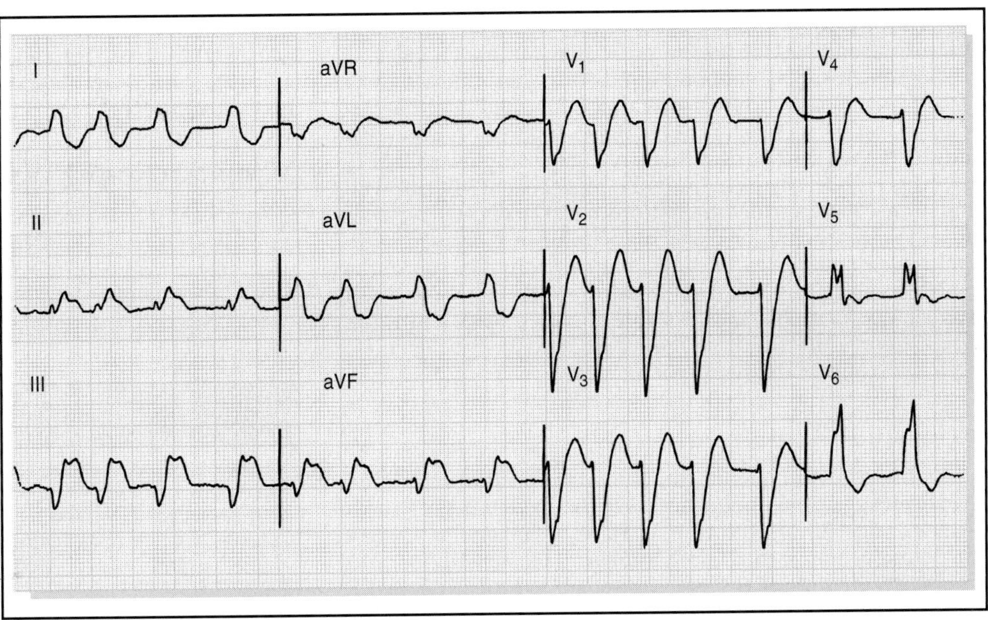

FIGURE 9–45 Complete left bundle branch block with acute inferior myocardial infarction. Note the prominent ST segment elevation in leads II, III, and aV_f, with reciprocal ST segment depression in I and aV_l superimposed on secondary ST-T changes. The underlying rhythm is atrial fibrillation.

Infarction of the left ventricular free (or lateral) wall ordinarily results in abnormal Q waves in the midprecordial to lateral precordial leads (and selected limb leads). However, the initial septal depolarization forces with LBBB are directed from right to left. These leftward forces produce an initial R wave in the midprecordial to lateral precordial leads, usually masking the loss of electrical potential (Q waves) caused by the infarction. Therefore, acute or chronic left ventricular free wall infarction by itself will not usually produce diagnostic Q waves in the presence of LBBB. Acute or chronic infarction involving both the free wall and the septum (or the septum itself) may produce abnormal Q waves (usually as part of QR-type complexes) in leads V_4 to V_6. These initial Q waves probably reflect posterior and superior forces from the spared basal portion of the septum (Fig. 9–46). Thus, a wide Q wave (≥40 msec) in one or more of these leads is a reliable sign of underlying infarction. The sequence of repolarization is also altered in LBBB, with the ST segment and T wave vectors being directed opposite the QRS complex. These changes can mask or simulate the ST segment changes of actual ischemia.

The following points summarize the ECG signs of myocardial infarction in LBBB: (1) ST segment elevation with tall positive T waves are frequently seen in the right precordial leads with uncomplicated LBBB. Secondary T wave inversions are characteristically seen in the lateral precordial leads. However, the appearance of ST elevations in the lateral leads or ST depressions or deep T wave inversions in leads V_1 to V_3 strongly suggests underlying ischemia. More marked ST elevations (≥0.5 mV) in leads with QS or rS waves may also be due to acute ischemia, but false-positive findings occur, especially with large-amplitude negative QRS complexes.[69] (2) The presence of QR complexes in leads I, V_5, or V_6 or in II, III, and aV_f with LBBB strongly suggests underlying infarction. (3) Chronic infarction is also suggested by notching of the ascending part of a wide S wave in the midprecordial leads or the ascending limb of a wide R wave in V_5 or V_6. Similar principles

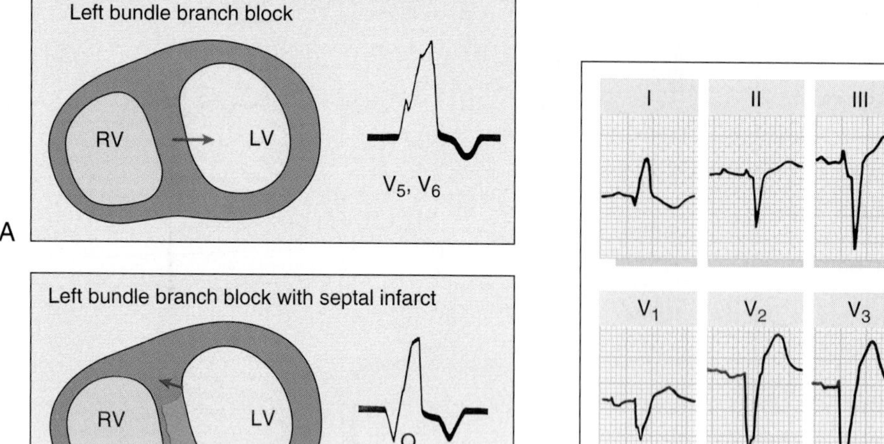

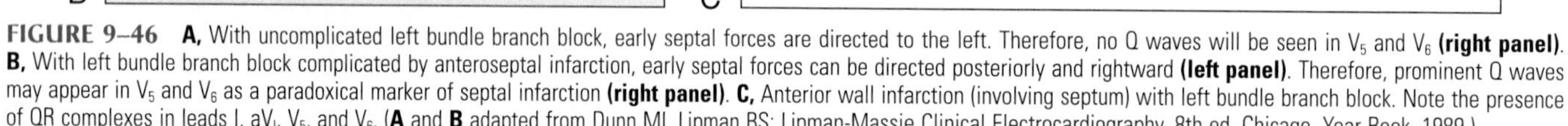

FIGURE 9–46 **A,** With uncomplicated left bundle branch block, early septal forces are directed to the left. Therefore, no Q waves will be seen in V_5 and V_6 **(right panel)**. **B,** With left bundle branch block complicated by anteroseptal infarction, early septal forces can be directed posteriorly and rightward **(left panel)**. Therefore, prominent Q waves may appear in V_5 and V_6 as a paradoxical marker of septal infarction **(right panel)**. **C,** Anterior wall infarction (involving septum) with left bundle branch block. Note the presence of QR complexes in leads I, aV_l, V_5, and V_6. (**A** and **B** adapted from Dunn MI, Lipman BS: Lipman-Massie Clinical Electrocardiography. 8th ed. Chicago, Year Book, 1989.)

can apply to the diagnosis of acute and chronic infarction in the presence of right ventricular pacing.[71] Comparison between an ECG exhibiting the LBBB prior to the infarction and the present ECG is often helpful to show these changes.

The diagnosis of concomitant LAFB and inferior wall infraction can also pose challenges. This combination can result in loss of the small r waves in the inferior leads, so that leads II, III, and aVF show QS, not rS, complexes. LAFB, however, will occasionally hide the diagnosis of inferior wall infarction. The inferior orientation of the initial QRS forces caused by the hemiblock can mask inferior Q waves, with resultant rS complexes in II, III, and aVF. In other cases, the combination of LAFB and inferior wall infarction will produce qrS complexes in the inferior limb leads, with the initial q wave the result of the infarct and the minuscule r wave the result of the hemiblock.

Atrial Infarction

A number of ECG clues to the diagnosis of atrial infarction have been suggested, including localized deviations of the PR segment (e.g., PR elevation in V_5 or V_6), changes in P wave morphology, and atrial arrhythmias. The sensitivity and specificity of these signs are limited, however. Diffuse PR segment changes (PR elevation in aV_r with depression in the inferolateral leads) with acute infarction usually indicate concomitant pericarditis (see later).

Electrocardiographic Differential Diagnosis of Ischemia and Infarction

The ECG has important limitations in both sensitivity and specificity in the diagnosis of coronary syndromes. An initially normal ECG does not exclude ischemia or even acute infarction.[72] However, a normal ECG throughout the course of an alleged acute infarct is distinctly uncommon. As a result, prolonged chest pain without diagnostic ECG changes should always prompt a careful search for noncoronary causes of chest pain (see Chap. 47). Pathological Q waves can be absent even in patients with depressed left ventricular function caused by severe coronary disease and a previous infarct. As noted, the diagnosis of acute or chronic infarction can be completely masked by ventricular conduction disturbances, especially those resulting from LBBB, as well as ventricular pacing and Wolff-Parkinson-White preexcitation. On the other hand, diagnostic confusion can arise because Q waves, ST elevation, ST depression, tall positive T waves, and deep T wave inversion can be seen in a wide variety of noncoronary settings.

Noninfarction Q Waves

Q waves simulating coronary artery disease can be related to one (or a combination) of the following four factors (Table 9–9): (1) physiological or positional variants, (2) altered ventricular conduction, (3) ventricular enlargement, and (4)

TABLE 9–9 Differential Diagnosis of Noninfarction Q Waves (with Selected Examples)
Physiological or positional factors
Normal-variant "septal" Q waves
Normal-variant Q waves in V_1-V_2, III, and aV_f
Left pneumothorax or dextrocardia: loss of lateral R wave progression
Myocardial injury or infiltration
Acute processes: myocardial ischemia without infarction, myocarditis, hyperkalemia (rare cause of transient Q waves)
Chronic myocardial processes: idiopathic cardiomyopathies, myocarditis, amyloid, tumor, sarcoid
Ventricular hypertrophy/enlargement
Left ventricular (poor R wave progression*)
Right ventricular (reversed R wave progression† or poor R wave progression, particularly with chronic obstructive lung disease)
Hypertrophic cardiomyopathy (can simulate anterior, inferior, posterior, or lateral infarcts) (see Fig. 9–47)
Conduction abnormalities
Left bundle branch block (poor R wave progression*)
Wolff-Parkinson-White patterns

Modified from Goldberger AL: Clinical Electrocardiography: A Simplified Approach. 6th ed. St Louis, CV Mosby, 1999.

*Small or absent R waves in the right precordial to midprecordial leads.

†Progressive decrease in R wave amplitude from V_1 to the midlateral precordial leads.

myocardial damage or replacement. Depending on the electrical axis, prominent Q waves (as part of QS- or QR-type complexes) can also appear in the limb leads (aV_l with a vertical axis and III and aV_f with a horizontal axis). A QS complex can appear in lead V_1 as a normal variant and rarely in leads V_1 and V_2. Prominent Q waves can be associated with a variety of other positional factors that alter the orientation of the heart vis-à-vis a given lead axis. Poor R wave progression, sometimes with actual QS waves, can be due solely to improper placement of chest electrodes above their usual position. In cases of dextrocardia, provided that no underlying structural abnormalities are present, normal R wave progression can be restored by recording leads V_2 to V_6 on the right side of the chest. A rightward mediastinal shift in left pneumothorax can contribute to the apparent loss of left precordial R waves. Other positional factors associated with poor R wave progression include pectus excavatum, congenitally corrected transposition of the great vessels, and congenital absence of the left pericardium.

An intrinsic change in the sequence of ventricular depolarization can lead to pathological, noninfarct Q waves. The two most important conduction disturbances associated with pseudoinfarct Q waves are LBBB and the Wolff-Parkinson-White preexcitation patterns. With LBBB, QS complexes can appear in the right precordial to midprecordial leads and occasionally in one or more of leads II, III, and aV_f. Depending on the location of the bypass tract, WPW preexcitation can mimic anteroseptal, lateral, or inferior-posterior infarction. LAFB is often cited as a cause of anteroseptal infarct patterns; however, LAFB has only minor effects on the QRS complex in horizontal plane leads. Probably the most common findings are relatively prominent S waves in leads V_5 and V_6. Poor R wave progression is not a routine feature of LAFB, although some authors have reported minuscule q waves in leads V_1 to V_3 in this setting. These small q waves can become more apparent if the leads are recorded one interspace above their usual position and disappear in leads one interspace below their usual position. As a general clinical rule, however, prominent Q waves (as part of QS or QR complexes) in the right precordial to midprecordial leads should *not* be attributed to LAFB alone.

Poor R Wave Progression. In contrast, poor R wave progression is commonly observed with LVH and with acute or chronic right ventricular overload. Q waves in such settings can reflect a variety of mechanisms, including a change in the balance of early ventricular depolarization forces and altered cardiac geometry and position. A marked loss of R wave voltage, sometimes with frank Q waves from V_1 to the lateral chest leads, can be seen with chronic obstructive pulmonary disease (see Fig. 9-23). The presence of low limb voltage and P pulmonale can serve as additional diagnostic clues. This loss of R wave progression may, in part, reflect right ventricular dilation. Furthermore, downward displacement of the heart in an emphysematous chest can play a major role in the genesis of poor R wave progression in this syndrome. Partial or complete normalization of R wave progression can be achieved in such cases simply by recording the chest leads an interspace lower than usual (see Fig. 9-23).

Other Pseudoinfarct Patterns in Ventricular Overload. A variety of pseudoinfarct patterns can occur with acute cor pulmonale caused by pulmonary embolism. Acute right ventricular overload in this setting can cause poor R wave progression and sometimes right precordial to midprecordial T wave inversion (right ventricular "strain"), mimicking anterior infarction. The classic $S_1Q_3T_3$ pattern can occur but is neither sensitive nor specific. A prominent Q wave (usually as part of a QR complex) can also occur in lead aV_f along with this pattern (see Fig. 9-24). However, acute right overload by itself does not cause a pathological Q wave in lead II. Right heart overload, acute or chronic, may also be associated with a QR complex in lead V_1 and simulate anteroseptal infarction.

Pseudoinfarct patterns are an important finding in patients with hypertrophic cardiomyopathy, and the ECG can simulate anterior, inferior, posterior, or lateral infarction. The pathogenesis of depolarization abnormalities in this cardiomyopathy is not certain. Prominent inferolateral Q waves (II, III, aV_f, and V_4 to V_6) and tall right precordial R waves are probably related to increased depolarization forces generated by the markedly hypertrophied septum (Fig. 9-47). Abnormal septal depolarization can also contribute to the bizarre QRS complexes.

Q Wave Pathogenesis with Myocardial Damage. Loss of electromotive force associated with myocardial necrosis contributes to R wave loss and Q wave formation in cases of myocardial infarction. This mechanism of Q wave pathogenesis, however, is not specific for coronary artery disease with infarction. Any process, acute or chronic, that causes sufficient loss of regional electromotive potential can result in Q waves. For example, replacement of myocardial tissue by electrically inert material such as amyloid or tumor can cause noninfarction Q waves. A variety of dilated cardiomyopathies associated with extensive myocardial fibrosis can be characterized by pseudoinfarct patterns. Ventricular hypertrophy can also contribute to Q wave pathogenesis in this setting. Finally, Q waves caused by myocardial injury, whether ischemic or nonischemic in origin, can appear transiently and do not necessarily signify irreversible heart muscle damage. Severe ischemia can cause regional loss of electromotive potential without actual cell death ("electrical stunning" phenomenon). Transient conduction disturbances can also cause alterations in ventricular activation and result in noninfarctional Q waves. In some cases, transient Q waves may represent unmasking of a prior Q wave infarct. New, but transient, Q waves have been described in patients with severe hypotension from a variety of causes, as well as with tachyarrhythmias, myocarditis, Prinzmetal angina, protracted hypoglycemia, phosphorus poisoning, and hyperkalemia.

ST-T Changes Simulating Ischemia

The differential diagnosis of ST segment elevation includes acute pericarditis (see Chap. 64) (Fig. 9–48), acute myocarditis (see Chap. 60), normal-variant "early repolarization" (see Fig. 9–16), and a number of other conditions[73,74] listed in Table 9–10. Acute pericarditis, in contrast to acute myocardial infarction, typically induces diffuse ST segment elevation, usually in most of the chest leads and also in leads I, aV_l, II, and aV_f. Reciprocal ST depression is seen in lead aV_r.

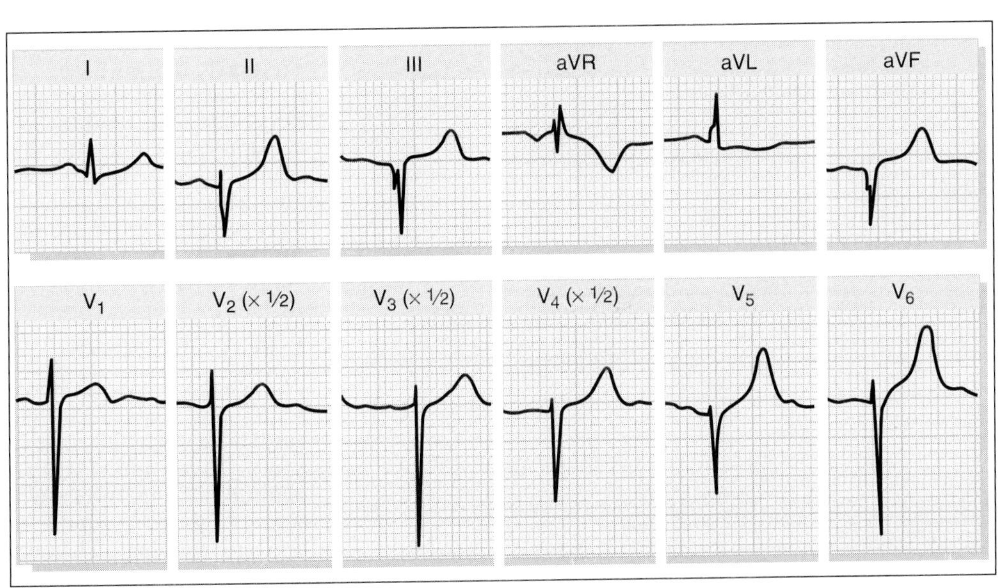

FIGURE 9–47 Hypertrophic cardiomyopathy simulating inferolateral infarction. This 11-year-old girl had a family history of hypertrophic cardiomyopathy. Note the W-shaped QS waves and the qrS complexes in the inferior and lateral precordial leads. (From Goldberger AL: Myocardial Infarction: Electrocardiographic Differential Diagnosis. 4th ed. St Louis, Mosby-Year Book, 1991.)

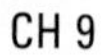

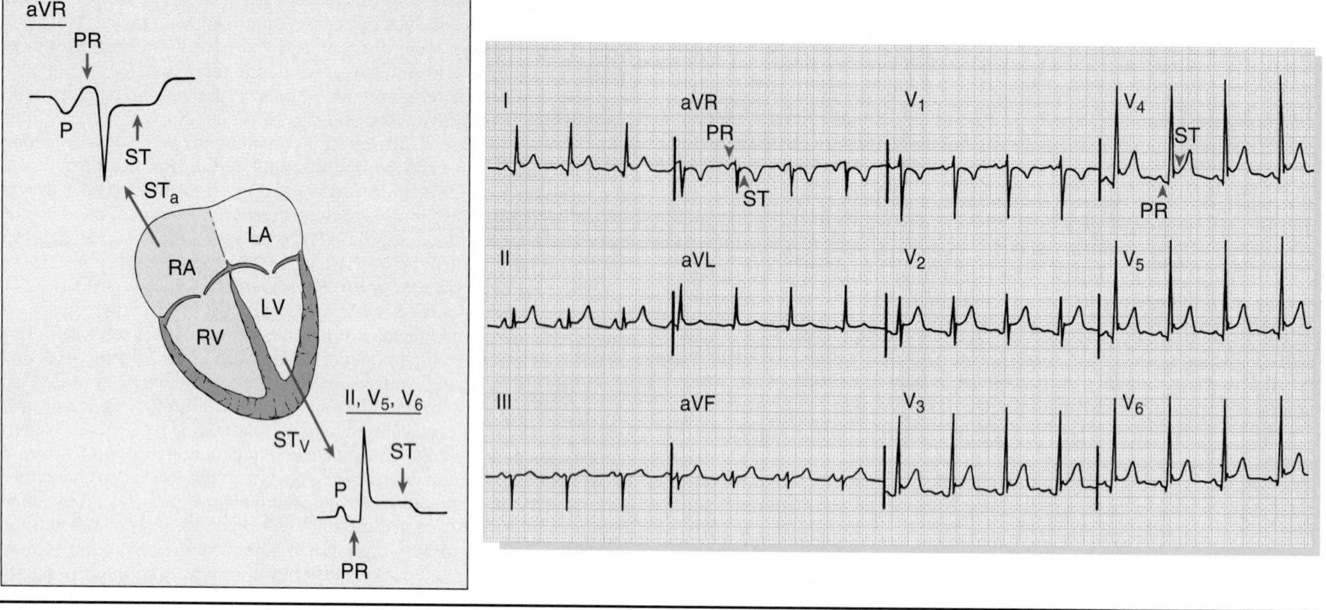

FIGURE 9–48 Acute pericarditis is often characterized by two apparent injury currents: one atrial, the other ventricular. The atrial injury current vector (ST_a) is usually directed upward and to the right and produces PR segment elevation in aV_r with reciprocal PR depression in II, V_5, and V_6. The ventricular injury current (ST_V) is directed downward and to the left, associated with ST elevation in II, V_5, and V_6 with reciprocal ST depression in aV. This characteristic PR-ST segment discordance is illustrated in the bottom-most tracing. Note the diffuse distribution of ST segment elevation in acute pericarditis (e.g., I, II, and V_2 through V_6, with reciprocal changes in aV_r and perhaps minimally in V_1). Note the PR segment elevation in aV. (From Goldberger AL: Myocardial Infarction: Electrocardiographic Differential Diagnosis. 4th ed. St Louis, Mosby-Year Book, 1991.)

TABLE 9–10 Differential Diagnosis of ST Segment Elevation
Myocardial ischemia/infarction Noninfarction, transmural ischemia (Prinzmetal angina pattern) (see Fig. 9–40) Acute myocardial infarction (see Fig. 9–37) Post myocardial infarction (ventricular aneurysm pattern)
Acute pericarditis (see Fig. 9–48)
Normal variant ("early repolarization" pattern) (see Fig. 9–16)
LVH/LBBB (V_1-V_2 or V_3 only)
Other (rarer) Myocardial injury Myocarditis (may look like myocardial infarction or pericarditis) Tumor invading the left ventricle Trauma to the ventricles
Hypothermia (J wave/Osborn wave) (see Fig. 9–53)
After DC-cardioversion
Intracranial hemorrhage
Hyperkalemia*
Brugada pattern (RBBB-like pattern and ST elevations in right precordial leads)*
Type 1C antiarrhythmic drugs*
Hypercalcemia*

LBBB = left bundle branch block; LVH = left ventricular hypertrophy; RBBB = right bundle branch block.
Modified from Goldberger AL: Clinical Electrocardiography: A Simplified Approach. 6th ed. St Louis, CV Mosby, 1999.
*Usually localized to V_1 to V_2.

An important clue to acute pericarditis, in addition to the diffuse nature of the ST elevation, is the frequent presence of PR segment elevation in aVR, with reciprocal PR segment depression in other leads, caused by a concomitant atrial current of injury[75] (see Fig. 9–48). Abnormal Q waves do not occur with acute pericarditis, and the ST elevation may be followed by T wave inversion after a variable period. Myocarditis can, in some patients, exactly simulate the ECG pattern of acute myocardial infarction, including ST elevation and Q waves. These pseudoinfarct findings can be associated with a rapidly progressive course and increased mortality.

A variety of factors such as digitalis, ventricular hypertrophy, hypokalemia, and hyperventilation can cause ST segment depression mimicking subendocardial ischemia. Similarly, tall positive T waves do not invariably represent hyperacute ischemic changes but can reflect normal variants, hyperkalemia, cerebrovascular injury, and left ventricular volume loads resulting from mitral or aortic regurgitation, among other causes. ST elevation and tall positive T waves are also common findings in leads V_1 and V_2 with LBBB or LVH patterns. In addition, tall T waves may be seen occasionally in the left chest leads with LVH, especially with volume (diastolic) overload syndromes (see Fig. 9–21).

T Wave Inversion

When caused by physiological variants, T wave inversion is sometimes mistaken for ischemia. T waves in the right precordial leads can be slightly inverted, particularly in leads V_1 and V_2. Some adults show persistence of the juvenile T wave pattern (see Fig. 9–15), with more prominent T wave inversion in right precordial to midprecordial leads showing an rS or RS morphology. The other normal variant that can be associated with prominent T wave inversion is the early repolarization pattern (see Fig. 9–16). Some subjects with this variant have prominent, biphasic T wave inversion in association with the ST elevation. This pattern, which may simulate the initial stages of an evolving infarct, is most prevalent in young adult black males and among athletes. These functional ST-T changes are probably due to regional disparities in repolarization and can be normalized by exercise.

PRIMARY AND SECONDARY T WAVE INVERSIONS. A variety of pathological factors can alter repolarization and cause prominent T wave inversion (Fig. 9–49). As noted earlier, T wave alterations are usefully classified as primary or secondary. Primary T wave changes are caused by alterations in the duration or morphology of ventricular action potentials in the absence of changes in the activation sequence. Examples include ischemia, drug effects, and metabolic factors. Prominent primary T wave inversion (or in some cases, tall positive T waves) is also a well-described feature of the ECG in cerebrovascular accidents, particularly with subarachnoid hemorrhage. The so-called cerebrovascular accident T wave pattern is characteristically diffuse, with a widely splayed appearance usually associated with marked QT prolongation (Fig. 9–49). Some studies have implicated structural damage (myocytolysis) in the hearts of patients with such T wave changes, probably induced by excessive sympathetic stimulation mediated via the hypothalamus. A role for concomitant vagal activation in the pathogenesis of such T wave changes, which are usually associated with bradycardia, has also been postulated. Similar T wave changes have been reported after truncal vagotomy, radical neck dissection, and bilateral carotid endarterectomy. In addition, the massive diffuse T wave inversion seen in some patients after Stokes-Adams syncope may be related to a similar neurogenic mechanism. Patients with subarachnoid hemorrhage can also show transient ST elevation, as well as arrhythmias, including torsades de pointes. Ventricular dysfunction can even occur.

In contrast to these primary T wave abnormalities, secondary T wave changes are caused by altered ventricular activation, without changes in action potential characteristics. Examples include bundle branch block, Wolff-Parkinson-White preexcitation, and ventricular ectopic or paced beats. In addition, altered ventricular activation (associated with QRS interval prolongation) can induce persistent T wave changes that appear after normal ventricular depolarization has resumed. The term *cardiac memory T wave changes* has been used in this context to describe repolarization changes subsequent to depolarization changes caused by ventricular pacing, intermittent LBBB, intermittent Wolff-Parkinson-White preexcitation, and other alterations of ventricular activation.[76] Finally, the designation *idiopathic global T wave inversion* has been applied in cases in which no identifiable cause for often marked, diffuse repolarization abnormalities can be found. An unexplained female preponderance has been reported. Major causes of prominent T wave inversion are summarized in Table 9–11, with selected examples in Figure 9–49.

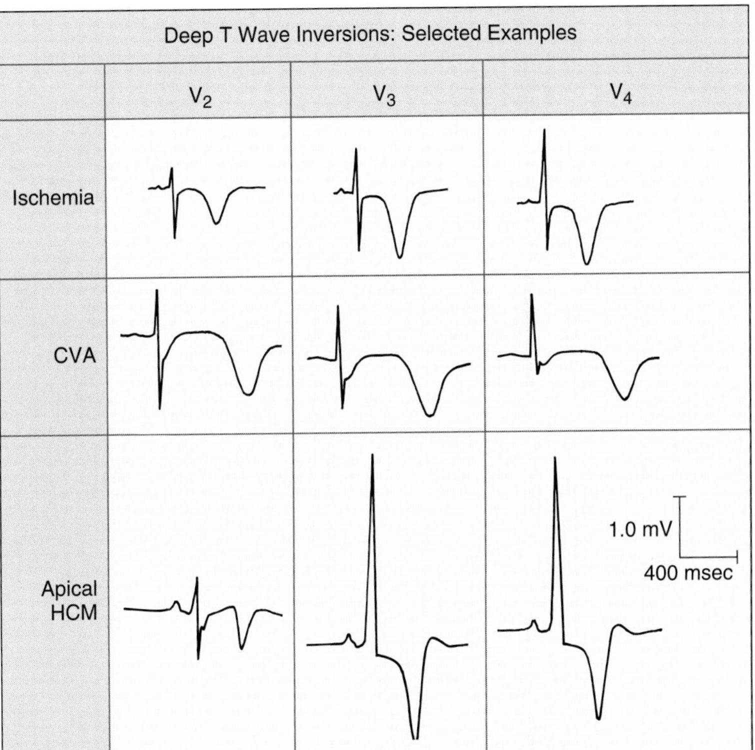

FIGURE 9–49 Deep T wave inversion can be due to a variety of causes (see Table 9–11). Note the marked QT prolongation in conjunction with the cerebrovascular accident (CVA) T wave pattern caused here by subarachnoid hemorrhage. Apical hypertrophic cardiomyopathy (HCM) is another cause of deep T wave inversion that can be mistaken for coronary disease. (From Goldberger AL: Deep T wave inversions. ACC Curr J Rev Nov/Dec:28, 1996.)

TABLE 9–11 Differential Diagnosis of Prominent T Wave Inversion

Normal variants Juvenile T wave pattern (see Fig. 9–15) Early repolarization
Myocardial ischemia/infarction (see Fig. 9–49)
Cerebrovascular accident (especially intracranial bleeding) and related neurogenic patterns (e.g., radical neck dissection, Stokes-Adams syndrome) (see Fig. 9–49)
Left or right ventricular overload Classic "strain" patterns Apical hypertrophic cardiomyopathy (Yamaguchi syndrome) (see Fig. 9–49)
Post-tachycardia T wave pattern
Idiopathic global T wave inversion syndrome
Secondary T wave alterations: bundle branch blocks, Wolff-Parkinson-White patterns
Intermittent left bundle branch block, preexcitation, or ventricular pacing ("memory T waves")

Modified from Goldberger AL: Clinical Electrocardiography: A Simplified Approach. 6th ed. St Louis, CV Mosby, 1999.

Drug Effects

Numerous drugs can affect the ECG, often in association with nonspecific ST-T alterations. More marked changes, as well as AV and intraventricular conduction disturbances, can occur with selected agents. The proarrhythmic effects of "antiarrhythmic" medications are described in Chapter 30.

Digitalis effect refers to the relatively distinctive "scooped" appearance of the ST-T complex and shortening of the QT interval, which correlates with abbreviation of the ventricular action potential duration (Fig. 9–50). Digitalis-related ST-T changes can be accentuated by an increased heart rate during exercise and result in false-positive stress test results[70] (see Chap. 10). Digitalis effect can occur with therapeutic or toxic doses of the drug. The term *digitalis toxicity* refers specifically to systemic effects (nausea and

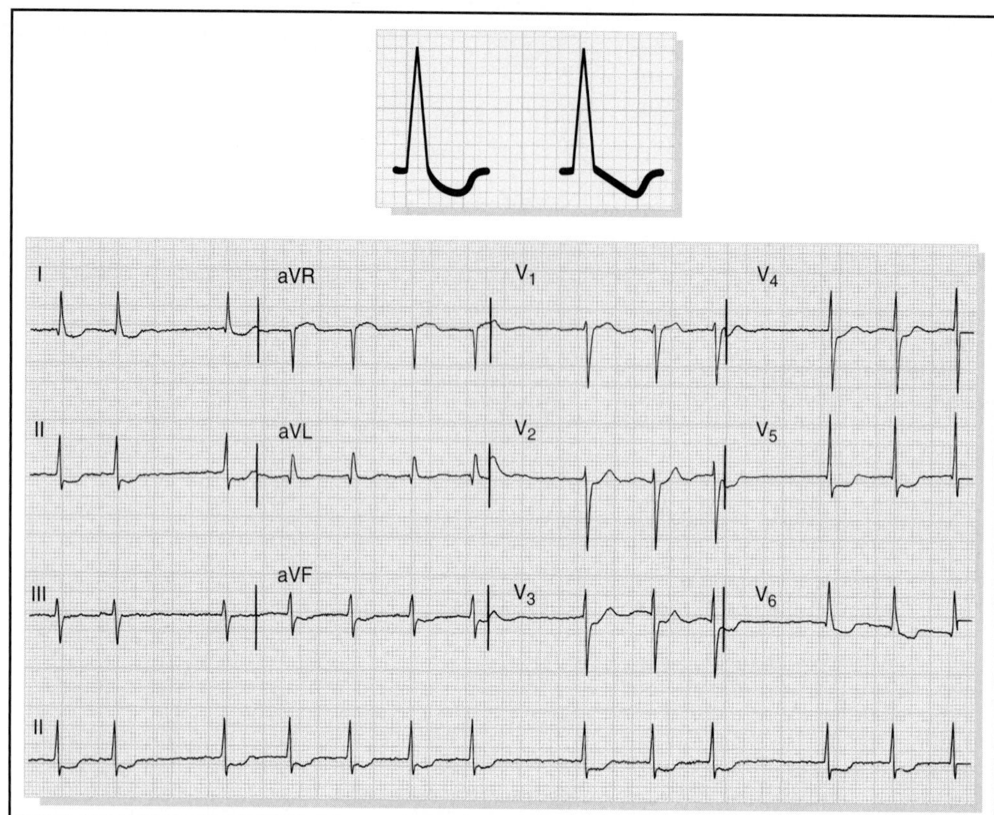

FIGURE 9–50 **Top,** Digitalis effect. Digitalis glycosides characteristically produce shortening of the QT interval with a "scooped" or downsloping ST-T complex. (From Goldberger AL: Clinical Electrocardiography: A Simplified Approach. 6th ed. St Louis, CV Mosby, 1999.) **Bottom,** Digitalis effect in combination with digitalis toxicity. The underlying rhythm is atrial fibrillation. A "group beating" pattern of QRS complexes with shortening of the R-R intervals is consistent with nonparoxysmal junctional tachycardia with exit (atrioventricular Wenckebach) block. ST segment depression and "scooping" (V_6) are consistent with digitalis effect, although ischemia or left ventricular hypertrophy cannot be excluded. Findings are strongly suggestive of digitalis excess; the serum digoxin level was greater than 3 ng/ml. Digitalis effect does not necessarily imply digitalis toxicity, however.

anorexia, among other effects) or conduction disturbances and arrhythmias caused by drug excess or increased sensitivity.

The ECG effects and toxicities of other cardioactive agents can be anticipated, in part, from ion channel effects (see Chap. 27). Inactivation of sodium channels by class 1 agents (e.g., quinidine, procainamide, disopyramide, flecainide) can cause QRS prolongation. Class 1A and class 3 agents (e.g., amiodarone, dofetilide, ibutilide, sotalol) can induce an acquired long QT(U) syndrome (see Chap. 30). Psychotropic drugs (e.g., tricyclic antidepressants and phenothiazines), which have class 1A-like properties, can also lead to QRS and QT(U) prolongation.[78] Toxicity can produce asystole or torsades de pointes. Right axis shift of the terminal 40 msec frontal plane QRS axis was reported to be a helpful marker of tricyclic antidepressant overdose.

Electrolyte and Metabolic Abnormalities

In addition to the structural and functional cardiac conditions already discussed, numerous systemic metabolic aberrations affect the ECG, including electrolyte abnormalities and acid-base disorders, as well as systemic hypothermia.

CALCIUM. Hypercalcemia and hypocalcemia predominantly alter the action potential duration. An increased extracellular calcium concentration shortens the ventricular action potential duration by shortening phase 2 of the action potential. In contrast, hypocalcemia prolongs phase 2 of the action potential. These cellular changes correlate with abbreviation and prolongation of the QT interval (ST segment portion) with hypercalcemia and hypocalcemia, respectively (Fig. 9–51). Severe hypercalcemia (e.g., serum Ca^{2+} >15 mg/dl) can also be associated with decreased T wave amplitude, sometimes with T wave notching or inversion. Hypercalcemia sometimes produces a high takeoff of the ST segment in leads V_1 and V_2 and can thus simulate acute ischemia (see Table 9–10).

POTASSIUM. Hyperkalemia is associated with a distinctive sequence of ECG changes (Fig. 9–52A). The earliest effect is usually narrowing and peaking (tenting) of the T wave. The QT interval is shortened at this stage, associated with decreased action potential duration. Progressive extracellular hyperkalemia reduces atrial and ventricular resting membrane potentials, thereby inactivating sodium channels, which decreases V_{max} and conduction velocity. The QRS begins to widen and P wave amplitude decreases. PR interval prolongation can occur, followed sometimes by second- or third-degree AV block. Complete loss of P waves may be associated with a junctional escape rhythm or so-called sinoventricular rhythm. In the latter instance, sinus rhythm persists with conduction between the SA and AV nodes and occurs without producing an overt P wave. Moderate to severe hyperkalemia occasionally induces ST elevations in the right precordial leads (V_1 and V_2) and simulates an ischemic current-of-injury pattern. However, even severe hyperkalemia can be associated with atypical or nondiagnostic ECG findings.[79] Very marked hyperkalemia leads to eventual asystole, sometimes preceded by a slow undulatory (sine-wave) ventricular flutter-like pattern. The ECG triad of

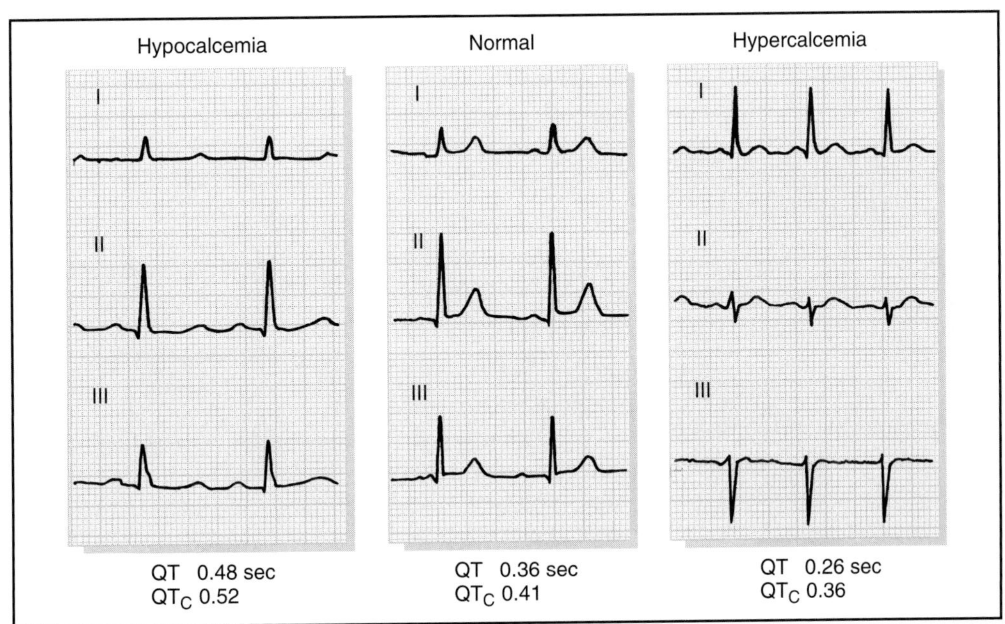

FIGURE 9–51 Prolongation of the QT interval (ST segment portion) is typical of hypocalcemia. Hypercalcemia may cause abbreviation of the ST segment and shortening of the QT interval. (From Goldberger AL: Clinical Electrocardiography: A Simplified Approach. 6th ed. St Louis, CV Mosby, 1999.)

(1) peaked T waves (from hyperkalemia), (2) QT prolongation (from hypocalcemia), and (3) LVH (from hypertension) is strongly suggestive of chronic renal failure.

The electrophysiological changes associated with hypokalemia, in contrast, include hyperpolarization of myocardial cell membranes and increased action potential duration. The major ECG manifestations are ST depression with flattened T waves and increased U wave prominence (Fig. 9–52B). The U waves can exceed the amplitude of T waves. Clinically, distinguishing T waves from U waves can be difficult or impossible from the surface ECG. Indeed, apparent "U" waves in hypokalemia and other pathologic settings may actually be part of T waves whose morphology is altered by the effects of voltage gradients between M, or midmyocardial cells, and adjacent myocardial layers.[80] The prolongation of repolarization with hypokalemia, as part of an acquired long QT(U) syndrome, predisposes to torsades de pointes. Hypokalemia also predisposes to tachyarrhythmias from digitalis.

MAGNESIUM. Specific ECG effects of mild to moderate isolated abnormalities in magnesium ion concentration are not well characterized. Severe hypermagnesemia can cause AV and intraventricular conduction disturbances that may culminate in complete heart block and cardiac arrest (Mg^{2+} >15 mEq/L). Hypomagnesemia is usually associated with hypocalcemia or hypokalemia. Hypomagnesemia can potentiate certain digitalis toxic arrhythmias. The role of magnesium deficiency in the pathogenesis and treatment of the acquired long QT(U) syndrome with torsades de pointes is discussed in Chapters 27 and 30.

OTHER FACTORS. Isolated hypernatremia or hyponatremia does not produce consistent effects on the ECG. Acidemia and alkalemia are often associated with hyperkalemia and hypokalemia, respectively. Systemic hypothermia may be associated with the appearance of a distinctive convex elevation at the junction (J point) of the ST segment and QRS complex (J wave or Osborn wave) (Fig. 9–53). The cellular mechanism of this type of pathological J wave appears to be related to an epicardial-endocardial voltage gradient associated with the localized appearance of a prominent epicardial action potential notch.

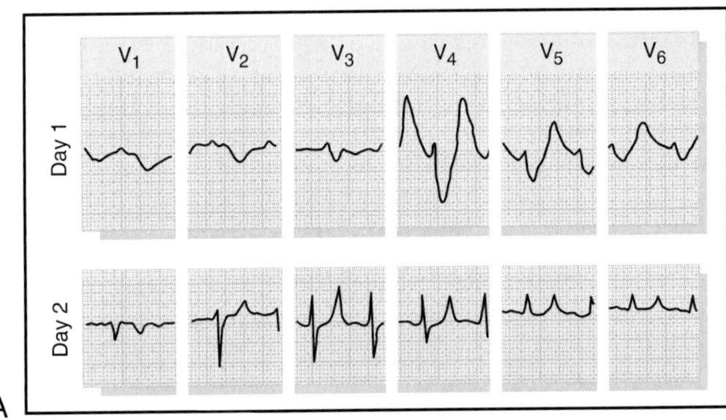

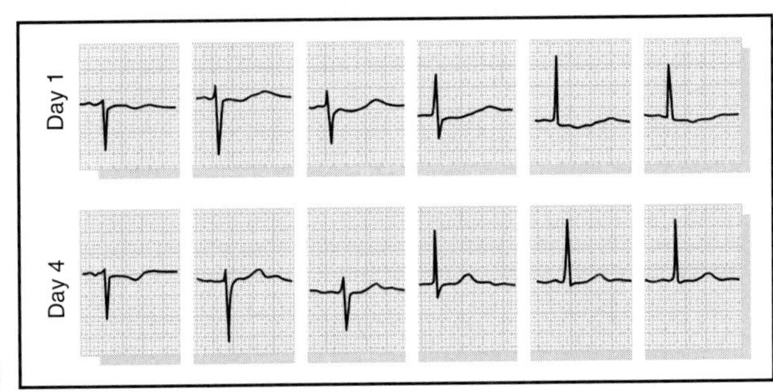

FIGURE 9–52 Electrocardiographic changes in hyperkalemia **(A)** and hypokalemia **(B)**. **A,** On day 1, at a K^+ level of 8.6 mEq/liter, the P wave is no longer recognizable and the QRS complex is diffusely prolonged. Initial and terminal QRS delay is characteristic of K^+-induced intraventricular conduction slowing and is best illustrated in leads V_2 and V_6. On day 2, at a K^+ level of 5.8 mEq/liter, the P wave is recognizable with a PR interval of 0.24 second, the duration of the QRS complex is approximately 0.10 second, and the T waves are characteristically "tented." **B,** On day 1, at a K^+ level of 1.5 mEq/liter, the T and U waves are merged. The U wave is prominent and the QU interval is prolonged. On day 4, at a K^+ level of 3.7 mEq/liter, the tracing is normal. (Courtesy of C. Fisch, M.D.)

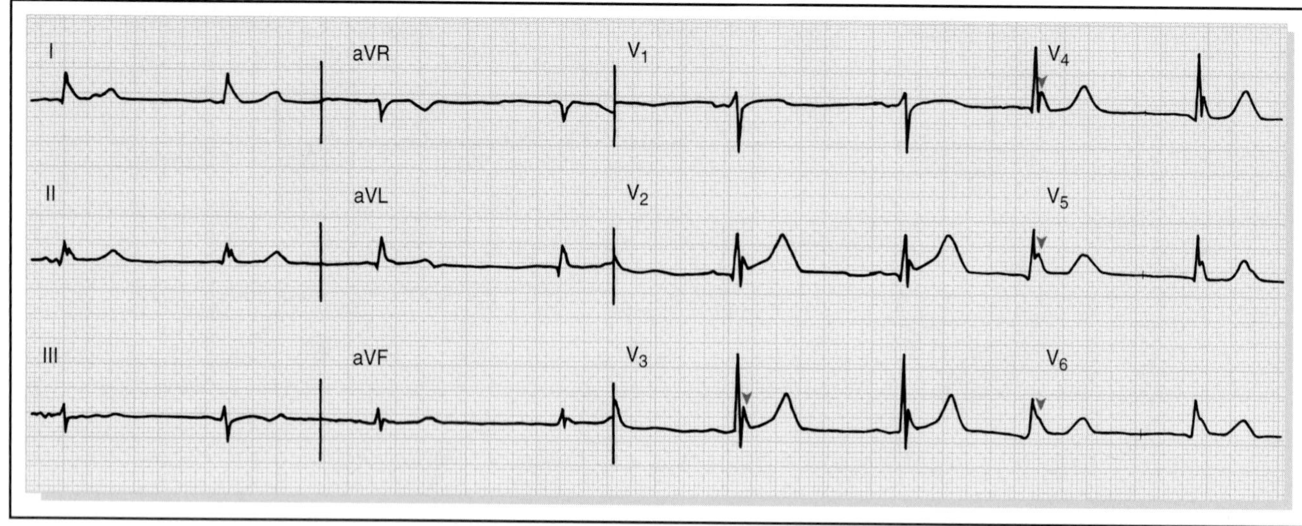

FIGURE 9–53 Systemic hypothermia. The arrows (V_3 through V_6) point to the characteristic convex J waves, termed *Osborn waves*. Prominent sinus bradycardia is also present. (From Goldberger AL: Clinical Electrocardiography: A Simplified Approach. 6th ed. St Louis, CV Mosby, 1999.)

Nonspecific QRS and ST-T Changes

Low QRS voltage is said to be present when the total amplitude of the QRS complexes in each of the six extremity leads is 0.5 mV or less or 1.0 mV or less in leads V_1 through V_6. Low QRS voltage can relate to a variety of mechanisms (Table 9–12), including increased insulation of the heart by air (chronic obstructive pulmonary disease) or adipose tissue (obesity); replacement of myocardium, for example, by fibrous tissue (ischemic or nonischemic cardiomyopathy), amyloid, or tumor; or short-circuiting (shunting) effects due to low resistance of the fluids (especially with pericardial or pleural effusions, or anasarca). The combination of relatively low limb voltage (QRS voltage ≤0.8 mV in each of the limb leads), relatively prominent QRS voltage in the chest leads (SV_1 or SV_2+RV_5 or RV_6 ≥3.5 mV), and poor R wave progression (R wave less than the S wave in V_1 through V_4) has been reported as a relatively specific, but not sensitive sign of dilated-type cardiomyopathies (ECG-congestive heart failure triad).

TABLE 9–12 Causes of Low-Voltage QRS Complexes
Adrenal insufficiency
Anasarca
Artifactual or spurious, e.g., unrecognized standardization of the electrocardiogram at half the usual gain (i.e., 5 mm/mV)
Cardiac infiltration or replacement (e.g., amyloidosis, tumor)
Cardiac transplantation, especially with acute or chronic rejection
Cardiomyopathies, idiopathic or secondary*
Chronic obstructive pulmonary disease constrictive pericarditis
Hypothyroidism (usually with sinus bradycardia)
Left pneumothorax (mid-left chest leads)
Myocardial infarction, extensive
Myocarditis, acute or chronic
Normal variant
Obesity
Pericardial effusion or tamponade (latter usually with sinus tachycardia)
Pleural effusions

*Dilated cardiomyopathies can be associated with a combination of relatively low limb lead voltage and prominent precordial voltage.

Many factors in addition to ischemia (e.g., postural changes, meals, drugs, hypertrophy, electrolyte and metabolic disorders, central nervous system lesions, infections, pulmonary diseases) can affect the ECG. Ventricular repolarization is particularly sensitive to these effects, which can lead to a variety of nonspecific ST-T changes. The term is usually applied to slight ST depression or T wave inversion or to T wave flattening without evident cause. Care must be taken to not overinterpret such changes, especially in subjects with a low prior probability of heart disease. At the same time, subtle repolarization abnormalities can be markers of coronary or hypertensive heart disease or other types of structural heart disease and probably account for the association of relatively minor but persistent nonspecific ST-T changes with increased cardiovascular mortality in middle-aged men and women.[81]

Alternans Patterns

The term *alternans* applies to conditions characterized by the sudden appearance of a periodic beat-to-beat change in some aspect of cardiac electrical or mechanical behavior. These abrupt changes (AAAA → ABAB pattern) are reminiscent of a generic class of subharmonic (period-doubling) bifurcation patterns observed in perturbed nonlinear control systems.[13,82] Many different examples of electrical alternans have been described clinically[83,84] (Table 9–13); a number of others have been reported in the laboratory.[85] Most familiar is total electrical alternans with sinus tachycardia, a specific but not highly sensitive marker of pericardial effusion with tamponade physiology (Fig. 9–54) (see Chap. 64). This finding is associated with an abrupt transition from a 1:1 to a 2:1 pattern in the "to-fro" swinging motion of the heart in the effusion. Other alternans patterns are due to primary electrical rather than mechanical causes. ST-T alternans has long been recognized as a marker of electrical instability in cases of acute ischemia, where it may precede ventricular tachyarrhythmia[86] (see Fig. 9–40). Considerable interest has recently been shown in the detection of microvolt T wave (or ST-T) alternans as a noninvasive marker of the risk of

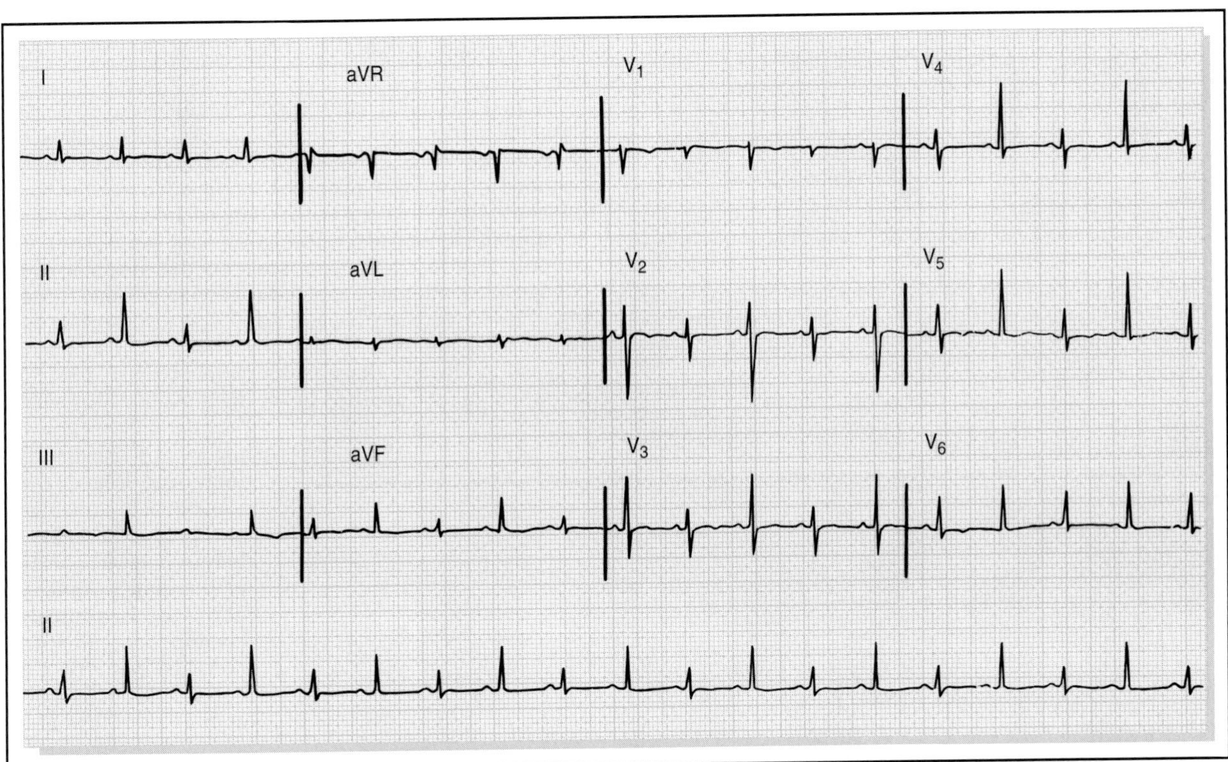

FIGURE 9–54 Total electrical alternans (P-QRS-T) caused by pericardial effusion with tamponade. This finding, particularly in concert with sinus tachycardia and relatively low voltage, is a highly specific, although not sensitive, marker of cardiac tamponade.

TABLE 9–13 Examples of Alternans Patterns in Electrocardiographic Diagnosis

Pattern	Comment
P wave alternans	Rarely reported; e.g., in pulmonary embolism
"Total" electrical alternans (P-QRS-T) with sinus tachycardia	Swinging-heart mechanism in pericardial effusion/tamponade* (see Fig. 9–54)
PR interval alternans	Dual AV nodal pathway physiology; alternating bundle branch block (see Fig. 9–30)
ST segment alternans	Can precede ischemic ventricular tachyarrhythmias (see Fig. 9–40)
T wave (or ST-T) alternans	Can precede nonischemic or ischemvc ventricular tachyarrhythmias
TU wave alternans	Can precede torsades de pointes in long QT(U) syndromes, congenital or acquired (see Fig. 9–55)
QRS alternans in supraventricular or ventricular tachycardias	Most common with AV reentrant tachycardias (concealed bypass tract)
R-R (heart rate) alternans	With sinus rhythm, e.g., in congestive heart failure With non–sinus rhythm tachyarrhythmias, e.g., PSVT
Bidirectional tachycardias	Usually ventricular in origin; may be caused by digitalis excess
Intermittent bundle branch/fascicular blocks or Wolff-Parkinson-White patterns	Rarely occur on beat-to-beat basis (see Fig. 9–31)

*Also case report of QRS-T alternans with sinus tachycardia in acute pulmonary embolism.
AV = atrioventricular; PSVT = paroxysmal supraventricular tachycardia.

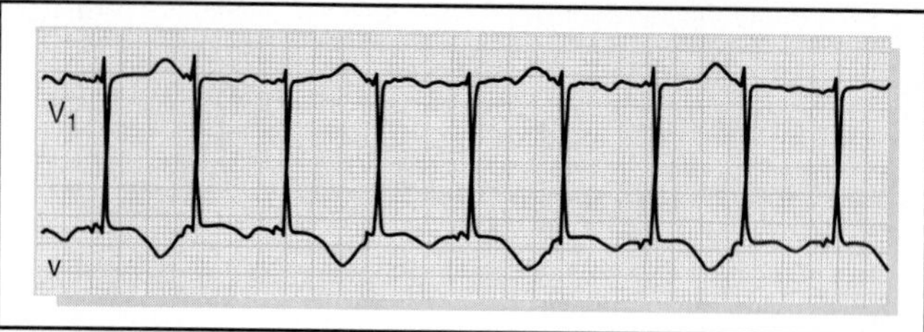

FIGURE 9–55 The QT(U) interval is prolonged (approximately 600 msec) with TU wave alternans. The tracing was recorded in a patient with chronic renal disease shortly following dialysis. This type of repolarization alternans may be a precursor to torsades de pointes. (Courtesy of C. Fisch, M.D.)

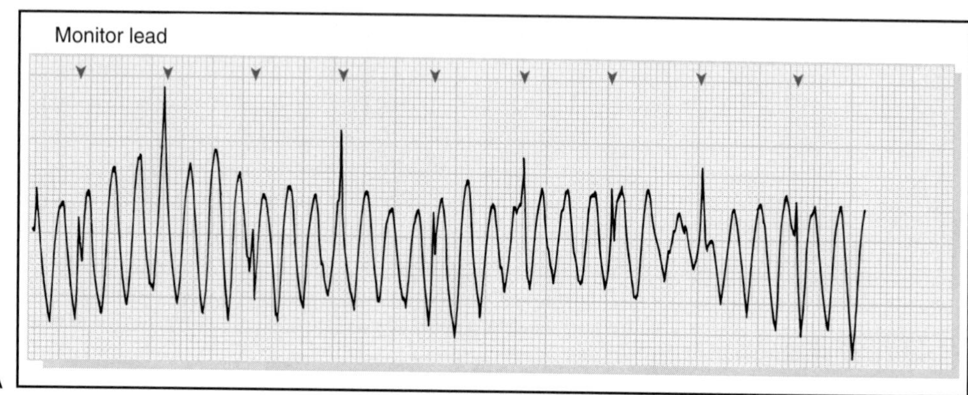

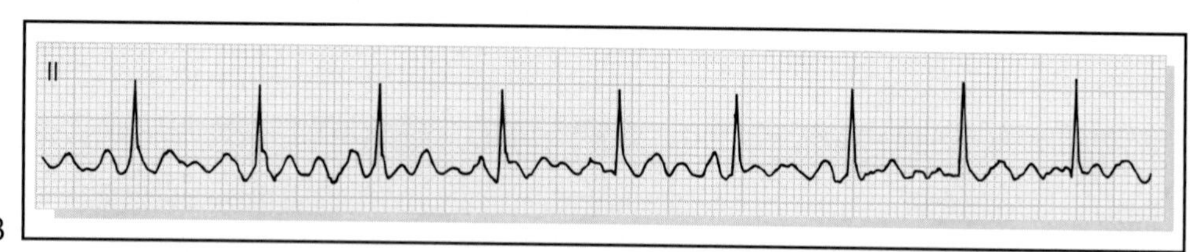

FIGURE 9–56 Artifacts simulating serious arrhythmias. **A,** Motion artifact mimicking ventricular tachyarrhythmia. Partly obscured normal QRS complexes (arrows) can be seen with a heart rate of about 100 beats/min. **B,** Parkinsonian tremor causing baseline oscillations mimicking atrial fibrillation. The regularity of QRS complexes may provide a clue to this artifact.

ventricular tachyarrhythmia in patients with chronic heart disease[87,88] (see Chap. 29). Similarly, TU wave alternans (Fig. 9–55) may be a marker of imminent risk of a ventricular tachyarrhythmia such as torsades de pointes in hereditary or acquired long QT syndromes.[89]

Clinical Issues in Electrocardiographic Interpretation

These principles and diagnostic ECG guidelines are, finally, subject to appropriate use in the clinical setting. Their effectiveness as a diagnostic tool depends on factors such as the indications for the procedure, the clinical context in which the ECG is used, and proper technique and skills of the ECG reader.

INDICATIONS FOR AN ECG. Limited attention has been paid to the indications for an ECG, probably because of its seeming simplicity and low cost. Because specific indications have not been accepted, there is wide variation in the use of the procedure.[90] However, the cumulative expense of low-cost tests performed at high volume is significant, and the risk to the patient of false diagnoses of cardiac disease can be damaging.

In patients with known cardiac disease, ECGs are warranted as part of a baseline examination; after therapy known to produce ECG changes that correlate with therapeutic responses, progression of disease, or adverse effects; and for intermittent follow-up with changes in signs or symptoms or relevant laboratory findings or after significant intervals (usually 1 year or longer), even in the absence of clinical changes. In patients suspected of having cardiac disease or at high risk for cardiac disease, an ECG is appropriate as part of an initial evaluation in the presence of signs or symptoms suggesting cardiac disease; in patients with important risk factors such as cigarette abuse, diabetes mellitus, peripheral vascular disease, or a family history of cardiac disease (including long QT interval syndromes and ventricular preexcitation); during therapy with cardioactive medications; and during follow-up if clinical events develop or at prolonged intervals (usually 1 year or more) if clinically stable. Preoperative tracings are appropriate for patients with known or suspected cardiac disease, although this application too may be questioned, especially if the cardiac condition is hemodynamically insignificant or the procedure is simple.

It has been common practice to include an ECG as part of routine health examinations, before any surgical procedure, and on any admission to a hospital in patients without current evidence of cardiac disease and without major risk factors. These ECGs are assumed to be of value in detecting any unknown abnormalities, serving as a baseline against which to compare later tracings, and assessing future risk of cardiovascular events. There is little evidence to support these practices. The overall sensitivity of the ECG for identifying specific patients who will have future events and the number of therapeutic or diagnostic changes provoked by routine ECG findings are too low to warrant universal screening.[91] The routine recording of the ECG before noncomplex surgery has also been questioned because of its limited value in risk stratification.[92] In these cases, use of the ECG should be based on clinical judgment rather than rigid protocol requirements. Flexible guidelines for ordering ECGs on general hospital admission and preoperatively have been proposed on the basis of age, gender, medical history, and physical examination.

KNOWLEDGE OF THE CLINICAL CONTEXT AND PRIOR ECG FINDINGS. Although most ECGs are read without a priori knowledge of the clinical condition of the patient, the accuracy and the value of the interpretation are enhanced by having clinical information about the patient. Such knowledge can include, for example, information about drug therapy, which can be a cause of observed ECG abnormalities, or prior myocardial infarction, which can produce ECG changes mimicking acute ischemia.[93]

Similarly, the availability of prior ECGs can improve the clinical value of the ECG. For example, knowledge of prior ECG patterns can improve diagnostic accuracy and triage decisions for patients with current ECG and clinical evidence of ischemia or infarction, as well as improve the proper interpretation of, for example, bundle branch block in the setting of acute infarction.[94]

TECHNICAL ERRORS AND ARTIFACTS. Technical errors can lead to significant diagnostic mistakes that can result in false diagnoses that place patients at risk for unneeded and potentially dangerous diagnostic tests and treatments and unnecessarily use limited health care resources.[95] Misplacement of one or more ECG electrodes is a common cause for errors in ECG interpretation. Some misplacements produce ECG patterns that can aid in identification of the error.[96,97] Reversal of the two arm electrodes, for example, results in an inverted P and QRS waveforms in lead I but not in lead V_6, two leads that would normally be expected to have similar polarities. Others are not as obvious. For example, placing the right precordial electrodes too high on the chest can yield patterns that mimic those produced by anterior myocardial infarction (poor R wave progression) or intraventricular conduction delay (rSr′ patterns). Electrical or mechanical artifacts such as produced by poor electrode contacts or tremors can simulate life-threatening arrhythmias[95] (Fig. 9–56), and excessive body motion can cause excessive baseline wander that may simulate an ST segment shift of myocardial ischemia or injury.

READING ERRORS. Errors in interpreting ECGs are common.[98-100] Studies assessing the accuracy of routine interpretations have demonstrated significant numbers of errors that can lead to clinical mismanagement, including failure to appropriately detect and triage patients with acute myocardial ischemia and other life-threatening situations. Organizations such as the American College of Cardiology have proposed minimal training and experience standards for electrocardiographers to help reduce these potentially serious errors.[100]

A final issue concerns overreliance on computerized interpretations. Computer systems have facilitated storage and retrieval of large numbers of ECGs and, as diagnostic algorithms have become more accurate, have provided important adjuncts to the clinical interpretation of ECGs. However, the current systems are not sufficiently accurate,[101] especially in the presence of rhythm disturbances or complex abnormalities, to be relied on in critical clinical environments without expert review. New analysis techniques based on artificial intelligence concepts may lead to future improvements,[102,103] and new hardware technology may result in expanded deployment of systems for prompt expert interpretation.[104]

ECGS FOR SELF-ASSESSMENT. A number of websites feature ECGs for self-assessment and clinical instruction. ECG Wave-Maven (http://ecg.bidmc.harvard.edu), for example, provides free access to more than 200 ECG case studies with answers and multimedia adjuncts.[105]

REFERENCES

Introduction and Fundamental Principles

1. Fisch C: Centennial of the string galvanometer and the electrocardiogram. J Am Coll Cardiol 26:1737, 2000.
2. Mirvis DM: Physiology and biophysics in electrocardiography. J Electrocardiol 29:175, 1996.
3. Ramanathan C, Rudy Y: Electrocardiographic imaging: I. Effect of torso inhomogeneities on body surface electrocardiographic potentials. J Cardiovasc Electrophysiol 12:229, 2001.
4. Madias JE, Bazaz B, Agarwal H, et al: Anasarca-mediated attenuation of the amplitude of electrocardiogram complexes: A description of a heretofore unrecognized phenomenon. J Am Coll Cardiol 38:756, 2001.
5. Novak PG, Davies C, Gin KG: Survey of British Columbia cardiologists' and emergency physicians: Practice of using nonstandard ECG leads (V_4R to V_6R and V_7 to V_9) in the diagnosis and treatment of acute myocardial infarction. Can J Cardiol 15:967, 1999.
6. Taccardi B, Punske BB, Lux RL, et al: Useful lessons from body surface mapping. J Cardiovasc Electrophysiol 9:773, 1998.
7. Horacek BM, Warren JW, Stovicek P, Feldman CL: Diagnostic accuracy of derived versus standard 12-lead electrocardiograms. J Electrocardiol 33(Suppl I):155, 2000.
8. Hurst JW: The use of the Grant method to interpret electrocardiograms. J Am Coll Cardiol 39:1878, 2002.

The Normal Electrocardiogram

9. Debbas NMG, Jackson SHD, de Jonghe D, et al: Human atrial depolarization: Effects of sinus rate, pacing and drugs on the surface electrocardiogram. J Am Coll Cardiol 33:358, 1999.
10. Markides V, Schilling RJ, Ho SY, et al: Characterization of left atrial activation in the intact human heart. Circulation 107:733, 2003.
11. Stovut DP, Wenstrom JC, Moeckel RB, et al: Respiratory sinus dysrhythmia persists in transplanted human hearts following autonomic blockade. Clin Exp Pharmacol Physiol 25:322, 1998.
12. Mietus JE, Peng CK, Henry I, Goldsmith RL, Goldberger AL: The pNNx-files: Re-examining a widely-used heart rate variability measure. Heart 88:378, 2002.
13. Goldberger AL, Amaral LAN, Hausdorff JM, et al: Fractal dynamics in physiology: Alterations with disease and aging. Proc Natl Acad Sci U S A 99(suppl 1):2466, 2002.
14. Mathew TC, Shankariah L, Spodick DH: Electrocardiographic correlates of absent septal q waves. Am J Cardiol 82:809, 1998.
15. Yotsukura M, Toyofuku M, Tajino K, et al: Clinical signifiicance of the disappearanc of septal Q wave after the onset of myocardial infarction: Correlation with location of responsible coronary lesions. J Electrocardiol 32:15, 1999.
16. MacAlpin RN: In search of left septal fascicular block. Am Heart J 144:948, 2002.
17. MacLeod RS, Ni Q, Erschler PR, et al: Effects of heart position on the body surface electrocardiogram. J Electrocardiol 33(Suppl):229, 2000.
18. Surawicz B: U wave: Facts, hypotheses, misconceptions, and misnomers. J Cardiovasc Electrophysiol 9:1117, 1998.
19. Wu J, Wu J, Zipes DP: Early afterdepolarizations, U waves and torsades de pointes. Circulation 105:675, 2002.
20. Bednar MM, Harrigan EP, Anziano RJ, et al: The QT interval. Prog Cardiovasc Dis 43(Suppl I):1-45, 2001.

20a. Molnar J, Zhang F, Weiss J, et al: Diurnal pattern of QTc interval: How long is prolonged? Possible relation to circadian triggers of cardiovascular events. J Am Coll Cardiol 27:76, 1996.

20b. Malik M: Is there a physiologic QT/RR relationship? J Cardiovasc Electrophysiol 13:1211, 2002.

21. Franz MR, Zabel M: Electrophysiological basis of QT dispersion measurements. Prog Cardiovasc Dis 47:311, 2000.
22. Pellicia A, Maron BJ, Culasso F, et al: Clinical signifiicance of abnormal electrocardigraphic patterns in trained athletes. Circulation 102:278, 2000.
23. Mehta M, Jain AC, Mehta A: Early repolarization. Clin Cardiol 27:59, 1999.
24. Surawicz B, Parikh SR: Prevalence of male and female patterns of early repolarization in the normal ECG of males and females from childhood to old age. J Am Coll Cardiol 40:1870, 2002.
25. Marcus RR, Kalisetti D, Raxwal V, et al: Early repolarization in patients with spinal cord injury: Prevalence and clinical signifiicance. J Spinal Cord Med 25:33, 2002.

Atrial Abnormalities; Ventricular Hypertrophy and Enlargement

26. Pinter A, Molin F, Savard P, et al: Body surface mapping of retrograde P waves in the intact dog by simulation of accessory pathway re-entry. Can J Cardiol 16:175, 2000.
27. Hazen MS, Marwick TH, Underwood DA: Diagnostic accuracy of the resting electrocardiogram in detection and estimation of left atrial enlargement: An echocardiographic correlation in 551 patients. Am Heart J 79:819, 1997.
28. Incalzi RA, Fuso L, De Rosa M, et al: Electrocardiographic signs of cor pulmonale: A negative prognostic fiinding in chronic obstructive pulmonary disease. Circulatio 99:1600, 1999.
29. Okin PM, Roman MJ, Devereux RB, et al: Time-voltage QRS area of the 12-lead electrocardiogram: Detection of left ventricular hypertrophy. Hypertension 31:937, 1998.
30. Okin PM, Devereux RB, Jern S, et al: Baseline characteristics in relation to electrocardiographic left ventricular hypertensive patients: The Losartan Intervention for Endpoint Reduction Study. Hypertension 36:766, 2000.
31. Okin PM, Devereux RB, Nieminen MS, et al: Relationship of the electrocardiographic strain pattern to left ventricular structure and function in hypertensive patients. Losartan Intervention For Endpoint. J Am Coll Cardiol 38:514, 2001.
32. Okin PM, Devereux RB, Fabsitz RR, et al: Quantitative assessment of electrocardiographic strain predicts increased left ventricular mass: The Strong Heart Study. J Am Coll Cardiol 40:1395, 2002.
33. Tomita S, Veno H, Takata M, et al: Relationship between electrocardiographic voltage and geometric patterns of left ventricular hypertrophy in patients with essential hypertension. Hypertens Res 21:259, 1998.
34. Rautaharju PM, Park LP, Gottdiener JS, et al: Race-and-sex-specifiic ECG models for lef ventricular mass in older populations. Factors inflluencing overestimation of left vetricular hypertrophy prevalence by ECG criteria in African-Americans. J Electrocardiol 33:205, 2000.
35. Okin PM, Jern S, Devereux RB, et al: Effect of obesity on electrocardiographic left ventricular hypertrophy in hypertensive patients: The losartan intervention for endpoint (LIFE) reduction in hypertension study. Hypertension 35:13, 2000.
36. Mirvis DM: The electrocardiogram as a prognostic tool. ACC Curr Rev J 4:181, 1999.
37. Menotti A, Seccareccia F: Electrocardiographic Minnesota code fiindings predictin short-term mortality in asymptomatic subjects. The Italian RIFLE Pooling Project (Risk Factors and Life Expectancy). G Ital Cardiol 27:40, 1997.
38. Sundstom J, Lind L, Arnlov J, et al: Echocardiographic and electrocardiographic diagnoses of left ventricular hypertrophy predict mortality independently of each other in a population of elderly men. Circulation 103:2346, 2001.

39. Jain A, Chandna H, Silber EN, et al: Electrocardiographic patterns of patients with echocardiographically determined biventricular hypertrophy. J Electrocardiol 32:269, 1999.

Intraventricular Conduction Delays and Preexcitation

40. Childers R, Lupovich S, Sochanski M, Knoarzewska H: Left bundle branch block and right axis deviation: A report of 36 cases. J Electrocardiol 33(Suppl):93, 2000.
41. Ducceschi V, Sarubbi B, D'Andrea A, et al: Electrophysiologic signifiicance of leftwar QRS axis deviation in bifascicular and trifascicular block. Clin Cardiol 21:597, 1998.
42. Mehdirad AA, Nelson SD, Love CJ, et al: QRS duration widening: Reduced synchronization of endocardial activation or transseptal conduction time? Pacing Clin Electrophysiol 21:1589, 1998.
43. Das MK, Cheriparambil K, Bedi A, et al: Prolonged QRS duration (QRS >/=170 ms) and left axis deviation in the presence of left bundle branch block: A marker for poor ventricular function? Am Heart J 142:756, 2001.
44. Skalidis EI, Kochiadakis GE, Koukouraki SI, et al: Phasic coronary flow pattern an flow reserve in patients with left bundle branch block and normal coronary arteries. J Am Coll Cardiol 33:1338, 1999.
45. Wagdy HM, Hodge D, Christian TF, et al: Prognostic value of vasodilator myocardial perfusion imaging in patients with left bundle branch block. Circulation 97:1563, 1998.
46. Peteiro J, Monserrat L, Martinez D, Castro-Beiras A: Accuracy of exercise echocardiography to detect coronary artery disease in left bundle branch block unassociated with either acute or healed myocardial infarction. Am J Cardiol 85:890, 2000.

Myocardial Ischemia and Infarction

47. Antzelevitch C, Brugada P, Brugada J, et al: Brugada syndrome: 1992-2003. A historical perspective. J Am Coll Cardiol 41:1665, 2003.
48. Zimetbaum PJ, Josephson ME: Use of the electrocardiogram in acute myocardial infarction. N Engl J Med 348:933, 2003.
49. Kleber AG: ST-segment elevation in the electrocardiogram: A sign of myocardial ischemia. Cardiovasc Res 45:111, 2000.
50. de Lemos JA, Antman EM, Giugliano RP, et al: ST-segment resolution and infarct-related artery patency and fllow after thrombolytic therapy. Am J Cardiol 85:299, 2000.
51. van't Hof AW, Liem A, de Boer MJ, et al: Clinical value of 12-lead electrocardiogram after successful reperfusion therapy for acute myocardial infarction. Zwolle Myocardial Infarction Study Group. Lancet 350:615, 1997.
52. Phibbs B, Marcus F, Marriott HJ, et al: Q-wave versus non-Q-wave myocardial infarction: A meaningless distinction. J Am Coll Cardiol 33:576, 1999.
53. Bosimini E, Giannuzzi P, Temporelli PL, et al: Electrocardiographic evolutionary changes and left ventricular remodeling after acute myocardial infarction: Results of the GISSI-3 Echo substudy. J Am Coll Cardiol 35:127, 2000.
54. Nagase K, Tamura A, Mikuriya Y, et al: Signifiicance of Q-wave regression after anterior wall acute myocardial infarction. Eur Heart J 19:742, 1998.
55. Chikamori T, Kitaoka H, Matsumura Y, et al: Clinical and electrocardiographic profiile producing exercise-induced U-wave inversion in patients with severe narrowing of the left anterior descending coronary artery. Am J Cardiol 80:628, 1997.
56. Hohnloser SH: Effect of coronary ischemia on QT dispersion. Prog Cardiovasc Dis 42:351, 2000.
57. Malik M: QT dispersion: time for an obituary? Eur Heart J 12:955, 2000.
58. Bogaty P, Boyer L, Rousseau L, Arsenault M: Is anteroseptal myocardial infarction an appropriate term? Am J Med 113:37, 2002.
59. Schmitt C, Lehman G, Schmieder S, et al: Diagnosis of acute myocardial infarction in angiographically documented occluded infarct vessel: Limitations of ST-segment elevation in standard and extended ECG leads. Chest 120:1540, 2001.
60. Matetzky S, Freimark D, Chouraqui P, et al: Signifiicance f ST segment elevations in posterior chest leads (V_7 to V_9) in patients with acute inferior myocardial infarction: Application for thrombolytic therapy. J Am Coll Cardiol 31:506, 1998.
61. Menown IBA, Allen J, Anderson JMcC, et al: Early diagnosis of right ventricular or posterior infarction associated with inferior wall left ventricular acute myocardial infarction. Am J Cardiol 85:934, 2000.
62. Porter A, Herz I, Strasberg B: Isolated right ventricular infarction presenting as anterior wall myocardial infarction on electrocardiography. Clin Cardiol 20:971, 1997.
63. Kosuge M, Kimura K, Ishikawa T, et al: New electrocardiographic criteria for predicting the site of coronary artery occlusion in inferior wall acute myocardial infarction. Am J Cardiol 82:1318, 1998.
64. Herz I, Assali AR, Adler Y, et al: New electrocardiographic criteria for predicting either the right or left circumfllex artery as the culprit coronary artery in inferior wall acut myocardial infarction. Am J Cardiol 80:1343, 1997.
65. Assali AR, Sclarovsky S, Herz I, et al: Comparison of patients with inferior wall acute myocardial infarction with versus without ST-segment elevation in leads V_5 and V_6. Am J Cardiol 81:81, 1998.
66. Arbane M, Goy JJ: Prediction of the site of total occlusion in the left anterior descending coronary artery using admission electrocardiogram in anterior wall acute myocardial infarction. Am J Cardiol 85:487, 2000.
67. Yamaji H, Iwasaki K, Kusachi S, et al: Prediction of acute left main coronary artery obstruction by 12-lead electrocardiography. ST segment elevation in lead aVR with less ST segment elevation in lead V1. J Am Coll Cardiol 38:1348, 2001.
68. Yip HK, Chen MC, Wu CJ, et al: Acute myocardial infarction with simultaneous ST-segment elevation in the precordial and inferior leads: Evaluation of anatomic lesions and clinical implications. Chest 123:1170, 2003.
69. Madias JE, Sinha A, Ashitani R, et al: A critique of the new ST-segment criteria for the diagnosis of acute myocardial infarction in patients with left bundle-branch block. Clin Cardiol 10:652, 2001.
70. Laham CL, Hammill SC, Gibbons RJ: New criteria for the diagnosis of healed inferior wall myocardial infarction in patients with left bundle branch block. Am J Cardiol 79:19, 1997.
71. Sgarbossa EB, Pinski SL, Gates KB, et al: Early electrocardiographic diagnosis of acute myocardial infarction in the presence of ventricular paced rhythm. GUSTO-1 investigators. Am J Cardiol 77:423, 1996.
72. Welch RD, Zalenski RJ, Frederick PD, et al: Prognostic value of a normal or nonspecifiic initial electrocardiogram in acute myocardial infarction. JAMA 286:1977, 2001.
73. Kok LC, Mitchell MA, Haines DE, et al: Transient ST elevation after transthoracic cardioversion in patients with hemodynamically unstable ventricular tachyarrhythmia. Am J Cardiol 85:878, 2000.
74. Krishnan SC, Josephson ME: ST segment elevation induced by class IC antiarrhythmic agents: Underlying electrophysiologic mechanisms and insights into drug-induced proarrhythmia. J Cardiovasc Electrophysiol 9:1167, 1998.
75. Baljepally R, Spodick DH: PR-segment deviation as the initial electrocardiographic response in acute pericarditis. Am J Cardiol 81:1505, 1998.

Drug Effects, Electrolyte and Metabolic Abnormalities; Nonspecific QRS and ST-T Abnormalities; Alternans Patterns

76. Shvilkin A, Danilo P, Wang J, et al: Evolution and resolution of long-time cardiac memory. Circulation 97:1810, 1998.
77. Sundqvist K, Jogestrand T, Nowak J: The effect of digoxin on the electrocardiogram of healthy middle-aged and elderly patients at rest and during exercise: A comparison with the ECG reaction induced by myocardial ischemia. J Electrocardiol 35:213, 2002.
78. Reilly JG, Ayis SA, Ferrier IN, et al: QT_C-interval abnormalities and psychotropic drug therapy in psychiatric patients. Lancet 355:1048, 2000.
79. Martinez-Vea A, Bardaji A, Garcia C, et al: Severe hyperkalemia with minimal electrocardiographic manifestations: A report of seven cases. J Electrocardiol 32:45, 1999.
80. Antzelevitch C, Shimizu W, Yan GX, et al: The M cell: Its contribution to the ECG and to normal and abnormal electrical function of the heart. J Cardiovasc Electrophysiol 10:1124, 1999.
81. Greenland P, Xie X, Liu K, et al: Impact of minor electrocardiographic ST-segment and/or T-wave abnormalities on cardiovascular mortality during long-term follow-up. Am J Cardiol 91:1068, 2003.
82. Ho KK, Moody GB, Pang CK, et al: Predicting survival in heart-failure case and control subjects by use of fully automated methods for deriving non-linear and conventional indices of heart rate dynamics. Circulation 96:442, 1997.
83. Fisch C, Mandrola JM, Rardon DP: Electrocardiographic manifestations of dual atrioventricular node conduction during sinus rhythm. J Am Coll Cardiol 29:1015, 1997.
84. Maury P, Racka F, Piot C, Davy JM: QRS and cycle length alternans during paroxysmal supraventricular tachycardia: what is the mechanism? J Cardiovasc Electrophysiol 13:92, 2002.
85. Hall K, Christini DJ, Tremblay M, et al: Dynamic control of cardiac alternans. Phys Rev Lett 78:4518, 1997.
86. Laguna P, Moody GB, Garcia J, et al: Analysis of the ST-T complex of the electrocardiogram using the Karhunen-Loève transform: Adaptive monitoring and alternans detection. Med Biol Eng Comput 37:175, 1999.
87. Pastore JM, Girouard SD, Laurita KR, et al: Mechanism linking T-wave alternans to the genesis of cardiac fiibrillation. Circulation 99:1385, 1999.
88. Gold MR, Bloomfiield DM, Anderson KP, et al: A comparison of T-wave alternans, signa averaged electrocardiography and programmed ventricular stimulation for arrhythmia risk stratifiication. J Am Coll Cardiol 36:2247, 2000.
89. Shimizu W, Antzelevitch C: Cellular and ionic basis for T-wave alternans under long Q-T conditions. Circulation 99:1499, 1999.

Clinical Issues in Electrocardiographic Interpretation

90. Stafford RS, Misra B: Variation in routine electrocardiogram use in academic primary care practice. Arch Intern Med 161:2351, 2001.
91. Ashley EA, Raxwal VK, Froelicher VF: The prevalence and prognostic signifiiance of electrocardiographic abnormalities. Curr Probl Cardiol 25:1, 2000.
92. Murdoch CJ, Murdoch DR, McIntyre P, et al: The preoperative ECG in day surgery: A habit? Anaesthesia 54:907, 1999.
93. Hatala R, Norman GR, Brooks LR: Impact of a clinical scenario on accuracy of electrocardiogram interpretation. J Gen Intern Med 14:126, 1999.
94. Pope JH, Aufderheide TP, Ruthazer R, et al: Missed diagnoses of cardiac ischemia in the emergency department. N Engl J Med 342:1163, 2000.
95. Knight BP, Michaud GF, Strickberger SA, et al: Clinical consequences of electrocardiographic artifact mimicking ventricular tachycardia. N Engl J Med 341:1270, 1999.
96. Ho KK, Ho SK: Use of the sinus P wave in diagnosing electrocardiographic limb lead misplacement not involving the right leg (ground) lead. J Electrocardiol 34:161, 2001.
97. Hurst JW: Electrocardiographic crotchets or common errors made in the interpretation of the electrocardiogram. Clin Cardiol 21:211, 1998.
98. Sur DK, Kaye L, Goad J, Morena A: Accuracy of electrocardiogram reading by family practice residents. Fam Med 32:315, 2000.
99. Goodacre S, Webster A, Morris F: Do computer generated ECG reports improve interpretation by accident and emergency room house offiicers? Postgrad Med J 7:455, 2001.
100. Kadish AH, Buxton AE, Kennedy HL, et al: ACC/AHA clinical competence statement on electrocardiography and ambulatory electrocardiography. Circulation 104:3169, 2001.
101. Spodick D: Computer treason: Intraobserver variability of an electrocardiographic computer system. Am J Cardiol 80:102, 1997.
102. Hedén B, Öhlin H, Rittner R, et al: Acute myocardial infarction detected in the 12-lead ECG by artifiicial neural networks. Circulation 96:1798, 1997.
103. Holst H, Ohlsson M, Peterson C, Edenbrandt L: A confiident decision support syste for interpreting electrocardiograms. Clin Physiol 19:410, 1999.
104. Pettis KS, Savona MR, Leibrandt PN, et al: Evaluation of the effiicacy of hand-held co-puter screens for cardiologists' interpretation of 12-lead electrocardiograms. Am Heart J 138:765, 1999.
105. McClennen S, Nathanson LA, Safran C, Goldberger AL: ECG Wave-Maven: An Internet-based electrocardiography self-assessment program for students and clinicians. Med Educ Online 8:2, 2003. (http://www.med-ed-online.org/issue2.htm#v8)

Electrocardiography

Guidelines for the performance of electrocardiograms (ECGs) have evolved little in recent years. The most widely cited guidelines were published by the American College of Cardiology and American Heart Association (ACC/AHA) in 1992.[1] These guidelines make recommendations on the use of ECGs in patients with and without cardiovascular disease. Other guidelines were published by the American Heart Association in 1987,[2] by a task force assembled by the Canadian government in 1991,[3] and by the US Preventive Task Force (USPTF) in 1996.[4] Standards for clinical competence were recommended more recently (in 2001) by an ACC/AHA task force.[5]

Patients with Known Cardiovascular Disease or Dysfunction

The ACC/AHA guidelines[1] endorse the use of ECGs in the baseline evaluation of all patients with known cardiovascular disease and for the evaluation of response to therapies likely to produce ECG changes (Table 9G–1). These guidelines use the older ACC/AHA convention of classifying indications according to one of three classes. Class I indications are conditions for which it is generally agreed that ECGs are useful. Class II indications are conditions for which opinions differ with

TABLE 9G–1 ACC/AHA Guidelines for Electrocardiography in Patients with Known Cardiovascular Disease or Dysfunction

Indication	Class I (appropriate)	Class II (equivocal)	Class III (inappropriate)
Baseline or initial evaluation	All patients	None	None
Response to therapy	Patients in whom prescribed therapy is known to produce ECG changes that correlate with therapeutic responses or progression of disease. Patients in whom prescribed therapy may produce adverse effects that may be predicted from or detected by ECG changes.	None	Patients receiving pharmacological or nonpharmacological therapy not known to produce ECG changes or to affect conditions that may be associated with such changes.
Follow-up	Patients with a change in symptoms, signs, or relevant laboratory findings. Patients with an implanted pacemaker or antitachycardia device. Patients with symptoms such as the following conditions, even in the absence of new symptoms or signs, after an interval of time appropriate for the condition or disease: Syncope and near-syncope Unexplained change in the usual pattern of angina pectoris Chest pain New or worsening dyspnea Extreme and unexplained fatigue, weakness, and prostration Palpitation New signs of congestive heart failure A new organic murmur or pericardial friction rub New findings suggesting pulmonary hypertension Accelerating or poorly controlled systemic arterial hypertension Evidence of a recent cerebrovascular accident Unexplained fever in patients with known valvular disease New onset of cardiac arrhythmia or inappropriate heart rate Chronic known congenital or acquired cardiovascular disease		Adult patients whose cardiovascular condition is usually benign and unlikely to progress (e.g., patients with asymptomatic mild mitral valve prolapse, mild hypertension, or premature contractions in the absence of organic heart disease) Adult patients with chronic stable heart disease seen at frequent intervals (i.e., 4 months) and who have no new or unexplained findings.
Before surgery	All patients with known cardiovascular disease or dysfunction except as noted under Class II.	Patients with hemodynamically insignificant congenital or acquired heart disease, mild systemic hypertension, or infrequent premature complexes in the absence of organic heart disease.	None

TABLE 9G–2 ACC/AHA Guidelines for Electrocardiography in Patients Suspected of Having or Who Are at Increased Risk for Cardiovascular Disease or Dysfunction

Setting	Class I (appropriate)	Class II (equivocal)	Class III (inappropriate)
Baseline or initial evaluation	All patients suspected of having or being at increased risk for cardiovascular disease. Patients who may have used cocaine, amphetamines, or other illicit drugs known to have cardiac effects. Patients who may have received an overdose of a drug known to have cardiac effects.	None	None
Response to therapy	To assess therapy with cardioactive drugs in patients with suspected cardiac disease. To assess the response to the administration of any agent known to result in cardiac abnormalities or ECG abnormalities (e.g., antineoplastic drugs, lithium, and antidepressant agents).	To assess the response to administration of any agent known to alter serum electrolyte concentrations.	To assess the response to administration of agents known not to influence cardiac structure or function.
Follow-up	The presence of any change in clinical status or laboratory findings suggesting interval development of cardiac disease or dysfunction. Periodic follow-up (e.g., every 1 to 5 yr) of patients known to be at increased risk for cardiac disease. Follow-up of patients after resolution of chest pain.	None	Follow-up ECGs more often than once yearly are not indicated in patients who remain clinically stable, who are not at increased risk for the development of cardiac disease, and who have not been demonstrated to have cardiac disease with previous studies.
Before surgery	As part of the preoperative evaluation of any patient with suspected, or at increased risk of developing, cardiac disease or dysfunction.	None	None

TABLE 9G–3 ACC/AHA Guidelines for Electrocardiography in Patients with No Apparent or Suspected Heart Disease or Dysfunction

Setting	Class I (appropriate)	Class II (equivocal)	Class III (inappropriate)
Baseline or initial evaluation	Persons aged 40 or more years undergoing physical examination. Before administration of pharmacological agents known to have a high incidence of cardiovascular effects (e.g., antineoplastic agents). Before exercise stress testing. People of any age who are in special occupations that require very high cardiovascular performance (e.g., fire fighters, police officers) or whose cardiovascular performance is linked to public safety (e.g., pilots, air traffic controllers, critical process operators, bus or truck drivers, and railroad engineers).	To evaluate competitive athletes	Routine screening or baseline ECGS in asymptomatic persons younger than 40 yr with no risk factors.
Response to therapy	To evaluate patients in whom prescribed therapy (e.g., doxorubicin) is known to produce cardiovascular effects.	None	To assess treatment that is known to not produce any cardiovascular effects.
Follow-up	To evaluate asymptomatic persons >40 yr of age.	None	To evaluate asymptomatic adults who have had no interval change in symptoms, signs, or risk factors and who have had a normal ECG within the recent past.
Before surgery	Patients >40 yr of age. Patients being evaluated as a donor for heart transplantation or as a recipient of a noncardiopulmonary transplant.	Patients 30–40 yr of age	Patients younger than 30 yr with no risk factors for coronary artery disease.

respect to the usefulness of ECGs. Class III indications are conditions for which it is generally agreed that ECGs have little or no usefulness.

The ACC/AHA guidelines do not comment on the frequency of follow-up ECGs but do endorse the use of serial ECGs for patients with known cardiovascular disease whenever there are changes in symptoms, signs, or laboratory findings. Even in the absence of such changes, follow-up ECGs are considered appropriate for patients with syndromes such as syncope, chest pain, and extreme fatigue. Follow-up ECGs are not considered appropriate for patients with mild chronic cardiovascular conditions that are not considered likely to progress (e.g., mild mitral valve prolapse). ECGs at each visit are considered inappropriate for patients with stable heart disease who are seen frequently (e.g., within 4 months) and have no evidence of clinical change.

Before surgical procedures, ECGs are considered appropriate for all patients with known cardiovascular disease or dysfunction, except those with insignificant or mild conditions such as mild systemic arterial hypertension.

Patients with Suspected Cardiovascular Disease or at High Risk for Cardiovascular Disease

The ACC/AHA guidelines make similar recommendations for patients with suspected cardiovascular disease and those who are at high risk for such conditions for the use of ECGs at baseline, for evaluation of the response to therapy, and before surgery (Table 9G–2). In the follow-up of patients at increased risk for heart disease, ECGs every 1 to 5 years are considered appropriate, but routine screening ECGs more frequently than yearly are not supported for patients who remain clinically stable, as long as they had not been previously demonstrated to have heart disease.

Patients without Known or Suspected Heart Disease

The various guidelines differ in their recommendations for the use of ECGs to screen for cardiovascular disease in healthy people. In the ACC/AHA guidelines, ECGs are considered appropriate screening tests in patients without apparent or suspected heart disease who are 40 years of age or older (Table 9G–3). Earlier guidelines from the AHA recommended that ECGs be obtained at ages 20, 40, and 60 years.[2] In contrast, the U.S. Preventive Services Task Force and the task force assembled by the Canadian government did not find evidence to support the use of screening ECG.[3,4]

The ACC/AHA guidelines recommend ECGs for patients for whom drugs with a high incidence of cardiovascular effects (e.g., chemotherapy) or exercise testing is planned and for people of any age in occupations with high cardiovascular demands or whose cardiovascular status might affect the safety of many other people (e.g., airline pilots). ECGs are considered appropriate before surgery in patients 40 of age or older and are equivocal in patients between the ages of 30 and 40 years in these guidelines. More recent guidelines from the ACC/AHA for perioperative evaluation[6] found good evidence for ECGs before noncardiac surgery in asymptomatic patients with diabetes (Table 76G–1), but otherwise do not strongly endorse routine preoperative ECG testing in patients without cardiovascular symptoms.

Clinical Competence

The ACC/AHA Clinical Competence Statement on electrocardiography[5] provides an overview for minimal standards for performance and interpretation of ECGs. In addition to making recommendations for the list of diagnoses with which ECG interpreters should be familiar, the Statement asserts that computer interpretations must be reviewed by an experienced electrocardiographer. The Task Force recommended a minimum of 100 ECG interpretations a year to maintain competence.

References

1. Schlant RC, Adolph RJ, DiMarco JP, et al: Guidelines for electrocardiography: A report of the American College of Cardiology/American Heart Association Task Force on Assessment of Diagnostic and Therapeutic Cardiovascular Procedures (Committee on Electrocardiography). J Am Coll Cardiol 19:473, 1992.
2. Grundy SM, Greenland P, Herd A, et al: Cardiovascular and risk factor evaluation of healthy American adults: A statement for physicians by an ad hoc committee appointed by the Steering Committee, American Heart Association. Circulation 75:1340A, 1987.
3. Hayward RSA, Steinberg EP, Ford DE, et al: Preventive care guidelines: 1991. Ann Intern Med 114:758, 1991.
4. US Preventive Task Force: Guide to Clinical Preventive Services. 2nd ed. Baltimore, Williams & Wilkins, 1996.
5. Kadish AH, Buxton AE, Kennedy HL, et al: ACC/AHA clinical competence statement on electrocardiography and ambulatory electrocardiography: A report of the American College of Cardiology/American Heart Association/American College of Physicians-American Society of Internal Medicine Task Force on Clinical Competence (ACC/AHA Committee to Develop a Clinical Competence Statement on Electrocardiography and Ambulatory Electrocardiography); Circulation104:3169, 2001.
6. Eagle KA, Berger PB, Calkins H, et al: ACC/AHA guideline update for perioperative cardiovascular evaluation for noncardiac surgery: A report of the American College of Cardiology/ American Heart Association Task Force on Practice Guidelines (Committee to Update the 1996 Guidelines on Perioperative Cardiovascular Evaluation for Noncardiac Surgery). 2002. American College of Cardiology Web site. (http:/www.acc.org/clinical/guidelines/perio/dirIndex.htm)

CHAPTER 10

Exercise Stress Testing

Bernard R. Chaitman

Exercise is a common physiological stress used to elicit cardiovascular abnormalities not present at rest and to determine the adequacy of cardiac function.[1-11] Exercise electrocardiography (ECG) is one of the most frequent noninvasive modalities used to assess patients with suspected or proven cardiovascular disease. The test is mainly used to estimate prognosis and to determine functional capacity, the likelihood and extent of coronary artery disease (CAD), and the effects of therapy. Hemodynamic and ECG measurements combined with ancillary techniques such as metabolic gas analysis, radionuclide imaging, and echocardiography enhance the information content of exercise testing in selected patients.[5]

Exercise Physiology

Anticipation of dynamic exercise results in an acceleration of ventricular rate due to vagal withdrawal, increase in alveolar ventilation, and increased venous return primarily as a result of sympathetic venoconstriction.[12] In normal persons, the net effect is to increase resting cardiac output before the start of exercise. The magnitude of hemodynamic response during exercise depends on the severity of the exercise and the amount of muscle mass involved. In the early phases of exercise in the upright position, cardiac output is increased by an augmentation in stroke volume mediated through the use of the Frank-Starling mechanism and heart rate; the increase in cardiac output in the latter phases of exercise is primarily due to a sympathetic-mediated increase in ventricular rate. At fixed submaximal workloads below anaerobic threshold, steady-state conditions are usually reached after the second minute of exercise, following which heart rate, cardiac output, blood pressure, and pulmonary ventilation are maintained at reasonably constant levels.[1,8] During strenuous exertion, sympathetic discharge is maximal and parasympathetic stimulation is withdrawn, resulting in vasoconstriction of most circulatory body systems, except for that in exercising muscle and in the cerebral and coronary circulations. Venous and arterial norepinephrine release from sympathetic postganglionic nerve endings, as well as plasma renin levels, are increased; the catecholamine release enhances ventricular contractility. As exercise progresses, skeletal muscle blood flow is increased, oxygen extraction increases by as much as threefold, total calculated peripheral resistance decreases, and systolic blood pressure, mean arterial pressure, and pulse pressure usually increase. Diastolic blood pressure does not change significantly. The pulmonary vascular bed can accommodate as much as a sixfold increase in cardiac output with only modest increases in pulmonary artery pressure, pulmonary capillary wedge pressure, and right atrial pressure; in normal individuals, this is not a limiting determinant of peak exercise capacity.

Cardiac output increases by four- to sixfold above basal levels during strenuous exertion in the upright position, depending on genetic endowment and level of training.[12] The maximum heart rate and cardiac output are decreased in older individuals, partly because of decreased beta-adrenergic responsivity.[13,14] Maximum heart rate can be estimated from the formula 220 − age in years, with a standard deviation of 10 to 12 beats per minute. The age-predicted maximum heart rate is a useful measurement for safety reasons. However, the wide standard deviation in the various regression equations used and the impact of drug therapy limit the usefulness of this parameter in estimating the exact age-predicted maximum for an individual patient.[15]

In the postexercise phase, hemodynamics return to baseline within minutes of termination of exercise. Vagal reactivation is an important cardiac deceleration mechanism after exercise and is accelerated in well-trained athletes but blunted in patients with chronic heart failure (see also section on heart rate). Intense physical work or significant cardiorespiratory impairment may interfere with achievement of a steady state, and an oxygen deficit occurs during exercise. The total oxygen uptake in excess of the resting oxygen uptake during the recovery period is the oxygen debt.

PATIENT'S POSITION

At rest, the cardiac output and stroke volume are higher when the person is in the supine position than when the person is in the upright position. With exercise in normal supine persons, the elevation of cardiac output results almost entirely from an increase in heart rate, with little augmentation of stroke volume. In the upright posture, the increase in cardiac output in normal individuals results from a combination of elevations in stroke volume and heart rate. A change from supine to upright posture causes a decrease in venous return, left ventricular end-diastolic volume and pressure, stroke volume, and cardiac index. Renin and norepinephrine levels are increased. End-systolic volume and ejection fraction are not significantly changed. In normal individuals, end-systolic volume decreases and ejection fraction increases to a similar extent from rest to exercise in the supine and upright positions. The magnitude and direction of change in end-diastolic volume from rest to maximum exercise in both positions are small and may vary according to the patient population studied. The net effect on exercise performance is an approximate 10 percent increase in exercise time, cardiac index, heart rate, and rate pressure product at peak exercise in the upright as compared with the supine position.

Cardiopulmonary Exercise Testing

Cardiopulmonary exercise testing involves measurements of respiratory oxygen uptake ($\dot{V}O_2$), carbon dioxide production ($\dot{V}CO_2$), and ventilatory parameters during a symptom-limited exercise test. During testing, the patient usually wears a nose clip and breathes through a nonrebreathing valve that separates expired air from room air. Important measurements of expired gas are PO_2, PCO_2, and air flow. Ventilatory measurements include respiratory rate, tidal volume, and minute ventilation ($\dot{V}e$). PO_2 and PCO_2 are sampled breath by breath or by use of a mixing chamber. The $\dot{V}O_2$ and $\dot{V}CO_2$ can be computed from ventilatory volumes and differences between inspired and expired gases.[4,5] Under steady-state conditions, $\dot{V}O_2$ and $\dot{V}CO_2$ measured at the mouth are equivalent to total-body oxygen consumption and carbon dioxide production. The relationship between work output, oxygen consumption, heart rate, and cardiac output during exercise is linear (Fig. 10–1). $\dot{V}O_2$max is the product of maximal arterial-venous oxygen difference and cardiac output and represents the largest amount of oxygen a person can use while performing dynamic exercise involving a large part of total muscle mass. The $\dot{V}O_2$max decreases with age, is usually less in women than in men, and can vary among individuals as a result of genetic factors.[4,5] $\dot{V}O_2$max is diminished by degree of cardiovascular impairment and by physical inactivity. In untrained persons, the arterial-mixed venous oxygen difference at peak exercise is relatively constant (14 to 17 volume-percent), and $\dot{V}O_2$max is an approximation of maximum cardiac output. Measured $\dot{V}O_2$max can be compared with predicted values from empirically derived formulas based on age, sex, weight, and height.[3-5] Most clinical studies that use exercise as a stress to assess cardiac reserve report peak $\dot{V}O_2$ that is the highest $\dot{V}O_2$ attained during graded exercise testing rather than $\dot{V}O_2$max. Peak exercise capacity is decreased when the ratio of measured to predicted $\dot{V}O_2$max is less than 85 to 90 percent. Oximetry, performed noninvasively, can be used to monitor arterial oxygen saturation, and the value normally does not decrease by more than 5 percent during exercise.[6] Estimates of oxygen saturation during strenuous exercise using pulse oximetry can be unreliable in some patients.

ANAEROBIC THRESHOLD. Anaerobic threshold is a theoretical point during dynamic exercise when muscle tissue switches over to anaerobic metabolism as an additional energy source. All tissues do not shift simultaneously, and there is a brief interval during which exercise muscle tissue shifts from predominantly aerobic to anaerobic metabolism.[4,5] Lactic acid begins to accumulate when a healthy untrained subject reaches about 50 to 60 percent of the maximal capacity for aerobic metabolism. The increase in lactic acid becomes greater as exercise becomes more intense, resulting in metabolic acidosis. As lactate is formed, it is buffered in the serum by the bicarbonate system, resulting in increased carbon dioxide excretion, which causes reflex hyperventilation. The gas exchange anaerobic threshold is the point at which $\dot{V}e$ increases disproportionately relative to $\dot{V}O_2$ and work; it usually occurs at 40 to 60 percent of $\dot{V}O_2$max in normal, untrained individuals with a wide range of normal values between 35 and 80 percent. Below the anaerobic threshold, carbon dioxide production is proportional to oxygen consumption. Above the anaerobic threshold, carbon dioxide is produced in excess of oxygen consumption. There are several methods to determine anaerobic threshold, which include (1) the V-slope method, the point at which the rate of increase in $\dot{V}CO_2$ relative to $\dot{V}O_2$ increases (see Fig. 10–1); (2) the point at which the $\dot{V}O_2$ and $\dot{V}CO_2$ slopes intersect; and (3) the point at which the ratio of $\dot{V}e/\dot{V}O_2$ and end-tidal oxygen tension begins to increase systematically without an immediate increase in the $\dot{V}e/\dot{V}O_2$ (see Fig. 10–1). The anaerobic threshold is a useful parameter because work below this level encompasses most activities of daily living. Anaerobic threshold is often reduced in patients with significant cardiovascular disease. An increase in anaerobic threshold with training can enhance an individual's capacity to perform sustained submaximal activities, with consequent improvement in quality of life and daily living. Changes in anaerobic

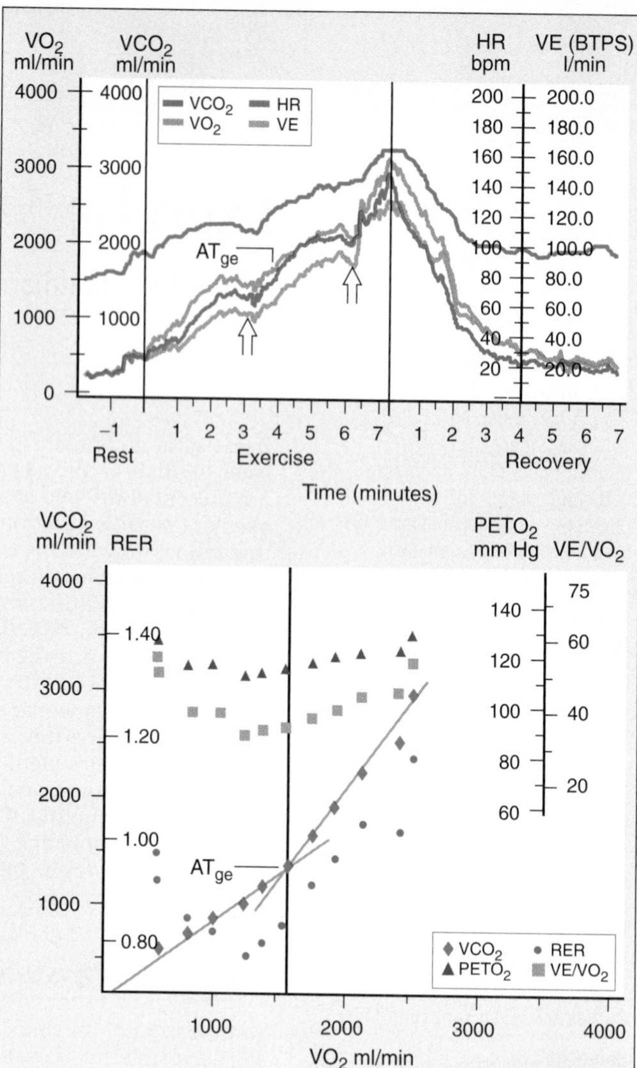

FIGURE 10–1 Cardiopulmonary exercise test in a healthy 53-year-old man using the Bruce protocol. The progressive linear increase in work output, heart rate (HR), and oxygen consumption ($\dot{V}O_2$) is noted, with steady-state conditions reached after 2 minutes in each of the first two stages **(top)**. Open arrows indicate the beginning of each new 3-minute stage. The subject completed 7 minutes and 10 seconds of exercise, and peak $\dot{V}O_2$ was 3.08 liters/min. The anaerobic threshold (AT_{ge}), determined by the V-slope method, is the point at which the slope of the relative rate of increase in $\dot{V}CO_2$ relative to $\dot{V}O_2$ changes; it occurred at a $\dot{V}O_2$ of 1.5 liters/min, or 49 percent of peak $\dot{V}O_2$, within predicted values for a normal sedentary population **(bottom)**. The AT_{ge} determined by the point at which the $\dot{V}O_2$ and $\dot{V}CO_2$ slopes intersect (1.8 liters/min) **(top)** is slightly greater than the AT_{ge} determined by the V-slope method **(bottom)**. The V-slope method usually provides a more reproducible estimate of AT_{ge}. $PETO_2$ = end-tidal pressure of oxygen; RER = respiratory exchange ratio; $\dot{V}e/\dot{V}O_2$ = ratio of ventilation to oxygen uptake.

threshold and peak $\dot{V}O_2$ with repeat testing can be used to assess disease progression, response to medical therapy, and improvement in cardiovascular fitness with training.

VENTILATORY PARAMETERS. In addition to peak $\dot{V}O_2$, minute ventilation and its relation to $\dot{V}CO_2$ and oxygen consumption are useful indices of cardiac and pulmonary function.[4,5,16,17] The respiratory exchange ratio represents the amount of carbon dioxide produced divided by the amount of oxygen consumed. The respiratory exchange ratio ranges from 0.7 to 0.85 at rest and is partly dependent on the predominant fuel used for cellular metabolism (e.g., the respiratory exchange rate for predominant carbohydrate use is 1.0, whereas the respiratory exchange ratio for predominant fatty acid use is 0.7). At high exercise levels, carbon dioxide production exceeds $\dot{V}O_2$, and a respiratory exchange ratio greater than 1.1 often indicates that the subject has performed at maximal effort.

METABOLIC EQUIVALENT. In current use, the term *metabolic equivalent* (MET) refers to a unit of oxygen uptake in a sitting, resting person; 1 MET is equivalent to 3.5 ml O_2/kg/min of body weight. Measured $\dot{V}O_2$ in ml O_2/min/kg divided by 3.5 ml O_2/kg/min determines the number of METs associated with activity. Work activities can be calculated in multiples of METs; this measurement is useful to determine exercise prescriptions, assess disability, and standardize the reporting of submaximal and peak exercise workloads when different protocols are used. An exercise workload of 3 to 5 METs is consistent with activities such as raking leaves, light carpentry, golf, and walking at 3 to 4 mph. Workloads of 5 to 7 METs are consistent with exterior carpentry, singles tennis, and light backpacking. Workloads in excess of 9 METs are compatible with heavy labor, handball, squash, and running at 6 to 7 mph. Estimating $\dot{V}O_2$ from work rate or treadmill time in individual patients may lead to misinterpretation of data if exercise equipment is not correctly calibrated, when the patient holds on to the front handrails, or if the patient fails to achieve steady state, is obese, or has peripheral vascular disease, pulmonary vascular disease, or cardiac impairment. $\dot{V}O_2$ does not increase linearly in some patients with cardiovascular or pulmonary disease as work rate is increased, and $\dot{V}O_2$ can thus be overestimated. The measurements obtained with cardiopulmonary exercise testing are useful in understanding an individual patient's response to exercise and can be useful in the diagnostic evaluation of a patient with dyspnea.[3-5,8]

Exercise Protocols

The main types of exercise are isotonic or dynamic exercise, isometric or static exercise, and resistive (combined isometric and isotonic) exercise. Dynamic protocols most frequently are used to assess cardiovascular reserve, and those suitable for clinical testing should include a low-intensity warm-up phase. In general, 6 to 12 minutes of continuous progressive exercise during which the myocardial oxygen demand is elevated to the patient's maximal level is optimal for diagnostic and prognostic purposes.[8] The protocol should include a suitable recovery or cool-down period. If the protocol is too strenuous for an individual patient, the test must be terminated early, and there is no opportunity to observe clinically important responses. If the exercise protocol is too easy for an individual patient, the prolonged procedure tests endurance and not aerobic capacity. Thus, exercise protocols should be individualized to accommodate a patient's limitations. Protocols may be set up at a fixed duration of exercise for a certain intensity to meet minimal qualifications for certain industrial tasks or sports programs.

STATIC EXERCISE. This form of isometric exercise generates force with little muscle shortening and produces a greater blood pressure response than dynamic exercise.11 Cardiac output does not increase as much as with dynamic exercise, because increased resistance in active muscle groups limits blood flow. In a common form of static exercise, the patient's maximal force on a hand dynamometer is recorded. The patient then sustains 25 to 33 percent of maximal force for 3 to 5 minutes while ECG and blood pressure are recorded. The increase in myocardial $\dot{V}O_2$ is often insufficient to initiate an ischemic response.

ARM ERGOMETRY. Arm crank ergometry protocols involve arm cranking at incremental workloads of 10 to 20 W for 2- or 3-minute stages. The heart rate and blood pressure responses to a given workload of arm exercise usually are greater than those for leg exercise. A bicycle ergometer with the axle placed at the level of the shoulders is used, and the subject sits or stands and cycles the peddles so that the arms are alternately fully extended. The most common frequency is 50 rpm. In normal individuals, maximal $\dot{V}O_2$ and $\dot{V}e$ for arm cycling approximates 50 to 70 percent of the same measures as leg cycling. Peak $\dot{V}O_2$ and peak heart rate are approximately 70 percent of the measures during leg testing. Arm ergometry exercise protocols for risk stratification of patients with suspected or documented CAD before noncardiac surgery can be used as a stressor when leg exercise is not possible or insufficient to test cardiac reserve.

BICYCLE ERGOMETRY. Bicycle protocols involve incremental workloads calibrated in watts or kilopond-meters per minute (kpm). One watt is equivalent to approximately 6 kpm. Because exercise on a cycle ergometer is not weight bearing, kpm or watts can be converted to oxygen uptake in milliliters per minute. In mechanically braked bicycles, work is determined by force and distance and requires a constant pedaling rate of 60 to 80 rpm, according to the patient's preference. Electronically braked bicycles provide a constant workload despite changes in pedaling rate and are less dependent on a patient's cooperation. They are more costly than a mechanically braked bicycle but are preferred for diagnostic and prognostic assessment. Most protocols start with a power output of 10 or 25 W/min (150 kpm), usually followed by increases of 25 W every 2 or 3 minutes until endpoints are reached. Younger subjects can start at 50 W, with increases in 50-W increments every 2 minutes. A ramp protocol differs from the staged protocols in that the patient starts at 3 minutes of unloaded pedaling at a cycle speed of 60 rpm. Work rate is increased by a uniform amount each minute, ranging from 5- to 30-W increments, depending on a patient's expected performance. Exercise is terminated if the patient is unable to maintain a cycling frequency above 40 rpm. In the cardiac catheterization laboratory, hemodynamic measurements can be made during supine bicycle ergometry at rest and at one or two submaximal workloads.

The bicycle ergometer is associated with a lower maximal $\dot{V}O_2$ and anaerobic threshold than the treadmill; maximal heart rate, maximal $\dot{V}e$, and maximal lactate values are often similar. The bicycle ergometer has the advantage of requiring less space than a treadmill; it is quieter and permits sensitive precordial measurements without much motion artifact. However, in North America, treadmill protocols are more widely used in the assessment of patients with coronary disease.

TREADMILL PROTOCOL. The treadmill protocol should be consistent with the patient's physical capacity and the purpose of the test. In healthy individuals, the standard Bruce protocol is popular, and a large diagnostic and prognostic data base has been published using this protocol.[1,2,7,8] The Bruce multistage maximal treadmill protocol has 3-minute periods to allow achievement of a steady state before workload is increased (Figs. 10–1 and 10–2). In older individuals or those whose exercise capacity is limited by cardiac disease, the protocol can be modified by two 3-minute warm-up stages at 1.7 mph and 0 percent grade and 1.7 mph and 5

Functional Class	Clinical Status	O_2 Cost ml/kg/min	METs
Normal and I	Healthy dependent on age, activity	56.0	16
		52.5	15
		49.0	14
		45.5	13
		42.0	12
		38.5	11
	Sedentary healthy	35.0	10
		31.5	9
	Limited	28.0	8
		24.5	7
II	Symptomatic	21.0	6
		17.5	5
III		14.0	4
		10.5	3
		7.0	2
IV		3.5	1

Bicycle Ergometer (1 watt = 6 kpds; for 70 kg body weight)

KPDS
1500
1350
1200
1050
900
750
600
450
300
150

Treadmill Protocols

Bruce (3-min stages) MPH	Bruce %GR	Cornell (2-min stages) MPH	Cornell %GR
5.5	20		
5.0	18	5.0	18
		4.6	17
4.2	16	4.2	16
		3.8	15
3.4	14	3.4	14
		3.0	13
2.5	12	2.5	12
		2.1	11
1.7	10	1.7	10
1.7	5	1.7	
1.7	0	1.7	0

Balke-Ware: % grad at 3.3 mph, 1-min stages: 26, 25, 24, 23, 22, 21, 20, 19, 18, 17, 16, 15, 14, 13, 12, 11, 10, 9, 8, 7, 6, 5, 4, 3, 2, 1

ACIP / mACIP (2-min stages; first 2 stages 1 min)

ACIP MPH	ACIP %GR	mACIP MPH	mACIP %GR
3.4	24	3.4	24
3.1	24	3.1	24
3	21	2.7	24
3	17.5	2.3	24
3	14	2	24
3	10.5	2	18.5
3.0	7.0	2	13.5
3.0	3.0	2	7
2.5	2.0	2	3.5
2.0	0	2	0

Naughton (2-min stages)

%GR 2 MPH	%GR 3 MPH	%GR 3.4 MPH
	32.5	
	30	24
	27.5	22
	25	20
	22.5	18
	20	16
	17.5	14
	15	12
	12.5	10
17.5	10	8
14	7.5	6
10.5	5	4
7	2.5	2
3.5	0	
0		

Weber (2-min stages)

MPH	%GR
3.4	14.0
3.0	15.0
3.0	12.5
3.0	10.0
3.0	7.5
2.0	10.5
2.0	7.0
2.0	3.5
1.5	
1.0	0

FIGURE 10–2 Estimated oxygen cost of bicycle ergometer and selected treadmill protocols. The standard Bruce protocol starts at 1.7 mph and 10 percent grade (5 METs), with a larger increment between stages than protocols such as the Naughton, ACIP, and Weber, which start at less than 2 METs at 2 mph and increase by 1- to 1.5-MET increments between stages. The Bruce protocol can be modified by two 3-minute warm-up stages at 1.7 mph and 0 percent grade and 1.7 mph and 5 percent grade. METs = metabolic equivalents. (Adapted from Fletcher GF, Balady G, Amsterdam EA, et al: Exercise Standards for Testing and Training. A statement for healthcare professionals from the American Heart Association. Circulation 104:1694, 2001. Copyright 2001 American Heart Association.)

percent grade. A limitation of the Bruce protocol is the relatively large increase in $\dot{V}O_2$ between stages and the additional energy cost of running as compared with walking at stages in excess of Bruce's stage III. The Naughton and Weber protocols use 1- to 2-minute stages with 1-MET increments between stages; these protocols may be more suitable for patients with limited exercise tolerance, such as patients with compensated congestive heart failure. The Asymptomatic Cardiac Ischemia Pilot (ACIP) trial and modified ACIP (mACIP) protocols use 2-minute stages with 1.5-MET increments between stages after two 1-minute warm-up stages with 1-MET increments. The ACIP protocols were developed to test patients with established CAD and result in a linear increase in heart rate and $\dot{V}O_2$, distributing the time to occurrence of ST segment depression over a wider range of heart rate and exercise time than protocols with more abrupt increments in workload between stages.[2] The mACIP protocol produces a similar aerobic demand as the standard ACIP protocol for each minute of exercise and is well suited for short or elderly individuals who cannot keep up with a walking speed of 3 mph (see Fig. 10–2).

Ramp protocols start the patient at relatively slow treadmill speed, which is gradually increased until the patient has a good stride. The ramp angle of incline is progressively increased at fixed intervals (e.g., 10 to 60 seconds), starting at zero grade with the increase in grade calculated on the basis of the patient's estimated functional capacity such that the protocol will be complete at 6 to 12 minutes.[8] In this type of protocol, the rate of work increase is continuous and steady-state conditions are not reached. A limitation of ramp protocols is the need to estimate functional capacity from an activity scale; underestimation or overestimation of functional capacity occasionally results in an endurance test or premature cessation. One formula for estimating $\dot{V}O_2$ from treadmill speed and grade is as follows:

$$\dot{V}O_2\ (\text{ml } O_2/\text{kg/min}) = (\text{mph} \times 2.68) + (1.8 \times 26.82 \times \text{mph} \times \text{grade} \div 100) + 3.5$$

The peak $\dot{V}O_2$ is usually the same regardless of treadmill protocol used; the difference is the rate of time at which the peak $\dot{V}O_2$ is achieved.

It is important to encourage patients not to grasp the handrails of the treadmill during exercise, particularly the front handrails. Functional capacity can be overestimated by as much as 20 percent in tests in which handrail support is permitted, and $\dot{V}O_2$ is decreased. Because the degree of handrail support is difficult to quantify from one test to another, more consistent results can be obtained during serial testing when handrail support is not permitted.

The 6-Minute Walk Test. The 6-minute walk test can be used for patients who have marked left ventricular dysfunction or peripheral arterial occlusive disease and who cannot perform bicycle or treadmill exercise. Patients are instructed to walk down a 100-foot corridor at their own pace, attempting to cover as much ground as possible in 6 minutes. At the end of the 6-minute interval, the total distance walked is determined and the symptoms experienced by the patient are recorded. The 6-minute walk test as a clinical measure of ambulatory function requires highly skilled personnel following a rigid protocol to elicit reproducible and reliable results. The coefficient of variation for distance walked during two 6-minute walk tests was 10 percent in one series of patients with peripheral arterial occlusive disease.[18]

TECHNIQUES. Patients should be instructed not to eat, drink caffeinated beverages, or smoke for 3 hours before testing and to wear comfortable shoes and loose-fitting clothes. Unusual physical exertion should be avoided before testing. A brief history and physical examination should be performed, and patients should be advised about the risks and benefits of the procedure. A written informed consent form is usually required. The indication for the test should be known. The supervising physician should be made aware of any recent deterioration in the patient's clinical status. The test should not be performed in subjects who are markedly hypertensive (e.g., >220/120 mm Hg) or who have unexplained hypotension (e.g., systolic blood pressure <80 mm Hg) or other contraindications to exercise testing (see section on safety and risks of exercise testing). In many laboratories, the presence or absence of atherosclerotic risk factors is noted and cardioactive medication recorded. A 12-lead ECG should be obtained with the electrodes at the distal extremities. The timing of cardioactive medication ingestion before testing depends on the test indication.

After the standard 12-lead ECG is recorded, torso ECGs should be obtained with the patient in the supine position and in the sitting or standing position. Postural changes can elicit labile ST-T wave abnormalities. Hyperventilation is not recommended before exercise. If a false-positive test result is suspected, hyperventilation should be performed after the test, and the hyperventilation tracing compared with the maximal ST segment abnormalities observed. The ECG and blood pressure should be recorded in both positions, and patients should be instructed on how to perform the test.

Adequate skin preparation is essential for high-quality recordings, and the superficial layer of skin needs to be removed to augment signal-to-noise ratio. The areas of electrode application are rubbed with an alcohol-saturated pad to remove oil and rubbed with free sandpaper or a rough material to reduce skin resistance to 5000 ohms or less. Silver chloride electrodes with a fluid column to avoid direct metal-to-skin contact produce high-quality tracings; these electrodes have the lowest offset voltage. The electrode fluid column can dry out over time and should be verified prior to application. This can be a cause of poor-quality tracings.

Cables connecting the electrodes and recorders should be light, flexible, and properly shielded. In a small minority of patients, a fishnet jersey may be required over the electrodes and cables to reduce motion artifact. The electrode-skin interface can be verified by tapping on the electrode and examining the monitor or by measuring skin impedance. Excessive noise indicates that the electrode needs to be replaced; replacement before the test rather than during exercise can save time. The ECG signal can be digitized systematically at the patient's end of the cable by some systems, reducing power line artifact. Cables, adapters, and the junction box have a finite life span and require periodic replacement to obtain the highest quality tracings. Exercise equipment should be calibrated regularly. Room temperature should be between 64° and 72°F (18° and 22°C) and humidity less than 60 percent.

Treadmill walking should be demonstrated to the patient. The heart rate, blood pressure, and ECG should be recorded at the end of each stage of exercise, immediately before and immediately after stopping exercise, at the onset of an ischemic response, and for each minute for at least 5 to 10 minutes in the recovery phase. A minimum of three leads should be displayed continuously on the monitor during the test. There is some controversy about optimal patient position in the recovery phase. In the sitting position, less space is required for a stretcher, and patients are more comfortable immediately after exertion. The supine position increases end-diastolic volume and has the potential to augment ST segment changes.[19]

Electrocardiographic Measurements

LEAD SYSTEMS. The Mason-Likar modification of the standard 12-lead ECG requires that the extremity electrodes be moved to the torso to reduce motion artifact. The arm electrodes should be located in the most lateral aspects of the infraclavicular fossae, and the leg electrodes should be in a stable position above the anterior iliac crest and below the rib cage. The Mason-Likar modification results in a right-axis shift and increased voltage in the inferior leads and may produce a loss of inferior Q waves and the development of new Q waves in lead aV_L. Thus, the body torso limb lead positions cannot be used to interpret a diagnostic resting 12-lead ECG. The more cephalad the leg electrodes are placed, the greater is the degree of change and the greater is the augmentation of R wave amplitude.

Bipolar lead groups place the negative, or reference, electrode over the manubrium (CM_5), right scapula (CB_5), RV_5 (CC_5), or on the forehead (CH_5), and the active electrode at V_5 or a proximate location to optimize R wave amplitude. In bipolar lead ML, which reflects inferior wall changes, the negative reference is at the manubrium and the active electrode in the left leg position. Bipolar lead groups may provide additional diagnostic information, and in some medical centers, lead CM_5 is substituted for lead aV in the Mason-Likar–modified lead system. Bipolar leads are frequently used when only a limited ECG set is required (e.g., in cardiac rehabilitation programs). The value of adding right precordial leads to improve test sensitivity is controversial.[20,21] The use of more elaborate lead set systems is usually reserved for research purposes.

Types of ST Segment Displacement

In normal persons, the PR, QRS, and QT intervals shorten as heart rate increases. P amplitude increases, and the PR segment becomes progressively more downsloping in the inferior leads. J point, or junctional, depression is a normal finding during exercise (Fig. 10–3). In patients with myocardial ischemia, however, the ST segment usually becomes more horizontal (flattens) as the severity of the ischemic response worsens. With progressive exercise, the depth of ST segment depression may increase, involving more ECG leads, and the patient may develop angina. In the immediate postrecovery phase, the ST segment displacement may persist, with downsloping ST segments and T wave inversion, gradually returning to baseline after 5 to 10 minutes (Figs. 10–4 and 10–5). Ischemic ST segment displacement may be seen only during exercise, emphasizing the importance of adequate skin preparation and electrode placement to capture high-quality recordings during maximum exertion (Fig. 10–6). In about 10 percent of patients, the ischemic response may appear only in the recovery phase. This is a relevant finding, and the prevalence of reversible perfusion defects by single-photon emission computed tomography criteria are comparable to those observed when the ischemic ST segment response occurs both during and after exercise.[22-24] Patients should not leave the exercise laboratory area until the postexercise ECG has returned to baseline. Figure 10–7 illustrates eight different ECG patterns seen during exercise testing.

Measurement of ST Segment Displacement

For purposes of interpretation, the PQ junction is usually chosen as the isoelectric point. The TP segment represents a true isoelectric point but is an impractical choice for most routine clinical measurements. The development of 0.10 mV (1 mm) or greater of J point depression measured from the PQ junction, with a relatively flat ST segment slope (e.g., <0.7 to

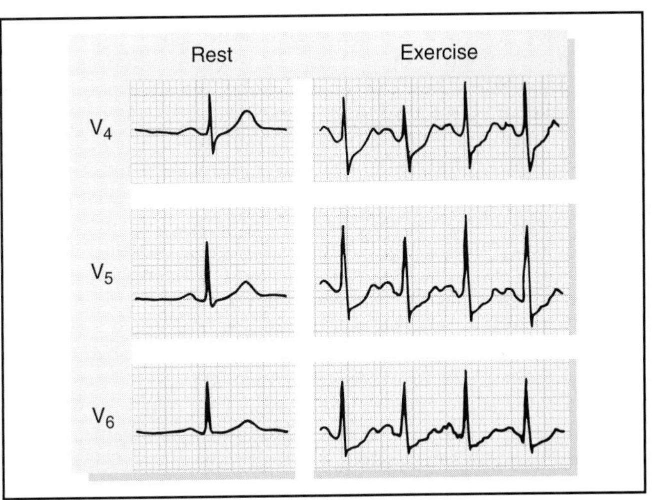

FIGURE 10–3 J point depression of 2 to 3 mm in leads V_4 to V_6 with rapid upsloping ST segments depressed approximately 1 mm 80 msec after the J point. The ST segment slope in leads V_4 and V_5 is 3.0 mV/sec. This response should not be considered abnormal.

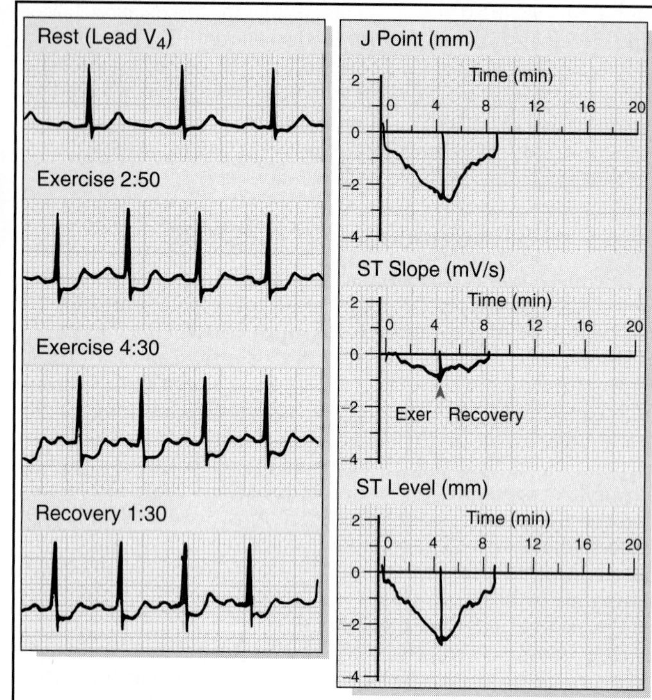

FIGURE 10–4 Bruce protocol. In lead V_4, the exercise electrocardiographic (ECG) result is abnormal early in the test, reaching 0.3 mV (3 mm) of horizontal ST segment depression at the end of exercise. The ischemic changes persist for at least 1 minute and 30 seconds into the recovery phase. The **right** panel provides a continuous plot of the J point, ST slope, and ST segment displacement at 80 msec after the J point (ST level) during exercise and in the recovery phase. Exercise ends at the vertical line at 4.5 minutes (red arrow). The computer trends permit a more precise identification of initial onset and offset of ischemic ST segment depression. This type of ECG pattern, with early onset of ischemic ST segment depression, reaching more than 3 mm of horizontal ST segment displacement and persisting several minutes into the recovery phase, is consistent with a severe ischemic response.

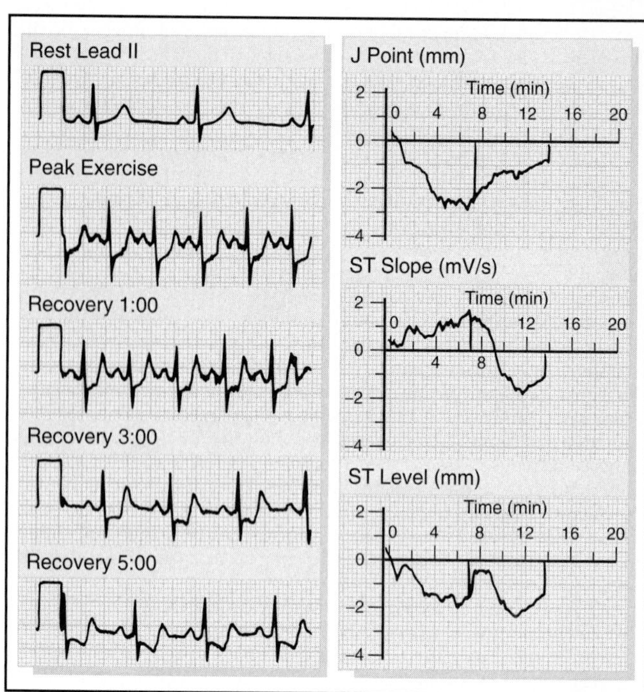

FIGURE 10–5 Bruce protocol. In this type of ischemic pattern, the J point at peak exertion is depressed 2.5 mm, the ST segment slope is 1.5 mV/sec, and the ST segment level at 80 msec after the J point is depressed 1.6 mm. This "slow upsloping" ST segment at peak exercise indicates an ischemic pattern in patients with a high pretest prevalence of coronary disease. A typical ischemic pattern is seen at 3 minutes of the recovery phase when the ST segment is horizontal and 5 minutes after exertion when the ST segment is downsloping. Exercise is discontinued at the vertical line in the **right** panels at 7.5 minutes.

1 mV/sec), depressed 0.10 mV or more 80 msec after the J point (ST 80) in three consecutive beats with a stable baseline is considered to be an abnormal response (Fig. 10–8). When the ST 80 measurement is difficult to determine at rapid heart rates (e.g., >130 beats/min), the ST 60 measurement should be used. The ST segment at rest may occasionally be depressed. When this occurs, the J point and ST 60 or ST 80 measurements should be depressed an additional 0.10 mV or greater to be considered abnormal.

When the degree of resting ST segment depression is 0.1 mV or greater, the exercise ECG becomes less specific, and myocardial imaging modalities should be considered.[1,2,8,25] In patients with early repolarization and resting ST segment elevation, return to the PQ junction is normal. Therefore, the magnitude of exercise-induced ST segment depression in a patient with early repolarization should be determined from the PQ junction and not from the elevated position of the J point before exercise. Exercise-induced ST segment depression does not localize the site of myocardial ischemia, nor does it provide a clue about which coronary artery is involved. For example, it is not unusual for patients with isolated right CAD to exhibit exercise-induced ST segment depression only in leads V_4 to V_6, nor is it unusual for patients with disease of the left anterior descending coronary artery to exhibit exercise-induced ST segment displacements in leads II, III, and aV_f. Exercise-induced ST segment elevation is relatively specific for the territory of myocardial ischemia and the coronary artery involved.

UPSLOPING ST SEGMENTS. Junctional or J point depression is a normal finding during maximal exercise, and

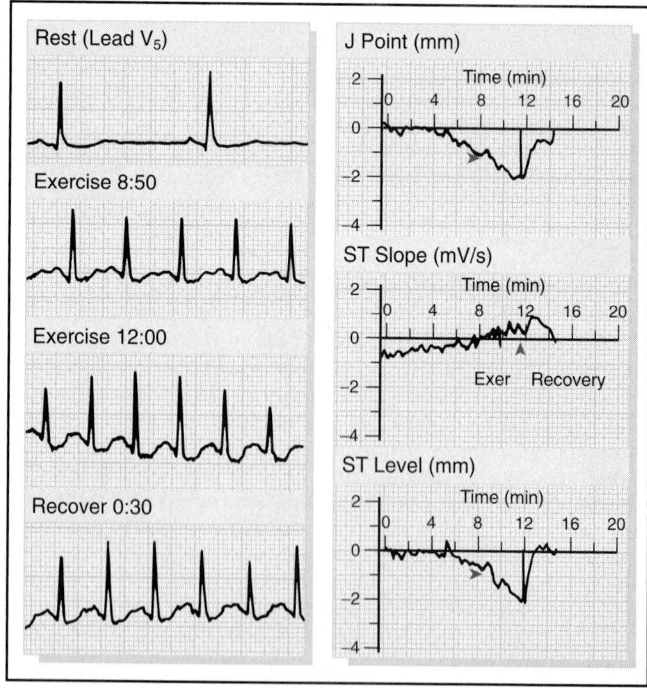

FIGURE 10–6 Bruce protocol. The exercise electrocardiographic (ECG) result is not yet abnormal at 8:50 minutes but becomes abnormal at 9:30 minutes (horizontal arrows, **right**) of a 12-minute exercise test and resolves in the immediate recovery phase. This ECG pattern in which the ST segment becomes abnormal only at high exercise workloads and returns to baseline in the immediate recovery phase may indicate a false-positive result in an asymptomatic individual without atherosclerotic risk factors. Exercise myocardial imaging would provide more diagnostic and prognostic information if this were an older person with several atherosclerotic risk factors. Vertical arrow indicates termination of exercise.

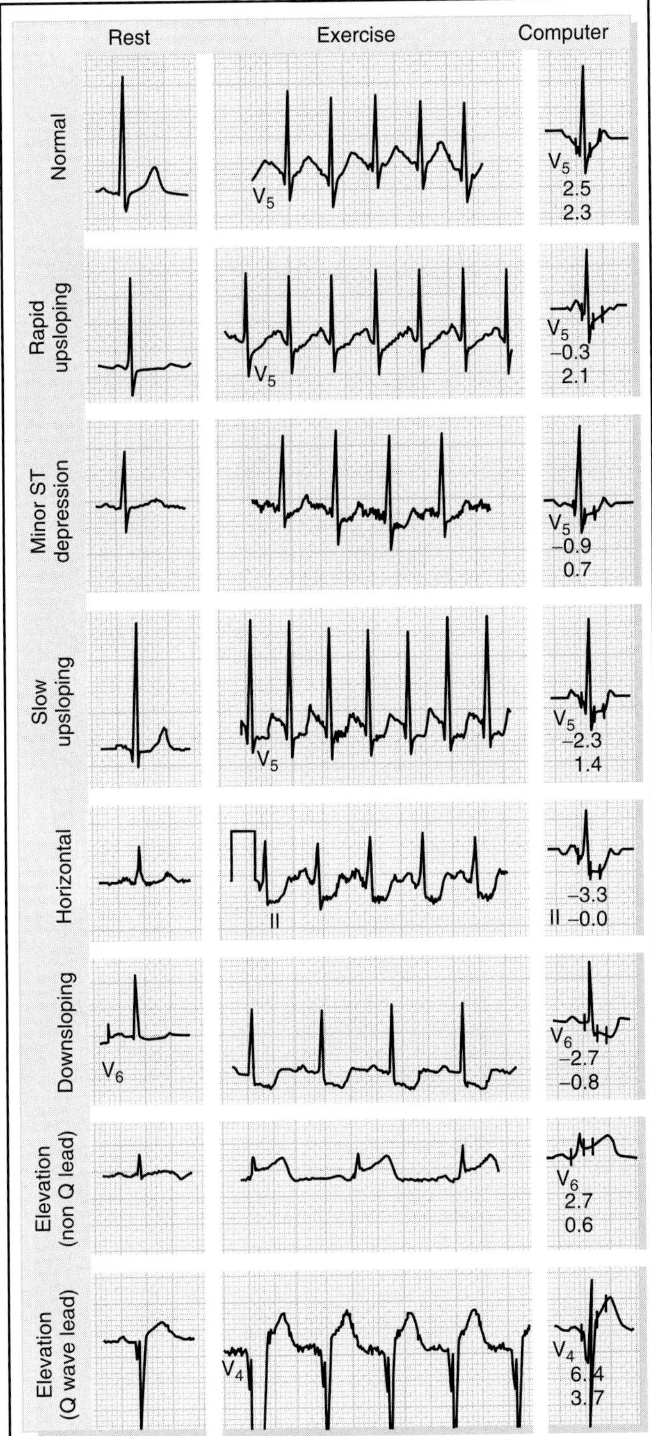

FIGURE 10–7 Illustration of eight typical exercise electrocardiographic (ECG) patterns at rest and at peak exertion. The computer-processed incrementally averaged beat corresponds with the raw data taken at the same time point during exercise and is illustrated in the last column. The patterns represent worsening ECG responses during exercise. In the column of computer-averaged beats, ST 80 displacement (top number) indicates the magnitude of ST segment displacement 80 msec after the J point relative to the PQ junction or E point. ST segment slope measurement (bottom number) indicates the ST segment slope at a fixed time point after the J point to the ST 80 measurement. At least three noncomputer average complexes with a stable baseline should meet criteria for abnormality before the exercise ECG result can be considered abnormal (see Fig. 10–9). The normal and rapid upsloping ST segment responses are normal responses to exercise. J point depression with rapid upsloping ST segments is a common response in an older, apparently healthy population. Minor ST depression can occur occasionally at submaximal workloads in patients with coronary disease; in this illustration, the ST segment is depressed 0.09 mV (0.9 mm) 80 msec after the J point. The slow upsloping ST segment pattern often demonstrates an ischemic response in patients with known coronary disease or those with a high pretest clinical risk of coronary disease. Criteria for slow upsloping ST segment depression include J point and ST 80 depression of 0.15 mV or more and ST segment slope of more than 1.0 mV/sec. Classic criteria for myocardial ischemia include horizontal ST segment depression observed when both the J point and ST 80 depression are 0.1 mV or more and ST segment slope is within the range of 1.0 mV/sec. Downsloping ST segment depression occurs when the J point and ST 80 depression are 0.1 mV and ST segment slope is −1.0 mV/sec. ST segment elevation in a non-Q wave noninfarct lead occurs when the J point and ST 60 are 1.0 mV or greater and represents a severe ischemic response. ST segment elevation in an infarct territory (Q wave lead) indicates a severe wall motion abnormality and in most cases is not considered an ischemic response. (From Chaitman BR: Exercise electrocardiographic stress testing. *In* Beller GA [ed]: Chronic Ischemic Heart Disease. *In* Braunwald E [series ed]: Atlas of Heart Diseases. Vol 5. Chronic Ischemic Heart Disease. Philadelphia, Current Medicine, 1995, pp 2.1-2.30.)

a rapid upsloping ST segment (>1 mV/sec) depressed less than 0.15 mV (1.5 mm) after the J point should be considered to be normal (see Fig. 10–3). Occasionally, however, the ST segment is depressed 0.15 mV (1.5 mm) or greater at 80 msec after the J point. This type of slow upsloping ST segment may be the only ECG finding in patients with well-defined obstructive CAD and may depend on the lead set used (see Figs. 10–5 and 10–7). In patient subsets with a high CAD prevalence, a slow upsloping ST segment depressed 0.15 mV or greater at 80 msec after the J point should be considered abnormal. The importance of this finding in asymptomatic individuals or those with a low CAD prevalence is less certain. Increasing the degree of ST segment depression at 80 msec after the J point to 0.20 mV (2.0 mm) or greater in patients with a slow upsloping ST segment increases specificity but decreases sensitivity.[1,2,7,8]

ST SEGMENT ELEVATION. Exercise-induced ST segment elevation may occur in an infarct territory where Q waves are present or in a noninfarct territory. The development of 0.10 mV (1 mm) or greater of J point elevation, persistently elevated greater than 0.10 mV at 60 msec after the J point in three consecutive beats with a stable baseline, is considered an abnormal response (see Fig. 10–7). This finding occurs in approximately 30 percent of patients with anterior myocardial infarctions and 15 percent of those with inferior ones tested early (within 2 weeks) after the index event and decreases in frequency by 6 weeks. As a group, postinfarct patients with exercise-induced ST segment elevation have a lower ejection fraction than those without, a greater severity of resting wall motion abnormalities, and a worse prognosis. Exercise-induced ST segment elevation in leads with abnormal Q waves is not a marker of more extensive CAD and rarely indicates myocardial ischemia. Exercise-induced ST

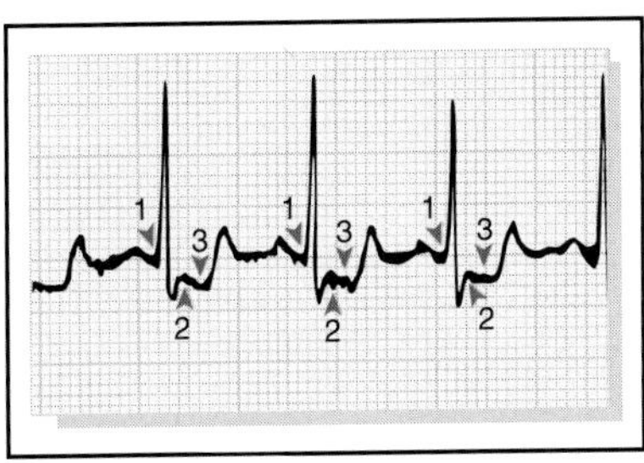

FIGURE 10–8 Magnified ischemic exercise–induced electrocardiographic pattern. Three consecutive complexes with a relatively stable baseline are selected. The PQ junction (1) and J point (2) are determined; the ST 80 (3) is determined at 80 msec after the J point. In this example, average J point displacement is 0.2 mV (2 mm) and ST 80 is 0.24 mV (24 mm). The average slope measurement from the J point to ST 80 is −1.1 mV/sec.

segment elevation may occasionally occur in a patient who has regenerated embryonic R waves after an acute myocardial infarction; the clinical significance of this finding is similar to that observed when Q waves are present.

When ST segment elevation develops during exercise in a non-Q wave lead in a patient without a previous myocardial infarction, the finding should be considered as likely evidence of transmural myocardial ischemia caused by coronary vasospasm or a high-grade coronary narrowing (Fig. 10–9). This finding is relatively uncommon, occurring in approximately 1 percent of patients with obstructive CAD. The ECG site of ST segment elevation is relatively specific for the coronary artery involved, and myocardial perfusion scintigraphy usually reveals a defect in the territory involved.

T WAVE CHANGES. The morphology of the T wave is influenced by body position, respiration, hyperventilation, drug therapy, and myocardial ischemia/necrosis. In patient populations with a low CAD prevalence, pseudonormalization of T waves (inverted at rest and becoming upright with exercise) is a nondiagnostic finding (Fig. 10–10). In rare instances, this finding may be a marker for myocardial ischemia in a patient with documented CAD, although it would need to be substantiated by an ancillary technique, such as the concomitant finding of a reversible myocardial perfusion defect.[26]

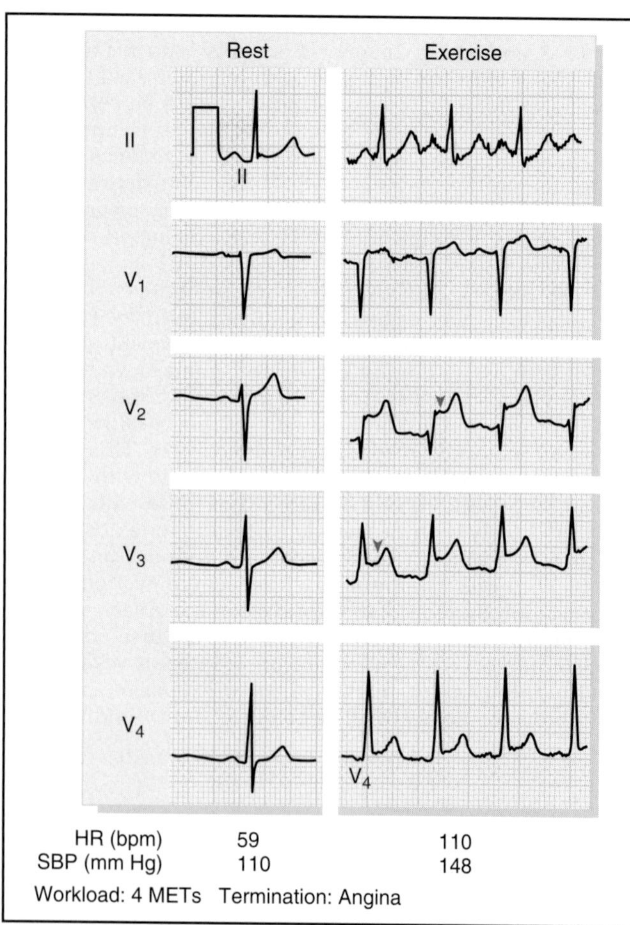

FIGURE 10–9 A 48-year-old man with several atherosclerotic risk factors and a normal resting electrocardiographic (ECG) result developed marked ST segment elevation (4 mm [arrows]) in leads V_2 and V_3 with lesser degrees of ST segment elevation in leads V_1 and V_4 and J point depression with upsloping ST segments in lead II, associated with angina. This type of ECG pattern is usually associated with a full-thickness, reversible myocardial perfusion defect in the corresponding left ventricular myocardial segments and high-grade intraluminal narrowing at coronary angiography. Rarely, coronary vasospasm produces this result in the absence of significant intraluminal atherosclerotic narrowing. HR = heart rate; METs = metabolic equivalents; SBP = systolic blood pressure. (From Chaitman BR: Exercise electrocardiographic stress testing. *In* Beller GA [ed]: Chronic Ischemic Heart Disease. *In* Braunwald E [series ed]: Atlas of Heart Diseases. Vol 5. Chronic Ischemic Heart Disease. Philadelphia, Current Medicine, 1995, pp 2.1-2.30.)

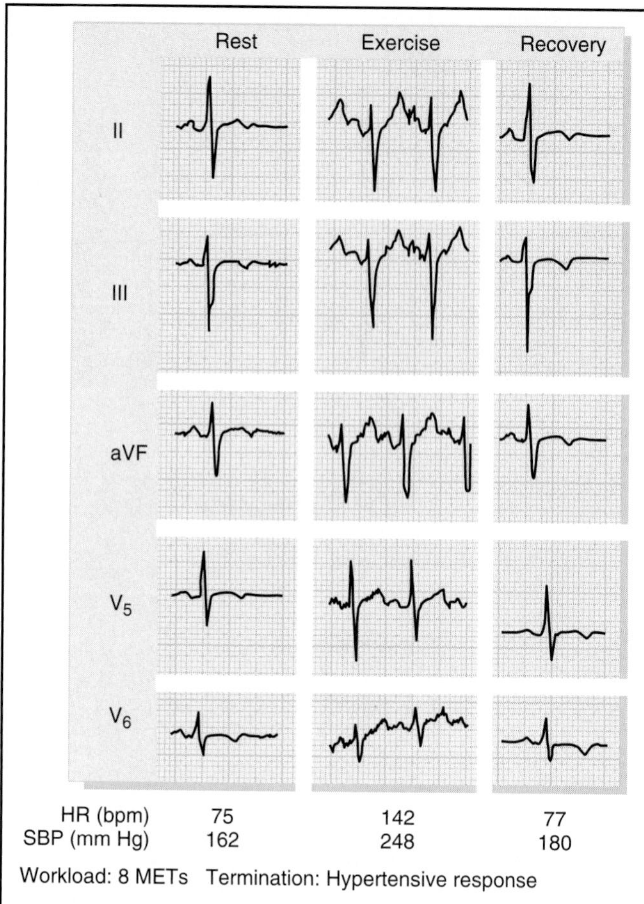

FIGURE 10–10 Pseudonormalization of T waves in a 49-year-old man referred for exercise testing. The patient had previously been seen for typical angina. The resting electrocardiogram in this patient with coronary artery disease shows inferior and anterolateral T wave inversion, an adverse long-term prognosticator. The patient exercised to 8 METs, reaching a peak heart rate of 142 beats/min and a peak systolic blood pressure of 248 mm Hg. At that point, the test was stopped because of hypertension. During exercise, pseudonormalization of T waves occurs, and it returns to baseline (inverted T wave) in the postexercise phase. The patient denied chest discomfort, and no arrhythmia or ST segment displacement was noted. Transient conversion of a negative T wave at rest to a positive T wave during exercise is a nonspecific finding in patients without prior myocardial infarction and does not enhance the diagnostic or prognostic content of the test; however, the ability to exercise to 8 METs without ischemic changes in the ST segment places this patient into a subset of lower risk. HR = heart rate; METs = metabolic equivalents; SBP = systolic blood pressure. (From Chaitman BR: Exercise electrocardiographic stress testing. *In* Beller GA [ed]: Chronic Ischemic Heart Disease. *In* Braunwald E [series ed]: Atlas of Heart Diseases. Vol 5. Chronic Ischemic Heart Disease. Philadelphia, Current Medicine, 1995, pp 2.1-2.30.

OTHER ELECTROCARDIOGRAPHIC MARKERS. Changes in R wave amplitude during exercise are relatively nonspecific and are related to the level of exercise performed. When the R wave amplitude meets voltage criteria for left ventricular hypertrophy, the ST segment response cannot be used reliably to diagnose CAD, even in the absence of a left ventricular strain pattern. Loss of R wave amplitude, commonly seen after myocardial infarction, reduces the sensitivity of the ST segment response in that lead to diagnose obstructive CAD. Adjustment of the extent of ST segment depression by R wave height in individual leads has not been consistently shown to improve the diagnostic value of the exercise ECG for CAD. U wave inversion can occasionally be seen in the precordial leads at heart rates of 120 beats/min. Although this finding is relatively specific for CAD, it is relatively insensitive.[27]

COMPUTER-ASSISTED ANALYSIS

The use of computers has facilitated the routine analysis and measurements required from exercise ECG and can be performed on-line as well as off-line. When the raw ECG data are of high quality, the computer can filter and average or select median complexes from which the degree of J point displacement, ST segment slope, and ST displacement 60 to 80 msec after the J point (ST 60 to 80) can be measured. The selection of ST 60 or ST 80 depends on the heart rate response. At ventricular rates greater than 130 beats/min, the ST 80 measurement may fall on the upslope of the T wave, and the ST 60 measurement should be used instead. In some computerized systems, the PQ junction or isoelectric interval is detected by scanning before the R wave for the 10-msec interval with the least slope. J point, ST slope, and ST levels are determined (see Figs. 10–4, 10–5, and 10–6); the ST integral can be calculated from the area below the isoelectric line from the J point to ST 60 or ST 80. Computerized treatment of ECG complexes permits reduction of motion and myographic artifacts. However, the averaged or median beats may occasionally be erroneous because of ECG signal distortion caused by noise, baseline wander, or changes in conduction, and identification of the PQ junction and ST segment onset can be imperfect. Therefore, it is crucial to ensure that the computer-determined averages or median complexes reflect the raw ECG data, and physicians should program the computer to print out raw data during exercise and inspect the raw data to be certain that the QRS template is accurately reproduced and the placement of the fiducial points are correctly placed at the PQ junction and J point before accepting the automatic measurements.

ST/HEART RATE SLOPE MEASUREMENTS. Heart rate adjustment of ST segment depression appears to improve the sensitivity of the exercise test, particularly the prediction of multivessel CAD.[28] The ST/heart rate slope depends on the type of exercise performed, number and location of monitoring electrodes, method of measuring ST segment depression, and clinical characteristics of the study population. Calculation of maximal ST/heart rate slope in mV/beats/min is performed by linear regression analysis relating the measured amount of ST segment depression in individual leads to the heart rate at the end of each stage of exercise, starting at the end of exercise. An ST/heart rate slope of 2.4 mV/beats/min is considered abnormal, and values that exceed 6 mV/beats/min are suggestive evidence of three-vessel CAD. The use of this measurement requires modification of the exercise protocol such that increments in heart rate are gradual, as in the Cornell protocol, as opposed to more abrupt increases in heart rate between stages, as in the Bruce or Ellestad protocols, which limit the ability to calculate statistically valid ST segment heart rate slopes. The measurement is not accurate in the early postinfarction phase. A modification of the ST segment/heart rate slope method is the ST segment/heart rate index calculation, which represents the average change of ST segment depression with heart rate throughout the course of the exercise test. The ST/heart rate index measurements are less than the ST/heart rate slope measurements, and a ST/heart rate index of 1.6 is defined as abnormal. A slight increase in the prognostic content of ST segment/heart rate slope measurements as compared with standard criteria was demonstrated in the Multiple Risk Factor Interventional Trial.[1,8]

Mechanism of ST Segment Displacement

PATHOPHYSIOLOGY OF THE MYOCARDIAL ISCHEMIC RESPONSE. Myocardial oxygen consumption (MO_2) is determined by heart rate, systolic blood pressure, left ventricular end-diastolic volume, wall thickness, and contractility (see Chap. 44).[1,2,7,8,12] The rate-pressure or double product (heart rate × systolic blood pressure) increases progressively with increasing work and can be used to estimate the myocardial perfusion requirement in normal persons and in many patients with coronary artery disease. The heart is an aerobic organ with little capacity to generate energy through anaerobic metabolism. Oxygen extraction in the coronary circulation is nearly maximal at rest. The only significant mechanism available to the heart to increase oxygen consumption is to increase perfusion, and there is a direct linear relationship between MO_2 and coronary blood flow in normal individuals. The principal mechanism for increasing coronary blood flow during exercise is to decrease resistance at the coronary arteriolar level. In patients with progressive atherosclerotic narrowing of the epicardial vessels, an ischemic threshold occurs, and exercise beyond this threshold can produce abnormalities in diastolic and systolic ventricular function, ECG changes, and chest pain. The subendocardium is more susceptible to myocardial ischemia than the subepicardium because of increased wall tension, causing a relative increase in myocardial oxygen demand in the subendocardium.

Dynamic changes in coronary artery tone at the site of an atherosclerotic plaque may result in diminished coronary flow during static or dynamic exercise instead of the expected increase that normally occurs from coronary vasodilation in a normal vessel; that is, perfusion pressure distal to the stenotic plaque actually falls as during exercise, resulting in reduced subendocardial blood flow (Fig. 10–11).[29,30] Thus, regional left ventricular myocardial ischemia may result not only from an increase in myocardial oxygen demand during exercise but also from a limitation of coronary flow as a result of coronary vasoconstriction, or inability of vessels to sufficiently vasodilate at or near the site of an atherosclerotic plaque.

Some patients with chronic angina have a warm-up phenomenon that can be demonstrated using sequential exercise testing.[31-33] Under these conditions, the time to angina and ischemic ST segment depression can be prolonged and can occur at a higher rate-pressure product on the second of two exercise tests performed within 10 to 30 minutes of each other. Improvement in performance on the second test is related to the magnitude of myocardial ischemia produced on the first test, and, usually, myocardial ischemia of more than moderate intensity is required to produce the warm-up response.

In normal persons, the action potential duration of the endocardial region is longer than that of the epicardial region,

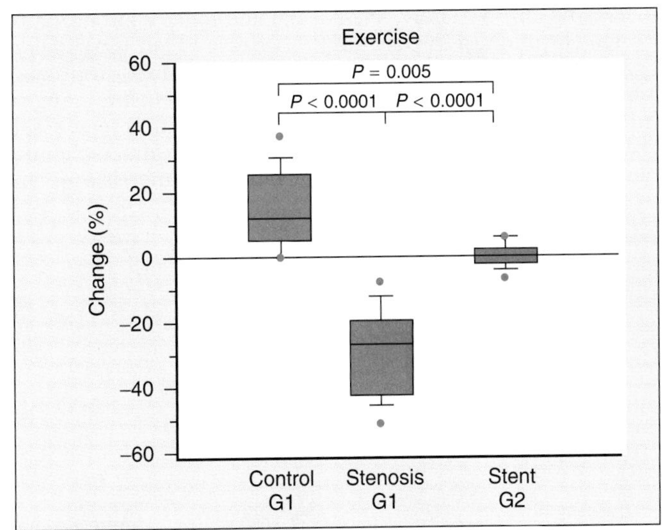

FIGURE 10–11 Box plot of exercise-induced changes of the left coronary artery in a control group of 12 patients with chronic angina and single vessel disease (G1) and results for 14 patients studied 10 months after coronary stenting (G2). In control group G1, the mean percentage diameter stenosis of the stenotic segment was 59 percent; during exercise, the stenotic segment exhibited coronary vasoconstriction (average –29 percent compared with rest) compared with a control segment in the same vessel that showed vasodilation (+15 percent compared with rest). Sublingual nitroglycerin induced maximal vasodilation in the nonstenotic segment (+36 percent) and mild vasodilation (+10 percent) in the stenotic segments (not shown). Exercise does not elicit any vasomotion in stent group G2, and vessel diameter remains unchanged. (From Maier W, Windecker S, Kung A, et al: Exercise-induced coronary artery vasodilation is not impaired by stent placement. Circulation 105:2373, 2002.)

and ventricular repolarization is from epicardium to endocardium. The action potential duration is shortened in the presence of myocardial ischemia, and electrical gradients are created, resulting in ST segment depression or elevation, depending on the surface ECG leads. At the molecular level, activation of sarcolemmal ATP-sensitive potassium (K_{ATP}) channels by ischemic ATP depletion may play a role. Transgenic mice with homozygous knockout of the Kir6-2 channel gene, which encodes the pore-forming subunit of cardiac surface K_{ATP} channels, lack the ability to generate an ST segment elevation response to acute coronary occlusion.[34] Increased myocardial oxygen demand associated with a failure to increase or an actual decrease in regional coronary blood flow usually causes ST segment depression; ST segment elevation may occasionally occur in patients with more severe coronary flow reduction.

Nonelectrocardiographic Observations

The ECG is only one part of the exercise response, and abnormal hemodynamics or functional capacity is just as important as, if not more important than, ST segment displacement.

BLOOD PRESSURE. The normal exercise response is to increase systolic blood pressure progressively with increasing workloads to a peak response ranging from 160 to 200 mm Hg, with the higher range of the scale in older patients with less compliant vascular systems.[1,7,8,35] As a group, black patients tend to have a higher systolic blood pressure response than white patients. At high exercise workloads, it is sometimes difficult to obtain a precise determination of systolic blood pressure by auscultation. In normal persons, the diastolic blood pressure does not usually change significantly. Failure to increase systolic blood pressure beyond 120 mm Hg, a sustained decrease greater than 10 mm Hg repeatable within 15 seconds, or a fall in systolic blood pressure below standing resting values during progressive exercise when the blood pressure has otherwise been increasing appropriately is abnormal and reflects either inadequate elevation of cardiac output because of left ventricular systolic pump dysfunction or an excessive reduction in systemic vascular resistance.[36] Exertional hypotension ranges from 3 to 9 percent and is higher in patients with three-vessel or left main CAD. Conditions other than myocardial ischemia that have been associated with a failure to increase or an actual decrease in systolic blood pressure during progressive exercise are cardiomyopathy, cardiac arrhythmias, vasovagal reactions, left ventricular outflow tract obstruction, ingestion of antihypertensive drugs, hypovolemia, and prolonged vigorous exercise.

It is important to distinguish between a decline in blood pressure in the postexercise phase and a decrease in or failure to increase systolic blood pressure during progressive exercise. The incidence of postexertional hypotension in asymptomatic subjects was 1.9 percent in 781 asymptomatic volunteers in the Baltimore Longitudinal Study on Aging, with a 3.1 percent incidence noted in subjects younger than 55 years and a 0.3 percent incidence in patients older than 55 years.[37] In this series, most hypotensive episodes were symptomatic, and only two patients had hypotension associated with bradycardia and vagal symptoms. Although ST segment abnormalities suggestive of ischemia occurred in one third of the patients with hypotension, none of the patients had a cardiac event during 4 years of follow-up. Rarely, in young patients, vasovagal syncope can occur in the immediate postexercise phase, progressing through sinus bradycardia to several seconds of asystole and hypotension before reverting to sinus rhythm. An abnormal hypertensive blood pressure response in patients with a high prevalence of CAD is associated with more extensive CAD and more extensive myocardial perfusion defects. Occasionally, a marked hypertensive response may cause new exercise-induced wall motion abnormalities in the absence of coronary disease.[38]

MAXIMAL WORK CAPACITY. This variable is one of the most important prognostic measurements obtained from an exercise test (Fig. 10–12).[1,2,7,8,10,39-41] Maximal work capacity in normal individuals is influenced by familiarization with the exercise test equipment, level of training, and environmental conditions at the time of testing. In patients with known or suspected CAD, a limited exercise capacity is associated with an increased risk of cardiac events, and, in general, the more severe the limitation, the worse the CAD extent and prognosis. In estimating functional capacity, the amount of work performed (or exercise stage achieved) expressed in METs, not the number of minutes of exercise, should be the parameter measured. Estimates of peak functional capacity for age and gender have been well established for most of the exercise protocols in common use, subject to the limitations described in the section on cardiopulmonary testing. Comparison of an individual's performance against normal standards provides an estimate of the degree of exercise impairment. There is a rough correlation between observed peak functional capacity during exercise treadmill testing and estimates derived from clinical data and specific activity questionnaires.

Serial comparison of functional capacity in individual patients to assess significant interval change requires a careful examination of the exercise protocol used during both tests, of drug therapy and time of ingestion, of systemic blood pressure, and of other conditions that might influence test performance. All these variables need to be considered before attributing changes in functional capacity to

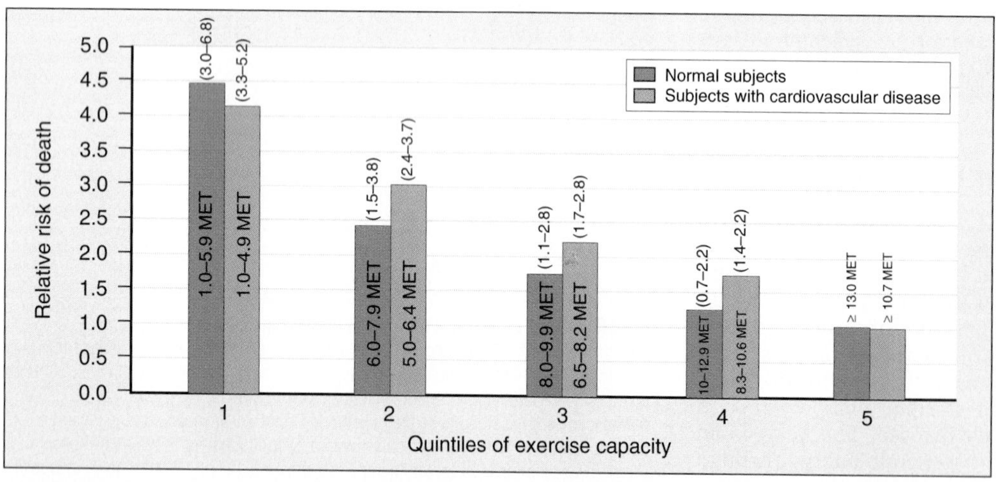

FIGURE 10–12 Age-adjusted relative risks of all-cause mortality by quintile of exercise capacity in 2534 subjects with a normal exercise test result and no history of cardiovascular disease and 3679 subjects with an abnormal exercise test result or history of cardiovascular disease. The mean duration of follow-up was 6.2 ± 3.7 years. Quintile 5 was used as the reference category. For each 1-MET increase in exercise capacity, the survival improved by 12 percent (From Myers J, Prakash M, Froelicher V, et al: Exercise capacity and mortality among men referred for exercise testing. N Engl J Med 346:793, 2002.)

progression of CAD or worsening of left ventricular function. Major reductions in exercise capacity usually indicate significant worsening of cardiovascular status; modest changes may not.[42]

SUBMAXIMAL EXERCISE. The interpretation of exercise test results for diagnostic and prognostic purposes requires consideration of maximal work capacity. When a patient is unable to complete moderate levels of exercise or reach at least 85 to 90 percent of age-predicted maximum, the level of exercise performed may be inadequate to test cardiac reserve. Thus, ischemic ECG, scintigraphic, or ventriculographic abnormalities may not be evoked and the test may be nondiagnostic. Nondiagnostic test results are more common in patients with peripheral vascular disease, orthopedic limitation, or neurological impairment and in patients with poor motivation. Pharmacological stress imaging studies should be considered in this setting.[1,2]

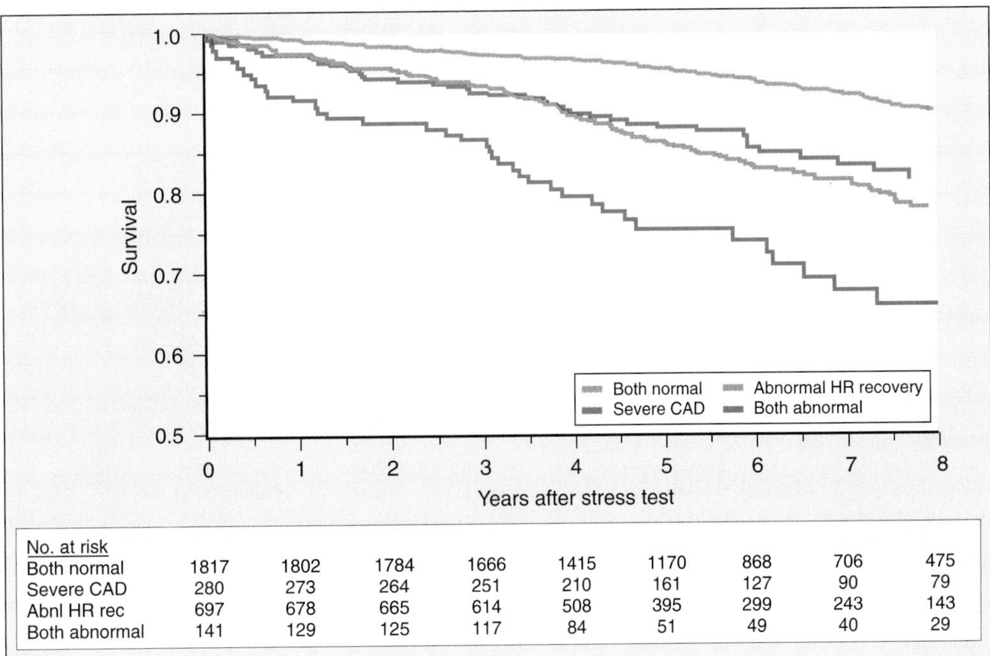

No. at risk									
Both normal	1817	1802	1784	1666	1415	1170	868	706	475
Severe CAD	280	273	264	251	210	161	127	90	79
Abnl HR rec	697	678	665	614	508	395	299	243	143
Both abnormal	141	129	125	117	84	51	49	40	29

FIGURE 10–13 Six-year follow-up in 2935 patients who underwent an exercise test and coronary angiography. After adjustment for age, gender, standard risk factors, medications, exercise capacity, coronary disease extent, and left ventricular function, abnormal heart rate recovery (Abnl HR rec) was an independent predictor of mortality. The survival plot illustrates a mortality gradient with the worst prognosis in patients with abnormal heart rate recovery and severe coronary artery disease (CAD). (From Vivekananthan DP, Blackstone EH, Poithier CE, et al: Heart rate recovery after exercise is a predictor of mortality, independent of the angiographic severity of coronary disease. J Am Coll Cardiol 42:831, 2003.)

HEART RATE RESPONSE. The sinus rate increases progressively with exercise, mediated in part through sympathetic and parasympathetic innervation of the sinoatrial node and circulating catecholamines. In some patients who may be anxious about the exercise test, there may be an initial overreaction of heart rate and systolic blood pressure at the beginning of exercise, with stabilization after approximately 30 to 60 seconds. An inappropriate increase in heart rate at low exercise workloads may occur in patients who are in atrial fibrillation, physically deconditioned, hypovolemic, or anemic or who have marginal left ventricular function; this increase may persist for several minutes in the recovery phase. In some patients, heart rate (HR) fails to increase appropriately with exercise and is associated with an adverse prognosis.[43-45] Chronotropic incompetence is determined by decreased heart rate sensitivity to the normal increase in sympathetic tone during exercise and is defined as inability to increase heart rate to at least 85 percent of age-predicted maximum or as an abnormal heart rate reserve. Heart rate reserve is calculated as follows:

$$\%HRR_{Used} = (HR_{peak} - HR_{rest})/(220 - \text{age} - HR_{rest})$$

The term *chronotropic index* refers to a heart rate increment per stage of exercise that is below normal or a peak heart rate below predicted at maximal workloads. It reflects an inability to use up all of the heart rate reserve. This finding may indicate autonomic dysfunction, sinus node disease, drug therapy such as beta blockers, or a myocardial ischemic response. When the chronotropic index is 80 percent or less, long-term mortality is increased. Chronotropic incompetence should not be used to estimate prognosis in patients on beta blocker therapy. Abnormal heart rate recovery (HRR) refers to a relatively slow deceleration of heart rate following exercise cessation. This type of response reflects decreased vagal tone and is associated with increased mortality.[46,47]

$$HRR = HR_{peak} - HR_{1\ \text{minute later}}$$

When the postexercise phase includes an upright cool down, a value 12 beats/min or less is abnormal. For patients undergoing stress echocardiography or otherwise assuming a supine position immediately after exercise, a value 18 beats/min or less is abnormal. When HRR is measured 2 minutes into recovery, a value 22 beats/min or less is abnormal. The prognostic value of abnormal HRR is independent of the exercise level attained, beta blocker usage, severity of coronary disease, left ventricular function, chronotropic incompetence, Duke treadmill score, and presence of exercise-induced angina or ischemic ECG abnormalities (Fig. 10–13). A submaximal heart rate response in a patient who is poorly motivated to complete the test or has a physical impairment that limits ability to perform sufficient exercise to test heart rate reserve (resulting in a nondiagnostic test, as described earlier) should be distinguished from a patient with chronotropic incompetence and an adequate test for prognostic estimates.

RATE-PRESSURE PRODUCT. The heart rate–systolic blood pressure product, an indirect measure of myocardial oxygen demand, increases progressively with exercise, and the peak rate-pressure product can be used to characterize cardiovascular performance. Most normal individuals develop a peak rate pressure product of 20 to 35 mm Hg × beats/min × 10^{-3}. In many patients with significant ischemic heart disease, rate-pressure products exceeding 25 mm Hg × beats/min × 10^{-3} are unusual. However, the cutpoint of 25 mm Hg × beats/min × 10^{-3} is not a useful diagnostic parameter; significant overlap exists between patients with disease and those without disease. Furthermore, cardioactive drug therapy significantly influences this measurement.

CHEST DISCOMFORT. Characterization of chest discomfort during exercise can be a useful diagnostic finding, particularly when the symptom complex is compatible with typical angina pectoris. In some patients, the exercise level during the test may exceed that which the patient exhibits in day-to-day activities. Exercise-induced chest discomfort usually occurs after the onset of ischemic ST segment abnormalities and may be associated with diastolic hypertension. In some patients, however, chest discomfort may be the only signal that obstructive CAD is present. In patients with chronic stable angina, exercise-induced chest discomfort occurs less frequently than ischemic ST segment depression. The severity of myocardial ischemia in a patient with exercise-induced angina and a normal ECG can often be assessed using a myocardial imaging technique.[1,2] The new development of an S_3, holosystolic apical murmur, or basilar rates in the early recovery phase of exercise enhances the diagnostic accuracy of the test.

EXERCISE TEST INDICATIONS

The most frequent indications for exercise testing are to aid in establishing the diagnosis of CAD, in determining functional capacity, and in estimating prognosis. The indications continue to evolve, with some that are uniformly accepted and others that are more controversial. The American Heart Association and American College of Cardiology Exercise Task Force determined several categories of test indications drawn from a large body of published literature on exercise testing[1] (see Guidelines section). Exercise testing should not be used to screen very low-risk, asymptomatic individuals because the test has limited diagnostic and prognostic value in this situation, and the resultant undesirable consequences of a false-positive exercise test result may be unnecessary follow-up, additional procedures, anxiety, and exercise restrictions.[7,8] Most asymptomatic subjects who are enrolled in an exercise screening program for CAD and who die suddenly of cardiac causes have had a previous normal exercise test result. In patients with established CAD, low-risk patients with an estimated annual mortality rate of less than 1 percent do not require repeat testing for several years after their initial evaluation. Higher risk patients (estimated annual mortality > 3%) might require more frequent follow-up testing on an annual basis in the absence of a change of symptoms.[48]

TABLE 10–1 Terms Useful in Evaluation of Test Results

Term	Definition
True positive (TP)	Abnormal test result in individual with disease
False positive (FP)	Abnormal test result in individual without disease
True negative (TN)	Normal test result in individual without disease
False negative (FN)	Normal test result in individual with disease
Sensitivity	Percentage of patients with CAD who have an abnormal result = TP/(TP + FN)
Specificity	Percentage of patients without CAD who have a normal result = TN/(TN + FP)
Predictive value	Percentage of patients with an abnormal result who have CAD = TN/(TN + FN)
Test accuracy	Percentage of true test results = (TP + TN)/total number tests performed
Likelihood ratio	Odds of a test result being true abnormal test result: sensitivity/(1 – specificity) normal test result: specificity/(1 – sensitivity)
Relative risk	Disease rate in persons with a positive test result/disease rate in persons with a negative test result

CAD = coronary artery disease.

Diagnostic Use of Exercise Testing

Appreciation of the noninvasive test literature to diagnose CAD requires an understanding of standard terminology such as *sensitivity*, *specificity*, and *test accuracy* (Table 10–1).[1,2,7,8] In patients selected for coronary angiography, the sensitivity of the exercise ECG in patients with CAD is approximately 68 percent, and specificity is 77 percent. In patients with single-vessel disease, the sensitivity ranges from 25 to 71 percent, with exercise-induced ST displacement most frequent in patients with left anterior descending CAD, followed by those with right CAD and those with isolated left circumflex CAD. In patients with multivessel CAD, sensitivity is approximately 81 percent and specificity is 66 percent. The sensitivity and specificity for left main or three-vessel CAD are approximately 86 percent and 53 percent, respectively. The exercise ECG tends to be less sensitive in patients with extensive anterior wall myocardial infarction and when a limited exercise ECG lead set is used. Approximately 75 to 80 percent of the diagnostic information on exercise-induced ST segment depression in patients with a normal resting ECG is contained in leads V_4 to V_6. Exercise ECG is less specific when patients in whom false-positive results are more common are included, such as those with valvular heart disease, left ventricular hypertrophy, marked resting ST segment depression, or digitalis therapy. Table 10–2 lists the more common causes of noncoronary exercise–induced ST segment depression.

The traditional reference standard against which the exercise ECG has been measured is a qualitative assessment of the coronary angiogram using 50 to 70 percent obstruction of the luminal diameter as the angiographic cutpoint. Limitations are inherent in angiographic classification of patients according to whether they have one-, two-, or three-vessel CAD, and the length of the coronary artery narrowing and the impact of serial lesions are not accounted for in correlative studies comparing diagnostic exercise testing with coronary angiographic findings. Other approaches, including intracoronary Doppler flow studies and quantitative coronary angiography, have been proposed to assess coronary vascular reserve; these may be more accurate than qualitative assessment of the angiogram.[49,50] The magnitude of coronary atherosclerosis in a coronary vessel is often underestimated on a luminal angiogram when intravascular ultrasonographic studies are performed.[51] A normal coronary angiogram does not eliminate the possibility that a patient's symptoms may be ischemic in origin. In a study of 20 patients with ischemic-appearing ST segment depression during exercise and normal findings on coronary angiography (syndrome X), intravenous adenosine infusion produced chest pain and subendocardial hypoperfusion detected with cardiac magnetic resonance

TABLE 10–2 Noncoronary Causes of ST Segment Depression

Severe aortic stenosis	Glucose load
Severe hypertension	Left ventricular hypertrophy
Cardiomyopathy	Hyperventilation
Anemia	Mitral valve prolapse
Hypokalemia	Intraventricular conduction disturbance
Severe hypoxia	Preexcitation syndrome
Digitalis use	Severe volume overload (aortic, mitral regurgitation)
Sudden excessive exercise	Supraventricular tachyarrhythmias

imaging in 95 percent of subjects, as compared with 40 percent in a control group.[52]

Selective referral of patients with a positive test result for further study both decreases the rate of detection of true-negative test results and increases the rate of detection of false-positive results, thus increasing sensitivity and decreasing specificity.[1,2,7,8] Froelicher and colleagues, in a study of 814 consecutive patients who presented with angina pectoris and agreed to undergo both exercise testing and coronary angiography, reported exercise ECG sensitivity of 45 percent and specificity of 85 percent for obstructive CAD using visual analysis in this population with reduced work-up bias.[53] Computerized ST segment measurements were similar to visual ST segment measurements in this study. A false-positive result is more common when only the inferior lead group (leads 2, 3, aV_f) is abnormal at high exercise workloads.

BAYES' THEOREM. The depth of exercise-induced ST-segment depression and the extent of the myocardial ischemic response can be thought of as continuous variables. Cutpoints such as 1 mm of horizontal or downsloping ST segment depression as compared with baseline cannot completely distinguish patients with disease from those without disease, and the requirement of more severe degrees of ST segment depression to improve specificity will decrease sensitivity. Sensitivity and specificity are inversely related, and false-negative and false-positive results are to be expected when ECG or angiographic cutpoints are selected to optimize the diagnostic accuracy of the test.

The use of Bayes' theorem incorporates the pretest risk of disease and the sensitivity and specificity of the test (likelihood ratio) to calculate the posttest probability of coronary disease. The patient's clinical information and exercise test results are used to make a final estimate about the probability of CAD. Atypical or probable angina in a 50-year-old man or a 60-year-old woman is associated with approximately 50 percent probability for CAD before exercise testing is performed. The diagnostic power of the exercise test is maximal when the pretest probability of CAD is intermediate (30 to 70 percent).

MULTIVARIATE ANALYSIS. Multivariate analysis of noninvasive exercise tests to estimate posttest risk also can provide important diagnostic information. Multivariate analysis offers the potential advantage that it does not require that the tests be independent of each other or that sensitivity and specificity remain constant over a wide range of disease prevalence rates (see section on prognosis). However, the multivariate technique depends critically on how patients are selected to establish the reference data base.[54,55] Both bayesian and multivariate approaches are commonly used to provide diagnostic and prognostic estimates of patients with CAD.

SEVERITY OF ELECTROCARDIOGRAPHIC ISCHEMIC RESPONSE. The exercise ECG result is more likely to be abnormal in patients with more severe coronary arterial obstruction, with more extensive CAD, and after more strenuous levels of exercise. Early onset of angina, ischemic ST segment depression, and fall in blood pressure at low exercise workloads are the most important exercise parameters associated with an adverse prognosis and multivessel CAD.[1,2,7,8] Additional adverse markers include profound ST segment displacement, ischemic changes in five or more ECG leads, and persistence of the changes late in the recovery phase of exercise (Table 10–3).

Exercise Testing in Determining Prognosis

Exercise testing provides not only diagnostic information but also, more importantly, prognostic data. The value of exercise testing to estimate prognosis must be considered in light of what is already known about a patient's risk status. Left ventricular dysfunction, CAD extent, electrical instability, and noncoronary comorbid conditions must be taken into consideration when estimating long-term outcome.

ASYMPTOMATIC POPULATION. The prevalence of an abnormal exercise ECG result in middle-aged asymptomatic men ranges from 5 to 12 percent. Rywik and colleagues studied 1083 volunteers from the Baltimore Longitudinal Study of Aging to determine the prognostic value of different types of exercise ECG response for cardiac events defined as onset of angina, myocardial infarction, or cardiac death. After a 7.9-year follow-up, horizontal or downsloping ST segment depression 1 mm or greater or intensification of minor pre-exercise ST segment depression to 1 mm or greater independently predicted cardiac events.[56] In earlier studies from other institutions, the risk of developing a cardiac event such as angina, myocardial infarction, or death in men was approximately nine times greater when the test result was abnormal than when it was normal; however, over 5 years of follow-up, only one in four men suffered a cardiac event, and this was most commonly the development of angina. The data illustrate the difficulty in identifying asymptomatic subjects destined to develop abrupt changes in plaque morphology based on an abnormal exercise electrocardiogram. The future risk of cardiac events is greatest if the test result is strongly positive or if an asymptomatic subject has atherosclerotic risk factors such as diabetes, hypertension, hypercholesterolemia, smoking history, or familial history of premature coronary disease (Fig. 10–14).[56-58] Target extracardiac end-organ damage such as peripheral vascular disease, proteinuria, or stroke further escalates the risk in accordance with bayesian

TABLE 10–3 Exercise Parameters Associated with an Adverse Prognosis and Multivessel Coronary Artery Disease

Duration of symptom-limiting exercise < 5 METs
Failure to increase systolic blood pressure ≥ 120 mm Hg, or a sustained decrease ≥ 10 mm Hg, or below rest levels, during progressive exercise
ST segment depression ≥ 2 mm, downsloping ST segment, starting at <5 METs, involving ≥5 leads, persisting ≥5 min into recovery
Exercise-induced ST segment elevation (aV excluded)
Angina pectoris at low exercise workloads
Reproducible sustained (>30 sec) or symptomatic ventricular tachycardia
Acute systemic illness (pulmonary embolism, aortic dissection)

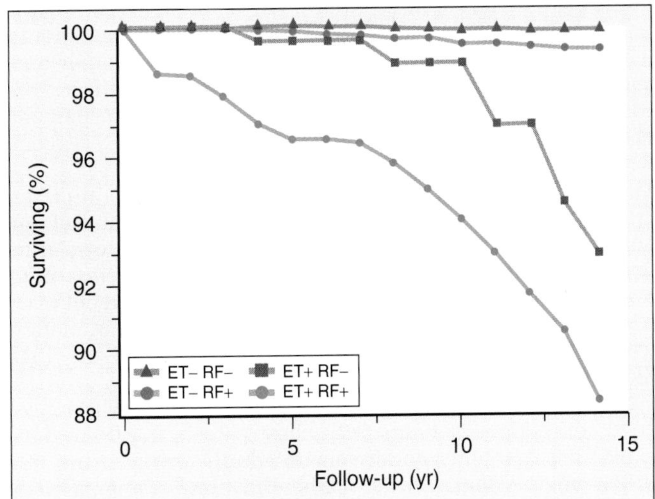

FIGURE 10–14 In 25,927 apparently healthy asymptomatic men 20 to 82 years of age followed for an average 8.4 years, cardiac event-free survival was worse in the patient subset with conventional atherosclerotic risk factors (RF+) and an abnormal exercise test (ET+). The age-adjusted relative risk (not shown) increased with the number of risk factors. In contrast, the event rate in subjects without risk factors (RF–) and an ET+ was not significantly different than in subjects with a normal exercise test (ET–) in the first 5 years of follow-up. (Gibbons LW, Mitchell TL, Wei M, et al: Maximal exercise test as a predictor of risk for mortality from coronary heart disease in asymptomatic men. Am J Cardiol 86:53, 2000.)

principles. Selection of asymptomatic subjects for an exercise test should be based on the atherosclerotic risk profile that can be used to provide a global risk estimate of the likelihood of death, myocardial infarction, or stroke. Appropriate asymptomatic subjects for exercise testing would be those with an estimated annual risk greater than 1 or 2 percent per year.[59] In asymptomatic middle-aged or older men with several atherosclerotic risk factors, a markedly abnormal exercise response is associated with a significantly increased risk of subsequent cardiac events, particularly when there is additional supporting evidence for underlying CAD (e.g., coronary calcification, abnormal results of thallium scan, and the like). Blumenthal and colleagues studied 734 asymptomatic siblings of persons with documented coronary disease and reported abnormal exercise perfusion results in 153 subjects, 95 percent of whom had mild to moderate atherosclerosis at angiography. Luminal narrowings of greater than 50 percent were found in 70 percent of subjects with an abnormal exercise ECG and scan.[58] Serial change of a negative exercise ECG result to a positive one in an asymptomatic person carries the same prognostic importance as an initially abnormal test result. However, when an asymptomatic individual with an initially abnormal test result has significant worsening of the ECG abnormalities at lower exercise workloads, this finding may indicate significant CAD progression and warrants a more aggressive diagnostic work-up. The prevalence of an abnormal exercise ECG result in middle-aged asymptomatic women ranges from 20 to 30 percent.[1,2,7,8] In general, the prognostic value of an ST segment shift in women is less than in men. Although the use of multivariate scores to predict CAD in women has improved diagnostic accuracy, false-positive results continue to be a problem in many patients, and supplemental imaging techniques are often necessary to enhance the diagnostic performance of the test.[1,2]

SYMPTOMATIC PATIENTS. Exercise testing should be routinely performed (unless this is not feasible or unless there are contraindications) before coronary angiography in patients with chronic ischemic heart disease. Patients who have excellent exercise tolerance (e.g., >10 METs) usually have an excellent prognosis regardless of the anatomical extent of CAD.[1,2,39-41] The test provides an estimate of the functional significance of angiographically documented coronary artery stenoses. The impact of exercise testing in patients with proven or suspected CAD was studied by Weiner and colleagues in 4083 medically treated patients in the CASS study.[60] A high-risk patient subset was identified (12 percent of the population), with an annual mortality rate of 5 percent when exercise workload was less than Bruce stage I (<4 METs) and the exercise ECG exhibited 0.1 mV (1 mm) or greater ST segment depression. A low-risk patient subset (34 percent of the population) who were able to exercise into Bruce stage III or higher and who had a normal exercise ECG result had an annual mortality rate of less than 1 percent over 4 years of follow-up. Similar ECG and workload parameters were useful in risk-stratifying patients with three-vessel CAD likely to benefit from coronary bypass grafting.

Mark and colleagues developed a treadmill score based on 2842 consecutive patients with chest pain in the Duke data bank; these patients underwent treadmill testing using the Bruce protocol and cardiac catheterization.[61] Patients with left bundle branch block (LBBB) or those with exercise-induced ST elevation in a Q wave lead were excluded. The treadmill (TM) score is calculated as follows:

$$\text{TM score} = \text{exercise time} - (5 \times \text{ST deviation}) - (4 \times \text{treadmill angina index})$$

Angina index was assigned a value of 0 if angina was absent, 1 if typical angina occurred during exercise, and 2 if angina was the reason the patient stopped exercising. Exercise-induced ST deviation was defined as the largest net ST displacement in any lead. The 13 percent of patients with a treadmill score of −11 or less had a 5-year survival rate of 72 percent, as compared with a 97 percent survival rate among the 34 percent of patients at low risk with a treadmill score of +5 or greater. The score added independent prognostic information to that provided by clinical data, coronary anatomy, and left ventricular ejection fraction. The stratified annual mortality rates predicted from the treadmill score were less in 613 outpatients referred for exercise testing from the same institution (Fig. 10–15).[62] The score worked equally well in men and women, although women had a lower overall risk than men for similar scores. The Duke treadmill score is not as effective in estimating risk in subjects 75 years of age or older (see section on elderly patients).[63] Exercise scoring systems can be used to identify prognostically intermediate- to high-risk patients in whom coronary angiography would be indicated to define coronary anatomy.[54,55,64] However, the decision to perform coronary revascularization should take into consideration the fact that in patients with less extensive CAD (e.g., one to two vessels narrowed and well-preserved left ventricular function), a similar degree of exercise-induced myocardial ischemia does not carry the same significant increased risk of cardiac events as in patients with more extensive disease (e.g., three vessels narrowed or impaired left ventricular function). When estimating prognosis in individual patients from the population-based data collected in the previous two decades, consideration should be given to the fact that actual survival rates in the current era are likely to be greater because of more aggressive treatment of atherosclerotic risk factors and use of noninvasive testing to identify the highest risk subjects that benefit from coronary revascularization.

SILENT MYOCARDIAL ISCHEMIA (see Chap. 50). In patients with documented CAD, the presence of exercise-induced ischemic ST segment depression confers increased risk of subsequent cardiac events regardless of whether angina occurs during the test.[65] The magnitude of the prognostic gradient in patients with an abnormal exercise ECG result with or without angina varies considerably in the published literature, most likely a feature of patient selection. In the CASS data bank, 7-year survival in patients with silent or symptomatic exercise-induced myocardial ischemia was similar in patients stratified by coronary anatomy and left ventricular function, with the worst survival in patients with the most extensive CAD. In the ACIP trial, coronary revascularization was a more effective treatment strategy to reduce exercise-induced myocardial ischemia than was medical therapy.

ACUTE CORONARY SYNDROMES (see Chaps. 47 and 49)

The incidence of exercise-induced angina or ischemic ST segment abnormalities in patients who have an acute coronary syndrome and who undergo a predischarge low-level protocol ranges from 30 to 40 percent. The finding of ischemic ST segment changes or limiting chest pain is associated with a significantly increased risk of subsequent cardiac events in men and postmenopausal women.[66-68] The absence of these findings identifies a low-risk patient subset. The prognostic risk assessment after an acute coronary syndrome should incorporate findings from the history, physical examination, resting 12-lead ECG, and level of serum markers to optimize mortality and morbidity estimates and to categorize patients into low-, intermediate-, and high-risk groups.[67] Exercise testing should be considered in the outpatient evaluation of low-risk patients with unstable angina (biomarker negative) who are free of active ischemic symptoms for a minimum of 8 to 12 hours, and in hospitalized low- to intermediate-risk ambulatory patients who are free of angina or heart failure symptoms for at least 48 hours.[69] In many intermediate- or high-risk patients, coronary angiography will have been performed during the acute phase of the illness; coronary disease extent, left ventricular function, and degree of coronary revascularization, if performed, should then be incorporated with the exercise test data to determine the overall predischarge prognostic risk estimate.

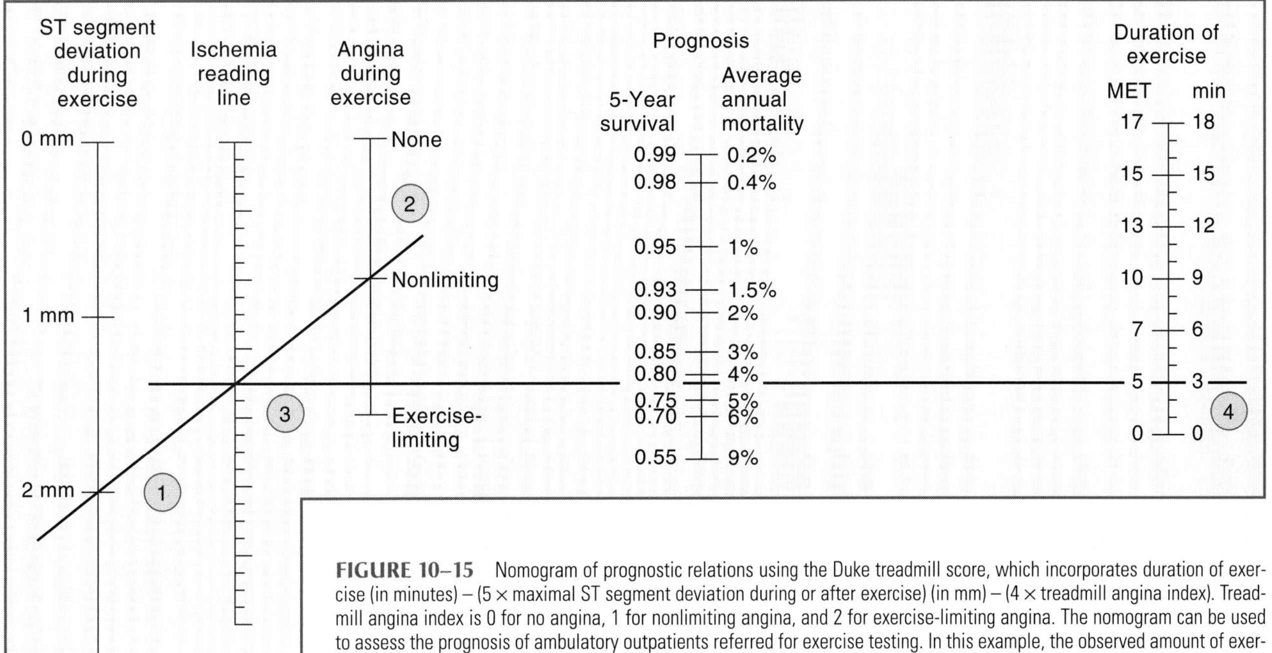

FIGURE 10–15 Nomogram of prognostic relations using the Duke treadmill score, which incorporates duration of exercise (in minutes) – (5 × maximal ST segment deviation during or after exercise) (in mm) – (4 × treadmill angina index). Treadmill angina index is 0 for no angina, 1 for nonlimiting angina, and 2 for exercise-limiting angina. The nomogram can be used to assess the prognosis of ambulatory outpatients referred for exercise testing. In this example, the observed amount of exercise-induced ST segment deviation (minus resting changes) is marked on the line for ST segment deviation during exercise (1). The degree of angina during exercise is plotted (2), and the points are connected. The point of intersection on the ischemic reading line is noted (3). The number of METs (or minutes of exercise if the Bruce protocol is used) is marked on the exercise duration line (4). The marks on the ischemia reading line and duration of exercise line are connected, and the intersection on the prognosis line determines 5-year survival rate and average annual mortality for patients with these selected specific variables. In this example, the 5-year prognosis is estimated at 78 percent in this patient with exercise-induced 2-mm ST depression, nonlimiting exercise angina, and peak exercise workload of 5 METs. MET = metabolic equivalent. (Adapted from Mark DE, Shaw L, Harrell FE Jr, et al: Prognostic value of a treadmill exercise score in outpatients with suspected coronary artery disease. N Engl J Med 325:849, 1991. Copyright Massachusetts Medical Society.)

MYOCARDIAL INFARCTION

Exercise testing after myocardial infarction (both non-ST and ST elevation) is useful to determine (1) risk stratification and assessment of prognosis, (2) functional capacity for activity prescription after hospital discharge, and (3) assessment of adequacy of medical therapy and need to use supplemental diagnostic or treatment options.[1,2,7,8] The incidence of fatal or nonfatal cardiac events associated with exercise testing after myocardial infarction is low. The risk of events is approximately twofold greater for symptom-limited protocols compared with submaximal tests, although the overall fatal event rate is extremely low with both types of exercise protocols. A low-level exercise test (achievement of 5 to 6 METs or 70 to 80 percent of age-predicted maximum) is frequently performed before hospital discharge to establish the hemodynamic response and functional capacity.[1,2,70] The ability to complete 5 to 6 METs of exercise or 70 to 80 percent of age-predicted maximum in the absence of abnormal ECG or blood pressure is associated with a 1-year mortality rate of 1 to 2 percent and may help guide the timing of early hospital discharge.[71] Parameters associated with increased risk include inability to perform or complete the low-level predischarge exercise test, poor exercise capacity, inability to increase or a decrease in exercise systolic blood pressure, and angina or exercise-induced ST segment depression at low workloads. Many postinfarct patients referred for exercise testing have been prescribed beta-adrenergic blocking agents and angiotensin-converting enzyme inhibitors. Although beta-adrenergic blocking drugs may attenuate the ischemic response, they do not interfere with poor functional capacity as a marker of adverse prognosis and should be continued in patients referred for testing. The relative prognostic value of a 3- to 6-week postdischarge exercise test is minimal once clinical variables and the results of the low-level predischarge test are adjusted for. For this reason, the timing of the exercise test after the infarct event favors predischarge exercise testing to allow implementation of a definitive treatment plan in patients in whom coronary anatomy is known as well as risk stratification of patients in whom coronary anatomy has not yet been determined. There is a trend toward early predischarge exercise testing (within 3 to 5 days) in uncomplicated cases after acute myocardial infarction.[71] A 3- to 6-week test is useful in clearing patients to return to work in occupations involving physical labor in which the MET expenditure is likely to be greater than that performed on a predischarge test.

The goals and basic principles of the predischarge evaluation have not been changed by the advent of reperfusion or direct percutaneous transluminal coronary angioplasty therapy for acute infarction. After receiving intravenous thrombolytic therapy or direct coronary angioplasty, patients with uncomplicated myocardial infarction tend to exhibit exercise-induced angina and ST segment depression less frequently than do consecutive postinfarct patients before these treatment strategies were widely applied. The occurrence of reciprocal ST segment depression associated with exercise-induced ST segment elevation in patients who undergo testing approximately 6 to 8 weeks after Q wave infarction with single-vessel disease may indicate residual tissue viability in the infarct-related area.[72] In patients with negative T waves after infarction, stress-induced normalization of the T waves may also indicate higher coronary flow reserve than in patients unable to normalize their T waves.[26]

RISK STRATIFICATION IN THE EMERGENCY DEPARTMENT. Patients who present to the emergency department are a heterogeneous population with a large range of pretest risk for CAD. Clinical algorithms can identify lower risk persons who can safely be further risk-stratified using exercise testing.[69,73,74] In one series of 1000 symptomatic low-risk patients with chest pain possibly of cardiac origin who presented to the emergency department, Amsterdam and colleagues reported a positive, intermediate, and nondiagnostic exercise test result in 13, 64, and 23 percent, respectively.[75] There were no adverse effects of exercise testing. The cost-effectiveness of this approach has been demonstrated in both low- and intermediate-risk patients. The accuracy of exercise testing in the emergency department setting follows bayesian principles, with the greatest diagnostic and prognostic estimates in intermediate-risk clinical patient subsets. Exercise testing in the emergency department should not be performed when (1) new or evolving ECG abnormalities are noted on the rest tracing, (2) the levels of cardiac enzymes are abnormal, (3) the patient cannot adequately perform exercise, (4) the patient reports worsening or persistent chest pain symptoms, or (5) clinical risk profiling indicates that imminent coronary angiography is likely. Several series of clinically low-risk subjects reported 6-month cardiac event rates less than 1 percent with a normal exercise test result.[76]

PREOPERATIVE RISK STRATIFICATION BEFORE NONCARDIAC SURGERY (see Chap. 77). Exercise ECG before elective noncardiac surgery provides an objective measurement of functional capacity and the potential to identify the likelihood of perioperative myocardial ischemia in patients with a low ischemic threshold.[77] In patients with intermittent claudication and no prior history of cardiac disease, approximately 20 to 25 percent will have an abnormal exercise ECG result. In patients with a prior history of myocardial infarction or an abnormal resting ECG, 35 to 50 percent will have an abnormal exercise ECG result. The risk of perioperative cardiac events and adverse long-term outcome is significantly increased in patients with abnormal exercise ECG results at low workloads. Coronary angiography with revascularization, when feasible, should be considered in such patients before noncardiac operative interventions that are considered high risk, such as aortic and other major vascular surgery and anticipated prolonged procedures associated with large fluid shifts or blood loss.[78-80]

CONGESTIVE HEART FAILURE. Cardiac and peripheral compensatory mechanisms are activated in patients with chronic congestive heart failure to partly or fully restore impaired left ventricular performance. Abnormal baroreflex function and increased norepinephrine spillover, sympathetic discharge, downregulation of beta-adrenergic receptors, and depletion of myocardial sympathetic stores characterize the disease process resulting in the hemodynamic response to exercise.[81-84] There is a wide range of exercise capacity in patients who have a markedly reduced ejection fraction, with some patients having near-normal peak exercise capacity. The magnitude of exercise capacity impairment is a function of the relative inability to augment stroke volume and abnormalities in skeletal muscle metabolism, which may be the predominant cause of functional limitation in a significant proportion of patients with heart failure. Fatigue may be related to altered skeletal muscle metabolism secondary to chronic physical deconditioning, impaired perfusion, and chronic anemia.[81,85-87] In a series of 26 heart failure patients with chronic anemia, peak $\dot{V}O_2$ was significantly increased when hemoglobin was increased from 11 to 14 g/dl with erythropoietin, iron, and folate administration.[86] Symptoms in patients with congestive heart failure are related to an excessive increase in blood lactate during low exercise levels, reduction in quantity of oxygen consumed at peak exertion, and disproportionate increase in ventilation at submaximal and peak workloads. The increased ventilatory requirement assessed by the hyperventilatory response to exercise and increase in pulmonary dead space leads to rapid, shallow breathing during exercise. Dyspnea and fatigue are the usual reasons for exercise termination.

Peak $\dot{V}O_2$ measurements in patients with compensated congestive heart failure are useful in risk-stratifying patients with congestive heart failure to determine the subsequent incidence of cardiac events (Fig. 10–16).[81,84,88-90] The ability to achieve a peak $\dot{V}O_2$ of greater than 20 ml O_2/kg/min and anaerobic threshold greater than 14 ml O_2/kg/min is associated with a relatively good long-term prognosis and maximal cardiac output greater than 8 liters/min/m^2. Patients who are unable to achieve a peak $\dot{V}O_2$ of 10 ml O_2/kg/min and anaerobic threshold of 8 ml O_2/kg/min have a poor prognosis, and their maximal exercise cardiac output is usually less than 4 liters/min/m^2. Failure of $\dot{V}O_2$ to decrease within 30 seconds after peak exertion is associated with more severe reductions in left ventricular ejection fraction and moderate to severe impairment of pulmonary gas exchange. Inability to increase oxygen pulse (milliliters of oxygen per beat) is related to a lack of or a minimal increase of stroke volume. A blunted heart rate response caused by postsynaptic desensitization of beta-adrenergic receptors is not uncommon in patients with congestive heart failure. Exercise protocols that limit exercise duration to 5 to 7 minutes are associated with the most reproducible peak $\dot{V}O_2$ measurements in patients with heart

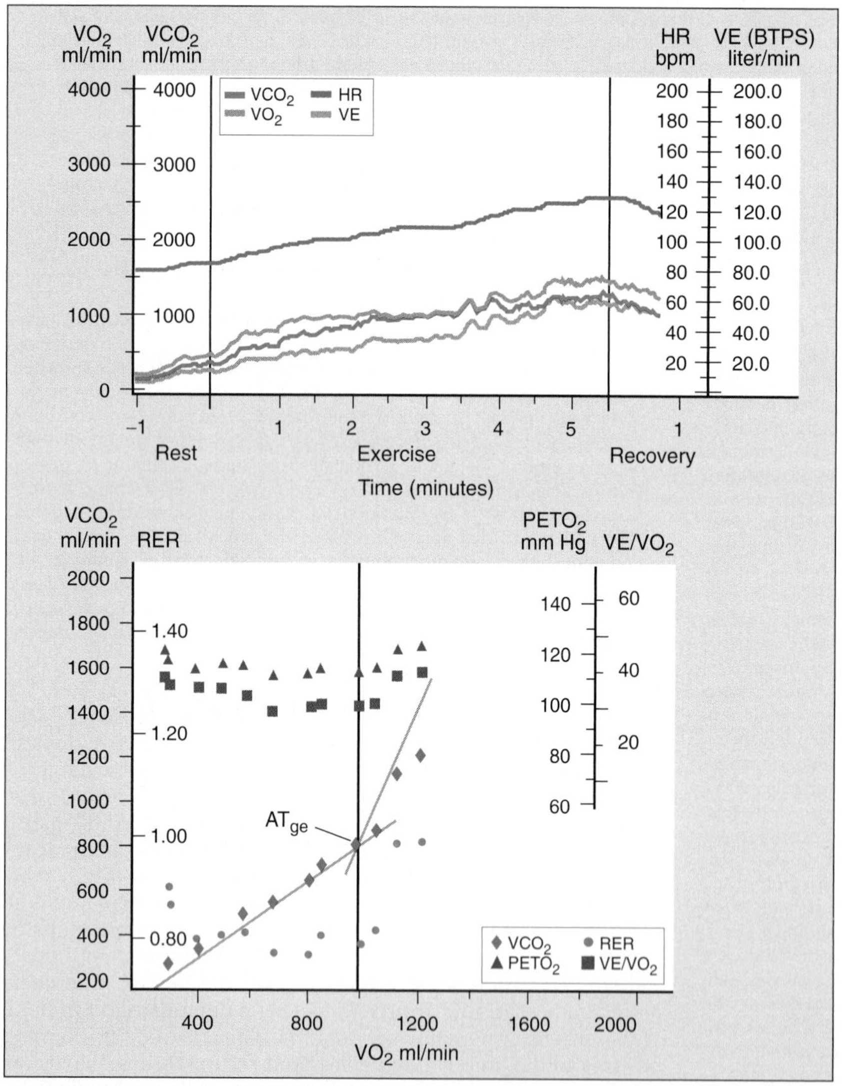

FIGURE 10–16 Cardiopulmonary exercise test in a 51-year-old man with cardiomyopathy in New York Heart Association Class III. A modified Bruce protocol was used. The patient reached a peak $\dot{V}O_2$ of 14 ml O_2/kg/min (4 METs), 44 percent of predicted for age, gender, and weight **(top)**. Anaerobic threshold (AT_{ge}) occurred at a $\dot{V}O_2$ of 977 ml/min **(bottom)**. The blunted cardiopulmonary response is typical for a patient with severe cardiomyopathy and marked impairment of cardiac reserve. This patient was listed for cardiac transplantation. METs = metabolic equivalents; $PETO_2$ = end-tidal pressure of oxygen.

failure. The interpretation of cardiopulmonary exercise test results in patients with heart failure can occasionally be difficult, because some patients hyperventilate during exercise, producing falsely low peak oxygen consumption, and it can be difficult to distinguish patients who are deconditioned from those who have impaired exercise performance and low peak $\dot{V}O_2$ due to cardiac pathology. Randomized controlled trials of long-term moderate exercise training in patients with chronic heart failure report a 15 to 20 percent improvement in peak $\dot{V}O_2$ and prolonged onset of anaerobic metabolism.[89] Thus, clinical decisions such as listing a patient for cardiac transplantation based on peak $\dot{V}O_2$ measurements need to take into consideration interval training effects.[89,90] The 6-minute walk test also can be used to evaluate functional capacity and to estimate prognosis in patients unable to exercise on a bicycle ergometer or treadmill.[91] However, in patients with moderate to severe heart failure, peak $\dot{V}O_2$ measurements are more reliable than the walking test for clinical decisions.[92]

Cardiac Arrhythmias and Conduction Disturbances

The genesis of cardiac arrhythmias includes reentry, triggered activity, and enhanced automaticity (see Chap. 27). Increased catecholamines during exercise accelerate impulse conduction velocity, shorten the myocardial refractory period, increase the amplitude of afterpotentials, and increase the slope of phase 4 spontaneous depolarization of the action potential. Other potentiators of cardiac rhythm disturbance include metabolic acidosis and exercise-induced myocardial ischemia. Ventricular premature complexes occur frequently during exercise testing and increase with age. Repetitive forms occur in 0 to 5 percent of asymptomatic subjects without suspected cardiac disease and are not associated with an increased risk of cardiac death. Exercise-induced ventricular ectopic activity is not a useful diagnostic marker of ischemic heart disease in the absence of ischemic ST segment depression. Suppression of ventricular ectopic activity during exercise is a nonspecific finding and may occur in patients with CAD as well as in normal subjects. The prognostic importance of ventricular arrhythmias in patients with chronic ischemic heart disease after adjustment for baseline, clinical, and left ventricular function characteristics is small. Approximately 20 percent of patients with known heart disease and 50 to 75 percent of sudden cardiac death survivors have repetitive ventricular beats induced by exercise. In patients with a recent myocardial infarction, the presence of exercise-induced repetitive forms is associated with an increased risk of subsequent cardiac events. Beta-adrenergic blocking drugs may suppress exercise-induced ventricular arrhythmias. Exercise-induced ventricular arrhythmias tend to be more frequent in the recovery phase of exercise because peripheral plasma norepinephrine levels continue to increase for several minutes after cessation of exercise, and vagal tone is high in the immediate recovery phase. Five-year all-cause mortality rates are significantly greater in patients who have frequent ventricular ectopy or repetitive ventricular beats in the recovery phase of exercise as compared with those who have ventricular arrhythmias that occur only during exercise.[93] The test is useful in evaluating the effects of antiarrhythmic drugs, detecting supraventricular arrhythmias, treating patients with chronic atrial fibrillation to test for ventricular rate control, and exposing possible drug toxicity in patients placed on antiarrhythmic drugs.

EVALUATION OF VENTRICULAR ARRHYTHMIAS. Exercise testing is useful in the assessment of patients with ventricular arrhythmias and has an important adjunctive role along with ambulatory monitoring and electrophysiological studies.[1,2,7,8,93,94] Exercise testing provokes repetitive ventricular premature beats in most patients with a history of sustained ventricular tachyarrhythmia, and in approximately 10 to 15 percent of such patients, spontaneously occurring arrhythmias are observed only during exercise testing (Fig. 10–17). Frequent ventricular ectopy that occurs in the early postexercise phase is associated with a worse long-term prognosis than ventricular ectopy that occurs only during exercise (Fig. 10–18). In patients with adrenergic-dependent rhythm disturbances (including monomorphic ventricular tachycardia and polymorphic ventricular tachycardia related to long-QT syndromes), ambulatory electrocardiography or event monitoring may fail to capture the arrhythmia, particularly if the patient is relatively sedentary.[95,96] Paradoxical prolongation of the QT_C interval greater than 10 msec with exercise identifies patients likely to develop a proarrhythmic effect on type 1A antiarrhythmic drugs. Exercise-induced widening of the QRS complex in patients using type 1C drugs may favor reentry induction of ventricular tachycardia. Amiodarone therapy increases the QRS duration during exercise by approximately 6 percent in patients with a QRS duration less than 110 msec, as compared with 15 percent in patients with a QRS duration longer than 110 msec.

SUPRAVENTRICULAR ARRHYTHMIAS. Supraventricular premature beats induced by exercise are observed in 4 to 10 percent of normal persons and up to 40 percent of patients with underlying heart disease. Sustained supraventricular tachyarrhythmias occur in only 1 to 2 percent of patients, although the frequency may approach as much as 10 to 15 percent in patients referred for management of episodic supraventricular arrhythmias. The presence of supraventricular arrhythmias is not diagnostic for ischemic heart disease.

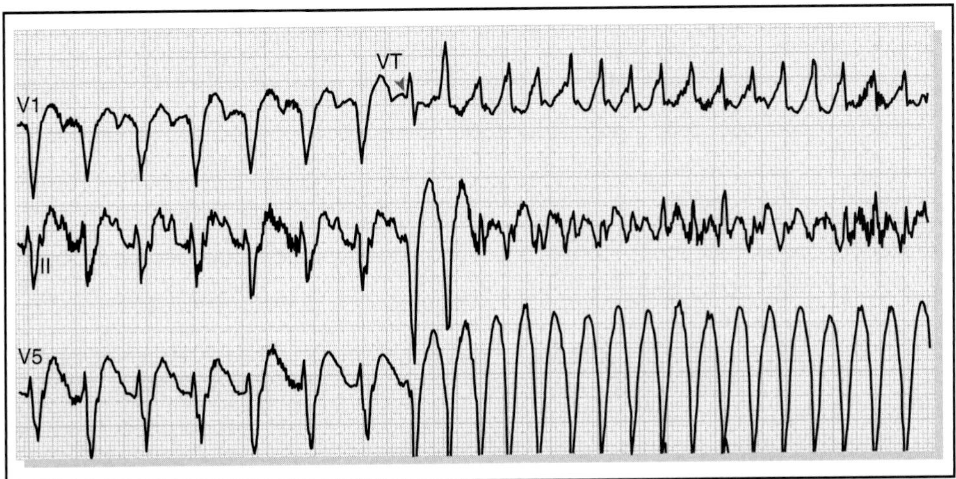

FIGURE 10–17 A 67-year-old man with ischemic cardiomyopathy referred for exercise testing had a left bundle branch block and first-degree atrioventricular (AV) block on the resting ECG. There was no worsening of the AV conduction disturbance immediately before onset of ventricular tachycardia (VT) (arrow). At 4:55 minutes into the test, a 27-beat run of VT was noted, reproducing the patient's symptoms of dizziness and chest pounding. The exercise test proved useful in directing subsequent patient management to treatment of the ventricular arrhythmia.

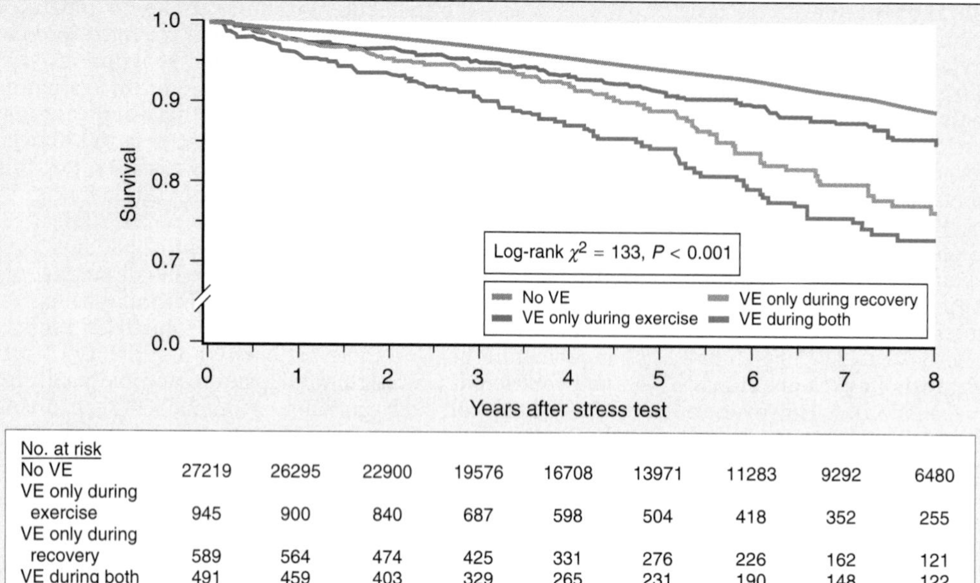

No. at risk									
No VE	27219	26295	22900	19576	16708	13971	11283	9292	6480
VE only during exercise	945	900	840	687	598	504	418	352	255
VE only during recovery	589	564	474	425	331	276	226	162	121
VE during both	491	459	403	329	265	231	190	148	122

FIGURE 10–18 In this series of 29,244 subjects, frequent ventricular ectopy occurred in 3 percent of subjects only during exercise, in 2 percent of subjects only during recovery from exercise, and in 2 percent of subjects during both exercise and recovery. The prognosis of patients who had postexercise-induced frequent ventricular ectopy was worse than the prognosis of subjects who had frequent ventricular ectopy only during exercise. The mean follow-up time was 5.3 years. (From Frolkis JP, Pothier CE, Blackstone EH, et al: Frequent ventricular ectopy after exercise as a predictor of death. N Engl J Med 348:781, 2003.)

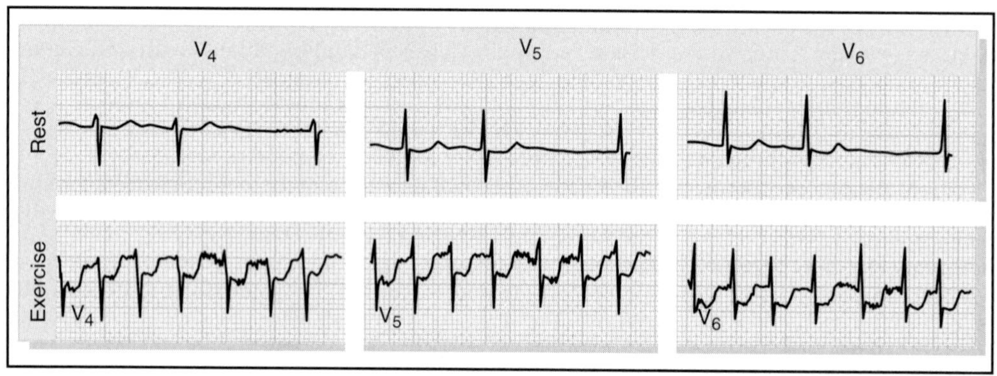

FIGURE 10–19 A 75-year-old woman with chronic atrial fibrillation and a 6-month history of atypical chest pain underwent mitral valve repair 1 year before testing, at which time nonobstructive coronary disease was noted. The patient exercised for 6 minutes, achieving a peak heart rate of 176 beats/min and peak blood pressure of 170/90 mm Hg. The resting electrocardiogram shows atrial fibrillation with a controlled ventricular response and minor ST segment depression. At peak exertion, marked ST segment depression is seen in the anterior leads, consistent with either digitalis effect or myocardial ischemia. In this type of patient, initial exercise testing with myocardial perfusion tracers or echocardiography would provide more useful diagnostic information than exercise testing alone.

ATRIAL FIBRILLATION. Patients with chronic atrial fibrillation tend to have a rapid ventricular response in the initial stages of exercise, and 60 to 70 percent of the total change in heart rate usually occurs within the first few minutes of exercise (Fig. 10–19). The effect of digitalis preparations and beta-adrenergic and selected calcium antagonists such as diltiazem on attenuating this rapid increase in heart rate for individual patients can be measured using exercise testing. Pharmacological control of the ventricular rate does not necessarily result in a significant increase in exercise capacity, which in many patients is related to the underlying cardiac disease process and not to adequacy of control of the ventricular rate.

SINUS NODE DYSFUNCTION. In general, patients with sinus node dysfunction have a lower heart rate at submaximal and maximal workloads compared with control subjects. However, as many as 40 to 50 percent of patients will have a normal exercise heart rate response.

ATRIOVENTRICULAR BLOCK. Exercise testing may help determine the need for atrioventricular (AV) sequential pacing in selected patients. In patients with congenital AV block, exercise-induced heart rates are low and some patients develop symptomatic rapid junctional rhythms that can be suppressed with DDD devices. In patients with acquired conduction disease, exercise can occasionally elicit advanced AV block.

LEFT BUNDLE BRANCH BLOCK. Exercise-induced ST segment depression is found in most patients with left bundle branch block (LBBB) and cannot be used as a diagnostic or prognostic indicator regardless of the degree of ST segment abnormality. In patients who are referred to a tertiary center and in whom exercise testing is carried out, the new development of exercise-induced transient left hemiblock is 0.3 percent and the new development of LBBB is 0.4 percent, with a slightly greater incidence in older patients.[97] The relative risk of death or other major cardiac events in patients with exercise-induced LBBB is increased approximately threefold over the risk in patients without this abnormality. In one series, permanent LBBB was reported in approximately half of patients who developed transient LBBB during exercise and who were monitored for an average of 6.6 years. High-grade AV block did not develop in any of the patients in this 15-patient series. The development of ischemic ST segment depression before the LBBB pattern appears or in the recovery phase after the LBBB has resolved does not attenuate the diagnostic yield of the ST segment shift. The ventricular rate at which the LBBB appears and disappears can be significantly different (Fig. 10–20).

RIGHT BUNDLE BRANCH BLOCK. The resting ECG in patients with right bundle branch block (RBBB) is frequently associated with T wave and ST segment changes in the early anterior precordial leads (V_1 to V_3). Exercise-induced ST depression in leads V_1 to V_4 is a common finding in patients with RBBB and is nondiagnostic (Fig. 10–21). The new development of exercise-induced ST segment depression in leads V_5 and V_6 or leads 2 and aV_f, reduced exercise capacity, and inability to adequately increase systolic blood pressure are useful in detecting patients who have CAD and a high clinical pretest risk of disease. The presence of RBBB decreases the sensitivity of the test. The new development of exercise-induced RBBB is relatively uncommon, occurring in approximately 0.1 percent of tests.

PREEXCITATION SYNDROME. The presence of Wolff-Parkinson-White syndrome invalidates the use of ST segment analysis as a diagnostic method for detecting CAD in preexcited as well as normally conducted beats; false-positive ischemic changes are frequently registered (Fig. 10–22).[98] In patients with persistent preexcitation, exercise may normalize the QRS complex, with disappearance of the delta wave in 20 to 50 percent of cases, depending on the series studied. Abrupt disappearance of the delta wave is presumptive evidence of a longer anterograde effective refractory period of the accessory pathway. Progressive disappearance of the delta wave is less reassuring and occurs when the improvement in AV node conduction is greater than in the accessory pathway; this finding does not preclude a possible significant or even critical shortening of the anterograde effective refractory period in the accessory pathway under the influence of sympathetic stimulation. Exercise-induced disappearance of the delta wave is more frequent with left-sided than right-sided accessory pathway positions. Although tachyarrhythmias appearing during an exercise test in patients with Wolff-Parkinson-White syndrome are rare, when they do occur, they provide an opportunity to evaluate AV conduction velocity. The presence of Wolff-Parkinson-White syndrome does not cause a limitation of physical work capacity.

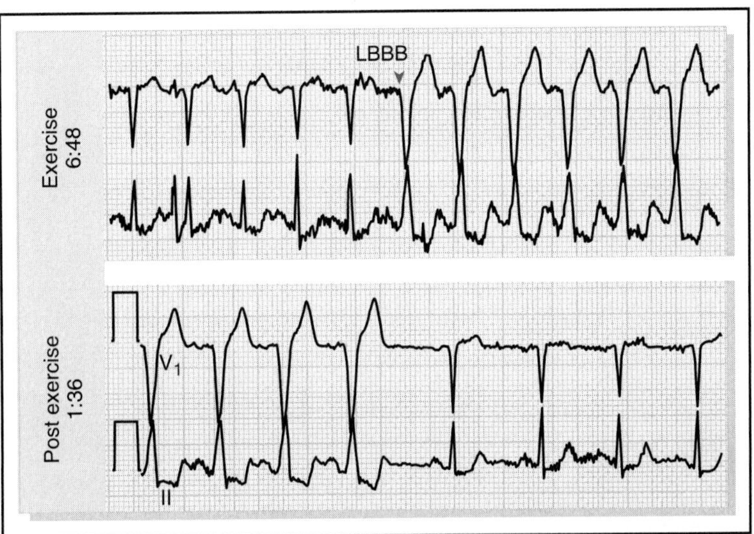

FIGURE 10–20 A 58-year-old hypertensive diabetic man with prior history of cigarette smoking was referred for evaluation of dyspnea and early fatigability during exercise. At 6:48 minutes into the test, the patient developed a rate-related left bundle branch block (LBBB) at a heart rate of 133 beats/min, which persisted during exercise and resolved at 1:36 minutes into the postexercise phase. The abnormal 2.5 to 3 mm downsloping ST segment depression in lead II during the LBBB is nondiagnostic for coronary artery disease because of the conduction disturbance. The test was stopped because of dyspnea at a peak heart rate of 138 beats/min (85 percent of predicted) and estimated workload of 6 METs. Peak blood pressure at the end of exercise was 174/94 mm Hg. Time to onset and offset of LBBB occurred at different ventricular rates related to fatigue in the left bundle, a common finding. METs = metabolic equivalents.

CARDIAC PACEMAKERS AND IMPLANTABLE CARDIOVERTER-DEFIBRILLATOR DEVICES. The exercise protocol used to assess chronotropic responsiveness in patients before and after cardiac pacemaker insertion should adjust for the fact that many patients with such devices are older individuals and may not tolerate high exercise workloads or abrupt and relatively large increments in work between stages of exercise. An optimal physiological cardiac pacemaker should normalize the heart rate response to exercise in proportion to oxygen uptake and should increase heart rate 2 to 4 beats/min for an increase in $\dot{V}O_2$ of 1 ml O_2/kg/min, with a slightly steeper slope for patients with severe left ventricular function impairment.[99] The exercise test can be particularly useful in evaluating sensor-triggered rate-adaptive pacing, in terms of both maximum heart rate achieved and rate of increase in heart rate during progressive exercise. Exercise testing can also be used to assess performance following cardiac resynchronization therapy in patients with heart failure and ventricular conduction delay.[100]

When testing patients with an implantable cardioverter-defibrillator device, the program detection interval of the device should be known. If the implantable cardioverter-defibrillator device is implanted for ventricular fibrillation or fast ventricular tachycardia, the rate will normally exceed that attainable during sinus tachycardia and the test can be terminated as the heart rate approaches 10 beats/min below the detection interval of the device. In patients with slower programmed detection rates, the implantable cardioverter-defibrillator can be reprogrammed to a faster rate to avoid accidental discharge during exercise testing or can be temporarily deactivated by a magnet. Exercise testing can be used to test the efficacy of tachycardic detection algorithms that apply criteria such as suddenness of onset and R-R variability.

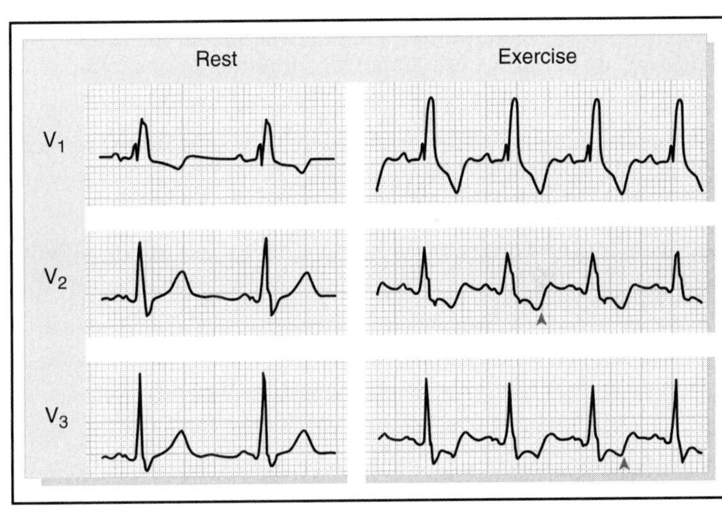

FIGURE 10–21 Exercise-induced ST segment depression is noted in leads V_2 to V_3 (arrows) in this patient with a resting right bundle branch block (RBBB) pattern. Exercise-induced horizontal or downsloping ST segment responses in the early anterior precordial leads (V_1 through V_4) are common in patients with RBBB and are secondary to the conduction disturbance. The presence of this finding in leads V_1 through V_4 is not diagnostic of obstructive coronary disease; however, if ischemic changes are seen in leads II, aV_F, or in leads V_5 or V_6, the specificity for coronary disease is improved.

Specific Clinical Applications

INFLUENCE OF DRUGS AND OTHER FACTORS. Patients with CAD demonstrate individual variability in time to onset of exercise-induced angina, time to onset of exercise-induced ischemic ST segment depression of 0.1 mV or greater, and cardiovascular efficiency during exercise testing.[7,8] The average individual variability in time to onset of exercise-induced myocardial ischemia or peak anaerobic capacity approximates as much as 20 percent in placebo-controlled trials of antianginal drugs. Average increases in exercise duration approach 40 to 60 seconds after 2 to 4 weeks and as much as 90 seconds after 12 weeks of placebo therapy.[101] Variability can be reduced by patients' familiarization with the exercise protocol and equipment, controlling for antianginal drug therapy at the time of testing, and stable test performance conditions. When two or three exercise tests are conducted within weeks of each other, the greatest increase in exercise time usually occurs between the first test and the second test. In one series of 24 subjects with stable

FIGURE 10–22 A 61-year-old man with atypical angina and a hiatal hernia was referred for diagnostic exercise testing. The test was stopped because of dyspnea. The standing resting ECG shows an intermittent Wolff-Parkinson-White pattern (arrows). In the nonpreexcited beats, ST segment depression does not occur either at peak exercise or in the postexercise phase. However, in the preexcited beats (arrows), an additional 1.3 mm of downsloping ST segment depression is noted as compared with baseline during and after exertion. METs = metabolic equivalents.

angina of less than class II, exercise time was increased by approximately 1 minute and time to onset of angina or ischemic ST segment depression by 3 minutes when two exercise tests were performed 15 minutes apart.[102] The mechanisms of the attenuation response with reexercise may be the results of ischemic preconditioning, familiarization with the exercise protocol, and improved musculoskeletal efficiency but do not appear to be dependent on exercise protocol intensity or downregulation of myocardial contractility induced by the initial ischemic stimulus.[31-33] In cold-sensitive individuals, exercise testing in a cooler environment results in onset of ischemic ST segment depression earlier than under normal temperature-controlled conditions. Conditions that increase carbon monoxide levels, such as chronic cigarette smoking, lower the ischemic response threshold.

Digitalis glycosides can produce exertional ST segment depression even if the effect is not evident on the resting ECG and can accentuate ischemic exercise-induced ST segment changes, particularly in older individuals. Absence of ST segment deviation during an exercise test in a patient receiving a cardiac glycoside is considered a valid negative response. Hypokalemia in patients on long-term diuretic therapy can be associated with exercise-induced ST segment depression. Antiischemic drug therapy with nitrates, beta-blocking drugs, or calcium channel blocking drugs prolongs the time to onset of ischemic ST segment depression, increases exercise tolerance, and, in a small minority of patients (10 to 15 percent), may normalize the exercise ECG response in patients with documented CAD.[7,8] The time and dose of drug ingestion may affect exercise performance. In some laboratories, cardioactive drug therapy is withheld for three to five half-lives and digitalis for 1 to 2 weeks before diagnostic testing. This is impractical in many cases, however.

WOMEN. The diagnostic accuracy of exercise-induced ST segment depression for obstructive CAD is less in women than in men. The decreased sensitivity results in part from a lower prevalence and extent of CAD in young and middle-aged women. Women tend to have a greater release of catecholamines during exercise, which could potentiate coronary vasoconstriction and augment the incidence of abnormal exercise ECG results, and false-positive results have been reported to be more common during menses or preovulation, or in postmenopausal women on isolated estrogen replacement therapy.[103,104] In a series of 976 symptomatic women referred for exercise testing and coronary angiography, low-, moderate-, and high-risk Duke treadmill scores were associated with CAD of 75 percent or greater luminal narrowing in 19.1, 34.9, and 89.2 percent of subjects, respectively. The frequency of three-vessel disease (75 percent or greater luminal narrowing) or left main CAD was 3.5, 12.4, and 46 percent, respectively. In a retrospective population-based cohort study of 1452 men and 741 women, exercise-induced angina, ischemic ECG changes, and workload were strongly associated with all-cause mortality and cardiac events in both sexes. The relationship between workload and outcome was linear, with an increment of 1 MET in workload associated with a 20 to 25 percent reduction in risk of death and cardiac events.[105] Alexander and colleagues compared the Duke treadmill score in 976 women and 2249 men; the 2-year mortality rate for women was 1, 2.2, and 3.6 percent for low-, moderate-, and high-risk scores, respectively, as compared with 1.7, 5.8, and 16.6 percent in men. In this report, women had a similar frequency of angina on the treadmill as men, but exertional angina in women was less often correlated with the presence of CAD.[106]

Morise and colleagues reported mortality rates ranging from 0.2 percent for a low-risk score to 7 percent for a high-risk score based on five clinical and three exercise test variables after an average 2.6-year follow-up in 442 symptomatic women referred for their first exercise test (Fig. 10–23).[55] Thus, in women with established CAD, exercise testing provides useful prognostic information for risk stratification and identification of low risk and higher risk patient subsets.

HYPERTENSION. Exercise testing has been used in an attempt to identify patients who have an abnormal blood pressure response and are destined subsequently to develop hypertension. In asymptomatic normotensive individuals, an exaggerated exercise systolic and diastolic blood pressure response during exercise or an exaggerated peak systolic

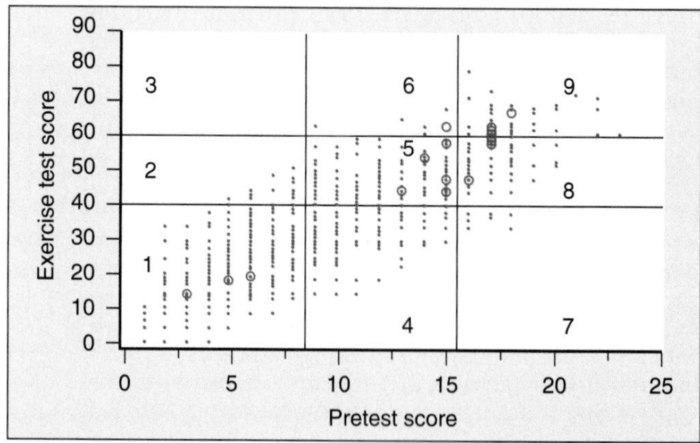

FIGURE 10–23 Scatter plot of exercise score as a function of pretest score for 1678 women referred for exercise testing. Points for those alive (closed circles) and dead (open circles) are shown. Heavy gridlines represent cutpoints for low-intermediate and intermediate-high risk groups for each score. Lowest risk patients (lowest pretest risk and lowest exercise score) are in sector 1 and highest risk patients (highest pretest risk and highest exercise score) in sector 9. Mortality after a mean 2.6-year follow-up was greatest in women with at least an intermediate pretest clinical score and exercise test score. Clinical variables include age, symptoms, diabetes, smoking, and estrogen status. Exercise ECG score variables include ST depression, peak heart rate, and Duke angina index. (From Morise AP, Lauer MS, Froelicher VF: Development and validation of a simple exercise test score for use in women with symptoms of suspected heart disease. Am Heart J 144:818, 2002.)

blood pressure response to 214 mm Hg or greater or an elevated systolic or diastolic blood pressure at the third minute of recovery is associated with significant increased long-term risk of hypertension (Fig. 10–24).[35,107,108] Severe systemic hypertension may interfere with subendocardial perfusion and cause exercise-induced ST segment depression in the absence of atherosclerosis, even when the resting ECG does not show significant ST or T wave changes. Beta- and calcium channel blocking drugs decrease submaximal and peak systolic blood pressure in many hypertensive patients. Exercise tolerance is decreased in patients with poor blood pressure control.

ELDERLY PATIENTS. Maximal aerobic capacity ($\dot{V}O_2max$) declines 8 to 10 percent per decade in sedentary men and women, with an approximately 50 percent reduction in exercise capacity between the ages of 30 and 80 years.[1,2,63] The exercise protocol in elderly patients should be selected according to estimated aerobic capacity. In patients with limited exercise tolerance, the test should be started at the slowest speed with a 0 percent grade and adjusted according to the patient's ability. Older patients may need to grasp the handrails for support. The frequency of abnormal exercise ECG patterns is greater in older than in younger individuals, and the risk of cardiac events is significantly increased because of a concomitant increase in prevalence of more extensive CAD.[1,2,40,109,110] The greater test sensitivity of the exercise ECG in elderly individuals is accompanied by a slight reduction in specificity. Cardiac arrhythmias, chronotropic incompetence, and hypertensive responses are more common in older individuals. The value of exercise testing to estimate prognosis in elderly subjects was evaluated in 3107 patients from Olmstead County, of whom 512 were 65 years of age or older. Workload expressed in METs was the only variable associated with all-cause mortality in subjects 65 years of age or older, whereas workload and exercise-induced angina were predictive of cardiac death or nonfatal myocardial infarction.[110] In elderly subjects 75 years of age or older, the Duke treadmill scoring system is less effective in estimating prognosis.[63] Most elderly patients tend to be categorized as intermediate risk, primarily because they cannot exercise long enough to be classified as low risk.

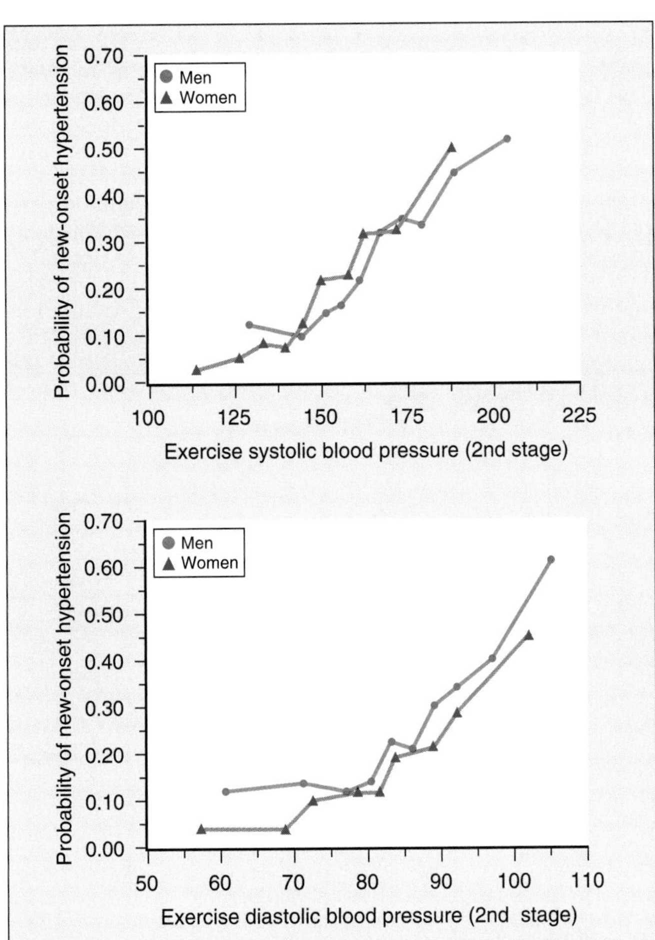

FIGURE 10–24 Probability of developing systemic hypertension within 8 years after exercise testing as a function of exercise-induced systolic **(top)** and diastolic **(bottom)** blood pressure responses in men and women. Crude probabilities of developing hypertension are displayed for mean systolic or diastolic blood pressure value for each exercise response during the second stage of treadmill testing. (From Singh JP, Larson MG, Manolio TA, et al: Blood pressure response during treadmill testing is a risk factor for new onset hypertension. The Framingham Heart Study. Circulation 99:1831, 1999.)

DIABETES MELLITUS. Coronary atherosclerosis and peripheral vascular disease are significantly increased in adult diabetic patients as compared with nondiabetic patients (see Chap. 51); the likelihood of atherosclerosis correlates closely with the duration of diabetes and the presence of microvascular disease, peripheral vascular disease, and autonomic neuropathy.[111] In patients with autonomic dysfunction and sensory neuropathy, anginal threshold may be increased, and abnormal exercise-induced heart rate and blood pressure responses are common. Once CAD is established, the incidence of exercise-induced ECG changes is similar to the incidence in nondiabetic persons.[112] The probability of an adverse cardiac outcome in a diabetic person as compared with a nondiabetic person for a similar abnormal exercise test result is likely to be increased because of the increased risk of dyslipidemia, impaired fibrinolysis, and hypertension associated with the diabetic process. Patients with diabetes who wish to enroll in a moderate- to high-intensity exercise program are considered to have a class IIa indication for exercise testing.[1] Further research is required to determine optimal noninvasive test procedures to diagnose early endothelial dysfunction and the presence and extent of obstructive CAD in patients with diabetes.

VALVULAR HEART DISEASE AND HYPERTROPHIC CARDIOMYOPATHY. The hemodynamics of exercise provide an excellent opportunity to measure gradients across stenotic valves, to assess ventricular function in patients with primary valvular regurgitation or mixed lesions, and to assess pulmonary and systemic vascular resistance (see Chap. 57).[113-115] The use of echocardiographic Doppler techniques (see Chap. 11) is particularly valuable in evaluating patients whose symptoms are out of proportion to the degree of hemodynamic abnormalities observed at rest and in assessing the results of valvulotomy or valve replacement. Clinical and exercise noninvasive assessment of patients with valvular heart disease can provide useful information on the timing of operative intervention and help achieve a more precise estimate of a patient's degree of incapacitation than can assessment of symptoms alone.[114] Studies of adults with moderate to severe aortic stenosis (e.g., valve area 0.5 to 1.5 cm^2 and mean gradients of 18 to 64 mm Hg) show that exercise testing can be safely performed when appropriate exercise protocols and precautions are used. Exercise testing is useful in evaluating aortic valve gradients during low-output flow states and with Doppler echocardiography provides important data on left ventricular functional reserve. Hypotension during exercise in asymptomatic patients with aortic stenosis may be a sufficient reason to consider valve replacement.[113] In patients with mitral stenosis, excessive heart rate response to relatively low levels of exercise, reduction of cardiac output with exercise (manifested by exercise-induced hypotension), and chest pain (ischemia secondary to low output or pulmonary hypertension) are indicators that favor earlier valve repair. In patients with mitral valve prolapse without regurgitation at rest, exercise-induced mitral regurgitation has been associated with the subsequent development of progressive mitral regurgitation, heart failure symptoms, or syncope.

Peak $\dot{V}O_2$ and anaerobic threshold are reduced in symptomatic patients with hypertrophic cardiomyopathy as compared with sedentary subjects (see Chap. 59). In a 50-patient series of hypertrophic cardiomyopathy, 59 percent of symptomatic subjects were unable to achieve a peak $\dot{V}O_2$ of 60 percent of predicted; only two patients achieved a peak $\dot{V}O_2$ greater than 80 percent of predicted.[116] Inability to increase blood pressure by 20 mm Hg during exercise may result from exercise-induced left ventricular systolic dysfunction and is associated with an adverse prognosis.[117] Abnormal blood pressure responses in patients with hypertrophic cardiomyopathy may normalize after transcoronary alcohol septal ablation, associated with only a slight increase in exercise time.[118]

CORONARY REVASCULARIZATION

CORONARY BYPASS GRAFTING (see Chap. 50). The degree of improvement in exercise-induced myocardial ischemia and aerobic capacity after coronary bypass grafting depends in part on the degree of revascularization achieved and on left ventricular function. Exercise-induced ischemic ST segment depression may persist when incomplete revascularization is achieved, albeit at higher exercise workloads. It also may persist in approximately 5 percent of patients in whom complete revascularization has been achieved. It usually takes at least 6 weeks of convalescence before maximum exercise can be performed. The natural history of saphenous vein grafts and internal mammary artery conduits is different, and serial conversion from an initially normal to an abnormal exercise ECG result over time depends in part on the type of conduit used and on CAD progression in nongrafted vessels. Stress imaging studies are likely to provide more useful information regarding the site and extent of myocardial ischemia after coronary revascularization procedures than the exercise electrocardiogram and are the preferred modality when noninvasive testing is performed for management decisions. The diagnostic and prognostic utility of exercise testing late after coronary revascularization (e.g., 5 to 10 years) is much greater than early (<1 year) testing, because a late abnormal exercise response is more likely to indicate graft occlusion, stenosis, or progression of CAD, particularly in the presence of typical angina or conditions of accelerated atherosclerosis such as diabetes mellitus, hemodialysis, or immunosuppressive therapy.[119] In selected patients with severe left ventricular dysfunction and symptomatic heart failure, coronary bypass surgery is associated with a significant increase in exercise capacity when a large amount of dysfunctional but viable myocardium (e.g., >25% of left ventricular mass) is revascularized.[120]

PERCUTANEOUS CORONARY INTERVENTION (see Chap. 52). The risk of restenosis after percutaneous coronary intervention (PCI) is time dependent; stent restenosis usually occurs within the first 12 months after PCI, and it is anticipated that rates of restenosis will be greatly reduced with the use of drug-eluting stents. In the early post-PCI phase (<1 month), an abnormal exercise ECG result may be secondary to a suboptimal result, impaired coronary vascular reserve in a successfully dilated vessel, or incomplete revascularization.[30,121-123] Thus, exercise electrocardiography has a low diagnostic accuracy to detect restenosis or an incomplete dilation in the periprocedural phase. The optimal time to perform an exercise test after PCI depends in part on the success of the procedure and the degree of revascularization obtained. In an otherwise asymptomatic patient, a 6- to 12-month postprocedure test allows sufficient time to document restenosis should it occur and allows the dilated vessel an opportunity to heal. Serial conversion of an initially normal exercise test result after PCI to an abnormal result in the initial 6 months after the procedure, particularly when it occurs at a lower exercise workload, is usually associated with restenosis. The use of exercise myocardial imaging in selected patients enhances the diagnostic content of the test and can help localize the territory of myocardial ischemia and guide indications for repeat coronary angiography in patients who have undergone multivessel/multilesion PCI. In general, routine periodic monitoring of asymptomatic patients after a coronary revascularization procedure (coronary artery bypass grafting or PCI) without a specific indication is not useful.

CARDIAC TRANSPLANTATION (see Chap. 26). Cardiopulmonary exercise testing is useful in selecting patients with end-stage heart failure for cardiac transplantation. A peak $\dot{V}O_2$ of less than 12 to 14 ml O_2/kg/min or 40 to 50 percent of predicted $\dot{V}O_2$ is associated with 2-year survival rates ranging from 30 to 50 percent (Fig. 10–25).[84] The use of percentage of predicted $\dot{V}O_2$, which adjusts an individual patient's peak $\dot{V}O_2$ for age, gender, and weight rather than weight alone, has been shown to further enhance prognostic estimates in patients who have a low peak exercise $\dot{V}O_2$. In patients with initial poor exercise capacity awaiting heart transplantation, the ability to increase peak oxygen uptake with increased peak oxygen pulse identifies a relatively lower risk group in whom cardiac transplantation may be able to be deferred if the patient's clinical status is stable.

Exercise performance in transplant recipients is influenced by the fact that the donor heart is surgically denervated without efferent parasympathetic or sympathetic innervation and by the occurrence of rejection and scar formation, systemic and pulmonary vascular resistance, level of training, and development of coronary atherosclerosis in the graft.[124] Maximal oxygen uptake and work capacity are reduced after cardiac transplantation compared with measures in age-matched control subjects but usually are markedly improved compared with preoperative findings.[125] Abnormalities of the ventricular rate response include a resting tachycardia due to parasympathetic denervation, a slow heart rate response during mild to moderate exercise, a more rapid response during more strenuous exercise, and a more prolonged time for the ventricular rate to return to baseline during recovery. The transplanted heart relies heavily on the Frank-Starling mechanism to increase cardiac output during mild to moderate exercise. Systemic vascular resistance may be increased because of cyclosporine therapy. Sympathetic reinnervation of the sinus node may occur after cardiac transplantation and partially restore a normal heart rate response to exercise, but in most patients will not return exercise capacity to normal.[126] The exercise ECG is relatively insensitive in detecting coronary artery vasculopathy after cardiac transplantation.

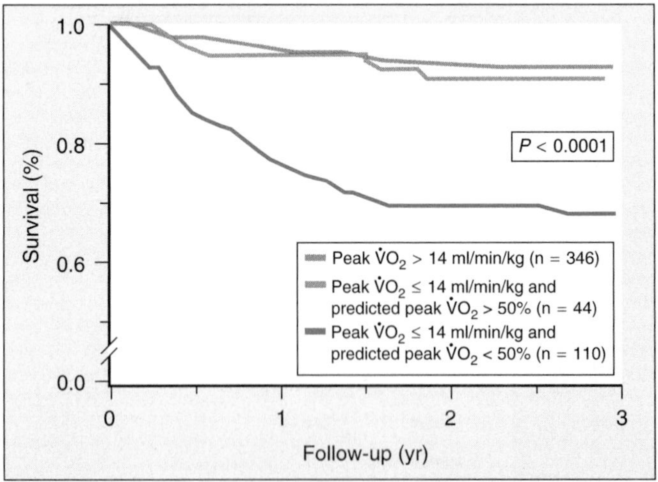

FIGURE 10–25 The 3-year survival of patients with congestive heart failure referred for cardiac transplant evaluation with a peak $\dot{V}O_2$ of 14 ml O_2/kg/min or less stratified according to predicted peak $\dot{V}O_2$ greater than 50 percent or less. The 91 ± 5 percent 3-year survival rate of the 44 patients with a predicted $\dot{V}O_2$ greater than 50 percent was similar to the survival rates of patients with a peak $\dot{V}O_2$ greater than 14 ml O_2/kg/min and significantly greater than the 61 ± 5 percent survival rate of the 110 patients with a peak $\dot{V}O_2$ of 50 percent or less. The data indicate that a low peak $\dot{V}O_2$ and percentage predicted $\dot{V}O_2$ identify high-risk patients with congestive heart failure whose survival may be improved by cardiac transplantation. (From Osada N, Chaitman BR, Miller LW, et al: Cardiopulmonary exercise testing identifies low risk patients with heart failure and severely impaired exercise capacity considered for heart transplantation. J Am Coll Cardiol 31:577, 1998.)

However, the new development of an abnormal exercise ECG result several years after cardiac transplantation may indicate focal intraluminal narrowing.

Safety and Risks of Exercise Testing

Exercise testing has an excellent safety record. The risk is determined by the clinical characteristics of the patient referred for the procedure. In nonselected patient populations, the mortality is less than 0.01 percent and morbidity is less than 0.05 percent.[127] The risk is greater when the test is performed soon after an acute ischemic event. In a survey of 151,941 tests conducted within 4 weeks of an acute myocardial infarction, mortality was 0.03 percent, and 0.09 percent of patients tested either had a nonfatal reinfarction or were resuscitated from cardiac arrest.[128] The relative risk of a major complication is about twice as great when a symptom-limited protocol is used as compared with a low-level protocol. Nevertheless, in the early postinfarction phase, the risk of a fatal complication during symptom-limited testing is only 0.03 percent. The risk is less for low-risk patients who are seen in the emergency department and who undergo exercise testing for risk stratification. Exercise testing can be safely performed in patients with compensated congestive heart failure, with no major complications reported in 1286 tests in which a bicycle ergometer was used.[129] The risk of exercise testing in patients referred for life-threatening ventricular arrhythmias was examined by Young and colleagues[130] in a series of 263 patients who underwent 1377 tests; 2.2 percent developed sustained ventricular tachyarrhythmias that required cardioversion, cardiopulmonary resuscitation, or antiarrhythmic drugs to restore sinus rhythm. The ventricular arrhythmias were more frequent in tests performed on antiarrhythmic drug therapy as compared with the baseline drug-free state. In contrast to the high risk in the aforementioned patient subsets, the risk of complications in asymptomatic subjects is extremely low, with no fatalities reported in several series.[1,7,8]

The risk of incurring a major complication during exercise testing can be reduced by performing a careful history and physical examination before the test and observing patients closely during exercise with monitoring of the ECG, arterial pressure, and symptoms. The standard 12-lead ECG should be verified before the test for any acute or recent changes. The contraindications to exercise testing are well defined (Table 10–4). Patients with critical obstruction to left ventricular outflow are at increased risk of cardiac events during exercise. In selected patients, low-level exercise can be useful in determining the severity of the left ventricular outflow tract obstruction. The cool-down period should be prolonged to at least 2 minutes in patients with left ventricular outflow tract obstruction or stenotic valves to avoid sudden pressure-volume shifts that occur in the immediate postexercise phase.

Uncontrolled systemic hypertension is a contraindication to exercise testing. Patients should continue antihypertensive drug therapy on the day of testing. Patients who present with systemic arterial pressure readings of 220/120 mm Hg or greater should rest for 15 to 20 minutes, and their blood pressure should be remeasured. If blood pressure remains at these levels, the test should be postponed until the hypertension is better controlled.

A resuscitator cart and defibrillator should be available in the room where the test procedure is carried out, and appropriate cardioactive medication should be available to treat cardiac arrhythmias, AV block, hypotension, and persistent chest pain. An intravenous line should be started in high-risk patients such as those being tested for adequacy of control of life-threatening ventricular arrhythmias. The equipment and supplies in the cart should be checked on a regular basis. A previously specified routine for cardiac emergencies needs to be determined; this includes patient transfer and admission to a coronary care unit if necessary.

Clinical judgment is required to determine which patients can be safely tested in an office as opposed to a hospital-based setting. The experience is acquired through training programs and maintenance of clinical competency.[131,132] High-risk patients, such as those with major left ventricular dysfunction, recent angina pectoris, cardiac syncope, or important ventricular ectopy on the pretest examination, should be tested in the hospital. Low-risk patients, such as asymptomatic individuals and those with a low pretest risk of disease, can be tested by specially trained nurses or physician assistants who have received advanced cardiac life support certification, with a physician in close proximity.

Termination of Exercise

The use of standard test indications to terminate an exercise test reduces risk (Table 10–5). Termination of exercise should be determined in part by the patient's recent activity level. The rate of perceived patient exertion can be estimated by the Borg scale. The scale is linear, with values of 9 for very light; 11 for fairly light; 13 for somewhat hard; 15 for hard; 17 for very hard; and 19 for very, very hard. Borg readings of 14 to 16 approximate anaerobic threshold, and readings of 18 or greater approximate a patient's maximum exercise capacity. It is helpful to grade exercise-induced chest discomfort on a 1 to 4 scale, with 1 indicating the initial onset of chest discomfort and 4 the most severe chest pain the patient has ever experienced. The exercise technician should note the onset of grade 1 chest discomfort on the work sheet, and the test should be stopped when the patient reports grade 3 chest pain. In the absence of symptoms, it is prudent to stop exercise when a patient demonstrates 0.3 mV (3 mm) or greater of ischemic ST segment depression or 0.1 mV (1 mm) or greater of ST segment elevation in a noninfarct lead without an abnormal Q wave. Significant worsening of ambient ventricular ectopy during exercise or the unsuspected appearance of ventricular tachycardia is an indication to terminate exercise. A progressive, reproducible decrease in systolic blood pressure of 10 mm Hg or more may indicate transient left ventricular dysfunction or an inappropriate decrease in systemic vascular resistance and is an indication to terminate exercise. The test should be stopped if the arterial blood pressure is 250 to 270/120 to 130 mm Hg or higher. Ataxia can indicate cerebral hypoxia.

The exercise test report should contain basic demographic data, the indication for testing, a brief description of the patient's profile, and exercise test results (Table 10–6).

TABLE 10–4 Absolute Contraindications to Exercise Testing
Acute myocardial infarction (<2 d)
High-risk unstable angina
Decompensated heart failure
Uncontrolled cardiac arrhythmias with symptoms or hemodynamic compromise
Advanced atrioventricular block
Acute myocarditis or pericarditis
Severe symptomatic aortic stenosis
Severe hypertrophic obstructive cardiomyopathy
Uncontrolled hypertension
Acute systemic illness (pulmonary embolism, aortic dissection)

TABLE 10–5 Indications for Terminating Exercise Testing

Absolute indications Drop in systolic blood pressure of >10 mm Hg from baseline blood pressure despite an increase in workload, when accompanied by other evidence of ischemia
Moderate to severe angina (grade 3/4)
Increasing nervous system symptoms (e.g., ataxia, dizziness, or near-syncope)
Signs of poor perfusion (cyanosis or pallor)
Technical difficulties in monitoring ECG or systolic blood pressure
Subject's desire to stop
Sustained ventricular tachycardia
ST elevation (≥1.0 mm) in noninfarct leads without diagnostic Q waves (other than V_1 or aV)
Relative indications Drop in systolic blood pressure of ≥10 mm Hg from baseline blood pressure despite an increase in workload, in the absence of other evidence of ischemia
ST or QRS changes such as excessive ST depression (>3 mm of horizontal or downsloping ST segment depression) or marked axis shift
Arrhythmias other than sustained ventricular tachycardia, including multifocal PVCs, triplets of PVCs, supraventricular tachycardia, heart block, or bradyarrhythmias
Fatigue, shortness of breath, wheezing, leg cramps, or claudication
Development of bundle branch block of intraventricular conduction delay that cannot be distinguished from ventricular tachyardia
Increasing chest pain
Hypertensive response

ECG = electrocardiogram; PVCs = premature ventricular contractions.
Modified from Fletcher GF: Exercise standards: A standard for healthcare professionals from the American Heart Association Writing Group. Circulation 91:580, 1995.

TABLE 10–6 Exercise Test Report Information

Demographic data: name, patient identifier, date of birth/age, gender, weight, height, test date
Indication(s) for test
Patient descriptors: atherosclerotic risk profile, drug usage, resting ECG findings
Exercise test results
Protocol used
Reason(s) for stopping exercise
Hemodynamic data: rest and peak heart rate, rest and peak blood pressure, percent maximum achieved heart rate, maximum rate of perceived exertion (Borg scale), peak workload, peak METs, total exercise duration in minutes
Evidence for myocardial ischemia: time to onset and offset of ischemic ST segment deviation or angina, maximum depth of ST segment deviation, number of abnormal exercise ECG leads, abnormal systemic blood pressure responses
General comments

ECG = electrocardiogram; METs = metabolic equivalents.

REFERENCES

1. Gibbons RJ, Balady GJ, Bricker JT, et al: ACC/AHA 2002 guideline update for exercise testing. Summary article: A report of the ACC/AHA Task Force on Practice Guidelines (Committee to Update the 1997 Exercise Testing Guidelines). J Am Coll Cardiol 40:1531, 2002.
2. Fletcher GF, Balady GJ, Amsterdam EA, et al: Exercise standards for testing and training: A statement for healthcare professionals from the American Heart Association. Circulation 104:1694, 2001.
3. Balady GJ, Berra KA, Golding LA, et al: ACSM's Guidelines for Exercise Testing and Prescription. 6th ed. Philadelphia, Lippincott Williams & Wilkins, 2000.
4. Wasserman K, Hansen JE, Sue DY, et al: Principles of Exercise Testing and Interpretation. 3rd ed. Philadelphia, Lippincott Williams & Wilkins, 1999.
5. American Thoracic Society/American College of Chest Physicians: Statement on cardiopulmonary exercise testing. Am J Respir Crit Care Med 167:211, 2003.
6. Hadeli KO, Siegel EM, Sherrill DL, et al: Predictors of oxygen desaturation during submaximal exercise in 8,000 patients. Chest 120:88, 2001.
7. Ellestad MH: Stress Testing: Principles and Practice. 4th ed. Philadelphia, FA Davis, 1996.
8. Froelicher VF, Myers J: Exercise and the Heart. 4th ed. Philadelphia, W.B. Saunders, 2000.
9. Fletcher GF, Flipse TR, Kligfield P, et al: Current status of ECG stress testing. Curr Probl Cardiol 23:353, 1998.
10. Fleg JL, Pina IL, Balady GJ, et al: Assessment of functional capacity in clinical and research applications: An advisory from the Committee on Exercise, Rehabilitation, and Prevention, Council on Clinical Cardiology, American Heart Association. Circulation 102:1591, 2000.
11. Pollock ML, Franklin BA, Balady GJ, et al: AHA Science Advisory. Resistance exercise in individuals with and without cardiovascular disease: Benefits, rationale, safety, and prescription. An advisory from the Committee on Exercise, Rehabilitation, and Prevention, Council on Clinical Cardiology, American Heart Association. Position paper endorsed by the American College of Sports Medicine. Circulation 101:828, 2000.

Exercise Physiology

12. Guyton AC, Hall JE: Textbook of Medical Physiology. 10th ed. Philadelphia, WB Saunders, 2000.
13. Correia LCL, Lakatta EG, O'Connor FC, et al: Attenuated cardiovascular reserve during prolonged submaximal cycle exercise in healthy older subjects. J Am Coll Cardiol 40:1290, 2002.
14. Williams MA, Fleg JL, Ades PA, et al: Secondary prevention of coronary heart disease in the elderly (with emphasis on patients ≥75 years of age): An American Heart Association scientific statement from the Council on Clinical Cardiology Subcommittee on Exercise, Cardiac Rehabilitation, and Prevention. Circulation 105:1735, 2002.
15. Tanaka H, Monahan KD, Seals DR: Age-predicted maximal heart rate revisited. J Am Coll Cardiol 37:153, 2001.
16. Gonzalez-Alonso J, Calbet JA: Reductions in systemic and skeletal muscle blood flow and oxygen delivery limit maximal aerobic capacity in humans. Circulation 107:824, 2003.
17. Hollenberg M, Tager IB: Oxygen uptake efficiency slope: An index of exercise performance and cardiopulmonary reserve requiring only submaximal exercise. J Am Coll Cardiol 36:194, 2000.
18. Montgomery PS, Gardner AW: The clinical utility of a six-minute walk test in peripheral arterial occlusive disease patients. J Am Geriatr Soc 46:706, 1998.
19. Badruddin SM, Ahmad A, Mickelson J, et al: Supine bicycle versus post-treadmill exercise echocardiography in the detection of myocardial ischemia: A randomized single-blind crossover trial. J Am Coll Cardiol 33:1485, 1999.

Electrocardiographic Measures

20. Michaelides AP, Psomadaki ZD, Dilaveris PE, et al: Improved detection of coronary artery disease by exercise electrocardiography with the use of right precordial leads. N Engl J Med 340:340, 1999.
21. Sabapathy R, Bloom HL, Lewis WR, Amsterdam EA: Right precordial and posterior chest leads do not increase detection of positive response in electrocardiogram during exercise treadmill testing. Am J Cardiol 91:75, 2003.
22. Rywik TM, Zink RC, Gittings NS, et al: Independent prognostic significance of ischemic ST segment response limited to recovery from treadmill exercise in asymptomatic subjects. Circulation 97:2117, 1998.
23. Soto JR, Watson DD, Beller GA.: Incidence and significance of ischemic ST-segment depression occurring solely during recovery after exercise testing. Am J Cardiol 88:670, 2001.
24. Akutsu Y, Shinozuka A, Nishimura H, et al: Significance of ST-segment morphology noted on electrocardiography during the recovery phase after exercise in patients with ischemic heart disease as analyzed with simultaneous dual-isotope single photon emission tomography. Am Heart J 144:335, 2002.
25. Fearon WF, Lee DP, Froelicher VF: The effect of resting ST segment depression on the diagnostic characteristics of exercise treadmill testing. J Am Coll Cardiol 35:1206, 2000.
26. Mobilia G, Zanco P, Desideri A, et al: T wave normalization in infarct-related electrocardiographic leads during exercise testing for detection of residual viability: Comparison with positron emission tomography. J Am Coll Cardiol 32:75, 1998.
27. Miwa K, Nakagawa K, Hirai T, Inoue H: Exercise-induced U-wave alterations as a marker of well-developed and well-functioning collateral vessels in patients with effort angina. J Am Coll Cardiol 35:757, 2000.
28. Okin PM, Prineas RJ, Grandits G, et al: Heart rate adjustment of exercise induced ST segment depression identifies men who benefit from a risk factor reduction program. Circulation 96:2899, 1997.

29. Julius BK, Vassalli G, Mandinov L, Hess OM: Alpha-adrenoreceptor blockade prevents exercise-induced vasoconstriction of stenotic coronary arteries. J Am Coll Cardiol 33:1499, 1999.
30. Maier W, Windecker S, Kung A, et al: Exercise-induced coronary artery vasodilation is not impaired by stent placement. Circulation 105:2373, 2002.
31. Kelion AD, Webb TP, Gardner MA, Ormerod OJM, Banning AP: The warm-up effect protects against ischemic left ventricular dysfunction in patients with angina. J Am Coll Cardiol 37:705, 2001.
32. Bogaty P, Poirier P, Boyer L, et al: What induces the warm-up ischemia/angina phenomenon: Exercise or myocardial ischemia? Circulation 107:1858, 2003.
33. Lambiase PD, Edwards RJ, Cusack MR, et al: Exercise-induced ischemia initiates the second window of protection in humans independent of collateral recruitment. J Am Coll Cardiol 41:1174, 2003.
34. Li RA, Leppo M, Miki T, et al: Molecular basis of electrocardiographic ST-segment elevation. Circ Res 87:837, 2000.

Nonelectrocardiographic Measures

35. Miyai N, Arita M, Miyashita K, et al: Blood pressure response to heart rate during exercise test and risk of future hypertension. Hypertension 39:761, 2002.
36. Reman A, Zelos G, Andrews NP, et al: Blood pressure changes during transient myocardial ischemia: Insights into mechanisms. J Am Coll Cardiol 30:1249, 1997.
37. Fleg JL, Lakatta EG: Prevalence and significance of postexercise hypotension in apparently healthy subjects. Am J Cardiol 57:1380, 1986.
38. Ha JW, Juracan EM, Mahoney DW, et al: Hypertensive response to exercise: A potential cause for new wall motion abnormality in the absence of coronary artery disease. J Am Coll Cardiol 39:323, 2002.
39. Myers J, Prakash M, Froelicher V, et al: Exercise capacity and mortality among men referred for exercise testing. N Engl J Med 346:793, 2002.
40. Spin JM, Prakash M, Froelicher VF, et al: The prognostic value of exercise testing in elderly men. Am J Med 112:453, 2002.
41. Florenciano-Sanchez R, Castillo-Moreno JA, Molina-Laborda E, et al: The exercise test that indicates a low risk of events. Differences in prognostic significance between patients with chronic stable angina and patients with unstable angina. J Am Coll Cardiol 38:1974, 2001.
42. Miller TD, Chaliki HP, Christian TF, et al: Usefulness of worsening clinical status or exercise performance in predicting future events in patients with coronary artery disease. Am J Cardiol 88:1294, 2001.
43. Lauer MS, Francis GS, Okin PM, et al: Impaired chronotropic response to exercise stress testing as a predictor of mortality. JAMA 281:524, 1999.
44. Elhendy A, Mahoney DW, Khandheria BK, et al: Prognostic significance of impairment of heart rate response to exercise: Impact of left ventricular function and myocardial ischemia. J Am Coll Cardiol 42:823, 2003.
45. Chaitman BR: Abnormal heart rate responses to exercise predict increased long-term mortality regardless of coronary disease extent. The question is why? J Am Coll Cardiol 42:2049, 2003.
46. Shetler K, Marcus R, Froelicher VF, et al: Heart rate recovery: Validation and methodologic issues. J Am Coll Cardiol 38:1980, 2001.
47. Vivekananthan DP, Blackstone EH, Pothier CE, Lauer MS: Heart rate recovery after exercise is a predictor of mortality, independent of the angiographic severity of coronary disease. J Am Coll Cardiol 42:831, 2003.

Diagnostic Applications

48. Gibbons RJ, Abrams J, Chatterjee K, et al: ACC/AHA 2002 guideline update for the management of patients with chronic stable angina: A report of the American College of Cardiology/American Heart Association Task Force on Practice Guidelines (Committee to update the 1999 Guidelines for the Management of Patients with Chronic Stable Angina). 2002. (http://www.acc.org/clinical/guidelines/stable/stable.pdf)
49. Danzi GB, Pirelli S, Mauri L, et al: Which variable of stenosis severity best describes the significance of an isolated left anterior descending artery lesion? Correlation between quantitative coronary angiography, intracoronary Doppler measurements and high dose dipyridamole echocardiography. J Am Coll Cardiol 31:526, 1998.
50. Schulman SP, Lasorda D, Farah T, et al: Correlations between coronary flow reserve measured with a Doppler guide wire and treadmill exercise testing. Am Heart J 134:99, 1997.
51. Nishioka T, Amanullah AM, Luo H, et al: Clinical validation of intravascular ultrasound imaging for assessment of coronary stenosis severity. J Am Coll Cardiol 33:1870, 1999.
52. Panting JR, Gatehouse PD, Yang GZ, et al: Abnormal subendocardial perfusion in cardiac syndrome X detected by cardiovascular magnetic resonance imaging. N Engl J Med 346:1948, 2002.
53. Froelicher VF, Lehmann KG, Thomas R: Veterans Affairs Cooperative Study in Health Services #016 (QUEXTA) Study Group. The electrocardiographic exercise test in a population with reduced workup bias: Diagnostic performance, computerized interpretation and multivariable prediction. Ann Intern Med 128:965, 1998.
54. Froelicher V, Shetler K, Ashley E: Better decisions through science: Exercise testing scores. Prog Cardiovasc Dis 44:395, 2002.
55. Morise AP, Lauer MS, Froelicher VF: Development and validation of a simple exercise test score for use in women with symptoms of suspected coronary artery disease. Am Heart J 144:818, 2002.

Prognostic Applications

56. Rywik TM, O'Connor FC, Gittings NS, et al: Role of nondiagnostic exercise-induced ST-segment abnormalities in predicting future coronary events in asymptomatic volunteers. Circulation 106:2787, 2002.
57. Laukkanen JA, Kurl S, Lakka TA, et al: Exercise-induced silent myocardial ischemia and coronary morbidity and mortality in middle-aged men. J Am Coll Cardiol 38:72, 2001.
58. Blumenthal RS, Becker DM, Yanek LR, et al: Detecting occult coronary disease in a high-risk asymptomatic population. Circulation 107:702, 2003.
59. Greenland P, Smith SC, Grundy SM: Improving coronary heart disease risk assessment in asymptomatic people: Role of traditional risk factors and noninvasive cardiovascular tests. Circulation 104:1863, 2001.
60. Weiner DH, Ryan T, McCabe CH, et al: Prognostic importance of a clinical profile and exercise test in medically treated patients with coronary artery disease. J Am Coll Cardiol 3:772, 1984.
61. Mark DB, Hlatky MA, Harrell FE, et al: Exercise treadmill score for predicting prognosis in coronary heart disease. Ann Intern Med 106:793, 1987.
62. Mark DB, Shaw L, Harrell FE Jr, et al: Prognostic value of a treadmill exercise score in outpatients with suspected coronary artery disease. N Engl J Med 325:849, 1991.
63. Kwok JMF, Miller TD, Hodge DO, Gibbons RJ: Prognostic value of the Duke treadmill score in the elderly. J Am Coll Cardiol 39:1475, 2002.
64. Morise AP, Haddad WJ, Beckner D: Development and validation of a clinical score to estimate the probability of coronary artery disease in men and women presenting with suspected coronary disease. Am J Cardiol 102:350, 1997.
65. Stone PH, Chaitman BR, Forman S, et al: Prognostic significance of myocardial ischemia detected by ambulatory electrocardiogram, exercise treadmill testing, and resting electrocardiogram to predict cardiac events by 1 year (the Asymptomatic Cardiac Ischemia Pilot [ACIP] Study). Am J Cardiol 80:1395, 1997.
66. Safstrom K, Nielsen NE, Bjorkholm A, et al: Unstable coronary artery disease in postmenopausal women: Identifying patients with significant coronary artery disease by basic clinical parameters and exercise test. Eur Heart J 19:899, 1998.
67. Braunwald E, Antman EM, Beasley JW, et al: ACC/AHA 2002 guideline update for the management of patients with unstable angina and non-ST-segment elevation myocardial infarction: A report of the American College of Cardiology/American Heart Association Task Force on Practice Guidelines (Committee on the Management of Patients With Unstable Angina). 2002. (http://www.acc.org/clnical/guidelines/unstable/unstable.pdf)
68. Goyal A, Samaha FF, Boden WE, et al: Stress test criteria used in the conservative arm of the FRISC-II trial underdetects surgical coronary artery disease when applied to patients in the VANQWISH trial. J Am Coll Cardiol 39:1601, 2002.
69. Stein RA, Chaitman BR, Balady GJ, et al: Safety and utility of exercise testing in emergency room chest pain centers: An advisory from the Committee on Exercise, Rehabilitation and Prevention, Council on Clinical Cardiology, American Heart Association. Circulation 102:1463, 2000.
70. Peterson ED, Shaw L, Califf RM, et al: Risk stratification after myocardial infarction. Ann Intern Med 126:561, 1997.
71. Senaratne MP, Smith G, Gulamhusein SS: Feasibility and safety of early exercise testing using the Bruce protocol after acute myocardial infarction. J Am Coll Cardiol 35:1212, 2000.
72. Nakano A, Lee JD, Shimizu H, et al: Reciprocal ST segment depression associated with exercise induced ST-segment elevation indicates residual viability after myocardial infarction. J Am Coll Cardiol 33:620, 1999.
73. de Filippi CR, Rosanio S, Tocchi M, et al: Randomized comparison of a strategy of predischarge coronary angiography versus exercise testing in low-risk patients in a chest pain unit: In-hospital and long-term outcomes. J Am Coll Cardiol 37:2050, 2001.
74. Diercks DB, Gibler B, Liu T, et al: Identification of patients at risk by graded exercise testing in an emergency department chest pain center. Am J Cardiol 86:289, 2000.
75. Amsterdam EA, Kirk JD, Diercks DB, et al: Immediate exercise testing to evaluate low-risk patients presenting to the emergency department with chest pain. J Am Coll Cardiol 40:251, 2002.
76. Farkouh ME, Smars PA, Reeder GS, et al: A clinical trial comparing a chest pain observation unit with routine admission in patients with unstable angina. N Engl J Med 339:1882, 1999.
77. Eagle KA, Berger PB, Calkins H, et al: ACC/AHA guidelines for perioperative cardiovascular evaluation for noncardiac surgery update: executive summary: A report of the American College of Cardiology/American Heart Association Task Force on Practice Guidelines (Committee to Update the 1996 Guidelines on Perioperative Cardiovascular Evaluation for Noncardiac Surgery). Circulation 105:1257, 2002.
78. Chaitman BR, Miller DD: Perioperative cardiac evaluation for noncardiac surgery noninvasive cardiac testing. Prog Cardiovasc Dis 40:405, 1998.
79. Best PJ, Tajik AJ, Gibbons RJ, et al: The safety of treadmill exercise stress testing in patients with abdominal aortic aneurysms. Ann Intern Med 129:628, 1998.
80. McGlade DP, Poon AB, Davies MJ: The use of a questionnaire and simple exercise test in the preoperative assessment of vascular surgery patients. Anaesth Intensive Care 29:520, 2001.
81. Pina IL, Apstein CS, Balady GJ, et al: Exercise and heart failure: A statement from the American Heart Association Committee on Exercise, Rehabilitation, and Prevention. Circulation 107:1210, 2003.
82. de Jonge N, Kirkels H, Lahpor JR, et al: Exercise performance in patients with end-stage heart failure after implantation of a left ventricular assist device and after heart transplantation: An outlook for permanent assisting? J Am Coll Cardiol 37:1794, 2001.
83. Wasserman K, Zhang YY, Gitt A, et al: Lung function and exercise gas exchange in chronic heart failure. Circulation 96:2221, 1997.
84. Osada N, Chaitman BR, Miller LW, et al: Cardiopulmonary exercise testing identifies low risk patients with heart failure and severely impaired exercise capacity considered for heart transplantation. J Am Coll Cardiol 31:582, 1998.
85. Duscha BD, Annex BH, Keteyian SJ, et al: Differences in skeletal muscle between men and women with chronic heart failure. J Appl Physiol 90:280, 2001.
86. Mancini DM, Katz SD, Lang CC, et al: Effect of erythropoietin on exercise capacity in patients with moderate to severe chronic heart failure. Circulation 107:294, 2003.
87. Duscha BD, Annex BH, Green HJ, Pikppen AM: Deconditioning fails to explain peripheral skeletal muscle alterations in men with chronic heart failure. J Am Coll Cardiol 39:1170, 2002.

88. Myers J, Gullestad L, Vagelos R, et al: Clinical, hemodynamic, and cardiopulmonary exercise test determinants of survival in patients referred for evaluation of heart failure. Ann Intern Med 129:293, 1998.
89. Belardinelli R, Georgiou D, Cianci G, et al: Randomized, controlled trial of long-term moderate exercise training in chronic heart failure. Effects on functional capacity, quality of life, and clinical outcome. Circulation 99:1173, 1999.
90. Metra M, Faggiano P, D'Aloia A, et al: Use of cardiopulmonary exercise testing with hemodynamic monitoring in the prognostic assessment of ambulatory patients with chronic heart failure. J Am Coll Cardiol 33:943, 1999.
91. Shah MR, Hasselblad V, Gheorghiade M, et al: Prognostic usefulness of the six-minute walk in patients with advanced congestive heart failure secondary to ischemic or nonischemic cardiomyopathy. Am J Cardiol 88:987, 2001.
92. Opasich C, Pinna GD, Mazza A, et al: Six-minute walking performance in patients with moderate-to-severe heart failure. Eur Heart J 22:488, 2001.

Arrhythmias and Conduction Disturbances

93. Frolkis JP, Pothier CE, Blackstone EH, Lauer MS: Frequent ventricular ectopy after exercise as a predictor of death. N Engl J Med 348:781, 2003.
94. Partington S, Myers J, Cho S, et al: Prevalence and prognostic value of exercise-induced ventricular arrhythmias. Am Heart J 145:139, 2003.
95. Takenaka K, Ai T, Shimizu W: Exercise stress test amplifies genotype-phenotype correlation in the LQT1 and LQT2 forms of the long-QT syndrome. Circulation 107:838, 2003.
96. Dillenburg RF, Hamilton RM: Is exercise testing useful in identifying congenital long QT syndrome? Am J Cardiol 89:233, 2002.
97. Grady TA, Chiu AC, Snader CE, et al: Prognostic significance of exercise-induced left bundle branch block. JAMA 279:153, 1998.
98. Shah PP, Nair M, Dhall A, et al: False-positive exercise stress electrocardiogram due to accessory pathway in the absence of manifest preexcitation. Pacing Clin Electrophysiol 23:1051, 2000.
99. Janosik DL: Effect of exercise on pacing hemodynamics. *In* Ellenbogen KA, Neal Kay G, Wilkoff BL (eds): Clinical Cardiac Pacing. 2nd ed. Philadelphia, WB Saunders, 1999.
100. Auricchio A, Kloss M, Trautmann SI, et al: Exercise performance following cardiac resynchronization therapy in patients with heart failure and ventricular conduction delay. Am J Cardiol 89:198, 2002.

Specific Clinical Applications

101. Chaitman BR: Measuring antianginal drug efficacy using exercise testing for chronic angina: Improved exercise performance with ranolazine, a pFOX inhibitor. Curr Probl Cardiol 27:527, 2002.
102. Bogaty P, Kingma JG Jr, Robitaille NM, et al: Attenuation of myocardial ischemia with repeated exercise in subjects with chronic stable angina: Relation to myocardial contractility, intensity of exercise and the adenosine triphosphate-sensitive potassium channel. J Am Coll Cardiol 32:1665, 1998.
103. Bokhari S, Bergmann SR: The effect of estrogen compared to estrogen plus progesterone on the exercise electrocardiogram. J Am Coll Cardiol 40:1092, 2002.
104. Henzlova MJ, Croft LB, Diamond JA: Effect of hormone replacement therapy on the electrocardiographic response to exercise. J Nucl Cardiol 9:385, 2002.
105. Roger VL, Jacobsen SJ, Pellika PA, et al: Gender differences in use of stress testing and coronary heart disease mortality: A population based study in Olmsted County, Minnesota. J Am Coll Cardiol 32:345, 1998.
106. Alexander KP, Shaw LJ, Delong ER, et al: Value of exercise treadmill testing in women. J Am Coll Cardiol 32:1657, 1998.
107. Singh JP, Larson MG, Manolio TA, et al: Blood pressure response during treadmill testing as a risk factor for new-onset hypertension. The Framingham Study. Circulation 99:1831, 1999.
108. Allison TG, Corderio MA, Miller TD, et al: Prognostic significance of exercise-induced systemic hypertension in healthy subjects. Am J Cardiol 83:371, 1999.
109. Era P, Schroll M, Hagerup L, Shult-Larsen Jurgensen K: Changes in bicycle ergometer test performance and survival in men and women from 50 to 60 and from 70 to 80 years of age: Two longitudinal studies in the Glostrup (Denmark) population. Gerontology 47:136, 2001.
110. Goraya TY, Jacobsen SJ, Pellikka PA, et al: Prognostic value of treadmill exercise testing in elderly persons. Ann Intern Med 132:862, 2000.
111. Rutter MK, McComb JM, Brady S, Marshall SM: Silent myocardial ischemia and microalbuminuria in asymptomatic subjects with non-insulin-dependent diabetes mellitus. Am J Cardiol 83:27, 1999.
112. Caracciolo EA, Chaitman BR, Forman SA, et al: Diabetics with coronary disease have a prevalence of asymptomatic ischemia during exercise treadmill testing and ambulatory ischemia monitoring similar to that of nondiabetic patients. An ACIP database study. Circulation 93:2097, 1996.
113. Bonow RO, Carabello B, deLeon AC Jr, et al: ACC/AHA guidelines for the management of patients with valvular heart disease: A report of the American College of Cardiology/American Heart Association Task Force on Practice Guidelines (Committee on Management of Patients with Valvular Heart Disease). J Am Coll Cardiol 32:1486, 1998.
114. Borer JS, Hockreiter C, Herrold EM, et al: Prediction of indications for valve replacement among asymptomatic or minimally symptomatic patients with chronic aortic regurgitation and normal left ventricular performance. Circulation 97:518, 1998.
115. Otto CM, Burwash IG, Legget ME, et al: Prospective study of asymptomatic valvular aortic stenosis: Clinical, echocardiographic, and exercise predictors of outcome. Circulation 95:2262, 1997.
116. Jones S, Elliott PM, McKenna WJ, et al: Cardiopulmonary responses to exercise in patients with hypertrophic cardiomyopathy. Heart 80:60, 1998.
117. Ciampi Q, Betocchi S, Lombardi R, et al: Hemodynamic determinants of exercise-induced abnormal blood pressure response in hypertrophic cardiomyopathy. J Am Coll Cardiol 40:278, 2002.
118. Kim JJ, Lee CW, Park SW, et al: Improvement in exercise capacity and exercise blood pressure response after transcoronary alcohol ablation therapy of septal hypertrophy in hypertrophic cardiomyopathy. Am J Cardiol 83:1220, 1999.
119. Krone RJ, Hardison RM, Chaitman BR, et al: Risk stratification after successful coronary revascularization: The lack of a role for routine exercise testing. J Am Coll Cardiol 38:136, 2001.
120. Marwick TH, Zuchowski C, Lauer MS, et al: Functional status and quality of life in patients with heart failure undergoing coronary bypass surgery after assessment of myocardial viability. J Am Coll Cardiol 33:750, 1999.
121. Ferrari M, Schnell B, Werner GS, et al: Safety of deferring angioplasty in patients with normal coronary flow velocity reserve. J Am Coll Cardiol 33:82, 1999.
122. Dagianti A, Rosanio S, Penco M, et al: Clinical and prognostic usefulness of supine bicycle exercise echocardiography in the functional evaluation of patients undergoing elective percutaneous transluminal coronary angioplasty. Circulation 95:1176, 1997.
123. Garzon P, Sheppard R, Eisenberg MJ, et al: Comparison of event and procedure rates following percutaneous transluminal coronary angioplasty in patients with and without previous coronary artery bypass graft surgery (the Routine versus Selective Exercise Treadmill Testing after Angioplasty [ROSETTA] Registry). Am J Cardiol 89:251, 2002.
124. Kavanagh T, Mertens DJ, Shephard RJ: Long-term cardiorespiratory results of exercise training following cardiac transplantation. Am J Cardiol 91:190, 2003.
125. Osada N, Chaitman BR, Donohue TJ, et al: Long-term cardiopulmonary exercise performance after heart transplantation. Am J Cardiol 79:451, 1997.
126. Wilson RF, Johnson TH, Haidet GC, et al: Sympathetic reinnervation of the sinus node and exercise hemodynamics after cardiac transplantation. Circulation 101:2727, 2000.

Safety and Risks of Exercise Testing

127. Stuart RJ, Ellestad MH: National survey of exercise stress testing facilities. Chest 77:94, 1980.
128. Hamm LF, Crow RS, Stull GA, Hannan P: Safety and characteristics of exercise testing early after acute myocardial infarction. Am J Cardiol 63:1193, 1989.
129. Tristani FE, Hughes CV, Archibald DG, et al: Safety of graded symptom-limited exercise testing in patients with congestive heart failure. Circulation 76:VI-54, 1987.
130. Young DZ, Lampert S, Graboys TB, Lown B: Safety of maximal exercise testing in patients at high risk for ventricular arrhythmia. Circulation 70:184, 1984.
131. Beller GA, Bonow RO, Fuster V, et al: ACC revised recommendations for training in adult cardiovascular medicine core cardiology training II (COCATS 2) (Revision of the 1995 COCATS Training Statement). J Am Coll Cardiol 39:1242, 2002.
132. Rodgers GP, Ayanian JZ, Balady G, et al: American College of Cardiology/American Heart Association clinical competence statement on stress testing. A report of the American College of Cardiology/American Heart Association/American College of Physicians—American Society of Internal Medicine Task Force on Clinical Competence. J Am Coll Cardiol 36:1441, 2000.

GUIDELINES *Thomas H. Lee*

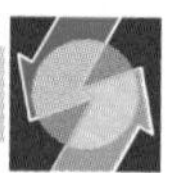

Exercise Stress Testing

Several sets of guidelines for the performance of exercise testing have been published by the American Heart Association and by committees commissioned jointly by the American College of Cardiology and the American Heart Association (ACC/AHA).[1-5] Use of exercise testing is addressed in guidelines for specific clinical syndromes, including acute myocardial infarction,[6] chronic stable angina,[7] valvular heart disease,[8] and congestive heart failure.[9] Recommendations for optimal use of treadmill exercise testing are also closely related to guidelines for use of nuclear cardiology tests for detection of myocardial ischemia.[10]

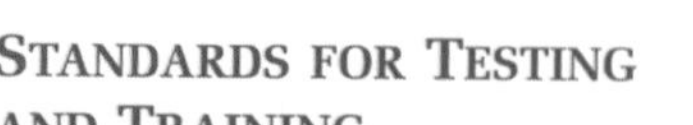

Standards for Testing and Training

The AHA published standards for performance of exercise testing in 2001,[1] which define absolute and relative contraindications to exercise testing; these recommendations were slightly modified in ACC/AHA guidelines published in 2002 (Table 10G–1). "Relative" contraindications are those that can be superseded if clinicians believe that the benefits of testing outweigh the risks of exercise. The AHA standards also provide recommendations for specific testing

TABLE 10G–1 ACC/AHA Guidelines: Absolute and Relative Contraindications to Exercise Testing

Absolute
Acute myocardial infarction (within 2 days)
High-risk unstable angina
Uncontrolled cardiac arrhythmias causing symptoms or hemodynamic compromise
Symptomatic severe aortic stenosis
Uncontrolled symptomatic heart failure
Acute pulmonary embolus or pulmonary infarction
Acute myocarditis or pericarditis
Acute aortic dissection
Relative
Left main coronary stenosis
Moderate stenotic valvular heart disease
Electrolyte abnormalities
Severe arterial hypertension (suggested definition: systolic blood pressure > 200 mm Hg and/or diastolic blood pressure > 100 mm Hg)
Tachyarrhythmias or bradyarrhythmias
Hypertrophic cardiomyopathy and other forms of outflow tract obstruction
Mental or physical impairment leading to inability to exercise adequately
High-degree atrioventricular block

From Gibbons RJ, Balady GJ, Bricker JT, et al: ACC/AHA 2002 guideline update for exercise testing: Summary article. A report of the ACC/AHA Task Force on Practice Guidelines (Committee to update the 1997 Exercise Testing Guidelines). Circulation 106:1883, 2002.

TABLE 10G–2 ACC/AHA Guidelines: Indications for Terminating Exercise Testing

Absolute
Drop in systolic blood pressure of >10 mm Hg from baseline blood pressure despite an increase in workload, when accompanied by other evidence of ischemia
Moderate to severe angina
Increasing nervous system symptoms (e.g., ataxia, dizziness, or near-syncope)
Signs of poor perfusion (cyanosis or pallor)
Technical difficulties in monitoring electrocardiogram or systolic blood pressure
Subject's desire to stop
Sustained ventricular tachycardia
ST elevation (≥1.0 mm) in leads without diagnostic Q waves (other than V_1 or aV_R)
Relative
Drop in systolic blood pressure of >10 mm Hg from baseline blood pressure despite an increase in workload, in the absence of other evidence of ischemia
ST or QRS changes such as excessive ST depression (>2 mm of horizontal or downsloping ST segment depression) or marked axis shift
Arrhythmias other than sustained ventricular tachycardia, including multifocal PVCs, triplets of PVCs, supraventricular tachycardia, heart block, or bradyarrhythmias
Fatigue, shortness of breath, wheezing, leg cramps, or claudication
Development of bundle-branch block or IVCD that cannot be distinguished from ventricular tachycardia
Increasing chest pain
Hypertensive response (suggested definition: systolic blood pressure > 250 mm Hg and/or a diastolic blood pressure of > 115 mm Hg)

ECG = electrocardiogram; ICD = implantable cardioverter-defibrillator discharge; IVCD = intraventricular conduction delay; PVCs = premature ventricular contractions.

From Gibbons RJ, Balady GJ, Bricker JT, et al: ACC/AHA 2002 guideline update for exercise testing: Summary article. A report of the ACC/AHA Task Force on Practice Guidelines (Committee to Update the 1997 Exercise Testing Guidelines). Circulation 106:1883, 2002.

procedures, such as patient instructions for preparation for the procedure. This Scientific Statement does not offer explicit recommendations on when and whether beta blockers or other drugs (e.g., vasodilators, digitalis, diuretics) should be discontinued before testing.

Indications for termination of exercise testing from this Scientific Statement were updated in the most recent ACC/AHA guidelines on exercise testing[4] and are summarized in Table 10G–2. Again, relative indications for termination of testing are those that can be superseded when the clinician considers the benefits of continued exercise to exceed the risks.

Exercise testing should be performed under the supervision of a physician, who should be in the vicinity and immediately available during all exercise tests. However, the Scientific Statement indicates that a properly trained nonphysician (i.e., a nurse, physician assistant, or exercise physiologist or specialist) can perform the direct supervision for healthy younger persons and those with stable chest pain syndromes.[1] An ACC/AHA Clinical Competence Statement on exercise testing published in 2000 describes a "majority opinion" of its authors that supervising physicians should participate in at least 50 exercise test procedures during training and perform at least 25 exercise tests per year.[2] This Statement also lists specific skills that are needed for competent test supervision and interpretation, and recommends that medical centers have a program of quality assurance to ensure systematic review and critique of a significant sample of exercise tests. Because computer processing can lead to an overestimation of ST depression, ACC/AHA guidelines recommend that the interpreting physician always be supplied with raw electrocardiographic (ECG) tracings in addition to any computerized summaries.[4]

Clinical Indications for Exercise Testing

Guidelines published by the ACC/AHA in 1997[3] and updated in 2002[4] assess the appropriateness of exercise testing in specific clinical settings. The complete guidelines are available at *www.americanheart.org* or *www.acc.org*. As with other ACC/AHA guidelines, these recommendations classify indications into one of three classes, including two levels of the intermediate group, as follows:

Class I: Conditions for which there is evidence and/or general agreement that exercise testing is useful and effective.

Class II: Conditions for which there is conflicting evidence and/or a divergence of opinion about the usefulness/efficacy of performing exercise testing.

Class IIa: Weight of evidence/opinion is in favor of usefulness/efficacy.

Class IIb: Usefulness/efficacy is less well established by evidence/opinion.

Class III: Conditions for which there is evidence and/or general agreement that exercise testing is not useful/effective and in some cases may be harmful.

Diagnosis of Obstructive Coronary Artery Disease

When the clinical question is whether obstructive coronary disease is present or absent in a patient (i.e., diagnosis), the ACC/AHA guidelines consider exercise testing most appropriate for patients with an "intermediate" pretest probability of coronary artery disease, such as patients with atypical or probable angina or younger patients with typical angina. Definitions of pretest risk status according to age, gender, and symptoms are summarized in Table 10G–3. Patients with high or low pretest probability of coronary disease are less likely to have their management altered by exercise testing; hence, exercise testing is not strongly supported by these guidelines in these populations (Table 10G–4). Exercise electrocardiography is considered appropriate in patients with complete right bundle branch block and less than 1 mm of resting ST depression, but not in patients with electrocardiographic patterns more likely to lead to uninterpretable tracings. The 2002 ACC/AHA guidelines lower the threshold for using an imaging technology in patients with minor ST depression. The prior ACC/AHA guidelines considered exercise electrocardiography "the first test option" in such patients,[3] whereas the 2002 update has changed this phrase to "a reasonable first test option."

Risk Assessment and Prognosis in Patients with Coronary Disease

The ACC/AHA guidelines emphasize that exercise testing should be used to improve risk stratification as part of a process that begins with assessment of routinely available data from the clinical examination and other laboratory tests. The decision of whether to order an exercise test should reflect the chances that test results might alter management, and the interpretation of the results should be considered in the context of the patient's overall clinical status.

The recommendations endorse routine use of exercise testing for risk stratification of patients with suspected or known coronary disease (Table 10G–5), whether stable or after a change in clinical status. The guidelines emphasize the importance of consideration of multiple types of data from the exercise test (e.g., exercise duration) and encourage use of tools such as the Duke Treadmill Score[11] to integrate these data into a risk prediction.

For patients with unstable angina, the guidelines support exercise testing early (8-12 hours) after presentation in patients with a low clinical risk of complications (Table 10G–6) if they have been free of active ischemic or heart failure symptoms. A longer delay (2-3 days) is recommended for patients with an intermediate risk of complications, although the guidelines indicate that there is good supportive evidence for earlier exercise testing as part of chest pain management protocols for stable patients from this population if there is no evidence of active ischemia (Class IIa indication). More detailed recommendations on exercise testing in chest pain centers were provided in a Science Advisory Statement from the American Heart Association in 2000.[5]

The guidelines discourage exercise testing for patients in whom the procedure would be dangerous (e.g., high-risk unstable angina patients); unlikely to add accurate information (e.g., patients with certain resting ECG abnormalities); or unlikely to change management

TABLE 10G–3 Pretest Probability of Coronary Artery Disease by Age, Gender and Symptoms

Age (yr)	Gender	Typical/Definite Angina Pectoris	Atypical/Probable Angina Pectoris	Nonanginal Chest Pain	Asymptomatic
30-39	Men	Intermediate	Intermediate	Low	Very low
	Women	Intermediate	Very low	Very low	Very low
40-49	Men	High	Intermediate	Intermediate	Low
	Women	Intermediate	Low	Very low	Very low
50-59	Men	High	Intermediate	Intermediate	Low
	Women	Intermediate	Intermediate	Low	Very low
60-69	Men	High	Intermediate	Intermediate	Low
	Women	High	Intermediate	Intermediate	Low

From Gibbons RJ, Balady GJ, Bricker JT, et al: ACC/AHA 2002 guideline update for exercise testing: Summary article. A report of the ACC/AHA Task Force on Practice Guidelines (Committee to Update the 1997 Exercise Testing Guidelines). Circulation 106:1883, 2002.

TABLE 10G–4 ACC/AHA Guidelines for Exercise Testing to Diagnose Obstructive Coronary Artery Disease

	Indication
Class I (indicated)	Adult patients (including those with complete right bundle branch block or less than 1 mm of resting ST depression) with an intermediate pretest probability of CAD on the basis of gender, age, and symptoms (specific exceptions are noted under Classes II and III below).
Class IIa (good supportive evidence)	Patients with vasospastic angina.
Class IIb (weak supportive evidence)	1. Patients with a high pretest probability of CAD by age, symptoms, and gender. 2. Patients with a low pretest probability of CAD by age, symptoms, and gender. 3. Patients with less than 1 mm of baseline ST depression and taking digoxin. 4. Patients with electrocardiographic criteria for left ventricular hypertrophy and less than 1 mm of baseline ST depression.
Class III (not indicated)	1. Patients with the following baseline ECG abnormalities: • Preexcitation (Wolff-Parkinson-White) syndrome • Electronically paced ventricular rhythm • Greater than 1 mm of resting ST depression • Complete left bundle branch block 2. Patients with a documented myocardial infarction or prior coronary angiography demonstrating significant disease who have an established diagnosis of CAD; however, ischemia and risk can be determined by testing.

CAD = coronary artery disease.

TABLE 10G–5 ACC/AHA Guidelines: Risk Assessment and Prognosis in Patients with Symptoms or a Prior History of Coronary Artery Disease

	Indication
Class I (indicated)	1. Patients undergoing initial evaluation with suspected or known CAD, including those with complete right bundle branch block or less than 1 mm of resting ST depression. Specific exceptions are noted below in Class IIb. 2. Patients with suspected or known CAD, previously evaluated, now presenting with significant change in clinical status. 3. Low-risk unstable angina patients 8 to 12 hours after presentation who have been free of active ischemic or heart failure symptoms. 4. Intermediate-risk unstable angina patients 2 to 3 days after presentation who have been free of active ischemic or heart failure symptoms.
Class IIa (good supportive evidence)	Intermediate-risk unstable angina patients who have initial cardiac markers that are normal, a repeat ECG without significant change, and cardiac markers 6 to 12 hours after the onset of symptoms that are normal and no other evidence of ischemia during observation.
Class IIb (weak supportive evidence)	1. Patients with the following resting ECG abnormalities: • Preexcitation (Wolff-Parkinson-White) syndrome • Electronically paced ventricular rhythm • 1 mm or more of resting ST depression • Complete left bundle branch block or any interventricular conduction defect with a QRS duration longer than 120 msec. 2. Patients with a stable clinical course who undergo periodic monitoring to guide treatment.
Class III (not indicated)	1. Patients with severe comorbidity likely to limit life expectancy and/or candidacy for revascularization. 2. High-risk unstable angina patients.

CAD = coronary artery disease; ECG = electrocardiogram.

TABLE 10G–6 ACC/AHA Classification System for Risk of Death or Nonfatal Myocardial Infarction in Patients with Unstable Angina

Feature	High Risk (at least one of the following features must be present)	Intermediate Risk (no high-risk feature but must have one of the following features)	Low Risk (no high- or intermediate-risk features, but may have any of the following features)
History		Prior MI, peripheral or cerbrovascular disease, or CABG, prior aspirin use	
Character of pain	Prolonged, ongoing (>20 min) pain at rest	Prolonged (>20 min) resting angina, now resolved, with moderate or high likelihood of CAD Rest angina (<20 min) or relieved with rest or sublingual NTG	New-onset or progressive CCSC III or IV angina in the past 2 weeks with moderate or high likelihood of CAD
Clinical findings	Pulmonary edema, most likely related to ischemia New or worsening MR murmur S3 or new/worsening rales Hypotension, bradycardia, tachycardia Age older than 75 years	Age older than 70 yr	
ECG findings	Angina at rest with transient ST changes ≥ 0.05 mV BBB, new or presumed new/sustained ventricular tachycardia	T-wave inversions greater than 0.2 mV Pathological Q waves	Normal or unchanged ECG during an episode of chest discomfort
Biochemical cardiac markers	Elevated (e.g., troponin T or I greater than 0.1 mg/ml)	Slightly elevated (e.g., troponin T > 0.01 but <0.1 mg/ml)	Normal

BBB = bundle branch block; CABG = coronary artery bypass graft; CAD = coronary artery disease; CCSC = Canadian Cardiovascular Society Classification; ECG = electrocardiogram; MI = myocardial infarction; MR = mitral regurgitation.

From Gibbons RJ, Balady GJ, Bricker JT, et al: ACC/AHA 2002 guideline update for exercise testing: Summary article. A report of the ACC/AHA Task Force on Practice Guidelines (Committee to update the 1997 Exercise Testing Guidelines). Circulation 106:1883, 2002.

(e.g., patients with stable clinical courses or who were poor candidates for revascularization) (see Table 10G–5).

After Acute Myocardial Infarction

Recommendations for the use of exercise testing after acute myocardial infarction (Table 10G–7) reflect an overall strategy for risk stratification and management that is described in ACC/AHA guidelines on acute myocardial infarction.[6] In this approach (Fig. 10G–1), if patients' clinical data suggest a high risk for complications, the patients should undergo invasive evaluation to determine whether they are candidates for coronary revascularization procedures (strategy I). For patients with apparently low risk for complications, two strategies for performing exercise testing are endorsed. One uses a symptom-limited exercise test at 14 to 21 days (strategy II). An alternative strategy for low-risk patients (strategy III) is to perform a submaximal exercise test at 4 to 7 days after myocardial infarction or just before hospital discharge. If the exercise test result is negative, a second

TABLE 10G–7 ACC/AHA Guidelines for Exercise Testing after Acute Myocardial Infarction

	Indication
Class I (indicated)	1. Before discharge for prognostic assessment, activity prescription, evaluation of medical therapy (submaximal at about 4 to 76 days).* 2. Early after discharge for prognostic assessment, activity prescription, evaluation of medical therapy, and cardiac rehabilitation if the predischarge exercise test was not done (symptom-limited; about 14 to 21 days).* 3. Late after discharge for prognostic assessment, activity prescription, evaluation of medical therapy, and cardiac rehabilitation if the early exercise test was submaximal (symptom-limited; about 3 to 6 weeks).*
Class IIa (good supportive evidence)	After discharge for activity counseling and/or exercise training as part of cardiac rehabilitation in patients who have undergone coronary revascularization.
Class IIb (weak supportive evidence)	1. Patients with the following electrocardiographic abnormalities: • Complete left bundle-branch block • Preexcitation syndrome • Left ventricular hypertrophy • Digoxin therapy • Greater than 1 mm of resting ST segment depression • Electronically paced ventricular rhythm 2. Periodic monitoring in patients who continue to participate in exercise training or cardiac rehabilitation.
Class III (not indicated)	1. Severe comorbidity likely to limit life expectancy and/or candidacy for revascularization. 2. At any time to evaluate patients with acute myocardial infarction who have uncompensated congestive heart failure, cardiac arrhythmia, or noncardiac conditions that severely limit their ability to exercise. 3. Before discharge to evaluate patients who have already been selected for, or have undergone, cardiac catheterization. Although a stress test may be useful before or after catheterization to evaluate or identify ischemia in the distribution of a coronary lesion of borderline severity, stress imaging tests are recommended.

*Exceptions are noted under Classes IIb and III.

TABLE 10G–8 ACC/AHA Guidelines for Exercise Testing with Ventilatory Gas Analysis

	Indication
Class I (indicated)	1. Evaluation of exercise capacity and response to therapy in patients with heart failure who are being considered for heart transplantation. 2. Assistance in the differentiation of cardiac versus pulmonary limitations as a cause of exercise-induced dyspnea or impaired exercise capacity when the cause is uncertain.
Class IIa (good supportive evidence)	Evaluation of exercise capacity when indicated for medical reasons in patients in whom the estimates of exercise capacity from exercise test time or work rate are unreliable.
Class IIb (weak supportive evidence)	1. Evaluation of the patient's response to specific therapeutic interventions in which improvement of exercise tolerance is an important goal or endpoint. 2. Determination of the intensity for exercise training as part of comprehensive cardiac rehabilitation.
Class III (not indicated)	Routine use to evaluate exercise capacity.

symptom-limited exercise test can be repeated at 3 to 6 weeks for patients undergoing vigorous activity during leisure time activities, at work, or exercise training as part of cardiac rehabilitation. Exercise imaging tests are reserved for patients with equivocal exercise electrocardiography tests or those with electrocardiography findings that preclude interpretation of ST changes. The extent of ischemia on noninvasive studies helps determine whether patients should undergo cardiac catheterization.

Exercise Testing with Ventilatory Gas Analysis

Although measurement of maximal oxygen uptake is the best index of aerobic capacity, the ACC/AHA guidelines do not support ventilatory gas analysis as part of routine exercise testing or for routine measurement of exercise capacity (Table 10G–8). Ventilatory gas analysis is recommended when it is most likely to change management, such as in patients being considered for transplantation or those in whom clinical differentiation between pulmonary and cardiac causes of exercise limitation is difficult. Some support is provided for ventilatory gas exchange for patients in whom estimates of exercise capacity from other sources (e.g., exercise test time) are unreliable, but the guidelines discourage use of this technology for assessment of response to therapy or as a routine part of cardiac rehabilitation.

Special Populations

Exercise electrocardiography has poorer overall test performance in women compared with men, but the ACC/AHA guidelines recommend that exercise electrocardiography be the first-choice noninvasive test for coronary disease in women.[4] This recommendation reflects the fact that stress imaging technologies also have poorer sensitivity and higher false-positive rates in women, leading to the conclusion that there was insufficient evidence to recommend them as the initial diagnostic test in women.

The ACC/AHA guidelines discourage routine exercise testing for asymptomatic persons without known coronary artery disease (Table 10G–9) and conclude that only weak evidence is available to support its appropriateness for asymptomatic patients with multiple risk factors or patients about to embark on an exercise program. The guidelines are more supportive of exercise testing of patients with diabetes who are about to start vigorous exercise programs, owing to the high risk for atherosclerotic disease in this population.

TABLE 10G–9 ACC/AHA Guidelines for Exercise Testing in Asymptomatic Persons without Known Coronary Artery Disease (CAD)

	Indication
Class I (indicated)	None
Class IIa (good supportive evidence)	Evaluation of asymptomatic persons with diabetes mellitus who plan to start vigorous exercise.
Class IIb (weak supportive evidence)	1. Evaluation of persons with multiple risk factors as a guide to risk reduction therapy.* 2. Evaluation of asymptomatic men older than 45 years and women older than 55 years: • Who plan to start vigorous exercise (especially if sedentary) or • Who are involved in occupations in which impairment might impact public safety or • Who are at high risk for CAD due to other diseases (e.g., peripheral vascular disease and chronic renal failure)
Class III (not indicated)	Routine screening of asymptomatic men or women.

*Multiple risk factors are defined as hypercholesterolemia (>240 mg/dl), hypertension (systolic blood pressure > 140 mm Hg or diastolic blood pressure > 90 mm Hg), smoking, diabetes, and family history of heart attack or sudden cardiac death in a first-degree relative younger than 60 years. An alternative approach might be to select patients with a Framingham risk score consistent with at least a moderate risk of serious cardiac events within 5 years.

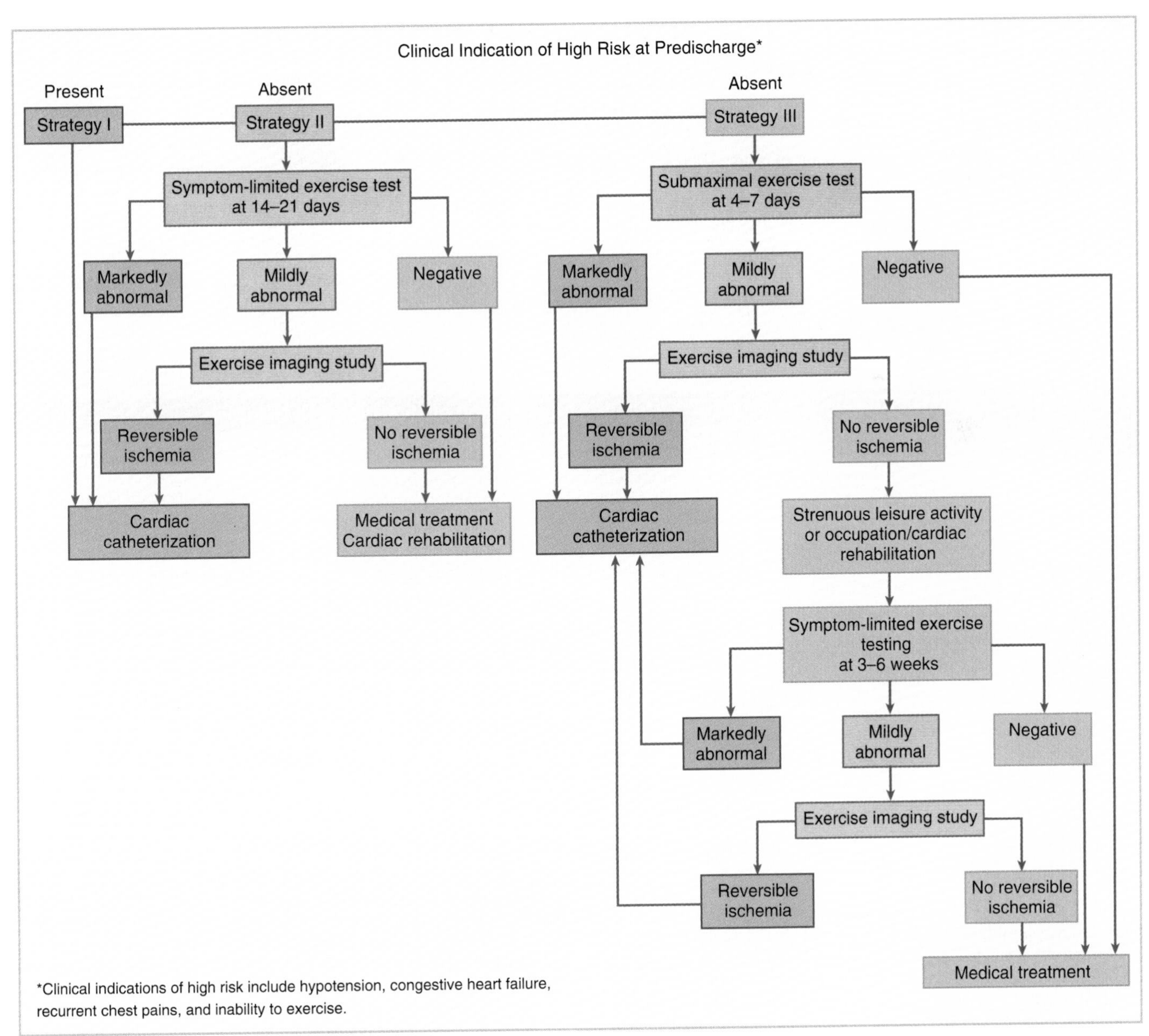

FIGURE 10G–1. Strategies for exercise test evaluation soon after myocardial infarction.

TABLE 10G–10 ACC/AHA Guidelines for Exercise Testing in Patients with Valvular Heart Disease

	Indication
Class I (indicated)	In chronic aortic regurgitation, assessment of functional capacity and symptomatic responses in patients with a history of equivocal symptoms.
Class IIa (good supportive evidence)	1. In chronic aortic regurgitation, evaluation of symptoms and functional capacity before participation in athletic activities. 2. In chronic aortic regurgitation, prognostic assessment before aortic valve replacement in asymptomatic or minimally symptomatic patients with left ventricular dysfunction.
Class IIb (weak supportive evidence)	Evaluation of exercise capacity in patients with valvular heart disease.
Class III (not indicated)	Diagnosis of coronary artery disease in patients with moderate to severe valvular disease or with the following baseline electrocardiographic abnormalities: • Preexcitation • Electronically paced ventricular rhythm • Greater than 1 mm ST depression • Complete left bundle branch block

TABLE 10G–11 ACC/AHA Guidelines for Exercise Testing Before and After Revascularization

	Indication
Class I (indicated)	1. Demonstration of ischemia before revascularization. 2. Evaluation of patients with recurrent symptoms that suggest ischemia after revascularization.
Class IIa (good supportive evidence)	After discharge for activity counseling and/or exercise training as part of cardiac rehabilitation in patients who have undergone coronary revascularization.
Class IIb (weak supportive evidence)	1. Detection of restenosis in selected, high-risk asymptomatic patients within the first 12 months after percutaneous coronary intervention. 2. Periodic monitoring of selected, high-risk asymptomatic patients for restenosis, graft occlusion, incomplete coronary revascularization, or disease progression.
Class III (not indicated)	1. Localization of ischemia for determining the site of intervention. 2. Routine, periodic monitoring of asymptomatic patients after percutaneous coronary intervention or coronary artery bypass grafting without specific indications.

TABLE 10G–12 ACC/AHA Guidelines for Exercise Testing for Investigation of Heart Rhythm Disorders

	Indication
Class I (indicated)	1. Identification of appropriate settings in patients with rate-adaptive pacemakers. 2. Evaluation of congenital complete heart block in patients considering increased physical activity or participation in competitive sports.
Class IIa (good supportive evidence)	1. Evaluation of patients with known or suspected exercise-induced arrhythmias. 2. Evaluation of medical, surgical, or ablative therapy in patients with exercise-induced arrhythmias (including atrial fibrillation).
Class IIb (weak supportive evidence)	1. Investigation of isolated ventricular ectopic beats in middle-aged patients without other evidence of coronary artery disease. 2. Investigation of prolonged first-degree atrioventricular block or type I second-degree Wenckebach block, left bundle branch block, right bundle branch block, or isolated ectopic beats in young patients considering participation in competitive sports.
Class III (not indicated)	Routine investigation of isolated ectopic beats in young patients.

Exercise testing is useful for assessing functional capacity in patients with valvular heart disease, particularly patients with regurgitant lesions (Table 10G–10). The guidelines note that exercise testing is usually not needed for symptomatic patients with stenotic valvular heart disease, and that severe aortic stenosis is classically considered a contraindication to exercise testing. However, the guidelines acknowledge that there are subsets of asymptomatic patients with stenotic valvular lesions in whom exercise testing may help assess functional capacity, for goals such as determination of whether they are truly asymptomatic.

The ACC/AHA guidelines support the use of exercise testing as part of the evaluation of patients before revascularization with coronary artery bypass grafting (CABG) or percutaneous coronary interventions and for evaluation of recurrent symptoms or part of the rehabilitation process. However, the guidelines do not support routine periodic exercise testing of asymptomatic patients after revascularization (Table 10G–11).

The guidelines endorse exercise testing for patients with heart rhythm disorders when the test is intended to diagnose exercise-induced arrhythmias or evaluate therapy (e.g., settings for rate-adaptive pacemakers, or impact of therapy for patients with exercise-induced arrhythmias). However, there is little support for exercise testing for heart rhythm abnormalities that, in isolation, are not associated with a higher risk of cardiovascular complications, such as isolated ventricular or atrial premature beats (Table 10G–12).

References

1. Fletcher GF, Balady GJ, Amsterdam EA, et al: Exercise standards for testing and training: A statement for healthcare professionals from the American Heart Association. Circulation 104:1694, 2001.
2. Rodgers GP, Ayanian JZ, Balady G, et al: American College of Cardiology/American Heart Association clinical competence statement on stress testing. Circulation 102:1726, 2000.
3. Gibbons RJ, Balady GJ, Beasley JW, et al: ACC/AHA guidelines for exercise testing: A report of the American College of Cardiology/American Heart Association Task Force on Practice Guidelines (Committee on Exercise Testing). J Am Coll Cardiol 30:260, 1997.
4. Gibbons RJ, Balady GJ, Bricker JT, et al: ACC/AHA 2002 guideline update for exercise testing: Summary article. A report of the ACC/AHA Task Force on Practice Guidelines (Committee to Update the 1997 Exercise Testing Guidelines). Circulation 106:1883, 2002.
5. Stein RA, Chaitman BR, Balady GJ, et al: Safety and utility of exercise testing in emergency room chest pain centers. An advisory from the Committee on Exercise, Rehabilitation, and Prevention, Council on Clinical Cardiology, American Heart Association. Circulation 102:1463, 2000.
6. Ryan TJ, Antman EM, Brooks NH, et al: ACC/AHA guidelines for the management of patients with acute myocardial infarction: 1999 update. A report of the American College of Cardiology/American Heart Association Task Force on Practice Guidelines (Committee on Management of Acute Myocardial Infarction). (http://www.acc.org)
7. Gibbons RJ, Abrams J, Chatterjee K, et al: ACC/AHA 2002 guideline update for the management of patients with chronic stable angina: Summary article. A report of the American College of Cardiology/American Heart Association Task Force on Practice Guidelines (Committee on the Management of Patents With Chronic Stable Angina). Circulation 107:149, 2003.
8. Bonow RO, Carabello B, de Leon AC Jr, et al: ACC/AHA guidelines for the management of patients with valvular heart disease: Executive summary. A report of the American College of Cardiology/American Heart Association Task Force on Practice Guidelines (Committee on Management of Patients With Valvular Heart Disease). Circulation 98:1949, 1998.
9. Hunt SA, Baker DW, Chin MH, et al: ACC/AHA guidelines for the evaluation and management of chronic heart failure in the adult: A report of the American College of Cardiology/American Heart Association Task Force on Practice Guidelines (Committee to Revise the 1995 Guidelines for the Evaluation and Management of Heart Failure). American College of Cardiology Web site, 2001. (http://www.acc.org/clinical/guidelines/failure/hf_index.htm)
10. Committee on Nuclear Imaging: Guidelines for Clinical Use of Cardiac Radionuclide Imaging. A Report of the American College of Cardiology/American Heart Association Task Force on the Assessment of Cardiovascular Procedures. J Am Coll Cardiol 25:521, 1995.
11. Mark DB, Shaw L, Harrell FE Jr, et al: Prognostic value of a treadmill exercise score in outpatients with suspected coronary artery disease. N Engl J Med 325:849, 1991.

CHAPTER 11

Echocardiography

William F. Armstrong

Principles of Cardiac Ultrasonography

Echocardiography is a group of interrelated applications of ultrasound including two-dimensional imaging, M-mode echocardiography, Doppler techniques, and contrast echocardiography. All of these techniques rely on sound in the frequency range of 2 to 10 MHz. Typically, adult imaging is performed at frequencies ranging from 2 to 5 MHz. For pediatric and specialized adult applications, higher frequencies of 7.5 and 10 MHz can also be used. This chapter deals with the clinical utility of echocardiographic techniques as they relate to the majority of forms of disease encountered in adult patient populations. It is important to have an understanding of the basic physical principles of ultrasound and image generation to understand the limitations and advantages of the technique.

Principles of Ultrasound Physics and Instrumentation

Cardiac ultrasonography relies on sound waves in the frequency of 2 to 10 MHz. Although typically displayed as a sine wave traveling through space, ultrasound actually consists of a pulsatile pressure phenomenon transmitted through a medium as alternating areas of pressure increase and pressure rarification. The periodicity of the pressure waveform, or its cycle, is expressed as frequency. A sound wave has several characteristics (Fig. 11–1), many of which are related. *Frequency* is the number of complete cycles occurring per second and is the inverse of *wavelength* (λ), which is the length of a single cycle. *Amplitude* is the power, or ability of the wave to transfer energy to the conducting medium or other insonated object. As the pressure wave propagates through a medium, the amplitude of the pressure change diminishes due to attenuation. The emitted sound wave is described as having an initial or fundamental frequency. This fundamental frequency is preserved during a propagation through a conducting medium, and a portion of the sound energy is reflected back at the same fundamental frequency.

A recent adaptation of cardiac ultrasonography relies on the generation of harmonic frequencies during transmission of the ultrasound beam. Traditionally, transducers have had narrow bandwidth elements that transmit and receive at narrowly defined frequencies. Modern transducers have a wide bandwidth that allows transmission and receipt of ultrasound over a broad range of frequencies. The traditional view of harmonics is that an insonated object may resonate and hence reflect back ultrasound not only at the fundamental, transmitted frequency but also at harmonics of that frequency. In the traditional view of harmonics, an object can be imaged at 2 MHz but reflect ultrasound back at 2 MHz and at 4 and 8 MHz harmonics (Fig. 11–2). Recently, it has been recognized that the transmission of ultrasound through tissue actually creates harmonic frequencies during propagation. Because the transmitted frequency is not a narrow discrete frequency but rather a broad range of frequencies, the full range of reflected frequencies and the resultant harmonics are likewise substantially broader than originally conceived. This is the premise for what has been termed *tissue harmonic imaging*. Harmonic frequencies increase in strength with depth of penetration but represent only a small portion of the total reflected ultrasound energy. The advantage of the reflected harmonic frequencies is that they are free of near-field reverberation and shadowing effect. This results in an increased signal-to-noise ratio of the harmonic signal.[1-3] This type of imaging shows tremendous promise for improved visualization of the myocardium but at the cost of a minor reduction in resolution. Additionally, tissue signature is brighter than usual, and there is loss of detail for evaluation of fine valvular structures.

For clinical imaging, the ultrasound energy is both generated and received by a transducer attached to an imaging platform. Ultrasound energy is generated by an electrically stimulated piezoelectric crystal. The ultrasound energy generated is modified by the physical elements of the transducer, which serves to provide damping functions as well as some focusing function. In its simplest application, a piezoelectric crystal emits ultrasound at a single discrete frequency that is not altered by either the transducer or during propagation. In modern scanners, broad-band technology is used such that the emitted ultrasound consists of not just a single frequency but a range of frequencies. For any given transducer, there is not only a center "fundamental" frequency but also a range of frequencies both greater and lesser than the fundamental frequency, each of which has less amplitude than the fundamental frequency. This results in the substantially greater ability to determine tissue signature than is possible with a single discrete fundamental frequency. The imaging beam is emitted as a series of pulses, each of which contains several cycles of ultrasound. The number of pulses emitted per second is the pulse repetition frequency.

The ultrasound beam has several characteristics that are determined by the

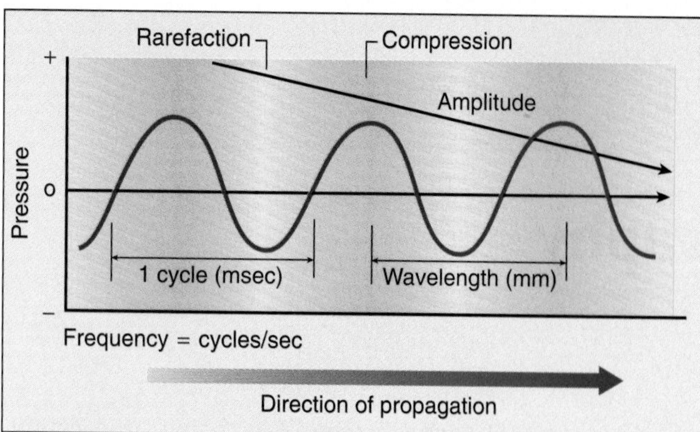

FIGURE 11–1 Schematic representation of a sound wave. The sound wave is typically described as a sine wave but actually represents alternating areas of pressure compression and rarification in a medium. Several characteristics that describe the sound wave, including amplitude, wavelength, and cycle, are schematized. Frequency is the number of cycles per second and, for clinical ultrasonography, ranges between 2.0 and 10 MHz. Amplitude (diagonal line) diminishes with distance from the sound source.

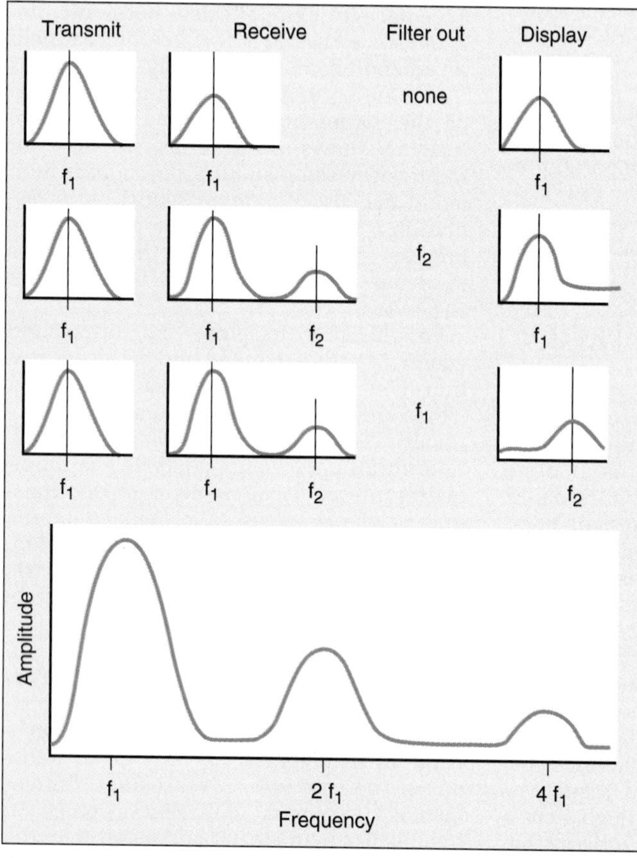

FIGURE 11–2 Schematic of second harmonics. A modern broadband transducer emits and receives ultrasound over a fairly broad range. Its central frequency is noted as the fundamental frequency (f_1). The frequency spectrum can also be described as a series of harmonics or multiples of that frequency, as noted. Harmonics are generated during transmission, with each successive harmonic being twice the preceding in frequency. Each successive harmonic has a substantially reduced amplitude, as noted. For detection of harmonics, selective filtering for receipt of the targeted frequency is employed, as is selective amplification of that frequency to enhance returning signals in the harmonic range. The bottom schematic depicts the phenomenon of multiple harmonics, each twice the frequency of the preceding, but with diminished amplitude. The top three schematics depict receiving and display characteristics of a narrow band (single frequency) transducer at the top and selective filtering to display either the fundamental (f_1) or harmonic (f_2) frequency.

transducer and that impact both its ability to penetrate a medium and its resolution for separating two objects in space. Low-frequency ultrasound provides a greater depth of penetration than does high-frequency ultrasound. Conversely, image resolution is greater with higher frequencies and less with low frequencies. Because ultrasound is propagated through tissue, it attenuates (loses energy) as well as losing the directional integrity of the beam. This results in far field dispersion of the ultrasound beam, so that it effectively images a larger area in the far field, more distant from the transducer face, than in the near field. It is within the near field that resolution is greatest. The distance of the near field from the transducer face can be calculated as outlined in Figure 11–3.

It should be emphasized that there are several forms of resolution, including axial, lateral, contrast, and temporal resolution (Fig. 11–4). ***Axial resolution*** refers to the ability to separate objects that fall in the direction of ultrasound propagation. ***Lateral resolution*** applies to the ability to detect objects that lie side by side within the ultrasound beam. ***Contrast resolution*** refers to the ability to detect objects of differing acoustic reflectivity, and ***temporal resolution*** refers to the ability to determine separation in time of events by ultrasound.

The amount of ultrasound energy delivered to the field can be controlled by the output of the transducer. For clinical

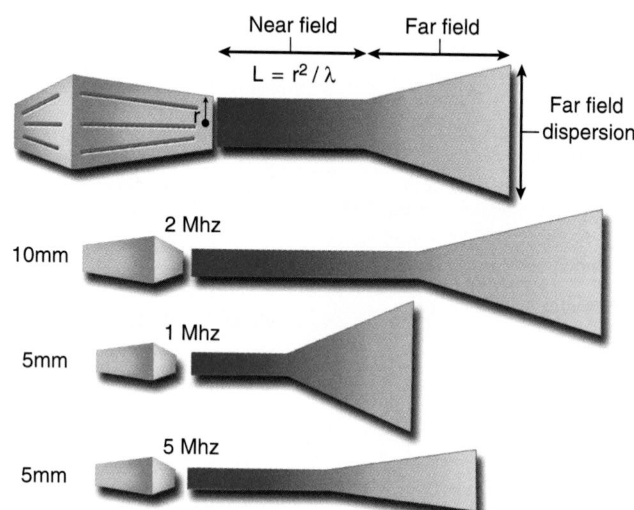

FIGURE 11–3 Schematic of a typical ultrasound transducer. The ultrasound transducer emits ultrasound from a series of piezoelectric crystals. The beam has several components, including a near field (Fresnel zone) with relatively narrow beam width and a far field where there is divergence of the ultrasound beam. Ultrasound intensity decreases with distance from the transducer face. The length of the near field can be calculated as $L = r^2/\lambda$. Changes in the transducer diameter and frequency have predictable effects on the near and far field characteristics, as is noted in the lower two illustrations. Higher frequencies preserve the length of the near field compared to lower frequencies, as do larger transducer diameters.

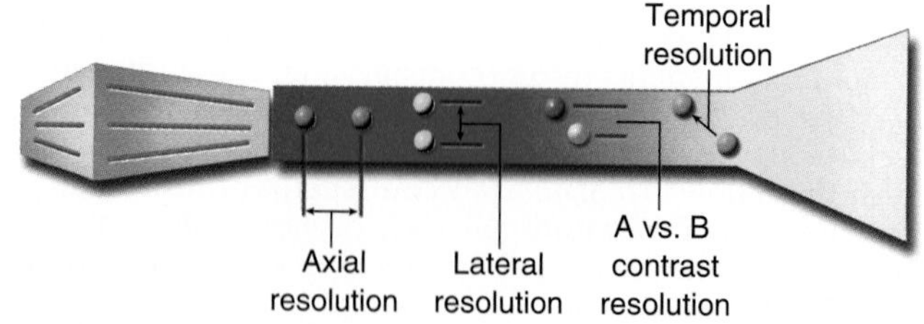

FIGURE 11–4 Schematic representation of different forms of ultrasound resolution. The four types of resolution—axial, lateral, temporal, and contrast—are all illustrated in the schematized ultrasound beam.

purposes, the delivered ultrasound power is typically described as a mechanical index. Mechanical index is defined as the peak negative acoustic pressure divided by the square root of the transmission frequency. For routine clinical imaging, a mechanical index of 1.0 to 1.6 is typically used. As the ultrasound energy delivered increases, it may result in destruction of microbubbles, so for contrast imaging a lower mechanical index is necessary.

THE DOPPLER PRINCIPLE

The Doppler principle states that the frequency of ultrasound reflected from a stationary object is identical to the transmitted frequency. If an object is moving toward the transducer, the reflected frequency will be higher than the transmitted frequency; and conversely, if an object is moving away from the transducer, the reflected frequency will be lower. The difference between the transmitted and received frequencies is the Doppler shift (Fig. 11-5). The magnitude of the Doppler shift is determined by the velocity and direction of the moving object and can be calculated by the Doppler equation. The Doppler equation relates the angle of interrogation, the Doppler shift, or change in frequency between the transmitted and reflected frequency, and a constant that is equal to the speed of sound in water to the velocity and direction of the moving object (Fig. 11-6). A major contributor to this equation is the angle θ, with which the interrogating beam intercepts flow. For maximum accuracy, interrogation should be directly in the line of flow, that is $\theta = 0$ degrees. Because the cosine of 0 degrees equals 1.0, solving the Doppler equation is a fairly straightforward process. With increasing angle of incidence (θ), cosine θ becomes progressively less than 1.0, and when incorporated into the equation results in a systematic and increasingly severe underestimation of the true velocity. For practical purposes, an angle of interrogation θ less than 20 degrees is essential to ensure clinically accurate information. The Doppler shift data that are generated are typically displayed as velocity rather than the actual frequency shift. By convention, motion toward the transducer is displayed above a "zero crossing line" and motion away from the transducer below the line (Fig. 11-7).

Pulsed versus Continuous-Wave Doppler. Doppler ultrasonography is used in two basic methods. The first is pulsed Doppler, which can be considered a "steerable stethoscope," in which a sample volume of variable size can be superimposed on the two-dimensional echocardiographic image. Range gating is used to ensure that only Doppler shifts from one discrete site are interpreted for velocity calculations. Thus, pulsed Doppler allows determination of direction and flow velocity at a precise point within the cardiac system. It is limited, however, in its maximum detectable velocity by the Nyquist limit. The Nyquist limit is defined as one-half of the pulse repetition frequency. For typical imaging systems, the maximum recordable velocity with pulsed Doppler is 1.5 to 2 m/sec. Many stenotic and regurgitant velocities exceed this limit, at which point the spectral display is paradoxically recorded as a velocity in the opposite direction of the moving target. This phenomenon is known as "aliasing" (Fig. 11-8).

Continuous-wave Doppler simultaneously and continuously transmits and interrogates the returning ultrasound beam for Doppler shifts. The line of interrogation is identifiable; however, the precise location of the maximum velocity must be deduced by integrating the interrogation line direction with known cardiac anatomy. Although continuous-wave Doppler imaging provides less precise localization of gradients, it is not constrained by velocity limits and hence can record velocities exceeding those that can be detected with pulsed Doppler.

Multigate Doppler. In an effort to increase the maximum velocity detectable with pulsed Doppler, a technique of multigating can be employed in which multiple pulsed gates are simultaneously employed, thus increasing the effective Nyquist limit. Multigate Doppler allows detection of velocities as high as 3.5 to 5 m/sec with the ability to identify one of the gates as the site of origin. In large part, multigate Doppler has been supplanted by steerable continuous wave Doppler methodology.

Color Flow Doppler. Color flow Doppler imaging represents a variation on multigate pulsed Doppler imaging and thus is subject to its velocity limitations. In color flow Doppler, instead of only a single site being interrogated for a Doppler shift, a variably sized matrix of sampling points can be created and used to simultaneously interrogate velocity over a large area of the heart. Because this represents multiple pulsed sample volumes, each of which must be independently interrogated, frame rates are relatively low for color Doppler flow imaging. Color flow imaging is the display solution for managing the data that are derived from thousands of sample sites simultaneously.[4,5] The typical color flow display algorithm involves displaying velocities toward the transducer in varying shades of red, and those heading away from the transducer in varying shades of blue with either the intensity or hue paralleling the actual velocity. If multiple velocity shifts are present at an interrogation point, this is defined as "variance" and may be colored in a yellow or green "confetti-like" image.

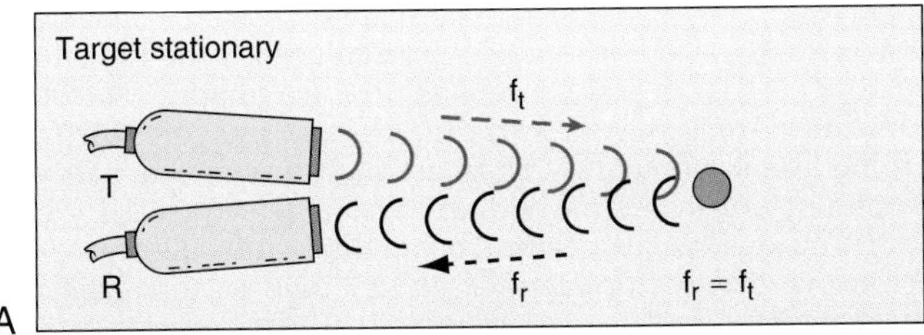

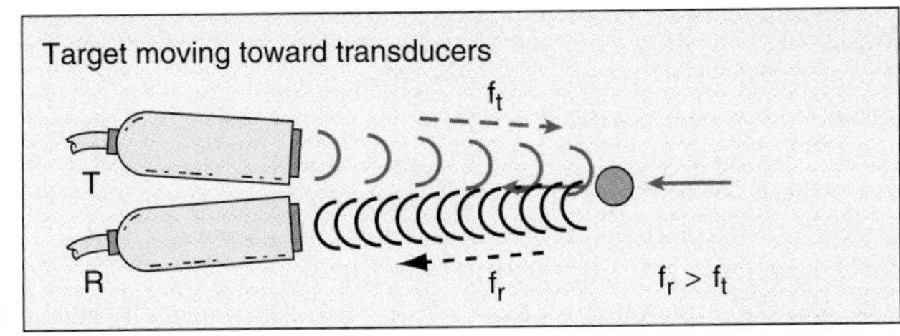

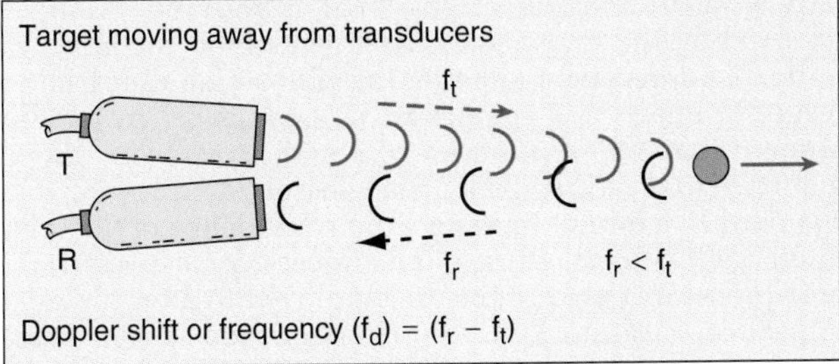

FIGURE 11-5 Demonstration of the Doppler effect. In each instance, the transmitted ultrasound beam is denoted emanating from the upper transducer and the returning beam off the reflecting object (orange circle) coming to the lower transducer. The upper panel depicts a stationary target in which the transmit frequency (f_t) is equal to the returning frequency (f_r) and there is no Doppler shift. The middle panel depicts an object moving toward the transducer in which the returning frequency (f_r) is greater than the transmit frequency (f_t). In the lower schematic, the object is moving away from the transducer, and the returning frequency (f_r) is less than the transmit frequency (f_t). The Doppler shift (f_d) equals the difference between these two frequencies. (From Feigenbaum H: Echocardiography. 4th ed. Malvern, PA, Lea & Febiger, 1986.)

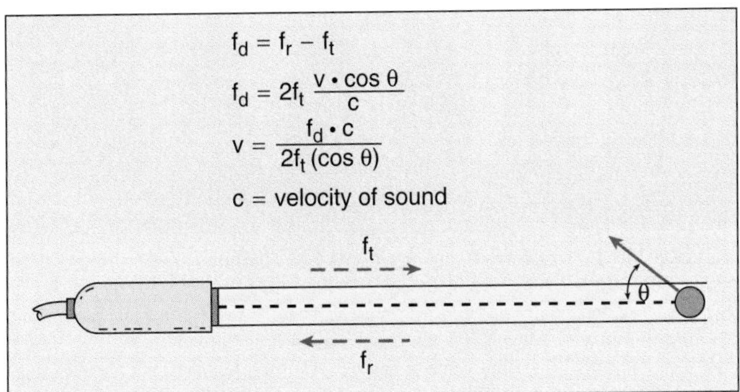

FIGURE 11-6 Demonstration of the Doppler equation for determining the velocity of a moving object. The Doppler shift (f_d) is calculated as the difference between the returning (f_r) and transmit (f_t) frequencies. The Doppler equation relates the Doppler shift (f_d) to the transmit frequency, the angle of interrogation (θ), the velocity of the moving object (V), and the speed of sound (C). The equation can be rearranged to solve for velocity as is noted in the third equation. (From Feigenbaum H: Echocardiography. 4th ed. Malvern, PA, Lea & Febiger, 1986.)

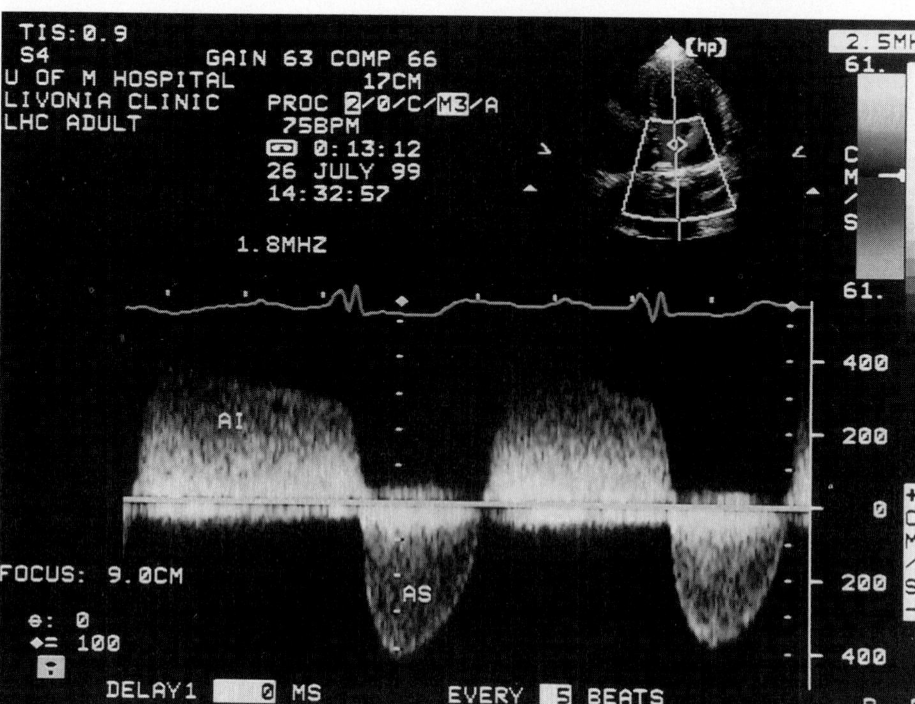

FIGURE 11–7 Combination of aortic stenosis (AS) and aortic insufficiency (AI), demonstrating the directional nature of spectral Doppler. The continuous-wave Doppler is recorded from the apex of the left ventricle along a line oriented through the aortic valve. Aortic stenosis is present with a peak velocity of 4 m/sec (400 cm/sec) that is directed away from the transducer and hence recorded below the zero crossing line. Aortic insufficiency is also present and is noted as a diastolic signal recorded above the zero crossing line.

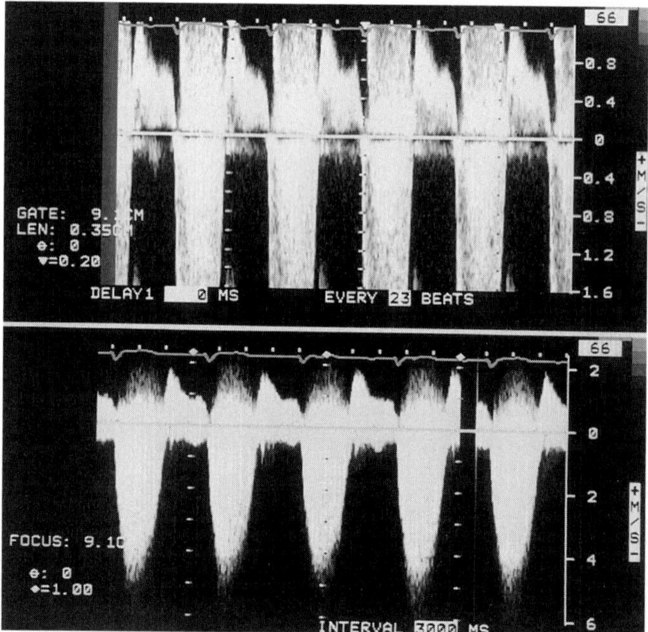

FIGURE 11–8 Pulsed **(top)** and continuous-wave **(bottom)** Doppler recording of mitral regurgitation. The lower panel recorded with continuous wave Doppler is free of the aliasing phenomenon, and the true peak velocity of the mitral regurgitation jet (5.5 m/sec) is fully displayed. The top panel was recorded in pulsed Doppler, which results in "aliasing." Once the velocity has exceeded the Nyquist limit (in this case, 1.6 m/sec) the signal is paradoxically displayed above the zero crossing line.

Image Generation

An ultrasound platform consists of several components. Modern scanners have highly computerized platforms for analog to digital conversion of returning ultrasound signals and then manipulation and display of the signal to provide either anatomical information (two-dimensional echocardiography) or information regarding velocity of motion (Doppler information) or other highly specialized applications such as tissue characterization.

An ultrasound transducer consists of a series of piezoelectric crystals, which when electrically activated, emit ultrasound energy. A transducer will be described by its frequency range as well as the number of crystals or channels incorporated in its face. This typically will range from 128 to 512 channels in modern scanners. Recently, scanners with a rectangular array of piezoelectric crystals (rather than a linear array) have been developed that allow a three-dimensional beam to be propagated in real time. Incorporated into the transducer construction is damping material to allow a crystal to be excited but then rapidly become quiescent, as well as filters to control the range of frequencies received and an effective "lens," which focuses the resulting ultrasound beam.

There are two basic mechanisms by which an ultrasound transducer creates the fan-shaped sector of ultrasound required for two-dimensional imaging. Virtually all modern scanners rely on phased array scan heads. In this technology, firing of individual crystals is sequentially controlled to steer the ultrasound beam through its 90-degree arc. A mechanical sector scanner utilizes one to three discrete piezoelectric crystals that are rotated at high velocity to then create an arc. In either instance, the piezoelectric crystals incorporated into the scan head serve the dual purpose of transmitting and receiving ultrasound energy.

Returning ultrasound energy is converted by the piezoelectric crystal into radiofrequency energy. This energy is in the analog domain. For processing purposes, it is converted to digital information by high-speed analog to digital converters within the ultrasound platform.

It should be emphasized that the resulting image that appears on the screen of the ultrasound platform contains only a small fraction of the total ultrasound information received by the transducer. Early-generation scanners transmitted and received a series of ultrasound lines and the resulting image was comprised of a series of "rastor lines." Modern scanners use a scan converter to convert the information being received along angles of interrogation into a standard X-Y format image devoid of evidence of the original interrogation lines. During the process of scan conversion, post-processing algorithms are employed to alter the relative impact of ultrasound in various amplitude ranges to create the aesthetically pleasing ultrasound image characteristic of current scanners.

Controls available for image manipulation include either enhancing or suppressing the signal from any given receipt depth. As the depth of imaging is directly related to the time of transit, this alteration is known as time-gain compensation. Current-generation scanners display images in 128 to 512 shades of gray, each of which can be assigned using a variety of post-processing algorithms designed for enhancement of myocardial texture, suppression of highly reflective objects or to enhance the ultrasound signature of faint objects. In an effort to enhance visual detection of anatomical boundaries and spectral Doppler signals, the fundamental gray scale image can be colorized. This has shown promise for detection and tracking of endocardial boundaries and for visualization of faint spectral Doppler signals.

When ultrasound interacts with a reflective surface, its interaction can be described as either specular or scattering. Specular reflectors generally reflect ultrasound energy back as a unified predictable beam. If the angle of the reflector is perpendicular to the beam, energy will be reflected back directly. If the reflector is tangential to the beam reflection can also be tangential to the original line of propagation. In any event, a portion of the ultrasound energy is reflected back as a discrete signal. Conversely, scattering reflectors tend to scatter the ultrasound beam and result in substantial lessening of its reflective amplitude. Biological examples of a specular reflector would be a bright pericardial echo or mechanical valve prosthesis. These objects reflect ultrasound back directly. Tissue tends to be a more scattering reflector that scatters the beam, which results in substantial dispersion of ultrasound energy, only a portion of which is reflected directly back to the transducer.

Ultrasound Image Formats

The simplest image to understand is the M-mode echocardiogram. An M-mode echocardiogram is acquired by interrogating returning ultrasound signals along a single line of interrogation. Each returning packet is analyzed for its round trip transit time, which is then converted to a distance from the transducer face. It is then displayed as a discrete point. The intensity of the point is directly related to the amplitude of the returning signal. Ultrasound reflected off of a highly reflective object such as a fibrotic or calcified structure has greater amplitude and hence is displayed as a brighter dot. Ultrasound reflected from a diffuse reflector such as myocardium is displayed as a fainter dot. This process is repeated at a frequency of 1000 to 3000 per second and then recorded. Early M-mode echocardiograms were recorded on a strip chart recorder at speeds of 25 to 100 mm/sec. Modern M-mode echocardiograms are recorded on a scrolling video screen. It is uncommon to use a dedicated M-mode transducer in contemporary practice. Using the electronic steering capability of a modern two-dimensional scanner, the operator can select a single line of interrogation within the 90-degree sector and obtain an M-mode interrogation line along that sector. The M-mode interrogation line can be "swept" over an area of cardiac anatomy and the image then displayed as a series of side-by-side M-mode interrogation lines (Fig. 11–9). M-mode echocardiography was once the mainstay of anatomical diagnosis but has been largely abandoned in favor of modern 90-degree two-dimensional sector scanning. M-mode echocardiography does confer substantially higher temporal resolution than two-dimensional echocardiography and in some instances may provide a higher degree of axial resolution than two-dimensional scanning. In general, however, its clinical role, especially as a stand-alone technique, has been largely supplanted by two-dimensional scanning.

Color M-Mode

Color M-mode echocardiography examines routine M-mode scanning with superimposed color Doppler information. As with M-mode echocardiography, the x axis represents time and the y axis represents distance from the transducer. Along the single line of interrogation, Doppler information is then color-encoded and superimposed on the M-mode display (Fig. 11–10). This technique provides high temporal resolution for timing intracardiac flow and can have particular value in determining the timing of a regurgitant valvular lesion and in determining the rate of inflow into the left ventricle. It is limited in that it provides information regarding velocity of flow in only one dimension.

THE ANATOMICAL ECHOCARDIOGRAPHIC EXAMINATION

The mainstay of the echocardiographic examination is transthoracic two-dimensional echocardiography. The fan-shaped scan plane is directed into the chest to provide tomographic imaging planes of the heart and great vessels (Figs. 11–11 to 11–17). Each returning ultrasound signal is then registered and converted to a two-dimensional image of the interrogated plane. This process is repeated 20 to 120 times per second, resulting in a frame rate of 20 to 120 Hz. The sequence of imaged frames results in a real-time moving image of the heart. The frame rate for two-dimensional imaging is dependent on line density and scanning depth. Smaller areas can be imaged at substantially higher (100-140 Hz) frame rates than larger sectors, which typically are imaged at 40 to 60 Hz.

For the transthoracic examination, patients are typically placed in a left lateral position and scanned from several different left intercostal spaces. The standard transthoracic views (Table 11–1) are recorded from parasternal and apical transducer positions. Subcostal and suprasternal transducer positions can also be used. From any transducer position, the Doppler modalities, including pulsed, continuous-wave, and color flow imaging, can be recorded. Other imaging windows, such as the right sternal border, can be used for specific examinations.

Traditionally, two-dimensional echocardiograms and Doppler echocardiograms have been recorded on videotape for subsequent analysis and activities. With modern ultrasonography equipment, the image is acquired in a digital format and stored as such. Digital images can be displayed side by side or as a quad screen containing multiple views for visualization simultaneously. Digital images can be transmitted to remote sites for review and are free from degradation seen when the source image is transferred to analog videotape.

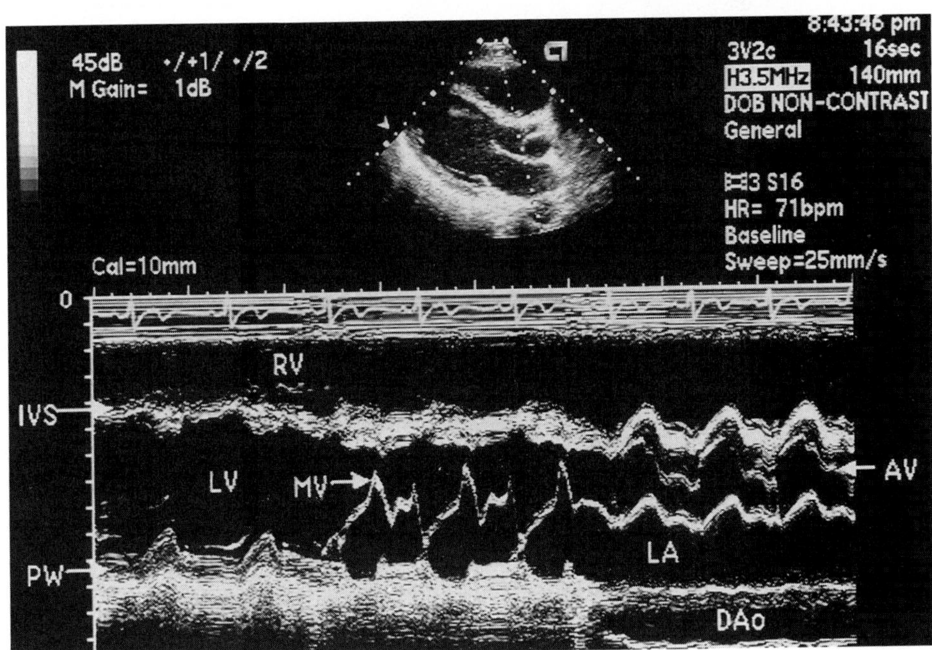

FIGURE 11–9 Normal M-mode echocardiogram in which the M-mode beam is swept from the aortic valve through the mitral valve and to the level of the papillary muscles. Note the normal box-like opening of the aortic valve and the biphasic, "M"-shaped opening pattern of the mitral valve. There is posterior motion of the ventricular septum synchronous with anterior motion of the posterior wall. AV = aortic valve; DAo = descending aorta; LA = left atrium; LV = left ventricle; MV = mitral valve; RV = right ventricle.

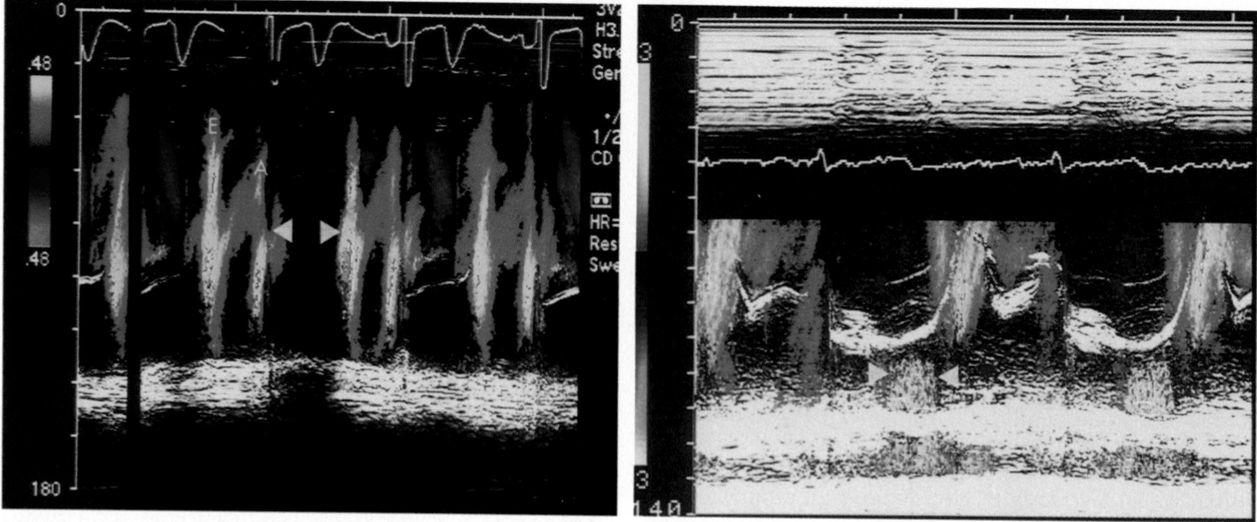

FIGURE 11–10 Color M-mode echocardiography. With this methodology, color flow imaging is superimposed on an M-mode echocardiogram. This provides excellent temporal resolution for timing intracardiac events. The **left panel** was recorded in a normal, disease-free individual from the apex of the left ventricle. Notice that both early and late (E and A) mitral inflow can be detected. The systolic interval (white arrowheads) is devoid of flow. The **right panel** was recorded in a patient with mitral valve prolapse and late systolic mitral regurgitation. Note the prominent early flow velocity through the mitral valve and a late systolic regurgitant flow (white arrowheads).

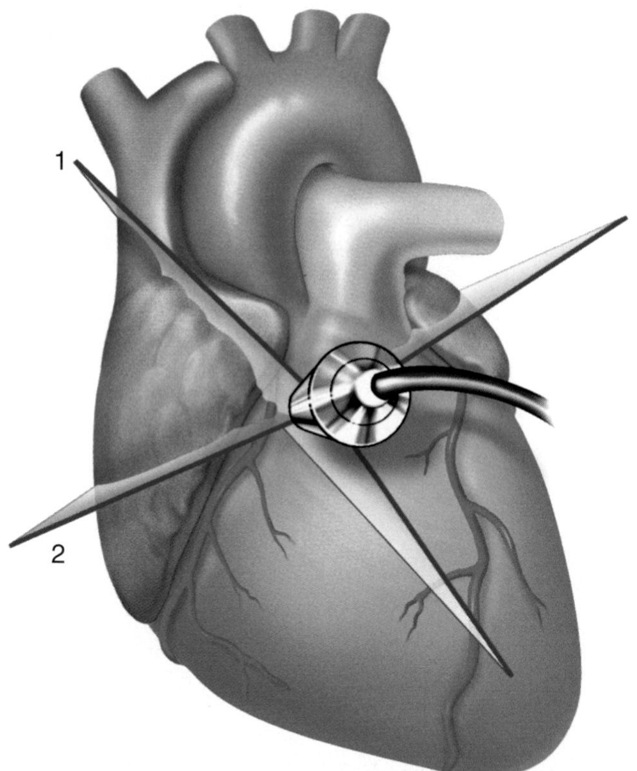

FIGURE 11–11 Schematic of the transducer orientation used for acquiring parasternal views. The scanning plane of the ultrasound beam is superimposed on a schematic of the heart. Plane 1 represents a parasternal long-axis view in which the right ventricular outflow tract, proximal portion of the aorta and aortic valve, anterior ventricular septum, cavity of the left ventricle containing the mitral valve, and inferoposterior wall of the left ventricle can be visualized. Scanning plane 1 results in an ultrasound image, as noted in Figure 11–12. Scanning plane 2 is obtained by rotating the transducer 90 degrees and can be used to obtain a family of short-axis views of the heart (see Fig. 11–14). (From Feigenbaum H: Echocardiography. 4th ed. Malvern, PA, Lea & Febiger, 1986.)

TABLE 11–1 Two-Dimensional Echocardiographic Examination

Parasternal Approach
Long-axis plane
Root of aorta—aortic valve, left atrium, left ventricular outflow tract
Body of left ventricle—mitral valve
Left ventricular apex
Right ventricular inflow tract—tricuspid valve
Short-axis plane
Root of the aorta—aortic valve, pulmonary valve, tricuspid valve, right ventricular outflow tract, left atrium, pulmonary artery, coronary arteries
Left ventricle—mitral valve
Left ventricle—papillary muscles
Left ventricle—apex
Apical Approach
Four-chamber plane
Four chambers
Four chambers with aorta
Long-axis plane
Two chambers—left ventricle, left atrium
Two chambers with aorta
Subcostal Approach
Four-chamber plane—all four chambers and both septa
Short-axis plane
Left ventricle
Right ventricle
Inferior vena cava
Suprasternal Approach
Four-chamber plane
Arch of aorta—descending aorta
Long-axis plane
Arch of aorta—pulmonary artery, left atrium

Examination and Appearance of the Normal Heart

PARASTERNAL LONG-AXIS VIEW. In this view (Fig. 11–12), the inferoposterior wall and interventricular septum are visualized, each of which is mildly concave toward the other. The normal ascending aorta is visualized, including its annulus, the sinuses of Valsalva, and the proximal portion of the ascending aorta. The anterior and posterior leaflets of the mitral valve can be visualized in the parasternal long-axis view, with the anterior leaflet appearing more elongated. Typically, the posterolateral papillary muscle is also visualized from this transducer position. Anterior to the aorta, a portion of the right ventricular outflow tract is visualized. By medially angulating the transducer, the right ventricular inflow tract can be visualized in which the inferior vena cava, right atrium, tricuspid valve, and right ventricle are visualized (Fig. 11–13). From the parasternal transducer position, a series of short-axis views can be obtained by rotating the transducer 90 degrees (Fig. 11–14). At the base of the heart, the circular aorta and the aortic valve with three equally sized leaflets are visualized, as well as the right ventricular outflow tract, which is seen as an inverted "U" overlying the aorta. By angling the transducer toward the apex, a short-axis view of the mitral valve can be visualized from which the actual orifice can be seen and its area measured. With further angulation, the circular cavity of the left ventricle is visualized, including the papillary muscles. The normal left ventricle has circular geometry, whether it is visualized at the level of the mitral valve, papillary muscles, or apex. In the short-axis projections at the level of the mitral valve and below, the right ventricle appears as a more trabeculated crescent-shaped structure.

APICAL VIEWS. From this transducer position, the normal left ventricle has a bullet-shaped geometry. The anterior and posterior mitral valve leaflets can be visualized. The left atrium and pulmonary veins are visualized as well (Fig. 11–15). In the four-chamber view, the right ventricle appears as a triangular structure. The tricuspid valve inserts into the annulus of the right ventricle at a position slightly more apical than the mitral valve. This results in a small portion of the ventricular septum (the atrioventricular septum) falling between the septal leaflets of the tricuspid and mitral valves. By rotating the transducer 90 degrees from the four-chamber view, a two-chamber view of the left ventricle and left atrium can be obtained (see Fig. 11–15).

SUBCOSTAL AND SUPRASTERNAL VIEWS. In addition to parasternal and apical transducer positions, subcostal and suprasternal positions also provide imaging windows in adult patients. The subcostal transducer position can be very effective in patients with chronic lung disease in whom parasternal and apical views are obscured by intervening lung tissue. For subcostal imaging, patients are placed in the supine position with the knees bent and the transducer placed in the subxiphoid position. Imaging during held inspiration often is effective at bringing the heart into optimal position. Views similar to a four-chamber view as well as a series of short-axis views can be obtained from this transducer position. The subcostal views also provide excellent visualization of the atrial septum and the connection between the inferior vena cava (IVC) and right atrium (Fig. 11–16).

SUPRASTERNAL VIEWS. These views are obtained by placing the transducer in the suprasternal notch. This transducer position may be somewhat uncomfortable for many patients. It provides a view of the arch and adjacent ascending and descending aorta. In the majority of patients, the great vessels and portions of the main pulmonary artery are also seen (Fig. 11–17).

Anatomic Variants

Several well-recognized anatomical and developmental variants can be seen with echocardiography. It is important to recognize these as normal variants to avoid confusion with pathological structures.

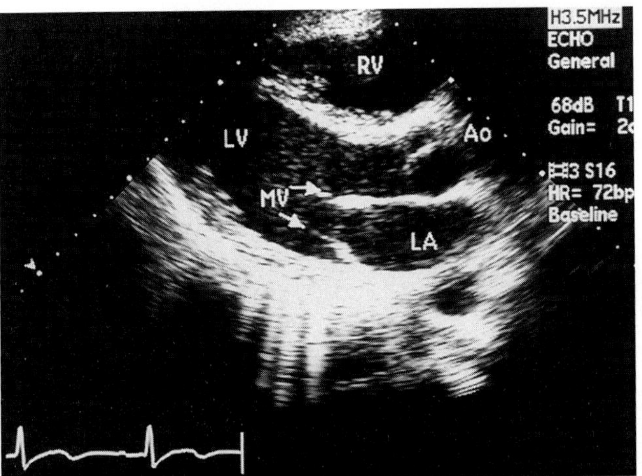

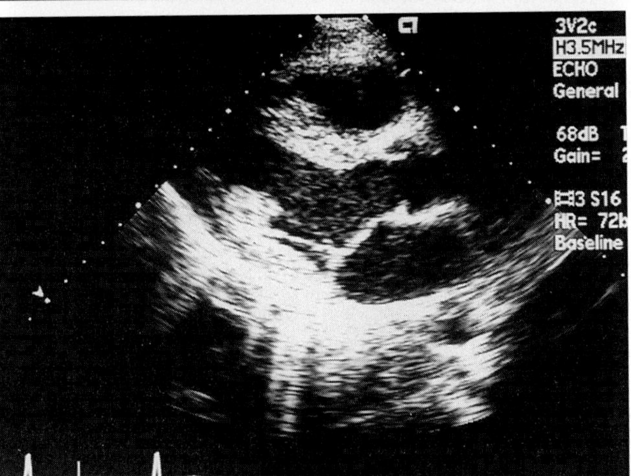

FIGURE 11–12 Parasternal long-axis view of the left ventricle in diastole **(top)** and systole **(bottom)**. Chambers and cardiac structures are as noted. This view corresponds to plane 1 of Figure 11–11. Ao = aorta; LA = left atrium; LV = left ventricle; MV = mitral valve; RV = right ventricular outflow tract.

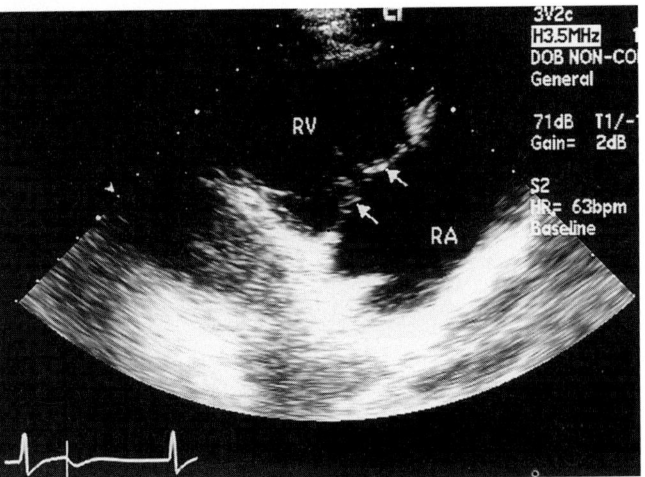

FIGURE 11–13 Two-dimensional echocardiogram of the right ventricular inflow tract, recorded from the parasternal transducer position. RA = right atrium; RV = right ventricle.

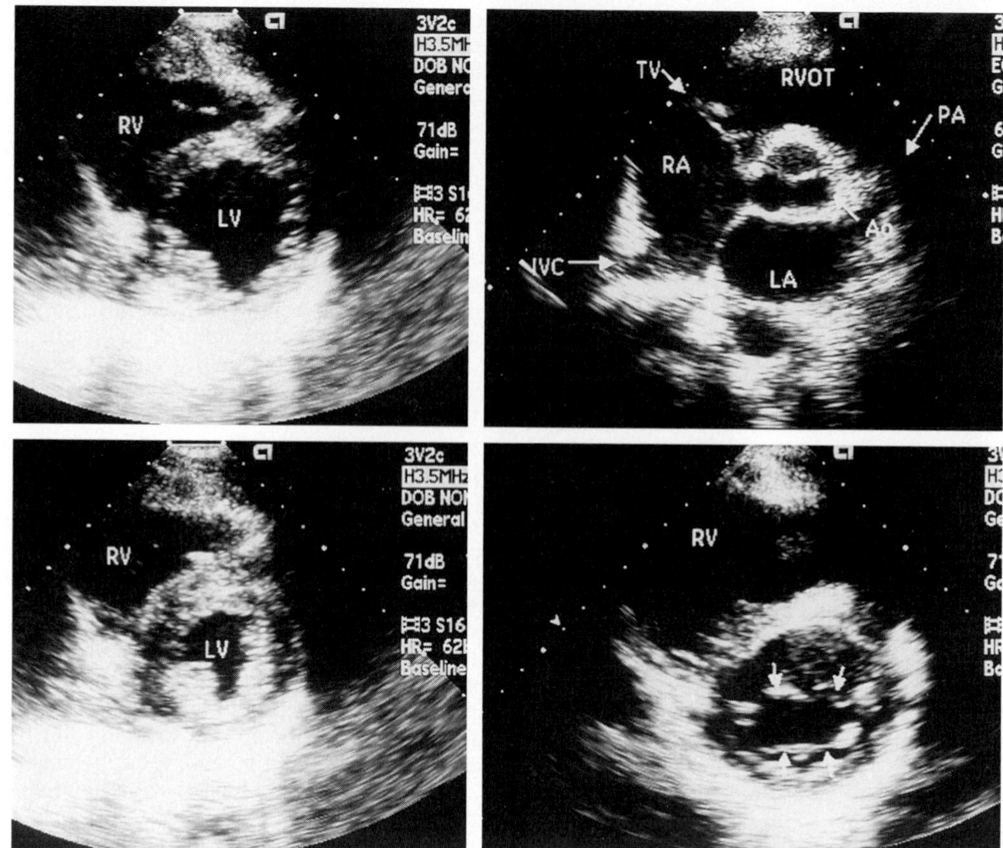

FIGURE 11–14 Short-axis two-dimensional echocardiograms, the two **left panels** are recorded at the level of the papillary muscles in diastole **(top)** and systole **(bottom)**. Note the symmetrical thickening of the myocardium and inward motion of the endocardium representing normal ventricular function in systole. The **top right panel** is recorded at the level of the aortic valve, and the **bottom right panel** is recorded at the level of the mitral valve in diastole. Ao = aorta; IVC = inferior vena cava; LA = left atrium; LV = left ventricle; PA = pulmonary artery; RA = right atrium; RV = right ventricle; RVOT = right ventricular outflow tract; TV = tricuspid valve.

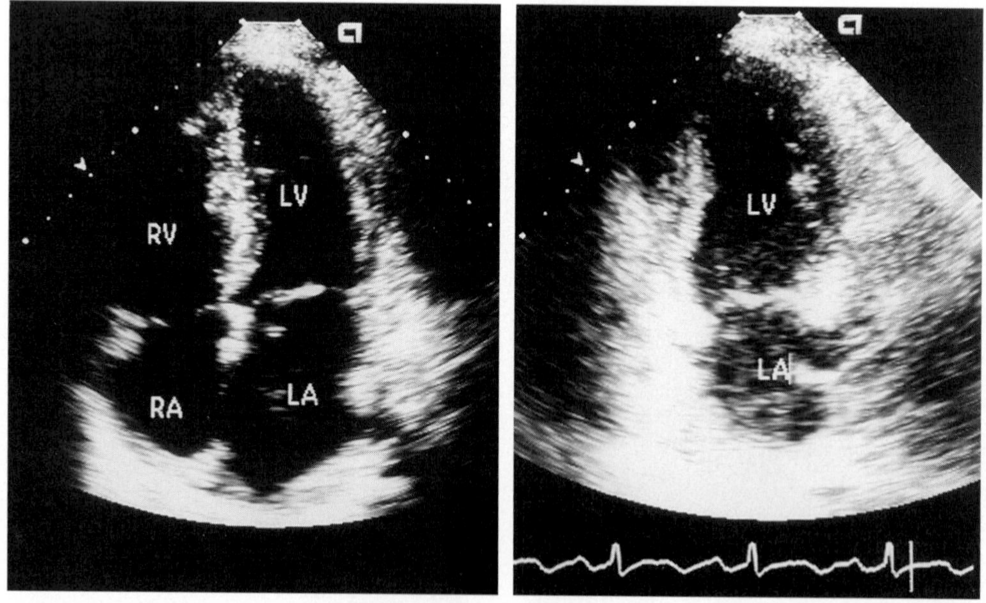

FIGURE 11–15 Apical four- and two-chamber views of the left ventricle. Note the normal "bullet-shaped" geometry of the left ventricle and the more triangular right ventricle. Note also the more apical insertion of the tricuspid valve compared with the mitral valve. LA = left atrium; LV = left ventricle; RA = right atrium; RV = right ventricle.

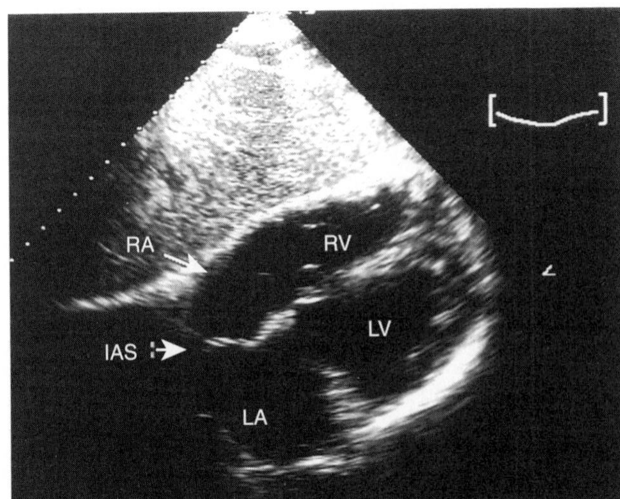

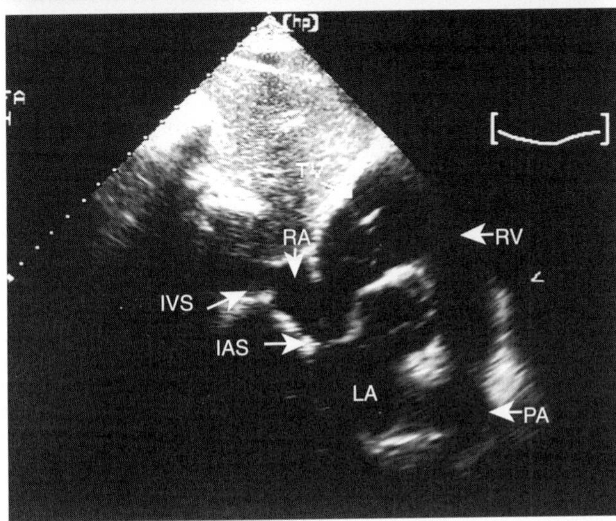

FIGURE 11–16 Two-dimensional echocardiograms recorded from the subcostal transducer position. The **upper panel** is a subcostal four-chamber view in which all four cardiac chambers are visualized as well as the plane of the mitral and tricuspid valves. The atrial septum is visualized in its entire length in this view. The **lower panel** was recorded in a short-axis view at the level of the aortic valve from the subcostal position. The right atrium (RA), tricuspid valve (TV), right ventricle (RV), and pulmonary artery (PA) are visualized as well as the circular aorta. The interatrial septum (IAS) and inferior vena cava (IVC) are both visualized in this view as well. LA = left atrium; LV = left ventricle.

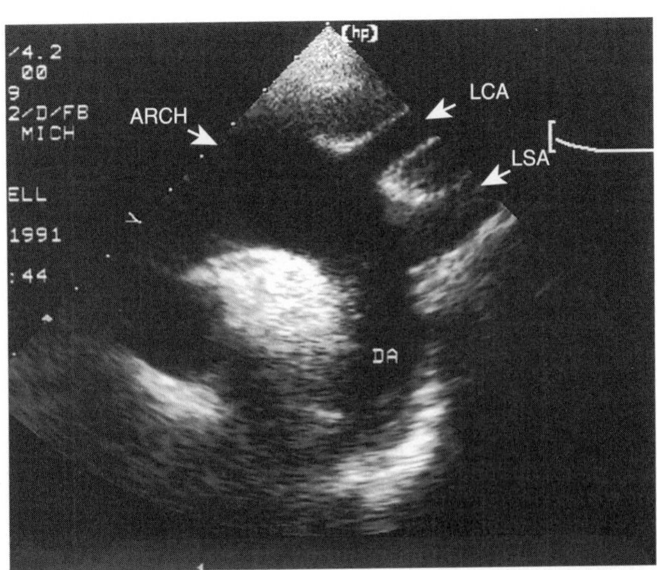

FIGURE 11–17 Two-dimensional echocardiogram recorded from a suprasternal transducer position. The arch of the aorta (ARCH) as well as a portion of the ascending and descending aorta can be visualized. Note also the great vessels arising from the arch (arrows). DA = descending aorta; LCA = left carotid artery; LSA = left subclavian artery.

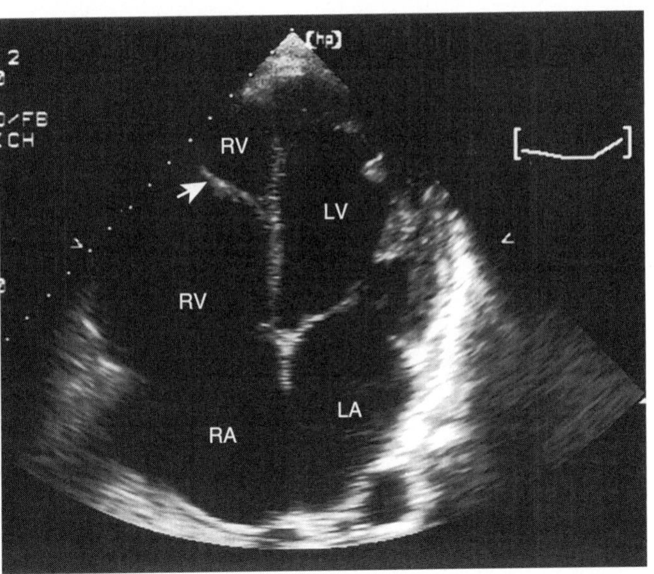

FIGURE 11–18 Apical four-chamber view of the heart revealing a prominent moderator band. The moderator band (arrow) appears as a muscle density structure traversing the apex of the right ventricle. This is a normal anatomical structure that should not be confused with a pathological process. LA = left atrium; LV = left ventricle; RA = right atrium; RV = right ventricle.

MUSCLE TRABECULATIONS. The right ventricle is more heavily trabeculated than the left, and, similarly, the right atrium is more trabeculated than the left atrium. High-resolution scanning virtually always detects multiple muscle trabeculations in the right ventricle, the most prominent of which is the moderator band, which is a muscular structure traversing from the lateral wall to the septum of the right ventricle near the apex (Fig. 11–18). On occasion, secondary muscle bundles are likewise noted. In any situation in which right ventricular hypertrophy occurs, the trabeculations become more prominent. It is important to recognize this phenomenon to avoid confusing a heavily trabeculated right ventricle with tumor, vegetation, thrombus, or other pathological mass.

The left ventricle is typically less trabeculated than the right, and other than the papillary muscles it is not common to note muscular tissue protruding into the left ventricle. Occasionally, a trabeculated left ventricular apex is encountered, the degree of which rarely approaches that seen in the right ventricle. Not infrequently, pseudochordae are seen in the left ventricular apex. Anatomically, these are structures similar to mitral valve chordae but that take an aberrant course, typically across the apex of the left ventricle. They are less often seen in the left ventricular outflow tract. They are more easily visualized in patients with cardiomyopathy and dilated hearts than in normal hearts, where they may lie against the endocardium and therefore not be visible.

RIGHT AND LEFT ATRIAL STRUCTURES. Several developmental remnants can be noted in the right atrium. These include the eustachian valve (Fig. 11–19) and Chiari network. In the embryo, a continuous membrane courses from the IVC to the coronary sinus to direct oxygenated blood from the IVC directly across the foramen ovale. During cardiac development, this membrane regresses. In the majority of patients, a small remnant known as the eustachian

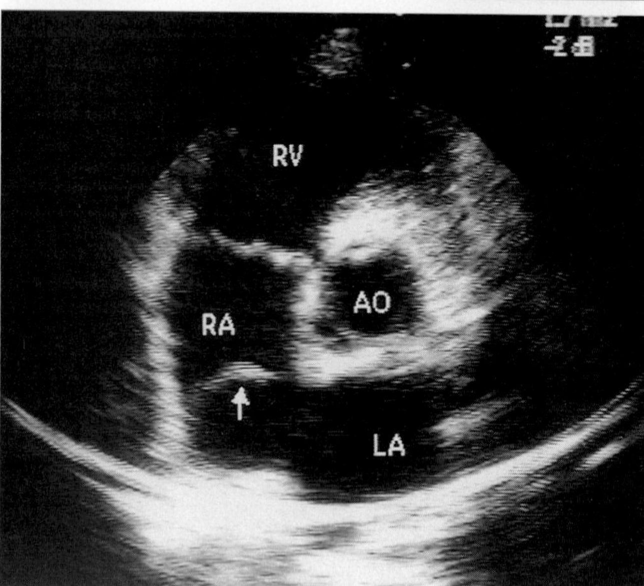

FIGURE 11–19 Transthoracic parasternal echocardiograms recorded in a patient with a prominent eustachian valve (EV). This is a normal anatomical variant that should not be confused for a mass, vegetation, or other pathological structure. The **top panel** is a right ventricular inflow tract view recorded from the left sternal border. Both the right atrium (RA) and right ventricle (RV) can be seen, and the tricuspid valve is closed. Note the linear echo arising from the junction of the right atrium and inferior vena cava coursing into the body of the right atrium. In real time this linear echo has highly mobile motion, mimicking valvular motion. The **bottom panel** is recorded in a parasternal short-axis view at the base of the heart. The same linear echo is noted in the bottom of the right atrium (arrow). AO = aorta.

valve can be seen at the right atrial–IVC junction. A second remnant is occasionally seen attached to the coronary sinus. This is known as a Chiari network and consists of a fine filamentous membrane with multiple perforations. On rare occasions, a "complete eustachian valve" is seen as a linear echo coursing from the IVC to the coronary sinus. In this instance, it has many perforations and rarely, if ever, is truly obstructive. Either the eustachian valve or a Chiari network can result in redirection of blood flow within the atrium and unusual patterns of blood flow noted with contrast echocardiography.

The right atrial appendage is typically visualized only with transesophageal echocardiography (TEE). It is a more trabeculated structure than the left atrial appendage, and, on occasion, trabeculae in the right atrial appendage have been confused for thrombi. Recognizing the full range of appearance of the right atrial appendage is essential to avoid this error.

The left atrium has a smoother wall than the right atrium. Using modern scanners, the left atrial appendage is often partially visualized with transthoracic imaging, either in the apical two-chamber view or in a parasternal short-axis view. It is optimally visualized with TEE, where it has the appearance of a "dog's ear" (Fig. 11–20). A substantial percentage of individuals have a multilobed left atrial appendage, which can result in a confusing appearance because the septation between the two lobes may be confused for thrombus.[6]

ATRIAL SEPTUM. The normal interatrial septum is visualized both in its primum and in its more superior portions, connected by the thin tissue of the foramen ovale. There is substantial variation in the thickness and prominence of the more muscular primum and superior portions of the atrial septum. A commonly encountered anomaly of the atrial septum is lipomatous atrial hypertrophy in which there is benign infiltration by lipomatous tissue of the primum and superior atrial septum (Fig. 11–21). The valve of the foramen ovale is spared, resulting in a "dumbbell" configuration of the atrial septum. The amount of infiltration is highly variable and can range from less than 1.0 cm to 5 cm or more. The tissue is homogeneous and somewhat brighter than the normal atrial septum. Because of its characteristic appearance, it should not be confused with intracardiac tumor or thrombus.

QUANTIFICATION OF VENTRICULAR PERFORMANCE

Echocardiography provides an excellent method for quantification of ventricular function. Linear measurements such as wall thickness, internal chamber dimension, and the derived parameters such as fractional shortening traditionally have been obtained from M-mode echocardiography. Normal values for adults and children are well established (Table 7–2).[7-11] Global ventricular function and cardiac volumes can be measured with a variety of algorithms using two-dimensional echocardiography. The most commonly employed method for quantitation of ventricular volume is Simpson's rule (Fig. 11–22). Once the chamber volumes have been determined, ejection fraction can be calculated. Calculation of ejection fraction represents only a small aspect of quantification of ventricular performance. Determination of left ventricular

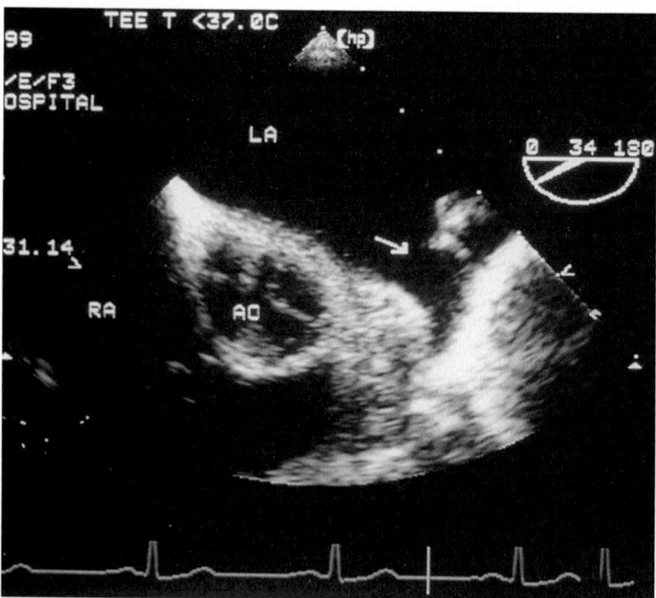

FIGURE 11–20 Transesophageal echocardiogram recorded at a 30-degree angle demonstrating the appearance of normal left atrial appendage. The body of the left atrium (LA) is at the apex of the scan and the normal "ear-shaped" left atrial appendage can be seen communicating with the body of the left atrium (arrow). AO = aorta; RA = right atrium.

TABLE 11–2 Normal Values of M-Mode Echocardiographic Measurements in Adults

	Range	Mean	No. of Subjects
Age (yrs)	13-54	26	134
Body surface area (M^2)	1.45-2.22	1.8	130
RVD—flat (cm)	0.7-2.3	1.5	84
RVD—left lateral (cm)	0.9-2.6	1.7	83
LVID—flat (cm)	3.7-5.6	4.7	82
LVID—left lateral (cm)	3.5-5.7	4.7	81
Posterior LV wall thickness (cm)	0.6-1.1	0.9	137
Posterior LV wall amplitude (cm)	0.9-1.4	1.2	48
IVS wall thickness (cm)	0.6-1.1	0.9	137
Mid IVS amplitude (cm)	0.3-0.8	0.5	10
Apical IVS amplitude (cm)	0.5-1.2	0.7	38
Left atrial dimension (cm)	1.9-4.0	2.9	133
Aortic root dimension (cm)	2.0-3.7	2.7	121
Aortic cusps' separation (cm)	1.5-2.6	2.9	93
Fractional shortening* (%)	34-44	36	20
Rate of circumferential shortening (Vcf)†or normalized shortening velocity (circ/sec)	1.02-1.94	1.3	38

d = end diastole; IVS = interventricular septum; LV = left ventricle; LVID = left ventricular internal dimension; RVD = right ventricular dimension; s = end systole.
*(LVIDd − LVIDs) ÷ LVIDd
†(LVIDd − LVIDs) ÷ (LVIDd × Ejection time)

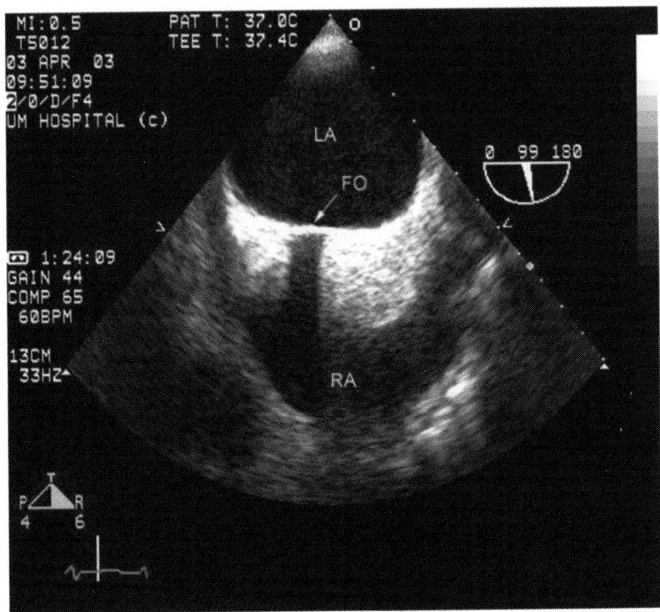

FIGURE 11–21 Transesophageal echocardiogram in a longitudinal view recorded in a patient with marked lipomatous atrial hypertrophy. Note the two large masses bulging off the atrial septum into the cavity of the right atrium, which represent lipomatous deposits. The foramen ovale (FO) is spared in the infiltrative process. LA = left atrium; RA = right atrium.

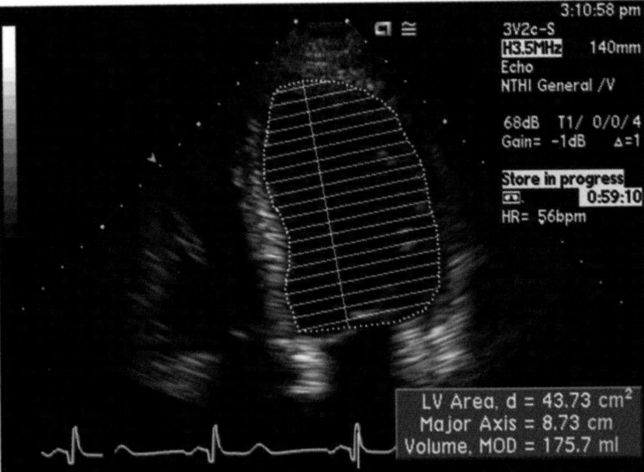

FIGURE 11–22 Apical four-chamber view from which left ventricular volume has been calculated using Simpson's rule. The endocardium has been traced and automatically subdivided into a series of discs. The volume of each of the discs is then calculated as disc area (πr^2) multiplied by the height of each disc. The volume of each separate disc is then summed to provide the volume of the ventricle (175.7 ml in this example).

volume requires manual tracings of the endocardial border in diastole and systole. Instrumentation exists that can automatically determine the endocardial border and calculate volumes and ejection fraction (Fig. 11-23).[12] Application of this technology requires high-quality images with a favorable signal-to-noise ratio. These automatically determined ventricular volumes can be combined with arterial pressure measurements to create pressure-volume loops for more sophisticated evaluation of ventricular performance.[13]

Left ventricular mass can be measured by several different methods.[14,15] One of the earliest was the "cube" method, which used M-mode septal, posterior wall, and left ventricular internal dimensions and assumed normal ventricular geometry. More recently, several two-dimensional methods have been shown to provide enhanced accuracy, especially in abnormally shaped ventricles.[15]

Normal wall motion consists of simultaneous myocardial thickening and inward motion of the endocardium toward the center of the chamber. In adults, the most common cause of a regional wall motion abnormality is myocardial ischemia or infarction. The extent of a wall motion abnormality can be measured in several different ways. Echocardiography is a tomographic technique that visualizes all of the cardiac walls. Traditionally, for quantitative purposes, the left ventricle is divided into 16 segments (Fig. 11-24). More recently, in an effort to provide better concordance with other imaging techniques, a 17-segment model has been proposed in which the true apex is considered the 17th segment.[16] Each segment can be attributed to one of the three major epicardial coronary arteries. There is substantial overlap in the posterior segments and inferior and lateral apical segments. For each of these segments, a wall motion score can be assigned (Fig. 11-25). This is a unitless hierarchical number in which 1 represents normal motion; 2, hypokinesis; 3, akinesis; and 4, dyskinesis. Each wall is then assigned a score, and the average score for the visualized segments is calculated. This number is directly proportional to the extent and severity of wall motion abnormalities.[17] There are several variations on a wall motion score, including addition of scores for aneurysm, mild hypokinesis, and hyperkinesis. The wall motion score can be calculated for all segments of the left ventricle or separately for anterior and posterior segments, representing the left anterior descending, right, and circumflex coronary artery territories. An M-mode interrogation line can be used to quantify endocardial excursion and myocardial thickening in any targeted segment (Fig. 11-26).

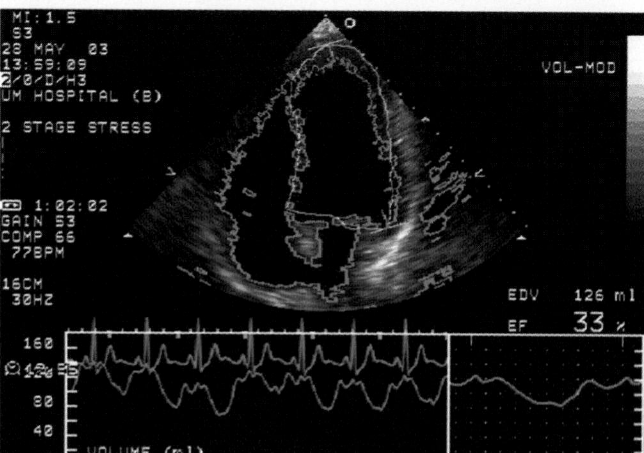

FIGURE 11–23 Apical four-chamber image in which an algorithm for automatic border detection has been used to determine instantaneous left ventricular volume. The white line outlining the endocardial border has been automatically drawn by the ultrasound machine. A graphic output of instantaneous ventricular volume (end diastolic volume = 126 ml) and ejection fraction (33%) is presented below the echocardiographic image.

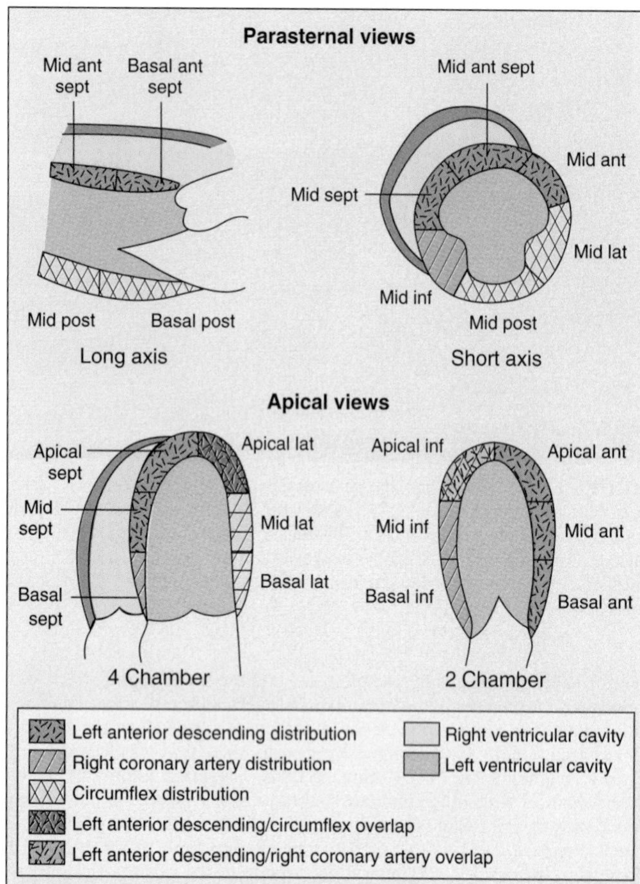

FIGURE 11–24 Schematic representation of a 16-segment model for segmenting the left ventricle. Each segment has been assigned to one of the three major coronary arteries with areas of overlap in the apex and posterior walls noted as well. ant = anterior; inf = inferior; lat = lateral; post = posterior; sept = septum.

There are several more complex methods for quantification of left ventricular function. Most rely on tracing the endocardial border in diastole and systole in either a short-axis or an apical view. Radians are then constructed from the center of mass, and either changes in radian length or changes in area subtended by an arc are then quantified.

Variants of Normal Wall Motion Patterns

ABNORMALITIES OF SEPTAL MOTION. The interventricular septum is a shared wall between the right and left ventricles, and thus its motion can be affected by processes in either ventricle. Myocardial ischemia and infarction cause a fairly characteristic absence of systolic thickening and dyskinesis of the septum. There are multiple nonischemic causes for septal wall motion abnormalities as well.

CONDUCTION DISTURBANCES. Both left bundle branch block and Wolff-Parkinson-White syndrome, with a septal pathway, can result in abnormalities of septal motion. Left bundle branch block characteristically causes an early systolic downward motion followed by relaxation of the ventricular septum and a secondary downward contraction. This is best appreciated with M-mode echocardiography. This phenomenon is most common in the proximal anterior septum and is less prominent in the distal septum. A similar pattern is seen in patients with ventricular pacing; however, the maximum location of abnormal motion is highly variable, depending on the location of the pacemaker lead.

Wolff-Parkinson-White syndrome results in ventricular preexcitation in a localized area of the left or right ventricle. The preexcited area contracts slightly earlier than the remainder of the heart and can be seen in the ventricular septal, posterior or lateral walls. The abnormality associated with Wolff-Parkinson-White syndrome is less dramatic than that seen with left bundle branch block. Although newer two-dimensional scanning instruments have temporal resolution sufficient to detect an abnormality of wall motion due to a conduction disturbance, the high temporal resolution of M-mode echocardiography may be necessary for precise identification of the wall motion abnormalities.

CONSTRICTIVE PERICARDITIS. Constrictive pericarditis interferes with the normal sequence of right and left ventricular filling and results in subtle septal wall motion abnormalities. This typically causes early downward motion of the septum, followed by paradoxical motion. Multiple patterns of septal motion abnormalities have been noted in constrictive pericarditis. As with electrical conduction disturbances, these may be best identified with M-mode echocardiography.

VENTRICULAR OVERLOAD. Either a volume or a pressure overload of the right ventricle results in a ventricular septal motion abnormality. In each instance, the right ventricle is dilated. In a pure volume overload, there is diastolic flattening of the ventricular septum so that the left ventricular geometry in diastole assumes a D shape rather than circular geometry. Because this is a low-pressure phenomenon, the left ventricle becomes circular in early systole before the onset of ventricular ejection (Fig. 11–27). A right ventricular pressure overload results in flattening of the septum not only in diastole but also in systole. The degree of flattening is directly proportional to the elevation in right ventricular systolic pressure. Frank reversal of septal curvature is seen in individuals with systemic level right-sided heart pressures.

A final septal motion abnormality that is commonly encountered is the "postoperative septum." This abnormality is characterized by paradoxical anterior motion of the septum in systole, with preserved myocardial thickening. Often posterior wall excursion appears exaggerated. This phenomenon may be seen in any form of cardiac surgery in which the pericardium has been opened. It often resolves 3 to 5 years after surgery.

Principles of the Doppler Examination

NORMAL FLOW PATTERNS. All four cardiac valves can be interrogated using either pulsed, continuous wave, or

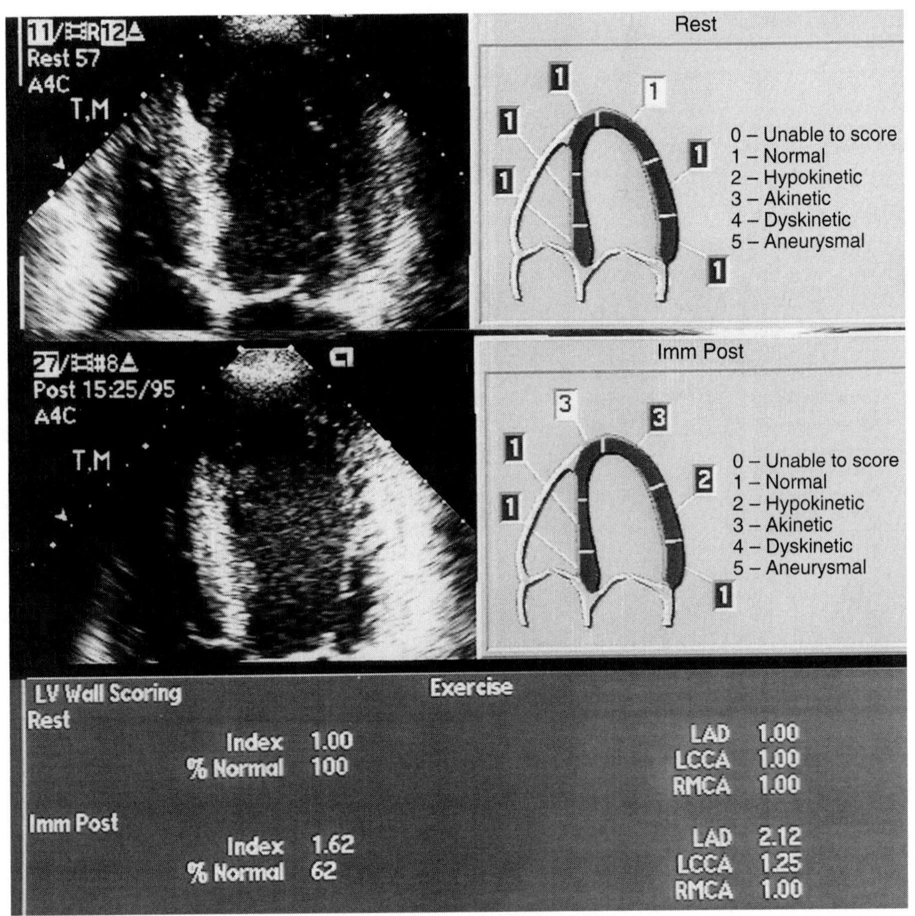

FIGURE 11–25 Wall motion score algorithm. For each of the predefined segments (typically 16), a score of 1 to 4 is assigned, with 1 representing normal motion and 4 representing dyskinetic motion. The wall motion score index equals the sum of these scores divided by the number of scored segments. Because each of the wall segments can be attributed to one of the coronary artery territories (see Fig. 11–24), wall motion scores can be calculated for the left anterior descending (LAD), left circumflex (LCCA), and right (RMCA) coronary arteries. The representative scores are as noted in the right-hand schematics, and both the global and regional wall motion scores at rest and with stress are noted in the bottom graphic.

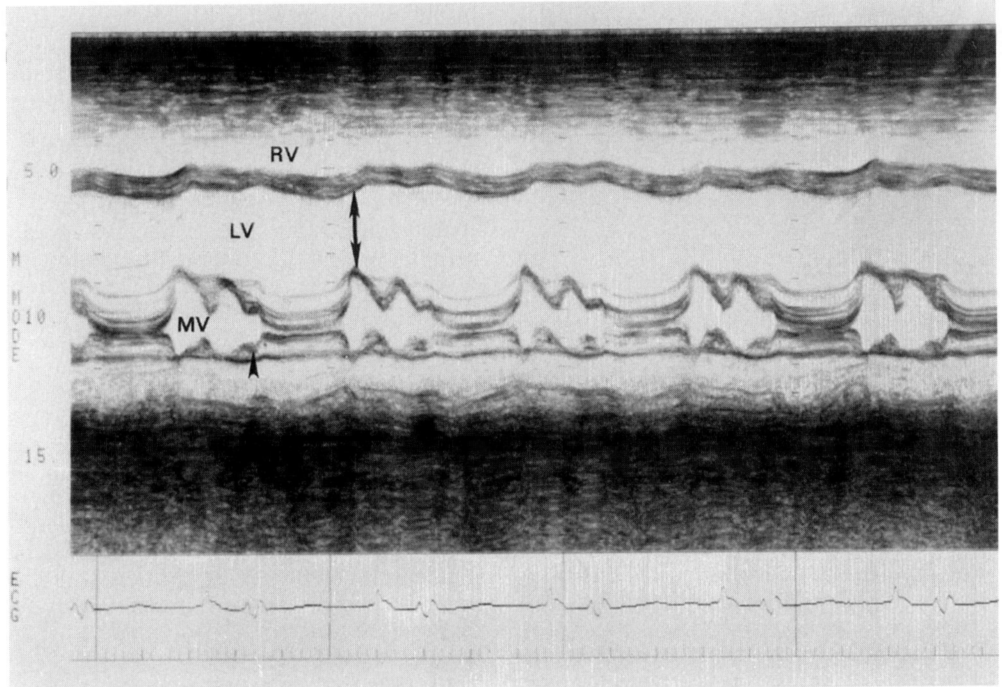

FIGURE 11–26 M-mode echocardiogram recorded in a patient with severe left ventricular systolic dysfunction. Note the dilated left ventricle (LV) and a decreased excursion of the septum and posterior wall compared with the normal example seen in Figure 11–9. There is additional evidence of left ventricular systolic dysfunction in that the mitral valve E point septal separation is increased (double-headed arrow). Evidence of elevated end-diastolic pressure is noted in the "B bump" (arrowhead), which delays final closure of the mitral valve (MV). RV = right ventricle.

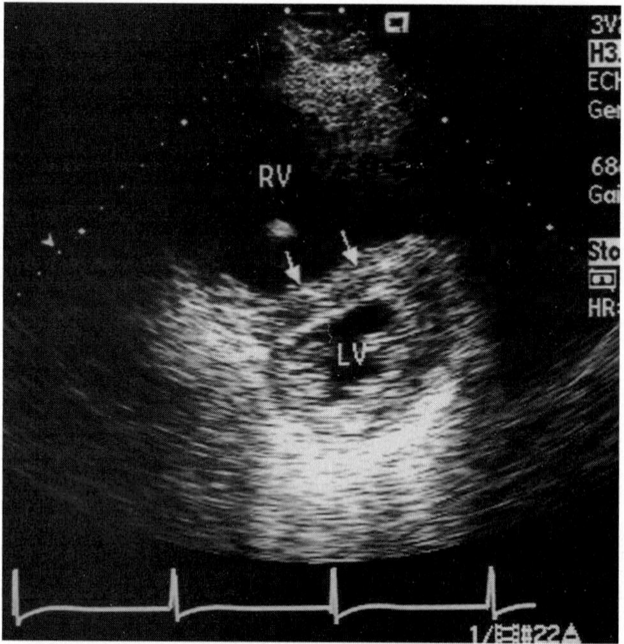

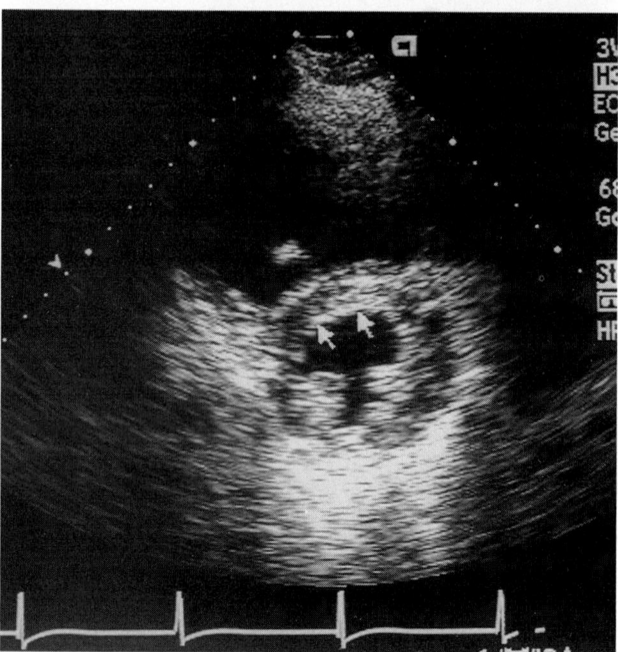

FIGURE 11–27 Short-axis two-dimensional echocardiogram depicting a right ventricular volume overload pattern. Compare the normal geometry of the left ventricle in a short-axis view (see Fig. 11–14) to that noted here. In the right ventricular volume overload pattern, there is dilation of the right ventricle (RV) and flattening of the ventricular septum (downward pointing arrows) so that in diastole the ventricle takes on a D-shaped configuration rather than circular geometry. With systole, there is restitution of normal circular geometry (upward arrows). LV = left ventricle.

color flow Doppler. Substantial physiological data can be derived from the recorded signals. Figure 11–28 is a representation of normal Doppler flow patterns across the four cardiac valves. Highly sensitive Doppler instrumentation frequently picks up mild amounts of physiological regurgitation, which is more common for the tricuspid and pulmonic than for the aortic and mitral valves. In the normal heart under physiological circumstances, the maximum velocity typically encountered is less than 1.5 m/sec. Pulmonary vein and hepatic vein flows can also be recorded in the majority of patients (Fig. 11–29).

Color flow Doppler provides the ability to track mitral and tricuspid inflow patterns and left and right ventricular outflow as well as to detect abnormal flow. Normal mitral inflow appears as a red encoded signal moving from the mitral orifice along the lateral wall to the left ventricular apex, where it reverses course and appears as a blue encoded signal along the septum. The flow profile accelerates with atrial systole. With systole, the organized flow in the left ventricular outflow tract appears as a series of color shifts as the accelerating flow exceeds the relatively low Nyquist limit of color Doppler imaging. Pathological flow will be detected either as turbulence due to a restricted orifice, such as flow through a stenotic valve, or as a regurgitant flow signal in a downstream chamber. The above scheme represents traditional color flow imaging algorithms. Many alternative color schemes and variance maps can be employed as well. It should be emphasized that the visualized jet area is heavily dependent on Doppler gain settings. At higher heart rates, the relatively low frame rate of color flow imaging also compromises accuracy. Substantial experience and attention to technical detail are essential to provide accurate clinical information from color flow Doppler imaging.

CALCULATION OF PRESSURE GRADIENTS. By interrogating the spectral Doppler profile, valuable physiological information can be derived. Once the velocity of the target has been determined, this information can be used to determine pressure gradients across an orifice using the Bernoulli equation. The Bernoulli equation contains many elements, including convective acceleration and viscous friction (Fig. 11–30). Of note, convective acceleration and viscous friction are relatively weak contributors in most biological systems and can be effectively ignored. The Bernoulli equation in its simplest form states that ΔP (the pressure gradient across a restrictive orifice) is $4V^2$, where V is the peak instantaneous velocity of flow through the restrictive orifice. In reality, the equation incorporates not only the peak instantaneous velocity at the restrictive orifice but also the velocity noted in the acceleration zone, V_1. For most clinically relevant conditions such as severe aortic stenosis, V_2 is substantially greater than V_1 and hence V_1 can effectively be ignored. There are several instances in which the V_1 velocity must be included. These include the obvious case of a serial obstruction, as well as situations in which V_1 is relatively large compared with V_2, such as in milder degrees of aortic stenosis and aortic stenosis combined with aortic insufficiency.

DOPPLER CALCULATION OF RIGHT VENTRICULAR SYSTOLIC PRESSURE. Obviously, application of the Bernoulli equation allows calculation of gradients across stenotic valves, but likewise it can be used to calculate a gradient between any high-pressure and low-pressure chambers. A commonly used application of the Bernoulli equation is the determination of the right ventricular systolic pressure.[18-20] Tricuspid regurgitation is very common in many disease states. By determining the peak velocity of a tricuspid regurgitation jet, one can then calculate the right ventricular–to–right atrial pressure gradient (Fig. 11–31). A key component of this is estimation of right atrial pressure. Approaches to this determination include assigning an empirical constant, assigning a floating constant of 5, 10, or 15 mm Hg (depending on the size of the right atrium, severity of regurgitation, and appearance of the inferior vena cava), or assigning a floating constant of 10 percent of the peak gradient. Each of these methods appears to result in satisfactory estimation of intercardiac pressure.

CALCULATION OF FLOW. Because the Doppler spectral profile provides a highly accurate measure of the velocity of the moving blood, this value, when combined with a measured or calculated area, can provide data regarding actual volumetric flow (Figs. 11–32 and 11–33). Multiplying the cross-sectional area of the flow times the velocity time integral

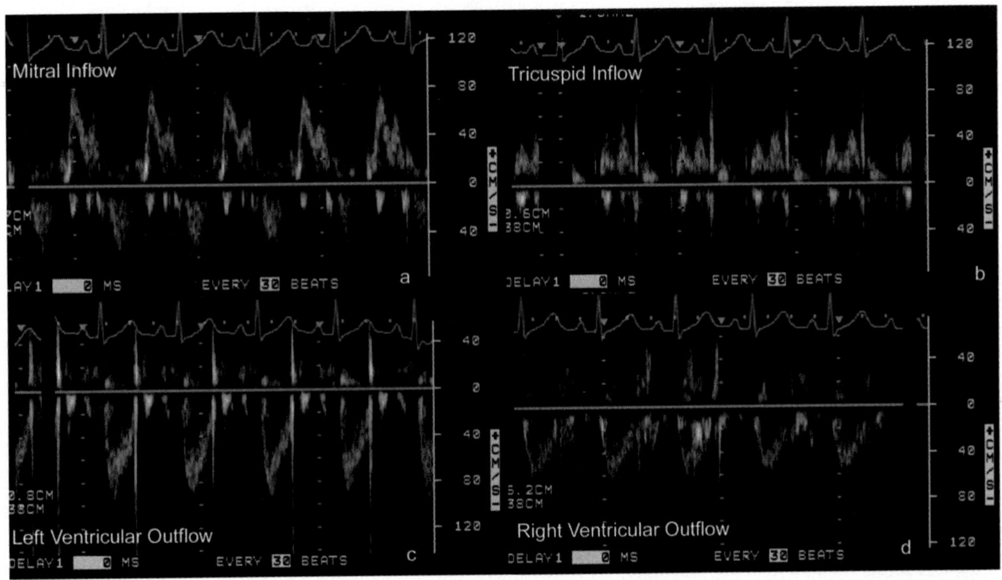

FIGURE 11–28 Composite pulsed Doppler tracings of normal flow in all four cardiac valves. Note the marked similarity between the aortic and pulmonary flow velocities, with a lower velocity in the pulmonary flow due to its larger diameter. Similarly, there is a lower velocity of tricuspid flow, but a similar relationship of early (e-wave) and atrial related (a-wave) flow when compared to mitral inflow.

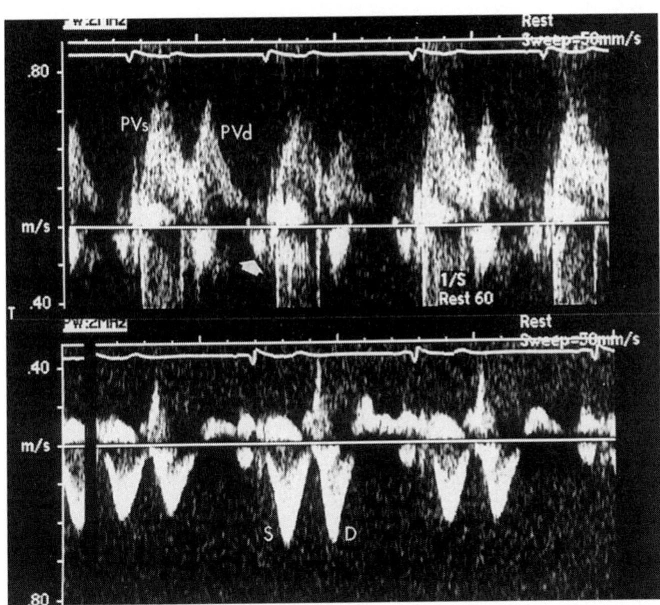

FIGURE 11–29 Normal pulmonary **(upper panel)** and hepatic **(lower panel)** vein flows. Nearly continuous, multiphasic flow is seen in the normal pulmonary and hepatic veins. Note that there is higher velocity of pulmonary vein inflow during ventricular systole then during diastole.

yields the actual volume of flow during that pulse interval. If the left ventricular outflow tract is interrogated, this value then represents the forward stroke volume of the left ventricle. This, in turn, can be used to calculate cardiac output.[21] The greatest source of error in this calculation is often determination of the cross-sectional area of the left ventricular outflow tract, which may not assume circular geometry. Additionally, because of the formula for determining area ($A = \pi r^2$), any error in measuring the diameter of the flow channel is squared. Thus, determination of stroke volume and cardiac output may have greater clinical value in following serial trends than in precise determination of volumetric flow. For clinical purposes, however, this remains a valuable technique. Similar calculations of flow volume can be performed for the pulmonic and mitral valves as well.

An expansion of volume flow calculation involves the "continuity equation" (Fig. 11-34).[22] The underlying principle of the continuity equation is that the volume of flow entering a channel must equal the volume of flow exiting that channel. If the cross-sectional area is equal at the entrance and exit points, then flow velocity will likewise be equal at those two points. If, however, the cross-sectional area decreases at the downstream site, then, of necessity, velocity must increase to maintain the same volumetric flow. The continuity equation can be applied for determination of aortic valve area in aortic stenosis and less often for mitral valve area or other conditions.

Color Doppler flow imaging can be used to determine volumetric flow as well. Flow converging on a relatively restrictive area will accelerate as it nears the downstream exit. Because of the relatively low Nyquist limit of color flow Doppler imaging, this results in a series of aliasing lines where the color flow signal will alternately change from blue to red. By purposely utilizing relatively low Nyquist limits, the echocardiographer can determine the distance from the actual flow exit point to one of the aliasing lines. Because the velocity at which flow aliases is known, the velocity of flow at that point is likewise known. If one assumes that flow converges at equal velocities symmetrically toward an orifice, then by applying the geometric formula for a hemisphere, one can determine the surface area of flow in motion at any of the aliasing points that represents an identifiable velocity (Fig. 11-35). From this, one can then calculate the actual volume of flow from this proximal isovelocity surface area as velocity times surface area.[23,24] In general terms, for any given Nyquist limit, the larger the proximal isovelocity surface area, the greater the amount of flow involved. Therefore, quantitation of proximal isovelocity surface area allows an additional clue as to the volume of regurgitant flow. Proximal isovelocity surface area calculations can be performed for any flow that accelerates toward a relatively restrictive orifice, including mitral regurgitation, aortic insufficiency, and shunt lesions. The major limitation of the use of proximal isovelocity surface area is the assumption that flow moves in a hemispherical manner. This assumption is true only for flow converging on a relatively flat surface. If flow is channeled through a funnel, corrections must be made for a surface area less than a full hemisphere.[25]

Close inspection of a regurgitant jet between either ventricle and its corresponding atrium can also provide clues to ventricular performance. In early systole, ventricular pressure exceeds atrial pressure by a wide margin and thus ejection of blood into the downstream atrium is at low resistance, resulting in a high dP/dt that corresponds to the forcefulness of ventricular contraction.[26] If myocardial failure occurs, the ability of the ventricle to eject forcefully is compromised and dP/dt decreases. This is also noted in spectral Doppler echocardiography of continuous-wave ejection parameters by a decrease in the ejection velocity slope (Fig. 11-36). Actual dP/dt can be calculated by determining the time in milliseconds between a regurgitant velocity of 1 and 3 m/sec. This corresponds to a pressure difference of 32 mm Hg. If the time over which this pressure difference is obtained is measured, a noninvasive dP/dt can be calculated.

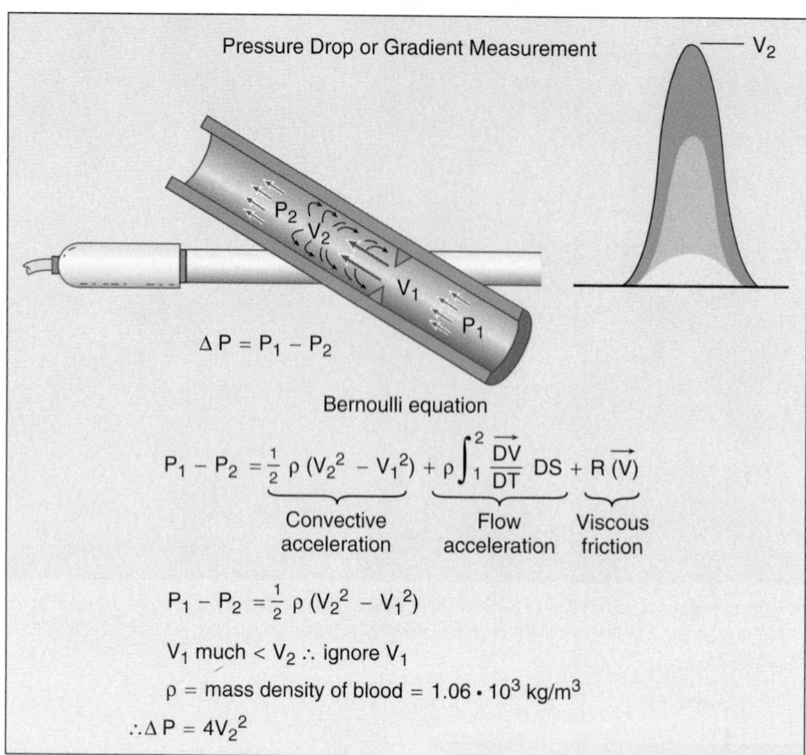

FIGURE 11–30 The Bernoulli equation can be used to calculate a pressure gradient across any restrictive orifice. The components of the Bernoulli equation are convective acceleration, flow acceleration, and viscous friction. The full equation can be modified to $P_1 - P_2 = (V_2^2 - V_1^2) \times 4$ and further simplified in the absence of a significant V_1 velocity to $\Delta P = 4V^2$. P_1 = pressure proximal to an obstruction; P_2 = pressure distal to an obstruction; V_1 = velocity proximal to an obstruction; V_2 = Doppler velocity distal to an obstruction. (From Feigenbaum H: Echocardiography. 4th ed. Malvern, PA, Lea & Febiger, 1986.)

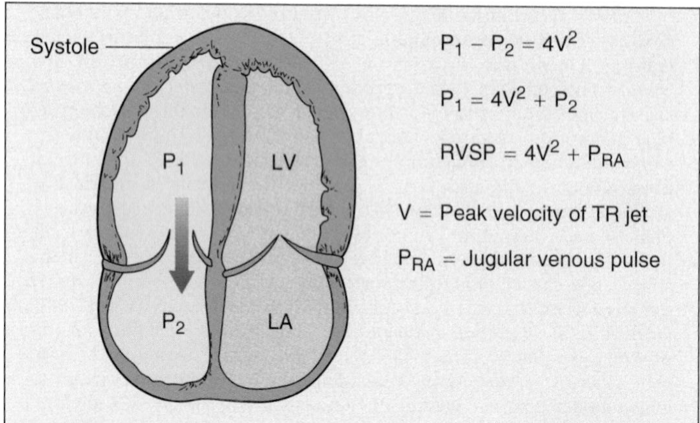

FIGURE 11–31 Measurement of right ventricular systolic pressure (RVSP) using the tricuspid regurgitation jet. The gradient between the right ventricle and right atrium ($P_1 - P_2$) can be calculated from the velocity of the tricuspid regurgitation jet using the modified Bernoulli equation ($\Delta P = 4V^2$). Actual right ventricular systolic pressure is then calculated as the sum of the pressure gradient between the two chambers and an assumed right atrial pressure (P_{RA}). Right atrial pressure can be estimated from examination of the jugular veins, by evaluation of the inferior vena cava for collapse during inspiration, or by using an empirical or floating constant (see text for further details). LA = left atrium; LV = left ventricle. (From Feigenbaum H: Echocardiography. 5th ed. Malvern, PA, Lea & Febiger, 1994.)

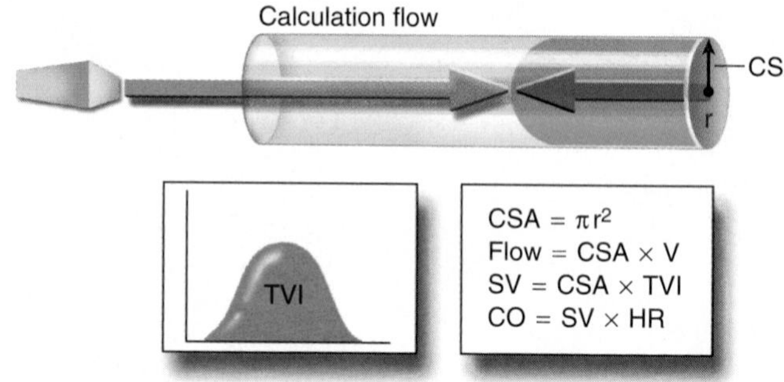

FIGURE 11–32 Schematic demonstration of the method for determining flow using a combination of Doppler and two-dimensional echocardiography. Flow can be calculated as the product of the cross-sectional area of the chamber or vessel through which flow is occurring (CSA) and the velocity of flow. The time-velocity integral (TVI) is used to calculate pulsatile flow. Cross-sectional areas are calculated as noted in the schematic, and cardiac output (CO) can then be calculated as the product of stroke volume (SV) and heart rate (HR).

The continuous-wave spectral profile can also provide clues as to the nature of obstruction in many disease states. The spectral profile provides high temporal resolution for determining the timing of pressure gradients. Thus, the contour of the spectral profile provides clues as to whether an obstruction is fixed or develops over time, in which case the peak gradient will occur late rather than early. The latter is classic for dynamic obstruction in cases of hypertrophic cardiomyopathy. Close examination of a regurgitant profile can also reveal evidence that atrial pressure has become acutely elevated toward the end of ejection when velocities taper off rapidly in the latter half of systole.

Much attention has been paid to mitral valve inflow patterns as they relate to diastolic function of the left ventricle.[27-30] This assessment must be done in patients who are in sinus rhythm, during which there are discrete E and A wave velocities of the mitral valve inflow. In normal individuals, early velocities exceed later velocities and the E to A ratio is typically greater than 1.2. With impaired relaxation of the left ventricle, this ratio declines and the rate of decay of the E wave velocity likewise decreases. Figure 11-37 schematizes several mitral valve Doppler inflow patterns. There are a number of other influences on the E to A ratio, including age and heart rate. With a pathological increase in left ventricular stiffness accompanied by excess volume, there is an augmentation of the normal E to A ratio. This increased E to A ratio is classic for a restrictive cardiomyopathy and constrictive pericarditis but is also typically seen in patients with end-stage heart disease of virtually any type who have markedly elevated diastolic pressures. It is imperative to incorporate the anatomical and other Doppler information into an assessment of mitral valve inflow patterns in an effort to provide clinically relevant information.

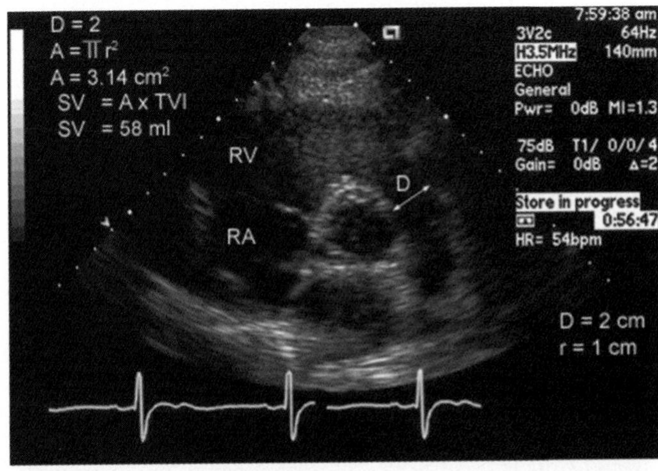

A

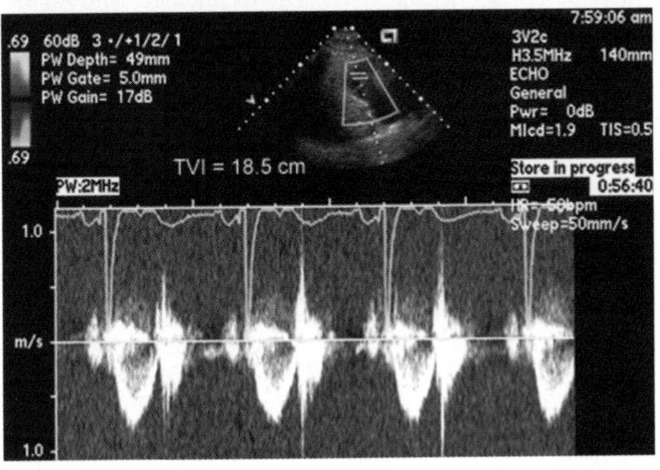

B

FIGURE 11–33 Demonstration of the calculation of stroke volume from a two-dimensional echocardiogram and pulsed wave Doppler in the right ventricular outflow tract. **A,** Recorded at the level of the aortic valve and right ventricular outflow tract, from which a proximal pulmonary artery diameter (D) of 2 cm can be measured. **B,** Pulsed wave Doppler at the same, from which a time velocity integral (TVI) of 18.5 cm can be determined. The calculations for determination of stroke volume are superimposed on the upper panel and result in a calculated stroke volume of 58 ml. RA = right atrium; RV = right ventricle.

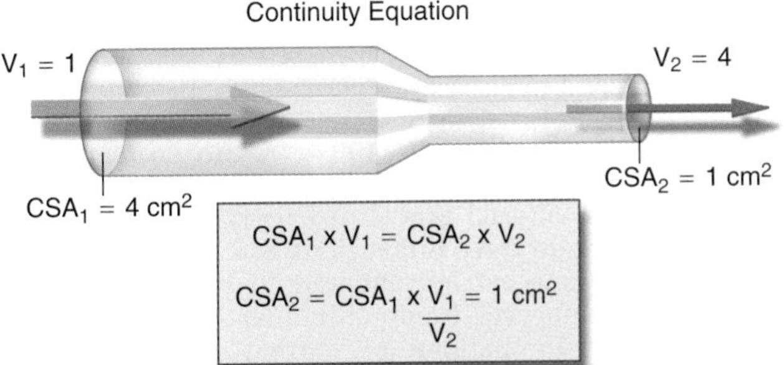

FIGURE 11–34 Schematic demonstration of the continuity equation. The continuity equation states that flow through a structure is equal at both the entrance and exit points. If there is a change in flow area, it must be accompanied by a directionally appropriate and proportionate change in velocity. In the example schematized, flow enters a chamber with a cross-sectional area (CSA_1) of 4 cm^2 and a velocity of 1, giving a flow of 4 ml. Downstream flow must also be 4 ml, but across the exiting cross-sectional area (CSA_2) has been reduced to 1 cm^2. Of necessity, the downstream velocity then must increase to 4. In clinical practice, the entrance cross-sectional area and entrance velocity are typically known, as is the exit velocity and the equation is solved for the exit cross-sectional area, as noted in the schematic.

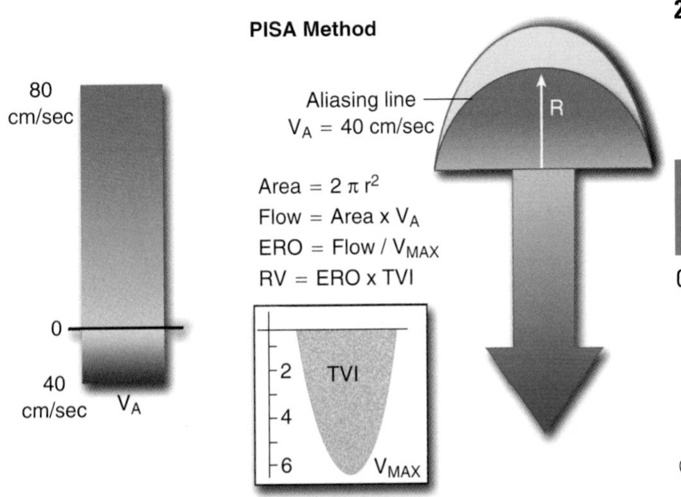

FIGURE 11–35 Demonstration of the proximal isovelocity surface area (PISA) method for determining flow. The figure on the **right** is a schematized color flow image of the acceleration of flow toward a regurgitant orifice in a patient with mitral regurgitation. The boundary between color shifts represents an aliasing line at which velocity has exceeded the Nyquist limit (V_A), which is displayed on the color bar (40 cm/sec). The calculations necessary to determine flow are as noted in the middle panel. For any given aliasing line, a hemisphere of flow is assumed. The surface area of a hemisphere is calculated as $2\pi r^2$. Flow is equal to the product of the surface area times the velocity, which is determined from the Nyquist limit. ERO = effective regurgitant orifice; TVI = time velocity integral.

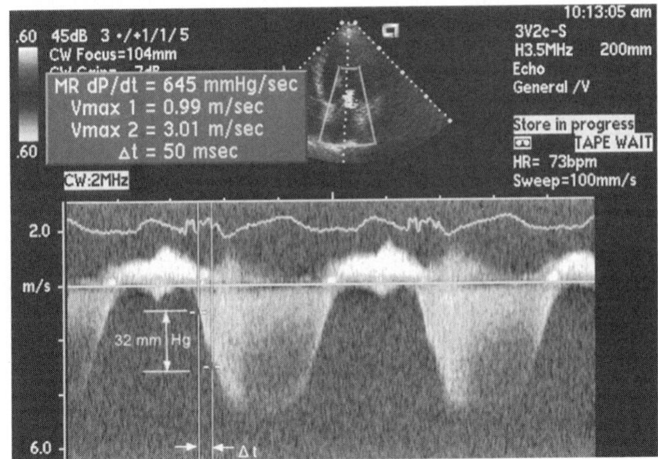

FIGURE 11–36 Use of the mitral regurgitation spectral display to determine positive and negative dP/dt of left ventricular contraction. The spectral mitral regurgitation jet is displayed at high sweep speed to maximize temporal resolution. The time in milliseconds (Δt) required for velocity to increase from 1 to 3 m/sec is then measured. This time is then divided into 32 mm Hg (the pressure difference between 1 and 3 m/sec) to determine dP/dt noninvasively (645 mm Hg/sec in this example).

Doppler can be used to evaluate the inflow patterns of the hepatic and pulmonary veins as well. Both hepatic and pulmonary vein inflow are biphasic with predominant flow in ventricular systole (see Fig. 11-29). Examination of the flow patterns can provide valuable clues in a variety of disease states, including mitral regurgitation, restrictive and constrictive processes, and other diseases that elevate right or left ventricular diastolic pressure.

Additional Imaging Formats and Techniques

Transesophageal Echocardiography

For this technique, the ultrasound transducer has been miniaturized and mounted on the tip of a flexible gastroscope-like instrument. The mechanics of the instrument allow both flexion and lateral motion of the tip to optimize views. Early transesophageal echocardiography (TEE) probes provided

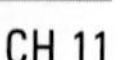

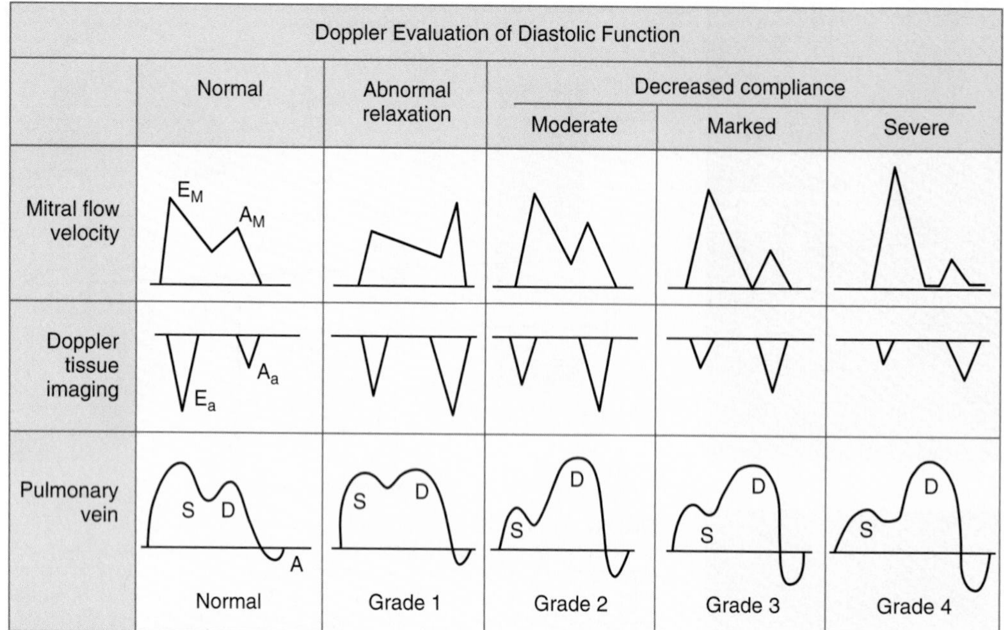

FIGURE 11–37 Schematic representation of mitral inflow, Doppler tissue imaging of the annulus, and pulmonary vein flow in normal and abnormal diastolic states. Normal mitral inflow is biphasic and consists of an early velocity (E_M) and a late flow velocity related to atrial contraction (A_M). Doppler tissue imaging of the annulus results in a similar pattern of early and late (E_A and A_A) annular velocities opposite in direction to the mitral inflow velocity. In patients with normal diastolic function, both E_M and E_A exceed A_M and A_A. In disease-free states, pulmonary vein flow is multiphasic, with roughly equal systolic and diastolic forward flow and a relatively narrow low velocity retrograde pulmonary vein a-wave. With varying degrees of diastolic dysfunction, there are predictable changes in mitral flow velocity, Doppler tissue annular velocities, and pulmonary vein velocities as noted in the schematic.

only a single plane of interrogation, with subsequent probes providing two perpendicularly oriented planes that could be viewed in alternate fashion. Modern TEE probes contain an array of ultrasound crystals at the tip of the probe that allow rotation of the ultrasound scanning plane through 360 degrees.

There are specific indications and contraindications to TEE as well as well-recognized inherent risks. TEE is indicated in patients in whom transthoracic echocardiography (TTE) is either unlikely to provide diagnostic information or has been nondiagnostic. Specific situations in which TEE is of proven incremental yield include detection of aortic dissection, evaluation of the mechanism of mitral regurgitation, evaluation of the left atrial appendage for thrombus prior to cardioversion of atrial fibrillation, and evaluation of patients for source of cardiac emboli. TEE is relatively contraindicated in individuals with significant esophageal pathology.

Transesophageal echocardiography is typically performed under intravenous conscious sedation after application of local anesthesia to the oropharynx. The exact choice of intravenous agents is institutionally dependent but frequently consists of a combination of narcotics and a benzodiazepine agent. Complications associated with TEE include those associated with the agents used for conscious sedation as well as complications related to the mechanical aspects of probe insertion. The latter can involve trauma to any aspect of the teeth, gums, oropharynx, or esophagus. Esophageal complications are most likely to arise in individuals with preexisting esophageal disorders. Trauma to the oropharynx, teeth, and gums is more likely in patients who are uncooperative.

There is a family of standardized views that are obtained during the TEE examination.[31] Most echocardiographers begin by examining the heart from behind the left atrium because this view provides a fairly rapid means for orienting the operator. Figures 11–38 and 11–39 outline views in the horizontal and longitudinal planes that correspond to 0- and 90-degree scanning planes using a multidirectional rotating transducer. Figures 11–40 and 11–41 are transesophageal echocardiograms recorded from several of the transducer positions schematized in Figures 11–38 and 11–39.

Three-Dimensional Echocardiography

Three-dimensional echocardiography remains a technique in evolution for which increases in image processing technology and speed have allowed substantial advancement in the last several years. There are two basic approaches to acquiring a three-dimensional data set. The first involves collection of the entire series of two-dimensional image planes. The location in space of each of these planes is known and registered for subsequent three-dimensional reconstruction. The localization of each plane can be performed by two methods. The first and oldest was by using a transducer positioning device which automatically recorded the precise location and angulation of the transducer from which the location and orientation of each acquired imaging plane could be determined. This resulted in collection of a data set composed of multiple two-dimensional images of known orientation and location that could then be compiled into a three-dimensional data set. Typically, this involved an external device that attached to the transducer for image localization. An advancement on this technique is available using a rotating scan head, as is found in multiplane transesophageal probes. The same technology has been adapted to TTE. With this technique, the imaging plane is rotated through 180 degrees while the transducer is held in a fixed position, thereby providing a 360-degree view around a point of reference. The location and orientation of each imaging plane is automatically known based on the angle of rotation of the transducer. Each individual image is then stored, and the three-dimensional data set can be derived.

The newest method for obtaining a three-dimensional echocardiogram involves transducers with a rectangular, rather than lineal, crystal array.[32-35] This type of transducer intrinsically scans in three dimensions and acquires a three-dimensional volume set, as opposed to creating a three-dimensional volume set from individual two-dimensional imaging planes. Limitations of current technology and processor capacity have limited three-dimensional echocardiography to structural imaging only in most systems. Increasing processor speed and computational capacity as well as transducer capability have allowed three-dimensional color reconstruction as well in select circumstances.

Once the three-dimensional data set is acquired with any of these techniques, there are several ways of displaying the information. These include identifying a desired two-dimensional plane in the three-dimensional data set and displaying it as a two-dimensional echocardiogram. This has

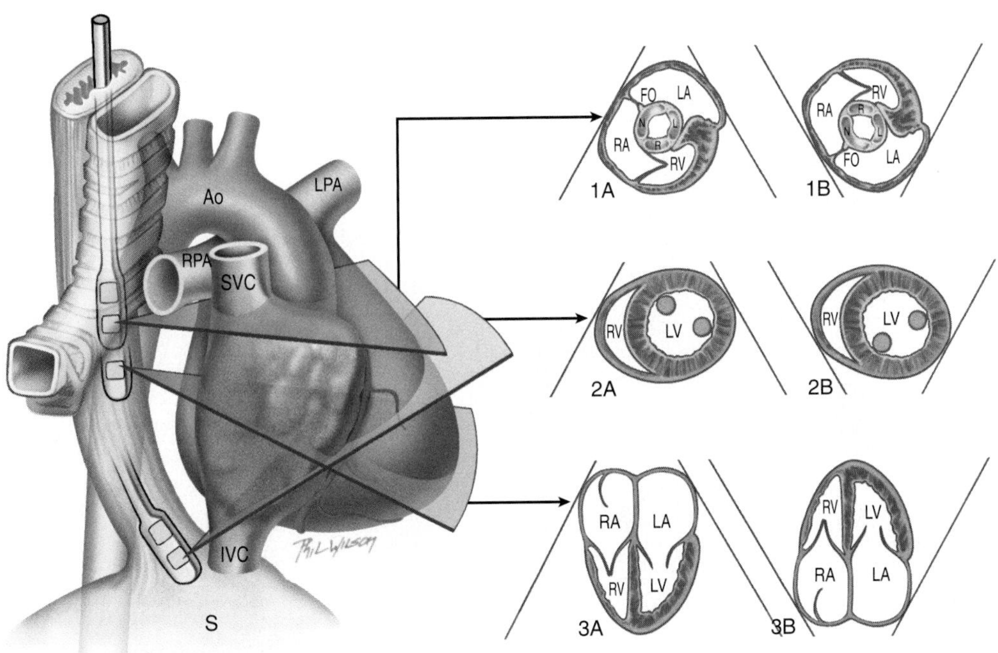

FIGURE 11–38 Schematic demonstrating the transesophageal echocardiographic images that can be obtained in a horizontal plane. Figures **2A** and **2B** are obtained from the transgastric location, **3A** and **3B** from the midesophageal position, and **1A** and **1B** from the upper esophageal position. (Images can be displayed with the apex of the sector either up [A figures] or the apex down [B figures].) Echocardiographic images corresponding to figures 1A, 2A, and 3A are presented in Figure 11–40. Ao = aorta; FO = fossa ovalis; IVC = inferior vena cava; LA = left atrium; LPA = left pulmonary artery; LV = left ventricle; RA; right atrium; RPA = right pulmonary artery; RV = right ventricle; S = stomach; SVC = superior vena cava. (From Feigenbaum H: Echocardiography. 5th ed. Malvern, PA, Lea & Febiger, 1994.)

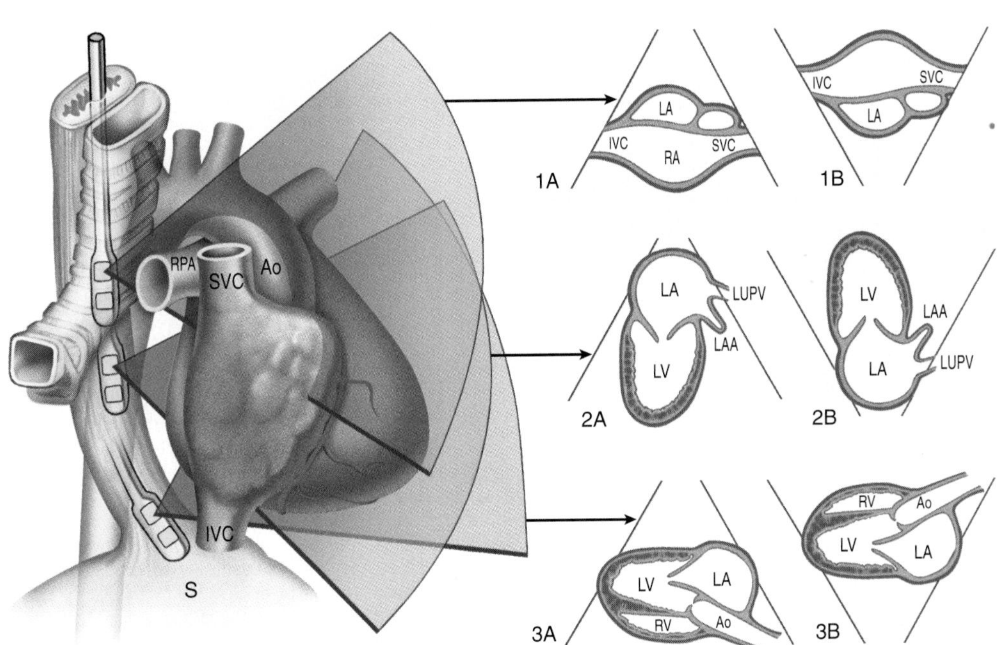

FIGURE 11–39 Transesophageal echocardiographic views obtained in the longitudinal transducer position. The **A** series of figures are recorded with the apex down and the **B** series with the apex up. **3A** and **3B** are recorded in the gastric position, **2A** and **2B** from the midesophagus, and **1A** and **1B** from the upper esophagus. Ao = aorta; IVC = inferior vena cava; LA = left atrium; LAA = left atrial appendage; LUPV = left upper pulmonary vein; LV = left ventricle; RA = right atrium; RPA = right pulmonary artery; RV = right ventricle; S = stomach; SVC = superior vena cava. (From Feigenbaum H: Echocardiography. 5th ed. Malvern, PA, Lea & Febiger, 1994.).

the advantage of allowing the operator to select a nontraditional imaging plane for precise quantitation or for viewing a structure that may lie in an off-axis position (Fig. 11–42). This technique has shown preliminary applicability in stress echocardiography, in which an entire three-dimensional data set can be rapidly acquired and then separate two-dimensional images extracted for subsequent analysis.

The second method for display of a three-dimensional data set is in a "surface-rendered" image in which the multiple two-dimensional planes are blended into a pseudo-three-dimensional image. Obviously, for display either as hard

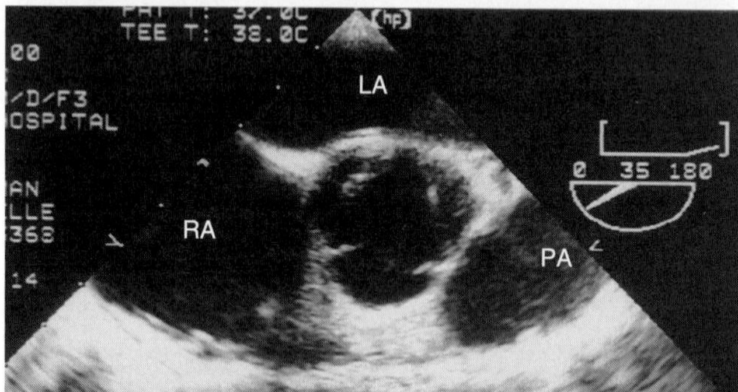

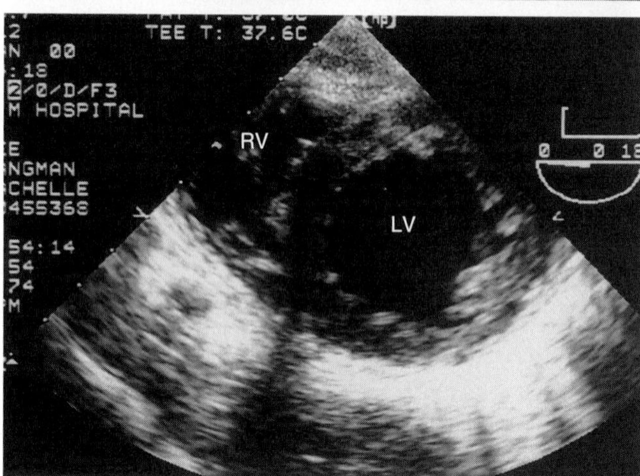

FIGURE 11–40 Transesophageal echocardiograms recorded in a horizontal plane. The **upper** and **lower panels** were recorded in a true 0-degree plane at a high level behind the left atrium and at a midesophageal level, respectively. In the left atrial view, a typical four-chamber view of the heart is obtained in which all four cardiac chambers as well as the mitral and tricuspid valves are clearly visualized. The lower panel was recorded at 0 degrees with the probe inserted deeper in the esophagus. A typical short-axis view of the left ventricle is obtained in which a circular left ventricle and crescent-shaped right ventricle are seen. This view is analogous to a parasternal short-axis view; however, the orientation is inverted such that the inferior wall is at the top of the image and the anterior wall at the bottom. The **middle panel** was recorded at 35 degrees and with pull back of the transducer slightly from the position needed for view in the upper panel. This provides a short-axis view at the base of the heart at which the circular aorta with an open aortic valve is clearly visualized. LA = left atrium, LV = left ventricle; PA = pulmonary artery; RA = right atrium; RV = right ventricle.

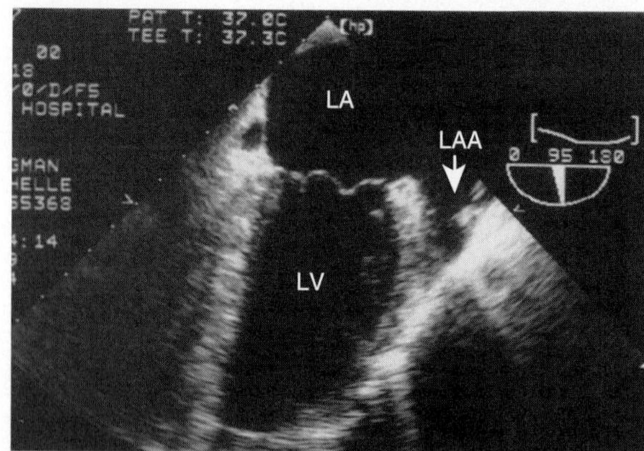

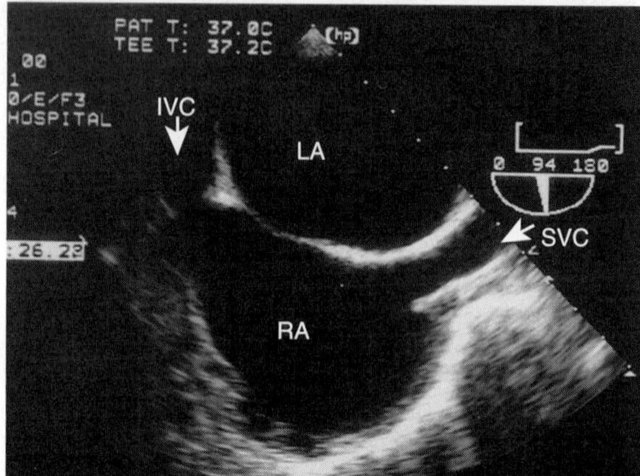

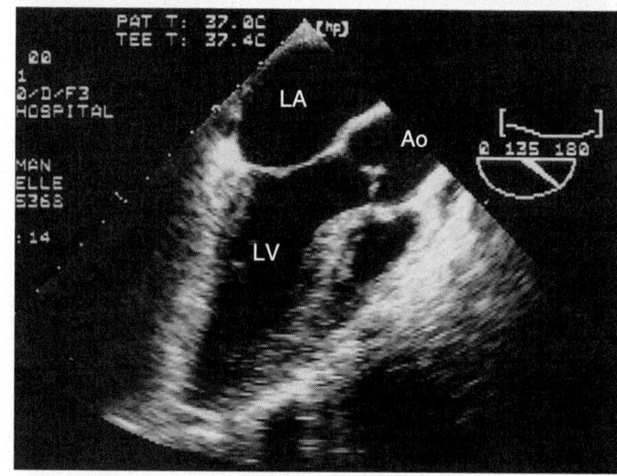

FIGURE 11–41 Transesophageal echocardiographic images recorded in view orthogonal to the horizontal images seen in Figure 11–40. The **top panel** is recorded at the same level in the esophagus as the top panel in Figure 11–40 at a 95-degree angle. In this view, the left atrium (LA) and left ventricle (LV) as well as left atrial appendage (LAA) are clearly visualized. Distinct scallops of the closed mitral valve are also well seen. The **middle panel** is likewise recorded at the same level in the esophagus with rotation of the probe clockwise. In this view, the left atrium and right atrium (RA) as well as inferior vena cava (IVC) and superior vena cava (SVC) are clearly visualized. The **bottom panel** was recorded at 135 degrees. This view provides excellent visualization of the left ventricular outflow tract and proximal aorta (Ao).

copy or on a video screen, no true third dimension is available; however, surface rendering adds depth to the apparent image (Fig. 11–43).

Proven advantages of three-dimensional echocardiography have been its ability to allow precise special characterization of complex lesions such as more complex forms of congenital heart disease,[36] more accurate identification of flail leaflets, and detection of complications of endocarditis. An additional advantage is in the quantitation of ventricular volumes, especially in irregularly shaped ventricles in which the ability to calculate precise volumes clearly exceeds that available from routine two-dimensional scanning.[37]

Intravascular Ultrasonography

Intracardiac ultrasonography is a discipline largely employed by the invasive cardiologist in the catheterization laboratory (see Chap. 18). This ultrasound technique relies on ultraminiaturization of ultrasound transducers that are then incorporated into the tip of intracardiac catheters. The catheters can be as small as 5 French for intracoronary work or as large as 10 or 12 French, which can be used inside cardiac chambers. Typically, either a phased array of crystals is placed circumferentially around the catheter tip or a single crystal, often reflected by a mirror, is mechanically rotated at the tip of a catheter. In either instance, high frequencies of 10 to 40 MHz are used. The smaller catheters can be placed, through a guiding catheter, into epicardial coronary arteries. They provide a high-resolution view of cardiac and intravascular anatomy (Fig. 11–44) and have provided previously unavailable visualization of morphology within the coronary artery and characterization of the intracoronary tissue.[38,39] Calcification and atherosclerosis can be identified and the eccentric or concentric nature of plaque likewise determined. Intracoronary ultrasonography has been instrumental in determining the success of interventions such as stent deployment in coronary artery disease.[40,41] Figure 11–45 depicts intracoronary ultrasound studies demonstrating increasing degrees of severity of atherosclerosis. A closely related technology is the use of miniaturized Doppler wires for monitoring intracoronary flow velocity.[42] Intravascular ultrasonography has also been used in the evaluation of patients with known or suspected aortic dissection, in which case it provides a high-resolution intraluminal view of dissection pathology and yields incremental information with respect to the origin of branch vessels. It has been instrumental in refining the techniques of emergent fenestration in stenting for acute type III dissections.

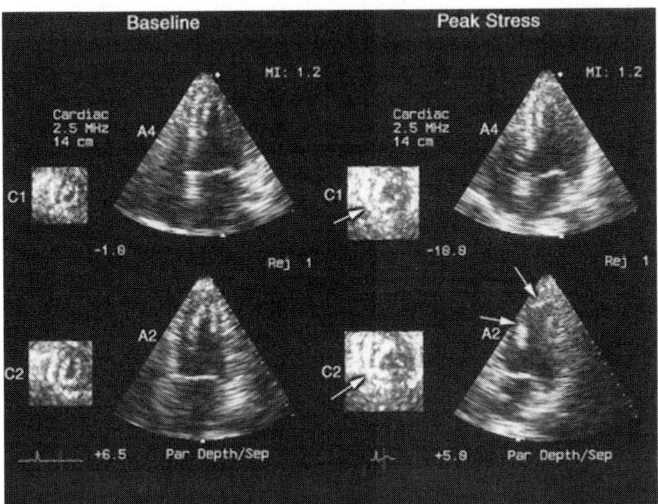

FIGURE 11–42 Apical real-time three-dimensional systolic frames at baseline and at peak stress in a patient with inducible ischemia. Arrows point to the inducible left ventricular wall motion abnormality at peak stress in A2, C1, and C2 images. (From Ahmad et al: Real-time three-dimensional dobutamine stress echocardiography in assessment of ischemia: Comparison with two-dimensional dobutamine stress echocardiography. J Am Coll Cardiol 37:1303, 2001; with permission from the American College of Cardiology Foundation.)

More recently, a 10 French catheter with a 64-element linear array (oriented along the long access of the catheter) was introduced for intracardiac use (Fig. 11–46).[43-45] This transducer provides steering in both anteroposterior and lateral directions and provides imaging for wide-angle two-dimensional real-time imaging, pulsed and continuous-wave Doppler, and color flow imaging. This device has shown tremendous promise for monitoring of interventional procedures such as atrial septostomy, mitral balloon valve valvotomy, and atrial septal defect closure.

Tissue Characterization

Tissue characterization refers to the detailed evaluation of the entire reflected ultrasound signal in an effort to extract information regarding actual tissue character. Typically, this has relied on evaluation of data in the radiofrequency signal component before processing into a diagnostic, visual image. One of the more promising applications has been in evaluating the cyclic variation in returning ultrasound signal intensity (cyclic variation in backscatter) as a marker of myocardial ischemia.[46,47]

Doppler Tissue Interrogation

The original application of Doppler echocardiography was for determination of the direction and velocity of blood flow.

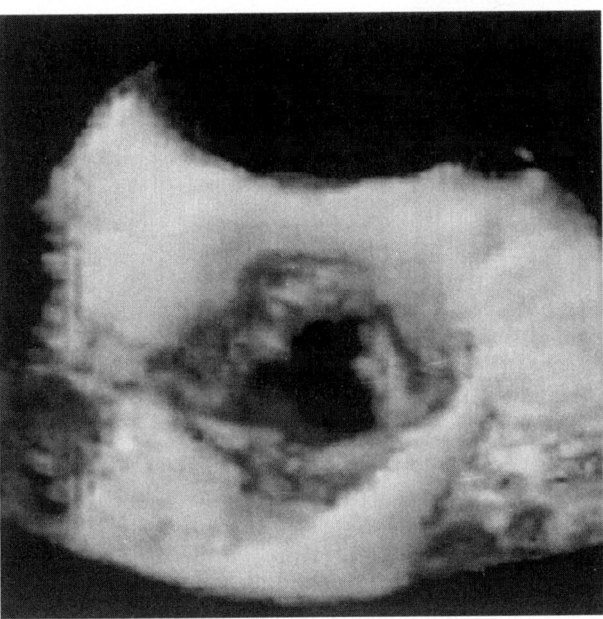

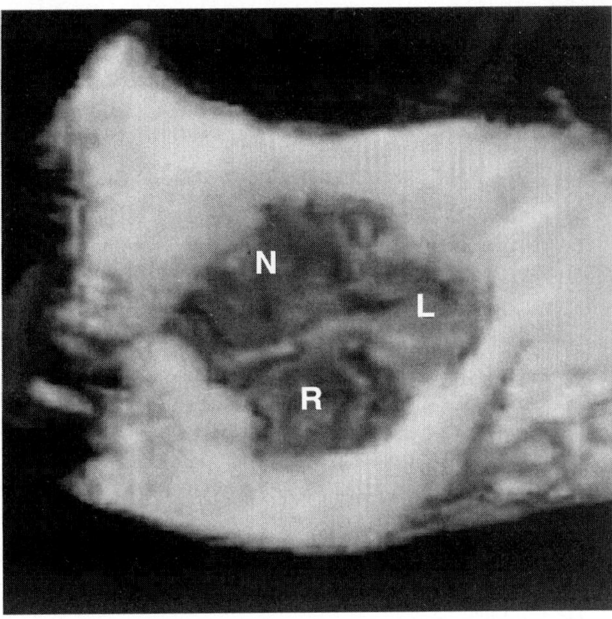

FIGURE 11–43 Surface-rendered three-dimensional echocardiogram showing a normal aortic valve. The panel on the **left** shows the valve in the open position, and a roughly triangular orifice is seen. The image has been captured at mid-opening. At the **right,** the valve is seen in the closed position and the right (R), left (L), and noncoronary (N) cusps are clearly visualized.

As such, original Doppler instrumentation provided filters to exclude highly reflective, slowly moving objects such as myocardium and to exclusively interrogate relatively rapid moving structures with faint reflectivity such as red blood cells. This resulted in the characteristic spectral profiles seen of moving blood in the cardiovascular system. By altering the amplitude and velocity filters, Doppler methodology can be used to determine the direction and velocity of motion of tissue such as left ventricular myocardium. All of the traditional Doppler display methods such as pulsed spectral displays or color encoding can be employed with this technique.

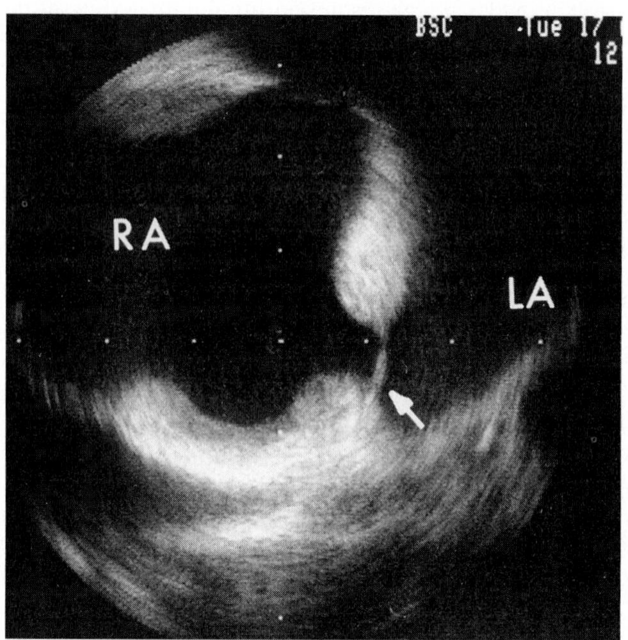

FIGURE 11–44 Intracardiac ultrasonographic image recorded from within the cavity of the right atrium (RA). Note the fairly thick tissue at the primum and more superior aspect of the atrial septum and the very thin valve of the foramen ovale (arrow). LA = left atrium.

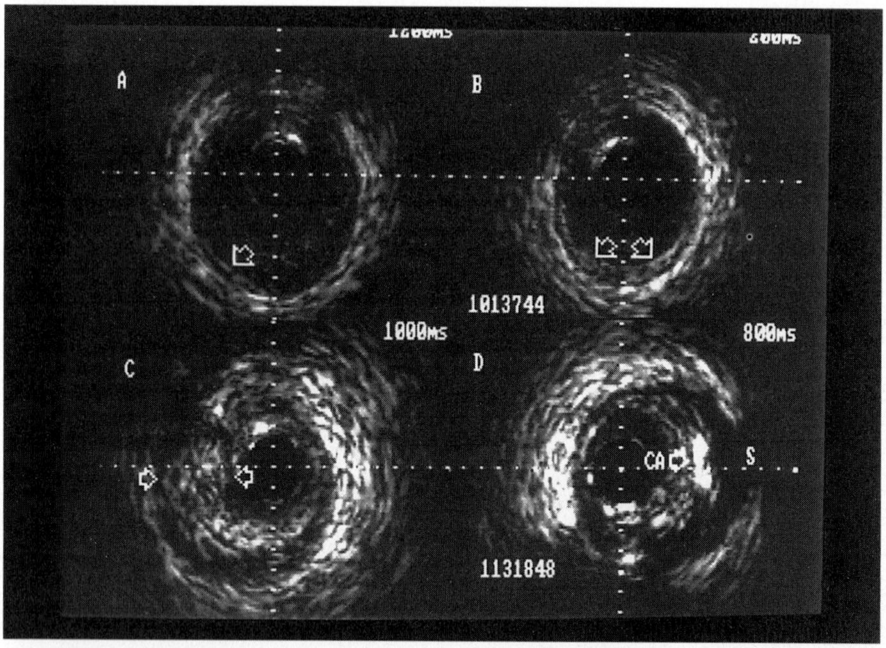

FIGURE 11–45 Intracoronary ultrasonographic images demonstrating the different severity of coronary atherosclerosis. **A,** Small rim of thickened intima (arrow). **B,** Larger amount of eccentric intimal thickening (arrows). **C,** Massive atherosclerotic plaque that is wider (arrows) than the residual lumen. **D,** Calcification in the plaque (CA) produces shadowing (S). (From Feigenbaum H: Echocardiography. 5th ed. Malvern, PA, Lea & Febiger, 1994.)

"Doppler Tissue Imaging" refers to the technique of determining directional velocity of tissue structures rather than the moving blood pool (Figs. 11–37 and 11–47). Doppler evaluation of annular motion has shown tremendous promise for the evaluation of diastolic function. When evaluated from an apical transducer, position annular motion is opposite in direction to the mitral inflow signal. The early annular velocity (Ea) exceeds late annular velocity (Aa) in a manner similar to the mitral valve E/A (see Fig. 11–37). This is a methodology that has shown tremendous promise and clinical applicability for characterizing detailed myocardial motion characteristics.[48-54]

Doppler tissue imaging records the velocity of motion of myocardium and can be targeted to discrete segments with sample volumes similar to that for routine Doppler interrogation. The information thus recorded is converted to velocity of tissue motion (centimeters per second). Several derivative calculations also provide valuable information. If both the velocity of motion and the duration of motion are known, then the absolute magnitude of motion can also be calculated.[54] Doppler tissue imaging can be used to calculate direction and velocity of motion in two adjacent myocardial segments of known distance of separation. From this strain, reflecting the relative velocity of either separation or closure between these two points can be calculated. This can further be developed into "strain rate imaging," which integrates the rate of distance change between two adjacent points over time, which in turn is a parameter that can be color-encoded over a segment of the myocardium. Both experimental animal and clinical data suggest that strain rate imaging can provide an increased level of resolution and accuracy for identification of subtle wall motion abnormalities in patients with ischemic and those with nonischemic heart disease.[55-61]

CONTRAST ECHOCARDIOGRAPHY

Contrast echocardiography is a rapidly evolving field that currently plays a number of routine clinical roles and has shown tremendous investigative promise for assessing myocardial perfusion.[62,63] All forms of contrast echocardiography rely on the fact that microbubbles, when injected into the blood pool, are intense echo reflectors. This pertains to the simplest contrast agent, agitated saline, as well as to the new, commercially available perfluorocarbon agents. Reflectivity of a microbubble is substantially greater than that of tissue, and as such in low concentration they create a highly reflective target. The interaction of the ultrasound beam with contrast is quite complex and occurs on three basic levels.

Depending on the power of the insonating ultrasound beam, the interaction may be simple reflection back at the fundamental frequency,[64,65] generation and reflection back of harmonic frequencies, or "stimulated acoustic omission."[66] The first and simplest interaction is pure reflection. This is characterized by reflection back of an intensive echo target from each individual microbubble. This was the phenomenon capitalized on for routine saline contrast echocardiography, which is used on a routine basis for detection of intracardiac shunts and enhancement of tricuspid regurgitation signals. Modern perfluorocarbon-based agents reflect back not only at the fundamental frequency but also at a harmonic of the insonating frequency. If these agents are insonated at a fundamental frequency and transducer receiving characteristics "tuned" to the harmonic frequency, the relative contribution of reflection from the oscillating microbubble (generating harmonic energy) is relatively greater than that from the sur-

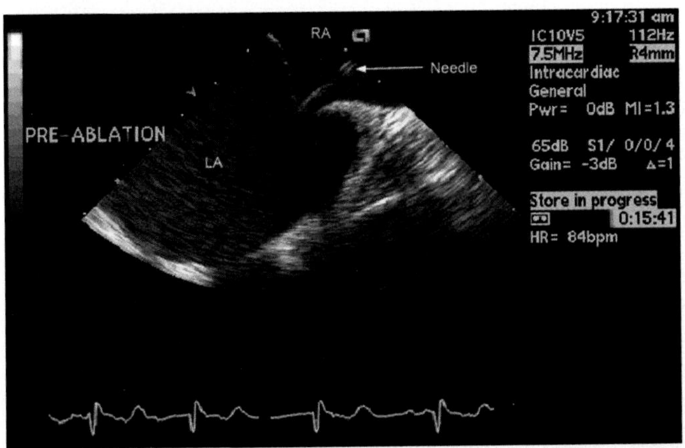

FIGURE 11–46 Image recorded from within the right atrium (RA) in a patient undergoing a transeptal puncture (needle) to gain access to a the left atrium (LA). Note the "tenting" of the atrial septum just prior to actual puncture.

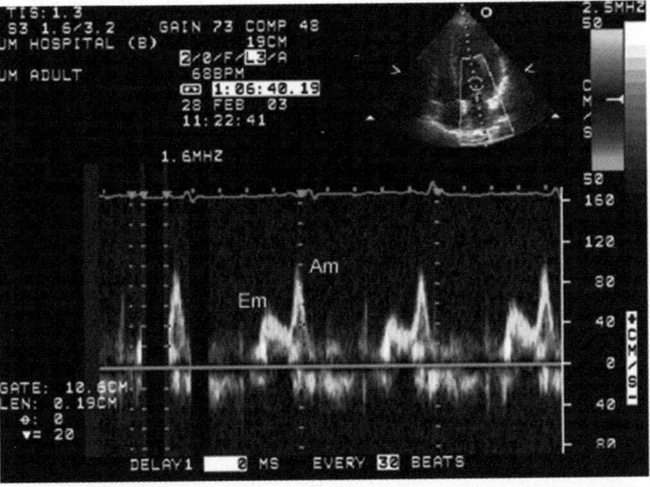

A

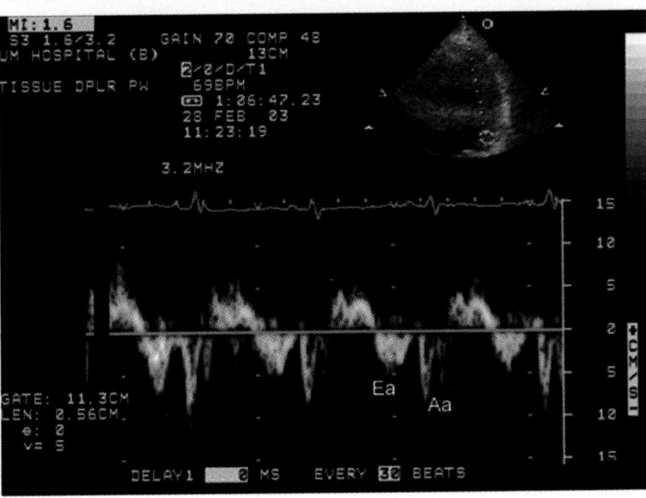

B

FIGURE 11–47 Mitral inflow velocity and Doppler tissue annular recording in a patient with diastolic dysfunction and impaired relaxation. Note the reversed E/A ratio, **(A)**, which is paralleled by a reduced annular E_A/A_A ratio.

rounding blood pool or tissue. This provides a *relatively* contrast-specific mode of imaging.

It has recently been recognized that interaction of bubbles with a ultrasound beam of significant amplitude results in actual disruption of the microbubble with subsequent loss of its reflectivity.[67-69] The initial interaction, however, results in an intense ultrasound signal emanating from the disrupted bubbles that contains an entire family of harmonic and subharmonic frequencies. Immediately following disruption of the microbubble in the blood pool, there is absence of any contrast-specific signal.

Microbubbles can be detected in the blood pool or tissue either using direct reflection in the fundamental or harmonic domains or by their creation of Doppler shifts after higher energy insonation. One of the more promising methods for contrast-specific imaging involves transmission of two sequential pulses that are 180 degrees out of phase with each other.[70] If these pulses reflect back in an unaltered manner and then are summed, the result is zero signal, as the sum of two waveforms 180 degrees out of phase results in cancellation of the signal. If, however, the signals interact with a microbubble capable of altering the insonating beam frequency, then each will be reflected back, no longer 180 degrees out of phase with the other, and the sum of the two signals results in the detectable ultrasound signal. Because tissue will not alter the frequency of the insonating beam, this results in a substantial degree of contrast specificity for this imaging modality. This type of phase shift analysis employs analysis in a Doppler domain rather than pure ultrasound reflection. A variation on this methodology is to emit two pulses of different amplitude and on receipt of the signal, amplify the weaker signal to match the transmitted amplitude of the stronger. This also, after subtraction of the two returning signals, results in a more contrast-specific imaging mode.

In clinical practice, contrast echocardiography is used on a daily basis for detection of shunts, typically using agitated saline. This can be accomplished easily in the clinical laboratory by vigorously agitating saline with a small amount of room air (typically 9.5 ml sterile saline plus 0.5 ml air) between two 10 ml syringes connected by a three-way stopcock. Vigorous agitation creates a population of microbubbles, 50 to 300 μm in diameter. These bubbles are relatively unstable and subject to rapid coalescence and should be injected quickly. After intravenous injection, they will appear in the right heart as a dense cloud of echoes, but because of their relatively large size, they are filtered by the pulmonary capillary bed. In the absence of a right-to-left shunt, these bubbles are confined to the right heart and cannot be used for visualization for left heart structures. Their appearance in the left heart is indirect evidence of a pathological right-to-left shunt.

The commercially developed perfluorocarbon agents contain populations of substantially smaller (typically 4-6 μm) microbubbles of near uniform size.[71] Because perfluorocarbons have low diffusibility, these microbubbles have substantial persistence after injection and because of their size can cross the pulmonary capillary bed and thus opacify left heart structures. They are currently approved for enhancing left heart border definition (Fig. 11–48). When used for this purpose, they have been shown to improve the ability to identify the left ventricular endocardial border in routine studies,[62,72,73] in the intensive care unit,[74,75] and during stress echocardiography,[76-78] and to enhance the accuracy of quantification.[79] They can also be used to enhance left-sided Doppler signals[80,81] and to improve detection of left ventricular thrombus.[82] Contrast agents currently in development use microbubbles that can be targeted to thrombus[83] or to endothelium.[84,85] When using these agents, it is important to recognize that they will be disrupted by high-amplitude ultrasound. For this reason, contrast-specific imaging algorithms utilize low mechanical index, typically less than 0.5, to provide smooth homogeneous imaging of the agent within the left ventricular cavity. Use of a higher mechanical index results in bubble destruction.

Because these new perfluorocarbon agents pass the pulmonary cavity bed, they will be present in all distally perfused tissues, including the myocardium, kidney, and liver. Their presence in the myocardium can be used as a marker of intact myocardial perfusion (to be discussed subsequently). Myocardial perfusion contrast echocardiography is a complex field currently in evolution that requires highly specific imaging formats and analysis algorithms.

ADVANTAGES AND LIMITATIONS OF ECHOCARDIOGRAPHY

As with any diagnostic technique, echocardiography has distinct advantages and disadvantages. Cardiac ultrasonography itself carries no risk to the patient, operator, bystanders, pregnant women, or fetus. Specialized examinations such as contrast echocardiography, TEE, and stress echocardiography carry the minimal additional risk associated with the procedural modifications necessary for their undertaking. Modern ultrasound instruments are capable of visualizing all four

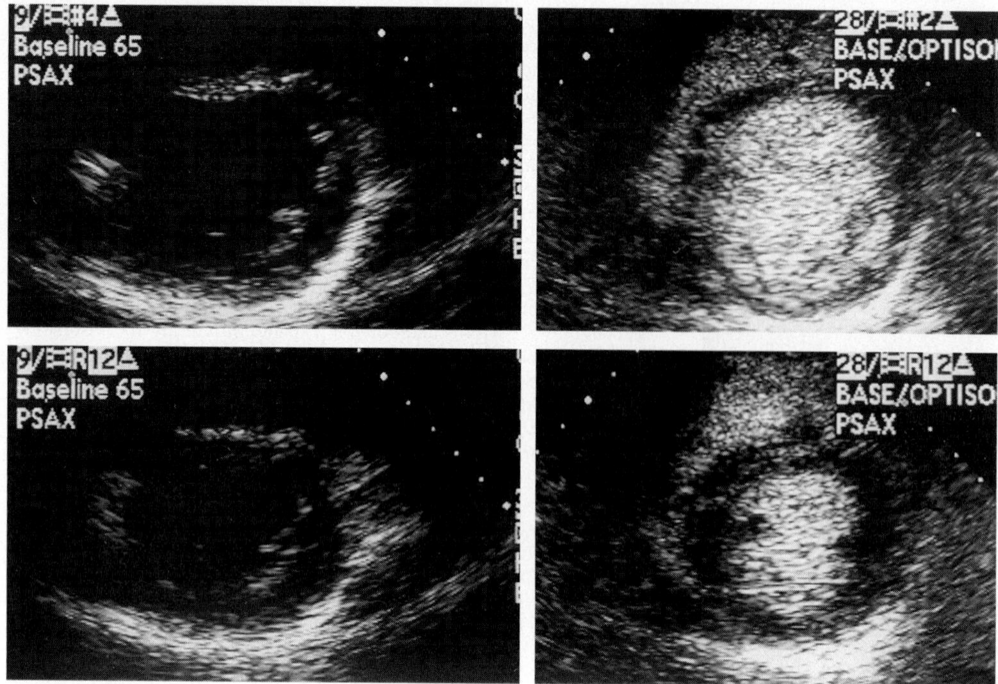

FIGURE 11–48 Demonstration of left ventricular cavity contrast enhancement after intravenous injection of a perfluorocarbon-based agent. The panels on the **left** were recorded before administration of contrast agent, and those on the **right** after opacification of the left ventricular cavity. Note the enhanced ability to identify the left ventricular cavity and distinguish it from the endocardial border after cavity opacification.

cardiac chambers, all four cardiac valves, and the great vessels. They provide high-resolution tomographic views in unlimited planes, which facilitates the ability to diagnose virtually all forms of anatomical cardiovascular disease. The addition of Doppler interrogation allows determination of physiological parameters as they relate to blood flow and myocardial velocities.

Echocardiography does have specific limitations because ultrasound does not transmit well through calcified structures such as bone, and an appropriate acoustic window is necessary for optimal visualization. In neonates and infants, ultrasound can pass through noncalcified cartilage and the windows available exceed those in adults. In the adult population, a noncalcified window must be obtained that typically is in the intercostal spaces or from the subxiphoid positions. In patients with narrow intercostal spaces, imaging can be problematic. A greater limitation is the degree to which the air-filled structures reflect ultrasound. Intervening lung tissue in patients with obstructive lung disease can result in suboptimal or even inadequate imaging.

Another area of concern for echocardiography is its potential for overuse. Because of the absence of risk from routine ultrasonography, overuse by less than adequately trained individuals has become a recent concern. The American College of Cardiology, American Heart Association, and American Society of Echocardiography have outlined recommendations for appropriate training in echocardiography and likewise recommendations on its appropriate clinical use.[86,87]

Clinical Applications of Echocardiography

Acquired Valvular Heart Disease (see Chap. 57)

Mitral Valve Disease

Virtually all types of mitral valve disease can be characterized anatomically using echocardiography. Doppler techniques provide accurate physiological information that complements the anatomical assessment. Figure 11–49 outlines the closure pattern of the normal mitral valve and the valve in multiple disease states, each of which are discussed.

MITRAL STENOSIS. Mitral stenosis was the first valvular lesion to be comprehensively evaluated with echocardiography. Two-dimensional echocardiography and Doppler ultrasonography remain the mainstay of diagnosis and characterization of this lesion. In the vast majority of adult patients, mitral stenosis is the result of rheumatic heart disease, with rarer cases of congenital mitral stenosis being encountered in adult patients. Rarely, heavy calcification of the mitral annulus results in functional restriction of the left ventricular inflow and can result in a left atrial to left ventricular gradient mimicking the physiological effects of valvular mitral stenosis.

The hallmark of mitral stenosis on two-dimensional echocardiography is thickening and restriction of motion of both mitral valve leaflets, with the predominant pathological process being fibrosis and fusion of the leaflet tips and proximal chordae (Fig. 11–50). In more advanced cases, the body of the leaflet itself may become involved and in even more advanced cases substantial calcification occurs within the leaflet and on the subvalvular apparatus, including the chordae and papillary muscle tips (Fig. 11–51). The earliest effect of rheumatic disease on the mitral valve is the result of inflammation and thickening of leaflet tips that restricts the motion of the tips while allowing free motion of the body of the leaflets. This results in a characteristic "doming" motion of the mitral valve in diastole. The appearance of the anterior leaflet in diastole has also been described as having a "hockey stick" configuration. Restriction of the tips results in a funnel-like mitral valve apparatus with the restrictive orifice being at the tips of the leaflets. This appearance is easily recognized from TTE in both the parasternal long-axis and apical four-chamber views. With careful attention to detail, the actual restrictive orifice of the mitral valve can be visualized and planimetered from a parasternal short-axis view (Fig. 11–52). This planimetered area correlates well with the area determined in the hemodynamic laboratory. M-mode echocardiography was the initial diagnostic tool for evaluation of mitral stenosis. By using this technique, the thickened leaflets could be identified as well as the restricted motion. The restricted motion pattern results in a flattening of the E-F slope of the mitral valve (Fig. 11–53). The E-F slope can be quantified and tracked as a measure of stenosis severity but provides no truly quantitative value by today's standards.

Assessment of Severity. In addition to determining the anatomical extent and severity of the stenotic lesion, assessment of physiological significance is made using Doppler echocardiography. Color flow imaging is instrumental in determining the degree of concurrent mitral regurgitation. Both continuous-wave and pulsed Doppler echocardiography can

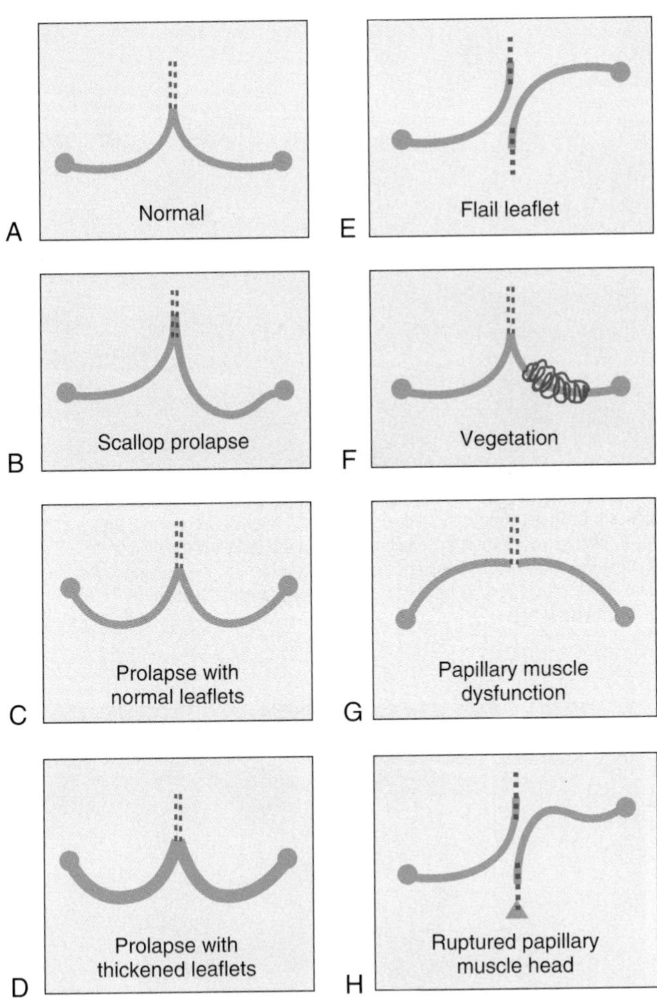

FIGURE 11–49 Schematic outlining both normal and abnormal mitral valve closure patterns in apical 4 chamber view. See text for details.

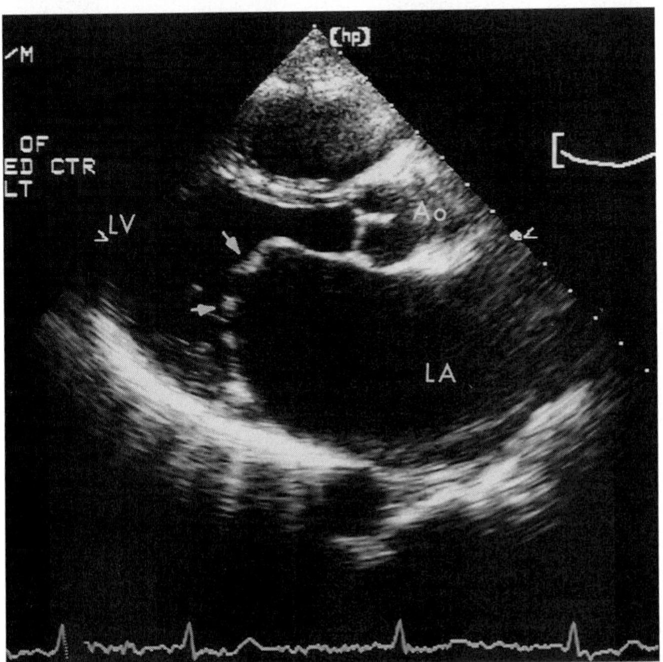

FIGURE 11–50 Parasternal long-axis view of a patient with mitral stenosis and a pliable noncalcified mitral valve leaflet. Note the "doming" motion of the mitral valve leaflets (arrowheads). Valves with these morphological features are excellent candidates for percutaneous balloon valvotomy. Ao = aorta; LA = left atrium; LV = left ventricle.

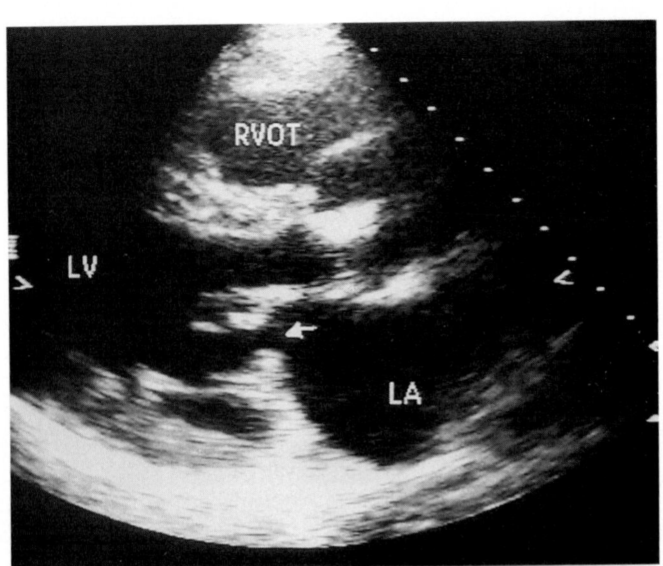

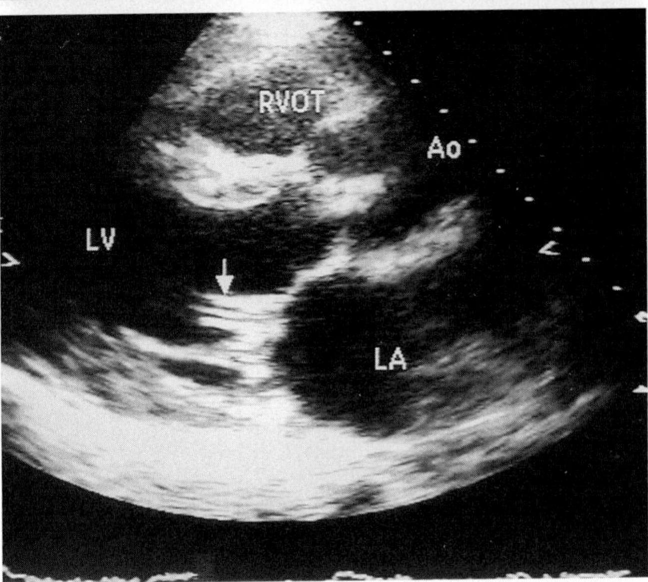

FIGURE 11–51 Parasternal long-axis view in diastole **(top)** and systole **(bottom)** in a patient with rheumatic heart disease and mitral stenosis. In the top panel, note the diffuse thickening of the mitral valve. The reduced orifice can be seen in this end-diastolic frame (arrow). The bottom panel was recorded in systole and provides a view of the chordal apparatus, which can be seen to be diffusely thickened and fibrotic. Valves with this appearance are less ideal candidates for percutaneous intervention than the valve presented in Figure 11–50. Ao = aorta; LA = left atrium; LV = left ventricle; RVOT = right ventricular outflow tract.

be obtained at rest and with exercise and provide accurate quantification of the transvalvular gradient (Fig. 11-54).[88-90] Determination of the transvalvular gradient should be performed in patients both at rest and with modest degrees of exercise. A population of symptomatic patients exists who have relatively unimpressive gradients at rest that increase dramatically with mild exercise.

A second Doppler method for determining the severity of mitral stenosis involves calculating the pressure half-time ($P_{1/2}t$), which is the time in milliseconds required for the peak pressure gradient to decline to one half of its original value.[91,92] The pressure half-time can be related to an anatomical valve area by the following formula:

$$\text{mitral valve area} = P_{1/2}t \div 220 \text{ msec}$$

This relationship is probably valid only for isolated mitral stenosis and is not accurate for quantitation of the mitral valve orifice if concurrent mitral regurgitation or significant aortic insufficiency is present. The relationship also has diminished accuracy in cases in which left ventricular diastolic compliance is markedly abnormal, such as in patients with

A

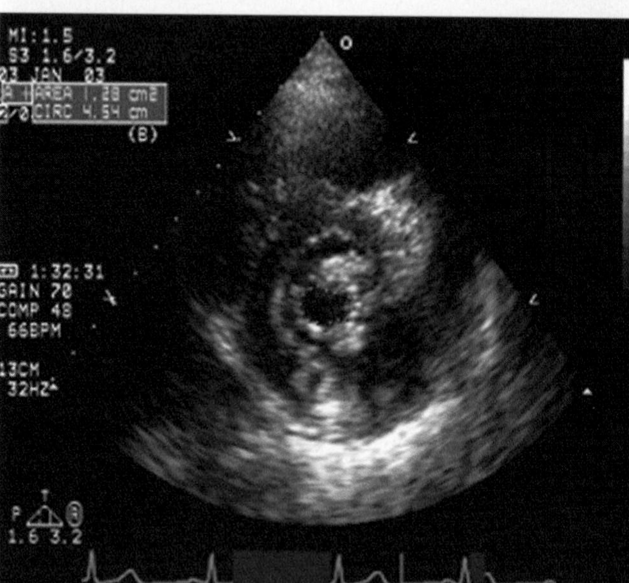

B

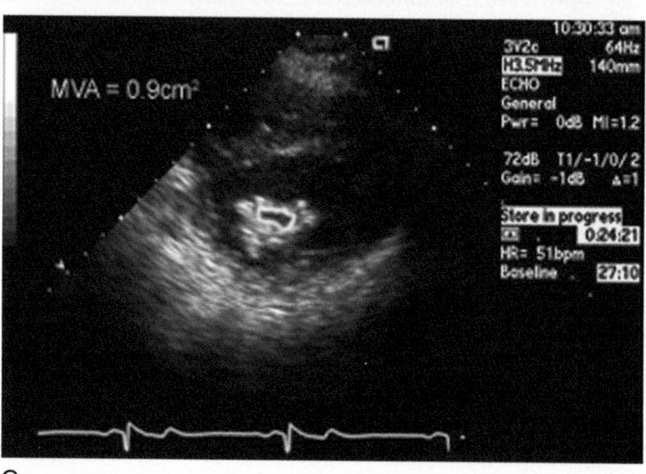

C

FIGURE 11–52 Mitral valve area. Three examples of planimetry of the stenotic mitral valve orifice. In each instance, a relatively regularly shaped mitral orifice can be planimetered. The planimetered values are superimposed in each figure.

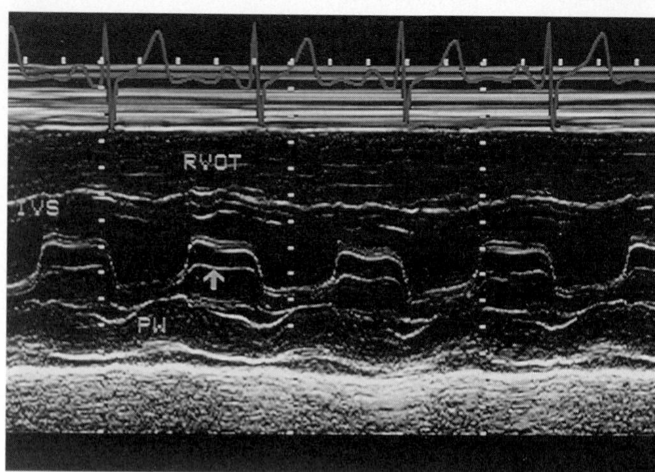

FIGURE 11–53 M-mode echocardiogram recorded in a patient with typical mitral stenosis. Compare this mitral valve opening pattern to the mitral valve motion in Figure 11–9. With mitral stenosis there is thickening of the leaflets, flattening of the E-F slope, and anterior motion of the posterior leaflet during mitral valve opening (arrow) in diastole. FW = left ventricular free wall; IVS = interventricular septum; RVOT = right ventricular outflow tract.

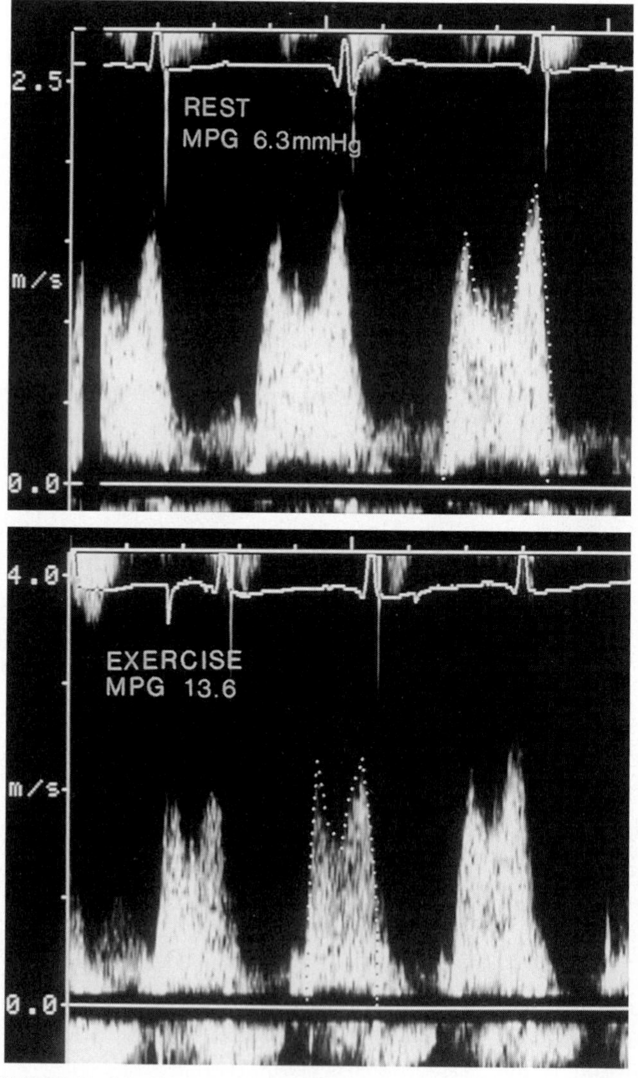

FIGURE 11–54 Transmitral Doppler recordings obtained in a patient with mitral stenosis at rest **(top)** and with exercise **(bottom)**. Heart rate has increased from 85 to 110 beats/min, resulting in an increase in the mean pressure gradient from 6.3 to 13.6 mm Hg.

severe hypertension or aortic stenosis and immediately after mitral balloon valvotomy.[93]

Other more detailed methods for determining the mitral valve area involve determination of quantitative mitral valve flow. This can be performed using the continuity equation in a manner analogous to that for aortic stenosis. Either flow and dimensions at the level of the mitral valve annulus or forward going flow in the left ventricular outflow tract can be used in this equation. Obviously, this approach has limitations in patients with concurrent regurgitation or multivalve disease.

Secondary effects of mitral stenosis include left atrial dilation with subsequent blood stasis and thrombus formation and secondary pulmonary hypertension. Evaluation of the left atrium for blood stasis and thrombus typically requires TEE (Fig. 11-55). The aortic, tricuspid, and pulmonic valves can likewise be directly interrogated for evidence of rheumatic involvement. The most common significant sequelae of mitral stenosis is development of secondary pulmonary hypertension with subsequent right heart dysfunction and tricuspid regurgitation. As with other diseases in which the right side of the heart is evaluated, the tricuspid regurgitation jet can be interrogated for determination of right ventricular systolic and pulmonary artery systolic pressures.

It is important to fully evaluate the anatomical features of mitral stenosis in patients in whom a mitral balloon valvotomy is contemplated. Four features of mitral valve anatomy have been identified that correlate with the success of this procedure. These include valve pliability, thickening, calcification, and subvalvular involvement. Each of these can be quantified on a score of 0 to 4 and a total score tabulated. Scores above 8 represent valves less likely to be successfully treated with a percutaneous approach.[94-96] More recent studies have suggested a disproportionate impact of calcification and subvalvular involvement on the likelihood of successful balloon valvotomy.

MITRAL REGURGITATION. Two-dimensional echocardiography and Doppler techniques can be used to detect the presence and severity of mitral regurgitation, to determine the cause of regurgitation and to look for secondary effects. Mitral regurgitation can be due to a wide variety of cardiac conditions, many of which are presented in schematic form in Figure 11–49. Often, mitral regurgitation will first be documented using Doppler color flow imaging. In the presence of significant mitral regurgitation, volume overload of left ventricle and left atrium occurs, resulting in dilation of these chambers, the degree of which is dependent on both the severity and duration of mitral regurgitation. The cause of mitral regurgitation is determined by assessing the anatomy of the left ventricle and the mitral valve apparatus. Many forms of mitral regurgitation are due to intrinsic disease of the mitral valve, such as mitral regurgitation concurrent with mitral stenosis, myxomatous degeneration with mitral valve prolapse, chordal rupture, endocarditis, and infarct-related papillary muscle rupture. Functional forms of mitral regurgitation also occur in which the mitral valve may be anatomically normal but fails to coapt because of dilation of the left ventricle. This can occur due to either cardiomyopathy or coronary artery disease. In the vast majority of instances, the anatomical and functional abnormality responsible for mitral regurgitation can be documented with TTE. On occasion, TEE is necessary to refine the anatomical assessment and may be particularly helpful in identifying rupture of a papillary muscle head and flail leaflets and in detecting smaller vegetations or perforations.[97,98]

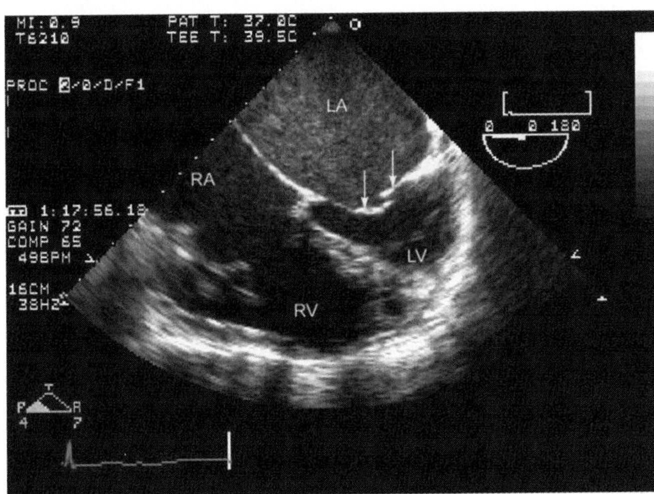

FIGURE 11–55 Transesophageal echocardiogram recorded in a patient with severe rheumatic mitral valvular stenosis and marked biatrial and right ventricular enlargement. This frame was recorded in diastole. Note the thickened immobile mitral leaflets, which have not appropriately separated in diastole. Note also the dense, spontaneous echo contrast in the body of the left atrium, which in real time appears as a mass of swirling echoes. LA = left atrium; LV = left ventricle; RA = right atrium; RV = right ventricle.

Assessment of Severity. Doppler color flow imaging is used to determine the severity of mitral regurgitation. The size of the regurgitant jet within the left atrium is directly proportional to the severity of mitral regurgitation. Multiple studies have confirmed the relationship between the size of the regurgitant jet and the severity of regurgitation determined with angiography or other techniques. Typically, the size of the jet is indexed to the size of the left atrium. Figure 11-56 demonstrates examples of mitral regurgitation. Jets that are peripheral or impinging on a wall, rather than central, cause predictable underestimation of severity. A regurgitant jet impinging on a wall results in a smaller color flow area than an equivalent central regurgitant volume.[99] The underlying mechanism of this phenomenon is that a regurgitant jet "recruits" the adjacent blood flow into motion. As color Doppler flow detects cells in motion, irrespective of their origin, the visualized regurgitant jet is the sum of the regurgitant volume and the recruited blood. A centrally oriented jet recruits in all of its dimensions, whereas a jet adjacent to a wall recruits only on its free surface, hence being relatively smaller than an equal volume of central regurgitation. A jet impinging on a wall underestimates the regurgitant volume by approximately 40 percent. In cases of moderate and severe mitral regurgitation, flow in the pulmonary veins may reverse direction in systole. A variation on this finding is attenuation of normal forward flow in the pulmonary vein during ventricular systole. More recently, three-dimensional reconstruction of mitral regurgitation jets has been shown to be feasible.[100,101] The incremental value of this method has not yet been shown.

Several characteristics of a regurgitant jet can give clues as to its origin. In the presence of normal ventricular function, an anatomically normal mitral valve closes along a 2- to 3-mm-long line of overlap of the leaflets (*zona coapta*). This overlap of leaflet tissue results in more efficient closure of the mitral valve than does tip-to-tip closure. With left ventricular dilatation, the papillary muscles are displaced apically and laterally, pulling the mitral valve leaflet toward the apex.[102,103] This results in a systolic doming of the leaflets and tip-to-tip closure of the mitral valve leaflet rather than overlapping in the *zona coapta* (Fig. 11-57). Tip-to-tip closure is inefficient and results in variable degrees of mitral regurgitation. In extreme examples, the leaflet tips may fail to coapt at all and the actual regurgitant orifice can be directly visualized. These jets are typically central in location. By using either color Doppler M-mode or careful interrogation of the spectral display, the timing of the mitral regurgitation jet can also be determined. Lesions such as mitral prolapse may result in regurgitant confined to midsystole and late systole.

Anatomical disruption of any portion of the mitral valve will result in regurgitation. This can range from a few ruptured chordae with isolated prolapse of a single scallop to disruption of an entire papillary muscle head with flail of an entire leaflet. TEE is often incrementally helpful in determining the precise degree of anatomical disruption of the valve (Fig. 11-58). Irrespective of the cause of a flail leaflet, the resultant jet is often highly eccentric and its flow is directed opposite the leaflet bearing the pathological lesion; that is, a flail posterior mitral valve leaflet results in an anteriorly directed jet. A highly eccentric jet should lead to a higher index of suspicion of a flail leaflet. Three-dimensional echocardiography has shown promise for detailed assessment of mitral valve pathology in mitral regurgitation (Fig. 11-59).

Quantitation of mitral regurgitation is heavily dependent on the color Doppler flow area. Other techniques for quantifying mitral regurgitation rely on determining the width of the jet at its origin (*vena contracta*) and on evaluation of the proximal isovelocity surface area. In general terms, for any given Nyquist limit, the larger the size is of the proximal isovelocity surface area, the greater the degree of regurgitation. Calcula-

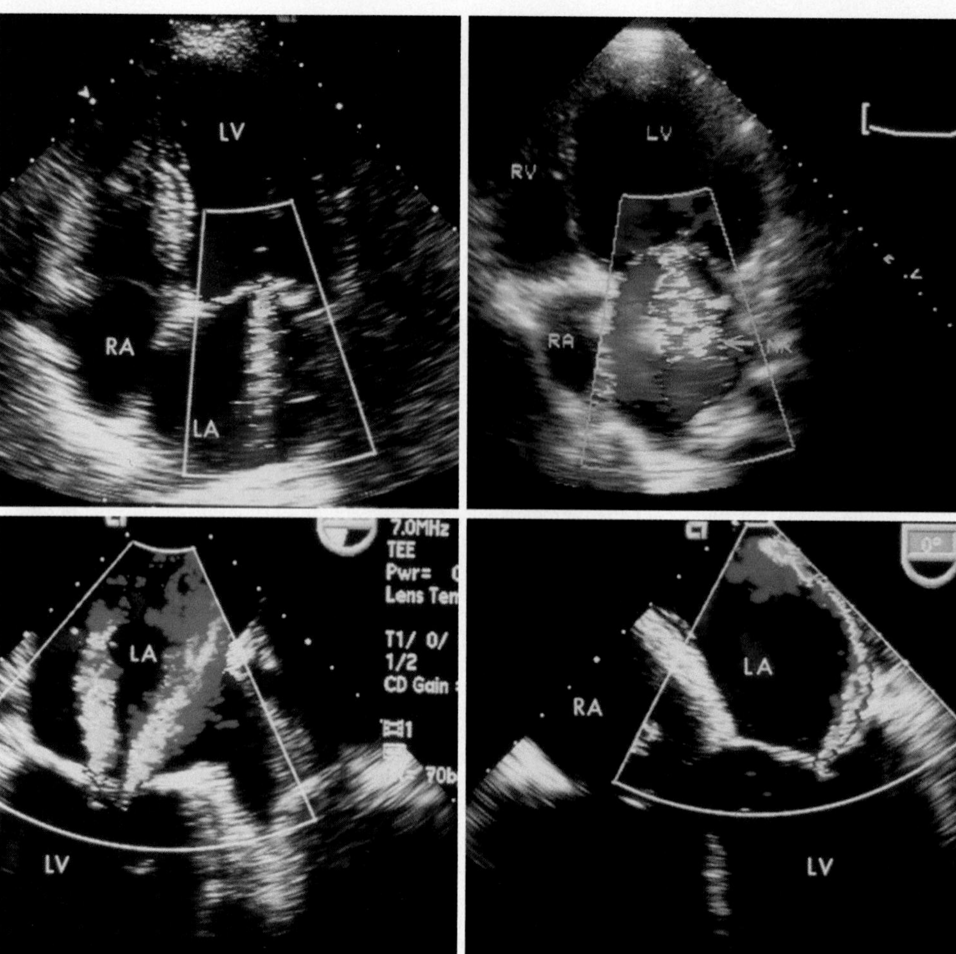

FIGURE 11–56 Four panels depicting varying degrees of mitral regurgitation; the two **top panels** are apical four-chamber transthoracic views showing, on the **left,** mild mitral regurgitation and, on the **right,** moderate to severe mitral regurgitation. On the left, note the relatively narrow jet directed from the tips of the mitral valve toward the posterior left atrial wall. On the right, note the larger jet, filling approximately 40 percent of the left atrial cavity. The two **bottom panels** are transesophageal echocardiograms. On the **left,** note the mitral regurgitation occurring in two discrete jets and, on the **right,** the highly eccentric jet, which courses along the extreme lateral wall of the left atrium. LA = left atrium; LV = left ventricle; RA = right atrium; RV = right ventricle.

tion of flow volume from proximal isovelocity surface area has already been discussed and can be applied to determine regurgitant volume. In addition to calculating flow volume using proximal isovelocity surface area, several derivative measurements can also be made (Fig. 11-60). The surface area of the isovelocity of flow represents the area of flow and, when multiplied by the aliasing velocity, results in regurgitant flow. This volume of regurgitant flow, when divided by the peak velocity, results in calculation of effective regurgitant orifice.[104,105] All of these measurements assume holosystolic mitral regurgitation. It should be emphasized that there are many instances in which mitral regurgitation may be confined to only a portion of systole. A classic example is mitral prolapse with regurgitation confined to the later half or third of systole. While there are no strict guidelines, when mitral regurgitation is identified as being confined to only a portion of systole, the assessment of severity whether based on the size of the regurgitant jet at one point in time or regurgitant flow must be adjusted accordingly for the partial duration of flow. A secondary finding seen in cases of moderate and severe mitral regurgitation is reversal of systolic flow in the pulmonary veins. In practice, combining observations from all these techniques is often beneficial for quantifying mitral regurgitation. Table 11-3 outlines the various criteria for determining severity of mitral regurgitation.

MITRAL VALVE PROLAPSE. The detection and characterization of mitral valve prolapse remains a common use of echocardiography. Early studies suggested a prevalence of prolapse of up to 21 percent in otherwise healthy young females. It should be emphasized that many individuals identified as having mitral prolapse in these earlier studies today are recognized to simply have normal bowing of the mitral valve. The normal mitral valve closure pattern is for the tips of the leaflets to point toward the left ventricular apex and for there to be gentle bowing of the leaflet with a concavity toward the apex of the left ventricle. Based largely on dimensional reconstruction techniques, the mitral valve annulus is known not to be a planar structure but rather to have complex three-dimensional geometry. Depending on the tomographic plane of interrogation, a portion of one or both leaflets may bow behind the imaginary annular line. In the presence of otherwise anatomically normal thin leaflets, this represents a variation of normal and does not represent pathological mitral valve prolapse.

The most extreme forms of mitral valve prolapse involve myxomatous degeneration of the valves with visible leaflet thickening (defined as greater than 3 to 5 mm in thickness) and either marked symmetrical bowing of the valve behind the majority of the annular plane or highly asymmetrical buckling of one or both leaflets into the plane of the left atrium (Figs. 11–61 and 11–62). This will be associated

TABLE 11–3 Mitral Regurgitation Severity*

	I (Mild)	II	III	IV (Severe)
MR = JET (% LA)	<15	15-30	35-50	>50
Spectral Doppler	Faint	—	—	Dense
Vena Contracta	<3 mm	—	—	>6 mm
Pulmonary vein flow	S > D	—	—	Systolic Reversed
RV (ml)	<30	30-44	45-59	≥60
ERO (cm²)	<0.2	0.2-0.29	0.3-0.39	30.40
PISA	Small	—	—	Large

D = antegrade flow in diastole; ERO = effective regurgitant orifice; % LA = percentage of left atrial area encompassed by the MR jet with color flow Doppler; MR = mitral regurgitation; PISA = proximal isovelocity surface area; RV = regurgitant volume; S = antegrade flow in systole.

*For some parameters, the observation is valid at the extremes of MR severity and there may be marked overlap in intermediate (grades II, III) MR. In these instances, no value is presented.

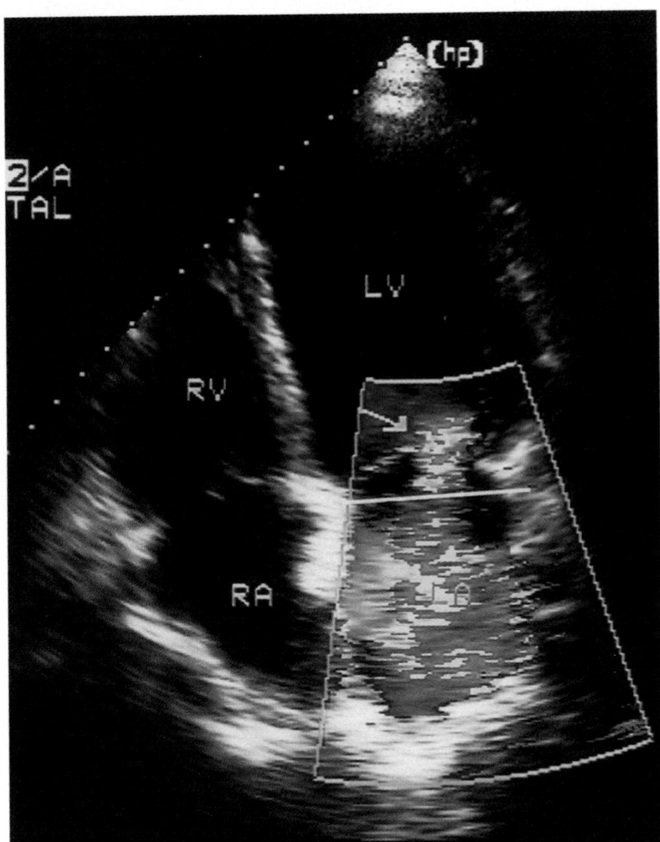

FIGURE 11–57 Apical four-chamber view in a patient with a dilated cardiomyopathy and severe mitral regurgitation due to a dilated annulus and abnormal mitral valve coaptation. The solid horizontal white line represents the plane of the mitral annulus. Note that the mitral valve closes well within the cavity of the left ventricle. The actual origin of the mitral regurgitation jet can be seen as it accelerates toward the regurgitant orifice (arrow) and is likewise displaced into the cavity of the left ventricle. LA = left atrium; LV = left ventricle; RA = right atrium; RV = right ventricle.

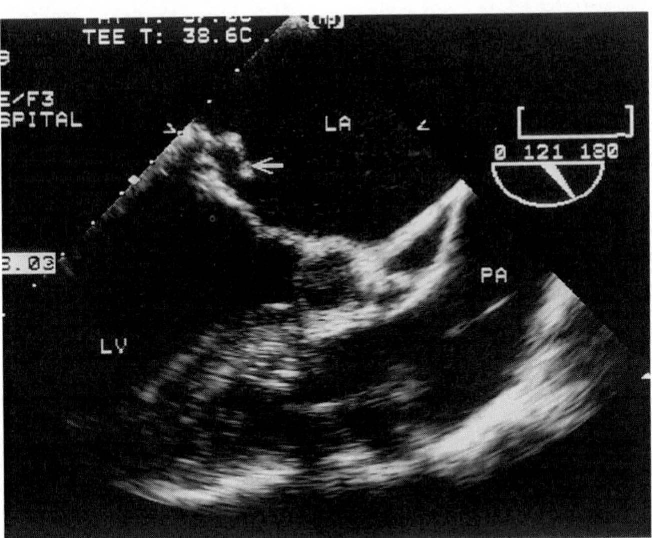

FIGURE 11–58 Transesophageal echocardiogram recorded in a patient with a flail posterior mitral valve leaflet. The echocardiogram is recorded in a longitudinal view in which the left atrium (LA), left ventricle (LV), and pulmonary artery (PA) are visualized. Because flail leaflets occur in atypical locations, it is often necessary to scan in unusual planes to identify the leaflet. In this projection, a substantial portion of the posterior leaflet (arrow) can be seen to protrude into the left atrium, with the tip of the leaflet no longer attached to the chordal apparatus.

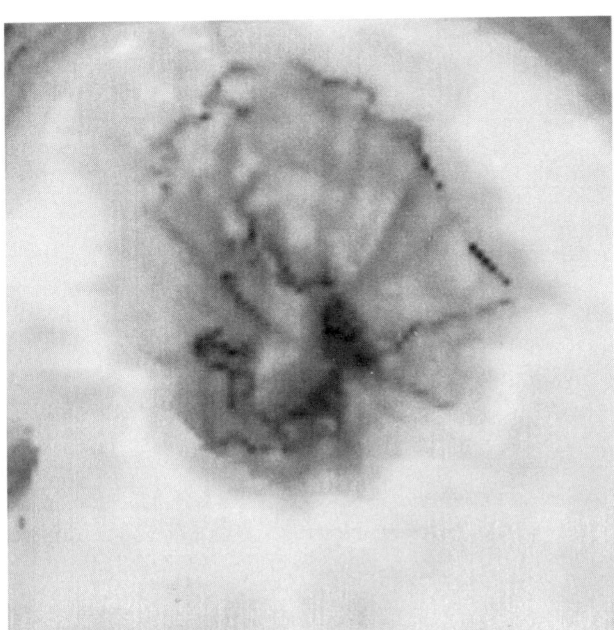

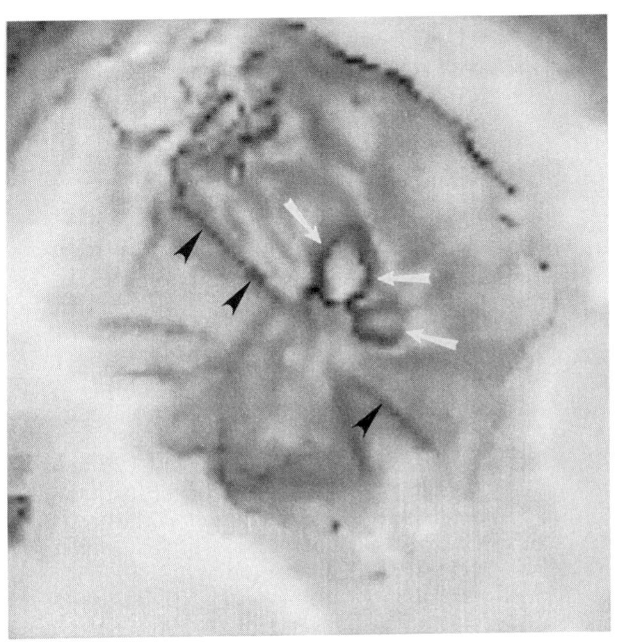

FIGURE 11–59 Three-dimensional echocardiogram recorded in a patient with a partial flail mitral anterior leaflet. For both panels, the orientation is a view of the mitral valve from within the left atrium. The left panel was recorded in diastole, and the unrestricted orifice can be seen. The right panel was recorded in mid-systole. Note the two scallops of the anterior leaflet that protrude into the left atrium (arrows).

A

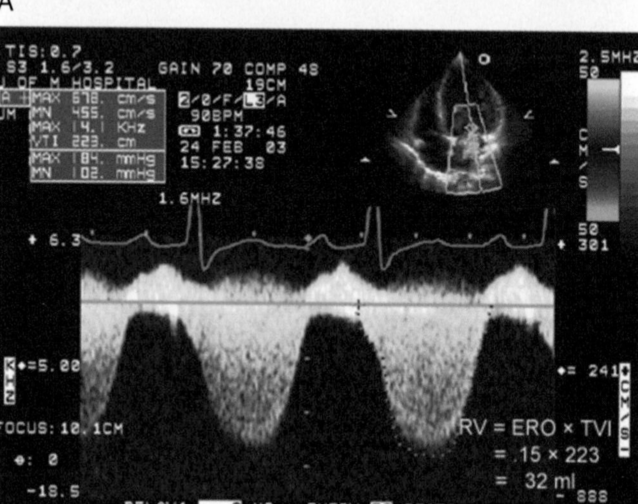

B

FIGURE 11–60 Example for calculation of regurgitant flow and effective regurgitant orifice (ERO) and regurgitant volume using the PISA technique. See Figure 11–35 for a schematic representation of these calculations as well. **A,** Color Doppler image from which the diameter of the convergence zone can be calculated as 0.67 cm. The aliasing limit is 35 cm^2. **B,** Continuous wave spectral display of the mitral regurgitation jet from which the VTI and V_{MAX} can be determined. From this, the regurgitant volume can be calculated as 32 ml. Using the calculation schematized in Figure 11–35, flow can be calculated as 98 ml/sec, and the effective regurgitant orifice as 0.15 cm^2.

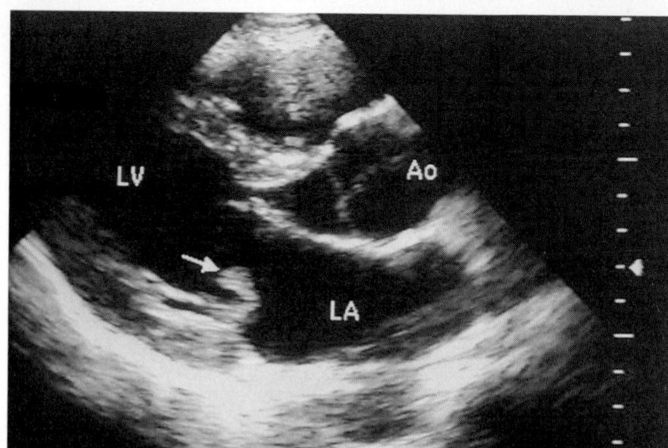

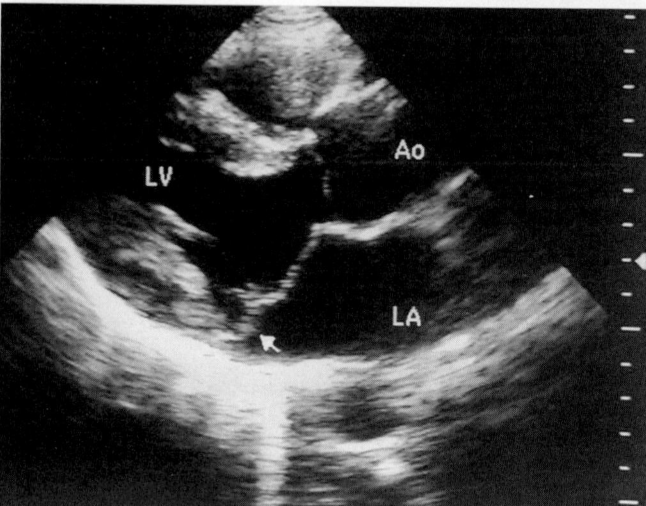

FIGURE 11–61 Parasternal long-axis view in diastole **(top)** and systole **(bottom)** in a patient with mitral valve prolapse and myxomatous changes. In the upper panel, note the open mitral valve and the diffuse thickening of the posterior mitral valve leaflet (arrow). The lower panel was recorded in systole. Note that both leaflets prolapse behind the plane of the mitral valve annulus. The prolapse of the posterior leaflet is somewhat more prominent (arrow). Ao = aorta; LA = left atrium; LV = left ventricle.

with variable degrees of mitral regurgitation, which may be either holosystolic or confined to middle to late systole. Because of the eccentric buckling of the myxomatous valve, the mitral regurgitation jet can be eccentric rather than central. The key aspects to the diagnosis of mitral valve prolapse rely not on the mere detection of a valve that buckles into the plane of the left atrium but on characterization of the valve morphology. As mentioned earlier, normal thin leaflets that bow gently into the left atrial plane probably represent a variation of normal closure patterns. Patients with thickened redundant valves and myxomatous changes of the leaflet have a true form of structural heart disease. It is these individuals who are most at risk for endocarditis, spontaneous rupture of chordae, and progressive mitral regurgitation (see Chap. 57). It also appears that there is a higher than usual incidence of ventricular arrhythmias and neurological events in this subset of patients.

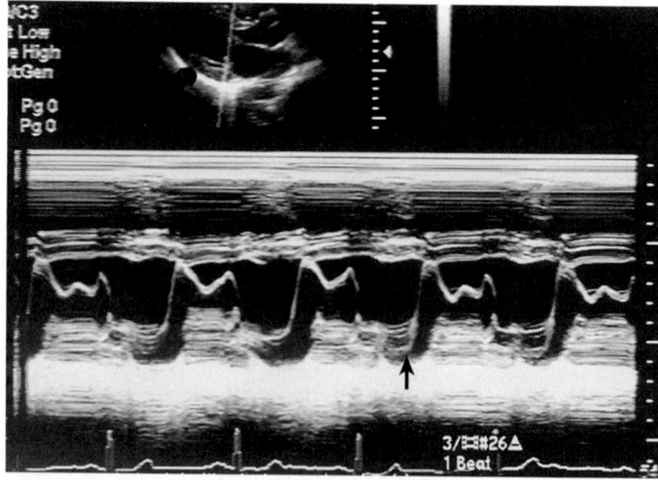

FIGURE 11–62 M-mode echocardiogram of the mitral valve recorded in the same patient noted in Figure 11–61. Note that the posterior leaflet is diffusely thickened and in systole prolapses posteriorly from the normal closure line (arrow).

Aortic Valve Disease

AORTIC STENOSIS. Aortic stenosis is most commonly due to one of three pathological processes: a bicuspid aortic valve, rheumatic heart disease, or degenerative aortic stenosis. On rare occasions, aortic stenosis can be the result of endocarditis or radiation heart disease. Bicuspid aortic valve typically manifests as a hemodynamically significant lesion in the fourth or fifth decade of life and calcific degenerative aortic stenosis in the seventh decade and beyond. Rheumatic aortic valve disease will virtually always be seen in patients who have concurrent rheumatic mitral valve disease.

The bicuspid aortic valve is the single most common congenital cardiac defect and occurs in approximately 2 percent of the population. There is a broad range of anatomical and physiological abnormalities associated with this condition. The bicuspid aortic valve is commonly thought of as a two-leaflet valve with roughly equal leaflet proportions. There is a range of abnormality in the "bicuspid valve" that includes nearly unicuspid valves and distribution of leaflet tissue other than 50/50 percent. Bicuspid aortic valves are commonly described as having either an anteroposterior or a lateral orientation of the leaflets. In reality, virtually any direction of the major coaptation can be seen. TTE is a reliable method for detecting the bicuspid aortic valve. With the use of this technique, the hallmark of the bicuspid valve will be eccentric closure of the leaflets within the aorta. In approximately 80 percent of cases, two rather than three leaflets can be directly visualized (Fig. 11–63). With closer scrutiny by way of TEE, what at first appears to be a true bicuspid valve often is found to represent a three-leaflet valve with unequal leaflet sizes and fusion of one of the three commissures, resulting in a functional bicuspid valve (Fig. 11–64). In this instance, there will be three coronary sinuses and normal orientation of the coronary arteries. In a true two-leaflet bicuspid aortic valve, there will be only two coronary sinuses and variable location of the coronary ostia. It is important to examine the opening pattern of the aortic valve to determine that it is functionally bicuspid. There is a strong association between coarctation of the aorta and bicuspid valve. When either of these conditions is clinically suspected, the other should also be considered.

Degenerative calcific valves appear as three-leaflet structures with marked thickening of the leaflets. Thickening and calcification may be more prominent at the base of the leaflets than at the tips. There is a broad range of immobility and stenosis, depending on the duration and severity of disease. In advanced cases, the degree of calcification may be so extensive that it is not possible to identify discrete valve cusps.

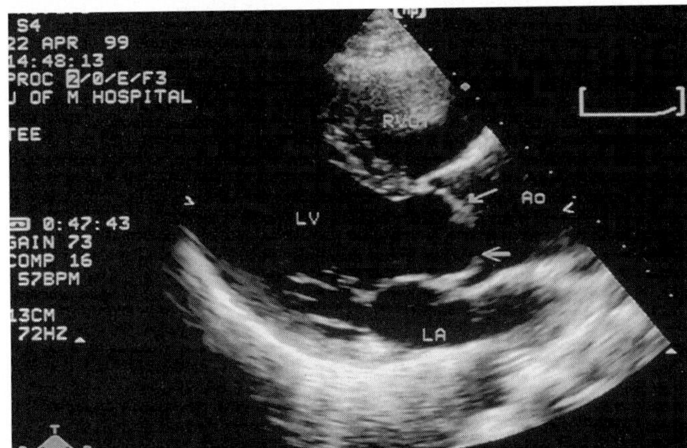

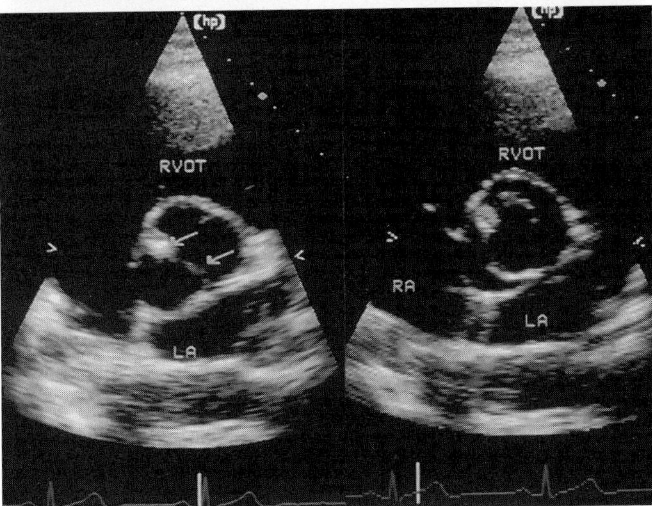

FIGURE 11–63 Transthoracic echocardiogram in a patient with bicuspid aortic valve. In the **upper panel,** note that the leaflets of the aortic valve do not open all the way to the margins of the aorta but are "tethered" in lumen of the proximal aorta. The two bottom panels are recorded in the short-axis view at the base of the heart. The **lower left panel** was recorded in diastole and reveals the closed bicuspid valve with a single commissure oriented from 10 o'clock to 4 o'clock (arrows). The **lower right panel** is recorded in systole, and the oval opening of the bicuspid valve can be appreciated within the circular aorta. Ao = aorta; LA = left atrium; LV = left ventricle; RA = right atrium; RVOT = right ventricular outflow tract.

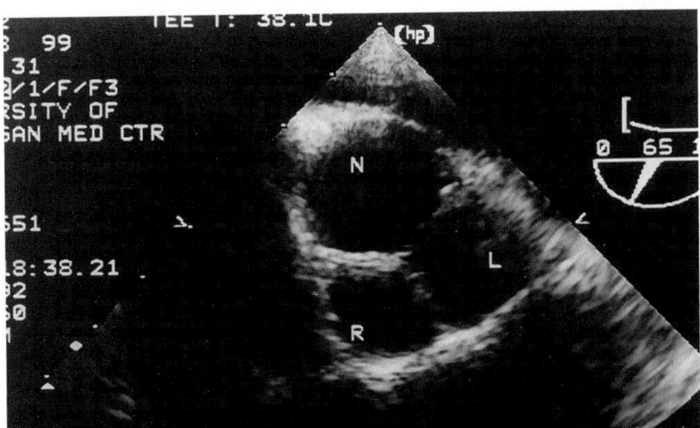

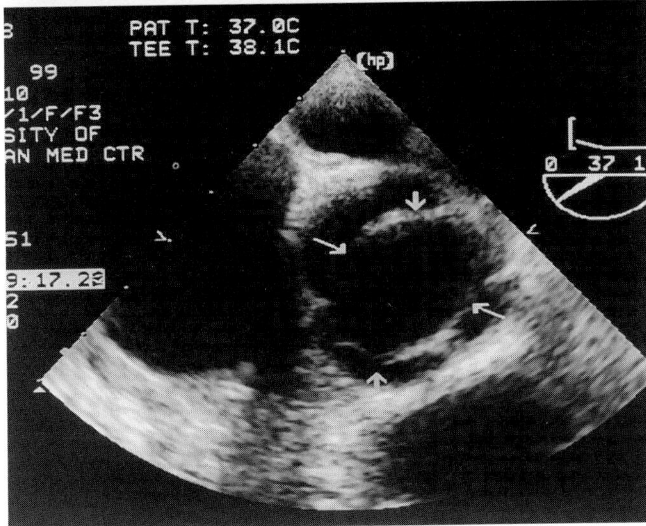

FIGURE 11–64 Transesophageal echocardiogram recorded in a patient with an anatomical three-leaflet valve with a fused commissure resulting in a functional bicuspid aortic valve. In the **top panel,** note the three cusps (N = noncoronary, L = left coronary, R = right coronary). The upper frame was recorded in diastole, and the closure lines would suggest the presence of three leaflets. The **lower panel** is recorded in systole, and instead of opening fully to the margins of the aorta with a circular orifice, the valve opens with an oval, fishmouth-shaped orifice. Note that the commissure between the right and left cusps is fused, resulting in a functionally bicuspid valve.

Rheumatic aortic stenosis typically results in leaflet thickening along the commissural edges. It will be seen almost exclusively in the presence of rheumatic mitral stenosis.

Once aortic stenosis is anatomically defined, secondary effects can also be evaluated. These include poststenotic dilation of the aorta and left ventricular hypertrophy. Assessment of left ventricular systolic function should also be undertaken.

Assessment of Severity. Doppler echocardiography is essential for assessment of the physiological significance of aortic stenosis (Fig. 11-65). In cases of clinically significant aortic stenosis, the gradient is likely to exceed 50 mm Hg. This corresponds to a Doppler velocity of approximately 3.5 m/sec, which is out of the range for accurate quantitation using pulsed-wave Doppler. For this reason, continuous-wave Doppler is essential for quantitation. From continuous-wave Doppler, both instantaneous peak and mean gradients can be determined using the Bernoulli equation. Either on-line or off-line outlining of the spectral display and automatic calculation of these values can be performed. In some instances, determination of the gradient at rest and with exercise may be beneficial. The gradients determined from Doppler echocardiography correlate very well with simultaneously determined invasive measurements. This correlation is maximal during simultaneous measurement and when micromanometer tip catheters are used (Fig. 11-66).[106] The commonly measured "peak to peak" gradient determined in the catheterization laboratory has no basis in physiological reality and will not correspond to either a peak instantaneous or a mean gradient determined by either micromanometer catheters or Doppler interrogation. In most instances, cardiac output and hence stroke volume are augmented in the catheterization laboratory compared with rest. For this reason, Doppler-determined gradients in the echocardiography laboratory may be lower than a catheterization-determined gradient. In asymptomatic patients, it may be beneficial to assess the aortic valve gradient at rest and with exercise.

On occasion, the Doppler gradient significantly underestimates the measured gradient. This is common with nonsimultaneous recordings, as noted earlier, but also occurs when the angle of interrogation (θ) exceeds 20 degrees. Off-angle interrogation is the single most common cause for underestimation of an aortic stenosis gradient. In instances in which there is a serial obstruction consisting of both valvular and subvalvular obstruction, both the V1 and the V2 component of the Bernoulli equation must be incorporated.

The actual valve orifice is usually not visualized to a reliable degree from TTE. TEE can be used to obtain a direct measurement of the aortic valve orifice in many patients with aortic stenosis. In cases of severe aortic stenosis, the orifice may be highly irregular and not all portions of it may lie in the same plane. With scrupulous attention to detail, it is possible in many instances to directly planimeter the area (Fig. 11-67).[107]

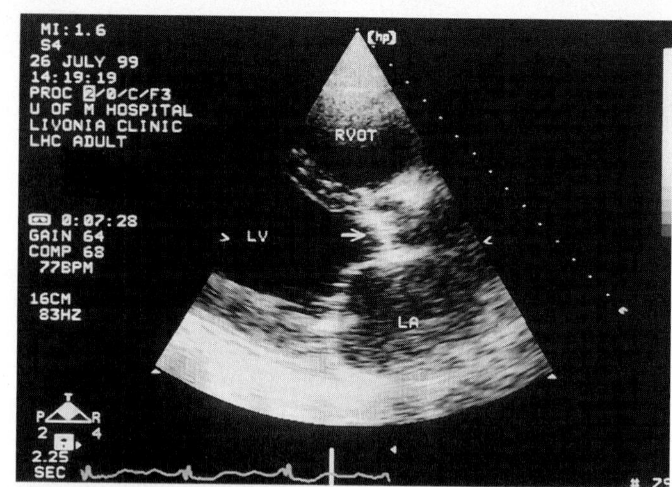

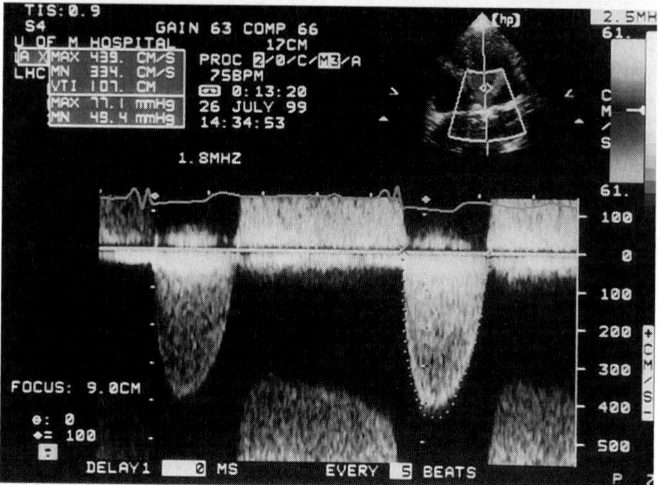

FIGURE 11–65 Echocardiogram recorded in a patient with severe aortic stenosis. The **top panel** is a parasternal long-axis view recorded in systole. Left ventricular function is diminished. The aortic valve is markedly thickened and partially calcified. Its motion is markedly reduced and in systole it appears that the valve occludes the orifice (arrow). The **lower panel** is a continuous-wave Doppler recorded from the apex of the left ventricle along a line aimed through the stenotic aortic valve. Note the aortic stenosis signal below the zero crossing line. The peak velocity is 430 cm/sec, which corresponds to a maximum gradient of 77 mm Hg and a mean gradient of 49.4 mm Hg. LA = left atrium; LV = left ventricle; RVOT = right ventricular outflow tract.

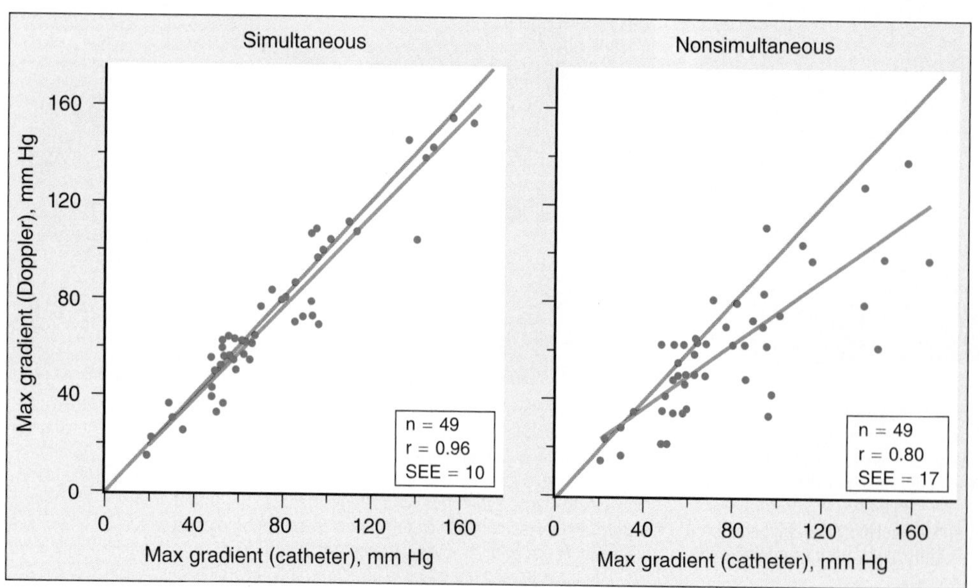

FIGURE 11–66 Graphic comparison of Doppler- and catheterization-determined gradients in patients with aortic stenosis. On the **left** are simultaneously recorded gradients and on the **right** are nonsimultaneous gradients. Note the stronger correlation between Doppler and catheterization when gradients are obtained in a simultaneous manner. (From Currie PJ, Hagler DJ, Seward JB, et al: Instantaneous pressure gradient: A simultaneous Doppler and dual catheter correlative study. J Am Coll Cardiol 7:800, 1986; with permission from the American College of Cardiology Foundation.)

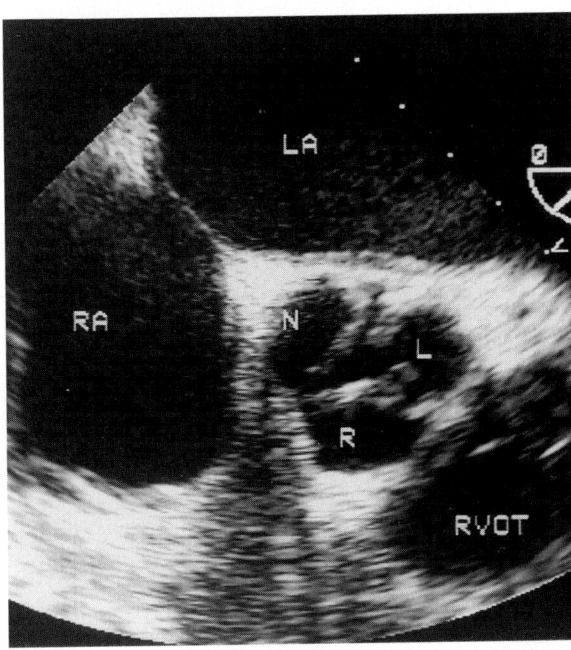

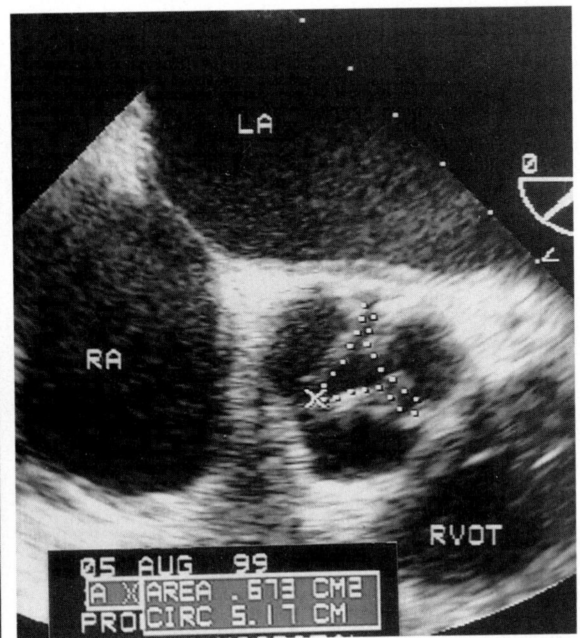

FIGURE 11–67 Transesophageal echocardiogram recorded in a patient with severe aortic stenosis. In the **left panel,** note the three aortic valve cusps (N = noncoronary, L = left coronary, R = right coronary). The leaflets are diffusely thickened and have restricted opening motion. The **right panel** is the same systolic frame in which the stenotic area of the aortic valve has been planimetered. Note that the area of the aortic valve is calculated as 0.67 cm^2, consistent with severe aortic stenosis. LA = left atrium; RA = right atrium; RVOT = right ventricular outflow tract.

An additional method for determining the aortic valve area relies on the continuity equation (Figs. 11-34 and 11-68).[108] Typically, in aortic stenosis, the left ventricular outflow tract area can be determined, assuming circular geometry. Pulsed Doppler is then used to determine the velocity of flow at that site. The product of the two is volumetric flow in the outflow tract. At the stenotic orifice, continuous-wave Doppler is used to determine the velocity integral. The algebraic equation can then be solved for the aortic valve area. A modification of this technique uses mitral valve flow instead of left ventricular outflow. Because the velocity of flow increases at the restrictive orifice, several investigators have suggested using the V1/V2 ratio as a marker of significant aortic stenosis. Other methods for determining the severity of aortic stenosis involve calculation of aortic valve resistance[109] and using echo-Doppler data in variations of the Gorlin formula.

From a practical standpoint, it is often not necessary to determine an aortic valve area. In a patient with thickened restricted leaflets and a mean gradient exceeding 50 mm Hg, the presence of severe aortic stenosis is clinically assured. Likewise, in a patient with normal ventricular function and a low peak gradient (20-25 mm Hg), the likelihood of significant aortic stenosis becomes negligible. Patients with reduced left ventricular function, typically with a left ventricular ejection fraction of 25 to 35 percent, and a modest transvalvular gradient of 25 to 30 mm Hg are problematic. This situation may either represent mild aortic valve disease and unrelated left ventricular dysfunction or, conversely, critical aortic stenosis with secondary left ventricular dysfunction. In the latter situation, patients will benefit from aortic valve replacement, whereas for the former situation, medical management is indicated. Dobutamine infusion, while monitoring left ventricular function and transvalvular gradients, can be a useful means for separating these two entities.[110] If left ventricular function augments with a dobutamine infusion and the gradient increases to clinically pertinent levels, the diagnosis is most likely severe aortic stenosis with secondary left ventricular dysfunction, and these patients will benefit from valve replacement. Conversely, if ventricular function improves without a change in the gradient, it is less likely that the aortic stenosis is the limiting factor.

AORTIC REGURGITATION. Detection and quantitation of aortic regurgitation rely predominantly on Doppler techniques. Using color flow imaging, the regurgitant jet can be visualized in the left ventricular outflow tract from several different planes (Fig. 11–69). In the majority of instances, there is an underlying anatomical abnormality of the aortic valve such as endocarditis, disease of the aortic root, rheumatic valve disease, or a bicuspid valve.

Several features of the regurgitant jet have been investigated as markers of the severity of aortic regurgitation.[111] Unlike mitral regurgitation, in which the overall jet size correlates well with regurgitation severity, neither the overall size nor the depth of penetration of the aortic regurgitation jet correlates strongly with the severity of aortic regurgitation. This is in large part due to the difficulty in separating the regurgitant flow stream from mitral valve inflow. A greater degree of success has been obtained by measuring either the width or the cross-sectional area of the regurgitant jet in the outflow tract and indexing this to the width or cross-sectional area of the outflow tract (Fig. 11–70). These measurements are dependent on imaging the jet in its true minor axis, and an eccentric jet, crossing tangentially across the outflow tract, will result in a disproportionately sized jet compared with its true dimension. TEE often provides more accurate visualization of the true direction and size of the regurgitant jet.

Assessment of Severity. By using continuous-wave Doppler from the apex, one can record the actual flow velocity profile of the regurgitant jet (Fig. 11-71). The velocity of the regurgitant jet is directly related to pressure gradient between the aorta and the left ventricle. If this gradient remains high throughout diastole, the slope of velocity and pressure decay is relatively flat. This implies a relatively mild degree of aortic regurgitation in which there has been little equilibration of aortic and left ventricular diastolic pressures. Conversely, with severe aortic regurgitation (especially if acute), there is a greater degree of equilibration of left ventricular and aortic diastolic pressures and the terminal aortic regurgitation velocities are relatively low, resulting in a fairly steep slope of velocity decay over the diastolic pressure curve. The pressure half-time of the regurgitant jet, defined as the time in milliseconds required for the initial transvalvular diastolic gradient to decline to one half of its peak value, can be calculated and is inversely related to the severity of aortic regurgitation. A pressure half-time less than 400 msec correlates with severe aortic regurgitation. In high-quality studies, the continuity equation can be used to calculate the aortic regurgitant volume. It should be noted that any concurrent disease that also increases left ventricular diastolic pressure will also cause a steeper slope of the aortic regurgitation flow signal. Quantitation of aortic regurgitation has also been performed using the proximal isovelocity surface area method.

Several secondary Doppler and anatomical features should also be noted in cases of aortic regurgitation. The proximal aorta often has progressive dilation with long-standing aortic regurgitation.[112] Left ventricu-

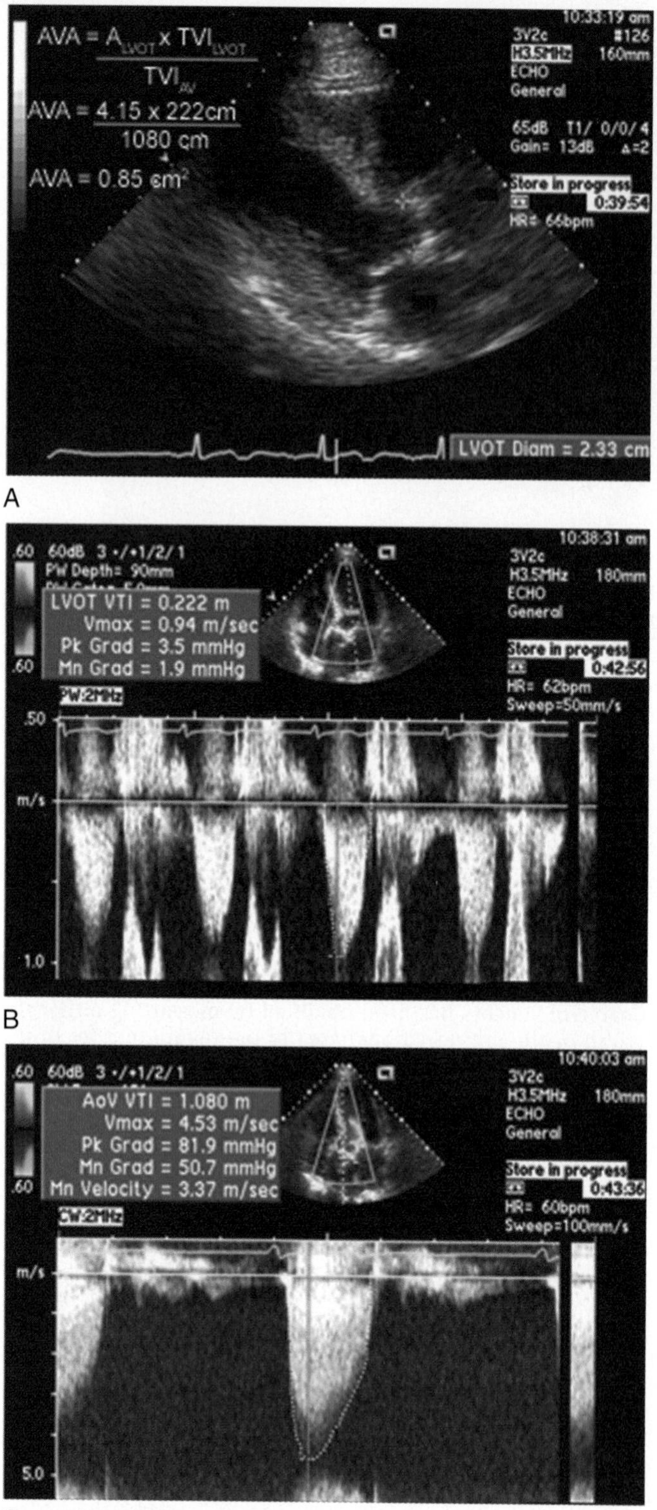

A

B

C

FIGURE 11–68 Transthoracic echocardiogram demonstrating the continuity equation for determining aortic valve area (AVA) in aortic stenosis. **A,** Parasternal long-axis view in which the thickened aortic valve can be appreciated; the left ventricular outflow tract diameter is measured as 2.33 cm. The overall calculations for AVA are presented in the text superimposed in the figure. **B,** Time-velocity integral (TVI) recorded from an apical four-chamber view with a sample volume in the left ventricular outflow tract (LVOT). The TVI is 222 cm. **C,** Spectral continuous wave Doppler of the aortic stenosis jet from which a peak gradient of 81.9 mm Hg and a TVI of 1080 cm are obtained. The calculation of aortic valve area is as noted in the text superimposed on the upper panel. In this instance, the aortic valve area calculates to 0.85 cm^2.

lar dilation is a natural consequence of long-standing hemodynamically significant aortic regurgitation. Left ventricular size can be normal in the acute phase. With moderate and severe aortic regurgitation, diastolic flow reversal in the descending thoracic aorta can frequently be detected from the suprasternal notch. Two-dimensional echocardiography often reveals an indentation of the anterior mitral valve leaflet during diastole. This is due to the impinging regurgitant jet that distorts the symmetrical opening pattern of the mitral leaflet. This is typically seen only in cases of moderate and severe aortic insufficiency. With M-mode echocardiography, fine high-velocity flutter of the anterior mitral leaflet and occasionally the septum can be appreciated (Fig. 11–72). Table 11–4 outlines many of these findings as they relate to the severity of aortic insufficiency.

Timing of Surgery. Aortic valve replacement is the most appropriate therapy in virtually all patients with symptomatic aortic regurgitation. Echocardiography also plays a significant role in the evaluation of these patients and in the timing of surgery in many asymptomatic patients. This decision is based largely on left ventricular size and performance rather than on the Doppler assessment of severity. Traditional echocardiographic findings that represent indications for surgery have included dilation of the left ventricle beyond 75 mm in diastole or beyond 55 mm in systole in association with fractional shortening or ejection fraction below the normal range (see Chap. 57). Additionally, a serial decline in left ventricular ejection fraction or progressive dilation of the left ventricle of 1.0 cm or more over a 12-month duration typically represents an indication for valve replacement.

Tricuspid Valve Disease

TRICUSPID REGURGITATION. Probably due to the complex closure pattern of the tricuspid valve, minimal and mild degrees of tricuspid regurgitation are commonly seen in normal disease-free individuals. The most common form of tricuspid valve disease is annular dilation due to right-sided heart overload, resulting in abnormal leaflet coaptation and tricuspid regurgitation. This is typically secondary to pulmonary hypertension, which most commonly is due to left-sided heart pathology. Tricuspid regurgitation due to annular dilation can be the result of virtually any form of heart disease that results in elevation of right ventricular pressure or volume. In these cases, the tricuspid valve typically appears anatomically normal but is found to be regurgitant. Quantitation of tricuspid regurgitation is done in a manner similar to that for mitral regurgitation and in clinical practice usually is a qualitative assessment (Fig. 11–73).[113] Minimal and mild degrees of tricuspid regurgitation are nearly ubiquitous in adult populations, even in the absence of identifiable structural heart disease. Moderate and severe tricuspid regurgitation and tricuspid regurgitation in association with elevated right ventricular systolic pressure are

TABLE 11–4 Aortic Insufficiency Severity*

	I	II	III	IV
Jet height (%LVOT)	<25	25-46	47-64	>65
Jet area/LVOT (short axis) (%)	<5	5-24	25-59	≥60
Reversal in descending aorta?	No	No	—	Yes
Spectral density	Faint	—	—	Dense
Pressure half-time (msec)	>400	—	—	≤250
Mitral preclosure?	No	—	—	Yes

LVOT = left ventricular outflow tract.

*For some parameters, the observation is valid at the extremes of mitral regurgitation severity and there may be marked overlap in intermediate (grades II, III) mitral regurgitation. In these instances, no value is presented.

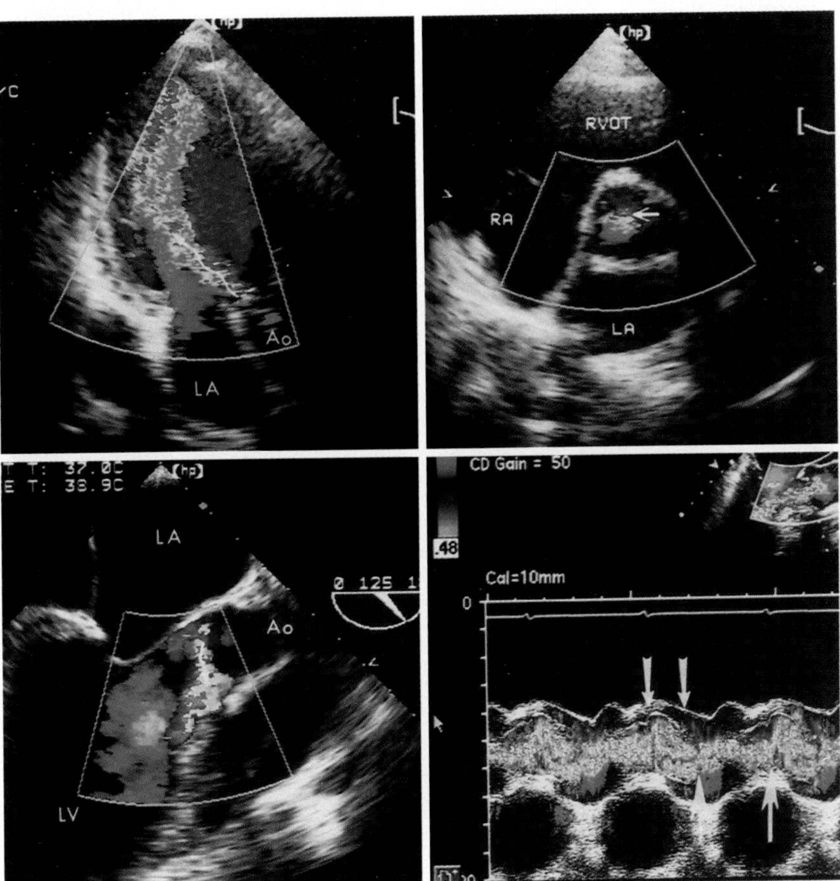

FIGURE 11–69 Composite of echocardiograms recorded in patients with aortic regurgitation. The two **top panels** were recorded in the same patient and show, on the left, an apical long-axis view and, on the right, a parasternal short-axis view. In the apical long-axis view, note the fairly extensive confetti-like aortic regurgitation jet arising from the proximal aorta and traversing to the left ventricular apex. Note also that the aortic regurgitation jet velocities merge with the mitral inflow velocities, rendering quantitation problematic. The **top right panel** is recorded in the same patient and shows a central aortic regurgitation jet. The **bottom left panel** is a transesophageal echocardiogram recorded in a longitudinal view. Note the highly eccentric aortic regurgitation jet that appears to fill the entire width of the left ventricular outflow tract. This apparent filling of the left ventricular outflow tract is due to the posterior to anterior jet direction (white arrow) rather than to a substantial true width of the jet. The **bottom right panel** is a color M-mode echocardiogram recorded in a patient with aortic insufficiency in which the normal systolic flow can be appreciated as well as a continuous diastolic flow in the lumen of the aorta that represents aortic insufficiency. The two downward pointing arrows denote the duration of systole, and the two upward pointing arrows indicate the duration of diastole. Ao = aorta; LA = left atrium; LV = left ventricle; RA = right atrium; RVOT = right ventricular outflow tract.

typically associated with cardiac pathology. Primary tricuspid valve disease can result in tricuspid regurgitation as well. Involvement by rheumatic heart disease, endocarditis, trauma with rupture of a papillary muscle, Ebstein anomaly, radiation heart disease, carcinoid heart disease, and tricuspid valve prolapse all have characteristic anatomical features that result in regurgitation. TEE can be useful in determining the feasibility of tricuspid valve repair. Carcinoid heart disease is a rare abnormality but has classic echocardiographic features (Fig. 11–74). In this syndrome, the leaflets appear stiffened and immobile. The annulus is secondarily dilated and the leaflets may fail to coapt. This lesion is typically associated with severe tricuspid regurgitation without elevation in right ventricular systolic pressure.

Irrespective of the cause of tricuspid regurgitation, one can capitalize on this lesion to calculate right ventricular systolic pressure, as noted in the section on Doppler calculations.[18-20] In the absence of obstruction to right ventricular outflow, this pressure equals pulmonary artery systolic pressure (see Fig. 11–31). Calculation of right ventricular systolic pressure can be measured both at rest and with exercise and is a valuable means of noninvasively determining pulmonary artery systolic pressures.

TRICUSPID STENOSIS. Isolated tricuspid stenosis is a very rare clinical entity. Tricuspid stenosis can be seen in individuals with rheumatic heart disease, in which case concurrent mitral stenosis will invariably be present. The carcinoid syndrome can result in tricuspid stenosis as well. Calculation of transvalvular gradients across the tricuspid valve is done in a manner identical to that for the mitral valve. In the majority of cases, tricuspid valve stenosis is associated with regurgitation.

Pulmonic Valve Disease

Primary disease of the pulmonic valve is uncommon in adult patients. Occasional patients with pulmonic stenosis (Fig. 11–75), either in isolation or in combination with other congenital lesions, may be encountered in the practice of adult cardiology. Congenital pulmonic stenosis results in thickening of the leaflets and restricted motion on two-dimensional echocardiography. Because the orientation of the pulmonary outflow tract is anterior to posterior, Doppler interrogation is quite easily performed within an angle of integration (θ) close to 0 degrees. The degree of stenosis and regurgitation across the pulmonic valve is determined in a manner analogous to that for the aortic valve. In the presence of pulmonic regurgitation, the pressure gradient between the pulmonary artery and right ventricle in diastole can be calculated, and from this an estimate of pulmonary artery diastolic pressure can be obtained.[114] This is done by calcu-

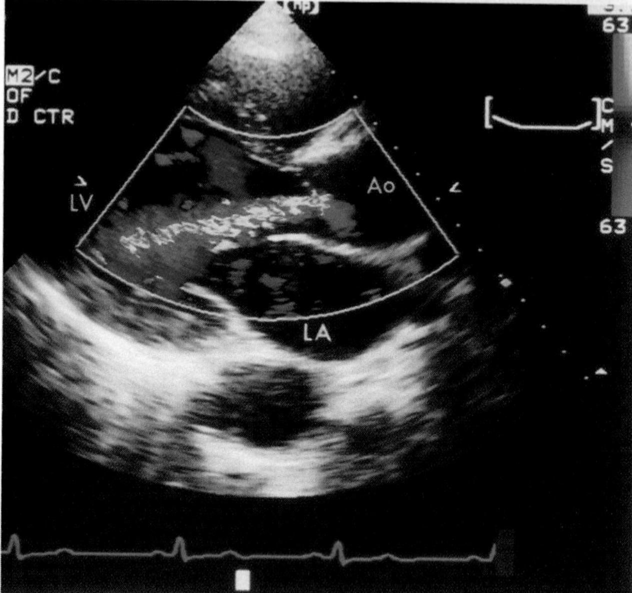

FIGURE 11–70 Parasternal long-axis two-dimensional echocardiograms in a patient with minimal **(top)** and a patient with moderate **(bottom)** aortic regurgitation. In the top panel, note the thin color jet of aortic regurgitation that fills less than 10 percent of the left ventricular outflow tract, compared with the wider aortic insufficiency profile, filling more than one third of the left ventricular outflow tract in the lower panel. Ao = aorta; LA = left atrium; LV = left ventricle.

lating the end-diastolic pulmonary artery–to–right ventricular gradient and adding an assumed right ventricular diastolic pressure.

Several characteristic patterns of pulmonary valve motion should be recognized on M-mode echocardiography. The first is that of pulmonic stenosis in which there is an augmented "a" wave but otherwise normal motion. In the presence of infundibular stenosis, coarse fluttering of the pulmonic valve is seen. In the presence of significant pulmonary hypertension, there is midsystolic notching of the pulmonic valve and loss of the pulmonary valve "a" wave. These findings are qualitative and may be seen only in the more advanced cases. In modern practice, determination of pulmonary artery hemodynamics relies heavily on Doppler interrogation.

Evaluation of the right ventricular outflow tract or pulmonary artery Doppler flow profile can provide valuable clues in patients with known or suspected pulmonary hypertension. Normally, after the onset of ejection, pulmonary artery flow reaches its maximum velocity 120 to 160 msec after the onset of ejection. In cases of pulmonary hypertension, this acceleration time is progressively shortened (Fig. 11–76). There is a linear and inverse correlation between the ejection time, defined as the time from onset of ejection to reaching peak velocity, and pulmonary artery systolic and mean pressures. In general, a pulmonary artery acceleration time less than 70 msec implies presence of a pulmonary artery systolic pressure exceeding 70 mm Hg. Other findings in pulmonary hypertension include notching of the pulmonary artery flow profile on spectral Doppler.

Miscellaneous Valvular Heart Diseases

Several miscellaneous forms of valvular heart disease deserve comment. Recently, attention has been drawn to the association between the use of anorectic drugs, particularly the combination of phentermine and fenfluramine (PhenFen), and development of valvular heart disease.[115,116] The exact incidence of diet drug–related valvular heart disease is unknown. Most studies have suggested that the predominant lesions are similar to that seen in carcinoid or ergot heart disease. The leaflets of the mitral valve and chordae appear thickened and immobile, and mitral regurgitation is present. Aortic insufficiency also has been noted in association with the use of these drugs, and it often appears out of proportion to the anatomical abnormalities noted on the aortic valve. Recent studies have suggested that these lesions may regress after exposure to the drugs has terminated.[117]

Radiation therapy can result in valvular dysfunction, most often thickening and insufficiency. The severity of the valvular insufficiency is dependent on the degree of anatomical damage to the valve, and the precise valves involved are dependent entirely on the radiation portal and dose. Typically, more anterior structures are involved and there may be concurrent myocardial dysfunction due to radiation myocarditis.

EVALUATION OF PROSTHETIC HEART VALVES

Modern echocardiographic techniques play a role in both preoperative and postoperative management of patients with prosthetic heart valves. Two-dimensional echocardiography can be used to determine the appropriate prosthesis size to implant in the aortic position and the need for additional procedures, such as aortic annuloplasty, to enlarge a pathologically small aortic root.[118-120] Evaluation of prosthetic heart valves can be a complex and time-consuming process. Prosthetic heart valves can be divided into three basic groups: mechanical prostheses, such as single or dual disc valves or ball and cage valves; stented bioprostheses, which use either porcine aortic valves or bovine pericardium for valve leaflets; and a newer generation of stentless porcine valves that at this time are approved for use only in the aortic position.[119] Each valve has unique echocardiographic characteristics, and different valves can be evaluated to varying degrees using TTE and TEE. Doppler echocardiography is obviously crucial for determining the presence of regurgitation and the flow characteristics of a valve. It is often not possible to fully evaluate a prosthetic valve with TTE, and TEE is often necessary. This is particularly true for visualization of mitral prostheses. Even with TEE, complete anatomical visualization of an aortic mechanical prosthesis can be problematic. For all but the new stentless aortic prosthesis, the sewing ring is characteristically visualized as an echo-dense circular structure within the appropriate annulus.

The ball and cage valve is typically visualized as an echo-dense sewing ring with three wire struts forming the cage and an echogenic ball moving within the cage. The ball itself may appear either as a spherical structure or as a single echo-dense line in motion. Single-disc mechanical prostheses are visualized as a sewing ring in which the disc can be seen to move. Typically, from the transthoracic route, all one sees is a single, bright echo-dense line with phasic motion during the cardiac cycle above and into the plane of the sewing ring. The discs of a two-disc valve cast a smaller echo signature, and actual disc motion can be difficult to discern from TTE. Using TEE, both leaflets of a two-disc valve are easily visualized in the mitral position and have a characteristic butterfly wing motion (Fig. 11–77). Identifying motion of both leaflets in the aortic position is more problematic. Stented porcine valves are visualized as a sewing ring in which three separate leaflets can be seen. These leaflets have the characteristics of a normal aortic valve. With fibrosis and degeneration or endocarditis, the leaflets may become thickened and brighter than usual (Fig. 11–78). The newer stentless prosthesis and aortic

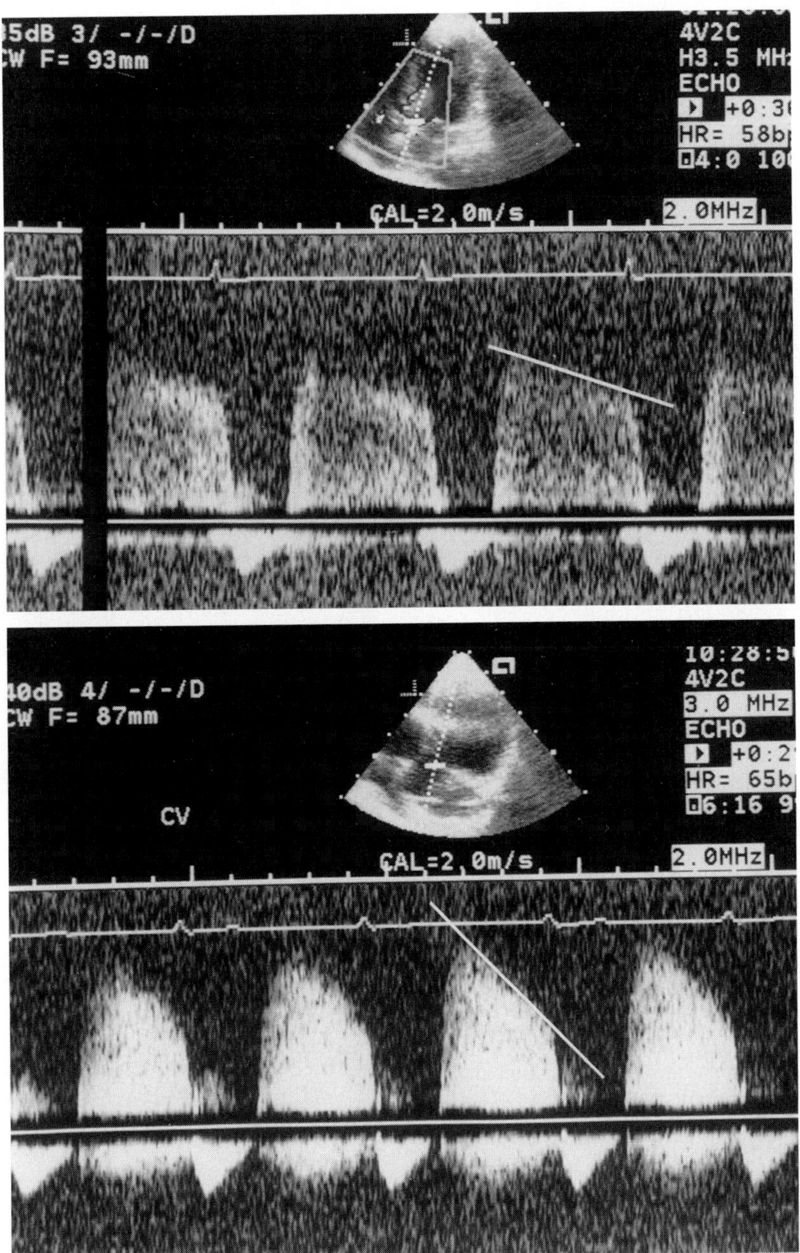

FIGURE 11–71 Continuous-wave spectral recordings of patients with mild **(top)** and severe **(bottom)** aortic insufficiency. Note the relatively flat slope pressure decay and faint spectral signal intensity in the mild insufficiency and a denser spectral signal and steeper slope of pressure decay, denoting near equalization of aortic and left ventricular diastolic pressures, seen in severe aortic insufficiency.

homograft valves can be difficult to distinguish from a native aortic valve. Depending on the implantation technique, there may be few clues as to the presence of a stentless prosthesis other than subtle echodensities at the line of attachment in the annulus or, if implanted within the native aorta, a double-density aortic wall can be seen.

Complete evaluation of prosthetic valves requires detailed Doppler assessment. Color flow imaging is used to determine the presence and severity of regurgitation. The combination of the sewing ring and/or the mechanical valve itself results in substantial reverberation and shadowing and dramatically reduces the ability to interrogate structures posterior to the mechanical prosthesis or sewing ring with Doppler. There is frequently a minimal amount of physiological regurgitation in mechanical prostheses that represents a combination of the closing velocity of the disc or ball and small physiological leaks at the closure lines. It is not uncommon to see minimal degrees of regurgitation in association with a stented or nonstented bioprosthesis. Valvular regurgitation in prosthetic valves can be quite eccentric, and one must use caution in applying rules for determining severity of regurgitation. This is particularly true for paravalvular regurgitation (Fig. 11–79). Three-dimensional echocardiography and Doppler have shown promise for providing incremental information regarding the location and size of a paravalvular leak.

Spectral Doppler is used to determine pressure gradients across prosthetic valves. Stentless bioprostheses behave in a manner nearly identical to native aortic valves and typically have a peak gradient of 10 to 15 mm Hg. Because of narrowing of the outflow tract by a sewing ring, a stented prosthesis often has a higher transvalvular gradient. The magnitude of this gradient is dependent on both flow and the size of the valve. Because of the wide range of anticipated gradients, it is crucial to establish a baseline for prosthetic valves at a time when they are known to be functioning normally. This avoids the problem of subsequent detection of a peak gradient that can be as high as 50 mm Hg. This may be due to the combination of a high flow state and a narrow orifice because of the sewing ring and may not represent valve deterioration. Doppler evaluation for the gradient across a mechanical prosthesis is complicated by several factors, including phenomena of localized gradients and pressure recovery.[121,122] As flow accelerates through the noncircular orifice of a mechanical prosthesis, there are areas of rapid flow acceleration that occur over very short distances. This acceleration results in instantaneous

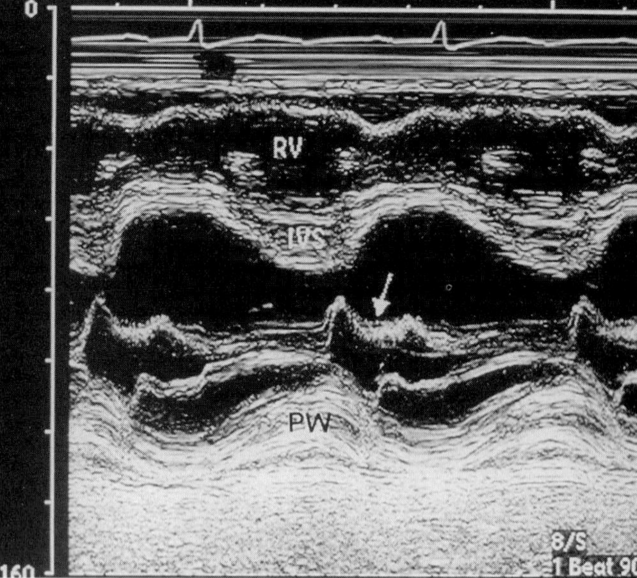

FIGURE 11–72 M-mode echocardiogram recorded in a patient with aortic insufficiency. Note the fine fluttering of the mitral valve leaflet secondary to impingement by the aortic insufficiency jet. IVS = interventricular septum; PW = posterior wall; RV = right ventricle.

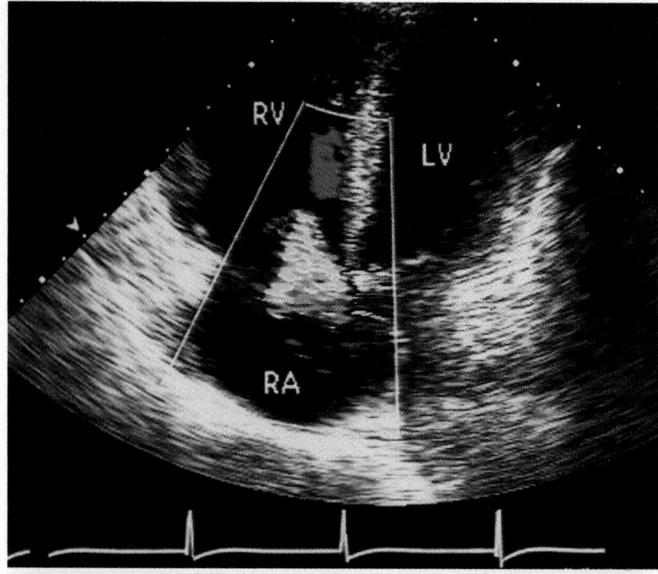

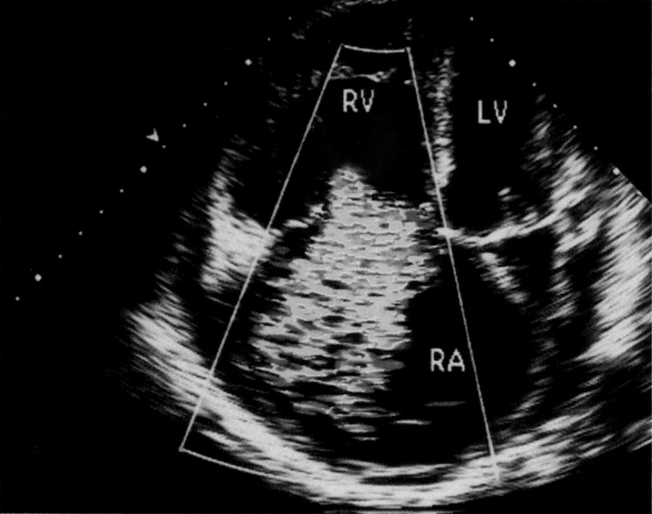

FIGURE 11–73 Two-dimensional echocardiograms with color flow imaging of patients with tricuspid regurgitation. **Top,** Echocardiogram is recorded in a patient with a mild degree of tricuspid insufficiency. **Bottom,** Echocardiogram of a patient with severe tricuspid regurgitation. LV = left ventricle; RA = right atrium; RV = right ventricle.

peak velocities of 3 to 4 m/sec, corresponding to gradients of 36 to 64 mm Hg. These pressure gradients occur over a very limited distance (1-2 mm) within the sewing ring and do not reflect the true left ventricular-to-proximal aorta pressure difference measured in the hemodynamic laboratory. As with a stented bioprosthesis, it is crucial to obtain an early baseline pressure gradient across a mechanical prosthesis at a time when it is known to function normally for subsequent comparison. This is best done by performing a full echocardiographic and Doppler examination at the time of the first follow-up visit after implantation.

Dysfunction of prosthetic valves occurs due to valvular dehiscence, in which case a paravalvular leak can be seen (see Fig. 11-79), or there may be endocarditis, thrombosis, or pannus interfering with motion of a mechanical valve. Typically, either stenosis or regurgitation can occur. If the mechanical valve becomes obstructed by pannus, vegetation, or thrombus, the transvalvular gradient typically will increase, although in some instances it may remain stable or even decline. Regurgitation is usually seen in conjunction with restriction of the leaflet unless the leaflet has been restricted in a fully closed position. In cases of suspected dysfunction of a prosthesis, TEE adds incremental value and is essential for complete evaluation.

ASSESSMENT OF MITRAL VALVE REPAIR

Transesophageal echocardiography has been instrumental in determining the success of mitral valve repair. The preoperative echocardiogram is highly reliable as a means for determining which patients are candidates for mitral valve repair, and intraoperative monitoring is an integral part of the surgical routine in determining success of repair. From a surgical perspective, the mitral valve is considered to have two leaflets, each with three scallops. The anterior leaflet scallops are designated A1, A2, A3 and the posterior scallops P1, P2, and P3. Each scallop can be viewed from many transesophageal imaging planes.[123,124] In general, patients with elongated redundant valves, those with pathological lesions of the posterior leaflet, and those with smaller vegetations or perforations are excellent candidates for mitral valve repair. Patients with a rheumatic origin of their condition and those with fibrotic leaflets are less likely to have good long-term results.

The postoperative transesophageal echocardiogram is used to determine transvalvular gradients to exclude iatrogenic mitral stenosis and determine the degree, if any, of residual mitral regurgitation. Other adverse sequelae of mitral valve repair include development of dynamic left ventricular outflow tract obstruction, which likewise can be assessed with TEE before the patient is removed from the operating room. Figures 11–58 and 11–80 are examples from a patient before and after successful mitral valve repair.

Infective Endocarditis (see Chap. 58)

Infective endocarditis represents an invasive infection, usually by a bacterial organism of the endothelial lining of the heart, most commonly on one of the four cardiac valves. Left-sided valves are more commonly involved than right-sided valves. The echocardiographic hallmark of bacterial endocarditis is formation of a vegetation on a valvular surface. Pathologically, a vegetation consists of a combination of thrombus, necrotic valvular debris, inflammatory material, and bacteria. Over time, a vegetation may become sterile, at which point only the residua of the inflammatory response with variable degrees of the thrombotic component persist. By echocardiography, a vegetation has the appearance of an irregularly shaped oscillating mass attached to a valve leaflet (Figs. 11–81 and 11–82). Classically, these are seen on the

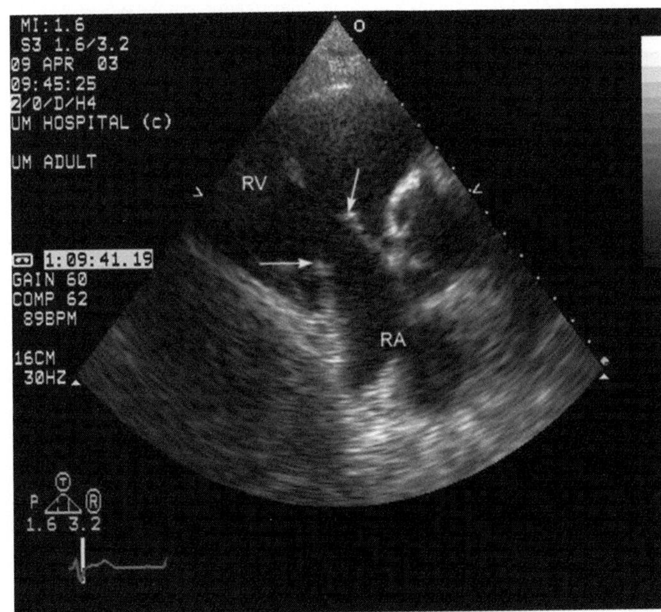

FIGURE 11–74 Right ventricular inflow tract view recorded in a patient with carcinoid disease and tricuspid regurgitation. The right atrium (RA) and right ventricle (RV) are both visualized in this systolic frame. The tricuspid valve leaflets are abnormally dense and immobile. In this systolic frame, the leaflets fail to coapt with the leaflet tip separated by approximately 2 cm. In real time, the leaflets are nearly immobile.

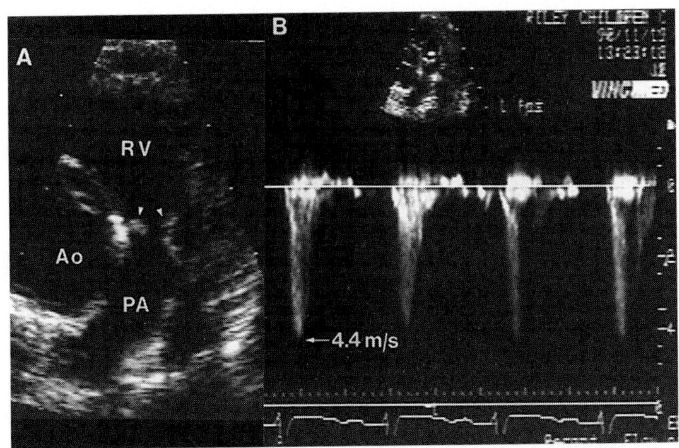

FIGURE 11–75 Two-dimensional **(A)** and continuous-wave Doppler **(B)** recorded in a patient with valvular pulmonic stenosis. The two-dimensional study shows a thickened pulmonic valve with restricted motion (arrowheads). The continuous-wave Doppler shows a peak velocity of 4.4 m/sec, which is consistent with a systolic gradient of approximately 78 mm Hg. Ao = aorta; PA = pulmonary artery; RV = right ventricle. (From Feigenbaum H: Echocardiography. 5th ed. Malvern, PA, Lea & Febiger, 1994.)

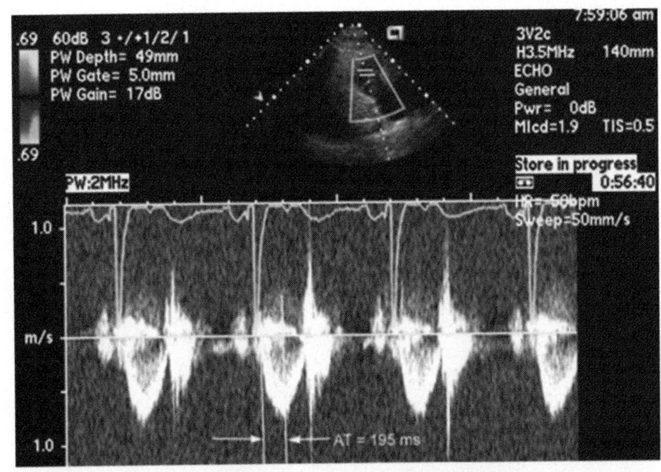

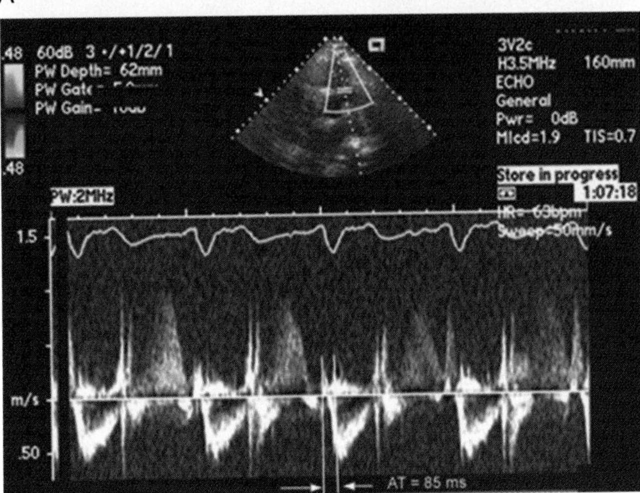

FIGURE 11–76 Pulsed-wave Doppler in the right ventricular outflow tract demonstrating the impact of pulmonary hypertension of the contour of the outflow tract signal. **A,** Signal from a normal individual. Note the normal acceleration time, defined as the time in milliseconds from onset of ejection to reaching peak velocity. In this instance, the acceleration time is approximately 200 msec. **B,** Recorded in a patient with pulmonary hypertension. Note the shortened acceleration time (85 msec).

downstream, low-pressure side of a valve. Therefore, one typically anticipates a vegetation on the left atrial side of the mitral valve and on the left ventricular outflow tract side of the aortic valve. In reality, larger vegetations can exist on both sides of a valve and atypical locations are not uncommon. In screening for vegetations, small unrelated masses or surface irregularities are not infrequently encountered, and thus the specificity for defining a vegetation is not 100 percent. Several large-scale studies have demonstrated that echocardiography may play an incremental role in rapidly establishing the diagnosis of endocarditis, and at least one algorithm for defining endocarditis has used echocardiography as an intrinsic component of the diagnosis.[125,126] Noninfectious vegetation, such as those seen in association with connective tissue disease, are also detected with echocardiographic imaging.

In addition to detection of a vegetation in patients with suspected endocarditis, echocardiography can be used to determine the functional significance and degree of anatomical impairment due to endocarditis and to evaluate complications of endocarditis. Typically, endocarditis results in valvular regurgitation and only rarely in significant valvular stenosis. Because of the variable location of vegetations and the highly variable degree to which the valvular surface may be interrupted, regurgitant lesions in patients with endocarditis are more often eccentric than seen in other forms of valvular heart disease.

Several studies have attempted to use echocardiographic features of vegetations as a marker for the likelihood of requiring surgery or progressing to heart failure. In general, larger and more mobile vegetations are more likely to be associated with embolic events than are smaller sessile vegetations.[127] Vegetations due to *Staphylococcus aureus* are more likely to result in abscess formation and less likely to be sterilized with antibiotics.

Complications of Endocarditis. Complications include progressive valvular regurgitation leading to congestive heart failure, abscess formation, failure to sterilize, and embolic phenomena. Intracardiac abscesses are most commonly

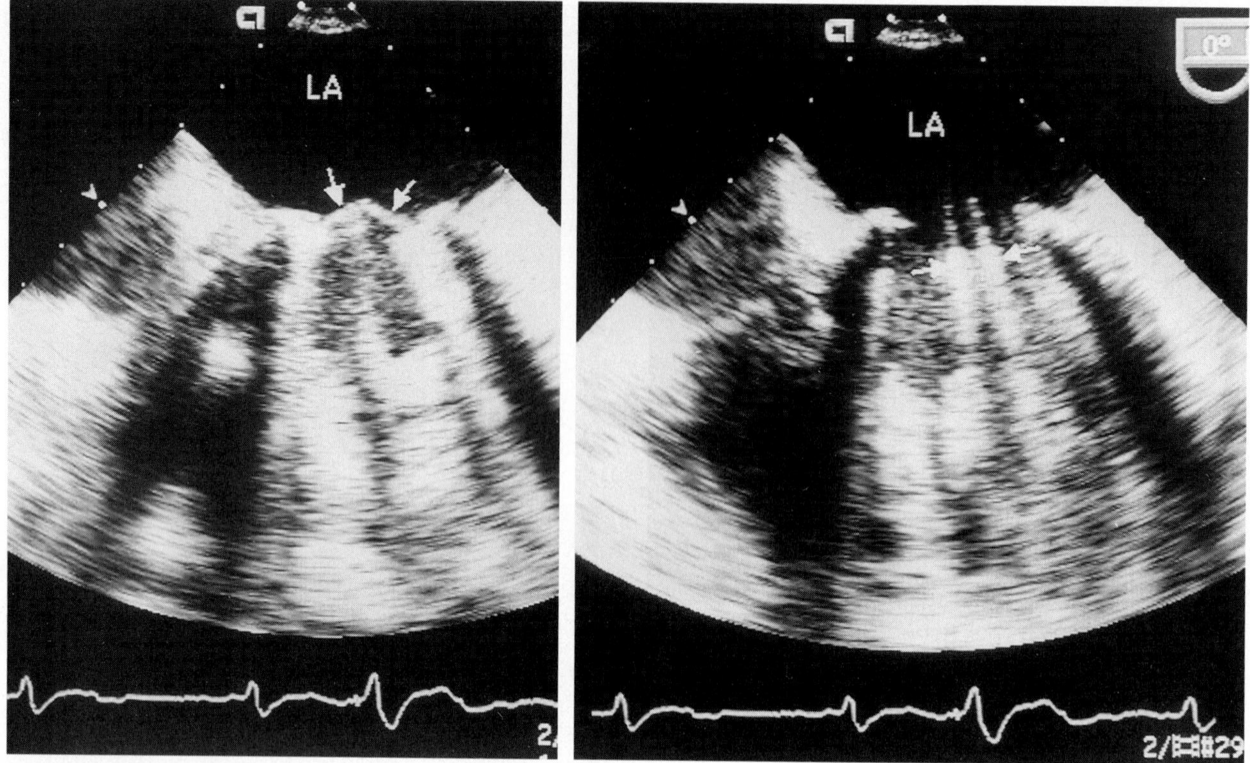

FIGURE 11–77 Transesophageal echocardiogram of a patient with a normally functioning St. Jude mitral valve prosthesis. The scans are recorded at 0 degrees from behind the left atrium. The **left panel** is recorded in systole. Note the two closed leaflets of the prosthetic valve (arrows). The **right panel** is recorded in diastole. Note that the two leaflets now have a parallel position, pointing into the cavity of the left ventricle (arrows). Note the substantial shadowing from the sewing ring and discs, which reduces the ability to visualize the left ventricular cavity. LA = left atrium.

encountered in the relatively avascular areas of the heart. For aortic valve endocarditis, this includes the aorta/mitral valve junction, and for mitral and tricuspid valve disease the annular structures. Less commonly, intramyocardial abscess or abscess within a papillary muscle is encountered.

TRANSESOPHAGEAL ECHOCARDIOGRAPHY. The relative diagnostic value of TTE and TEE has been evaluated in several studies. Because of the higher quality, higher resolution imaging afforded by TEE, virtually all studies have demonstrated an increased sensitivity for detection of vegetations with TEE (see Fig. 11–82). Often the clinical diagnosis of endocarditis has included detection of vegetations, and, thus, many of these studies tend to overstate the sensitivity of TEE. Most studies have also suggested that when a high-quality, entirely normal transthoracic echocardiogram has been obtained in which there is no evidence of valvular mass or thickening and no evidence of pathological regurgitation, the yield in proceeding to TEE is relatively low. Because TEE provides a high-resolution view of the heart, it also detects many limited areas of valvular thickening that are not related to an infectious process. Thus, its specificity for excluding the diagnosis of endocarditis may be less than optimal.

There are several situations in which there is a proven advantage to TEE in patients with endocarditis. Perhaps the most well established is the detection of abscesses, particularly in the aortic root (Fig. 11–83).[128] Data suggest that detection rates from the transthoracic approach are less than 30 percent, whereas sensitivity for detecting an abscess in the aortic root with TEE exceeds 95 percent. Additionally, TEE provides more accurate characterization of the size and mobility of vegetations and detection of multiple vegetations in endocarditis. Finally, TEE is more accurate for determining the cause of valvular regurgitation than is TTE. TEE can identify valvular perforations, ruptured chordae, and flail leaflets with a higher degree of reliability than can TTE.

CALCIFICATION OF THE MITRAL ANNULUS

Fibrosis and calcification of the mitral annulus are common findings with increasing age and can be seen in younger patients with renal disease and other metabolic abnormalities that result in abnormal calcium metabolism (Fig. 11–84). The degree of calcification can range from limited, focal deposits in the annulus to larger deposits resulting in a mass effect. In advanced degrees, the basal aspects of the posterior mitral valve leaflet may be involved. In rare situations, annular calcification can result in functional restriction of the mitral valve orifice and a left atrial–left ventricular pressure gradient. Only in advanced and rare cases does the degree of obstruction result in pressure gradients likely to cause symptoms or result in secondary pulmonary hypertension. More commonly, mitral annular calcification is associated with varying degrees of mitral regurgitation. Heavy annular calcification may result in a lower likelihood of successful valve replacement and is a situation in which paravalvular regurgitation is not uncommon after mitral valve replacement. Statistically, it also has been associated with embolic events and other adverse cardiovascular outcomes.[129]

Congenital Heart Disease (see Chap. 56)

Modern two-dimensional echocardiographic techniques provide a comprehensive means for evaluating virtually all forms of congenital heart disease found in both adults and children. Additionally, echocardiography can be used to evaluate repaired and palliated congenital heart disease. In the modern era, it is unusual for cardiac catheterization or other techniques to be necessary for defining the anatomical anomaly in congenital heart disease. Cardiac magnetic resonance imaging (MRI) may provide incremental information regarding pulmonary artery anatomy and complex venous and great artery connections. Doppler echocardiography often provides the majority of physiological information necessary for the clinical decision-making.

It has become increasingly uncommon to make the diagnosis of congenital heart disease de novo in adult

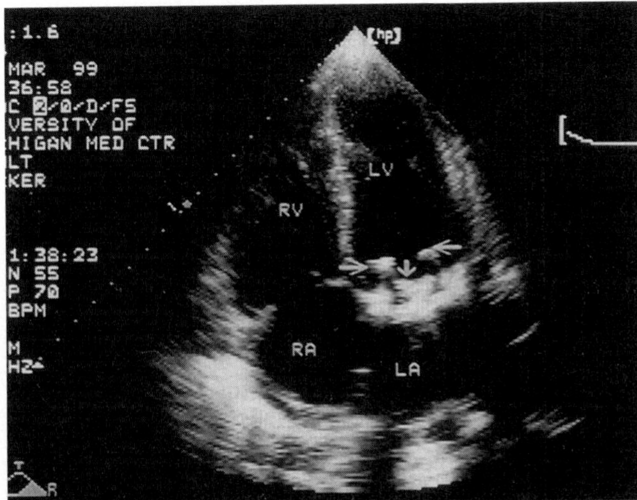

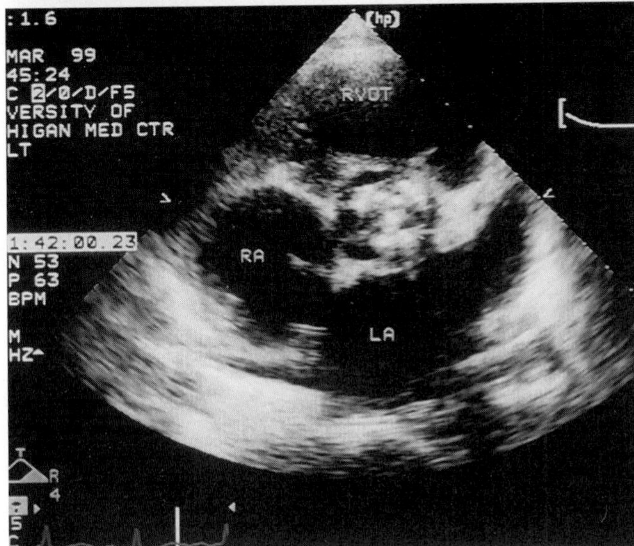

FIGURE 11–78 Apical four-chamber **(top)** and parasternal short-axis views **(bottom)** recorded in a patient with stented porcine bioprostheses in the mitral **(top)** and aortic **(bottom)** positions. In the **top panel,** the horizontally oriented arrows denote the struts of the stented porcine valve that protrude in the cavity of the left ventricle. Within the struts note the echo-dense mass that represents vegetation. In the **lower panel,** the three struts of the porcine bioprosthesis can be visualized at 2, 6, and 10 o'clock positions. Within the sewing ring of the bioprosthesis are noted several echo densities that represent vegetations. LA = left atrium; LV = left ventricle; RA = right atrium; RV = right ventricle; RVOT = right ventricular outflow tract.

populations. Because of the increased access to well-trained pediatricians, family practitioners, and pediatric cardiologists, the majority of "significant" congenital heart lesions are detected in childhood and adolescence. Thus, the number and nature of lesions "escaping" detection until adulthood has changed over the past several decades. The single most common congenital lesion to be detected in adulthood, other than the bicuspid aortic valve, is the atrial septal defect. There are infrequent cases of ventricular septal defect and other anomalies that escape detection to adulthood. This section deals only with the more common entities likely to be encountered in adult populations and evaluation of the more common repaired and palliated lesions.

Intracardiac Shunts

ATRIAL SEPTAL DEFECT. The most common shunt lesion to be detected de novo in adulthood is the atrial septal defect. Because atrial septal defects result in a relatively innocent murmur, they are often overlooked in childhood and may escape detection until adolescence or adulthood. Atrial septal defects result in a left-to-right shunt at a level of the atrium and, consequently, a diastolic volume overload of the right ventricle. The volume overload pattern of the right ventricle is manifest as dilation of the right ventricle and usually the right atrium. Additionally, the septum is "flattened" and the left ventricle, rather than assuming circular geometry, has a D-shaped geometry (see Fig. 11–27). This septal flattening is present predominantly in diastole, and during systole the septum assumes its normal circular geometry. This right ventricular volume overload pattern, which is typically seen in atrial septal defects, is also seen in any other lesion resulting in right ventricular diastolic volume overload, including significant pulmonary insufficiency, tricuspid regurgitation, and anomalous pulmonary venous return. On M-mode echocardiography, the right ventricular volume overload pattern is characterized as paradoxical septal motion. It is now recognized that this "paradoxical" septal motion actually represents restitution of normal circular geometry with the onset of ventricular systole.

Detection of a right ventricular volume overload pattern may be the first clue to the presence of an atrial septal defect, after which further interrogation of the atrial septum should be undertaken to identify the location of the defect. The three most common locations of an atrial septal defect are secundum, primum, and sinus venosus, representing approximately 70 percent, 15 percent, and 15 percent of atrial septal defects, respectively. Rarer forms of atrial septal defect, including the unroofed coronary sinus, are also encountered.

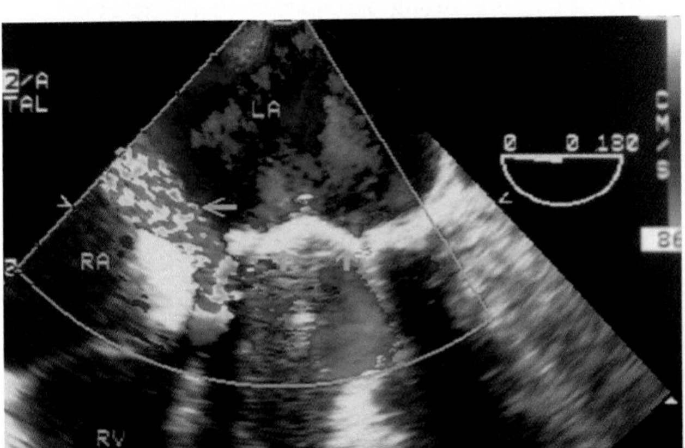

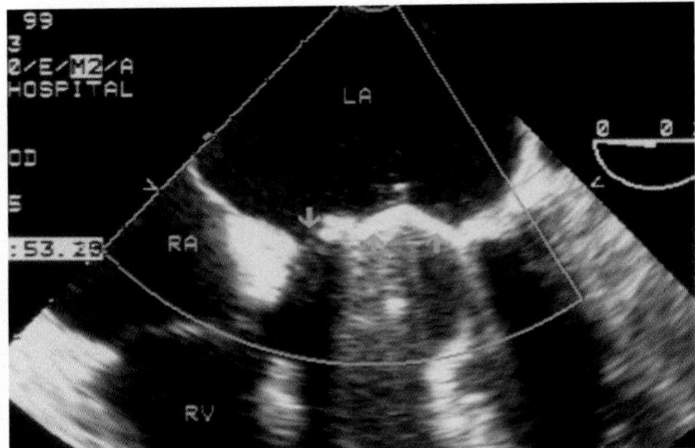

FIGURE 11–79 Transesophageal echocardiogram recorded in a patient with a St. Jude mitral valve replacement and a paravalvular leak, resulting in moderate mitral regurgitation. **Left,** Recorded in systole. Note the two discs of the St. Jude prosthesis in their closed position (up-pointing arrows). Immediately outside the boundary of the sewing ring is a distinct color jet (horizontal arrow) representing an eccentric mitral regurgitation jet arising from outside the border of the sewing ring. **Right,** The same image with color suppressed. Again note the closed leaflets of the St. Jude valve. With the color suppressed, a distinct gap between the sewing ring and tissue (down-pointing arrow) can be seen, representing partial valve dehiscence. LA = left atrium; RA = right atrium; RV = right ventricle.

FIGURE 11–80 Two-dimensional echocardiogram recorded in a patient after mitral valve repair and annuloplasty ring. The ring is seen as an echo-dense structure in the annulus (arrows). DA = descending aorta; LA = left atrium; LV = left ventricle; PV = pulmonary vein; RA = right atrium; RV = right ventricle.

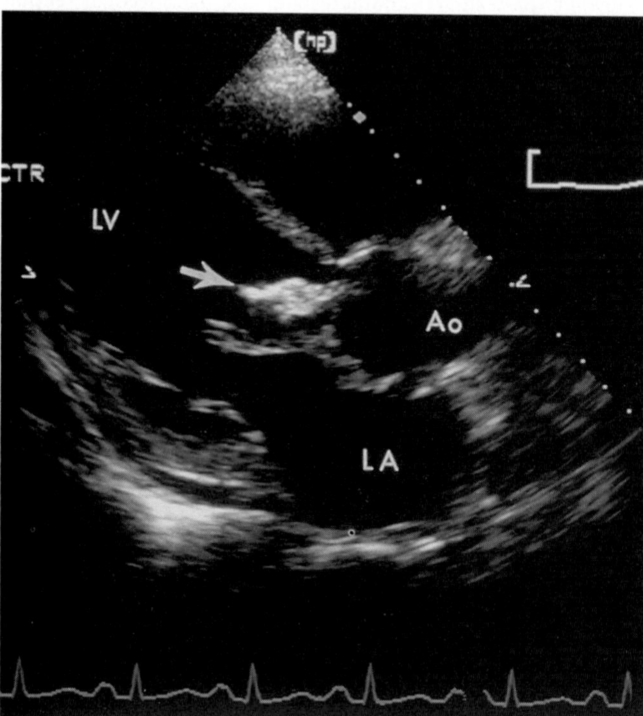

FIGURE 11–81 Parasternal long-axis view of patient with aortic valve vegetation. Note the relatively echo-dense, irregular mass prolapsing into the left ventricular outflow tract in this diastolic frame (arrow). Ao = aorta; LA = left atrium; LV = left ventricle.

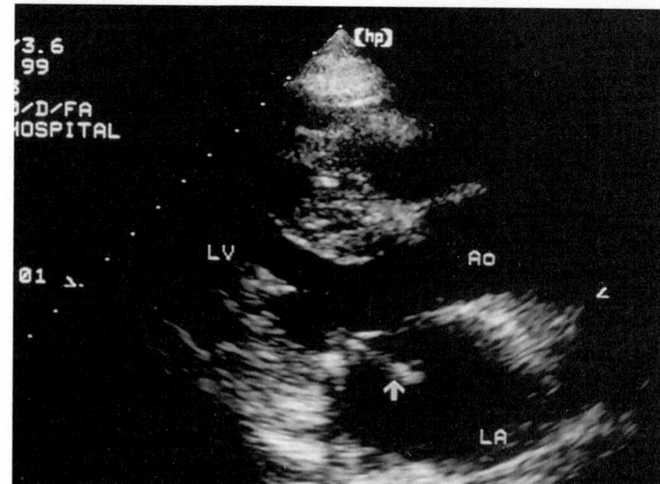

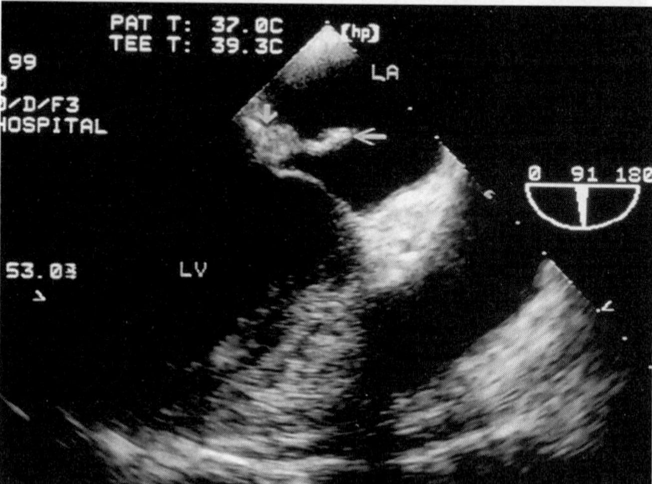

FIGURE 11–82 Transthoracic **(top)** and transesophageal echocardiogram **(bottom)** recorded in a patient with a mitral valve vegetation. In the transthoracic parasternal long-axis view, a highly mobile filamentous echo can be seen prolapsing into the left atrium (LA) during systole. This is consistent with a highly mobile vegetation. A systolic frame from the transesophageal echocardiogram is presented in the bottom panel. Again, the highly filamentous mobile echo is noted (horizontal arrow). In addition, there is a more sessile 8 mm diameter mass attached to the mitral valve (downward pointing arrow). Ao = aorta; LV = left ventricle.

Whereas the secundum atrial septal defect is an isolated entity, there are strong associations between sinus venosus atrial septal defect and malalignment of the pulmonary veins, resulting in functional anomalous pulmonary venous return. A primum atrial septal defect is a variant of endocardial cushion defect in which a small, perimembranous ventricular septal defect and anomalies of the mitral valve may also be encountered. The classic mitral valve abnormality associated with a primum defect is a cleft mitral valve with varying degrees of mitral regurgitation.

On occasion, a right ventricular volume overload pattern is encountered but no anatomical defect can be visualized. In these instances, contrast echocardiography using agitated saline can be a valuable means of detecting the right-to-left component of interatrial shunting. Of the three common types of atrial septal defect, the sinus venosus defect is most likely to escape direct visualization on a transthoracic echocardiogram. TEE is nearly 100 percent specific and sensitive in detection of all types of atrial septal defects, including sinus venosus defects (Fig. 11–85).[130,131] With TEE, the atrial septal defect is visualized as a loss of tissue. The size of the defect can be accurately measured, and color flow

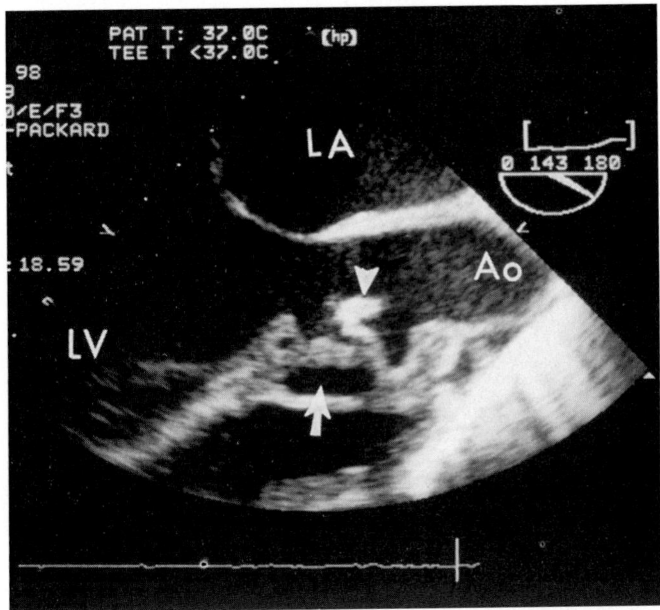

FIGURE 11–83 Transesophageal echocardiogram recorded in a patient with an aortic root abscess, obtained in a longitudinal orientation. Note the thickened aortic valve with superimposed vegetation (arrowhead) and the echo-free space (arrow) between the wall of the aorta and the right ventricular outflow tract, which represents a periaortic abscess. Ao = aorta; LA = left atrium; LV = left ventricle.

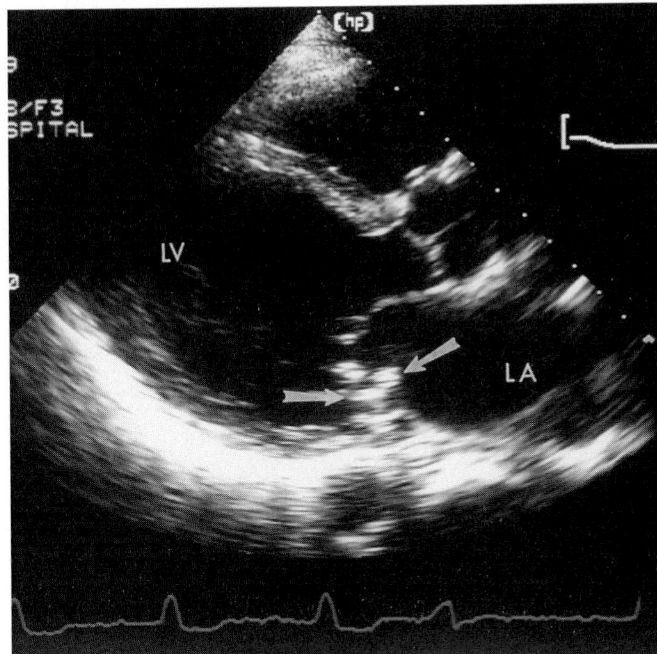

FIGURE 11–84 Two-dimensional echocardiogram recorded in a patient with renal insufficiency and calcification of the mitral annulus. Mitral annular calcium appears as an echo-dense mass in the mitral annulus (arrows). LA = left atrium; LV = left ventricle.

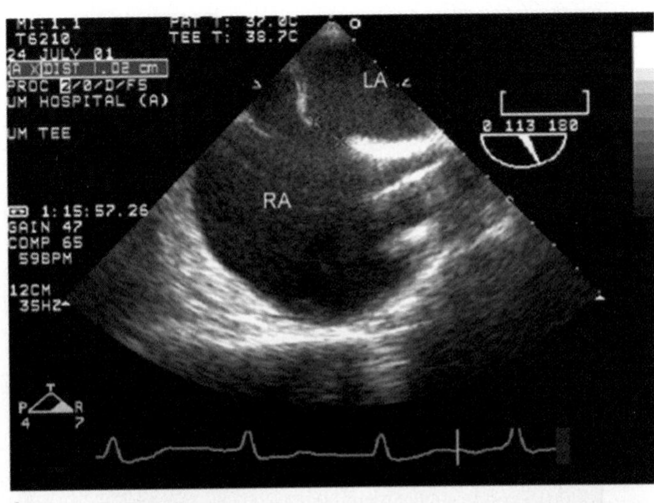

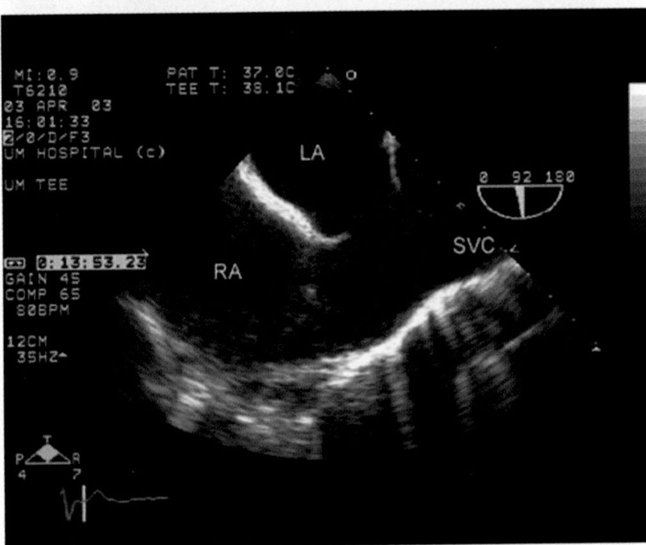

FIGURE 11–85 Transesophageal echocardiograms in a patient with a secundum atrial septal defect **(A)** and a sinus venosus defect **(B)**. The margins of the secundum defect are easily seen and the defect can be measured approximately 1 cm in maximum dimension. In panel B, there is a larger defect at the junction of the atrial septum and superior vena cava (SVC). LA = left atrium; RA = right atrium.

imaging can be used to identify abnormal transatrial flow patterns (Fig. 11–86). Often the diagnosis can be established with a degree of accuracy and confidence so that catheterization is not necessary before surgical repair or percutaneous closure.

Once identified, further characterization of the atrial septal defect can be undertaken using two-dimensional echocardiography and Doppler techniques. Three-dimensional echocardiography can provide valuable clues as to the complex shape of an atrial septal defect.[132] TEE can be an invaluable technique for determining the integrity of the tissues surrounding the atrial septal defect and plays a valuable role in determining the feasibility of percutaneous closure.[133,134] Defects less than 2 cm in diameter and with relatively firm tissue at the margins are more likely to be successfully closed, compared with large defects and those with fairly thin tissue at the margin or multiple perforations.

Numerous attempts have been made to quantify the ratio of pulmonary and systemic flow in intracardiac shunt lesions, including atrial septal defect. The majority of these attempts have been by calculating the instantaneous stroke volume of the pulmonary outflow tract and left ventricular outflow tract (see section on Doppler calculations). This calculation has been fairly reproducible and has correlated with hemodynamic assessment in the animal laboratory and in children. Because of the margin of error for measuring the dimension of the outflow tract, it has seen less use in adult patients. In general, the threshold for recommending closure of an atrial septal defect has diminished to a Qp/Qs (pulmonary/systemic flow ratio) of 1.5 or less. Detection of a right

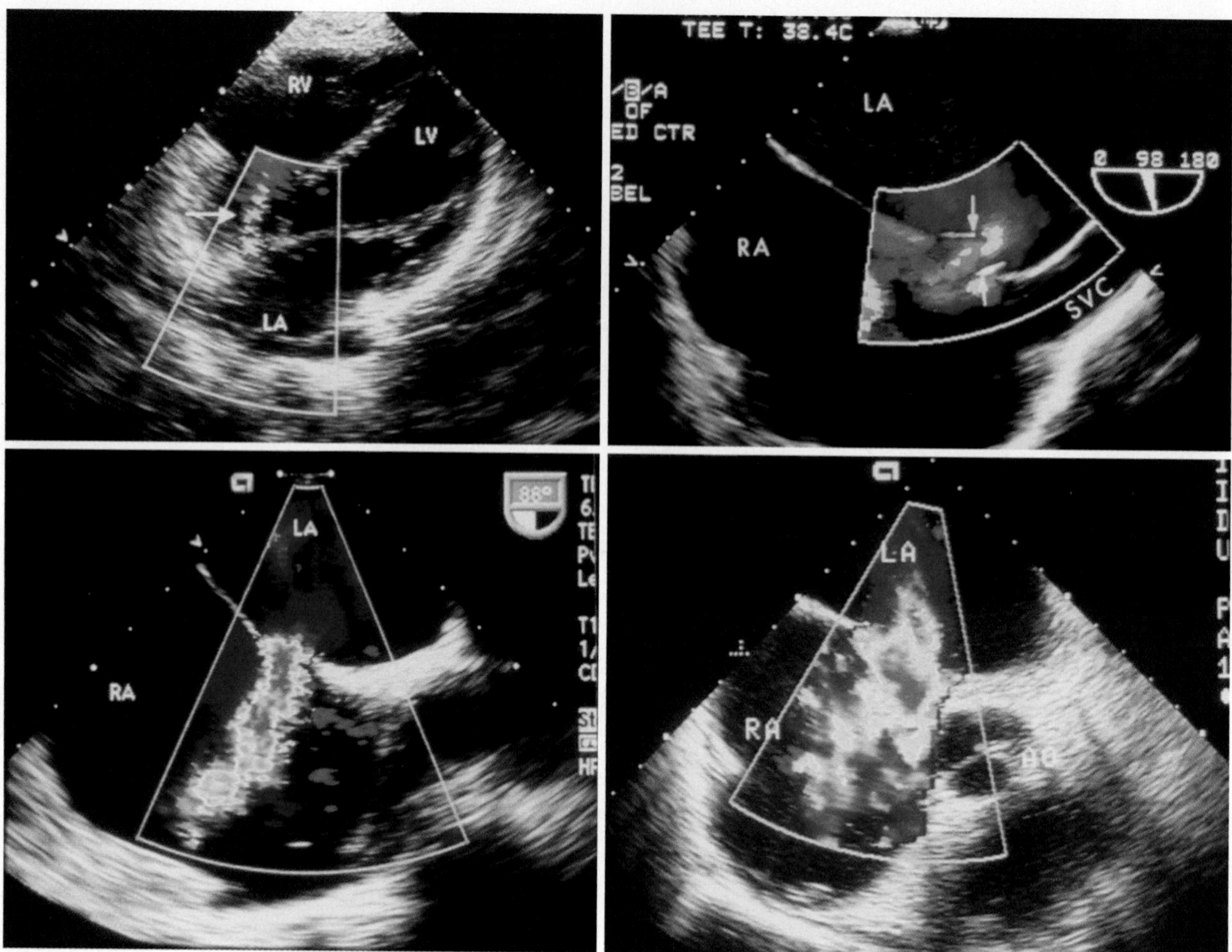

FIGURE 11–86 Four illustrations of patients with atrial septal defects. **Top left,** Recorded from a subcostal transducer position in a patient with a small atrial septal defect (also illustrated in the lower left panel). From the subcostal transducer position, the entire length of the atrial septum can be visualized. There is a defect approximately 7 mm in diameter in the secundum portion of the atrial septum with a color flow signal coursing from the left atrium into the right atrium (arrow), consistent with secundum septal defect. **Bottom left,** Transesophageal echocardiogram from the same patient presented on the top left. The size of the defect can be more accurately appreciated, and again there is a distinct color flow image coursing from the left atrium into the right atrium. **Top right,** Longitudinal view of the atrial septum showing a large patent foramen. Note the margins of the atrial septal tissue (arrows). The atrial septal tissue does not oppose, in this case leaving a 1 cm defect, through which flow shunts from the left atrium to the right atrium. **Bottom right,** Recorded in a patient with a large secundum defect. Note the color flow image denoting a substantial flow from left atrium to right atrium. The defect is approximately 2 cm in diameter. AO = aorta; LA = left atrium; LV = left ventricle; RA = right atrium; RV = right ventricle; SVC = superior vena cava.

ventricular volume overload pattern denotes a shunt of at least this level, and thus the majority of detected atrial septal defects fall into the range that warrant closure.

Repaired Atrial Septal Defect. Depending on the magnitude of the initial shunt and the age at which an atrial septal defect is repaired, the two-dimensional echocardiogram may revert to normal with respect to chamber sizes or show evidence of residual right-sided heart dilation. In instances in which the defect was large and repaired only late, residual right ventricular dysfunction, varying degrees of pulmonary hypertension, and right ventricular hypertrophy may persist throughout adulthood. Depending on the nature of the repair technique, the atrial septum can appear anatomically normal or can reveal areas of echo density consistent with the type of patch material used. In general, the right ventricular volume overload pattern resolves but can be replaced by a postoperative septal motion pattern.

Other Abnormalities of the Atrial Septum. In addition to atrial septal defect, anomalies such as aneurysm of the atrial septum, lipomatous atrial hypertrophy, and patent foramen ovale[135] can be detected. The aneurysmal atrial septum is not infrequently associated with small perforations and minor degrees of either right-to-left or left-to-right atrial shunting (Fig. 11–87). Contrast echocardiography can detect minor degrees of right-to-left shunting in both of these situations.

Anomalous Pulmonary Venous Return. A final congenital lesion that results in a right ventricular volume overload pattern is anomalous pulmonary venous return. A variation on anomalous return is seen in patients with sinus venosus atrial septal defects who have functional anomalous return due to malalignment of the right superior pulmonary vein such that its flow is directed into the superior vena cava and right atrium. True anomalous pulmonary venous return often results in creation of a venous chamber posterior to the left atrium, which then drains to the right atrium.

VENTRICULAR SEPTAL DEFECT. Although the ventricular septal defect represents the most common congenital intracardiac shunt encountered in infants and children, it accounts for a small percentage of defects detected de novo in adults. A substantial number of small ventricular septal defects close spontaneously during childhood and thus are not present in adults, whereas the larger defects result in symptoms and are detected in childhood. Furthermore, the smaller persistent defects are associated with prominent pathological murmurs and unlikely to be confused for a flow murmur, and therefore these individuals come to medical attention promptly. On occasion, patients with small ventricular septal defects escape detection to adulthood, when the defects are found on the basis of a pathological murmur. Ventricular septal defects occur

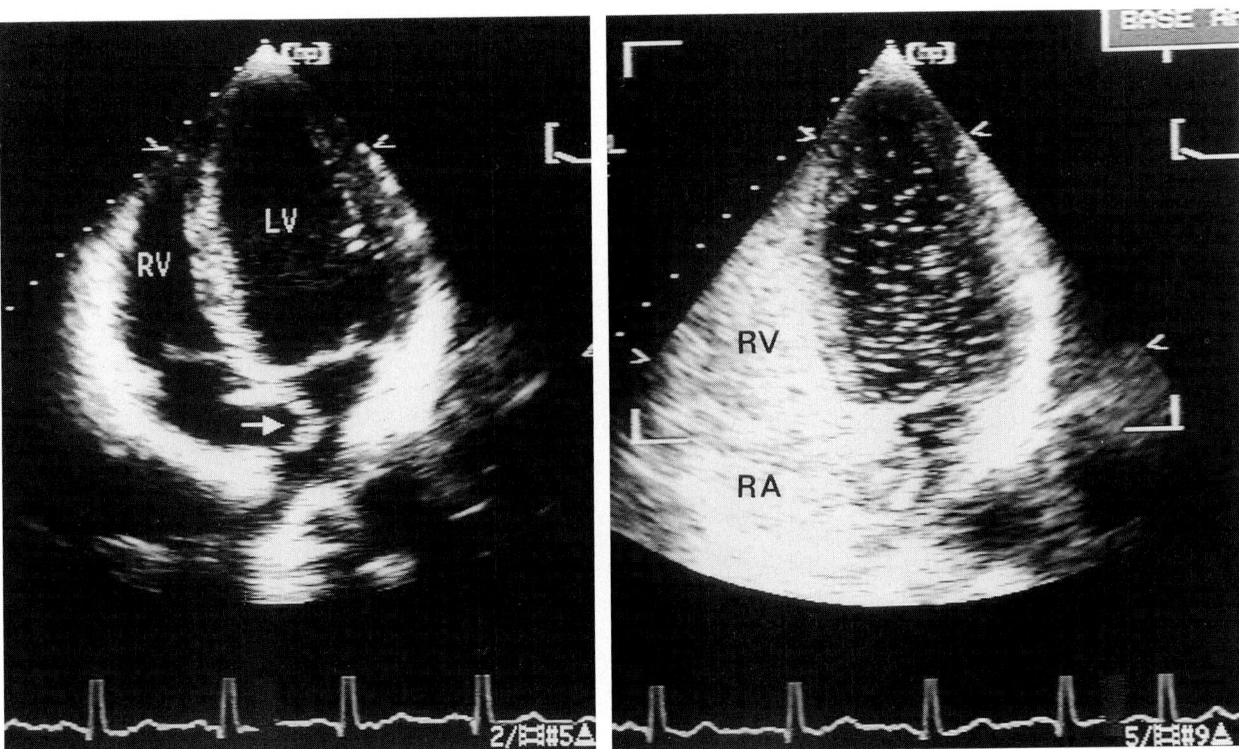

FIGURE 11–87 Apical four-chamber view recorded in a patient with an atrial septal aneurysm. Note the marked bulging of the atrial septum into the cavity of the left atrium **(A)**. **B,** Recorded after injection of saline contrast medium. Note that the contrast medium has filled the right ventricular cavity, and numerous individual microbubbles are seen in the cavity of both the left atrium and left ventricle, consistent with a right-to-left shunt through fenestrations in the atrial septal aneurysm. LV = left ventricle; RA = right atrium; RV = right ventricle.

in several different locations, which are denoted echocardiographically in Figure 11–88. The most common location is a small perimembranous septal defect; however, other locations, including supracristal, are not uncommonly encountered. Muscular defects can occur anywhere within the muscular septum and may take a serpiginous route through the septal myocardium. Small apical defects are frequently multiple.

A ventricular septal defect can be visualized as a dropout of myocardial tissue with communication between the left and right ventricles. The resolution of TTE, using 3- and 5-MHz transducers, is such that most defects below a 3 mm size may not be directly visualized. It is uncommon to directly visualize small muscular defects that may take an angulated or serpiginous course through the ventricular septum. Color Doppler imaging over areas of the septum is a reliable means for detecting the abnormal transseptal flow (Fig. 11–89). It is often necessary to scan in unusual and atypical planes to identify flow through the septum, especially when searching for a muscular defect. For the isolated small perimembranous defect, continuous-wave Doppler can be used to determine the velocity of flow from the left ventricle to the right ventricle and hence the transventricular pressure gradient. This can then be subtracted from arm blood pressure to estimate right ventricular systolic pressure. With the use of this methodology, the small restrictive ventricular septal defect can be characterized as a defect resulting in little or no chamber dilation, having small anatomical extent on two-dimensional scanning, and associated with a high transventricular gradient.

The magnitude of shunting through a ventricular septal defect can be calculated using several Doppler techniques. Larger ventricular septal defects may be associated with substantial left-to-right shunts and development of secondary pulmonary hypertension. In this instance, the right ventricle will be dilated and hypertrophied. By using the tricuspid regurgitation signal, right ventricular systolic pressure can be calculated. In the presence of a ventricular septal defect, it is important to look for associated anomalies of the right ventricular outflow tract and pulmonary valve. Pulmonic stenosis and right ventricular outflow tract obstruction are both protective of the pulmonary circuit and will lead to the scenario of elevated right ventricular systolic pressure with elevation or even normal pulmonary artery pressures. This has obvious clinical implications with respect to surgical intervention.

Closed and Repaired Ventricular Septal Defect. As noted earlier, many small ventricular septal defects close spontaneously in infancy and

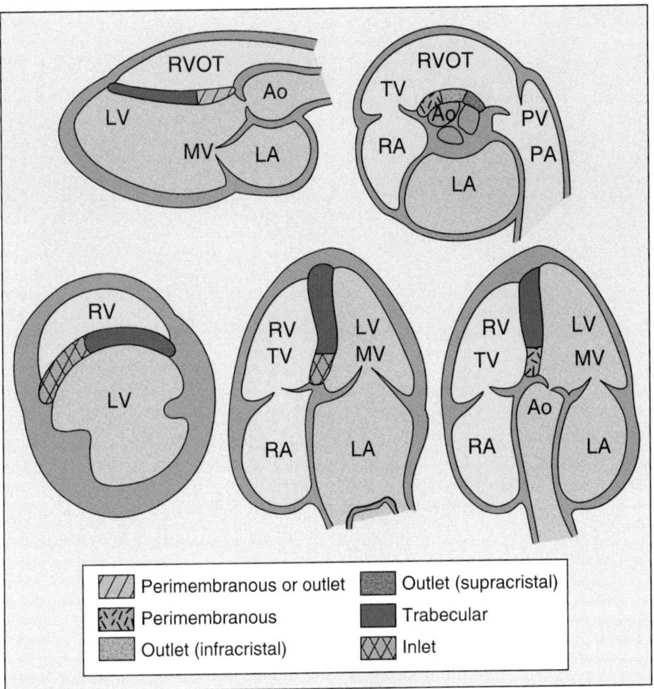

FIGURE 11–88 Schematic depicting the location of different ventricular septal defects compared with the different echocardiographic views. Ao = aorta; LA = left atrium; LV = left ventricle; MV = mitral valve; PV = pulmonary vein; RA = right atrium; RV = right ventricle; RVOT = right ventricular outflow tract; TV = tricuspid valve. (From Feigenbaum H: Echocardiography. 5th ed. Malvern, PA, Lea & Febiger, 1994.)

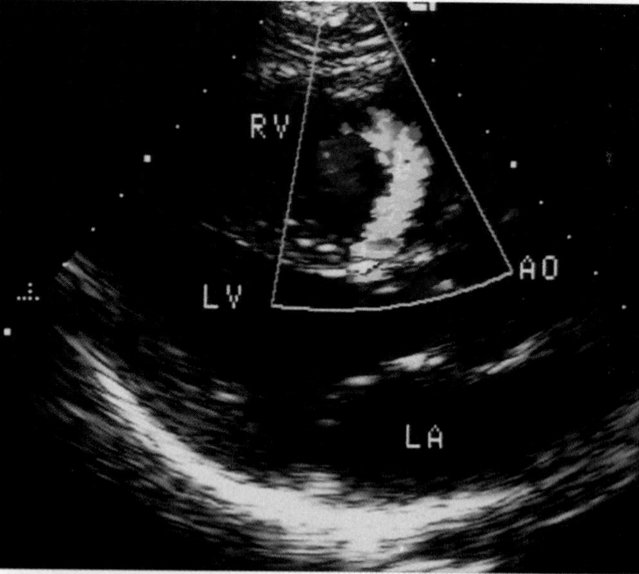

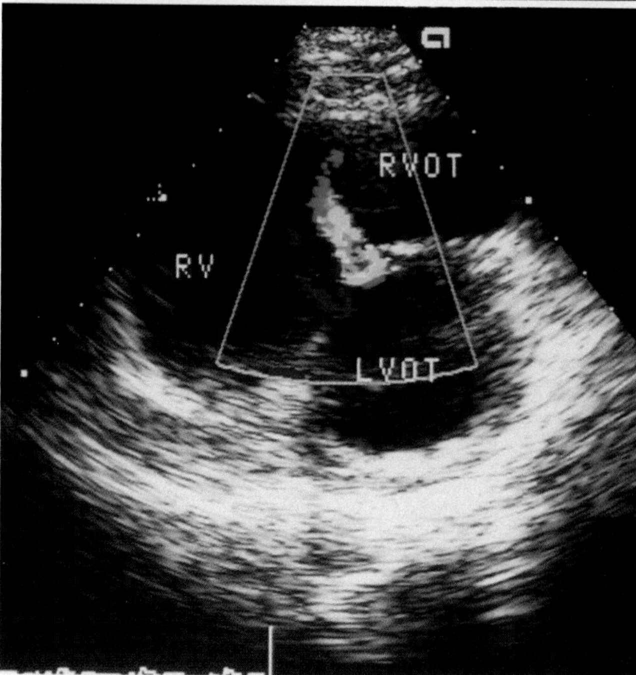

FIGURE 11–89 Parasternal two-dimensional echocardiographic views in a patient with a moderate-sized perimembranous ventricular septal defect. The **upper panel** is recorded in a parasternal long-axis view and shows the proximal anterior septum. The **lower panel** is recorded in a short-axis view at the base of the heart. Note in each instance the distinct color jet arising on the left ventricular side of the ventricular septum and coursing in the right ventricular outflow tract. This is consistent with left-to-right ventricular septal defect flow. AO = aorta; LA = left atrium; LV = left ventricle; LVOT = left ventricular outflow tract; RV = right ventricle; RVOT = right ventricular outflow tract.

childhood. This occurs by way of two basic mechanisms. The first is fusion of a portion of the tricuspid leaflet to the ventricular septal defect. In this case, one may visualize a very thin membrane closing the actual ventricular septal defect. The second mechanism appears to be growth of additional tissue from the margins of the ventricular septal defect. In this instance, there may be irregular tissue closing the ventricular septal defect, the extent of which can be highly variable. In many instances, a thin-walled aneurysm may be noted in the area of the previous ventricular septal defect. The aneurysm typically bows into the right ventricular outflow tract. A small residual left-to-right shunt may be encountered that often is of little hemodynamic significance but that may result in a murmur and pose a risk for endocarditis.

Other Congenital Disorders

TETRALOGY OF FALLOT. Tetralogy of Fallot represents a constellation of lesions, including a ventricular septal defect with overriding aorta, obstruction to right ventricular outflow tract at either the infundibular or valvular level, and right ventricular hypertrophy (Fig. 11–90). The fourth component is a right-sided aortic arch. Before correction, the lesion is characterized by a ventricular septal defect in which the tip of the ventricular septum is directed not at the anterior wall of the aorta but at the aortic lumen. Varying degrees of right ventricular outflow tract obstruction, including true valvular stenosis and infundibular muscular stenosis, can be seen. Tetralogy of Fallot represents the most common cyanotic congenital lesion to be encountered that is likely to result in survival to adulthood and, furthermore, the most common complex lesion to be encountered in the adult population after repair.

Preoperatively, tetralogy of Fallot represents a broad spectrum of ventricular septal defect size and outflow tract obstruction. Postoperatively, varying degrees of residual abnormalities can be encountered, ranging from a nearly normal-appearing heart to one in which there are substantial degrees of right ventricular dysfunction and residual right ventricular outflow tract obstruction. Two-dimensional echocardiography and Doppler techniques can be a definitive means for following these individuals with respect to recovery of right ventricular function and development of complications such as recurrent right ventricular outflow tract obstruction and residual ventricular septal defect.

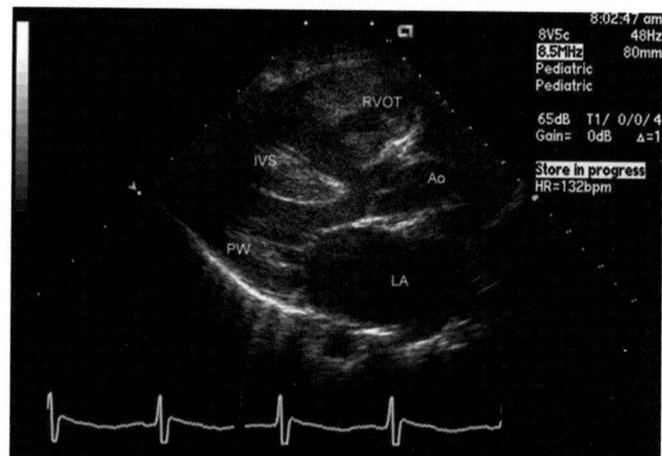

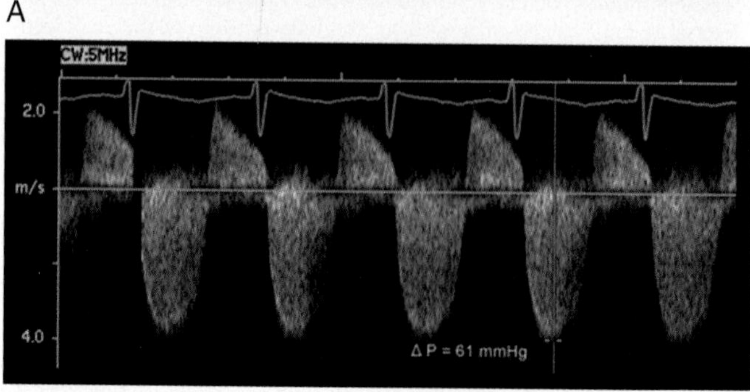

FIGURE 11–90 **A,** Two-dimensional echocardiogram recorded in a patient with an unrepaired tetralogy of Fallot. Note the large ventricular septal defect and the overriding aorta. Because of the overriding aorta, both right and left ventricular outflow is directed toward the aorta. **B,** Continuous wave Doppler recorded through the right ventricular outflow tract. Note the peak gradient of 61 mm Hg. Ao = aorta; IVS = interventricular septum; LA = left atrium; PW = posterior wall; RVOT = right ventricular outflow tract.

PULMONIC STENOSIS. Isolated pulmonic stenosis is a relatively common congenital lesion. As with the bicuspid aortic valve, its hemodynamic severity ranges from negligible to severe and life threatening early in infancy. Because of the orientation of the proximal pulmonary artery and pulmonic valve, it is easily interrogated with Doppler. Underestimation of pulmonic valve gradients due to off-angle interrogation is uncommon. Anatomically, the stenotic pulmonary valve appears somewhat thickened and has "doming" motion (see Fig. 11–75). On M-mode echocardiography, there may be an accentuation of the pulmonic valve "a" wave. In adult patients, it is not uncommon for valvular pulmonic stenosis to be associated with secondary infundibular hypertrophy with concurrent right ventricular outflow tract obstruction. Thus, it is important to evaluate both the subvalvular and valvular aspects of the pulmonary valve in adult patients. Less frequently, peripheral pulmonic stenosis will be encountered. Identification and characterization of the peripheral pulmonary arteries in adult populations can be quite problematic and constitute an area in which MRI can play an incremental and valuable role.

ABNORMALITIES OF THE LEFT VENTRICULAR OUTFLOW TRACT. The most common abnormality of left ventricular outflow is the bicuspid aortic valve, which has been discussed previously. Additionally, both tunnel and discrete subaortic stenosis are occasionally encountered in adult patients. Tunnel aortic stenosis is visualized as a diffuse narrowing of the left ventricular outflow tract and more often is identified in children. Discrete, membranous subvalvular stenosis occasionally escapes detection until adulthood and is characterized by the presence of a thin membrane or ridge that encircles the left ventricular outflow tract (Fig. 11–91). Components of the membrane may be attached to the ventricular septum and to the anterior mitral valve leaflet. The membrane itself can be difficult to visualize from TTE positions and may require TEE for complete visualization. The obstructing membrane results in turbulence in the left ventricular outflow tract, which can be detected with color Doppler flow imaging and eventually results in secondary pathology of the aortic valve with subsequent aortic insufficiency. M-mode echocardiography often reveals characteristic coarse systolic fluttering of the aortic valve leaflets. This finding can help distinguish valvular from subvalvular obstruction. This should be contrasted to hypertrophic cardiomyopathy, in which anatomical abnormalities of the aortic valve and aortic insufficiency are uncommon and a single notch representing valve preclosure may be noted.

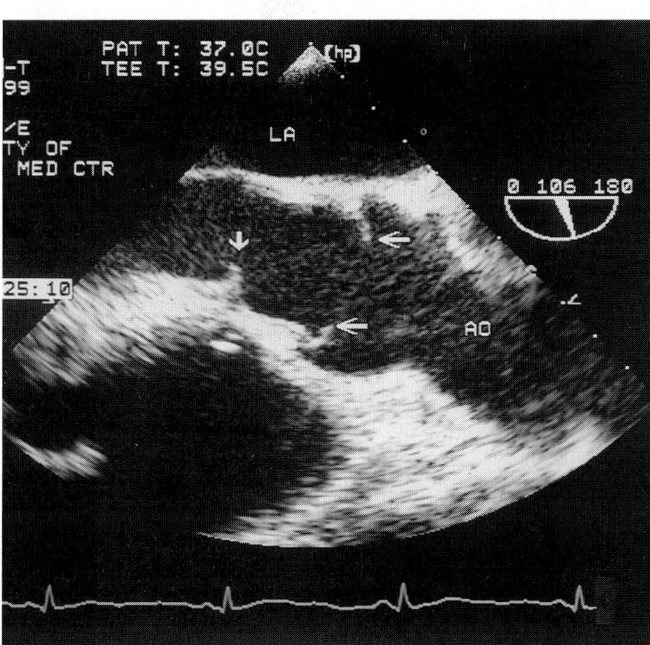

FIGURE 11–91 Transesophageal echocardiogram in a longitudinal plane of the left ventricular outflow tract demonstrating a small, discrete subaortic membrane (downward pointing arrow). The aortic leaflets are mildly thickened (horizontal arrows). This small membrane was not visualized from the transthoracic echocardiogram. AO = aorta; LA = left atrium.

CONGENITAL ABNORMALITIES OF THE MITRAL VALVE. Congenital abnormalities of the mitral valve, likely to be encountered in adult populations, include the previously mentioned cleft mitral valve, seen in association with a primum atrial septal defect as well as congenital mitral stenosis. The latter can occur either in the presence of a single papillary muscle, in which all chordae attach to a central point, rendering an otherwise unremarkable valve functionally stenotic, or in a valve that is intrinsically stenotic but with two papillary muscle attachments. Functionally, these patients present in a manner nearly identical to that of patients with rheumatic mitral stenosis. Awareness of the anatomical features of congenital mitral stenosis is necessary to separate it from rheumatic causes. In many instances, the congenital lesion will be characterized by an obstructive but eccentrically directed mitral valve orifice without the characteristic chordal and leaflet thickening. Transvalvular gradients can be measured across the congenitally stenotic mitral valve but may require unusual transducer angulations and lines of interrogation.

Cor triatriatum represents a membrane within the body of the left atrium that likewise may be obstructive. Transthoracic imaging may suffice for identification of the membrane (Fig. 11-92), but in many instances TEE, which affords a more accurate view of the left atrium, is necessary. A final congenital abnormality of the mitral valve is the submitral ring or web. This represents a membrane attached near the mitral annulus within the left atrium that is variably obstructive to flow.

ANOMALIES OF THE TRICUSPID VALVE. The most common congenital tricuspid valve anomaly to escape detection to adulthood is Ebstein anomaly. In this situation, the lateral leaflet is elongated and tethered to the lateral wall of the right ventricle and the septal leaflet is relatively small and apically displaced. This results in conversion of a portion of the right ventricle to an "atrialized" right ventricle (Figs. 11-93 and 11-94). Tricuspid regurgitation is invariably present and results in dilation of the right side of the heart in general but predominantly of the right atrium and atrialized right ventricle. Atrial septal defect is a common association with Ebstein anomaly and should be considered in all instances. Because the coaptation of the tricuspid valve is displaced toward the apex of the right ventricle, the apical location of the convergence zone of the tricuspid regurgitation jet may be one of the clues to the presence of this anomaly.

Once identified, it is important to characterize several features of Ebstein anomaly that have direct relevance to the feasibility of surgical repair. Surgical repair can be undertaken in individuals with a relatively large functional right ventricle, compared with the atrialized portion, and in whom there is not extensive tethering of the lateral leaflet.

Tricuspid Atresia. Tricuspid atresia is usually detected in infancy and after palliation may allow survival to adulthood. In patients with tricuspid atresia, there is no functional tricuspid valve tissue, although the tricuspid annulus may be closed by a thin membrane with small perforations. Because of the atretic tricuspid valve, right ventricular hypoplasia coexists. Obviously, a complete form of tricuspid atresia is incompatible with life unless a concurrent atrial or ventricular septal defect is present.

PERSISTENT DUCTUS ARTERIOSUS. Persistent ductus arteriosus represents persistence of the normal communication between the descending thoracic aorta and the left pulmonary artery. The size of the communication varies from 1 or 2 mm to a centimeter or more. The magnitude of left-to-right shunting is dependent on the size of the defect. Initially, persistent ductus rsults in a continuous left-to-right shunt at the great artery level that may result in left-sided heart volume overload early in childhood and adolescence. Because of the increased pulmonary flow, pulmonary hypertension may develop, in which case only the systolic component of the shunt persists. Echocardiographic detection of persistent ductus arteriosus is dependent on detection of left-sided heart enlargement and/or an abnormal pulmonary artery flow pattern. With the use of suprasternal notch views, it is occasionally possible to directly visualize the ductus. More commonly, Doppler interrogation of the proximal pulmonary artery is the initial clue to the presence of a persistent ductus. By using either color Doppler flow imaging or pulsed Doppler, one can detect continuous turbulent flow in the proximal pulmonary artery (Fig. 11–95). Further careful interrogation will frequently identify the origin of the abnormal flow from the descending aorta into the left main pulmonary artery.

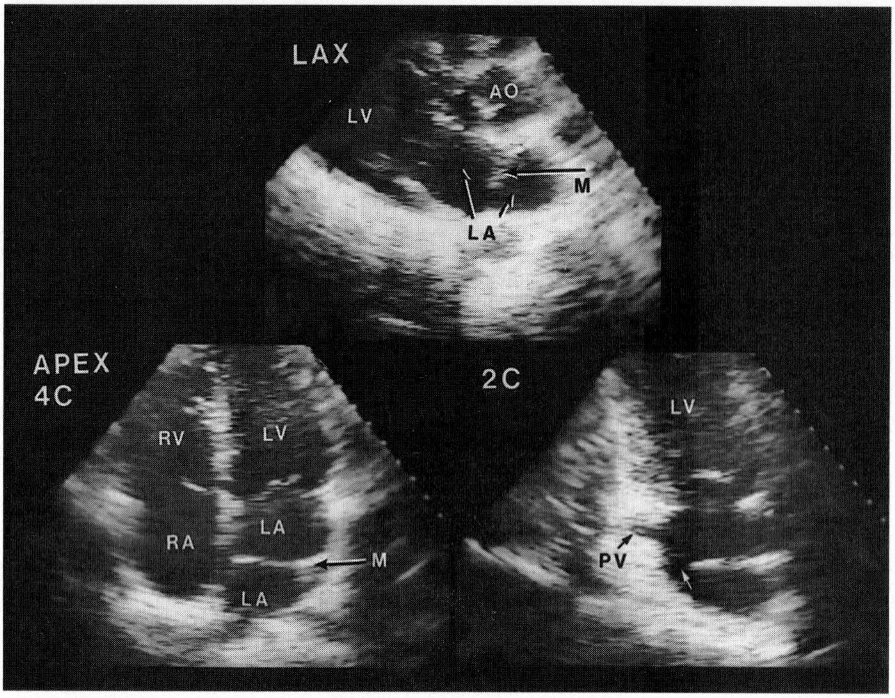

COARCTATION OF THE AORTA. Narrowing or coarctation of the aorta occurs after the takeoff of the left subclavian artery. It results in reduction of systolic pressure distally and may present in adulthood as a secondary cause of systemic hypertension. The anatomical extent of coarctation may be visualized from the suprasternal notch, and continuous-flow Doppler can be used to determine the coarctation gradient (Fig. 11–96). There is a strong association between coarctation and bicuspid aortic valve; and whenever coarctation is discovered, efforts should be made to define the aortic valve anatomy.

FIGURE 11–92 Transthoracic echocardiogram recorded in a patient with *cor triatriatum* in the parasternal long-axis view **(top)** and apical views **(bottom)**. A linear echo courses posteriorly from the area of the aorta (AO). From the apical views, the membrane (M) can be seen to divide the left atrium (LA) into two chambers. LV = left ventricle; PV = pulmonary vein; RA = right atrium; RV = right ventricle. (From Feigenbaum H: Echocardiography. 5th ed. Malvern, PA, Lea & Febiger, 1994.)

TRANSPOSITION OF THE GREAT ARTERIES. *Transposition* refers to the situation in which there is ventricular-arterial discordance. This is defined as a connection of the left ventricle to the pulmonary artery and the right ventricle to the aorta. Two forms of transposition may be encountered. D-Transposition is an isolated malposition of the great vessels due to failure of the conotruncos to appropriately coil. In this situation, the pulmonary artery is attached to the left ventricle, which receives blood from the left atrium. The aorta is attached to the right ventricle, which receives blood from the right atrium. This results in two parallel circulations and is obviously not compatible with life in the absence of an intracardiac shunt such as a persistent ductus or large ventricular or atrial septal defect. This lesion is invariably detected in infancy and is not encountered in adult patients, other than in surgically corrected or palliated forms. Previously, surgical correction of transposition consisted of creation of an atrial septal defect early and subsequent surgical creation of a baffle that directed right atrial blood into the left ventricle and left atrial blood flow into the right ventricle. Currently, an anatomical switch of the great arteries is the preferred surgical procedure. L-Transposition occurs when there is both inversion of the ventricles and transposition of the great arteries (Fig. 11–97). In this situation, blood flows from the anatomical right atrium through an anatomical mitral valve into the anatomical left ventricle and then into the pulmonary artery. Blood returning to the left atrium flows through an anatomical tricuspid valve into an anatomical right ventricle and then to the aorta. This results in "corrected" transposition, in which physiological blood flow is maintained.

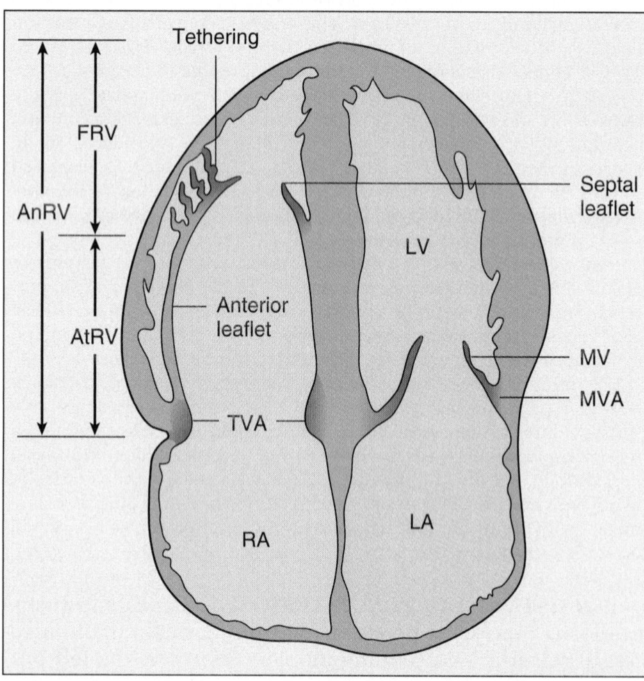

FIGURE 11–93 Schematic of the anatomical and echocardiographic abnormalities seen in Ebstein anomaly, including apical displacement of the septal leaflet and elongation and tethering of the lateral leaflet. Both the functional (FRV) and atrialized right ventricle (AtRV) are noted. AnRV = anatomic right ventricle; LA = left atrium; LV = left ventricle; MV = mitral valve; MVA = mitral valve annulus; RA = right atrium; TVA = tricuspid valve annulus. (From Feigenbaum H: Echocardiography. 5th ed. Malvern, PA, Lea & Febiger, 1994.)

In either type of transposition, the great arteries no longer have the circular and crescent orientation but rather arise from the heart in a parallel fashion. In adult patients, it can be difficult to directly visualize the parallel nature of the great vessels. Clues to the presence of congenitally "corrected" transposition include the presence of a trabeculated ventricle with a more apically placed valve in a left and posterior position. L-Transposition is compatible with survival into the fourth and fifth decade. After this period of time, substantial hypertrophy of the anatomical right ventricle occurs and right ventricular dysfunction is not uncommon. Regurgitation of the anatomical tricuspid valve in the systemic circuit is also quite common in adult patients.

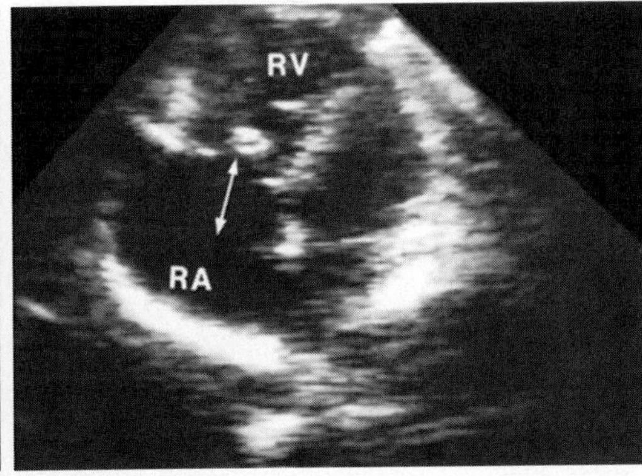

FIGURE 11–94 Two-dimensional echocardiogram recorded in a patient with Ebstein anomaly. Note the small, apically displayed septal leaflet and the elongated lateral leaflet that is tethered to the myocardium of the right ventricular lateral wall. LA = left atrium; LV = left ventricle; MV = mitral valve; RA = right atrium; RV = right ventricle; TV = tricuspid valve. (From Feigenbaum H: Echocardiography. 5th ed. Malvern, PA, Lea & Febiger, 1994.)

COMPLEX CONGENITAL HEART DISEASE. The echocardiographic and clinical evaluation of complex congenital heart disease is best undertaken by individuals with specific interest and training in the area and is beyond the scope of this chapter. Three-dimensional echocardiography has been a valuable adjunct in evaluating the complex anatomy seen in complex lesions (Fig. 11–98).

Diseases of the Pericardium (see Chap. 64)

Pericardial Effusion

Detection of pericardial effusion was one of the earliest uses of echocardiography, and modern ultrasonographic techniques remain the predominant diagnostic tool for detection, quantitation, and determination of the physiological significance of pericardial effusion. A pericardial effusion is viewed as an echo-free space surrounding the heart, most commonly seen posteriorly (Fig. 11–99). Most clinical laboratories document the presence of pericardial effusion and quantify it as minimal, small, moderate, or large. A minimal effusion represents the 5 to 20 ml of normal pericardial fluid seen in disease-free individuals. This is most frequently noted as an echo-free space, confined to the posterior atrioventricular

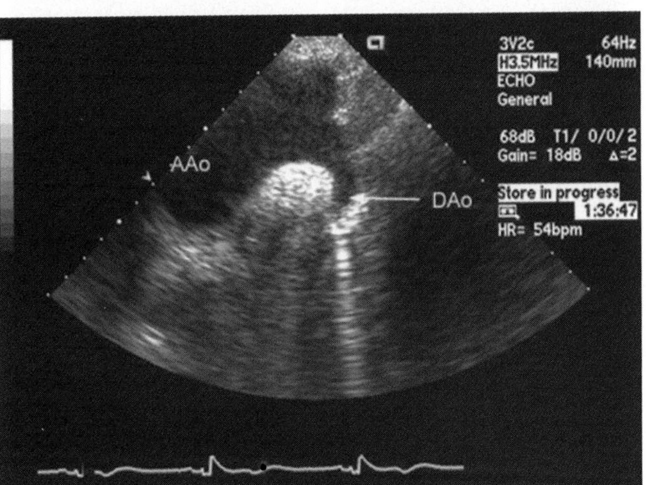

A

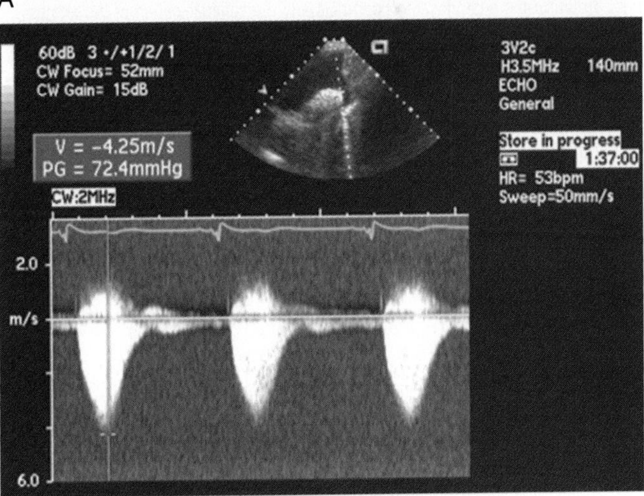

B

FIGURE 11–96 Coarctation of the aorta. **A,** Suprasternal two-dimensional echocardiogram revealing a dilated ascending aorta (AAo) and a markedly narrowed descending aorta (DAo). The actual tissue of the coarctation is not easily visualized in this image. **B,** Continuous-wave Doppler through the descending thoracic aorta, revealing a peak pressure gradient across the area of narrowing of 72 mm Hg.

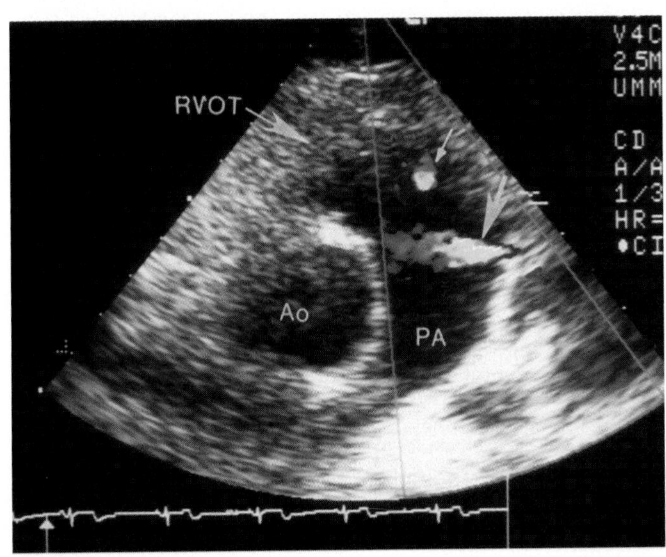

FIGURE 11–95 Parasternal short-axis view at the level of the great vessels recorded in a patient with persistent ductus arteriosus. Note the dilated pulmonary artery (PA) and the abnormal color flow signal (large arrow) that originates from the area of the descending thoracic aorta and flows into the pulmonary artery distal to the pulmonary valve. In this diastolic frame, note the small pulmonic insufficiency jet (small white arrow). Ao = aorta; RVOT = right ventricular outflow tract.

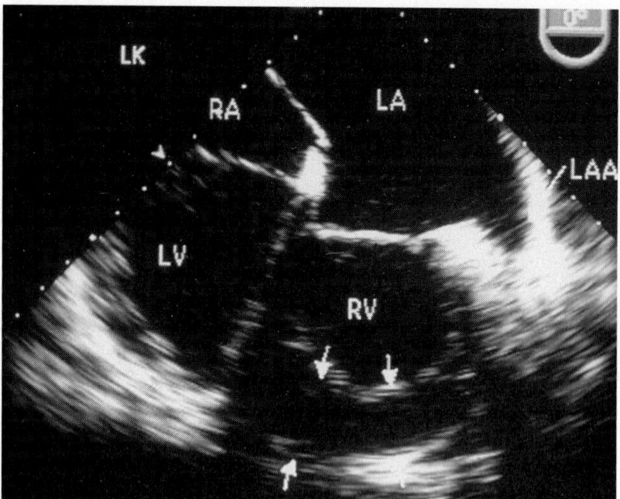

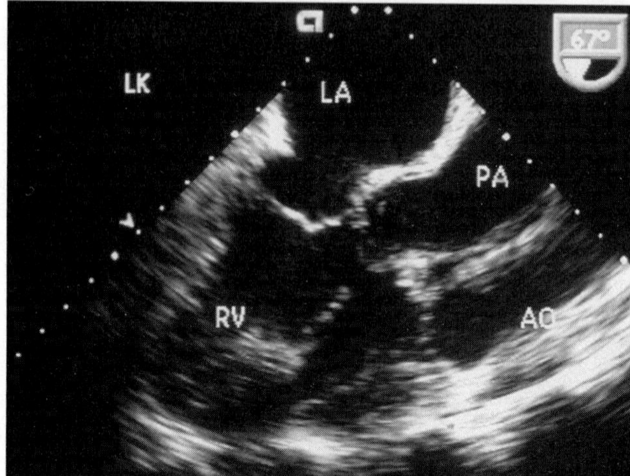

FIGURE 11–97 Transesophageal echocardiogram in an adult patient with L-transposition of the great vessels. In the **top panel,** the connection of the anatomical right atrium to the anatomical left ventricle and the communication of the anatomical left atrium, through an anatomical tricuspid valve, into an anatomical right ventricle can be appreciated. Note the normal-appearing left atrial appendage (LAA). Note also the marked hypertrophy of the right ventricular trabeculations, which nearly obliterate the apex of the anatomical right ventricle (RV) (arrows). There is apical displacement of the atrioventricular valve contained within the anatomical right ventricle, compared with the atrioventricular (mitral) valve connecting the right atrium (RA) to the left ventricle (LV). The **lower panel** depicts the parallel orientation of the pulmonary artery (PA) and aorta (AO). The more anteriorly placed aorta is in communication with the anatomical right ventricle.

groove often only in systole. A small pericardial effusion is defined as less than 5 mm in maximum dimension, which is visualized throughout the cardiac cycle. Moderate pericardial effusions typically are 15 to 20 mm in dimension and tend to be more circumferential. Large effusions are defined as those larger than 20 mm. Because patients are scanned in a supine or left lateral position, the fluid tends to pool and to be mostly visible in the posterior aspects of the imaging planes. Numerous attempts have been made to quantify the amount of pericardial fluid but have not seen uniform acceptance. The majority of laboratories use the semiquantitative scheme noted earlier. Three-dimensional echocardiography has shown some promise for enhanced localization and quantitation of pericardial effusion. The most commonly employed technique for quantifying the volume of effusion is to image the effusion in orthogonal planes and determine the intrapericardial volume using Simpson's rule. The entire cardiac silhouette can then likewise be traced and the total cardiac volume determined. The difference between the pericardial and cardiac volumes represents the volume of pericardial fluid. Although theoretically accurate, there are practical limitations to tracing both the cardiac and pericardial volumes that render this technique less than optimal and of little true clinical utility.

Other aspects of a pericardial effusion also can be noted with echocardiography. Soft tissue density masses, thickening of the visceral pericardium, and presence of fibrinous strands can all be identified. All of these features are more common in patients with marked inflammatory or malignant causes for pericardial effusion. Additionally, the nature of the fluid can be further characterized as clear or "cloudy." The hallmark of the benign, idiopathic effusion is a clear echo-free space, whereas malignancy, bacterial infection, and hemorrhagic effusions are more likely to have solid components or stranding.

Cardiac Tamponade

Several echocardiographic findings are reliable indicators of elevated intrapericardial pressure, which in turn correlate with hemodynamic compromise or clinical tamponade. One of the earliest described was collapse of the right ventricular outflow tract during early diastole. This is best visualized in the parasternal views but can also be appreciated in the four-chamber view. The precise timing and duration of right ventricular collapse can best be determined with M-mode echocardiography. Cardiac tamponade occurs when pericardial effusion of sufficient magnitude has accumulated to result in equilibration of intrapericardial and passively determined intracardiac pressures. Immediately after mechanical systole, the ventricle begins to relax, with a greater degree of active relaxation attributed to the left ventricle compared with the right. This results in disproportionate or favored filling of the left ventricle with a transient elevation in intrapericardial pressure, which results in turn in early diastolic collapse of the highly compliant right ventricular outflow tract (Figs. 11–100 and 11–101). Detection of transient outflow tract collapse is a reliable marker that intrapericardial pressure is elevated and hemodynamic compromise is present. It is correlated with the presence of overt tamponade but also has been seen in patients who subsequently developed tamponade. The atrial corollary of this phenomenon is exaggerated atrial emptying. Because of elevated intrapericardial pressures, filling of the right ventricle is impeded in early diastole (a manifestation of which is early diastolic right ventricular collapse) and occurs to an exaggerated degree with atrial systole. This results in a delayed and exaggerated contraction of the right atrium with actual invagination of the atrial wall in late diastole (Fig. 11–102). This echocardiographic sign of hemodynamic compromise is more sensitive than right ventricular diastolic collapse but less specific, because it occurs earlier in the course of intrapericardial pressure elevation. Right ventricular collapse may be absent even in the presence of elevated pericardial pressures in patients with right ventricular hypertrophy or significant pulmonary hypertension. In the presence of loculated effusion or in complex situations, either right- or left-sided chambers may be differentially compressed.

Doppler echocardiography can also provide valuable clues as to the hemodynamic significance of pericardial effusions. In patients with hemodynamically significant effusions, there is exaggerated interplay between right and left ventricular filling, occurring with phases of the respiratory cycle. Clinically, this is manifest as an exaggerated pulsus paradoxus. Echocardiographically exaggerated respiratory variation can be documented by examining the left ventricular and right ventricular outflow tract flows in systole and noting exaggerated phasic variation in velocities and time velocity integrals (Fig. 11–103). Similarly, in patients with a hemodynamically significant effusion, ventricular filling is impeded. The normal respiratory variation of the tricuspid valve is 25 percent, with a greater velocity in inspiration than expiration, and the normal mitral valve shows the opposite pattern with a variation of approximately 15 percent. In patients with hemodynamically significant effusions, there is a greater than usual variation in this respiratory pattern (Fig. 11–104).

Constrictive Pericarditis

Although chronic constrictive pericarditis remains an elusive diagnosis, echocardiography and Doppler evaluation can provide valuable clues as to its presence. The classic form of constrictive pericarditis is calcific constrictive pericarditis after tuberculosis infection. In contemporary times, constric-

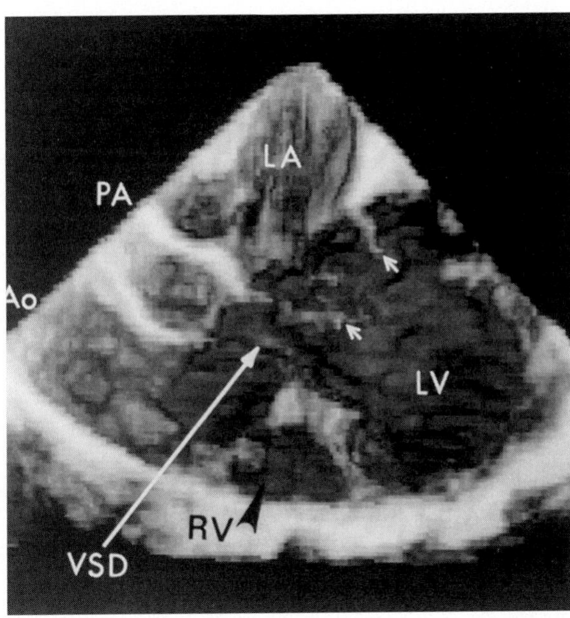

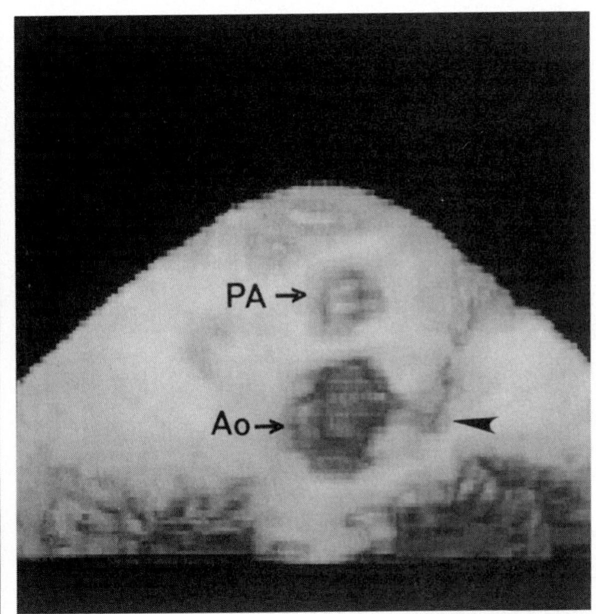

FIGURE 11–98 Three-dimensional echocardiogram of a patient with a ventricular septal defect, transposition, and double outlet right ventricle. Note the small right ventricular cavity and the parallel orientation of the two great vessels. Ao = aorta; LA = left atrium; LV = left ventricle; PA = pulmonary artery; RV = right ventricle; VSD = ventricular septal defect.

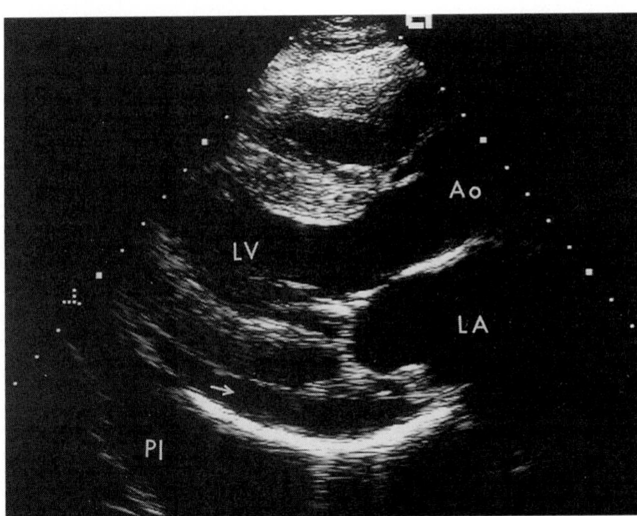

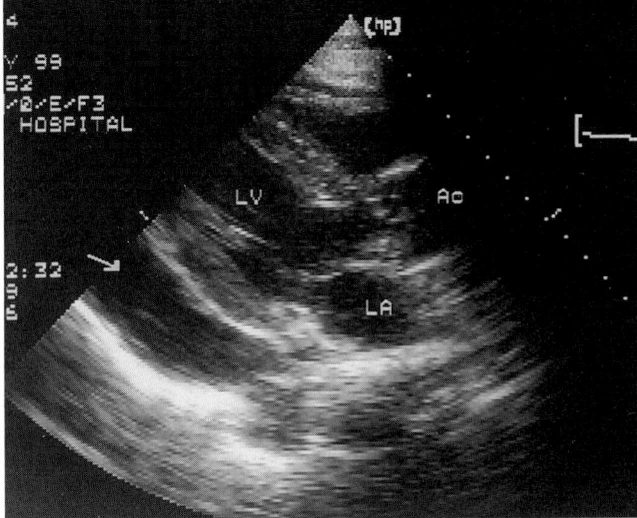

FIGURE 11–99 Transthoracic parasternal long-axis echocardiograms recorded in a patient with a small **(top)** pericardial effusion. Note the echo-free space confined to the area posterior to the heart (arrow). The **bottom panel** reveals a similar pattern but with a larger echo-free space (arrow). Ao = aorta; LA = left atrium; LV = left ventricle; PI = pleural effusion.

tion is more likely to be related to nontuberculous infections, hemorrhagic effusions, cardiac surgery, or irradiation. The clinical presentation and echocardiographic appearance often vary from those classically described with calcific constriction. Numerous attempts have been made to quantify pericardial thickness using echocardiography. Routine transthoracic imaging has not been an accurate means for detecting pericardial thickening. TEE has shown more promise but has not seen clinical acceptance. Intracardiac ultrasonography does provide a high-resolution view of the pericardium but is an invasive procedure and has been validated in only a small number of patients. Determination of pericardial thickening is probably more accurately done with computed tomography (CT) or MRI.

In the absence of direct ultrasonographic documentation of thickened pericardium, there are indirect signs of pericardial constriction that should be evaluated in suspected cases, including abnormalities of ventricular septal motion. The abnormalities of septal motion that occur are an exaggerated respiratory variation in septal position with marked bowing of the ventricular septum toward the left ventricle during inspiration. Additionally, when viewed from the parasternal long-axis position, an abnormality of septal motion is often detected. This frequently is seen as a downward motion of the ventricular septum in early systole, followed by a brief anterior motion, which can be confused with a conduction disturbance and is best detected with M-mode scanning.

The Doppler hallmarks of cardiac constriction include exaggerated respiratory variation of mitral and tricuspid inflows with a pathologically elevated E/A ratio (Fig. 11–105).[136,137] Additionally, deceleration time is abnormally short and may vary to a disproportionate degree during the respiratory cycle. Examination of the IVC frequently reveals dilation. The normal multiphasic hepatic vein flow is replaced by monophasic flow, occurring predominantly in systole.

The diagnosis of constrictive pericarditis in large part remains one of exclusion. From an echocardiographic standpoint, this diagnosis should be suspected in individuals with symptoms consistent with that diagnosis (i.e., edema, fatigue, and apparent low output state), normal left ventricular systolic function, and no valvular heart disease. Detection of

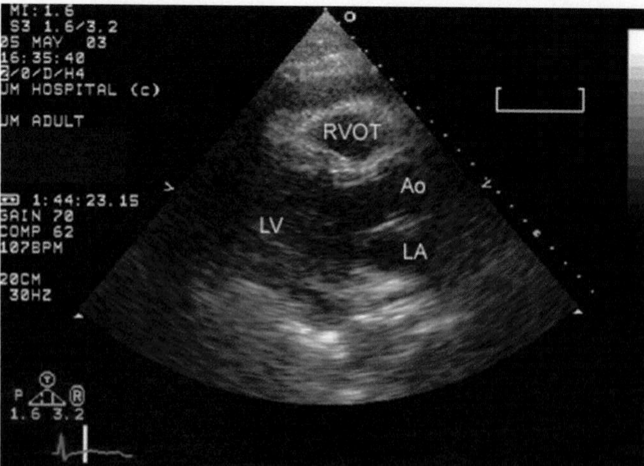

A

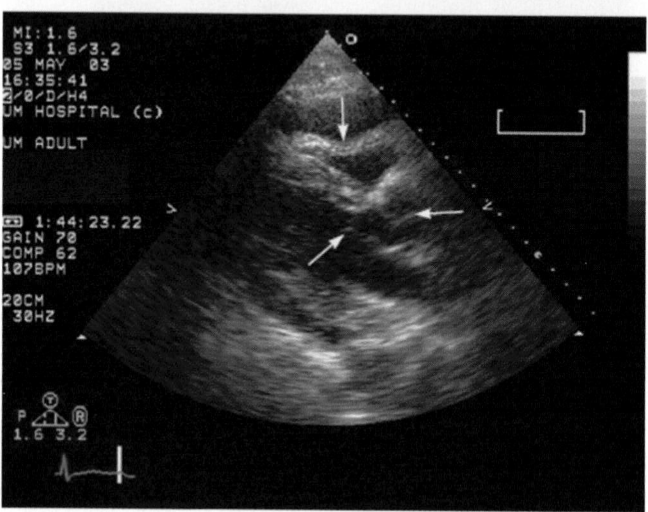

B

FIGURE 11–100 Parasternal long-axis view of a patient with a moderate pericardial effusion and collapse of the right ventricular outflow tract in early diastole. **A,** Recorded in midsystole to late systole (see electrocardiogram in lower left of figure). The right ventricular outflow tract (RVOT) has a normal configuration. **B,** Recorded in early diastole; note the open mitral valve and closed aortic valve (arrows). There is distinct inward collapse of the RVOT (downward pointing arrow) at this point in the cardiac cycle. Ao = aorta; LA = left atrium; LV = left ventricle.

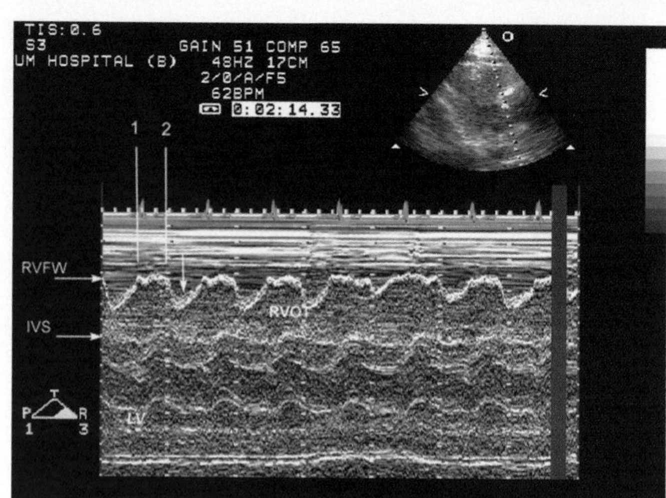

FIGURE 11–101 M-mode echocardiogram recorded in a patient with evidence of hemodynamic compromise. The M-mode beam traverses the right ventricular outflow tract (RVOT), right ventricular free wall (RVFW), and interventricular septum (IVS). Note the distinct diastolic collapse of the right ventricular free wall. Point 1 represents end diastole and the right ventricle is fully expanded. Point 2 represents end systole, at which point the right ventricle has remained expanded. Note that following end systole, there is a dramatic downward motion of the RVFW (arrow), representing collapse of the RVFW, which is indicative of elevated intrapericardial pressure.

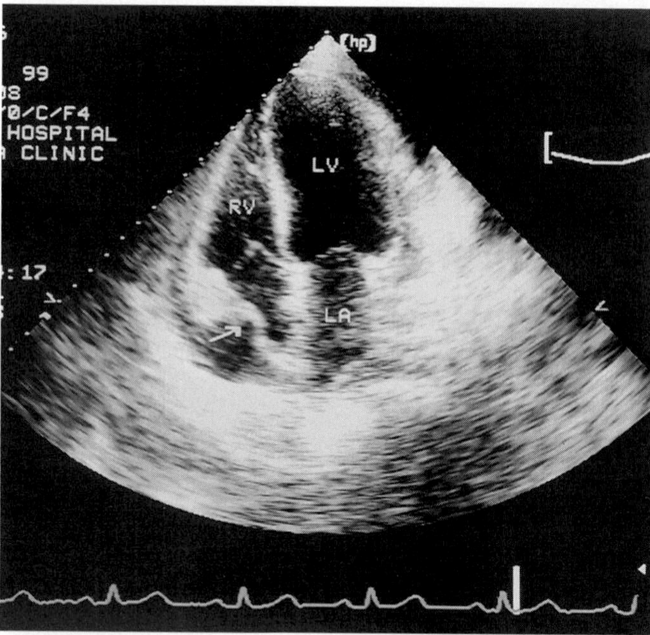

FIGURE 11–102 Apical four-chamber view recorded in a patient with a moderate pericardial effusion and evidence of hemodynamic compromise. The frame is recorded in early ventricular systole, immediately after atrial contraction. Note that the right atrial wall is indented inward and its curvature is frankly reversed (arrow), implying elevated intrapericardial pressure above right atrial pressure. LA = left atrium; LV = left ventricle; RV = right ventricle.

abnormal septal motion, exaggerated respiratory variation, and an elevated E/A ratio provide the majority of the confirmatory evidence of this diagnosis.

MISCELLANEOUS CONDITIONS OF THE PERICARDIUM. Congenital absence of the pericardium occurs in both partial and complete forms. In the complete form, there is a marked abnormality of septal motion with exaggerated intracardiac motion within the thorax. In the partial form, varying degrees of septal motion abnormality can be detected, depending on the degree to which the pericardium is anatomically deficient. Pericardial cysts are detected as echo-free spaces adjacent to the heart. The diagnosis should probably be confirmed by CT or MRI as well.

Cardiomyopathies (see Chap. 59)

Cardiomyopathies can be divided into three basic types: dilated cardiomyopathy of any cause, hypertrophic cardiomyopathy, and restrictive cardiomyopathy.

Dilated Cardiomyopathy

Irrespective of the cause of a dilated cardiomyopathy, left ventricular dilation with global systolic dysfunction is noted (Figs. 11–106 and 11–107). Depending on the duration of the disease, left atrial dilation likewise occurs; if significant mitral regurgitation is present, secondary pulmonary hypertension with right-sided heart dilation is common. The range of systolic dysfunction in patients with dilated cardiomyopathy is quite broad, and ejection fraction ranges from less

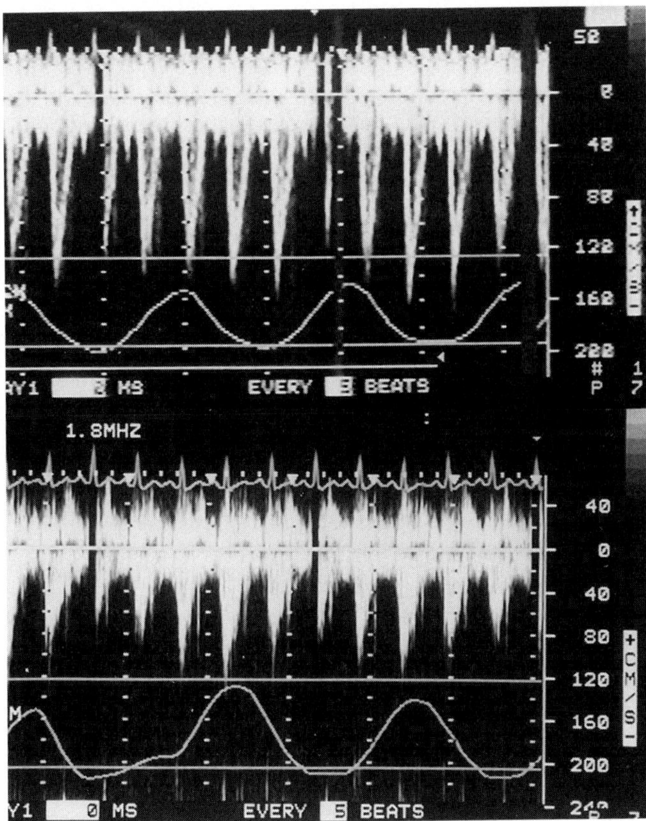

FIGURE 11–103 Pulsed-wave spectral Doppler recorded through the left ventricular outflow tract **(top)** and right ventricular outflow tract **(bottom)** in a patient with hemodynamic compromise due to pericardial effusion. Note the respirometry line on the bottom of each tracing. There is exaggerated respiratory velocity of flow in both the left ventricular and right ventricular outflow tracts. Note the reciprocal nature of the flow variation, with flow increasing during expiration and decreasing in early inspiration for the left ventricular outflow tract and the opposite pattern seen in the right ventricular outflow tract.

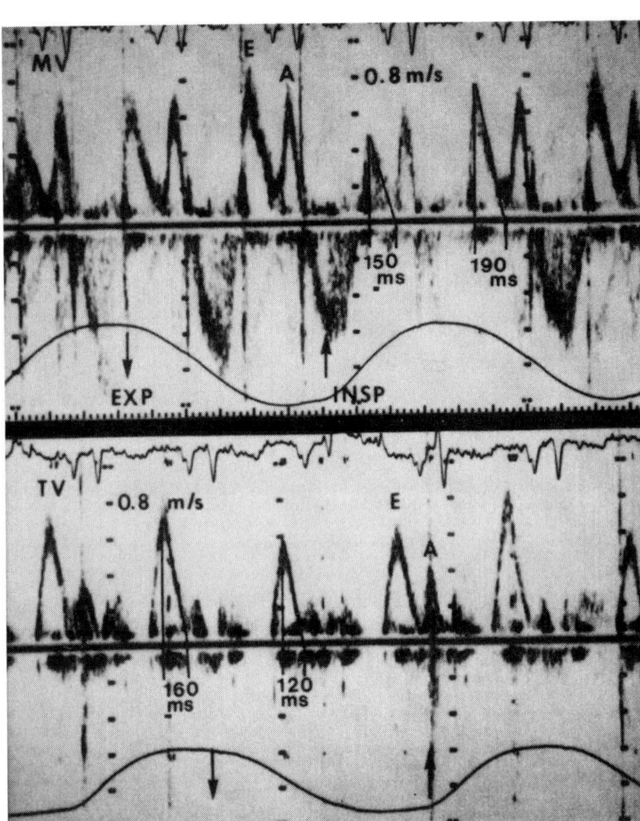

FIGURE 11–105 Pulsed Doppler recording through the mitral valve **(top)** and tricuspid **(bottom)** in a patient with constrictive pericarditis. Note the respirometer tracing for each. There is exaggerated respiratory variation in inflow velocities in both the mitral and tricuspid valves. Note also that the deceleration time is shorter with inspiration (150 msec) than with expiration in the mitral tracing. Reciprocal changes are noted in the tricuspid valve flow patterns. (From Oh JK, Hatle LK, Seward JB, et al: Diagnostic role of Doppler echocardiography in constrictive pericarditis. J Am Coll Cardiol 23:154, 1994; with the permission of the American College of Cardiology Foundation.)

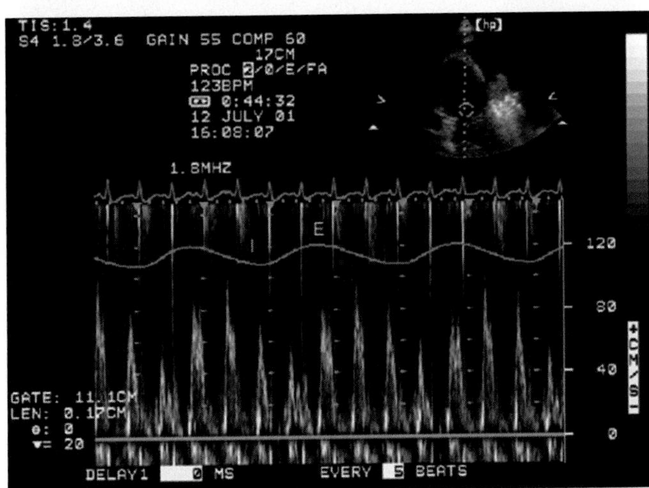

FIGURE 11–104 Pulsed Doppler of the mitral valve inflow in a patient with hemodynamically significant pericardial effusion. Note the exaggerated respiratory variation of inflow with greater than 25 percent variation in e-wave velocity. A respirometer tracing is superimposed on the pulsed Doppler flow velocity. E = expiration; I = inspiration.

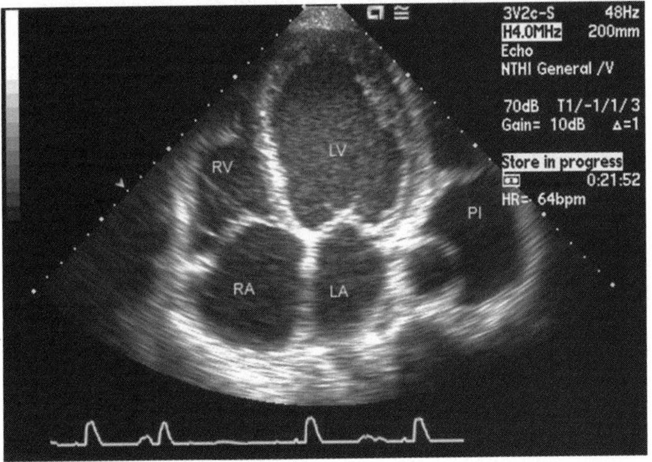

FIGURE 11–106 Apical four-chamber view of a patient with a dilated cardiomyopathy. Note the dilation of all four chambers and the relatively spherical geometry of the left ventricular cavity. Incidental note is made of a pleural effusion (PI). LA = left atrium; LV = left ventricle; RA = right atrium; RV = right ventricle.

than 10 percent to only mildly diminished. Although dilated cardiomyopathy is a global process, because of regional wall stress and loading conditions, regional heterogeneity of function is seen.[138] Typically, the proximal portions of the infero-posterior and posterolateral walls have relatively preserved systolic function, whereas the more distal walls, the ventricular septum, and apex appear more severely compromised. This pattern of wall motion may initially be confused with ischemic heart disease. The absence of frank scar or aneurysm and the absence of any truly normally functioning segments

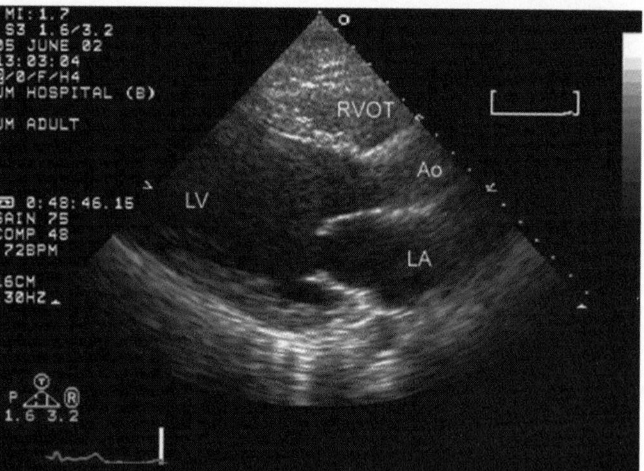

A

B

FIGURE 11–107 Parasternal long-axis views of a patient with a dilated cardiomyopathy recorded in diastole **(A)** and systole **(B)**. Note in the lower panel, the mitral valve is now closed (arrow), however, there is little visible change in the size of the left ventricular cavity. Ao = aorta; LA = left atrium; LV = left ventricle; RVOT = right ventricular outflow tract.

should lead the observer to appropriately make a diagnosis of nonischemic cardiomyopathy. The echocardiographic appearance of nonischemic cardiomyopathy is not dependent on its cause, and patients with alcoholic, doxorubicin (Adriamycin)–induced, idiopathic, or postviral causes all have a similar echocardiographic appearance.

As a consequence of left ventricular dilation, the bullet-shaped geometry of the left ventricle is often distorted and the left ventricle becomes more spherical. This has the effect of drawing the papillary muscles away from the mitral valve annulus and results in functional mitral regurgitation due to abnormal coaptation of the mitral valve (see Fig. 11–57).[102,103] Mitral regurgitation severity may range from mild to severe, and, as a consequence, left atrial dilation to some degree is invariably present. Because of the diffuse nature of the initial insult, the right ventricle can be primarily affected with dilation and hypokinesis and also secondarily affected due to subsequent pulmonary hypertension. Other complications of dilated cardiomyopathy that should be evaluated include the presence of left ventricular thrombus and, in certain circumstances, development of left atrial thrombi. Detection of the latter requires TEE. The magnitude of secondary tricuspid regurgitation and pulmonary hypertension can be reliably determined from Doppler evaluation of the tricuspid valve. Evaluation of diastolic properties of the left ventricle may provide valuable prognostic information. Generally, mitral valve inflow patterns showing a "restrictive pattern" with a high E/A ratio or pseudonormalization confer a substantially worse prognosis.[139-141] Other echocardiographic features associated with a worse prognosis include increased left atrial size[142] and mitral and tricuspid regurgitation.[143]

HYPERTROPHIC CARDIOMYOPATHY

Hypertrophic cardiomyopathy is a heterogeneous disease in which there is inappropriate, pathological hypertrophy of the left ventricle and, less commonly, the right ventricle. The classic form of hypertrophic cardiomyopathy was previously termed *idiopathic hypertrophic subaortic stenosis*. In this entity, there is characteristic disproportionate hypertrophy of the proximal ventricular septum with dynamic left ventricular outflow tract obstruction (Fig. 11–108). Because hypertrophic cardiomyopathy is a heterogeneous disease, the preferred terminology is *hypertrophic cardiomyopathy*, secondarily described as focal, concentric, apical, and with or without obstruction.

From an echocardiographic perspective, outflow obstructive hypertrophic cardiomyopathy is associated with systolic anterior motion of the mitral valve. This results in development of a dynamic systolic gradient that develops in the left ventricular outflow tract over the course of systole (Fig. 11–109). Thus, the maximum gradient is in late systole as opposed to early or midsystole, which is characteristic of a fixed valvular or other discrete obstruction. Systolic anterior motion of the mitral valve can be detected with two-dimensional echocardiography, typically from the parasternal long-axis view, and also with M-mode echocardiography (Fig. 11–110). Although Doppler echocardiography remains the definitive examination for detection and quantification of outflow tract obstruction, secondary evidence of outflow tract obstruction can be

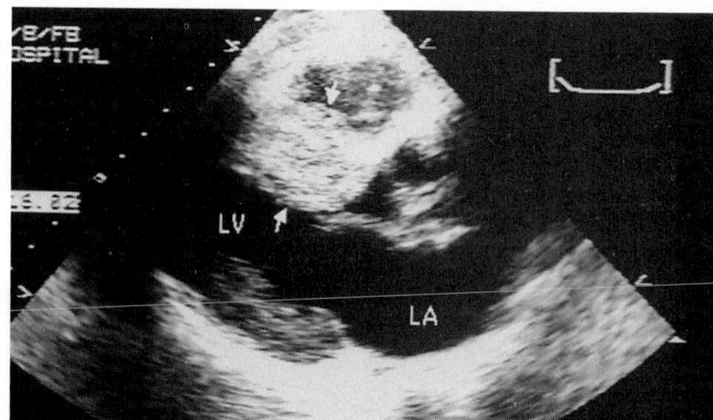

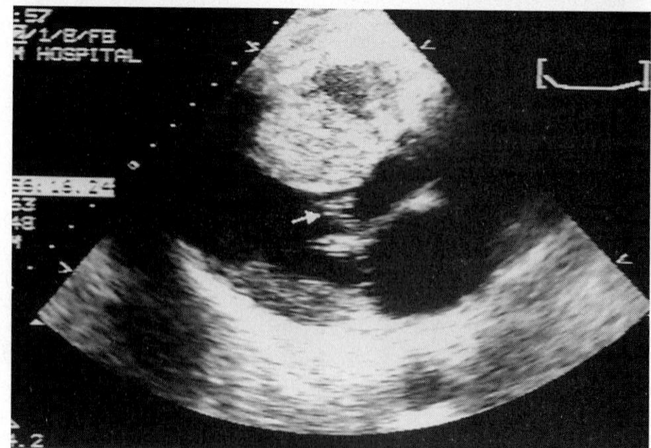

FIGURE 11–108 Parasternal long-axis views recorded in a patient with a hypertrophic cardiomyopathy. The **top panel** is diastole and the **bottom panel** is systole. (Note this image has been recorded in tissue harmonic imaging and therefore myocardial signatures and brightness are increased. No assumptions regarding tissue characterization should be made from a tissue harmonic image.) In the top panel, note the marked thickening of the ventricular septum (white arrows), which measures approximately 3 cm in thickness. The posterior wall was only mildly hypertrophied. The bottom panel was recorded in systole, and systolic anterior motion of the mitral valve (arrow) is clearly seen. LA = left atrium; LV = left ventricle.

obtained from the M-mode echocardiogram. Systolic anterior motion of the mitral valve that remains in contact with the septum for 40 percent of the systolic cycle is more likely to be associated with significant hemodynamic obstruction. Additionally, the outflow tract obstruction results in a characteristic systolic notching pattern on the aortic valve that is best visualized with M-mode echocardiography.

Mitral regurgitation is common in patients with obstructive hypertrophic cardiomyopathy, and the continuous wave of Doppler spectral profile of the mitral regurgitation may occasionally be confused with outflow tract obstruction. It should be kept in mind that the mitral regurgitation velocity will peak relatively early, whereas the outflow tract obstruction has a characteristic late-peaking "dagger-like" appearance.

Other variants of hypertrophic cardiomyopathy include mid-cavity obstruction, in which case the maximum gradient is typically at the papillary muscle level. An additional form of hypertrophy includes concentric left ventricular hypertrophy that may have no associated outflow tract obstruction. In this instance, patients can be highly symptomatic because of a relatively small left ventricular cavity with markedly elevated diastolic pressures. Additionally, the small cavity, even with supernormal systolic functions, results in a low stroke volume and cardiac output. Occasionally, patients are encountered who have isolated hypertrophy of the lateral or inferior walls (Fig. 11-111). A final variant of hypertrophic cardiomyopathy is the apical variant, which is more common in Asian populations. Deep T-wave inversions across the precordium are seen in this variant. By definition, it is not obstructive.

Two-dimensional echocardiography and Doppler imaging can be used to follow the status of outflow tract gradients at rest or exercise and after either pharmacological, surgical, or, more recently, catheter-based septal reduction therapy.[144] A reduction in both the outflow tract gradient and the severity of mitral regurgitation can be documented after successful therapy. On occasion, patients present with what appears to be a "burned-out" hypertrophic cardiomyopathy. In this instance, unexplained pathological hypertrophy is present with a relatively normal-sized left ventricle that is diffusely hypokinetic. Frequently, systolic function has deteriorated to the point that there is no longer an outflow tract gradient. Any of the forms of hypertrophic cardiomyopathy can result in long-standing elevation of diastolic pressure and secondary pulmonary hypertension.

Restrictive and Infiltrative Cardiomyopathy

Restrictive cardiomyopathies are a family of diseases in which systolic function is relatively preserved until very late stages but the ventricular myocardium is pathologically stiff, leading to chronic elevation of diastolic pressure. Symptoms result because of the elevated diastolic pressures. By definition, obstruction is not present, nor is there a primary cause for abnormal myocardial relaxation. The most common form of restrictive cardiomyopathy is the idiopathic restrictive cardiomyopathy most often seen in the elderly. In this disease, both atria are dilated, wall thickness tends to be at the upper normal limit or mildly hypertrophied, systolic function is within normal limits or only mildly depressed, and there is Doppler evidence of abnormal ventricular filling. Typically, this is manifest as an elevated E/A ratio without exaggerated respiratory variation.

Other causes of restrictive physiology include infiltrative cardiomyopathies, the most common of which is cardiac amyloidosis. Other rarer causes include the glycogen storage diseases and association with other systemic diseases.

Cardiac amyloidosis can manifest as either a primary or a secondary entity and is often associated with amyloid deposits in other organs. Amyloid deposition in the myocardium results in hypertrophy in the absence of hypertension and abnormal myocardial texture, which is noted as a bright "speckling" appearance (Fig. 11–112). Caution is advised when using second harmonic imaging, because this type of instrumentation leads to the appearance of an abnormal myocardial signature as well. There is often evidence of diastolic dysfunction. In the early phases, a reduced E/A ratio with a flat deceleration slope is seen. Later, an elevated E/A ratio occurs, associated with a short deceleration time. This pattern has been associated with a worse prognosis.[145] In patients with advanced amyloid, virtually all cardiac structures, including valve leaflets, are involved. In late phases, systolic dysfunction is seen.

DISTINCTION OF RESTRICTIVE AND CONSTRICTIVE PHYSIOLOGY. The distinction between constrictive pericarditis and a restrictive cardiomyopathy is often clinically problematic. Echocardiography can play several valuable roles in this clinical situation. The first is in the exclusion of primary valvular disease, left ventricular dysfunction, and pulmonary hypertension, which may have resulted in the clinical presentation. Typically, patients in whom this dilemma arises have preserved right and left ventricular systolic function with signs and symptoms of heart failure. Signs and symptoms of right-sided failure often predominate. Other than detection of cardiac amyloid or in patients in whom there are classic findings of constriction, the separation of these two entities relies heavily on Doppler echocardiography. In both cases, the E/A ratio is elevated, but in cases of constriction there is a greater than usual respiratory variation

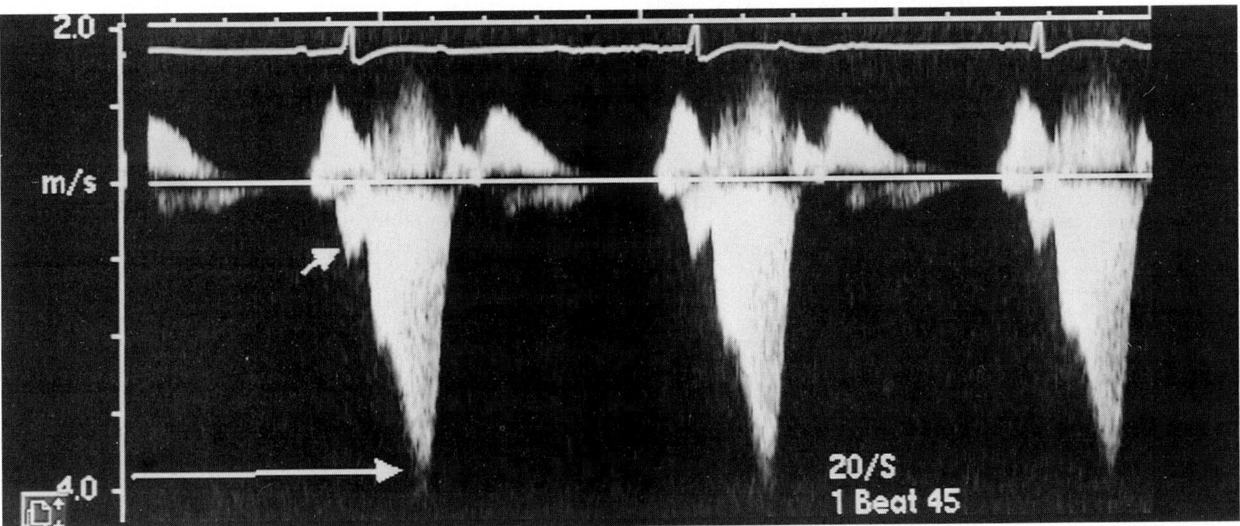

FIGURE 11–109 Continuous-wave Doppler recorded from the apex of the left ventricle with the interrogation being directed through the left ventricular outflow tract in a patient with an obstructive hypertrophic cardiomyopathy. Note the late peaking systolic gradient with a peak velocity of approximately 3.8 m/sec (corresponding to a peak pressure gradient of 58 mm Hg). Additionally (small arrow), there is evidence of presystolic forward flow in the left ventricular outflow tract, following atrial systole. This is consistent with a hypertrophied and noncompliant ventricle in which atrial contraction results in presystolic flow in the outflow tract.

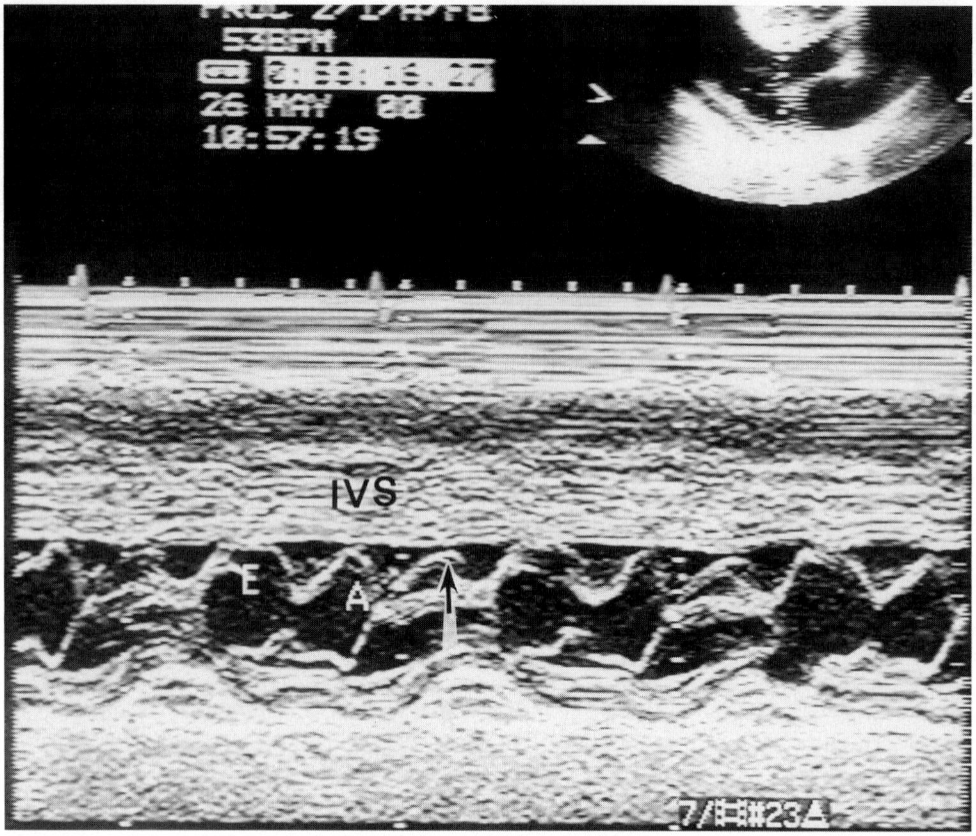

FIGURE 11–110 M-mode echocardiogram recorded in the same patient depicted in Figure 11–108. Note the markedly thickened ventricular septum. The mitral valve as seen directly below the ventricular septum and the E and A waves in diastole are noted. Note in systole there is anterior motion of the mitral valve (black/white arrow).

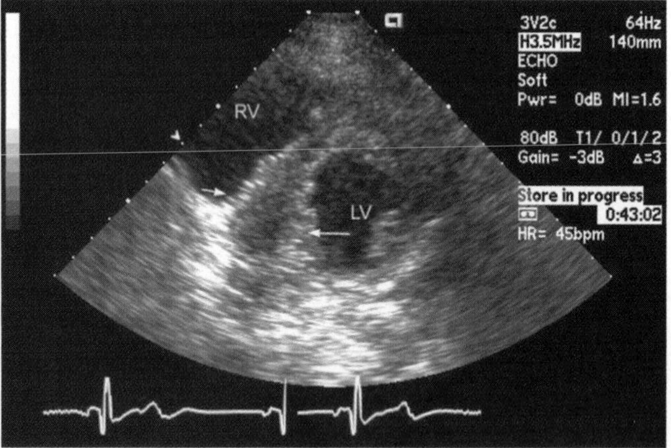

FIGURE 11–111 Transthoracic two-dimensional echocardiogram in a short axis at the midventricular level in a patient with hypertrophic cardiomyopathy. This is a variant of hypertrophic cardiomyopathy in which the predominant hypertrophy is in the true inferior wall and inferior septum. The full thickness of the inferior septum and wall are as noted by the arrows. LV = left ventricle; RV = right ventricle.

in inflow velocities.[146,147] Deceleration time is short in both but varies to a greater degree in restrictive than in constrictive processes. Examination of pulmonary and hepatic vein flow can be helpful as well. In both instances, vein flow is monophasic, but in cases of restriction, there is a greater degree of flow reversal in late diastole coincident with inspiration. Doppler tissue imaging to interrogate the velocity of myocardial relaxation can also play a role. Most patients with restrictive disease have delayed relaxation and delayed motion of the annulus compared with patients with constrictive pericarditis.[148] The diagnosis of constrictive pericarditis and its separation from restrictive diseases remains problematic even in experienced hands, and many atypical cases of each process exist. Both processes can also coexist, and this combination is not uncommon after radiation therapy, in which there may be a constrictive component in the pericardium but a restrictive component to the right ventricle due to radiation injury.

Ischemic Heart Disease

BASIC PRINCIPLES. Myocardial ischemia and infarction result in regional disturbances of ventricular contraction. After acute reduction in coronary flow, both diastolic and systolic dysfunction occur. Normal systolic contraction consists of both myocardial thickening and inward motion of the endocardium (see Figs. 11–12 and 11–14). Immediately after the onset of ischemia, myocardial thickening ceases and, depending on the size of the anatomical area and the severity of ischemia, the wall can become frankly dyskinetic (Figs. 11–113 and 11–114). If blood flow is not restored, myocardial necrosis results and the wall motion abnormality persists. Over a period of approximately 6 weeks, actual tissue loss occurs, and there is replacement by fibrous tissue and a scar forms.

Myocardial Infarction (see Chap. 46)

As noted earlier, myocardial necrosis, once established, results in a permanent wall motion abnormality. The degree of transmural involvement required before wall motion becomes abnormal is approximately 20 percent. The implication of this is that nontransmural myocardial infarction will result in hypokinesis or akinesis of the wall, even though the majority of the myocardial mass may still be perfused and viable. A tethering effect of nontransmural infarction or ischemia results in dysfunction of the entire wall thickness. Because the balance of the myocardium is intrinsically normal, it is capable of overriding this effect during either pharmacological stimulation or stress, therefore resulting in substantial cardiovascular reserve in segments that may be akinetic at rest. The regional wall motion score is directly related to the size of the myocardial infarction; however, because of the tethering phenomenon, wall motion abnormalities overestimate the true anatomical extent.[149]

Tethering occurs in several different forms. The most common occurs in substantial size myocardial infarction where the infarcted area may be frankly dyskinetic. During systole, the dyskinetic segment drags the normal myocardium outward. Thus, this normal myocardium, which intrinsically has the capacity to contract, is tethered to the abnormal myocardium and is functionally abnormal. The opposite phenomenon can occur in patients with relatively small infarctions in whom, during cardiovascular stress, the normal

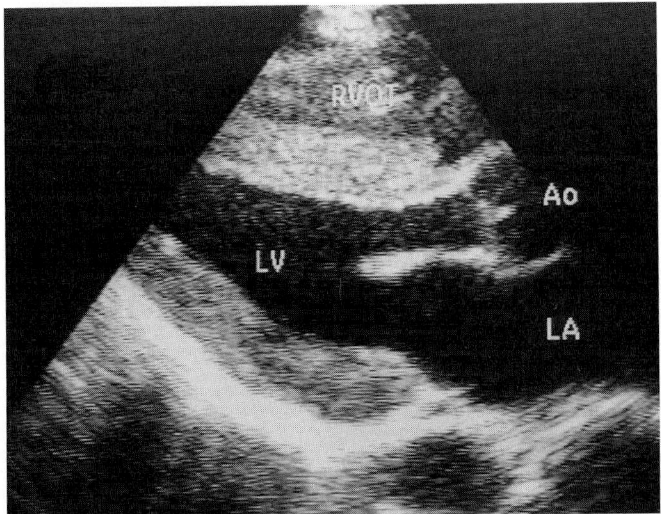

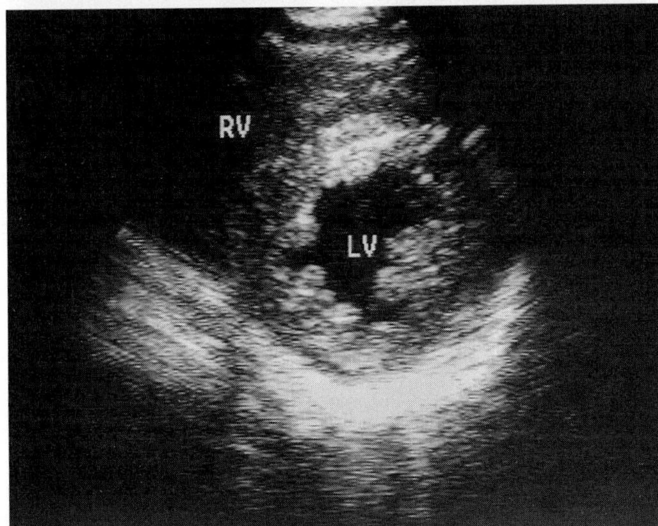

FIGURE 11–112 Two-dimensional echocardiogram recorded in a patient with cardiac amyloid. In both the parasternal long-axis view **(top)** and short-axis view **(bottom)**, note the homogeneous echo intensity of the myocardium. Both the mitral and aortic valves are also thickened. In real time, the myocardium takes on a speckled appearance. Ao = aorta; LA = left atrium; LV = left ventricle; RV = right ventricle.

healthy adjacent myocardium contracts more vigorously and drags the abnormal segment with it, thus masking the wall motion abnormality. A final form of tethering is "vertical" tethering, in which ischemic or infarcted subendocardial layers exert a disproportionate effect on overall myocardial contractility. Because only 20 percent of the myocardium needs to be involved in the ischemic or infarction process for the entire wall to become dysfunctional, nontransmural (non-Q-wave myocardial infarction) results in a wall motion abnormality that is indistinguishable from that of transmural infarction.

More recently advanced Doppler-based methods have been used to detect and quantify wall motion abnormalities. Both Doppler tissue imaging and strain rate imaging have shown promise as a sensitive means for detecting systolic and diastolic abnormalities during ischemia.[150,151]

Depending on the location and size of the necrotic area, ventricular remodeling will also occur. Remodeling takes several forms and ranges from formation of a frank aneurysm (Figs. 11–115 and 11–116) to progressive left ventricular dilation. Echocardiographically, an aneurysm is defined as a noncontracting area of myocardium with abnormal geometry in both diastole and systole.

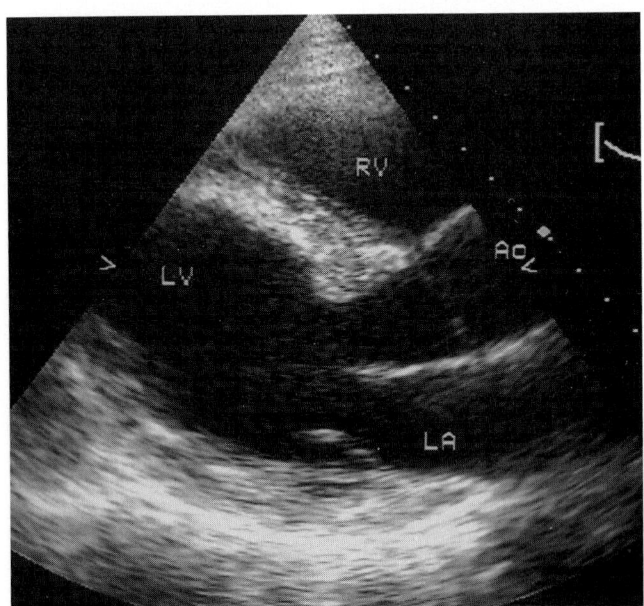

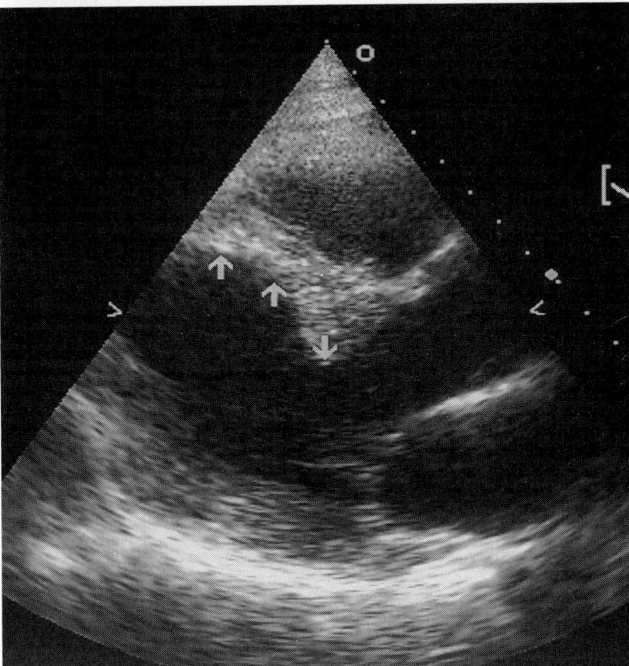

FIGURE 11–113 Transthoracic echocardiogram recorded in a patient with an acute anterior anteroseptal myocardial infarction. This tracing was recorded in a parasternal long-axis view, in diastole **(top)** and in systole **(bottom)**. In the lower panel, note the normal downward motion of the proximal portion of the ventricular septum and the dyskinesis of the more distal portions of the anterior septum (upward arrows). Ao = aorta; LA = left atrium; LV = left ventricle; RV = right ventricle.

In clinical echocardiography, a regional wall motion abnormality, conforming to a known coronary distribution, is the hallmark of acute ischemia or myocardial infarction. Detection of a wall motion abnormality with echocardiography can be a valuable adjunct in the diagnosis of ischemia in patients who are presenting with chest pain.[152-154] After successful reperfusion, wall motion abnormalities typically will resolve. The time course over which they resolve is variable and may range from 12 hours to 2 weeks. Typically, wall motion abnormalities recover within 72 hours if blood flow has been restored in a timely fashion.

At the time of a patient's presentation with acute myocardial infarction, there are several echocardiographic findings that relate to prognosis. As with all imaging techniques, the

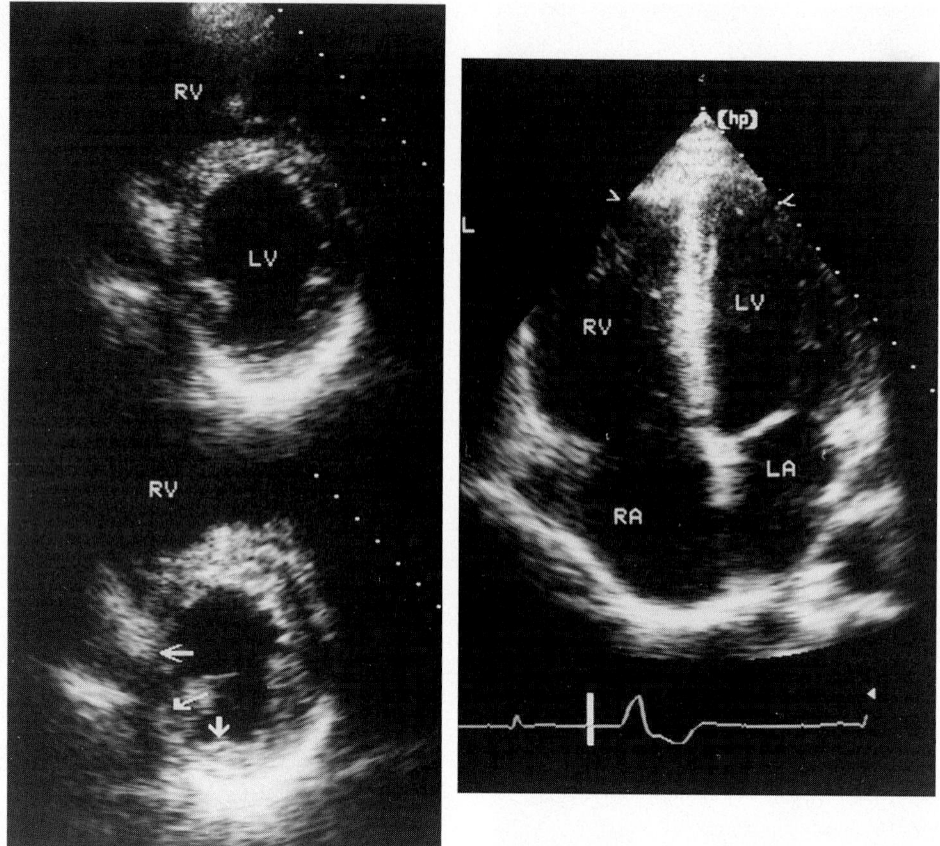

FIGURE 11–114 Two-dimensional echocardiogram recorded in a patient with an inferior myocardial infarction complicated by right ventricular infarction. The **left panel** shows two parasternal short-axis views recorded at the level of the papillary muscles. The **top left** is recorded in diastole. Note the full-thickness myocardium and the circular geometry of the left ventricle (LV). In systole **(bottom left)**, the inferior wall (arrows) becomes frankly dyskinetic and fails to show normal systolic thickening, whereas the remaining walls thickened appropriately and moved inward. The **right panel** is an apical four-chamber view demonstrating a dilated right ventricle (RV) that is globally hypokinetic in real time. This is consistent with right ventricular involvement. LA = left atrium; RA = right atrium.

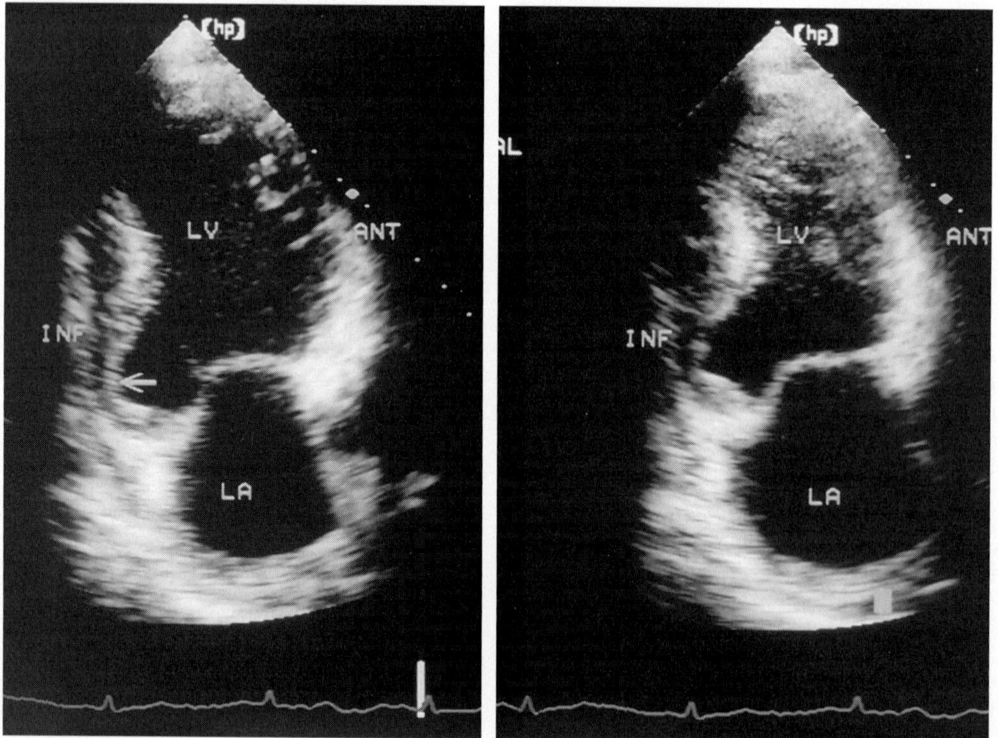

FIGURE 11–115 Apical two-chamber view of a patient with a remote inferior myocardial infarction. The proximal third of the inferior wall (INF) is thin, with distorted geometry consistent with a basilar aneurysm. The **right panel** was recorded in systole, and this area can be seen to bulge further compared with the remaining ventricular walls, which contract normally. ANT = anterior; INF = inferior; LA = left atrium; LV = left ventricle.

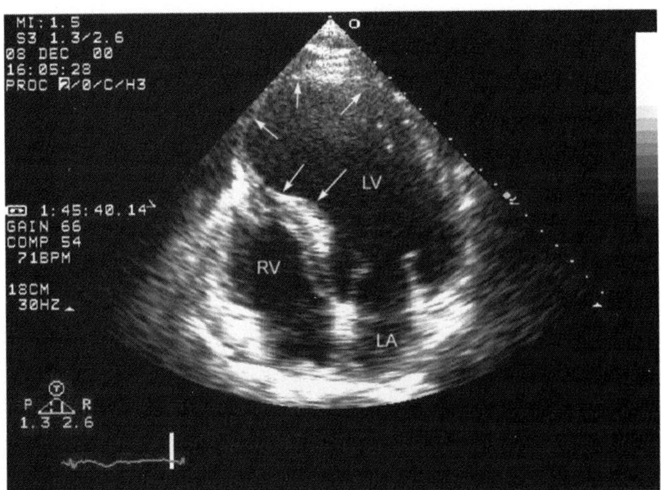

FIGURE 11–116 Apical four-chamber view recorded in a patient with a large anteroapical aneurysm. Note the marked distortion in geometry seen in this diastolic frame with marked aneurysmal bulging of the distal septum and apex (arrows). LA = left atrium; LV = left ventricle; RV = right ventricle.

greater the degree of left ventricular dysfunction found, the greater the likelihood is of complications such as the development of heart failure and death.[155] The size of the myocardial infarction can be approximated with echocardiography by calculating a wall motion score or by calculation of an ejection fraction. Both of these values can be tracked over time to determine the recovery of function. Evaluation of the mitral valve inflow with Doppler echocardiography provides valuable prognostic information as well. Because myocardial ischemia causes immediate diastolic abnormalities, mitral valve inflow patterns become abnormal early in the course of myocardial infarction. One can anticipate an abnormal (typically reduced) E/A ratio in patients with myocardial ischemia. With more substantial areas of ischemia and greater degrees of diastolic dysfunction, an increased E/A ratio, suggesting restrictive physiology, can be seen. This is of more ominous prognostic significance.[156,157] Additionally, development of mitral regurgitation in association with myocardial infarction confers a worse prognosis.

COMPLICATIONS OF MYOCARDIAL INFARCTION. Table 11-5 outlines the complications of myocardial infarction that can be reliably detected using two-dimensional echocardiography. Virtually all mechanical complications are accurately identified.

Left ventricular thrombi may form in the first 24 hours after myocardial infarction and are most commonly seen in anterior infarctions with large areas of apical dyskinesis. They are far less common in cases of inferior wall myocardial infarction. Thrombi can present either as laminar, pedunculated, or mobile masses (Fig. 11-117). There is a substantially greater likelihood of subsequent embolization in mobile and pedunculated thrombi than in sessile and laminar thrombi.

Infarct expansion is defined as progressive dilation of the infarct zone without recurrent myocardial necrosis.[158] This can occur either acutely, after myocardial infarction, in which case it can be confused with reinfarction, or more chronically over the first 3 to 6 months. When infarct expansion (remodeling) occurs acutely it is seen in the substrate of necrotic and highly friable myocardium. Acute infarct expansion manifests as an aneurysm appearing in the first 72 hours, is the anatomical precursor of free wall rupture and ventricular septal defect, and carries a grave prognosis. Chronic infarct expansion occurs over several months, and the likelihood of mechanical complications is low. It results in tethering of normal walls and progressive chamber dilation with reduction in overall systolic performance. It has been linked to development of both arrhythmias and progressive congestive heart failure.

Pericardial effusion occurs in approximately 40 percent of patients with transmural myocardial infarction. It is often asymptomatic and detected only with echocardiographic scanning. A pericardial effusion

TABLE 11–5 Complications of Myocardial Infarction Detected by Echocardiography

EARLY
Pericardial effusion
Infarct expansion
Thrombus formation
Myocardial rupture
Free wall
Ventricular septal defect
Papillary muscle
Functional mitral regurgitation
Right ventricular infarction
LATE
Infarct expansion
Left ventricular aneurysm
Left ventricular thrombus
Pericardial effusion
Functional mitral regurgitation

occurring in the presence of acute infarct expansion is far more worrisome and may be one of the earlier signs of partial myocardial rupture.

Myocardial Rupture. The myocardium can rupture in one of three locations. In each case, infarct expansion usually precedes rupture. Free wall rupture complicates approximately 3 percent of unintervened acute myocardial infarction and is usually not a survivable event. Clinically, patients with myocardial rupture present with recurrent pain and rapidly develop pericardial effusion and tamponade, and death results. In rare instances, echocardiography has been used to document the presence of free wall rupture and allow emergency corrective surgery. A pseudoaneurysm forms when a partial rupture spontaneously seals off, resulting in an extra cardiac chamber, the walls of which consist of pericardium and thrombus. It typically connects to the left ventricle with a narrow mouth, distinguishing it from a true aneurysm, which communicates with the left ventricular cavity by way of a wide opening.

Rupture of either a papillary muscle or the ventricular septum results in signs and symptoms of heart failure and a prominent holosystolic murmur, owing to acute mitral regurgitation or ventricular septal defect (Figs. 11-118, 11-119, and 11-120). Two-dimensional echocardiography is a highly accurate technique for separating the two entities. Because of the critically ill nature of these individuals, many of them are intubated and TEE may be necessary to establish the diagnosis. Once the diagnosis is established, the degree of mechanical disruption can be determined. Additionally, echocardiography can be used to assess left and right ventricular function. Both of these are critical components of risk assessment when planning surgical intervention. Ventricular septal defect with concurrent right ventricular dysfunction carries a substantially greater risk of mortality.

RIGHT VENTRICULAR INFARCTION. Some degree of right ventricular dysfunction accompanies a large proportion of patients with inferior infarction due to occlusion of the proximal right coronary artery. Both systolic and diastolic dysfunction occur, and variable degrees of tricuspid regurgitation are common. Depending on which right ventricular branches are involved, the right ventricular wall motion abnormality can be either apical or more laterally located. Frequently, all that is noted is right ventricular dilation with fairly uniform hypokinesis of the right ventricle (see Fig. 11-114).[159] In many instances, right ventricular ischemia is a transient phenomenon and there is fairly rapid recovery of function. An additional complication of right ventricular infarction is the opening of a patent foramen ovale with subsequent right-to-left shunting. Shunts of significant size can result in arterial oxygen desaturation. The presence of a right-to-left shunt can be reliably documented with saline contrast echocardiography.

In patients with severe multivessel disease, an ischemic cardiomyopathy can develop. This term refers to diffuse global left ventricular systolic dysfunction as a consequence of severe, multivessel coronary artery disease. In many cases, there have been multiple, unrecognized acute myocardial infarctions. This type of cardiomyopathy presents as a nearly globally hypokinetic ventricle, often with patchy areas of wall thinning but without distinct aneurysm. Secondary mitral regurgitation is common and is due to papillary muscle dysfunction and dilation of the mitral valve annulus.

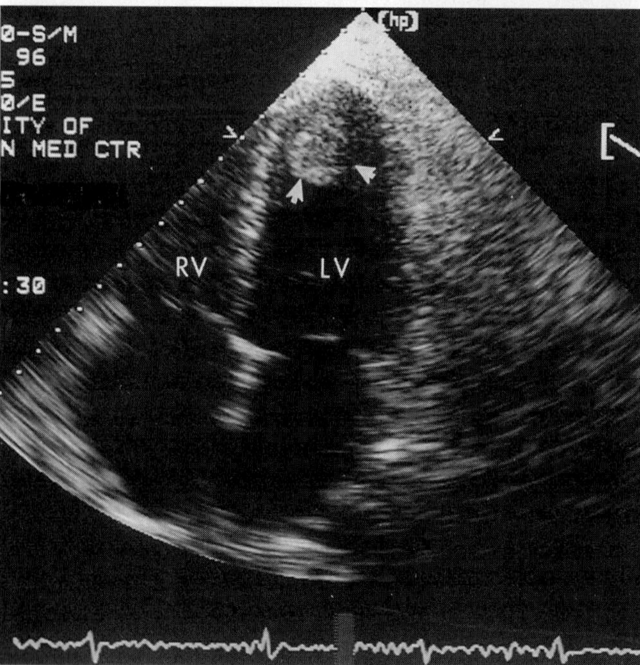

FIGURE 11–117 Apical four-chamber views recorded in two different patients with anterior infarct and left ventricular thrombus. The **top panel** denotes a large laminar thrombus filling a substantial portion of the apex and adherent to the ventricular septum (arrows). The **bottom panel** denotes a smaller, more spherical thrombus in the apex of the patient with a more limited apical myocardial infarction (arrows). LA = left atrium; LV = left ventricle; RA = right atrium; RV = right ventricle.

Myocardial Stunning and Hibernation (see Chap. 44)

There are two phenomena that result in potentially reversible myocardial dysfunction.[160] The first of these is myocardial stunning, which occurs after a severe acute ischemic insult. In this scenario, flow is restored and there is no myocardial necrosis. The exact physiological causes of myocardial stunning are not fully understood, but the syndrome results in spontaneous recovery of myocardial function after restitution of blood flow. Typically, myocardial function recovers in 1 to 7 days. Echocardiography can be used to track recovery of function in patients with this syndrome, and dobutamine stress echocardiography is an excellent means of predicting viability.

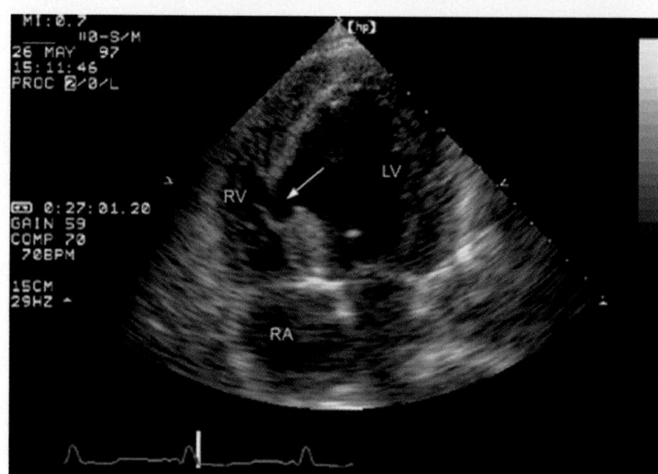

A

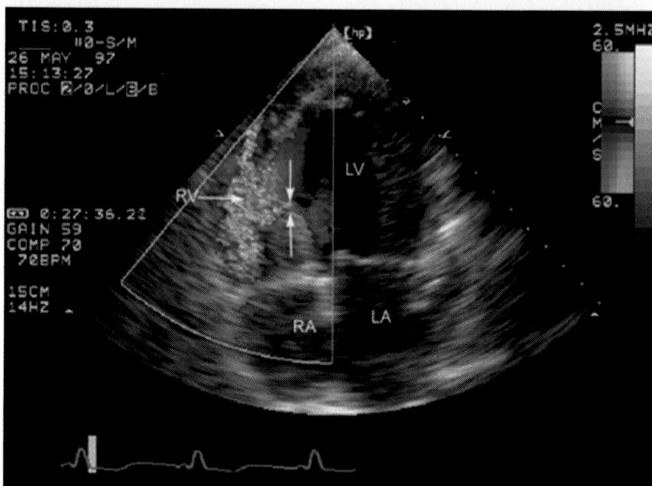

B

FIGURE 11–118 Apical four-chamber views in a patient with an acute anteroseptal myocardial infarction and a postinfarct ventricular septal defect. **A,** Routine two-dimensional image; **B,** accompanying color Doppler image. In panel **A**, there is a distinct break in the continuity of the ventricular septum (arrow) representing the ventricular septal defect with communication between the left and right ventricle. In panel **B**, color Doppler flow imaging has been used to demonstrate the high-velocity turbulent flow from the left ventricle to the right ventricle. LA = left atrium; LV = left ventricle; RA = right atrium; RV = right ventricle.

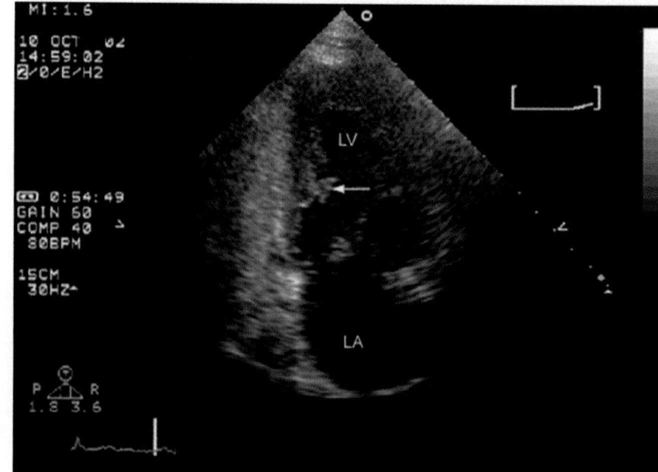

FIGURE 11–119 Transthoracic apical view demonstrating a ruptured papillary muscle in a patient with an acute myocardial infarction. Significant mitral regurgitation was present in this patient, in whom a remnant of the papillary muscle head (arrow) can be seen along the inferior wall. LA = left atrium; LV = left ventricle.

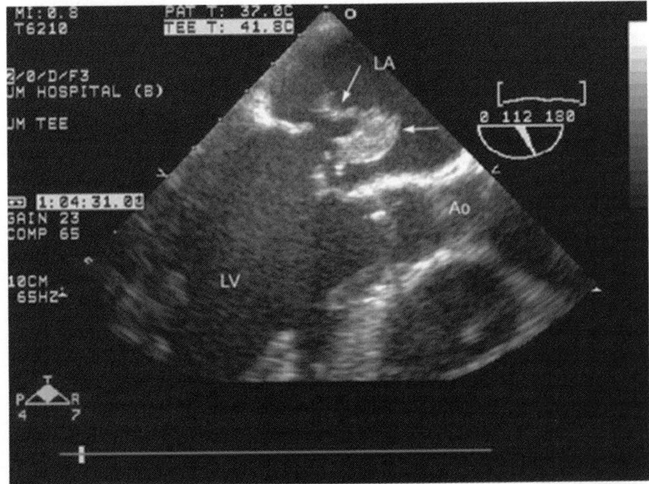

A

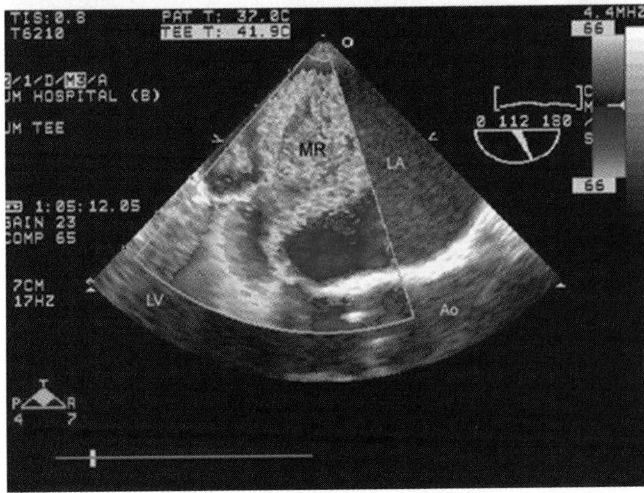

B

FIGURE 11–120 Transesophageal echocardiogram recorded in a patient with an acute myocardial infarction and complete rupture of a papillary muscle. **A,** Recorded in a longitudinal view in systole; a large, bulky muscular mass can be seen prolapsing into the left atrium (arrows). This represents the body of a papillary muscle. **B,** Recorded in the same view, using color flow imaging; demonstrates the presence of severe mitral regurgitation. Ao = aorta; LA = left atrium; LV = left ventricle.

Myocardial hibernation is a similar phenomenon usually encountered in a chronic case. Conceptually, hibernation represents myocardial dysfunction related to reduced coronary blood flow with no identifiable acute event. In many instances, what has been termed "myocardial hibernation" may represent repetitive stunning. In either scenario, functional recovery of the myocardium occurs after successful revascularization. As in cases of stunning, dobutamine stress echocardiography is an excellent means for detecting hibernation myocardium.[161-164]

Stress Echocardiography

Stress echocardiography is a family of examinations in which two-dimensional echocardiographic monitoring is undertaken before, during, and after cardiovascular stress. It has been shown to be a cost-effective means for evaluating patients presenting with chest pain. The form of cardiovascular stress can include exercise with treadmill or bicycle ergometry. By evaluating wall motion at rest and then comparing myocardial performance at stress, one obtains indicators of inducible ischemia that can be assigned to specific coronary territory (Figs. 11–25 and 11–121). Although treadmill exercise is often more familiar to patients, it is limited by the need to image only at rest and after exercise. It is not possible to successfully image an upright walking individual. Bicycle exercise provides the opportunity to image at each sequential stage of stress, and therefore peak exercise images are available.

For patients incapable of physical exercise, pharmacological stress, most commonly employing a dobutamine infusion, can be used. These protocols typically rely on an incremental infusion protocol of 10, 20, 30, and 40 μg/kg/min, augmented by atropine to obtain an adequate heart rate response when necessary. Images can be obtained at each stage of dobutamine infusion. Patients with significant obstructive coronary disease develop regional wall motion abnormalities identical to those seen during physical stress. The safety record of dobutamine has been excellent, and its accuracy appears equivalent to that of exercise echocardiography. An alternative to dobutamine is dipyridamole infusion, which relies on provocation of ischemia by differential vasodilation in normal and diseased arteries.

All of the different exercise echocardiography modalities have been validated against coronary arteriography as a standard and appear to have accuracy equivalent to the competing radionuclide procedures (Table 11–6; see also Chap. 13).[165-179] In general, the sensitivity of thallium scintigraphy tends to be slightly higher than that of exercise echocardiography, whereas the specificity of exercise echocardiography typically has been higher than that of thallium. As with all other forms of cardiovascular stress, exercise echocardiography has distinct advantages and disadvantages. Even in experienced laboratories, there may be a 5 percent failure rate due to suboptimal imaging. Patients in whom adequate levels of cardiovascular stress have not been obtained will not have positive study findings, even in the presence of coronary disease. The clinical utility and value of stress echocardiography has been specifically evaluated in female populations. In female populations, it appears to be an effective clinical tool for diagnosis and prognosis, but with a slightly lower overall accuracy than seen in male patients. Accuracy also appears to be preserved in the elderly and in hypertensive patients. Accuracy can be reduced in patients with left bundle branch block, who have a septal wall motion abnormality due to the conduction disturbance.

In addition to the diagnosis of coronary disease, stress echocardiography has been used extensively for determining patient prognosis in general populations[180-187] and after myocardial infarction[188,189] as well as in tracking results of percutaneous interventions. It plays a major role in determining myocardial viability in suspected cases of stunning or hibernation.[161-164] Dobutamine stress echocardiography has seen substantial success in determining preoperative risk assessment in patients undergoing noncardiac surgery.[190] Its accuracy for predicting cardiac events of myocardial infarction and death after major vascular surgery is equivalent to or greater than that of competing thallium scintigraphic techniques.

Myocardial Contrast Echocardiography

Myocardial contrast echocardiography is a field in evolution that shows tremendous promise for providing information about myocardial perfusion from contrast enhanced echocardiograms.[191-194] It should be emphasized that its utilization remains investigational, and a substantial amount of technical skill and expertise as well as specialized imaging equipment may be required for its appropriate utilization. As noted in the section on contrast echocardiography, modern perfluorocarbon-based agents are capable of transpulmonary passage, after which they perfuse virtually all organs, including the ventricular myocardium (Fig. 11-122). The appearance of contrast in the myocardium parallels the distribution of myocardial blood flow, and parameters of its appearance in the myocardium parallel actual coronary flow.

In the simplest analysis, the absence of contrast in the ventricular myocardium implies the absence of significant capillary level flow, whereas homogeneous opacification of the myocardium implies normal capillary flow. Intermediate levels of contrast appearance suggest delayed capillary flow and suggest the presence of underlying obstructive coronary artery disease. Animal experimentation has demonstrated that the presence of contrast in the ventricular myocardium is a highly accurate marker of perfused versus nonperfused myocardium and accurately identifies infarct areas following total coronary occlusion. Similarly, total absence of contrast in the myocardium in human clinical studies has been correlated with the presence of myocardium infarction (Fig. 11-123). Preserved capillary flow as demonstrated by myocardial contrast echocardiography is also an accurate predictor of myocardial viability.[195,196]

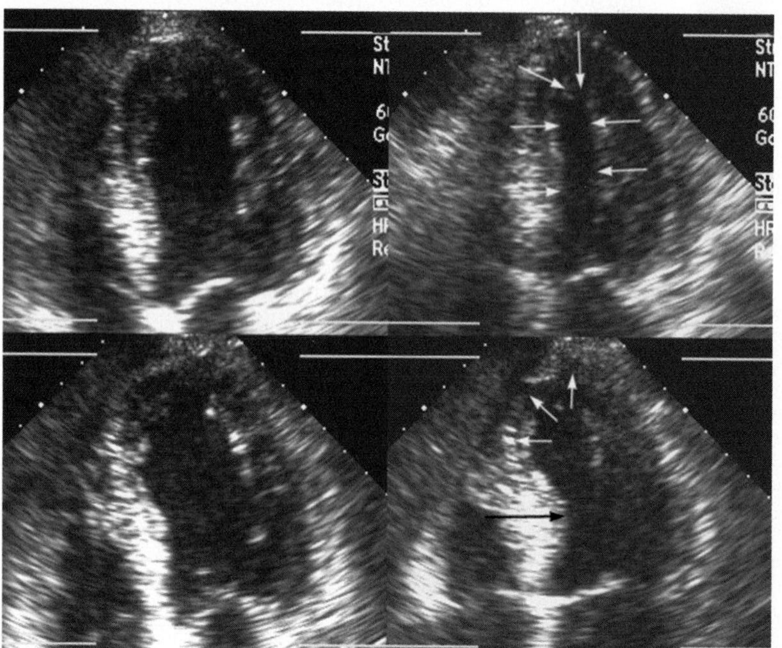

FIGURE 11–121 Stress echocardiogram in a patient with an obstructive lesion of the left anterior descending coronary artery. All four panels are four-chamber views. The **upper panels** were recorded at rest and reveal normal motion of all walls (white arrows); the **lower panels** were recorded immediately following stress. The **right lower panel** is an end-systolic frame immediately following exercise in which normal appropriate motion of the proximal septum (black arrow) is noted. The more distal portions of the septum and apex, however, were frankly dyskinetic (white arrows) indicating ischemia in the left anterior descending artery distribution.

In an effort to refine the technique, it is important to determine the time-of-appearance curve contrast in the myocardium. To create a time-activity curve of contrast in the myocardium requires creation of "a bolus effect" in which contrast flows into a previously unopacified myocardium. The most effective method for creating a bolus effect is to use a myocardial perfusion agent as a continuous infusion in which its presence in the bloodstream can be considered constant and therefore, its presence in the coronary bed stable. To create a bolus effect the mechanical index of the ultrasound beam is transiently increased to acutely destroy all of the contrast in the myocardium, after which the myocardium refills with contrast and its appearance time and intensity can then be tracked.[191] This maneuver can be repeated on multiple occasions to create several different time-activity curves, either under basal conditions or during pharmacological vasodilation. Figure 11-124 is an example of using this technique in which four different bolus effects have been created by transient bubble destruction and then tracking the appearance of contrast. In each example, baseline and vasodilation contrast has been destroyed, leaving a relatively dark appearance to the myocardium. The contrast-enhanced frames for each were recorded five cardiac cycles after bubble destruction. Under basal circumstances, there is definite visible contrast in the myocardium. However, during pharmacological vasodilation, at the same point after destruction, there is a more dramatic contrast effect in the myocardium, implying faster refill time.

Two different characteristics of the appearance curve have relevance for coronary disease. The actual intensity of contrast in the myocardium is directly related to capillary volume (as opposed to being related to actual flow). The plateau level of myocardial intensity is referred to as alpha (α) and the appearance rate or time constant of appearance as beta (β). The product of the two is directly proportional to myocardial blood flow.[191] In the

TABLE 11–6 Accuracy of Stress Echocardiography for Detection of Coronary Artery Disease

Study	Stress	No. of Patients	Sensitivity %	Sensitivity No.	Specificity %	Specificity No.
Armstrong et al.[165]	Treadmill	123	88		86	
Crouse et al.[166]	Treadmill	228	97	170/175	64	34/35
Marwick et al.[167]	Treadmill	150	84	96/114	86	31/36
Roger et al.[168]	Treadmill	150	83	50/60	62	56/90
Beleslin et al.[169]	Treadmill	136	88	105/119	82	14/17
Quinones et al.[170]	Treadmill	112	74	64/86	88	22/26
Ryan et al.[171]	Bike	309	91	193/211	77	76/98
Cohen et al.[172]	Bike	52	78	29/37	87	13/15
Hecht et al.[173]	Bike	180	93	127/137	86	37/43
Luotolahti et al.[174]	Bike	118	93	101/108	70	7/10
Marwick et al.[175]	DSE	217	72	102/142	83	62/75
Ling et al.[176]	DSE	183	93	151/162	62	13/21
Marcovitz and Armstrong[177]	DSE	141	96	105/109	66	21/32
Beleslin et al.[169]	DSE	136	82	98/119	77	13/17
Takeuchi et al.[178]	DSE	120	85	63/74	93	43/46

DSE = dobutamine stress echocardiography.

presence of significant coronary stenosis, the time constant of appearance (β) will be reduced; however, the actual eventual intensity (α) will be equivalent to that in a nondisease state. Creation of time-activity curves such as depicted in Figure 11–124 can provide valuable information regarding the presence of a flow-limiting obstructive coronary lesion. Myocardial contrast echocardiography can be recorded either in real time or using intermittent imaging at variable imaging intervals (1:1, 1:2, 1:4, 1:8, etc.) from which time-intensity curves can be developed.

It should be emphasized that detection of contrast within the myocardium requires highly specialized imaging algorithms, typically relying on analysis of sequential pulses. Much of the contemporary analysis of myocardial contrast cardiograms occurs in a Doppler domain rather than the gray-scale imaging domain. Limitations of the technique include the substantial learning curve, the requirement for highly specialized imaging platforms, and the tendency for more distal structures to be shadowed and thus mimic absence of perfusion. With continued development of agents and imaging platforms as well as experience, myocardial contrast echocardiography has shown tremendous promise as a technique that can give information similar to that provided by competing rate radionuclide perfusion methodologies.

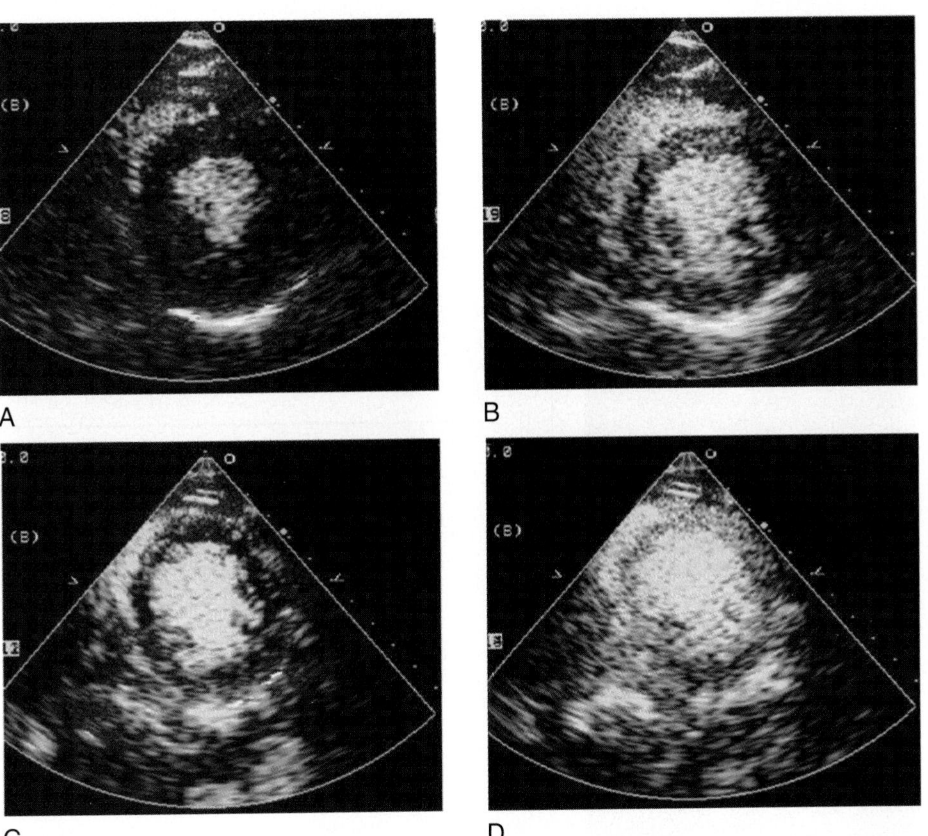

FIGURE 11–122 Myocardial contrast echocardiogram recorded in a patient without obstructive coronary disease. **A** and **B**, Recorded under basal conditions; **C** and **D**, recorded during dipyridamole infusion. Panels **A** and **C** were recorded immediately after a burst of high-intensity ultrasound intended to destroy contrast. Note the relatively dark appearance of the myocardium. Panels **B** and **D** were recorded five cardiac cycles after purposeful microbubble destruction. Under basal conditions **(B)**, note the definite but relatively faint opacification of the myocardium. Panel **D** was recorded five cardiac cycles after purposeful destruction but during infusion of dipyridamole to create a hyperemic response. The intensity of contrast at an equivalent time point after purposeful destruction is substantially greater during dipyridamole infusion than under basal conditions.

DIRECT VISUALIZATION OF CORONARY ARTERIES

Using high-frequency transducers, it is possible to directly visualize the proximal portions of the left main and right coronary arteries (Fig. 11–125). This can be done to identify their takeoff and to exclude anomalous origin of a coronary artery.[197] With scrupulous attention to detail, one can visually characterize the wall of the left main and proximal left interior descending coronary artery and detect areas of atherosclerotic involvement and calcification. Detection of calcification within the proximal left anterior descending coronary artery appears to be a potentially reliable marker that significant obstructive coronary artery disease is present.[198] Proximal coronary artery aneurysms can also be detected in children with Kawasaki disease. Either from the transesophageal or the transthoracic approach, it is also possible to place a Doppler sample volume in the coronary artery lumen and to quantify phasic flow in the coronary artery.[199] It is also possible to use Doppler echocardiography to determine the velocity of flow in the coronary sinus. This can be done both under basal conditions and after vasodilation.

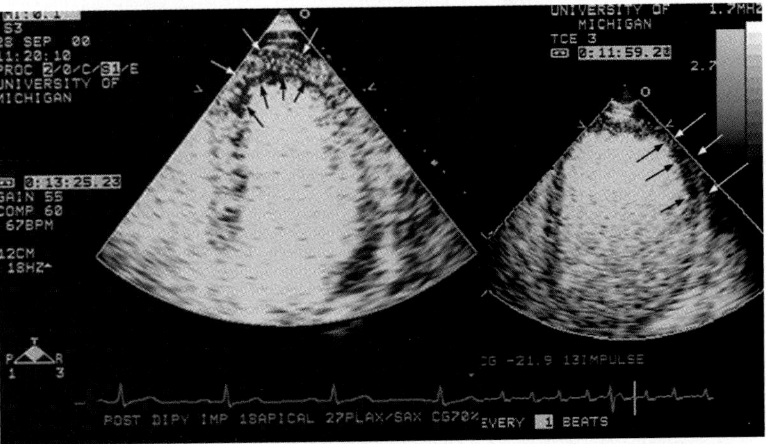

FIGURE 11–123 Myocardial contrast echocardiograms recorded in patients with disease of the mid-left anterior descending coronary artery. Both were recorded using a technique similar to that used for Figure 11–122. **Left,** Selective lack of myocardial contrast in the subendocardium at the apex (black arrows), indicative of absent perfusion in that territory. **Right,** Recorded in a patient with prior lateral wall infarction and reveals transmural loss of contrast effect in the area between the black and white arrows.

Diseases of the Aorta (see Chap. 53)

Transthoracic echocardiography visualizes the proximal 3 to 5 cm of the ascending aorta and portions of the descending thoracic aorta behind the left atrium from parasternal positions. In the majority of patients, a portion of the aortic arch can be visualized from the suprasternal transducer position. The sensitivity for detecting aortic disease is relatively poor from the transthoracic approach. If disease of the aorta is suspected, TEE is usually necessary. TEE provides a high-resolution view of the ascending aorta and descending thoracic aorta as far as the gastroesophageal junction but does not

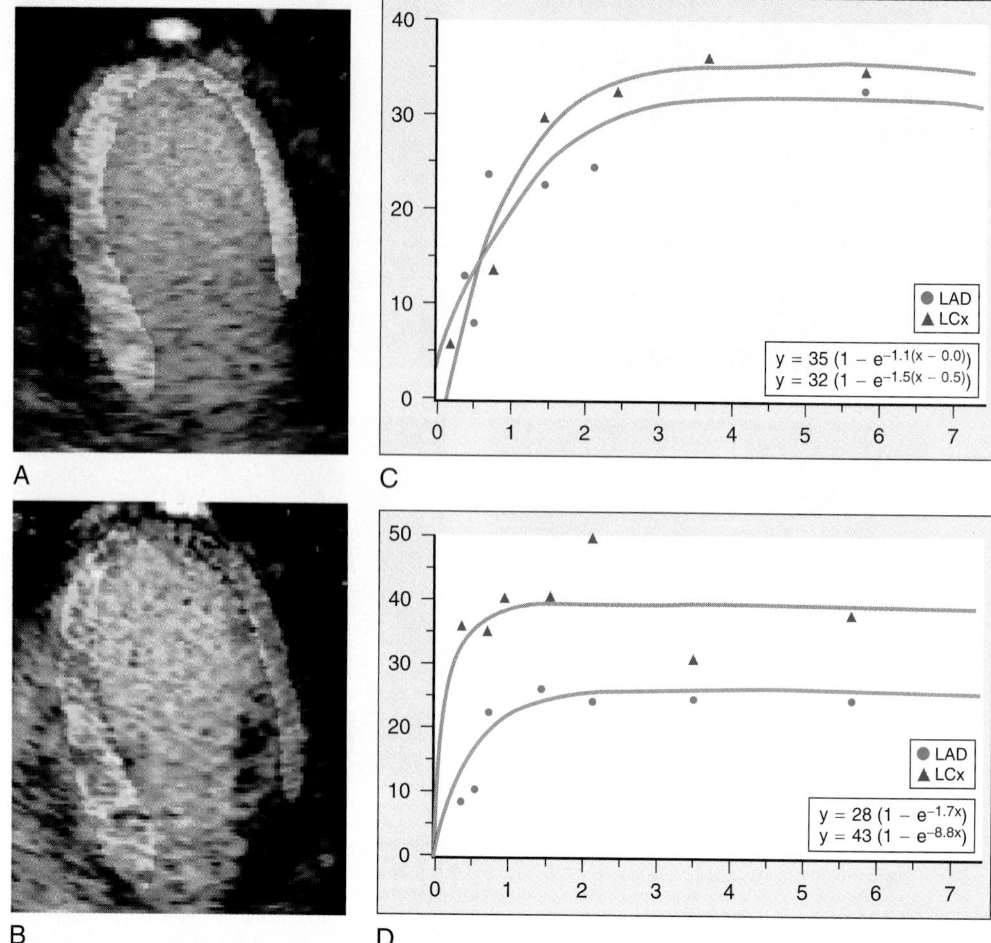

FIGURE 11–124 **A** and **B,** Background subtracted color-coded images from an apical two-chamber view from a patient with a 60 percent left anterior descending artery stenosis. Panel A represents the contrast appearance (contrast minus baseline) at baseline and panel B during hyperemia induced by intravenous adenosine infusion. **C,** Graph representing the time-intensity curve in the left anterior descending (LAD) and left circumflex (LCx) distributions. Note the similar appearance of the curves with respect to their peak video intensity and rate of rise of contrast intensity. **D,** Note the dramatic difference of appearance curves in the LAD and circumflex territories with a substantially reduced video intensity and slower rate of rise to a plateau in a diseased LAD artery, versus the normal circumflex territory. (From Wei K, Ragosta M, Thorpe J, et al: Noninvasive quantification of coronary blood flow reserve in humans using myocardial contrast echocardiography. Circulation. 103:2560, 2001; with permission from the American Heart Association.)

visualize the abdominal aorta. Additionally, there is a very limited area of the aortic arch that may be suboptimally viewed. In many centers, TEE has become the preferred and standard examination for evaluation of patients with suspected aortic disease.

AORTIC DISSECTION. Acute aortic dissection is a life-threatening disease requiring emergency surgical intervention. TTE can be used for early screening and is valuable for detecting aortic dilation, determining whether secondary aortic insufficiency is present, and assessing left ventricular function. Its accuracy for actual detection of the aortic dissection flap and determining its extent is not adequate as a stand-alone technique. TEE has proven to be a highly accurate and reliable technique for diagnosing and excluding aortic dissection, determining its extent, identifying communication points, assessing the severity of aortic insufficiency, and obviously determining complications such as rupture and adventitial hematoma. The accuracy for detection of acute aortic dissection is equivalent to that of CT and MRI (Table 11–7).[200-203]

Aortic dissection is classified by several schemes, all of which are designed to distinguish dissection of the ascending aorta from that confined to the descending thoracic aorta. A dissection flap appears as a thin linear echo within the lumen of the aorta (Fig. 11–126). In patients with connective tissue disease and relatively nonatherosclerotic aortas, the intimal flap is frequently highly mobile. It may take a spiral course as it courses through the descending thoracic aorta. More chronic dissections appear as a linear echo dividing the aorta into two or more lumens. In this instance, the intimal flap may appear thicker and less mobile than in the acute setting. In cases of acute dissection of the ascending aorta, dilation of the ascending aorta is seen in virtually all instances. Other echocardiographic findings of acute aortic dissection include presence of pleural effusion and of adventitial hematoma, which appears as a homogeneous echo-dense mass outside the wall of the aorta tracking along its course.

Specific cardiac features to be noted in aortic dissection include the presence or absence of pericardial effusion and of aortic insufficiency. Aortic insufficiency can be due either to sinotubular dilation with abnormal aortic cusp coaptation, direct extension of the dissection into the annulus, disruption of the support for the aortic valve, or, less commonly, prolapse of a portion of the intimal flap through the aorta, resulting in a conduit for insufficiency.[204]

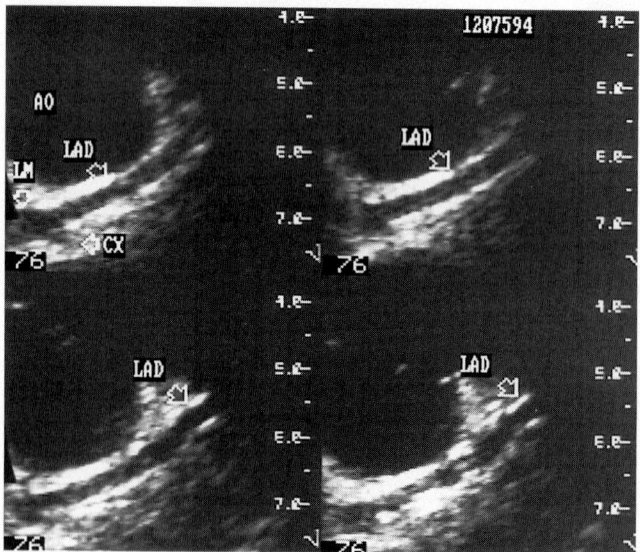

FIGURE 11–125 Transthoracic echocardiogram of the left coronary artery. The left main (LM), left anterior descending (LAD), and a proximal portion of the circumflex (CX) coronary artery are clearly visualized.

TABLE 11–7 Accuracy of Transesophageal Echocardiography for Detection of Aortic Dissection

Study	Year	No. of Patients	No. with Dissection	Sensitivity (n [%])	Specificity (n [%])
Erbel et al.[200]	1989	164	82	81/82 (99)	80/82 (98)
Hashimoto et al.[201]	1989	22	22	22/22 (100)	N/A
Ballal et al.[202]	1991	61	34	33/34 (97)	27/27 (100)
Nienaber et al.[203]	1993	110	44	43/44 (98)	20/26 (77)

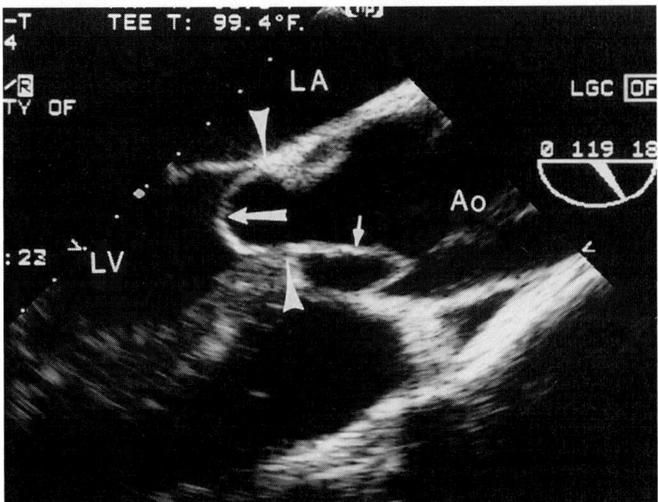

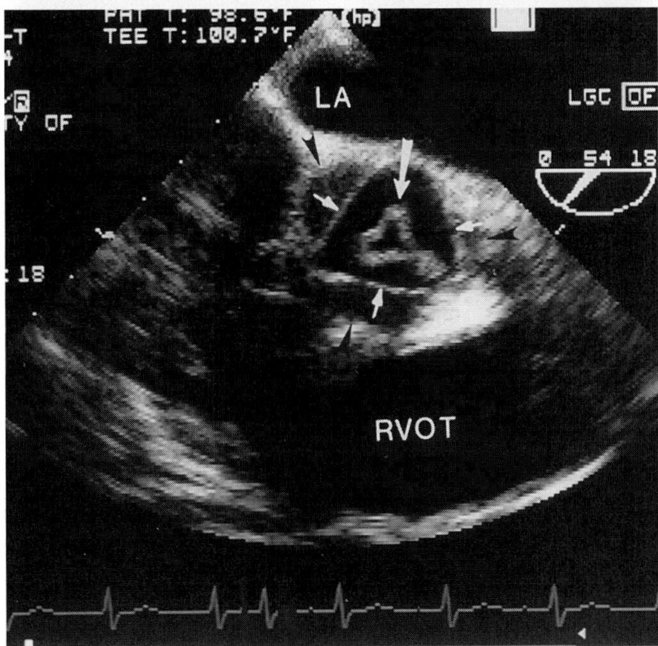

FIGURE 11–126 Transesophageal echocardiogram recorded in a patient with an acute type A dissection of the aorta. The **top panel** is a longitudinal view of the ascending aorta. Note the dilation of the proximal aorta and the thin linear echo present in both in the lumen of the aorta, a portion of which prolapses through the aortic valve into the left ventricular outflow tract (arrows). The white arrowheads denote the actual margins of the aortic annulus. The **bottom panel** is recorded in a view orthogonal to the upper panel and reveals the external diameter of the aorta (black arrowheads) as well as the open three-leaflet aortic valve (small white arrows). Within the actual orifice of the aortic valve is a portion of the dissection tear (large white arrow). Ao = aorta; LA = left atrium; LV = left ventricle; RVOT = right ventricular outflow tract.

The phenomenon of intramural hematoma has recently received much attention. Intramural hematoma often occurs in the setting of underlying atherosclerotic disease and is the result of spontaneous rupture and hemorrhage in the medial layers of the aorta.[205] The syndrome of acute intramural hemorrhage is virtually identical to acute dissection from the standpoint of clinical presentation. Intramural hemorrhage may be a focal process resulting in local breakdown in the medial layers or can result in creation of a dissection plane through the media. By definition, there is no communication between the lumen and the medial space.

AORTIC ANEURYSM. Aneurysm of the ascending aorta, arch, and descending thoracic aorta can be diagnosed and characterized with TEE. Characteristics of the aneurysm as fusiform or discrete and the extent of atherosclerotic involvement and secondary thrombus formation can all be determined. Because thoracic aneurysm without dissection is a chronic process requiring serial evaluation, most centers rely more heavily on CT or MRI for elective follow-up of chronic thoracic aortic aneurysms.

ATHEROSCLEROTIC DISEASE. The transesophageal echocardiogram is an excellent tool for determining the extent and nature of atherosclerotic involvement of the thoracic aorta (Fig. 11–127).[206,207] Atherosclerotic disease can be characterized as focal or diffuse and further characterized as mild, moderate, and severe. Complex and mobile components likewise can be noted and have relevance for embolic phenomena.

MARFAN SYNDROME AND DISEASE OF THE PROXIMAL AORTA. Marfan syndrome is a heritable disorder of connective tissue that results in abnormalities in the proximal aorta. The underlying pathological condition is cystic medial necrosis, which results in characteristic dilation of the proximal aorta, most prominent in the sinuses of Valsalva. There is secondary effacement of the sinotubular junction and dilation of the ascending aorta. Because the predominant area of dilation is in the proximal aorta, TTE often suffices for screening (Fig. 11–128). Complications of the aortic process in patients with Marfan syndrome include progressive dilation with secondary aortic insufficiency and development of aortic dissection. Echocardiography has seen tremendous success in the serial evaluation of these individuals and in the timing of elective surgery.

SINUS OF VALSALVA ANEURYSM. In addition to the characteristic symmetrical dilation seen in patients with Marfan syndrome, aneurysms can arise in the sinus of Valsalva. These range from relatively small and discrete to large "windsock" aneurysms that protrude into the right ventricular outflow tract. On occasion, rupture occurs, leading to a continuous shunt from the aorta into the downstream chamber. The most common site for a sinus of Valsalva aneurysm to rupture is into the right atrium or the right ventricular outflow tract. In this instance, remnants of the aneurysm can be seen prolapsing into the right ventricular outflow tract and high-velocity turbulent flow is noted in the downstream chamber. Because of the rupture, coarse fluttering of the right coronary cusp of the aortic valve may be noted.

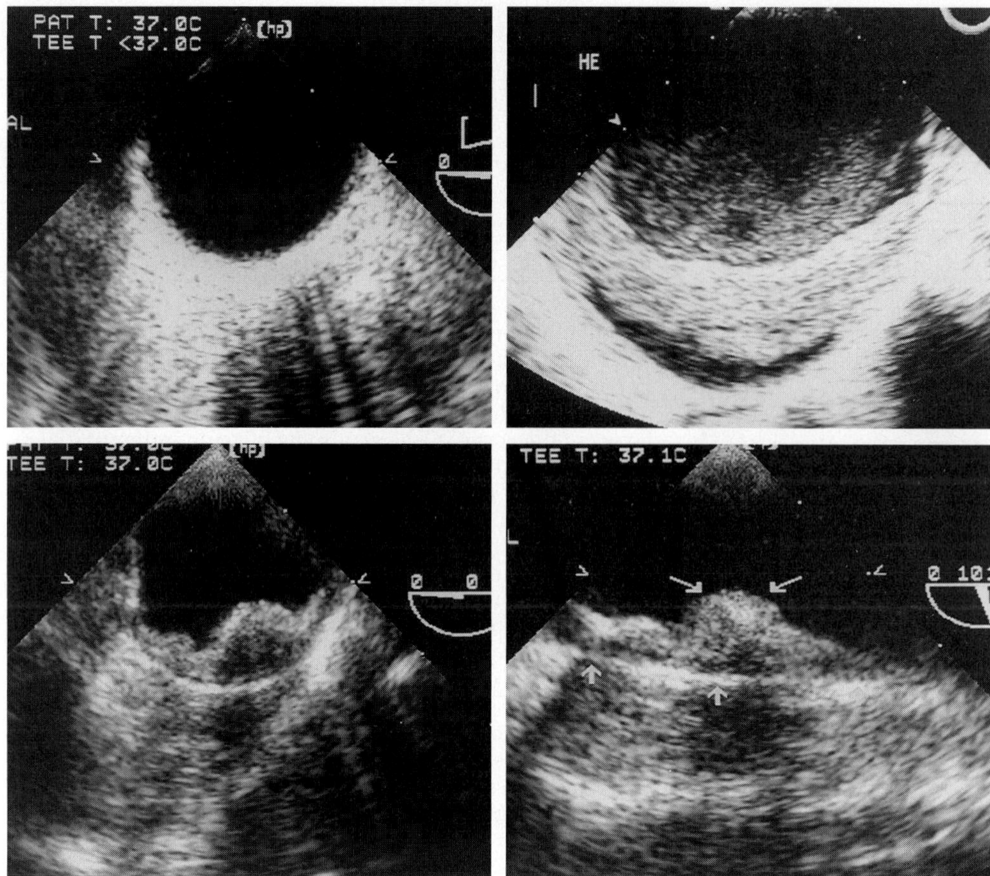

FIGURE 11–127 Transesophageal echocardiograms recorded in three different patients, visualizing the descending thoracic aorta. The **upper left panel** is recorded in a normal, disease-free aorta. Notice the circular geometry and the lack of any thickening or irregularity in the wall of the aorta. The **upper right panel** was recorded in a patient with a large descending thoracic aortic aneurysm measuring approximately 6 cm in its greatest dimension. Note the substantial atherosclerosis present as well as the vague, smoke-like echoes in the lumen of the aorta representing stagnant blood. There is also a lucency posterior to the wall representing spontaneous intramural hemorrhage. The **lower panels** were recorded in a patient with moderately severe atherosclerotic disease of the thoracic aorta. The panel on the **left** was recorded in the transverse view of the aorta. Note the irregular contour of the lumen, which is due to atherosclerotic involvement of the wall. The panel on the **right** was recorded at the same level of the aorta but in a longitudinal projection. The up-pointing arrows denote the outer wall of the aorta. Note the irregularity in the aortic lumen and the protruding atheroma (arrows).

CARDIAC MASSES AND TUMORS (see Chap. 63)

Echocardiography is the primary screening tool for patients with known or suspected intracardiac tumors. Cardiac tumors can be divided into those that are primary to the heart and those that are secondary or metastatic. They can be further divided into benign and malignant types.

Atrial Myxoma. The most common benign primary tumor of the heart is the atrial myxoma. Approximately 75 percent of atrial myxomas are isolated, pedunculated tumors in the left atrium attached to the area of the foramen ovale by a stalk (Fig. 11-129). Less common locations include the right atrium and either ventricle, pulmonary vein, or vena cava. The classic left atrial myxoma is a smooth, relatively homogeneously echo-dense mass with substantial mobility. It moves into the orifice of the mitral valve in diastole and prolapses back into the left atrium in systole. Depending on its size, it may result in functional obstruction of the mitral valve, thereby mimicking mitral stenosis. Concurrent mitral regurgitation is not uncommon. In the presence of a typical appearance of a myxoma, the diagnosis is virtually certain from an echocardiographic standpoint, and no further evaluation may be necessary. Because of the tendency to cause obstruction of the mitral valve, secondary pulmonary hypertension can occur. Additionally, emboli from the surface of the myxoma are not uncommon.

Other Primary Cardiac Tumors. Cardiac lipomas are benign primary cardiac tumors with a broad range of appearances. They are most common in the body of the left ventricle and occasionally may be present as pedunculated masses. Although unlikely to embolize, they can be associated with superimposed thrombus, which can embolize. Echocardiography is useful for identification of the mass but is unable to precisely identify it as lipomatous tissue. MRI has substantially succeeded in tissue characterization of these masses.

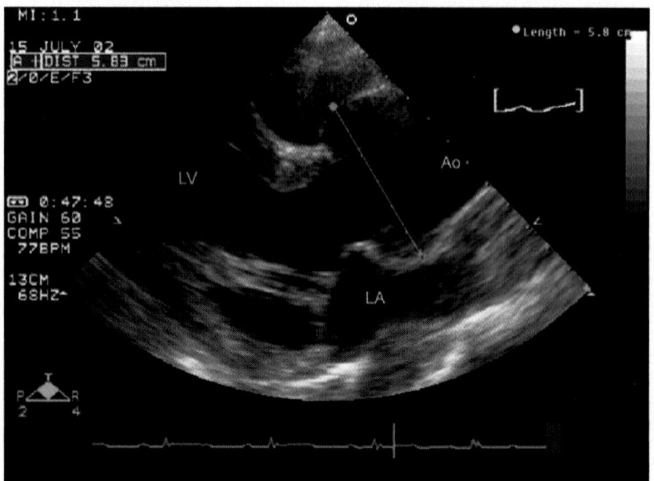

FIGURE 11–128 Transthoracic echocardiogram in a patient with Marfan syndrome. Note the marked dilation of the sinuses of proximal aorta (arrow). Ao = aorta; LA = left atrium; LV = left ventricle.

Papilloma. Benign papillomas occasionally occur on valvular structures. These appear as homogeneous, usually spherical masses, typically less than 1 cm in diameter.[208] They may appear on the mitral valve chordae and occasionally on the aortic valve. As with other cardiac tumors, they have been associated with emboli. The main differential diagnosis is between benign papilloma and vegetation.

Cardiac Malignancies. The majority of cardiac malignancies represent metastatic disease, most commonly from esophagus, lung, or breast. Diffuse malignancy, such as lymphoma, can also involve the heart either primarily or secondarily. Metastatic disease of the heart is virtually always associated with pericardial involvement as well. The appearance of metastatic disease in the heart is typically of mobile echo-dense masses attached to the endothelium (Fig. 11-130), although isolated intramural masses and diffuse myocardial invasion have also been noted.

There are several primary malignant tumors of the heart, including angiosarcoma and rhabdomyoma. Rhabdomyoma is more common in children. Cardiac malignancies are relatively rare and can appear in virtually any chamber in adults. There is a greater prevalence of sarcoma and rhabdomyoma in the right atrium (Fig. 11-131) and right ventricle and involving the veins or great vessels than in the actual body of the heart.

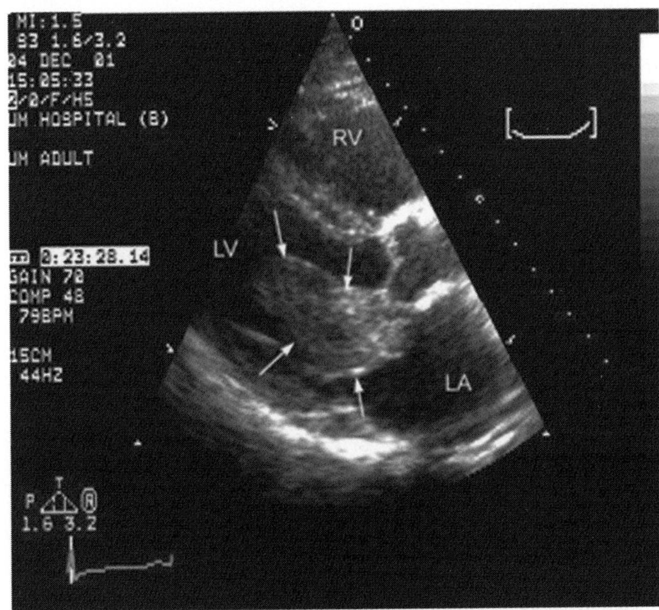

A

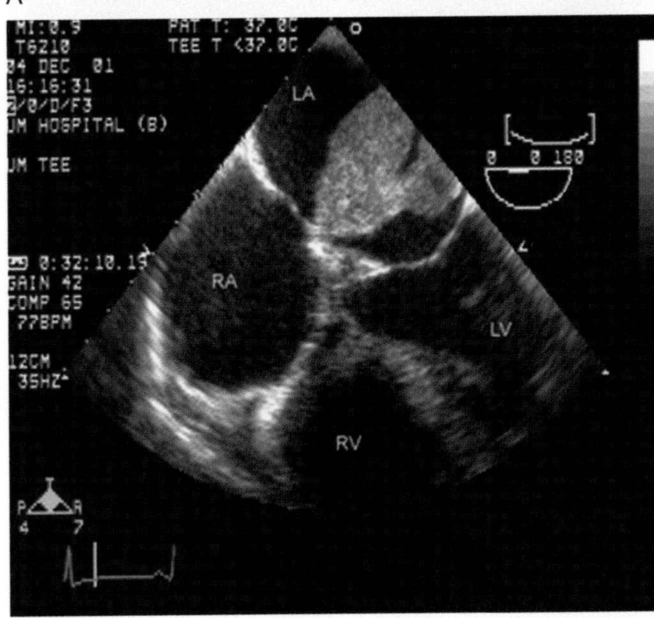

B

FIGURE 11–129 Transthoracic **(A)** and transesophageal **(B)** echocardiograms recorded in a patient with a large left atrial myxoma. Panel **A** is recorded in diastole. Note the large bulky mass (white arrows) essentially filling the entire mitral orifice. Panel **B** is recorded in the same patient. Note the irregular bilobed appearance of the mass and its attachment to the atrial septum by a relatively narrow stalk. LA = left atrium; LV = left ventricle; RA = right atrium; RV = right ventricle.

Intracardiac Thrombus. Thrombi can occur in any chamber of the heart but are most common in the left ventricular apex (see Fig. 11-117) after myocardial infarction or in the setting of cardiomyopathy, and in the left atrium in the setting of mitral stenosis or atrial fibrillation. Ventricular thrombi have been discussed previously.

Atrial thrombi appear as echo-dense masses within the body of the left atrium but more commonly in the left atrial appendage. The left atrial appendage has a fine muscular ridge-like network (pectinate muscles) that can be confused with small thrombi. Because thrombi occur in the presence of stasis, spontaneous contrast with "smoke-like" echoes is frequently seen in the left atrium and left atrial appendage as well.

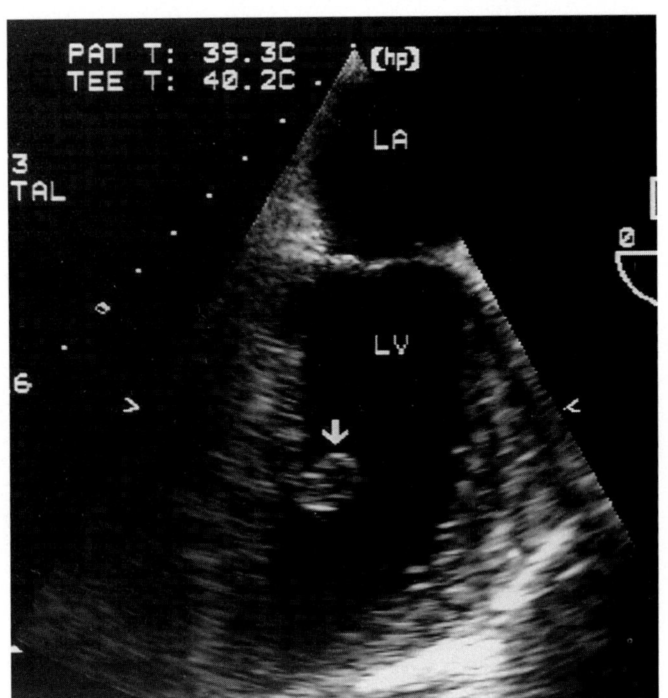

FIGURE 11–130 Transesophageal echocardiogram recorded in a long-axis view of the left atrium (LA) and left ventricle (LV) in a patient with an intracardiac tumor. Note the approximately 1 cm diameter, spherical mass attached to the posterior wall of the left ventricle by a thin stalk (arrow).

Specific Clinical Utilization of Echocardiography

The previous discussion represents an outline of the diagnostic capabilities of echocardiography. There are several specific clinical situations in which echocardiography can be used and that should be understood by the clinician. Table 11–8 outlines the role of different echocardiographic modalities in clinical problem-solving.

EVALUATION OF DYSPNEA AND CONGESTIVE HEART FAILURE. Two-dimensional echocardiography is recommended as an initial part of the evaluation in patients with known or suspected congestive heart failure (see Chap. 24). Evaluation of ventricular function can be undertaken, and determination of both primary and secondary valvular abnormalities can likewise be accurately assessed. Doppler echocardiography can play a valuable role with respect to determining diastolic function and establishing the diagnosis of diastolic heart failure. Heart failure with normal systolic function but abnormal diastolic relaxation accounts for 30 to 40 percent of patients presenting with congestive heart failure. Because the therapy of this condition is distinctly different from that of systolic dysfunction, establishing the appropriate cause and diagnosis is essential. This can be effectively done with the combination of two-dimensional echocardiography and Doppler echocardiography.

CARDIAC SOURCE OF EMBOLUS. It has become increasingly recognized that many neurological events and large artery occlusions are the result of embolization from the heart or other major vascular structures. Identifying patients who are most likely to have a cardiac source of embolus has been problematic, but in general, any patient with abrupt occlusion of a major vessel or younger individual (typically younger than 45 years of age) with a neurological event should be suspected of having a potential cardiac

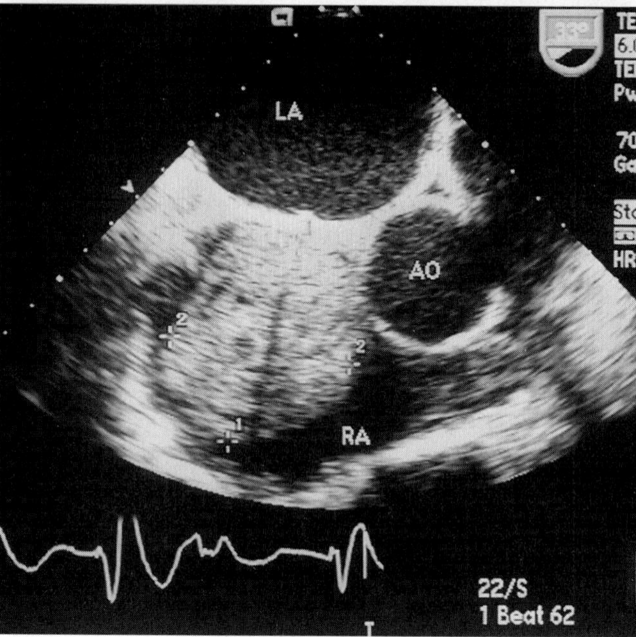

FIGURE 11–131 Apical four-chamber view **(top)** and transesophageal echocardiogram **(bottom)** in a patient with a large right atrial mass. In the top panel, the mass can be seen arising from the area of the inferior vena cava and essentially filling the right atrium (RA). A similar appearance is seen in the transesophageal echocardiogram **(bottom)**, where the mass appears adjacent to the atrial septum. AO = aorta; LA = left atrium; LV = left ventricle; RV = right ventricle.

cause. Additionally, older individuals with neurological events but who do not have identifiable vascular disease require screening for a cardiac cause. Several large-scale surveillance studies have demonstrated prevalence and range of abnormalities associated with neurological and embolic events.[209-211]

One of the more common abnormalities to identify in this situation is a patent foramen ovale with or without a right-to-left shunt identified by contrast echocardiography (see Fig. 11–87).[212,213] TEE is often required for complete evaluation because TTE is not sufficient to exclude left atrial thrombus or evaluate the thoracic aorta for atherosclerotic degree. A potential cardiac source of embolus will be identified in many patients with neurological and other embolic events, but the identification of such a lesion does not necessarily prove cause and effect. The degree to which atherosclerotic disease of the aorta and patent foramen ovale are causative rather than coexistent with other causes often remains unproven. In a substantial number of patients, highly mobile strands and areas of fibrosis may be noted on either the aortic or the mitral valve. The clinical implication of these anomalies is unknown.

ATRIAL FIBRILLATION. Echocardiography plays a crucial role in the evaluation of patients with atrial fibrillation (see Chap. 30). Patients with atrial fibrillation should be characterized as having underlying heart disease or having a structurally normal heart, in which case a diagnosis of lone atrial fibrillation can be made. Determination of the underlying cardiac anatomy is essential for decision-making regarding the likelihood of conversion to and maintenance of

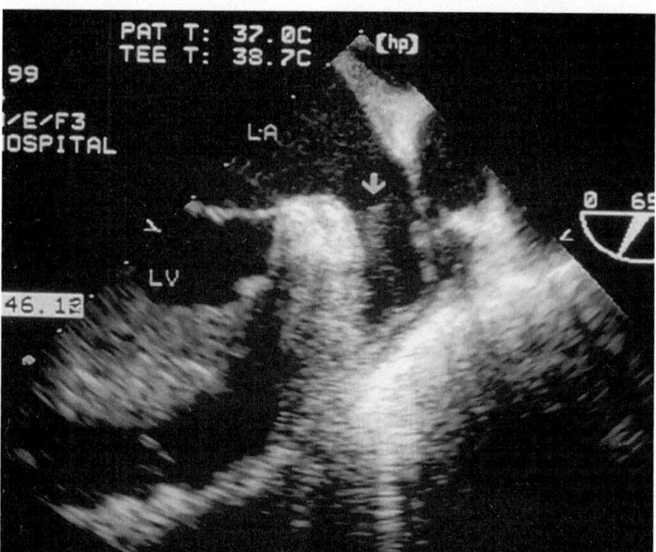

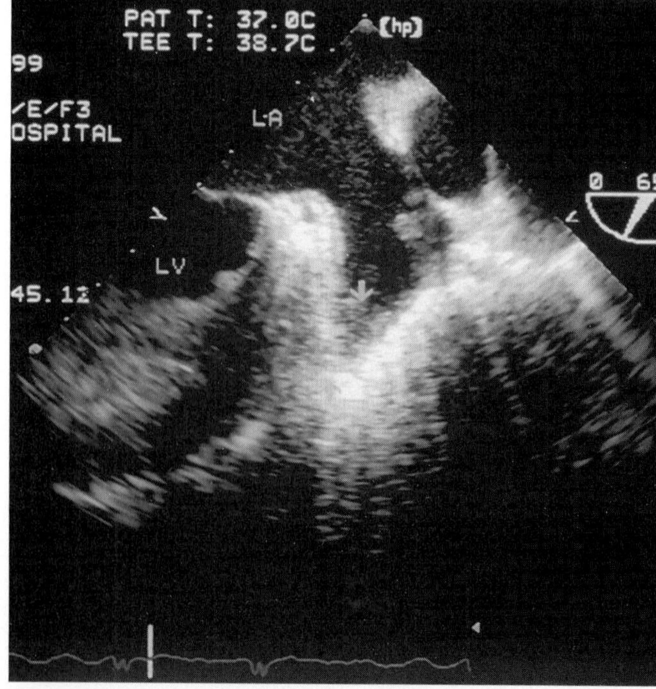

FIGURE 11–132 Transesophageal echocardiogram recorded in a patient with a recent neurological event. There is vague echo mass **(top),** which in real time has a swirling smoke-like appearance (downward pointing arrow). At a slightly different transducer position, the actual apex of the left atrial appendage can be seen to contain a filling defect consistent with thrombus, noted between the two vertically oriented arrows. LA = left atrium; LV = left ventricle.

TABLE 11–8 Clinical Utility of Echocardiography

Situation	2D	Doppler	CFD	Continuous Wave	TEE	Stress
Pericardial disease	1	2	3	4	4	N/A
Valvular heart disease						
Murmur	1	1	1	3	4	N/A
Mitral stenosis	1	1	1	—	3	3
Mitral regurgitation	1	1	1	—	3	N/A
Aortic stenosis/regurgitation	1	1	1	—	3	3
Prosthetic heart valve dysfunction	1	1	1	—	2	N/A
Coronary artery disease						
Chest pain syndrome	1	3	3	4	4	1
Rule out coronary artery disease	1	3	3	4	4	1
Diagnose acute myocardial infarction	1	3	3	4	4	N/A
Complications of infarction						
Aneurysm	1	3	3	4	4	N/A
Thrombus	1	3	3	4	4	N/A
Ventricular septal defect/papillary muscle rupture	1	1	1	3	2	N/A
Assess left ventricular function	1	1	2	4	4	3
Congenital heart disease	1	1	1	3	3	3
Atrial septal defect	1	1	1	2	2	4
Cardiomyopathy						
Dilated	1	1	1	4	4	3
Hypertrophic	1	1	1	4	4	3
Endocarditis	1	1	1	4	2	N/A
Pulmonary hypertension						
Known	1	1	1	2	3	3
Occult	1	1	1	2	3	2
Congestive heart failure	1	1	1	4	4	3
Stroke/source of embolus	1	2	2	1	2	N/A
Aortic dissection	2	2	1	4	1	N/A
Dyspnea evaluation	1	1	1	1	4	1

1 = Indicated and essential; 2 = often required—may add, informative; 3 = necessary in select instances for specific question; 4 = rarely necessary; 2D = two-dimensional; CFD = color flow Doppler; TEE = transesophageal echocardiography; N/A = not available.
From Armstrong WF: Echocardiography. *In* Kelly's Textbook of Medicine. 4th ed. Philadelphia, Lippincott Williams & Wilkins, 2000.

sinus rhythm and for determining the embolic potential and hence the need for long-term anticoagulation. In general, patients with normal cardiac anatomy are unlikely to sustain an embolic event and highly likely to revert to sinus rhythm and have sinus rhythm maintained. Conversely, patients with cardiomyopathy and severe mitral stenosis are less likely to be maintained in sinus rhythm and have a higher likelihood of embolic events. Thus, these individuals are candidates for long-term anticoagulation. TEE has also been proposed as a management tool in determining the timing for elective cardioversion.[214-216] Immediately after electrical cardioversion, there is an increased likelihood of embolization. Embolization in this setting arises either from a preexisting thrombus or, more likely, from atrial stunning with subsequent thrombus formation (Fig. 11–132). A strategy of TEE to exclude left atrial thrombus, followed immediately by cardioversion, has been demonstrated to be an efficient means of restoring sinus rhythm without requiring long-term pre-cardioversion anticoagulation. After cardioversion, atrial stunning occurs and the likelihood of new thrombus formation is actually transiently enhanced. For this reason, anticoagulation is indicated in virtually all patients after cardioversion for 6 weeks to 6 months. Although TEE-guided cardioversion has been demonstrated to be a safe alternative to the standard approach of 3 weeks of aortic coagulation followed by cardioversion, it has not been shown to result in a higher success rate for either initial conversion to sinus rhythm or maintenance of sinus rhythm at 1 year.

PULMONARY EMBOLUS (see Chap. 66). Patients with pulmonary embolus may present with atypical symptoms. In this instance, TEE and TTE can provide valuable clinical information.[217-219] In a patient presenting with a combination of chest pain and dyspnea, with or without evidence of venous stasis, detection of right heart dilation and dysfunction and/or elevation of pulmonary artery pressures can be valuable clues to the nature of the underlying process. Direct visualization of large pulmonary emboli is occasionally possible with either TTE or TEE, but more usually with TEE. Additionally, by using either technique, embolus in transit can be detected as a highly mobile serpiginous mass, typically entrapped in the tricuspid valve apparatus and less commonly spanning a patent foramen ovale. Detection of a typical serpiginous mass in the right atrium identifies a patient at substantial risk for further embolization and is a clinical situation requiring emergency therapy (Fig. 11–133).

PULMONARY HYPERTENSION (see Chap. 67). Pulmonary hypertension represents an elusive diagnosis. Clinically, pulmonary hypertension can occur either as a primary phenomenon or secondary to a variety of either cardiac or pulmonary processes. The majority of patients with established pulmonary hypertension have identifiable abnormalities on echocardiography, including variable degrees of right ventricular enlargement and hypertrophy (Fig. 11–134).[220,221] As noted earlier, pulmonary artery pressures can be estimated from the velocity of the tricuspid regurgitation jet (see Fig. 11–31). In patients with only mild elevation of pulmonary

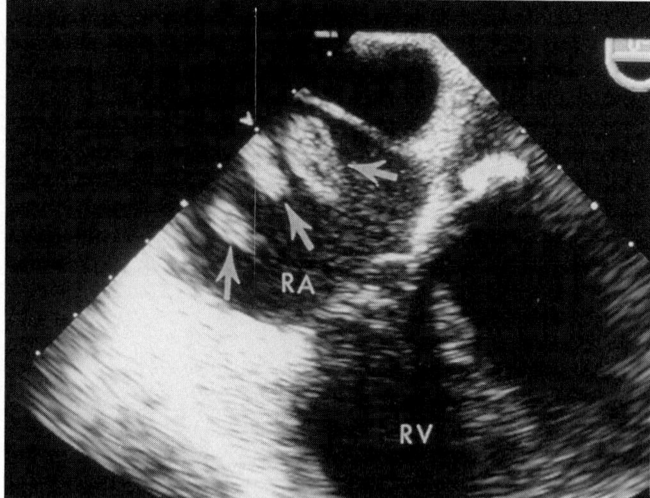

FIGURE 11–133 Transesophageal echocardiogram recorded in a patient with pulmonary embolus, found to have "thromboembolism in transit." Image was recorded at 0 degrees. The dilated right atrium and right ventricle are obvious. Three highly mobile components of a long serpiginous thrombus can be seen in the right atrium (arrows). RA = right atrium; RV = right ventricle.

pressure, exercise echocardiography can be used to track pulmonary artery pressures with stress and provides valuable information regarding the presence of occult, exercise-induced pulmonary hypertension.[222] Doppler echocardiography can also be used to follow pulmonary artery pressures during therapy.

FETAL ECHOCARDIOGRAPHY. Because cardiac ultrasonography carries no risk to the pregnant woman or fetus and is fully noninvasive, it can be used to make the antepartum diagnosis of congenital heart disease. This should be undertaken only by pediatric echocardiographers with appropriate experience in the technique. Many major intracardiac abnormalities can be detected at the end of the first trimester, and the majority of physiologically significant abnormalities can be detected in utero in the second trimester. This technique has seen substantial use in identifying fetuses with congenital heart defects who may warrant urgent transfer to a neonatal intensive care unit or an emergency intervention for life-threatening cardiac problems immediately after birth.

EVALUATION AND MONITORING OF INVASIVE AND INTERVENTIONAL PROCEDURES. Two-dimensional echocardiography, often using TEE, has seen substantial success as a means of monitoring invasive procedures. This includes direct online monitoring of pericardiocentesis and assistance in localization and placement of catheters for electrophysiological ablation as well as online monitoring of endomyocardial biopsy. Additionally, TEE is an instrumental component of transcatheter closure of atrial septal defects in the catheterization laboratory[223,224] and often used in other

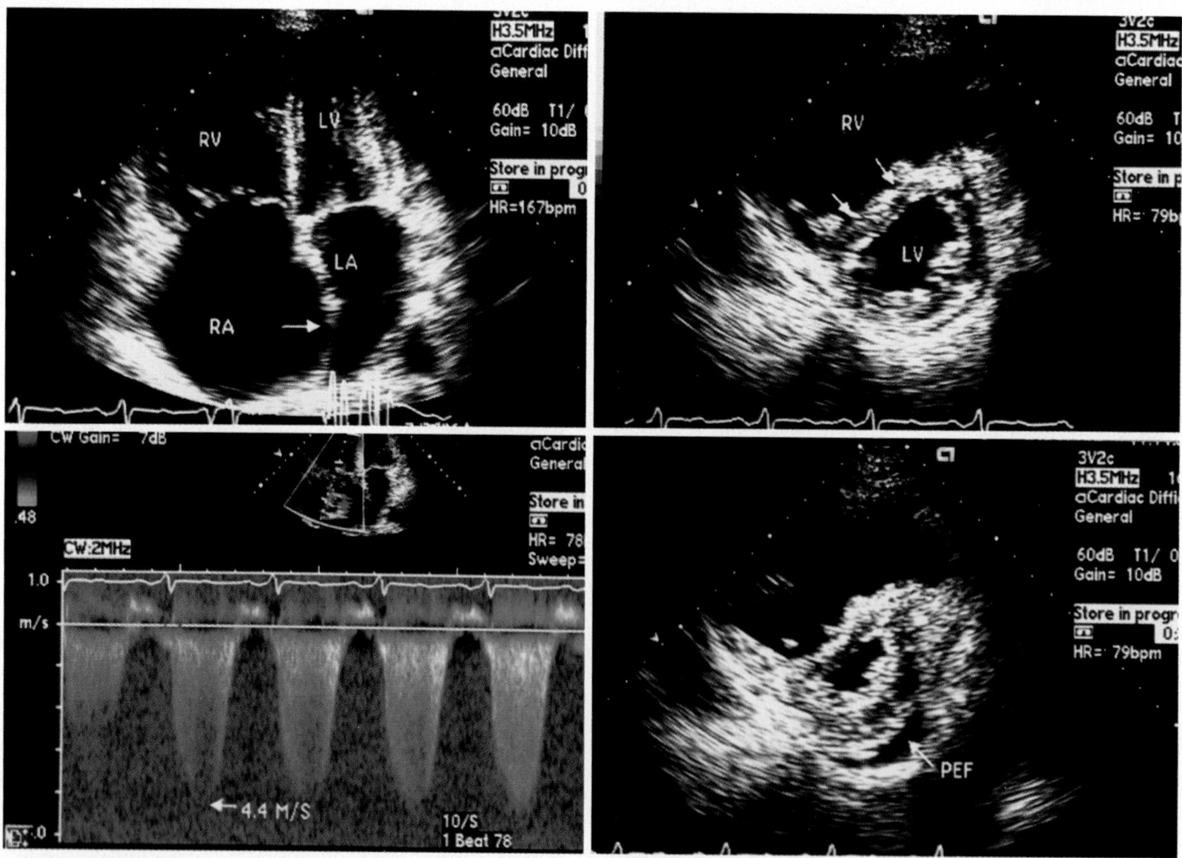

FIGURE 11–134 Composite images recorded in a patient with severe pulmonary hypertension. The **upper left panel** is an apical four-chamber view in which marked dilation of the right ventricle (RV) and right atrium (RA) can be appreciated. Notice the bowing of the atrial septum from right to left, implying that right atrial pressure exceeds left atrial pressure. The two **right panels** are recorded in a parasternal short-axis view and demonstrate a classic right ventricular pressure in volume overload pattern with flattening of the ventricular septum in both diastole and systole. The **lower left panel** is a continuous-wave Doppler recording of the tricuspid regurgitation jet, from which a peak velocity of 4.4 m/sec, corresponding to a right ventricular-right atrial pressure gradient of 77 mm Hg, can be calculated. Addition of right atrial pressure (assumed to be 15 mm Hg) results in an estimated right ventricular systolic pressure of 92 mm Hg in this instance. LA = left atrium; LV = left ventricle; PEF = pericardial effusion.

procedures where a transatrial approach is necessary for therapy, such as mitral balloon valvotomy.

REFERENCES

Principles of Cardiac Ultrasonography

1. Senior R, Soman P, Khattar RS, et al: Improved endocardial visualization with second harmonic imaging compared with fundamental two-dimensional echocardiographic imaging. Am Heart J 138:163, 1999.
2. Skolnick DG, Sawada SG, Feigenbaum H, et al: Enhanced endocardial visualization with noncontrast harmonic imaging during stress echocardiography. J Am Soc Echocardiogr 12:559, 1999.
3. Sozzi FB, Poldermans D, Bax JJ, et al: Second harmonic imaging improves sensitivity of dobutamine stress echocardiography for the diagnosis of coronary artery disease. Am Heart J 142:153, 2001.
4. Stevenson JG: Appearance and recognition of basic Doppler concepts in color flow imaging. Echocardiography 6:451, 1989.
5. Ritter SB: Red, green and blue: The flag of Doppler color flow mapping: Flow mapping. Echocardiography 6:369, 1989.
6. Veinot JP, Harrity PJ, Gentile F, et al: Anatomy of the normal left atrial appendage: A quantitative study of age-related changes in 500 autopsy hearts: Implications for echocardiographic examination. Circulation 96:3112, 1997.

Quantification of Ventricular Function

7. Huwez FU, Houston AB, Watson J, et al: Age and body surface area related normal upper and lower limits of M mode echocardiographic measurements and left ventricular volume and mass from infancy to early adulthood. Br Heart J 72:276, 1994.
8. Chuang ML, Hibberd MG, Salton CJ, et al: Importance of imaging method over imaging modality in noninvasive determination of left ventricular volumes and ejection fraction: Assessment by two- and three-dimensional echocardiography and magnetic resonance imaging. J Am Coll Cardiol 35:477, 2000.
9. Marcus R, Krause L, Weder AB, et al: Sex-specific determinants of increased left ventricular mass in the Tecumseh Blood Pressure Study. Circulation 90:928, 1994.
10. Pearlman JD, Triulzi MO, King ME, et al: Limits of normal left ventricular dimensions in growth and development: Analysis of dimensions and variance in the two-dimensional echocardiograms of 268 normal healthy subjects. J Am Coll Cardiol 12:1432, 1988.
11. Weyman AE: Appendix A: Normal Cross-Sectional Echocardiographic Measurements. *In* Principles and Practice of Echocardiography. Philadelphia, Lea & Febiger, 1994.
12. Yvorchuk KJ, Davies RA, Chan KL: Measurement of left ventricular ejection fraction by acoustic quantification and comparison with radionuclide angiography. Am J Cardiol 74:1052, 1994.
13. Gorcsan J 3rd, Romand JA, Mandarino WA, et al: Assessment of left ventricular performance by on-line pressure-area relations using echocardiographic automated border detection. J Am Coll Cardiol 23:242, 1994.
14. Devereux RB, Alonso DR, Lutas EM, et al: Echocardiographic assessment of left ventricular hypertrophy: Comparison to necropsy findings. Am J Cardiol 57:450, 1986.
15. Byrd BF 3rd, Finkbeiner W, Bouchard A, et al: Accuracy and reproducibility of clinically acquired two-dimensional echocardiographic mass measurements. Am Heart J 118:133, 1989.
16. Cerqueira MD, Weissman NJ, Dilsizian V, et al: Standardized myocardial segmentation and nomenclature for tomographic imaging of the heart: A statement for healthcare professionals from the Cardiac Imaging Committee of the Council on Clinical Cardiology of the American Heart Association. Circulation 105:539, 2002.
17. Bourdillon PD, Broderick TM, Sawada SG, et al: Regional wall motion index for infarct and noninfarct regions after reperfusion in acute myocardial infarction: Comparison with global wall motion index. J Am Soc Echocardiogr 2:398, 1989.

Doppler Examination

18. Chan KL, Currie PJ, Seward JB, et al: Comparison of three Doppler ultrasound methods in the prediction of pulmonary artery pressure. J Am Coll Cardiol 9:549, 1987.
19. McQuillan BM, Picard MH, Leavitt M, et al: Clinical correlates and reference intervals for pulmonary artery systolic pressure among echocardiographically normal subjects. Circulation 104:2797, 2001.
20. Scapellato F, Temporelli PL, Eleuteri E, et al: Accurate noninvasive estimation of pulmonary vascular resistance by Doppler echocardiography in patients with chronic heart failure. J Am Coll Cardiol 37:1813, 2001.
21. Moulinier L, Venet T, Schiller NB, et al: Measurement of aortic blood flow by Doppler echocardiography: Day to day variability in normal subjects and applicability in clinical research. J Am Coll Cardiol 17:1326, 1991.
22. Taylor R: Evolution of the continuity equation in the Doppler echocardiographic assessment of the severity of valvular aortic stenosis. J Am Soc Echocardiogr 3:326, 1990.
23. Recusani F, Bargiggia GS, Yoganathan AP, et al: A new method for quantification of regurgitant flow rate using color Doppler flow imaging of the flow convergence region proximal to a discrete orifice: An in vitro study. Circulation 83:594, 1991.
24. Shiota T, Jones M, Teien DE, et al: Evaluation of mitral regurgitation using a digitally determined color Doppler flow convergence "centerline" acceleration method: Studies in an animal model with quantified mitral regurgitation. Circulation 89:2879, 1994.
25. Pu M, Vandervoort PM, Griffin BP, et al: Quantification of mitral regurgitation by the proximal convergence method using transesophageal echocardiography: Clinical validation of a geometric correction for proximal flow constraint. Circulation 92:2169, 1995.
26. Kolias TJ, Aaronson KD, Armstrong WF: Doppler-derived dP/dt and -dP/dt predict survival in congestive heart failure. J Am Coll Cardiol 36:1594, 2000.
27. Oh JK, Appleton CP, Hatle LK, et al: The noninvasive assessment of left ventricular diastolic function with two-dimensional and Doppler echocardiography. J Am Soc Echocardiogr 10:246, 1997.
28. Nishimura RA, Tajik AJ: Evaluation of diastolic filling of left ventricle in health and disease: Doppler echocardiography is the clinician's Rosetta Stone. J Am Coll Cardiol 30:8, 1997.
29. Wachtell K, Smith G, Gerdts E, et al: Left ventricular filling patterns in patients with systemic hypertension and left ventricular hypertrophy (the LIFE study). Losartan Intervention For Endpoint. Am J Cardiol 85:466, 2000.
30. Firstenberg MS, Levine BD, Garcia MJ, et al: Relationship of echocardiographic indices to pulmonary capillary wedge pressures in healthy volunteers. J Am Coll Cardiol 36:1664, 2000.

Transesophageal and Three-Dimensional Imaging

31. Seward JB, Khandheria BK, Freeman WK, et al: Multiplane transesophageal echocardiography: Image orientation, examination technique, anatomic correlations, and clinical applications. Mayo Clin Proc 68:523, 1993.
32. Takuma S, Zwas DR, Fard A, et al: Real-time, 3-dimensional echocardiography acquires all standard 2-dimensional images from 2 volume sets: A clinical demonstration in 45 patients. J Am Soc Echocardiogr 12:1, 1999.
33. Collins M, Hsieh A, Ohazama CJ, et al: Assessment of regional wall motion abnormalities with real-time 3-dimensional echocardiography. J Am Soc Echocardiogr 12:7, 1999.
34. Balestrini L, Fleishman C, Lanzoni L, et al: Real-time 3-dimensional echocardiography evaluation of congenital heart disease. J Am Soc Echocardiogr 13:171, 2000.
35. Ahmad M, Xie T, McCulloch M, et al: Real-time three-dimensional dobutamine stress echocardiography in assessment stress echocardiography in assessment of ischemia: Comparison with two-dimensional dobutamine stress echocardiography. J Am Coll Cardiol 37:1303, 2001.
36. Salustri A, Spitaels S, McGhie J, et al: Transthoracic three-dimensional echocardiography in adult patients with congenital heart disease. J Am Coll Cardiol 26:759, 1995.
37. Schmidt MA, Ohazama CJ, Agyeman KO, et al: Real-time three-dimensional echocardiography for measurement of left ventricular volumes. Am J Cardiol 84:1434, 1999.

Intravascular Imaging

38. Pinto FJ, Chenzbraun A, Botas J, et al: Feasibility of serial intracoronary ultrasound imaging for assessment of progression of intimal proliferation in cardiac transplant recipients. Circulation 90:2348, 1994.
39. de Feyter PJ, Kay P, Disco C, et al: Reference chart derived from post-stent-implantation intravascular ultrasound predictors of 6-month expected restenosis on quantitative coronary angiography. Circulation 100:1777, 1999.
40. Schiele F, Meneveau N, Gilard M, et al: Intravascular ultrasound-guided balloon angioplasty compared with stent: Immediate and 6-month results of the multicenter, randomized Balloon Equivalent to Stent Study (BEST). Circulation 107:545, 2003.
41. Oemrawsingh PV, Mintz GS, Schalij MJ, et al: Intravascular ultrasound guidance improves angiographic and clinical outcome of stent implantation for long coronary artery stenoses: Final results of a randomized comparison with angiographic guidance (TULIP Study). Circulation 107:62, 2003.
42. Di Mario C, Krams R, Gil R, et al: Slope of the instantaneous hyperemic diastolic coronary flow velocity-pressure relation: A new index for assessment of the physiological significance of coronary stenosis in humans. Circulation 90:1215, 1994.
43. Fu M, Hung JS, Lo PH, et al: Intracardiac echocardiography via the transvenous approach with use of 8F 10-MHz ultrasound catheters. Mayo Clin Proc 74:775, 1999.
44. Bruce CJ, Packer DL, Seward JB: Transvascular imaging: Feasibility study using a vector phased array ultrasound catheter. Echocardiography 16:425, 1999.
45. Packer DL, Stevens CL, Curley MG, et al: Intracardiac phased-array imaging: Methods and initial clinical experience with high resolution, under blood visualization: Initial experience with intracardiac phased-array ultrasound. J Am Coll Cardiol 39:509, 2002.

Tissue Characterization and Doppler Tissue Imaging

46. Milunski MR, Mohr GA, Perez JE, et al: Ultrasonic tissue characterization with integrated backscatter: Acute myocardial ischemia, reperfusion, and stunned myocardium in patients. Circulation 80:491, 1989.
47. Iwakura K, Ito H, Kawano S, et al: Detection of TIMI-3 flow before mechanical reperfusion with ultrasonic tissue characterization in patients with anterior wall acute myocardial infarction. Circulation 107:3159, 2003.
48. Garcia MJ, Rodriguez L, Ares M, et al: Myocardial wall velocity assessment by pulsed Doppler tissue imaging: Characteristic findings in normal subjects. Am Heart J 132:648, 1996.
49. Derumeaux G, Ovize M, Loufoua J, et al: Assessment of nonuniformity of transmural myocardial velocities by color-coded tissue Doppler imaging: Characterization of normal, ischemic, and stunned myocardium. Circulation 101:1390, 2000.
50. Pasquet A, Armstrong G, Beachler L, et al: Use of segmental tissue Doppler velocity to quantitate exercise echocardiography. J Am Soc Echocardiogr 12:901, 1999.
51. Wang M, Yip GW, Wang AY, et al: Peak early diastolic mitral annulus velocity by tissue Doppler imaging adds independent and incremental prognostic value. J Am Coll Cardiol 41:820, 2003.
52. Waggoner AD, Bierig SM: Tissue Doppler imaging: A useful echocardiographic method for the cardiac sonographer to assess systolic and diastolic ventricular function. J Am Soc Echocardiogr 14:1143, 2001.
53. Kukulski T, Jamal F, D'Hooge J, et al: Acute changes in systolic and diastolic events during clinical coronary angioplasty: A comparison of regional velocity, strain rate, and strain measurement. J Am Soc Echocardiogr 15:1, 2002.
54. Cain P, Baglin T, Khoury V, et al: Automated regional myocardial displacement for facilitating the interpretation of dobutamine echocardiography. Am J Cardiol 89:1347, 2002.

55. Stoylen A, Slordahl S, Skjelvan GK, et al: Strain rate imaging in normal and reduced diastolic function: Comparison with pulsed Doppler tissue imaging of the mitral annulus. J Am Soc Echocardiogr 14:264, 2001.
56. D'Hooge J, Heimdal A, Jamal F, et al: Regional strain and strain rate measurements by cardiac ultrasound: Principles, implementation and limitations. Eur J Echocardiogr 1:154, 2000.
57. Edvardsen T, Gerber BL, Garot J, et al: Quantitative assessment of intrinsic regional myocardial deformation by Doppler strain rate echocardiography in humans: Validation against three-dimensional tagged magnetic resonance imaging. Circulation 106:50, 2002.
58. Hoffmann R, Altiok E, Nowak B, et al: Strain rate measurement by Doppler echocardiography allows improved assessment of myocardial viability inpatients with depressed left ventricular function. J Am Coll Cardiol 39:443, 2002.
59. Belohlavek M, Pislaru C, Bae RY, et al: Real-time strain rate echocardiographic imaging: Temporal and spatial analysis of postsystolic compression in acutely ischemic myocardium. J Am Soc Echocardiogr 14:360, 2001.
60. Pislaru C, Belohlavek M, Bae RY, et al: Regional asynchrony during acute myocardial ischemia quantified by ultrasound strain rate imaging. J Am Coll Cardiol 37:1141, 2001.
61. Kukulski T, Jamal F, Herbots L, et al: Identification of acutely ischemic myocardium using ultrasonic strain measurements: A clinical study in patients undergoing coronary angioplasty. J Am Coll Cardiol 41:810, 2003.

Contrast Echocardiography

62. Mulvagh SL, DeMaria AN, Feinstein SB, et al: Contrast echocardiography: Current and future applications. J Am Soc Echocardiogr 13:331, 2000.
63. Kaul S: Myocardial contrast echocardiography: 15 years of research and development. Circulation 96:3745, 1997.
64. Becher H, Tiemann K, Schlief R, et al: Harmonic power Doppler contrast echocardiography: Preliminary clinical results. Echocardiography 14:637, 1997.
65. Senior R, Kaul S, Soman P, et al: Power doppler harmonic imaging: A feasibility study of a new technique for the assessment of myocardial perfusion. Am Heart J 139:245, 2000.
66. Tiemann K, Becher H, Bimmel D, et al: Stimulated acoustic emission nonbackscatter contrast effect of microbubbles seen with harmonic power Doppler imaging. Echocardiography 14:65, 1997.
67. Villarraga HR, Foley DA, Aeschbacher BC, et al: Destruction of contrast microbubbles during ultrasound imaging at conventional power output. J Am Soc Echocardiogr 10:783, 1997.
68. Wei K, Skyba DM, Firschke C, et al: Interactions between microbubbles and ultrasound: In vitro and in vivo observations. J Am Coll Cardiol 29:1081, 1997.
69. Skyba DM, Price RJ, Linka AZ, et al: Direct in vivo visualization of intravascular destruction of microbubbles by ultrasound and its local effects on tissue. Circulation 98:290, 1998.
70. Simpson DH: Pulse inversion Doppler: A new method for detecting nonlinear echoes from microbubble contrast agents. IEEE Trans Ultrasonics Ferroelectrics Frequency Control 20:16, 1998.
71. Goldberg BB, Liu JB, Forsberg F: Ultrasound contrast agents: A review. Ultrasound Med Biol 20:319, 1994.
72. Cohen JL, Cheirif J, Segar DS, et al: Improved left ventricular endocardial border delineation and opacification with OPTISON (FS069), a new echocardiographic contrast agent: Results of a phase III multicenter trial. J Am Coll Cardiol 32:746, 1998.
73. Main ML, Grayburn PA: Clinical applications of transpulmonary contrast echocardiography. Am Heart J 137:144, 1999.
74. Reilly JP, Tunick PA, Timmermans RJ, et al: Contrast echocardiography clarifies uninterpretable wall motion in intensive care unit patients. J Am Coll Cardiol 35:485, 2000.
75. Yong Y, Wu D, Fernandes V, et al: Diagnostic accuracy and cost-effectiveness of contrast echocardiography on evaluation of cardiac function in technically very difficult patients in the intensive care unit. Am J Cardiol 89:711, 2002.
76. Dolan MS, Riad K, El-Shafei A, et al: Effect of intravenous contrast for left ventricular opacification and border definition on sensitivity and specificity of dobutamine stress echocardiography compared with coronary angiography in technically difficult patients. Am Heart J 142:908, 2001.
77. Rainbird AJ, Mulvagh SL, Oh JK, et al: Contrast dobutamine stress echocardiography: Clinical practice assessment in 300 consecutive patients. J Am Soc Echocardiogr 14:378, 2001.
78. Shimoni S, Zoghbi WA, Xie F, et al: Real-time assessment of myocardial perfusion and wall motion during bicycle and treadmill exercise echocardiography: Comparison with single photon emission computed tomography. J Am Coll Cardiol 37:741, 2001.
79. Thomson HL, Basmadjian AJ, Rainbird AJ, et al: Contrast echocardiography improves the accuracy and reproducibility of left ventricular remodeling measurements: A prospective, randomly assigned, blinded study. J Am Coll Cardiol 38:867, 2001.
80. von Bibra H, Becher H, Firschke C, et al: Enhancement of mitral regurgitation and normal left atrial color Doppler flow signals with peripheral venous injection of a saccharide-based contrast agent. J Am Coll Cardiol 22:521, 1993.
81. von Bibra H, Sutherland G, Becher H, et al: Clinical evaluation of left heart Doppler contrast enhancement by a saccharide-based transpulmonary contrast agent. The Levovist Cardiac Working Group. J Am Coll Cardiol 25:500, 1995.
82. Thanigaraj S, Schechtman KB, Perez JE: Improved echocardiographic delineation of left ventricular thrombus with the use of intravenous second-generation contrast image enhancement. J Am Soc Echocardiogr 12:1022, 1999.
83. Takeuchi M, Ogunyankin K, Pandian NG, et al: Enhanced visualization of intravascular and left atrial appendage thrombus with the use of a thrombus-targeting ultrasonographic contrast agent (MRX-408A1): In vivo experimental echocardiographic studies. J Am Soc Echocardiogr 12:1015, 1999.
84. Lindner JR, Dayton PA, Coggins MP, et al: Noninvasive imaging of inflammation by ultrasound detection of phagocytosed microbubbles. Circulation 102:531, 2000.
85. Leong-Poi H, Christiansen J, Klibanov AL, et al: Noninvasive assessment of angiogenesis by ultrasound and microbubbles targeted to alpha(v)-integrins. Circulation 107:455, 2003.
86. Cheitlin MD, Alpert JS, Armstrong WF, et al: ACC/AHA Guidelines for the Clinical Application of Echocardiography. A report of the American College of Cardiology/American Heart Association Task Force on Practice Guidelines (Committee on Clinical Application of Echocardiography). Developed in collaboration with the American Society of Echocardiography. Circulation 95:1686, 1997.
87. Quinones MA, Douglas PS, Foster E, et al: American College of Cardiology/American Heart Association clinical competence statement on echocardiography: A report of the American College of Cardiology/American Heart Association/American College of Physicians—American Society of Internal Medicine Task Force on Clinical Competence. Circulation 107:1068, 2003.

Acquired Valvular Heart Disease

88. Nishimura RA, Rihal CS, Tajik AJ, et al: Accurate measurement of the transmitral gradient in patients with mitral stenosis: A simultaneous catheterization and Doppler echocardiographic study. J Am Coll Cardiol 24:152, 1994.
89. Wang A, Ryan T, Kisslo KB, et al: Assessing the severity of mitral stenosis: Variability between noninvasive and invasive measurements in patients with symptomatic mitral valve stenosis. Am Heart J 138:777, 1999.
90. Leavitt JI, Coats MH, Falk RH: Effects of exercise on transmitral gradient and pulmonary artery pressure in patients with mitral stenosis or a prosthetic mitral valve: A Doppler echocardiographic study. J Am Coll Cardiol 17:1520, 1991.
91. Fredman CS, Pearson AC, Labovitz AJ, et al: Comparison of hemodynamic pressure half-time method and Gorlin formula with Doppler and echocardiographic determinations of mitral valve area in patients with combined mitral stenosis and regurgitation. Am Heart J 119:121, 1990.
92. Loperfido F, Laurenzi F, Gimigliano F, et al: A comparison of the assessment of mitral valve area by continuous wave Doppler and by cross sectional echocardiography. Br Heart J 57:348, 1987.
93. Thomas JD, Wilkins GT, Choong CY, et al: Inaccuracy of mitral pressure half-time immediately after percutaneous mitral valvotomy: Dependence on transmitral gradient and left atrial and ventricular compliance. Circulation 78:980, 1988.
94. Hernandez R, Banuelos C, Alfonso F, et al: Long-term clinical and echocardiographic follow-up after percutaneous mitral valvuloplasty with the Inoue balloon. Circulation 99:1580, 1999.
95. Palacios IF, Sanchez PL, Harrell LC, et al: Which patients benefit from percutaneous mitral balloon valvuloplasty? Prevalvuloplasty and postvalvuloplasty variables that predict long-term outcome. Circulation 105:1465, 2002.
96. Wang A, Krasuski RA, Warner JJ, et al: Serial echocardiographic evaluation of restenosis after successful percutaneous mitral commissurotomy. J Am Coll Cardiol 39:328, 2002.
97. Himelman RB, Kusumoto F, Oken K, et al: The flail mitral valve: Echocardiographic findings by precordial and transesophageal imaging and Doppler color flow mapping. J Am Coll Cardiol 17:272, 1991.
98. Shyu KG, Lei MH, Hwang JJ, et al: Morphologic characterization and quantitative assessment of mitral regurgitation with ruptured chordae tendineae by transesophageal echocardiography. Am J Cardiol 70:1152, 1992.
99. Chao K, Moises VA, Shandas R, et al: Influence of the Coanda effect on color Doppler jet area and color encoding: In vitro studies using color Doppler flow mapping. Circulation 85:333, 1992.
100. De Simone R, Glombitza G, Vahl CF, et al: Three-dimensional color Doppler: A clinical study in patients with mitral regurgitation. J Am Coll Cardiol 33:1646, 1999.
101. Sugeng L, Spencer K, Mor-Avi V, et al: Dynamic three-dimensional color flow Doppler: An improved technique for the assessment of mitral regurgitation. Echocardiography 20:265, 2003.
102. Kwan J, Shiota T, Agler DA, et al: Geometric differences of the mitral apparatus between ischemic and dilated cardiomyopathy with significant mitral regurgitation: Real-time three-dimensional echocardiography study. Circulation 107:1135, 2003.
103. Otsuji Y, Handschumacher MD, Liel-Cohen N, et al: Mechanism of ischemic mitral regurgitation with segmental left ventricular dysfunction: Three-dimensional echocardiographic studies in models of acute and chronic progressive regurgitation. J Am Coll Cardiol 37:641, 2001.
104. Vandervoort PM, Rivera JM, Mele D, et al: Application of color Doppler flow mapping to calculate effective regurgitant orifice area: An in vitro study and initial clinical observations. Circulation 88:1150, 1993.
105. Rodriguez L, Thomas JD, Monterroso V, et al: Validation of the proximal flow convergence method: Calculation of orifice area in patients with mitral stenosis. Circulation 88:1157, 1993.
106. Currie PJ, Hagler DJ, Seward JB, et al: Instantaneous pressure gradient: A simultaneous Doppler and dual catheter correlative study. J Am Coll Cardiol 7:800, 1986.
107. Tribouilloy C, Shen WF, Peltier M, et al: Quantitation of aortic valve area in aortic stenosis with multiplane transesophageal echocardiography: Comparison with monoplane transesophageal approach. Am Heart J 128:526, 1994.
108. Ray R: Evolution of the continuity equation in the Doppler echocardiographic assessment of the severity of valvular aortic stenosis. J Am Soc Echocardiogr 3:326, 1990.
109. Ford LE, Feldman T, Carroll JD: Valve resistance. Circulation 89:893, 1994.
110. Lin SS, Roger VL, Pascoe R, et al: Dobutamine stress Doppler hemodynamics in patients with aortic stenosis: Feasibility, safety, and surgical correlations. Am Heart J 136:1010, 1998.
111. Evangelista A, del Castillo HG, Calvo F, et al: Strategy for optimal aortic regurgitation quantification by Doppler echocardiography: Agreement among different methods. Am Heart J 139:773, 2000.
112. Padial LR, Oliver A, Sagie A, et al: Two-dimensional echocardiographic assessment of the progression of aortic root size in 127 patients with chronic aortic regurgitation: Role of the supraaortic ridge and relation to the progression of the lesion. Am Heart J 134:814, 1997.

113. Mugge A, Daniel WG, Herrmann G, et al: Quantification of tricuspid regurgitation by Doppler color flow mapping after cardiac transplantation. Am J Cardiol 66:884, 1990.
114. Stephen B, Dalal P, Berger M, et al: Noninvasive estimation of pulmonary artery diastolic pressure in patients with tricuspid regurgitation by Doppler echocardiography. Chest 116:73, 1999.
115. Jollis JG, Landolfo CK, Kisslo J, et al: Fenfluramine and phentermine and cardiovascular findings: Effect of treatment duration on prevalence of valve abnormalities. Circulation 101:2071, 2000.
116. Gardin JM, Schumacher D, Constantine G, et al: Valvular abnormalities and cardiovascular status following exposure to dexfenfluramine or phentermine/fenfluramine. JAMA 283:1703, 2000.
117. Gardin JM, Weissman NJ, Leung C, et al: Clinical and echocardiographic follow-up of patients previously treated with dexfenfluramine or phentermine/fenfluramine. JAMA 286:2011, 2001.
118. Abraham TP, Kon ND, Nomeir AM, et al: Accuracy of transesophageal echocardiography in preoperative determination of aortic annulus size during valve replacement. J Am Soc Echocardiogr 10:149, 1997.
119. Bridgman PG, Bloomfield P, Reid JH, et al: Prediction of stentless aortic bioprosthesis size with transesophageal echocardiography and magnetic resonance imaging. J Heart Valve Dis 6:487, 1997.
120. Oh CC, Click RL, Orszulak TA, et al: Role of intraoperative transesophageal echocardiography in determining aortic annulus diameter in homograft insertion. J Am Soc Echocardiogr 11:638, 1998.
121. Vandervoort PM, Greenberg NL, Powell KA, et al: Pressure recovery in bileaflet heart valve prostheses. Localized high velocities and gradients in central and side orifices with implications for Doppler-catheter gradient relation in aortic and mitral position. Circulation 92:3464, 1995.
122. Baumgartner H, Khan S, DeRobertis M, et al: Effect of prosthetic aortic valve design on the doppler-catheter gradient correlation. J Am Coll Cardiol 19:324, 1992.
123. Kodavatiganti R: Intraoperative assessment of the mitral valve by transoesophageal echocardiography: An overview. Ann Cardiac Anaesth 5:127, 2002.
124. Shanewise JS, Cheung AT, Aronson S, et al: ASE/SCA guidelines for performing a comprehensive intraoperative multiplane transesophageal echocardiography examination: Recommendations of the American Society of Echocardiography Council for Intraoperative Echocardiography and the Society of Cardiovascular Anesthesiologists Task Force for Certification in Perioperative Transesophageal Echocardiography. Anesth Analg 89:870, 1999.
125. Yvorchuk KJ, Chan KL: Application of transthoracic and transesophageal echocardiography in the diagnosis and management of infective endocarditis. J Am Soc Echocardiogr 7:294, 1994.
126. Durack DT, Lukes AS, Bright DK: New criteria for diagnosis of infective endocarditis: Utilization of specific echocardiographic findings. Duke Endocarditis Service. Am J Med 96:200, 1994.
127. Heinle S, Wilderman N, Harrison JK, et al: Value of transthoracic echocardiography in predicting embolic events in active infective endocarditis. Duke Endocarditis Service. Am J Cardiol 74:799, 1994.
128. Leung DY, Cranney GB, Hopkins AP, et al: Role of transoesophageal echocardiography in the diagnosis and management of aortic root abscess. Br Heart J 72:175, 1994.
129. Fox CS, Vasan RS, Parise H, et al: Mitral annular calcification predicts cardiovascular morbidity and mortality: The Framingham Heart Study. Circulation 107:1492, 2003.

Congenital Heart Disease

130. Watanabe F, Takenaka K, Suzuki J, et al: Visualization of sinus venosus-type atrial septal defect by biplane transesophageal echocardiography. J Am Soc Echocardiogr 7:179, 1994.
131. Hausmann D, Daniel WG, Mugge A, et al: Value of transesophageal color Doppler echocardiography for detection of different types of atrial septal defect in adults. J Am Soc Echocardiogr 5:481, 1992.
132. Dall'Agata A, McGhie J, Taams MA, et al: Secondum atrial septal defect is a dynamic three-dimensional entity. Am Heart J 137:1075, 1999.
133. Mazic U, Gavora P, Masura J: The role of transesophageal echocardiography in transcatheter closure of secundum atrial septal defects by the Amplatzer septal occluder. Am Heart J 142:482, 2001.
134. Mullen MJ, Dias BF, Walker F, et al: Intracardiac echocardiography guided device closure of atrial septal defects. J Am Coll Cardiol 41:285, 2003.
135. Kerut EK, Norfleet WT, Plotnick GD, et al: Patent foramen ovale: A review of associated conditions and the impact of physiological size. J Am Coll Cardiol 38:613, 2001.

Pericardial and Myocardial Disease

136. Oh JK, Hatle LK, Seward JB, et al: Diagnostic role of Doppler echocardiography in constrictive pericarditis. J Am Coll Cardiol 23:154, 1994.
137. Myers RB, Spodick DH: Constrictive pericarditis: Clinical and pathophysiologic characteristics. Am Heart J 138:219, 1999.
138. Bach DS, Beanlands RS, Schwaiger M, et al: Heterogeneity of ventricular function and myocardial oxidative metabolism in nonischemic dilated cardiomyopathy. J Am Coll Cardiol 25:1258, 1995.
139. Hansen A, Haass M, Zugck C, et al: Prognostic value of Doppler echocardiographic mitral inflow patterns: Implications for risk stratification in patients with chronic congestive heart failure. J Am Coll Cardiol 37:1049, 2001.
140. Yong Y, Nagueh SF, Shimoni S, et al: Deceleration time in ischemic cardiomyopathy: Relation to echocardiographic and scintigraphic indices of myocardial viability and functional recovery after revascularization. Circulation 103:1232, 2001.
141. Whalley GA, Doughty RN, Gamble GD, et al: Pseudonormal mitral filling pattern predicts hospital re-admission in patients with congestive heart failure. J Am Coll Cardiol 39:1787, 2002.
142. Rossi A, Cicoira M, Zanolla L, et al: Determinants and prognostic value of left atrial volume in patients with dilated cardiomyopathy. J Am Coll Cardiol 40:1425, 2002.
143. Koelling TM, Aaronson KD, Cody RJ, et al: Prognostic significance of mitral regurgitation and tricuspid regurgitation in patients with left ventricular systolic dysfunction. Am Heart J 144:524, 2002.
144. Faber L, Seggewiss H, Ziemssen P, et al: Intraprocedural myocardial contrast echocardiography as a routine procedure in percutaneous transluminal septal myocardial ablation: Detection of threatening myocardial necrosis distant from the septal target area. Catheter Cardiovasc Interv 47:462, 1999.
145. Klein AL, Hatle LK, Taliercio CP, et al: Prognostic significance of Doppler measures of diastolic function in cardiac amyloidosis: A Doppler echocardiography study. Circulation 83:808, 1991.
146. Tabata T, Kabbani SS, Murray RD, et al: Difference in the respiratory variation between pulmonary venous and mitral inflow Doppler velocities in patients with constrictive pericarditis with and without atrial fibrillation. J Am Coll Cardiol 37:1936, 2001.
147. Garcia MJ, Rodriguez L, Ares M, et al: Differentiation of constrictive pericarditis from restrictive cardiomyopathy: Assessment of left ventricular diastolic velocities in longitudinal axis by Doppler tissue imaging. J Am Coll Cardiol 27:108, 1996.
148. Palka P, Lange A, Donnelly JE, et al: Differentiation between restrictive cardiomyopathy and constrictive pericarditis by early diastolic doppler myocardial velocity gradient at the posterior wall. Circulation 102:655, 2000.

Acute Myocardial Infarction

149. Force T, Kemper A, Perkins L, et al: Overestimation of infarct size by quantitative two-dimensional echocardiography: The role of tethering and of analytic procedures. Circulation 73:1360, 1986.
150. Derumeaux G, Loufoua J, Pontier G, et al: Tissue Doppler imaging differentiates transmural from nontransmural acute myocardial infarction after reperfusion therapy. Circulation 103:589, 2001.
151. Gotte MJ, van Rossum AC, Twisk JWR, et al: Quantification of regional contractile function after infarction: Strain analysis superior to wall thickening analysis in discriminating infarct from remote myocardium. J Am Coll Cardiol 37:808, 2001.
152. Sabia P, Abbott RD, Afrookteh A, et al: Importance of two-dimensional echocardiographic assessment of left ventricular systolic function in patients presenting to the emergency room with cardiac-related symptoms. Circulation 84:1615, 1991.
153. Elhendy A, van Domburg RT, Bax JJ, et al: Significance of resting wall motion abnormalities in 2-dimensional echocardiography in patients without previous myocardial infarction referred for pharmacologic stress testing. J Am Soc Echocardiogr 13:1, 2000.
154. Kontos MC, Kurdziel K, McQueen R, et al: Comparison of 2-dimensional echocardiography and myocardial perfusion imaging for diagnosing myocardial infarction in emergency department patients. Am Heart J 143:659, 2002.
155. Burns RJ, Gibbons RJ, Yi Q, et al: The relationships of left ventricular ejection fraction, end-systolic volume index and infarct size to six-month mortality after hospital discharge following myocardial infarction treated by thrombolysis. J Am Coll Cardiol 39:30, 2002.
156. Moller JE, Sondergaard E, Poulsen SH, et al: Pseudonormal and restrictive filling patterns predict left ventricular dilation and cardiac death after a first myocardial infarction: A serial color M-mode Doppler echocardiographic study. J Am Coll Cardiol 36:1841, 2000.
157. Moller JE, Egstrup K, Kober L, et al: Prognostic importance of systolic and diastolic function after acute myocardial infarction. Am Heart J 145:147, 2003.
158. Picard MH, Wilkins GT, Gillam LD, et al: Immediate regional endocardial surface expansion following coronary occlusion in the canine left ventricle: Disproportionate effects of anterior versus inferior ischemia. Am Heart J 121:753, 1991.
159. Mehta SR, Eikelboom JW, Natarajan MK, et al: Impact of right ventricular involvement on mortality and morbidity in patients with inferior myocardial infarction. J Am Coll Cardiol 37:37, 2001.

Myocardial Stunning and Hibernation

160. Kloner RA, Bolli R, Marban E, et al: Medical and cellular implications of stunning, hibernation, and preconditioning: An NHLBI workshop. Circulation 97:1848, 1998.
161. Bax JJ, Poldermans D, Elhendy A, et al: Improvement of left ventricular ejection fraction, heart failure symptoms and prognosis after revascularization in patients with chronic coronary artery disease and viable myocardium detected by dobutamine stress echocardiography. J Am Coll Cardiol 34:163, 1999.
162. Bonow RO: Identification of viable myocardium. Circulation 94:2674, 1996.
163. Bolognese L, Buonamici P, Cerisano G, et al: Early dobutamine echocardiography predicts improvement in regional and global left ventricular function after reperfused acute myocardial infarction without residual stenosis of the infarct-related artery. Am Heart J 139:153, 2000.
164. Allman KC, Shaw LJ, Hachamovitch R, et al: Myocardial viability testing and impact of revascularization on prognosis in patients with coronary artery disease and left ventricular dysfunction: A meta-analysis. J Am Coll Cardiol 39:1151, 2002.

Stress Echocardiography

165. Armstrong WF, O'Donnell J, Ryan T, et al: Effect of prior myocardial infarction and extent and location of coronary disease on accuracy of exercise echocardiography. J Am Coll Cardiol 10:531, 1987.
166. Crouse LJ, Harbrecht JJ, Vacek JL, et al: Exercise echocardiography as a screening test for coronary artery disease and correlation with coronary arteriography. Am J Cardiol 67:1213, 1991.
167. Marwick TH, Nemec JJ, Pashkow FJ, et al: Accuracy and limitations of exercise echocardiography in a routine clinical setting. J Am Coll Cardiol 19:74, 1992.
168. Roger VL, Pellikka PA, Oh JK, et al: Identification of multivessel coronary artery disease by exercise echocardiography. J Am Coll Cardiol 24:109, 1994.
169. Beleslin BD, Ostojic M, Stepanovic J, et al: Stress echocardiography in the detection of myocardial ischemia: Head-to-head comparison of exercise, dobutamine, and dipyridamole tests. Circulation 90:1168, 1994.

170. Quinones MA, Verani MS, Haichin RM, et al: Exercise echocardiography versus 201Tl single-photon emission computed tomography in evaluation of coronary artery disease. Analysis of 292 patients. Circulation 85:1026, 1992.
171. Ryan T, Segar DS, Sawada SG, et al: Detection of coronary artery disease with upright bicycle exercise echocardiography. J Am Soc Echocardiogr 6:186, 1993.
172. Cohen JL, Ottenweller JE, George AK, et al: Comparison of dobutamine and exercise echocardiography for detecting coronary artery disease. Am J Cardiol 72:1226, 1993.
173. Hecht HS, DeBord L, Shaw R, et al: Digital supine bicycle stress echocardiography: A new technique for evaluating coronary artery disease. J Am Coll Cardiol 21:950, 1993.
174. Luotolahti M, Saraste M, Hartiala J: Exercise echocardiography in the diagnosis of coronary artery disease. Ann Med 28:73, 1996.
175. Marwick T, D'Hondt AM, Baudhuin T, et al: Optimal use of dobutamine stress for the detection and evaluation of coronary artery disease: Combination with echocardiography or scintigraphy, or both? J Am Coll Cardiol 22:159, 1993.
176. Ling LH, Pelikka PA, Mahoney DW: Atropine augmentation in dobutamine stress echocardiography. J Am Coll Cardiol 28:551, 1996.
177. Marcovitz PA, Armstrong WF: Accuracy of dobutamine stress echocardiography in detecting coronary artery disease. Am J Cardiol 69:1269, 1992.
178. Takeuchi M, Araki M, Nakashima Y, et al: Comparison of dobutamine stress echocardiography and stress thallium-201 single-photon emission computed tomography for detecting coronary artery disease. J Am Soc Echocardiogr 6:593, 1993.
179. Kwok Y, Kim C, Grady D, et al: Meta-analysis of exercise testing to detect coronary artery disease in women. Am J Cardiol 83:660, 1999.
180. Chuah SC, Pellikka PA, Roger VL, et al: Role of dobutamine stress echocardiography in predicting outcome in 860 patients with known or suspected coronary artery disease. Circulation 97:1474, 1998.
181. Poldermans D, Fioretti PM, Boersma E, et al: Long-term prognostic value of dobutamine-atropine stress echocardiography in 1737 patients with known or suspected coronary artery disease: A single-center experience. Circulation 99:757, 1999.
182. Marwick TH, Case C, Sawada S, et al: Prediction of mortality using dobutamine echocardiography. J Am Coll Cardiol 37:754, 2001.
183. Bholasingh R, Cornel JH, Kamp O, et al: Prognostic value of predischarge dobutamine stress echocardiography in chest pain patients with a negative cardiac troponin T. J Am Coll Cardiol 41:596, 2003.
184. Kamalesh M, Matorin R, Sawada S: Prognostic value of a negative stress echocardiographic study in diabetic patients. Am Heart J 143:163, 2002.
185. Elhendy A, Mahoney DW, Khandheria BK, et al: Prognostic significance of the location of wall motion abnormalities during exercise echocardiography. J Am Coll Cardiol 40:1623, 2002.
186. McCully RB, Roger VL, Mahoney DW, et al: Outcome after abnormal exercise echocardiography for patients with good exercise capacity: Prognostic importance of the extent and severity of exercise-related left ventricular dysfunction. J Am Coll Cardiol 39:1345, 2002.
187. Arruda-Olson AM, Juracan EM, Mahoney DW, et al: Prognostic value of exercise echocardiography in 5,798 patients: Is there a gender difference? J Am Coll Cardiol 39:625, 2002.
188. Carlos ME, Smart SC, Wynsen JC, et al: Dobutamine stress echocardiography for risk stratification after myocardial infarction. Circulation 95:1402, 1997.
189. Shaw LJ, Peterson ED, Kesler K, et al: A metaanalysis of predischarge risk stratification after acute myocardial infarction with stress electrocardiographic, myocardial perfusion, and ventricular function imaging. Am J Cardiol 78:1327, 1996.
190. Shaw LJ, Eagle KA, Gersh BJ, et al: Meta-analysis of intravenous dipyridamole-thallium-201 imaging (1985 to 1994) and dobutamine echocardiography (1991 to 1994) for risk stratification before vascular surgery. J Am Coll Cardiol 27:787, 1996.

Myocardial Contrast Echocardiography

191. Wei K, Jayaweera AR, Firoozan S, et al: Quantification of myocardial blood flow with ultrasound-induced destruction of microbubbles administered as a constant venous infusion. Circulation 97:473, 1998.
192. Heinle SK, Noblin J, Goree-Best P, et al: Assessment of myocardial perfusion by harmonic power Doppler imaging at rest and during adenosine stress: Comparison with (99m)Tc-sestamibi SPECT imaging. Circulation 102:55, 2000.
193. Porter TR, Xie F, Silver M, et al: Real-time perfusion imaging with low mechanical index pulse inversion Doppler imaging. J Am Coll Cardiol 37:748, 2001.
194. Masugata H, Peters B, Lafitte S, et al: Quantitative assessment of myocardial perfusion during graded coronary stenosis by real-time myocardial contrast echo refilling curves. J Am Coll Cardiol 37:262, 2001.
195. Balcells E, Powers ER, Lepper W, et al: Detection of myocardial viability by contrast echocardiography in acute infarction predicts recovery of resting function and contractile reserve. J Am Coll Cardiol 41:827, 2003.
196. Shimoni S, Frangogiannis NG, Aggeli CJ, et al: Identification of hibernating myocardium with quantitative intravenous myocardial contrast echocardiography: Comparison with dobutamine echocardiography and thallium-201 scintigraphy. Circulation 107:538, 2003.
197. Angelini P, Velasco JA, Flamm S: Coronary anomalies: Incidence, pathophysiology, and clinical relevance. Circulation 105:2449, 2002.
198. Gradus-Pizlo I, Sawada SG, Wright D, et al: Detection of subclinical coronary atherosclerosis using two-dimensional, high-resolution transthoracic echocardiography. J Am Coll Cardiol 37:1422, 2001.
199. Watanabe N, Akasaka T, Yamaura Y, et al: Noninvasive detection of total occlusion of the left anterior descending coronary artery with transthoracic Doppler echocardiography. J Am Coll Cardiol 38:1328, 2001.

Disease of the Aorta

200. Erbel R, Engberding R, Daniel W, et al: Echocardiography in diagnosis of aortic dissection. Lancet 1:457, 1989.
201. Hashimoto S, Kumada T, Osakada G, et al: Assessment of transesophageal Doppler echography in dissecting aortic aneurysm. J Am Coll Cardiol 14:1253, 1989.
202. Ballal RS, Nanda NC, Gatewood R, et al: Usefulness of transesophageal echocardiography in assessment of aortic dissection. Circulation 84:1903, 1991.
203. Nienaber CA, von Kodolitsch Y, Nicolas V, et al: The diagnosis of thoracic aortic dissection by noninvasive imaging procedures. N Engl J Med 328:1, 1993.
204. Keane MG, Wiegers SE, Yang E, et al: Structural determinants of aortic regurgitation in type A dissection and the role of valvular resuspension as determined by intraoperative transesophageal echocardiography. Am J Cardiol 85:604, 2000.
205. Song JK, Kim HS, Kang DH, et al: Different clinical features of aortic intramural hematoma versus dissection involving the ascending aorta. J Am Coll Cardiol 37:1604, 2001.
206. Di Tullio MR, Sacco RL, Savoia MT, et al: Aortic atheroma morphology and the risk of ischemic stroke in a multiethnic population. Am Heart J 139:329, 2000.
207. Tunick PA, Kronzon I: Atheromas of the thoracic aorta: Clinical and therapeutic update. J Am Coll Cardiol 35:545, 2000.

Specific Clinical Applications

208. Sun JP, Asher CR, Yang XS, et al: Clinical and echocardiographic characteristics of papillary fibroelastomas: A retrospective and prospective study in 162 patients. Circulation 103:2687, 2001.
209. Labovitz AJ: Transesophageal echocardiography and unexplained cerebral ischemia: A multicenter follow-up study. The STEPS Investigators. Significance of Transesophageal Echocardiography in the Prevention of Recurrent Stroke. Am Heart J 137:1082, 1999.
210. McNamara RL, Lima JA, Whelton PK, et al: Echocardiographic identification of cardiovascular sources of emboli to guide clinical management of stroke: A cost-effectiveness analysis. Ann Intern Med 127:775, 1997.
211. Meissner I, Whisnant JP, Khandheria BK, et al: Prevalence of potential risk factors for stroke assessed by transesophageal echocardiography and carotid ultrasonography: The SPARC study. Stroke Prevention: Assessment of Risk in a Community. Mayo Clin Proc 74:862, 1999.
212. Homma S, Di Tullio MR, Sacco RL, et al: Characteristics of patent foramen ovale associated with cryptogenic stroke: A biplane transesophageal echocardiographic study. Stroke 25:582, 1994.
213. Steiner MM, Di Tullio MR, Rundek T, et al: Patent foramen ovale size and embolic brain imaging findings among patients with ischemic stroke. Stroke 29:944, 1998.
214. Klein AL, Grimm RA, Black IW, et al: Cardioversion guided by transesophageal echocardiography: The ACUTE Pilot Study. A randomized, controlled trial. Assessment of Cardioversion Using Transesophageal Echocardiography. Ann Intern Med 126:200, 1997.
215. Silverman DI, Manning WJ: Role of echocardiography in patients undergoing elective cardioversion of atrial fibrillation. Circulation 98:479, 1998.
216. Klein AL, Murray RD, Grimm RA: Role of transesophageal echocardiography-guided cardioversion of patients with atrial fibrillation. J Am Coll Cardiol 37:691, 2001.
217. Grifoni S, Olivotto I, Cecchini P, et al: Short-term clinical outcome of patients with acute pulmonary embolism, normal blood pressure, and echocardiographic right ventricular dysfunction. Circulation 101:2817, 2000.
218. Ribeiro A, Lindmarker P, Johnsson H, et al: Pulmonary embolism: One-year follow-up with echocardiography Doppler and five-year survival analysis. Circulation 99:1325, 1999.
219. Miniati M, Monti S, Pratali L, et al: Value of transthoracic echocardiography in the diagnosis of pulmonary embolism: Results of a prospective study in unselected patients. Am J Med 110:528, 2001.
220. Bossone E, Duong-Wagner TH, Paciocco G, et al: Echocardiographic features of primary pulmonary hypertension. J Am Soc Echocardiogr 12:655, 1999.
221. Raymond RJ, Hinderliter AL, Willis PW, et al: Echocardiographic predictors of adverse outcomes in primary pulmonary hypertension. J Am Coll Cardiol 39:1214, 2002.
222. Bossone E, Rubenfire M, Bach DS, et al: Range of tricuspid regurgitation velocity at rest and during exercise in normal adult men: Implications for the diagnosis of pulmonary hypertension. J Am Coll Cardiol 33:1662, 1999.
223. Ewert P, Berger F, Daehnert I, et al: Diagnostic catheterization and balloon sizing of atrial septal defects by echocardiographic guidance without fluoroscopy. Echocardiography 17:159, 2000.
224. Cooke J, Gelman J, Harper R: Echocardiologists' role in the deployment of the Amplatzer atrial septal occluder device in adults. J Am Soc Echocardiogr 14:588, 2001.

Use of Echocardiography

Jointly, the American College of Cardiology and the American Heart Association (ACC/AHA) published guidelines for the use of echocardiography in 1997,[1] and, in collaboration with several other professional societies, issued recommendations regarding standards of clinical competence in 2003.[2] Recommendations regarding the use of echocardiography are also included in guidelines for specific clinical syndromes, such as management of heart failure (see Chap. 24), valvular heart disease (see Chap. 57), and suspected endocarditis (see Chap. 58). These recommendations are included in appendices for chapters devoted to those syndromes.

The 1997 guidelines provide recommendations for the use of echocardiography in various clinical settings, using the standard three-class system of ACC/AHA guidelines. The guidelines specify situations in which echocardiography is considered likely or unlikely to contribute information that improves the management of patients. They also make recommendations on the frequency with which Doppler echocardiography should be repeated for some clinical issues. In general, the guidelines urge restraint in the use of echocardiography for patients whose initial evaluations indicated minimal or mild abnormalities, unless there is a change in clinical status.

Murmurs and Valvular Heart Disease

The ACC/AHA guidelines for use of echocardiography in patients with known or suspected valvular heart disease reflect the critical role of this test in assessing cardiac structure and function (Table 11G–1). Accordingly, echocardiography is considered appropriate in any patient with cardiorespiratory symptoms and a heart murmur, and any asymptomatic patient with a murmur in whom there is a reasonable probability of structural heart disease. However, the guidelines also emphasize that echocardiography is not a substitute for a careful clinical evaluation. The guidelines repeatedly state that this test is not appropriate in patients with murmurs or other clinical findings that an experienced observer identifies as functional or innocent. Serial or follow-up testing is discouraged in the absence of any change in symptoms or signs.

For patients with known or suspected valvular stenosis, the guidelines support the use of echocardiography for assessing severity of valvular stenosis and ventricular dysfunction. Reevaluation with echocardiography is considered appropriate with changing symptoms or signs, and also for patients with severe valvular stenosis even if asymptomatic. Pregnancy in a patient with valvular stenosis is considered a sufficient change in clinical status to justify echocardiographic evaluation.

Doppler echocardiography is the test of choice to evaluate valvular regurgitation and assess the need for surgical intervention. Because left ventricular dysfunction is such a critical issue in the management of such patients, serial use of echocardiography is appropriate in asymptomatic patients with severe regurgitation or with left ventricular dilatation, as well as in those with changes in symptoms or signs or who have become pregnant. The guidelines were less supportive of routine serial echocardiography for patients with mild to moderate valvular regurgitation without chamber dilatation or clinical symptoms.

The guidelines emphasize that diagnosis of mitral valve prolapse should be made on the basis of the physical examination, in part due to the high rates of false-positive results with echocardiography. Specifically discouraged is the use of echocardiography to exclude mitral valve prolapse in patients with ill-defined symptoms but no other clinical evidence for this condition.

Echocardiography is strongly supported in virtually all patients with known or suspected infective endocarditis. (ACC/AHA guidelines on the use of echocardiography in this setting are discussed in the Guidelines in Chap. 58). Similarly, the guidelines support the use of echocardiography before and after operative interventions for valvular heart disease. The incremental value of transesophageal echocardiography over transthoracic echocardiography is acknowledged for several clinical issues related to patients for whom procedures are contemplated or have been performed. Specific recommendations about the ideal interval for repeat evaluations in patients without changes in symptoms or signs are not made.

Chest Pain and Ischemic Heart Disease

Ischemic heart disease and other cardiac conditions (e.g., pericarditis and acute aortic dissection) are major diagnostic considerations in the evaluation of acute chest pain; accordingly, the ACC/AHA guidelines support the use of echocardiography when routinely available clinical data, including the electrocardiogram, are not diagnostic and in patients with suspected aortic dissection or severe hemodynamic instability (Table 11G–2). This test was not considered necessary for routine use in patients with a high likelihood of myocardial ischemia or infarction.

For patients with suspected acute myocardial ischemic syndromes, echocardiography is considered an appropriate tool for detection of ischemia or injury when other data are not conclusive; for evaluations of left and right ventricular function; and for detection of mechanical complications such as ruptured papillary muscles or a mural thrombus. Once the diagnosis of acute ischemic heart disease is established, the ACC/AHA guidelines support the use of echocardiography to assess the extent of myocardial injury and assess ventricular function, and to help assess prognosis as part of pharmacological or exercise stress testing. The guidelines were less certain but generally supportive of the use of echocardiography for assessment of the location and severity of disease in patients with ongoing ischemia, or for assessment of myocardial viability when patients were candidates for coronary revascularization (Class IIa).

For patients with chronic ischemic heart disease, the guidelines support echocardiography as appropriate for assessment of ventricular function and as a method for assessing myocardial viability and jeopardy through exercise or pharmacological stress testing. However, the guidelines explicitly state that echocardiography should not be routinely substituted "for treadmill exercise testing in patients for whom electrocardiographic (ECG) analysis is expected to suffice" (see Table 11G–2).

Cardiomyopathy and Assessment of Left Ventricular Function

Echocardiography is the ideal first test for assessment of global and regional left ventricular function and is therefore the preferred first-line test for patients with symptoms or signs consistent with left ventricular dysfunction (Table 11G–3). Transesophagealechocardiography (TEE) is recommended when transthoracic echocardiography (TTE) is not diagnostic. Echocardiography is also recommended for assessment of left ventricular hypertrophy, restrictive cardiomyopathy, and heart failure due to diastolic dysfunction. Use of this test is discouraged for routine evaluation of clinically stable patients in whom no change in management is contemplated and in patients with edema but normal venous pressures and no evidence of heart disease.

Pericardial Disease

Echocardiography remains the test of choice for detection of pericardial effusion, and an appropriate test for diagnosis of other pericardial disease (see Table 11G–3). The guidelines discourage the use of

TABLE 11G–1 ACC/AHA Guidelines for Use of Echocardiography in the Evaluation of Patients with Murmurs or Valvular Heart Disease

Indication	Class I (Indicated)	Class IIa (Good Supportive Evidence)	Class IIb (Weak Supportive Evidence)	Class III (Not Indicated)
Evaluation of heart murmurs	1. A murmur in a patient with cardiorespiratory symptoms. 2. A murmur in an asymptomatic patient if the clinical features indicate at least a moderate probability that the murmur is reflective of structural heart disease.	1. A murmur in an asymptomatic patient in whom there is a low probability of heart disease but in whom the diagnosis of heart disease cannot be reasonably excluded by the standard cardiovascular clinical evaluation.		1. In an adult, an asymptomatic heart murmur that has been identified by an experienced observer as functional or innocent.
Valvular stenosis	1. Diagnosis; assessment of hemodynamic severity. 2. Assessment of LV and RV size, function, and/or hemodynamics. 3. Reevaluation of patients with known valvular stenosis with changing symptoms or signs. 4. Assessment of changes in hemodynamic severity and ventricular compensation in patients with known valvular stenosis during pregnancy. 5. Reevaluation of asymptomatic patient with severe stenosis.	1. Assessment of the hemodynamic significance of mild to moderate valvular stenosis by stress Doppler echocardiography. 2. Reevaluation of patients with mild to moderate aortic stenosis with LV dysfunction or hypertrophy even without clinical symptoms.	1. Reevaluation of patients with mild to moderate aortic valvular stenosis with stable signs and symptoms.	1. Routine reevaluation of asymptomatic adult patients with mild aortic stenosis having stable physical signs and normal LV size and function. 2. Routine reevaluation of asymptomatic patients with mild to moderate mitral stenosis and stable physical signs.
Native valvular regurgitation	1. Diagnosis; assessment of hemodynamic severity. 2. Initial assessment and reevaluation (when indicated) of LV and RV size, function, and/or hemodynamics. 3. Reevaluation of patients with mild to moderate valvular regurgitation with changing symptoms. 4. Reevaluation of asymptomatic patient with severe regurgitation. 5. Assessment of changes in hemodynamic severity and ventricular compensation in patients with known valvular regurgitation during pregnancy. 6. Reevaluation of patients with mild to moderate regurgitation with ventricular dilation without clinical symptoms. 7. Assessment of the effects of medical therapy on the severity of regurgitation and ventricular compensation and function.		1. Reevaluation of patients with mild to moderate mitral regurgitation without chamber dilation and without clinical symptoms. 2. Reevaluation of patients with moderate aortic regurgitation without chamber dilation and without clinical symptoms.	1. Routine reevaluation in asymptomatic patients with mild valvular regurgitation having stable physical signs and normal LV size and function.
Mitral valve prolapse (MVP)	1. Diagnosis; assessment of hemodynamic severity, leaflet morphology, and/or ventricular compensation in patients with physical signs of MVP.	1. To exclude MVP in patients who have been diagnosed but without clinical evidence to support the diagnosis. 2. To exclude MVP in patients with first-degree relatives with known myxomatous valve disease. 3. Risk stratification in patients with physical signs of MVP or known MVP.		1. Exclusion of MVP in patients with ill-defined symptoms in the absence of a constellation of clinical symptoms or physical findings suggestive of MVP or a positive family history. 2. Routine repetition of echocardiography in patients with MVP with no or mild regurgitation and no changes in clinical signs or symptoms.

TABLE 11G–1 ACC/AHA Guidelines for Use of Echocardiography in the Evaluation of Patients with Murmurs or Valvular Heart Disease—cont'd

Indication	Class I (Indicated)	Class IIa (Good Supportive Evidence)	Class IIb (Weak Supportive Evidence)	Class III (Not Indicated)
Interventions for valvular heart disease and prosthetic valves	1. Assessment of the timing of valvular intervention based on ventricular compensation, function, and/or severity of primary and secondary lesions. 2. Selection of alternative therapies for mitral valve disease (such as balloon valvuloplasty, operative valve repair, valve replacement).* 3. Use of echocardiography (especially TEE) in performing interventional techniques (eg, balloon valvotomy) for valvular disease. 4. Postintervention baseline studies for valve function (early) and ventricular remodeling (late). 5. Reevaluation of patients with valve replacement with changing clinical signs and symptoms; suspected prosthetic dysfunction (stenosis, regurgitation) or thrombosis.*	1. Routine reevaluation study after baseline studies of patients with valve replacements with mild to moderate ventricular dysfunction without changing clinical signs or symptoms.	1. Routine reevaluation at the time of increased failure rate of a bioprosthesis without clinical evidence of prosthetic dysfunction.	1. Routine reevaluation of patients with valve replacement without suspicion of valvular dysfunction and unchanged clinical signs and symptoms. 2. Patients whose clinical status precludes therapeutic interventions.

*TEE may provide incremental value in addition to information obtained by TTE.
LV = left ventricular; MVP = mitral valve prolapse; RV = right ventricular; TEE = transesophageal echocardiography; TTE = transthoracic echocardiography.

TABLE 11G–2 ACC/AHA Guidelines for Use of Echocardiography in the Evaluation of Patients with Chest Pain and Known or Suspected Ischemic Heart Disease

Indication	Class I (Indicated)	Class IIa (Good Supportive Evidence)	Class IIb (Weak Supportive Evidence)	Class III (Not Indicated)
Patients with chest pain	1. Diagnosis of underlying cardiac disease in patients with chest pain and clinical evidence of valvular, pericardial, or primary myocardial disease. 2. Evaluation of chest pain in patients with suspected acute myocardial ischemia, when baseline ECG is nondiagnostic and when study can be obtained during pain or soon after its abatement. 3. Evaluation of chest pain in patients with suspected aortic dissection. 4. Chest pain in patients with severe hemodynamic instability.			1. Evaluation of chest pain for which a noncardiac cause is apparent. 2. Diagnosis of chest pain in a patient with electrocardiographic changes diagnostic of myocardial ischemia/infarction.
Diagnosis of acute myocardial ischemic syndromes	1. Diagnosis of suspected acute ischemia or infarction not evident by standard means. 2. Measurement of baseline LV function. 3. Patients with inferior myocardial infarction and bedside evidence suggesting possible RV infarction. 4. Assessment of mechanical complications and mural thrombus (TEE is indicated when TTE studies are not diagnostic).	1. Identification of location/severity of disease in patients with ongoing ischemia.		1. Diagnosis of acute myocardial infarction already evident by standard means.

TABLE 11G–2 ACC/AHA Guidelines for Use of Echocardiography in the Evaluation of Patients with Chest Pain and Known or Suspected Ischemic Heart Disease—cont'd

Indication	Class I (Indicated)	Class IIa (Good Supportive Evidence)	Class IIb (Weak Supportive Evidence)	Class III (Not Indicated)
Risk assessment, prognosis, and assessment of therapy in acute myocardial ischemic syndromes	1. Assessment of infarct size and/or extent of jeopardized myocardium 2. In-hospital assessment of ventricular function when the results are used to guide therapy. 3. In-hospital or early postdischarge assessment of the presence/extent of inducible ischemia whenever baseline abnormalities are expected to compromise electrocardiographic interpretation.*	1. In-hospital or early postdischarge assessment of the presence/extent of inducible ischemia in the absence of baseline abnormalities expected to compromise ECG interpretation.* 2. Assessment of myocardial viability when required to define potential efficacy of revascularization (dobutamine stress echocardiography). 3. Reevaluation of ventricular function during recovery when results are used to guide therapy. 4. Assessment of ventricular function after revascularization.	1. Assessment of long-term prognosis (≥2 years after acute myocardial infarction).	1. Routine reevaluation in the absence of any change in clinical status.
Diagnosis and prognosis of chronic ischemic heart disease	1. Diagnosis of myocardial ischemia in symptomatic individuals.* 2. Assessment of global ventricular function at rest. 3. Assessment of myocardial viability (hibernating myocardium) for planning revascularization. (dobutamine stress echocardiography) 4. Assessment of functional significance of coronary lesions (if not already known) in planning percutaneous transluminal coronary angioplasty.*		1. Diagnosis of myocardial ischemia in selected patients with an intermediate or high pretest likelihood of coronary artery disease.* 2. Assessment of an asymptomatic patient with positive results from a screening treadmill test. 3. Assessment of global ventricular function with exercise.*	1. Screening of asymptomatic persons with a low likelihood of coronary artery disease. 2. Routine periodic reassessment of stable patients for whom no change in therapy is contemplated. 3. Routine substitution for treadmill exercise testing in patients for whom ECG analysis is expected to suffice.
Assessment of interventions in chronic ischemic heart disease	1. Assessment of LV function when needed to guide institution and modification of drug therapy in patients with known or suspected LV dysfunction. 2. Assessment for restenosis after revascularization in patients with atypical recurrent symptoms.*	1. Assessment for restenosis after revascularization in patients with typical recurrent symptoms.*		1. Routine assessment of asymptomatic patients after revascularization.

*Exercise or pharmacological stress echocardiogram.
ECG = electrocardiogram; LV = left ventricular; RV = right ventricular; TEE = transesophageal echocardiography; TTE = transthoracic echocardiography.

echocardiography when findings are unlikely to change management and note that pericardial friction rubs are common after acute myocardial infarction and the early postoperative period after cardiac surgery, and echocardiography is not routinely needed in such settings. Echocardiographic assessment of pericardial thickness to assess the diagnosis of constrictive pericarditis is not supported by these guidelines, which note that other technologies (computed tomography or magnetic resonance imaging) provide more accurate data.

Cardiac Masses and Tumors

Echocardiography is also the first-line test for detection of cardiac masses and tumors and is therefore considered appropriate in patients with syndromes suggestive of such abnormalities (e.g., patients with arterial emboli of unknown origin or patients with auscultatory findings suggesting intermittent obstruction of intracardiac flow) (see Table 11G–3). Other candidates include patients with malignancies with a high incidence of cardiovascular involvement, such as hypernephroma, metastatic melanoma, or malignancies of intrathoracic organs.

Diseases of the Great Vessels

Transthoracic echocardiography is often adequate for detection of abnormalities of the aortic root and proximal pulmonary vasculature, but TEE is a far more sensitive tool for evaluation of most conditions affecting the great vessels. Therefore, TEE is the procedure of choice for evaluation of possible aortic dissection or rupture (see Table

TABLE 11G–3 ACC/AHA Guidelines for Use of Echocardiography in the Evaluation of Left Ventricular Function and Other Cardiovascular Anatomy

Indication	Class I (Indicated)	Class IIa (Good Supportive Evidence)	Class IIb (Weak Supportive Evidence)	Class III (Not Indicated)
Patients with dyspnea, edema, or cardiomyopathy	1. Assessment of LV size and function in patients with suspected cardiomyopathy or clinical diagnosis of heart failure.* 2. Edema with clinical signs of elevated central venous pressure when a potential cardiac cause is suspected or when central venous pressure cannot be estimated with confidence and clinical suspicion of heart disease is high.* 3. Dyspnea with clinical signs of heart disease. 4. Patients with unexplained hypotension, especially in the intensive care unit.* 5. Patients exposed to cardiotoxic agents, to determine the advisability of additional or increased dosages. 6. Reevaluation of LV function in patients with established cardiomyopathy when there has been a documented change in clinical status or to guide medical therapy.		1. Reevaluation of patients with established cardiomyopathy when there is no change in clinical status. 2. Reevaluation of patients with edema when a potential cardiac cause has already been demonstrated.	1. Evaluation of LV ejection fraction in patients with recent (contrast or radionuclide) angiographic determination of ejection fraction. 2. Routine reevaluation in clinically stable patients in whom no change in management is contemplated. 3. In patients with edema, normal venous pressure, and no evidence of heart disease.
Pericardial disease	1. Patients with suspected pericardial disease, including effusion, constriction, or effusive-constrictive process. 2. Patients with suspected bleeding in the pericardial space, e.g., trauma, perforation. 3. Follow-up study to evaluate recurrence of effusion or to diagnose early constriction. Repeat studies may be goal directed to answer a specific clinical question. 4. Pericardial friction rub developing in acute myocardial infarction accompanied by symptoms such as persistent pain, hypotension, and nausea.	1. Follow-up studies to detect early signs of tamponade in the presence of large or rapidly accumulating effusions. A goal-directed study may be appropriate. 2. Echocardiographic guidance and monitoring of pericardiocentesis.	1. Postsurgical pericardial disease, including postpericardiotomy syndrome, with potential for hemodynamic impairment. 2. In the presence of a strong clinical suspicion and nondiagnostic TTE, TEE assessment of pericardial thickness to support a diagnosis of constrictive pericarditis.	1. Routine follow-up of small pericardial effusion in clinically stable patients. 2. Follow-up studies in patients with cancer or other terminal illness for whom management would not be influenced by echocardiographic findings. 3. Assessment of pericardial thickness in patients without clinical evidence of constrictive pericarditis. 4. Pericardial friction rub in early uncomplicated myocardial infarction or early postoperative period after cardiac surgery.
Cardiac masses and tumors	1. Evaluation of patients with clinical syndromes and events suggesting an underlying cardiac mass. 2. Evaluation of patients with underlying cardiac disease known to predispose to mass formation for whom a therapeutic decision regarding surgery or anticoagulation will depend on the results of echocardiography. 3. Follow-up or surveillance studies after surgical removal of masses known to have a high likelihood of recurrence (i.e., myxoma). 4. Patients with known primary malignancies when echocardiographic surveillance for cardiac involvement is part of the disease staging process.		1. Screening persons with disease states likely to result in mass formation but for whom no clinical evidence for the mass exists.	1. Patients for whom the results of echocardiography will have no impact on diagnosis or clinical decision-making.

TABLE 11G–3 ACC/AHA Guidelines for Use of Echocardiography in the Evaluation of Left Ventricular Function and Other Cardiovascular Anatomy—cont'd

Indication	Class I (Indicated)	Class IIa (Good Supportive Evidence)	Class IIb (Weak Supportive Evidence)	Class III (Not Indicated)
Suspected thoracic aortic disease	TEE: 1. Aortic dissection. 2. Aortic aneurysm. 3. Aortic rupture. 4. Degenerative or traumatic aortic disease with clinical atheroembolism. 5. Follow-up of aortic dissection, especially after surgical repair when complications or progression is suspected. TTE: 1. Aortic aneurysm (especially for aortic root aneurysm). 2. Aortic root dilation in Marfan or other connective tissue syndromes. 3. Follow-up of aortic dissection, especially after surgical repair without suspicion of complication or progression. 4. First-degree relative of a patient with Marfan syndrome or other connective tissue disorder.			

LV = left ventricular; TEE = transesophageal echocardiography; TTE = transthoracic echocardiography.

11G–3). Because TTE is a less invasive and expensive procedure than TEE, it is recommended for follow-up of patients after repair of aortic dissection who do not have suspicion of complications or progression and of first-degree relatives of patients with Marfan syndrome or other connective tissue disorders.

Pulmonary Disease

Primary pulmonary disease often compromises the quality of TTE, but echocardiography can be an appropriate test for evaluation of the right ventricle and right-sided heart pressures that may be abnormal in patients with conditions such as pulmonary hypertension and pulmonary emboli (Table 11G–4). When other clinical data were not diagnostic, the ACC/AHA guidelines considered echocardiography appropriate for attempts to distinguish cardiac and noncardiac causes of dyspnea. However, echocardiography was not considered necessary for routine evaluation of patients with pulmonary disease or patients with pulmonary disease without changes in clinical status.

Systemic Hypertension

Use of echocardiography in patients with hypertension is supported by the ACC/AHA guidelines when the assessment of left ventricular function or hypertrophy is likely to influence management. An example of such a case would be a patient with mild hypertension in whom the detection of left ventricular hypertrophy would lead to initiation of drug therapy. The guidelines explicitly state that not every patient with hypertension should have a left ventricular function assessment and discourage serial echocardiograms to assess changes in left ventricular mass as patients are treated.

Neurological Disease and Other Cardioembolic Disease

The ACC/AHA guidelines support the use of echocardiography for evaluation of patients with embolic events affecting any major peripheral or visceral artery (see Table 11G–4). Echocardiography was considered clearly appropriate in patients with neurological events without evidence of cerebrovascular disease; its appropriateness in patients with neurological events and known intrinsic cerebrovascular disease was less clear (Class IIb). Echocardiography was discouraged when results would not influence management, such as in patients in whom anticoagulation was absolutely discouraged.

Arrhythmias and Palpitations

Because arrhythmias can be a manifestation of underlying structural heart disease, the ACC/AHA guidelines consider echocardiography appropriate in several subsets of patient with arrhythmias and palpitations (see Table 11G–4). However, echocardiography is discouraged in most patients with palpitations or isolated ventricular premature complexes if they do not have other evidence for structural or arrhythmic cardiac disease. The guidelines support the use of echocardiography as an adjunct to some advanced electrophysiological procedures.

The 1997 ACC/AHA guidelines support the use of TEE to assess risk of thromboembolic events in patients under atrial fibrillation if the need to proceed to cardioversion is urgent and an extended course of anticoagulation is not desirable (see Table 11G–4). There is also limited support for this strategy if the duration of atrial fibrillation is less than 48 hours. However, these guidelines were written before more recent research demonstrating the safety of using TEE to assess risk for thromboembolic events for patients undergoing elective cardioversion of atrial fibrillation of more than 48 hours' duration.[3] Therefore, future revisions of these guidelines can be expected to provide even more support for the use of TEE as an alternative to conventional management with several weeks of anticoagulation.

The ACC/AHA guidelines discourage the routine use of echocardiography for the evaluation of classic neurogenic syncope or for patients in whom there was no suspicion of cardiac disease (see Table 11G–4). Echocardiography is considered appropriate for patients with clinical evidence of cardiac disease or periexertional syncope. The guidelines are somewhat supportive of the use of echocardiography in patients with syncope who are in high-risk professions, such as airline pilots (Class IIa).

Text continued on page 270.

TABLE 11G–4 ACC/AHA Guidelines for Use of Echocardiography in the Evaluation of Other Clinical Syndromes

Indication	Class I (Indicated)	Class IIa (Good Supportive Evidence)	Class IIb (Weak Supportive Evidence)	Class III (Not Indicated)
Pulmonary disease	1. Suspected pulmonary hypertension. 2. Pulmonary emboli and suspected clots in the right atrium or ventricle or main pulmonary artery branches.* 3. For distinguishing cardiac versus noncardiac cause of dyspnea in patients in whom all clinical and laboratory clues are ambiguous.* 4. Follow-up of pulmonary artery pressures in patients with pulmonary hypertension to evaluate response to treatment. 5. Lung disease with clinical suspicion of cardiac involvement (suspected cor pulmonale).	1. Measurement of exercise pulmonary artery pressure. 2. Patients being considered for lung transplantation or other surgical procedure for advanced lung disease.*		1. Lung disease without any clinical suspicion of cardiac involvement. 2. Reevaluation studies of RV function in patients with chronic obstructive lung disease without a change in clinical status.
Hypertension	1. When assessment of resting LV function, hypertrophy, or concentric remodeling is important in clinical decision-making (see LV function). 2. Detection and assessment of functional significance of concomitant coronary artery disease (stress echocardiography). 3. Follow-up assessment of LV size and function in patients with LV dysfunction when there has been a documented change in clinical status or to guide medical therapy.	1. Identification of LV diastolic filling abnormalities with or without systolic abnormalities. 2. Assessment of LV hypertrophy in a patient with borderline hypertension without LV hypertrophy on ECG to guide decision-making regarding initiation of therapy. A limited goal-directed echocardiogram may be indicated for this purpose.	1. Risk stratification for prognosis by determination of LV performance.	1. Reevaluation to guide antihypertensive therapy based on LV mass regression. 2. Reevaluation in asymptomatic patients to assess LV function.
Neurological events or other vascular occlusive events	1. Patients of any age with abrupt occlusion of a major peripheral or visceral artery. 2. Younger patients (typically <45 years) with cerebrovascular events. 3. Older patients (typically >45 years) with neurological events without evidence of cerebrovascular disease or other obvious cause. 4. Patients for whom a clinical therapeutic decision (e.g., anticoagulation) will depend on the results of echocardiography.	1. Patients with suspicion of embolic disease and with cerebrovascular disease of questionable significance.	1. Patients with a neurological event and intrinsic cerebrovascular disease of a nature sufficient to cause the clinical event.	1. Patients for whom the results of echocardiography will not impact a decision to institute anticoagulant therapy or otherwise alter the approach to diagnosis or treatment.
Arrhythmias and palpitations	1. Arrhythmias with clinical suspicion of structural heart disease. 2. Arrhythmia in a patient with a family history of a genetically transmitted cardiac lesion associated with arrhythmia such as tuberous sclerosis, rhabdomyoma, or hypertrophic cardiomyopathy. 3. Evaluation of patients as a component of the work-up before electrophysiological ablative procedures.	1. Arrhythmia requiring treatment. 2. TEE guidance of transseptal catheterization and catheter placement during ablative procedures.	1. Arrhythmias commonly associated with, but without clinical evidence of, heart disease. 2. Evaluation of patients who have undergone radiofrequency ablation in the absence of complications. (In centers with established ablation programs, a postprocedural echocardiogram may not be necessary.)	1. Palpitation without corresponding arrhythmias or other cardiac signs or symptoms. 2. Isolated premature ventricular contractions for which there is no clinical suspicion of heart disease.
Before cardioversion	1. Evaluation of patient for whom a decision concerning cardioversion will be impacted by knowledge of prognostic factors (e.g., LV function, coexistent mitral valve disease).	1. Patients with atrial fibrillation of <48 hours duration and other heart disease (TEE only)	1. Patients with atrial fibrillation of <48 hours duration and no other heart disease (TEE only). 2. Patients with mitral valve disease or hypertrophic	1. Patients requiring emergent cardioversion. 2. Patients who have been on long-term anticoagulation at therapeutic levels and

Continued

TABLE 11G–4 ACC/AHA Guidelines for Use of Echocardiography in the Evaluation of Other Clinical Syndromes–cont'd

Indication	Class I (Indicated)	Class IIa (Good Supportive Evidence)	Class IIb (Weak Supportive Evidence)	Class III (Not Indicated)
	TEE only: 1. Patients requiring urgent (not emergent) cardioversion for whom extended precardioversion anticoagulation is not desirable.* 2. Patients who have had prior cardioembolic events thought to be related to intraatrial thrombus.* 3. Patients for whom anticoagulation is contraindicated and for whom a decision about cardioversion will be influenced by TEE results.* 4. Patients for whom intraatrial thrombus has been demonstrated in previous TEE.*		cardiomyopathy who have been on long-term anticoagulation at therapeutic levels before cardioversion (TEE only). 3. Patients undergoing cardioversion from atrial flutter.	who do not have mitral valve disease or hypertrophic cardiomyopathy before cardioversion. 3. Precardioversion evaluation of patients who have undergone previous TEE and with no clinical suspicion of a significant interval change.
Patients with syncope	1. Syncope in a patient with clinically suspected heart disease. 2. Periexertional syncope.	1. Syncope in a patient in a high-risk occupation (e.g., pilot).	1. Syncope of occult origin with no findings of heart disease on history or physical examination.	1. Recurrent syncope in a patient in whom previous echocardiographic or other testing demonstrated a cause of syncope. 2. Syncope in a patient for whom there is no clinical suspicion of heart disease. 3. Classic neurogenic syncope.
Screening	1. Patients with a family history of genetically transmitted cardiovascular disease. 2. Potential donors for cardiac transplantation. 3. Patients with phenotypic features of Marfan syndrome or related connective tissue diseases. 4. Baseline and reevaluations of patients undergoing chemotherapy with cardiotoxic agents.		1. Patients with systemic disease that may affect the heart.	1. The general population. 2. Competitive athletes without clinical evidence of heart disease.
Critically ill	1. The hemodynamically unstable patient 2. Suspected aortic dissection (TEE)			1. The hemodynamically stable patient not expected to have cardiac disease. 2. Reevaluation follow-up studies on hemodynamically stable patients.
Critically injured	1. Serious blunt or penetrating chest trauma (suspected pericardial effusion or tamponade). 2. Mechanically ventilated multiple-trauma or chest trauma patient. 3. Suspected preexisting valvular or myocardial disease in the trauma patient. 4. The hemodynamically unstable multiple-injury patient without obvious chest trauma but with a mechanism of injury suggesting potential cardiac or aortic injury (deceleration or crush). 5. Widening of the mediastinum, postinjury suspected aortic injury (TEE). 6. Potential catheter, guidewire, pacer electrode, or pericardiocentesis needle injury with or without signs of tamponade.	1. Evaluation of hemodynamics in multiple-trauma or chest trauma patients with pulmonary artery catheter monitoring and data disparate with clinical situation. 2. Follow-up study on victims of serious blunt or penetrating trauma.		1. Suspected myocardial contusion in the hemodynamically stable patient with a normal ECG.

TABLE 11G–4 ACC/AHA Guidelines for Use of Echocardiography in the Evaluation of Other Clinical Syndromes—cont'd

Indication	Class I (Indicated)	Class IIa (Good Supportive Evidence)	Class IIb (Weak Supportive Evidence)	Class III (Not Indicated)
Adult patient with congenital heart disease	1. Patients with clinically suspected congenital heart disease, as evidenced by signs and symptoms such as a murmur, cyanosis, or unexplained arterial desaturation, and an abnormal ECG or x-ray suggesting congenital heart disease. 2. Patients with known congenital heart disease on follow-up when there is a change in clinical findings. 3. Patients with known congenital heart disease for whom there is uncertainty as to the original diagnosis or when the precise nature of the structural abnormalities or hemodynamics is unclear. 4. Periodic echocardiograms in patients with known congenital heart lesions and for whom ventricular function and atrioventricular valve regurgitation must be followed (e.g., patients with a functionally single ventricle after Fontan procedure, transposition of the great vessels after Mustard procedure, L-transposition and ventricular inversion, and palliative shunts). 5. Patients with known congenital heart disease for whom following pulmonary artery pressure is important (e.g., patients with moderate or ventricular septal defects, atrial septal defects, single ventricle, or any of the above with an additional risk factor for pulmonary hypertension). 6. Periodic echocardiography in patients with surgically repaired (or palliated) congenital heart disease with the following: change in clinical condition or clinical suspicion of residual defects, LV or RV function that must be followed, or when there is a possibility of hemodynamic progression or a history of pulmonary hypertension. 7. To direct interventional catheter valvotomy, radiofrequency ablation valvotomy interventions in the presence of complex cardiac anatomy.		1. A follow-up Doppler echocardiographic study, annually or once every 2 years, in patients with known hemodynamically significant congenital heart disease without evident change in clinical condition.	1. Multiple repeat Doppler echocardiography in patients with repaired patent ductus arteriosus, atrial septal defect, ventricular septal defect, coarctation of the aorta, or bicuspid aortic valve without change in clinical condition. 2. Repeat Doppler echocardiography in patients with known hemodynamically insignificant congenital heart lesions (e.g., small atrial septal defect, small ventricular septal defect) without a change in clinical condition.

*TEE is indicated when TTE studies are not diagnostic.

ECG = electrocardiogram; LV = left ventricular; RV = right ventricular; TEE = transesophageal echocardiography; TTE = transthoracic echocardiography.

Screening

The ACC/AHA guidelines do not support using echocardiography to screen for heart disease in the general population or asymptomatic athletes (see Table 11G–4). Examples of settings in which screening echocardiography may be appropriate include those involving patients with a family history of genetically transmitted cardiovascular diseases, those involving potential donors for heart transplantation, and serial evaluation of patients receiving potentially cardiotoxic chemotherapy.

Critically Ill and Injured Patients

Echocardiography is often useful for establishing the diagnosis in hemodynamically unstable, critically ill and injured patients (see Table 11G–4). TEE is particularly useful if injury to the aorta or spontaneous dissection is suspected.

Adult Patients with Congenital Heart Disease

Echocardiography is useful for diagnosis of congenital heart disease in adults, and for follow-up of manifestations of disease such as ventricular function and hemodynamically significant shunts. The guidelines discourage the overuse of serial echocardiography in patients without changes in clinical status, particularly if they are known to have lesions of minor hemodynamic significance, such as small atrial or ventricular septal defects.

Standards for Clinical Competence

A joint statement on standards for Clinical Competency was issued in 2003 by the ACC/AHA and other professional societies. It described three levels of expertise and standards for the duration and depth of training. Level I training (3 months, 75 examinations performed, 150 examinations interpreted) constitutes the minimum amount of training that must be achieved by all trainees in adult cardiovascular medicine. Level II training (6 months, 150 cases performed, 300 cases interpreted) is the minimum training for physicians who perform and interpret echocardiograms independently. Level III training (12 months, 300 cases performed, 750 cases interpreted) is appropriate for physicians who direct echocardiography laboratories and supervise quality control systems for interpretation of tests. Different criteria are recommended for experienced echocardiographers who completed training before these guidelines were established.

For competence in TEE, trainees in cardiovascular medicine should perform at least 25 esophageal intubations with an echocardiographic probe and perform approximately 50 TEEs under the supervision of a level III trained echocardiographer. To maintain competence in TEE, the task force recommends a minimum of 25 to 50 cases per year.

References

1. Cheitlin MD, Alpert JS, Armstrong WF, et al: ACC/AHA guidelines for the clinical application of echocardiography: A report of the American College of Cardiology/American Heart Association Task Force on Practice Guidelines (Committee on Clinical Application of Echocardiography). Circulation 95:1686, 1997.
2. Douglas PS, Foster E, Gorcsan J, et al: ACC/AHA clinical competence statement on echocardiography: A report of the American College of Cardiology/American Heart Association/American College of Physicians-American Society of Internal Medicine Task Force on Clinical Competence (Committee on Echocardiography). J Am Coll Cardiol 41:687, 2003.
3. Klein AL, Grimm RA, Murray RD, et al: Use of transesophageal echocardiography to guide cardioversion in patients with atrial fibrillation. N Engl J Med 344:1411, 2001.

CHAPTER 12

The Chest Radiograph in Cardiovascular Disease

Michael A. Bettmann

The chest radiograph was one of the first types of x-ray films to be used clinically.[1] It remains the most common x-ray examination and one of the most difficult examinations to interpret. It contains a large amount of anatomical and physiological information, but it is difficult and sometimes even impossible to interpret objectively. There are major variations in information as a function of radiographic technique, body habitus, age, underlying physiological status, and training and focus of the interpreter. The aims of this chapter are to review the way chest radiographs are obtained, to present a basic approach to how to interpret them, and to discuss and illustrate common as well as characteristic findings that are relevant to cardiovascular disease.

Technical Considerations

The usual chest radiograph consists of a frontal and a lateral view. The frontal is a posteroanterior (PA) view, with the patient standing with the chest toward the film. The lateral is also taken with the patient standing, with the left side toward the film. For both, the x-ray tube is kept at a distance of 6 feet from the film. The rationale for these conventions is based on simple physics. X-rays are created by first inducing a high current across a diode, thereby generating electrons. These electrons are aimed at a metal target, the rotating anode, which gives off the x-rays. The x-rays are allowed to emerge only through a small opening in the tube, the focal spot. The ability of the x-rays to penetrate structures is determined by the combination of kilovoltage, milliamperage, and time used to produce them. These factors also determine the exposure to the patient.[2,3]

In theory, x-rays emerge from the x-ray tube as a point source, remain parallel, and do not diverge from each other, and there is no geometrical distortion of structures as they pass through the body and are recorded on film. In practice, the x-rays diverge from the focal spot and are not parallel. As a result, when they are captured on film there is geometrical distortion as a function of the distance from the midline of the x-ray beam and the distance of the structures from the film. The farther from the tube an object is, the more parallel are the x-rays that penetrate it. Conversely, the closer to the tube the object and the film are, the more the incident x-rays must diverge to cover the edges of the object. Thus, the farther an object is from the source, the less geometrical distortion is encountered. The greater the distance from the source, however, the more energy must be applied to penetrate the object to be imaged and expose the x-ray film. That is, in simple terms, resolution is improved by increasing the source-image distance (SID) but tube energy and thus exposure to the patient must also be increased with increasing SID. As a result, a standard convention has been developed: standard chest radiographs are obtained with an SID of 6 feet. X-rays are blocked from the film to varying degrees by various structures, leading to shades of gray that allow discrimination between the heart, which is fluid filled and is relatively impervious to x-rays, and the air-filled lung parenchyma, which blocks few x-rays.

Several practical observations result from the physics of chest radiographs. If patients are unable to stand, chest radiographs are not generally obtained with the chest toward the film (PA). With the standard PA view, the heart appears smaller and its size and contour are more accurately depicted than on a portable film, which is usually an anteroposterior (AP) view (i.e., the tube is in front of the patient and the film is behind) with resultant greater divergence of x-rays because the heart lies relatively anteriorly and the SID is short. Similarly, on a standard lateral film, the right ribs appear larger than the left (Fig. 12–1). In both cases, this effect occurs because a structure is further from the film. As a result, there is increased divergence of the x-rays from the midline point source, and relative magnification. The side of an effusion, therefore, can generally be delineated on a lateral radiograph.

There are several inherent practical limitations to portable chest radiographs. Most are obtained with patients positioned either supine or semisupine. The degree of inspiration is therefore likely to be substantially less than with an erect film. Further, portable radiographs are invariably taken as AP views and the SID is less than 6 feet, of necessity, because of the nature of the portable x-ray machine and also because of the usual position of the patient, sitting or lying in a bed. Most portable x-ray units are not able to generate sufficient energy to penetrate a patient adequately and expose the film from 6 feet. Space constraints and the patient's position are additional hurdles. Also, because exposure time must usually be longer than with fixed units, edge definition is compromised. For all these reasons, the inherent resolution is poorer with portable radiographs, and the accuracy is limited. Because of the lower available kilovoltage with portable x-ray units and the longer exposure time that is necessary, radiation exposure to the patient is also greater than with a standard PA film. Portable films are most useful for answering relatively simple questions, such as whether the pacemaker or implantable cardioverter-defibrillator (ICD) is properly positioned, whether the endotracheal tube is in the correct location, and whether the mediastinum is midline (Fig. 12–2).[2,4,5]

Other questions cannot be answered accurately from a portable chest x-ray film. If the film is obtained with the patient in a less than upright position, it is impossible to exclude even a sizable pneumothorax or pleural effusion. Because of the patient's

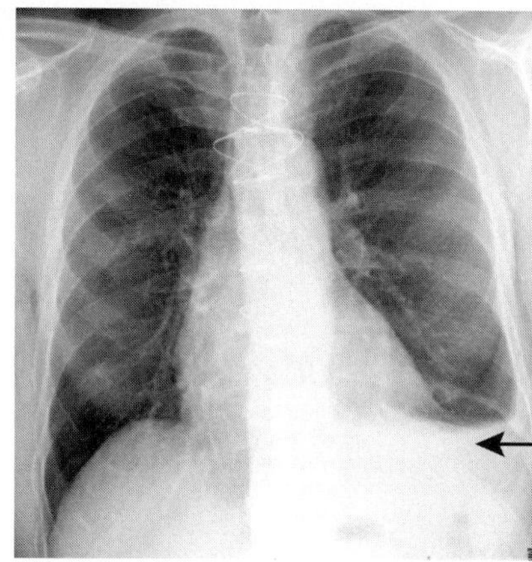

A

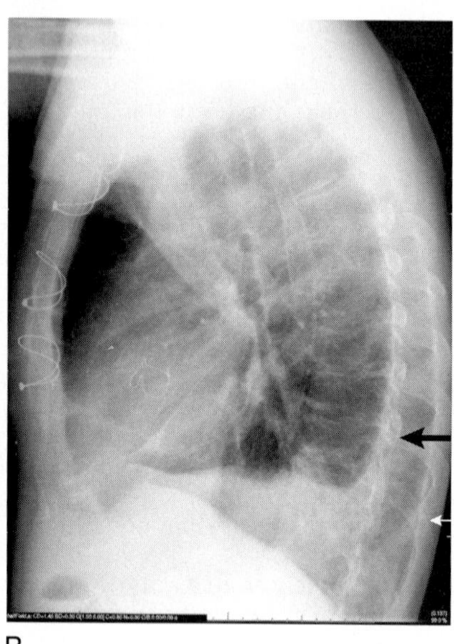

B

FIGURE 12–1 Standard upright chest radiographs of a 74-year-old man who has undergone aortic valve replacement. **A,** Posteroanterior view shows median sternotomy wires, a left pleural effusion (arrow), and normal pulmonary vascular pattern. **B,** Lateral view. Note that the right ribs (small arrow) are magnified compared with the left (large arrow), and the effusion can be localized to the left.

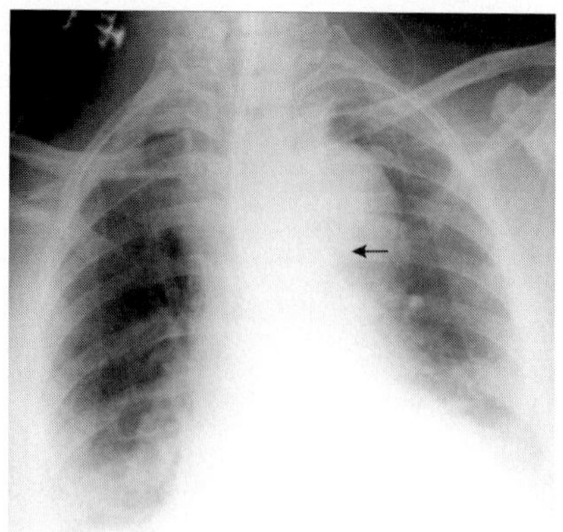

A

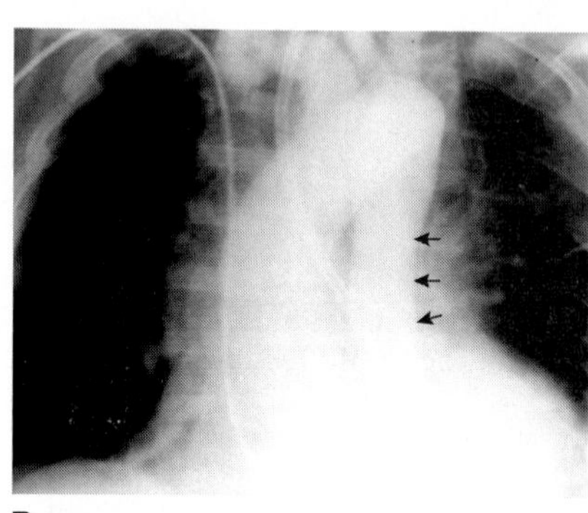

B

FIGURE 12–2 **A,** Portable chest radiograph of a 70-year-old man with spontaneous dissection of the thoracic aorta. Portable frontal view cannot accurately demonstrate heart size or pulmonary vascularity but shows a double density (arrow) at the level of the descending aorta. Note also widened superior mediastinum, with nasogastic tube deviated toward the right. **B,** Levo phase of a right-heart angiogram shows an evident Stanford type B dissection, with a flap (arrows) beginning at the level of the left subclavian artery, and filling of the true (but not the false) lumen of the descending aorta.

position, conventional SID, and the limited tube output, it is impossible to evaluate heart size and contour or status of pulmonary vascularity. It may be possible to say that there is or is not acute pulmonary edema, but it is not possible to judge whether or not there is cardiomegaly, mild to moderate congestive heart failure, or the presence or absence of a small infiltrate.

Digital Imaging

Chest radiographs have generally been recorded on high-resolution x-ray film. With optimal technique and a cooperative patient who can hold a deep inspiration, the result is a study that clearly and accurately depicts very small structures, such as the contour of small pulmonary arteries. With the advent of digital radiography (DR), a filmless form of radiography, chest radiographs are increasingly stored on digital media. There are two principal ways to do this. The first is computed radiography (CR), which is widely available. It is essentially a digital conversion of conventionally obtained chest radiographs. The second method, DR, is the direct recording of images by digital means, without conversion of analog to digital information. There is, then, an inherent difference, with the elimination of added noise and lost information that occurs with this conversion. CR is accomplished with a reusable plate to record the images, which are then converted to a digital format. True DR can be accomplished in many ways. The most promising is "flat plate" technology, for reasons of resolution, utility, and (in the long term) cost. It involves the use of an image-sensing plate that directly converts the incident photons into a digital signal rather than producing a transient conversion as with an image intensifier, producing a reusable CR plate, or altering a silver iodide crystal in a film emulsion, as in standard film radiography. DR is truly "filmless"; CR can be either, and the classic chest radiograph relies on film that is exposed and developed.[6-11]

Resolution with DR may be marginally decreased because the pixel size is larger than that of the silver iodide crystals in the emulsion on x-ray film.[6,9,11] Such a decrease, however, is generally below the ability of the eye to detect. At this time, DR equipment is more costly than either standard radiographic rooms or CR rooms. Both DR and CR have significant advantages for several reasons. First, with the widespread adoption of picture archiving and communication systems (PACSs), films that are obtained digitally or are directly converted to digital format are immediately available for review at any location where there is a PACS-enabled workstation. This system obviates the problem of lost films (all films are digitally archived) and the need to go to a remote location to review a film.[12,13] Also, each film is available for review immediately after it is obtained and stored. In addition, the exposure dose is generally lower, and the need to repeat films because of inadequacy is limited if not eliminated. There is less need to repeat films because of the inherent ability to manipulate the image after it is obtained; the relative density (window and level), magnification, and even area included can be altered without reexposure. Most PACSs now utilize the Internet for gaining access to images, further simplifying availability.

There are several additional basic considerations. The first is radiation exposure. The radiation necessary for PA and lateral chest films is usually minimal in terms of radiation effects, regarding both the dose of a single study and the cumulative dose of repeated chest x-ray studies. Radiation dose is always a consideration in the pediatric age group, however, for obvious reasons.[2] It is also a consideration in patients who undergo interventional cardiology procedures.[3-5] Excluding oncological radiology, the majority of recently reported cases of radiation skin damage have occurred in patients who have undergone repeated prolonged interventional procedures. In this setting, it is important to be alert to any additional radiation exposure. Consequently, each extra chest film should be ordered with care. DR is important in this regard, because it generally provides a lower radiation dose to the patient.

The Normal Chest Radiograph

Reading standard PA and lateral chest radiographs is a daunting task. The amount of information present is huge, and there are countless relevant variables. It is imperative to have a systematic approach, based on an assessment first of anatomy and then of physiology. This approach, of course, is based on an understanding of what is normal.[14,15]

In the standard PA chest study, the overall heart diameter is normally less than half the transverse diameter of the thorax (Fig. 12–3). The heart overlies the thoracic spine, roughly three-fourths to the left of the spine and one-fourth to the right. The mediastinum is narrow superiorly, and normally the descending aorta can be defined from the arch to the dome of the diaphragm, on the left. Below the aortic arch, the pulmonary hila are seen, slightly higher on the left than the right. On the lateral film (Fig. 12–4), the left main pulmonary artery can be seen coursing superiorly and posteriorly compared with the right. On both frontal and lateral views, the ascending aorta (aortic root) is normally obscured by the main pulmonary artery and both atria. The location of the pulmonary outflow tract is usually clear on the lateral film.

Cardiac Chambers and Aorta

On the normal chest film, it is not usually possible to define individual cardiac chambers. It is imperative, however, both to know their normal position and to examine the film to determine whether the size and location of each are within the normal range. On the PA view, the right contour of the mediastinum contains the right atrium but also the ascending aorta and the superior vena cava. The right ventricle, as is clear on echocardiography, is located partially overlying the left ventricle on both frontal and lateral views.[16] The left atrium is located just inferior to the left pulmonary hilum. In normal persons, there is a concavity at this level, the location of the left atrial appendage. The atrium constitutes the upper portion of the posterior contour of the heart on the lateral film but cannot be separated from the left ventricle. The left ventricle constitutes the prominent, rounded apex of the heart on the frontal view as well as the sloping inferior portion of the mediastinum on the lateral (see Fig. 12–4B).

The apex is often not clearly delineated for a reason related to x-ray attenuation. The heart is evident and distinguishable from the lungs because it contains water-density blood rather than air. Because blood attenuates x-rays to a greater extent than air, the heart appears relatively white (less so than bones) and the lungs relatively black (less so than the edges of the film where there is no interposed tissue). A fat pad of varying thickness surrounds the apex of the heart (Fig. 12–5). Fat has a density greater than that of air and marginally less than that of blood. As it covers the ventricular apex, the fat pad is relatively thick and dense. As it thins out toward the left lateral chest wall, it is progressively less dense—hence the hazy, poorly marginated appearance of the apex. Similarly, a fat pad may be seen on the lateral chest film as a wedge-shaped density overlying the anterior aspect of the left ventricle. The pericardial sac cannot normally be defined (Fig. 12–6). The borders of the cardiac silhouette are normally moderately but not completely sharp in contour. Even though the exposure time for a chest x-ray is very short (less than 100 milliseconds), there is usually sufficient cardiac motion to cause minor haziness of the silhouette. If a portion of the heart border does not move, as in the case of a left ventricular aneurysm, the border is unusually sharp (Fig. 12–7). The aortic arch, however, is usually visible, as the aorta courses posteriorly and is surrounded by air. Most of the descending aorta is also visible. The position and the size of each can be easily evaluated (Fig. 12–8) using the frontal and lateral views.

Lungs and Pulmonary Vasculature

Lung size varies as a function of inspiratory effort, age, body habitus, water content, and intrinsic pathological processes. For example, because lung distensibility decreases with age, the lungs appear subtly but progressively smaller with advancing age, even with maximal inspiratory effort. Also, with increasing left ventricular dysfunction, the interstitial fluid in the lungs increases and lung expansion decreases. On the other hand, the lungs appear both larger and blacker in the presence of chronic obstructive lung disease with bulla formation (Fig. 12–9). As lung expansion decreases, the heart appears relatively slightly larger even though it does not

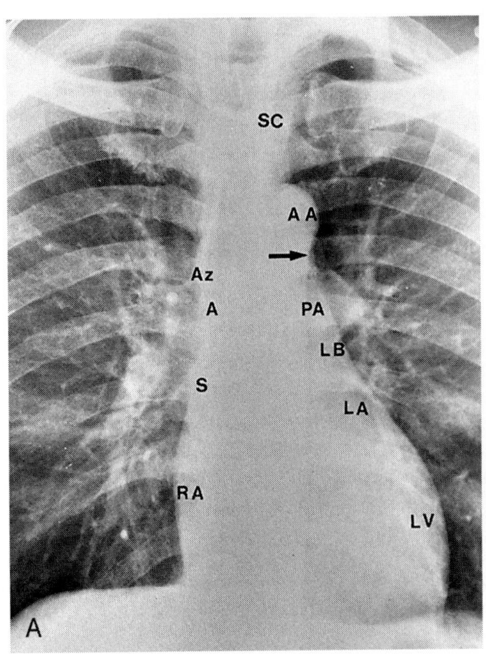

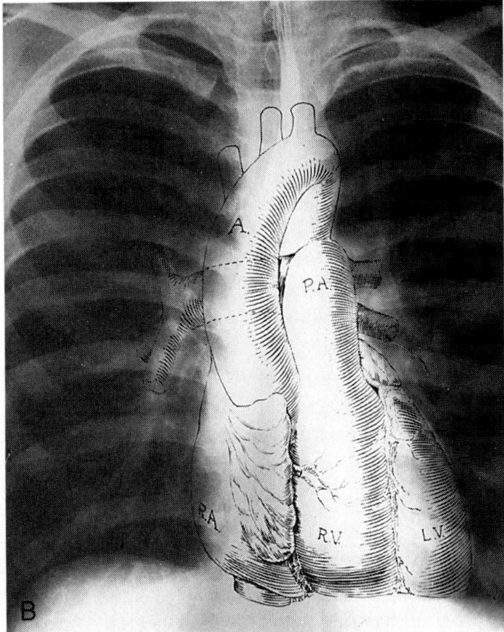

FIGURE 12–3 Frontal projection of the heart and great vessels. **A,** Left and right heart borders in the frontal projection. **B,** A line drawing in the frontal projection demonstrates the relationship of the cardiac valves, rings, and sulci to the mediastinal borders. A = ascending aorta; AA = aortic arch; Az = azygous vein; LA = left atrial appendage; LB = left lower border of pulmonary artery; LV = left ventricle; PA = main pulmonary artery; RA = right atrium; S = superior vena cava; SC = subclavian artery.

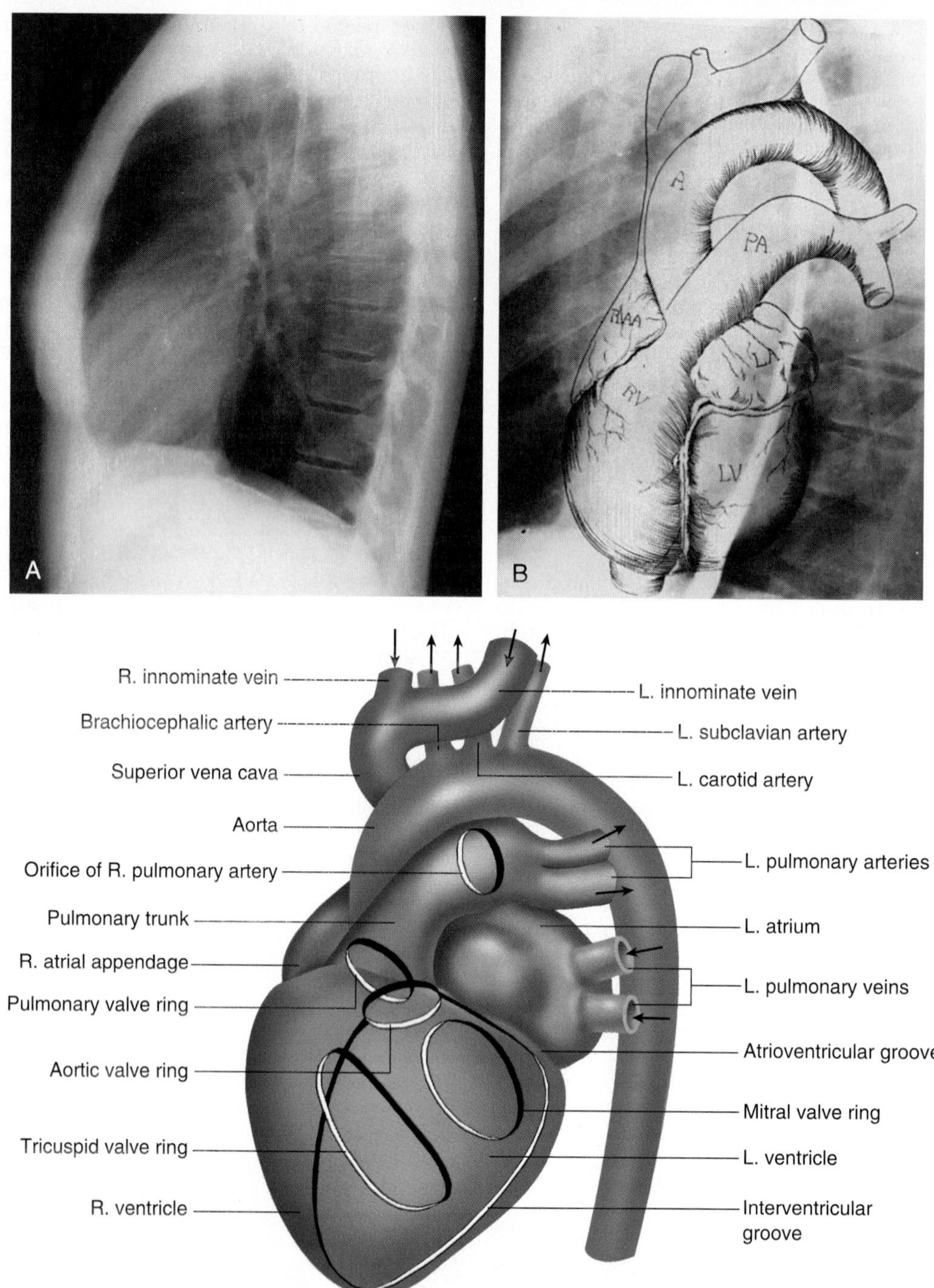

FIGURE 12–4 **A,** Lateral chest radiograph. **B,** Superimposed anatomical drawing of the cardiac chambers and great vessels. **C,** Diagram of the lateral projection of the heart showing the position of the cardiac chambers, valve rings, and sulci. Arrows indicate direction of blood flow.

change in size. However, the heart does not exceed half the transverse diameter of the chest in a good-quality PA film unless there is true cardiomegaly. It is important to keep in mind that evident enlargement may be due to enlargement of the heart overall, to dilation of one or more chambers, or to pericardial fluid (Fig. 12–10). In patients with chronic obstructive pulmonary disease, the heart often appears small or normal in size even in the presence of cardiac dysfunction (see Fig. 12–9).

In normal subjects, pulmonary vascularity has a predictable pattern.[17] Pulmonary arteries are usually easily visible centrally in the hila and progressively less so more peripherally. The central main right and left pulmonary arteries are usually not individually identifiable, as they lie within the mediastinum (see Figs. 12–3 and 12–4). If the lung is thought of in three zones, the major arteries are central, the clearly distinguishable small arteries in the middle zone, and the small arteries and arterioles that are normally below the limit of resolution in the outer zone. The visible small arteries have sharp, easily defined margins. As noted earlier, this is because of the sharp border between water-density and air-density structures. In the standard, standing frontal view, the arteries in the lower zone are larger than those in the upper zone, at an equal distance from the hila. This

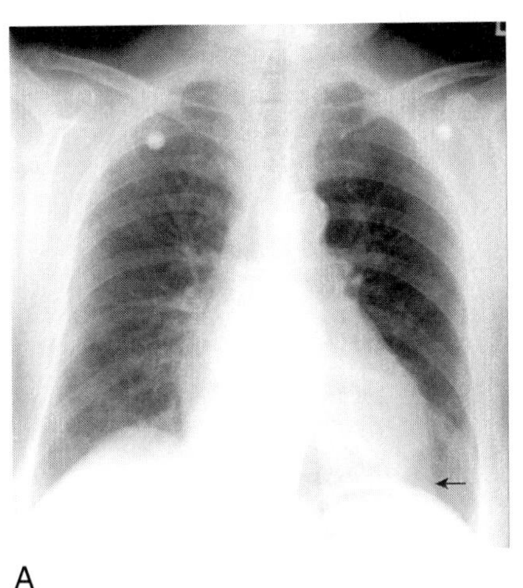

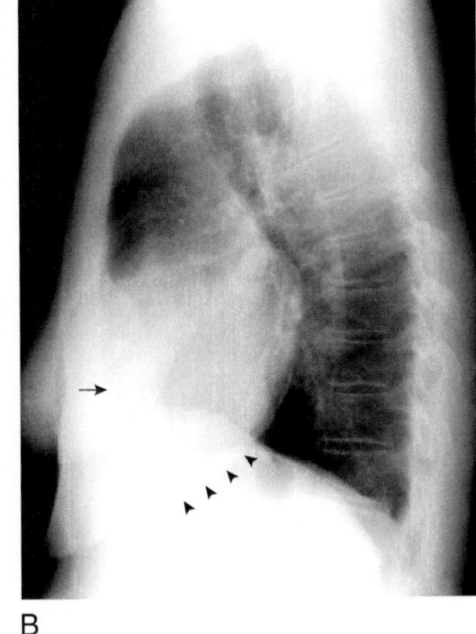

A B

FIGURE 12–5 Chest radiographs of a 70-year-old woman with rheumatic heart disease and combined aortic stenosis and mitral stenosis. Her pulmonary capillary wedge pressure is 30 mm Hg. **A,** Posteroanterior view. There is evidence of chronically elevated pulmonary venous pressures with moderate (not marked) pulmonary vascular redistribution. There is moderate left ventricular enlargement and prominence of the left atrial appendage. **B,** Lateral view. Note enlargement of the left ventricle, extending below the diaphragm and compressing the gastric bubble (arrowheads).

Also note the apical fat pad, seen as the hazy density on the frontal view (**A,** arrow), and the anterior, retrosternal, well-delineated, wedge-shaped density on the lateral view (**B,** arrow).

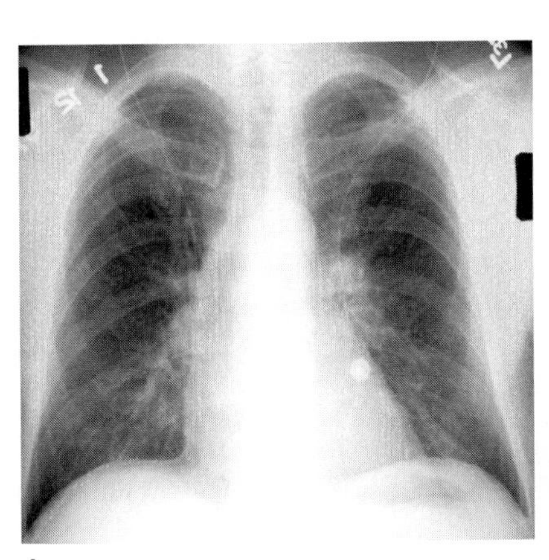

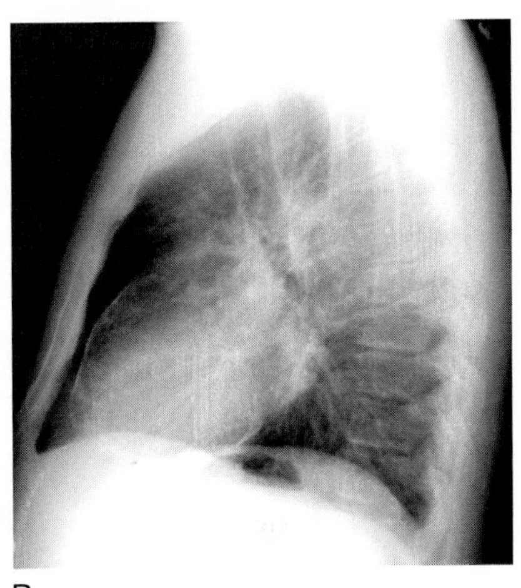

A B

FIGURE 12–6 Chest radiographs of a 45-year-old man with calcific pericarditis. **A,** Posteroanterior view is essentially normal. **B,** Lateral view demonstrates thin, irregular calcification of pericardium around the left ventricular contour.

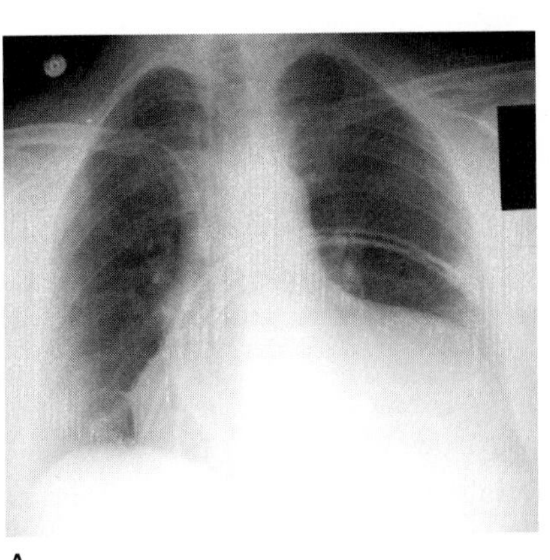

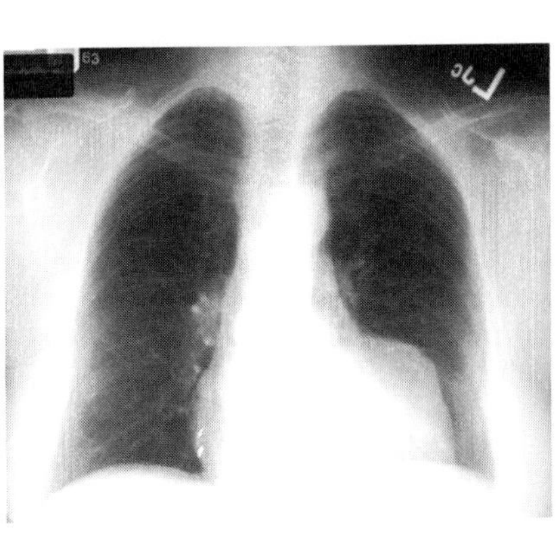

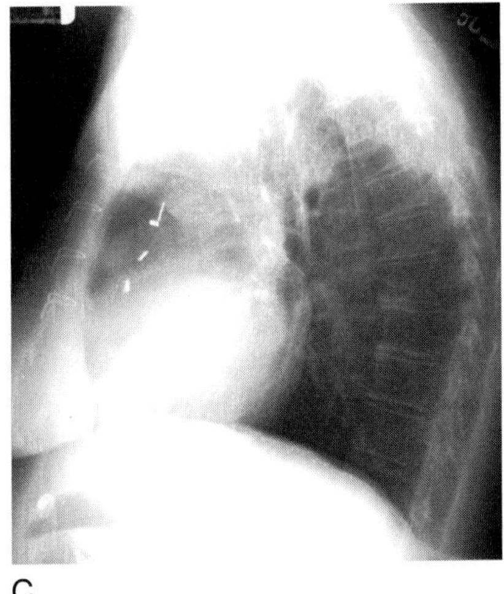

A B C

FIGURE 12–7 Chest radiographs of a 53-year-old woman with coronary artery disease and heart failure following a large anterolateral myocardial infarction. **A,** Frontal, portable view suggests cardiomegaly and heart failure. Sharp, horizontal contour of the left ventricle is suggestive of anterior wall aneurysm. **B** and **C,** Posteroanterior and lateral views after revascularization and aneurysmectomy demonstrate persistence of an abnormal contour of the left ventricle, consistent with recurrent aneurysm, and clips on side branches of saphenous vein graft to right coronary artery.

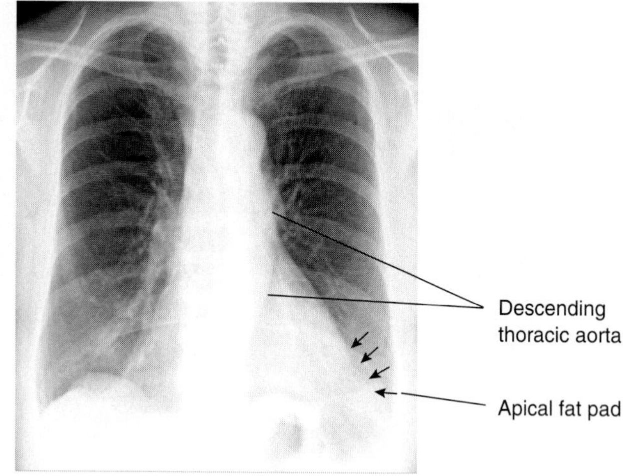

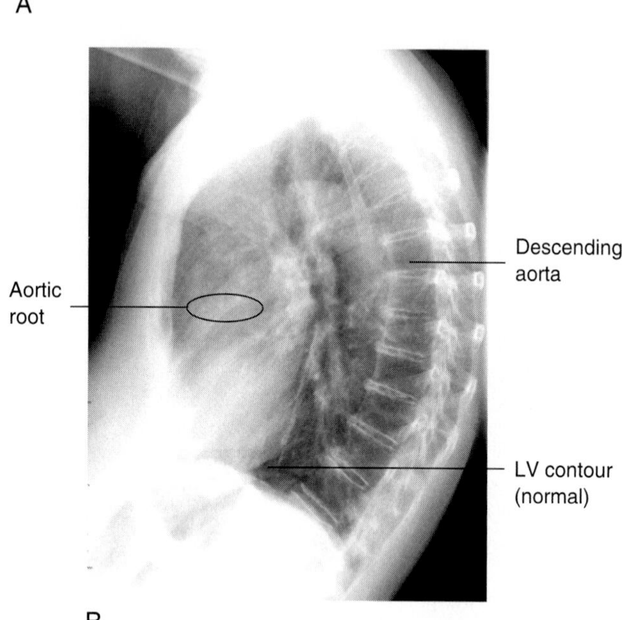

FIGURE 12–8 Chest radiographs of a 67-year-old woman with aortic stenosis. **A,** The posteroanterior view shows a normal cardiac size and pulmonary vascular pattern and enlargement of the aortic root. Note also prominence of the apical fat pad (arrows) on the left and no real cardiomegaly. Note also moderate pectus excavatum (causing blurring of the right heart border). **B,** The lateral view shows normal pulmonary vasculature and enlargement of the aortic root. There is moderate pectus excavatum. There is no visible aortic valve calcification or left ventricular enlargement.

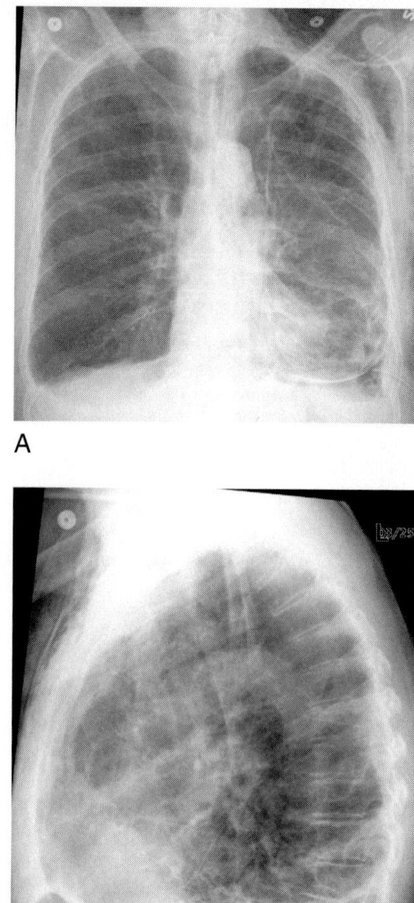

FIGURE 12–9 Patient with severe bullous chronic obstructive lung disease (COPD), spontaneous pneumothorax, and subcutaneous emphysema. Posteroanterior **(A)** and lateral **(B)** views of the chest show loculation of the left-sided pneumothorax to the inferior lateral region because of bullae and fibrosis. Note small cardiac silhouette, secondary to severe COPD.

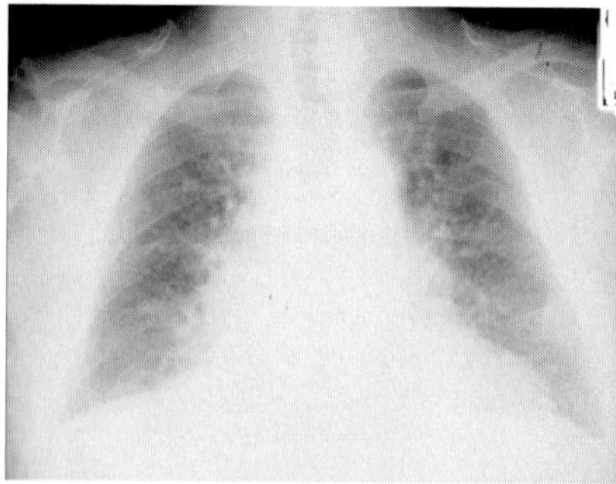

FIGURE 12–10 Chest film of a 63-year-old man with end-stage renal disease. There is marked enlargement of the cardiac silhouette secondary to pericardial effusion associated with renal failure. Note also marked pulmonary vascular redistribution.

appearance is related to the effect of gravity on the normal, low-pressure lung circulation. That is, gravity leads to slightly greater intravascular volume at the lung bases than in the upper zones. This effect is also seen in a normal perfusion lung scan. Because the radionuclide is generally administered with the patient supine, there is a greater concentration posteriorly than anteriorly, as confirmed in the count rates. If the patient is sitting or standing when the radionuclide is injected, the count rate is greater at the lung base than at the apices.

The angles that the lungs make with the diaphragm are normally very sharp and can be delineated bilaterally on both frontal and lateral views. The pleura is usually tightly applied, not separated from the ribs on the PA or lateral view. The contour that the inferior vena cava (IVC) makes with the heart is clearly seen on the lateral film (see Fig. 12–1B). Its relationship to the cardiac contour varies markedly, depending on minor degrees of rotation of the patient. That is, the IVC lies on the right of the mediastinum and posterior to the contour of the heart. This contour is made up of the left atrium and ventricle, which lie toward the left side of the thorax. If the patient is placed laterally with the left side against the film, the right is relatively slightly magnified compared with the left (see Fig. 12–1B). If the patient rotates minimally anterior or posterior to true lateral, the relationship between the IVC and the left-sided contours changes substantially. This change is worth noting, as in the past a formula has been employed (using the "Riegler sign") to determine left ventricular enlargement as a function of its relationship to the IVC.[18] This sign, although sometimes still used, is not accurate and should not be used.[19,20]

Normal Variations

Anatomical variables and aging present challenges in the evaluation of chest radiographs in addition to those posed by decreased lung compliance. The aorta and great vessels normally dilate and become more tortuous and prominent with increasing age, leading to widening of the superior mediastinum. As noted, the heart appears larger because of decreasing lung compliance, although unless there is true cardiac disease it is less than half the transverse diameter of the chest on a PA view. There are additional important anatomical considerations. Patients who are obese are likely to have a degree of inhibition of maximal lung expansion that may make a normal heart appear slightly larger. Patients with pectus excavatum have a narrowed AP diameter of the chest, increasing the transverse diameter (Fig. 12–11; see Fig. 12–8). Consequently, the heart may appear enlarged on the frontal view but the narrow AP diameter seen on the lateral view explains this. There may also be lack of definition of the right heart border on the frontal view because of compression by the sternum. Marked kyphosis or scoliosis can also cause the heart or mediastinum to look abnormal. It is thus important to examine the spine and other bone structures systematically when looking at a chest radiograph. Delineation of all anatomical abnormalities is beyond the scope of this chapter. For an in-depth discussion, *Fraser and Pare's Diagnosis of Diseases of the Chest*[21] is a useful reference.

Evaluating the Chest Radiograph in Heart Disease

Cardiovascular disease states cause various and complex changes in the appearance of the chest radiograph. Overall cardiomegaly can be judged with reasonable accuracy on the frontal view by noting whether or not the diameter of the heart exceeds half the diameter of the thorax. Cardiomegaly is probably most often seen as a result of ischemic cardiomyopathy following one or more myocardial infarctions (Fig. 12–12). Cardiomegaly is a common finding but a nonspecific one (Fig. 12–13; see Fig. 12–10).[22-26] A systematic approach to the evaluation of a chest radiograph is imperative, to distinguish normal from abnormal and to define the underlying pathology and pathophysiology. The first step is to decide what type of film is being evaluated—PA and lateral, PA alone, or AP (either portable or one obtained in the AP view because the patient is unable to stand). The next step is to determine whether prior films are available for comparison.[27] Many abnormalities are put into appropriate perspective by determining whether or not they are new. Common examples are a prominent aortic arch, a visible major fissure related to prior inflammatory process, or a widened superior mediastinum related to substernal thyroid.

There are many ways of proceeding, and it is most appropriate that each person develop his or her own system. Any system should include a routinely utilized, deliberate attempt to look at areas that are easily ignored. These include the thoracic spine, the neck (for masses and tracheal position), the costophrenic angles, the lung apices, the retrocardiac space, and the retrosternal space. Looking at these areas allows definition of mediastinal position and cardiac and aortic situs and the presence of pleural effusions, scarring, or diaphragmatic elevation. Next, the lung fields are evaluated. This evaluation should involve a careful search for infiltrates or masses even when looking at a chest radiograph for cardiovascular abnormalities, keeping in mind that many people with coronary artery disease have a history of tobacco abuse and are, therefore, at increased risk for lung malignancies. The overall size of the cardiac silhouette, its position, and the location of the ascending and descending aorta are then evaluated. Dextrocardia and a right descending aorta are rare, particularly in adults, but are easy to check for. They are important to recognize because of their association with congenital cardiac and abdominal situs abnormalities. It is also important to look at the site and the position of the stomach. This information can be used to differentiate between a high diaphragm and a pleural effusion (see Fig. 12–1). It can also provide information about other pathological processes (see Fig. 12–13).

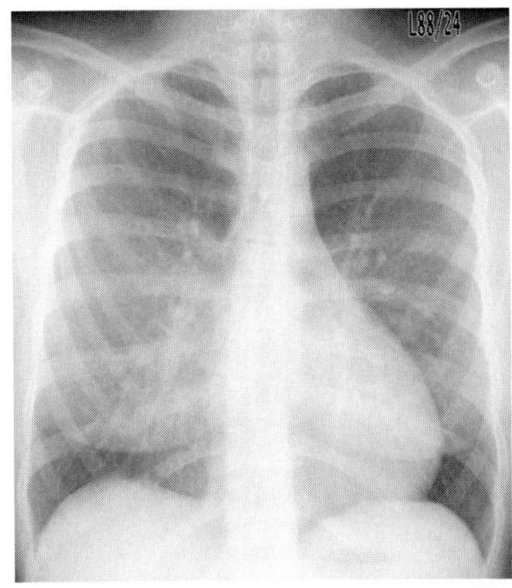

A

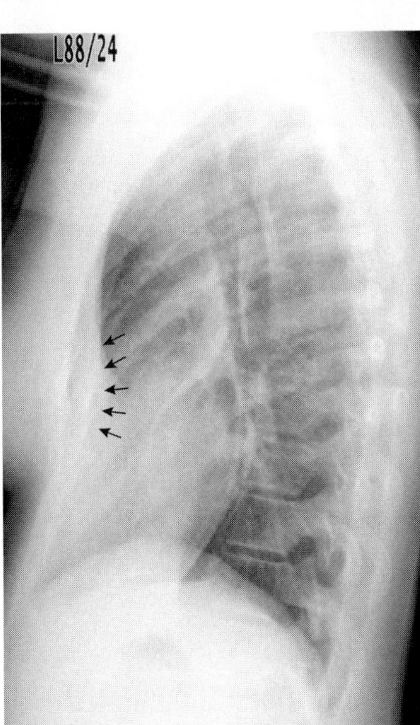

B

FIGURE 12–11 Chest radiographs of a 12-year-old girl with marked pectus excavatum. **A,** The posteroanterior (PA) view shows suggestion of mild cardiomegaly and haziness of the right heart border. Note sharp contour of cardiac apex related to absence of a fat pad. **B,** Lateral view confirms pectus deformity (arrows) and narrow anteroposterior diameter of the chest, explaining the appearance on the PA film.

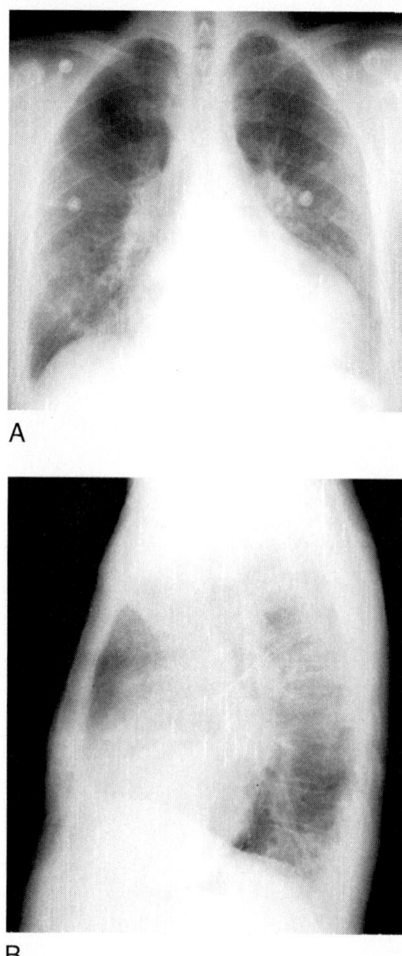

FIGURE 12–12 Chest radiographs of a 53-year-old man with severe ischemic cardiomyopathy and marked cardiomegaly. Frontal **(A)** and lateral **(B)** views show markedly enlarged cardiac silhouette, without clear enlargement of individual chambers, and marked pulmonary vascular redistribution.

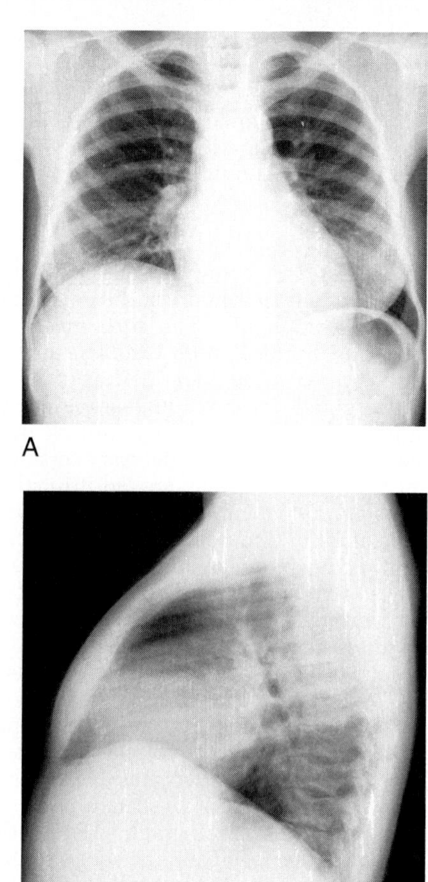

FIGURE 12–13 Chest radiographs of a 22-year-old woman with sickle cell disease. There is mild cardiomegaly and plethoric pulmonary vascularity secondary to anemia with a resultant high-output state. **A,** Gastric bubble is lateral in position related to autosplenectomy. **B,** "Fish mouth" vertebral bodies, characteristic of sickle cell disease.

Lungs and Pulmonary Vasculature

Evaluation of the pulmonary vascular pattern is difficult and imprecise but very important. As noted earlier, it varies with the patient's position (erect versus supine) and is altered substantially by underlying pulmonary disease. It is best to define pulmonary vascularity by looking at the middle zone of the lungs (i.e., the third of the lungs between the hilar region and the peripheral region laterally) and comparing a region in the upper lung field with a region in the lower at equal distances from the hilum.[17] Vessels should be larger in the lower lung but sharply marginated in both upper and lower zones. In normal persons, the vessels taper and bifurcate and are difficult to define in the outer third of the lung. They normally cannot be seen near the pleura (see Fig. 12–8).

Two distinct patterns of abnormality are recognizable. In patients with a high-output state (e.g., pregnancy, severe anemia as in sickle cell disease, hyperthyroidism) or left-to-right shunt, because pulmonary arterial flow is increased, the pulmonary vessels are seen more prominently than usual in the periphery of the lung (Fig. 12–14; see Fig. 12–13). They are uniformly enlarged, but their margins remain clear. In situations with elevated pulmonary artery pressure, the vessel borders become hazy, the lower zone vessels constrict and the upper zone vessels enlarge, and vessels become visible farther toward the pleura, in the outer third of the lungs (see Fig. 12–12). With increasing left ventricular end-diastolic pressure (LVEDP) or left atrial pressure, interstitial edema increases and ultimately pulmonary edema occurs. There is usually a reasonable correlation between the pulmonary vascular pattern and pulmonary capillary wedge pressure (PCWP). At a PCWP of less than 8 mm Hg, the vascular pattern is normal. As the PCWP increases to 10 to 12 mm Hg, the lower zone vessels appear equal in diameter to or smaller than the upper zone vessels. At pressures of 12 to 18 mm Hg, the vessel borders become progressively hazier because of increasing extravasation of fluid into the interstitium. This effect is sometimes evident as *Kerley B lines*, which are horizontal, pleural-based, peripheral linear densities. As PCWP increases above 18 to 20 mm Hg, pulmonary edema occurs, with interstitial fluid present in sufficient amounts to cause a perihilar "bat wing" appearance (Fig. 12–15).

Again, these typical appearances may be altered for various reasons. In patients with extensive pulmonary fibrosis or multiple bullae, the vascular pattern is abnormal at baseline, and as the PCWP increases, it does not change in predictable ways as definable on a chest radiograph. In patients with chronic congestive heart failure, there are chronic changes in the pulmonary vascular pattern that do not correlate with the changes that occur in patients with normal left ventricular pressure at baseline. For example, a patient with a chronic elevation of LVEDP to 25 to 30 mm Hg resulting from ischemic myopathy or other cause may have a normal

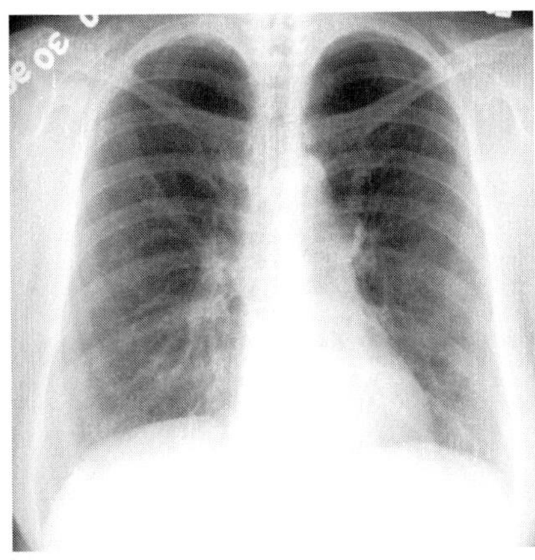
A

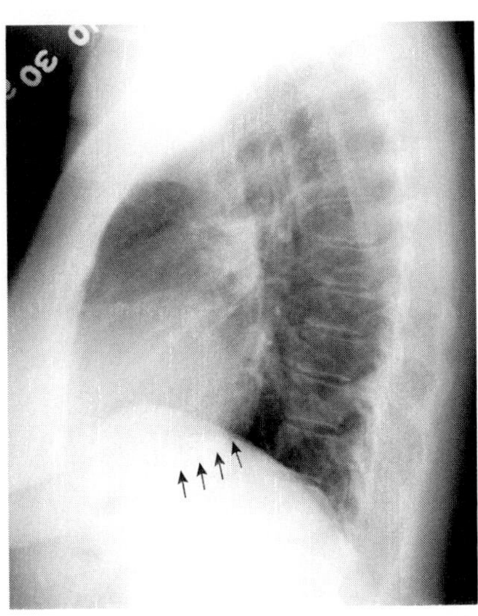
B

FIGURE 12–14 Chest radiographs of a 47-year-old asymptomatic woman with a small atrial septal defect. **A,** The posteroanterior view shows a normal cardiac contour, with mild pulmonary vascular plethora. at the periphery of the lung fields. **B,** Lateral view shows mild prominence of the left ventricle (arrows).

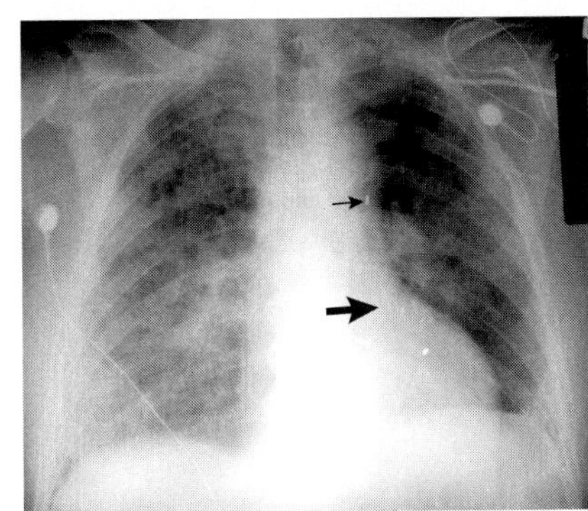

FIGURE 12–15 Patient with acute pulmonary edema. Note engorged hila bilaterally, with typical pattern of pulmonary edema on the right. Also note intraaortic counterpulsation balloon with radiopaque tip at the top of the descending aorta (arrow) and the balloon expanded in the aorta below it (large arrow).

pulmonary vascular pattern or moderate rather than marked redistribution (see Fig. 12–5). Characteristically, heart size increases with increasing pulmonary vascular redistribution. If pulmonary edema is independent of left ventricular dysfunction, however, as may occur at high altitude or following cerebral trauma, the heart size may remain normal. Despite these limitations, it is important to evaluate the pulmonary vascular pattern routinely, as it does provide relevant information.

Cardiac Chambers and Great Vessels

Evaluation of the heart must also be done systematically. After assessing overall size and pulmonary vascular pattern—as a reflection of left-heart physiological status—the individual chambers should be examined. As noted, it is not possible to define clearly individual chambers in a normal chest radiograph (see Figs. 12–3 and 12–4). Furthermore, when the cardiac silhouette is enlarged, it is most often related to biventricular failure, and, again, individual chamber enlargement is not visible (see Fig. 12–12). In acquired valvular disease and in many types of congenital heart disease, however, individual chamber enlargement is present and crucial to plain film (and often clinical) diagnosis.[14,22,28] This information is now readily available with other, more expensive imaging modalities, namely cardiac echocardiography, magnetic resonance imaging (MRI), and computed tomography (CT) (see also Chaps. 11, 14, and 15).[29] Plain films remain important nonetheless as they allow fairly straightforward and inexpensive assessment of changes over time and are routinely and quickly available.[30-33]

RIGHT ATRIUM. Right atrial enlargement is essentially never isolated except in the presence of congenital tricuspid atresia or Ebstein anomaly, both rarely encountered even in the pediatric age group. The right atrium may dilate in the presence of pulmonary hypertension or tricuspid regurgitation, but right ventricular dilation usually predominates and prevents definition of the atrium. The right atrial contour blends with that of the superior vena cava, right main pulmonary artery, and right ventricle. In adults, therefore, it is virtually impossible to define, and in fact it is pointless to try.

RIGHT VENTRICLE. The classic signs of right ventricular enlargement are a "boot-shaped" heart and filling in of the retrosternal airspace.[16] The former is due to transverse displacement of the apex of the right ventricle as it dilates (Fig. 12–16A). Because in adults it is rare for the right ventricle to dilate without left ventricular dilation, this boot shape is not often obvious. It is most commonly seen in congenital heart disease, classically in tetralogy of Fallot. As the right ventricle dilates, it expands superiorly as well as laterally and posteriorly, filling in the retrosternal airspace (Fig. 12–17; see Fig. 12–16B). The classic teaching is that in a lateral chest radiograph in normal patients the soft tissue density is confined to less than one-third of the distance from the suprasternal notch to the tip of the xyphoid. If the soft tissue fills in more than half of this distance, it is a reliable indication of right ventricular enlargement.

There are other causes of increased soft tissue density in this region, and history and other findings must be considered. Common causes that are generally easy to distinguish from right ventricular enlargement include retrosternal adenopathy, midmediastinal mass (e.g., lymphoma or thymoma), marked dilation of the main pulmonary artery (Fig. 12–18A and B), and marked aortic root dilation (see Fig. 12–8). By far the most common cause of increased retrosternal soft tissue, however, is prior median sternotomy with resultant scarring (see Fig. 12–7C). Right ventricular enlargement is most often seen in mitral valve disease, secondary to pulmonary hypertension (see Fig. 12–17A and B). Less commonly, it is the result of primary pulmonary hypertension.

LEFT ATRIUM. Several classic signs define left atrial enlargement.[14,34] First is dilation of the left atrial appendage,

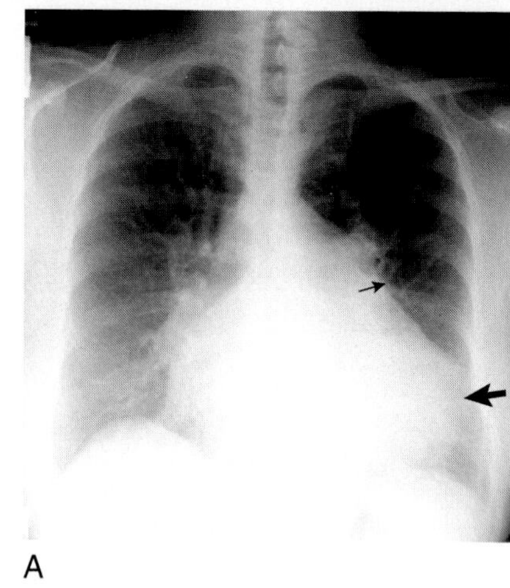

A

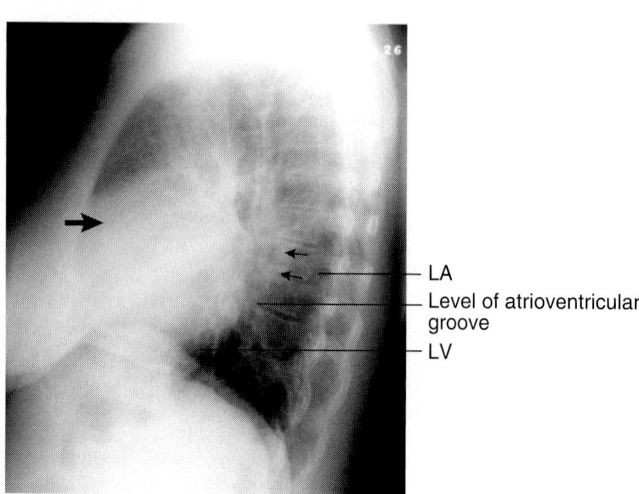

B

FIGURE 12–16 Chest radiographs of a 59-year-old woman with history of rheumatic heart disease and mitral stenosis. **A,** The posteroanterior view demonstrates enlarged cardiac silhouette, with suggestion of a double density seen through the heart (left atrial enlargement), prominent convexity of the left atrial appendage (arrow), and slightly elevated cardiac apex (large arrow), suggestive of right ventricular (rather than left ventricular) enlargement. There is significant elevation of the pulmonary venous pressures. **B,** The lateral view confirms marked right ventricular (arrow) and left atrial (small arrows) enlargement. Note filling in of the retrosternal airspace. LA = left atrium; LV = left ventricle.

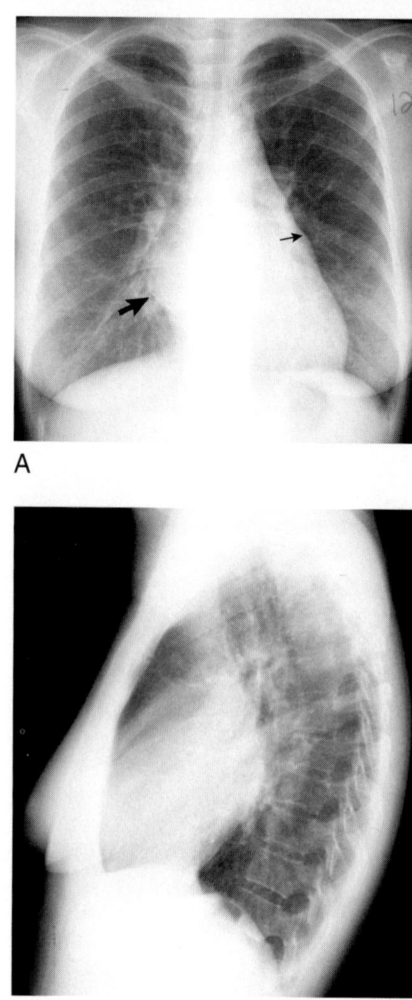

A

B

FIGURE 12–17 Chest radiographs of a 39-year-old Asian woman with rheumatic mitral stenosis. **A,** Frontal view shows normal heart size, mild vascular redistribution, and marked, focal enlargement of the left atrium (small arrow), which extends to the right of the midline (large arrow). There is elevation of the left main stem bronchus. **B,** Lateral view shows dilated right ventricle, with filling in of the retrosternal airspace. The left ventricle is normal in size and contour.

which is seen as a focal convexity where there is normally a concavity between the left main pulmonary artery and the left border of the left ventricle on the frontal view (Fig.12–19A). Second, because of its location, as the left atrium enlarges, it elevates the left main stem bronchus. In so doing, it widens the angle of the carina (see Fig. 12–19A).[35] Third, as the left atrium enlarges posteriorly, it may cause focal bowing of the middle to low thoracic aorta toward the left. This bowing is distinguishable from the tortuosity seen with progressive atherosclerosis, which involves the descending thoracic aorta either in its upper portion or throughout. Next, with marked left atrial enlargement, a double density can be seen on the frontal view, as the left atrium projects laterally toward the right as well as posteriorly and is surrounded by lung (see Figs.12–17A and 12–19A). Finally, on the lateral film, left atrial enlargement appears as a focal, posteriorly directed bulge (see Fig. 12–19B).

Isolated left atrial enlargement in the adult is most often seen in mitral stenosis, and definable left atrial enlargement is the hallmark of mitral valve disease (see Chap. 57). In mitral stenosis, the left atrium is enlarged, there is progressive evidence of pulmonary vascular redistribution (often with Kerley B lines), and there is ultimately enlargement of the right ventricle. The left ventricle, however, remains normal in size (see Figs. 12–17 and 12–19). In mitral regurgitation, the left atrium and ventricle both enlarge because of increased flow (Fig. 12–20). The pulmonary vascular redistribution is more variable in mitral regurgitation than in mitral stenosis, as is right ventricular dilation. It is also important to note mitral annulus calcification: it is common but does not have a strong association with valvular dysfunction. It does, however, have an association with premature coronary artery disease (Fig. 12–21).[36]

LEFT VENTRICLE. Left ventricular enlargement is characterized by a prominent, downwardly directed contour of the apex, as distinguished from the transverse displacement seen with right ventricular enlargement. The overall cardiac contour is also usually enlarged, although this is nonspecific. It is also important to evaluate the left ventricle on the lateral film. Here, it is seen as a posterior bulge, below the level of the mitral annulus (Fig. 12–22). It may also be seen inferiorly, pushing the gastric bubble (see Fig. 12–14B). Enlargement in this way is an illustration of findings that lie outside the usual confines of the chest. This is another example of the value of looking at the entire chest radiograph. Focal left ventricular enlargement in adults is most commonly seen in the presence of aortic insufficiency (with aortic root dilation; see Fig. 12–22) or mitral regurgitation (with left atrial dilation; see Fig. 12–19). Left ventricular dilation is less common with aortic stenosis, although it can occur, accompanied by congestive heart failure.[18-20,28,37]

PULMONARY ARTERIES. The main pulmonary artery can appear abnormal in many situations. In the presence of pulmonic stenosis, the main pulmonary artery and the left pulmonary artery dilate (see Fig. 12–18A and B). This dilation is thought to be due to the jet effect through the stenotic valve, coupled with the anatomy. That is, the main pulmonary artery continues straight into the left main pulmonary artery, but the right comes off at a fairly sharp angle and is not generally affected by the jet. This enlargement can be seen with a prominent left hilum on the frontal view and a prominent pulmonary outflow tract on the lateral. It is important to remember that the pulmonic valve lies higher than and more peripherally in the outflow tract than the aortic valve (see Fig. 12–4). It is also located anterior to the aortic valve on the lateral view.

AORTA. The aorta dilates in different ways as a function of the underlying pathology. It is often possible to define the pathology not only by the pattern of aortic dilation but also by associated cardiac abnormalities.[38] On the frontal chest radiograph, aortic dilation is seen as a prominence to the right of the middle mediastinum (Fig. 12–23A). There is also a prominence in the anterior mediastinum on the lateral view, behind and superior to the pulmonary outflow tract (see Figs. 12–5, 12–8, and 12–23B). Dilation of the aortic root is probably most commonly seen in the presence of long-term, poorly controlled systemic hypertension. Enlargement of the aortic root is also seen in the presence of aortic valve disease.

In aortic valve stenosis (see Chap. 57), there is usually focal dilation of the aortic root, often subtle, and often without left ventricular enlargement (see Figs. 12–8 and 12–23). It is important to look for this, as there are often no other signs on the chest radiograph, even in the presence of a very small valve area.[37] The left ventricle generally hypertrophies in response to increased resistance to outflow rather than dilating as it does in response to the increased flow volume that occurs with aortic insufficiency. This wall thickening with hypertrophy is seen with echocardiography, CT, or MRI, but the ventricle may appear entirely normal on the chest radiograph despite tight aortic valve stenosis. Aortic valve calcification is pathognomonic of significant aortic valve disease (see Fig. 12–23B), but it is usually difficult to see on a chest radiograph because of the overlying soft tissue densities and the minimal blurring caused by cardiac motion, even with a

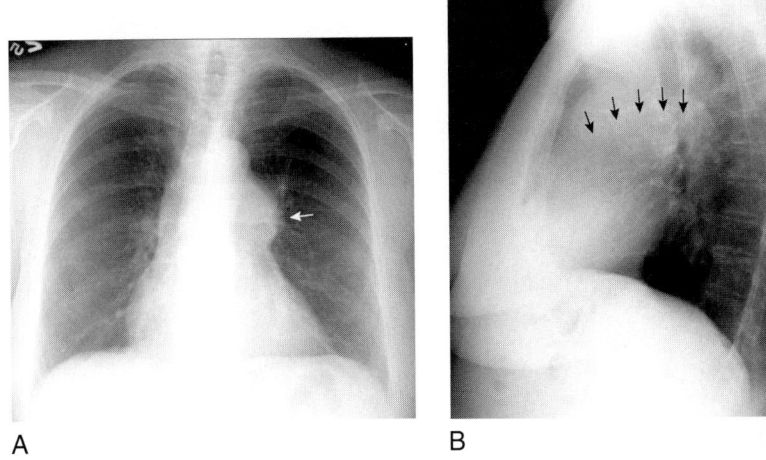

FIGURE 12–18 Chest radiographs of a 56-year-old asymptomatic woman with incidentally discovered pulmonic stenosis. **A,** Posteroanterior view shows marked enlargement of the main pulmonary trunk extending into the left main pulmonary artery (arrow). **B,** Lateral view confirms prominence of the pulmonary outflow tract and main and left pulmonary arteries (arrows).

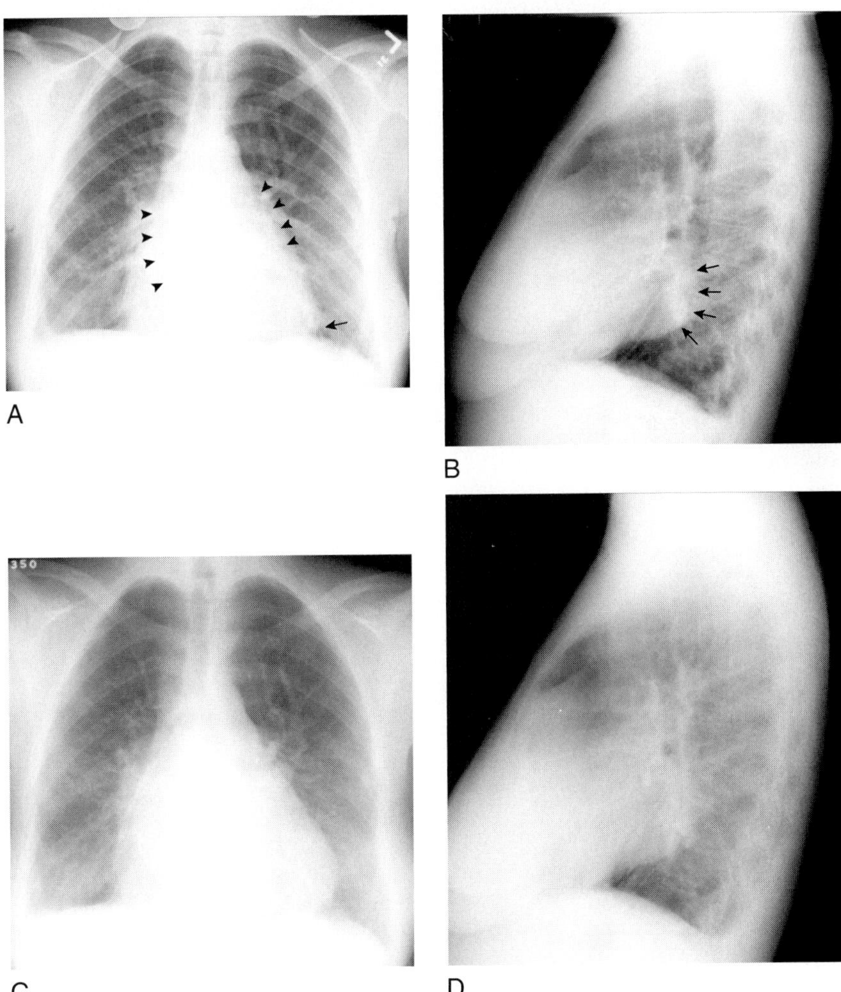

FIGURE 12–19 Chest radiographs of a 60-year-old woman with severe progressive mitral stenosis, with serial films spanning 4 years. **A,** Initial posteroanterior (PA) view shows enlargement of the left atrium (arrowheads), prominence of the hilar vessels, and pulmonary venous redistribution. Transverse angle of the apex suggests right ventricular enlargement (arrow). **B,** Initial lateral view confirms this, with filling in of the retrosternal airspace. Note also severe left atrial enlargement (arrows). **C** and **D,** PA and lateral views 4 years later show progressive left atrial and right ventricular enlargement, with increased double density of the left atrium on the frontal view with prominent focal bulge on the lateral view above the level of the left ventricular contour. There is increased density in the retrosternal airspace.

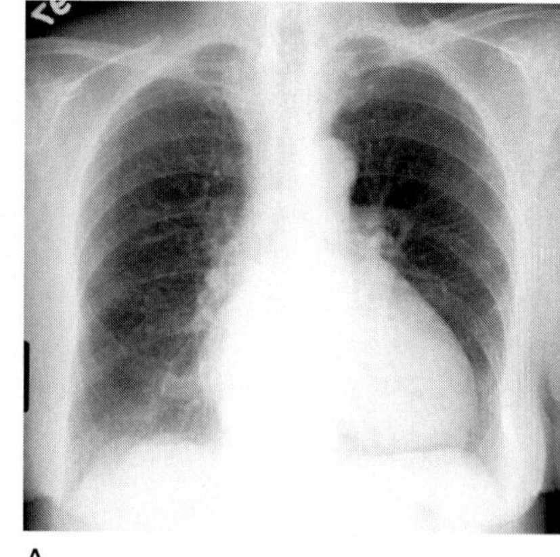

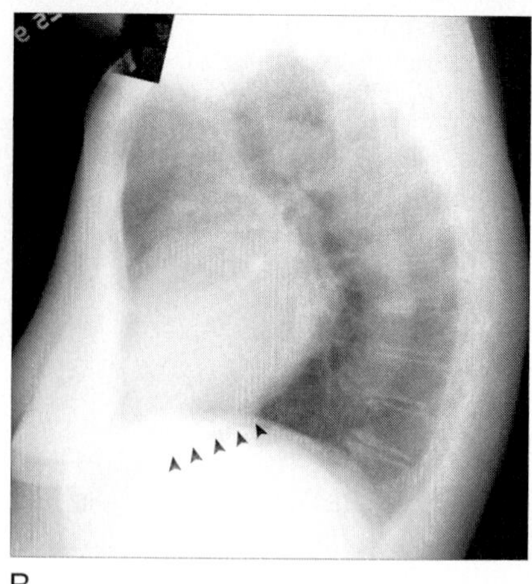

FIGURE 12–20 Chest films of a 78-year-old woman with pure mitral regurgitation and atrial fibrillation. **A,** Posteroanterior view shows enlargement of the left atrium and left ventricle with mild pulmonary vascular redistribution. **B,** Lateral view confirms these findings. Arrowheads indicate prominent left ventricular contour.

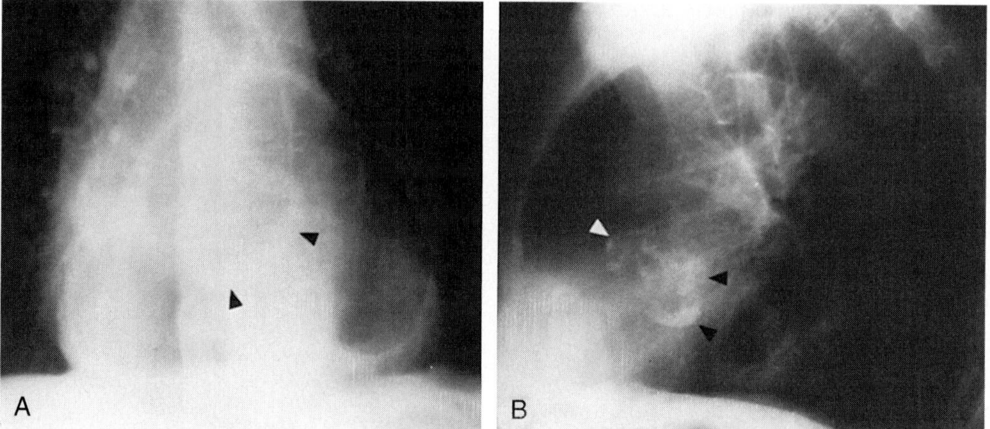

FIGURE 12–21 **A,** Mitral valve calcification in the posteroanterior projection. **B,** Mitral valve calcification in the lateral projection. Valve calcification (black arrows) lies below the line drawn from the left main bronchus to the anterior costophrenic sulcus, which localizes it to the mitral valve. The aortic valve in this projection lies more anteriorly and above the line (white arrows).

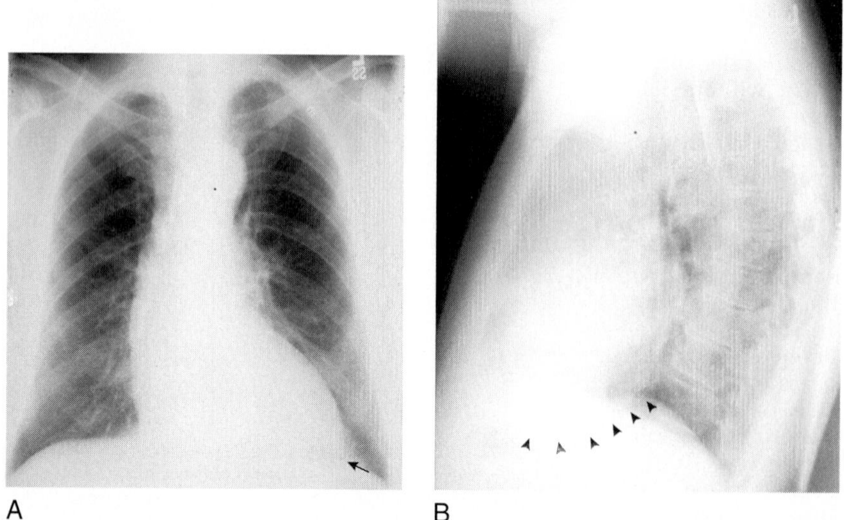

FIGURE 12–22 Chest radiographs of a 63-year-old man with chronic aortic regurgitation. **A,** Posteroanterior view shows downward displacement of the apex (arrow), suggestive of left ventricular enlargement. There is prominence and enlargement of the ascending aorta, creating a convex right border of the mediastinum. **B,** Lateral view shows prominent left ventricular enlargement (arrowheads). The aortic root is markedly enlarged in the retrosternal airspace but is separate from the sternum (in contrast to findings in right ventricular enlargement; see Figs. 12–16B and 12–17B).

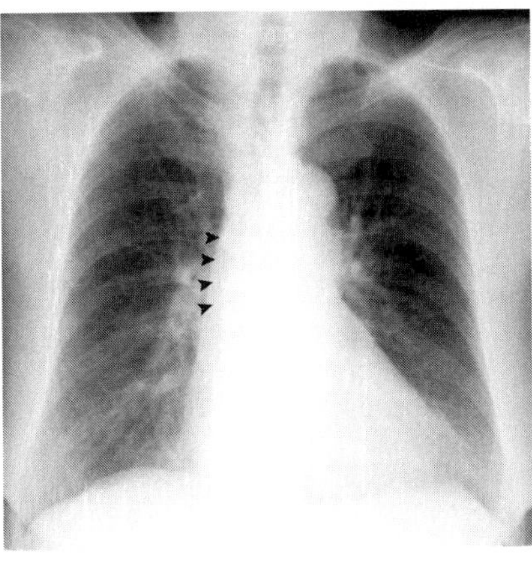

A

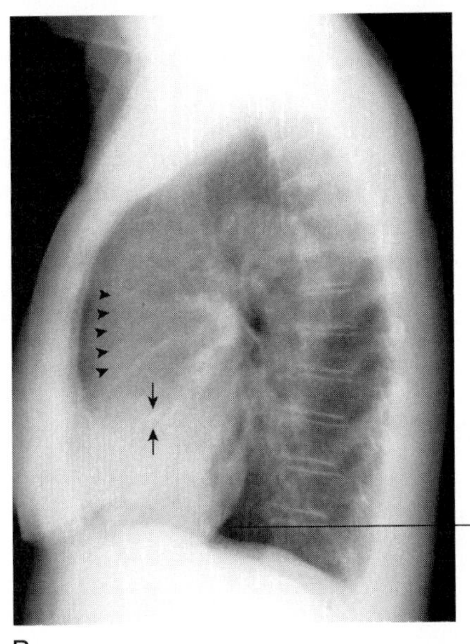

B

FIGURE 12–23 Chest radiographs of a 65-year-old woman with severe aortic stenosis. **A,** Frontal view shows prominent aortic root, to the right of the midline (arrowheads). Note absence of cardiomegaly and presence of normal pulmonary vascular pattern. **B,** Lateral view demonstrates calcification of the aortic valve leaflets (arrows), suggestive of a bicuspid valve. There is a prominent, mildly dilated aortic root (arrowheads).

very stenotic valve. Calcification, if present, is much more easily seen with fluoroscopy. Despite the decreased resolution of fluoroscopy compared with a standard chest radiograph, real-time visualization facilitates definition of calcification.[39-41]

It is important to remember that there is a subset of patients with aortic stenosis who present with left ventricular decompensation. In these patients, there is left ventricular and aortic root enlargement, and to distinguish this from aortic regurgitation it is important to look carefully for aortic valve calcification. It is not possible on a chest radiograph to establish definitively the etiology of aortic stenosis: rheumatic versus bicuspid valve versus degenerative. It can be helpful, however, to remember that rheumatic disease essentially always involves the mitral valve (see Chap. 57), and the absence of signs of mitral stenosis generally indicates that the etiology is not rheumatic (see Fig. 12–5).

In aortic regurgitation, aortic involvement is usually more diffuse than in aortic stenosis and more easily seen (see Chap. 57). In pure aortic regurgitation, the left atrium is not usually enlarged. Over time, however, dilation of the mitral annulus may occur secondary to the left ventricular dilation with resultant mitral regurgitation and left atrial dilation. Although aortic regurgitation classically occurs secondary to rheumatic fever (with associated mitral valve disease), congenital defects, or degenerative valve disease, it may also be caused by disease of the aortic root, including cystic medial necrosis, with or without Marfan syndrome. In cystic medial necrosis, the involvement is diffuse, and there is generally dilation of the aorta from the level of the valve at least through the arch (see Chap. 53). In tertiary syphilis, now rarely seen, the characteristic finding is marked dilation of the aorta from the root to the arch, with abrupt return to normal diameter at this level. With cystic medial necrosis, the transition of diameter is gradual. Aneurismal dilation of the ascending aorta also occurs in cystic medial necrosis and may be hard to define as distinct from the heart itself. Other aortic abnormalities, such as acute (see Fig. 12–2B) or chronic dissection and traumatic rupture or pseudoaneurysm, are better defined with CT. A chest radiograph may delay appropriate diagnosis and intervention in acute trauma, for example, in the case of suspected aortic rupture. The findings on the chest films are generally nonspecific indirect ones, such as the presence of mediastinal widening, blood at the left apex or a large left effusion (presumably blood), or rib fractures. Spiral or multislice CT can provide a rapid and accurate answer (see Chap. 15).

Pleura and Pericardium

The pleura and pericardium also require systematic evaluation (see Chap. 64). The pericardium is rarely distinctly definable on plain films of the chest (see Fig. 12–10).[42] There are two situations, however, in which it can be seen. In the presence of a large pericardial effusion, the visceral and the parietal pericardium separate. Because there is a fat pad associated with each, it is sometimes possible on the lateral film to make out two parallel lucent lines, usually in the area of the cardiac apex, with density (fluid) between them. Echocardiography, MRI, and CT, however, are all far more reliable for defining a pericardial effusion (see Chaps. 11, 14, and 15). Nonetheless, if the cardiac silhouette is enlarged on the chest radiograph is important to look for specific explanations. Although cardiac dilation and valvular disease are more common causes, the presence of an unsuspected effusion is worth considering. Classically, the cardiac silhouette has a "water bottle" shape in the presence of a pericardial effusion, but such a shape is not in itself diagnostic.

Both pleural and pericardial calcification can occur, but they are often not obvious (see Fig.12–6). Pericardial calcification is associated with a history of pericarditis, most often related to tuberculosis but also with other etiologies, such as a viral process. It is usually thin and linear and follows the contour of the pericardium. Because the calcification is thin, it is often seen only on one view, as in Figure 12–6. Myocardial calcification secondary to a large myocardial infarction with transmural necrosis is rare but can generally be distinguished from pericardial calcification. It tends to appear thicker, more focal, and less in conformance with the outer contour of the heart. Pleural calcification is essentially pathognomonic for asbestos exposure. It is associated with a high risk of malignant mesothelioma but is not diagnostic of such a tumor. It is generally easy to distinguish from pericardial calcification by its location.

Specific Conditions

The multitude of findings associated with cardiac disease are beyond the scope of this chapter, but several entities and situations are worth considering as they are either common or characteristic of certain disease states. As noted, the most common explanation for cardiomegaly and pulmonary vascular redistribution is ischemic heart disease.[20,23,24] In most patients with an acute myocardial infarction, the cardiac silhouette is not enlarged but there is pulmonary vascular redistribution, consistent with an acute increase in LVEDP. This condition is most easily defined when the chest radiograph is compared with a prior or subsequent one. After infarction, a variety of alterations can occur. Left ventricular aneurysms, either true (generally in the distribution of the left anterior descending artery) (see Fig. 12–7A) or false (usually involving the base or the posterior wall) are uncommon.[43,44] Although the location usually differs, the appearance of both is similar; there is focal prominence (of the anterolateral cardiac contour with true aneurysms), there may be linear myocardial calcification, and the margin is unusually sharp because the area of the aneurysm does not have normal cardiac motion. Again, this is best seen in comparison with prior chest radiographs.

It is impossible to define a postinfarction ventricular septal defect on the chest radiograph because the presentation is usually characterized by cardiac dilation and failure. On presentation, there is generally enlargement of the cardiac silhouette and evidence of heart failure, both nonspecific findings. After percutaneous repair, however, the septal repair device can often be identified (Fig. 12–24).[45]

Chest radiographs provide a wealth of physiological and anatomical information. As such, they play a central role in the evaluation and management of patients with a wide variety of cardiovascular and other disorders. Portable chest films should be used as infrequently as possible because the information they provide is limited and may even be misleading (for example, in defining cardiomegaly or in ruling out a pneumothorax or effusion). Standard 6-foot frontal and lateral chest films, on the other hand, are almost always of value. Whether recorded conventionally or digitally, if they are evaluated carefully using a systematic approach and when possible are compared with prior chest radiographs, it is hard to overestimate their importance.

Implantable Devices

A final important and broad area concerns the chest radiograph following surgery or other procedures. In these situations, it is crucial to recognize devices that have been implanted and changes that may occur. Devices include various valve prostheses,[46] pacemakers[47] and ICDs (Fig. 12-25), and intraaortic counterpulsation balloons (see Fig. 12-15). There are also clear changes that occur after surgery, such as the presence of clips on the side branches of saphenous veins used for coronary artery bypass grafting (see Fig. 12-7B and C) and retrosternal blurring (Fig. 12-26) and effusions (see Fig. 12-1).[48] Some such findings may be temporary, such as lines and tubes associated with surgery and effusions. Pacers and ICDs present specific questions. The first is the patency of the leads,[49,50] and the second is the position of the tip. Although course and tip position are generally confirmed fluoroscopically at the time of placement, malposition can occur. The ends of the wires (if there are two

A

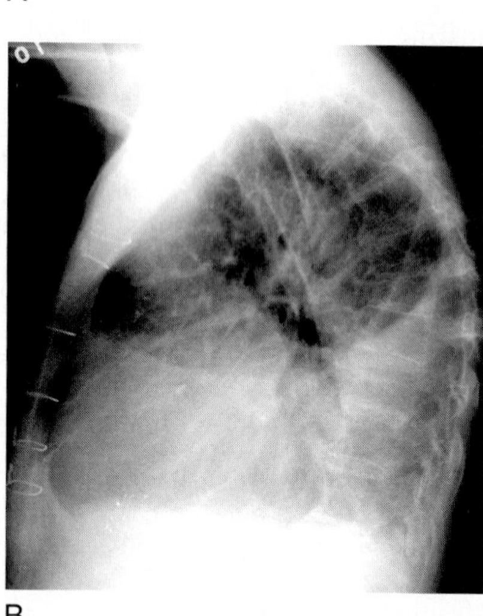

B

FIGURE 12–24 Radiographs of an elderly man after acute myocardial infarction complicated by ventricular septal defect (VSD) and heart failure, who has undergone a percutaneous closure. **A,** Posteroanterior view demonstrates cardiomegaly, marked pulmonary vascular redistribution, and a large left pleural effusion. Note effusion outlining left major fissure. **B,** Lateral view shows left (versus right) effusion and the VSD repair device at the level of the right diaphragm.

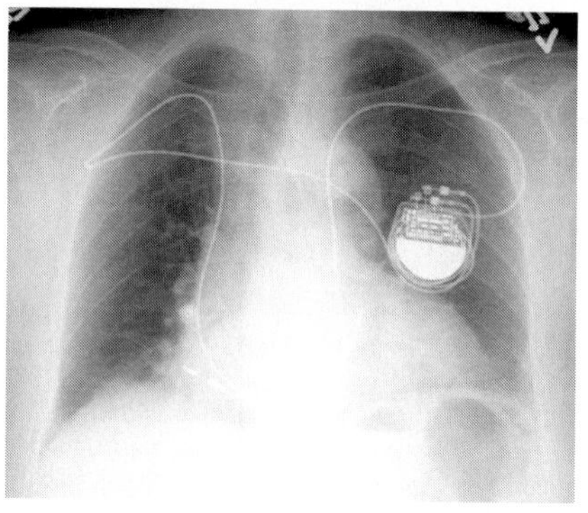

A

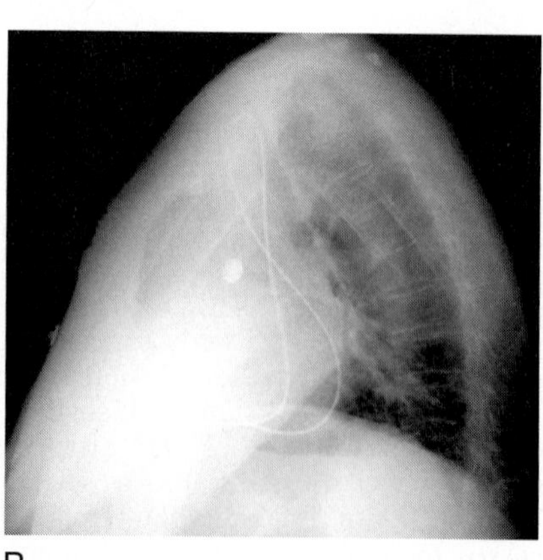

B

FIGURE 12–25 Chest radiographs of a 62-year-old woman with two pacemakers, with left-sided pacemaker implanted because of failure of the right. As seen on frontal **(A)** and lateral **(B)** views, the right-sided wire traverses the right superior vena cava and the right atrium and its tip lies superiorly and anteriorly in the pulmonary outflow tract. The left-sided wire traverses a persistent left superior vena cava (a normal anatomical variant) and the coronary sinus, and its tip, the lower of the two, is in the right atrium.

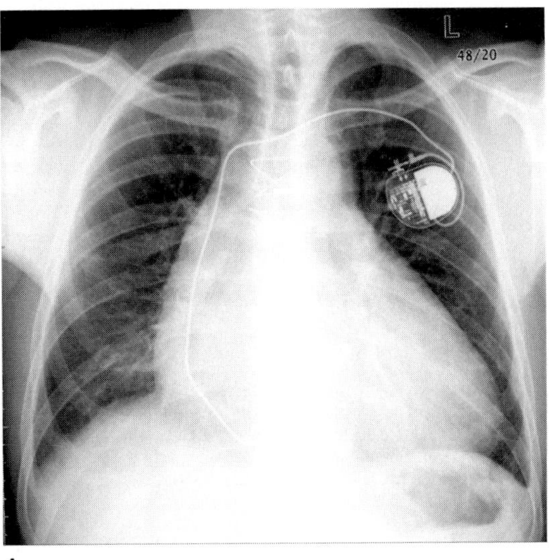

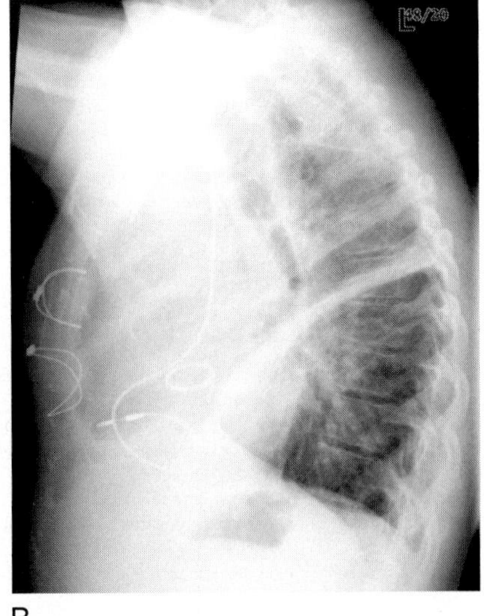

FIGURE 12–26 Chest radiographs of a 28-year-old man who has undergone aortic valve replacement with a porcine bioprosthesis. **A,** Posteroanterior view. There is marked left ventricular (LV) enlargement with downwardly displaced apex. Note pacemaker wire with tip in the right ventricular (RV) apex. **B,** Lateral view confirms primary LV dilation, shows position of the aortic valve, and also shows the tip of the pacing wire in the RV apex. This confirms LV versus RV dilation.

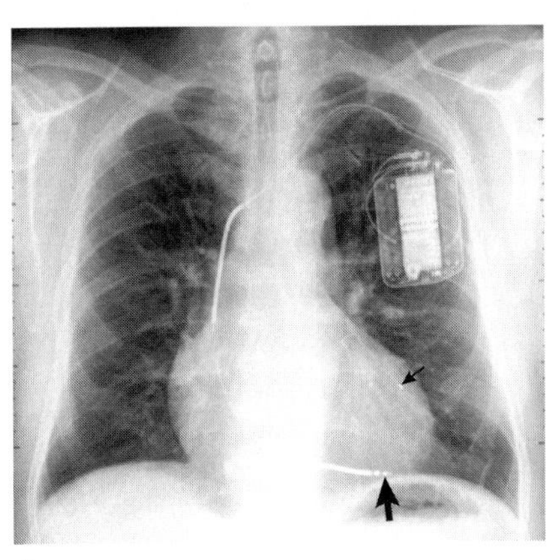

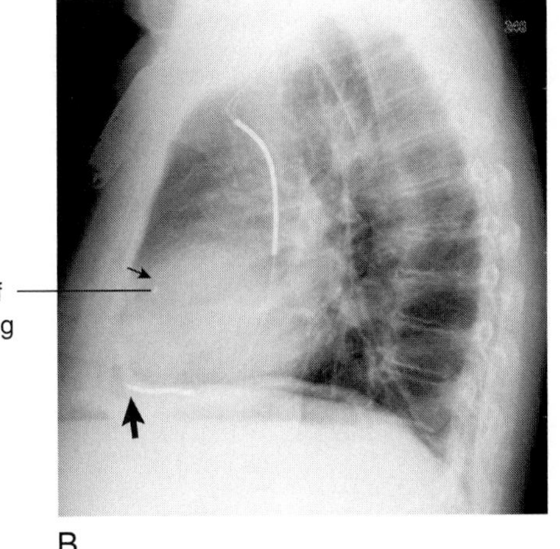

FIGURE 12–27 **A** and **B,** Chest radiographs of a 78-year-old man after aortic valve replacement. Note wire position (arrow), through coronary sinus into great coronary vein (running parallel to the left anterior descending coronary artery), and biventricular enlargement. Also note position of AICD tip in right ventricular apex (large arrow).

leads) should be in the anterolateral wall of the right atrium and the apex of the right ventricle. If the leads are not so positioned, the reasons should be carefully determined (Fig. 12–27). That is, are they positioned because of error or because of anatomical variants, such as a persistent left superior vena cava that empties into the coronary sinus and then the right atrium (see Fig. 12–25)?[51] The position of the wires and of valve prostheses can help in the definition of specific chamber enlargement (see Fig. 12–27).

REFERENCES

1. Williams FH: A method for more fully determining the outline of the heart by means of a flluoroscope together with other uses of the instrument in medicine. Boston Me Surg J 135:335, 1896.

Technical Considerations

2. Hintenlang KM, Williams JL, Hintenlang DE: A survey of radiation dose associated with pediatric plain-fiilm chest X-ray examinations. Pediatr Radiol 32:771, 2002.
3. Wagner LK, Eifel PJ, Geise RA: Potential biological effects following high x-ray dose interventional procedures. J Vasc Intervent Radiol 5:71, 1994.
4. Krivopal M, Shlobin OA, Schwartzstein RM: Utility of daily routine portable chest radiographs in mechanically ventilated patients in the medical ICU. Chest 123:1607, 2003.
5. Shiralkar S, Rennie A, Snow M, et al: Doctors' knowledge of radiation exposure: Questionnaire study. BMJ 327:371, 2003.
6. Rong XJ, Shaw CC, Liu X, et al: Comparison of an amorphous silicon/cesium iodide fllat-panel digital chest radiography system with screen/fiilm and computed radiogrhy systems: A contrast-detail phantom study. Med Phys 28:2328, 2000.
7. Garmer M, Hennigs SP, Jäger HJ, et al: Digital radiography versus conventional radiography in chest imaging: Diagnostic performance of a large area fllat-panel detector in clinical CT-controlled study. AJR 174:75, 2000.
8. Chotas HG, Dobbins JT, Ravin CE: Principles of digital radiography with large-area electronically readable detectors: A review of the basics. Radiology 210:595, 1999.
9. Bacher K, Smeets P, Bonnarens K, et al: Dose reduction in patients undergoing chest imaging: Digital amorphous silicon fllat-panel detector radiography versus conventiona fiilm-screen radiography and phosphor-based computed radiography. AJR 181:923, 2003.
10. Schaefer-Prokop C, Uffmann M, Eisenhuber E, et al: Digital radiography of the chest: Detector techniques and performance parameters. J Thorac Imaging 18:124, 2003.
11. Ganten M, Radeleff B, Kampschulte A, et al: Comparing image quality of fllat-panel ches radiography with storage phosphor radiography and fiilm-screen radiography. AJ 181:171, 2003.
12. Honeyman-Buck J: PACS adoption. Semin Roentgenol 38:256, 2003.
13. Weatherburn GC, Ridout D, Strickland NH, et al: A comparison of conventional film CR hard copy and PACS soft copy images of the chest: Analyses of ROC curves and inter-observer agreement. Eur J Radiol 47:206, 2003.

The Normal Chest Radiograph

14. Baron MG: The cardiac silhouette. J Thorac Imaging 15:230, 2000.
15. Ohye RG, Kulik TA: Images in cardiovascular medicine. Normal chest x-ray. Circulation 105:2455, 2002.
16. Boxt LM: Radiology of the right ventricle. Radiol Clin North Am 37:379, 1999.

17. Sharma S, Bhargave A, Krishnakumar R, et al: Can pulmonary venous hypertension be graded by the chest radiograph? Clin Radiol 53:899, 1998.
18. Hoffman RB, Rigler LG: Evaluation of left ventricular enlargement in the lateral projection of the chest. Radiology 85:93, 1965.
19. Freeman V, Mutatiri C, Pretorius M, et al: Evaluation of left ventricular enlargement in the lateral position of the chest using the Hoffman and Rigler sign. Cardiovasc J S Afr 14:134, 2003.
20. Jung G, Landwehr P, Schanzenbacher G, et al: Value of thoracic radiography in the assessment of cardiac size. A comparison with left ventricular cardiography. Rofo Fortschr Geb Rontgenstr Neuen Bildgeb Verfahr 162:368, 1995.
21. Fraser RS, Muller NL, Colman N, et al (eds): Fraser and Pare's Diagnosis of Diseases of the Chest. 4th ed. Philadelphia, WB Saunders, 1999.

Evaluating the Chest Radiograph in Heart Disease

22. Satou GM, Lacro RV, Chung T, et al: Heart size on chest x-ray as a predictor of cardiac enlargement by echocardiography in children. Pediatr Cardiol 22:218, 2001.
23. Thomas JT, Kelly RF, Thomas SJ, et al: Utility of history, physical examination, electrocardiogram, and chest radiograph for differentiating normal from decreased systolic function in patients with heart failure. Am J Med 112:437, 2002.
24. Ernst ER, Shub C, Bailey KR, et al: Radiographic measurements of cardiac size as predictors of outcome in patients with dilated cardiomyopathy. J Card Fail 7:13, 2001.
25. Petrie MC: It cannot be cardiac failure because the heart is not enlarged on the chest X-ray. Eur J Heart Fail 5:117, 2003.
26. Perez AA, Ribeiro AL, Barros MV, et al: Value of the radiological study of the thorax for diagnosing left ventricular dysfunction in Chagas' disease. Arq Bras Cardiol 80:208, 2003.
27. Berbaum KS, Smith WL: Use of reports of previous radiologic studies. Acad Radiol 5:111, 1998.
28. Murphy ML, Blue LR, Thenabadu PN, et al: The reliability of the routine chest roentgenogram for determination of heart size based on specifiic ventricular chambe evaluation at postmortem. Invest Radiol 20:21, 1985.
29. Schmermund A, Rensing BJ, Sheedy PF, et al: Reproducibility of right and left ventricular volume measurements by electron-beam CT in patients with congestive heart failure. Int J Card Imaging 14:201, 1998.
30. Ferri C, Emdin M, Nielsen H, et al: Assessment of heart involvement. Clin Exp Rheumatol 21:S24, 2003.
31. Rothrock SG, Green SM, Costanzo KA, et al: High yield criteria for obtaining non-trauma chest radiography in the adult emergency department population. J Emerg Med 23:117, 2002.
32. Oeppen RS, Fairhurst JJ, Argent JD: Diagnostic value of the chest radiograph in asymptomatic neonates with a cardiac murmur. Clin Radiol 57:736, 2002.
33. Gardiner S: Are routine chest x ray and ECG examinations helpful in the evaluation of asymptomatic heart murmurs? Arch Dis Child 88:638, 2003.
34. Lipton MJ, Coulden R: Valvular heart disease. Radiol Clin North Am. 37:319, 1999.
35. Murray JG, Brown AL, Anagnostou EA, et al: Widening of the tracheal bifurcation on chest radiographs: Value as a sign of left atrial enlargement. AJR 164:1089, 1995.
36. Atar S, Jeon DS, Luo H, et al: Mitral annular calcifiication: A marker of severe coronar artery disease in patients under 65 years old. Heart 89:161, 2003.
37. Rodan BA, Chen JT, Halber MD, et al: Chest roentgenographic evaluation of the severity of aortic stenosis. Invest Radiol 17:453, 1982.
38. Yamamoto H, Shavelle D, Takasu J, et al: Valvular and thoracic aortic calcium as a marker of the extent and severity of angiographic coronary artery disease. Am Heart J 146:153, 2003.
39. Cook C, Styles C, Hopkins R: Calcifiication on the chest X-ray: A pictorial rview. Hosp Med 62:210, 2001.
40. Li J, Galvin HK, Johnson SC, et al: Aortic calcifiication on plain chest radiograph increases risk for coronary artery disease. Chest 121:1468, 2002.
41. Kiryu S, Raptopoulos V, Baptista J, et al: Increased prevalence of coronary artery calcifiication in patients with suspected pulmonary embolism. Acad Radiol 10:840, 2003.
42. Wang ZJ, Reddy GP, Gotway MB, et al: CT and MR imaging of pericardial disease. Radiographics 23:S167, 2003.
43. Kao CL, Chang JP: Left ventricular pseudoaneurysm secondary to left ventricular apical venting. Tex Heart Inst J 30:162, 2003.
44. Brown SL, Gropler RJ, Harris KM: Distinguishing left ventricular aneurysm from pseudoaneurysm. A review of the literature. Chest 111:1403, 1997.
45. Kim JH, Siegel MJ, Goldstein JA, et al: Radiologic fiindings of 2 commonly used cardia septal occluders with clinical correlation. J Thorac Imaging 18:183, 2003.
46. Bordlee RP: Cardiac valve reconstruction and replacement: A brief review. Radiographics 12:659, 1992.
47. Bejvan SM, Ephron JH, Takasugi JE, et al: Imaging of cardiac pacemakers. AJR 169:1371, 1997.
48. Kurihara Y, Yakushiji YK, Nakajima Y, et al: The vertical displacement sign: A technique for differentiating between left and right ribs on the lateral chest radiograph. Clin Radiol 54:367, 1999.
49. Morishima I, Sone T, Tsuboi H, et al: Follow-up X rays play a key role in detecting implantable cardioverter defiibrillator lead fracture: A case of incessant inappropriat shocks due to lead fracture. Pacing Clin Electrophysiol 26:911, 2003.
50. Drucker EA, Brooks R, Garan H, et al: Malfunction of implantable cardioverter defiibrilators placed by a nonthoracotomy approach: Frequency of malfunction and value of chest radiography in determining cause. AJR 165:275, 1995.
51. Schummer W, Schummer C, Frober R: Persistent left superior vena cava and central venous catheter position: Clinical impact illustrated by four cases. Surg Radiol Anat 25:315, 2003.

CHAPTER 13

Nuclear Cardiology

James E. Udelson • Vasken Dilsizian • Robert O. Bonow

The era of noninvasive radionuclide cardiac imaging in humans began in the early 1970s, with the first reports of noninvasive evaluation of resting myocardial blood flow. Since that time, there have been major advances in the technical ability to image cardiac physiology and pathophysiology, including that of myocardial blood flow, myocardial metabolism, and ventricular function. Just as important has been a major growth in the understanding of how to apply the image information to care of patients and the effect of that information on clinical decision-making. Ultimately, the role of information derived from any imaging procedure is to enhance the clinician's decision-making process to improve symptoms or clinical outcomes, or both.

Technical Aspects of Image Acquisition, Display, and Interpretation

Single-Photon Emission Computed Tomography Imaging of Perfusion and Function

The most commonly performed imaging procedure in nuclear cardiology is single-photon emission computed tomography (SPECT) imaging of myocardial perfusion. Following injection of the chosen radiotracer, the isotope is extracted from the blood by viable myocytes and retained within the myocyte for some period of time. Photons are emitted from the myocardium in proportion to the magnitude of tracer uptake, in turn related to perfusion. The standard camera used in nuclear cardiology studies, a gamma camera, captures the gamma ray photons and converts the information into digital data representing the *magnitude of uptake* and the *location of the emission*. The photoemissions collide along their flight path with a detector crystal. There, the gamma photons are absorbed and converted into visible light events (a "scintillation event"). Emitted gamma rays are selected for capture and quantitation by a *collimator* attached to the face of the camera-detector system. Most often, parallel hole collimators are used so that only photon emissions coursing perpendicular to the camera head and parallel to the collimation holes are accepted (Fig. 13–1). This arrangement allows better appropriate *localization of the source* of the emitted gamma rays. Photomultiplier tubes, the final major component in the gamma camera, sense the light-scintillation events and convert the events into an electrical signal to be further processed (see Fig. 13–1). The final result of SPECT imaging is the creation of multiple tomograms, or slices, of the organ of interest, comprising a digital display representing radiotracer distribution throughout the organ.[1] With SPECT myocardial perfusion imaging (MPI), the display represents the distribution of perfusion throughout the myocardium.

SPECT Image Acquisition

In order to construct the three-dimensional model of the heart from which tomograms are created, the myocardial perfusion data must be sampled from multiple angles over 180 or 360 degrees around the patient (Fig. 13–2A). Multiple images, each comprising 20 to 25 seconds of emission data, are collected. Each one of the separate "projection" images constitutes a two-dimensional snapshot of myocardial perfusion from the angle at which the projection was acquired. Then, the imaging information from each of the angles is *back projected* onto an imaging matrix, creating a reconstruction of the organ of interest (see Fig. 13–2B). The reader is referred to detailed reviews for more extensive information on the technical aspects of SPECT imaging and image reconstruction.[2,3]

SPECT Image Display

From the three-dimensional reconstruction of the heart, computer processing techniques are used to identify the long axis of the left ventricle, and standardized tomographic images in three standard planes are derived. *Short-axis* images, representing "donut-like" slices of the heart cut perpendicular to the long axis of the heart, are displayed beginning toward the apex and moving toward the base. This tomographic orientation is similar to the short-axis view in two-dimensional echocardiography, although shifted counterclockwise (Fig. 13–3A). Tomographic slices cut parallel to the long axis of the heart and also parallel to the long axis of the body are termed *vertical long-axis* tomograms (see Fig. 13–3B), and slices also cut parallel to the long axis of the heart but perpendicular to the vertical long axis slices are known as *horizontal long-axis* tomograms (see Fig. 13–3C). From all of these tomographic planes, the entire three-dimensional myocardium is sampled and displayed, minimizing overlap of structures.

Basics of Quality Control

The quality of SPECT MPI and the "accuracy" of the representation of regional myocardial perfusion are dependent on multiple quality control issues. These issues include the stability of the tracer distribution in the organ of interest during the acquisition interval, the absence of motion of the patient or organ of interest or both during the acquisition, and the absence of overlying structures that would attenuate the photon emissions from one region relative to another region across the different projection images. Those issues are related to the patient and the organ being imaged, and other quality control issues involve the camera and detector system, including the uniformity of photon detection efficiency across the camera face as well as the stability of the camera across the entire orbit of acquisition.[4]

It is important when interpreting SPECT images to be aware of possible sources of image artifacts.[5] Discrete motion of the patient (and thus motion of the heart outside its original field) causes an abnormality in the final images that may be corrected with motion correction software. Imaging artifacts commonly occur because of the effects of overlying structures that attenuate photon emissions. These include breast attenuation in women and attenuation of the inferobasal wall related to the diaphragm, most commonly seen in men. Strategies to overcome quality problems such as attenuation are described subsequently.

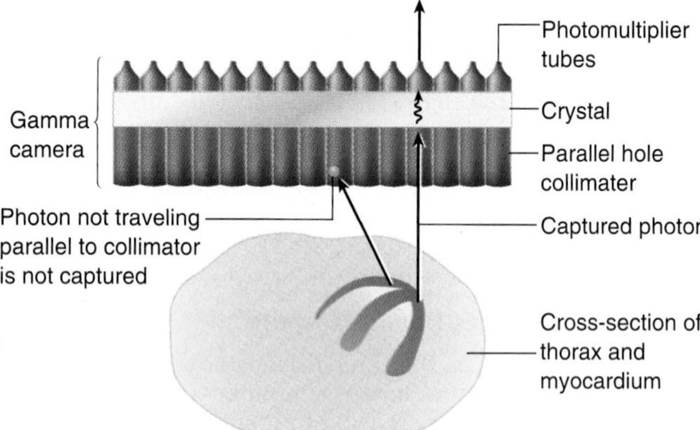

FIGURE 13–1 Capture of emitted photons by a gamma camera. Emissions are captured by a parallel hole collimator, allowing photons to interact with a detector crystal, and are recorded as scintillation events. The event is localized on the basis of where the photon interacts with the crystal.

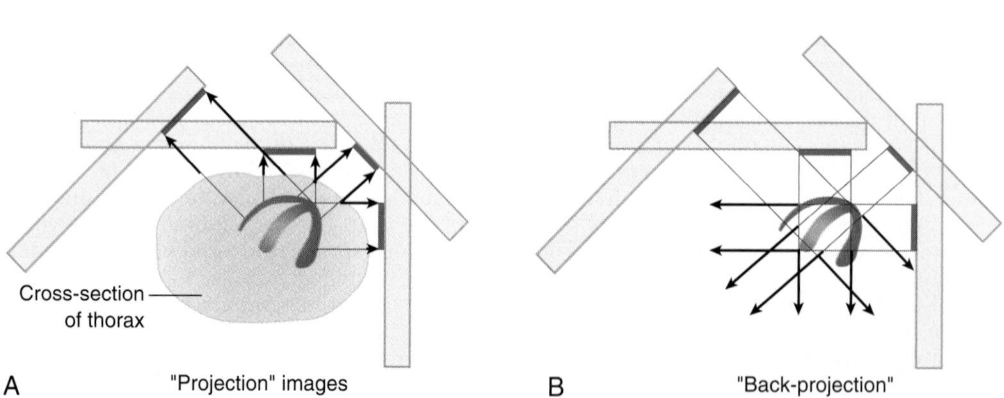

FIGURE 13–2 **A,** Single-photon emission computed tomography imaging technique. The gamma camera collects photon emission information from multiple angles around the body in order to reconstruct a three-dimensional image of the organ of interest. **B,** Back-projection technique during computer processing. Scintillation events as seen by the camera are back projected onto a matrix to reconstruct an image of the organ of interest.

SPECT Perfusion Tracers and Protocols

Thallium-201. Thallium-201 was introduced in the 1970s and propelled the clinical application of MPI as an adjunct to exercise treadmill testing. Thallium-201 is a monovalent cation with biological properties similar to those of potassium. As potassium is the major intracellular cation in muscle and is virtually absent in scar tissue, thallium-201 is a well-suited radionuclide for differentiating normal and ischemic from scarred myocardium.[6] Thallium-201 emits 80 keV of photon energy and has a physical half-life of 73 hours. The initial myocardial uptake early after intravenous injection of thallium is proportional to regional blood flow. First-pass extraction fraction (the proportion of tracer extracted from the blood as it passes through the myocardium) is high, in the range of 85 percent. It is transported across the myocyte cell membrane by the Na^+,K^+-adenosine triphosphatase (ATPase) transport system and by facilitative diffusion. Peak myocardial concentration of thallium occurs within 5 minutes of injection, with rapid clearance from the intravascular compartment. Although the initial uptake and distribution of thallium are primarily a function of blood flow, the subsequent *redistribution* of thallium, which begins within 10 to 15 minutes after injection, is unrelated to flow but is related to the rate of thallium clearance from myocardium, linked to the concentration gradient between myocytes and the blood levels of thallium (Fig. 13–4A). Thallium clearance is more rapid from normal myocardium with high thallium activity compared with myocardium with reduced thallium activity (ischemic myocardium), a process termed "differential washout" (see Fig. 13–4B).

Thallium studies can be divided into protocols in which thallium-201 is administered during stress or at rest.[6] Following stress, the reversal of a thallium defect from the initial peak stress to delayed 3- to 4-hour or 24-hour redistribution images is a marker of reversibly ischemic, viable myocardium. When thallium is injected at *rest*, the extent of thallium defect reversibility from the initial rest images to delayed redistribution images (at 3 to 4 hours) reflects viable myocardium with resting hypoperfusion. When scarred myocardium is present, the initial rest or stress thallium defect persists over time, termed an "irreversible" or "fixed" defect. However, in some patients with coronary artery disease (CAD), the initial uptake of thallium during stress may be severely decreased, and tracer accumulation from the recirculating thallium in the blood during the redistribution phase may be slow or even absent because of rapid decline of thallium levels in the blood. The result is that some severely ischemic but viable regions may show no redistribution on either early (3- to 4-hour) or late (24-hour) imaging, *even if viable myocardium is present*. Viable myocardium in this situation can be revealed by raising blood levels of thallium by reinjecting a small dose (1 mCi) of thallium at rest. Thus, in some patients, thallium reinjection is necessary to identify viable myocardium when there are irreversible defects on stress-redistribution images.

Technetium-99m–Labeled Tracers. Tc 99m–labeled myocardial perfusion tracers were introduced in the clinical arena in the 1990s.[7] Technetium-99m emits 140 keV of photon energy and has a physical half-life of 6 hours. Despite the excellent myocardial extraction and flow kinetics properties of thallium, its energy spectrum of 80 keV is suboptimal for conventional gamma cameras (ideal photopeak in the 140-keV range). In addition, thallium's long physical half-life (73 hours) limits the amount of thallium that may be administered in order to stay within acceptable radiation exposure parameters. Thus, Tc 99m–labeled tracers improve on these two limitations of thallium. Although three Tc 99m–labeled tracers (sestamibi, teboroxime, and tetrofosmin) have received U.S. Food and Drug Administration approval for detection of CAD, only sestamibi and tetrofosmin are available for clinical use at present.

Sestamibi and tetrofosmin are lipid-soluble cationic compounds with first-pass extraction fraction in the range of 60 percent. Myocardial uptake and clearance kinetics of both tracers are similar. They cross the sarcolemmal and mitochondrial membranes of myocytes by passive distribution, driven by the transmembrane electrochemical gradient, and they are retained within the mitochondria.[7] There is minimal redistribution with these

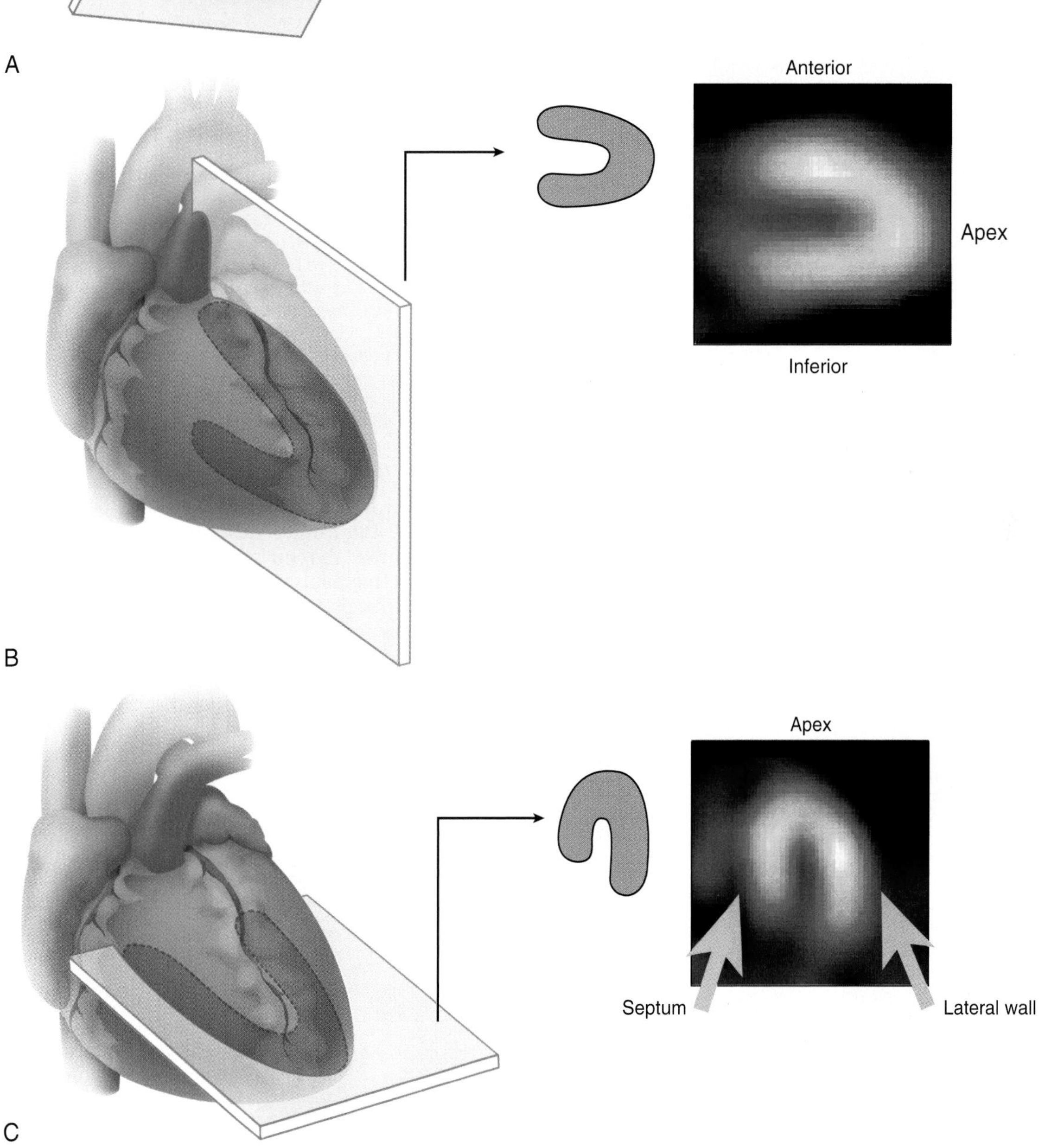

FIGURE 13–3 Standard single-photon emission computed tomography imaging tomographic display. **A,** The short-axis images each represent a portion of the anterior, lateral, inferior, and septal walls. **B,** Vertical long-axis images are displayed from left to right from the septal edge to the lateral wall and represent the anterior wall, apex, and inferior wall. **C,** Horizontal long-axis images are displayed from left to right from inferior to superior, representing the septum, apex, and lateral walls.

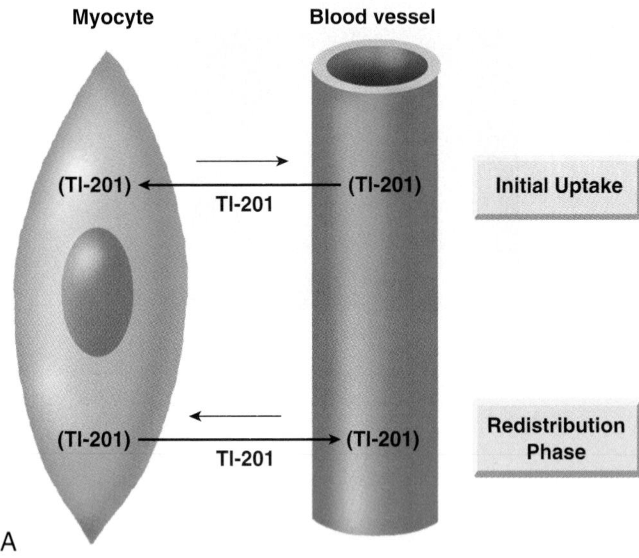

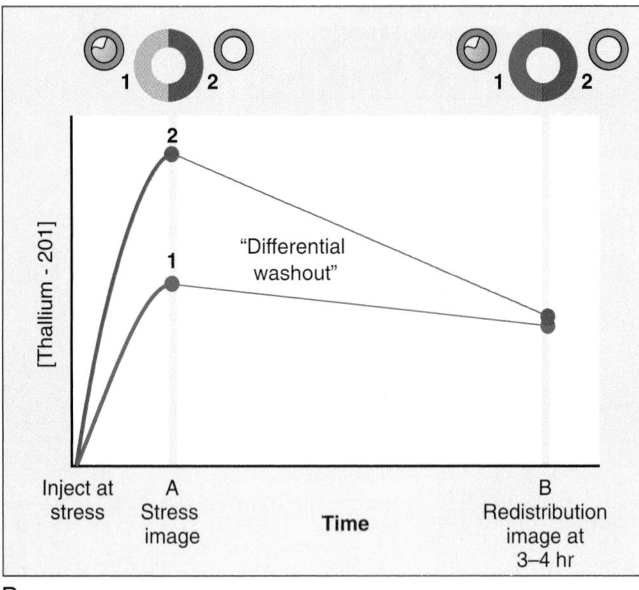

FIGURE 13–4 Thallium-201 redistribution. **A,** After initial uptake into the myocyte, an equilibrium is created between the intracellular and extracellular concentrations of thallium. After blood levels diminish during the redistribution phase, the equilibrium favors egress of thallium out of the myocyte. **B,** On the basis of that equilibrium, thallium concentration diminishes over time in zones of normal uptake, while diminishing more slowly in zones with less initial thallium uptake, i.e., those with diminished flow reserve or ischemia. In this example, segment 1 of the myocardial schematic is supplied by an artery with an 80 percent stenosis and segment 2 is supplied by a normal artery. During peak stress, normal blood flow reserve is present in segment 2; blunted flow reserve, based on the presence of stenosis, is present in segment 1, and there is less initial thallium uptake into segment 1 (time point A). Thallium washout is more rapid from the territory with initially normal uptake and slower from the ischemic zone, creating the phenomenon of differential washout. When redistribution imaging is done 3 to 4 hours later, (time point B), thallium concentrations are equal in segments 1 and 2. Thus, a reversible stress defect is seen in segment 1, based on the redistribution properties and differential washout. (Adapted from Dilsizian V: SPECT and PET techniques. *In* Dilsizian V, Narula J [eds]: Atlas of Nuclear Cardiology. Braunwald E (series ed). Philadelphia. Current Medicine, 2003, pp 19-46.)

tracers compared with thallium. Thus, myocardial perfusion studies with Tc 99m-labeled tracers require *two separate injections, one at peak stress and the second at rest.*

There are three basic protocols[8] with Tc 99m-labeled tracers: (1) a single-day study, in which myocardial blood flow is interrogated at rest and at peak stress, or in the reverse order, as long as the first injected dose is low (8 to 10 mCi) and the second injected dose is high (22 to 30 mCi); (2) a 2-day study, (commonly performed in patients with large body habitus) in which higher doses of the tracer are injected (20 to 30 mCi) both at rest and at peak stress in order to optimize myocardial count rate; and (3) a dual-isotope technique, which combines injection of thallium at rest followed by injection of a Tc 99m tracer at peak stress. The last approach takes advantage of the favorable properties of each of the two tracers, including high-quality gated SPECT images from Tc-99m and the potential of acquiring redistribution images from thallium (either at 4 hours prior to the stress study or at 24 hours after the Tc 99m activity has decayed).

A comparison of the properties of the available isotopes for perfusion imaging is shown in Table 13–1.

SPECT Image Interpretation

SPECT myocardial perfusion images may be evaluated visually, with the interpreter describing the perfusion pattern findings. Because the imaging data are digital, computer-aided quantitative analysis may also be used.[9]

For visual interpretation, the key elements to be reported include the *presence and location of perfusion defects* and whether defects on stress images are *reversible* on the rest images (implying stress-induced ischemia) or whether stress perfusion defects are *irreversible or "fixed"* (often implying myocardial infarction [MI]). Moreover, substantial literature has documented that the *extent* and the *severity* of the perfusion abnormality are independently associated with clinical outcomes.[10] Extent of perfusion abnormality refers to the amount of myocardium or vascular territory that is abnormal, and the severity refers to the magnitude of reduction in tracer uptake in abnormal zone relative to normal. Examples of stress and rest SPECT myocardial perfusion abnormalities of varying extents and severity are shown in Figure 13–5.

To minimize subjectivity in image interpretation,

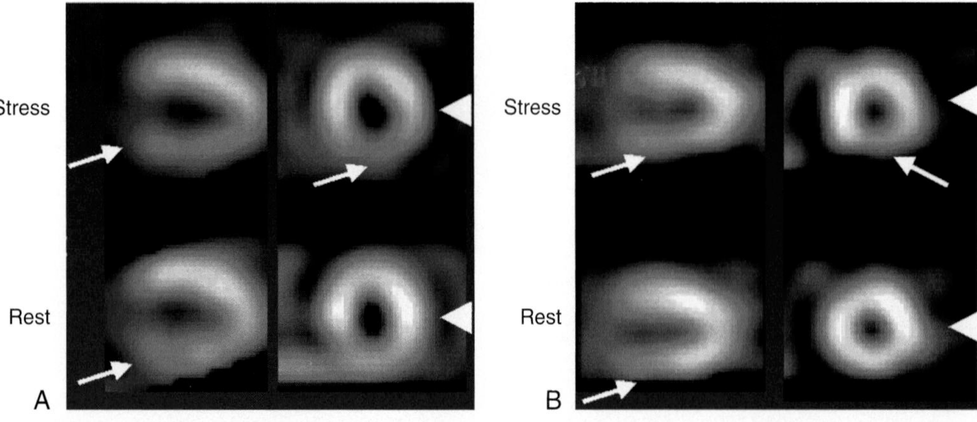

FIGURE 13–5 Abnormal single-photon emission computed tomography images of different extent and severity. **A,** A large, moderately severe, reversible inferior wall defect (arrows) reflecting a severe flow reserve abnormality. **B,** A milder reversible inferior wall defect (arrows) reflecting a less severe stenosis or a more severe stenosis with well-developed collaterals minimizing the defect severity. In both patients, there is also a mild lateral wall reversible defect (arrowheads). Note how the lateral wall brightens relative to the septum on the rest images compared with the stress images.

TABLE 13–1 Properties of SPECT Tracers

Tracer	Physical Half-Life (hr)	Uptake	Myocardial Clearance	"Differential Washout"	Maximum Extraction Fraction
Thallium-201	73	Active	~50% at 6 hr	Yes	~0.70
Tc 99m sestamibi	6	Passive	Minimal	Minimal	0.39
Tc 99m tetrafosmin	6	Passive	Minimal	Minimal	0.24
Tc 99m teboroxime	6	Passive	~50% at 10 min	Yes	0.72

SPECT = single-photon emission computed tomography.

From Gerson MC, McGoron A, Roszell N, et al: Myocardial perfusion imaging: Radiopharmaceuticals and tracer kinetics. *In* Gerson MC (ed): Cardiac Nuclear Medicine. New York, McGraw Hill, 1997, pp 3-27.

semiquantitative visual analysis or fully quantitative computer analysis may be applied to MPI data.[11] With semiquantitative visual analysis, a score is assigned to represent perfusion for each of multiple segments of the myocardium. A segmentation model has been standardized for this approach by dividing the myocardium into 17 segments[12] on the basis of three short-axis slices and a representative long-axis slice to depict the apex (Fig. 13–6). Perfusion is graded on a scale of 0 to 4, with 0 representing normal perfusion and 4 representing a very severe perfusion defect. Scores for all 17 segments are added to create the "summed" score. The summed score from the stress images (summed stress score, SSS) represents the extent and severity of stress perfusion abnormality, the magnitude of perfusion defect related to *both ischemia and infarction*. The sum of the 17 segmental scores from the rest image (the summed rest score, SRS) represents the *extent of infarction*. The summed difference score (SDS) is derived by subtracting SRS from the SSS and represents the extent and severity of *stress-induced ischemia*. As discussed subsequently, a substantial literature has validated these scores as predictors of natural history outcomes.

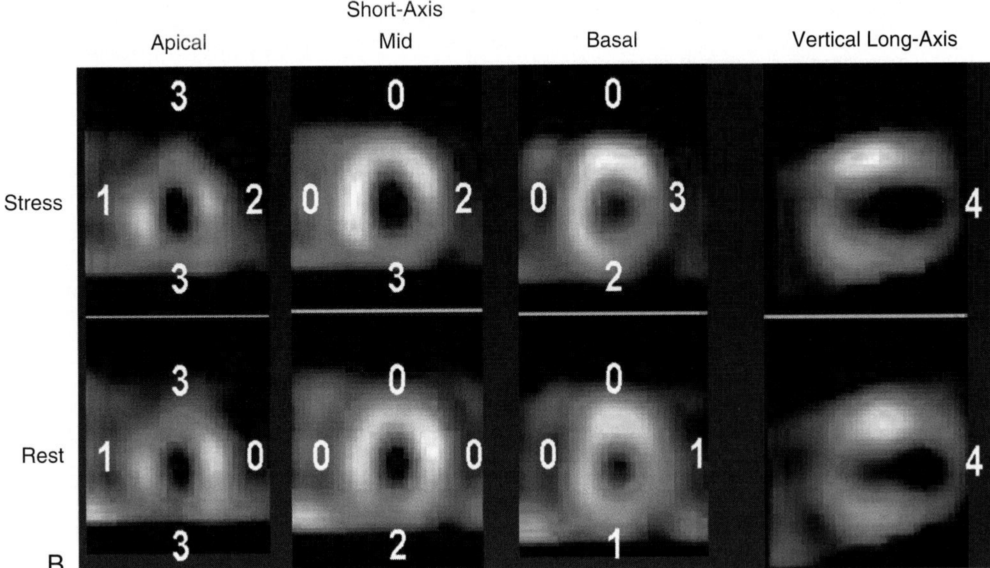

FIGURE 13–6 **A,** Standard segmental myocardial display for semiquantitative visual analysis in a 17-segment model. **B,** Segmental scoring of a patient whose stress and rest single-photon emission computed tomography perfusion images show a severe apical fixed defect (in the vertical long axis), extending into the inferoapical and anteroapical walls (in the apical short axis), with evidence of reversible defects in the inferior and lateral walls (in the middle and short axis). The summed stress score (SSS) represents extensive perfusion abnormality at stress (reflecting ischemia and infarct), the summed rest score (SRS) represents the extent of infarct, and the summed difference score (SDS) represents the extent of ischemia. LAD = left anterior descending (artery); LCX = left circumflex (coronary artery); RCA = right coronary artery.

Because SPECT MPI data are a digital representation of radiotracer distribution, the data can be analyzed quantitatively. The most common technique involves creation of a *circumferential profile* of relative tracer activity around the tomogram of interest, such as a short-axis tomogram.[13] With this technique, the 360 degrees around the tomogram are sampled at every 3 to 6 degrees, along a ray extending from the center of the image. The maximum counts at a picture element ("pixel") along the ray, usually occurring in the midportion of the myocardium, are recorded for each angle. The data may be plotted to create a profile of the perfusion pattern of that tomogram relative to the most "normal" area of uptake, which is assigned a value of 100 percent uptake (Fig. 13–7A). Circumferential profiles for an individual patient can be compared directly with a composite profile representing normal perfusion.[13,14] The

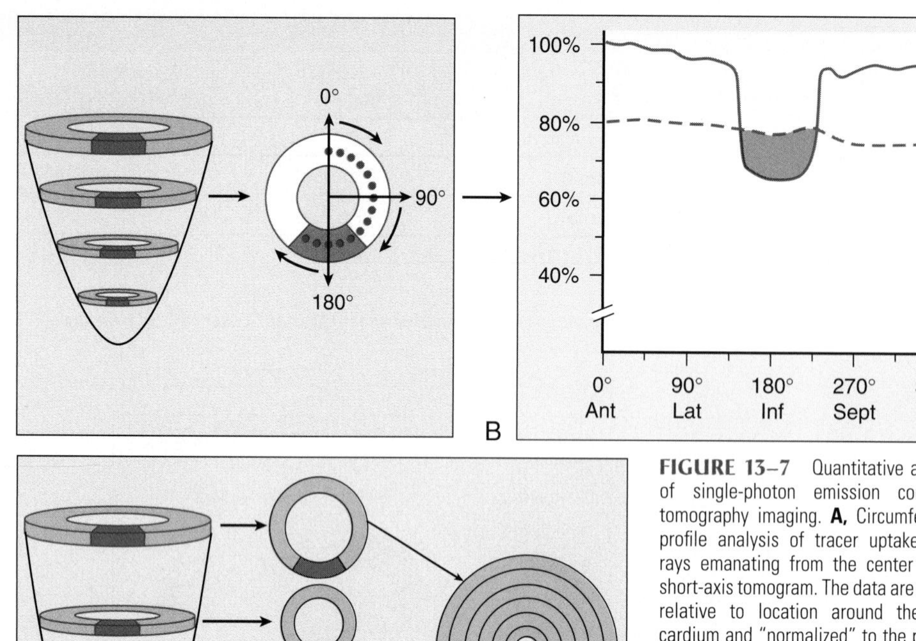

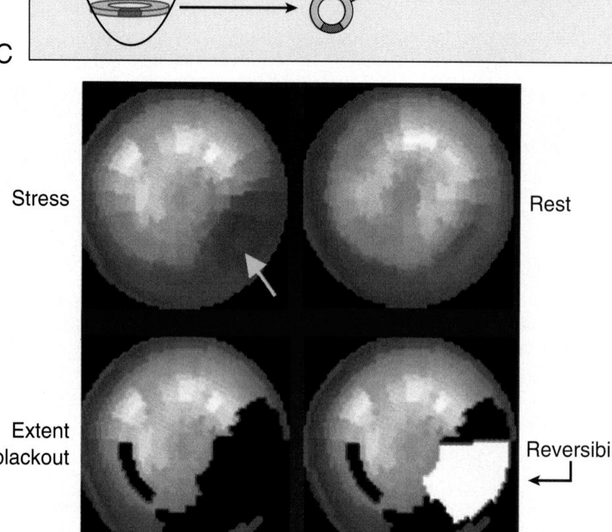

FIGURE 13–7 Quantitative analysis of single-photon emission computed tomography imaging. **A,** Circumferential profile analysis of tracer uptake along rays emanating from the center of the short-axis tomogram. The data are plotted relative to location around the myocardium and "normalized" to the point of peak uptake, which is assigned a value of 100 percent. From this procedure, a circumferential profile of tracer uptake around the myocardium is developed for each short-axis tomogram. In this example, there is a perfusion defect in the inferior wall (purple area). **B,** The patient's data are compared with lower limits of normal (dashed line) derived from a group of subjects without coronary artery disease of the same gender. From this comparison, the quantitative extent and severity of the perfusion abnormality can be derived (orange area). **C,** Data from the individual short-axis tomograms can be combined to create a bull's-eye polar plot, representing a two-dimensional compilation of all of the three-dimensional short-axis perfusion data. The inferior wall perfusion defect (gray area) is seen on the two-dimensional map. **D,** Example of a bull's-eye polar plot for a patient with a reversible defect of the inferolateral wall (yellow arrow on the stress bull's-eye plot, upper left). The "blackout" area (on the extent blackout plot, lower left) represents the myocardium that falls below the lower limits of normal, and in the reversibility plot (lower right) the white area represents the extent of that abnormality that is reversible (ischemic) on rest imaging. (Images courtesy of Ernest Garcia, Ph.D.)

normal perfusion data are often created from studies performed in normal subjects with a very low clinical probability of CAD or in those with known normal coronary arteries (see Fig. 13–7B). A quantitative extent of abnormality can be derived (the total amount of myocardium that falls below the lower limit of normal) as well as a derivation of the severity of the perfusion abnormality (the depth of the patient's perfusion abnormality relative to the lower limit of normal).

Most contemporary computer systems and analysis programs have the ability to create "bull's-eye" or "polar" maps representing perfusion of the entire three-dimensional myocardium in a two-dimensional plot (see Fig. 13–7C). Quantitative data may be derived on the extent of global perfusion abnormality, abnormality within vascular territories, as well as the extent of reversible and fixed defects (see Fig. 13–7D).

ADDITIONAL IMPORTANT SIGNS IN SPECT IMAGING ANALYSIS BEYOND MYOCARDIAL PERFUSION. There are other abnormal findings that provide additional information beyond that provided by the perfusion pattern alone, including lung uptake of tracer (particularly thallium-201) and transient ischemic dilation of the left ventricle.

Lung Uptake. In some patients, substantial tracer uptake is apparent throughout the lung fields following stress that is not present at rest (Fig. 13–8A). Patients with lung uptake often have severe multivessel disease, elevation of pulmonary capillary wedge pressure during exercise, and decreases in ejection fraction (EF) during exercise, all implying extensive myocardial ischemia.[15] It is likely that elevation in left atrial and pulmonary pressures slows pulmonary transit of the tracer, allowing more time for extraction or transudation into the interstitial spaces of the lung, accounting for this imaging sign.

Lung uptake of thallium-201 has been more extensively validated than lung uptake of the technetium-99m tracers sestamibi and tetrofosmin. There is minimal splanchnic or background activity after thallium stress injection, allowing image acquisition earlier after stress. In addition, the redistribution properties of thallium mandate that imaging begin relatively early after stress, and thus lung uptake may be more apparent.

With the technetium-99m perfusion tracers, liver uptake is more prominent than the heart immediately after injection; thus, image acquisition should begin 15 to 30 minutes after exercise stress injection and 30 to 60 minutes after pharmacological stress.[8] Thus, lung uptake, even if it had been present early after stress, may be missed with technetium-99m tracers because of the more delayed onset of imaging compared with thallium.

Transient Ischemic Dilation of the Left Ventricle. Transient ischemic dilation (TID) refers to an imaging pattern in which the left ventricle or left ventricular (LV) cavity appears larger on the stress images than at rest (see Fig. 13–8B).[16] For patients in whom the entire left ventricle appears larger during stress, the pathophysiology is probably related to extensive ischemia and prolonged postischemic systolic dysfunction, resulting in a dilated, dysfunctional left ventricle during the stress acquisition relative to the rest acquisition. In other patients, the epicardial silhouette appears similar at stress and rest, but there is apparent dilation in the LV cavity. This probably represents diffuse subendocardial ischemia (relatively less tracer uptake in the subendocardium creating the appearance of an enlarged cavity) and is also associated with severe and extensive CAD. Contemporary processing systems can automatically quantify TID.[17]

Both lung uptake and TID provide clues to more extensive CAD than may have been suspected from the perfusion pattern alone. Both signs have been associated with angiographically extensive and severe CAD and with unfavorable long-term outcomes and thus are considered "high-risk" findings.

COMMON NORMAL VARIATIONS IN SPECT IMAGING

Normal variations in perfusion images can be falsely interpreted as a defect. These perturbations from a completely homogeneous tracer pattern throughout the myocardium are related to structural variations of the myocardium as well as technical factors associated with image acquisition.

One example is the "drop-out" of the upper septum because of the muscular septum merging with the membranous septum (Fig. 13–9A). Apical thinning is another variation of normal that can be mistaken for a perfusion defect (see Fig. 13–9B). The apex is anatomically thinner than other myocardial regions, creating this appearance. In normal SPECT images, the lateral wall may often appear brighter than the contralateral septum (see Fig. 13–9C). This is not due to a difference in lateral versus septal wall myocardial blood flow. Rather, during a SPECT acquisition, the camera is physically closer to the lateral myocardial wall (in close proximity to the lateral chest wall) than to the septum, thus subject to less soft tissue attenuation and associated with more efficient count capture. A careful review of a series of normal volunteers or subjects with a low probability of CAD with one's own equipment is an important step in minimizing the influence of these normal variations on the sensitivity and specificity for detecting CAD.[9]

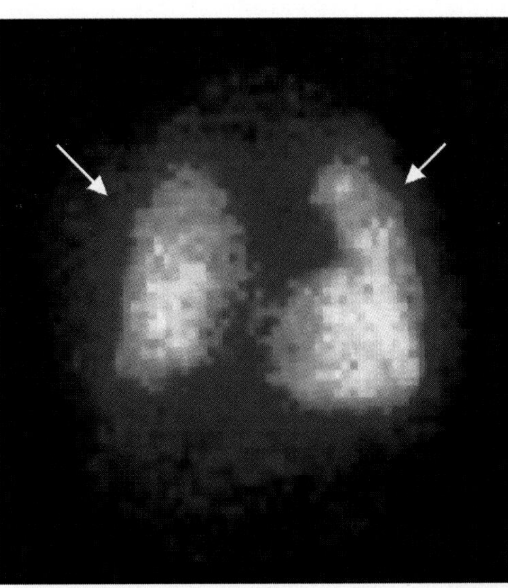

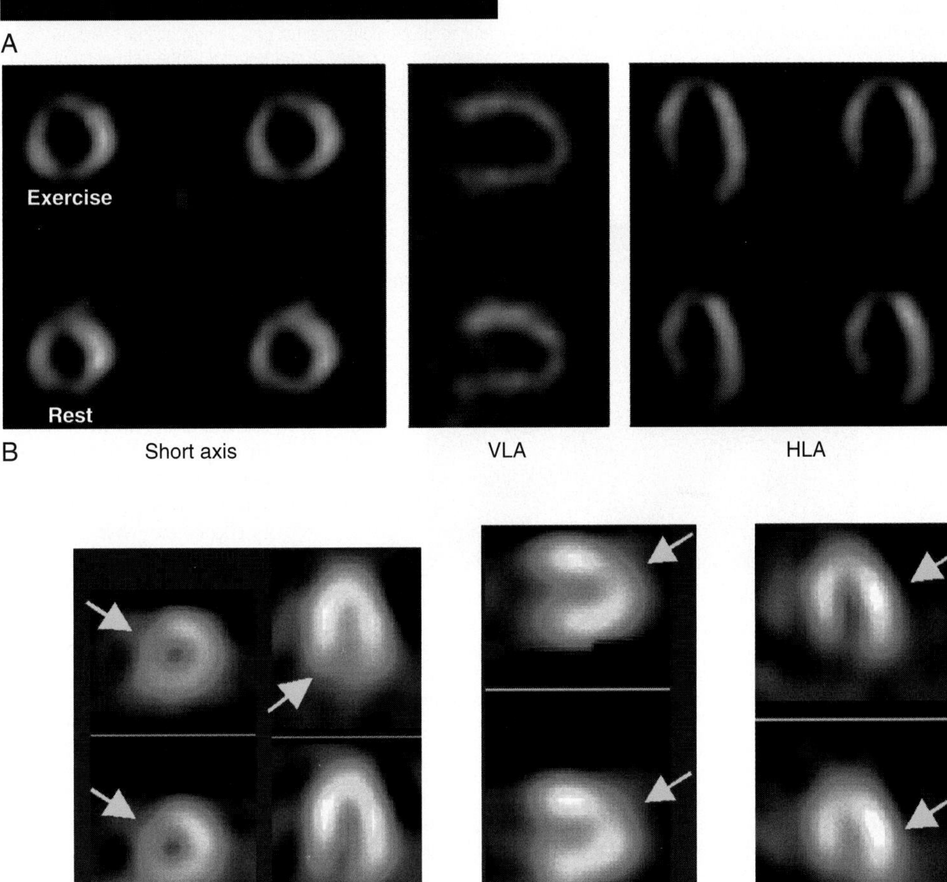

FIGURE 13–8 **A,** Increased lung uptake of thallium-201, imaged in the anterior projection. Lung uptake such as this is associated with extensive coronary artery disease and an adverse prognosis. **B,** Transient ischemic dilation of the left ventricle after stress. In the stress images, the apparent size of the left ventricular cavity is larger compared with the rest images, i.e., transiently dilated. HLA = horizontal long axis; VLA = vertical long axis.

A B C

FIGURE 13–9 Normal variations in single-photon emission computed tomography perfusion imaging. **A,** Normal "dropout" of the basal septum. **B,** Normal apical thinning. **C,** The lateral wall is often slightly "hotter" than the septum, another normal variation.

Technical Artifacts Affecting Image Interpretation

Breast Attenuation. In patients with large or dense breasts, significant attenuation may create artifacts varying considerably in their appearance and location (Fig. 13–10A and B). A review of the cine display of the raw projection images may reveal the presence of potential breast attenuation.[5] Gender-matched quantitative data bases have had a favorable although modest impact on this issue, as such data bases generally consist of subjects who are of average body and breast size.

Several approaches toward minimizing the impact of breast tissue have been taken in order to improve specificity (lowering the false-positive rate) in women. Most well documented is the use of technetium-99m–based agents with SPECT imaging with electrocardiographic (ECG) gating. In the setting of a mild to moderately severe fixed defect, most often of the anterior or anterolateral wall, that may represent breast attenuation artifact versus nontransmural MI, the *presence of preserved wall motion suggests the absence of infarct* and supports the interpretation of attenuation artifact (see Fig. 13–10A, bottom). Specificity for ruling out CAD in women has been improved significantly with this technique,[18] as discussed subsequently.

Inferior Wall Attenuation. Inferior wall attenuation artifacts are commonly encountered in SPECT imaging. This

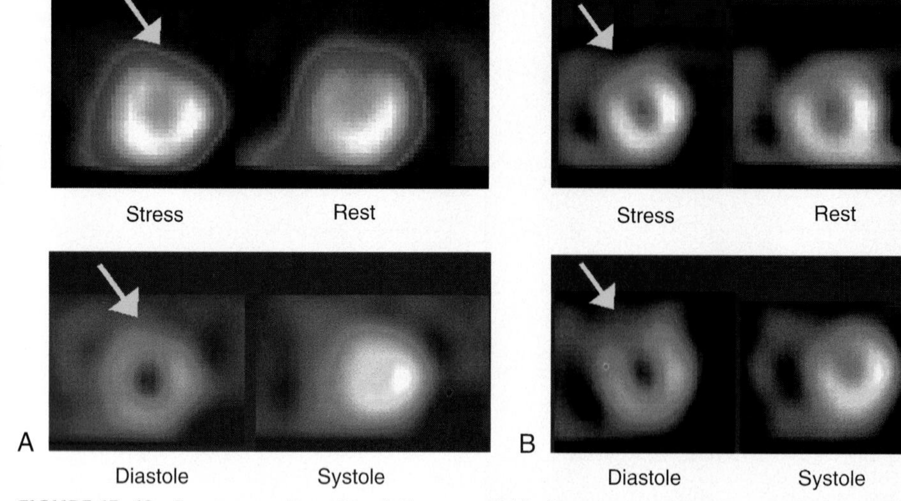

FIGURE 13–10 Breast attenuation artifact. **A,** Top row: a mild fixed anterior defect related to a possible breast attenuation artifact. In the bottom row, diastolic and systolic frames from an electrocardiographic-gated single-photon emission computed tomography (SPECT) acquisition demonstrating preserved wall thickening in the territory of the mild anterior fixed defect. The preserved wall thickening supports the conclusion that the mild defect is an attenuation artifact. **B,** A more severe anterior fixed defect is unlikely to represent an artifact on the basis of the severity and is more likely to represent myocardial infarction. In the bottom row, diastolic and systolic frames from the gated SPECT acquisition demonstrate abnormal thickening, supporting the interpretation of infarct rather than artifact.

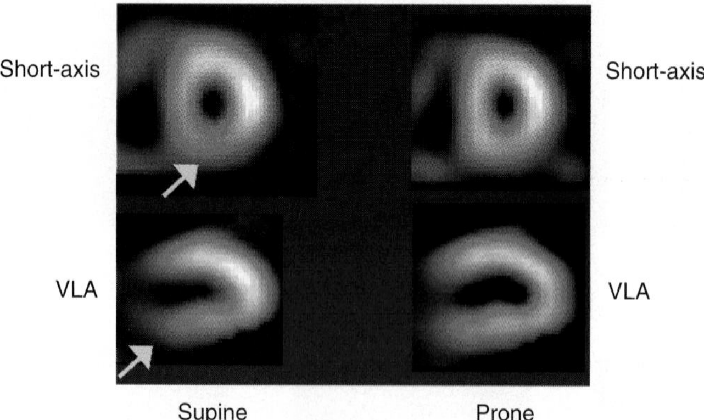

FIGURE 13–11 **Left,** Attenuation of the inferior basal wall (yellow arrows) possibly related to attenuation by overlying left hemidiaphragm. Most commonly, this appears as a tapering of the inferior wall seen best on the vertical long-axis (VLA) image. **Right,** One solution to the problem of inferior wall attenuation is reimaging the patient in the prone position.

artifact may be caused by extracardiac structures such as the diaphragm overlapping the inferior wall (Fig. 13–11). In addition, during a SPECT acquisition, the longer distance from the inferior wall to the camera means that photons must traverse a greater degree of tissue before reaching the detectors, which may increase the degree of scatter and attenuation.

As with breast attenuation artifact detection, the demonstration of preserved wall thickening by gated SPECT imaging may be helpful in distinguishing attenuation artifact from infarct. The patient's positioning may also minimize the degree of attenuation. When patients are imaged in the *prone* position,[19] the inferior wall is brought closer to the detector, although sometimes at the expense of image quality for the anterior wall (see Fig. 13–11).

Artifacts Related to Extracardiac Tracer Uptake. Tracer in extracardiac structures can cause artifacts in SPECT images. When such a structure is near the heart, increased counts may reach the detector. This may falsely elevate the number of counts the system assigns to the nearby cardiac wall, so that the cardiac region is displayed as falsely "hotter." A second possibility occurs when a nearby hot extracardiac structure causes a "ramp filter" or "negative lobe" artifact.[20] This artifact is due to a hot extracardiac structure "stealing" counts from the heart during the calculation of the summed SPECT images. The adjacent myocardium appears falsely "cool." If substantial extracardiac uptake is noted, image acquisition may be repeated after waiting a longer period of time before imaging. Having the patient drink cold water may enhance clearance of tracer from visceral organs, particularly bowel.

Attenuation Correction

Advances in camera hardware and computer software have led to new methods of *correcting for attenuation,* with the goal of reducing false-positive scans stemming from attenuation artifacts. Attenuation correction techniques use an associated transmission scan of an isotope distinct from the perfusion tracer to create a patient-specific "attenuation map." This map is then used to "correct" the patient's emission data (the perfusion images) for tissue attenuation specific to the patient. There are several methodologies for attenuation correction, reviewed in detail elsewhere.[21]

Although attenuation correction is a relatively new technique, there is now substantial validation of its effectiveness in improving the specificity of SPECT imaging for CAD.[22] At this writing, the hardware and software required for attenuation correction are not yet widely available, although its use is likely to grow given the published data. When such attenuation correction algorithms are used, it is important to interpret the original, uncorrected images as well as the corrected images.

Gated SPECT Display, Interpretation, and Quantitation

An important advance in the use and application of SPECT MPI has been the incorporation of ECG-gated SPECT perfusion imaging for *simultaneous assessment of LV function as well as perfusion.* Prior to the use of gated SPECT, comprehensive information on both perfusion and function required separate testing modalities, such as SPECT MPI and a separate radionuclide ventriculogram or echocardiogram

Electrocardiographically Gated Radionuclide Techniques to Assess the Physiology of Ventricular Function

To assess parameters of cardiac function with echocardiography, LV endocardial borders are drawn over several beats to derive parameters such as EF. With contrast left ventriculography, endocardial borders are drawn for either one beat or an average of several beats to calculate EF. In contrast, the commonly used radionuclide techniques to assess ventricular function create *one cardiac cycle for analysis that represents an average of several hundred beats* acquired over a period of 8 to 15 minutes, using a technique known as ECG gating (Fig. 13–12).

During an ECG-gated image acquisition, the patient's ECG is monitored simultaneously with the image.[23] As the peak of an R wave is detected, the "gate" opens and a set number of milliseconds of imaging information is stored in a "frame." For a typical gated SPECT acquisition, each R-R interval is divided into eight frames. For example, if the patient's resting heart rate is 60 beats/min (1000 milliseconds per beat), an eight-

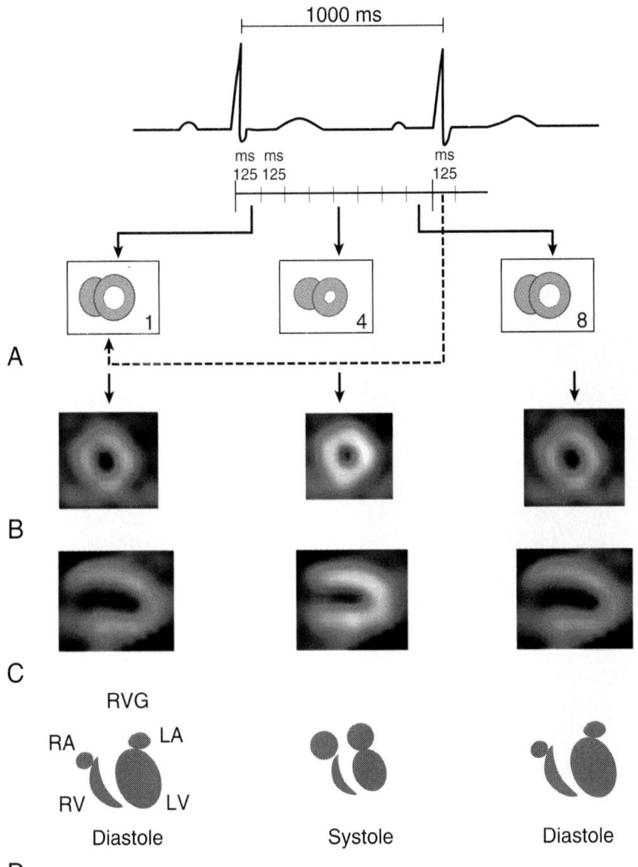

FIGURE 13–12 Basis for the technique of electrocardiographic (ECG) gating. **A,** The scintigraphic acquisition data are collected in conjunction with the electrocardiogram. The R-R interval is divided into a prespecified number of frames (in this example eight frames). At a heart rate of 60 beats/min (1000 msec/beat), each of the eight frames would comprise 125 milliseconds. For the first 125 milliseconds after the peak of the initial R wave, all imaging data are recorded in frame 1; the second 125 milliseconds are recorded in frame 2 and so on until the peak of the next R wave is detected, and this is repeated for each beat in the acquisition. Frame 1 thus represents the end-diastolic events, and one of the frames in the middle of the acquisition (frame 4 in this example) represents end-systolic events. **B,** Examples of gated single-photon emission computed tomography perfusion imaging. Short-axis images are seen at end diastole and at end systole. **C,** Similar timing with images displayed from the vertical long-axis orientation. Visually, wall thickening and brightening are seen across the course of systole. These events represent regional wall thickening and changes in global function across the cardiac cycle. **D,** ECG-gated equilibrium radionuclide ventriculographic (RVG) images are shown at diastole and at end systole. LA = left atrium; LV = left ventricle; RA = right atrium; RV = right ventricle. (Adapted from Germano G, Berman DS: Acquisition and processing for gated SPECT: Technical aspects. *In* Germano G, Berman DS [eds]: Clinical gated cardiac SPECT. Armonk, NY, Futura Publishing, 1999, pp 93-114.)

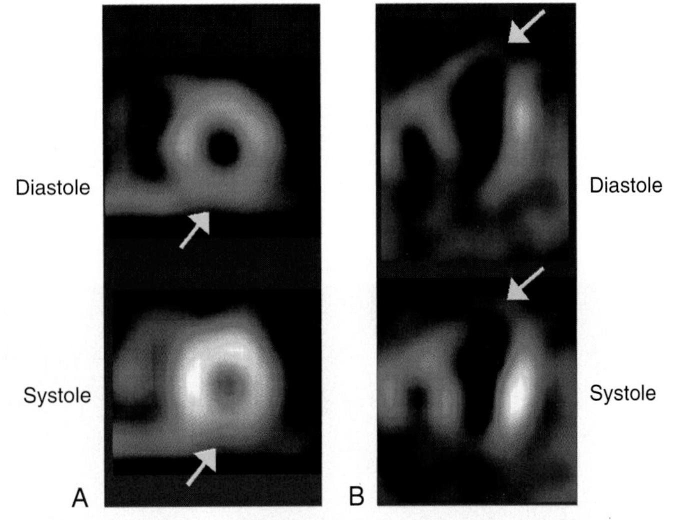

FIGURE 13–13 Examples of regional dysfunction detected by ECG-gated single-photon emission computed tomography perfusion imaging. **A,** The *hypokinetic* inferior region appears to brighten less (arrows) than the other regions from diastole to systole. **B,** The *akinetic* apex in the horizontal long axis (arrows) appears to have no change from diastole to systole, in contrast to the normally thickening (brightening) lateral walls.

frame acquisition across the cardiac cycle comprises 125 milliseconds per frame. After the first 125 milliseconds of imaging data have been recorded in frame 1, the gate closes and then instantly reopens, allowing the second 125 milliseconds of information to be recorded in frame 2 (see Fig. 13-12). This sequence continues through the prespecified number of frames throughout the cardiac cycle. When the R wave of the next beat is detected by the ECG-gated system, the sequence is repeated for each beat that occurs throughout the image acquisition.

The number of counts recorded during any individual cardiac cycle is insufficient to create an interpretable image. When several hundred beats have been recorded, an average cardiac cycle representing all the recorded beats can be reconstructed by redisplaying the frames sequentially in a cine or movie format. The first few frames represent systolic events, and the latter frames represent diastolic events (see Fig. 13-12).

High-quality ECG-gated images require that included cardiac cycles have reasonably homogeneous beat lengths. This is usually accomplished by "beat-length windowing," whereby the computer acquisition system is programmed to accept beats into the acquisition of only certain cycle lengths. Typically, the beat length represented by the average heart rate of the patient (1000 milliseconds in the preceding example) along with beat lengths of ±10 to 15 percent around the average length is allowed into the acquisition. Cardiac cycles with cycle lengths above or below that limit are rejected. For example, the short cardiac cycle from the R wave of a normal beat to the R wave of a premature ventricular contraction (PVC) would not be allowed into the acquisition, nor would the long cycle representing the post-PVC pause. This makes physiological sense; the short pre-PVC beat and the more prolonged post-PVC beat have distinctly different systolic and diastolic characteristics than the beats during normal sinus rhythm.

ECG-Gated SPECT Imaging. The technique most commonly used to assess ventricular function clinically is ECG-gated SPECT imaging.[23] Normal regional systolic function is depicted as brightening of the wall during systole (see Fig. 13-12B). The wall appears to thicken, and there is apparent endocardial excursion. Assessment of regional LV function by gated SPECT imaging is based on an effect known in imaging physics as the *partial volume effect*, sometimes referred to as the *recovery coefficient* effect. When objects being imaged fall below a certain thickness threshold, count (or photon) recovery from the object is related not only to the tracer concentration within that object but also to the thickness of the object.[24] For the myocardium, usually all thicknesses fall below that threshold for SPECT imaging. Although tracer concentration within the myocardium is constant during a gated SPECT image acquisition, the recovery of counts (and thus the brightness of the object being imaged) is related to wall thickness. Hence, during systolic wall thickening, it appears that the LV wall is becoming brighter and thicker, even though the isotope concentration per gram of myocardial tissue is actually unchanged. This principle forms the basis for gated SPECT imaging.

Regional myocardial function is usually assessed visually, in a manner similar to the analysis performed in echocardiography. Regions that brighten normally have normal regional systolic performance, and those with diminished but apparent brightening are labeled hypokinetic. Regions with slight brightening are interpreted as severely hypokinetic and regions with no apparent brightening as akinetic (Fig. 13-13). Regional function can also be analyzed by quantitative techniques and displayed in a polar map format.

Quantitative Analysis of Global Left Ventricular Function by Gated SPECT Imaging

All contemporary camera-computer systems have software capable of quantitative analysis of global LV function. These computer-based methodologies are fully automated and thus extremely reproducible. The most common method involves automated interrogation of the apparent epicardial and endocardial borders of all of the tomograms in all three orthogonal planes (Fig. 13–14A). These multiple two-dimensional contours are then reconstructed to create a surface-rendered three-dimensional display representing global LV function across a typical cardiac cycle (see Fig. 13–14B) that can be viewed from any direction by simple maneuvering of the computer display screen or cursor.[23] The three-dimensional display is accompanied by automated calculation of EF and LV volumes.

EF measurements from automated analysis of ECG-gated SPECT perfusion imaging have been extensively validated against other quantitative techniques assessing LV function, such as equilibrium radionuclide ventriculography (RVG), invasive measures of contrast left ventriculography, and cardiac magnetic resonance imaging.[23] Across a wide range of ventricular function, and even in the setting of severe perfusion defects, ECG-gated SPECT imaging provides robust, highly reproducible estimates of LVEF.

The incorporation of ECG-gated SPECT imaging into a SPECT acquisition is now routine in MPI and is recommended as standard by contemporary guidelines.[25] As discussed subsequently, the addition of LV function data to the perfusion information provides incremental and independent prognostic information as well as being of practical importance in management decisions. Gated SPECT imaging has also been an important advance in helping to differentiate attenuation artifacts from infarct, as regions with persistent low counts that show normal motion and thickening represent soft tissue artifacts rather than scar. Thus, gated SPECT has improved the specificity of perfusion imaging for ruling out CAD, particularly in women.[18]

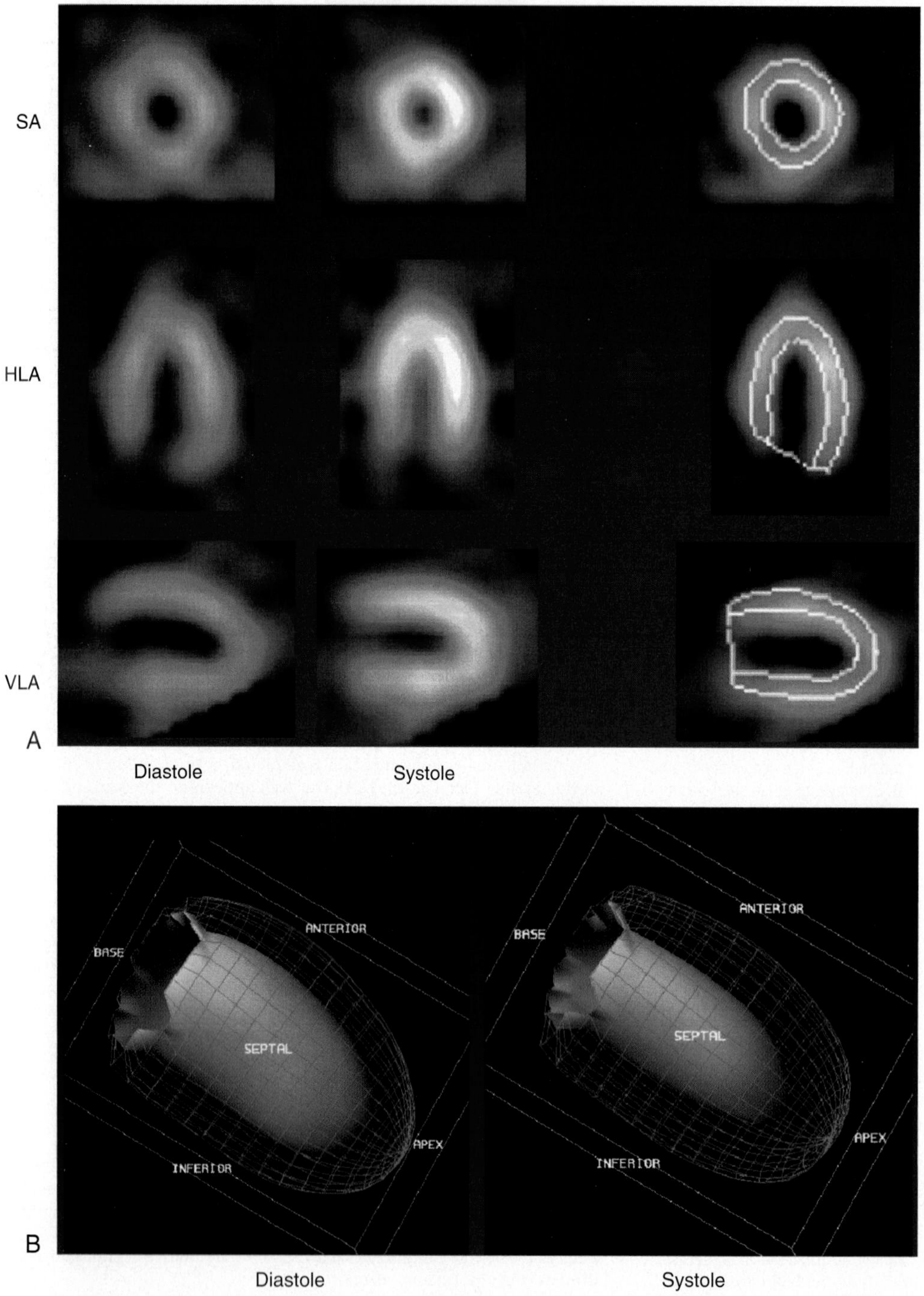

FIGURE 13–14 **A,** ECG-gated single-photon emission computed tomography (SPECT) perfusion images in short axis (SA), vertical long axis (VLA), and horizontal long axis (HLA), shown frozen at diastole (left column) and at end systole (middle column). Endocardial and epicardial borders are shown on the diastolic frames as automatically assigned by the software analysis program (right column). **B,** From the contours that are created from all of the two-dimensional tomograms, a three-dimensionally surface-rendered image of the left ventricle can be created and displayed in multiple orientations here frozen at end diastole (left) and end systole (right). The green "mesh" represents the epicardium, and the gray surface represents the endocardium. Ejection fraction is quantitated from the volume change. During image interpretation, gated SPECT images are displayed in the cine format, as an endless loop movie rather than as the still frames depicted here.

Planar Myocardial Perfusion Imaging

Prior to the widespread application of tomographic (SPECT) perfusion imaging techniques, planar imaging was the standard acquisition and display methodology. In planar imaging, three separate two-dimensional images are obtained with the gamma camera following radiotracer injection and uptake into the myocardium.[26] The three standard views are an anterior, a left anterior oblique, and a more lateral view (Fig. 13–15).

Using planar imaging, the imaging views are standard and the reader must account for the different orientations of the heart in assignng regional abnormalities. In contrast, because the tomographic slices of SPECT imaging are constructed perpendicular and parallel to an assigned long axis, SPECT images are oriented in a uniform manner for display and interpretation without influence by the individual patient's cardiac orientation.

An advantage of planar imaging over SPECT imaging is its simplicity. Each of the three views can be acquired

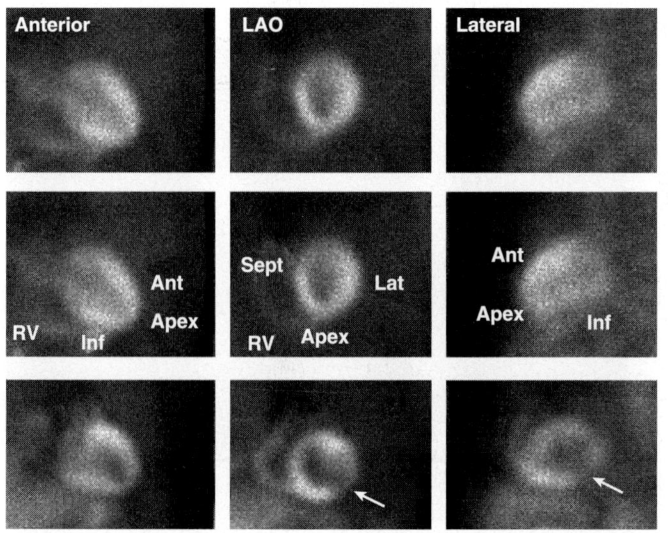

FIGURE 13–15 Examples of planar myocardial perfusion imaging. **Top row:** A normal stress planar perfusion study in the anterior, shallow left anterior oblique (LAO), and more lateral views. Tracer uptake is uniform throughout the myocardial walls. **Middle row:** The same normal planar stress perfusion images are shown, with the myocardial walls that are seen in each view labeled. The anterior wall (ant), apex, and inferior (inf) walls are seen in the anterior view as well as the right ventricle (RV). The septum (sept), apex, and lateral walls (lat) and the RV are seen in the shallow LAO view, and the anterior wall, apex, and inferior walls are seen in the lateral view. **Bottom row:** Example of an abnormal planar study showing a lateral wall stress perfusion defect in the shallow LAO view (arrow), extending into the inferior wall in the lateral view (arrow). Rest images are not shown. (Courtesy of Kim A. Williams, M.D.)

over 5 to 8 minutes with patients lying on a table with their arms by their side. Planar imaging is less affected by patients' motion than is SPECT imaging. With planar imaging, there is no extensive image processing as with SPECT, which creates many more sources of potential error and artifact. However, given the two-dimensional nature of planar imaging, in each of the standard views there is substantial overlap of myocardial regions and less ability to differentiate smaller and particularly milder perfusion abnormalities. The more standard orientation of SPECT imaging lends itself to easier understanding of the localization of perfusion abnormalities.

The original data on the sensitivity and specificity of perfusion imaging for CAD, as well as the prognostic value of perfusion imaging, were developed using planar imaging and later revalidated using SPECT imaging. In contemporary practice, planar imaging may be used for patients who do not tolerate the position that must be maintained during a SPECT acquisition, those who have difficulty coping with the larger SPECT camera being so close to the body, or those with large body habitus that surpasses the weight and size limits of SPECT systems.[10]

Quantitative analytical techniques such as the circumferential profile technique were originally developed using planar perfusion imaging.[2] A substantial literature has documented that when quantitative analysis is applied to planar perfusion imaging, there is an improvement in the sensitivity to detect multivessel CAD.

Radionuclide Angiography or Ventriculography

Radionuclide angiography (RNA), also known as RVG or blood pool imaging, may be performed by *first-pass* or by *equilibrium gated* techniques.[27,28] The equilibrium technique is often referred to as multiple gated acquisition (MUGA) scanning. Although the two techniques use distinct tracers and data recording, they provide similar results for global EF and chamber volumes. Both techniques provide a highly reproducible means to quantify global LV and right ventricular (RV) EF.

Equilibrium Radionuclide Angiography or Ventriculography (Gated Blood Pool Imaging)

In equilibrium RVG studies, data are recorded in a computer system synchronized with the R wave of the patient's ECG, similar to ECG-gated SPECT (see Fig. 13–12). Most commonly, technetium-99m labeling is applied to red blood cells or albumin. Image contrast is usually better with ^{99m}Tc-labeled red blood cells, but ^{99m}Tc-labeled albumin is preferable in patients in whom red blood cell labeling may be difficult. Labeling of red blood cells with ^{99m}Tc pertechnetate requires a reducing agent, stannous pyrophosphate, which is administered 15 to 30 minutes prior to pertechnetate injection. The reader is referred to reviews of red blood cell labeling techniques for additional detail.[29]

Image Acquisition. Although few counts are recorded during a single ECG-gated cardiac cycle, the summation of counts from 800 to 1000 cardiac cycles produces an average cardiac cycle with high resolution. Images of the heart are usually acquired in three standard projections: anterior, left anterior oblique (best separation of the left and right ventricles), and left lateral (or left posterior oblique). The minimum framing rate for a resting RVG study is 16 frames/cycle (about 50 msec/frame).[27] For quantitative assessment of diastolic indices and regional EF, the framing rate should be increased to 32 frames/cycle (about 25 msec/frame). For adequate counting statistics, images are acquired for a preset count of at least 250,000 per frame or count density of 300 counts per pixel, which corresponds to an acquisition time of 5 to 10 minutes per projection. For exercise studies, adequate counts can be obtained in the best septal view with a 2-minute acquisition using a high-sensitivity collimator. Arrhythmias such as multiple PVCs can adversely affect the study if these beats account for more than 10 percent of the total. In patients with atrial fibrillation, there may be considerable beat-to-beat variability, and the mean EF obtained over the period of acquisition may underestimate the actual LVEF.[27]

Image Display and Analysis. Qualitative inspection of equilibrium studies as an endless cinematic loop of the cardiac cycle (see Fig. 13–12D) allows assessment of (1) the size of heart chambers and great vessels; (2) regional wall motion; (3) global function (qualitative assessment) (Fig. 13–16A and B); (4) ventricular wall thickness, pericardial effusion, or paracardiac pericardial fat pad or mass; and (5) extracardiac uptake (such as splenomegaly). Quantification of systolic and diastolic indices and volumes is derived from the ventricular time-activity curve,[30] which is analogous to the angiographic time-volume curve (Fig. 13–17). In addition to the time-activity curve, functional images, such as amplitude and phase images, can be produced that have been useful in characterizing regional asynergy and asynchrony.

First-Pass Radionuclide Angiography or Ventriculography

In first-pass RVG studies, the bolus of radioactivity passes initially through the right chambers of the heart, then through the lungs, and finally through the left-sided chambers of the heart. Radiopharmaceuticals used for this purpose must produce adequate counts in a short period of time at an acceptably low radiation dose to the patient.[28] Although both technetium-99m diethylenetriaminepentaacetic acid (DTPA) and ^{99m}Tc pertechnetate have short intravascular residence time, ^{99m}Tc-DTPA is the recommended radionuclide of choice because the DTPA salt enhances renal excretion.

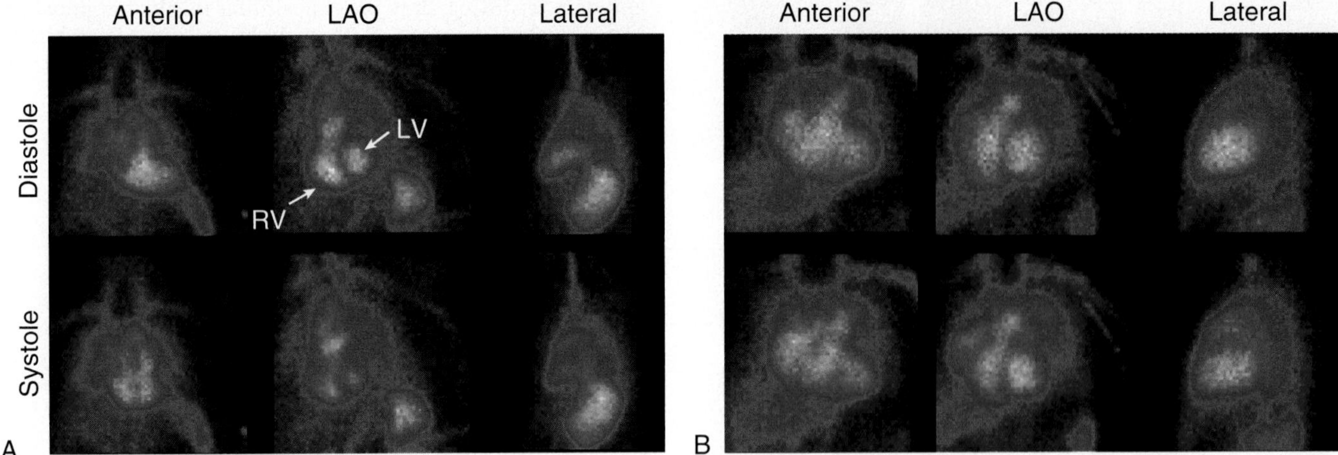

FIGURE 13–16 Equilibrium radionuclide ventriculography (RVG). The isotope (Tc99m) is labeled to red blood cells, and hence the images represent the blood "pools" in the left ventricle (LV), the right ventricle (RV), the other cardiac chambers and the great vessels, as well as the spleen. Typically, three views are obtained, as shown. **A,** Normal left ventricular function, with end-diastolic images in the top row and end-systolic images in the bottom row. LV and RV volumes diminish from diastole to systole. **B,** Images obtained in a patient with LV dysfunction. There is significant LV and RV dilatation at both end diastole (top) and end systole (bottom), and severely dimished LV systolic function (i.e., much less volume change from end diastole to end systole compared to the study in panel A). LAO = left anterior oblique projection.

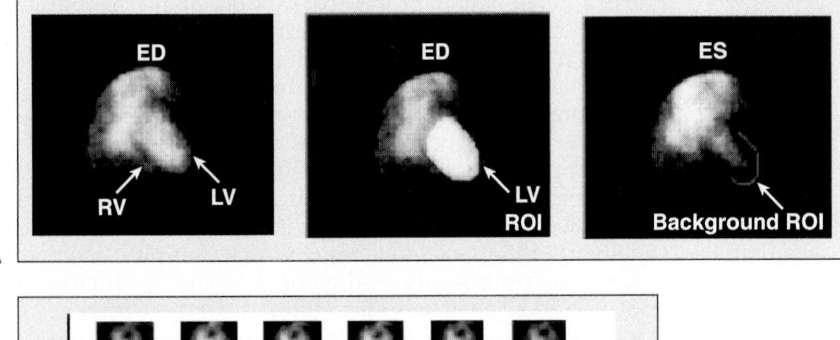

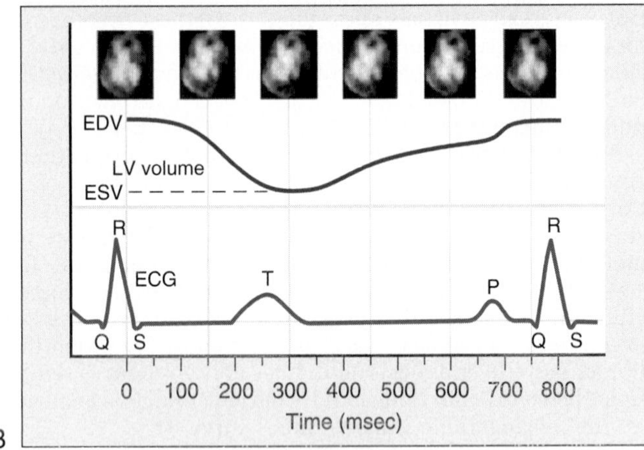

FIGURE 13–17 Quantitative analysis of equilibrium ECG-gated radionuclide ventriculography. **A,** The left anterior oblique view of the left ventricle (LV) and right ventricle (RV) is shown at end diastole (ED) **(left)**, with a region of interest (ROI) identifying the LV contour at end diastole **(middle)** and a "background" ROI drawn at end systole (ES) **(right)**, used to correct for count activity in front of and behind the LV. In **B,** a time-activity curve is demonstrated that illustrates the change in counts within the regions of interest shown in A across a cardiac cycle. Because count activity is related to LV chamber volume, the time-activity curve represents the relative volume change of the LV chamber across a cardiac cycle, from end diastole to end systole and back to end diastole. EDV = end-diastolic volume; ESV = end-systolic volume. (From Green MV, Bacharach SL, Douglas MA, et al: The measurement of left ventricular function and the detection of wall motion abnormalities with high temporal resolution ECG-gated scintigraphic angiocardiography. IEEE Trans Nucl Sci NS-23, 1976.)

Image Acquisition. Images are acquired very rapidly as the tracer passes through the heart chambers. Separation of the right and left ventricles is achieved because of the temporal separation of the bolus. Image quality is related to the injection technique, which should be rapid (over 2 to 3 seconds) in order to achieve an uninterrupted bolus (Fig. 13–18). Images are acquired in the supine position following the rapid injection of 25 mCi of tracer through an 18-gauge or larger intravenous catheter placed in the medial antecubital or external jugular vein. The shallow (20 to 30 degree) right anterior oblique projection is used to optimize separation of the atria and great vessels from the ventricles and to view the ventricles parallel to their long axes. Although the right anterior oblique view maximizes overlap of the right and left ventricles, this is not a problem in most patients because the timing of tracer appearance reliably identifies each chamber sequentially. A 1-mCi tracer dose may be used to ensure proper positioning so that the right and left ventricles are in the field of view.

Image Analysis. To identify the RV and LV phases, regions of interest are drawn around the right and left ventricles at end diastole.[28] Time-activity curves are generated, and cycles around and including the peak time-activity curve are used to calculate EFs. In general, two to five cardiac cycles are summed for the RV phase, and five to seven cycles are summed for the LV phase. From these data, quantitative analysis of LV and RV EF is performed.

COMPARISON OF EQUILIBRIUM AND FIRST-PASS TECHNIQUES

Advantages of the first-pass technique are the high target-to-background ratio, more distinct temporal separation of the cardiac chambers, and rapidity of imaging. RV EF may be more readily assessed using the first-pass technique because of the more distinct separation of this structure from the other chambers with that technique. Advantages of equilibrium technique are the potential for repeated assessment of cardiac function during rapidly varying physiological conditions, high count density, and acquisition of images in multiple projections. In contemporary practice, the equilibrium technique is performed more commonly.[10]

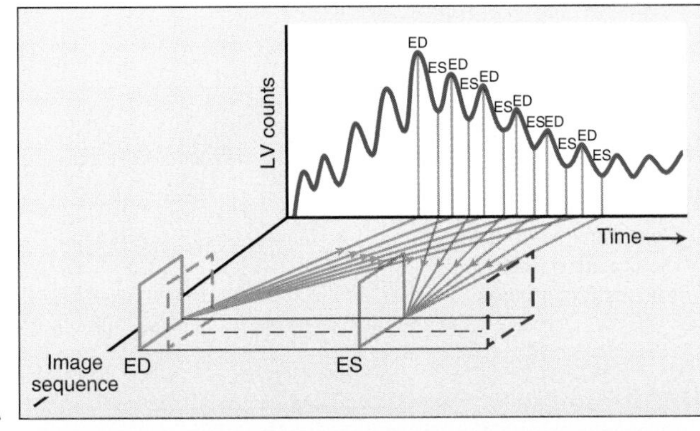

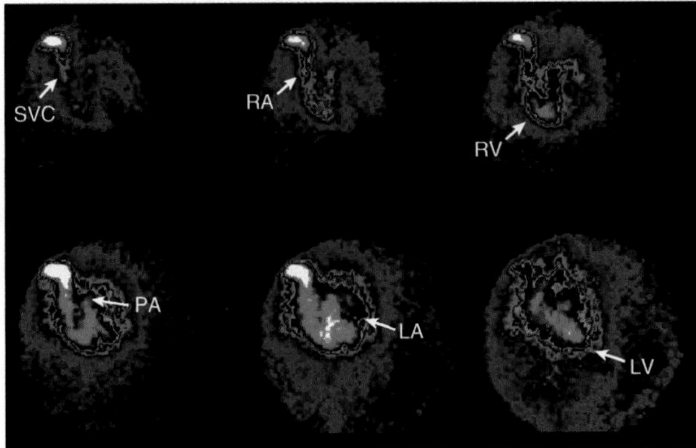

FIGURE 13–18 First-pass radionuclide ventriculography. **A,** First-pass image acquisition and analysis. ED = end diastole; ES = end systole. (From Bacharach SL, Green MV, Borer JS: Instrumentation and data processing in cardiovascular nuclear medicine: Evaluation of ventricular function. Semin Nucl Med 9:257-274, 1979.) **B,** Individual frames from a first-pass radionuclide ventriculography acquisition, illustrating the path of the bolus isotope through the superior vena cava (SVC), the right atrium (RA), the right ventricle (RV), the pulmonary outflow tract and lungs (pulmonary artery, PA), the left atrium (LA), and the left ventricular (LV) phase, from which the isotope bolus is then distributed systemically.

POSITRON-EMISSION TOMOGRAPHY

Because of the quantitative capabilities of positron-emission tomography (PET), measurement of myocardial perfusion and metabolism can be obtained with PET in absolute quantitative terms, a potential advantage compared with SPECT imaging. The radiotracers used in PET are labeled with positron-emitting isotopes that have chemical and physical properties identical to those of naturally occurring elements, such as carbon, oxygen, nitrogen, and fluorine. *Incorporating such elements allows interrogation of physiologically relevant processes in normal and diseased states.*[31] Although most positron-emitting radiotracers are cyclotron produced with short half-lives, the development of *generator-produced* positron-emitting isotopes, such as rubidium, makes it feasible for laboratories to perform cardiac PET studies without an on-site cyclotron.

Clinically available cardiac PET radiotracers fall within two broad categories: those that evaluate myocardial perfusion and those that evaluate myocardial metabolism (Table 13–2).[10] The perfusion tracers, rubidium-82 and [^{13}N]ammonia, and the myocardial metabolic tracer ^{18}F-labeled 2-fluoro-2-deoxyglucose (FDG) have received U.S. Food and Drug Administration approval.

Image Acquisition. PET employs camera systems designed to optimize the detection of positron-emitting radioisotopes. The process by which a positron-emitting radionuclide attempts to stabilize over time is termed beta decay, which occurs when the nucleus of an atom emits a positron, a positively charged beta particle. A negatively charged beta particle represents an electron (Fig. 13–19A). After a high-energy positron is emitted from a nucleus, it travels a few millimeters in tissue and collides with an electron. This collision results in complete annihilation of both the positron and the electron, with conversion to energy in the form of electromagnetic radiation composed of two high-energy gamma rays, each with 511-keV energy. The discharged gamma rays travel in perfectly opposite directions (180 degrees from each other). PET detectors can be programmed to register only events with temporal *coincidence* of photons that strike at directly opposing detectors (see Fig. 13–19B). The outcome of such selective *coincidence detection* is an improvement in spatial and temporal resolution of PET compared with SPECT imaging.[32] Unlike the procedure in SPECT, in which an extrinsic collimator is used to limit the direction at which photons enter the detector, the coincidence detection with PET provides intrinsic collimation and improves the sensitivity of the camera. An attenuation scan is acquired (using a rod source or external ring of radioactivity) before emission data collection in order to measure photon attenuation correction factors.

In addition, an important distinction between PET and SPECT is in the ease of labeling primary substrates for energy metabolism and membrane receptor subtypes in the heart, allowing the interrogation of such pathways in vivo. Moreover, dynamic mode with PET scanning allows potential analysis of the *change in tracer content* in a specific region of interest in the heart with time.

Image Analysis. Emission data are displayed as tomograms in the horizontal and vertical long-axis and short-axis views.[32] If the data are acquired in dynamic mode, with appropriate mathematical modeling, myocardial perfusion and metabolic data can be displayed in absolute terms: in milliliters per gram per minute for blood flow and moles per gram per minute for metabolism.

PET Perfusion Tracers. PET perfusion tracers can be divided into two types: (1) freely diffusible tracers, which accumulate and wash out from myocardial tissue as a function of blood flow, and (2) nondiffusible tracers, characterized by retention in myocardial tissue as a function of blood flow.[31] The rapid physiological washout of the freely diffusible tracers, such as ^{15}O-labeled water, makes it possible to repeat studies in rapid sequence. The images of the distribution of such tracers are usually not visually meaningful; mathematical modeling is done to arrive at flow values at each pixel. An advantage of freely diffusible tracers is that they do not depend on a metabolic trapping mechanism that might change as a function of a changing metabolic environment.

The nondiffusible flow tracers are easier to image as the tracer is retained in myocardium for a reasonable length of time. Rubidium-82 and [^{13}N]ammonia fall into this second category of flow tracers—the more microsphere-like flow tracers. Rubidium-82 is a cation, with biological properties similar to those of potassium and thallium. Uptake across the sarcolemmal membrane reflects active transport by the Na^+,K^+-ATPase pump. In experimental studies, its extraction fraction does not change significantly over a wide range of metabolic conditions. However, the very short half-life of 75 seconds for ^{82}Rb means that any trapped ^{82}Rb quickly disappears from the myocardium by physical decay. Despite its short half-life, ^{82}Rb is easily obtained as it is generator produced, and it can be used clinically without the need for an on-site cyclotron.

[^{13}N]Ammonia is an extractable perfusion tracer, with a physical half-life of 10 minutes. Its transport across cell membranes may occur by passive diffusion or by the active Na-K transport mechanism. Retention of [^{13}N]ammonia in the myocyte involves metabolic trapping. As with rubidium-82, myocardial uptake of ammonia reflects absolute blood flows up to 2 to 3 ml/gm/min and plateaus at more hyperemic flows. The use of this tracer to assess myocardial blood flow has been extensively validated in both experimental and clinical studies.[32]

TABLE 13–2 Properties of Selected Positron-Emission Tomography Tracers

Tracer	Produced	Half-Life	Compound
Perfusion			
Oxygen-15	Cyclotron	2.1 min	H_2O
Nitrogen-13	Cyclotron	10 min	NH_3
Rubidium-82	Generator	76 sec	RbCl
Metabolism			
Carbon-11	Cyclotron	20.4 min	Acetate Palmitate
Fluorine-18	Cyclotron	110 min	Deoxyglucose

Adapted from Bergmann SR: Positron emission tomography of the heart. *In* Gerson MC (ed): Cardiac Nuclear Medicine. New York, McGraw-Hill, 1997, pp 267-300.

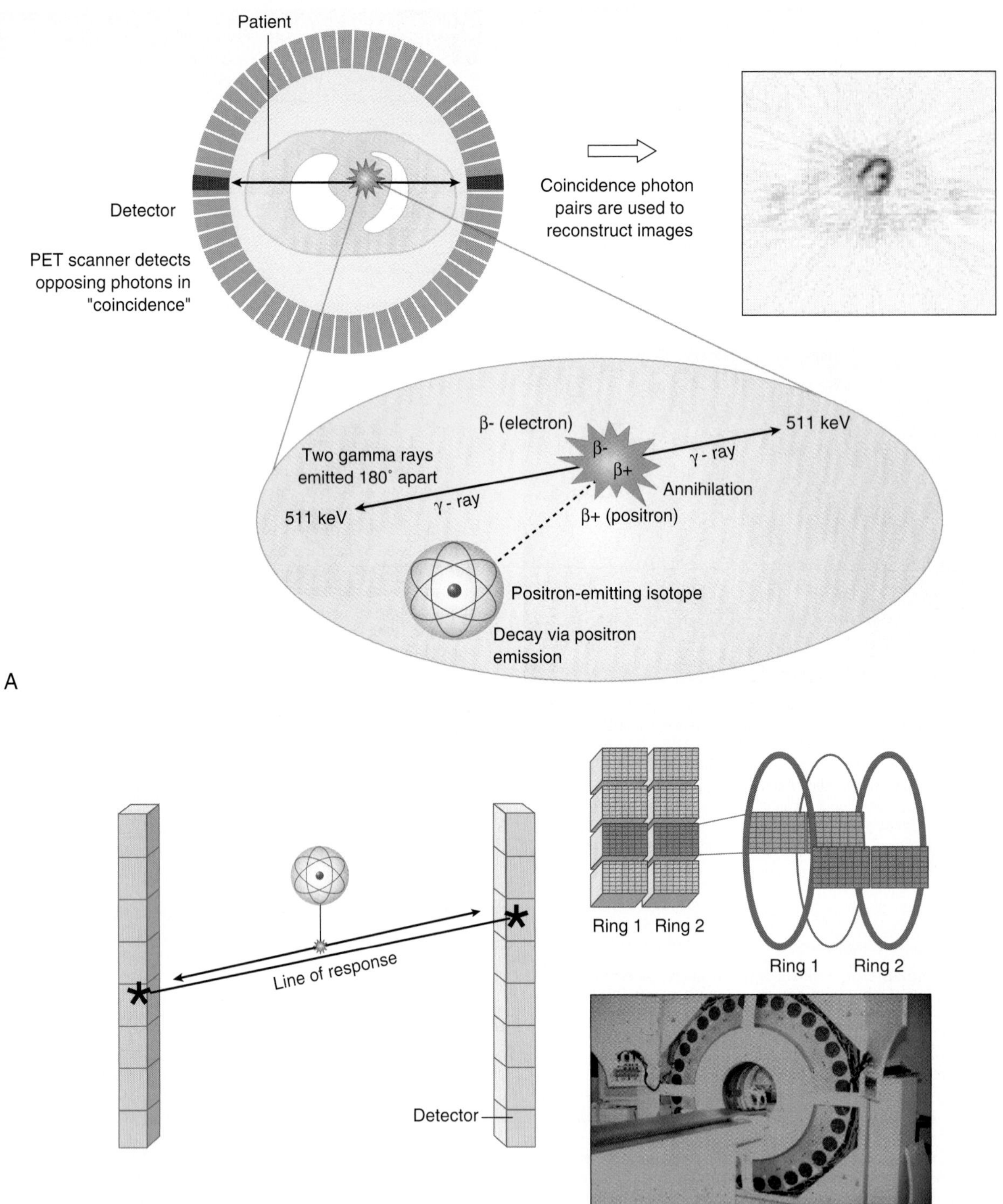

FIGURE 13–19 **A,** Schematic of positron and electron beta particle emission as the basis of positron-emission tomography (PET) imaging. **B,** Schematic of PET camera coincidence detection. (Courtesy of Martin Logde and Bruce Line.)

Assessment of the Physiology and Pathophysiology of Myocardial Blood Flow, Myocardial Metabolism, and Ventricular Function

Assessment of Myocardial Blood Flow by Radionuclide Imaging

Resting Myocardial Blood Flow

Myocardial blood flow at rest is tightly regulated in order to provide nutritive perfusion to viable, contractile myocytes. SPECT tracers to image myocardial blood flow are commonly referred to as "perfusion tracers," that is, *the magnitude of regional tracer uptake is proportional to the magnitude of regional myocardial blood flow.* However, although these tracers are delivered to regions of myocardium by perfusion, they require viable myocyte cell membranes for uptake and retention in order to be visualized.[33] Thus, the uptake and retention of the tracers reflect regional flow differences, with myocyte cell membrane integrity being a prerequisite. Although visualization of myocardial regions suggests the presence of working, viable cell membranes, lack of visualization of myocardium does not necessarily suggest the absence of viable cells. Decreased regional myocardial tracer uptake at rest could reflect either lack of cell membrane integrity in an area of infarcted myocardium or reduced blood flow secondary to hibernating but viable myocardium. A severe reduction in tracer activity usually signifies infarction, and a more moderate reduction in regional activity of a blood flow tracer *alone* cannot always differentiate hibernating from partially scarred myocardium in patients with ischemic LV dysfunction. In that setting, techniques that assess intact cellular metabolic processes, e.g., FDG, or myocardial potassium space, e.g., thallium-201 redistribution, are sometimes used as an adjunct to resting myocardial blood flow.[34]

Imaging Myocardial Infarction. In patients with prior MI, blood flow to the infarcted region is usually diminished, often severely, and there are few viable myocytes within the scarred territory.[10] Thus, severely reduced uptake of a radionuclide perfusion tracer in a resting study is a good marker of presence, location, and extent of MI (Fig. 13–20).

Assessment of Infarct Size. Contemporary studies have used ^{99m}Tc sestamibi to provide an assessment of infarct size.[35] As there is minimal clearance out of the myocardium following initial uptake, images acquired even hours after initial injection represent a "snapshot" of blood flow conditions and tracer uptake at the time of injection.

Infarct size as assessed by quantitative analysis of resting sestamibi uptake has been validated against many other measures of infarct size.[36] Moreover, a significant association between sestamibi infarct size and mortality over long-term follow-up has been demonstrated. Many clinical trials now use final infarct size by sestamibi SPECT imaging as an early post-MI surrogate endpoint to assess new agents to reduce infarct size.

When a tracer such as sestamibi is injected *during acute infarction* in the setting of an occluded infarct-related artery *before reperfusion therapy*, the resulting defect, even when imaged hours later after successful reperfusion, represents the *risk area* of the occluded artery.[35] A second injection of sestamibi at rest with subsequent imaging can be done at a later time during the post-MI course and represents *final infarct size*. The change in defect size between the initial image acquired in the acute stage and the later image represents the *magnitude of salvaged myocardium from reperfusion*. Hence, SPECT imaging at rest in the early postinfarct period can provide important information regarding final infarct size and infarct zone viability.

Coronary blood flow must respond rapidly to changing metabolic conditions and oxygen demand in order to meet the nutrient needs of myocytes being called on to contract more quickly and with more force. Oxygen extraction by the myocardium is near maximum at rest; thus, any increase in oxygen demand can be met only through increasing coronary blood flow to deliver more oxygen per unit time. The major determinants of coronary blood flow include the perfusion pressure at the head of the system (principally aortic diastolic pressure) and the downstream resistance, residing predominantly in the coronary *arteriolar* bed. Because aortic diastolic pressure during exercise varies little from the resting value, the major mechanism responsible for increasing coronary blood flow during stress involves a reduction in coronary vascular resistance. During *exercise* stress, coronary blood flow can increase approximately two to three times over resting levels. During *pharmacological* stress to minimize coronary arteriolar resistance, with intravenous coronary arteriolar vasodilator agents such as dipyridamole or adenosine (discussed further later), coronary blood flow can increase up to four to five times over resting levels. The magnitude of blood flow increase secondary to any stress relative to resting flow values is termed *coronary blood flow reserve*.[37]

PERFUSION TRACERS AND CORONARY BLOOD FLOW RESERVE. The ideal perfusion tracer should track myocardial blood flow across the entire physiologically relevant range of blood flow achievable in animal models and in humans (Fig. 13-21). It should be taken up rapidly, as the hemodynamic conditions during peak stress are not maintained for long periods of time. The ideal tracer should be taken up (extracted) as completely as possible out of the bloodstream, and it should be retained in myocardium for a sufficient period to be imaged. Moreover, perturbations in metabolic conditions, such as ischemia, or commonly used cardioactive drugs should neither influence nor interfere with uptake so that the resulting regional tracer concentrations primarily reflect myocardial perfusion.[33]

Despite the excellent first-pass myocardial extraction (85 percent), the energy spectrum of thallium is lower (69 to 80 keV) than optimum for current gamma cameras. The 140-keV energy spectrum of ^{99m}Tc perfusion tracers results in less scatter and soft tissue attenuation, with improved spatial resolution compared with thallium.[8] However, the first-pass myocardial extraction of both sestamibi and tetrofosmin is only in

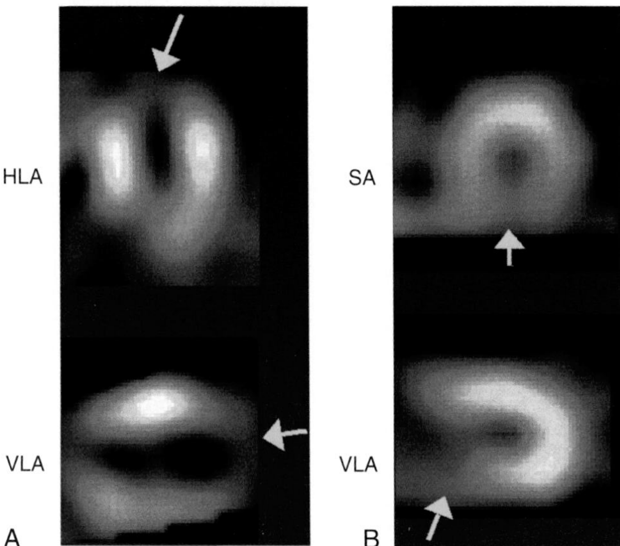

FIGURE 13–20 Single-photon emission computed tomography perfusion images demonstrating myocardial infarction in different locations. **A,** An apical infarction (arrow) in the horizontal long-axis (HLA) and vertical long-axis (VLA) views. **B,** An inferior infarction in the short-axis (SA) and VLA views. In both studies, the *severity* of the defect suggests minimal myocyte viability within those territories.

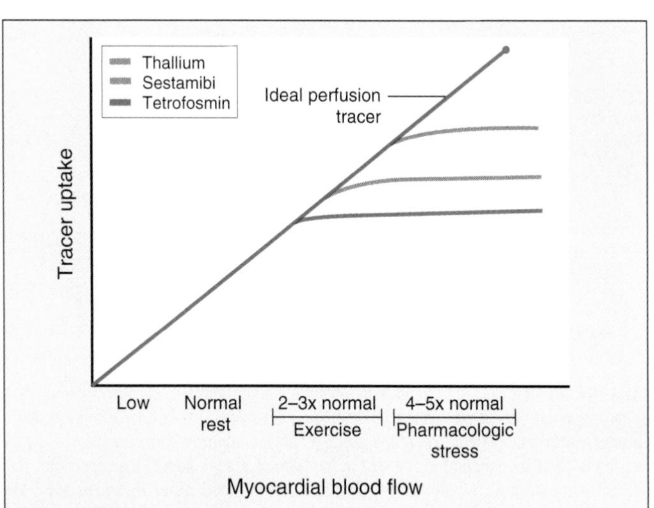

FIGURE 13–21 The relation between myocardial blood flow and perfusion tracer uptake. The ideal perfusion tracer would track myocardial blood flow across the entire range of physiologically relevant flows. However, the available perfusion tracers "roll off" at higher levels of flow. The different tracers begin to reach a plateau at different levels of myocardial blood flow, as demonstrated in this schematic example based on multiple studies in animal models.

the 60 percent range with nonlinear extraction at high flows. Thus, none of the clinically available SPECT perfusion tracers have all of the properties of an ideal perfusion tracer (see Fig. 13–21). Nonetheless, regional differences in myocardial tracer uptake during exercise or pharmacological stress have provided important diagnostic as well as prognostic information.[10]

The PET perfusion tracer [^{13}N]ammonia displays an extraction fraction exceeding 90 percent; rubidium-82 has a lower extraction fraction and reaches a plateau more rapidly at hyperemic range of flow. In the clinical setting, the evaluation of regional myocardial blood flow and flow reserve with [^{13}N]ammonia and rubidium-82 has also been validated for detecting and localizing CAD.[10] Because exercise studies are difficult to perform in the PET scanner and attenuation correction with PET requires close alignment of transmission and emission data, most PET studies evaluating coronary flow reserve use pharmacological rather than exercise stress.

EFFECT OF A CORONARY STENOSIS ON CORONARY BLOOD FLOW RESERVE. In animal models in which discrete coronary stenoses of varying degrees were induced, *resting* coronary blood flow was maintained by autoregulatory dilation of the downstream arteriolar resistance vessels until a stenosis between 80 and 90 percent diameter was reached (Fig. 13–22). As stenosis severity increases further, the arteriolar vasodilatory capacity to maintain resting flow is exhausted, at which point resting coronary blood flow diminishes.[38]

In contrast, *maximum coronary blood flow reserve* begins to decrease when the upstream coronary stenosis reaches 50 percent diameter. There are three levels of resistance that influence coronary blood flow: that provided by the large conductance epicardial vessels (R1), the coronary arteriolar resistance (R2), and the resistance in the subendocardium by wall tension from the ventricular chamber (R3) (see Fig. 13–22). Under normal conditions, most of the resistance at rest is provided by R2, and most of the increase in coronary flow during heightened demand occurs through reduction of resistance at this level, potentially increasing flow as much as four times as demand increases. Normal epicardial vessels dilate slightly (R1 decreases slightly) in response to increased coronary flow as a consequence of normal endothelial cell function. Depending on the type of exercise that is performed, the R3 component may remain unchanged or may increase, with an increase in chamber radius and wall tension. Achieving maximal flow is predominantly dependent on the vasodilatory capacity of the downstream resistance vessels.[37,38] With a coronary stenosis, in which some vasodilatory reserve has been used to maintain resting flow, less vasodilatory reserve is available to minimize resistance during stress. Thus, in a vessel with a moderate stenosis, *coronary blood flow reserve* is blunted and detectable by a perfusion tracer (see Fig. 13–22).

In contrast to animal models, human CAD is more complex. Stenoses may not be discrete, the length and complexity of the stenosis may affect the coronary reserve, and impaired endothelial function plays a role.[39] In subjects with preserved endothelial function, the increased coronary flow during stress leads to coronary arterial and arteriolar vasodilation, contributing to maximal coronary flow reserve. Endothelial function is often abnormal with early atherosclerosis, or risk factors for atherosclerosis, contributing to the blunting of coronary flow reserve.[40] The development of collaterals to the distal perfusion bed of a myocardial territory with a severe upstream coronary stenosis also influences blood flow at rest and during stress.[41]

With SPECT imaging, *relative* regional differences of tracer uptake can be detected and quantified (Fig. 13–23), whereas with PET imaging, *absolute* regional coronary blood flow at rest and during stress (in milliliters per gram per minute) can be quantified.[32]

Detecting Stress-Induced Ischemia Versus Infarct with Myocardial Perfusion Imaging. In standard practice, stress and rest myocardial perfusion images are compared in order to determine the presence, extent, and severity of stress-induced perfusion defects and to determine whether such defects represent regions of myocardial ischemia or infarction.[8,9,10] *Regions with stress-induced perfusion abnormalities, which have normal perfusion at rest, are termed reversible perfusion defects and represent viable regions with blunted coronary blood flow reserve* (Fig. 13–24). Strictly speaking, SPECT MPI is demonstrating stress induced reversible abnormalities in perfusion reserve, although these findings are often referred to as "ischemia." Regional myocardial *tissue ischemia* per se is not being demonstrated, although it is indeed often present, based on a mismatch between oxygen supply and demand. Perfusion abnormalities at stress that are *irreversible*, or *fixed*, as seen on resting images (unchanged from stress to rest) most often represent infarction, particularly if the defect is severe (see Fig. 13–24). When both viable myocardium and scarred myocardium are present, thallium redistribution or technetium 99m tracer reversibility is incomplete, giving the appearance of

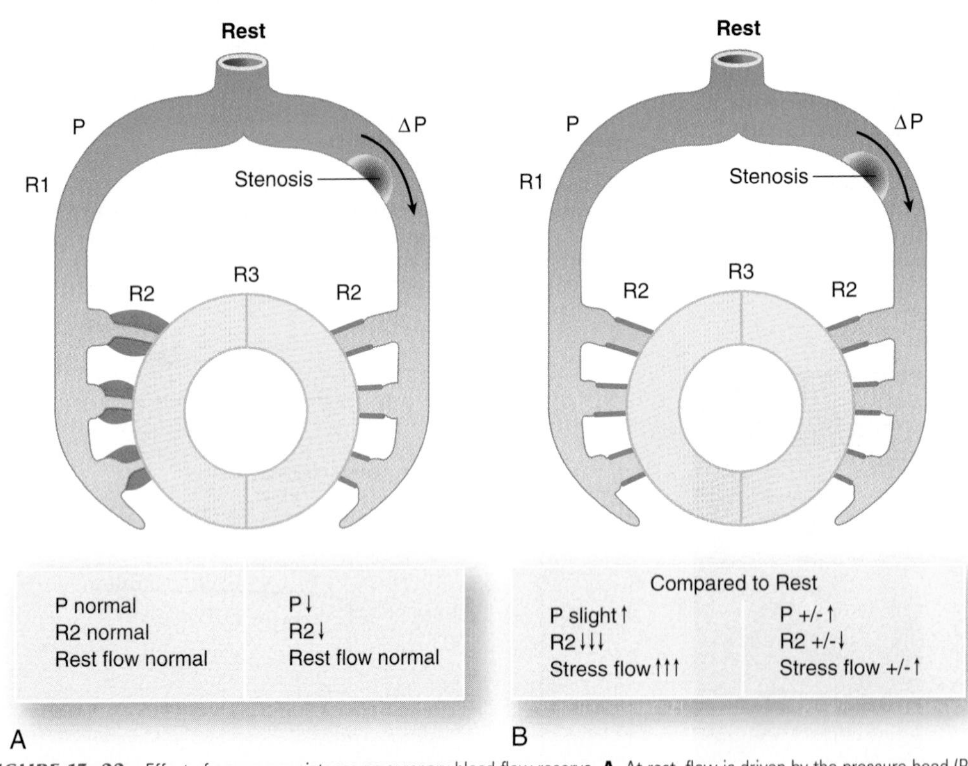

FIGURE 13–22 Effect of coronary resistance on coronary blood flow reserve. **A,** At rest, flow is driven by the pressure head (P) at the proximal end of the system. R1 refers to resistance offered by the large epicardial conductance vessels. R2 represents the coronary arteriolar resistance, which predominantly regulates coronary blood flow. R3 represents the resistance provided by wall tension in the subendocardium. At rest in the normal vessel, some vasoconstrictor resistance is present. In the setting of an epicardial coronary stenosis, blood flow at rest can be maintained, as coronary resistance can be lowered downstream (R2 decreased) by autoregulatory dilation. Thus, with lower resistance, flow may be maintained despite the lower pressure head at the distal end of stenosis. **B,** With a demand stress or with the administration of coronary arteriolar vasodilators, perfusion increases substantially in the area supplied by the normal epicardial artery as R2 decreases. However, there is blunted flow reserve in the area supplied by the stenosis because most vasodilator reserve at the R2 level has been used to maintain resting flow. (Adapted from Follansbee WP: Alternatives to leg exercise in the evaluation of patients with coronary artery disease: Functional and pharmacologic stress modalities. *In* Gerson MC [ed]: Cardiac Nuclear Medicine. New York, McGraw-Hill, 1997, pp 193-236.)

partial reversibility on the delayed thallium or rest technetium 99m images.

Exercise Stress to Induce Coronary Hyperemia

SPECT MPI is commonly performed with exercise stress to induce coronary hyperemia, particularly suitable for patients with exertional symptoms, as this provides the opportunity to link the *symptoms* induced during exercise to the location, extent, and severity of abnormal perfusion patterns.[10] Moreover, performing exercise stress in conjunction with MPI allows the opportunity to incorporate additional information on functional capacity, stress-induced ECG changes or arrhythmias, and utilization of heart rate reserve and heart rate recovery in the assessment of CAD probability or prognosis.[42]

Physiology of Exercise Stress–Induced Coronary Hyperemia. During exercise, systolic pressure rises but diastolic pressure usually changes little. Thus, the driving pressure for coronary perfusion is relatively unchanged, and increases in flow necessary to match increased demand occur predominantly by reducing arteriolar resistance. In the presence of coronary stenosis, if a degree of downstream resistance has been reduced to maintain resting flow, coronary flow reserve during exercise stress is blunted.[37,38]

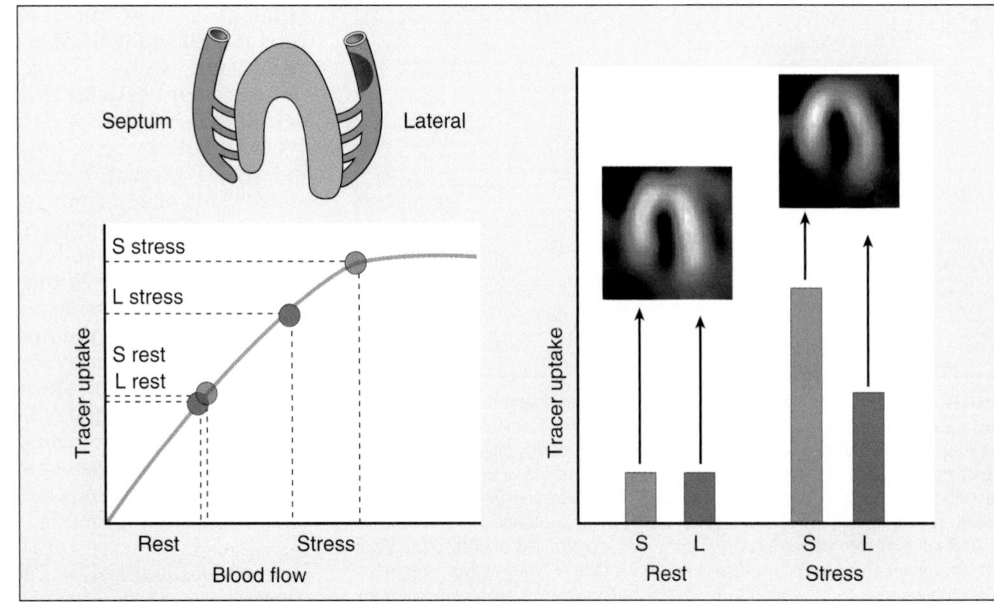

FIGURE 13–23 Illustration of coronary blood flow reserve abnormalities, the concomitant perfusion tracer concentration differences, and the resulting tomographic images. **Left,** The myocardial blood flow profiles at rest and stress of two myocardial regions are shown, with region S (septum) supplied by a normal epicardial artery and region L (lateral wall) supplied by an artery with a significant epicardial coronary stenosis. Blood flow at stress is diminished in region L compared with S. **Right,** The perfusion tracer uptake profile is demonstrated with myocardial blood flow on the y-axis. Tracer uptake is diminished in region L relative to S during stress. In the resulting perfusion images, a relative "defect" of tracer uptake is seen in the lateral wall compared with the septum, whereas at rest both regions demonstrate similar tracer uptake. The lateral wall thus demonstrates a reversible perfusion defect, reflecting the blunted coronary blood flow reserve and indirectly reflecting the presence of the coronary stenosis.

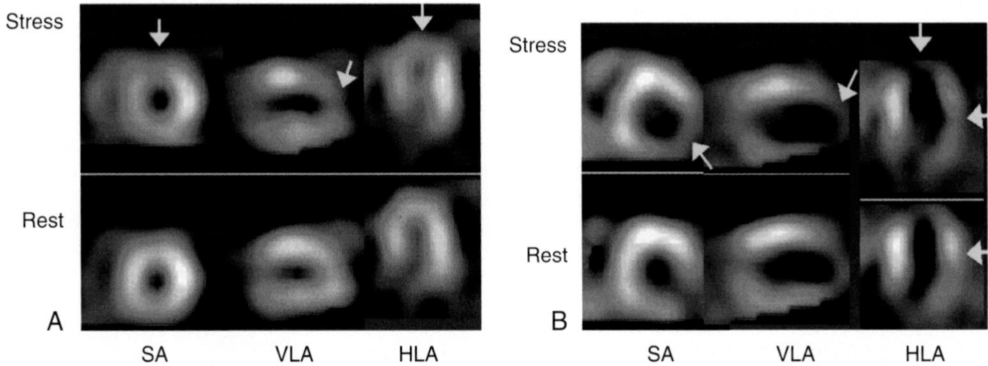

FIGURE 13–24 **A,** Example of single-photon emission computed tomography anterior and apical reversible perfusion defects (arrows), representing inducible regional myocardial ischemia in the short axis (SA), vertical long axis (VLA), and horizontal long axis (HLA). **B,** Example of irreversible or fixed defects of the inferolateral wall in the SA and of the apex in the VLA image (arrows), representing predominant myocardial infarction. There is also evidence of a reversible lateral wall defect (arrowhead) in the HLA image representing lateral wall ischemia.

Pharmacological Stress to Induce Coronary Hyperemia

Exercise stress is the preferred modality for inducing coronary hyperemia as it allows a correlation between exertional symptoms and the perfusion pattern and provides information on exercise duration, workload achieved, and the presence and extent of ischemic ECG changes, all of which provide important diagnostic and prognostic information.[10] However, a substantial proportion of patients are incapable of attaining a sufficient level of exercise. Patients with exertional symptoms may not exercise adequately to reproduce these symptoms, and patients may not achieve more than 85 percent of the maximum predicted heart rate for age (see Chap. 10), considered the optimal level of exertion to achieve coronary hyperemic responses.[10,42] As the population ages and comorbid disease states such as peripheral vascular disease and diabetes increase, the proportion of patients referred for stress testing who are unable to achieve adequate levels of exercise will increase.

In such patients, *pharmacological stress testing* can be used to induce coronary hyperemia. The most widely used agents for pharmacological stress testing can be divided into those that act as coronary arteriolar vasodilators, adenosine and dipyridamole, and adrenergic agents such as dobutamine.[43]

Mechanism of Coronary Arteriolar Vasodilator Pharmacological Stress. Stimulation of adenosine A_{2a} receptors on the smooth muscle cells leads to enhanced production of adenylate cyclase, increased intracellular cyclic adenosine monophosphate, and other effects that produce vasorelaxation. With maximal arteriolar vasodilation (maximal decrease in coronary resistance), coronary blood flow increases to near-maximum levels.

Adenosine is a powerful, endogenous molecule that acts as a regulator of blood flow in many organ beds, including the coronary circulation. It has many other effects mediated by different receptor subtypes (Fig. 13–25). Adenosine A_1 recep-

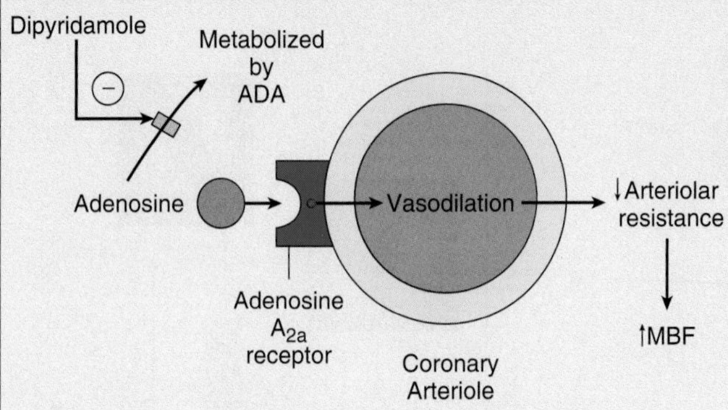

FIGURE 13–25 Schematic of the mechanism of action of dipyridamole and adenosine. Exogenously administered adenosine acts directly on its receptor to result in coronary arteriolar vasodilation and thus an increase in myocardial blood flow (MBF) as resistance is minimized. The adenosine A_{2a} receptor mediates coronary arteriolar vasodilation, which is the basis for pharmacological stress testing. Dipyridamole blocks the intracellular retransport of adenosine and also inhibits adenosine deaminase (ADA), resulting in increased intracellular and interstitial concentrations of adenosine, which then interacts with its receptor. (Adapted from Follansbee WP: Alternatives to leg exercise in the evaluation of patients with coronary artery disease: Functional and pharmacologic stress modalities. *In* Gerson MC [ed]: Cardiac Nuclear Medicine. New York, McGraw-Hill, 1997, pp 193-236.)

tors are present in the sinus node and atrioventricular (AV) node and mediate diminished heart rate and AV nodal conduction. Adenosine A_{2b} receptors are present in bronchioles and the peripheral vasculature, and stimulation may result in bronchial constriction and peripheral vasodilation. Adenosine A_3 receptors are less well characterized but appear to be important in the preconditioning response.

Initial studies of adenosine demonstrated that a dose of 140 µg/kg/min induced maximal coronary hyperemia, with no further increase in maximum coronary blood flow at higher doses.[44] Following the onset of intravenous adenosine infusion, maximum coronary flow occurs at an average of 84 seconds with a range of up to 125 seconds. Dipyridamole blocks the intracellular retransport of adenosine and inhibits adenosine deaminase, responsible for the intracellular breakdown of adenosine.[44] Thus, dipyridamole acts as an indirect coronary arteriolar vasodilator, increasing intracellular and interstitial concentrations of adenosine (see Fig. 13–25).

Heterogeneity of Coronary Hyperemia with Pharmacological Stress. With the administration of dipyridamole or adenosine, the resistance vessels in the area subtended by a normal epicardial vessel dilate, diminishing coronary resistance and resulting in an increment in coronary blood flow four to five times above normal. Coronary resistance in a bed supplied by a stenotic epicardial vessel is diminished at rest (i.e., coronary vasodilator reserve has been utilized), and only minor or no further reductions can take place. Thus, myocardial blood flow in that territory does not change or may even decrease slightly because of the peripheral vasodilation and drop in diastolic blood pressure characteristic of pharmacological stress. The net result of these changes is heterogeneity in myocardial blood flow (increased in the normal territory and relatively unchanged in the territory supplied by the stenotic epicardial vessel). Perfusion tracer administration in this setting demonstrates a defect in the area supplied by the stenotic vessel (see Fig. 13–22).[44,45]

During exercise stress, the increase in myocardial oxygen demand and limitation of oxygen supply create a supply-demand mismatch often resulting in cellular ischemia. With pharmacological stress, the perfusion defect may represent merely the heterogeneity in coronary flow reserve. "Demand" may change little during pharmacological stress; there is often a reduction in blood pressure accompanied by a reflex although modest increase in heart rate, so that double product, reflecting oxygen demand, changes little during the vasodilator "stress." Thus, a supply-demand mismatch may not occur and cellular ischemia may not be present despite vasodilator-induced perfusion defects.[44]

Under certain conditions, true myocardial ischemia may indeed be present, related to development of a *coronary steal*.[38] This phenomenon appears to occur when the myocardial perfusion bed supplied by a severe epicardial stenosis is also dependent on collateral vessels from remote coronary arteries. Blood flow through coronary collaterals is dependent on perfusion pressure, particularly if the collaterals are jeopardized; that is, their parent blood vessel is compromised by a moderate coronary stenosis. In this setting, administration of a vasodilator stress agent diminishes the perfusion pressure supplying the collaterals, and collateral flow diminishes. Flow to the bed supplied by a severe epicardial stenosis may then *decrease* compared with resting flow, and the diminished supply may create supply-demand mismatch and true myocardial ischemia.

Hemodynamic Effects of Vasodilator Pharmacological Stress. Dipyridamole and adenosine both result in adenosine receptor–mediated systemic as well as coronary vasodilation, resulting in an average 8 to 10 mm Hg reduction in systolic and diastolic blood pressure, often accompanied by a reflex increase in heart rate.[44] The magnitude of the heart rate increase is variable, usually between 10 and 20 beats/min. A blunted heart rate response may be observed in patients who are taking beta blockers or in diabetic patients with underlying autonomic insufficiency.

Side Effects and Symptoms Associated with Vasodilator Pharmacological Stress. The symptoms and side effects associated with pharmacological vasodilator stress are the result of stimulation of the adenosine A_1, A_{2b}, and A_3 receptors and are common.[43-46] Following dipyridamole stress, approximately 50 percent of patients experience some side effect. In a large registry study, more than 80 percent of patients undergoing adenosine stress experienced untoward symptoms or side effects, or both, most commonly flushing, chest pain, or shortness of breath.[43-45]

As a result of adenosine's effect on the conduction system, AV block may develop during adenosine administration. Approximately 10 percent of patients manifest first-degree AV block, with 5 percent developing either second- or third-degree AV block. AV block is more common in patients who are studied while taking beta blockers or heart rate–lowering calcium channel blockers. Patients with baseline evidence of second- or third-degree AV block in the absence of a pacemaker should not receive adenosine. However, patients with first-degree AV block or left bundle branch block (LBBB) appear to tolerate adenosine infusion well, without an exacerbation of conduction abnormalities.[8,10]

Ischemic ST depression is observed in 10 to 15 percent of patients undergoing pharmacological vasodilator stress, probably representing the physiological consequence of induction of a coronary steal and regional myocardial ischemia. Such patients often have extensive and severe perfusion defects on imaging and more often have collateralized multivessel disease on angiography.

Chest pain, even typical angina pectoris, develops commonly during pharmacological vasodilator stress testing. Although it may reflect regional myocardial ischemia based on a coronary steal, chest pain may also occur in patients with no ischemic ECG changes and with normal perfusion studies because of involvement of adenosine A_1 receptors in the nociceptive pathway influencing the sensation of chest pain.[43-46] Thus, chest pain by itself is a nonspecific finding during vasodilator pharmacological stress.

In early reports of dipyridamole testing, infrequent but severe episodes of bronchospasm occurred, probably related to a nonspecific adenosine receptor–mediated mechanism. Thus, patients with a significant history of reactive airways disease should not undergo vasodilator stress testing.[8,10] However, patients with obstructive lung disease without a reactive airways component generally tolerate the procedure well.

Reversing the Effects of Vasodilator Pharmacological Stress. Methylxanthine compounds such as theophylline and caffeine act as competitive antagonists of adenosine at the receptor level, and infusion of intravenous aminophylline antagonizes the effects of dipyridamole or adenosine.[8,10] As adenosine has a very short half-life (~20 to 30 seconds), administration of aminophylline is rarely required during adenosine testing, as simply stopping the infusion results in cessation of symptoms within 20 to 30 seconds. Following intravenous dipyridamole, infusion of aminophylline at approximately 1 to 2 mg/kg, given over 30 seconds, reverses side effects (as well as the coronary vasodilator effects), usually within 1 to 2 minutes. As the coronary vasodilator effects are reversed as well, reversal of the dipyridamole effect should be delayed until at least 1 to 2 minutes after radionuclide administration if clinically safe, or the true stress perfusion pattern may not be manifest. Generally, side effects from vasodilator pharmacological stress, although common, may be tolerated for this period of time. However, with more severe side effects such as severe shortness of breath or bronchospasm or with more dramatic ST segment abnormalities, reversal of the dipyridamole effect more quickly is prudent. As caffeine is a methylxanthine compound and antagonizes the effect of adenosine at its receptor, it is critical that patients be instructed to withhold caffeine, ideally for 24 hours prior to vasodilator pharmacological stress testing.

In some patients, myocardial ischemia provoked during vasodilator stress testing triggers a cascade of events that maintains ischemia even after reversal of the vasodilator effect with aminophylline. The sensation of chest pain may drive a heightened sympathetic response, with an elevation of heart rate and blood pressure. In that setting, when aminophylline has been given to reverse the effects of the vasodilator, it is safe to administer sublingual nitroglycerin or other measures to relieve myocardial ischemia. It is *not safe* to give sublingual nitroglycerin *prior to* aminophylline to treat signs of myocardial ischemia. Because systemic vasodilation is present during vasodilator stress testing, administration of nitroglycerin prior to aminophylline may result in substantial systemic hypotension. Thus, aminophylline should always be given first to reverse the effect of the vasodilator, after which it is safe to pursue other anti-ischemic measures.

In contemporary practice, a small number of patients may be encountered who are taking oral dipyridamole preparations for their antiplatelet effects. As dipyridamole is an adenosine deaminase inhibitor and prevents the usual rapid breakdown of adenosine, infusion of intravenous adenosine in patients receiving oral dipyridamole may be accompanied by a far more prolonged adenosine effect than usual. Thus, for adenosine testing, oral dipyridamole compounds must be stopped at an appropriate period of time before testing. Oral dipyridamole as background therapy does not complicate the performance of intravenous dipyridamole testing.

Protocols for Pharmacological Stress Testing. The accepted protocols for performing vasodilator pharmacological stress testing are listed in Table 13–3.[8,10] Since the original descriptions of these protocols, iterations have been studied, with the goal of shortening the test procedure or minimizing side effects, or both,[47,48] by shortening the duration of the adenosine infusion or adding low-level exercise.

Handgrip exercise may be used in order to raise peripheral blood pressure and thus coronary perfusion pressure. Reports are mixed on whether image quality is improved. This approach may be useful in patients with borderline low blood pressure prior to the test to avoid significant hypotension.

Low-level treadmill exercise has been increasingly applied in combination with vasodilator stress testing. Although no clear advantage in diagnostic performance has been demonstrated, a reduction in side effects of pharmacological stress testing has been demonstrated, as well as a reduction in extracardiac tracer uptake that improves image quality.[47,48]

TABLE 13–3 Pharmacological Stress Protocols

	Dose (μg/kg/min)	Duration	Isotope Injection
Dipyridamole	142	4 min by hand infusion or pump	3 min after completion of infusion
Adenosine	140	6-min infusion by pump	At 3 min into infusion

Initial reports of intravenous adenosine testing described a protocol in which the dose was progressively increased. More commonly, adenosine is given now as an infusion starting with the maximum dose. This allows a shortened total infusion period of 4 minutes rather than 6 minutes, with radionuclide injected at 3 minutes into the 4-minute infusion. Published data (with thallium imaging) suggest that diagnostic sensitivity is maintained while decreasing the overall time of testing.[44]

Specific agonists of the adenosine A_{2a} receptor are under development to achieve arteriolar vasodilation and thus myocardial perfusion images similar to those obtained with adenosine or dipyridamole, accompanied by fewer or less severe side effects, because of lack of stimulation of the A_1, A_{2b}, and A_3 receptors. A bolus injection of the specific A_{2a} receptor agonist binodenoson achieves myocardial perfusion images that are concordant with adenosine MPI, with a significant reduction in the incidence and severity of side effects.[46]

DIFFERENCES BETWEEN VASODILATOR AND EXERCISE STRESS. The perfusion images obtained using vasodilator pharmacological stress are generally concordant with those obtained with maximal exercise stress in the same patient, but there are several important differences. *Higher levels of coronary flow are achieved during vasodilator pharmacological stress compared with exercise,* possibly because of the increased resistance to flow with exercise caused by higher subendocardial pressures (i.e., at the R3 level of resistance). Although theoretically this should result in increased sensitivity for detecting CAD with pharmacological stress, that has not been clearly demonstrated. The failure to demonstrate increased sensitivity may be due to the inability of the radionuclide tracers to reflect myocardial blood flow adequately at the highest levels of flow.[43-45]

Vasodilator pharmacological stress is less "physiological" than exercise, and symptoms during testing cannot be as clearly linked to the perfusion pattern. Optimal diagnostic performance of MPI during exercise is often dependent on the patient achieving a maximal level of stress, which does not always occur. In contrast, vasodilator pharmacological stress affords generally predictable coronary flow responses.[8,10,44]

Antiischemic medications may significantly affect the results of MPI during exercise.[10] The effect of background antiischemic medications on the results of pharmacological stress imaging is not as certain. Reports have now suggested that the extent and severity of myocardial perfusion defects may be affected in an important way by background medication during pharmacological stress.[49-51] Thus, antianginal medications should be withheld if possible prior to the study.

Dobutamine Stress to Induce Coronary Hyperemia

In some patients, vasodilator pharmacological stress is contraindicated because of reactive bronchospastic airways disease or background methylxanthines. In such situations, intravenous dobutamine hydrochloride may be used to induce coronary hyperemia.[8,10] Dobutamine has a relatively rapid onset of action, with a half-life of approximately 2 minutes. This agent is given starting at a dose of 5 μg/kg/min and increased in a stepwise fashion by 5 μg/kg/min every 3 minutes, to a maximum dose of 40 μg/kg/min. Dobutamine is a broad adrenergic receptor agonist, at varying doses stimulating the $beta_1$, $beta_2$, and $alpha_1$ receptors. At relatively low doses, the predominant effect is an increase in contractility through adrenergic receptors. As the dose is increased beyond 10 μg/kg/min, heart rate rises steadily, and the increase in oxygen demand stimulates an increase in myocardial blood flow.

The hemodynamic response to dobutamine generally involves a modest increase in systolic blood pressure with a modest decrease in diastolic blood pressure through doses up to 20 μg/kg/min, with only small further changes after that point. As the increase in myocardial blood flow is dependent on the increase in oxygen demand, optimal sensitivity for MPI based on optimizing heterogeneity of flow is dependent on achieving a high dose of dobutamine.

The increment in myocardial blood flow during maximal doses of dobutamine appears to be less than achieved during vasodilator pharmacological stress, and hence the degree of heterogeneity of coronary flow with a coronary stenosis is also less. Thus, vasodilator stress is the preferred pharmacological modality for MPI in patients who cannot exercise adequately. Dobutamine stress is reserved for cases in which vasodilator stress is contraindicated or cannot be performed because of background medications.[8,10,52]

Side effects during dobutamine are frequent and can be bothersome.[52] The most common side effects include palpitations and chest pain, and arrhythmias including ventricular extrasystoles and nonsustained ventricular tachycardia may be encountered. Hypotension occurs in approximately 10 percent of patients, possibly as a result of myocardial mechanoreceptor stimulation during increased contractility with resulting withdrawal of peripheral constrictor tone. Hypotension during dobutamine stress does not have the same prognostic implications as exercise-induced hypotension. Because of the relatively short half-life, side effects generally resolve within a few minutes of stopping the infusion and can be aborted more quickly with intravenous beta blockade.[8,10,52]

Assessment of Myocardial Cellular Metabolism and Physiology by Radionuclide Imaging

Myocardial Ischemia and Viability

Programmed Cell Survival. Imbalance between oxygen supply and demand results in myocardial ischemia. If the imbalance is transient (i.e., triggered by exertion), it represents reversible ischemia. However, if supply-demand imbalance is prolonged, high-energy phosphates are depleted, and regional contractile function progressively deteriorates. If the supply-demand balance is sufficiently prolonged, cell membrane rupture with cell death follows.

The myocardium has several mechanisms of acute and chronic adaptation to a temporary or sustained reduction in coronary blood flow (Fig. 13–26), known as stunning, hibernation, and ischemic preconditioning.[53] These responses to ischemia preserve sufficient energy to protect the structural and functional integrity of the cardiac myocyte. In contrast to programmed cell death, or apoptosis, the term "programmed cell survival" has been used to describe the commonality between myocardial stunning, hibernation, and ischemic preconditioning despite their distinct pathophysiology.[54] Radionuclide imaging has played an important role in understanding the changes in blood flow and metabolism in these states and clinically distinguishing their presence from regional infarct.[34]

Stunned and Hibernating Myocardium. In stunned and hibernating myocardium, *myocardial function is depressed at rest but myocytes remain viable.* Although LV dysfunction may be reversible in both stunning and hibernation, these states differ in the relationship between myocardial perfusion and function. *Stunned myocardium* is most commonly observed after a *transient period of ischemia followed by reperfusion* (depressed function at rest but preserved perfusion).[55] The ischemic episodes can be single or multiple, brief or prolonged, but never severe enough to result in injury. *Hibernating myocardium* refers to an adaptive response of the myocardium to *prolonged myocardial hypoperfusion at rest* (depressed function and perfusion at rest).[56] In the clinical setting, it is likely that the adaptive responses of hibernation and stunning coexist.

Myocardial Viability. Requirements for cellular viability include (1) sufficient myocardial blood flow, (2) cell membrane integrity, and (3) preserved metabolic activity. Myocardial blood flow has to be adequate to deliver substrate to the myocyte for metabolic processes and to remove the end products of metabolism.[57] If blood flow is severely reduced, metabolites accumulate, causing inhibition of the enzymes of the metabolic pathway, depletion of high-energy phosphates, cell membrane disruption, and cell death. Thus, with severe reduction in blood flow, perfusion tracers alone provide information regarding myocardial viability.[10] However, in regions in which the reduction in blood flow is of less severity, perfusion information alone may be an insufficient signal to identify clinically relevant viability, and additional data, such as metabolic indices, would be important.[10,57]

Membrane integrity to maintain electrochemical gradients across the myocyte is also a requirement for cell survival. Because cell membrane integrity is dependent on preserved intracellular metabolic activity to generate high-energy phosphates, tracers that reflect cation flux (thallium-201), electrochemical gradients (sestamibi or tetrofosmin), or metabolic processes (FDG) provide insight into myocardial viability (Fig. 13–27).[8,34,57]

Major Myocardial Fuels and Energetics in Normal and Ischemic Myocardium

High-energy phosphates, such as adenosine triphosphate (ATP), provide the fuel that powers the contractile proteins of the myocytes. ATP is generated in the myocardium by two different but integrated metabolic processes: *oxidative phosphorylation* and *glycolysis.*[58] Fatty acids, glucose, and lactate are the major sources of energy in the heart, and depending on the arterial concentration of each and the physiological condition, any one of these three substrates can be the principal provider of energy (Fig. 13–28). Increased uptake and utilization of one substrate leads to a decreased contribution by the others.

In the fasting state, long-chain free fatty acids are the preferred source of energy in the heart, with glucose accounting for only 15 to 20 percent of the total energy supply. The ATP yield is 130 per mole of free fatty acid and 38 per mole of glucose. When the oxygen supply is *normal,* high levels of ATP and tissue citrate formed by breakdown of fatty acids suppress the oxidation of glucose. When the oxygen supply is *decreased,* ATP and citrate levels fall, and the rate of glycolysis is accelerated. Anaerobic glycolysis can be maintained only if lactate and hydrogen ion (the byproducts of glycolysis) are removed and do not accumulate. In the setting of *severe* hypoperfusion, these end products of the glycolytic pathway accumulate, causing inhibition of the glycolytic enzymes and depletion of high-energy phosphates, resulting in cell membrane disruption and cell death.[59] Thus, to maintain anaerobic glycolysis, minimally sufficient blood flow is necessary.

IMAGING ALTERATIONS IN MYOCARDIAL METABOLISM

Imaging Fatty Acid Metabolism

[^{11}C]Palmitate. Because fatty acids are the primary source of myocardial energy production in the fasting state, early PET studies focused on characterizing the kinetics of long-chain fatty acids, such as [^{11}C]palmitate.[60] Measurement by dynamic PET imaging allows the observation of tracer inflow (by regional perfusion), peak accumulation, and release of the tracer within a region of interest. Once the tracer is in the cell, it either (1) enters the endogenous lipid pool or (2) moves to the mitochondria, where rapid degradation by beta-oxidation results in the generation of carbon dioxide. Depending on demand, about 80 percent of the extracted [^{11}C]palmitate is activated for transport from the lipid pool into the mitochondria for breakdown by beta-oxidation. Because of its complicated kinetic modeling and numerous confounding effects, [^{11}C]palmitate imaging has not gained wide clinical acceptance.

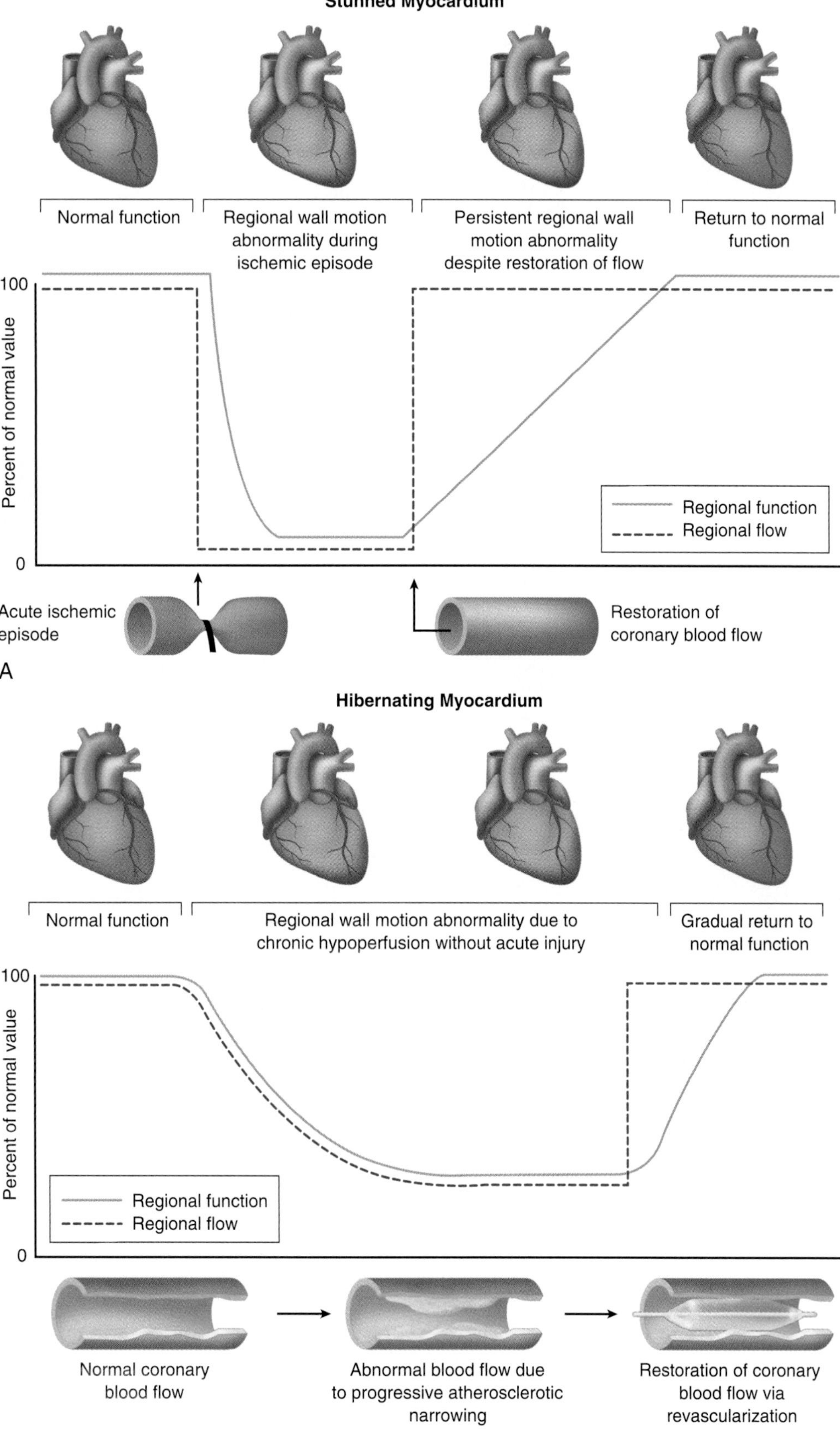

FIGURE 13–26 Pathophysiology of stunning and hibernation, representing different mechanisms of acute and chronic reversible left ventricular dysfunction. (Adapted from Dilsizian V: Myocardial viability: Reversible left ventricular dysfunction. *In* Dilsizian V, Narula J, Braunwald E [eds]: Atlas of Nuclear Cardiology. Philadelphia, Current Medicine, 2003, pp 131-145.)

[^{123}I]BMIPP. Fatty acid imaging with radioiodine-labeled fatty acid analogs such as iodine-123-beta-methyliodopentadecanoic acid (BMIPP) using SPECT is an investigational area for the assessment of *ischemic memory*.[61] After an ischemic episode, fatty acid metabolism may be suppressed for a prolonged time, and BMIPP imaging can demonstrate a regional metabolic defect even if perfusion has returned to normal.[62,63] This metabolic signal of recent ischemia has been termed "ischemic memory" and may be clinically useful, for example, in patients who report to an emergency department (ED) with chest pain that resolved hours earlier.[63] Although BMIPP is approved for clinical use in Japan, it has not yet received approval by the U.S. Food and Drug Administration.

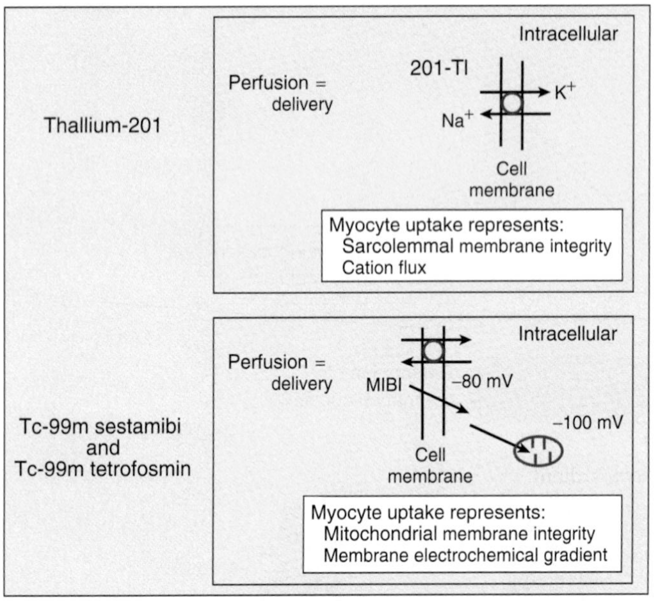

FIGURE 13–27 Mechanisms of uptake and retention of thallium-201 and technetium-99m perfusion tracers.

Imaging Glucose Metabolism

Whereas fatty acids are the primary source of fuel in the *fasting state*, increased arterial glucose concentration in the *fed state* results in an increase in insulin levels, stimulating glucose metabolism while inhibiting lipolysis.[31,32,64] The result is a switch in myocardial metabolism from predominantly fatty acid utilization to glucose utilization.

The principle of using a metabolic tracer that tracks glycolysis is based on the concept that glucose utilization may be preserved or increased relative to flow in hypoperfused but viable (hibernating) myocardium, termed *metabolism-perfusion mismatch*.[31,32,34,65] Myocardial glucose utilization is absent in scarred or fibrotic tissue, termed *metabolism-perfusion match* (Fig. 13–29). Although the amount of energy produced by glycolysis may be adequate to maintain myocyte viability and preserve the electrochemical gradient across the cell membrane, it may not be sufficient to sustain contractile function. This is the conceptual basis for hibernation, an adaptive response preserving myocardial viability in the absence of clinically evident ischemia.[34,53]

2-[^{18}F]Fluoro-2-Deoxyglucose. FDG is a glucose analog used to image myocardial glucose utilization with PET.[31,32,34,64,65] Following injection of 5 to 10 mCi, FDG rapidly exchanges across the capillary and cellular membranes. It is phosphorylated by hexokinase to FDG-6-phosphate (see Fig. 13–28) and not metabolized further or used in glycogen synthesis. Because the dephosphorylation rate of FDG is slow, it becomes trapped in the myocardium, permitting PET or SPECT imaging of regional glucose utilization (see Fig. 13–28). FDG uptake may be increased in hibernating but viable myocardium, and FDG uptake in asynergic myocardial regions with reduced blood flow at rest has become a scintigraphic marker of hibernation.

Diagnostic quality of FDG imaging is critically dependent on hormonal milieu and substrate availability. Most FDG clinical studies are performed after 50 to 75 gm of glucose loading in the form of oral dextrose approximately 1 to 2 hours before the FDG injection to increase glucose metabolism, increase FDG uptake, and improve image quality.[31,32] Although 90 percent of FDG images are of diagnostic quality in nondiabetic patients, the quality of FDG images after glucose loading alone is less certain in patients with clinical or subclinical diabetes, as the increase in plasma insulin levels may be attenuated, tissue lipolysis may not be inhibited, and free fatty acid levels may remain high. Standardization schemes to optimize FDG image quality in diabetic patients include[31,32] (1) intravenous insulin injections after glucose loading, (2) hyperinsulinemic-euglycemic clamping, and (3) use of nicotinic acid derivative.

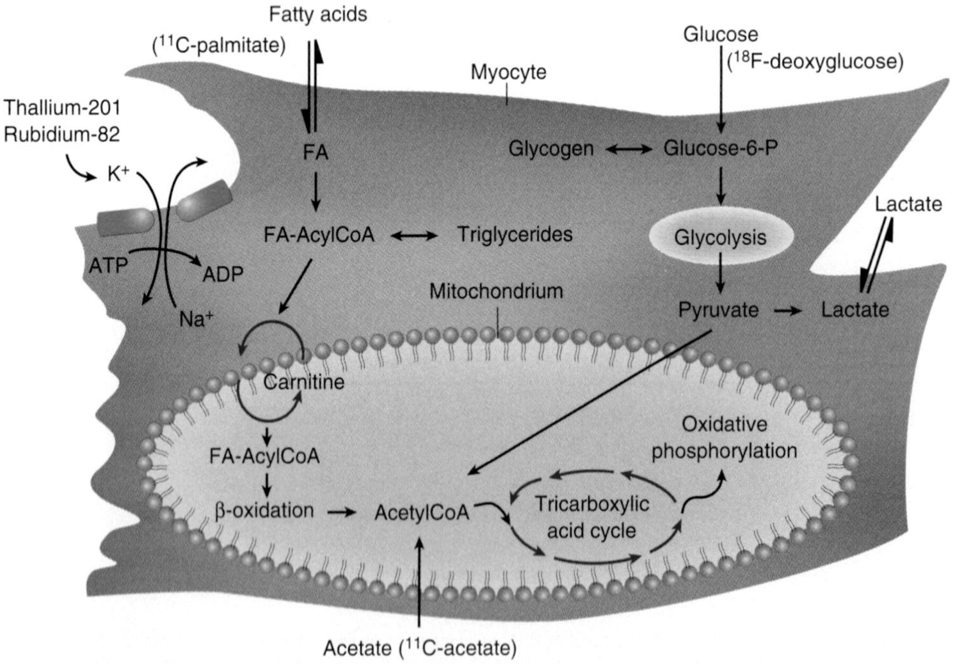

FIGURE 13–28 Mechanism of uptake and retention of positron-emission tomography agents tracing perfusion (rubidium-82) and oxidative and anaerobic metabolism (^{11}C-acetate, ^{11}C-palmitate, and ^{18}F-deoxyglucose). ADP = adenosine diphosphate; ATP = adenosine triphosphate; CoA = coenzyme A; FA = fatty acid. (Adapted from Dilsizian V: SPECT and PET techniques. *In* Dilsizian V, Narula J, Braunwald E [eds]: Atlas of Nuclear Cardiology. Philadelphia, Current Medicine, 2003, pp 19-46.)

Imaging Oxidative Metabolism and Mitochondrial Function

[^{11}C]Acetate. All oxidative fuels are metabolized in the tricarboxylic acid (TCA) cycle after conversion to acetyl coenzyme A (CoA). [^{11}C] Acetate is avidly extracted by the myocardium and metabolized predominantly by conversion to [^{11}C]acetyl-CoA in the cytosol and oxidation by the TCA cycle in the mitochondria to [^{11}C]carbon dioxide and water. Hence, the rapid myocardial turnover and clearance of [^{11}C]acetate in the form of [^{11}C]carbon dioxide may reflect myocardial oxidative metabolism and provide insight into mitochondrial function. In patients with recent MI and chronic stable angina, clearance rates of [^{11}C]acetate predict myocardial viability and functional recovery after revascularization. Despite encouraging data in the literature, [^{11}C]acetate remains an investigational tracer.[66]

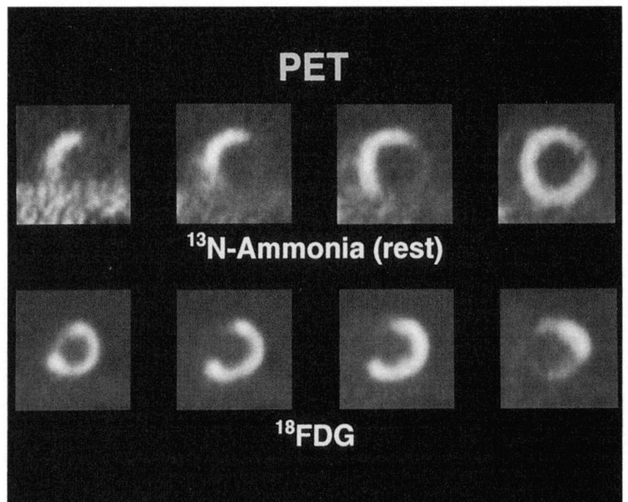

FIGURE 13–29 Assessment of viability by PET imaging. In the **top row,** ^{13}N-ammonia is used as a tracer of myocardial blood flow at rest in these short-axis images starting toward the apex (left) and moving toward the base of the heart (right). There is reduced resting blood flow in the anterolateral, lateral, and inferior walls (defects best seen on the first three images from the left). In the **bottom row,** ^{18}F-fluorodeoxyglucose (FDG) is used as a tracer of myocardial glucose metabolism. There is *enhanced* FDG uptake relative to blood flow in the anterolateral, lateral, and inferior walls, referred to as the "PET mismatch" pattern, indicative of viable myocardium in areas with diminished resting flow, or hibernation. (Adapted from Dilsizian V: Myocardial viability: Reversible left ventricular dysfunction. *In* Dilsizian V, Narula J, Braunwald E [eds]: Atlas of Nuclear Cardiology. Philadelphia, Current Medicine, 2003, pp 131-145.)

Assessment of Ventricular Function by Radionuclide Imaging

Assessing the Physiology of Ventricular Function

The EF is an index of global systolic LV performance influenced by many factors, including the intrinsic state of contractility, preload, and afterload as well as neurohormonal and inotropic influences. Despite its load dependence, EF as an index of ventricular performance has proved clinically quite useful. In the aftermath of acute MI, the postinfarction EF is among the most powerful indices predictive of subsequent mortality.[10,67] The radionuclide techniques used to image ventricular function, RVG and gated SPECT imaging, have provided substantial insight into the physiology of LV function and the response to disease states.

Assessing the Left Ventricular Response to Exercise. Equilibrium gated RVG and first-pass RVG are among the few noninvasive imaging techniques that can evaluate ventricular performance *during exercise.*[27,28] Most often, this is accomplished by imaging the patient during bicycle exercise, supine or semisupine for equilibrium RVG and upright for first-pass RVG bicycle exercise. EF measurements during exertion can then be compared with the resting EF.[27,28]

This technique has been used to study the response of LV function and volumes to exercise. For example, in younger normal subjects, the normal increase in EF and cardiac output is accomplished by decreasing end-systolic volume. In contrast, among older normal subjects, the increase in EF and cardiac output during exercise is accomplished by increasing end-diastolic volume (utilizing preload reserve). In healthy subjects, the normal EF response to exercise is an increase of more than five EF units. The underlying physiology of this increase changes as normal subjects age.[68]

The relative ease by which the EF response to exercise may be studied with RVG techniques led to many reports in the late 1970s and throughout the 1980s. However, evaluation of LV function during exercise by RVG has now been largely replaced by exercise echocardiography (see Chap. 11).

Evaluation of Left Ventricular Volumes. With the RVG technique, the counts detected from the LV region of interest are proportional to ventricular volume. The proportional relation can be estimated from a blood sample of known volume, in which the quantitative relationship between counts and volume can be determined after correction for attenuation.[69] The reader is referred to seminal publications for details.[70,71]

The major advantage of the RVG technique for evaluation of ventricular volumes (and function) over contrast ventriculographic and echocardiographic methods is that the radionuclide techniques *do not require assumptions about ventricular geometry.* Among patients with dilated left ventricles, particularly in the presence of multiple regional wall motion abnormalities, assumptions of ventricular shape, usually that of a prolate ellipsoid, may not be valid. Using RVG techniques, volumes are calculated from count rates over a region of interest involving the left or right ventricle, or both, and are based on photon emissions from the region of interest.[27] Thus, the radionuclide techniques are *not dependent on any assumption of ventricular geometry* and are suitable for the study of ventricular volumes when ventricular geometry is abnormal.

Serial studies of ventricular volumes have been useful in evaluating the process of LV remodeling after MI and in chronic heart failure,[72] in which there is a progressive increase in LV volume in the absence of neurohormonal blockade. Serial RVG studies have shown that the effect of angiotensin-converting enzyme (ACE) inhibition is an early reduction in LV volume, which is maintained over follow-up.[72]

LV volumes may also be calculated using *gated SPECT perfusion imaging,* and volumetric data have been validated against other quantitative techniques.[73,74] At this time, there is less experience using gated SPECT perfusion imaging for serial evaluation of LV volumes compared with equilibrium RVG volumetric techniques. Nonetheless, the ability to evaluate simultaneously LV function, perfusion, and volumes with gated SPECT perfusion imaging suggests that this technique will be increasingly used to study pathophysiological changes.

SERIAL EVALUATION OF LEFT VENTRICULAR FUNCTION

The quantitative nature of radionuclide analysis of ventricular function and the high reproducibility of the measurement make ECG-gated RVG or ECG-gated SPECT imaging well suited for serial follow-up of changes in LV systolic performance. There are many clinical situations in which serial changes in LV function are clinically relevant, such as in patients with heart failure,[75] those observed with valvular heart disease,[76,77] and those being treated with cardiotoxic chemotherapy.[78] Serial RVG studies demonstrating diminution in EF suggesting the early onset of myocardial dysfunction can herald the onset of a higher risk clinical course directing clinical management decisions.

The accuracy and reproducibility of the RVG technique for assessment of LV function make this technique particularly suitable for serial follow-up assessment of patients with regurgitant valvular heart disease. As an example, studies using RVGs have shown that patients being followed up with asymptomatic chronic severe aortic regurgitation who demonstrate the onset of LV dysfunction during follow-up, even when remaining asymptomatic, are at higher risk for adverse clinical outcomes than those with preserved LV performance.[76,77] On the basis of such RVG data, the onset of LV dysfunction in an asymptomatic patient with aortic regurgitation is an indication for surgery. Similarly, serial RVG follow-up of patients undergoing cardiotoxic chemotherapy[78] has demonstrated that a decline in EF as detected by RVG of 10 percent to a final level less than 50 percent indicates high risk for the development of subsequent heart failure.

EVALUATION OF DIASTOLIC FUNCTION WITH RADIONUCLIDE TECHNIQUES

Although the most important quantitative variable derived from RVG evaluation of LV function in the majority of cardiac diseases is the EF, numerous other quantitative variables, including indices describing LV diastolic performance, may also be derived.

Left Ventricular Diastolic Filling. Radionuclide assessment of LV filling properties is based on analysis of the LV time-activity curve, usually obtained using equilibrium RVG techniques,[68] which represents relative volume changes throughout the cardiac cycle (Fig. 13-30). With appropriate data acquisition methods and attention to technical considerations, several parameters of diastolic function may be computed from the time-activity curve, including the peak rate of rapid diastolic filling, the time to peak filling rate, and the relative contributions of the rapid filling period and of atrial systole to total LV stroke volume. Several studies have shown good correlation between various radionuclide and Doppler echocardiographic measures of filling, as both techniques assess physiological events during the filling period.[79]

COMBINED PRESSURE-VOLUME ANALYSIS OF LEFT VENTRICULAR FUNCTION. The influence of LV relaxation and distensibility on the rate, magnitude, and timing of diastolic filling may be studied in the context of the instantaneous relation between LV pressure and volume throughout the cardiac cycle. It is possible with equilibrium RVG techniques to obtain ventricular volume data in the catheterization laboratory, along with simultaneous acquisition of ventricular pressure measurements, to study the interplay between LV relaxation, filling, and pressure-volume relations (Fig. 13-31). LV distensibility or compliance may be studied by the contour, location, and slope of the pressure-volume relation during the filling phase of diastole.[68]

Evaluation of Diastolic Filling by Equilibrium Radionuclide Ventriculography Techniques in Disease States

Hypertrophic Cardiomyopathy. Abnormal diastolic properties of the hypertrophied ventricle are a characteristic feature of hypertrophic cardiomyopathy (HCM), contributing notably to clinical manifestations.[80] Studies using RVG evaluation of diastolic filling have demonstrated that the rate and extent of rapid filling are reduced in HCM, that the time to peak filling rate is prolonged, and that the contribution of atrial systole to total LV stroke volume is increased.[81]

Combined radionuclide and hemodynamic measurements indicate that enhanced LV filling after verapamil in HCM (effective in relieving symptoms in many patients) is associated with improved indices of LV relaxation and favorable shift in the diastolic pressure-volume relations (see Fig. 13-31).[68] Radionuclide studies have also demonstrated that enhanced LV filling after verapamil in HCM correlates with objective symptomatic improvement as measured by exercise treadmill time, suggesting that reversal of LV filling abnormalities is an important mechanism by which patients experience reduction of symptoms.[82]

Heart Failure. Radionuclide studies have provided evidence of an abnormal end-diastolic volume response to exercise in patients with heart failure and *preserved* systolic performance, supporting the concept of diastolic dysfunction as an underlying cause for symptoms.[83] Patients with heart failure but preserved systolic performance do not increase end-diastolic volume during exercise, associated with a substantial increase in wedge pressure (Fig. 13-32). In contrast, normal subjects demonstrate an increase in end-diastolic volume associated with no change in wedge pressure, recruiting preload despite no change in left atrial driving pressure. Patients with heart failure and normal systolic performance require higher filling pressures to maintain stroke volume, at the cost of an increased pulmonary wedge pressure, resulting in shortness of breath. Thus, abnormal diastolic performance, manifested by an ***impaired ability to recruit end-diastolic volume (preload reserve)***, as demonstrated by equilibrium RVG techniques, results in physiological abnormalities leading to heart failure in these patients with normal systolic function.

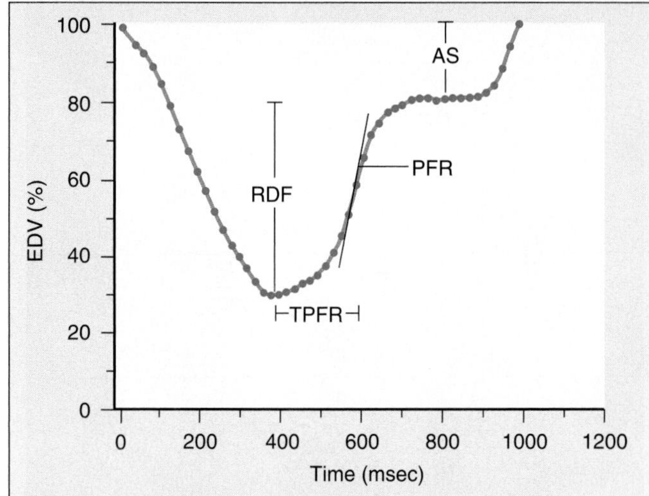

FIGURE 13–30 Quantitative analysis of systolic and diastolic events by radionuclide ventriculography. The x-axis represents time across one average cardiac cycle, and the y-axis represents count activity within the left ventricular region of interest, which is expressed as a percentage of end-diastolic volume (% EDV). The time-activity curve represents the relative change in volume within the ventricle during the cardiac cycle. In this high-temporal-resolution example, each point represents 20 milliseconds. Indices of diastolic function may be computed from analysis of the filling portion of the curve, including the peak rate of rapid filling (PFR), the time from end systole at which peak filling occurs (TPFR), and the relative contribution of rapid diastolic filling (RDF) and of atrial systole (AS) to total stroke volume. (Adapted from Udelson JE, Bonow RO: Radionuclide ventriculography in left ventricular diastolic dysfunction. *In* Gaasch WH, LeWinter M [eds]: Heart Failure and Diastolic Dysfunction. Philadelphia, Lea & Febiger, 1994, pp 167-191.)

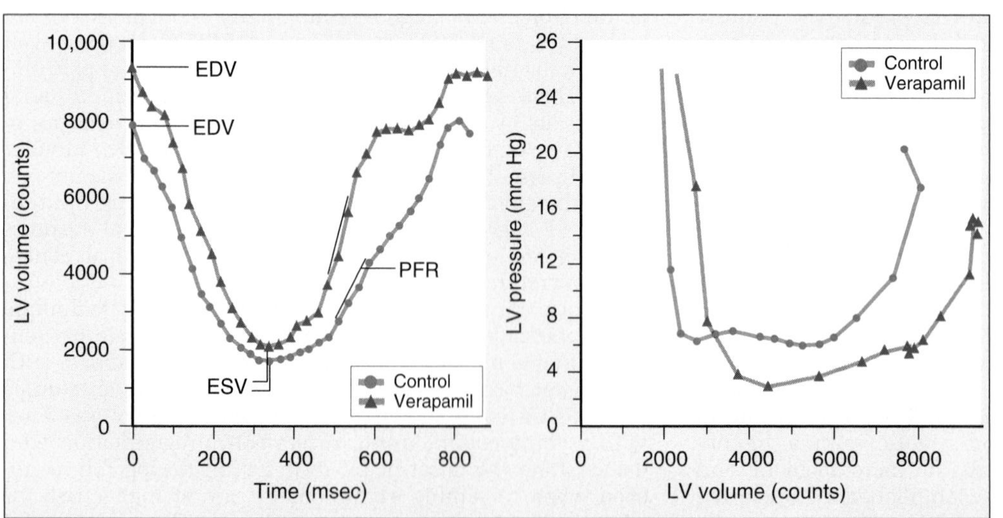

FIGURE 13–31 Pressure-volume analysis to study the effect of drug intervention in diastolic dysfunction. **Left,** Time-activity (volume) curves from a patient with hypertrophic cardiomyopathy under control conditions (magenta line) and after intravenous verapamil (blue line). There is an increase in left ventricular (LV) end-diastolic volume (EDV) and end-systolic volume (ESV) and an increase in peak filling rate (PFR) following verapamil administration. **Right,** Diastolic pressure-volume curves. Following verapamil, there is a favorable downward and rightward shift in diastolic pressure-volume relation, suggesting improved diastolic distensibility, as left ventricular volume is higher at any given pressure. In this example, volume data were acquired with radionuclide analysis of LV count changes and pressure data with a micronanometer catheter. (Adapted from Udelson JE, Bonow RO: Left ventricular diastolic function and the use of calcium channel blockers in hypertrophic cardiomyopathy. *In* Gaasch WH, LeWinter M [eds]: Heart Failure and Diastolic Dysfunction. Philadelphia, Lea & Febiger, 1994, pp 462-489.)

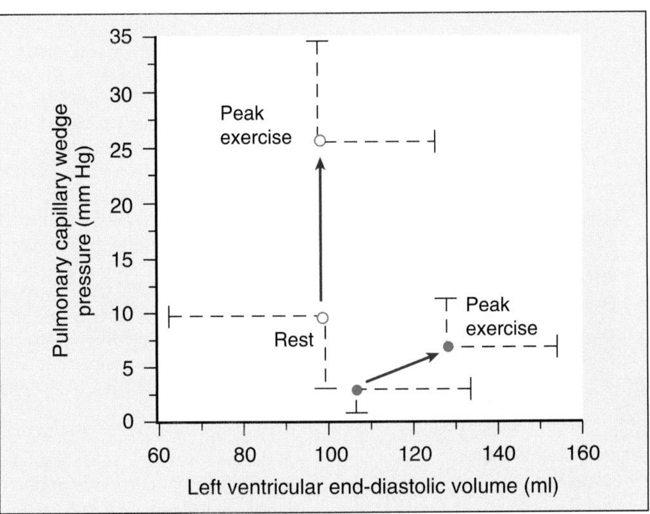

FIGURE 13–32 Use of radionuclide ventriculography to evaluate changes in end-diastolic volume (EDV) during exercise. In normal subjects (closed symbols), there is an increase in EDV during exercise (recruitment of preload reserve) with only minor change in pulmonary capillary wedge (PCW) pressure. In contrast, patients with heart failure and preserved systolic function (open symbols) manifest no change in EDV during exercise despite substantial increase in PCW pressure, to levels that would be associated with symptoms such as shortness of breath. (Adapted from Kitzman DW, Higginbotham MB, Cobb FR, et al: Exercise intolerance in patients with heart failure and preserved left ventricular systolic function: Failure of the Frank-Starling mechanism. J Am Coll Cardiol 17:1065, 1991.)

Disease Detection, Risk Stratification, and Clinical Decision-Making

Stable Chest Pain Syndromes

Application of Radionuclide Imaging: Answering the Clinical Questions

For patients with stable symptoms of suspected CAD who are referred for noninvasive testing, the two major goals of testing are (1) determination of whether CAD is present or absent (the "diagnostic" construct) and (2) determination of the longer term prognosis or risk of an adverse outcome over time (the "prognostic" construct). These goals of testing are linked to the treatment goals for any patients with suspected or known CAD. The two main goals of treatment are (1) minimization of symptoms in everyday life and (2) improvement in natural history.

Establishing the presence of or ruling out CAD is an important goal of testing. The performance characteristics of radionuclide imaging for this purpose are based on the detection of CAD, usually defined as greater than or equal to 50 or 70 percent stenosis in an individual epicardial vessel. This definition of CAD is in part based on seminal studies in animal models showing that a 50 percent stenosis begins to blunt coronary flow reserve.[84] However, over time a view has emerged that CAD is a more complex process than can be defined dichotomously by a 50 percent or even a 70 percent luminal stenosis. Throughout the progression of plaque growth, there is a risk of transformation from a stable plaque to an unstable plaque, with the potential for an acute coronary syndrome (ACS) that abruptly alters the natural history of the patient.[85] Plaque encroachment of the lumen occurs later in the process but has a potentially important impact on the patient's everyday quality of life by causing symptoms related to exertional ischemia.

PATIENT-RELATED OUTCOMES AS A "GOLD STANDARD." The evolution of preventive therapies, such as 3-hydroxy-3-methylglutaryl (HMG) CoA reductase inhibitors, to reduce cardiovascular risk has focused attention on the ability of global risk scores or noninvasive testing to *assess risk of future events* in order to best target strategies to reduce risk.[86,87] Thus, from the perspective of improving natural history, knowledge of whether or not a greater than 50 percent stenosis is present in a patient with stable anginal symptoms becomes less important than *knowledge of the patient's risk of a cardiovascular event, i.e., cardiac death or nonfatal MI.* After initial investigations of the performance of radionuclide imaging to detect or rule out CAD (sensitivity and specificity), the trajectory of the literature has been toward gaining more understanding of how noninvasive imaging results assess prognosis and stratify the risk of future cardiac events.[88] This has occurred in parallel with similar directions in primary prevention efforts, such as the use of a Framingham risk score, with a goal of life-style and treatment interventions to lower that risk.[86] In much the same way, risk stratification and assessment of prognosis by noninvasive imaging will inform clinical management decisions geared toward reducing risk of MI and cardiac death, and optimizing the selection of patients for revascularization and medical therapies.

Risk Stratification in Stable Chest Pain Syndromes

Definitions for Understanding the Literature. For prognostic assessment, an important goal is to detect patients at risk for "hard" cardiac events. This definition includes *nonfatal MI* as well as *cardiac death* or *all-cause mortality*, irreversible events that it is important to prevent.[89] "Soft" cardiac events include revascularization and hospital admission for unstable angina or heart failure. Such events occur more often than the hard cardiac events and thus contribute to a larger number of endpoints for data analysis. However, these events are not as important in terms of natural history and may be driven by subjective changes in symptoms and, in the case of revascularization, by the results of the imaging tests themselves.

Risk categories as described in the American College of Cardiology/American Heart Association (ACC/AHA) stable angina guidelines include (1) low risk, defined as a less than 1 percent per year risk of hard event; (2) intermediate risk, defined as a 1 to 3 percent per year risk, and (3) high risk, defined as a greater than 3 percent per year risk of hard cardiac events.[90] These definitions are conceptually linked to implied treatment strategies. Patients with greater than 3 percent per year risk would be most likely to benefit from a revascularization strategy, whereas those at low risk would be least likely to benefit from revascularization, in terms of natural history, and thus could be treated medically, with treatment directed against symptoms as well as risk factor modification.

The Relation Between the Extent of Perfusion Defect and Natural History Outcomes. Seminal studies in the 1980s demonstrated that the *extent of perfusion abnormality* by stress MPI has an important relationship with the *subsequent likelihood of an adverse natural history outcome* (cardiac death or nonfatal MI).[91,92] Among patients presenting with chest pain and *suspected* CAD (without any prior known CAD history, such as an MI or revascularization), the risk of cardiac death or MI increased as the number of reversible perfusion defects, i.e., the extent of inducible ischemia, increased (Fig. 13–33).

This concept has been confirmed many times by investigators around the world. Moreover, this robust concept not only applies to *exercise* stress MPI but also extends across the spectrum of procedural variation in nuclear cardiology, including different stressors (vasodilator pharmacological stress, dobutamine stress), isotopes (thallium-201 and ^{99m}Tc agents), and imaging protocols (including dual-isotope imaging).[10] An example of data on risk stratification implying therapeutic management strategies is demonstrated by the images shown in Figure 13–34A and B. In two older men with

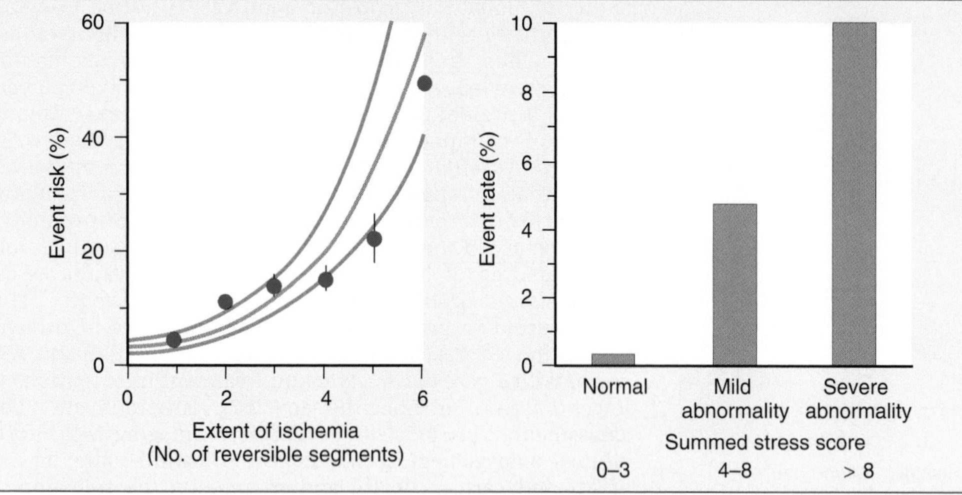

FIGURE 13–33 Prognostic implications of myocardial perfusion imaging. **A,** Cardiac event rate (risk of cardiac death or myocardial infarction [MI]) over long-term follow-up plotted as a function of the extent of inducible ischemia (the number of reversible perfusion defects). There is an exponential relationship between the extent of ischemia and the risk of a cardiac event (brown line = modeling of data points; magenta lines = confidence limits). **B,** Extent and severity of perfusion abnormality, expressed as the summed stress score, are related to the risk of subsequent cardiac death or MI. As the extent and severity of the perfusion abnormality increase, the event risk increases as well. (A, Adapted from Ladenheim ML, Pollock BH, Rozanski A, et al: Extent and severity of myocardial hypoperfusion as predictors of prognosis in patients with suspected coronary artery disease. J Am Coll Cardiol 7:464, 1986; B, adapted from Hachamovitch R, Berman DS, Kiat H, et al: Exercise myocardial perfusion SPECT in patients without known coronary artery disease: Incremental prognostic value and use in risk stratification. Circulation 93:905, 1996.)

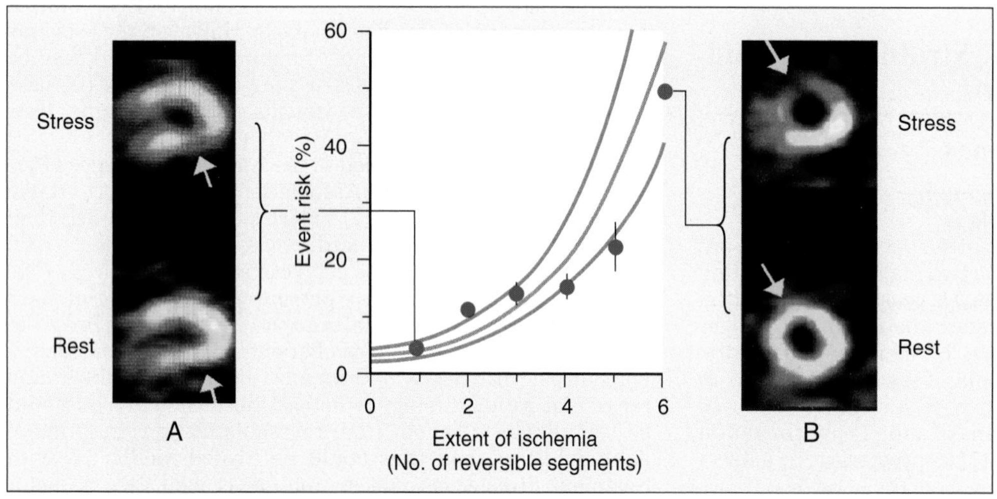

FIGURE 13–34 Single-photon emission computed tomography perfusion images in two patients with stable anginal symptoms. **A,** Small area of inferoapical ischemia (arrows). When this extent of ischemia is plotted on the graph from Figure 13–33A (line to red circle), the patient is placed in a low-risk category. **B,** In contrast, the large, severe area of anterior and septal ischemia in this patient places him in a high-risk group (line to red circle).

typical exertional angina, it would be predicted that the probability of CAD is very high, according to established guidelines. However, what is *not* established from that clinical information is the *natural history risk*. These examples demonstrate that patients presenting with similar symptoms might be identified as having distinct natural histories on the basis of perfusion imaging data, with distinct implications for subsequent management.

THE INCREMENTAL VALUE OF PERFUSION IMAGING. The term "incremental value" implies that perfusion imaging data provide information on natural history risk and outcomes that are *additive to* (incremental to) information from more available or less expensive tests, such as clinical data and stress ECG findings.[93,94]

Stress MPI data have been shown to have incremental prognostic value when added to prognostic stress ECG instruments such as the Duke Treadmill Score (DTS), a well-validated instrument incorporating symptoms, treadmill performance, and stress ECG findings to predict natural history outcomes (see Chap. 10). In a group of 2200 patients with suspected CAD referred for nuclear testing, the DTS was used to place patients in subgroups according to the risk of a hard event (Fig. 13-35).[95] When information from stress MPI studies was incorporated, incremental value to predict outcome was demonstrated within each of the three DTS risk categories.

The importance of this information in driving management decisions for patients can be illustrated by considering how clinicians would manage patients given certain amounts of information. Given the DTS information alone, the management of low-risk patients would probably be conservative and the management of high-risk patients would probably involve revascularization. The optimal management of intermediate-risk patients is unclear, but many would probably be referred for catheterization. However, almost 80 percent of the patients in the intermediate DTS category had a *normal* stress perfusion study (see Fig. 13-35A), associated with a very low risk natural history, implying that conservative management would be a safe and effective strategy.

These findings have been confirmed by other studies. In a large population of more than 4000 patients with an intermediate-risk DTS, normal stress MPI was associated with a very low risk of a hard cardiac event over multiple years of follow-up.[96]

Another method used to demonstrate the incremental value of MPI data over clinical, stress, and even angiographic data involves the creation of a multivariable model to measure the strength of association of individual factors with the natural history outcomes.[94,97,98] This is often illustrated by assessing the incremental chi-square value measuring the strength of the association of the factor with subsequent cardiac death and nonfatal MI (see Fig. 13-35B).

Identification of Treatment Benefit Following Risk Stratification. Although numerous studies have suggested that the extent and severity of perfusion abnormality are related to subsequent natural history risk, few studies have documented *reduction* in that risk associated with a particular therapy. Information is now available suggesting that more extensive ischemia determined by MPI identifies patients in whom revascularization would lead to an improvement in outcome. In a group of more than 10,000 patients with suspected CAD studied by stress MPI, the extent of ischemic myocardium predicted reduction in the risk of death with revascularization compared with medical therapy (Fig.

13–36), beginning at just over 10 percent of ischemic myocardium.[99] As the percentage of ischemic myocardium increased, the magnitude of benefit of revascularization increased as well. Thus, MPI data can predict the magnitude of a potential treatment benefit from revascularization, helping to guide management decisions.

The Prognostic Value of Normal Myocardial Perfusion Imaging. A consistent finding in studies assessing progno-sis has been the benign prognosis associated with a normal stress myocardial perfusion study. As summarized in the ACC/AHA/American Society for Nuclear Cardiology (ASNC) Radionuclide Imaging Guidelines,[10] data on outcomes associated with a normal stress MPI SPECT study now involve almost 21,000 patients. In patients with a normal study, the hard event rate occurring over an average follow-up of 2 years is 0.7 percent per year. This concept applies across a broad spectrum of isotopes, protocols, and stressors.[10,100] The prediction of low-risk outcome following a normal MPI extends approximately 2 years after testing (i.e., the "warranty period").[101] Patients who at baseline represent higher risk subsets (i.e., those with diabetes) have a slightly higher risk of an adverse outcome after a normal stress MPI,[102] consistent with Bayes' theorem; that is, given a certain MPI finding, the posttest probability (outcome risk) is related in part to the pretest risk.

Even when angiographic CAD is present with a stable symptom complex, a normal stress MPI study is associated with a low-risk outcome (~0.9 percent per year).[103] The mechanism for a normal MPI despite established CAD has not been conclusively demonstrated but may involve preserved endothelial function, allowing appropriate flow-mediated vasodilation during stress, reducing the impact of an angiographic stenosis on downstream myocardial perfusion. If this is true, such preserved endothelial function may identify a patient less susceptible to plaque fissuring or rupture and more likely to have a stable clinical course.

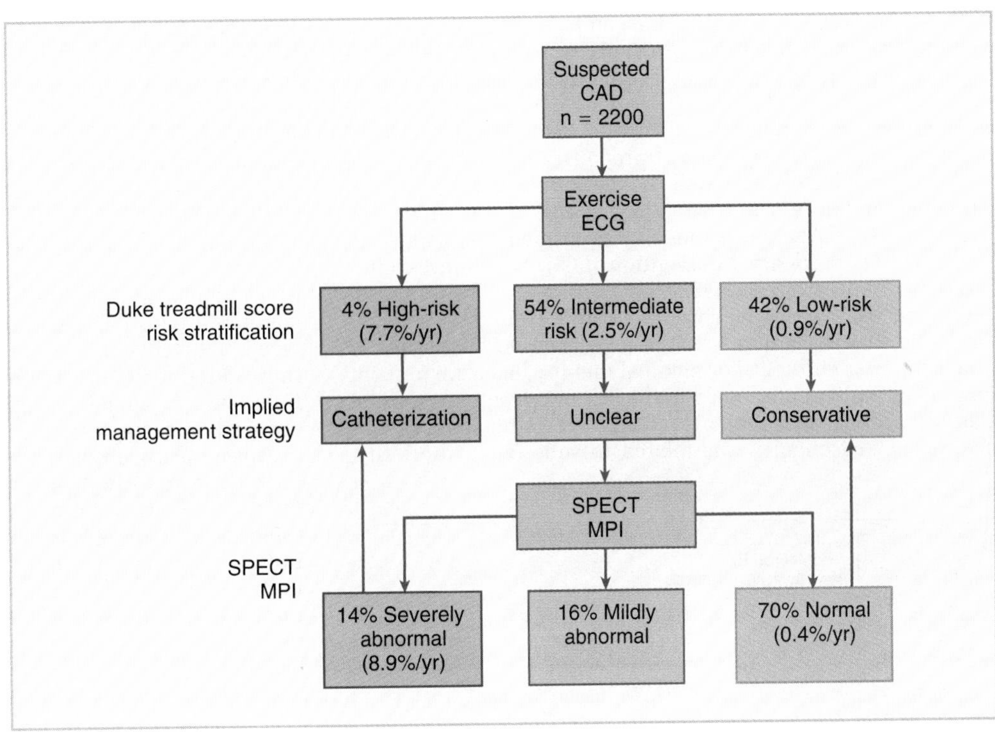

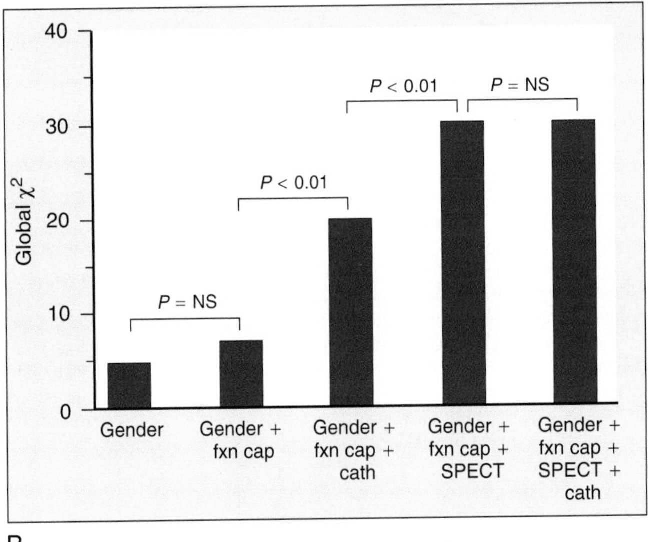

FIGURE 13–35 Incremental value of single-photon emission computed tomography (SPECT) perfusion imaging. **A,** Comparison with the Duke Treadmill Score (DTS). A large group of patients with suspected coronary artery disease (CAD) was initially risk stratified by the well-validated DTS. Figures in parentheses are the observed annual event rates. The majority of the population is classified as "intermediate risk" by DTS, and management strategy is not clear. High-risk patients may be managed aggressively, and low-risk patients may be managed conservatively. Among patients originally categorized as intermediate risk by the DTS, almost 70 percent had a normal SPECT perfusion study, associated with a very low event rate. Following SPECT myocardial perfusion imaging (MPI), more patients are classified at the "extremes" of risk (low or high), where management is more clearly implied by the risk prediction. Thus, the imaging data allowed further stratification and thus had incremental value over the DTS information. **B,** The incremental value of imaging data may be expressed as the incremental chi-square value, a statistical measure of the strength of the association of clinical, demographic, stress, or imaging factors to risk stratification. Among patients with known CAD who had undergone catheterization (cath), clinical information is added on the x-axis, with the global chi-square value associated with the information depicted on the y-axis. The larger the chi-square value, the stronger the relation between the combination of factors on the x-axis and the natural history outcome of cardiac death or myocardial infarction. Even when anatomical information is available, the physiological information provided by SPECT MPI adds significantly to risk prediction ability. fxn cap = functional capacity. (A, Adapted from Hachamovitch R, Berman DS, Kiat H, et al: Exercise myocardial perfusion SPECT in patients without known coronary artery disease: Incremental prognostic value and use in risk stratification. Circulation 93:905, 1996; B, adapted from Beller GA: First annual Mario S. Verani, MD, Memorial Lecture: Clinical value of myocardial perfusion imaging in coronary artery disease. J Nucl Cardiol 10:529, 2003.)

Dynamic Assessment of Prognosis by Serial Scintigraphic Studies: A New Paradigm?

Although there is an important correlation between the extent of ischemia and subsequent outcome, the specificity of such determinations is low. That is, among patients with high-risk scintigraphic signs, only a minority suffer an important cardiac event during follow-up and the majority of "high-risk" patients remain event-free. As most of these high-risk patients undergo catheterization and intervention, many patients who will not have an event are receiving interventions in order to prevent such events in the minority. Clinicians accept this trade-off, but evolving data suggest that the response of scintigraphic ischemia to medical therapy may allow more precise estimates of prognosis.

The Angioplasty Compared to Medicine (ACME) investigators[104] randomly assigned 328 patients with single- or double-vessel CAD and stable angina to medical therapy or percutaneous coronary intervention (PCI). Six months after randomization, exercise MPI was performed. The 6-month MPI data were strongly correlated with subsequent 5-year cardiac events.[104] Patients with a reversible perfusion defect 6 months after *either* PCI or medical therapy had a 3.6 percent annual mortality rate, compared with a 1.6 percent annual mortality rate among patients with no reversible defects, and the extent of ischemia was related to subsequent mortality.

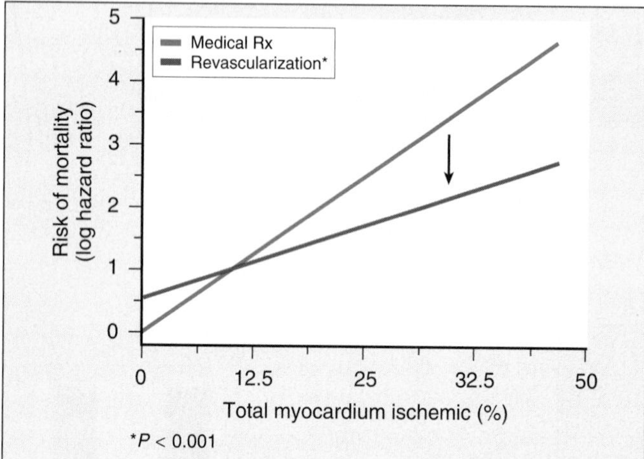

FIGURE 13–36 Predicting the magnitude of treatment benefit by revascularization. Risk of death is plotted as a function of the percent ischemic myocardium by single-photon emission computed tomography perfusion imaging. The solid lines represent patients treated with medical therapy (medical Rx, magenta) or revascularization (blue). When the magnitude of ischemia exceeds approximately 12 percent, there is a potential survival benefit with revascularization. (Adapted from Hachamovitch R, Hayes SW, Friedman JD, et al: Comparison of the short-term survival benefit associated with revascularization compared with medical therapy in patients with no prior coronary artery disease undergoing stress myocardial perfusion single photon emission computed tomography. Circulation 107:2900, 2003.)

Exercise ECG data were not predictive of late outcomes. Even if the 6-month MPI study was performed in patients receiving medical therapy alone in the absence of prior PCI, the outcome prediction was similar. These data suggest that follow-up MPI to assess the effect of medical therapy on the extent of ischemia may help to predict late outcomes more precisely and subcategorize patients more precisely within risk groups.

Similar results have been reported for patients who underwent PCI or medical therapy early after acute MI.[49] The extent of ischemia was similarly reduced with medical therapy compared with PCI on a follow-up SPECT perfusion study 6 weeks later. Event-free survival was significantly related to the reduction in perfusion defect size, independent of the intervention. Ongoing trials are testing this concept using contemporary aggressive secondary prevention therapies.

Studies using either PET or SPECT assessment of perfusion have concordantly demonstrated improvement in stress perfusion following statin therapy (Fig. 13–37).[105,106] As such therapy is unlikely to affect significantly the degree of luminal encroachment by a plaque, the data suggest that improvement in perfusion may be a result of statin-mediated improvement in endothelial function. Favorable changes in perfusion may identify cohorts of patients gaining most benefit from statin therapy in terms of vascular stability, a concept that requires longer term follow-up of such patients.

Detecting the Presence and Extent of Coronary Artery Disease

Noninvasive testing in patients with suspected CAD is commonly performed to determine the presence or absence of CAD. In this diagnostic construct, CAD is usually defined dichotomously, by a threshold degree of coronary stenosis in a major epicardial vessel, usually greater than or equal to 50 or 70 percent stenosis by angiography. In this paradigm, angiography is the gold standard to define the presence or absence of CAD, and performance of the noninvasive test is measured by its *sensitivity* (percentage of true-positive tests among those with CAD as defined by angiography) as well as its *specificity* (percentage of true-negative tests among those without CAD).[107] Published values of sensitivity for detecting CAD and specificity for ruling out CAD vary widely.[10] There are many factors influencing these performance characteristics that should be understood in order to incorporate imaging data appropriately into clinical decision-making. These include either methodological or physiological factors.

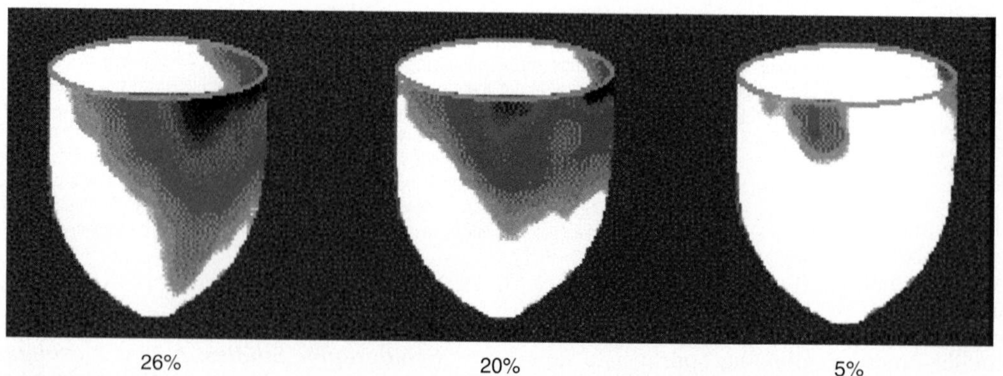

FIGURE 13–37 Improvement in perfusion after statin therapy. Three-dimensional surface-rendered models of myocardial perfusion before statin therapy (**left**) and after 6 weeks (**middle**) and 6 months (**right**) of therapy, viewed from the inferior surface of the heart. White areas represent normal perfusion, with red, blue, and black representing increasingly severe degrees of ischemia. The extent of ischemia is below each image, expressed as a percentage of total myocardium. There is a substantial improvement in the degree of inferior wall ischemia over the course of statin therapy. (Adapted from Schwartz RG, Pearson TA, Kalaria VG, et al: Prospective serial evaluation of myocardial perfusion and lipids during the first six months of pravastatin therapy: Coronary artery disease regression single photon emission computed tomography monitoring trial. J Am Coll Cardiol 42:600, 2003.)

METHODOLOGICAL INFLUENCES ON SENSITIVITY AND SPECIFICITY

Referral Bias. The *apparent* accuracy of any noninvasive test to detect CAD depends on the indications for coronary angiography. Accuracy of a new diagnostic test is usually determined initially in patients who are undergoing coronary angiography. As the test becomes implemented in routine diagnostic strategies, its results determine which patients are to be referred for coronary angiography (Fig. 13-38). For example, patients with abnormal MPI are more likely to undergo coronary angiography than those with normal MPI. This results in a phenomenon termed "posttest referral bias," in which the specificity of a diagnostic test declines over time as it is accepted into clinical practice and plays a gatekeeper role in determining which patients undergo angiography.[10,108] In its extreme form, in which only patients with an abnormal test are referred for angiography, the posttest referral bias drives the specificity to zero (all patients with normal coronary arteriograms have false-positive MPI results and there are no true-negatives). The same phenomenon artificially increases the sensitivity of the test and in its extreme drives the sensitivity to 100 percent (all patients with abnormal coronary arteriograms have true-positive MPI, with no false-negatives). This concept holds not only for MPI but also for any diagnostic test that might determine the indications for angiography.

The concept of "normalcy rate" has been developed in an attempt to compensate for this referral bias.[10] Normalcy is calculated in the same manner as specificity but includes only the imaging test results of patients with a clinically low or very low pretest likelihood of CAD, whether or not they are referred for cardiac catheterization. Normalcy rates tend to be greater than specificity.

Angiography as the Gold Standard. In humans, coronary atherosclerosis is a complex disease most often involving the coronary arteries diffusely and not merely focally. Moreover, whether a given discrete stenosis, imaged at rest during coronary angiography, results in a perfusion abnormality during stress is dependent on a number of factors besides the percent degree of stenosis. These factors include the dilatory or constrictor response of the vessel during stress (mediated by endothelial function) and the presence or absence of collaterals.[107,109] For example, a vessel with 70 percent stenosis but with preserved endothelial function and a well-developed collateral supply may *not* be associated with an abnormality on stress perfusion. In a diagnostic construct, such a result would be categorized as false-negative, reducing MPI sensitivity. However, the MPI data may be providing the *correct physiological information* regarding the functional significance of the angiographic finding, demonstrating that collateral flow during exercise or normal endothelial function or both were associated with preserved coronary blood flow reserve despite the coronary stenosis. This example illustrates the limitation of using angiography as a gold standard in evaluating a physiological modality.

Many published studies define CAD as greater than or equal to 50 percent stenosis, whereas others use a threshold of greater than or equal to 70 percent stenosis.[8,10] Using the former would decrease sensitivity (as some 50 to 70 percent stenoses are not hemodynamically significant) and increase specificity. In contrast, using the latter threshold would increase sensitivity, as more such stenoses are likely to be associated with perfusion abnormality, but decrease specificity, as any positive scan result with 50 to 70 percent stenosis would be considered false-positive.

PHYSIOLOGICAL INFLUENCES ON SENSITIVITY AND SPECIFICITY

A number of disease processes involving the coronary vasculature or the myocardium may result in abnormalities in myocardial perfusion in the *absence of a discrete coronary stenosis*. In a diagnostic construct for CAD, such abnormalities would be labeled false-positive, reducing specificity (i.e., the test is positive in the absence of epicardial CAD). However, MPI may actually be providing correct information regarding perfusion physiology.

Left Bundle Branch Block. Isolated reversible perfusion defects of the septum in patients with LBBB may be seen in the absence of stenosis of the left anterior descending (LAD) coronary artery.[8,10] This phenomenon may represent true heterogeneity of flow between the LAD and left circumflex territories, related to delayed relaxation of the septum in LBBB leading to reduced coronary flow reserve in early diastole, or reduced oxygen demand as a result of late septal contraction when wall stress is decreasing. The specificity and predictive value of a septal perfusion defect with LBBB are thus low. However, apical or anterior involvement in septal perfusion defects increases the specificity for CAD.[110] As a septal defect in LBBB is most commonly seen at high heart rates, pharmacological stress improves specificity, and vasodilator stress is recommended in the setting of LBBB.[10,110]

Hypertrophic Cardiomyopathy. The asymmetrical septal hypertrophy in many patients with HCM can lead to the appearance of a greater amount of tracer uptake in the hypertrophied septum relative to the lateral wall, creating the impression of a mild lateral wall perfusion defect, especially when polar maps are employed.

Many reports have demonstrated myocardial perfusion abnormalities in patients with HCM in the absence of epicardial CAD.[111,112] Such findings have important pathophysiological relevance: patients with fixed perfusion defects are likely to have thinned akinetic walls on echocardiography and diminished EF (Fig. 13-39).[113] Of asymptomatic patients

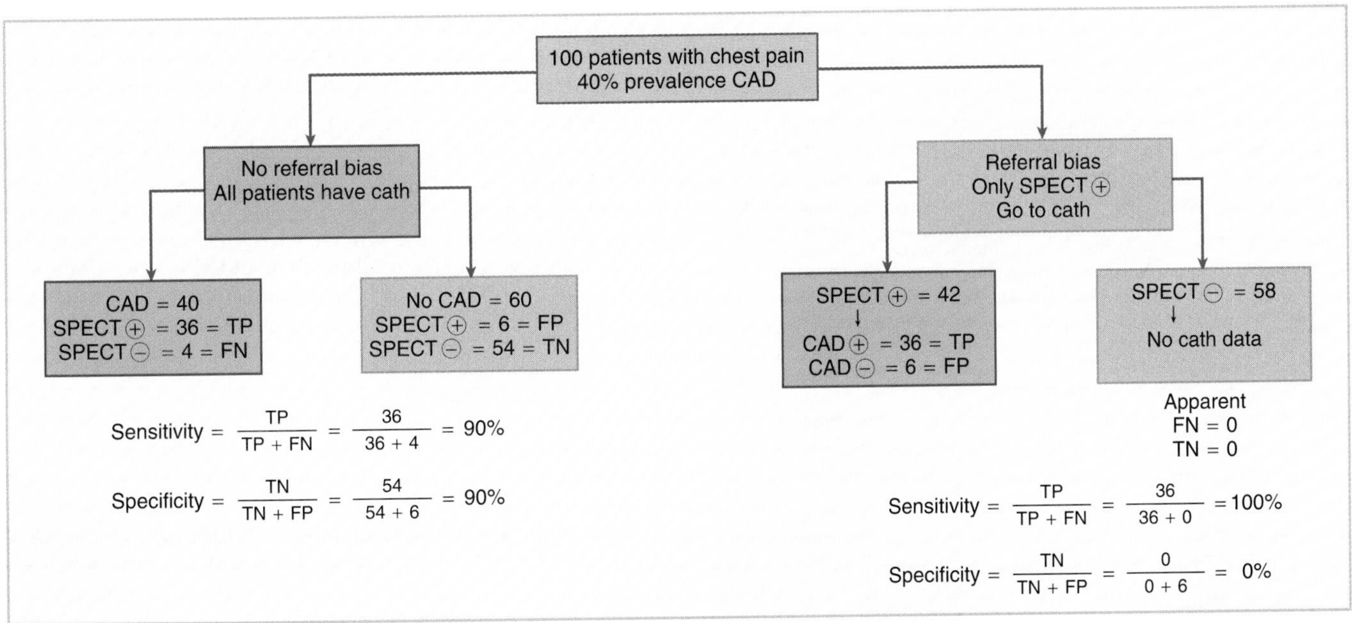

FIGURE 13-38 The effect of referral bias on specificity calculation. If the test being evaluated is used as the "gatekeeper" to coronary angiography, many patients who are true negatives (i.e., have a normal test and do not have coronary disease) will not undergo angiography and thus will not be included in the specificity calculations (right). This has an effect of artificially reducing the apparent specificity of the noninvasive test in question. CAD = coronary artery disease; FN = false negative; FP = false positive; TN = true negative; TP = true positive. (Adapted from Rozanski A, Diamond GA, Berman D, et al: The declining specificity of exercise radionuclide ventriculography. N Engl J Med.309:518, 1983.)

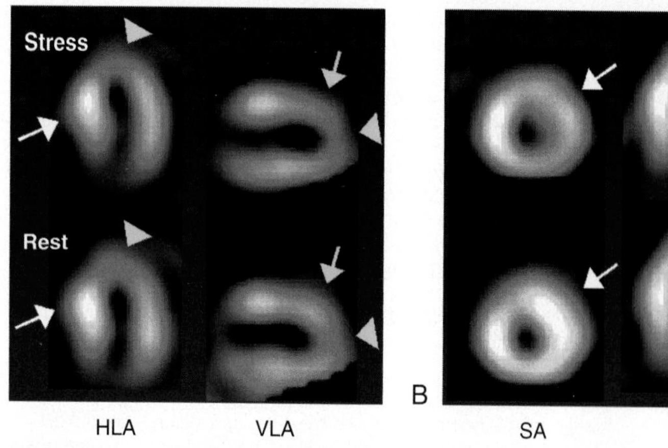

FIGURE 13–39 Single-photon emission computed tomography perfusion imaging in hypertrophic cardiomyopathy (HCM) in young asymptomatic patients with normal coronary arteries. **A,** Fixed perfusion defect of the apex consistent with infarction, indicated by yellow arrowheads in the horizontal (HLA) and vertical (VLA) long-axis images, with a reversible defect of the anterior wall (yellow arrows in the VLA images). The hypertrophied septum is evident (white arrows in the HLA images). **B,** Extensive inducible silent ischemia in the anterior, lateral, and inferior walls (white arrows). Transient ischemic cavity dilation is also present, possibly related to subendocardial ischemia.

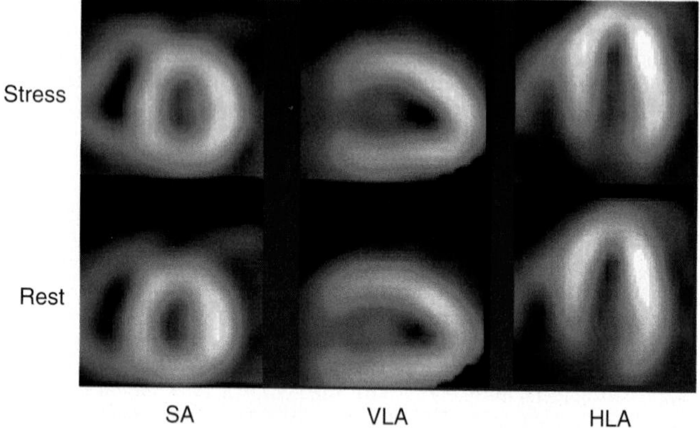

FIGURE 13–40 Single-photon emission computed tomography perfusion images at stress and rest from a patient with heart failure. The images depict a dilated left ventricle but with normal perfusion patterns, suggesting a low likelihood that coronary artery disease is the etiology of heart failure. HLA = horizontal long axis; SA = short axis; VLA = vertical long axis.

with HCM, approximately 50 percent have inducible, reversible perfusion abnormalities in the absence of CAD, typically involving the septum.[114] Such patients have more abnormal indices of diastolic function and demonstrate hemodynamic and metabolic abnormalities consistent with ischemia during atrial pacing tachycardia.[115] Thus, inducible perfusion defects in HCM represent inducible myocardial ischemia, possibly related to microvascular abnormalities, and as such have low specificity for CAD in patients with HCM. The blunted coronary flow reserve in patients with HCM is associated with a more unfavorable natural history.[112]

Left Ventricular Hypertrophy. As with the experience in HCM, inducible perfusion abnormalities may develop in patients with pressure overload LV hypertrophy (LVH) related to either hypertension or aortic stenosis.[116,117] In the absence of CAD, it is presumed that these abnormalities represent regional myocardial ischemia based on abnormal microcirculation and limited vasodilator reserve in patients with LVH. However, studies in patients with LVH by ECG criteria have generally demonstrated an accuracy of MPI for detecting CAD that is comparable to that in patients without LVH.[10] On the basis of such data, MPI is a class I indication for CAD detection when LVH is present on ECG according to ACC/AHA guidelines.[10] SPECT imaging data in patients with LVH also have a risk stratification value similar to that in patients without LVH.[118]

Dilated Cardiomyopathy. Abnormalities in myocardial perfusion are common in patients with dilated cardiomyopathy (DCM) despite normal epicardial coronary arteries.[119] Several studies have demonstrated abnormal coronary flow reserve in these patients, and as with data in HCM, blunted flow reserve identifies a cohort of patients with DCM with a more unfavorable natural history.[120,121] Such data support the relevance of the perfusion abnormalities rather than simply classifying them as false-positive if epicardial CAD is not present.

An important diagnostic consideration in patients with LV systolic dysfunction involves distinguishing those whose cardiomyopathy may be primarily due to CAD (many of whom have potentially reversible LV dysfunction) from those with idiopathic DCM. Although many patients with DCM may have perfusion abnormalities detected on MPI, the *absence* of perfusion abnormalities virtually excludes CAD as the etiology of the cardiomyopathy (Fig. 13-40).[122] *Extensive* perfusion abnormalities in the setting of LV dysfunction are virtually always associated with CAD rather than DCM, especially when the perfusion defects are segmental.

Endothelial Dysfunction. Abnormalities in myocardial perfusion detected by SPECT MPI in patients with coronary endothelial dysfunction, in the absence of "significant" epicardial vessel stenosis, have been demonstrated.[40] That these perfusion findings represent true abnormalities in coronary flow reserve is supported by studies showing *improvement* in perfusion on follow-up MPI after treatment with medical therapies directed at improving endothelial function.[123] Further support for this concept comes from cardiac magnetic resonance imaging studies demonstrating blunted subendocardial coronary flow reserve in patients with angina and normal coronary arteries.[124]

SENSITIVITY AND SPECIFICITY OF MYOCARDIAL PERFUSION IMAGING. The 2003 ACC/AHA/ASNC Radionuclide Imaging Guidelines summarize sensitivity and specificity data from 33 studies involving 4480 patients undergoing exercise SPECT imaging.[10] Sensitivity to detect CAD was 87 percent (range 71 to 97 percent) in this pooled analysis, and specificity to rule out CAD was 73 percent (range 36 to 100 percent). Few if any of these studies incorporated ECG-gated SPECT imaging of regional function or attenuation correction, techniques that appear to enhance specificity.[21] For example, in one study of women undergoing coronary angiography, specificity was improved from 76 to 96 percent when gated SPECT Tc 99m sestamibi imaging was used compared with non-gated SPECT thallium-201.[125]

Influence of Perfusion Tracer on Detection of Coronary Artery Disease. Despite the expectation of improved diagnostic accuracy with use of ^{99m}Tc-based agents, based on more favorable attributes as a radioisotope for gamma camera imaging compared with ^{201}Tl, studies comparing the widely used agents have not shown significant improvement in sensitivity or specificity. An exception is the demonstration of improved specificity in women with the use of ^{99m}Tc sestamibi compared with thallium,[125] as noted earlier. Thus, the choice of radiotracer for MPI does not notably affect the discrimination between the presence and absence of CAD. It is important to recognize that published studies often involve subjects who may not fully represent those who are most challenging to image. It would be expected that the ^{99m}Tc-based agents, with their greater photon energy, would offer improved performance in obese patients and those with large breasts as well as allow the option of higher quality gated images.

Influence of Automated Quantitation of Myocardial Perfusion Images in Detection of Coronary Artery Disease. There may be significant intra- and interobserver variability in the visual analysis of myocardial perfusion images. Several methods of quantitative analysis of MPI have been developed[10] to reduce the variability in reading by "objectifying" image analysis, by comparing regional uptake values with a normal data base.

Automated quantitative analysis systems are incorporated into most SPECT camera-computer equipment. Some of the most common are Emory Toolbox,[126] Cedars QPS,[127] and 4D MSPECT (Fig. 13–41).[128] Although published data do not clearly demonstrate improved sensitivity or specificity of these programs over visual analysis for CAD detection, such data arise from expert centers, often where the quantitative software was developed, and the visual analysis data are derived from experienced readers in laboratories with excellent quality control.

In practice, the use of contemporary quantitative programs can improve image acquisition quality as well as interpretation. Some programs incorporate motion-sensing algorithms that interrogate the raw data and alert the technologist that motion correction may be needed.

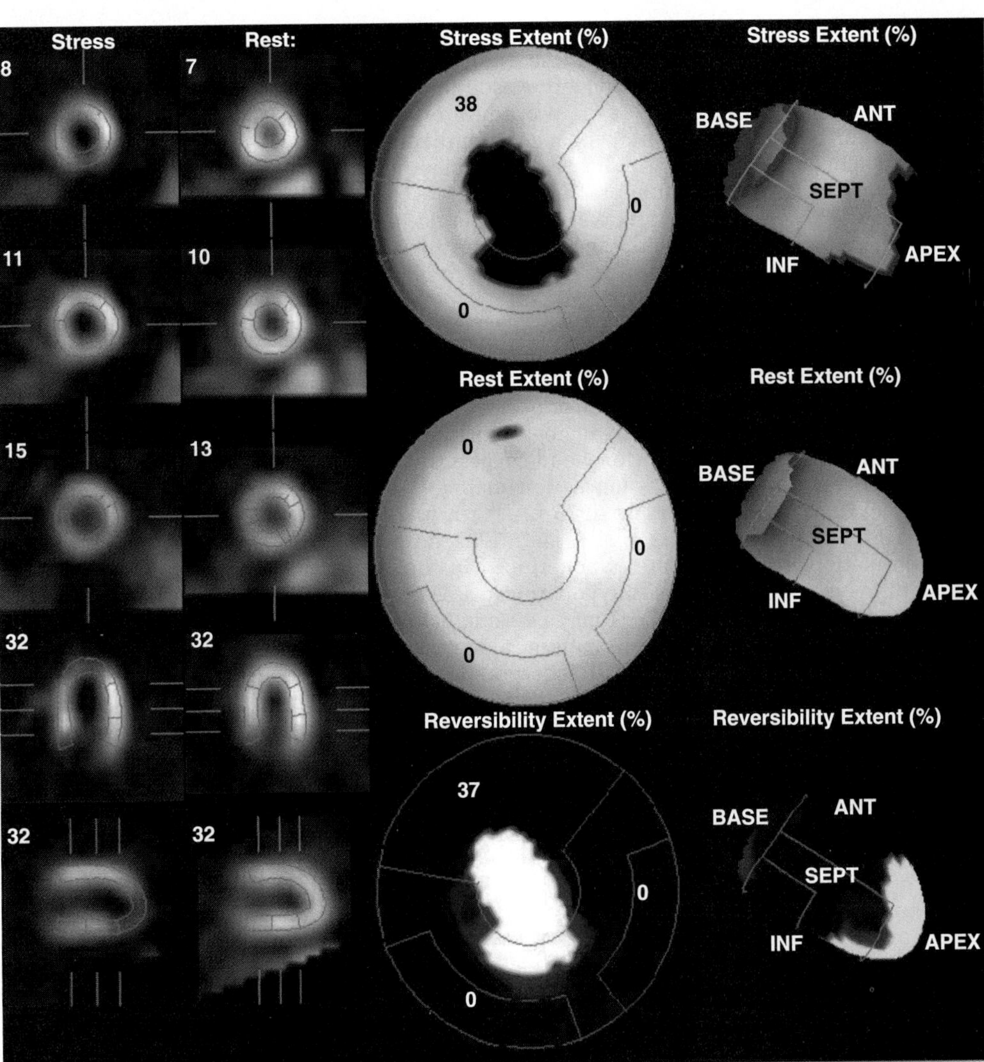

FIGURE 13–41 Automated quantitative analysis software. Selected short- and long-axis tomograms from stress and rest studies (two left columns) are automatically segmented and scored. Bull's-eye plots are created (third column) representing the stress (top) and rest (middle) data and demonstrate a large apical reversible defect. The bottom bull's-eye plot displays the extent of ischemic myocardium (white area), which measures 23 percent of the total myocardium. The bull's-eye information is also displayed in a three-dimensional format (right column, top, middle, and bottom, respectively). (Images courtesy of Guido Germano, Ph.D.)

PHARMACOLOGICAL STRESS TESTING FOR DETECTION OF CORONARY ARTERY DISEASE. Reports examining the sensitivity and specificity of vasodilator pharmacological stress combined with MPI for the detection of CAD have achieved results similar to those reported with exercise stress. A pooled analysis from the 2003 ACC/AHA/ASNC Radionuclide Imaging Guidelines involving 2465 catheterized patients in 17 studies[10] demonstrated sensitivity of 89 percent and specificity of 75 percent, similar to values from exercise SPECT MPI studies.

The more powerful hyperemic stress response achieved with vasodilator stress compared with exercise might be expected to result in improved sensitivity to detect CAD, particularly more moderate stenoses. This has not been demonstrated, possibly because of the "roll off" property of the common perfusion tracers, caused by diffusion limitation at hyperemic blood flow levels.[7] Thus, the more favorable hyperemic stress achieved with pharmacological stress is offset by the lack of linear tracer uptake in the areas with the highest flow.

The diagnostic ability of dobutamine stress imaging appears to be generally similar to that of other pharmacological and exercise stress modalities for the detection of CAD.[52] Relative to adenosine and dipyridamole, dobutamine results in a reduced hyperemic flow response, which may be exacerbated by an inadequate heart rate response. One study demonstrated that there is an increase in false-negative scans when patients with known positive dobutamine MPI are retested after receiving intravenous propranolol.[52] On the basis of these considerations, dobutamine is used only when adenosine or dipyridamole is contraindicated, such as in a patient with reactive airways disease.

EFFECT OF SUBMAXIMAL EXERCISE PERFORMANCE ON CORONARY ARTERY DISEASE DETECTION. The sensitivity of MPI to detect CAD is optimized by achieving the highest possible level of oxygen demand to stimulate the greatest increment in coronary flow reserve. In exercise ECG testing, sensitivity to detect CAD falls significantly if greater than 85 percent of maximum predicted heart rate for age is not achieved.[129] Because perfusion heterogeneity usually develops at a lower degree of supply-demand mismatch than ECG changes, the sensitivity of MPI to detect CAD is maintained at somewhat lower workloads. In one study, patients with CAD were stressed with MPI at a maximal workload and then again at a less than maximal workload.[130] There was no difference in sensitivity between the maximal and the submaximal tests. However, the extent and severity of reversible perfusion defects appear to be less at submaximal compared with maximal workloads, which may affect the prognostic value of the test.

Thus, the selection of a stress protocol can be summarized as follows[8,10]: exercise is the preferred stressor, as it allows the optimal potential association of symptoms with perfusion abnormalities. The use of exercise also allows incorporation of validated stress test criteria such as the DTS, heart rate reserve, or heart rate recovery with the MPI data.[42] For patients who cannot exercise adequately, vasodilator stress with adenosine or dipyridamole is the procedure of choice, with dobutamine used for patients with a contraindication to the vasodilators.[8,10] For patients who begin exercise but do not reach 85 percent of maximum predicted heart rate for age *or* who do not reach an appropriate symptomatic endpoint, isotope injection can be withheld, the exercise portion of the test terminated, and vasodilator stress performed to optimize diagnostic and risk stratification information.

DETECTING AND DEFINING THE EXTENT OF CORONARY ARTERY DISEASE. In formulating a management strategy for patients, it is important to determine the *extent* of disease rather than just the *presence or absence* of disease. The term "extensive CAD" refers to angiographic patterns of CAD that have prognostic significance and suggest treatment benefit from revascularization, such as left main or severe three-vessel CAD involving the proximal LAD artery.

SPECT MPI is limited by the relative nature of the perfusion information; if all areas are hypoperfused in the presence of three-vessel CAD, the least hypoperfused area appears normal and the true extent of CAD may be underestimated. However, although the perfusion pattern alone may not directly suggest the full extent of CAD, incorporation of other findings, including regional functional abnormalities, can be used to estimate more correctly the probability of disease extent.

Wall motion abnormalities on poststress gated SPECT imaging may be of benefit in the detection of extensive CAD. In one study,[131] incorporating the finding of poststress wall motion abnormality on gated SPECT imaging along with the degree of perfusion abnormality allowed improved sensitivity (85 to 91 percent) for detecting proximal 90 percent LAD lesions or multivessel disease related to 90 percent or greater proximal lesions. Similar findings have been reported for improving detection of three-vessel CAD.[132]

As noted previously, TID of the LV cavity and increased lung uptake of the perfusion tracer on poststress SPECT images have also been shown to enhance detection of multivessel CAD (see Fig. 13–8). Numerous reports suggest that the presence of TID raises the probability of multivessel CAD for any given extent of perfusion abnormality.[8,10]

Findings unrelated to imaging are also useful in enhancing the diagnosis of left main or three-vessel CAD. The development of greater than 2 mm of ST depression or hypotension on ECG treadmill testing increases the likelihood of left main or three-vessel CAD.[129]

DETECTION OF CORONARY ARTERY DISEASE IN WOMEN. The detection of CAD using exercise ECG testing is problematic in women.[90,129] A meta-analysis of 19 studies of exercise ECG testing in women revealed sensitivity and specificity of only 61 percent and 68 percent, respectively.[133] The use of ^{201}Tl for detecting CAD in women is limited by problems associated with breast attenuation. The use of ^{99m}Tc-labeled tracers should improve specificity as there is slightly less tissue attenuation, as demonstrated in a study comparing ^{201}Tl SPECT with ^{99m}Tc sestamibi gated SPECT for the detection of angiographic CAD.[125] With the incorporation of gated SPECT sestamibi imaging, a specificity of 92 percent was achieved compared with 67 percent with ^{201}Tl (see Fig. 13–10). A similar study confirmed these data in women, in whom a specificity of 91 percent was achieved using ^{99m}Tc sestamibi.[134]

DETECTION OF CORONARY ARTERY DISEASE IN VALVULAR HEART DISEASE. Several studies have evaluated the use of MPI in the assessment of the possible copresence of CAD in patients with valvular heart disease; most of the published studies involved patients with aortic stenosis. Sensitivity of MPI has ranged from 61 to 100 percent, with specificity 64 to 77 percent.[10] Although it is potentially useful in selected cases to assist in symptom evaluation, these performance characteristics are not sufficient to preclude the use of coronary angiography to define the presence of CAD in patients being considered for surgery.

RADIONUCLIDE ANGIOGRAPHY OR VENTRICULOGRAPHY FOR DETECTION OF CORONARY ARTERY DISEASE. Early reports of exercise RVG to detect CAD included predominantly patients with extensive CAD, resulting in high sensitivity. As the test was more widely applied to populations with less extensive disease, sensitivity values were lower. However, although the EF response to exercise may be a relatively insensitive marker of CAD, it is a powerful prognostic marker.[10,135]

As the LVEF response to exercise may be normal in many patients with less extensive CAD, a regional wall motion abnormality during exercise may be more sensitive for identifying CAD.[136] Radionuclide ventricular function data during exercise are usually acquired in only one view, the left anterior oblique "best septal" view.[27,28,135] Thus, the view of the inferior wall is limited, and regional wall motion abnormalities are insensitive for disease of the right coronary artery.

The normal range for an exercise EF response was initially defined by a group of young normal volunteers, a population that differs from those with chest pain and normal coronary arteriograms.[136] Posttest referral bias has also been invoked to explain the decline in specificity in exercise RVG.[137] However, as with a normal MPI study, a preserved ventricular response to exercise is associated with a good prognosis,[27,28,135] despite the presence of CAD.

In contrast to studies of MPI demonstrating little change in the ability to detect CAD at slightly submaximal workloads,[130] the sensitivity for detecting CAD by exercise RVG is impaired at submaximal workloads[137] A similar problem would be expected with stress echocardiographic studies of inducible regional wall motion abnormalities.

Exercise RVG is rarely used in contemporary practice for CAD detection. Sensitivity and specificity are modest, and visual image analysis of regional wall motion abnormalities is challenging. Nonetheless, the EF response to exercise or the absolute value of the exercise EF is a powerful prognostic indicator in suspected or known CAD, and these data have informed the contemporary use of poststress ECG-gated SPECT imaging as well as stress echocardiography.

Imaging in Patients with Established Coronary Artery Disease

There are several potential roles for SPECT MPI in patients who are known to have established CAD. Clinical questions may remain after angiography regarding the "physiological significance" of stenoses. The results of stress-rest SPECT MPI correlate generally with invasive measures of coronary flow reserve. Moreover, improvement of SPECT evidence of ischemia has been commonly documented after successful PCI, suggesting that SPECT MPI can identify the "culprit" ischemic lesion.[10]

Imaging after Coronary Artery Bypass Surgery. Studies of patients who develop recurrent symptoms after coronary artery bypass graft (CABG) surgery have demonstrated that SPECT MPI can accurately detect the presence and location of graft stenoses, even if the symptoms are atypical for ischemia.

A number of studies have concordantly demonstrated the risk stratification value of SPECT MPI in patients after CABG, especially late after CABG, even if symptoms are not present.[10] The extent of perfusion abnormality is related to the subsequent risk of cardiac death and nonfatal MI, and SPECT information has incremental predictive value over clinical and stress data (Fig. 13–42). As the outcome risk is generally low in the early years after CABG, *routine* assessment for the presence and extent of ischemia in an asymptomatic patient is not recommended by current guidelines. Nonetheless, in a study of almost 900 asymptomatic patients studied with SPECT MPI after CABG,[138] perfusion defects were common and were associated with significantly increased relative risk of death or

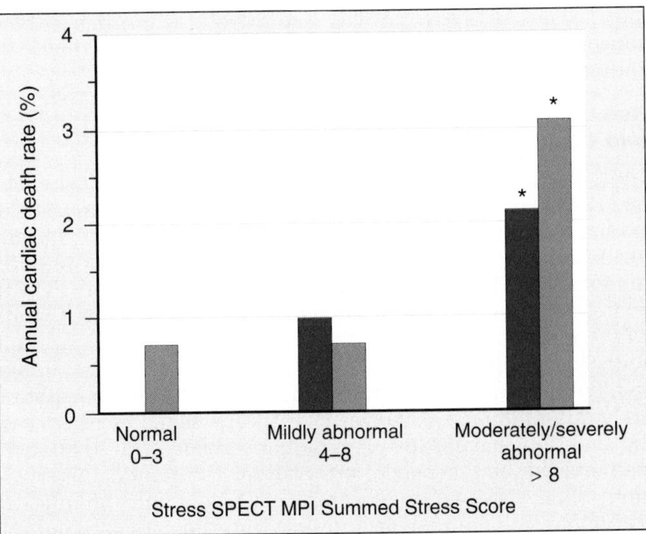

FIGURE 13–42 Annual cardiac death rate as a function of the extent of perfusion abnormality (as the summed stress score) in patients having coronary artery bypass graft (CABG) surgery within 5 years of testing (purple bars) or more than 5 years after CABG (blue bars). The risk of cardiac death increases significantly in both groups as the perfusion images become more abnormal, particularly with a moderate or severe abnormality (* $p < 0.05$ compared with other groups). MPI = myocardial perfusion imaging; SPECT = single-photon emission computed tomography. (Adapted from Zellweger M, Lewin H, Shenghan L, et al: When to stress patients after coronary artery bypass surgery? Risk stratification in patients early and late post-CABG using stress myocardial perfusion SPECT: Implications of appropriate clinical strategies. J Am Coll Cardiol 37:144, 2001.)

major events (as was impaired exercise capacity), even when controlling for time after CABG. In *symptomatic* post-CABG patients, such information can guide the need for catheterization and intervention. In *asymptomatic* patients, in whom aggressive secondary prevention strategies should be in place, the implications for clinical decision-making are less clear. In this situation, the *extent* of SPECT abnormality is important, as a more extensive perfusion abnormality is associated with a progressively higher risk of subsequent cardiac death or MI[139] and at some threshold would justify an invasive approach.

Imaging after Percutaneous Coronary Intervention. Exercise MPI is superior in detecting the presence and location of restenosis after PCI compared with exercise ECG, and current guidelines recommend stress imaging in symptomatic post-PCI patients.[10] In studies similar in concept to studies of patients with suspected CAD and those studied after CABG, the extent of SPECT MPI abnormality in patients studied after PCI is correlated with the subsequent risk of cardiac death or MI on long-term follow-up, even late after PCI, and this appears to hold true in patients even in the absence of symptoms.[140] Thus, although *routine* assessment of patients after PCI with SPECT MPI is not currently recommended, important information may be gleaned by imaging of symptomatic patients to guide decisions regarding reintervention and in selected high-risk asymptomatic patients late after PCI, to assess subsequent risk.[10]

Reports have suggested that very early after PCI, SPECT MPI may demonstrate a mild reversible defect in the territory of the treated vessel (although less severe than before PCI).[10] This may be due to delayed return of full coronary flow reserve after PCI, thus representing a true physiological phenomenon.

Left Ventricular Function During Exercise in Patients with Known Coronary Artery Disease. The EF response to exercise (as determined by exercise RVG) can be considered a reflection of the impact of regional ischemia on global ventricular performance. Even among patients with three-vessel disease by angiography, the EF response to exercise may be maintained.[136] This finding may be due to the possibility that only small areas of the LV become ischemic if some of the stenoses are not physiologically significant or if distal vessels are well collateralized. Patients with three-vessel disease who have an abnormal exercise EF response are at high risk for adverse events over follow-up and thus are more likely to benefit from revascularization.[136,141] In contrast, patients who manifest a more normal EF response to exercise have a more favorable natural history and thus are less likely to benefit from revacularization in terms of natural history.

Detection of Preclinical Coronary Artery Disease and Risk Stratification in Asymptomatic Subjects

As sudden cardiac death is too often the first manifestation of CAD, there is interest in screening populations for CAD or for CAD risk. On the basis of Bayesian principles, the low prevalence of CAD in the general asymptomatic population results in low predictive value of a positive test (for detection of CAD or determining risk of events), although negative predictive value is high. Current guidelines do not recommend routine stress MPI in asymptomatic populations.[10]

There may be circumstances, however, in which the baseline risk of a specific asymptomatic population may warrant testing with MPI. In a study of asymptomatic siblings of patients with known CAD, an abnormal SPECT MPI was associated with a fivefold increase in risk for cardiac events, with higher relative risk if both stress MPI and ECG were abnormal.[142] A key question in considering the use of testing such as SPECT MPI in asymptomatic populations is how the information will be used to manage or reduce risk. Current guidelines suggest aggressive risk factor reduction in those at high clinical risk for the development of vascular disease.[143] Whether further intensification of risk factor reduction in the setting of an abnormal imaging test, or diminished aggressiveness of risk factor reduction in the setting of a normal MPI study, results in improved outcomes is unproved and worthy of study.

Patients with diabetes are at significant risk for CAD development and cardiac events. An emerging literature suggests that a substantial proportion of *asymptomatic* diabetic patients have abnormal SPECT MPI studies and that such patients may be at even higher risk for events over time. Studies have suggested that 20 to 40 percent of asymptomatic diabetic patients have abnormal SPECT MPI studies, often with evidence of inducible, silent ischemia.[144-146] SPECT MPI has substantial risk stratification value in patients with diabetes, with risk being higher for any given perfusion abnormality than in nondiabetic patients. Moreover, similar risk stratification value has been demonstrated for diabetic patients who are *asymptomatic and without known CAD*.[146] Although guidelines at present do not suggest routine screening of asymptomatic diabetic patients with stress SPECT MPI, ongoing studies of prognosis and randomized trials in asymptomatic diabetic patients should clarify the role of SPECT MPI in diabetes.

Radionuclide Imaging in Acute Coronary Syndromes

Application of Radionuclide Imaging: Answering the Clinical Questions

For patients with *suspected* acute coronary syndromes (ACSs), radionuclide imaging techniques can both play a diagnostic role (is the clinical syndrome due to ischemia and CAD?) and provide prognostic information. Among patients who present with an ACS and ST segment depression or elevation, the typical role for imaging is in the stabilized patient, to provide risk stratification information to drive a management strategy aimed at improving natural history.

Acute Coronary Syndromes in the Emergency Department

Many patients present to EDs with symptoms suggestive of ACS but with nondiagnostic ECG findings and are often admitted to an observation unit for serial biomarker studies and possible stress testing. ^{99m}Tc- based perfusion agents may be administered to a patient in the ED with images acquired 45 to 60 minutes later,[147] and as there is minimal redistribution, images reflect myocardial blood flow *at the time of injection*.

In this setting, negative predictive value for ruling out MI has equaled or exceeded 99 percent in all observational series.[147] Patients with positive MPI have a higher risk of cardiac events during the index hospitalization as well as during follow-up (Fig. 13–43A and B). Thus, rest SPECT MPI provides information to assist triage decisions (admit or not admit) in the ED.

One study[148] found SPECT sestamibi imaging performed in the ED 92 percent sensitive for detecting acute MI, whereas

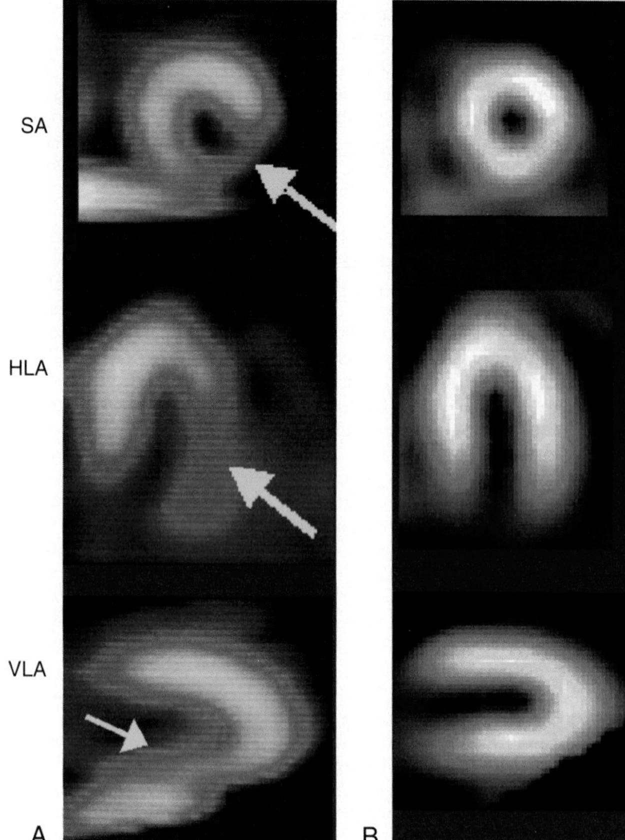

FIGURE 13–43 Examples of resting single-photon emission computed tomography (SPECT) images in patients evaluated in the emergency department with chest pain and nondiagnostic initial electrocardiographic findings. **A,** Patient with a severe inferolateral resting perfusion defect (arrows) suggestive of resting ischemia or infarction in that territory. Subsequent emergent angiography demonstrated an occluded left circumflex artery. **B,** Normal resting SPECT myocardial perfusion imaging study in a patient presenting with atypical chest pain and a nondiagnostic initial electrocardiogram in the emergency department. This normal study is associated with a very high negative predictive value for ruling out an acute coronary syndrome. HLA = horizontal long axis; SA = short axis; VLA = vertical long axis.

initial troponin I values in samples drawn at the same time had a sensitivity of only 39 percent. The maximum troponin I over the first 24 hours had a sensitivity similar to that of rest sestamibi imaging but at a distinctly later time point. Thus, acute MPI has the potential to identify ACS *earlier* than biomarkers. SPECT perfusion imaging data have been shown to provide incremental risk stratification value over clinical data for predicting unfavorable cardiac events.[149] One randomized study[150] of 46 ED patients with ongoing chest pain and a nondiagnostic ECG test found that an MPI-guided strategy incurred lower costs and resulted in shorter lengths of stay.

The Emergency Room Assessment of Sestamibi for Evaluation of (ERASE) Chest Pain Trial[151] randomly assigned 2475 patients with symptoms suggestive of ACS to a usual evaluation strategy or a strategy including acute rest SPECT MPI information. There was a significant 20 percent relative reduction in unnecessary admissions of patients ultimately found *not to have* ACS for those randomly assigned to the MPI strategy. The imaging data were among the most powerful factors associated with the decision to discharge the patient appropriately from the ED.

Thus, evidence from controlled, randomized trials suggests that incorporating SPECT MPI in ED patients with suspected ACS but no definitive ECG changes can improve triage decisions. The ACC/AHA/ASNC Radionuclide Imaging Guidelines classify MPI in this setting as a class I, level A indication.

Non-ST-Segment Elevation Myocardial Infarction and Unstable Angina

Guidelines suggest that patients with high-risk clinical characteristics in the setting of unstable angina (UA) should undergo direct catheterization.[89] Contemporary clinical trials suggest that patients with positive biomarkers, or those with a high-risk Thrombolysis in Myocardial Infarction (TIMI) score, benefit in terms of outcomes from an "invasive" strategy.[152] For patients with intermediate or low clinical risk, i.e., with "medically stabilized" UA, stress MPI has been shown to have substantial risk stratification value.[10] Patients without ischemia or infarct, especially in the presence of preserved LV function, have a low-risk outcome, suggesting that such patients can be managed conservatively without catheterization (Fig. 13–44),[153] whereas patients with significant inducible ischemia are at high-risk and thus are selected for intervention (see Fig. 13–44). The ACC/AHA/ASNC Radionuclide Imaging Guidelines[10] classify the use of stress MPI for detecting residual ischemia and the use of RVG or gated SPECT to assess LV function as class I indications.

Although the results of randomized clinical trials such as Treat Angina with Aggrastat and determine Cost of Therapy with an Invasive or Conservative Strategy (TACTICS)-TIMI 18 and others suggest slight superiority of an invasive approach in patients with UA or non–ST segment elevation MI (NSTEMI), subgroup analyses suggest that an important proportion of patients may be well managed by the conservative strategy of risk stratification by MPI followed by more selective catheterization and intervention. A retrospective analysis of the TIMI-III-B trial data has shown that by using a simple clinical score (based on age, creatine kinase with muscle and brain subunits, history of accelerated angina, and ST depression on the electrocardiogram), more than half of the population could be classified as at low risk with no outcome benefit after an early invasive strategy.[154] In TACTICS-TIMI 18, the troponin-positive subgroup, constituting 60 percent of the total population, had a larger reduction in death or MI with the early invasive strategy.[152] Therefore, patients of the TACTICS type without elevation of troponin or high TIMI risk score[155] may be optimally managed by a more conservative approach with risk stratification by using imaging techniques.

ST Segment Elevation Myocardial Infarction

Clinical variables such as recurrent ischemia, heart failure, and nonacute arrhythmias during hospitalization for acute ST segment elevation MI (STEMI) identify a subgroup of patients at high risk in whom early catheterization and intervention are indicated.[156] However, patients surviving the initial acute period may have a relatively stable course, and current guidelines suggest that noninvasive risk stratification prior to hospital discharge is appropriate.[10,156]

ASSESSMENT OF INDUCIBLE ISCHEMIA AFTER ACUTE MYOCARDIAL INFARCTION. Three major determinants of natural history risk following an acute MI include residual resting LV function; the extent of ischemic, jeopardized myocardium; and the susceptibility to ventricular arrhythmias. Thus, measures of LV function and the extent of inducible ischemia would be expected to provide important prognostic information in the aftermath of acute STEMI. Gated SPECT MPI, on the basis of the comprehensive ability to provide this information, has the potential to be the single most important test in the stable patient following STEMI.

In one of the earliest studies to examine the relation of MPI data to outcomes in stable patients following MI, thallium-

201 scintigraphic data contained the most robust information on stratifying post-MI risk. A "low-risk" thallium-201 image (no reversible defects and no lung uptake) was associated with a very low risk natural history outcome after MI.[157]

An important proportion of patients following uncomplicated MI are not able to exercise, even to a submaximal workload. Using pharmacological stress MPI in the post-MI setting, the presence of reversible defects has been reported as the only significant predictor of cardiac events on multivariable analysis,[158] whereas the absence of reversible defects identified a low-risk cohort. Subsequent reports[159] confirmed these findings.

Studies in the reperfusion era have reported generally similar results regarding the relation of stress-induced ischemia to post-MI outcomes. In a study of 134 consecutive patients within 14 days of an uncomplicated MI,[160] the extent of ischemia on the SPECT MPI was the only significant correlate of a future cardiac event on Cox regression analysis (Fig. 13–45). The extent of SPECT ischemia remained a strong correlate of a cardiac event in those who received thrombolytic therapy. The *quantitated* extent of ischemia on adenosine SPECT MPI was reported as an important predictor of post-MI cardiac events in another large study of post-MI risk stratification.[161]

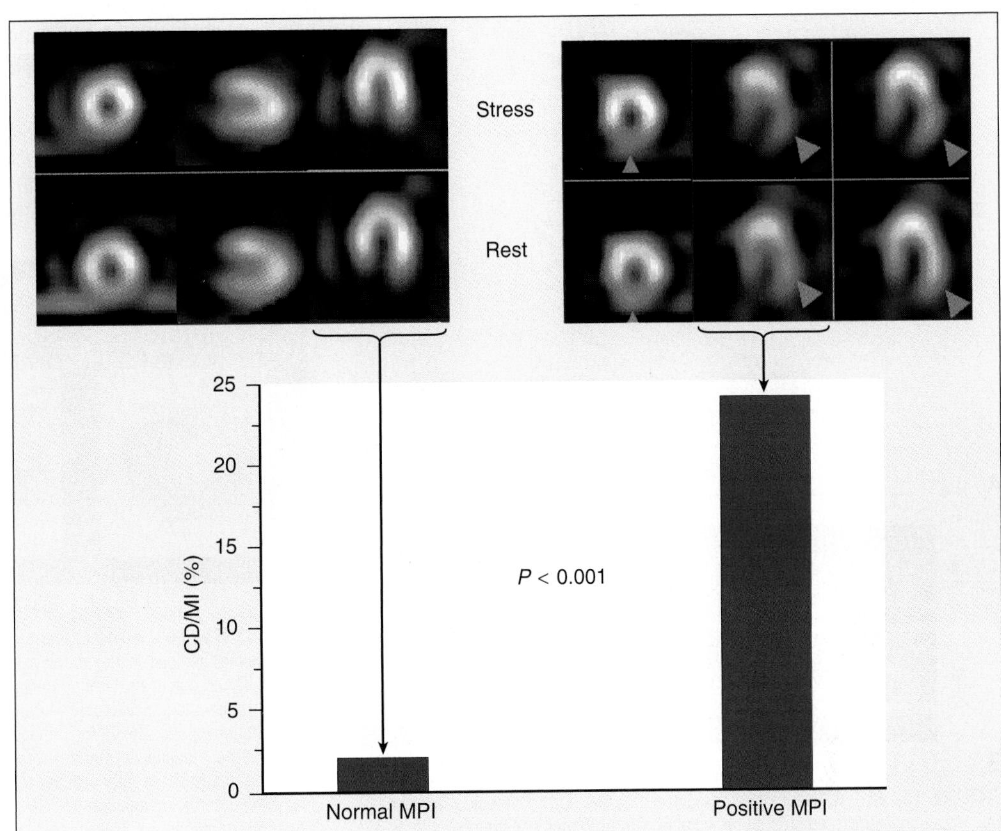

FIGURE 13–44 Single-photon emission computed tomography (SPECT) perfusion imaging in patients after medical stabilization of unstable angina. **Upper left,** Normal study, associated with a low risk of cardiac events during follow-up, suggesting that such a patient can be managed conservatively without catheterization, but with aggressive secondary preventive strategies. The bottom graph is a summary of predictive values of SPECT imaging in the aftermath of unstable angina from multiple studies. Similar to the concepts in populations with stable chest pain, the presence of abnormal perfusion imaging after unstable angina is associated with a substantial increase in the risk of cardiac death or myocardial infarction (CD/MI) during follow-up. **Upper right,** An example of a high-risk stress-rest SPECT myocardial perfusion imaging (MPI) study in the aftermath of unstable angina. Despite the stabilization of symptoms, extensive reversible perfusion abnormalities in the inferior and lateral walls suggest high risk of cardiac death or myocardial infarction, or both, during follow-up. Thus, this patient would be managed more aggressively with catheterization and intervention. (Adapted in part from Brown KA: Management of unstable angina: The role on noninvasive risk stratification. J Nucl Cardiol 4:S164,1997.)

These data are representative of the contemporary management of MI in large populations and suggest that there is an important role for post-MI gated SPECT MPI in the current era. By analogy with the data for stable outpatient populations, post-MI patients with extensive inducible ischemia are at high risk for future cardiac events, and interventional management is likely to result in improved outcome.

Clinical Trials Incorporating Results of Stress Testing Following Myocardial Infarction. The true utility of a risk-predictive test is best demonstrated insofar as it can be used not only to *predict* outcomes but also for clinical decision-making to *improve* outcomes. In this regard, several studies have been reported in which the presence of inducible ischemia following MI was used to guide clinical decisions.

The TIMI phase II trial[162] randomly assigned 3339 patients who received intravenous tissue plasminogen activator for acute MI to either an invasive strategy (catheterization at 18 to 48 hours after MI with angioplasty or CABG on the basis of angiographic findings) or a conservative arm in which catheterization was performed only in response to spontaneous or inducible ischemia (by stress RVG). The 1-year outcomes were similar with the two strategies, suggesting that a noninvasive strategy is associated with *similar outcomes* with less need for catheterization and revascularization compared with a direct catheterization strategy, implying cost-effectiveness.

The *absence* of scintigraphic ischemia has also been investigated for its influence on clinical decision-making after MI. In a study involving patients who had received thrombolytic therapy and had a *negative* functional test for ischemia in the setting of a residual infarct artery stenosis, patients were randomly assigned to medical therapy or to angioplasty of the residual stenosis.[163] Infarct-free survival was 98 percent at 12 months in the conservative therapy group and 91 percent in the group randomly assigned to PCI. These data suggest that patients with *no evidence of scintigraphic ischemia within the infarct zone on stress MPI,* even in the setting of a residual stenosis of the infarct-related artery, derive no benefit from angioplasty of the infarct-related artery.

These results suggest that testing for the presence and extent of myocardial ischemia in the aftermath of an acute MI can play an important role in clinical decision-making regarding the need for, and benefit of, catheterization and revascularization and can also identify a cohort of patients whose outcome is favorable *without* catheterization.

VERY EARLY POST-MYOCARDIAL INFARCTION RISK STRATIFICATION. Because pharmacological stress with

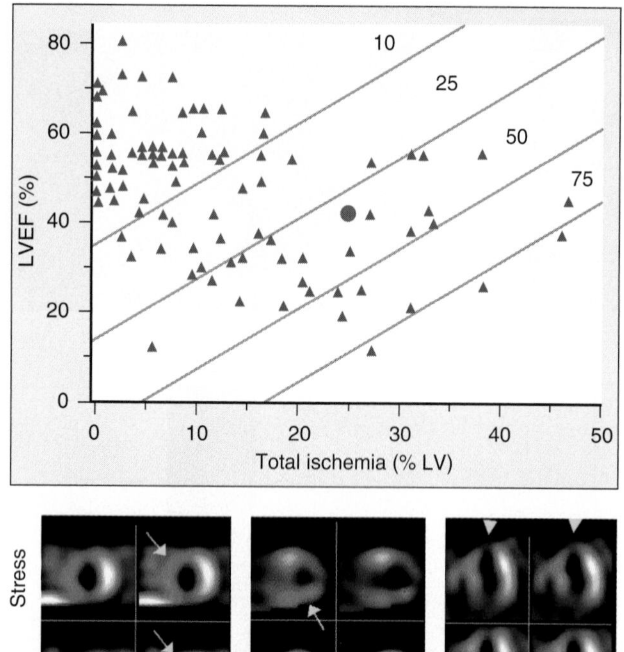

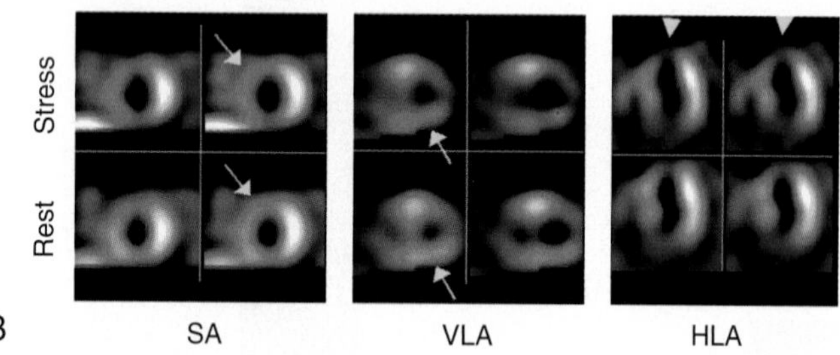

FIGURE 13–45 **A,** Risk of cardiac event during long-term follow-up after myocardial infarction (MI) is predicted by the combination of infarct size (represented by left ventricular ejection fraction [LVEF]) and the extent of reversible ischemia. As the extent of inducible ischemia increases (x-axis), and the LVEF decreases (y-axis), the outcome risk increases. The blue lines represent isobars of 10, 25, 50, and 75 percent risk of an adverse event during post-MI follow-up. The large red symbol refers to the images in panel B. **B,** Example of a patient studied several days after acute ST segment elevation MI and medical stabilization. Besides the fixed defect representing the MI in the anterior wall and apex (arrowhead), there is extensive inducible ischemia both within and remote from the infarct territory (septum and inferior walls, arrows), involving 25 percent of the ventricle. Gated single-photon emission computed tomography EF was 38 percent. On the basis of the data in A, there is an approximately 25 percent risk of post-MI adverse event (large red circle in A). HLA = horizontal long axis; SA = short axis; VLA = vertical long axis. (Adapted from Mahmarian JJ, Mahmarian AC, Marks GF, et al: Role of adenosine thallium-201 tomography for defining long term risk in patients after acute myocardial infarction. J Am Coll Cardiol 25:1333, 1995.)

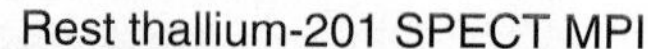

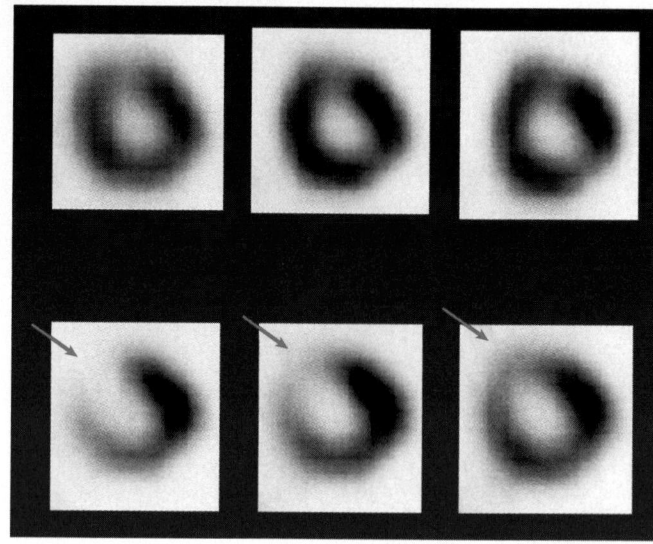

FIGURE 13–46 Iodine-123-beta-methyliodopentadecanoic acid (BMIPP) imaging of ischemic memory. In the top row, multiple short-axis tomograms of thallium-201 uptake at rest demonstrate near-homogeneous resting perfusion in a patient who presented to an emergency department and whose symptoms of chest pain had resolved many hours earlier. The BMIPP images in the same short-axis tomographic planes demonstrate a significant anteroseptal defect (arrows), suggesting prolonged postischemic suppression of fatty acid metabolism, referred to as "ischemic memory." MPI = myocardial perfusion imaging; SPECT = single-photon emission computed tomography. (Adapted from Kawai Y, Tsukamoto E, Nozaki Y, et al: Significance of reduced uptake of iodinated fatty acid analogues for the evaluation of patients with acute chest pain. J Am Coll Cardiol 38:1888, 2001.)

adenosine or dipyridamole induces coronary hyperemia with only minimal increments in oxygen demand, it may potentially be performed safely even very early after MI. This concept was examined[164] in a study of 451 patients randomly assigned to a standard post-MI evaluation strategy or to a strategy incorporating dipyridamole SPECT MPI *2 to 3 days* after uncomplicated MI. The testing was safe, and MPI supplied better risk stratification data predicting outcomes than the submaximal stress MPI data. Thus, pharmacological stress can safely allow management decisions to be made earlier in the post-MI course.

STUDIES EXAMINING BOTH PERFUSION IMAGING AND LEFT VENTRICULAR FUNCTION AFTER ACUTE MYOCARDIAL INFARCTION. As post-MI EF falls, there is a progressive increase in mortality risk. The availability of gated SPECT imaging to evaluate myocardial perfusion and LV function simultaneously raises an important question regarding the incremental information provided by combining the analysis of perfusion and function information within one test.

One study[165] comprehensively evaluated LV function and adenosine SPECT MPI in patients in relation to long-term cardiac events. Both the extent of perfusion defect and LVEF provided superior risk categorization compared with either variable alone. These data strongly suggest that perfusion abnormalities and LVEF following MI have complementary roles, and their measurement together powerfully categorizes patients' risk in the post-MI setting.

Radionuclide Imaging for Acute Coronary Syndromes: Research Directions

Imaging Ischemic Memory. A possible future approach to risk stratification in patients with *suspected* ACS involves the imaging of fatty acid metabolism. As noted earlier, following a regional ischemic insult, abnormalities in fatty acid metabolism may persist long after perfusion has returned to normal, a finding termed ischemic memory. Imaging fatty acid metabolism may therefore allow assessment of *recent* ischemia. The radiolabeled fatty acid analog 15-(*p*-[iodine-123] iodophenyl)-3-(*R,S*) methylpentadecanoic acid (BMIPP) was imaged with SPECT 1 to 5 days after presentation in patients with suspected ACS. The BMIPP images showed greater sensitivity than did rest MPI in identifying the presence and site of the culprit coronary stenosis (Fig. 13–46).[166] Future studies will determine whether such techniques can help guide management decisions.

Imaging of Potentially Unstable Atherosclerotic Plaques and Platelet Activation. Plaque rupture exposes the lipid core to platelet activation. ^{125}I-labeled low-density lipoprotein has been used to image atherosclerotic disease in carotid arteries. A radionuclide target for macrophages, ^{131}I-labeled monocyte chemoattractant protein-1, has been shown to accumulate in lipid-rich, macrophage-rich regions in animal models of atherosclerosis.[167,168] Whether these favorable results in animals can be translated to the clinical setting of patients with potentially unstable atherosclerosis is a subject of ongoing study.

Assessment of Heart Failure with Radionuclide Imaging

Is Coronary Artery Disease the Etiology of Heart Failure?

Determining whether LV dysfunction is due predominantly to the consequences of CAD or to one of the many other etiologies included in the term "nonischemic" cardiomyopathy is a critical early step in the management of patients with heart failure. Because CAD is the most common cause of heart failure in developed countries, noninvasive assessment of myocardial ischemia and viability would identify the subgroup of patients with heart failure who have a potentially *reversible* degree of LV dysfunction and may benefit from revascularization. Therapeutic interventions that improve dysfunctional but viable myocardium may significantly affect global LVEF, LV remodeling, and patients' survival. Furthermore, the identification of CAD in patients with heart failure has implications in secondary prevention strategies, as acute MI is a common mechanism of death in patients with heart failure.

A *normal* stress MPI scan in a patient with heart failure and LV dysfunction is highly predictive for the *absence* of CAD. Studies of MPI for detecting CAD in patients with LV dysfunction have shown high sensitivity but modest specificity (Fig. 13–47; see Fig. 13–40).[122] The modest specificity of MPI to rule out CAD is explained in part by pathological as well as cardiac magnetic resonance imaging studies[169] demonstrating that patients with "nonischemic" cardiomyopathy may have patchy or larger confluent territories of fibrosis or scarring, manifest as fixed defects on SPECT MPI. Invasive studies as well as PET imaging have demonstrated attenuated coronary blood flow at rest and during hyperemic stress in nonischemic cardiomyopathy,[121,170] which could be manifest as reversible defects. Hence, both fixed and reversible perfusion defects have been observed in patients with nonischemic cardiomyopathy, with important prognostic implications.[122,170]

Although the presence of *any* perfusion abnormality is not specific for ruling out CAD, the *pattern* of perfusion abnormality may assist in the differentiation between CAD and "nonischemic" etiology of heart failure. *More extensive* or *more severe* perfusion defects, or both, are more likely to represent CAD, whereas smaller and milder defects are more likely in patients with nonischemic cardiomyopathy.[10,122,171]

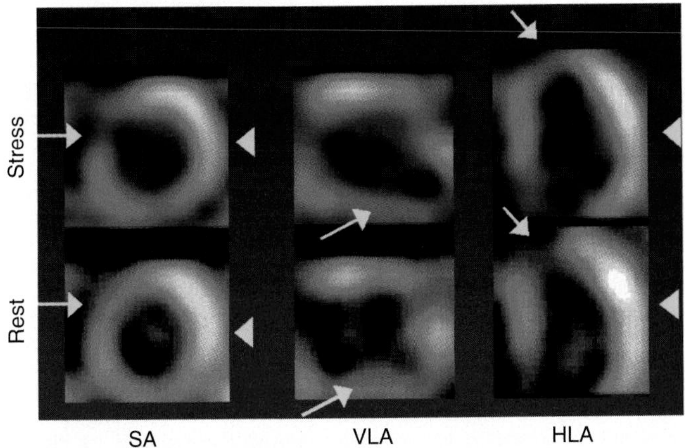

FIGURE 13–47 Single-photon emission computed tomography perfusion imaging demonstrating extensive severe fixed defects of the septum, apex, and inferior wall (arrows) suggestive of extensive prior myocardial infarction, as well as extensive inducible ischemia of the lateral wall (arrowheads). This strongly suggests that coronary artery disease is the etiology of the heart failure syndrome in this patient. HLA = horizontal long axis; SA = short axis; VLA = vertical long axis.

Hence, comprehensive early evaluation of patients with heart failure and LV systolic dysfunction includes an assessment of the underlying etiology (CAD or noncoronary causes). If CAD is identified as a causative factor in the heart failure syndrome, assessment of the extent of inducible ischemia and preserved viability within dysfunctional myocardium aids in determining the potential for reversal of LV dysfunction following revascularization.

Assessment of Myocardial Viability and the Potential Benefit of Revascularization

The goal of assessing viability is to optimize selection of patients with heart failure whose symptoms and natural history may improve following revascularization. Data suggest that hibernation and stress-induced ischemia are common in patients with stable heart failure, even in the absence of angina.[172] In a clinical trial of stable community-based patients with heart failure of whom only a minority had angina, hibernation or stress-induced ischemia, or both, were demonstrated by SPECT imaging in approximately 70 percent of patients, suggesting that an important subpopulation of patients with heart failure may benefit from a noninvasive search for viability and ischemia.

Studies have demonstrated that the *potential for improved heart failure symptoms* following revascularization correlates with the magnitude of the PET "mismatch" pattern (i.e., enhanced FDG uptake relative to perfusion).[173] In a meta-analysis of outcome studies after viability imaging, patients with evidence of preserved myocardial viability[174] who underwent revascularization had a substantial reduction in the *risk of cardiac death* during long-term follow-up (Fig. 13–48). Revascularization conferred no natural history advantage in patients without substantial myocardial viability. These data suggest that noninvasive imaging of viability and ischemia can play an important role in selecting patients for revascularization, with the expectation of improving symptoms and natural history.

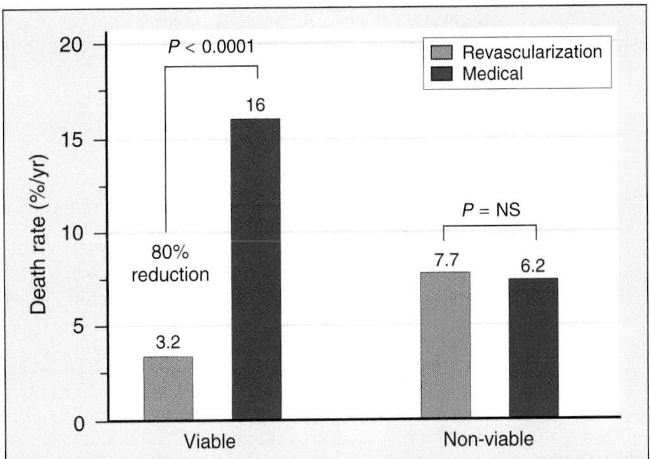

FIGURE 13–48 Outcome of patients with ischemic left ventricular dysfunction after viability testing. Among patients determined to have predominantly viable myocardium, treatment with medical therapy is associated with a 16 percent annual risk of cardiac death. Similar patients treated with revascularization have only a 3.2 percent annual risk of cardiac death, representing an 80 percent reduction in risk with revascularization. In contrast, patients with predominantly nonviable myocardium have no difference in outcome whether they are treated with medical therapy or revascularization. These data suggest that noninvasive interrogation of myocardial viability can identify treatment strategies associated with more favorable long-term outcomes. (Adapted from Allman K, Shaw L, Hachamovitch R, Udelson JE: Myocardial viability testing and impact of revascularization on prognosis in patients with coronary artery disease and left ventricular dysfunction: A meta-analysis. J Am Coll Cardiol 39:1151, 2002.)

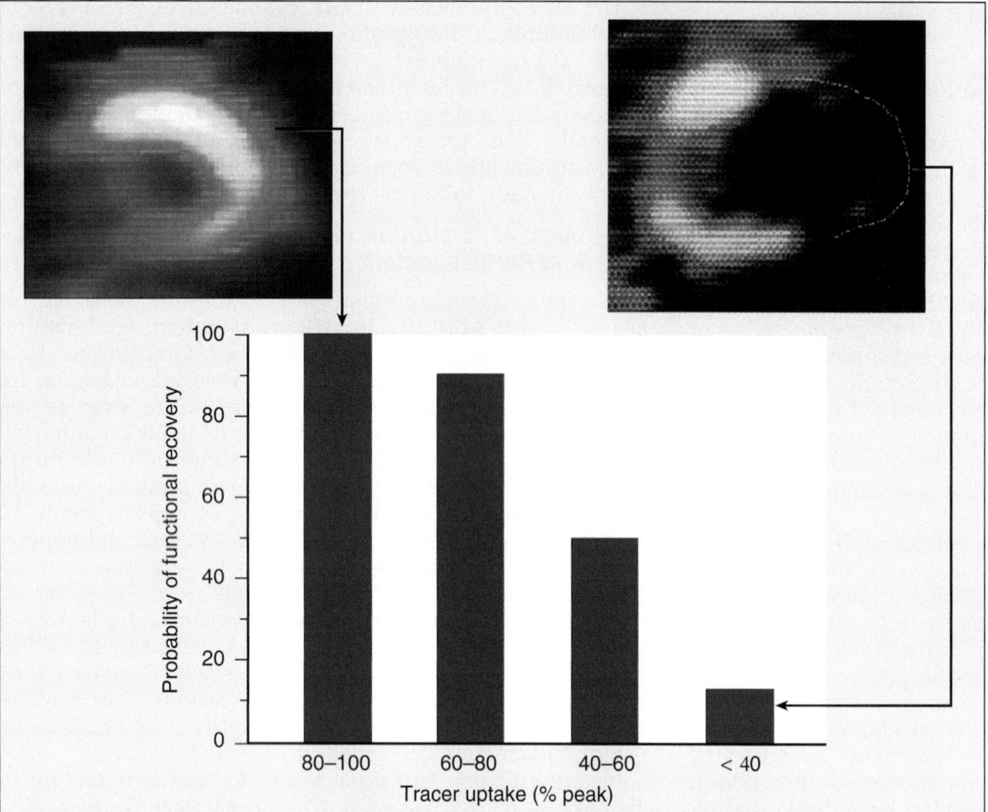

FIGURE 13–49 Relation between tracer uptake in a dysfunctional territory and the subsequent probability of functional recovery after revascularization. The probability of improved regional left ventricular function after revascularization is significantly related to the quantitative degree of tracer uptake. **Upper right,** A patient with a large, severe defect in the anterior and apical walls. The severity of the defect suggests that significant functional recovery would not be expected with revascularization. **Upper left,** Extensive myocardial viability in a patient with left ventricular dysfunction (ejection fraction 30 percent) and severe three-vessel coronary disease. There is substantial tracer uptake throughout the anterior wall and apex (arrow), territories with significant regional dysfunction. The retained degree of tracer uptake suggests extensive myocardial (myocyte) viability and high probability of functional recovery after revascularization. (Adapted from Bonow RO: Assessment of myocardial viability with thallium-201. *In* Zaret BL, Beller GA [eds]: Nuclear Cardiology: State of the Art and Future Directions. St. Louis, Mosby, 1999, pp 503-512; and Udelson JE: Assessment of myocardial viability with technetium-99m-labeled agents. *In* Zaret BL, Beller GA [eds]: Nuclear Cardiology: State of the Art and Future Directions. St. Louis, Mosby, 1999, pp 513-533.)

PRINCIPLES OF ASSESSING MYOCARDIAL VIABILITY BY RADIONUCLIDE TECHNIQUES

The radionuclide tracers and techniques most often used to assess viability have been evaluated for their relation to preserved tissue viability directly by correlating tracer uptake with histologically confirmed extent of tissue viability.[34] Quantitative analysis of tracer uptake correlates directly with the magnitude of preservation of tissue viability, and tracer uptake represents a *continuous variable*; i.e., the magnitude of tracer uptake directly reflects the magnitude of preserved tissue viability.[175,176] For a dysfunctional segment or territory, the probability of functional recovery after revascularization is related to the magnitude of tracer uptake, representing the degree of preserved myocardial viability (extent of hibernation or stunning) within that territory. A dysfunctional territory with normal or only mildly reduced tracer uptake thus has a high likelihood of improved function after revascularization. In contrast, a territory with a severe reduction in tracer uptake would represent predominant infarction, and the likelihood of improved function after revascularization would be low (Fig. 13–49). The magnitude of potential improvement of *global LV function* after revascularization is in turn determined by the extent of viable dysfunctional myocardium.

Imaging Protocols for Assessing Myocardial Viability

Thallium-201. The presence of thallium-201 after redistribution implies preserved myocyte cellular viability. However, as the *absence* of thallium-201 uptake on the redistribution images is not a sufficient sign of the *absence* of regional viability, iterations of the standard thallium-201 protocol have been investigated[175,177] in order to optimize the assessment of regional viability (Fig. 13–50A and B). After thallium-201 *reinjection*, approximately 50 percent of regions with "fixed" defects on stress-redistribution imaging show significant enhancement of thallium-201 uptake, predictive of improvement in regional LV function (see Fig. 13–50A). The presence of a severe thallium-201 defect after reinjection identifies areas with a very low probability of improvement in function.

Late redistribution imaging, 24 to 48 hours after the initial stress thallium-201 injection, allows more time for redistribution to occur and has good positive predictive value for improvement in function. The negative predictive value is suboptimal, as redistribution does not take place in some patients even after a prolonged time, and image quality may be suboptimal.[10,175]

With *rest-redistribution thallium-201 imaging*, images are obtained 15 to 20 minutes after tracer injection at rest, reflecting resting regional blood flow, and images obtained 3 to 4 hours following redistribution reflect preserved viability. The finding of a *reversible resting defect* may identify areas of myocardial hibernation (see Fig. 13–50B). This finding appears to be an insensitive although specific sign of potential improvement in regional function.[10,175,177]

Technetium 99m Sestamibi and Tetrofosmin. Studies have demonstrated that the performance of these agents for predicting improvement in regional function after revascularization is similar to that of thallium-201.[10,176] Administration of nitrates to improve resting blood flow prior to injection of sestamibi appears to improve slightly the ability of these tracers to detect myocardial viability.[10,176]

Positron-Emission Tomography. The extent of the PET mismatch pattern (enhanced FDG uptake relative to blood flow) correlates with improvement in LV function after revascularization as well as with the clinical course, magnitude of improvement in heart failure symptoms, and survival after revascularization (see Fig. 13–29).[10,32,173] Patients with heart failure and extensive PET match pattern (diminished blood flow and severe reduction in FDG uptake), representing predominant infarction, are unlikely to benefit clinically from revascularization.[173]

Comparison of Imaging Techniques for Viability Assessment. On the basis of a meta-analysis evaluating the ability of the various radionuclide techniques to predict improvements in regional function, all the radionuclide techniques (as well as low-dose dobutamine echocardiography) perform in a relatively similar manner regarding positive and negative predictive values for improvements in regional function.[178] SPECT techniques appear to be slightly more sensitive, dobutamine echocardiography slightly more specific, and PET techniques appear to have better accuracy. A randomized trial of patients with moderate LV dysfunction being considered for revascularization randomly allocated to have viability information supplied by either PET imaging or SPECT stress-rest sestamibi imaging found no difference in outcomes over long-term follow-up.[179] As noted previously, a meta-analysis of observational outcome studies related to myocardial viability demonstrated no difference between the techniques commonly used to assess viability (PET versus SPECT versus dobutamine echocardiography) with regard to reduction of mortality after revascularization.[174]

Selection of Patients with Heart Failure for Viability Assessment

Guidelines suggest that patients with heart failure *and* active angina benefit in terms of natural history from revascularization and thus should be referred directly for angiography.[180] In some situations, subsequent noninvasive definition of regional viability and ischemia may be important for planning the revascularization strategy when the anatomy is known.

For patients with heart failure and *no angina*, recommendations are less clear. Studies suggest that ischemia and viability may be present in a significant proportion of such patients, who have potential benefit from revascularization,[172] and for most patients with heart failure, a search for underlying ischemia and viability would be an appropriate clinical strategy at some point in their evaluation. If substantial ischemia or viability of dysfunctional territories is found in the setting of vessels technically amenable to revascularization, the literature would suggest a *clinical benefit* from revascularization.[10] In the *absence* of substantial ischemia or viability, such a benefit is less likely. The imaging data can be used in decision-making to help balance the *risks and benefits* of revascularization in a patient with heart failure and LV dysfunction, by supplying information on potential *benefit* of a revascularization strategy.

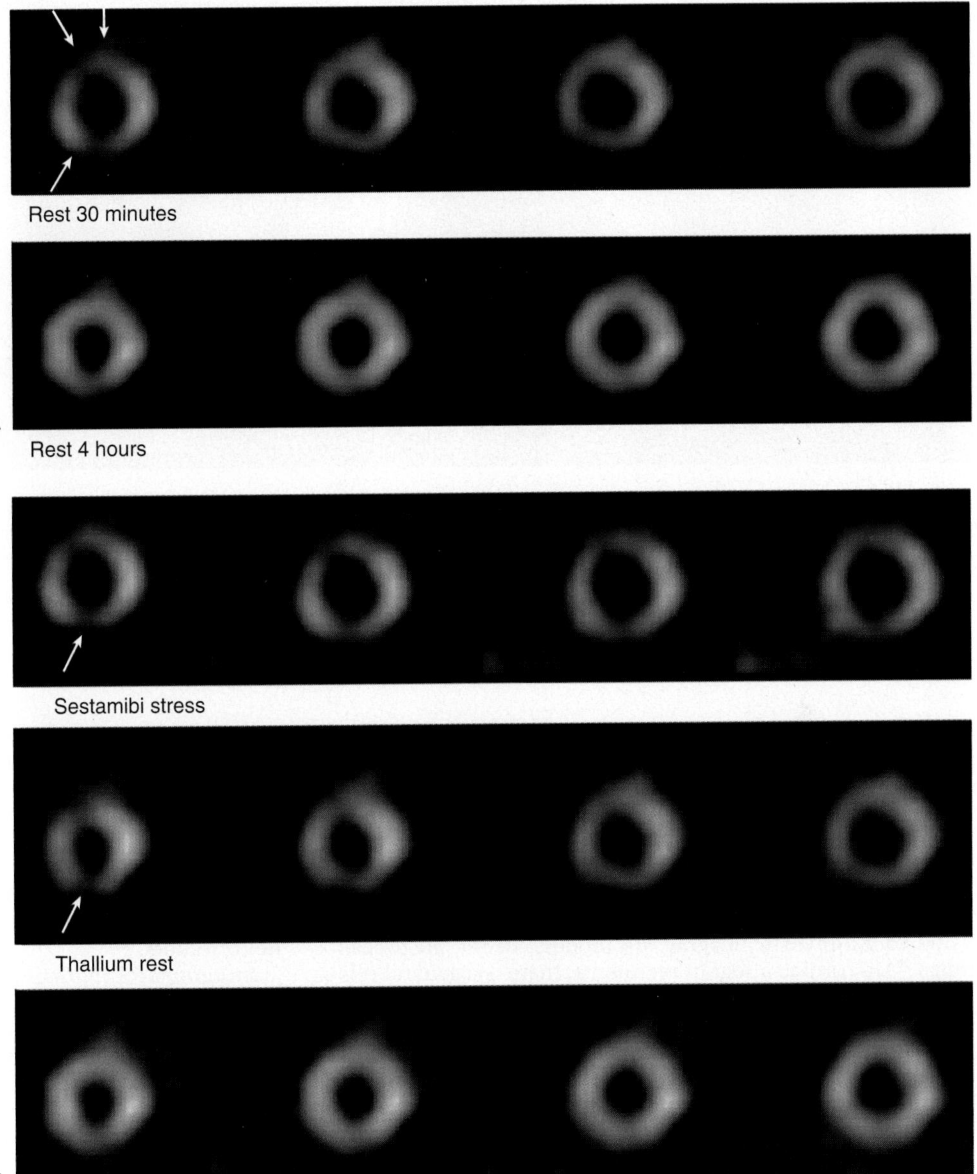

FIGURE 13–50 Myocardial viability imaging with single-photon emission computed tomography. **A,** Rest-redistribution thallium imaging, demonstrating redistribution in regions with initial reductions in thallium uptake, particularly the anterior wall, septum, and inferior walls (arrows), indicating resting hypoperfusion. **B,** Incorporation of rest-redistribution thallium imaging as part of a dual-isotope protocol using sestamibi with stress and thallium at rest. The irreversible defect of the inferior wall (arrow) between stress and rest images can be evaluated further by late imaging after decay of sestamibi to evaluate thallium redistribution kinetics.

Assessment of Left Ventricular Function in Heart Failure

For patients with the clinical syndrome of heart failure, the distinction between those with preserved and those with impaired systolic function has important clinical relevance. Clinical trials evaluating the use of such therapies as ACE inhibitors, angiotensin receptor blockers, and beta blockers have focused on the subpopulation of heart failure patients with impaired systolic function.[180] Less information is available from randomized trials for heart failure patients with preserved ventricular function, many of whom have abnormalities of diastolic function as the basis for symptoms. Thus, accurate determination of LV function in a patient with heart failure defines the evidence-based therapeutic approach that should be undertaken.

On the basis of the quantitative and reproducible nature of the EF results, equilibrium RVG techniques have been used in large clinical trials to identify systolic dysfunction.[10,180] In contemporary practice, the ECG-gated SPECT technique is often used for determination of systolic function. The *simultaneous* assessment of LV systolic function as well as stress and rest perfusion by gated SPECT imaging can provide a range of information relevant to the care and clinical decision-making for patients with heart failure, including the state of LV function, the probability of CAD as the etiology of heart failure, and the presence and extent of viability and ischemia.

Imaging in Inflammatory and Infiltrative Cardiomyopathies

MYOCARDITIS. Inflammatory injury to the myocardium by infective agents, postinfective immune processes (i.e., Chagas disease, rheumatic carditis), hypersensitivity, and autoimmune conditions can cause myocardial dysfunction. The clinical manifestation of such an inflammatory process is acute myocarditis and cardiac allograft rejection. As myocyte necrosis is an obligatory component of myocarditis (cellular infiltrates, predominantly lymphocytes and

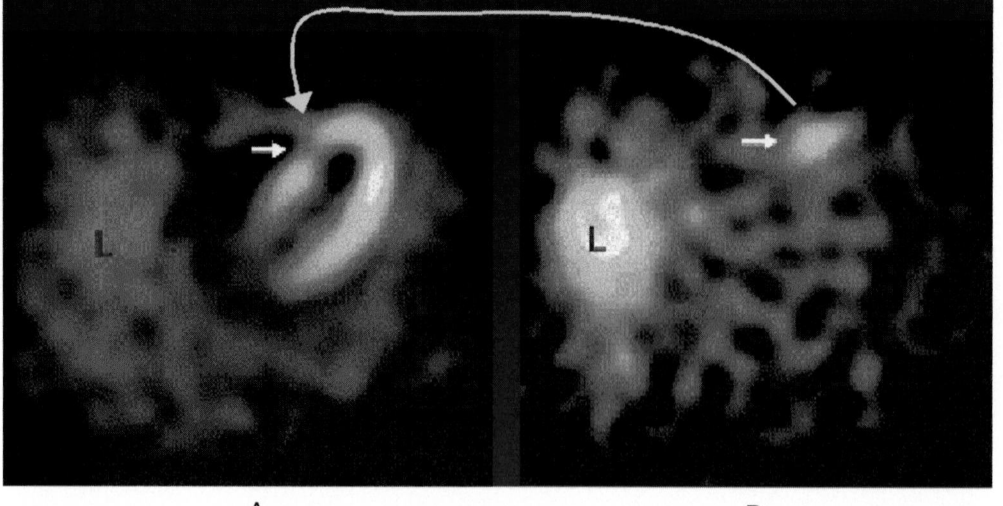

FIGURE 13–51 Example of annexin imaging of apoptosis. **A,** Resting sestamibi study in a patient several days after myocardial infarction (MI), showing a defect in the septum, identifying the territory of the MI (white arrow). **B,** ^{99m}Tc-annexin imaging of apoptosis in the same tomographic plane. The area of uptake (white arrow) corresponds to the area of resting perfusion defect (yellow arrow), suggesting the presence of apoptosis in the MI territory. L = liver. (Adapted from Hofstra L, Liem IH, Dumont EA, et al: Visualization of cell death in vivo in patients with acute myocardial infarction. Lancet 356:209, 2000.)

macrophages, clustered around necrotic myocytes), ^{111}In-labeled antimyosin antibody, which specifically targets myosin heavy chain, has been used for the detection of necrosis associated with myocarditis and heart transplant rejection. In patients with biopsy-positive myocarditis, the sensitivity of an antimyosin scan is approximately 95 percent, with a negative predictive value of approximately 95 percent. However, the specificity and positive predictive value of antimyosin imaging are modest, in the 50 percent range.[181] In cardiac allograft recipients, there is a general relationship between the severity of transplant rejection by biopsy and the magnitude of antimyosin uptake by scintigraphy. However, the highly variable antimyosin uptake across the severity range of rejection precludes antimyosin imaging as a sufficiently reliable noninvasive test for detection of transplant rejection.[182] Observational studies with myocardial perfusion, gated blood pool, and ^{123}I metaiodobenzylguanidine (MIBG) imaging have reported regional perfusion defects, wall motion abnormalities, and sympathetic denervation in patients who present with myocarditis, in the absence of significant CAD.[10]

SARCOID HEART DISEASE. Cardiac involvement occurs in about 20 percent of patients with sarcoidosis. In patients presenting with advanced AV block, myocardial perfusion SPECT or gallium-67 imaging (a nonspecific indicator of inflammation) along with magnetic resonance imaging or chest computed tomography can localize myocardial involvement of sarcoidosis.[10] Focal fibromuscular dysplasia found in the small coronary arteries may provide an explanation for focal ischemic injuries and reversible defects described on myocardial perfusion SPECT. Perfusion defects involving the left ventricle have been associated with AV block and heart failure, and defects involving the right ventricle on SPECT have been associated with ventricular tachycardia of right ventricular origin.[183]

CARDIAC AMYLOIDOSIS. Cardiac involvement of amyloidosis involves the deposition of light chain amino acids into the myofibrils, which leads to impaired relaxation. Patients with amyloidosis may demonstrate abnormally prolonged LV diastolic filling and an increased atrial contribution to the total diastolic filling. These indices of abnormal diastolic filling pattern can be obtained from RNA as well as echocardiography. Although the hallmark of the clinical presentation is dyspnea and heart failure symptoms, advanced AV block can also be a presenting feature in cardiac amyloidosis. ^{123}I MIBG imaging has shown marked cardiac sympathetic denervation, providing insight into the pathogenesis of cardiac conduction disturbances in amyloidosis.[184] ^{99m}Tc pyrophosphate scintigraphy may be useful in identifying patients with cardiac amyloidosis, demonstrating diffuse uptake throughout the myocardium.[10]

Radionuclide Imaging in Heart Failure and Left Ventricular Dysfunction: Research Directions

Assessment of Cardiac Sympathetic Innervation. An emerging area of risk stratification involves the use of ^{123}I MIBG imaging of cardiac sympathetic innervation. In the post-MI setting, the territory of abnormal MIBG uptake (corresponding to sympathetic *denervation*) often exceeds the final infarct size, and such patients are at higher risk for subsequent ventricular arrhythmias.[122,185,186] Should this finding prove prognostic for outcomes in patients with LV dysfunction, as suggested by earlier studies, MIBG imaging may have a role in selecting post-MI patients who may optimally benefit from defibrillators.[186]

Imaging of Apoptosis. Another potential approach to evaluating patients with LV dysfunction after MI is the visualization of apoptosis, or programmed cell death, in humans using ^{99m}Tc-labeled annexin V, which localizes to apoptotic cells. In one study, positive uptake of this agent was seen in six of seven post-MI patients, localized to areas of resting perfusion defects (Fig. 13–51).[187] This agent may herald the onset of the ability to track this process noninvasively in syndromes such as heart failure and to study approaches to attenuate the unfavorable pathophysiology of apoptosis.

Radionuclide Imaging of Cell- or Gene-Based Regenerative Therapy. Local targeted gene delivery or implantation of autologous skeletal myoblasts, bone marrow stromal cells, or hematopoietic stem cells may functionally revitalize scarred, noncontractile myocardial regions. Noninvasive assessment of the fate of myogenic cell grafts and therapeutic genes in vivo may provide insight into the mechanism by which they improve cardiac function or prevent remodeling. In animal studies, transplanted cardiomyoblasts expressing a PET reporter gene have been imaged longitudinally to gain insight into the pattern of cell survival.[188] Using cardiac micro-PET imaging, detailed tomographic locations of transplanted cells were obtained (Fig. 13–52). This may become an important method to study regenerative therapies in human studies.

Imaging the Tissue Angiotensin-Converting Enzyme Receptor System. Radionuclide imaging has been used in experimental systems to study the tissue ACE receptor system directly. Using the radiotracer [^{18}F]fluorobenzyl-lisinopril,[189] preliminary observations have shown a relationship between ACE and collagen replacement, as ACE was absent in the collagen-stained areas and was increased in the juxtaposed areas of replacement fibrosis.[190,191] These data suggest that

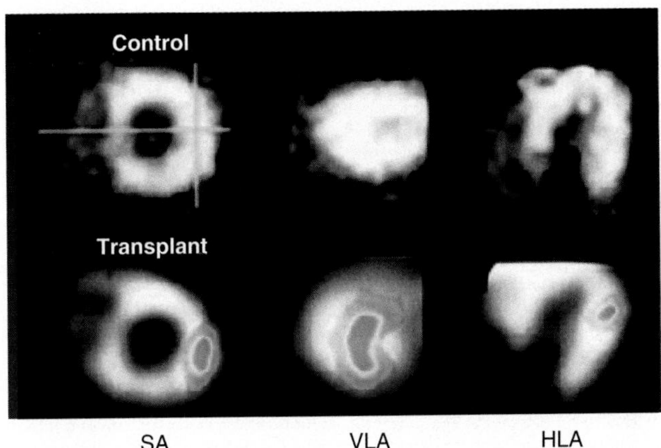

FIGURE 13–52 Cardiac micro-positron-emission tomography (PET) images in the short-axis (SA), vertical long-axis (VLA), and horizontal long-axis (HLA) views of a rat heart transplanted with cardiomyoblasts expressing a PET reporter gene. The gray/white uptake represents homogeneous perfusion by $^{13}N\text{-}NH_3$, and the color uptake in the lateral wall represents the viable transplanted cardiomyoblasts studied in vivo (bottom row). There is no uptake in the control heart, with normal perfusion (top row). (Adapted from Wu JC, Chen IY, Sundaresan G, et al: Molecular imaging of cardiac cell transplantation in living animals using optical bioluminescence and positron emission tomography. Circulation 108:1302, 2003.)

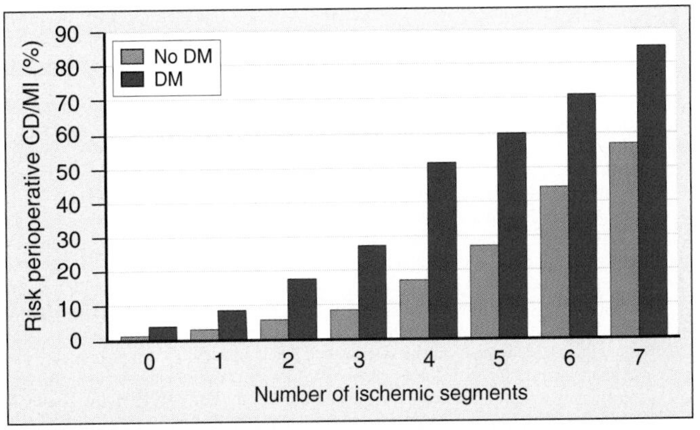

FIGURE 13–53 Relation between the extent of inducible ischemia (as the number of segments with ischemic defects, x-axis) and the risk of perioperative cardiac death (CD) or myocardial infarction (MI) in patients following peripheral vascular surgery undergoing preoperative pharmacological stress myocardial perfusion imaging. As the extent of preoperative reversible defect increases, the risk of a major perioperative event increases as well. Moreover, the presence of diabetes mellitus (DM) confers additional risk: for any given extent of preoperative ischemia, the event risk is higher if DM is present. (Adapted from Brown K: Prognostic value of myocardial perfusion imaging: State of the art and new developments. J Nucl Cardiol 3:516, 1996.)

increased ACE may be a stimulus for collagen replacement and remodeling. In the future, noninvasive imaging with PET in patients with heart failure may allow monitoring of changes in ACE patterns in vivo, possibly reflecting progression of disease and the effect of therapies before collagen replacement ensues.

Imaging to Assess Cardiac Risk Prior to Noncardiac Surgery

The clinical role of MPI for evaluating patients prior to elective noncardiac surgery has grown, as CAD represents an important perioperative and long-term risk in such patients. The ischemic burden from the stress of surgery and postoperative recovery can result in MI or cardiovascular death. Prospective identification of such patients has important prognostic and preventive implications.

Initial cardiac assessment of patients undergoing noncardiac surgery should be based on (1) the prevalence of CAD in a given surgical population, (2) the type of the surgical procedure and the institutional event rate, (3) cardiac history and risk factors, and (4) functional capacity.[192] Surgical procedures can be classified as high-risk procedures (cardiac risk of >5 percent), such as major vascular surgery, emergent major operations, and prolonged surgical procedures with large fluid shifts or blood loss. Intermediate-risk procedures have cardiac risks of 1 to 5 percent and include carotid endarterectomy, intraperitoneal and intrathoracic operations, and orthopedic operations. Low-risk (<1 percent) procedures include endoscopic procedures, cataract surgery, and breast surgery. If the institutional event rate for an elective operation is less than 2 to 3 percent, most screening studies are inefficient with regard to lowering the cardiac event rate in the perioperative period.

Clinical parameters of increased risk include advanced age (older than 70 years), diabetes, history of angina or recent ACS, heart failure, and ventricular arrhythmias. When added to the type of surgery and clinical parameters, the findings of exercise duration of less than 3 minutes and ST segment depression of greater than 1.5 to 2.0 mm indicate significant and independent risk for an adverse cardiac outcome.[192,193]

Patients with known prior CAD may be considered to have a low perioperative cardiac risk on the basis of their functional capacity and symptoms. Asymptomatic patients with known CAD who have had revascularization within the past 5 years require no further evaluation.[192] Patients with intermediate risk on the basis of clinical predictors, functional capacity, and type of surgery are optimal candidates for further stratification by imaging procedures.

Studies of MPI using pharmacological stress have uniformly shown that a normal MPI study predicts a low likelihood (~1 percent) for perioperative or longer term postoperative cardiac events.[193] Reversible perfusion defects predict an increased risk of cardiac events, and the magnitude of risk is related to the extent of ischemia (Fig. 13–53). Although fixed perfusion defects (infarct) portend a lower risk for perioperative cardiac events than ischemia, the risk is higher than that with a normal scan, and patients with infarct or LV dysfunction are at higher *long-term* risk for death or heart failure.[193]

In clinical practice, most patients in whom extensive ischemia is demonstrated preoperatively undergo catheterization with expectation of revascularization. Clinical trial evidence supporting this point is lacking, and the threshold of ischemia extent above which revascularization might *reduce* short- or long-term cardiac risk is not known. Clinical studies suggest that beta blockers, if appropriately administered, reduce perioperative ischemia and may reduce the risk for MI and death in high-risk patients.[194]

REFERENCES

Technical Aspects of Image Acquisition, Display, and Interpretation

1. Jain D, Strauss HW: Principles of cardiovascular nuclear imaging. *In* Dilsizian V, Narula J, Braunwald E (eds): Atlas of Nuclear Cardiology. Philadelphia, Current Medicine, 2003, pp 1-18.
2. Garcia EV: Physics and instrumentation of radionuclide imaging. *In* Braunwald E (ed): Cardiac Imaging: A Companion to Braunwald's Heart Disease. Philadelphia, WB Saunders, 1991, pp 977-1005.
3. Faber TL: Tomographic imaging: Methods. *In* Gerson MC (ed): Cardiac Nuclear Medicine. New York, McGraw-Hill, 1997.
4. Garcia E, Berman DS, Port SC, et al: American Society of Nuclear Cardiology. Imaging guidelines for nuclear cardiology procedures. Part 2. J Nucl Cardiol 6:G53, 1999.
5. Links JM, Becker LC, Rigo P, et al: Combined corrections for attenuation, depth-dependent blur, and motion in cardiac SPECT: A multicenter trial. J Nucl Cardiol 7:414, 2000.
6. Dilsizian V: SPECT and PET techniques. *In* Dilsizian V, Narula J, Braunwald E (eds): Atlas of Nuclear Cardiology. Philadelphia, Current Medicine, 2003, pp 19-46.

7. Kailasnath P, Sinusas AJ: Comparison of Tl-201 with Tc-99m-labeled myocardial perfusion agents: Technical, physiologic, and clinical issues. J Nucl Cardiol 8:482, 2001.
8. American Society of Nuclear Cardiology: Updated imaging guidelines for nuclear cardiology procedures, part 1. J Nucl Cardiol 8:G5, 2001.
9. DePuey EG: A stepwise approach to myocardial perfusion SPECT interpretation. *In* Gerson MC (ed): Cardiac Nuclear Medicine. New York, McGraw-Hill, 1997, pp 81-142.
10. Klocke FJ, Baird MG, Bateman TM, et al: ACC/AHA/ASNC guidelines for the clinical use of cardiac radionuclide imaging: A report of the American College of Cardiology/American Heart Association Task Force on Practice Guidelines (ACC/AHA/ASNC Committee to Revise the 1995 Guidelines for the Clinical Use of Radionuclide Imaging). 2003. American College of Cardiology Web Site. Available at: http://www.acc.org/clinical/ guidelines/radio/rni_fulltext.pdf.
11. Berman DS, Hachamovitch R, Germano G: Risk stratification and patient management. *In* Dilsizian V, Narula J, Braunwald E (eds): Atlas of Nuclear Cardiology. Philadelphia, Current Medicine, 2003, pp 97-114.
12. Cerqueira MD, Weissman NJ, Dilsizian V, et al: Standardized myocardial segmentation and nomenclature for tomographic imaging of the heart: A statement for healthcare professionals from the cardiac imaging committee of the council on clinical cardiology of the American Heart Association. Circulation 105:539, 2002.
13. Garcia EV, Van Train K, Maddahi J, et al: Quantification of rotational thallium-201 myocardial tomography. J Nucl Med 26:17, 1985.
14. Liu YH, Sinusas AJ, Deman P, et al: Quantification of SPECT myocardial perfusion images: Methodology and validation of the Yale-CQ method. J Nucl Cardiol 6:190, 1999.
15. Beller GA: Radionuclide perfusion imaging techniques for evaluation of patients with known or suspected coronary artery disease. Adv Intern Med 42:139, 1997.
16. McLaughlin MG, Danias PG: Transient ischemic dilation: A powerful diagnostic and prognostic finding of stress myocardial perfusion imaging. J Nucl Cardiol 9:663, 2002.
17. Mazzanti M, Germano G, Kiat H, et al: Identification of severe and extensive coronary artery disease by automatic measurement of transient ischemic dilation of the left ventricle in dual-isotope myocardial perfusion SPECT. J Am Coll Cardiol 27:1612, 1996.
18. Taillefer R, DePuey EG, Udelson JE, et al: Comparative diagnostic accuracy of Tl-201 and Tc-99m sestamibi SPECT imaging (perfusion and ECG-gated SPECT) in detecting coronary artery disease in women. J Am Coll Cardiol 29:69, 1997.
19. Kiat H, Van Train KF, Friedman JD, et al: Quantitative stress redistribution thallium-201 SPECT using prone imaging: Methodologic development and validation. J Nucl Med 33:1509, 1992.
20. DePuey EG: Artifacts clarified and caused by gated myocardial perfusion SPECT. *In* Germano G, Berman DS (eds): Clinical Gated Cardiac SPECT. Armonk, NY, Futura Publishing, 1999, pp 183-238
21. King MA, Tsui BMW, Pan T: Attenuation compensation for cardiac single-photon emission computed tomographic imaging: Part 2. Attenuation compensation algorithms. J Nucl Cardiol 3:55, 1996.
22. Hendel RC, Corbett JR, Cullom SJ, et al: The value and practice of attenuation correction for myocardial perfusion SPECT imaging: A joint position statement from the American Society of Nuclear Cardiology and the Society of Nuclear Medicine. J Nucl Cardiol 9:135, 2002.
23. Germano G, Berman DS: Acquisition and processing for gated SPECT: Technical aspects. *In* Germano G, Berman DS (eds): Clinical Gated Cardiac SPECT. Armonk, NY, Futura Publishing, 1999, pp 93-114.
24. Smith WH, Kastener RJ, Calnon DA, et al: Quantitative gated SPECT imaging: A counts-based method for display and measurement of regional and global ventricular systolic function. J Nucl Cardiol 4:451, 1997.
25. Bateman TM, Berman DS, Heller GV, et al: American Society of Nuclear Cardiology position statement on electrocardiographic gating of myocardial perfusion SPECT scintigrams. J Nucl Cardiol 6:470, 1999.
26. Gerson MC: Myocardial perfusion imaging: Planar methods. *In* Gerson MC (ed): Cardiac Nuclear Medicine. New York, McGraw-Hill, 1997, pp 29-52.
27. Wackers FJ: Equilibrium radionuclide angiography. *In* Gerson MC (ed): Cardiac Nuclear Medicine. New York, McGraw-Hill, 1997, pp 315-346.
28. Borer JS: First pass and equilibrium radionuclide angiography. *In* Dilsizian V, Narula J, Braunwald E (eds): Atlas of Nuclear Cardiology. Philadelphia, Current Medicine, 2003, pp 147-166.
29. Arrighi JA, Dilsizian V: Radionuclide angiography in coronary and noncoronary heart disease: Technical background and clinical applications. *In* Harbert JC, Eckelman WC, Neumann RD (eds): Nuclear Medicine. New York, Thieme Medical Publishers, 1996, pp 501-531.
30. Aggarwal, A, Brown KA, LeWinter MM: Diastolic dysfunction: Pathophysiology, clinical features, and assessment with radionuclide methods. J Nucl Cardiol 8:98, 2001.
31. Dilsizian V: SPECT and PET techniques. *In* Dilsizian V, Narula J, Braunwald E (eds): Atlas of Nuclear Cardiology. Philadelphia, Current Medicine, 2003, pp 131-146.
32. Bacharach SL, Bax JJ, Case J, et al: PET myocardial glucose metabolism and perfusion imaging: Part I—Guidelines for patient preparation and data acquisition. J Nucl Cardiol 10:543, 2003.

Assessment of the Physiology and Pathophysiology of Myocardial Blood Flow, Myocardial Metabolism, and Ventricular Function

33. Watson DD, Glover DK: Overview of kinetics and modeling. *In* Zaret BL, Beller GA (eds): Nuclear Cardiology: State of the Art and Future Directions. St. Louis, Mosby, 1999, pp 3-12.
34. Shirani J, Lee J, Quigg RJ, et al: Relation of thallium uptake to morphologic features of chronic ischemic heart disease: Evidence for myocardial remodeling in non-infarct myocardium. J Am Coll Cardiol 38:84, 2001.
35. Gibbons RJ, Miller TD, Christian TF: Infarct size measured by single photon emission computed tomographic imaging with ^{99m}Tc-sestamibi: A measure of the efficacy of therapy in acute myocardial infarction. Circulation 101:101, 2000.
36. Christian TF: The use of perfusion imaging in acute myocardial infarction. Application for clinical trials and clinical care. J Nucl Cardiol 2:423, 1995.
37. Kern MJ, Meier B: Evaluation of the culprit plaque and the physiological significance of coronary atherosclerotic narrowings. Circulation 103:3142, 2001.
38. Follansbee WP: Alternatives to leg exercise in the evaluation of patients with coronary artery disease: Functional and pharmacologic stress modalities. *In* Gerson MC (ed): Cardiac Nuclear Medicine. New York, McGraw-Hill, 1997, pp 193-236.
39. Gould KL, Nakagawa Y, Nakagawa K, et al: Frequency and clinical implications of fluid dynamically significant diffuse coronary artery disease manifest as graded, longitudinal, base-to-apex myocardial perfusion abnormalities by noninvasive positron emission tomography. Circulation 101:1931, 2000.
40. Hasdai D, Gibbons RJ, Holmes DR Jr, et al: Coronary endothelial dysfunction in humans is associated with myocardial perfusion defects. Circulation 96:3390, 1997.
41. He Z, Mahmarian JJ, Verani MS: Myocardial perfusion in patients with total occlusion of a single coronary artery with and without collateral circulation. J Nucl Cardiol 8:452, 2001.
42. Mark DB, Lauer MS: Exercise capacity: The prognostic variable that doesn't get enough respect. Circulation 108:1534, 2003.
43. Hendel RC: Diagnostic and prognostic applications for vasodilator stress myocardial perfusion imaging and the importance of radiopharmaceutical selection. J Nucl Cardiol 8:523, 2001.
44. Miller DD: Pharmacologic stressors in coronary artery disease. *In* Dilsizian V, Narula J, Braunwald E (eds): Atlas of Nuclear Cardiology. Philadelphia, Current Medicine, 2003, pp 47-62.
45. Verani MS: Pharmacologic stress myocardial perfusion imaging. Curr Probl Cardiol 18:481, 1993.
46. Udelson JE, Heller GV, Wackers FJ, et al: A randomized, controlled dose-ranging study of the selective adenosine A_{2A} receptor agonist binodenoson for pharmacologic stress as an adjunct to myocardial perfusion imaging. Circulation 109:457, 2004.
47. Thomas GS, Prill NV, Majmundar H, et al: Treadmill exercise during adenosine infusion is safe, results in fewer adverse reactions, and improves myocardial perfusion imaging quality. J Nucl Cardiol 7:439, 2000.
48. Elliott MD, Holly TA, Leonard SM, Hendel RC: Impact of abbreviated adenosine protocol incorporating adjunctive treadmill exercise on adverse effects and image quality in patients undergoing stress myocardial perfusion imaging. J Nucl Cardiol 7:584, 2000.
49. Dakik HA, Kleiman NS, Farmer JA, et al: Intensive medical therapy versus coronary angioplasty for suppression of myocardial ischaemia in survivors of acute myocardial infarction: A prospective randomized pilot study. Circulation 98:2017, 1998.
50. Sharir T, Rabinowitz B, Livschitz S, et al: Underestimation of extent and severity of coronary artery disease by dipyridamole stress thallium-201 single-photon emission computed tomographic myocardial perfusion imaging in patients taking antianginal drugs. J Am Coll Cardiol 31:1540, 1998.
51. Taillefer R, Ahlberg AW, Masood Y, et al: Acute beta-blockade reduces the extent and severity of myocardial perfusion defects with dipyridamole Tc-99m sestamibi SPECT imaging. J Am Coll Cardiol 42:1475, 2003.
52. Geleijnse M, Elhendy A, Fioretti P, et al: Dobutamine stress myocardial perfusion imaging. J Am Coll Cardiol 36:2017, 2000.
53. Wijns W, Vatner SF, Camici PG: Mechanisms of disease: Hibernating myocardium. N Engl J Med 339:173, 1998.
54. Taegtmeyer H: Modulation of responses to myocardial ischemia: Metabolic features of myocardial stunning, hibernation, and ischemic preconditioning. *In* Dilsizian V (ed): Myocardial Viability: A Clinical and Scientific Treatise. Armonk, NY, Futura Publishing, 2000, pp 25-36.
55. Braunwald E, Kloner RA: The stunned myocardium: Prolonged, postischemic ventricular dysfunction. Circulation 66:1146, 1982.
56. Rahimtoola SH: A perspective on the three large multicenter randomized clinical trials of coronary bypass surgery for chronic stable angina. Circulation 72(Suppl V):V-123, 1985.
57. Dilsizian V, Arrighi JA: Myocardial viability in chronic coronary artery disease: Perfusion, metabolism, and contractile reserve. *In* Gerson MC (ed): Cardiac Nuclear Medicine. New York, McGraw-Hill, 1997, pp 143-192.
58. Schelbert HR: Measurements of myocardial metabolism in patients with ischemic heart disease. Am J Cardiol 82:61K, 1998.
59. Tawakol A, Skopicki HA, Abraham SA, et al: Evidence of reduced resting blood flow in viable myocardial regions with chronic asynergy J Am Coll Cardiol 36:2146, 2000.
60. Feinendegen LE: Myocardial imaging of lipid metabolism with labeled fatty acids. *In* Dilsizian V (ed): Myocardial Viability: A Clinical and Scientific Treatise. Armonk, NY, Futura Publishing Company, 2000, pp 349-389.
61. Kudoh T, Tamaki N, Magata Y, et al: Metabolism substrate with negative myocardial uptake of iodine-123-BMIPP. J Nucl Med 38:548, 1997.
62. Hansen CL: Myocardial metabolic imaging with radiolabeled fatty acids. *In* Gerson MC (ed): Cardiac Nuclear Medicine. New York, McGraw-Hill, 1997, pp 239-258.
63. Udelson JE, Dilsizian V, Bateman TM, et al: Proof of principle study of β-methyl-*p*-[^{123}I]-iodophenyl-pentadecanoic acid (BMIPP) for ischemic memory following demand ischemia [abstract]. Circulation 108:IV-405, 2003.
64. Schelbert HR: Principles of positron emission tomography. *In* Skorton DJ, Schelbert HR, Wolf GL, Brundage BH (eds): Marcus Cardiac Imaging: A Companion to Braunwald's Heart Disease. 2nd ed. Philadelphia, WB Saunders, 1996, pp 1063-1092.
65. Dilsizian V, Bacharach SL, Maung KM, Smith MF: Fluorine-18-deoxyglucose SPECT and coincidence imaging for myocardial viability: Clinical and technological issues. J Nucl Cardiol 8:75, 2001.
66. Gropler RJ, Siegel BA, Sampathkumaran K, et al: Dependence of recovery of contractile function on maintenance of oxidative metabolism after myocardial infarction. J Am Coll Cardiol 19:989, 1992.
67. Jafary F, Udelson JE: Assessment of myocardial perfusion and left ventricular function in acute coronary syndromes: Implications for gated SPECT imaging. In Germano G,

Berman DS (eds): Clinical Gated Cardiac SPECT. Armonk, NY, Futura Publishing, 1999, pp 259-306.
68. Udelson JE, Bonow RO: Radionuclide ventriculography in left ventricular diastolic dysfunction. *In* Gaasch WH, LeWinter M (eds): Heart Failure and Diastolic Dysfunction. Philadelphia, Lea & Febiger, 1994, pp 167-191.
69. Gerson MC, Rohe R: Radionuclide ventriculography: Left ventricular volumes and pressure-volume relations. *In* Gerson MC (ed): Cardiac Nuclear Medicine. New York, McGraw-Hill, 1997, pp 347-370.
70. Links JM, Becker LC, Shindledecker JG, et al: Measurement of absolute left ventricular volumes from gated blood pool studies. Circulation 65:82, 1982.
71. Verani MS, Gaeta J, LeBlanc AD, et al: Validation of left ventricular volume measurements by radionuclide angiography. J Nucl Med 26:1394, 1985.
72. Anand IS, Florea VG, Solomon SD, et al: Noninvasive assessment of left ventricular remodeling: Concepts, techniques, and implications for clinical trials. J Card Fail 8:S452, 2002.
73. Iskandrian AE, Germano G, VanDecker W, et al: Validation of left ventricular volume measurements by gated SPECT 99mTc-labeled sestamibi imaging. J Nucl Cardiol 5:574, 1998.
74. Germano G, Berman DS: Quantitative gated perfusion SPECT. *In* Germano G, Berman DS (eds): Clinical Gated Cardiac SPECT. Armonk, NY, Futura Publishing, 1999, pp 115-146.
75. Metra M, Giubbini R, Nodari S, et al: Differential effects of ß-blockers in patients with heart failure: A prospective, randomized, double-blind comparison of the long-term effects of metoprolol versus carvedilol. Circulation 102:546, 2000.
76. Borer JS, Bonow RO: Contemporary approach to aortic and mitral regurgitation. Circulation 108:2432, 2003.
77. Bonow RO, Carabello B, de Leon AC Jr, et al: ACC/AHA guidelines for the management of patients with valvular heart disease: A report of the American College of Cardiology/American Heart Association Task Force on Practice Guidelines (Committee on Management of Patients with Valvular Heart Disease). J Am Coll Cardiol 32:1486, 1998.
78. Imitani I, Jain D, Joska TM, et al: Doxorubicin cardiotoxicity: Prevention of congestive heart failure with serial cardiac function monitoring with equilibrium radionuclide angiocardiography in the current era. J Nucl Cardiol 10:132, 2003.
79. Spirito P, Maron BJ, Bonow RO: Noninvasive assessment of left ventricular diastolic function: Comparative analysis of Doppler echocardiographic and radionuclide angiographic techniques. J Am Coll Cardiol 7:518, 1986.
80. Maron BJ: Hypertrophic cardiomyopathy: A systematic review. JAMA 287:1308, 2002.
81. Udelson JE, Bonow RO: Left ventricular diastolic function and the use of calcium channel blockers in hypertrophic cardiomyopathy. *In* Gaasch WH, LeWinter M (eds): Heart Failure and Diastolic Dysfunction. Philadelphia, Lea & Febiger, 1994, pp 462-489.
82. Bonow RO, Dilsizian V, Rosing DR, et al: Verapamil-induced improvement in left ventricular diastolic filling and increased exercise tolerance in patients with hypertrophic cardiomyopathy: Short- and long-term effects. Circulation 72:853, 1985.
83. Kitzman DW, Higginbotham MB, Cobb FR, et al: Exercise intolerance in patients with heart failure and preserved left ventricular systolic function: Failure of the Frank-Starling mechanism. J Am Coll Cardiol 17:1065, 1991.

Disease Detection, Risk Stratification, and Clinical Decision-Making

84. Gould KL: Noninvasive assessment of coronary stenoses by myocardial perfusion imaging during pharmacologic coronary vasodilatation: I. Physiologic basis and experimental validation. Am J Cardiol 41:267, 1978.
85. Libby P, Ridker PM, Maseri A: Inflammation and atherosclerosis Circulation 105:1135, 2002.
86. Expert Panel on Detection, Evaluation, and Treatment of High Blood Cholesterol in Adults: Executive Summary of the Third Report of the National Cholesterol Education Program (NCEP) Expert Panel on Detection, Evaluation and Treatment of High Blood Cholesterol in Adults (Adult Treatment Panel III). JAMA 285:2486, 2001.
87. Fletcher GF, Balady GJ, Vogel RA: Preventive cardiology: How can we do better? 33rd Bethesda Conference. J Am Coll Cardiol 40:579, 2002.
88. Gibbons RJ: Nuclear cardiology in hospital-based practice. J Nucl Cardiol 4:179, 1997.
89. Braunwald E, Antman EM, Beasley JW, et al: ACC/AHA 2002 guideline update for the management of patients with unstable angina and non-ST-segment elevation myocardial infarction: A report of the American College of Cardiology/American Heart Association Task Force on Practice Guidelines (Committee on the Management of Patients with Unstable Angina). 2002. Available at: http://www.acc.org/clinical/guidelines/unstable/incorporated/index.htm.
90. Gibbons RJ, Abrams J, Chatterjee K, et al: ACC/AHA 2002 guideline update for the management of patients with chronic stable angina—Summary article: A report of the American College of Cardiology/American Heart Association Task Force on Practice Guidelines (Committee on the Management of Patients with Chronic Stable Angina). Circulation 107:149, 2003.
91. Brown K: Prognostic value of myocardial perfusion imaging: State of the art and new developments. J Nucl Cardiol 3:516, 1996.
92. Ladenheim ML, Pollock BH, Rozanski A, et al: Extent and severity of myocardial hypoperfusion as predictors of prognosis in patients with suspected coronary artery disease. J Am Coll Cardiol 7: 464, 1986.
93. Shaw LJ, Hachamovitch R, Eisenstein EL: A primer of biostatistic and economic methods for diagnostic and prognostic modeling in nuclear cardiology: Part I. J Nucl Cardiol 3:538, 1996.
94. Pollock SG, Abbott RD, Boucher CA, et al: Independent and incremental prognostic value of tests performed in hierarchical order to evaluate patients with suspected coronary artery disease: Validation of models based on these tests. Circulation 85:237, 1992.
95. Hachamovitch R, Berman DS, Kiat H, et al: Exercise myocardial perfusion SPECT in patients without known coronary artery disease: Incremental prognostic value and use in risk stratification. Circulation 93:905, 1996.
96. Gibbons RJ, Hodge DO, Berman DS, et al: Long-term outcome of patients with intermediate-risk exercise electrocardiograms who do not have myocardial perfusion defects on radionuclide imaging. Circulation 100:2140, 1999.
97. Beller GA: First Annual Mario S. Verani, MD, Memorial Lecture: Clinical value of myocardial perfusion imaging in coronary artery disease. J Nucl Cardiol 10:529, 2003.
98. Vanzetto G, Ormezzano O, Fagret D, et al: Long-term additive prognostic value of thallium-201 myocardial perfusion imaging over clinical and exercise stress test in low to intermediate risk patients. Study in 1137 patients with 6-year follow-up. Circulation 100:1521, 1999.
99. Hachamovitch R, Hayes SW, Friedman JD, et al: Comparison of the short-term survival benefit associated with revascularization compared with medical therapy in patients with no prior coronary artery disease undergoing stress myocardial perfusion single photon emission computed tomography. Circulation 107: 2900, 2003.
100. Shaw LJ, Hendel R, Borges-Neto S, et al, for the Myoview Multicenter Registry: Prognostic value of normal exercise and adenosine 99mTc-tetrofosmin SPECT imaging: Results from the multicenter registry of 4,728 patients. J Nucl Med 44:134, 2003.
101. Hachamovitch R, Hayes S, Friedman JD, et al: Determinants of risk and its temporal variation in patients with normal stress myocardial perfusion scans. What is the warranty period of a normal scan? J Am Coll Cardiol 41:1329, 2003.
102. Giri S, Shaw LJ, Murthy DR, et al: Impact of diabetes on the risk stratification using stress single-photon emission computed tomography myocardial perfusion imaging in patients with symp toms suggestive of coronary artery disease. Circulation 105:32, 2002.
103. Brown K: Prognostic value of myocardial perfusion imaging: State of the art and new developments. J Nucl Cardiol 3:516, 1996.
104. Parisi AF, Hartigan PM, Folland ED, for the ACME Investigators: Evaluation of exercise thallium-201 scintigraphy versus exercise electrocardiography in predicting survival outcomes and morbid cardiac events in patients with single- and double-vessel disease. Findings from the angioplasty compared to medicine study. J Am Coll Cardiol 30:1256, 1997.
105. Schwartz RG, Pearson TA, Kalaria VG, et al: Prospective serial evaluation of myocardial perfusion and lipids during the first six months of pravastatin therapy: Coronary artery disease regression single photon emission computed tomography monitoring trial. J Am Coll Cardiol 42:600, 2003.
106. Baller D, Notohamiprodjo G, Gleichmann U, et al: Improvement in coronary flow reserve determined by positron emission tomography after 6 months of cholesterol-lowering therapy in patients with early stages of coronary atherosclerosis. Circulation 99:2871, 1999.
107. Beller GA, Zaret BL: Contributions of nuclear cardiology to diagnosis and prognosis of patients with coronary artery disease. Circulation 101:1465, 2000.
108. Rozanski A, Diamond GA, Berman D, et al: The declining specificity of exercise radionuclide ventriculography. N Engl J Med 309:518, 1983.
109. Gerson MC: Test accuracy, test selection, and test result interpretation in chronic coronary artery disease. *In* Gerson MC (ed): Cardiac Nuclear Medicine. New York, McGraw-Hill, 1997, pp 527-580.
110. Matzer L, Kiat H, Friedman JD, et al: A new approach to the assessment of tomographic thallium-201 scintigraphy in patients with left bundle branch block. J Am Coll Cardiol 17:1309, 1991.
111. Dilsizian V, Bonow RO, Epstein SE, Fananapazir L: Myocardial ischemia detected by thallium scintigraphy is frequently related to cardiac arrest and syncope in young patients with hypertrophic cardiomyopathy. J Am Coll Cardiol 22:796, 1993.
112. Cecchi F, Olivotto I, Gistri R, et al: Coronary microvascular dysfunction and prognosis in hypertrophic cardiomyopathy. N Engl J Med 349:1027, 2003.
113. O'Gara PT, Bonow RO, Maron BJ, et al: Myocardial perfusion abnormalities in patients with hypertrophic cardiomyopathy: Assessment with thallium-201 emission computed tomography. Circulation 76:1214, 1987.
114. Udelson JE, Bonow RO, O'Gara PT, et al: Verapamil prevents silent myocardial perfusion abnormalities during exercise in asymptomatic patients with hypertrophic cardiomyopathy. Circulation 79:1052, 1989.
115. Cannon RO, Dilsizian V, O'Gara PT, et al: Myocardial metabolic, hemodynamic, and electrocardiographic significance of reversible thallium-201 abnormalities in hypertrophic cardiomyopathy. Circulation 83:1660, 1991.
116. Schulman DS, Francis CK, Black HR, Wackers FJ: Thallium-201 stress imaging in hypertensive patients. Hypertension 10:16, 1987.
117. Tubau JF, Szlachcic J, Hollenberg M, Massie BM: Usefulness of thallium-201 scintigraphy in predicting the development of angina pectoris in hypertensive patients with left ventricular hypertrophy. Am J Cardiol 64:45, 1989.
118. Amanullah AM, Berman DS, Kang X, et al: Enhanced prognostic stratification of patients with left ventricular hypertrophy with the use of single-photon emission computed tomography. Am Heart J 140:3456, 2000.
119. Yamaguchi S, Tsuiki K, Hayasaka M, Yasui S: Segmental wall motion abnormalities in dilated cardiomyopathy: Hemodynamic characteristics and comparison with thallium-201 myocardial scintigraphy. Am Heart J 113:1123, 1987.
120. Doi YL, Chikamori T, Takata J, et al: Prognostic value of thallium-201 perfusion defects in idiopathic dilated cardiomyopathy. Am J Cardiol 67:188, 1991.
121. Neglia D, Michelassi C, Trivieri MG, et al: Prognostic role of myocardial blood flow impairment in idiopathic left ventricular dysfunction. Circulation 105:186, 2002.
122. Udelson JE, Shafer CD, Carrio I: Radionuclide imaging in heart failure: Assessing etiology and outcomes and implications for management. J Nucl Cardiol 9:S40, 2002.
123. Masoli O, Perez Baliño N, Sabaté D, et al: Effect of endothelial dysfunction on regional perfusion in myocardial territories supplied by normal and diseased vessels in patients with coronary artery disease. J Nucl Cardiol 7:199, 2000.
124. Panting JR, Gatehouse PD, Yang GZ, et al: Abnormal subendocardial perfusion in cardiac syndrome X detected by cardiovascular magnetic resonance imaging. N Engl J Med 346:1948, 2002.
125. Taillefer R, DePuey EG, Udelson JE, et al: Comparative diagnostic accuracy of Tl-201 and Tc-99m sestamibi SPECT imaging (perfusion and ECG-gated SPECT) in detecting coronary artery disease in women. J Am Coll Cardiol 29:69, 1997.

126. Faber TL, Cooke CD, Peifer JW, et al: Three-dimensional displays of left ventricular epicardial surface from standard cardiac SPECT perfusion quantification techniques. J Nucl Med 36:697, 1995.
127. Germano G, Berman DS: Quantitative gated SPECT. J Nucl Med 42:528, 2001.
128. Ficaro EP, Quaife RA, Kitzman JN, Corbett JR: Accuracy and reproducibility of 3D-MSPECT for estimating left ventricular ejection fraction in patients with severe perfusion abnormalities [abstract]. Circulation 100:I-26, 1999.
129. Gibbons RJ, Balady GJ, Timothy B, et al: ACC/AHA 2002 guideline update for exercise testing: Summary article. A report of the American College of Cardiology/American Heart Association Task Force on Practice Guidelines (Committee to Update the 1997 Exercise Testing Guidelines). J Am Coll Cardiol 40:1531, 2002.
130. Heller GV, Ahmed I, Tilkemeier PL, et al: Comparison of chest pain, electrocardiographic changes and thallium-201 scintigraphy during varying exercise intensities in men with stable angina pectoris. Am J Cardiol 68:569, 1991.
131. Sharir T, Bacher-Stier C, Dhar S, et al: Identification of severe and extensive coronary artery disease by postexercise regional wall motion abnormalities in Tc-99m sestamibi gated single-photon emission computed tomography. Am J Cardiol 86:1171, 2000.
132. Lima RSL, Watson, DD, Goode AR, et al: Incremental value of combined perfusion and function over perfusion alone by gated SPECT myocardial perfusion imaging for detection of severe three-vessel coronary artery disease. J Am Coll Cardiol 42:64, 2003.
133. Kwok Y, Kim C, Grady D, et al: Meta-analysis of exercise testing to detect coronary artery disease in women. Am J Cardiol 83:660, 1999.
134. Santana-Boado C, Candell-Riera J, Castell-Conesa J, et al: Diagnostic accuracy of technetium-99m-MIBI myocardial SPECT in women and men. J Nucl Med 39:751, 1998.
135. Garcia E, Berman DS, Port SC, et al: American Society of Nuclear Cardiology. Imaging guidelines for nuclear cardiology procedures. Part 2. J Nucl Cardiol 6:G53, 1999.
136. Borer JS: Measurement of ventricular volume and function. *In* Zaret BL, Beller GA (eds): Nuclear Cardiology: State of the Art and Future Directions. St. Louis, Mosby, 1999, pp 201-215.
137. Udelson JE, Rajendran V, Leppo JA: Detection of coronary disease by SPECT imaging and radionuclide angiography. *In* Murray IPC, Ell PJ, Van der Wall H (eds): Nuclear Medicine in Clinic Diagnosis and Treatment. 2nd ed. Edinburgh, Churchill Livingstone, 1998, pp 1389-1414.
138. Lauer MS, Lytle B, Pashkow F, et al: Prediction of death and myocardial infarction by screening with exercise-thallium testing after coronary-artery-bypass grafting. Lancet 351:615, 1998.
139. Zellweger M, Lewin H, Shenghan L, et al: When to stress patients after coronary artery bypass surgery? Risk stratification in patients early and late post-CABG using stress myocardial perfusion SPECT: Implications of appropriate clinical strategies. J Am Coll Cardiol 37:144, 2001.
140. Acampa W, Petretta M, Florimonte L, et al: Prognostic value of exercise cardiac tomography performed late after percutaneous coronary intervention in symptomatic and symptom-free patients. Am J Cardiol 9:259, 2003.
141. Bonow RO, Kent KM, Rosing DR: Exercise-induced ischemia in mildly symptomatic patients with coronary-artery disease and preserved left ventricular function. Identification of subgroups at risk of death during medical therapy. N Engl J Med 311:1339, 1984.
142. Blumenthal RS, Becker DM, Moy TF, et al: Exercise thallium tomography predicts future clinically manifest coronary heart disease in a high-risk asymptomatic population. Circulation 93:915, 1996.
143. Smith SC, Greenland P, Grundy SM: Prevention Conference V: Beyond secondary prevention: Identifying the high-risk patient for primary prevention: Executive summary. Circulation 101:111, 2000.
144. Wackers F, Young L, Inzucchi S, et al, and the DIAD Investigators: The prevalence of silent myocardial ischemia in asymptomatic patients with type 2 diabetes mellitus: Results of the DIAD study. Detection of Ischemia in Asymptomatic Diabetics [abstract]. Diabetes 52(Suppl 1):A56. 2003.
145. Miller TD, Rajagopalan N, Hodge DO, et al: The yield of screening stress myocardial perfusion imaging in asymptomatic diabetics [abstract]. J Am Coll Cardiol 39:163A, 2002.
146. De Lorenzo A, Lima RS, Siqueira-Filho AG, Pantoja MR: Prevalence and prognostic value of perfusion defects detected by stress technetium-99m sestamibi myocardial perfusion single-photon emission computed tomography in asymptomatic patients with diabetes mellitus and no known coronary artery disease. Am J Cardiol 90:827, 2002.
147. Wackers FJ, Brown KA, Heller GV, et al: American Society of Nuclear Cardiology position statement on radionuclide imaging in patients with suspected acute ischemic syndromes in the emergency department or chest pain center. J Nucl Cardiol 9:246, 2002.
148. Kontos MC, Jesse RL, Anderson P, et al: Comparison of myocardial perfusion imaging and cardiac troponin I in patients admitted to the emergency department with chest pain. Circulation 99:2073, 1999.
149. Heller GV, Stowers SA, Hendel RC, et al: Clinical value of acute rest technetium-99m tetrofosmin tomographic myocardial perfusion imaging in patients with acute chest pain and non diagnostic electrocardiogram. J Am Coll Cardiol 31:1011, 1998.
150. Stowers SA, Eisenstein EL, Wackers FJ, et al: An economic analysis of an aggressive diagnostic strategy with single photon emission computed tomography myocardial perfusion imaging and early exercise stress testing in emergency department patients who present with chest pain but non diagnostic electrocardiograms: Results from a randomized trial. Ann Emerg Med 35:17, 2000.
151. Udelson JE, Beshansky JR, Ballin DS, et al: Myocardial perfusion imaging for evaluation and triage of patients with suspected acute cardiac ischemia: A randomized controlled trial. JAMA 288:2693, 2002.
152. Cannon CP, Weintraub WS, Demopoulos LA, et al: Comparison of early invasive and conservative strategies in patients with unstable coronary syndromes treated with the glycoprotein IIb/IIIa inhibitor tirofiban. N Engl J Med 344:1879, 2001.
153. Brown KA: Management of unstable angina: The role of noninvasive risk stratification. J Nucl Cardiol 4:S164, 1997.
154. Solomon DH, Stone PH, Glynn RJ, et al: Use of risk stratification to identify patients with unstable angina likeliest to benefit from an invasive versus conservative management strategy. J Am Coll Cardiol 38:969, 2001.
155. Antman EM, Cohen M, Bernink PJ, et al: The TIMI risk score for unstable angina/non-ST elevation MI: A method for prognostication and therapeutic decision making. JAMA 284:835, 2000.
156. Ryan TJ, Antman EM, Brooks NH, et al: ACC/AHA guidelines for the management of patients with acute myocardial infarction. Circulation 100:1016, 1999.
157. Gibson RS, Watson DD, Craddock GB, et al: Prediction of cardiac events after uncomplicated myocardial infarction: Prospective study comparing predischarge exercise thallium-201 scintigraphy and coronary angiography. Circulation 68:321, 1983.
158. Leppo JA, O'Brien J, Rothendler JA, et al: Dipyridamole-thallium-201 scintigraphy in the prediction of future cardiac events after acute myocardial infarction. N Engl J Med 310:1014, 1984.
159. Miller DD, Stratman HG, Shaw LJ, et al: Dipyridamole technetium 99m sestamibi myocardial tomography as an independent predictor of cardiac event-free survival after acute ischemic events. J Nucl Cardiol 1:72, 1994.
160. Travin MI, Dessovki A, Cameron T, et al: Use of exercise technetium-99m sestamibi SPECT imaging to detect residual ischaemia and for risk stratification after acute myocardial infarction. Am J Cardiol 75:665, 1995.
161. Mahmarian JJ, Mahmarian AC, Marks GF, et al: Role of adenosine thallium-201 tomography for defining long term risk in patients after acute myocardial infarction. J Am Coll Cardiol 25:1333, 1995.
162. TIMI Study group: Comparison of invasive and conservative strategies after treatment with intravenous tPA in acute myocardial infarction: Results of the Thrombolysis in MI (TIMI) phase II trial. N Eng J Med 320:618, 1989:
163. Ellis SG, Mooney MR, George BS, et al: Randomised trial of late elective angioplasty versus conservative management for patients with residual stenoses after thrombolytic treatment for myocardial infarction (TOPS trial). Circulation 86:1400, 1992.
164. Brown KA, Heller GV, Landin RS, et al: Early dipyridamole ^{99m}Tc-sestamibi single photon emission computed tomographic imaging 2 to 4 days after acute myocardial infarction predicts in-hospital and postdischarge cardiac events: Comparison with submaximal exercise imaging. Circulation 100:2060, 1999.
165. Mahmarian JJ, Mahmarian AC, Marks GF, et al: Role of adenosine thallium-201 tomography for defining long-term risk in patients after acute myocardial infarction. J Am Coll Cardiol 25:1333, 1995.
166. Kawai Y, Tsukamoto E, Nozaki Y, et al: Significance of reduced uptake of iodinated fatty acid analogues for the evaluation of patients with acute chest pain. J Am Coll Cardiol 38:1888, 2001.
167. Narula J, Virmani R, Zaret BL: Radionuclide imaging of atherosclerotic lesions. *In* Dilsizian V, Narula J, Braunwald E (eds): Atlas of Nuclear Cardiology. Philadelphia, Current Medicine, 2003, pp 217-236.
168. Ohtsuki K, Hayase M, Akashi K, et al: Detection of monocyte chemoattractant protein-1 receptor expression in experimental atherosclerotic lesions: An autoradiographic study. Circulation 104:203, 2001.
169. McCrohon JA, Moon JCC, Prasad SK, et al: Differentiation of heart failure related to dilated cardiomyopathy and coronary artery disease using gadolinium-enhanced cardiovascular magnetic resonance. Circulation 108:54, 2003.
170. Bennett SK, Smith MF, Gottlieb SS, et al: Effect of metoprolol on absolute myocardial blood flow in patients with heart failure secondary to ischemic or non-ischemic cardiomyopathy. Am J Cardiol 89:1431, 2002.
171. Danias PG, Ahlberg AW, Clark BE 3rd, et al: Combined assessment of myocardial perfusion and left ventricular function with exercise technetium-99m sestamibi gated single-photon emission computed tomography can differentiate between ischemic and nonischemic dilated cardiomyopathy. Am J Cardiol 82:1253, 1998.
172. Cleland JG, Pennell DJ, Ray SG, et al: Myocardial viability as a determinant of the ejection fraction response to carvedilol in patients with heart failure (CHRISTMAS trial): Randomised controlled trial. Lancet 362:14, 2003.
173. Di Carli MF, Asgarzadie F, Schelbert HR, et al: Quantitative relation between myocardial viability and improvement in heart failure symptoms after revascularization in patients with ischemic cardiomyopathy. Circulation 92:3436, 1995.
174. Allman K, Shaw L, Hachamovitch R, Udelson JE: Myocardial viability testing and impact of revascularization on prognosis in patients with coronary artery disease and left ventricular dysfunction: A meta-analysis. J Am Coll Cardiol 39:1151, 2002.
175. Bonow RO: Assessment of myocardial viability with thallium201. *In* Zaret BL, Beller GA (eds): Nuclear Cardiology: State of the Art and Future Directions. St. Louis, Mosby, 1999, pp 503-512.
176. Udelson JE: Assessment of myocardial viability with technetium-99m-labeled agents. *In* Zaret BL, Beller GA (eds): Nuclear Cardiology: State of the Art and Future Directions. St. Louis, Mosby, 1999, pp 513-533.
177. Kitsiou AN, Srinivasan G, Quyyumi AA, et al: Stress-induced reversible and mild-to-moderate irreversible thallium defects: Are they equally accurate for predicting recovery of regional left ventricular function after revascularization? Circulation 98:501, 1998.
178. Bax JJ, Wijns W, Cornel JH, et al: Accuracy of currently available techniques for prediction of functional recovery after revascularization in patients with left ventricular dysfunction due to chronic coronary artery disease: Comparison of pooled data. J Am Coll Cardiol 30:1451, 1997.
179. Siebelink HM, Blanksma P, Crijns H, et al: No difference in cardiac event-free survival between positron emission tomography and single-photon emission computed tomography-guided patient management. J Am Coll Cardiol 37:81, 2001.
180. Hunt SA, Baker DW, Chin MH: ACC/AHA guidelines for the evaluation and management of chronic heart failure in the adult: Executive summary. J Am Coll Cardiol 38:2101, 2001.

181. Narula J, Khaw BH, Dec GW: Diagnostic accuracy of antimyosin scintigraphy in suspected myocarditis. J Nucl Cardiol 3:371, 1996.
182. Ballester M, Bordes R, Tazelaar HD, et al: Evaluation of biopsy classification for rejection: Relation to detection of myocardial damage by monoclonal antimyosin antibody imaging. J Am Coll Cardiol 31:1357, 1998.
183. Eguchi M, Tsuchihashi K, Hotta D, et al: Technetium-99m sestamibi/tetrofosmin myocardial perfusion scanning in cardiac and noncardiac sarcoidosis. Cardiology 94:193, 2000.
184. Hongo M, Urushibata K, Kai R, et al: Iodine-123 metaiodobenzylguanidine scintigraphic analysis of myocardial sympathetic innervation in patients with AL (primary) amyloidosis. Am Heart J 144:122, 2002.
185. Carrio I: Cardiac neurotransmission imaging. J Nucl Med 42:1062, 2001.
186. Arora R, Ferrick KJ, Nakata T, et al: 123-metaiodobenzylguanidine (MIBG) imaging and heart rate variability analysis to predict the need for an implantable cardioverter defibrillator. J Nucl Cardiol 10:121, 2003.
187. Hofstra L, Liem IH, Dumont EA, et al: Visualization of cell death in vivo in patients with acute myocardial infarction. Lancet 356:209, 2000.
188. Wu JC, Chen IY, Sundaresan G, et al: Molecular imaging of cardiac cell transplantation in living animals using optical bioluminescence and positron emission tomography. Circulation 108:1302, 2003.
189. Lee YHC, Kiesewetter DO, Lang L, et al: Synthesis of 4-[^{18}F]fluorobenzoyllisinopril: A radioligand for angiotensin converting enzyme (ACE) imaging with positron emission tomography. J Labelled Cpd Radiopharm 44:S268, 2001.
190. Dilsizian V, Shirani J, Lee YHC, et al: Specific binding of [^{18}F] fluorobenzoyl-lisinopril to angiotensin converting enzyme in human heart tissue of ischemic cardiomyopathy. Circulation 104:II-694, 2001.
191. Dilsizian V, Loredo ML, Ferrans VJ, et al: Evidence for increased angiotensin II type I receptor immunoreactivity in peri-infarct myocardium of human explanted hearts. J Am Coll Cardiol 39:365A, 2002.
192. Eagle KA, Berger PB, Calkins H, et al: ACC/AHA guideline update for perioperative cardiovascular evaluation for noncardiac surgery: Executive summary: A report of the American College of Cardiology/American Heart Association Task Force on Practice Guidelines (Committee to Update the 1996 Guidelines on Perioperative Cardiovascular Evaluation for Noncardiac Surgery). Circulation 105:1257, 2002.
193. Cohen MC, Eagle KA: Preoperative risk stratification: An overview. *In* Zaret BL, Beller GA (eds): Nuclear Cardiology: State of the Art and Future Directions. St. Louis, Mosby, 1999, pp 346-367.
194. Poldermans D, Boersma E, Bax JJ, et al: The effect of bisoprolol on perioperative mortality and myocardial infarction in high-risk patients undergoing vascular surgery. N Engl J Med 341:1789, 1999.

GUIDELINES *Thomas H. Lee and James E. Udelson*

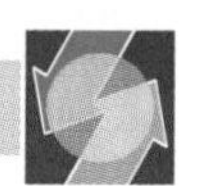

Nuclear Cardiology

Guidelines for the use of cardiac radionuclide imaging were published by the American Heart Association (AHA), the American College of Cardiology (ACC), and the American Society of Nuclear Cardiology (ASNC) in 2003.[1] Other recent commentaries on the role of nuclear cardiology tests are included under guidelines for exercise testing published in 2002[2] and for the management of acute myocardial infarction in 1999.[3] These guidelines reaffirm the fundamental theme and recommendations of the 1995 ACC/AHA radionuclide imaging guidelines.[4] The consistent message is that radionuclide imaging should be used in situations in which the history, electrocardiographic changes, and other laboratory measurements do not provide reliable information to guide management.

As with most ACC/AHA guidelines, the indications for use of nuclear cardiology tests are classified into one of four classes:

Class I: Conditions for which there is evidence and/or general agreement that testing is useful and effective.

Class II: Conditions for which there is conflicting evidence and/or a divergence of opinion about the usefulness/efficacy of performing testing.

Class IIa: Weight of evidence/opinion is in favor of usefulness/efficacy.

Class IIb: Usefulness/efficacy is less well established by evidence/opinion.

Class III: Conditions for which there is evidence and/or general agreement that testing is not useful/effective and in some cases may be harmful.

Acute ST Segment Elevation Myocardial Infarction

The ACC/AHA/ASNC guidelines indicate that radionuclide imaging should have a limited role in the diagnosis of acute myocardial infarction. These technologies are not appropriate for routine diagnosis and should be used only when information from the history, electrocardiogram, and laboratory tests is not sufficient. The task force considered evidence to be supportive of the use of radionuclide imaging for the assessment of infarct size, for the diagnosis of right ventricular infarction, or for cases in which the diagnosis of myocardial infarction was unclear and the patient presented late (more than 24 hours and less than 7 days) after the onset of symptoms (Table 13G–1).

For evaluation of prognosis after acute myocardial infarction, stress myocardial perfusion imaging was considered appropriate to assess the presence and extent of stress-induced ischemia. The guidelines do not address settings in which radionuclide imaging is preferable to exercise electrocardiography, but the 1999 guidelines on care of acute myocardial infarction indicate that exercise electrocardiography should be the first test used for risk stratification after acute myocardial infarction; imaging studies should be reserved for cases in which the electrocardiogram is likely to be uninterpretable or when the exercise electrocardiograph is equivocal.[3] Radionuclide angiography was considered useful for assessment of ventricular function after acute myocardial infarction, but echocardiography is cited as a low-cost, convenient, widely accessible alternative technology for this purpose.[3]

Unstable Angina/Non-ST Segment Elevation Myocardial Infarction

The ACC/AHA/ASNC guidelines consider radionuclide imaging to be potentially useful for diagnosis and assessment of severity of ischemia in patients with unstable angina and for assessment of left ventricular function when angina is satisfactorily stabilized with medical therapy. Myocardial perfusion imaging was also considered potentially useful (class IIa) for patients with ongoing ischemia who undergo imaging at rest. For patients presenting to emergency departments with a possible acute coronary syndrome but with nondiagnostic initial ECG and biomarkers, the guidelines recommend perfusion imaging at rest as a class I indication, based in part on a randomized controlled trial that found that sestamibi imaging can improve emergency department triage decision making for patients with suspected acute cardiac ischemia.[5]

Chronic Ischemic Heart Disease

The ACC/AHA/ASNC guidelines consider exercise or pharmacological myocardial perfusion imaging to be appropriate (class I) for evaluation of the extent and severity of coronary artery disease in patients with chronic ischemic heart disease. The guidelines consider thallium-201 and technetium-99m to be sufficiently similar to be used interchangeably in this population. Review of data on the three most commonly used agents in pharmacological perfusion imaging (dipyridamole, adenosine, and dobutamine) led the task force to conclude that adenosine or dipyridamole is preferred for patients who cannot exercise adequately. The ACC/AHA guidelines

TABLE 13G–1 American College of Cardiology/American Heart Association/American Society of Nuclear Cardiology Guidelines for the Clinical Use of Cardiac Radionuclicle Imaging*

Indication	Class I (Indicated)	Class IIa (Good Supportive Evidence)	Class IIb (Weak Supportive Evidence)	Class III (Not Indicated)
Diagnosis of STE acute myocardial infarction		Right ventricular infarction Infarction not diagnosed by standard means—late presentation		Routine diagnosis with ischemia/necrosis already documented clinically
Risk assessment, prognosis, and assessment of therapy after STE acute myocardial infarction	Rest RV/LV function Presence/extent of stress-induced ischemia Detection of infarct size and residual viable myocardium			
Diagnosis, prognosis, and assessment of therapy in patients with unstable angina/NSTEMI	Identification of ischemia in the distribution of the culprit lesion or in remote areas Measurement of baseline LV function Identification of the severity/extent of disease in patients whose angina is satisfactorily stabilized with medical therapy	Identification of the severity/extent of disease in patients with ongoing ischemia but nondiagnostic ECG	Diagnosis of myocardial ischemia in patients when the combination of history and ECG changes is unreliable	
Suspected ACS in the emergency department with nondiagnostic ECG and initial biomarkers	Assessment of risk with rest MPI Stress MPI for diagnosis of CAD after negative biomarkers or normal rest MPI			
Diagnosis of chronic ischemic heart disease	Diagnosis of symptomatic and selected patients with asymptomatic myocardial ischemia Assessment of ventricular performance (rest or exercise) Planning PTCA—identifying lesions causing myocardial ischemia, if not otherwise known Risk stratification before noncardiac surgery in select patients			Screening of asymptomatic patients with low likelihood of disease
Assessment of severity/prognosis/risk stratification of chronic ischemic heart disease	Assessment of LV performance Identification of extent and severity of ischemia and localization of ischemia† Risk stratification in patients with an intermediate risk Duke Treadmill Score Assessment of functional significance of intermediate coronary stenosis	MPI as the initial test in patients with diabetes or with >20% 10-yr CHD risk	Redefining risk 1-3 yr after initial MPI in patients with stable symptoms	
Assessment of interventions in chronic ischemic heart disease	Assessment for restenosis after PCI (symptomatic) Assessment of ischemia in symptomatic patients after CABG	Assessment 3-5 yr after CABG or PCI in select, high-risk asymptomatic patients	Assessment of drug therapy for myocardial perfusion	Routine assessment of asymptomatic patients after PTCA or CABG
Heart failure	Determination of initial LV and RV performance in heart failure Initial evaluation of LV function in patients receiving chemotherapy with doxorubicin Assessment of myocardial viability in patients with CAD and LV dysfunction without angina	Assessment of the co-presence of CAD in patients without angina	Routine serial assessment of LV and RV function Detection of myocarditis Diagnosis of CAD in hypertrophic cardiomyopathy	
After cardiac transplantation	Assessment of ventricular performance		Detection and assessment of coronary angiopathy	
Valvular heart disease	Initial and serial assessment of LV and RV function		Detection and assessment of function significance of concomitant coronary artery disease	

*Table represents a compilation of recommendations from the 1995 and 2003 guidelines.

†Exercise MPI in patients with baseline ECG abnormalities, vasodilator pharmacologic stress MPI in patients who cannot exercise adequately or who have LBBB or paced rhythm.

ACS = acute coronary syndrome; CABG = coronary artery bypass graft; CAD = coronary artery disease; CHD = coronary heart disease; ECG = electrocardiographic; LBBB = left bundle branch block; LV = left ventricular; MPI = myocardial perfusion imaging; NSTEMI = non-ST segment elevation myocardial infarction; PCI = percutaneous coronary intervention; PTCA = percutaneous transluminal coronary angioplasty; RV = right ventricular; STE = ST segment elevation.

on exercise testing continue to assert that exercise electrocardiography remains the first-choice test for women as well as men, and the imaging technologies should be used when patients cannot exercise or when the electrocardiogram is likely to be uninterpretable.[2]

Asymptomatic Patients

The ACC/AHA/ASNC guidelines do not consider cardiac radionuclide imaging an appropriate routine test for diagnosis of coronary artery disease in patients who are not symptomatic. However, radionuclide imaging is considered potentially useful for determining the need for coronary angiography in patients with positive exercise electrocardiography tests.

Before Noncardiac Surgery

Most studies of the radionuclide imaging in patients undergoing noncardiac surgery have been performed in patients undergoing major vascular procedures. Such testing was considered appropriate (class I) in patients with chronic ischemic heart disease (see Table 13G–1). However, the guidelines discourage use of radionuclide imaging before noncardiac surgery in most patients undergoing nonvascular surgery because of the lower cardiac risk of these procedures.

Before and After Revascularization Procedures

Myocardial perfusion imaging is appropriate for planning for coronary revascularization procedures and for detection of ischemia in patients who are symptomatic after these procedures (see Table 13G–1). However, the guidelines discourage routine assessment of patients who are asymptomatic after revascularization because of lack of data supporting interventions in such patients. These conclusions are consistent with recent guidelines for exercise testing.[2]

Heart Failure

The ACC/AHA/ASNC guidelines consider radionuclide assessment of left and right ventricular function to be useful in the initial work-up for heart failure, although echocardiography provides additional information on valvular disease. The noninvasive assessment of the co-presence of coronary artery disease (CAD) by myocardial perfusion imaging in patients with heart failure without angina is considered a class IIa indication. The guidelines recommend radionuclide assessment of myocardial viability as a class I indication for consideration of revascularization in patients with known CAD and left ventricular systolic dysfunction who do not have active angina.

Other Conditions

Radionuclide angiography is considered to be useful for assessment of ventricular function in patients who have undergone cardiac transplantation or who have valvular heart disease. It is also considered to be useful for baseline and serial monitoring of left ventricular function during therapy with cardiotoxic drugs.

References

1. Klocke FJ, Baird MG, Bateman TM, et al: ACC/AHA/ASNC Guidelines for the Clinical Use of Cardiac Radionuclide Imaging: A Report of the American College of Cardiology/American Heart Association Task Force on Practice Guidelines, 2003. (http://www.acc.org/clinical/guidelines/radio/index.pdf)
2. Gibbons RJ, Balady GJ, Bricker JT, et al: ACC/AHA 2002 guideline update for exercise testing: Summary article: A report of the ACC/AHA Task Force on Practice Guidelines (Committee to Update the 1997 Exercise Testing Guidelines). Circulation 106:1883, 2002.
3. Ryan TJ, Antman EM, Brooks NH, et al: ACC/AHA guidelines for the management of patients with acute myocardial infarction: 1999 update: A report of the American College of Cardiology/American Heart Association Task Force on Practice Guidelines (Committee on Management of Acute Myocardial Infarction). (http:www.acc.org)
4. Guidelines for Clinical Use of Cardiac Radionuclide Imaging. A Report of the American College of Cardiology/American Heart Association Task Force on the Assessment of Cardiovascular Procedures (Committee on Nuclear Imaging). J Am Coll Cardiol 25:521, 1995.
5. Udelson JE, Beshansky JR, Ballis DS, et al: Myocardial perfusion imaging for evaluation and triage of patients with suspected acute cardiac ischemia: A randomized controlled trial. JAMA 288:2693, 2002.

CHAPTER 14

Cardiovascular Magnetic Resonance

Dudley Pennell

Introduction to Cardiovascular Magnetic Resonance

Magnetic resonance (MR) applied to the cardiovascular system has been termed *cardiovascular magnetic resonance*, or *CMR*, by the international scientific community. CMR has grown considerably in recent years and is now firmly established in clinical and research cardiovascular medicine in the larger centers. This growth and acceptance stem from a number of factors, including technical advancements (speed, reliability, ease of use, new applications), superb image quality and field of view, and the reporting of CMR-derived new insights into entrenched problem areas in cardiology. In addition, a recognition of the excellent reproducibility of CMR images has encouraged widespread adoption of its use by academic medicine and the pharmaceutical industry so that trials can be completed with considerable power but substantially reduced sample sizes, which hastens results and lower costs. It is also worth noting that in the modern climate of safety priority, radiowave technology shares with ultrasound an inescapable advant-age over x-ray and gamma-ray modalities, which suggests that these nonionizing technologies may be preferred in the future. Further strengthening this perspective is the appreciation that echocardiography is the faster and more portable modality, whereas CMR typically provides superior image quality at a higher entry price. Echocardiography and CMR are therefore powerful and complementary partners (see Chap. 11).

Fundamental Principles of Magnetic Resonance

This abbreviated physics background to MR is included to facilitate understanding of the technical terms used throughout this chapter; greater detail can be found in more specialized texts.[1] The physical interaction required for MR is at the level of the atomic nucleus and was first described in 1946, when it was also found that the frequency of radiowave absorption depends on the strength of the external magnetic field. These two key findings form the basis for modern clinical MR imaging. Because MR does not therefore interfere with electrons in the outer atomic shell, which are responsible for chemical binding, it is fundamentally safe, unlike ionizing radiation such as x-rays, which may interact with electron binding, damaging molecules such as DNA. MR occurs only in atomic nuclei with unpaired spin (nucleons). In clinical practice, this means hydrogen-1, which is abundant in water and fat. Since hydrogen is abundant in the human body and has good sensitivity to the phenomenon of magnetic resonance, images with a high signal-to-noise ratio can be obtained. Other important elements are useful for investigation in the laboratory to characterize biochemical processes (^{13}C, ^{17}O, ^{19}F, ^{23}Na, ^{39}K), but these are not used clinically. Human spectroscopy usually makes use of the phosphorus-31 nucleus, which is important because this occurs in compounds involved in energy metabolism, such as adenosine triphosphate (ATP) and phosphocreatine (PCr). MR spectra are rarely used to construct images, however; the data are usually used to quantify metabolite concentrations.

Hydrogen nuclei behave like magnets and align to an external magnetic field. At baseline, the nuclei precess randomly about a 1.5-T magnetic field at a resonance frequency of 63 MHz, which is in the radiowave range. A body region can be excited by a pulse of radiowaves at this frequency, which has the effect of causing all the excited hydrogen nuclei to rotate away from the direction of the main magnetic field axis (the flip angle) and precess in a coordinated manner, which causes a net magnetization. After the excitation pulse is finished, the net magnetization decays to its former position (relaxation), and energy is transmitted as a radio signal. Typically, this signal is formed into a radiowave echo by the scanner such that it can be used to form an image by a receiver antenna. The contrast between different tissues in the image depends on the delay between excitation and the signal read-out (TE, or echo time) and the time between repetitive radiowave excitations (TR, or repeat time). The different forms of contrast are derived from two principal relaxation processes that affect the net magnetization, which are decay in the longitudinal axis (T1) and the transverse plane (T2). Additional magnetic fields (gradient fields), which can be rapidly switched on and off, are required to localize the radiowaves coming from the body. An MR image therefore represents a spatially resolved map of radio signals.

THE CMR SCANNER. A modern CMR scanner consists of major components of hardware. The superconducting magnet produces the static magnetic field, which is highly homogeneous, stable over time, and large enough for chest examinations. The gradient fields are generated by gradient amplifiers with ultrafast capability, which rapidly drive large currents at high voltages through the resistive gradient coils within the bore of the magnet. The radiofrequency amplifier generates the excitation pulses, and a radiofrequency antenna receives the radio signals coming from the patient. A computer controls all the scanner components with complex software. It is also used to perform the Fourier transformation and other complex mathematical processes on the raw radio signal data matrix (known as k-space), which ultimately generates the images.

SEQUENCES

A CMR scanner can only generate useful images if the various component pieces of hardware are intricately coordinated. The timing and magnitude of radiowave and magnetic field pulses along with data collection form MR sequences, which are controlled by the scanner computer. Sequences have various components such as *preparation pulses* (used to alter contrast between tissues), *excitation pulses* (shape and location of the area of the body to be excited by radiowaves), *gradient* and *magnetic field pulses* (formation of a radiowave echo to generate a useful signal for image formation), and *signal read-out* (filling of the raw data matrix or k-space). There are a large variety of sequences, which can appear daunting at first. Fundamentally, however, it is a knowledge of the properties of the sequences rather than their exact nature that is required for medical interpretation.

For CMR, the majority of imaging is performed using two basic sequences known as *spin echo* and *gradient echo*. Spin-echo sequences are also known as "black blood" and gradient-echo sequences as "white blood," although this terminology is a simplification. Spin-echo sequences are routinely used for multislice anatomical imaging, whereas gradient-echo sequences are used for physiological assessment of function through cine acquisitions. The most common prepulse is known as *inversion recovery*, and this gives strong T1 weighting, which is valuable for infarct/viability imaging. Alternatively, T2 preparation is used for coronary imaging. The read-out of the signal can be achieved in many ways, leading to sequences with other names. Usually the read-out is modified for CMR to be as fast as possible so that images, or cines, can be acquired within single breath-holds, and the faster schemes include fast low angle shot (FLASH), steady state with free precession (SSFP, also known as FISP and FIESTA), spiral imaging, and echo-planar imaging (EPI). These fast sequences yield images during a 4- to 20-second breath-hold, which substantially reduces artifact from respiratory motion and also allows three-dimensional acquisitions.

Some other sequences are also very useful in examination of the cardiovascular system. *Velocity mapping* displays each pixel in the image as a pixel velocity rather than a signal magnitude.[2] This is derived from encoding of the phase of the radio signal by using modified gradient profiles. Higher pixel velocities cause a higher phase shift, and this information can be recovered during Fourier transformation of the signal read-out. This is invaluable for measurement of peak velocities through stenosis and true flow for shunt assessment, which is calculated from the integral over time throughout the cardiac cycle of the product of mean velocity and area of a vessel. For coronary CMR, some high resolution acquisitions cannot be completed within one breath-hold, and a specialized sequence called a *navigator echo* is used to greatly reduce respiratory motion. The diaphragm movement is monitored in real time and the scanning computer calculates the coronary position, corrected for the position in the breathing cycle. A sequence called *tagging* is being increasingly used to study myocardial contraction. In this sequence, a grid of dark lines is laid across the image in diastole. The lines of altered magnetization persist and deform throughout the cardiac cycle. Using computer analysis, the intersections of the lines can be used to calculate myocardial strain, which is a quantitative and observer-independent measure of myocardial contractility. CMR angiography is a rapidly growing technique in which three- or four-dimensional visualization of a vessel lumen is achieved, usually after intravenous injection of an MR contrast agent based on the element gadolinium.

CONTRAST AGENTS

A number of classes of contrast agents are used for MR, but for the cardiovascular system, only the gadolinium agents are currently in clinical use. Gadolinium has seven unpaired electrons in its outer shell, which allows it to couple efficiently with excited water spins such that their relaxation is hastened. This predominantly results in a shortening of T1, which increases signal on T1-weighted images. Gadolinium is a toxic element and is therefore chelated to other molecules for clinical use. The properties of the chelator determine the distribution of the gadolinium, and all current gadolinium contrast agents remain in the extracellular compartment. These agents have proven invaluable for arterial angiography and viability imaging. Many other MR contrast agents exist, and some are based on other elements such as iron, manganese, or dysprosium, which have dominant effects on shortening T2, thereby reducing the MR signal. Iron-based contrast agents have been evaluated in humans for angiography and perfusion and for showing macrophage activity in atherosclerotic plaque. Finally, a class of targeted contrast agents has been described that links large number of gadolinium atoms through an intermediary compound to antibody fragments, which in principle allows any biological epitope to be selectively imaged. This has been demonstrated for thrombus and may become a powerful CMR tool of the future.

Gating and Safety

All cardiac and many vascular CMR sequences rely on cardiac gating to prevent artifact from the periodic cardiac contraction cycle. In nearly all current scanners, this is achieved through gating to the R wave of the electrocardiogram. In some CMR scanners, gating is linked to the vector electrocardiogram (two-dimensional electrical activation over time), which may have advantages of reliability, more consistent timing to the R wave peak, and more effective arrhythmia rejection. Older scanners also used gating to the peripheral pulse, but this is now largely abandoned. Most recently, cardiac gating has been achieved without the electrocardiogram by gating the CMR image acquisition directly to bulk cardiac motion detected directly during imaging.

The safety of CMR is well described, and in comparison with x-ray–based techniques there are obvious advantages. However, there are two main problems with MR that must be considered. The first is the issue of flying projectiles in the magnet room, which have the potential to strike the patient. The problem items are iron-based with ferromagnetic properties. These include scissors, electrical items with power transformers such as injection pumps, and oxygen cylinders. Strict adherence to protocols restricting access into the magnet room to only fully trained staff is essential. The second major issue involves metallic implants or implanted electronic devices. Most metallic implants are MR compatible, including all prosthetic cardiac valves, vascular stents, and orthopedic implants. Although some stent manufacturers suggest abstinence from MR for a period after implantation, there are no published data to support this recommendation, and several reports concur with clinical experience that MR can be performed at any time after implantation with absence at 1.5 T of magnetic attraction,[3] heating,[4] or adverse clinical risk.[5] Problems remain with some neurological devices such as cerebrovascular clips, and a specialist's neurological advice is required in these patients. Electronic implants are more problematic for MR, and in principle the high magnetic field of MR will interfere with the electronics and programming of such devices. For CMR, the main implants in question are pacemakers and cardioverter-defibrillators, and their presence is a strong relative contraindication for CMR. An extra reason for caution is that the pacing wires can couple to the radiofrequency waves and heat significantly. Recent work, however, shows that there are strategies that will allow CMR in these patients, in particular if the device can be turned off for the duration of the scan, but until further evidence is available, this can only be considered in patients for whom benefit exceeds risk.

Clinical Applications

Coronary Artery Disease (see Chap. 50)

ASSESSMENT OF VENTRICULAR VOLUMES, MASS, AND FUNCTION. CMR is well validated for quantifying the volumes and mass of the ventricles, and it has become the clinical gold standard against which other techniques are measured because of its three-dimensional nature, which is not reliant on geometric assumptions. Comparisons with other techniques show wide variability in individual patients and are not greatly instructive, other than illustrating the difficulties of comparison of clinical techniques.[6] The accuracy and reproducibility of the measurements make CMR useful for the longitudinal follow-up of patients and for research using small sample sizes in hemodynamic and remodeling research.

The accuracy of CMR for measurement of global left ventricular volume has been established by comparing CMR images of ex vivo ventricles with the water displacement volume of casts of the ventricles.[7] In vivo, volume validation is more difficult to achieve, but the grounds for determining accuracy depend on comparing left ventricular stroke volume with the stroke volume of the right ventricle,[7] or with aortic flow measured using velocity mapping,[2] and showing their equivalence in normal human subjects. Right ventricular volumes have also been validated against water displacement of casts[8] and by comparing the right ventricular stroke volume with pulmonary artery flow. Left ventricular mass measurements have been validated against human autopsy hearts and in animals.[9] Right ventricular mass measurements have been validated against ex vivo animal hearts.[10]

An important feature of CMR is the excellent interstudy reproducibility of volume and mass measurements. Although other forms of reproducibility are often quoted for functional techniques (interobserver, intraobserver), they have little statistical import, whereas interstudy reproducibility can be directly used to quantify sample sizes in research studies and the minimum clinical difference observable, which represents a true clinical change. Interstudy reproducibility is measured as the standard deviation (SD) of the differences in two measurements of a parameter over a reasonable time period in which no clinical change is expected, but no substantial recollection is expected by the operator of patient positioning and other procedural factors. The SD is often expressed as a coefficient of variability by division into the parameter mean value. Sample sizes for trials are easily calculated from the technique interstudy SD, and low SDs are important because a reduction in SD between techniques leads to a squared reduction in sample size (i.e., half the SD equals one quarter the sample size). The interstudy SD for volumes and mass by CMR is excellent for both the left ventricle[11] and the right ventricle,[12] and is considerably superior to that of two-dimensional echocardiography.[11] Several drug trials have now used CMR as a primary or major endpoint.[13]

CMR is valuable for assessment of regional contractile function; clinically, this is usually achieved by visual inspection of cines in standard imaging planes. Quantification of wall motion and thickening using conventional techniques is possible for both the left ventricle and the right ventricle but is not widely used. A preferable CMR technique is tagging, which directly assesses myocardial strain and other deformations as a measure of contractility. Tagging CMR has been validated using sonomicrometer studies and can be applied for full three-dimensional myocardial analysis by collective modeling of the numerous small individual myocardial elements.[14] Recently, advanced tagging CMR acquisitions have greatly increased the spatial and temporal resolution and considerably simplified postprocessing. Clinical applications are just starting to emerge.

ASSESSMENT OF MYOCARDIAL INFARCTION AND VIABILITY. Myocardial infarction (MI) can be detected with high resolution using a protocol known as late gadolinium enhancement CMR. Gadolinium is given intravenously and CMR is performed after a delay using an inversion recovery sequence. Little gadolinium enters areas of normal myocardium, because there is uniform tightly packed muscle and gadolinium is an extracellular contrast agent. However, the extracellular compartment is expanded in areas of MI due to cellular rupture, and therefore differential distribution occurs. The kinetics of entry of gadolinium into the MI territory is delayed and the optimal time for imaging of the distribution of gadolinium is after 10 to 15 minutes. By nulling (forcing to near-zero) of the normal myocardial signal with adjustment of the inversion time, the area of infarction can be shown with extremely high contrast relative to the black normal myocardium. A simple but helpful mnemonic is that "bright is dead." The transmural distribution of MI can be visualized in vivo for the first time using this technique because of its high resolution. Validation has been performed in animal models (Fig. 14-1).[15] In humans, late gadolinium enhancement CMR detects Q wave and non-Q wave MI accurately[16] and with such high sensitivity that small MIs can be demonstrated that are not apparent using gated perfusion single-photon emission computed tomography (SPECT) (Fig. 14-2),[17] and microinfarcts can be shown after percutaneous coronary intervention.[18] In the acute setting, the extent of late gadolinium enhancement is related to the magnitude of cardiac enzyme release and the functional outcome after recovery. Late gadolinium enhancement CMR reveals a permanent record of MI (both acute and chronic) and is proving very useful clinically for the diagnosis of MI in cases of doubt, or when other techniques for detection are inconclusive. The technique has clarified the pathological significance of Q waves after MI.[19] It has good interstudy reproducibility,[20] suggesting a useful role in studies of therapies for limiting MI in the acute setting (see Chap. 47).

In the assessment of myocardial viability to determine the likely benefit from coronary bypass surgery, both conventional and late gadolinium CMR images are useful, and studies are ongoing to determine which technique yields more optimal results. An established approach is to measure myocardial wall thickness in areas of chronic transmural MI, using the premise from pathological studies that preserved thickness (>5 mm) indicates preserved viability. This simple criterion shows good correlation in cases of chronic MI to fluorodeoxyglucose positron emission tomography (FDG-PET).[21] In dysfunctional myocardium, improved thickening shown by low-dose dobutamine CMR is also in good agreement with FDG-PET findings.[21] More recently, the simple morphological measure of the transmural extent of late gadolinium enhancement by CMR has been shown to be highly predictive of viability,[22] with high likelihood of recovery when the transmural extent of infarction is less than 50 percent (Fig. 14-3).[23] Unlike wall thickness measurements, however, which can only be applied in cases of chronic MI, late gadolinium enhancement is also useful for prediction of functional recovery in cases of acute MI.[24] There is high concordance of late gadolinium enhancement CMR with PET,[25] and superior results have been shown in comparison with thallium 201 SPECT[26] (see Chap. 13).

STRESS VENTRICULOGRAPHY. Stress CMR using dobutamine is now clinically established for diagnosing obstructive coronary artery disease (CAD) through induction of new wall motion abnormalities (Fig. 14–4).[27] Pharmacological stress is preferred to dynamic exercise within the magnet to prevent motion artifacts. Stress CMR is superior to dobutamine stress echocardiography (see Chap. 11),[28] which is a function of higher image quality. Stress CMR is effective in the diagnosis of CAD in patients who are unsuitable for dobutamine echocardiography.[29] Outcome studies following normal stress CMR are limited but show a low event rate.[29-31] CMR has been used for preoperative risk assessment, and higher risk has been shown with demonstration of ischemia.[30] Real-time stress CMR may hasten the acquisition and make the study easier for the patient by eliminating the need for breath-holding.

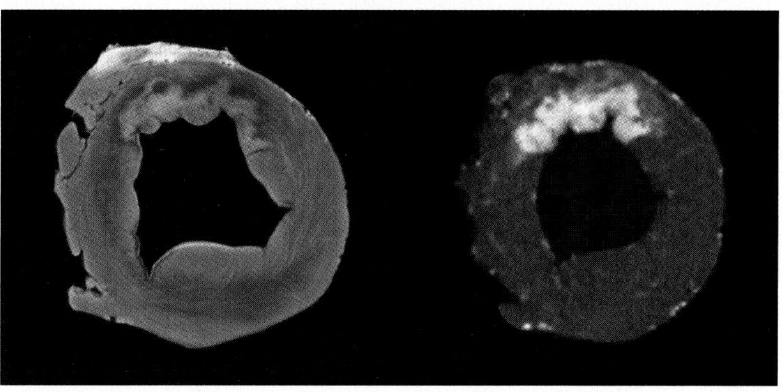

FIGURE 14–1 Validation of late gadolinium-enhanced cardiovascular magnetic resonance (Gd-CMR). A subendocardial infarct has been produced by ligation of a coronary artery in a dog, and gadolinium was injected shortly before sacrifice. On the **left,** the triphenyltetrazolium chloride (TTC)–negative area indicates the extent and shape of the infarct that is closely matched by the ex vivo CMR scan **(right).** Studies such as this have shown increased gadolinium concentration within the infarct zone and close correlation between the total infarct size by histology and CMR. Note the transmural resolution of the CMR scan and the similarity in shape of the infarctions. (Courtesy of Drs. R.J. Kim and R.M. Judd.)

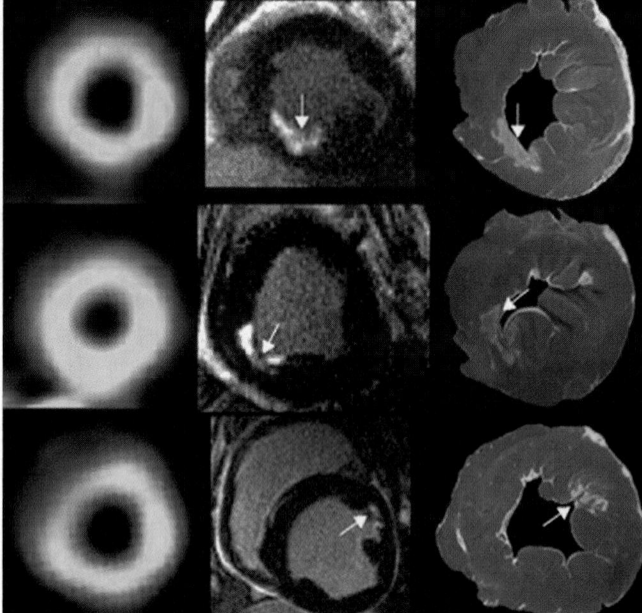

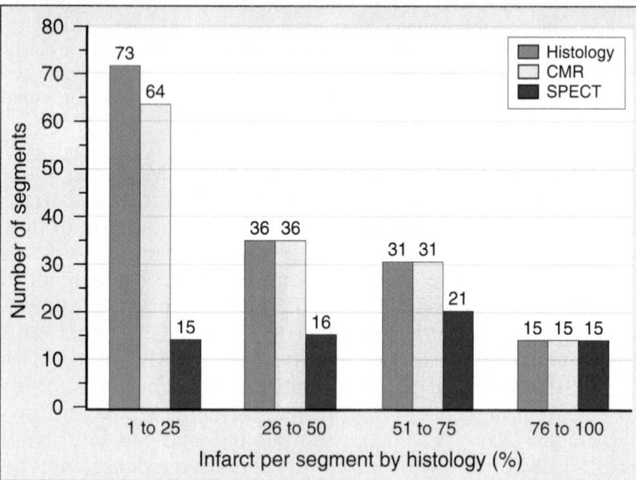

FIGURE 14–2 Comparison of cardiovascular magnetic resonance (CMR), ^{99m}Tc-sestamibi single-photon emission computed tomography (SPECT), and histologic findings in patients with subendocardial infarction. This figure shows a comparison between SPECT **(left),** late gadolinium-enhanced CMR **(middle),** and triphenyltetrazolium chloride histology **(right)** in three different dogs with experimentally induced subendocardial infarction. There is close similarity between histological and CMR findings, but in all three cases SPECT fails to demonstrate the infarction because of inadequate resolution. The effects of this are summarized in the graph, which shows excellent agreement between histology and CMR between the number of segments with infarction categorized by the percentage of infarction per segment. The agreement with SPECT, however, is only satisfactory in segments with greater than 75 percent infarction per segment. This shows that CMR is significantly more accurate in identifying small infarctions and the extent of infarction than SPECT. (From Wagner A, Mahrholdt H, Holly TA, et al: Contrast-enhanced MRI and routine single photon emission computed tomography [SPECT] perfusion imaging for detection of subendocardial myocardial infarcts: an imaging study. Lancet 361:374, 2003.)

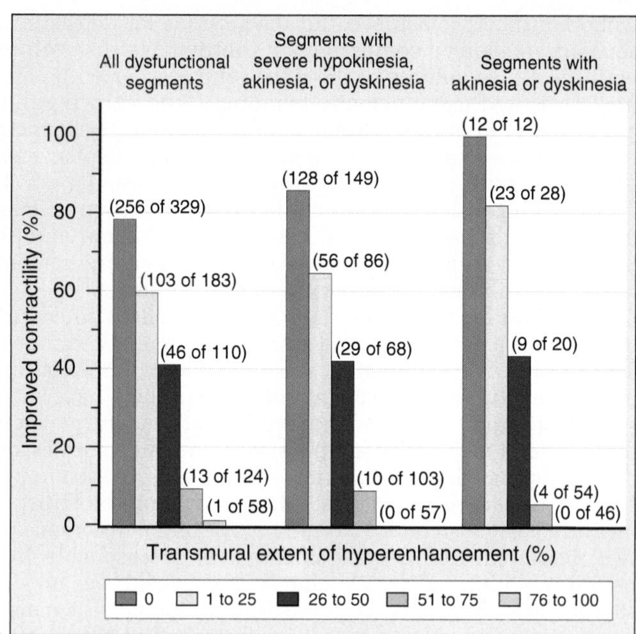

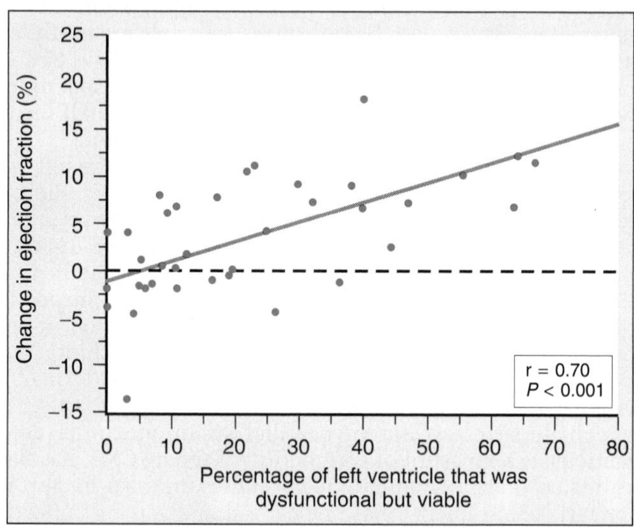

FIGURE 14–3 Assessment of myocardial hibernation by late gadolinium-enhanced cardiovascular magnetic resonance (CMR). There is a significant relationship between the likelihood of improvement of contraction in a segment that is dysfunctional, and the preoperative transmural extent of late gadolinium enhancement. **A,** Relation for all dysfunctional segments, those with at least severe hypokinesis, and those with at least akinesis. The discrimination is greatest for the most dysfunctional segments. The change in left ventricular ejection fraction was directly related to the percentage of the left ventricle, which was dysfunctional but viable using the late gadolinium-enhancement technique **(B)**. (From Kim RJ, Wu E, Rafael A, et al: The use of contrast-enhanced magnetic resonance imaging to identify reversible myocardial dysfunction. N Engl J Med 16:1445, 2000.)

A valuable adjunct to stress CMR would be the quantification of wall motion assessment, which would reduce the observer variability encountered with dobutamine-enhanced echocardiography. This has been approached in several ways, with early results. A center line method for assessing wall thickening during dobutamine-enhanced echocardiography, with comparison to normal ranges, improved the accuracy for detection of CAD in patients with single-vessel disease. Tagging CMR has also been applied, and this is expected to be more useful because of the independence of intrinsic strain measurements from endocardial motion.[32] Increased sensitivity with tagging has been shown,[31] but larger clinical trials and improved post-processing are needed to demonstrate clinical applicability. Other work in quantification has included assessment of stress diastolic function and stress global ventricular function measured with velocity mapping of aortic flow.[33] Further work is required to determine the clinical role of these techniques.

MYOCARDIAL PERFUSION. Myocardial perfusion CMR is in development but is close to achieving clinical utility. This has the potential for significant impact because of the combination of greatly enhanced resolution with no ionizing radiation. Full ventricular segmental coverage is achieved by using multiple contiguous short-axis slices or mixed short- and long-axis planes. A fast intravenous bolus (typically 5 to 7 ml/sec) of gadolinium contrast agent is given using a power injector, and the myocardial signal changes during the first pass are measured. Ideally, each slice is imaged with each cardiac cycle to maximize the quality of the analysis, although imaging on alternate cycles has been performed with good results.[34] Low signal areas representing reduced perfusion can be visualized directly. Alternatively, computer quantification of parameters such as the signal upslope can be used to generate parametric relative perfusion maps (Fig. 14–5)[34] or measures of perfusion index at rest and stress.[35] More complex analysis for quantification of myocardial perfusion or perfusion reserve includes preprocessing to remove respiratory motion and deconvolution of the myocardial signal curve with the input function taken from the left ventricular blood pool.[36] Perfusion CMR has been validated using microspheres in animal models[37,38] and in humans using PET.[34]

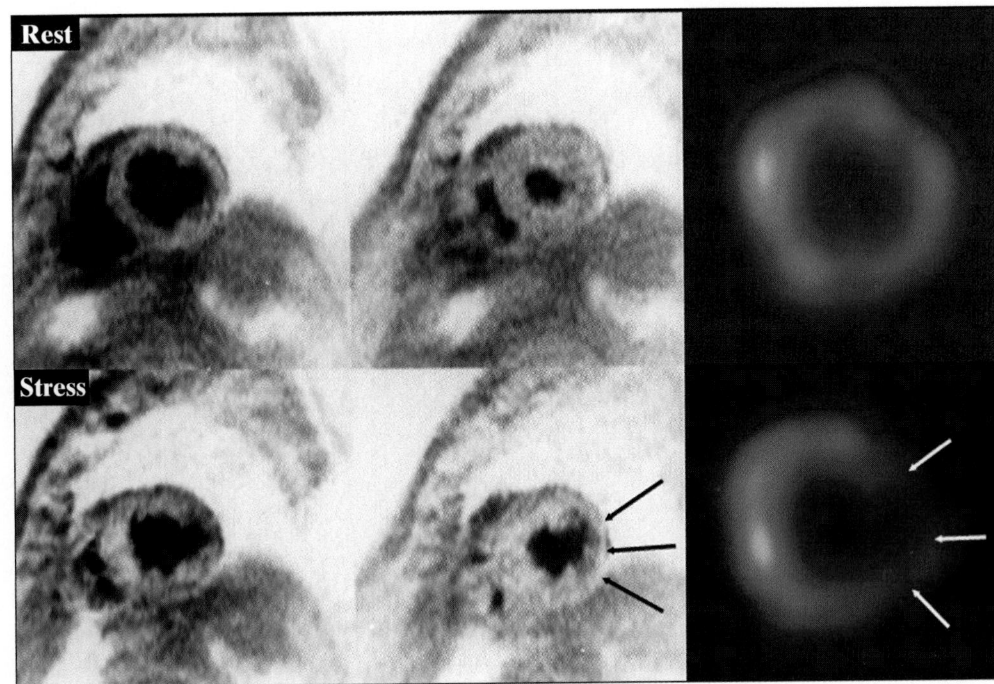

FIGURE 14–4 Cardiovascular magnetic resonance (CMR) stress ventriculography in a patient with left circumflex stenosis. The **left** and **middle panels** show end-diastolic and end-systolic frames, respectively, from CMR cines (the video scale is inverted, and blood therefore appears black), and the **right panels** show the corresponding slice by thallium single-photon emission computed tomography. The **upper row** is images taken at rest and the **lower row** is images taken during dobutamine stress. There is stress-induced wall motion abnormality; this is well shown in the end-systolic stress image (black arrows), which is similar in location and extent to the ischemia shown on the stress thallium scan (white arrows). (From Pennell DJ, Underwood SR, Manzara CC, et al: Magnetic resonance imaging during dobutamine stress in coronary artery disease. Am J Cardiol 70:34, 1992.)

For clinical application, several perfusion CMR protocols are being tested using adenosine as a pharmacological stress agent. One approach is to assess stress myocardial perfusion only[34] and define areas of nonviability using late gadolinium enhancement. A more conventional approach is to perform both stress and resting myocardial perfusion CMR to produce perfusion reserve measurements.[39] When both stress and resting studies are performed, however, the optimal order has not yet been defined, because residual gadolinium from the first injection has the potential to interfere with the subsequent study. The ideal CMR sequence is also not fully resolved, because superior coverage is obtained with a hybrid gradient-echo–echo-planar imaging sequence but higher signal is obtained with SSFP. Both techniques appear to give good results. A technique that does not require ultrafast imaging or gadolinium contrast has also been described called T2* blood oxygen level dependent (BOLD),[40] but the sensitivity of T2* to perfusion change may be quite low and its clinical role is not yet defined. There is general consensus that fast gadolinium injection is desirable for quantification, although for purely qualitative analysis this is not necessary. There is little difference among gadolinium contrast agents for perfusion CMR, because all currently distribute into the extracellular space, although those with lower viscosity can be injected at lower pressures, which has some patient safety advantages.

Myocardial perfusion CMR has shown very good results for the detection of CAD, in comparison with coronary angiography (see Chap. 18),[34] PET,[34] and SPECT (see Chap. 13). Improvements in myocardial perfusion reserve have been shown after coronary angioplasty.[41] The excellent resolution of perfusion CMR has also allowed visualization of perfusion abnormality not related to epicardial coronary artery in other conditions such as cardiac syndrome X (Fig. 14–6),[35] which agrees with results of CMR spectroscopy.[42] Perfusion CMR is likely to improve our understanding of the pathophysiology of these types of conditions and may have significant clinical application if the findings have diagnostic, therapeutic, or prognostic value.

CORONARY ANGIOGRAPHY AND FLOW. Coronary CMR angiography is still technically difficult for confident assignment of both presence and severity of coronary stenosis owing to small arterial size, tortuosity, complex anatomy, and cardiac and respiratory motion. Using highly optimized three-dimensional acquisitions, there has been gradual improvement in resolution and clinical robustness using both breath-hold and navigator techniques. The most significant clinical study, with multicenter participation, showed good results for the exclusion of multivessel proximal CAD requiring operative intervention.[43] However, current limitations of spatial resolution and rapid coronary motion during the acquisition allow only broad categorization of diameter stenosis, and distal run-off assessment is difficult for surgical planning.

These limitations of luminal stenosis imaging are not problematic, however, for the assessment of the course of anomalous coronary arteries, in which CMR plays a significant clinical role. The malignant course of some coronary arteries between the aorta and pulmonary artery is significantly better depicted by CMR than by x-ray coronary angiography because of the three-dimensional CMR tomograms in comparison with two-dimensional x-ray projections with overlapping structures.[44] Coronary CMR sequences can image coronary vein bypass grafts. Black and white blood approaches are approximately 90 percent accurate for identifying graft patency. This may prove useful in postoperative chest pain syndromes, but vein graft stenoses and the distal anastomoses cannot be assessed directly by luminal assessment. Although coronary imaging for luminal stenosis remains very challenging, some technical advances may prove valuable, such as high magnetic field scanners (Fig. 14–7),[45] intravascular contrast agents,[46] preoxygenation, and novel sequences.

Assessment of coronary function can also be achieved by measuring coronary flow velocities using CMR images. Adenosine stress coronary flow has been reported in animals and in humans, and the coronary flow

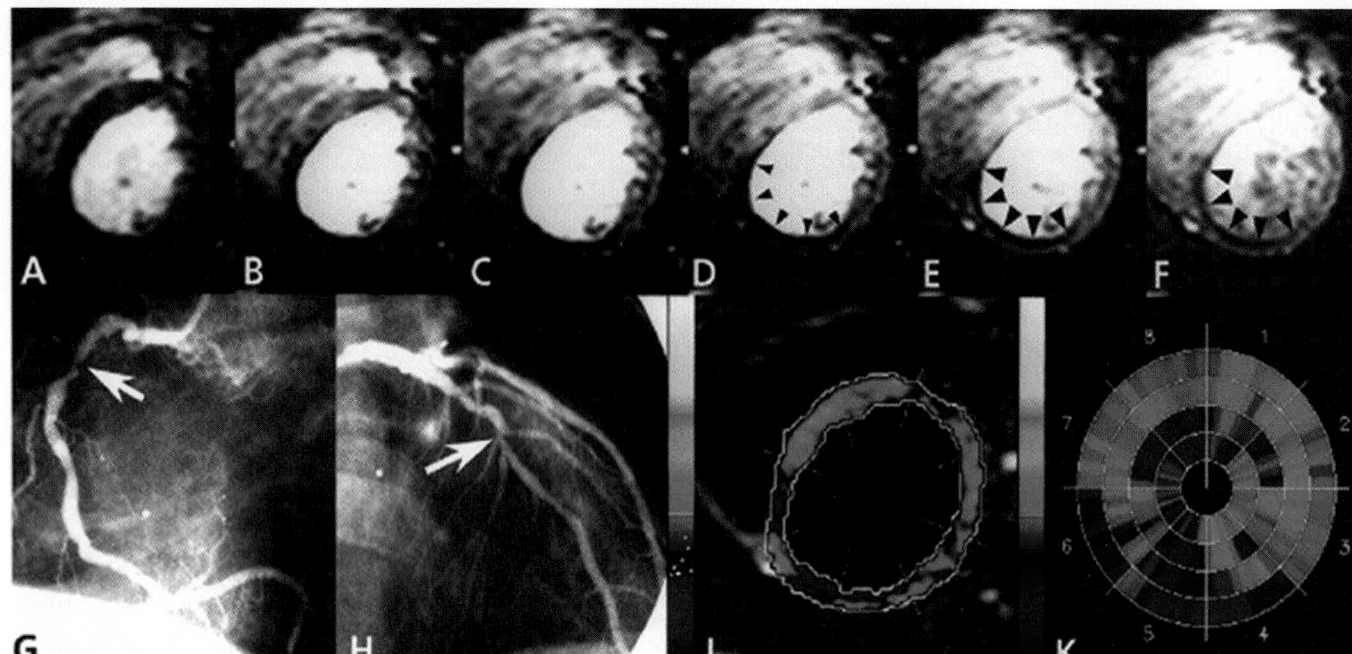

FIGURE 14–5 Perfusion cardiovascular magnetic resonance (CMR) images and parametric maps in a patient with stenosis of the right coronary and left anterior descending arteries (arrows in panels **G** and **H**). A single slice shown in panels **A** through **F** shows delayed wash-in the inferior wall of gadolinium-enhanced images during first pass (arrows). The parametric map in panel **I** shows this abnormality in blue. The polar map shown in panel **K** indicates areas of abnormal perfusion in blue in both the inferoseptal and the anteroseptal regions, corresponding to the right coronary and left anterior descending artery stenoses, respectively. (From Schwitter J, Nanz D, Kneifel S, et al: Assessment of myocardial perfusion in coronary disease by magnetic resonance: A comparison with positron emission tomography and coronary angiography. Circulation 103:2230, 2001.)

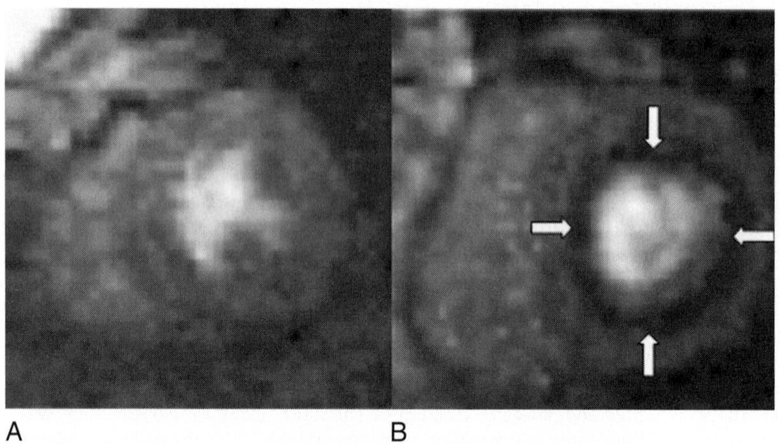

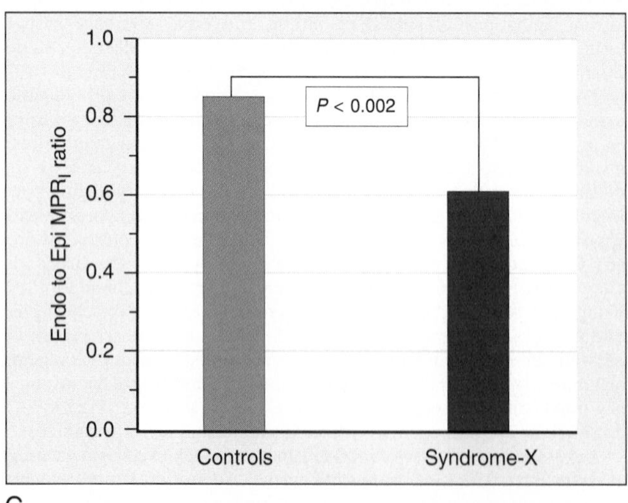

FIGURE 14–6 Perfusion cardiovascular magnetic resonance (CMR) in a patient with syndrome X. The high resolution of CMR allows the in vivo visualization of subendocardial perfusion defects for the first time. A perfusion CMR study at rest **(A)** and during adenosine stress **(B)** is shown in a patient with syndrome X (typical angina, greater than 2-mm ST segment depression during exercise electrocardiography, and normal coronary arteries). The two CMR images are from peak enhancement during the first pass of gadolinium enhancement. The image at baseline is normal but the image during adenosine enhancement shows subendocardial hypoperfusion. The graph **(C)** shows the myocardial perfusion reserve ratio between the endocardium and the epicardium in a group of syndrome X patients and control subjects. The ratio is significantly lower in patients with syndrome X, indicating reduced endocardial perfusion reserve. (From Panting JR, Gatehouse PD, Yang GZ, et al: Abnormal subendocardial perfusion in cardiac syndrome-X detected by cardiovascular magnetic resonance imaging. N Engl J Med 346:1948, 2002.)

reserve has been used to identify stenosis of the left anterior descending artery[47] and in-stent restenosis.[48] It has also been shown that reduced baseline flow and flow reserve in vein grafts are useful in identifying significant stenosis.[49]

ARTERIAL WALL: FUNCTION AND STRUCTURE. The arterial wall offers opportunities for assessment of atherosclerosis by CMR that have the potential to yield important additional information compared to luminal imaging, from endothelial dysfunction to arterial mechanical properties, total plaque burden, and plaque characterization, including vulnerability. Most CMR data are derived from work on the aorta and carotid and brachial arteries, but more recently coronary wall studies have been published (Fig. 14–8).

Endothelial function is considered one of the earliest triggers of atherosclerosis (see Chap. 35). As with ultrasonography, endothelial function can be examined noninvasively by CMR using stimuli that cause arterial vasodilation, such as flow-mediated dilation (endothelium dependent) and direct-acting drugs such as nitroglycerin (endothelium independent). Flow-mediated dilation is assessed by forearm cuff occlusion for a standard time period, followed by release, which induces increased endothelial shear, the release of nitric oxide, and arterial dilation. This technique has been performed using CMR on the brachial artery, but unlike ultrasonography, which measures arterial diameter, CMR measures arterial area and thus has significant advantages.[50] These include improved determination that the imaging is perpendicular to the vessel, greater immunity to arterial shape changes with transducer application and patient movement during the procedure, and increased sensitivity. Validation studies have been performed in humans using invasive techniques, and repeated measurements by CMR appear to have greater reproducibility than measurements by ultrasonography, suggesting smaller sample sizes for trials using CMR.[50] An additional advantage of CMR is that flow changes can also be measured directly in response to the standard stimuli.[51] Arterial dilation measurements have also been performed by CMR in the proximal coronary arteries, but more experience is needed in this area.

The mechanical properties of the arterial wall are significantly affected by sclerosis, and in the aorta this increases pulse pressure, afterload, and cardiac workload, resulting in reduced organ perfusion. Sclerosis of the vessel wall can be assessed in a number of ways, but CMR has usually been used to measure compliance in the ascending aorta (change of aortic sectional volume normalized to pulse pressure in μl/mm Hg) and pulse wave velocity around the aortic arch (rate of propagation of the flow wave in early systole in meters/sec). These measures have an age-dependent normal range, are abnormal in early atherosclerosis, and have been shown to be predictive of cardiac events.

Arterial wall CMR can also be used to identify total plaque burden within an imaging volume. Plaque burden is usually assessed on T1-weighted images with double or triple inversion to suppress blood signal in the lumen. Quantification of the vessel wall volume over the imaging stack is achieved by summation by planimetry of the difference in each image between the outer and inner vessel boundary.[52] This total vessel volume includes normal vessel wall and the atherosclerotic burden, which is dominant in cases of disease and dynamic for longitudinal studies of natural history and treatment. CMR studies show sufficient sensitivity to measure the effectiveness of antiatheroma therapy such as statin treatment over 12 months, showing a reduction in total wall volume.[53] More recently, the technique has been extended to the coronary wall, and wall thickening has been identified.[54]

Plaque constituents can be assessed using a combination of T1-, T2-, and proton density–weighted images, which allows assessment of plaque vulnerability.[55] Cholesterol pools are identified from low signal on T1 and T2 images,[56] and the fibrous cap can be identified overlying this.[57] Thin or disrupted caps on CMR have been strongly linked with cerebrovascular events.[58] Contrast agents have been used to further characterize plaque and show inflammation,[59] neovasculature,[60] and the fibrous cap.[61] Longitudinal study by CMR has followed the lipid pool.[62] Coronary plaque constituents have also been identified, but improved resolution would improve assessment in these small vessels.[54]

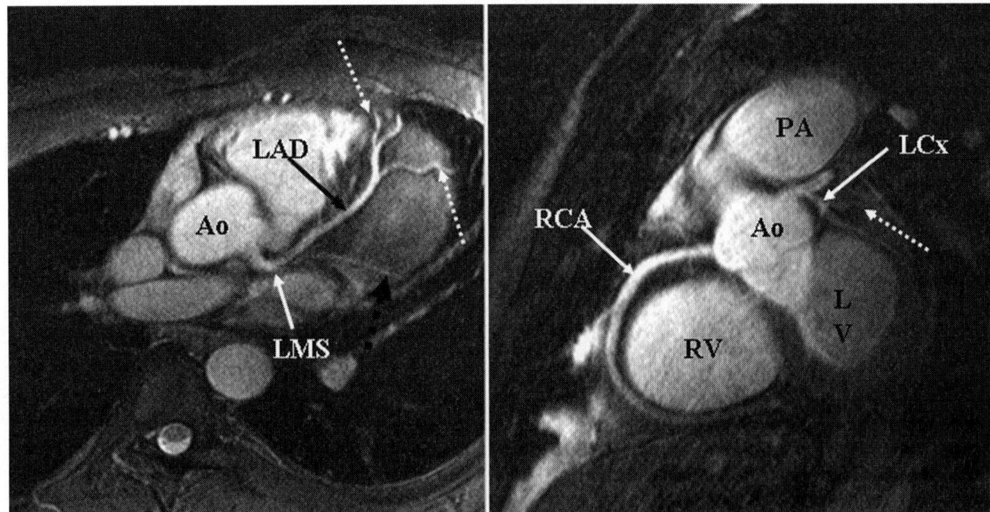

FIGURE 14–7 Coronary cardiovascular magnetic resonance (CMR) at 3 T. The **left panel** shows the left coronary artery and branches (dotted arrows) and the **right panel** shows the right coronary artery (RCA). Ao = aorta; LAD = left anterior descending artery; LMS = left main stem; LCx = left circumflex artery; LV = left ventricle; PA = pulmonary artery; RV = right ventricle. (From Stuber M, Botnar RM, Fischer SE, et al: Preliminary report on in vivo coronary MRA at 3 Tesla in humans. Magn Reson Med 48:425, 2002.)

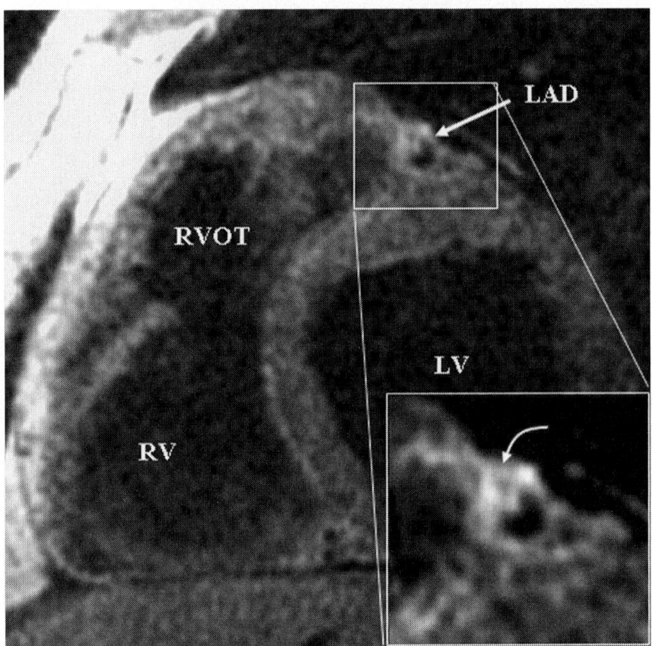

FIGURE 14–8 Coronary wall cardiovascular magnetic resonance (CMR). The **main panel** shows a short-axis cut of the ventricles at the base of the heart, and in the interventricular groove lies the left anterior descending artery (LAD). This is enlarged in the **inset** and a substantial eccentric plaque is identified (curved arrow). The lumen is still widely patent. RV = right ventricle; RVOT = right ventricular outflow tract; LV = left ventricle. (From Fayad ZA, Fuster V, Fallon JT, et al: Noninvasive in vivo human coronary artery lumen and wall imaging using black-blood magnetic resonance imaging. Circulation 102:506, 2000.)

Evaluation of Acute Coronary Syndromes

(see Chaps. 47 and 49)

Cardiac myocardial resonance has been used for the assessment of acute chest pain.[63] CMR showed a sensitivity of 84 percent and a specificity of 85 percent, was the strongest predictor of an acute coronary syndrome, and added diagnostic value over the usual clinical parameters, including the electrocardiogram, troponin, and TIMI risk score. CMR also can be used to identify microvascular obstruction in cases of acute MI.[64] This is demonstrated approximately 1 to 2 minutes after intravenous injection of gadolinium during the vascular distribution phase of the contrast agent and well before late gadolinium-enhancement CMR is performed. Areas within the MI that have severely compromised perfusion appear black, indicating microvascular collapse. Microvascular obstruction detected by CMR is associated with ventricular remodeling[65] and an increased likelihood of cardiovascular events that is independent of the size of the MI.[66]

Cardiomyopathy (see Chap. 59)

DILATED CARDIOMYOPATHY. CMR clearly demonstrates the functional abnormalities associated with dilated cardiomyopathy (DCM), and ventricular volumetric analysis is useful for follow-up. The right ventricle is usually involved in DCM, which may be a useful diagnostic marker. The quantitative effects of therapy can be assessed.[13,67] A key clinical question in the diagnosis of DCM is its differentiation from heart failure resulting from CAD. In many centers, coronary angiography is routinely performed for this task. In those patients with unobstructed coronary arteries and no other etiological factor, the diagnosis of DCM is usually made. This differentiation is important clinically for several reasons in patients with CAD: they have a worse prognosis; they may benefit from revascularization and/or aneurysmectomy; and secondary preventive pharmacotherapy with statins and aspirin are typically used. Conversely, in DCM patients, secondary causes, such as excess alcohol ingestion or myocardial iron overload,[68] need to be excluded; as genetic studies of DCM begin to identify inherited abnormalities, accurate phenotyping and family screening are important for early diagnosis. Late gadolinium-enhanced CMR has been shown to be very useful in this respect. In a study of patients with the clinical label of DCM following normal coronary angiography, 59 percent showed no gadolinium enhancement, 28 percent showed patchy or longitudinal striae of midwall enhancement, clearly different than the distribution in CAD patients, and 13 percent had gadolinium enhancement indistinguishable from patients with CAD (Fig. 14–9).[69] These data suggest that using the coronary angiogram as the arbiter for the presence of left ventricular dysfunction due to CAD could have led to an incorrect assignment of DCM etiology in 13 percent of patients, possibly because of coronary recanalization after infarction. The midwall myocardial enhancement in DCM patients is similar to the fibrosis found at autopsy and has not been visualized in vivo with other techniques; it may have prognostic importance as a source of reentrant tachyarrhythmias. CMR may therefore become a useful alternative to routine coronary angiography in the diagnostic work-up of DCM by allowing direct and highly sensitive assessment of the myocardial substrate for CAD, rather than relying on the coronary angiogram, which yields problems with false-positive results (coincidental coronary disease in DCM that has not caused myocardial infarction) and false-negative results (normal coronary arteries despite previous myocardial damage due to arterial recanalization). Such accurate phenotyping is particularly useful for genotyping. Another CMR technique for assessing prognosis in DCM is spectroscopy, in which adverse outcomes are predicted by a low PCr/ATP ratio.[70]

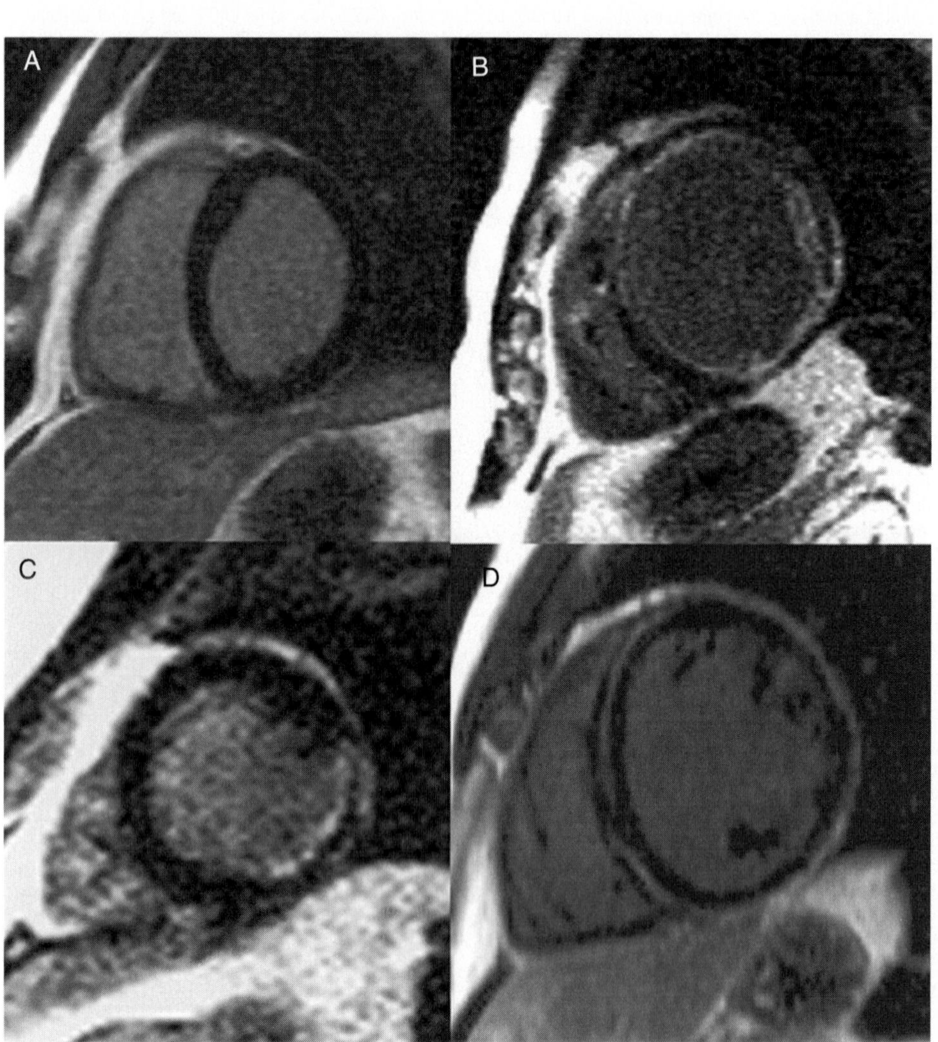

FIGURE 14–9 Late gadolinium-enhanced cardiovascular magnetic resonance (CMR) in patients with dilated cardiomyopathy (DCM). **A,** Patient with DCM and no gadolinium enhancement. **B,** Patient with known previous myocardial infarction resulting in heart failure in which late gadolinium enhancement is seen throughout the subendocardium causing thinning, particularly in the septum and inferolateral wall. **C,** Patient with the presumed clinical diagnosis of DCM because of the presence of a dilated heart with symptoms of heart failure but with normal coronary arteries by coronary angiography. Late gadolinium-enhanced CMR clearly shows an inferolateral infarction despite the normal coronary arteries, and it is likely that this patient's heart failure relates to coronary disease and not DCM. **D,** Patient with DCM who has late gadolinium enhancement of the midwall of the septum in the ventricular longitudinal fibers. This pattern of fibrosis is recognized by pathologists but has not been previously visualized in vivo. (From McCrohon JA, Moon JC, Prasad SK, et al: Differentiation of heart failure related to dilated cardiomyopathy and coronary artery disease using gadolinium-enhanced cardiovascular magnetic resonance. Circulation 108:54, 2003.)

HYPERTROPHIC CARDIOMYOPATHY. CMR is very useful in the diagnosis and assessment of hypertrophic cardiomyopathy (HCM), with ideal image quality covering both ventricles completely for localization of hypertrophy. CMR is used when echocardiography is questionable, particularly with apical hypertrophy.[71] Cines oriented in the plane of the left ventricular outflow tract show obstruction, and velocity mapping can be used to assess peak velocities. Systolic anterior motion of the mitral valve is also clearly seen. Improvement in obstruction after septal ablation or resection can be demonstrated, as can the location and size of the associated infarction, which are helpful for planning of repeat procedures. CMR myocardial tagging identifies abnormal patterns of strain, shear, and torsion in cases of HCM, demonstrating significant dysfunction in hypertrophic areas. CMR spectroscopy shows bioenergetic defects in HCM patients with varying genetic mutations, which supports the hypothesis that the underlying substrate for HCM might be inefficient energy utilization.[72] The accuracy of the phenotypic determination of HCM by CMR is helpful for family screening, and genetic linkage studies for causative mutations are improved in power. Late gadolinium enhancement occurs in HCM, which represents myocardial fibrosis.[73] Most patients have no gadolinium enhancement, and a common benign pattern is two stripes running along the junction of the right ventricular insertion into the left ventricle. More extensive gadolinium enhancement can be dense and plaque-like or diffuse. The greater the gadolinium enhancement, the higher the risk of heart failure or sudden death, presumably because of reentrant tachycardias and systolic failure from myocyte replacement (Fig. 14–10).[74] More work needs to be done in this promising area. CMR has also proved useful in differentiating causes of hypertrophy, which can mimic HCM. This includes Fabry disease (α-galactoside deficiency), which occurs in 4 percent of HCM populations and is an X-linked genetic disorder causing accumulation of glycosphingolipid in myocytes and endothelium, in which CMR shows unusual lateral wall gadolinium enhancement.[75] Other differential diagnoses, including amyloidosis and athletic heart, can be distinguished by CMR.

IRON OVERLOAD CARDIOMYOPATHY. Iron overload, or siderotic cardiomyopathy, occurs in patients with severe inherited anemia requiring regular blood transfusions from birth. The iron load of the transfusions can be combined with increased intestinal iron absorption, leading to iron deposition in the tissues because the body has no mechanism for iron excretion. The iron is toxic and causes oxidative cellular damage and organ dysfunction. The most important of these conditions is beta-thalassemia major; 71 percent of these patients die from heart failure at a young age. Beta-thalassemia major is a substantial worldwide health problem, with 60,000 affected children born annually who require long-term treatment. It has not been possible to measure cardiac iron except by myocardial biopsy, which is usually compromised because of sampling error due to patchy iron distribution. This has led to the usual clinical management being based on blood ferritin and liver iron levels, which is clearly not ideal because of the ongoing incidence of heart failure. Recently, CMR has been shown to be useful, with measurement of the myocardial relaxation parameter T2*. A low myocardial T2* indicates iron overload[68] and is related to left ventricular dysfunction and increased ventricular volumes and mass, providing clinical validation of the technique (Fig. 14–11). Further evidence for the value of the myocardial T2* measurement has come from evidence that T2* increases with left ventricular function recovery in thalassemia patients undergoing intensive iron chelation treatment for heart failure.[76] CMR has also shown the effects of different chelation regimens on myocardial

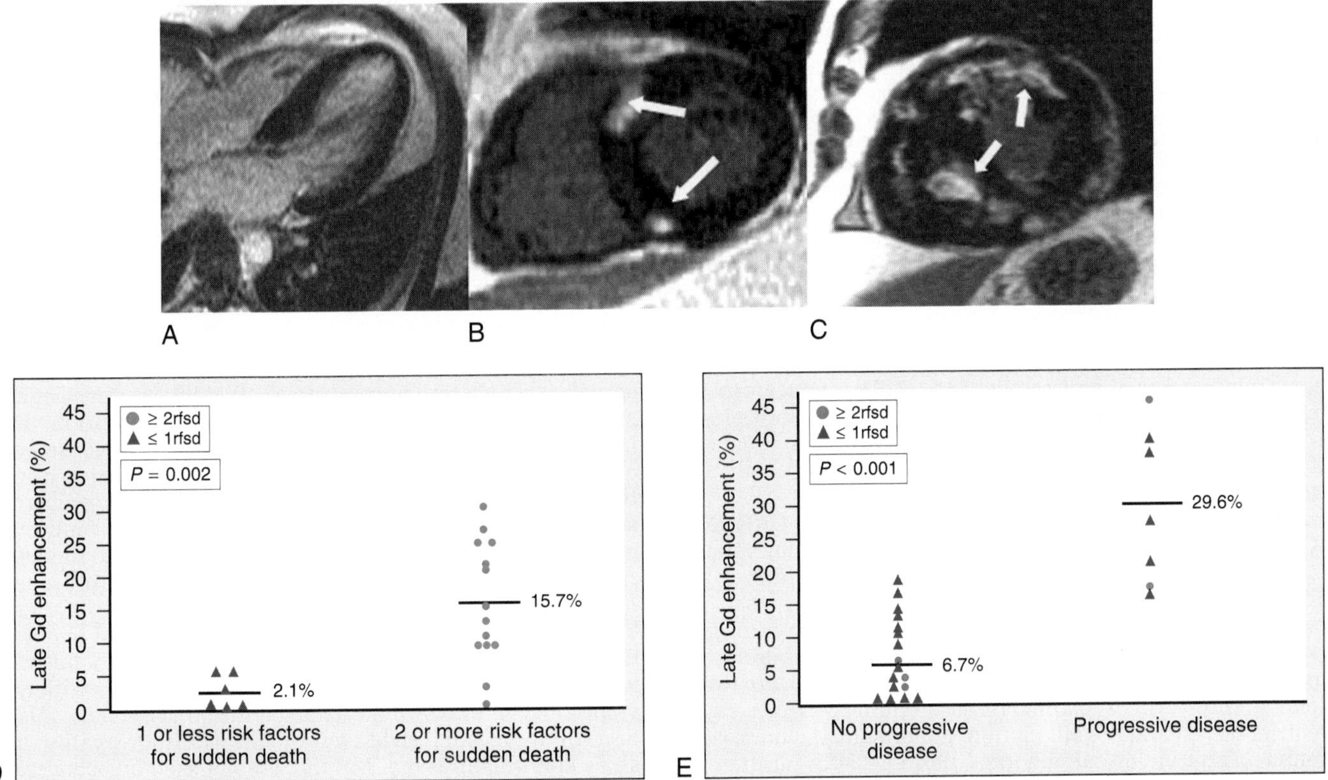

FIGURE 14–10 Late gadolinium enhancement and risk assessment in patients with hypertrophic cardiomyopathy (HCM). **A,** HCM patient with no gadolinium enhancement. **B,** HCM patient with longitudinal striae of late gadolinium enhancement at the insertion points of the right ventricle into the left ventricle (arrows). **C,** HCM patient with extensive plaque-like fibrosis (arrows). The relationship between the extent of late gadolinium enhancement and the number of risk factors for sudden death (rfsd) is shown in **D,** and documented progression of ventricular dilation toward heart failure is shown in **E.** In both cases, extensive gadolinium enhancement indicated a poor prognosis. (From Moon JCC, McKenna WJ, McCrohon JA, et al: Toward clinical risk assessment in hypertrophic cardiomyopathy with gadolinium cardiovascular magnetic resonance. J Am Coll Cardiol 41:1561, 2003.)

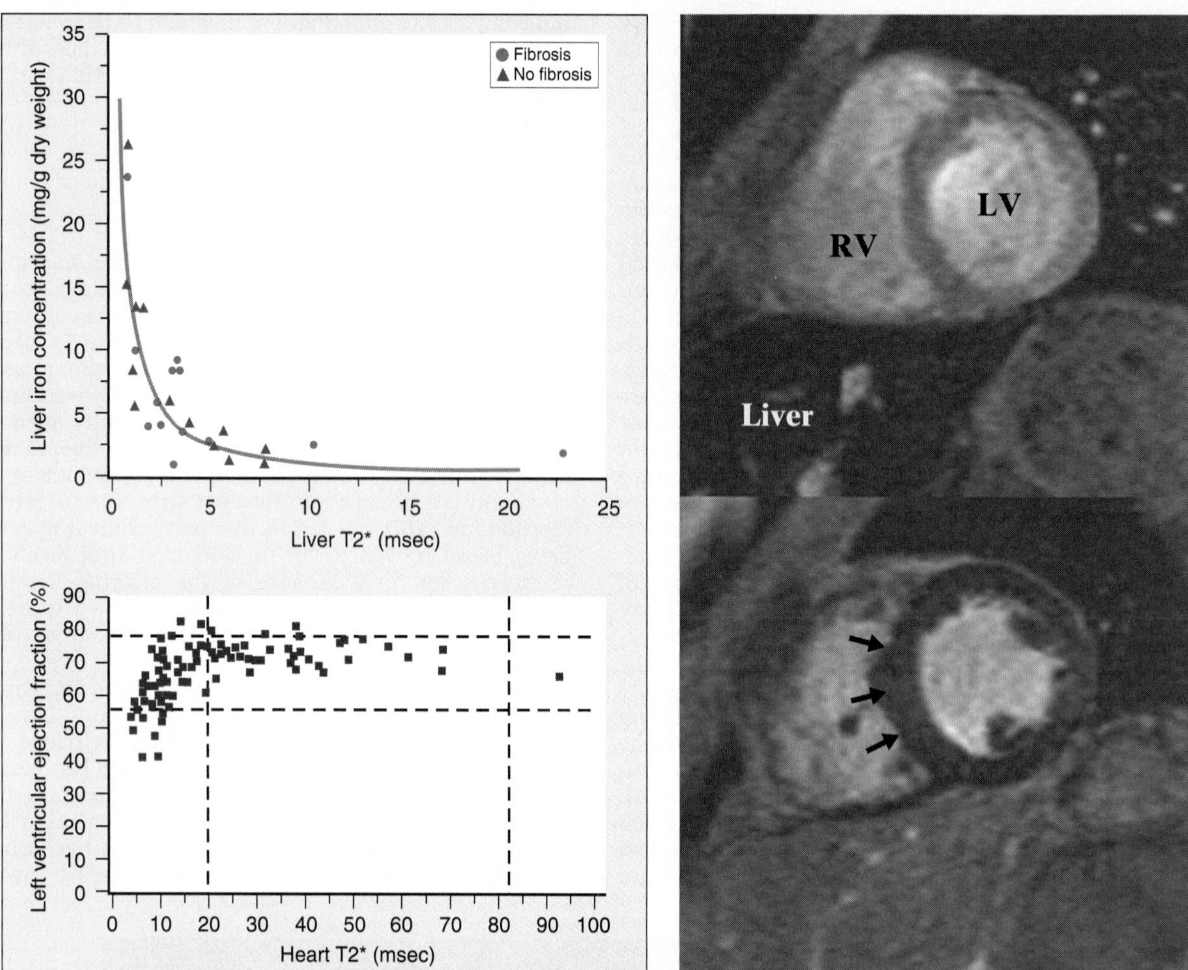

FIGURE 14–11 T2* cardiovascular magnetic resonance (CMR) in patients with iron overload cardiomyopathy. The **upper graph (left)** shows the tissue calibration between T2* of the liver and liver biopsy. The fit is best for the nonfibrotic liver samples, as expected. The curvilinear relationship is transformed into a linear relationship with a log-log plot. The **lower graph** shows the relationship between myocardial T2* and the left ventricular ejection fraction. Normal values for heart T2* are greater than 20 msec, and in this range the ejection fraction is normal. Below this range, there is a marked fall in ejection fraction related to iron toxicity. The two CMR scans **(right)** are short-axis cuts showing both the ventricular myocardium and the liver. The **upper panel** shows an iron-loaded liver (dark) but a normal heart appearance. If there were concern about this patient's heart iron status, liver biopsy would suggest iron loading, which could lead to an increase in chelation therapy with desferrioxamine and the risk of significant side effects. The **lower panel** shows the opposite scenario in which the liver has normal signal, but the heart is iron loaded (dark, arrows). Should this patient have a liver biopsy, the result would be falsely reassuring and chelation therapy would not be increased, and the patient would be at risk of death from heart failure and arrhythmias. These disparities in iron between the heart and liver help to explain why heart failure is the biggest cause of mortality in thalassemia patients. LV = left ventricle; RV = right ventricle. (From Anderson LJ, Holden S, Davies B, et al: Cardiovascular T2* (T2 star) magnetic resonance for the early diagnosis of myocardial iron overload. Eur Heart J 22:2171, 2001.)

iron.[77] On modern scanners, the T2* CMR sequence can be completed in a single breath-hold and may therefore prove to be cost-effective in areas of the world with large numbers of beta-thalassemia patients, such as in Asia and the Mediterranean.

ARRHYTHMOGENIC RIGHT VENTRICULAR CARDIOMYOPATHY. CMR depicts well the structural and functional abnormalities of the right ventricle, with no limitation from its retrosternal location. CMR is therefore widely used in expert centers for the investigation of arrhythmogenic right ventricular cardiomyopathy.[78] The diagnostic criteria of arrhythmogenic right ventricular cardiomyopathy are well defined, and CMR is helpful in ascertaining whether right ventricular regional wall motion abnormalities, increased volumes, morphological abnormalities, and fatty infiltration are present. Follow-up of the quantitative parameters over time can also be useful clinically. Problems occur if the scans are overinterpreted, because the right ventricle shows substantial normal variations, including reduced regional wall motion in the region of the moderator band insertion, highly variable trabeculation, and substantial fat around the coronary vessels and epicardium. Sufficient experience of the normal variants is therefore important. In addition, it is important to recognize the limitations of CMR, because poor-quality breath-holds with fast spin-echo images may lead to the misinterpretation of wall thinning, because epicardial fat may not be distinguished clearly from right ventricular myocardium, and artifacts may give rise to an increased right ventricular wall signal that mimics fat. Fatty infiltration is not considered a definitive sign of disease in any case, because it can occur in other circumstances.[79] An abnormal CMR scan has been linked to an adverse prognosis, but more work needs to be done in this area. Finally, patients with right ventricular outflow tract tachycardia that is not related to arrhythmogenic right ventricular cardiomyopathy may show abnormalities by CMR that are not seen by echocardiography,[80]

MYOCARDIAL SARCOIDOSIS. Myocardial sarcoidosis is relatively uncommon, but sudden death may be its initial clinical presentation. Standard imaging techniques suffer from low diagnostic accuracy, and the clinical diagnosis is difficult.[81] CMR may be of value, with gadolinium enhancement occurring in presumed areas of fibrosis.[82] Enhancement may reduce after steroid treatment and is therefore a potential therapeutic marker of myocardial activity. The use of T2-weighted sequences may also be helpful in identifying active myocardial inflammation. CMR requires further assessment in this area.

MYOCARDIAL AMYLOIDOSIS. CMR is useful in cases of restrictive cardiomyopathy, such as amyloidosis, which can be recognized by typical diastolic dysfunction, ventricular hypertrophy, and interatrial septum thickening.[83] Amyloid infiltration of the myocardium may show increased signal with late gadolinium enhancement. CMR can exclude with reasonable accuracy the differential diagnosis of constriction when the pericardial thickness is normal.

MYOCARDITIS (see Chap. 60). The diagnosis and investigation of myocarditis are often difficult. CMR shows focal increases of myocardial signal in patients with acute myocarditis using gadolinium-enhanced T1-weighted spin-echo CMR images with early imaging at 1 to 2 minutes and measurement of relative myocardial enhancement compared with skeletal muscle.[84] Abnormal myocardial signal is also seen with T2-weighted spin-echo CMR images. Normalization of signal intensity occurs with healing, unless cell death has occurred, in which case late gadolinium imaging may show patchy enhancement. Contrast enhancement 4 weeks after the onset of symptoms has been predictive for the functional and clinical long-term outcomes.[85] Although promising clinically, more experience is needed with this technique on various CMR scanners. A similar technique has been shown to predict anthracycline toxicity.[86]

HEART TRANSPLANTATION (see Chap. 26). Acute rejection results in an increase in myocardial mass, reduction in ventricular function, high myocardial signal intensity, and increased T2, which occur with myocardial edema or cellular infiltration. These changes are not reliable indicators of acute rejection, particularly in the early stages. In cases of early rejection, decreased PCr/ATP ratios are evident by CMR spectroscopy, although this has to be distinguished from ischemia. CMR can assess medical treatment on the remodeling process associated with long-term use of cyclosporine.[87]

Valvular Heart Disease (see Chap. 57)

CMR is useful in cases of valve disease but often plays a secondary role to echocardiography. However, in cases of difficulty in obtaining adequate echocardiography examinations, and for valvular regurgitation in particular, CMR has significant clinical utility.[88]

VALVE MORPHOLOGY. Normal heart valves are thin and rapidly moving, and only with the use of breath-hold sequences have the leaflets become well defined on CMR images on a routine basis. Abnormal valves are thicker and less mobile and are thus more easily visualized, but calcification causes local signal loss that may obscure valve pathology on black-blood images. Valve leaflet function throughout the cardiac cycle is well assessed using gradient-echo cines, especially with the latest SSFP techniques. Valve area can be assessed by direct planimetry using a cross-sectional plane immediately downstream from the valve, and plane-following techniques can be used to ensure tracking of the valve movement throughout the cycle, to eliminate through-plane motion errors.[89] Calcification has the potential to increase valve area on direct planimetry, but this is uncommon because calcifications are mainly located within the cusps. Bicuspid aortic valves or fused valve leaflets can be readily identified.

ASSESSMENT OF TURBULENCE AND JETS. Turbulence causes intravoxel dephasing with gradient-echo CMR cines, and this is useful clinically for the identification of regurgitation with signal loss in the receiving chamber (Fig. 14-12). The length and area of the signal loss are only semiquantitive measures of severity, however, because these measures depend on hemodynamic variables such as size and shape of the valve orifice, the pressure gradient, and technical parameters of the pulse sequence. Modern CMR systems now typically acquire cines using the SSFP technique, which is less sensitive to turbulence-related signal loss, so that comparison between cine types for the area of signal loss is not clinically useful. Real-time color flow CMR has been implemented, but its clinical utility has not yet been assessed. Therefore, flow and volumetric techniques are used to quantify regurgitation. For quantification of regurgitation, flow in the aorta and pulmonary artery at each time point through the cardiac cycle are measured by multiplying the vessel cross-sectional area by the mean flow; the results are displayed as flow curves. For stenotic jets, the peak velocity can be measured in plane or through plane using velocity mapping and related to the peak pressure gradient by the modified Bernoulli equation in the normal way. Using short echo time sequences, the jets appear coherent with high signal, although surrounding turbulence may cause signal loss (Fig. 14-13). The velocity-sensitivity should be set above the expected peak velocity, to avoid aliasing.

QUANTIFICATION OF REGURGITATION. Quantitative assessment of regurgitation can be obtained in a number of ways. If a single valve is affected on either side of the heart, the regurgitant volume can be calculated from the difference of right ventricular and left ventricular stroke volumes using the volumetric technique of contiguous short-axis cine slices spanning the ventricles.[90] If single valves on both sides of the heart are regurgitant, the method can be extended by subtracting great vessel flow, measured by CMR velocity mapping, from the ventricular stroke volumes measured with the volumetric technique. This method compares favorably with catheterization and Doppler echocardiography (see Chaps. 11 and 17).[91] Reversal of pulmonary vein flow indicates severe mitral regurgitation, as with echocardiography. Direct methods for measuring systolic regurgitant flow and ventricular inflow at the mitral annulus level are less satisfactory because of annulus motion and jet eccentricity. An alternative technique for pulmonary or aortic regurgitation is the direct assessment of regurgitation using flow mapping immediately downstream of the valve by measuring the retrograde volume flow after valve closure. This diastolic backflow is divided into the systolic forward flow to derive a regurgitant fraction. This simple technique has been used to identify responses to angiotensin-converting enzyme inhibition[92] and vasodilation.[93] It has high interstudy reproducibility, suggesting that it may be valuable for longitudinal follow-up of regurgitation severity over time.[94]

QUANTIFICATION OF STENOSIS. To quantify the velocity of a jet through a valve stenosis, it is necessary to adjust the imaging parameters so that signal is present in the jet core. For higher velocities, this requires a very short TE to prevent signal loss or other artifacts interfering with the measurement. Turbulence around the jet core is usual, appears dark on the cine, and does not interfere with measurements within the jet. There is good agreement between CMR and other techniques in evaluating mitral and aortic valve stenosis.[95] The valve area can also be directly

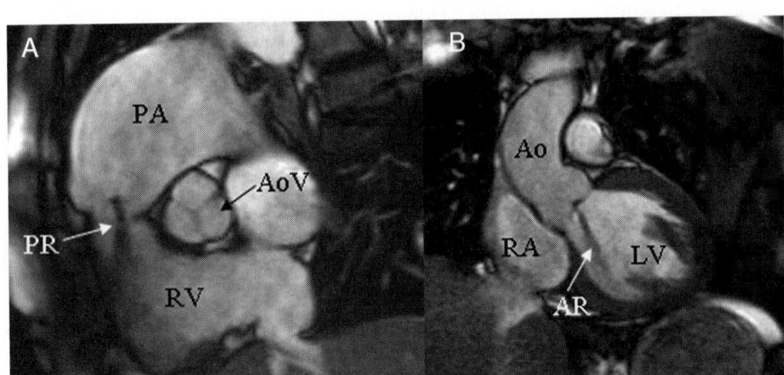

FIGURE 14–12 Cardiovascular magnetic resonance (CMR) of patients with valvular regurgitation. **A,** Patient with pulmonary hypertension with a dilated pulmonary artery. The images are from a steady state with free precession (SSFP) cine in diastole, and the aortic valve (AoV) is seen to be closed. A jet of pulmonary regurgitation (PR) can be seen entering the right ventricle. **B,** Patient with aortic regurgitation (AR) in the coronal plane. Ao = aorta; LV = left ventricle; PA = pulmonary artery; RA = right atrium; RV = right ventricle.

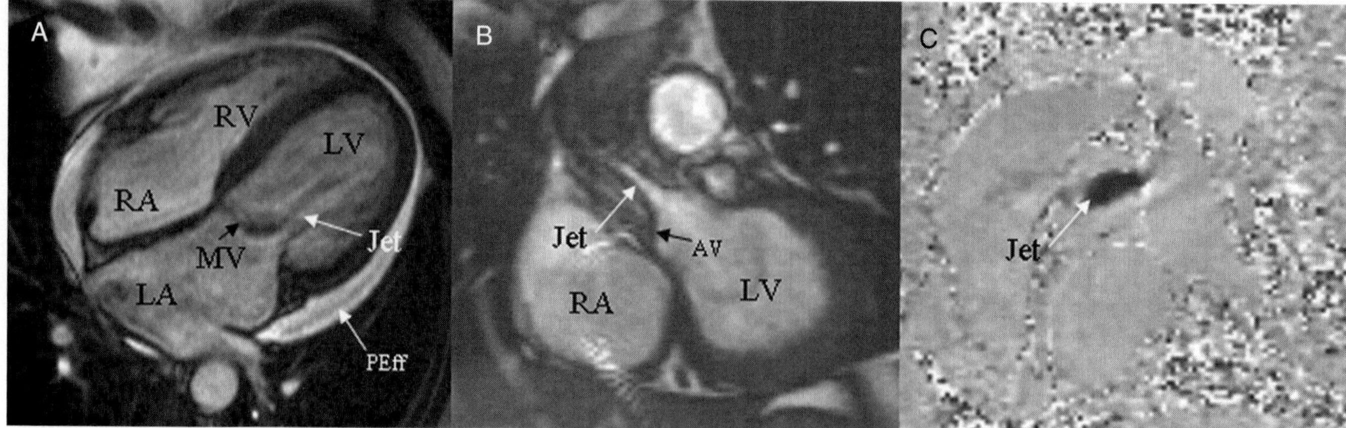

FIGURE 14–13 Cardiovascular magnetic resonance (CMR) of patients with valvular stenosis. **A,** Diastolic frame from a four-chamber steady state with free precession (SSFP) cine. The mitral valve (MV) is thickened, and there is poor opening with jet formation and surrounding signal loss from turbulence (Jet). The left atrium (LA) is enlarged and there is pericardial effusion (PEff). **B,** Aortic stenosis, with central bright jet formation and surrounding signal loss from turbulence. **C,** Velocity map taken through the aortic stenotic jet, with a measured velocity of 4.3 meters/sec, equal to a calculated pressure drop of 74 mm Hg. AV = aortic valve; LV = left ventricle; RA = right atrium; RV = right ventricle.

planimetered in patients with aortic stenosis.[96] Because echocardiography is the first-line clinical test to investigate valve stenosis, CMR is used when acoustic windows are poor or when discordant imaging and invasive results occur. Improved left ventricular and microvascular function and reduced hypertrophy,[97] as well as myocardial metabolism and diastolic function,[98] have been shown by CMR after aortic valve replacement for stenosis.

PROSTHETIC VALVES. CMR of all prosthetic heart valves at 1.5 T is safe, because there is no substantial magnetic interaction and heating is negligible.[99] Metallic valve components produce artifacts and signal loss, however, which are mild on spin-echo images but more apparent on gradient-echo cines. Small paravalvular jets can be obscured by the artifact, but velocity profiles close to aortic valve prostheses have been measured using valve tracking techniques.

Diseases of the Pericardium (see Chap. 64)

CMR is well suited to defining functional and anatomical abnormalities associated with the pericardium[100] but is mainly used when echocardiography yields incomplete information. CMR is very sensitive in the detection of pericardial effusion, which has high signal intensity with SSFP cine imaging and has clinical value when the effusion is loculated or complex. Signal from effusion is usually low on spin-echo images. Pericardial constriction is usually, but not invariably, associated with pericardial thickening, which is well depicted with both spin-echo and gradient-echo imaging (Fig. 14–14). The signal of the normal pericardium is low and appears as a thin dark line between fat outside the visceral and parietal layers. The thickness in normal subjects is 1 to 2 mm, but the upper range of normal for CMR is usually taken as 4 mm, which allows for chemical shift signal cancellation effects at the fat-pericardium border. Pericardial thickening is often inhomogeneous in cases of acute and chronic pericardial disease, and the signal characteristics can be variable. Acute inflammation may give rise to a pericardium with increased signal on spin-echo images, which enhances early after gadolinium administration. It is important to distinguish pericardial thickening from pericardial effusion, as both may appear dark on spin-echo images. The distinction is achieved by using cine sequences. Calcium is not seen directly by CMR but appears dark, and computed tomography should be used if information on calcium is clinically required. Other pericardial abnormalities can also be identified by CMR. Cysts have characteristic signal intensity, with low signal on T1-weighted spin-echo images but high signal with T2 weighting. Complete absence of the pericardium is indicated by a leftward shift of the long axis of the heart, and partial absence is seen as a protrusion of a portion of the heart.

Cardiac Tumors (see Chaps. 63 and 83)

Cardiac tumors are usually first diagnosed or suspected after transthoracic echocardiography, often as an incidental finding. Information can be obtained by echocardiography on the tumor localization, origin, extent, and resectability, but characterization may well be incomplete. CMR can then be very helpful.[101] The wide field of view of CMR allows significantly improved determination of the relationship of the tumor to adjacent structures for surgical planning, as well as identifying infiltration into the pericardium. CMR also offers a number of means of tumor characterization, which may have important clinical value. The most obvious example is that of a well-circumscribed, high signal intensity lesion that shows complete signal suppression using fat saturation techniques, which is diagnostic of lipoma (Fig. 14–15). A variant of this diagnosis, which is also very well demonstrated by CMR, is atrial lipomatous hypertrophy. Alternatively, an irregular tumor that shows signal increase during the first-pass bolus of

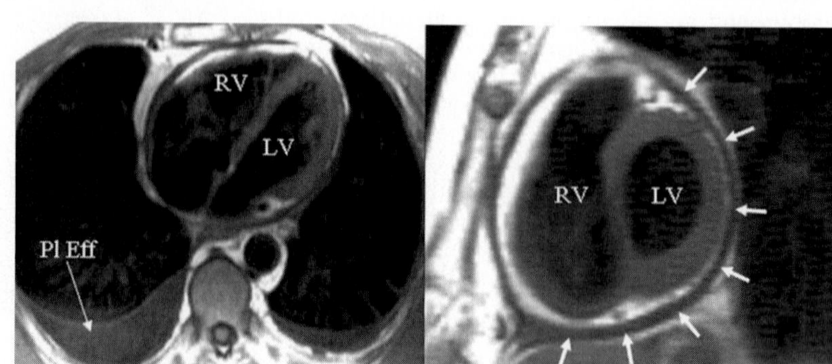

FIGURE 14–14 Cardiovascular magnetic resonance in a patient with constrictive pericarditis. On the **right** is a basal short-axis view of the ventricles showing a thickened pericardium encasing the heart (arrows). On the **left** is a transaxial view, again showing the thickened pericardium, particularly over the right heart, but also a pleural effusion (Pl Eff). LV = left ventricle; RV = right ventricle.

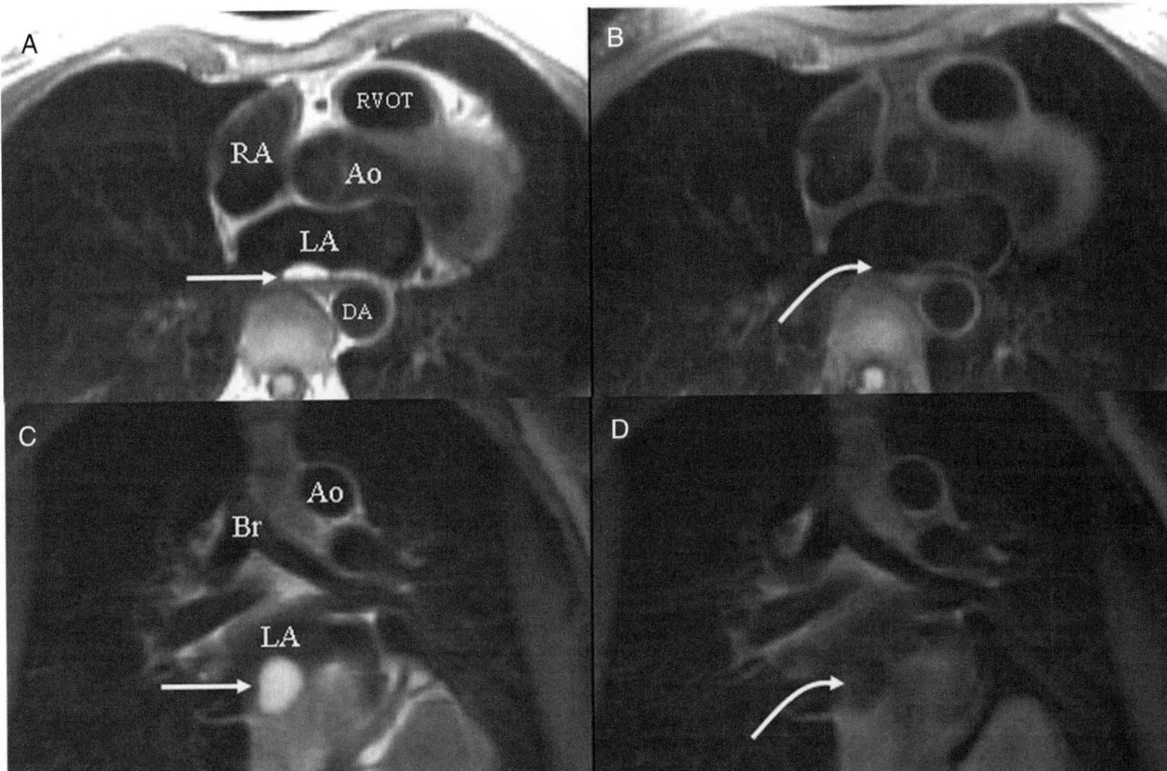

FIGURE 14–15 Cardiovascular magnetic resonance of a patient with retroatrial lipoma. **A** and **B,** Transaxial cuts through the heart. **C** and **D,** Coronal cuts posteriorly. A tumor is present posterior to the left atrium (straight arrow) in panels **A** and **C.** Panels **B** and **D** show the equivalent images with fat suppression turned on and abolition of signal within the tumor (curved arrows), therefore confirming the diagnosis of lipoma. Ao = aorta; Br = bronchus; DA = descending aorta; LA = left atrium; RA = right atrium; RVOT = right ventricular outflow tract.

gadolinium (perfusion), significant early tissue enhancement (increased vascularity), and significant late enhancement (fibrosis or necrosis) is typically an angiosarcoma (Fig. 14–16). Other useful signal characteristics include high T1-weighted signal in recent hemorrhage (due to the paramagnetic effects of the breakdown of hemoglobin), cysts with high protein content, and melanoma; low T1-weighted signal in low protein content cysts, calcified lesions, or air; high T2-weighted signal in cysts; high signal during the first pass of gadolinium in hemangioma (noninvasive) and angiosarcoma (invasive); necrotic areas highlighted against surrounding enhancement in malignant tumors 1 to 2 minutes after the intravenous administration of gadolinium; absence of early gadolinium enhancement in most benign tumors, with the exclusion of hemangioma and myxoma; and late gadolinium enhancement in fibrosis and its absence in cysts. The clinical setting and location of the tumor also yield important diagnostic information. Finally, CMR is excellent at identifying thrombus. Thrombus is usually hypointense on SSFP cines. On spin-echo images, thrombus is usually visible against the black blood pool and in the subacute phase may have areas of high signal intensity due to the paramagnetic effect of hemoglobin breakdown products. Thrombus is also identified with high accuracy using an inversion recovery technique with an inversion time 2 minutes after gadolinium injection. The thrombus has low vascularity and appears as a dark area surrounded by intense blood and myocardial signal.

Congenital Heart Disease (see Chap. 56)

CMR is ideally suited to the evaluation of congenital heart disease for several reasons: three-dimensional contiguous data sets are very effective for the complete depiction of anatomy; functional assessments are readily combined with the anatomical data; and CMR is less operator dependent than echocardiography. In addition, long-term follow-up is greatly facilitated by good reproducibility, noninvasiveness, access to relatively unrestricted fields of view, and freedom from ionizing radiation. The combination of CMR with transesophageal echocardiography has been particularly effective in patient evaluation because the two investigations often yield complementary information (see Chap. 11),[102] and the need, duration, and risks of invasive catheterization have diminished in recent years. However, the ease of use and value of CMR depend on the age and clinical condition of the patient. For small children, anesthesia or sedation is required for CMR, and monitoring may be demanding; for these patients, echocardiography is usually adequate. The contributions of CMR tend to increase in older children and adults. CMR is also relatively more effective in evaluating more complex anatomy and after surgery in the many patients now surviving to adult life, because scar tissue and limitations of acoustic access are increasing problems for echocardiography. CMR is thus the preferred technique for the serial evaluation of right ventricular volumes, mass, and function,[12,103] valvular regurgitation,[103] the pulmonary arteries, and extracardiac conduits. Expertise in CMR is highly recommended in centers specializing in the care of patients with congenital heart disease.[102] The range of congenital abnormalities is large, and a summary follows, but more detail can be found in specialized texts.[104,105]

GREAT VESSEL ABNORMALITIES. Coarctation usually occurs in the proximal descending aorta opposite the ductus arteriosus, just distal to the left subclavian artery. CMR is the optimal technique for assessment of coarctation (Fig. 14–17), especially in adults and after operative repair. CMR identifies the coarctation site and extent, any involvement of arch vessels, and poststenotic dilation. Velocity

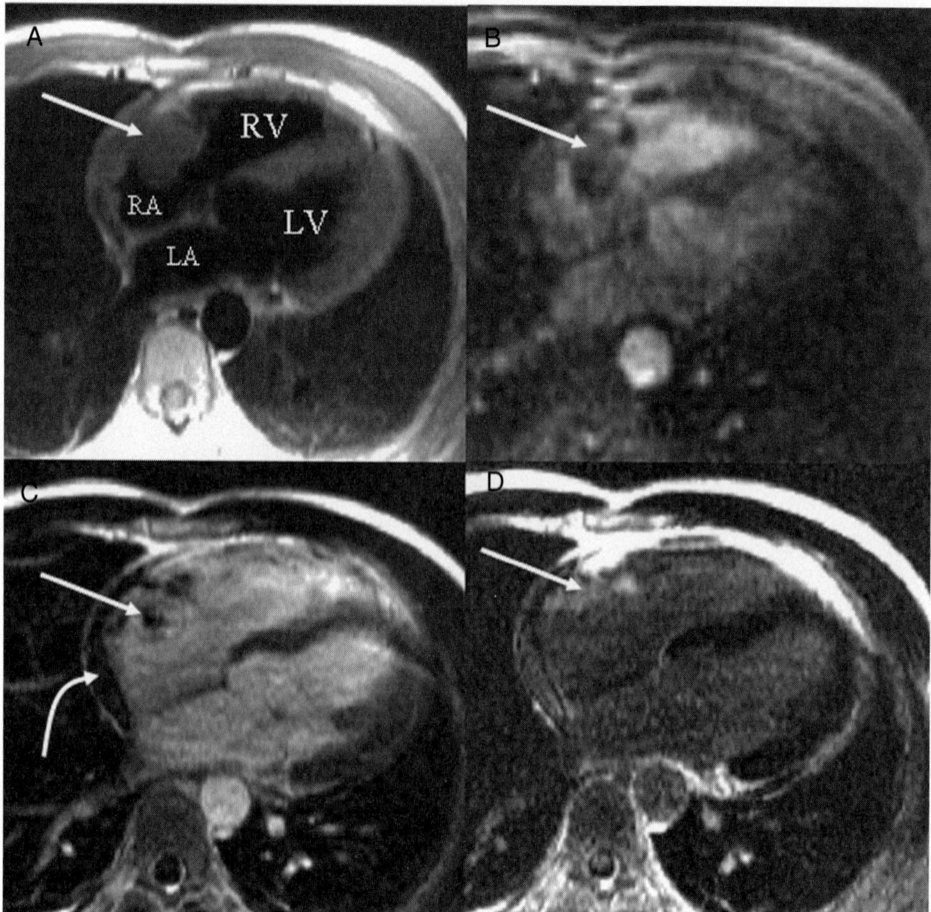

FIGURE 14–16 Cardiovascular magnetic resonance (CMR) of patients with right atrial angiosarcoma. All images are in the transaxial plane at the same level. **A,** T1-weighted spin-echo image showing a tumor (straight arrow) in the right atrial wall. For characterization, gadolinium was given intravenously as a bolus. **B,** CMR image taken during the first pass of gadolinium, showing considerable signal within the tumor, which indicates high vascularity (arrow). **C,** Inversion recovery image taken 1 to 2 minutes after injection, showing areas of absent signal within the tumor compatible with microvascular obstruction (straight arrow). There is also a pericardial effusion best seen in this image (curved arrow). **D,** Late gadolinium enhancement. The tumor has high signal, indicating fibrosis. All these feature taken together indicate a likely diagnosis of angiosarcoma, which was confirmed at surgery. LA = left atrium; LV = left ventricle; RA = right atrium; RV = right ventricle.

mapping of the coarctation jet yields a pressure gradient in most cases, and the jet duration into diastole is a useful guide to severity. Typically, CMR angiography is also performed to assess the size of collateral vessels, but flow mapping of upper and lower sites in the descending aorta can also be used to assess the volume of collateral flow. Long-term follow-up is advised in these patients because of the complications of restenosis and repair site aneurysms. Tortuosity of the isthmal region without significant obstruction has been termed *pseudocoarctation*. No significant narrowing or jet formation is present, however, and there is no collateral flow.

CMR displays vascular rings in detail, including the relationship between aortic arch anomalies and other structures. A double aortic arch may cause compression from encirclement of the trachea and esophagus. A vascular sling is also well demonstrated by CMR, in which an anomalous left pulmonary artery arises from the right pulmonary artery and courses between the trachea and esophagus back to the left lung, which can result in airway compression. In infants, patent ductus arteriosus is usually visualized by echocardiography, but CMR has a role in older patients. CMR is also useful for visualizing the aortopulmonary window. CMR is valuable for assessing anomalous pulmonary venous drainage, in which some or all of the pulmonary veins do not enter the left atrium. Anomalous pulmonary veins can be missed with conventional cardiological investigations, but the anatomy is easily visualized with standard CMR sequences or, more commonly, CMR angiography.[106] CMR correctly identifies anomalies of the systemic venous system (bilateral superior cava, interrupted inferior cava), including connection to the left heart in patients with occult arterial desaturation. Finally, pulmonary artery anatomy is very well depicted by CMR, including the presence of pulmonary arteries and their size, confluence, and relationship to other structures. Main and branch vessel stenosis can be detected, the pressure gradient assessed, and differential pulmonary flow measured. CMR angiography is very effective for demonstrating systemic to pulmonary collateral vessels.[107]

ATRIAL AND VENTRICULAR MORPHOLOGY. The morphological right atrium has a broad-based and triangular appendage, whereas the morphological left atrium has a narrow entrance to the appendage, with a tubular configuration. The right atrium is also connected to the inferior vena cava in virtually all cases. Furthermore, atrial situs is nearly always concordant with the visceral situs, and therefore the morphological right atrium is on the side of the short main bronchus and the liver. The morphological left atrium likewise is on the side of the long main bronchus and the aorta, spleen, and stomach. The morphological right ventricle is characterized by a prominent moderator band, a more apical insertion point of the tricuspid valve into the ventricular septum, and an infundibulum or conus separating the tricuspid and pulmonary valves. The morphological left ventricle is more smoothly contoured toward the apex and lacks a muscular infundibulum; therefore, it has a fibrous continuity between the mitral and aortic valves. In situs solitus, the normal atrial arrangement applies; the left pulmonary artery passes over the left main bronchus and the right pulmonary artery runs anterior and slightly inferior to the right bronchus. The atrial arrangement is reversed in cases of situs inversus. In atrial isomerism, both atria are alike and develop sidedness according to the thoracic and abdominal viscera. Left-sided isomerism is associated with polysplenia and right-sided isomerism with asplenia. Because CMR provides anatomical data that are easily related to the surrounding structures of the body, reliable diagnosis of situs is possible even in difficult cases.

ATRIOVENTRICULAR CONNECTION ABNORMALITIES. Because of the excellent ability to define the atrial and ventricular morphology, CMR demonstrates atrioventricular discordance well. Atrioventricular discordance is present in congenitally corrected transposition (combined with ventriculoarterial discordance), in which the left atrium drains into the right ventricle, which supplies the systemic arterial circulation. Other abnormalities of atrial connection include atrioventricular valve atresia, connection of both atria to a single ventricle, and connection of one valve to both ventricles. CMR also provides excellent visualization of crisscrossed atrioventricular connections, conditions in which ventricular positions are rotated with respect to the atria, with connections being either concordant or discordant.

VENTRICULOARTERIAL CONNECTION ABNORMALITIES. CMR demonstrates the anatomy of transposition of the great arteries (discordant ventriculoarterial connections) very well, with the connections between the ventricles and great vessels showing an anterior aorta arising from the morphological right ventricle and the posterior pulmonary artery arising from the morphological left ventricle. CMR is effective for assessing intraatrial baffles after atrial repair of transposition of the great arteries (Fig. 14–18).[108] After arterial switch repair, which has now become the operation of choice, CMR provides good views of the right ventricular outflow tract and pulmonary arteries, which may be stenosed. Double-outlet right ventricle is defined as an abnormal ventriculoarterial connection in which more than half of both the aorta and pulmonary artery arise from the morphological right ventricle. This condition typically presents with the aorta to the right of the pulmonary artery at the semilunar valve level. An additional feature is a complete muscle rim separating both semilunar valves from the anterior leaflet of the mitral valve. Truncus arteriosus is a failure of the embryonic truncus to separate into an individual aorta and a pulmonary artery. A single large artery arises above a ventricular septal defect from which the aorta, pulmonary, and coronary arteries arise, and this is well shown by CMR. Because of the problem with graft degeneration, CMR is valuable for assessing long-term postoperative conduit patency and stenosis, regurgitation, or aneurysm formation. Echocardiography can be limited in evaluating conduits by their retrosternal position and calcification.

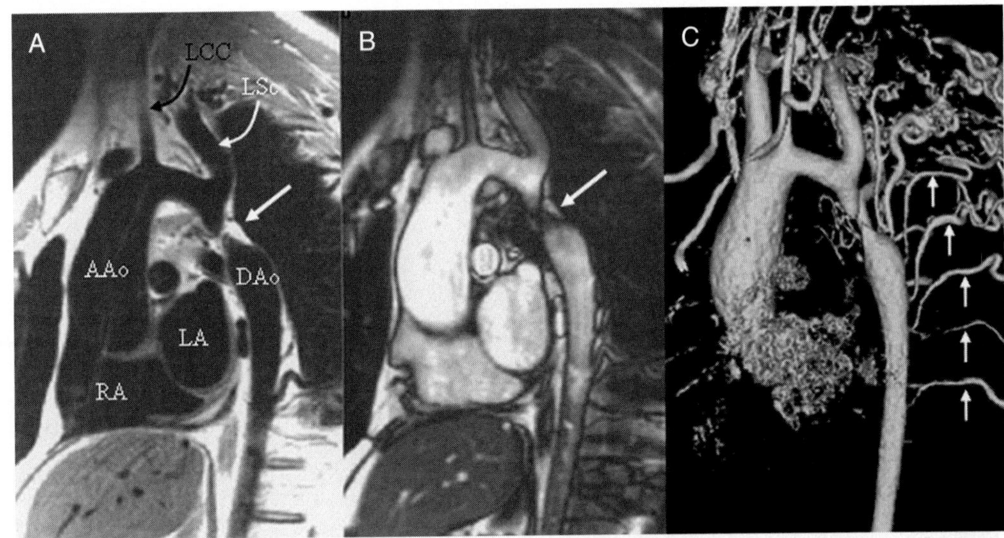

FIGURE 14–17 Cardiovascular magnetic resonance (CMR) in a patient with aortic coarctation. **A,** Oblique sagittal view showing the ascending aorta (AAo), which is dilated, giving rise to dilated left common carotid (LCC) and left subclavian (LSc) arteries. Immediately distal to the left subclavian artery is the coarctation (straight arrow), after which the descending aorta (DAo) is formed. **B,** Similar findings are seen in this image, one frame from a steady state with free precession (SSFP) cine. **C,** Projection from a three-dimensional CMR angiogram, showing multiple intercostal collateral arteries joining the descending aorta (small arrows), which can be responsible for rib notching on the chest x-ray. LA = left atrium; RA = right atrium. (From Babu-Narayan SV, Kilner PJ, Gatzoulis MA: When to order cardiovascular magnetic resonance in adults with congenital heart disease. Curr Cardiol Rep 5:324, 2003.)

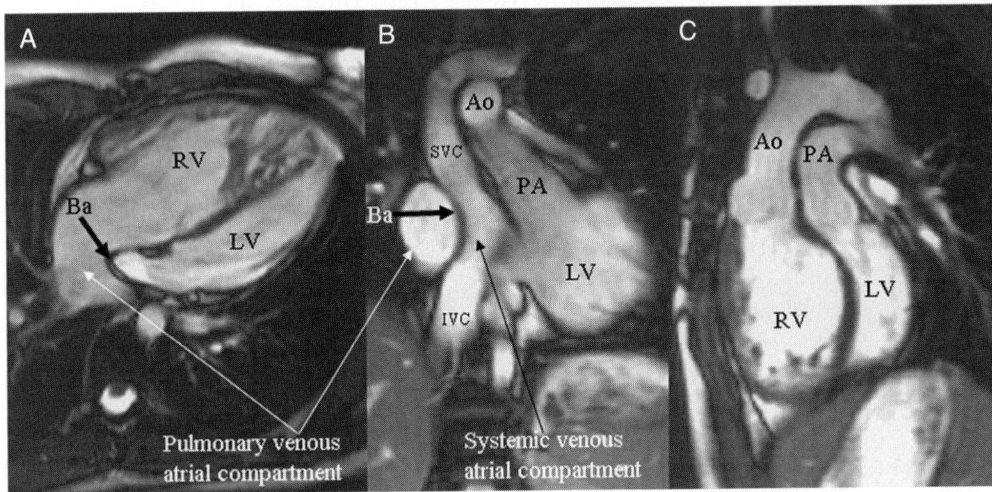

FIGURE 14–18 Cardiovascular magnetic resonance (CMR) in a patient with transposition of the great arteries following a Senning procedure, with insertion of atrial baffle, showing single frames from steady state with free precession (SSFP) cines. **A,** Oblique transaxial plane. **B,** Oblique coronal plane. **C,** Oblique sagittal plane. The atrial baffle (Ba) is seen in panels **A** and **B.** The pulmonary venous atrial compartment is unobstructed, as seen in panels **A** and **B,** and the systemic venous atrial compartment is likewise unobstructed, as seen in panel **B.** Panel **C** shows the aorta (Ao) arising from the right ventricle (RV) and the pulmonary artery (PA) arising from the left ventricle (LV). This is a good late postoperative result. IVC = inferior vena cava; SVC = superior vena cava.

SEPTAL DEFECTS. The anatomy of atrial and ventricular septal defects is usually well delineated using CMR, especially using SSFP sequences. The defect location and size can be determined directly and the systemic-to-pulmonary flow ratio measured,[109] all of which are useful for planning of intervention. The effects on right ventricular function can also be quantified. CMR is relatively more valuable than echocardiography in patients with more complex anatomy, especially those with additional abnormalities. In addition, CMR is valuable for excluding shunting from other sources, such as anomalous pulmonary venous drainage, in which echocardiography is problematic (Fig. 14–19).[110] This is important because partial anomalous venous return may coexist with atrial septal defect.

VALVULAR ABNORMALITIES. Simple (e.g., mitral stenosis) and complex (e.g., Ebstein anomaly of the tricuspid valve) congenital valve abnormalities can be assessed by CMR, but echocardiography has the significant primary role. CMR is particularly helpful in the assessment of valve regurgitation and the effects of valve pathology on the volumes and function of the associated ventricle. This has proved particularly useful for assessment of pulmonary regurgitation in patients with Fallot tetralogy[111] and surgical right ventricular to pulmonary artery conduits.[112]

TETRALOGY OF FALLOT. Tetralogy of Fallot is well assessed by CMR, both before intervention and in long-term follow-up. The full tetralogy includes an over-riding aorta with membranous ventricular septal defect, infundibular or pulmonary stenosis, and right ventricular hypertrophy, but additional features are common, such as stenosis of the pulmonary arteries and, in severe cases, aortopulmonary collateral vessels. As adults, most patients will have undergone corrective surgery, and CMR is ideal for monitoring right ventricular volumes and function as well as pulmonary regurgitation, which is common after correction. Right ventricular

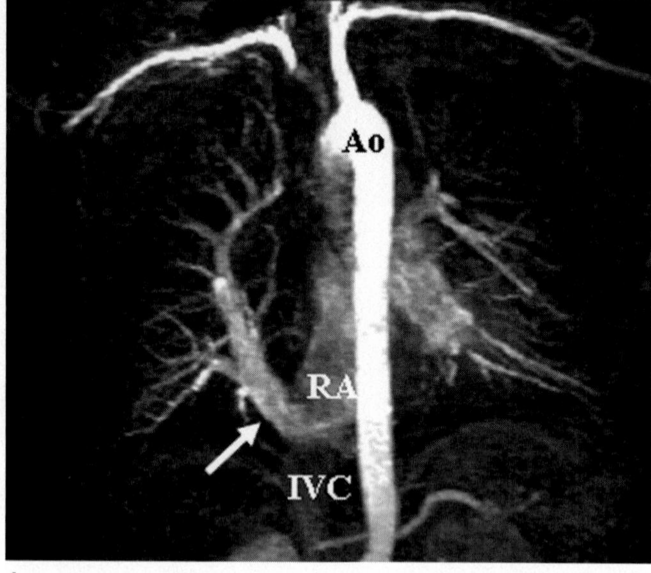

FIGURE 14–19 Cardiovascular magnetic resonance angiography in a patient with anomalous pulmonary venous drainage. **A,** The pulmonary venous angiogram showed the right upper and lower pulmonary veins draining into a common trunk (arrow) and into the inferior vena cava (IVC) and right atrium (RA). **B,** Direct flow measurements of the pulmonary artery and aorta (Ao) are shown in this graph, which yielded a Qp:Qs ratio of 2.7. (From Tan RS, Behr ER, McKenna WJ, Mohiaddin RH: Images in cardiovascular medicine. Occult anonymous pulmonary venous drainage: The clinical value of cardiac magnetic resonance imaging. Circulation 105:e25, 2002.)

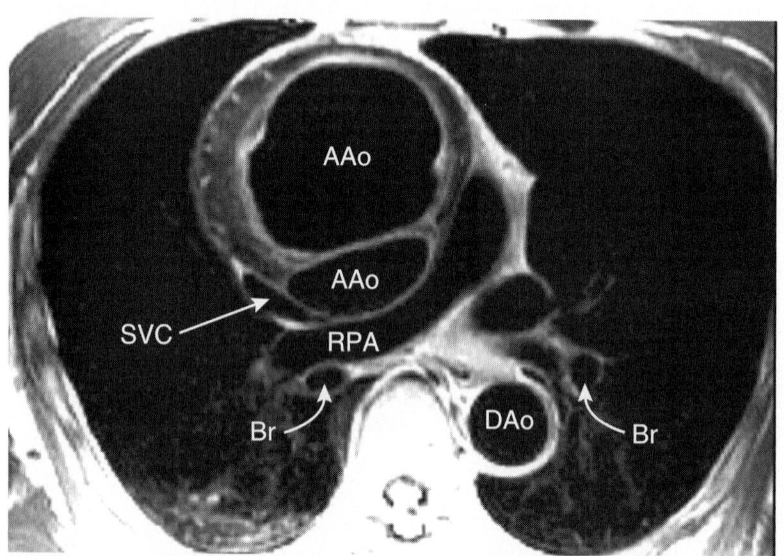

FIGURE 14–20 Cardiovascular magnetic resonance in a patient with type A aortic dissection. This transaxial spin-echo image shows a very dilated ascending aorta (AAo) with two lumina, intramural hematoma, and a compressed superior vena cava (SVC) and right pulmonary artery (RPA). Br = bronchus; Dao = descending aorta.

arrhythmias and failure are the most important causes of mortality.

SINGLE VENTRICLE. CMR is useful in determining the anatomical features of this condition, including the ventricular morphology, the atrioventricular and ventriculoarterial connections, situs, and the presence of associated anomalies. Compared with the dominant ventricle, a rudimentary right ventricle is usually anterosuperior and a rudimentary left ventricle is usually posteroinferior. In adults, a dominant left ventricle is most common. Some single ventricles have no characteristic morphological features and are termed *indeterminate*.

CORONARY ARTERY ANOMALIES. CMR is useful in defining congenital or inflammatory changes of the coronary arteries, as in Kawasaki disease.[113] In adults, the course of congenitally anomalous coronary arteries can be reliably depicted by CMR in patients with otherwise normal anatomy and in those with other congenital heart disease, in whom the prevalence of anomalies reaches 30 percent.[44] CMR has significant advantages over x-ray angiography in clarifying the spatial relationship of these arteries, most importantly whether the proximal portion runs between the aorta and the pulmonary artery, which is associated with sudden death. In other forms of congenital heart disease, the course and location of the coronary arteries can be important for surgical planning.

Acquired Disease of the Major Arteries

CMR angiography of the major central arteries has advanced rapidly in recent years and in experienced centers is replacing invasive x-ray techniques.[114] Substantial diagnostic information can often be gained in the larger vessels from conventional CMR images, but gadolinium-enhanced three-dimensional CMR angiography can now be completed in a few seconds and is now routinely used for large and small vessels. The older nongadolinium CMR angiographic techniques, such as time-of-flight angiography, are not commonly used in the central circulation but do have application elsewhere.

GREAT VESSELS. CMR is an ideal technique for assessing the aorta, because of the large field of view and ability of CMR angiography to image obliquely and in three dimensions. CMR accurately depicts aortic aneurysms showing cross-sectional diameter, the relation to branch vessels, and associated thrombus. Additional CMR angiography shows associated branch vessel occlusive disease and is useful to define the relationship of the aneurysm to smaller vessels. Inflammatory abdominal aortic aneurysms show enhancement with gadolinium. CMR can be used for stent planning and follow-up. Aortic dissection is a well-established indication for CMR,[115] and the diagnosis can be made rapidly (Fig. 14–20). The associated complications of dissection, such as extent, aortic regurgitation, pericardial effusion, and branch vessel involvement are all readily assessed by CMR. Other techniques, however, can be used in the acute setting, which largely reflects availability (see Chaps 11 and 15). In the chronic follow-up setting, CMR is the technique of choice. CMR is also useful for depiction of intramural hematoma and penetrating ulcer. CMR is ideal in the assessment and long-term follow-up of patients with Marfan syndrome. CMR angiography is also useful in the pulmonary arteries. Reasonable results have been obtained in patients with pulmonary embolism using three-dimensional contrast-enhanced CMR angiography,[116] but computed tomography remains the study of choice because of superior spatial resolution and a shorter breath-hold requirement (see Chap. 15). Pulmonary artery aneurysms and dissections are well evaluated by CMR.

ARTERIAL BRANCHES OF THE AORTA. CMR angiography of the internal carotid artery has proved valuable, and both three-dimensional time-of-flight and gadolinium-enhanced techniques have similar accuracy to invasive x-ray techniques,[117] although the gadolinium technique is faster and has improved coverage in the superior-inferior direction. Gadolinium CMR angiography is used for the renal (Fig. 14–21)[118] and mesenteric vessels. The lower spatial resolution of CMR compared with x-ray angiography limits quantitative assessment of the degree of stenosis and evaluation of accessory or branch vessels. For the arteries to the leg, three-dimensional gadolinium CMR angiography is very useful diagnostically[119] and has been used for interventional planning of limb-threatening ischemia. For the arms, there is less clinical experience, but gadolinium CMR angiography has been used with good results.

Intravascular and Interventional CMR

There is active research into the use of CMR for intravascular and interventional applications because of the whole-body imaging capability in any plane without exposure to x-rays. This requires the combination of a number of techniques, including real-time image acquisition and reconstruction, angiography, and image guidance. In addition, the instruments required must be safe to use in the MR environment, and magnet designs must allow sufficient patient access for the operator. For the cardiovascular system, a key component is the tracking of the catheter and guidewire. This can be achieved by incorporating a small receive-only coil in the tip of the device. The coil generates a signal that can be rapidly localized in three dimensions and shown on a previously acquired MR image, and different coils and receivers can be used for multiple devices. Technical advances are still in progress. Results have been reported for renal angiography,[120] femoral angioplasty, wall imaging, placement of stents, coronary angiography,[121] and assessment of radiofrequency ablation procedures.[122] Dual x-ray and CMR facilities have been proposed for more efficient diagnostic and interventional procedures during a single anesthesia session.[123] The future of this technology in uncertain at present, but there is considerable interest in its development.

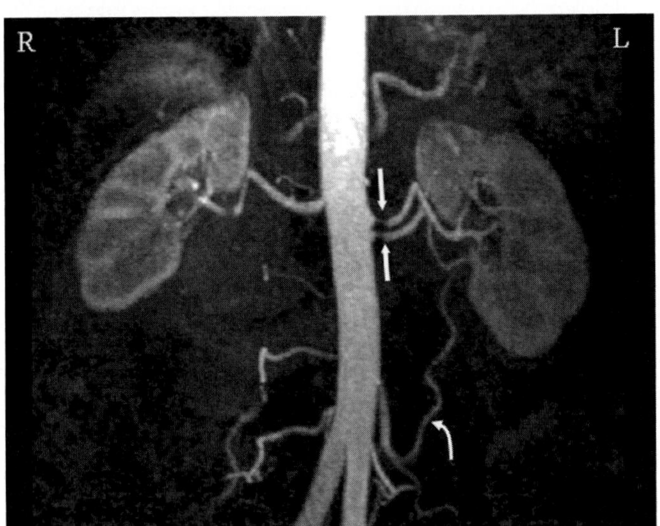

FIGURE 14–21 Cardiovascular magnetic resonance (CMR) renal angiography. The panels show a projection of a three-dimensional CMR angiogram of both kidneys from the thoracic aorta to beyond the bifurcation into the iliac arteries. The right kidney and renal artery are normal. There are three renal arteries supplying the left kidney. The upper pair, which are opposite the right renal artery, are both stenosed (straight arrows). Shortly before the bifurcation of the aorta, an accessory renal artery is seen, which is not stenosed (curved arrow).

REFERENCES

Properties of Magnetic Resonance

1. Manning WJ, Pennell DJ: Cardiovascular Magnetic Resonance. Philadelphia, Churchill Livingstone, 2002.
2. Firmin DN, Nayler GL, Klipstein RH, et al: In vivo validation of magnetic resonance velocity imaging. J Comput Assist Tomogr 11:751, 1987.
3. Scott NA, Pettigrew RI: Absence of movement of coronary stents after placement in a magnetic resonance imaging field. Am J Cardiol 73:900, 1994.
4. Strohm O, Kivelitz D, Gross W, et al: Safety of implantable coronary stents during H-1 magnetic resonance imaging at 1.0 and 1.5 T. J Cardiovasc Magn Reson 1:239, 1999.
5. Schroeder AP, Houlind K, Pedersen EM, et al: Magnetic resonance imaging seems safe in patients with intracoronary stents. J Cardiovasc Magn Reson 2:43, 2000.

Ventricular Volumes, Mass, and Function

6. Bellenger NG, Burgess M, Ray SG, et al, on behalf of the CHRISTMAS Steering Committee and Investigators: Comparison of left ventricular ejection fraction and volumes in heart failure by two-dimensional echocardiography, radionuclide ventriculography and cardiovascular magnetic resonance: Are they interchangeable? Eur Heart J 21:1387, 2000.
7. Longmore DB, Klipstein RH, Underwood SR, et al: Dimensional accuracy of magnetic resonance in studies of the heart. Lancet 1:1360, 1985.
8. Jauhainen T, Jarvinen VM, Hekali PE, et al: MR gradient echo volumetric analysis of human cardiac casts: Focus on the right ventricle. J Comput Assist Tomogr 22:899, 1998.
9. Myerson SG, Bellenger NG, Pennell DJ: Assessment of left ventricular mass by cardiovascular magnetic resonance. Hypertension 39:750, 2002.
10. Bloomgarden DC, Fayad ZA, Ferrari VA, et al: Global cardiac function using breath-hold MRI: Validation of new acquisition and analysis techniques. Magn Reson Med 37:683, 1997.
11. Grothues F, Smith GC, Moon JCC, et al: Comparison of interstudy reproducibility of cardiovascular magnetic resonance with two-dimensional echocardiography in normal subjects and in patients with heart failure or left ventricular hypertrophy. Am J Cardiol 90:29, 2002.
12. Grothues F, Moon JCC, Bellenger NG, et al: Interstudy reproducibility of right ventricular volumes, function and mass with cardiovascular magnetic resonance. Am Heart J 147:218, 2004.
13. Osterziel KJ, Strohm O, Schuler J, et al: Randomised, double-blind, placebo-controlled trial of human recombinant growth hormone in patients with chronic heart failure due to dilated cardiomyopathy. Lancet 351:1233, 1998.
14. Young AA, Axel L: Three dimensional motion and deformation of the heart wall: Estimation with spatial modulation of magnetisation—A model based approach. Radiology 185:241, 1992.

Myocardial Infarction and Viability

15. Kim RJ, Fieno DS, Parrish RB, et al: Relationship of MRI delayed contrast enhancement to irreversible injury, infarct age, and contractile function. Circulation 100:185, 1999.
16. Wu E, Judd RM, Vargas JD, et al: Visualisation of presence, location and transmural extent of healed Q-wave and non-Q-wave myocardial infarction. Lancet 357:21, 2001.
17. Wagner A, Mahrholdt H, Holly TA, et al: Contrast-enhanced MRI and routine single photon emission computed tomography (SPECT) perfusion imaging for detection of subendocardial myocardial infarcts: An imaging study. Lancet 361:374, 2003.
18. Ricciardi MJ, Wu E, Davidson CJ, et al: Visualization of discrete microinfarction after percutaneous coronary intervention associated with mild creatine kinase-MB elevation. Circulation 103:2780, 2001.
19. Moon JCC, Perez de Arenaza D, Elkington AG, et al: The pathological basis of Q wave and non-Q wave myocardial infarction: A cardiovascular magnetic resonance study. J Am Coll Cardiol 2003, in press.
20. Mahrholdt H, Wagner A, Holly TA, et al: Reproducibility of chronic infarct size measurement by contrast-enhanced magnetic resonance imaging. Circulation 106:2322, 2002.
21. Baer FM, Voth E, Schneider CA, et al: Comparison of low-dose dobutamine-gradient-echo magnetic resonance imaging and positron emission tomography with [18F]fluorodeoxyglucose in patients with chronic coronary artery disease. A functional and morphological approach to the detection of residual myocardial viability. Circulation 91:1006, 1995.
22. Ramani K, Judd RM, Holly TA, et al: Contrast magnetic resonance imaging in the assessment of myocardial viability in patients with stable coronary artery disease and left ventricular dysfunction. Circulation 98:2687, 1998.
23. Kim RJ, Wu E, Rafael A, et al: The use of contrast-enhanced magnetic resonance imaging to identify reversible myocardial dysfunction. N Engl J Med 16:1445, 2000.
24. Gerber BL, Garot J, Bluemke DA, et al: Accuracy of contrast-enhanced magnetic resonance imaging in predicting improvement of regional myocardial function in patients after acute myocardial infarction. Circulation 106:1083, 2002.
25. Klein C, Nekolla SG, Bengel FM, et al: Assessment of myocardial viability with contrast-enhanced magnetic resonance imaging: Comparison with positron emission tomography. Circulation 105:162, 2002.
26. Kitagawa K, Sakuma H, Hirano T, et al: Acute myocardial infarction: Myocardial viability assessment in patients early thereafter—Comparison of contrast enhanced MR imaging with resting 201-Tl SPECT. Radiology 226:138, 2003.
27. Nagel E, Lorenz C, Baer F, et al: Stress cardiovascular magnetic resonance: Consensus panel report. J Cardiovasc Magn Reson 3:267, 2001.
28. Nagel E, Lehmkuhl HB, Bocksch W, et al: Noninvasive diagnosis of ischemia induced wall motion abnormalities with the use of high dose dobutamine stress MRI. Comparison with dobutamine stress echocardiography. Circulation 99:763, 1999.

29. Hundley WG, Hamilton CA, Thomas MS, et al: Utility of fast cine magnetic resonance imaging and display for the detection of myocardial ischemia in patients not well suited for second harmonic stress echocardiography. Circulation 100:1697, 1999.
30. Hundley WG, Morgan TM, Neagle CM, et al: Magnetic resonance imaging determination of cardiac prognosis. Circulation 106:2328, 2002.
31. Kuijpers D, Ho KY, van Dijkman PR, et al: Dobutamine cardiovascular magnetic resonance for the detection of myocardial ischemia with the use of myocardial tagging. Circulation 107:1592, 2003.
32. Scott CH, St. John Sutton MG, Gusani N, et al: Effect of dobutamine on regional left ventricular function measured by tagged magnetic resonance imaging in normal subjects. Am J Cardiol 83:412, 1999.

Myocardial Perfusion

33. Pennell DJ, Firmin DN, Burger P, et al: Assessment of magnetic resonance velocity mapping of global ventricular function during dobutamine infusion in coronary artery disease. Br Heart J 74:163, 1995.
34. Schwitter J, Nanz D, Kneifel S, et al: Assessment of myocardial perfusion in coronary artery disease by magnetic resonance: A comparison with positron emission tomography and coronary angiography. Circulation 103:2230, 2001.
35. Panting JR, Gatehouse PD, Yang GZ, et al: Abnormal subendocardial perfusion in cardiac syndrome-X detected by cardiovascular magnetic resonance imaging. N Engl J Med 346:1948, 2002.
36. Jerosch-Herold M, Wilke N, Stillman AE, Wilson RF: Magnetic resonance quantification of the myocardial perfusion reserve with a Fermi function model for constrained deconvolution. Med Phys 25:73, 1998.
37. Wilke N, Simm C, Zhang J, et al: Contrast enhanced first pass myocardial perfusion imaging: Correlation between myocardial blood flow in dogs at rest and during hyperemia. Magn Reson Med 29:485, 1993.
38. Epstein FH, London JF, Peters DC, et al: Multislice first pass cardiac perfusion MRI: Validation in a model of myocardial infarction. Magn Reson Med 47:482, 2002.
39. Al-Saadi N, Nagel E, Gross M, et al: Noninvasive detection of myocardial ischemia from perfusion reserve based on cardiovascular magnetic resonance. Circulation 101:1379, 2000.
40. Wacker CM, Hartlep AW, Pfleger S, et al: Susceptibility-sensitive magnetic resonance imaging detects human myocardium supplied by a stenotic coronary artery without a contrast agent. J Am Coll Cardiol 41:834, 2003.
41. Al-Saadi N, Nagel E, Gross M, et al: Improvement of myocardial perfusion reserve early after coronary intervention: Assessment with cardiac magnetic resonance imaging. J Am Coll Cardiol 36:1557, 2000.
42. Buchtal SD, den Hollander JA, Merz NB, et al: Abnormal myocardial phosphorus-31 nuclear magnetic resonance spectroscopy in women with chest pain but normal coronary angiograms. N Engl J Med 342:829, 2000.

Imaging the Coronary Arteries

43. Kim WY, Danias PG, Stuber M, et al: Coronary magnetic resonance angiography for the detection of coronary stenosis. N Engl J Med 345:1863, 2001.
44. Taylor AM, Thorne SA, Rubens MB, et al: Coronary artery imaging in grown-up congenital heart disease: Complementary role of MR and x-ray coronary angiography. Circulation 101:1670, 2000.
45. Stuber M, Botnar RM, Fischer SE, et al: Preliminary report on in vivo coronary MRA at 3 Tesla in humans. Magn Reson Med 48:425, 2002.
46. Li D, Carr JC, Shea SM, et al: Coronary arteries: Magnetization-prepared contrast-enhanced three-dimensional volume-targeted breath-hold MR angiography. Radiology 219:270, 2001.
47. Hundley WG, Hamilton CA, Clarke GD, et al: Visualisation and functional assessment of proximal and middle left anterior descending coronary stenosis in humans with magnetic resonance imaging. Circulation 99:3248, 1999.
48. Nagel E, Thouet T, Klein C, et al: Noninvasive determination of coronary blood flow velocity with cardiovascular magnetic resonance in patients after stent deployment. Circulation 107:1738, 2003.
49. Langerak SE, Vliegen HW, Jukema JW, et al: Value of magnetic resonance imaging for the noninvasive detection of stenosis in coronary artery bypass grafts and recipient coronary arteries. Circulation 107:1502, 2003.
50. Sorenson MB, Collins P, Ong PJL, et al: Long term use of contraceptive depot medroxyprogesterone acetate in young women impairs arterial endothelial function assessed by cardiovascular magnetic resonance. Circulation 106:1646, 2002.
51. Silber HA, Bluemke DA, Ouyang P, et al: The relationship between vascular wall shear stress and flow-mediated dilation: Endothelial function assessed by phase-contrast magnetic resonance angiography. J Am Coll Cardiol 38:1859, 2001.
52. Yuan C, Beach KW, Smith LH, Hatsukami TS: Measurement of atherosclerotic carotid plaque size in-vivo using high resolution magnetic resonance imaging. Circulation 98:2666, 1998.
53. Corti R, Fuster V, Fayad ZA, et al: Lipid lowering by simvastatin induces regression of human atherosclerotic lesions: Two years' follow-up by high-resolution noninvasive magnetic resonance imaging. Circulation 106:2884, 2002.
54. Fayad ZA, Fuster V, Fallon JT, et al: Noninvasive in vivo human coronary artery lumen and wall imaging using black-blood magnetic resonance imaging. Circulation 102:506, 2000.

Acute Coronary Syndromes

55. Cai JM, Hatsukami TS, Ferguson MS, et al: Classification of human carotid atherosclerotic lesions with in vivo multicontrast magnetic resonance imaging. Circulation 106:1368, 2002.
56. Yuan C, Mitsumori LM, Ferguson MS, et al: In vivo accuracy of multispectral magnetic resonance imaging for identifying lipid-rich necrotic cores and intraplaque hemorrhage in advanced human carotid plaques. Circulation 104:2051, 2001.
57. Mitsumori LM, Hatsukami TS, Ferguson MS, et al: In vivo accuracy of multisequence MR imaging for identifying unstable fibrous caps in advanced human carotid plaques. J Magn Reson Imaging 17:410, 2003.
58. Yuan C, Zhang SX, Polissar NL, et al: Identification of fibrous cap rupture with magnetic resonance imaging is highly associated with recent transient ischemic attack or stroke. Circulation 105:181, 2002.
59. Ruehm SG, Corot C, Vogt P, et al: Magnetic resonance imaging of atherosclerotic plaque with ultrasmall superparamagnetic particles of iron oxide in hyperlipidemic rabbits. Circulation 103:415, 2001.
60. Kerwin W, Hooker A, Spilker M, et al: Quantitative magnetic resonance imaging analysis of neovasculature volume in carotid atherosclerotic plaque. Circulation 107:851, 2003.
61. Wasserman BA, Smith WI, Trout HH 3rd, et al: Carotid artery atherosclerosis: In vivo morphologic characterization with gadolinium-enhanced double-oblique MR imaging initial results. Radiology 223:566, 2002.
62. Zhao XQ, Yuan C, Hatsukami TS, et al: Effects of prolonged intensive lipid-lowering therapy on the characteristics of carotid atherosclerotic plaques in vivo by MRI: A case-control study. Arterioscler Thromb Vasc Biol 21:1623, 2001.
63. Kwong RY, Schussheim AE, Rekhraj S, et al: Detecting acute coronary syndrome in the emergency department with cardiac magnetic resonance imaging. Circulation 107:531, 2003.
64. Wu KC, Kim RJ, Bluemke DA, et al: Quantification and time course of microvascular obstruction by contrast-enhanced echocardiography and magnetic resonance imaging following acute myocardial infarction and reperfusion. J Am Coll Cardiol 32:1756, 1998.
65. Gerber BL, Rochitte CE, Melin JA, et al: Microvascular obstruction and left ventricular remodeling early after acute myocardial infarction. Circulation 101:2734, 2000.
66. Wu KC, Zerhouni EA, Judd RM, et al: Prognostic significance of microvascular obstruction by magnetic resonance imaging in patients with acute myocardial infarction. Circulation 97:765, 1998.

Cardiomyopathy

67. Groenning BA, Nilsson JC, Sondergaard L, et al: Antiremodeling effects on the left ventricle during beta-blockade with metoprolol in the treatment of chronic heart failure. J Am Coll Cardiol 36:2072, 2000.
68. Anderson LJ, Holden S, Davies B, et al: Cardiovascular T2* (T2 star) magnetic resonance for the early diagnosis of myocardial iron overload. Eur Heart J 22:2171, 2001.
69. McCrohon JA, Moon JC, Prasad SK, et al: Differentiation of heart failure related to dilated cardiomyopathy and coronary artery disease using gadolinium-enhanced cardiovascular magnetic resonance. Circulation 108:54, 2003.
70. Neubauer S, Horn M, Cramer M, et al: Myocardial phosphocreatine to ATP ratio is a predictor of mortality in patients with dilated cardiomyopathy. Circulation 96:2190, 1997.
71. Moon JCC, Fisher NG, McKenna WJ, Pennell DJ: Detection of apical hypertrophic cardiomyopathy by cardiovascular magnetic resonance in patients with non-diagnostic echocardiography. Heart 2004, in press.
72. Crilley JG, Boehm EA, Blair E, et al: Hypertrophic cardiomyopathy due to sarcomeric gene mutations is characterized by impaired energy metabolism irrespective of the degree of hypertrophy. J Am Coll Cardiol 41:1776, 2003.
73. Moon JCC, Reed E, Sheppard M, et al: The histological basis of myocardial enhancement by gadolinium cardiovascular magnetic resonance in hypertrophic cardiomyopathy. J Am Coll Cardiol 2004, in press.
74. Moon JCC, McKenna WJ, McCrohon JA, et al: Toward clinical risk assessment in hypertrophic cardiomyopathy with gadolinium cardiovascular magnetic resonance. J Am Coll Cardiol 41:1561, 2003.
75. Moon JCC, Sachdev B, Elkington AG, et al: Gadolinium enhanced cardiovascular magnetic resonance in Anderson-Fabry disease: Evidence for a disease specific abnormality of the myocardial interstitium. Eur Heart J 24:2151, 2003.
76. Anderson LJ, Bunce N, Davis B, et al: Reversal of siderotic cardiomyopathy: A prospective study with cardiac magnetic resonance. Heart 85(Suppl 1):33, 2001.
77. Anderson LJ, Wonke B, Prescott E, et al: Comparison of effects of oral deferiprone and subcutaneous desferrioxamine on myocardial iron levels and ventricular function in beta thalassemia. Lancet 360:516, 2002.
78. Blake LM, Scheinman MM, Higgins CB: MR features of arrhythmogenic right ventricular dysplasia. Am J Roentgenol 162:809, 1994.
79. Burke AP, Farb A, Tashko G, Virmani R: Arrhythmogenic right ventricular cardiomyopathy and fatty replacement of the right ventricular myocardium: Are they different diseases? Circulation 97:1571, 1998.
80. Proclemer A, Basadonna PT, Slavich GA, et al: Cardiac magnetic resonance imaging findings in patients with right ventricular outflow tract premature contractions. Eur Heart J 18:2002, 1997.
81. Danias PG: Gadolinium-enhanced cardiac magnetic resonance imaging: Expanding the spectrum of clinical applications. Am J Med 110:591, 2001.
82. Vignaux O, Dhote R, Duboc D, et al: Clinical significance of myocardial magnetic resonance abnormalities in patients with sarcoidosis: A 1-year follow-up study. Chest 122:1895, 2002.
83. Fattori R, Rocchi G, Celletti F, et al: Contribution of magnetic resonance imaging in the differential diagnosis of cardiac amyloidosis and symmetric hypertrophic cardiomyopathy. Am Heart J 136:824, 1998.
84. Friedrich MG, Strohm O, Schulz-Menger J, et al: Contrast media enhanced magnetic resonance imaging visualises myocardial changes in the course of viral myocarditis. Circulation 97:1802, 1998.
85. Wagner A, Schulz-Menger J, Dietz R, Friedrich MG: Long-term follow-up of patients with acute myocarditis by magnetic resonance imaging. MAGMA 16:17, 2003.
86. Wassmuth R, Lentzsch S, Erdbruegger U, et al: Subclinical cardiotoxic effects of anthracyclines as assessed by magnetic resonance imaging—A pilot study. Am Heart J 141:1007, 2001.

87. Schwitter J, De Marco T, Globits S, et al: Influence of felodipine on left ventricular hypertrophy and systolic function in orthotopic heart transplant recipients: Possible interaction with cyclosporine medication. J Heart Lung Transplant 18:1003, 1999.

Valvular Heart Disease

88. Mohiaddin RH, Kilner PJ: Valvular heart disease. *In* Manning WJ, Pennell DJ (eds): Cardiovascular Magnetic Resonance. Philadelphia, Churchill Livingstone, 2002, pp 387-404.
89. Kozerke S, Schwitter J, Pedersen EM, Boesiger P: Aortic and mitral regurgitation quantification using moving slice velocity mapping. J Magn Reson Imaging 14:106, 2001.
90. Globits S, Frank H, Mayr H, et al: Quantitative assessment of aortic regurgitation by magnetic resonance imaging. Eur Heart J 13:78, 1992.
91. Kizilbash AM, Hundley WG, Willett DL, et al: Comparison of quantitative Doppler with magnetic resonance imaging for assessment of the severity of mitral regurgitation. Am J Cardiol 81:792, 1998.
92. Globits S, Blake L, Bourne M, et al: Assessment of hemodynamic effects of ACE inhibitor therapy in chronic aortic regurgitation by using velocity encoded cine magnetic resonance imaging. Am Heart J 131:289, 1996.
93. Hoffmann U, Frank H, Stefenelli T, et al: Afterload reduction in severe aortic regurgitation. J Magn Reson Imaging 14:693, 2001.
94. Dulce MC, Mostbeck GH, O'Sullivan M, et al: Severity of aortic regurgitation: Interstudy reproducibility of measurements with velocity-encoded cine MR imaging. Radiology 185:235, 1992.
95. Kilner PJ, Manzara CC, Mohiaddin RH, et al: Magnetic resonance jet velocity mapping in mitral and aortic valve stenosis. Circulation 87:1239, 1993.
96. Friedrich MG, Schulz-Menger J, Poetsch T, et al: Quantification of valvular aortic stenosis by magnetic resonance imaging. Am Heart J 144:329, 2002.
97. Rajappan K, Rimoldi OE, Camici PG, et al: Functional changes in coronary microcirculatory function after valve replacement in patients with aortic stenosis. Circulation 107:3170, 2003.
98. Beyerbacht HP, Lamb HJ, van der Laarse A, et al: Aortic valve replacement in patients with aortic valve stenosis improves myocardial metabolism and diastolic function. Radiology 219:637, 2001.
99. Edwards MB, Taylor KM, Shellock FG: Prosthetic heart valves: Evaluation of magnetic field interactions, heating, and artifacts at 1.5 T. J Magn Reson Imaging 12:363, 2000.

Pericardial Disease and Cardiac Tumors

100. Vick GW, Rokey R: CMR evaluation of the pericardium in health and disease. *In* Manning WJ, Pennell DJ (eds): Cardiovascular Magnetic Resonance. Philadelphia, Churchill Livingstone, 2002, pp 355-363.
101. Frank H: Cardiac masses. *In* Manning WJ, Pennell DJ (eds): Cardiovascular Magnetic Resonance. Philadelphia, Churchill Livingstone, 2002, pp 342-354.

Congenital Heart Disease

102. Hirsch R, Kilner PJ, Connelly MS, et al: Diagnosis in adolescents and adults with congenital heart disease: Prospective assessment of indi-vidual and combined roles of magnetic resonance imaging and transesophageal echocardiography. Circulation 90:2937, 1994.
103. Niezen RA, Helbing WA, van der Wall EE, et al: Biventricular systolic function and mass studied with MR imaging in children with pulmonary regurgitation after repair for tetralogy of Fallot. Radiology 201:135, 1996.
104. Kilner PJ: Adult congenital heart disease. *In* Higgins CB, de Roos A (eds): Cardiovascular MRI and MRA. Philadelphia, Lippincott Williams & Wilkins, 2003, pp 353-366.
105. Higgins CB, Silverman NH, Kersting-Sommerhoff BA, Schmidt K: Congenital Heart Disease: Echocardiography and Magnetic Resonance Imaging. New York, Raven Press, 1990.
106. Prasad SK, Soukias N, Hornung T, et al: Role of MRA in the diagnosis of major aortopulmonary collateral arteries and partial anomalous pulmonary venous drainage. Circulation 109:207, 2004.
107. Geva T, Greil GF, Marshall AC, et al: Gadolinium-enhanced 3-dimensional magnetic resonance angiography of pulmonary blood supply in patients with complex pulmonary stenosis or atresia: Comparison with x-ray angiography. Circulation 106:473, 2002.
108. Chung KJ, Simpson IA, Glass RF, et al: Cine magnetic resonance imaging after surgical repair in patients with transposition of the great arteries. Circulation 77:104, 1988.
109. Hundley WG, Li HF, Lange RA, et al: Assessment of left-to-right intracardiac shunting by velocity-encoded, phase-difference magnetic resonance imaging: A comparison with oximetric and indicator dilution techniques. Circulation 91:2955, 1995.
110. Greil GF, Powell AJ, Gildein HP, Geva T: Gadolinium-enhanced three-dimensional magnetic resonance angiography of pulmonary and systemic venous anomalies. J Am Coll Cardiol 39:335, 2002.
111. Rebergen SA, Chin JG, Ottenkamp J, et al: Pulmonary regurgitation in the late postoperative follow-up of tetralogy of Fallot: Volumetric quantitation by nuclear magnetic resonance velocity mapping. Circulation 92:1123, 1993.
112. Holmqvist C, Oskarsson G, Stahlberg F, et al: Functional evaluation of extracardiac ventriculopulmonary conduits and of the right ventricle with magnetic resonance imaging and velocity mapping. Am J Cardiol 83:926, 1999.
113. Greil GF, Stuber M, Botnar RM, et al: Coronary magnetic resonance angiography in adolescents and young adults with Kawasaki disease. Circulation 105:908, 2002.

Diseases of the Major Arteries

114. Prince MR, Grist TM, Debatin JF (eds): 3D Contrast-Enhanced MR Angiography. Berlin, Springer-Verlag, 1997.
115. Nienaber CA, von Kodolitsch Y, Nicolas V, et al: The diagnosis of thoracic aortic dissection by noninvasive imaging procedures. N Engl J Med 328:1, 1993.
116. Oudkerk M, van Beek EJ, Wielopolski P, et al: Comparison of contrast-enhanced magnetic resonance angiography and conventional pulmonary angiography for the diagnosis of pulmonary embolism: A prospective study. Lancet 359:1643, 2002.
117. Fellner FA, Fellner C, Wutke R, et al: Fluoroscopically triggered contrast-enhanced 3D MR DSA and 3D time-of-flight turbo MRA of the carotid arteries: First clinical experiences in correlation with ultrasound, x-ray angiography, and endarterectomy findings. Magn Reson Imaging 18:575, 2000.
118. Schenberg SO, Rieger J, Johannson LO, et al: Diagnosis of renal artery stenosis with magnetic resonance angiography: Update 2003. Nephrol Dial Transplant 18:1252, 2003.
119. Ruehm SG, Goyen M, Barkhausen J, et al: Rapid magnetic resonance angiography for detection of atherosclerosis. Lancet 357:1086, 2001.

Intravascular and Interventional CMR

120. Wildermuth S, Debatin JF, Leung DA, et al: MR imaging-guided intravascular procedures: Initial demonstration in a pig model. Radiology 202:578, 1997.
121. Serfaty JM, Yang X, Foo TK, et al: MRI-guided coronary catheterization and PTCA: A feasibility study on a dog model. Magn Reson Med 49:258, 2003.
122. Lardo AC, McVeigh ER, Jumrussirikul P, et al: Visualization and temporal/spatial characterization of cardiac radiofrequency ablation lesions using magnetic resonance imaging. Circulation 102:698, 2000.
123. Kuehne T, Saeed M, Higgins CB, et al: Endovascular stents in pulmonary valve and artery in swine: Feasibility study of MR imaging-guided deployment and postinterventional assessment. Radiology 226:475, 2003.

CHAPTER 15

Computed Tomography of the Heart

Stephan Achenbach • Werner G. Daniel

Principles of Computed Tomography

Computed tomography (CT) imaging was introduced in 1972. The ability to obtain cross-sectional images of the body revolutionized medicine, and for the development of computer assisted tomography, Sir Geoffrey N. Hounsfield and Allan M. Cormack were awarded the Nobel Prize in Medicine in 1979. CT is an x-ray–based technique. An x-ray source that rotates on a circular path around the patient emits a fan-shaped beam of x-rays that passes through the body. Collimators are used to confine the x-ray beam to the slice that shall be imaged; its thickness can vary from less than one to several millimeters. Opposite to the x-ray source, extremely sensitive detectors record the intensity of x-rays that have passed through the body. Based on the x-ray attenuations obtained from a multitude of angles, a cross-sectional image of the body can be calculated. Each pixel of the reconstructed image is assigned an x-ray attenuation value (also called *CT number*), which is expressed in Hounsfield Units (HU). The Hounsfield scale is calibrated in a way that yields 0 HU for water and −1000 HU for air. CT numbers within one cross section of the body can thus range from close to −1000 HU (e.g., the lungs) to several thousand HU (e.g., bone or metal). Since the human eye cannot distinguish a gray scale over such a wide range, adjustments (window "width" and window "level" or "center") are made when displaying the reconstructed images. The width value represents the range of CT numbers that are displayed on a gray scale. Each value below that range will be displayed black, each value exceeding the range will be displayed white. The "level" or "center" value determines the CT number around which the "window" is centered (e.g., in an image displayed with a center of 500 HU and width of 400 HU, each pixel with a density of less than 300 HU will displayed black, and each pixel with a density greater than 700 HU will be displayed white). By convention, body images obtained by CT are displayed as if looking upward from the patient´s feet (Fig. 15–1).

Special Considerations for Cardiac Imaging

Due to technical limitations, the clinical value of cardiac CT has, for a long time, been very limited. Cardiac imaging requires a very high temporal resolution, because the heart is in constant, rapid motion. Conventional CT imaging, on the other hand, is an imaging modality with low temporal resolution: the heavy x-ray tube and the detector array must very accurately be moved in a circular pattern around the body, so centrifugal forces and the need to keep the geometry of source and detectors exactly aligned limit the rotation speed. Dedicated scanner designs therefore needed to be developed to increase acquisition speed.

Cardiac CT imaging requires one further prerequisite: to provide continuous cross-sectional images of the heart, every displayed image must be of the same heart phase. Otherwise, gaps may occur if adjacent images depict the heart in different phases of the cardiac cycle. Data acquisition must therefore either be triggered by the patient´s electrocardiogram (ECG) or, in case of continuous acquisition of x-ray data, image reconstruction must be synchronized to a function that is correlated to cardiac motion, such as the simultaneously recorded ECG ("retrospective ECG gating")

Lastly, the heart is subjected not only to intrinsic motion due to cardiac contraction, but also to motion caused by breathing. To avoid artifacts, CT imaging of the complete heart thus has to be performed within one single breath-hold and CT scanners have to provide for sufficiently fast volume coverage. In practice, image acquisition times of up to 35 seconds are usually tolerated by a cooperative patient.

The availability of CT techniques with high temporal resolution, the ability to obtain images in defined phases of the cardiac cycle, and progressive improvements in spatial resolution have continuously increased the clinical utility of cardiac CT imaging in recent years.

Electron Beam Tomography

The electron beam tomography (EBT) scanner was developed specifically for cardiac imaging. In contrast to conventional ("mechanical") CT scanners, x-rays are not created by a mechanically moving tube. Instead, a stationary high-voltage electron gun produces a beam of electrons at a substantial distance from the anode (Fig. 15–2). Within a large vacuum tube, a system of electromagnetic deflection coils focuses and steers the electron beam to sweep over tungsten targets, which constitute the anode and are arranged in a semicircular array under the patient table. Where the electron beam hits the anode, a fan of x-rays is created that penetrates the patient. Stationary detector arrays are mounted opposite the targets. Because of this design, cross-sectional images can be acquired without the constraints of mechanical motion: The electron beam can sweep across the target rings in as little as 33 msec. Typical scan speeds are 33, 50, or 100 msec for the newest generation of EBT scanners and 100 msec for previous generations of scanners. The two detector arrays permit simultaneous acquisition of two contiguous images of 1.5 mm, 3 mm, or 7 mm thickness. If desired, the electron beam can sweep up to four parallel targets in short succession. By combination of four targets with two detectors, up to eight images of 7 mm thickness each can be acquired without table motion.

Image acquisition by EBT can be prospectively triggered to the patient's ECG. X-rays

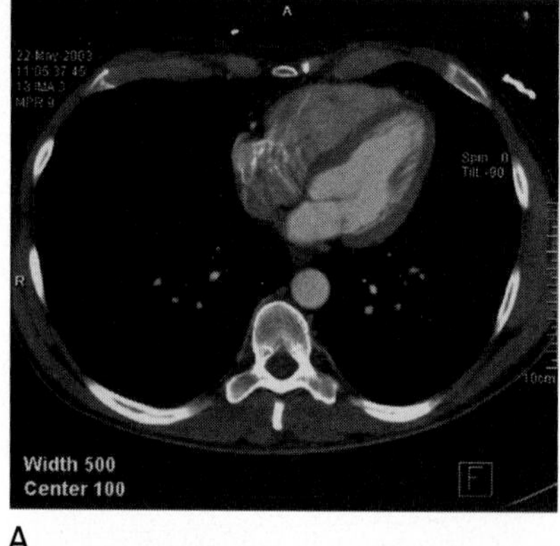

A

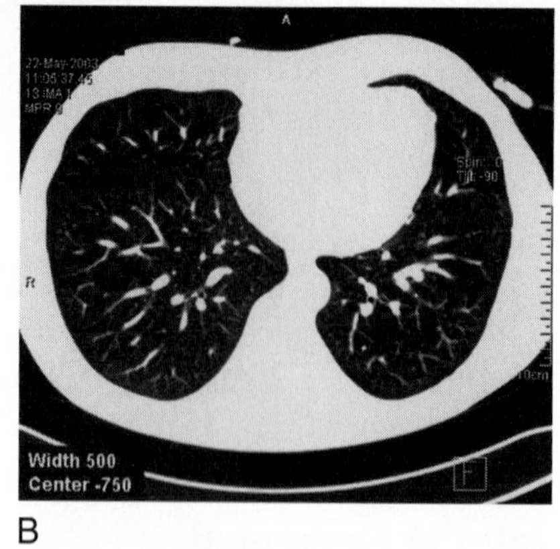

B

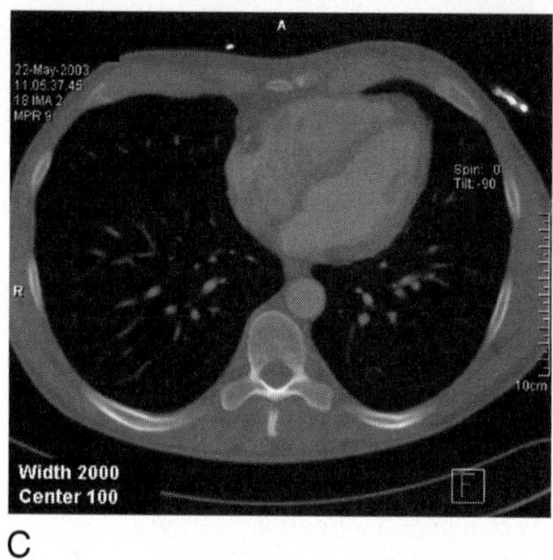

C

FIGURE 15–1 Display of computed tomography (CT) images. The same contrast-enhanced cross-sectional image of the chest is displayed in three different settings of window and level. **A,** Window width of 500 HU and center of 100 HU provides good soft-tissue contrast. Lungs (low CT attenuation) are displayed black, and bones (high attenuation) are displayed white. **B,** Same image, displayed with a window width of 500 HU and center of −750 HU. All structures with a CT number of −500 HU or more are now displayed in white, and low-density structures (e.g., the lungs) are displayed with good contrast. **C,** Window width of 2000 HU and center of 100 HU. The image has low contrast but displays all structures from very low (lungs) to high density (bones). By convention in CT, images are displayed as if looking up from the patient's feet.

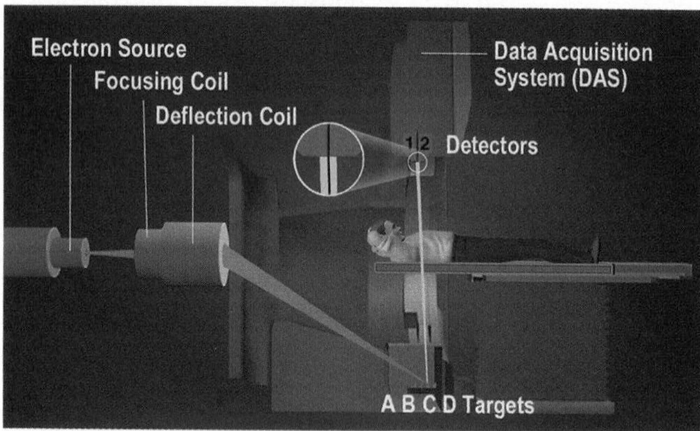

FIGURE 15–2 Principle of electron beam tomography (EBT). An electron beam is created by a high-voltage electron gun. In a large vacuum chamber, the electron beam is focused and deflected by electromagnetic coils to sweep over an anode that is arranged in a semicircular fashion below the patient. Where the electron beam hits the anode, x-rays are created. They penetrate the patient and are received by an array of detectors arranged on the opposite side. To create one image, the electron beam needs to perform a 210-degree sweep over the anodes, which in the usual scan modes requires 50 to 100 msec. By combining four parallel anode rings and two detector arrays, up to eight images can be obtained in rapid succession without movement of the patient table.

TABLE 15–1 Sample Image Acquisition Protocols for Cardiac Imaging by Electron Beam Tomography*

	Coronary Arteries	Coronary Calcium
Number of images	80	40
Slice collimation	2 × 1.5 mm	2 × 3.0 mm
Tube voltage	140 kV	130 kV
Electrocardiographic trigger	Prospective, one acquisition per cardiac cycle	Prospective, one acquisition per cardiac cycle
Temporal resolution	50 msec	50 msec
Contrast enhancement	Intravenous, iodinated contrast (~160 ml)	—
Approximate radiation dose†	~1.5-2.0 mSv[2] ~1.1 mSv[3]	~1.0-1.3 mSv[2] ~0.7 mSv[3]

*(The protocols are given for the newest generation of electron beam tomography scanners. Settings may vary for older generation scanners).
†Radiation doses are effective doses. As they are approximations and partly obtained from different sources than in Table 15–2, they are therefore not immediately comparable.

are emitted only at one or several predefined time points in the cardiac cycle. Table 15–1 lists typical image acquisition protocols for cardiac imaging by EBT.

Mechanical Computed Tomography

To use mechanical CT scanners for cardiac imaging, special measures had to be undertaken to improve temporal resolution. Modern multidetector CT (MDCT) scanners permit image acquisition in several parallel cross-sections (4 to 16) with slice collimations as low as 0.5 mm. Also, the time for one 360-degree tube rotation has been decreased to 500 msec or less. The scanners can be operated either in sequential ("step and shoot") mode or in spiral (or heli-cal) mode.

SEQUENTIAL AND SPIRAL SCAN MODES. In sequential mode, images are acquired at one level, and after enough data have been collected for image reconstruction, the table is advanced so that data can be acquired at another level (usually in the next cardiac cycle) (Fig. 15–3). Spiral mode offers faster coverage of large volumes. While the gantry is rotating and data are acquired continuously, the table is advanced at a constant speed. After the x-ray data set has been collected, images can retrospectively be reconstructed at any desired level. To reconstruct an image at a given level, a set of projections from numerous angles has to be obtained at that very plane. Since the tube does not perform a full rotation in any given plane, x-ray data for every projection angle are interpolated from the preceding and following tube rotation (see Fig. 15–3).

PARTIAL SCAN RECONSTRUCTION. One of the major prerequisites for cardiac imaging is high temporal resolution (short image acquisition times). Modern scanners have gantry rotation times of 500 msec or less, but due to the rapid cardiac motion, even reconstructing images with an acquisition window of 500 msec will not be fast enough to reliably suppress cardiac motion artifacts. However, it is not necessary to use x-ray data from a full rotation (360 degrees) to reconstruct one image. Parts of the data are redundant (for example, attenuation will be the same when an x-ray beam passes through the body from back to front or from front to back).

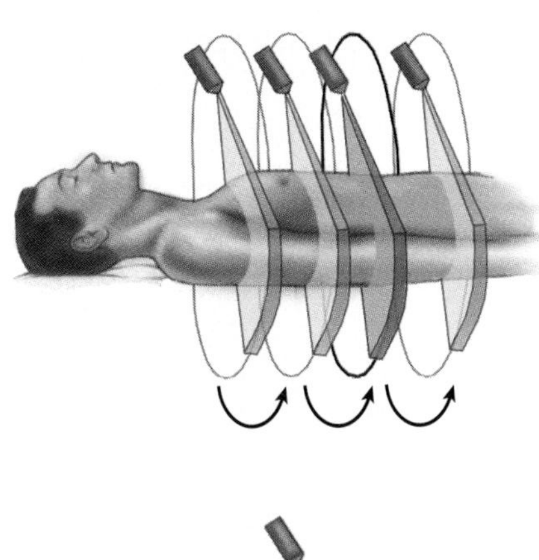
A

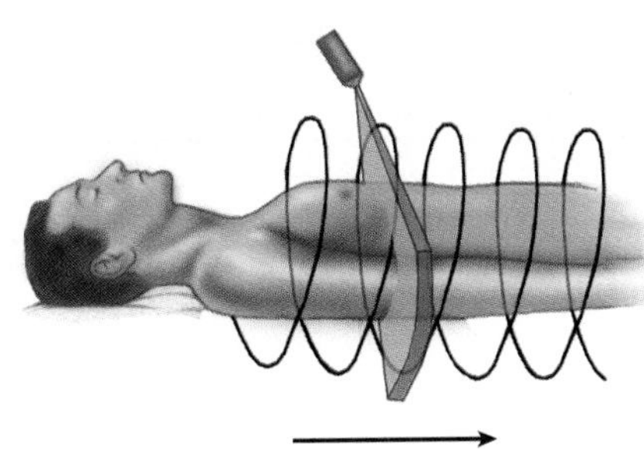
B

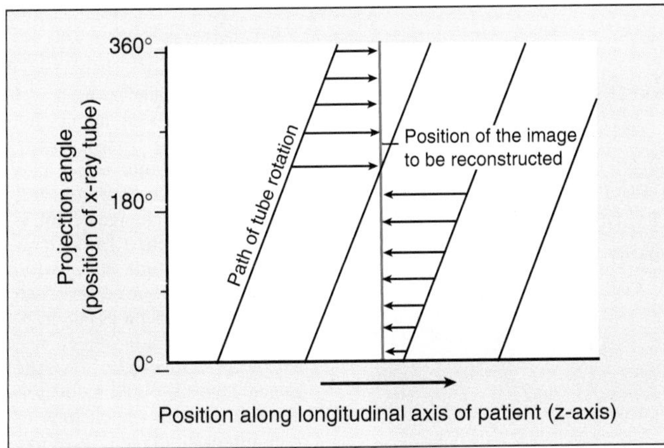

C

FIGURE 15–3 Principle of sequential and spiral scan modes. **A,** Sequential scanning. X-ray data are acquired at one table position with the x-ray source and detectors on a circular path. After enough data have been collected for image reconstruction, the x-ray tube is switched off and the table is advanced so that data can be acquired in another level. With multidetector computed tomography (CT), several (4 to 16) image slices can be acquired at each table position. Usually, table movement and image acquisition are triggered to the electrocardiogram so that every acquisition will be performed at the same instant in the cardiac cycle. **B,** Spiral scanning. X-ray data are continuously acquired with the x-ray tube and detectors in constant circular motion. Simultaneously, the patient table is advanced at a constant speed. The x-ray tube and detectors thus move on a spiral (or "helical") path relative to the patient. **C,** Image reconstruction in spiral CT. To reconstruct an image at a given level, a set of projections from numerous angles has to be obtained at that very plane. Since the tube does not perform a full rotation at any given imaging plane, x-ray data for every projection angle are interpolated from the preceding and following tube rotation.

To reconstruct one complete cross-sectional image, it is only necessary to use data from projections over 180 degrees plus the width of the fan angle emitted by the x-ray tube (approximately 50 degrees for most manufacturers). Image reconstruction algorithms that use projections covering less than 360 degrees are called *partial scan reconstruction algorithms.* The most commonly used algorithms for cardiac imaging use x-ray data from a single sweep over 180 degrees (plus the fan angle) and are usually referred to as *half-scan reconstruction algorithms.* With this reconstruction technique, a temporal resolution of half the gantry rotation time can be achieved in the center of the scan field.

For multidetector systems, more advanced partial scan reconstruction algorithms are available that make use of less than 180 degrees of tube rotation. To fill gaps and provide missing projection angles for reconstruction of an image at a given level, data are used that are acquired during a later heart beat by another detector and assigned to the correct heart phase by means of the simultaneously recorded ECG. Even though, theoretically, a better temporal resolution can be achieved by confining image reconstruction to shorter segments of the cardiac cycle, the necessity to combine data from several successive heart beats constitutes a major disadvantage. Since the heart may not return to exactly the same position from heart beat to heart beat, this may reduce image quality. A clear advantage of these techniques over half-scan reconstruction has so far not been shown.

ELECTROCARDIOGRAPHIC GATING. Another prerequisite for cardiac imaging by CT is the ability to synchronize the obtained images to the cardiac cycle. To achieve this, image acquisition can be triggered by the patient's ECG in sequential scan modes. In spiral scan mode, x-ray data are continuously acquired and modern CT systems permit simultaneous recording of the patient's ECG with the x-ray data. Using the partial scan reconstruction methods described earlier, it is thus possible to reconstruct cross-sectional images at any given instant in the cardiac cycle. This technique can be used to minimize motion artifacts (by retrospectively selecting the cardiac phase with the fewest artifacts) or to provide data sets during systole and diastole, which permits dynamic analysis of cardiac function. Although the availability of data throughout the cardiac cycle thus represents an advantage of continuous data acquisition and retrospective ECG gating, this scanning mode is associated with a higher radiation dose than sequential scan modes.[1-4] Table 15–2 lists typical scan parameters for multidetector spiral CT of the heart.

VISUALIZATION OF THE HEART IN COMPUTED TOMOGRAPHY

NONENHANCED IMAGING. CT imaging of the heart can be performed with and without injection of a contrast agent. The x-ray attenuation of soft tissue (e.g., myocardium) and blood is almost identical. In cardiac images obtained without injection of contrast agent, it is therefore not possible to discern structures within the heart (Fig. 15–4). Epicardial fat has a lower CT attenuation value, so that the proximal coronary arteries, which are frequently surrounded by fat, can often be recognized (see Fig. 15–4). Nonenhanced CT studies of the heart are almost exclusively performed to assess calcified structures within the heart, most notably coronary artery calcification.

CONTRAST-ENHANCED IMAGING. To increase the CT attenuation of the blood pool, an iodinated contrast agent can be injected. During the time of CT data acquisition (15 to 35 seconds for a high-resolution MDCT or EBT scan, depending on scanner type and scan parameters), maximum enhancement of the blood pool should be maintained. To limit the amount of contrast agent that needs to be injected and to achieve good contrast, the correct timing of the actual CT scan relative to contrast injection is important. The CT scan should start when the contrast agent arrives in the ascending aorta. This is usually 15 to 25 seconds after the start of contrast injection into a peripheral vein. Individual determination of the contrast agent transit time is recommended for each patient. If only arterial structures (left ventricle, coronary arteries) are to be investigated, the duration of contrast injection should be approximately the same as the duration of the scan. If structures of the right heart and pulmonary circulation are also to be analyzed, contrast injection must be longer to maintain enhancement in the right heart until the end of the scan.

Contrast-enhanced CT studies permit delineation of the cardiac chambers, valves, great cardiac vessels, and, under the prerequisite of sufficient spatial resolution and successful suppression of motion artifacts, the coronary artery lumen (Fig. 15–5). Contrast enhancement in the right atrium is often inhomogeneous because blood saturated with contrast material from the superior vena cava mixes with nonenhanced blood

TABLE 15–2 Sample Image Acquisition Protocols for Cardiac Imaging by Multidetector Spiral Computed Tomography*

	Coronary Arteries	Coronary Calcium, Retrospective	Coronary Calcium, Prospective
Slice collimation	16 × 0.75 mm	16 × 1.5 mm	16 × 1.5 mm
Rotation time	420 ms	420 ms	420 ms
Tube voltage	120 kV	120 kV	120 kV
Electrocardiographic (ECG) gating†	Retrospective, half-scan reconstruction (temporal resolution 210 ms in center of scan field), individual positioning of reconstruction window in cardiac cycle	Retrospective, half-scan reconstruction (temporal resolution 200-250 ms in center of scan field), individual positioning of reconstruction window in cardiac cycle	Prospective, half-scan reconstruction (temporal resolution 210 ms in center of scan field)
Image reconstruction	1.0 mm slice thickness in 0.5 mm increments (~240 images)	3.0 mm slice thickness in 1.5 mm increments (~80 images)	3.0 mm slice thickness in 1.5 mm increments (~80 images)
Contrast enhancement	Intravenous, iodinated contrast (~80 ml)	—	—
Approximate radiation dose‡	~5-10 mSv[1]	~1-3 mSv [1]	~0.5-0.7 mSv[1] ~1.5-1.8 mSv[2] ~1.0 mSv[3]

*The protocols represent examples for a 16-slice scanner with 0.75 mm collimation (Siemens Sensation 16). Settings may vary for other manufacturers or older scanner generations.

†For retrospective ECG gated acquisitions, ECG-correlated tube current modulation may lead to a dose reduction of 30-50%[1,4].

‡Radiation doses represent effective doses. As they are approximations and partly obtained from different sources than in Table 15–1, they are not immediately comparable.

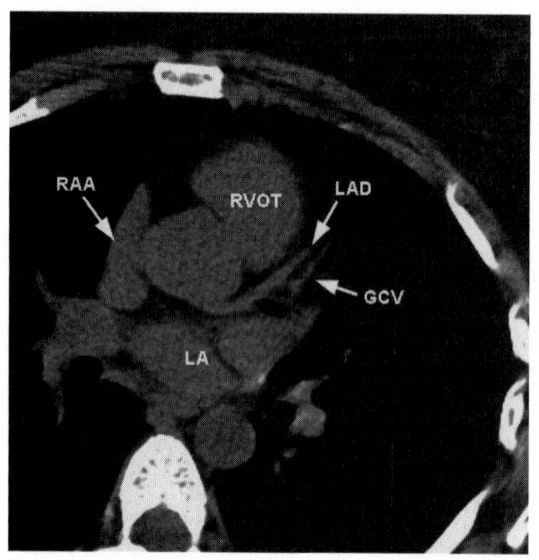

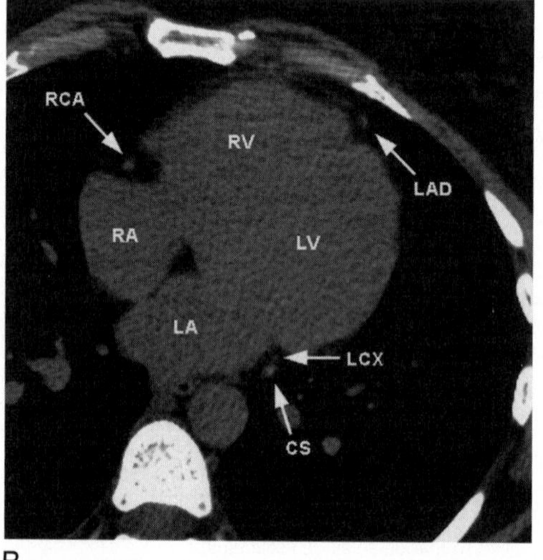

FIGURE 15–4 Normal cardiac anatomy as depicted by nonenhanced computed tomography (CT). Images are in the axial (transverse) plane and displayed as if looking up from the patient's feet. Blood has a similar CT attenuation as connective tissue (e.g., the myocardium). It is therefore not possible to delineate the ventricular cavities or other structures within the heart. **A,** Level of the left coronary artery ostium from the aortic root. **B,** Level of the mid right coronary artery (RCA). CS = coronary sinus, GCV = great cardiac vein, LA = left atrium, LAD = left anterior descending coronary artery, LCX = left circumflex coronary artery, LV = left ventricle; RA = right atrium, RV = right ventricle, RVOT = right ventricular outflow tract.

from the inferior vena cava. The resulting artifacts can frequently impair visualization of structures in the right atrium, the interatrial septum, and the tricuspid valve.

TYPICAL ARTIFACTS. CT imaging of the heart is prone to artifacts, since it stretches the temporal and spatial resolution of CT scanners to their limits, and additional artifacts can be introduced by the partial scan reconstruction algorithms. It is important to recognize typical artifacts to avoid misinterpretation. Motion artifacts will typically blur the contours of the heart, especially of the coronary arteries (Fig. 15-6). Inconsistent triggering or arrhythmias may cause misalignment of adjacent slices (see Fig. 15-6). In combination with motion, partial scan reconstruction can cause streaks and low-density artifacts adjacent to regions of very high CT density (e.g., metal or calcium). Edge-enhancing reconstruction filters can lead to artifacts along borders between very low and high density (e.g., the interface between lung and cardiac tissue) by assigning artificially high CT numbers to pixels along that border (see Fig. 15-6). Finally, the partial volume effect is a general phenomenon in CT imaging: if an image pixel is only partially filled by a structure of very high attenuation (e.g., metal or bone), a very high CT number will be assigned to the complete pixel, which will thus appear bright on the image. This may lead to overestimation of the dimensions of high-intensity objects (e.g., calcifications within coronary arteries) and may cause difficulties in image interpretation.

Clinical Applications

Cardiac Morphology

Computed tomography imaging has a relatively high spatial resolution, and a high contrast between the blood pool and other tissues can be achieved after injection of contrast agent. CT imaging therefore has the ability to provide high-resolution morphologic imaging of the heart. Clinically, however, CT imaging does not play a very prominent role in evaluating cardiac morphology, because echocardiography or magnetic resonance imaging can provide all relevant information in most clinical situations (see Chaps. 11 and 14). Since echocardiography and magnetic resonance imaging neither expose the patient to radiation nor require the injection of potentially nephrotoxic contrast agents, echocardiography, possibly followed by magnetic resonance imaging, will usually be the preferred approach to imaging for assessment of cardiac morphology. However, cardiac CT imaging can be clinically helpful in a variety of situations, including the need for cross-sectional

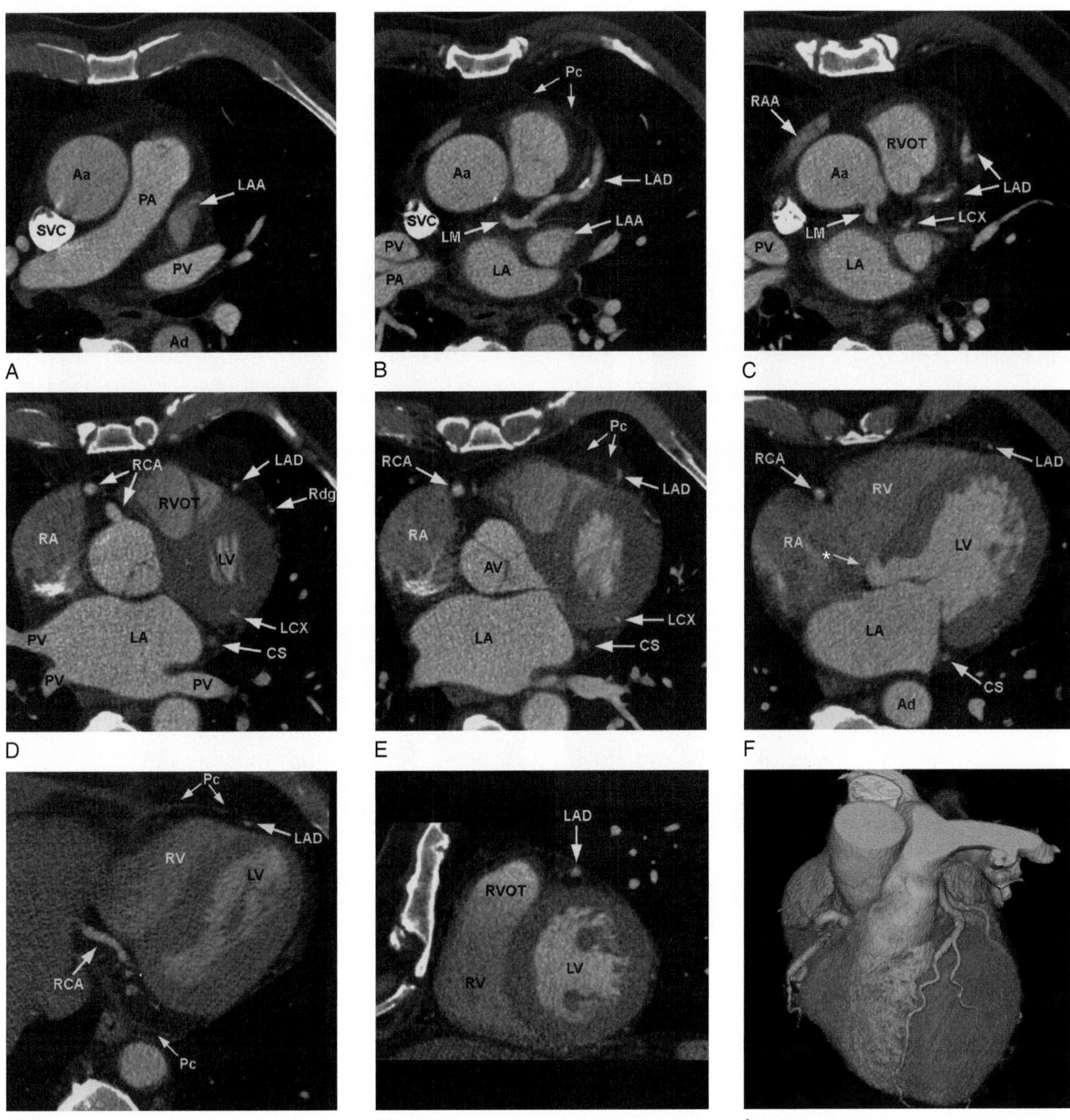

FIGURE 15–5 Normal cardiac anatomy as depicted by contrast-enhanced multidetector computed tomography (MDCT). **A** to **G** represent axial (transverse) cross sections acquired with 210 msec temporal resolution. A craniocaudal sequence of noncontiguous cross sections is shown. **A,** Level of the ascending aorta (Aa). Bright contrast is seen in the superior vena cava, since contrast material is injected into a cubital vein. **B,** Visualization of a long segment of the proximal left anterior descending artery (LAD), with some calcification. **C,** Level of the left main coronary artery (LM) ostium. **D,** Level of the right coronary artery (RCA) ostium. **E,** Level of the aortic valve (AV). **F,** Level of the mid-right coronary artery. All four cardiac chambers are displayed. Note the membranous part of the interventricular septum (asterisk and arrow). **G,** Level of the distal right coronary artery. **H,** Multiplanar reconstruction orthogonal to the axial imaging plane to create a "short axis" view of the left ventricle (LV). **I,** Three-dimensional surface reconstruction of the heart, shown from an anterior view. The coronary arteries can be recognized on the surface of the heart. Ad = descending aorta; CS = coronary sinus; LA = left atrium; LAA = left atrial appendage; LCX = left circumflex coronary artery; Pc = pericardium; PA = pulmonary artery; PV = pulmonary vein; RA = right atrium; RAA = right atrial appendage; Rdg = diagonal branch; RV = right ventricle; RVOT = right ventricular outflow tract; SVC = superior vena cava.

imaging after echocardiography in patients with pacemakers or other devices that preclude magnetic resonance imaging. Also, CT techniques have an extremely high accuracy for the depiction of calcified structures. Finally, cardiac CT imaging is increasingly applicable for coronary artery visualization.

Pericardial Disease (see Chap. 64)

Since the pericardium is usually embedded in epicardial and pericardial fat, it can, in most cases, be delineated in CT images. It usually appears as a thin line (see Fig. 15–5) and is best delineated on the anterior face of the heart. Congenital absence of the pericardium can be complete or partial. This condition is infrequent, and patients are usually asymptomatic. CT can be helpful in establishing the absence or presence of a segment of pericardium, but lack of visualization, especially on the posterior surface, is not a sufficient criterion to make the diagnosis.[5] Recent studies found the normal thickness of pericardium on high-resolution scans to

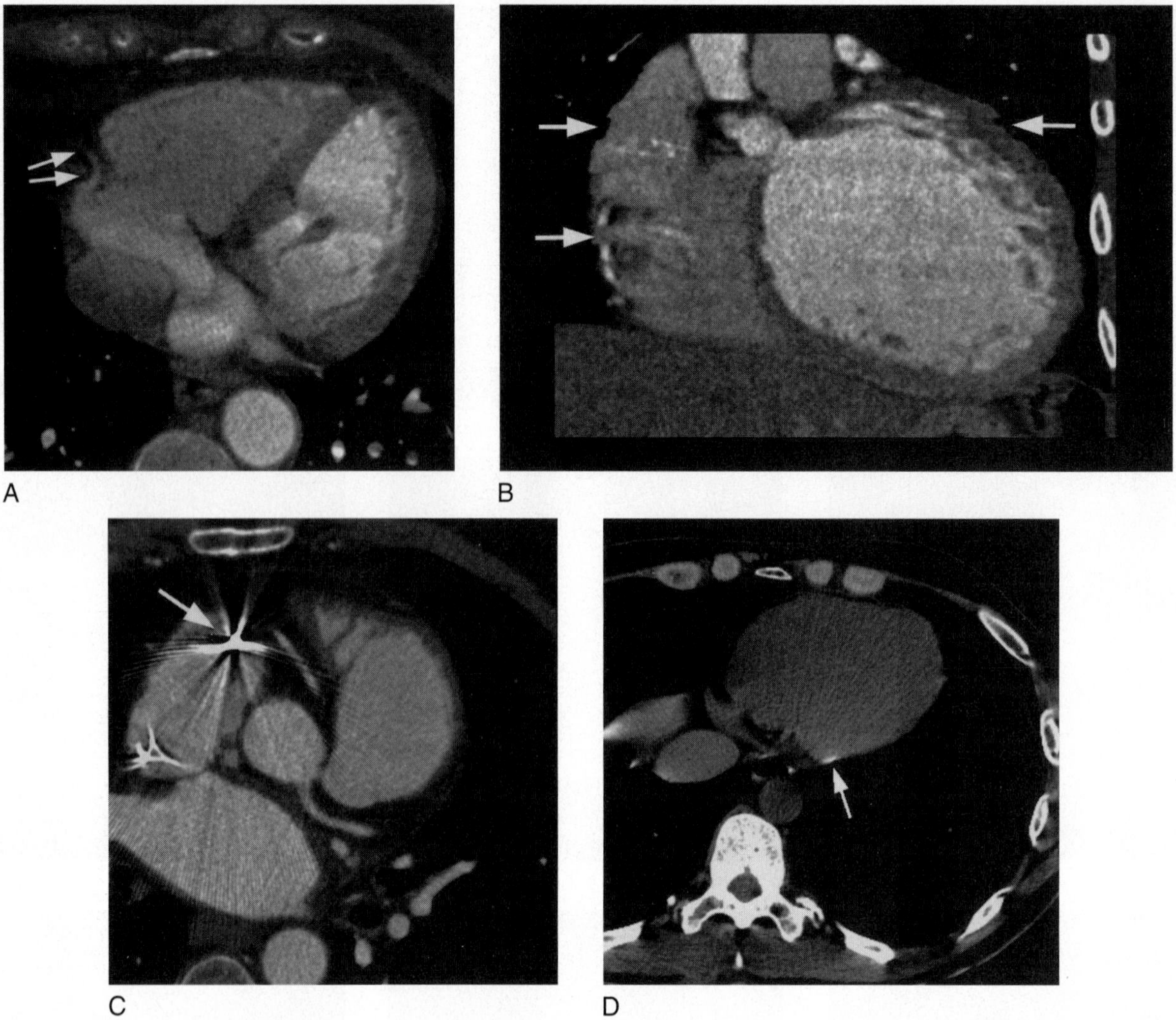

A B C D

FIGURE 15–6 Examples of typical artifacts encountered in cardiac computed tomography (CT) imaging. Most artifacts are related to limited temporal resolution and partial scan reconstruction. **A,** Motion artifact of the right coronary artery. **B,** Trigger artifacts caused by irregular (ectopic) heart beats. Coronal multiplanar reconstruction of the heart. Arrows point at artifacts caused by ectopic beats, which result in parts of the imaging volume being acquired in an offset cardiac phase. **C,** Streaks and low-density artifacts caused by objects of very high density (here: pacemaker lead in right atrium). **D,** Edge-enhancement can cause artifacts at interfaces between tissues with a high difference in CT attenuation (here: interface of pericardium and lung; see arrow). Pixels along that interface may be assigned a higher intensity value than corresponds to their actual attenuation. In this case, this artifact could be misinterpretated as calcification.

range between 1 and 2 mm.[6] Pericardial thickening can be a helpful finding in cases of suspected constriction, but it does not prove any hemodynamic relevance. Thickened pericardium can be found in a multitude of situations, including the early postoperative period, uremia, rheumatic heart disease, and sarcoidosis or as a consequence of radiation therapy, and per se does not constitute proof of constriction. Similarly, a normal pericardial thickness can not rule out constriction.[5] CT imaging can clearly delineate pericardial calcification (Fig. 15–7) and in the clinical setting of suspected constriction, it should be considered a significant finding.[5]

PERICARDIAL FLUID. Pericardial fluid can reliably be detected by CT, and small amounts of fluid in pericardial recesses can frequently be observed in healthy individuals.[7] Although echocardiography has an excellent sensitivity to detect relevant pericardial effusion in the majority of clinical situations (see Chap. 11), its application can be limited in postoperative patients, and some localized effusions may be outside the echocardiographic acoustic windows. CT can clearly delineate the anatomical distribution of pericardial fluid (Fig. 15–8). CT attenuation numbers measured in the pericardial fluid may give some indication as to the genesis of the effusion. Densities higher than water (above approximately 10 HU) suggest high protein content (e.g., blood).

PERICARDIAL CYSTS AND NEOPLASMS. Pericardial cysts appear on CT images as paracardiac masses, typically in the right cardiophrenic angle. The cysts have a thin capsule that is not always visualized but that may occasionally be calcified. The cysts are usually filled with fluid of water-equivalent density (Fig. 15–9). Bronchiogenic cysts or teratomas may mimic pericardial cysts in location and appearance. Primary neoplasms of the pericardium are infrequent but can be the reason for thickened pericardium on CT scans. Both primary neoplasms and secondary involvement of the pericardium can be accompanied by hemorrhagic pericardial effusions.[8]

Myocardial Disease (see Chap. 59)

The role of CT in the assessment of myocardial disease is limited. Even though CT can clearly show left ventricular geometry, wall thickness, and also function, the diagnosis of dilated or hypertrophic cardiomyopathy does not require cross-sectional imaging. Except for occasional case reports, little is known about the value of CT in assessing infiltrative myocardial disease.[9,10] Typical findings in arrhythmogenic

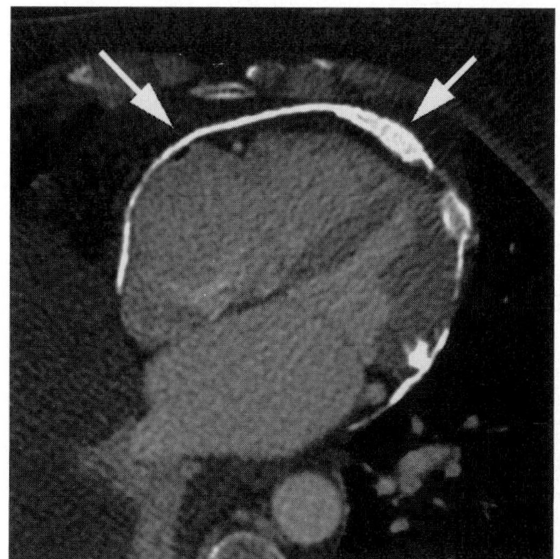

FIGURE 15–7 Severe pericardial calcification. (Courtesy of R. Rienmüller, MD, Interdisciplinary Cardiac Imaging Center, University Graz.)

right ventricular dysplasia include dilation of the right ventricle, infiltration of the myocardium with fatty tissue of low CT attenuation, and aneurysms and local bulging of the right ventricular free wall (Fig. 15–10).[11]

Valvular Disease (see Chap. 57)

Although visualization of the tricuspid and pulmonary valves is inconsistent, the mitral and aortic valves can reliably be depicted in contrast-enhanced cardiac CT scans (Fig. 15–11). Functional analysis is not possible, however, and CT plays no relevant role in the work-up of valvular lesions concerning their hemodynamic relevance. However, the unique ability of CT to detect and quantify calcification has recently been applied, especially to aortic valve disease (see Fig. 15–11). CT has shown high accuracy and reproducibility in quantifying aortic valve calcification and its progression.[12-15] This may develop into clinically relevant applications with respect to the prognostic relevance of aortic valve sclerosis[16] as well as the problem of bioprosthesis calcification.

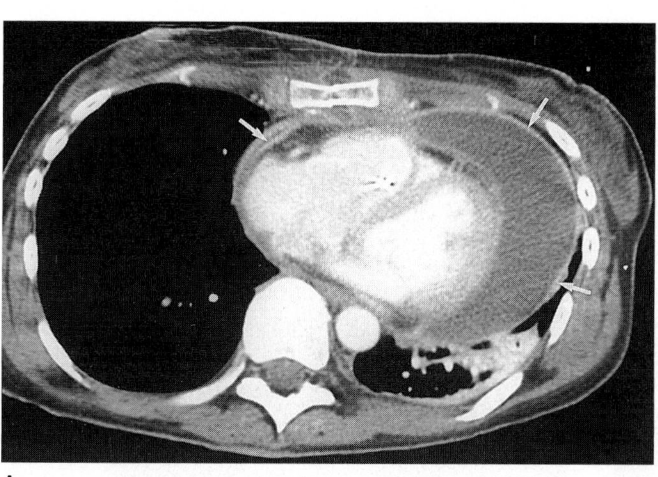

A

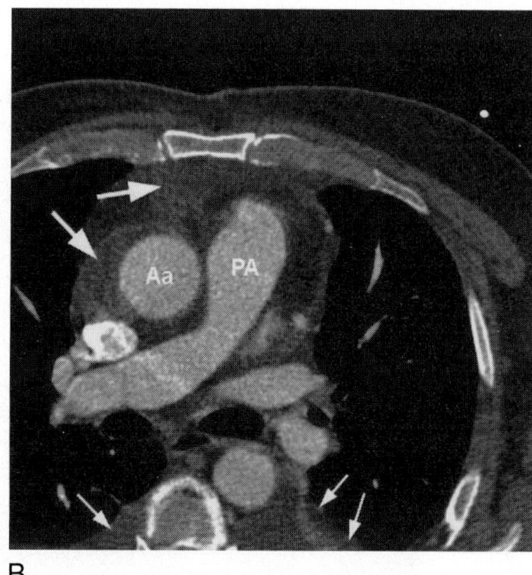

B

FIGURE 15–8 Pericardial effusion. **A,** Large pericardial effusion with contrast enhancement of the pericardium (arrows), suggesting pericardial inflammation (Courtesy of GE Imatron). **B,** Localized pericardial effusion in the superior aortic recess in a patient 4 days after bypass surgery (large arrows). Bilateral pleural effusion is also present (small arrows). Aa = ascending aorta, PA = pulmonary artery.

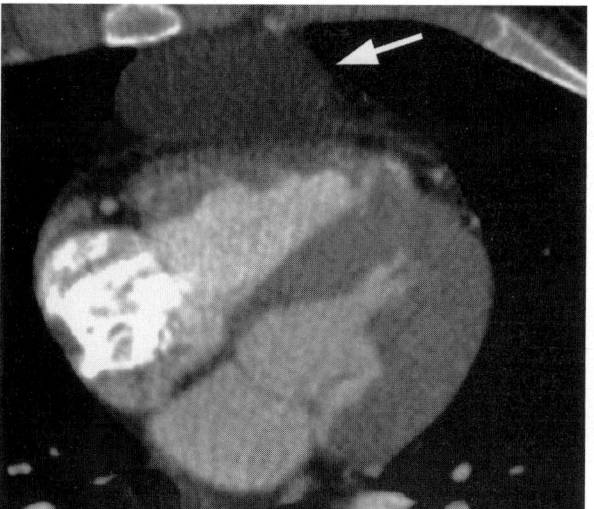

FIGURE 15–9 Pericardial cyst located anterior to the right ventricle in a contrast-enhanced scan (arrow).

Coronary Artery Disease (see Chap. 50)

Cardiac CT has several potential applications in patients with coronary artery disease. CT can demonstrate the morphological consequences of ischemic heart disease (Figs. 15–12 and 15–13),[17] can assess ventricular function and perfusion, and is applied with increasing success to visualizing coronary arteries. In addition, the assessment of coronary artery calcification, especially with EBT, has received considerable attention with respect to its potential role in the early detection of subclinical atherosclerosis. In the diagnostic work-up of coronary artery disease, the emerging abilities of CT imaging compete with a multitude of other well-established and readily available diagnostic modalities. In this context, the most appropriate clinical use of CT is made when limiting its application to situations in which clinical evidence shows advantages over other modalities.

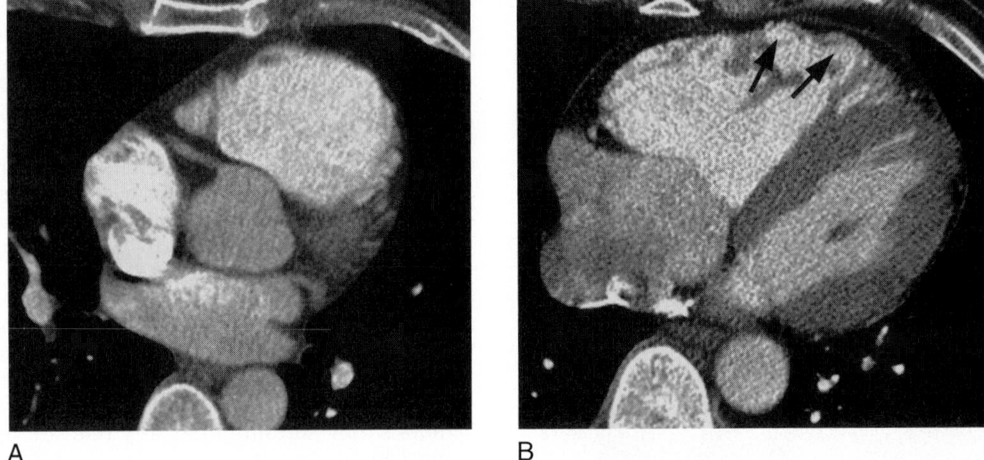

FIGURE 15–10 Dilated right ventricle and aneurysmal bulging of the right ventricular free wall (arrows) in a patient with arrhythmogenic right ventricular dysplasia. (Courtesy of J. F. Breen, MD, Mayo Clinic, Rochester, MN.)

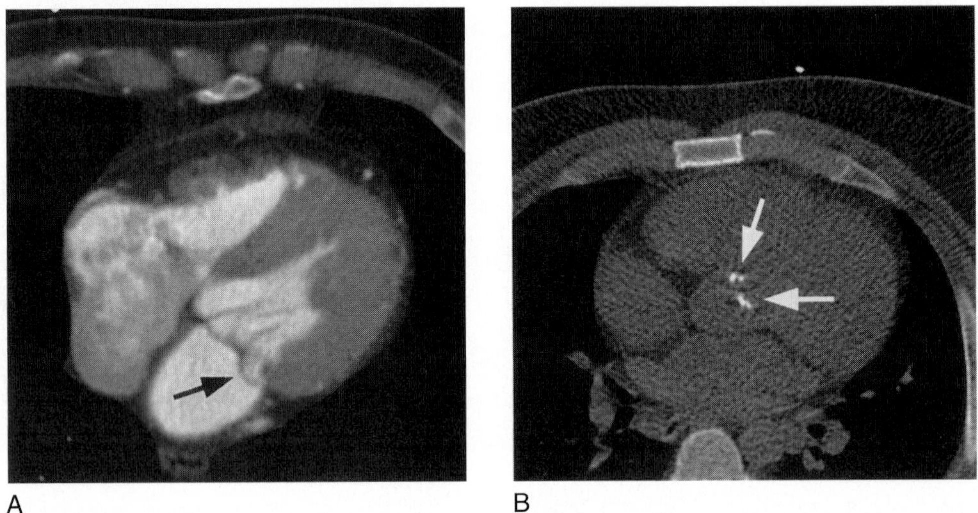

FIGURE 15–11 Visualization of cardiac valves by computed tomography. **A,** Prolapse of the posterior mitral leaflet in a contrast-enhanced systolic image (arrow). **B,** Calcifications of the aortic valve (arrows) detected in a nonenhanced scan.

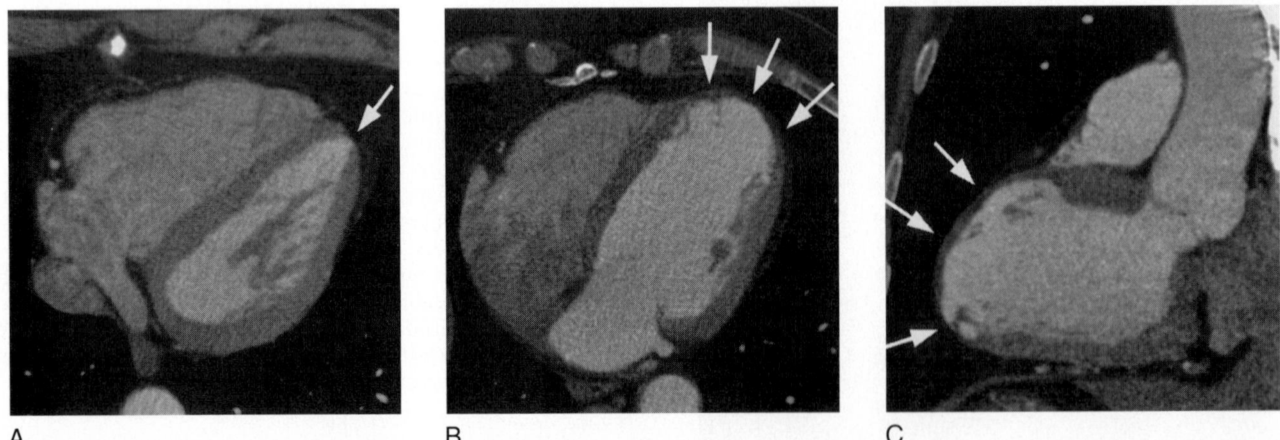

FIGURE 15–12 Computed tomography (CT) clearly depicts regional wall thinning as a consequence of myocardial infarction. It is important to note that in healthy subjects, the left ventricular wall in the very apical region can be paper-thin, which constitutes a frequent normal finding.[17] **A,** Normal tapering of the left ventricular apex as frequently observed in high-resolution CT scans (arrow). **B and C,** Infarction of the anterior wall (arrows) in an axial cross section **(B)** and multiplanar reformat **(C).**

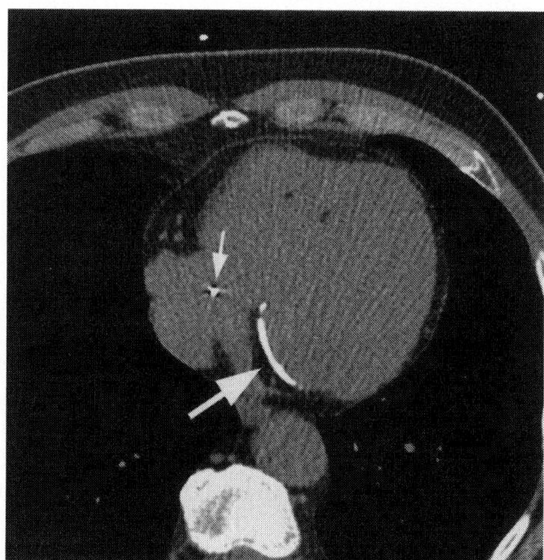

FIGURE 15–13 Calcified left ventricular aneurysm (large arrow) as a consequence of posterior myocardial infarction in a nonenhanced scan (small arrow = pacemaker lead).

CORONARY ARTERY CALCIFICATION

PATHOLOGY. Coronary calcium is a surrogate marker for coronary atherosclerotic plaque. In the coronary arteries, calcifications occur almost exclusively in the context of atherosclerotic changes.[18,19] Medial (nonatherosclerotic) calcification of the coronary artery wall is exceedingly rare. Within a coronary vessel or larger segment of the vessel, the quantity of coronary calcium correlates moderately closely with the extent of atherosclerotic plaque burden.[18,19] On the other hand, not every atherosclerotic coronary plaque is calcified. The presence or absence of calcium is not closely associated with the propensity of an individual atherosclerotic plaque to rupture, and calcification is a sign of neither stability nor instability of an individual plaque.[18] Plaques with healed ruptures almost invariably contain calcium, whereas plaque erosions are frequently not calcified. In the vast majority of patients with acute coronary syndromes, coronary calcium can be detected, and the amount of calcium in these patients is substantially greater than in matched control subjects without coronary artery disease.[20-22]

Although there is a strong quantitative relationship between coronary calcification and coronary plaque burden, there is only a weak, nonlinear correlation between the amount of coronary calcium and the angiographic severity of obstructive coronary artery disease.[19] The complete absence of coronary calcium makes the presence of significant coronary luminal obstruction highly unlikely, however.[19,23]

In patients with end-stage renal disease, the prevalence and extent of coronary calcification are high. However, the relationship of coronary calcium to coronary atherosclerosis is less well established in this patient group.[18,24]

DETECTION OF CORONARY CALCIUM. Electron beam tomography and ECG-gated spiral CT with subsecond rotation permit detection and quantification of coronary artery calcium.[25] Mechanical CT without ECG gating is unsuited for the reliable detection of coronary calcium.[26] The vast majority of existing data concerning histopathological validation and clinical evaluation of coronary calcium assessment has been obtained using EBT.

The usual protocol to detect and quantify coronary calcification by EBT consists of the acquisition of high-resolution axial cross-sections of the heart with a 100-msec acquisition time per image, 3.0 mm slice thickness, and no overlap (see Table 15–1). Some investigators propose a 0.5 mm overlap of consecutive images. The presence of calcifications is assumed if contiguous pixels with a density exceeding 130 HU are found within the coronary artery system (Fig. 15–14).[19] The so-called Agatston score has most frequently been used to quantify the amount of coronary calcium in EBT. The Agatston score is derived by measuring the area of each calcified coronary lesion and multiplying it by a coefficient that has a value of 1 to 4, depending on the maximum CT attenuation within the lesion. The sum of all lesions represents the Agatson score for the patient. Several large reference data sets are available that describe the distribution of Agatston scores found in the respective (usually self-referred) population, stratified by age and gender.[21,27]

By MDCT, prospectively triggered sequential scanning or retrospectively ECG-gated continuous spiral scanning can be applied for the detection of coronary calcium (see Table 15–2). Scan parameters have not been standardized and vary substantially according to scanner type and manufacturer. The best image quality is usually obtained with retrospectively gated scans and thin slice collimation, albeit at the expense of high radiation exposure.[28] Motion artifacts, especially in sequential scan mode, are more frequent than in EBT (Fig. 15–15). Similar to EBT, the presence of calcium is usually assumed if pixels above 130 HU are observed within the coronary arteries, and modified versions of the Agatston score are used for quantification.

The analysis of coronary calcification in coronary CT images is usually straightforward. Difficulties in interpretation can arise in the presence of motion artifacts (see Fig. 15–15). The close proximity of the left circumflex coronary artery to the mitral valve and annulus can sometimes lead to misinterpretation of mitral calcification as coronary calcium (see Fig. 15–15). The interobserver variability of coronary calcium quantification is low. Interscan variability can be high for patients with small amounts of calcium, but on average the latest technology provides for interscan variability of less than 10%. Alternative scoring methods, such as volumetric scores or determination of the calcium mass, have been proposed but have not been validated on a large scale.

CLINICAL SIGNIFICANCE OF CORONARY CALCIUM. Coronary calcium correlates with the presence and extent of coronary atherosclerosis. The absence of coronary calcium thus rules out the presence of significant coronary artery stenoses with high predictive value.[19,23] However, since even pronounced coronary atherosclerotic plaque burden is not necessarily associated with hemodynamically relevant luminal narrowings, the detection even of large amounts of calcium does not imply the presence of significant stenoses. Thus, the finding of pronounced calcifications by itself does not necessitate invasive coronary angiography.

Several cohort studies have shown that the presence of coronary calcium demonstrated by EBT in asymptomatic individuals is a prognostic parameter with high predictive power regarding the development of hard cardiac events during the following 3 to 5 years.[21,29-33] A meta-analysis demonstrated that a calcium score higher than the median was associated with an unadjusted odds ratio of 4.2 (95% CI, 1.6-11.3) for myocardial infarction or death.[34] It is currently assumed that individuals who seem to be at intermediate risk for coronary events (0.6-2.0 percent annual risk) based on traditional risk factor analysis will be most likely

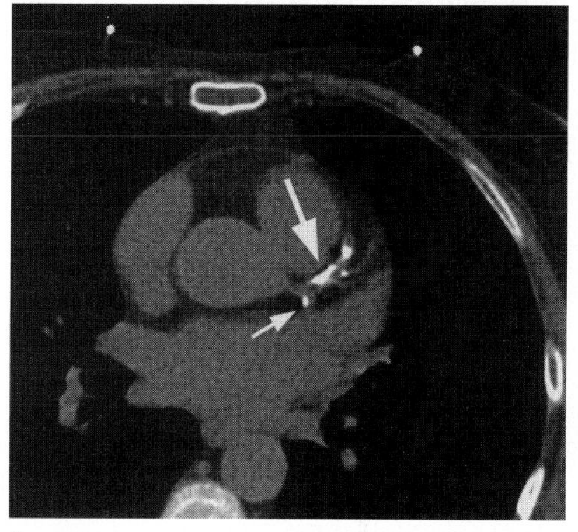

A

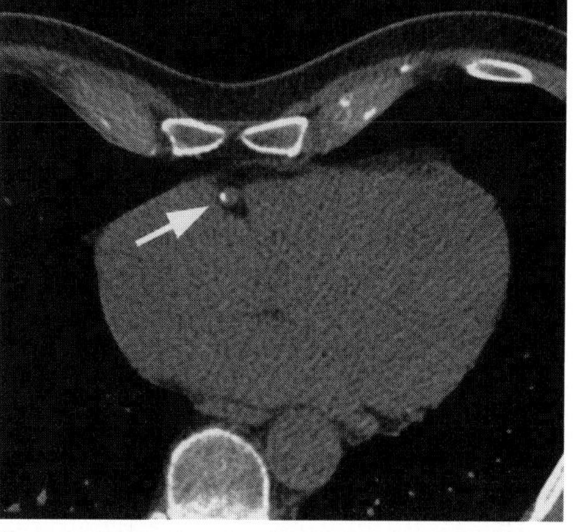

B

FIGURE 15–14 Examples of coronary calcification. **A,** Calcification of the left anterior descending coronary artery (large arrow) and left circumflex coronary artery (small arrow). **B,** Calcification of the right coronary artery (arrow).

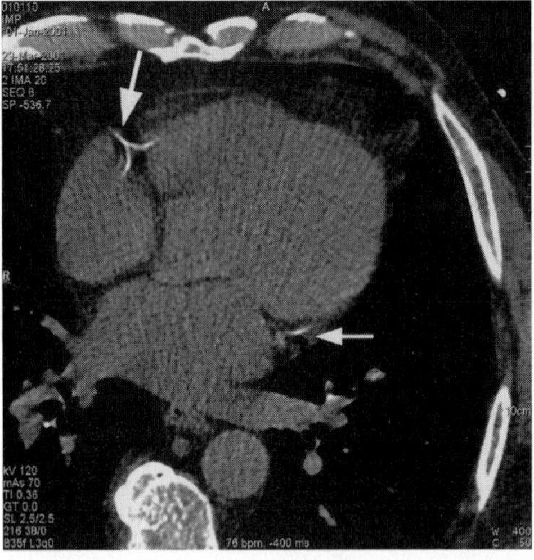

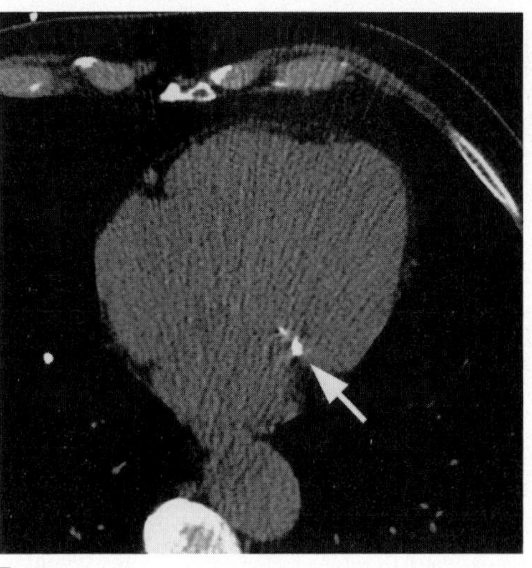

A B

FIGURE 15–15 Interpretation problems in coronary calcium scans. **A,** Motion artifacts of the right coronary artery (large arrow) and, to a lesser extent, of the left circumflex coronary artery (small arrow) in prospectively electrocardiographically triggered sequential multidetector computed tomography (four-slice scanner, 500 msec rotation, patient with a heart rate of 75/min). **B,** Calcification of the mitral annulus (arrow). Owing to the proximity of the course of the left circumflex coronary artery, mitral calcification can be misinterpreted as calcium in the left circumflex coronary artery.

to profit from noninvasive testing for subclinical atherosclerosis, such as the assessment of coronary calcification. Unselected "screening" or patient self-referral is uniformly not recommended.[19,35]

Coronary calcification has been found to be progressive over time.[36] Several studies have reported an influence of lipid levels and lipid-lowering therapy on the rate of progression of calcification.[37-39] Little is known, however, concerning the relationship between calcium progression and clinical events. Thus, recommendations for repeat scanning can currently not be made.[25]

VISUALIZATION OF THE CORONARY LUMEN. Electron beam tomography and multidetector spiral CT have been applied for visualization of the coronary artery lumen after intravenous injection of a contrast agent. Based on the axial cross sections of the heart, two- or three-dimensional reconstructions of the coronary arteries can be rendered (Figs. 15–16 and 15–17). Concerning the detection of coronary stenoses, two-dimensional "maximum intensity projections" provide the highest diagnostic accuracy. Three-dimensional reconstruction usually adds no further information but may be useful to document findings. Several investigators have compared the accuracy of EBT[40] and MDCT[41-45] for coronary stenosis detection to invasive coronary angiography. Given the small dimensions of the coronary arteries, it is obvious that high spatial resolution is critical for reliable assessment of the coronary lumen. Consequently, the best results so far have been obtained by 16-slice MDCT, with a sensitivity ranging from 92 to 95 percent and specificity of 86 to 93 percent for the detection of coronary stenoses of more than 50 percent diameter reduction.[44,45] However, MDCT is limited by its lower temporal resolution as compared to EBT, and several reports have shown that the patient should have a heart rate of 60 beats/min or less during the MDCT scan for good image quality to be reliably achieved. Hence, most investigators propose the administration of short-acting beta-blockers prior to the MDCT scan.[44,45] Heart rate is no limitation for the faster EBT scanner. Accurate grading of the severity of a coronary lesion (percentage of stenosis) is currently not possible, and even in optimally prepared patients, pronounced coronary calcifications, trigger artifacts due to arrhythmias, or high image noise can prevent analysis of coronary segments concerning the presence of stenoses. Owing to these limitations and the lack of larger clinical trials, EBT and MDCT coronary angiography currently cannot be considered routine clinical tools with broad applicability. However, clinical application, especially to rule out coronary stenoses in patients with low pretest likelihood of disease, is conceivable.

Imaging of coronary stents has been demonstrated (Fig. 15–18), but partial volume effects and artifacts caused by metal frequently prevent adequate visualization of the coronary lumen inside stents. Therefore, clinical application of CT for reliable assessment of in-stent restenosis is currently not possible. Patency and occlusion of bypass grafts can be established with very high accuracy[46,47] (Fig. 15–19), but limitations exist concerning the detection of stenoses at the site of the anastomosis to the coronary artery and in the peripheral run-off vessels. Clinical situations that may benefit from noninvasive assessment of bypass patency by CT are therefore limited.

The image quality of noninvasive coronary and bypass angiography by CT has rapidly improved during the last years. Technical developments toward faster

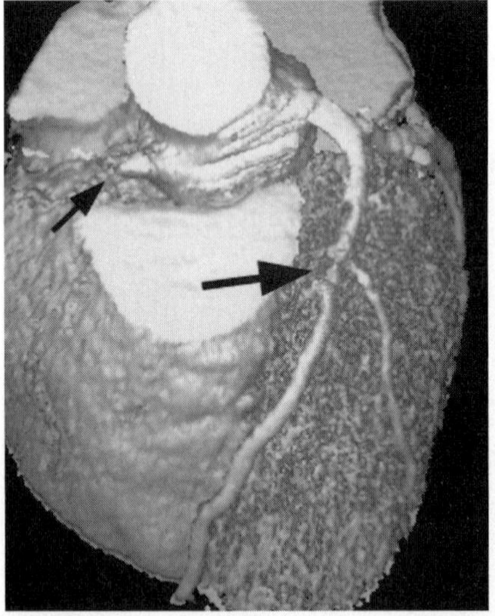

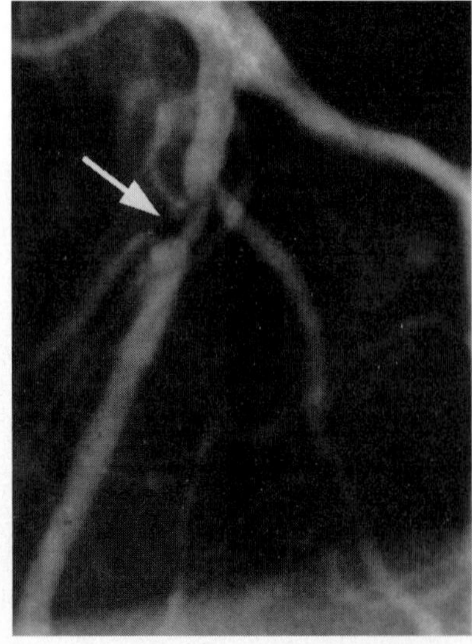

A B

FIGURE 15–16 Noninvasive coronary angiography by cardiac computed tomography. **A,** Three-dimensional reconstruction obtained by electron beam tomography in a patient with a high-grade stenosis of the left anterior descending coronary artery (large arrow). The right coronary artery is occluded (small arrow). **B,** Corresponding invasive angiogram of the left coronary artery.

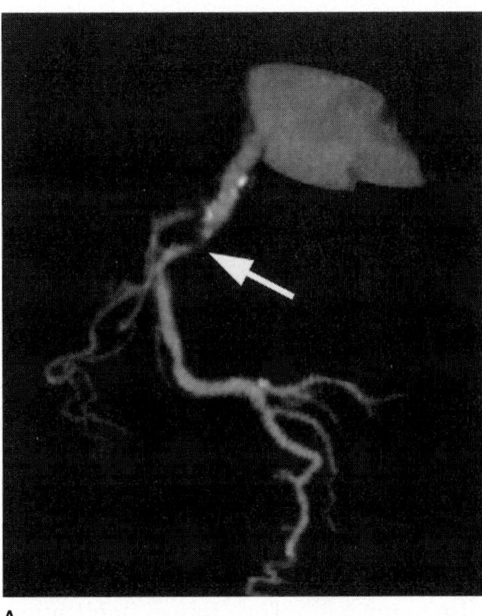

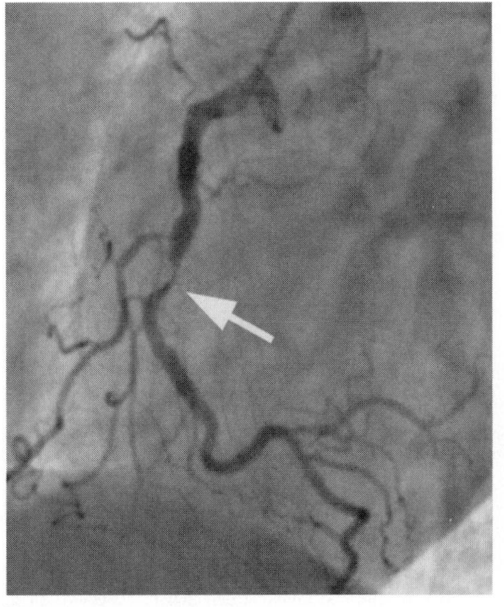

A B

FIGURE 15–17 Patient with a high-grade right coronary artery stenosis (arrows). **A,** Two-dimensional reconstruction (maximum intensity projection) obtained by multidetector computed tomography. **B,** Corresponding invasive coronary angiogram.

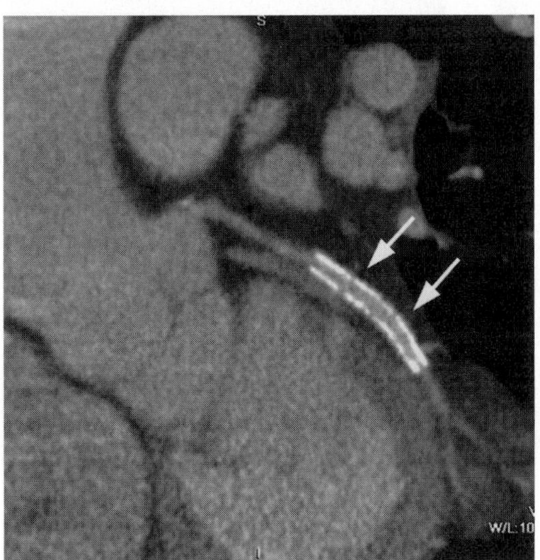

FIGURE 15–18 Visualization of a patent stent (arrows) in the left circumflex coronary artery. (Courtesy of M. Grover-McKay, MD, and S. Lipson, MD, Long Beach Memorial Medical Center, Long Beach, CA.)

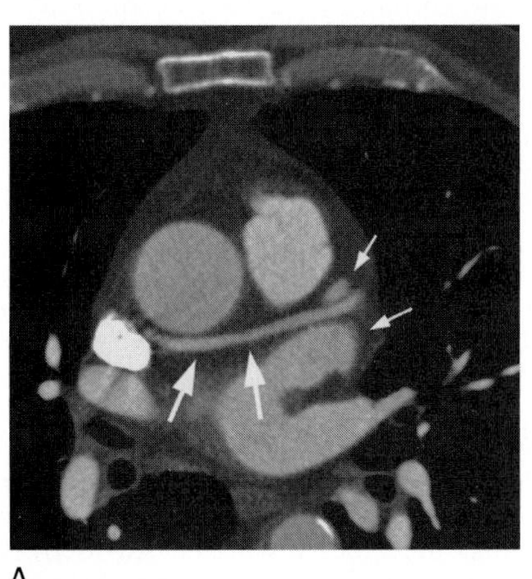

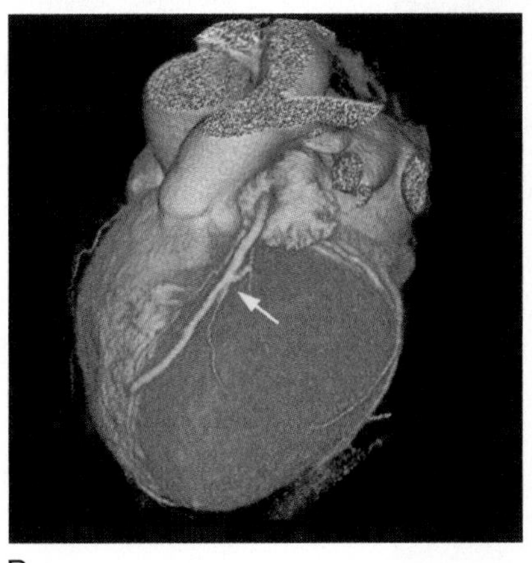

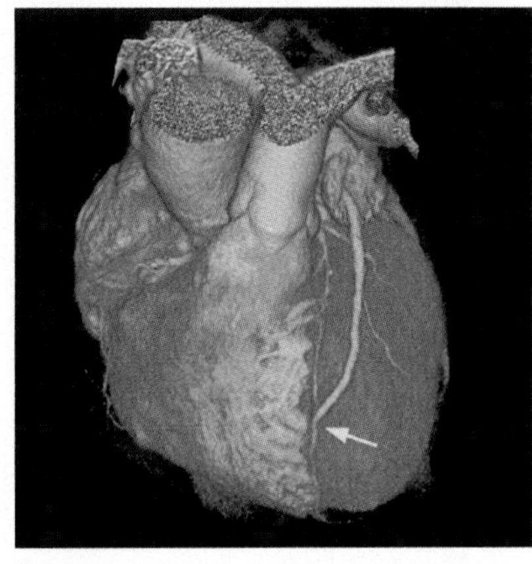

A B C

FIGURE 15–19 Patient with a single venous bypass graft to the diagonal branch and left anterior descending coronary artery. **A,** Axial contrast-enhanced image showing the bypass graft (large arrows), which follows a retroaortic course (small arrows = left atrial appendage). **B and C,** Three-dimensional reconstructions that show the bypass grafts and anastomoses to the diagonal branch and left anterior descending coronary artery (arrows).

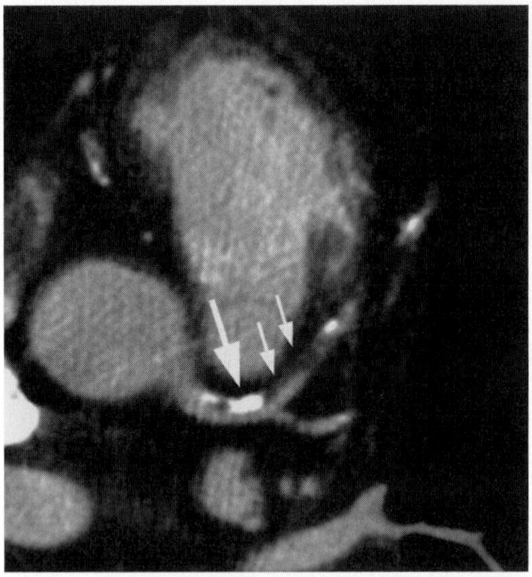

scanners with higher resolution will continue. With increasing image quality, it can thus be anticipated that accuracy and clinical applicability of "noninvasive coronary angiography" by EBT and MDCT will continue to improve.

VISUALIZATION OF NONCALCIFIED CORONARY ARTERY PLAQUE. The observation that noncalcified coronary atherosclerotic plaque can be visualized in high-resolution, contrast-enhanced CT scans of the coronary arteries[48] has sparked intense interest in using CT imaging for the detection, quantification, and characterization of coronary plaque in the context of risk assessment (Fig. 15–20). A comparison of 21 patients with acute myocardial infarction to 19 patients with stable angina found that MDCT detected noncalcified coronary atherosclerotic plaque significantly more frequently in patients with acute infarction.[49] Sensitivity and specificity for plaque detection as well as the ability to quantify noncalcified plaque by CT have so far not been investigated systematically. Under the assumption that lipid-rich plaques have a higher risk of rupture with consequent thrombosis than fibrotic plaques, researchers have tried to use measurements of CT attenuation values to differentiate plaque types.[50-52] The clinical implications of these interesting initial findings, however, are currently unclear.[53]

FIGURE 15–20 Visualization of calcified (large arrow) and noncalcified (small arrows) coronary atherosclerotic plaque by contrast-enhanced computed tomography.

A

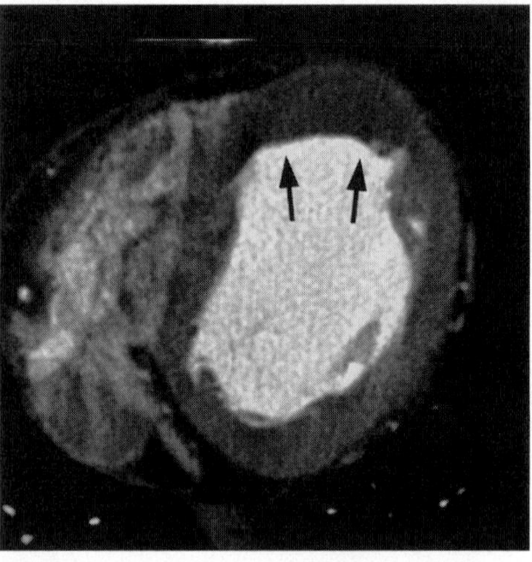

B

FIGURE 15–21 Left ventricular thrombi in contrast-enhanced computed tomography (CT) images. **A,** Spherical apical thrombus after myocardial infarction (arrows). **B,** Large mural thrombus (arrows) in a patient with a large anterior infarction. The CT attenuation of the thrombus is only a little less than the density of the adjacent myocardium.

Cardiac Masses (see Chap. 63)

Although echocardiography is the first-line diagnostic tool for cardiac masses, CT can provide helpful additional information due its high resolution and ability to clearly visualize cardiac morphology without the restriction of acoustic windows. CT provides less information concerning the tissue type than magnetic resonance imaging but may provide limited insight into the nature of a mass through measurement of the x-ray attenuation (CT numbers).[54] Lipomas have low CT numbers (typically <50 HU), whereas cysts have water-like density (0-10 HU). The CT numbers of intracardiac thrombi usually range from 20 to 90 HU,[55] but their density values may overlap with those of myocardium, and great care may thus be necessary to correctly delineate the extent of mural thrombi (Fig. 15–21). As they age, hematomas may develop calcifications or even take up contrast agent. Atrial myxomas are the most frequent primary intracardiac tumor. They have an average CT number of approximately 30 HU and may also contain calcification (Fig. 15–22).[56] Neoplasms can have an attenuation close to that of myocardium and if displaying a diffusely infiltrative pattern of growth, such as cardiac lymphoma, may be difficult to outline in CT images (Fig. 15–23). Both in primary cardiac neoplasms and in metastatic cardiac or pericardial involvement, pericardial effusion (often with above-water CT numbers) may be the only finding in CT.[8,54]

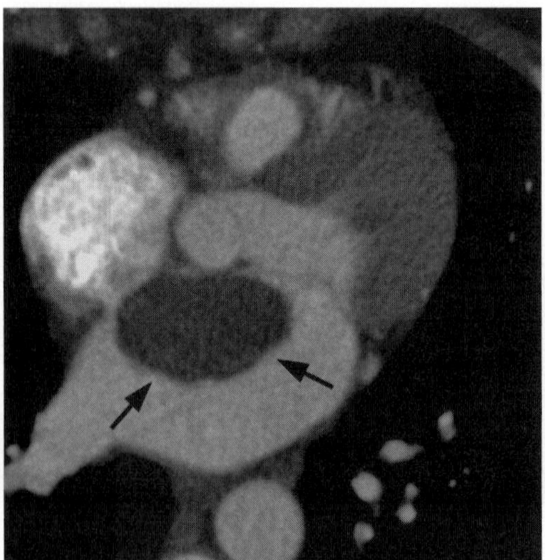

FIGURE 15–22 Left atrial myxoma (arrows) in typical position with attachment to the interatrial septum.

Congenital Heart Disease (see Chap. 56)

Although echocardiography constitutes the first-line diagnostic modality for patients with congenital heart disease, cross-sectional imaging may be warranted to delineate cardiac morphology and especially the anatomy of the great arteries, pulmonary veins, and anomalous coronary arteries. Newer EBT and MDCT scanner generations have the ability to cover a large imaging volume within one breath-hold and

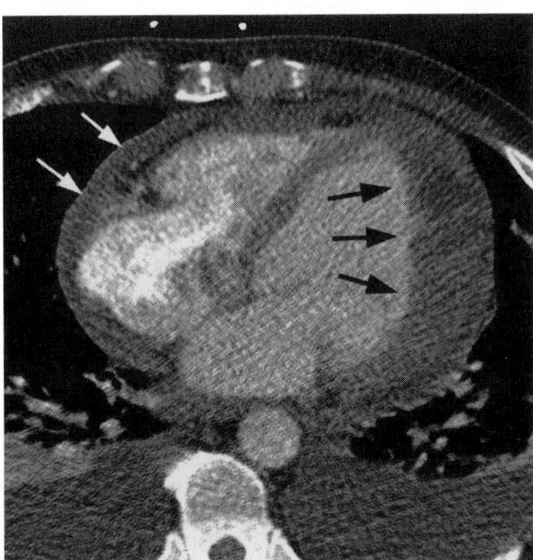

FIGURE 15–23 Primary cardiac lymphoma in a patient who presented with ventricular arrhythmias. Inhomogeneous thickening of the lateral left ventricular wall (black arrows) is caused by infiltrative growth of the lymphoma. Pericardial effusion (white arrows) and bilateral pleural effusion are present.

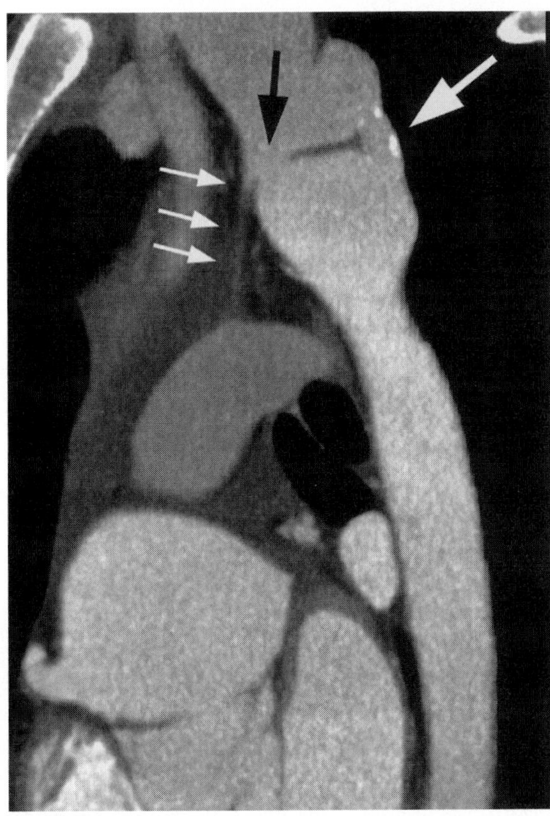

FIGURE 15–24 A 31-year-old patient with aortic coarctation. A sagitally reformatted multidetector computed tomography scan shows the descending aorta (black arrow = coarctation). A partly calcified, patent bypass conduit that was implanted at the age of 9 years can be seen (large white arrow). Note obliterated ductus arteriosus (small white arrows).

to acquire thin transaxial cross-sections that permit reformatting in any desired plane. This has substantially increased the diagnostic value of CT imaging in the setting of congenital heart disease. Limitations in obtaining information about flow or shunts and the necessity for contrast injection and radiation exposure constitute disadvantages of CT over magnetic resonance imaging (see Chap. 14). However, CT provides morphological analysis with very high resolution and is not limited by the presence of implanted devices such as pacemakers or ICDs, which are encountered with increasing frequency in adults with congenital heart disease. The systematic use of EBT and MDCT imaging has been described, especially for analysis of great vessels and pulmonary venous return[57,58] and for the exact delineation of the course of anomalous coronary arteries (Figs. 15–24 and 15–25).[59] The fact that detailed information about the dimensions and function of both ventricles can be obtained by CT may be important in the follow-up of adults with surgically corrected disease, since right ventricular assessment may be especially problematic by echocardiography.

Function and Perfusion

Computed tomography permits detailed and accurate analysis of left and right ventricular function. Using retrospective ECG gating, spiral CT data sets can be reconstructed at any desired phase of the cardiac cycle. EBT provides the option of prospectively acquiring high-resolution data sets at several predefined instances in the cardiac cycle. The high contrast between the ventricular cavity and myocardium in contrast-enhanced scans permits accurate measurements of ventricular volumes at systole and diastole, thus enabling exact analysis of global function and regional wall motion.[60,61] Thus, information about ventricular function can be obtained as a byproduct of contrast-enhanced data sets acquired for other reasons, such as coronary artery visualization or cardiac morphology in cases of congenital heart disease. In clinical reality, however, it is seldom necessary to resort to CT imaging to obtain information about global or regional wall motion.

Electron beam tomography is well suited to analyze myocardial perfusion after bolus injection of contrast agent with high resolution.[62] Studies can be performed at rest and during exercise. In fact, wall motion and perfusion analysis can be combined into one single scan. Owing to the ready availability of alternative imaging modalities (see Chap. 13), however, clinical applications have so far been limited.

Great Vessels

THORACIC AORTA. Computed tomography is extremely accurate for the diagnosis of aortic disease, including aneurysms, dissection, and intramural hematoma. Demonstration of the intimal flap (low CT attenuation within contrast-enhanced aortic lumen) is required for the diagnosis of aortic dissection (Fig. 15–26). A dissection with complete thrombosis of the false lumen may be difficult to differentiate from an aortic aneurysm with mural thrombus. Inward displacement of calcium toward the aortic lumen may help indicate dissection in this case. Higher temporal resolution and the availability of ECG triggering have substantially reduced pulsation artifacts that could cause misdiagnosis of dissection, especially in the ascending aorta,[63] and the accuracy of CT for establishing the diagnosis of dissection, assuming optimal technology, is close to 100 percent.[64,65] The individual clinical situation must dictate whether transesophageal echocardiography, magnetic resonance imaging, or computed tomography constitutes the optimal approach in a given patient (see Chaps. 11 and 14). Detailed visualization of the aorta and branch vessels and ready availability represent the advantages of CT, whereas the need for contrast injection is a drawback. The ability of CT to depict the lumen of metallic stents in the aorta and to detect leaks by demonstrating extravasation of contrast agent makes it a useful follow-up tool after interventional treatment of aortic aneurysms.[65]

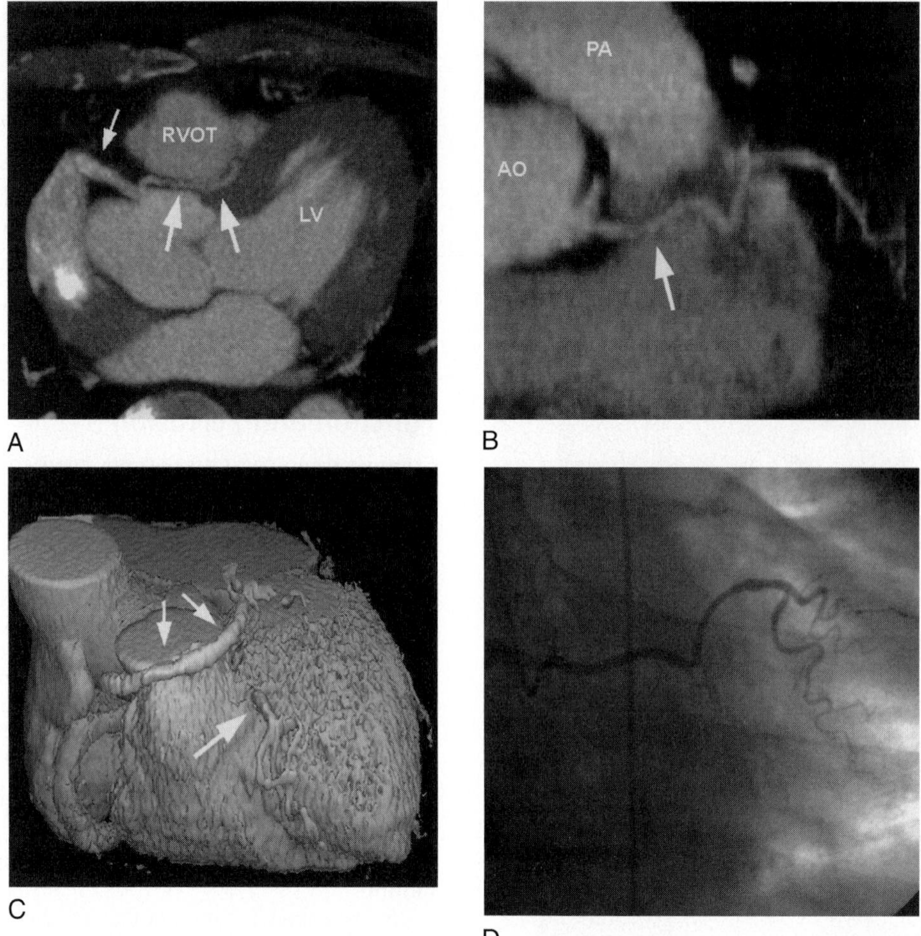

FIGURE 15–25 Patient with a complex anomaly of the coronary arteries. **A,** Axial maximum intensity projection shows the origin of the left anterior descending coronary artery (large arrows) from the right coronary ostium and course between the aortic root and right ventricular outflow tract (RVOT) toward the interventricular septum (small arrow = right coronary artery). **B,** Multiplanar reformat (sagittal view) shows passage of the left anterior descending coronary artery (arrow) through the interventricular septum. **C,** Three-dimensional reconstruction shows left anterior descending coronary artery surfacing in the anterior interventricular groove (large arrow). The left circumflex coronary artery also has an anomalous origin from the right sinus valsalvae and follows a course anterior to the pulmonary trunk (small arrows). **D,** Invasive angiogram of the left anterior descending coronary artery. AO = aortic root; LV = left ventricle; PA = pulmonary artery.

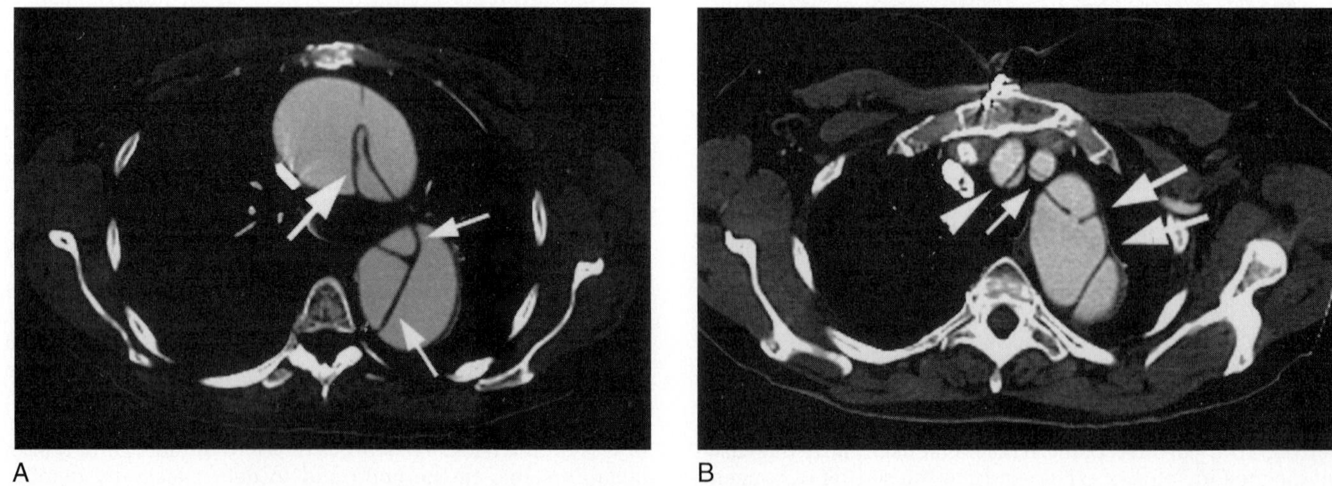

FIGURE 15–26 Aortic dissection. **A,** Dissection membranes clearly visualized in the ascending aorta (large arrow) and descending aorta (small arrows). **B,** Same patient. Dissection membrane, partially fenestrated, in the aortic arch (large arrows). The dissection extends into the left common carotid artery (small arrow) and innominate artery (arrowhead). (Courtesy of R. C. Gilkeson, MD, Case Western Reserve University, Cleveland, OH.)

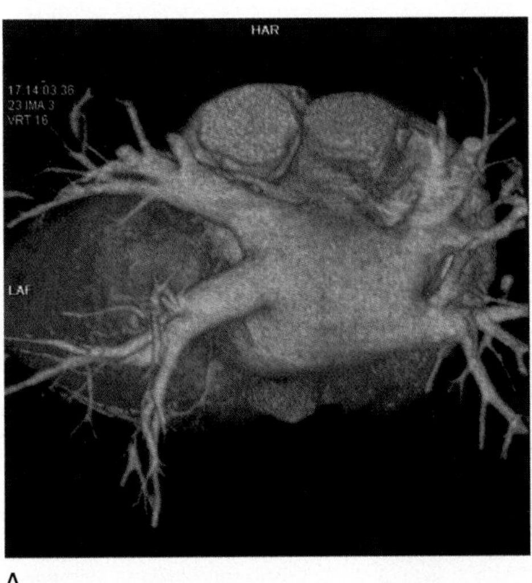

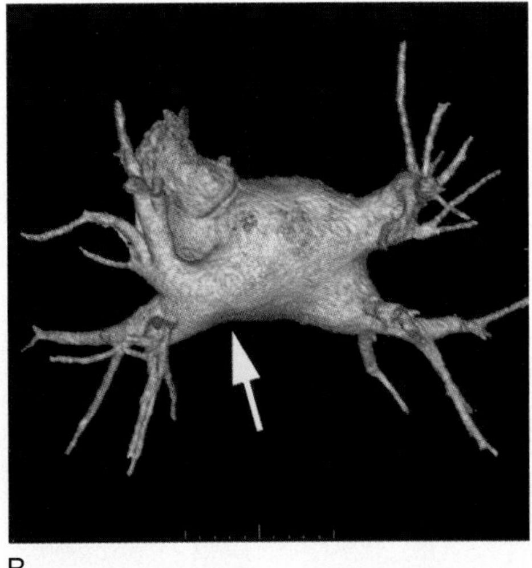

A B

FIGURE 15–27 Three-dimensional visualization of pulmonary vein anatomy by computed tomography. **A,** Normal anatomy of the four pulmonary veins draining into the left atrium in a three-dimensional reconstructional view of the posterior face of the heart. **B,** Common ostium of the left inferior and superior pulmonary vein (arrow). (Courtesy of J. Lacomis, MD, University of Pittsburgh Medical Center, Pittsburgh, PA.)

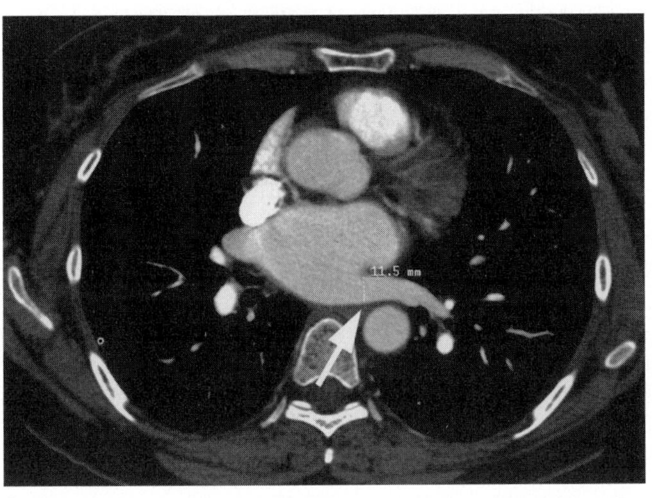

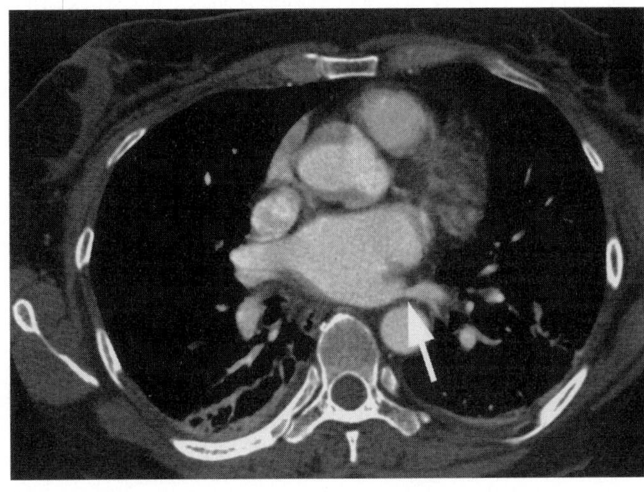

A B

FIGURE 15–28 Visualization of pulmonary veins before and after ablation of the pulmonary vein ostium for atrial fibrillation. **A,** Transaxial cross section at the ostium of the left inferior pulmonary vein (arrow). Normal anatomy prior to ablation. **B,** Same patient 6 weeks after ablation. Severe stenosis can be seen at the ostium of the pulmonary vein (arrow). (Courtesy of J. F. Breen, MD, Mayo Clinic, Rochester, MN.)

PULMONARY VEINS. In the context of electrophysiology interventions, for example to electrically isolate the pulmonary veins for prevention of atrial fibrillation, visualization of the exact anatomy of pulmonary veins and detection of supernumerary veins are of clinical importance. Suitable imaging information can reduce the duration of the interventional procedure. In addition, pulmonary vein stenosis is a possible consequence of ablation and difficult to assess with echocardiography. Similar to magnetic resonance imaging, CT can provide two-dimensional and three-dimensional images that show the exact anatomy of pulmonary veins (Figs. 15–27 and 15–28).[66] Image quality may be degraded if the CT examination is performed during atrial fibrillation but usually remains sufficiently high. Anomalous pulmonary venous return can be present in congenital heart disease and is also clearly depicted by CT.

PULMONARY EMBOLISM (see Chap. 66). EBT[67] and MDCT[68] have been demonstrated to provide high diagnostic accuracy for the detection of pulmonary embolism. In contrast-enhanced scans, the thrombi appear as filling defects in the pulmonary arteries (Fig. 15–29). Approximately 60 to 120 ml of contrast agent are necessary to provide enhancement of the pulmonary vasculature during the scan. There is consensus that a thin-collimation CT scan of the thorax with 1 to 2 mm image reconstruction can be used as an alternative to $\dot{V}/\dot{Q}$ scan during the diagnostic evaluation of patients with suspected pulmonary embolism[69,70] and that a normal CT scan, possibly in combination with ultrasonography or CT venography of the lower extremity veins or other clinical findings, is sufficient to withhold anticoagulation therapy.[68-71] Current recommendations are based on the results of single-slice spiral CT. The accuracy of MDCT can be expected to be higher.[72-74] In patients with suspected pulmonary embolism, the individual clinical situation will drive the decision toward appropriate testing. In patients with acute right heart failure, the need to inject a relatively large amount of contrast

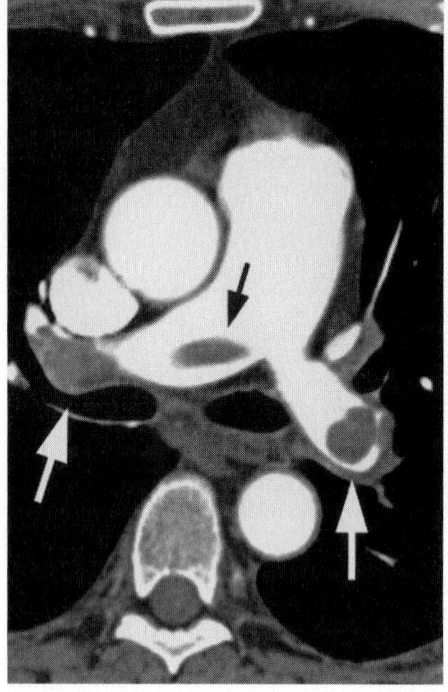

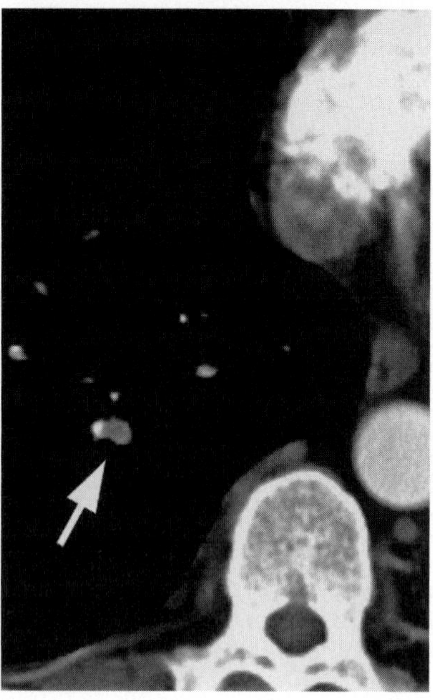

FIGURE 15–29 Visualization of pulmonary embolism by contrast-enhanced computed tomography in central pulmonary arteries (**A,** arrows), and peripheral arteries (**B,** arrow). (Courtesy of U.J. Schoepf, MD, Brigham and Women's Hospital, Boston, MA.)

material constitutes a limitation of CT, but echocardiography will usually be sufficient to reach a treatment decision in these cases (see Chap. 11).

REFERENCES

Technical Principles

1. Flohr TG, Schoepf JU, Kuettner A, et al: Advances in cardiac imaging with 16-section CT systems. Acad Radiol 10:366, 2003.
2. Hunoldt P, Vogt FM, Schmermund A, et al: Radiation exposure during cardiac CT: Effective doses at multi-detector-row CT and electron beam CT. Radiology 226:145, 2003.
3. Morin RL, Gerber TC, McCollough CH: Radiation dose in computed tomography of the heart. Circulation 107:917, 2003.
4. Jakobs TF, Becker CR, Ohnesorge B, et al: Multislice helical CT of the heart with retrospective ECG gating: Reduction of radiation exposure by ECG-controlled tube current modulation. Eur Radiol 12:1081, 2002.

Diseases of the Pericardium and Myocardium

5. Breen JF: Imaging of the pericardium. J Thorac Imaging 16:47, 2001.
6. Bull RK, Edwards PD, Dixon AK: CT dimensions of the normal pericardium. Br J Radiol 71:923, 1998.
7. Groell R, Schaffler GJ, Rienmueller R: Pericardial sinuses and recesses: Findings at electrocardiographically triggered electron-beam CT. Radiology 212:69, 1999.
8. Chiles C, Woodard P, Gutierrez FR, et al: Metastatic involvement of the heart and pericardium: CT and MR imaging. Radiographics 21:439, 2001.
9. Funabashi N, Toyozaki T, Matsumoto Y, et al: Myocardial fibrosis in Fabry disease demonstrated by multislice computed tomography. Circulation 107:2519, 2003.
10. Scatarige JC, Fishman EK: Interventricular septal mass: An unusual manifestation of sarcoidosis demonstrated on helical computed tomography. Clin Imaging 24:344, 2000.
11. Kimura F, Sakai F, Sakomura Y, et al: Helical CT features of arrhythmogenic right ventricular cardiomyopathy. Radiographics 22:1111, 2002.

Valvular Heart Disease

12. Willmann JK, Weishaupt D, Lachat M, et al: Electrocardiographically gated multi-detector row CT for assessment of valvular morphology and calcification in aortic stenosis. Radiology 225:120, 2002.
13. Pohle K, Maffert R, Ropers D, et al: Progression of aortic valve calcification: Association with coronary atherosclerosis and cardiovascular risk factors. Circulation 104:1927, 2001.
14. Budoff MJ, Mao S, Takasu J, et al: Reproducibility of electron-beam CT derived measures of aortic valve calcification. Acad Radiol 9:1122, 2002.
15. Melina G, Scott MJ, Cunanan CM, et al: In-vitro verification of the electron beam tomography method for measurement of heart valve calcification. J Heart Valve Dis 11:402, 2002.
16. Otto CM, Lind BK, Kitzman DW, et al: Association of aortic-valve sclerosis with cardiovascular mortality and morbidity in the elderly. N Engl J Med 341:142, 1999.
17. Bradfield JW, Beck G, Vecht RJ: Left ventricular apical thin point. Br Heart J 39:806, 1977.

Coronary Artery Calcification

18. Burke AP, Virmani R, Galis Z, et al: Task Force #2—What is the pathologic basis for new atherosclerosis imaging techniques? J Am Coll Cardiol 41:1874, 2003.
19. O'Rourke RA, Brundage B, Froelicher VF, et al: ACC/AHA Expert Consensus Document on electron-beam computed tomography for the diagnosis and prognosis of coronary artery disease. Circulation 102:126, 2000.
20. Pohle K, Ropers D, Mäffert R, et al: Coronary calcifications in young patients with first, unheralded myocardial infarction: A risk factor matched analysis by electron beam tomography. Heart 89:625, 2003.
21. Raggi P, Callister TQ, Cooil B, et al: Identification of patients at increased risk of first unheralded acute myocardial infarction by electron-beam computed tomography. Circulation 101:850, 2000.
22. Schmermund A, Schwartz RS, Adamzik M, et al: Coronary atherosclerosis in unheralded sudden coronary death under age fifty: Histopathologic comparison with "healthy" subjects dying out of hospital. Atherosclerosis 155:499, 2001.
23. Haberl R, Becker A, Leber A, et al: Correlation of coronary calcification and angiographically documented stenoses in patients with suspected coronary artery disease: Results of 1,764 patients. J Am Coll Cardiol 37:451, 2001.
24. Schoenhagen P, Tuczu M: Coronary artery calcification and end-stage renal disease: Vascular biology and clinical implications. Cleve Clin J Med 69(Suppl 3):S12, 2002.
25. Redberg RF, Vogel RA, Criqui MH, et al: Task Force #3—What is the spectrum of current and emerging techniques for the noninvasive measurement of atherosclerosis? J Am Coll Cardiol 41:1886, 2003.
26. Goldin JG, Yoon HC, Greaser LE 3rd, et al: Spiral versus electron-beam CT for coronary artery calcium scoring. Radiology 221:213, 2001.
27. Hoff JA, Chomka EV, Krainik AJ, et al: Age and gender distribution of coronary artery calcium detected by electron beam tomography in 35246 adults. Am J Cardiol 87:1335, 2001.
28. Ulzheimer S, Kalender WA: Assessment of calcium scoring performance in cardiac computed tomography. Eur Radiol 13:484, 2003.
29. Arad Y, Spadaro LA, Goodman K, et al: Prediction of coronary events with electron beam computed tomography. J Am Coll Cardiol 36:1253, 2000.
30. Park R, Detrano R, Xiang M, et al: Combined use of computed tomography coronary calcium scores and C-reactive protein levels in predicting cardiovascular events in nondiabetic individuals. Circulation 106:2073, 2002.
31. Vliegenthart R, Oudkerk M, Song B, et al: Coronary calcification detected by electron-beam computed tomography and myocardial infarction. The Rotterdam Coronary Calcification Study. Eur Heart J 23:1596, 2002.
32. Wong ND, Hsu JC, Detrano RC, et al: Coronary artery calcium evaluation by electron beam computed tomography and its relation to new cardiovascular events. Am J Cardiol 86:495, 2000.
33. Kondos GT, Hoff JA, Sevrukov A, et al: Electron-beam tomography coronary artery calcium and coronary events: A 37-month follow-up of 5635 initially asymptomatic low- to intermediate-risk adults. Circulation 107:2571, 2003.
34. O'Malley PG, Taylor AJ, Jackson JL, et al: Prognostic value of coronary electron-beam computed tomography for coronary heart disease events in asymptomatic patients. Am J Cardiol 85:945, 2000.
35. Taylor AJ, Bairey Merz CN, Udelson JE: 34th Bethesda Conference. Executive Summary—Can atherosclerosis imaging techniques improve the detection of patients at risk for ischemic heart disease? J Am Coll Cardiol 41:1860, 2003.
36. Schmermund A, Baumgart D, Möhlenkamp S, et al: Natural history and topographic pattern of progression of coronary calcification in symptomatic patients. Arterioscler Thromb Vasc Biol 21:421, 2001.
37. Callister TQ, Raggi P, Cooil B, et al: Effect of HmG-CoA reductase inhibitors on coronary artery disease as assessed by electron-beam computed tomography. N Engl J Med 339:1972, 1998.
38. Achenbach S, Ropers D, Pohle K, et al: Influence of lipid-lowering therapy on the progression of coronary artery calcification: a prospective evaluation. Circulation 106:1077, 2002.
39. Budoff MJ, Lane KL, Bakhsheshi H, et al: Rates of progression of coronary calcium by electron beam tomography. Am J Cardiol 86:8, 2000.

Imaging the Coronary Artery Lumen

40. Achenbach S, Moshage W, Ropers D, et al: Value of electron-beam computed tomography for the detection of high-grade coronary artery stenoses and occlusions. N Engl J Med 339:1964, 1998.
41. Nieman K, Oudkerk M, Rensing BJ, et al: Coronary angiography with multi-slice computed tomography. Lancet 357:599, 2001.
42. Achenbach S, Giesler T, Ropers D, et al: Detection of coronary artery stenoses by contrast-enhanced, retrospectively ECG-gated, multi-slice spiral CT. Circulation 103:2535, 2001.
43. Kopp AF, Schroeder S, Kuettner A, et al: Non-invasive coronary angiography with high resolution multidetector-row computed tomography. Results in 102 patients. Eur Heart J 23:1714, 2002.

44. Nieman K, Cademartiri F, Lemos PA, et al: Reliable noninvasive coronary angiography with fast submillimeter multislice spiral computed tomography. Circulation 106:2051, 2002.
45. Ropers D, Baum U, Pohle K, et al: Detection of coronary artery stenoses with thin-slice multi-detector row spiral computed tomography and multiplanar reconstruction. Circulation 107:664, 2003.
46. Achenbach S, Moshage W, Ropers D, et al: Noninvasive, three-dimensional visualization of coronary artery bypass grafts by electron beam tomography. Am J Cardiol 79:856, 1997.
47. Ropers D, Ulzheimer S, Wenkel E, et al: Investigation of aortocoronary bypass grafts by multislice spiral computed tomography with electrocardiographic-gated image reconstruction. Am J Cardiol 88:792, 2001.

Coronary Artery Plaque Imaging

48. Becker CR, Knez A, Ohnesorge B, et al: Imaging of noncalcified coronary plaques using helical CT with retrospective ECG gating. AJR 175:423, 2000.
49. Leber AW, Knez A, White CR, et al: Composition of coronary atherosclerotic plaque in patients with acute myocardial infarction and stable angina pectoris determined by contrast-enhanced multislice computed tomography. Am J Cardiol 91:714, 2003.
50. Estes JM, Quist WC, Lo Gerfo FW, et al: Noninvasive characterization of plaque morphology using helical computed tomography. J Cardiovasc Surg (Torino) 39:527, 1998.
51. Schroeder S, Kopp AF, Baumbach A, et al: Noninvasive detection and evaluation of atherosclerotic coronary plaques with multislice computed tomography. J Am Coll Cardiol 37:1430, 2001.
52. Becker CR, Nikolaou K, Muders M, et al: Ex vivo coronary atherosclerotic plaque characterization with multi-detector-row CT. Eur Radiol 13:2094, 2003.
53. Fayad ZA, Fuster V, Nikolaou K, et al: Computed tomography and magnetic resonance imaging for noninvasive coronary angiography and plaque imaging: Current and potential future concepts. Circulation 106:2026, 2002.

Other Cardiac Applications

54. Araoz PA, Eklund HE, Welch TJ, et al: CT and MR imaging of primary cardiac malignancies. Radiographics 19:1421, 1999.
55. Kirchhof K, Welzel T, Mecke C, et al: Differentiation of white, mixed, and red thrombi: Value of CT in estimation of the prognosis of thrombolysis-Phantom study. Radiology 228:126, 2003.
56. Grebenc ML, Rosado-de-Christenson ML, Green CE, et al: Cardiac myxoma: Imaging features in 83 patients. Radiographics 22:673, 2002.
57. Gilkeson RC, Ciancibello L, Zahka K: Multidetector CT evaluation of congenital heart disease in pediatric and adult patients. AJR 180:973, 2003.
58. Haramati LB, Glickstein JS, Issenberg HJ, et al: MR imaging and CT of vascular anomalies and connections in patients with congenital heart disease: Significance in surgical planning. Radiographics 22:337, 2002.
59. Ropers D, Moshage W, Daniel WG, et al: Visualization of coronary artery anomalies and their course by contrast-enhanced electron beam tomography and three-dimensional reconstruction. Am J Cardiol 87:193, 2001.
60. Halliburton SS, Petersilka M, Schvartzman PR, et al: Evaluation of left ventricular dysfunction using multiphasic reconstructions of coronary multi-slice computed tomography data in patients with chronic ischemic heart disease: Validation against cine magnetic resonance imaging. Int J Cardiovasc Imaging 19:73, 2003.
61. Gerber TC, Behrenbeck T, Allison T, et al: Comparison of measurement of left ventricular ejection fraction by Tc-99m sestamibi first-pass angiography with electron beam computed tomography in patients with anterior wall acute myocardial infarction. Am J Cardiol 83:1022, 1999.
62. Mohlenkamp S, Lerman LO, Lerman A, et al: Minimally invasive evaluation of coronary microvascular function by electron beam computed tomography. Circulation 102:2411, 2000.

Great Vessels and the Pulmonary Circulation

63. Batra P, Bigoni B, Manning J, et al: Pitfalls in the diagnosis of thoracic aortic dissection at CT angiography. Radiographics 20:309, 2000.
64. Hartnell GG: Imaging of aortic aneurysms and dissection: CT and MRI. J Thorac Imaging 16:35, 2001.
65. Erbel R, Alfonso F, Boileau C, et al: Diagnosis and management of aortic dissection. Recommendations of the Task Force on Aortic Dissection, European Society of Cardiology. Eur Heart J 22:1642, 2001.
66. Schwartzman D, Lacomis J, Wigginton WG: Characterization of left atrium and distal pulmonary vein morphology using multidimensional computed tomography. J Am Coll Cardiol 41:1349, 2003.
67. Teigen CL, Maus TP, Sheedy PF, et al: Pulmonary embolism: Diagnosis with contrast-enhanced electron beam CT and comparison with pulmonary angiography. Radiology 194:313, 1995.
68. van Strijen MJ, de Monye W, Schiereck J, et al: Single-detector helical computed tomography as the primary diagnostic test in suspected pulmonary embolism: A multicenter clinical management study of 510 patients. Ann Intern Med 138:307, 2003.
69. American College of Chest Physicians: Clinical policy: Critical issues in the evaluation and management of adults presenting with suspected pulmonary embolism. Ann Emerg Med 41:257, 2003.
70. Kruip MJ, Leclercq MG, Heul CV, et al: Diagnostic strategies for excluding pulmonary embolism in clinical outcome studies: A systematic review. Ann Intern Med 138:941, 2003.
71. Katz DS, Loud PA, Bruce D, et al: Combined CT venography and pulmonary angiography: a comprehensive review. Radiographics 22:S3, 2002.
72. Raptopoulos V, Boiselle PM: Multi-detector row spiral CT pulmonary angiography: Comparison with single-detector row spiral CT. Radiology 221:606, 2001.
73. Schoepf JU, Holzknect N, Helmberger TK, et al: Subsegmental pulmonary emboli: Improved detection with thin-collimation multi-detector row spiral CT. Radiology 222:483, 2002.
74. Patel S, Kazerooni EA, Cascade PN: Pulmonary embolism: Optimization of small pulmonary artery visualization at multi-detector row CT. Radiology 227:455, 2003.

CHAPTER 16

Relative Merits of Cardiac Diagnostic Techniques

George A. Beller

The Spectrum of Cardiovascular Diagnostic Procedures

Noninvasive cardiovascular imaging can be used for the diagnostic and prognostic assessment of patients with suspected or known cardiovascular disease. The technologies supporting these techniques vary widely, are in constant evolution, and require significant training of physicians who supervise and interpret test results. The clinical indications for these imaging modalities are guided by practice guidelines emanating predominantly from specialty and subspecialty societies. Emerging technologies are initially evaluated in small single-center studies and later in multicenter trials. Use of technology in the practice setting is not only governed by evidence-based clinical science but also by reimbursement policies. Widespread clinical application of a given imaging technique is dependent on both evidence-based guidelines and reimbursement consideration by payers such as CMS. The confidence of requesting physicians who order tests based on these imaging technologies also relates to their own experience regarding the accuracy of test results in their patient populations from the laboratories to which such patients are referred. Although one test modality may have higher specificity for the detection of disease than a competing test aimed at identifying the same pathophysiology as reported from specialized centers of excellence, the specificity advantage may not apply in local settings because of issues related to quality control and/or experience of the test interpreter. It is always difficult to definitively declare superiority of one diagnostic test over another, since local instrumentation and expertise can substantially influence test results.

Most of the diagnostic imaging tests currently available are based on assessment of regional and global function (echocardiography [see Chap. 11], radionuclide angiography [see Chap. 13], magnetic resonance imaging [MRI] [see Chap. 14]), myocardial perfusion (single-photon emission computed tomography [SPECT], positron emission tomography [PET], contrast echocardiography, contrast-enhanced MRI), myocardial metabolism (PET [see Chap. 13]), or coronary anatomy (computed tomography [CT] angiography, magnetic resonance angiography, coronary angiography [see Chaps. 14, 15, and 18]) under resting conditions, stress conditions, or both. The cardiovascular system can be stressed by either exercise or pharmacological means, such as the infusion of a vasodilator or an inotropic agent. Combining low-level exercise with vasodilator stress for myocardial perfusion imaging enhances the quality of the images and reduces side effects of the vasodilator. The principle underlying nuclear and echocardiographic stress tests is uncovering abnormal flow reserve or an ischemic response in patients with physiologically significant luminal narrowing of one or more coronary arteries. The ischemic response can be identified as flow heterogeneity represented by a "defect" on a perfusion scan, abnormal regional systolic thickening or abnormal wall motion, or abnormal regional metabolism. Regional myocardial perfusion and metabolism are simultaneously assessed for the detection of myocardial viability in ischemic cardiomyopathy using nuclear techniques, particularly PET. Various other techniques used to distinguish viable from nonviable myocardium are inotropic reserve as assessed with dobutamine echocardiography or MRI, determination of the integrity of the microcirculation as evaluated with contrast echocardiography, evaluation of myocardial membrane transport as determined from imaging a radiolabeled monovalent cation such as thallium-201 (^{201}Tl), or delineation of the transmural extent of scar by contrast-enhanced MRI.

Diagnostic techniques such as electron beam CT (EBCT),[1] multislice cardiac CT scanning, and measurement of carotid intimal-medial thickness have emerged in recent years for detecting asymptomatic coronary or carotid atherosclerosis, respectively. These technologies are not aimed at identifying an ischemic response but at detecting occult vascular disease in the coronary or peripheral circulation.

SOURCES OF BIAS WHEN EVALUATING AND COMPARING DIAGNOSTIC TECHNIQUES

The "gold standard" used for comparing the sensitivity and specificity of the various noninvasive techniques for detecting coronary artery disease (CAD) remains the coronary angiogram, which can be obtained only with invasive means (see Chap. 18). However, the coronary angiogram can at times be misleading, and it often underestimates disease severity, particularly in segments with crescentic lumina and in the presence of diffuse disease rendering the reference diameter misleading. A high degree of intraobserver and interobserver variability in visually interpreting the degree and significance of coronary stenosis is well known. Quantitative angiography for measuring the minimal luminal diameter of a coronary lesion has greater predictive physiological significance with less intraobserver and interobserver variability. In recent years, the amount of information that can be obtained at the time of coronary angiography regarding the extent and severity of CAD has increased (see Chap. 18). Assessment of coronary flow reserve with Doppler-tipped catheters in conjunction with adenosine infusion adds value to the mere identification of coronary obstructive lesions. The use of intravascular ultrasonography has also provided important additional diagnostic and prognostic information in comparison with contrast angiography alone. Currently, the noninvasive techniques aimed at diagnosing CAD and assessing its functional and prognostic severity are being compared with physiological data obtained at cardiac catheterization using the flow wire or pressure wire and not with the degree of coronary anatomical narrowing alone.

Another significant limitation in determining the specificity of noninvasive techniques for detection of CAD is that most patients with normal noninvasive study findings (e.g., a normal stress perfusion scan or normal stress echocardiogram) are not referred for coronary angiography. Patients are referred for coronary angiography most often because of abnormal noninvasive test results, which leads to a *posttest referral bias,* whereby predominantly patients with true-positive or false-positive noninvasive test results (an abnormal perfusion scan or abnormal echocardiogram and normal coronary arteries) undergo angiography. Patients with true-negative noninvasive test results are usually not sent to cardiac catheterization. This trend has led to use of the normalcy rate as a surrogate for specificity in evaluating the accuracy of a noninvasive test for CAD diagnosis (see Chap. 13). The normalcy rate represents the percentage of normal scans in patients who have less than a 5 percent posttest likelihood of CAD when taking into account clinical information, the resting electrocardiogram (ECG), and exercise treadmill test results. When reviewing the literature, one should keep in mind this tendency of the posttest referral bias to lower the specificity if a normal coronary angiogram is required as the gold standard for a normal test result, particularly with reports following the introduction of a new test.

A critical observer should bear in mind that the sensitivity and specificity of a test for detecting a cardiovascular abnormality (e.g., significant CAD, resting left ventricular dysfunction) are always very high in the first few reports that are published for a newly introduced imaging methodology. These initial good results relate to many variables, including the inclusion of a highly selected patient population that may include normal volunteers on one end of the spectrum and patients with severe disease at the other end.

When evaluating the worth of a test for diagnosing cardiovascular disease or a complication of disease, cost should now also be considered.[2,3] One test may have a sensitivity that is a few percentage points higher than another test to which it is being compared, but the cost may be twice as high. Thus, the cost/benefit ratio should also be weighed when comparing the worth of two or more tests that are developed for the same clinical application.[4]

Table 16–1 summarizes the major clinical indications for noninvasive and invasive testing and lists various techniques applicable to each of these clinical indications. The remainder of this chapter sequentially addresses the headings provided in this table.

TABLE 16–1 Clinical Applications of Noninvasive and Invasive Techniques in Cardiovascular Disease

Assessment of left ventricular function
Two-dimensional or three-dimensional echocardiography
Contrast echocardiography
Radionuclide angiography
Gated SPECT
Gated MRI
Contrast ventriculography
Detection of coronary artery disease and assessment of prognosis
Exercise electrocardiographic stress testing
Exercise or pharmacological stress SPECT myocardial perfusion imaging
Exercise or dobutamine echocardiography
Contrast echocardiography with vasodilator stress
Pharmacological stress magnetic resonance perfusion imaging
Dobutamine stress MRI
Contrast-enhanced MRI
Magnetic resonance angiography
Magnetic resonance coronary lumen and plaque imaging
Electron beam computed tomography for calcium scoring and angiography
Multislice computed tomography angiography for calcium scoring and angiography
Selective intracoronary angiography, intravascular ultrasonography, and measurement of flow reserve
Assessment of myocardial viability
Resting SPECT perfusion imaging
Low-dose dobutamine echocardiography
Positron emission tomography
Contrast-enhanced MRI
Low-dose dobutamine MRI

MRI = magnetic resonance imaging; SPECT = single-photon emission computed tomography.

Assessment of Left Ventricular Function at Rest

Echocardiography (see Chap. 11)

Of all the noninvasive techniques available for the assessment of regional and global left ventricular function at rest, echocardiography is the most versatile overall, provides the most ancillary information, and has the lowest cost.[5] Two-dimensional echocardiography provides excellent images of the heart and great vessels, but it depends on obtaining satisfactory windows from the body surface to the area of interest in the heart. When good windows are obtained, echocardiography is superbly well suited for the evaluation of global and regional left ventricular systolic function because of its high spatial and temporal resolution and its ability to define both regional wall thickening and inward endocardial excursion. When compared with all other techniques, it should be the preferred initial test to diagnose heart muscle diseases of as yet unknown origin. These disease entities include ischemic cardiomyopathy, nonischemic dilated cardiomyopathy, hypertrophic cardiomyopathy, and restrictive myocardial disease (see Chap. 59). Resting echocardiographic technology not only allows a thorough assessment of cardiac morphology and function but also permits the simultaneous assessment of valvular, pericardial, intramyocardial, and extracardiac abnormalities.

Regional myocardial wall thickening is a better marker of regional function than is regional wall motion, and it is not influenced by either cardiac translation or the center of reference used. Regional thickening abnormalities cannot be well identified by radionuclide angiography or contrast ventriculography. The only other technique that perhaps permits a more accurate assessment of regional systolic thickening than echocardiography is gated MRI. This technique, however, is currently more expensive than two-dimensional echocardiography and cannot be performed at the bedside in critically ill patients. The advent of small portable echocardiographic apparatus could enhance only the bedside utility of this technique. A limitation of resting echocardiography in gauging the severity of regional or global left ventricular dysfunction is the lack of a reproducible quantitative technique to measure the left ventricular ejection fraction. A quantitative ejection fraction is better obtained by using alternative approaches such as left ventricular contrast angiography, radionuclide angiography, MRI, and quantitative gated SPECT imaging.

Echocardiography is invaluable in assisting in the detection of acute myocardial infarction and such mechanical complications as right ventricular infarction, acute mitral regurgitation from papillary muscle rupture or dysfunction, ventricular septal defect, a true or false left ventricular aneurysm, or pericardial effusion (see Chap. 11).[5] Thus, it is the noninvasive technique of choice for the comprehensive evaluation of regional and global left ventricular dysfunction and associated abnormalities in the setting of acute myocardial infarction. Transesophageal echocardiography can be performed at the bedside in an acutely ill patient with shock in the intensive care unit setting to help identify the cause of the hemodynamic disturbance. Echocardiography can also be performed in the emergency room in patients with chest pain and a possible acute ischemic syndrome. A defined regional wall motion abnormality in the absence of prior history of myocardial infarction lends support to a presumptive diagnosis that regional ischemia may be the cause of the chest pain syndrome.

Echocardiography is more sensitive than ECG for detecting left ventricular hypertrophy[6] and is an excellent technique for estimating left ventricular mass, which has been shown to independently predict cardiovascular morbidity and mortality.[7,8] The variability in left ventricular mass measurements and the reliability of serial measurements to assess regression of hypertrophy[9] have been reduced by the substitution of linear measurements of left ventricular wall thickness and internal dimension from the two-dimensional parasternal long-axis view whenever the two-dimensional directed M-mode beam is not ideally oriented for measuring thickness and cavity dimensions (see Chap. 11).[10] Further improvements in the echocardiographic measurement of left ventricular mass may be offered by three-dimensional localization of imaging slices.[11] Three-dimensional echocardiography with automatic edge detection software to identify endocardial borders permits measurement of left ventricular volumes with left ventricular ejection fraction calculated from volume-time loop curves for each frame. Tissue Doppler measurement of myocardial velocity displacement is another approach to better quantifying regional cardiac function.[12] Diastolic function can be evaluated by assessing transmitral flow velocities. Restrictive left ventricular filling patterns can be identified using pulsed Doppler echocardiography. Increased left atrial pressure from an increased left ventricular filling pressure can be assessed by measures of isovolumic relaxation time, E/A ratio, E-wave deceleration time, the ratio of systolic to diastolic pulmonary venous flow, and E/E′ ratio.[13]

Radionuclide Angiography (see Chap. 13)

First-pass radionuclide angiography and gated equilibrium blood pool radionuclide angiography are nuclear cardiology techniques that use a gamma camera and ECG gating for determining the changes in radioactivity in the left and right ventricular chambers over the cardiac cycle by generating time-activity curves. Quantitative ejection fraction measurements from both the right and left ventricles are highly accurate. Ventricular and pulmonary blood volumes and regional ventricular wall motion can also be assessed. As with echocardiography, resting radionuclide angiography is clinically useful for prognostication: the lower the resting left ventricular ejection fraction or the more global the left ventricular dysfunction, the worse the subsequent outcome with respect to survival. An advantage of radionuclide angiography over echocardiography is its ability to accurately quantitate the left and right ventricular ejection fractions by using a "count-based" technique and to obtain data in virtually all patients. Patients with arrhythmias can undergo radionuclide angiography, since windows for cycle length can be preset and all beats falling outside the window are rejected.

Chemotherapy with anthracycline agents can result in a dose-dependent deterioration in left ventricular function because of the toxic effects of the drug on cardiac myocytes (see Chap. 83). Radionuclide angiography is ideally suited to provide serial quantitative left ventricular ejection fraction measurements in patients who have received or are receiving doxorubicin therapy.[14] If doxorubicin administration is continued after objective evidence of reduced systolic function, significant symptomatic congestive heart failure and irreversible left ventricular dysfunction may ensue. Resting radionuclide angiography may provide a more quantitative assessment of left ventricular dysfunction after myocardial infarction, but it cannot provide other important information, such as the extent of infarction expansion, presence of left ventricular thrombus, development of mitral regurgitation, and extent of regional systolic thickening abnormalities. Radionuclide angiography provides significant prognostic information in patients with severe arrhythmias arising from the right ventricle in the setting of arrhythmogenic right ventricular cardiomyopathy.[15] Gated blood-pool imaging of left ventricular function can also be accomplished using SPECT technology, and left ventricular ejection fraction measurements using gated blood-pool SPECT correlate well with left ventricular ejection fraction measured by the standard planar technique.[16]

Gated Spect Imaging (see Chap. 13)

The emergence of technetium-99m (^{99m}Tc)-labeled myocardial perfusion agents led to the development of gated ^{99m}Tc-SPECT imaging, which permits simultaneous evaluation of regional systolic thickening, left ventricular volumes, global left ventricular function, and myocardial perfusion.[17,18] The introduction of gated ^{99m}Tc-SPECT imaging significantly enhanced the specificity of SPECT for the detection of CAD in patients with chest pain,[19,20] permitted measurement of regional wall thickening and detection of postischemic stunning,[21,22] and improved the ability to risk-stratify patients by providing information relevant to the global left ventricular ejection fraction.[23] New techniques using technology similar to that used for gated equilibrium blood pool imaging allow for automated determination of the left ventricular ejection fraction.[24] Thus, a quantitative global ejection fraction and percentage of thickening in various regions of the left ventricle can be reported with results of myocardial perfusion analysis under resting and stress conditions.

Severe perfusion abnormalities can limit quantitation of the left ventricular ejection fraction by the gated SPECT technique by interfering with detection of endocardial edges along the whole left ventricular volume on SPECT images. Manrique and colleagues found that gated SPECT underestimated the left ventricular ejection fraction when compared with equilibrium radionuclide angiography in patients with left ventricular dysfunction and large perfusion defects.[25] Other authors have reported accurate left ventricular ejection fraction measurements by gated SPECT in the presence of large perfusion defects.[26] Count-based techniques for assessing regional systolic thickening are not as adversely influenced by low regional radioactive counts in areas of severe defects.[24] Gated ^{99m}Tc-tetrofosmin SPECT imaging compared favorably with cine-MRI with respect to grading regional wall motion abnormalities in patients with an acute myocardial infarction.[27] Two methods of measuring left ventricular volumes by gated SPECT correlated well with MRI volumes, although the QGS (Quantitative Gated SPECT) technique underestimated the MRI values.[28] MRI cardiac images provide a complete three-dimensional portrayal of the heart with high spatial and temporal resolution.

Gated SPECT can also be performed with ^{201}Tl. He and associates[26] reported similar left ventricular ejection fraction measurements for ^{201}Tl-gated SPECT (54 ± 15 percent) and ^{99m}Tc-gated SPECT (54 ± 16 percent) in 63 patients who had left ventricular ejection fractions also determined by first-pass radionuclide angiography (54 ± 12 percent).

Gated fluorine-18 fluorodeoxyglucose (FDG) PET can accurately measure global left ventricular function and evaluate regional wall motion.[29] Global ejection fractions from FDG-PET were 29.3 ± 11.5 percent versus 31.1 ± 10.4 percent for radionuclide angiography.

Magnetic Resonance Imaging (see Chap. 14)

Cardiac MRI has emerged as a superb noninvasive technique for assessing left ventricular and right ventricular function.[30-32] Regional and global cardiac function can be evaluated at rest and under pharmacological stress with MRI, and high-speed MRI techniques allow for the simultaneous assessment of myocardial perfusion with magnetic resonance contrast agents. MRI is superior to other noninvasive imaging modalities in diagnosing congenital heart disease,[31,32] aortic disease, anomalous coronary arteries, and right ventricular dysplasia. At present, echocardiographic techniques appear to still have cost/benefit characteristics superior to those of MRI for assessing regional and global function. The major strength of MRI is its ability to provide high-resolution detail of cardiovascular anatomy. It can yield three-dimensional information on anatomy, function, and blood flow. It is accurate in determining wall thickness and may be the best technique for quantitating overall left ventricular mass. MRI tagging is an imaging modality that uses a grid overlying the full thickness of the myocardium on tomographic slices for assessment of progressive thickening of endocardial, midwall, and epicardial layers during the cardiac cycle. This technique measures intramyocardial function, which enhances measurement of the degree of regional myocardial dysfunction. Cardiac MRI is an excellent method for distinguishing ischemic from nonischemic cardiomyopathy and the assessment of patients with heart failure.[33] Serial assessment of left ventricular mass and volume is important in monitoring left ventricular remodeling after myocardial infarction, and this technique is being used in clinical trials to test certain pharmacological interventions for their effect on remodeling.

Contrast Left Ventriculography (see Chap. 17)

Left ventriculography has been available for many years for the assessment of left ventricular function in patients with a variety of pathological disorders. It has been used as the gold standard to which noninvasive techniques have been compared. Abnormal wall motion, but not abnormal thickening, can be assessed by contrast left ventriculography and quantitative measurements of left ventricular ejection fraction, and absolute volumes are highly reproducible and perhaps yield the most precise quantitative measurements of global function of all the noninvasive techniques discussed earlier. Limitations of contrast ventriculography include its invasive nature, high cost, potential nephrotoxicity of the dye, and the need to trace endocardial contours to quantitate ejection fraction and volume. Left ventricular hypertrophy and left ventricular mass are better quantitated by echocardiography or MRI. An advantage of contrast ventriculography is its ability to simultaneously measure intracavitary pressure and other hemodynamic variables such as stroke and end-diastolic volume, as well as performance of coronary angiography during the same cardiac catheterization procedure. Differentiation between dilated and ischemic cardiomyopathy can easily be made, and associated valvular lesions such as mitral or aortic regurgitation can be simultaneously diagnosed and semiquantitated. Left-to-right shunts at the atrial and ventricular levels are most accurately quantitated by cardiac catheterization measurements, although echocardiography and MRI can precisely localize atrial and ventricular septal defects.

THE UTILITY OF DIFFERENT APPROACHES TO THE ASSESSMENT OF LEFT VENTRICULAR FUNCTION

Overall, when all factors are considered, two-dimensional echocardiography with Doppler remains the most useful and convenient approach to assessment of resting left ventricular function. Its major limitation is an inability to visualize all regions of the left ventricle in every patient, and poor-quality images are acquired in certain patients, such as those with severe chronic obstructive pulmonary disease. The lack of a highly accurate and reproducible method for deriving a quantitative measurement of left ventricular ejection fraction also limits the utility of echocardiography. Contrast echocardiography improves visualization of myocardial walls and shows promise for the simultaneous assessment of regional perfusion at rest and during stress.[34] Echocardiographic contrast agents are capable of producing left ventricular cavity opacification, which helps in delineating endocardial borders, particularly in patients with poor acoustic windows.[35] Gated ^{99m}Tc-SPECT and gated MRI provide precise determinations of regional myocardial thickening and left ventricular ejection fraction, and MRI also allows for simultaneous assessment of perfusion and viability by using a contrast agent. Of course, patients with implanted pacemakers or automatic defibrillators are not candidates for MRI. Table 16–2 summarizes the strengths and limitations of the various techniques for assessment of regional and global left ventricular function.

Detection of Coronary Artery Disease

A number of noninvasive techniques are available to the clinician for detection of CAD in patients with chest pain. The techniques vary greatly in methodology but have as a fundamental principle the detection of myocardial ischemia or flow heterogeneity with exercise or pharmacological stress. The variables indicative of myocardial ischemia differ considerably and are specific for the test under consideration. The advent of myocardial imaging techniques using radionuclide tracers, echocardiography, or MRI methodology has provided enhanced accuracy for detection of CAD but at a higher cost than for the standard exercise treadmill test. Soon, noninvasive coronary angiography with multislice CT may become feasible, and plaque detection and characterization by MRI is on the horizon.[30,36,37] The strengths and limitations of the various noninvasive techniques used for the detection of CAD are described in the sections to follow.

Exercise Electrocardiography (see Chap. 10)

A review of the literature concerning the diagnostic accuracy of the standard exercise test was published by Gibbons and colleagues[38] and used as a basis for formulating guidelines for exercise testing by the American College of Cardiology/American Heart Association Practice Guidelines Task Force. Meta-analysis showed that the sensitivity and specificity of the exercise ECG stress test for the detection of CAD were 68 and 77 percent, respectively, in 147 consecutively published reports of patients who underwent both angiography and exercise testing.[39] However, bias from the selection of patients who agreed to undergo both treadmill testing and coronary angiography at the outset led to a 45 percent sensitivity for 1.0 mm of horizontal or downward ST segment depression but an 85 percent specificity.[40] Even when studies that included patients with resting ST segment depression were excluded, the sensitivity and specificity of the exercise test were only 67 and 84 percent, respectively.[38]

SENSITIVITY. The sensitivity of exercise ECG is very dependent on the level of exercise achieved. Sensitivity is reduced in patients who fail to achieve 85 percent of the age-adjusted maximum predicted heart rate or greater. Specificity of the ST segment depression response is markedly affected by variables such as left ventricular hypertrophy, hyperventilation, digoxin therapy, intraventricular conduction disturbances, preexcitation syndrome, hypokalemia, severe hypertension, and resting ST segment depression from a variety of causes. Many patients are precluded from undergoing treadmill testing alone because of nonspecific resting ST or T wave abnormalities, conduction abnormalities, or claudication. Interestingly, however, the specificity of the exercise test was only 69 percent in an analysis of 10 studies totaling 3548 patients who underwent exercise testing without digitalis therapy. Similarly, the specificity of the exercise test in studies excluding left ventricular hypertrophy only increased to 77 percent, which was just 8 percent higher than the 69 percent specificity of the ST segment response for CAD detection when studies including left ventricular hypertrophy were analyzed.

SPECIFICITY. The specificity of the exercise ECG response is also suboptimal in women, particularly those who are in the premenopausal age group with a low to intermediate pretest likelihood of CAD.[41] In contrast, the negative predictive value of a normal exercise ECG response in women

TABLE 16–2 Strengths and Limitations of the Various Diagnostic Techniques for Assessment of Left Ventricular Function

Technique	Strengths	Limitations
Echocardiography	Portability, immediate availability, versatility, repeatability Provides ancillary structural and physiological information High spatial and temporal resolution Accurately measures regional systolic thickening Sensitive for detecting LV hypertrophy and measuring LV mass Good for RV function assessment Excellent for detection of diastolic dysfunction LV volume with three-dimensional technique No ionizing radiation or contrast material needed Low cost	Poor acoustic windows in some patients Lack of quantitative ejection fraction High operator dependence
Radionuclide angiography	Accurate measurement of LV and RV ejection fractions Reproducibility Little operator dependency Serial monitoring of patients receiving cancer chemotherapy Quantitation of diastolic filling abnormalities	Regional systolic thickening not evaluated Radiation exposure Ancillary anatomical information not obtained Difficult to detect LV hypertrophy
Gated ^{99m}Tc SPECT imaging	Assessment of systolic thickening and wall motion Global LV ejection fraction and LV volumes accurately measured Simultaneous evaluation of perfusion and function Viability assessment Postischemic stunning identified	Decreased accuracy of LV ejection fraction assessment with large defects Lack of portability LV hypertrophy and mass not measured No ancillary structural information obtained Lower spatial resolution than ultrasonography and MRI
Magnetic resonance imaging	Absence of ionizing radiation Contrast agents not nephrotoxic Best technique for diagnosing congenital heart disease High-resolution anatomical detail Excellent for measuring wall thickness and LV mass Provides functional images in any desired imaging plane Can accurately assess regional and global LV function Gives three-dimensional information Proximal coronary arteries visualized Myocardial tagging permits analysis of subendocardial, midwall, and subepicardial function High-speed conrast-enhanced MRI permits perfusion imaging and viability assessment (delayed hyperenhancement)	Lack of portability Causes claustrophobia in some patients Need to correct for cardiac and respiratory motion Patients with metallic objects, pacemakers, and other devices excluded

LV = left ventricular; MRI = magnetic resonance imaging; RV = right ventricular; SPECT = single-photon emission computed tomography.

for excluding CAD is high. Women with a normal baseline resting ECG who achieve greater than 85 percent of the maximum predicted heart rate for age and have a normal peak stress ECG have an excellent prognosis and a low prevalence of underlying CAD. The negative predictive value of the exercise ECG response appears to be lower in men than in women, whereas the positive predictive value of the ST segment depression response is higher in men than women. Heart rate adjustment for the ST segment response may improve diagnostic accuracy of the exercise ECG.

EXTENT OF CAD. The extent of CAD affects the sensitivity of the exercise ECG. Its sensitivity is less than 50 percent for patients with single-vessel disease but exceeds 85 percent for patients with three-vessel disease. Horizontal or downsloping ST segment depression at low exercise heart rates has a higher positive predictive accuracy for CAD than does ST segment depression at very high heart rates or workloads. The administration of beta-blocking drugs certainly influences exercise test results, since these drugs prevent the patient from attaining the desired heart rate–blood pressure product at which ischemic ST segment depression would appear. This effect leads to an increased prevalence of false-negative responses. In addition, other antianginal drugs, such as nitrates given before testing, may prevent the appearance of abnormal ST segment changes. Slow upsloping ST segment depression has occasionally been used to increase the criteria for a positive test. Although such responses may enhance the sensitivity of the exercise ECG, specificity is lowered.[42]

In summary, although the exercise ECG is the least expensive of the noninvasive tests for detecting CAD, it has limited sensitivity and specificity in certain patient populations. Its main value may be as the initial test for excluding CAD in patients with a low pretest likelihood of CAD based on age and gender, in those who have a normal resting ECG, and in patients with nonanginal or very atypical chest pain.[43] If such patients achieve their maximum exercise heart rates with no ST segment depression and with normal hemodynamic responses, significant stenoses would not be likely to be the cause of their atypical chest pain syndrome. However, in most other populations, the exercise ECG is limited by suboptimal sensitivity and specificity for diagnosing CAD for the reasons outlined earlier.

Stress Radionuclide Myocardial Perfusion Imaging (see Chap. 13)

Exercise or pharmacological stress ^{201}Tl or ^{99m}Tc-sestamibi SPECT imaging in patients with chest pain yields a sensitivity for detecting CAD in the 85 to 90 percent range.[44,45] Specificity for excluding CAD is in the 90 percent range when gated SPECT imaging is used.[19] Exercise SPECT imaging and pharmacological SPECT imaging both yield sensitivities and specificities for CAD detection that are superior to those of exercise ECG testing alone.[44] Radionuclide stress perfusion imaging has particular value when compared with exercise ECG testing alone in (1) patients with resting ECG abnormalities, such as those seen with left ventricular hypertrophy, digitalis effect, preexcitation, and intraventricular conduction abnormalities, and (2) patients who fail to achieve greater than 85 percent of the maximum predicted heart rate and have no ST segment depression. Patients who fail to achieve a target heart rate and stop exercising at submaximal exercise levels demonstrate a higher sensitivity for CAD detection than when exercise ECG testing is performed alone because flow heterogeneity in response to stress appears earlier during the course of graded exercise stress. The ST segment depression response appears to require a higher rate-pressure product than that required to induce flow heterogeneity, which is demonstrated as a perfusion defect on scintigraphy.

The addition of stress perfusion imaging to the exercise ECG stress test greatly assists in differentiating true-positive from false-positive exercise ST segment depression responses. In patients with a low to intermediate pretest likelihood of CAD, approximately 40 percent with ST segment depression have no evidence of CAD (false-positive findings). Quantitative analysis of SPECT has resulted in a higher sensitivity and specificity than merely visual evaluation of SPECT images. The single-vessel disease detection rate with stress SPECT imaging is approximately 25 percent higher than the rate achieved with exercise ECG testing alone. The sensitivity for detecting three-vessel disease with exercise SPECT is in the range of 95 to 100 percent. A low percentage of patients with three-vessel disease, however, have inducible defects in all three vascular regions.[21,46]

LIMITATIONS OF PERFUSION IMAGING. A limitation of myocardial perfusion imaging is the difficulty in distinguishing false-positive defects due to attenuation artifacts from defects related to myocardial ischemia or scar. This high rate is predominantly attributed to image attenuation artifacts that are interpreted as defects secondary to CAD. Although quantitation of SPECT images improves specificity, the false-positive rate is higher than desirable, particularly with imaging of obese persons and women, who may demonstrate defects reflecting breast attenuation artifacts. Such artifacts are sometimes difficult to distinguish from myocardial perfusion abnormalities caused by inducible ischemia or from myocardial scarring (see Chap. 13). In the past decade, gated SPECT using ^{99m}Tc-labeled perfusion agents such as sestamibi and tetrofosmin has enhanced the specificity of SPECT. The quality of images obtained with ^{99m}Tc-labeled radionuclides is superior to that of images obtained with ^{201}Tl because of the more favorable physical characteristics of ^{99m}Tc for imaging with a gamma camera. The feasibility of using ^{99m}Tc doses approximately 10 to 20 times higher than the doses used with ^{201}Tl permits the acquisition of images with higher count density, less scatter and attenuation, and fewer artifacts than seen with ^{201}Tl imaging. Another limitation of exercise SPECT for detecting CAD is the influence of antiischemic medications administered at the time of testing.[47]

Electrocardiography-gated SPECT yields important information about regional and global left ventricular function that could previously be obtained only with a second test, such as radionuclide angiography, echocardiography, or contrast ventriculography. The ability to accurately measure the resting left ventricular ejection fraction with ^{99m}Tc-sestamibi or ^{99m}Tc-tetrofosmin adds supplementary value to the detection of reversible perfusion abnormalities alone.[23]

Since soft tissue attenuation causes nonuniformity of photon activity in the myocardium that results in artifacts often perceived as perfusion defects, attempts have been made to correct for attenuation by using certain algorithms emerging from advances in gamma camera instrumentation and software development.[48] Attenuation-corrected SPECT identified more left main CAD patterns (64 percent) than detected from uncorrected SPECT (7 percent) in a group of patients with 50 percent or greater left main stenoses.[49] Improvement in the normalcy rate can also be achieved by using attenuation/scatter-corrected images, thereby reducing the false-positive rate for CAD detection.[50] Attenuation correction and ECG gating in combination seems to provide the highest diagnostic accuracy for myocardial perfusion SPECT and enhance both sensitivity for multivessel disease detection and specificity for CAD detection.[51]

Some patients are less than ideal candidates for treadmill testing alone, and pharmacological stress with vasodilators such as dipyridamole or adenosine[52] or an inotropic agent such as dobutamine[53] is an alternative to exercise for detecting physiologically significant coronary artery stenosis. The basis for vasodilator perfusion imaging relates to the concept of coronary flow reserve (see Chap. 13). When coronary blood flow is maximally increased with an intravenously administered vasodilator, an impairment in flow reserve capacity in a stenotic artery simultaneous with a large flow increase in a normal vascular bed results in relative inhomogeneity of myocardial perfusion between normal and stenotic beds. If tracers such as ^{201}Tl or ^{99m}Tc-sestamibi are injected during peak vasodilation in the presence of a hemodynamically significant coronary stenosis with reduced flow reserve, heterogeneity in tracer uptake will be observed as defects on poststress images acquired soon after tracer injection. Sensitivity and specificity for CAD detection are comparable for dipyridamole and adenosine.[44] Dobutamine stress is preferred in patients who have bronchospasm or a history of asthma or in those who have consumed caffeine before testing. Dipyridamole or adenosine administration in these patients could result in severe bronchospasm. Vasodilator imaging is the scintigraphic method of choice for detection of CAD in patients with complete left bundle branch block. These patients are not candidates to undergo diagnostic exercise ECG testing alone.

Today, most laboratories use ^{99m}Tc perfusion imaging agents for detection of CAD in conjunction with exercise or pharmacological stress because of enhanced specificity for CAD detection and the ability to gate the images to the ECG to view regional systolic thickening. Mild nonreversible defects that represent attenuation artifacts usually show preserved systolic thickening, whereas if such areas of diminished tracer uptake represent scar, abnormal systolic thickening is observed. The dual-imaging approach involves performing rest ^{201}Tl imaging and stress imaging with one of the ^{99m}Tc-labeled perfusion agents.

Exercise and Dobutamine Stress Echocardiography (see Chap. 11)

Stress echocardiography can be performed with treadmill, upright bicycle, or supine bicycle exercise or by using pharmacological stressors such as dobutamine or dipyridamole.[5,54] Dobutamine stress has a higher sensitivity than does vasodilator stress. In a pooled analysis of data in the literature,[5] the weighted mean sensitivity, specificity, and overall accuracy for exercise echocardiography were 86 percent, 81 percent, and 85 percent, respectively. For dobutamine stress echocardiography, these values were 82 percent, 84 percent, and 83 percent, respectively. For the same reasons as outlined for SPECT perfusion imaging, stress echocardiography is more sensitive and specific for detecting inducible ischemia than is exercise ECG testing alone. Sensitivity is higher in multivessel-disease patients than in single-vessel disease patients and in patients with greater than 70 percent stenoses versus 50 percent to 70 percent stenoses.[5]

Variability exists in the literature with respect to sensitivity for CAD detection for stress echocardiography[5,55] and may be related to patient selection, including the percentage of patients in each study with previous infarction and/or multivessel disease, the definition of what constitutes a new stress-induced wall motion abnormality (a new wall motion abnormality versus failure to demonstrate hyperkinesis), the use of beta-blockers during testing, and pretest referral bias. The sensitivity of exercise echocardiography may be diminished if submaximal exercise heart rates are attained. Marwick and coauthors reported that when exercise heart rates were less than 85 percent of the maximum predicted heart rate, the sensitivity of exercise echocardiographic tests was only 42 percent.[56] The sensitivity of stress echocardiography in women is less than in men. Weighted mean sensitivity was 81 percent in 1000 women with suspected CAD, with a specificity of 86 percent.[5] Sensitivity was 89 percent in women with multivessel disease.

Digital imaging is advantageous for stress echocardiography for side-by-side comparison of regional function at rest and stress and for reviewing progression of contraction on a frame-by-frame basis.[54]

Side effects can be quite bothersome for patients undergoing dobutamine stress echocardiography. Secknus and Marwick reported premature termination of dobutamine stress echocardiography in 15 percent of 3000 patients.[57] Most of the episodes of premature test termination were due to cardiovascular side effects, including ventricular and supraventricular arrhythmias, severe hypertension, hypotension, severe ischemia by echocardiography, or severe chest pain.

COMPARISON OF EXERCISE SPECT PERFUSION IMAGING AND EXERCISE ECHOCARDIOGRAPHY

Stress echocardiography and stress perfusion imaging share common positive features that deserve emphasis before the value and limitations of each technique are compared. First, both are associated with a higher sensitivity and specificity for CAD detection than is exercise ECG testing alone. Second, both noninvasive techniques provide functional information for risk stratification, assessment of the area at risk, and determination of myocardial viability that is superior to that obtained with coronary angiography (see later).

Advantages of Stress Echocardiography. When compared with radionuclide perfusion imaging, advantages of stress echocardiography include the following: (1) The technique is totally noninvasive, safe, and repeatable; (2) no radiation exposure is involved; (3) the time to complete a full examination is short; (4) the technique is portable and requires no highly sophisticated instrumentation; (5) the cost is relatively low; (6) it has the ability to identify structural abnormalities of the heart, including coexisting valvular disease, left ventricular hypertrophy, and pericardial abnormalities; and (7) imaging quality is increased using contrast echocardiography versus conventional stress echocardiography to allow for simultaneous assessment of regional myocardial perfusion and regional systolic function. Contrast echocardiography with microbubbles performed in association with vasodilator stress permits the assessment of myocardial perfusion and can delineate the spatial extent and magnitude of stress-induced ischemia.[34,58]

Limitations of Stress Echocardiography. Limitations include the following: (1) Images are difficult to acquire at peak exercise because of exertional hyperapnea and cardiac excursion. (2) An ischemic response is required for the elucidation of regional abnormal wall motion, and inadequate heart rate responses, particularly with dobutamine echocardiography, reduce sensitivity. Atropine is often given to elevate the heart rate. (3) Rapid recovery of wall motion abnormalities can be seen with mild ischemia, particularly with single-vessel disease, which may lead to a false-negative test result if the images are not acquired rapidly after exercise. (4) Detection of residual ischemia within an infarct zone is difficult because of resting akinesis. (5) The technique is highly operator dependent for data collection and image analysis, and considerable interindividual variability in interpreting stress echocardiograms has been reported.[59] (6) Good-quality, complete images are acquired in only 70 percent of patients. An inability to image all of the left ventricular myocardium occurs in approximately 15 percent of patients. (7) A long training period is required to gain experience. (8) Quantitative assessment of inducible wall motion abnormalities and left ventricular ejection fraction is operator dependent. And (9), at present, myocardial contrast echocardiography can be difficult and is not ready for routine use. Intermittent imaging, in which microbubbles are destroyed and the time required for replenishment is measured by number of cardiac cycles, enhances the detection of flow heterogeneity using this technique.[58] Harmonic imaging has also increased the sensitivity of the technique. One multicenter phase II study showed a 93 percent concordance between dipyridamole ^{99m}Tc-sestamibi SPECT and dipyridamole stress myocardial contrast echocardiography for classifying patients as normal or abnormal and 74 percent concordance for location of perfusion defects.[60] For this study, intermittent harmonic power Doppler was performed to quantitate myocardial blood flow velocity. A limitation of assessment of myocardial perfusion imaging for CAD detection using this technique is the number of falsely abnormal results in the circumflex territory compared with ^{99m}Tc-sestamibi SPECT.[61]

Advantages of Stress Perfusion Imaging. When compared with conventional exercise echocardiography, the following advantages of exercise myocardial perfusion imaging for detection of CAD can be listed: (1) myocardial perfusion imaging detects abnormal flow reserve and does not require an ischemic response for a positive test result; (2) data relevant to abnormal myocardial perfusion are obtained at peak stress with treadmill exercise rather than after exercise, as required for echocardiography; (3) the sensitivity for detecting CAD is slightly higher (8 to 10 percent) with exercise perfusion imaging, chiefly because the sensitivity for detecting single-vessel disease and mild stenoses of 50 to 70 percent narrowing is lower with exercise echocardiography; (4) perfusion imaging appears to identify more ischemic regions than stress echocardiography does, perhaps because mere flow heterogeneity and not true ischemia causing systolic myocardial dysfunction produces defects on stress scintigrams; (5) infarct zone ischemia is more easily identified with perfusion imaging by demonstration of a partial reversible defect in an area that contains a mixture of scar and viable myocardium; (6) operator dependency is not nearly as much a factor with SPECT perfusion imaging for the acquisition of images as it is with echocardiography; (7) virtually 100 percent of patients can undergo adequate SPECT perfusion imaging in which all areas of the myocardium are visualized; (8) with ^{99m}Tc-sestamibi or ^{99m}Tc-tetrofosmin, simultaneous assessment of myocardial perfusion and function can be obtained, and the resting left ventricular ejection fraction, regional wall thickening, and ventricular volumes can be accurately measured from gated ^{99m}Tc SPECT; and (9) vasodilator stress SPECT imaging has a significantly higher sensitivity for CAD detection than does vasodilator stress echocardiography.

Limitations of Stress Perfusion Imaging. When compared with stress echocardiography, the limitations of stress SPECT imaging are (1) longer imaging protocols, which may take many hours; (2) greater equipment expense and the necessity of injecting radiopharmaceuticals with exposure to radiation; (3) less than desirable specificity for CAD detection in many laboratories because of failure to distinguish attenuation artifacts (e.g., breast, diaphragmatic) from scarring; (4) inability to visualize the heart in a real-time approach; (5) lower spatial resolution than seen with echocardiography; (6) higher cost to patients; (7) lower detection rate of three-vessel disease patients who have balanced ischemia or diffusely abnormal flow reserve yielding perfusion images with homogeneous tracer uptake; and (8) often difficulty in evaluating the inferior wall because of high visceral uptake of the ^{99m}Tc-labeled tracers.

COMPARATIVE STUDIES OF STRESS ECHOCARDIOGRAPHY VERSUS PERFUSION IMAGING

In seven comparative studies,[62] the overall sensitivity of myocardial perfusion imaging was 80 percent versus 74 percent for stress echocardiography. In contrast, the specificity for stress echocardiography was higher than that of myocardial perfusion imaging (88 percent versus 78 percent). When single-vessel disease detection was analyzed separately, the sensitivity of myocardial perfusion imaging was 76 percent, as compared with 67 percent for stress echocardiography. Another review of the literature by O'Keefe and colleagues that involved 11 studies and 808 patients reported an overall sensitivity and specificity for stress echocardiography of 78 and 86 percent, respectively, as compared with 83 and 77 percent for myocardial perfusion imaging.[63] Schinkel and colleagues[64] reviewed 17 direct comparisons comprising 1405 patients and confirmed a slightly higher overall sensitivity (84 percent versus 80 percent) for stress radionuclide perfusion imaging, but specificity was higher for echocardiography (86 percent versus 77 percent). Most of the nuclear studies analyzed did not employ gated SPECT, which enhances specificity.[65]

Fleischmann and associates reviewed 44 articles to compare the diagnostic performance of exercise echocardiography and exercise SPECT imaging for CAD detection.[66] These authors concluded that when exercise echocardiography was compared with exercise SPECT via a receiver operating characteristic model, exercise echocardiography yielded significantly better discriminatory power when adjusted for age, publication year, and a setting including known CAD than did SPECT studies. This review did not include some of the more recent studies using gated ^{99m}Tc SPECT in which the specificity for detection of CAD is higher than the specificity with ^{201}Tl.[19] Also, in the SPECT cohort, combination of different radionuclide imaging agents and reading techniques and inclusion of studies utilizing experimental techniques resulted in significant heterogeneity of sensitivity and specificity value.[55] A high prevalence of CAD in studies reported enhanced sensitivity in the meta-analysis.[67]

Few studies have compared multiple diagnostic techniques for CAD detection in the same patient population. In one study, 60 patients being evaluated for the first time for chest pain underwent exercise stress testing, dipyridamole and dobutamine stress echocardiography, and dipyridamole and dobutamine ^{99m}Tc-sestamibi imaging.[68] With greater than 70 percent coronary stenosis used as the criteria for CAD, the sensitivity was 58 percent for exercise ECG testing, 55 percent for dipyridamole echocardiography, 61 percent for dobutamine echocardiography, 97 percent for dipyridamole ^{99m}Tc-sestamibi, and 91 percent for dobutamine ^{99m}Tc-sestamibi. The specificities for these tests were 67, 96, 96, 89, and 81 percent, respectively. All tests yielded higher sensitivity values for multivessel disease than for single-vessel disease. Although dobutamine echocardiography had a lower sensitivity than reported by other groups, this result agrees with the observation in another study that approximately 25 percent of patients manifested dobutamine-induced perfusion abnormalities without reversible wall motion abnormalities on dobutamine echocardiography.[69] Smart and colleagues[70] reported comparable sensitivity (87 percent) for dobutamine-atropine echocardiography and dobutamine ^{99m}Tc-sestamibi SPECT, but dobutamine echocardiography was more specific (95 percent versus 76 percent). Gated SPECT was not performed, which may have influenced specificity. Diagnostic accuracy for single-vessel disease detection was not improved when dobutamine ^{99m}Tc-sestamibi imaging and dobutamine echocardiography were combined.[71] Quantitative gated SPECT correlates well with echocardiography for assessment of left ventricular volumes and left ventricular ejection fraction.

Magnetic Resonance Coronary Angiography
(see Chap. 14)

Magnetic resonance coronary angiography (MRCA) is a developing technique and can depict the major coronary arteries.[30,32,72,73] Obstacles to its clinical use include need for correction for cardiac and respiratory motion, for millimeter spatial resolution, and for suppression of signal from adjacent epicardial fat and myocardium. Avoiding the need for breath-holding with real-time tracking of diaphragmatic motion would be advantageous. Three-dimensional navigator-gated (to compensate for respiratory motion in the foot-to-head direction) and prospectively corrected free-breathing MRCA can provide more favorable signal-to-noise ratios but is limited by poor contrast between coronary blood and myocardium. Kim and colleagues[74] performed MRCA during free breathing and could evaluate 84 percent of proximal and middle coronary artery segments and found an accuracy of 72 percent in diagnosing CAD. It was highly accurate in ruling out left main CAD. Yang and colleagues[72] have reported the ability of a spiral high-resolution coronary imaging sequence for MRCA with rapid real-time localization. This technique achieved 0.7 to 0.9 mm resolution with 14-heartbeat breath-holds, good image quality in 78 percent of coronary segments, and a 76 percent sensitivity and a 91 percent specificity for CAD detection compared with x-ray angiography. Cardiac MRI can noninvasively measure coronary flow velocity reserve after stent deployment with values similar to those obtained with invasive intracoronary Doppler.[75] This method had an 83 percent sensitivity and 94 percent specificity for detecting restenosis (75 percent or greater stenoses). MRCA, using a high-resolution navigator-gated three-dimensional technique, was highly accurate in detecting vein graft disease.[76] The receiver-operating characteristic curve for detecting graft occlusion was 0.89.

Magnetic Resonance Perfusion Imaging
(see Chap. 14)

Magnetic resonance perfusion imaging can be used for CAD detection employing bolus injection of gadolinium after dipyridamole or adenosine administration. In 84 patients who also underwent coronary angiography, this technique employing a turbogradient echo/echo-planar imaging-hybrid sequence yielded a sensitivity of 88 percent, specificity of 90 percent, and accuracy of 89 percent.[77] A myocardial blood flow reserve index can be determined with vasodilator gadolinium MRI, which can assist in the identification of patients with abnormal flow reserve in areas remote from stenotic regions.[78] Resting MRI has been evaluated for detecting acute coronary syndromes in the emergency room and yields a sensitivity of 84 percent and a specificity of 85 percent.[79] This approach includes assessment of both perfusion and regional systolic function.

Dobutamine MRI is another approach to detecting myocardial ischemia. When used with myocardial tagging, dobutamine cardiac MRI was performed at rest and during increasing doses of dobutamine in 211 consecutive patients with chest pain. Patients with new wall motion abnormalities underwent coronary angiography, of whom 96 percent had significant CAD on angiography.[80] Compared with resting PET imaging, flow reserve indices by first-pass perfusion MRI underestimate flow reserve values but could represent a useful semiquantitative technique for detection and severity of regional stenotic lesions.[81] Myocardial perfusion imaging with cardiac MRI hypothetically should be more sensitive for detecting subendocardial ischemia compared with exercise or vasodilator SPECT imaging because of its enhanced resolution. Subendocardial ischemia can be separated from subepicardial ischemia with contrast MRI performed with hyperemia following vasodilator stress. In one study, receiver-operating characteristic analysis of subendocardial upslope data revealed a sensitivity of 91 percent and a specificity of 94 percent for detection of CAD as defined by PET and 87 percent and 85 percent, respectively, in comparison with quantitative coronary angiography.[82] Abnormal subendocardial perfusion has been detected in patients with cardiac syndrome X employing MRI with perfusion imaging.

Magnetic resonance imaging offers the potential of examining the atheromatous lesion as well as the lumen.[73] However, traditional selective x-ray coronary angiography currently offers higher resolution (0.1 mm). Arteries can be viewed by MRI in cross section, and plaques can be visualized and characterized.[83-85] High spatial resolution black-blood MRI, a method free of motion and blood flow artifacts, provides noninvasive images of the coronary artery lumen and wall. This technique might be useful for identifying asymptomatic coronary atherosclerosis.[86,87] Figure 16–1 shows an example of lipid-rich plaque identified by MRI.[87] Macrophages that accumulate in atherosclerotic plaques in carotid arteries have been detected with MRI enhanced by injection of ultrasmall superparamagnetic particles of iron oxide.[88] This may be a promising MRI approach for identifying rupture-prone atherosclerotic lesions in humans. In the future, real-time MRI-guided catheterization of coronary arteries using dilute contrast agents will be feasible.[89]

Noninvasive Intravenous Coronary Angiography Using Computed Tomography (see Chap. 15)

A new generation of multislice CT systems permits the simultaneous acquisition of up to 16 submillimeter slices with fast rotation, yielding

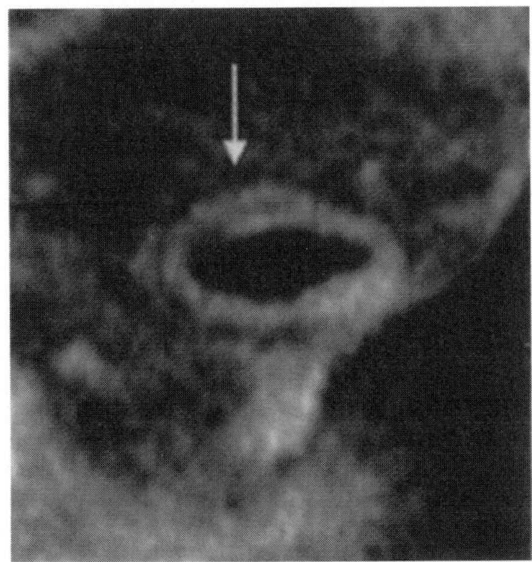

A

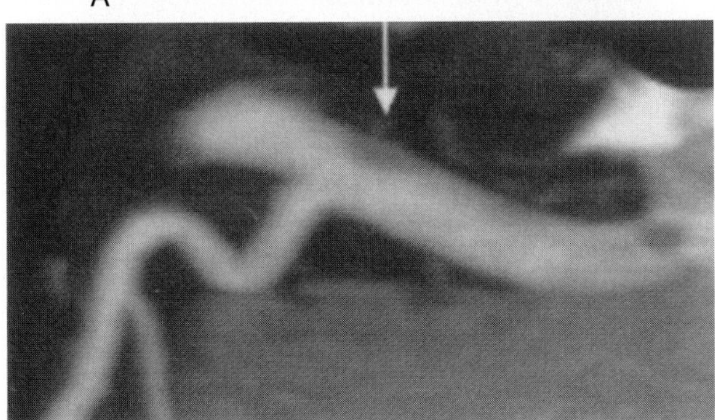

B

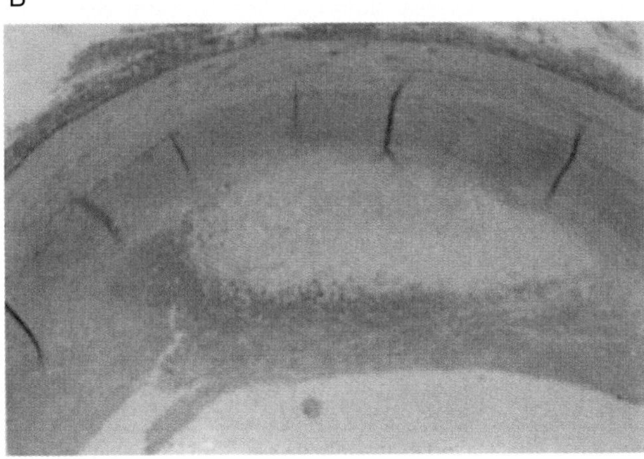

C

FIGURE 16–1 Magnetic resonance imaging and computed tomography (CT) plaque characterization. **A,** Cross-sectional ex vivo T2-weighted magnetic resonance image of the human left anterior descending artery with a lipid-rich lesion (arrow). **B,** Multislice CT image of the same lesion (arrow) showing a low-density area containing lipid-rich tissue. **C,** Corresponding histopathological section showing a significant lipid containing plaque. (From Fayad ZA, Fuster V, Nikolaou K, Becker C: Computed tomography and magnetic resonance imaging for noninvasive coronary angiography and plaque imaging: Current and potential future concepts. Circulation 106:2026, 2002.)

coronary CT angiograms of good quality when the heart rate is initially lowered to 60 beats/min employing beta blockade.[36] Figure 16–2 shows an example of a CT coronary angiogram showing an ostial stenosis of the left main coronary artery.[36] In comparison with invasive coronary angiography, multidetector spiral CT scanning correctly classified 85 percent of patients as having at least one coronary stenosis and correctly detected 73 percent of all coronary lesions. After excluding coronary arteries that were classified as unevaluable by noninvasive CT angiography, 57 of 62 lesions were detected, and absence of significant stenoses was correctly identified in 194 of 208 vessels. This yielded a 92 percent sensitivity and 93 percent specificity for detection of coronary artery stenoses. A limitation of contrast-enhanced, ECG-gated multislice spiral CT is that about 30 percent of coronary arteries are unevaluable, mainly because of artifacts caused by coronary motion. When only evaluable arteries are considered, this technique had a 91 percent sensitivity and an 84 percent specificity for detecting stenoses of 70 percent or greater.[90] EBCT can also be used for noninvasive coronary angiography.[91] Multislice CT angiography provides better image quality in more coronary segments than EBCT angiography because of its better contrast-to-noise ratio and higher spatial resolution.[91] One main reason for unevaluable arteries by multislice CT angiography is heavy coronary calcification that is seen in approximately 10 percent of plaques. Fortunately, breath-holding is reduced to 20 seconds in the 16-slice per second CT scanners. For the future, multislice CT must be done in real time with fast postprocessing techniques. Ultimately, its value could be greatest in imaging patients with a low probability of CAD to exclude a significant coronary stenosis.

Multidetector CT scanners or EBCT scanners can detect coronary atherosclerosis by the demonstration of coronary calcification (see Chap. 15).[1,92] Because the presence of coronary calcium is very specific for presence of atherosclerosis, any identifiable calcium on CT scanning is considered as evidence for CAD. The specificity of coronary calcification, however, for identifying flow-limiting stenoses is limited, since many patients can have a high coronary calcium score but no obstructive coronary stenoses that would produce an ischemic response on stress testing using other modalities. Sensitivity is, of course, very high, although some patients have lipid-laden, noncalcified plaques causing angina without demonstration of coronary calcification on scanning. Coronary calcification imaging with CT scanning has been chiefly employed for risk assessment in asymptomatic patients with data showing that the higher the calcium score, the greater the risk for subsequent coronary events. The relative risk of coronary events is in the range of 4.0 for patients with calcium scores above a certain threshold compared with those with scores below that threshold.[93] Figure 16–3 shows the risk of cardiac events relative to tertiles of calcium scores and low or high C-reactive protein values from the work of Park and associates.[94]

Assessment of Prognosis of Patients Evaluated for Coronary Artery Disease (see Chap. 50)

One of the chief applications of noninvasive stress testing in patients with suspected or known CAD is the identification of patients at either high or low risk for future ischemic cardiac events.[5,38] Prognostication using noninvasive stress ECG testing or stress imaging technology is based on the rationale that physiological alterations under stress conditions predict events better than does knowledge of coronary artery anatomy. Accurate risk stratification contributes importantly to clinical decision-making. For example, patients who are identified as being at low risk for future cardiac events on the basis of noninvasive test variables can be spared unnecessary or premature referral for invasive strategies unless symptoms are not adequately alleviated by antiischemic drugs. Conversely, patients with high-risk ECG stress test and/or imaging variables may benefit from early referral for invasive strategies, including revascularization, even if symptoms are mild.

Treadmill ECG Stress Testing for Evaluation of Prognosis (see Chap. 10)

Treadmill exercise ECG stress testing alone without the addition of an imaging procedure is useful for differentiating low- and high-risk patients with chest pain. The demonstration of 1.0 mm or more of horizontal or downsloping ST segment depression at low exercise heart rates or workloads is a significant predictor of an adverse outcome when using exercise ECG testing for prognostication. Perhaps the most powerful predictive variable on treadmill testing for identifying high-risk patients is functional capacity reflected by workload

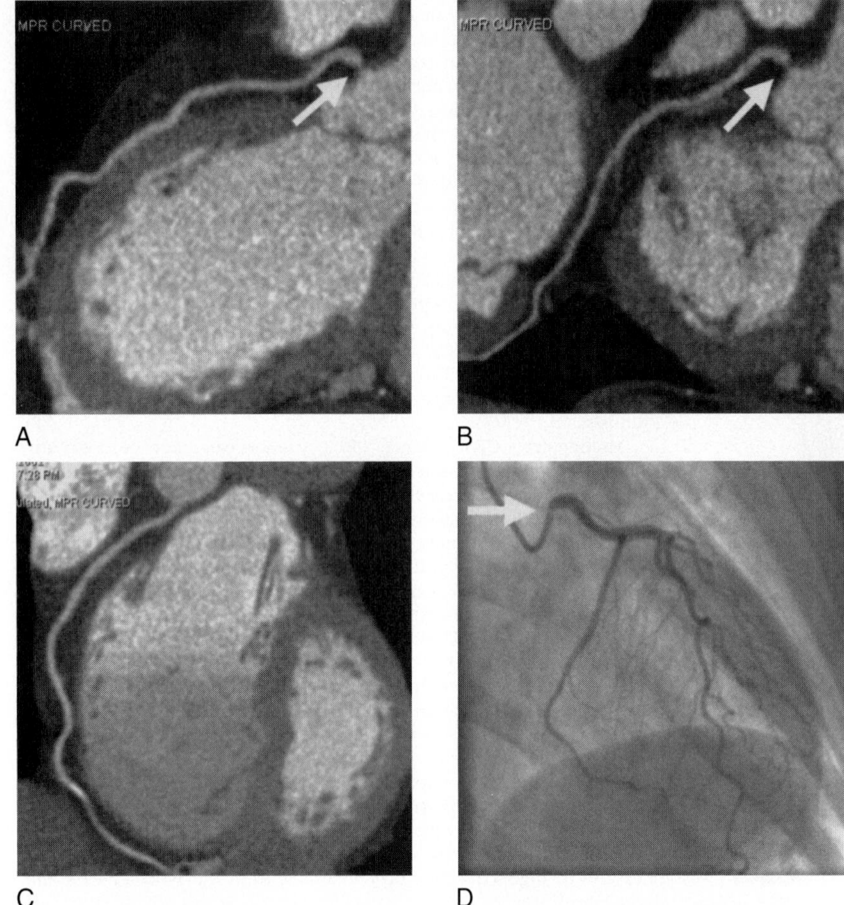

FIGURE 16–2 Thin-slice multidetector row spiral computed tomography scan showing an ostial stenosis of the left main coronary artery. **A,** Curved multiplanar reconstruction of the left main and left anterior descending coronary arteries showing the osteostenosis (arrow). **B,** Curved multiplanar reconstruction of the left main and circumflex coronary arteries with the same left main osteostenosis shown (arrow). **C,** Curved multiplanar reconstruction of the right coronary artery with no stenoses present. **D,** Contrast invasive coronary angiogram showing the severe left main osteostenosis (arrow). (From Ropers D, Baum U, Pohle K, et al: Detection of coronary artery stenoses with thin-slice multi-detector row spiral computed tomography and multiplanar reconstruction. Circulation 107:664, 2003.)

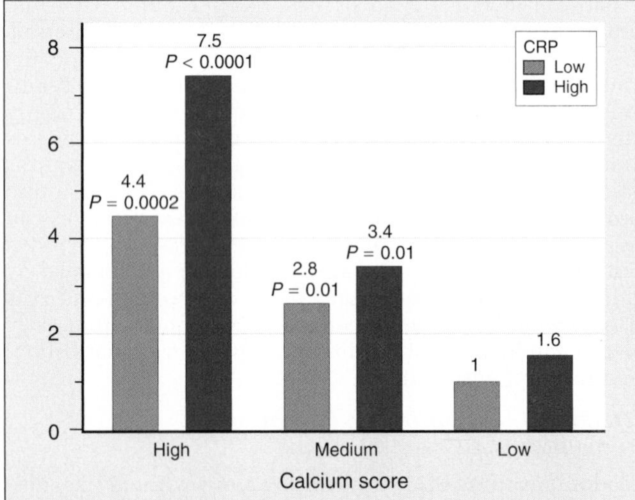

FIGURE 16–3 Risk ratios of nonfatal myocardial infarction, coronary death, percutaneous transluminal coronary angioplasty, coronary artery bypass grafting, or stroke associated with high (±75th percentile) and low levels of C-reactive protein (CRP) and high (>142.1), medium (3.7 to 142.1), and low (<3.7) tertiles of calcium scores. The highest risk of an event is in the patient group with a high calcium score and high CRP. (From Park R, Detrano R, Xiang M, et al: Combined use of computed tomography coronary calcium scores and C-reactive protein levels in predicting cardiovascular events in nondiabetic individuals. Circulation 106:2073, 2002.)

achieved.[95] Absolute peak exercise capacity is a stronger predictor of death than the percentage of age-predicted maximum heart rate achieved.[95] Each one metabolic equivalent (MET) increase in exercise capacity was associated with a 12 percent improvement in survival. Figure 16–4 shows the risk of death related to workload achieved on exercise testing in groups of patients with various risk factors.[95] Chronotropic incompetence, identified as an attenuated heart rate response to exercise, predicts increased mortality. A very rapid heart rate recovery immediately after exercise was associated with a lower risk of cardiovascular disease events in the Framingham study.[96] Poor exercise tolerance can be observed in patients with depressed resting left ventricular function with or without superimposed transient exercise-induced ischemia.

A treadmill score has been proposed for better separating high- and low-risk patients undergoing ECG stress testing (see Chap. 10). Perhaps the most popular of these scores, derived by the Duke University group, relies on the duration of exercise, the maximal ST segment deviation, and a treadmill angina index.[97] In a follow-up study from the Duke group,[98] patients with a low-risk Duke treadmill score who were treated medically had a 3.1 percent 5-year mortality rate, whereas those deemed at high risk had a 35 percent 5-year mortality rate. The low-risk group, which represented 36 percent of the cohort, had a 40 percent prevalence of any CAD and a 9 percent prevalence of severe CAD determined angiographically. The high-risk group, which represented only 9 percent of the entire cohort, had a 74 percent incidence of severe CAD, and all patients had at least one or more coronary stenoses.

The practical problem with the Duke treadmill score is that a substantial proportion of patients are classified as having intermediate or moderate risk after exercise ECG treadmill testing. In a study by Shaw and associates, 55 percent of the patients were classified as having moderate risk by the Duke treadmill score, and they had a 9.5 percent 5-year mortality rate and a 31 percent prevalence of severe CAD.[98] Perfusion imaging variables are useful in further risk-stratifying patients with intermediate-risk Duke treadmill scores.[99,100] A substantial number of these patients can be deemed to be at low risk if they show normal perfusion or only a mild postexercise defect.

LIMITATIONS. Exercise ECG stress tests have other important limitations in assessing prognosis. First, a strongly positive exercise ECG, which is defined as an early or low ischemic threshold, significant horizontal ST segment depression, and a prolonged ST depression recovery time, does not necessarily signify more severe CAD by either angiographic or scintigraphic criteria.[101] The extent of exercise ST segment depression poorly predicts the extent of CAD, and the maximum ST segment depression achieved at peak exercise correlates poorly with the extent of stress-induced hypoperfusion by scintigraphy. Also, a considerable portion of patients have an uninterpretable exercise ECG response.[102] For these patients, imaging variables provided substantial supplementary prognostic information over ECG stress test variables. Patients with normal exercise perfusion scans or exercise echocardiograms have an excellent outcome even if the ECG stress test is nondiagnostic or abnormal.

Exercise ECG testing alone has particular utility in the risk assessment of patients with a normal resting ECG who have nonanginal or very atypical chest pain. If these patients achieve an adequate exercise heart rate or workload without significant ST segment depression, the prognosis during follow-up is excellent. Stress imaging is not cost effective in patients with low-risk Duke treadmill scores unless they have a significant number of high-risk clinical variables (e.g., advanced age, diabetes). However, for improved diagnostic and prognostic value, an imaging technique should be performed in conjunction with treadmill testing in patients with an intermediate or a high pretest likelihood of CAD on the basis of age, gender, and type of chest pain.

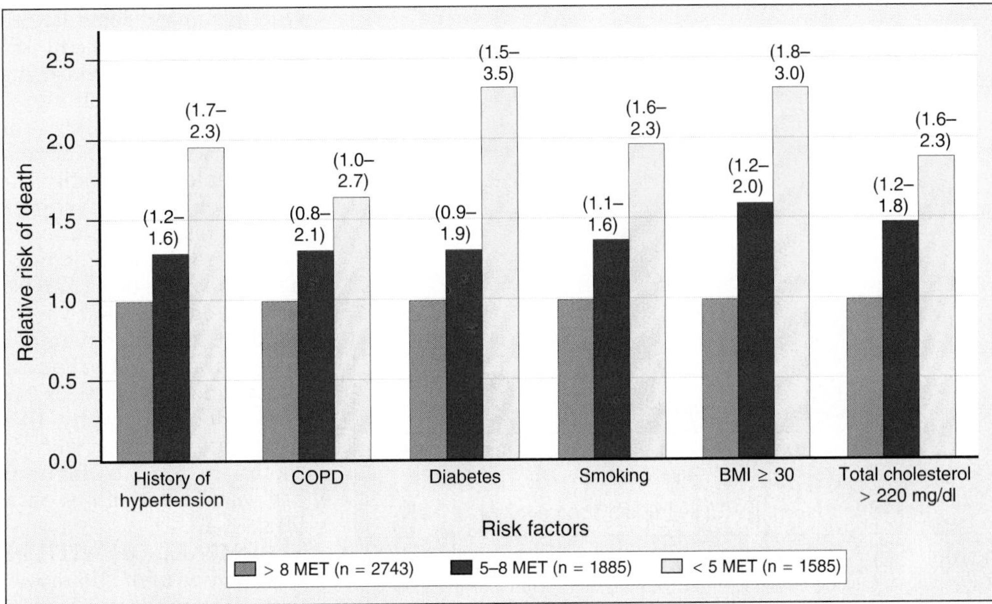

FIGURE 16–4 Relative risks of death from any cause among subjects with various risk factors who achieved exercise workloads of either less than 5 METs or 5 to 8 METs compared with subjects whose exercise capacity was more than 8 METs (first bar of each triad normalized to 1.0). The numbers within parentheses above the bars are 95% confidence intervals. BMI = body mass index; COPD = chronic obstructive pulmonary disease. (From Myers J, Prakash M, Froelicher V, et al: Exercise capacity and mortality among men referred for exercise testing. N Engl J Med 346:793, 2002. Copyright © 2002 Massachusetts Medical Society. All rights reserved.)

Stress Myocardial Perfusion Imaging for Evaluation of Prognosis (see Chap. 13)

The prognostic value of exercise and pharmacological stress myocardial perfusion imaging has been established in thousands of patients evaluated in multiple clinical studies.[44,45,103] The major prognostic variables on stress perfusion images predictive of future cardiac events are (1) a large defect size (>20 percent of the left ventricle); (2) multiple perfusion abnormalities in two or more coronary supply regions suggestive of multivessel CAD; (3) defect reversibility reflective of inducible ischemia in multiple myocardial segments, even in the distribution of one major coronary artery; (4) a large number of nonreversible defects; (5) transient left ventricular cavity dilation from stress to rest images; (6) increased ^{201}Tl lung uptake best assessed by quantitating the lung/heart ^{201}Tl ratio; and (7) a resting left ventricular ejection fraction of less than 40 percent measured on gated SPECT.[44,45] One of the most valuable features of exercise or pharmacological stress perfusion imaging with ^{201}Tl, ^{99m}Tc-sestamibi, or ^{99m}Tc-tetrofosmin is the ability to predict a low combined mortality and nonfatal myocardial infarction rate in patients with a totally normal scan. In a pooled analysis of 20,963 patients from 16 published studies in the literature with a follow-up of slightly more than 2 years, the combined annual cardiac death or nonfatal infarction rate in those with normal perfusion scans was 0.7 percent per year.[44] The annual hard cardiac event rate is in the range of 7.0 percent in patients with abnormal scans.[104]

INCREMENTAL VALUE OF PERFUSION IMAGING OVER ECG STRESS TESTING. Numerous published studies have demonstrated the incremental value of stress myocardial perfusion imaging over clinical and ECG treadmill stress test variables for prognostication. The event rate increases in proportion to the extent of stress-induced hypoperfusion or the extent or severity of reversible defects reflective of ischemia. With gated SPECT, the extent of regional wall motion or thickening abnormalities, the ejection fraction and end-systolic and end-diastolic volumes, and the extent of reversible regional dysfunction on poststress images indicative of stunning add to the high-risk assessment.[21-23,46,105,106] Patients at the highest risk for subsequent cardiac death or infarction are those with baseline left ventricular dysfunction with moderate to severe stress-induced reversible perfusion defects.[23] Patients at the lowest risk for subsequent cardiac events are those who demonstrate good exercise tolerance (e.g., achieving 85 percent or greater of maximum predicted heart rate) with normal perfusion on SPECT images.[107] As mentioned earlier, imaging variables on stress/rest SPECT imaging provide incremental prognostic information over clinical and exercise stress test variables, including the Duke treadmill score.[100,108] Figure 16-5 shows the death or myocardial infarction rate per year in patients with low, intermediate, or high Duke treadmill scores further risk stratified by the extent of the stress defect on exercise SPECT images.[100] It appears that variables on stress perfusion imaging might identify patients who have an excellent outcome with medical therapy even with the demonstration of mild ischemia.[109] In contrast, patients with extensive stress-induced hypoperfusion may have a better outcome with respect to cardiac mortality with revascularization strategies.[109]

COST-EFFECTIVENESS OF SPECT IMAGING. The use of myocardial perfusion imaging as an initial evaluation in patients with stable chest pain is highly cost-effective when compared with an initial invasive strategy. A large observational study consisting of 11,372 consecutive stable angina patients referred for stress myocardial perfusion SPECT imaging or direct catheterization revealed that costs were higher for the initial invasive strategy in clinical subsets with a low, intermediate, or high pretest likelihood of disease.[110] Diagnostic and follow-up costs of care were 30 to 41 percent higher for patients undergoing direct cardiac catheterization without any reduction in mortality or infarction. The diagnostic costs were, respectively, \$1320, \$1275, and \$1229 greater for low-, intermediate-, and high-risk patients undergoing initial cardiac catheterization than for those having stress perfusion imaging as the initial test for CAD detection. The cardiac death rate and nonfatal infarction rate in the 5826 patients undergoing initial stress perfusion imaging for assessment of stable angina were both 2.8 percent as compared with 3.3 and 3.0 percent, respectively, for the 5423 patients who were referred directly for cardiac catheterization as the initial diagnostic strategy. The cost of screening women with myocardial perfusion imaging was shown in a separate analysis to be considerably lower than the cost of direct coronary angiography in a similar type of analysis.[111] Thus, stress myocardial perfusion imaging undertaken as the initial step in diagnosis and assessment of prognosis yields comparable outcomes at a lower cost than does direct referral for cardiac catheterization. This noninvasive strategy

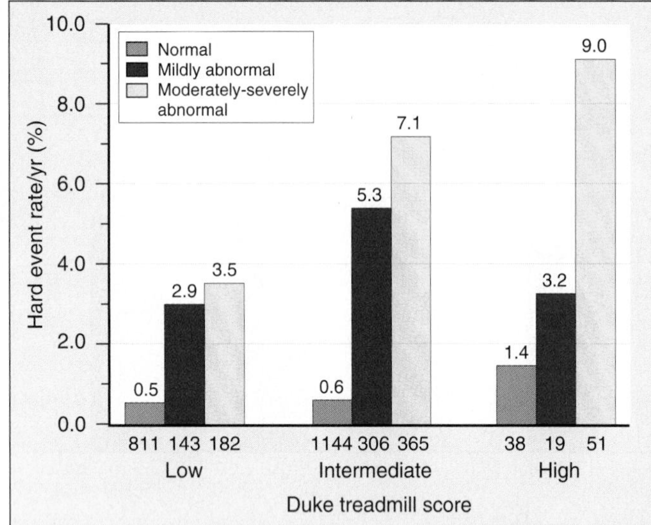

FIGURE 16–5 Rates of hard cardiac events per year as a function of the results of stress single-photon emission tomography (SPECT) in patients with low, intermediate, or high Duke treadmill scores; $P < 0.05$ across SPECT categories in all Duke treadmill score subgroups. (From Hachamovitch R, Berman DS, Kiat H, et al: Value of stress myocardial perfusion single photon emission computed tomography in patients with normal resting electrocardiograms: An evaluation of incremental prognostic value and cost-effectiveness. Circulation 105:823, 2002.)

is "ischemia driven" and should be applicable even to patients with angiographic disease and normal scans, since this group also has an excellent prognosis.[112]

CONCLUSIONS. Thus, taken together, data reported from the literature demonstrate that patients with normal regional myocardial perfusion and normal left ventricular function on gated SPECT scans have an excellent prognosis, whereas patients with abnormal scans have an increased rate of cardiac death and nonfatal infarction during follow-up. The greater the extent of stress-induced hypoperfusion and reversibility, the greater the probability of an event. It is apparent from the many studies cited that myocardial perfusion imaging variables provide supplementary prognostic information to exercise ECG testing alone, particularly in patients who have an intermediate risk of an adverse outcome estimated by clinical variables and exercise stress testing. Diabetic patients seem to significantly benefit from stress perfusion imaging for separating high and lower risk subsets.[113,114] Stress perfusion imaging variables appear to be equal or even superior to mere knowledge of coronary anatomical variables for assessing prognosis because the extent of hypoperfusion during stress and the magnitude and extent of stress-induced ischemia better predict subsequent cardiac death than does demonstration of the presence of one-, two-, or three-vessel disease alone. In fact, patients with three-vessel disease on angiography can be further risk-stratified by myocardial perfusion imaging performed after catheterization into low-, intermediate-, and high-risk groups.

Echocardiographic Assessment of Prognosis (see Chap. 11)

Evaluation of left ventricular function on the resting echocardiogram obtained before commencing the stress portion of the protocol offers considerable prognostic information by itself. A large area of asynergy is predictive of future cardiac events. The sensitivity of stress echocardiography to identify patients with severe CAD is good.

Heupler and coauthors reported that detection of exercise-induced wall motion abnormalities independently predicted cardiac events in 508 women monitored for 41 ± 10 months after exercise echocardiography.[115] Evidence of ischemia by echocardiography foretold future cardiac events better than did exercise capacity or inducible ST segment depression. The prognostic data provided by the exercise echocardiogram added to that provided by clinical and exercise ECG variables in patients with both undiagnosed and known CAD. In a study from the same institution consisting of both men and women, the presence of ischemia on exercise echocardiography predicted future cardiac events well and, in a multivariate model, was the strongest independent predictor of cardiac death, myocardial infarction, or unstable angina.[116]

Exercise echocardiography has been reported to provide incremental prognostic information in patients 65 years of age or older.[117] An abnormal left ventricular end-systolic volume response and exercise left ventricular ejection fraction were independent predictors of cardiac events. In patients with good exercise capacity, extent and severity of exercise-induced left ventricular dysfunction provided independent and incremental prognostic value.[118] Incremental values of exercise echocardiography are comparable in men and women.[119] Marwick and associates[120] showed that exercise echocardiography, like exercise SPECT, is particularly useful in patients with intermediate-risk Duke treadmill scores. In 5375 patients, the mortality rate was 1 percent per year in patients with normal exercise echocardiograms (Fig. 16–6).

COMPARISON WITH PERFUSION IMAGING

Few studies in the literature have compared exercise echocardiography with exercise perfusion imaging for long-term prediction of prognosis. Olmos and colleagues compared clinical, exercise, echocardiographic, and SPECT ^{201}Tl variables in 248 patients who underwent both stress imaging modalities simultaneously.[121] The clinical models characterized by exercise echocardiography with exercise ECG testing and ^{201}Tl SPECT with exercise ECG were comparable in the prediction of cardiac events. For the exercise echocardiography model, the exercise wall motion score index and induction of ischemia were the strongest predictors of events. For the model with exercise ^{201}Tl SPECT, the strongest predictor was the extent of the ischemic perfusion defect. Of interest, for the prediction of ischemic events and/or cardiac death, echocardiographic and ^{201}Tl variables were the only predictive variables.

One reason for the failure to predict some events by stress echocardiography is the inability to attain an adequate heart rate response. This limitation agrees with the finding of compromised sensitivity of stress echocardiography for detecting ischemia in the setting of inadequate heart rate responses.[56] Therefore, patients who are deemed unable to exercise

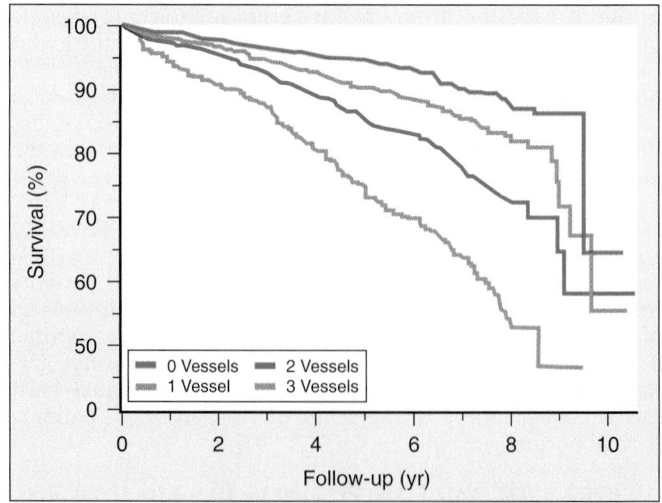

FIGURE 16–6 Survival free of death according to total extent of wall motion abnormalities at peak stress on exercise echocardiography. The extent of wall motion abnormality is reflected as a one-vessel, two-vessel, or three-vessel disease pattern. (From Marwick TH, Case C, Vasey C, et al: Prediction of mortality by exercise echocardiography: A strategy for combination with the Duke treadmill score. Circulation 103:2566, 2001.)

adequately should undergo dobutamine stress echocardiography for both diagnosis and prognosis indications.

With respect to the comparison of dobutamine echocardiography and simultaneously performed ^{99m}Tc-sestamibi SPECT imaging, Geleijnse and coauthors reported that any abnormality or ischemia on echocardiography or scintigraphy was associated with cardiac events.[122] Dobutamine-atropine echocardiography and ^{99m}Tc-sestamibi imaging provided comparable prognostic information. With respect to the negative predictive value of a normal study, patients with normal study results had equally very low event rates (0.4 percent by echocardiography and 0.5 percent by ^{99m}Tc-sestamibi). As with exercise perfusion imaging, patients with a normal exercise echocardiogram have a very low cardiac event rate.[5,123]

Dobutamine echocardiography also provides prognostic value in patients with suspected or known CAD. In the study by Poldermans and colleagues of 1737 patients with known or suspected CAD who underwent dobutamine-atropine stress echocardiography, a normal echocardiographic study was associated with an annual event rate of cardiac death or infarction of 1.3 percent over a 5-year period.[124] In that study, the rate of cardiac death or myocardial infarction in patients with new wall motion abnormalities or extensive resting wall motion abnormalities increased 3.6-fold and 2.5-fold, respectively. A negative echocardiographic response to pharmacological stress in women was associated with a less than 1 percent hard cardiac event rate over 3 years of follow-up.[125] Echocardiographic evidence of ischemia was found as the only independent predictor of hard cardiac events (odds ratio, 27.5) in this study. Marwick and colleagues[126] showed that dobutamine echocardiography is an independent predictor of death, and a normal study finding is associated with a 1 percent annual mortality risk. In a multicenter trial comprising 7333 patients who underwent either high-dose dipyridamole echocardiography or high-dose dobutamine echocardiography, Kaplan-Meier survival estimates showed a significantly better outcome for patients with normal pharmacological stress echocardiograms compared with those with abnormal studies during a mean follow-up of 2.6 years.[127]

Few studies have directly compared vasodilator stress and inotropic stress with echocardiography for prognostication.

Prediction of Perioperative Ischemic Events

A meta-analysis of 15 studies demonstrated the prognostic value of dipyridamole ^{201}Tl imaging and dobutamine echocardiography for predicting perioperative ischemic events in patients undergoing risk stratification before vascular surgery (see Chap. 77).[128] For dipyridamole ^{201}Tl studies, the cardiac death rate or myocardial infarction rate was 1, 7, and 9 percent for normal results, fixed defects, and reversible defects, respectively. For patients with a dobutamine-induced new or worsening wall motion response, 23.1 percent had a perioperative ischemic event as compared with 0.4 percent of patients with a normal stress echocardiographic response. Summary odds ratios were greater for dobutamine echocardiography than for dipyridamole ^{201}Tl, but the 95 percent confidence intervals were wider with echocardiography because of a smaller sample size. Late cardiac events after vascular surgery (average 19 ± 11 months) can also be predicted by stress-induced ischemia on dobutamine echocardiography.[129]

CONCLUSIONS: STRESS PERFUSION IMAGING VERSUS STRESS ECHOCARDIOGRAPHY

In summary, both stress perfusion imaging and stress echocardiography provide prognostic information supplemental to that of clinical and exercise ECG stress test variables. Both techniques have excellent negative predictive value for identifying low-risk patients. Such patients with either a normal perfusion study finding at peak stress or normal regional function have an excellent outcome with a cardiac death or infarction rate of less than 1 percent per year. The negative predictive value of a normal study result is perhaps slightly better with perfusion imaging than echocardiography because of its slightly higher sensitivity for identifying mild CAD. Patients with high-risk stress imaging findings on either perfusion imaging or echocardiography have a worse outcome with medical therapy, and the greater the degree of regional abnormalities (either perfusion or function), the higher the event rate. Either technique is superior to exercise ECG test variables alone. An abnormal workload and a suboptimal heart rate response are excellent prognostic variables derived from the ECG stress test for identifying high-risk patients. Ischemia occurring at low exercise heart rates and workloads should prompt evaluation with coronary angiography. Pharmacological stress imaging provides comparable prognostic information to exercise imaging for both nuclear cardiology and echocardiographic techniques, and either can be used for preoperative risk stratification in intermediate- or high-risk patients scheduled for vascular surgical procedures. Patients with normal vasodilator stress or dobutamine stress perfusion scans have a higher event rate than patients with normal exercise images. Improvement in ischemic perfusion abnormalities is observed with medical therapy for CAD, which improves endothelial function. Advances in contrast echocardiography and attenuation- and scatter-corrected SPECT with quantitation will improve accuracy of these imaging techniques.

MAGNETIC RESONANCE PERFUSION AND FUNCTION IMAGING (see Chap. 14)

Magnetic resonance perfusion imaging performed with gadolinium-based contrast agents and a stressor such as adenosine and assessment of regional left ventricular function with MRI during dobutamine stress are alternative approaches to detecting CAD and assessing prognosis. Few data are available with respect to the prognostic value of vasodilator stress myocardial perfusion MRI or dobutamine stress MRI. In one study, the cardiac event-free survival rate was 98.2 percent for patients with negative dobutamine cardiac MRI study at an average follow-up of 17.3 months.[80] The presence of inducible ischemia or a left ventricular ejection fraction of less than 40 percent on dobutamine/atropine MRI was associated with future cardiac death or myocardial infarction at 20 months of follow-up (hazard ratio 3.3).[130] Dipyridamole stress MRI had 85 percent agreement with ^{201}Tl scintigraphy in detection of CAD and a correlation of 0.86 in sizing perfusion defects.[131]

Stress MRI with contrast may ultimately be very clinically useful in that the technique provides high spatial resolution and has the capability of imaging in any desired plane without ionizing radiation. Images can be acquired with reproducible quality that is operator independent. Since no imaging window is required, images can be obtained in virtually all patients, including those with emphysema. The endocardial border can easily be defined and separated from the cavity blood volume.

Disadvantages of stress MRI techniques are an inability to image patients with pacemakers and implanted cardioverter-defibrillators and the need for prolonged breath-holding.

Table 16-3 summarizes the major strengths and limitations of the various techniques used for detection of CAD and assessment of prognosis.

Noninvasive Assessment of Myocardial Viability

Regional and global left ventricular dysfunction leading to depressed left ventricular ejection fractions in patients with CAD can result from myocardial necrosis or scarring, postischemic stunning, or myocardial hibernation (see Chaps. 44 and 50). *Hibernation* is defined as the state in which myocytes are chronically hypoperfused or repetitively

TABLE 16–3 Major Strengths and Limitations of Various Techniques for Detecting Coronary Artery Disease and Assessing Prognosis

Technique	Strengths	Limitations
Exercise ECG	Low cost, short duration Functional status evaluated High sensitivity in three-vessel or left main CAD Provides useful prognostic information (e.g., ischemia at low workload) Indicated as first test for patients at low probability of CAD	Suboptimal sensitivity Low detection rate of one-vessel disease Nondiagnostic with abnormal baseline ECG Poor specificity in certain patient populations (e.g., premenopausal women) Need to achieve ≥85 percent of maximum heart rate for maximizing accuracy
Exercise or pharmacological SPECT perfusion imaging	Simultaneous evaluation of perfusion and function with gated SPECT Higher sensitivity and specificity than exercise ECG High specificity with ^{99m}Tc-labeled agents Studies can be performed in almost all patients Significant additional prognostic value Comparable accuracy with pharmacological stress Viability and ischemia simultaneously assessed Quantitative image analysis	Suboptimal specificity because of artifacts Long procedure time when rest and stress both performed with ^{99m}Tc-labeled agents No standardized correction for attenuation and scatter Higher cost than exercise ECG Radiation exposure Poor-quality images in obese patients Absolute flow reserve not quantitated May underestimate three-vessel disease because of "balanced ischemia"
PET perfusion imaging	Accurate quantitation of blood flow in ml/g/min secondary to tracer kinetic modeling and attenuation correction using either rubidium-82 or nitrogen-13 ammonia	Use restricted to pharmacological stress High cost Low availability
Exercise or pharmacological stress echocardiography	Higher sensitivity and specificity than exercise ECG Additional prognostic value Comparable value with dobutamine stress Short time to complete examination Identification of coexisting structural cardiac abnormalities (e.g., valvular disease) Simultaneous evaluation of perfusion with contrast agents Relatively lower cost than other techniques No radiation	Decreased sensitivity for detection of one-vessel disease or mild stenosis with postexercise imaging Inability to image all of the left ventricle in some patients Highly operator dependent for image analysis No quantitative image analysis Poor acoustic window in some patients (e.g., chronic obstructive lung disease) Infarct zone ischemia less well detected False-positive defects in posterolateral wall with contract echo
Magnetic resonance imaging	High spatial resolution MRI coronary angiography promising Bypass grafts well seen Imaging of arterial wall and plaque Flow mapping with contrast Visualization of subendocardial perfusion Pharmacological stress procedure short No radiation	Inability to image patients with metal devices Difficult to image in setting of irregular heart rhythm Motion artifacts in absence of good breath-hold and respiratory gating Coronary motion No large clinical studies yet published
EBCT angiography and MSCT angiography	Noninvasive coronary angiography to rule out significant coronary stenoses	Radiation exposure Cardiac motion artifacts Beta blockers often required to reduce heart rate to <60 beats/min Artifacts caused by coronary motion Unevaluable arteries for lumen assessment with heavy calcification Prolonged breath-holding for scanners with <16-slice per sec Images not generated in real time MSCTA better contrast-to-noise ratio and spatial resolution compared with EBCTA but 3.5 times higher radiation exposure Slow acquisition time for MSCTA

CAD = coronary artery disease; EBCT = electron beam computed tomography; ECG = electrocardiogram; MSCT = multislice computed tomography; PET = positron emission tomography; SPECT = single-photon emission computed tomography; VD = vessel disease.

stunned but in which flow is sufficient to sustain structural integrity. Hibernating myocardium, by definition, demonstrates improved systolic function with improved resting perfusion after coronary revascularization.

An accurate noninvasive determination of myocardial viability that is capable of distinguishing irreversible myocardial cellular injury from hibernation is critically important for the clinical decision-making process. It allows for improved selection of patients with CAD and resting left ventricular dysfunction who will benefit most from revascularization strategies.[132] Patients with substantial zones of myocardial viability in asynergic myocardium reflective of hibernation demonstrate better function and overall improved outcomes after revascularization than do patients with left ventricular dysfunction predominantly caused by myocardial scarring. Such patients with extensive areas of viability have a better survival rate with revascularization than medical therapy (Fig. 16–7).[132]

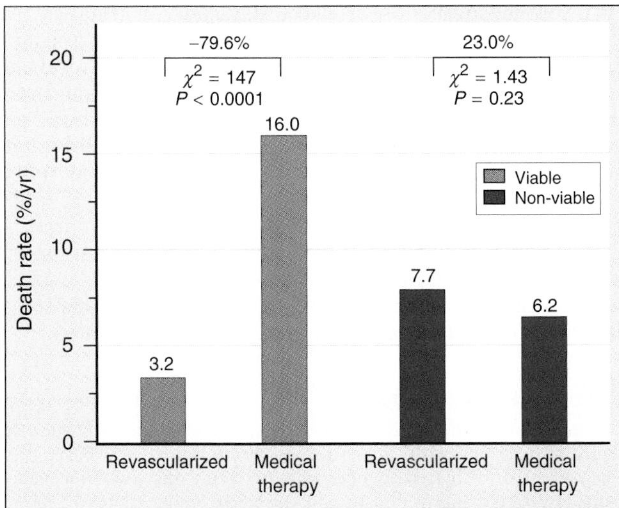

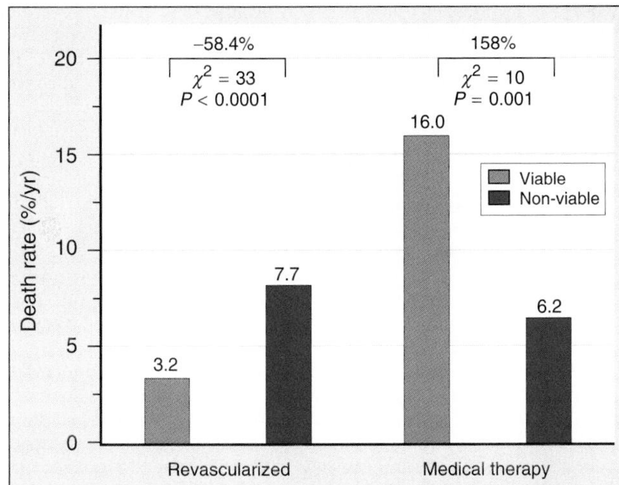

FIGURE 16–7 **A,** Death rates for patients with and without myocardial viability treated by revascularization or medical therapy. There is a 79.6 percent reduction in mortality for patients with viability treated by revascularization ($P < 0.001$). No significant difference in mortality with revascularization versus medical therapy was observed in patients with predominantly nonviable myocardium. **B,** Same data as in part A with comparison made on treatment strategy in patients with and without viability. Annual mortality was significantly higher in medically treated patients when viability was present versus absent. (From Allman KC, Shaw LJ, Hachamovitch R, Udelson JE: Myocardial viability testing and impact of revascularization on prognosis in patients with coronary artery disease and left ventricular dysfunction: A meta-analysis. J Am Coll Cardiol 39:1151, 2002. Copyright 2002, with permission from American College of Cardiology Foundation.)

Techniques Used for Myocardial Viability Assessment

Thallium-201 Imaging (see Chap. 13)

Thallium-201 rest and delayed redistribution imaging is the most commonly used radionuclide imaging modality for the assessment of myocardial viability. It is used for this purpose because the initial uptake of ^{201}Tl is related to both blood flow and myocardial membrane integrity. Several groups have shown that approximately 60 to 70 percent of asynergic myocardial segments showing greater than 50 or 60 percent ^{201}Tl uptake on resting ^{201}Tl scintigraphy will show improved systolic function after revascularization.[133] The most likely reason for the lack of enhanced systolic function after revascularization in zones judged to be viable before revascularization is the presence of subendocardial scar. That is, certain segments showing 20 to 30 percent subendocardial scarring may not demonstrate improved systolic thickening after revascularization, even if greater than 50 percent ^{201}Tl uptake is seen in those regions. However, such patients may benefit from revascularization by reducing stress-induced ischemic dysfunction or reinfarction. Other problems with ^{201}Tl include poor-quality images in obese patients, difficulty in distinguishing attenuation artifacts from scar, and the long imaging time to perform rest-redistribution studies (e.g., 4 hours).

Technetium-99m-Labeled Agents (see Chap. 13)

Technetium-99m-labeled perfusion agents do not show significant redistribution over time after being injected intravenously at rest. Nevertheless, several studies have shown comparable sensitivity and specificity for viability detection between these agents and ^{201}Tl.[134,135] The advantage of ^{99m}Tc-labeled agents is less attenuation and less scatter than noted with ^{201}Tl, which produces higher quality images. In addition, gated SPECT imaging can be undertaken with ^{99m}Tc-sestamibi or ^{99m}Tc-tetrofosmin to allow for simultaneous assessment of regional systolic thickening in myocardial perfusion. Demonstration of intact thickening at rest or when images are acquired during dobutamine infusion indicates viability. The detection of viability in asynergic regions is enhanced with nitrates given prior to ^{99m}Tc-sestamibi administration, as demonstrated by Sciagra and associates.[136] This study showed the prognostic value of nitrate ^{99m}Tc-sestamibi perfusion imaging in relation to medical versus revascularization therapy.

Positron Emission Tomography (see Chap. 13)

Positron emission tomography is considered by many to be the standard of reference for the noninvasive detection of myocardial viability by nuclear cardiology techniques because PET imaging can simultaneously assess myocardial perfusion and metabolism.[137] Nitrogen-13-labeled ammonia is the most often used perfusion tracer, and FDG is the metabolic tracer for assessing glucose utilization. Patients with a mismatch pattern, with reduced perfusion but preserved FDG uptake, will show improved regional and global left ventricular function after revascularization, whereas patients demonstrating a concordant reduction in perfusion and FDG uptake (a "match" pattern) have predominantly myocardial scar as the cause of asynergy, and segments showing this pattern have a significantly lower chance of improved function after revascularization. Preserved myocardial oxygen consumption estimated by carbon 11 (^{11}C)-acetate PET imaging is found in myocardial regions that are hibernating. Hence, ^{11}C-acetate PET imaging[138] is an alternative to FDG-PET imaging for detection of viability. From the practical standpoint relevant to clinical decision-making, no difference in cardiac event-free survival between PET-guided and SPECT-guided patient management has been observed.[139] Both techniques are associated with comparable outcomes with respect to patient survival after revascularization (Fig. 16–8).[132,139]

Dobutamine Echocardiography (see Chap. 11)

Low-dose dobutamine echocardiography is another useful modality for assessment of viability.[5,133] The rationale for inotropic stress is the identification of contractile reserve in zones of severe myocardial asynergy. This technique furnishes an alternative noninvasive approach to resting SPECT perfusion imaging or PET imaging. Enhanced systolic thickening with low-dose dobutamine predicts functional recovery well. A biphasic response in which systolic thickening increases at low doses and then deteriorates at high doses indicates both viability and ischemia and is the most sensitive criterion for improved function after revascularization.[140] End-diastolic wall thickness is also an important marker of

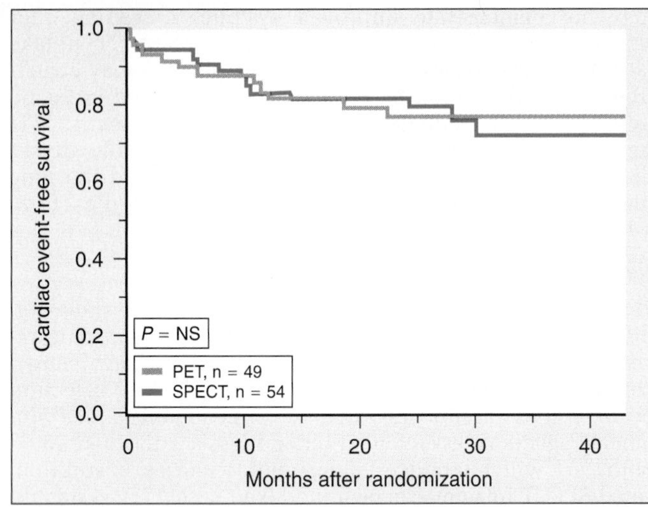

FIGURE 16–8 Cardiac event-free survival curves for patients randomized to ^{13}N-ammonia/^{18}FDG-PET or stress/rest ^{99m}Tc-sestamibi SPECT-based management (revascularization or medical therapy). All patients were potential candidates for revascularization. Note that there was no difference in survival with either the PET or the SPECT strategy in patient evaluation. (From Siebelink H-MJ, Blanksma PK, Crijns HJGM, et al: No difference in cardiac event-free survival between positron emission tomography-guided and single-photon emission computed tomography-guided patient management: A prospective, randomized comparison of patients with suspicion of jeopardized myocardium. J Am Coll Cardiol 37:81, 2001. Copyright 2001, with permission from American College of Cardiology Foundation.)

myocardial viability in patients with suspected hibernation and has been shown to predict recovery of function in a manner similar to that of ^{201}Tl scintigraphy after revascularization. The greater the number of viable segments detected by dobutamine echocardiography, the greater the chance is of survival after revascularization in patients with ischemic cardiomyopathy.

Contrast echocardiography with microbubbles for assessment of myocardial perfusion is a complementary technique to evaluating inotropic reserve for viability assessment in CAD patients with severe left ventricular dysfunction. This may be beneficial in predicting left ventricular contractile recovery in patients with acute myocardial infarction who have undergone reperfusion therapy.[141] The presence of preserved myocardial perfusion by myocardial contrast echocardiography before primary coronary stenting in acute myocardial infarction patients is associated with maintained or improved perfusion at 3 to 5 days and eventual recovery of resting wall motion of the infarct zone.[142] The greater the improvement in microcirculatory perfusion by intravenous contrast echocardiography, the greater the functional recovery in the zone of infarction. Myocardial contrast echocardiography can also be used to identify hibernating myocardium. In one study in 20 patients, the sensitivity of contrast echocardiography for prediction of recovery of function after revascularization was 90 percent, compared with 92 percent for ^{201}Tl SPECT and 80 percent for demonstration of dobutamine-induced contractile reserve.[143] A drawback of the contrast echocardiographic technique is artifacts in basal inferior segments, limiting interpretation in this area.[144]

Magnetic Resonance Imaging (see Chap. 14)

Contrast-enhanced MRI can accurately distinguish normal myocardium from myocardium with subendocardial or transmural scar based on the spatial extent of hyperenhancement.[145,146] With this technique, gadolinium is injected intravenously, and the agent concentrates in necrotic tissue in patients with acute infarction or in scar tissue 10 minutes later, whereas it has washed out of normally perfused and viable myocardium. The scarred area appears bright, and there is a close correlation between the volume of the signal enhancement and the transmural extent of nonviability. Wagner and colleagues reported that resting SPECT and contrast-enhanced MRI detect transmural myocardial infarctions at similar rates (Fig. 16–9), but MRI has significantly higher sensitivity for detecting subendocardial infarcts that are missed by SPECT.[147] In this study, cardiac MRI identified 92 percent of segments with subendocardial infarction characterized by less than 50 percent transmural extent of the full thickness of the left ventricular wall, whereas SPECT identified only 28 percent of these areas. Both techniques show comparable specificity (97 to 98 percent). MRI hyperenhancement, as a detector of myocardial scar, seems to identify scar tissue more frequently than PET (Fig. 16–10),[148] and MRI also differentiates between subendocardial scar and transmural scar better than PET.

The clinical reproducibility of contrast-enhanced MRI for infarct size assessment is excellent and compares favorably with that of clinical SPECT.[149] McCrohon and associates demonstrated that gadolinium-enhanced cardiac MRI may be a very useful technique to distinguish ischemic cardiomyopathy causing left ventricular dysfunction from dilated cardiomyopathy.[150] In that study, CAD patients had contrast enhancement primarily with a subendocardial or transmural pattern, whereas patients with dilated cardiomyopathy had either no enhancement (59 percent), patchy or midwall enhancement different from the distribution in CAD patients (28 percent), or enhancement patterns indistinguishable from those of patients with ischemic cardiomyopathy (13 percent). Finally, in a study looking at the ability of contrast MRI to predict improvement in left ventricular function after revascularization, Kim and associates[151] showed that the likelihood of improvement in regional contractility after revascularization decreased progressively as the transmural extent of hyperenhancement observed before revascularization increased. Approximately 80 percent of segments with no hyperenhancement improved function after revascularization, whereas if only 25 percent of the transmural tissue was normal, only a small percentage improved with revascularization.

Dobutamine MRI may also be employed for the assessment of viability and predicting myocardial functional recovery after revascularization.[152] Dobutamine-induced systolic wall thickening in zones of severe myocardial asynergy has an approximately 70 percent to 90 percent sensitivity and specificity for predicting functional recovery after revascularization. Dobutamine MRI with tagging and contrast-enhanced MRI have been shown to be complementary in assessing functional recovery after reperfused myocardial infarction.[153] A reduction in the transmural extent of a hyperenhancement by contrast-enhanced MRI early after myocardial infarction is associated with early restoration of flow and subsequent improvement in regional function.[154]

As previously cited for other applications with cardiac MRI, problems include patient claustrophobia in the closed scanner-designed instruments; inability to scan patients with implantable devices such as pacemakers, defibrillators, and cerebral aneurysm clips; and

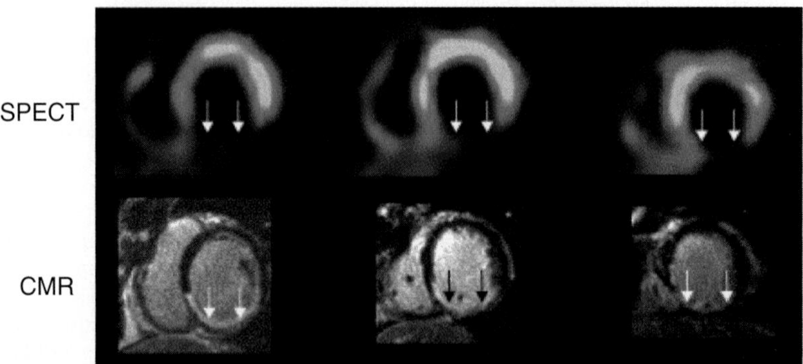

FIGURE 16–9 Short-axis views of resting thallium-201 single-photon emission computed tomography (^{201}Tl-SPECT) (top row) and contrast-enhanced cardiac magnetic resonance imaging (MRI) in a patient with a nearly transmural inferior wall infarction. Note that an area of delayed hyperenhancement on MRI scans (arrows) correlates well with the region of the severe perfusion abnormality on SPECT scan. (From Wagner A, Mahrholdt H, Holly TA, et al: Contrast-enhanced MRI and routine single photon emission computed tomography (SPECT) perfusion imaging for detection of subendocardial myocardial infarcts: An imaging study. Lancet 361:374, 2003.)

inability to obtain adequate images in patients with significantly irregular rhythms such as atrial fibrillation. Image artifact emanating from excessive respiratory motion may be a problem without good respiratory gating techniques such as navigator imaging. Long-term outcome studies in large numbers of patients with respect to the capability of contrast-enhanced MRI techniques to identify which patients have the best prognosis with revascularization versus medical therapy have not been undertaken as have been for the more conventional techniques employing radionuclide imaging or echocardiography.

STRENGTHS AND WEAKNESSES OF VARIOUS MODALITIES FOR ASSESSING VIABILITY

When compared with ^{201}Tl or ^{99m}Tc-sestamibi, dobutamine echocardiography is more specific but less sensitive. The positive predictive value of inotropic reserve for predicting improved regional systolic function with dobutamine echocardiography after revascularization is higher than that of ^{201}Tl scintigraphy when greater than 50 percent ^{201}Tl uptake is used as the criterion for myocardial viability. The number of asynergic segments exhibiting preserved ^{201}Tl uptake or showing rest ^{201}Tl redistribution exceeds the number of segments with residual capacity for systolic thickening as determined by dobutamine infusion.[155] Similarly, the number of severely asynergic segments with preserved FDG uptake significantly on PET imaging exceeds the number of segments with residual inotropic reserve on dobutamine echocardiography.[156]

The sensitivity of dobutamine echocardiography is lower than the sensitivity of SPECT imaging because certain regions that are severely underperfused and are akinetic at rest with no flow reserve can be viable but not demonstrate enhanced systolic thickening, even with the lowest doses of dobutamine.[157] Thus, SPECT imaging has a higher negative predictive value in terms of predicting which segments will *not* improve after revascularization. The combination of ^{201}Tl SPECT and dobutamine echocardiography provided higher accuracy than either technique alone for prediction of recovery of function after revascularization.[158]

Dobutamine echocardiography shows reduced sensitivity in predicting recovery of dysfunctional myocardium supplied by totally occluded vessels.[159] Despite the differences in sensitivity and specificity between SPECT or PET and dobutamine echocardiography for viability detection, the meta-analysis by Allman and associates[132] indicates that there is no measurable performance difference for predicting survival benefit from revascularization between the three imaging techniques. The decrease in mortality with revascularization of viable myocardium was 42.8 percent for ^{201}Tl and 40.5 percent for dobutamine echocardiography (see Fig. 16–7).[132] The lower the resting left ventricular ejection fraction is in patients with viable myocardium, the greater the survival benefit is after revascularization.

Summary of Approaches to Assessment of Viability

Taken together, all of the techniques for the assessment of myocardial viability have high accuracy in the noninvasive detection of viable but dysfunctional myocardium. All provide value in decision-making that is supplementary to clinical and coronary angiographic information alone with respect to the benefit of coronary revascularization in patients with ischemic cardiomyopathy. All the techniques show that the greater the number of viable segments preoperatively, the greater the improvement in ejection fraction and exercise tolerance after revascularization. A limitation of the published studies in the literature regarding the value of viability imaging is that patients were not randomized to medical therapy versus revascularization.[160] Referral bias may have been prevalent in the allocation of patients to either medical therapy or revascularization. Thus, the studies showing better outcomes with revascularization for patients with viability should be considered observational. A note of caution regarding viability imaging, in general, deserves mention. Increased left ventricular volumes and cavity size are predictors of poor prognosis in patients with ischemic cardiomyopathy even when viability is evident.[161] Progressive remodeling after infarction limits the value of revascularization in enhancing left ventricular function.

Table 16–4 summarizes the strengths and limitations of the various noninvasive techniques for the detection of myocardial viability. All have been shown to be clinically useful in identifying which patients with ischemic cardiomyopathy have the greatest chance of enhancement of regional and global left ventricular function, as well as improved survival, after revascularization. Contrast-enhanced MRI is emerging as one of the most promising techniques for assessment of myocardial viability and currently exhibits the greatest sensitivity for detecting subendocardial scar because of its superior spatial resolution compared with nuclear and echocardiographic techniques.

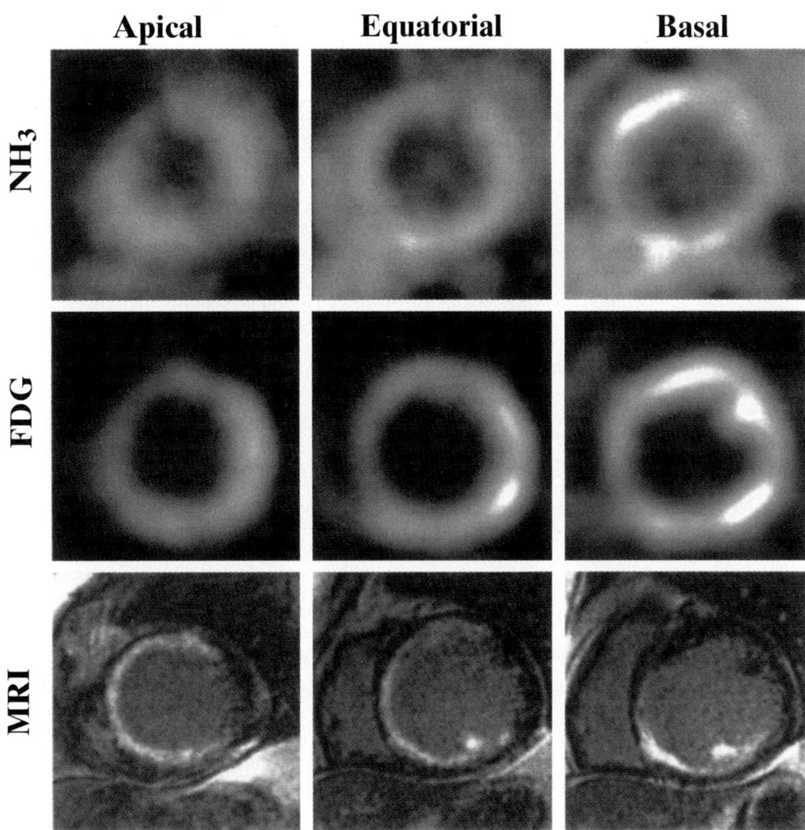

FOIGURE 16–10 Short-axis positron emission tomography (PET) images as part of a viability study employing nitrogen-13 ammonia (NH_3) for perfusion and fluorodeoxyglucose-18 (FDG) for metabolism compared with contrast magnetic resonance imaging (MRI) with evidence for delayed hyperenhancement shown on the bottom row. Note that in the areas showing reduced perfusion and metabolism, a corresponding increased MRI signal is observed. Because of better spatial resolution with MRI than with PET, the differentiation between subendocardial and transmural scans can be better identified. Often the border between hyperenhanced regions and normal areas is well delineated (see comparisons above). (From Klein C, Nekolla SG, Bengel FM, et al: Assessment of myocardial viability with contrast-enhanced magnetic resonance imaging: Comparison with positron emission tomography. Circulation 105:162, 2002.)

TABLE 16–4 Strengths and Limitations of Noninvasive Techniques for Assessment of Myocardial Viability

Technique	Strengths	Limitations
SPECT imaging	High sensitivity for predicting improved function after revascularization Uses quantitative objective criteria (e.g., ≥60 percent segmental uptake) FDG imaging with special collimator LVEF quantitated on ^{99m}Tc-sestamibi or ^{99m}TC-tetrofosmin imaging Predictive of clinical outcomes in a large number of studies	Reduced spatial resolution and sensitivity in comparison to PET Less quantitative than PET Areas of attenuation (e.g., inferior wall on ^{99m}Tc-sestamibi scans) misconstrued as nonviability Cannot differentiate endocardial from epicardial viability Lower specificity than dobutamine echocardiography for predicting improved function after revascularization but higher sensitivity
PET imaging	Simultaneous assessment of perfusion and metabolism More sensitive than other techniques Good specificity No attenuation problems Absolute blood flow can be measured Predictive of outcomes	Lower specificity than dobutamine echocardiography or MRI Cannot separate endocardial from epicardial viability High cost and highly sophisticated technology Limited availability
Dobutamine echocardiography	Higher specificity than nuclear techniques Viability assessed at low doses and ischemia at higher doses Evaluation of mitral regurgitation on baseline echocardiography Good spatial resolution Predictive of clinical outcomes Widely available Lower cost than dobutamine MRI	Poor windows in 30 percent of patients Lower sensitivity than nuclear techniques Viable regions with absent flow reserve will not show increased thickening during dobutamine stimulation Reliance on visual assessment of wall thickening
Contrast echocardiography	Microcirculatory integrity evaluated as well as systolic thickening Better estimation of extent of viability than functional assessment alone Precise delineation of area of necrosis Viability assessed in presence of total coronary occlusion Use of very long pulsing intervals Pulse inversion, power pulse inversion, and power modulation reduce attenuation artifacts	Difficult windows in 30 percent of patients Attenuation problems Scant clinical data available
Contrast-enhanced MRI and dobutamine MRI	Delayed hyperenhancement accurate for measuring extent of transmural scar Superior spatial resolution compared with nuclear and echo techniques More accurate detection of subendocardial infarction than echo or nuclear techniques Can evaluate inotropic reserve with tagging Measurement of wall thickness more accurate than with TEE Simultaneous assessment of perfusion, function, and viability Good imaging windows in all patients	Higher cost than echocardiography Limited availability Need better, faster automated techniques Imaging information not available in real time Patients with pacemakers or ICDs cannot be imaged No large outcome studies reported

FDG = ^{18}F-fluorodeoxyglucose; ICDs = implantable cardioverter-defibrillators; LVEF = left ventricular ejection fraction; MRI = magnetic resonance imaging; PET = positron emission tomography; SPECT = single-photon emission computed tomography; TEE = transesophageal echocardiography.

A PERSPECTIVE ON THE FUTURE OF CARDIAC IMAGING

The future appears bright for further progress in technology and clinical application of noninvasive imaging techniques. Advances in instrumentation and the emergence of new imaging agents will permit enhanced diagnostic and prognostic value of the methodologies reviewed in this chapter. With respect to nuclear cardiology, the widespread introduction of attenuation- and scatter-correction reconstruction algorithms with quantitative SPECT will be associated with fewer imaging artifacts and enhanced specificity and sensitivity for CAD detection. New SPECT camera design may provide higher resolution and sensitivity and ultimately the ability to measure absolute coronary flow reserve.[162] New radiopharmaceuticals on the horizon may allow molecular imaging of apoptosis, inflammation, and gene expression. Imaging of vulnerable atherosclerotic plaques and angiogenesis may soon be feasible. Receptor imaging of the adrenergic nervous system in the heart may have clinical utility in patients with heart failure.

With respect to contrast echocardiography, progress with microbubble contrast agents and imaging technology to enhance the microbubble signal-to-noise ratio will enable better assessment of myocardial perfusion and viability with intravenous injection of contrast material. Imaging of myocardial inflammation after ischemia-reperfusion, imaging with microbubbles targeted to *d*-integrins for evaluation of angiogenesis, detection of inflamed plaques, and imaging of acute cardiac transplant rejection have been shown to be feasible.[163-167] Microbubbles adhere to damaged endothelial cells and may thus furnish a way to assess areas of microvascular endothelial dysfunction in vivo. Microbubbles may ultimately prove useful for local drug delivery, since such bubbles can be destroyed in tissue by ultrasound in vivo.

We can expect continued advances in the field of cardiac MRI in the ensuing years. In addition to the noninvasive assessment of regional and global function, myocardial perfusion with first-pass gadolinium contrast with rest and stress, and viability assessment by quantitating the transmural extent of delayed hyperenhancement, cardiac magnetic resonance looks promising for imaging atherosclerotic plaques and determining its constituents, MRCA for detection of coronary stenoses, and molecular imaging using targeted contrast agents as with labeling of stem cells or macrophages with superparamagnetic iron oxide particles. In vivo characterization of molecular processes using nanoscale paramagnetic targeting agents (nanoparticles) for "hot spot" MRI has proved feasible.[168] Spectroscopic imaging using carbon-13-enhanced compounds may permit imaging of biochemical pathways in the heart.[30] The ability to visualize and track catheters will allow invasive MRCA that could replace x-ray angiography in the future.

Multislice CT is being perfected to achieve improved resolution and shorter acquisition times, which should allow for routine coronary lumen imaging and defining plaque composition. EBCT allows for rapid image acquisition in the time of 50 msec to 100 msec per slice and also has been used to perform contrast-enhanced coronary angiography. Its disadvantages compared with multislice CT are the poor signal-to-noise ratio and increased slice thickness, as well as the lack of general availability of EBCT. Compared with cardiac MRI, the radiation dose is a factor. With multislice CT, new scanners now permit 16 slices per rotation, which allows for greater coverage for a given acquisition time. The whole heart can be scanned with one breath-hold with a slice thickness of 1 mm.

REFERENCES

1. O'Rourke RA, Brundage BH, Froelicher VF, et al: American College of Cardiology/American Heart Association expert consensus document on electron beam computed tomography for the diagnosis and prognosis of coronary artery disease. J Am Coll Cardiol 36:326, 2000.
2. Maddahi J, Gambhir SS: Cost-effective selection of patients for coronary angiography. J Nucl Cardiol 4(Suppl):141, 1997.
3. Gibbons R: Nuclear cardiology in hospital-based practice. J Nucl Cardiol 4(Suppl):179, 1997.
4. Bax JJ, Wijns W, Cornel JH, et al: Accuracy of currently available techniques for prediction of functional recovery after revascularization in patients with left ventricular dysfunction due to chronic coronary artery disease: Comparison of pooled data. J Am Coll Cardiol 30:1451, 1997.

Assessment of Left Ventricular Function at Rest

5. Cheitlin MD, Armstrong WF, Aurigemma GP, et al: ACC/AHA/ASE 2003 guideline update for the clinical application of echocardiography: Summary article. A report of the American College of Cardiology/American Heart Association Task Force on Practice Guidelines (ACC/AHA/ASE Committee to Update the 1997 Guidelines on the Clinical Application of Echocardiography). J Am Coll Cardiol 42:954, 2003. Available at: www.acc.org/clinical/guidelines/echo/index.pdf.
6. Levy D, Labib SB, Anderson KM, et al: Determinants of sensitivity and specificity of electrocardiographic criteria for left ventricular hypertrophy. Circulation 81:815, 1990.
7. Bikkina M, Levy D, Evans JC, et al: Left ventricular mass and risk of stroke in an elderly cohort. The Framingham Heart Study. JAMA 272:33, 1994.
8. Quiñones MA, Greenberg BH, Kopelen HA, et al: Echocardiographic predictors of clinical outcome in patients with left ventricular dysfunction enrolled in the SOLVD registry and trials: Significance of left ventricular hypertrophy. J Am Coll Cardiol 35:1237, 2000.
9. Gardin J: How reliable are serial echocardiographic measurements in detecting regression in left ventricular hypertrophy and changes in function? J Am Coll Cardiol 34:1633, 1999.
10. Palmieri V, Dahlöf B, DeQuattro V, et al: Reliability of echocardiographic assessment of left ventricular structure and function: The PRESERVE study. J Am Coll Cardiol 34:1625, 1999.
11. Gopal AS, Schnellbaecher MJ, Shen Z, et al: Freehand three-dimensional echocardiography for determination of left ventricular volume and mass in patients with abnormal ventricles: Comparison with magnetic resonance imaging. J Am Soc Echocardiogr 10:853, 1997.
12. Cain P, Khoury V, Short L, et al: Usefulness of quantitative echocardiographic techniques to predict recovery of regional and global left ventricular function after acute myocardial infarction. Am J Cardiol 91:391, 2003.
13. Gibson DG, Francis DP: Clinical assessment of left ventricular diastolic function. Heart 89:231, 2003.
14. Mitani I, Jain D, Joska TM, et al: Doxorubicin cardiotoxicity: Prevention of congestive heart failure with serial cardiac function monitoring with equilibrium radionuclide angiocardiography in the current era. J Nucl Cardiol 10:132, 2003.
15. Le Guludec D, Gauthier H, Porcher R, et al: Prognostic value of radionuclide angiography in patients with right ventricular arrhythmias. Circulation 103:1972, 2001.
16. Groch MW, DePuey EG, Belzberg AC, et al: Planar imaging versus gated blood-pool SPECT for the assessment of ventricular performance: a multicenter study. J Nucl Med 42:1773, 2001.
17. Sharir T, Berman DS, Waechter PB, et al: Quantitative analysis of regional motion and thickening by gated myocardial perfusion SPECT: normal heterogeneity and criteria for abnormality. J Nucl Med 42:1630, 2001.
18. Nichols K, Santana CA, Folks R, et al: Comparison between ECTb and QGS for assessment of left ventricular function from gated myocardial perfusion SPECT. J Nucl Cardiol 9:285, 2002.
19. Taillefer R, DePuey EG, Udelson JE, et al: Comparative diagnostic accuracy of Tl-201 and Tc-99m sestamibi SPECT imaging (perfusion and ECG-gated SPECT) in detecting coronary artery disease in women. J Am Coll Cardiol 29:69, 1997.
20. Smanio PEP, Watson DD, Segalla DL, et al: Value of gating of technetium-99m sestamibi single-photon emission computed tomographic imaging. J Am Coll Cardiol 30:1687, 1997.
21. Shirai N, Yamagishi H, Yoshiyama M, et al: Incremental value of assessment of regional wall motion for detection of multivessel coronary artery disease in exercise ^{201}Tl gated myocardial perfusion imaging. J Nucl Med 43:443, 2002.
22. Emmett L, Iwanochko RM, Freeman MR, et al: Reversible regional wall motion abnormalities on exercise technetium-99m-gated cardiac single photon emission computed tomography predict high-grade angiographic stenoses. J Am Coll Cardiol 39:991, 2002.
23. Sharir T, Germano G, Kang X, et al: Prediction of myocardial infarction versus cardiac death by gated myocardial perfusion SPECT: Risk stratification by the amount of stress-induced ischemia and the poststress ejection fraction. J Nucl Med 42:831, 2001.
24. Calnon DA, Kastner RJ, Smith WH, et al: Validation of a new counts-based gated single photon emission computed tomography method for quantifying left ventricular systolic function: Comparison with equilibrium radionuclide angiography. J Nucl Cardiol 4:464, 1997.
25. Manrique A, Faraggi M, Vera P, et al: ^{201}Tl and ^{99m}Tc-MIBI gated SPECT in patients with large perfusion defects and left ventricular dysfunction: Comparison with equilibrium radionuclide angiography. J Nucl Med 40:805, 1999.
26. He ZX, Cwajg E, Preslar JS, et al: Accuracy of left ventricular ejection fraction determined by gated myocardial perfusion SPECT with Tl-201 and Tc-99m sestamibi: Comparison with first-pass radionuclide angiography. J Nucl Cardiol 6:412, 1999.
27. Vaduganathan P, He ZX, Vick GW 3rd, et al: Evaluation of left ventricular wall motion, volumes, and ejection fraction by gated myocardial tomography with technetium 99m-labeled tetrofosmin: A comparison with cine magnetic resonance imaging. J Nucl Cardiol 6:3, 1999.
28. Faber TL, Vansant JP, Pettigrew RI, et al: Evaluation of left ventricular endocardial volumes and ejection fractions computed from gated perfusion SPECT with magnetic resonance imaging: comparison of two methods. J Nucl Cardiol 8:645, 2001.
29. Saab G, Dekemp RA, Ukkonen H, et al: Gated fluorine 18 fluorodeoxyglucose positron emission tomography: determination of global and regional left ventricular function and myocardial tissue characterization. J Nucl Cardiol 10:297, 2003.
30. Forder JR, Pohost GM: Cardiovascular nuclear magnetic resonance: Basic and clinical applications. J Clin Invest 111:1630, 2003.
31. Manning WJ, Stuber M, Danias PG, et al: Coronary magnetic resonance imaging: Current status. Curr Probl Cardiol 27:275, 2002.
32. Pennell D: Cardiovascular magnetic resonance. Heart 85:581, 2001.
33. Prasad S, Pennell DJ: Magnetic resonance imaging in the assessment of patients with heart failure. J Nucl Cardiol 9:S60, 2002.
34. Lindner JR, Wei K: Contrast echocardiography. Curr Probl Cardiol 27:454, 2002.
35. Lang RM, Mor-Avi V, Zoghbi WA, et al: The role of contrast enhancement in echocardiographic assessment of left ventricular function. Am J Cardiol 90(suppl 10A):28J, 2002.

Detection of Coronary Artery Disease: General and Exercise ECG

36. Ropers D, Baum U, Pohle K, et al: Detection of coronary artery stenoses with thin-slice multi-detector row spiral computed tomography and multiplanar reconstruction. Circulation 107:664, 2003
37. de Feyter PJ, Nieman K, van Ooijen P, et al: Non-invasive coronary artery imaging with electron beam computed tomography and magnetic resonance imaging. Heart 84:442, 2000.
38. Gibbons RJ, Balady GJ, Bricker JT, et al: ACC/AHA 2002 guideline update for exercise testing: summary article: A report of the ACC/AHA Task Force on Practice Guidelines (Committee to Update the 1997 Exercise Testing Guidelines). Circulation 106:1883, 2002. Available at: www.acc.org/clinical/guidelines/exercise/dirIndex.htm.
39. Gianrossi R, Detrano R, Mulvihill D, et al: Exercise-induced ST depression in the diagnosis of coronary artery disease. A meta-analysis. Circulation 80:87, 1989.
40. Froelicher VF, Lehmann KG, Thomas R, et al: The electrocardiographic exercise test in a population with reduced workup bias: Diagnostic performance, computerized interpretation, and multivariable prediction. Veterans Affairs Cooperative Study in Health Services: 016 (QUEXTA) Study Group. Qualitative Exercise Testing and Angiography. Ann Intern Med 128:965, 1998.
41. Alexander KP, Shaw LJ, Shaw LK, et al: Value of exercise treadmill testing in women. J Am Coll Cardiol 32:1657, 1998 (published erratum appears in J Am Coll Cardiol 33:289, 1999).
42. Sansoy V, Watson DD, Beller GA: Significance of slow upsloping ST-segment depression on exercise stress testing. Am J Cardiol 79:709, 1997.
43. Gibbons RJ, Abrams J, Chatterjee K, et al: ACC/AHA 2002 guideline update for the management of patients with chronic stable angina-summary article: A report of the American College of Cardiology/American Heart Association Task Force on Practice Guidelines (Committee on the Management of Patients With Chronic Stable Angina). J Am Coll Cardiol 41:159, 2003.

Detection of Coronary Artery Disease: Perfusion Imaging

44. Klocke FJ, Baird MG, Bateman TM, et al: ACC/AHA/ASNC guidelines for the clinical use of cardiac radionuclide imaging: A report of the American College of Cardiology/American Heart Association Task Force on Practice Guidelines (ACC/AHA/ASNC Committee to Revise the 1995 Guidelines for the Clinical Use of Radionuclide Imaging). 2003. American College of Cardiology Web Site. Available at: http://www.acc.org/clinical/guidelines/radio/rni_fulltext.pdf.
45. Beller GA, Zaret BL: Contributions of nuclear cardiology to diagnosis and prognosis of patients with coronary artery disease. Circulation 101:1465, 2000.

46. Lima RSL, Watson DD, Goode AR, et al: Incremental value of combined perfusion and function over perfusion alone by gated SPECT myocardial perfusion imaging for detection of severe three-vessel coronary artery disease. J Am Coll Cardiol 42:64, 2003.
47. Berman DS, Kang X, Schisterman EF, et al: Serial changes on quantitative myocardial perfusion SPECT in patients undergoing revascularization or conservative therapy. J Nucl Cardiol 8:428, 2001.
48. Hendel RC, Corbett JR, Cullom SJ, et al: The value and practice of attenuation correction for myocardial perfusion SPECT imaging: A joint position statement from the American Society of Nuclear Cardiology and the Society of Nuclear Medicine. J Nucl Cardiol 9:135, 2002.
49. Duvernoy CS, Ficaro EP, Karabajakian MZ, et al: Improved detection of left main coronary artery disease with attenuation-corrected SPECT. J Nucl Cardiol 7:639, 2000.
50. Hendel RC, Berman DS, Cullom SJ, et al: Multicenter clinical trial to evaluate the efficacy of correction for photon attenuation and scatter in SPECT myocardial perfusion imaging. Circulation 99:2742, 1999.
51. Links JM, DePuey EG, Taillefer R, et al: Attenuation correction and gating synergistically improve the diagnostic accuracy of myocardial perfusion SPECT. J Nucl Cardiol 9:183, 2002.
52. Hendel RC: Diagnostic and prognostic applications for vasodilator stress myocardial perfusion imaging and the importance of radiopharmaceutical selection. J Nucl Cardiol 8:523, 2001.
53. Elhendy A, Bax JJ, Poldermans D: Dobutamine stress myocardial perfusion imaging in coronary artery disease. J Nucl Med 43:1634, 2002.

Detection of Coronary Artery Disease: Echocardiography

54. Marwick T: Stress echocardiography. Heart 89:113, 2003.
55. Kymes SM, Bruns DE, Shaw LJ, et al: Anatomy of a meta-analysis: A critical review of "exercise echocardiography or exercise SPECT imaging? A meta-analysis of diagnostic test performance." J Nucl Cardiol 7:599, 2000.
56. Marwick TH, Nemec JJ, Pashkow FJ, et al: Accuracy and limitations of exercise echocardiography in a routine clinical setting. J Am Coll Cardiol 19:74, 1992.
57. Secknus MA, Marwick TH: Evolution of dobutamine echocardiography protocols and indications: Safety and side effects in 3,011 studies over 5 years. J Am Coll Cardiol 29:1234, 1997.
58. Stewart MJ: Contrast echocardiography. Heart 89:342, 2003.
59. Hoffman R, Lethen H, Marwick T, et al: Analysis of interinstitutional observer agreement in interpretation of dobutamine stress echocardiograms. J Am Coll Cardiol 27:330, 1996.
60. Wei K, Crouse L, Weiss J, et al: Comparison of usefulness of dipyridamole stress myocardial contrast echocardiography to technetium-99m sestamibi single-photon emission computed tomography for detection of coronary artery disease (PB127 Multicenter Phase 2 Trial results). Am J Cardiol 91:1293, 2003.
61. Heinle SK, Noblin J, Goree-Best P, et al: Assessment of myocardial perfusion by harmonic power Doppler imaging at rest and during adenosine stress: Comparison with ^{99m}Tc-sestamibi SPECT imaging. Circulation 102:55, 2000.
62. Brown K: Diagnostic and prognostic use of noninvasive imaging in patients with known or suspected coronary artery disease. Comparison of stress myocardial perfusion imaging and echocardiography. Cardiol Rev 6:90, 1998.
63. O'Keefe JH Jr, Barnhart CS, Bateman TM: Comparison of stress echocardiography and stress myocardial perfusion scintigraphy for diagnosing coronary artery disease and assessing its severity. Am J Cardiol 75:25D, 1995.
64. Schinkel AF, Bax JJ, Geleijnse ML, et al: Noninvasive evaluation of ischaemic heart disease: Myocardial perfusion imaging or stress echocardiography? Eur Heart J 24:789, 2003.
65. Smanio PEP, Watson DD, Segalla DL, et al: Value of gating of technetium-99m sestamibi single-photon emission computed tomographic imaging. J Am Coll Cardiol 30:1687, 1997.
66. Fleischmann KE, Hunink MG, Kuntz KM, et al: Exercise echocardiography or exercise SPECT imaging? A meta-analysis of diagnostic test performance. JAMA 280:913, 1998.
67. Jacobs M: Review: Exercise ECHO is a more specific and discriminatory test than exercise SPECT for coronary artery disease. (Diagnosis.) ACP Journal Club 130:45, 1999. (Abstract and commentary for: Fleischmann KE, Hunink MG, Kuntz KM, et al: Exercise echocardiography or exercise SPECT imaging? A meta-analysis of diagnostic test performance. JAMA 280:913, 1998.)
68. Santoro GM, Sciagra R, Buonamici P, et al: Head-to-head comparison of exercise stress testing, pharmacologic stress echocardiography, and perfusion tomography as first-line examination for chest pain in patients without history of coronary artery disease. J Nucl Cardiol 5:19, 1998.
69. Elhendy A, Geleijnse ML, Roelandt JR, et al: Dobutamine-induced hypoperfusion without transient wall motion abnormalities: Less severe ischemia or less severe stress? J Am Coll Cardiol 27:323, 1996.
70. Smart SC, Bhatia A, Hellman R, et al: Dobutamine-atropine stress echocardiography and dipyridamole sestamibi scintigraphy for the detection of coronary artery disease: Limitations and concordance. J Am Coll Cardiol 36:1265, 2000.
71. Elhendy A, van Domburg RT, Bax JJ, et al: Accuracy of dobutamine technetium 99m sestamibi SPECT imaging for the diagnosis of single-vessel coronary artery disease: Comparison with echocardiography. Am Heart J 139:224, 2000.

Detection of Coronary Artery Disease: MRI and CT

72. Yang PC, Meyer CH, Terashima M, et al: Spiral magnetic resonance coronary angiography with rapid real-time localization. J Am Coll Cardiol 41:1134, 2003.
73. Worthley SG, Helft G, Fuster V, et al: Noninvasive in vivo magnetic resonance imaging of experimental coronary lesions in a porcine model. Circulation 101:2956, 2000.
74. Kim WY, Danias PG, Stuber M, et al: Coronary magnetic resonance angiography for the detection of coronary stenoses. N Engl J Med 345:1863, 2001.
75. Nagel E, Thouet T, Klein C, et al: Noninvasive determination of coronary blood flow velocity with cardiovascular magnetic resonance in patients after stent deployment. Circulation 107:1738, 2003.
76. Langerak SE, Vliegen HW, de Roos A, et al: Detection of vein graft disease using high-resolution magnetic resonance angiography. Circulation 105:328, 2002.
77. Nagel E, Klein C, Paetsch I, et al: Magnetic resonance perfusion measurements for the noninvasive detection of coronary artery disease. Circulation 108:432, 2003.
78. Doyle M, Fuisz A, Kortright E, et al: The impact of myocardial flow reserve on the detection of coronary artery disease by perfusion imaging methods: An NHLBI WISE study. J Cardiovasc Magn Reson 5:475, 2003.
79. Kwong RY, Schussheim AE, Rekhraj S, et al: Detecting acute coronary syndrome in the emergency department with cardiac magnetic resonance imaging. Circulation 107:531, 2003.
80. Kuijpers D, Ho KY, van Dijkman PR, et al: Dobutamine cardiovascular magnetic resonance for the detection of myocardial ischemia with the use of myocardial tagging. Circulation 107:1592, 2003.
81. Ibrahim T, Nekolla SG, Schreiber K, et al: Assessment of coronary flow reserve: Comparison between contrast-enhanced magnetic resonance imaging and positron emission tomography. J Am Coll Cardiol 39:864, 2002.
82. Schwitter J, Nanz D, Kneifel S, et al: Assessment of myocardial perfusion in coronary artery disease by magnetic resonance: A comparison with positron emission tomography and coronary angiography. Circulation 103:2230, 2001.
83. Murphy RE, Moody AR, Morgan PS, et al: Prevalence of complicated carotid atheroma as detected by magnetic resonance direct thrombus imaging in patients with suspected carotid artery stenosis and previous acute cerebral ischemia. Circulation 107:3053, 2003.
84. Kramer CM: Magnetic resonance imaging to identify the high-risk plaque. Am J Cardiol 90(suppl 3):15L, 2002.
85. Yuan C, Zhang SX, Polissar NL, et al: Identification of fibrous cap rupture with magnetic resonance imaging is highly associated with recent transient ischemic attack or stroke. Circulation 105:181, 2002.
86. Fayad ZA, Fuster V, Fallon JT, et al: Noninvasive in vivo human coronary artery lumen and wall imaging using black-blood magnetic resonance imaging. Circulation 102:506, 2000.
87. Fayad ZA, Fuster V, Nikolaou K, et al: Computed tomography and magnetic resonance imaging for noninvasive coronary angiography and plaque imaging: Current and potential future concepts. Circulation 106:2026, 2002.
88. Kooi ME, Cappendijk VC, Cleutjens KB, et al: Accumulation of ultrasmall superparamagnetic particles of iron oxide in human atherosclerotic plaques can be detected by in vivo magnetic resonance imaging. Circulation 107:2453, 2003.
89. Omary RA, Green JD, Schirf BE, et al: Real-time magnetic resonance imaging-guided coronary catheterization in swine. Circulation 107:2656, 2003.
90. Achenbach S, Giesler T, Ropers D, et al: Detection of coronary artery stenoses by contrast-enhanced, retrospectively electrocardiographically-gated, multislice spiral computed tomography. Circulation 103:2535, 2001.
91. Leber AW, Knez A, Becker C, et al: Non-invasive intravenous coronary angiography using electron beam tomography and multislice computed tomography. Heart 89:633, 2003.
92. Greenland P, Gaziano JM: Clinical practice. Selecting asymptomatic patients for coronary computed tomography or electrocardiographic exercise testing. N Engl J Med 349:465, 2003.
93. O'Malley PG, Taylor AJ, Jackson JL, et al: Prognostic value of coronary electron-beam computed tomography for coronary heart disease events in asymptomatic populations. Am J Cardiol 85:945, 2000.
94. Park R, Detrano R, Xiang M, et al: Combined use of computed tomography coronary calcium scores and C-reactive protein levels in predicting cardiovascular events in nondiabetic individuals. Circulation 106:2073, 2002.

Assessment of Prognosis of Patients Evaluated for Coronary Artery Disease

95. Myers J, Prakash M, Froelicher V, et al: Exercise capacity and mortality among men referred for exercise testing. N Engl J Med 346:793, 2002.
96. Morshedi-Meibodi A, Larson MG, Levy D, et al: Heart rate recovery after treadmill exercise testing and risk of cardiovascular disease events (The Framingham Heart Study). Am J Cardiol 90:848, 2002.
97. Mark DB, Shaw L, Harrell FE Jr, et al: Prognostic value of a treadmill exercise score in outpatients with suspected coronary artery disease. N Engl J Med 325:849, 1991.
98. Shaw LJ, Peterson ED, Shaw LK, et al: Use of a prognostic treadmill score in identifying diagnostic coronary disease subgroups. Circulation 98:1622, 1998.
99. Hachamovitch R, Berman DS, Kiat H, et al: Exercise myocardial perfusion SPECT in patients without known coronary artery disease: Incremental prognostic value and use in risk stratification. Circulation 93:905, 1996.
100. Hachamovitch R, Berman DS, Kiat H, et al: Value of stress myocardial perfusion single photon emission computed tomography in patients with normal resting electrocardiograms: An evaluation of incremental prognostic value and cost-effectiveness. Circulation 105:823, 2002.
101. Bogaty P, Guimond J, Robitaille NM, et al: A reappraisal of exercise electrocardiographic indexes of the severity of ischemic heart disease: Angiographic and scintigraphic correlates. J Am Coll Cardiol 29:1497, 1997 (published erratum appears in J Am Coll Cardiol 30:1416, 1997).
102. Berman DS, Hachamovitch R, Kiat H, et al: Incremental value of prognostic testing in patients with known or suspected ischemic heart disease: A basis for optimal utilization of exercise technetium-99m sestamibi myocardial perfusion single-photon emission computed tomography. J Am Coll Cardiol 26:639, 1995 (published erratum appears in J Am Coll Cardiol 27:756, 1996).

103. Beller GA: First Annual Mario S. Verani, MD, Memorial Lecture: Clinical value of myocardial perfusion imaging in coronary artery disease. J Nucl Cardiol 10:529, 2003.
104. Iskander S, Iskandrian AE: Risk assessment using single-photon emission computed tomographic technetium-99m sestamibi imaging. J Am Coll Cardiol 32:57, 1998.
105. Sharir T, Bacher-Stier C, Dhar S, et al: Identification of severe and extensive coronary artery disease by postexercise regional wall motion abnormalities in Tc-99m sestamibi gated single-photon emission computed tomography. Am J Cardiol 86:1171, 2000.
106. Yamagishi H, Shirai N, Yoshiyama M, et al: Incremental value of left ventricular ejection fraction for detection of multivessel coronary artery disease in exercise ^{201}Tl gated myocardial perfusion imaging. J Nucl Med 43:131, 2002.
107. Chatziioannou SN, Moore WH, Ford PV, et al: Prognostic value of myocardial perfusion imaging in patients with high exercise tolerance. Circulation 99:867, 1999.
108. Hachamovitch R, Berman DS, Shaw LJ, et al: Incremental prognostic value of myocardial perfusion single photon emission computed tomography for the prediction of cardiac death: Differential stratification for risk of cardiac death and myocardial infarction. Circulation 97:535, 1998 (published erratum appears in Circulation 98:190, 1998).
109. Hachamovitch R, Hayes SW, Friedman JD, et al: Comparison of the short-term survival benefit associated with revascularization compared with medical therapy in patients with no prior coronary artery disease undergoing stress myocardial perfusion single photon emission computed tomography. Circulation 107:2900, 2003.
110. Shaw LJ, Hachamovitch R, Berman DS, et al: The economic consequences of available diagnostic and prognostic strategies for the evaluation of stable angina patients: An observational assessment of the value of precatheterization ischemia. The Economics of Noninvasive Diagnosis (END) Multicenter Study Group. J Am Coll Cardiol 33:661, 1999.
111. Shaw LJ, Heller GV, Travin MI, et al: Cost analysis of diagnostic testing for coronary artery disease in women with stable chest pain. Economics of Noninvasive Diagnosis (END) study group. J Nucl Cardiol 6:559, 1999.
112. Brown KA, Rowen M: Prognostic value of a normal exercise myocardial perfusion imaging study in patients with angiographically significant coronary artery disease. Am J Cardiol 71:865, 1993.
113. Giri S, Shaw LJ, Murthy DR, et al: Impact of diabetes on the risk stratification using stress single-photon emission computed tomography myocardial perfusion imaging in patients with symptoms suggestive of coronary artery disease. Circulation 105:32, 2002.
114. Berman DS, Kang X, Hayes SW, et al: Adenosine myocardial perfusion single-photon emission computed tomography in women compared with men. Impact of diabetes mellitus on incremental prognostic value and effect on patient management. J Am Coll Cardiol 41:1125, 2003.

Assessment of Prognosis: Stress Echocardiography

115. Heupler S, Mehta R, Lobo A, et al: Prognostic implications of exercise echocardiography in women with known or suspected coronary artery disease. J Am Coll Cardiol 30:414, 1997.
116. Marwick TH, Mehta R, Arheart K, et al: Use of exercise echocardiography for prognostic evaluation of patients with known or suspected coronary artery disease. J Am Coll Cardiol 30:83, 1997.
117. Arruda AM, Das MK, Roger VL, et al: Prognostic value of exercise echocardiography in 2,632 patients ≥65 years of age. J Am Coll Cardiol 37:1036, 2001.
118. McCully RB, Roger VL, Mahoney DW, et al: Outcome after abnormal exercise echocardiography for patients with good exercise capacity: Prognostic importance of the extent and severity of exercise-related left ventricular dysfunction. J Am Coll Cardiol 39:1345, 2002.
119. Arruda-Olson AM, Juracan EM, Mahoney DW, et al: Prognostic value of exercise echocardiography in 5,798 patients: is there a gender difference? J Am Coll Cardiol 39:625, 2002.
120. Marwick TH, Case C, Vasey C, et al: Prediction of mortality by exercise echocardiography: A strategy for combination with the Duke treadmill score. Circulation 103:2566, 2001.

Comparison with Perfusion Imaging

121. Olmos LI, Dakik H, Gordon R, et al: Long-term prognostic value of exercise echocardiography compared with exercise ^{201}Tl, ECG, and clinical variables in patients evaluated for coronary artery disease. Circulation 98:2679, 1998.
122. Geleijnse ML, Elhendy A, van Domburg RT, et al: Cardiac imaging for risk stratification with dobutamine-atropine stress testing in patients with chest pain. Echocardiography, perfusion scintigraphy, or both? Circulation 96:137, 1997.
123. McCully RB, Roger VL, Mahoney DW, et al: Outcome after normal exercise echocardiography and predictors of subsequent cardiac events: Follow-up of 1,325 patients. J Am Coll Cardiol 31:144, 1998.
124. Poldermans D, Fioretti PM, Boersma E, et al: Long-term prognostic value of dobutamine-atropine stress echocardiography in 1737 patients with known or suspected coronary artery disease: A single-center experience. Circulation 99:757, 1999.
125. Cortigiani L, Dodi C, Paolini EA, et al: Prognostic value of pharmacological stress echocardiography in women with chest pain and unknown coronary artery disease. J Am Coll Cardiol 32:1975, 1998.
126. Marwick TH, Case C, Sawada S, et al: Prediction of mortality using dobutamine echocardiography. J Am Coll Cardiol 37:754, 2001.
127. Sicari R, Pasanisi E, Venneri L, et al: Echo Persantine International Cooperative (EPIC) Study Group; Echo Dobutamine International Cooperative (EDIC) Study Group: Stress echo results predict mortality: A large-scale multicenter prospective international study. J Am Coll Cardiol 41:589, 2003.
128. Shaw LJ, Eagle KA, Gersh BJ, et al: Meta-analysis of intravenous dipyridamole-thallium-201 imaging (1985 to 1994) and dobutamine echocardiography (1991 to 1994) for risk stratification before vascular surgery. J Am Coll Cardiol 27:787, 1996.
129. Poldermans D, Arnese M, Fioretti PM, et al: Sustained prognostic value of dobutamine stress echocardiography for late cardiac events after major noncardiac vascular surgery. Circulation 95:53, 1997.
130. Hundley WG, Morgan TM, Neagle CM, et al: Magnetic resonance imaging determination of cardiac prognosis. Circulation 106:2328, 2002.
131. Lauerma K, Virtanen KS, Sipila LM, et al: Multislice MRI in assessment of myocardial perfusion in patients with single-vessel proximal left anterior descending coronary artery disease before and after revascularization. Circulation 96:2859, 1997.

Noninvasive Assessment of Myocardial Viability

132. Allman KC, Shaw LJ, Hachamovitch R, et al: Myocardial viability testing and impact of revascularization on prognosis in patients with coronary artery disease and left ventricular dysfunction: A meta-analysis. J Am Coll Cardiol 39:1151, 2002.
133. Bax JJ, Poldermans D, Elhendy A, et al: Sensitivity, specificity, and predictive accuracies of various noninvasive techniques for detecting hibernating myocardium. Curr Probl Cardiol 26:141, 2001.
134. Udelson JE, Coleman PS, Metherall J, et al: Predicting recovery of severe regional ventricular dysfunction: Comparison of resting scintigraphy with ^{201}Tl and ^{99m}Tc-sestamibi. Circulation 89:2552, 1994.
135. Cuocolo A, Acampa W, Nicolai E, et al: Quantitative thallium-201 and technetium 99m sestamibi tomography at rest in detection of myocardial viability in patients with chronic ischemic left ventricular dysfunction. J Nucl Cardiol 7:8, 2000.
136. Sciagra R, Pellegri M, Pupi A, et al: Prognostic implications of Tc-99m sestamibi viability imaging and subsequent therapeutic strategy in patients with chronic coronary artery disease and left ventricular dysfunction. J Am Coll Cardiol 36:739, 2000.
137. Camici PG: Imaging techniques: Positron emission tomography and myocardial imaging. Heart 83:475, 2000.
138. Wolpers HG, Burchert W, van den Hoff J, et al: Assessment of myocardial viability by use of ^{11}C-acetate and positron emission tomography: Threshold criteria of reversible dysfunction. Circulation 95:1417, 1997.
139. Siebelink HM, Blanksma PK, Crijns HJ, et al: No difference in cardiac event-free survival between positron emission tomography-guided and single-photon emission computed tomography-guided patient management: A prospective, randomized comparison of patients with suspicion of jeopardized myocardium. J Am Coll Cardiol 37:81, 2001.
140. Rizzello V, Schinkel AF, Bax JJ, et al: Individual prediction of functional recovery after coronary revascularization in patients with ischemic cardiomyopathy: The scar-to-biphasic model. Am J Cardiol 91:1406, 2003.
141. Bandano LP, Werren M, Di Chiara A, et al: Contrast echocardiographic evaluation of early changes in myocardial perfusion after recanalization therapy in anterior wall acute myocardial infarction and their relation with early contractile recovery. Am J Cardiol 91:532, 2003.
142. Balcells E, Powers ER, Lepper W, et al: Detection of myocardial viability by contrast echocardiography in acute infarction predicts recovery of resting function and contractile reserve. J Am Coll Cardiol 41:827, 2003.
143. Shimoni S, Fragogiannis NG, Aggeli CJ, et al: Identification of hibernating myocardium with quantitative intravenous myocardial contrast echocardiography: Comparison with dobutamine echocardiography and thallium-201 scintigraphy. Circulation 107:538, 2003.
144. Senior R, Swinburn JM: Incremental value of myocardial contrast echocardiography for the prediction of recovery of function in dobutamine nonresponsive myocardium early after acute myocardial infarction. Am J Cardiol 91:397, 2003.
145. Ramani K, Judd RM, Holly TA, et al: Contrast magnetic resonance imaging in the assessment of myocardial viability in patients with stable coronary artery disease and left ventricular dysfunction. Circulation 98:2687, 1998.
146. Kim RJ, Fieno DS, Parrish TB, et al: Relationship of MRI delayed contrast enhancement to irreversible injury, infarct age, and contractile function. Circulation 100:1992, 1999.
147. Wagner A, Mahrholdt H, Holly TA, et al: Contrast-enhanced MRI and routine single photon emission computed tomography (SPECT) perfusion imaging for detection of subendocardial myocardial infarcts: An imaging study. Lancet 361:374, 2003.
148. Klein C, Nekolla SG, Bengel FM, et al: Assessment of myocardial viability with contrast-enhanced magnetic resonance imaging: Comparison with positron emission tomography Circulation 105:162, 2002.
149. Mahrholdt H, Wagner A, Holly TA, et al: Reproducibility of chronic infarct size measurement by contrast-enhanced magnetic resonance imaging. Circulation 106:2322, 2002.
150. McCrohon JA, Moon JC, Prasad SK, et al: Differentiation of heart failure related to dilated cardiomyopathy and coronary artery disease using gadolinium-enhanced cardiovascular magnetic resonance. Circulation 108:54, 2003.
151. Kim RJ, Wu E, Rafael A, et al: The use of contrast-enhanced magnetic resonance imaging to identify reversible myocardial dysfunction. N Engl J Med 343:1445, 2000.
152. Trent RJ, Waiter GD, Hillis GS, et al: Dobutamine magnetic resonance imaging as a predictor of myocardial functional recovery after revascularization. Heart 83:40, 2000.
153. Kramer CM, Rogers WJ Jr, Mankad S, et al: Contractile reserve and contrast uptake pattern by magnetic resonance imaging and functional recovery after reperfused myocardial infarction. J Am Coll Cardiol 36:1835, 2000.
154. Hillenbrand HB, Kim RJ, Parker MA, et al: Early assessment of myocardial salvage by contrast-enhanced magnetic resonance imaging. Circulation 102:1678, 2000.

Strengths and Weaknesses of Various Modalities for Assessing Viability

155. Perrone-Filardi P, Pace L, Prastaro M, et al: Assessment of myocardial viability in patients with chronic coronary artery disease: Rest-4-hour-24-hour ^{201}Tl tomography versus dobutamine echocardiography. Circulation 97:2712, 1996.

156. Bax JJ, Cornel JH, Visser FC, et al: Prediction of recovery of myocardial dysfunction after revascularization: Comparison of fluorine-18 fluorodeoxyglucose/thallium-201 SPECT, thallium-201 stress-reinjection SPECT and dobutamine echocardiography. J Am Coll Cardiol 28:558, 1996.
157. Skopicki HA, Abraham SA, Weissman NJ, et al: Factors influencing regional myocardial contractile response to inotropic stimulation: Analysis in humans with stable ischemic heart disease. Circulation 94:643, 1996.
158. Dellegrottaglie S, Perrone-Filardi P, Pace L, et al: Prediction of long-term effects of revascularization on regional and global left ventricular function by dobutamine echocardiography and rest Tl-201 imaging alone and in combination in patients with chronic coronary artery disease. J Nucl Cardiol 9:174, 2002.
159. Piscione F, Perrone-Filardi P, De Luca G, et al: Low dose dobutamine echocardiography for predicting functional recovery after coronary revascularisation. Heart 86:679, 2001.
160. Bourque JM, Velazquez EJ, Borges-Neto S, et al: Radionuclide viability testing: Should it affect treatment strategy in patients with cardiomyopathy and significant coronary artery disease? Am Heart J 145:758, 2003.
161. DiCarli MF, Hachamovitch R, Berman DS: The art and science of predicting postrevascularization improvement in left ventricular (LV) function in patients with severely depressed LV function. J Am Coll Cardiol 40:1744, 2002.

A Perspective on the Future of Cardiac Imaging

162. Schwaiger M: Future perspectives and conclusions. Eur Heart J Suppl 3(Suppl F):F, 2001.
163. Lindner JR, Coggins MP, Kaul S, et al: Microbubble persistence in the microcirculation during ischemia/reperfusion and inflammation is caused by integrin- and complement-mediated adherence to activated leukocytes. Circulation 101:668, 2000.
164. Lindner JR, Dayton PA, Coggins MP, et al: Noninvasive imaging of inflammation by ultrasound detection of phagocytosed microbubbles. Circulation 102:531, 2000.
165. Leong-Poi H, Christiansen J, Klibanov AL, et al: Noninvasive assessment of angiogenesis by ultrasound and microbubbles targeted to alpha(v)-integrins. Circulation 107:455, 2003.
166. Lindner JR: Detection of inflamed plaques with contrast ultrasound. Am J Cardiol 90(10C):32L, 2002.
167. Weller GE, Lu E, Csikari MM, et al: Ultrasound imaging of acute cardiac transplant rejection with microbubbles targeted to intercellular adhesion molecule-1. Circulation 108:218, 2003.
168. Wickline SA, Lanza GM: Molecular imaging, targeted therapeutics, and nanoscience. J Cell Biochem Suppl 39:90, 2002.

CHAPTER 17

Cardiac Catheterization

Charles J. Davidson • Robert O. Bonow*

Indications for Diagnostic Cardiac Catheterization

As with any procedure, the decision to recommend cardiac catheterization is based on an appropriate risk-benefit ratio. In general, diagnostic cardiac catheterization is recommended whenever it is clinically important to define the presence or severity of a suspected cardiac lesion that cannot be adequately evaluated by noninvasive techniques. Because the risk of a major complication from cardiac catheterization is less than 1 percent with a mortality of less than 0.08 percent, there are few patients who cannot be studied safely in an active laboratory. Intracardiac pressure measurements and coronary arteriography are procedures that can be performed with reproducible accuracy only by invasive catheterization. Noninvasive estimation of intracardiac pressures can be achieved with echocardiography (see Chap. 11), and magnetic resonance imaging and computed tomography show promise for assessment of coronary anatomy (see Chaps. 14 and 15).

The guidelines for diagnostic coronary angiography have been developed by a joint task force of the American College of Cardiology and the American Heart Association.[1] These guidelines describe a three-tiered priority classification for specific disease states. Class I indications apply to conditions in which there is general agreement that coronary angiography is justified, although this may not be the only appropriate diagnostic procedure. Class II indications apply to conditions in which coronary angiography is frequently performed but about which there is a divergence of opinion with respect to justification of the usefulness or efficacy of the procedure. Class IIa applies to situations in which the weight of evidence is in favor of usefulness. Class IIb indications are less well established by evidence or opinion. Class III conditions are those about which there is general agreement that cardiac catheterization is not ordinarily useful or effective and in some cases may be harmful. Diseases are grouped under several categories: known or suspected coronary heart disease, atypical chest pain, acute myocardial infarction, valvular heart disease, congenital heart disease, and other conditions. Table 17–1 summarizes the class I and IIa recommendations of the task force.

The indications for cardiac catheterization are likely to continue to evolve. Expansion of indications has been in two divergent directions. At one extreme, many critically ill and hemodynamically unstable patients are evaluated during acute myocardial ischemia, severe heart failure, or cardiogenic shock. At the other end of the spectrum, an increasing number of procedures are being performed in an outpatient setting. These settings include hospitals with or without cardiac surgery capability and freestanding or mobile laboratories.[2] The result has been the expansion of traditional indications for cardiac catheterization to include both critically ill patients and ambulatory patients.

Cardiac catheterization should be considered to be a diagnostic test used in combination with complementary noninvasive tests. For example, cardiac catheterization in patients with valvular or congenital heart disease is best done with full echocardiographic knowledge and any other functional information. The catheterization can be directed and simplified without obtaining redundant anatomical information.

Identification of coronary artery disease and assessment of its extent and severity are the most common indications for cardiac catheterization in adults (see Chap. 18). The information obtained by catheterization is crucial to optimize therapy for patients with various chest pain syndromes. In addition, the presence of dynamic coronary vascular lesions, such as spasm or thrombosis, can be identified. The consequences of coronary heart disease, such as ischemic mitral regurgitation or left ventricular dysfunction, can be defined. In the current era of acute percutaneous catheter intervention for acute coronary syndromes, patients are often studied during evolving acute myocardial infarction, unstable angina, or in the early period after acute myocardial injury (see Chaps. 48 and 49). The approach of individual centers in evaluating such patients often depends on local facilities and treatment philosophies as well as the availability of surgical support.

In patients with myocardial disease, cardiac catheterization may provide critical information (see Chap. 59). It can exclude coronary artery disease as the cause of symptoms and evaluate left ventricular dysfunction in patients with cardiomyopathy. Cardiac catheterization also permits quantification of the severity of both diastolic and systolic dysfunction, differentiation of myocardial restriction from pericardial constriction, assessment of the extent of valvular regurgitation, detection of active myocarditis by endomyocardial biopsy, and observation of the cardiovascular response to acute pharmacological intervention.

In patients with valvular heart disease, cardiac catheterization provides data both confirmatory and complementary to noninvasive echocardiography, magnetic resonance, and nuclear studies (see Chap. 57). The risk-benefit ratio of cardiac

*The authors would like to thank Robert Fishman, MD, for his contribution to a previous edition of this chapter.

TABLE 17–1 Indications for Coronary Angiography

Known or Suspected* Coronary Disease in Patients Who Are Currently Asymptomatic or Have Stable Angina (Known: Previous myocardial infarction, coronary bypass surgery, or PTCA. Suspected: Rest- or exercise-induced ECG abnormalities suggesting silent ischemia)

Asymptomatic or Stable Angina

Class I

1. Evidence of high risk on noninvasing testing.
2. Canadian Cardiovascular Society (CSS) class III or IV angina on medical treatment.
3. Patients resuscitated from sudden cardiac death or with sustained monomorphic VT or nonsustained polymorphic VT.

Class IIa

1. CCS class III or IV angina that improves to class I or II on medical therapy.
2. Serial noninvasive testing showing progressive abnormalities.
3. Patient with disability or illness that cannot be stratified by other means.
4. CCS class I or II with intolerance or failure to respond to medical therapy.
5. Individuals whose occupation involves safety of others (e.g., pilots, bus drivers) with abnormal stress test results or high-risk clinical profile.

Nonspecific Chest Pain

Class I

High-risk findings on noninvasive testing.

Class IIa

None.

Unstable Coronary Syndromes

Class I

1. High or intermediate risk for adverse outcome in patients with unstable angina refractory to initial adequate medical therapy or recurrent symptoms after initial stabilization. Emergent catheterization is recommended.
2. High risk for adverse outcome in patients with unstable angina. Urgent catheterization is recommended.
3. High- or intermediate-risk unstable angina that stabilizes after initial treatment.
4. Initially low short-term risk unstable angina that is subsequently high risk on noninvasive testing.
5. Suspected Prinzmetal variant angina.

Class IIa

None.

Patients with Postrevascularization Ischemia

Class I

1. Suspected abrupt closure or subacute stent thrombosis after percutaneous revascularization.
2. Recurrent angina or high-risk criteria on noninvasive evaluation within 9 mo of percutaneous revascularization.

Class IIa

1. Recurrent symptomatic ischemia within 12 mo of CABG.
2. Noninvasive evidence of high-risk criteria occurring at any time postoperatively.
3. Recurrent angina inadequately controlled by medical means after revascularization.

During the Initial Management of Acute MI (MI Suspected and ST Segment Elevation or Bundle Branch Block Present)

Coronary Angiography Coupled with the Intent to Perform Primary PTCA

Class I

1. As an alternative to thrombolytic therapy in patients who can undergo angioplasty of the infarct-related artery within 12 hr of the onset of symptoms or beyond 12 hr if ischemic symptoms persist, *if performed in a timely fashion by individuals skilled in the procedure and supported by experienced personnel in an appropriate laboratory environment.*
2. In patients who are within 36 hr of an acute ST elevation Q or new LBBB MI who develop cardiogenic shock, who are younger than 75 years, and in whom revascularization can be performed within 18 hr of the onset of the shock.

Class IIa

As a reperfusion strategy in patients who are candidates for reperfusion but who have a contraindication to fibrinolytic therapy, if angioplasty can be performed as outlined earlier in class I.

Early Coronary Angiography in the Patient with Suspected MI (ST Segment Elevation or Bundle Branch Block Present) Who Has Not Undergone Primary PTCA

Class I

None.

Class IIa

Cardiogenic shock or persistent hemodynamic instability.

Early Coronary Angiography in Acute MI (MI Suspected but No ST Segment Elevation)

Class I

1. Persistent or recurrent (stuttering) episodes of symptomatic ischemia, spontaneous or induced, with or without associated ECG changes.
2. The presence of shock, severe pulmonary congestion, or continuing hypotension.

Class IIa

None.

Coronary Angioplasty During the Hospital Management Phase (Patients with Q Wave and Non-Q-Wave Infarction)

Class I

1. Spontaneous myocardial ischemia or myocardial ischemia provoked by minimal exertion, during recovery from infarction.
2. Before definitive therapy of a mechanical complication of infarction such as acute mitral regurgitation, ventricular septal defect, pseudoaneurysm, or left ventricular aneurysm.
3. Persistent hemodynamic instability.

TABLE 17–1 Indications for Coronary Angiography—cont'd

Class IIa
1. When MI is suspected to have occurred by a mechanism other than thrombotic occlusion at an atheroslcerotic plaque (e.g., coronary embolism, arteritis, trauma, certain metabolic or hematological diseases or coronary spasm).
2. Survivors of acute MI with left ventricular EF < 0.40, CHF, prior revascularization, or malignant ventricular arrhythmias.
3. Clinical heart failure during the acute episode, but subsequent demonstration of preserved left ventricular function (left ventricular EF > 0.40).

During the Risk Stratification Phase (Patients with All Types of MI)

Class I

Ischemia at low levels of exercise with ECG changes (≥1-mm ST segment depression or other predicators of adverse outcome) and/or imaging abnormalities.

Class IIa
1. Clinically significant CHF during the hospital course.
2. Inability to perform an exercise test with left ventricular EF ≤ 0.45.

Perioperative Evaluation Before (or After) Noncardiac Surgery

Class I: Patients with suspected or known CAD
1. Evidence for high risk of adverse outcome based on noninvasive test results.
2. Angina unresponsive to adequate medical therapy.
3. Unstable angina, particularly when facing intermediate- or high-risk noncardiac surgery.
4. Equivocal noninvasive test result in high clinical risk patient undergoing high-risk surgery.

Class IIa
1. Multiple intermediate clinical risk markers and planned vascular surgery.
2. Ischemia on noninvasive testing but without high-risk criteria.
3. Equivocal noninvasive test result in intermediate clinical risk patient undergoing high-risk noncardiac surgery.
4. Urgent noncardiac surgery while convalescing from acute MI.

Patients with Valvular Heart Disease

Class I
1. Before valve surgery or balloon valvotomy in an adult with chest discomfort, ischemia by noninvasive imaging, or both.
2. Before valve surgery in an adult free of chest pain but with many risk factors for CAD.
3. Infective endocarditis with evidence of coronary embolization.

Class IIa

None.

Patients with Congenital Heart Disease

Class I
1. Before surgical correction of congenital heart disease when chest discomfort or noninvasive evidence is suggestive of associated CAD.
2. Before surgical correction of suspected congenital coronary anomalies such as congenital coronary artery stenosis, coronary arteriovenous fistula, and anomalous origin of the left coronary artery.
3. Forms of congenital heart disease frequently associated with coronary artery anomalies that may complicate surgical management.
4. Unexplained cardiac arrest in a young patient.

Class IIa

Before corrective open-heart surgery for congenital heart disease in an adult whose risk profile increases the likelihood of coexisting CAD.

Patients with Congestive Heart Failure

Class I
1. CHF due to systolic dysfunction with angina or with regional wall motion abnormalities and/or scintigraphic evidence or reversible myocardial ischemia when revascularization is being considered.
2. Before cardiac transplantation.
3. CHF secondary to postinfarction ventricular aneurysm or other mechanical complications of MI.

Class IIa
1. Systolic dysfunction with unexplained cause despite noninvasive testing.
2. Normal systolic function, but episodic heart failure raises suspicion if ischemically mediated left ventricular dysfunction.

Other Conditions

Class I
1. Diseases affecting the aorta when knowledge of the presence of extent of coronary artery involvement is necessary for management (e.g., aortic dissection or aneurysm with known CAD).
2. Hypertrophic cardiomyopathy with angina despite medical therapy when knowledge of coronary anatomy might affect therapy.
3. Hypertrophic cardiomyopathy with angina when heart surgery is planned.

Class IIa
1. High risk for CAD when other cardiac surgical procedures are planned (e.g., pericardiectomy or removal of chronic pulmonary emboli).
2. Prospective immediate cardiac transplant donors whose risk profile increases the likelihood of CAD.
3. Asymptomatic patients with Kawasaki disease who have coronary artery aneurysms on echocardiography.
4. Before surgery for aortic aneurysm/dissection in patients without known CAD.
5. Recent blunt chest trauma and suspicion of acute MI, without evidence of preexisting CAD.

CABG = coronary artery bypass graft; CAD = coronary artery disease; CHF = congestive heart failure; ECG = electrocardiographic; EF = ejection fraction; LBBB = left bundle branch block; MI = myocardial infarction; PTCA = percutaneous transluminal coronary angioplasty; VT = ventricular tachycardia.

From Scanlon PJ, Faxon DF, Auden AM, et al: ACC/AHA guidelines for coronary angiography: A report of the American College of Cardiology/American Heart Association Task Force on practice guidelines (Committee on Coronary Angiography). Developed in collaboration with the Society for Cardiac Angiography and Interventions. J Am Coll Cardiol 33:1756, 1999.

catheterization prior to valvular surgery is weighted heavily in favor of the cardiac catheterization. However, catheterization may be unnecessary in some preoperative situations, such as patients with an atrial myxoma or young patients with endocarditis or acute valvular regurgitation. Nevertheless, additional confirmation of the severity of the valvular lesion, identification of associated coronary disease or anomalies, quantification of the hemodynamic consequences of the valvular lesions (such as pulmonary hypertension), and occasionally quantification of the acute hemodynamic response to pharmacological therapy all provide useful preoperative information that fully defines the operative risk and permits a more directed surgical approach.

The current role of cardiac catheterization in certain congenital disease states is less well defined. Echocardiography with Doppler and cardiac magnetic resonance imaging often provides adequate information. Because gross cardiac anatomy can generally be well defined by these methods, catheterization is required only if certain hemodynamic information (e.g., shunt size or pulmonary vascular resistance) is important in determining the indications for surgical procedures, if percutaneous interventional methods are contemplated, or if coronary anomalies are suspected (see Chap. 56).

Technical Aspects of Cardiac Catheterization

CATHETERIZATION LABORATORY FACILITIES

Cardiac catheterization facilities have evolved to include traditional hospital-based laboratories with in-house cardiothoracic surgical programs, hospital-based laboratories without on-site surgical programs, freestanding laboratories, and mobile laboratories. The relative merits of each type of facility have been discussed in detail by a task force of the American College of Cardiology and Society for Cardiac Angiography and Interventions.[2] At present, about three quarters of cardiac catheterization laboratories have on-site surgical backup. The goals of the freestanding and mobile cardiac catheterization facilities are to reduce cost while offering services in a convenient location for low-risk patients. In one study evaluating the safety of mobile catheterization involving 1001 low-risk patients, no patient died, 0.9 percent required urgent referral for clinical instability, 0.6 percent had major complications, and 27 percent required further referral to a tertiary site for additional diagnostic or therapeutic procedures.[3] Recommendations for groups of patients who should be excluded from invasive procedures in settings without cardiac surgery are given in Table 17–2.

Because of cost containment considerations and the documented safety of diagnostic cardiac catheterization, there has been increasing utilization of catheterization on an outpatient basis.[2] Medicare data indicate that in 1986, catheterization was performed on an outpatient basis in 5 percent of total cases. This rate rose to 23 percent in 1993 and has increased further to 40 to 50 percent in most hospital-based practices today. In general, patients who require preprocedural hospitalization are uncommon. These cases include patients receiving continuous anticoagulation therapy in order to switch from warfarin to heparin, those with severe congestive heart failure, and those with renal insufficiency requiring prehydration. Noninvasive testing can identify patients who would be more appropriately evaluated in a setting where cardiac surgery is available, including those with severe ischemia discovered during stress testing, ischemia at rest, known or highly suspected severe left main or proximal three-vessel disease, critical aortic stenosis, and severe comorbid disease. Most patients can be discharged on the same day within 2 to 6 hours of their procedure.

The most common procedure-related complication necessitating hospitalization is hematoma formation requiring prolonged bed rest and observation. Also, findings from the procedures may require hospitalization, including left main or severe three-vessel coronary artery disease. Other considerations for hospitalization include New York Heart Association Class III or IV heart failure, unstable ischemic symptoms, recent myocardial infarction, severe aortic stenosis with left ventricular dysfunction, severe aortic insufficiency, renal insufficiency, or need for continuous anticoagulation.[2]

PERSONNEL

Personnel in the catheterization laboratory include the medical director, physicians, nurses, cardiology trainees (fellows), physician extenders including nurse practitioners and physician assistants, and radiological technologists. All members should be trained in cardiopulmonary resuscitation and preferably in advanced cardiac life support. It is desirable for facilities to be associated with a cardiothoracic surgical program. In

TABLE 17–2 General Exclusion Criteria for Invasive Cardiac Procedures in Settings Without Cardiac Surgery

Setting	Type of Patient	Diagnostic Procedures	Therapeutic Procedures
Hospital	Adult	• Age > 75 yr • NYHA Class III or IV heart failure • Acute, intermediate- or high-risk ischemic syndromes • Recent MI with postinfarction ischemia • Pulmonary edema thought to be caused by ischemia • Markedly abnormal noninvasive test indicating a high likelihood of left main or severe multivessel coronary disease • Known left main coronary artery disease • Severe valvular dysfunction, especially in the setting of depressed left ventricular performance • Patients at increased risk for vascular complications • Complex adult congenital heart disease	• All valvuloplasty procedures • Diagnostic pericardiocentesis when the effusion is small or moderate in size and there is no tamponade • Elective coronary interventions • Therapeutic procedures in adult congenital heart disease
	Pediatric	• No procedures approved	• No therapeutic procedures approved
Freestanding laboratory	Adult	• All of the above • Patients at high risk because of the presence of comorbid conditions, including the need for anticoagulation therapy, poorly controlled hypertension or diabetes, contrast agent allergy, or renal insufficiency	• No therapeutic procedures approved
	Pediatric	• No procedures approved	• No therapeutic procedures approved

NYHA = New York Heart Association.

From Bashore TM, Bates ER, Berger PB, et al: ACC/SCAI clinical expert consensus document on cardiac catheterization laboratory standards. J Am Coll Cardiol 37:2179, 2001.

general, high-risk diagnostic studies and all elective percutaneous interventions should be performed in laboratories with on-site surgical facilities. However, the American College of Cardiology/American Heart Association task force assessment of diagnostic and therapeutic cardiovascular procedures suggested that percutaneous coronary intervention in high-risk patients with acute myocardial infarction may be performed by trained physicians without on-site surgical backup if the patient cannot be transferred to a more traditional setting without additional risk.[4]

In order to maintain proficiency, laboratories for adult studies should perform a minimum of 300 procedures per year. Physicians training for diagnostic catheterization should perform a minimum of 300 procedures per year with 200 as a primary operator during 12 months of fellowship. However, the minimum caseload for established physicians in practice has not been established.[2,5] Regular evaluation with quality indicator assessment of laboratory and physician, nurse, and technology performance and outcomes is mandatory.[2]

EQUIPMENT

The physical requirements for the catheterization facility have been described in detail elsewhere.[2] Necessary equipment includes the radiographic system, physiological data monitoring and acquisition instrumentation, sterile supplies, and an emergency cart. Also included is support equipment consisting of a power injector, cineangiographic film with processing or digital archiving, and viewing equipment.

RADIOGRAPHIC EQUIPMENT. High-resolution x-ray imaging is required for optimal performance of catheterization procedures.The necessary equipment includes a generator, x-ray tube, image intensifier, video system, and either digital archiving or a cine camera.[6] Virtually all new facilities have made the transition from traditional film-based cineangiography to digital angiography, thus becoming "cinefilm-less" laboratories. There are many advantages of digital acquisition and archiving, including the ability to have immediate on-line review, elimination of film development, quantitative computer analysis, image manipulation capabilities, freeze frames, and flicker-free images at low frame rates, minimizing radiation exposure. With these technologies, transfer of images among cardiac catheterization laboratories, hospitals, and physician offices can be accomplished using a common network.[7,8] The development of Digital Imaging and Communications in Medicine (DICOM) standards for cardiac angiography has allowed compatibility among different systems. Compact disc read-only memory (CD-ROM) technology has been utilized to exchange information between providers. Digital image quality is superior to that of cinefilm and allows a telemedicine approach to cardiac catheterization. Increased computer storage capabilities have allowed storage and easy access to thousands of cases.

PHYSIOLOGICAL MONITORS. Continuous monitoring of blood pressure and the electrocardiogram (ECG) are required during cardiac catheterization. Systemic, pulmonary, and intracardiac pressures are generally recorded using fluid-filled catheters connected to strain-gauge pressure transducers and then transmitted to a monitor. Equipment for determination of thermodilution and Fick cardiac output and blood gas determination, as well as a standard 12-lead ECG machine, are necessary.

RADIATION SAFETY

The patient and catheterization laboratory personnel must be protected from the harmful effects of radiation. Installing and maintaining optimal x-ray imaging equipment reduce unnecessary radiation exposure. The amount of radiation exposure to the patient can be reduced by limiting fluoroscopic and image acquisition time, collimation of the beam to the anatomical region of interest, using low-intensity fluoroscopy, acquiring images at lower frame rates (i.e., 15 frames/sec), maintaining a minimum distance between the image intensifier and the x-ray tube, and using lead shielding when appropriate. Personnel in the laboratory can limit radiation exposure by minimizing acquisition and fluoroscopy times by using low-dose fluoroscopy and acquisition rates of 15 frames/sec. The most important factors are maximizing distance from the source of x-rays and using appropriate shielding (lead aprons, lead thyroid collars, lead eyeglasses, and movable leaded glass barriers). Severely angulated views, especially the left anterior oblique view, substantially increase the radiation exposure of the operators.

A method for measuring radiation exposure for personnel is required. It is recommended that two film badges be worn, one on the outside of the apron at the neck and another under the apron at the waist.[9] The latter monitors the effectiveness of the lead apron. The maximum allowable whole-body radiation dose per year for those working with radiation is 5 roentgen-equivalent-man (rem). A full discussion of radiation safety has been presented by the Society for Cardiac Angiography and Interventions and others.[2,9]

Catheterization Laboratory Protocol

PREPARATION OF THE PATIENT FOR CARDIAC CATHETERIZATION. Before arrival in the catheterization laboratory, the cardiologist responsible for the procedure should explain the procedure fully to patients, including the risks and benefits, and answer questions that the patient or family may have. Precatheterization evaluation includes the patient's history, physical examination, ECG, and laboratory evaluation (complete blood count, platelet count, and determinations of serum creatinine, serum electrolytes, blood glucose, prothrombin time, and partial thromboplastin time [in patients receiving heparin]). Important components of the history that need to be addressed include diabetes mellitus (insulin or non–insulin requiring), renal insufficiency, anticoagulation status, and peripheral vascular disease, as well as previous contrast medium or latex allergy. Full knowledge of any prior procedures, including cardiac catheterizations, percutaneous interventions, peripheral arterial interventions or surgery, and cardiac surgery, is necessary before the procedure. Patients should be fasting, and an intravenous line should be established.

Oral or intravenous sedation is usually administered (e.g., benzodiazepine). Pulse oximetry should be used to monitor respiratory status when these agents are used. Some laboratories routinely premedicate patients with antihistamines such as diphenhydramine (25 mg intravenous push) for its antiallergic properties and to prolong sedation. Oral anticoagulants should be discontinued and the prothrombin time international normalized ratio should be less than 1.8 to avoid increased risk of bleeding. Aspirin is not stopped prior to the procedure. Patients with diabetes receiving metformin should have the medication discontinued the morning of the procedure and not restarted until the creatinine is stable at least 48 hours after the procedure.[10] All patients should receive pre- and postprocedural hydration. The amount of hydration is dependent on the cardiac function but, if tolerated, at least 1 liter is recommended.

Those with a known history of contrast medium allergy need either oral or intravenous prophylaxis before the procedure.[11] A recommended regimen is administration of either prednisone 60 mg by mouth or hydrocortisone 100 mg intravenous push given 12 hours and immediately prior to the procedure. Cimetidine, a nonselective histamine antagonist, and diphenhydramine may also be given. A history of shellfish allergy does not predispose the patient to contrast medium reactions.

CATHETERIZATION PROTOCOL. Each physician should develop a routine for performing diagnostic catheterization to ensure efficient acquisition of all pertinent data. The particular technical approach and necessary procedures should be established individually for each patient so that the specific clinical questions can be addressed (Table 17–3). In general, hemodynamic measurements and cardiac output determination should be made before angiography to reflect basal conditions most accurately and to guide angiography. When angiography is performed, the vessel or chamber with most clinical importance should be visualized first in case an untoward reaction to the contrast medium or another complication of the procedure occurs.

Right-heart catheterization should not be performed in all patients undergoing routine coronary angiography. Despite limited risks, right-heart catheterization including screening oximetric analysis, measurement of pressures, and determination of cardiac output has a low yield in patients with suspected coronary artery disease without other known cardiac disease.[2] Right-heart catheterization is indicated when the clinical question cannot be answered by isolated left-heart catheterization or when a patient has left ventricular dysfunction, congestive heart failure, complicated acute myocardial infarction, valvular disease, suspected pulmonary

TABLE 17–3 Catheterization Protocol

Clinical Issue	LHC	RHC	CORO	LV	AO	RV	PA	BX	PROVO	IABP	PCI
Known or suspected coronary artery disease											
Stable angina	✓		✓	✓							
Positive stress test result	✓		✓	✓							
Preoperative evaluation	✓		✓	✓							
Atypical chest pain	✓		✓	✓					±		
Unstable or new-onset angina	✓		✓	✓							±
Acute myocardial infarction	✓	✓	✓	±						±	±
Failed thrombolysis	✓	✓	✓	±						±	±
Postinfarction angina	✓		✓	±						±	±
Cardiogenic shock	✓	✓	✓	±						±	±
Mechanical complications	✓	✓	✓	✓						±	±
Sudden cardiac death	✓	✓	✓	✓							
Valvular heart disease	✓	✓	✓	✓	✓						
Myocardial disease	✓	✓	✓	✓	✓			±			
Pericardial disease	✓	✓	✓	✓							
Congenital heart disease	✓	✓	✓	✓	±	±	±				
Aortic dissection	✓	±	✓	±	✓						
Pulmonary disease	✓	✓	✓	✓		±	±				

AO = aortogram; BX = biopsy; CORO = coronary angiography; IABP = intraaortic balloon pump; LHC = left-heart catheterization, including measurement of left ventricular end-diastolic pressure and aortic valve gradient; LV = left ventriculography; PA = pulmonary angiography or wedge pulmonary angiography; PROVO = provocative challenge (i.e., ergot alkaloids, acetylcholine); PCI = percutaneous coronary intervention; RHC = right-heart catheterization including pressure measurement, determination of cardiac output, oximetric analysis; RV = right ventriculography; ✓ = appropriate; ± = may be appropriate in certain clinical circumstances.

hypertension, a congenital anomaly, intracardiac shunts, or pericardial disease.

Although the use of a temporary pacemaker is not indicated for routine cardiac catheterization, operators should understand the techniques for proper insertion and setting of the pacemaker if needed. Even in patients with isolated left bundle branch block, right-heart catheterization can generally be safely performed with balloon flotation catheters without causing additional conduction disturbance.

CATHETERS AND ASSOCIATED EQUIPMENT. Physicians performing cardiac catheterization should be familiar with technical aspects of the equipment used during the procedure.[12] Catheters used for cardiac catheterization are available in various lengths, sizes, and shapes. The widely used balloon flotation catheter (Swan-Ganz) is shown in Figure 17–1. Typical catheter lengths vary between 50 and 125 cm, with 100 cm being the most commonly used length for adult left-heart catheterization by the femoral approach. The outer diameter of the catheter is specified using French units, where one French unit (F) = 0.33 mm. The inner diameter of the catheter is smaller than the outside diameter owing to the thickness of the catheter material. Guidewires used during the procedure must be small enough to pass through the inner diameters of both the introducer needle and the catheter. Guidewires are described by their length in centimeters, diameter in inches, and tip conformation. A commonly used wire is a 150-cm, 0.035-inch J-tipped wire. The introducer sheaths are specified by the French number of the largest catheter that passes freely through the inner diameter of the sheath, rather than its outer diameter. Therefore, a 7F introducer sheath accepts a 7F catheter but has an outer diameter of more than 7F or 2.31 mm.

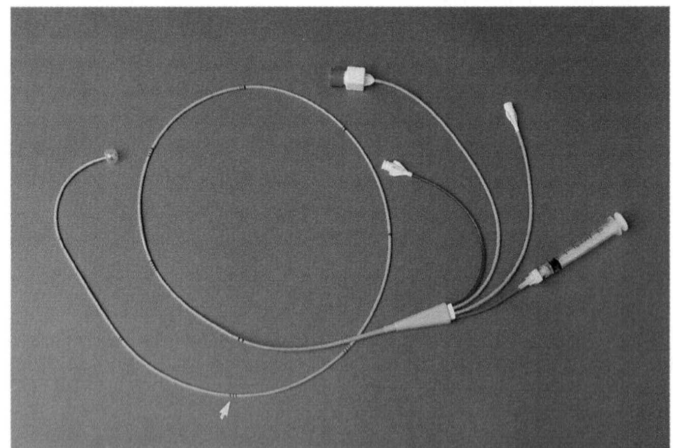

FIGURE 17–1 Typical Swan-Ganz catheter. Proximal ports, left to right, are proximal injection hub, thermistor connector, distal lumen hub, and balloon inflation valve with syringe. The distal end of the catheter has a balloon and a distal end-hole. The proximal injectate port exits at 30 cm from the distal lumen (arrow). The thermistor lies just proximal to the balloon.

The choice of the size of the catheters to be used is made by balancing the needs to opacify the coronary arteries and cardiac chambers adequately, to have adequate catheter manipulation, to limit vascular complications, and to permit early ambulation. Although the larger catheters (7 and 8F) allow greater catheter manipulation and excellent visualization, the smaller catheters (4 to 6F) permit earlier ambulation after catheterization. Catheter technology has advanced such that 4 to 6F systems are used for routine angiography without significant compromise of angiographic quality. The smaller catheters require greater technical skill of manipulation and have lower flow rates. Thus, their use in tortuous anatomy or patients with large body habitus is limited. The 6F diagnostic catheter is most widely used for routine angiography because this size appears to balance most appropriately the needs outlined earlier. The relationship between sheath size and vascular complications is not clear. Rather, anticoagulation status and operator experience are more important factors related to vascular complications.[13]

Techniques

Right-Heart Catheterization

Right-heart catheterization allows measurement and analysis of right-heart, pulmonary artery, and pulmonary capillary wedge pressures; measurement of cardiac output by thermodilution; screening for intracardiac shunts; temporary ventricular pacing; assessment of arrhythmias; and pulmonary wedge angiography. Right-heart catheterization is performed antegrade through either the inferior vena cava (IVC) or superior vena cava (SVC). Percutaneous entry is achieved through the femoral, subclavian, jugular, or antecubital vein. The anatomy of the major arteries and veins used for cardiac catheterization is shown in Figures 17–2 and 17–3. In the cardiac catheterization laboratory, the femoral venous access is used most often because the Judkins technique of left-heart catheterization is performed concurrently. However, when the catheter is to be left in place following the procedure, the internal jugular approach may be preferable. This approach allows the patient to sit up in bed rather than lying flat.

BALLOON FLOTATION CATHETERS. Balloon flotation catheters are the simplest and most widely used (see Fig. 17–1). If thermodilution cardiac outputs must be determined, catheters that contain thermistors, such as Swan-Ganz catheters, should be used. These catheters have balloon tips, proximal and distal ports, and thermistors. Therefore, both intracardiac pressures and oxygen saturation to evaluate intracardiac shunts can be obtained. They are both flexible and flow directed, but when the femoral approach is used, fluoroscopic guidance is almost always necessary to cannulate the pulmonary artery and to obtain pulmonary capillary wedge position. Although most right-heart catheters have a J-shaped curvature distally to facilitate passage from the SVC to the pulmonary artery, a catheter with an S-shaped distal end has been designed for femoral insertion. Despite limited manipulation, the balloon flotation catheters are the safest and most rapid method for obtaining right-heart pressures and blood samples. Other right-heart balloon flotation end-hole catheters are stiffer and allow passage of conventional 0.035- or 0.038-inch guidewires to improve manipulation. Although these lack the ability to obtain thermodilution cardiac outputs, they yield better pressure fidelity owing to less catheter whip artifact and a larger end hole.

There are two methods for advancing a balloon flotation catheter from the femoral vein. On many occasions, the catheter can be advanced directly through the right atrium and across the tricuspid valve. Once in the right ventricle, the catheter is manipulated to point superiorly and directly into the right ventricular outflow tract. This orientation can usually be achieved while the catheter is advanced with slight clockwise rotation. Once in the outflow tract, the balloon tip should allow flotation into the pulmonary artery and wedge positions (Fig. 17–4). When necessary, deep inspiration or cough can facilitate this maneuver and assist in crossing the pulmonic valve. If the catheter continues to point inferiorly toward the right ventricular apex, another technique should be used because further advancement can risk perforation of the right ventricular apex.

One such additional technique for performing right-heart catheterization with a balloon flotation catheter is shown in Figure 17–4. A loop is formed in the right atrium, with the catheter tip directed laterally. The loop can be created by hooking the catheter tip on the hepatic vein or by advancing the catheter while it is directed laterally in the right atrium. Once the loop is formed, the catheter should be advanced further, which directs the tip inferiorly and then medially across the tricuspid valve. Antegrade blood flow should then direct the catheter into the pulmonary artery. After the catheter is placed into the wedge position, the redundant loop should be removed by slow withdrawal.

Screening blood samples for oximetric analysis should be obtained from the SVC and the pulmonary artery to evaluate

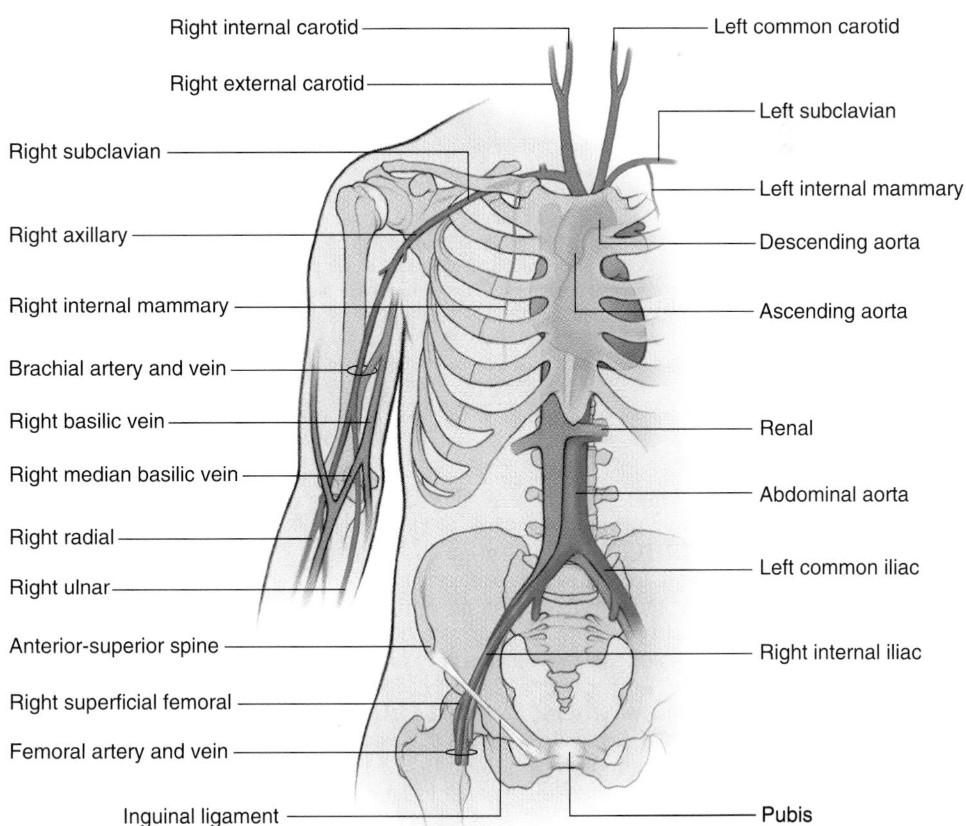

FIGURE 17–2 Principal arteries used for access during cardiac catheterization. Only the superficial veins are shown on the forearm. (Modified from Thibodeau GA, Patton KT [eds]: Anthony's Textbook of Anatomy and Physiology. 17th ed. St. Louis, CV Mosby, 2002.)

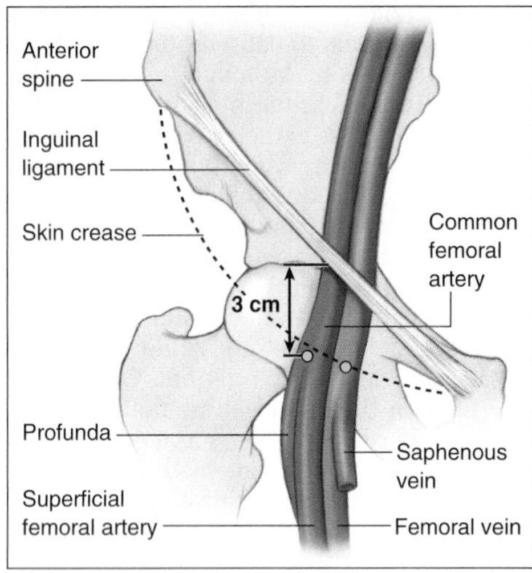

B

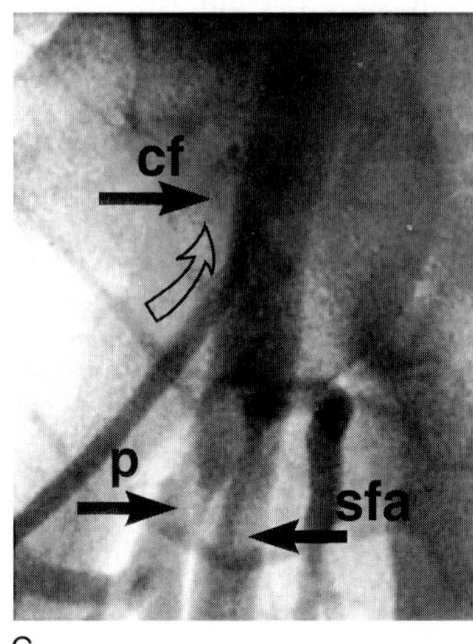

FIGURE 17–3 Regional anatomy relevant to percutaneous femoral arterial and venous catheterization. **A,** Schematic diagram showing the right femoral artery and vein coursing underneath the inguinal ligament, which runs from the anterior superior iliac spine to the pubic tubercle. The arterial skin nick should be placed approximately 3 cm below the ligament and directly over the femoral arterial pulsation, and the venous skin nick should be placed at the same level but approximately one fingerbreadth more medial. Although this level corresponds roughly to the skin crease in most patients, anatomical localization relative to the inguinal ligament provides a more constant landmark. **B,** Fluoroscopic localization of skin nick (marked by clamp tip) to the inferior border of the femoral head (ibfh). **C,** Catheter (open arrow) inserted through this skin nick has entered the common femoral artery (cf), above its bifurcation into the superficial femoral artery (sfa) and profunda (p) branches. (From Baim DS, Grossman W: Percutaneous approach, including transseptal and apical puncture. *In* Baim DS, Grossman W [eds]: Cardiac Catheterization, Angiography, and Intervention. 6th ed. Philadelphia, Lea & Febiger, 2000, p 71.)

for intracardiac shunts. Cardiac output can also be determined by thermodilution techniques.

NONFLOTATION CATHETERS. When an end-hole catheter (e.g., Cournand or multipurpose) that does not have a balloon tip is used, the technique for cannulating the pulmonary artery is markedly different. Manipulation and torquing of the nonflotation catheter are necessary to advance into the pulmonary artery. The catheter should be directed inferiorly across the tricuspid valve and then superiorly into the right ventricular outflow tract. It is generally recommended that one attempt be made to form a loop in the right atrium before advancement into the right ventricle in order to lessen the risk of perforation.

A probe-patent foramen ovale is present in about 30 percent of adult patients that allows access to the left atrium. It can be entered using a multipurpose catheter with the tip directed medially and slightly posterior. The catheter is withdrawn slowly from the SVC or high right atrium until a slight forward and medial motion is observed. The catheter then prolapses into the left atrium with mild pressure against the interatrial septum in patients with a probe-patent foramen ovale. Left atrial position can be verified by the pressure waveform, by blood samples demonstrating arterial saturation, or by hand contrast medium injection. If left atrial access is necessary and cannot be obtained with this technique, a transseptal catheterization should be undertaken (see Transseptal Catheterization).

COMPLICATIONS. The most common complications of right-heart catheterization are nonsustained atrial and ventricular arrhythmias. Major complications associated with right-heart catheterization are infrequent. These include pulmonary infarction, pulmonary artery or right ventricular perforation, and infection. Pulmonary artery rupture can be avoided by combined use of fluoroscopic guidance and constant evaluation of the pressure waveform. Confusion about the location of the distal end of the catheter may arise in the setting of large v waves in the pulmonary capillary wedge pressure tracing. The operator may mistake this waveform as a pulmonary artery waveform (Fig. 17–5). Careful attention to the timing of the peak pulmonary artery systolic pressure and the v wave with respect to the ECG, along with the use of fluoroscopy, prevents inadvertent inflation of the balloon in the wedged position, which can cause pulmonary artery rupture.

Left-Heart Catheterization and Coronary Arteriography

THE JUDKINS TECHNIQUE. Because of its relative ease, speed, reliability, and low complication rate,[1,2] the Judkins technique has become the most widely used method of left-heart catheterization and coronary arteriography. After local anesthesia with 1 percent lidocaine (Xylocaine), percutaneous entry of the femoral artery is achieved by puncturing the vessel 1 to 3 cm (or one to two fingerbreadths) below the inguinal ligament. The ligament can be palpated as it courses from the anterior superior iliac spine to the superior pubic ramus. This ligament, not the inguinal crease, should be used as the landmark. The inguinal crease can be misleading, particularly in the obese patient. A transverse skin incision is made over the femoral artery with a scalpel. A hemostatic clamp can be used under fluoroscopy to verify that the nick is made over the inferior edge of the femoral head. Using a modified Seldinger technique (Fig. 17–6), an 18-gauge thin-

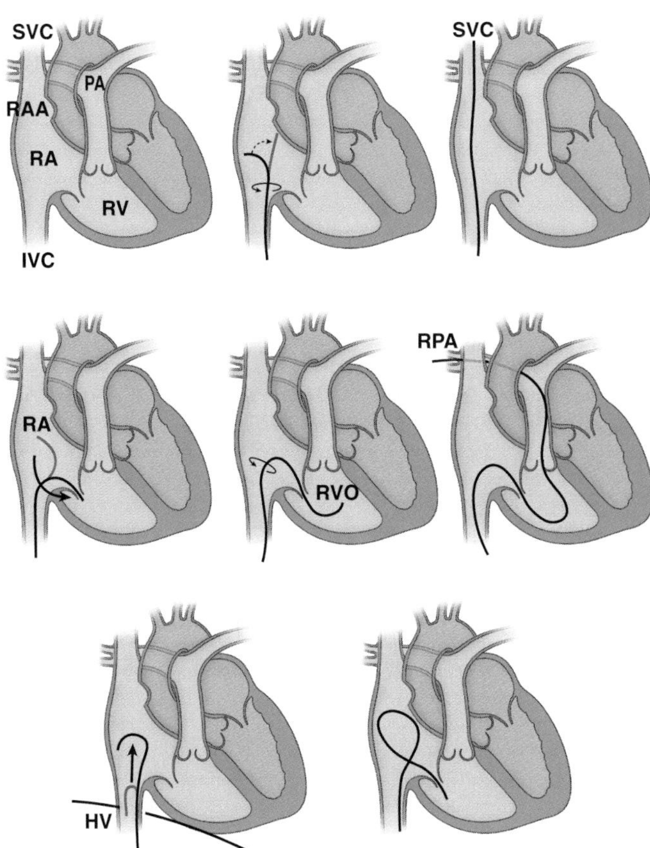

FIGURE 17–4 Right-heart catheterization from the femoral vein, shown in cartoon form. **Top row,** The right-heart catheter is initially placed in the right atrium (RA) aimed at the lateral atrial wall. Counterclockwise rotation aims the catheter posteriorly and allows advancement into the superior vena cava (SVC). Although not evident in the figure, clockwise catheter rotation into an anterior orientation would lead to advancement into the right atrial appendage (RAA), precluding SVC catheterization. **Center row,** The catheter is then withdrawn back into the right atrium and aimed laterally. Clockwise rotation causes the catheter tip to sweep anteromedially and cross the tricuspid valve. With the catheter tip in a horizontal orientation just beyond the spine, it is positioned below the right ventricular outflow (RVO) tract. Additional clockwise rotation causes the catheter to point straight up, allowing advancement into the main pulmonary artery and from there into the right pulmonary artery (RPA). **Bottom row,** Two maneuvers useful in catheterization of a dilated right heart. A larger loop with a downward-directed tip may be required to reach the tricuspid valve and can be formed by catching the catheter tip in the hepatic vein (HV) and advancing the catheter quickly into the right atrium. The reverse loop technique (bottom right) gives the catheter tip an upward direction, aimed toward the outflow tract. IVC = inferior vena cava; PA = pulmonary artery; RV = right ventricle. (From Baim DS, Grossman W: Percutaneous approach, including transseptal and apical puncture. *In* Baim DS, Grossman W [eds]: Cardiac Catheterization, Angiography, and Intervention. 6th ed. Philadelphia, Lea & Febiger, 2000, p 78.)

walled needle (Fig. 17–7) is inserted at a 30- to 45-degree angle into the femoral artery, and a 0.035- or 0.038-inch J-tip polytetrafluoroethylene (Teflon)-coated guidewire is advanced through the needle into the artery. The wire should pass freely up the aorta. After arterial access is obtained, a sheath at least equal in size to the coronary catheter is usually inserted into the femoral artery. Although it is generally recommended that the patient receive approximately 3000 U of heparin after access is obtained, its benefit has not been well proven. In patients receiving heparin prior to arrival in the laboratory, an activated clotting time should be obtained following access. Sheath removal is usually not recommended until the activated clotting time is less than 175 seconds unless a vascular closure device is being utilized.

Left ventricular systolic and end-diastolic pressures can be obtained by advancing a pigtail catheter into the left ventricle (Fig. 17–8). In assessing valvular aortic stenosis, left ventricular and aortic or femoral artery pressures should be recorded simultaneously. In suspected mitral stenosis, left ventricular and wedge or left atrial pressures should be obtained simultaneously. Left ventriculography is performed in the 30-degree right anterior oblique and 45- to 50-degree left anterior oblique views. A pigtail catheter is most commonly used for this purpose. Power injection of 30 to 40 ml of contrast medium into the ventricle is used to assess left ventricular function and the severity of mitral regurgitation. After ventriculography, left ventricular systolic and end-diastolic pressure measurements may be repeated and the systolic pressure recorded as the catheter is withdrawn from the left ventricle into the aorta. If an aortic transvalvular gradient is present, recording these pressures can detect it. For measurement of suspected intraventricular gradients, a multipurpose catheter with an end hole is desirable to localize the gradient in the left ventricle. Pigtail catheters contain side holes, which obscure the capacity to define whether the gradient is intraventricular, subvalvular, or transvalvular.

After coronary arteriography and left-heart catheterization have been completed, the catheters are removed and firm pressure is applied to the femoral area for 15 to 20 minutes, either by hand or by a mechanical clamp. The patient should be instructed to lie in bed for several hours, with the leg remaining straight to prevent hematoma formation. With 4 or 5F catheters, 2 hours of bed rest is usually sufficient, whereas use of 6F catheters usually involves at least 3 to 4 hours.

Alternatively, vascular closure devices may be used. Three types are currently available: collagen plugs, suture closure, and hemostatic patches. Each allows earlier ambulation of the patients, within 1 to 2 hours after the procedure.[14,15] They also permit early sheath removal in patients receiving anticoagulation. However, none has been shown to lower vascular complication rates compared with conventional hand compression.[16] The ultimate success of any means of achieving hemostasis relies on a single front wall puncture of the common femoral artery.

The main advantage of the Judkins technique is speed and ease of selective catheterization. These attributes do not, however, preclude the importance of extensive operator experience to ensure quality studies with acceptable safety. The main disadvantage of this technique is its use in patients with severe iliofemoral atherosclerotic disease, in whom retrograde passage of catheters through areas of extreme narrowing or tortuosity may be difficult or impossible. However, even passage through synthetic aortofemoral grafts has a low complication rate.[17]

BRACHIAL ARTERY TECHNIQUE—SONES TECHNIQUE. Sones and colleagues introduced the first technique for coronary artery catheterization by means of a brachial artery cutdown. The Sones technique is still popular in many centers and is described in Chapter 18.

PERCUTANEOUS BRACHIAL ARTERY TECHNIQUE

A modification of the Sones technique is the percutaneous brachial artery technique using preformed Judkins catheters. This technique uses the Seldinger method of percutaneous brachial artery entry. A 4 to 6F sheath is placed into the brachial artery, and 3000 to 5000 U of heparin is infused into the side port. A guidewire is then advanced to the ascending aorta under fluoroscopic control. Judkins left, right, and pigtail catheters are passed over the guidewire for routine arteriography and ventriculography. The guidewire may occasionally be necessary to direct the left coronary catheter into the left sinus of Valsalva and the ostium of the left main coronary artery. Alternatively, an Amplatz left 1 or 2 is used to intubate the coronary ostium. Following removal of the sheath, the arm should be maintained straight with an armband for 4 to 6 hours with observation of radial and brachial pulses.

The main advantage of the percutaneous brachial technique is that it avoids a brachial artery cutdown and repair. The main disadvantage is that manipulation of catheters can be difficult. When this technique was

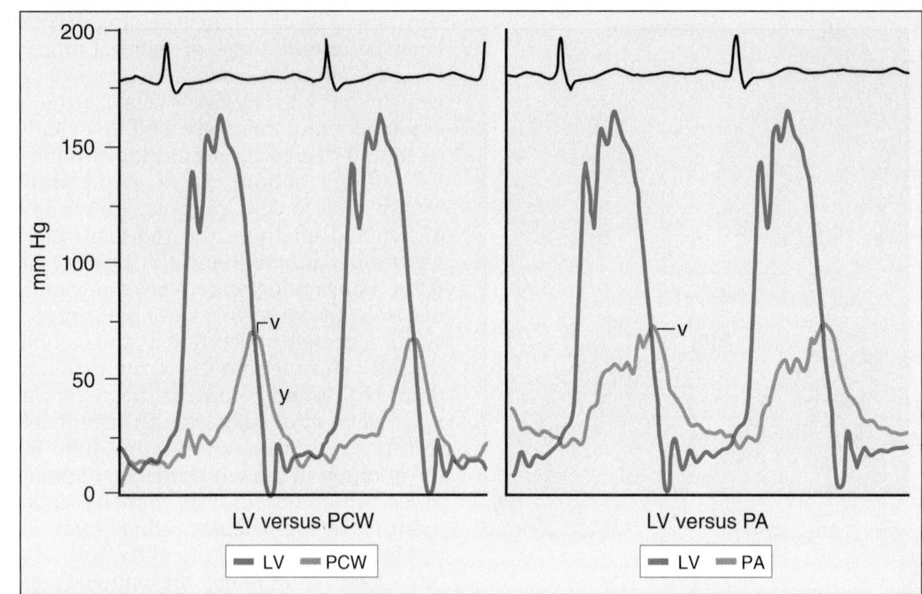

FIGURE 17–5 Acute mitral regurgitation with poor left atrial compliance. The left ventricle (LV) pressure versus the pulmonary capillary wedge (PCW) pressure is shown on the left. A large regurgitant v wave is seen. This v wave is transmitted through the pulmonary bed to the pulmonary arterial (PA) tracing and is superimposed in the right panel. (From Bashore TM, Harrison JK, Davidson CJ: Cardiac catheterization, angiography, and interventional techniques in valvular and congenital heart disease. *In* Sabiston DC, Spencer FC [eds]: Surgery of the Chest. 6th ed. Philadelphia, WB Saunders, 1995, p 1144.)

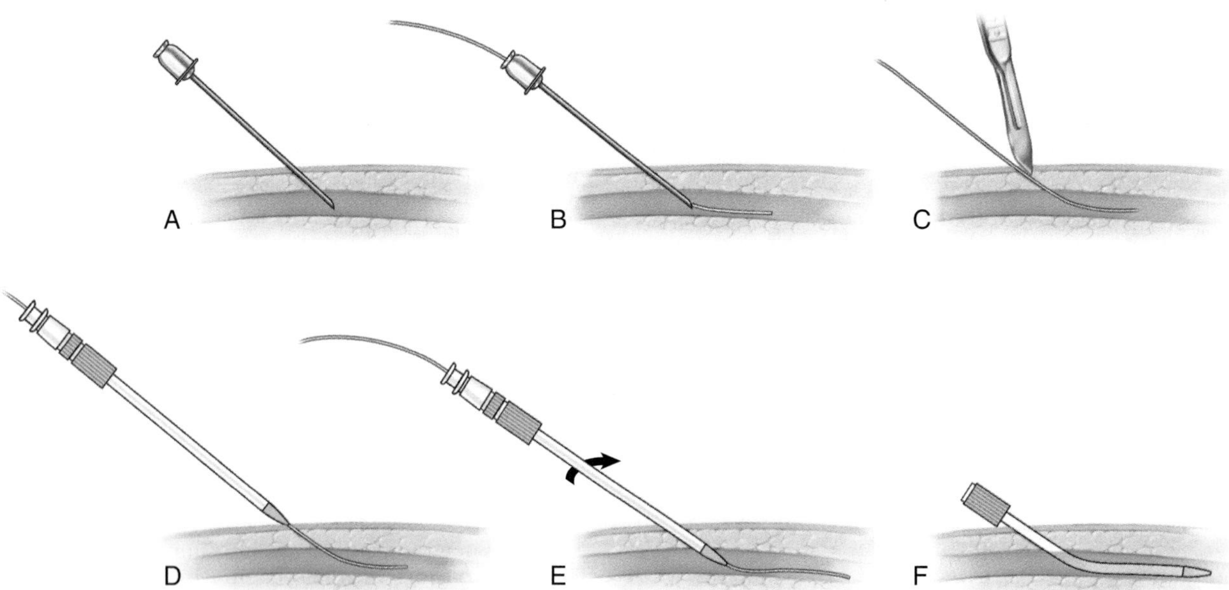

FIGURE 17–6 Modified Seldinger technique for percutaneous catheter sheath introduction. **A,** Vessel punctured by needle. **B,** Flexible guidewire placed into the vessel through the needle. **C,** Needle removed, guidewire left in place, and the hole in the skin around the wire enlarged with a scalpel. **D,** Sheath and dilator placed over the guidewire. **E,** Sheath and dilator advanced over the guidewire and into the vessel. **F,** Dilator and guidewire removed while the sheath remains in the vessel. (From Hill JA, Lambert CR, Vlietstra RE, Pepine CJ: Review of general catheterization techniques. *In* Pepine CJ, Hill JA, Lambert CR [eds]: Diagnostic and Therapeutic Cardiac Catheterization. 3rd ed. Baltimore, Williams & Wilkins, 1998, p 107.)

compared with the femoral technique, patients' comfort, hemostasis time, and time to ambulation favored the brachial technique, whereas procedural efficiency, time of radiation exposure, and diagnostic film quality were more favorable with the femoral approach.[18] Complication rates appear similar.

PERCUTANEOUS RADIAL ARTERY TECHNIQUE

Left-heart catheterization by the radial artery approach was developed as an alternative to the percutaneous transbrachial approach in an attempt to limit vascular complications. The inherent advantages of the transradial approach are that the hand has a dual arterial supply connected through the palmar arches and that there are no nerves or veins at the site of puncture. In addition, bed rest is unnecessary after the procedure, allowing more efficient outpatient angiography.

The procedure requires a normal Allen test result. After manual compression of both the radial and ulnar arteries during fist clenching, normal color returns to the opened hand within 10 seconds after releasing pressure over the ulnar artery, and significant reactive hyperemia is absent on releasing pressure over the radial artery.

The arm is abducted and the wrist hyperextended over a gauze roll. Routine skin anesthesia is used, a small incision is made just proximal to the styloid process of the radius, and the subcutaneous tissue is tunneled

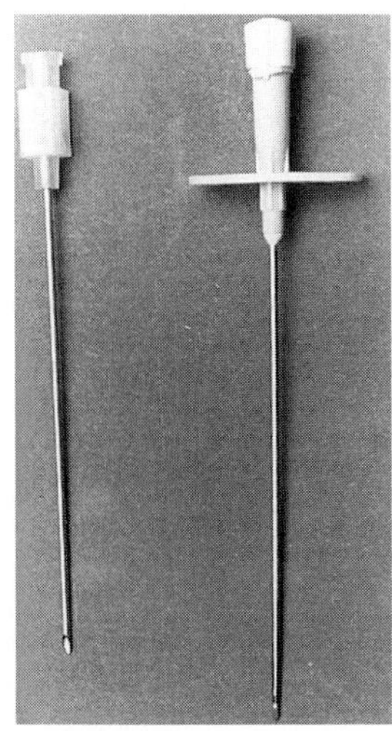

FIGURE 17–7 Two most commonly used needle types for vascular access. On the left, a single-piece, thin-walled "front-wall needle"; on the right, a two-component, thin-walled Seldinger needle. (From MacDonald RG: Catheters, sheaths, guidewires, needles, and related equipment. *In* Pepine CJ, Hill JA, Lambert CR [eds]: Diagnostic and Therapeutic Cardiac Catheterization. 3rd ed. Baltimore, Williams & Wilkins, 1998, p 130.)

using forceps. An 18-gauge needle is introduced at a 45-degree angle and an exchange-length 0.035- or 0.038-inch J-tip guidewire is inserted. A 23-cm-long 4 or 5F sheath is then introduced. Heparin, 5000 U, is administered through the side arm of the sheath. Coronary catheters are then advanced over the exchange wire into the ascending aorta. The left coronary artery is intubated in a manner similar to the brachial approach using either a left 4- or 5-cm tip Judkins (JL 4.0, 5.0), a left Amplatz, or a brachial Castillo type II catheter. The right coronary artery is intubated using a 4-cm right Judkins (JR 4.0), a left Amplatz, or a multipurpose catheter. Left ventriculography can be performed using a standard pigtail catheter. Hemostasis is obtained at the end of the procedure after sheath removal using direct pressure. It is recommended that the arterial puncture site be allowed to bleed for several beats before maintaining direct pressure. The radial pulse should be monitored regularly for several hours after the procedure.

The potential limitations of this procedure include the inability to cannulate the radial artery owing to its smaller size and propensity to develop spasm, poor visualization of the coronary arteries resulting from the small-caliber catheters with limited manipulation potential, and risk of radial arterial occlusion caused by dissection or thrombus formation. In addition, when right-heart catheterization is required, additional approaches are necessary. If intervention is contemplated, device selection may be limited by guide catheter size. Although there is little debate that the femoral approach is the simplest and probably the safest technique for left-heart catheterization, the transradial approach for left-heart catheterization has gained in popularity.[19]

Transseptal Catheterization

Transseptal left-heart catheterization has received renewed interest with the advent of percutaneous balloon mitral commissurotomy as a viable option to surgical commissurotomy, with electrophysiological procedures requiring access to pulmonary veins, and with increasing use of disc-type prosthetic valves in the aortic position. This type of mechanical prosthetic valve cannot be crossed safely and prohibits retrograde left-heart catheterization. When performed by experienced operators, the technique has a low complication rate of less than 2 percent.[20]

The transseptal catheter is a short, curved catheter with a tapered tip (Fig. 17–9). Alternatively, an 8F Mullins sheath and dilator combination is used. The Brockenbrough needle is 18 gauge that tapers to 21 gauge at the distal tip. One commonly used approach is to place a 0.032-inch guidewire through the femoral vein, through the right atrium, and into the SVC. The Mullins transseptal sheath and dilator are then advanced over the wire into the SVC. The guidewire is removed and replaced with a Brockenbrough needle, and the distal port is connected to a pressure manifold. With the needle tip just proximal to the Mullins sheath tip, the entire catheter system is withdrawn. The catheter is simultaneously rotated from a 12 o'clock to a 5 o'clock position. The operator observes two abrupt rightward movements. The first occurs as the catheter descends from the SVC to the right atrium. The second occurs as the Mullins dilator tip passes over the limbic edge into the fossa ovalis. The curve of the sheath and needle should be oriented slightly anteriorly. The dilator and needle can then be advanced gently as a unit. Steady gentle pressure is often adequate to advance the system through the fossa ovalis into the left atrium. If not, the needle should be advanced across the interatrial septum while holding the Mullins sheath in place. In cases in which transseptal puncture is technically difficult because of a large right atrium, postsurgical condition, or anatomical variant, intracardiac echocardiography can be useful to localize the fossa ovalis and interatrial septum. (See Intracardiac Echocardiography.)

Left atrial position can be confirmed by the overall increase in pressure with left atrial a and v waveforms, hand injection of contrast medium, or measurement of arterial oxygen saturation. When the position is confirmed, the catheter should be rotated toward 3 o'clock and the dilator and sheath safely advanced 2 to 3 cm into the left atrium. The sheath is held firmly, and the dilator and needle are removed. Left atrial pressure measurements should then be repeated. If measurement of left ventricular pressure or left ventriculography, or both, is necessary, the catheter can usually be advanced easily into the left ventricle after slight counterclockwise rotation. The major risk of transseptal catheterization lies in inadvertent puncture of atrial structures, such as the atrial free wall, left atrial appendage, or coronary sinus, or entry into the aortic root or pulmonary artery.

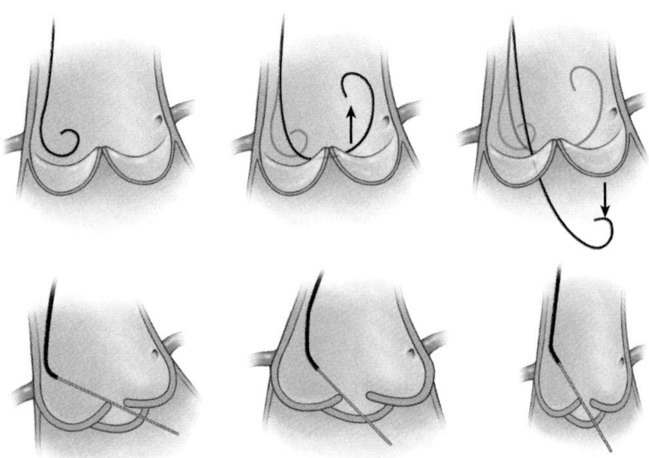

FIGURE 17–8 Technique for retrograde crossing of an aortic valve using a pigtail catheter. The upper row shows the technique for crossing a normal aortic valve. In the bottom row, the use of a straight guidewire and pigtail catheter in combination is shown. Increasing the length of protruding guidewire straightens the catheter curve and causes the wire to point more toward the right coronary ostium; reducing the length of protruding wire restores the pigtail contour and deflects the guidewire tip toward the left coronary artery. When the correct length of wire and the correct rotational orientation of the catheter have been found, repeated advancement and withdrawal of catheter and guidewire together allow retrograde passage across the valve. In a dilated aortic root, the angled pigtail catheter is preferable. In a small aortic root (bottom row, right), a right coronary Judkins catheter may have advantages. In patients with bicuspid valves, an Amplatz left catheter is often used as it directs the wire more superiorly. (From Baim DS, Grossman W: Percutaneous approach including transseptal and apical puncture. *In* Baim DS, Grossman W [eds]: Cardiac Catheterization, Angiography, and Intervention. 6th ed. Philadelphia, Lea & Febiger, 2000, p 86.)

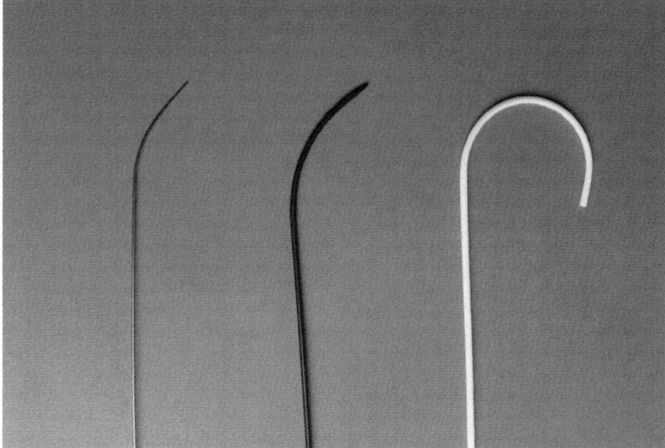

A

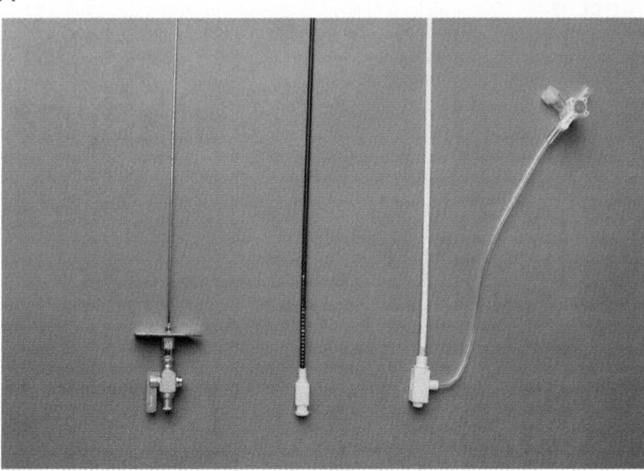

B

FIGURE 17–9 Transseptal catheters. **A,** Distal catheter. **B,** Proximal catheter. Left, Mullins transseptal sheath. Middle, Introducer (dilator) that is placed inside sheath to add stiffness to the catheter. Right, Brockenbrough transseptal needle that is placed inside the sheath and is used to penetrate the septum.

Direct Transthoracic Left Ventricular Puncture

The sole indication for direct left ventricular puncture is to measure left ventricular pressure and to perform ventriculography in patients with mechanical prosthetic valves in both the mitral and aortic positions, preventing retrograde arterial and transseptal catheterization. Crossing tilting-disc valves with catheters should be avoided because it may result in catheter entrapment, occlusion of the valve, or possible dislodgment of the disc with embolization.

The procedure is performed after localizing the left ventricular apex by palpation or, preferably, by using echocardiography.[21] After local anesthesia is administered, an 18- or 21-gauge 6-inch Teflon catheter system is inserted at the upper rib margin and directed slightly posteriorly and toward the right second intercostal space until the impulse is encountered. The needle and sheath are advanced into the left ventricle The stylet and needle are removed, and the sheath is connected for pressure measurement.

The risks of this procedure include cardiac tamponade, hemothorax, pneumothorax, laceration of the left anterior descending coronary artery, embolism of left ventricular thrombus, vagal reactions, and ventricular arrhythmias. The risk of pericardial tamponade, however, is limited in patients who have undergone prior cardiac surgery because mediastinal fibrosis is present. However, with current noninvasive imaging techniques including transesophageal echocardiography, this procedure is infrequently indicated.

ENDOMYOCARDIAL BIOPSY

Endomyocardial biopsy can be performed using various disposable or reusable bioptomes. Disposable bioptomes have become the more commonly used devices because of the difficulty in maintaining and adequately resterilizing the reusable varieties.The most popular devices used for the internal jugular vein approach include the reusable stiff-shaft Caves-Schulz Stanford bioptome and the floppy-shaft King bioptome. Right ventricular biopsy may be performed using the internal jugular vein,[22] the subclavian vein, or the femoral vein. Left ventricular biopsy may be performed using the femoral arterial approach.

When performing right ventricular biopsy through the right internal jugular vein, a 7 to 9F sheath is introduced using the usual Seldinger technique. A 7 to 9F bioptome is advanced under fluoroscopic guidance to the lateral wall of the right atrium. Using counterclockwise rotation, the device is advanced across the tricuspid valve and toward the interventricular septum. Position of the bioptome against the interventricular septum is confirmed using 30-degree right anterior oblique and 60-degree left anterior oblique fluoroscopic projections. Alternatively, two-dimensional echocardiography has been used to guide the position of the bioptome with good results. Contact with the myocardium is confirmed by the presence of premature ventricular contractions, lack of further advancement, and transmission of the ventricular impulse to the operator. The bioptome is then slightly withdrawn from the septum, the forceps jaws are opened, the bioptome is readvanced to make contact with the myocardium, and the forceps closed. A slight tug is felt on removal of the device. Approximately four to six samples of myocardium are required for adequate pathological analysis. Consultation with a pathologist should be obtained to ensure appropriate specimen collection and processing.

Right ventricular biopsy from the femoral vein requires insertion of a long 6 or 7F sheath directed toward the portion of the ventricle to be sampled. Various configurations of sheaths are used for right ventricular biopsy. The conventional sheath has a 45-degree angle on its distal end to allow access to the right ventricle. However, newer designs including the Daig biopsy sheath have dual curves. This catheter possesses the usual 180-degree Mullins curve and an additional distal perpendicular septal plane curve of 90 degrees, which allows improved manipulation and positioning toward the interventricular septum.

An angled pigtail or balloon flotation catheter and long guidewire system can be used to enter the right ventricle. The sheath is then advanced over the pigtail catheter into the right ventricle, the catheter is withdrawn, the sheath is flushed, and pressure is measured. The bioptome is advanced through the sheath. The biopsy sheath should be visualized in both the 30-degree right anterior oblique and 40-degree left anterior oblique views. The right anterior oblique view ensures that the catheter is in the midventricle away from the apex. The left anterior oblique view verifies that the sheath tip is oriented toward the interventricular septum. Contrast medium infusion through the side port of the sheath can be confirmatory. Samples of myocardium are taken in a manner similar to that described earlier.

If left ventricular biopsy is to be performed, the biopsy sheath is generally inserted through the femoral artery and positioned over a multipurpose or pigtail catheter that has been placed in the ventricle. The sheath is advanced below the mitral apparatus and away from the posterobasal wall. The catheter is then withdrawn, and either a long King bioptome or the Stanford left ventricular bioptome is inserted. Care must be taken when left ventricular biopsy is performed to prevent air embolism while introducing the bioptome into the sheath. A constant infusion of flush solution through the sheath minimizes the risk of air or thrombus embolism.

Complications of endomyocardial biopsy include cardiac perforation with cardiac tamponade, emboli (air, tissue, or thromboembolus), arrhythmias, electrical conduction disturbances, injury to heart valves, vasovagal reactions, and pneumothorax. The overall complication rate is between 1 and 2 percent, with the risk of cardiac perforation with tamponade generally reported as less than 0.05 percent.[23] Systemic embolization and ventricular arrhythmias are more common with left ventricular biopsy. Left ventricular biopsy should generally be avoided in patients with right bundle branch block because of the potential for developing complete atrioventricular block as well as in patients with known left ventricular thrombus.

The indications for endomyocardial biopsy remain controversial.[24] Generally agreed is that endomyocardial biopsy is indicated to monitor cardiac allograft rejection and that it may also be useful to monitor for anthracycline cardiotoxicity. However, considerable persistent controversy surrounds the use of endomyocardial biopsy to evaluate the cause of dilated cardiomopathy.[24] Other possible indications for endomyocardial biopsy include differentiation between restrictive and constrictive myopathies,[25] determination of whether myocarditis is the cause of ventricular arrhythmias, and assessment of patients with left ventricular dysfunction associated with human immunodeficiency virus infection.[26]

Percutaneous Intraaortic Balloon Pump Insertion

The intraaortic balloon counterpulsation devices available for adults are positioned in the descending thoracic aorta. They have a balloon volume of 30 to 50 ml, use helium as the inflation gas, and are timed to inflate during diastole and deflate during systole. Details of the technique of balloon insertion have been well described.[27] Briefly, the device is inserted through the femoral artery using the standard Seldinger technique. The device is placed so that the tip is just below the level of the left subclavian artery. Optimal positioning requires fluoroscopic guidance. Timing of the balloon is adjusted during 1:2 (one inflation for each two beats) pumping so that inflation of the balloon occurs at the aortic dicrotic notch and deflation occurs immediately before systole. This timing ensures maximal augmentation of diastolic flow and maximal systolic unloading.

Favorable hemodynamic effects include reduction in left ventricular afterload and improvement in myocardial oxygenation.[28] Intraaortic balloon pump (IABP) insertion is indicated for patients with angina refractory to medical therapy, cardiogenic shock, or mechanical complications of myocardial infarction (including severe mitral regurgitation, ventricular septal defect) or for those who have severe left main coronary artery stenosis and will be undergoing cardiac surgery. IABP may also be valuable in patients undergoing high-risk percutaneous coronary intervention or after primary angioplasty in the setting of acute myocardial infarction.[29,30] IABP insertion is contraindicated in patients with moderate or severe aortic regurgitation, aortic dissection, aortic aneurysm, patent ductus arteriosus, severe peripheral vascular disease, bleeding disorders, or sepsis.

Complications of IABP insertion include limb ischemia requiring early balloon removal or vascular surgery, balloon rupture, balloon entrapment, hematomas, and sepsis.[29] The incidence of vascular complications ranges from 12 to greater than 40 percent.[29] Most patients in whom limb ischemia develops after insertion of a balloon pump device have resolution of the ischemia on balloon removal and do not require surgical intervention (thrombectomy, vascular repair, fasciotomy, or amputation). The risk of limb ischemia is heightened in patients with diabetes or peripheral vascular disease, in women, and in patients with a postinsertion ankle-brachial index of less than 0.8. However, with the development of smaller catheters (8 to 9.5F) and the advent of the sheathless insertion techniques, vascular complications have been reduced.[29-31]

Hemodynamic Data

The hemodynamic component of the cardiac catheterization procedure focuses on pressure measurements, the measurement of flow (e.g., cardiac output, shunt flows, flow across a stenotic orifice, regurgitant flows, and coronary blood flow), and the determination of vascular resistances. Simply stated, flow through a blood vessel is determined by the pressure difference within the vessel and the vascular resistance as described by Ohm's law: $Q = \Delta P/R$.

Pressure Measurements

Accurate recording of pressure waveforms and correct interpretation of physiological data derived from these waveforms are major goals of cardiac catheterization. A pressure wave is the cyclical force generated by cardiac muscle contraction, and its amplitude and duration are influenced by various mechanical and physiological parameters. The pressure waveform from a particular cardiac chamber is influenced by the force of the contracting chamber and its surrounding structures, including the contiguous chambers of the heart, the pericardium, the lungs, and the vasculature. Physiological variables of heart rate and the respiratory cycle also influence the pressure waveform. An understanding of the components of the cardiac cycle is essential to the correct interpretation of hemodynamic data obtained in the catheterization laboratory.

Pressure Measurement Systems

FLUID-FILLED SYSTEMS. Intravascular pressures are typically measured using a fluid-filled catheter that is attached to a pressure transducer. The pressure wave is transmitted from the catheter tip to the transducer by the fluid column within the catheter. The majority of pressure transducers used currently are disposable electrical strain gauges. The pressure wave distorts the diaphragm or wire within the transducer. This energy is then converted to an electrical signal proportional to the pressure being applied using the principle of the Wheatstone bridge. This signal is then amplified and recorded as an analog signal.[32]

There are a number of sources of error when pressures are measured using a fluid-filled catheter-transducer system. Distortion of the output signal occurs as a result of the frequency response characteristics and damping characteristics of the system. The frequency response of the system is the ratio of the output amplitude to input amplitude over a range of frequencies of the input pressure wave. The natural frequency is the frequency at which the system oscillates when it is shock-excited in the absence of friction. Dissipation of the energy of the system, such as by friction, is called *damping*. To ensure a high-frequency response range, the pressure measurement system should have the highest possible natural frequency and optimal damping. With optimal damping the energy is dissipated gradually, thus maintaining the frequency response curve as close as possible to an output/input ratio of 1 as it approaches the system's natural frequency. Optimal damping is achieved by using a short, wide-bore, noncompliant catheter-tubing system that is directly connected to the transducer using a low-density liquid from which all air bubbles have been removed.[32]

The pressure transducer must be calibrated against a known pressure, and the establishment of a zero reference must be undertaken at the start of the catheterization procedure. To "zero" the transducer, the transducer is placed at the level of the atria, which is approximately midchest. If the transducer is attached to the manifold and is therefore at variable positions during the procedure, a second fluid-filled catheter system should be attached to the transducer and positioned at the level of the midchest. All transducers being used during the procedure should be zeroed and calibrated simultaneously. Because of possible variable drift during the procedure, all transducers should be rebalanced immediately prior to obtaining simultaneous recordings for transvalvular gradient determinations.

Potential sources of error include catheter whip artifact (motion of the tip of the catheter within the measured chamber), end-pressure artifact (an end-hole catheter measures an artificially elevated pressure because of streaming or high velocity of the pressure wave), catheter impact artifact (when the catheter is struck by the walls or valves of the cardiac chambers), and catheter tip obstruction within small vessels or valvular orifices occurring because of the size of the catheter itself. The operator must be aware of the many sources of potential error, and when there is a discrepancy between the observed data and the clinical scenario, the system should be examined for errors or artifacts.

MICROMANOMETER CATHETERS. The use of these catheters, which have the pressure transducer mounted at their tip, greatly reduces many of these errors in measurement. However, their utility is limited by the additional cost and time needed for properly calibrating and using the system. These catheters have higher natural frequencies and more optimal damping characteristics because the interposing fluid column is eliminated. In addition, there is a decrease in catheter whip artifact. The pressure waveform is less distorted and is without the 30- to 40-millisecond delay seen in the fluid-filled catheter-transducer system. Commercially available high-fidelity micromanometer systems have both an end hole and side holes to allow over-the-wire insertion into the circulation while also permitting angiography. Catheters that have two transducers separated by a short distance are useful for accurate measurement of gradients across valvular structures and within ventricular chambers. The micromanometer system has been used for research purposes to assess the rate of ventricular pressure rise (dP/dt), wall stress, the rate of ventricular pressure decay (–dP/dt), the time constant of relaxation, and ventricular pressure-volume relationships (see Chap. 20).

The micromanometer catheter systems have several disadvantages, including their expense, fragility, and added procedural time. In addition, the zero level of these systems may drift after the pressure is zeroed to the fluid-filled lumen within the catheter.

Normal Pressure Waveforms

An understanding of the normal pressure waveform morphologies is necessary for comprehending the abnormalities that characterize certain pathological conditions. Normal pressures in the cardiac chambers and great vessels are listed in Table 17–4. Simply stated, whenever fluid is added to a chamber or compressed within a chamber, the pressure usually rises; conversely, whenever fluid exits from a chamber or the chamber relaxes, the pressure usually falls. One exception to this rule is the early phase of ventricular diastolic filling, when ventricular volume increases after mitral valve opening but ventricular pressure continues to decrease because of active relaxation.[33] Examples of normal pressure waveforms are shown in Figure 17–10.

TABLE 17–4 Normal Pressures and Vascular Resistances

Pressures	Average (mm Hg)	Range (mm Hg)
Right atrium		
a wave	6	2-7
v wave	5	2-7
mean	3	1-5
Right ventricle		
peak systolic	25	15-30
end-diastolic	4	1-7
Pulmonary artery		
peak systolic	25	15-30
end-diastolic	9	4-12
mean	15	9-19
Pulmonary capillary wedge		
mean	9	4-12
Left atrium		
a wave	10	4-16
v wave	12	6-21
mean	8	2-12
Left ventricle		
peak systolic	130	90-140
end-diastolic	8	5-12
Central aorta		
peak systolic	130	90-140
end-diastolic	70	60-90
mean	85	70-105
Vascular Resistances	**Mean (dyne-sec · cm^{-5})**	**Range (dyne-sec · cm^{-5})**
Systemic vascular resistance	1100	700-1600
Total pulmonary resistance	200	100-300
Pulmonary vascular resistance	70	20-130

ATRIAL PRESSURE. The *right atrial pressure waveform* has three positive deflections, the a, c, and v waves. The a wave is due to atrial systole and follows the P wave of the ECG. The height of the a wave depends on atrial contractility and the resistance to right ventricular filling. The *x* descent follows the a wave and represents relaxation of the atrium and downward pulling of the tricuspid annulus by right ventricular contraction. The *x* descent is interrupted by the c wave, which is a small positive deflection caused by protrusion of the closed tricuspid valve into the right atrium. Pressure in the atrium rises after the *x* descent owing to passive atrial filling. The atrial pressure then peaks as the v wave, which represents right ventricular systole. The height of the v wave is related to atrial compliance and the amount of blood returning to the atrium from the periphery. The right atrial v wave is generally smaller than the a wave. The *y* descent occurs after the v wave and reflects tricuspid valve opening and right atrial emptying into the right ventricle. During spontaneous respiration, right atrial pressure declines during inhalation as intrathoracic pressure falls. Right atrial pressure rises during exhalation as intrathoracic pressures increase. The opposite effect is seen when patients are mechanically ventilated.

The *left atrial pressure waveform* is similar to that of the right atrium, although normal left atrial pressure is

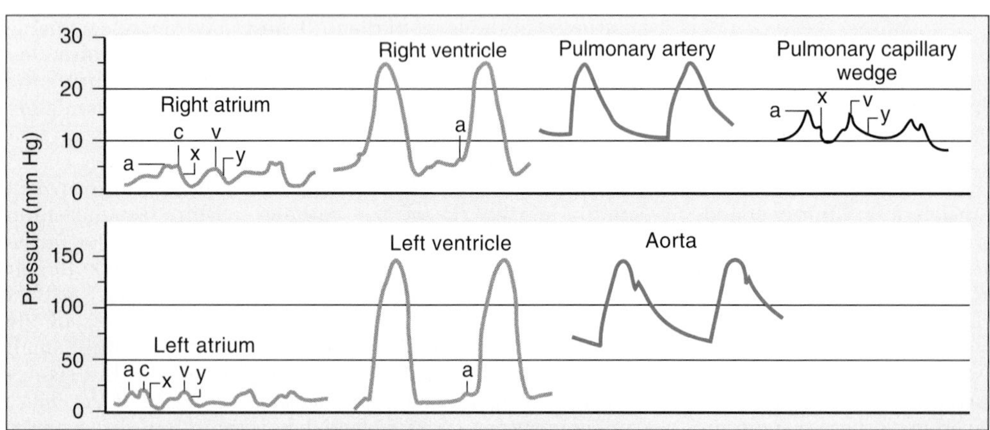

FIGURE 17–10 Normal right- and left-heart pressures recorded from fluid-filled catheter systems in a human. (From Pepine C, Hill JA, Lambert CR [eds]: Diagnostic and Therapeutic Cardiac Catheterization. 3rd ed. Baltimore, Williams & Wilkins, 1998.)

higher, reflecting the high-pressure system of the left side of the heart. In the left atrium, as opposed to the right atrium, the v wave is generally higher than the a wave. This difference occurs because the left atrium is constrained posteriorly by the pulmonary veins, whereas the right atrium can easily decompress throughout the IVC and SVC. The height of the left atrial v wave most accurately reflects left atrial compliance.

PULMONARY CAPILLARY WEDGE PRESSURE. The pulmonary capillary wedge pressure waveform is similar to the left atrial pressure waveform but is slightly damped and delayed as a result of transmission through the lungs. The a and v waves with both *x* and *y* descents are visible, but c waves may not be seen. In the normal state, the pulmonary artery diastolic pressure is similar to the mean pulmonary capillary wedge pressure because the pulmonary circulation has low resistance. In certain disease states that are associated with elevated pulmonary vascular resistance (hypoxemia, pulmonary embolism, and chronic pulmonary hypertension), and occasionally after mitral valve surgery, the pulmonary capillary wedge pressure may overestimate true left atrial pressure. In this circumstance, accurate measurement of the mitral valve gradient may require obtaining direct left atrial pressure.[34,35]

VENTRICULAR PRESSURE. Right and left ventricular waveforms are similar in morphology. They differ mainly with respect to their magnitudes. The durations of systole and isovolumic contraction and relaxation are longer and the ejection period shorter in the left than in the right ventricle. There may be a small (5 mm Hg) systolic gradient between the right ventricle and the pulmonary artery. Ventricular diastolic pressure is characterized by an early rapid filling wave during which most of the ventricle fills, a slow filling phase, and the a wave denoting atrial systolic activity. End-diastolic pressure is generally measured at the C-point, which is the rise in ventricular pressure at the onset of isovolumic contraction. When the C-point is not well seen, a line is drawn from the R wave on the simultaneous ECG to the ventricular pressure waveform, and this is used as the end-diastolic pressure.

GREAT VESSEL PRESSURES. The contour of the *central aortic pressure* and the *pulmonary artery pressure* tracing consists of a systolic wave, the incisura (indicating closure of the semilunar valves), and a gradual decline in pressure until the following systole. The pulse pressure reflects the stroke volume and compliance of the arterial system. The mean aortic pressure more accurately reflects peripheral resistance. As the systemic pressure wave is transmitted through the length of the aorta, the systolic wave increases in amplitude and becomes more triangular, and the diastolic wave decreases until it reaches the midthoracic aorta and then increases. The mean aortic pressures, however, are usually similar, with the mean *peripheral arterial pressure* typically equal to or less than 5 mm Hg lower than the mean central aortic pressure. The difference in systolic pressures between the central aorta and the periphery (femoral, brachial, or radial arteries) is greatest in younger patients owing to their increased vascular compliance. These potential differences between proximal aorta and peripheral artery must be considered in order to measure and interpret the peak systolic pressure gradient between the left ventricle and systemic arterial system in patients with suspected aortic stenosis. When a transvalvular gradient is present, the most accurate measure of the aortic pressure is obtained at the level of the coronary arteries. This measurement avoids the effect of pressure recovery, which is defined as the variable increase in lateral pressure downstream from a stenotic orifice (see Chap. 57). This approach can become clinically important in cases of mild to moderate aortic stenosis, particularly when the aorta is small.[36,37]

ABNORMAL PRESSURE CHARACTERISTICS. Abnormal pressure waveforms may be diagnostic of specific pathological conditions. Table 17–5 summarizes the more commonly encountered waveforms.

Cardiac Output Measurements

There is no totally accurate method of measuring cardiac output, but it can be estimated on the basis of various assumptions. The two most commonly used methods are the Fick method and thermodilution method. For comparison among patients, cardiac output is often corrected for the patient's size on the basis of the body surface area and expressed as cardiac index.

INDICATOR-DILUTION TECHNIQUES. The indicator-dilution method was the original clinical method used to measure cardiac output since its introduction by Stewart in 1897 and subsequent modification by Hamilton in 1932. The basic equation, commonly referred to as the Stewart-Hamilton equation, follows:

$$\text{Cardiac output (liter/min)} = \frac{\text{amount of indicator injected (mg)} \cdot 60\ \text{sec/min}}{\text{mean indicator concentration (mg/ml)} \cdot \text{curve duration}}$$

The assumption is made that after the injection of a certain quantity of an indicator into the circulation, the indicator appears and disappears from any downstream point in a manner commensurate with the cardiac output. For example, if the indicator rapidly appears at a specific location downstream and then washes out quickly, the assumption is that the cardiac output is high. Although variation can occur, the site of injection is usually a systemic vein or the right side of the heart, and the sampling site is generally a systemic artery. The normal curve itself has an initial rapid upstroke followed by a slower downstroke and eventual appearance of recirculation of the tracer. In practice, this recirculation creates some uncertainty on the tail of the curve, and assumptions are required to correct for this distortion.

There are several sources of error in this determination. Because the dye is unstable over time and can be affected by light, fresh preparations of indocyanine green dye are necessary. The exact amount of dye must be accurately measured. After injection, the indicator must mix well before reaching the sampling site, and the dilution curve must have an exponential decay over time so that extrapolation can be performed. If, for example, there is severe valvular regurgitation or a low cardiac output state in which the washout of the indicator is prolonged and recirculation begins well before an adequate decline in the indicator curve occurs, determinations are erroneous. Intracardiac shunts may also greatly affect the shape of the curve.

THERMODILUTION TECHNIQUES. Because of the rather tedious and time-consuming nature of the indicator-dilution method, it has been replaced by thermodilution techniques in many laboratories. The development of balloon flotation (e.g., Swan-Ganz) catheters with a proximal port and distal thermistor (see Fig. 17–1) has greatly expanded the ability to obtain thermodilution cardiac outputs in many clinical settings.

The thermodilution procedure requires injection of a bolus of liquid (saline or dextrose) into the proximal port of the catheter. The resultant change in temperature in the liquid is measured by a thermistor mounted in the distal end of the catheter. The change in temperature versus time can be plotted in a manner similar to that in the dye-dilution method described earlier (in which the indicator is now the cooler liquid). The cardiac output is then calculated using an equation that considers the temperature and specific gravity of the injectate and the temperature and specific gravity of the blood

TABLE 17–5 Pathological Waveforms

I. Right atrial pressure waveforms
  A. Low mean atrial pressure
    1. Hypovolemia
    2. Improper zeroing of the transducer
  B. Elevated mean atrial pressure
    1. Intravascular volume overload states
    2. Right ventricular failure due to valvular disease (tricuspid or pulmonic stenosis or regurgitation)
    3. Right ventricular failure due to myocardial disease (right ventricular ischemia, cardiomyopathy)
    4. Right ventricular failure due to left-sided heart failure (mitral stenosis/regurgitation, aortic stenosis/regurgitation, cardiomyopathy, ischemia)
    5. Right ventricular failure due to increased pulmonary vascular resistance (pulmonary embolism, chronic obstructive pulmonary disease, primary pulmonary hypertension)
    6. Pericardial effusion with tamponade physiology
    7. Obstructive atrial myxoma
  C. Elevated a wave (any increase to ventricular filling)
    1. Tricuspid stenosis
    2. Decreased ventricular compliance due to ventricular failure, pulmonic valve stenosis, or pulmonary hypertension
  D. Cannon a wave
    1. Atrial-ventricular asynchrony (atria contract against a closed tricuspid valve, as during complete heart block, following premature ventricular contraction, during ventricular tachycardia, with ventricular pacemaker)
  E. Absent a wave
    1. Atrial fibrillation or atrial standstill
    2. Atrial flutter
  F. Elevated v wave
    1. Tricuspid regurgitation
    2. Right ventricular heart failure
    3. Reduced atrial compliance (restrictive myopathy)
  G. a wave equal to v wave
    1. Tamponade
    2. Constrictive pericardial disease
    3. Hypervolemia
  H. Prominent *x* descent
    1. Tamponade
    2. Subacute constriction and possibly chronic constriction
    3. Right ventricular ischemia with preservation of atrial contractility
  I. Prominent *y* descent
    1. Constructive pericarditis
    2. Restrictive myopathies
    3. Tricuspid regurgitation
  J. Blunted *x* descent
    1. Atrial fibrillation
    2. Right atrial ischemia
  K. Blunted *y* descent
    1. Tamponade
    2. Right ventricular ischemia
    3. Tricuspid stenosis
  L. Miscellaneous abnormalities
    1. Kussmaul sign (aspiratory rise or lack of decline in right atrial pressure): constrictive pericarditis, right ventricular ischemia
    2. Equalization (≤5 mm Hg) of mean right atrial ventricular diastolic, pulmonary artery diastolic, pulmonary capillary wedge, and pericardial pressures in tamponade
    3. M or W patterns: right ventricular ischemia, pericardial constriction, congestive heart failure
    4. Ventricularization of the right atrial pressure: severe tricuspid regurgitation
    5. Sawtooth pattern: atrial flutter
    6. Dissociation between pressure recording and intracardiac electrocardiogram: Ebstein anomaly

II. Left atrial pressure/pulmonary capillary wedge pressure waveforms
  A. Low mean pressure
    1. Hypovolemia
    2. Improper zeroing of the transducer
  B. Elevated mean pressure
    1. Intravascular volume overload states
    2. Left ventricular failure due to valvular disease (mitral or aortic stenosis or regurgitation)
    3. Left ventricular failure due to myocardial disease (ischemia or cardiomyopathy)
    4. Left ventricular failure due to systemic hypertension
    5. Pericardial effusion with tamponade physiology
    6. Obstructive atrial myxoma
  C. Elevated a wave (any increase to ventricular filling)
    1. Mitral stenosis
    2. Decreased ventricular compliance due to ventricular failure, aortic valve stenosis, or systemic hypertension
  D. Cannon a wave
    1. Atrial-ventricular asynchrony (atria contract against a closed mitral valve, as during complete heart block, following premature ventricular contraction, during ventricular tachycardia, or with ventricular pacemaker)
  E. Absent a wave
    1. Atrial fibrillation or atrial standstill
    2. Atrial flutter

TABLE 17–5 Pathological Waveforms—cont'd

F. Elevated v wave
  1. Mitral regurgitation
  2. Left ventricular heart failure
  3. Ventricular septal defect
G. a wave equal to v wave
  1. Tamponade
  2. Constrictive pericardial disease
  3. Hypervolemia
H. Prominent *x* descent
  1. Tamponade
  2. Subacute constriction and possibly chronic constriction
I. Prominent *y* descent
  1. Constrictive pericarditis
  2. Restrictive myopathies
  3. Mitral regurgitation
J. Blunted *x* descent
  1. Atrial fibrillation
  2. Atrial ischemia
K. Blunted *y* descent
  1. Tamponade
  2. Ventricular ischemia
  3. Mitral stenosis
L. Pulmonary capillary wedge pressure not equal to left ventricular end-diastolic pressure
  1. Mitral stenosis
  2. Left atrial myxoma
  3. Cor triatriatum
  4. Pulmonary venous obstruction
  5. Decreased ventricular compliance
  6. Increased pleural pressure
  7. Placement of catheter in a nondependent zone of the lung

III. Pulmonary artery pressure waveforms
  A. Elevated systolic pressure
    1. Primary pulmonary hypertension
    2. Mitral stenosis or regurgitation
    3. Congestive heart failure
    4. Restrictive myopathies
    5. Significant left-to-right shunt
    6. Pulmonary disease (pulmonary embolism, hypoxemia, chronic obstructive pulmonary disease)
  B. Reduced systolic pressure
    1. Hypovolemia
    2. Pulmonary artery stenosis
    3. Subvalvular or supravalvular stenosis
    4. Ebstein anomaly
    5. Tricuspid stenosis
    6. Tricuspid atresia
  C. Reduced pulse pressure
    1. Right-heart ischemia
    2. Right ventricular infarction
    3. Pulmonary embolism
    4. Tamponade
  D. Bifid pulmonary artery waveform
    1. Large left atrial v wave transmitted backward (i.e., mitral regurgitation)
  E. Pulmonary artery diastolic pressure greater than pulmonary capillary wedge pressure
    1. Pulmonary disease
    2. Pulmonary embolus
    3. Tachycardia

IV. Ventricular pressure waveforms
  A. Systolic pressure elevated
    1. Pulmonary or systemic hypertension
    2. Pulmonary valve or aortic stenosis
    3. Ventricular outflow tract obstruction
    4. Supravalvular obstruction
    5. Right ventricular pressure elevation with significant:
      a. Atrial septal defect
      b. Ventricular septal defect
    6. Right ventricular pressure elevation due to factors that increase pulmonary vascular resistance (see factors that increase right atrial pressure)
  B. Systolic pressure reduced
    1. Hypovolemia
    2. Cardiogenic shock
    3. Tamponade
  C. End-diastolic pressure elevated
    1. Hypervolemia
    2. Congestive heart failure
    3. Diminished compliance
    4. Hypertrophy
    5. Tamponade
    6. Regurgitant valvular disease
    7. Pericardial constriction
  D. End-diastolic pressure reduced
    1. Hypovolemia
    2. Tricuspid or mitral stenosis
  E. Diminished or absent a wave
    1. Atrial fibrillation or flutter
    2. Tricuspid or mitral stenosis
    3. Tricuspid or mitral regurgitation when ventricular compliance is increased
  F. Dip and plateau in diastolic pressure wave
    1. Constrictive pericarditis
    2. Restrictive myopathies
    3. Right ventricular ischemia
    4. Acute dilation associated with:
      a. Tricuspid regurgitation
      b. Mitral regurgitation
  G. Left ventricular end-diastolic pressure > right ventricular end-diastolic pressure
    1. Restrictive myopathies

V. Aortic pressure waveforms
  A. Systolic pressure elevated
    1. Systemic hypertension
    2. Arteriosclerosis
    3. Aortic insufficiency
  B. Systolic pressure reduced
    1. Aortic stenosis
    2. Heart failure
    3. Hypovolemia
  C. Widened pulse pressure
    1. Systemic hypertension
    2. Aortic insufficiency
    3. Significant patent ductus arteriosus
    4. Significant ruptures of sinus of Valsalva aneurysm
  D. Reduced pulse pressure
    1. Tamponade
    2. Congestive heart failure
    3. Cardiogenic shock
    4. Aortic stenosis
  E. Pulsus bisferiens
    1. Aortic insufficiency
    2. Obstructive hypertrophic cardiomyopathy
  F. Pulsus paradoxus
    1. Tamponade
    2. Chronic obstructive airway disease
    3. Pulmonary embolism
  G. Pulsus alternans
    1. Congestive heart failure
    2. Cardiomyopathy
  H. Pulsus parvus et tardus
    1. Aortic stenosis
  I. Spike-and-dome configuration
    1. Obstructive hypertrophic cardiomyopathy

along with the injectate volume. A calibration factor is also used. The cardiac output is inversely related to the area under a thermodilution curve, plotted as a function of temperature versus time, with a smaller area indicative of a higher cardiac output. The use of two thermistors can significantly improve the accuracy of this technique.[38]

The thermodilution method has several advantages. It obviates the need for withdrawal of blood from an arterial site and is less affected by recirculation. Perhaps its greatest advantage is the rapid display of results using computerized methods (Fig. 17–11). However, a significant error occurs in patients with severe tricuspid regurgitation. Also, in patients with low outputs (especially <2.5 liter/min), thermodilution tends to overestimate the cardiac output.

FICK METHOD

The Fick principle assumes that the rate at which oxygen is consumed is a function of the rate of blood flow times the rate of oxygen pickup by the red blood cells. The basic assumption is that the flow of blood in a given period of time is equal to the amount of substance entering the stream of flow in the same period of time divided by the difference between the concentrations of the substance in the blood upstream and downstream from its point of entry into the circulation (Fig. 17–12). The same number of red blood cells that enter the lung must leave the lung if no intracardiac shunt is present. Thus, if certain parameters were known (the number of oxygen molecules that were attached to the red blood cells entering the lung, the number of oxygen molecules that were attached to the red blood cells leaving the lung, and the number of oxygen molecules consumed during travel through the lung), the rate of flow of these red blood cells as they pass through the lung could be determined. This can be expressed in the following terms:

$$\text{Cardiac output (liter/min)} = \frac{O_2 \text{ consumption (ml/min)}}{\text{A-V}O_2 \text{ difference (vol \%)} \cdot 10}$$

where A-VO_2 is the arteriovenous oxygen difference.

Measurements must be made in the steady state. Automated methods can accurately determine the oxygen content within the blood samples. Thus, the greatest source of measurement variability is the oxygen consumption. In traditional Fick determinations, expiratory gas samples were collected in a large bag over a specified period. By measuring the expiratory oxygen concentration and by knowing the concentration of oxygen in room air, the quantity of oxygen consumed over time could be determined. Techniques that allow measurement of the expired oxygen concentration are quantified by using a polarograph. This device can be connected to the patient by use of a plastic hood or by a mouthpiece and tubing.

The advantage of the Fick method is that it is the most accurate method in patients with low cardiac output and thus is preferred over the thermodilution method in these circumstances. It is also independent of the factors that affect curve shape and cause errors in thermodilution cardiac output. The Fick method suffers primarily from the difficulty in obtaining accurate oxygen consumption measurements and the inability to obtain a steady state under certain conditions. Because the method assumes mean flow over a period of time, it is not suitable during rapid change in flow. It requires additional time and effort in the catheterization laboratory to obtain the appropriate data. Many laboratories use an "assumed" Fick method in which the oxygen consumption index is assumed on the basis of the patient's age, gender, and body surface area or an estimate is made (125 ml/m^2) on the basis of body surface area. The inaccuracy of oxygen consumption measurements results in up to 10 percent variability in the calculated cardiac output, which may be even greater when assumed oxygen consumption, rather than measured oxygen consumption, is used.

ANGIOGRAPHIC CARDIAC OUTPUT. Angiographic stroke volume can be calculated by tracing the end-diastolic and end-systolic images. Stroke volume is the quantity of blood ejected with each beat. End-diastolic volume is the maximum left ventricular volume and occurs immediately before the onset of systole. It occurs immediately after atrial contraction in patients in sinus rhythm. End-systolic volume is the minimum volume during the cardiac cycle. Calibration of the images with grids or ventricular phantoms is necessary to obtain accurate ventricular volumes. Angiographic cardiac output and stroke volume are derived from the following equations:

$$\text{Stroke volume} = \text{EDV} - \text{ESV}$$
$$\text{Cardiac output} = (\text{EDV} - \text{ESV}) \cdot \text{heart rate}$$

where EDV = end-diastolic volume and ESV = end-systolic volume. The inherent inaccuracies of calibrating angiographic volumes often make this method of measurement unreliable. In cases of valvular regurgitation or atrial fibrillation, angiographic cardiac output does not accurately measure true systemic outputs. However, the angiographic or thermodilution cardiac output is preferred over the Fick or thermodilution output for calculation of stenotic valve areas in patients with significant aortic or mitral regurgitation.

Determination of Vascular Resistance

Vascular resistance calculations are based on hydraulic principles of fluid flow, in which resistance is defined as the ratio of the decrease in pressure between two points in a vascular

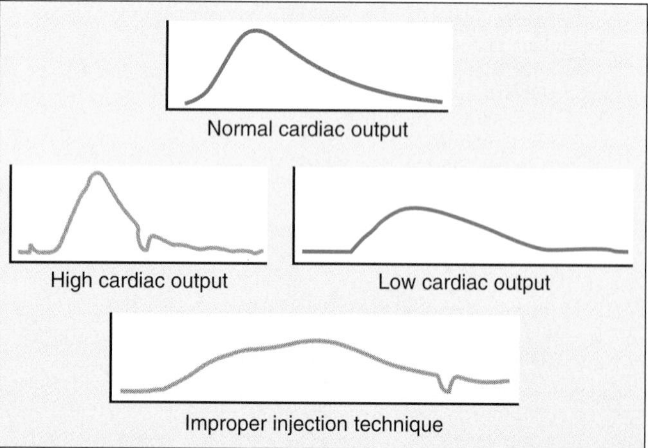

FIGURE 17–11 Thermodilution cardiac output curves. A normal curve has a sharp upstroke following an injection of saline. A smooth curve with a mildly prolonged downslope occurs until it is back to baseline. The area under the curve is inversely related to the cardiac output. At low cardiac output, a prolonged period is required to return to baseline. Therefore, there is a larger area under the curve. In a high cardiac output state, the cooler saline injectate moves faster through the right side of the heart and temperature returns to baseline more quickly. The area under the curve is smaller and the output is higher.

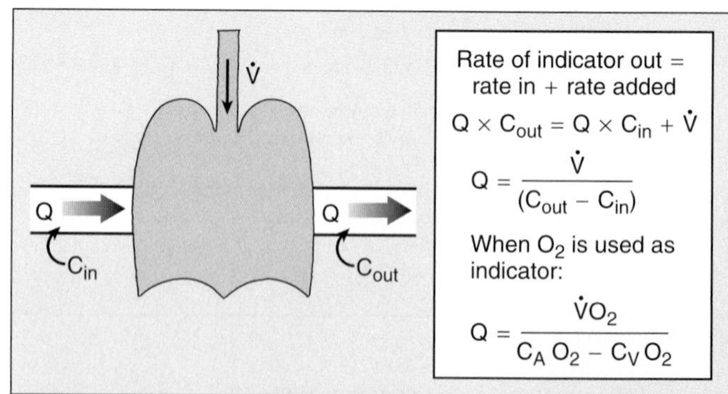

FIGURE 17–12 Schematic illustration of flow measurement using the Fick principle. Fluid containing a known concentration of an indicator (C_{in}) enters a system at flow rate Q. As the fluid passes through the system, indicator is continuously added at rate $\dot{V}$, raising the concentration in the outflow to C_{out}. In a steady state, the rate of indicator leaving the system (QC_{out}) must equal the rate at which it enters (QC_{in}) plus the rate at which it is added ($\dot{V}$). When oxygen is used as the indicator, cardiac output can be determined by measuring oxygen consumption ($\dot{V}O_2$), arterial oxygen content (C_AO_2), and mixed venous oxygen content (C_VO_2). (From Winniford MD, Kern MJ, Lambert CR: Blood flow measurement. *In* Pepine CJ, Hill JA, Lambert CR [eds]: Diagnostic and Therapeutic Cardiac Catheterization. 3rd ed. Baltimore, Williams & Wilkins, 1998, p 400.)

segment and the blood flow through the segment. Although this straightforward analogy to Ohm's law represents an oversimplification of the complex behavior of pulsatile flow in dynamic and diverse vascular beds, the calculation of vascular resistance based on these principles has proven to be of value in a number of clinical settings.

Determination of the resistance in a vascular bed requires measurement of the mean pressure of the proximal and distal ends of the vascular bed and accurate measurement of cardiac output. Vascular resistance (R) is usually defined in absolute units (dyne-sec · cm^{-5}) and is defined as R = [mean pressure gradient (dyne/cm^2)]/[mean flow (cm^3/sec)]. Hybrid units (Wood units) are less often used.[39]

Systemic vascular resistance in absolute units is calculated using the following equation:

$$SVR = 80(Ao_m - RA_m)/Q_s$$

where Ao_m and RA_m are the mean pressures (in mm Hg) in the aorta and right atrium, respectively, and Q_s is the systemic cardiac output (in liter/min). The constant 80 is used to convert units from mm Hg/liter/min (Wood units) to the absolute resistance units dyne-sec · cm^{-5}. If the right atrial pressure is not known, the term RA_m can be dropped, and the resulting value is called the *total peripheral resistance* (TPR).

$$TPR = 80(Ao_m)/Q_s$$

Similarly, the pulmonary vascular resistance is derived from the following equation:

$$PVR = 80(PA_m - LA_m)/Q_p$$

where PA_m and LA_m are the pulmonary artery and left atrial pressures, respectively, and Q_p is the pulmonary blood flow. Mean pulmonary capillary wedge pressure is commonly substituted for mean left atrial pressure if the latter has not been measured directly, although errors can occur because of this substitution. In the absence of an intracardiac shunt, Q_p is equal to the systemic cardiac output. Normal values are listed in Table 17–4.

Elevated resistances in the systemic and pulmonary circuits may represent reversible abnormalities or may be fixed owing to irreversible anatomical changes. In several clinical situations, such as congestive heart failure, valvular heart disease, primary pulmonary hypertension, and congenital heart disease with intracardiac shunting, determination of whether elevated systemic or pulmonary vascular resistance can be lowered transiently in the catheterization laboratory may provide important insights into potential management strategies. Interventions that may be used in the laboratory for this purpose include administration of vasodilating drugs (e.g., sodium nitroprusside), exercise, and (in patients with pulmonary hypertension) oxygen inhalation or intravenous epoprostenol (Flolan), a pulmonary and systemic vasodilator (see Chap. 67).

Vascular impedance measurements account for blood viscosity, pulsatile flow, reflected waves, and arterial compliance. Hence, vascular impedance has the potential to describe the dynamic relation between pressure and flow more comprehensively than is possible using the simpler calculations of vascular resistance. However, because the simultaneous pressure and flow data required for the calculation of impedance are complex and difficult to obtain, the concept of impedance has failed to gain widespread acceptance, and vascular impedance has not been adopted as a routine clinical index.

Evaluation of Valvular Stenosis (see Chap. 57)

Determining the severity of valvular stenosis on the basis of the pressure gradient and flow across the valve is one of the most important aspects of evaluation of patients with valvular heart disease. In many patients, the magnitude of the pressure gradient alone is sufficient to distinguish clinically significant from insignificant valvular stenosis.

DETERMINATION OF PRESSURE GRADIENTS

In patients with *aortic stenosis*, the transvalvular pressure gradient is best measured with a catheter in the left ventricle and another in the proximal aorta. Although it is convenient to measure the gradient between the left ventricle and the femoral artery, downstream augmentation of the pressure signal and delay in pressure transmission between the proximal aorta and femoral artery may alter the pressure waveform substantially and introduce errors into the measured gradient.[37,38]

Left ventricular-femoral artery pressure gradients may suffice in many patients as an estimate of the severity of aortic stenosis to confirm the presence of a severely stenotic valve. If the side port of the arterial introducing sheath is used to monitor femoral pressure, the inner diameter of the sheath should be at least 1F size larger than the outer diameter of the left ventricular catheter.

The operator should obtain simultaneous ascending aortic and femoral artery pressures in order to verify similarity between the two sites. The left ventricular-femoral artery pressure gradient may not always be relied on in the calculation of valve orifice area in patients with moderate valve gradients. A careful single catheter pull-back from left ventricle to aorta is often preferable to simultaneous measurement of left ventricular and femoral artery pressures. Alternatively, a single catheter with distal and proximal lumen or a micromanometer catheter with distal and proximal transducers may be used for simultaneous measurement of left ventricular pressure and central aortic pressure. Another method is to place two arterial catheters, one in the aorta and the second in the left ventricle. However, this requires punctures of both femoral arteries and is rarely used.

In patients with very severe aortic stenosis, the left ventricular catheter itself may reduce the effective orifice area, resulting in an artifactual increase in the measured pressure gradient. This overestimation of the severity of aortic stenosis is rarely an important clinical issue because the diagnosis of severe aortic stenosis is already apparent in such patients.

The mean pressure gradient across the aortic valve is determined by planimetry of the area separating the left ventricular and aortic pressures using multiple beats (Fig. 17-13), and it is this gradient that is applied to calculation of the valve orifice area. The peak-to-peak gradient, measured as the difference between peak left ventricular pressure and peak aortic pressure, is commonly used to quantify the valve gradient because this measurement is rapidly obtained and can be estimated visually. However, there is no physiological basis for the peak-to-peak gradient because the maximum left ventricular and aortic pressures rarely occur

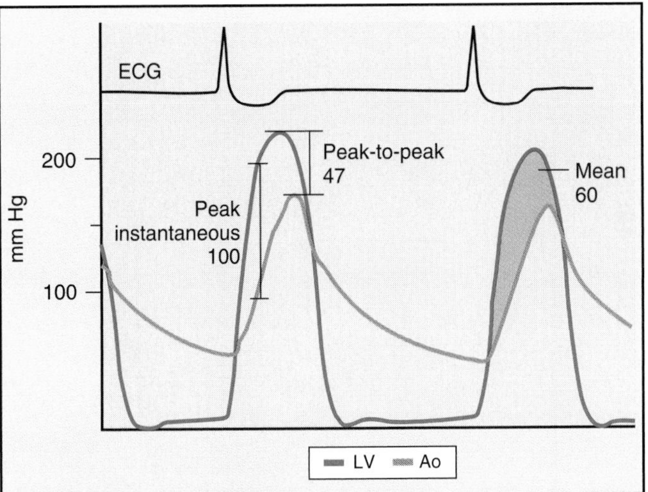

FIGURE 17–13 Various methods of describing an aortic transvalvular gradient. The peak-to-peak gradient (47 mm Hg) is the difference between the maximal pressure in the aorta (Ao) and the maximal left ventricle (LV) pressure. The peak instantaneous gradient (100 mm Hg) is the maximal pressure difference between the Ao and LV when the pressures are measured in the same moment (usually during early systole). The mean gradient (green shaded area) is the integral of the pressure difference between the LV and Ao during systole (60 mm Hg). ECG = electrocardiogram. (From Bashore TM: Invasive Cardiology: Principles and Techniques. Philadelphia, BC Decker, 1990.)

simultaneously. The peak-to-peak gradient measured in the catheterization laboratory is generally lower than the peak instantaneous gradient measured in the echocardiography laboratory. It is lower because the peak instantaneous gradient represents the maximum pressure difference between the left ventricle and aorta when measured simultaneously. This maximum pressure difference occurs on the upslope of the aortic pressure tracing (see Fig. 17–13). Mean aortic transvalvular gradient and aortic valve area are well correlated with both techniques.[40]

In patients with *mitral stenosis,* the most accurate means of determining the mitral valve gradient is measurement of left atrial pressure using the transseptal technique with simultaneous measurement of left ventricular pressure and with planimetry of the area bounded by the left ventricular and left atrial pressures in diastole using several cardiac cycles (Fig. 17–14). In most laboratories, the pulmonary capillary wedge pressure is substituted for the left atrial pressure, as the pulmonary wedge pressure is more readily obtained. The pulmonary wedge pressure tracing must be realigned with the left ventricular tracing for accurate mean gradient determination. Although it has been generally accepted that pulmonary capillary wedge pressure is a satisfactory estimate of left atrial pressure, some studies indicate that the pulmonary wedge pressure may systematically overestimate the left atrial pressure by 2 to 3 mm Hg, thereby increasing the measured mitral valve gradient.[34] In addition, accurate wedge tracings may be difficult to obtain in patients with mitral stenosis because of pulmonary hypertension or dilated right-sided heart chambers. Improperly wedged catheters, resulting in damped pulmonary artery pressure recordings, further overestimate the severity of mitral stenosis. If there is doubt about accurate positioning of the catheter in the wedge position, the position can be confirmed by slow withdrawal of blood for oximetric analysis. An oxygen saturation equal to that of the systemic circulation confirms the wedge position.

In *pulmonic stenosis,* the valve gradient is usually obtained by a catheter pull-back from the pulmonary artery to the right ventricle or by placing separate catheters in the right ventricle and pulmonary artery. Multilumen catheters are also available for simultaneous pressure recordings. *Tricuspid valve gradients* should be assessed with simultaneous recording of right atrial and right ventricular pressures.

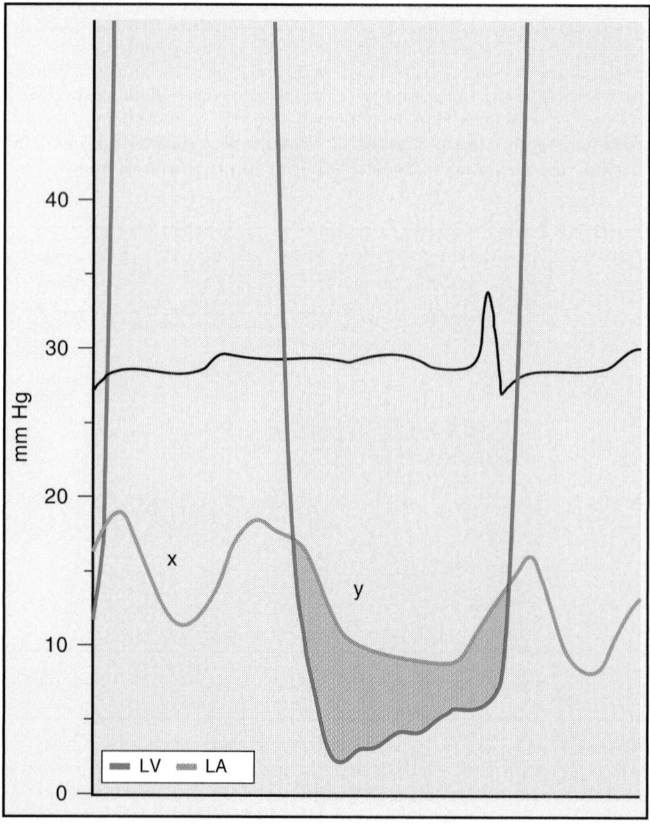

FIGURE 17–14 Pressure gradient in a patient with mitral stenosis. The pressure in the left atrium (LA) exceeds the pressure in the left ventricle (LV) during diastole, producing a diastolic pressure gradient (green shaded area). (From Bashore TM: Invasive Cardiology: Principles and Techniques. Philadelphia, BC Decker, 1990.)

CALCULATION OF STENOTIC VALVE ORIFICE AREAS. The stenotic orifice area is determined from the pressure gradient and cardiac output using the formula developed by Gorlin and Gorlin from the fundamental hydraulic relationships linking the area of an orifice to the flow and pressure drop across the orifice. Flow (F) and orifice area (A) are related by the fundamental formula

$$F = cAV$$

where V is velocity of flow and c is a constant accounting for central streaming of fluid through an orifice, which tends to reduce the effective orifice size. Hence,

$$A = F/cV$$

Velocity is related to the pressure gradient through the relation $V = k\sqrt{(2g\Delta P)}$, where k is a constant accounting for frictional energy loss, g is the acceleration due to gravity (980 cm/sec^2), and ΔP is the mean pressure gradient (mm Hg). Substituting for V in the orifice area equation and combining c and k into one constant C,

$$A = FC\sqrt{(1960\Delta P)} = F\ 44.3C\sqrt{\Delta P}$$

Gorlin and Gorlin determined the value of the constant C by comparing the calculated valve area with actual valve area measured at autopsy or at surgery in 11 mitral valves. The maximal discrepancy between the actual mitral valve area and calculated values was only 0.2 cm^2 when the constant 0.85 was used. No data were obtained for aortic valves, a limitation noted by the Gorlins, and a constant of 1.0 was assumed. Because flow across the aortic valve occurs only in systole, the flow value for calculating aortic valve area (cm^2) is the cardiac output in milliliters per minute divided by the systolic ejection period (SEP) in seconds per beat times the heart rate (HR) in beats per minute. The systolic ejection period is defined from aortic valve opening to closure. Hence, the aortic valve area is calculated from the Gorlin formula using the following equation:

$$\text{Aortic value area} = \frac{\text{cardiac output}}{44.3(\text{SEP})(\text{HR})\sqrt{\text{mean gradient}}}$$

Similarly, as mitral flow occurs only in diastole, the cardiac output is corrected for the diastolic filling period (DFP) in seconds per beat in the equation for mitral valve area, where the diastolic filling period is defined from mitral valve opening to mitral valve closure:

$$\text{Mitral valve area} = \frac{\text{cardiac output}}{37.7(\text{DFP})(\text{HR})\sqrt{\text{mean gradient}}}$$

The normal aortic valve area is 2.6 to 3.5 cm^2 in adults. Valve areas of 0.8 cm^2 or less represent severe aortic stenosis. The normal mitral valve area is 4 to 6 cm^2, and severe mitral stenosis is present with valve areas less than 1.3 cm^2.

The calculated valve area is often crucial in management decisions for patients with aortic stenosis or mitral stenosis. Hence, it is essential that accurate and simultaneous pressure gradient and cardiac output determinations be made, especially in patients with borderline or low pressure gradients.

Limitations of the Orifice Area. As the square root of the mean gradient is used in the Gorlin formula, the valve area calculation is more strongly influenced by the cardiac output than the pressure gradient. Thus, errors in measuring cardiac output may have profound effects on the calculated valve area, particularly in patients with low cardiac outputs, in whom the calculated valve area is often of greatest importance.

The Fick method of determining cardiac output is the most accurate for assessing cardiac output, especially in low-output states. As noted previously, both the dye-dilution technique and the thermodilution technique may provide inaccurate cardiac output data when cardiac output is reduced or when concomitant aortic, mitral, or tricuspid regurgitation is present. In patients with mixed valvular disease (stenosis and regurgitation) of the same valve, the use of forward flow as determined by the Fick method or thermodilution technique overestimates the severity of the valvular stenosis. This overestimation occurs because the Gorlin formula depends on total forward flow across the stenotic valve, not net forward flow. If valvular regurgitation is present, the angiographic cardiac output is the most appropriate measure of flow. If both aortic and mitral regurgitation are present, flow across a single valve cannot be determined and neither aortic valve area nor mitral valve area can be assessed accurately.

Other potential errors and limitations are inherent in the use of the Gorlin formula, related both to inaccuracies in measurement of valve gradients and to more fundamental issues regarding the validity of the assumptions underlying the formula. In low-output states, the Gorlin formula may systematically predict smaller valve areas than are actually present. Several lines of evidence indicate that the aortic valve area from the Gorlin formula increases with increases in cardiac output.[41] Although this may represent an actual greater opening of stenotic valves by the higher proximal opening pressures that result from increases in transvalvular flow, the flow dependence of the calculated valve area may also reflect inherent errors in the assumptions underlying the Gorlin formula, particularly with respect to the aortic valve.[41,42] Tricuspid aortic valve stenosis determinations appear particularly influenced by flow.[42]

A study was performed to compare simultaneous aortic valve area determinations by transesophageal echocardiographic planimetry and the Gorlin formula.[43] The study demonstrated that with increases in transvalvular flow, the Gorlin valve area also increased. This finding was not associated with alterations in direct planimetry of the aortic valve area. These results suggest that flow-related variation in the Gorlin aortic valve area is due to disproportional flow dependence of the formula and not a true change in the valve area.

An alternative simplified formula for determining valve areas has been proposed but is not well validated. The effects of the systolic ejection period and the diastolic filling period are relatively constant at normal heart rates, and these terms can be eliminated from the equation. This assumes that (HR · SEP · 44.3) ≈ 1000 in most circumstances. In this modified approach, the aortic valve area can be quickly estimated from the following formula:

$$\text{Aortic valve area} = \frac{\text{cardiac output (liter/min)}}{\sqrt{\text{mean gradient (mm Hg)}}}$$

One approach to patients with a low aortic transvalvular gradient and low cardiac output is to calculate the aortic valve resistance using the following formula:

$$\text{Aortic valve resistance} = \frac{\text{mean gradient}}{\text{flow}} = \frac{1.33(\text{mean gradient})(\text{HR})(\text{SEP})}{\text{cardiac output}}$$

where HR is heart rate, SEP is systolic ejection period, and valve resistance is expressed in dyne-sec · cm^{-5}.[41,44] The limited data available using aortic valve resistance suggest that this measure may be a helpful adjunct in distinguishing the patients with borderline aortic valve areas (0.8 to 1.0 cm^2) who have severe versus mild aortic stenosis. Despite its theoretical limitations, however, the Gorlin formula has proved to be an excellent clinical determination for evaluating patients with suspected aortic stenosis.[45]

Measurement of Intraventricular Pressure Gradients

The demonstration of an intracavitary pressure gradient is among the most interesting and challenging aspects of diagnostic catheterization. Simultaneous pressure measurements are usually obtained in either the central aorta or femoral artery and from within the ventricular cavity. Pull-back of the catheter from the ventricular apex to a posterior position just beneath the aortic valve demonstrates an intracavitary gradient. An erroneous intracavitary gradient may be seen if the catheter becomes entrapped by the hypertrophic myocardium.

The intracavitary gradient is distinguished from aortic valvular stenosis related to the loss of the aortic–left ventricular gradient when the catheter is still within the left ventricle yet proximal to the myocardial obstruction. In addition, careful analysis of the upstroke of the aortic pressure waveform distinguishes a valvular from a subvalvular stenosis, as the aortic pressure waveform demonstrates a slow upstroke in aortic stenosis. Other methods for localizing intracavitary gradients include the use of a dual-lumen catheter, a double-sensor micromanometer catheter, or placement of an end-hole catheter in the left ventricular outflow tract while a transseptal catheter is advanced into the left ventricle, with pressure measured simultaneously. An intracavitary gradient may be increased by various provocative maneuvers including the Valsalva maneuver, inhalation of amyl nitrate, introduction of a premature ventricular beat, or isoproterenol infusion (see Physiological and Pharmacological Maneuvers).

ASSESSMENT OF VALVULAR REGURGITATION

The severity of valvular regurgitation is generally graded by visual assessment, although calculation of the regurgitant fraction is used occasionally.

VISUAL ASSESSMENT OF REGURGITATION. Valvular regurgitation may be assessed visually by determining the relative amount of radiographic contrast medium that opacifies the chamber proximal to its injection. The estimation of regurgitation depends on the regurgitant volume as well as the size and contractility of the proximal chamber. The original classification scheme devised by Sellers and colleagues remains the standard in most catheterization laboratories:

- \+ Minimal regurgitant jet seen. Clears rapidly from proximal chamber with each beat.
- ++ Moderate opacification of proximal chamber, clearing with subsequent beats.
- +++ Intense opacification of proximal chamber, becoming equal to that of the distal chamber.
- ++++ Intense opacification of proximal chamber, becoming more dense than that of the distal chamber. Opacification often persists over the entire series of images obtained.

REGURGITANT FRACTION. A gross estimate of the degree of valvular regurgitation may be obtained by determining the regurgitant fraction (RF). The difference between the angiographic stroke volume and the forward stroke volume can be defined as the regurgitant stroke volume. The RF is that portion of the angiographic stroke volume that does not contribute to the net cardiac output.

$$\text{Regurgitant stroke volume} = \text{angiographic stroke volume} - \text{forward stroke volume}$$

$$\text{RF} = \frac{(\text{angiographic stroke volume} - \text{forward stroke volume})}{\text{angiographic stroke volume}}$$

Forward stroke volume is the cardiac output determined by the Fick or thermodilution method divided by the heart rate. Thermodilution cardiac output cannot be used if there is significant concomitant tricuspid regurgitation.

As detected visually, 1+ regurgitation is roughly equivalent to an RF less than or equal to 20 percent, 2+ regurgitation to an RF of 21 to 40 percent, 3+ to an RF of 41 to 60 percent, and 4+ to an RF of more than 60 percent.

The assumption underlying the determination of RF is that the angiographic and forward cardiac outputs are accurate and comparable, a state requiring similar heart rates, stable hemodynamic states between measurements, and only a single regurgitant valve. Given these conditions, the equation yields only a gross approximation of regurgitant flow.

Shunt Determinations

Normally, pulmonary blood flow and systemic blood flow are equal. With an abnormal communication between intracardiac chambers or great vessels, blood flow is shunted either from the systemic circulation to the pulmonary circulation (left-to-right shunt), from the pulmonary circulation to the systemic circulation (right-to-left shunt), or in both directions (bidirectional shunt). Although many shunts are suspected before cardiac catheterization, physicians performing the procedure should be vigilant in determining the cause of unexpected findings. For example, an unexplained pulmonary artery oxygen saturation exceeding 80 percent should raise the operator's suspicion of a left-to-right shunt, whereas unexplained arterial desaturation (<93 percent) may indicate a right-to-left shunt.[46] Arterial desaturation commonly results from alveolar hypoventilation and associated "physiological shunting," the causes of which include oversedation from premedication, pulmonary disease, pulmonary venous congestion, pulmonary edema, and cardiogenic shock. If arterial desaturation persists after the patient takes several deep breaths, coughs, or after administration of 100 percent oxygen, a right-to-left shunt must be highly suspected.

Several noninvasive and invasive methods are available for detection of intracardiac shunts. Noninvasive methods include echocardiographic, radionuclide, and magnetic resonance imaging techniques. The most commonly used method in the cardiac catheterization laboratory is the oximetric method.

OXIMETRIC METHOD. The oximetric method is based on blood sampling from various cardiac chambers for the determination of oxygen saturation. A left-to-right shunt is detected when a significant increase in blood oxygen saturation is found between two right-sided vessels or chambers.

A screening oxygen saturation measurement for any left-to-right shunt is often performed with right-heart catheterization by sampling blood in the SVC and the pulmonary artery. If the difference in oxygen saturation between these samples is 8 percent or more, a left-to-right shunt may be present, and an oximetry "run" should be performed. This run includes obtaining blood samples from all right-sided locations including the SVC, IVC, right atrium, right ventricle, and pulmonary artery. In cases of interatrial or interventricular shunts, it may be helpful to obtain multiple samples from the high, middle, and low right atrium or the right ventricular inflow tract, apex, and outflow tract in order to localize the level of the shunt. One may miss a small left-to-right shunt using the right atrium for screening purposes rather than the SVC because of incomplete mixing of blood in the right atrium, which receives blood from the IVC, SVC, and coronary sinus. Oxygen saturation in the IVC is higher than in the SVC because the kidneys use less oxygen relative to their blood flow than do other organs, whereas coronary sinus blood has very low oxygen saturation. Mixed venous saturation is most accurately measured in the pulmonary artery after complete mixing has occurred.

A full saturation run involves obtaining samples from the high and low IVC; high and low SVC; high, middle, and low right atrium; right ventricular inflow and outflow tracts and midcavity; main pulmonary artery; left or right pulmonary artery; pulmonary vein and left atrium if possible; left ventricle; and distal aorta. When a right-to-left shunt must be localized, oxygen saturation samples must be taken from the pulmonary veins, left atrium, left ventricle, and aorta. Although the major weakness of the oxygen step-up method is its lack of sensitivity, clinically significant shunts are generally detected by this technique. Obtaining multiple samples from each chamber can improve sampling error and variability. Most instruments analyze samples with a measurement error ranging from 2.5 to 1 percent saturation or better.[47] Another method of oximetric determination of intracardiac shunts uses a balloon-tipped fiberoptic catheter that allows continuous registration of oxygen saturation as it is withdrawn from the pulmonary artery through the right-heart chambers into the SVC and IVC.

Shunt Quantification. The principles used to determine Fick cardiac output are also used to quantify intracardiac shunts. To determine the size of a left-to-right shunt, pulmonary blood flow (PBF) and systemic blood flow (SBF) determinations are required. PBF is simply oxygen consumption divided by the difference in oxygen content across the pulmonary bed, whereas SBF is oxygen consumption divided by the difference in oxygen content across the systemic bed. The effective blood flow (EBF) is the fraction of mixed venous return received by the lungs without contamination by the shunt flow. In the *absence* of a shunt, PBF, SBF, and EBF all are equal. These equations are as follows:

$$\text{PBF} = \frac{\text{O}_2 \text{ consumption (ml/min)}}{(\text{P}\bar{\text{v}}\text{O}_2 - \text{PaO}_2)}$$

$$\text{SBF} = \frac{\text{O}_2 \text{ consumption (ml/min)}}{(\text{SaO}_2 - \text{M}\bar{\text{v}}\text{O}_2)}$$

$$\text{EBF} = \frac{\text{O}_2 \text{ consumption (ml/min)}}{(\text{P}\bar{\text{v}}\text{O}_2 - \text{M}\bar{\text{v}}\text{O}_2)}$$

where $\text{P}\bar{\text{v}}\text{O}_2$, PaO_2, SaO_2, and $\text{M}\bar{\text{v}}\text{O}_2$ are the oxygen contents (in milliliters of oxygen per liter of blood) of pulmonary venous, pulmonary arterial, systemic arterial, and mixed venous bloods, respectively. The oxygen content is determined as outlined in the section on Fick cardiac output.

If a pulmonary vein is not sampled, systemic arterial oxygen content may be substituted, assuming systemic arterial saturation is 95 percent or more. As discussed earlier, if systemic arterial saturation is less than 95 percent, a right-to-left shunt may be present. If arterial desaturation is present but not secondary to a right-to-left shunt, systemic arterial oxygen content is used. If a right-to-left shunt is present, pulmonary venous oxygen content is calculated as 98 percent of the oxygen capacity.

The mixed venous oxygen content is the average oxygen content of the blood in the chamber proximal to the shunt. When assessing a left-to-right shunt at the level of the right atrium, one must calculate mixed venous oxygen content on the basis of the contributing blood flow from the IVC, SVC, and coronary sinus. The most common method used is the Flamm formula:

$$\text{Mixed venous oxygen content} = \frac{3(\text{SVC O}_2 \text{ content}) + 1(\text{IVC O}_2 \text{ content})}{4}$$

Assuming conservation of mass, the size of a left-to-right shunt, when there is no associated right-to-left shunt, is simply

$$\text{L}\rightarrow\text{R shunt} = \text{PBF} - \text{SBF}$$

When there is evidence of a right-to-left shunt in addition to a left-to-right shunt, the approximate left-to-right shunt size is

$$\text{L}\rightarrow\text{R shunt} = \text{PBF} - \text{EBF}$$

and the approximate right-to-left shunt size is

$$\text{R}\rightarrow\text{L shunt} = \text{SBF} - \text{EBF}$$

The flow ratio PBF/SBF (or Q_p/Q_s) is used clinically to determine the significance of the shunt. A ratio of less than 1.5 indicates a small left-to-right shunt, and a ratio of 1.5 to 2.0, a moderate-sized shunt. A ratio of 2.0 or more indicates a large left-to-right shunt and generally requires percutaneous or surgical repair to prevent future pulmonary or right ventricular complications, or both. A flow ratio of less than 1.0 indicates a net right-to-left shunt. If oxygen consumption is not measured, the pulmonic/systemic blood flow ratio may be calculated as follows:

$$\frac{PBF}{SBF} = \frac{(SaO_2 - M\bar{v}O_2)}{(P\bar{v}O_2 - PaO_2)}$$

where SaO_2, $M\bar{v}O_2$, $P\bar{v}O_2$, and PaO_2 are systemic arterial, mixed venous, pulmonary venous, and pulmonary arterial blood oxygen saturations, respectively.

INDICATOR-DILUTION METHOD

Although the indicator-dilution method is more sensitive than the oximetric method in detection of small shunts, it cannot be used to localize the level of a left-to-right shunt (Fig. 17–15). An indicator such as indocyanine green dye is injected into a proximal chamber while a sample is taken from a distal chamber using a densitometer, and the density of dye is displayed over time. To detect a left-to-right shunt, dye is injected into the pulmonary artery and sampling is performed in a systemic artery. Presence of a shunt is indicated by early recirculation of the dye on the downslope of the curve. The presence of aortic or mitral regurgitation may distort the downslope of the curve, yielding a false-positive result. In adults, the indocyanine green method provides estimates of shunt magnitude that are somewhat smaller than those of the oximetric method, although they are in general agreement with one another concerning the PBF/SBF.[48,49] To detect a right-to-left shunt, dye is injected into the right side of the heart proximal to the presumed shunt and sampling is performed in a systemic artery. If there is a right-to-left shunt, a distinct early peak is seen on the upslope of the curve. The level of the right-to-left shunt may be localized by injecting more distally until the early peak disappears. Shunts may also be quantified using this technique.

MISCELLANEOUS TECHNIQUES

A sensitive method for detection and localization of a left-to-right shunt is to check systematically within the various right-heart chambers for the early appearance of an indicator that is injected distal to the presumed shunt. Indicators that have been used for this purpose include indocyanine green dye, inhaled hydrogen, hydrogen dissolved in saline, and ascorbic acid. Platinum-tipped electrodes are used for detection when hydrogen and ascorbic acid are used. These techniques may also be used to detect small right-to-left shunts by altering the sites of injection and sampling.

Selective injection of radiographic contrast medium (angiocardiography) can detect both left-to-right and right-to-left shunts, although these cannot be quantified. Angiocardiography is a useful adjunct to transesophageal echocardiography as part of a preoperative evaluation. It is also useful in detecting pulmonary arteriovenous fistulas that may not be detected by other methods.

Physiological and Pharmacological Maneuvers

Potentially significant cardiac abnormalities may be absent in the resting condition but may be unmasked by stress. Therefore, if the physician performing a cardiac catheterization procedure cannot elucidate the cause of a patient's symptoms at rest, various physiological and pharmacological maneuvers can be considered.

DYNAMIC EXERCISE

Dynamic exercise in the catheterization laboratory is most commonly performed using supine bicycle ergometry, although straight leg raises or arm or upright bicycle exercise may be used. Upright treadmill exercise may also be performed outside the catheterization laboratory, using a balloon flotation catheter inserted through an antecubital vein to measure pulmonary artery and wedge pressures and cardiac output. The associated changes in the heart rate, cardiac output, oxygen consumption, and intracardiac pressures are monitored at steady state during progressive stages of exercise. Normally, the increased oxygen requirements of exercise are met by an increase in cardiac output and an increase in oxygen extraction from arterial blood. Patients with cardiac dysfunction are unable to increase their cardiac output appropriately in response to exercise and must meet the demands of the exercising muscle groups by increasing the extraction of oxygen from arterial blood, thereby increasing the arteriovenous oxygen difference. The relationship between cardiac output and oxygen consumption is linear, and a regression formula can be used to calculate the predicted cardiac index at a given level of oxygen consumption. The actual cardiac index divided by the predicted cardiac index is defined as the *exercise index*. A value of 0.8 or more indicates a normal cardiac output response to exercise. The *exercise factor* is another method of describing the same relationship

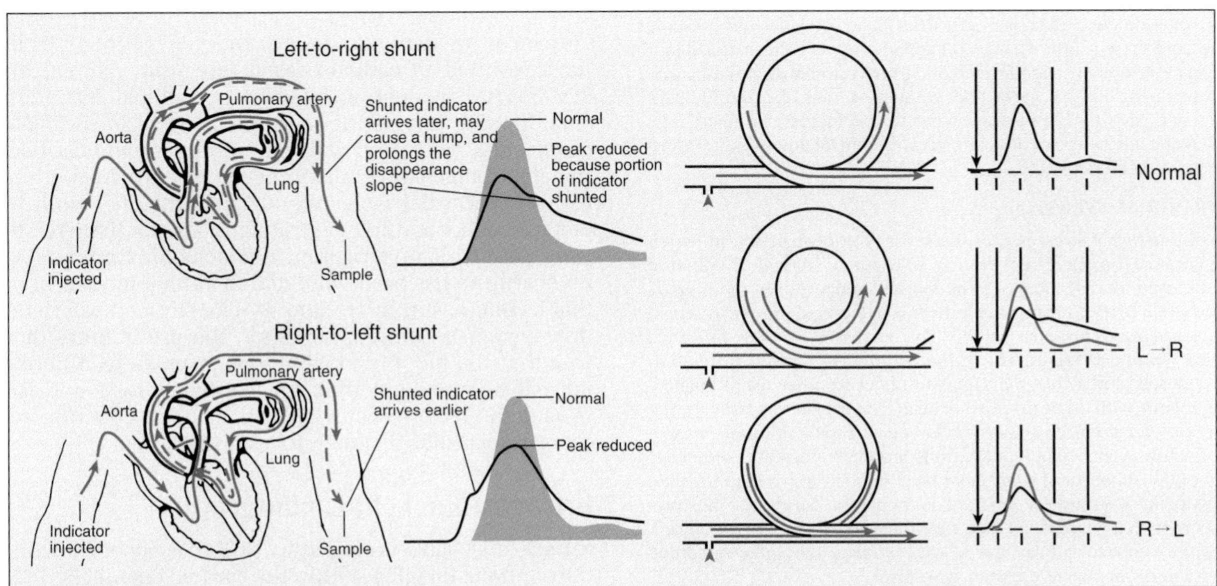

FIGURE 17–15 **Top,** Left-to-right shunt (increased pulmonic flow). Indicator is not cleared rapidly but recirculates through the central circulation through a defect. Depending on the magnitude of the shunt, a constant fraction leaves the central pool with each circulation. Maximal deflection is reduced, and the disappearance is prolonged as a result of slow clearance. **Bottom,** Right-to-left shunt (decreased pulmonic flow). A portion of the indicator passes directly to the arterial circulation through the defect without passing through the lungs and arrives at the arterial sampling site before the portion that did traverse the pulmonary circulation. (From Kern MJ, Deligonul U, Donohue T, et al: Hemodynamic data. *In* Kern MJ [ed]: The Cardiac Catheterization Handbook. 2nd ed. St. Louis, Mosby–Year Book, 1995, p 142.)

between the cardiac output and oxygen consumption. The exercise factor is the increase in cardiac output divided by the increase in oxygen consumption. Normally, for every 100 ml/min increase in oxygen consumption with exercise, the cardiac output should increase by at least 600 ml/min. Therefore, a normal exercise factor should be 0.6 or more.[50]

Supine exercise normally causes a rise in mean arterial and pulmonary pressures. There is a proportionately greater decrease in systemic vascular resistance compared with pulmonary vascular resistance and an increase in heart rate. Myocardial contractility increases owing to both increased sympathetic tone and the increase in heart rate. Left ventricular ejection fraction rises. During early levels of exercise, increased venous return augments left ventricular end-diastolic volume, leading to an increase in stroke volume. At progressively higher levels of exercise, both left ventricular end-systolic and end-diastolic volumes decrease so that there is a negligible rise in stroke volume. Thus, the augmentation in cardiac output during peak supine exercise in the catheterization laboratory is generally caused by an increase in heart rate. For this reason, all agents that may impair the chronotropic response should be discontinued before catheterization if exercise is contemplated during the procedure.

Exercise may provoke symptoms in a patient who had been found to have valvular disease of borderline significance in the resting state (see Chap. 57). Exercise increases the gradient across the mitral valve and pulmonary artery pressures in mitral stenosis and may provoke symptoms not experienced at rest. The hemodynamic response to exercise is also useful in evaluating regurgitant valvular lesions. Clinically important valvular regurgitation exists if an increase occurs in left ventricular end-diastolic pressure, pulmonary capillary wedge pressure, and systemic vascular resistance, in conjunction with a reduced exercise index and abnormal exercise factor. Simultaneous echocardiographic data may also be useful in equivocal cases. Patients with myocardial disease, ischemic or otherwise, may have pronounced increases in left ventricular end-diastolic pressure with exercise.

ISOMETRIC EXERCISE

Isometric handgrip exercise causes an increase in heart rate, mean arterial pressure, and cardiac output. Because the systemic vascular resistance does not increase, the elevation in arterial pressure is due to the rise in cardiac output rather than a vasoconstrictor response. Patients with left ventricular dysfunction respond abnormally to isometric exercise (i.e., significant increase in left ventricular end-diastolic pressure, a failure to increase stroke work appropriately, and a blunted rise in left ventricular peak dP/dT).[50]

PACING TACHYCARDIA

Rapid atrial or ventricular pacing increases myocardial oxygen consumption and myocardial blood flow. With pacing, in contradistinction to dynamic or isometric exercise, left ventricular end-diastolic volume decreases and there is little change in cardiac output.[51] This method may be used to determine the significance of coronary artery disease or valvular abnormalities. For example, the gradient across the mitral valve increases with rapid atrial pacing owing to the increase in heart rate. Pacing has the advantage of allowing greater control and rapid termination of the induced stress.

PHYSIOLOGICAL STRESS

Various physiological stresses alter the severity of obstruction in hypertrophic cardiomyopathy. The *Valsalva maneuver* (forcible expiration against a closed glottis) increases the systolic subaortic pressure gradient in the strain phase, during which there is a decrease in venous return and decreased left ventricular volume. This maneuver is often abnormal in patients with heart failure. The *Müller maneuver* (forced inspiration against a closed glottis) has the opposite effect. Another useful maneuver in patients with hypertrophic obstructive cardiomyopathy is the introduction of a *premature ventricular beat* (Brockenbrough maneuver). Premature ventricular contractions normally increase the pulse pressure of the subsequent ventricular beat. In obstructive hypertrophic cardiomyopathy, the outflow gradient is increased during the postpremature beat with a decrease in the pulse pressure of the aortic contour. A premature ventricular beat may also accentuate the spike-and-dome configuration of the aortic pressure waveform.

Rapid volume loading may reveal occult pericardial constriction, when atrial and ventricular filling pressures are relatively normal under baseline conditions owing to hypovolemia, and may help distinguish pericardial constriction from myocardial restriction. The *Kussmaul sign* occurs in pericardial constriction. It is demonstrated when, with inspiration, right atrial pressure fails to decrease or actually increases in relation to impaired right ventricular filling.[52]

PHARMACOLOGICAL MANEUVERS

Isoproterenol infusion may be used to simulate supine dynamic exercise, although untoward side effects may limit its applicability. This drug's positive inotropic and chronotropic effects may increase the gradients in obstructive hypertrophic cardiomyopathy and mitral stenosis. *Nitroglycerin* and *amyl nitrate* decrease preload and accentuate the systolic gradient in patients with obstructive hypertrophic cardiomyopathy. Amyl nitrate is generally inhaled, and its onset and offset of action are very rapid. Agents that increase systemic vascular resistance, such as *phenylephrine,* reduce the gradient in obstructive hypertrophic cardiomyopathy. Afterload reduction or an intravenous inotropic agent may clarify the precise severity of aortic stenosis in patients with low cardiac outputs and low transvalvular gradients.[53] Infusion of *sodium nitroprusside* may improve the cardiac output and filling pressures in patients with dilated cardiomyopathies and in patients with mitral regurgitation by lowering systemic and pulmonary vascular resistances. A favorable response to sodium nitroprusside infusion may predict a good clinical outcome.

Methylergonovine maleate has replaced ergonovine as a safer and more specific provocation test for coronary artery spasm. Small intracoronary increments of 5 to 10 μg are given. Total dose should not exceed 50 μg. Intracoronary acetylcholine is also as effective and safe as methylergonovine.[54]

Adjunctive Diagnostic Techniques

Coronary Pressure and Blood Flow Determinations

Five methods are available for measuring human coronary blood flow in the cardiac catheterization laboratory: thermodilution, digital subtraction angiography, electromagnetic flowmeters, Doppler velocity probes, and pressure wires.[55] Although most current methods measure relative changes in coronary blood flow, useful information about the physiological significance of stenosis, cardiac hypertrophy, and pharmacological interventions can be obtained. Doppler FloWires and translesional gradients are the most commonly used clinical techniques (see Chap. 44).

Left Ventricular Electromechanical Mapping

Advances in catheter design and navigational technology have resulted in catheter-based three-dimensional mapping systems for evaluating regional and global left ventricular function. By integrating measurements of local endocardial electrical activity and wall motion during the cardiac cycle, the electromechanical mapping system provides information about myocardial ischemia and viability. The ability of the electromechanical left ventricular maps to distinguish viable from nonviable myocardium and ischemic from nonischemic myocardium has been validated in animal models of myocardial ischemia and infarction.[56,57] The clinical experience with this system is limited. However, the preliminary data indicate that the mapping system has promise in differentiating normal myocardium from myocardial fibrosis and ischemic from infarcted myocardium and has the potential to guide transendocardial therapeutic administration.[58-60]

Intracardiac Echocardiography

Intracardiac echocardiography (ICE) has become available for transvenous imaging within the cardiac chambers. It consists of a 10F, 90-cm-long device that permits two planes of bidirectional steering in the anterior-posterior and left-right direction. The transducers have variable frequencies of 5 to 10 MHz with multiple phased array features including two-dimensional imaging, color, and spectral Doppler.

ICE can provide imaging of interatrial or interventricular septum and left-heart structures from either the right atrium or ventricle, with penetration up to 15 cm. Current applications include guidance of percutaneous atrial septal defect and patent foramen ovale closures, thus mitigating the need for transesophageal echocardiography and anesthesia (Fig. 17–16). In patients undergoing transseptal puncture, ICE can facilitate localization of the fossa ovalis. ICE can also be used to guide electrophysiological procedures with identification of anatomical structures difficult to view by fluoroscopy (e.g., pulmonary veins or fossa ovalis for transseptal puncture).

Complications Associated with Cardiac Catheterization (Table 17–6)

Cardiac catheterization is a relatively safe procedure but has a well-defined risk of morbidity and mortality.[1,61,62] The potential risk of major complications during cardiac catheterization may be difficult to ascertain owing to the confounding aspects of comorbid disease and disparities in methods used to collect complication data. Advances including the use of low-osmolar and isosmolar contrast media, lower profile diagnostic catheters, and extensive operator experience all serve to reduce further the incidence of complications. Several large studies provide insight into the incidence of major events and delineate cohorts of patients that are at increased risk.[1,61-63]

Death related to diagnostic cardiac catheterization occurs in 0.08 to 0.75 percent of patients, depending on the population studied. Data from the Society for Cardiac Angiography identified subsets of patients with an increased mortality rate.[62] In an analysis of 58,332 patients, multivariate predictors of significant complications were moribund status, advanced New York Heart Association functional class, hypertension, shock, aortic valve disease, renal insufficiency, unstable angina, mitral valve disease, acute myocardial infarction within 24 hours, congestive heart failure, and cardiomyopathy. The risk of cardiac catheterization appears to be further increased in octogenarians.[63] Although the overall mortality is approximately 0.8 percent in this cohort, the risk of nonfatal major complications, which are primarily peripheral vascular, is about 5 percent.

The risk of myocardial infarction varies from 0.03 to 0.06 percent, of neurological complications from 0.03 to 0.2 percent, and of significant bradyarrhythmias or tachyarrhythmias from 0.56 to 1.3 percent.[62] One study utilizing serial cranial magnetic resonance imaging demonstrated a 22 percent incidence of focal acute cerebral embolic events following retrograde crossing of stenotic aortic valves. Three percent demonstrated clinically apparent neurological deficits.[64] This preliminary study is in direct contradistinc-

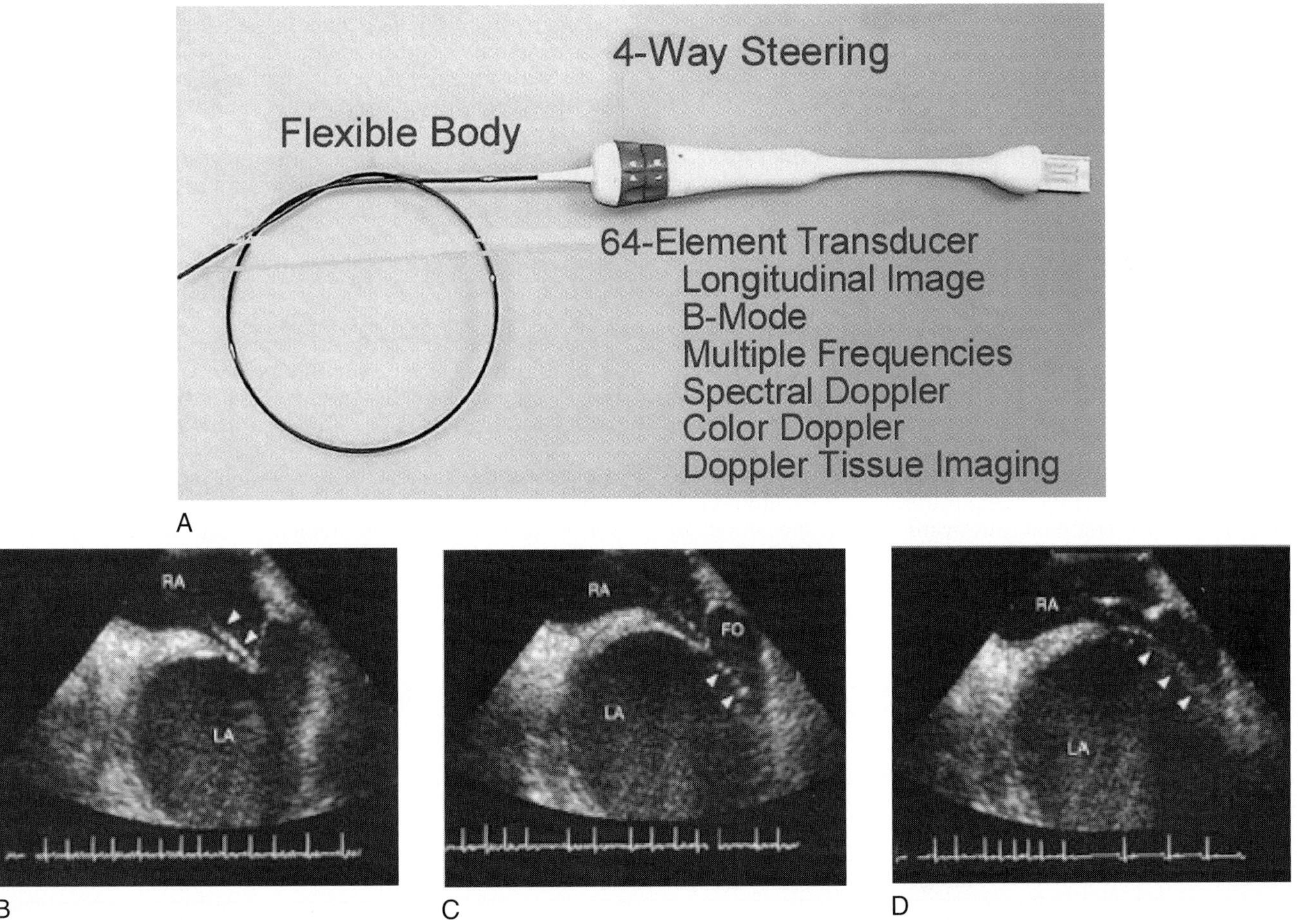

FIGURE 17–16 **A,** Intracardiac echo disposable transducer (Acuson, Inc.). Steering apparatus on proximal end and flexible body with transducer on distal tip of catheter. **B,** Tenting of the membranous fossa by the dilator-needle assembly. The transseptal needle assembly (arrowheads) is advanced to indent the fossal membrane. **C,** Advancements of the transseptal needle across the membranous fossa. Here the needle (arrowheads) is seen near the posterosuperior left atrial wall. The membrane remains tented because the dilator has not yet crossed the septum. **D,** Dilator and sheath passage across the interatrial septum. The dilator and sheath assembly has now advanced into the left atrium, releasing the tenting of the membranous fossa. FO = fossa ovalis; LA = left atrium; RA = right atrium. (From Johnson SB, Seward JB, Packer DL. Phased-array intracardiac echocardiography for guiding transseptal catheter placement: Utility and learning curve. Pacing Clin Electrophysiol 25:402, 2002.)

TABLE 17–6 Risk of Cardiac Catheterization and Coronary Angiography*

Complication	Risk (%)
Mortality	0.11
Myocardial infarction	0.05
Cerebrovascular accident	0.07
Arrhythmia	0.38
Vascular complications	0.43
Contrast reaction	0.37
Homodynamic complications	0.26
Perforation of heart chamber	0.03
Other complications	0.28
Total of major complications	1.70

From Scanlon PJ, Faxon DP, Audet AM, et al: ACC/AHA guidelines for coronary angiography: A report of the American College of Cardiology/American Heart Association Task Force on Practice Guidelines (Committee on Coronary Angiography). J Am Coll Cardiol 33:1760, 1999.
*No. of patients = 59,792.

tion to previously published large clinical series and requires additional validation.

Reports of the incidence of major vascular complications have varied widely, with most series suggesting a slightly higher frequency when the Sones brachial approach is used. The incidence of major vascular complications has been reported as approximately 0.40 percent.[62] Major vascular complications include occlusion requiring arterial repair or thrombectomy, retroperitoneal bleeding, hematoma formation, pseudoaneurysm, arteriovenous fistula formation, and infection. The risk of requiring surgical repair for vascular injury is related to advanced age, congestive heart failure, and larger body surface area.[65]

Systemic complications can vary from mild vasovagal responses to severe vagal reactions that lead to cardiac arrest. Prolonged hypotension during the procedure may also occur as a result of various mechanisms that include the vasodepressor vagal response, contrast medium–induced vasodilation or osmotic diuresis, cardiac tamponade caused by myocardial perforation or coronary laceration, myocardial infarction, and an acute anaphylactoid reaction to the contrast medium. Minor complications occur in approximately 4 percent of patients undergoing routine cardiac catheterization.[66] The most common untoward effects are transient hypotension and brief episodes of angina lasting less than 10 minutes. With the use of low-osmolar contrast media, however, bradycardia is infrequent and usually responds to cough. Rarely, administration of intravenous atropine is necessary.

Contrast Media–Induced Nephropathy

After the procedure, diuresis from the radiographic contrast load and subsequent hypotension can occur. Intravenous hydration given before and after the procedure can usually restore the intravascular volume to compensate for the anticipated diuresis. A prospective trial evaluated the effects of saline, mannitol, and furosemide in preventing nephropathy induced by contrast media.[67] It was concluded that saline hydration alone without forced diuresis was the most effective in reducing nephropathy. The incidences of acute renal dysfunction in patients with baseline renal insufficiency were 28 and 40 percent with mannitol and furosemide, respectively, compared with 11 percent with saline hydration alone.

The various classes of contrast agents are given in Table 17–7. High-osmolar ionic contrast media produce various adverse hemodynamic and electrophysiological effects during coronary angiography. Most of these adverse events are clearly related to the osmolality, sodium content, and calcium-binding characteristics of the ionic contrast solutions. Low-osmolar contrast agents clearly reduce acute adverse hemodynamic and electrophysiological reactions. The selection of contrast media, particularly for high-risk patients including those with preexisting renal impairment, is unsettled. Several studies have demonstrated that contrast media–related toxicity occurs in 1.4 to 2.3 percent of patients receiving ionic contrast media.[66,68] Patients with diabetes and those with preexisting renal insufficiency are at higher risk, with up to 48 percent of patients experiencing an increase in creatinine greater than 0.5 mg/dL.[68]

Clinical studies reveal no advantage of low-osmolar contrast over ionic contrast media in the prevention of nephrotoxicity in patients with normal renal function.[66,69] However, the risk of contrast media–induced nephropathy is significantly reduced in patients with baseline renal insufficiency with or without diabetes mellitus if nonionic low-osmolar contrast medium is used (odds ratio = 3.3 [1.6 to 6.6]).[68]

Baseline renal insufficiency has been consistently shown to be the most important independent predictor of subsequent contrast media–induced nephrotoxicity.[69] Contrast media–induced renal dysfunction can be minimized if the dose of contrast medium is kept below 30 ml for the entire study. Several studies have suggested that acetylcysteine, an antioxidant, can be orally administered in the periprocedural period to reduce the incidence of contrast media–induced nephropathy.[70,71] However, other investigators have not confirmed this effect.[72,73] Larger trials are necessary to define the potential role of this agent.

TABLE 17–7 Classification of Contrast Media

	Osmolality (mOsm/kg)			
Property	*High osmolar (1800-2100)*	*Low osmolar (600)*	*Low osmolar (700-840)*	*Isosmolar (280)*
Ionicity	Ionic	Ionic	Nonionic	Nonionic
Benzene rings	Monomer	Dimer	Monomer	Dimer
Iodine-to-particle ratio	1.5	3	3	6
Generic names (brand names)	Diatrizoate (Renografin, Hypaque)	Ioxaglate (Hexabrix)	Iohexol (Omnipaque) Iopamidol (Isovue) Ioversol (Optiray)	Iodixanol (Visipaque)
Viscosity at 37°C	8.4	7.5	8-10.5	12

TABLE 17–8 Recommendations for Management of Patients with Renal Insufficiency

1. Administer at least 1 liter of 0.9% NS over 12-24 hr before and after the procedure.[67] Adjust for patients with history of CHF. *Avoid dehydration.*
2. Limit contrast dose to <30 ml for diagnostic studies and <100 ml for PCI. Use biplane angiography if available.
3. If PCI is complex, stage PCI at least 48 hr after diagnositic procedure.
4. Administer low osmolar contrast media.[68] Consider isosmolar contrast media.[75]
5. Discontinue nonsteroidal antiinflammatory medications, if possible.
6. Discontinue metformin for at least 48 hr after procedure or until creatinine returns to baseline.[10]
7. Avoid repeated contrast exposure during the recovery phase of acute tabular necrosis.
8. Consider administering acetylcysteine 300 mg PO b.i.d. × 2 d.[70-73]

NS = normal saline; PCI = percutaneous coronary intervention.

A prospective multicenter trial has demonstrated that an isosmolar nonionic contrast agent, iodixanol, produced fewer major adverse cardiac events during percutaneous coronary interventions than the low-osmolar ionic contrast medium ioxaglate.[74] Data also indicate that the isosmolar agent can reduce the incidence of contrast media–induced nephropathy in patients with preexisting renal insufficiency (3 percent versus 26 percent, $p = 0.002$).[75] Thus, clinical studies evaluating both cardiovascular and renal effects of contrast media indicate that the pharmacological properties can have a salutary effect on local thrombogenicity and nephrotoxicity within the coronary vasculature, particularly in high-risk patients. Table 17–8 outlines clinical recommendations for prevention of contrast media–induced nephropathy in patients with renal impairment presenting for invasive cardiac procedures.

REFERENCES

Indications for Cardiac Catheterization

1. Scanlon PJ, Faxon DP, Audet AM, et al: ACC/AHA guidelines for coronary angiography: A report of the American College of Cardiology/American Heart Association Task Force on Practice Guidelines (Committee on Coronary Angiography). J Am Coll Cardiol 33:1756, 1999.
2. Bashore, TM, Bates ER, Berger PB, et al: ACC/SCAI clinical expert consensus document on cardiac catheterization laboratory standards. J Am Coll Cardiol 37:2170, 2001.

Technical Aspects of Cardiac Catheterization

3. Bersin RM, Elliott CM, Fedor JM, et al: Mobile cardiac catheterization registry: Report of the first 1,001 patients. Cathet Cardiovasc Diagn 31:1, 1994.
4. Smith SC, Dove JT, Jacobs AK, et al: ACC/AHA Guidelines for percutaneous coronary intervention—Executive summary. J Am Coll Cardiol 37:2215, 2001.
5. Jacobs AK, Faxon DP, Hirshfeld JW, Holmes DR: Task force 3: Training in diagnostic cardiac catheterization and interventional cardiology. Revision of the 1995 COCATS training statement. J Am Coll Cardiol 39:1242, 2002.
6. Holmes DR Jr, Wondrow MS, Tulsrud PR: Radiographic techniques used in cardiac catheterization. *In* Pepine CJ, Hill JA, Lambert CR (eds): Diagnostic and Therapeutic Cardiac Catheterization. 2nd ed. Baltimore, Williams & Wilkins, 1998, p 162.
7. Cusma JT, Wondrow MA, Holmes DR: Replacement of cinefilm with a digital archive and review network. Int J Card Imaging 14:293,1998.
8. American College of Cardiology, American College of Radiology and industry develop standard for digital transfer of Angiographic images. ACC/ACR/NEMA Ad Hoc Group. J Am Coll Cardiol 25:800,1995.
9. Limacher MC, Douglas PS, Germano G, et al: Radiation safety in the practice of cardiology. J Am Coll Cardiol 31:892, 1998.
10. Heupler FA Jr: Guidelines for performing angiography in patients taking metformin. Members of the Laboratory Performance Standards Committee of the Society for Cardiac Angiography and Interventions. Cathet Cardiovasc Diagn 43:121, 1998.
11. Goss JE, Chambers CE, Heupler FA: Systemic anaphylactoid reactions to iodinated contrast media during cardiac catheterization procedures: Guidelines for prevention, diagnosis, and treatment. Laboratory Performance Standards Committee for the Society for Cardiac Angiography and Interventions. Cathet Cardiovasc Diagn 34:99, 1995.
12. Baim DS: Percutaneous approach, including transseptal and apical puncture. *In* Baim DS, Grossman W (eds). Cardiac Catheterization, Angiography, and Intervention. 6th ed. Philadelphia, Lippincott Williams & Wilkins, 2000, p 69.
13. Piper WD, Malenka DJ, Ryan TR Jr: Predicting vascular complications in percutaneous coronary interventions. Am Heart J 145:1022, 2003.
14. Kussmaul WG, Buchbinder M, Whitlow P, et al: Rapid arterial hemostasis after cardiac catheterization and percutaneous transluminal angioplasty—Results of a randomized trial of a novel hemostatic device. J Am Coll Cardiol 25:1685, 1995.
15. Baim DS, Knopf WDD, Hinohara T, et al: Suture mediated closure of the femoral access site after cardiac catheterization. Am J Cardiol 85:864, 2000.
16. Ward SR, Casale P, Raymond R, et al: Efficacy and safety of a hemostatic puncture closure device with early ambulation after coronary angiography. Am J Cardiol 81:569, 1998.
17. Lesnefsky EJ, Carrea FP, Groves BM: Safety of cardiac catheterization via peripheral vascular grafts. Cathet Cardiovasc Diagn 29:113, 1993.
18. Lefevre T, Morice MC, Bonan R, et al: Coronary angiography using 4 or 6 French diagnostic catheters: A prospective, randomized study. J Invasive Cardiol 13:674, 2001.
19. Kiemeneij F, Laarman GH, Odekerken D, et al: A randomized comparison of percutaneous transluminal coronary angioplasty by the radial, brachial, and femoral approaches: The ACCESS study. J Am Coll Cardiol 29:1269, 1997.
20. Roelke M, Smith AJC, Palacios IF: The technique and safety of transseptal left heart catheterization—The Massachusetts General Hospital experience with 1279 procedures. Cathet Cardiovasc Diagn 32:332, 1994.
21. Ommen SR, Higano ST, Nishimura RA, Holmes DR: Summary of the Mayo Clinic experience with direct left ventricular puncture. Cathet Cardiovasc Diagn 44:175, 1998.
22. Anderson AS, Levin TN, Feldman T: External jugular vein approach for percutaneous right ventricular biopsy. J Heart Lung Transplant 16:576, 1997.
23. Wu LA, Lapeyre AC 3rd, Cooper LT: Current role of endomyocardial biopsy in the management of dilated cardiomyopathy and myocarditis. Mayo Clin Proc 76:1030, 2001.
24. Hunt SA, Baker DW, Chin MH: ACC/AHA Guidelines for the evaluation and management of chronic heart failure in the adult. J Am Coll Cardiol 38:2101, 2001.
25. Mehta A, Mehta M, Jain AC: Constrictive pericarditis. Clin Cardiol 22:334, 1999.
26. Barbaro G, DiLorenzo G, Grisorio B, et al: Incidence of dilated cardiomyopathy and detection of HIV in myocardial cells in HIV-positive patients. N Engl J Med 339:1093, 1998.
27. Cohen M, Ferguson JJ 3rd, Freedman RJ Jr, et al: Comparison of outcomes after 8 vs. 9.5 French size intra-aortic balloon counterpulsation catheters based on 9,332 patients in the prospective Benchmark registry. Cathet Cardiovasc Interv 56:200, 2002.
28. O'Rourke MF: Augmentation of coronary blood flow with intra-aortic balloon pump counter-pulsation. Circulation 103:E129, 2001.
29. Ferguson JJ, Cohen M, Freedman RJ: The current practice of intra-aortic balloon counterpulsation: Results from the Benchmark registry. J Am Coll Cardiol 38:1456, 2001.
30. Stone GW, Ohman EM, Miller MF: Contemporary utilization and outcomes of intra-aortic balloon counterpulsation in acute myocardial infarction: The Benchmark registry. J Am Coll Cardiol 41:1940, 2003.
31. Winters KJ, Smith SC, Cohen M: Reduction in ischemic vascular complications with a hydrophilic-coated intra-aortic balloon catheter. Cathet Cardiovasc Interv 46:357, 1999.

Hemodynamic Data

32. Grossman W: Pressure measurement. *In* Grossman W, Baim DS (eds): Cardiac Catheterization, Angiography, and Intervention. 6th ed. Philadelphia, Lea & Febiger, 2000, p 139.
33. Ruzumna P, Gheorghiade M, Bonow RO: Mechanisms and management of heart failure due to diastolic dysfunction. Curr Opin Cardiol 11:269, 1996.
34. Nishimura RA, Rihal CS, Tajik AJ, Holmes DR: Accurate measurements of the transmitral gradient in patients with mitral stenosis: A simultaneous catheterization and Doppler echocardiographic study. J Am Coll Cardiol 24:152, 1994.
35. Hildick-Smith DJ, Walsh JT, Shapiro LM: Pulmonary capillary wedge pressure in mitral stenosis accurately reflects mean left atrial pressure but overestimates transmitral gradient. Am J Cardiol 85:512, 2000.
36. Schobel WA, Voelker W, Haase KK: Extent, determinants and clinical importance of pressure recovery in patients with aortic valve stenosis. Eur Heart J 20:1355, 1999.
37. Niederberger J, Schima H, Maurer G, Baumgartner H: Importance of pressure recovery for the assessment of aortic stenosis by Doppler ultrasound. Circulation 94:1934, 1996.
38. Lehmann, KG, Platt MS: Improved accuracy and precision of thermodilution cardiac output measurement using a dual thermistor catheter system. J Am Coll Cardiol 33:883, 1999.
39. Nichols WW, O'Rourke MF (eds): McDonald's Blood Flow in Arteries. 4th ed. New York, Oxford University Press, 1998.
40. Otto CM: Cardiac catheterization and angiography. *In* Otto CM (ed): Valvular Heart Disease. Philadelphia, WB Saunders, 1999, pp 87-92.
41. Tardif JC, Rodrigues AG, Hardy JF: Simultaneous determination of aortic valve area by the Gorlin formula and by transesophageal echocardiography under different transvalvular flow conditions. Evidence that anatomic aortic valve area does not change with variations in flow in aortic stenosis. J Am Coll Cardiol 29:1296, 1997.
42. Shively BK, Charlton GA, Crawford MH, Chaney RK: Flow dependence of valve area in aortic stenosis: Relation to valve morphology. J Am Coll Cardiol 31:654, 1998.
43. Tardif JC, Rodrigues AG, Hardey JF, et al: Simultaneous determination of aortic valve area by the Gorlin formula and by transesophageal echocardiography under different transvalvular flow conditions. J Am Coll Cardiol 29:1296, 1997.
44. ACC/AHA guidelines for the management of patients with valvular heart disease. A report of the American College of Cardiology/American Heart Association Task Force on Practice Guidelines (Committee on Management of Patients with Valvular Heart Disease). J Am Coll Cardiol 32:1486, 1998.

45. Voelker W, Reul H, Nienhaus G, et al: Comparison of valvular resistance, stroke work loss, and Gorlin valve area for quantification of aortic stenosis. Circulation 91:1196, 1995.
46. Grossman W: Shunt detection and measurement. *In* Grossman W, Baim DS (eds): Cardiac Catheterization, Angiography, and Intervention. 6th ed. Philadelphia, Lea & Febiger, 2000, p 179.
47. Shepherd AP, McMahon CA: Role of oximeter error in the diagnosis of shunts. Cathet Cardiovasc Diagn 37:435, 1996.
48. Daniel WC, Lange RA, Willard JE, et al: Oximetric versus indicator dilution techniques for quantitating intracardiac left-to-right shunting in adults. Am J Cardiol 75:199, 1995.
49. Dehmer GJ, Rutala WA: Current use of green dye curves. Am J Cardiol 75:170, 1995.
50. Grossman W: Stress testing during cardiac catheterization: Exercise and pacing tachycardia. *In* Grossman W, Baim DS (eds): Cardiac Catheterization, Angiography, and Intervention. 6th ed. Philadelphia, Lea & Febiger, 2000, p 325.
51. Udelson JE, Bacharach SL, Cannon RO, Bonow RO: Minimum left ventricular pressure during beta-adrenergic stimulation in human subjects: Evidence for elastic recoil and diastolic "suction" in the normal heart. Circulation 82:1174, 1990.
52. Higano ST, Azrak E, Tahirkheli NK, Kern MJ: Hemodynamic rounds series II: Hemodynamics of constrictive physiology: Influence of respiratory dynamics on ventricular pressures. Cathet Cardiovasc Interv 46:473, 1999.
53. Carabello BA, Crawford FA: Valvular heart disease. N Engl J Med 337:32, 1997.
54. Baim DS, Grossman W: Coronary angiography. *In* Grossman W, Baim DS (eds): Cardiac Catheterization, Angiography, and Intervention. 6th ed. Philadelphia, Lea & Febiger, 2000, p 211.

Adjunctive Diagnostic Techniques

55. Kern MJ: Curriculum in interventional cardiology: Coronary pressure and flow measurements in the cardiac catheterization laboratory. Cathet Cardiovasc Interv 54:378, 2001.
56. Kornowski R, Hong MK, Gepstein L, et al: Preliminary animal and clinical experiences using an electro-mechanical endocardial mapping procedure to distinguish infarcted from healthy myocardium. Circulation 98:1116, 1998.
57. Gepstein L, Goldin A, Lessick I, et al: Electromechanical characterization of chronic myocardial infarction in the canine coronary occlusion model. Circulation 98:2055, 1998.
58. Kornowski R, Hong MK, Leon MB: Comparison between left ventricular electromechanical mapping and radionuclide perfusion imaging for detection of myocardial viability. Circulation 98:1837, 1998.
59. Kornowski R, Baim DS, Moses JW: Short and intermediate term clinical outcomes from direct myocardial laser revascularization guided by biosense left ventricular electromechanical mapping. Circulation 102:1120, 2000.
60. Vale PR, Losordo DW, Milliken CE, et al: Left ventricular electromechanical mapping to assess efficacy of $phVEGF_{165}$ gene transfer for therapeutic angiogenesis in chronic myocardial ischemia. Circulation 102:965, 2000.

Complications Associated with Cardiac Catheterization

61. Davidson CJ, Mark DB, Pieper KS, et al: Thrombotic and cardiovascular complications related to nonionic contrast media during cardiac catheterization. Analysis of 8517 patients. Am J Cardiol 65:1481, 1990.
62. Laskey W, Boyle J, Johnson LW, and the Registry Committee of the Society for Cardiac Angiography and Interventions: Multivariable model for prediction of risk of significant complication during diagnostic cardiac catheterization. Cathet Cardiovasc Diagn 30:185, 1993.
63. Clark VL, Khaja F: Risk of cardiac catheterization in patients aged >80 years without previous cardiac surgery. Am J Cardiol 74:1076, 1994.
64. Omran H, Schmidt H, Hackenbroch M, et al: Silent and apparent cerebral embolism after retrograde catheterisation of the aortic valve in valvular stenosis: A prospective, randomised study. Lancet 361:1241, 2003.
65. McCann RL, Schwartz LB, Pieper KS: Vascular complications of cardiac catheterization. J Vasc Surg 14:375, 1991.
66. Davidson CJ, Hlatky M, Morris GG, et al: Cardiovascular and renal toxicity of a nonionic radiographic contrast agent after cardiac catheterization. Ann Intern Med 110:119, 1989.

Contrast Media–Induced Nephropathy

67. Solomon R, Werner C, Mann D, et al: Effects of saline, mannitol, and furosemide on acute decreases in renal function induced by radiocontrast agents. N Engl J Med 331:1416, 1994.
68. Rudnick MR, Goldfarb S, Wexler L, et al: Nephrotoxicity of ionic and nonionic contrast media in 1,196 patients: A randomized trial. The Iohexol Cooperative Study. Kidney Int 47:254, 1995.
69. Erdogan A, Davidson CJ: Recent trials with iodixanol. Rev Cardiovasc Med 4:543, 2003.
70. Tepel M, Von Der Giet M, Schwarzfeld C, et al: Prevention of radiographic contrast agent induced reactions in renal function by acetylcysteine. N Engl J Med 343:180, 2000.
71. Kay J, Chow W, Chan TM, et al: Acetylcysteine for prevention of acute deterioration of renal function following elective coronary angiography and intervention. JAMA 289:553, 2003.
72. Briguori C, Maganelli F, Scarpato P, et al: Acetylcysteine and contrast agent–associated nephrotoxicity. J Am Coll Cardiol 40:298, 2002.
73. Durham JD, Caputo C, Dokko J, et al: A randomized controlled trial of *N*-acetylcysteine to prevent contrast nephropathy in cardiac angiography. Kidney Int 62:2202, 2002.
74. Davidson CJ, Laskey WK, Hermiller JB, et al: Randomized trial of contrast media utilization in high-risk PTCA: The COURT Trial. Circulation 101:2172, 2000.
75. Aspelin P, Aubry P, Fransson SG, et al, the NEPHRIC study investigators: Nephrotoxic effects in high-risk patients undergoing angiography. N Engl J Med 348:491, 2003.

CHAPTER 18

Coronary Angiography and Intravascular Ultrasound Imaging

Jeffery J. Popma*

Coronary arteriography remains the "gold standard" for identifying the presence or absence of arterial narrowings related to atherosclerotic coronary artery disease (CAD) and provides the most reliable anatomical information for determining the appropriateness of medical therapy, percutaneous coronary intervention (PCI), or coronary artery bypass graft (CABG) surgery in patients with ischemic CAD. First performed by Sones in 1959, coronary arteriography has subsequently become one of the most widely used invasive procedures in cardiovascular medicine. It is performed by directly injecting radiopaque contrast material into the coronary arteries and recording radiographic images on 35-mm cinefilm or digital recordings. More than 2 million patients will undergo coronary arteriography in the United States this year alone, and coronary arteriography is now available in 25 percent of acute care hospitals in this country.

The methods used to perform coronary arteriography have evolved substantially since 1959. Smaller (5 to 6 French [5 to 6F]), high-flow injection catheters have replaced larger (8F), thick-walled catheters, and the reduced sheath size has allowed same-day coronary arteriography, ambulation, and discharge. Complication rates associated with coronary arteriography have fallen due to a better understanding of the periprocedural management of patients undergoing cardiac catheterization. The number of "filmless" digital laboratories increases steadily because of advances in digital image acquisition, storage, and data transfer.[1] New adjunct invasive imaging modalities that can be performed at the time of coronary arteriography, such as intravascular ultrasonography (IVUS), can now provide the clinician with more precise characterization of the vessel wall and extent of atherosclerosis.

This chapter reviews the indications for and techniques of coronary arteriography, the normal coronary anatomy and pathological coronary variants, the qualitative and quantitative angiographic methods for assessing severity of stenoses, and the advantages and limitations of IVUS for characterizing atherosclerotic plaque.

Indications for Coronary Arteriography

Coronary arteriography can establish the presence or absence of coronary stenoses, define therapeutic options, and determine the prognosis of patients with symptoms or signs of ischemic CAD.[2] Coronary arteriography can also be utilized as a research tool to evaluate serial changes that occur after PCI or pharmacological therapy. The American College of Cardiology/American Heart Association (ACC/AHA) Task Force has established indications for coronary arteriography in patients with known or suspected CAD (Table 18–1).[2]

Patients with suspected CAD who have severe stable angina (Canadian Cardiovascular Society [CCS] class III or IV) or those who have less severe symptoms or are asymptomatic but demonstrate "high-risk" criteria for an adverse outcome on noninvasive testing should undergo coronary arteriography. High-risk features include resting or exercise-induced left ventricular dysfunction (left ventricular ejection fraction [LVEF] < 35 percent) or a standard exercise treadmill test demonstrating hypotension or 1 to 2 mm or more ST segment depression associated with decreased exercise capacity.[2] Stress imaging that demonstrates a moderate or large perfusion defect (particularly in the anterior wall), multiple defects, a large fixed perfusion defect with left ventricular dilation or increased lung uptake, or extensive stress or dobutamine-induced wall motion abnormalities also indicate high risk for an adverse outcome. Patients resuscitated from sudden cardiac death, particularly those with residual ventricular arrhythmias, are also candidates for coronary arteriography, given the favorable outcomes associated with revascularization in these patients. In the absence of symptoms and signs of ischemia, the presence of coronary calcification on fluoroscopy and a high calcium score by ultrafast computed tomographic scanning are not indications for coronary arteriography.

Patients with unstable angina who develop recurrent symptoms despite medical therapy or who are at intermediate or high risk for subsequent death or myocardial infarction (MI) are also candidates for coronary arteriography.[2,3] High-risk features include prolonged ongoing (>20 minutes) chest pain, pulmonary edema, worsening mitral regurgitation, dynamic ST segment depression of 1 mm or more, and hypotension.[2] Intermediate-risk features include

*The author acknowledges the contributions of Dr. John Bittl, a coauthor of this chapter in previous editions of this book.

TABLE 18–1 Indications for Coronary Arteriography

Class I	Class IIa	Class IIb	Class III
Asymptomatic or stable angina			
CCS class III and IV on medical therapy High-risk criteria on noninvasive testing irrespective of angina Successfully resuscitated from sudden cardiac death with sustained monomorphic VT or nonsustained polymorphic VT	CCS class III or IV which improves to class I or II with medical therapy Worsening noninvasive testing Patients with angina and severe illness that precludes risk stratification CCS class I or II angina with intolerance to medical therapy Individuals whose occupation affects the safety of others	CCS class I or II angina with demonstrable ischemia but no high-risk criteria on noninvasive testing Asymptomatic men or postmenopausal women with > two major clinical risks with low-risk noninvasive testing and no prior CAD Asymptomatic patients with prior MI, normal LV function, and not-high-risk noninvasive testing	Angina in patients who prefer to avoid revascularization Angina in patients who are not candidates for revascularization or in whom it will not improve QOL As a screening test for CAD After CABG when there is no evidence of ischemia on noninvasive testing Coronary calcification on fluoroscopy or EBCT
Unstable angina			
High or intermediate risk for adverse outcome in patients refractory to medical therapy High or intermediate risk that stabilizes after initial treatment Initially low short-term risk that is high risk on noninvasive testing Suspected Prinzmetal variant angina	None	Low short-term risk unstable angina without high-risk criteria on noninvasive testing	Recurrent chest discomfort suggestive of unstable angina but without objective signs of ischemia and with a normal coronary angiogram within the past 5 years Unstable angina in patients who are not candidates for revascularization
Postrevascularization ischemia			
Suspected abrupt closure or subacute stent thrombosis after PCI Recurrent angina and high-risk criteria on noninvasive evaluation within 9 months of PCI	Recurrent symptomatic ischemia within 12 months of CABG Noninvasive evidence of high-risk criteria occurring anytime after CABG Recurrent angina inadequately controlled by medications	Asymptomatic post-PCI patient suspected of having restenosis within the first months after PCI because of an abnormal but not high-risk noninvasive test Recurrent angina without high-risk criteria on noninvasive testing occurring >1 year postoperatively Asymptomatic post-CABG patient in whom a deteriorating noninvasive test is found	Symptoms in a post-CABG patient who is not a candidate for revasascularization Routine angiography after PCI or CABG unless part of an approved research protocol
After QWMI or NQWMI			
Spontaneous myocardial ischemia or ischemia provoked with minimal exertion Before surgical therapy for acute MR, VSD, true or pseudoaneurysm Persistent hemodynamic instability	Suspected MI due to coronary embolism, arteritis, trauma, certain metabolic diseases, or coronary spasm Survivors of acute MI with LVEF < 0.40, CHF, prior PCI or CABG, or malignant ventricular arrhythmias	For a suspected persistent occlusion of the IRA to perform delayed PCI Coronary arteriography performed without risk stratification to identify the presence of left main or three-vessel CAD All patients after NQWMI Recurrent ventricular tachycardia despite antiarrhythmic therapy without ongoing ischemia	Patients who are not a candidate for or refuse revascularization
Nonspecific chest pain			
High-risk features on noninvasive testing	None	Patients with recurrent hospitalizations for chest pain who have abnormal or equivocal findings on noninvasive testing	All other patients with nonspecific chest pain

Class I: Conditions for which there is agreement that the procedure is useful and effective; Class IIa: Weight of the evidence is in favor of usefulness and efficacy; Class IIb: Weight of the evidence is less well established by evidence and opinion; Class III: Conditions for which there is general agreement that the procedure is not useful and effective and in some cases may be harmful.

CABG = coronary artery bypass graft surgery; CAD = coronary artery disease; CCS = Canadian Cardiovascular Society; CHF = congestive heart failure; EBCT = electron beam computed tomography; IRA = infarct-related artery; LV = left ventricular; MI = myocardial infarction; MR = mitral regurgitation; NQWMI = non-Q-wave MI; PCI = percutaneous coronary intervention; QOL = quality of life; VSD = ventricular septal defect; VT = ventricular tachycardia.

From Scanlon P, Faxon D, Audet A, et al: ACC/AHA guidelines for coronary angiography. J Am Coll Cardiol 33:1756, 1999.

angina at rest (>20 minutes) relieved with rest or sublingual nitroglycerin, angina associated with dynamic electrocardiographic changes, recent-onset angina with a high likelihood of CAD, pathological Q waves or ST segment depression less than 1 mm in multiple leads, and age older than 65 years.[2]

Patients with an ST segment elevation myocardial infarction (STEMI), a non-ST segment elevation myocardial infarction (NSTEMI), or unstable angina who develop spontaneous ischemia; or with ischemia at a minimal workload; or who have MI complicated by congestive heart failure (CHF), hemodynamic instability, cardiac arrest, mitral regurgitation, or ventricular septal rupture should undergo coronary arteriography. Patients with angina or provocable ischemia after MI should also undergo coronary arteriography because revascularization may reduce the high risk of reinfarction in these patients.

Patients who present with chest pain of unclear etiology, particularly those who have high-risk criteria on noninvasive testing, may benefit from coronary arteriography to diagnose or exclude the presence of significant CAD.[2,4] Patients who have undergone prior revascularization should undergo coronary arteriography if there is suspicion of abrupt vessel closure or when recurrent angina develops that meets high-risk noninvasive criteria.

Coronary arteriography should also be performed in patients scheduled to undergo noncardiac surgery who demonstrate high-risk criteria on noninvasive testing, have angina unresponsive to medical therapy, develop unstable angina, or have equivocal noninvasive test results and are scheduled to undergo high-risk surgery (see also Chap. 77). Coronary arteriography is also recommended for patients scheduled to undergo surgery for valvular heart disease or congenital heart disease, particularly those with multiple cardiac risk factors and those with infective endocarditis and evidence of coronary embolization.[2]

Coronary arteriography should be performed annually in patients after cardiac transplantation in the absence of clinical symptoms because of the characteristically diffuse and often asymptomatic nature of graft atherosclerosis. Coronary arteriography is useful in potential donors for cardiac transplantation whose age or cardiac risk profile increases the likelihood of CAD. The arteriogram often provides important diagnostic information about the presence of CAD in patients with intractable arrhythmias before electrophysiological testing or in patients who present with a dilated cardiomyopathy of unknown etiology.

CONTRAINDICATIONS. Although there are no absolute contraindications for coronary arteriography, relative contraindications include unexplained fever, untreated infection, severe anemia with hemoglobin less than 8 gm/dl, severe electrolyte imbalance, severe active bleeding, uncontrolled systemic hypertension, digitalis toxicity, previous contrast reaction but no pretreatment with corticosteroids, and ongoing stroke.[2] Other disease states that are relative contraindications to coronary arteriography include acute renal failure; decompensated CHF; severe intrinsic or iatrogenic coagulopathy (international normalized ratio [INR] > 2.0); and active endocarditis.[2] Risk factors for significant complications after catheterization include advanced age as well as several general medical, vascular, and cardiac characteristics (Table 18–2).

Given that the majority of these conditions are self-limited, deferral of coronary arteriography until important comorbidities have been stabilized is generally preferred unless there is evidence of ongoing myocardial necrosis. It is recognized that coronary arteriography performed under emergency conditions is associated with a higher risk of procedural complications, and the risks and benefits of the procedure and its alternatives should be carefully reviewed with the patient and family in all circumstances before undertaking coronary arteriography in the presence of relative contraindications.

TABLE 18–2 Patients at Increased Risk for Complications after Coronary Arteriography

Increased general medical risk
Age > 70 years
Complex congenital heart disease
Morbid obesity
General debility or cachexia
Uncontrolled glucose intolerance
Arterial oxygen desaturation
Severe chronic obstructive lung disease
Renal insufficiency with creatinine greater than 1.5 mg/dl
Increased cardiac risk
Three-vessel coronary artery disease
Left main coronary artery disease
Functional class IV
Significant mitral or aortic valve disease or mechanical prosthesis
Ejection fraction less than 35%
High-risk exercise treadmill testing (hypotension or severe ischemia)
Pulmonary hypertension
Pulmonary artery wedge pressure greater than 25 mm Hg
Increased vascular risk
Anticoagulation or bleeding diathesis
Uncontrolled systemic hypertension
Severe peripheral vascular disease
Recent stroke
Severe aortic insufficiency

Adapted from Scanlon P, Faxon D, Audet A, et al: ACC/AHA guidelines for coronary angiography. J Am Coll Cardiol 33:1756, 1999.

Complications of Coronary Arteriography

Major complications are uncommon (<1 percent) after coronary arteriography (Table 18–3)[5] and include death (0.10 to 0.14 percent), MI (0.06 to 0.07 percent), contrast agent reactions (0.23 percent), and local vascular complications (0.24 to 0.1 percent).[6,7] More recent series have shown no change in the major complication rates associated with coronary arteriography, despite increased morbidity of patients and lesion complexity.[5,8,9]

The incidence of death during coronary arteriography is higher in the presence of left main coronary artery (LMCA) disease (0.55 percent), with LVEF less than 30 percent (0.30 percent), and with New York Heart Association functional Class IV disease (0.29 percent). Stroke is uncommon (0.07 to 0.14 percent) after coronary arteriography[10] but may develop due to embolization of atherosclerotic debris into the cerebral circulation or embolization of clot that formed on the injection catheters, particularly in patients with prior CABG who have a diseased ascending aorta.[9,11] Embolic stroke related to atherothrombotic embolization is generally reversible.

Air embolus is an uncommon occurrence (0.1 percent) during diagnostic coronary arteriography and is generally preventable with meticulous flushing and elimination of air within the manifold. If an air embolus and air lock do occur, 100 percent oxygen should be administered, which allows resorption of smaller amounts of air within 2 to 4 minutes. Morphine sulfate may be given for pain relief. Ventricular arrhythmias associated with air embolus can be treated with lidocaine and direct-current cardioversion. Cholesterol embolization is a rare but important complication that can occur during coronary arteriography.[12] Cholesterol embolization occurs more often in the presence of catheter manipulation within an abdominal aortic aneurysm that has diffuse atherosclerosis (see also Chap. 54).[13] Nerve pain after diagnostic catheterization occurs rarely.[14,15] Although there was initial concern about the occurrence of lactic acidosis after coronary angiography in diabetic patients taking metformin, this complication has been minimized when metformin is discontinued after coronary arteriography until renal function has recovered.[16]

With the expanded use of complex PCI, patients may now return for multiple procedures over their lifetime that may subject them to the risk of cumulative radiation injury. Scattered reports of radiodermatitis related to prolonged x-ray exposure[17,18] have led to the recommendation that patients who receive fluoroscopy for more than 60 minutes be counseled about the delayed effects of radiation injury to the skin. Radiation-induced lesions are generally identified by their location in the region of the x-ray tube and are manifest by an acute erythema, delayed pigmented telangiectasia, and indurated or ulcerated plaques in the upper back or below the axilla.[17]

TABLE 18–3 Risk of Cardiac Catheterization

Complication	SCAI Registry (%)
Mortality	0.11
Myocardial infarction	0.05
Cerebrovascular accident	0.07
Arrhythmias	0.38
Vascular complications	0.43
Contrast reaction	0.37
Hemodynamic complications	0.26
Perforation of heart chamber	0.03
Other complications	0.28
Total of major complications	1.70

SCAI = Society for Cardiac Angiography and Intervention.
Adapted from Scanlon P, Faxon D, Audet A, et al: ACC/AHA guidelines for coronary angiography. J Am Coll Cardiol 33:1756, 1999.

Technique of Coronary Arteriography

PREPARATION OF THE PATIENT. Elective coronary arteriography should be performed alone or in conjunction with right-heart catheterization or contrast left ventriculography (see Chap. 17) when comorbid conditions, such as CHF, diabetes mellitus, or renal insufficiency, are stable. A baseline electrocardiogram (ECG), electrolyte and renal function tests, complete blood cell count, and coagulation panel should be reviewed before coronary arteriography. Patients who may undergo PCI should receive aspirin, 80 to 325 mg, at least 2 hours before the procedure if PCI is planned. Warfarin should be discontinued 2 days before elective coronary arteriography, and the INR should be less than 2.0 before arterial puncture. Patients at increased risk for systemic thromboembolism on withdrawal of warfarin, such as those with atrial fibrillation, mitral valve disease, or a prior history of systemic thromboembolism, may be treated with intravenous unfractionated heparin or subcutaneous low-molecular-weight heparin in the periprocedural period.

VASCULAR ACCESS. A variety of vascular approaches are available for coronary arteriography. The selection of the vascular access depends on the operator's and patient's preferences, anticoagulation status, and presence of peripheral vascular disease.

Femoral Artery Approach. The right or left femoral arteries are the most commonly used access sites for coronary arteriography. The common femoral artery courses medially to the femoral head and the bifurcation of the common femoral artery into its branches is generally distal to the middle third of the femoral head, which can be localized by fluoroscopy before arterial puncture (Fig. 18–1A). The anterior wall of the common femoral artery should be punctured several centimeters below the inguinal ligament but proximal to the bifurcation of the superficial femoral and profunda arterial branches (see Fig. 18–1B). If the puncture site is proximal to the inguinal ligament, hemostasis after the procedure may be difficult with manual compression, leading to an increased risk of retroperitoneal hemorrhage. If the puncture site is at or distal to the femoral bifurcation, there is a higher risk of pseudoaneurysm formation after sheath removal. Ipsilateral cannulation of the femoral artery and femoral vein also increases the risk of arteriovenous fistula formation.

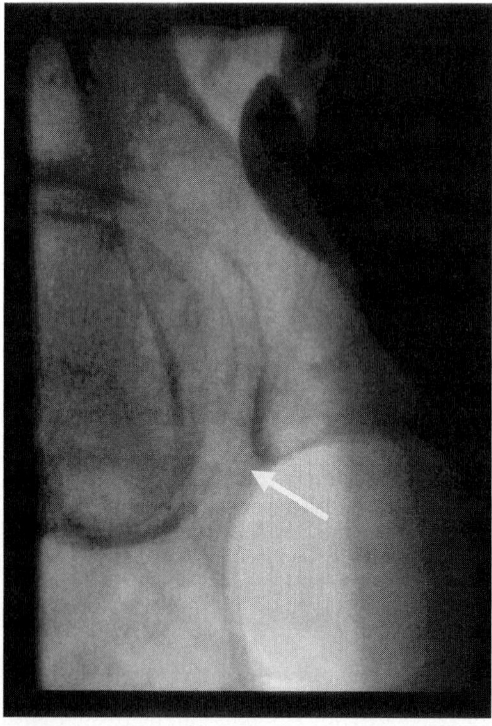
A

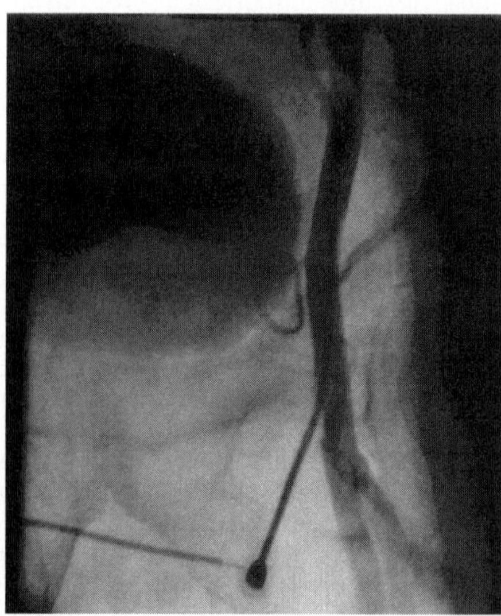
B

FIGURE 18–1 Radiographic landmarks can be used to identify the course of the common femoral artery. **A,** The middle third of the right femoral head identifies the usual course of the common femoral artery (arrow). **B,** The arterial sheath is shown placed proximally to the bifurcation of the femoris superficial femoral artery and the profunda femoris.

Brachial and Radial Artery Approaches. Although Sones first introduced the cutdown approach to the brachial artery for coronary arteriography, access to the brachial and radial arteries is now most often obtained percutaneously. These approaches are preferred to the femoral approach in the presence of severe peripheral vascular disease[19] and morbid obesity.[20] Systemic anticoagulation with intravenous heparin, use of hydrophilic sheath, and administration of intraarterial verapamil and nitroglycerin have reduced the occurrence of vascular complications with the radial approach. Saphenous vein grafts (SVGs) can be engaged using either brachial or radial artery, but cannulation of the internal mammary artery (IMA) is best performed from the left brachial or radial artery. Engagement of the left IMA from the right brachial or radial artery is technically challenging but may be performed using a "headhunter" or another shaped catheter for selective entry into the left subclavian artery. A 0.035-inch angled hydrophilic guidewire is the most useful guidewire for access to the subclavian artery.

The brachial artery easily accommodates an 8F (1 French = 0.33 mm in diameter) sheath, whereas the radial artery is smaller and generally limited to 6 or 7F catheters. Before radial artery access is attempted, an Allen test should be carried out to ensure that the ulnar artery is patent in the event of radial artery occlusion.

Catheters

A number of injection catheters have been developed for coronary arteriography. Diagnostic catheters are generally constructed of polyethylene or polyurethane with a fine wire braid within the wall to allow advancement and directional control (torquability) and to prevent kinking. The outer diameter size of the catheters ranges from 4 to 8F, but 5 and 6F catheters are used most commonly for diagnostic arteriography.

JUDKINS CATHETERS. The left Judkins catheter is preshaped to allow entry into the left coronary ostium from the femoral approach with minimal catheter manipulation (Figs. 18-2 and 18-3). A preformed left Judkins catheter can also be used from the left brachial or radial artery, but a catheter with 0.5 cm less curvature than required for the femoral approach is generally better suited for coronary cannulation. The right Judkins catheter is shaped to permit entry into the right coronary artery (RCA) with a small amount of rotational (clockwise) catheter manipulation from any vascular approach.

Selection of Judkins catheter shape is based on the body habitus of the patient and size of the aortic root. The left coronary artery (LCA) is easily engaged with the Judkins left 4.0 catheter from the femoral approach in most patients, whereas patients with a dilated ascending aorta (e.g., in the setting of congenital aortic stenosis and poststenotic dilation) may require the use of a Judkins left 5.0 or 6.0 catheter. Patients with large ascending aortic aneurysms may require arteriography with heat-modified catheters to achieve Judkins left 7.0 to 10.0 shapes. Use of a Judkins shape that is too small for the ascending aorta often leads to folding of the catheter within the aortic root. The best technique for removing a folded Judkins left catheter from the body involves withdrawing the folded catheter into the descending aorta and advancing a guidewire anterograde in the contralateral common iliac artery. On withdrawal of the catheter and guidewire together, the catheter straightens and can be removed safely from the body without disrupting the arterial access site.

AMPLATZ CATHETERS. Amplatz catheters can be used for the femoral or brachial approach to coronary arteriography (Fig. 18-4). The Amplatz catheters are an excellent alternative in cases in which the Judkins catheter is not appropriately shaped to enter the coronary arteries. The Amplatz L-1 or L-2 catheter may be used for coronary angiography from the right brachial or radial approach. A modified right Amplatz catheter (AR-1 or AR-2) can be used for engagement of a horizontal or upward takeoff RCA or SVG.

OTHER CATHETERS. Other catheters used for coronary arteriography include the left IMA catheter with an angulated tip that allows engagement of the IMA or an upward takeoff RCA. Catheter shapes that permit engagement of SVGs include the multipurpose catheter (Fig. 18-5), right Judkins, modified right Amplatz, and hockey stick catheters. Specially designed catheters for engagement of the coronary arteries from the radial artery have also been developed.

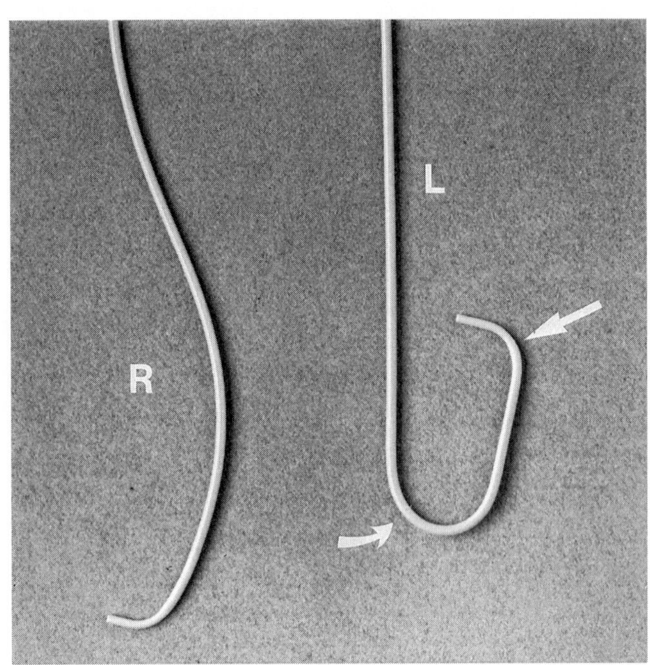

FIGURE 18–2 Right (R) and left (L) Judkins catheters. The primary (straight arrow) and secondary (curved arrow) curves of the left Judkins catheter are shown. (Courtesy of Cordis Corporation.)

Drugs Used During Coronary Arteriography

ANALGESICS. The goal of analgesic use is to achieve a state of conscious sedation, defined by a minimally depressed level of consciousness that allows a patient to respond appropriately to verbal commands and to maintain a patent airway.[21-23] Several different sedation regimens are recommended, but depending on the patient's comorbid conditions, most use diazepam, 2.5 to 10 mg orally, and diphenhydramine, 25 to 50 mg orally, 1 hour before the procedure. Intravenous midazolam, 0.5 to 2 mg, and fentanyl, 25 to 50 µg, are useful agents to provide sedation during the procedure. Patients undergoing conscious sedation should have continuous hemodynamic, ECG, and oximetry monitoring and access to oxygen and suction ports and a resuscitation cart.

ANTICOAGULANTS. Intravenous unfractionated heparin is no longer required during routine coronary arteriography. Patients at increased risk for thromboembolic complications, including those with severe aortic stenosis, critical peripheral arterial disease, or arterial atheroembolic disease or those undergoing procedures in which there is a need for prolonged (>1 to 2 minutes) use of guidewires in the central circulation may be given intravenous heparin, 2000 to 5000 units. Patients undergoing brachial or radial artery catheterization should also receive systemic anticoagulation with unfractionated heparin or bivalirudin. Frequent flushing of all diagnostic and guiding catheters with heparinized saline prevents the formation of microthrombi within the catheter tip. A continuous flush through the arterial access sheath may also lower the occurrence of distal thromboembolism.

The anticoagulant effect of unfractionated heparin can be reversed with protamine, 1 mg for every 100 units of heparin. Protamine causes anaphylaxis or serious hypotensive episodes in approximately 2 percent of patients, and protamine should not be administered to patients with prior exposure to NPH insulin, in those with a history of unstable angina or high-risk coronary anatomy, or in patients who have undergone coronary arteriography by means of the brachial or radial arteries. Femoral sheaths can be removed

CH 18

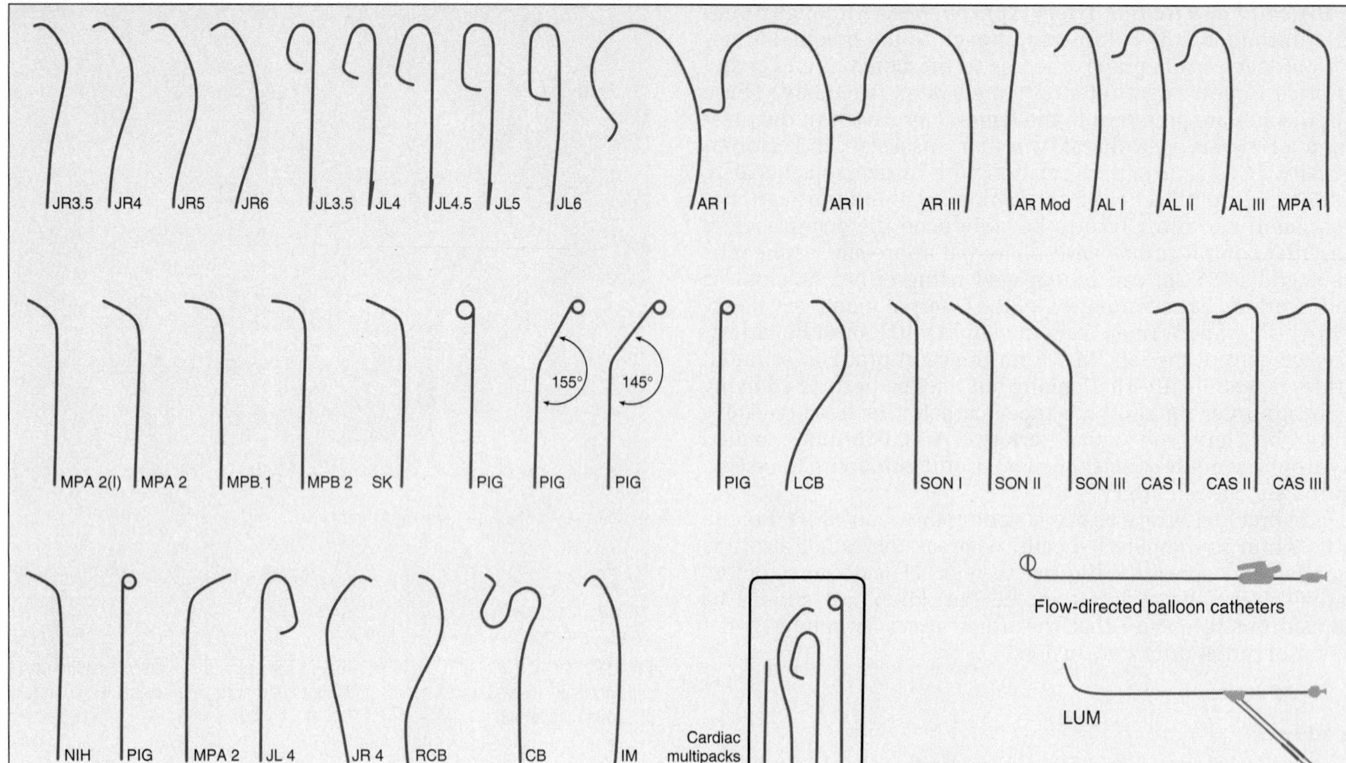

FIGURE 18–3 Tip configurations for several catheters useful in coronary arteriography. JR = Judkins right; JL = Judkins left; AR = Amplatz right; Mod = modified; AL = Amplatz left; MP = multipurpose; PIG = pigtail; LCB = left coronary bypass graft; SON = Sones; CAS = Castillo; NIH = National Institutes of Health; RCB = right coronary bypass graft; CB = coronary bypass catheter; IM = internal mammary; LUM = lumen. (Courtesy of Cordis Corporation.)

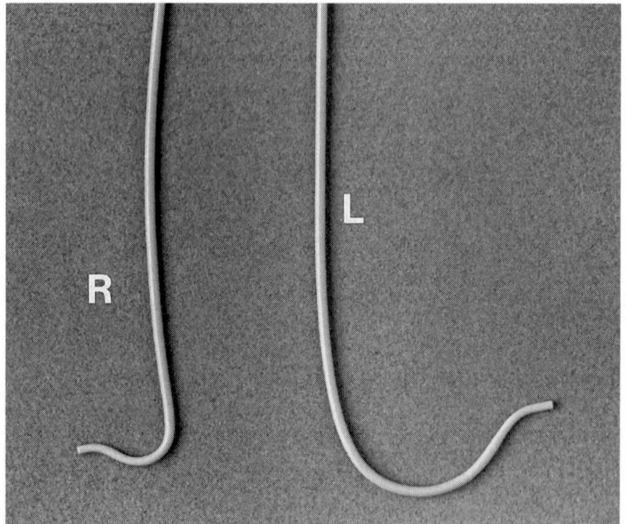

FIGURE 18–4 Right (R) and left (L) Amplatz catheters. (Courtesy of Cordis Corporation.)

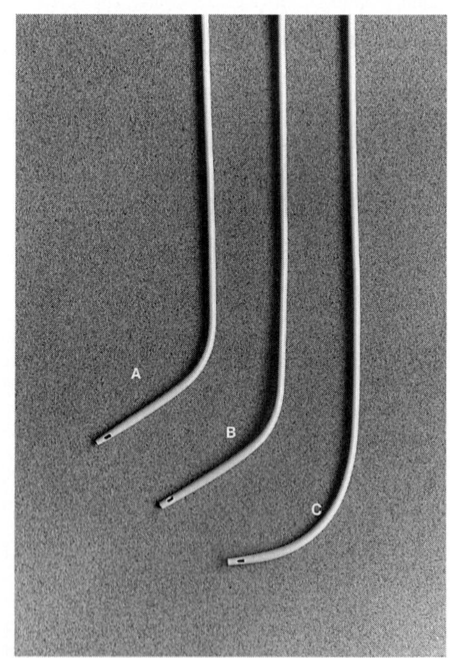

FIGURE 18–5 Multipurpose A, B, and C type catheters. (Courtesy of Cordis Corporation.)

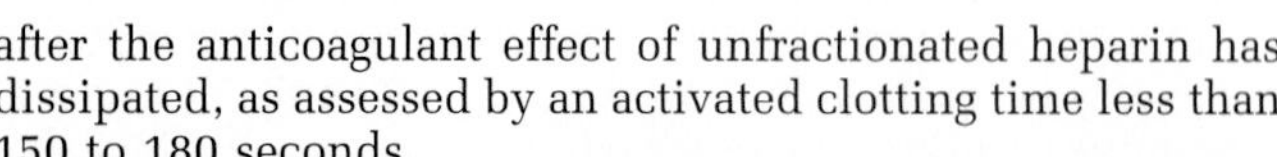

after the anticoagulant effect of unfractionated heparin has dissipated, as assessed by an activated clotting time less than 150 to 180 seconds.

TREATMENT OF PERIPROCEDURAL ISCHEMIA. Patients may develop angina during coronary arteriography because of ischemia induced by tachycardia, hypertension, contrast agents, microembolization, coronary spasm or enhanced vasomotor tone, or dynamic platelet aggregation. Sublingual (0.3 mg), intracoronary (50 to 200 μg), or intravenous (10 to 25 μg/min) nitroglycerin can be given in patients with a systolic blood pressure greater than 100 mm Hg. Patients without contraindications to beta blockers, such as bradycardia, bronchospasm, or left ventricular dysfunction, can be given intravenous metoprolol, 2.5 to 5.0 mg, or

TABLE 18–4 Characteristics of Radiocontrast Agents

Compound	Brand Name	Osmolality mOsm/kg H_2O	Viscosity at 37°C	Iodine (mg/ml)	Sodium (mEq/liter)	Additives	Side Effects Profile
High osmolar ionic agents							
Sodium diatrizoate	Hypaque	1690	9.0	370	160	Calcium disodium EDTA	Electophysiologic (++++) Hemodynamic (++++) Anticoagulant (++++) Nephrotoxicity (+++) Allergic (+++)
Sodium meglumine diatrizoate	Renografin	1940	8.4	370	160	Sodium citrate, disodium EDTA	
Nonionic or low osmolar							
Ioxaglate	Hexabrix	600	7.5	320	150	Calcium disodium EDTA	Electophysiologic (+) Hemodynamic (+) Anticoagulant (+) Nephrotoxicity (++) Allergic (+)
Iohexol	Omnipaque	844	10.4	350	5	Tromethamine calcium disodium EDTA	
Iopamidol	Isovue	790	9.4	370	2	Tromethamine calcium disodium EDTA	
Ioversol	Optiray	702	5.8	320	2	Tromethamine calcium disodium EDTA	
Iodixanol	Visipaque	290	11.8	320	19	Tromethamine calcium disodium EDTA + 0.15 mEq/liter calcium	

++++ = common; +++ = occasional; ++ = infrequent; + = rare; EDTA = ethylene diaminetetraacetic acid (a divalent cation chelating agent).

Modified from Hill J, Lambert C, Pepine C: Radiographic contrast agents. *In* Pepine C, Hill J, Lambert C (eds): Diagnostic and Therapeutic Cardiac Catheterization. Baltimore, Williams & Wilkins, 1994, pp 182-194.

propranolol, 1 to 4 mg. Intraaortic balloon counterpulsation is also a useful adjunct in patients with coronary ischemia and left main CAD, cardiogenic shock, or refractory pulmonary edema.

Contrast Agents

All radiographic contrast agents contain iodine, which effectively absorbs x-rays in the energy range of the angiographic imaging system. Radiographic contrast agents currently used for coronary arteriography may also produce a number of adverse hemodynamic, electrophysiological, and renal effects. The frequency of these side effects varies among the different radiocontrast agents because of differences in their ionic content, osmolality, and viscosity (Table 18–4).

IONIC CONTRAST AGENTS. The monomeric ionic contrast agents initially used for coronary arteriography were the high-osmolar meglumine and sodium salts of diatrizoic acid. These substances dissociated into cations and iodine-containing anions that have a higher serum osmolality (>1500 mOsm) than human plasma (300 mOsm). The hypertonicity of these compounds produced sinus bradycardia, heart block, QT interval and QRS prolongation, ST segment depression, giant T wave inversion, decreased left ventricular contractility, decreased systolic pressure, and increased left ventricular end-diastolic pressure, owing, in part, to the calcium-chelating properties of these agents. Ventricular tachycardia and fibrillation occurred in 0.5 percent of cases and developed more often when ionic contrast agents were injected into a damped coronary catheter, were given too rapidly, or were administered in too great a volume. Because of the availability of other less toxic contrast agents, ionic contrast agents are now rarely used for coronary arteriography. When ionic agents are selected, additional precautions are needed to avoid complications. Patients should be counseled about coughing, which helps clear contrast material from within the coronary artery, before the first selective coronary arteriogram is performed and the minimal amount of contrast agent needed to fill the entire coronary artery should be given.

NONIONIC AND LOW-OSMOLAR CONTRAST AGENTS. Nonionic agents do not ionize in solution and provide more iodine-containing particles per milliliter of contrast material than ionic agents. Their osmolality is substantially reduced (<850 mOsm) because these agents exist in solution as single neutral molecules and do not chelate calcium, potentially leading to fewer side effects.

Side Effects. Unwanted reactions may also occur after use of nonionic radiocontrast agents, related in part to the hyperosmolality of these agents (Table 18–5). These reactions include hot flushing, nausea, vomiting, and arrhythmia. Hypotension after contrast medium administration may be due to an anaphylactoid reaction, a direct toxic effect, or a vasovagal reaction. Ionic radiocontrast agents may inhibit clot formation when mixed with blood. Although nonionic agents exhibit less of an anticoagulant effect, potentially leading to clots within the manifold where low-osmolar and nonionic contrast agents and blood are in direct contact with one another, the clinical effects of this finding related to embolization of thrombus into the coronary arteries are not known. The low-osmolality ionic dimer methylglucamine-sodium ioxaglate retains most of the anticoagulant properties of diatrizoate sodium, but has more complications than the

TABLE 18–5 Toxicities Associated with Radiocontrast Agents

Side Effect
Allergic (anaphylactoid) reactions Grade I: Single episode of emesis, nausea, sneezing, or vertigo Grade II: Hives, multiple episodes of emesis, fevers, or chills Grade III: Clinical shock, bronchospasm, laryngospasm or edema, loss of consciousness, hypotension, hypertension, cardiac arrhythmia, angioedema, or pulmonary edema
Cardiovascular toxicity Electrophysiologic Bradycardia (asystole, heart block) Tachycardia (sinus, ventricular) Ventricular fibrillation Hemodynamic Hypotension (cardiac depression, vasodilation) Heart failure (cardiac depression, increased intravascular volume)
Nephrotoxicity
Discomfort Nausea, vomiting Heat and flushing
Hyperthyroidism

isosmolar, nonionic dimer contrast agent iodixanol.[24] Iodixanol may also be the preferred contrast agent in diabetic patients with underlying renal insufficiency.[25]

CONTRAST-INDUCED NEPHROPATHY (see also Chap. 86). Worsening of renal function may occur after contrast agent administration in 13 to 20 percent of patients, particularly in those with prior renal insufficiency, diabetes mellitus, dehydration before the procedure, CHF, larger volumes of contrast material, and recent (<48 hour) contrast exposure.[26-30] The incidence, pathogenesis, and preventive measures for the treatment of contrast-induced nephropathy are reviewed in detail in Chapter 86. Fluid administration is recommended in all patients.[31-34] Periprocedural aminophylline appears to be of limited value.[35] Although the clinical data have been mixed,[36] a weighted analysis of the preprocedural use of *N*-acetylcysteine, particularly in patients with underlying renal insufficiency, appears to indicate a benefit for reduction of the occurrence of contrast-induced nephropathy (see Chap. 86).[37-42] Despite encouraging initial results,[43-45] use of felodipine does not appear to lessen the occurrence of nephropathy after contrast agent administration.[46] Randomized trials have shown a benefit with hemofiltration[47,48] but not hemodialysis[49] for the prevention of contrast-induced renal insufficiency in high-risk patients.

CONTRAST REACTION PROPHYLAXIS. Reactions to radiocontrast agents are classified as mild (grade I: single episode of emesis, nausea, sneezing, or vertigo), moderate (grade II: hives, multiple episodes of emesis, fevers, or chills), or severe (grade III: clinical shock, bronchospasm, laryngospasm or edema, loss of consciousness, hypotension, hypertension, cardiac arrhythmias, angioedema, or pulmonary edema). Although mild or moderate reactions occur in approximately 9.0 percent of patients, severe reactions are uncommon (0.15 to 0.7 percent). Contrast reactions may be more difficult to manage in patients receiving beta blocker therapy. Recurrence rates may approach 50 percent on reexposure to contrast agents, and prophylactic use of H_1 and H_2 histamine blocking agents and aspirin therapy has been advocated. Patients treated with corticosteroids (methylprednisolone, 32 mg) 12 hours and 2 hours before contrast agent exposure had a lower (6.4 percent) incidence of allergic reactions than patients treated with a single dose of methylprednisolone 2 hours before contrast agent exposure (9.4 percent) or placebo (9.0 percent) ($p < 0.001$).[50] On the basis of these findings, patients with a prior history of radiocontrast reactions should receive two doses of prednisone, 60 mg (or its equivalent) the night before and again at 2 hours before the procedure. Diphenhydramine, 50 mg, and cimetidine, 300 mg, may also be given before the procedure.

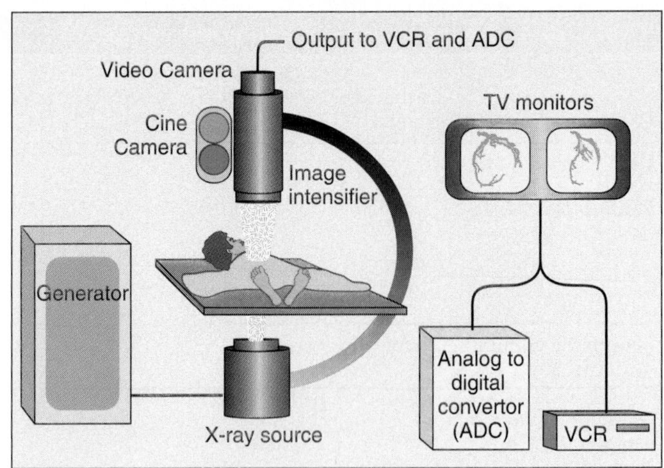

FIGURE 18–6 Cineangiographic equipment. The major components include a generator, x-ray tube, image intensifier attached to a positioner such as a C-arm, optical system, cine camera, video camera, videocassette recorder (VCR), analog-to-digital converter (ADC), and television monitors. The x-ray tube is the source of the x-ray beam, which passes superiorly through the patient.

Anatomy and Variations of the Coronary Arteries

The basic principle of radiographic coronary imaging is that radiation produced by the x-ray tube is attenuated as it passes through the body and detected by the image intensifier (Fig. 18–6). Iodinated contrast medium injected into the coronary arteries enhances the absorption of x-rays and produces a sharp contrast with the surrounding cardiac tissues. The x-ray shadow is then converted into a visible light image by an image intensifier, displayed on fluoroscopic monitors, and stored on 35-mm cinefilm or digital storage systems. Although 35-mm cinefilm has better image resolution (4 line pairs/mm) than digital imaging (2.5 line pairs/mm) archived in a standard DICOM3 512 × 512 × 8 bit pixel matrix format, digital imaging has largely replaced 35-mm cinefilm for coronary angiography due to its versatility with respect to image transfer, low-cost acquisition and storage, and capability for image enhancement after image acquisition.

The major epicardial branches and their second- and third-order branches can be visualized using coronary arteriography. The network of smaller intramyocardial branches generally are not seen because of their size, cardiac motion, and limitations in resolution of cineangiographic systems. These fourth-order and higher "resistance" vessels play a major role in autoregulation of coronary blood flow, may limit myocardial perfusion during stress, and contribute to ischemia in patients with left ventricular hypertrophy or systemic hypertension. Coronary perfusion within these smaller branch vessels can be quantitatively assessed using the myocardial blush score.[51]

ARTERIAL NOMENCLATURE AND EXTENT OF DISEASE. The Coronary Artery Surgery Study (CASS) inves-

TABLE 18–6 Classification System for Coronary Segments

Number	Map Location	Number	Map Location	Number	Map Location
Right coronary artery		**Left main coronary artery**		**Left circumflex**	
1	Proximal RCA	11	Left main coronary artery	18	Proximal LCx
2	Mid RCA	**Left anterior descending**		19	Distal LCx
3	Distal RCA	12	Proximal LAD	20	1st obtuse marginal
4	Right posterior descending branch	13	Mid LAD	21	2nd obtuse marginal
5	Right posterior atrioventricular	14	Distal LAD	22	Third obtuse marginal
6	First right posterolateral	15	1st diagonal	23	LCx atrioventricular groove
7	Second right posterolateral	16	2nd diagonal	24	1st left posterolateral branch
8	Third right posterolateral	17	LAD septal perforators	25	2nd left posterolateral branch
9	Posterior descending septals	29	3rd diagonal	26	3rd left posterolateral branch
10	Acute marginal segment			27	Left posterior descending branch
				28	Ramus intermedium branch

LAD = left anterior descending; LCx = left circumflex; RCA = right coronary artery.

From CASS Principal Investigators and their Associates: Coronary Artery Surgery Study (CASS): A randomized trial of coronary artery surgery: Survival data. Circulation 68:939, 1983.

tigators established the nomenclature most commonly used to describe the coronary anatomy, defining 27 segments in three major coronary arteries (Table 18–6). The Bypass Angioplasty Revascularization Investigators (BARI) modified these criteria by addition of two segments for the ramus intermedius and the third diagonal branch. In this system, the three major coronary arteries include the left anterior descending (LAD), left circumflex (LCx), and RCA with a right-dominant, balanced, or left-dominant circulation (see later). CAD is defined as a more than 50 percent diameter stenosis in one or more of these vessels, although it is clear that stenoses of less than 50 percent have major prognostic implications because these lesions most commonly lead to plaque rupture and acute MI. Subcritical stenoses of less than 50 percent are best characterized as nonobstructive CAD; obstructive CAD is classified as one-, two-, or three-vessel disease.

A number of "jeopardy scores" were developed to quantitate plaque burden, predict patient-based clinical outcomes, and identify risk factors for the presence of atherosclerosis and its progression. The Califf scoring system divided the coronary circulation into six segments with two points allotted for each coronary stenosis of 75 percent or more (score range: 0 to 12). The Gensini scoring system used an ordinal ranking based on stenosis severity in 11 coronary segments (score range: 0 to 72). The Candell-Riera scoring system used an ordinal ranking (from 1 to 5) of 13 coronary segments (score range: 0 to 65). Differences between these scoring systems were primarily related to definitions rather than to their ability to provide unique prognostic information, as one comparative study found that 80 percent of the prognostic information in one jeopardy index was obtained with other indices using subtly different methodologies. In CASS, the major determinants of 6-year outcome included the number of diseased vessels, the number of diseased proximal segments, and the global left ventricular function; these three factors alone accounted for 80 percent of the prognostic information.

ANGIOGRAPHIC PROJECTIONS. The major coronary arteries traverse the interventricular and atrioventricular grooves, aligned with the long and short axes of the heart, respectively. Because the heart is oriented obliquely in the thoracic cavity, the coronary circulation is generally visualized in the right anterior oblique (RAO) and left anterior oblique (LAO) projections to furnish true posteroanterior and lateral views of the heart (Figs. 18–7 and 18–8), but these views are limited by vessel foreshortening and superimposition of branches. Simultaneous rotation of the x-ray beam in the sagittal plane provides a better view of the major coronary arteries and their branches. A simple nomenclature has evolved for the description of these sagittal views, which characterizes the relationship between the image intensifier and the patient. Assuming that the x-ray tube is under the patient's table and the image intensifier is over the patient's table, the projection is referred to as the "cranial" view if the image intensifier is tilted toward the head of the patient. The projection is referred to as "caudal" if the image intensifier is tilted down toward the feet of the patient.

It is difficult to predict which angulated views will be most useful for any particular patient because the "optimal" angiographic projection depends largely on body habitus, variation in the coronary anatomy, and location of the lesion. It is recommended that the coronary arteries be visualized in both the LAO and RAO projections using both cranial and caudal angulation.

Left Coronary Artery

CANNULATION. The Judkins left 4.0 coronary catheter is used most often to engage the LCA (Fig. 18–9). If the Judkins left catheter begins to turn out of profile (so that one or both curves of the catheter are no longer visualized en face), it can be rotated clockwise very slightly and advanced slowly to enter the left sinus of Valsalva, permitting the catheter tip to engage the ostium of the LCA. When the ascending aorta is dilated or the aortic arch is unfolded, advancement of the Judkins left 4.0 coronary catheter may result in the formation of an acute secondary angle of the catheter, pointing the tip of the catheter upward, away from the left coronary ostium. Further advancement of the left Judkins catheter in this position should be avoided because the catheter then prolapses upon itself and becomes folded in the ascending aortic arch. In the event this occurs, a guidewire can be temporarily reinserted into the catheter to straighten the secondary bend and permit the catheter to be advanced to the left sinus of Valsalva. If the ascending aorta is significantly dilated, the Judkins left 4.0 catheter should be exchanged for a larger size (e.g., Judkins left 5.0 or 6.0). If the tip of the Judkins left catheter advances beyond the ostium of the LCA without engagement, the primary bend of the catheter can be reshaped within the patient's body by further careful advancement and prompt withdrawal of the catheter, allowing the tip to "pop into" the ostium of the LCA. This maneuver, along with gentle clockwise or counterclockwise rotation, frequently permits selective engagement of the LCA when the initial attempt has failed. If the catheter tip is located below the origin of the LCA, as in the case of a smaller aortic root, a shorter Judkins 3.5 catheter can be used to allow coaxial engagement of the LCA.

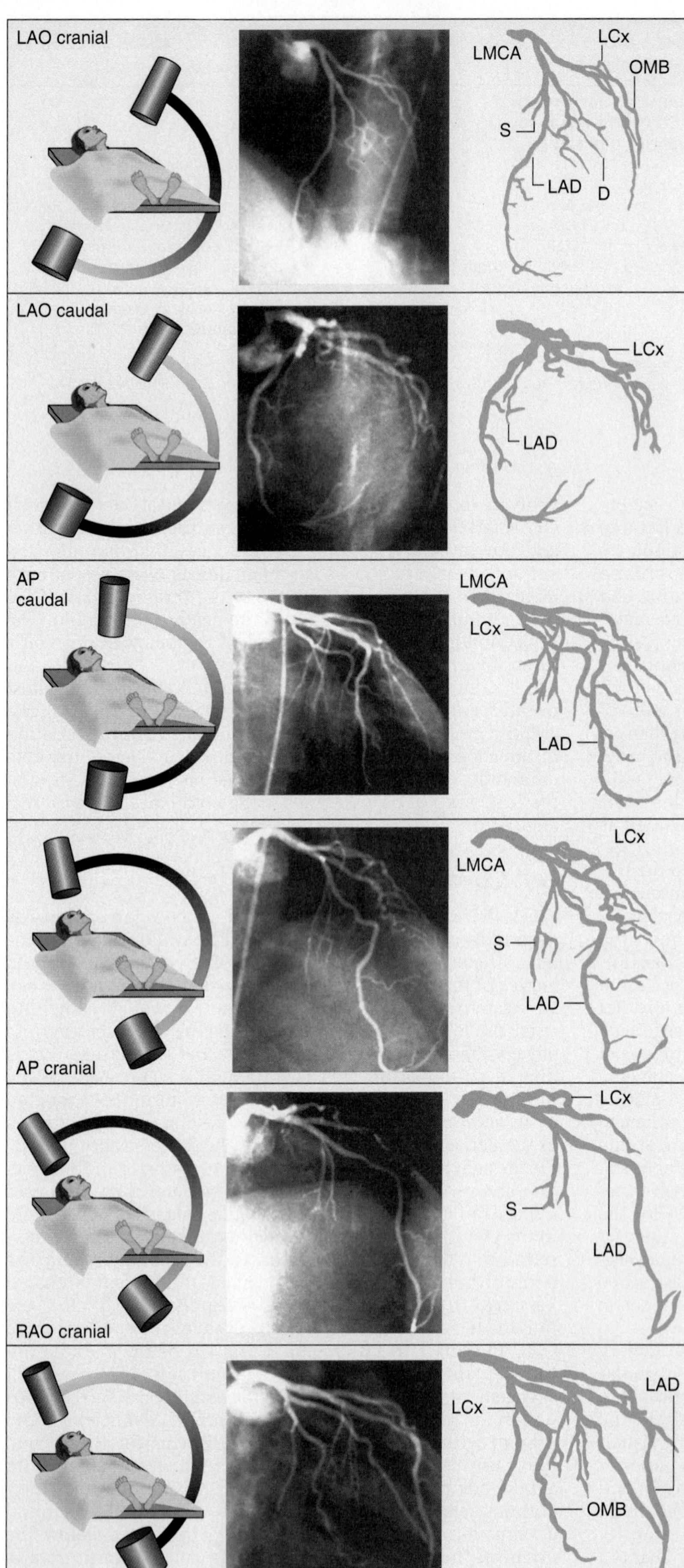

FIGURE 18–7 Angiographic views of the left coronary artery. The approximate positions of the x-ray tube and image intensifier are shown for each of the commonly used angiographic views. The 60-degree left anterior oblique view with 20 degrees of cranial angulation (LAO cranial) shows the ostium and distal portion of the left main coronary artery (LMCA), the middle and distal portions of the left anterior descending artery (LAD), septal perforators (S), diagonal branches (D), and the proximal left circumflex (LCx) and superior obtuse marginal branch (OMB). The 60-degree left anterior oblique view with 25 degrees of caudal angulation (LAO caudal) shows the proximal LMCA and the proximal segments of the LAD and LCx. The anteroposterior projection with 20 degrees of caudal angulation (AP caudal) shows the distal LMCA and proximal segments of the LAD and LCx. The anteroposterior projection with 20 degrees of cranial angulation (AP cranial) also shows the midportion of the LAD and its septal (S) branches. The 30-degree right anterior oblique projection with 20 degrees of cranial angulation (RAO cranial) shows the course of the LAD and its septal (S) and diagonal branches. The 30-degree right anterior oblique projection with 25 degrees of caudal angulation (RAO caudal) shows the LCx and obtuse marginal branches (OMB).

Use of the Amplatz left catheters to cannulate the LCA requires more catheter manipulation than with the standard Judkins left catheter. In this circumstance, the broad secondary curve of the Amplatz left 1 or 2 catheter is positioned so that it rests on the right aortic cusp with its tip pointing toward the left aortic cusp. Alternating advancement and retraction of the catheter with slight clockwise rotation allows the catheter tip to advance slowly and superiorly along the left sinus of Valsalva to enter the left coronary ostium. When the tip enters the ostium, the position of the catheter can usually be stabilized with slight retraction of the catheter. After the left coronary ostium has been cannulated, the pressure at the tip of the catheter should be checked immediately to ensure that there is no damping or "ventricularization" of the pressure contour. If a damped or ventricularized pressure tracing is obtained, the catheter should be removed immediately from the LCA and an attempt at repositioning should be made. If abnormal pressure recording persists, the catheter should be withdrawn from the coronary artery and a nonselective injection of contrast medium into the LCA should be performed in the anteroposterior (AP) view to evaluate the LMCA. If the pressure measured at the catheter tip is normal and a test injection of contrast agent suggests the absence of LMCA disease, left coronary arteriography is then performed using standard techniques. To remove the Amplatz left catheter from the coronary artery, the catheter should be advanced forward in the body to disengage the catheter tip superiorly from the coronary ostium. Simply withdrawing the Amplatz left catheter results in deep seating of the catheter tip within the coronary artery, potentially resulting in catheter-induced arterial dissection.

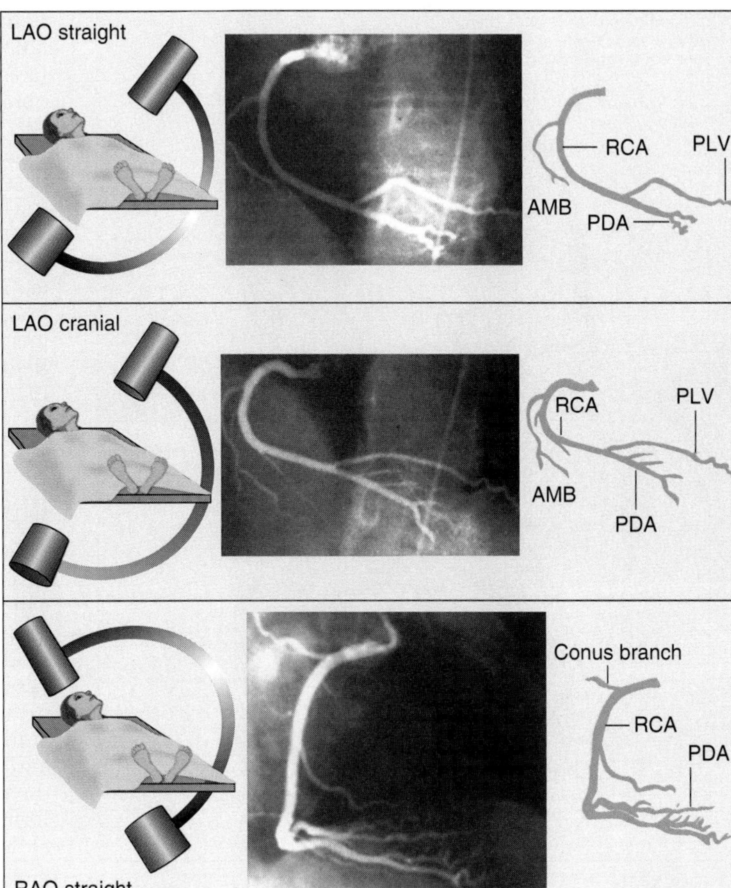

FIGURE 18–8 Angiographic views of the right coronary artery. The approximate positions of the x-ray tube and image intensifier are shown for each of the commonly used angiographic views. The 60-degree left anterior oblique view (LAO straight) shows the proximal and midportions of the right coronary artery (RCA) as well as the acute marginal branches (AMB) and termination of the RCA in the posterior left ventricular branches (PLV). The 60-degree left anterior oblique view with 25 degrees of cranial angulation (LAO cranial) shows the midportion of the RCA and the origin and course of the posterior descending artery (PDA). The 30-degree right anterior oblique view (RAO) shows the midportion of the RCA, the conus branch, and the course of the PDA.

LEFT MAIN CORONARY ARTERY. The LMCA arises from the superior portion of the left aortic sinus, just below the sinotubular ridge of the aorta, which defines the border separating the left sinus of Valsalva from the smooth (tubular) portion of the aorta. The LMCA ranges from 3 to 6 mm in diameter and may be up to 10 to 15 mm in length. The LMCA courses behind the right ventricular outflow tract and usually bifurcates into the LAD artery and LCx branches. Rarely, the LMCA is absent, and there are separate ostia of the LAD and LCx arteries. The LMCA is best visualized in the AP projection with slight (0 to 20 degrees) caudal angulation, but it should be viewed in several projections with the vessel off the spine to exclude LMCA stenosis (Figs. 18–10 to 18–12).

LEFT ANTERIOR DESCENDING ARTERY. The LAD courses along the epicardial surface of the anterior interventricular groove toward the cardiac apex. In the RAO projection, it extends along the anterior aspect of the heart; in the LAO projection, it passes down the cardiac midline, between the right and left ventricles (see Fig. 18–7).

The major branches of the LAD are the septal and diagonal branches. The septal branches arise from the LAD at approximately 90-degree angles and pass into the interventricular septum, varying in size, number, and distribution. In some cases there is a large first septal branch that is vertically oriented and divides into a number of secondary "pitch forking" branches that ramify throughout the septum. In other cases, a more horizontally oriented, large first septal branch is present that passes parallel to the LAD itself within the myocardium. In still other cases, a number of septal arteries are roughly comparable in size. These septal branches interconnect with similar septal branches passing upward from the posterior descending branch of the RCA to produce a network of potential collateral channels. The interventricular septum is the most densely vascularized area of the heart.

The diagonal branches of the LAD pass over the anterolateral aspect of the heart. Although virtually all patients have a single LAD in the anterior interventricular groove, there is wide variability in the number and size of diagonal branches. Most patients (90 percent) have one to three diagonal branches, and acquired atherosclerotic occlusion of the diagonal branches should be suspected if no diagonal branches are seen, particularly if there are unexplained contraction abnormalities of the anterolateral left ventricle. Visualization of the origin of the diagonal branches often requires very steep (50 to 60 degrees) LAO and angulated cranial (20 to 40 degrees) skews.

In some patients, the LMCA trifurcates into the LAD, LCx, and ramus intermedius. When present, the ramus intermedius arises between the LAD and LCx arteries. This vessel is analogous to either a diagonal branch or an obtuse marginal branch, depending on its anterior or posterior course along the lateral aspect of the left ventricle. In most patients (80 percent), the LAD courses around the left ventricular apex and terminates along the diaphragmatic aspect of the left ventricle. In the remaining patients, the LAD fails to reach the diaphragmatic surface, terminating instead either at or before the cardiac apex. In this circumstance, the posterior descending branch (PDA) of the RCA or LCx is larger and longer than usual and supplies the apical portion of the ventricle.

The best angiographic projections for viewing the course of the LAD are the cranially angulated LAO, AP, and RAO views. The LAO cranial view displays the midportion of the LAD and separates the diagonal and septal branches. The RAO cranial view displays the proximal, middle, and distal segment of the LAD and allows separation of the diagonal branches superiorly and the septal branches inferiorly. The AP view requiring cranial (20 to 40 degrees) skew often projects the midportion of the LAD,

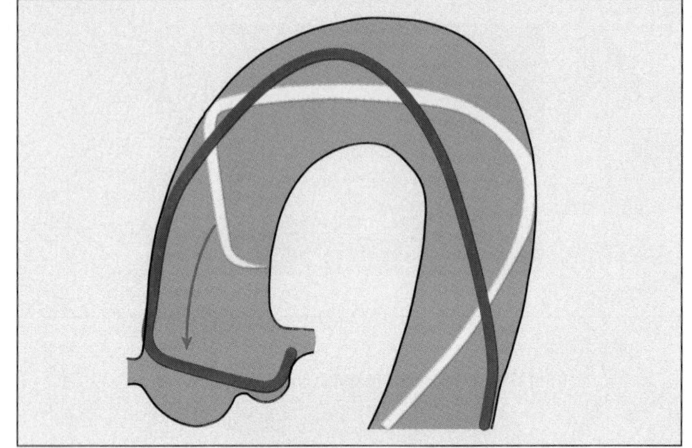

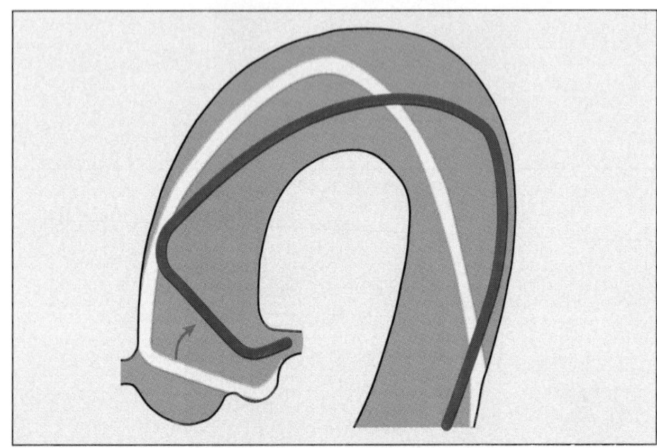

FIGURE 18–9 Push-pull technique for catheterizing the left coronary artery with the Judkins left catheter. In the left anterior oblique view, the coronary catheter is positioned in the ascending aorta over a guidewire and the guidewire is removed. The catheter is advanced so that the tip enters the left sinus of Valsalva. If the catheter does not selectively engage the ostium of the left coronary artery, further slow advancement into the left sinus of Valsalva imparts a temporary acute angle at the catheter. Prompt withdrawal of the catheter allows easy entry into the left coronary artery.

separating the vessel from its diagonal and septal branches. The LAO caudal view also displays the origin of the LAD in a horizontally oriented heart, and the AP caudal or shallow RAO caudal view visualizes the proximal LAD as it arises from the LMCA. The RAO caudal projection is also useful for visualizing the distal LAD and its apical termination.

In some patients with no LMCA but separate ostia for the LAD and LCx, the LAD generally has a more anterior origin than the LCx. The LAD can be engaged with the left Judkins catheter in this setting with paradoxical counterclockwise rotation, which rotates the secondary bend of the catheter to a posterior position in the aorta and turns the primary bend and tip of the catheter to an anterior position. The opposite maneuver may be used to engage the LCx selectively in the setting of separate LAD and LCx ostia. A Judkins catheter, such as a Judkins left 5.0 with a larger curve, selectively engages the downward coursing LCx, and a catheter with shorter curve, such as a Judkins left 3.5, tends to engage selectively the more anterior and superior LAD.

LEFT CIRCUMFLEX ARTERY. The LCx artery originates from the LMCA and courses within the posterior (left) atrioventricular groove toward the inferior interventricular groove (see Fig. 18–7). The LCx artery is the dominant vessel in 15 percent of patients, supplying the left PDA from the distal continuation of the LCx. In the remaining vessels, the distal LCx varies in size and length, depending on the number of posterolateral branches supplied by the distal RCA. The LCx usually gives off one to three large obtuse marginal branches as it passes down the atrioventricular groove. These are the principal branches of the LCx because they supply the lateral free wall of the left ventricle. Beyond the origins of the obtuse marginal branches, the distal LCx tends to be small. The actual position of the LCx can be determined on the late phase of a left coronary injection when the coronary sinus becomes opacified with diluted contrast material.

The RAO caudal and LAO caudal projections are best for visualizing the proximal and middle LCx and obtuse marginal branches. The AP (or 5- to 15-degree RAO) caudal projections also show the origins of the obtuse marginal branches. More severe rightward angulation often superimposes the origins of the obtuse marginal branches on the LCx. If the LCA is dominant, the optimal projection for the left PDA is the LAO cranial view. The LCx also gives rise to one or two left atrial circumflex branches. These branches supply the lateral and posterior aspects of the left atrium.

Right Coronary Artery

Cannulation of the origin of the RCA is also performed in the LAO position but requires different maneuvers than cannulation of the LCA. Whereas the left Judkins catheter naturally seeks the ostium of the LCA, the right Judkins or modified Amplatz catheters must be rotated to engage the vessel. This is usually accomplished by first passing the catheter to a point just superior to the aortic valve in the left sinus of Valsalva with the tip of the catheter facing rightward and then rotating the catheter clockwise while withdrawing the catheter slightly, which forces the tip to move anteriorly from the left sinus of Valsalva to the right sinus of Valsalva along the sinotubular ridge (Fig. 18–13). Sudden rightward and downward movement of the catheter tip signifies the entry into the right coronary ostium. If the ostium of the RCA is not easily located, the most common reason is that the ostium has a more superior and anterior origin than anticipated. Repeated attempts to engage the RCA should be made at a level slightly more distal to the aortic valve. Nonselective contrast agent injections in the right sinus of Valsalva may reveal the site of the origin of the RCA. Positioning a left Amplatz catheter in the ostium of the RCA requires a technique similar to that used with the right Judkins catheter. If a gentle attempt to withdraw the Amplatz catheter results in paradoxical deep entry into the coronary artery, removal of the catheter can be achieved by clockwise or counterclockwise rotation and advancement to prolapse the catheter into the aortic sinus.

An abnormal pressure tracing showing damping or ventricularization may suggest the presence of an ostial stenosis or spasm, selective engagement of the conus branch, or deep intubation of the RCA. If an abnormal pressure tracing has been encountered, the catheter tip should be gently rotated counterclockwise and withdrawn slightly in an effort to free the tip of the catheter. If persistent damping occurs, a very small amount of contrast medium (<1 ml) can be injected carefully and the catheter immediately withdrawn in a "shoot-and-run" maneuver, which may allow the cause of damping to be identified. The frequency of ventricular fibrillation and iatrogenic coronary dissection are higher when the RCA is injected in the presence of a damped pressure tracing. If the pressure tracing is normal on entry into the RCA, the vessel should be imaged in at least two projections. The initial injection should be gentle because of the possibility that forceful injection through a catheter whose tip is immediately adjacent to the vessel wall may also lead to dissection. Coronary spasm of the RCA ostium may also occur as a result of catheter intubation. When an ostial stenosis of the RCA is seen, intracoronary nitroglycerin or calcium channel antagonists may be useful in excluding catheter-induced spasm as a cause of the coronary artery narrowing.

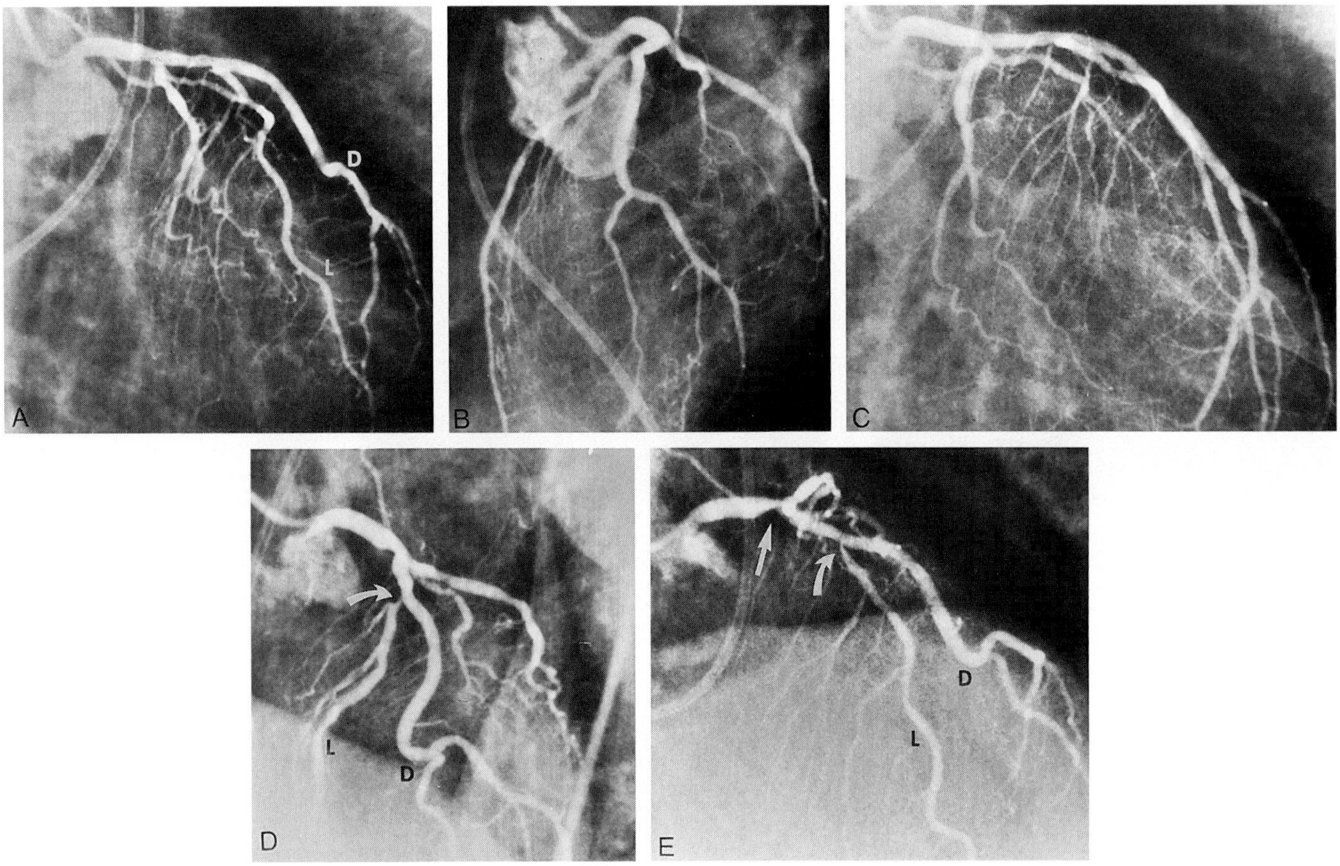

FIGURE 18–10 Missed left main coronary artery (LMCA) stenosis. **A** to **C,** Left coronary arteriography in the standard right anterior oblique, left anterior oblique, and right anterior oblique caudal views fails to demonstrate significant stenoses of the LMCA or left anterior descending (LAD) artery. **D,** Left anterior oblique cranial view shows severe stenosis (curved arrow) for the LAD (L) immediately beyond the origin of the diagonal branch. **E,** Right anterior oblique cranial view shows the LAD stenosis (curved arrow) but also shows a severe stenosis of the LMCA (straight arrow) at its bifurcation.

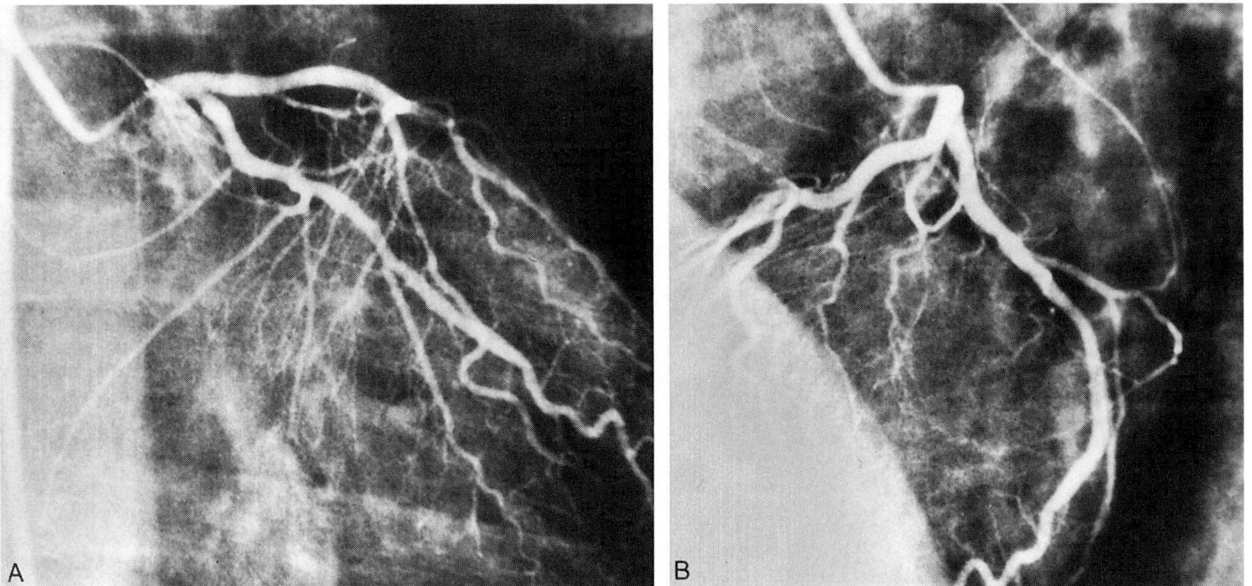

FIGURE 18–11 Difficulty in detecting ostial left main coronary artery (LMCA) stenosis. **A,** Shallow right anterior oblique view of the left anterior descending artery with the catheter not well seated in the vessel results in poor visualization of the ostial stenosis of the LMCA. **B,** Left anterior oblique cranial view shows the catheter tip selectively positioned in the LMCA without reflux of contrast medium around the tip.

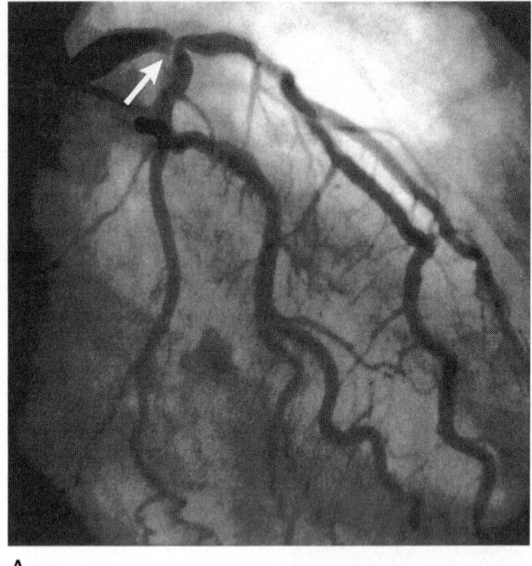

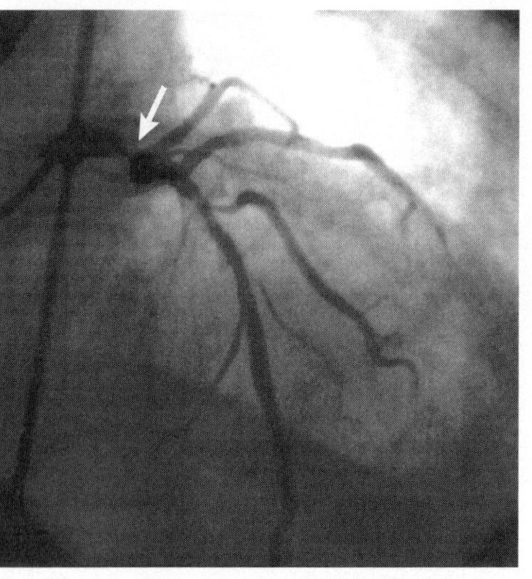

A B

FIGURE 18–12 Severe stenosis of the distal left main coronary artery. **A,** Right anterior oblique projection with caudal angulation demonstrates a severe ulcerated stenosis in the distal portion of the left main coronary artery (arrow). **B,** An anteroposterior view with cranial angulation demonstrates this stenosis in a second view. Limited coronary arteriography should be performed when severe left main stenosis (arrow) has been demonstrated.

The RCA originates from the right anterior aortic sinus somewhat inferior to the origin of the LCA (see Fig. 18–8). It passes along the right atrioventricular groove toward the crux (a point on the diaphragmatic surface of the heart where the anterior atrioventricular, the posterior atrioventricular groove, and the inferior interventricular groove coalesce. The first branch of the RCA is generally the conus artery, which arises at the right coronary ostium or within the first few millimeters of the RCA in about 50 percent of patients. In the remaining patients, the conus artery arises from a separate ostium in the right aortic sinus just above the right coronary ostium. The second branch of the RCA is usually the sinoatrial node artery. It has been found that this vessel arises from the RCA in just under 60 percent of patients, from the LCx in just under 40 percent, and from both arteries with a dual blood supply in the remaining cases. The midportion of the RCA usually gives rise to one or several medium-sized acute marginal branches. These branches supply the anterior wall of the right ventricle and may provide collateral circulation in patients with LAD occlusion. The RCA terminates in a PDA and one or more right posterolateral branches.

Because the RCA traverses both the atrioventricular and the interventricular grooves, multiple angiographic projections are needed to visualize each segment of the RCA. The ostium of the RCA is best evaluated in the LAO views, with or without cranial or caudal angulation. The left lateral is also useful for visualizing the ostium of the RCA in difficult cases. The ostium is identified by the reflux of contrast material from the RCA that also delineates the aortic root with swirling of contrast in the region of the ostium. The proximal RCA is generally evaluated in the LAO cranial or LAO caudal projections but is markedly foreshortened in the RAO projections. The midportion of the RCA is best seen in the LAO cranial, RAO, and left lateral projections. The origin of the PDA and the posterolateral branches are best evaluated in the LAO cranial or AP cranial views, whereas the midportion of the PDA can be shown in the AP cranial or RAO projection.

RIGHT CORONARY ARTERY DOMINANCE. The RCA is dominant in 85 percent of patients, supplying the PDA and at least one posterolateral branch (right dominant) (Figs. 18–14 to 18–16). The PDA courses in the inferior interventricular groove and gives rise to a number of small inferior septal branches, which pass upward to supply the lower portion of the interventricular septum and interdigitate with superior septal branches passing down from the LAD. After giving rise to the PDA, the dominant RCA continues beyond the crux cordis (the junction of the atrioventricular and interventricular grooves) as the right posterior atrioventricular branch along the distal portion of the posterior (left) atrioventricular groove, terminating in one or several posterolateral branches that supply the diaphragmatic surface of the left ventricle. The RCA is nondominant in 15 percent of patients. One-half of these patients have a left PDA and left posterolateral branches that are provided by the distal LCx artery (left dominant circulation). In these cases, the RCA is very small, terminates before reaching the crux, and does not supply any blood to the left ventricular myocardium. The remaining patients have an RCA that gives rise to the PDA with the LCx artery providing all the posterolateral branches (balanced or codominant circulation). In about 25 percent of patients with RCA dominance, there are significant anatomical variations in the origin of the PDA. These variations include partial supply of the PDA territory by acute marginal branches, double PDA, and early origin of the PDA proximal to the crux. At or near the crux, the dominant artery gives rise to a small atrioventricular node artery, which passes upward to supply the atrioventricular node.

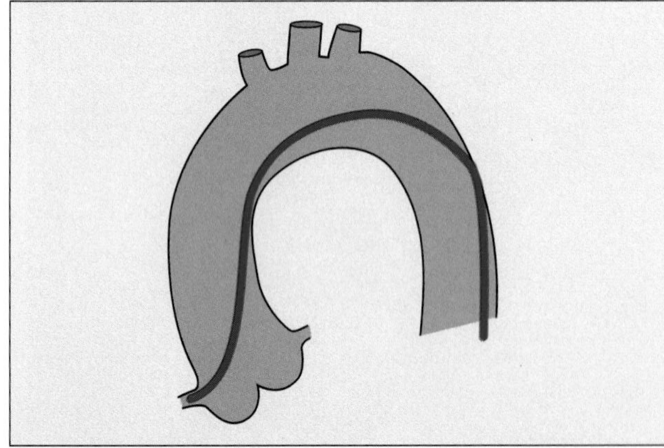

FIGURE 18–13 Cannulation of the right coronary artery using the right Judkins catheter. **A,** The catheter is advanced to a point just superior to the aortic valve in the left sinus of Valsalva with the tip of the catheter facing rightward, and then the catheter is rotated clockwise while withdrawing the catheter slightly. **B,** Sudden rightward and downward movement of the catheter tip signifies the entry into the right coronary ostium.

CORONARY BYPASS GRAFTS. Selective cannulation of bypass grafts may be more challenging than cannulation of

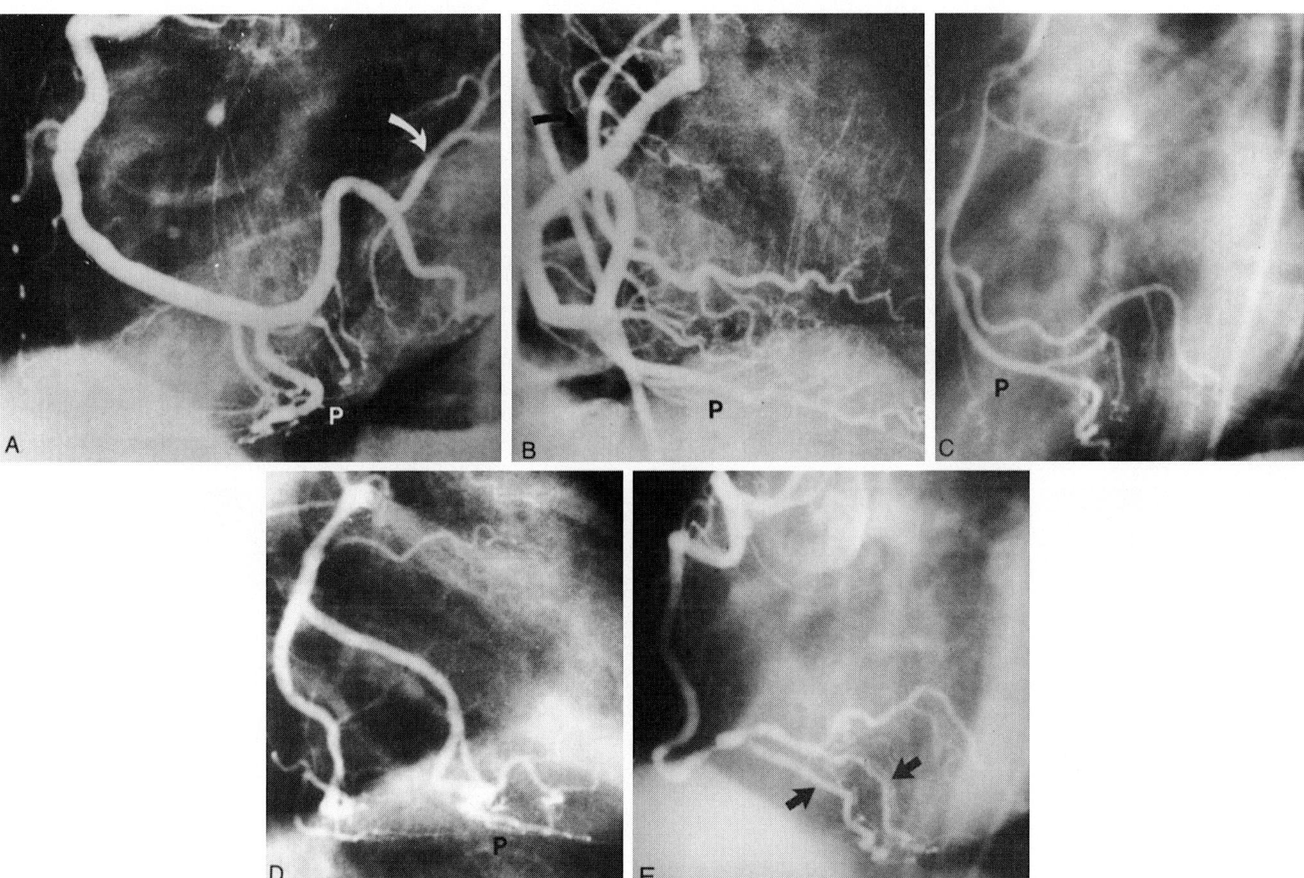

FIGURE 18–14 Strongly dominant right coronary artery (RCA). **A** and **B,** Left anterior oblique and right anterior oblique views of the RCA show that the distal segment (arrows) extends to the left atrioventricular groove. After giving rise to the posterior descending artery, the RCA gives rise to multiple posterior left ventricular branches. **C,** A variation in the origin of the posterior descending artery, which originates early from the RCA, runs parallel to it, and enters the posterior interventricular groove. **D,** Right anterior oblique right coronary arteriogram showing the posterior descending artery (P) arising from a right ventricular branch of the RCA. **E,** Left anterior oblique right coronary arteriogram showing duplicated posterior descending arteries (arrows). (From Levin DC, Baltaxe HA: Angiographic demonstration of important anatomic variations of the posterior descending artery. AJR 116:41, 1972.)

the native coronary arteries because the locations of graft ostia are more variable, even when surgical clips or ostia markers are used. Knowledge of the number, course, and type of bypass grafts obtained from the operative report is invaluable for the identification of the location of the bypass grafts during arteriography.

SAPHENOUS VEIN GRAFTS. SVGs from the aorta to the distal RCA or PDA originate from the right anterolateral aspect of the aorta approximately 5 cm superior to the sinotubular ridge. SVGs to the LAD originate from the anterior portion of the aorta about 7 cm superior to the sinotubular ridge. SVGs to the obtuse marginal branches arise from the left anterolateral aspect of the aorta 9 to 10 cm superior to the sinotubular ridge. In most patients, all SVGs can be engaged with a single catheter, such as a Judkins right 4.0 or a modified Amplatz right 1 or 2. Other catheters useful for engaging SVGs include the right and left bypass graft catheters. Amplatz left 1 to 2 catheters are useful for superiorly oriented SVGs (see Fig. 18–4). A multipurpose catheter may also be useful for the cannulation of the downward takeoff SVG to the RCA or PDA.

Viewed in the LAO projection, the Judkins right 4 or Amplatz right 2 catheters rotate anteriorly from the leftward position as the catheter is rotated in a clockwise direction. The relation between the movement of catheter shaft at the femoral artery and the response of catheter tip on fluoroscopy immediately indicates whether the catheter tip is anteriorly positioned in the aorta and likely to enter an SVG ostium or posteriorly positioned and unlikely to engage an SVG. Steady advancement and withdrawal of the catheter tip proximal and distal in the ascending aorta, 5 to 10 cm above the sinotubular ridge, with varying degrees of rotation, usually result in entry into the SVG. Entry into the SVG is associated with abrupt outward motion of the tip of the catheter. When this occurs, a small test injection of contrast material verifies that the catheter is in the SVG. A well-circumscribed "stump" is almost always present if the SVG is occluded. Each SVG or stump must be viewed in nearly orthogonal views. The relation between the origin of the SVGs and surgical clips confirms whether all targeted SVGs have been visualized. If neither a patent SVG nor a stump can be located, it may be necessary to perform an ascending aortogram (preferably in biplane) in an attempt to visualize all SVGs and their course to the coronary arteries.

The goal of SVG angiography is to assess the ostium of the SVG, its entire course, and the distal insertion ("touchdown") site at the anastomosis between the bypass SVG and the native coronary vessel. The ostium of a SVG must be evaluated by achieving a coaxial engagement of the catheter tip and the origin of the SVG. The midportion (body) of the SVG must be evaluated with complete contrast filling of the SVG because inadequate opacification produces an angiographic artifact suggestive of friable filling defects. It is critical to assess the SVG insertion or anastomotic site in full profile without any overlap of the distal SVG or the native vessel. Angiographic assessment of the native vessels beyond SVG

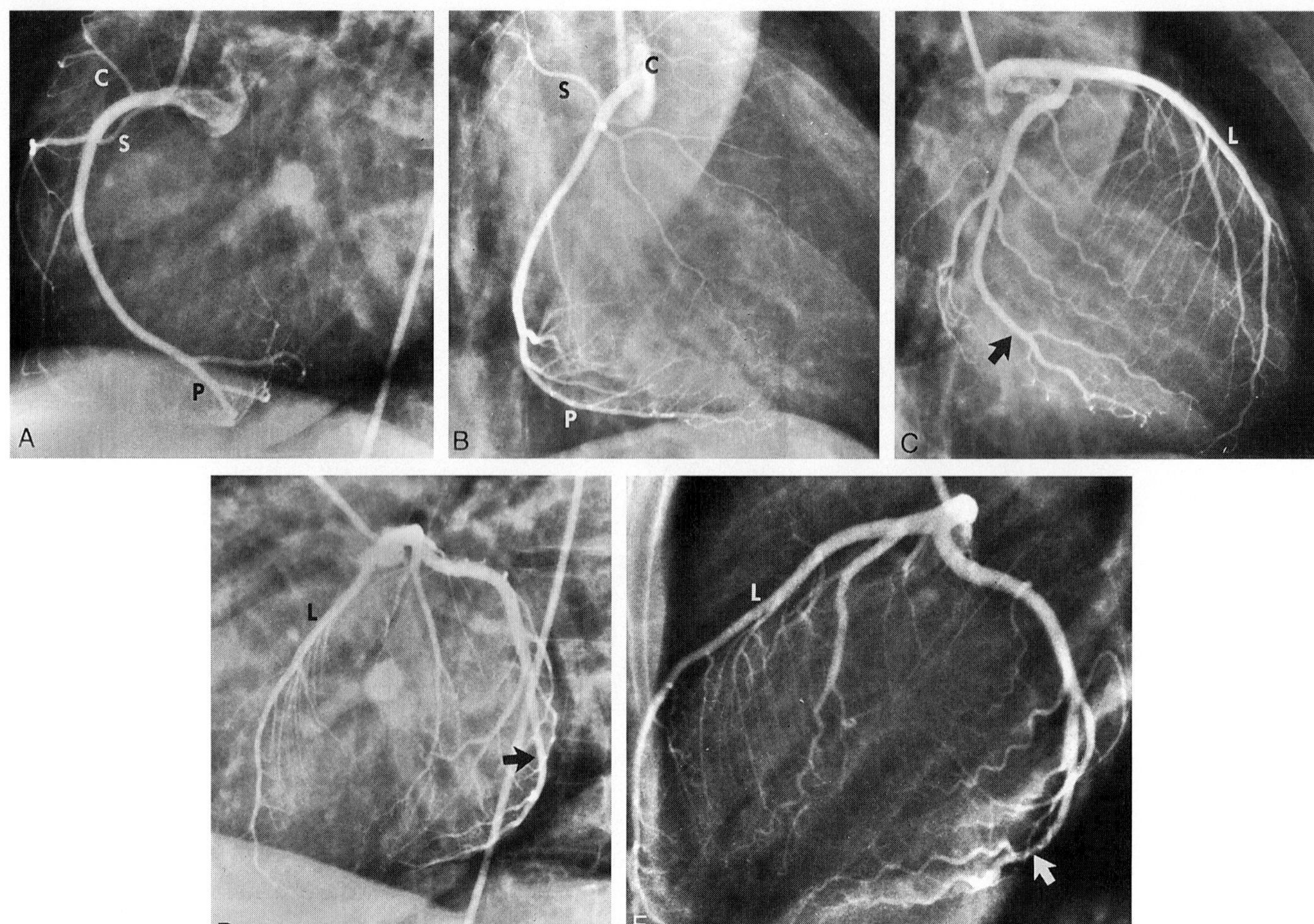

FIGURE 18–15 Weakly dominant right coronary artery (RCA). **A** and **B,** Left anterior oblique and right anterior oblique views of the RCA. Both the conus and sinoatrial node artery arise from the RCA. The distal portion of the RCA beyond the origin of the posterior descending artery is short and gives rise to a single small posterior left ventricular branch. **C** to **E,** Left coronary artery in the right anterior oblique, left anterior oblique, and left lateral projections. Note that the circumflex artery gives rise to four obtuse marginal branches, the most distal of which (arrow) supplies some of the diaphragmatic surface of the left ventricle. The left anterior descending artery gives rise to two small and one medium-sized diagonal branches. C = conus branch; L = left anterior descending artery; P = posterior descending artery; S = sinoatrial nodal artery.

anastomotic sites requires views that are conventionally used for the native segments themselves.

INTERNAL MAMMARY ARTERY. The left IMA arises inferiorly from the left subclavian artery approximately 10 cm from its origin. Catheterization of the left IMA is performed with a specially designed J-tip IMA catheter (see Fig. 18–3, bottom row). The catheter is advanced into the aortic arch distal to the origin of the left subclavian artery in the LAO projection and then rotated counterclockwise and is gently withdrawn with the tip pointing in a cranial direction, allowing entry into the left subclavian artery (Fig. 18–17). A 0.035 J or angled Terumo guidewire is advanced to the left subclavian artery under fluoroscopy, and the catheter is advanced into the subclavian artery. The RAO or AP projections then can be used to cannulate the IMA selectively by withdrawing and slightly rotating the catheter anteriorly (counterclockwise) with tip down. The right IMA can also be cannulated with the IMA catheter. The innominate artery is entered in the LAO projection, and the guidewire is advanced cautiously to avoid entry into the right common carotid artery. When the guidewire is positioned in the distal right subclavian artery, the IMA catheter is advanced to a point distal to the expected origin of the right IMA. The catheter is withdrawn in the LAO view and rotated to cannulate the right IMA.

The IMA itself is rarely affected by atherosclerosis. Angiographic studies of the IMAs should assess not only the patency of the graft itself but also the distal anastomosis, where most IMA graft compromise occurs. Although the LAO cranial view may be limited in its ability to demonstrate the anastomosis of the IMA and the LAD because of vessel overlap, the left lateral or AP cranial projection usually provides adequate visualization of the LIMA-LAD anastomotic site. The risk of catheter-induced dissection of the origin of the IMA can be reduced by careful manipulation of the catheter tip and avoidance of forceful advancement without the protection of the guidewire. If the IMA cannot be selectively engaged because of tortuosity of the subclavian artery, nonselective arteriography can be enhanced by placing a blood pressure cuff on the ipsilateral arm and inflating it to a pressure above systolic arterial pressure. Alternatively, the ipsilateral brachial or radial artery may be used to facilitate coaxial IMA engagement. IMA spasm can be treated with 50 to 200 μg of intraarterial nitroglycerin or 50 to 100 μg of intraarterial verapamil. The patient may feel chest warmth or discomfort with contrast injection due to injection into small IMA branches supplying the chest wall.

GASTROEPIPLOIC ARTERY. The right gastroepiploic artery (GEA) is the largest terminal artery of the gastroduodenal artery and was briefly used as an alternative in situ

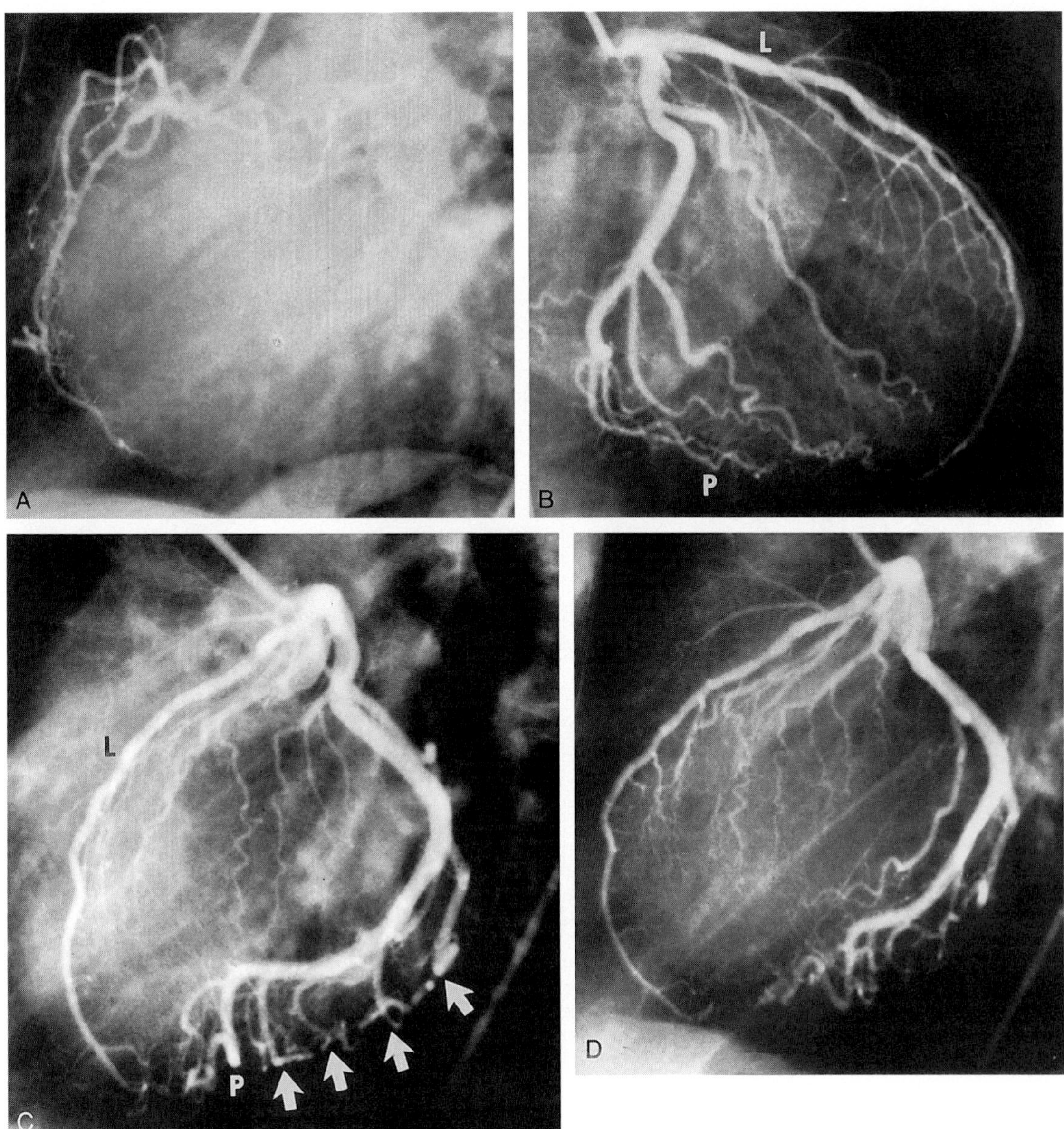

FIGURE 18–16 Dominant left coronary system. **A,** The left anterior oblique projection shows that the right coronary artery is small and terminates before reaching the crux. **B** to **D,** The right anterior oblique, left anterior oblique, and left lateral projections show that the left circumflex artery is large and gives rise to the posterior descending artery (PDA) at the crux of the heart and to several posterior descending arteries. L = left anterior descending coronary artery; P = posterior descending artery.

arterial conduit to the PDA in patients undergoing CABG. The gastroduodenal artery arises from the common hepatic artery in 75 percent of cases, but it may also arise from the right or left hepatic artery or the celiac trunk. Catheterization of the right GEA is carried out by first entering the common hepatic artery with a cobra catheter (Fig. 18–18). A torquable, hydrophilic-coated guidewire is advanced to the gastroduodenal artery and then to the right GEA. The cobra catheter is then exchanged for a multipurpose or Judkins right coronary catheter, which then permits selective arteriography of the right GEA.

STANDARDIZED PROJECTION ACQUISITION. Although general recommendations can be made for sequences of angiographic image acquisition that are applicable to most patients, tailored views may be needed to accommodate individual variations in anatomy. As a general rule, each coronary artery should be visualized with a number of different projections that minimize vessel foreshortening and overlap (Figs. 18–19 to 18–21). An AP view with shallow caudal angulation is often performed first to evaluate the possibility of LMCA disease. Other important views include (1) the LAO cranial view used to evaluate the middle and distal LAD, which should have sufficient leftward positioning of the image intensifier to allow separation of the LAD, diagonal, and septal branches; (2) the LAO caudal view to evaluate the LMCA, origin of the LAD, and proximal segment of the LCx; (3) the RAO caudal view to assess the LCx and marginal branches; and (4) a shallow RAO or AP cranial view to evaluate the midportion and distal portion of the LAD. The RCA should be visualized in at least two views, including an LAO cranial view that demonstrates the RCA and origin of the PDA and posterolateral branches and an RAO view that demonstrates the mid-RCA and proximal, middle, and distal termination of the PDA. An AP cranial projection may also be useful for the demonstration of the distal termination of the RCA, and a left lateral view is useful to visual the ostium of the RCA and midportion of the RCA with separation of the RCA and its right ventricular branches.

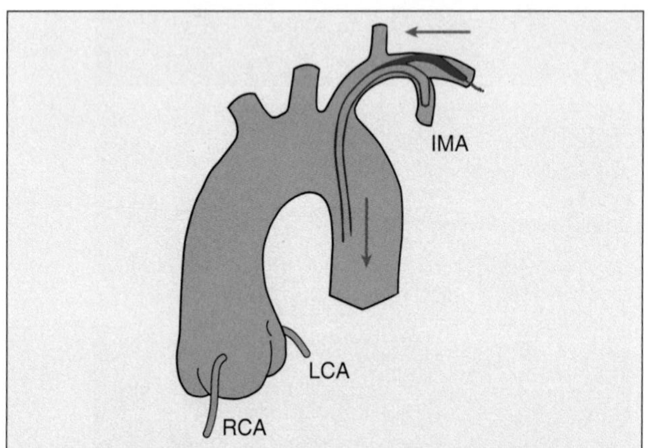

FIGURE 18–17 Catheterization of the left internal mammary artery (IMA). The internal mammary catheter is positioned in the aortic arch and visualized in the left anterior oblique position. The catheter tip is rotated so that it engages the origin of the left subclavian artery immediately subjacent to the head of the clavicle **(A)**. This is followed by gentle advancement of the guidewire into the left subclavian artery to a point distal to the origin of the left internal mammary artery. After the guidewire is removed, the left subclavian artery is visualized in the right anterior oblique projection, the catheter is withdrawn, and the catheter tip engages the ostium of the left internal mammary artery selectively **(B)**. (From Judkins MW: Coronary arteriography. *In* Douglas JS Jr, King SB III [eds]: Coronary Arteriography and Intervention. New York, McGraw-Hill, 1985, p 231.)

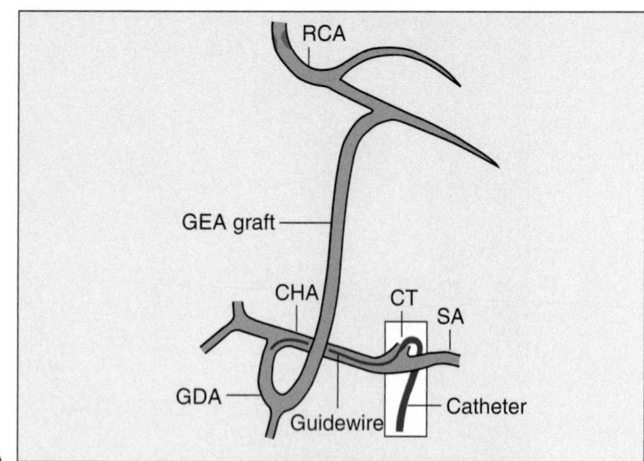

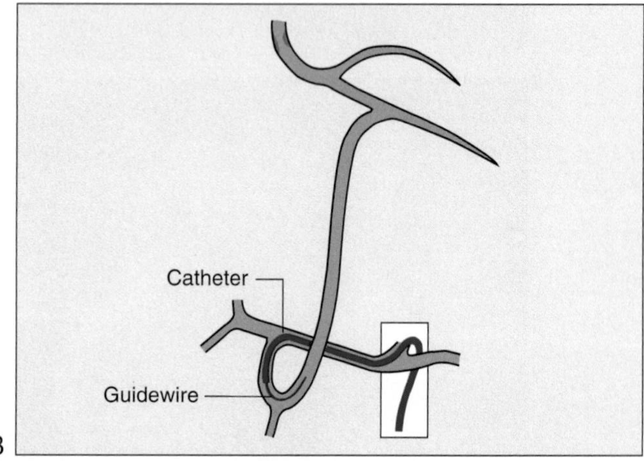

FIGURE 18–18 Catheterization of the right gastroepiploic artery (GEA) graft. The celiac trunk (CT) is selectively engaged with a cobra catheter, and a guidewire is gently advanced to the gastroduodenal artery (GDA) and the GEA. The catheter is advanced over the guidewire for selective arteriography of the GEA graft. CHA = common hepatic artery; RCA = right coronary artery; SA = splenic artery.

Congenital Anomalies of the Coronary Circulation

Anomalous origins of the coronary arteries are present in approximately 0.5 percent of patients undergoing coronary arteriography.[52] The most common anomaly is a separate origin of the LAD and LCx coronary arteries (35.3 percent), followed by an origin of the RCA from the left coronary sinus (20.6 percent) and origin of the LCx from the right coronary sinus (20 percent). A single coronary artery was seen in fewer cases (8.8 percent).[52] Other anomalies occurred much less commonly. Coronary artery anomalies are divided into those that cause and those that do not cause myocardial ischemia.[53,54]

ANOMALIES THAT CAUSE MYOCARDIAL ISCHEMIA

CORONARY ARTERY FISTULAS. Coronary artery fistulas are a common hemodynamically significant abnormality of the coronary arteries.[55] Although half of the patients with a coronary artery fistula remain asymptomatic, the other half develop CHF, infective endocarditis, myocardial ischemia, or rupture of an aneurysm. Fistulas arise from the RCA or its branches in about half of the cases; the remaining fistulas arise from the LAD or LCx arteries or their branches, or they have multiple origins (Fig. 18–22). Drainage occurs into the right ventricle in 41 percent, right atrium in 26 percent, pulmonary artery in 17 percent, left ventricle in 3 percent, and superior vena cava in 1 percent. A left-to-right shunt exists in more than 90 percent. Coronary arteriography is the best method for demonstrating the origin of these fistulas.

ORIGIN OF THE LEFT CORONARY ARTERY FROM THE PULMONARY ARTERY. Most infants with the origin of the LCA from the main pulmonary artery manifest CHF and myocardial ischemia in the first 4 months of life.[56] About 25 percent survive to adolescence or adulthood but develop mitral regurgitation, angina, or CHF. Aortography typically shows a large RCA with absence of a left coronary ostium in the left aortic sinus. During the late phase of the aortogram, patulous LAD and LCx branches fill by means of collateral circulation from RCA branches. Still later in the filming sequence, retrograde flow from the LAD and LCx opacifies the LMCA and its origin from the main pulmonary artery (Fig. 18–23). The clinical course of the patient tends to be more favorable if extensive collateral circulation exists. In rare instances, the RCA rather than the LCA may arise from the pulmonary artery.

CONGENITAL CORONARY STENOSIS OR ATRESIA. Congenital stenosis or atresia of a coronary artery can occur as an isolated lesion or in association with other congenital diseases, such as calcific coronary sclerosis, supravalvular aortic stenosis, homocystinuria, Friedreich ataxia, Hurler syndrome, progeria, and rubella syndrome. In these cases, the atretic vessel usually fills by means of collateral circulation from the contralateral side.[57]

ANOMALOUS ORIGIN OF EITHER CORONARY ARTERY FROM THE CONTRALATERAL SINUS. Origin of the LCA from the proximal RCA or the right aortic sinus with subsequent passage between the aorta and the right ventricular outflow tract has been associated with

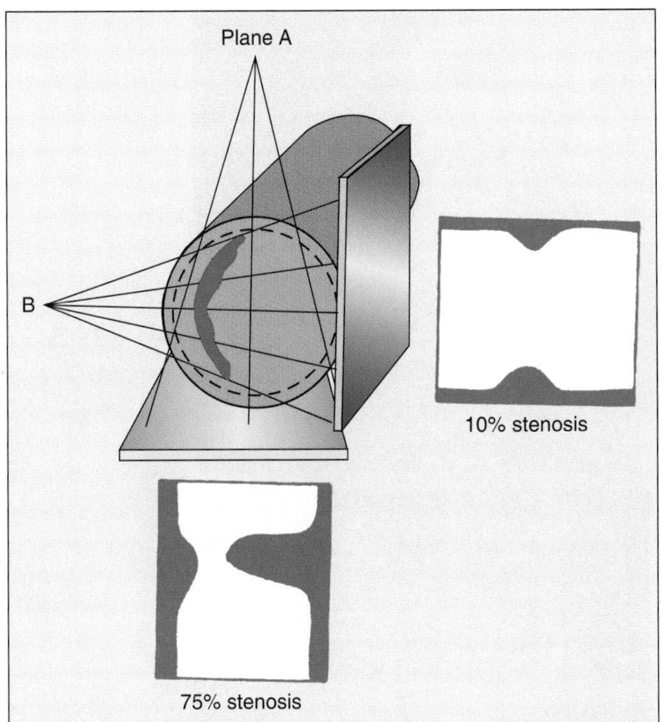

FIGURE 18–19 Importance of orthogonal projections. Each vascular segment of the coronary artery must be recorded in two orthogonal or nearly orthogonal views to avoid missing important diagnostic information about eccentric stenoses. In plane A the image is associated with 75 percent stenosis, but in plane B the image results in 10 percent stenosis.

sudden death during or shortly after exercise in young persons (see Fig. 18-23).[58-60] The increased risk of sudden death may be due to a slit-like ostium with acute takeoff angles of the aberrant coronary arteries or possible compression between the pulmonary trunk and aorta. After its aberrant origin, the LCA takes an abrupt leftward turn and tunnels between the aorta and the right ventricular outflow tract. Sudden death is thought to result from transient occlusion of the anomalous LCA, caused by an increase in blood flow through the aorta and pulmonary artery that occurs during exercise and creates either a kink at the sharp leftward bend or a pinchcock mechanism in the tunnel. Origin of the RCA from the LCA or left aortic sinus with passage between the aorta and the right ventricular outflow tract is somewhat less dangerous (Figs. 18-24 and 18-25).[61-63] This anomaly, however, has also been associated with myocardial ischemia or sudden death, presumably through the same mechanism. In rare cases of anomalous origin of the LCA from the right aortic sinus, myocardial ischemia may occur even if the LCA passes anterior to the right ventricular outflow tract or posterior to the aorta (i.e., not through a tunnel between the two great vessels).

The course of the anomalous coronary arteries is easily assessed by angiography in the RAO view (Fig. 18-26). The four common courses for the anomalous LCA arising from the right sinus of Valsalva include a septal, anterior, interarterial, or posterior course.[64,65] The posterior course of the anomalous LCA arising from the left sinus of Valsalva is similar to the course of the anomalous LCx arising from the right sinus of Valsalva (Fig. 18-27), whereas the common interarterial course of the anomalous RCA from the left sinus of Valsalva is similar to the interarterial course of the anomalous LCA arising from the right sinus of Valsalva.

When either the LCA or the LAD arises anomalously from the right aortic sinus, another angiographic method to identify the course of the anomalous vessel is to pass a catheter into the main pulmonary artery and then perform an arteriogram of the aberrant coronary artery in the steep AP caudal projection. This places the aberrant coronary artery, the rightward and anterior pulmonary valve, and the leftward and posterior aortic valve all in one plane (see Fig. 18-27). From this "laid-back" aortogram, which can be used even in mapping the course of anomalous coronary arteries in transposition of the great vessels, it is usually possible to confirm whether the course of the aberrant coronary artery is between the great vessels. Although angiography is useful for establishing the presence of anomalous coronary arteries, transesophageal echocardiography may also be an important adjunctive diagnostic tool for establishing the course of the vessels.

SINGLE CORONARY ARTERY. Although there are numerous variations of this anomaly, it assumes hemodynamic significance when a major branch passes between the aorta and the right ventricular outflow tract.[66]

ANOMALIES NOT CAUSING MYOCARDIAL ISCHEMIA

In this category of anomalies, the coronary arteries originate from the aorta, but their origins are in unusual locations. Although myocardial perfusion is normal, cannulation of the origin of these vessels may be problematic. These anomalies occur in about 0.5 to 1.0 percent of adult patients undergoing coronary arteriography.

ORIGIN OF THE LEFT CIRCUMFLEX ARTERY FROM THE RIGHT AORTIC SINUS. Anomalous origin of the circumflex artery from the right aortic sinus is the most common of these anomalies (see Fig. 18-27). In a series of nearly 3000 patients, this anomaly was found in 0.67 percent. The anomalous LCx generally arises posterior to the RCA and courses inferiorly and posteriorly to the aorta to enter the left atrioventricular groove. An interarterial course for an anomalous LCx originating from the right sinus of Valsalva is extremely uncommon.

HIGH ANTERIOR ORIGIN OF THE RIGHT CORONARY ARTERY. This anomaly is commonly encountered but of no hemodynamic significance. The inability to engage the ostium of the RCA selectively by conventional catheter manipulation raises the question of this superior origin of the RCA above the sinotubular ridge. Forceful, nonselective injection of contrast medium into the right sinus of Valsalva may reveal the anomalous takeoff of the RCA, which can then be selectively engaged with a Judkins right 5.0 catheter or Amplatz left 1.0 or 2.0 catheter.

Coronary Artery Spasm (see also Chap. 50)

Coronary artery spasm is defined as a dynamic and reversible occlusion of an epicardial coronary artery because of focal constriction of the smooth muscle cells within the arterial wall.[67] It was first described as a clinical syndrome in 1959 by Prinzmetal and colleagues ("Prinzmetal" or "variant" angina), who described an unusual or variant form of angina in which the onset of chest pain was not provoked by the usual factors, such as exercise, emotional upset, cold, or ingestion of a meal. Patients considered to have variant angina are those in whom chest pain commences at rest or both at rest and during exertion, occurs in a cyclical pattern at the same time every day, and is accompanied by ST segment elevation if an ECG is recorded. Coronary artery spasm can be invoked by cigarette smoking, cocaine use, alcohol, intracoronary radiation, and administration of catecholamines during general anesthesia. Although the ST segment elevation is often striking, it rapidly reverts to normal when the pain disappears spontaneously or is terminated by the administration of nitroglycerin. Coronary artery spasm may be accompanied by atrioventricular block, ventricular ectopic activity, ventricular tachycardia, or ventricular fibrillation. MI and death are rare manifestations of coronary artery spasm. Coronary artery spasm can be superimposed on the presence of an intramyocardial bridge.[68]

Coronary arteriography is useful in patients with suspected coronary artery spasm, both to exclude the presence of concomitant CAD and to document an episode of coronary artery spasm using provocative intravenous medications. Angiographic studies have shown that coronary spasm is superimposed on areas of fixed stenosis in about 60 percent of patients, and it occurs in segments of coronary arteries that appear angiographically normal in about 40 percent of patients. MI in the presence of normal epicardial coronary arteries is often attributed to the presence of coronary artery spasm, but other conditions such as cocaine abuse, coronary embolism, hypercoagulable states, coronary trauma, and anemia must first be excluded.

Three provocative tests can be performed to detect the presence of coronary artery spasm. Intravenous ergonovine maleate was introduced in the late 1970s to provoke spasm

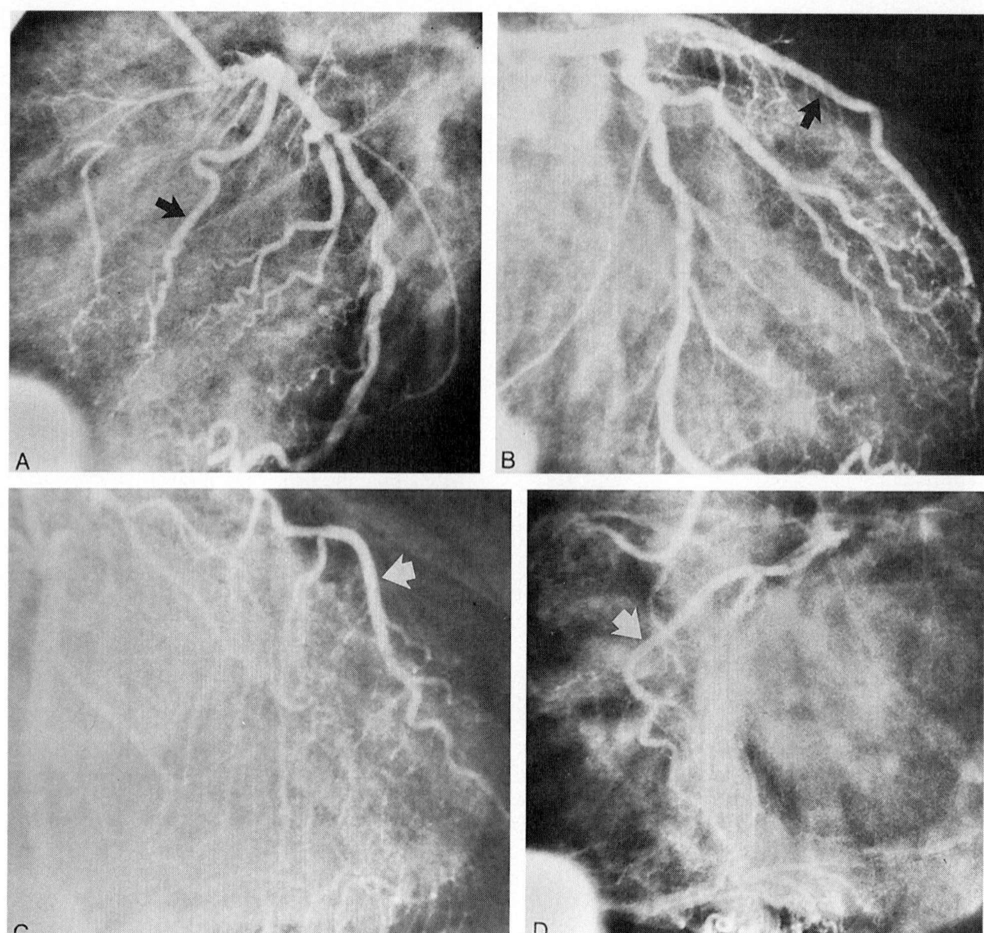

FIGURE 18–20 Superimposition of branches. **A** and **B,** Left anterior oblique and right anterior oblique views of the left coronary arteriogram show that the left anterior descending artery (LAD) is totally occluded, although the point of occlusion is not visualized. There is a large diagonal branch (black arrows) that closely parallels the LAD in both projections and could be mistaken for the LAD. Late-phase frames from a right anterior oblique **(C)** and left anterior oblique **(D)** right coronary arteriogram show filling of the LAD (white arrows) by means of septal collaterals.

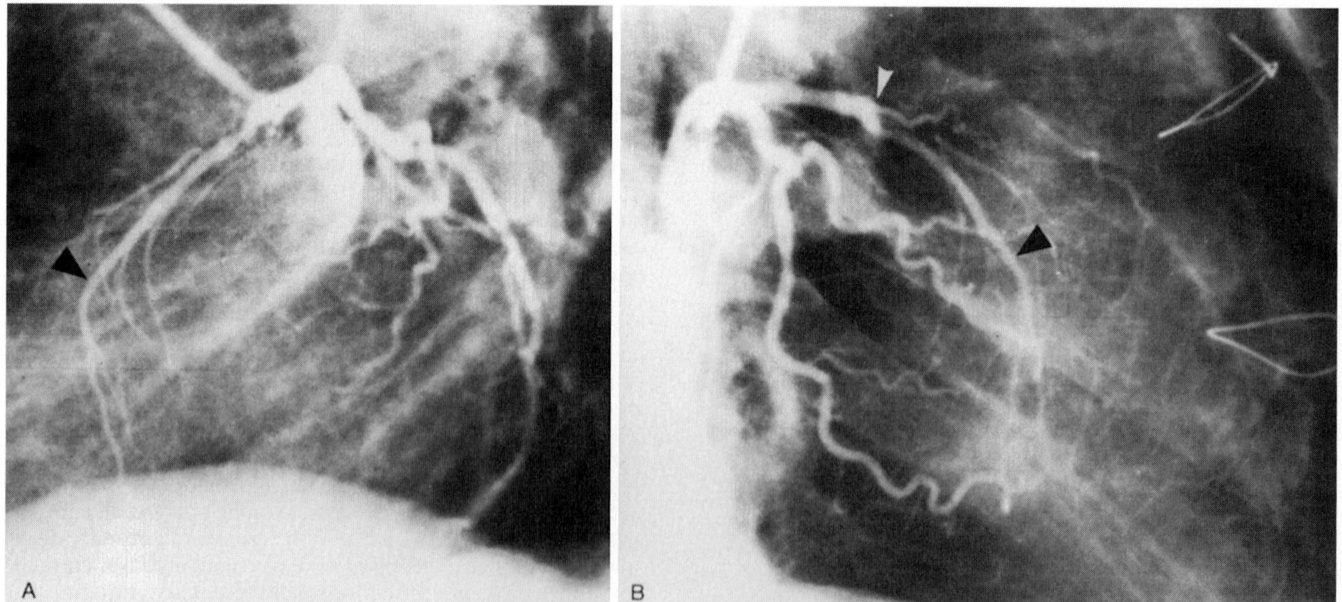

FIGURE 18–21 Septal branch mimicking the left anterior descending artery (LAD). **A,** Left anterior oblique left coronary arteriogram shows an enlarged septal branch (arrowhead) occupying the expected course of the LAD. **B,** The right anterior oblique view shows that the LAD is totally occluded (white arrowhead). The septal branch (black arrowhead) runs in a course approximately parallel to the LAD but below it and within the interventricular septum. (From Levin DC, Baltaxe HA, Sos TA: Potential sources of error in coronary arteriography: II. Interpretation of the study. AJR 124:386, 1975.)

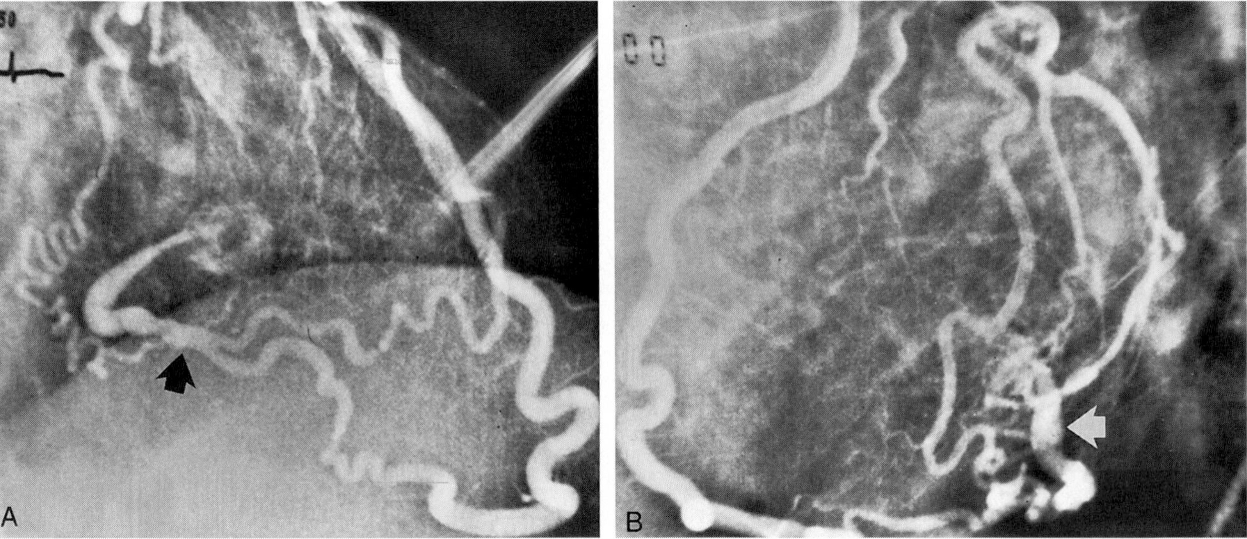

FIGURE 18–22 Congenital fistula. **A,** Right anterior oblique cranial view of the left coronary arteriogram shows a congenital fistula (arrow) arising from branches of both the left anterior descending and left circumflex arteries and draining into the left ventricle. **B,** Left anterior oblique view of the left coronary arteriogram shows the fistula (arrow).

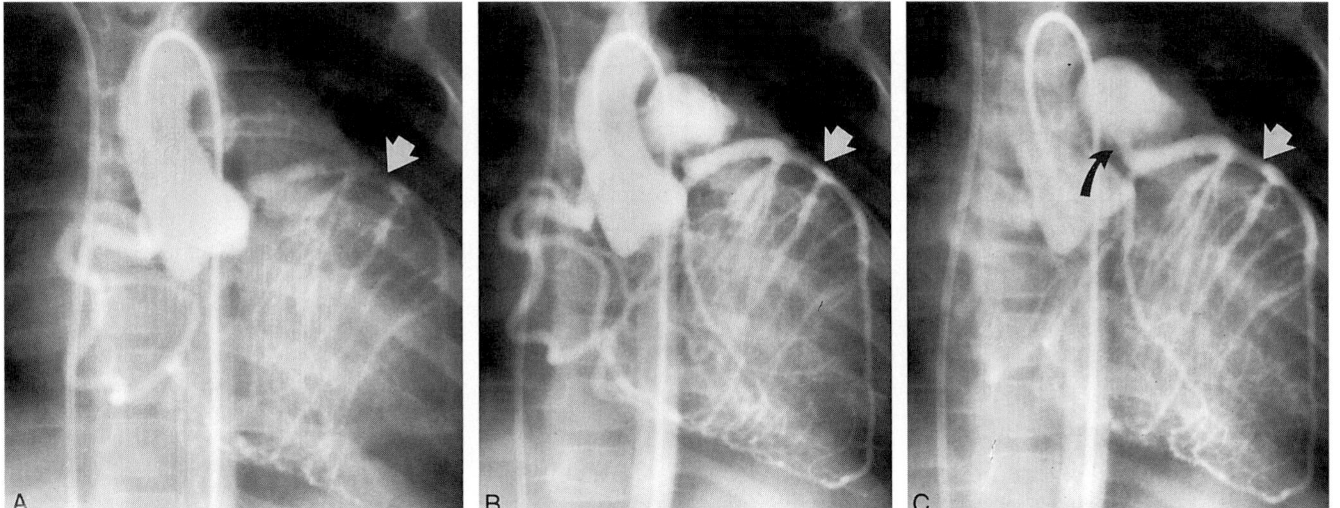

FIGURE 18–23 Anomalous origin of the left coronary artery (LCA) from the pulmonary artery. **A** to **C,** The thoracic aortogram shows a large right coronary artery (RCA) and no antegrade filling of the LCA. The LCA fills primarily through extensive collaterals from the RCA to the LAD (white arrows). The anomalous origin of the LCA from the pulmonary artery is demonstrated in late phases of the aortogram (**C,** curved arrow).

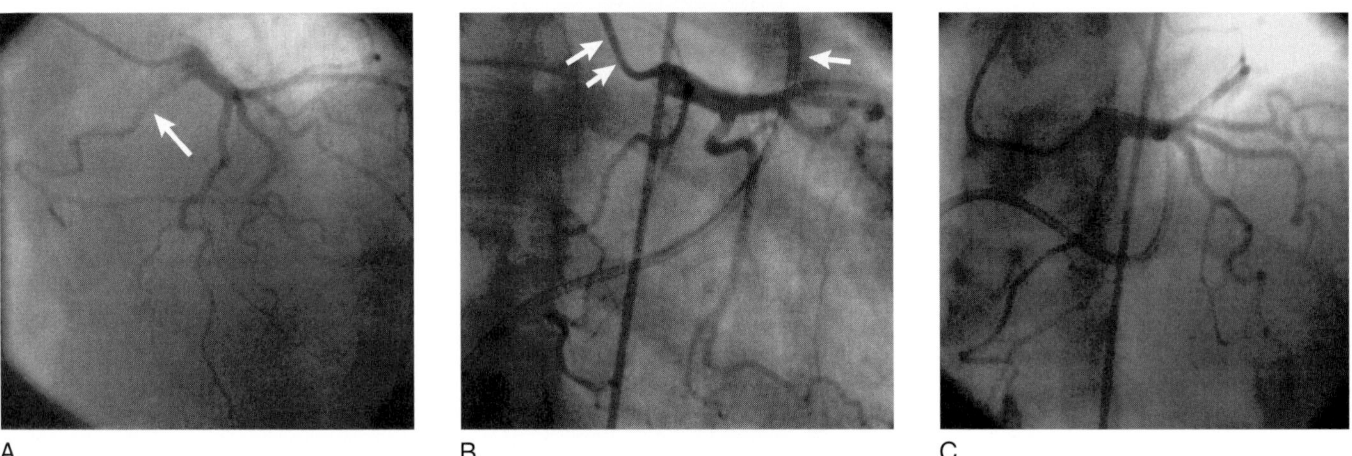

FIGURE 18–24 Anomalous origin of the RCA from the left main coronary artery. **A,** A left anterior oblique view with cranial angulation demonstrates the origin of the anomalous RCA from the left main coronary artery (arrow). **B,** A right anterior oblique view with caudal angulation demonstrates the right coronary artery coursing between the pulmonary artery (noted by the arrow with the pulmonary artery catheter) and aorta (noted by the double arrow of the injection catheter). **C,** The relationship of the RCA to the pulmonary artery and aorta is confirmed in the anteroposterior view with cranial angulation.

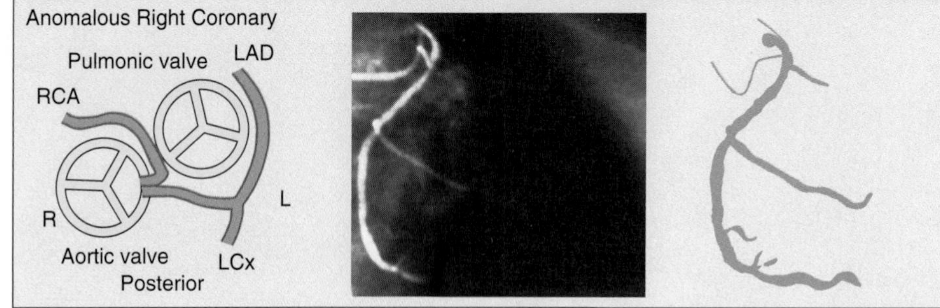

FIGURE 18–25 Anomalous origin of the right coronary artery (RCA). Right anterior oblique coronary arteriogram shows an anomalous RCA arising from the left sinus of Valsalva. The origin of the aberrantly arising artery, which is engaged with a left Judkins catheter, arises immediately anterior to the origin of the left coronary artery (not shown in the arteriogram). The anomalous right coronary follows an interarterial course opposite but analogous to that for the anomalous left coronary artery arising from the right sinus of Valsalva.

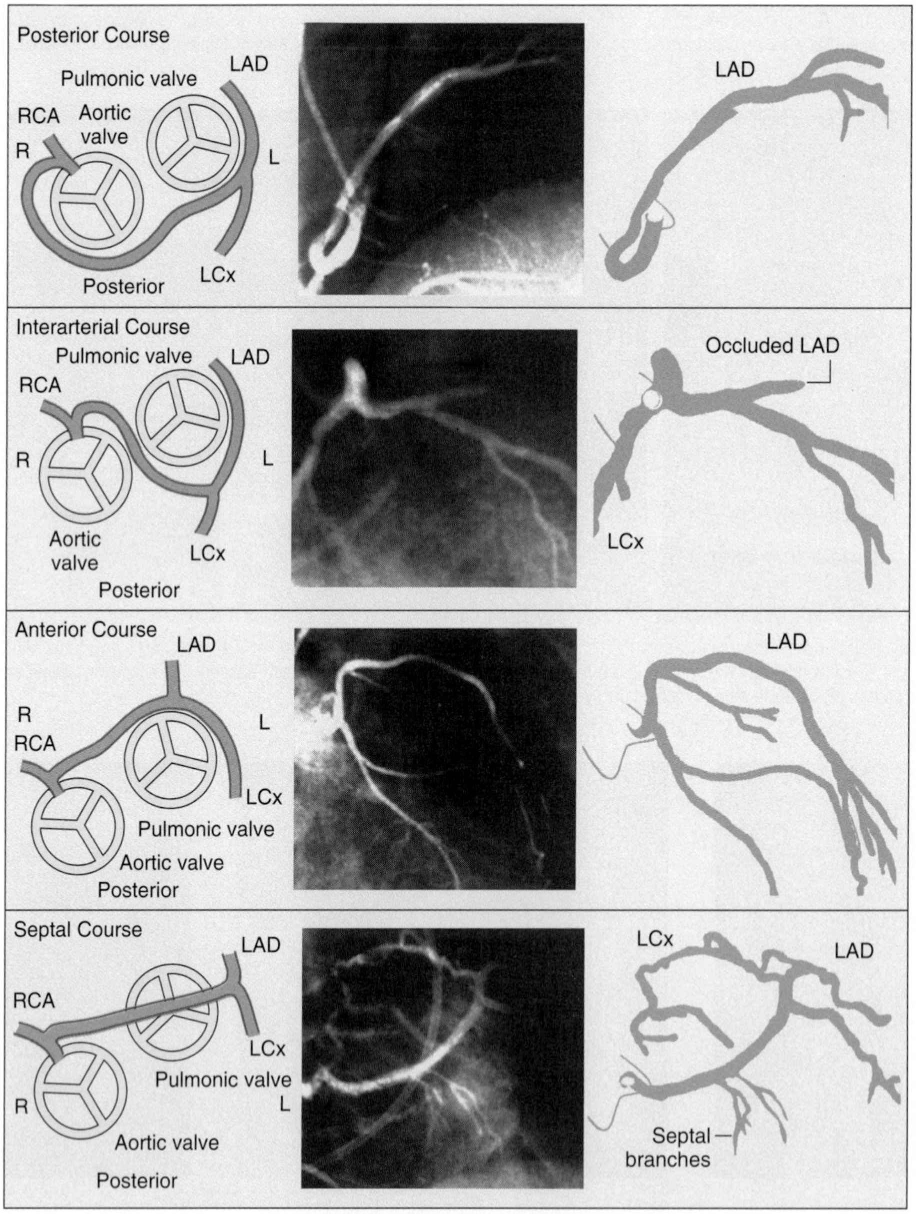

FIGURE 18–26 Anomalous origin of the left coronary artery from the right sinus of Valsalva. Each panel includes a caudocranial cross-sectional schematic representation at the level of the semilunar valves, showing the course of the anomalous coronary. The right anterior oblique angiograms and bitmaps show examples of each of the four most common courses of the anomalous left coronary artery aberrantly arising from the right sinus of Valsalva: posterior (retroaortic), interarterial, anterior, and septal (subpulmonic) courses. LAD = left anterior descending; LCx = left circumflex; RCA = right coronary artery.

in patients with suspected variant angina who were undergoing coronary arteriography.[69] Two types of angiographic responses can be expected with escalating dosages of intravenous ergonovine. A diffuse coronary vasoconstriction may occur in all the epicardial arteries that may be associated with angina symptoms. This physiological response to ergonovine is not diagnostic of coronary artery spasm. The second response to ergonovine is a focal, occlusive spasm of the epicardial artery that is associated with chest pain and ST segment elevation. Nitroglycerin should be administered directly into the coronary artery to relieve the coronary spasm. This response is diagnostic for coronary artery spasm. Ergonovine-induced coronary spasm may be found in 85 percent of patients with primarily rest angina who are observed to have spontaneous episodes of ST segment elevation. Intravenous acetylcholine may also be used to detect the presence of coronary artery spasm.[70] Although it is more sensitive, it may be less specific because of the positive response in patients with atherosclerotic CAD. In a study of 685 consecutive patients who were injected with incremental doses of acetylcholine, 20, 50, and 80 μg into the RCA and 20, 50, and 100 μg into the LCA, coronary vasospasm was found in 32.3 percent of patients.[70] Coronary artery spasm occurred in 49 percent of patients with effort and rest angina, in 34 percent of patients with exertional angina, and in 67 percent of patients with rest angina. It also occurred in 9 percent of patients with nonischemic heart disease. The third test is hyperventilation during coronary arteriography, which is less sensitive but highly specific for the presence of coronary artery spasm.

In the absence of a positive stimulation test, the diagnosis of coronary artery spasm must rely instead on clinical features and response to treatment with nitrates and calcium channel blockers. Sole therapy with beta blockers should be avoided because it can worsen the occurrence of coronary artery spasm. Coronary artery spasm that is refractory to conventional therapy with long-acting calcium channel blockers and nitrates can be treated with coronary stenting.[71]

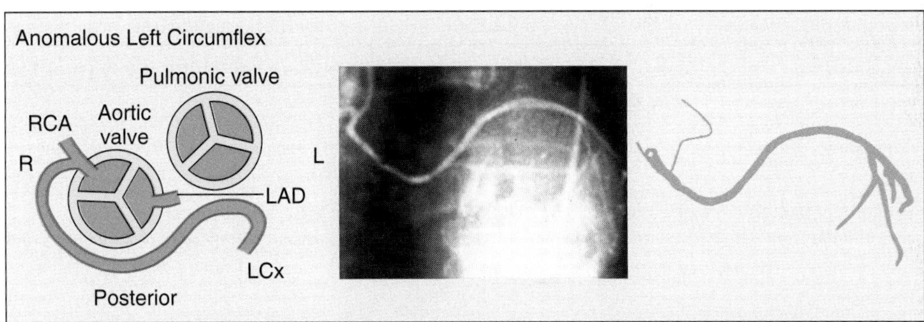

FIGURE 18–27 Anomalous origin of the left circumflex artery. The caudocranial cross-sectional view at the level of the semilunar valves shows the common course of the left circumflex coronary artery aberrantly arising from the right sinus of Valsalva. The left circumflex artery passes behind the aortic root and runs to the left atrioventricular groove following an initial course identical to that for the anomalous left coronary artery arising from the right sinus of Valsalva that follows a posterior, retroaortic course. LAD = left anterior descending; LCx = left circumflex; RCA = right coronary artery.

Angiographic Morphology of Atherosclerotic Lesions

Heterogeneity of the composition, distribution, and location of atherosclerotic plaque within the native coronary artery results in unique patterns of stenosis morphology in patients with CAD. These unique atherosclerotic patterns have been used to identify risk factors for procedural outcome and complications after PCI and to assess the risk for recurrent events in patients who present with an acute coronary syndrome.[72,73] Criteria established by a joint ACC/AHA task force (Table 18–7) were prospectively tested in a series of 350 patients undergoing multivessel PCI; it was found that procedural success and complication rates after balloon angioplasty were 92 and 2 percent, respectively, for type A lesions; 76 and 10 percent, respectively, for type B lesions; and 61 and 21 percent, respectively, for type C lesions. Lesions with two or more type B lesion characteristics (modified ACC/AHA B2) had a risk intermediate between those of lesions with one type B characteristic (modified ACC/AHA B1) and type C lesions.[74] Certain lesion characteristics were associated with

TABLE 18–7 Characteristics of Type A, B, and C Coronary Lesions

Lesion-Specific Characteristics	
Type A lesions (high success, > 85%; low risk)	
Discrete (<10 mm)	Little or no calcium
Concentric	Less than totally occlusive
Readily accessible	Not ostial in locations
Nonangulated segment, < 45 degree	No major side branch involvement
Smooth contour	Absence of thrombus
Type B lesions (moderate success, 60-85%; moderate risk)	
Tubular (10 to 20 mm length)	Moderate to heavy calcification
Eccentric	Total occlusions < 3 mo old
Moderate tortuosity of proximal segment	Ostial in location
Moderately angulated segment, ≥ 45 degrees, < 90 degrees	Bifurcation lesion requiring double guidewire
Irregular contour	Some thrombus present
Type C lesions (low success, < 60%; high risk)	
Diffuse (≥2 cm length)	Total occlusion > 3 mo old
Excessive tortuosity of proximal segment	Inability to protect major side branches
Extremely angulated segments, ≥ 90 degrees	Degenerated vein grafts with friable lesions

From Ryan TJ, Bauman WB, Kennedy JW, et al: Guidelines for percutaneous coronary angioplasty. A report of the American Heart Association/American College of Cardiology Task Force on Assessment of Diagnostic and Therapeutic Cardiovascular Procedures (Subcommittee on Percutaneous Transluminal Coronary Angioplasty). Circulation 88:2987, 1993.

TABLE 18–8 Definitions of Preprocedural Lesion Morphology

Feature	Frequency (%)	Definition
Eccentricity	48.0	Stenosis that is noted to have one of its luminal edges in the outer one-quarter of the apparent normal lumen.
Irregularity	17.9	Characterized by lesion ulceration, intimal flap, aneurysm, or sawtooth pattern
Ulceration	12.1	Lesions with a small crater consisting of a discrete luminal widening in the area of the stenosis
Intimal flap	3.22	A mobile, radiolucent extension of the vessel wall into the arterial lumen
Aneurysm	5.49	Segment of arterial dilation larger than the dimensions of the normal arterial segment
"Sawtooth"	0.84	Multiple, sequential stenosis irregularities
Length		Measured "shoulder to shoulder" in an unforeshortened view
Discrete	55.0	Lesion length < 10 mm
Tubular	34.8	Lesion length 10-20 mm
Diffuse	10.2	Lesion length ≥ 20 mm
Ostial location	10.0	Origin of the lesion within 3 mm of the vessel origin
Angulation		Vessel angle formed by the centerline through the lumen proximal and distal to the stenosis
Moderate	15.3	Lesion angulation ≥ 45 degrees
Severe	0.93	Lesion angulation ≥ 90 degrees
Bifurcation stenosis	6.05	Stenosis involving the parent and daughter branch if a medium or large branch (>1.5 mm) originates within the stenosis and if the side branch is completely surrounded by stenotic portions of the lesion to be dilated
Proximal tortuosity		
Moderate	15.3	Lesion is distal to two bends ≥ 75 degrees
Severe	NR	Lesion is distal to three bends ≥ 75 degrees
Degenerated SVG	7.1	Graft characterized by luminal irregularities or ectasia constituting > 50% of the graft length
Calcification	34.3	Readily apparent densities noted within the apparent vascular wall at the site of the stenosis
Total occlusion	6.4	TIMI 0 or 1 flow
Thrombus	3.4	Discrete, intraluminal filling defect is noted with defined borders and is largely separated from the adjacent wall. Contrast staining may or may not be present.

NR = not reported; SVG = saphenous vein graft; TIMI = Thrombolysis in Myocardial Infarction.
Data obtained from 846 lesions undergoing qualitative angiographic analysis at the Washington Hospital Center Angiographic Core Laboratory.

higher risk, including chronic total occlusions, high-grade stenoses, stenoses on a bend of 60 degrees or more, and lesions located in vessels with proximal tortuosity.

Specific Lesion Characteristics

Estimation of procedural risk may be more usefully based on the presence of one or more specific adverse morphological features rather than use of a composite scoring system (see Chap. 52) (Table 18–8).

IRREGULAR LESIONS. Lesion irregularity, including lesions with ulceration, aneurysm formation, a "sawtooth" pattern, or an intimal flap, suggests a friable surface, correlating pathologically with plaque fissuring, rupture, and platelet and fibrin aggregation. Complex, irregular plaques have been associated with unstable coronary syndromes and progression to total occlusion, whereas smooth lumen contours are more suggestive of stable angina. Other surface morphology features associated with unstable angina and infarction include lesions with sharply angulated leading or trailing borders, multiple serpiginous channels, and discrete intraluminal filling defects.

LESION LENGTH. Estimates of axial lesion length have been obtained using a number of methods, including measurement of the "shoulder-to-shoulder" extent of atherosclerotic narrowing greater than 20 percent and determination of the lesion length with a more than 50 percent visual diameter stenosis. In clinical practice, the lesion length is often estimated by the distance between the proximal and distal angiographically "normal" segments. The ACC/AHA criteria categorize lesions as discrete (<10 mm), tubular (10 to 20 mm), and diffuse (>20 mm). Diffuse lesions are associated with reduced procedural success. Lesion length is also an important predictor of restenosis after PCI, potentially related to the more extensive plaque burden in long lesions. The prognosis of patients with long lesions has been markedly improved with the availability of drug-eluting stents (see Chap. 52).

OSTIAL LOCATION. Ostial lesions are defined as those arising within 3 mm of origin of the vessel or branch. Balloon angioplasty of aortoostial lesions and ostial lesions of LAD or LCx coronary arteries has been associated with reduced procedural success and high recurrence rates owing to smooth muscle and eccentric intimal proliferation noted pathologically in ostial lesions. Technical factors may also account for the suboptimal success rates, such as difficulty with guide catheter support, lesion inelasticity precluding maximal balloon inflation, and the need for multiple balloon exchanges.

ANGULATED LESIONS. Balloon angioplasty of highly angulated (>45 degrees) lesions carries an increased risk of procedural complications (13 versus 3.5 percent in nonangulated stenoses; $p < 0.001$). Complications are most often due to coronary dissection, with the risk of dissection related to the severity of the angulation.[75] Vessel curvature should be measured in the most unforeshortened projection using a length of curvature that approximates the balloon or stent length used for coronary dilation. Devices that are relatively rigid (e.g., directional atherectomy) are less useful in angulated lesions. Coil stents appear better able to conform to an angulated segment than tubular slotted or multicellular designs.

BIFURCATION LESIONS. The risk of side branch occlusion ranges from 14 to 27 percent in bifurcation lesions, related to the extent of atherosclerotic involvement within the origin of the side branch. The risk of side branch compromise has been reduced using advanced angioplasty methods, including guidewire protection, "kissing balloon" techniques, branch vessel stent placement, and lesion angulation, but calcification or vessel size may preclude adequate side branch protection in some cases. Side branch occlusion during PCI is a frequent cause of periprocedural cardiac enzyme elevation.

DEGENERATED SAPHENOUS VEIN GRAFTS. The procedural success rate after balloon angioplasty of SVG lesions ranges from 84 to 92 percent, depending, in part, on the presence of SVG friability or degeneration, lesion location, and SVG age of 36 months or more. Few criteria have been proposed for classifying the degree of SVG degeneration, although such a definition should include an estimate of the percentage of SVG irregularity and ectasia, friability, presence of thrombus, and number of discrete or diffuse lesions (>50 percent stenosis) located within the SVG. The major periprocedural risk for PCI is the occurrence of distal embolization of thrombus and plaque contents, often associated with the "no-reflow" phenomenon.

LESION CALCIFICATION. Coronary artery calcium is an important marker for coronary atherosclerosis. With IVUS as a reference standard, conventional angiography is moderately sensitive for the detection of extensive lesion calcium (sensitivity 60 and 85 percent for three- and four-quadrant calcium, respectively) but is less sensitive for the presence of milder degrees of lesion calcification. The presence of angiographic coronary artery calcium has also been related to reduced procedural success rates after balloon angioplasty and directional coronary atherectomy (DCA). Higher (90 percent) procedural success rates have been reported after rotational atherectomy in heavily calcified lesions.

THROMBUS. Conventional angiography is a relatively insensitive method for detecting coronary thrombus, although complex lesion morphology has been associated with clinical findings of "high-risk" unstable angina. When it is present, angiographic thrombus, defined as discrete, intraluminal filling defects within the arterial lumen, has also been associated with a variably higher (range: 6 to 73 percent) incidence of ischemic complications after PCI. Large, intracoronary thrombi may be treated with a combination of pharmacological agents (e.g., glycoprotein IIb/IIIa inhibitors) and mechanical devices (e.g., rheolytic thrombectomy) (see Chap. 52).

TOTAL OCCLUSION. Total coronary occlusion is identified on the cineangiogram as an abrupt termination of the epicardial vessel; anterograde and retrograde collaterals may be present and are helpful in quantifying the length of the totally occluded segment. Primary success rates for balloon angioplasty of total occlusions remain suboptimal (66 to 83 percent), lower than the 94.2 percent primary success rates for subtotal occlusions. The risk of an unsuccessful procedure depends on the duration of the occlusion and certain lesion morphological features, such as bridging collaterals, occlusion length greater than 15 mm, and the absence of a "nipple" to guidewire advancement.

CORONARY PERFUSION. Perfusion distal to a coronary stenosis can occur anterograde by means of the native vessel, retrograde through collaterals, or through a coronary bypass graft. The rate of anterograde coronary flow is influenced by both the severity and complexity of the stenosis and the status of the microvasculature. The Thrombolysis in Myocardial Infarction (TIMI) study group established criteria to assess the degree of anterograde coronary reperfusion in patients with acute MI (Table 18–9). Successful reperfusion was present with TIMI flow 2 or 3, whereas TIMI 0 or 1 flow was deemed failed reperfusion. It is now clear that TIMI 2 flow may also be insufficient for myocardial perfusion, associated with increased mortality in patients with acute MI compared with those with normal TIMI 3 perfusion.[51] The TIMI frame count was subsequently introduced to quantify the coronary artery perfusion rates in patients with acute MI that have been correlated with mortality rates.[51] With this method, the number of cinefilm frames required for opacification of the involved vessel is counted by means of an automated frame counter, which is present on most cine projectors. Flow delayed more than 60 frames (approximately two cardiac cycles at 30 frames/sec) and 90 frames (approximately three cardiac cycles at 30 frames/sec) may be associated with increased risks for cardiac morbidity.

Coronary Collateral Circulation

In the normal human heart, networks of tiny anastomotic branches interconnect the major coronary arteries and are precursors for the development of a collateral circulation.[76] These anastomotic arteries cannot be visualized in patients with normal or mildly diseased coronary arteries because they carry only minimal flow and their small (<200 μm) caliber is well beyond the spatial resolution capabilities of coronary imaging systems, yet recruitable collaterals can be identified in up to 30 percent of patients with nonobstructive CAD or normal coronary arteries.[77] As atherosclerosis progresses and coronary artery obstructions develop, a pressure

TABLE 18–9 Thrombolysis in Myocardial Infarction (TIMI) Flow

TIMI Flow	
Grade 3 (complete reperfusion)	Anterograde flow into the terminal coronary artery segment through a stenosis is as prompt as anterograde flow into a comparable segment proximal to the stenosis. Contrast material clears as rapidly from the distal segment as from an uninvolved, more proximal segment.
Grade 2 (partial reperfusion)	Contrast material flows through the stenosis to opacify the terminial artery segment. However, contrast material enters the terminal segment perceptibly more slowly than more proximal segments. Alternatively, contrast material clears from a segment distal to a stenosis noticeably more slowly than from a comparable segment not preceded by a significant stenosis.
Grade 1 (penetration with minimal perfusion)	A small amount of contrast material flows through the stenosis but fails to opacity fully the artery beyond.
Grade 0 (no perfusion)	No contrast flow through the stenosis.

Modified from Sheehan F, Braunwald E, Canner P, et al: The effect of intravenous thrombolytic therapy on left ventricular function: A report on the tissue-type plasminogen activator and streptokinase from the Thrombolysis in Myocardial Infarction (TIMI) phase 1 trial. Circulation 72:817, 1989.

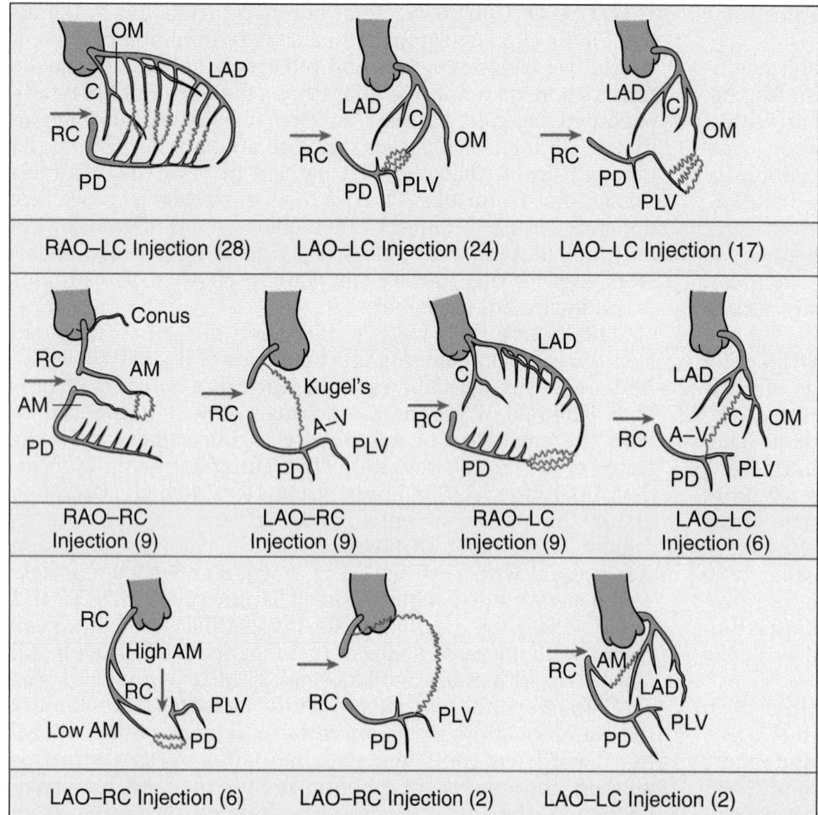

FIGURE 18–28 Coronary collaterals seen with right coronary artery occlusion and common collateral pathways seen with right coronary artery occlusion. The arrows point to the site of obstruction. The small tortuous channels represent the collateral connections. Numbers in parentheses refer to the frequency with which each pathway was visualized in a series of 200 patients with significant coronary disease. AM = acute marginal branch of the right coronary artery; A-V = artery to the atrioventricular node; C = circumflex artery; LAD = left anterior descending; LAO = left anterior oblique; OM = obtuse marginal branch of the circumflex artery; PD = posterior descending branch of the RCA; RAO = right anterior oblique; RC = right coronary artery. (From Levin DC: Pathways and functional significance of the coronary collateral circulation. Circulation 50:831, 1974. Copyright 1974, American Heart Association.)

gradient is generated within anastomotic vessels connecting the distal hypoperfused segment with the proximal artery or the adjacent anastomotic channels of other vessels. The transstenosis pressure gradient facilitates blood flow through the anastomotic vessels, which progressively dilate and eventually become visible as collateral channels.

Angiographically apparent coronary collaterals are usually not seen until the coronary obstruction is greater than 90 percent, at which point the coronary perfusion pressure falls substantially and the blood flow through the collateral increases. A number of collateral pathways exist in patients with severe CAD (Figs. 18–28 to 18–30). The visible collateral channels arise either from the contralateral coronary artery or from the ipsilateral coronary artery through intracoronary collateral channels or through "bridging" channels that have a serpiginous course from the proximal coronary artery to the coronary artery distal to the occlusion. The collateral circulation may provide up to 50 percent of anterograde coronary flow in chronic total occlusions. A considerable fraction of collateral flow is immediately lost after recanalization, indicating that chronic occlusion may not remain protected from future ischemic events by a well-developed collateral function.[78]

It is not entirely clear why some patients develop effective collateral vessels distal to a severe stenosis and others do not; a gradual rate of obstruction formation may allow enlargement of preexisting channels or growth of new ones by angiogenesis.[79] This may allow the development of a "protected" region of myocardial perfusion that does not develop ischemia during enhanced myocardial oxygen demands. Collateral circulation may be severely compromised in patients who have a limited degree of spontaneous myocardial angiogenesis and arteriogenesis, resulting in ischemia during stress in the compromised zone. One study identified the clinical characteristics associated with angiographically apparent collaterals and myocardial blush score in a consecutive group of 112 patients with a native artery chronic total coronary occlusion.[80] Ejection fraction tended to be higher in patients with better collateral grades (grades 1 to 4: 46, 48, 51, and 54 percent, respectively; $p = 0.052$). Hypercholesterolemia was a predictor of a better angiographic collateral grade (odds ratio = 1.3), and diabetes mellitus was correlated with a lower perfusion grade (odds ratio = 0.72).[80]

Recruitment of collateral channels may occur quickly in patients who develop an acute ST segment elevation MI because of a sudden thrombotic occlusion. Among patients studied within 6 hours of MI, about half show angiographically visible collateral vessels. When angiography was performed more than 24 hours after MI, virtually all patients had visible collaterals. This suggests that recruited collateral flow may develop rapidly, potentially within hours after an abrupt vessel occlusion. Accordingly, it appears that collateral circulation results from the utilization of already existing vessels that carried little blood flow because of adequate distal perfusion before the occlusion rather than from the formation of new blood vessels after the occlusion occurs. Other factors that affect collateral development are patency of the arteries supplying the collateral and the size and vascular resistance of the segment distal to the stenosis. A classification system is used for the grading of coronary collaterals (Table 18–10).[81]

Coronary collateral vessels have a number of functional roles. In patients with total occlusions, regional left ventricular contraction is better in segments supplied by adequate collateral circulation than in segments supplied by inadequate or no collateral circulation. In patients with acute MI undergoing emergency coronary arteriography without antecedent thrombolytic therapy, those with adequate collaterals had significantly lower left ventricular end-diastolic pressures, higher cardiac index, higher ejection fraction, and lower percentage of area dyssynergy than patients without collaterals.[79] Patients with stress-induced myocardial perfusion defects have insufficient collaterals more often than those with an intact collateral circulation. During balloon occlusion, patients with well-developed collateral vessels experience less pain, have better distal coronary perfusion pressures, and have less left ventricular asynergy and summed ST segment elevation than those with poorly developed collateral vessels. The presence of well-developed coronary collaterals reduced the risk for subsequent unstable cardiac events.[82] In a series of 403 patients with stable angina pectoris undergoing PCI and quantitative collateral assessment using Doppler measurements, the occurrence of cardiac death, MI, unstable angina pectoris, and stable angina pectoris was only 2.2 percent in patients with good collateral flow compared with 9.0 percent in patients with poorly developed collaterals ($p = 0.01$).[82] The incidence of stable angina pectoris (compared with unstable angina) was

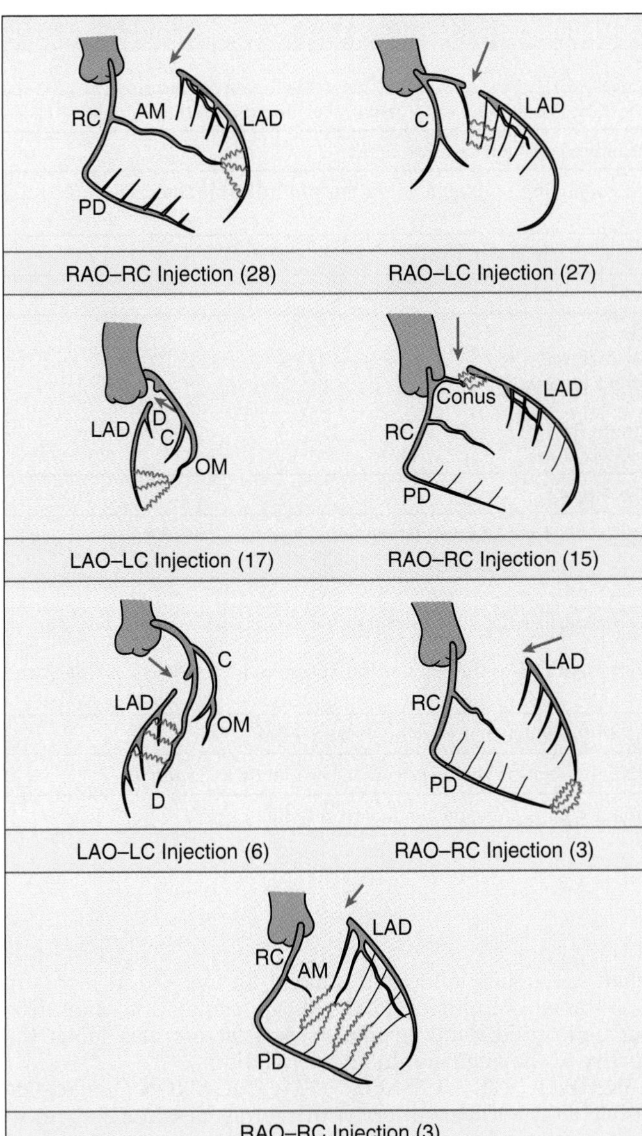

FIGURE 18–29 Common collateral pathways seen with left anterior descending artery occlusion. AM = acute marginal branch of the right coronary artery; A-V = artery to the atrioventricular node; C = circumflex artery; LAO = left anterior oblique; OM = obtuse marginal branch of the circumflex artery; PD = posterior descending branch of the RCA; RAO = right anterior oblique; RC = right coronary artery. (From Levin DC: Pathways and functional significance of the coronary collateral circulation. Circulation 50:831, 1974. Copyright 1974, American Heart Association.)

significantly higher in patients with well-developed collaterals than in those with poorly developed collaterals (21 versus 12 percent; $p = 0.01$).[82]

QUANTITATIVE ANGIOGRAPHY

Both qualitative and quantitative angiographic measures can be used to assess procedural outcome after PCI (Table 18-11). The development of quantitative angiography as a research tool emerged from the recognized limitations of visual estimation of stenosis severity, which include observer variability, overestimation of the stenosis severity before PCI and underestimation of the stenosis severity after PCI, and provision of some visual estimates (>90 percent) that are physiologically untenable. It does seem clear that once the inherent limitations of visual estimation

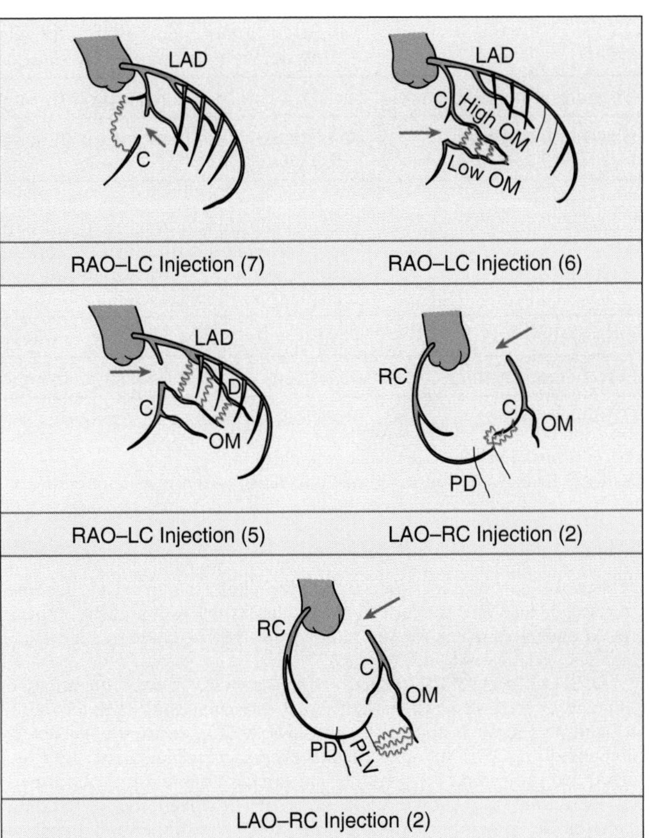

FIGURE 18–30 Common collateral pathways seen with left circumflex artery occlusion. AM = acute marginal branch of the right coronary artery; A-V = artery to the atrioventricular node; C = circumflex artery; LAO = left anterior oblique; OM = obtuse marginal branch of the circumflex artery; PD = posterior descending branch of the RCA; RAO = right anterior oblique; RC = right coronary artery. (From Levin DC: Pathways and functional significance of the coronary collateral circulation. Circulation 50:831, 1974. Copyright 1974, American Heart Association.)

TABLE 18–10 Perfusion Grades Distal to a Coronary Stenosis

Grade	TIMI	Collateral Flow	Rentrop Collateral Grade
3	Prompt anterograde flow and rapid clearing	Excellent	Complete perfusion. Contrast material enters and completely opacifies the target epicardial vessel.
2	Slow distal filling but full opacification of distal vessel	Good	Partial collateral flow. Contrast material enters but fails to opacify the target epicardial vessel completely.
1	Small amount of flow but incomplete opacification of distal vessel	Poor	Barely detectable collateral flow. Contrast medium passes through collateral channels but fails to opacify the epicardial vessel at any time.
0	No contrast flow	No visible flow	No collaterals present

Modified from Alderman E, Stadius M: The angiographic definitions of the Bypass Angioplasty Revascularization Investigation. Coron Artery Dis 3:1189, 1992.

TABLE 18–11 Standardized Criteria for Postprocedural Lesion Morphology

Feature	Definition
Abrupt closure	Obstruction of contrast flow (TIMI 0 or 1) in a dilated segment with previously documented anterograde flow.
Ectasia	A lesion diameter greater than the reference diameter in one or more areas.
Luminal irregularities	Arterial contour that has a "sawtooth" pattern consisting of opacification but not fulfilling the criteria for dissection or intracoronary thrombus
Intimal flap	A discrete filling defect in apparent continuity with the arterial wall
Thrombus	Discrete, mobile angiographic filling defect with or without contrast staining
Dissection,* A	Small radiolucent area within the lumen of the vessel
B	Linear, nonpersisting extravasation of contrast material
C	Extraluminal, persisting extravasation of contrast material
D	Spiral-shaped filling defect
E	Persistent lumen defect with delayed anterograde flow
F	Filling defect accompanied by total coronary occlusion
Dissection, length (in mm)	Measure end to end for type B through F dissections
Dissection, staining	Persistence of contrast within the dissection after washout of contrast material from the remaining portion of the vessel
Perforation	
Localized	Extravasation of contrast material confined to the pericardial space immediately surrounding the artery and not associated with clinical tamponade
Nonlocalized	Extravasation of contrast material with a jet not localized to the pericardial space, potentially associated with clinical tamponade
Side branch loss	TIMI 0, 1, or 2 flow in a side branch > 1.5 mm in diameter that previously had TIMI 3 flow
Distal embolization	Migration of a filling defect or thrombus to distally occlude the target vessel or one of its branches
Coronary spasm	Transient or permanent narrowing > 50% when a < 25% stenosis has been previously noted

TIMI = Thrombolysis in Myocardial Infarction.
*National Heart, Lung and Blood Institute classification system for coronary dissection.

of stenosis severity are understood, the clinician's eye can become "retrained," and one series has shown that visual estimates by experienced observers may correlate more closely with quantitative measurements.

DIGITAL CALIPERS. Digital calipers provide a more quantitative estimate of stenosis severity than visual estimates, and, when properly applied, this method appears to correlate with automated edge detection algorithms. With the use of digital calipers, cineangiograms are magnified and projected onto a wall or flat surface. Calibration is performed by measuring the known dimensions of the diagnostic or guiding catheter. The lumen border is measured using the caliper, and a calibration factor is obtained to determine quantitative dimensions.

AUTOMATED EDGE DETECTION ALGORITHMS. On the basis of early work using hand-drawn arterial contours that corrected for pincushion distortion and reconstructed a three-dimensional representation of the arterial contour, computer-assisted methods for automated arterial contour detection were developed. Quantitative angiographic analysis is divided into several distinct processes, including film digitization, image calibration, and arterial contour detection. The contrast agent–filled diagnostic or guiding catheter can be used as a scaling device for determining absolute vessel dimensions, yielding a calibration factor in millimeters per pixel. Catheter and arterial contours are obtained by drawing a centerline through the segment of interest. Linear density profiles are then constructed perpendicular to the centerline, and a weighted average of the first and second derivative function is used to define the catheter or arterial edges. Individual edge points are then connected using an automated algorithm, and outliers are discarded and the edges smoothed. The automated algorithm is then applied to a selected arterial segment, and absolute coronary dimensions and percent diameter stenosis are obtained.

Pitfalls of Coronary Arteriography

Errors in image acquisition and interpretation can have a profound impact on management strategies, particularly when the angiographic and clinical findings are discordant. A systematic approach to the image acquisition should be pursued, understanding that several factors may affect the quality of the angiographic interpretation.

INADEQUATE VESSEL OPACIFICATION. Inadequate filling of the coronary artery with contrast medium may result in streaming of contrast medium and give the impression of ostial stenoses, missing side branches, or thrombus. Superselective injection of contrast medium into the LCx through a short LMCA may give the impression of total occlusion of the LAD. Adequate filling of the coronary arteries and bypass grafts is required to overcome the native flow of unopacified blood and produce high-quality coronary arteriograms. Streaming of contrast medium, admixed with unopacified blood, leads to an artifactual impression of filling defects and incomplete assessment of stenosis severity. The causes of incomplete filling include competition from increased native coronary blood flow in the setting of left ventricular hypertrophy associated with aortic insufficiency or anemia and inadequate placement of the diagnostic catheter with subselection of the LCx through a short LCMA. The problem of underfilling can be overcome by more forceful contrast agent injection as long as catheter tip position and pressure recording confirm the safety of such a maneuver. Under some conditions, switching to an angioplasty-guiding catheter with a soft, short tip and a larger lumen than a diagnostic catheter may allow more complete opacification of the target coronary artery or bypass graft.

ECCENTRIC STENOSES. Coronary atherosclerosis more often leads to eccentric or slit-like atherosclerotic narrowings than concentric narrowings. If the long axis of the lumen is projected, the vessel may appear to have a normal or near-normal caliber. Only if the short axis of the stenotic lumen is projected is the narrowing visible. For this reason, coronary arteries must be viewed in at least two projections approximately 90 degrees apart.

A related problem is that of the band-like or membranous stenosis. Such lesions may be exceedingly difficult to detect. It is not clear whether these peculiar lesions represent pure atherosclerotic stenosis or are caused in some instances by congenital membranous bands. Aside from the difficulty in detecting these lesions, it is difficult to ascertain their hemodynamic significance. Measurement of the pressure gradient across the lesion using a micromanometer-tip guidewire during intracoronary or intravenous adenosine may be useful to identify significant narrowings.

UNRECOGNIZED OCCLUSIONS. Flow disturbances associated with branch points predispose to the development of atherosclerosis and total occlusions of major arteries at this location. Because of this fact and the variability of the number and distribution of side branches in the normal coronary circulation, it is possible for flush occlusions at branch origins to escape detection. In some cases, occlusion of a branch can be recognized only by late filling of the distal segment of this branch by means of collateral circulation.

SUPERIMPOSITION OF BRANCHES. Superimposition of major branches of the left coronary tree in the LAO and RAO projections can result in failure to detect stenoses or total occlusions of these branches. Although this problem most commonly affects the LAD and parallel diagonal branches, it is alleviated by the use of cranial and caudal angulation. Septal branches may mimic the LAD in the LAO cranial projection. When the LAD is occluded beyond the origin of the first septal branch, this branch often becomes quite enlarged in an attempt to provide collateral circulation to the vascular bed of the distal LAD.

MYOCARDIAL BRIDGING. The major coronary arteries generally pass over the epicardial surface of the heart. In some cases, however, short segments descend into the myocardium for a variable distance. This occurs in 5 to 12 percent of patients and is almost always confined to the LAD. Because a "bridge" of myocardial fibers passes over the involved segment of the LAD, each systolic contraction of these fibers can cause narrowing of the artery. Myocardial bridging has a characteristic appearance on cineangiography. The bridged segment is of normal caliber during diastole but abruptly narrows with each systole. Systolic narrowing caused by myocardial bridging should not be confused with an atherosclerotic plaque. Although bridging is not thought to have any hemodynamic significance in most cases, some have suggested that when it produces severe systolic narrowing, ischemia or infarction may result. The presence of myocardial bridging has important implications for interventional cardiovascular therapy because bridges do not respond to balloon dilation or other interventions.

RECANALIZATION. Although a narrowed segment of a coronary artery seen on arteriography is usually considered a "stenosis," such lesions may actually be a segment that was once totally occluded but has recanalized. Pathological studies suggest that approximately one-third of totally occluded coronary arteries ultimately recanalize. The arteriographic appearances of stenosis and recanalization may be indistinguishable. Recanalization usually results in the development of multiple tortuous channels, which are quite small and close to one another, creating an impression on cineangiography of a single, slightly irregular channel. Cineangiography lacks sufficient spatial resolution to demonstrate this degree of detail in most patients with recanalized total occlusions, but this has important implications for interventional cardiovascular treatments because they are unlikely to be successful in the setting of multiple microscopic channels.

Intravascular Ultrasonography

(see also Chap. 11)

Contrast coronary arteriography is limited in its ability to quantify the extent or distribution of atherosclerosis or to identify changes within the vessel wall over time. IVUS is a safe, accurate, and reproducible method of detecting vessel wall structure and disease and lends insight into the dynamic changes before, after, and late after PCI. The two-dimensional tomographic images provided by IVUS also permit 360-degree characterization of arterial lumen dimensions in regions that are difficult to assess using conventional angiography, such as the LMCA and the ostia of the LAD, LCx, and RCA. When a mechanized pullback of the IVUS catheter is performed at a fixed rate, a three-dimensional reconstruction of the arterial wall and its lumen can be obtained.

TECHNICAL ISSUES. IVUS has evolved substantially since the early 1990s, resulting in the commercial availability of rapid exchange, mechanical, or dynamic array imaging catheters, ranging in size from 2.6 to 3.2F, compatible with 6 to 7F guiding catheters, and yielding a 30-MHz imaging frequency for enhanced tissue characterization. Longitudinal or three-dimensional display of the arterial wall is best performed using an automated pullback device, which uses side branches and other anatomical landmarks to ascertain the plaque location along the axial length of the vessel.

VESSEL WALL COMPOSITION. In nondiseased arteries, IVUS differentiates the vessel wall into three components: (1) the intima, which is composed of endothelial cells, subjacent smooth muscle cells, and extracellular matrix, is 150 to 200 μm in diameter and partitioned from the media by the internal elastic lamina; (2) the media, which is composed of smooth muscle cells, elastin, and collagen, is 100 to 350 μm in diameter and encircled by the external elastic membrane (EEM); and (3) the adventitia, which contains fibrous tissue, is 300 to 500 μm in diameter and encased by perivascular stroma and epicardial fat.[83] Differences in acoustic impedance between the cell layers generally account for the "three-layer" appearance seen in the normal vessel wall of most patients by IVUS. A "two-layer" coronary artery is seen in some patients, depending on the IVUS transducer frequency (<30 MHz), intimal thickness (<160 μm), and collagen content of the media.

In diseased arteries, the differentiation between vessel wall components becomes more obscure and, depending on the cellular composition of the atherosclerotic plaque, at least three plaque types can be described.[83] Hypoechoic, or soft, plaques are echolucent compared with the EEM and indicate a high lipid content present in a pool (Fig. 18–31).[83] IVUS has also been used to assess the changes in plaque volume after lipid-lowering therapy[84] and has demonstrated that multiple plaques may develop simultaneous rupture in patients with acute MI.[85]

Thrombus within the vessel lumen often can be mistaken for soft plaque, but it can be distinguished from soft plaque by its mobility, lobular edges, and movement away from the vessel wall during the cardiac cycle.[83] Fibrous plaques have brightness similar to that of the adventitia and consistent with a higher content of collagen and elastin.[83] Calcified plaques are identified by their bright, echogenic components with acoustic shadowing of the underlying vascular structures.[83] A calcified plaque may be characterized as superficial or deep and quantified by its circumferential extent (from 0 to 360 degrees) and by its axial length (in millimeters).[83] Comparative studies with IVUS show that fluoroscopy is relatively insensitive for the detection of vessel wall calcium. In one study of 110 patients undergoing PCI, IVUS detected calcium in 76 percent of target lesions, whereas fluoroscopy identified calcium in only 48 percent ($p < 0.001$).

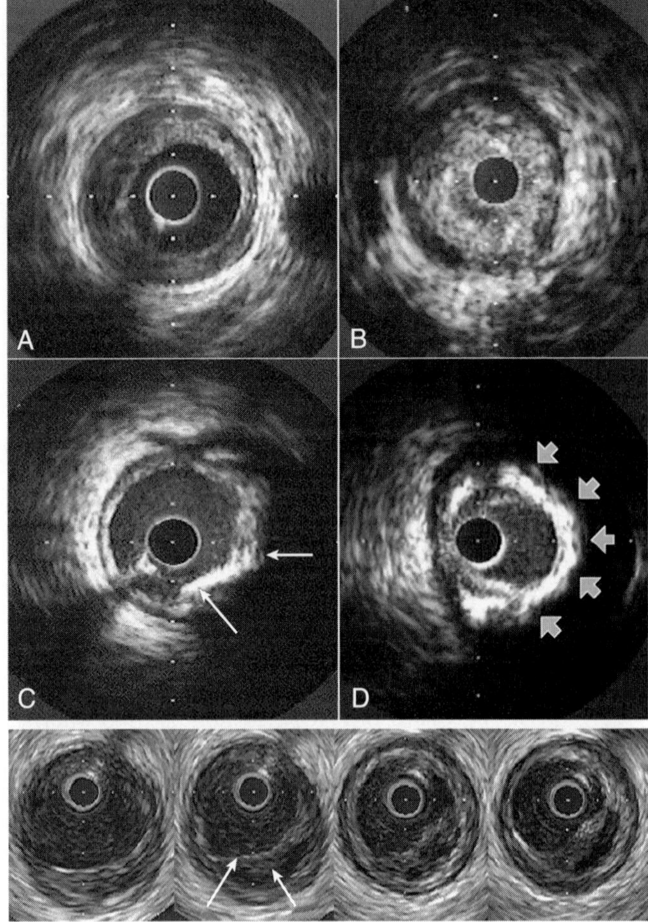

FIGURE 18–31 Intravascular ultrasound (IVUS) characterization of plaque morphology. **A,** A concentric "soft" plaque with concentric vessel wall involvement is less echogenic than a fibrous plaque that presumably contains more collagenous components. **B,** Calcification within the vessel is characterized by a bright leading edge with echo dropout (acoustic shadowing) behind the calcification, and may be focal **(C)** (arrows) or extensive **(D)** (arrows). (Courtesy of Steven Nissen, MD.) **E,** Adjacent IVUS cross sections of a "vulnerable" plaque show a thin fibrous cap (thick arrow) and a large lipid core (thin arrow). (Courtesy of Gary Mintz, MD.)

Fluoroscopic detection of calcium increased to 74 percent in lesions with two or more quadrants of calcium by IVUS and 86 percent in lesions with calcium 6 mm or more in length or with a circumferential arc of calcium of 180 degrees or more by IVUS. The presence of lesion calcification has also been correlated with the overall plaque burden.

IVUS studies in patients undergoing PCI have also demonstrated that coronary atherosclerosis is more diffuse than appreciated using conventional angiography (Fig. 18–32). In an IVUS series of 884 angiographically "normal" reference segments, only 6.8 percent were free of atherosclerosis, with an average 51 percent cross-sectional plaque area found proximal or distal to the target lesion. IVUS studies have also confirmed an earlier pathological finding of Glagov and colleagues, suggesting that the coronary artery undergoes "adaptive" remodeling, or vessel expansion, in most patients in the early stages of atherosclerosis, maintaining a nonobstructive coronary lumen diameter (Figs. 18–33 and 18–34; see also Chap. 35). Once the EEM has expanded by 40 percent, further accumulation of plaque encroaches on the arterial lumen. Arterial constriction does occur in some patients, particularly diabetic patients, owing to "negative" arterial remodeling.[86]

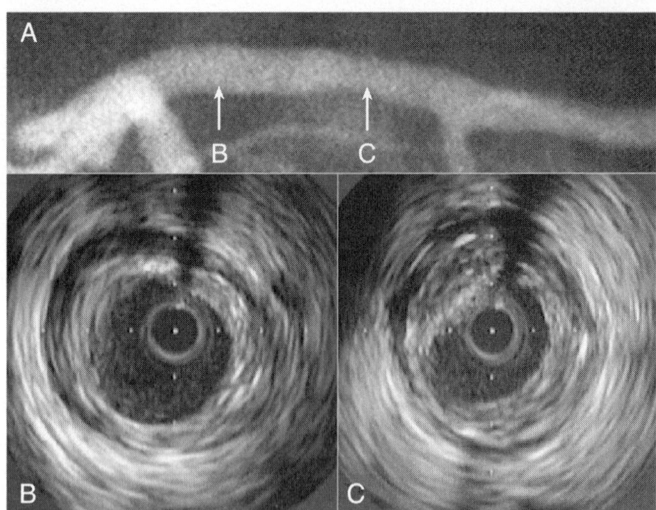

FIGURE 18–32 Discordance between angiographic and intravascular ultrasound (IVUS) findings. **A,** Angiographic imaging of the midportion of the LAD shows only minor lumen irregularities within the vessel. The arrows show the sites imaged in cross section by IVUS below. IVUS imaging of the angiographically normal site **(B)** and the most normal aspect **(C)** of the LAD. Note the substantial atherosclerotic plaque within the wall of the coronary artery that is not appreciated by angiography. (Courtesy of Steven Nissen, MD.)

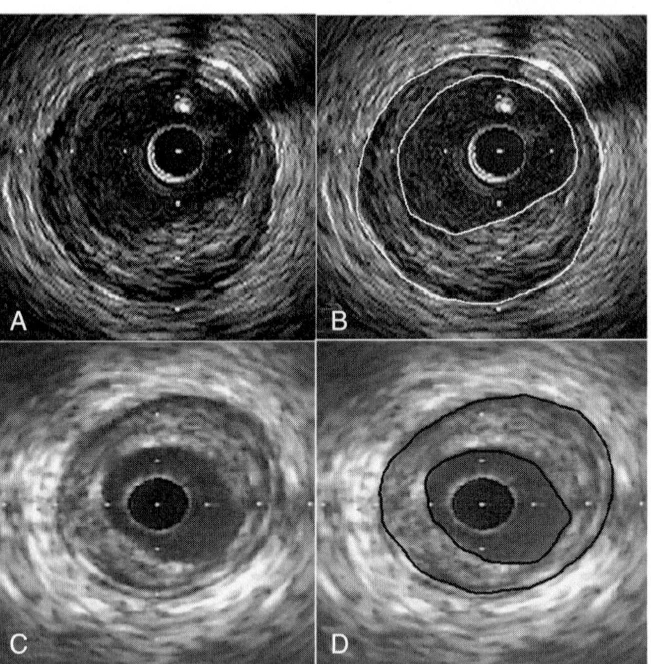

FIGURE 18–33 Quantitative intravascular ultrasound (IVUS) measurements. **A,** IVUS image obtained using a mechanical imaging transducer. **B,** The external elastic membrane is identified by the outer circle and the lumen cross-sectional area is demonstrated by the inner circle. (Courtesy of Gary Mintz, MD.) **C,** IVUS cross-sectional image obtained using a phased-array catheter. **D,** The external elastic membrane is identified by the outer circle and the lumen cross-sectional area is demonstrated by the inner circle. (Courtesy of Steven Nissen, MD.)

USE OF INTRAVASCULAR ULTRASONOGRAPHY DURING PERCUTANEOUS CORONARY INTERVENTION. IVUS may be used for several purposes during PCI: (1) to characterize baseline plaque composition, vessel size, and lesion accessibility to select the best single device or combination of devices for PCI; (2) to confirm (or refute) angiographic estimates of stenosis severity, particularly in regions

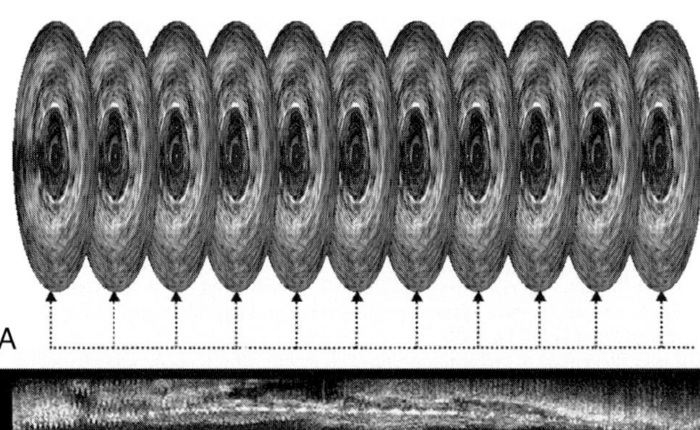

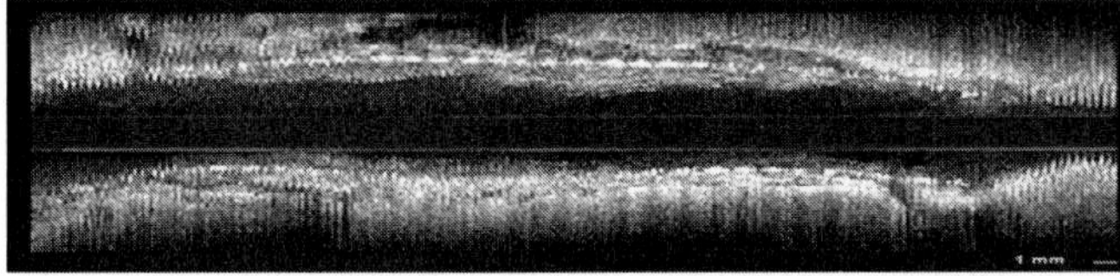

FIGURE 18–34 Longitudinal intravascular ultrasound (IVUS) imaging. Motorized "pullback" IVUS allows reconstruction of the individual two-dimensional cross-sectional images **(A)** into a longitudinal display that characterizes the coronary artery in three dimensions **(B)**. (Courtesy of Peter Fitzgerald, MD.)

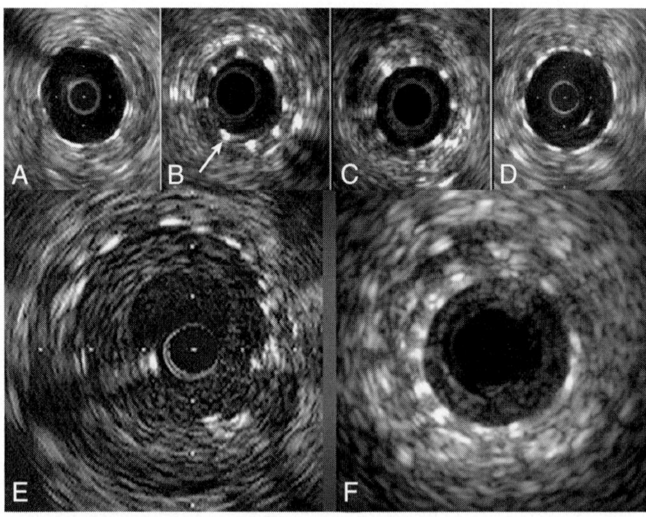

FIGURE 18–35 Stent deployment and in-stent restenosis assessed by intravascular ultrasound (IVUS). **A–D,** Coronary stent apposed against the vessel wall (**B,** arrow). **E,** Obtained in a patient who developed in-stent restenosis, as assessed by the soft-shadowed intimal hyperplasia that obstructs the lumen. **F,** Complete catheter entrapment with the soft intimal hyperplasia that results in stent restenosis. (Courtesy of Gary Mintz, MD, and Neil Weissman, MD.)

difficult to visualize using conventional methods; and (3) to assess anatomical results and detect complications, including dissections and residual minimal cross-sectional area, after PCI.[87] One study of 144 patients with long lesions found that IVUS guidance resulted in lower restenosis rates (23 percent) than in patients treated with angiography alone (45 percent; $p = 0.008$).[88] At 12 months, target lesion revascularization and the combined endpoint occurred in 10 and 12 percent of the IVUS group and 23 and 27 percent of the angiography group ($p = 0.018$ and $p = 0.026$), respectively.[88]

VESSEL WALL CHANGES AFTER PERCUTANEOUS CORONARY INTERVENTION. IVUS provides unique insight into the dynamic changes that occur within the vessel wall after PCI.[89] Sequential IVUS studies show that lumen renarrowing after balloon angioplasty and atherectomy is related to both arterial remodeling and, to a lesser extent, intimal hyperplasia. In the Serial Ultrasound Restenosis (SURE) trial involving a registry of 61 lesions treated with balloon angioplasty or DCA, performing angiography and IVUS at baseline, after PCI, and 24 hours, 1 month, and 6 months later. Lumen cross-sectional area by IVUS improved from 6.81 mm^2 after PCI to 8.22 mm^2 at 1 month ($p = 0.0001$) but decreased to 4.88 mm^2 6 months later ($p = 0.0001$). Vessel, or EEM, cross-sectional area enlarged from 17.32 mm^2 after PCI to 19.39 mm^2 at 1 month ($p = 0.0001$) but decreased to 16.33 mm^2 at 6 months ($p = 0.0001$). Intimal hyperplasia, as assessed by the plaque plus media cross-sectional area, increased from 10.51 mm^2 after PCI to 10.96 mm^2 at 24 hours ($p = 0.001$) and 11.45 mm^2 ($p = 0.03$) 6 months later. Changes in lumen cross-sectional area in each study interval correlated more closely with changes in vessel cross-sectional area than with changes in intimal hyperplasia cross-sectional area. In contrast to these findings, IVUS studies have also shown that lumen renarrowing after stent implantation is virtually all due to intimal hyperplasia within the axial length of the stent or its border.

IVUS has also been used to evaluate the magnitude of intimal hyperplasia in patients treated with drug-eluting stents (Fig. 18–35).[90] In the RAndomized study with the sirolimus-eluting VElocity balloon-expandable stent in the treatment of patients with de novo native coronary artery Lesions (RAVEL) trial, 238 patients were randomly assigned to receive either an 18-mm sirolimus-eluting or an uncoated

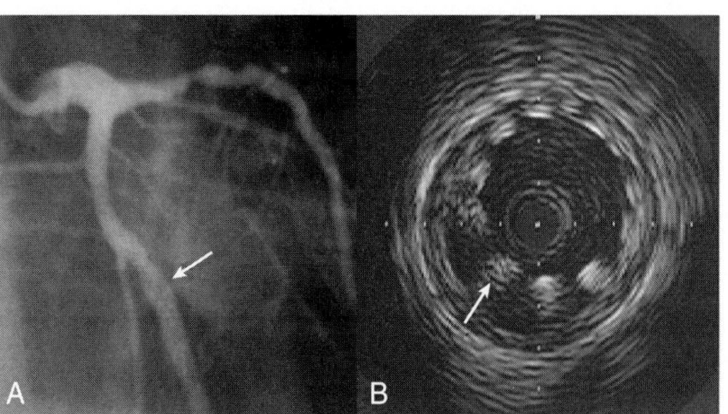

FIGURE 18–36 Incomplete stent apposition. Intravascular ultrasound (IVUS) imaging after coronary stent deployment. **A,** Excellent angiographic result after stent deployment (arrow). **B,** Despite this initial angiographic result, the stent struts are not completely apposed against the vessel wall (arrow). (Courtesy of Peter Fitzgerald, MD.)

stent.[90] In a subset of 95 patients, IVUS was performed after the procedure and at a 6-month follow-up. The difference in neointimal hyperplasia (2 versus 37 mm^3) and percentage of volume obstruction (1 versus 29 percent) at 6 months between the two groups was highly significant ($p < 0.001$), emphasizing the nearly complete abolition of the proliferative process inside the drug-eluting stent.[90] Although there was a higher incidence of incomplete stent apposition in the sirolimus group compared with the uncoated stent group ($p < 0.05$), it was not associated with any adverse clinical events at 1 year (Fig. 18–36).[90]

LIMITATIONS OF INTRAVASCULAR ULTRASONOGRAPHY. A number of factors have limited the widespread use of IVUS during PCI, including its cost, its cumbersome setup for occasional IVUS users, the steep "learning curve" for "online" IVUS interpretation, and the improved outcomes associated with routine use of stents. Current catheter-based IVUS systems are also limited by their inability to assess lumen diameters less than 1.0 mm owing to the catheter size and "ring-down" artifact, and the limited spatial resolution of a 30-MHz imaging transducer (theoretical spatial resolution, 80 μm; usual spatial resolution, 120 to 150 μm) makes IVUS detection of a "vulnerable" plaque somewhat problematic. Radiofrequency backscatter analysis may provide better insights into plaque morphology than standard IVUS image analysis.[91,92] Other invasive imaging techniques, such as optical coherence tomography, may provide higher spatial resolution (20 to 50 μm) for the characterization of vulnerable plaque.[93] Nevertheless, IVUS will remain useful for lesions difficult to assess using conventional angiography as these limitations are addressed with newer IVUS designs. Nonetheless, IVUS provides a powerful research tool for clinical trials, taking advantage of its ability to visualize the vessel wall as well as the lumen. Insights into the efficacy of therapeutic interventions have already emerged from application of this tool to clinical trials.

REFERENCES

Guidelines for Coronary Arteriography

1. Oetgen M, New G, Moussa I, et al: Procedural costs of digital vs. analog archiving of diagnostic cardiac catheterizations. Catheter Cardiovasc Interv 49:246, 2000.
2. Scanlon P, Faxon D, Audet A, et al: ACC/AHA guidelines for coronary angiography. J Am Coll Cardiol 33:1756, 1999.
3. Braunwald E, Antman E, Beasley J, et al: ACC/AHA 2002 guideline update for the management of patients with unstable angina and non-ST-segment elevation myocardial infarction—Summary article: A report of the American College of Cardiology/American Heart Association task force on practice guidelines (Committee on the Management of Patients With Unstable Angina). J Am Coll Cardiol 40:1366, 2002.
4. Wright R, Monnahan R, Kopecky S, et al: Cardiac catheterization reduces resource utilization in patients with chronic chest pain. Catheter Cardiovasc Interv 49:363, 2000.

Complications

5. Ammann P, Brunner-La Rocche HP, Angehrn W, et al: Procedural complications following diagnostic coronary angiography are related to the operator's experience and the catheter size. Catheter Cardiovasc Interv 59:13, 2003.
6. Samal A, White C: Percutaneous management of access site complications. Catheter Cardiovasc Interv 57:12, 2002.
7. Witz M, Cohen Y, Lehmann J: Retroperitoneal haematoma—A serious vascular complication of cardiac catheterisation. Eur J Vasc Endovasc Surg 18:364, 1999.
8. Chandrasekar B, Doucet S, Bilodeau L, et al: Complications of cardiac catheterization in the current era: A single-center experience. Catheter Cardiovasc Interv 52:289, 2001.
9. Jackson J, Meyer G, Pettit T: Complications from cardiac catheterization: Analysis of a military database. Mil Med 165:298, 2000.
10. Segal A, Abernethy W, Palacios I, et al: Stroke as a complication of cardiac catheterization: Risk factors and clinical features. Neurology 56:975, 2001.
11. Hinchey J, Sweeney P: Transient cortical blindness after coronary angiography. Lancet 351:1513,. 1998.
12. Fukumoto Y, Tsutsui H, Tsuchihashi M, et al: The incidence and risk factors of cholesterol embolization syndrome, a complication of cardiac catheterization: A prospective study. J Am Coll Cardiol 42:211, 2003.
13. Blanco V, Moris C, Barriales V, et al: Retinal cholesterol emboli during diagnostic cardiac catheterization. Catheter Cardiovasc Interv 51:323, 2000.
14. Butler R, Webster M: Meralgia paresthetica: An unusual complication of cardiac catheterization via the femoral artery. Catheter Cardiovasc Interv 56:69, 2002.
15. Kuruvilla A, Kuruttukulam G, Francis B: Femoral neuropathy following cardiac catheterization for balloon mitral valvotomy. Int J Cardiol 71:197, 1999.
16. Heupler F: Guidelines for performing angiography in patients taking metformin. Members of the Laboratory Performance Standards Committee of the Society for Cardiac Angiography and Interventions. Cathet Cardiovasc Diagn 43:121, 1998.
17. Dehen L, Vilmer C, Humiliere C, et al: Chronic radiodermatitis following cardiac catheterisation: A report of two cases and a brief review of the literature. Heart 81:308, 1999.
18. Schecter A, Lewis M, Robinson-Bostom L, et al: Cardiac catheterization–induced acute radiation dermatitis presenting as a fixed drug eruption. J Drugs Dermatol 2:425, 2003.
19. Cooper C, El-Shiekh R, Cohen D, et al: Effect of transradial access on quality of life and cost of cardiac catheterization: A randomized comparison. Am Heart J 138:430, 1999.
20. McNulty P, Ettinger S, Field J, et al: Cardiac catheterization in morbidly obese patients. Catheter Cardiovasc Interv 56:174, 2002.

Conscious Sedation

21. Scheinman M, Calkins H, Gillette P, et al: NASPE policy statement on catheter ablation: Personnel, policy, procedures, and therapeutic recommendations. Pacing Clin Electrophysiol 26:789, 2003.
22. Goodwin S: Pharmacologic management of patients undergoing conscious sedation. Clin Nurse Spec 15:269, 2001.
23. Venneman I, Lamy M: Sedation, analgesia and anesthesia for interventional radiological procedures in adults. Part II. Recommendations for interventional radiologists. JBR-BTR 83:116, 2000.

Radiocontrast Agents

24. Davidson CJ, Laskey WK, Hermiller JB, et al: Randomized trial of contrast media utilization in high-risk PTCA: The Court Trial. Circulation 101:2172, 2000.
25. Aspelin P, Aubry P, Fransson S-G, et al: Nephrotoxic effects in high-risk patients undergoing angiography. N Engl J Med 348:491, 2003.
26. Agrawal M, Stouffer G: Cardiology grand rounds from The University of North Carolina at Chapel Hill. Contrast induced nephropathy after angiography. Am J Med Sci 323:252, 2002.
27. Curhan G: Prevention of contrast nephropathy. JAMA 289:606, 2003.
28. Gomes V, Blaya P, de Figueiredo, CE, et al: Contrast-media induced nephropathy in patients undergoing coronary angiography. J Invasive Cardiol 15:304, 2003.
29. Huber W, Schipek C, Ilgmann K, et al: Effectiveness of theophylline prophylaxis of renal impairment after coronary angiography in patients with chronic renal insufficiency. Am J Cardiol 91:1157, 2003.
30. Solomon R: Radiocontrast-induced nephropathy. Semin Nephrol 18:551, 1998.
31. Bailey S: Past and present attempts to prevent radiocontrast nephropathy. Rev Cardiovasc Med 2(Suppl 1):S14, 2001.
32. Baker C: Prevention of radiocontrast-induced nephropathy. Catheter Cardiovasc Interv 58:532, 2003.
33. Stevens M, McCullough P, Tobin K, et al: A prospective randomized trial of prevention measures in patients at high risk for contrast nephropathy: Results of the P.R.I.N.C.E. Study. Prevention of Radiocontrast Induced Nephropathy Clinical Evaluation. J Am Coll Cardiol 33:403, 1999.
34. Mueller C, Buerkle G, Buettner H, et al: Prevention of contrast media–associated nephropathy: Randomized comparison of 2 hydration regimens in 1620 patients undergoing coronary angioplasty. Arch Intern Med 162:329, 2002.
35. Shammas N, Kapalis M, Harris M, et al: Aminophylline does not protect against radiocontrast nephropathy in patients undergoing percutaneous angiographic procedures. J Invasive Cardiol 13:738, 2001.
36. Allaqaband S, Tumuluri R, Malik A, et al: Prospective randomized study of *N*-acetylcysteine, fenoldopam, and saline for prevention of radiocontrast-induced nephropathy. Catheter Cardiovasc Interv 57:279, 2002.
37. Baker C, Wragg A, Kumar S, et al: A rapid protocol for the prevention of contrast-induced renal dysfunction: The RAPPID study. J Am Coll Cardiol 41:2114, 2003.
38. Diaz-Sandoval L, Kosowsky B, et al: Acetylcysteine to prevent angiography-related renal tissue injury (the APART trial). Am J Cardiol 89:356, 2002.
39. Durham J, Caputo C, Dokko J, et al: A randomized controlled trial of *N*-acetylcysteine to prevent contrast nephropathy in cardiac angiography. Kidney Int 62:2202, 2002.
40. Kay J, Chow W, Chan T, et al: Acetylcysteine for prevention of acute deterioration of renal function following elective coronary angiography and intervention: A randomized controlled trial. JAMA 289:553, 2003.
41. Shyu K, Cheng J, Kuan P: Acetylcysteine protects against acute renal damage in patients with abnormal renal function undergoing a coronary procedure. J Am Coll Cardiol 40:1383, 2002.
42. Vaitkus P: Does *N*-acetylcysteine prevent contrast-induced nephropathy? Am J Cardiol 90:1424; author reply 1424, 2002.
43. Kini A, Sharma S: Managing the high-risk patient: Experience with fenoldopam, a selective dopamine receptor agonist, in prevention of radiocontrast nephropathy during percutaneous coronary intervention. Rev Cardiovasc Med 2(Suppl 1):S19, 2001.
44. Madyoon H: Clinical experience with the use of fenoldopam for prevention of radiocontrast nephropathy in high-risk patients. Rev Cardiovasc Med 2(Suppl 1):S26, 2001.
45. Mathur V: Pathophysiology of radiocontrast nephropathy and use of fenoldopam for its prevention. Rev Cardiovasc Med 2(Suppl 1):S4, 2001.
46. Stone GW, McCullough PA, Tumlin JA, et al: Fenoldopam mesylate for the prevention of contrast-induced nephropathy: A randomized controlled trial. JAMA 290:2284, 2003.
47. Marenzi G, Bartorelli A, Lauri G, et al: Continuous veno-venous hemofiltration for the treatment of contrast-induced acute renal failure after percutaneous coronary interventions. Catheter Cardiovasc Interv 58:59, 2003.
48. Marenzi G, Marana I, Lauri G, et al: The prevention of radiocontrast-agent-induced nephropathy by hemofiltration. N Engl J Med 349:1333, 2003.
49. Frank H, Werner D, Lorusso V, et al: Simultaneous hemodialysis during coronary angiography fails to prevent radiocontrast-induced nephropathy in chronic renal failure. Clin Nephrol 60:176, 2003.
50. Lasser ED, Berry CC, Talner LB, et al: Participants. Pretreatment with corticosteroids to alleviate reactions to intravenous contrast material. N Engl J Med 317:845, 1987.
51. Gibson C, Cannon C, Murphy S, et al: Relationship of TIMI myocardial perfusion grade to mortality after administration of thrombolytic drugs. Circulation 101:125, 2000.

Coronary Anomalies

52. Harikrishnan S, Jacob S, Tharakan J, et al: Congenital coronary anomalies of origin and distribution in adults: A coronary arteriographic study. Indian Heart J 54:271, 2002.
53. Angelini P: Coronary artery anomalies—Current clinical issues: definitions, classification, incidence, clinical relevance, and treatment guidelines. Tex Heart Inst J 29:271, 2002.
54. Rapp A, Hillis L: Clinical consequences of anomalous coronary arteries. Coron Artery Dis 12:617, 2001.
55. Burma O, Rahman A, Ilkay E: Coronary arteriovenous fistulas from both coronary arteries to pulmonary artery. Eur J Cardiothorac Surg 21:86, 2002.
56. Kandzari D, Harrison J, Behar V: An anomalous left coronary artery originating from the pulmonary artery in a 72-year-old woman: Diagnosis by color flow myocardial blush and coronary arteriography. J Invasive Cardiol 14:96, 2002.
57. McConnell S, Collins K: Sudden unexpected death resulting from an anomalous hypoplastic left coronary artery. J Forensic Sci 43:708, 1998.
58. Altun A, Erdogan O: Stent implantation to the stenosed right coronary artery in a patient whose right and left coronary arteries originate from a single ostium in the right sinus of Valsalva. Cardiol Rev 11:101, 2003.
59. Fineschi M, Del SM, Leosco D, et al: A rare anatomic variation of the anomalous origin of all three major coronary arteries from the right sinus of Valsalva. G Ital Cardiol 28:564, 1998.

60. Wong C, Schreiber T: Stenting of an anomalous left circumflex coronary artery arising from the right sinus of Valsalva. Tex Med 94:64, 1998.
61. Cohen M, Tolleson T, Peter R, et al: Successful percutaneous coronary intervention with stent implantation in anomalous right coronary arteries arising from the left sinus of Valsalva: A report of two cases. Catheter Cardiovasc Interv 55:105, 2002.
62. Doorey A: Anomalous origin of the right coronary artery from the left coronary sinus. Tex Heart Inst J 29:232, 2002.
63. Garcia-Rinaldi R: Right coronary arteries that course between aorta and pulmonary artery. Ann Thorac Surg 74:973; author reply 974, 2002.
64. Serota H, Barth CW III, Seuc CA, et al: Rapid identification of the course of anomalous coronary arteries in adults: The "dot and eye" method. Am J Cardiol 65:891, 1990.
65. Rentoukas E, Alpert M, Deftereos S, et al: Anomalous left coronary artery arising from the right sinus of Valsalva in a man with unstable angina pectoris and right coronary artery stenosis. Am J Med Sci 323:223, 2002.
66. Turkay C, Golbasi I, Bayezid O: A single coronary artery from the right sinus of Valsalva associated with atherosclerosis. Acta Cardiol 57:377, 2002.

Coronary Artery Spasm

67. Auch-Schwelk W: [Coronary spasm—A clinically relevant problem?]. Herz 23:106, 1998.
68. Rozenberg V, Nepomnyashchikh L: Pathomorphology of myocardial bridges and their role in the pathogenesis of coronary disease. Bull Exp Biol Med 134:593, 2002.
69. Yoshitomi Y, Kojima S, Sugi T, et al: Coronary vasoreactivity to ergonovine after angioplasty: Difference between the infarct-related coronary artery and the noninfarct-related coronary artery. Coron Artery Dis 9:105, 1998.
70. Sueda S, Ochi N, Kawada H, et al: Frequency of provoked coronary vasospasm in patients undergoing coronary arteriography with spasm provocation test of acetylcholine. Am J Cardiol 83:1186, 1999.
71. Jeong M, Park J, Rhew J, et al: Successful management of intractable coronary spasm with a coronary stent. Jpn Circ J 64:897, 2000.

Lesion Morphology

72. Krone R, Kimmel S, Laskey W, et al: Evaluation of the Society for Coronary Angiography and Interventions' lesion classification system in 14,133 patients with percutaneous coronary interventions in the current stent era. Catheter Cardiovasc Interv 55:1, 2002.
73. Krone R, Laskey W, Johnson C, et al: A simplified lesion classification for predicting success and complications of coronary angioplasty. Registry Committee of the Society for Cardiac Angiography and Intervention. Am J Cardiol 85:1179, 2000.
74. Smith S, Dove J, Jacobs A, et al: ACC/AHA guidelines of percutaneous coronary interventions (revision of the 1993 PTCA guidelines)—Executive summary. A report of the American College of Cardiology/American Heart Association Task Force on Practice Guidelines (committee to revise the 1993 guidelines for percutaneous transluminal coronary angioplasty). J Am Coll Cardiol 37:2215, 2001.
75. Ellis SG, Vandormael MG, Cowley MJ, et al, for the Multivessel Angioplasty Prognosis Study Group: Coronary morphologic and clinical determinants of procedural outcome with angioplasty for multivessel coronary disease: Implications for patient selection. Circulation 82:1193, 1990.
76. Koerselman J, van der Graaf Y, de Jaegere PP, et al: Coronary collaterals: An important and underexposed aspect of coronary artery disease. Circulation 107:2507, 2003.
77. Wustmann K, Zbinden S, Windecker S, et al: Is there functional collateral flow during vascular occlusion in angiographically normal coronary arteries? Circulation 107:2213, 2003.
78. Werner GS, Richartz BM, Gastmann O, et al: Immediate changes of collateral function after successful recanalization of chronic total coronary occlusions. Circulation 102:2959, 2000.
79. Werner GS, Ferrari M, Betge S, et al: Collateral function in chronic total coronary occlusions is related to regional myocardial function and duration of occlusion. Circulation 104:2784, 2001.
80. Kornowski R: Collateral formation and clinical variables in obstructive coronary artery disease: The influence of hypercholesterolemia and diabetes mellitus. Coron Artery Dis 14:61, 2003.
81. Werner GS, Ferrari M, Heinke S, et al: Angiographic assessment of collateral connections in comparison with invasively determined collateral function in chronic coronary occlusions. Circulation 107:1972, 2003.
82. Billinger M, Kloos P, Eberli FR, et al: Physiologically assessed coronary collateral flow and adverse cardiac ischemic events: A follow-up study in 403 patients with coronary artery disease. J Am Coll Cardiol 40:1545, 2002.

Intravascular Ultrasound

83. Uren N, Yock P, Fitzgerald P: Intravascular ultrasound image interpretation: Normal arteries, abnormal vessels, and atheroma types pre- and post-intervention. *In* Siegel R (ed): Intravascular Ultrasound Imaging in Coronary Artery Disease. New York, Marcel Dekker, 1998, pp 19-37.
84. Matsuzaki M, Hiramori K, Imaizumi T, et al: Intravascular ultrasound evaluation of coronary plaque regression by low density lipoprotein-apheresis in familial hypercholesterolemia: The Low Density Lipoprotein-Apheresis Coronary Morphology and Reserve Trial (LACMART). J Am Coll Cardiol 40:220, 2002.
85. Mintz G, Maehara A, Bui A, et al: Multiple versus single coronary plaque ruptures detected by intravascular ultrasound in stable and unstable angina pectoris and in acute myocardial infarction. Am J Cardiol 91:1333, 2003.
86. Kornowski R, Mintz GS, Lansky AJ, et al: Paradoxic decreases in atherosclerotic plaque mass in insulin-treated diabetic patients. Am J Cardiol 81:1298, 1998.
87. Dangas G, Ambrose J, Rehmann D, et al: Balloon optimization versus stent study (BOSS): Provisional stenting and early recoil after balloon angioplasty. Am J Cardiol 85:957, 2000.
88. Oemrawsingh P, Mintz G, Schalij M, et al: Intravascular ultrasound guidance improves angiographic and clinical outcome of stent implantation for long coronary artery stenoses: Final results of a randomized comparison with angiographic guidance (TULIP Study). Circulation 107:62, 2003.
89. Ahmed J, Mintz G, Castagna M, et al: Intravascular ultrasound assessment of the mechanism of lumen enlargement during cutting balloon angioplasty treatment of in-stent restenosis. Am J Cardiol 88:1032, 2001.
90. Serruys P, Degertekin M, Tanabe K, et al: Intravascular ultrasound findings in the multicenter, randomized, double-blind RAVEL (RAndomized study with the sirolimus-eluting VElocity balloon-expandable stent in the treatment of patients with de novo native coronary artery Lesions) trial. Circulation 106:798, 2002.
91. Stahr P, Hofflinghaus T, Voigtlander T, et al: Discrimination of early/intermediate and advanced/complicated coronary plaque types by radiofrequency intravascular ultrasound analysis. Am J Cardiol 90:19, 2002.
92. Nair A, Kuban B, Tuzcu E, et al: Coronary plaque classification with intravascular ultrasound radiofrequency data analysis. Circulation 106:2200, 2002.
93. MacNeill BD, Hayase M, Jang I: The comparison between optical coherence tomography and intravascular ultrasound. Minerva Cardioangiol 50:497, 2002.

PART III

Heart Failure

CHAPTER 19

Mechanisms of Cardiac Contraction and Relaxation

Lionel H. Opie

Microanatomy of Contractile Cells and Proteins

Ultrastructure of Contractile Cells

The major function of myocardial muscle cells *(cardiomyocytes* or *myocytes)* is to execute the cardiac contraction-relaxation cycle. The contractile proteins of the heart lie within these myocytes, which constitute about 75 percent of the total volume of the myocardium although only about one-third in number of all the cells. About half of each ventricular cell is occupied by myofibers and about one-quarter to one-third by mitochondria (Table 19–1). A *myofiber* is a group of myocytes (Fig. 19–1) held together by surrounding collagen connective tissue, the latter being the major component of the extracellular matrix. Further strands of collagen connect myofibers to each other. Excess collagen, one cause of left ventricular (LV) diastolic dysfunction, accumulates as part of the growth response to LV pressure overload.

The individual contractile myocytes that account for more than half of the heart's weight are roughly cylindrical in shape. Those in the atrium are quite small, being less than 10 μm in diameter and about 20 μm in length. Relative to atrial cells, human ventricular myocytes are large, measuring about 17 to 25 μm in diameter and 60 to 140 μm in length (see Table 19–1).

When examined under the light microscope, the atrial and ventricular myocytes have cross striations and are branched. Each myocyte is bounded by a complex cell membrane, the *sarcolemma* (*sarco* = flesh; *lemma* = thin husk), and is filled with rod-like bundles of *myofibrils* (see Fig. 19–1). The latter are the contractile elements. The sarcolemma of the myocyte invaginates to form an extensive tubular network (the *T tubules*) that extends the extracellular space into the interior of the cell (Fig. 19–2; see Fig. 19–1). The nucleus, which contains almost all of the cell's genetic information, is often centrally located. Some myocytes have several nuclei. Interspersed between the myofibrils and immediately beneath the sarcolemma are many mitochondria, the main function of which is to generate the energy in the form of adenosine triphosphate (ATP) needed to maintain the heart's contractile function and the associated ion gradients. Of the other organelles, the *sarcoplasmic reticulum* (SR) is most important (see Fig. 19–1).

When the wave of electrical excitation reaches the closely approximated T tubules, the tubular calcium channels open to admit a relatively small amount of calcium to trigger the release of much more calcium from the calcium release channels of the SR. This is the calcium that initiates myocardial contraction. When the calcium is once again taken up into the SR, relaxation ensues.

Anatomically, the SR is a fine network spreading throughout the myocytes, demarcated by its lipid bilayer, which is rather similar to that of the sarcolemma. The *calcium release channels* (also called the *ryanodine receptors*) are found in the expanded parts of the SR that lie in very close apposition to the T tubules. These are called *subsarcolemmal cisternae* (boxes or baskets, Latin) or the *junctional SR.* The second part of the SR, the *longitudinal or network SR*, consists of ramifying tubules (see Fig. 19–1) and is concerned with the uptake of calcium that initiates relaxation. This uptake is achieved by the ATP-requiring calcium pump, also called *SERCA* (sarcoendoplasmic reticulum Ca^{2+}-adenosine triphosphatase [ATPase]), which increases its activity in response to beta-adrenergic stimulation. Calcium taken up into the SR is then stored at high concentration in a number of storage proteins including *calsequestrin* before being released again in response to the next wave of depolarization.

TABLE 19–1 Characteristics of Cardiac Cells, Organelles, and Contractile Proteins

	Microanatomy of Heart Cells		
Characteristic	***Ventricular Myocyte***[a]	***Atrial Myocyte***	***Purkinje Cells***
Shape	Long and narrow	Elliptical	Long and broad
Length, µm	60-140	About 20	150-200
Diameter, µm	About 20	5-6	35-40
Volume, μm^3	15,000-45,000	About 500	135,000-250,000
T-tubules	Plentiful	Rare or none	Absent
Intercalated disc	Prominent end-to-end transmission	Side-to-side as well as end-to-end transmission	Very prominent abundant gap junctions. Fast; end-to-end transmission
General appearance	Mitochondria and sarcomeres very abundant. Rectangular branching bundles with little interstitial collagen	Bundles of atrial tissue separated by wide areas of collagen	Fewer sarcomeres, paler

	Composition and Function of Ventricular Cell	
Organelle	***% of Cell Volume***	***Function***
Myofibril	About 50-60	Interaction of thick and thin filaments during contraction cycle
Mitochondria	16 in neonate 33 in adult rat 23 in adult human	Provide adenosine triphosphate chiefly for contraction
T system	About 1	Transmission of electrical signal from sarcolemma to cell interior
Sarcoplasmic reticulum (SR)	33 in neonate 2 in adult	Takes up and releases Ca^{2+} during contraction cycle
Terminal cisternae of SR	0.33 in adult	Site of calcium storage and release
Rest of network of SR	Rest of volume	Site of calcium uptake en route to cisternae
Sarcolemma	Very low	Control of ionic gradients; channels for ions (action potential); maintenance of cell integrity; receptors for drugs and hormones
Nucleus	About 5	Protein synthesis
Lysosomes	Very low	Intracellular digestion and proteolysis
Sarcoplasm (= cytoplasm) (+ nuclei + other structures)	About 12 in adult rat 18 in humans	Provides cytosol in which rise and fall of ionized calcium occur; contains other ions and small molecules

The *cytoplasm* is the intracellular fluid and proteins therein, contained within the sarcolemma but excluding the contents of organelles such as mitochondria and the SR. The fluid component of the cytoplasm, minus the proteins, is called the *cytosol*. It is in the cytosol that the concentrations of calcium ions rise and fall to cause cardiac contraction and relaxation. The proteins of the sarcoplasm include myriads of specialized molecules, the *enzymes* that accelerate the conversion of one chemical form to another, thereby stimulating crucial metabolic or signaling paths and eventually promoting energy production.

SUBCELLULAR MICROARCHITECTURE. The molecular signal systems that convey messages from surface receptors to intracellular organelles may be directed to specific sites by molecules that "anchor" components of the internal messenger chain to specific organelles, as when the beta-adrenergic chain must link up with the calcium pump of the SR (see later). *Scaffolding proteins* bring interacting molecules closely together as in the case of the signaling chain leading to myocyte growth. An example of physiological subcellular compartmentation is the local unloading of ATP where it is needed by the exact location of the enzyme creatine kinase, which converts creatine phosphate to ATP. "In the world of intracellular real estate, location, location, and location are the key determinants of in vivo function."[1]

Contractile Proteins

The major molecules involved in the contraction-relaxation cycle are the two chief contractile proteins, the thin actin filament and the thick myosin filament (see Fig. 19–1). Calcium ions initiate the contraction cycle by interacting with troponin C to relieve the inhibition otherwise exerted by troponin I (Fig. 19–3). Titin is a newly discovered large elastic molecule that supports myosin (Fig. 19–4). During contraction, the filaments slide over each other without the individual molecules of actin or myosin actually shortening. As they slide, they pull together the two ends of the fundamental contractile unit called the *sarcomere*. On electron microscopy, the sarcomere is limited on either side by the *Z line* (Z, abbreviation for German *Zückung*, contraction) to which the actin filaments are attached (see Fig. 19–2). Conversely, the myosin filaments extend from the center of the sarcomere in either direction toward but not actually reaching the Z lines (see Fig. 19–1).

The interaction of the myosin heads with actin filaments when sufficient calcium arrives from the SR (see Fig. 19–1) is called *cross-bridge cycling*. As the actin filaments move inward toward the center of the sarcomere, they draw the Z lines closer together so that the sarcomere shortens. The energy for this shortening is provided by the breakdown of ATP, chiefly made in the mitochondria.

TITIN AND LENGTH SENSING. Titin is a giant molecule, the largest protein yet described. It is an extraordinarily long, flexible, and slender myofibrillar protein (see Fig. 19–4). Titin acts as a third filament to provide elasticity. Being between 0.6 and 1.2 mm in length, the titin molecule extends from the Z line stopping just short of the M line (see Fig. 19–1). It has two distinct segments: an inextensible anchoring segment and an extensible elastic segment that stretches as sarcomere length increases.

Titin has multiple functions. First, it tethers the myosin molecule to the Z line (see Fig. 19–2), thereby stabilizing the contractile proteins. Second, as it stretches and relaxes, its elasticity explains the stress-strain relation of cardiac and skeletal muscle. At short sarcomere lengths, the elastic domain is folded on itself to generate restoring forces (see Fig. 19–4). These changes in titin help to explain the *series elastic element*, the postulate being that there is elasticity in series between the contractile elements and the ends of the muscle. Third, increased diastolic stretch of titin as the sarcomere length of cardiac muscle is increased causes the enfolded part of the titin molecule to straighten. This stretched molecular spring then contracts more vigorously in systole.[2] Such enhanced systolic contraction helps to explain the Frank-Starling mechanism (see later). Fourth, titin may transduce mechanical stretch into growth signals. In sustained diastolic stretch as in volume overload, the elastic segment of titin is constantly under strain and transmits this mechanical signal to the muscle LIM (Lin-11 and mec-3) protein (MLP) that is attached to the terminal part of titin that forms part of the Z disc complex.[3] The MLP is proposed as the stretch sensor that transmits the signals that result in the myocyte growth pattern characteristic of volume overload.[3] This signal system may be defective in a subset of human dilated cardiomyopathy.[3]

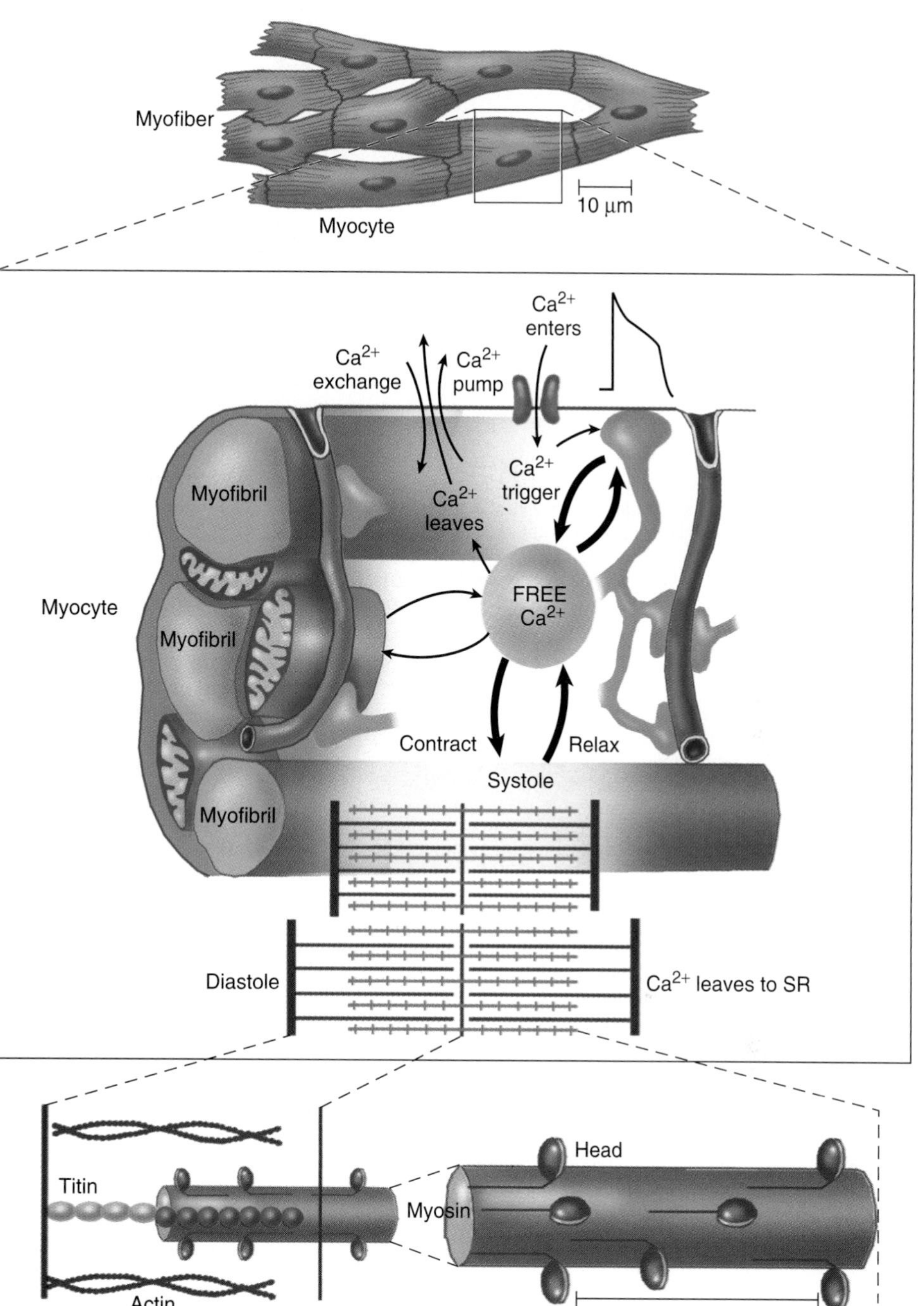

FIGURE 19–1 The crux of the contractile process lies in the changing concentrations of Ca^{2+} ions in the myocardial cytosol. Ca^{2+} ions are schematically shown as entering through the calcium channel that opens in response to the wave of depolarization that travels along the sarcolemma. These Ca^{2+} ions "trigger" the release of more calcium from the sarcoplasmic reticulum (SR) and thereby initiate a contraction-relaxation cycle. Eventually, the small amount of calcium that has entered the cell leaves predominantly through an Na^+/Ca^{2+} exchanger with a lesser role for the sarcolemmal calcium pump. The varying actin-myosin overlap is shown for systole, when calcium ions arrive, and diastole, when calcium ions leave. The myosin heads, attached to the thick filaments, interact with the thin actin filaments, as shown in Figure 19–6. For the role of titin, see Figure 19–4. The upper panel shows the difference between the myocardial cell or myocyte and the myofiber, composed of many myocytes. MITO = mitochondria. (The upper panel is from Braunwald E, Ross J, Sonnenblick EH: Mechanisms of Contraction of the Normal and Failing Heart. 2nd ed. Boston, Little Brown, 1976. The other panels are from Opie LH: Heart Physiology, from Cell to Circulation. Philadelphia, Lippincott Williams & Wilkins, 2004. Copyright L. H. Opie, © 2004.)

STRONG AND WEAK BINDING STATES. Although at a molecular level the events underlying the cross-bridge cycle are exceedingly complex, one simple current hypothesis is that the cross bridges exist in either a strong or a weak binding state.[4] The arrival of calcium ions at the contractile proteins is a crucial link in the series of events known as *excitation-contraction coupling.* The ensuing interaction of calcium with troponin C and the deinhibition of troponin I put the cross bridges in the strong binding state. As long as enough calcium ions are present, the strong binding state potentially dominates. If, however, the strong binding state were continuously present, the contractile proteins could never relax. Thus, the proposal is that the binding of ATP to the myosin head puts the cross bridges into a weak binding state even when calcium is high.[4]

Conversely, when ATP is hydrolyzed to adenosine diphosphate (ADP) and inorganic phosphate (P_i), the strong binding state again predominates (Fig. 19–5). Thus, the ATP-induced changes in the molecular

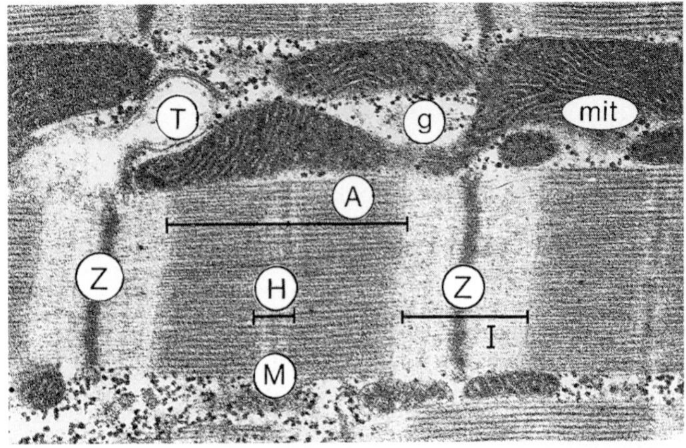

FIGURE 19–2 The sarcomere is the distance between the two Z lines. Note the presence of numerous mitochondria (mit) sandwiched between the myofibrils and the presence of T tubules (T), which penetrate into the muscle at the level of the Z lines. This two-dimensional picture should not disguise the fact that the Z line is really a "Z disc," as is the M line (M), also shown in Figure 19–1. A = band of actin-myosin overlap; g = glycogen granules; H = central clear zone containing only myosin filament bodies and the M line; I = band of actin filaments, titin, and Z line. Rat papillary muscle, ×32,000. (Courtesy of Dr. J. Moravec, Dijon, France.)

configuration of the myosin head result in corresponding variations in the physical properties (a similar concept is common in metabolic regulation). Length activation also promotes the strong binding state (see Length-Dependent Activation). Conversely, the weak binding state predominates when cytosolic calcium levels fall at the start of diastole. As the calcium ions leave troponin C, a master switch is turned off and tropomyosin again assumes the inhibitory configuration.

ACTIN AND TROPONIN COMPLEX. Although calcium ions provide the essential switch-on signal to the cross-bridge cycle by binding to troponin C, current evidence suggests more than an "on-off" signaling process. Rather, the arrival of calcium initiates a series of interactions between the troponin components of the thin filament to allow movement of the tropomyosin molecule, which in turn promotes the strong binding state so that contraction takes place. To understand the role of calcium first requires a brief description of the molecular structure of actin and the troponin complex. Thin filaments are composed of two actin units, which intertwine in a helical pattern, both being carried on a heavier tropomyosin molecule that functions as a "backbone" (see Fig. 19-5A). At regular intervals of 38.5 nm along this twisting structure is a closely bound group of three regulatory proteins called the *troponin complex*. Of these three, it is troponin C that responds to the calcium ions that are released in large amounts from the SR to start the cross-bridge cycle.

Schematically, when the cytosolic calcium level is low, the tropomyosin molecule is twisted in such a way that the myosin heads cannot interact with actin (see Fig. 19-3D). Thereby most cross bridges are in the "blocked position," although some are still in the weakly binding state.[5] As calcium ions increasingly arrive at the start of the contractile cycle and interact with troponin C, the activated troponin C binds tightly to the inhibitory molecule, troponin I. The latter moves to a new position on the thin filament, thereby weakening the interaction between troponin T and tropomyosin (see Fig. 19-3D). Ultimately, tropomyosin is repositioned on the thin filament,[5] thereby removing most of the inhibition exerted by tropomyosin on the actin-myosin interaction. Thus, weakly bound or blocked cross bridges enter the strongly bound state, and the cross-bridge cycle is initiated. As the strong cross bridges form, they activate "near neighbors" and thereby spread the activation process.[5] They also promote further tropomyosin movement to cause more forceful cross-bridge interaction.

MYOSIN AND MOLECULAR BASIS OF MUSCULAR CONTRACTION. Each myosin head is the terminal part of a heavy chain. The bodies of two of these chains intertwine, and each terminates in a short "neck" that carries the elongated myosin head (see Fig. 19–3B). According to the model of Rayment and colleagues,[6] it is the base of the head, also sometimes called the neck, that changes configuration in the contractile cycle. Together with the "bodies" of all the other heads, the myosin thick filament is formed. Each lobe of the bilobed head has an *ATP-binding pocket* (also called nucleotide pocket) and a narrow cleft that extends from the base of this pocket to the actin-binding face.[6] ATP and its breakdown products ADP and P_i bind to the nucleotide pocket in close proximity to the myosin ATPase activity that breaks down ATP to its products (see Fig. 19–3B).

Currently, there is controversy about the role in the contractile cycle of the narrow *actin-binding cleft* that splits the central 50-kDa segment of the myosin head. According to the revised Rayment model,[7] this cleft responds to the binding of ATP or its breakdown products to the nucleotide pocket in such a way that the conformational changes necessary for movement of the head are produced. According to Dominguez and colleagues,[8] the cleft is closed in the weakly attached states before the power stroke (see Fig. 19–5) but opens when P_i is released through the cleft, whereupon the myosin head attaches strongly to actin to induce the power stroke (see Fig. 19–5D and E).

Starting with the rigor state (see Fig. 19–5A), the binding of ATP to its pocket changes the molecular configuration of the myosin head so that the head detaches from actin to terminate the rigor state (see Fig. 19–5B). Next, the ATPase activity of the myosin head splits ATP into ADP and P_i and the head flexes (see Fig. 19–5C). As ATP is hydrolyzed, the myosin head binds to an adjacent actin unit. Then P_i is released from the head through the cleft, and there is strong binding of the myosin head to actin (see Fig. 19–5D). Next, the head extends, i.e., straightens. A power stroke takes place, the actin molecule moves by about 10 nm,[8] and the myosin head is now in the rigor state. The pocket then releases ADP, ready for acceptance of ATP and repetition of the cycle.

The Rayment model[6] postulates straightening and not flexion of the light chain region of the head (i.e., the neck) that produces the power stroke. The lever-arm model[9] is more applicable to many cells and organelles that depend on movement of myosin rather than of actin, for example, for intracellular transport. By contrast, in contracting cardiomyocytes, myosin is fixed and tethered by titin and myosin binding protein C. The lever-arm model proposes that movements of the neck, which is the lever arm, produce large displacements that translate into movement of the whole myosin molecule. This model provides evolutionary data that reinforce the crucial nature of movements of the myosin neck (shown as the flexible domain in Fig. 19–5C).

MYOSIN ATPase ACTIVITY. This activity normally responds to calcium in such a way that increases in calcium concentrations that are associated with the contraction cycle in the whole heart result in a severalfold increase in the myosin ATPase activity besides increasing calcium binding to troponin C and force development.[10]

MYOSIN HEAVY CHAIN ISOFORMS. These isoforms help regulate myosin ATPase activity. Each myosin filament consists of two heavy chains, the bodies of which are intertwined and each ending in one head, and four light chains, two in apposition to each head. The heavy chains, containing the myosin ATPase activity on the heads, occur in two isoforms, beta and alpha, of the same molecular weight but with substantially different ATPase activities. The beta myosin heavy chain (beta-MHC) isoform has lower ATPase activity and is the predominant form in the adult human. The faster alpha-MHC component decreases and the slower beta-MHC pattern increases in human heart failure.[11]

MYOSIN HEADS: TWO ARE BETTER THAN ONE. The double-headed structure is required to produce the full displacement of actin, about 10 nm, versus only 6 nm with single-headed myosin.[12]

THE MYOSIN NECK. The myosin neck is chiefly formed by long alpha helix (see Fig. 19-3B), surrounded by two *light chains* (four per bilobed head) that act as a cervical collar. The light chain that is more proximal to the myosin head, the *essential light chain* (myosin light chain-1 [MLC-1]), may inhibit the contractile process by interaction with actin. The other *regulatory light chain* (MLC-2) is a potential site for phosphorylation, for example, in response to beta-adrenergic stimulation. Such phosphorylation (i.e., the gaining of a phosphate grouping) may promote cross-bridge cycling by increasing the affinity of myosin for actin.[13] Mutation of this light chain in one type of human cardiomyopathy impairs the contractile response to tachycardia.[14] In vascular smooth muscle, the phosphorylation that occurs under the influence of the enzyme myosin light chain kinase (MLCK) is an obligatory step in the initiation of the contractile process.

MYOSIN BINDING PROTEIN C. This protein runs at approximate right angles to the myosin molecules to tether myosin molecules by linking the structures that lie around subfragments of the myosin heads. This binding protein stabilizes the myosin head as it flexes and extends at the level of the light chains. Defects in binding protein C may be involved in some types of hypertrophic cardiomyopathy.

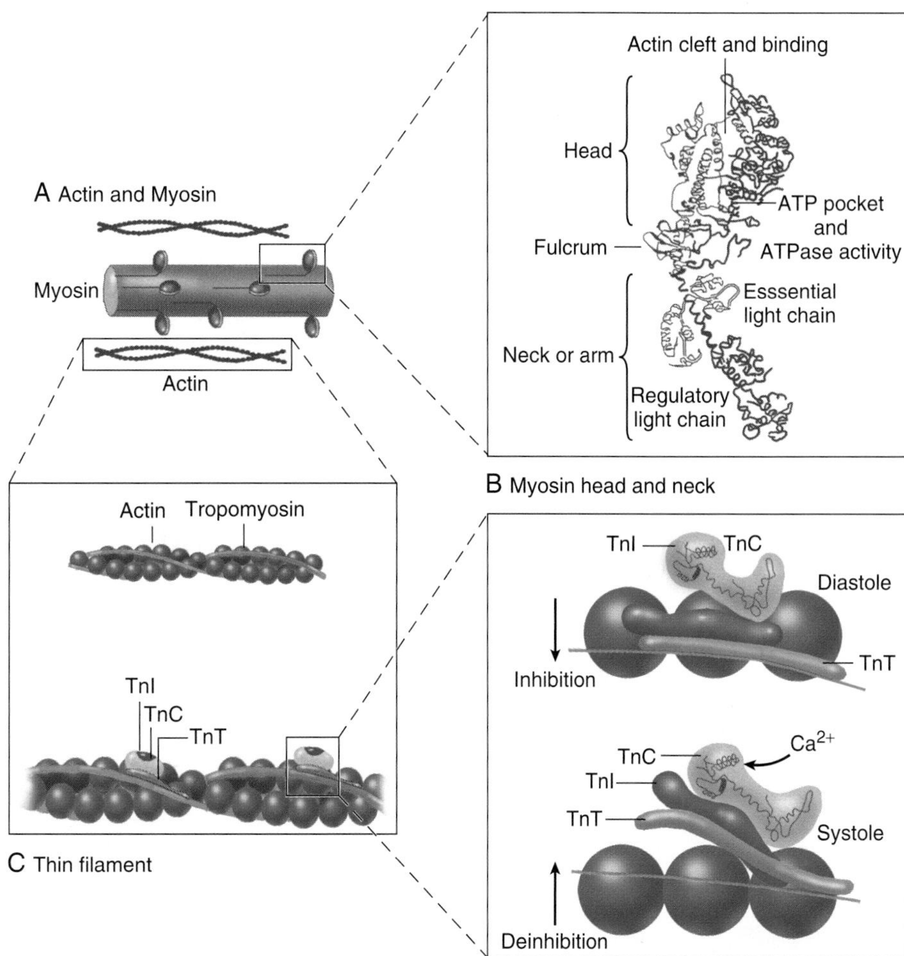

FIGURE 19–3 The major molecules of the contractile system. The thin actin filament **(A)** interacts with the myosin head **(B)** when Ca^{2+} ions arrive at troponin C (TnC) **(C)**. A complex interaction between TnC and the other troponins moves tropomyosin to "uncover" an actin site to which a myosin head can attach (see Fig. 19–5). The molecular aspects are as follows. **A,** The thin actin filament contains TnC and its Ca^{2+} binding sites. When TnC is not activated by Ca^{2+}, troponin I (TnI) inhibits the actin-myosin interaction. Troponin T (TnT) may also participate in the activation cycle **(D)**. **B,** Myosin head molecular structure, based on Rayment and colleagues,[6] is composed of heavy and light chains. The heavy head chain in turn has two major domains: one of 70 kDa (i.e., molecular weight 70,000) that interacts with actin at the actin cleft and has an ATP-binding pocket. The "neck" domain of 20 kDa, also called the "lever," is an elongated alpha helix that extends and bends and has two light chains surrounding it as a collar. The essential light chain is part of the structure. The other regulatory light chain may respond to phosphorylation to influence the extent of the actin-myosin interaction. **C,** TnC with sites in the regulatory domain for activation by calcium and for interaction with TnI. **D,** Calcium binding to TnC induces a conformational change in TnC that elongates (compare systole with diastole). TnI closes up to TnC, and the normal inhibition of TnI on actin-tropomyosin is lessened. There is a strengthening of the interaction between TnC and TnT. These changes allow repositioning of tropomyosin in relation to actin, with lessening of its normal inhibitory effects, as shown in the bottom panel. Now the contractile cycle can start. ATP = adenosine triphosphate; ATPase = adenosine triphosphatase. (Modified from Opie LH: Heart Physiology, from Cell to Circulation. Philadelphia, Lippincott Williams & Wilkins, 2004. Copyright L. H. Opie, © 2004. **D,** Modified from Solaro RJ, Van Eyk J: Altered interactions among thin filament proteins modulate cardiac function. J Mol Cell Cardiol 28:217, 1999.)

GRADED EFFECTS OF INCREASED CYTOSOLIC CALCIUM LEVELS ON THE CROSS-BRIDGE CYCLE. Calcium ions play a crucial role in linking external neurohumoral control of the heart to stimulation of the contractile process by acting at multiple control sites[5,10]; calcium interaction with troponin C is essential for cross-bridge cycling. Does calcium act as an on-off switch to regulate the total number of cycling cross bridges? According to this proposal, the enhanced force development in response to a greater calcium ion concentration must be due to recruitment of additional cross bridges. Alternatively, to explain the graded model, there may be (1) a graded response of troponin C to calcium ions, including altered rates of calcium binding and release; (2) a graded response of myosin ATPase to calcium; (3) near-neighbor self-activation whereby the actin-myosin interaction activates additional cross bridges even in the absence of increased binding of calcium to the troponin C of those cross bridges[5]; or (4) alterations in the extent of myosin light chain phosphorylation.[13] Of specific interest is the proposal that tightly bound cross bridges act to spread activation to near-neighbor units to achieve full activation.[5] By such mechanisms, one calcium-troponin complex could turn on as many as 14 actin molecules.

LENGTH-DEPENDENT ACTIVATION. Besides the cytosolic calcium concentration, the other major factor influencing the strength of contraction is the length of the muscle fiber at the end of diastole, just before the onset of systole. Starling observed that the greater the volume of the heart in diastole, the more forceful the contraction. The increased heart volume translates into an increased muscle length, which acts by a length-sensing mechanism (Fig. 19–6). Previously, this relation was ascribed to a more optimal overlap between actin and myosin. The current view is that an increased sarcomere length leads to greater sensitivity of the contractile apparatus to the prevailing cytosolic calcium ion concentration.[5] A plausible mechanism for this regulatory change may reside in the decreasing interfilament spacing as the heart muscle is stretched.[5] This rather satisfactory lattice-dependent explanation for the Frank-Starling relationship has been dealt a setback by the careful x-ray diffraction studies of de Tombe's group.[15] Reducing sarcomere lattice spacing by osmotic compression failed to influence calcium sensitivity. Alternatively, sarcomere stretch increases the passive forces built up by titin,[16] which could in turn hypothetically influence the position of myosin heads. Another proposal, that troponin C is the length sensor, is currently less favored.[5] Probably several mechanisms are at work.

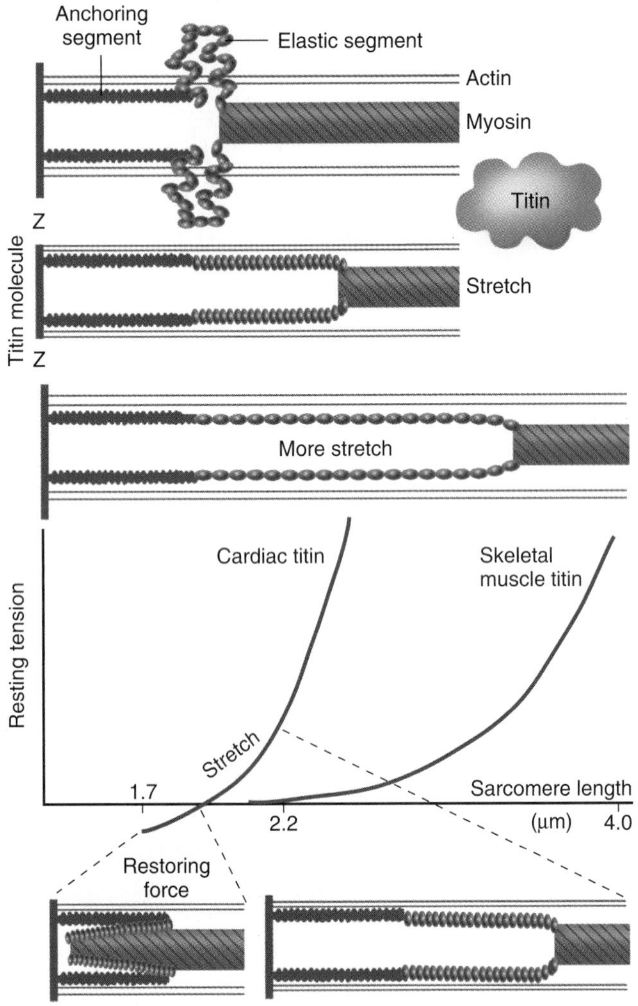

FIGURE 19–4 Titin, a very large elongated protein with elasticity, binds myosin to the Z line. It may act as a bidirectional spring that develops passive forces in stretched sarcomeres and resting forces in shortened sarcomeres. As the sarcomere is stretched to its maximum physiological diastolic length of 2.2 mm (Fig. 19–23), titin first undergoes straightening (up to 2 μm) and then elongation, the latter rapidly increasing the passive forces generated. At low sarcomere lengths, when sarcomeres are slack at about the diastolic limit of 1.85 mm (Fig. 19–23), the mechanically active elastic domain is folded on top of itself. At even shorter lengths, which may not be physiological in the intact heart, substantial restoring forces are generated. (Modified with permission of the American Heart Association from Trombitas K, Jian-Ping J, Granzier H: The mechanically active domain of titin in cardiac muscle. Circ Res 77:856, 1995, and Helmes M, Trombitas K, Granzier H: Titin develops restoring force in rat cardiac myocytes. Circ Res 79:619, 1996.)

CROSS-BRIDGE CYCLING DIFFERS FROM CARDIAC CONTRACTION-RELAXATION CYCLE. The cardiac cycle of Wiggers (see Fig. 19-19) must be distinguished from the cross-bridge cycle. The former reflects the overall pressure changes in the left ventricle, whereas the latter cycle is the repetitive interaction between myosin heads and actin. According to the Rayment model, the binding of ATP or ADP regulates in part whether the cross bridges are weak or strong in nature (see Fig. 19-5). As long as enough calcium ions are bound to troponin C, many repetitive cycles of this nature occur. Thus, at any given moment, some myosin heads are flexing or flexed, some are extending or extended, and some are attached to actin and some detached from actin. Numerous such cross-bridge cycles, each lasting only a few microseconds, actively move the thin actin filaments toward the central bare area of the thick myosin filaments, thereby shortening the sarcomere. The sum total of all the shortening sarcomeres leads to systole, which is the contraction phase of the cardiac cycle. When calcium ions depart from their binding sites on troponin C, cross-bridge cycling cannot occur, and the diastolic phase of the cardiac cycle sets in.

MYOFILAMENT RESPONSE TO HEMODYNAMIC DEMANDS. Solaro and Rarick[5] hypothesized that myofilament activity is coupled to the prevailing hemodynamic demands of the circulation. Besides length-dependent activation, there are two chief mechanisms. First, there may be variable rates of calcium binding and release from troponin C (as discussed in a previous section). Second, phosphorylation and dephosphorylation of the contractile proteins may help to control the extent of activation of the myofilaments. Thus, increased beta-adrenergic-dependent phosphorylation of troponin I *reduces* the myofilament sensitivity to calcium and thereby leads to an *increased* rate of relaxation during beta-adrenergic stimulation.[13] Hypothetically, this mechanism enhances the relaxant (lusitropic) effect of increased uptake rates of calcium into the SR. The effects of phosphorylation of other proteins such the myosin essential light chains and C protein, still imperfectly understood, may also be important.[5]

FORCE TRANSMISSION. Volume overload and pressure overload may owe their different effects on myocardial growth to different patterns of force transmission. Whereas increased diastolic forces are transmitted longitudinally through titin to reach the postulated sensor, the MLP (see earlier, Titin and Length Sensing), increased systolic forces may be transmitted laterally (that is, at right angles) through the Z disc and cytoplasmic actin to reach the proteins of the cell-to-matrix junctions such as the focal adhesion complex. How these mechanical forces become translated into signals that activate the growth pathways such as those leading to mitogen-activated protein (MAP) kinase still remains to be discovered.

CONTRACTILE PROTEINS AND CARDIOMYOPATHY (see Chap. 59). The concept is that genetically based hypertrophic and dilated cardiomyopathies not only produce hearts that look and behave very differently but also have diverse molecular etiologies. Hypertrophic cardiomyopathy is, in general, linked to mutant genes that cause abnormalities in the force-generating system, such as beta-MHC. Less commonly, there may be defects in the genes encoding troponin T, myosin light chain isoforms, troponin I and C isoforms, myosin binding protein C, and alpha-tropomyosin. In some human familial cases, there are abnormalities in the enzyme that functions as the "fuel gauge of the cell," adenosine monophosphate (AMP)-activated protein kinase, giving rise to the current hypothesis that the mutations all impair the contractile response, with less force generated per ATP expenditure. This defect is postulated to induce a compensatory hypertrophy in the remaining fibers.[17]

In contrast, dilated cardiomyopathy can be related to mutations in non-force-generating cytoskeletal proteins, such as dystrophin, nuclear lamin, cytoplasmic actin, and titin. This distinction between the two types of cardiomyopathy remains useful but not totally true. For example, abnormal actin and titin have been found in hypertrophic cardiomyopathy and abnormal myosin in dilated cardiomyopathy. Chien's group postulated that at least in some cases of dilated cardiomyopathy, there is a defect of the length sensor.[3] The Seidman group found a family with dilated cardiomyopathy and early death from heart failure related to enhanced activity of phospholamban, the proposed mechanism being inhibition of the calcium uptake pump of the SR and limitation of normal calcium cycling.[18]

Calcium Ion Fluxes in Cardiac Contraction-Relaxation Cycle

Calcium Movements and Excitation-Contraction Coupling

Calcium has a crucial role in regulating the contraction and relaxation phases of the cardiac cycle. The details of the associated calcium ion fluxes that link contraction to the wave of excitation (*excitation-contraction coupling*) are now reasonably well clarified.[19] The generally accepted hypothesis is based on the crucial role of *calcium-induced calcium release* from the SR. Relatively small amounts of calcium ions, the *trigger calcium ions*, actually enter and leave the cardiomyocyte during each cardiac cycle, whereas much larger amounts move in and out of the SR (Fig. 19–7). The basic proposal is that each wave of depolarization traveling down the T tubules opens the L-type calcium channels that are physically closely approximated to the part of the SR lying close to the T tubule to activate the calcium release channels, collectively called the *ryanodine receptors*. Depolarization thereby releases relatively large amounts of calcium ions into the cytosol in response to the much smaller amounts entering the cardiomyocyte.[19] This process elevates by about 10-fold the concentration of calcium ions in the cytosol. The result is the increasing interaction of calcium ions with troponin C to trigger the contractile process.

This theory has received strong support from several sources: (1) the tight proximity of the ryanodine receptors on the SR to the L-type calcium channels of the T tubules; (2) the molecular characterization of the calcium-releasing ryanodine receptor on the SR (Fig. 19–8); (3) proof of the control of this receptor not only by calcium ions but also by beta-adrenergic-mediated phosphorylation and by binding proteins of the FK506 binding protein (FKBP) family[20]; and (4) electrophysiological evidence closely linking the duration of the action potential with the extent of Ca^{2+} release.[19]

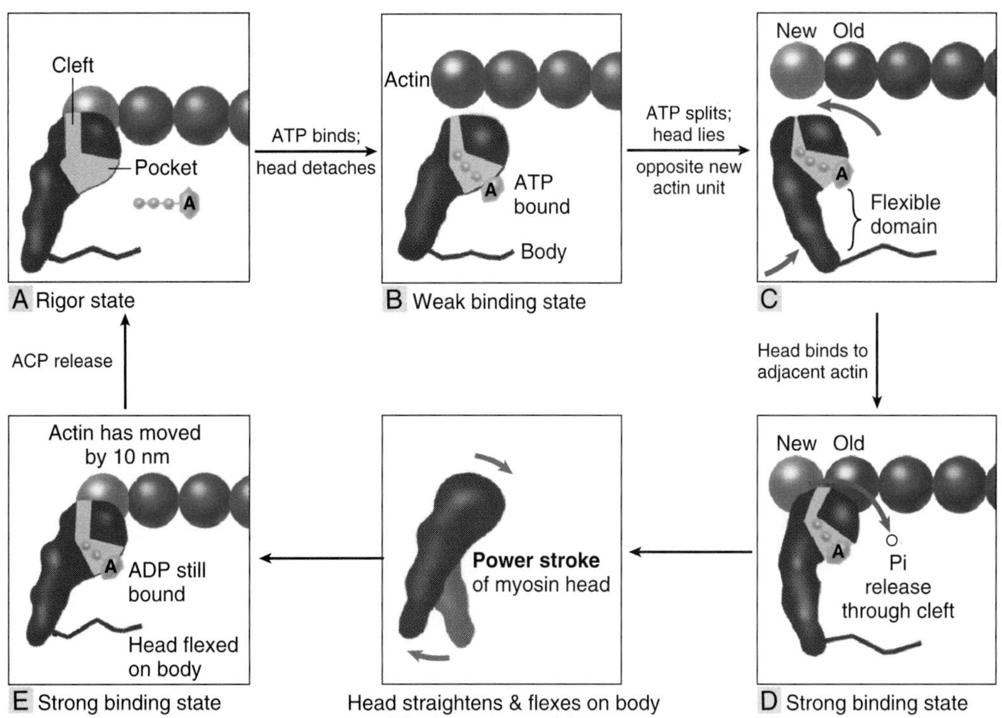

FIGURE 19–5 Cross-bridge cycling molecular model updated by the present author from the five-step model of Rayment and colleagues[6] for interaction between the myosin head and the actin filament, taking into account other models.[8,139,140] The cross bridge (only one myosin head depicted) is pear shaped and consists of the catalytic motor domain that interacts with the actin molecule and an extended alpha helical "neck region" acting as a lever arm.[8] The nucleotide pocket receiving and binding adenosine triphosphate (ATP) is a depression near the center of the catalytic domain. The actin-binding cleft bisects the catalytic motor domain. During the cross-bridge cycle, the width of the actin-binding cleft changes in size, although details remain controversial. Starting with the rigor state **(A)**, the binding of ATP to the pocket **(B)** is followed by ATP hydrolysis **(C)** that partly closes the actin-binding cleft. The cleft opens when phosphate is released (through the cleft rather than through the pocket) and the myosin head strongly attaches to actin to induce the power stroke **(D, E)**. During the power stroke, the latter rotates about a fulcrum in the region where the helix terminates within the catalytic motor domain.[8] As the head flexes, the actin filament is displaced by about 10 nm **(E)**. In the process adenosine diphosphate is also released so that the binding pocket becomes vacant. Finally, the rigor state is reached again **(A)** when the myosin head is again ready to receive ATP to reinitiate the cross-bridge cycle. Throughout, the actin monomer with which the myosin head is interacting is shown in orange. Pi = inorganic phosphate. (Professor J. C. Rüegg of Heidelberg University, Germany, is thanked for valuable comments.)

Calcium Release Channels of the Sarcoplasmic Reticulum

RYANODINE RECEPTORS. Each L-type calcium channel of the sarcolemma controls a cluster of possibly 6 to 20 SR release channels by virtue of close anatomical proximity of the calcium channels on the T tubules to the calcium release channels, situated on the SR. The calcium release channel is part of the complex structure known as the *ryanodine receptor*, so called because it coincidentally binds the potent insecticide ryanodine and is often abbreviated to RyR2 to indicate the cardiac isoform.

Ryanodine receptors have a dual function, containing the calcium release channels of the SR and acting as scaffolding proteins that localize numerous key regulatory proteins to the junctional complexes.[19] These proteins include those that respond to phosphorylation by protein kinase A (PKA) and its anchoring protein, AKAP, to enhance channel opening (see Figs. 19-8 and 19-11), phosphatases that work in the opposite direction, and binding proteins (technical term: FKBP-506 and others) that are thought to coordinate opening of neighboring ryanodine calcium channels by the process of *coupled gating*.

The anatomical basis of the scaffolding function is that part of the ryanodine receptor extends from the membrane of the SR toward the T tubule to constitute the *junctional calcium release complex* that bridges the gap between the SR and the T tubule. Here the ryanodine receptors are packed in large organized arrays of perhaps 50 to 300 per junction. The ryanodine receptor is very large, and four of them link to form a megacomplex containing one calcium release channel (see Fig. 19-8) Added to this are all the proteins adhering to the complex through their binding sites so that the total megacomplex has a molecular weight approximating that of titin. After the wave of depolarization has reached the T tubule and opened the voltage-operated L-type calcium channels, the trigger calcium ions enter the cardiomyocyte to reach the junctional regions of the SR with their ryanodine receptors. The result is a change in the molecular configuration of the ryanodine receptor that opens the calcium release channel of the SR to discharge calcium ions into the subsarcolemmal space between the foot and the T tubule and thence into the cytosol.

TURN-OFF OF CALCIUM RELEASE. The rise of cytosolic calcium that triggers contraction comes to an end as the wave of excitation passes, no more calcium ions enter, and the release of calcium from the SR ceases. This turn-off of release is not as well understood as control of calcium release from the SR but is important in avoiding cytosolic calcium overload with potentially serious consequences such as arrhythmias and impaired contraction-relaxation cycles. There are several proposals to explain turn-off, as follows: (1) the rising cytosolic calcium ion concentration inhibits the release process; (2) the rising cytosolic calcium ion concentration can activate the calcium uptake pump of the SR; (3) the SR becomes locally depleted of calcium; or (4) the ryanodine receptor is inactivated so that it becomes resistant to the prevailing calcium concentration.[19] The overall effect of these mechanisms is that the cytosolic calcium ion concentration starts to fall and diastole is initiated. As the cytosolic calcium decreases, calcium binding to troponin C lessens, tropomyosin again starts to inhibit the interaction between actin and myosin, and relaxation proceeds.

CALCIUM SPARKS. These are the very small amounts of calcium spontaneously and locally released from the SR even in the absence of L-channel opening. Hypothetically, the spark represents the spontaneous opening of one or at the most a cluster of calcium release channels. There is so little calcium diffusing away from a spark, that it fails to activate the neighboring calcium release channels and contraction is not initiated. When the calcium channels of the T tubules open, several thousand

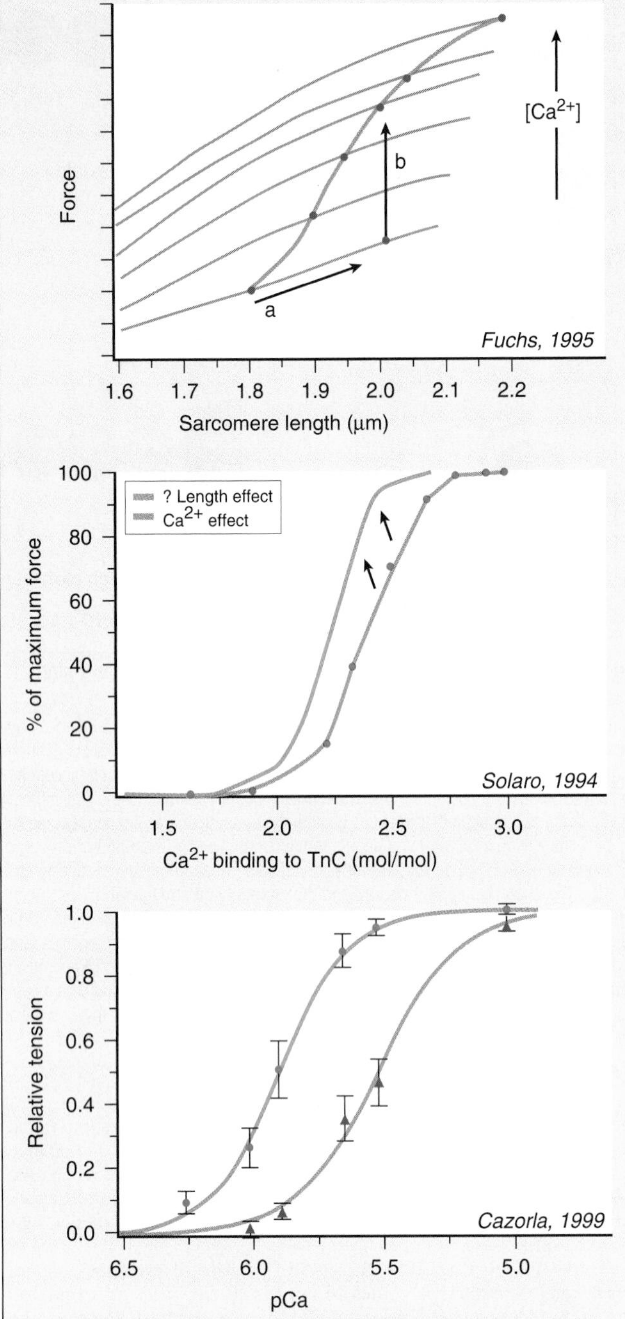

FIGURE 19–6 The proposed explanation for the Starling effect, whereby a greater end-diastolic fiber length develops a greater force. **Top,** How the steep ascending limb of the cardiac force-length curve is explained by an interaction between sarcomere length and calcium ions. Light lines show a family of hypothetical force-length curves for increasing free Ca^{2+} concentrations, each drawn on the assumption that the shape of the curve is determined solely by the degree of overlap of thin and thick filaments (see Fig. 19–1). It is postulated that an increase in end-diastolic fiber length (a) at any given free Ca^{2+} concentration would increase force by a small amount on the basis of the change in filament overlap. In addition, length-dependent activation explains how the sarcomere can "upgrade itself" (b) to a higher force-length curve. **Middle,** Proposal that the effects of Ca^{2+} and length can be explained by the properties of troponin C (TnC) and the binding of calcium to TnC. As more Ca^{2+} ions bind to TnC in a skinned-fiber preparation, more force is developed. There is a steep relation, similar to that shown in the top panel. When the fiber is stretched and the sarcomere length increased, it is postulated that for any given number of Ca^{2+} ions binding to TnC there is greater force development. **Bottom,** How the Ca^{2+} concentration influences the development of tension at long (filled circles) and shorter (open circles) sarcomere lengths. (**Top,** Modified from Fuchs F: Mechanical modulation of the Ca^{2+} regulatory protein complex in cardiac muscle. News Physiol Sci 10:6, 1995; **Middle,** modified from Solaro RJ, Wolska BM, Westfall M: Regulatory proteins and diastolic relaxation. *In* Lorell BH, Grossman W [eds]: Diastolic Relaxation of the Heart. Norwell, Mass, Kluwer Academic Publishers, 1994, pp 53-53; **Bottom,** modified from Cazorla O, Vassort G, Garnier D, LeGuennec J-Y: Length modulation of active force in rat cardiac myocytes: Is titin the sensor? J Mol Cell Cardiol 31:1215, 1995.)

calcium sparks can unite in time and space to become a subsarcolemmal calcium wave that triggers excitation-contraction coupling.[21] This model predicts that the graded response in calcium release can be explained by both an increased number of channels that are opened and an increased amount of calcium released by each channel. When the SR is overloaded with calcium as in pathological conditions such as catecholamine toxicity or during early reperfusion, calcium sparks can lead to propagated calcium waves with risk of serious arrhythmias or impaired contractile activity.

CALCIUM UPTAKE BY THE CALCIUM ATPASE OF THE SARCOPLASMIC RETICULUM (see also Chap. 21). Calcium ions are taken up into the SR by the activity of the calcium pump called SERCA that constitutes nearly 90 percent of the protein component of the SR. Its molecular weight is about 115 kDa, and it straddles the SR membrane in such a way that part of it actually protrudes into the cytosol. It exists in several isoforms, of which the dominant cardiac form is SERCA2a. For each mole of ATP hydrolyzed by this enzyme, two calcium ions are taken up to accumulate within the SR (Fig. 19–9). The source of the energy is at least in part cytosolic generation of ATP through glycolysis.[22] Important links between SERCA and cardiac contractile activity are found in a variety of genetic models. For example, in heart failure the activity of SERCA is decreased, whereas gene transfer of SERCA2a improves survival and high-energy phosphate metabolism.[23]

Phospholamban was so named by its discoverers, Tada and Katz, to mean "phosphate receiver."[24] The activity of phospholamban is governed by a state of phosphorylation, a process that alters the molecular configuration of SERCA to promote its activity (see Fig. 19–9). Two major protein kinases are involved, one activated by PKA in response to beta-adrenergic stimulation and cyclic AMP and the other by calcium ions and calmodulin, and these act at two different phosphorylation sites.[25] When phospholamban responds to beta-adrenergic stimulation of the cardiomyocyte by enhancing the uptake of calcium by SERCA into the SR, thus increasing the rate of relaxation,[19] the major activation is phosphorylation of the PKA site.[25] A further proposal is that the enhanced store of calcium in the SR correspondingly increases the amount of calcium released by the ryanodine receptor in response to subsequent waves of depolarization to give an increased rate and force of contraction.[26] This sequence is strongly supported by a model of transgenic mice, totally deficient in phospholamban, with hyperdynamic hearts in which rates of contraction and relaxation are maximal with attenuated responses to added beta-adrenergic stimulation by isoproterenol.[25] Conversely, in hearts overexpressing phospholamban, cardiac function is depressed.[25]

Calcium, taken up into the SR by the calcium uptake pump, is stored within the SR prior to further release. The highly charged storage protein, *calsequestrin*, is found in the part of the SR that lies near the T tubules. Calcium stored with calsequestrin becomes available for the release process as calsequestrin discharges Ca^{2+} into the inner mouth of the calcium release channel. This process replaces the calcium ions liberated from the outer mouth into the cytosol. *Calreticulin* is another Ca^{2+}-storing protein, similar in structure to calsequestrin and probably similar in function. Hypothetically, calsequestrin and two other proteins located in the SR

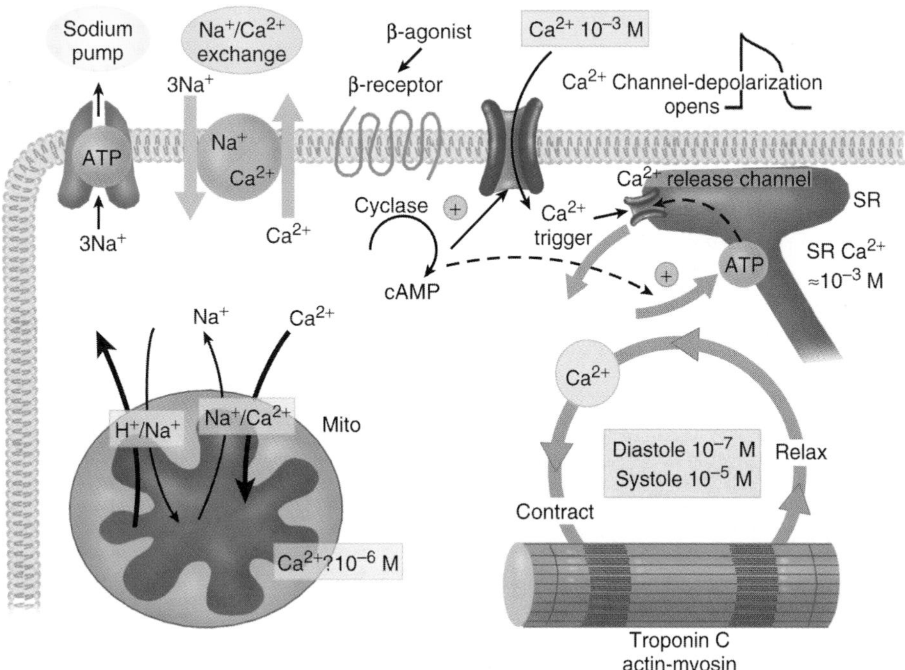

FIGURE 19–7 Calcium fluxes in the myocardium. Crucial features are (1) entry of Ca^{2+} ions through the voltage-sensitive L-type Ca^{2+} channels, acting as a trigger for the release of Ca^{2+} ions from the sarcoplasmic reticulum (SR); (2) the effect of beta-adrenergic stimulation with adenylate cyclase forming cyclic adenosine monophosphate (cAMP), the latter helping both to open the Ca^{2+} channel and to increase the rate of uptake of Ca^{2+} into the SR; and (3) exit of Ca^{2+} ions chiefly through Na^+/Ca^{2+} exchange, with the sodium pump thereafter extruding the Na^+ ions thus gained. The latter process requires adenosine triphosphate. Note the much higher extracellular (10^{-3} M) than intracellular cytosolic Ca^{2+} values, with much higher calcium values in the SR because of its storage function, and a hypothetical mitochondrial value of about 10^{-6} M. The mitochondria can act as a buffer against excessive changes in the free cytosolic calcium concentration. MITO = mitochondria. (From Opie LH: Heart Physiology, from Cell to Circulation. Philadelphia, Lippincott Williams & Wilkins, 2004. Copyright L. H. Opie, © 2004.)

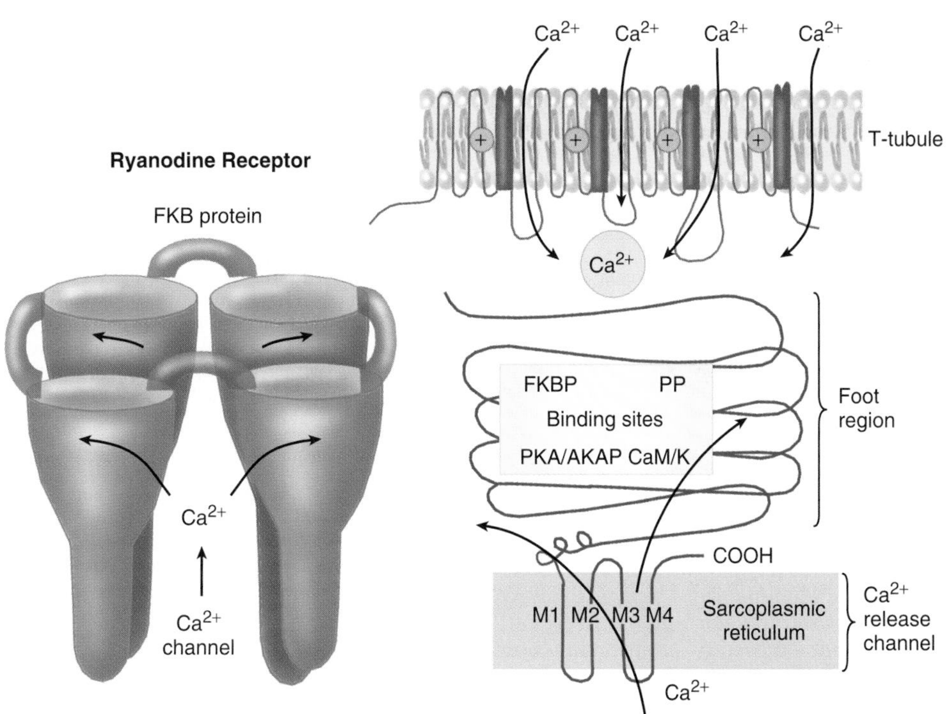

FIGURE 19–8 Role of ryanodine receptor (RyR) in calcium-induced calcium release. The RyR protein forms a link between the T tubule and the SR and is a scaffolding protein (which binds other proteins such as kinases and phosphatases). The result is a macromolecular complex, also called the "foot" region. One high-affinity RyR is composed of four RyR monomer proteins. The molecular model of one RyR is shown schematically at the right. The four RyR proteins make a single calcium release channel, in a manner similar to the formation of some other ion channels (schematic, left). Depolarization stimulates the L-type calcium channel of the T tubule to allow calcium ion entry. The incoming calcium binds to the RyR to cause molecular conformational changes that result in opening of the calcium release channel and calcium release from the SR. AKAP = anchoring protein for PKA; CaM/K = calmodulin or calmodulin kinase; FKBP = FK506 binding protein; PKA = protein kinase A; PP = protein phosphatases. (From Opie LH: Heart Physiology, from Cell to Circulation. Philadelphia, Lippincott Williams & Wilkins, 2004. Copyright L. H. Opie, © 2004.)

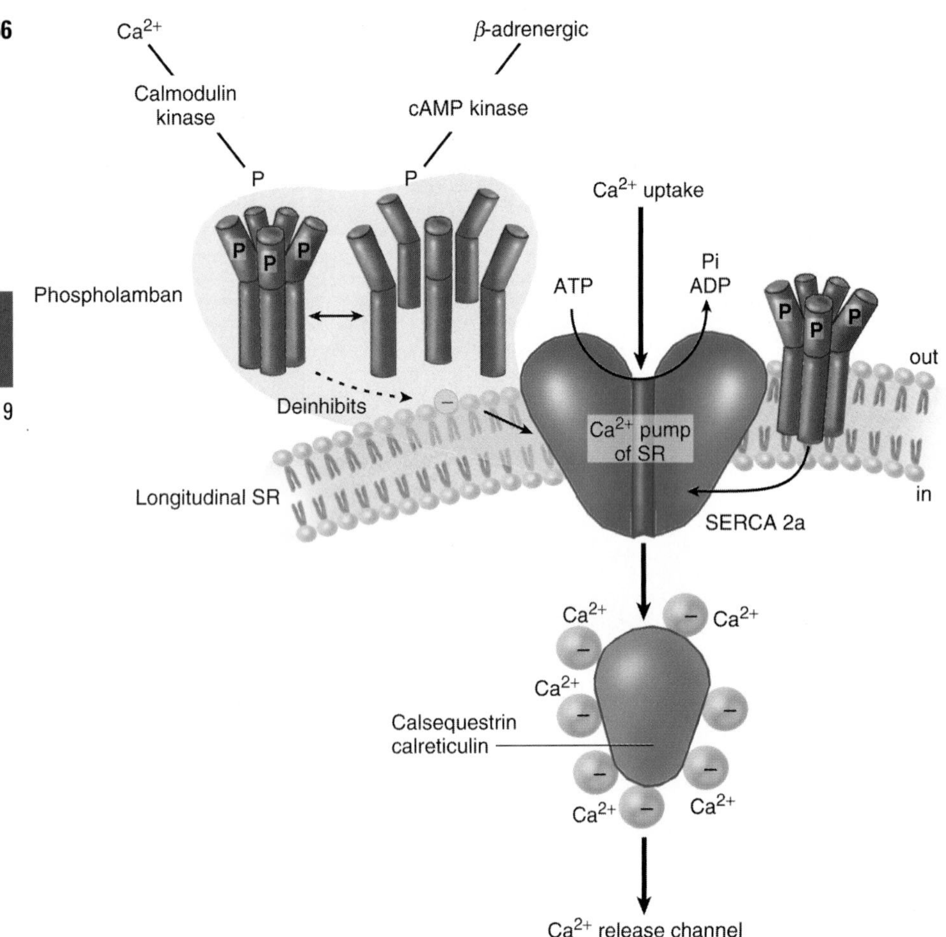

FIGURE 19–9 Lusitropic mechanism of calcium uptake into the sarcoplasmic reticulum (SR) by the energy-requiring calcium pump sarcoendoplasmic reticulum Ca^{2+}-adenosine triphosphatase ($SERCA_{2a}$). Phospholamban can be phosphorylated (P) to remove the inhibition exerted by its dephosphorylated form (positive charges) on the calcium pump. Thereby, calcium uptake is increased in response to either enhanced cytosolic calcium or beta-adrenergic stimulation. Thus, there are two phosphorylations activating phospholamban at two distinct sites and their effects are additive. An increased rate of uptake of calcium into the SR enhances the rate of relaxation (*lusitropic effect*). cAMP = cyclic adenosine monophosphate; P_i = inorganic phosphate. (Modified from Opie LH: Heart Physiology, from Cell to Circulation. Philadelphia, Lippincott Williams & Wilkins, 2004. Copyright L. H. Opie, © 2004.)

membrane (junctin and triadin) may help regulate the properties of the ryanodine receptor.[27]

Sarcolemmal Control of Calcium and Sodium Ions

Calcium Channels

All current models of excitation-contraction coupling ascribe a crucial role to the voltage-induced opening of the sarcolemmal L-type calcium channels in the initiation of the contractile process. Channels are pore-forming macromolecular proteins that span the sarcolemmal lipid bilayer to allow a highly selective pathway for ion transfer into the heart cell when the channel changes from a closed to an open state. Ion channels have two major properties: gating and permeation. Guarding each channel are two or more hypothetical gates that control its opening. Ions can permeate through the channel only when both gates are open. In the case of the sodium and calcium channels, which are best understood, the activation gate is shut at the normal resting membrane potential and the inactivation gate is open so that the channels are *voltage gated.* Depolarization opens the activation gate.

MOLECULAR STRUCTURE OF L-TYPE CALCIUM CHANNELS. There is a superfamily of voltage-gated ion channels that includes both the sodium and calcium channels and some of the potassium channels.[27] The potassium channels have a simpler structure from which it is thought that the more complex sodium and calcium channels evolved. Both sodium and calcium channels contain a major alpha subunit with four transmembrane subunits or domains that are similar to each other in structure. In addition, both sodium and calcium channels include in their overall structure a number of other subunits whose function is less well understood, such as the alpha subunit. Each of the four transmembrane domains of the alpha subunit is made up of six helices and is folded in on itself so that the four S5-S6 spans combine structurally to form the single functioning *pore* of each calcium channel (Fig. 19-10).[28]

Activation is now understood in molecular terms as the change in charge on the fourth transmembrane segment, S4, called the *voltage sensor,* of each of the four subunits of the sodium or calcium channel.[28] *Inactivation* is the process whereby the current initially elicited by depolarization decreases with time despite continuation of the original stimulus. Channels are not simply open or closed. Rather, the open state is the last of a sequence of many molecular states, varying from a fully closed to a fully open configuration. Therefore, it is more correct to speak of the *probability of channel opening.*

CURRENT ACTIVATION AND DEACTIVATION. Having been activated by depolarization, the L-type calcium current is inactivated by (1) the rising voltage during depolarization, at a more positive potential than for activation; and (2) the rising internal calcium ion concentration. Especially the calcium flowing from the ryanodine receptor pushes up the subsarcolemmal internal calcium ion concentration near the mouth of the L channels of the T tubules to help terminate current flow.[29]

CALCIUM CHANNEL PHOSPHORYLATION. The $alpha_1$ subunit (the organ-specific subunit) of the sarcolemmal calcium channel can be phosphorylated at several sites especially in the C-terminal tail.[27] During beta-adrenergic stimulation, cyclic AMP increases within the cell and phosphate groups are transferred from ATP to the $alpha_1$ subunit. Thereby, the electrical charges near the inner mouth of the nearby pores are altered to induce changes in the molecular conformation of the pores so that there is an increased probability of opening of the calcium channel.

T- AND L-TYPE CALCIUM CHANNELS. There are two major subpopulations of sarcolemmal calcium channels relevant to the cardiovascular system, namely the T channels and the L channels. The T (transient) channels open at a more negative voltage, have short bursts of opening, and do not interact with conventional calcium antagonist drugs.[28] The T channels presumably account for the earlier phase of the opening of the calcium channel, which may also give them a special role in the early electrical depolarization of the sinoatrial node and hence initiation of the heartbeat. Although T channels are found in atrial cells, their existence in normal ventricular cells is controversial. T channels are not found in T tubules despite the coincidental sharing of the T.[19] Rather, the sarcolemmal L (long-lasting) channels are the standard calcium channels found in the myocardium and the T tubules; they are involved in calcium-induced calcium release and are inhibited by calcium channel blockers such as verapamil, diltiazem, and the dihydropyridines.

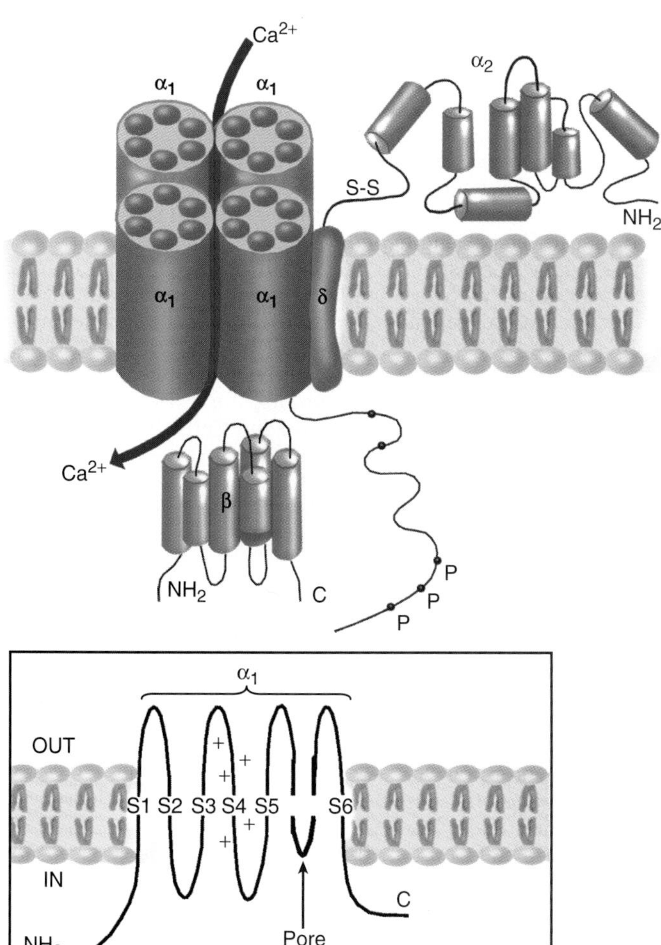

FIGURE 19–10 Simplified model of Ca^{2+} channel showing the alpha$_1$ subunit (α_1) forming the central pore, the regulatory beta-subunit (β), and alpha$_2$ and delta subunits of unknown function. Beta-adrenergic stimulation, by means of cyclic adenosine monophosphate, promotes phosphorylation (P) and the opening probability of the Ca^{2+} channel. The proposal is that four domains, each similar to that shown at the bottom and composed of six spanning segments, combine to form the alpha$_1$ subunit. Segment S4 is thought to respond to voltage depolarization (+ = positive charges) by altering the molecular configuration of the loop between S5 and S6 (part of the pore) so that there is a greater probability of Ca^{2+} ions entering (channel opens). (**Top,** modified from Varadi G, Mori Y, Mikala G, Schwartz A: Molecular determinants of Ca^{2+} channel function and drug action. Trends Pharmacol Sci 16:43, 1995; **Bottom,** modified from Tomaselli GF, Backx PH, Marban E: Molecular basis of permeation in voltage-rated ion channels. Circ Res 72:491, 1993. Copyright 1993, American Heart Association.)

Ion Exchangers and Pumps

To balance the small amount of calcium ions entering the heart cell with each depolarization, a similar quantity must leave the cell by one of two processes. First, calcium can be exchanged for sodium ions entering by Na^+/Ca^{2+} exchange, and, second, an ATP-consuming sarcolemmal calcium pump can transfer calcium into the extracellular space against a concentration gradient.

SODIUM-CALCIUM EXCHANGER. During relaxation, the sarcoplasmic calcium uptake pump and the Na^+/Ca^{2+} exchanger compete for the removal of cytosolic calcium, with the SR pump normally being dominant.[19] Restitution of calcium balance takes place by the activity of a series of transsarcolemmal exchangers, the chief of which is the Na^+/Ca^{2+} exchanger (see Fig. 19–17). The exchanger (molecular weight 108 kDa) consists of 970 amino acids and does not have substantial homology to any other known protein. The direction of ion exchange is responsive to the membrane potential and to the concentrations of sodium and calcium ions on either side of the sarcolemma. Because sodium and calcium ions can exchange either inward or outward in response to the membrane potential, there must be a specific membrane potential, called the *reversal* or *equilibrium potential*, at which the ions are so distributed that they can move as easily one way as the other. The reversal potential may lie about halfway between the resting membrane potential and the potential of the fully depolarized state.

The other major factor influencing the exchanger is the concentration of sodium and calcium ions on either side of the sarcolemma. Changing the membrane potential from the resting value of, say, −85 mV to +20 mV in the phase of rapid depolarization of the action potential and entry of sodium ions therefore briefly reverse the direction of Na^+/Ca^{2+} exchange. Thus, the sodium ions that have just entered during the opening of the sodium channel tend to leave, and calcium ions tend to enter. This process, thought to occur more in larger mammals with slow heart rates and long action potential durations, contrasts with the standard "forward mode" (Na^+ in, Ca^{2+} out) and is called "reverse mode" exchange. Such transsarcolemmal calcium entry may participate in calcium-induced calcium release.[19] In myocytes from the failing human heart, enhanced reversed exchange contributes to the slow decline of the Ca^{2+} transient,[30] which may explain delayed diastolic relaxation (see Impaired Relaxation and Cytosolic Calcium). Prolongation of the action potential duration also provokes reverse mode exchange, with risk of ventricular arrhythmias.[19]

Heart Rate and Na^+/Ca^{2+} Exchange. This exchanger may participate in the force-frequency relationship (treppe or Bowditch phenomenon). According to the "sodium pump lag" hypothesis, the rapid accumulation of calcium ions during fast stimulation of the myocardium outstrips the ability of the Na^+/Ca^{2+} exchanger and the sodium pump to achieve return to ionic normality. The result is an accumulation of calcium ions within the SR and an increased force of contraction.

SODIUM PUMP (Na^+,K^+-ATPase). The sarcolemma becomes highly permeable to Na^+ only during the opening of the Na^+ channel during early depolarization, and Na^+ also enters during the exit of Ca^{2+} by Na^+/Ca^{2+} exchange. Most of this influx of Na^+ across the sarcolemma must be corrected by the activity of the Na^+/K^+ pump, also called the Na^+, K^+-ATPase pump or simply the Na^+ pump. The pump is activated by internal Na^+ or external K^+.[31] One ATP molecule is used per transport cycle. The ions are first secluded within the pump protein and then extruded to either side. Although there has been some dispute about the exact ratio of Na^+ to K^+ ions that are pumped, a generally accepted model is that for each three Na^+ exported, two K^+ are imported. During this process, one positive charge must leave the cell. Hence, the pump is electrogenic and is also called the electrogenic Na^+ pump.[31] The current induced by sustained activity of the pump may contribute about −10 mV to the resting membrane potential.[28] Because the pump must extrude Na^+ ions entering by either Na^+/Ca^{2+} exchange or by the Na^+ channel, its sustained activity is essential for the maintenance of normal ion balance.

Beta-Adrenergic Signal Systems

Families of Receptors Coupled to G Proteins

The autonomic nervous system can initiate signal systems that profoundly alter the fluxes of calcium and other ions. Both adrenergic and cholinergic receptors belong to the family of seven transmembrane-spanning receptors, also called the G protein–coupled receptors.[32] The sum total of these processes converting an extracellular hormonal or neural stimulus to an intracellular physiological change is called *signal transduction*, which typically starts with the agonist binding to a receptor site. Thus, adrenergic or cholinergic stimulation of the sarcolemmal receptors inaugurates the activity of a complex system of sarcolemmal and cytosolic messengers. Occupancy of the beta-adrenergic receptor is coupled by a G protein complex (Figs. 19–11 and 19–12) to activation of a sarcolemmal enzyme, *adenylyl cyclase* (also called adenylate cyclase or shortened to adenyl cyclase), that sets in motion a series of signals that terminate with activation by phosphorylation of certain crucial proteins, such as those of the calcium channel (see Fig. 19–12).

Other cardiac receptors, such as the alpha-adrenergic receptor, have an alternative dual messenger system involving inositol triphosphate (IP_3) and diacylglycerol, with the latter activating protein kinase C (PKC). Such signals are of established importance in controlling calcium flux in vascular smooth muscle, thereby regulating vascular tone and indirectly the blood pressure. In the case of cardiac myocytes, it is now appreciated that receptors coupled to PKC, such as angiotensin II, may play a major role in the regulation of cardiac myocyte growth and sometimes may have inotropic effects. Yet other messenger systems exist to convey different signals. For example, in blood vessels, nitric oxide (NO) formed in the inner endothelial layer stimulates the formation of cyclic guanosine monophosphate (GMP) in the smooth muscle layer, thereby causing relaxation (vasodilation).

Beta-Adrenergic Receptor Subtypes

Cardiac beta-adrenergic receptors are chiefly the $beta_1$ subtype, whereas most noncardiac receptors are $beta_2$. There are also $beta_2$ receptors in the human heart, about 20 percent of the total beta receptor population in the left ventricle and about twice as high a percentage in the atria. $Beta_3$ receptors have also been identified and are probably of major importance only in heart failure. Whereas the $beta_1$ receptors are linked to the stimulatory G protein, G_s, component of the G protein–adenylyl cyclase system, $beta_2$ receptors are linked to both G_s and the inhibitory G_i, so that controversially their signaling pathway bifurcates at the first postreceptor step.[33] Hypothetically, $beta_2$ receptors are normally more strongly coupled to G_s, but in heart failure this coupling is weakened and that to G_i is strengthened.[33] The beta-adrenergic receptor site is highly stereospecific, the best fit among catecholamines being obtained with the synthetic agent isoproterenol (ISO) rather than with the naturally occurring catecholamines norepinephrine (NE) and epinephrine (E). In the case of $beta_1$ receptors, the order of agonist activity is ISO > E = NE, whereas in the case of $beta_2$ receptors, the order is ISO > E > NE. Human $beta_1$ and $beta_2$ receptors have now been cloned.[34] The transmembrane domains are held to be the site of agonist and antagonist binding, whereas the cytoplasmic domains interact with G proteins. One of the phosphorylation sites on the terminal COOH tail may be involved in desensitization (see next section).

G Proteins

THE STIMULATORY G PROTEIN G_S. G proteins are a superfamily of proteins that bind guanosine triphosphate (GTP) and other guanine nucleotides. G proteins are crucial in carrying the signal onward from the first messenger and its receptor to the activity of the membrane-bound enzyme system that produces the second messenger (see Fig. 19–12).[35] The triple combination of the beta receptor, the G protein complex, and adenylate cyclase is termed the *beta-adrenergic system*. The G protein itself is a heterotrimer composed of G_α, G_β, and G_γ, which upon receptor stimulation splits into the alpha subunit that is bound to GTP and the beta-gamma subunit. Either of these subunits may regulate different effectors such as adenylate cyclase, phospholipase C, and ion channels. The activity of adenylate cyclase is controlled by two different G protein complexes, namely G_s, which stimulates, and G_i, which inhibits. The alpha subunit of G_s ($alpha_s$) combines with GTP and then separates off from the other two subunits to enhance the activity of adenylate cyclase. The beta and gamma subunits (beta-gamma) appear to be linked structurally and in function.

THE INHIBITORY G PROTEIN, G_I. In contrast, a second trimeric GTP-binding protein, G_i, is responsible for inhibition of adenylate cyclase.[35] During cholinergic signaling, the muscarinic receptor is stimulated and GTP binds to the inhibitory alpha subunit ($alpha_i$). The latter then dissociates from the other two components of the G protein complex, which are, as in the case of G_s, the combined beta-gamma subunits.

The beta-gamma subunits act as follows. By stimulating the enzyme GTPase, they

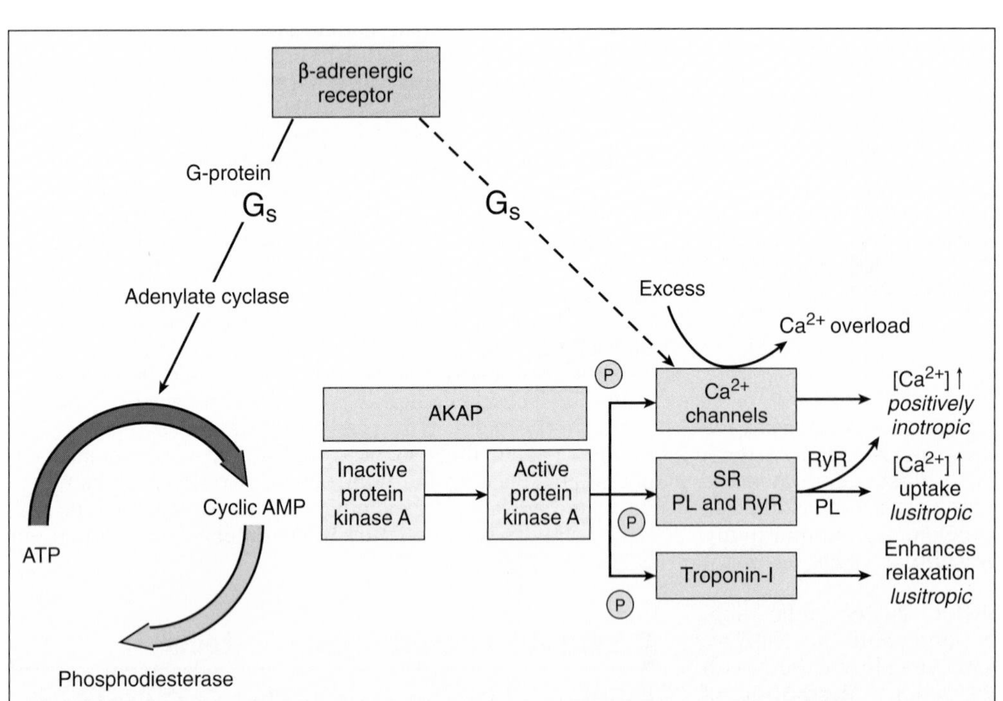

FIGURE 19–11 Key role of protein kinase A (PKA) in the beta-adrenergic response. The major intracellular effects of beta-agonist catecholamines occur by formation of cyclic adenosine monophosphate (Cyclic AMP), which increases the activity of the cAMP-dependent PKA. The latter achieves its optimal intracellular site by localizing to the scaffolding protein, A-kinase anchoring protein (AKAP), whereupon PKA phosphorylates various proteins concerned with contraction and relaxation. PL = phospholamban; RyR = ryanodine receptor; SR = sarcoplasmic reticulum. For inotropic and lusitropic mechanisms, see Figure 19–12. (Modified from Opie LH: Heart Physiology, from Cell to Circulation. Philadelphia, Lippincott Williams & Wilkins, 2004. Copyright L. H. Opie, © 2004.)

break down the active alpha$_s$ subunit (alpha$_s$-GTP) so that the activation of adenylate cyclase in response to alpha stimulation becomes less. Furthermore, the beta-gamma subunit activates the K_{ACh} channel, which, in turn, can inhibit the sinoatrial node to contribute to the bradycardiac effect of cholinergic stimulation. The alpha$_i$ subunit activates another potassium channel (K_{ATP}) whose physiological function in the myocardium is still unclear. Pathophysiologically, preconditioning may link to this channel (see later).

THE THIRD G PROTEIN, G_Q. G_q links a group of heptahelical (*hepta* = seven) myocardial receptors, including the alpha-adrenergic receptor and those for angiotensin II and endothelin, to another membrane-associated enzyme, phospholipase C, and thence to PKC (see later). G_q has at least four isoforms, of which two have been found in the heart. This G protein, unlike G_i, is not susceptible to inhibition by the pertussis toxin. Overexpression of G_q in mice induced a dilated cardiomyopathy,[36] which is of interest because angiotensin II and endothelin, which act through Gq, are overactive in human heart failure. Conversely, when the activity of G_q is genetically inhibited, the hypertrophic response to pressure overload is attenuated, and wall stress increases, but cardiac function is relatively well maintained.[37]

CYCLIC ADENOSINE MONOPHOSPHATE AND PROTEIN KINASE A

Adenylyl Cyclase. Adenylyl cyclase is a transmembrane enzyme system, also called adenylate or adenyl cyclase, that responds to input from G proteins. When stimulated by G_s, adenylyl cyclase produces the second messenger cyclic AMP, which then acts through a further series of intracellular signals and specifically the third messenger PKA to increase cytosolic calcium transients. In contrast, cholinergic stimulation exerts inhibitory influences, largely on the heart rate but also on contraction, acting at least in part by decreasing the rate of formation of cyclic AMP.

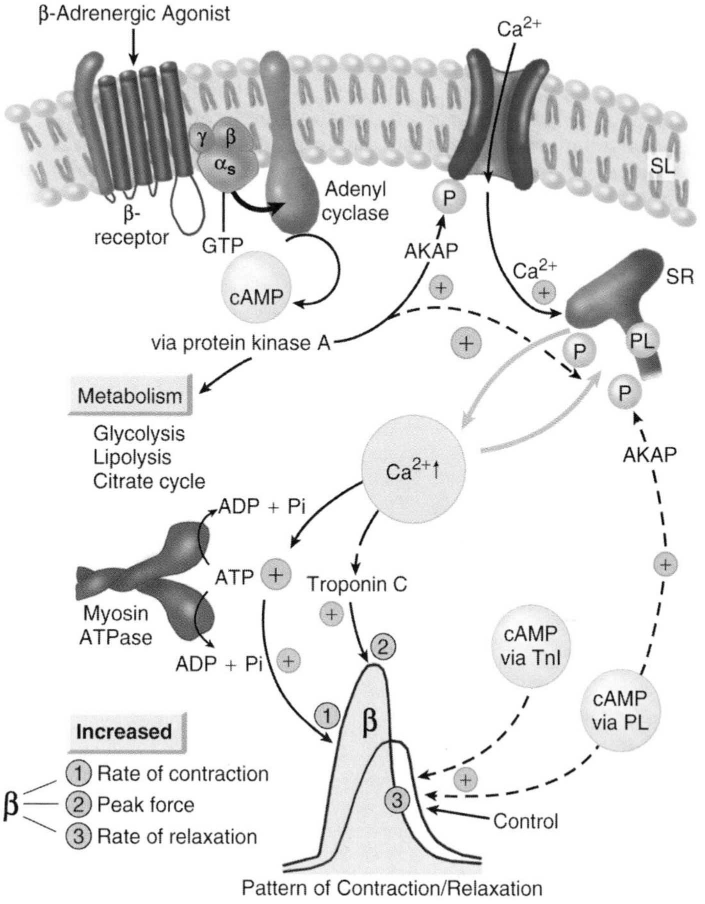

FIGURE 19–12 Signal systems involved in positive inotropic and lusitropic (enhanced relaxation) effects of beta-adrenergic stimulation. When the beta-adrenergic agonist interacts with the beta receptor, a series of G protein–mediated changes (see Fig. 19–11) lead to activation of adenylate cyclase and formation of cyclic adenosine monophosphate (cAMP). The latter acts through protein kinase A to stimulate metabolism (on the left) and to phosphorylate the calcium channel protein. The result is an enhanced opening probability of the calcium channel, thereby increasing the inward movement of Ca^{2+} ions through the sarcolemma (SL) of the T tubule. These Ca^{2+} ions release more calcium from the sarcoplasmic reticulum (SR) (see Fig. 19–7) to increase cytosolic calcium and to activate troponin C. Calcium ions also increase the rate of breakdown of ATP to ADP and inorganic phosphate (P_i). Enhanced myosin adenosine triphosphatase (ATPase) activity explains the increased rate of contraction with increased activation of troponin C explaining increased peak force development. An increased rate of relaxation is explained because cAMP also activates the protein phospholamban, situated on the membrane of the SR that controls the rate of uptake of calcium into the SR (see Fig. 19–9). The latter effect explains enhanced relaxation (lusitropic effect). AKAP = A-kinase anchoring protein; P = phosphorylation; PL = phospholamban. For TnI see Fig. 19–3. (Modified from Opie LH: Heart Physiology, from Cell to Circulation. Philadelphia, Lippincott Williams & Wilkins, 2004. Copyright L. H. Opie, © 2004.)

Adenylyl cyclase is the only enzyme system producing cyclic AMP and specifically requires low concentrations of ATP (and magnesium) as substrate. Surprisingly, the proposed molecular structure resembles that of certain channel proteins, such as that of the calcium channel. Most of the protein is located on the cytoplasmic side, the presumed site of interaction with the G protein. Another cyclic nucleotide, cyclic GMP, acts as a second messenger for some aspects of vagal activity. In vascular smooth muscle, cyclic GMP is the second messenger of the NO messenger system. These messenger chemicals are present in the heart cell in minute concentrations, that of cyclic AMP being roughly about 10^{-9} M and that of cyclic GMP about 10^{-11} M.

Cyclic AMP has very rapid turnover as a result of a constant dynamic balance between its formation by adenylate cyclase and removal by another enzyme, phosphodiesterase. In general, directional changes in the tissue content of cyclic AMP can be related to directional changes in cardiac contractile activity. For example, beta-adrenergic stimulation increases both, whereas beta blockade inhibits the increases induced by beta agonists. *Forskolin*, a direct stimulator of adenylate cyclase, increases cyclic AMP and contractile acivity. Adenosine, acting through A_1 receptors, inhibits adenylate cyclase, decreases cyclic AMP, and lessens contractile activity. A number of hormones or peptides can couple to myocardial adenylate cyclase independently of the beta-adrenergic receptor. These are glucagon, thyroid hormone, prostacyclin (prostaglandin I_2), and the calcitonin gene-related peptide.

INHIBITION OF ADENYLYL CYCLASE. The major physiological stimulus to G_i is thought to be vagal muscarinic receptor stimulation. In addition, adenosine, by interaction with A_1 receptors, couples to G_i to inhibit contraction and heart rate. The adenosine A_2 receptor paradoxically increases cyclic AMP. The latter effect, only of ancillary significance in the myocardium, is of major importance in vascular smooth muscle, where it induces vasorelaxation. Pathologically, inhibitory G_i is increased in experimental postinfarct heart failure[38] and in donor hearts prior to cardiac transplantation.[39]

CYCLIC AMP–DEPENDENT PROTEIN KINASES. It is now clear that most, if not all, of the effects of cyclic AMP are ultimately mediated by PKA, which phosphorylates various key proteins and enzymes (see Fig. 19–11).[40] *Phosphorylation* is the donation of a phosphate group to the enzyme concerned, acting as a fundamental metabolic switch that can extensively amplify the signal.

Each protein kinase is composed of two subunits, regulatory (R) and catalytic (C). When cyclic AMP (cAMP) interacts with the inactive protein kinase, it binds to the R subunit to liberate the active kinase, which is the C subunit:

$$(R_2 + C_2) + 2cAMP \rightarrow 2RcAMP + 2C$$

At a molecular level, this active kinase catalyzes the transfer of the terminal phosphate of ATP to serine and threonine residues of the protein substrates, leading to phosphorylation and modification of the properties of the proteins concerned and thereby promoting further key reactions. PKA occurs in different cells in two isoforms: PKA-II predominates in cardiac cells. The proposed anchorage of this kinase by *A-kinase anchoring proteins* (AKAPs) to specific organelles such as the SR explains the phenomenon of cyclic AMP compartmentation[40] because anchored PKA requires focal elevation of cyclic AMP even at an unchanged cytosolic concentration. In addition, the G protein system may not be evenly spread throughout the sarcolemma but may be localized to certain focal areas. Thus, it is likely that there is only a specific subcompartment of cyclic AMP available to increase contractile activity.

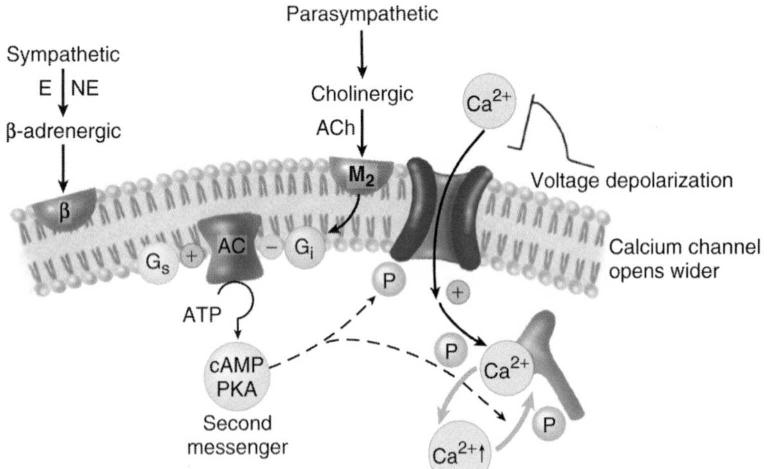

PHYSIOLOGICAL BETA$_1$-ADRENERGIC EFFECTS. The probable sequence of events describing the positive inotropic effects of catecholamines is as follows (Fig. 19–13).

> Catecholamine stimulation → beta receptor → molecular changes → binding of GTP to alpha$_s$ subunit of G protein → GTP alpha$_s$ subunit stimulates adenylyl cyclase → formation of cyclic AMP from ATP → activation of cyclic AMP-dependent protein kinase (PKA), locally bound by an A-kinase anchoring protein (AKAP) → phosphorylation of a sarcolemmal protein p27 → increased entry of calcium ion through increased opening of the voltage-dependent L-type calcium channels → greater calcium-induced calcium release through ryanodine receptor of SR, coupled with phosphorylation of the ryanodine receptor → greater and more rapid rise of intracellular free calcium ion concentration → increased calcium–troponin C interaction with deinhibition of tropomyosin effect on actin-myosin interaction → increased rate and number of cross bridges interacting with increased myosin ATPase activity → increased rate and peak of force development.

FIGURE 19–13 Interaction between sympathetic and parasympathetic systems could best be explained by the inhibitory effect on the formulation of cyclic adenosine monophosphate (cAMP), including formation of inhibitory G protein G_i in response to M_2 receptor stimulation. AC = adenylyl cyclase; ACh = acetylcholine; E = epinephrine; NE = norepinephrine; PKA = protein kinase A. (Modified from Opie LH: Heart Physiology, from Cell to Circulation. Philadelphia, Lippincott Williams & Wilkins, 2004. Copyright L. H. Opie, © 2004.)

The increased *lusitropic (relaxant)* effect is the consequence of increased PKA-mediated phosphorylation of phospholamban (see Fig. 19–12). Also, increased phosphorylation of troponin I may help to desensitize the contractile apparatus to calcium ions.

Physiological Switch-Off, Beta-Agonist Receptor Kinase, and Arrestin

There is a potent feedback mechanism whereby the degree of postreceptor response to a given degree of beta-adrenergic receptor stimulation can be muted (Fig. 19–14). Sustained beta-agonist stimulation rapidly induces the activity of the beta-agonist receptor kinase (βARK) that is involved in the transfer of the phosphate group to the phosphorylation site on the terminal COOH tail of the receptor, a process that of itself does not markedly affect the signaling properties. Rather, βARK increases the affinity of the beta receptor for another protein family, the *arrestins*, which cause the uncoupling. Beta-arrestin is a scaffolding protein that links to one of the cytoplasmic loops of the G protein–coupled beta-adrenergic receptor,[41] thus uncoupling receptor occupancy from G_s and activation of adenylyl cyclase, and thereby inhibiting the functioning of this receptor. Resensitization of the receptor occurs if the phosphate group is split off by a phosphatase and the receptor may then be more readily linked to G_s.

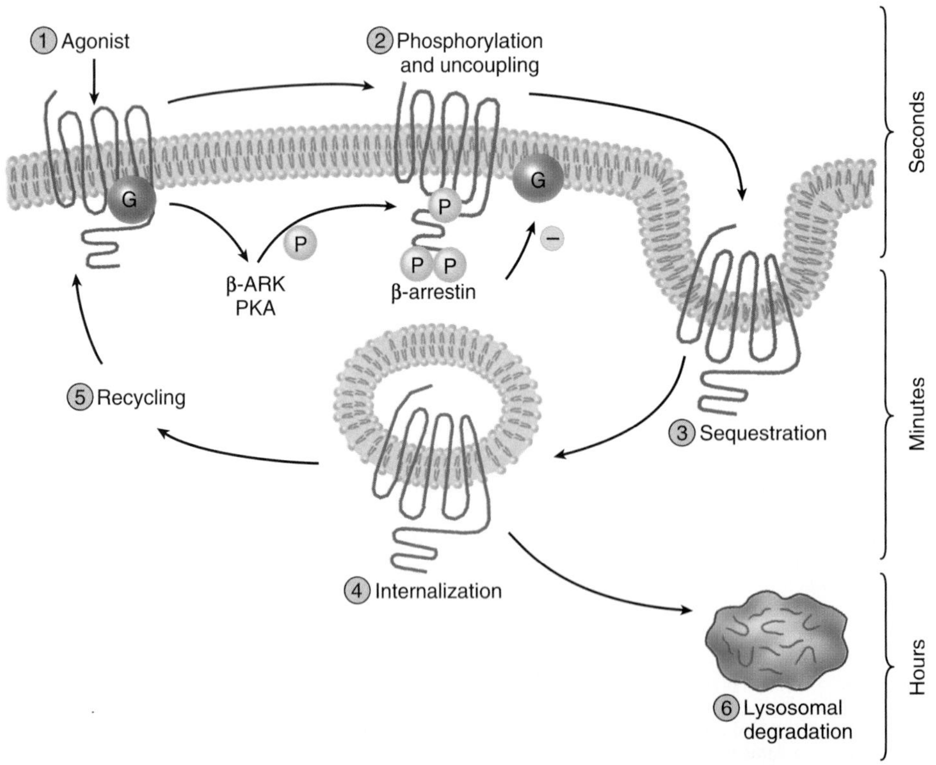

FIGURE 19–14 Mechanisms of beta-adrenergic receptor desensitization and internalization. Note links between the internalized receptor complex with growth stimulation through mitogen-activated protein (MAP) kinase. βARK = beta-agonist receptor kinase; PKA = protein kinase A. (Modified from Hein L, Kobilka BK: Adrenergic receptors. From molecular structures to in vivo function. Trends Cardiovasc Med 7:137, 1997.)

> Physiologically, the βARK-arrestin mechanism helps to terminate the beta receptor signal by a rapid *desensitization of the beta receptor* within minutes to seconds (see Fig. 19–14). This mechanism also plays a role in long-term desensitization of the beta-adrenergic receptor

in heart failure. Because beta-arrestin is a scaffolding protein, it simultaneously activates other systems[41] such as the tyrosine kinases, leading to growth by ultimately linking to MAP kinase.[42] Thus, prolonged beta receptor stimulation may have growth as an end result rather than conventional inotropic and lusitropic endpoints. Although the βARK-arrestin effects are best described for the $beta_2$ receptor, they also occur to a lesser extent with the $beta_1$ receptor.[43] These changes in postreceptor signaling may help to explain some of the harm of excess beta stimulation and relative upregulation of the $beta_2$ receptor in heart failure.

ISCHEMIC INACTIVATION OF βARK. As outlined, βARK regulates beta-adrenergic activity by phosphorylation of the target receptor. Following ischemia, there is a decrease in βARK activity and loss of the ability of increased beta stimulation to be desensitized.[44] Following coronary ligation, this loss of regulatory ability coincides with a phase of increased fatal ventricular arrhythmias,[44] presumably the result of increased beta-adrenergic activity.

$BETA_2$ AND $BETA_3$ ADRENERGIC EFFECTS. In the normal ventricle, about 20 percent of the receptors are $beta_2$ in nature; yet in heart failure this percentage of the whole can double because of $beta_1$ receptor downregulation (see Heart Failure). The $beta_2$ postreceptor signaling involves both the stimulatory and the inhibitory G proteins.[45] In humans, the positive inotropic response to $beta_2$ stimulation by salbutamol occurs, at least in part, through $beta_2$ receptors on the terminal neurons of the cardiac sympathetic nerves, thereby releasing norepinephrine, which in turn exerts dominant $beta_1$ effects.[46] Indirect evidence suggests that the G_i inhibitory path is relatively augmented in heart failure, whereas the strength of the stimulatory G_s path is lessened because of uncoupling of G_s from the $beta_2$ receptor.

Regarding *$beta_3$-adrenergic receptors*, their stimulation results in a negative inotropic effect through NO and formation of inhibitory cyclic GMP.[47] These effects resemble those of cholinergic stimulation (see next section). Physiologically, the role of the $beta_3$ receptor system could be pictured as opposing adverse effects of excess $beta_1$ stimulation such as too rapid a heart rate. In heart failure the $beta_3$ receptors are relatively upregulated (see later) and may contribute to the overall spectrum of adversely altered beta-adrenergic stimulation rather than promoting contraction (Fig. 19–15).

Cholinergic and Nitric Oxide Signaling

Cholinergic Signaling

Parasympathetic stimulation reduces heart rate and is negatively inotropic. The key features of its signaling system are similar to that of the $beta_1$-adrenergic system. There are again an extracellular first messenger (acetylcholine), a receptor system (the cholinergic muscarinic receptor), a sarcolemmal signaling system (the G protein system, specifically the inhibitory G_i), and a second messenger (cyclic GMP). The myocardial *muscarinic receptor* (M_2) is associated specifically with the activity of the vagal nerve endings. Receptor stimulation produces a negative chronotropic response that is inhibited by atropine. NO facilitates cholinergic signaling at two levels, the nerve terminal and the activity of the enzyme system that produces cyclic GMP.

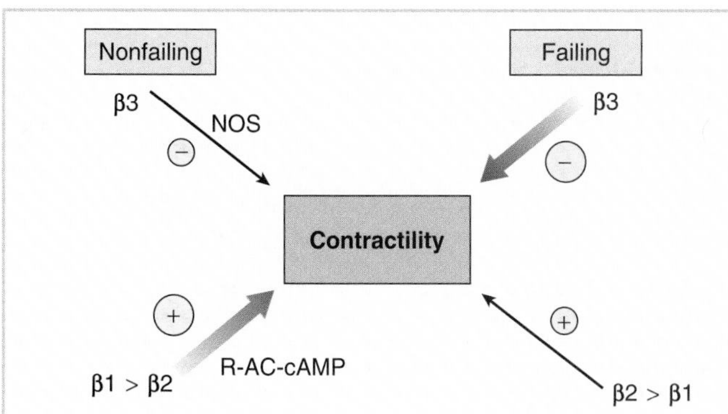

FIGURE 19–15 Proposed role of $beta_3$-adrenergic receptors. Normally, beta-adrenergic stimulation increases contractility, acting largely through the $beta_1$ receptors with backup from the $beta_2$ receptors. The $beta_3$-adrenergic receptors mediate cardioinhibitory signals that may counterbalance excess adrenergic stimulation, through nitric oxide and cyclic guanosine monophosphate (see Fig. 19–17), according to the proposals of Moniotte and colleagues.[120] In heart failure, the $beta_1$ receptors are downregulated (see Fig. 19–34) and the $beta_2$ receptors uncoupled so that their combined inotropic input is diminished. Conversely, $beta_3$ receptors are upregulated with a manifest negative inotropic effect despite some nitric oxide downregulation.[120] AC = adenylyl cyclase; cAMP = cyclic adenosine monophosphate; NOS = endothelial nitric oxide synthase; R = receptor.

THE MECHANISM OF VAGAL HEART RATE LOWERING. Cyclic GMP acts as a second messenger to vagal stimulation just as cyclic AMP does to beta-adrenergic stimulation. Of note, cell-permeable analogs of cyclic GMP have antiadrenergic effects. Cholinergic stimulation of the M_2 receptor activates guanylyl (= guanylate = guanyl) cyclase to form cyclic GMP, with consequent stimulation of protein kinase G that results in inhibitory cardiac effects such as a decreased heart rate and negative inotropic response.[48] These effects are largely achieved by modulation of calcium ion entry through the L calcium channel and through inhibition of internal calcium cycling.[49] In addition, muscarinic M_2 stimulation acts through G_i to lessen the G_s activation that results from beta receptor occupation. Thus, the vagus has a dual effect on second messengers, inhibiting the formation of cyclic AMP and increasing that of cyclic GMP, thereby providing one of several explanations for *sympathetic-parasympathetic interaction.*

Regarding the *negative inotropic effect of vagal stimulation* (see Fig. 19–16), the mechanism includes (1) heart rate slowing (negative treppe phenomenon), (2) inhibition of the formation of cyclic AMP, and (3) a direct negative inotropic effect mediated by cyclic GMP. It has been controversial whether ventricular tissue is as responsive to muscarinic agonists as atrial tissue, although the receptor populations are similar in density. However, using pressure-volume loops and the slope of the pressure-volume relationship (see E_s in Fig. 19–26) as an index of contractility, vagal stimulation in humans markedly decreased this load-independent measure.[50]

The sympathetic terminal neurons are another site of parasympathetic-sympathetic interaction (see Fig. 19–17). There the presynaptic muscarinic M_2 receptor inhibits the release of norepinephrine. In addition, both adrenergic and cholinergic stimuli exert important and often opposing effects on ion channels and cardiac function (Table 19–2). The presence of such multiple mechanisms for the inhibitory effects of vagal stimulation on the heart rate, the inotropic state, and arrhythmogenicity, suggests that "braking" of beta-adrenergic stimulation is desirable. Otherwise, the risk may be that intense beta-adrenergic stimulation would excessively increase the heart rate or inotropic state or provoke potentially fatal arrhythmias.

Nitric Oxide, the Ubiquitous Messenger
(Figs. 19–16, 19–17)

NO, the focus of a Nobel Prize for 1998, is a unique messenger in that it is formed in so many tissues, is a gas, and is a physiological free radical that should more correctly (but infrequently) be written as •NO. Nonetheless, the standard abbreviation is NO. It is generated in the heart by one of three isoenzymes.[49] Vasodilatory NO is generated in the vascular endothelium by endothelial nitric oxide synthase (eNOS, also called NOS-3) in response to increased blood flow, increased cardiac load, or bradykinin. It is induced in cardiomyocytes in disease states such as cardiogenic or septic shock by the inducible enzyme (iNOS, also called NOS-2). Generation of NO by neuronal NOS (nNOS, also called NOS-1), the form of the synthase found in vagal nerve terminals, enhances the release of acetylcholine.[51] Exercise training leads to increased formation of NO through iNOS in animals[51] and through

TABLE 19–2 Ionic Effects of Adrenergic and Cholinergic Stimulation: Relation to Heart Rate and Contractile Activity

Agonist	Ionic Current	Effect
Beta-adrenergic stimulation*,†	I_{Ca} increased I_K increased I_{Ks} increased‡ I_{to} increased I_f increased I_{Na} increased	+Inotropic ↓APD, ↑filling time ↓APD, ↑filling time ↓APD, ↑filling time ↑Heart rate ↑Contraction, ↑conduction
Acetylcholine (ACh) during beta stimulation*,§	I_{Ca} decreased I_{Na} decreased I_f decreased	–Inotropic –Dromotropic –Chronotropic
ACh direct effect on K^+ currents‖	I_{kACh} and I_{kATP} increased	Heart rate↓
Alpha-adrenergic stimulation¶	I_{to} decreased I_k decreased I_{kACh} decreased	+Inotropic +Inotropic Atrial current, effects not clear

*Data from Matsuda et al.[130]
†Data from Matsuda et al.[131]
‡Data from Volders et al.[135]
§Data from Chang and Cohen[132]
‖Data from Kurachi.[133]
¶Data from Fedida.[134]
– = negative; + = positive; ↑ = increased; ↓ = decreased; APD = action potential duration; ATP = adenosine triphosphate.

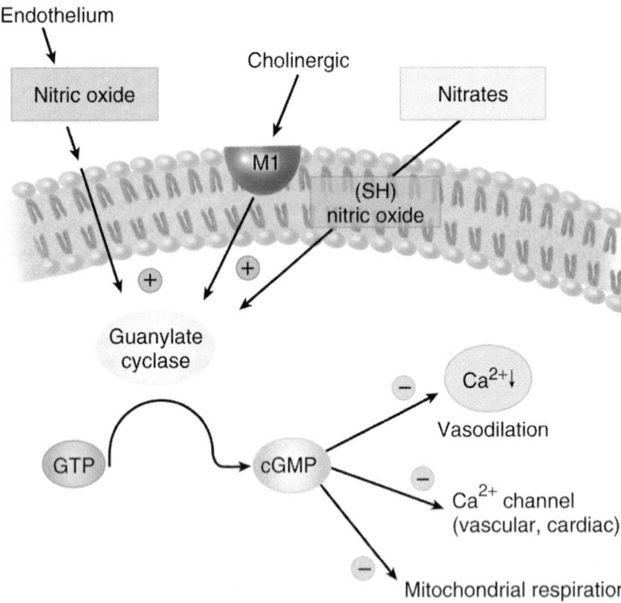

FIGURE 19–16 Nitric oxide messenger system. Proposed role of nitric oxide in stimulating soluble guanylate cyclase to form cyclic guanosine monophosphate (cGMP) to cause vasodilation and a negative inotropic effect. Antianginal nitrates also cause coronary vasodilation by this mechanism. GTP = guanosine triphosphate; M1 = muscarinic receptor, subtype 1. (Modified from Opie LH: Heart Physiology, from Cell to Circulation. Philadelphia, Lippincott Williams & Wilkins, 2004. Copyright L. H. Opie, © 2004.)

eNOS in humans with coronary disease.[52] Because the activity of guanylyl cyclase, promoted by cholinergic stimulation, is sensitive to and enhanced by NO,[48] previous concepts are revised in that NO is now seen as augmenting parasympathetic simulation both upstream and downstream from acetylcholine.

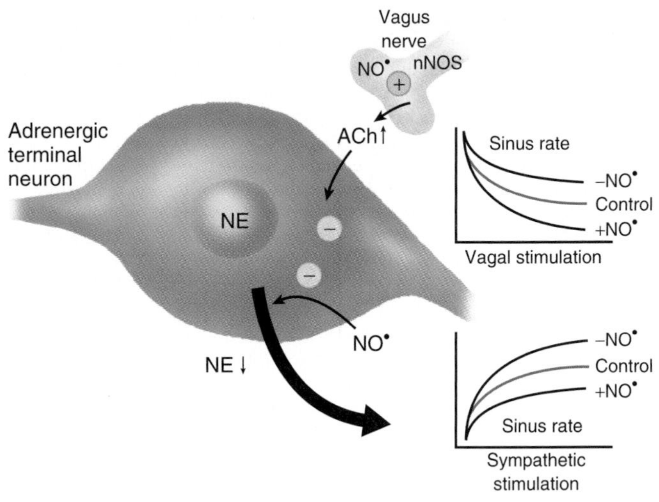

FIGURE 19–17 Nitric oxide (NO) mediates release of acetylcholine (ACh) from vagal nerve terminals. NO, produced in the terminal vagal nerve endings, increases the release of ACh and decreases that of norepinephrine (NE). Thus, the sinus rate response to either vagal or sympathetic stimulation is changed accordingly. For concept, see Paterson.[51] nNOS = neuronal nitric oxide synthase. (Modified from Opie LH: Heart Physiology, from Cell to Circulation. Philadelphia, Lippincott Williams & Wilkins, 2004. Copyright L. H. Opie, © 2004.)

Protective Role of Nitric Oxide. NO contributes to both early and late phases of preconditioning (see later), either as part of the protective messenger systems invoked by ischemia or by inhibition of mitochondrial calcium uptake.[53]

Adverse Effects of Excess Nitric Oxide. Whereas physiological amounts of NO are cardioprotective, substantial evidence indicates that excess NO is harmful. The free radical peroxynitrite ($ONOO^-$), formed from NO and superoxide, leads to the conversion product nitrotyrosine, both with toxic myocardial effects. Examples occur in septic or cardiogenic shock[54] or during prolonged nitrate therapy when peroxynitrite inhibits the formation of cyclic GMP to contribute to nitrate tolerance. Whereas physiological NO suppresses cell death through apoptosis, higher levels promote it.

Does Nitric Oxide Regulate Contractility? This role of NO is controversial. "Puffs" of NO may be formed in diastole to prolong diastole and ventricular filling.[55] Yet any effects on contractility are probably not direct but occur through the autonomic modulation of heart rate.[56]

Other Inhibitory Signal Systems

ADENOSINE SIGNALING. Adenosine, like NO, is a physiological vasodilator. It is formed from the breakdown of ATP both physiologically (as during an increased heart load) and pathologically (as in ischemia). Adenosine can diffuse from myocardial cells to act on coronary arterial smooth muscle to cause vasodilation. The mechanism of the latter effect is reasonably well understood and involves the stimulation of vascular adenylate cyclase and cyclic AMP formation. A_2 receptors mediate such vasodilation. Although A_2 receptors have also been identified in cardiomyocytes, stimulation of such receptors does not have functional consequences.[57] Therefore, it is only the A_1 receptors that are coupled to adenylate cyclase by the inhibitory G protein (alpha$_i$ subunit) that are functional in the myocardium.

Other signal systems and other receptor subtypes are also involved. First, A_1 receptors couple to the acetylcholine-sensitive potassium channel (current I_{KACh}) to stimulate channel opening and thereby to exert inhibitory effects on the sinus and atrioventricular nodes. The latter inhibition is the basis for the use of adenosine in the treatment of supraventricular nodal reentry arrhythmias. Second, A_1 receptors may couple to the PKC system, and thence to the ATP-sensitive potassium channel, thereby hypothetically explaining their role in preconditioning (see Preconditioning). Third, A_3 receptors also precondition through PKC but without the obvious hemodynamic effects of A_1 receptor stimulation.[58]

OPIOID RECEPTORS. Opioids released in the central nervous system are known to participate in cardiovascular regulation by inhibiting sympathetic and promoting parasympathetic outflow. Such endogenous opiates, called *endorphins*, may be involved in the benefits of cardiovascular training. In congestive heart failure, opioid activity may limit adrenergic activation. In animals, opioid receptor stimulation may help to explain the phenomenon of hibernation.[59] In addition, opioid drugs such as morphine are often used in cardiovascular medicine and may have effects beyond pain relief. Opioid effects may be mediated, in part, through local cardiovascular opioid receptors that respond to stimulation of the opioid system in response to conditions of physiological or psychosocial stress. There are three opioid receptors, delta, kappa, and mu, of which the first two are found in the human heart, whereas the mu receptors mediate signals that dampen the pain response. In the heart, the delta receptors inhibit the adrenergic system by coupling to G_i to inhibit the activation of adenylyl cyclase by beta-adrenergic stimulation. In addition, by stimulation of the PKC pathway (see later), they mediate preconditioning.[60]

Vasoconstrictive Signaling

VASCULAR G PROTEIN–COUPLED RECEPTORS. Agonists with vasoconstriction as their major physiological role are $alpha_1$-adrenergic catecholamines, angiotensin II, and endothelin (Fig. 19–18). By regulating the degree of vasoconstriction, the peripheral vascular resistance can be tuned to the needs of the circulation, with, for example, vasoconstriction occurring in response to $alpha_1$-adrenergic stimulation during the stress of blood loss. Each of these agonists is coupled to its appropriate seven-transmembrane-spanning receptor, linked through the G protein G_q to effectors different from those of adrenergic and cholinergic signaling. Specifically, a different calcium release signal system is involved to achieve vasoconstrictive calcium release in vascular tissue. The myocardial ryanodine receptor is replaced by that for IP_3. This IP_3 receptor has a high degree of molecular homology with the ryanodine receptor but is only about half its size. The IP_3 messenger system is of fundamental importance in regulating the release of calcium from the SR and thereby regulating arterial tone and hence the afterload against which the heart must work. In cardiac muscle, the role of IP_3 is still sufficiently controversial to question its role in the inotropic response.

VASOCONSTRICTIVE PATHS AND MYOCARDIAL GROWTH. IP_3 is one of two major signaling molecules produced by the G_q-mediated activation of phospholipase C that converts phosphatidylinositol to IP_3 and diacylglycerol. The latter activates PKC, once PKC has been translocated from the cytosol to the sarcolemma, for example, during the preconditioning sequence (see later). PKC is also implicated as a key activator of the MAP kinase path that leads to increased myocardial growth and LV hypertrophy, especially in response to receptor stimulation by angiotensin II. In addition, mechanically induced cytoskeletal distortion, acting through integrins and other structural proteins, can activate the MAP kinase cascade.[61] Whether the vasoconstrictive agonists can also act as backup positive inotropic agents for the myocardium remains controversial.

Cytokine Signaling

TUMOR NECROSIS FACTOR-ALPHA. Tumor necrosis factor-alpha (TNF-α) is one of the family of peptide cytokines that form part of the innate immune system. Such cytokines mediate local events and are distinct from circulating neurotransmitters or hormones. TNF-α stimulation has bifunctional effects, mediating both protective signals as a component of preconditioning[62] and adverse cardiodepressant signaling in response to diffuse myocardial ischemia as in embolization.[63] The signaling paths involved are complex, starting with two surface receptors for TNF-α leading through sphingolipids to apparently bifurcating paths. One path is adaptive and sends further signals through nuclear factor kappa B to the nucleus for the manufacture of protective molecules. The other maladaptive path leads to apoptosis through activation of caspases. These paths are neither simple nor well understood. For example, NO can act both upstream and downstream from TNF-α.[63] Currently, it is not known why the intracellular signaling paths activated by TNF-α sometimes lead to beneficial effects such as preconditioning and cell survival and at other times lead to depressed myocardial function and apoptosis. Two proposals are (1) that there are short-term adaptive and long-term maladaptive effects of TNF-α and (2) that low concentrations are adaptive and high concentrations maladaptive.[64]

Contractile Performance of the Intact Heart

There are three main determinants of myocardial mechanical performance, namely the Frank-Starling mechanism, the contractile state, and the heart rate. This section describes the cardiac cycle and then the determinants of LV function.

The Cardiac Cycle

The cardiac cycle, fully assembled by Lewis[65] but first conceived by Wiggers,[66] yields important information on the temporal sequence of events in the cardiac cycle. The three basic events are (1) LV contraction, (2) LV relaxation, and (3) LV filling (Table 19–3). Although similar mechanical events occur in the right side of the heart, it is those on the left side that are focused on.

LEFT VENTRICULAR CONTRACTION. LV pressure starts to build up when the arrival of calcium ions at the contractile proteins starts to trigger actin-myosin interaction (Fig. 19–19). On the electrocardiogram, the advance of the wave of depolarization is indicated by the peak of the R wave. Soon after, LV pressure in the early contraction phase builds up and exceeds that in the left atrium (normally 10 to 15 mm Hg) followed about 20 milliseconds later by M_1, the mitral component of the first heart sound. The exact relation of M_1 to mitral valve closure is open to dispute. Although mitral valve closure is often thought to coincide with the crossover point at which the LV pressure starts to exceed the left atrial pressure,[67] in reality mitral valve closure is delayed because the valve is kept open by the inertia of the blood flow. Shortly thereafter, pressure changes in the right ventricle, similar in pattern to those in the left ventricle but of lesser magnitude, cause the tricuspid valve to close, thereby creating T_1, which is the second component of the first heart sound. During this phase of contraction between mitral valve and aortic valve opening, the LV volume is fixed (*isovolumic contraction*) because both aortic and mitral valves are shut. As more and

TABLE 19–3 The Cardiac Cycle

Left Ventricular Contraction
Isovolumic contraction (b)
Maximal ejection (c)
Left Ventricular Relaxation
Start of relaxation and reduced ejection (d)
Isovolumic relaxation (e)
LV filling: rapid phase (f)
Slow LV filling (diastasis) (g)
Atrial systole or booster (a)

The letters a to g refer to the phases of the cardiac cycle shown in Wiggers' diagram (Fig. 19–19). These letters are arbitrarily allocated so that atrial systole (a) coincides with the A wave and (c) with the C wave of the jugular venous pressure.

LV = left ventricular.

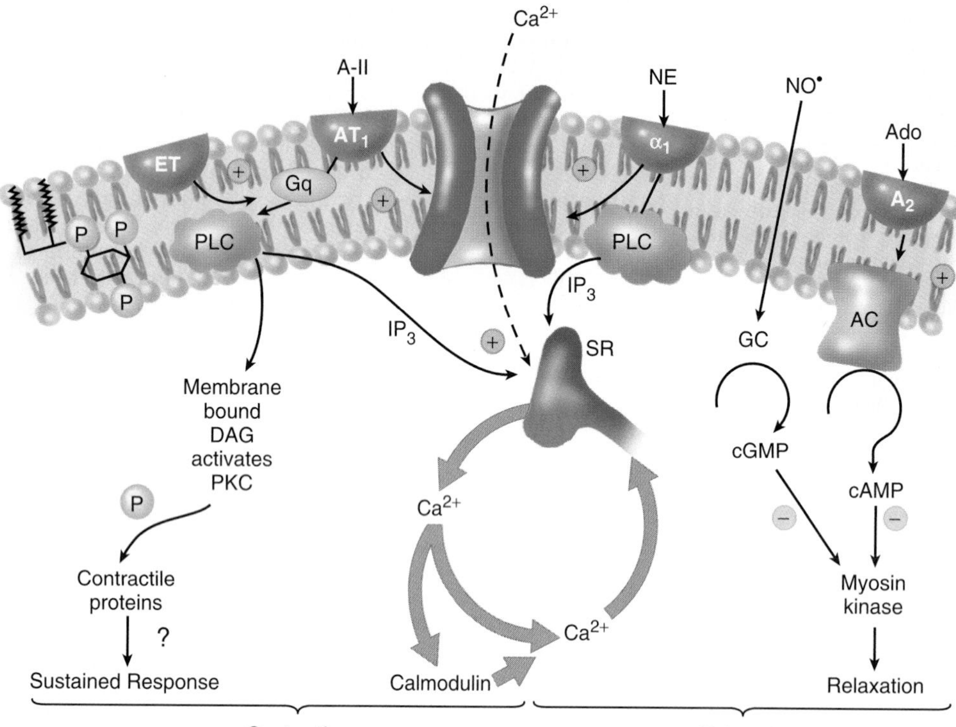

FIGURE 19–18 Patterns of contraction and relaxation in vascular smooth muscle. For example, the angiotensin II (A-II) signaling system is coupled through a G protein to phospholipase C (PLC), which breaks down phosphatidylinositol (PIP_2) to 1,2-diacylglycerol (DAG) and inositol triphosphate (IP_3). DAG translocates protein kinase C from cytosol to the sarcolemma, thereby activating PKC. Signals beyond PKC are not clear. It may phosphorylate ion channels to give the sustained vasoconstrictive response. IP_3 releases calcium from the sarcoplasmic reticulum to initiate vascular smooth muscle contraction. Other vasoconstrictors such as endothelin (ET receptor) act by the same signal system. In response to norepinephrine (NE), an alpha$_1$-agonist, a similar sequence of events occurs to promote contraction. Relaxation is achieved by inhibition of myosin kinase when either cyclic guanosine monophosphate (cGMP) or cyclic adenosine monophosphate (cAMP) is formed in response, respectively, to nitric oxide (NO•) or adenosine (A). AC = adenylyl cyclase; GC = guanylyl cyclase. (Modified from Opie LH: Heart Physiology, from Cell to Circulation. Philadelphia, Lippincott Williams & Wilkins, 2004. Copyright L. H. Opie, © 2004.)

more myofibers enter the contracted state, pressure development in the left ventricle proceeds. The interaction of actin and myosin increases, and cross-bridge cycling is augmented. When the pressure in the left ventricle exceeds that in the aorta, the aortic valve opens, usually a clinically silent event. Opening of the aortic valve is followed by the phase of *rapid ejection*. The rate of ejection is determined not only by the pressure gradient across the aortic valve but also by the elastic properties of the aorta and the arterial tree, which undergoes systolic expansion. LV pressure rises to a peak and then starts to fall.

LEFT VENTRICULAR RELAXATION. As the cytosolic calcium ion concentration starts to decline because of uptake of calcium into the SR under the influence of activated phospholamban, more and more myofibers enter the state of relaxation and the rate of ejection of blood from the left ventricle into the aorta falls (*phase of reduced ejection*). During this phase, blood flow from the left ventricle to the aorta rapidly diminishes but is maintained by aortic recoil—the Windkessel effect. The pressure in the aorta exceeds the falling pressure in the left ventricle. The aortic valve closes, creating the first component of the second sound, A_2 (the second component, P_2, results from closure of the pulmonary valve as the pulmonary artery pressure exceeds that in the right ventricle). Thereafter, the ventricle continues to relax. Because the mitral valve is closed during this phase, the LV volume cannot change (*isovolumic relaxation*). When the LV pressure falls to below that in the left atrium, the mitral valve opens (normally silent) and the filling phase of the cardiac cycle restarts (see Fig. 19–19).

LEFT VENTRICULAR FILLING PHASES. As LV pressure drops below that in the left atrium, just after mitral valve opening, the *phase of rapid or early filling* occurs to account for most of ventricular filling.[68] Active diastolic relaxation of the ventricle may also contribute to early filling (see section on ventricular suction). Such rapid filling may cause the physiological third heart sound (S_3), particularly when there is a hyperkinetic circulation.[69] As pressures in the atrium and ventricle equalize, LV filling virtually stops (*diastasis*, separation). Renewed filling requires that the pressure gradient from the atrium to the ventricle increase. This is achieved by *atrial systole* (or the *left atrial booster*), which is especially important when a high cardiac output is required as during exercise or when the left ventricle fails to relax normally as in LV hypertrophy.[68]

Definitions of Systole and Diastole

In Greek, *systole* means contraction and *diastole* means "to send apart." The start of systole can be regarded as either (1) the beginning of isovolumic contraction when LV pressure exceeds the atrial pressure or (2) mitral valve closure (M_1). These correspond reasonably well because mitral valve closure actually occurs only about 20 milliseconds after the crossover point of the pressures. Thus, in practice the term isovolumic contraction often also includes this brief period of early systolic contraction even before the mitral valve shuts, when the heart volume does not change substantially. *Physiological systole* lasts from the start of isovolumic contraction (at which LV pressure crosses over atrial pressure, see Fig. 19–19) to the peak of the ejection phase, so that physiological diastole commences as the LV pressure starts to fall (Table 19–4).

TABLE 19–4 Physiological Versus Cardiologic Systole and Diastole

Physiological Systole Isovolumic contraction Maximal ejection	**Cardiologic Systole** From M_1 to A_2, including: Major part of isovolumic contraction* Maximal ejection Reduced ejection
Physiological Diastole Reduced ejection Isovolumic relaxation Filling phases	**Cardiologic Diastole** A_2-M_1 interval (filling phases included)

*Note that M_1 occurs with a definite albeit short delay after the start of LV contraction.

This concept fits well with the standard pressure-volume curve. *Physiological diastole* commences as calcium ions are taken up into the SR, so that myocyte relaxation dominates over contraction, and the LV pressure starts to fall as shown on the pressure-volume curve. In contrast, *cardiological systole* is demarcated by the interval between the first and second heart sounds, lasting from the first heart sound (M_1) to the closure of the aortic valve (A_2). The remainder of the cardiac cycle automatically becomes *cardiological diastole*. Thus, cardiological systole, demarcated by heart sounds rather than physiological events, starts fractionally later than physiological systole and ends significantly later. For the cardiologist, *protodiastole* is the early phase of rapid filling, the time when the third heart sound (S_3) can be heard. This sound probably reflects ventricular wall vibrations during rapid filling and becomes audible with an increase in LV diastolic pressure or wall stiffness or rate of filling.

In contrast stands another physiological concept, promulgated by Brutsaert and colleagues,[70] who argued that diastole starts much later, only when the whole of the contraction-relaxation cycle is over. According to this minority view, diastole would occupy only a short portion of the cardiac cycle.[70] This definition of diastole, although seldom used in cardiological practice, does give a reminder that abnormalities of LV contraction often underlie defective relaxation.

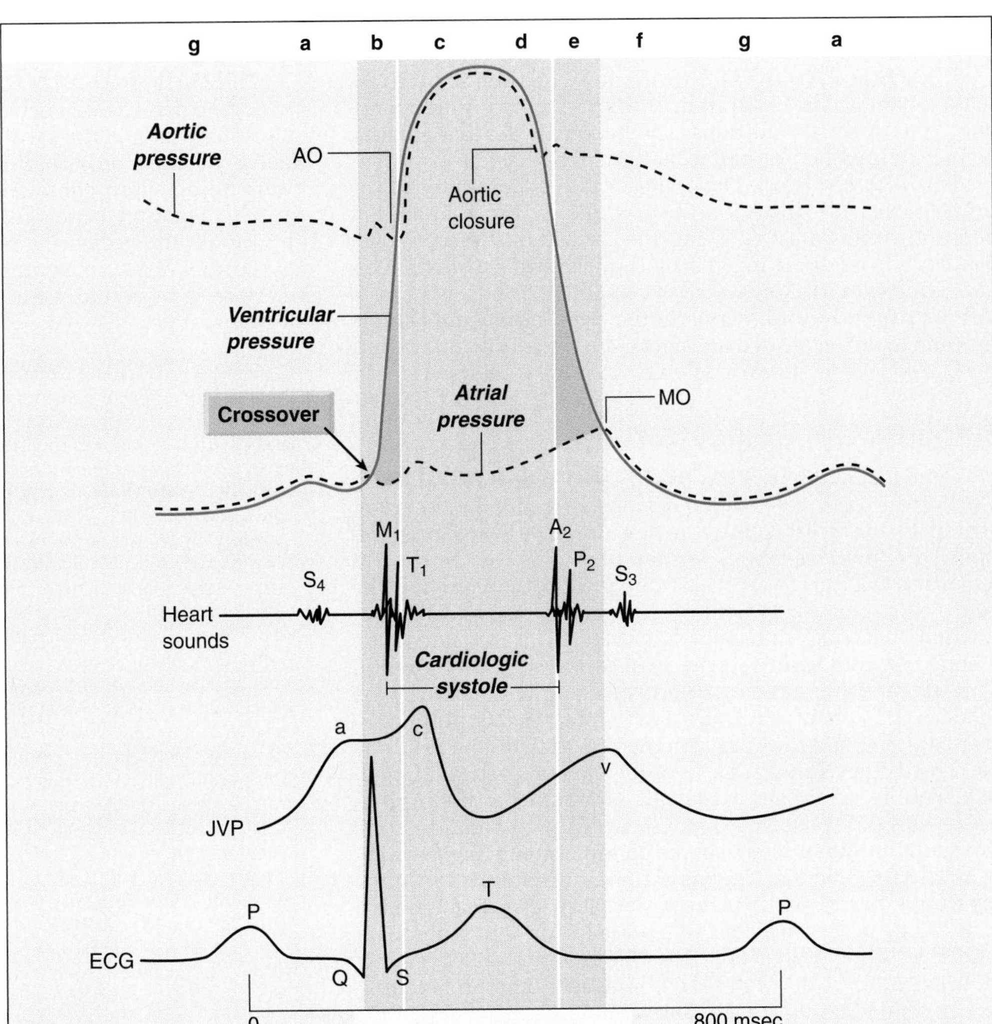

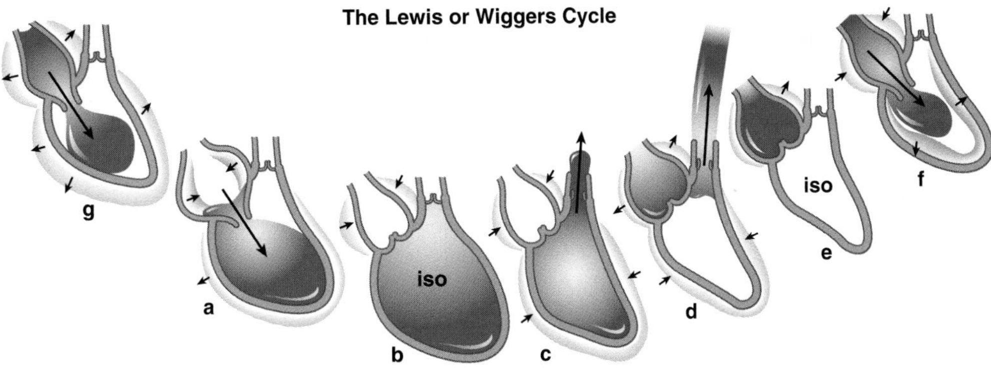

FIGURE 19–19 The mechanical events in the cardiac cycle, first assembled by Lewis in 1920[65] but first conceived by Wiggers in 1915.[66] Note that mitral valve closure occurs *after* the crossover point of atrial and ventricular pressures at the start of systole. For an explanation of phases a to g, see Table 19–3. Cycle length of 800 milliseconds for 75 beats/min. A_2 = aortic valve closure, aortic component of second sound; AO = aortic valve opening, normally inaudible; ECG = electrocardiogram; JVP = jugular venous pressure; M_1 = mitral component of first sound at time of mitral valve closure; MO = mitral valve opening, may be audible in mitral stenosis as the opening snap; P_2 = pulmonary component of second sound, pulmonary valve closure; S_3 = third heart sound; S_4 = fourth heart sound; T_1 = tricuspid valve closure, second component of first heart sound; a = wave produced by right atrial contraction; c = carotid wave artifact during rapid left ventricular ejection phase; v = venous return wave, which causes pressure to rise while tricuspid valve is closed. (Visual phases of the ventricular cycle at the bottom modified from Shepherd JT, Vanhoutte PM: The Human Cardiovascular System. New York: Raven Press, 1979, p 68. Modified from Opie LH: Heart Physiology, from Cell to Circulation. Philadelphia, Lippincott Williams & Wilkins, 2004.)

Contractility Versus Loading Conditions

CONTRACTILITY. *Contractility is the inherent capacity of the myocardium to contract independently of changes in the preload or afterload.* It is a key word in our cardiological language. At a molecular level, an increase in contractility can be explained by enhanced interaction between calcium ions and the contractile proteins. Increased contractility means a greater rate of contraction to reach a greater peak force. Often, an increased contractility is associated with enhanced rates of relaxation, called the *lusitropic effect*. Alternative names for contractility are the *inotropic state* (*ino*, fiber; *tropos*, to move) and the *contractile state*. Contractility is an important regulator of the myocardial oxygen uptake. Factors that increase contractility include exercise, adrenergic stimulation, digitalis, and other inotropic agents.

PRELOAD AND AFTERLOAD. It is important to stress that any change in the contractile state should be independent of the loading conditions. The *preload* is the load present before contraction has started, at the end of diastole (the afterload is discussed later). The preload reflects the venous filling pressure that fills the left atrium, which in turn fills the left ventricle during diastole. When the preload increases, the left ventricle distends during diastole, and the stroke volume rises according to Starling's law (see next section). The heart rate is also increased by stimulation of the atrial mechanoreceptors that enhance the rate of discharge of the sinoatrial node. Thus, the cardiac output (stroke volume times heart rate) rises.

Starling's Law of the Heart

VENOUS FILLING PRESSURE AND HEART VOLUME. Starling in 1918 related the venous pressure in the right atrium to the heart volume in the dog heart-lung preparation.[28] He proposed that, within physiological limits, the larger the volume of the heart, the greater the energy of its contraction and the amount of chemical change at each contraction. Starling did not, however, measure sarcomere length. He could only relate *LV volume* to cardiac output. This relationship holds in normal, compliant hearts. One modern version of Starling's law is that stroke volume is related to the end-diastolic volume. The LV volume can now be directly measured with two-dimensional echocardiography. Yet the value found depends on a number of simplifying assumptions such as a spherical LV shape and neglects the confounding influence of the complex anatomy of the left ventricle. In practice, therefore, the LV volume is not often measured; rather, use is made of a variety of surrogate measures such as LV end-diastolic pressure or the pulmonary capillary wedge pressure. Yet the relation between LV end-diastolic volume and LV end-diastolic pressure is curvilinear depending on the LV compliance.

The venous filling pressure can be measured in humans albeit indirectly by the technique of *Swan-Ganz catheterization*, as can the stroke volume. The LV pressure and volume are, however, not linearly related because of variations in the compliance of the myocardium. Therefore, a jump from pressure to volume is required to apply the Starling concept to the hemodynamic management of those who are critically ill and receiving a Swan-Ganz catheter.

FRANK AND ISOVOLUMIC CONTRACTION. If a larger heart volume increases the initial length of the muscle fiber, to increase the stroke volume and hence the cardiac output, then diastolic stretch of the left ventricle actually increases contractility. Frank in 1895 had already reported that the greater the initial LV volume, the more rapid the rate of rise, the greater the peak pressure reached, and the faster the rate of relaxation.[28] He described both a positive *inotropic effect* and an increased lusitropic effect. These complementary findings of Frank and Starling are often combined into the *Frank-Starling law*. Between them, they could account for two of the mechanisms underlying the increased stroke volume of exercise, namely both the increased diastolic filling (Starling's law) and the increased inotropic state (Frank's findings).

AFTERLOAD. The afterload is the systolic load on the left ventricle after it has started to contract. In the nonfailing heart, the left ventricle can overcome any physiological acute increase in load. Chronically, however, the left ventricle must hypertrophy to overcome sustained arterial hypertension or significant aortic stenosis. In clinical practice, the arterial blood pressure is often taken to be synonymous with the afterload while ignoring the *aortic compliance*—the extent to which the aorta can "yield" during systole. A stiff aorta, as in isolated systolic hypertension of elderly people, increases the afterload.

PRELOAD AND AFTERLOAD ARE INTERLINKED. The preceding distinctions between preload and afterload do not allow for the situations in which the two change concurrently. By the Frank-Starling law, an increased LV volume leads to increased contractility, which in turn increases the systolic blood pressure and hence the afterload. Nonetheless, in general, the preload is related to the degree to which the myocardial fibers are stretched at the end of diastole, and the afterload is related to the wall stress generated by those fibers during systole.

FORCE-LENGTH RELATIONSHIPS AND CALCIUM TRANSIENTS. Proof that there is no increase in the calcium transient as the sarcomere length increases is provided by direct measurements (Fig. 19-20). The favored explanation for the steep length-tension relation of cardiac muscles is *length-dependent activation*, whereby an increase in calcium sensitivity is the major factor explaining the steep increase of force development as the initial sarcomere length increases. This change may be explained by stretch of the titin molecule (see Fig. 19-4). Is the degree of overlap of actin and myosin also involved? Whereas the overlap theory explains the force-length relationship in skeletal muscle, in cardiac muscle the situation is different (Fig. 19-21). In cardiac muscle, even at 80 percent of the maximal length, only 10 percent or less of the maximal force is developed. Thus, it can be predicted that cardiac sarcomeres must function near the upper limit of their maximal length (L_{max}). Rodriguez and colleagues[71] have tested this prediction by relating sarcomere length changes to volume changes of the intact heart. By implanting small radiopaque beads in only about 1 cm^3 of the LV free wall and using biplane cineradiography, the motion of the markers could be tracked through various cardiac cycles with allowances made for local myocardial deformation. Thus, the change in sarcomere length from approximately 85 percent of L_{max} to L_{max} itself is able to effect physiological LV volume changes (Fig. 19-22). This estimate is remarkably close to the normal fiber shortening of 15 percent in the human heart in situ.[72]

ANREP EFFECT: ABRUPT INCREASE IN AFTERLOAD. When the aortic pressure is elevated abruptly, a positive inotropic effect follows within 1 or 2 minutes. This effect used to be called homeometric autoregulation (*homeo*, the same; *metric*, length) because it was apparently independent of muscle length and by definition a true inotropic effect. A reasonable speculation would be that increased LV wall tension could act on myocardial stretch receptors to increase cytosolic sodium and then, by Na^+/Ca^{2+} exchange, the cytosolic calcium. Thus, this effect would be different from that of an increase in preload (which acts by length activation).

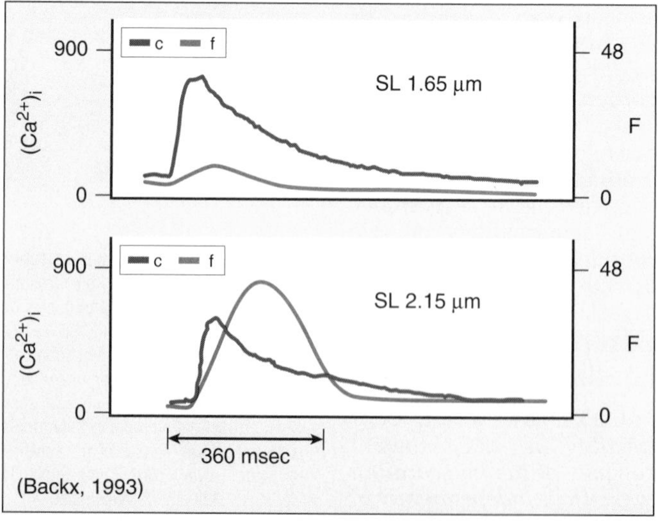

FIGURE 19–20 Length sensitization of the sarcomere. **Top,** The sarcomere length (SL) is 1.65 μm, which gives very little force (f) development (see Fig. 19–7). **Bottom,** At a near-maximum sarcomere length (see Fig. 19–7), the same Ca^{2+} transient (c) with the same peak value and overall pattern causes much greater force development. Therefore, there has been length-induced calcium sensitization. (Modified from Backx PH, ter Keurs HEDJ: Fluorescent properties of rat cardiac trabeculae microinjected with fura-2 salt. Am J Physiol 264:H1098, 1993.)

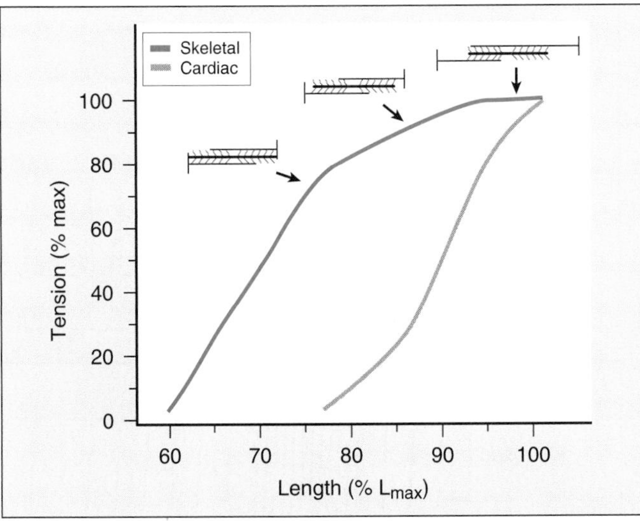

FIGURE 19–21 Force-length relationship. Schematic drawing illustrating general shape of ascending limb in skeletal (A) and cardiac (B) muscle. Normalized force is plotted as a function of normalized length, that is, length relative to the length at which maximum force is generated (L_{max}). Also shown is the approximate disposition of thick and thin filaments at different points along the physiologically relevant portion of the ascending limb. The maximum length (L_{max} 100%) corresponds to the situation at maximum sarcomere lengths, 2.2 mm (Fig. 19–22) or 2.15 mm (Fig. 19–20). (Modified from Fuchs F: Mechanical modulation of the Ca^{2+} regulatory protein complex in cardiac muscle. News Physiol Sci 10:6, 1995.)

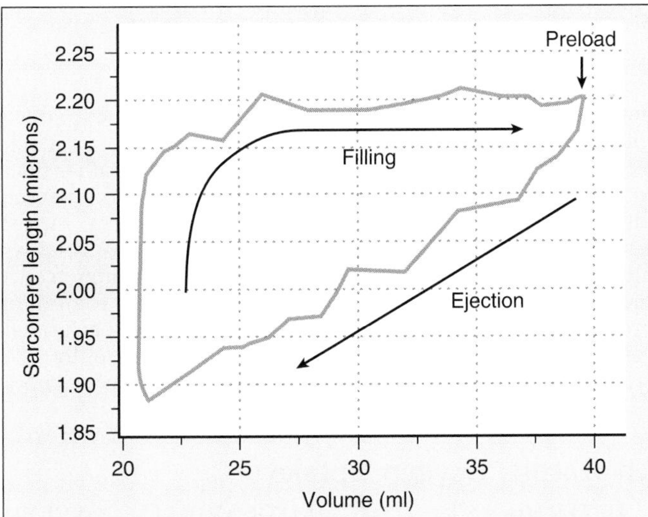

FIGURE 19–22 Changes in sarcomere length during a typical cardiac contraction-relaxation cycle. During diastole the sarcomere length is 2.2 μm, decreasing to 1.90 μm during systole in the intact dog heart. Starting at the top right, the *preload* is the maximum sarcomere length just before the onset of contraction. As ejection decreases the left ventricular volume, by somewhat more than half, sarcomere length falls from 2.20 to 1.90 μm. Then, during the rapid phase of filling (see Fig. 19–19), the sarcomere length increases from 1.90 to 2.15 mm to be followed by the phase of constant sarcomere length (diastasis). (Modified from Rodriguez EK, Hunter WC, Royce MJ, et al: A method to reconstruct sarcomere lengths and orientations to transmural sites in beating canine hearts. Am J Physiol 263:H293, 1992, with permission of the American Physiological Society.)

Wall Stress

Stress develops when tension is applied to a cross-sectional area, and the units are force per unit area. According to the Laplace law (Fig. 19–23):

$$\text{Wall stress} = \frac{\text{pressure} \times \text{radius}}{2 \times \text{wall thickness}}$$

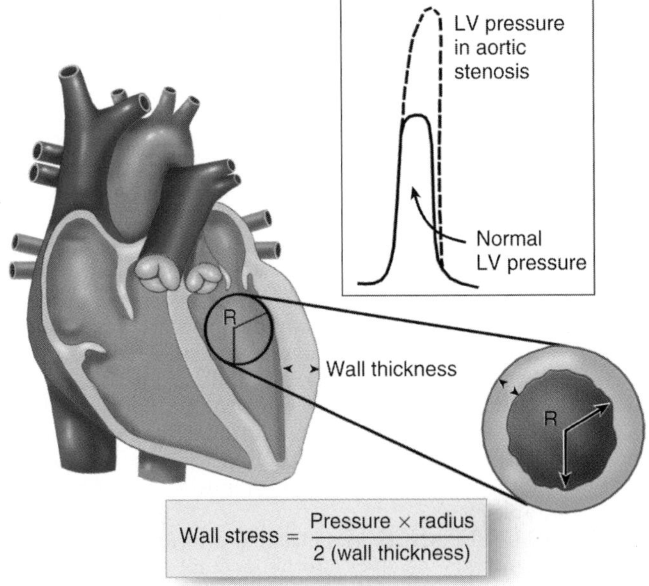

FIGURE 19–23 Wall stress increases as the afterload increases. The formula shown is derived from the Laplace law. The increased left ventricular (LV) pressure in aortic stenosis is compensated for by LV wall hypertrophy, which decreases the denominator on the right side of the equation. (Modified from Opie LH: Heart Physiology, from Cell to Circulation. Philadelphia, Lippincott Williams & Wilkins, 2004. Copyright L. H. Opie, © 2004.)

This equation, although an oversimplification, emphasizes two points. First, the bigger the left ventricle and the greater its radius, the greater the wall stress. Second, at any given radius (LV size), the greater the pressure developed by the left ventricle, the greater the wall stress. An increase in wall stress achieved by either of these two mechanisms (LV size or intraventricular pressure) increases myocardial oxygen uptake because a greater rate of ATP use is required as the myofibrils develop greater tension.

In cardiac hypertrophy, Laplace's law explains the effects of changes in wall thickness on wall stress (see Fig. 19–23). The increased wall thickness related to hypertrophy balances the increased pressure, and the wall stress remains unchanged during the phase of compensatory hypertrophy. This change, previously regarded as compensatory and beneficial, has been seriously challenged by a mouse model in which the process of hypertrophy was genetically inhibited so that wall stress increased in response to a pressure load, yet these mice had better cardiac mechanical function than the wild type that developed compensatory hypertrophy (see Chap. 21).[37] Despite this "mighty mouse" challenge, it is difficult to see how a patient with significant aortic stenosis could develop the intraventricular pressure required to eject blood through the stenosed valve without the development of LV hypertrophy. Another clinically useful concept is that in congestive heart failure, the heart dilates so that the increased radius elevates wall stress. Furthermore, because ejection of blood is inadequate, the radius stays too large throughout the contractile cycle, and both end-diastolic and end-systolic tensions are higher. Reduction of heart size decreases wall stress and improves LV function.

WALL STRESS, PRELOAD, AND AFTERLOAD. *Preload* can now be defined more exactly as the wall stress at the end of diastole and therefore at the maximal resting length of the sarcomere (see Fig. 19–22). Measurement of wall stress in vivo is difficult because the radius of the left ventricle (see preceding sections) neglects the confounding influence of the complex anatomy of the left ventricle. Surrogate measurements of the indices of preload include LV end-diastolic pressure or dimensions (the latter being the major and minor axes of the heart in a two-dimensional echocardiographic view). The *afterload*, being the load on the contracting myocardium, is also the wall stress during LV ejection. Increased afterload means that an increased intraventricular pressure has to be generated first to open the aortic valve and then during the ejection phase. These increases translate into an increased myocardial wall stress, which can be measured either as an average value or at end systole. *End-systolic wall stress* reflects the three major components of the afterload, namely the peripheral resistance, the arterial compliance, and the peak intraventricular pressure. Decreased arterial compliance and increased afterload can be anticipated when there is aortic dilation as in severe systemic hypertension or in elderly persons. Generally, in clinical practice, it is a sufficient approximation to take the systolic blood pressure as an indirect measure of the afterload (reflecting both peripheral resistance and peak intraventricular pressure), provided there is neither significant aortic stenosis nor change in arterial compliance.

AORTIC IMPEDANCE. Also termed *arterial input impedance*, aortic impedance gives another accurate measure of the afterload. The aortic impedance is the aortic pressure divided by the aortic flow at that instant, so that this index of the afterload varies at each stage of the contraction cycle. Factors that reduce aortic flow, such as high arterial blood pressure or aortic stenosis or loss of aortic compliance, increase impedance and hence the afterload. During systole, when the aortic valve is open, an increased afterload communicates itself to the ventricles by increasing wall stress. In LV failure, aortic impedance is augmented not only by peripheral vasoconstriction but also by decreases in aortic compliance. The problem with the clinical measurement of aortic impedance is that invasive instrumentation is required. An approximation can be found by using transesophageal echocardiography to determine aortic blood flow at, for example, the time of maximal increase of aortic flow just after aortic valve opening.

Heart Rate And Force-Frequency Relation

TREPPE OR BOWDITCH EFFECT. An increased heart rate progressively enhances the force of ventricular contraction, even in an isolated papillary muscle preparation (Bowditch staircase phenomenon). Alternative names are the *treppe* (steps, German) phenomenon or positive inotropic effect of activation or force-frequency relationship (Fig. 19–24). Conversely, a decreased heart rate has a negative staircase effect. When stimulation becomes too rapid, force decreases. The proposal is that during rapid stimulation, more sodium and calcium ions enter the myocardial cell than can be handled by the sodium pump and the mechanisms for calcium exit. Opposing the force-frequency effect is the negative contractile influence of the decreased duration of ventricular filling at high heart rates. The longer the filling interval, the better the ventricular filling and the stronger the subsequent contraction. This phenomenon can be shown in patients with atrial fibrillation with a variable filling interval.

Post-extrasystolic potentiation and the inotropic effect of paired pacing can be explained by the same model, again assuming an enhanced contractile state after the prolonged interval between beats. Nonetheless, the exact cellular mechanism remains to be clarified.

FORCE-FREQUENCY RELATIONSHIP AND OPTIMAL HEART RATE. Normally, peak contractile force at a fixed muscle length (isometric contraction) increases and a peak is reached at about 150 to 180 stimuli per minute.[73] This is the human counterpart of the treppe phenomenon. In situ, the optimal heart rate not only is the rate that would give maximal mechanical performance of an isolated muscle strip but also is determined by the need for adequate time for diastolic filling. In normal humans, it is not possible to attach exact values to the heart rate required to decrease rather than to increase cardiac output or to keep it steady. Atrial pacing rates of up to 150 per minute can be tolerated, whereas higher rates cannot because of the development of atrioventricular block. In contrast, during exercise, indices of LV function still increase up to a maximum heart rate of about 170 per minute, presumably because of enhanced contractility and peripheral vasodilation.[74] In patients with severe LV hypertrophy, the critical heart rate is between 100 and 130 per minute, with a fall-off in LV function at higher rates.[75]

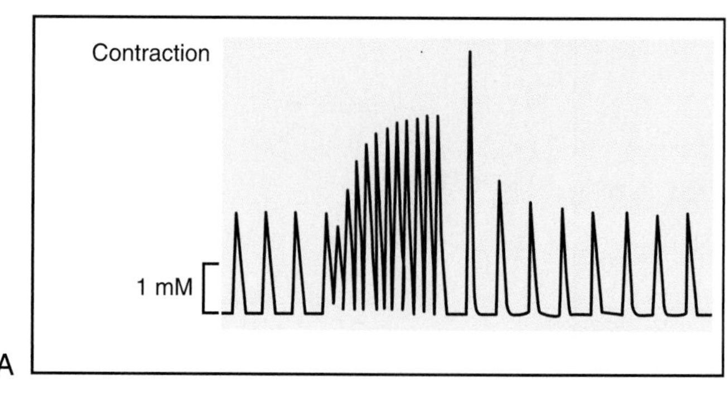

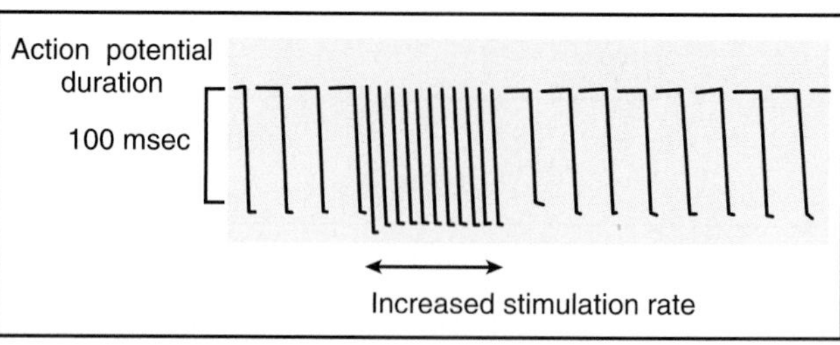

FIGURE 19–24 Bowditch or treppe phenomenon. An increased stimulation rate **(B)** increases the force of contraction **(A)**. The stimulus rate is shown as the action potential duration on an analog analyzer where ms equals milliseconds. The tension developed by papillary muscle contraction is shown in mN (millinewtons). On cessation of rapid stimulation, the contraction force gradually declines. Hypothetically, the explanation for the increased contraction during the increased stimulation is repetitive Ca^{2+} entry with each depolarization and, hence, an accumulation of cytosolic calcium. (From Noble MIM: Excitation-contraction coupling. *In* Drake-Holland AJ, Noble MIM [eds]: Cardiac Metabolism. Chichester, England, John Wiley, 1983, pp 49-71.)

Myocardial Oxygen Uptake

DETERMINANTS OF MYOCARDIAL OXYGEN DEMAND. Myocardial oxygen demand can be increased by heart rate, preload, or afterload (Fig. 19–25), factors that can all precipitate myocardial ischemia in those with coronary artery disease. The O_2 uptake can be augmented by increased contractility as during beta-adrenergic stimulation. Because myocardial O_2 uptake ultimately reflects the rate of mitochondrial metabolism and of ATP production, any increase of ATP requirement is reflected in increased O_2 uptake. In general, factors that increase wall stress increase the O_2 uptake. An increased afterload causes an increased systolic wall stress, which requires greater O_2 uptake. An increased diastolic wall stress, resulting from an increased preload, also requires more O_2 because the greater stroke volume must be ejected against the afterload. In states of enhanced contractility, the rate of change of wall stress is increased. Thus, thinking in terms of wall stress provides a comprehensive approach to the problem of myocardial O_2 uptake. Because the systolic blood pressure is an important determinant of the afterload, a practical index of the O_2 uptake is systolic blood pressure × heart rate, the *double product*. In addition, there

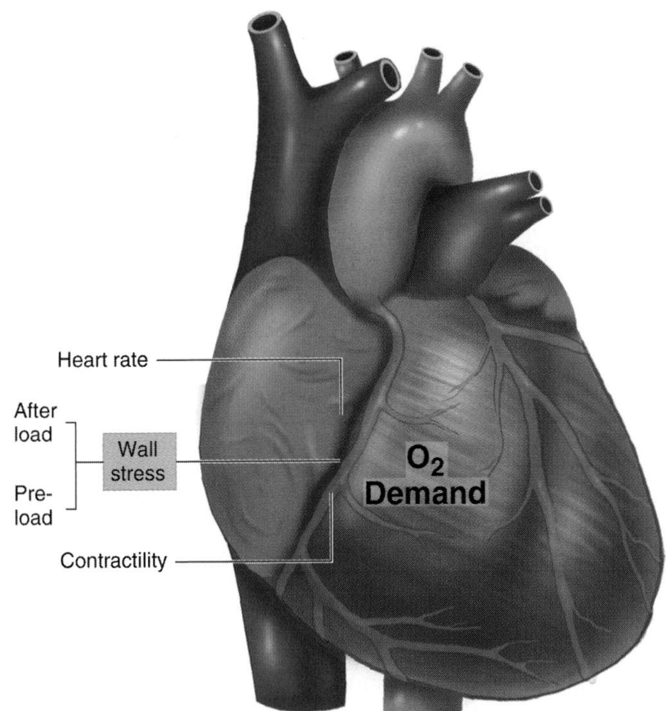

FIGURE 19–25 Major determinants of the oxygen demand of the normal heart. These are heart rate, wall stress, and contractility. For use of pressure-volume area as index of oxygen uptake, see Figure 19–26. (Modified from Opie LH: The Heart, Physiology, from Cell to Circulation. Philadelphia, Lippincott Raven, 1998. Copyright L. H. Opie, © 1998.)

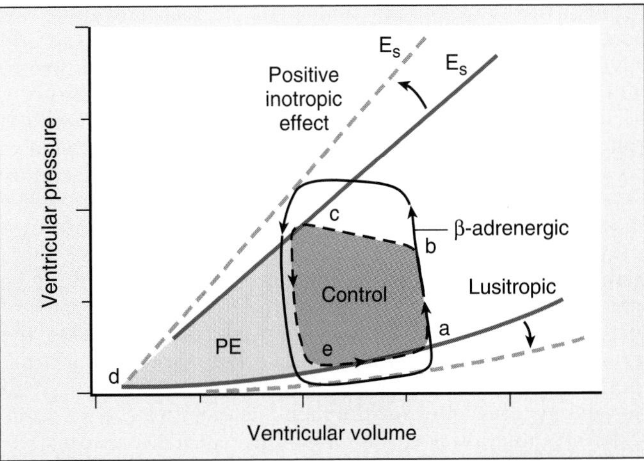

FIGURE 19–26 Pressure-volume loop of left ventricle. Note the effects of beta-adrenergic catecholamines with both positive inotropic (increased slope of line E_s) and increased lusitropic (relaxant) effects. E_s is the slope of the pressure-volume relationship. The total pressure-volume area (for control area, see a, b, c, d) is closely related to the myocardial oxygen uptake. The area c, d, e is the component of work spent in generating potential energy (PE). (Modified from Opie LH: Heart Physiology, from Cell to Circulation. Philadelphia, Lippincott Williams & Wilkins, 2004. Copyright L. H. Opie, © 2004.)

may be a metabolic component of the oxygen uptake that is usually small but may be prominent in certain special conditions, such as the "oxygen wastage" found with abnormally high circulating free fatty acid values. The concept of wall stress in relation to O_2 uptake also explains why heart size is such an important determinant of the myocardial O_2 uptake (because a larger radius increases wall stress).

WORK OF THE HEART. External work is done when, for example, a mass is lifted a certain distance. In terms of the heart, the cardiac output is the mass moved, and the resistance against which it is moved is the blood pressure. Because volume work requires less oxygen than pressure work, it might be supposed that external work is not an important determinant of the myocardial O_2 uptake. However, three determinants of the myocardial O_2 uptake are involved: preload (because it helps determine the stroke volume), afterload (in part determined by the blood pressure), and heart rate, as can be seen from the following formula:

$$\text{Minute work} = \text{SBP} \times \text{SV} \times \text{heart rate}$$

where SBP = systolic blood pressure and SV = stroke volume. Thus, it is not surprising that heart work is related to oxygen uptake. The *pressure-work index* takes into account both the double product (SBP × HR) and the HR × stroke volume, i.e., cardiac output. The *pressure-volume area* is another index of myocardial O_2 uptake, requiring invasive monitoring for accurate measurements. External cardiac work can account for up to 40 percent of the total myocardial O_2 uptake.

Internal Work (Potential Energy). The total oxygen consumption is related to the total work of the heart (area a, b, c, d in Fig. 19–26), meaning both the external work (the area a, b, c, e) and the volume-pressure triangle joining the end-systolic volume-pressure point to the origin (the area c, d, e; marked PE).[76] Although this area has been called internal work, more strictly it should be called *potential energy* that is generated within each contraction cycle but not converted to external work. Such potential energy at the end of systole (point c) may be likened to the potential energy of a compressed spring.

Kinetic Work. In strict terms, the work performed *(power production)* needs to take into account not only pressure but also kinetic components. It is the pressure work that has been discussed (product of cardiac output and peak systolic pressure). The kinetic work is the component required to move the blood against the afterload. Normally, kinetic work is less than 1 percent of the total. In aortic stenosis, kinetic work increases sharply as the cross-sectional area of the aortic valve narrows, whereas pressure work increases as the gradient across the aortic valve rises. Noninvasive measures of peak power production are being assessed as indices of cardiac contractility.

Efficiency of Work. The efficiency of work is the relation between the work performed and the myocardial oxygen uptake. Exercise increases the efficiency of external work, an improvement that offsets any metabolic cost of the increased contractility.[77] Metabolically, efficiency is increased by promotion of glucose rather than fatty acids as the major myocardial fuel.[78] Conversely, heart failure decreases the efficiency of work, possibly by beta-adrenergically promoted fatty acid metabolism.[79] The subcellular basis for changes in efficiency of work is not fully understood. Because as little as 12 to 14 percent of the oxygen uptake may be converted to external work,[77] it is probably the "internal work" that becomes more or less demanding. Internal ion fluxes ($Na^+/K^+/Ca^{2+}$) account for about 20 to 30 percent of the ATP requirement of the heart, so that most ATP is spent on actin-myosin interaction and much of that on generation of heat rather than on external work. An increased initial muscle length sensitizes the contractile apparatus to calcium (see Fig. 19–20), thereby theoretically increasing the efficiency of contraction by diminishing the amount of calcium flux required.

Measurements of Contractility

(see also Chap. 20)

FORCE-VELOCITY RELATIONSHIP AND MAXIMUM CONTRACTILITY IN MUSCLE MODELS. If the concept of contractility is truly independent of the load and the heart rate, unloaded heart muscle stimulated at a fixed rate should have a maximum value of contractility for any given magnitude of the cytosolic calcium transient. This value, the V_{max} of muscle contraction, is defined as the *maximal velocity of contraction* when there is no load on the isolated muscle or no afterload to prevent maximal rates of cardiac ejection. Beta-adrenergic stimulation increases V_{max}, and converse changes are found in the failing myocardium. V_{max} is also termed V_0 (the maximum velocity at zero load). The problem with this relatively simple concept is that V_{max} cannot be measured directly but is extrapolated from the peak rates of force development in unloaded muscle obtained from the intercept on the velocity axis. In another extreme condition, there is no muscle shortening at all (zero shortening), and all the energy goes into development of pressure (P_0) or force (F_0). This situation is an example of *isometric shortening* (*iso*, the same; *metric*, length). Because the peak velocity is obtained at zero load when there is no external force development, the relationship is usually termed the *force-velocity relationship*.

The concept of V_{max} has been subject to much debate over many years, chiefly because of the technical difficulties in obtaining truly unloaded conditions. Braunwald and coworkers[80] used cat papillary muscle to define a hyperbolic force-velocity curve, with V_{max} relatively independent of the initial muscle length but increased by the addition of norepinephrine. Another preparation used to examine force-velocity relations involves single cardiac myocytes isolated by enzymatic digestion of the rat myocardium and then permeabilized with a staphylococcal toxin. Again, the force-velocity relation is hyperbolic, suggesting the existence of intracellular *passive elastic elements* that contribute to the load on the isolated myocyte. In fact, the more hyperbolic and increased curvilinear nature of the force-velocity relationship in isolated myocytes than in the papillary muscle suggests that internal passive forces such as those generated by titin (see Fig. 19–4) are greater than expected in the isolated myocytes. In the intact heart, the noncontractile components contribute relatively little to overall mechanical behavior, at least in physiological circumstances.[81] Data from both papillary muscle and sarcomeres suggest that in unloaded conditions the intrinsic contractility as assessed by V_{max} does not change with initial fiber or sarcomere length.

MECHANISM OF BETA-ADRENERGIC EFFECTS ON FORCE-VELOCITY RELATIONSHIP. The data on papillary muscles showing that norepinephrine can increase V_{max} could be explained by either an effect of beta-adrenergic stimulation on enhancing calcium ion entry or a direct effect on the contractile proteins, or both. Strang and coworkers[82] showed that either isoproterenol (beta stimulant) or PKA (intracellular messenger) increased V_{max} by about 40 percent concurrently with phosphorylation of troponin I and of C protein in an isolated ventricular myocyte preparation. The overall concept would be that beta-adrenergic stimulation mediates the major component of its inotropic effect through increasing the cytosolic calcium transient and the factors controlling it, such as the rate of entry of calcium ions through the sarcolemmal L-type channels, the rate of calcium uptake under the influence of phospholamban into the SR, and the rate of calcium release from the ryanodine receptor in response to calcium entry in association with depolarization.

ISOMETRIC VERSUS ISOTONIC CONTRACTION. Despite the similarities in the force-velocity patterns in the data obtained on papillary muscle and isolated myocytes, it should be considered that a number of different types of muscular contraction may be involved. For example, data for P_0 are obtained under isometric conditions (length unchanged). When muscle is allowed to shorten against a steady load, the conditions are *isotonic* (*iso*, same; *tonic*, contractile force). Thus, the force-velocity curve may be a combination of initial isometric conditions followed by isotonic contraction and then followed by the abrupt and total unloading to measure V_{max}. Although isometric conditions can be found in the whole heart as an approximation during isovolumic contraction, isotonic conditions cannot prevail because the load is constantly changing during the ejection period, and complete unloading is impossible. Therefore, the application of force-velocity relations to the heart in vivo is limited.

PRESSURE-VOLUME LOOPS. Accordingly, measurements of pressure-volume loops are among the best of the current approaches to the assessment of the contractile behavior of the intact heart. Major criticisms arise when it is assumed that E_s is necessarily linear (it may be curvilinear) or when E_s is used as an index of "absolute" contractility (for E_s, see Fig. 19–26). Also, in clinical practice, the need to change the loading conditions and the requirement for invasive monitoring, required for the full loop, lessen the usefulness of this index. To measure LV volume adequately and continuously throughout the cardiac cycle is not easy. During a positive inotropic intervention, the pressure-volume loop reflects a smaller end-systolic volume and a higher end-systolic pressure, so that the slope of the pressure-volume relationship (E_s) has moved upward and to the left (see Fig. 19–26). When the positive inotropic intervention is by beta-adrenergic stimulation, enhanced relaxation (lusitropic effect) results in a lower pressure-volume curve during ventricular filling than in controls.

CONTRACTILITY

Defects in the Concept. Despite all the foregoing procedures that can be adopted to attempt to measure true contractility, the concept has at least two serious defects: (1) the absence of any potential index that can be measured in situ and that is free of significant criticism and, in particular, the absence of any acceptable noninvasive index, and (2) the impossibility of separating the cellular mechanisms of contractility changes from those of load or heart rate. Thus, an increased heart rate through the sodium pump lag mechanism gives rise to increased cytosolic calcium, which is thought to explain the treppe phenomenon. An increased preload involves increased fiber stretch, which in turn causes length activation, explicable by sensitization of the contractile proteins to the prevailing cytosolic calcium concentration. An increased afterload may increase cytosolic calcium through stretch-sensitive channels. Thus, there is a clear overlap between contractility, which should be independent of load or heart rate, and the effects of load and heart rate on the cellular mechanisms. Hence, the traditional separation of inotropic state from load or heart rate effects as two independent regulators of cardiac muscle performance is no longer simple now that the underlying cellular mechanisms have been uncovered. An example of this dilemma arises in humans with atrial fibrillation and a constantly varying force-frequency relationship. Contractility as measured in situ by pressure-volume loops constantly changes from beat to beat, and the explanation could be either a "true" change in contractility or the operation of the Frank-Starling mechanism because of varying diastolic filling times.[83]

The Concept Is Essential and the Search Continues. Whatever the defects of the concept and the problems of measuring it, contractility remains an essential cardiac concept to separate the effects of a primary change in loading conditions or heart rate from an intrinsic change in the force of contraction. An analogy could be that the rate at which a truck travels is determined not only by external "loading" factors such as the weight of the goods carried on the back and the slope of the road but also by "internal" factors such as the horsepower of the engine and the gear used. Hence, the quest for the perfect index of contractility continues. Currently, tissue Doppler imaging is being assessed to provide indices such as the rate of myocardial acceleration during the phase of isovolumic contraction.[84]

Ventricular Relaxation and Diastolic Dysfunction (see also Chaps. 20 and 21). Diastolic dysfunction and diastolic heart failure are frequently discussed but controversial topics.[85,86] Among the many complex physiological and pathological factors influencing relaxation, four are of chief interest. First, the cytosolic calcium level must fall to cause the relaxation phase, a process requiring ATP and phosphorylation of phospholamban for uptake of calcium into the SR (see Fig. 19–27). Second, the inherent viscoelastic properties of the myocardium are of importance. In the hypertrophied heart with increased fibrosis, relaxation occurs more slowly. Particularly in the early stages of the hypertrophied heart of hypertension and aortic stenosis, a situation arises in which systolic function is relatively well preserved but diastolic relaxation is impaired. The probable explanation is that hypertrophy is accompanied by increasing fibrosis.[87] Third, increased phosphorylation of troponin I enhances the rate of relaxation.[88] Fourth, relaxation is influenced by the systolic load.[86] Thus, the history of contraction affects cross-bridge relaxation. Within limits, the greater the systolic load, the faster the rate of relaxation.

This complex relationship has been explored in detail by Brutsaert and colleagues[70] but could perhaps be simplified as follows. When the workload is high, peak cytosolic calcium is also high. Thus, the rate of fall of calcium is also greater provided that the diastolic uptake mechanisms function effectively. In this way, a systolic pressure load and the rate of diastolic relaxation can be related. Furthermore, a greater muscle length (when the workload is high) at the end of systole should produce a more rapid rate of relaxation by the opposite of length-dependent sensitization. When the afterload exceeds a certain limit, relaxation is delayed[86] with diastolic dysfunction. Thus, in congestive heart failure caused by an excess systolic load, relaxation becomes increasingly afterload dependent, so that therapeutic reduction of the systolic load should improve LV relaxation.

IMPAIRED RELAXATION AND CYTOSOLIC CALCIUM. For these purposes, this chapter uses the clinical definition of diastole according to which diastole extends from aortic valve closure to the start of the first heart sound. The first phase of diastole is the isovolumic phase, which, by definition, does not contribute to ventricular filling. The second phase of rapid filling provides most of ventricular filling. The third phase of slow filling or diastasis accounts for only 5 percent of the total filling. The final atrial booster phase accounts for the remaining 15 percent.

Isovolumic relaxation is energy dependent, requiring ATP for the uptake of calcium ions by the SR (Fig. 19–27), which is an active, not a passive process. Impaired relaxation is an early event in angina pectoris. A proposed metabolic explanation is that there is impaired generation of energy, which diminishes the supply of ATP required for the early diastolic uptake of calcium by the SR. The result is that the cytosolic calcium level, at a peak in systole, has a delayed return to normal in the early diastolic period. In other conditions, too, there is a relationship between the rate of diastolic decay of the calcium transient and diastolic relaxation, with a relation to impaired function of the SR.[89] When the relaxation is prolonged by hypothyroidism, the return of the systolic calcium elevation is likewise delayed, whereas opposite changes occur in hyperthyroidism. In congestive heart failure, diastolic relaxation is also delayed and irregular, as is the rate of decay of the cytosolic calcium elevation. Most patients with coronary artery disease have a variety of abnormalities of diastolic filling, probably related to those also found in angina pectoris. Theoretically, such abnormalities of relaxation are potentially reversible because they depend on changes in patterns of calcium ion movement. Indices of the

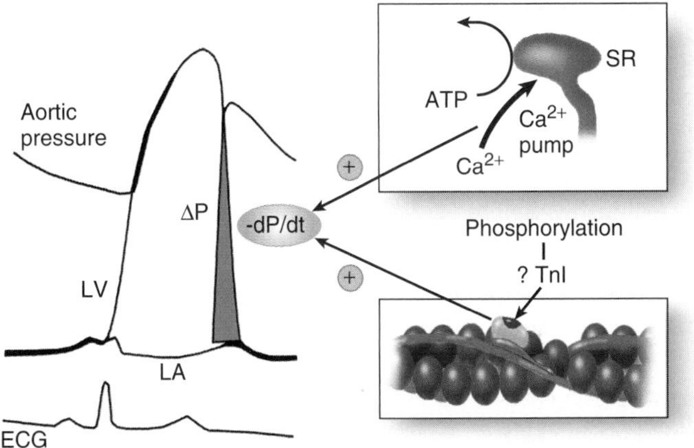

FIGURE 19–27 Factors governing the isovolumic relaxation phase of the cardiac cycle. This period of the cycle extends from the aortic second sound (A_2) to the crossover point between the left ventricular and left atrial pressures (see Fig. 19–20). The maximum negative rate of pressure development ($-dP/dt_{max}$), which gives the isovolumic relaxation rate, is measured either invasively or by a continuous-wave Doppler velocity spectrum in aortic regurgitation. Isovolumic relaxation is increased (+ sign) when the rate of calcium uptake into the sarcoplasmic reticulum (SR) is enhanced, for example during beta-adrenergic stimulation (see Fig. 19–15). Isovolumic relaxation may also be enhanced when phosphorylation of troponin I (TnI), as in response to beta-adrenergic stimulation, may decrease the affinity of the contractile system for calcium. ECG = electrocardiogram; LA = left atrium; LV = left ventricle. (Modified from Opie LH: Heart Physiology, from Cell to Circulation. Philadelphia, Lippincott Williams & Wilkins, 2004. Copyright L. H. Opie, © 2004.)

isovolumic phase and other indices of diastolic function are shown in Table 19–5.

IS THERE VENTRICULAR SUCTION DURING EARLY FILLING? Whether the LV suction by active relaxation could increase the pressure gradient from left atrium to left ventricle during the early filling phase remains controversial although well supported by data. An LV suction effect can be found by carefully comparing LV and left atrial pressures, and it occurs especially in the early diastolic phase of rapid filling. The sucking effect may be of most importance in mitral stenosis when the mitral valve does not open as it otherwise should in response to diastolic suction. During catecholamine stimulation, the rate of relaxation may increase to enhance the sucking effect and to prolong the period of filling. The currently proposed mechanism of sucking is as follows. In early diastole, myosin is pulled into the space between the two anchoring segments of titin (see Fig. 19–4) to lower the intraventricular pressure to below that in the atrium.[90]

ATRIAL FUNCTION. The left atrium, besides its well-known function as a blood-receiving chamber, helps to complete LV filling by presystolic contraction and the atrial booster function. The atrial pressure-volume loop is very different in shape from that of the ventricles. There are two parts, the overall loop somewhat resembling a figure of 8. The first phase of volume increase (v loop) reflects atrial filling and passive emptying, followed by atrial work (a loop) done during presystolic atrial contraction.[91] During atrial pacing, the preload is increased and the atria are distended so that the volume part of the loop is small and the contraction part of the loop is much enlarged.[91]

Two additional functions of the atria are as follows. First, it is the volume sensor of the heart, releasing atrial natriuretic peptide in response to intermittent stretch and several other stimuli including angiotensin II and endothelin. Second, the atrium contains receptors for the afferent arms of various reflexes including mechanoreceptors that increase the sinus discharge rate, thereby contributing to the tachycardia of exercise as the venous return increases (Bainbridge reflex). The atria have a number of differences in structure and function from the ventricles, having smaller myocytes with a shorter action potential duration as well as a more fetal type of myosin (in both heavy and light chains). The more rapid atrial repolarization is thought to be due to increased outward potassium currents, such as I_{to} and I_{kACh}. In general, these histological and physiological changes can be related to the decreased need for the atria to generate high intrachamber pressures, rather being sensitive to volume changes, while retaining enough contractile action to help with LV filling and to respond to inotropic stimuli.

MEASUREMENT OF ISOVOLUMIC RELAXATION. The rate of isovolumic relaxation is best measured by negative

TABLE 19–5 Some Indices of Diastolic Function

Isovolumic Relaxation
(−)dP/dt$_{max}$ (Fig. 19–28)
Aortic closing–mitral opening interval
Peak rate of LV wall thinning
Time constant of relaxation (τ)
Early Diastolic Filling
Relaxation kinetics on ERNA (rate of volume increase)
Early filling phase (E phase) on Doppler transmitral velocity trace
Diastasis
Pressure-volume relation indicates compliance
Atrial Contraction
Invasive measurement of atrial and ventricular pressures
Doppler transmitral pattern (E to A ratio)

A = atrial contraction phase; E = early filling phase; ERNA = equilibrated radionuclide angiography; LV = left ventricular.

dP/dt$_{max}$ at invasive catheterization. *Tau*, the time constant of relaxation, describes the rate of fall of LV pressure during isovolumic relaxation and also requires invasive techniques for precise determination. Tau is increased as the systolic LV pressure rises. Other indices of isovolumic relaxation can be obtained echocardiographically or from tissue Doppler measurements to monitor the peak rate of wall thinning.

DIASTOLIC DYSFUNCTION AND MYOCARDIAL MECHANICAL PROPERTIES. In hypertrophic hearts, as in chronic hypertension or severe aortic stenosis, abnormalities of diastole are common and may precede systolic failure (see Chap. 21). But the existence of "pure" diastolic dysfunction and heart failure is challenged by tissue Doppler measurements that show subtle but evident systolic abnormalities.[92,93] Experimentally, there are several defects in early hypertensive hypertrophy, including decreased rates of contraction and relaxation and decreased peak force development. The mechanism of diastolic dysfunction is not clear, although it is thought to be related to the fibrosis that occurs with ventricular hypertrophy or indirectly to a stiff left atrium. Impaired relaxation is associated with an increase of the late (atrial) filling phase so that E/A ratios (see Table 19–5) on the mitral Doppler pattern decline (see also Chap. 20).

Effects of Ischemia and Reperfusion on Contraction and Relaxation

Contractile Impairment in Ischemia

HIGH-ENERGY PHOSPHATES. These are reviewed by Opie and Heusch.[94] Early contractile failure (Fig. 19–28) can occur even when calcium transients are normal or even increased; therefore, a metabolic cause must be sought. The latter could be either decreased sensitivity of the contractile proteins to calcium, such as caused by acidosis, or inhibition of the cross-bridge cycle, such as from the early rise in P_i. As creatine phosphate falls, the activity of the creatine phosphate shuttle decreases so that "local" ATP, required for calcium movements in the contractile cycle, falls. In addition, the free energy of hydrolysis of ATP decreases during ischemia. The large increase in P_i that results from creatine phosphate breakdown decreases the free energy of hydrolysis, as do the smaller decreases in ATP and increases in ADP. The creatine phosphate decrease can also indirectly inhibit contractility by accumulation of P_i, which decreases the contractile effects of any given cytosolic calcium level. P_i may act by promotion of formation of weak rather than strong cross bridges. *Accumulation of neutral lactate* can promote mitochondrial damage, decrease the action potential

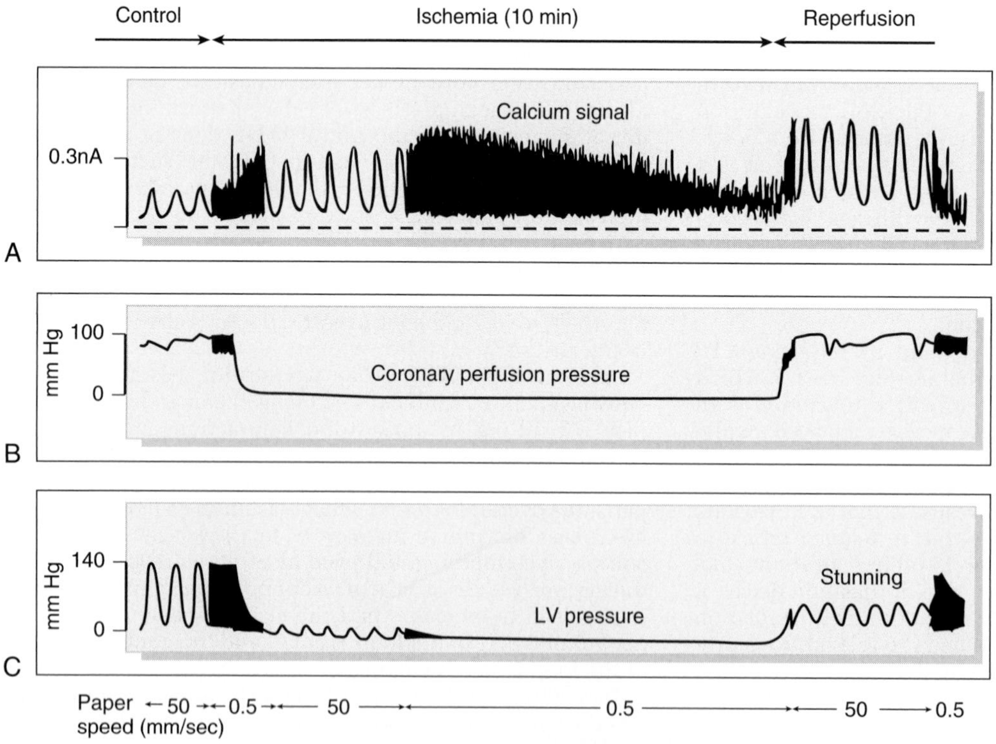

FIGURE 19–28 Can left ventricular (LV) mechanical failure during severe ischemia be explained by changes in the cytosolic calcium? These data show that when there is abrupt ischemic LV failure (LV pressure falls to zero in **C**), the calcium signal **(A)** increases before it falls. Ischemia is designated by the abrupt fall of coronary perfusion pressure to zero in this isolated rat heart preparation **(B)**. During reperfusion there is also a dissociation between the cytosolic calcium oscillations, which are augmented (right side of **A**), in contrast to LV contraction, which is decreased (right side of **C**), so that there is mechanical stunning. It is thought that excess calcium oscillations damage the contractile proteins. (From Meisner A, Morgan JP: Contractile dysfunction and abnormal Ca^{2+} modulation during postischemic reperfusion in rat heart. Am J Physiol. 268:H100, 1995.)

during balloon angioplasty the manifestations of ischemia including chest pain become less with repeated balloon inflations.[98] Early preconditioning may be part of the explanation for the phenomenon of "walk-through" or "warm-up" angina, in which the severity of the initial anginal attack is lessened during subsequent exercise.[98] Exercise can also induce late preconditioning in those with coronary artery disease.[106] This effect could contribute to the clinical benefit of exercise training. Patients with preinfarction angina may suffer from a less severe infarct than those thought to undergo sudden coronary occlusion without the opportunity for preconditioning.[98] Pharmacologically, a number of adenosine analogs have been used to test the effects of preconditioning in humans but thus far without consistent success. One antianginal compound, nicorandil, besides having nitrate-like qualities, opens the mitochondrial ATP-dependent potassium channel and thereby potentially invokes preconditioning in humans. Whether this property expands the antianginal protection is not clear.

Hibernation

The hibernating myocardium, like the hibernating animal, is temporarily asleep and can wake up to function normally when the blood supply is fully restored (Table 19–6). Rahimtoola[107] proposed that the fall of myocardial function to a lower level copes with the reduced myocardial oxygen supply and leads to self-preservation so that the myocardium is "exquisitely regulated" and successfully adapted to the prevailing circumstances. The alternative and now dominant point of view is that hibernation can occur even when the resting coronary flow is normal or low normal despite the presence of coronary disease. The basic problem lies in a critical stenosis that limits coronary vascular reserve[108] so that episodes of tachycardia must precipitate ischemia. Such recurrent episodes of ischemia would then leave behind a repetitively stunned myocardium. Thus, chronic hibernation, according to this proposal, is no more than cumulative stunning. The mandatory need for revascularization remains.

CELLULAR EVENTS IN HIBERNATION. Heusch and Schulz[108] related the loss of contractile function to signaling by inflammatory-like processes involving TNF-α, known to depress myocardial function.[109] In humans, too, there is increased gene expression of both TNF-α and NOS, both inhibitory to contraction.[110] In addition, there are complex defects in calcium cycling and excitation-contraction coupling[108] and decreased beta-adrenergic receptor density.[110] The hypocontractile segments that still have sustained glucose extraction, as shown by positron-emission tomography (PET), have a high chance of recovery after coronary artery bypass surgery. "Mismatch" refers to the increased glucose extraction of the viable myocardium that can be visibly contrasted with the poor coronary blood flow (ammonia signal on PET). In one series, up to 27 percent of patients with ischemic cardiomyopathy could have enough viable segments to benefit from revascularization.[111] Postoperative recovery of contractile function may vary from rapid, within hours or even minutes, to long delays over weeks or even months. Thus, hibernation, like stunning, is a "syndrome."

Stunning

The first observation was that the recovery of mechanical function following transient coronary occlusion was not instant but delayed. Thereafter, Braunwald and Kloner[112] defined the "stunned myocardium" as one characterized by prolonged postischemic myocardial dysfunction with eventual return of normal contractile activity. Stunning is now thought to occur in many clinical situations,[113] including hibernation, delayed recovery from effort angina, unstable angina, early thrombolytic reperfusion, ischemic cardioplegia, cardiac transplantation, cardiac arrest, and coronary angioplasty. Interactive mechanisms are increased cytosolic calcium (Fig. 19–31; see Fig. 19–28) and the formation of oxygen-derived free radicals upon reperfusion.[113] The hydroxyl ion is "one of the most aggressive species of oxygen free radicals"[114] and is the key mediator of stunning.[115] Direct measurements of cytosolic calcium in stunned myocardium show that antioxidants decrease cytosolic calcium levels and increase the force of contraction.[116]

TUMOR NECROSIS FACTOR-ALPHA AND POSTISCHEMIC CONTRACTILE DEPRESSION. Following ischemia, production of TNF-α by both interstitial cells and human cardiomyocytes increases.[109] Theoretically, TNF-α may promote stunning by several mechanisms such as desensitization of the contractile proteins to calcium, induction of other cardiodepressant agents such as NO or interleukin-1, or formation of free radicals.

TABLE 19–6 Characteristics of Stunning, Hibernation, and Ischemia

Parameter	Stunning	Hibernation	True Ischemia
Myocardial mechanical function	Reduced	Reduced	Reduced
Coronary blood flow	Postischemic: normal/high	Modestly reduced or low normal; reduced coronary vascular reserve	Most severely reduced
Myocardial energy metabolism	Harmful effects of fatty acid fuels versus glucose	Reduced or low normal; in steady state with intermittent ischemia-reperfusion	Reduced; increasingly severe as ischemia proceeds
Duration	Hours to days; merges with delayed recovery from ischemia over weeks	Days to hours to months; occasionally longer	Minutes to hours; then lethal
Outcome	Full spontaneous recovery	Variable recovery if revascularized	Myocyte necrosis if severe ischemia persists
Proposed change in metabolic regulation of calcium	Cytosolic overload of calcium in early reperfusion with damage to contractile proteins	Hypothetically enough glycolytic ATP to prevent contracture (glucose mismatch)	Insufficient glycolytic ATP to prevent calcium overload and irreversibility

ATP = adenosine triphosphate.

Modified from Opie L, Heusch G: Lack of blood flow: Ischemia and angina. *In* Opie LH (ed): Heart Physiology, from Cell to Circulation. 4th ed. Philadelphia, Lippincott Williams & Wilkins, 2004, pp 525-552.

duration, and inhibit glyceraldehyde-3-phosphate dehydrogenase. The mechanism of these lactate effects may include extracellular acidosis with Na^+/H^+ exchange, a subsequent gain in cell Na^+, and then Na^+/Ca^{2+} exchange with gain of harmful Ca^{2+}.

POTASSIUM EFFLUX. Major early potassium efflux in ischemia occurs as the ATP-inhibited potassium channel (K_{ATP}) opens, as shown in a mouse model in which this channel is genetically inactivated.[95] In addition, other potassium channels such as those activated by sodium or by fatty acids may play a role. Second, inhibition of the sodium-potassium pump has long been suspected; the onset of such inhibition is probably too late to explain early potassium egress, although it probably contributes to the later phase of potassium loss. The importance of potassium loss is that because the action potential duration is shortened, calcium influx diminishes, which is one of the several factors causing early loss of contractile function after the onset of ischemia.

Response to Ischemia

The myocardium is now known to have a diverse and flexible response to ischemia, varying from rapid contractile arrest to delayed stimulation of potentially protective synthetic pathways involving signals similar to those inducing growth. Three specific new entities identified are preconditioning, hibernation, and stunning. All three have in common that they are different responses to ischemia and reperfusion. Ischemia-reperfusion injury is a well-recognized experimental entity, varying from reversible damage with mild transient ischemia to irreversible cell death with severe ischemia followed by reperfusion. Adverse effects associated with reperfusion include arrhythmias, mechanical dysfunction, degradation of contractile proteins such as troponin I, and apoptosis.[96] The proposal is that these adverse effects are at least to some extent offset by *a repertoire of myocardial protective events resulting from activation of a variety of signaling and metabolic pathways.*

Preconditioning

Preconditioning is the chief among these protective mechanisms. Contrary to expectations, many repetitive episodes of ischemia do not produce cumulative damage if each is short lived and followed by reperfusion. Rather, an endogenous myocardial protective mechanism is invoked, namely, preconditioning as first described by Jennings and colleagues in a seminal paper.[97] The final result is that when a prolonged ischemic episode occurs that would normally give rise to lethal myocardial damage, the heart is largely, but not totally, protected. This protection comes in two phases; the first window of early or "classical" preconditioning lasts only a few hours, whereas the second window of protection lasts for several days.

MECHANISMS OF PRECONDITIONING. Even after extensive research, the full mechanism of preconditioning is not clarified, and several different paths appear to be involved. The current consensus of opinion[98] is that the first window results from the liberation of a number of compounds from the ischemic myocardium, including adenosine, bradykinin, and opioids. Adenosine preconditioning is best understood and involves the A_1 and A_3 receptors acting through the inhibitor G_i protein to increase the activity of PKC (Fig. 19-29). Further signaling steps are not clear but might involve activation of MAP kinase. The mitochondria also play an important role with increased activity of the ATP-dependent potassium channel (K_{ATP}), which in turn decreases the calcium load of the ischemic mitochondria and increases ATP production. Mitochondria also produce reactive oxygen species that help to activate PKC. NO may play a role by generation of free radicals but is not a direct activator of preconditioning.[99]

SECOND WINDOW OF PROTECTION. This phase may be a "universal response of the heart to stress in general."[100] The mechanism involves at least two pathways leading to nuclear protein synthesis (Fig.

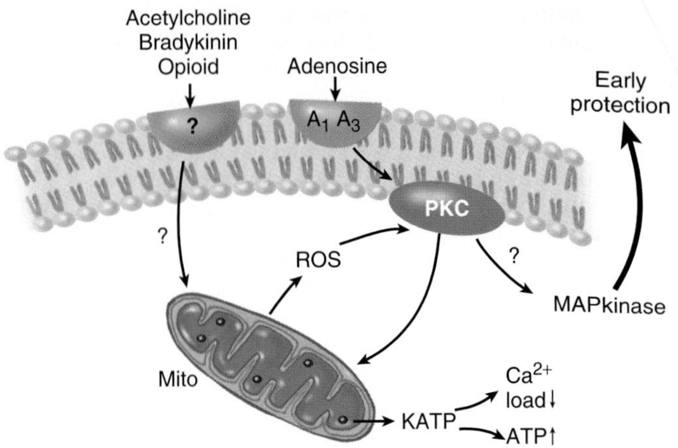

FIGURE 19–29 Early phase preconditioning. Adenosine, liberated during the brief ischemic period that triggers preconditioning and acting chiefly by myocardial A_1 and A_3 receptors, is thought to play a crucial role. A crucial event is activation of protein kinase C (PKC), particularly the epsilon isoform. Further steps leading to opening of the mitochondrial ATP-sensitive potassium channel (KATP) are not clear. Other effects could occur through the inhibitory protein G_i or the mitogen-activated protein (MAP) kinase cascade. In response to other mediators of preconditioning such as acetylcholine, liberation of reactive oxygen species (ROS), possibly from the mitochondria, is a key event and probably upstream from PKC. (Modified from Opie LH: Heart Physiology, from Cell to Circulation. Philadelphia, Lippincott Williams & Wilkins, 2004. Copyright L. H. Opie, © 2004.)

19-30) One involves the epsilon isoform of PKC (PKC-ε) that activates nuclear factor kappa B, which in turn increases nuclear synthesis of a variety of protective proteins such as cyclooxygenase-2 and iNOS. At present, much attention has been focused on the role of the mitochondria in both windows of preconditioning.[101] The mitochondrial permeability transition pore (PTP) is activated by ischemia-reperfusion injury and mitochondrial calcium overload results. Bcl-2 is an antiapoptotic protein found in the outer mitochondrial membrane that inhibits PTP opening and the release of cytochrome *c* that promotes apoptotic cell death. The second window of protection may be associated with increased Bcl-2 expression and, hence, with closing of the PTP.[102] Clearly, much more work needs to be done before the mechanisms underlying preconditioning, a powerful protective mechanism, have definite clinical application.

PRECONDITIONING VERSUS CARDIOPROTECTION

Protein Kinase C Isoforms. These are not the same entities in that preconditioning is only one form of cardioprotection. PKC is a key kinase with multiple functions and plays an important role in both. First, it is linked to the phospholipase signaling system, which is of prime importance in vascular contraction and possibly acts as an inotropic backup system in the myocardium (see Fig. 19-18). Second, PKC may be a key molecular switch in the "hypertrophic signal system," responding to stretch and to neurohormonal input[103] such as the angiotensin II released during stretch. Third, it plays a pivotal role in preconditioning, receiving stimuli from a number of G protein–linked receptors and ultimately activating the mitochondrial ATP-sensitive potassium channels (see Fig. 19-29). Such multiple functions may be mediated by different isoforms of PKC, of which there are at least 10, the functions of which are still poorly understood. The isoforms are divided into three groups, the conventional (which respond to calcium in vitro), the novel (which respond to diacylglycerol but not to calcium), and the atypical isoforms (which respond to neither calcium nor diacylglycerol but rather to phospholipids). The conventional beta isoforms, increased in the failing human heart, may be linked to enhanced growth.[103]

Current attention is focused on the delta and epsilon isoforms.[104] Each isoform becomes active when localized to a specific subcellular site by binding to its selective anchoring protein or RACK (receptor for activated C kinase). By inhibiting and activating, respectively, delta- and epsilon-specific forms of RACK, infarct size in rat hearts was markedly reduced,[104] showing that these two isoforms have opposite effects in this model. Concordant studies with overexpression of activated PKC-ε also showed cardioprotection.[105] In preconditioning, PKC-ε is translocated, consonant with its cardioprotective role.

PRECONDITIONING IN HUMANS. Does preconditioning occur in humans? Early preconditioning explains why

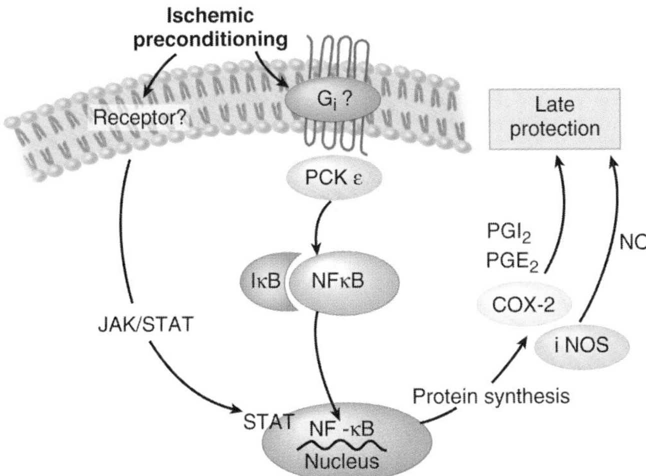

FIGURE 19–30 Late phase preconditioning. Note that preconditioning occurs in two phases, early and late, the latter probably involving nuclear protein synthesis. Figure based on the concepts of Bolli and colleagues.[141] COX-2 = cyclooxygenase-2; IκB = inhibitor of nuclear factor kappa B; iNOS = inducible nitric oxide synthase; JAK = Janus kinase; NFκB = nuclear factor kappa B; NO = nitric oxide; PG = prostaglandin; STAT = signal transducer and activator of transcription. (Modified from Opie LH: Heart Physiology, from Cell to Circulation. Philadelphia, Lippincott Williams & Wilkins, 2004. Copyright L. H. Opie, © 2004.)

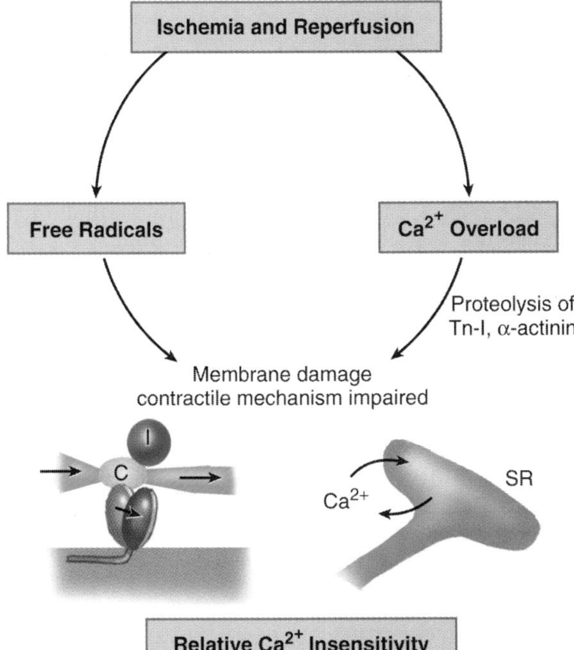

FIGURE 19–31 Mechanisms of ischemic reperfusion damage. The major three, probably with interactive effects, involve oxygen-derived free radicals, calcium overload, and relative insensitivity of the contractile protein troponin C (C) to calcium released from the sarcoplasmic reticulum (SR). For role of proteolysis of troponin I (Tn-I), see Bolli and Marban.[113] (Copyright L.H. Opie © 2001.)

ATRIAL STUNNING. After cessation of atrial fibrillation, atrial contractility may be reduced or absent up to several weeks despite normal electrical activity. Such stunning is clinically relevant and potentially harmful because it predisposes to the formation of atrial thrombosis with risk of stroke. Atrial stunning is part of the complex process of atrial remodeling that occurs during and after atrial fibrillation.[91]

CONCURRENT ISCHEMIA-RELATED EVENTS. Because the human heart with advanced coronary artery disease is known to suffer from intermittent ischemia, ischemia-reperfusion injury and its consequences may all be occurring at the same time. Thus, the same heart may concurrently manifest one or more components of the newly emphasized ischemic syndromes, namely stunning, hibernation, and preconditioning, as well as ischemic damage. When one episode of severe ischemia is followed by clinical reperfusion, as in thrombolysis, the extent of postischemic dysfunction could be determined by a combination of ischemic and reperfusion pathology, the former depending on how long the myocardium has been ischemic and the latter potentially causing a spectrum of ischemic syndromes.

Heart Failure (see also Chap. 21)

Human heart failure is a complex phenomenon at both clinical and cellular levels, the end result of several disparate disease processes that have been subject to a variety of therapies. There is poor contractile performance with systolic impairment and delayed diastolic relaxation. In human tissue obtained at cardiac transplantation, there are major disturbances in the force-frequency relationship, in gene programming, in beta-adrenergic activity, and in calcium cycling.

Force-Frequency Relationship

Muscle strips prepared from patients with severe LV failure behave very differently from normal muscle in that there is hardly any response to an increased stimulation frequency (Fig. 19–32). Whereas in strips from normal hearts, optimal force development is reached at rates of about 150 to 180 beats/min, in patients with cardiomyopathy an increased heart rate produces a decreased twitch tension (Fig. 19–33) In addition, the diastolic tension rises markedly with the stimulation frequency,[117] compatible with a rate-induced cytosolic calcium overload causing diastolic dysfunction. This complex picture is at least in part related to changes in gene expression and to downregulated beta-adrenergic receptor activity.

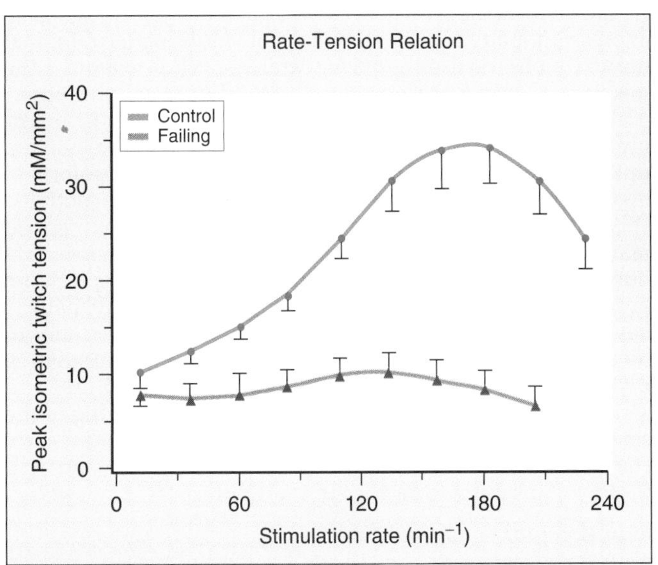

FIGURE 19–32 Force-frequency relationship in humans, comparing nonfailing control hearts with failing hearts with mitral regurgitation. Plots of average steady-state isometric twitch tension versus stimulation frequency. Each point represents the mean ± standard error of the mean of eight control or mitral regurgitation preparations at 37°C. (Data from Mulieri LA, Leavitt BJ, Martin BJ: Myocardial force-frequency defect in mitral regurgitation heart failure is reversed by forskolin. Circulation 88:2700, 1993. Copyright 1993, American Heart Association.)

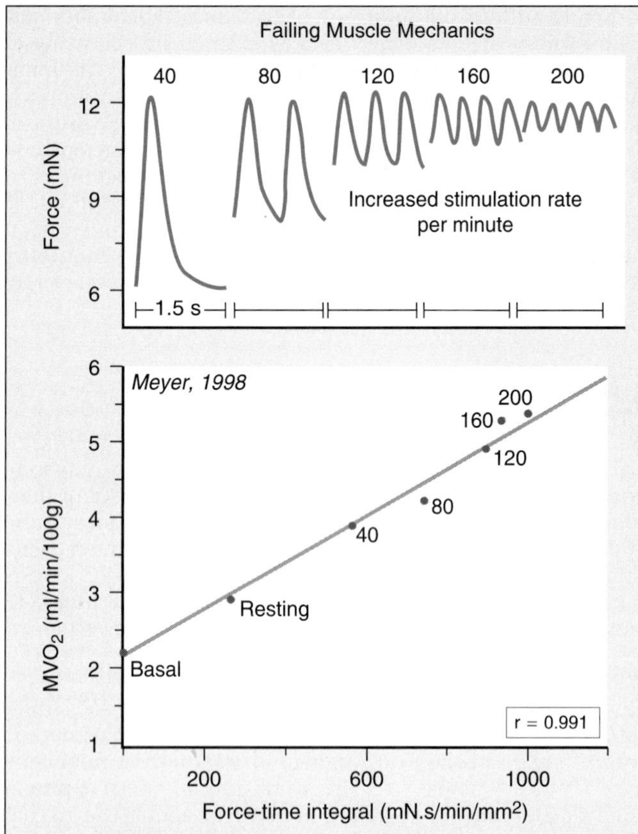

FIGURE 19–33 Diastolic tension markedly increased during pacing of a muscle strip from a patient with advanced heart failure. Note, at the bottom, the increased myocardial oxygen uptake (MVO_2) with increased force (measured as the force-time integral). The combination of decreased cardiac force development and increased oxygen uptake indicates decreased efficiency of cardiac work. (Modified from Meyer M, Keweloh B, Guth K, et al: Frequency-dependence of myocardial energetics in failing human myocardium as quantified by a new method for the measurement of oxygen consumption in muscle strip preparations. J Mol Cell Cardiol 30:1459, 1998.)

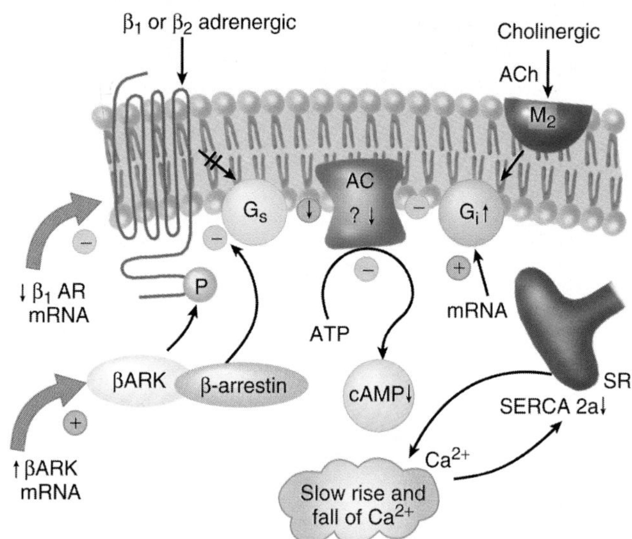

FIGURE 19–34 Proposed changes in beta-adrenergic receptor signal system and sarcoplasmic reticulum (SR) in severe congestive heart failure (CHF). AC = adenylate cyclase; ACh = acetylcholine; β_1AR = beta$_1$-adrenergic receptor; β_2AR = beta$_2$-adrenergic receptor; βARK = beta-adrenergic receptor kinase; G_i = inhibitory G protein; G_s = stimulatory G protein; M_2 = muscarinic receptor; mRNA = messenger ribonucleic acid. For SERCA2, see Figure 19–9. (From Opie LH: Heart Physiology, from Cell to Circulation. Philadelphia, Lippincott Williams & Wilkins, 2004. Copyright L. H. Opie, © 2004.)

Fetal Gene Program

As the ventricle fails, there is a change in the ventricular gene expression pattern from the normal adult pattern to that normally observed only during fetal life.[11] For example, the mechanical forces associated with LV failure lead to myocardial expression of atrial natriuretic peptide and brain natriuretic peptide (BNP). There is downregulation of the calcium uptake pump (SERCA2) and of the fast-contracting isoform of myosin heavy chain that has the greater ATPase activity. What activates the fetal program? Cytosolic calcium overload may be basic, by adding phosphate groups to enzymes that normally inhibit the fetal program.[118] There is, as yet, no known means of reverting a fetal to a normal adult pattern besides nonspecific treatment of heart failure with relief of biomechanical stress on the left ventricle. Thus, circulating BNP levels drop during the treatment of heart failure, and serial decreases of BNP levels should mirror lessening of the severity of LV failure. Metabolic therapies, as yet at an early stage, include inhibition of fatty acid metabolism and will probably be explored further in the future.[11]

Beta Receptor Abnormalities

BETA-ADRENERGIC SIGNALING IN HEART FAILURE. In congestive heart failure (Fig. 19–34), changes in the beta-adrenergic system include downregulation of the receptors and G proteins that stimulate the contraction cycle (beta$_1$ and beta$_2$, both through G_s) and upregulation of the inhibitory paths (beta$_2$ through G_i and beta$_3$ through NO). In more detail, (1) there is major beta$_1$ receptor downregulation[119] with moderate uncoupling from the stimulatory G protein, (2) beta$_2$ receptor density is unchanged but modestly uncoupled from G_s, and (3) inhibitory beta$_3$ receptors, linked to NO, are upregulated.[120] Adenylate cyclase activity decreases and levels of the inhibitory G_i proteins increase.[120] *Uncoupling* of the beta$_1$ and beta$_2$ receptors from the G_s signaling system may be explained by the increased activity of the βARK mechanism and of arrestin (see Fig. 19–14). Note the dual effect of beta$_2$ receptors on both stimulatory and inhibitory G proteins. The downregulation of G_s should decrease the stimulatory effect of beta$_2$ receptors through G_s on formation of cyclic AMP, yet the effect of arrestin is to uncouple these receptors from adenyl cyclase. Thus, overall, the upregulated G_i gives an increased inhibitory effect. According to this scheme, beta blockade can be expected to lessen the degree of hyperphosphorylation of the ryanodine receptor, thereby improving calcium channel release function toward normal.[121] The consequence would be improved calcium cycling as reflected in the better calcium transients found in transplant recipients who received prior beta blockade.[122] In addition, some nonselective blockers could be expected to block the beta$_3$-mediated inhibitory stimuli.

METABOLIC EFFECTS OF BETA-BLOCKADE ON MYOCARDIAL OXYGEN UPTAKE. Beta blockade might also be beneficial in heart failure by increasing the efficiency of work. This measure compares the myocardial oxygen uptake with the work performance. In experimental heart failure there is a marked fall-off in myocardial efficiency, which can be remedied by inhibition of fatty acid metabolism.[123] The hypothesis may be that excess fatty acid mobilization occurs as part of the increased catecholamine stimulation in heart failure and that this mobilization increases the uptake of fatty acids by the myocardium with a detrimental uncoupling effect on the mitochondria. The increased efficiency of work achieved when beta blockade is given to patients with heart failure may be related to inhibition of fatty acid oxidation.[79,124]

Calcium Cycling, Contractile Heart Failure, and Arrhythmias

CALCIUM CYCLING. Changes in the calcium cycle are fundamental to the impaired contractile performance of the

TABLE 19–7 Abnormalities of Calcium Cycling in Heart Failure

Subcellular	Organelle	Whole Heart	Reference
SERCA2a↓	SR Ca depleted	Negative FFR	127
RyR hyperphosphorylated	SR Ca release↓ Diastolic leak	Rate of contraction↓ Diastolic tension↑	126 136
Na/Ca exchange ↑	Released Ca extruded	Negative FFR	137
Prolonged APD and RyR changes	Cytosolic Ca↑	Diastolic tension↑ with pacing	138

APD = action potential duration; FFR = force-frequency relationship; RyR = ryanodine receptor; SERCA = sarcoendoplasmic reticulum Ca^{2+}-adenosine triphosphatase; SR = sarcoplasmic reticulum.

failing heart (Table 19–7). The SR calcium stores are severely depleted because of the combined effects of (1) depressed calcium uptake into the SR resulting from decreased SERCA activity, both downregulated and inhibited,[125] and (2) the diastolic calcium leak associated with hyperphosphorylation and abnormal functioning of the ryanodine receptor.[126] Thus, the calcium ions entering with depolarization are unable to trigger release of enough calcium to generate a normal calcium transient (see Fig. 19–34). There is a close relationship between the depression of SERCA in human heart failure and the depressed force-frequency relationship.[127] Paradoxically, the diastolic calcium level is higher than normal, a probable result of the diastolic leak through the defective ryanodine receptor and the prolonged action potential. Starting from this higher level, the proposed events as the heart rate increases could be that calcium ions enter more rapidly through the calcium channels of the T tubules than can be extruded through the Na/Ca exchange so that the diastolic levels rise, as does the diastolic tension.

ELECTRICAL ALTERNANS IN HEART FAILURE AND MYOCARDIAL ISCHEMIA. Ventricular fibrillation is probably the major cause of sudden death in patients with severe heart failure. An important mechanism of ventricular fibrillation is the subcellular phenomenon of *cardiac transient alternans,*[128] which is increased in cardiovascular disease and particularly in ischemic or failing hearts, or both. Alternans describes a fluctuation in any signal from beat to beat. Electrical alternans is the beat-to-beat variation in the electrocardiographic pattern. Calcium transient alternans is the fluctuation in peak amplitude of the cytosolic calcium transient from beat to beat. Such transient alternans is the cause of mechanical alternans.[128] Transient alternans may not be uniform throughout the cell but may occur in different subcellular patterns.[129] Such subcellular alternans appears to be commonly associated with depressed RyR function, even before measurable electrical or mechanical alternans occurs. In heart failure, the RyR is abnormal with dissociation of the binding protein FKBP12.6 that increases the diastolic calcium leak from the SR and depresses the triggered release of calcium from the SR. Conversely, genetic overexpression of this protein improves calcium handling and keeps the RyR in the closed stable conformation.[129]

Defective RyR function predisposes to calcium transient alternans in a manner not fully clarified. Hypothetically, cytosolic calcium overload and SR calcium "underload" mean that the trigger calcium is unable to elicit more than feeble calcium release from the SR. However, more calcium has entered the cytosol with the wave of depolarization and more is taken up by the SR. Thus, the next wave of depolarization elicits more calcium release from the SR with a larger calcium transient. Thereafter the pattern is repeated, with electrical inhomogeneity and risk of ventricular tachycardia and fibrillation. Thus, a currently provocative hypothesis is that abnormal subcellular patterns of calcium ion movement are found in both myocardial ischemia and heart failure and predispose to serious ventricular arrhythmias.[129]

REFERENCES

Microanatomy of Contractile Cells and Proteins

1. Zuker CZ, Ranganathan R: The path to specificity. Science 283:650, 1999.
2. Sutko JL, Publicover NG, Moss RL: An elastic link between length and active force production in myocardium. Circulation 104:1585, 2001.
3. Knoll R, Hoshijima M, Hoffman HM, et al: The cardiac mechanical stretch sensor machinery involves a Z disc complex that is defective in a subset of human dilated cardiomyopathy. Cell 111:943, 2002.
4. Solaro RJ, Wolska BM, Westfall M: Regulatory proteins and diastolic relaxation. *In* Lorell BH, Grossman W (eds): Diastolic Relaxation of the Heart. Boston, Kluwer Academic Publishers, 1994, pp 43-53.
5. Solaro RJ, Rarick HM: Troponin and tropomyosin: Proteins that switch on and tune in the activity of cardiac myofilaments. Circ Res 83:471, 1998.
6. Rayment I, Holden HM, Whittaker M: Structure of the actin-myosin complex and its implications for muscle contraction. Science 261:58, 1993.
7. Fisher AJ, Smith CA, Thoden J: Structural studies of myosin: A revised model for the molecular basis of muscle contraction. Biophys J 68:19s, 1995.
8. Dominguez R, Freyzon Y, Trybus KM, Cohen C: Crystal structure of a vertebrate smooth muscle myosin motor domain and its complex with the essential light chain: Visualization of the prepower stroke state. Cell 94:559, 1998.
9. Geeves M: Stretching the lever-arm theory. Nature 415:129, 2002.
10. Bers DM: Calcium fluxes involved in control of cardiac myocyte contraction. Circ Res 87:275, 2000.
11. Bristow M: Etomoxir: A new approach to treatment of chronic heart failure. Lancet 356:1621, 2000.
12. Tyska MJ, Dupuis DE, Guilford WH, et al: Two heads of myosin are better than one for generating force and motion. Proc Natl Acad Sci U S A 96:4402, 1999.
13. Solaro RJ: Modulation of cardiac myofilament activity by protein phosphorylation. *In* Fozzard H, Solaro RJ (eds): Handbook of Physiology. Sec 2: The Cardiovascular System. New York, Oxford University Press, 2002, pp 264-300.
14. Vemuri R, Lankford EB, Poetter K, et al: The stretch-activation response may be critical to the proper functioning of the mammalian heart. Proc Natl Acad Sci U S A 96:1048, 1999.
15. Konhilas JP, Irving TC, de Tombe PP: Myofilament calcium sensitivity in skinned rat cardiac trabeculae. Role of interfilament spacing. Circ Res 90:59, 2002.
16. Cazorla O, Vassort G, Garnier D, Le Guennec J-Y: Length modulation of active force in rat cardiac myocytes: Is titin the sensor? J Mol Cell Cardiol 31:1215, 1999.
17. Blair E, Redwood C, Ashrafian H, et al: Mutations of the G_2 subunit of AMP-activated protein kinase cause familial hypertrophic cardiomyopathy: Evidence for the central role of energy compromise in disease pathogenesis. Hum Mol Genet 10:1215, 2001.
18. Schmitt JP, Kamisago M, Asahi M, et al: Dilated cardiomyopathy and heart failure caused by a mutation in phospholamban. Science 299:1410, 2003.

Calcium Ion Fluxes in Cardiac Contraction-Relaxation Cycle

19. Bers DM: Cardiac excitation-contraction coupling. Nature 415:198, 2002.
20. Marx SO, Reiken S, Hisamatsu Y, et al: PKA phosphorylation dissociates FKBP12.6 from the calcium release channel (ryanodine receptor): Defective regulation in failing hearts. Cell 101:365, 2000.
21. Wier WG, Balke CW: Ca^{2+} release mechanisms, Ca^{2+} sparks, and local control of excitation-contraction coupling in normal heart muscle. Circ Res 85:770, 1999.
22. Boehm E, Ventua-Clapier R, Mateo P, et al: Glycolysis supports calcium uptake by the sarcoplasmic reticulum in skinned ventricular fibres of mice deficient in mitochondrial and cytosolic creatinine kinase. J Mol Cell Cardiol 32:891, 2000.
23. del Monte F, Williams E, Lebeche D, et al: Improvement in survival and cardiac metabolism after gene transfer of sarcoplasmic reticulum Ca^{2+}- ATPase in a rat model of heart failure. Circulation 104:1424, 2001.
24. Tada M, Katz AM: Phosphorylation of the sarcoplasmic reticulum and sarcolemma. Annu Rev Physiol 44:401, 1982.
25. Brittsan AG, Kranias EG: Phospholamban and cardiac contractile function. J Mol Cell Cardiol 32:2131, 2000.
26. Li Y, Kranias EG, Mignery GA, Bers DM: Protein kinase A phosphorylation of the ryanodine receptor does not affect calcium sparks in mouse ventricular myocytes. Circ Res 90:309, 2002.
27. Bers DM, Perez-Reyes E: Ca channels in cardiac myocytes: Structure and function in Ca influx and intracellular Ca release. Cardiovasc Res 42:339, 1999.
28. Opie LH: Heart Physiology, from Cell to Circulation. 4th ed. Philadelphia, Lippincott Williams & Wilkins, 2004.
29. Carmeliet E: Cardiac ionic currents and acute ischemia: from channels to arrhythmias. Physiol Rev 79:917, 1999.
30. Dipla K, Mattiello JA, Margulies KB, et al: The sarcoplasmic reticulum and the Na^+/Ca^{2+} exchanger both contribute to the Ca^{2+} transient of failing human ventricular myocytes. Circ Res 84:435, 1999.
31. Glitsch HG: Electrophysiology of the sodium-potassium-ATPase in cardiac cells. Physiol Rev 81:1781, 2001.

32. Rockman HA, Koch WJ, Lefkowitz RJ: Seven-transmembrane-spanning receptors and heart function. Nature 415:206, 2002.
33. Xiao RP, Cheng H, Zhou YY, et al: Recent advances in cardiac β_2-adrenergic signal transduction. Circ Res 85:1092, 1999.
34. Smith C, Teitler M: Beta-blocker selectivity at cloned human beta$_1$- and beta$_2$-adrenergic receptors. Cardiovasc Drugs Ther 13:123, 1999.
35. Lefkowitz RJ: Clinical implications of basic research. G proteins in medicine. N Engl J Med 332:186, 1995.
36. Roth DM, Gao MH, Lai C, et al: Cardiac-detected adenylyl cyclase expression improves heart function in murine cardiomyopathy. Circulation 99:3099, 1999.
37. Esposito G, Rapacciuolo A, Prasad SVN, et al: Genetic alterations that inhibit in vivo pressure-overload hypertrophy prevent cardiac dysfunction despite increased wall stress. Circulation 105:85, 2002.
38. Kompa AR, Gu X-H, Evans BA, Summers RJ: Desensitization of cardiac β-adrenoreceptor signaling with heart failure produced by myocardial infarction in the rat. Evidence for the role of G_i but not G_s phosphorylating proteins. J Mol Cell Cardiol 31:1185, 1999.
39. Owen VA, Burton PBJ, Michel MC, et al: Myocardial dysfunction in donor hearts. A possible etiology. Circulation 99:2565, 1999.
40. Bers DM, Ziolo M: When is cAMP not cAMP? Effects of compartmentalization [editorial]. Circ Res 89:373, 2001.
41. Hall RA, Lefkowitz RJ: Regulation of G protein–coupled receptor signaling by scaffold proteins. Circ Res 91:672, 2002.
42. Luttrell LM, Ferguson SSG, Kaaka Y, et al: β-Arrestin-dependent formation of β_2 adrenergic receptor–Src protein kinase complexes. Science 283:655, 1999.
43. Rohrer DK: Molecular organisation of the β-adrenergic system. *In* Böhm M, Laragh J, Zehender M (eds): From Hypertension to Heart Failure. Berlin, Springer, 1998, pp 129-158.
44. Yu X, Zhang M, Kyker K, et al: Ischemic inactivation of G protein–coupled receptor kinase and altered desensitization of canine cardiac β-adrenergic receptors. Circulation 102:2535, 2000.
45. Xiao R-P, Avdonin P, Zhou U-Y, et al: Coupling of β_2-adrenoreceptor to G_i proteins and its physiological relevance in murine cardiac myocytes. Circ Res 84:43, 1999.
46. Newton GE, Azevedo ER, Parker JD: Inotropic and sympathetic responses to the intracoronary infusion of a β_2-receptor agonist. A human in vivo study. Circulation 99:2402, 1999.
47. Varghese P, Harrison RW, Lofthouse RA, et al: β_3-Adrenorecptor deficiency blocks nitric oxide–dependent inhibition of myocardial contractility. J Clin Invest 106:697, 2000.

Cholinergic and Nitric Oxide Signaling

48. Friebe A, Koesling D: Regulation of nitric oxide–sensitive guanylyl cyclase. Circ Res 93:96, 2003.
49. Ziolo MT, Bers DM: The real estate of NOS signaling. Location, location, location. Circ Res 92:1279, 2003.
50. Lewis ME, Al-Khalidi AH, Bonser RS, et al: Vagus nerve stimulation decreases left ventricular contractility in vivo in the human and pig heart. J Physiol (Lond) 534:547, 2001.
51. Paterson DJ: Nitric oxide and the autonomic regulation of cardiac excitability. Exp Physiol 86:1, 2001.
52. Hambrecht R, Adams V, Erbs S, et al: Regular physical activity improves endothelial function in patients with coronary artery disease by increasing phosphorylation of endothelial nitric oxide synthase. Circulation 107:3152, 2003.
53. Rakhit RD, Mojet MH, Marber MS, Duchen MR: Mitochondria as targets for nitric oxide–induced protection during simulated ischemia and reoxygenation in isolated neonatal cardiomyocytes. Circulation 103:2617, 2001.
54. Hochman JS: Cardiogenic shock complicating acute myocardial infarction. Expanding the paradigm. Circulation 107:2998, 2003.
55. Pinsky DJ, Patton S, Mesaros S, et al: Mechanical transduction of nitric oxide synthesis in the beating heart. Circ Res 81:372, 1997.
56. Chowdhary S, Nuttall SL, Coote JH, Townend JN: L-Arginine augments cardiac vagal control in healthy human subjects. Hypertension 39:51, 2002.
57. Shyrock J, Song Y, Wang D, et al: Selective A_2-adenosine receptor agonists do not alter action potential duration, twitch shortening, or cAMP accumulation in guinea pig, rat or rabbit isolated ventricular myocytes. Circ Res 72:194, 1993.
58. Tracey WR, Magee W, Masamune H, et al: Selective activation of adenosine A_3 receptors with N^6-(3-chlorobenzyl)-5′-*N*-methylcarboxamidoadenosine (CB-MECA) provides cardioprotection via K_{ATP} channel activation. Cardiovasc Res 40:138, 1998.
59. Kevelaitis E, Peynet J, Mouas C, et al: Opening of potassium channels. The common cardioprotective link between preconditioning and natural hibernation. Circulation 99:3079, 1999.
60. Gross GJ: Role of opioids in acute and delayed preconditioning. J Mol Cell Cardiol 35:709, 2003.
61. Bishop JE, Lindahl G: Regulation of cardiovascular synthesis by mechanical load. Cardiovasc Res 42:27, 1999.
62. Lecour S, Smith RM, Woodward B, et al: Identification of a novel role for sphingolipid signalling in TNF-α and ischemic preconditioning mediated protection. J Mol Cell Cardiol 34:509, 2002.
63. Thielmann M, Dorge H, Martin C, et al: Myocardial dysfunction with coronary microembolization. Signal transduction through a sequence of nitric oxide, tumour necrosis factor-α, and sphingosine. Circ Res 90:807, 2002.
64. Sack MN, Smith RM, Opie LH: Tumour necrosis factor in myocardial hypertrophy and ischaemia—An anti-apoptotic perspective. Cardiovasc Res 45:688, 1999.

Contractile Performance of the Intact Heart

65. Lewis T: The Mechanism and Graphic Registration of the Heart Beat. London, Shaw and Sons, 1920.
66. Wiggers CJ: Modern Aspects of Circulation in Health and Disease. Philadelphia, Lea & Febiger, 1915.
67. Rhodes J, Udelson JE, Marx GR, et al: A new noninvasive method for the estimation of peak dP/dt. Circulation 88:2693, 1993.
68. Ohno M, Cheng CP, Little WC: Mechanism of altered patterns of left ventricular filling during the development of congestive heart failure. Circulation 89:2241, 1994.
69. Glower DD, Murrah RL, Olsen CO, et al: Mechanical correlates of the third heart sound. J Am Coll Cardiol 19:450, 1992.
70. Brutsaert DL, Sys SU, Gilbert TC: Diastolic failure: Pathophysiology and therapeutic implications. J Am Coll Cardiol 22:318, 1993.
71. Rodriguez EK, Hunter WC, Royce MJ: A method to reconstruct myocardial sarcomere lengths and orientations at transmural sites in beating canine hearts. Am J Physiol 263:H293, 1992.
72. MacGowan GA, Shapiro EP, Azhari H, et al: Noninvasive measurement of shortening in the fiber and cross-fiber directions in the normal human left ventricle and in idiopathic dilated cardiomyopathy. Circulation 96:535, 1997.
73. Mulieri LA, Leavitt BJ, Martin BJ: Myocardial force-frequency defect in mitral regurgitation heart failure is reversed by forskolin. Circulation 88:2700, 1993.
74. Pierard LA, Serruys PW, Roelandt J, Melzer RS: Left ventricular function at similar heart rates during tachycardia induced by exercise and atrial pacing: An echocardiographic study. Br Heart J 57:154, 1987.
75. Inagaki M, Yokota M, Izawa H, et al: Impaired force-frequency relations in patients with hypertensive left ventricular hypertrophy. Circulation 99:1822, 1999.
76. Suga H, Hisano R, Hirata S, et al: Mechanism of higher oxygen consumption rate: Pressure-loaded vs volume-loaded heart. Am J Physiol 242:H942, 1982.
77. Nozawa T, Cheng C-P, Noda T, Little WC: Effect of exercise on left ventricular mechanical efficiency in conscious dogs. Circulation 90:3047, 1994.
78. Chavez PN, Stanley WC, McElfresh TA, et al: Effect of hyperglycemia and fatty acid oxidation inhibition during aerobic conditions and demand-induced ischemia. Am J Physiol 284:H1521, 2003.
79. Beanlands RSB, Nahmias C, Gordon E, et al: The effects of β_1-blockade on oxidative metabolism and the metabolic cost of ventricular work in patients with left ventricular dysfunction. Circulation 102:2070, 2000.
80. Braunwald E, Sonnenblick EH, Ross J: Normal and abnormal circulatory function. *In* Braunwald E (ed): Heart Disease. A Textbook of Cardiovascular Medicine. 4th ed. Philadelphia, WB Saunders, 1992, pp 351–392.
81. Campbell KB, Kirkpatrick RD, Tobias AH: Series coupled non-contractile elements are functionally unimportant in the isolated heart. Cardiovasc Res 28:242, 1994.
82. Strang KT, Sweitzer NK, Greaser ML, Moss RL: β-Adrenergic receptor stimulation increases unloaded shortening velocity of skinned single ventricular myocytes from rats. Circ Res 74:542, 1994.
83. Brookes CIO, White PA, Staples M, et al: Myocardial contractility is not constant during spontaneous atrial fibrillation in patients. Circulation 98:1762, 1998.
84. Vogel M, Cheung MH, Li J, et al: Noninvasive assessment of left ventricular force-frequency relationships using tissue Doppler-derived isovolumic acceleration. Circulation 107:1647, 2003.
85. Zile MR, Brutsaert DL: New concepts in diastolic dysfunction and diastolic heart failure: Part 1. Circulation 105:1387, 2002.
86. Leite-Moreira AF, Correia-Pinto J, Gillebert TC: Afterload induced changes in myocardial relaxation: A mechanism for diastolic dysfunction. Cardiovasc Res 43:344, 1999.
87. Hein S, Amon E, Kostin S, et al: Progression from compensated hypertrophy to failure in the pressure-overloaded human heart. Structural deterioration and compensatory mechanisms. Circulation 107:984, 2003.
88. Zhang R, Zhao J, Mandveno A, Potter JD: Cardiac troponin I phosphorylation increases the rate of cardiac muscle relaxation. Circ Res 76:1028, 1995.
89. Cory CR, Grange RW, Houston ME: Role of sarcoplasmic reticulum in loss of load-sensitive relaxation in pressure overload cardiac hypertrophy. Am J Physiol 266:H68, 1994.
90. Bell SP, Nyland L, Tischler MD, et al: Alterations in the determinants of diastolic suction during pacing tachycardia. Circ Res 87:235, 2000.
91. Schotten U, Duytschaever M, Ausma J, et al: Electrical and contractile remodeling during the first days of atrial fibrillation go hand in hand. Circulation 107:1433, 2003.
92. Yu C-M, Lin H, Yang H, et al: Progression of systolic abnormalities in patients with "isolated" diastolic heart failure and diastolic dysfunction. Circulation 105:1195, 2002.
93. Nagueh SF, Middleton KJ, Kopelen HA, et al: Doppler tissue imaging: A noninvasive technique for evaluation of left ventricular relaxation and estimation of filling pressures. J Am Coll Cardiol 30:1527, 1997.

Effects of Ischemia and Reperfusion on Contraction and Relaxation

94. Opie L, Heusch G: Lack of blood flow: Ischemia and angina. *In* Opie LH (ed): Heart Physiology, from Cell to Circulation. 4th ed. Philadelphia, Lippincott Williams & Wilkins, 2004, pp 525–552.
95. Li RA, Leppo M, Miki T, et al: Molecular basis of electrocardiographic ST-segment elevation. Circ Res 87:837, 2000.
96. McDonough JL, Arrell K, Van Eyk JE: Troponin I degradation and covalent complex formation accompanies myocardial ischemia/reperfusion injury. Circ Res 84:9, 1999.
97. Murry CE, Jennings RB, Reimer KA: Preconditioning with ischemia: A delay of lethal cell injury in ischemic myocardium. Circulation 74:1124, 1986.
98. Yellon DM, Downey JM: Preconditioning the myocardium: From cellular physiology to clinical cardiology. Physiol Rev 83:1113, 2003.
99. Nakano A, Liu GS, Heusch G, et al: Exogenous nitric oxide can trigger a preconditioned state through a free radical mechanism, but endogenous nitric oxide is not a trigger of classical ischemic preconditioning. J Mol Cell Cardiol 32:1159, 2000.
100. Bolli R: Cardioprotective function of inducible nitric oxide synthase and role of nitric oxide in myocardial ischemia and preconditioning: An overview of a decade of research. J Mol Cell Cardiol 33:1897, 2001.

101. Minners J, McLeod C, Sack MN: Mitochondrial plasticity in classical ischemic preconditioning—Moving beyond the mitochondrial K_{ATP} channel. Cardiovasc Res 59:1, 2003.
102. Rajesh KG, Sasaguri S, Zhitian Z, et al: Second window of ischemic preconditioning regulates mitochondrial permeability transition pore by enhancing Bcl-2 expression. Cardivasc Res 59:297, 2003.
103. Simpson PC: β-Protein kinase C and hypertrophic signaling in human heart failure. Circulation 99:334, 1999.
104. Inagaki K, Hahn HS, Dorn GW 2nd, Mochly-Rosen D: Additive protection of the ischemic heart ex vivo by combined treatment with δ-protein kinase C inhibitor and ε-protein kinase C activator. Circulation 108:869, 2003.
105. Cross HR, Murphy E, Bolli R, et al: Expression of activated PKC epsilon (PKC_ε) protects the ischemic heart, without attenuating ischemic H^+ production. J Mol Cell Cardiol 34:361, 2002.
106. Lambiase PD, Edwards RJ, Cusack MR, et al: Exercise-induced ischemia initiates the second window of protection in humans independent of collateral recruitment. J Am Coll Cardiol 41:1174, 2003.
107. Rahimtoola S: Myocardial hibernation: Current clinical perspectives. *In* Yellon DM, Rahimtoola SH, Opie LH (eds): New Ischemic Syndromes. New York, Lippincott-Raven, 1997, pp 215-234.
108. Heusch G, Schulz R: Hibernating myocardium. New answers, still more questions! Circ Res 91:863, 2002.
109. Cain BS, Harken AH, Meldrum DR: Therapeutic strategies to reduce TNF-α medicated cardiac contractile depression following ischemia and reperfusion. J Mol Cell Cardiol 31:931, 1999.
110. Kalra DK, Zhu X, Ranchandani MK, et al: Increased myocardial gene expression of tumour necrosis factor-alpha and nitric oxide synthase-2: A potential mechanism for depressed myocardial function in hibernating myocardium in humans. Circulation 105:1537, 2002.
111. Auerbach MA, Scholder H, Hoh C, et al: Prevalence of myocardial viability as detected by position emission tomography in patients with ischemic cardiomyopathy. Circulation 99:2921, 1999.
112. Braunwald E, Kloner RA: The stunned myocardium: Prolonged, postischemic ventricular dysfunction. Circulation 66:1146, 1982.
113. Bolli R, Marban E: Molecular and cellular mechanisms of myocardial stunning. Physiol Rev 79:609, 1999.
114. Zeitz O, Maass E, Van Nguyen P, et al: Hydroxyl radical–induced acute diastolic dysfunction is due to calcium overload via reverse-mode Na^+-Ca^{2+} exchange. Circ Res 90:988, 2002.
115. Kloner RA, Jennings RB: Consequences of brief ischemia: Stunning, preconditioning, and their clinical implications. Part 1. Circulation 104:2981, 2001.
116. Perez NG, Gao WD, Marban E: Novel myofilament Ca^{2+}-sensitizing property of xanthine oxidase inhibitors. Circ Res 83:423, 1998.

Heart Failure

117. Meyer M, Keweloh B, Guth K, et al: Frequency-dependence of myocardial energetics in failing human myocardium as quantified by a new method for the measurement of oxygen consumption in muscle strip preparations. J Mol Cell Cardiol 30:1459, 1998.
118. Marx J: How to subdue a swelling heart. Science 300:1492, 2003.
119. Maurice JP, Shah AS, Kypson AP, et al: Molecular beta-adrenergic signaling abnormalities in failing rabbit hearts after infarction. Am J Physiol 276:H1853, 1999.
120. Moniotte S, Kobzik L, Feron O, et al: Upregulation of $beta_3$-adrenoreceptors and altered contractile response to inotropic amines in human failing myocardium. Circulation 103:1649, 2001.
121. Reiken S, Wehrens XHT, Vest JA, et al: β-Blockers restore calcium release channel function and improve cardiac muscle performance in human heart failure. Circulation 107:2459, 2003.
122. Kubo H, Margulies K, Piacentino V 3rd, et al: Patients with end-stage congestive heart failure treated with β-adrenergic receptor antagonists have improved ventricular myocyte calcium regulatory protein abundance. Circulation 104:1012, 2001.
123. Chandler MP, Stanley WC, Morita H, et al: Short-term treatment with ranolazine improves mechanical efficiency in dogs with chronic heart failure. Circ Res 91:278, 2002.
124. Wallhaus TR, Taylor M, Degrado TR, et al: Myocardial free fatty acid and glucose use after carvedilol treatment in patients with congestive heart failure. Circulation 103:2441, 2001.
125. Münch G, Bolck B, Karczewski P, Schwinger RHG: Evidence for calcineurin-mediated regulation of SERCA 2a activity in human myocardium. J Mol Cell Cardiol 34:321, 2002.
126. Marks AR, Reiken S, Marx SO: Progression of heart failure: Is protein kinase a hyperphosphorylation of the ryanodine receptor a contributing factor. Circulation 105:272, 2002.
127. Münch G, Bolck B, Brixius K, et al: SERCA2a activity correlates with the force-frequency relationship in human myocardium. Am J Physiol 278:H1924, 2000.
128. Clusin WT: Calcium and cardiac arrhythmias: DADs, EADs and alternans. Crit Rev Clin Lab Sci 40:337, 2003.
129. Pieske B, Kockskämper J: Alternans goes subcellular. A "disease" of the ryanodine receptor? Circ Res 91:553, 2002.
130. Matsuda JJ, Lee H-C, Shibata EF: Acetylcholine reversal of isoproterenol-stimulated sodium currents in rabbit ventricular myocytes. Circ Res 72:517, 1993.
131. Matsuda JJ, Lee H, Shibata EF: Enhancement of rabbit cardiac sodium channels by β-adrenergic stimulation. Circ Res 74:369, 1992.
132. Chang F, Cohen IS: Mechanism of acetylcholine action on pacemaker current (I_f) in canine Purkinje fibers. Pflugers Arch 420:389, 1992.
133. Kurachi Y: G-protein control of cardiac potassium channels. Trends Cardiovasc Med 4:64, 1994.
134. Fedida D: Modulation of cardiac contractility by α_1-adrenoreceptors. Cardiovasc Res 27:1735, 1993.
135. Volders PGA, Stengl M, van Opstal JM, et al: Probing the contribution of I_{KS} to canine ventricular repolarization. Circulation 107:2753, 2003.
136. Shannon TR, Ginsburg KS, Bers DM: Quantitative assessment of the SR Ca^{2+} leak-load relationship. Circ Res 91:594, 2002.
137. Pieske B, Maier LS, Bers DM, Hasenfuss G: Ca^{2+} handling and sarcoplasmic reticulum Ca^{2+} content in isolated failing and nonfailing human myocardium. Circ Res 85:38, 1999.
138. Piacentino V 3rd, Weber CR, Chen X, et al: Cellular basis of abnormal calcium transients of failing human ventricular myocytes. Circ Res 92:651, 2003.
139. Cooke R: Actomyosin interactions in striated muscle. Physiol Rev 77:671, 1997.
140. Holmes KC: The swinging lever-arm hypothesis of muscle contraction. Curr Biol 7:R112, 1997.
141. Bolli R, Shinmura K, Tang X-L, et al: Discovery of a new function of cyclooxygenase (COX)-2: COX-2 is a cardioprotective protein that alleviates ischemia/reperfusion injury and mediates the late phase of preconditioning. Cardiovasc Res 55:506, 2002.

CHAPTER 20

Assessment of Normal and Abnormal Cardiac Function

John D. Carroll • Otto M. Hess

The history of the study of cardiac function has been a progression from a description of cardiac anatomy, from this deducing function, to quantifying physiology, and now to the unraveling of molecular pathways.[1] The phenotype and genotype of disease states in patients provide a comprehensive understanding of pathophysiology, yielding answers to the question of why alterations in cardiac function occur. On the other hand, it is the clinical assessment of cardiac function that is necessary to determine the prognosis and the impact of therapy (Table 20–1).

New Relevance of Assessment of Cardiac Function

The rapid introduction and dissemination of novel therapies for cardiac dysfunction (see Chaps. 23 and 24) have characterized clinical cardiology in the last decade. Many of these new approaches and therapies have called on, resurrected, and extended a large reservoir of prior art in the field of assessment of cardiac function. The five examples that follow illustrate how contemporary investigators and clinicians require an in-depth understanding of the assessment of the relations between cardiac function, the quantification of reverse remodeling, and clinical outcomes.

RESYNCHRONIZATION THERAPY (see Chaps. 24 and 31). The mechanical and metabolic inefficiencies consequent to the loss of synchronous contraction and relaxation were topics confined to laboratory investigators of ventricular function until the advent of resynchronization therapy in heart failure with biventricular pacing.[2] Now there is a broad need for tools to quantify asynchrony and its modification by various modes of pacing (see Fig. 20–5).

VENTRICULAR ASSIST DEVICES (see Chap. 25). New mechanical cardiac assist devices may be implanted surgically or placed percutaneously and require a high level of sophistication in assessing cardiac function.[3] Distinguishing between the right and left ventricular components of a clinical syndrome of severe heart failure is important for proper patient selection. Management issues that involve assessment of preload and afterload in a two-pump environment, i.e., the native heart and the mechanical assist device, are common. Finally, the evaluation of therapeutic endpoints including reverse remodeling, as well as the serial assessment of cardiac function during weaning from the ventricular assist device, are critical to patient management.

ANGIOGENESIS AND STEM CELL TRANSPLANTATION (see Chap. 69). Transplantation of skeletal myoblasts and hematopoietic stem cells into regions of damaged myocardium is currently a field of active investigation.[4] Some cell lines enhance angiogenesis with the potential for ending the hibernating status of native myocytes. Others may become functional components of the myocardial syncytium. Both approaches present investigators with challenges in clarifying mechanisms of altered cardiac mechanical function and bring the need to assess serially regional and global chamber function.

PERCUTANEOUS VALVE REPAIR AND REPLACEMENT (see Chap. 57). Percutaneous approaches to reducing mitral regurgitation by either a coronary venous approach of annular reduction or a leaflet attachment approach provide a more comprehensive understanding of the complexities of valvular function that are linked to chamber size and function. Instantaneous changes in annular size, the severity of mitral regurgitation, and left ventricular function need to be assessed acutely and followed serially noninvasively.

VENTRICULAR PASSIVE CONSTRAINT DEVICES. Another novel therapeutic approach is the surgical or percutaneous insertion of passive ventricular restraining devices that prevent ventricular distention.[5] This approach focuses on prevention of deleterious remodeling after acute events such as large myocardial infarctions. A large body of knowledge on pericardial mechanics and restraining forces on the normal heart has now become timely to understand device design and to anticipate the changes of systolic and diastolic function occurring after implantation. As shown in Figure 20–1, a variety of tools is needed to evaluate the therapeutic effect of a restraining device as well as to monitor for unwanted effects.

Left Ventricular Systolic Function

Concepts

The fundamental task of the cardiovascular system is to supply adequate quantities of oxygenated blood to the peripheral tissues. The performance of the heart that is required to perform this task requires the complex interplay between the properties of the myocardium, the influences of neural and humoral factors, the circulating blood volume, and peripheral vascular compliance and resistance. An important determinant of cardiac performance is left ventricular systolic function, which in turn is determined by (1) preload, (2) afterload, (3) myocardial contractility, and (4) heart rate.

These four determinants allow the heart to adapt its performance to the changing requirements of the peripheral organs, as well as to compensate for a loss of myocardial mass and/or function. Cardiac performance is evaluated primarily by assessing left ventricular systolic function. Systole begins with the onset of depolarization and contraction and ends at the cessation of muscle contraction (Fig. 20–2).

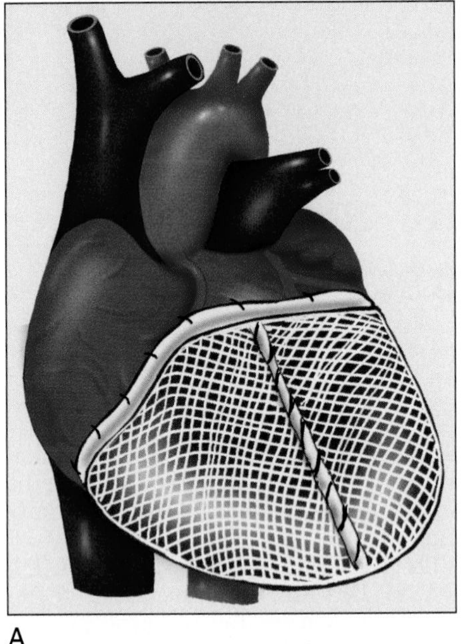

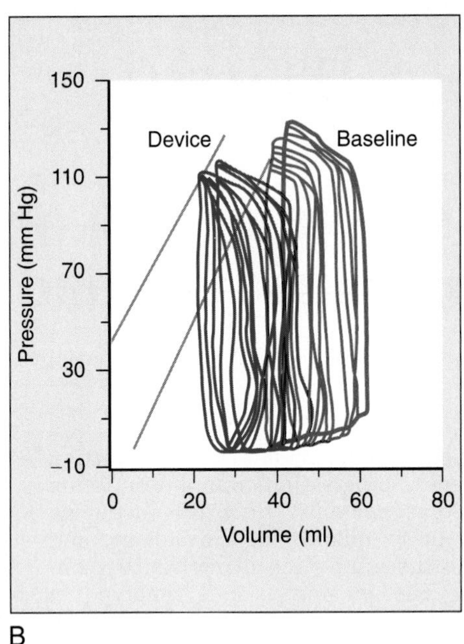

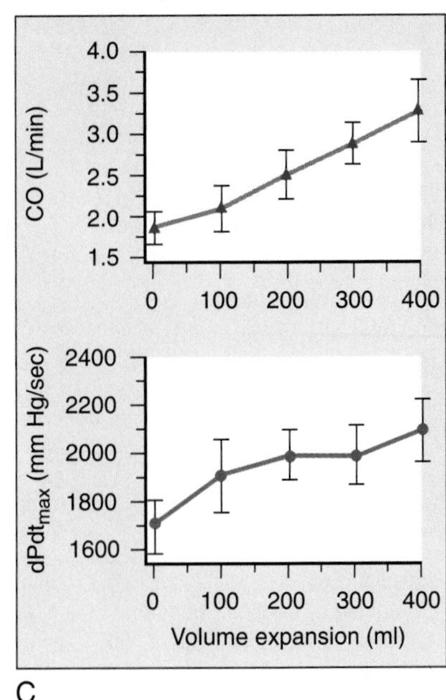

A B C

FIGURE 20–1 **A,** Passive ventricular restraining device. **B,** Device-induced reduction in chamber size and enhanced systolic performance accompanying this reverse remodeling. **C,** Preservation of recruitable preload with volume expansion. The pressure-volume loops generated under different loading states **(B)** demonstrate end-systolic pressure-volume relationships as well as diastolic chamber properties. Data in **C** show the systolic augmentation with volume expansion that was not compromised by the device. These data were obtained in an animal model. (Adapted from Saavedra WF, Tunin RS, Paolocci N, et al: Reverse remodeling and enhanced adrenergic reserve from passive external support in experimental dilated heart failure. J Am Coll Cardiol 39:2069, 2002.)

TABLE 20–1 Uses of Cardiac Function Assessment
Diagnosis
Prognostication
Timing of intervention
Mechanism of therapy
Assessment of therapy
Detection of complications
Surrogate for clinical outcomes

Definitions (Table 20–2)

PRELOAD. The stretch of the individual sarcomere regulates the performance of the heart. In the words of physiologists in the 19th century, preload is the property of cardiac muscle such that "the larger the quantity of blood which reaches the ventricles . . . the larger the quantity will be which it throws out."[6] Surrogates of the degree of sarcomere stretch at the onset of contraction include the ventricular end-diastolic volume, diameter, and end-diastolic pressure. Table 20–2 contrasts the differences between acute and chronic alterations in ventricular end-diastolic volume and pressure. The former enhance cardiac performance (adaptive mechanisms), whereas the latter ultimately impair performance (maladaptive mechanisms) (Table 20–3).

AFTERLOAD. This is the force against which muscle contracts. It is more challenging to quantify afterload in the intact circulation than in isolated cardiac muscle. Two approaches have been followed. The first focuses on the vascular load and uses descriptors such as peripheral vascular resistance or the more complex input impedance (see later) that includes the pulsatile load. The second focuses on the tension in the ventricular wall and considers pressure and cavity size in a more complex formulation, Laplace's law, which considers wall tension to be the product of pressure and radius, whereas the force (or tension) per unit of muscle is expressed in three dimensions, i.e., circumferential, meridional, and radial (Fig. 20–3).

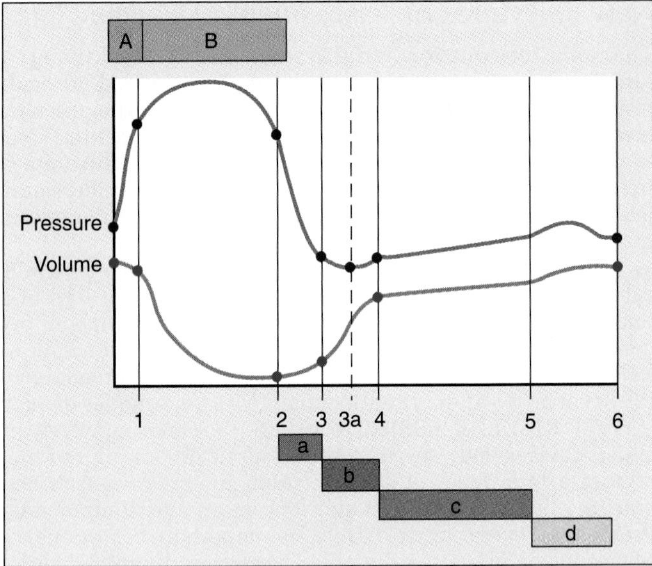

FIGURE 20–2 The cardiac cycle is shown in this schematic with both the left ventricular pressure waveform and a plot of left ventricular volume. The time landmarks during the cardiac cycle include the following: 1, aortic valve opening and the beginning of ejection; 2, aortic valve closure; 3, mitral valve opening; 3a, pressure nadir; 4, end of rapid early diastolic filling; 5, onset of atrial contraction; and 6, end-diastole. The phases of the cardiac cycle are denoted with the shaded rectangles displaying the timing of each phase. The two systolic phases are noted above the waveforms, where A = isovolumic contraction and B = ejection. The four diastolic phases are noted below the waveforms, where a = isovolumic relaxation; b = early diastolic filling; c = diastasis; and d = atrial filling.

CONTRACTILITY. This is the intrinsic ability of heart muscle to generate force and to shorten. In the intact circulation it is manifest as the rate of pressure development and of shortening from any given preload. Contractility is normally modulated by a variety of factors including the neurohumoral milieu. Measures of systolic function and

TABLE 20–2 Definitions of Terms Used to Describe Systolic and Diastolic Function

Term	Definition
Preload	Distending force of the ventricular wall, which is highest at end-diastole and is responsible for sarcomere length at the beginning of systolic contraction
Afterload	Resisting force of the ventricular wall during systolic ejection, which is necessary to overcome peripheral vascular resistance or impedance; measures of afterload are peak-systolic, mean-systolic, or end-systolic wall stress
Contractility	Intrinsic ability of the myocardium to generate force at a certain rate and time (controlled for loading conditions)
Cardiac output	Stroke volume multiplied by heart rate
Stroke work	Mean systolic blood pressure multiplied by stroke volume
Stroke force	Stroke work per ejection time
Stress	Force per area
Wall stress	Pressure multiplied by radius, divided by wall thickness × 2
Compliance or distensibility	Change in volume per change in pressure (dV/dP)
Elastance	Slope of the end-systolic pressure-volume relation
Elasticity	Property of a material to restore its initial length or geometry after distending force has been removed
Strain	Length change in percent of initial length; two definitions are used: LaGrangian strain $e = (l - l_o)l_o$ and natural strain $e = \ln(l/lo)$
Stiffness	Pressure per volume change (dP/dV). *Ventricular stiffness* is a measure for changes of the ventricle as a whole; *myocardial stiffness* is a measure for changes of the myocardium itself. Ventricular properties are characterized by instantaneous pressure-volume relations, whereas myocardial properties are best described by stress-strain relations.
Creep	Time-dependent lengthening of a material in the presence of a constant force
Stress relaxation	Time-dependent decrease of stress in the presence of a constant length
Viscoelasticity	Resistance of a material to length changes (strain) or the velocity of length changes (strain rate)

TABLE 20–3 Two Pathways of Ventricular Dilation and Increased Filling Pressure

Hemodynamic (Acute) Dilation and increased end-diastolic pressure caused when increased venous return or decreased ejection increases end-diastolic volume. This form of dilation occurs when physiological (functional) signaling increases sarcomere length, which increases the heart's ability to perform work (Starling law of the heart)
Architectural (Chronic) Dilation and increased filling pressures caused when hypertrophy increases cardiac myocyte length and alters passive muscle properties. By increasing wall stress, this growth response increases the energy demands of the heart and decreases cardiac efficiency, initiating a vicious circle that worsens heart failure. This form of dilation occurs when abnormal transcriptional (proliferative) signaling causes eccentric hypertrophy (systolic dysfunction), and it tends to progress (remodeling)

Adapted from Katz A: Ernest Henry Starling, his predecessors, and the "law of the heart." Circulation 106:2986, 2002.

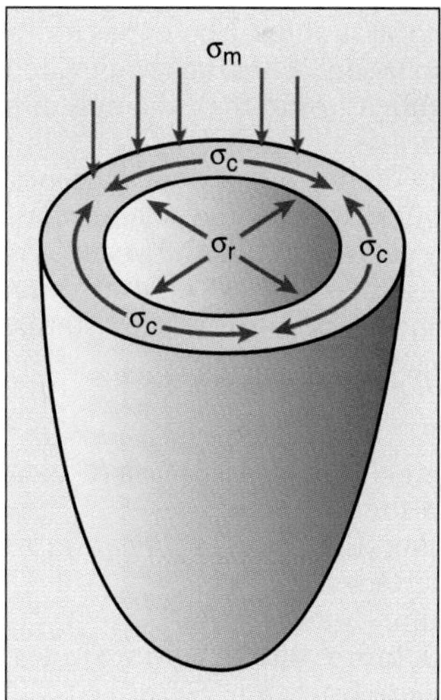

FIGURE 20–3 Circumferential (σ_c), meridional (σ_m), and radial (σ_r) components of left ventricular wall stress from an ellipsoid model. The three components of wall stress are mutually perpendicular. (From Fifer MA, Grossman W: Measurement of ventricular volumes, ejection fraction, mass, and wall stress. In Grossman W [ed]: Cardiac Catheterization and Angiography. 5th ed. Philadelphia, Lea & Febiger, 1996, p 34.)

contractility are often considered together and include stroke volume, ejection fraction, the maximum rate of pressure increases during isovolumic contraction, and a variety of more sophisticated measurements that attempt to control for loading conditions (Table 20–4).[1]

FILLING PRESSURES. The determination of systolic function should be placed in the framework of the ventricular filling pressure that reflects preload; the latter, in turn, is influenced importantly by the status of the circulating blood volume. Filling pressures are also related to both the contractility and diastolic properties of the ventricle (see later). Filling pressures such as ventricular end-diastolic pressure, atrial pressure, and pulmonary capillary wedge pressure (for the left ventricle) and central venous pressure (for the right

TABLE 20–4 Characteristics of Selected Indices of Global Ventricular Function

Index	Sensitive to Inotropic Changes	Dependence On Preload	Dependence On Afterload	Dependence On Ventricular Volume or Mass	Ease of Application
Ejection fraction; fractional shortening	++	++	+++	++	++++
End-systolic volume or dimension	+	0	+++	++	++++
VCF	+++	0	+++	++	+++
Afterload-corrected VCF	+++	0	0	0	+
ESPVR	++++	0	0	+++	+
End-systolic stiffness	++++	0	0	0	+
Preload recruitable stroke work	+++	0	0	++	+
Left ventricular dP/dt	++++	++	++	++	++

ESPVR = slope of end-systolic pressure-volume relation; VCF = velocity of circumferential fiber shortening; dP/dt = rate of ventricular pressure rise.
Adapted from Carabello B: Evolution of the study of left ventricular function: Everything old is new again. Circulation 105:2701, 2002.

ventricle) provide valuable clinical information that aids in the differentiation between disparate conditions causing hypotension, e.g., hypovolemia versus myocardial failure.

Left ventricular end-diastolic pressure (LVEDP) is measured routinely in the cardiac catheterization laboratory during retrograde left heart catheterization (see Chap. 17). It may be difficult to measure LVEDP precisely at rapid heart rates using fluid-filled catheters, especially when there is not a distinctive plateau after atrial contraction. The measurement of LVEDP during invasive and interventional procedures provides a simple and often useful indicator of cardiac function. Several common clinical examples demonstrate the utility of this measurement. An elevated LVEDP in the presence of a normal left ventricular ejection fraction (LVEF) suggests the presence of diastolic dysfunction (see later). A low LVEDP after a percutaneous coronary intervention suggests volume depletion that should be corrected before the development of hypotension. A markedly elevated LVEDP may be a strong contraindication to the injection of contrast dye and suggests that diuresis is needed.

Central venous pressure is a poor indicator of left ventricular filling pressure, since it may be normal in the presence of an abnormally elevated LVEDP. Tricuspid regurgitation and pericardial disease may elevate central venous pressure and confound it as an indicator of volume status.

Calculations and Measurements of Systolic Function

Clinical parameters for assessing left ventricular systolic function include the following:

- Cardiac index (liter/min/m^2): heart rate × stroke volume per body surface area
- Stroke volume index (ml/m^2)
- Stroke work index: stroke volume index × mean systolic blood pressure (ml × mm Hg/m^2)
- Stroke force index: stroke work index per ejection period in seconds
- Preload recruitable stroke work = relationship between stroke work and end-diastolic volume

CARDIAC OUTPUT AND RELATED MEASURES. Cardiac output is commonly measured by the thermodilution technique (see Chap. 17). Saline injected into the right atrium is detected as a temperature change at a thermistor at the tip of a catheter in the pulmonary artery. The thermodilution catheter transmits the temperature data to a small computer that calculates cardiac output. To improve accuracy, the determination is usually repeated several times and the results are averaged. This technique is less accurate when flow is severely reduced, especially in the presence of tricuspid regurgitation, which leads to dissipation of the "temperature bolus." The presence of intracardiac shunts also introduces potential errors and misinterpretation since right- and left-sided flows are not equal. The Fick method of measuring cardiac output has greater accuracy than the thermodilution method when oxygen consumption is actually measured, rather than assumed. However measured, cardiac output is usually expressed relative to body size, i.e., cardiac index, which is calculated as cardiac output divided by body surface area, expressed in square meters.

Cardiac output (and index) can be divided by the heart rate to yield stroke volume (and index). An alternative method of deriving stroke volume is by calculating the difference between left ventricular volume at end-diastole and end-systole. This approach is limited by the accuracy of the imaging modality in determining chamber volumes. Accuracy is greatest with a three-dimensional (3D) determined volume with high-resolution imaging, but it may be impaired by the normal beat-to-beat variation in chamber size that occurs during respiration and is accentuated in atrial fibrillation and other arrhythmias. The product of pressure generation and stroke volume equals stroke work; when related to the time interval during which the stroke volume is ejected from the left ventricle (i.e., the ejection time) stroke force may be derived.

VENTRICULAR FUNCTION CURVES. Reduced values of stroke parameters (volume, work, force, and their indices, i.e., corrected for body surface area) are often associated with depressed myocardial contractility, but since these parameters are highly dependent on the loading conditions (preload and afterload), these two variables must also be assessed. The dependency of stroke volume on preload was described more than 100 years ago by Otto Frank and E. H. Starling, and since then has been called the Frank-Starling mechanism.[6] Using this relationship between preload and stroke volume or stroke work, a *ventricular function curve* can be constructed by plotting stroke work at various levels of preload; the latter may be expressed as ventricular end-diastolic volume, end-diastolic pressure, or end-diastolic wall stress. Preload can be altered by volume loading (leg elevation, volume infusion) and unloading (vena caval balloon occlusion). Left ventricular afterload can be estimated from the mean or end systolic arterial or ventricular pressure or, more accurately, by calculating mean systolic, peak systolic, or end-systolic wall stress. The most reliable method for determination of left ventricular contractility represents the end-systolic pressure-volume relationship (ESPVR; maximum elastance), which is nearly

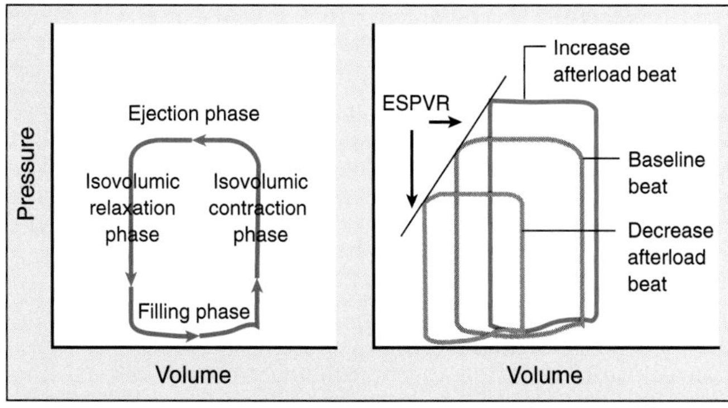

FIGURE 20–4 **Left,** Left ventricular pressure-volume relationship is shown, with the four phases of the cardiac cycle. **Right,** The graph shows how two additional pressure-volume loops appear with an acute increase and decrease in afterload. Changes in preload can also be used to generate the coordinates. In the clinical setting it is difficult to generate the end-systolic pressure-volume relationship (ESPVR) free of changes in reflex-mediated variations in contractility. It also requires a means to measure pressure and volume accurately and simultaneously. The end-systolic pressure-volume coordinates form a linear relationship, ESPVR. The slope of the ESPVR line is end-systolic elastance.

independent of preload and afterload. The slope of this relationship is a measure of left ventricular contractility (Figs. 20–4 and 20–5; see also Fig. 20–1).

The use of ventricular function curves in assessing left ventricular function is limited by variability dependent on gender, age, and afterload. Furthermore, changes in right ventricular filling pressure can affect the position of the interventricular septum and thereby alter left ventricular diastolic pressure and thereby alter the position of the ventricular function curve as well.

Specific Indices

There are several indices of global left ventricular systolic function and contractility.[1] As shown in Table 20–4, each index is variably dependent on preload and afterload and can be modified by ventricular volume and myocardial mass. The ease of application to the clinical setting is an important feature.

EJECTION FRACTION. The *ejection fraction* is defined as the ratio of stroke volume to end-diastolic volume. It is most often computed as follows:

$$EF = EDV - ESV/EDV \times 100\ (\%)$$

where EF = ejection fraction, EDV = end-diastolic volume, and ESV = end-systolic volume.

Normal values of LVEF are 0.55 to 0.75 when determined by angiocardiography and echocardiography but may be lower when determined by radionuclide angiography (0.50 to 0.65). There are no gender differences, but ejection fraction normally declines with age. An acute increase in afterload, such as occurs during acute pressure loading, may decrease ejection fraction to 0.45 or 0.50 in normal subjects. However, a reduction of LVEF below 0.45 indicates impaired myocardial function, independent of loading conditions.

The widespread utility of the ejection fraction in clinical practice is a result of multiple factors including the conceptual simplicity of its derivation, the ability to determine it easily and reproducibly, using a variety of different imaging techniques, and an extensive documentation of its clinical utility.[1] This parameter has been shown to be of great prognostic value both short-term and long-term in patients with a variety of heart diseases. However, its limitation is its dependency not only on myocardial contractility but also on preload and afterload, as well as heart rate and synchronicity of contraction. Therefore, it measures much more than contractility.

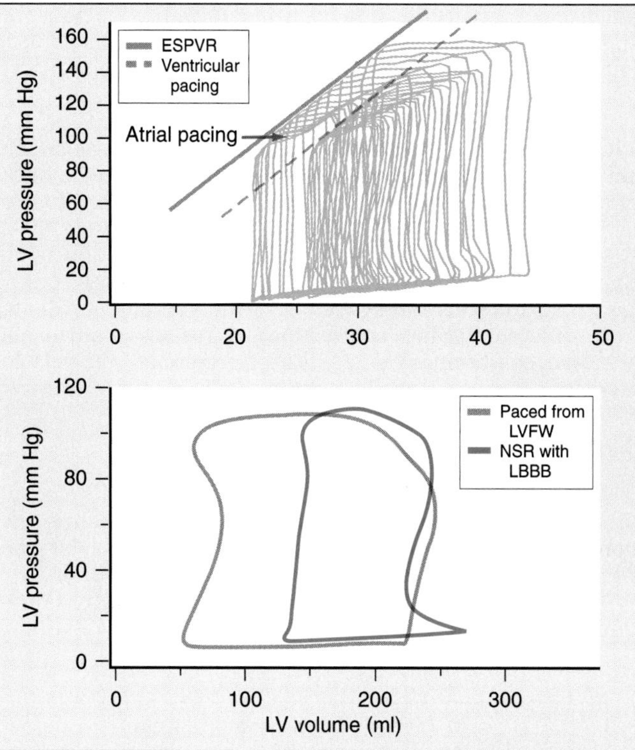

FIGURE 20–5 **Top,** Left ventricular (LV) pressure-volume loops in an experimental animal during transient caval occlusions. The upper left corners of the loops define the LV end-systolic pressure-volume relation (ESPVR). During atrial pacing producing normal LV activation, the ESPVR is shifted leftward in a parallel fashion, compared with ventricular pacing that produces dyssynchronous LV activation and contraction. **Bottom,** Steady-state LV pressure-volume loop recorded using the conductance catheter in a patient with dilated cardiomyopathy and dyssynchronous LV activation due to left bundle branch block (LBBB). A decrease in dyssynchronous contraction produced by LV free wall (LVFW) pacing produced loops with greater width (stroke volume) as the end-systolic pressure-volume point shifted toward the left. NSR = normal sinus rhythm. (**Top,** From Park RC, Little WC, O'Rourke RA: Effect of alteration of left ventricular activation sequence on the left ventricular end-systolic pressure-volume relation in closed-chest dogs. Circ Res 57:711, 1985; and **Bottom,** Kass DA, Chen DH, Curry C, et al: Improved left ventricular mechanics from acute VDD pacing in patients with dilated cardiomyopathy and ventricular conduction delay. Circulation 99:1570, 1999.)

END-SYSTOLIC VENTRICULAR VOLUME OR DIMENSION. The clinical utility of end-systolic volume or dimension is its relative *independence* of preload. Although strongly afterload dependent, it is of particular value in assessing left ventricular function in patients with valvular regurgitation.

VELOCITY OF CIRCUMFERENTIAL FIBER (VCF) SHORTENING. This ejection phase index of systolic function has been used primarily in research studies. Typically, the changes in the left ventricular volume or circumference during systole (corrected to the end-diastolic value) are divided by ejection time to yield the mean velocity of ejection or fiber shortening.

AFTERLOAD-CORRECTED VCF. Since ejection phase indices such as VCF are highly afterload dependent, they become more accurate indicators of ventricular function by correcting with some measure of afterload. Further correction for left ventricular geometry is made by using stress instead of pressure. There are several methods for calculating wall stress; the most common model of Sandler and Dodge has been used (circumferential wall stress):

$$P \times b/h \times (1 - b^2/[a^2 + 2b + h])$$

where P = pressure, h = left ventricular wall thickness, b = short half-axis, and a = long half-axis. Patients with reduced left ventricular contractility have a downward shift of the systolic shortening–mean systolic wall stress relationship.

SLOPE OF END-SYSTOLIC PRESSURE-VOLUME RELATIONSHIP (END SYSTOLIC ELASTANCE). The most reliable index for assessing myocardial contractility in the intact circulation is the ESPVR, which is almost *insensitive* to changes in preload, afterload, and heart rate (see Figs. 20–1, 20–4, and 20–5). This is widely used in animal studies and occasionally clinically. This relationship can be determined from instantaneous end-systolic pressure-volume coordinates from different cardiac contractions at varying preload and afterload conditions. Using a linear regression analysis for assessing the end-systolic pressure-volume curve, the following equation is used:

$$E(t) = P(t)/V(t) - V_o(t)$$

where E = maximum elastance, P = pressure, V = volume, and V_o = extrapolated volume at pressure 0. The slope of this relationship represents the end-systolic elastance, which is a sensitive parameter for assessing myocardial contractility.

Assessment of elastance is difficult under clinical conditions, because it requires simultaneous pressure-volume relations, as well as changes in preload or afterload for construction of the ESPVR. However, this measurement is facilitated by the use of techniques such as radionuclide angiography or the use of conductance catheters, which allow continuous measurements of left ventricular volume while left ventricular volume is changed, e.g., by caval occlusion.

END-SYSTOLIC STIFFNESS. This index of contractile function is derived from the exponential constant of the end-systolic relation between wall stress and the natural logarithm of the reciprocal of wall thickness.[1]

PRELOAD RECRUITABLE STROKE WORK. The relation between left ventricular stroke work and left ventricular end-diastolic volume is a representation of systolic function.[7] Like the end-systolic elastance, it is difficult to assess this parameter in patients because preload needs to be varied to generate this parameter.

MAXIMUM RATE OF PRESSURE RISE. The maximal rate of ventricular pressure rise (maximum dP/dt) is analogous to the maximal rate of tension development of isolated cardiac muscle, a well-established index of myocardial contractility. However, the concept of a true isovolumic contraction period in the intact heart is no longer correct, since it has been shown with myocardial tagging that during isovolumic contraction there is systolic rotation (reflecting myocardial shortening) without a change in volume (see Fig. 20–12). As a further limitation, maximum dP/dt is dependent not only on left ventricular contractility but also on heart rate, preload, and afterload (Fig. 20–6), synchronicity of contraction, and myocardial hypertrophy. Since this isovolumic index of systolic function is preload dependent, the relationship between ventricular end-diastolic volume and dP/dt is a more accurate index of contractility than dP/dt alone.

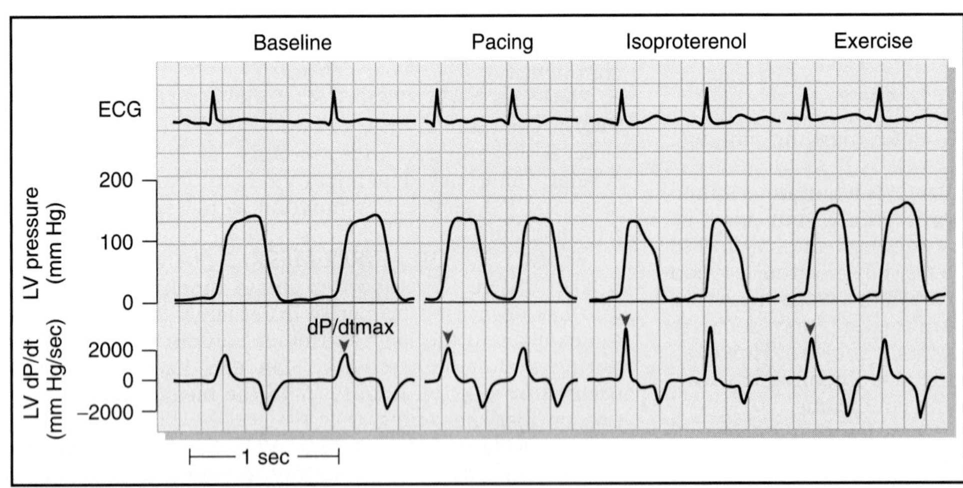

FIGURE 20–6 **A,** Recording of left ventricular pressure (LVP), the rate of change of left ventricular pressure (dP/dt), and left ventricular volume (LVV). The maximum value of dP/dt (dP/dt_{max}) increases in response to dobutamine; however, dP/dt_{max} also increases when left ventricular end-diastolic volume is increased by infusing dextran. This demonstrates the sensitivity of dP/dt_{max} to both contractility and left ventricular end-diastolic volume (preload). **B,** Recordings in a normal subject demonstrating increase in dP/dt_{max} during increases in contractility produced by pacing tachycardia, isoproterenol, and exercise. ECG = electrocardiogram. (**A,** Data from Little WC: The left ventricular dP/dt_{max} end-diastolic volume relation in closed-chest dogs. Circ Res 56:808, 1985; and **B,** Modified from Inagaki M, Yokota M, Izawa H, et al: Impaired force-frequency relations in patients with hypertensive left ventricular hypertrophy. Circulation 99:1826, 1999.)

Regional Indices of Left Ventricular Function

Global measures of left ventricular function, such as those described earlier, lose accuracy when the disease process affects regions of the ventricle differentially; this occurs most notably in coronary artery disease. Chronic myocardial ischemia, i.e., stunning or hibernation (see Chap. 19), and acute or old myocardial infarction may be associated with regional wall motion abnormalities with hypokinesis (reduced shortening) and akinesis (absent shortening) or dyskinesis (systolic elongation or bulging). Often the nonischemic portion of the ventricle is hypercontractile, leading to a normal *global* left ventricular function in the presence of impairment of regional function.

The most widely used technique for assessing regional wall motion is the centerline method (Fig. 20–7), which demonstrates that shortening at the apex normally is less than at the base. For normalization, systolic shortening may be divided by ejection time. This approach to quantifying regional left ventricular function was initially used in contrast angiograms and then extended to echocardiograms. These measures of endocardial motion and

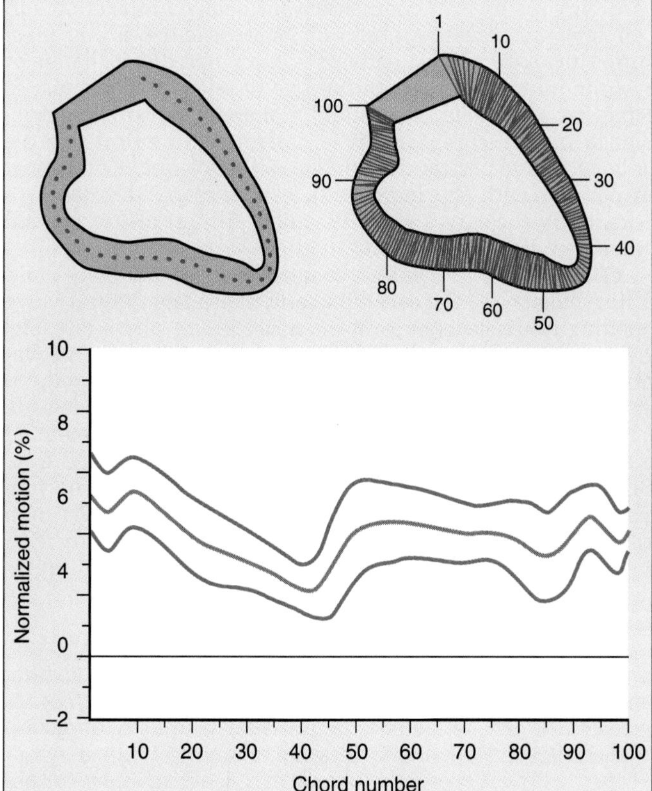

FIGURE 20–7 Assessment of regional left ventricular function using the centerline method. Regional wall motion is determined along 100 chords drawn perpendicular to a centerline constructed midway between the end-diastolic and end-systolic contours. Calculated wall motion of the 100 chords **(bottom)** is normalized for heart size by dividing each chord by the length of the end-diastolic perimeter. The normal range is indicated by the dotted lines (mean ± 1 SD). (From Sheehan FH, Bolson EL, Dodge HT, et al: Advantages and applications of the centerline method for characterizing regional ventricular function. Circulation 74:293, 1986.)

changes in wall thickness are afterload dependent but do allow comparisons of different regions of the ventricle. As discussed later, nuclear magnetic resonance imaging with tagging provides the most comprehensive assessment of regional wall motion, and more recently tissue Doppler strain rates (see Chap. 11) have been used experimentally and clinically.

Diastolic Function

(see Chaps. 19, 21, and 22)

Assessment of cardiac performance has focused traditionally on systolic function, whereas diastole was considered of secondary importance. More recently, however, diastolic function has been found to play an important role in cardiac morbidity and mortality and to influence both preload and afterload. Diastolic function is influenced importantly by ventricular structure and composition.[8-10] Diastole begins with the isovolumic relaxation period that starts after aortic valve closure (see Fig. 20–2). Because relaxation is an active, energy-consuming process, some authors consider relaxation in a strict sense to be a part of systole.[9,10] However, from a clinical standpoint, four separate phases of diastole need to be distinguished: (1) isovolumic relaxation; (2) early (rapid) diastolic filling; (3) slow ventricular filling (diastasis); and (4) atrial filling.

Definitions (see Table 20–2)

Diastolic function is influenced by several factors, e.g., myocardial relaxation, ventricular filling, and the ventricle's passive elastic properties, but one of the major determinants is heart rate, which determines how much time is available for ventricular filling. An increase in heart rate shortens the diastolic filling time interval disproportionately. This reduction must be compensated for by an increase in the rate of relaxation and an augmentation of elastic recoil with enhanced diastolic suction. Thus, impaired diastolic function can be aggravated by tachycardia and can be improved simply by a reduction in heart rate, which allows the heart to fill over a longer period.

In the normal left ventricle, the end-systolic volume is smaller than its elastic equilibrium and it thus generates *elastic recoil,* which varies inversely with the end-systolic volume. The elastic recoil causes diastolic suction that fills the ventricle at a low pressure and induces a potential for negative left ventricular pressure in early diastole. This filling mechanism is important during exercise and allows the normal ventricle to reduce minimal diastolic pressure and to maintain end-diastolic pressure constant despite a threefold to fivefold increase in cardiac output.[8-10] A loss of elastic recoil occurs during acute ischemia with a reduction in early diastolic filling accompanied by an increase in left atrial filling pressure and heart rate.[11,12]

Another important determinant of diastolic function is the *atrioventricular pressure gradient,* which is dependent on atrial pressure, relaxation rate, viscous forces in the myocardium, and ventricular filling rates.[8-11] An increase in the rate of relaxation can maintain left atrial pressure at normal levels, despite an increase in cardiac output. However, a reduction in ventricular filling rate can be compensated for by an increase in left atrial pressure, as occurs in patients with left ventricular hypertrophy or myocardial infarction.

ABNORMALITIES OF DIASTOLIC FUNCTION. From a clinical standpoint, a number of abnormalities of diastolic function have been described.[13-17] They are variously termed *diastolic abnormalities, diastolic dysfunction,* and *diastolic heart failure,* in ascending order of severity.

Diastolic abnormalities are characterized by abnormal filling indices, are commonly identified by echocardiography, and known to have a reduced early diastolic filling rate or a prolonged isovolumic relaxation period, but without clinical symptoms. In this situation the ventricle is able to compensate for abnormal diastolic function and to maintain a normal level of left ventricular filling pressure. *Diastolic dysfunction* is characterized by an increase in diastolic filling pressure, which may be responsible for the occurrence of dyspnea. This symptom may occur during exercise ("latent" diastolic dysfunction) or may be present also at rest ("manifest" diastolic dysfunction). Many patients with moderate to severe left ventricular hypertrophy may suffer from diastolic dysfunction. *Diastolic heart failure* is associated with the clinical signs of heart failure, such as paroxysmal nocturnal dyspnea, orthopnea, and edema. The clinical differentiation between systolic and diastolic dysfunction is important, because prognosis and therapeutic interventions are different in these two forms of heart failure (see Chap. 22).[9,10,13-17]

RELAXATION. Isovolumic relaxation begins with aortic valve closure and ends with mitral valve opening. The timing and the rate of relaxation are dependent on preload and afterload, myocardial inactivation, and synchrony of cardiac contraction.[8-10] The important determinants of relaxation are maximal systolic pressure, end-systolic fiber stretch, coronary flow ("erectile effect"), and stored energy (elastic recoil). A delayed or incomplete relaxation (>3.5 time constants) can retard and/or delay the onset of diastolic filling (Fig. 20–8).

This is typically the case in patients with left ventricular hypertrophy or myocardial ischemia and, when sufficiently severe, leads to an increase in diastolic filling pressure. An increase in myocardial contractility and an augmentation of elastic recoil, as occurs in patients with hypertrophic cardiomyopathy, can compensate for delayed relaxation and can prevent excessive elevation of ventricular filling pressure. However, in most patients with myocardial ischemia or systolic pump failure, both the rate of relaxation and elastic recoil are decreased in parallel,[18,19] thereby elevating ventricular filling pressure. Finally, in patients with mitral stenosis or constrictive pericarditis, the rate of relaxation is enhanced in parallel with the increase in elastic recoil that leads to potentially negative early diastolic filling pressures and enhanced diastolic suction.

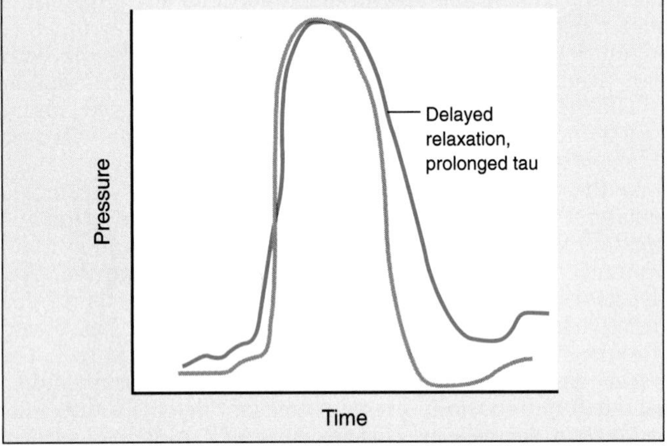

FIGURE 20–8 Two left ventricular pressure waveforms show a normal contour and then a waveform with delayed relaxation producing a prolonged time constant of relaxation (tau). The pressure coordinates from aortic valve closing to mitral valve opening, i.e., during the isovolumic relaxation period, can be plotted and the negative reciprocal of the log plot is the calculated relation value (tau).

FILLING. In the normal ventricle there are two rapid filling phases: (1) the early diastolic phase from mitral valve opening to diastasis and (2) the atrial filling phase (see Fig. 20–2).[8-10] Rapid diastolic filling is dependent on four mechanisms: (1) rate of relaxation, (2) elastic ventricular recoil, (3) atrioventricular pressure gradient, and (4) passive elastic properties of the atrium and the ventricle. Assessment of diastolic filling can be obtained most conveniently from Doppler echocardiography (see Chap. 11), which allows an assessment of maximal filling velocities as well as the ratio between early (E wave) and late (A wave) filling velocity (E/A ratio) (Fig. 20–9) (see Chap. 21). Late diastolic filling is dependent on the strength of left atrial contraction and the diastolic stiffness of the left ventricle.

PASSIVE ELASTIC PROPERTIES. It is necessary to distinguish between ventricular (chamber) and myocardial (muscle) properties (Fig. 20–10).[8-10,20] *Ventricular stiffness* is determined and defined by the pressure-volume relationship of the left ventricle and is directly related to clinical symptoms, whereas *myocardial stiffness* is determined by the stress-strain relationship of the left ventricle, which is a function of the structural composition of the myocardium.[8-10,21-25] Ventricular stiffness reaches its nadir at the lowest diastolic pressure but increases progressively during diastolic filling and is maximal at end-diastole. Myocardial stiffness impedes myocardial lengthening. Since wall stress and myocardial fiber length increase during diastolic filling, they reach maximal levels at end-diastole (i.e., the preload), which according to the Frank-Starling principle is an important determinant of the extent of systolic myocardial fiber shortening.

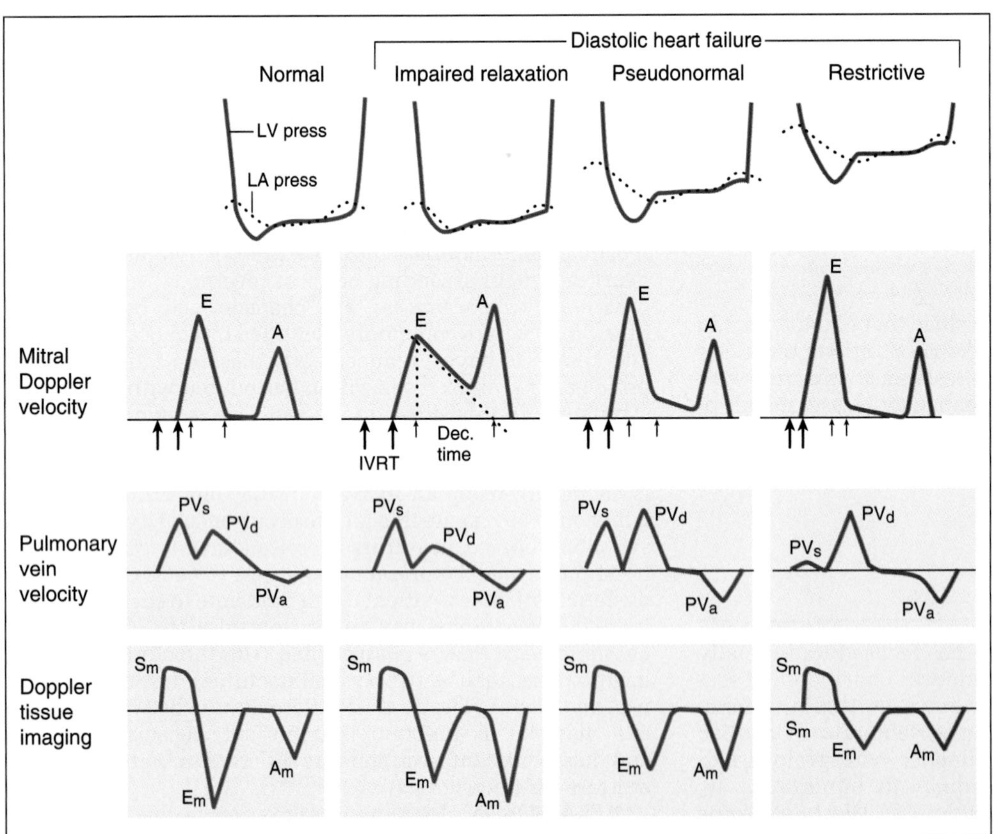

FIGURE 20–9 The techniques of assessing diastolic function include direct pressure measurement of the small diastolic, physiological gradients between the left atrium (LA) and the left ventricle (LV) (**first panel** [top]), transmitral inflow Doppler velocity profile (**second panel,** IVRT = isovolumic relaxation time; Dec. time = deceleration time of e wave; E = early LV filling velocity; A = velocity of LV filling contributed by atrial contraction), pulmonary vein Doppler velocity (**third panel,** PV_s = systolic pulmonary vein velocity; PV_d = diastolic pulmonary vein velocity; PV_a = pulmonary vein velocity resulting from atrial contraction), and Doppler tissue velocity (**fourth panel,** S_m = myocardial velocity during systole; E_m = myocardial velocity during early filling; A_m = myocardial velocity during filling produced by atrial contraction). (Adapted from Zile M, Brutsaert D: New concepts in diastolic dysfunction and diastolic heart failure: I. Diagnosis, prognosis, and measurements of diastolic function. Circulation 105:1387, 2002.)

CHAMBER PROPERTIES. The diastolic properties of the left ventricle can be described by the diastolic pressure-volume or pressure-dimension relationships (Fig. 20–11; see also Fig. 20–10). These relations can be described mathematically by an exponential equation, the constant of chamber stiffness, defined by the slope of this relationship. The slope and position of the pressure-volume relationship represent *ventricular stiffness,*

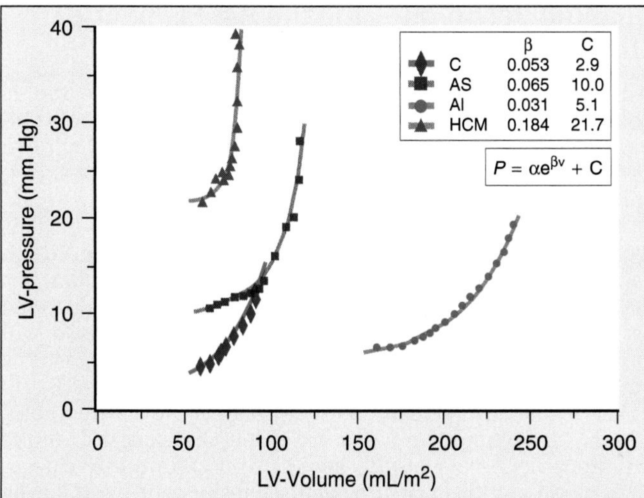

FIGURE 20–10 Left ventricular (LV) pressure-volume relationship during diastole in a control subject (C) and patients with aortic stenosis (AS), aortic regurgitation (AI), and hypertrophic cardiomyopathy (HCM). There is a parallel upward shift in the HCM and a small upward shift in the AS patient due to the increase in diastolic stiffness. The constant of chamber stiffness (β) is 0.184 in HCM and 0.065 in AS compared with 0.053 in the control patient. However, there is a rightward shift in the AI patient due to the increase in LV diastolic volume with a minimal increase in diastolic filling pressure (i.e., due to a low diastolic chamber stiffness). β is 0.031 in this patient. (From Mandinov L, Eberli FR, Seiler C, Hess OM: Diastolic heart failure. Cardiovasc Res 45:814, 2000.)

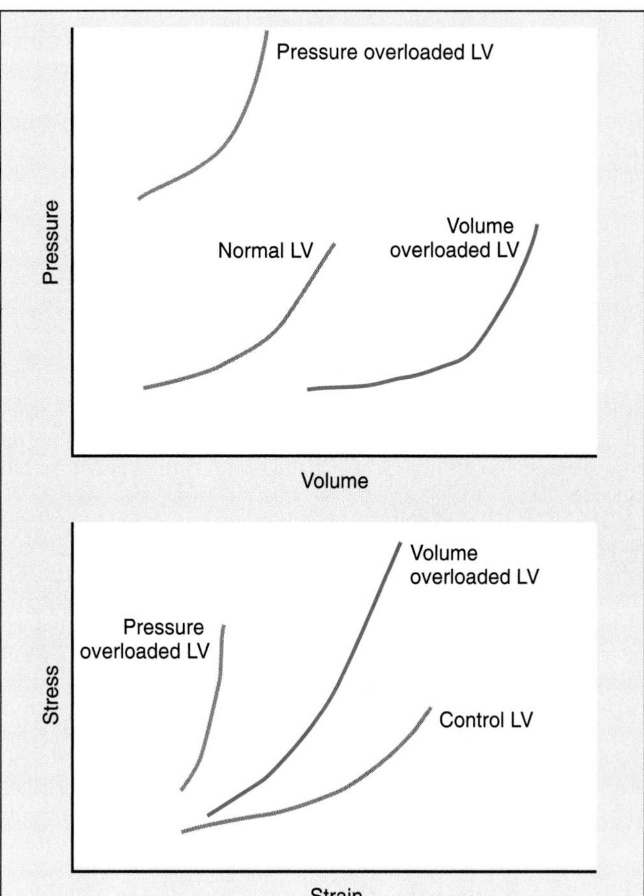

FIGURE 20–11 Schematic representation of the diastolic left ventricular (LV) pressure-volume **(top)** and LV stress-strain relationship **(bottom)**. The pressure-volume relationship is dependent on changes of the left ventricle as a whole associated with chronic pressure (upward shift) or volume-overload (rightward shift), whereas the LV stress-strain relationship represents changes of the myocardium. The slope of the stress-strain relationship has been called *stiffness constant of the myocardium*, i.e., the steeper the slope, the stiffer the muscle. Muscle stiffness is influenced by the composition of the myocardium, i.e., the ratio of the muscular tissue to the extracellular matrix.

which is dependent on intrinsic and extrinsic factors.[8-10] The intrinsic factors include left ventricular chamber size, left ventricular muscle mass, coronary perfusion, collagen tissue, and collagen orientation. The extrinsic factors include right/left ventricular interaction, pericardial pressure, intrathoracic pressure, and intravascular volume.

MYOCARDIAL PROPERTIES. Myocardial stiffness is represented by the passive elastic properties of the myocardium that are influenced by the cardiac interstitium and by the structural composition of the myocytes themselves.[20,21,24] Histomorphometric examinations have shown that disorientation of the collagen fibers in experimental heart failure contributes to the increase in myocardial stiffness. The slope of the diastolic stress-strain relationship has been termed the *constant of myocardial stiffness* (see Figs. 20–10 and 20–11). This constant is dependent on the properties, quantity, and orientation of the collagen fibers, as well as on myocardial perfusion and temperature.[8-10,20-25]

PERICARDIAL PROPERTIES. The pericardium forms a strong, purely elastic sac with extensions that enclose the origins of the ascending aorta, venae cavae, as well as the proximal and distal ends of the pulmonary artery and veins (see Chap. 64). The pericardium consists of two layers—the fibrous outer and the serous inner—with up to 30 ml of fluid normally. The pericardium acts as a barrier to reduce friction between the heart and the surrounding organs. The normal pericardium is relatively stiff,[26,27] and the relationship between intrapericardial volume and pressure is a steep, monoexponential curve. A small increase in intrapericardial volume leads to a rapid augmentation of intrapericardial pressure and, thereby, intracavitary diastolic pressures. Normal intrapericardial pressure is zero or negative. However, when the volume of the heart increases and exceeds the elastic limit of the pericardial sac, intracavitary pressures in all four chambers of the heart increase. An acute increase in the right- or left-sided volume affects the filling of the contralateral chamber by increasing its diastolic pressure (i.e., through ventricular interaction). The pericardium contributes to diastolic coupling of the atria and ventricles such that right and left ventricular filling pressures are closely correlated in the presence of an intact pericardium but are lower in the absence of the pericardium. Cardiac distensibility without the pericardium is influenced primarily by the properties of the myocardium. Chronic elevations of intrapericardial volume lead to an increase in the volume of the pericardial sac. If the intrapericardial volume increases slowly and persists over days or weeks, the pericardium slowly stretches and pericardial constraint may remain.[26,27] The volume of intrapericardial fluid may be as high as 1000 to 1200 ml in chronic pericardial effusion with little constraint on cardiac chambers.

Assessment

Several noninvasive techniques may be useful tools for the diagnosis of diastolic dysfunction, but cardiac catheterization with simultaneous pressure and volume measurements still represents the gold standard for quantitative studies.

LEFT VENTRICULAR RELAXATION. The most commonly used parameter to evaluate left ventricular relaxation is the time constant of isovolumic pressure decay (τ, expressed in milliseconds), which has been shown to be exponential under most circumstances but may deviate from a true monoexponential decay in the presence of aortic regurgitation or myocardial ischemia. Originally, a logarithmic pressure-time relation was used with the assumption that the asymptote of the pressure decline is zero. However, recently it has been shown that, in the transiently nonfilling ventricle, left ventricular pressure declines to negative values. Thus, a nonzero asymptote was added to the monoexponential model or a two-sequential monoexponential, polynomial or logistic model has been proposed[18]:

$$P = Ae^{-\alpha t} + Pb$$

where P = pressure, A = pressure at peak negative dP/dt, e = base of natural logarithm, α = slope of pressure time relationship, t = time, and Pb = pressure asymptote.

The time constant τ is calculated as

$$\tau = -1/\alpha$$

In normal subjects, τ averages 48 milliseconds, with a range from 40 to 60 milliseconds.[8-10] Relaxation is defined as being complete at 3.5 times the time constant τ after aortic valve closure.[18]

DIASTOLIC FILLING. The left ventricular chamber can be assessed angiographically from a frame-by-frame analysis, which may be accurate but has a lower temporal resolution (20 to 40 milliseconds) in comparison to Doppler echocardiography. Several indices of diastolic filling can be calculated, including the instantaneous filling rate, time to peak filling rate (PFR) (i.e., the time from end-systole to peak positive dV/dt), the fraction of filling that occurs during the rapid filling phase, as well as acceleration and deceleration of early diastolic filling. The most rapid rate of filling occurs during the first half of diastole and is termed the *early PFR* (normal value 300 ± 70 ml/sec). This index and the ratio of early to late diastolic filling (PFR1/PFR2 or E/A ratio) are the most commonly used parameters to describe left ventricular filling. Filling parameters calculated using a conductance catheter may be more useful than angiographic filling parameters due to their higher temporal resolution.

PASSIVE ELASTIC PROPERTIES. Calculation of *left ventricular chamber stiffness* is carried out by plotting left ventricular diastolic filling pressure against left ventricular diastolic volume from the minimal diastolic pressure to the end-diastolic pressure (see Figs. 20-10 and 20-11).

The most commonly used equation for assessing chamber stiffness is

$$P = \alpha e^{\beta V} + C$$

where P = pressure, α = intercept, e = base of the natural logarithm, β = slope of the pressure-volume relationship (chamber stiffness constant), V = volume, and C = pressure asymptote. A nonlinear curve-fitting procedure is employed. Normal values for the chamber stiffness constant average 0.05 ml^{-1}, and they range between 0.01 and 0.09 ml^{-1}.[8-10,12,19]

Left ventricular myocardial stiffness is calculated by plotting instantaneous left ventricular wall stress against left ventricular midwall strain from the lowest diastolic to end-diastolic pressure or from the end of the rapid filling phase to the peak of the a wave (see Fig. 20–11). The calculation of stress involves a geometric model of the left ventricle, whereas the calculation of strain requires some assumption of the unstressed left ventricular volume. The most commonly used equation for assessing myocardial stiffness is

$$S = \alpha e^{\beta V} + C$$

where S = wall stress, α = intercept, e = base of the natural logarithm, β = slope of the stress-strain relationship (muscle stiffness constant), V = strain, and C = stress asymptote. Again, a nonlinear curve-fitting procedure is employed. *Muscle stiffness* is the slope of the myocardial stress-strain relation. Average normal values for the muscle stiffness constant are 12, ranging between 5 and 20.

Imaging Techniques for the Assessment of Diastolic Function

Although the intraventricular pressure and angiographic volume measurements remain the gold standard, a number of noninvasive techniques have been used for the clinical assessment of diastolic function in patients with coronary, valvular, or myocardial heart disease.

DOPPLER ECHOCARDIOGRAPHY (Table 20–5). This technique (see Chap. 11) has emerged as an important clinical tool that provides reliable and useful data on diastolic function. Three different approaches are used routinely in the assessment of diastolic function: measurement of transmitral and pulmonary venous flow as well as intraventricular flow patterns (Doppler-flow propagation) (see Fig. 20–9).[28-31]

The *transmitral velocity pattern* remains the starting point of echocardiographic assessment of left ventricular diastolic function, since it is easy to acquire and can rapidly categorize patients with normal or abnormal diastolic function by E/A ratio (early to late filling velocity). In healthy young individuals, most diastolic filling occurs in early diastole so that the E/A ratio exceeds 1.0.[4] When relaxation is impaired, early diastolic filling decreases progressively and a vigorous compensatory atrial contraction ("atrial kick") occurs. This results in a reversed E/A ratio (E/A < 1 = *delayed relaxation pattern*), increased deceleration time, and increased isovolumic relaxation time (IVRT).[8-10] With further disease progression, left ventricular compliance becomes reduced and filling pressures begin to increase, leading to compensatory augmentation of left atrial pressure with increase in early filling despite impaired relaxation, so that the filling pattern becomes relatively normal (*pseudonormalization pattern* = E/A ratio > 1). This pattern, however, represents abnormalities of both relaxation and compliance and is distinguished from normal filling by a shortened early deceleration time. Finally, in patients with severe decrease in left ventricular compliance, left atrial pressure is markedly elevated and drives vigorous early diastolic filling despite impaired relax-

TABLE 20–5 Normal Values of Parameters of Left Ventricular Diastolic Filling Measured by Doppler Echocardiography

Parameters	Adults <41 yr	Adults >55 yr
Peak mitral flow velocity (E) (cm/sec)	76 ± 13	63 ± 11
Peak mitral filling rate (A) (cm/sec)	38 ± 8	52 ± 9
Mitral E/A	2.1 ± 0.6	1.3 ± 0.3
Mitral E deceleration time	184 ± 24	—
Mitral E deceleration rate (m/sec²)	5.6 ± 2.7	—
Isovolumetric relaxation time (msec)	74 ± 26	—
Peak pulmonary venous AR wave (cm/sec)	18 ± 3	25 ± 5
Peak pulmonary venous S wave (cm/sec)	41 ± 10	60 ± 10
Peak pulmonary venous D wave (cm/sec)	53 ± 10	38 ± 10

E/A = E wave/A wave ratio.

Data from Little WC. Downes TR: Clinical evaluation of left ventricular diastolic performance. Prog Cardiovasc Dis 32:273, 1990; and Rakowski H, et al: Canadian consensus recommendations for the measurements and reporting of diastolic dysfunction by echocardiography. J Am Soc Echocardiogr 9:745, 754, 1996.

TABLE 20–6 Left Atrial and Ventricular Function Influences on the Pulmonary Venous Flow Velocity Profile

Pulmonary Venous Wave	Left Atrial Function	LV Function
First systolic wave	Atrial relaxation	
Second systolic wave	Reservoir function Atrial compliance	LV contraction RV contraction
Early diastolic wave	Conduit function	Ventricular relaxation Ventricular chamber stiffness
Atrial reversal wave	Booster pump function Atrial compliance	Ventricular chamber stiffness

LV = left ventricular; RV = right ventricular.
Adapted from Tabata T, Thomas JD, Klein AL: Pulmonary venous flow by Doppler echocardiography: Revisited 12 years later. J Am Coll Cardiol 41:1243-1250, 2003.

ation. This *restrictive filling pattern* (E/A >> 1) is consistent with an abnormal rise in left ventricular diastolic pressure and an abrupt deceleration of flow with little additional filling during mid-diastole and atrial contraction. In extreme cases the dP/dT overshoots left atrial pressure so that mitral regurgitation in mid-diastole may occur.

The *IVRT* represents the time interval from closure of the aortic to opening of the mitral valve (see Fig. 20–2). The IVRT (normal range, 60 to 90 milliseconds) reflects the rate of myocardial relaxation but is dependent on afterload and heart rate.[8-10] It is probably the most sensitive Doppler index to detect impaired relaxation because it is the first to become abnormal. The deceleration time (see Fig. 20–9), which is affected by ventricular stiffness and atrial and ventricular pressure, can be used to derive the rapid filling rate. The normal value of this parameter is 193 ± 23 milliseconds; when prolonged, this index permits distinction between a normal and pseudonormal E/A ratio.[28]

Analysis of the *pulmonary venous filling patterns* (Table 20–6) provides a second window into left ventricular diastolic function.[29,30] The S wave, occurring during systole, depends on atrial relaxation and mitral annular motion. The D wave occurring during diastole reflects left ventricular filling, and the A wave, which is opposite to the other waves and occurs during atrial contraction, reflects left ventricular compliance. One indication for examining the pulmonary venous flow pattern is to distinguish the truly normal filling pattern from pseudonormalization. The main difference between these is the forward A wave of the transmitral flow and the reversed A wave in the pulmonary veins (see Fig. 20–9). In the presence of pseudonormalization, the atrium contracts against an increased afterload due to an elevated diastolic filling pressure or a stiff left ventricle. Accordingly, blood is preferentially ejected into the pulmonary veins, resulting in a high and prolonged pulmonary venous A wave.

Color M-mode Doppler echocardiography is a useful technique for examining the dynamics of blood flow across the mitral valve.[31] The velocity of inflow is enhanced with rapid relaxation and left ventricular suction. Clinical and experimental studies have demonstrated that the inverse correlation to τ (the time constant of relaxation [see earlier]) is relatively independent of left atrial pressure. Furthermore, combined evaluation of flow propagation velocity and early diastolic annular velocity can be used for estimation of filling pressure.[32] In normal persons the mitral annular motion is almost a mirror image of the transmitral flow pattern, but in patients with a pseudonormal or restrictive filling pattern, annular motion is abnormally low, implying that it is relatively independent of preload.[33-36]

Doppler tissue imaging (see Chap. 11) yields information on intramyocardial velocity, providing a unique insight into left ventricular mechanics during isovolumic contraction and relaxation (see Fig. 20–9).[9,37,38] It has been shown that relaxation velocities in the myocardium are inversely correlated with τ, so that calculation of the time constant of relaxation may be possible. Furthermore, this preload-independent peak negative myocardial velocity gradient may be used as a noninvasive index of left ventricular diastolic function.

Through the integrated use of Doppler echocardiography and Doppler tissue imaging, it is possible to obtain a fairly precise picture of left ventricular systolic and diastolic function. However, atrial fibrillation or frequent ectopic beats introduce major limitations of these techniques.

MAGNETIC RESONANCE IMAGING (see Chap. 14). This technique has been shown to be of considerable use in the morphological and functional assessment of the heart. Additional information may be gained from newer techniques such as magnetic resonance (MR) myocardial tagging, which allows the labeling of specific myocardial regions (Fig. 20–12).[39-43] From these tags the rotational and translational motion of the left ventricle can be determined; it is characterized by a systolic twisting motion with a clockwise rotation at the base and a counterclockwise rotation at the apex during systole. This motion can best be described by the wringing out of a wet towel. The untwisting motion occurs very early in diastole and is directly related to myocardial relaxation. Untwisting may be used as a measure of the rate and completeness of relaxation and may serve as an estimate of early diastolic filling. In the normal left ventricle, systolic rotation commences during isovolumic contraction (see Fig. 20–12) and continues during systolic ejection after the aortic valve has opened. Diastolic back rotation starts at end-systole and continues during isovolumic relaxation, whereas diastolic lengthening begins with mitral valve opening and ends with the next end-diastole.

Thus, the normal left ventricle performs a rectangular twisting-shortening (i.e., systole) and untwisting-lengthening (i.e., diastole) loop that occurs in opposite directions at the apex and base (Fig. 20–13) and is determined by the orientation of the muscle fibers within the myocardium. The relationship between myocardial rotation or twisting and changes in chamber size provide a unique insight into left ventricular systolic and diastolic function and their interaction.

A loss of myocardial tissue, as in myocardial infarction, or the occurrence of left ventricular asynchrony, as occurs in left bundle branch block, leads to a loss of the normal rotation-relaxation pattern that is associated with an increase in myocardial energy requirements. The normal systolic wringing motion allows the heart to work economically at a low-energy threshold because the wringing motion requires less energy than the "squeezing" motion. The traditional physiological concept of an isovolumic contraction and relaxation period has to be revised because the concept of an isometrically contracting or isometrically relaxing muscle is no longer valid. The shortening of the muscle fibers within the left ventricular wall induces systolic rotation during isovolumic contraction and diastolic untwisting during isovolumic relaxation. Athletes (with physiological hypertrophy) have a normal rotation–diastolic relaxation pattern, whereas patients with aortic stenosis (with pathologic hypertrophy) show a delayed systolic rotation–diastolic relaxation pattern (Fig. 20–14).

RADIONUCLIDE ANGIOGRAPHY (see Chap. 13). This technique may be used to study the rapid filling phase of diastole, the duration of the isovolumic relaxation phase, the relative contribution of rapid filling to total diastolic filling, and

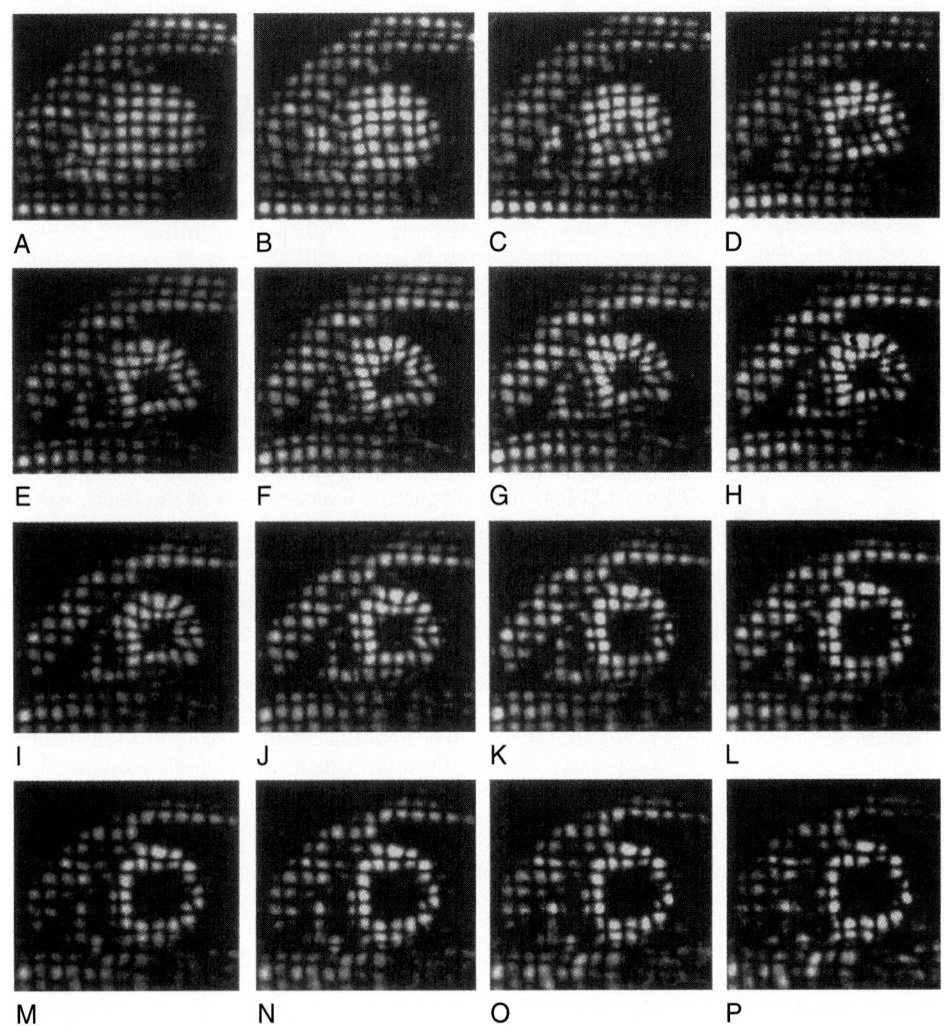

FIGURE 20–12 **A-P,** Series of MR images in a control patient with normal left ventricular function (temporal resolution 35 milliseconds). The MR images show horizontal and vertical lines (myocardial tags) that are superimposed on the conventional MR image. From the movement of the grid crossing points, the contraction and relaxation behavior of the left ventricle can be determined. During isovolumic contraction there is a counterclockwise rotation at the apex followed by systolic shortening. During isovolumic relaxation there is a clockwise rotation ("untwisting") followed by diastolic lengthening. This systolic-diastolic contraction-relaxation behavior is altered in patients with diastolic dysfunction with prolongation of diastolic back-rotation. (From Lazar-Mandinov L, Eberli F, Seiler C, Hess OM: Diastolic heart failure. Cardiovasc Res 45:813-825, 2000.)

the relation between regional nonuniformity of left ventricular function and global filling properties.[44] However, radionuclide angiography does *not* permit assessment of the left atrial–left ventricular pressure gradient or the simultaneous evaluation of changes in left ventricular pressure and volume during relaxation and filling. Therefore, complete clinical interpretation of "abnormal" left ventricular filling indices or changes in these indices after interventions is not possible. However, despite its inherent limitations, radionuclide evaluation of left ventricular filling may provide clinically useful insights.

COMPUTED TOMOGRAPHY (see Chap. 15). Computed tomography (CT) scanning of the heart permits rapid and accurate investigation of the heart and the adjacent vessels. Three techniques are currently used to evaluate cardiac anatomy and function.

Spiral CT scanning uses multiple rotations of the CT gantry while the table is moved continuously through the x-ray source. Computer reconstructions allow determination of multiple transaxial scans, 4 to 10 mm in thickness, of the entire heart and the adjacent vessel during a single breath-hold period. Usually, 80 to 100 ml of contrast medium is injected intravenously to study intravascular volumes and myocardial perfusion.

Ultrafast electron-beam tomography uses an electron gun that produces a stream of electrons that are magnetically focused and directed into different target rings, each of which emits two x-ray beams. This technology allows complete cardiac imaging in 50 milliseconds without the need for electrocardiographic gating or breath-holding. Contrast enhancement by intravenous injection of contrast medium permits accurate delineation of intracardiac chambers and vessels at end-diastole and end-systole. However, the infrastructure of this technique is expensive and radiation exposure is relatively high. Therefore, electron-beam tomography has not gained wide application.

Multislice CT scanning has gained a lot of interest in the recent years. This technique uses 8 to 64 image planes for assessing cardiac dimensions and function. Quantification of regional myocardial wall thickening and noninvasive representation of the coronary arteries have been done in normal patients and in patients with coronary artery disease.

Right Ventricular Function

PATHOPHYSIOLOGY. Right ventricular function plays a central role in the clinical outcome in a wide variety of cardiopulmonary disorders. The right ventricle is pivotal in many specific congenital cardiac malformations, and this importance continues into adulthood. Examples are the adaptation to chronic volume overloading from residual pulmonary regurgitation in repaired tetralogy of Fallot and to left-to-right shunting from an untreated atrial septal defect. In addition, acquired diseases such as primary and secondary pulmonary hypertension produce a remodeling of the right ventricle that resembles the remodeling of the left ventricle with pressure overload.

The right ventricle differs from the left ventricle regarding the type of work performed. Stroke volume is, of course, equal for the two ventricles, but the left ventricle must generate a high pressure to overcome gravitation effects and allow appropriate distribution of flow to multiple beds with differences in local resistance. The right ventricle, on the other hand, ejects into a more uniform and compliant pulmonary vascular bed and, therefore, has a thinner wall than the left ventricle to generate this lower pressure. The right ventricle also fills differently. It takes in systemic venous return at very low pressures, including the inspiratory creation of negative intrathoracic pressures that further sucks venous return into this chamber.

Although the prognostic significance of right ventricular adaptation to pressure or volume overload is widely recognized, the methods for studying this chamber have been slow to develop. A central problem has been in the imaging of this unusually shaped chamber that normally wraps around the interventricular septum, which functions primarily as a component of the left ventricle (Fig. 20–15). The thin-walled right ventricular free wall reduces the feasibility of studying wall thickening during systole and thinning during diastole, as is done in the assessment of left ventricular function.

ASSESSMENT OF RIGHT VENTRICULAR FUNCTION. Traditional 2D echocardiography allows assessment of right ventricular shape, size, and changes in size during the cardiac cycle. More recently, MR imaging has advanced the study of right ventricular function by providing images of this eccentric chamber and information on blood flow, regional function, and wall characteristics. A summary of the parameters assessed by MR imaging and ultrasonography is provided in Table 20–7. Contrast angiography, nuclear angiography, and the conductance catheter have their roles in special focused applications in assessing right ventricular function.

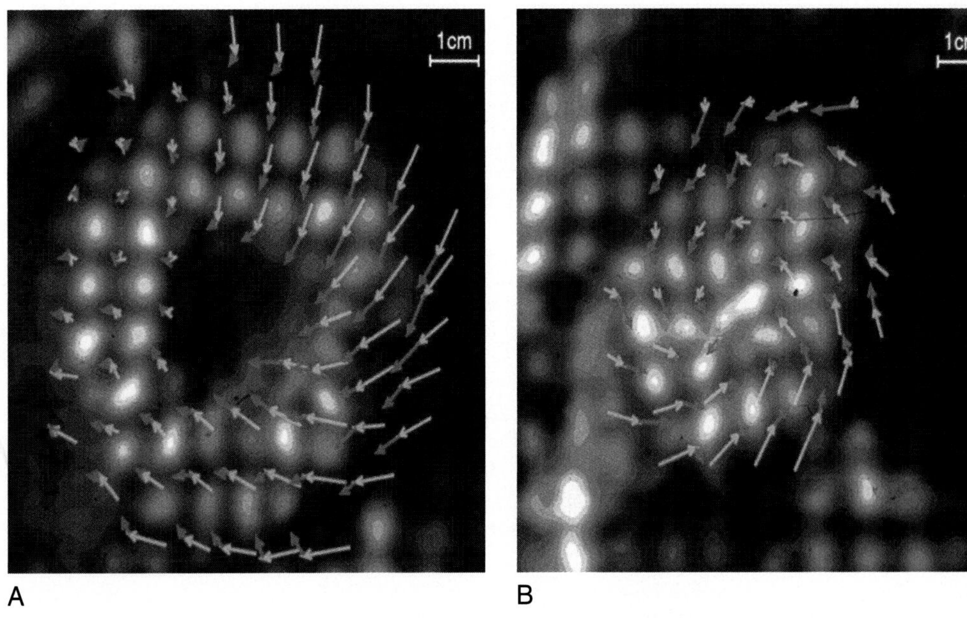

FIGURE 20–13 Ejection phase of the left ventricle at the apex **(A)** and at the base **(B)** of a healthy subject. End-systolic acquisitions are overlaid with corresponding local trajectories. There is a clockwise rotation at the base and counterclockwise rotation at the apex. This motion pattern has been described as a systolic wringing motion and provides a more sophisticated approach to quantifying regional left ventricular systolic function versus the traditional methods of endocardial shortening and simple wall thickening. (From Stuber M, Schedegger MB, Fischer SE, et al: Alterations in the local myocardial motion pattern in patients suffering from pressure overload due to aortic stenosis. Circulation 100:361-368, 1999.)

Function and Remodeling of the Right Ventricle: Four Paradigms

An understanding of right ventricular function is best illustrated by considering four examples of the response of this chamber to different pathophysiological conditions, as discussed in the following sections.

CHRONIC VOLUME OVERLOAD. Tricuspid regurgitation from damage to the valve apparatus by frequent endomyocardial biopsy in heart transplantation patients provides a model of the evolution of right ventricular volume overload.[45] Two-dimensional echocardiography (see Fig. 20–15) allows quantification of the progressive enlargement of the right ventricular end-diastolic cavity area with a change toward a more spherical chamber as reflected in an increased ratio of midchamber minor dimension to long axis of 0.5 to 0.7.

Atrial septal defect before and after closure provides another example of the chronic remodeling of the right ventricle and the extent of reversal following percutaneous closure.[46] Within 1 month of closure, the right ventricle undergoes important electrical-mechanical remodeling with a subsequent plateau at 6 months. The four-chamber 2D echocardiographic views of the right ventricular inflow and outflow tracts demonstrate that all patients have a decrease in chamber size, but 29 percent have some residual chamber enlargement at 1 year. Accompanying this structural remodeling is a significant reduction in QRS duration.[46]

Both right ventricular and left ventricular function, including chamber compliance, are major determinants of the degree and direction of shunting through the atrial septal defect and ultimately may influence right ventricular remodeling after closure.[47] Left-to-right shunting may increase in adulthood as the left ventricle becomes less compliant from acquired diseases. Shunting can, on the other hand, become bidirectional as the right ventricle loses its more compliant nature or develops frank failure.

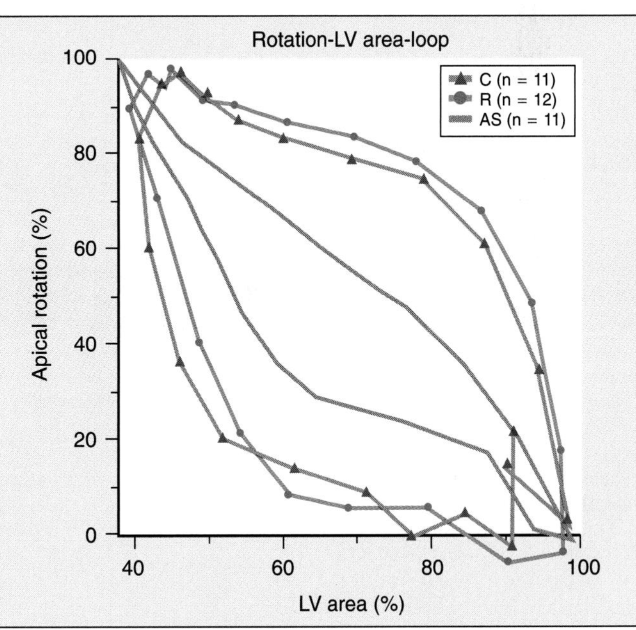

FIGURE 20–14 Tagged MR imaging–derived averaged patient data presented as rotation-area loop in controls (C; $n = 11$), professional rowers (R; $n = 12$), and patients with severe aortic stenosis (AS; $n = 11$). In the rowing athletes the rotation-area loop has a rectangular shape, as in controls, but in patients with severe hypertrophy (AS), delayed systolic rotation and relaxation are observed. This abnormal rotation-relaxation behavior in pathologic hypertrophy reflects changes in left ventricular (LV) afterload and myocardial hypertrophy. (From Stuber M, Schedegger MB, Fischer SE, et al: Alterations in the local myocardial motion pattern in patients suffering from pressure overload due to aortic stenosis. Circulation 100:361-368, 1999.)

CHRONIC PRESSURE OVERLOAD. The right ventricle undergoes extensive hypertrophy in primary pulmonary hypertension and leads to progressive right ventricular dilation, reduced systolic performance, secondary tricuspid regurgitation, and overt right ventricular failure with

TABLE 20–7 Echo/Doppler Assessment and MR Imaging of Right Ventricular Size, Shape, and Function

Parameter	Echo/Doppler	MR imaging
RV volume	Standard 2D views allow measurement of multiple dimensions (Fig. 20-15). The parasternal long-axis view shows the outflow tract diameter	Segmentation of individual slices provides chamber size. Adjacent areas are then summated to provide volume and shape measurements
Regional wall motion	Free RV wall and interventricular septum are imaged and paradoxical motion can easily be detected	Cine MR imaging provides contrast between the blood pool and the myocardial wall. RV wall motion is assessed using RVOT cines in the sagittal and short-axis cine images
RV mass	Approximated by wall thickness determinations along with chamber size measurements	Myocardium from the junction between the RV free wall and the interventricular septum can be traced on each slice from the base to the apex, including trabeculations. Myocardial volume computed from summated multiple slices is multiplied by 1.05 to give the mass in grams
RV wall composition	Not well studied in transthoracic images. Intracardiac ultrasound provides higher resolution data	MR imaging is potentially useful to distinguish fat from muscle
Regurgitant fraction	Doppler profiles provide semiquantitative approach	True regurgitant volumes can be measured from phase velocity maps in the main pulmonary artery and aortic root

RV = right ventricular; RVOT = RV outflow tract; 2D = two-dimensional.

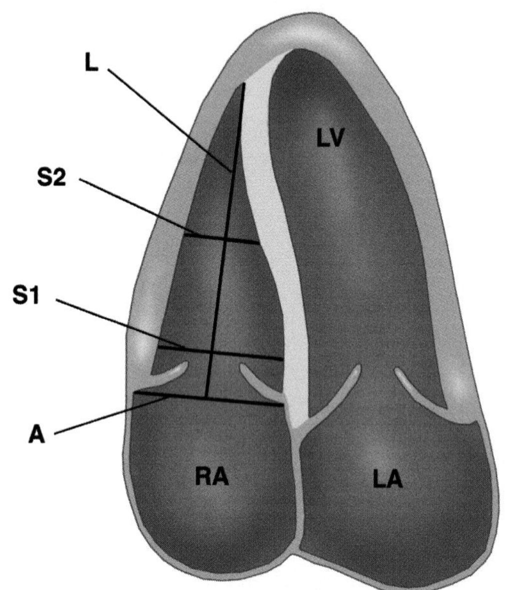

FIGURE 20–15 The right ventricle is schematically illustrated as seen in the echocardiographic apical four-chamber view. From this view right ventricular size can be quantified along its major axis (L) and two minor axes (S1 and S2) of the right ventricle. Tricuspid annular diameter (A) may also be measured. The important additional measurements of the outflow tract are not shown. The two-dimensional images of the right ventricle from echocardiography are suboptimal in assessing chamber volume and function and provide an impetus for three-dimensional techniques based on ultrasound or other modalities such as MR imaging and CT scanning. LV = left ventricle; RA = right atrium; LA = left atrium. (From Reynertson S, Kundur R, Mullen G, et al: Asymmetry of right ventricular enlargement in response to tricuspid regurgitation. Circulation 100:465, 1999.

peripheral edema and ascites (see Chap. 67).[48] Although regression of right ventricular hypertrophy has been described as a result of vasodilator therapy, the progressive nature of the primary disease process is unremitting. Direct (catheter-based) measurement of pressure and cardiac output is an important complement to noninvasive imaging.

A more reversible form of pressure overload hypertrophy of the right ventricle is seen in pulmonary hypertension secondary to chronic thromboembolism.[49] After surgical thromboembolectomy, 2D echocardiography quantified a significant reduction in end-diastolic (30 ± 7 to 21 ± 5 cm^2) and end-systolic (24 ± 6 to 14 ± 4 cm^2) cavity area in the four-chamber view.[50] Right ventricular fractional shortening increased and tricuspid regurgitation decreased. Furthermore, there was a resultant normalization of interventricular septal motion, improved diastolic filling, and rise in cardiac output.

Valvular pulmonic stenosis produces right ventricular hypertrophy that appears reversible after successful balloon valvuloplasty.[47] The secondary relief of a subvalvular pressure gradient in the right ventricular outflow tract also occurs, presumably from regression of infundibular hypertrophy.[51]

ACUTE ISCHEMIC DYSFUNCTION (see Chap. 46). The acute deterioration in right ventricular function during acute myocardial infarction has been studied by 2D echocardiography and invasively determined pressures and cardiac output.[52,53] Motion of the right ventricular free wall may be dramatically decreased with chamber dilation and an acute elevation of right-sided filling pressures resulting from increased chamber stiffness, mediated in part by an acute pericardial restraining influence. Enlargement of the right ventricular cavity may develop rapidly with a reversal of septal curvature and paradoxical movement during systole. The derangement of right ventricular function, if severe enough, can result in right-sided heart failure, clear lung fields, and a low cardiac output despite nearly normal left ventricular function.

CHRONIC VENTRICULAR DYSFUNCTION. Preliminary studies have shown that resynchronization with right ventricular pacing improves function in patients with chronic right ventricular dysfunction, as reflected in right ventricular maximum positive dP/dt and cardiac output.[1,54]

THE LEFT ATRIUM

In the last decade Doppler echocardiography has provided a large experience in functional assessment of the left atrium while MR imaging and CT scanning now provide in-depth 3D anatomical assessment of this chamber. A variety of new interventional techniques require more intensive study of the left atrium. For example, catheter-based treatment of atrial fibrillation, left atrial appendage occlusion devices, atrial septal closure devices, and a variety of emerging mitral valve interventions have stimulated an interest in the left atrium, whereas there also has been a new appreciation of the importance of left atrial size and function in a broad spectrum of cardiac disease states.[55-57]

LEFT ATRIAL APPENDAGE. Pulsed-Doppler interrogation of left atrial appendage flow is a major component of the functional assessment of this chamber. The function of the left atrial appendage is determined by factors well studied in the past for left ventricular function.[58-61] Removal of the appendage as well as insertion of devices into the left atrial appendage to block thrombus formation may make the remaining left atrial chamber less compliant.[60]

LEFT ATRIAL CHAMBER SIZE AND SHAPE. The relations between body size, gender, age, and left atrial volume have been detailed in a reference population using ultrasound techniques.[62] The normal left atrial volume is 42 ± 12 ml. The 3D reconstruction of the left atrium has been developed with ultrasound.[63] CT scanning and MR imaging have been applied to both left atrial size and shape. Images of the left atrium and distal pulmonary veins using multidetector helical CT with multidimensional reconstruction provide accurate, detailed information of these structures.[64]

LEFT ATRIAL FUNCTION. Conceptually, left atrial function can be described as having three components: (1) a distensible reservoir during ventricular systole as blood enters this chamber from the pulmonary veins, while the mitral valve is closed; (2) a passive conduit of blood in early ventricular diastole after mitral valve opening; and (3) a booster pump function occurring during late ventricular diastole and involving atrial contraction.

To understand its function, the volume of the left atrium is determined at three points in time during the cardiac cycle. Immediately before mitral valve opening the left atrium is at its maximal volume, reflecting its reservoir function. With mitral valve opening, the left atrium decompresses rapidly, in part due to a suction effect from the normal left ventricle during early diastole. The second time point is reached immediately before atrial systole, when the left atrial pre-A volume is determined. With subsequent atrial contraction there is further emptying of the left atrium until ventricular end-diastole is reached, and this minimum left atrial volume is measured immediately after atrial contraction. Hoit and Gabel have shown that left atrial conduit function represented 35 percent of all flow through the chamber.[65] The relative roles of active atrial contraction versus atrial conduit function have been clarified in animal studies demonstrating that the conduit function can compensate for atrial myocardial failure as long as left ventricular function is normal.

Left atrial function studied by transmitral flow as well as pulmonary venous flow patterns and left atrial appendage emptying flow are Doppler-based techniques that are widely available and can be applied clinically. Multiple factors influence the triphasic and quadriphasic pattern of pulmonary venous flow pattern (see Table 20-6).[29] The systolic or booster pump function of the left atrium can be characterized in many ways that are parallel to left ventricular systolic function assessment.[66-70]

CLINICAL APPLICATIONS OF ASSESSMENTS OF THE LEFT ATRIUM. Doppler-based techniques have been applied to understand better the timing and extent of left atrial myocardial dysfunction, or stunning, after conversion to sinus rhythm from atrial fibrillation[71] and the return of left atrial contractile function following the Maze operation.[72] Pharmacological modification of left ventricular diastolic properties that enhance chamber distensibility can augment the atrial contribution to left ventricular filling.[73] A reduction in left atrial size and an increase in left atrial-mediated passive filling of the left ventricle have been observed after modification of left ventricular systolic and diastolic properties following alcohol septal ablation in obstructive hypertrophic cardiomyopathy.[74]

Exercise (see Chap. 17)

Physical exercise is associated with increases in heart rate, venous return, cardiac output, stroke volume, and systolic pressure. Arterial diastolic pressure remains relatively unchanged or decreases slightly and, thus, pulse pressure increases during exercise, while the ejection period shortens. Hemodynamic adaptation depends largely on the type of exercise, i.e., dynamic or isometric exercise, as well as the severity of exercise and the mass of exercising muscles. Exercise capacity is determined by many factors, such as body position; gender; age; body mass; level of exercise training; and environmental factors, such as temperature, humidity, and ambient oxygen concentration. Adaptation of cardiac function is largely dependent on the level of exercise and the response of the cardiovascular system as well as the magnitude of adrenergic stimulation. For instance, dynamic exercise (e.g., running, swimming, cycling) is associated with a large increase in cardiac output achieved mainly by increases in heart rate and in stroke volume,[75] whereas isometric exercise (e.g., handgrip, weight lifting, bodybuilding) is associated with a moderate increase in cardiac output but a large increase in arterial pressure consequent to enhanced sympathetic stimulation (*pressure loading*). In daily living, both forms of exercise are frequently used.

Definition of Abnormal Cardiac Function During Exercise

Most noninvasive exercise studies are carried out in the upright position (treadmill, bicycle ergometer), but invasive (catheter-based) studies are usually performed in the supine position. Since venous return is increased in the supine position, diastolic filling pressure, stroke volume, and cardiac output in the resting state are higher in the supine than in the upright position. Assessment of cardiac function during dynamic or isometric exercise has been carried out by hemodynamic monitoring of the right heart using Swan-Ganz catheters or with fluid-filled catheters in the left heart and left ventricular angiography. However, most data on exercise have been obtained from right heart catheterization in the supine position. However, higher cardiac outputs are reached during maximal exercise in the erect position, but due to technical limitations of most measuring techniques, submaximal exercise has been preferred, to allow a short steady state for measuring hemodynamic data. Increasingly, noninvasive techniques, including 2D echocardiography, radionuclide angiography, and MR imaging, have been employed to study the response to exercise.

Abnormal cardiac function during *maximal* exercise has been based on pulmonary capillary wedge pressure or LVEDP exceeding 20 mm Hg, the cardiac output failing to reach 15 liters per minute, and the ejection fraction failing to rise.

SYSTOLIC FUNCTION. Hemodynamic adaptation of the ventricles to exercise is regulated by the increase in sympathetic activity and the resultant increases in heart rate and cardiac contractility. In the normal heart, when exercise is carried out in the supine position, both left and right ventricular end-diastolic volumes increase slightly, whereas end-systolic volumes decrease significantly. Both stroke volume and systolic ejection fraction increase and contribute to the augmentation of cardiac output. Since end-diastolic volume exhibits little change during exercise, the Frank- Starling mechanism does not play a major role in cardiac adaptation during exercise in the healthy heart. Increases in the ventricular filling pressures during exercise and volume occur only when the increase in the heart rate rise during exercise is blunted, as occurs in patients with atrioventricular block or in those treated with a beta-adrenergic blocker.

The increase in cardiac output during mild exercise is achieved by an augmentation of both stroke volume and heart rate, whereas the further increases in output during severe exercise result primarily from an increase in heart rate. Normal aging is associated with a decline in cardiac output that is mainly due to the reduction in the maximal heart rate.

DIASTOLIC FUNCTION. Most studies of the effects of exercise have focused on systolic function; less is known about diastolic function of the normal heart during exercise. There is general agreement that left ventricular end-systolic volume is smaller during exercise due to the enhanced contractile state. At the same time, the rate of relaxation is increased, which allows more rapid filling. These two mechanisms lead to an increase in elastic recoil that enhances ventricular filling at high heart rates when diastolic filling time is abbreviated.[76] These mechanisms maintain stroke volume and prevent undue elevation of ventricular diastolic pressures even at very high workloads and, thus, preload reserve is not needed in the normal heart to achieve maximal cardiac output.

In summary, left ventricular diastolic function during exercise is characterized by the following:

1. Enhanced elastic recoil with a small left ventricular end-systolic volume
2. Rapid left ventricular relaxation due to enhanced inotropic stimulation
3. Low early diastolic pressures (even negative pressures may occur) due to enhanced diastolic suction
4. Rapid diastolic filling that starts after mitral valve opening; one third of the stroke volume enters the left ventricle when its pressure is still falling

COUPLING OF CARDIAC CHAMBERS AND THE VASCULAR SYSTEM (Table 20–8)

The interplay between the left ventricle and the properties of the vascular bed is described by the term *ventriculoarterial coupling* and has been studied with a variety of tools such as Fourier analysis of arterial waveforms, ESPVRs, and calculations of power.[77] An additional form of analysis can be applied to the vascular systems themselves.[78] The computation of vascular resistance is commonly performed (see Chap. 17) and is clinically useful for a variety of purposes. More sophisticated measurements of vascular properties involve assessments of the pressure and vessel size, including the impact of different degrees of vascular tone. The measurement of pulse wave velocity provides insight into vascular properties, including the composition of the vessel wall and vascular tone and the relationships between wave velocity and distending pressure. With normal aging, arterial pulse pressure and pulse wave velocity rise while arterial compliance falls. Age-related differences in pulse wave velocity are differentially modified by vasodilators such as nitroprusside.

The arterial system has been traditionally modeled using a Windkessel model with the more recent addition of wave reflections into the conceptual framework. Total arterial compliance is calculated from the arterial diastolic pressure decay either measured directly or estimated from tonometry. Estimated arterial compliance, C, can be calculated by the formula

$$C = A_d/R(P_s - P_d)$$

where A_d = area under the diastolic pressure waveform computed from P_s (the maximum pressure after the dicrotic notch) to P_d (minimum pressure near end-diastole), and R = the systemic vascular resistance calculated from cardiac output and mean aortic pressure.

TABLE 20–8 Age-Related Differences in LV and Arterial Coupling in Patients with Dilated Cardiomyopathy

Parameters	Young Patients <35 yr	Intermediate-Aged Patients 35-50 yr	Older Patients >50 yr
Maximum + dP/dt (mm Hg/sec)	1011 ± 160	1170 ± 159	1147 ± 374
Stroke work (g-m/m²)	19 ± 10	20 ± 10	19 ± 10
Pulse pressure (mm Hg)	26 ± 8	30 ± 11	38 ± 10
Pulse wave velocity (m/sec)	4.7 ± 0.4	6.5 ± 0.9	7.9 ± 0.6
Systemic vascular resistance (dyn-sec · cm⁻⁵)	1872 ± 789	2373 ± 762	2440 ± 770
Arterial compliance (ml/mm Hg)	1.33 ± 0.63	0.72 ± 0.40	0.51 ± 0.17

LV = left ventricular.

Adapted from Carroll JD, Shroff S, Arand P, et al: Arterial mechanical properties in dilated cardiomyopathy. J Clin Invest 87:1002-1009, 1991.

NEUROHUMORAL ASSESSMENT OF CARDIAC FUNCTION (see Chap. 21)

The use of neurohumoral assays to complement and potentially replace direct assessment of cardiac function has emerged in the last decade.[79,80] This development follows our understanding of the neurohumoral response as an important part of the pathophysiology of cardiovascular dysfunction as well as a target of treatment. The activation of the neurohumoral system occurs in a variety of forms of heart failure including systolic and diastolic dysfunction but also in patients with valvular disease. Activation of the adrenergic and renin-angiotensin systems have been well characterized. Theoretically whenever a cardiac condition produces elevated pressures, activation of intramyocardial stretch receptors and other hemodynamic and mechanical perturbations may lead to a release of natriuretic peptides. The results of these assays can provide insights and direction for the clinician in a broad range of circumstances, including the differential diagnosis of dyspnea as being of cardiac or noncardiac origin, as an early warning sign of disease progression, as a correlate of functional class, as a surrogate of the magnitude of the cardiac function abnormality, and as an independent determinant of the patient's prognosis and response to therapy.[81,82]

The complex interplay between cardiac mechanical function, neurohumoral function, and modification in hemostatic control is also apparent in the left atrium. Left atrial mechanical function is specifically linked to the release of atrial natriuretic peptide release. This interplay is illustrated in patients converted from atrial fibrillation.[83] Left atrial enlargement is also an independent risk factor for the development of left atrial thrombi. The reduced velocity of blood motion within the fibrillating, dilated left atrium is suggested by the presence of "smoke" on transesophageal and intracardiac echocardiographic visualization of the left atrium.[84]

Abnormal hemodynamics may cause other biochemical effects. Recent attention has been given to understanding how von Willebrand factor circulating in the blood as a large protein is altered by cardiac conditions with pathologically high fluid shear stress such as aortic stenosis, ventricular septal defect, and patent ductus arteriosus.[85] Acquired defects occur as a consequence of damage to von Willebrand factor during passage through the stenotic orifice and then contribute to the known association of severe aortic stenosis and bleeding, especially from preexisting lesions such as gastrointestinal angiodysplasia. The correlation between the hemostatic defect and the hemodynamic severity of aortic stenosis is strong and may in the future help determine the timing of valve intervention.

These recent insights emphasize that cardiac function can be quantified from different perspectives. The biology of cardiac function is an area that will advance rapidly during the next decade.

REFERENCES

1. Carabello B: Evolution of the study of left ventricular function: Everything old is new again. Circulation 105:2701, 2002.
2. Abraham WT, Fisher WG, Smith AL, et al: Cardiac resynchronization in chronic heart failure. N Engl J Med 346:1845, 2002.
3. Delgado D, Rao V, Ross H, et al: Mechanical circulatory assistance: State of art. Circulation 106:2046, 2002.
4. Perin E, Geng Y, Willerson J: Adult stem cell therapy in perspective. Circulation 107:935, 2003.
5. Sabbah H: The cardiac support device and the Myosplint: Treating heart failure by targeting left ventricular size and shape. Ann Thorac Surg 75:S13, 2003.
6. Katz A: Ernest Henry Starling: His predecessors, and the "law of the heart." Circulation 106:2986, 2002.
7. Karunanithi M, Feneley M: Single-beat determination of preload recruitable stroke work relationship: Derivation and evaluation in conscious dogs. J Am Coll Cardiol 35:502, 2000.

Diastolic Function

8. Hess OM: Diastolic Function of the Left Ventricle. Stuttgart, Georg Thieme Verlag, 1982.
9. Zile M, Brutsaert D: New concepts in diastolic dysfunction and diastolic heart failure: I. Diagnosis, prognosis, and measurements of diastolic function. Circulation 105:1387, 2002.
10. Zile M, Brutsaert D: New concepts in diastolic dysfunction and diastolic heart failure: II. Causal mechanisms and treatment. Circulation 105:1503, 2002.
11. Bell SP, Nyland L, Tischler MD, et al: Alterations in the determinants of diastolic suction during pacing tachycardia. Circ Res 87:235, 2000.
12. Hess OM, Osakada G, Lavelle J, et al: Diastolic myocardial wall stiffness and ventricular relaxation during partial and complete coronary occlusion in the conscious dog. Circ Res 52:387, 1983.
13. Angeja B, Grossmann W: Evaluation and management of diastolic heart failure. Circulation 107:659, 2003.
14. Zile MR, Gaasch WH, Carroll JD, et al: Heart failure with a normal ejection fraction: Is measurement of diastolic function necessary to make the diagnosis of diastolic heart failure? Circulation 104:779-782, 2001.

15. Paulus WJ, for the European Study Group on Diastolic Heart Failure: How to diagnose diastolic heart failure. European Study Group on Diastolic Heart Failure. Eur Heart J 19:990-1003, 1998.
16. Kass DA: Assessment of diastolic dysfunction: Invasive modalities. Cardiol Clin 18:571-586, 2000.
17. Paulus WJ, Vantrimpont PJ, Rousseau MF: Diastolic function of nonfilling human left ventricle. J Am Coll Cardiol 20:1524, 1992.
18. Mandinov L, Eberli FR, Seiler C, Hess OM: Diastolic heart failure. Cardiovasc Res 45:813, 2000.
19. Carroll JD, Hess OM, Hirzel HO, Krayenbuehl HP: Exercise-induced ischemia: The influence of altered relaxation on early diastolic pressures. Circulation 67:521, 1983.
20. Nagel E, Hess OM: Ventrikelfunktion: Systolische und diastolische funktion. *In* Hess OM, Simon RWR (eds): Herzkatheter-Einsatz in Diagnostik und Therapie. Berlin, Springer Verlag 2000.
21. Neumann T, Vollmer A, Schaffner T, et al: Diastolic dysfunction and collagen structure in canine pacing-induced heart failure. J Am Coll Cardiol 31:179, 1999.
22. Spinale FG, Coker ML, Thomas CV, et al: Time-dependent changes in matrix metalloproteinase activity and expression during the progression of congestive heart failure: Relation to ventricular and myocyte function. Circ Res 82:482, 1998.
23. Javier Díez J, Querejeta R, López B, et al: Losartan-dependent regression of myocardial fibrosis is associated with reduction of left ventricular chamber stiffness in hypertensive patients. Circulation 105:2512, 2002.
24. Hein S, Gaasch W, Schaper J: Giant molecule titin and myocardial stiffness. Circulation 106:1303, 2002.
25. Weber KT: Targeting pathological remodeling: Concepts of cardioprotection and reparation. Circulation 102:1342, 2000.
26. Hess OM, Bhargava V, Ross J, Shabetai R: The role of the pericardium in interactions between the cardiac chambers. Am Heart J 106:1377, 1983.
27. Hoit B: Management of effusive and constrictive pericardial heart disease. Circulation 105:2939, 2002.
28. Rakowski H, Appleton C, Chan KL, et al: Canadian consensus recommendations for the measurement and reporting of diastolic dysfunction by echocardiography. The Investigators of Consensus on Diastolic Dysfunction by Echocardiography. J Am Soc Echocardiogr 9:736, 1999.
29. Tabata T, Thomas JD, Klein AL: Pulmonary venous flow by Doppler echocardiography: Revisited 12 years later. J Am Coll Cardiol 41:1243, 2003.
30. Jensen JL, Williams FE, Beilby BJ, et al: Feasibility of obtaining pulmonary venous flow velocity in cardiac patients using transthoracic pulsed wave Doppler technique. J Am Soc Echocardiogr 10:60, 1997.
31. Takatsuji H, Mikami T, Urasawa K, et al: A new approach for evaluation of left ventricular diastolic function: Spatial and temporal analysis of left ventricular filling flow propagation by color M-mode Doppler echocardiography [see comments]. J Am Coll Cardiol 27:365, 1996.
32. Nagueh SF, Lakkis NM, Middleton KJ, et al: Doppler estimation of left ventricular filling pressure in patients with hypertrophic cardiomyopathy. Circulation 99:254, 1999.
33. Sohn DW, Chai IH, Lee DJ, et al: Assessment of mitral annulus velocity by Doppler tissue imaging in the evaluation of left ventricular diastolic function. J Am Coll Cardiol 30:474, 1997.
34. Lindstrom L, Wranne B: Pulsed tissue Doppler evaluation of mitral annulus motion: A new window to assessment of diastolic function. Clin Physiol 19:1, 1999.
35. Sohn DW, Kim YJ, Kim HC, et al: Evaluation of left ventricular diastolic function when mitral E and A waves are completely fused: role of assessing mitral annulus velocity. J Am Soc Echocardiogr 12:203, 1999.
36. Blomstrand P, Kongstad O, Broqvist M, et al: Assessment of left ventricular diastolic function from mitral annulus motion: A comparison with pulsed Doppler measurements in patients with heart failure. Clin Physiol 16:483, 1996.
37. Oki T, Tabata T, Yamada H, et al: Clinical application of pulsed Doppler tissue imaging for assessing abnormal left ventricular relaxation .Am J Cardiol 79:921, 1997.
38. Shimizu Y, Uematsu M, Shimizu H, et al: Peak negative myocardial velocity gradient in early diastole as a noninvasive indicator of left ventricular diastolic function: Comparison with transmitral flow velocity indices. J Am Coll Cardiol 32:1418, 1998.
39. Kudelka AM, Turner DA, Liebson PR, et al: Comparison of cine magnetic resonance imaging and Doppler echocardiography for evaluation of left ventricular diastolic function. Am J Cardiol 80:384, 1997.
40. Stuber M, Schedegger MB, Fischer SE, et al: Alterations in the local myocardial motion pattern in patients suffering from pressure overload due to aortic stenosis. Circulation 100:361, 1999.
41. Maier SE, Fischer SE, McKinnon GC, et al: Evaluation of left ventricular segmental wall motion in hypertrophic cardiomyopathy with myocardial tagging. Circulation 86:1919, 1992.
42. Fischer SE, McKinnon GC, Maier SE, Boesiger P: Improved myocardial tagging contrast. Magn Reson Med 31:401, 1994.
43. Briguori C, Betocchi S, Losi MA, et al: Noninvasive evaluation of left ventricular diastolic function in hypertrophic cardiomyopathy. Am J Cardiol 81:180, 1998.
44. Bonow RO: Radionuclide angiographic evaluation of left ventricular diastolic function. Circulation 84:I208, 1991.

Right Ventricular Function

45. Reynertson S, Kundur R, Mullen G, et al: Asymmetry of right ventricular enlargement in response to tricuspid regurgitation. Circulation 100:465, 1999.
46. Veldtman G, Razack V, Siu S, et al: Right ventricular form and function after percutaneous atrial septal defect device closure. J Am Coll Cardiol 37:2108, 2001.
47. Brickner M, Hillis L, Lang R: Congenital heart disease in adults: I. N Engl J Med 342:256, 2000.
48. Rubin L: Primary pulmonary hypertension. N Engl J Med 336:111, 1997.
49. Fedullo P, Auger W, Kerr K, Rubin L: Chronic thromboembolic pulmonary hypertension. N Engl J Med 345:1465, 2001.
50. Menzel T, Wagner S, Kramm T, et al: Pathophysiology of impaired right and left ventricular function in chronic embolic pulmonary hypertension: Changes after pulmonary thromboendarterectomy. Chest 118:897, 2000.
51. Chen C, Cheng T, Huang T, et al: Percutaneous balloon valvuloplasty for pulmonic stenosis in adolescents and adults. N Engl J Med 335:21, 1996.
52. Goldstein J: Pathophysiology and management of right heart ischemia. J Am Coll Cardiol 40:841, 2002.
53. Bowers T, O'Neill W, Pica M, Goldstein J: Patterns of coronary compromise resulting in acute right ventricular ischemic dysfunction. Circulation 106:1104, 2002.
54. Dubin A, Feinstein J, Reddy M, et al: Electrical resynchronization: A novel therapy for the failing right ventricle. Circulation 107:2287, 2003.
55. Grigioni F, Avierinos JF, Ling LH, et al: Atrial fibrillation complicating the course of degenerative mitral regurgitation. J Am Coll Cardiol 40:84-92, 2002.
56. Rossi A, Cicoira M, Zanolla L, et al: Determinants and prognostic value of left atrial volume in patients with dilated cardiomyopathy. J Am Coll Cardiol 40:142, 2002.
57. Moller J, Hillis GS, Oh JK, et al: Left atrial volume: A powerful predictor of survival after acute myocardial infarction. Circulation 107:2207, 2003.
58. Hoit BD, Shao Y, Gabel M: Influence of acutely altered loading conditions on left atrial appendage flow velocities. J Am Coll Cardiol 24:1117, 1994.
59. Hondo T, Okamoto M, Yamane T, et al: The role of the left atrial appendage: A volume loading study in open-chest dogs. Jpn Heart J 36:225, 1995.
60. Hoit BD, Shao Y, Tsai LM, et al: Altered left atrial compliance after atrial appendectomy: Influence on left atrial and ventricular filling. Circ Res 72:167, 1993.
61. Agmon Y, Khanderia K, Gentile F, Seward JB: Echocardiographic assessment of the left atrial appendage. J Am Coll Cardiol 34:1867, 1999.
62. Pritchett AM, Jacobsen SJ, Mahoney DW, et al: Left atrial volume as an index of left atrial size: A population-based study. J Am Coll Cardiol 41:1036, 2003.
63. Szili-Torok T, Kimman GJ, Scholten HF, et al: Interatrial septum pacing guided by three-dimensional intracardiac echocardiography. J Am Coll Cardiol 40:2139, 2002.
64. Schwartzman D, Lacomis J, Wigginton W: Characterization of left atrium and distal pulmonary vein morphology using multidimensional computed tomography. J Am Coll Cardiol 41:1349, 2003.
65. Hoit BD, Gabel M: Influence of left ventricular dysfunction on the role of atrial contraction: An echocardiographic-hemodynamic study in dogs. J Am Coll Cardiol 36:1713, 2000.
66. Manning WJ, Silverman DI, Katz SE, Douglas PS: Atrial ejection force: A noninvasive assessment of atrial systolic function. J Am Coll Cardiol 22:221, 1993.
67. Alexander J Jr, Sunagawa K, Chang N, Sagawa K: Instantaneous pressure-volume relation of the ejecting canine left atrium. Circ Res 61:209 , 1987.
68. Hoit BD, Shao Y, Gabel M, Walsh RA: In vivo assessment of left atrial contractile performance in normal and pathological conditions using a time-varying elastance model. Circulation 89:1829, 1994.
69. Stefanadis C, Dernellis J, Tsiamis E, Toutouza P: Effects of pacing-induced and balloon coronary occlusion ischemia on left atrial function in patients with coronary artery disease. J Am Coll Cardiol 33:687, 1999.
70. Nakatani S, Garcia MJ, Firstenberg MS, et al: Noninvasive assessment of left atrial maximum dP/dt by a combination of transmitral and pulmonary venous flow. J Am Coll Cardiol 34:795, 1999.
71. Sparks P, Jayaprakash S, Mond Hg, et al: Left atrial mechanical function after brief duration atrial fibrillation. J Am Coll Cardiol 33:342, 1999.
72. Yuda S, Nakatani S, Kosakai Y, et al: Long-term follow-up of atrial contraction after the Maze procedure in patients with mitral valve disease. J Am Coll Cardiol 37:1622, 2001.
73. Sakai H, Kunichika H, Murata K, et al: Improvement of afterload mismatch of left atrial booster pump function with positive inotropic agent. J Am Coll Cardiol 37:270, 2001.
74. Nagueh S, Lakkis NM, Middleton KJ, et al: Changes in left ventricular filling and left atrial function six months after nonsurgical septal reduction therapy for hypertrophic obstructive cardiomyopathy. J Am Coll Cardiol 34:1123, 1999.

Exercise

75. Weber KT, Janicki JS, McElroy PA, Reddy HK: Concepts and applications of cardiopulmonary exercise testing. Chest 93:843, 1988.
76. Nonogi H, Hess OM, Ritter M, Krayenbuehl HP: Diastolic properties of the normal left ventricle during supine exercise. Br Heart J 60:30-38, 1988.
77. Kawaguchi M, Hay I, Fetics B, Kass D: Combined ventricular systolic and arterial stiffening with heart failure and preserved ejection fraction: Implications for systolic and diastolic reserve. Circulation 107:714, 2003.
78. Nichols WW, O'Rourke W: McDonald's Blood Flow in Arteries. 4th ed. London, Arnold, 1998.
79. Francis GS, Cohn JN, Johnson G, et al. Plasma norepinephrine, plasma renin activity, and congestive heart failure: Relations to survival and the effects of therapy in V-HeFT II. Circulation 87:V140, 1993.
80. Lubien E, DeMaria A, Krishnaswamy P, et al: Utility of B-natriuretic peptide in detecting diastolic dysfunction: Comparison with Doppler velocity recordings. Circulation 105:595, 2002.
81. de Lemos JA, McGuire DK, Drazner MH: B-type natriuretic peptide in cardiovascular disease. Lancet 362:316, 2003.
82. Bozkurt B, Mann DL: Use of biomarkers in the management of heart failure: Are we there yet? Circulation 107:1231, 2003.
83. Wozÿkowska-Kaplon B, Opolski G: Concomitant recovery of atrial mechanical and endocrine function after cardioversion in patients with persistent atrial fibrillation. J Am Coll Cardiol 41:1716 , 2003.
84. Peverill RE, Harris G, Gelman J, et al: Effect of warfarin on regional left atrial coagulation activity in mitral stenosis. Am J Cardiol 79:339, 1997.
85. Vincentelli A, Susen S, Le Tourneau T, et al: Acquired von Willebrand syndrome in aortic stenosis. N Engl J Med 349:343, 2003.

CHAPTER 21

Pathophysiology of Heart Failure

Wilson S. Colucci • Eugene Braunwald

Heart (or cardiac) failure is the pathophysiological state in which the heart is unable to pump blood at a rate commensurate with the requirements of the metabolizing tissues or can do so only from an elevated filling pressure. The American College of Cardiology/American Heart Association Guidelines for the Evaluation and Management of Chronic Heart Failure in the Adult defined heart failure as a "complex clinical syndrome that can result from any structural or functional cardiac disorder that impairs the ability of the ventricle to fill with or eject blood."[1] It is often, but not always, caused by a defect in myocardial contraction, that is, by *myocardial failure.*[2,3] However, in some patients with heart failure a similar clinical syndrome is present without a detectable abnormality of *myocardial* function. In many such cases, heart failure is caused by conditions in which the normal heart is suddenly presented with a load that exceeds its capacity[4] or in which ventricular filling is impaired.[1]

Heart failure may be caused by myocyte death, myocyte dysfunction, ventricular remodeling, or some combination. Abnormal energy utilization, ischemia, and neurohormonal disturbances can lead to the progression of heart failure (see also Chap. 23).[2,5-8] *Heart failure* should be distinguished from *circulatory failure,* in which an abnormality of some component of the circulation—the heart, the blood volume, the concentration of oxygenated hemoglobin in the arterial blood, or the vascular bed—is responsible for the inadequate cardiac output.

Thus, the terms myocardial failure, heart failure, and circulatory failure are *not* synonymous but refer to progressively more inclusive entities. Myocardial failure, when sufficiently severe, always causes heart failure, but the converse is not necessarily the case because a number of conditions in which the heart is suddenly overloaded (e.g., acute aortic regurgitation secondary to acute infective endocarditis) can cause heart failure in the presence of normal myocardial function, at least early in the course of the illness. Myocardial failure may be associated with systolic dysfunction, diastolic dysfunction, or most commonly both. Also, conditions such as tricuspid or mitral stenosis and constrictive pericarditis, which interfere with cardiac filling, can cause heart failure without myocardial failure. Heart failure, in turn, always causes circulatory failure, but again the converse is not necessarily the case because a variety of noncardiac conditions (e.g., hypovolemic shock) can produce circulatory failure at a time when cardiac function is normal or only modestly impaired.

The hemodynamic, contractile, and wall motion disorders in heart failure are discussed in the chapters on echocardiography (see Chap. 11), cardiac catheterization (see Chap. 17), radionuclide imaging (see Chap. 13), assessment of cardiac function (see Chap. 20), and clinical features (see Chap. 22). In this chapter, we focus on the physiological, neurohumoral, biochemical, molecular, and cellular changes characteristic of heart failure.

Short-Term Adaptive Mechanisms

In the presence of a primary disturbance in myocardial contractility or an excessive hemodynamic burden placed on the ventricle, or both, the heart depends on a number of adaptive mechanisms for maintenance of its pumping function (Fig. 21–1, Table 21–1).[9] Most important among these are (1) the Frank-Starling mechanism, in which an increased preload helps to sustain cardiac performance; (2) activation of neurohumoral systems, especially the release of the neurotransmitter norepinephrine (NE) by adrenergic cardiac nerves, which augments myocardial contractility, and activation of the renin-angiotensin-aldosterone system as well as other neurohumoral adjustments that act to maintain arterial pressure and perfusion of vital organs; and (3) myocardial remodeling with or without cardiac chamber dilatation, in which the mass of contractile tissue is augmented. The first two of these adaptations occur rapidly, within several cardiac cycles after the onset of severe myocardial dysfunction, and may be adequate to maintain the overall pumping performance of the heart at relatively normal levels. Myocardial remodeling and hypertrophy develop more slowly, over weeks to months, and play an important role in long-term adaptation to hemodynamic overload. However, each of these mechanisms has a finite capacity to sustain cardiac performance in the presence of hemodynamic overload and, when chronically maintained, becomes maladaptive.

HEMODYNAMIC AND CIRCULATORY CONSEQUENCES OF HEART FAILURE. *Cardiac output* is often depressed, and the arterial–mixed venous oxygen difference is widened in the basal state in patients with the common forms of chronic heart failure secondary to ischemic heart disease, hypertension, primary myocardial disease, valvular disease, and pericardial disease (so-called low-output, systolic heart failure). Arterial pressure is maintained and systemic vascular resistance is elevated. In mild heart failure, the cardiac output may be normal at rest but fails to rise normally

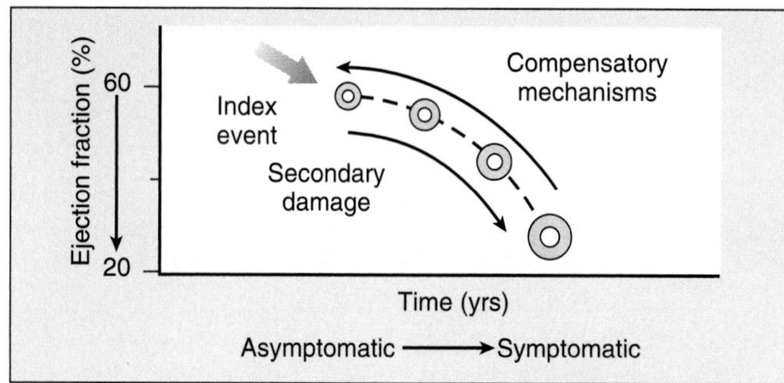

FIGURE 21–1 Pathogenesis of heart failure. Heart failure begins after an "index event" produces an initial decline in pumping capacity of the heart. After this initial decline in pumping capacity of the heart, a variety of compensatory mechanisms are activated, including the adrenergic nervous system, the renin-angiotensin system, and the cytokine system. In the short term, these systems are able to restore cardiovascular function to a normal hemostatic range and the patient remains asymptomatic. However, with time the sustained activation of these systems can lead to secondary end-organ damage within the ventricle, with worsening left ventricular remodeling and subsequent cardiac decompensation. As a result of worsening left ventricular remodeling and cardiac decompensation, patients undergo the transition from asymptomatic to symptomatic heart failure. (From Mann DL: Mechanisms and models in heart failure: A combinatorial approach. Circulation 100:99, 1999.)

during exercise. When the volume of blood delivered into the systemic arterial bed is chronically reduced or when one or both ventricles have an elevated filling pressure, or both, a complex sequence of adjustments occurs that ultimately results in the *retention of sodium and water* in the intravascular and interstitial compartments. Many of the clinical manifestations of heart failure such as dyspnea and edema are secondary to this excessive retention of fluid in the pulmonary and systemic venous beds (see Chap. 22).

Interaction Between the Frank-Starling Mechanism and the Adrenergic Nervous System

It is useful to consider the function of the normal and failing heart within the framework of the Frank-Starling mechanism, in which an increase in preload, reflected in an elevation of end-diastolic volume, augments ventricular performance.[4] The normal relationship between ventricular end-diastolic volume and performance is shown in Figure 21–2, curve 1. During exercise and other stresses, the increases in adrenergic nerve impulses to the myocardium, increases in the concentration of circulating catecholamines, and tachycardia all augment myocardial contractility with a shift from curve 1 to curve 2. Ventricular performance, as reflected in stroke work or cardiac output, increases with little change in end-diastolic pressure and volume. This is represented by a shift from point A to point B in Figure 21–2. Vasodilation occurs in the exercising skeletal muscles as a consequence of their heightened metabolism, reducing peripheral vascular resistance and aortic impedance. This combination of augmented myocardial contractility and vasodilatation enhances ventricular emptying and allows achievement of a greatly elevated cardiac output during exercise, at an arterial pressure only slightly higher than in the resting state. During intense exercise in a normal subject, cardiac output can rise 5-fold (and total body O_2 10-fold) if use is also made of the Frank-Starling mechanism, as reflected in modest increases in the left ventricular end-diastolic volume and pressure (point B to point C).

In moderately severe systolic heart failure, as represented by curve 3, cardiac output and external ventricular performance at rest are within normal limits but are maintained at these levels only because the end-diastolic fiber length and the ventricular end-diastolic volume (ventricular preload) are elevated (i.e., through the operation of the Frank-Starling mechanism). The elevations of left ventricular diastolic pressure are associated with abnormally high levels of pulmonary capillary pressure, contributing to the dyspnea experienced by patients with heart failure, sometimes even at rest (point D).

Heart failure is characterized by generalized adrenergic activation and parasympathetic withdrawal (Fig. 21–3).[4,10,11] This condition leads to stimulation of myocardial contractility, tachycardia, sodium retention, activation of the renin-angiotensin-aldosterone system, and generalized systemic vasoconstriction. Heart failure is frequently accompanied by

TABLE 21–1 Short-Term and Long-Term Responses to Impaired Cardiac Performance

Response	Short-Term Effects*	Long-Term Effects†
Salt and water retention	Augments preload	Causes pulmonary congestion, anasarca
Vasoconstriction	Maintains blood pressure for perfusion of vital organs (brain, heart)	Exacerbates pump dysfunction (after-load mismatch); increases cardiac energy expenditure
Sympathetic stimulation	Increases heart rate and ejection	Increases energy expenditure
Sympathetic desensitization		Spares energy
Hypertrophy	Unloads individual muscle fibers	Leads to deterioration and death of cardiac cells; cardiomyopathy of overload
Capillary deficit		Leads to energy starvation
Mitochondrial density	Increase in density helps meet energy demands	Decrease in density leads to energy starvation
Appearance of slow myosin		Increases force, decreases shortening velocity and contractility; is energy sparing
Prolonged action potential		Increases contractility and energy expenditure
Decreased density of sarcoplasmic reticulum calcium pump sites		Slows relaxation; may be energy sparing
Increased collagen	May reduce dilatation	Impairs relaxation

From Katz AM: Cardiomyopathy of overload: A major determinant of prognosis in congestive heart failure. N Engl J Med 322:100, 1990. Copyright 1990, Massachusetts Medical Society.

*Short-term effects are mainly adaptive and occur after hemorrhage and in acute heart failure.

†Long-term effects are mainly deleterious and occur in chronic heart failure.

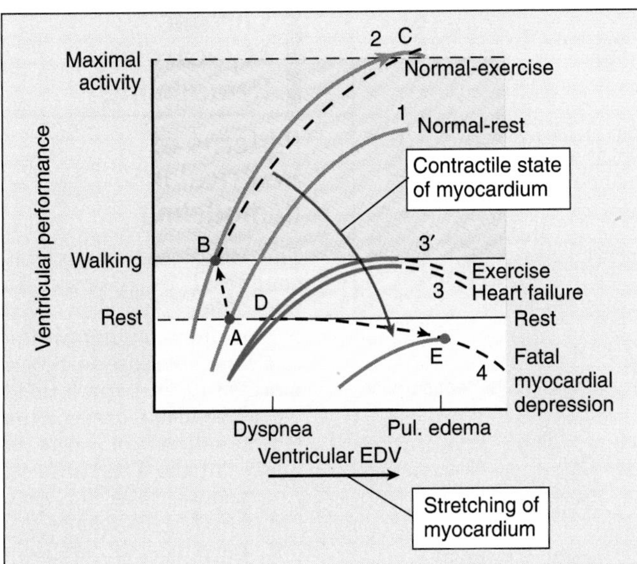

FIGURE 21–2 Diagram showing the interrelationship of influences on ventricular end-diastolic volume (EDV) through stretching of the myocardium and the contractile state of the myocardium. Levels of ventricular EDV associated with filling pressures that result in dyspnea and pulmonary edema are shown on the abscissa. Levels of ventricular performance required during rest, walking, and maximal activity are designated on the ordinate. The dashed lines are the descending limbs of the ventricular performance curves, which are rarely seen during life but that show what the level of ventricular performance would be if EDV could be elevated to very high levels. (Modified from Braunwald E, Ross J Jr, Sonnenblick EH: Mechanisms of Contraction of the Normal and Failing Heart. Boston, Little, Brown, 1979.)

reductions in NE stores and myocardial beta adrenoceptor density. As a consequence, ventricular function (performance) curves cannot be elevated to normal levels by the adrenergic nervous system and the normal enhancement of contractility that takes place during physical activity is attenuated (see Fig. 21–2, curves 3 to 3′). The factors that tend to augment ventricular filling during exertion push the failing ventricle even farther along its flattened, depressed function curve. There are marked elevations of ventricular end-diastolic volume and pressure and therefore of pulmonary capillary pressure. The elevation of the latter intensifies dyspnea and plays an important role in limiting the intensity of exertion that can be performed. Left ventricular failure becomes fatal when the left ventricular function curve becomes depressed (curve 4) to the point at which either cardiac output is insufficient to satisfy the requirements of the peripheral tissue at rest or the left ventricular end-diastolic and pulmonary capillary pressures are elevated to levels that result in pulmonary edema or both (point E).

Vascular Redistribution of Left Ventricular Output

Maintenance of arterial pressure in the presence of a reduced cardiac output is a primitive but effective compensatory mechanism. In both hypovolemia and severe heart failure, this important mechanism is brought into play to allow the limited cardiac output to be most useful for survival. Thus, vasoconstriction occurs earliest and is most intense in areas that are not vital for immediate survival, such as the skin, skeletal muscle, gut, and kidney.

INCREASED VASOCONSTRICTOR ACTIVITY

The major mechanism of increased vascular tone is an increase in the activity of vasoconstrictor systems, in particular the sympathetic nervous system, the renin-angiotensin-aldosterone system, and endothelin. In patients with moderately severe heart failure, in whom the cardiac output at rest is normal, abnormal vasoconstriction in selected vascular beds occurs when an additional burden (such as exertion) is imposed on the circulation and the cardiac output fails to rise normally to meet the peripheral demands. As cardiac performance declines, left ventricular output is ultimately redistributed, even at rest. This redistribution maintains the delivery of oxygen to vital organs such as the brain and heart, whereas blood flow to less critical areas is reduced.[12,13]

This underperfusion of skeletal muscle leads to anaerobic metabolism,[14] lactic acidosis, an excess oxygen debt, weakness, and fatigue. Occasionally, serious complications can result from the redistribution of cardiac output and the resulting regional reductions of blood flow. These include marked sodium and nitrogen retention as a consequence of diminished renal perfusion, hepatic dysfunction, and, in extreme cases, gangrene of the tips of the phalanges and mesenteric infarction.

With heart failure there is a generalized increase in sympathetic activity. Neurograms obtained from adrenergic nerves to the limbs display increased traffic in patients with heart failure.[11] Substantial changes also occur in the function of the adrenergic nerves that innervate splanchnic and renal vessels.[15] Although direct neurograms of the nerves to these beds are not feasible in humans, it has been shown that exercise induces a much more marked reduction in mesenteric blood flow and elevation of mesenteric vascular resistance in dogs with experimental heart failure than in normal dogs.[16] Similar changes during exercise were observed in other major visceral vascular beds, such as the renal bed. Evidence that this intense vasoconstriction during exercise is mediated by the adrenergic nervous system is provided by observations on dogs with experimentally produced heart failure in which one kidney was denervated. Blood flow through the innervated kidney declined precipitously during exercise, and calculated renal vascular resistance increased markedly. In contrast, little change in renal blood flow and calculated renal vascular resistance occurred in the denervated kidney.[16] This intense visceral vasoconstriction during exercise helps to divert the limited cardiac output to exercising muscle but contributes to hypoperfusion of the gut and kidneys.

The renin-angiotensin system and endothelin also contribute to the increased systemic vascular tone in heart failure. These potent vasoconstrictor systems are activated in patients with heart failure (see Renin-Angiotensin-Aldosterone System, later), in whom their contribution to systemic vasoconstriction has been demonstrated by the ability of specific inhibitors for angiotensin[17] and endothelin[18] receptors to cause vasodilation in patients with heart failure. Vasopressin is released in very advanced stages.

ENDOTHELIAL DYSFUNCTION. Both ischemia-induced and exercise-induced vasodilations in the extremities are attenuated in patients with heart failure, and this attenuation impairs the normal exercise-induced blood flow response.[19] The attenuation is related in part to endothelial dysfunction. The response of blood flow to infused acetylcholine and methacholine, which are endothelium-dependent vasodilators, is reduced in heart failure. The vasodilator response can be restored by the administration of L-arginine, a precursor of endothelium-derived nitric oxide (NO), which is synthesized in vascular endothelial cells by endothelial cell NO synthase (eNOS). These findings suggest that defective endothelial function contributes to the impaired vasodilator capacity in heart failure. The mechanisms potentially responsible include impaired endothelial cell receptor function, deficiency of L-arginine substrate, and abnormal expression of eNOS resulting in the impaired release and rapid degradation of NO by superoxide anion.[20] Activation of the renin-angiotensin-aldosterone system may contribute to endothelial dysfunction as well. Impaired endothelial function is improved in patients by regular exercise.[21]

CHANGES IN THE VASCULAR WALL. The sodium content of the vascular wall is increased in heart failure, and this contributes to the stiffening, thickening, and compression of blood vessel walls, which raises vascular resistance and also prevents normal vasodilation during exercise. It has been postulated that angiotensin II causes proliferation of smooth muscle and other elements of the vascular wall, causing vascular stiffening. Reduced density of skeletal muscle capillaries may contribute as well. The venous system in the extremities of patients with heart failure is also constricted by the activity of the adrenergic nervous system as well as by circulating and locally acting venoconstrictors (NE, angiotensin, and endothelin). This venoconstriction results in displacement of blood to the heart and lungs.

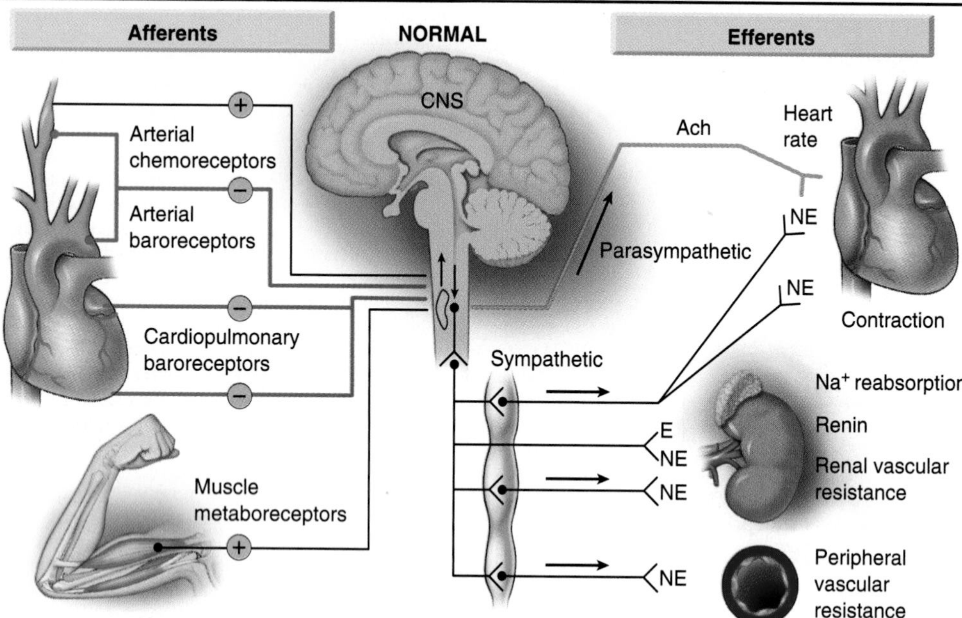

FIGURE 21–3 Mechanisms for generalized sympathetic activation and parasympathetic withdrawal in heart failure. **A,** Under normal conditions, inhibitory (–) inputs from arterial and cardiopulmonary baroreceptor afferent nerves are the principal influence on sympathetic outflow. Parasympathetic control of heart rate is also under potent arterial baroreflex control. Efferent sympathetic traffic and arterial catecholamines are low, and heart rate variability is high. **B,** As heart failure progresses, inhibitory input from arterial and cardiopulmonary receptors decreases and excitatory (+) input increases. The net response to this altered balance includes a generalized increase in sympathetic nerve traffic, blunted parasympathetic and sympathetic control of heart rate, and impairment of the reflex sympathetic regulation of vascular resistance. Anterior wall ischemia has additional excitatory effects on efferent sympathetic nerve traffic. See text for details. Ach = acetylcholine; CNS = central nervous system; E = epinephrine; Na^+ = sodium; NE = norepinephrine. (From Floras JS: Alterations in the sympathetic and parasympathetic nervous system in heart failure. *In* Mann DL [ed]: Heart Failure: A Companion to Braunwald's Heart Disease. Philadelphia, Elsevier, 2004, pp 247-278.)

2,3-DIPHOSPHOGLYCERATE. A progressive decline in the affinity of hemoglobin for oxygen caused by an increase in 2,3-diphosphoglycerate (DPG) also occurs in heart failure.[22] The rightward shift in the oxygen-hemoglobin dissociation curve represents a compensatory mechanism that facilitates oxygen transport; the increased DPG, tissue acidosis, and slowed circulation characteristic of heart failure act synergistically to maintain the delivery of oxygen to the metabolizing tissues in the presence of reduced cardiac output.

Chronic Myocardial Remodeling

Patterns of Ventricular Remodeling

The classical experiments conducted by Meerson in the 1960s[23] showed that immediately on imposition of a large pressure load, the increase in work performed by the ventricle exceeds the augmentation of cardiac mass and the heart dilates. As discussed earlier (see Fig. 21–1), a compensatory phase sets in as the ventricle remodels and the contractile function returns to approximately normal levels. If the compensatory response is adequate to "match" the work demands, a period of relative stability ensues. However, if the extent or form of myocardial remodeling is insufficient or if the magnitude of the overload increases further, regardless of the initial cause, there is further deterioration in myocardial function as a consequence of "afterload mismatch"; that is, the hypertrophy is insufficient to normalize mechanical stress on the myocyte and a vicious circle is created. Later, in what Meerson termed the "exhaustion" phase, several macroscopic events take place; there may be myofibrillar lysis, an increase in the number of lysosomes (presumably to digest worn-out cell constituents), distortion of the sarcoplasmic reticulum (SR), a reduction in the surface density of the key tubular system, and fibrous replacement of cardiac cells. This combination of changes leads to failure of the cardiac pump.

Ventricular remodeling, comprising changes in mass, volume, shape, and composition, constitutes one of the principal mechanisms by which the heart compensates for an increased load (Fig. 21–4).[24] Grossman and associates examined systolic and diastolic wall stresses in normal subjects and in patients with chronic pressure- and volume-overloaded left ventricles who were compensated and not in heart failure.[25] Left ventricular mass was increased approximately equally in both the pressure- and volume-overloaded groups. There was a substantial

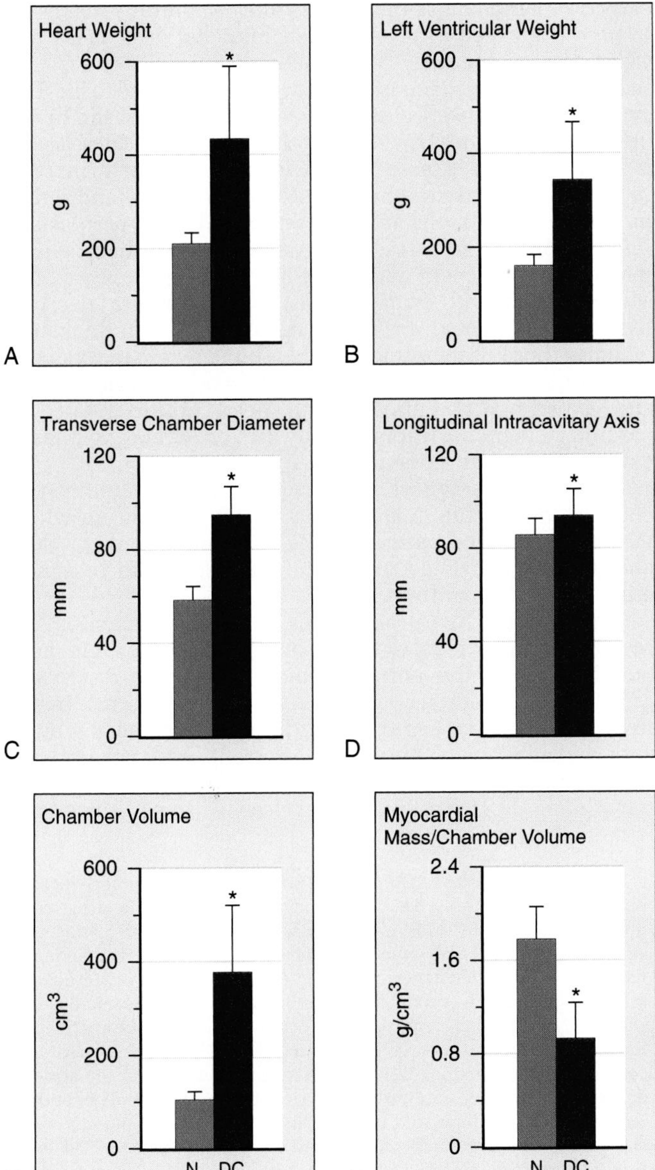

FIGURE 21–4 Cardiac characteristics of human dilated cardiomyopathy. Results are presented as mean + SD. N = normal hearts; DC = dilated cardiomyopathy; $*p < 0.05$) (From Mann DL [ed]: Heart Failure: A Companion to Braunwald's Heart Disease: A Textbook of Cardiovascular Medicine. Philadelphia, Elsevier, 2004. Data adapted from Beltrami CA, Finato N, Roco M, et al: The cellular basis of dilated cardiomyopathy in humans. J Mol Cell Cardiol 27:291, 1995.)

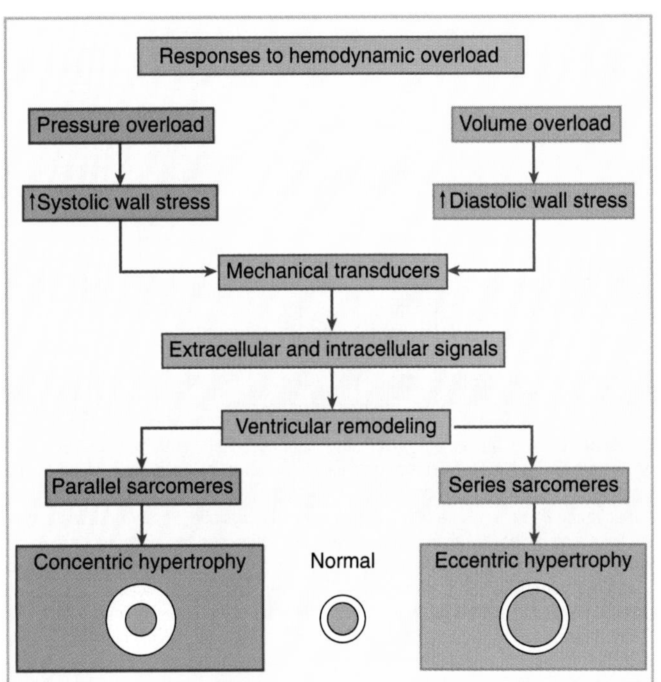

FIGURE 21–5 The morphological response to a hemodynamic overload depends on the nature of the stimulus. When the overload is predominantly due to an increase in pressure (e.g., with systemic hypertension or aortic stenosis), the increase in systolic wall stress leads to the parallel addition of sarcomeres and widening of the cardiac myocytes, resulting in concentric hypertrophy of the ventricle. When the overload is predominantly due to an increase in ventricular volume, the increase in diastolic wall stress leads to the series addition of sarcomeres, lengthening of cardiac myocytes, and eccentric chamber hypertrophy. (From Colucci WS [ed]: Heart Failure: Cardiac Function and Dysfunction. 2nd ed. Philadelphia, Current Medicine, 1999, p 4.2.)

increase in wall thickness in the pressure-overloaded ventricles but only a mild increase in wall thickness in the volume-overloaded ventricles (Fig. 21–5). The latter was just sufficient to counterbalance the increased radius so that the ratio of wall thickness to radius remained normal for the patients with volume-overload hypertrophy. However, this ratio was substantially increased in patients with pressure-overload hypertrophy, in whom there was disproportionate thickening of the ventricular wall.

These observations suggest that myocardial hypertrophy develops in a manner that maintains or returns systolic stress to normal limits. Thus, when the primary stimulus to hypertrophy is *pressure overload*, the resultant increase in systolic wall stress leads to parallel replication of myofibrils, thickening of individual myocytes, which at the organ level is referred to as "concentric" hypertrophy. A small increase in cell number (hyperplasia) has also been documented.[26] On the other hand, when the primary stimulus is ventricular *volume overload*, increased diastolic wall stress leads to replication of sarcomeres in series, elongation of myocytes, and ventricular dilatation. This effect, in turn, results in a modest increase in systolic stress (by the Laplace relationship), which causes proportional wall thickening that (as in pressure overload) returns systolic stress toward normal (Fig. 21–6). The chronically volume-overloaded ventricle becomes more spherical, and this change in shape can distort papillary muscle geometry and thereby cause functional mitral regurgitation.

In compensated subjects, both volume overload and pressure overload alter ventricular geometry and wall thickness so that systolic stress does not change greatly. Pressure overload and volume overload result in distinct cellular phenotypes at the molecular level with different patterns of activation of genes for several peptide growth factors.[27] This heterogeneity at the molecular level presumably reflects differences in the way the two types of hemodynamic overload activate signaling pathways.

Left ventricular wall thickness is a critical determinant of ventricular performance in patients with pressure overload hypertrophy related to aortic stenosis or hypertension. Impaired performance in such patients may be secondary to inadequate hypertrophy, leading to increased wall stress (afterload), which in turn may be responsible for inadequate muscle shortening. This condition has been termed afterload mismatch by Ross,[28] whose group found that when the aorta in conscious dogs was suddenly constricted and left ventricular systolic pressure rose, the left ventricle dilated and the left ventricular wall thinned; this effect was associated with a large increase in wall stress and a reciprocal reduction in the extent and velocity of shortening. During the next few weeks, the left ventricle became hypertrophied and left ventricular wall stress and shortening both returned toward normal. When the constriction was

	Normal	Acute load	Compensatory hypertrophy	Cardiac failure
LV systolic pressure	N	+	+	+
LV radius	N	+	+	+
LV wall thickness	N	N	+	+
LV diastolic volume	N	+	±	++
Systolic wall stress	N	+	N	+
Diastolic wall stress	N	+	N	+

FIGURE 21–6 The normal (N) relationship between left ventricular wall thickness (h) and chamber radius (r) is shown (first panel). An acute increase in systolic pressure (acute load) causes an increase in systolic wall stress, which can be approximated by the equation $P \times r/h$, where P is left ventricular (LV) systolic pressure. Diastolic wall stress is also increased when there is chamber dilation or when diastolic pressure is elevated (second panel). If sufficient compensatory hypertrophy occurs, the increase in ventricular wall thickness may normalize the systolic and diastolic wall stresses (third panel). However, if additional chamber dilation occurs or the increase in wall thickness is insufficient, systolic and diastolic wall stresses remain abnormally elevated. In this situation, further chamber dilation may occur in association with hemodynamic failure (fourth panel). (From Colucci WS [ed]: Heart Failure: Cardiac Function and Dysfunction. 2nd ed. Philadelphia, Current Medicine, 1999, p 4.2.)

suddenly released, wall stress declined and shortening became supernormal. (More recent experiments have challenged these traditional concepts but require confirmation.)

Prolonged athletic training causes a moderate increase in myocardial mass (see also Chap. 75). Isotonic exercise, such as long-distance running or swimming, resembles volume overload and causes an increase in left ventricular diastolic volume with only mild thickening of the wall. Isometric exercise, such as weightlifting or wrestling, causes intermittent pressure overload and can result in an increase in wall thickness. Neither form of hypertrophy appears to be deleterious in the absence of heart disease, and the hypertrophy rapidly disappears when training is discontinued.

CELLULAR CHANGES IN MYOCARDIAL REMODELING. The synthesis of additional mitochondria is one of the early cellular changes that occurs after a stimulus for hypertrophy is applied. The expanded mitochondrial mass provides the high-energy phosphates required to meet the increased energy demands of the hypertrophied cell. This synthesis is followed closely by an expansion of the myofibrillar mass. After the neonatal period, the increase in myocardial mass is associated with a proportional increase in the size of individual cells (i.e., hypertrophy) and only a minor increase in the number of cells (i.e., hyperplasia).[26] Intense, prolonged stress can cause some cardiac cells to reenter the cell cycle and replicate (see Chaps. 69 and 71). Myocytes isolated from animals with pressure overload hypertrophy related to aortic constriction are thickened, whereas those from animals with volume overload related to an aortocaval fistula are elongated.[29] Myocytes from patients and experimental animals with heart failure related to chronic ischemic cardiomyopathy are longer and, to a lesser extent, wider than normal cells (Fig. 21–7).

These changes within the myocyte are accompanied by changes in both the quantity and quality of collagen within the extracellular matrix (ECM).[30] Taken together, these changes in myocyte geometry and the ECM result in remodeling of the myocardium.

Hemodynamic overload causes gene reprogramming that reactivates growth factors present in the embryonic heart but dormant in the normal adult heart. These reactivated growth factors are responsible for stimulating the hypertrophy of cardiac myocytes and regulating the synthesis and degradation of the ECM. Current understanding of the funda-mental mechanisms responsible for myocardial remodeling is described earlier (see Chronic Myocardial Remodeling).

ULTRASTRUCTURAL CHANGES. Structural features of hypertrophied human myocytes (Fig. 21-8) include abnormal Z-band patterns, multiple intercalated discs, and prominent collagen fibrils connecting adjacent myocardial cells. Nuclei are enlarged and lobulated and contain well-developed nucleoli; there is an abundance of ribosomes, presumably reflecting enhanced protein synthesis. However, electron microscopic studies of myocardium removed from overloaded, dilated hearts fixed at the elevated filling pressures that existed during life have revealed sarcomere lengths averaging 2.2 μm—no longer than those at the apex of the length-active tension curve of normal cardiac muscle. This finding indicates that the depressed contractility of failing heart muscle is *not* due to the disengagement of actin and myosin filaments, as had once been suggested.

Sham

2 weeks post MI

4 weeks post MI

6 weeks post MI

MI

100 μm

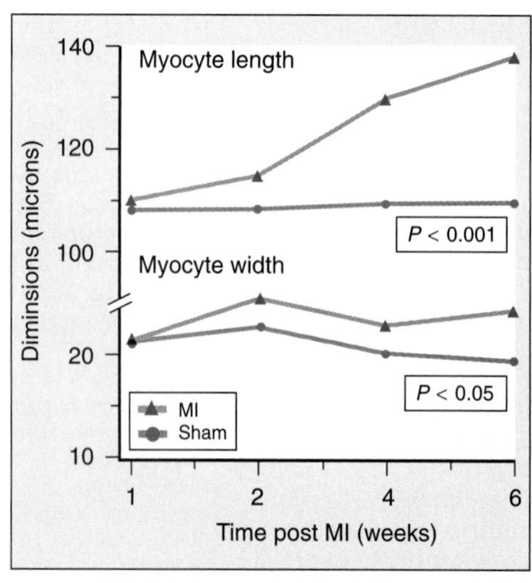

FIGURE 21–7 Cardiac myocyte remodeling in the rat infarct model. Myocyte length and width from rats at 2, 4, and 6 weeks after myocardial infarction are compared with those from a sham-operated animal. Note the predominant increase in myocyte length as the major determinant of the increase in ventricular volume. MI = myocardial infarction. (From Anand IS, Liu D, Chugh SS, et al: Isolated myocyte contractile function is normal in postinfarct remodeled rat heart with systolic dysfunction. Circulation 96:3974, 1997.)

Mechanical Performance of Remodeled Myocardium

Myocardial remodeling provides one of the aforementioned key compensatory mechanisms that permits the ventricle to sustain an increased load (as in hypertension or valvular disease) or to sustain a normal load in the presence of a loss of myocytes (as following myocardial infarction). However, as described later, a ventricle subjected to an abnormally elevated load for a prolonged period may fail to maintain compensation despite the presence of remodeling, and pump failure may ultimately occur. The widely held notion that hypertrophy is a compensatory, albeit insufficient, response to hemodynamic overload has been challenged by exper-

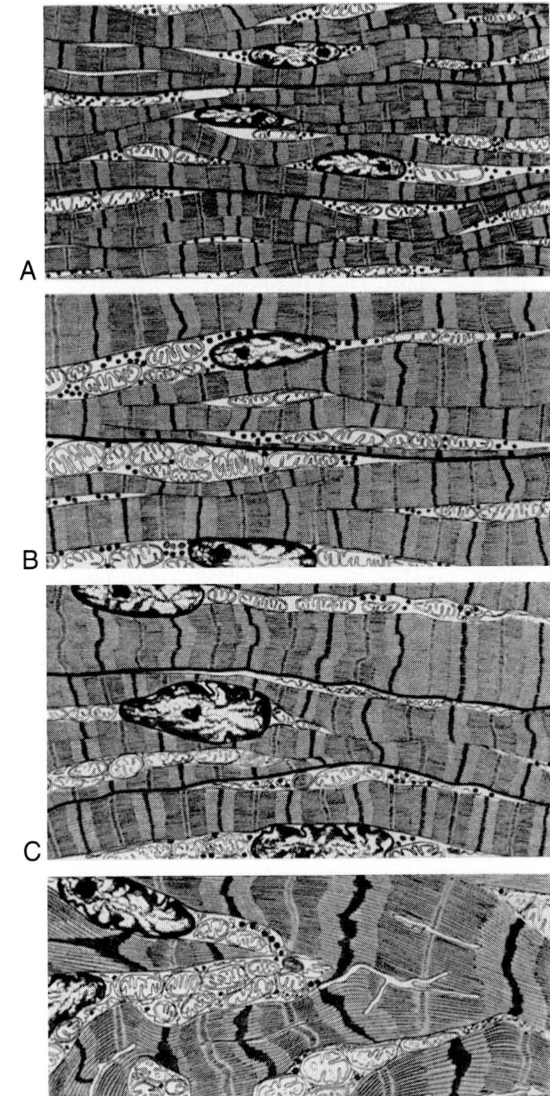

FIGURE 21–8 The early stage of cardiac hypertrophy **(A)** is characterized morphologically by increases in the number of myofibrils and mitochondria as well as enlargement of mitochondria and nuclei. Muscle cells are larger than normal, but cellular organization is largely preserved. At a more advanced stage of hypertrophy **(B)**, preferential increases in the size or number of specific organelles, such as mitochondria, as well as irregular addition of new contractile elements in localized areas of the cell, result in subtle abnormalities of cellular organization and contour. Adjacent cells may vary in their degree of enlargement. Cells subjected to longstanding hypertrophy **(C)** show more obvious disruptions in cellular organization, such as markedly enlarged nuclei with highly lobulated membranes, which displace adjacent myofibrils and cause breakdown of normal Z-band registration. The early preferential increase in mitochondria is supplanted by a predominance by volume of myofibrils. The late stage of hypertrophy **(D)** is characterized by loss of contractile elements with marked disruption of Z bands, severe disruption of the normal parallel arrangement of the sarcomeres, deposition of fibrous tissue, and dilation and increased tortuosity of T tubules. (From Ferrans VJ: Morphology of the heart in hypertrophy. Hosp Pract 18:69, 1983. Copyright 1983, McGraw-Hill Companies, Inc.)

iments in which transgenic mice that overexpress an inhibitor to G_q were exposed to pressure overload caused by aortic constriction.[31] In these mice, the usual hypertrophic response did *not* occur, and yet the progression to failure was delayed, suggesting that the hypertrophic response to a pathological stimulus need not be compensatory. These new ideas require confirmation.

ISOLATED CARDIAC MUSCLE. Cardiac muscle isolated from animals in which the heart had been subjected to a controlled stress has been studied by many investigators. One convenient experimental model of ventricular pressure overload is the cat (or ferret) with pulmonary artery constriction. Papillary muscles are then removed from the right ventricles in which either hypertrophy or overt failure has developed, and the excised muscles are studied in vitro. Both right ventricular hypertrophy and failure reduce the maximum velocity of (unloaded) shortening (V_{max}) of excised muscle below the values observed in muscles obtained from normal cats.[32-34] These changes are more marked in animals in which heart failure has been present than in those with hypertrophy alone (Fig. 21–9). Because the depression of myocardial contractility is evident in vitro and when the muscle's physical and chemical milieu is controlled, it is considered to be *intrinsic* and not the result of any humoral or neural stimuli or abnormal loading conditions that are present in vivo.

In this model, the depression of contractility in hypertrophied myocardium is less marked or even absent when the stress is imposed slowly and when the measurements are made during a stable phase of the ventricular response to overload. The force and rate of force development are also

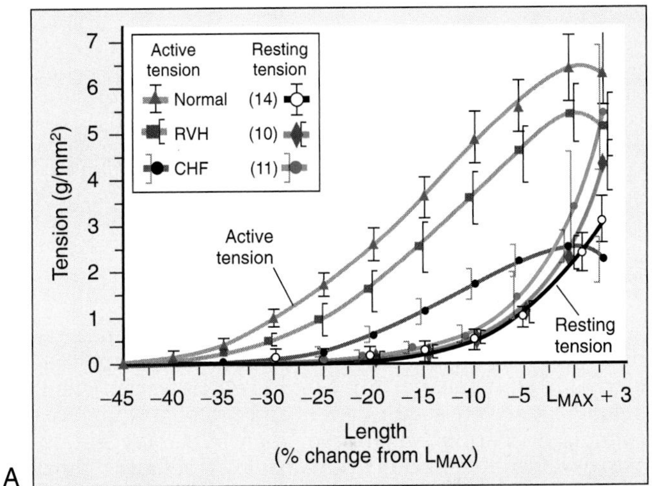

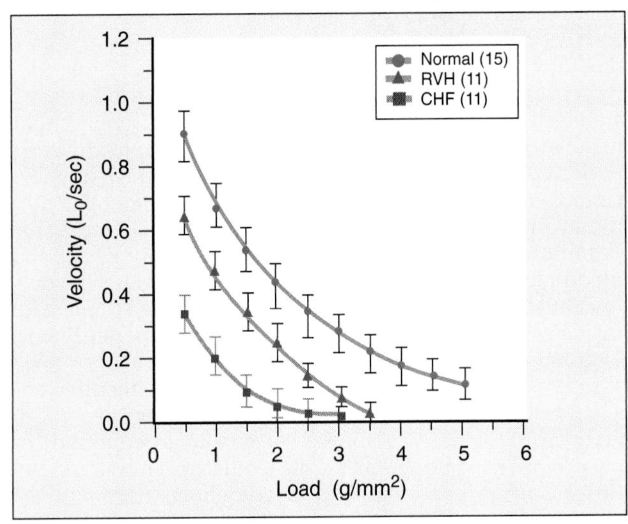

FIGURE 21–9 **A,** Relation between muscle length and tension of papillary muscles from normal (blue), hypertrophied (RVH, brown), and failing (CHF, black) right ventricles. Resting tension and actively developed tension is shown. Tension is corrected for cross-sectional area (g/mm²). Numbers in parentheses = number of animals. **B,** Force-velocity relations of the three groups of cat papillary muscles. Average values ± SEM are given for each point. Velocity has been corrected to muscle lengths per second (L_0/sec). RVH = right ventricular hypertrophy; CHF = congestive heart failure. (From Spann JF Jr, Buccino RA, Sonnenblick EH, Braunwald E: Contractile state of cardiac muscle obtained from cats with experimentally produced ventricular hypertrophy and heart failure. Circ Res 21:341, 1967. Copyright 1967, American Heart Association.)

depressed in isometrically contracting myocardium obtained from hearts with totally different forms of heart failure (e.g., Syrian hamsters with hereditary cardiomyopathy) as well as papillary muscles removed from the left ventricles of patients with heart failure related to chronic valvular disease. Also in the failing heart, the inotropic effects of adrenergic stimulation are reduced.[34,35] Thus, the "contractile reserve" of the failing heart is usually greatly reduced.

INTACT HEART. Changes in performance of the intact heart subjected to abnormal hemodynamic loads are, in general, similar to those in isolated cardiac tissue. Thus, the right ventricles of cats with pulmonary artery constriction exhibit a marked depression paralleling that observed in the isolated papillary muscles removed from these ventricles. When compared with normal values, the active tension developed by the right ventricle at equivalent end-diastolic fiber lengths is markedly reduced in cats with heart failure produced by pressure overload.[36]

Immediately after the imposition of a *volume* overload (e.g., the opening of a large arteriovenous fistula), the contractility of the ventricle, as reflected in the end-systolic stress-circumference relationship, may actually increase, perhaps as a consequence of adrenergic stimulation. However, it then declines while overall hemodynamic performance (i.e., cardiac work) is sustained. Later in the course of a large volume overload, overt clinical heart failure develops, accompanied by increases in left ventricular end-diastolic volume and in the ratio of left ventricular weight to body weight and by depressed indices of left ventricular contractility (see Chap. 19). As the ventricle fails, it moves to the right along a depressed performance (function) curve (see Fig. 21-2) so that it requires an abnormally elevated end-diastolic volume (and often an elevation of end-diastolic pressure as well) to generate a level of tension equal to that achieved by the normal heart at a normal end-diastolic volume.[36]

Transition to Heart Failure

When the ventricle is stressed, cardiac performance is initially maintained by the acute adaptive (compensatory) mechanisms summarized in Table 21–1. However, when the hemodynamic overload is severe and prolonged, myocardial contractility becomes depressed. In an animal model of pressure overload hypertrophy produced by gradually tightening a hydraulic constrictor around the ascending aorta, there was depression of myocardial contractility, as assessed by *load-independent* contractility indices, suggesting that the cardiac dysfunction in this model was due not entirely to insufficient hypertrophy causing afterload mismatch but also to a depression of the myocardium's *intrinsic* contractility.[37] Impaired myocardial contractility has also been observed in patients with hypertension and fully compensatory ventricular hypertrophy, normal myocardial stress, and apparently normal pump function. Such patients have displayed reduction of intramural myocardial shortening, as determined by spatial modulation of magnetization, using magnetic resonance imaging techniques[38]; this reduction indicates a depression of myocardial contractility in the presence of apparently normal loading conditions.

In its mildest form, this depression is manifested by a reduction in the velocity of shortening of unloaded myocardium (V_{max}) (see Fig. 21–9)[32] or by a reduction in the rate of force development during isometric contraction but by little if any reduction in the development of maximal isometric force or in the extent of shortening of afterloaded isotonic contractions. As myocardial contractility becomes further depressed, V_{max} is further reduced, now accompanied by a decline in isometric force development and shortening. At this point, circulatory compensation may still be provided by ventricular remodeling, dilation, and an increase in muscle mass—which tend to maintain systolic tension development while maintaining wall stress at normal levels. Although cardiac output and stroke volume are sustained in the resting state, the ejection fraction at rest as well as the maximal cardiac output that can be attained during stress decline. As contractility falls farther, overt congestive heart failure, reflected in a depression of cardiac output and work or an elevation of ventricular end-diastolic volume and pressure at rest, or both, supervenes.

Molecular Mechanisms of Myocardial Remodeling and Failure

Myocardial remodeling and the transition from compensated hypertrophy to failure of the myocardium involve a complex of events at the molecular and cellular level.[37-41] These events include (1) myocyte growth or hypertrophy; (2) changes in myocyte phenotype resulting from reexpression of fetal gene programs and decreased expression of adult gene programs; (3) alterations in the expression or function, or both, of proteins involved in excitation-contraction coupling and contraction; (4) myocyte death caused by necrosis and apoptosis; (5) changes in the ECM; and (6) abnormalities in energetics (Fig. 21–10). Together, these events result in changes in myocardial structure (e.g., increase in myocardial mass, chamber dilation, greater sphericity) and function (e.g., impaired systolic or diastolic function, or both) that often lead to further pump dysfunction and hemodynamic overload. Stimuli for these changes include mechanical strain on the myocyte, neurohormones (e.g., NE, angiotensin II), inflammatory cytokines (e.g., tumor necrosis factor-alpha [TNF-α]), other peptides and growth factors (e.g., endothelin), and reactive oxygen species (e.g., superoxide, NO).[41-44] These stimuli occur both systemically and in the myocardium in response to circulatory failure and hemodynamic overload. They serve as an important link between pathological factors in the environment and the inter- and intracellular signaling pathways that mediate changes in the structure and function of the cellular elements in the myocardium.[41,45]

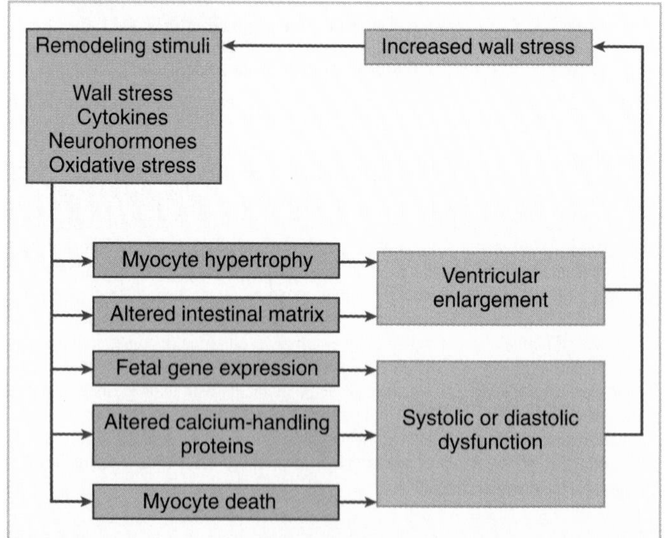

FIGURE 21–10 Overview of the pathophysiology of myocardial remodeling. Remodeling stimuli such as increased mechanical wall stress and neuroendocrine activation lead to a complex of molecular and cellular events, including hypertrophy of cardiac myocytes, changes in gene expression with a reexpression of fetal programs and decreased expression of adult programs, changes in the quantity and nature of the interstitial matrix, and cell death. These events lead to changes in the structure and function of the ventricle, which may result in further pump dysfunction and increased wall stresses, thereby promoting further pathological remodeling. (From Sawyer DB, Colucci WS: Molecular and cellular events in myocardial hypertrophy and failure. *In* Colucci WS [ed]: Heart Failure: Cardiac Function and Dysfunction. Vol 4. Philadelphia, Current Medicine, 1999, p 4.2.)

Myocyte Loss

Impaired myocardial contractile function may reflect a decrease in the number of viable, fully functional myocytes, a decrement in the function of viable myocytes, or a combination of these mechanisms. Myocyte loss may occur by one of two major mechanisms—necrosis or apoptosis. In most instances, myocyte death is caused by a (variable) combination of these two mechanisms.

NECROSIS. Necrosis occurs when myocytes are deprived of oxygen or energy, leading to the loss of cellular membrane integrity, the influx of extracellular fluid, cellular swelling, and the release of proteolytic enzymes that cause cellular disruption. Myocyte necrosis may be localized, as in myocardial infarction, or diffuse, as in dilated cardiomyopathy (see Chap. 59), myocardial damage by toxic agents such as daunorubicin (see Chap. 62), or myocarditis (see Chap. 60). In addition, capillary density and coronary reserve are reduced in remodeled myocardium and may result in diffuse ischemia, which is most severe in the subendocardium. Thus, a diminished response of endocardial blood flow to adenosine and exercise-induced vasodilation has been demonstrated in dogs with pressure overload hypertrophy. This diminished response is caused in part by hypertrophy and in part by an exercise-induced increase in left ventricular subendocardial wall stress. The reduced subendocardial perfusion in turn may cause subendocardial ischemic cell death and replacement fibrosis, which impair both systolic and diastolic function, accelerating the development of heart failure (see Chap. 44)

APOPTOSIS (see Chap. 71). In contrast to necrosis, apoptosis (programmed cell death) is an energy-dependent process in which a specific genetic program leads to the activation of a molecular cascade that causes the degradation of nuclear deoxyribonucleic acid (DNA) (Fig. 21–11). Also in contrast to necrosis, apoptosis is marked by the involution of the myocyte, resulting in phagocytosis by neighboring cells (Fig. 21–12).[46] Apoptosis is a common cellular mechanism during organogenesis and in adult cells that have rapid turnover, such as blood cells and gut epithelium. Because cardiac myocytes were uniformly considered to be terminally differentiated, it was not generally believed that they would undergo apoptosis. However, there have now been several reports demonstrating the presence of apoptotic myocytes in failing human myocardium (Fig. 21–13)[46] as well as in models of myocardial failure, hemodynamic overload, and myocardial infarction.[47,48]

Several factors known to be present or increased in the failing myocardium have been shown to cause apoptosis of

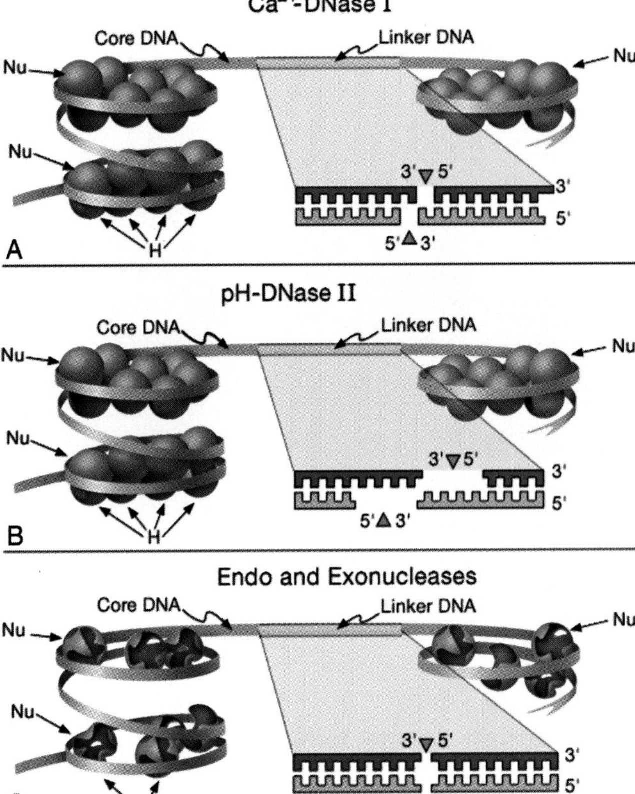

FIGURE 21–12 Schematic representation of chromatin structure and DNA damage associated with apoptosis (**A** and **B**) and necrosis (**C**). Panels **A** to **C** each illustrate three nucleosomes (Nu) connected by linker DNA. Each nucleosome consists of a histone (H) core surrounded by two full turns of double-stranded DNA (Core DNA). A sequence of nucleotides present in the linker DNA is shown in the lower part of **A** and **B.** A similar sequence of nucleotides pertaining to the linker or core DNA is depicted in the lower part of **C. A,** DNA damage mediated by activation of Ca^{2+}-dependent DNase I characterized by staggered ends in the DNA with single-base 3′ overhangs (solid arrows in the sequence of the nucleotides). This type of DNA injury is identified by a polymerase chain reaction (PCR)–generated *Taq* polymerase probe, which processes complementary structures; this probe interacts only with damaged DNA exhibiting single-base 3′ overhangs. **B,** DNA damage mediated by activation of pH-dependent DNase II characterized by staggered ends in the DNA with one or more, up to four, base 3′ overhangs (solid arrows in the sequence of nucleotides). This type of DNA injury is identified by the terminal deoxynucleotidyl transferase (TdT) assay that links labeled nucleotides to 3′ overhangs, and the generated sequence can be visualized by fluorescence. **C,** DNA damage associated with cell necrosis. Loss of plasma membrane integrity and the release of lysosomal proteases lead to degradation of histones in the nucleosomes (Nu), which results in the loss of DNA protection and its exposure to endonucleases and exonucleases. Endonucleases produce double-strand cleavage of the DNA with recessed 3′ ends or 3′ overhangs, whereas exonucleases remove terminal nucleotides leading to a form of damage with blunt DNA ends (solid arrows in the sequence of nucleotides). This type of DNA injury is identified by a PCR-generated *Pfu* polymerase probe, which possesses complementary structures; this probe interacts only with damaged DNA exhibiting blunt ends. (From Anversa P: Myocyte apoptosis in the development of heart failure. *In* Braunwald E [ed]: Harrison's Advances in Cardiology. New York, McGraw Hill, 2003, pp 446-450.)

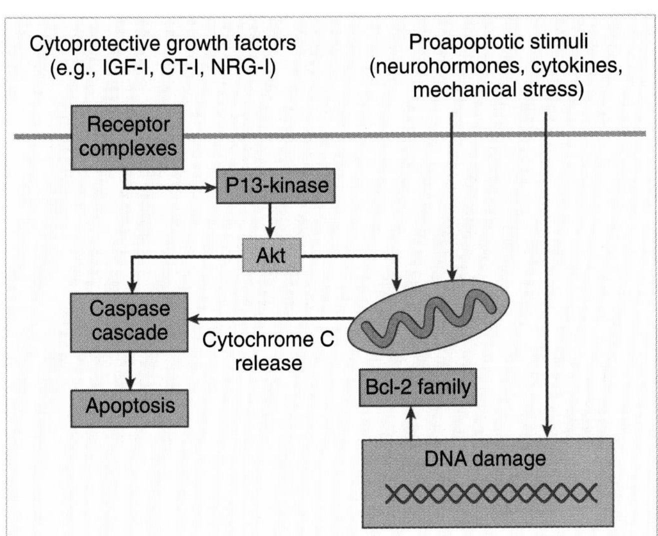

FIGURE 21–11 Regulation of myocyte survival in heart failure. The proapoptotic effects of chronic neurohormonal, inflammatory cytokine, mechanical stress, and other stimuli are counterbalanced by prosurvival pathways. The fate of any single myocyte is a function of the *net* effect of these influences. Antiapoptotic influences in the myocardium are mediated in part by cytoprotective growth factors, including insulin-like growth factor-1 (IGF-1), cardiotrophin-1 (CT-1), and neuregulin-1 (NRG-1), that suppress the apoptotic cascade at multiple levels at least in part through the activation of phosphoinositol-3kinase and Akt as depicted. (From Sawyer DB, Colucci WS: Molecular and cellular events in myocardial hypertrophy and failure. *In* Colucci WS [ed]: Atlas of Heart Failure: Cardiac Function and Dysfunction. 3d ed. Philadelphia, Current Medicine, 2002.)

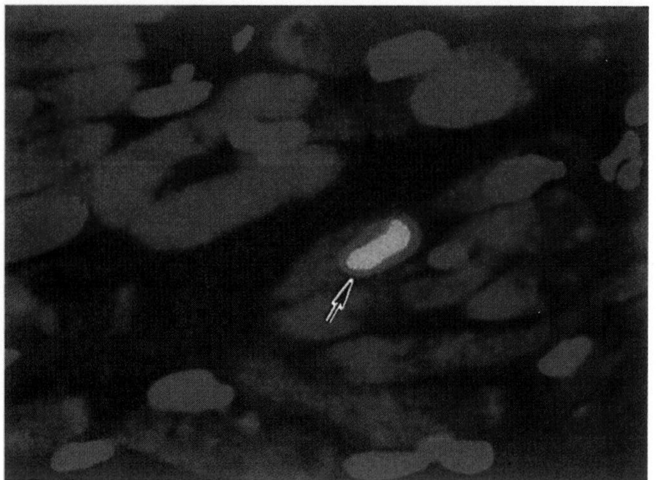

FIGURE 21–13 Human heart affected by end-stage ischemic cardiomyopathy. Confocal image illustrating an apoptotic myocyte by yellow fluorescence (arrow). The myocyte nucleus shows positive staining for terminal deoxynucleotidyl transferase assay. Red fluorescence of nuclei corresponds to propidium iodide staining, and red fluorescence of the myocyte cytoplasm corresponds to sarcomeric actin antibody labeling. Confocal microscopy, 800×. (From Anversa P: Myocyte apoptosis in the development of heart failure. *In* Braunwald E [ed]: Harrison's Advances in Cardiology. New York, McGraw Hill, 2003, pp 446-450.)

cardiac myocytes in vitro, including catecholamines acting through beta-adrenergic receptors,[49,50] angiotensin II,[51] reactive oxygen species (Fig. 21–14),[52] NO,[53] inflammatory cytokines, and mechanical strain.[54] Although the role of apoptosis in the transition to heart failure is not known, it appears likely that it represents an important cause of cell death in the failing heart.[9] Because both angiotensin II and catecholamines promote apoptosis, the therapeutic success of angiotensin-converting enzyme (ACE) inhibitors and beta-adrenergic antagonists in the treatment of heart failure suggests that this may be an important mechanism for myocardial failure.

Dropout of individual myocytes has also been observed in the senescent rat and human heart.[55] Olivetti and colleagues reported a loss of an average of 38 million nuclei per year in aging persons without cardiovascular disease. This loss in myocyte number was accompanied by a reciprocal increase in myocyte cell volume per nucleus, thereby preserving ventricular wall thickness.[56] This process, which appears to reflect myocyte death by both necrosis and apoptosis, may contribute to cardiac dysfunction and, when there is an additional stress such as hypertension, to the development of heart failure in elderly persons.

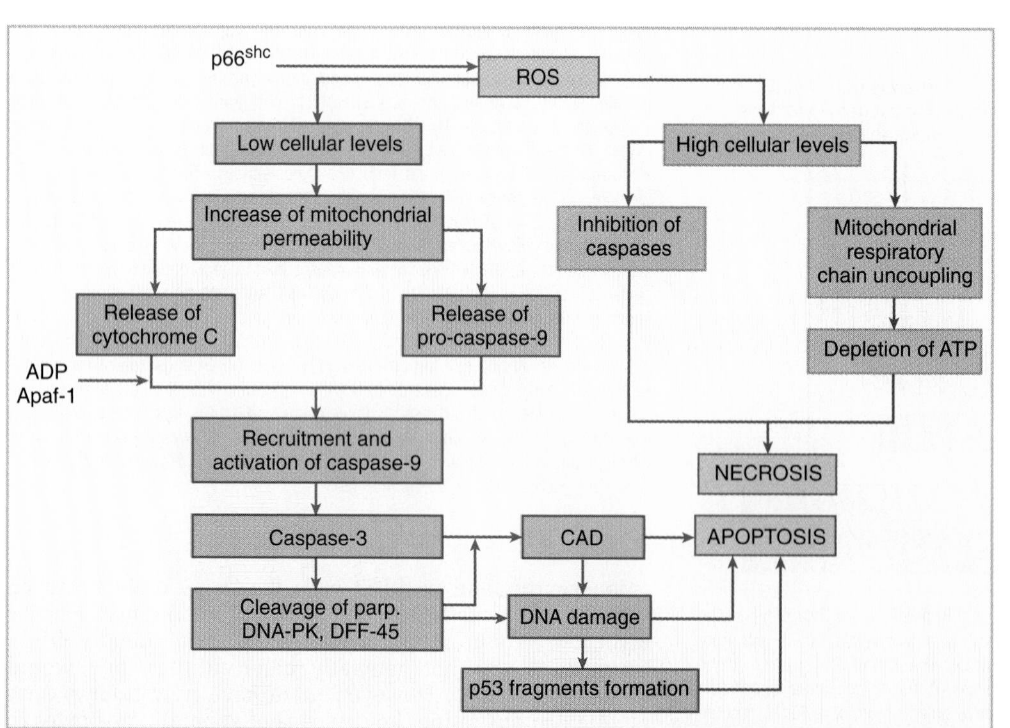

FIGURE 21–14 Scheme illustrating the effects of different levels of reactive oxygen species (ROS) on the activation of cell apoptosis and necrosis. Apaf-1 = apoptotic protease activating factor; ADP = adenosine diphosphate; ATP = adenosine triphosphate; CAD = caspase-activated deoxyribonuclease; DFF-45 = DNA fragmentation factor; DNA-PK = DNA-dependent protein kinase; parp = poly(ADP-ribose) polymerase. (From Anversa P: Myocardial basis for heart failure. Role of cell death. *In* Mann DL [ed]: Heart Failure: A Companion to Braunwald's Heart Disease. Philadelphia, Elsevier, 2004.)

Alterations in Excitation-Contraction Coupling (see Chap. 20)

In addition to reducing the absolute number of myocytes, as already described, hemodynamic overload may cause a decrease in the *intrinsic* contractility of individual myocytes.[2] Several functional abnormalities involving excitation-contraction coupling, contractile proteins, and energetics have been identified in hypertrophied and failing myocardium.

Role of Calcium in Excitation-Contraction Coupling

Ca^{2+} plays a central role in the regulation of myocardial contraction and relaxation,[2,3,9,34,39] and there is increasing evidence that disturbances in Ca^{2+} handling play a central role in the disturbed contractile function in myocardial failure. Hypocalcemia, secondary to hypoparathyroidism and to a variety of other conditions, can cause heart failure that is responsive to the infusion of calcium. Elevation of serum ionized Ca^{2+} has been shown to augment contractility in patients with renal failure undergoing dialysis and in patients with severe heart failure secondary to cardiomyopathy who have downregulation of beta-adrenergic receptors.

Myocardium obtained at the time of cardiac transplantation from patients with end-stage heart failure exhibits abnormal prolongation of the action potential and developed force and impaired relaxation.[34] Observations using the Ca^{2+} indicator aequorin in myocardium have shown that these alterations in electrical and contractile properties are associated with a prolonged elevation of the intracellular Ca^{2+} transient during relaxation. Likewise, in myocytes obtained from patients with end-stage heart failure, the action potential is prolonged. The intracellular Ca^{2+} transient, as assessed by the fluorescent indicator fura-2, demonstrates a blunted rise with depolarization, reflecting slower delivery of Ca^{2+} to the contractile apparatus (causing slower activation) and a slowed rate of fall during repolarization (causing slowed relaxation) (Fig. 21–15).[57] These two abnormalities could explain both systolic and diastolic dysfunction.

Additional evidence of abnormal myocardial Ca^{2+} handling is provided by the observation that there is a reduction in the amount of tension-independent heat produced in myocardium from patients with heart failure.[58] Tension-independent heat, which is believed to reflect the energy expended for Ca^{2+} transport, can be used to estimate the amount of Ca^{2+} cycled per heartbeat. With this approach, it was shown that Ca^{2+} cycling is reduced by approximately 50 percent in failing human myocardium.[58]

FORCE-FREQUENCY RELATIONSHIP. In nonfailing myocardium, the force of contraction and rate of tension development rise with increased stimulation frequency, the so-called *positive force-frequency relationship* (see Chap. 19). However, there is evidence of an abnormal (negative) force-frequency relationship in failing human myocardium.[2] The mechanism responsible for this response appears to be impaired reuptake of calcium into the SR because of a decrease in Ca^{2+} adenosine triphosphatase (ATPase) (SERCA2) activity in failing myocardium.[34,39] Excitation-contraction coupling can also be assessed by examination of the force-frequency response. In normal myocardium, contractile force increases with increasing rates of stimulation, whereas in myocardium obtained from patients with end-stage heart failure the force-frequency response is markedly attenuated.[2,33] A similar phenomenon is observed in intact patients with heart failure studied at the time of catheterization. In patients with normal ventricular function, left ventricular contractility (as measured by +dP/dt or the end-systolic pressure-volume ratio) increases progressively as heart rate is increased by atrial pacing. By comparison, in patients with severe heart failure there is little or no increase in either contractile index. The normal force-frequency relationship depends on the cycling of Ca^{2+} between the SR and cytoplasm with each beat, an event that is accomplished by several enzymes and channels located in the sarcolemma, and SR (see Chap. 19). The expression or function, or both, of a number of these proteins may be altered in hypertrophied and failing myocardium,[59,60] leading to dysfunction of otherwise viable myocytes. Observations on the altered force-frequency relation in failing heart muscle are consistent with the suggestion that the quantity of Ca^{2+} released from the SR is reduced at more rapid heart rates.[61] There is evidence that Ca^{2+} release from the SR by the inward Ca^{2+} current during depolarization is reduced.

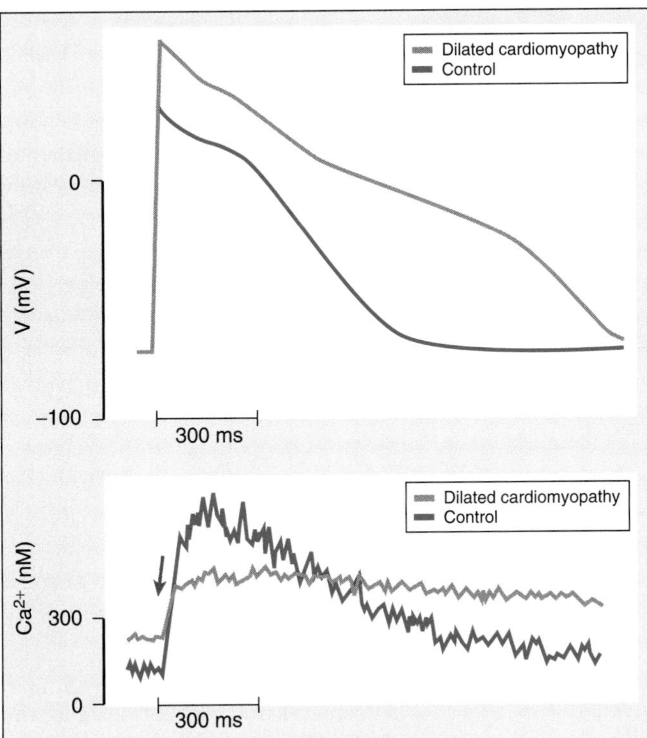

FIGURE 21–15 Abnormal action potential and intracellular calcium transient in failing cardiac myocytes. **Top,** The action potential recorded in a myocyte isolated from the heart of a patient with dilated cardiomyopathy is markedly prolonged compared with that in a myocyte from a normal heart (control). Such abnormalities could contribute to both the generation of arrhythmias and the abnormal diastolic relaxation. **Bottom,** The intracellular calcium transient measured with the fluorescent calcium indicator fura-2 is also markedly abnormal in myocytes isolated from the myocardium of patients with dilated cardiomyopathy. Compared with a normal myocyte (control), the myocyte from a patient with dilated cardiomyopathy shows an attenuated rise with depolarization (arrow) and a markedly delayed return to baseline. These abnormalities reflect the altered expression or function of key calcium-handling proteins (e.g., Ca^{2+}-adenosine triphosphatase) and probably contribute to the abnormal action potential in the top illustration. (Modified from Beuckelmann DJ, Nabauer M, Erdmann E: Intracellular calcium handling in isolated ventricular myocytes from patients with terminal heart failure. Circulation 85:1046, 1992. Copyright 1992, American Heart Association.)

SARCOPLASMIC RETICULUM Ca^{2+}-ATPASE AND PHOSPHOLAMBAN. A number of alterations in the SR in the failing heart have been described (Table 21–2). Ca^{2+} reuptake by the SR is mediated primarily by SERCA2. The activity of SERCA2 is inhibited by the associated protein phospholamban, and this inhibition is relieved by cyclic adenosine monophosphate (AMP)–mediated (e.g., by beta-adrenergic receptor stimulation) phosphorylation of phospholamban, thereby resulting in increased Ca^{2+} reuptake into the SR and the acceleration of diastolic relaxation (see Fig. 19–10). The reuptake of Ca^{2+} by the SR is equally important for normal systolic function, which requires that ample SR Ca^{2+} be available for release during systole to mediate contraction.

Several (but not all) reports indicate that the levels of SERCA2 messenger ribonucleic acid (mRNA) and protein are reduced in myocardium obtained from patients with end-stage heart failure as well as in the animal model of tachycardia-induced heart failure.[60] The decrease in SERCA2, which is part of an "adult" gene program in cardiac muscle, correlates inversely with the reexpression of fetal genes such as atrial natriuretic peptide (ANP) (Fig. 21–16). This shift in SERCA2 expression was associated with a corresponding

TABLE 21–2 Sarcoplasmic Reticulum Alterations in the Failing Heart

Protein	Change in Human Heart Failure
Sarcoplasmic Reticulum	
Calcium pump ATPase (SERCA)	Normal or decreased
Phospholamban	Normal or decreased
Calcium release channel (ryanodine receptor)	Normal or decreased
Calsequestrin	Normal
Calreticulin	Normal
Plasma Membrane	
L-type calcium channels	?Increased channel opening
Sodium/calcium exchanger	Increased
Sodium pump	Reexpression of fetal isoforms

ATPase = adenosine triphosphatase.

From Katz AM: Heart Failure. Philadelphia, Lippincott Williams & Wilkins, 2000.

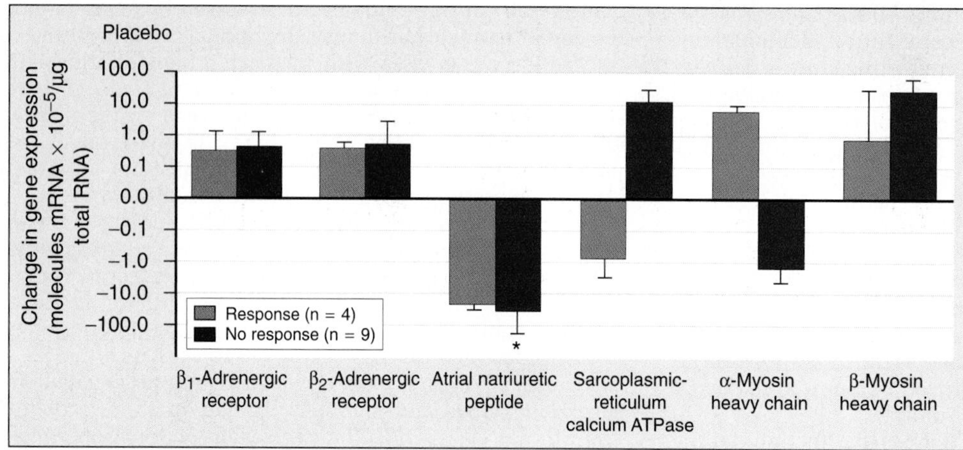

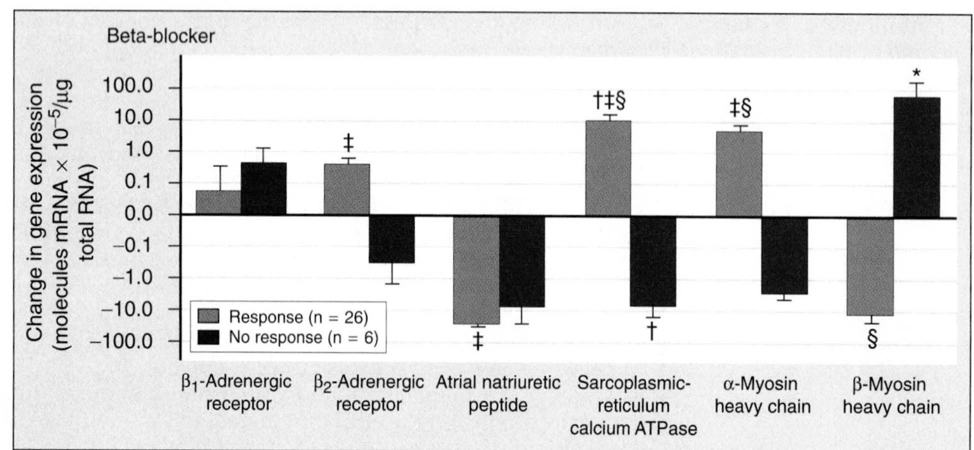

FIGURE 21–16 Changes in myocardial messenger RNA (mRNA) expression and beta-adrenergic receptor protein levels. **A** and **B,** Changes between baseline and the end of the 6-month study in the abundance of myocardial mRNA for six contractility-regulating or hypertrophy-regulating proteins in patients who received placebo or a beta blocker. The changes in patients who had an improvement in left ventricular ejection fraction (a "response," defined as an increase by at least five ejection fraction [EF] units) were compared with the changes in patients who did not have such a response. Gene expression is shown as molecules of mRNA per microgram of total RNA on a logarithmic scale; The asterisk indicates $p < 0.10$ for the change between the baseline value and the value measured at 6 months by the paired t-test, the daggers $p < 0.05$ for the comparison with the placebo group by the test for interaction, the double daggers $p < 0.05$ for the change between the baseline value and the value measured at 6 months by the paired t-test, and the section marks $p < 0.05$ for the comparison with patients who did not have a response. Each panel shows results for patients with complete data for the indicated mRNA and receptor protein measurements. (From Lowes BD, Gilbert EM, Abraham WT, et al: Myocardial gene expression in dilated cardiomyopathy treated with beta blocking agents. N Engl J Med 346:1357, 2002.)

reduction in SR Ca^{2+} reuptake in some[62-64] (but not all) studies of human myocardium from patients with severe failure. Furthermore, the decreases in SERCA2 protein and Ca^{2+}-ATPase activity have been shown to correlate inversely with the force-frequency relationship,[63] suggesting that reduced expression of SERCA2 contributes to intrinsic myocyte dysfunction. In vitro, mechanical strain and several agonists such as NE and angiotensin II downregulate the expression of SERCA2 in cardiac myocytes. It has been proposed that the reduced activity of SERCA2 alters Ca^{2+} release from the SR; this alteration impairs both contraction and relaxation and is responsible for the transition from compensation to heart failure.[65]

Because phospholamban activity inhibits SERCA2, the net activity of SERCA2 depends on the ratio of SERCA2 to phospholamban.[66] The expression of phospholamban is decreased in failing human myocardium,[62] as is its phosphorylation,[2,3,9] and this may interfere with SR function. Viral expression vectors have been used to express SERCA2 and phospholamban in cultured cardiac myocytes.[67] SERCA2 has also been expressed in transgenic mice[68] and in rat hearts after direct injection of an adenovirus carrying the gene.[69] These or similar approaches might allow the use of SERCA2 or inhibitors of phospholamban to augment myocyte function in patients. It has been suggested that induced changes in the ratio of SERCA2 to its inhibitor phospholamban can alter Ca^{2+} handling by the failing heart.

Na^+/Ca^{2+} EXCHANGER. The Na^+/Ca^{2+} exchanger in the cell membrane accounts for approximately 20 percent of the removal of Ca^{2+} from the cytoplasm during diastole. Abnormalities in Na^+/Ca^{2+} exchange have been demonstrated in heart failure.[2,3,9] The mRNA and protein levels of the Na^+/Ca^{2+} exchanger were found to be increased in myocardium obtained from patients with heart failure related to both ischemic and idiopathic dilated cardiomyopathy and correlated inversely with the decrease in SERCA2 mRNA levels.[69] This augmentation in Na^+/Ca^{2+} exchange activity might be a compensatory response to the reduction in Ca^{2+} reuptake caused by a decrease in SERCA2. In animals with experimental heart failure, impaired cytosolic Ca^{2+} removal caused by reduced SERCA2 was partially compensated for by an increase in the Na^+/Ca^{2+} exchanger.[69,70] Although this compensation would facilitate diastolic Ca^{2+} removal, it might do so at the expense of increased arrhythmogenicity because Ca^{2+} efflux by this mechanism is associated with an influx of Na^+ that can prolong depolarization and cause afterdepolarizations.

THE Ca^{2+} RELEASE CHANNEL. The Ca^{2+} release channel (CRC), located on the SR, mediates the release of Ca^{2+} from the SR into the myoplasm during systole and is therefore critical to the activation of the contractile elements of the myocyte. Some[71] (but not all[72]) studies of failing human myocardium have shown decreases in the mRNA level for the CRC. In addition, in myocardium from patients with heart failure the CRC is hyperphosphorylated by protein kinase A, resulting in a high rate of Ca^{2+} "leakage" from the SR. This leakage can reduce the SR Ca^{2+} content, release, and net uptake,[2,73-75] and treatment with beta blockers has been shown to restore CRC function toward normal[76]

VOLTAGE-DEPENDENT Ca^{2+} CHANNEL. The mRNA and protein levels of the voltage-dependent Ca^{2+} channel have also been shown to be decreased in failing human myocardium obtained from patients with both ischemic heart disease and dilated cardiomyopathy, which may contribute to a depressed calcium transient[77] leading to impaired excitation-contraction coupling.

CALSEQUESTRIN. This is the major protein in the SR that binds Ca^{2+} and thereby serves a storage function. Several studies have found calsequestrin mRNA levels to be unchanged in failing human myocardium.

Alterations in the Contractile Apparatus

Patients with aortic stenosis without heart failure exhibit a normal fraction of myofibrils per cell, whereas those with left ventricular failure show a significant reduction in cell volume occupied by myofibrils, suggesting that this reduction in the quantity of the contractile machinery may play a role in the development of cardiac decompensation. In end-stage heart failure in the human, electron microscopic observations likewise show a reduction of ventricular myofibrillar protein (Table 21–3).

Reduction of Myosin Adenosine Triphosphatase Activity

Considerable data suggest that qualitative, as well as quantitative, alterations of contractile proteins occur in heart failure. First, the finding that the reduced velocity of contraction of failing myocardium occurs in chemically skinned ventricular fibers suggests that this change reflects intrinsic alterations in the contractile apparatus. Early studies showed that the activity of myofibrillar ATPase was reduced in the hearts of patients who died of heart failure.[9,78] Furthermore, reductions in the activities of myofibrillar ATPase, actomyosin ATPase, or myosin ATPase have been demonstrated in several animal models of heart failure. These depressions of enzymatic activity could occur if an altered subunit of the myosin molecule (i.e., the portion of the molecule responsible for the ATPase activity) were produced in the overloaded heart and reduced contractility by lowering the rate of interaction between actin and myosin filaments. A reduction in the Mg^{2+}-ATPase activity (which expresses the response of myofibrils to Ca^{2+}) has been demonstrated in myofibrils obtained from patients with end-stage heart failure at the time of transplantation and in less sick patients undergoing valve replacement.[79]

MYOSIN ISOFORM CHANGES. Animal studies have indicated that when the adult heart hypertrophies, fetal and neonatal forms of contractile proteins (termed isoforms) and other proteins (such as ANP) reappear, signifying reexpression of the genes for these fetal and neonatal isoforms.[80] Thus, hemodynamic overload leads to enhanced overall protein synthesis[9] and alters the proteins qualitatively as well (i.e., it leads to the synthesis of protein isoforms that were present during fetal and neonatal life when protein synthesis in the heart was also rapid).

TABLE 21–3 Contractile Protein Alterations in the Failing Heart

Protein	Experimental Heart Failure	Human Heart Failure
Myosin heavy chain	Reversion to fetal phenotype	Reversion to fetal phenotype
Myosin light chains	Reversion to fetal phenotype	Reversion to fetal phenotype
Actin	Reversion to fetal phenotype	No change
Troponin I	Reversion to fetal phenotype	Reversion to fetal phenotype
Troponin T	Reversion to fetal phenotype	Reversion to fetal phenotype
Troponin C	No change	No change
Tropomyosin	No change	No change

From Katz AM: Heart Failure. Philadelphia, Lippincott Williams & Wilkins, 2000.

Altered isoforms of cardiac proteins may arise from the expression of different members of a multigene family or from the assembly of the same gene in a different pattern. In rodents the predominant myosin heavy chain (MHC) is the "fast" V_1 isoform (high ATPase activity, encoded by the alpha-MHC gene). With pressure-induced hypertrophy or myocardial failure after myocardial infarction in the rat, there is reexpression of the "slow" V_3 isoform (low ATPase activity, encoded by the beta-MHC gene) and deinduction of the V_1 isoform.[80] A shift in MHC isoforms would provide an attractive explanation for the reduction in myofibrillar ATPase activity observed in failing human myocardium. However, the predominant MHC isoform in humans is the slower V_3 isoform (encoded by the beta-MHC gene) and the V_1 isoform (encoded by the alpha-MHC mRNA) has been difficult to detect, making it appear unlikely that a shift in myosin isoforms is responsible for the observed decrease in myosin ATPase activity in failing human myocardium. However, the use of more refined methodology has demonstrated that alpha-MHC accounts for about 33 percent of MHC mRNA in normal human myocardium and is markedly reduced to about 2 percent in failing myocardium.[81,82] It remains to be determined whether the decrease in alpha-MHC mRNA translates into a comparable decrease in the ratio of the beta- to alpha-MHC protein isoforms and, thus, a decrease in ATPase activity.

Bristow and colleagues measured the expression of mRNA for alpha- and beta-MHC in right ventricular biopsy specimens from patients with idiopathic dilated cardiomyopathy at 6-month intervals.[80,83] In patients with an improvement in left ventricular function there were reciprocal changes in the levels of alpha-MHC (increase) and beta-MHC (decrease) mRNA but no consistent changes in the mRNA levels for SERCA2, the $beta_1$- or $beta_2$-adrenergic receptors, or ANP. They further showed that patients who had a good hemodynamic response to beta blocker therapy had a similar increase in the alpha-/beta-MHC ratio. These observations support the thesis that a decrease in the expression of alpha-MHC plays a significant role in the pathophysiology of dilated cardiomyopathy.

ALTERED REGULATORY PROTEINS. Another possible cause of a decrease in cardiac contractile function is an alteration in the expression or activity, or both, of regulatory proteins. In animals with experimental heart failure, there are changes in the myosin light chain and the troponin-tropomyosin complex.[84] Changes in myosin light chain isoforms have been observed in the atria and ventricles of patients whose hearts have been subjected to mechanical overload; and the expression of troponin T, a component of the troponin complex that regulates the interaction of myosin and actin, was found to be altered in failing human myocardium. In normal myocardium, troponin T is expressed as a single isoform (T_1), which accounts for approximately 98 percent of the troponin T. In myocardium from patients with end-stage heart failure, a second isoform (T_2) was found to be expressed at increased levels, and its level of expression was related to the severity of heart failure.[85]

Mice with deletion of the troponin I gene are born normally but express a fetal isoform of troponin that takes the place of the absent adult isoform. Over time, the expression of the fetal isoform decreases and the mice develop lethal heart failure.[86] Likewise, the transgenic overexpression of a mutant tropomyosin results in increased calcium sensitivity and decreased rate of relaxation.[87] Although the clinical significance of changes in the expression of troponin and other regulatory proteins remains to be determined, these observations suggest that important functional changes in contractile proteins could be due to changes in regulatory proteins and need not reflect alterations in the contractile proteins themselves.[88]

Alterations in the Cardiac Matrix

The structural properties of the ventricle are determined not only by its myocytes but also by the interstitial connective tissue, which is rich in type I and type III fibrillar collagen (Fig. 21–17).[89,90] The latter provides struts along which the myocytes are aligned. Branches of collagen fibers course at right angles to connect and align muscle bundles. A depletion of these struts may lead to chamber dilation, and an excess may interfere with ventricular relaxation and filling. Thus, the quantity and type of ECM can have profound effects on the diastolic properties of the myocardium by affecting its elasticity and physical disposition.[90,91]

REGULATION OF INTERSTITIAL COLLAGEN. The quantity and nature of the collagen in the ECM are determined by the balance between synthesis and degradation. The latter is regulated by the opposing actions of matrix metalloproteinases (MMPs), a family of enzymes that degrade matrix proteins, and tissue inhibitors of metalloproteinases (TIMPs), a family of enzymes that inhibit the activity of MMPs (Fig. 21–18).[91] The ECM is a dynamic system. It changes with and contributes to ventricular remodeling in the presence of pressure and volume overload, myocardial infarction, and cardiomyopathy (Table 21–4).[89]

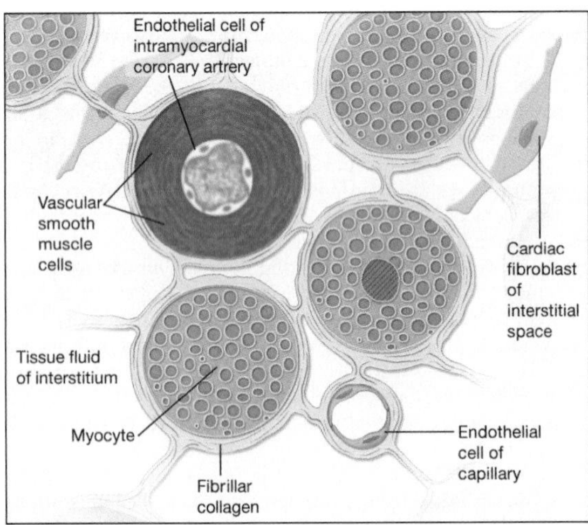

FIGURE 21–17 Myocyte and nonmyocyte constituents of the heart. Although myocytes are the major components of the heart on the basis of mass, they represent only a minority of the cells on the basis of number. Nonmyocyte cellular constituents of the myocardium include fibroblasts, smooth muscle cells, and endothelial cells. Myocytes and nonmyocytes are interconnected by a complex of connective tissue and extracellular matrix. Components of the extracellular matrix include collagens, proteoglycans (such as fibronectin), several peptide growth factors, and proteases (such as plasminogen activators). There is increasing appreciation that by regulating the nature and quantity of the extracellular matrix, nonmyocytes in the heart play an important role in determining the response of the myocardium to pathologic stimuli, such as hemodynamic overload. (From Colucci WS [ed]: Atlas of Heart Failure: Cardiac Function and Dysfunction. 3rd ed. Philadelphia, Current Medicine, 2002, p 7.7. Adapted from Weber KT, Brilla CG: Pathological hypertrophy and cardiac interstitium. Fibrosis and renin-angiotensin-aldosterone system. Circulation 83:1849, 1991.)

COLLAGEN STRUT DEPLETION. In myocardium from humans and animal models of systolic failure, ultrastructural observations have shown a depletion of the fibrillar collagen struts that help to maintain the alignment of myocytes. It has been proposed that *depletion* of the collagen struts may contribute to chamber dilation by allowing "slippage" of myocytes.[91] This thesis is consistent with the observation that the activity of MMPs is increased in myocardium obtained from patients with end-stage heart failure[92] and in animal models of heart failure.[93] Likewise, the activity of TIMPs is decreased in myocardium from patients with end-stage heart failure.[94] A role for MMPs is supported by the demonstration that an MMP inhibitor partially protected against the loss of collagen struts in an animal model of heart failure.[95] It has been shown that post-myocardial infarction remodeling is exacerbated in mice deficient in TIMP-1,[96] whereas it is ameliorated in mice with the targeted deletion of MMP9.[97] In patients with dilated cardiomyopathy, reduced fibrillar collagen and its cross-linking have been reported.

INTERSTITIAL MATRIX ACCUMULATION. On the other hand, in experimentally induced chronic pressure overload hypertrophy, as well as in patients with hypertension, there is an *increase* in the quantity of interstitial collagen, which may contribute to the characteristic abnormalities of diastolic function.[91] The spontaneously hypertensive rat develops progressive myocardial hypertrophy and failure with age. Papillary muscles from these animals have increased passive stiffness that is associated with increased left ventricular collagen concentration, interstitial fibrosis,[98] and expression of mRNAs for collagen and transforming growth factor-alpha (TGF-α).[99] Treatment with an ACE inhibitor prevented the increases in muscle stiffness, interstitial fibrosis, and the induction of collagen and TGF-α mRNAs.[100] Thus, it seems likely that pathways leading to increased collagen accumulation are involved in the pathogenesis of diastolic dysfunction.

Myocardial Energetics in Heart Failure

The heart is an aerobic organ requiring substantial energy. Energy is required for myofibrillar contraction and relaxation, the uptake (against a concentration gradient) of Ca^{2+} into the SR, and the restoration of ion concentrations between the

TABLE 21–4 Extracellular Myocardial Remodeling Events During the Progression of Heart Failure: A Summary of Potential Global Extracellular Matrix Changes in the Left Ventricular Remodeling Process

Disease Process	Myocardial Infarction	Hypertrophy	Cardiomyopathy
Early adaptive phase	ECM proteolysis in MI region Activation of MMPs Rapid ECM turnover MI scar formation	ECM turnover to facilitate myocyte growth ECM biosynthesis rates favor accumulation Diminished MMP activity	Biophysical stress induces MMPs Proteolysis of normal ECM
Compensatory phase	Scar maturation ECM accumulation in viable myocardium Persistent ECM turnover in MI border zone	ECM reaches steady state Continued downregulation of MMPs	Induction of "MMP portfolio" and continued ECM turnover Diminished ECM support of myocytes
Transition to failure	Continued ECM proteolysis in MI border and infarct expansion LV wall remodeling and dilation Increased MMPs and acceleration of LV remodeling and dilation	Increased myocardial stiffness due to ECM accumulation and impairment of diastolic function	Increased MMP activation and reduced inhibitory control Accelerated proteolysis of normal ECM structure and loss of structural support LV dilation and diminished transduction of myocyte shortening

ECM = extracellular matrix; LV = left ventricular; MI = myocardial infarction; MMP = matrix metalloproteinase.
From Gunasinghe SK, Spinale FG: Myocardial basis for heart failure. *In* Mann DL (ed): Heart Failure. Philadelphia, Elsevier, 2004, p 66.

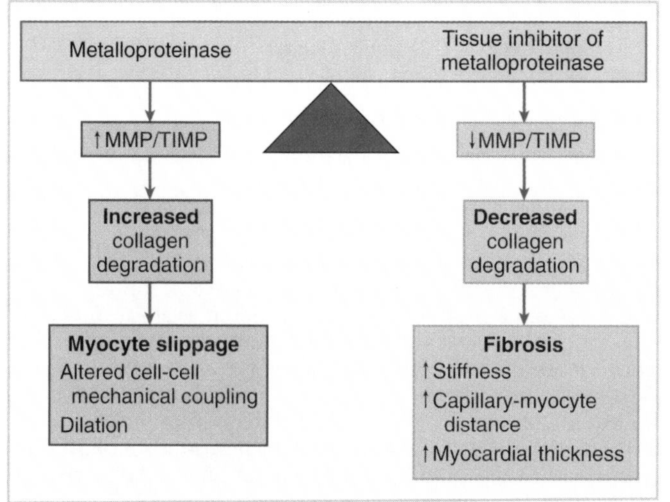

FIGURE 21–18 The regulation of extracellular matrix degradation is determined by the balance between the activity of matrix metalloproteinases (MMPs) and their tissue inhibitors (TIMPs). Both an increase in MMP activity and a decrease in TIMP activity have been observed in failing myocardium from patients. Theoretically, such an increase in the MMP/TIMP ratio could contribute to depletion of the fibrillar collagen struts that tether myocytes together and might thus contribute to chamber dilation. Conversely, an increase in extracellular matrix accumulation, which might occur as the result of a decrease in the MMP/TIMP ratio or an increase in matrix synthesis, could contribute to chamber stiffness and abnormal relaxation. (From Sawyer DB, Colucci WS: Molecular and cellular events in myocardial hypertrophy and failure. *In* Colucci WS [ed]: Atlas of Heart Failure: Cardiac Function and Dysfunction. 3rd ed. Philadelphia, Current Medicine, 2002, p 7.8.)

extracellular and intracellular spaces in diastole. Although acutely induced energy deficiency, as occurs in severe ischemia, can interfere with cardiac contraction and relaxation, heart failure frequently occurs in the presence of adequate myocardial perfusion, oxygen, and substrate. When contractility is acutely depressed in experimental preparations, myocardial oxygen consumption of the intact ventricle also declines.[101] However, in chronic heart failure myocardial O_2 consumption is normal or increased.[102]

MYOCARDIAL ENERGY PRODUCTION. Lactate is a more important fuel for energy generation in heart failure than in the normal state.[102] Considerable dispute has centered on the question of whether mitochondrial oxidative phosphorylation (i.e., ATP production) is abnormal in heart failure. The cytochromes are located in the inner mitochondrial membrane and are constituents of the respiratory chain that couples oxidation to the synthesis of chemical energy. In one study in human dilated cardiomyopathy, a reduction in cytochrome *a* content and in cytochrome-dependent enzyme activity was reported.[103] Mitochondria obtained from failing human cardiac muscle have also shown reduced oxygen consumption during active phosphorylation and reduced rates of reduced nicotinamide adenine dinucleotide (NADH)–linked respiratory activity. These and other observations have led to the thesis that myocardial failure in the setting of hemodynamic overload may be related to an inability of oxidative phosphorylation (i.e., ATP production by mitochondria) to keep pace with the needs of the contractile apparatus. Katz has proposed that the mitochondrial abnormalities observed in the failing heart may be the result of damage to these structures and that the resultant mitochondrial abnormalities reduce the high-energy phosphates available for contraction and thereby contribute to the development of heart failure.[9]

The nucleotide-transporting protein located on the inner mitochondrial membrane, the so-called adenosine diphosphate (ADP)-ATP carrier, has been identified as an autoantigen in viral myocarditis and in dilated cardiomyopathy. In guinea pigs immunized to this carrier protein, both myocardial oxygen flux (i.e., O_2 production and consumption) and cardiac work fell.[104] These findings are compatible with the hypothesis that the impaired cardiac performance in some cases of myocarditis (and dilated cardiomyopathy) may be secondary to an imbalance between energy delivery and demand.

MYOCARDIAL ENERGY RESERVES. Observations on myocardial ATP concentration in compensated *hypertrophy* have shown no consistent change.[105] However, in myocardium from dogs with heart failure related to rapid pacing or chronic ischemia and from humans with end-stage cardiomyopathy, ATP, the total adenine nucleotide pool (ATP, AMP, and AMP), creatine kinase (CK) activity (required for synthesis of ATP), the concentrations of creatine phosphate (CrP), and the CPr/ATP ratio were all decreased[102,105-107] whereas the ATP/AMP and ATP/ADP ratios were maintained as the total adenine pool declined.[102] ATP synthesis and utilization were both reduced and, because the latter may exceed the former, ATP concentration declined. These observations have led to the hypothesis that myocardial failure may be the consequence of decreased energy reserve or at least that such decreased reserve contributes to the development of heart failure (Fig. 21–19). The measurement of CK flux provides a sensitive measure of myocardial energy reserves and may detect abnormalities in the absence of changes in ATP and CrP concentrations. By studying high-energy flux in vivo using nuclear magnetic resonance (NMR) technology, it has been demonstrated that CK activity is markedly reduced in the myopathic Syrian hamster. This abnormality was almost completely corrected by treatment with an ACE inhibitor. Likewise, in turkeys with furazolidone-induced heart failure, contractile failure was associated with a reduction in ATP, CrP, and CK activity.[102]

The mechanism responsible for the decrease in CK activity is not understood, but it is associated with alterations in the isoforms of CK. In failing myocardium, there was a decrease in the adult (MM) isoform and an increase or no change in the fetal isoform (MB).[105] The effect of

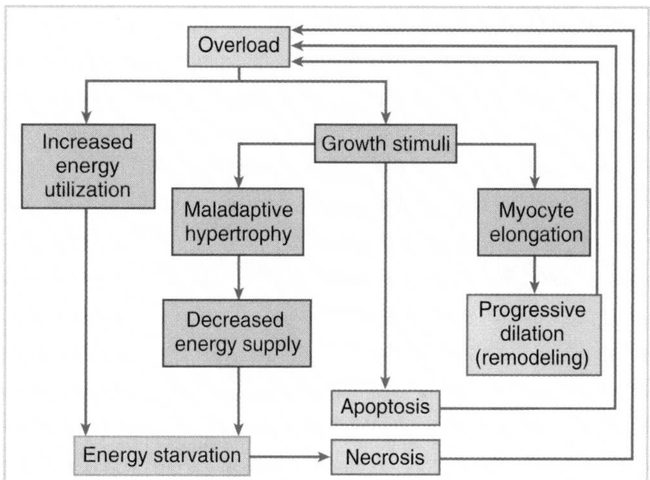

FIGURE 21–19 Some of the vicious circles that operate in the overloaded heart. Overload both increases energy utilization and stimulates growth. The former contributes directly to a state of energy starvation, which is made worse by several consequences of maladaptive hypertrophy that decrease energy supply. The latter include myocyte elongation, which causes remodeling, a progressive dilation that increases wall tension so as to increase the overload. Growth stimuli also promote apoptosis, which by decreasing the number of viable cardiac myocytes increases the load on those that survive. Hypertrophy also causes architectural changes that reduce the energy supply to working cardiac myocytes. (From Katz AM: Heart Failure. Philadelphia, Lippincott Williams & Wilkins, 2000.)

decreased CK activity on myocardial function and energetics was tested in mice with genetic deficiencies of the CK M isoform, the mitochondrial isoform, or both. The mice lacking both isoforms had a greater increase in ADP and a more pronounced decrease in the free energy released from ATP, suggesting that cardiac work was more costly energetically. In studies of rat hearts hypertrophied consequent to aortic bounding, increase in ADP and inorganic phosphate (P_i) were associated with slowing of cross-bridge cycling as well as cardiac relaxation.[102]

NMR spectroscopy with phosphorus-31, a noninvasive technique (see Chap. 13), has been employed to study the CrP-to-ATP ratio (CrP/ATP) in normal subjects and in patients. Reductions have been described in patients with severe aortic valve disease, cardiomyopathy, and myocardial ischemia.[108,109] In patients with chronic mitral regurgitation, the reduction in CrP/ATP has been found to be related to the severity of the hemodynamic impairment as reflected in the left ventricular end-systolic diameter. The extent of reduction of the ratio has been shown to correlate with the clinical severity of the heart failure and with the prognosis (Fig. 21-20).[110] These changes in CrP/ATP may be caused by the previously mentioned reduction in the phosphorylation of creatine and of CK activity.[102,105-107,111]

One unusual form of heart failure that is primarily related to a reduction of myocardial energy stores is that caused by phosphate deficiency. Chronic hypophosphatemia induced by dietary means is associated with reversible depression of myocardial performance in isolated muscle as well as in the intact heart of animals and humans, presumably as a consequence of reduced ATP stores.[112]

In the final analysis, the reduction of high-energy phosphates in the failing heart results in a decrease in the quantity of energy made available by the hydrolysis of ATP. When severe, the reduction in the energy available to the SR for Ca^{2+} uptake impairs relaxation (diastolic failure) and in that available to the contractile apparatus impairs cross-bridge cycling (systolic failure).[102]

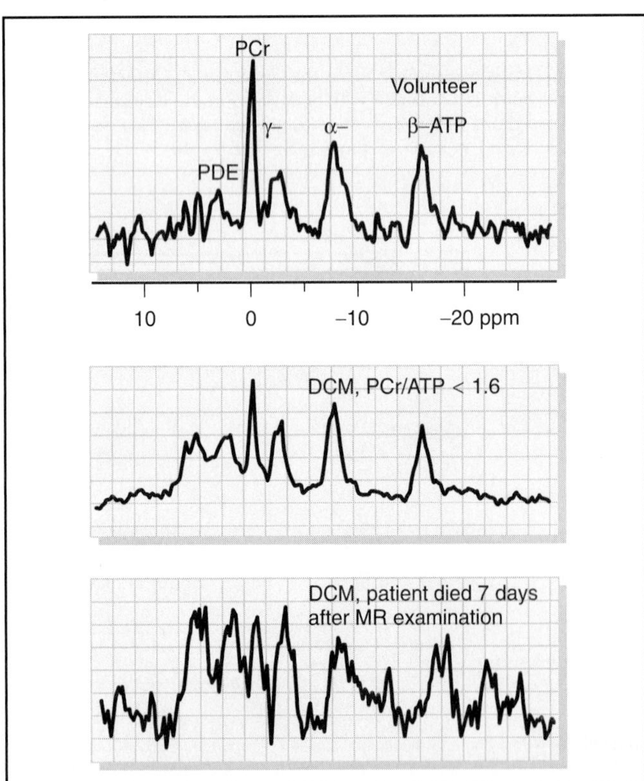

FIGURE 21–20 Cardiac ^{31}P magnetic resonance spectra. From top to bottom: spectra from volunteer patients with dilated cardiomyopathy (DCM) with normal phosphocreatine/ATP ratio and severely reduced phosphocreatine/ATP ratio; the latter patient died 7 days after the magnetic resonance examination. (From Neubauer S, Horn M, Cramer M, et al: Myocardial phosphocreatine-to-ATP ratio is a predictor of mortality in patients with dilated cardiomyopathy. Circulation 96:2190, 1997. Copyright 1997, American Heart Association.)

Pathophysiology of Diastolic Heart Failure (see also Chaps. 19 and 20)

Alterations in Diastolic Properties

Approximately one-third of patients with heart failure have predominantly diastolic heart failure (see Chap. 22), which may be defined as pulmonary (or systemic) venous congestion, and the symptoms consequent thereto in the presence of normal or almost normal systolic function.[113-116] Several mechanisms may be operative (Fig. 21–21). Approximately one third have predominantly disordered systolic function, and the remainder exhibit impairment of both systolic and diastolic function. Left ventricular pressure-volume loops displaying the difference between systolic and diastolic heart failure are shown in Figure 22–3. Among patients with the clinical diagnosis of congestive heart failure in the Framingham Heart Study population, 51 percent had a left ventricular ejection fraction greater than or equal to 0.50.[115]

ALTERED VENTRICULAR RELAXATION (see also Sarcoplasmic Reticulum Ca^{2+}-ATPase and Phospholamban, earlier). Although two aspects of the heart's diastolic characteristics (i.e., relaxation and wall stiffness) are often considered together, they actually describe two different properties.[113,114] Relaxation (inactivation of contraction) is a dynamic process that begins at the termination of contraction and occurs during isovolumetric relaxation and early ventricular filling (Fig. 21–22; see Fig. 19–19). The rate of ventricular relaxation is controlled primarily by the uptake of Ca^{2+} by the SR but also by the efflux of Ca^{2+} from the myocyte. These processes are regulated by SERCA2 as well as by sarcolemmal calcium pumps (see Table 21–2). Because these Ca^{2+} movements are against concentration gradients, they are energy consuming. Therefore, reductions in ATP concentration due to ischemia-induced ATP depletion interfere with these processes and slow myocardial relaxation (see Fig. 21–22A). Increases in cytoplasmic P_i contribute to this effect.[102] On the other hand, beta-adrenergic receptor stimulation, by increasing cyclic AMP and cyclic AMP–dependent protein kinase activity, causes the phosphorylation of phospholamban (see Chap. 19), which accelerates Ca^{2+} uptake by the SR and thereby enhances relaxation.

Impaired relaxation can also be caused by abnormalities in the sarcolemmal channels through which Ca^{2+} is extruded from the cytoplasm, in the Na^+/Ca^{2+} exchanger (see Na^+/Ca^{2+} Exchanger, earlier), as well as in the phosphorylation of proteins that affect SERCA2 such as phospholamban.[116] Cardiac relaxation requires hydrolysis of ATP for detachment of

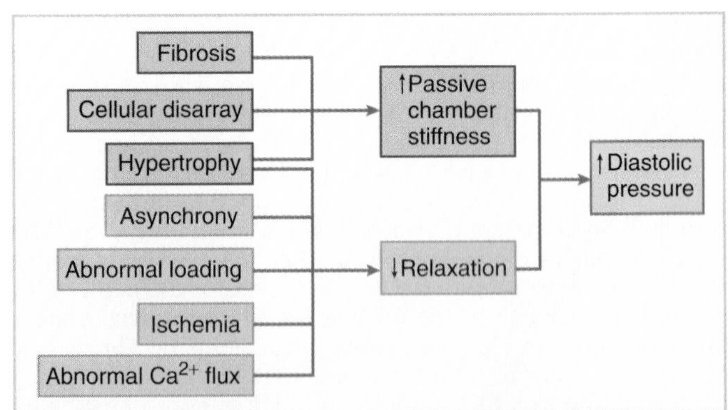

FIGURE 21–21 Factors responsible for diastolic dysfunction and increased left ventricular diastolic pressure. (From Gaasch WH, Izzi G: Clinical diagnosis and management of left ventricular diastolic dysfunction. *In* Hori M, Suga H, Baan J, Yellin EL [eds]: Cardiac Mechanics and Function in the Normal and Diseased Heart. New York, Springer-Verlag, 1989, p 296.)

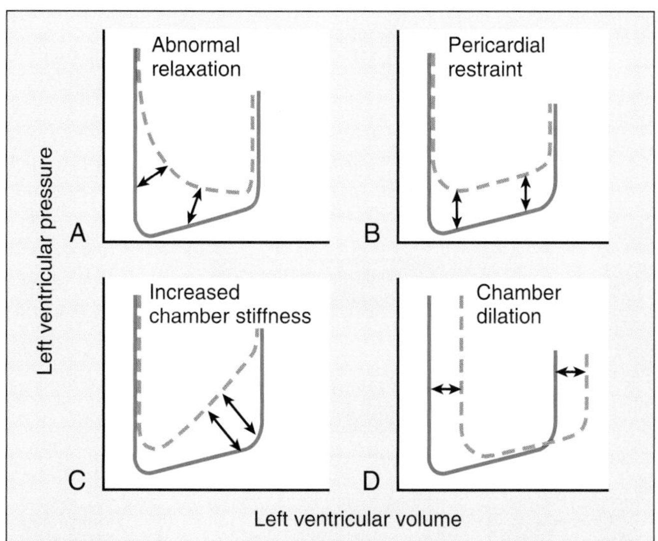

FIGURE 21–22 Mechanisms that cause diastolic dysfunction. Only the bottom half of the pressure-volume loop is depicted. Solid lines represent normal subjects; dashed lines represent patients with diastolic dysfunction. (From Zile MR: Diastolic dysfunction: Detection, consequences, and treatment: II. Diagnosis and treatment of diastolic function. Mod Concepts Cardiovasc Dis 59:1, 1990. Copyright 1990, American Heart Association.)

myosin from actin. Ischemia (or any process including heart failure; see earlier) that reduces myocyte ATP concentration can interfere with this process as well.

ALTERED VENTRICULAR FILLING. During early ventricular filling, the myocardium normally lengthens rapidly and homogeneously. Regional variation in the onset, rate, and extent of myocardial lengthening is referred to as *ventricular heterogeneity* or *diastolic asynergy.* Temporal dispersion of relaxation, with some fibers lengthening later than others, is referred to as *diastolic asynchrony.*[117] Both diastolic asynergy and asynchrony interfere with early diastolic filling. In contrast to these early diastolic events, myocardial *elasticity* (i.e., the change in muscle length for a change in force), ventricular *compliance* (i.e., the change in ventricular volume for a given change in pressure), and ventricular *stiffness* (i.e., the inverse of compliance) are generally measured in the relaxed ventricle at end diastole.

These diastolic properties of the ventricle are described by its curvilinear pressure-volume relation (see Fig. 21–22D). The slope of a tangent to this curvilinear relation (dP/dv) defines the chamber compliance at any level of filling pressure. An increase in chamber stiffness may occur secondary to any one or a combination of these three mechanisms:

1. *A rise in filling pressure* (i.e., movement of the ventricle up along its pressure-volume [stress-strain] curve to a steeper portion) (see Fig. 21–22D). This rise may occur in conditions such as volume overload secondary to acute valvular regurgitation and in acute left ventricular failure caused by myocarditis.
2. *A shift to a steeper ventricular pressure-volume* (see Fig. 21–22C) *or stress-strain curve.* Such an increase in stiffness results most commonly from an increase in ventricular mass and wall thickness. Thus, although hypertrophy constitutes a principal compensatory mechanism to sustain systolic emptying of the overloaded ventricle, it may simultaneously interfere with the ventricle's diastolic properties and impair ventricular filling. This shift to a steeper pressure-volume curve can also be caused by an increase in *intrinsic* myocardial stiffness (the stiffness of a unit of the cardiac wall regardless of the total mass or thickness of the myocardium), as occurs with disorders in which there is myocardial infiltration (e.g., amyloidosis), myocardial or endomyocardial fibrosis, or myocardial ischemia.
3. *A parallel upward displacement of the diastolic pressure-volume curve.* This effect is generally referred to as a *decrease in ventricular distensibility* and is usually caused by extrinsic compression of the ventricles, as occurs in cardiac tamponade or constrictive pericarditis (see Chap. 64) (see Fig. 21–22B).

Chronic Changes in Ventricular Diastolic Pressure-Volume Relationships

The compliance (inverse of stiffness) of the ventricle, reflected in the end-diastolic pressure-volume relationship, is altered in a variety of cardiac disorders, reflecting one or more basic mechanisms (see Fig. 21–21) (see Chap. 20). Substantial shifts in the diastolic pressure-volume curve of the left ventricle can be demonstrated during sustained volume overload.[118] For example, dogs with large chronic arteriovenous fistulas exhibit a rightward displacement of the entire diastolic pressure-volume curve, whereby ventricular volume is greater at any end-diastolic pressure but the slope of this curve is steeper, indicating increased chamber stiffness.[119] Patients with severe volume overloading related to chronic aortic or mitral regurgitation, or both, demonstrate similar shifts of the diastolic left ventricular pressure-volume relationship. Similar changes frequently occur in patients with dilated or ischemic cardiomyopathy or after large transmural myocardial infarction (see later).

In contrast, concentric left ventricular hypertrophy, as occurs in aortic stenosis, hypertension, and hypertrophic cardiomyopathy, shifts the pressure-volume relation of the ventricle to the left along its volume axis so that at any diastolic volume ventricular diastolic pressure is abnormally elevated (see Fig. 21–22C).[113,114] In contrast to the changes in the diastolic properties of the ventricular *chamber,* the stiffness of *each unit of myocardium* may or may not be altered in the presence of myocardial hypertrophy secondary to pressure overload. In the presence of concentric left ventricular hypertrophy, there is an inverse relationship between the thickness of the posterior wall of the ventricle and its peak thinning rate during early diastole; a higher than normal diastolic ventricular pressure is required to fill the hypertrophied ventricle. Patients with hypertension have demonstrated slowing of ventricular filling even when systolic function is normal.

Chronic changes in ventricular diastolic pressure-volume relations can also result from alterations in the cytoskeleton of the myocyte. For example, experimental cardiomyopathy with an increase in ventricular stiffness has been found to be associated with changes in titin isoforms and their distribution.[120] Changes in the *extracellular* matrix, especially in fibrillar collagen, can affect ventricular stiffness.[121] Collagen synthesis can be influenced by preload and afterload, as well as by activation of the adrenergic nervous system and of the renin-angiotensin-aldosterone system, and by the activities of MMPs and their inhibitors.[121]

ISCHEMIC HEART DISEASE. Marked changes in the diastolic properties of the left ventricle can occur in the presence of ischemic heart disease. First, acute myocardial ischemia slows ventricular relaxation (see Fig. 21–22A) and increases myocardial wall stiffness.[122] Myocardial infarction causes more complex changes in ventricular pressure-volume relationships, depending on the size of the infarct and the time after infarction at which the measurements are made. Infarcted muscle tested very early exhibits reduced stiffness. Subsequently, the development of myocardial contracture, interstitial edema, fibrocellular infiltration, and scar contributes to increased chamber stiffness, with a steeper ventricular pressure-volume curve (a greater increase in pressure for any increase in volume).[123] Later still, in the case of large infarcts, left ventricular remodeling and dilatation cause a rightward displacement of the pressure-volume curve,[124] resembling that observed in volume overload.

The subendocardial ischemia that is characteristic of severe concentric hypertrophy (even in the presence of a normal coronary circulation) intensifies the failure of relaxation; and when coronary artery obstruction accompanies severe hypertrophy, this abnormality may be particularly severe. Tachycardia, by reducing the duration of diastole and thereby intensifying ischemia, exaggerates this diastolic abnormality and may raise ventricular diastolic pressure even while reducing diastolic ventricular volume, whereas bradycardia has the opposite effect. Successful treatment of ischemia improves diastolic relaxation and lowers ventricular diastolic and pulmonary venous pressures, thereby reducing dyspnea.

CARDIOMYOPATHY AND PERICARDIAL DISEASE. The restrictive cardiomyopathies, especially those such as amyloid heart disease with intracardiac infiltration, the transplanted heart during rejection, and endomyocardial fibrosis (see Chap. 59), are all characterized by upward and leftward displacement of the diastolic pressure-volume relation, with a higher pressure at any volume and a greater increase in diastolic pressure for any increase in volume. Pericardial tamponade and constrictive pericarditis also change the apparent diastolic properties of the heart (see Chap. 50). Early filling is unimpaired because the myocardium is normal. However, filling is abruptly halted in mid-diastole by the constricted or tamponading pericardium, which imposes its mechanical properties on those of the ventricle in the latter half of diastole (see Fig. 21–22B).

Neurohormonal, Autocrine, and Paracrine Adjustments

In response to the reduction of cardiac output, the inadequate arterial volume that is characteristic of systolic heart failure, and atrial hypertension, a complex series of neurohormonal changes takes place (see Table 21–1). In the early stages of severe, acute systolic failure, these changes—heightened adrenergic drive, activation of the renin-angiotensin-aldosterone axis, and augmented release of vasopressin and endothelin—compensate and act to maintain perfusion to vital organs and to expand the inadequate arterial blood volume and via renal retention of sodium and water (Figs. 21–23 and 21–24). However, each of these mechanisms may be thought of as a "double-edged sword." As heart failure becomes chronic, several of these compensatory mechanisms can cause undesirable effects, such as excessive vasoconstriction, increased afterload, excessive retention of salt and water,[125] electrolyte abnormalities, arrhythmias, and direct effects on cardiac myocytes leading to cell death or changes in protein expression and functions (see Table 21–1). In contrast, other responses, such as the release of ANP and brain natriuretic peptide (BNP) in response to distention of the atria and ventricles, may oppose these adverse effects by causing vasodilation, increased excretion of salt and water, and inhibition of sympathetic activity.[126]

Several mediators are involved in control of the cardiovascular system in heart failure. Some are circulating hormones (endocrine effect). Some act on neighboring cells of another type (paracrine effect) or on the cell of origin (autocrine effect). These include peptides that act primarily locally in the vicinity of their production, such as endothelin, peptide growth factors (e.g., TGF-α), and inflammatory cytokines (e.g., interleukin-1 beta [IL-1β] and TNF-α). These and other local mediators act in concert with the autonomic nervous system and circulating hormones to modulate cardiovascular organ function. In addition, many if not all of these mediators have effects on the growth, death, and phenotype of cardiovascular tissues and may thereby play an important role in the remodeling of myocardium and its progression to failure (see Fig. 21–10).[41]

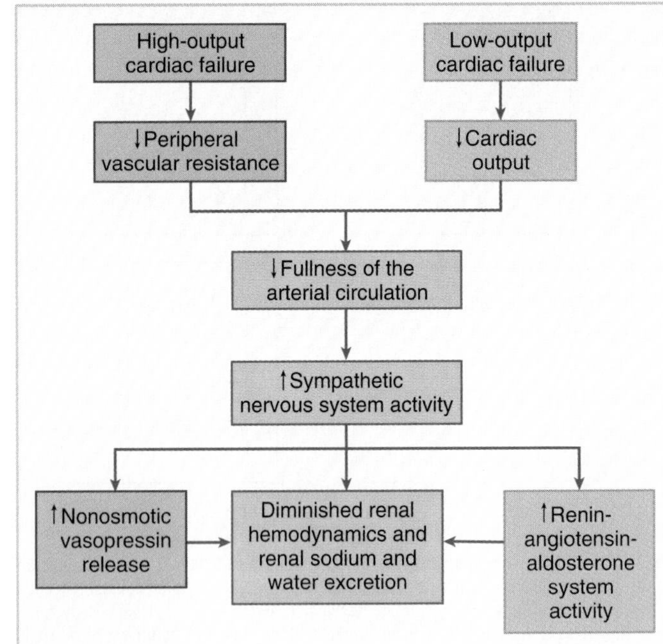

FIGURE 21–23 Mechanisms by which high-output or low-output heart failure leads to the activation of neurohumoral vasoconstrictor systems and renal sodium and water retention. (From Schrier RW, Abraham WT: Hormones and hemodynamics in heart failure. N Engl J Med 341:577, 1999; adapted from Schrier RW: Pathogenesis of sodium and water retention in high-output and low output cardiac failure, nephrotic syndrome, cirrhosis, and pregnancy. N Engl J Med 319:1065, 1988.)

Autonomic Nervous System

INCREASED SYMPATHETIC ACTIVITY (see Figs. 21–23 and 21–24). Activation of the sympathetic (adrenergic) nervous system is a hallmark of heart failure. Measurements of the concentration of the adrenergic neurotransmitter NE in arterial blood provide a crude index of the activity of this system, which is critical to the normal regulation of cardiac performance. At rest, in patients with advanced heart failure, the circulating NE concentration is elevated, generally two to three times the level found in normal subjects,[127] and this elevation is accompanied by elevation of circulating dopamine and sometimes by epinephrine as well; the latter reflects increased adrenomedullary activity. Measurement of 24-hour urinary NE excretion also reveals marked elevations in patients with heart failure.[128] Plasma NE may be elevated, even in asymptomatic patients with left ventricular dysfunction, and is a predictor of mortality in heart failure. During comparable levels of exercise, much greater elevations in circulating NE occur in patients with heart failure than in normal subjects, presumably reflecting greater activation of the adrenergic nervous system during exercise in these patients.

The elevation of circulating NE may result from a combination of increased release of NE from adrenergic nerve endings and its consequent "spillover" into the plasma as well as reduced uptake of NE by adrenergic nerve endings.[129] Patients with heart failure demonstrate increased adrenergic nerve outflow, as measured by microneurography of the peroneal nerve, and the level of nerve activity correlates with the concentration of plasma NE.[130] The level of adrenergic nerve activity also correlates directly with the levels of left and right ventricular filling pressures. Whereas the normal heart usually extracts NE from the arterial blood, in patients with heart failure the coronary sinus NE concentration exceeds the arterial concentration, indicating increased adrenergic activation of the heart. Drugs such as the alpha$_2$-agonist moxonidine (which reduces adrenergic nerve impulse traffic) reduce plasma NE, indicating that presynaptic control of adrenergic nervous activity is intact in patients with heart failure.[131] It has been suggested that treatment with such agents might be useful in the treatment of heart failure. However, this general concept has been challenged by the results of a large clinical trial in which moxonidine was associated with a substantial decrease in plasma NE but an *increase* in morbidity and mortality.[132] Perhaps in this trial the dose of the drug was too high and the reduction in adrenergic support too profound, analogous to the hazardous effects of rapidly escalating doses of beta-adrenergic blockers in patients with advanced heart failure.

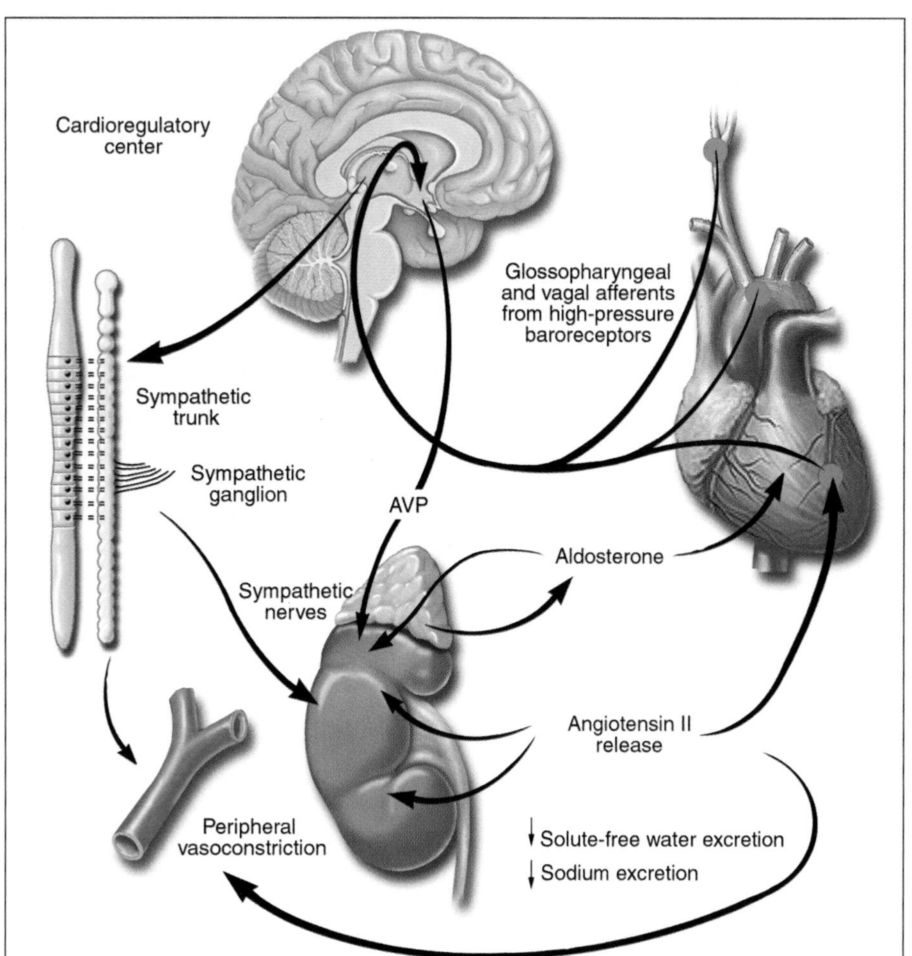

FIGURE 21–24 Unloading of high-pressure baroceptors (circles) in the left ventricle, carotid sinus, and aortic arch generates afferent signals that stimulate cardioregulatory centers in the brain, resulting in the activation of efferent pathways in the sympathetic nervous system. The sympathetic nervous system appears to be the primary integrator of the neurohumoral vasoconstrictor response to arterial underfilling. Activation of renal sympathetic nerves stimulates the release of arginine vasopressin (AVP). Sympathetic activation also causes peripheral and renal vasoconstriction, as does angiotensin II. Angiotensin II constricts blood vessels and stimulates the release of aldosterone from the adrenal gland, and it also increases tubular sodium reabsorption and causes remodeling of cardiac myocytes. Aldosterone may also have direct cardiac effects, in addition to increasing the reabsorption of sodium and the secretion of potassium and hydrogen ions in the collecting duct. The lines designate circulating hormones. (Modified from Schrier RW, Abraham WT: Hormones and hemodynamics in heart failure. N Engl J Med 341:577, 1999.)

Increased adrenergic activation results in an increase in Ca^{2+} influx into the myocytes, an increase in Ca^{2+} storage (and release) by the SR, phosphorylation and therefore reduced inhibition of SERCA2 by phospholamban, as well as a decreased Ca^{2+} binding affinity of troponin.[2] Although NE enhances both contraction and relaxation, myocardial energy requirements are augmented, which could intensify ischemia when myocardial O_2 delivery is restricted. The augmented adrenergic outflow from the central nervous system in patients with heart failure may trigger ventricular tachycardia or even sudden cardiac death, particularly in the presence of myocardial ischemia, as well as myocyte apoptosis.

In addition to activation of beta-adrenergic receptors in the heart, the heightened activity of the adrenergic nervous system leads to stimulation of myocardial $alpha_1$-adrenergic receptors, which elicits a modest positive inotropic effect.[133] Stimulation of myocardial $alpha_1$-adrenergic receptors may also cause myocyte hypertrophy, changes in phenotype characterized by the reexpression of a fetal gene program, and the induction of peptide growth factors.[134] $Alpha_1$-adrenergic receptors are of low density in the human heart; however, in contrast to $beta_1$-adrenergic receptors, which are downregulated, $alpha_1$-adrenergic receptors appear to be unchanged in number in failing human myocardium.

CARDIAC NOREPINEPHRINE DEPLETION. The concentration of NE in atrial and ventricular tissue removed at operation from patients with heart failure is extremely low.[127,128,134] In patients, cardiac NE content determined from endomyocardial biopsies correlates directly with the ejection fraction and inversely with plasma epinephrine concentration. NE concentrations are also markedly depressed in the ventricles of dogs with right ventricular failure produced by the creation of pulmonary stenosis and tricuspid regurgitation.[135] Local cardiac NE stores do not appear to play any role in the *intrinsic* contractile state of cardiac muscle. Thus, no differences were found in the length-tension or force-velocity relationships displayed by papillary muscles removed from normal cats and from cats with NE depletion produced by chronic cardiac denervation or reserpine pretreatment.[136] However, the reduction in cardiac NE stores represents a depletion of the adrenergic neurotransmitter in adrenergic nerve endings, and, as a consequence, the response to activation of the sympathetic nervous system is blunted (see Fig. 21-2).

The mechanism responsible for cardiac NE depletion in severe heart failure is not clear; it may be an "exhaustion" phenomenon resulting from the prolonged adrenergic activation of the cardiac adrenergic nerves in heart failure. Reductions in the activity of tyrosine hydroxylase, which catalyzes the rate-limiting step in the biosynthesis of NE, and in the rate at which noradrenergic vesicles can take up dopamine have also been incriminated. In patients with cardiomyopathy, iodine-131-labeled metaiodobenzylguanidine (MIBG), a radiopharmaceutical that is taken up by adrenergic nerve endings, is not taken up normally,[137] suggesting that NE reuptake is impaired in heart failure. Treatment with the beta-adrenergic antagonist metoprolol was associated with correction of MIBG uptake.[138]

ABNORMAL BAROREFLEX CONTROL IN HEART FAILURE. Increased adrenergic activity in heart failure is due, in part, to abnormal baroreflex control of adrenergic outflow from the central nervous system (see Fig. 21-24). In dogs with experimental heart failure, carotid occlusion elicited a blunted reflex response of heart rate, arterial pressure, and vascular resistance.[139]

The possibility of defective adrenergic control of heart rate in patients with heart failure has been studied by observing the reflex hemodynamic responses to stimuli such as upright tilt and vasodilator-induced hypotension. An inadequate increase in heart rate in patients with heart failure was observed when arterial pressure was reduced by a vasodilator.[140] Although the changes in mean arterial pressure

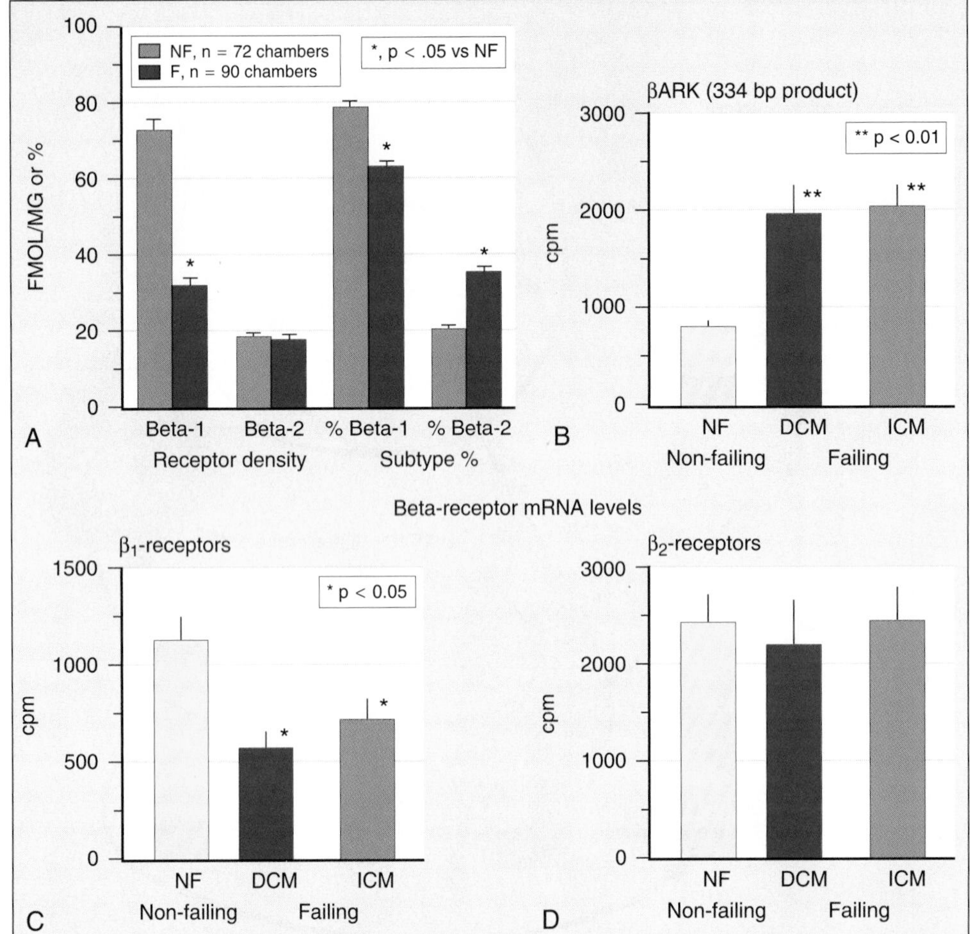

FIGURE 21–25 Downregulation of beta-adrenergic receptors in myocardium from patients with heart failure. Although human ventricular myocardium expresses both beta$_1$- and beta$_2$-adrenergic receptor subtypes, only the beta$_1$ subtype is significantly downregulated in failing myocardium **(A)**. Downregulation of beta$_1$ receptors is associated with upregulation of beta-adrenergic receptor kinase (βARK), an enzyme that phosphorylates beta-adrenergic receptors and thereby contributes to their uncoupling from second messenger pathways **(B)**. In addition, the messenger RNA (mRNA) level for beta$_1$-, but not beta$_2$-, adrenergic receptors is decreased in failing human myocardium **(C** and **D)**. NF = nonfailure; F = congestive heart failure; DCM = dilated cardiomyopathy; ICM = ischemic cardiomyopathy. (Data from Bristow MR: Changes in myocardial and vascular receptors in heart failure. J Am Coll Cardiol 22:61A, 1993; and Ungerer M, Bohm M, Elce JS, et al: Altered expression of beta-adrenergic receptor kinase and beta$_1$-adrenergic receptors in the failing human heart. Circulation 87:454, 1993. Copyright 1993, American Heart Association.)

observed in response to the vasodilators were similar in patients with heart failure and in normal subjects, the changes in heart rate after vasodilators correlated significantly with the changes in concentration of circulating NE and with the sum of circulating NE and epinephrine. In normal individuals, both heart rate and NE concentrations rose, whereas in patients with heart failure, in whom resting catecholamine levels were already increased, cardiac acceleration was blunted and NE concentration failed to rise normally. Similarly, during upright tilt, patients with heart failure exhibited a blunting of the normal increases in plasma NE and forearm vascular resistance.[141]

Some patients with heart failure exhibit a major reduction in arterial pressure during tilting, analogous to what is observed in idiopathic orthostatic hypotension. Further evidence for impairment of baroreflex control of the systemic circulation comes from investigations in which lower body negative pressure failed to cause normal reflex augmentation of forearm vascular resistance.[142]

ATRIAL STRETCH RECEPTORS. Abnormal baroreflex control of the circulation also contributes to the reduced ability of patients with heart failure to excrete salt and water. Under normal circumstances, elevated left atrial pressure stimulates atrial stretch receptors. The increased activity of both myelinated and nonmyelinated (C-fiber) afferents inhibits the release of antidiuretic hormone, thereby increasing water excretion, which in turn reduces plasma volume and thereby restores left atrial pressure to normal. In addition, enhanced activation of left atrial stretch receptors depresses renal efferent sympathetic nerve activity and increases renal blood flow and glomerular filtration rate, thereby enhancing the ability of the kidney to reduce plasma volume.

With the prolonged elevation of left atrial pressure in heart failure, there is desensitization of atrial (and arterial) baroreceptors. This desensitization may be responsible for the inappropriately high plasma antidiuretic hormone levels in severe heart failure and may contribute to the renal vasoconstriction, peripheral edema, ascites, and hyponatremia characteristic of this condition. With chronic heart failure and its attendant cardiac distention and decreased sensitivity of cardiac receptors, the reflex inhibition of adrenergic activity disappears. The adrenergic drive to the peripheral vascular bed and the adrenal medulla is enhanced, contributing to the vasoconstriction, tachycardia, and sodium retention state characteristic of heart failure.

There is evidence that blunted baroreflex responsiveness is associated with increased activity of Na^+,K^+-ATPase in the baroreceptors; digitalis glycosides, which inhibit Na^+,K^+-ATPase, can partially correct this abnormality. This ability of digitalis to correct baroreflex function and thereby suppress adrenergic nerve activity may play a significant role in its clinical efficacy (see Chap. 23). NO also increases baroreflex sensitivity, whereas angiotensin II decreases it, and exogenous NO and blockade of angiotensin receptors can correct the reduced baroreceptor sensitivity characteristic of experimental heart failure.[143]

Beta-Adrenergic Receptor–G Protein–Adenylyl Cyclase Pathway

BETA-ADRENERGIC RECEPTORS (see also Chap. 19). Ventricles obtained from patients with heart failure demonstrate a marked reduction in NE content, beta-adrenergic receptor density, isoproterenol-mediated adenylyl cyclase stimulation, and the contractile response to beta-adrenergic agonists.[144] It is generally believed that the downregulation of beta-adrenergic receptors is mediated by increased levels of NE in the vicinity of the receptor. In patients with dilated cardiomyopathy, this reduction in receptor density is proportional to the severity of heart failure and involves primarily beta$_1$, but not beta$_2$, receptors, thus reducing the ratio of beta$_1$ to beta$_2$ receptors (Fig. 21–25A). The beta$_2$ receptor, although not downregulated, becomes partially "uncoupled" from its effector enzyme (adenylyl cyclase), producing a similar effect.

In isolated cardiac myocytes, the proapoptotic effect of beta-adrenergic receptor stimulation is mediated by the beta$_1$

receptor subtype, whereas the beta$_2$ subtype exerts an opposing antiapoptotic effect.[145] Although this observation might lead to the prediction that clinically beta$_1$-selective blockade would be superior to nonselective blockade in the treatment of heart failure, such superiority has not been observed in clinical trials,[146] probably reflecting other adverse actions of the beta$_2$ subtype such as facilitation of NE release from presynaptic sympathetic neuron.

In myocardium from patients with heart failure the level of beta$_1$-adrenergic receptor mRNA is decreased, indicating that the downregulation of beta$_1$-adrenergic receptors is mediated, at least in part, by a decrease in receptor synthesis, whereas the level of beta$_2$-adrenergic receptor mRNA is unchanged (see Fig. 21–25). In addition, there are increases in the expression of beta-adrenergic receptor kinase (βARK) and its mRNA level in failing human myocardium (see Fig. 21–25B). βARK is an enzyme that phosphorylates both beta$_1$- and beta$_2$-adrenergic receptors and thereby plays a central role in uncoupling of the receptor from its G protein (Fig. 21–26).[147] Increased βARK activity may therefore contribute to the uncoupling of both beta$_1$- and beta$_2$-adrenergic receptors in patients with heart failure.

Downregulation of beta$_1$ receptors in patients with heart failure may be reversed by the administration of metoprolol, a relatively specific beta$_1$ antagonist. The long-term clinical benefit of beta blockade in heart failure (see Chap. 23) has been reported to be associated with both a restoration of myocardial beta receptor density and the contractile response to administered catecholamines.[148]

The relative importance of beta-adrenergic receptor downregulation versus receptor uncoupling may depend on the cause of heart failure. In myocardium obtained from patients with heart failure secondary to ischemic heart disease, there is a relatively greater degree of receptor desensitization than in myocardium from patients with dilated cardiomyopathy. This observation, together with apparent differences in the regulation of G protein function, has led to the suggestion that there are differences in the behavior of the beta-adrenergic receptor–G protein complex in these two forms of heart failure.

Genetic differences related to polymorphisms or mutations that affect the function of beta- or alpha-adrenergic receptors may contribute to the pathophysiology of myocardial failure. Patients with heart failure with a Thr-to-Ile polymorphism at amino acid 164 of the beta$_2$ receptor have a decrease in receptor function that is associated with a decrease in survival.[149] Likewise, black patients who have a polymorphism in the beta$_1$ receptor resulting in increased function combined with a polymorphism in the alpha$_{2C}$ receptor resulting in decreased function were found to have an increased risk of heart failure (Fig. 21–27).[150] Because the alpha$_2$ receptor inhibits NE release from sympathetic nerve endings, whereas the beta$_1$ receptor mediates the proapoptotic effect on the cardiac myocyte, these polymorphisms may exert synergistic adverse effects by providing higher levels of NE to a hyperresponsive beta$_1$ receptor on the cardiac myocyte.

G PROTEINS AND ADENYLYL CYCLASE (see also Chap. 20). G proteins play a critical role in coupling receptors, including beta-adrenergic receptors, to effector enzymes such as adenylyl cyclase (see Fig. 19–12).[151] Cardiac cells contain at least three types of G proteins: (1) G_s, which mediates the *stimulation of adenylyl cyclase* (and thereby causes a rise in intracellular cyclic AMP, which in turn stimulates Ca^{2+} influx into the myocyte through Ca^{2+} channels in the sarcolemmal membrane and accelerates the uptake of Ca^{2+} by the SR); (2) G_i, which mediates the *inhibition of adenylyl cyclase* and has the opposite effect on the movements of Ca^{2+}; and (3) G_q, which mediates the *stimulation of phospholipase C,* thereby leading to an activation of protein kinase C by several receptors generally associated with myocyte hypertrophy including those for angiotensin II, alpha-adrenergic receptors for NE, and endothelin.[152]

Heart failure secondary to dilated cardiomyopathy is associated with an increase in G_i activity and protein level in heart muscle, which appears to be mediated at the posttranscriptional level. G_s appears normal in failing human myocardium. However, the functional consequences of an increase in G_i activity remain to be established. In mice, the cardiac-specific overexpression of G_s led to cardiac failure that was associated with apoptosis of cardiac myocytes and with myocardial fibrosis and hypertrophy.[153] Mice with overexpression of cardiac G_q exhibited myocardial hypertrophy and, with higher levels of G_q expression, developed dilated cardiomyopathy associated with myocyte apoptosis.[154] Although the effects of overexpression studies such as

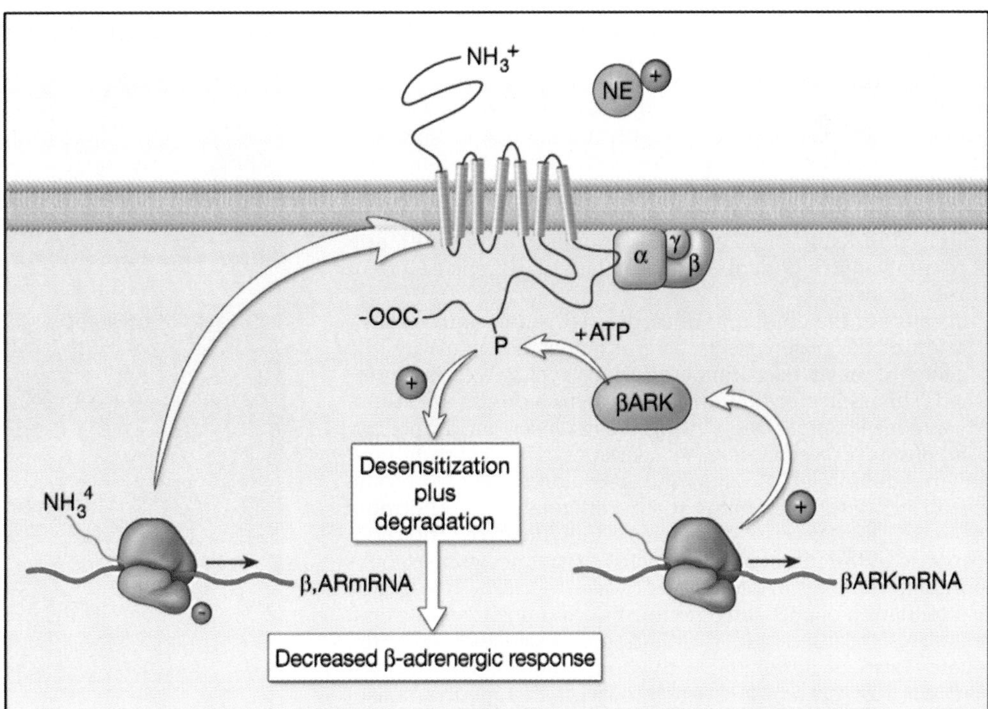

FIGURE 21–26 Alterations in beta-adrenergic pathways in the failing heart. A characteristic physiological abnormality in patients with heart failure is a reduction in the inotropic and chronotropic responses to exercise and other types of sympathetic stimulation. The molecular basis for this appears to involve multiple changes in the beta$_1$-adrenergic receptor coupling that are a response to the chronic increase in adrenergic stimulation. In myocardium from patients with end-stage heart failure, compared with control tissue from patients without failure, the level of beta-adrenergic receptor kinase (ßARK) messenger RNA (mRNA) is increased and the level of beta$_1$-adrenergic receptor mRNA is reduced. This leads not only to reduction in transcription of new beta$_1$-adrenergic receptors but also to increased phosphorylation of receptors leading to desensitization and degradation of receptors. (From Colucci WS [ed]: Atlas of Heart Failure: Cardiac Function and Dysfunction. 3rd ed. Philadelphia, Current Medicine, 2002, p 7.9.)

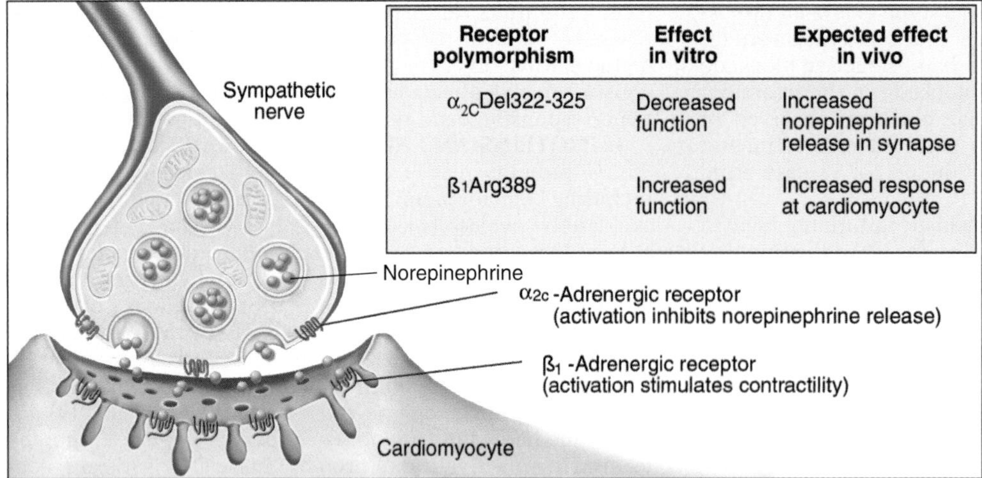

FIGURE 21–27 Basis of the hypothesis that the α_{2c}Del322-325 and β_1Arg389 receptors act synergistically as risk factors for heart failure. The α_{2c}-adrenergic receptor (along with the α_{2a}-adrenergic receptor) inhibits norepinephrine release at cardiac presynaptic nerve endings through negative feedback. The presence of the dysfunctional α_{2c}Del322-325 receptor would be expected to result in enhanced norepinephrine release. The β_1-adrenergic receptor is the receptor for norepinephrine on the cardiomyocyte, and the presence of the hyperfunctional β_1Arg389 receptor would be expected to increase contractile response at the myocytes. The combination of increased norepinephrine release and increased responsiveness of the receptor was hypothesized to be a risk factor for heart failure. (From Small KM, Wagoner LE, Levin AM, et al: Synergistic polymorphisms of β_1 and α_{2c}-adrenergic receptors and the risk of congestive heart failure. N Engl J Med 347:1135, 2002.)

these need to be interpreted with caution, they suggest that receptors coupled to G_s and G_q play an important role in the pathophysiology of myocardial hypertrophy and failure.

REDUCED ADRENERGIC SUPPORT OF THE FAILING HEART. The importance of the adrenergic nervous system in maintaining ventricular contractility when myocardial function is depressed in heart failure is demonstrated by the effects of adrenergic blockade. *Acute* pharmacological blockade of the adrenergic nervous system may cause intensification of heart failure as well as sodium and water retention.[155,156] The *acute* administration of beta blockers to patients with heart failure results in reductions in both systolic and diastolic myocardial function. Despite the long-term very salutary effects of beta-blocker therapy in patients with heart failure (see Chaps. 23 and 24), caution should be exercised in using these agents, particularly at the initiation of therapy and in patients in whom heart failure is severe or of recent onset.

Because of the depletion of cardiac NE stores and desensitization of the postsynaptic beta adrenoceptor pathway, the capacity of the myocardium to produce cyclic AMP is diminished, sometimes profoundly, in patients with heart failure. As a consequence, the failing heart loses an important compensatory mechanism. In patients with heart failure, downregulation of postsynaptic beta adrenoceptors in the sinoatrial node contributes to the attenuated chronotropic response to exercise. Likewise, the positive inotropic response to the infusion of the beta-adrenergic agonist dobutamine is reduced in patients with heart failure. The degree of attenuation of both the chronotropic and positive inotropic responses to adrenergic stimulation is correlated with the level of baseline adrenergic activation as reflected by the concentration of plasma NE. An important therapeutic consequence of the alterations of the beta-adrenergic pathway described earlier is that the positive inotropic response to beta adrenoceptor agonists, and to a lesser extent to phosphodiesterase inhibitors, is reduced in myocardium obtained from patients with end-stage heart failure.

ADVERSE EFFECTS OF ADRENERGIC STIMULATION. Increased adrenergic nerve activity may influence the chronic remodeling of the myocardium by affecting the progression of myocardial failure through direct harmful effects of NE on adrenergic receptors located on several cardiac cell types, including cardiac myocytes and fibroblasts. The tonic stimulation of beta-adrenergic receptors, or the downstream cyclic AMP pathway to which they are coupled, resulted in death of cardiac myocytes by apoptosis.[157] In vitro, tonic exposure to NE caused apoptosis of adult rat cardiac myocytes that was mediated through the beta-adrenergic receptor adenylyl cyclase and cyclic AMP (Fig. 21–28).[49] A similar effect was seen in neonatal rat cardiomyocytes.[49] Likewise, the chronic infusion of isoproterenol to rats caused myocardial failure associated with apoptosis,[158] and transgenic mice that overexpressed either the beta_1-adrenergic receptor or G_s[153,154,159] developed myocardial failure associated with myocyte

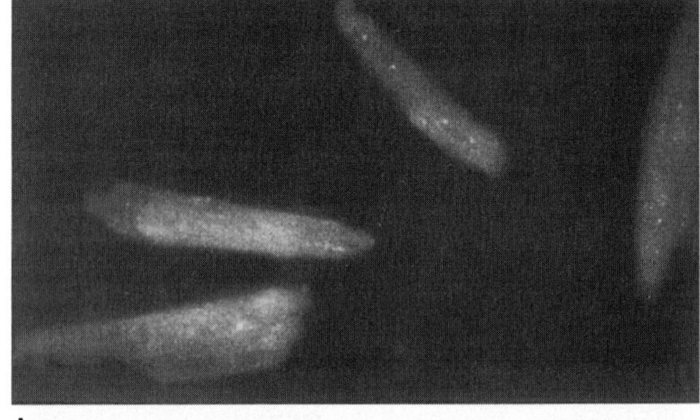

A

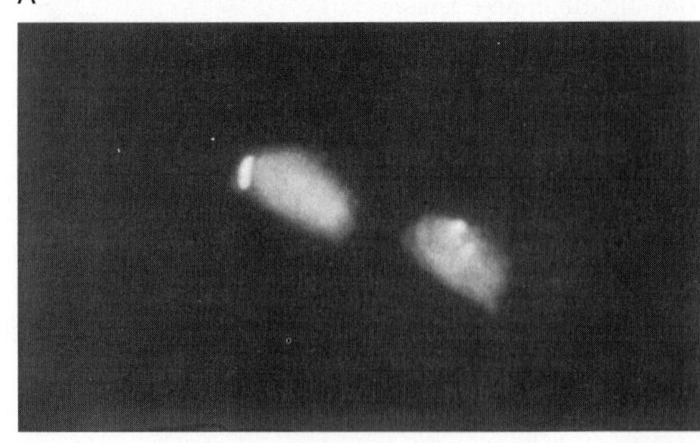

B

FIGURE 21–28 Effect of norepinephrine (NE) on myocyte apoptosis. Adult rat cardiac myocytes in tissue culture were exposed to control media **(A)** or NE **(B)** for 24 hours and apoptosis was measured by the terminal deoxynucleotidyl transferase-mediated-VTP nick end labeling (TUNEL) staining for fragmented DNA shown in two nuclei in this panel. NE caused an approximately fourfold increase in TUNEL-positive myocytes (From Sawyer DB, Colucci WS: Molecular and cellular events in myocardial hypertrophy and failure. *In* Colucci WS [ed]: Heart Failure: Cardiac Function and Dysfunction. 3rd ed. Philadelphia, Current Medicine, 2002, p 4.12.)

apoptosis. When viewed from this perspective, the desensitization of the beta-adrenergic pathway, although impairing short-term myocardial function, may protect the myocardium from excessive adrenergic activation.

In addition, NE, acting on both alpha$_1$-adrenergic and beta-adrenergic receptors located on cardiac myocytes and fibroblasts, can increase and alter the composition of the interstitial matrix, which may play an important role in the pathophysiology of myocardial dysfunction (see Interstitial Matrix Accumulation, earlier).

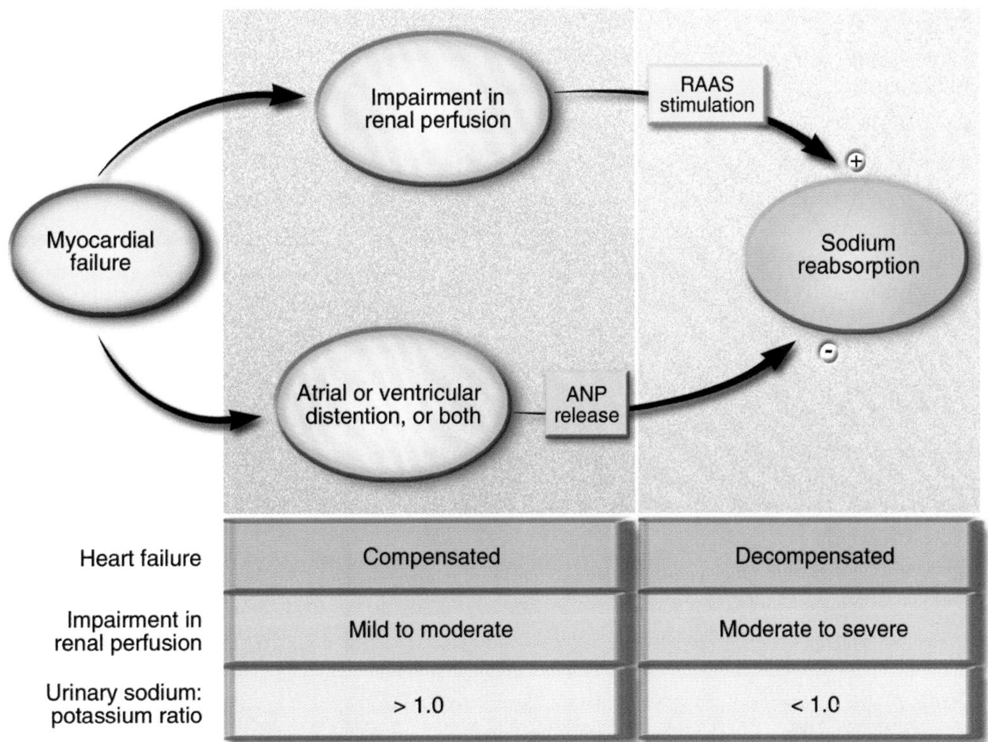

FIGURE 21–29 Compensated and decompensated heart failure, as indicated by the presence or absence of urinary sodium retention, together with symptoms and signs of expanded intravascular and extravascular volume. In compensated heart failure with mild to moderate reductions in renal perfusion, natriuretic peptides, such as atrial natriuretic peptide (ANP) released by distended atria, stimulate sodium excretion (decreasing reabsorption, minus sign) so that the urinary sodium/potassium ratio is greater than 1.0. In decompensated heart failure, moderate to severe reductions in renal perfusion activate the renin-angiotensin-aldosterone system (RAAS), overriding the action of natriuretic peptides to stimulate nearly complete urinary sodium reabsorption (plus sign), resulting in a urinary sodium/potassium ratio less than 1.0. (From Weber KT: Aldosterone in congestive heart failure. N Engl J Med 345:1689, 2001, and Weber KT, Villareal D: Aldosterone and antialdosterone therapy in congestive heart failure. Am J Cardiol 71[Suppl 3A]:11A, 1993.)

PARASYMPATHETIC FUNCTION IN HEART FAILURE

Cardiac enlargement, with or without heart failure, is associated with marked disturbances of parasympathetic as well as sympathetic function. The parasympathetic restraint on sinoatrial node automaticity was markedly reduced in patients with heart failure (see Fig. 21–3), who exhibited less heart rate slowing for any given elevation of systemic arterial pressure than did normal subjects.[160] The aforementioned reduction in the sensitivity of the baroreceptor reflex, which is notably dependent on parasympathetic outflow, has also been shown to be significantly reduced in dogs with heart failure. Measurements of heart rate variability, which indirectly reflect autonomic nervous system function, indicated that parasympathetic activity in patients with heart failure is abnormal both at rest and in response to exercise.[161]

Abnormal parasympathetic function may also be altered at the level of the peripheral nerve and the postsynaptic receptor. Cardiomyopathic hamster hearts display a reduction in the activity of choline acetyltransferase, an enzyme that provides an estimate of the density of parasympathetic innervation, and there is evidence that the density of high-affinity muscarinic receptors is reduced in the hearts of dogs with experimental heart failure.

Renin-Angiotensin-Aldosterone System

In low–cardiac output states, there is activation of the renin-angiotensin-aldosterone system, which operates in concert with the activated adrenergic nervous–adrenal medullary system to maintain arterial pressure and to retain sodium and water (Figs. 21–24 and 21–29). These two systems are clearly coupled. Heightened adrenergic drive stimulates beta$_1$ adrenoceptors in the juxtaglomerular apparatus of the kidneys. This process is a principal mechanism responsible for the release of renin in acute heart failure. Activation of the baroreceptors in the renal vascular bed by a reduction of renal blood flow is also responsible for the release of renin, and in patients with severe chronic heart failure after salt restriction and diuretic treatment, reduction of the sodium presented to the macula densa contributes to the release of renin. Elevated plasma renin activity is a common, although not universal, finding in heart failure. In the Studies of Left Ventricular Dysfunction (SOLVD) study of heart failure, plasma angiotensin II was significantly elevated even in asymptomatic patients and was further elevated in patients with symptomatic heart failure.[162]

ADVERSE EFFECTS OF RENIN-ANGIOTENSIN-ALDOSTERONE SYSTEM ACTIVATION. Angiotensin II is a potent peripheral vasoconstrictor and contributes, along with increased adrenergic activity, to the excessive elevation of systemic vascular resistance and the vicious circle already referred to (see Increased Vasoconstrictor Activity, earlier) in patients with heart failure. Angiotensin II also enhances the adrenergic nervous system's release of NE as well as the release of aldosterone from the adrenal cortex. Aldosterone has potent sodium-retaining properties and contributes to the development of edema (see later). Therefore, it is not surprising that interruption of the renin-angiotensin-aldosterone axis by means of ACE inhibition reduces system vascular resistance, diminishes afterload, and thereby elevates cardiac output in heart failure. In some patients ACE inhibitors also exert a mild diuretic action, presumably by lowering the angiotensin II–stimulated production of aldosterone.[163-165]

Angiotensin II may also play a direct role in modifying myocardial structure and function.[166] Angiotensin II has been shown to cause cellular hypertrophy, the induction of fetal gene programs, and apoptosis in cultured cardiac myocytes (Fig. 21–30).[167] Angiotensin II also appears to play a role in mediating the apoptotic effect of mechanical strain on the myocardium and is a potent stimulator of several signaling pathways, including those involved in oxidative stress, inflammation, and the regulation of the ECM.[168]

TISSUE RENIN-ANGIOTENSIN SYSTEM. The major portion (90 to 99 percent) of ACE in the body is found in tissues, and the remaining 1 to 10 percent circulates. All of

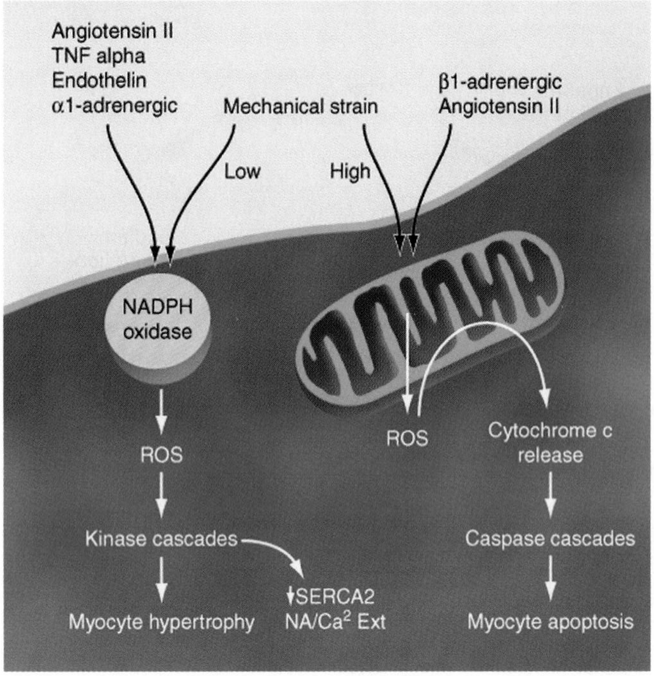

FIGURE 21–30 Schematic of the effects of reactive oxygen species (ROS) on myocyte phenotype. Through activation of kinase cascades such as mitogen activated protein kinase (MAPK), ROS can induce myocyte hypertrophy. ROS can also alter the activity and expression of Ca^{2+}-handling proteins including SERCA2 and the Na^+/Ca^{2+} exchanger to alter myocardial contractility. Mitochondrial ROS may be particularly prone to induce apoptosis by stimulating the mitochondrial release of cytochrome *c*, which is necessary for the activation of caspase cascades. NADPH = reduced nicotinamide adenine dinucleotide phosphate; TNF = tumor necrosis factor. (From Mann DL [ed]: Heart failure: A Companion to Braunwald's Heart Disease. Philadelphia, Elsevier, 2004. Adapted from Sawyer DB, Siwik DA, Xiao L, et al: Role of oxidative stress in myocardial hypertrophy and failure. J Mol Cell Cardiol 34:379, 2002.)

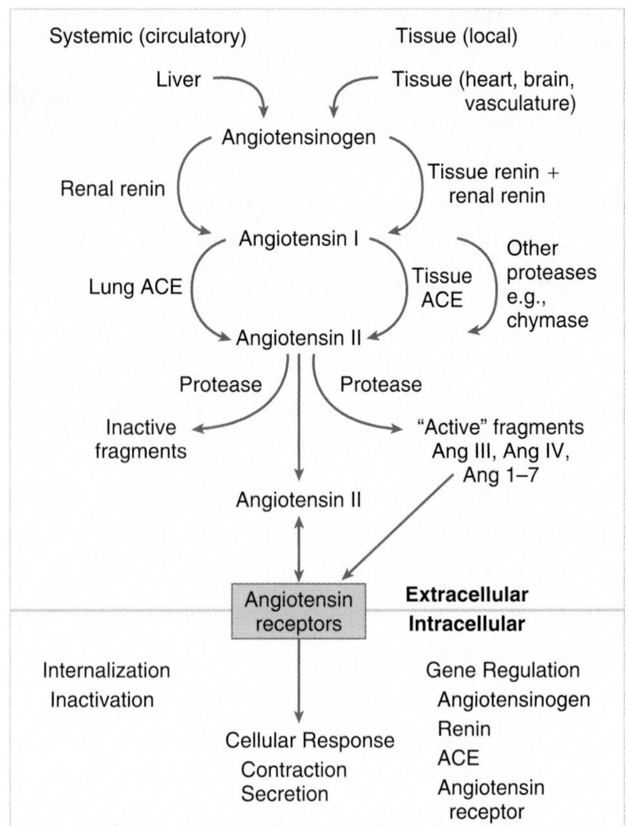

FIGURE 21–31 The systemic and tissue components of the renin-angiotensin system. Several tissues, including myocardium, vasculature, kidney, and brain, have the capacity to generate angiotensin II independent of the circulating renin-angiotensin system. Angiotensin II produced at the tissue level may play an important role in the pathophysiology of heart failure. ACE = angiotensin-converting enzyme. (Modified from Timmermans PB, Wong PC, Chiu AT, et al: Angiotensin II receptors and angiotensin II receptor antagonists. Pharmacol Rev 45:205, 1993.)

the necessary components of the renin-angiotensin system (RAS) (Fig. 21–31) are likewise present in several organs and tissues, including the vasculature, heart, and kidneys. In myocardium from animals with experimental myocardial hypertrophy or failure, there is increased expression of ACE and angiotensinogen, the substrate for angiotensin I production by renin. It has been suggested that the tissue RAS may be activated during compensated heart failure at a time when activity of the circulating system can be relatively normal (Fig. 21–32). The tissue production of angiotensin II may also occur by a pathway not dependent on ACE (the chymase pathway). This pathway may be of major importance in the myocardium, particularly when the levels of renin and angiotensin I are increased by the use of ACE inhibitors. The density of ACE binding sites is increased in myocardium from patients with end-stage heart failure related to idiopathic cardiomyopathy.[169]

ANGIOTENSIN RECEPTORS. The predominant angiotensin receptor in the vasculature is the angiotensin$_1$ subtype (AT_1). Both AT_1 and AT_2 receptor subtypes are present in human myocardium with the AT_2 receptor predominating in a ratio of 2:1. The number of AT_1 and AT_2 receptors is normal in patients with moderate heart failure, but both are downregulated in patients with end-stage heart failure. Downregulation of the AT_1 subtype has been observed in myocardium from patients with both ischemic and idiopathic dilated cardiomyopathy and is associated with a decrease in the mRNA level for the receptor.[9]

Aldosterone

Beyond its action to increase renal sodium retention, aldosterone may exert direct adverse effects on both the vascula-

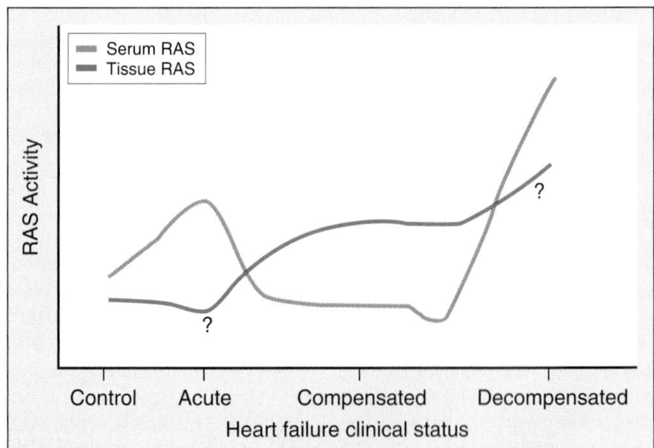

FIGURE 21–32 Relative roles of the circulating and tissue renin-angiotensin systems (RASs) postulated in patients with heart failure. The tissue system may have alternative pathways for the production of angiotensin II that do not depend on converting enzyme (e.g., chymase) and that therefore are not suppressed by converting enzyme inhibitors. It has been proposed that activation of the tissue RAS may follow a different time course than that of the circulating system, particularly during the compensated phase of heart failure when the circulating RAS may be relatively quiescent and during treatment with converting enzyme inhibitors that may increase the activity of the tissue system by elevating circulating renin levels. (Modified from Dzau VJ: Tissue renin-angiotensin system in myocardial hypertrophy and failure. Arch Intern Med 153:937, 1993. Copyright 1993, American Medical Association.)

ture and myocardium (Fig. 21–33) leading to hypertrophy and fibrosis and thereby contribute to reduced vascular compliance and ventricular diastolic dysfunction.[170] These direct effects on the cardiovascular system appear to involve inflammation and oxidative stress in target tissues.[171] Transgenic mice with a selective increase in activation of the aldosterone receptors in cardiac myocytes develop myocardial hypertrophy and interstitial fibrosis leading to progressive left ventricular dilation, heart failure, and death: All of these events are prevented by treatment with the aldosterone receptor antagonist eplerenone.[172]

The importance of aldosterone, independent of angiotensin II, was demonstrated by two large clinical trials. The randomized aldactone evaluation study (RALES) trial found that low-dose spironolactone increased the survival of patients with chronic heart failure related to systolic dysfunction.[173] This effect could not be attributed to changes in volume or electrolyte status. The EPlerenone's neuroHormonal Efficacy and SUrvival Study (EPHESUS) trial likewise found that early administration of the selective aldosterone receptor antagonist eplerenone improved survival after myocardial infarction.[174]

ARGININE VASOPRESSIN

Arginine vasopressin (AVP) is a pituitary hormone that plays a central role in the regulation of free water clearance and plasma osmolality (see Fig. 21-24). Circulating AVP is elevated in many patients with heart failure, even after correction for plasma osmolality. Patients with acute heart failure secondary to massive myocardial infarction may have particularly elevated levels, which are usually associated with elevated concentrations of catecholamines and renin. The plasma AVP concentration was significantly elevated in asymptomatic patients in the prevention arm of the SOLVD study and was elevated further in patients with symptomatic heart failure.[162] Control of circulating AVP concentration is abnormal in patients with heart failure who fail to show the normal reduction of AVP with a reduction of osmolality. This abnormal control may contribute to their inadequate ability to excrete free water and hence to the plasma hypoosmolarity in some patients with heart failure. Decreased sensitivity of atrial stretch receptors, which normally inhibit AVP release with atrial distention, may contribute to the elevation of circulating AVP. In addition, patients with heart failure exhibit failure of the normal suppression of AVP after administration of ethanol.

Two types of AVP receptors (V_1 and V_2) have been identified in a variety of tissues. In dogs with pacing-induced heart failure, the selective inhibition of V_1 receptors increased cardiac output without affecting electrolytes or hormone levels.[175] In contrast, inhibition of V_2 receptors increased serum sodium concentration, plasma renin activity, and plasma AVP levels but did not affect hemodynamics. When the two inhibitors were combined, the hemodynamic effects were potentiated. These results suggest that in heart failure, in addition to regulating free water clearance through the V_2 receptor, AVP may contribute to systemic vasoconstriction through the V_1 receptor.

Natriuretic Peptides

Three natriuretic peptides—ANP, BNP, and C-natriuretic peptide (CNP)—have been identified. ANP is stored mainly in the right atrium and is released in response to an increase in atrial distending pressure. This peptide causes vasodilation and natriuresis and counteracts the water-retaining effects of the adrenergic, renin-angiotensin-aldosterone, and AVP systems. BNP is stored mainly in cardiac ventricular myocardium and may be responsive—albeit less so than ANP—to changes in ventricular filling pressures. BNP has a high level of homology with ANP at the structural level and, like ANP, causes natriuresis and vasodilation. CNP is located primarily in the vasculature. Although the physiological role of CNP is not yet clarified, it appears to play an important regulatory role in juxtaposition to the RAS system.

At least three receptors for natriuretic peptides (A, B, and C) have been identified. The A and B receptors mediate the vasodilatory and natriuretic effects of the peptides. The C-type receptor appears to act primarily as a clearance receptor, which, along with neutral endopeptidase, regulates available levels of the peptides.

Circulating levels of both ANP and BNP are elevated in the plasma of patients with heart failure.[176] In normal human hearts, ANP predominates in the atria, where there is also a low level of expression of BNP and CNP. In patients with heart failure, the atrial content of ANP is unchanged and the contents of BNP and CNP increase 10-fold and 2- to 3-fold, respectively.[176] In the SOLVD study, the level of plasma ANP was elevated even in asymptomatic patients and was further elevated in patients with symptoms.[162] Although the atrial peptides are present only in very low levels in normal ventricular myocardium, in patients with heart failure all three peptides are markedly elevated, and ventricular production contributes significantly to the circulating levels.[177] The secretion of ANP and BNP appears to be regulated mainly by wall tension. The N-terminal of the ANP free hormone (N-terminal pro-ANP) has a longer half-life and greater stability than ANP and has been shown to be a powerful and independent predictor of cardiovascular mortality and the development of heart failure. ANP levels become normal after cardiac transplantation.

Because plasma BNP release is less affected by atrial filling pressures, it provides a better reflection of myocardial disease. Plasma BNP has been shown to be useful in distinguishing cardiac from noncardiac causes of dyspnea[178] and provides prognostic information in patients with chronic heart failure[179] and following acute coronary syndromes.[180] Changes in plasma BNP may also reflect beneficial effects of drug therapy.[181] As with ANP, the N-terminal peptide frag-

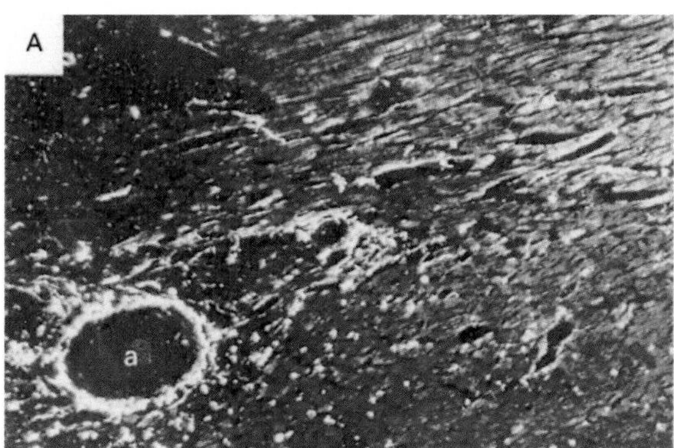

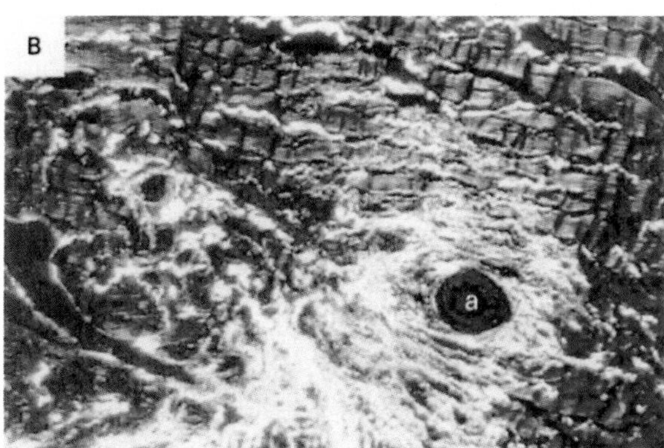

FIGURE 21–33 Coronary vascular remodeling caused by hyperaldosteronism in rats. **A,** A section from a normal heart with a normal intramural coronary artery (a) surrounded by yellow-stained fibrillar collagen. A small amount of collagen is also present between the muscle fibers. **B,** A section from the heart of a rat given aldosterone (plus salt) shows marked perivascular fibrosis of coronary vessels (a) and the contiguous interstitial space between muscle fibers. (Sirius red staining and polarized light, 40×). (From Weber KT: Aldosterone in congestive heart failure. N Engl J Med 345:1689, 2001.)

ment (N-terminal pro-BNP), which is cleaved to form the active hormone, may be more stable than BNP and thus provide more reliable information.

Studies using an ANP receptor antagonist in dogs with pacing-induced heart failure showed that despite attenuated hemodynamic and renal effects, the peptide continues to exert an important suppressive effect on the activity of the RAS and NE levels.[182] One approach that attempts to capitalize on the beneficial effects of the natriuretic peptides is to inhibit their degradation through the use of neutral endopeptidase inhibitors. The infusion of the endopeptidase inhibitor candoxatrilat into patients with heart failure mimics the action of infused ANP; it causes a reduction in left- and right-sided filling pressures associated with suppression of plasma NE levels and a transient reduction in plasma vasopressin, aldosterone, and renin activity. Likewise, the infusion of a human BNP exerts beneficial hemodynamic effects characterized by decreases in arterial and venous pressures, an increase in cardiac output, and suppression of neurohormonal activation,[183] and it has been approved by the Food and Drug Administration for the short-term treatment of patients with decompensated heart failure (see Chap. 23). In addition to the beneficial effect of natriuretic peptides on neurohormones, renal function, and hemodynamics, there is evidence that the natriuretic peptides may directly inhibit myocyte and vascular smooth muscle hypertrophy and interstitial fibrosis.

Natriuretic peptides are degraded by neutral endopeptidase. Vasopeptidase inhibitors such as omapatrilat inhibit both neutral endopeptidase and ACE and thereby combine the effects of ACE inhibition with increased levels of natriuretic peptides chronically. Although some early trials suggested that neutral endopeptidase inhibition would have a greater benefit than ACE inhibition, more recent trials have found the two classes of drug to exert similar effects on survival.[184]

ENDOTHELIN AND OTHER PEPTIDES

Endothelin is a potent peptide vasoconstrictor released by endothelial cells throughout the circulation. Like angiotensin II, endothelin can also be synthesized and released by a variety of other cell types such as cardiac myocytes. Three endothelin peptides (endothelin-1, endothelin-2, and endothelin-3), all of which are potent constrictors, have been identified.[185] At least two subtypes of endothelin receptors (types A and B) have been identified in human myocardium.[186]

The release of endothelin from endothelial cells in vitro can be enhanced by several vasoactive agents (e.g., NE, angiotensin II, thrombin) and cytokines (e.g., TGF-β and IL-1β). Several reports have documented an increase in circulating levels of endothelin-1 in patients with heart failure.[187] Plasma endothelin concentration correlates directly with pulmonary artery pressure, pulmonary vascular resistance, and the ratio of pulmonary to systemic vascular resistance. This has led to the suggestion that endothelin plays a pathophysiological role in mediating pulmonary hypertension in patients with heart failure. In normal subjects, plasma endothelin levels rise with orthostatic stress. However, in patients with heart failure, endothelin levels are already elevated and show no further increase with orthostatic stress, similar to the pattern of response seen with a variety of other vasoconstrictor substances, including angiotensin II and NE. Plasma endothelin levels have been shown to be increased in patients with acute myocardial infarction and to correlate with the Killip class in these patients.

Antagonists of endothelin receptors have been used to demonstrate the physiological effects of endothelin. When administered to rats with heart failure after myocardial infarction, the endothelin antagonist bosentan, which blocks both endothelin$_A$ and endothelin$_B$ receptors, decreased arterial pressure and exerted an effect additive to that of an ACE inhibitor.[188] Endothelin causes hypertrophy of cardiac myocytes in vitro, and the endothelin$_A$ receptor antagonist BQ123 inhibited myocardial hypertrophy in rats with pressure overload–induced hypertrophy caused by aortic banding. In rats with myocardial infarction, chronic administration of endothelin antagonists resulted in a reduction in left ventricular chamber remodeling and enlargement; it also improved hemodynamic function and improved survival.[189] This beneficial effect of endothelin receptor blockade on left ventricular dilation is associated with inhibition of MMPs, which may be involved in chamber dilation.[190] Likewise, endothelin$_A$ receptor blockade improved hemodynamic function in pigs with rapid pacing-induced heart failure.[191] These observations suggest that endothelin receptor antagonists may be of value in both the acute and chronic treatment of patients with heart failure.[192] Although administration of endothelin antagonists to patients has been shown to improve hemodynamic function,[193,194] long-term clinical beneficial effects on disease progression and survival have not been shown.

Several other peptides, including acidic fibroblast growth factor, basic fibroblast growth factor, TGF-β1, and platelet-derived growth factor, have been shown to affect the growth and phenotype of cardiac myocytes or fibroblasts in vitro. The expression of these and other peptides is increased in myocardium after myocardial infarction[195] or with hemodynamic overload, suggesting that they play a role in the orchestration of myocardial remodeling.

INFLAMMATORY CYTOKINES, INCLUDING TNF-α. Inflammatory cytokines, including TNF-α and IL-1β, may play an important role in the pathogenesis of myocardial failure.[196,197] In vitro, these and other inflammatory cytokines can regulate growth and gene expression in cardiac myocytes and other cells present in the myocardium. The circulating levels of proinflammatory cytokines including TNF-α and interleukin-6 (IL-6) are increased in patients with heart failure. The level of TNF-α correlated with depressed heart rate variability, an index of integrated autonomic nervous system function.[198] Conversely, the plasma concentrations of antiinflammatory cytokines such as IL-10 are reduced in patients with heart failure and are decreased more in patients with severe than with mild disease.[199] The failing myocardium, itself, may be a source of inflammatory cytokines, which might thus be present in high concentrations locally.[200]

Inflammatory cytokines have protean effects on the myocardium (Table 21–5). TNF-α can induce immediate myocardial dysfunction and has been shown to attenuate intracellular calcium transients in vitro.[201] In cultured cardiac myocytes, TNF-α and IL-1β can stimulate hypertrophy and

TABLE 21–5 Inflammatory Mediators

Cardiac Pathophysiologic Conditions Associated with Inflammatory Mediators
Acute viral myocarditis
Cardiac allograft rejection
Myocardial infarction
Unstable angina
Myocardial reperfusion injury
Hypertrophic cardiomyopathy*
Heart failure*
Cardiopulmonary bypass*
Magnesium deficiency*
Pressure overload*
Effects of Inflammatory Mediators on Left Ventricular Remodeling
Alterations in the biology of the myocyte
Myocyte hypertrophy
Contractile abnormalities
Fetal gene expression
Alteration in the extracellular matrix
MMP activation
Degradation of the matrix
Fibrosis
Progressive myocyte loss
Necrosis
Apoptosis

MMP = matrix metalloproteinase.

From Mann DL: Activation of inflammatory mediators in heart failure. *In* Mann DL (ed): Heart Failure. Philadelphia, Elsevier, 2004, pp 159, 164.

*Indicates conditions not traditionally associated with immunologiclly mediated inflammation.

reexpression of a fetal gene program[202] and can cause apoptosis,[203] which may be mediated, in part, by NO.[53] The chronic systemic infusion of TNF-α in rats resulted in left ventricular failure,[204] and mice that overexpressed TNF-α in the myocardium developed a dilated cardiomyopathy that was associated with increased myocyte apoptosis. Although pilot clinical trials with soluble TNF-α receptors that reduce the level of TNF-α available to the tissues have suggested that this may a feasible form of therapy for patients,[205] the results of a large clinical trial failed to demonstrate benefit with regard to hospitalization and survival.[206] The results of another trial that used infliximab, an antibody directed against TNF-α, found an increase in hospitalizations and mortality.[207] Likewise, observations from the Food and Drug Administration MedWatch program have suggested that the use of anti-TNF-α therapy may be associated with the new onset of heart failure.[208] It remains to be determined whether this lack of benefit is a reflection of the basic premise, the mode of drug action, or the complexity of the immune response. Other drugs that decrease plasma TNF-α levels, thalidomide[209] and pentoxifylline,[210] have shown promise in small clinical trials.

Nitric Oxide

At least two of the three known isoforms of nitric oxide synthase (NOS), termed NOS1, NOS2, and NOS3, are expressed in human myocardium. NOS2 is an inducible isoform that is not normally expressed in the myocardium but is synthesized de novo in response to inflammatory cytokines, thereby causing high levels of NO production. The expression and activity of NOS2 are increased in myocardium from animals with experimental heart failure[211] and patients with severe heart failure,[211] possibly as a result of stimulation by inflammatory cytokines.

The actions of NO on the myocardium are complex, involving both short-term alterations in function and energetics and longer term effects on structure.[212,213] It has been shown that NO mediates the inhibitory effect of inflammatory cytokines on the contractile response to beta-adrenergic stimulation in cardiac myocytes and myocardium by the induction of NOS2.[212-214] In normal human subjects, intracoronary infusion of nitroprusside, an NO donor, improved left ventricular distensibility,[215] whereas inhibition of NO synthesis by intracoronary infusion of an NOS inhibitor potentiated the positive inotropic response to dobutamine in patients with left ventricular dysfunction.[216] NO also appears to play a role in the regulation of myocardial energetics.[217] In addition to these short-term effects on myocardial function, NO may lead to longer term alterations in myocardial structure and function through its direct actions on myocytes to cause apoptosis[53,218] and modulate the response to hypertrophic stimuli such as NE and angiotensin. In transgenic mice deficient in NOS2, left ventricular remodeling was ameliorated and survival improved after myocardial infarction,[219] and beta-adrenergic responsiveness was improved in mice with dilated cardiomyopathy related to cardiac-specific overexpression of TNF-α.[213] Conversely, overexpression of NOS3 resulted in improved remodeling after myocardial infarction.[220] These contrasting effects of NOS2 (inducible) and NOS3 (endothelial) may reflect the differences in amount of NO produced, which is much higher with NOS2.

Oxidative Stress

There is evidence that oxidative stress is increased both systemically and in the myocardium of patients with heart failure.[221] Increased oxidative stress may be due to reduced antioxidant capacity or the increased production of reactive oxygen species, which may be a consequence of mechanical strain on the myocardium or stimulation by neurohormones and inflammatory cytokines. Possible sources of increased production of reactive oxygen species include the mitochondria, xanthine oxidase, and NADPH oxidase.[222] Reactive oxygen species can stimulate myocyte hypertrophy (see Fig. 21–30), reexpression of fetal gene programs, and apoptosis in cardiac myocytes in culture.[223] Mice with knockout of the antioxidant enzyme manganese superoxide dismutase (MnSOD) developed dilated cardiomyopathy and died at a young age.[224] Conversely, in animal models of hemodynamic overload–induced remodeling and failure, treatment with antioxidants prevented the progression to myocardial failure.[224-226] Although these observations have led to the suggestion that antioxidants might be of therapeutic value in patients, clinical trials to test this thesis are not available.

REFERENCES

Short-Term Adaptive Mechanisms

1. Hunt SA, Baker, DW, Chin ML, et al: Report of the ACC/AHA Guidelines for the Evaluation and Management of Chronic Heart Failure in the Adult. Circulation 104:2996, 2001.
2. Houser SR, Margulies KB: Is depressed myocyte contractility centrally involved in heart failure? Circ Res 92:350, 2003.
3. Hasenfuss G, Pieske B: Calcium cycling in congestive heart failure. J Mol Cell Cardiol 34:951, 2002.
4. Braunwald E, Ross J Jr, Sonnenblick EH: Mechanisms of Contraction of the Normal and Failing Heart. 2nd ed. Boston, Little, Brown, 1976, p 417.
5. Francis GS: Pathophysiology of chronic heart failure. Am J Med 110:37S, 2001.
6. Braunwald E, Bristow MR: Congestive heart failure: Fifty years of progress. Circulation 102:IV-14, 2000.
7. Konstam MA, Mann DL: Contemporary medical options for treating patients with heart failure. Circulation 105:2244, 2002.
8. Alpert NR, Mulieri LA, Warshaw D: The failing human heart. Cardiovasc Res 54:1, 2002.
9. Katz AM: Heart Failure. Philadelphia, Lippincott Williams & Wilkins, 2000.
10. Floras JS: Alterations in the sympathetic and parasympathetic nervous system in heart failure. *In* Mann DL (ed): Heart Failure: A Companion to Braunwald's Heart Disease: A Textbook of Cardiovascular Medicine. Philadelphia, WB Saunders, 2004, pp 247-278.
11. Leier CV, Brinkley PF, Cody RJ: Alpha adrenergic component of the sympathetic nervous system in congestive heart failure. Circulation 82:168, 1990.
12. Zelis R, Mason DT, Braunwald E: A comparison of the effects of vasodilator stimuli on peripheral resistance vessels in normal subjects and in patients with congestive heart failure. J Clin Invest 47:960, 1968.
13. Zelis R, Mason DT, Braunwald E: Partition of blood flow to the cutaneous and muscular beds of the forearm at rest and during leg exercise in normal subjects and in patients with heart failure. Circ Res 24:799, 1969.
14. Mancini DM, Coyle E, Coggan A, et al: Contribution of intrinsic skeletal muscle changes to ^{31}P NMR skeletal muscle metabolic abnormalities in patients with chronic heart failure. Circulation 80:1338, 1989.
15. Leier CV, Binkley PF, Cody RJ: Alpha-adrenergic component of the sympathetic nervous system in congestive heart failure. Circulation 82:168, 1990.
16. Higgins CB, Vatner SF, Millard RW, et al: Alterations in regional hemodynamics in experimental heart failure in conscious dogs. Trans Assoc Am Physicians 85:267, 1972.
17. Newby DE, Goodfield NE, Flapan AD, et al: Regulation of peripheral vascular tone in patients with heart failure: Contribution of angiotensin II. Heart 80:134, 1998.
18. Muders F, Luchner A, Friedrich EB, et al: Modulation of renal blood flow by endogenous endothelin-1 in conscious rabbits with left ventricular dysfunction. Am J Hypertens 12:835, 1999.
19. Wilson JR, Mancini DM: Factors contributing to the exercise limitation of heart failure. J Am Coll Cardiol 22(Suppl A):93a, 1993.
20. Hirooka Y, Imaizumi T, Tagawa T, et al: Effects of L-arginine on impaired acetylcholine-induced and ischemic vasodilation of the forearm in patients with heart failure. Circulation 90:658, 1994.
21. Hambrecht R, Fiehn E, Weigl C, et al: Regular physical exercise corrects endothelial dysfunction and improves exercise capacity in patients with chronic heart failure. Circulation 98:2709, 1998.
22. Bersin RM, Kwasman M, Lau D, et al: Importance of oxygen-haemoglobin binding to oxygen transport in congestive heart failure. Br Heart J 70:443, 1993.

Chronic Myocardial Remodeling

23. Meerson FZ: The myocardium in hyperfunction, hypertrophy, and heart failure. Circ Res 25(Suppl 2):1, 1969.
24. Cohn JN, Ferrari R, Sharpe N: Cardiac remodeling—Concepts and clinical implications: A consensus paper from an international forum on cardiac remodeling. J Am Coll Cardiol 35:569, 2000.
25. Grossman W, Jones D, McLaurin LP: Wall stress and patterns of hypertrophy in the human left ventricle. J Clin Invest 56:56, 1975.
26. Anversa P, Kajstura J: Ventricular myocytes are not terminally differentiated in the adult mammalian heart. Circ Res 83:1, 1998.
27. Calderone A, Takahashi N, Izzo NJ Jr, et al: Pressure- and volume-induced left ventricular hypertrophies are associated with distinct myocyte phenotypes and differential induction of peptide growth factor mRNAs. Circulation 92:2385, 1995.

28. Ross J Jr: Afterload mismatch and preload reserve: A conceptual framework for the analysis of ventricular function. Prog Cardiovasc Dis 18:255, 1976.
29. Gerdes AM: Cardiac myocyte remodeling in hypertrophy and progression to failure. J Card Fail 8:S264, 2002.
30. Spinale FG: Matrix metalloproteinases: Regulation and dysregulation in the failing heart. Circ Res 90:520, 2002.
31. Esposite G, Rapacciuolo A, Naga PSV, et al: Genetic alterations that inhibit in vivo pressure-overload hypertrophy prevent cardiac dysfunction despite increased wall stress. Circulation 105:85, 2002.
32. Spann JF Jr, Buccino RA, Sonnenblick EH, Braunwald E: Contractile state of cardiac muscle obtained from cats with experimentally produced ventricular hypertrophy and heart failure. Circ Res 21:341, 1987.
33. Pieske B, Maier LS, Piacentino V 3rd, et al: Rate dependence of $[Na^+]_i$ contractility in nonfailing and failing human myocardium. Circulation 106:447, 2002.
34. Piacentino V III, Weber CR, Chen X, et al: Cellular basis of abnormal calcium transients of failing human ventricular myocytes. Circ Res 92:651, 2003.
35. Lefkowitz RJ, Rockman HA, Koch WJ: Catecholamines, cardiac β adrenergic receptors, and heart failure. Circulation 101:1634, 2000.
36. Spann JF Jr, Covell JW, Eckberg DL et al: Contractile performance of the hypertrophied and chronically failing cat ventricle. Am J Physiol 223:1150, 1972.
37. Aoyagi T, Fujii AM, Flanagan MF, et al: Transition from compensated hypertrophy to intrinsic myocardial dysfunction during development of left ventricular pressure-overload hypertrophy in conscious sheep: Systolic dysfunction precedes diastolic dysfunction. Circulation 88:2415, 1993.
38. Palmon LC, Reichek N, Yeon SB, et al: Intramural myocardial shortening in hypertensive left ventricular hypertrophy with normal pump function. Circulation 89:122, 1994.

Molecular Mechanisms of Myocardial Remodeling and Failure

39. Monte FD, Hajjar RJ: Targeting calcium cycling proteins in heart failure through gene transfer. J Physiol (Lond) 546:49, 2003.
40. Sawyer DB, Colucci WS: Molecular and cellular events in myocardial hypertrophy and failure. *In* Colucci WS (ed): Atlas of Heart Failure: Cardiac Function and Dysfunction. 3rd ed. Philadelphia, Current Medicine, 2002, pp 65-85.
41. Maytin M, Colucci WS: Molecular and cellular mechanisms of myocardial remodeling. J Nucl Cardiol 9:319, 2002.
42. Givertz MM, Colucci WS: New targets for heart-failure therapy: Endothelin, inflammatory cytokines, and oxidative stress. Lancet 352(Suppl 1):SI34, 1998.
43. Hunter JJ, Chien KR: Signaling pathways for cardiac hypertrophy and failure. N Engl J Med 341:1276, 1999.
44. Sawyer DB, Siwik DA, Xiao L, et al: Role of oxidative stress in myocardial hypertrophy and failure. J Mol Cell Cardiol 34:379, 2002.
45. Dorn GW, Mann DL: Signaling pathways involved in left ventricular remodeling: Summation. J Card Fail 8:S387, 2002.
46. Kang PM, Yue P, Izumo S: New insights into the role of apoptosis in cardiovascular disease. Circ J 66:1, 2002.
47. Olivetti G, Abbi R, Quaini F, et al: Apoptosis in the failing human heart. N Engl J Med 336:1131, 1997.
48. Kajstura J, Liu Y, Baldini A, et al: Coronary artery constriction in rats: Necrotic and apoptotic myocyte death. Am J Cardiol 82(5A):30K, 1998.
49. Communal C, Singh K, Pimentel DR, Colucci WS: Norepinephrine stimulates apoptosis in adult rat ventricular myocytes by activation of the β-adrenergic pathway. Circulation 98:1329, 1998.
50. Iwai-Kanai E, Hasegawa K, Araki M, et al: Alpha- and beta-adrenergic pathways differentially regulate cell type–specific apoptosis in rat cardiac myocytes. Circulation 100:305, 1999.
51. Leri A, Claudio PP, Li Q, et al: Stretch-mediated release of angiotensin II induces myocyte apoptosis by activating p53 that enhances the local renin-angiotensin system and decreases the Bcl-2-to-Bax protein ratio in the cell. J Clin Invest 101:1326, 1998.
52. Siwik DA, Tzortzis JD, Pimental DR, et al: Inhibition of copper-zinc superoxide dismutase induces cell growth, hypertrophic phenotype, and apoptosis in neonatal rat cardiac myocytes in vitro. Circ Res 85:147, 1999.
53. Ing DJ, Zang J, Dzau VJ, et al: Modulation of cytokine-induced cardiac myocyte apoptosis by nitric oxide, Bak, and Bcl-x. Circ Res 84:21, 1999.
54. Pimentel DR, Amin JK, Xiao L, et al: Reactive oxygen species mediate amplitude-dependent hypertrophic and apoptotic responses to mechanical stretch in cardiac myocytes. Circ Res 89:453, 2001.
55. Pollack M, Phaneuf S, Dirks A, Leeuwenburgh C: The role of apoptosis in the normal aging brain, skeletal muscle, and heart. Ann NY Acad Sci 959:93, 2002.
56. Olivetti G, Melissari M, Capasso JM, Anversa B: Cardiomyopathy of the aging human heart: Myocyte loss and reactive cellular hypertrophy. Circ Res 68:1560, 1991.

Role of Calcium in Excitation-Contraction Coupling

57. Beuckelmann DJ, Nabauer M, Erdmann E: Intracellular calcium handling in isolated ventricular myocytes from patients with terminal heart failure. Circulation 85:1046, 1992.
58. Hasenfuss G, Mulieri LA, Leavitt BJ, et al: Alteration of contractile function and excitation-contraction coupling in dilated cardiomyopathy. Circ Res 70:1225, 1992.
59. Shorofsky SR, Aggarwal R, Corretti M, et al: Cellular mechanisms of altered contractility in the hypertrophied heart: Big hearts, big sparks. Circ Res 84:424, 1999.
60. Winslow RL, Rice J, Jafri S, et al: Mechanisms of altered excitation-contraction coupling in canine tachycardia-induced heart failure: II. Model studies. Circ Res 84:571, 1999.
61. Margulies KB, Houser SR: Myocyte abnormalities in human heart failure. *In* Mann DL (ed): Heart Failure: A Companion to Braunwald's Heart Disease: A Textbook of Cardiovascular Medicine. Philadelphia, WB Saunders, 2004, pp 41-56.
62. Flesch M, Schwinger RH, Schnabel P, et al: Sarcoplasmic reticulum Ca^{2+} ATPase and phospholamban mRNA and protein levels in end-stage heart failure due to ischemic or dilated cardiomyopathy. J Mol Med 74:321, 1996.
63. Frank K, Bolck B, Bavendiek U, Schwinger RH: Frequency dependent force generation correlates with sarcoplasmic calcium ATPase activity in human myocardium. Basic Res Cardiol 93:405, 1998.
64. Hobai IA, O'Rourke B: Decreased sarcoplasmic reticulum calcium content is responsible for defective excitation-contraction coupling in canine heart failure. Circulation 103:1577, 2001.
65. Li S, Margulies KB, Cheng H, Houser SR: Calcium current and calcium transients are depressed in failing human ventricular myocytes and recover in patients supported with left ventricular assist devices [abstract]. Circulation 100:160, 1999.
66. Meyer M, Bluhm WF, He H, et al: Phospholamban-to-SERCA2 ratio controls the force-frequency relationship. Am J Physiol 276:H779, 1999.
67. Giordano FJ, He H, McDonough P, et al: Adenovirus-mediated gene transfer reconstitutes depressed sarcoplasmic reticulum Ca^{2+}-ATPase levels and shortens prolonged cardiac myocyte Ca^{2+} transients. Circulation 96:400, 1997.
68. He H, Giordano FJ, Hilal-Dandan R, et al: Overexpression of the rat sarcoplasmic reticulum Ca^{2+} ATPase gene in the heart of transgenic mice accelerates calcium transients and cardiac relaxation. J Clin Invest 100:380, 1997.
69. Studer R, Reinecke H, Bilger J, et al: Gene expression of the cardiac Na^+-Ca^{2+} exchanger in end-stage human heart failure. Circ Res 75:443, 1994.
70. Weber CR, Piacentino V III, Margulies KB, et al: Calcium influx via I(NCX) is favored in failing human ventricular myocytes. Ann NY Acad Sci 976:478, 2002.
71. Brillantes A-M, Allen P, Takahasi T, et al: Differences in cardiac calcium release channel (ryanodine receptor) expression in myocardium from patients with end-stage heart failure caused by ischemic versus dilated cardiomyopathy. Circ Res 71:18, 1992.
72. Schumacher C, Konigs B, Sigmund M, et al: The ryanodine binding sarcoplasmic reticulum calcium release channel in nonfailing and in failing human myocardium. Naunyn Schmiedebergs Arch Pharmacol 353:80, 1995.
73. Marks AR, Reiken S, Marx SO: Progression of heart failure: Is protein kinase a hyperphosphorylation of the ryanodine receptor a contributing factor? Circulation 105:272, 2002.
74. Prestle J, Janssen PM, Janssen AP, et al: Overexpression of FK506-binding protein FKBP12.6 in cardiomyocytes reduces ryanodine receptor-mediated Ca^{2+} leak from the sarcoplasmic reticulum and increased contractility. Circ Res 88:188, 2001.
75. Marx SO, Marks AR. Regulation of the ryanodine receptor in heart failure. Basic Res Cardiol 97(Suppl 1):I49, 2002.
76. Reiken S, Wehrens XH, Vest JA, et al: Beta-blockers restore calcium release channel function and improve cardiac muscle performance in human heart failure. Circulation 107:2459, 2003.
77. Chen X, Piacentino V III, Furukawa S, et al: L-type Ca^{2+} channel density and regulation are altered in failing human ventricular myocytes and recover after support with mechanical assist devices. Circ Res 91:517, 2002.

Reduction of Myosin ATPase Activity

78. Izumo S, Pu WT: The molecular basis of heart failure. *In* Mann DL (ed): Heart Failure: A Companion to Braunwald's Heart Disease: A Textbook of Cardiovascular Medicine. Philadelphia, Saunders, 2004, pp 10-40.
79. Solaro RJ, Powers FM, Gao L, Gwathmey JK: Control of myofilament activation in heart failure. Circulation 87:VII-38, 1993.
80. Abraham WT, Gilbert EM, Lowes BD, et al: Coordinate changes in myosin heavy chain isoform gene expression are selectively associated with alterations in dilated cardiomyopathy phenotype. Mol Med 8:750, 2002.
81. Nakao K, Minobe W, Roden R, et al: Myosin heavy chain gene expression in human heart failure. J Clin Invest 100:2362, 1997.
82. Lowes BD, Minobe W, Abraham WT, et al: Changes in gene expression in the intact human heart: Downregulation of alpha myosin heavy chain in hypertrophied, failing ventricular myocardium. J Clin Invest 100:2315, 1997.
83. Lowes BD, Gilbert EM, Abraham WT, et al: Myocardial gene expression in dilated cardiomyopathy treated with beta-blocking agents. N Engl J Med 346:1357, 2002.
84. Solaro RJ, Rarick HM: Troponin and tropomyosin: Proteins that switch on and tune in the activity of cardiac myofilaments. Circ Res 83:471, 1998.
85. Anderson PA, Malouf NN, Oakeley AE, et al: Troponin T isoform expression in the normal and failing human left ventricle: A correlation with myofibrillar ATPase activity. Basic Res Cardiol 87:117, 1992.
86. Huang X, Pi Y, Lee KJ, et al: Cardiac troponin I gene knockout: A mouse model of myocardial troponin I deficiency. Circ Res 84:1, 1999.
87. Fatkin D, McConnell BK, Mudd JO, et al: An abnormal Ca^{2+} response in mutant sarcomere protein-mediated familial hypertrophic cardiomyopathy. J Clin Invest 106:1351, 2000.
88. Kamisago M, Sharman SD, DePalma SR, et al: Mutations in sarcomere protein genes as a cause of dilated cardiomyopathy. N Engl J Med 343:1688, 2000.
89. Gunasinghe SK, Spinale FG: Myocardial basis for heart failure: Role of cardiac interstitium. *In* Mann DL (ed): Heart Failure: A Companion to Braunwald's Heart Disease: A Textbook of Cardiovascular Medicine. Philadelphia, WB Saunders, 2004, pp 57-70.
90. Mann DL, Spinale FG: Activation of matrix metalloproteinases in the failing human heart: Breaking the tie that binds [editorial]. Circulation 98:1699, 1998.
91. Burlew BS, Weber KT: Cardiac fibrosis as a cause of diastolic dysfunction. Herz 27:92, 2002.
92. Thomas CV, Coker ML, Zellner JL, et al: Increased matrix metalloproteinase activity and selective upregulation in LV myocardium from patients with end-stage dilated cardiomyopathy. Circulation 97:1708, 1998.
93. Coker ML, Thomas CV, Clair MJ, et al: Myocardial matrix metalloproteinase activity and abundance with congestive heart failure. Am J Physiol 274:H1516, 1998.
94. Li YY, Feldman AM, Sun Y, McTiernan CF: Differential expression of tissue inhibitors of metalloproteinases in the failing human heart. Circulation 98:1728, 1998.

95. Spinale FG, Coker ML, Krombach SR, et al: Matrix metalloproteinase inhibition during the development of congestive heart failure: Effects on left ventricular dimensions and function. Circ Res 85:364, 1999.
96. Creemers EE, Davis JN, Parkhurst AM, et al: Deficiency of TIMP-1 exacerbates LV remodeling after myocardial infarction in mice. Am J Physiol 284:H364, 2003.
97. Ducharme A, Frantz S, Aikawa M, et al: Targeted deletion of matrix metalloproteinase-9 attenuates left ventricular enlargement and collagen accumulation after experimental myocardial infarction. J Clin Invest 106:55, 2000.
98. Conrad CH, Brooks WW, Hayes JA, et al: Myocardial fibrosis and stiffness with hypertrophy and heart failure in the spontaneously hypertensive rat. Circulation 91:161, 1995.
99. Boluyt MO, O'Neill L, Meredith AL, et al: Alterations in cardiac gene expression during the transition from stable hypertrophy to heart failure: Marked upregulation of genes encoding extracellular matrix components. Circ Res 75:23, 1994.
100. Brooks WW, Bing OH, Robinson KG, et al: Effect of angiotensin-converting enzyme inhibition on myocardial fibrosis and function in hypertrophied and failing myocardium from the spontaneously hypertensive rat. Circulation 96:4002, 1997.
101. Graham TP Jr, Ross J Jr, Covell JW: Myocardial oxygen consumption in acute experimental cardiac depression. Circ Res 21:123, 1967.
102. Ingwall JS: Energetic basis for heart failure. *In* Mann DL (ed): Heart Failure: A Companion to Braunwald's Heart Disease: A Textbook of Cardiovascular Medicine. Philadelphia, WB Saunders, 2004, pp 91-108.
103. Buchwald A, Till H, Unterberg C, et al: Alterations of the mitochondrial respiratory chain in human dilated cardiomyopathy. Eur Heart J 11:509, 1990.
104. Schulze K, Becker BF, Schauer R, Schultheiss HP: Antibodies to ADP-ATP carrier—An autoantigen in myocarditis and dilated cardiomyopathy impairs cardiac function. Circulation 81:959, 1990.
105. Ingwall JS: Is cardiac failure a consequence of decreased energy reserve? Circulation 87:VII-58, 1993.
106. Conway MA, Allis J, Ouwerkerk R, et al: Detection of low phosphocreatine to ATP ratio in failing hypertrophied human myocardium by ^{31}P magnetic resonance spectroscopy. Lancet 338:973, 1991.
107. Hardy CJ, Weiss RG, Bottomley PA, Gerstenblith G: Altered myocardial high-energy phosphate metabolites in patients with dilated cardiomyopathy. Am Heart J 122:795, 1991.
108. Bottomley PA: NMR spectroscopy of the human heart: The status and the challenges. Radiology 191:593, 1994.
109. Conway MA, Bottomley PA, Ouwerkerk R, et al: Mitral regurgitation: Impaired systolic function, eccentric hypertrophy, and increased severity are linked to lower phosphocreatine/ATP ratios in humans. Circulation 97:1716, 1998.
110. Neubauer S, Horn M, Cramer M, et al: Myocardial phosphocreatine-to-ATP ratio is a predictor of mortality in patients with dilated cardiomyopathy. Circulation 96:2190, 1997.
111. Liao R, Nascimben L, Friedrich J, et al: Decreased energy reserve in an animal model of dilated cardiomyopathy: Relationship to contractile performance. Circ Res 78:893, 1996.
112. Davis SV, Olichwier KK, Chakko SC: Reversible depression of myocardial performance in hypophosphatemia. Am J Med Sci 295:183, 1988.

Pathophysiology of Diastolic Heart Failure

113. Zile MR, Brutsaert DL: New concepts in diastolic dysfunction and diastolic heart failure: Part I: Diagnosis, prognosis, and measurements of diastolic function. Circulation 105:1387, 2002.
114. Zile MR, Brutsaert DL: New concepts in diastolic dysfunction and diastolic heart failure: Part II: Causal mechanisms and treatment. Circulation 105:1503, 2002.
115. Vasan RS, Larson MG, Benjamin EJ, et al: Congestive heart failure in subjects with normal versus reduced left ventricular ejection fraction: Prevalence and mortality in a population-based cohort. J Am Coll Cardiol 33:1948, 1999.
116. Zile MR, Baicu CF: Alterations in ventricular function: Diastolic heart failure. *In* Mann DL (ed): Heart Failure: A Companion to Braunwald's Heart Disease: A Textbook of Cardiovascular Medicine. Philadelphia, WB Saunders, 2004, pp 209-228.
117. Heyndrickx GR, Paulus WJ: Effect of asynchrony on left ventricular relaxation. Circulation 81(Suppl III):41, 1990.
118. Corin WJ, Murakami T, Monrad ES, et al: Left ventricular passive diastolic properties in chronic mitral regurgitation. Circulation 83:797, 1991.
119. McCullagh WH, Covell JW, Ross J Jr: Left ventricular dilatation and diastolic compliance changes during chronic volume overloading. Circulation 45:943, 1972.
120. Cazolla O, Freiburg A, Helmes M, et al: Differential expression of cardiac titin isoforms and modulation of cellular stiffness. Circ Res 86:59, 2000.
121. Burlew BS, Weber KT: Connective tissue and the heart. Functional significance and regulatory mechanisms. Cardiol Clin 18:435, 2000.
122. Hess OM, Osakada G, Lavelle JF, et al: Diastolic myocardial wall stiffness and ventricular relaxation during partial and complete coronary occlusions in the conscious dog. Circ Res 52:387, 1983.
123. Diamond C, Forrester JS: Effect of coronary artery disease and acute myocardial infarction on left ventricular compliance in man. Circulation 45:11, 1972.
124. Fletcher PJ, Pfeffer JM, Pfeffer MA, Braunwald E: Left ventricular diastolic pressure-volume relations in rats with healed myocardial infarction: Effects on systolic function. Circ Res 49:618, 1981.

Neurohormonal, Autocrine, and Paracrine Adjustments

125. Schrier RW, Abraham WT: Hormones and hemodynamics in heart failure. N Engl J Med 341:577, 1999.
126. Abramson BL, Ando S, Notarius CF, et al: Effect of atrial natriuretic peptide on muscle sympathetic activity and its reflex control in human heart failure. Circulation 99:1810, 1999.
127. Chidsey CA, Harrison DC, Braunwald E: Augmentation of plasma norepinephrine response to exercise in patients with congestive heart failure. N Engl J Med 267:650, 1962.
128. Chidsey CA, Braunwald E, Morrow AG: Catecholamine excretion and cardiac stores of norepinephrine in congestive heart failure. Am J Med 39:442, 1965.
129. Esler M, Kaye D, Lambert G, et al: Adrenergic nervous system in heart failure. Am J Cardiol 80:71, 1997.
130. Leimbach WN, Wallin BG, Victor HG, et al: Direct evidence from intraneural recordings for increased central sympathetic outflow in patients with heart failure. Circulation 73:913, 1986.
131. Swedberg K, Bristow MR, Cohn JN, et al: Effects of sustained-release moxonidine, an imidazoline agonist, on plasma norepinephrine in patients with chronic heart failure. Circulation 105:1797, 2002.
132. Jones CG, Cleland JG: Meeting report—The LIDO, HOPE, MOXCON and WASH studies. Heart Outcomes Prevention Evaluation. The Warfarin/Aspirin Study of Heart Failure. Eur J Heart Fail 1:425, 1999.
133. Landzberg JS, Parker JD, Gauthier DF, Colucci WS: Effects of myocardial alpha$_1$-adrenergic receptor stimulation and blockade on contractility in humans. Circulation 84:1608, 1991.
134. Satoh N, Suter TM, Liao R, Colucci WS: Chronic alpha-adrenergic receptor stimulation modulates the contractile phenotype of cardiac myocytes in vitro. Circulation 102:2249, 2000.
135. Chidsey CA, Sonnenblick EH, Morrow AG, Braunwald E: Norepinephrine stores and contractile force of papillary muscle from the failing human heart. Circulation 33:43, 1966.
136. Spann JF Jr, Sonnenblick E, Cooper EH, Braunwald E: Cardiac norepinephrine stores and the contractile state of heart muscle. Circ Res 19:317, 1966.
137. Merlet P, Benvenuti C, Moyse D, et al: Prognostic value of MIBG imaging in idiopathic dilated cardiomyopathy. J Nucl Med 40:917, 1999.
138. Merlet P, Pouillart F, Dubois-Rande JL, et al: Sympathetic nerve alterations assessed with ^{123}I-MIBG in the failing human heart. J Nucl Med 40:224, 1999.
139. Higgins CB, Vatner SF, Eckberg DL, Braunwald E: Alterations in the baroreceptor reflex in conscious dogs with heart failure. J Clin Invest 51:715, 1972.
140. Levine TB, Francis GS, Goldsmith SR, Cohn JN: The neurohumoral and hemodynamic response to orthostatic tilt in patients with congestive heart failure. Circulation 67:1070, 1983.
141. Goldsmith SR, Francis GS, Levine TB, Cohn JN: Regional blood flow response to orthostasis in patients with congestive heart failure. J Am Coll Cardiol 1:1391, 1983.
142. Kubo SH, Cody RJ: Circulatory autoregulation in chronic congestive heart failure: Responses to head-up tilt in 41 patients. Am J Cardiol 52:512, 1983.
143. Liu JL, Zucker IH: Regulation of sympathetic nerve activity in heart failure: A role for nitric oxide and angiotensin II. Circ Res 84:417, 1999.
144. Bristow MR: Beta adrenergic receptor blockade in chronic heart failure. Circulation 101:558, 2000.
145. Communal C, Singh K, Sawyer DB, Colucci WS: Opposing effects of beta (1)- and beta (2)-adrenergic receptors on cardiac myocyte apoptosis: Role of pertussis toxin–sensitive G protein. Circulation 100:2210, 1999.
146. Poole-Wilson PA, Swedberg K, Cleland JG, et al: A comparison of carvedilol and metoprolol on clinical outcomes in patients with chronic heart failure in the Carvedilol Or Metoprolol European Trial (COMET): Randomised controlled trial. Lancet 362:7, 2003.
147. Eckhart AD, Ozaki T, Tevaearai H, et al: Vascular-targeted overexpression of G protein–coupled receptor kinase-2 in transgenic mice attenuates beta-adrenergic receptor signaling and increases resting blood pressure. Mol Pharmacol 61:749, 2002.
148. Gilbert EM, Abraham WT, Olsen S, et al: Comparative hemodynamic, left ventricular functional, and antiadrenergic effects of chronic treatment with metoprolol versus carvedilol in the failing heart. Circulation 94:2817, 1996.
149. Ligett SB, Wagoner LE, Craft LL, et al: The Ile164 beta2-adrenergic receptor polymorphism adversely affects the outcome of congestive heart failure. J Clin Invest 102:1534, 1998.
150. Small KM, Wagoner LE, Levin AM, et al: Synergistic polymorphisms of beta1- and alpha2C-adrenergic receptors and the risk of congestive heart failure. N Engl J Med 347:1135, 2002.
151. Zolk O, Kouchi I, Schnabel P, Bohm M: Heterotrimeric G proteins in heart disease. Can J Physiol Pharmacol 78:187, 2000.
152. Dorn GW, Brown JH: Gq signaling in cardiac adaptation and maladaptation. Trends Cardiovasc Med 9:26, 1999.
153. Geng YJ, Ishikawa Y, Vatner DE, et al: Apoptosis of cardiac myocytes in Gs-alpha transgenic mice. Circ Res 84:34, 1999.
154. Iwase M, Uechi M, Vatner DE, et al: Cardiomyopathy induced by cardiac Gs alpha overexpression. Am J Physiol 272:H585, 1997.
155. Gaffney TE, Braunwald E: Importance of the adrenergic nervous system in the support of circulatory function in patients with congestive heart failure. Am J Med 34:320, 1963.
156. Epstein SE, Braunwald E: The effect of beta-adrenergic blockade on patterns of urinary sodium excretion: Studies in normal subjects and in patients with heart disease. Ann Intern Med 75:20, 1966.
157. Singh K, Xiao L, Remondino A, et al: Adrenergic regulation of cardiac myocyte apoptosis. J Cell Physiol 189:257, 2001.
158. Shizukuda Y, Buttrick PM, Geenen DL, et al: Beta-adrenergic stimulation causes cardiocyte apoptosis: Influence of tachycardia and hypertrophy. Am J Physiol 275:H961, 1998.
159. Bisognano JD, Weinberger HD, Bohlmeyer TJ, et al: Myocardial-directed overexpression of the human beta$_1$-adrenergic receptor in transgenic mice. J Mol Cell Cardiol 32:817, 2000.
160. Eckberg DL, Drabinsky M, Braunwald E: Defective cardiac parasympathetic control in patients with heart disease. N Engl J Med 285:877, 1971.

161. Grassi G, Esler M: How to assess sympathetic activity in humans. J Hypertens 17:719, 1999.
162. Francis GS, Benedict C, Johnstone DE, et al: Comparison of neuroendocrine activation in patients with left ventricular dysfunction with and without congestive heart failure: A substudy of the Studies of Left Ventricular Dysfunction (SOLVD). Circulation 82:1724, 1990.
163. Yusuf S, Sleight P, Pogue J, et al: Effects of an angiotensin-converting-enzyme inhibitor, ramipril, on cardiovascular events in high-risk patients. The Outcomes Prevention Evaluation Study. N Engl J Med 342:145, 2000.
164. Farquharson CA, Struthers AD: Spironolactone increases nitric oxide bioactivity, improves endothelial vasodilator dysfunction, and suppresses vascular angiotensin I/angiotensin II conversion in patients with chronic heart failure. Circulation 101:1594, 2000.
165. van Veldhuisen DJ, Voors AA: Blockade of the renin angiotensin system in heart failure: The potential place of angiotensin II receptor blockers. Eur Heart J 21:14, 2000.
166. Kim S, Iwao H: Molecular and cellular mechanisms of angiotensin II–mediated cardiovascular and renal diseases. Pharmacol Rev 52:11, 2000.
167. Kajstura J, Cigola E, Malhotra A, et al: Angiotensin II induces apoptosis of adult ventricular myocytes in vitro. J Mol Cell Cardiol 29:859, 1997.
168. Kawano H, Do YS, Kawano Y, et al: Angiotensin II has multiple profibrotic effects in human cardiac fibroblasts. Circulation 101:1130, 2000.
169. Zisman LS, Asano K, Dutcher DL, et al: Differential regulation of cardiac angiotensin converting enzyme binding sites and AT1 receptor density in the failing human heart. Circulation 98:1735, 1998.
170. Weber KT: Aldosterone in congestive heart failure. N Engl J Med 345:1689, 2001.
171. Sun Y, Zhang J, Lu L, et al: Aldosterone-induced inflammation in the rat heart: Role of oxidative stress. Am J Pathol 161:1773, 2002.
172. Qin W, Rudolph AE, Bond BR, et al: Transgenic model of aldosterone-driven cardiac hypertrophy and heart failure. Circ Res 93:69, 2003.
173. Pitt B, Zannand F, Remme WJ, et al: The effect of spironolactone on morbidity and mortality in patients with severe heart failure. Randomized Aldactone Evaluation Study Investigators. N Engl J Med 341:709, 1999.
174. Pitt B, Remme W, Zannad F, et al: Eplerenone, a selective aldosterone blocker, in patients with left ventricular dysfunction after myocardial infarction. N Engl J Med 348:1309, 2003.
175. Naitoh M, Suzuki H, Murakami M, et al: Effects of oral AVP receptor antagonists OPC-21268 and OPC-31260 on congestive heart failure in conscious dogs. Am J Physiol 267:H2245, 1994.
176. Talwar S, Siebenhofer A, Williams B, Ng L: Influence of hypertension, left ventricular hypertrophy, and left ventricular systolic dysfunction on plasma N terminal proBNP. Heart 83:278, 2000.
177. Wei CM, Heublein DM, Perrella MA, et al: Natriuretic peptide system in human heart failure. Circulation 88:1004, 1993.
178. Morrison LK, Harrison A, Krishnaswamy P, et al: Utility of rapid B-natriuretic peptide assay in differentiating congestive heart failure from lung disease in patients presenting with dyspnea. J Am Coll Cardiol 39:202, 2002.
179. Sugimoto Y, Kinoshita M: Attenuation of compensation of endogenous cardiac natriuretic peptide system in chronic heart failure: Prognostic role of plasma brain natriuretic peptide concentration in patients with chronic symptomatic left ventricular dysfunction. Circulation 96:509, 1997.
180. Morrow DA, deLemos JA, Sabatine MS, et al: Evaluation of B-type natriuretic peptide for risk assessment in unstable angina/non-ST-elevation myocardial infarction: B-type natriuretic peptide and prognosis in TACTICS-TIMI 18. J Am Coll Cardiol 41:1264, 2003.
181. Anand IS, Fisher LD, Chiang YT, et al: Changes in brain natriuretic peptide and norepinephrine over time and mortality and morbidity in the Valsartan Heart Failure Trial (Val-HeFT). Circulation 107:1278, 2003.
182. Wada A, Tsutamoto T, Matsuda Y, Kinoshita M: Cardiorenal and neurohumoral effects of endogenous atrial natriuretic peptide in dogs with severe congestive heart failure using a specific antagonist for guanylate cyclase–coupled receptors. Circulation 89:2232, 1994.
183. Colucci WS: Nesiritide for the treatment of decompensated heart failure. J Card Fail 7:92, 2001.
184. Packer M, Califf RM, Konstam MA, et al: Comparison of omapatrilat and enalapril in patients with chronic heart failure: The Omapatrilat Versus Enalapril Randomized Trial of Utility in Reducing Events (OVERTURE). Circulation 106:920, 2002.
185. Sam F, Colucci WS: Role of endothelin-1 in myocardial failure. Proc Assoc Am Physicians 111:417, 1999.
186. Zolk O, Quattek J, Sitzler G, et al: Expression of endothelin-1, endothelin-converting enzyme, and endothelin receptors in chronic heart failure. Circulation 99:2118, 1999.
187. Serneri GG, Cecioni I, Vanni S, et al: Selective upregulation of cardiac endothelin system in patients with ischemic but not idiopathic dilated cardiomyopathy: Endothelin-1 system in the human failing heart. Circ Res 86:377, 2000.
188. Teerlink JR, Loffler BM, Hess P, et al: Role of endothelin in the maintenance of blood pressure in conscious rats with chronic heart failure: Acute effects of the endothelin receptor antagonist Ro 47-0203 (bosentan). Circulation 90:2510, 1994.
189. Fraccarollo D, Hu K, Galuppo P, et al: Chronic endothelin receptor blockade attenuates progressive ventricular dilation and improves cardiac function in rats with myocardial infarction: Possible involvement of myocardial endothelin system in ventricular remodeling. Circulation 96:3963, 1997.
190. Podesser BK, Siwik DA, Eberli FR, et al: ET(A)-receptor blockade prevents matrix metalloproteinase activation late postmyocardial infarction in the rat. Am J Physiol 280:H984, 2001.
191. Saad D, Mukherjee R, Thomas PB, et al: The effects of endothelin-A receptor blockade during the progression of pacing-induced congestive heart failure. J Am Coll Cardiol 32:1779, 1998.
192. Colucci WS: Myocardial endothelin: Does it play a role in myocardial failure? Circulation 93:1069, 1996.
193. Kiowski W, Sutsch G, Hunziker P, et al: Evidence for endothelin-1–mediated vasoconstriction in severe chronic heart failure. Lancet 346:732, 1995.
194. Sutsch G, Bertel O, Kiowski W: Acute and short-term effects of the nonpeptide endothelin-1 receptor antagonist bosentan in humans. Cardiovasc Drugs Ther 10:717, 1997.
195. Ono K, Matsumori A, Shioi T, et al: Cytokine gene expression after myocardial infarction in rat hearts: Possible implication in left ventricular remodeling. Circulation 98:149, 1998.
196. Mann DL: Inflammatory mediators and the failing heart: Past, present, and the foreseeable future. Circ Res 91:988, 2002.
197. Mann DL: Activation of cytokine systems in heart failure. *In* Mann DL (ed): Heart Failure: A Companion to Braunwald's Heart Disease: A Textbook of Cardiovascular Medicine. Philadelphia, Elsevier, 2004, pp 159-180.
198. Malave HA, Taylor AA, Nattama J, et al: Circulating levels of tumor necrosis factor correlate with indexes of depressed heart rate variability: A study in patients with mild-to-moderate heart failure. Chest 123:716, 2003.
199. Stumpf C, Lehner C, Yilmaz A, et al: Decrease of serum levels of the anti-inflammatory cytokine interleukin-10 in patients with advanced chronic heart failure. Clin Sci (Lond) 105:45, 2003.
200. Torre-Amione G, Kapadia S, Lee J, et al: Tumor necrosis factor-alpha and tumor necrosis factor receptors in the failing human heart. Circulation 93:704, 1996.
201. Janczewski AM, Kadokami T, Lemster B, et al: Morphological and functional changes in cardiac myocytes isolated from mice overexpressing TNF-alpha. Am J Physiol 284:H960, 2003.
202. Thaik CM, Calderone A, Takahashi N, Colucci WS: Interleukin-1 beta modulates the growth and phenotype of neonatal rat cardiac myocytes. J Clin Invest 96:1093, 1995.
203. Krown KA, Page MT, Nguyen C, et al: Tumor necrosis factor alpha–induced apoptosis in cardiac myocytes: Involvement of the sphingolipid signaling cascade in cardiac cell death. J Clin Invest 98:2854, 1996.
204. Bozkurt B, Kribbs SB, Clubb FJ Jr, et al: Pathophysiologically relevant concentrations of tumor necrosis factor-alpha promote progressive left ventricular dysfunction and remodeling in rats. Circulation 97:1382, 1998.
205. Deswal A, Bozkurt B, Seta Y, et al: Safety and efficacy of a soluble P75 tumor necrosis factor receptor (Enbrel, etanercept) in patients with advanced heart failure. Circulation 99:3224, 1999.
206. Krum H: Tumor necrosis factor-alpha blockade as a therapeutic strategy in heart failure (RENEWAL and ATTACH): Unsuccessful, to be specific. J Card Fail 8:365, 2002.
207. Chung ES, Packer M, Lo KH, et al: Randomized, double-blind, placebo-controlled, pilot trial of infliximab, a chimeric monoclonal antibody to tumor necrosis factor-alpha, in patients with moderate-to-severe heart failure: Results of the anti-TNF Therapy Against Congestive Heart Failure (ATTACH) trial. Circulation 107:3133, 2003.
208. Kwon HJ, Cote TR, Cuffe MS, et al: Case reports of heart failure after therapy with a tumor necrosis factor antagonist. Ann Intern Med 138:807, 2003.
209. Gullestad L, Semb AG, Holt E, et al: Effect of thalidomide in patients with chronic heart failure. Am Heart J 144:847, 2002.
210. Sliwa K, Woodiwiss A, Candy G, et al: Effects of pentoxifylline on cytokine profiles and left ventricular performance in patients with decompensated congestive heart failure secondary to idiopathic dilated cardiomyopathy. Am J Cardiol 90:1118, 2002.
211. Orus J, Heras M, Morales-Ruiz M, et al: Nitric oxide synthase II mRNA expression in cardiac tissue of patients with heart failure undergoing cardiac transplantation. J Heart Lung Transplant 19:139, 2000.
212. Hare JM, Colucci WS: Role of nitric oxide in the regulation of myocardial function. Prog Cardiovasc Dis 38:155, 1995.
213. Funakoshi H, Kubota T, Kawamura N, et al: Disruption of inducible nitric oxide synthase improves beta-adrenergic inotropic responsiveness but not the survival of mice with cytokine-induced cardiomyopathy. Circ Res 90:959, 2002.
214. Gealekman O, Abassi Z, Rubinstein I, et al: Role of myocardial inducible nitric oxide synthase in contractile dysfunction and beta-adrenergic hyporesponsiveness in rats with experimental volume-overload heart failure. Circulation 105:236, 2002.
215. Paulus WJ, Vantrimpont PJ, Shah AM: Acute effects of nitric oxide on left ventricular relaxation and diastolic distensibility in humans: Assessment by bicoronary sodium nitroprusside infusion. Circulation 89:2070, 1994.
216. Hare JM, Loh E, Creager MA, Colucci WS: Nitric oxide inhibits the positive inotropic response to beta-adrenergic stimulation in humans with left ventricular dysfunction. Circulation 92:2198, 1995.
217. Chen Y, Traverse JH, Du R, et al: Nitric oxide modulates myocardial oxygen consumption in the failing heart. Circulation 106:273, 2002.
218. Bishopric NH: A thousand times NO. J Mol Cell Cardiol 34:601, 2002.
219. Sam F, Sawyer DB, Xie Z, et al: Mice lacking inducible nitric oxide synthase have improved left ventricular contractile function and reduced apoptotic cell death late after myocardial infarction. Circ Res 89:351, 2001.
220. Scherrer-Crosbie M, Ullrich R, Bloch KD, et al: Endothelial nitric oxide synthase limits left ventricular remodeling after myocardial infarction in mice. Circulation 104:1286, 2001.
221. Mallat Z, Philip I, Lebret M, et al: Elevated levels of 8-iso-prostaglandin F2alpha in pericardial fluid of patients with heart failure: A potential role for in vivo oxidant stress in ventricular dilatation and progression to heart failure. Circulation 97:1536, 1998.
222. Li JM, Gall NP, Grieve DJ, et al: Activation of NADPH oxidase during progression of cardiac hypertrophy to failure. Hypertension 40:477, 2002.
223. Hare JM: Oxidative stress and apoptosis in heart failure progression. Circ Res 89:198, 2001.
224. Li Y, Huang T-T, Carlson EJ, et al: Dilated cardiomyopathy and neonatal lethality in mutant mice lacking manganese superoxide dismutase. Nat Genet 11:376, 1995.
225. Dhalla AK, Hill MF, Singal PK: Role of oxidative stress in transition of hypertrophy to heart failure. J Am Coll Cardiol 28:506, 1996.
226. Kinugawa S, Tsutsui H, Hayashidani S, et al: Treatment with dimethylthiourea prevents left ventricular remodeling and failure after experimental myocardial infarction in mice: Role of oxidative stress. Circ Res 87:392, 2000.

CHAPTER 22

Clinical Aspects of Heart Failure; Pulmonary Edema, High-Output Failure

Michael M. Givertz • Wilson S. Colucci • Eugene Braunwald

Definition

Heart failure is a principal complication of virtually all forms of heart disease. An American College of Cardiology/American Heart Association (ACC/AHA) Task Force on Practice Guidelines described this condition as follows.

Heart failure is a complex clinical syndrome that can result from any structural or functional cardiac disorder that impairs the ability of the ventricle to fill with or eject blood. The cardinal manifestations of heart failure are dyspnea and fatigue, which may limit exercise tolerance, and fluid retention, which may lead to pulmonary congestion and peripheral edema. Both abnormalities can impair the functional capacity and quality of life of affected individuals, but they do not necessarily dominate the clinical picture at the same time. Because not all patients have volume overload at the time of initial or subsequent evaluation, the term "heart failure" is preferred over the older term "congestive heart failure."[1]

Myocardial failure, a term used to denote abnormal systolic or diastolic function, may be asymptomatic or progress to heart failure. *Circulatory failure* is not synonymous with heart failure because a variety of noncardiac conditions (e.g., hemorrhagic shock) can lead to circulatory collapse while cardiac function is preserved. *Cardiomyopathy* and *left ventricular dysfunction* are more general terms that describe abnormalities of cardiac structure or function, or both, which may lead to heart failure.

The clinical manifestations of heart failure vary enormously and depend on a variety of factors, including the age of the patient, the extent and rate at which cardiac performance becomes impaired, and the ventricle initially involved in the disease process. A broad spectrum of severity of impairment of cardiac function is ordinarily included within the definition of heart failure, ranging from the mildest, which is manifest clinically only during stress, to the most advanced form, in which cardiac pump function is unable to sustain life without external support. Useful criteria for the diagnosis of heart failure, which emerged from the Framingham Study (Table 22–1),[2] emphasize that heart failure is, in the final analysis, a clinical diagnosis.

To emphasize the evolution and progression of heart failure, the ACC/AHA guidelines on the evaluation and management of heart failure set forth a staging system (Table 22–2).[1] This staging system recognizes that there are established risk factors and structural prerequisites for the development of heart failure, that therapeutic interventions that are initiated before the onset of left ventricular dysfunction or symptoms can reduce morbidity and mortality, that patients generally progress from one stage to the next unless disease progression is slowed or stopped by treatment, and that all patients benefit from risk factor modification including blood pressure control, lipid management, exercise training, and smoking and alcohol cessation.

Prevalence and Incidence

Heart failure is a relatively common disorder. It is estimated that 4.9 million persons in the United States are being treated for heart failure, with 550,000 new cases diagnosed each year.[3,4] The prevalence of heart failure increases dramatically with age, occurring in 1 to 2 percent of persons aged 45 to 54 years and up to 10 percent of individuals older than 75 years (Fig. 22–1).[2,3] For individuals free of heart failure at age 40, the remaining lifetime risk for developing heart failure is 21 percent for men and 20.3 percent for women.[5] Approximately 80 percent of all heart failure admissions occur in patients older than 65; as a result, heart failure is the leading discharge diagnosis in persons aged 65 years or older in the United States with an average length of stay of 5.3 days.[6] Between 1979 and 2000, the number of heart failure hospitalizations rose from 377,000 to 999,000, an increase of 165 percent (Fig. 22–2).[3] In the United States, approximately 56,000 deaths each year are primarily caused by heart failure and heart failure was listed as a contributing cause in 262,000 deaths.[7] The U.S. mortality rate related to heart failure is estimated at 20.2 deaths per 100,000 population. The trend toward increased morbidity and mortality related to heart failure may be due in part to the aging of the population and in part to the improved survival of patients with cardiovascular disease.

Heart failure has an enormous economic impact on the U.S. health care system, owing to direct medical costs, disability, and loss of employment. In 2000, $3.5 billion was spent on Medicare beneficiaries for the in-hospital management of heart failure.[8] Estimated treatment costs for all inpatients with heart failure in 2003 were $24.3 billion. The cost of hospitalizations for heart failure is twice that for all forms of cancer and myocardial infarctions combined.[9]

Forms and Causes of Heart Failure

Forward Versus Backward Heart Failure

Focusing on cardiovascular hemodynamics, early investigators postulated that the

TABLE 22–1 Framingham Criteria for Heart Failure*

Major Criteria
Paroxysmal nocturnal dyspnea
Neck vein distention
Rales
Radiographic cardiomegaly
Acute pulmonary edema
S_3 gallop
Increased central venous pressure > 16 cm H_2O
Circulation time ≥ 25 sec
Hepatojugular reflux
Pulmonary edema, visceral congestion, or cardiomegaly at autopsy
Weight loss ≥ 4.5 kg in 5 days in response to treatment of heart failure
Minor Criteria
Bilateral ankle edema
Nocturnal cough
Dyspnea on ordinary exertion
Hepatomegaly
Pleural effusion
Decrease in vital capacity by one third from maximal value recorded
Tachycardia (rate ≥ 120 beats/min)

From Ho KL, Pinsky JL, Kannel WB, Levy D: The epidemiology of heart failure: The Framingham Study. J Am Coll Cardiol 22(Suppl A):6A, 1993.

*The diagnosis of heart failure in this study required that two major or one major and two minor criteria be present concurrently. Minor criteria were acceptable only if they could not be attributed to another medical condition.

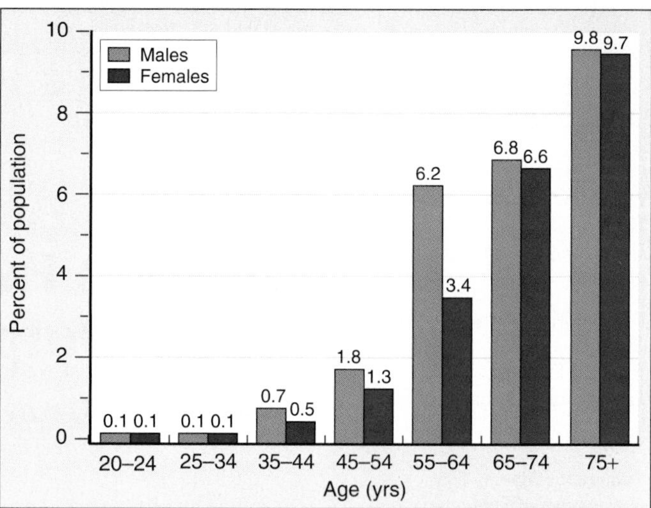

FIGURE 22–1 Prevalence rates of heart failure by gender and age in the United States between 1988 and 1994: the Third National Health and Nutrition Examination Survey (NHANES III). Among men (blue), the prevalence increased from 18 cases per 1000 in those aged 45 to 54 years to 98 cases per 1000 in those aged 75 years and older. Among women (purple), the prevalence increased from 13 cases per 1000 in those aged 45 to 54 years to 97 cases per 1000 in those aged 75 years and older. (Data from American Heart Association: Heart Disease and Stroke Statistics—2003 Update. Dallas, American Heart Association, 2002.)

clinical manifestations of heart failure arose as a consequence of inadequate cardiac output or damming up of blood behind one or both ventricles, or both. These two principal mechanisms were the basis of the forward and backward pressure theories of heart failure. The *backward failure hypothesis*, first proposed by James Hope in 1832, contends that when the ventricle fails to discharge its contents, blood accumulates and pressure rises in the atrium and the venous system emptying into it. As discussed in Chapter 19, the inability of cardiac muscle to shorten against a load alters the relationship between ventricular end-systolic pressure and volume so that end-systolic volume rises. The following sequence then occurs, which at first maintains cardiac output at a normal level but ultimately leads to clinical decompensation: (1) ventricular end-diastolic volume and pressure increase, (2) the volume and pressure rise in the atrium behind the failing ventricle, (3) the atrium contracts more vigorously (a manifestation of Starling's law, operating on the atrium), (4) the pressure in the venous and capillary beds behind the failing ventricle rises, and (5) transudation of fluid from the capillary bed into the interstitial space (pulmonary or systemic) increases. Many of the symptoms characteristic of heart failure can be traced to this sequence of events and the resultant increase in fluid in the interstitial spaces of the lungs, liver, subcutaneous tissues, and serous cavities.

An important extension of the backward failure theory is the development of right ventricular failure as a consequence of left ventricular failure. According to this concept, the

TABLE 22–2 Stages of Heart Failure

Stage	Description	Examples
A	At high risk for developing HF because of the presence of conditions that are strongly associated with the development of HF No identified structural or functional abnormalities of the pericardium, myocardium, or cardiac valves No history of signs or symptoms of HF	Systemic hypertension Coronary artery disease Diabetes mellitus History of cardiotoxic drug therapy History of alcohol abuse Family history of cardiomyopathy
B	Presence of structural heart disease that is strongly associated with the development of HF No history of signs or symptoms of HF	Left ventricular hypertrophy or fibrosis Left ventricular dilation or dysfunction Asymptomatic valvular heart disease Previous myocardial infarction
C	Current or prior symptoms of HF associated with underlying structural heart disease	Dyspnea or fatigue due to left ventricular systolic dysfunction Asymptomatic patients receiving treatment for prior symptoms of HF
D	Advanced structural heart disease and marked symptoms of HF at rest despite maximal medical therapy Require specialized interventions	Frequent HF hospitalizations and cannot be discharged In the hospital awaiting heart transplant At home with continuous inotropic or mechanical support In hospice setting for management of HF

HF = heart failure.

Adapted from Hunt SA, Baker DW, Chin MH, et al: ACC/AHA guidelines for the evaluation and management of chronic heart failure in the adult: Executive summary. A report of the American College of Cardiology/American Heart Association Task Force on Practice Guidelines (Committee to Revise the 1995 Guidelines for the Evaluation and Management of Heart Failure). Circulation 104:2996, 2001.

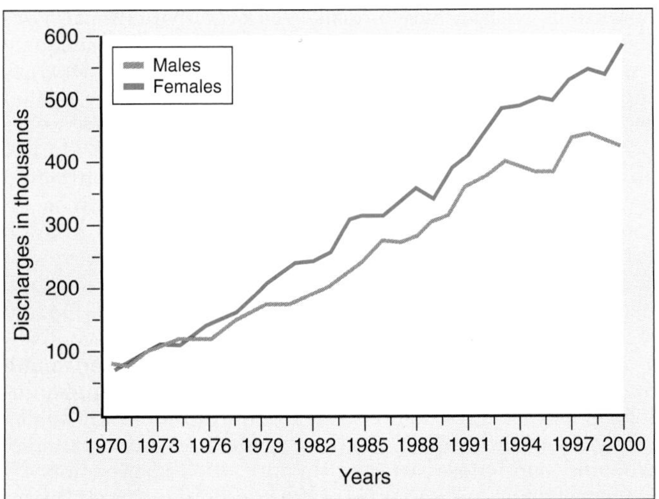

FIGURE 22–2 Hospital discharges for heart failure by gender in the United States between 1970 and 2000. Among men (blue), the number of discharges increased from 90,000 per year in 1970 to 410,000 per year in 2000. Among women (magenta), the number of discharges increased from 90,000 per year in 1970 to 580,000 per year in 2000. Source: Centers for Disease Control and Prevention, National Center for Health Statistics. (Data from American Heart Association: Heart Disease and Stroke Statistics—2003 Update. Dallas, American Heart Association, 2002.)

elevation of left ventricular diastolic, left atrial, and pulmonary venous pressures results in backward transmission of pressure into the pulmonary arterial circulation and leads to pulmonary hypertension, which ultimately causes right ventricular failure. It is now recognized that changes in the structure and function of the pulmonary vasculature play an important role in the development of secondary pulmonary hypertension associated with heart failure.[10]

Eighty years after the publication of Hope's work, Mackenzie proposed the *forward failure hypothesis*, which relates clinical manifestations of heart failure to inadequate delivery of blood into the arterial system. According to this hypothesis, the principal clinical manifestations of heart failure are due to reduced cardiac output, which results in diminished perfusion of vital organs, including the brain, leading to mental confusion; skeletal muscles, leading to weakness; and kidneys, leading to sodium and water retention. Sodium and water retention occurring through a series of complex neurohormonal mechanisms[11,12] in turn augment extracellular fluid volume and ultimately lead to symptoms of heart failure.

Although these two seemingly opposing views concerning the pathogenesis of heart failure led to lively controversy during the first half of the 20th century, neither theory takes into account the full spectrum of pathophysiological changes that contribute to ventricular remodeling and disease progression in patients with chronic heart failure.

RIGHT-SIDED VERSUS LEFT-SIDED HEART FAILURE

Implicit in the backward failure theory is the idea that fluid localizes behind the specific cardiac chamber that is *initially* affected. Thus, symptoms secondary to pulmonary congestion initially predominate in patients with left ventricular infarction, hypertension, or aortic or mitral valve disease; that is, they manifest *left-sided heart failure*. With time, however, fluid accumulation becomes generalized, and ankle edema, congestive hepatomegaly, ascites, and pleural effusion occur; thus, the patients subsequently exhibit *right-sided heart failure* as well.

FLUID RETENTION

Fluid retention in heart failure is due in part to reduction in glomerular filtration rate and in part to activation of neurohormonal systems, including the renin-angiotensin-aldosterone system and sympathetic nervous system.[12] Reduced cardiac output is associated with a lowered glomerular filtration rate and an increased elaboration of renin, which, through the activation of angiotensin, results in the release of aldosterone (see Chap. 21). The combination of impaired hepatic function, owing to hepatic venous congestion, and reduced hepatic blood flow interferes with the metabolism of aldosterone, further raising its plasma concentration and augmenting the retention of sodium and water. Arginine vasopressin is also elevated in patients with chronic heart failure and contributes to systemic vasoconstriction and free water retention.

Cardiac output (and glomerular filtration rate) may be normal in many patients with heart failure, particularly when they are at rest. However, during stress, such as physical exercise, the cardiac output fails to rise normally, the glomerular filtration rate declines, and the renal mechanisms for salt and water retention described earlier come into play. In addition, ventricular filling pressure and therefore pressures in the atrium and systemic veins behind the ventricle may be normal at rest, only to rise abnormally during stress. This effect, in turn, may cause transudation and symptoms of tissue congestion (e.g., pulmonary congestion in the case of the left ventricle) during exercise. For this reason, rest may induce diuresis and relieve symptoms in many patients with mild to moderate heart failure.

ACUTE VERSUS CHRONIC HEART FAILURE

The clinical manifestations of heart failure depend importantly on the *rate* at which the syndrome develops and specifically on whether sufficient time has elapsed for compensatory mechanisms to become operative and for fluid to accumulate in the interstitial space. For example, when a previously normal individual suddenly develops a serious anatomical or functional abnormality of cardiac function, such as a massive myocardial infarction, tachyarrhythmia with a very rapid rate, or rupture of a valve secondary to infective endocarditis, a marked reduction in cardiac output occurs, associated with symptoms related to inadequate organ perfusion or acute congestion of the venous bed behind the affected ventricle, or both. If the same anatomical abnormality develops gradually, or if the patient survives the acute insult, a number of adaptive mechanisms become operational, including cardiovascular remodeling and neurohormonal activation (see Chap. 21), and these allow the patient to adjust to and tolerate not only the anatomical abnormality but also a reduction in cardiac output with less difficulty.

LOW-OUTPUT VERSUS HIGH-OUTPUT HEART FAILURE

Low cardiac output at rest, or in milder cases during exertion and other stresses, characterizes heart failure occurring in many forms of cardiovascular disease (i.e., congenital, valvular, rheumatic, hypertensive, coronary, and cardiomyopathic). A variety of high-cardiac output states, including thyrotoxicosis, arteriovenous fistulas, beriberi, Paget disease of bone, and anemia (discussed later in this chapter), may lead to heart failure as well. Low-output heart failure is characterized by clinical evidence of systemic vasoconstriction with cold, pale, and sometimes cyanotic extremities. In advanced forms of low-output failure, marked reduction in the stroke volume is reflected by a narrowing of the pulse pressure.[13] In contrast, in high-output heart failure, the extremities are usually warm and flushed and the pulse pressure is widened or at least normal.

The ability of the heart to deliver the oxygen required by the metabolizing tissues is reflected in the arterial-mixed venous oxygen difference, which is abnormally widened (i.e., >50 ml/liter in the resting state) in patients with systemic hypoperfusion or low-output heart failure. This difference may be normal or even reduced in high-output states owing to elevation of the mixed venous oxygen saturation by the admixture of blood that has been shunted away from metabolizing tissues.

Systolic Versus Diastolic Heart Failure

Heart failure has been defined in physiological terms to occur when an abnormality of cardiac function causes the heart to fail to pump blood at a rate required by the metabolizing tissues or to do so only with an elevated filling pressure.[14] Implicit in this definition is the observation that heart failure can be caused by an abnormality in systolic function leading to a defect in the expulsion of blood (i.e., *systolic heart failure*) or by an abnormality in diastolic function leading to a defect in ventricular filling (i.e., *diastolic heart failure*) (Fig. 22–3). The former is the classic form of heart failure associated with an impaired inotropic state. Equally important is diastolic heart failure (also termed heart failure with normal

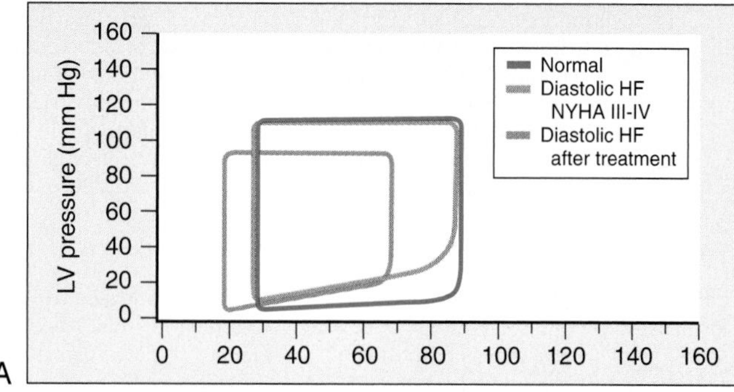

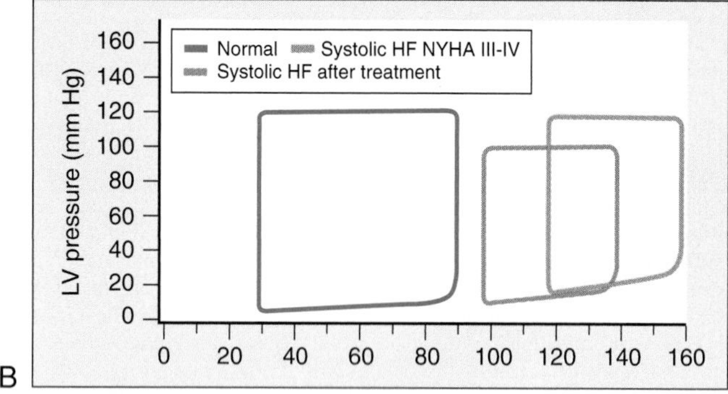

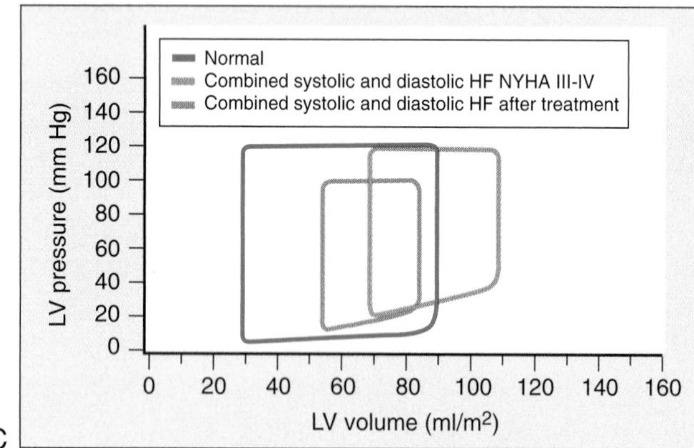

FIGURE 22–3 Pressure-volume loops contrasting isolated diastolic heart failure **(A)** with systolic heart failure **(B)** and combined systolic and diastolic heart failure **(C)**. In each panel, a normal subject (magenta) is compared with a patient with heart failure before (gold) and after (blue) treatment. **A,** Isolated diastolic heart failure is characterized by increased diastolic pressures with normal diastolic volumes (i.e., an upward shift of the diastolic pressure-volume relationship). Contractile performance is normal. When diastolic pressures are markedly elevated, patients are symptomatic with minimal exertion or at rest. With treatment, diastolic volumes and pressures can be reduced and the patient is less symptomatic, but the diastolic pressure-volume relationship remains abnormal. **B,** Systolic heart failure is characterized by abnormalities of the systolic pressure-volume relationship with decreases in ejection fraction and stroke volume. In addition, the diastolic pressure-volume relationship is shifted to the right. The increase in diastolic pressures and abnormal relaxation reflect diastolic dysfunction. With treatment, systolic and diastolic pressures are reduced, resulting in either no change or an increase in stroke volume. **C,** Combined systolic and diastolic heart failure typical of patients with ischemic heart disease is characterized by a modest decrease in contractile function and a modest increase in end-diastolic volume but a marked increase in end-diastolic pressure reflecting decreased left ventricular compliance. HF = heart failure; LV = left ventricular; NYHA = New York Heart Association. (From Zile MR, Brutsaert DL: New concepts in diastolic dysfunction and diastolic heart failure: Part I. Circulation 105:1387, 2002.)

systolic function or preserved ejection fraction), in which the ability of the ventricle or ventricles to accept blood is impaired.[15-18] This may be due to slowed or incomplete ventricular relaxation, which may be transient, as occurs in acute ischemia, or sustained, as in myocardial hypertrophy or restrictive cardiomyopathy secondary to infiltrative conditions such as amyloidosis. The principal clinical manifestations of systolic heart failure result from an inadequate cardiac output or salt and water retention, or both, whereas the major consequences of diastolic heart failure are related to elevation of the ventricular filling pressure leading to pulmonary or systemic venous congestion, or both. Studies also suggest that systolic ventricular and arterial stiffening beyond that associated with aging or hypertension is an important contributor to heart failure with normal systolic function.[19,20]

There are many examples of isolated systolic or diastolic heart failure. Examples of the former are patients with acute massive myocardial infarction or pulmonary embolism, whereas examples of the latter are patients with hypertrophic or restrictive cardiomyopathy. Community-based epidemiological studies have demonstrated that diastolic heart failure is common and is particularly prevalent in older patients, women, and those with a history of hypertension.[21-23] However, in many patients, systolic heart failure and diastolic heart failure coexist. The most common form of heart failure, that caused by chronic ischemic heart disease, is an example of combined systolic and diastolic heart failure. In this condition, systolic heart failure is caused by both the chronic loss of contracting myocardium secondary to prior myocardial infarction and the acute loss of myocardial contractility induced by transient ischemia. Diastolic heart failure is due to the ventricle's reduced compliance caused by replacement of normal, distensible myocardium with nondistensible fibrous scar tissue and by the acute reduction of diastolic distensibility during ischemia. A number of clinical features and laboratory findings characterize these two forms of heart failure (Table 22–3). However, it is important to recognize that the clinical features of heart failure may be similar whether left ventricular systolic function is normal or depressed, underscoring the need for evaluation of ventricular function in all patients with heart failure. Vasan and Levy have proposed diagnostic criteria for diastolic heart failure (Table 22–4) that consider the clinical presentation as well as documentation of systolic and diastolic function.[24]

Underlying Causes of Heart Failure

From a clinical viewpoint, it is useful to classify the causes of heart failure into two broad categories: (1) *underlying causes*, comprising the structural abnormalities—congenital or acquired—that affect the peripheral and coronary vessels, pericardium, myocardium, or cardiac valves and lead to the increased hemodynamic burden, increased myocardial stress, or coronary insufficiency responsible for heart failure (see Fig. 22–4), and (2) *precipitating causes*, including the specific causes or incidents that precipitate worsening heart failure in 50 to 90 percent of episodes of clinical heart failure.[25,26] *Underlying mechanisms* comprise the neurohormonal, biochemical, and genetic pathways through which either an increased hemodynamic burden or a reduction in myocardial oxygen delivery results in abnormal myocardial structure and function (see Chap. 21). Population-based epidemiological studies have also recognized *risk factors* for the development of heart failure,[27,28] including hypertension, smoking, diabetes mellitus, and obesity (Fig. 22–4).

It is helpful for the clinician to identify both the underlying and the precipitating causes of heart failure. Appropriate management of the underlying heart disease (e.g., surgical correction of a congenital defect or an acquired valvular abnormality or pharmacological management of hypertension) may prevent the development or progression of heart failure. Similarly, treatment of a precipitating cause such as an infection often results in a significant improvement in the clinical status of a patient with heart failure and may be life

TABLE 22–3 Systolic Versus Diastolic Heart Failure*

Parameters	Systolic	Diastolic
History		
Coronary artery disease	+++[†]	++
Hypertension	++	++++
Diabetes	++	++
Valvular heart disease	++++	+
Paroxysmal dyspnea	++	+++
Physical Examination		
Cardiomegaly	+++	+
Soft heart sounds	++++	+
S_3 gallop	+++	+
S_4 gallop	+	+++
Hypertension	++	++++
Mitral regurgitation	+++	+
Rales	++	+
Edema	+++	+
Jugular venous distention	+++	+
Chest Radiograph		
Cardiomegaly	+++	+
Pulmonary congestion	+++	+++
Electrocardiogram		
Left ventricular hypertrophy	++	++++
Q waves	++	+
Low voltage	+++	–
Echocardiogram		
Left ventricular hypertrophy	++	++++
Left ventricular dilation	++	–
Left atrial enlargement	++	++
Reduced ejection fraction	++++	–

Adapted from Young JB: Assessment of heart failure. *In* Colucci WS (ed): Heart Failure: Cardiac Function and Dysfunction. 3rd ed. *In* Braunwald E (series ed): Atlas of Heart Diseases. Philadelphia, Current Medicine, 2002, pp 127–143.

*Certain aspects of the history and physical examination, along with clinical measurements, may help to distinguish diastolic from systolic heart failure. For example, patients with hypertensive heart disease and severe left ventricular hypertrophy often experience heart failure because of diastolic dysfunction.

†*Plus signs* indicate "suggestive" (the number reflects relative weight). *Minus signs* indicate "not very suggestive."

saving. More important, *avoidance* of a precipitating cause can *prevent* worsening heart failure.

Decompensated heart failure may also be precipitated by the progression of the underlying heart disease. A previously stable, compensated patient may develop heart failure that is apparent clinically for the first time when the intrinsic process has advanced to a critical point, such as with further narrowing of a stenotic aortic valve or progressive obliteration of the pulmonary vascular bed in a patient with cor pulmonale. Alternatively, decompensation may occur as a result of failure or exhaustion of the compensatory mechanisms, but without any change in the load on the heart, in patients with chronic severe pressure or volume overload.

Precipitating Causes of Heart Failure

In one study of 435 patients admitted nonelectively to an urban university hospital with the diagnosis of heart failure, precipitating factors could be identified in 66 percent.[25]

INAPPROPRIATE REDUCTION OF THERAPY. Perhaps the most common cause of decompensation in a previously compensated patient with heart failure is inappropriate reduction in the intensity of treatment, be it dietary sodium and fluid restriction, pharmacological therapy, or both. *Dietary excesses of sodium*, incurred frequently on vacations or holidays or during any change in home cooking routine, are frequent causes of cardiac decompensation. Education of the patient and family, including referral to a nutritionist when indicated, is a simple and effective measure to prevent this common clinical problem. Self-discontinuation or physician withdrawal of effective pharmacotherapy such as angiotensin-converting enzyme (ACE) inhibitors, diuretics, or digoxin can precipitate heart failure.[26]

ARRHYTHMIAS. Cardiac arrhythmias are common in patients with underlying structural heart disease and commonly precipitate or worsen heart failure. The development of arrhythmias may precipitate heart failure through several mechanisms:

1. *Tachyarrhythmias,* most commonly atrial fibrillation, reduce the time available for ventricular filling. When there is already an impairment of ventricular filling, as in mitral stenosis, or reduced ventricular compliance, as in left ventricular hypertrophy, tachycardia raises atrial pressure and reduces cardiac output further. In addition, tachyarrhythmias increase myocardial oxygen demands and, in a patient with obstructive coronary artery disease, may induce or intensify myocardial ischemia, thereby raising left atrial pressure and causing pulmonary congestion. Tachycardia may also directly impair contractility in failing human myocardium, owing in part to a negative force-frequency relationship (see Chap. 19), and, if persistent, may cause a reversible dilated cardiomyopathy.[29]
2. *Marked bradycardia* in a patient with underlying heart disease usually depresses cardiac output because stroke volume may already be maximal and cannot rise further to maintain cardiac output.
3. *Dissociation between atrial and ventricular contraction*, which occurs in many arrhythmias, results in loss of the atrial booster pump mechanism, which impairs ventricular filling, lowers cardiac output, and raises atrial pressure. This loss is particularly deleterious in patients with impaired ventricular filling related to cardiac hypertrophy (e.g., in systemic hypertension, aortic stenosis, and hypertrophic cardiomyopathy).
4. *Abnormal intraventricular conduction*, which occurs in many arrhythmias such as ventricular tachycardia, impairs myocardial performance because of loss of the normal mechanical synchrony of ventricular contraction. In addition to precipitating heart failure, arrhythmias, which may be fatal, may be *caused* by heart failure.

TABLE 22–4 Diagnostic Criteria for Diastolic Heart Failure

Criterion	Possible Diastolic Heart Failure	Probable Diastolic Heart Failure	Definite Diastolic Heart Failure
Definitive evidence of HF	Signs and symptoms of HF, supporting laboratory tests,* and response to diuretics	Signs and symptoms of HF, supporting laboratory tests,* and response to diuretics	Signs and symptoms of HF, supporting laboratory tests,* and response to diuretics
Objective evidence of normal LV systolic function	LVEF ≥ 50% but not at the time of HF event	LVEF ≥ 50% within 72 hr of HF event	LVEF ≥ 50% within 72 hr of HF event
Objective evidence of LV diastolic dysfunction	No conclusive information	No conclusive information	Abnormal LV relaxation, filling, and/or distensibility at cardiac catheterization

*Chest radiograph, B-type natriuretic peptide level.
HF = heart failure; LV = left ventricular; LVEF = LV ejection fraction.
Adapted from Vasan RS, Levy D: Defining diastolic heart failure: A call for standardized diagnostic criteria. Circulation 101:2118, 2000.

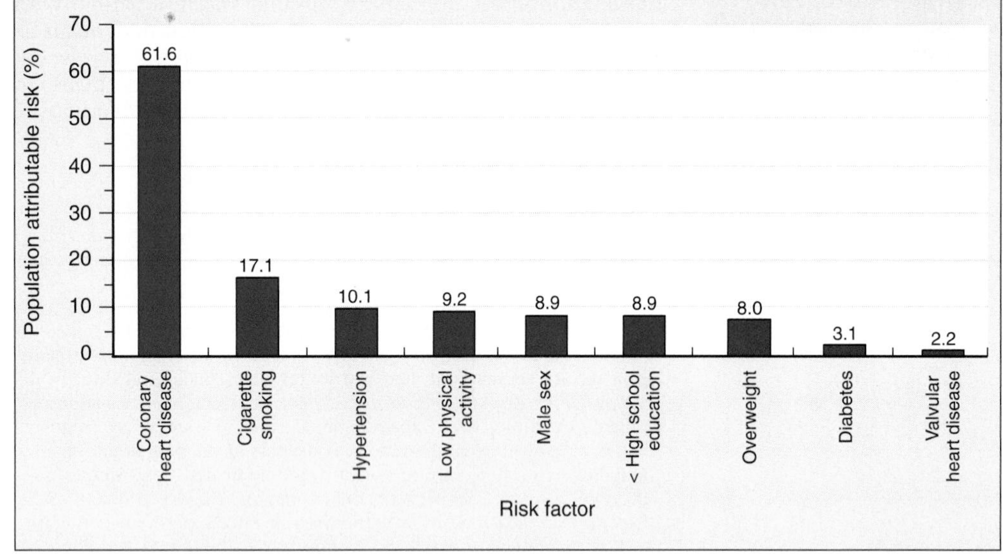

FIGURE 22–4 Estimates of the population attributable risk of heart failure related to various risk factors in 5545 men and 8098 women participating in the First National Health and Nutrition Examination Survey (NHANES I) Epidemiologic Follow-up Study. In the general population, coronary heart disease was the major cause of heart failure in 61.6 percent of all cases, followed by cigarette smoking (17.1 percent) and hypertension (10.1 percent). Obesity accounted for 8.0 percent of cases, and diabetes accounted for only 3.1 percent. (From He J, Ogden LG, Bazzano LA, et al: Risk factors for congestive heart failure in US men and women: NHANES I Epidemiologic Follow-up Study. Arch Intern Med 161:996, 2001.)

MYOCARDIAL ISCHEMIA OR INFARCTION. In patients with ischemic heart disease, acute myocardial infarction (see Chap. 46), unstable angina (see Chap. 49), or silent ischemia (see Chap. 50) can precipitate heart failure. Reduced myocardial oxygen delivery may be exacerbated by the increase in myocardial oxygen demand resulting from tachycardia and hypertension. Mitral regurgitation related to ischemic papillary muscle dysfunction may contribute to heart failure and lead to acute pulmonary edema.[30]

SYSTEMIC INFECTION. Any serious infection may precipitate cardiac failure. The mechanisms include increased total body metabolism as a consequence of fever, discomfort, and cough, which increases the hemodynamic burden on the heart; the accompanying sinus tachycardia plays an additional adverse role. Patients with advanced heart failure are particularly susceptible to pulmonary infections,[26] presumably because of the diminished ability of congested lungs to expel respiratory secretions. Furthermore, it is postulated that increased circulating levels of proinflammatory cytokines, such as tumor necrosis factor-α and interleukin-1β, which impair myocardial function in sepsis, may precipitate heart failure in the setting of non–life-threatening bacterial or viral infections.[31]

PULMONARY EMBOLISM (see also Chap. 66)**.** Patients with heart failure, particularly when confined to bed, are at high risk for the development of venous thromboembolism. Other thromboembolic risk factors in heart failure include low cardiac output with intracardiac stasis and atrial fibrillation.[32] Pulmonary emboli may increase the hemodynamic burden on the right ventricle by elevating pulmonary artery pressure and pulmonary vascular resistance further and may cause fever, tachypnea, hypoxemia, and tachycardia.

PHYSICAL, EMOTIONAL, AND ENVIRONMENTAL STRESS. Intense, prolonged exertion or marked fatigue, such as may result from prolonged travel or emotional crises, are relatively common precipitants of cardiac decompensation. Severe climatic change (e.g., to a hot, humid environment) may also precipitate worsening heart failure.

CARDIAC INFECTION AND INFLAMMATION. Myocarditis as a consequence of a variety of inflammatory, allergic, or infectious processes, including viral myocarditis (see Chap. 60), may impair myocardial function directly and exacerbate existing heart disease. The anemia, fever, and tachycardia that frequently accompany these processes are also deleterious. In patients with infective endocarditis (see Chap. 58), valvular damage may also precipitate cardiac decompensation.

DEVELOPMENT OF AN UNRELATED ILLNESS. Heart failure may be precipitated in patients with compensated cardiovascular disease when an unrelated illness develops. For example, the development of acute or acute-on-chronic renal failure[33] may further impair the ability of patients with heart failure to excrete sodium or free water and thus may exacerbate fluid retention (see Chap. 86). Similarly, blood transfusion or the administration of sodium-containing fluid during and after noncardiac surgery may result in acute heart failure in patients with underlying structural heart disease.

ADMINISTRATION OF MYOCARDIAL DEPRESSANT OR SALT-RETAINING DRUGS. A number of drugs depress myocardial function; among these are nondihydropyridine calcium antagonists (verapamil and diltiazem), many antiarrhythmic agents, inhalation and intravenous anesthetics (see Chap. 50), and antineoplastic drugs such as doxorubicin and cyclophosphamide (see Chap. 83). Beta-adrenergic antagonists, which are now mainstays of therapy for chronic heart failure (see Chap. 23), can decrease cardiac contractility and must be initiated at low doses and titrated slowly in patients with heart failure. Other medications, such as estrogens, corticosteroids, and nonsteroidal antiinflammatory agents,[34] may cause salt and water retention. Cyclooxygenase-2 (COX-2)-specific inhibitors have been implicated in causing renal insufficiency and fluid retention.[35] Any of these drugs, when administered to a patient with already impaired cardiac function, can precipitate or worsen heart failure.

CARDIAC TOXINS. Alcohol is a potent myocardial depressant and may be responsible for the development of cardiomyopathy (see Chap. 59), arrhythmias, and sudden death.[36] In patients with asymptomatic or mildly symptomatic left ventricular dysfunction, excessive alcohol consumption may precipitate heart failure, either directly by an acute depression of myocardial contractility or indirectly through the development of tachyarrhythmias. Illicit use of cocaine may precipitate acute heart failure by a number of mechanisms, including myocardial ischemia or infarction (see Chap. 62), severe hypertension, arrhythmias, myocarditis, or, in the case of injection drug users, acute infective endocarditis.

HIGH-OUTPUT STATES. Acute heart failure may be precipitated in patients with underlying heart disease, such as valvular heart disease, or by the development of one of the hyperkinetic circulatory states, such as pregnancy or anemia (see High-Output Heart Failure). Anemia may also contribute to disease progression and clinical decompensation in patients with chronic heart failure.[37]

It is essential to search for these precipitating causes systematically in all patients with heart failure. In most instances, the precipitant can be treated effectively, after which appropriate measures should be instituted to avoid recurrence.

Clinical Manifestations

Symptoms

Respiratory Distress

Breathlessness, a cardinal manifestation of left ventricular failure, may arise with progressively increasing severity as (1) exertional dyspnea, (2) orthopnea, (3) paroxysmal nocturnal dyspnea, (4) dyspnea at rest, and (5) acute pulmonary edema.

EXERTIONAL DYSPNEA (see also Chap. 7)**.** The principal difference between exertional dyspnea in normal subjects and that in patients with heart failure is the degree of activity necessary to induce the symptom. As left ventricular failure progresses, the intensity of exercise resulting in breathlessness declines progressively. However, there is no close correlation between subjective exercise tolerance and objective measures of left ventricular performance.[38] Exertional dyspnea may be absent in patients with heart failure who are sedentary for a variety of reasons, such as angina pectoris, intermittent claudication, or a noncardiovascular condition (e.g., osteoarthritis).

ORTHOPNEA. This symptom may be defined as dyspnea that develops in the recumbent position and is relieved by elevation of the head with pillows or by use of an electric adjustable bed. In the recumbent position, blood is displaced from the extrathoracic to the thoracic compartment. The failing left ventricle cannot accept and pump out the extra blood volume delivered to it by the competent right ventricle without dilating. Pulmonary venous and capillary pressures rise further, causing interstitial pulmonary edema, reduced pulmonary compliance, increased airway resistance, and dyspnea.[39] Orthopnea occurs rapidly, often within a minute or two of assuming recumbency, and develops when the patient is awake. It is a nonspecific symptom and may occur in *any* condition in which vital capacity is low. Marked ascites or a large pleural effusion, for example, whatever their cause, may cause orthopnea. *Trepopnea* is a rare form of orthopnea limited to one lateral decubitus position. In patients with advanced heart failure, trepopnea is related to impaired left ventricular filling and may explain the preference for sleeping in the right lateral decubitus position.[40]

The patient with orthopnea generally elevates his or her head and chest on several pillows to prevent nocturnal breathlessness and subsequently the development of paroxysmal nocturnal dyspnea. In advanced left ventricular failure, orthopnea may be so severe that the patient cannot lie down and must spend the night in the sitting position.

COUGH. Cough may be caused by pulmonary congestion, occurs under the same circumstances as dyspnea (i.e., during exertion or on recumbency), and is relieved by treatment of heart failure. Thus, a nonproductive cough in patients with heart failure is often a "dyspnea equivalent," whereas a cough on recumbency may be considered an "orthopnea equivalent."

PAROXYSMAL NOCTURNAL DYSPNEA. Attacks of paroxysmal dyspnea in resting patients usually occur at night. The patient awakens, often quite suddenly and with a feeling of severe anxiety and suffocation, sits bolt upright, and gasps for breath. Bronchospasm, which may be caused by congestion of the bronchial mucosa and by interstitial pulmonary edema compressing the small airways, increases ventilatory difficulty and the work of breathing and is a common complicating factor. The associated wheezing is responsible for the alternative name of this condition, *cardiac asthma.* In contrast to orthopnea, which may be relieved immediately by sitting upright at the side of the bed with the legs dependent, attacks of paroxysmal nocturnal dyspnea may require 30 minutes or longer in this position for relief.

Paroxysmal nocturnal dyspnea is a common clinical feature associated with Cheyne-Stokes respiration in patients with heart failure (see later).[41] Cardiac asthma may be exacerbated by downregulation of pulmonary beta receptors leading to attenuation of cyclic adenosine monophosphate–mediated airway relaxation.

MECHANISMS OF DYSPNEA

Increased awareness of respiration or difficulty in breathing is commonly associated with pulmonary venous hypertension caused by an elevation of left atrial or left ventricular filling pressure. This is particularly true in patients with acute heart failure in whom activation of J receptors in the lung by elevated pulmonary pressures and hypoxemia is the main stimulus for dyspnea.[42] Patients with chronic left ventricular failure typically exhibit a restrictive ventilatory defect, characterized by a reduction of vital capacity as a consequence of the replacement of the air in the lungs with blood or interstitial fluid or both. Consequently, the lungs become stiffer, air trapping occurs because of earlier than normal closure of dependent airways, and the work of breathing is increased because higher intrapleural pressures are needed to distend the stiff lungs.[39] Tidal volume is reduced, and respiratory frequency rises in a compensatory fashion. Engorgement of blood vessels may reduce the caliber of the peripheral airways, increasing airway resistance.

Thus, dyspnea and orthopnea in heart failure are clinical expressions of pulmonary venous and capillary congestion. In addition, there are alterations in the distribution of ventilation and perfusion, resulting in widened alveolar-arterial differences for oxygen, hypoxemia, and an increased ratio of dead space to tidal volume. Paroxysmal nocturnal dyspnea reflects the presence primarily of *interstitial* edema, whereas pulmonary edema, in which there is transudation and expectoration of blood-tinged fluid, is often a manifestation of *alveolar* edema.

There is an increased ventilatory drive as a consequence of the stimulation of stretch receptors in the pulmonary vessels and interstitium as well as of hypoxemia and metabolic acidosis. The increased work of breathing, combined with a low cardiac output and resulting impaired perfusion of the respiratory muscles, causes fatigue and ultimately the sensation of dyspnea.[43]

Dyspnea at rest may also occur in end-stage heart failure when low cardiac output, hypoxemia, and acidosis combine to reduce the delivery of oxygen to the respiratory and peripheral muscles.

Differentiation Between Cardiac and Pulmonary Dyspnea

In most patients with dyspnea there is obvious clinical evidence of disease of either the heart *or* the lungs, but in some the differentiation between cardiac and pulmonary dyspnea may be difficult. Like patients with heart failure, those with chronic obstructive pulmonary disease also may awaken at night with dyspnea, but it is usually associated with sputum production; the dyspnea is relieved after patients rid themselves of secretions by coughing rather than specifically by sitting up. When the dyspnea arises after a history of intensified cough and expectoration, it is often primarily pulmonary in origin. *Acute cardiac asthma* (paroxysmal nocturnal dyspnea with prominent wheezing) usually occurs in patients who have obvious clinical evidence of heart disease and may be further differentiated from acute bronchial asthma by diaphoresis and bubblier airway sounds and the more common occurrence of cyanosis.

Airway obstruction and dyspnea that respond to bronchodilators or smoking cessation favor a pulmonary origin of the dyspnea, whereas symptomatic improvement with diuretics or nitrates supports heart failure as the cause of dyspnea. The availability of a rapid point-of-care assay for measuring plasma levels of B-type natriuretic peptide (BNP), a cardiac neurohormone that is elevated in heart failure (see Chap. 21), may help to differentiate heart failure from lung disease in patients presenting with dypnea.[44] Dyspnea that persists despite appropriate cardiovascular or respiratory pharmacotherapy may be related to psychosocial factors (e.g., anxiety, emotional stress).[45]

Pulmonary Function Testing

Pulmonary function testing should be carried out in patients in whom the etiology of dyspnea is unclear despite detailed clinical evaluation. The major alterations in pulmonary function in heart failure are reductions of vital capacity, total lung capacity, pulmonary diffusion capacity, and pulmonary compliance; resistance to air flow is moderately increased; residual volume and functional residual volume are normal.[46] Expiratory flows are further reduced by smoking.[46] Often there is hyperventilation at rest and during exercise, an increase in dead space, and some abnormalities of ventilation-perfusion relations with slight reductions in arterial carbon dioxide partial pressure (P_{CO_2}) and P_{O_2}. With pulmonary capillary hypertension, pulmonary compliance decreases and there is air trapping because of earlier than normal closure of dependent airways.

Rarely, it may be difficult, on clinical examination, to differentiate between cardiac dyspnea, dyspnea based on *malingering,* and dyspnea caused by *anxiety.*[47,48] Careful observation for the appearance of effortless or irregular respiration during exercise testing often helps to identify the patient in whom dyspnea is related to the latter two noncardiac causes. Patients whose anxiety focuses on the heart may exhibit sighing respiration and difficulty in taking a deep breath as well as dyspnea at rest. Their breathing patterns are not rapid and shallow, as in cardiac dyspnea. Rarely a "therapeutic test" is helpful, and amelioration of dyspnea, accompanied by a weight loss exceeding 2 kg induced by administration of a diuretic, supports a cardiac origin for the dyspnea. Conversely, failure of these measures to achieve such weight reduction and to diminish dyspnea argues against a cardiac origin. Other noninvasive tools to assess cardiac size, such as echocardiography, and cardiac filling pressures in heart failure, such as thoracic bioimpedance[49] and BNP levels,[50] may help to clarify the cause of dyspnea in some patients.

Reduced Exercise Capacity

MECHANISMS OF EXERCISE INTOLERANCE. Exercise capacity may be limited for a variety of reasons in patients with heart failure, including abnormalities in central and peripheral cardiovascular function.[51] The primary central limitations to exercise in patients with heart failure include the development of dyspnea related to pulmonary vascular congestion and the failure of the cardiovascular system to provide sufficient blood flow to exercising muscles. The latter reflects primarily an inadequate cardiac output response to exercise[52] and in some instances worsening functional mitral regurgitation (Fig. 22–5).[53] Secondary pulmonary hypertension[54] and right ventricular dysfunction may also contribute to the reduced cardiac output response to exercise in patients with advanced heart failure.

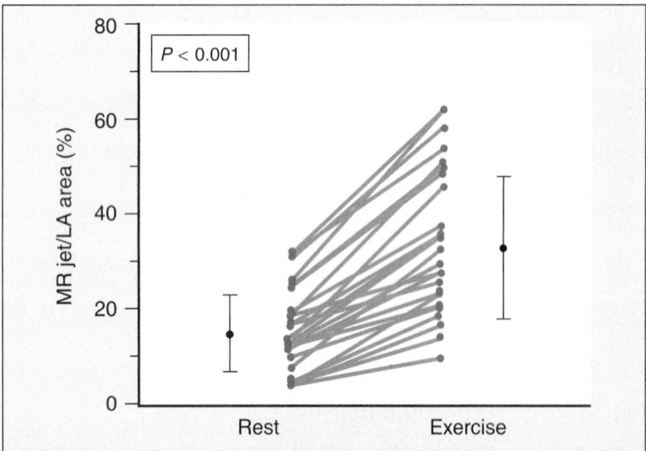

FIGURE 22–5 Functional mitral regurgitation increases with dynamic exercise in heart failure. In this study, 25 patients with chronic heart failure (mean age 53 ± 12 years; New York Heart Association Class 2.6 ± 0.6; left ventricular end-diastolic dimension 73 ± 7 mm; fractional shortening 17 ± 4 percent) underwent symptom-limited bicycle exercise testing with gas-exchange analysis and echocardiography. Individual changes in mitral regurgitation (MR) jet/left atrium (LA) areas are shown. On average, MR was mild to moderate at baseline (MR jet/LA area 15 ± 8 percent) and increased with exercise (MR jet/LA area 33 ± 15 percent). (Data from Lapu-Bula R, Robert A, Van Craeynest D, et al: Contribution of exercise-induced mitral regurgitation to exercise stroke volume and exercise capacity in patients with left ventricular dysfunction. Circulation 106:1342, 2002.)

Other factors that may contribute to reduced exercise capacity in patients with heart failure[51] include anemia,[55] attenuated peripheral vascular response,[56] abnormal skeletal muscle metabolism,[57] and deconditioning of skeletal and respiratory muscles.[58] A rapid improvement in the peripheral vascular response to exercise after intensive, hemodynamically guided therapy has been demonstrated.[59]

There is evidence that the judicious use of cardiac rehabilitation can improve functional capacity,[60] quality of life,[60] and clinical outcomes[61] in patients with heart failure, possibly by (1) improving chronotropic responsiveness, diastolic function, autonomic control of the circulation, and peripheral blood flow[62,63]; (2) reducing neurohormonal activation,[64] proinflammatory cytokines[65] and oxidative stress[66]; (3) reversing abnormalities of skeletal muscle metabolism[67] and respiratory muscle function; and (4) improving patients' perceptions of their quality of life and symptom severity.

To determine the long-term safety and efficacy of exercise training in heart failure,[68] the National Heart, Lung and Blood Institute has initiated a large, multicenter randomized controlled trial of exercise training in patients with New York Heart Association (NYHA) functional Class II to IV heart failure (HF-ACTION).

Exercise Testing (see also Chap. 10)

MAXIMAL EXERCISE CAPACITY. Exercise stress testing may be an exceedingly useful adjunct in the *clinical assessment* of patients with suspected or known heart failure. With use of a bicycle ergometer or treadmill and a progressively increasing load, the maximum level of exercise that can be achieved can be determined; the latter correlates closely with the total oxygen uptake ($\dot{V}O_2$). Close observation of the patient during an exercise test may disclose obvious difficulty in breathing at a low level of exercise (or the opposite). Thus, this simple test may be considered an extension of the clinical examination.

A more formal assessment, in which $\dot{V}O_2$ is measured at each stage of exercise or preferably in which $\dot{V}O_2$ and $\dot{V}CO_2$ are measured continuously, allows determination of maximum $\dot{V}O_2$. It also permits measurement of the anaerobic threshold (i.e., the point during the exercise test at which the respiratory quotient rises as a consequence of the production of excess lactate). A progressive exercise test is carried out until (1) $\dot{V}O_2$ fails to rise with further increases in activity or (2) the patient is limited by severe dyspnea or fatigue, or both. When the $\dot{V}O_2$ is less than 25 ml/kg/min and the reduction is caused by a cardiac abnormality (rather than by pulmonary disease, anemia, peripheral vascular disease, osteoarthritis, an orthopedic disability, marked obesity, or severe deconditioning), it may be used to classify the severity of heart failure. It may also be used to follow the progress of the patient, assess the efficacy of therapeutic maneuvers, and determine prognosis.[69,70] The percentage achieved of predicted maximum $\dot{V}O_2$,[71] the hyperventilatory response to exercise as measured by the $\dot{V}e/\dot{V}CO_2$ slope,[72] and the cardiac output response to exercise measured directly with a pulmonary artery catheter[52] also provide important independent prognostic information in ambulatory patients with heart failure.

SUBMAXIMAL EXERCISE CAPACITY. Because usual daily activities generally require much less than maximal exercise capacity, the measurement of submaximal exercise capacity may provide information that is complementary to that provided by maximal exercise testing.[73] Submaximal exercise capacity can be assessed by measuring the duration of exercise at a constant workload that is generally chosen to be at or below the patient's anaerobic threshold.[74] The 6-minute walk test, most common of the fixed-time tests, measures the distance walked on level ground in 6 minutes.[75] In this test, the patient is asked to walk along a level corridor as far as he or she can in 6 minutes. The patient can slow down or even stop, may be given a carefully controlled level of encouragement, and is told when 3 and 5 minutes have elapsed. The 6-minute walk test and other similar submaximal tests are moderately predictive of maximal oxygen consumption, and, as noted later, the 6-minute walk test independently predicts morbidity and mortality in heart failure.[75,76]

OTHER SYMPTOMS

FATIGUE AND WEAKNESS. These symptoms, which are often accompanied by a feeling of heaviness in the limbs, are generally related to poor perfusion of the skeletal muscles in patients with a reduced cardiac output. They may be associated with impaired flow-mediated vasodilation and altered metabolism in skeletal muscle,[56,57] activation of inflammatory cytokines, and poor nutrition.[77] However, fatigue and weakness are nonspecific symptoms and may be caused by a variety of noncardiopulmonary diseases.

URINARY SYMPTOMS. *Nocturia* may occur relatively early in the course of heart failure. Urine formation is suppressed during the day when the patient is upright and active. When the patient rests in the recumbent position at night, renal vasoconstriction diminishes, and urine formation increases. Nocturia may be troublesome in that it prevents the patient with heart failure from obtaining much-needed rest. *Oliguria* is a sign of advanced heart failure and is related to the suppression of urine formation as a consequence of severely reduced cardiac output.

CEREBRAL SYMPTOMS. Confusion, memory loss, anxiety, headache, insomnia, nightmares, and, rarely, psychosis with disorientation, delirium, and even hallucinations may occur in elderly patients with advanced heart failure,[78] particularly in those with underlying cerebrovascular disease.

SYMPTOMS OF PREDOMINANT RIGHT-SIDED HEART FAILURE. Breathlessness is not as prominent in isolated right ventricular failure as it is in left-sided heart failure because pulmonary congestion is usually absent. Congestive hepatomegaly may produce discomfort, generally described as a dull ache or heaviness, in the right upper quadrant or epigastrium. This discomfort, which is caused by stretching of the hepatic capsule, may be severe when the liver enlarges rapidly, as in *acute* right-sided heart failure. Other gastrointestinal symptoms, including anorexia, nausea, bloating, a sense of fullness after meals, and constipation, are due to congestion of the liver and gastrointestinal tract.

Functional Classification

A classification of patients with heart disease on the basis of the relation between symptoms and the amount of effort required to provoke them was developed by the NYHA.[79] Although there are obvious limitations to assigning numerical values to subjective findings, this classification is nonetheless useful in comparing groups of patients as well as the same patient at different times. In addition, NYHA class has proved to be a strong, independent predictor of survival in patients with chronic heart failure.[80]

As discussed in Chapter 7, the accuracy and reproducibility of this classification are limited. To overcome these limitations, Goldman and associates developed a useful classification based on the estimated metabolic cost of various activities (see Table 7–7). This Specific Activity Scale (SAS) has been used in chronic heart failure trials to assess clinical response to pharmacotherapy.[81]

QUALITY OF LIFE. The three main goals of treatment for heart failure are to reduce symptoms, prolong survival, and improve quality of life. A good "quality of life" implies the ability to live as one wants, free of physical, social, emotional, and economic limitations. Heart failure can have an enormous deleterious impact on the quality of life. Although a number of generic instruments are available to assess health-related quality of life,[82,83] the Minnesota Living with Heart Failure (MLHF) questionnaire[83] and the Kansas City Cardiomyopathy Questionnaire (KCCQ)[84] were designed specifically for use in these patients.

The MLHF consists of 21 brief questions, each of which is answered on a scale of 0 to 5. Eight questions have a strong relationship to the symptoms of dyspnea and fatigue and are referred to as *physical dimension measures.* Five other questions that are strongly related to emotional issues are referred to as *emotional dimension measures.* The test is self-administered and takes only 5 to 10 minutes to complete. For each question, the patient selects a number from 0 to 5. Zero indicates that heart failure had no effect, and 5 indicates a very large effect.

The KCCQ is a self-administered, 23-item questionnaire developed to provide a better description of health-related quality of life in patients with heart failure. It quantifies physical limitation, symptoms, quality of life, social interference, and self-efficacy. The survey requires 4 to 6 minutes to complete and is scored by assigning each response an ordinal value, beginning and summing items within each domain. A clinical summary score is calculated by combining the functional status with the quality of life and social limitation domains.

Although such questionnaires have little role in routine clinical management of patients, they have provided valuable information in clinical investigation by providing prognostic information independent of clinical variables[85] and allowing the response to various pharmacological and device therapies to be quantified.[86] Quality of life instruments have also been used to assess response to cardiac rehabilitation (Fig. 22-6) and multidisciplinary, disease management programs.[87]

Physical Findings (see also Chap. 8)

GENERAL APPEARANCE. Patients with mild or moderate heart failure appear to be in no distress after a few minutes of rest. However, they may be obviously dyspneic during and immediately after moderate activity. Patients with left ventricular failure may become uncomfortable if they lie flat without elevation of the head for more than a few minutes. Those with severe heart failure appear anxious and may exhibit signs of air hunger in this position. Patients with heart failure of recent onset appear acutely ill but are usually well nourished, whereas those with chronic heart failure often appear malnourished and sometimes even cachectic. Chronic, marked elevation of systemic venous pressure may produce severe tricuspid regurgitation and may lead to visible systolic pulsation of the eyes and of the neck veins. Cyanosis, icterus, a malar flush, and abdominal distention caused by ascites may be evident in patients with severe heart failure or adults with chronic heart failure related to uncorrected congenital heart disease.

In *severe* heart failure, stroke volume is reduced, which is reflected in a diminished pulse pressure and dusky discoloration of the skin. With severe unstable heart failure,

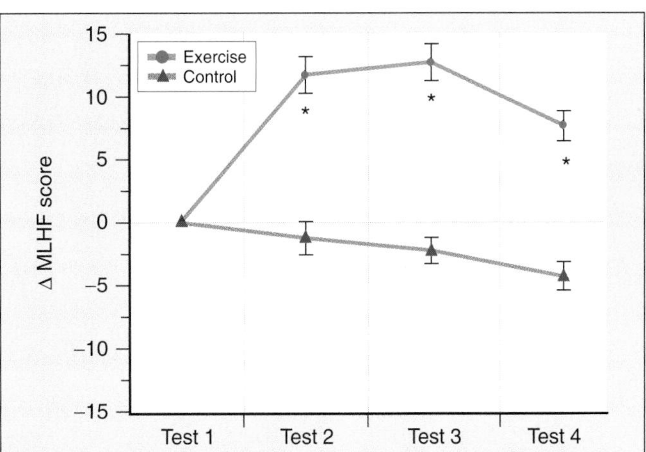

FIGURE 22–6 Changes in the Minnesota Living with Heart Failure (MLHF) questionnaire scores for stable heart failure patients enrolled in a 14-month exercise training program (magenta) compared with untrained control subjects (blue) at baseline (test 1) and after 2, 14, and 24 months (tests 2, 3, and 4). MLHF scores improved significantly in trained patients after 2 months and remained stable after the subsequent 12-month exercise-training program and during follow-up (*$P < 0.001$ for all comparisons). Exercise training was associated with an increase in peak total oxygen uptake ($\dot{V}O_2$) and reductions in both mortality and hospital readmission for heart failure. (Data from Belardinelli R, Georgiou D, Cianci G, Purcaro A: Randomized, controlled trial of long-term moderate exercise training in chronic heart failure: Effects on functional capacity, quality of life, and clinical outcome. Circulation 99:1173, 1999.)

particularly if the cardiac output has declined acutely, systolic arterial pressure may be reduced. The pulse may be rapid, weak, and thready. The proportional pulse pressure (pulse pressure/systolic pressure) shows some correlation with the cardiac output, especially in patients with pulmonary congestion.[88] In one study, when the proportional pulse pressure was less than 25 percent, it usually reflected a cardiac index of less than 2.2 liters/min/m^2.

INCREASED ADRENERGIC ACTIVITY. This is responsible for pallor and coldness of the extremities and cyanosis of the digits, diaphoresis, sinus tachycardia, and distention of the peripheral veins secondary to venoconstriction. Diastolic arterial pressure may be slightly elevated.

PULMONARY RALES. Moist rales result from the transudation of fluid into the alveoli and then into the airways. Rales heard over the lung bases are characteristic of left ventricular failure of at least moderate severity. They are usually heard at both lung bases, but if unilateral they occur more commonly on the right side and may be related to unilateral pleural effusion.[89] In acute pulmonary edema, coarse, bubbling rales and wheezes are heard over both lung fields and are accompanied by the expectoration of frothy, blood-tinged sputum (see Cardiogenic Pulmonary Edema). However, the absence of rales does not exclude considerable elevation of pulmonary capillary pressure. With congestion of the bronchial mucosa, excessive bronchial secretions or bronchospasm or both may give rise to rhonchi and wheezes.

SYSTEMIC VENOUS HYPERTENSION. This can be detected more readily by inspection of the jugular veins, which provides a useful index of right atrial pressure.[90] The upper limit of normal of the jugular venous pressure is approximately 4 cm above the sternal angle when the patient is examined at a 45-degree angle, corresponding to a right atrial pressure of less than 10 cm H_2O. When tricuspid regurgitation is present, the v wave and y descent are most prominent. The jugular venous pressure normally declines on inspiration, but in patients with heart failure (and in those with constrictive pericarditis; see Chap. 64) it rises, a finding known as the *Kussmaul sign*. Elevated jugular venous pressure independently predicts adverse outcomes including death or hospitalization for heart failure.[91]

HEPATOJUGULAR REFLUX. In patients with mild right-sided heart failure, the jugular venous pressure may be normal at rest but rises to abnormal levels with compression of the right upper quadrant, a sign known as the *hepatojugular (or abdominojugular) reflux*.[92] To elicit this sign, the right upper quadrant or epigastrium should be compressed firmly, gradually, and continuously for up to 1 minute while the veins of the neck are observed. The patient should be advised to avoid straining, holding the breath, or carrying out a Valsalva maneuver. A positive test (i.e., expansion of the jugular veins, or increase in jugular venous pressure greater than 3 cm, during and immediately after compression) usually reflects the combination of a congested abdomen and inability of the right side of the heart to accept or eject the transiently increased venous return.

CONGESTIVE HEPATOMEGALY. The liver often enlarges *before* overt edema develops, and it may remain so even after other symptoms of right-sided heart failure have disappeared. If hepatomegaly has occurred rapidly and relatively recently, the liver is usually tender owing to rapid stretching of its capsule. In longstanding heart failure this tenderness disappears, even though the liver remains enlarged. In patients with advanced heart failure, hepatomegaly has been associated with systemic hypoperfusion in the absence of congestion (e.g., the "cold/dry" hemodynamic profile).[88]

Splenomegaly may also occur in severe chronic heart failure or in the presence of severe congestive hepatomegaly in patients with tricuspid valve disease or constrictive pericarditis.[93]

EDEMA. Although a cardinal manifestation of heart failure, edema does not correlate well with the level of systemic venous pressure. In patients with chronic left ventricular failure and a low cardiac output, extracellular fluid volume may be sufficiently expanded to cause edema in the presence of only slight elevations of systemic venous pressure. A substantial gain of extracellular fluid volume, a minimum of 4 liters in adults, must usually take place before peripheral edema is manifested.

Edema in heart failure is usually symmetrical and pitting and generally occurs first in the dependent portions of the body. Accordingly, cardiac edema in ambulatory patients is usually first noted in the feet or ankles at the end of the day and generally resolves overnight. In bedridden patients it is most commonly found over the sacrum. Late in the course of heart failure, edema may become massive and generalized (anasarca), and weight gain associated with anasarca correlates with attenuation of electrocardiographic (ECG) voltage.[94] Longstanding edema results in pigmentation, reddening, and induration of the skin of the lower extremities, usually the dorsum of the feet and the pretibial areas.

HYDROTHORAX (PLEURAL EFFUSION). Because the pleural veins drain into both the systemic and the pulmonary venous beds, hydrothorax is observed most commonly in patients with hypertension involving both venous systems; it may also occur when there is marked elevation of pressure in either venous bed.[95] Effusions occur as increased amounts of fluid in the lung interstitial spaces exit across the visceral pleura, which in turn overwhelm the capacity of the lymphatics in the parietal pleura to resorb the fluid. An increase in capillary permeability probably also plays a role in the pathogenesis of cardiac hydrothorax. Hydrothorax is usually bilateral, but when unilateral it is usually confined to the right side.[89,96] When hydrothorax develops, dyspnea usually intensifies, owing to a further reduction in vital capacity and stimulation of J receptors. Although the excess fluid in hydrothorax is usually resorbed as heart failure improves, loculated interlobar effusions may persist and may require therapeutic thoracentesis.

ASCITES. This finding occurs in patients with increased pressure in the hepatic veins and in the veins draining the peritoneum. Ascites usually reflects longstanding systemic venous hypertension. In patients with organic tricuspid valve disease and chronic constrictive pericarditis,[97] ascites may be more prominent than subcutaneous edema. As in the case of hydrothorax, there is increased capillary permeability because the protein content is similar to that of hepatic lymph (i.e., four to six times that of edema fluid). Protein-losing enteropathy may rarely occur in patients with visceral congestion[98] or end-stage congenital heart disease, and the resultant reduced plasma oncotic pressure may lower the threshold for the development of ascites.

Cardiac Findings (see also Chap. 8)

The presence of cardiac disease is usually readily evident on clinical examination of patients with chronic heart failure.

CARDIOMEGALY. This finding is nonspecific and occurs in the majority of patients with chronic systolic heart failure. Notable exceptions include diastolic heart failure, heart failure associated with chronic constrictive pericarditis or restrictive cardiomyopathy, and acute forms of heart failure.

GALLOP SOUNDS. Protodiastolic sounds, generally emanating from the left ventricle (but occasionally from the right) and occurring 0.13 to 0.16 second after the second heart sound, are common findings in healthy children and young adults. Such physiological sounds are seldom audible in healthy persons after age 40 but occur in patients of all ages with heart failure and are referred to as *protodiastolic*, or *S_3, gallops*.[90] A study showed that the third heart sound is an independent predictor of death and heart failure hospitalizations.[91]

PULSUS ALTERNANS. This sign is characterized by a regular rhythm with alternating strong and weak ventricular contractions.[99] It should be distinguished from the alternation of strong and weak beats that occurs in pulsus bigeminus, in which the weak beat follows the strong beat by a shorter time interval than the strong beat follows the weak. In pulsus alternans, the beats are equally spaced. Severe pulsus alternans may be detected either by palpation of the peripheral pulses (the femoral more readily than the brachial, radial, or carotid) or by sphygmomanometry. As the cuff is slowly deflated, only alternate beats are audible for a variable number of millimeters of mercury below the systolic level, depending on the severity of the alternans, and then all beats are heard. Rarely, the weak beat is so small that the aortic valve is not opened, and this results in an apparent halving of the pulse rate, a condition referred to as *total alternans*. Pulsus alternans may be accompanied by alternation in the intensity of the heart sounds and of existing heart murmurs.

Pulsus alternans occurs most commonly in systolic heart failure and is usually associated with a ventricular protodiastolic gallop sound (S_3). It signifies advanced myocardial disease and often disappears with treatment of heart failure. Pulsus alternans can often be elicited by assumption of the erect posture, tends to be present during tachycardia, and is often initiated by a premature beat.

Pulsus alternans is attributed to an alternation in the stroke volume ejected by the left ventricle and, ultimately, to a deletion in the number of contracting cells in every other cycle, presumably owing to incomplete myocardial recovery. Rarely, pulsus alternans is accompanied by *electrical alternans;* however, the latter condition is usually due not to mechanical alternans but to alternating positions of the heart within the fluid-filled pericardial sac.

ACCENTUATION OF P_2 AND SYSTOLIC MURMURS. With the development of left ventricular failure, pulmonary artery pressure rises and P_2 becomes accentuated (often louder than A_2) and more widely transmitted. *Systolic murmurs* are common in heart failure owing to the functional mitral or tricuspid regurgitation that may occur secondary to ventricular and annular dilation. Often, these murmurs diminish or disappear when compensation is restored with pharmacological[100] or device therapies.[101]

ABNORMAL RESPONSE TO THE VALSALVA MANEUVER. Performance of this maneuver—forced expiration against a closed glottis—is helpful in the diagnosis of heart failure. The test has been standardized as follows. The patient is asked to blow against an aneroid manometer and to maintain a pressure of 40 mm Hg for 30 seconds. Intrathoracic pressure rises, venous return to the heart diminishes, stroke volume falls, and venous pressure rises. Arterial pressure tracings normally show four distinct phases: (1) an initial rise in arterial pressure, which represents transmission to the periphery of the increased intrathoracic pressure; (2) with continuation of the strain and the accompanying reduction of venous return, reductions in systolic, diastolic, and pulse pressures accompanied by a reflex increase in heart rate; (3) on release of the strain, a sudden drop of arterial pressure equivalent to the fall in intrathoracic pressure; and (4) an overshoot of arterial pressure to above control levels, with a wide pulse pressure and bradycardia, caused by a transient rise in cardiac output as blood pooled in the venous system returns to the heart with the release of the strain.

In heart failure, phases 1 and 3 are normal; that is, there is normal transmission of the elevated intrathoracic pressure into the arterial tree during phase 1 and sudden loss of this with the release of the strain during phase 3. However, because the heart operates on the flat portion of its Starling curve, the impedance of venous return during phase 2 does not affect stroke volume. Therefore, the baroreceptor reflex is not activated, and there is no overshoot on release of the strain. This results in a "square-wave" appearance of the tracing. An intermediate response (the so-called absent overshoot response) to the Valsalva maneuver has been demonstrated in patients with moderate depression of left ventricular systolic function.

Experienced clinicians may use bedside sphygmomanometric determination of arterial blood pressure with the Valsalva maneuver to detect elevated left-sided filling pressure.[102] Automated devices are being developed for the same purpose.[103]

FEVER. A low-grade fever (38°C), which results from cutaneous vasoconstriction and therefore impairment of heat loss, may occur in severe heart failure. Fever usually subsides when compensation is restored. Greater elevations of temperature usually signify the presence of infection, pulmonary infarction, or infective endocarditis.

CARDIAC CACHEXIA. Long-standing severe heart failure, particularly right ventricular failure, may lead to anorexia as a consequence of hepatic and intestinal congestion and mesenteric hypoperfusion. Occasionally, there is impaired intestinal absorption of fat[104] and, rarely, protein-losing enteropathy.[98] An association between celiac disease and cardiac cachexia has been described.[105]

Patients with heart failure may also exhibit increased total metabolism secondary to (1) an augmentation of myocardial oxygen consumption, as occurs in patients with aortic stenosis and hypertension; (2) excessive work of breathing; (3) low-grade fever; (4) increased activity of the sympathetic nervous system; and (5) elevated levels of circulating tumor necrosis factor-α.[106] This proinflammatory cytokine is produced by monocytes and contributes to cachexia and anorexia. There is also evidence that inflammatory cytokines, including tumor necrosis factor-α, may depress myocardial contractility and contribute to ventricular remodeling by stimulating myocyte apoptosis and turnover of the extracellular matrix.[107,108]

Other metabolic pathways that cause catabolic-anabolic imbalance and that have been implicated in wasting associated with heart failure include the growth hormone–insulin-like growth factor-1 system and the pituitary-thyroid hormone axis.[109] The combination of reduced caloric intake and increased caloric expenditure may lead to a reduction of tissue mass and, in severe cases, to cardiac cachexia. In some patients, the cachexia may be severe enough to suggest the presence of disseminated malignant disease. In others, the loss of lean body mass may be masked by the accumulation of edema. Cardiac cachexia is an independent risk factor for increased mortality in heart failure.[110]

CHEYNE-STOKES RESPIRATION. Also known as *periodic* or *cyclic respiration,* Cheyne-Stokes respiration is characterized by the combination of depression in the sensitivity of the respiratory center to carbon dioxide and left ventricular failure (Fig. 22-7).[41,111] During the apneic phase, arterial Po_2 falls and Pco_2 rises; this combination excites the depressed respiratory center, resulting in hyperventilation and, subsequently, hypocapnia, followed by another period of apnea. The principal causes of depression of the respiratory center in patients with Cheyne-Stokes respiration are cerebral arteriosclerosis, stroke, and head injury. These causes are often exaggerated by sleep, barbiturates, and narcotics, all of which further depress the sensitivity of the respira-

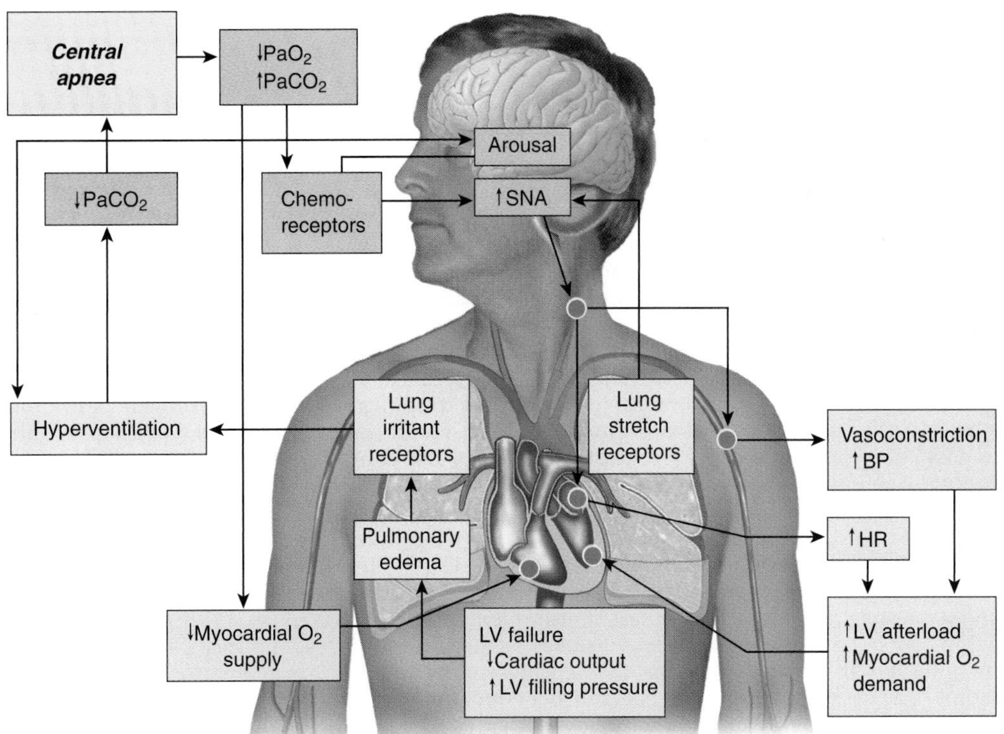

FIGURE 22–7 Pathophysiology of central sleep apnea and Cheyne-Stokes respiration in heart failure (HF). HF leads to increased left ventricular (LV) filling pressure. The resulting pulmonary congestion activates lung vagal irritant receptors, which stimulate hyperventilation and hypocapnia. Superimposed arousals cause further abrupt increases in ventilation and drive the partial pressure of carbon dioxide in arterial blood ($Paco_2$) below the threshold for ventilation, triggering a central apnea. Central sleep apneas are sustained by recurrent arousal resulting from apnea-induced hypoxia and the increased effort to breathe during the ventilatory phase because of pulmonary congestion and reduced lung compliance. Increased sympathetic activity causes increases in blood pressure (BP) and heart rate (HR) and increases myocardial oxygen (O_2) demand in the presence of reduced supply. SNA = sympathetic nervous system activity; PaO_2 = partial pressure of oxygen in arterial blood. (Redrawn from Bradley TD, Floras JS: Sleep apnea and heart failure. Part II: Central sleep apnea. Circulation 107:1822, 2003.)

tory center. Left ventricular failure, which prolongs the circulation time from the lung to the brain, results in a sluggish response of the system and is responsible for the oscillations between apnea and hyperpnea that prevent return to a steady state of ventilation and blood gases. Cheyne-Stokes respiration is also associated with enhanced cardiac sympathetic activity,[112] decreased heart rate variability, and increased peripheral chemosensitivity.[111]

Cheyne-Stokes respiration is seen in up to 40 percent of patients with heart failure and is typically associated with more advanced symptoms.[111] Usually, patients are not aware of Cheyne-Stokes respiration. However, it can be readily observed in a sleeping patient or a history can be elicited from the patient's bed partner. Cheyne-Stokes respiration may contribute to daytime sleepiness, insomnia, and snoring.

PATHOLOGICAL FINDINGS

LUNGS. In patients who have died of left ventricular failure, the lungs are enlarged, firm, and dark and may be filled with bloody fluid. With longstanding pulmonary congestion, they are brown with deposition of hemosiderin and usually do not seep edematous fluid. On microscopic examination, the capillaries are engorged, and there is thickening of the alveolar septa as well as extravasation of large mononuclear cells containing red blood cells or hemosiderin granules or both. Often, the pulmonary vessels show medial hypertrophy and intimal hyperplasia.

LIVER. In acute right-sided heart failure, the liver is slightly enlarged, tense, and cyanotic with rounded edges. On microscopic examination, the central hepatic veins and sinusoids are dilated. With chronic right-sided heart failure, the liver returns to normal size, subsequently atrophies, and becomes "nutmeg" in appearance as a consequence of the dark red areas of central venous congestion and the lighter, fatty area in the periphery of the lobule. Cardiac cirrhosis, also termed *cardiac sclerosis*, is a result of sustained, chronic severe heart failure and is characterized by centrilobular necrosis and atrophy as well as extensive or patchy fibrous retraction. In addition, there may be fibrosis and thrombosis of the hepatic veins.[113]

Liver biopsy specimens of patients with acute cardiomyopathy and fulminant hepatic failure show bridging centrilobular necrosis. Presumably, the hypoxia caused by hypoperfusion produces hepatocyte necrosis; erythrocytes may then enter the space of Disse between damaged endothelial cells.

Laboratory Findings

SERUM ELECTROLYTES. In severe heart failure, prolonged sodium restriction, coupled with intensive diuretic therapy and the inability to excrete free water, may lead to dilutional hyponatremia.[12] Hypervolemic hyponatremia occurs because of substantial expansion of extracellular fluid volume and a normal or only slightly increased level of total body sodium. It may be accompanied by, and presumably is caused in part by, elevated circulating levels of arginine vasopressin.[114] Serum potassium levels are usually normal, although prolonged administration of kaliuretic diuretics, such as the thiazides or loop diuretics, may result in hypokalemia.[115] Secondary hyperaldosteronism may also contribute to hypokalemia. Hyperkalemia may occur in patients with severe heart failure who show marked reductions in glomerular filtration rate and inadequate delivery of sodium to the distal tubular sodium-potassium exchange sites,[116] particularly if they are also receiving ACE inhibitors,[117] potassium-sparing diuretics,[117,118] or potassium supplements. Other common electrolyte abnormalities observed in heart failure include hypophosphatemia and hypomagnesemia[119] (commonly associated with alcohol use and poor nutrition) and hyperuricemia,[120] which may precipitate gout.

RENAL FUNCTION. Proteinuria and a high urine specific gravity are common findings in heart failure. Blood urea nitrogen and creatinine levels are often moderately elevated secondary to reductions in renal blood flow and glomerular filtration rate.[121] Other contributing factors include altered balance of vasoconstrictor and vasodilating hormones and comorbidities such as diabetes and hypertension. In patients with advanced heart failure, the *cardiorenal syndrome*[13] may be exacerbated by several commonly used classes of drugs including ACE inhibitors, angiotensin receptor antagonists, diuretics, nonsteroidal antiinflammatory agents, and COX-2 inhibitors.

LIVER FUNCTION TESTS. Congestive hepatomegaly and cardiac cirrhosis are often associated with impaired hepatic function, characterized by abnormal values of aspartate aminotransferase (AST), alanine aminotransferase (ALT), lactate dehydrogenase (LDH), and other liver enzymes.[122,123] Hyperbilirubinemia, both direct and indirect, is common, and in severe cases of acute (right or left) ventricular failure, frank jaundice may occur. *Acute* hepatic venous congestion can result in severe jaundice with a bilirubin level as high as 15 to 20 mg/dl, elevation of AST to more than 10 times the upper limit of normal, and elevation of the serum alkaline phosphatase level, as well as prolongation of the prothrombin time. The impairment of hepatic function is rapidly ameliorated by successful treatment of heart failure.[124] In patients with longstanding cardiac cirrhosis, albumin synthesis may be impaired, with resultant hypoalbuminemia intensifying the accumulation of fluid. In advanced heart failure, hypoalbuminemia may contribute to and be exacerbated by cardiac cachexia.[77]

HEMATOLOGICAL STUDIES. Anemia is common in heart failure[37,125] and may be due to increased plasma volume (hemodilution) or decreased red cell mass (true anemia). Contributing factors include malnutrition with iron deficiency, bone marrow suppression from activation of proinflammatory cytokines or ACE inhibitors, and chronic renal insufficiency. In a population-based cohort of over 12,000 patients with heart failure, 17 percent had anemia, 58 percent of whom had anemia of chronic disease.[126] Anemia may contribute to ventricular remodeling and disease progression in heart failure by stimulating neurohormonal and cytokine activation and promoting left ventricular hypertrophy.[127] When moderate to severe anemia is present, it may exacerbate underlying ischemic heart disease by causing myocardial and peripheral hypoxia. Rarely, severe anemia may cause high-output failure. Erythropoietin may improve symptoms, exercise tolerance, and cardiac function in anemic patients with chronic heart failure,[55] although the effect of erythropoietin on morbidity and mortality remains to be determined.[128]

Leukocytosis may occur following acute myocardial infarction. In patients presenting with acute heart failure or hemodynamic instability, leukocytosis may suggest the presence of infective endocarditis (see Chap. 58) or pulmonary embolism (see Chap. 66). The erythrocyte sedimentation rate may be low or normal in advanced heart failure because of impaired fibrinogen synthesis and decreased fibrinogen concentration, but more commonly it is elevated because of cytokine activation.[129] A marked increase in sedimentation rate, when present with fever or leukocytosis, should prompt an investigation for infective endocarditis or Takayasu or giant cell arteritis (see Chap. 54).

Chest Radiography (see also Chap. 12)

Two principal features of the chest radiograph are useful in the evaluation of patients with heart failure.[130] The *size and shape of the cardiac silhouette* provide important information concerning the precise nature of the underlying heart disease. Both the cardiothoracic ratio and the heart volume determined on the plain film are relatively specific but insensitive indicators of increased left ventricular end-diastolic volume.

In the presence of normal pulmonary capillary and venous pressure, the lung bases are better perfused than the apices in the erect position, and the vessels supplying the lower lobes are significantly larger than those supplying the upper lobes. With elevation of left atrial and pulmonary capillary pressures, interstitial and perivascular edema develops and is most prominent at the lung bases because hydrostatic pressure is greater there. When pulmonary capillary pressure is slightly elevated (i.e., 13 to 17 mm Hg), the resultant compression of pulmonary vessels in the lower lobes causes equalization in size of the vessels at the apices and bases. With greater pressure elevation (18 to 23 mm Hg), actual pulmonary vascular redistribution occurs (i.e., further constriction of vessels leading to the lower lobes and dilation of vessels leading to the upper lobes) (see Figs. 12–5A and 12–17A). When pulmonary capillary pressures exceed 20 to 25 mm Hg, interstitial pulmonary edema occurs. This edema may be of several varieties: (1) *septal,* producing Kerley lines (i.e., sharp, linear densities of interlobular interstitial edema); (2) *perivascular,* producing loss of sharpness of the central and peripheral vessels; and (3) *subpleural,* producing spindle-shaped accumulations of fluid between the lung and adjacent pleural surface. When pulmonary capillary pressure exceeds 25 mm Hg, alveolar edema, with a cloud-like appearance and concentration of the fluid around the hili in a "butterfly" pattern, and large pleural effusions may occur (see Fig. 12–15). With elevation of systemic venous pressure, the azygos vein and superior vena cava may enlarge.

In patients with *chronic* left ventricular failure, higher pulmonary capillary pressures can be accommodated with fewer clinical and radiological signs of congestion, presumably because of enhanced lymphatic drainage. Pleural effusions are also commonly seen on the chest radiograph in patients with chronic heart failure and, if necessary, can be better defined by thoracic ultrasonography.[131]

Prognosis

Survival is markedly shortened in patients with heart failure, which accounts for a substantial portion of all deaths from cardiovascular diseases. The overall 5-year mortality for all patients with heart failure is approximately 50 percent,[3,132] and the 1-year mortality in patients with end-stage heart failure may be as high as 75 percent.[133] In the United States alone, approximately 260,000 patients die of heart failure each year.[7] The Framingham Heart Study found that between the years 1948 and 1988, patients with a diagnosis of heart failure had a median survival of 1.7 years for men and 3.2 years for women despite the fact that the patients with the poorest prognosis—that is, those dying within 90 days of the diagnosis—were excluded from the analysis.[134] More recent data from the Framingham Study looking at long-term trends in the survival of patients with heart failure demonstrate improved survival in both men and women.[132] Survival of patients with heart failure and preserved systolic function may be better than that of patients with reduced systolic function.[21] More than 90 percent of deaths of patients with heart failure are due to cardiovascular causes, most commonly progressive heart failure and sudden cardiac death.

A large number of factors have been found to correlate with mortality in patients with heart failure.[80,135,136] These fall into four major categories, as follows.

CLINICAL. In general, male gender,[132,137] the presence of coronary artery disease as the etiology of heart failure,[138] the presence of an audible S_3 or elevated jugular venous pressure (Fig. 22–8),[91] low pulse and systolic arterial pressures, a high NYHA class (Fig. 22–9), and reduced exercise capacity (Fig. 22–10)[52,70,139] have each been shown to be associated with increased mortality. When the NYHA class is integrated with the maximal O_2 consumption ($\dot{V}O_{2max}$) determined during exercise, the mortality is 20 percent per year in patients in Class III with a $\dot{V}O_{2max}$ of 10 to 15 ml/kg/min and rises to 60 percent in patients in Class IV with a $\dot{V}O_{2max}$ of less than 10 ml/kg/min. Submaximal exercise also carries important prognostic information in ambulatory patients with heart failure.[75] The distance walked in 6 minutes predicted both morbidity and mortality in the Studies of Left Ventricular Dysfunction (SOLVD) trial (Fig. 22–11)[76] and the Digitalis Investigation Group (DIG) trial. Other exercise parameters associated with impaired survival in heart failure include enhanced ventilatory response to exercise,[140] reduced anaerobic threshold,[141] inspiratory muscle dysfunction,[142] and impaired peripheral chemosensitivity.[143] Additional clinical predictors of mortality in chronic heart failure include important comorbidities such as diabetes mellitus[144] and chronic renal insufficiency (Fig. 22–12),[33] Cheyne-Stokes respiration,[145] sleep apnea,[146,147] cardiac cachexia,[110] and depression.[148] Obesity may confer a more favorable prognosis in patients with advanced heart failure.[149]

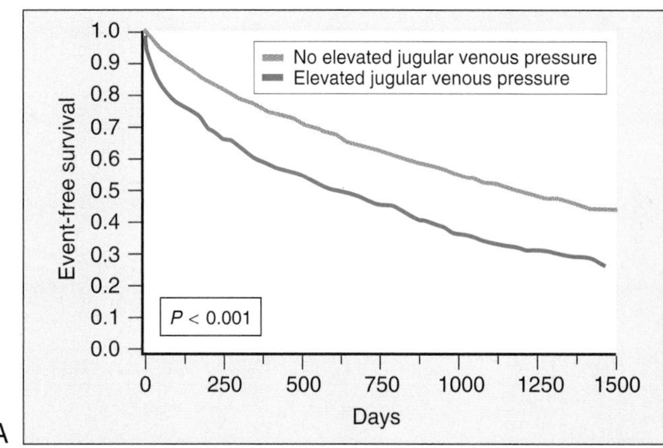

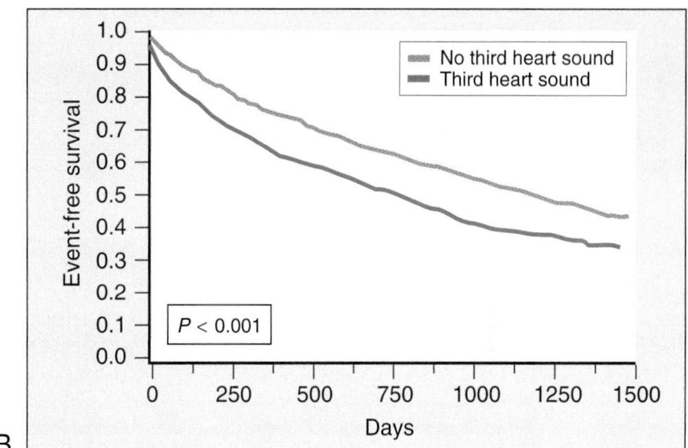

FIGURE 22–8 Event-free survival according to the presence or absence of elevated jugular venous pressure **(A)** and a third heart sound **(B)** in 2569 patients with heart failure enrolled in the Studies of Left Ventricular Dysfunction (SOLVD) treatment trial. **A,** The 280 patients with an elevated jugular venous pressure had a rate of death or hospitalization for heart failure significantly higher than that of the 2199 patients without elevated jugular venous pressure (38.1 events per 100 person-years versus 22.0 events per 100 person-years, $P < 0.001$ by the log rank test). **B,** The 597 patients with a third heart sound had a rate of death or hospitalization for heart failure significantly higher than that of the 1882 patients without a third heart sound (30.9 events per 100 person-years versus 21.4 events per 100 person-years, $P < 0.001$ by log rank test). (From Drazner MH, Rame JE, Stevenson LW, Dries DL: Prognostic importance of elevated jugular venous pressure and a third heart sound in patients with heart failure. N Engl J Med 345:574, 2001.)

STRUCTURAL. The cardiothoracic ratio as measured by chest radiography carries strong independent prognostic information. Other structural variables that can be assessed by two-dimensional echocardiography and that have been associated with increased risk of arrhythmias or death include left ventricular volumes, ventricular mass and sphericity index,[150] secondary mitral or tricuspid regurgitation[151] and left atrial enlargement.[152]

HEMODYNAMIC. Variables such as cardiac index, stroke work index, and both left and right ventricular ejection fractions[153-155] have been shown to correlate directly with survival in patients with heart failure, whereas heart rate, systemic and pulmonary vascular resistances, pulmonary artery pressures, and pulmonary capillary wedge pressure correlate inversely.[156] Combinations of hemodynamic abnormalities, such as depression of stroke work associated with elevation of filling pressure and systemic vascular resistance, are associated with a poor prognosis. Studies have examined the impact of exercise hemodynamics on survival and found that the stroke work index[139] and cardiac output[52] responses to

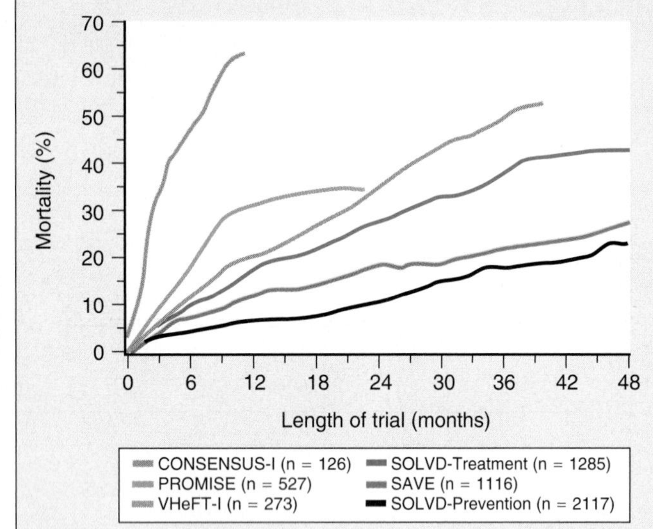

FIGURE 22–9 Clinical correlates of survival in heart failure. On the basis of data from several contemporary, placebo-controlled clinical trials, it can be estimated that the 1-year mortality is on the order of 50 to 60 percent in patients with New York Heart Association (NYHA) functional Class IV symptoms, 15 to 30 percent in patients with Class II to III symptoms, and 5 to 10 percent in asymptomatic patients with left ventricular dysfunction. Patients in CONSENSUS I were in NYHA Class IV and were treated with digitalis and diuretics; patients in SOLVD (Prevention) and SAVE had reduced left ventricular ejection fractions (35 and 40 percent, respectively) but no or mild limitation (NYHA Classes I or II). Patients in PROMISE, SOLVD (Treatment), and VHeFT-I had moderate heart failure (NYHA Class II or III). CONSENSUS = Cooperative North Scandinavian Enalapril Survival Study; PROMISE = Prospective Randomized Milrinone Survival Evaluation; SAVE = Survival And Ventricular Enlargement; SOLVD = Studies of Left Ventricular Dysfunction; VHeFT = Vasodilator Heart Failure Trial. (From Young JB: Assessment of heart failure. *In* Colucci WS [ed]: Heart Failure: Cardiac Function and Dysfunction. 3rd ed. *In* Braunwald E [series ed]: Atlas of Heart Diseases. Philadelphia, Current Medicine, 2002, pp 127-143.)

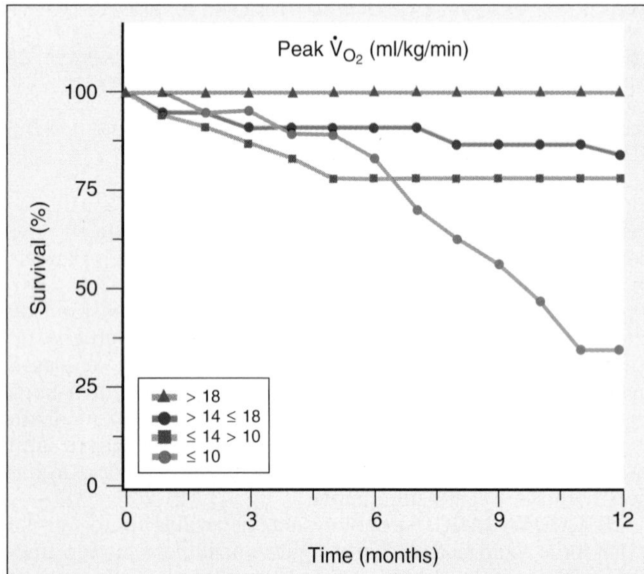

FIGURE 22–10 Kaplan-Meier survival analysis in patients with severe left ventricular dysfunction stratified by peak oxygen consumption ($\dot{V}O_2$) as measured by cardiopulmonary exercise testing during evaluation for cardiac transplantation. Patients with a peak $\dot{V}O_2$ of 10 ml/kg/min or less had significantly reduced survival rates compared with patients with peak $\dot{V}O_2$ greater than 14 ml/kg/min. (From Mancini DM, Eisen H, Kussmaul W, et al: Value of peak exercise oxygen consumption for optimal timing of cardiac transplantation in ambulatory patients with heart failure. Circulation 83:778, 1991.)

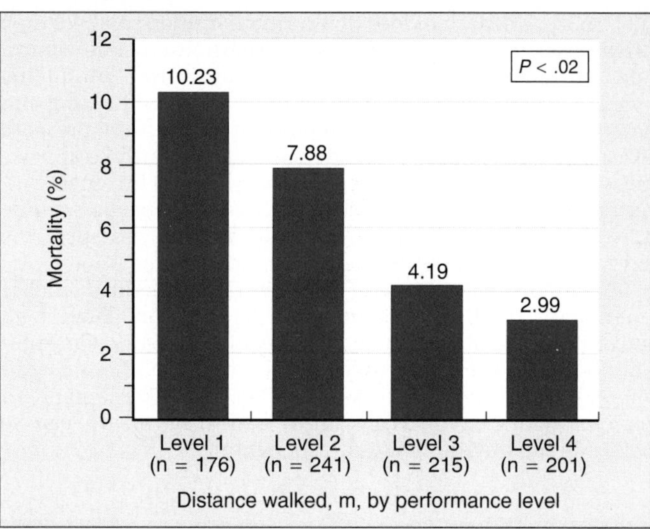

FIGURE 22–11 Mortality (percent) as a function of performance level (based on distance walked in 6 minutes). Mortality decreased as performance on the 6-minute walk test improved. (From Bittner V, Weiner DH, Yusuf S, et al: Prediction of mortality and morbidity with a 6-minute walk test in patients with left ventricular dysfunction. JAMA 270:1702, 1993.)

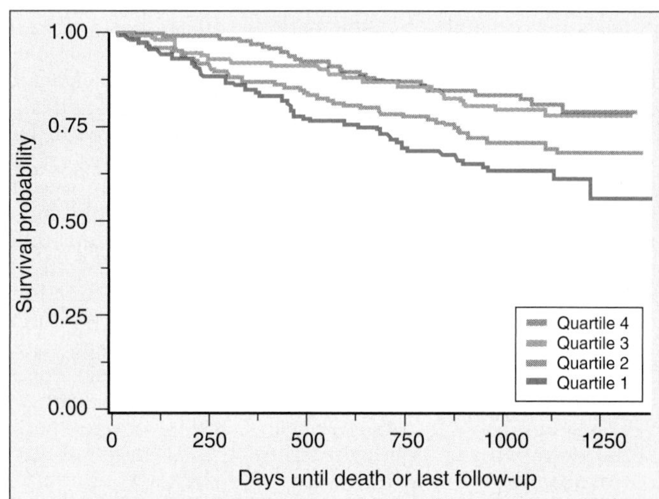

FIGURE 22–12 The prognostic value of baseline renal function was determined in 585 participants in an exercise substudy of the Digitalis Investigation Group (DIG) trial. Baseline characteristics of these patients were similar to those of the main trial (age 65 ± 12 years, ejection fraction 35 ± 13 percent). Mortality by increasing quartiles of estimated creatinine clearance using the Cockcroft-Gault equation was 37 percent (18 to 48 ml/min), 29 percent (47 to 64 ml/min), 18 percent (64 to 86 ml/min), and 21 percent (86 to 194 ml/min) with corresponding hazard ratios relative to the top quartile of 2.1, 1.6, and 0.9, respectively. (From Mahon NG, Blackstone EH, Francis GS, et al: The prognostic value of estimated creatinine clearance alongside functional capacity in ambulatory patients with chronic congestive heart failure. J Am Coll Cardiol 40:1106, 2002.)

exercise provide valuable independent prognostic information. In one study, patients with reduced cardiac output response to exercise and $\dot{V}O_{2max}$ less than or equal to 10 ml/kg/min had an extremely poor prognosis (i.e., 1-year survival rate of 38 percent).[52] Others have shown that $\dot{V}O_{2max}$ is superior to hemodynamic measurements in predicting outcome in severe heart failure.[157] In patients with idiopathic dilated cardiomyopathy, a significant reduction in myocardial blood flow as assessed by positron emission tomography was associated with an increased risk of death or progression of heart failure.[154]

Studies using Doppler echocardiography to assess the pattern of mitral valve inflow have demonstrated an association between *diastolic* dysfunction and impaired survival in patients with chronic *systolic* heart failure.[158] In a prospective study of 331 patients with impaired left ventricular function (ejection fraction < 40 percent), a restrictive filling pattern added incremental value to $\dot{V}O_{2max}$ in determining the risk of death or transplantation.[158]

BIOCHEMICAL. The observation that there is activation of the neurohormonal axis in heart failure has prompted examination of the relationships between a variety of biochemical measurements and clinical outcome. Strong inverse correlations have been reported between survival and plasma levels of norepinephrine (Fig. 22–13),[159,160] renin,[159] arginine vasopressin,[161] aldosterone,[162] atrial and B-type natriuretic peptides (Fig. 22–14),[160,163-165] and endothelin-1.[166] The concentrations of these substances reflect the severity of the underlying impairment of cardiovascular function. In addition, some may exert adverse hemodynamic effects; norepinephrine, angiotensin II, arginine vasopressin, and endothelin-1 are potent vasoconstrictors, augmenting ventricular afterload and thereby reducing the shortening of myocardial fibers. Furthermore, they may be directly responsible for adverse biochemical effects on the myocardium. For example, the elevated norepinephrine concentration may be responsible for ventricular tachyarrhythmias, as may hypokalemia and reduction of total-body potassium stores

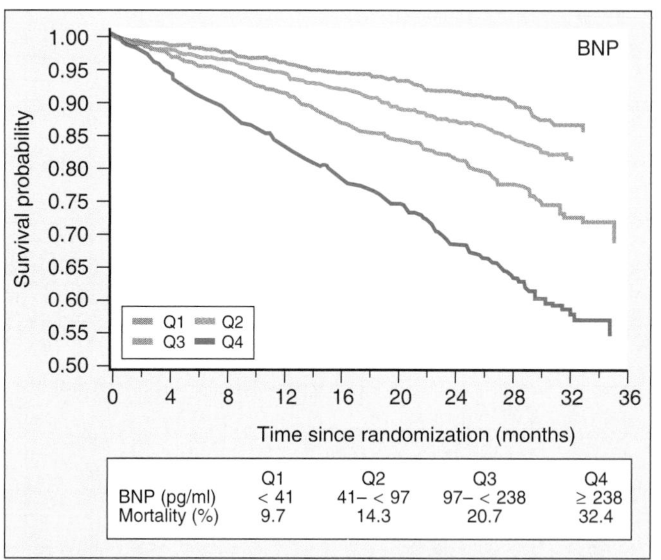

FIGURE 22–14 Plasma B-type natriuretic peptide (BNP) was measured before randomization and during follow-up in approximately 4300 patients in the Valsartan Heart Failure Trial. The baseline values for BNP in quartiles were less than 41, 41 to less than 97, 97 to less than 238, and greater than or equal to 238 pg/ml. Kaplan-Meier curves show a significant quartile-dependent increase in mortality and first morbid events. (From Anand IS, Fisher LD, Chiang YT, et al: Changes in brain natriuretic peptide and norepinephrine over time and mortality and morbidity in the Valsartan Heart Failure Trial (Val-HeFT). Circulation 107:1278, 2003.)

resulting from the activation of the renin-angiotensin-aldosterone system (and the administration of potassium-losing diuretics). Norepinephrine also exerts direct toxic effects on the myocardium, including stimulation of cellular hypertrophy, apoptosis, and changes in extracellular matrix regulation, and thus contributes directly to ventricular remodeling and disease progression.[167] Like norepinephrine, endothelin-1 is a potent vasoconstrictor peptide that exerts growth-promoting effects on the myocardium and vascular smooth muscle cells.[10,31] Hyponatremia also correlates well with increased mortality,[168] but it is likely that this variable reflects activation of the renin-angiotensin-aldosterone axis.

MULTIVARIATE ANALYSIS. In many studies, the aforementioned variables have been assessed in a univariate manner (i.e., independently of one another) and there is disagreement regarding which provides *independent* prognostic information. However, Rector and Cohn have shown that although left ventricular function appears to have the most profound effect on survival in patients with advanced heart failure, exercise tolerance (as reflected in peak oxygen consumption during a progressive exercise test) and activation of the sympathetic nervous system (as reflected in the plasma norepinephrine concentration) *each* provide important independent information.[135] More recent studies of patients with heart failure receiving neurohormonal antagonists (e.g., ACE inhibitors and beta blockers) have identified pro-BNP and BNP levels as strong independent predictors of sudden cardiac death[169] and all-cause mortality.[80,160,163,164]

It is important to note that most of these studies measured biomarkers at baseline and assessed their relationship to subsequent clinical events. Only recently have investigators sought to determine the relationship between the *change* in biomarkers over time and outcomes. An analysis of more than 4000 patients observed in the Valsartan Heart Failure Trial (Val-HeFT) demonstrated that the percentage changes in norepinephrine and BNP over 12 months are independently associated with corresponding changes in morbidity and mortality.[160] Data such as these may allow clinicians to use biomarkers to manage chronic heart failure.[170]

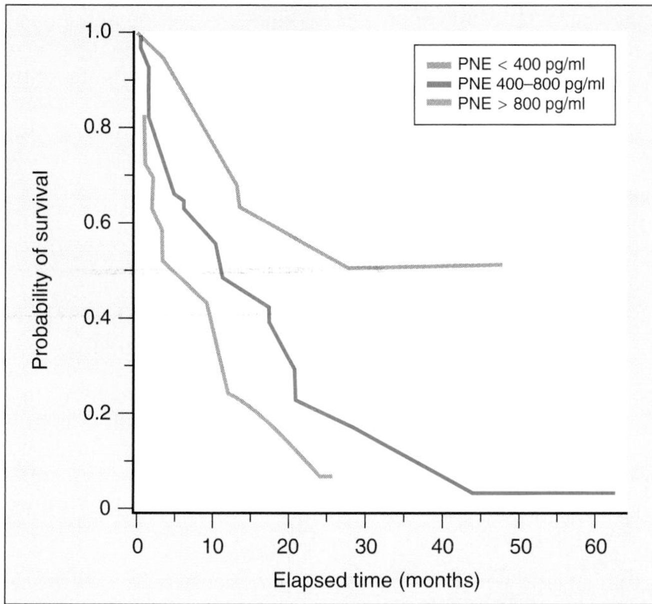

FIGURE 22–13 Activation of the sympathetic nervous system is a marker of impaired survival in heart failure. Life table analysis of survival, according to tercile, based on level of plasma norepinephrine (PNE). Group 1 (<400 pg/ml) contained 27 patients, group 2 (400 to 800 pg/ml) had 49 patients, and group 3 (>800 pg/ml) had 30 patients. The probability of survival in each group was significantly different from the probabilities in the other two groups. (From Cohn JN, Levine TB, Olivari MT, et al: Plasma norepinephrine as a guide to prognosis in patients with chronic congestive heart failure. N Engl J Med 311:819, 1984.)

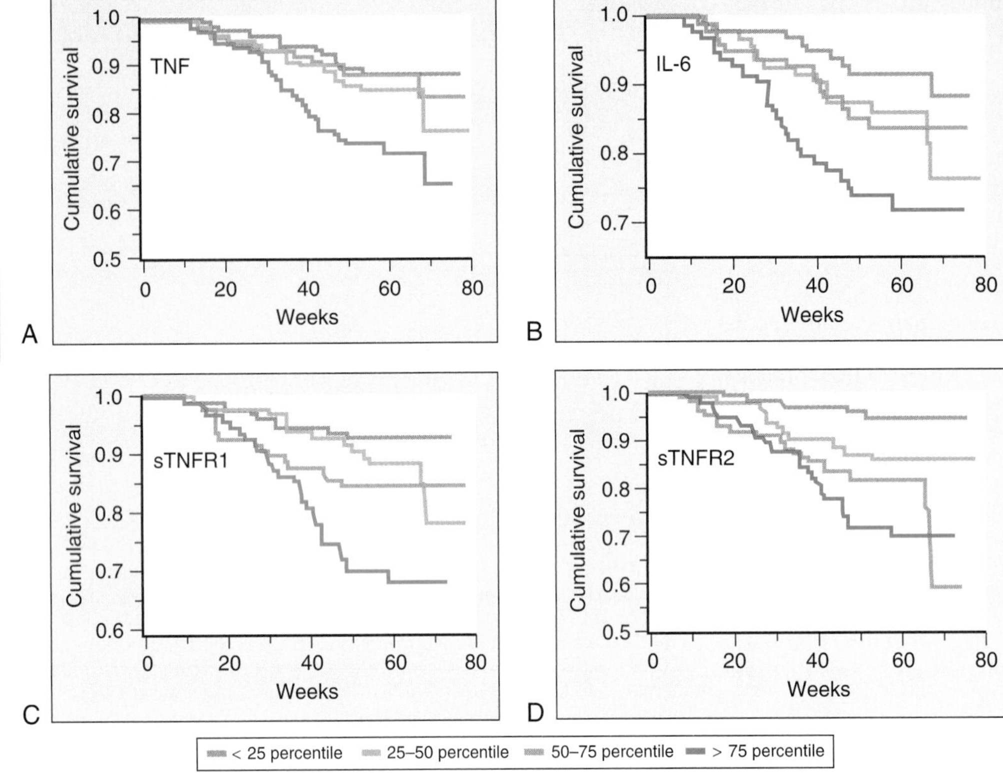

FIGURE 22–15 Kaplan-Meier survival analysis in 1200 consecutive subjects who were enrolled in a multicenter, randomized, placebo-controlled trial of vesnarinone in patients with advanced heart failure (VEST study). Circulating levels of **(A)** tumor necrosis factor (TNF), **(B)** interleukin-6 (IL-6), **(C)** soluble TNF receptor 1 (sTNFR1), and **(D)** soluble TNF receptor 2 (sTNFR2) were examined in relation to patients' survival during a mean follow-up of 55 weeks. Plasma levels of cytokines and cytokine receptors were divided into quartiles, with increasing levels associated with worse survival. (From Deswal A, Petersen NJ, Feldman AM, et al: Cytokines and cytokine receptors in advanced heart failure: an analysis of the cytokine database from the Vesnarinone Trial (VEST). Circulation 103:2055, 2001.)

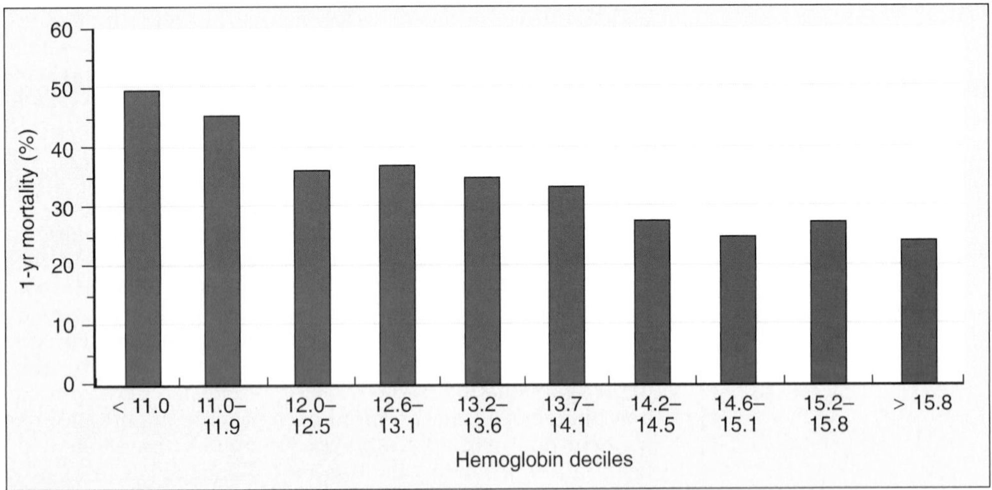

FIGURE 22–16 Anemia is associated with increased mortality in heart failure. In this single-center study, 1061 patients with advanced heart failure were evaluated for cardiac transplantation between 1983 and 1999. At initial presentation, mean hemoglobin (Hb) was 13.5 ± 1.9 gm/dl, and Hb ranged from 7.1 to 19.0 gm/dl. Lower hemoglobin levels were associated with greater symptoms, reduced exercise capacity, and impaired renal function. One-year mortality rates in the entire cohort divided by decile of Hb level are shown. (From Horwich TB, Fonarow GC, Hamilton MA, et al: Anemia is associated with worse symptoms, greater impairment in functional capacity and a significant increase in mortality in patients with advanced heart failure. J Am Coll Cardiol 39:1780, 2002.)

OTHER MARKERS OF PROGNOSIS. In addition to traditional neurohormones, several other biological mediators have been shown to carry important prognostic information in heart failure. Plasma levels of proinflammatory cytokines, including tumor necrosis factor-α[171,172] and interleukin-6[165,173] and their cognate receptors (Fig. 22–15), are elevated in relation to disease severity and predict adverse outcomes. Cytokines exert direct negative effects on cardiac myocytes and the extracellular matrix and have been implicated in ventricular remodeling and disease progression.[107] Markers of oxidative stress, such as oxidized low-density lipoprotein[174] and serum uric acid,[175] have also been associated with worsening clinical status and impaired survival in patients with chronic heart failure. Like inflammation, oxidative stress probably plays an important role in the pathophysiology of heart failure. In patients with stable chronic heart failure, the erythrocyte sedimentation rate correlates with inflammatory cytokines, and high erythrocyte sedimentation rates indicate a poor prognosis independent of NYHA class, ejection fraction, and $\dot{V}O_{2max}$.[129] Cardiac troponin T, a sensitive marker of myocyte damage (see Chap. 46), may be elevated in patients with nonischemic heart failure and predict adverse cardiac outcomes.[176]

A strong association between chronic heart failure and anemia has been demonstrated that carries important prognostic implications (see Laboratory Findings).[125] In a study of 1061 patients with NYHA Class III or IV heart failure and ejection fraction less than 40 percent, lower hemoglobin quartiles were associated with worse symptoms, lower $\dot{V}O_{2max}$, and increased mortality (Fig. 22–16).[125]

ELECTROPHYSIOLOGICAL. Death in patients with severe heart failure occurs either by progressive pump failure or, in as many as one half of all patients, suddenly and unexpectedly, presumably from an arrhythmia. When present, a variety of arrhythmias, especially frequent ventricular extrasystoles,[177] ventricular tachycardia,[178] left bundle branch block[179] and atrial fibrillation,[180] have been shown to be predictors of mortality and sudden death. What is not yet clear is whether these arrhythmias are simply indicators of the severity of left ventricular dysfunction or whether they are responsible for and trigger fatal arrhythmias. Although there is some evidence that ventricular arrhythmias confer independent adverse prognostic effects,[177] this may not hold true after adjusting for other variables, especially ejection fraction.[178] Furthermore, the routine treatment of patients with heart failure–associated arrhythmias with antiarrhythmic drugs has not been shown to exert a protective effect and reduce mortality.[181] Preliminary data from a large trial of cardiac resynchronization therapy (see Chap. 24) suggest a significant survival benefit when biventricular pacing is combined with an implantable cardioverter-defibrillator in patients with ischemic or nonischemic cardiomyopathy.[182]

Other electrophysiological parameters that have been associated with increased mortality or sudden death in heart failure, or both, include increased QT interval[183] and QT dispersion,[184] T wave alternans,[185] abnormal signal-averaged ECG, and decreased heart rate variability.[177]

Pulmonary Edema

Mechanism of Pulmonary Edema

ALVEOLAR-CAPILLARY MEMBRANE. Pulmonary edema develops when the movement of liquid from the blood to the interstitial space, and in some instances to the alveoli, exceeds the return of liquid to the blood and its drainage through the lymphatics.[186] The barrier between pulmonary capillaries and alveolar gas, the alveolar-capillary membrane, consists of three anatomical layers with distinct structural characteristics: (1) cytoplasmic projections of the capillary endothelial cells that join to form a continuous cytoplasmic tube; (2) the interstitial space, which varies in thickness and may contain connective tissue fibrils, fibroblasts, and macrophages between the capillary endothelium and the alveolar epithelium, terminal bronchioles, small arteries and veins, and lymphatic channels; and (3) the lining of the alveolar wall, which is continuous with the bronchial epithelium and is composed predominantly of large squamous cells (type I) with thin cytoplasmic projections.

There is normally a continuous exchange of liquid, colloid, and solutes between the vascular bed and interstitium.[187] A pathological state exists only when there is an increase in the net flux of liquid, colloid, and solutes from the vasculature into the interstitial space. Experimental studies have confirmed that the basic principles outlined in the classic Starling equation apply to the lung as well as to the systemic circulation.

$$Q_{(iv\text{-}int)} = K_f[(P_{iv} - P_{int}) - \sigma_f(\Pi_{iv} - \Pi_{int})]$$

where $Q_{iv\text{-}int}$ = net rate of transudation (flow of liquid from blood vessels to interstitial space), P_{int} = interstitial hydrostatic pressure, P_{iv} = intravascular hydrostatic pressure, Π_{int} = interstitial colloid osmotic pressure, Π_{iv} = intravascular colloid osmotic pressure, σ_f = reflection coefficient for proteins, and K_f = filtration coefficient.

LYMPHATICS. These vessels serve to remove solutes, colloid, and liquid derived from the blood vessels. Because of a more negative pressure in the peribronchial and perivascular interstitial spaces and the increased compliance of this nonalveolar interstitium, liquid is more likely to increase here when the pumping capacity of the lymphatic channels is exceeded. As a consequence of the development of interstitial edema, small airways and blood vessels may become compressed.

The lymphatics play a key role in removing liquid from the interstitial space, and if the pumping capacity of the lymphatic channels is exceeded, pulmonary edema occurs. With chronic elevations of left atrial pressure, the pulmonary lymphatic system hypertrophies and is able to transport greater quantities of capillary filtrate, thereby protecting the lungs from edema. By contrast, a sudden marked increase in pulmonary capillary pressure can be rapidly fatal in a patient not preconditioned by growth of the lymphatic drainage system.

SEQUENCE OF FLUID ACCUMULATION DURING PULMONARY EDEMA. Whether initiated by an imbalance of Starling forces or by primary damage to the various components of the alveolar-capillary membranes, the sequence of liquid exchange and accumulation in the lungs is the same and can be represented in three stages. In *stage 1,* there is an increase in mass transfer of liquid and colloid from blood capillaries through the interstitium. Despite the increased filtration, there is no measurable increase in interstitial volume because there is an equal increase in lymphatic outflow. *Stage 2* occurs when the filtered load from the pulmonary capillaries is sufficiently large that the pumping capacity of the lymphatics is approached or exceeded, and liquid and colloid begin to accumulate in the more compliant interstitial compartment surrounding bronchioles, arterioles, and venules. In *stage 3,* further increments in filtered load exceed the volume limits of the loose interstitial spaces, causing distention of the less compliant interstitial space of the alveolar-capillary septum and resulting in alveolar flooding.

Classification of Pulmonary Edema

The two most common forms of pulmonary edema are those initiated by an imbalance of Starling forces and those initiated by disruption of one or more components of the alveolar-capillary membrane (Table 22–5).[186,188] Less often, lymphatic insufficiency can be involved as a predisposing, if not initiating, factor in the genesis of edema.

IMBALANCE OF STARLING FORCES

INCREASED PULMONARY CAPILLARY PRESSURE. Pulmonary edema occurs only when the pulmonary capillary pressure rises to values exceeding the plasma colloid osmotic pressure, which is approximately 28 mm Hg in the human. Because the normal pulmonary capillary pressure is 8 to 12 mm Hg, there is a substantial margin of safety in the development of pulmonary edema. Although pulmonary capillary pressures must be abnormally high to increase the flow of interstitial fluid, at a time when edema is clearly present these pressures may not correlate with the severity of pulmonary edema. In fact, pulmonary capillary wedge pressures may have returned to normal at a time when there is still considerable pulmonary edema because time is required for removal of both interstitial and alveolar edema. Other factors obscure the relationship between the severity of edema and measured pulmonary capillary pressures in addition to slower rates of removal after edema has collected. The rate of increase in lung liquid at any given elevation of capillary pressure is related to the functional capacity of lymphatics, which may vary from patient to patient, and to variations in interstitial oncotic and hydrostatic pressures.

HYPOALBUMINEMIA. Pulmonary edema does not develop with hypoalbuminemia alone. However, hypoalbuminemia may alter the fluid conductivity of the interstitial space so that liquid moves more easily between capillaries and lymphatics. Therefore, in addition to hypoalbuminemia, there must be some elevations of pulmonary capillary pressure, but only small increases are necessary before pulmonary edema ensues in the presence of hypoalbuminemia.

INCREASED NEGATIVE INTERSTITIAL PRESSURE. Pulmonary edema may result from the rapid removal of pleural air to relieve a pneumothorax—so-called reexpansion pulmonary edema. Risk factors include young age and a large pneumothorax.[189] Usually, the pneumothorax has been present for several hours to days, allowing time for alterations in surfactant so that large negative pressures are necessary to open collapsed alveoli. In these instances, the edema is unilateral and is most often only a radiographic finding, with few clinical findings. In rare cases, reexpansion pulmonary edema may be severe and require rapid and extensive clinical treatment. Studies using radiolabeled transferrin suggest that an abnormality in microvascular permeability contributes to the development of localized pulmonary edema, possibly related to hypoxic injury[190] and local production of proinflammatory cytokines.[191] Hemodynamic studies have also demonstrated an increase in cardiac output immediately prior to the development of pulmonary edema.[192]

PRIMARY ALVEOLAR-CAPILLARY BARRIER DAMAGE

Many diverse medical and surgical conditions are associated with pulmonary edema that is due to damage of the alveolar-capillary barrier rather than to a primary alteration in Starling forces.[186] These conditions include acute pulmonary infections and pulmonary effects of gram-negative sepsis and nonthoracic trauma, as well as any condition associated with disseminated intravascular coagulation. Despite the diversity of underlying causes, when diffuse alveolar-capillary injury has occurred, the pathophysiological and clinical sequence of events are quite similar in most patients. Because of the resemblance of the clinical picture to that seen with respiratory distress of the neonate, these conditions have been referred to as the *acute respiratory distress syndrome* (ARDS).[193,194]

TABLE 22–5 Classification of Pulmonary Edema on the Basis of Initiating Mechanism

Imbalance of Starling Forces
Increased pulmonary capillary pressure
1. Increased pulmonary venous pressure without left ventricular failure (e.g., mitral stenosis)
2. Increased pulmonary venous pressure secondary to left ventricular failure
3. Increased pulmonary capillary pressure secondary to increased pulmonary arterial pressure (so-called overperfusion pulmonary edema)*

Decreased plasma oncotic pressure: hypoalbuminemia secondary to renal, hepatic, protein-losing enteropathic, or dermatological disease or nutritional causes†
Increased negativity of interstitial pressure
1. Rapid removal of pneumothorax with large applied negative pressures
2. Large negative pressures due to acute airway obstruction along with increased end-expiratory volumes (asthma)*

Increased interstitial oncotic pressure: no known clinical or experimental example

Alveolar-Capillary Barrier Damage (Acute Respiratory Distress Syndrome)
Direct lung injury
1. Pneumonia—bacterial, viral, parasitic
2. Aspiration of gastric contents
3. Inhaled toxins (e.g., phosgene, ozone, chlorine, nitrogen dioxide, smoke)
4. Pulmonary contusion
5. Fat emboli
6. Near-drowning
7. Radiation pneumonitis

Indirect lung injury
1. Sepsis
2. Nonthoracic trauma with shock and multiple transfusions
3. Disseminated intravascular coagulation
4. Hypersensitivity pneumonitis due to drugs (e.g., nitrofurantoin), leukoagglutinins
5. Acute pancreatitis
6. Endogenous vasoactive substances (e.g., histamine, kinins*)
7. Circulating foreign substances (e.g., snake venom, alloxan,† alpha-naphthyl thiourea‡)

Lymphatic Insufficiency
After lung transplantation
Lymphangitic carcinomatosis
Fibrosing lymphangitis (e.g., silicosis)

Unknown or Incompletely Understood
High-altitude pulmonary edema
Neurogenic pulmonary edema
Narcotic overdose
Pulmonary embolism
Preeclampsia-eclampsia
After cardioversion
After anesthesia
After cardiopulmonary bypass

*Not certain to exist as a clinical entity.
† Not certain that this, as a single factor, leads to pulmonary edema.
‡ Predominantly an experimental technique.

Direct evidence for increased permeability of the alveolar-capillary barrier in ARDS, leading to influx of protein-rich fluid into the air spaces,[195] has come mainly from experimental studies. It is likely that epithelial injury leading to increased permeability of the alveolar-capillary barrier is a critical initiating event in most cases of ARDS.[193] The loss of integrity of the alveolar epithelium results in impaired removal of edema fluid from the alveolar space, reduced production of surfactant, increased risk of septic shock, and disorganized epithelial repair. Although it remains unclear whether neutrophil-mediated inflammation is a cause or the result of lung injury, evidence suggests that an imbalance between proinflammatory cytokines and antiinflammatory mediators contributes to both the initiation and amplification of injury.[186]

Cardiogenic Pulmonary Edema

PATHOPHYSIOLOGY. Cardiogenic pulmonary edema is characterized by the transudation of protein-poor fluid into the lungs secondary to an increase in left atrial and subsequently pulmonary capillary pressure. This transudation occurs in the absence of an alteration in the permeability or integrity of the alveolar-capillary membrane and results in decreased diffusing capacity, hypoxemia, and shortness of breath.

During *stage 1*, the distention and recruitment of small pulmonary vessels secondary to elevation of left atrial pressure may actually improve gas exchange in the lung and augment slightly the diffusing capacity for carbon monoxide. Exertional dyspnea accompanies these abnormalities, and inspiratory rales related to opening of closed airways may be present.

With progression to *stage 2, interstitial edema* attributable to increased liquid in the loose interstitial space contiguous with the perivascular tissue of larger vessels may cause a loss of the normally sharp radiographic definition of pulmonary vascular markings, haziness and loss of demarcation of hilar shadows, and thickening of interlobular septa (Kerley B lines). Competition for space between vessels, airways, and increased liquid within the loose interstitium may compromise small airway lumina, particularly in the dependent portions of the lungs, and there may be reflex bronchoconstriction. A mismatch exists between ventilation and perfusion that results in hypoxemia and more wasted ventilation. Indeed, in the setting of acute myocardial infarction, the degree of hypoxemia correlates with the degree of elevation of the pulmonary capillary wedge pressure. Tachypnea is a frequent finding with interstitial edema and has been attributed to stimulation of J-type receptors or stretch receptors in the interstitium rather than to hypoxemia, which is rarely of sufficient magnitude to stimulate breathing. There are few changes in the standard spirometric indices.

With the development of alveolar flooding, or *stage 3* edema, gas exchange is quite abnormal, with severe hypoxemia and often hypocapnia. Alveolar flooding can proceed to such a degree that many large airways are filled with blood-tinged foam that may be expectorated. Vital capacity and other lung volumes are markedly reduced. A right-to-left intrapulmonary shunt develops as a consequence of perfusion of the flooded alveoli. Although hypocapnia is the rule, hypercapnia with acute respiratory acidemia can occur in more severe cases or in patients with concomitant chronic obstructive pulmonary disease. It is in such instances that morphine, with its well-known respiratory depressant effects, should be used with caution.

ROLE OF LYMPHATICS. As discussed earlier, the rate of accumulation of lung liquid at a given elevation in pulmonary capillary pressure is related to the functional capacity of the pulmonary lymphatic vessels to remove excess fluid. With acute increases in pulmonary capillary pressure, lymphatic vessels in the lungs lack the capacity to increase rapidly the rate of fluid removal. As a result, patients with acute heart failure develop pulmonary edema at pulmonary capillary pressures as low as 18 mm Hg. In contrast, patients with chronic heart failure usually do not develop pulmonary edema until pulmonary capillary pressures have increased to 25 mm Hg or higher, presumably because of increased lymphatic capacity.

ETIOLOGY AND DIAGNOSIS. Acute cardiogenic pulmonary edema is the most dramatic symptom of left-sided heart failure.[196,197] It may be caused by impairment of left atrial outflow, left ventricular systolic or diastolic dysfunction, left ventricular volume overload, or left ventricular outflow obstruction. Elevated left atrial and pulmonary capillary wedge pressures lead to cardiogenic pulmonary edema, which, in turn, interferes with oxygen transfer in the lungs and depresses arterial oxygen tension. Simultaneously, the sensation of suffocation and oppression in the chest intensifies the patient's fright, elevates heart rate and blood pressure, and further restricts ventricular filling. The increased discomfort and work of breathing place an additional load on the heart, and cardiac function becomes depressed further by the hypoxia. If this vicious circle is not interrupted, it may lead rapidly to death.

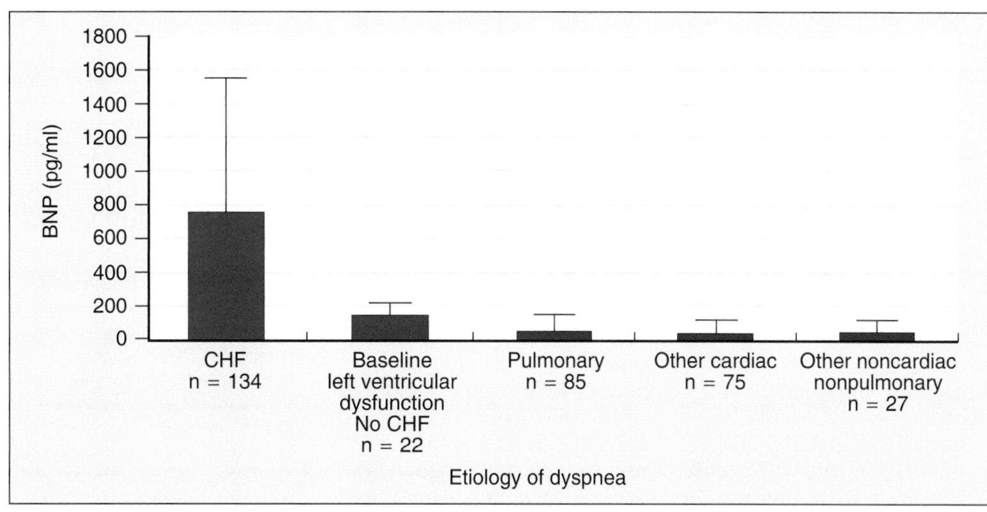

FIGURE 22–17 B-type natriuretic peptide (BNP) levels in 321 patients presenting to the emergency room with acute dyspnea and diagnosed with congestive heart failure (CHF), left ventricular dysfunction without CHF, pulmonary disease, other cardiac disease (e.g., angina, atypical chest pain), or other noncardiac nonpulmonary disease (e.g., anxiety, gastroesophageal reflux). In patients with pulmonary disease ($n = 85$), BNP levels were highest in the small groups of patients with pulmonary embolism or lung cancer. (From Morrison LK, Harrison A, Krishnaswamy P, et al: Utility of a rapid B-natriuretic peptide assay in differentiating congestive heart failure from lung disease in patients presenting with dyspnea. J Am Coll Cardiol 39:202, 2002.)

CLINICAL MANIFESTATIONS. Acute cardiogenic pulmonary edema differs from orthopnea and paroxysmal nocturnal dyspnea in the more rapid and extreme development of pulmonary capillary hypertension. Acute pulmonary edema is a terrifying experience for the patient and often the bystander as well. Usually, extreme breathlessness develops suddenly and the patient becomes extremely anxious, coughs, and expectorates pink, frothy liquid with a feeling of drowning. The patient sits bolt upright or may stand, exhibits air hunger, and may thrash about. The respiratory rate is elevated, the alae nasi are dilated, and there is inspiratory retraction of the intercostal spaces and supraclavicular fossae that reflects the large negative intrapleural pressures required for inspiration. The patient often grasps the sides of the bed to allow use of the accessory muscles of respiration. Respiration is noisy, with loud inspiratory and expiratory gurgling sounds that are often easily audible across the room. Sweating is profuse, and the skin is usually cold, ashen, and cyanotic, reflecting low cardiac output and increased sympathetic drive.

On *auscultation*, there are many adventitious lung sounds, with rhonchi, wheezes, and moist and fine crepitant rales that appear at first over the lung bases but then extend upward to the apices as the condition worsens. Cardiac auscultation may be difficult because of the respiratory sounds, but a third heart sound and an accentuated pulmonic component of the second heart sound are frequently present. In patients with ischemic heart disease, a holosystolic murmur of mitral regurgitation may also be heard at the cardiac apex or axilla.

The patient may suffer from intense precordial pain if the pulmonary edema is secondary to acute myocardial infarction (see Chap. 46). Unless cardiogenic shock is present, arterial pressure is usually elevated above the patient's baseline as a result of anxiety and discomfort, which cause adrenergically mediated vasoconstriction. Because of the presence of systemic hypertension, it may be suspected (inappropriately) that the pulmonary edema is due to hypertensive heart disease. However, it should be noted that hypertensive crises[198] are now uncommon (Chap. 37), and if arterial pressure is elevated, funduscopic examination usually indicates whether or not hypertensive heart disease is actually present.

DIFFERENTIATION FROM ASTHMA. It may be difficult to differentiate severe asthma[199] from acute pulmonary edema because both conditions may be associated with extreme dyspnea, pulsus paradoxus, demands for an upright posture, and diffuse wheezes that interfere with cardiac auscultation. In asthma, there is usually a history of previous similar episodes and the patient is aware of the diagnosis. During the acute attack, the asthmatic patient does not usually sweat profusely, and arterial hypoxemia, although present, is not usually of sufficient magnitude to cause cyanosis. In addition, the chest is hyperexpanded and hyperresonant and use of accessory muscles is most prominent during expiration. Although nonspecific, wheezes are higher pitched and more musical than in pulmonary edema, and other adventitious sounds such as rhonchi and rales are less prominent.

The patient with acute cardiogenic pulmonary edema usually perspires profusely and is frequently cyanotic owing to desaturation of arterial blood and decreased cutaneous blood flow. The chest is often dull to percussion, there is no hyperexpansion, accessory muscle use is less prominent than in asthma, and moist, bubbly rales and rhonchi are heard in addition to wheezes. Chest radiography shows interstitial or alveolar edema. As the patient recovers, the radiological appearance of pulmonary edema usually resolves more slowly than the elevated pulmonary capillary wedge pressure.

Other diagnostic tests have been evaluated in this setting. Rapid measurement of plasma BNP levels may help to distinguish acute cardiogenic pulmonary edema from severe asthma in patients presenting to an emergency room with dyspnea (Fig. 22–17).[44,50] Alternatively, in patients with intermediate BNP levels and nonspecific radiological findings, a "restrictive" pattern of mitral valve inflow as assessed by Doppler echocardiography may suggest the diagnosis of heart failure.[200]

PULMONARY CAPILLARY WEDGE PRESSURE. Measurement of pulmonary capillary wedge pressure by means of a flow-directed catheter (see Chap. 17) may be critical in distinguishing between pulmonary edema secondary to an imbalance of Starling forces (i.e., cardiogenic pulmonary edema) and that secondary to alterations of the alveolar-capillary barrier. Specifically, a pulmonary capillary wedge or pulmonary artery diastolic pressure greater than 20 mm Hg in a patient without previous pulmonary capillary pressure elevation (or greater than 30 mm Hg in a patient with chronic pulmonary capillary hypertension) and with the clinical features of pulmonary edema strongly suggests that the edema is cardiogenic. However, the use of a pulmonary artery catheter to measure pulmonary capillary wedge pressure is generally reserved for hospitalized patients with decompensated heart failure, leaving only noninvasive means of estimating left heart pressures in the majority of patients. Unfortunately, the routine clinical evaluation of patients with chronic systolic heart failure lacks the sensitivity and specificity needed for accurate assessment of left atrial pressure. Noninvasive methods that can reliably predict left-sided filling pressures and may have clinical application in the ambulatory setting are being investigated.[102] These include newer echocardiographic techniques such as Doppler tissue imaging and measurement of pulmonary venous inflow, thoracic bioimpedence, and a noninvasive Valsalva response recorder.

ELECTROCARDIOGRAPHIC CHANGES. ECG changes of myocardial ischemia or infarction (see Chap. 9) are commonly seen in patients with acute cardiogenic pulmonary edema. In patients presenting with hypertensive crises, the electrocardiogram may reveal left ventricular hypertrophy with a "strain" pattern that is exaggerated compared with the baseline tracing. In patients with cardiogenic but nonischemic pulmonary edema, large inverted T waves with marked QT prolongation may evolve within 24 hours of clinical stabilization and resolve within 1 week.[201] The cause of these "nonischemic" changes is unknown but may include subendocardial ischemia related to increased wall stress, acute increase in cardiac sympathetic tone, or increased electrical heterogeneity exacerbated by metabolic changes or catecholamines.

PROGNOSIS. After effective treatment of the pulmonary edema (see Chaps. 23 and 24), patients are often restored rapidly to the condition that existed before the attack, although they usually feel exhausted. Between attacks of pulmonary edema, there may be few symptoms or signs of heart failure. The long-term prognosis after an episode of acute pulmonary edema depends on the underlying cause of pulmonary edema (e.g., acute myocardial infarction) and the presence of comorbidities such as diabetes or end-stage renal disease. In a study of 150 consecutive patients hospitalized with acute pulmonary edema, the in-hospital mortality rate was 12 percent, with more than 80 percent of deaths attributed to cardiac failure.[202] Predictors of in-hospital mortality included diabetes, left ventricular dysfunction, hypotension or shock, and need for mechanical ventilation.

Pulmonary Edema of Unknown or Incompletely Defined Pathogenesis

HIGH-ALTITUDE PULMONARY EDEMA. High-altitude pulmonary edema (HAPE) is a noncardiogenic pulmonary edema that occurs most commonly in healthy young adults who ascend rapidly to altitudes in excess of 2500 meters and who then engage in strenuous exercise at those altitudes before they have become acclimated.[203,204] Estimates place the incidence of HAPE at 6.4 clinically apparent cases per 100 exposures to high altitude in persons younger than 21 years of age and 0.4 cases per 100 exposures in those older than 21 years. In addition to age, the major factors that determine the occurrence of HAPE are the altitude achieved (although HAPE may occur at altitudes of less than 2400 meters[205]), the speed of ascent, the level of exertion, and individual susceptibility. Affected individuals complain of dry cough, exertional dyspnea, and fatigue, usually within 1 to 2 days of ascent. As pulmonary edema worsens, these symptoms may progress rapidly (i.e., to dyspnea at rest) and may be associated with chest pain, orthopnea, and pink frothy sputum. Headache, drowsiness, and confusion may occur secondary to hypoxemia and the development of acute mountain sickness or high-altitude cerebral edema. Clinical evaluation reveals tachypnea, tachycardia, bilateral moist rales, and cyanosis, accompanied by marked arterial hypoxemia and respiratory alkalosis. Fever may also be present. The electrocardiogram reveals sinus tachycardia and evidence of right heart strain, and the chest radiograph shows discrete, patchy pulmonary infiltrates. As HAPE progresses and then resolves, pulmonary infiltrates often become diffuse and homogeneous.

A central abnormality in the pathophysiology of HAPE is an abnormal rise in pulmonary artery pressures and pulmonary vascular resistance in response to hypoxia (Fig. 22–18).[206] Possible mechanisms underlying the exaggerated hypoxic pulmonary vascular response in susceptible individuals include a decreased hypoxic ventilatory response, exaggerated sympathetic activation,[207] and endothelial dysfunction related to decreased pulmonary production of nitric oxide,[208] augmented release or decreased clearance of endothelin-1, or both.[209] The association of HAPE with the major histocompatibility human leukocyte antigens HLA-DR6 and HLA-DQ4 also suggests an immunogenetic susceptibility.[210] Uneven pulmonary vasoconstriction during hypoxia or exercise,[206] resulting in overperfused areas and "stress failure" of the pulmonary capillaries,[211] is believed to contribute to the development of pulmonary edema. Analysis of bronchoalveolar lavage fluid from subjects with HAPE revealed normal levels of leukocytes and proinflammatory cytokines, suggesting that inflammation does not play a primary role in the pathogenesis of HAPE.[212]

TREATMENT. Early recognition of this syndrome is critical. HAPE is reversed rapidly (i.e., in less than 48 hours) by returning the patient to a lower altitude or by administering a high inspiratory concentration of oxygen, or both. Bed rest, fluid restriction, and continuous positive airway pressure should also be considered.[205] Sleeping below 2500 meters, slow ascent with gradual acclimatization, and avoidance of heavy exertion for the first 2 or 3 days at high altitude are thought to be preventive. Nifedipine has been used successively both in

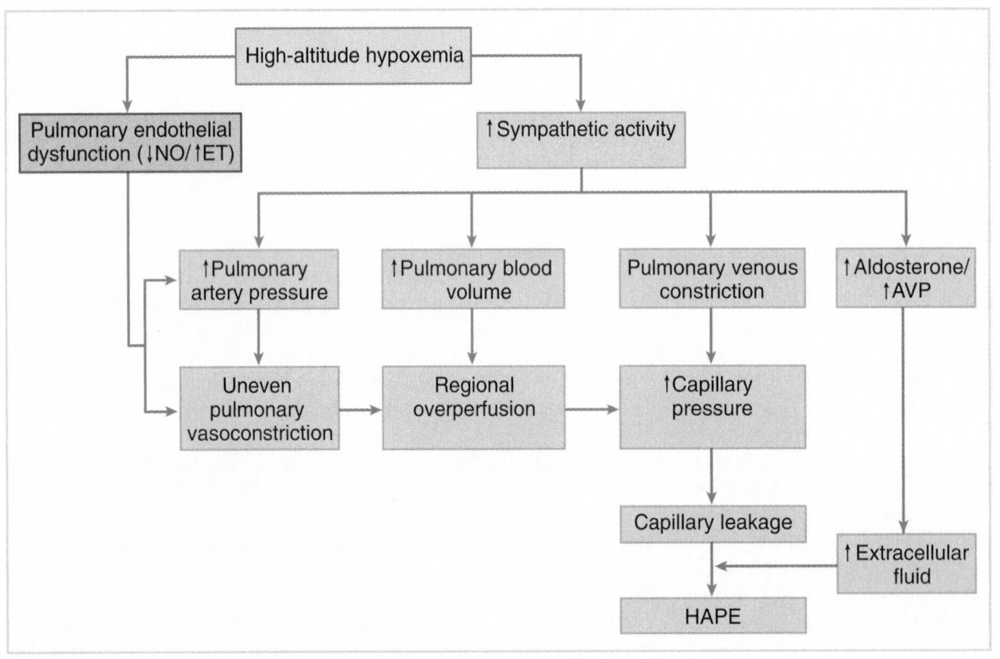

FIGURE 22–18 Diagram showing the sequence of events in the pathogenesis of high-altitude pulmonary edema (HAPE). AVP = arginine vasopressin; ET = endothelin-1; NO = nitric oxide. (Modified from Hackett PH, Roach RC: High-altitude illness. N Engl J Med 345:107, 2001.)

the treatment of HAPE and as prophylaxis[203,213] but is necessary only when oxygen is unavailable or descent is impossible. Prophylactic inhalation of salmeterol, a beta-adrenergic agonist, has been shown to reduce the incidence of HAPE by about 50 percent in susceptible individuals.[214] When HAPE has developed, inhaled nitric oxide, either alone or in combination with supplemental oxygen, can lower pulmonary vascular resistance and improve arterial oxygenation, although its availability is limited.[215] The improvement in gas exchange with inhaled NO may be due to a shift in blood flow away from edematous segments of the lung toward nonedematous segments. Although death caused by HAPE is rare, HAPE is responsible for the majority of deaths related to high-altitude illness.

NEUROGENIC PULMONARY EDEMA. A variety of central nervous system disorders including head trauma, seizures, stroke, and subarachnoid hemorrhage can be associated with acute pulmonary edema (without detectable left ventricular dysfunction).[216,217] Neurogenic pulmonary edema can also occur after surgical craniotomy. It is believed that sympathetic overactivity with massive catecholamine surges shifts blood from the systemic to the pulmonary circulation, with secondary elevations of left atrial and pulmonary capillary pressures. The resulting imbalance of Starling forces (i.e., a hydrostatic mechanism[218]) may therefore be the basis for this form of pulmonary edema. Pulmonary capillary leak caused by pressure-induced mechanical injury or direct nervous system control over capillary permeability, or both, may also play a contributory role. Although inhibition of nitric oxide production in the central nervous system has been shown to worsen neurogenic pulmonary edema in a rat model, the therapeutic implications of this finding remain unclear.[219] Symptom onset tends to be rapid (i.e., within 4 hours of the neurological event), and chest radiography shows diffuse bilateral infiltrates.

Treatment of neurogenic pulmonary edema, usually in an intensive care setting, consists of ventilatory support and maneuvers to reduce intracranial pressure. A reversible impairment in left ventricular systolic function resulting in hypotension may accompany neurogenic pulmonary edema. Mortality rates of 10 percent have been reported, but surviving patients usually recover quickly.

NARCOTIC OVERDOSE PULMONARY EDEMA. First described by Osler in 1880, acute pulmonary edema is a well-recognized sequela of heroin overdose.[220,221] Risk factors include male gender and shorter duration of heroin use, and concomitant use of cocaine and alcohol is common.[221] The onset of dyspnea and hypoxemia is usually rapid, occurring immediately or within hours of heroin overdose. Chest radiography typically shows diffuse fluffy infiltrates, although unilateral or patchy lung involvement has been described. Treatment consists of naloxone, supplemental oxygen, and in approximately one third of patients temporary mechanical ventilatory support.[220] Complete resolution of hypoxemia in 1 to 2 days is the rule. Because of the illicit traffic in this drug, which is given by the intravenous route, the syndrome was initially thought to be due to injected impurities rather than to the heroin itself. However, because oral methadone and dextropropoxyphene can also be associated with pulmonary edema, the syndrome cannot be attributed entirely to injected impurities. The fact that edema fluid contains protein concentrations nearly identical to those found in plasma and that pulmonary capillary wedge pressures, when measured, are normal argues for an alveolar-capillary membrane leak as the initiating cause.

PULMONARY EMBOLISM (see Chap. 66). Acute pulmonary edema in association with either a massive embolus or multiple smaller emboli has been well described and most often attributed to concomitant left ventricular dysfunction related to a combination of hypoxemia and encroachment of the interventricular septum on the left ventricular cavity.[222] It has been suggested that in the pulmonary edema related to pulmonary microthrombi an increase in permeability of the alveolar-capillary membrane occurs.

ECLAMPSIA (see Chap. 74). Acute pulmonary edema is a well-recognized complication of preeclampsia-eclampsia, occurring with an overall frequency of 3 to 5 percent.[223] In a retrospective review of 16,800 deliveries at a large, urban medical center, pulmonary edema occurred in 0.5 percent of all obstetrical cases.[224] The incidence of pulmonary edema is higher in women who are older, who are multiparous, and who have preexisting chronic hypertension. The majority of cases, approximately 70 percent, occur post partum. Multiple factors including cerebral dysfunction with massive sympathetic discharge, left ventricular dysfunction secondary to acute systemic hypertension, hypervolemia caused by excessive colloid and crystalloid infusions or transfusions, hypoalbuminemia secondary to renal losses, and disseminated intravascular coagulation may play a role in the pathogenesis.

Patients present with acute dyspnea and arterial hypoxemia, and chest radiography reveals extensive airspace consolidation. The average time to resolution of pulmonary edema is 2 to 3 days, and a minority of patients (approximately 15 percent) require mechanical ventilatory support. Risk factors for prolonged intubation include infection and fetal surgery.[224] Pulmonary artery catheterization is safe and commonly reveals elevated right- and left-sided cardiac filling pressures, elevated cardiac index, and normal systemic vascular resistance, although hemodynamics consistent with pulmonary capillary leak have also been reported.[225] Echocardiography may show normal, hyperdynamic, or depressed left ventricular systolic function with or without diastolic filling abnormalities.[226] The occurrence of pulmonary edema in obstetrical patients is associated with high maternal and perinatal morbidity and mortality.

AFTER CARDIOVERSION. Acute pulmonary edema is an uncommon albeit well-recognized complication of cardioversion, occurring in less than 0.5 percent of cases.[227] The mechanisms underlying postcardioversion pulmonary edema are poorly understood. Ineffective left atrial function immediately after cardioversion resulting in decreased cardiac output has been suggested as a contributing factor,[227] yet left ventricular diastolic dysfunction related to direct current shock and neurogenic mechanisms are also possible. Additional contributory factors may include underlying cardiac disease, cardiodepressant anesthetic agents, and pulmonary or cardiac emboli or both. One half of cases occur within 3 hours after cardioversion.

AFTER ANESTHESIA. Pulmonary edema has been described in the early postoperative period in previously healthy subjects, without a clear relationship to fluid overload or any subsequent evidence of left ventricular dysfunction.[228] The basis for this disorder is unknown, but proposed mechanisms include postanesthesia laryngospasm with marked negative intrathoracic pressure ("postobstructive" or "negative pressure" pulmonary edema), hypoxia, and a hyperadrenergic state. In a retrospective analysis of 8195 major operations, pulmonary edema occurred in 7.6 percent of cases, with a mortality rate of 12 percent.[228] Patients with fatal postoperative pulmonary edema retained an average of 67 ml/kg of fluid within the first 24 hours following surgery and presented with cardiopulmonary arrest, arterial hypoxemia, and metabolic acidosis. Pulmonary artery pressures were normal.

AFTER CARDIOPULMONARY BYPASS. Although all patients who undergo cardiopulmonary bypass have significant heart disease, the development of pulmonary edema has been associated with normal left atrial pressures.[229] Alterations of surfactant related to prolonged collapse of the lung during the procedure, with subsequent need to apply high negative intrapleural pressures for reexpansion, and release of toxic substances including thromboxane have been suggested as mechanisms. Increased pulmonary vascular resistance and intrapulmonary shunting contribute to hypoxemia. Cardiopulmonary bypass also causes a systemic inflammatory response[229] with activation of complement, cytokines, and reactive oxygen species, which may contribute to the development of noncardiogenic pulmonary edema. Some data suggest that allergic reactions to fresh frozen plasma or protamine may account for some episodes. The increasing use of off-pump coronary artery bypass (OPCAB)[230] in high-risk elderly patients with reduced left ventricular function or chronic renal insufficiency would be expected to reduce the incidence of this already rare entity.

TRANSFUSION-RELATED ACUTE LUNG INJURY. A clinical syndrome that includes fever, dyspnea, hypotension, and bilateral pulmonary edema may occur following transfusion of blood products.[231] The pathogenesis is poorly understood, and affected individuals often have other acute or chronic illnesses that may contribute to the development of cardiogenic or noncardiogenic pulmonary edema. Data suggest that this syndrome is underdiagnosed and underreported.[231]

HANTAVIRUS PULMONARY SYNDROME. In Asia, hantaviruses are associated with hemorrhagic fever and renal disease. In 1993, an outbreak of severe respiratory illness occurred in the southwestern United States and was attributed to a newly described hantavirus.[232] The majority of patients affected were Native American. Prodromal symptoms included fever, myalgia, cough, dyspnea, and gastrointestinal symptoms. Most infected patients developed rapidly progressive noncardiogenic pulmonary edema associated with profound hypotension, with a case-fatality rate of 76 percent. The pathogenesis of hantavirus pulmonary syndrome remains unknown. It has been suggested that local T cells acting on the infected pulmonary vascular endothelium result in the production of cytokines, including interferon-gamma and tumor necrosis factor-α, which may play an important role in the reversible increase in vascular permeability.[233]

OTHER VIRAL INFECTIONS. Enteroviruses can cause outbreaks of hand-foot-and-mouth disease or herpangina, which are usually self-limiting. In 1998, an outbreak of enterovirus 71 infection in Taiwan

TABLE 22–6 Initial Differentiation of Cardiogenic from Noncardiogenic Pulmonary Edema

Parameters	Cardiogenic Pulmonary Edema	Noncardiogenic Pulmonary Edema
History		
Acute cardiac event	Usually present	Uncommon (but possible)
Physical Examination		
Cardiac output state	Low-flow state (cool periphery)	High-flow state (warm periphery, bounding pulses)
S_3 gallop	Present	Absent
Jugular venous distention	Present	Absent
Crackles	Wet	Dry
Underlying noncardiac disease (e.g., sepsis)	Usually absent	Present
Laboratory Tests		
Electrocardiogram	Ischemia/infarction	Usually normal
Chest radiograph	Perihilar distribution	Peripheral distribution
Cardiac enzymes	May be elevated	Usually normal
Pulmonary capillary wedge pressure	≥18 mm Hg	<18 mm Hg
Intrapulmonary shunting	Small	Large
Edema fluid/serum protein	<0.5	>0.7

From Sibbald WJ, Cunningham DR, Chin DN: Noncardiac or cardiac pulmonary edema? A practical approach to clinical differentiation in critically ill patients. Chest 84:460, 1983.

resulted in severe infection in more than 400 patients with a case-fatality rate of 19 percent.[234] Complications of severe disease, which were commonly seen in children younger than 6 years, included meningoencephalitis, flaccid paralysis, pulmonary edema or hemorrhage, and myocarditis. Of the patients who died, 83 percent had pulmonary edema or hemorrhage.

Several outbreaks of severe acute respiratory syndrome (SARS) have been reported in China, Vietnam, Canada, and Germany.[235,236] Common symptoms include fever, chills, myalgias, and cough. Peripheral airspace consolidation leading to respiratory failure and death have occurred, and postmortem examination of the lungs revealed pulmonary edema with hyaline membrane formation suggestive of the early phase of ARDS.[235] Using virus isolation techniques, electron microscopic and histological studies, and molecular and serological assays, investigators have identified a novel coronavirus as the causative agent.[236]

Differential Diagnosis of Pulmonary Edema

The differentiation between the two principal forms of pulmonary edema—that is, cardiogenic (hemodynamic) and noncardiogenic (caused by alterations in the alveolar-capillary barrier)—can usually be made through assessment of the clinical context in which it occurs and through examination and consideration of the clinical data as shown in Table 22–6. Although this approach suggests an either/or situation, this may not be the case in clinical practice. For example, sudden and large increases in intravascular pressure may disrupt the capillary and alveolar membranes, leading to interstitial edema and alveolar loading with macromolecules that produce an edema liquid more compatible with noncardiogenic causes.[188] Thus, a primary hemodynamic event can cause "stress failure" of the alveolar-capillary barrier. Furthermore, only mild elevations in capillary hydrostatic pressures in the presence of alveolar capillary damage can cause an increase in the rate and extent of edema formation. Therefore, hemodynamic factors can and do play a role in increasing and perpetuating increased permeability.

High-Output Heart Failure

High–cardiac output states (Table 22–7) by themselves are seldom responsible for heart failure, but their development in the presence of underlying heart disease often precipitates heart failure. In these conditions, which are often characterized by arteriovenous shunting, the requirements of the peripheral tissues for oxygen can be met only by an increase in cardiac output. Although the normal heart is capable of augmenting its output on a long-term basis, this may not be true of the diseased heart.

TABLE 22–7 High-Cardiac Output States

Anemia

Acquired arteriovenous fistulas
  Traumatic
  Iatrogenic
  Infectious
  Surgical (hemodialysis)
  Atherosclerotic
  Malignancy

Congenital arteriovenous fistulas
  Hemangiomas
  Hereditary hemorrhagic telangiectasia
  Hepatic hemangioendothelioma

Thyrotoxicosis
Beriberi heart disease
Paget disease of bone
Fibrous dysplasia
Multiple myeloma
Polycythemia vera
Carcinoid syndrome
Acromegaly
Pregnancy

Anemia

Chronic anemia is associated with high cardiac output when hemoglobin is equal to or less than approximately 8 gm/dl. Reduced systemic vascular resistance, which results from decreased arteriolar tone and decreased blood viscosity, plays an important role in the pathophysiology of this high-output state (Fig. 22–19). Enhanced basal production of endothelium-derived nitric oxide may be responsible, in part, for the low systemic vascular resistance in patients with anemia.[237] Impaired renal excretion of sodium and water leading to volume overload may be due to decreased renal blood flow,

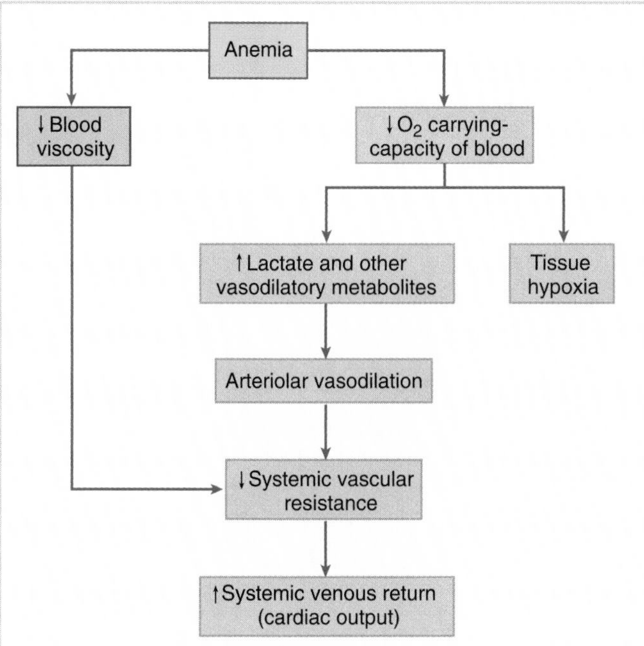

FIGURE 22–19 Diagram showing the pathophysiological mechanisms underlying the high–cardiac output state associated with anemia. Decreased blood viscosity and a reduction in arteriolar tone resulting from tissue hypoxia and lactic acidosis contribute to reduced systemic vascular resistance, which in turn increases cardiac output. In addition, chronic anemia is associated with increased endothelium-derived nitric oxide, which contributes to enhanced vasodilation. O_2 = oxygen. (From Hassapoyannes CA, Nelson WP, Hopkins CB, et al: Other causes and contributing factors to congestive heart failure. *In* Hosenpud JD, Greenberg BH [eds]: Congestive Heart Failure. New York, Springer-Verlag, 1994, pp 281-300.)

reduced glomerular filtration rate, and neurohormonal activation.[238] In animal models of high-output heart failure, blunted cardiac secretion of natriuretic peptides in response to a volume challenge and decreased renal responsiveness to their actions have also been demonstrated.[239]

Anemia, even when severe, rarely causes heart failure or angina pectoris in patients with normal hearts; when these problems occur, it is likely that the high cardiac output is superimposed on some specific cardiac abnormality, such as valvular or ischemic heart disease.

PHYSICAL EXAMINATION. Physical findings secondary to anemia are often superimposed on those of an underlying cardiovascular disorder. The anemic patient often has a pale, "pasty" appearance; in blacks, the findings of paleness of the conjunctivae, mucous membranes, and palmar creases are helpful. Arterial pulses are bounding, "pistol shot" sounds can be heard over the femoral arteries (Traube sign), and subungual capillary pulsations (Quincke pulse) are present, as in patients with aortic regurgitation (see Chap. 57). A medium-pitched, midsystolic murmur along the left sternal border, generally grade 1/6 to 3/6 in intensity (seldom accompanied by a thrill), is common. Heart sounds are accentuated, and the pulmonic component of the second heart sound may be particularly prominent in patients with sickle cell anemia and pulmonary hypertension; in such patients, a right ventricular lift can usually be palpated. A mid-diastolic flow murmur secondary to augmented blood flow across the mitral orifice, holosystolic murmurs resulting from tricuspid and mitral regurgitation secondary to ventricular dilation, and, rarely, diastolic murmurs resulting from aortic and pulmonic valve incompetence secondary to dilation of these vessels may be heard. A protodiastolic gallop sound (S_3) is frequently audible at the cardiac apex. Jugular venous distention is uncommon and, although peripheral edema and hepatomegaly are occasionally present, they may be due not only to heart failure but also to accompanying abnormalities such as hypoalbuminemia and nutritional deficiency.

DIAGNOSTIC TESTING. In patients with severe chronic anemia without underlying heart disease, the chest radiograph usually demonstrates mild to moderate cardiomegaly. The electrocardiogram often does not show any specific changes but may reveal tachycardia and T wave inversions in the lateral precordial leads. The echocardiogram generally shows a modest and symmetrical increase in the size of all chambers, with large systolic excursions of the septal and posterior left ventricular walls. In addition, an attenuated increase in the fractional shortening in response to exercise, abnormal ventricular filling, valvular regurgitation, pericardial thickening with or without effusion, and pulmonary hypertension may be seen.[240] These findings are superimposed on those resulting from the underlying heart disease. Hematological and blood chemistry findings reflect the specific type of anemia present.

MANAGEMENT. Treatment of heart failure associated with severe anemia should be specific for the anemia (e.g., iron, folate, vitamin B_{12}). When heart failure is present, diuretics and cardiac glycosides are advisable, although some believe that the latter drugs are not helpful in this condition. ACE inhibitors or angiotensin receptor antagonists may improve the renal response to natriuretic peptides and facilitate diuresis[239] but may cause systemic hypotension from excessive vasodilation.

When both heart failure and anemia are severe, treatment must be carried out on an urgent basis and presents a difficult challenge. On the one hand, correction of the anemia is desirable to increase oxygen delivery to metabolizing tissues and thereby decrease the need for a sustained high cardiac output. On the other hand, rapid expansion of the blood volume may intensify the manifestations of heart failure.

The diagnostic steps for determining the etiology of the anemia should be taken immediately (e.g., blood drawn for serum iron, folate, and vitamin B_{12} and reticulocyte count, review of peripheral smear, and stool guaiac). The patient should be placed at bed rest and given supplementary oxygen. *Packed red blood cells* should then be transfused slowly (250 to 500 ml per 24 hours), preceded or accompanied, or both, by vigorous diuretic therapy (e.g., furosemide, 40 mg intravenously every 8 to 12 hours), and the patient should be observed closely for the development or exacerbation of dyspnea and pulmonary rales. If worsening heart failure occurs, the transfusion should be discontinued or slowed to avoid precipitating pulmonary edema. Vasodilator therapy is seldom helpful because impedance to left ventricular emptying is already markedly reduced in most cases.

Systemic Arteriovenous Fistulas

Systemic arteriovenous fistulas may be congenital or acquired; the latter are usually posttraumatic or iatrogenic. Increased cardiac output associated with such fistulas depends on the size of the communication and the magnitude of the resultant reduction in systemic vascular resistance.

The *physical findings* depend on the underlying disease and the location and size of the shunt. In general, a widened pulse pressure, brisk carotid and peripheral arterial pulsations, and mild tachycardia are present. The extremities are often warm and flushed. The *Branham sign* (also called the *Nicoladoni-Branham sign*), which consists of slowing of the heart rate after manual compression of the fistula,[241] is present in the majority of cases; this maneuver also raises arterial and lowers venous pressure. It appears to result from the operation of a cardioaccelerator reflex with both afferent and efferent pathways in the vagus nerves. The decrease in heart rate after fistula occlusion correlates with the flow in the fistula.

The skin overlying the fistula is warmer than normal, and a continuous "machinery" murmur and thrill are usually present over the lesion. Third and fourth heart sounds are commonly heard, as well as a precordial midsystolic murmur secondary to increased cardiac output. The ECG changes of left ventricular hypertrophy are often seen. Rarely, the fistula may become infected, leading to bacterial endarteritis, or cause major bleeding.

ACQUIRED ARTERIOVENOUS FISTULAS. These occur most frequently after such injuries as gunshot wounds and stab wounds and may involve any part of the body, most frequently the thigh.[242] Blood flow in the affected limb distal to the fistula diminishes after the creation of the fistula but then returns to normal and often increases with the passage of time. As a consequence, the affected limb is usually larger than its opposite member and the overlying skin is warmer. Cellulitis, venostasis, edema, and dermatitis with pigmentation frequently occur, in part as a consequence of chronically elevated venous pressure. Surgical repair or excision is generally advisable in fistulas that develop after gunshot wounds or trauma.[242]

Femoral arteriovenous fistulas following diagnostic or interventional cardiac catheterization are uncommon (0.11 to 0.16 percent of cases) but may result in high-output cardiac failure.[243,244] These may occur when a needle track crosses both the femoral artery and vein and is then dilated during the catheterization. Although the traditional approach to management of catheterization-related femoral artery injuries has been surgical repair,[245] newer techniques include ultrasound-guided compression and percutaneous stent placement or coil embolization.[243,246] Late stent thrombosis has been reported.

A rare form of acquired arteriovenous fistula results from spontaneous rupture of an aortic aneurysm into the inferior vena cava.[247] This event usually produces an enormous arteriovenous shunt, renal insufficiency, and rapidly progressive left ventricular failure. On physical examination, a pulsating mass can be readily palpated superficially in the abdomen and a continuous bruit is audible. Severe lower extremity and scrotal edema may be present. Survival depends on prompt diagnosis by ultrasonography or angiography and surgical closure with aortic reconstruction. Aortocaval fistulas may rarely occur after blunt or penetrating abdominal trauma.[248] Massive arteriovenous fistulas have been associated with Wilms tumors of the kidney and can cause high-output cardiac failure in children. Renal arteriovenous fistulas complicating pregnancy have also been reported.[249]

High-output heart failure resulting from the arteriovenous shunts surgically constructed for vascular access in patients undergoing long-term hemodialysis is uncommon.[250] Cardiac outputs as high as 10 liters/min, which decrease substantially during temporary occlusion of the shunt, are found. These values also reflect the chronic anemia present in many of these patients, but it is clear that it is the added hemodynamic burden[251] imposed by the shunt that precipitates heart failure in patients who had previously tolerated chronic anemia without apparent impairment of cardiac function. It is usually possible to revise or band the fistula to reduce it to the appropriate size for dialysis without compromising cardiac function. If this approach is ineffective, the shunt should be surgically closed and a new arteriovenous fistula created.

CONGENITAL ARTERIOVENOUS FISTULAS

Congenital arteriovenous fistulas result from arrest of the normal embryonic development of the vascular system and are structurally similar to embryonic capillary networks. When fistulas are large, patients generally complain of disfigurement as well as swelling and pain in the limb. On physical examination, erythema and cyanosis are often present, as are venous varices, a continuous murmur, and thrill. Examination also shows hemangiomatous changes associated with venous distention, deformity, and increased limb length. The fistulous connection may involve any vascular bed, including an internal mammary artery–pulmonary artery connection. *Left-sided heart failure* occurs particularly in patients with larger lesions that involve the pelvis as well as the extremities. Angiography is useful in confirming the diagnosis and in determining the physical extent of the anomaly.

Surgical excision is the ideal treatment,[252] but in many instances the lesions are not sufficiently localized to permit this. Embolization of absorbable gelatin (Gelfoam) pellets delivered through a catheter has been reported to obliterate multiple systemic arteriovenous fistulas and thereby diminish high-output heart failure.

HEREDITARY HEMORRHAGIC TELANGIECTASIA. Also known as *Osler-Weber-Rendu disease,* this autosomal dominant disorder is characterized by angiodysplastic lesions involving the skin, gastrointestinal tract, and brain. In addition, in 15 to 30 percent of cases, arteriovenous fistulas are present in the lungs[253] or liver.[254] Involvement of the liver, in particular, can produce a hyperdynamic circulation, with heart failure as well as hepatomegaly, liver bruits, manifestations of severe portal hypertension such as ascites and variceal bleeding, or biliary disease.

The congenital arteriovenous communications resulting from *infantile hepatic hemangioendothelioma* are commonly associated with marked increases in cardiac output, sometimes as high as 10 liters/min, and heart failure.[255] Other common presenting features include an abdominal mass, coagulopathy, and anemia. The hepatic lesions may be quite large, increase in size with time, and lead to heart failure, even in infancy. Treatment strategies include medical management with corticosteroids or interferon alfa or, in cases of failed medical therapy, use of percutaneous or surgical intervention, including hepatic artery ligation or embolization, surgical resection, or orthotopic liver transplantation.

Hyperthyroidism (see also Chap. 79)

In addition to enhancing sympathetic activation, increased circulating levels of thyroid hormone exert direct effects on the cardiovascular system including an increase in heart rate and cardiac contractility and a reduction in systemic vascular resistance. The principal findings on the physical examination of the cardiovascular system are resting tachycardia, systolic hypertension with a widened pulse pressure, brisk carotid and peripheral arterial pulsations, a hyperkinetic cardiac apex, and loud first heart sound. A midsystolic murmur along the left sternal border, secondary to increased flow, is common; occasionally, this murmur has an unusual scratchy component (the so-called Means-Lerman scratch), thought to be due to the rubbing together of normal pleural and pericardial surfaces by the hyperdynamic heart. Rarely, systolic murmurs of mitral and tricuspid regurgitation, secondary to papillary muscle dysfunction or ventricular dilation, may occur.

As in many other high-output states, the hyperkinetic state of hyperthyroidism does not usually lead to heart failure in the absence of underlying cardiovascular disease.[256] The normal heart appears capable of tolerating the burden imposed by hyperthyroidism simply by means of dilation and hypertrophy. However, heart failure may be precipitated when the elevated flow load of hyperthyroidism is superimposed on a reduced cardiovascular reserve (i.e., a patient with heart disease who is compensated).[257] Similarly, in patients with ischemic heart disease who are asymptomatic or who have only mild evidence of ischemia in the euthyroid state, the demand for increased coronary blood flow with hyperthyroidism frequently leads to an exacerbation of angina, often with the sensation of palpitations. The high-output cardiac failure of hyperthyroidism is frequently accompanied by and exacerbated by atrial fibrillation and a rapid ventricular rate.[258] Atrial fibrillation occurs in about 10 percent of hyperthyroid patients. In addition, respiratory muscle weakness may contribute to exertional dyspnea.

It is particularly important to recognize *apathetic hyperthyroidism,*[259] a condition in elderly people in which the usual clinical manifestations of thyrotoxicosis, such as palpitations, tachycardia, and moist skin, are not present. In such patients, the first clinical signs of hyperthyroidism may be unexplained heart failure, an exacerbation of angina, or new-onset atrial fibrillation,[260] usually but not always with a rapid ventricular rate.

BERIBERI HEART DISEASE

PATHOGENESIS AND CLINICAL CONSIDERATIONS. Thiamine pyrophosphate (TPP), the most abundant thiamine ester found in tissues, is essential for carbohydrate metabolism. Deficiency leads to impaired oxidative metabolism through inhibition of the citric acid cycle and the hexose monophosphate shunt and results in lactic acidosis.[261] Beriberi heart disease is due to severe thiamine deficiency persisting for at least 3 months.[262-264] Clinical beriberi is found most frequently in the Far East,[263,264] although even in that part of the world it is far less prevalent now than in the past. It occurs predominantly in individuals whose staple diet consists of polished rice, which is deficient in thiamine but high in carbohydrates, or foods containing thiaminases. The presence of thiamine in the enriched flour used in white bread has virtually eradicated this disease in the United States and Western Europe, where beriberi is found most commonly in diet faddists and alcoholics. Like polished rice, alcohol is low in vitamin B_1 but has a high carbohydrate content. In the West, alcoholics may become thiamine deficient not only because of low intake and impaired absorption and storage of the vitamin but also because they eat "junk" foods or drink large quantities of beer. The high carbohydrate content of these foods leads to a greater requirement for thiamine. Beriberi heart disease has also been reported in Western countries in elderly persons and in patients with malnutrition associated with advanced human immunodeficiency virus disease or those receiving total parenteral nutrition.[265]

Patients in Asia present with edema, ranging from peripheral edema to anasarca, as well as general malaise and fatigue. The elevation of cardiac output[263,266] is presumably secondary to the reduced systemic vascular resistance and augmented venous return (Fig. 22-20).

PHYSICAL FINDINGS. In most cases in Western countries, physical findings of the high-output state and usually of severe generalized malnutrition and vitamin deficiency are present. Evidence of peripheral polyneuropathy with sensory and motor deficits is common ("dry beriberi"), as is the presence of nutritional "cirrhosis" characterized by paresthesias of the extremities, absent or decreased knee and ankle jerks, painful glossitis, the anemia of combined iron and folate deficiency, and hyperkeratinized skin lesions.

Beriberi heart disease[262,263] is characterized by biventricular heart failure, sinus rhythm, and marked edema ("wet beriberi"). There is arteriolar vasodilation and the cutaneous vessels may be dilated, or in later cases with heart failure they may be constricted. A third heart sound and an apical systolic murmur are heard almost invariably, and there is a wide pulse pressure characteristic of the hyperkinetic state.

Heart failure may develop explosively in beriberi, and some patients succumb to the illness within 48 hours of the onset of symptoms. *Shoshin* (Japanese for "acute damage to the heart") *beriberi,* found most frequently in Asia and Africa, is a fulminant form of thiamine deficiency[267] characterized by hypotension, tachycardia, and lactic acidosis. If left untreated, patients with this disorder die within hours of cardiogenic shock and pulmonary edema. Thus, because the course of the disease may advance rapidly, treatment must be begun immediately once the diagnosis has been established. In the Western world, this fulminant form of the disease is uncommon.

LABORATORY FINDINGS. The electrocardiogram characteristically exhibits low voltage of the QRS complex, prolongation of the QT interval, and low voltage or inversion of T waves, most commonly in the right precordial leads. The chest radiograph usually shows cardiomegaly, pulmonary vascular congestion, and pleural effusions. In alcoholics with beriberi heart disease, the left ventricular ejection fraction and peak rate of rise of left ventricular pressure are usually reduced. The role played by alcoholic cardiomyopathy[36] (see Chap. 59) in this hemodynamic picture is not clear. The cardiac output falls, and the peripheral resistance rises acutely when thiamine is administered in the catheterization laboratory (see Fig. 22-20).[263]

Laboratory diagnosis of thiamine deficiency can be made by demonstration of increased serum pyruvate and lactate levels in the presence of a low red blood cell transketolase level.[262] Enhancement in transketolase activity resulting from added TPP is referred to as the TPP effect. A TPP effect greater than 15 percent suggests thiamine deficiency. The thiamine concentration may be determined in biological fluids to confirm the diagnosis. If specific laboratory tests are unavailable or impractical, an objective clinical and hemodynamic response to thiamine administration (see later) is considered diagnostic.

At *postmortem examination,* the heart usually shows chamber dilation without other changes. On microscopic examination, there is sometimes edema and fatty degeneration of the muscle fibers. Nonspecific histological and electron microscopic abnormalities have been found in cardiac biopsy specimens.

TREATMENT. Patients with beriberi heart disease fail to respond adequately to digitalis and diuretics alone. However, improvement after the administration of thiamine (up to 100 mg intravenously followed by 25 mg/d orally for 1 to 2 weeks) may be dramatic (see Fig. 22-20). Marked diuresis, decreases in heart rate and left ventricular size, and clearing of pulmonary congestion may occur within 12 to 48 hours. However, acute reversal of vasodilation induced by correction of the deficiency may cause the unprepared left ventricle to go into low-output failure. Therefore, patients should receive a glycoside and diuretic therapy along with thiamine. Thiamine replacement also results in improvement in the polyneuropathy caused by thiamine deficiency.

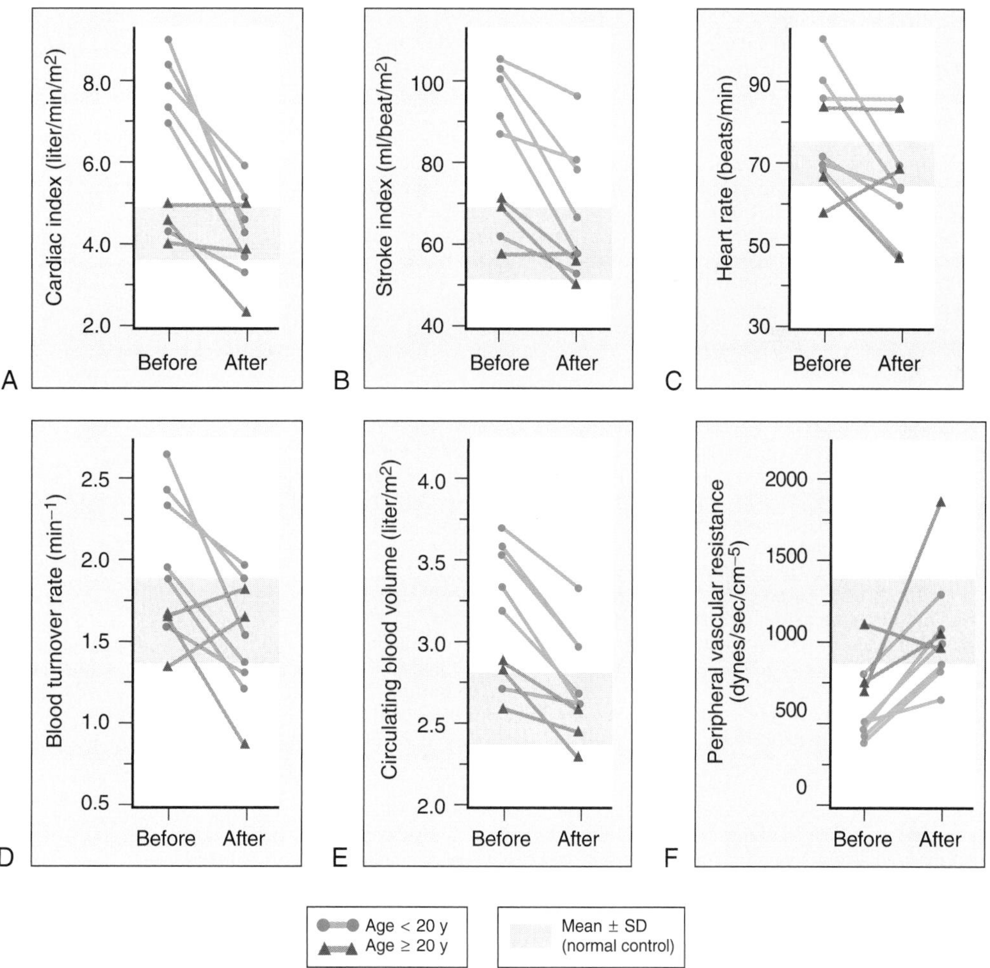

FIGURE 22-20 Hemodynamic changes in beriberi heart disease before and after treatment with intravenous thiamine in patients younger than or older than or equal to 20 years of age. Wet beriberi is characterized by increases in cardiac index **(A)**, stroke index **(B)**, heart rate **(C)**, blood turnover rate **(D)**, and circulating blood volume **(E)** and a decrease in peripheral vascular resistance **(F)**, particularly in younger patients. Thiamine replacement results in a rapid reversal of the high-output state. (From Kawai C, Nakamura Y: The heart in nutritional deficiencies. *In* Abelmann WH [ed]: Cardiomyopathies, Myocarditis, and Pericardial Disease. *In* Braunwald E [series ed]: Atlas of Heart Diseases. Vol 2. Philadelphia, Current Medicine, 1995, pp 7.1-7.18.)

In endemic areas, effective management of beriberi heart disease also involves disease prevention. Recommendations include (1) ingestion of germ-retaining polished rice, undermilled rice, or rice enriched with thiamine; (2) avoidance of excessive intake of carbonated beverages and strenuous exercise during hot summer months; (3) baking or boiling foods that contain thiaminase, such as clams or raw fish; and (4) avoidance of chronic diuretic therapy.

PAGET DISEASE

PATHOGENESIS. Paget disease of bone (osteitis deformans) is an asymmetrical skeletal disorder characterized by excessive resorption of bone followed by replacement of normal marrow with vascular, fibrous connective tissue and of resorbed bone with coarse, trabecular bone.[268] The cause of Paget disease is unknown, although genetic factors or viral infection, or both, may play an important role. Paget disease is most commonly asymptomatic and is diagnosed on a plain radiograph obtained for other reasons or because of a high serum alkaline phosphatase level noted on a routine chemistry screen.

CLINICAL FINDINGS. The two main clinical manifestations of Paget disease are pain and skeletal deformities most commonly affecting the pelvis, skull, spine, and long bones. Traumatic and pathological fractures, bone tumors including malignant osteosarcomas and benign giant cell tumors, and cranial neuropathies may also occur. There appears to be a linear relationship between the amount of skeletal involvement and the increase in cardiac output. Involvement of at least 15 percent of the skeleton by Paget disease in an active stage, accompanied by a high alkaline phosphatase level, is necessary before a clinically significant augmentation of cardiac output is observed.[269] Such a high-output state may be well tolerated for years with the patient remaining asymptomatic. However, if a specific cardiac disorder (e.g., valvular or ischemic heart disease) is present, the combination may cause rapid clinical deterioration.

The cardiovascular findings are not distinguishable from those in other conditions with high-output states. However, metastatic calcifications are characteristic and, if they involve the heart, may lead to sclerosis and calcification of the valve rings, with extension into the interventricular septum. The electrocardiogram may show atrioventricular conduction disturbance or bundle branch block. Echocardiograms often demonstrate aortic sclerosis or stenosis as well as left ventricular dilation, hypertrophy, and mild systolic dysfunction.[270] Successful treatment of the underlying bone disease with bisphosphonates or calcitonin,[271] as reflected by decreases in serum alkaline phosphatase levels or the urinary excretion of hydroxyproline, may normalize the cardiac output over several months.

OTHER CAUSES OF HIGH-OUTPUT CARDIAC FAILURE

FIBROUS DYSPLASIA. This condition, in which there is proliferation of fibrous tissue in bone, may also be associated with an elevated cardiac output, especially when multiple bones are involved.[272] Approximately one quarter of patients with polyostotic fibrous dysplasia have more than half the skeleton affected by disease, most commonly the limbs and craniofacial bones. Calcitonin may be an effective treatment in widespread disease. Bisphosphonates (e.g., pamidronate) have also been used to decrease bone pain and serum alkaline phosphatase levels.

MULTIPLE MYELOMA. Increased cardiac output and less commonly high-output heart failure have been described in this condition.[273,274] The mechanism is not clear, but it may be due to the associated anemia or hyperperfusion of the neoplastic tissue, or both, especially in patients with extensive bone disease.[275] Arteriovenous shunting has been demonstrated in involved bones, especially the femur, using intraarterial injection of radiolabeled albumin, and correlates with cardiac index.[273]

OTHER CONDITIONS. During normal pregnancy (see Chap. 74), cardiac output is elevated secondary to increases in blood volume, heart rate, and metabolic demands as well as the presence of the placenta acting as an arteriovenous shunt. If pregnancy is complicated by marked anemia, high-output heart failure may rarely develop, requiring bed rest and diuretic therapy in addition to transfusions. High-output heart failure also occurs in renal disease, especially glomerulonephritis (see Chap. 86), cor pulmonale (see Chap. 67), polycythemia vera (see Chap. 83), the carcinoid syndrome,[276] acromegaly[277] and marked obesity.[278] In patients with widespread psoriasis or exfoliative dermatitis, increased cardiac output related to marked cutaneous dilation may precipitate heart failure when underlying structural heart disease is present.

REFERENCES

Forms and Causes of Heart Failure

1. Hunt SA, Baker DW, Chin MH, et al: ACC/AHA guidelines for the evaluation and management of chronic heart failure in the adult: Executive summary. A Report of the American College of Cardiology/American Heart Association Task Force on Practice Guidelines (Committee to Revise the 1995 Guidelines for the Evaluation and Management of Heart Failure). Circulation 104:2996, 2001.
2. Ho KK, Pinsky JL, Kannel WB, Levy D: The epidemiology of heart failure: The Framingham Study. J Am Coll Cardiol 22:6A, 1993.
3. American Heart Association: Heart Disease and Stroke Statistics—2004 Update. Dallas, American Heart Association, 2003.
4. Massie BM, Shah NB: Evolving trends in the epidemiologic factors of heart failure: Rationale for preventive strategies and comprehensive disease management. Am Heart J 133:703, 1997.
5. Lloyd-Jones DM, Larson MG, Leip EP, et al: Lifetime risk for developing congestive heart failure: The Framingham Heart Study. Circulation 106:3068, 2002.
6. Rich MW, Nease RF: Cost-effectiveness analysis in clinical practice: The case of heart failure. Arch Intern Med 159:1690, 1999.
7. Minino AM, Arias E, Kochanek KD, et al: Deaths: Final Data for 2000. National Vital Statistics Reports. Vol 50, No 15. Hyattsville, Md, National Center for Health Statistics, 2002.
8. Centers for Medicare and Medicaid Services: 2002 Data Compendium. Baltimore, 2002.
9. O'Connell JB, Bristow MR: Economic impact of heart failure in the United States: Time for a different approach. J Heart Lung Transplant 13:S107, 1994.
10. Moraes DL, Colucci WS, Givertz MM: Secondary pulmonary hypertension in chronic heart failure: The role of the endothelium in pathophysiology and management. Circulation 102:1718, 2000.
11. Winaver J, Abassi Z, Green J, Skorecki KL: Control of extracellular fluid volume and the pathophysiology of edema formation. *In* Brenner BM, Rector FC (eds): Brenner and Rector's The Kidney. Philadelphia, WB Saunders, 2000, pp 795-865.
12. Schrier RW, Abraham WT: Hormones and hemodynamics in heart failure. N Engl J Med 341:577, 1999.
13. Nohria A, Lewis E, Stevenson LW: Medical management of advanced heart failure. JAMA 287:628, 2002.
14. Braunwald E: Report of the Task Force on Research in Heart Failure. Bethesda, Md, National Heart, Lung and Blood Institute, 1994.
15. Hogg K, Swedberg K, McMurray J: Heart failure with preserved left ventricular systolic function: Epidemiology, clinical characteristics, and prognosis. J Am Coll Cardiol 43:317, 2004.
16. Zile MR, Brutsaert DL: New concepts in diastolic dysfunction and diastolic heart failure: Part II: Causal mechanisms and treatment. Circulation 105:1503, 2002.
17. Zile MR, Brutsaert DL: New concepts in diastolic dysfunction and diastolic heart failure: Part I: Diagnosis, prognosis, and measurements of diastolic function. Circulation 105:1387, 2002.
18. Angeja BG, Grossman W: Evaluation and management of diastolic heart failure. Circulation 107:659, 2003.
19. Hundley WG, Kitzman DW, Morgan TM, et al: Cardiac cycle–dependent changes in aortic area and distensibility are reduced in older patients with isolated diastolic heart failure and correlate with exercise intolerance. J Am Coll Cardiol 38:796, 2001.
20. Kawaguchi M, Hay I, Fetics B, Kass DA: Combined ventricular systolic and arterial stiffening in patients with heart failure and preserved ejection fraction: Implications for systolic and diastolic reserve limitations. Circulation 107:714, 2003.
21. Vasan RS, Larson MG, Benjamin EJ, et al: Congestive heart failure in subjects with normal versus reduced left ventricular ejection fraction: Prevalence and mortality in a population- based cohort. J Am Coll Cardiol 33:1948, 1999.
22. Senni M, Redfield MM: Heart failure with preserved systolic function. A different natural history? J Am Coll Cardiol 38:1277, 2001.
23. Masoudi FA, Havranek EP, Smith G, et al: Gender, age, and heart failure with preserved left ventricular systolic function. J Am Coll Cardiol 41:217, 2003.
24. Vasan RS, Levy D: Defining diastolic heart failure: A call for standardized diagnostic criteria. Circulation 101:2118, 2000.
25. Chin MH, Goldman L: Factors contributing to the hospitalization of patients with congestive heart failure. Am J Public Health 87:643, 1997.
26. Tsuyuki RT, McKelvie RS, Arnold JM, et al: Acute precipitants of congestive heart failure exacerbations. Arch Intern Med 161:2337, 2001.
27. He J, Ogden LG, Bazzano LA, et al: Risk factors for congestive heart failure in US men and women: NHANES I epidemiologic follow-up study. Arch Intern Med 161:996, 2001.
28. Levy D, Larson MG, Vasan RS, et al: The progression from hypertension to congestive heart failure. JAMA 275:1557, 1996.
29. Shinbane JS, Wood MA, Jensen DN, et al: Tachycardia-induced cardiomyopathy: A review of animal models and clinical studies. J Am Coll Cardiol 29:709, 1997.
30. Bentancur AG, Rieck J, Koldanov R, Dankner RS: Acute pulmonary edema in the emergency department: Clinical and echocardiographic survey in an aged population. Am J Med Sci 323:238, 2002.
31. Givertz MM, Colucci WS: New targets for heart-failure therapy: Endothelin, inflammatory cytokines, and oxidative stress. Lancet 352(Suppl 1):S134, 1998.
32. Koniaris LS, Goldhaber SZ: Anticoagulation in dilated cardiomyopathy. J Am Coll Cardiol 31:745, 1998.
33. Dries DL, Exner DV, Domanski MJ, et al: The prognostic implications of renal insufficiency in asymptomatic and symptomatic patients with left ventricular systolic dysfunction. J Am Coll Cardiol 35:681, 2000.
34. Page J, Henry D: Consumption of NSAIDs and the development of congestive heart failure in elderly patients: An underrecognized public health problem. Arch Intern Med 160:777, 2000.

35. Brater DC: Anti-inflammatory agents and renal function. Semin Arthritis Rheum 32:33, 2002.
36. Piano MR: Alcohol and heart failure. J Card Fail 8:239, 2002.
37. Felker GM, Gattis WA, Leimberger JD, et al: Usefulness of anemia as a predictor of death and rehospitalization in patients with decompensated heart failure. Am J Cardiol 92:625, 2003.

Clinical Manifestations

38. Wilson JR, Rayos G, Yeoh TK, et al: Dissociation between exertional symptoms and circulatory function in patients with heart failure. Circulation 92:47, 1995.
39. Duguet A, Tantucci C, Lozinguez O, et al: Expiratory flow limitation as a determinant of orthopnea in acute left heart failure. J Am Coll Cardiol 35:690, 2000.
40. Leung RS, Bowman ME, Parker JD, et al: Avoidance of the left lateral decubitus position during sleep in patients with heart failure: Relationship to cardiac size and function. J Am Coll Cardiol 41:227, 2003.
41. Quaranta AJ, D'Alonzo GE, Krachman SL: Cheyne-Stokes respiration during sleep in congestive heart failure. Chest 111:467, 1997.
42. Mancini DM: Pulmonary factors limiting exercise capacity in patients with heart failure. Prog Cardiovasc Dis 37:347, 1995.
43. Nanas S, Nanas J, Kassiotis C, et al: Respiratory muscles performance is related to oxygen kinetics during maximal exercise and early recovery in patients with congestive heart failure. Circulation 100:503, 1999.
44. Morrison LK, Harrison A, Krishnaswamy P, et al: Utility of a rapid B-natriuretic peptide assay in differentiating congestive heart failure from lung disease in patients presenting with dyspnea. J Am Coll Cardiol 39:202, 2002.
45. Rietveld S, van Beest I, Everaerd W: Stress-induced breathlessness in asthma. Psychol Med 29:1359, 1999.
46. Johnson BD, Beck KC, Olson LJ, et al: Pulmonary function in patients with reduced left ventricular function: Influence of smoking and cardiac surgery. Chest 120:1869, 2001.
47. Weisman IM, Zeballos RJ: Clinical evaluation of unexplained dyspnea. Cardiologia 41:621, 1996.
48. Coats AJ: Origin of symptoms in patients with cachexia with special reference to weakness and shortness of breath. Int J Cardiol 85:133, 2002.
49. Rosenberg P, Yancy CW: Noninvasive assessment of hemodynamics: An emphasis on bioimpedance cardiography. Curr Opin Cardiol 15:151, 2000.
50. Maisel AS, Krishnaswamy P, Nowak RM, et al: Rapid measurement of B-type natriuretic peptide in the emergency diagnosis of heart failure. N Engl J Med 347:161, 2002.
51. Pina IL, Apstein CS, Balady GJ, et al: Exercise and heart failure: A statement from the American Heart Association Committee on exercise, rehabilitation, and prevention. Circulation 107:1210, 2003.
52. Chomsky DB, Lang CC, Rayos GH, et al: Hemodynamic exercise testing. A valuable tool in the selection of cardiac transplantation candidates. Circulation 94:3176, 1996.
53. Lapu-Bula R, Robert A, Van Craeynest D, et al: Contribution of exercise-induced mitral regurgitation to exercise stroke volume and exercise capacity in patients with left ventricular systolic dysfunction. Circulation 106:1342, 2002.
54. Butler J, Chomsky DB, Wilson JR: Pulmonary hypertension and exercise intolerance in patients with heart failure. J Am Coll Cardiol 34:1802, 1999.
55. Mancini DM, Katz SD, Lang CC, et al: Effect of erythropoietin on exercise capacity in patients with moderate to severe chronic heart failure. Circulation 107:294, 2003.
56. Shoemaker JK, Naylor HL, Hogeman CS, Sinoway LI: Blood flow dynamics in heart failure. Circulation 99:3002, 1999.
57. Mancini DM, Wilson JR, Bolinger L, et al: In vivo magnetic resonance spectroscopy measurement of deoxymyoglobin during exercise in patients with heart failure. Demonstration of abnormal muscle metabolism despite adequate oxygenation. Circulation 90:500, 1994.
58. Cicoira M, Zanolla L, Franceschini L, et al: Skeletal muscle mass independently predicts peak oxygen consumption and ventilatory response during exercise in noncachectic patients with chronic heart failure. J Am Coll Cardiol 37:2080, 2001.
59. Johnson W, Lucas C, Stevenson LW, Creager MA: Effect of intensive therapy for heart failure on the vasodilator response to exercise. J Am Coll Cardiol 33:743, 1999.
60. Gottlieb SS, Fisher ML, Freudenberger R, et al: Effects of exercise training on peak performance and quality of life in congestive heart failure patients. J Card Fail 5:188, 1999.
61. Belardinelli R, Georgiou D, Cianci G, Purcaro A: Randomized, controlled trial of long-term moderate exercise training in chronic heart failure: Effects on functional capacity, quality of life, and clinical outcome. Circulation 99:1173, 1999.
62. Keteyian SJ, Brawner CA, Schairer JR, et al: Effects of exercise training on chronotropic incompetence in patients with heart failure. Am Heart J 138:233, 1999.
63. Linke A, Schoene N, Gielen S, et al: Endothelial dysfunction in patients with chronic heart failure: Systemic effects of lower-limb exercise training. J Am Coll Cardiol 37:392, 2001.
64. Braith RW, Welsch MA, Feigenbaum MS, et al: Neuroendocrine activation in heart failure is modified by endurance exercise training. J Am Coll Cardiol 34:1170, 1999.
65. Adamopoulos S, Parissis J, Karatzas D, et al: Physical training modulates proinflammatory cytokines and the soluble Fas/soluble Fas ligand system in patients with chronic heart failure. J Am Coll Cardiol 39:653, 2002.
66. Ennezat PV, Malendowicz SL, Testa M, et al: Physical training in patients with chronic heart failure enhances the expression of genes encoding antioxidative enzymes. J Am Coll Cardiol 38:194, 2001.
67. Pu CT, Johnson MT, Forman DE, et al: Randomized trial of progressive resistance training to counteract the myopathy of chronic heart failure. J Appl Physiol 90:2341, 2001.
68. Whellan DJ, O'Connor CM: The state of exercise training: A need for action. Am Heart J 144:1, 2002.
69. Wasserman K, Hansen JE, Sue D, et al: Principles of Exercise Testing and Interpretation. 3rd ed. Philadelphia, Lippincott Williams & Wilkins, 1999.
70. Pardaens K, Van Cleemput J, Vanhaecke J, Fagard RH: Peak oxygen uptake better predicts outcome than submaximal respiratory data in heart transplant candidates. Circulation 101:1152, 2000.
71. Stelken AM, Younis LT, Jennison SH, et al: Prognostic value of cardiopulmonary exercise testing using percent achieved of predicted peak oxygen uptake for patients with ischemic and dilated cardiomyopathy. J Am Coll Cardiol 27:345, 1996.
72. Arzt M, Harth M, Luchner A, et al: Enhanced ventilatory response to exercise in patients with chronic heart failure and central sleep apnea. Circulation 107:1998, 2003.
73. Larsen AI, Aarsland T, Kristiansen M, et al: Assessing the effect of exercise training in men with heart failure; comparison of maximal, submaximal and endurance exercise protocols. Eur Heart J 22:684, 2001.
74. Faggiano P, D'Aloia A, Gualeni A, Giordano A: Hemodynamic profile of submaximal constant workload exercise in patients with heart failure secondary to ischemic or idiopathic dilated cardiomyopathy. Am J Cardiol 81:437, 1998.
75. Cahalin LP, Mathier MA, Semigran MJ, et al: The six-minute walk test predicts peak oxygen uptake and survival in patients with advanced heart failure. Chest 110:325, 1996.
76. Bittner V, Weiner DH, Yusuf S, et al: Prediction of mortality and morbidity with a 6-minute walk test in patients with left ventricular dysfunction. SOLVD Investigators. JAMA 270:1702, 1993.
77. Anker SD, Rauchhaus M: Insights into the pathogenesis of chronic heart failure: Immune activation and cachexia. Curr Opin Cardiol 14:211, 1999.
78. Zuccala G, Cattel C, Manes-Gravina E, et al: Left ventricular dysfunction: A clue to cognitive impairment in older patients with heart failure. J Neurol Neurosurg Psychiatry 63:509, 1997.
79. The Criteria Committee of the New York Heart Association: Nomenclature and Criteria for Diagnosis of Diseases of the Heart and Great Vessels. 9th ed. Boston, Little, Brown, 1994.
80. Bettencourt P, Ferreira A, Dias P, et al: Predictors of prognosis in patients with stable mild to moderate heart failure. J Card Fail 6:306, 2000.
81. Australia/New Zealand Heart Failure Research Collaborative Group: Randomised, placebo-controlled trial of carvedilol in patients with congestive heart failure due to ischaemic heart disease. Lancet 349:375, 1997.
82. Bennet SJ, Oldridge NB, Eckert GJ, et al: Discriminant properties of commonly used quality of life measures in heart failure. Qual Life Res 11:349, 2002.
83. al Kaade S, Hauptman PJ: Health-related quality of life measurement in heart failure: Challenges for the new millennium. J Card Fail 7:194, 2001.
84. Green CP, Porter CB, Bresnahan DR, Spertus JA: Development and evaluation of the Kansas City Cardiomyopathy Questionnaire: A new health status measure for heart failure. J Am Coll Cardiol 35:1245, 2000.
85. Konstam V, Salem D, Pouleur H, et al: Baseline quality of life as a predictor of mortality and hospitalization in 5,025 patients with congestive heart failure. SOLVD Investigations. Studies of Left Ventricular Dysfunction Investigators. Am J Cardiol 78:890, 1996.
86. Abraham WT, Fisher WG, Smith AL, et al: Cardiac resynchronization in chronic heart failure. N Engl J Med 346:1845, 2002.
87. Kasper EK, Gerstenblith G, Hefter G, et al: A randomized trial of the efficacy of multidisciplinary care in heart failure outpatients at high risk of hospital readmission. J Am Coll Cardiol 39:471, 2002.
88. Shah MR, Hasselblad V, Stinnett SS, et al: Hemodynamic profiles of advanced heart failure: Association with clinical characteristics and long-term outcomes. J Card Fail 7:105, 2001.
89. Kataoka H: Pericardial and pleural effusions in decompensated chronic heart failure. Am Heart J 139:918, 2000.
90. Perloff JK: The jugular venous pulse and third heart sound in patients with heart failure. N Engl J Med 345:612, 2001.
91. Drazner MH, Rame JE, Stevenson LW, Dries DL: Prognostic importance of elevated jugular venous pressure and a third heart sound in patients with heart failure. N Engl J Med 345:574, 2001.
92. Wiese J: The abdominojugular reflux sign. Am J Med 109:59, 2000.
93. O'Reilly RA: Splenomegaly in 2,505 patients at a large university medical center from 1913 to 1995. 1963 to 1995: 449 patients. West J Med 169:88, 1998.
94. Madias JE, Bazaz R, Agarwal H, et al: Anasarca-mediated attenuation of the amplitude of electrocardiogram complexes: A description of a heretofore unrecognized phenomenon. J Am Coll Cardiol 38:756, 2001.
95. Light RW: Clinical practice. Pleural effusion. N Engl J Med 346:1971, 2002.
96. Johnson JL: Pleural effusions in cardiovascular disease. Pearls for correlating the evidence with the cause. Postgrad Med 107:95, 2000.
97. Van der Merwe S, Dens J, Daenen W, et al: Pericardial disease is often not recognised as a cause of chronic severe ascites. J Hepatol 32:164, 2000.
98. Chan FK, Sung JJ, Ma KM, et al: Protein-losing enteropathy in congestive heart failure: Diagnosis by means of a simple method. Hepatogastroenterology 46:1816, 1999.
99. Kodama M, Kato K, Hirono S, et al: Mechanical alternans in patients with chronic heart failure. J Card Fail 7:138, 2001.
100. Capomolla S, Pozzoli M, Opasich C, et al: Dobutamine and nitroprusside infusion in patients with severe congestive heart failure: Hemodynamic improvement by discordant effects on mitral regurgitation, left atrial function, and ventricular function. Am Heart J 134:1089, 1997.
101. Linde C, Leclercq C, Rex S, et al: Long-term benefits of biventricular pacing in congestive heart failure: Results from the MUltisite STimulation in cardiomyopathy (MUSTIC) study. J Am Coll Cardiol 40:111, 2002.
102. Sanders GP, Mendes LA, Colucci WS, Givertz MM: Noninvasive methods for detecting elevated left-sided cardiac filling pressure. J Card Fail 6:157, 2000.
103. Givertz MM, Slawsky MT, Moraes DL, et al: Noninvasive determination of pulmonary artery wedge pressure in patients with chronic heart failure. Am J Cardiol 87:1213, 2001.
104. King D, Smith ML, Chapman TJ, et al: Fat malabsorption in elderly patients with cardiac cachexia. Age Ageing 25:144, 1996.
105. Peracchi M, Trovato C, Longhi M, et al: Tissue transglutaminase antibodies in patients with end-stage heart failure. Am J Gastroenterol 97:2850, 2002.

106. Torre-Amione G, Kapadia S, Benedict C, et al: Proinflammatory cytokine levels in patients with depressed left ventricular ejection fraction: A report from the studies of left ventricular dysfunction (SOLVD). J Am Coll Cardiol 27:1201, 1996.
107. Feldman AM, Combes A, Wagner D, et al: The role of tumor necrosis factor in the pathophysiology of heart failure. J Am Coll Cardiol 35:537, 2000.
108. Mann DL, Spinale FG: Activation of matrix metalloproteinases in the failing human heart: Breaking the tie that binds. Circulation 98:1699, 1998.
109. Anker SD, Chua TP, Ponikowski P, et al: Hormonal changes and catabolic/anabolic imbalance in chronic heart failure and their importance for cardiac cachexia. Circulation 96:526, 1997.
110. Anker SD, Negassa A, Coats AJ, et al: Prognostic importance of weight loss in chronic heart failure and the effect of treatment with angiotensin-converting enzyme inhibitors: An observational study. Lancet 361:1077, 2003.
111. Ponikowski P, Anker SD, Chua TP, et al: Oscillatory breathing patterns during wakefulness in patients with chronic heart failure: Clinical implications and role of augmented peripheral chemosensitivity. Circulation 100:2418, 1999.
112. Mansfield D, Kaye DM, Brunner La Rocca H, et al: Raised sympathetic nerve activity in heart failure and central sleep apnea is due to heart failure severity. Circulation 107:1396, 2003.
113. Giallourakis CC, Rosenberg PM, Friedman LS: The liver in heart failure. Clin Liver Dis 6:947, 2002.
114. Palm C, Reimann D, Gross P: The role of V2 vasopressin antagonists in hyponatremia. Cardiovasc Res 51:403, 2001.
115. Laragh JH, Sealey JE: K(+) depletion and the progression of hypertensive disease or heart failure. The pathogenic role of diuretic-induced aldosterone secretion. Hypertension 37:806, 2001.
116. Obialo CI, Ofili EO, Mirza T: Hyperkalemia in congestive heart failure patients aged 63 to 85 years with subclinical renal disease. Am J Cardiol 90:663, 2002.
117. Schepkens H, Vanholder R, Billiouw JM, Lameire N: Life-threatening hyperkalemia during combined therapy with angiotensin-converting enzyme inhibitors and spironolactone: An analysis of 25 cases. Am J Med 110:438, 2001.
118. Bozkurt B, Agoston I, Knowlton AA: Complications of inappropriate use of spironolactone in heart failure: When an old medicine spirals out of new guidelines. J Am Coll Cardiol 41:211, 2003.
119. Milionis HJ, Alexandrides GE, Liberopoulos EN, et al: Hypomagnesemia and concurrent acid-base and electrolyte abnormalities in patients with congestive heart failure. Eur J Heart Fail 4:167, 2002.
120. Doehner W, Schoene N, Rauchhaus M, et al: Effects of xanthine oxidase inhibition with allopurinol on endothelial function and peripheral blood flow in hyperuricemic patients with chronic heart failure: Results from 2 placebo-controlled studies. Circulation 105:2619, 2002.
121. Ruilope LM, van Veldhuisen DJ, Ritz E, Luscher TF: Renal function: The Cinderella of cardiovascular risk profile. J Am Coll Cardiol 38:1782, 2001.
122. Batin P, Wickens M, McEntegart D, et al: The importance of abnormalities of liver function tests in predicting mortality in chronic heart failure. Eur Heart J 16:1613, 1995.
123. Naschitz JE, Slobodin G, Lewis RJ, et al: Heart diseases affecting the liver and liver diseases affecting the heart. Am Heart J 140:111, 2000.
124. Wiesen S, Reddy KR, Jeffers LJ, Schiff ER: Fulminant hepatic failure secondary to previously unrecognized cardiomyopathy. Dig Dis 13:199, 1995.
125. Horwich TB, Fonarow GC, Hamilton MA, et al: Anemia is associated with worse symptoms, greater impairment in functional capacity and a significant increase in mortality in patients with advanced heart failure. J Am Coll Cardiol 39:1780, 2002.
126. Ezekowitz JA, McAlister FA, Armstrong PW: Anemia is common in heart failure and is associated with poor outcomes: Insights from a cohort of 12 065 patients with new-onset heart failure. Circulation 107:223, 2003.
127. Levin A, Thompson CR, Ethier J, et al: Left ventricular mass index increase in early renal disease: Impact of decline in hemoglobin. Am J Kidney Dis 34:125, 1999.
128. SoRelle R: Erythropoietin—Not at the Olympics but maybe for anemic heart failure patients. Circulation 107:e9004, 2003.
129. Sharma R, Rauchhaus M, Ponikowski PP, et al: The relationship of the erythrocyte sedimentation rate to inflammatory cytokines and survival in patients with chronic heart failure treated with angiotensin-converting enzyme inhibitors. J Am Coll Cardiol 36:523, 2000.
130. Davidson C: Can heart failure be diagnosed in primary care? Chest radiography is still useful. BMJ 321:1414, 2000.
131. Kataoka H, Takada S: The role of thoracic ultrasonography for evaluation of patients with decompensated chronic heart failure. J Am Coll Cardiol 35:1638, 2000.

Prognosis

132. Levy D, Kenchaiah S, Larson MG, et al: Long-term trends in the incidence of and survival with heart failure. N Engl J Med 347:1397, 2002.
133. Rose EA, Gelijns AC, Moskowitz AJ, et al: Long-term mechanical left ventricular assistance for end-stage heart failure. N Engl J Med 345:1435, 2001.
134. Ho KK, Anderson KM, Kannel WB, et al: Survival after the onset of congestive heart failure in Framingham Heart Study subjects. Circulation 88:107, 1993.
135. Rector TS, Cohn JN: Prognosis in congestive heart failure. Annu Rev Med 45:341, 1994.
136. Deedwania PC: The key to unraveling the mystery of mortality in heart failure: An integrated approach. Circulation 107:1719, 2003.
137. Simon T, Mary-Krause M, Funck-Brentano C, Jaillon P: Sex differences in the prognosis of congestive heart failure: Results from the Cardiac Insufficiency Bisoprolol Study (CIBIS II). Circulation 103:375, 2001.
138. Bart BA, Shaw LK, McCants CB Jr, et al: Clinical determinants of mortality in patients with angiographically diagnosed ischemic or nonischemic cardiomyopathy. J Am Coll Cardiol 30:1002, 1997.
139. Metra M, Faggiano P, D'Aloia A, et al: Use of cardiopulmonary exercise testing with hemodynamic monitoring in the prognostic assessment of ambulatory patients with chronic heart failure. J Am Coll Cardiol 33:943, 1999.
140. Ponikowski P, Francis DP, Piepoli MF, et al: Enhanced ventilatory response to exercise in patients with chronic heart failure and preserved exercise tolerance: Marker of abnormal cardiorespiratory reflex control and predictor of poor prognosis. Circulation 103:967, 2001.
141. Gitt AK, Wasserman K, Kilkowski C, et al: Exercise anaerobic threshold and ventilatory efficiency identify heart failure patients for high risk of early death. Circulation 106:3079, 2002.
142. Meyer FJ, Borst MM, Zugck C, et al: Respiratory muscle dysfunction in congestive heart failure: Clinical correlation and prognostic significance. Circulation 103:2153, 2001.
143. Ponikowski P, Chua TP, Anker SD, et al: Peripheral chemoreceptor hypersensitivity: An ominous sign in patients with chronic heart failure. Circulation 104:544, 2001.
144. Dries DL, Sweitzer NK, Drazner MH, et al: Prognostic impact of diabetes mellitus in patients with heart failure according to the etiology of left ventricular systolic dysfunction. J Am Coll Cardiol 38:421, 2001.
145. Sin DD, Logan AG, Fitzgerald FS, et al: Effects of continuous positive airway pressure on cardiovascular outcomes in heart failure patients with and without Cheyne-Stokes respiration. Circulation 102:61, 2000.
146. Bradley TD, Floras JS: Sleep apnea and heart failure: Part I: Obstructive sleep apnea. Circulation 107:1671, 2003.
147. Bradley TD, Floras JS: Sleep apnea and heart failure: Part II: Central sleep apnea. Circulation 107:1822, 2003.
148. Vaccarino V, Kasl SV, Abramson J, Krumholz HM: Depressive symptoms and risk of functional decline and death in patients with heart failure. J Am Coll Cardiol 38:199, 2001.
149. Horwich TB, Fonarow GC, Hamilton MA, et al: The relationship between obesity and mortality in patients with heart failure. J Am Coll Cardiol 38:789, 2001.
150. Naqvi TZ, Goel RK, Forrester JS, et al: Usefulness of left ventricular mass in predicting recovery of left ventricular systolic function in patients with symptomatic idiopathic dilated cardiomyopathy. Am J Cardiol 85:624, 2000.
151. Koelling TM, Aaronson KD, Cody RJ, et al: Prognostic significance of mitral regurgitation and tricuspid regurgitation in patients with left ventricular systolic dysfunction. Am Heart J 144:524, 2002.
152. Dini FL, Cortigiani L, Baldini U, et al: Prognostic value of left atrial enlargement in patients with idiopathic dilated cardiomyopathy and ischemic cardiomyopathy. Am J Cardiol 89:518, 2002.
153. Cohn JN, Johnson GR, Shabetai R, et al: Ejection fraction, peak exercise oxygen consumption, cardiothoracic ratio, ventricular arrhythmias, and plasma norepinephrine as determinants of prognosis in heart failure. The V-HeFT VA Cooperative Studies Group. Circulation 87:VI-5, 1993.
154. Neglia D, Michelassi C, Trivieri MG, et al: Prognostic role of myocardial blood flow impairment in idiopathic left ventricular dysfunction. Circulation 105:186, 2002.
155. Zornoff LA, Skali H, Pfeffer MA, et al: Right ventricular dysfunction and risk of heart failure and mortality after myocardial infarction. J Am Coll Cardiol 39:1450, 2002.
156. Rickenbacher PR, Trindade PT, Haywood GA, et al: Transplant candidates with severe left ventricular dysfunction managed with medical treatment: Characteristics and survival. J Am Coll Cardiol 27:1192, 1996.
157. Myers J, Gullestad L, Vagelos R, et al: Clinical, hemodynamic, and cardiopulmonary exercise test determinants of survival in patients referred for evaluation of heart failure. Ann Intern Med 129:286, 1998.
158. Hansen A, Haass M, Zugck C, et al: Prognostic value of Doppler echocardiographic mitral inflow patterns: Implications for risk stratification in patients with chronic congestive heart failure. J Am Coll Cardiol 37:1049, 2001.
159. Francis GS, Cohn JN, Johnson G, et al: Plasma norepinephrine, plasma renin activity, and congestive heart failure. Relations to survival and the effects of therapy in V-HeFT II. The V-HeFT VA Cooperative Studies Group. Circulation 87:VI-40, 1993.
160. Anand IS, Fisher LD, Chiang YT, et al: Changes in brain natriuretic peptide and norepinephrine over time and mortality and morbidity in the Valsartan Heart Failure Trial (Val-HeFT). Circulation 107:1278, 2003.
161. Goldsmith SR: Vasopressin: A therapeutic target in congestive heart failure? J Card Fail 5:347, 1999.
162. Jessup M: Aldosterone blockade and heart failure. N Engl J Med 348:1380, 2003.
163. Stanek B, Frey B, Hulsmann M, et al: Prognostic evaluation of neurohumoral plasma levels before and during beta-blocker therapy in advanced left ventricular dysfunction. J Am Coll Cardiol 38:436, 2001.
164. Berger R, Stanek B, Frey B, et al: B-type natriuretic peptides (BNP and PRO-BNP) predict longterm survival in patients with advanced heart failure treated with atenolol. J Heart Lung Transplant 20:251, 2001.
165. Maeda K, Tsutamoto T, Wada A, et al: High levels of plasma brain natriuretic peptide and interleukin-6 after optimized treatment for heart failure are independent risk factors for morbidity and mortality in patients with congestive heart failure. J Am Coll Cardiol 36:1587, 2000.
166. Hulsmann M, Stanek B, Frey B, et al: Value of cardiopulmonary exercise testing and big endothelin plasma levels to predict short-term prognosis of patients with chronic heart failure. J Am Coll Cardiol 32:1695, 1998.
167. Cohn JN, Ferrari R, Sharpe N: Cardiac remodeling—Concepts and clinical implications: A consensus paper from an international forum on cardiac remodeling. Behalf of an International Forum on Cardiac Remodeling. J Am Coll Cardiol 35:569, 2000.
168. Saxon LA, Stevenson WG, Middlekauff HR, et al: Predicting death from progressive heart failure secondary to ischemic or idiopathic dilated cardiomyopathy. Am J Cardiol 72:62, 1993.
169. Berger R, Huelsman M, Strecker K, et al: B-type natriuretic peptide predicts sudden death in patients with chronic heart failure. Circulation 105:2392, 2002.
170. Bozkurt B, Mann DL: Use of biomarkers in the management of heart failure: Are we there yet? Circulation 107:1231, 2003.
171. Deswal A, Petersen NJ, Feldman AM, et al: Cytokines and cytokine receptors in advanced heart failure: An analysis of the cytokine database from the vesnarinone trial (VEST). Circulation 103:2055, 2001.

172. Rauchhaus M, Doehner W, Francis DP, et al: Plasma cytokine parameters and mortality in patients with chronic heart failure. Circulation 102:3060, 2000.
173. Tsutamoto T, Hisanaga T, Wada A, et al: Interleukin-6 spillover in the peripheral circulation increases with the severity of heart failure, and the high plasma level of interleukin-6 is an important prognostic predictor in patients with congestive heart failure. J Am Coll Cardiol 31:391, 1998.
174. Tsutsui T, Tsutamoto T, Wada A, et al: Plasma oxidized low-density lipoprotein as a prognostic predictor in patients with chronic congestive heart failure. J Am Coll Cardiol 39:957, 2002.
175. Hare JM, Johnson RJ: Uric acid predicts clinical outcomes in heart failure: Insights regarding the role of xanthine oxidase and uric acid in disease pathophysiology. Circulation 107:1951, 2003.
176. Sato Y, Yamada T, Taniguchi R, et al: Persistently increased serum concentrations of cardiac troponin t in patients with idiopathic dilated cardiomyopathy are predictive of adverse outcomes. Circulation 103:369, 2001.
177. La Rovere MT, Pinna GD, Maestri R, et al: Short-term heart rate variability strongly predicts sudden cardiac death in chronic heart failure patients. Circulation 107:565, 2003.
178. Singh SN, Fisher SG, Carson PE, Fletcher RD: Prevalence and significance of nonsustained ventricular tachycardia in patients with premature ventricular contractions and heart failure treated with vasodilator therapy. Department of Veterans Affairs CHF STAT Investigators. J Am Coll Cardiol 32:942, 1998.
179. Iuliano S, Fisher SG, Karasik PE, et al: QRS duration and mortality in patients with congestive heart failure. Am Heart J 143:1085, 2002.
180. Dries DL, Exner DV, Gersh BJ, et al: Atrial fibrillation is associated with an increased risk for mortality and heart failure progression in patients with asymptomatic and symptomatic left ventricular systolic dysfunction: A retrospective analysis of the SOLVD trials. Studies of Left Ventricular Dysfunction. J Am Coll Cardiol 32:695, 1998.
181. Moss AJ, Zareba W, Hall WJ, et al: Prophylactic implantation of a defibrillator in patients with myocardial infarction and reduced ejection fraction. N Engl J Med 346:877, 2002.
182. Bristow MR, Feldman AM, Saxon LA: Heart failure management using implantable devices for ventricular resynchronization: Comparison of Medical Therapy, Pacing, and Defibrillation in Chronic Heart Failure (COMPANION) trial. COMPANION Steering Committee and COMPANION Clinical Investigators. J Card Fail 6:276, 2000.
183. Vrtovec B, Delgado R, Zewail A, et al: Prolonged QTc interval and high B-type natriuretic peptide levels together predict mortality in patients with advanced heart failure. Circulation 107:1764, 2003.
184. Pinsky DJ, Sciacca RR, Steinberg JS: QT dispersion as a marker of risk in patients awaiting heart transplantation. J Am Coll Cardiol 29:1576, 1997.
185. Klingenheben T, Zabel M, D'Agostino RB, et al: Predictive value of T-wave alternans for arrhythmic events in patients with congestive heart failure. Lancet 356:651, 2000.

Pulmonary Edema

186. Flick MR, Matthay MA: Pulmonary edema and acute lung injury. *In* Murray JF, Nadel JA (eds): Textbook of Respiratory Medicine. Philadelphia, WB Saunders, 2000, pp 1575-1629.
187. Guyton AC, Hall JE: Pulmonary circulation; pulmonary edema; pleural fluid. Textbook of Medical Physiology. Philadelphia, WB Saunders, 2000, pp 444-451.
188. West JB, Mathieu-Costello O: Structure, strength, failure, and remodeling of the pulmonary blood-gas barrier. Annu Rev Physiol 61:543, 1999.
189. Sherman SC: Reexpansion pulmonary edema: A case report and review of the current literature. J Emerg Med 24:23, 2003.
190. Woodring JH: Focal reexpansion pulmonary edema after drainage of large pleural effusions: Clinical evidence suggesting hypoxic injury to the lung as the cause of edema. South Med J 90:1176, 1997.
191. Nakamura M, Fujishima S, Sawafuji M, et al: Importance of interleukin-8 in the development of reexpansion lung injury in rabbits. Am J Respir Crit Care Med 161:1030, 2000.
192. Tan HC, Mak KH, Johan A, et al: Cardiac output increases prior to development of pulmonary edema after re-expansion of spontaneous pneumothorax. Respir Med 96:461, 2002.
193. Ware LB, Matthay MA: The acute respiratory distress syndrome. N Engl J Med 342:1334, 2000.
194. Herridge MS, Cheung AM, Tansey CM, et al: One-year outcomes in survivors of the acute respiratory distress syndrome. N Engl J Med 348:683, 2003.
195. Pugin J, Verghese G, Widmer MC, Matthay MA: The alveolar space is the site of intense inflammatory and profibrotic reactions in the early phase of acute respiratory distress syndrome. Crit Care Med 27:304, 1999.
196. Edoute Y, Roguin A, Behar D, Reisner SA: Prospective evaluation of pulmonary edema. Crit Care Med 28:330, 2000.
197. Gandhi SK, Powers JC, Nomeir AM, et al: The pathogenesis of acute pulmonary edema associated with hypertension. N Engl J Med 344:17, 2001.
198. Phillips RA, Greenblatt J, Krakoff LR: Hypertensive emergencies: Diagnosis and management. Prog Cardiovasc Dis 45:33, 2002.
199. McFadden ER Jr, Warren EL: Observations on asthma mortality. Ann Intern Med 127:142, 1997.
200. Logeart D, Saudubray C, Beyne P, et al: Comparative value of Doppler echocardiography and B-type natriuretic peptide assay in the etiologic diagnosis of acute dyspnea. J Am Coll Cardiol 40:1794, 2002.
201. Littmann L: Large T wave inversion and QT prolongation associated with pulmonary edema: A report of nine cases. J Am Coll Cardiol 34:1106, 1999.
202. Roguin A, Behar D, Ben Ami H, et al: Long-term prognosis of acute pulmonary oedema—An ominous outcome. Eur J Heart Fail 2:137, 2000.
203. Hackett PH, Roach RC: High-altitude illness. N Engl J Med 345:107, 2001.
204. Bartsch P, Swenson ER, Maggiorini M: Update: High altitude pulmonary edema. Adv Exp Med Biol 502:89, 2001.
205. Gabry AL, Ledoux X, Mozziconacci M, Martin C: High-altitude pulmonary edema at moderate altitude (<2,400 m; 7,870 feet): A series of 52 patients. Chest 123:49, 2003.
206. Grunig E, Mereles D, Hildebrandt W, et al: Stress Doppler echocardiography for identification of susceptibility to high altitude pulmonary edema. J Am Coll Cardiol 35:980, 2000.
207. Duplain H, Vollenweider L, Delabays A, et al: Augmented sympathetic activation during short-term hypoxia and high-altitude exposure in subjects susceptible to high-altitude pulmonary edema. Circulation 99:1713, 1999.
208. Busch T, Bartsch P, Pappert D, et al: Hypoxia decreases exhaled nitric oxide in mountaineers susceptible to high-altitude pulmonary edema. Am J Respir Crit Care Med 163:368, 2001.
209. Sartori C, Vollenweider L, Loffler BM, et al: Exaggerated endothelin release in high-altitude pulmonary edema. Circulation 99:2665, 1999.
210. Hanaoka M, Tanaka M, Ge RL, et al: Hypoxia-induced pulmonary blood redistribution in subjects with a history of high-altitude pulmonary edema. Circulation 101:1418, 2000.
211. West JB: Invited review: Pulmonary capillary stress failure. J Appl Physiol 89:2483, 2000.
212. Swenson ER, Maggiorini M, Mongovin S, et al: Pathogenesis of high-altitude pulmonary edema: Inflammation is not an etiologic factor. JAMA 287:2228, 2002.
213. Hackett P, Rennie D: High-altitude pulmonary edema. JAMA 287:2275, 2002.
214. Sartori C, Allemann Y, Duplain H, et al: Salmeterol for the prevention of high-altitude pulmonary edema. N Engl J Med 346:1631, 2002.
215. Scherrer U, Vollenweider L, Delabays A, et al: Inhaled nitric oxide for high-altitude pulmonary edema. N Engl J Med 334:624, 1996.
216. Ayus JC, Varon J, Arieff AI: Hyponatremia, cerebral edema, and noncardiogenic pulmonary edema in marathon runners. Ann Intern Med 132:711, 2000.
217. Fontes RB, Aguiar PH, Zanetti MV, et al: Acute neurogenic pulmonary edema: Case reports and literature review. J Neurosurg Anesthesiol 15:144, 2003.
218. Smith WS, Matthay MA: Evidence for a hydrostatic mechanism in human neurogenic pulmonary edema. Chest 111:1326, 1997.
219. Hamdy O, Maekawa H, Shimada Y, et al: Role of central nervous system nitric oxide in the development of neurogenic pulmonary edema in rats. Crit Care Med 29:1222, 2001.
220. Sporer KA, Dorn E: Heroin-related noncardiogenic pulmonary edema: A case series. Chest 120:1628, 2001.
221. Sterrett C, Brownfield J, Korn CS, et al: Patterns of presentation in heroin overdose resulting in pulmonary edema. Am J Emerg Med 21:32, 2003.
222. Goldhaber SZ, Elliott CG: Acute pulmonary embolism: Part I: Epidemiology, pathophysiology, and diagnosis. Circulation 108:2726, 2003.
223. Mattar F, Sibai BM: Eclampsia. VIII. Risk factors for maternal morbidity. Am J Obstet Gynecol 182:307, 2000.
224. DiFederico EM, Burlingame JM, Kilpatrick SJ, et al: Pulmonary edema in obstetric patients is rapidly resolved except in the presence of infection or of nitroglycerin tocolysis after open fetal surgery. Am J Obstet Gynecol 179:925, 1998.
225. Gilbert WM, Towner DR, Field NT, Anthony J: The safety and utility of pulmonary artery catheterization in severe preeclampsia and eclampsia. Am J Obstet Gynecol 182:1397, 2000.
226. Desai DK, Moodley J, Naidoo DP, Bhorat I: Cardiac abnormalities in pulmonary oedema associated with hypertensive crises in pregnancy. Br J Obstet Gynaecol 103:523, 1996.
227. Upshaw CB Jr: Hemodynamic changes after cardioversion of chronic atrial fibrillation. Arch Intern Med 157:1070, 1997.
228. Arieff AI: Fatal postoperative pulmonary edema: Pathogenesis and literature review. Chest 115:1371, 1999.
229. Asimakopoulos G, Smith PL, Ratnatunga CP, Taylor KM: Lung injury and acute respiratory distress syndrome after cardiopulmonary bypass. Ann Thorac Surg 68:1107, 1999.
230. Nathoe HM, van Dijk D, Jansen EW, et al: A comparison of on-pump and off-pump coronary bypass surgery in low-risk patients. N Engl J Med 348:394, 2003.
231. Kopko PM, Marshall CS, MacKenzie MR, et al: Transfusion-related acute lung injury: Report of a clinical look-back investigation. JAMA 287:1968, 2002.
232. Duchin JS, Koster FT, Peters CJ, et al: Hantavirus pulmonary syndrome: A clinical description of 17 patients with a newly recognized disease. The Hantavirus Study Group. N Engl J Med 330:949, 1994.
233. Peters CJ, Khan AS: Hantavirus pulmonary syndrome: The new American hemorrhagic fever. Clin Infect Dis 34:1224, 2002.
234. Ho M, Chen ER, Hsu KH, et al: An epidemic of enterovirus 71 infection in Taiwan. Taiwan Enterovirus Epidemic Working Group. N Engl J Med 341:929, 1999.
235. Lee N, Hui D, Wu A, et al: A major outbreak of severe acute respiratory syndrome in Hong Kong. N Engl J Med 348:1986, 2003.
236. Ksiazek TG, Erdman D, Goldsmith CS, et al: A novel coronavirus associated with severe acute respiratory syndrome. N Engl J Med 348:1947, 2003.

High-Output Heart Failure

237. Anand IS, Chandrashekhar Y, Wander GS, Chawla LS: Endothelium-derived relaxing factor is important in mediating the high output state in chronic severe anemia. J Am Coll Cardiol 25:1402, 1995.
238. Anand IS, Chandrashekhar Y, Ferrari R, et al: Pathogenesis of oedema in chronic severe anaemia: Studies of body water and sodium, renal function, haemodynamic variables, and plasma hormones. Br Heart J 70:357, 1993.
239. Willenbrock R, Scheuermann M, Thibault G, et al: Angiotensin inhibition and atrial natriuretic peptide release after acute volume expansion in rats with aortocaval shunt. Cardiovasc Res 42:733, 1999.
240. Aessopos A, Farmakis D, Karagiorga M, et al: Cardiac involvement in thalassemia intermedia: A multicenter study. Blood 97:3411, 2001.
241. Wattanasirichaigoon S, Pomposelli FB Jr: Branham's sign is an exaggerated Bezold-Jarisch reflex of arteriovenous fistula. J Vasc Surg 26:171, 1997.

242. Ilijevski N, Radak D, Radevic B, et al: Popliteal traumatic arteriovenous fistulas. J Trauma 52:739, 2002.
243. Thalhammer C, Kirchherr AS, Uhlich F, et al: Postcatheterization pseudoaneurysms and arteriovenous fistulas: Repair with percutaneous implantation of endovascular covered stents. Radiology 214:127, 2000.
244. Nasser TK, Mohler ER III, Wilensky RL, Hathaway DR: Peripheral vascular complications following coronary interventional procedures. Clin Cardiol 18:609, 1995.
245. Toursarkissian B, Allen BT, Petrinec D, et al: Spontaneous closure of selected iatrogenic pseudoaneurysms and arteriovenous fistulae. J Vasc Surg 25:803, 1997.
246. Waigand J, Uhlich F, Gross CM, et al: Percutaneous treatment of pseudoaneurysms and arteriovenous fistulas after invasive vascular procedures. Catheter Cardiovasc Interv 47:157, 1999.
247. Davidovic LB, Kostic DM, Cvetkovic SD, et al: Aorto-caval fistulas. Cardiovasc Surg 10:555, 2002.
248. Sigler L, Gutierrez-Carreno R, Martinez-Lopez C, et al: Aortocava fistula: Experience with five patients. Vasc Surg 35:207, 2001.
249. Korn TS, Thurston JM, Sherry CS, Kawalsky DL: High-output heart failure due to a renal arteriovenous fistula in a pregnant woman with suspected preeclampsia. Mayo Clin Proc 73:888, 1998.
250. Young PR Jr, Rohr MS, Marterre WF Jr: High-output cardiac failure secondary to a brachiocephalic arteriovenous hemodialysis fistula: Two cases. Am Surg 64:239, 1998.
251. Ori Y, Korzets A, Katz M, et al: Haemodialysis arteriovenous access—A prospective haemodynamic evaluation. Nephrol Dial Transplant 11:94, 1996.
252. McCarthy RE, Lytle JO, Van Devanter S: The use of total circulatory arrest in the surgery of giant hemangioma and Klippel-Trenaunay syndrome in neonates. Clin Orthop (289):237, 1993.
253. Pollak Y, Katzen BT, Pollak W: High-output congestive failure in a patient with pulmonary arteriovenous malformations. Cardiol Rev 10:188, 2002.
254. Hisamatsu K, Ueeda M, Ando M, et al: Peripheral arterial coil embolization for hepatic arteriovenous malformation in Osler-Weber-Rendu disease; useful for controlling high output heart failure, but harmful to the liver. Intern Med 38:962, 1999.
255. Daller JA, Bueno J, Gutierrez J, et al: Hepatic hemangioendothelioma: Clinical experience and management strategy. J Pediatr Surg 34:98, 1999.
256. Kahaly GJ, Kampmann C, Mohr-Kahaly S. Cardiovascular hemodynamics and exercise tolerance in thyroid disease. Thyroid 12:473, 2002.
257. Biondi B, Palmieri EA, Lombardi G, Fazio S: Effects of subclinical thyroid dysfunction on the heart. Ann Intern Med 137:904, 2002.
258. Shimizu T, Koide S, Noh JY, et al: Hyperthyroidism and the management of atrial fibrillation. Thyroid 12:489, 2002.
259. Kahaly GJ, Nieswandt J, Mohr-Kahaly S: Cardiac risks of hyperthyroidism in the elderly. Thyroid 8:1165, 1998.
260. Krahn AD, Klein GJ, Kerr CR, et al: How useful is thyroid function testing in patients with recent-onset atrial fibrillation? The Canadian Registry of Atrial Fibrillation Investigators. Arch Intern Med 156:2221, 1996.
261. Witte KK, Clark AL, Cleland JG: Chronic heart failure and micronutrients. J Am Coll Cardiol 37:1765, 2001.
262. Blanc P, Boussuges A: Cardiac beriberi. Arch Mal Coeur Vaiss 93:371, 2000.
263. Kawai C, Wakabayashi A, Matsumura T, Yui Y: Reappearance of beriberi heart disease in Japan. A study of 23 cases. Am J Med 69:383, 1980.
264. Chen KT, Chiou ST, Chang YC, et al: Cardiac beriberi among illegal mainland Chinese immigrants. J Int Med Res 29:37, 2001.
265. Kitamura K, Yamaguchi T, Tanaka H, et al: TPN-induced fulminant beriberi: A report on our experience and a review of the literature. Surg Today 26:769, 1996.
266. Gabrielli A, Caruso L, Stacpoole PW: Early recognition of acute cardiovascular beriberi by interpretation of hemodynamics. J Clin Anesth 13:230, 2001.
267. Shivalkar B, Engelmann I, Carp L, et al: Shoshin syndrome: Two case reports representing opposite ends of the same disease spectrum. Acta Cardiol 53:195, 1998.
268. Reddy SV, Kurihara N, Menaa C, Roodman GD: Paget's disease of bone: A disease of the osteoclast. Rev Endocr Metab Disord 2:195, 2001.
269. Lyles KW, Siris ES, Singer FR, Meunier PJ: A clinical approach to diagnosis and management of Paget's disease of bone. J Bone Miner Res 16:1379, 2001.
270. Hultgren HN: Osteitis deformans (Paget's disease) and calcific disease of the heart valves. Am J Cardiol 81:1461, 1998.
271. Roux C, Dougados M: Treatment of patients with Paget's disease of bone. Drugs 58:823, 1999.
272. Krane SM, Shiller AL: Paget's disease and other dysplasias of bone. *In* Braunwald E, Fauci AS, Kasper DL, et al (eds): Harrison's Principles of Internal Medicine. New York, McGraw-Hill, 2001, pp 2237-2245.
273. Inanir S, Haznedar R, Atavci S, Unlu M: Arteriovenous shunting in patients with multiple myeloma and high-output failure. J Nucl Med 39:1, 1998.
274. Kuribayashi N, Matsuzaki H, Hata H, et al: Multiple myeloma associated with serum amino acid disturbance and high output cardiac failure. Am J Hematol 57:77, 1998.
275. McBride W, Jackman JD Jr, Grayburn PA: Prevalence and clinical characteristics of a high cardiac output state in patients with multiple myeloma. Am J Med 89:21, 1990.
276. Yun D, Heywood JT: Metastatic carcinoid disease presenting solely as high-output heart failure. Ann Intern Med 120:45, 1994.
277. Damjanovic SS, Neskovic AN, Petakov MS, et al: High output heart failure in patients with newly diagnosed acromegaly. Am J Med 112:610, 2002.
278. Alpert MA, Terry BE, Mulekar M, et al: Cardiac morphology and left ventricular function in normotensive morbidly obese patients with and without congestive heart failure, and effect of weight loss. Am J Cardiol 80:736, 1997.

CHAPTER 23

Drugs in the Treatment of Heart Failure

Michael R. Bristow • Stuart Linas • J. David Port

Pharmacological therapy for heart failure (HF) is divided into two distinct settings and approaches: treatment of *decompensated HF* and treatment of *chronic stable HF* (Table 23–1). The goals of these two types of treatment are different, and part of the challenge of treating individual patients with HF is the art of converting patients in the former category to the latter. In the treatment of patients with decompensated HF, the goals are to stabilize the patient, restore organ perfusion, return filling pressure to optimal levels, and begin the conversion to chronic therapy. In contrast, the goals of treatment of patients with chronic stable HF are to enhance survival, minimize symptoms and disability, improve functional capacity, and delay disease progression. As discussed here, diuretics, vasodilators, and positive inotropic agents are used to minimize symptoms and improve functional capacity, and neurohormonal inhibitors are used primarily to enhance survival and delay disease progression.

Diuretics

The importance of diuretics in the treatment of HF is related to the central role of the kidney as the target organ of many of the neurohumoral and hemodynamic changes that occur in response to a failing heart.[1–4] The net effect of these physiological responses is an increase in salt and water retention, which results in expansion of the extracellular fluid volume. This effect is highlighted in Figure 23–1, where the adrenergic system and the renin-angiotensin-aldosterone system (RAAS), two important compensatory neurohormonal mechanisms that are activated in concert early in the course of HF, produce volume expansion. In the case of adrenergic mechanisms, volume expansion may occur through adrenergic receptor (alpha and beta)[5]-mediated nonosmotic release or beta receptor-mediated increase in gene expression of vasopressin. For RAAS mechanisms, volume expansion occurs through angiotensin II-mediated increases in aldosterone and vasopressin secretion and stimulation of thirst.[5] In the short term, volume expansion serves to sustain cardiac output and tissue perfusion by allowing the heart to operate higher on its ventricular function (Frank-Starling) curve (Fig. 23–2). However, these physiological adaptations also result in higher end-diastolic filling pressure and increased wall stress in diastole and systole, which contributes to hypertrophy and remodeling (see Chap. 21) and may cause dyspnea or even pulmonary edema.

With the exception of the aldosterone antagonists, diuretics do not influence the natural history of chronic HF. However, diuretics improve congestive symptoms and may also slow the progression of ventricular remodeling by reducing ventricular filling pressure and wall stress. The acute effect of diuretics in patients with HF-related volume overload is to decrease left ventricular (LV) filling pressure without much change in cardiac output because of the depressed and flat Frank-Starling curve in these subjects as depicted in Figure 23–2. However, it should also be emphasized that in situations of very high filling pressures diuretics can actually increase organ perfusion, because decreasing markedly elevated venous pressures can increase flow across capillary beds.

Renal Adaptation to Heart Failure (see also Chap. 86)

Increased salt and water retention by the kidney is due primarily to characteristic alterations in intrarenal hemodynamics that occur in response to decreased cardiac output. In addition, salt and water retention activates the adrenergic nervous system and several hormonal and cytokine systems (see Chap. 21). A decrease in cardiac output results in increased peripheral and intrarenal vascular resistance, activation of intrarenal and other tissue vasoconstrictor systems such as angiotensin II and endothelin-1, and release of vasopressin from the posterior pituitary gland. Angiotensin II-mediated increased adrenal cortical activity promote aldosterone synthesis and release, and increased intraatrial and intraventricular pressure promote the production and secretion of atrial natriuretic peptide (ANP) and brain natriuretic peptide (BNP) in cardiac muscle.

INTRARENAL HEMODYNAMICS IN HEART FAILURE. The changes in intrarenal hemodynamics that occur early in the course of HF result in preservation of the glomerular filtration rate (GFR) despite a decline in cardiac output and renal blood flow.[1–4] Although increases in adrenergic activity and local release of angiotensin II act to increase resistance in both the afferent and efferent glomerular arterioles, preservation of the GFR is due in large part to a greater increase in efferent than in afferent arteriolar tone. Pressure differences across the glomerulus (P_{GC}) and across the glomerular capillary membrane and Bowman's space (P_t) are two major determinants of single-nephron GFR. The other main determinants of single-nephron GFR are the glomerular membrane ultrafiltration coefficient (K_f), which tends to decline in HF, and differences between glomerular capillary and proximal tubular colloid osmotic pressure, which are usually unchanged in HF.

NEUROHORMONAL ACTIVATION. In addition to hemodynamic changes in the proximal nephron, increased renal sympathetic nerve activity activates the intrarenal renin-angiotensin system (RAS) and has direct tubular effects that result in augmented salt retention along the nephron.[2] Activation of a local endothelin-1 generating system also occurs.[6]

TABLE 23–1 Classes of Drugs (Noninvestigational Agents Only) Used to Treat Heart Failure

Drug Class	Use
Diuretics	
"Loop" diuretics ($Na^+/K^+/2Cl^-$ cotransporter inhibitors)	DHF (IV); CSHF (PO) stage 2-4*
Thiazides (Na^+/Cl^- cotransporter inhibitors)	DHF (IV); CSHF (PO) stage 2-4
K^+ sparing (epithelial Na^+ channel inhibitors)	CSHF (PO) stage 2-4
Type I (mineralocorticoid) receptor antagonists	CSHF (PO) stage 3, 4
Carbonic anhydrase inhibitors (acetazolamide)	DHF (IV)
Vasodilators	
Nitrovasodilators	DHF (IV); CSHF (PO) stage 2-4
"Direct-acting" or unknown mechanism vasodilators	DHF (IV); CSHF (PO) stage 2-4
Calcium channel blockers (vasoselective agents only)	Angina or persistent HTN in setting of HF DHF (IV)
Natriuretic peptides (nesiritide)	
Positive Inotropic Agents	
Digitalis derivatives	CSHF (PO), stage 2-4
Beta-adrenergic receptor agonists	DHF (IV), stage 4
Phosphodiesterase inhibitors	DHF (IV)
Phosphodiesterase inhibitors with calcium sensitizer action	DHF (IV)
Neurohormonal Inhibitors	
Angiotensin-converting enzyme inhibitors (ACEIs)	CSHF (PO) stage 1-4
Angiotensin receptor blockers (ARBs)	CSHF (PO) stage 2, 3
Beta-adrenergic receptor blocking compounds	CSHF (PO) stage 2, 3

CSHF = chronic stable heart failure; DHF = decompensated heart failure; HTN = hypertension.

*For definitions of the stages of heart failure, see Table 24–3.

As a result of renal vasoconstrictor influences, renal blood flow is directed away from superficial cortical nephrons to the more efficient solute-resorbing juxtamedullary nephrons. These nephrons rely on the high capacity of the ion transport carriers in the loop of Henle and the countercurrent mechanism of the medulla to allow the formation of concentrated urine. Elevated arginine vasopressin (AVP) levels cause further reductions in free water clearance by the kidney. This reduced clearance of free water, coupled with the increased thirst of many patients with advanced HF (perhaps caused by higher intracerebral angiotensin II levels), often leads to a hypotonic edematous state. As with other complex biological systems, countervailing intrarenal and humoral responses also occur, including increased prostaglandin E_2 and prostacyclin levels within the kidney and the release of humoral natriuretic factors, including ANP and BNP.[1,4]

Mechanisms of Action of Diuretics

By definition, a diuretic is any drug that increases urine flow. However, the term "diuretic" is commonly used to refer to agents that enhance the delivery of sodium chloride, other small ions, and water into urine. In this context, agents such as cardiac glycosides and dopamine may indirectly increase urine production by enhancing renal blood flow and the GFR, which promotes a fall in the glomerular filtration fraction and thereby diminishes water and solute resorption by the proximal tubule. Furthermore, endogenous substances such as ANP or BNP, when administered as drugs, may have salutary effects on cardiovascular function as well as on intrarenal hemodynamics and tubular sodium resorption.

Most diuretics, however, act directly on the kidney to inhibit solute and water reabsorption. A number of classification schemes for diuretics have been proposed on the basis of their mechanism of action, their anatomical locus of action within the nephron, and the form of diuresis that they elicit. Diuretics can be classified according to whether they induce a "solute" or "water" diuresis. Of the latter ("aquaretics"), only three agents are of clinical relevance: demeclocycline, lithium, and vasopressin V_2 receptor antagonists, each of which, by different mechanisms, inhibits the action of AVP on the collecting duct, thereby increasing free water clearance. Drugs that cause solute diuresis are subdivided into two types: osmotic diuretics, which are nonresorbable solutes that osmotically retain water and other solutes in the tubular lumen, and drugs that selectively inhibit ion transport pathways across tubular epithelia, which constitute the majority of potent, clinically useful diuretics.

Now that many of the specific ion transport proteins that are the molecular targets for diuretics have been cloned and their intrarenal distribution characterized, a new classification of these drugs on the basis of their molecular pharmacology has been advocated. However, a more traditional and familiar scheme of classification, employing a combination of chemical (e.g., "thiazide" diuretic), site of action (e.g., "loop" diuretics), or clinical outcome (e.g., "potassium-sparing" diuretics), is used throughout this chapter. The sites of action of commonly used diuretics and those in clinical development are given in Table 23–2.

Classes of Diuretics

Classes of diuretics and individual class members are listed in Table 23–2, and their renal sites of action are depicted in Figure 23–3.

Loop Diuretics

The agents traditionally classified as loop or high-ceiling diuretics, including furosemide, bumetanide, and torsemide, have been known for more than a decade to inhibit reversibly the $Na^+/K^+/2Cl^-$ symporter (cotransporter) when applied to the luminal but not the basolateral membranes of epithelial cells of the thick ascending limb of the loop of Henle (Fig. 23–3; see Table 23–2). Agents in a second functional class of these drugs, typified by ethacrynic acid, are also effective only from the tubular lumen but exhibit a slower onset of action and delayed and only partial reversibility. Individual agents that act as $Na^+/K^+/2Cl^-$ cotransporter inhibitors[7] are listed in Table 23–2.

MECHANISMS OF ACTION. The molecular targets of these drugs have been cloned and sequenced and were found to encompass a family of cation chloride symporters that have now been described in a number of cell types and tissues.[7] Inhibition of this cotransporter results in a marked increase in the fractional excretion of Na^+ and Cl^- and indirectly results in the fractional excretion of Ca^{2+} and Mg^{2+}. By inhibiting the concentration of solute within the medullary interstitium, these drugs also reduce the driving force for water resorption in the collecting duct, regardless of the presence of AVP; the decreased resorption of water in turn results in the production of urine that is nearly isotonic with plasma at the height of the diuresis. The delivery of large amounts of Na^+ and fluid to the distal nephron increases both K^+ and H^+ secretion, a process that is accelerated by aldosterone and that results in hypokalemia and metabolic alkalosis.

HEMODYNAMIC EFFECTS. Loop diuretics also exhibit several characteristic effects on intracardiac pressure and systemic hemodynamics. An increase in venous capacitance and lowering of pulmonary capillary wedge pressure within minutes of a bolus infusion of intravenous furosemide (0.5 to 1.0 mg/kg) have been well documented in patients with congestive symptoms following acute myocardial infarction or in those with valvular heart disease.[8] Some increase in pulmonary venous compliance probably occurs as well. Similar data, although not as extensive, have accumulated for bumetanide and torsemide.[9] Despite the fall in LV end-diastolic filling pressure, systemic vascular resistance often increases acutely in response to loop diuretics, an effect that has been attributed to transient activation of the systemic or intravascular RAS. The net effect of these actions on cardiac function may contribute to some improvement in HF symptoms. However, the potentially deleterious rise in LV afterload reinforces the importance of initiating vasodilator therapy with diuretics in patients with acute pulmonary edema and adequate blood pressure.

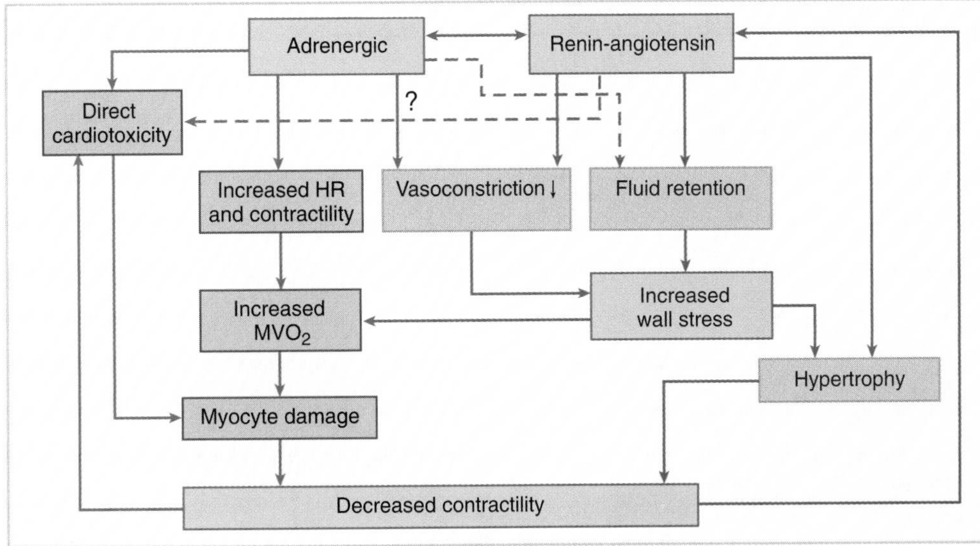

FIGURE 23–1 Hemodynamic and biological consequences of coordinated activation of the adrenergic and renin-angiotensin systems in heart failure. HR = heart rate; MVO_2 = myocardial oxygen consumption. Solid lines = established mechanisms.

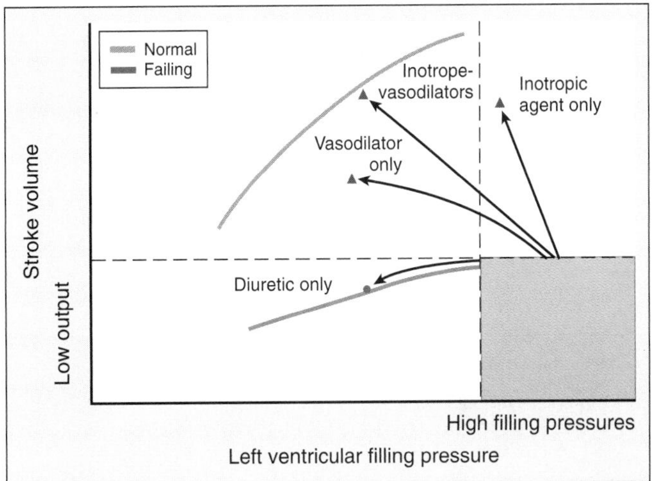

FIGURE 23–2 Frank-Starling relationship for ventricular function in heart failure. In patients with heart failure, the normal relationship between cardiac output (y-axis) and filling pressure (x-axis) is shifted lower and to the right such that a low-output state and congestive symptoms may be coincident. At one extreme, the addition of a pure inotropic agent, such as digoxin, primarily increases stroke volume with minimal impact on filling pressure. Conversely, the addition of a diuretic primarily decreases filling pressure without having an impact on cardiac output. Clinically, it is common to use multiple classes of agents, or agents with combined effects, to produce both increased cardiac output and decreased filling pressure. (Adapted from Cohn JN, Franciosa JA: Vasodilator therapy of cardiac failure [first of two parts]. N Engl J Med 297:27, 1977.)

All the rapid hemodynamic actions of loop diuretics are attenuated in patients with chronic HF. Although most of these effects have been attributed in the past to activation of the RAS by the kidney in response to loop diuretics, with subsequent release of renal and intravascular prostaglandins, more recent evidence indicates that these drugs have direct effects on endothelial cells and vascular smooth muscle. In in vitro experiments, furosemide stimulated the release of prostacyclin and nitric oxide by increasing the release of vasoactive kinins, presumably after inhibition of $Na^+/K^+/2Cl^-$ cotransporter function in endothelial cells in vitro.[10] Furosemide has also been shown to relax precontracted pulmonary venous rings by a direct effect on smooth muscle that was dependent on inhibition of vascular smooth muscle $Na^+/K^+/2Cl^-$ cotransporter function in these cells.[11]

Thiazide and Thiazide-Like Diuretics

This class of diuretic, of which chlorothiazide is the prototype, includes the first effective orally bioavailable diuretics with acceptable safety profiles to become widely used in clinical practice, supplementing the much more toxic mercurial diuretics of the 1950s. A number of these agents are available for clinical use in the United States (Table 23–2). Although not all are technically benzothiadiazine derivatives, they are often collectively referred to as "thiazide" diuretics. The site of action of these drugs within the distal convoluted tubule has been identified at a molecular level as being the Na^+/Cl^- cotransporter of the distal convoluted tubule. This cotransporter has 12 membrane-spanning domains and shares 60 percent amino acid homology with the $Na^+/K^+/2Cl^-$ cotransporter of the ascending limb of the loop of Henle; however, it is insensitive to the effects of furosemide. This cotransporter (or related isoforms) is also present on cells within the vasculature and many cell types within other organs and tissues and may contribute to some of the other actions of these agents, such as their utility as antihypertensive agents.

By blocking solute uptake in the distal convoluted tube, Na^+/Cl^- cotransporter inhibitors prevent maximal dilution of urine, decrease the kidney's ability to increase free water clearance, and may contribute to the development of hyponatremia. Thiazides increase Ca^{2+} resorption in the distal nephron (Fig. 23–3) by several mechanisms, occasionally resulting in a small increase in serum Ca^{2+} levels. In contrast, Mg^{2+} resorption is diminished and hypomagnesemia may occur with prolonged use. Increased delivery of NaCl and fluid into the collecting duct directly enhances K^+ and H^+

TABLE 23–2 Diuretic Classes Used in the Treatment of Chronic Heart Failure

Diuretic	Brand Name	Principal Site and Mechanism of Action	Effects on Urinary Electrolytes	Effects on Blood Electrolytes and Acid-Base Balance	Extrarenal Effects	Usual Dosage*	Drug Interactions
Loop Diuretics ($Na^+/K^+/2Cl^-$/ Cotransporter Inhibitors)							
Furosemide	Lasix	Thick ascending limb of the loop of Henle; inhibition of the $Na^+/K^+/2Cl^-$ cotransporter	↑Na^+ ↑Cl^- ↑K^+	Hypochloremic alkalosis ↑HCO_3^- ↓K^+, ↓Na^+ ↓Cl^- ↑Uric acid	Acute: ↑venous capacitance ↑Systemic vascular resistance when given IV, secondary to neurohormonal activation Chronic: ↓cardiac preload, ototoxicity	10-360 mg/d	Tubular secretion delayed by competing organic acids (renal failure) and some drugs Effectiveness reduced by prostaglandin inhibitors Additive ototoxicity with aminoglycosides Longer duration of action that furosemide
Bumetanide	Bumex					0.5-20 mg/d	
Piretanide[†]	Arelix, Diumax, Tauliz					6-20 mg/d	
Ethacrynic acid	Edecrin					50-200 mg/d	
Torsemide	Demadex					2.5-200 mg/d	
Thiazide and Thiazide-like Diuretics (Na^+/Cl^- Cotransporter Inhibitors)							
Chlorothiazide	Diuril	Distal tubule: inhibits Na^+/Cl^- cotransporter	↑Na^+, ↑Cl^-, ↑K^+ ↑Mg^{2+}, ↓Ca^{2+}	↓Na^+, particularly in elderly patients ↓Cl^-, ↑HCO_3^- (mild alkalosis) ↑Uric acid, ↑Ca^{2+} ↓K^+, ↓Mg^{2+}	↑Glucose ↑LDL/triglycerides (may be dose related) Extrarenal effects less marked with indapamide	50-100 mg/d	Efficacy reduced by prostaglandin inhibitors Reduces renal lithium clearance Additive effect on NaCl and K^+ excretion with loop diuretics
Hydroclorothiazide	HydroDIURIL					25-50 mg/d	
Trichlormethiazide	Metahydrin					2-8 mg/d	
Chlorthalidone	Hygroton					25-100 mg/d	
Metolazone	Mykrox, Zaroxolyn					0.5-10 mg/d 5-10 mg/d	
Quinethazone	Hydromox					50-100 mg/d	
Indapamide	Lozol					2.5-5 mg/d	
K^+-Sparing Diuretics (Epithelial Na^+ Channel Inhibitors)							
Triamterene	Dyrenium	Collecting duct; inhibits apical membrane Na^+ conductance	↓K^+ ↑Na^+	Metabolic acidosis ↑Mg^{2+}		100-300 mg/d	Useful when used with K^+ wasting diuretics; may induce hyperkalemia with ACE inhibitors/ARBs
Amiloride	Midamor					5-10 mg/d	
Type I Mineralocorticoid Receptor Antagonists (also K^+-Sparing Diuretics)							
Spironolactone	Aldactone	Collecting duct: aldosterone antagonists	↓K^+, ↑Na^+, ↑Cl^-	↑K^+, metabolic acidosis	Gynecomastia for spironolactone, not for eplerenone	12.5-25 mg/d	Useful adjunct to K^+ wasting diuretics; ↑K^+ may be worse in presence of other RAAS inhibitors
Eplerenone	Inspra					25-50 mg/d	
Carbonic Anhydrase Inhibitors							
Acetazolamide	Diamox	Proximal tubule Carbonic anhydrase inhibition	↑Na^+, ↑K^+, ↑HCO_3^-	Metabolic acidosis	↑Ventilatory drive ↓Intraocular pressure	250-500 mg/d	May be useful in alkalemia related to other diuretics; may cause severe K^+ wasting
Dichlorphenamide	Doranide					10-20 mg/d	
Methazolamide	Neptazane					25-100 mg/d	
Vasopressin Antagonists							
Tolvaptan (V_2 RA)[†]	TBD	Collecting duct, inhibits recruitment of aquaporin H_2O channels	↓Na^+, ↑free H_2O	Hypernatremia, ↑ osmolarity	?	TBD	May cause diabetes insipidus
Lixivaptan (V_2 RA)[†]							
Conivaptan (V_1/V_2 RA)[†]							

ACE = angiotensin-converting enzyme; ARB = angiotensin receptor blocker; LDL = low-density lipoprotein; RA = receptor antagonist; TBD = to be determined; RAAS = renin-angiotensin-aldosterone system.

*Dosages are approximate (PO).

[†]Not yet approved in the United States.

secretion by this segment of the nephron and may lead to clinically important hypokalemia.

Potassium-Sparing Diuretics

The apical (luminal) membranes of the principal cells of the late distal convoluted tubule and the cortical collecting duct contain Na^+-selective channels that permit Na^+ entry from within the tubular lumen, driven by the electrochemical gradient established by Na^+,K^+-adenosine triphosphatase (ATPase) in the basolateral membranes of these cells (Fig. 23–3).[12] The number of epithelial Na^+ channels available for entry into tubular epithelial membranes is regulated in part by mineralocorticoid levels. The activity (conductance) of these Na^+ channels appears to be regulated by both protein kinase A-mediated phosphorylation and guanosine triphosphate (GTP) binding proteins (i.e., $G_{\alpha i}$). Na^+ conductance by these channels is inhibited by *amiloride* and by *triamterene* (Table 23–2), which subsequently diminishes the electrochemical potential for K^+ secretion into the urine. Thus, these agents, along with mineralocorticoid inhibitors (see later), are commonly referred to as "potassium-sparing" diuretics.

Because Na^+ retention in HF occurs in more proximal nephron sites, neither amiloride nor triamterene is effective in achieving a net negative Na^+ balance when given alone. Amiloride and its congeners also inhibit Na^+/H^+ antiporters in renal epithelial cells and in many other cell types, but only at concentrations that are higher than those used clinically. Both amiloride and triamterene affect cardiac repolarization, possibly by inhibiting delayed rectifier K^+ currents (I_K), and may exaggerate the prolonged repolarization observed with Na^+ channel blocker antiarrhythmics (e.g., quinidine).[13,14]

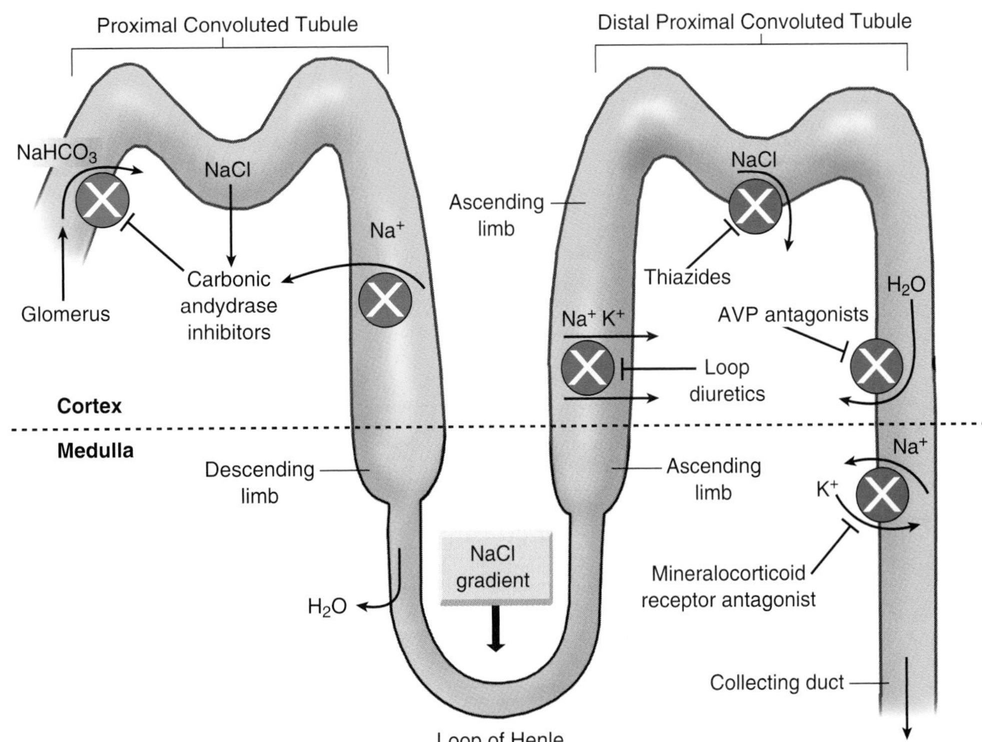

FIGURE 23–3 Sites of action of diuretics in the kidney. AVP = arginine vasopressin.

Aldosterone Type I or Mineralocorticoid Receptor Antagonists

Spironolactone (see Table 23–2) and its active metabolites canrenone and potassium canrenoate have been known for more than two decades to inhibit competitively the binding of aldosterone to mineralocorticoid or type I receptors in many tissues, including epithelial cells of the distal convoluted tubule and collecting duct. These cytosolic receptors are members of a "superfamily" of cytosolic proteins that are ligand-dependent transcription factors, which upon ligand binding translocate to the cell nucleus, where they bind to specific DNA sequences and regulate the transcription and synthesis of a number of gene products, including apical membrane Na^+ channels, H^+,K^+-ATPase, and Na^+,K^+-ATPase, among others.[15] The spironolactone-bound type I receptor complex is inactive and prevents Na^+ resorption as well as K^+ and H^+ secretion by this portion of the nephron, particularly in patients with high plasma aldosterone levels, as in HF.[16] Hyperkalemia and metabolic acidosis may result from the use of these drugs. The molecular pharmacology of steroid receptors is complex and relatively poorly understood. Endogenous glucocorticoids appear to be the principal ligand for the type I "mineralocorticoid" receptor in most cell types,[17] but in the cortical collecting tubule, the enzyme 11β-hydroxysteroid dehydrogenase protects the receptor from contact with high circulating levels of glucocorticoids so that aldosterone binding is facilitated. As discussed in Chapter 24, and shown in Table 23–7, spironolactone reduces mortality in patients with Class III and IV (stage 3) HF when administered on a background of angiotensin-converting enzyme (ACE) inhibition.[18] However, spironolactone or its metabolites, or both, have antiandrogenic and progestational activities, which may cause side effects that include gynecomastia or impotence in men and menstrual irregularities in women.

Eplerenone is another competitive inhibitor of the mineralocorticoid receptor. It was developed by replacing the 17α-thioacetyl group of spironolactone with a carbomethoxy group.[19] Because of this modification, eplerenone has greater selectivity for the mineralocorticoid receptor than for steroid receptors.[20] The sex hormone side effects associated with spironolactone are not observed with eplerenone.[21] Eplerenone has been shown to lower mortality when administered after myocardial infarction in patients with LV dysfunction when added to background therapy of ACE inhibition and beta blockers (Fig. 23–4).[21] Eplerenone is also an effective antihypertensive agent and produces regression of LV hypertrophy that is additive with ACE inhibitors (ACEIs).[22]

VASOPRESSIN ANTAGONISTS

Increased levels of circulating vasopressin (AVP, antidiuretic hormone) contribute to the increased systemic vascular resistance and positive solute and water balance in patients with advanced HF.[23] Physiologically, the primary site of action of vasopressin is the renal collecting duct (see Fig. 23–3), where it acts to increase water permeability (see later); however, it is clear that vasopressin has a number of nonrenal effects on the cardiovascular and central nervous system and on blood coagulation.

VASOPRESSIN RECEPTORS. These have been divided into V_1 and V_2 receptor subtypes, which exhibit different ligand-binding specificities. V_{1a} (vascular/hepatic/myocardial) and V_{1b} (pituitary) receptors, like angiotensin II (AT_1) and alpha$_1$-adrenergic receptors, are coupled through the $G_{\alpha q}$ subtype of G proteins to activation of phospholipase C in the plasma membranes of vascular smooth muscle cells and other tissues. Stimulation of V_1 receptors results in vasoconstriction, platelet activation, glycogenolysis, and adrenocorticotropic hormone release as well as stimulation of the transcription factors c-fos and c-jun, which ultimately results in cell growth. In contrast, V_2 receptors, found largely in distal nephron segments within the kidney, are coupled through stimulatory $G_{\alpha s}$ proteins to the stimulation of adenylyl cyclase activity, increased production of the second messenger cyclic adenosine monophosphate (cAMP), and activation of protein kinase A. By interrupting this phosphorylation cascade, V_2-selective receptor antagonists inhibit recruitment of aquaporin-CD water channels,[24] amiloride-sensitive Na^+ channels, and urea transporters into the apical membranes of collecting duct epithelial cells. Therefore, the ability of the collecting duct to resorb water is reduced.

The prototypical orally bioavailable nonpeptide V_2-selective antagonist is OPC-31260.[24] In general, this agent increases free water clearance, thereby increasing plasma osmolality as well as increasing the serum Na^+ concentration. A general consensus from studies in animal models with both the V_1-selective antagonist, OPC-21268,[25] and OPC-31260[26] suggests that vasopressin contributes to the development of HF more through the actions of V_2 receptor-mediated fluid retention and less so through alterations in systemic hemodynamics.[27] An analog of OPC-31260, OPC-41061 (tolvaptan),[27] is in clinical development and has shown efficacy as an aquaretic in HF.[28] Another V_2-selective antagonist, WAY-VPA-985 (lixivaptan),[29] has also shown dose-related aquaretic efficacy in HF. In addition, nonselective vasopressin antagonists such as YM087 (conivaptan)[30] have been developed. In a clinical trial in patients with HF, conivaptan, a V_{1a}/V_2 antagonist delivered intravenously, acutely reduced pulmonary wedge

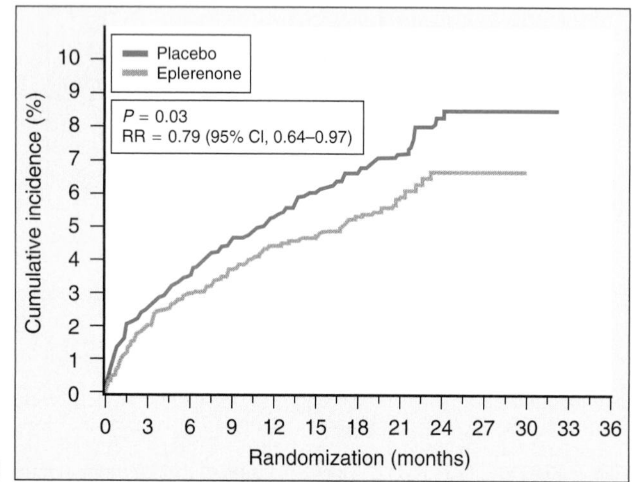

FIGURE 23–4 Kaplan-Meier estimates of the rate of death from any cause **(A)** and the rate of sudden death from cardiac causes **(B)** in the Eplerenone Post-Acute Myocardial Infarction Heart Failure Efficacy and Survival Study (EPHESUS) trial. This trial involved 6632 patients with acute myocardial infarction complicated by heart failure and left ventricular systolic dysfunction. CI = confidence interval; RR = relative risk. (Modified from Pitt B, Remme W, Zannad F, et al, Eplerenone Post-Acute Myocardial Infarction Heart Failure Efficacy and Survival Study Investigators: Eplerenone, a selective aldosterone blocker, in patients with left ventricular dysfunction after myocardial infarction. N Engl J Med 348:1309, 2003.)

and right atrial mean pressures while increasing free water excretion,[31] and this agent is undergoing additional testing in the setting of chronic HF.[32] This agent could have an advantage in long-term use in view of the fact that V_{1a} antagonism but not V_2 prevented remodeling in the infarct rat model.[33]

Although the use of these drugs (see Table 23-2) will undoubtedly present challenges in patients with HF, most of whom receive other vasodilators and natriuretic aquatic drugs and in whom vasopressin levels vary as a function of plasma osmolality and cardiac output, among other factors, vasopressin antagonists may ultimately prove to be valuable adjuncts to the treatment of HF.

CARBONIC ANHYDRASE INHIBITORS

At least two isoenzymes (types II and IV) of carbonic anhydrase are abundantly expressed in proximal tubular epithelial cells, in the luminal and basolateral membranes (see Fig. 23-3). These isoforms are inhibited by acetazolamide, whose use as a diuretic in patients with HF is confined to temporary administration to correct the metabolic alkalosis that occurs as a "contraction" phenomenon in response to the administration of other diuretics. When used repeatedly, acetazolamide (see Table 23-2) can cause metabolic acidosis as well as severe hypokalemia. The latter effect may occur in HF because increases in distal nephron HCO_3^- delivery favor K^+ secretion when aldosterone levels are elevated.

Diuretic Resistance and Management

Loop diuretics are the only class of diuretics that are effective as single agents in moderate and advanced HF. The rationale for this assumption was the magnitude of their maximal ("ceiling") natriuretic effect and the fact that the natriuretic effect of more distally acting drugs may be limited by the increased resorption of solute and water by proximal nephron segments in individuals with HF. However, even the effectiveness of potent loop diuretics can decrease with worsening HF. Although the bioavailability of these drugs is not generally decreased in HF, the potential delay in their rate of absorption may result in peak drug levels within the tubular lumen in the ascending loop of Henle that are insufficient to induce maximal natriuresis.[34] Resorting to an intravenous formulation typically obviates this problem. However, even with intravenous dosing, a rightward shift of the dose-response curve is observed between the diuretic concentration in the tubular lumen and its natriuretic effect in HF; in addition, the maximal effect or ceiling is lower. This rightward shift has been termed "diuretic resistance" and can be due to several contributing factors. A point of distinction is that diuretic resistance should be distinguished from "diuretic adaptation" or the "braking" phenomenon that is observed even in normal subjects given multiple doses of a short-acting loop diuretic.[35]

Mechanisms

Diuretic-induced alterations in intrarenal hemodynamics, caused by tubuloglomerular feedback and increased sympathetic nerve activity, among other possible mechanisms (see later), result in avid renal sodium retention by all nephron segments as intraluminal drug levels decline. If dietary salt intake is sufficiently high, as in many Western diets, a daily net negative sodium balance may not be achieved despite several daily intravenous doses of a loop diuretic. These data imply that salt intake must be restricted in normal subjects and particularly in patients with HF to obtain a negative sodium balance. They also indicate that short-acting diuretics, particularly furosemide and bumetanide, must be administered several times per day to obtain consistent daily salt and water loss unless dietary sodium intake is severely restricted.

An alternative strategy in hospitalized patients is to administer the same daily parenteral dose of a loop diuretic by continuous intravenous infusion, which leads to sustained natriuresis because of the continuous presence of high drug levels within the tubular lumen. This approach requires the use of a constant-infusion pump but permits more precise control of the natriuretic effect achieved over time, particularly in carefully monitored patients. It also diminishes the potential for a too rapid decline in intravascular volume and hypotension as well as the risk of ototoxicity in patients given large bolus intravenous doses of a loop diuretic. A typical continuous furosemide infusion is initiated with a 20- to 40-mg intravenous loading dose as a bolus injection, followed by a continuous infusion of 5 to 10 mg/hr for a patient who had been receiving 200 mg of oral furosemide (or 100 mg of intravenous drug) per day in divided doses.

Even in normal subjects with an Na^+-restricted diet, the natriuretic effect of diuretics declines with time; that is, a rightward and downward shift is seen in the sigmoidal concentration-effect relationship as a result of the braking phenomenon. This effect is now known to be due in large part to compensatory hypertrophy of the tubular epithelium distal to the site of action of the $Na^+/K^+/2Cl^-$ cotransporter inhibitor, which increases the solute resorptive capacity of the kidney, as well as other adaptive mechanisms.[36] In this context,

Morsing and colleagues[36] demonstrated that chronic and perhaps even acute treatment with loop diuretics causes rapid (within 60 minutes) upregulation of the thiazide-sensitive Na^+/Cl^- cotransporter in the distal tubule (as measured by increased ^{3}H-metolazone binding). In addition, many patients with HF manifest some degree of renal impairment, which also shifts the diuretic concentration-effect relationship downward and to the right. Although the maximum effect expressed as the fractional excretion of sodium may be unchanged in patients with some degree of intrinsic renal disease, the absolute natriuretic effect is limited by the reduced filtered load of sodium into the remaining functional nephrons.

The cause of apparent resistance to diuretics in patients who initially achieve an acceptable natriuretic and diuretic response may be multifactorial, as indicated. In the absence of an abrupt decline in cardiac or renal function or noncompliance with either the drug regimen or dietary salt restriction, the usual reason for diuretic resistance is the concurrent administration of other drugs. In this regard, one of the biggest offending classes of agents is nonsteroidal antiinflammatory drugs (NSAIDs), which reduce renal function by decreasing the renal synthesis of vasodilator prostaglandins.[36] The same effects occur with cyclooxygenase-2 inhibitors. All NSAIDs, including aspirin, can diminish diuretic efficacy. Rarely, drugs such as probenecid or high plasma concentrations of some antibiotics may compete with the organic ion transporters in the proximal tubule responsible for the transfer of most diuretics from the recirculation into the tubular lumen.

The use of increasing doses of vasodilators, with or without a marked decline in intravascular volume as a result of concomitant diuretic therapy, is a common cause of diuretic resistance. It is often difficult to distinguish clinically between intravascular volume depletion following aggressive diuretic and vasodilator therapy and a decrease in cardiac output caused by primary HF, although a more marked decline in urea clearance than in creatinine clearance suggests intravascular volume depletion. Pulmonary arterial and venous or left atrial pressure monitoring may be required to make this distinction. In addition, all vasodilators commonly used as afterload-reducing agents in HF dilate a number of central and peripheral vascular beds. Therefore, renal blood flow may be reduced despite an increase in cardiac output, and the effectiveness of the diuretic declines. Vasodilator therapy also may lower renal perfusion pressure below that necessary to maintain normal autoregulation and glomerular filtration in patients with renal artery stenosis from atherosclerotic disease.

Management

Among the vasodilators, RAS antagonists can uniquely augment the effectiveness of diuretics by mechanisms that are independent of their ability to reduce systemic vascular resistance (see later).[38] However, by reducing efferent arteriolar tone, these drugs may also diminish diuretic effectiveness by reducing the transglomerular perfusion pressure to the point that the GFR declines abruptly. This response is most commonly observed in patients with decreased renal arterial perfusion pressure caused either by renal artery stenosis or by limited cardiac output; in these patients, high efferent arteriolar tone mediated by angiotensin II is necessary to maintain glomerular filtration. This cause of diuretic resistance is usually characterized by an abrupt rise in the serum creatinine concentration and should be distinguished from the more common, limited increases in serum creatinine levels that often accompany initiation of ACEI therapy. In addition to ACEIs, the alpha$_1$-adrenergic antagonist prazosin has been shown to have direct tubular action in reducing sodium resorption at doses below those necessary to lower arterial pressure (e.g., 0.50 mg).

With a cardiac output and mean arterial pressure adequate to sustain autoregulation of glomerular filtration, diuretic resistance can be managed by increasing the frequency of loop diuretic dosing or by switching to a continuous intravenous infusion. If this treatment is ineffective, concomitant administration of a more distally acting diuretic, usually an Na^+/Cl^- symport inhibitor (e.g., a thiazide or thiazide-like diuretic such as intravenous chlorothiazide or oral metolazone), usually results in substantial natriuresis.[39] Although effective, this diuretic combination may cause profound intravascular volume depletion, hypotension, renal potassium wasting, hyponatremia, and eventually a fall in cardiac output and GFR. Accordingly, this combination should be used cautiously and with careful monitoring of renal function and serum potassium and sodium, especially in outpatients. A mineralocorticoid receptor antagonist (e.g., spironolactone) may also increase diuretic effectiveness of more proximally acting diuretics, although patients are at increased risk for hyperkalemia if they concomitantly receive another RAAS antagonist. Despite this possibility, most subjects receiving large doses of loop diuretics or loop diuretics plus thiazides benefit from a potassium-sparing diuretic. If tolerated, spironolactone or eplerenone should be the potassium-sparing diuretics used because of their mortality-reducing effects.

In hospitalized patients, dopamine administered at doses that cause selective dopaminergic receptor stimulation may increase renal blood flow and decrease tubular solute resorption (i.e., ≤2 μg/kg/min, based on estimated lean body weight). In some subjects, a short-term infusion of nesiritide (human BNP [hBNP]) may be beneficial in improving renal hemodynamics and enhancing the effects of diuretics (see Natriuretic Peptides). In addition, selective V_1 and V_2 vasopressin receptor antagonists, once approved, may individually or in combination increase the efficacy of $Na^+/K^+/2Cl^-$ symporter inhibitors as indicated by experimental animal data and preliminary evidence in humans. Finally, mechanical circulatory support may become necessary in patients with marginal cardiac output for diuretics to be effective, particularly in patients recovering from cardiac surgery or myocarditis or as a "bridge" to transplantation. Discrete renal arterial stenoses that limit renal blood flow and systemic vasodilator therapy may be amenable to percutaneous angioplasty in patients with adequate cardiac output and diuretic resistance from marginal renal perfusion.

Electrolyte and Metabolic Disorders in Heart Failure: Complications of Diuretic Therapy

POTASSIUM HOMEOSTASIS. All of the diuretics discussed in this chapter, with the exceptions of V_2 vasopressin receptor antagonists and hBNP, affect renal K^+ handling.[39] In patients with chronic HF, both hypokalemia caused by K^+-wasting diuretics and hyperkalemia caused by K^+ supplements administered with a K^+-sparing diuretic or an RAS antagonist may contribute to morbidity and mortality. Renal K^+ losses from diuretic use can be exacerbated by the hyperaldosteronism characteristic of patients with untreated HF and by the marked increases in distal nephron Na^+ delivery that follow use of either loop or distal nephron diuretics. The level of dietary salt intake may also contribute to the extent of renal K^+ wasting with diuretics. High-salt diets increase delivery of NaCl to distal tubular K^+ secretory sites, and very low-salt diets may stimulate aldosterone-induced K^+ secretion. Extrarenal regulators of the serum K^+ concentration may also produce effects additive to renal loss of K^+. K^+ is shifted from extra- to intracellular sites after the release of epinephrine in response to stress, myocardial ischemia, pulmonary edema, or the administration of insulin. Long-term infusion of either low-molecular-weight or unfractionated heparin, conversely, reduces aldosterone synthesis and may cause hyperkalemia, particularly in patients with insulin-dependent diabetes and in patients receiving potassium replacement or potassium-sparing drugs, or both.[51] Any beta-agonist or phosphodiesterase inhibitor (PDEI) lowers potassium levels by shifting potassium into skeletal muscle through a beta$_2$-adrenergic or cAMP pathway effect.[40,41]

Despite the absence of conclusive data to determine whether routine administration of K supplements or K-sparing diuretics, or both, reduces serious morbidity or mortality in the treatment of patients with primary hypertension, it is recommended that serum K^+ be maintained between 3.5 and 5.0 mEq/liter.[42] However, for patients with HF, the recommendation is to maintain serum K^+ between 4.3 and 5.0 mEq/liter. One of the reasons for the higher serum K^+ is that subjects with HF are often being treated with agents in which the proarrhythmic effects are exacerbated by hypokalemia, including digoxin, type III antiarrhythmics, beta-agonists, or PDEIs. Because patients with chronic HF are at a much higher risk for malignant ventricular arrhythmias and sudden death than patients with hypertension, it is sound clinical practice to monitor K^+ levels frequently and maintain them well up in the normal range.

If supplementation is necessary, oral K supplements in the form of KCl extended-release tablets or liquid concentrate should be used whenever possible. Intravenous K is potentially hazardous and should be avoided except in emergencies. The routine use of "sliding scales" for intravenous K administration in hospitalized patients is also potentially dangerous and should be discouraged.

OTHER METABOLIC AND ELECTROLYTE DISTURBANCES. Diuretics may be associated with multiple other metabolic and electrolyte disturbances, including hypomagnesemia, hyponatremia, metabolic alkalosis, hyperglycemia, hyperlipidemia, and hyperuricemia.[43] None of these disturbances are limiting in the usual patient with HF. Hypomagnesemia can be caused by both loop and thiazide diuretics, but its detection (because of the poor correlation of total serum magnesium levels with either ionized levels or total-body stores) is difficult and its impact is uncertain. Magnesium replacement should be given for signs or symptoms that could be due to hypomagnesemia (arrhythmias, muscle cramps), and it can be routinely given (with uncertain benefit) to all subjects receiving large doses of diuretics or requiring large amounts of K^+ replacement.

Hyponatremia. This is usually a manifestation of advanced HF with very high degrees of activation of the vasopressin system or inadequate RAS inhibition, or both. Hyponatremia can typically be treated by more stringent water restriction or an increase in RAS inhibition. When V_2 receptor antagonists are available as diuretics, this problem will probably be eliminated.

Metabolic Alkalosis. This complication can generally be treated by increasing KCl supplementation, lowering diuretic doses, or transiently treating with acetazolamide, as discussed earlier. The small level of glucose intolerance or hyperlipidemia produced by thiazide diuretics is not usually clinically important, and blood glucose and lipids should be controlled according to standard guidelines regardless of the presence of any perceived diuretic effect. Hyperuricemia from thiazide diuretics is occasionally a problem and may precipitate gout, particularly in predisposed subjects or in the presence of renal dysfunction. If a thiazide diuretic is absolutely necessary in such patients, allopurinol can be administered to reduce uric acid synthesis.

Vasodilators

Rationale and Mechanism of Action

The rationale for the use of vasodilators grew out of experience with parenteral sympatholytic agents and nitroprusside in patients with severe HF. Cohn and Franciosa, in an influential article in 1977, reviewed the evidence and advocated the use of these drugs in decompensated HF.[44] As originally conceived, the pharmacological rationale for the use of vasodilators in HF was purely hemodynamic and based on the application of Ohm's law to blood flow: flow = $\Delta P/R$, where ΔP is the difference between arterial and venous pressure and R is resistance across the vascular bed. Because systemic vascular resistance is usually increased in HF as a result of neurohormonal activation, vasodilation of resistance vessels increases central cardiac output and flow to some organs. Figure 23–1 illustrates this point: activation of the adrenergic and RAS systems results in multiple effects that are detrimental to the natural history of HF, including vasoconstriction. The hemodynamic consequences of alterations in preload and afterload by vasodilators are shown in Figure 23–2, and the vasodilator profiles of individual agents or classes are given in Table 23–3.

TABLE 23–3 Profile of Various Vasodilator Classes for Producing Venous or Arteriolar Dilation

Class/Compound	Venodilation	Arteriolar Dilation
Nitrovasodilators	+++	+
Direct acting (hydralazine)	+	+++
Flosequinan	++	+++
Calcium channel blockers	+	+++
K^+ channel activators (e.g., diazoxide, minoxidil)	++	+++
Vasodilator prostaglandins (prostacyclin)	+++	++
Natriuretic peptides (BNP)	+++	+
ACEIs, ARBs	++	+

ACEI = angiotensin-converting enzyme inhibitor; ARB = angiotensin receptor blocker; BNP = brain natriuretic peptide.

VENTRICULAR-VASCULAR COUPLING. As described in Chapters 19 and 20, myocardial function is dependent on loading conditions. From the point of view of the ventricles, *afterload* is the force opposing contraction and *preload* is the amount of stretch applied to ventricular myocardium before contraction. Vasodilator-mediated arteriolar relaxation reduces vascular resistance, which is a major component of afterload.[44] From a biomechanical point of view, the circulatory system is defined by *ventricular-vascular coupling*.[45] The force ejecting blood from the ventricle is known as end-systolic elastance, a load-independent measure of contractility, and the force resisting ejection of blood is termed vascular elastance. When end-systolic elastance overcomes vascular elastance, blood is ejected as stroke volume. For a given end-diastolic volume, the major determinants of the size of the stroke volume are the velocity of shortening of ventricular contraction and the amount of vascular elastance.[45] For the left ventricle, systemic vascular resistance is a major component of vascular elastance.[44,45] From these relationships it is clear that stroke volume can be increased by increasing the velocity of shortening (positive inotropic effect) or by decreasing systemic vascular resistance (vasodilator effect) to overcome the abnormal respective decreases and increases in these parameters inherent in HF resulting from systolic dysfunction.

EFFECTS ON DIFFERENT VASCULAR BEDS. An important aspect of vasodilator use in chronic HF is that the potential exists to affect different types of vascular beds. The original concept of vasodilator use was based on small arteriolar dilation because this is the biggest contribution to systemic vascular resistance. However, perhaps even more important is the ability of certain classes of agents to effect venodilation of "capacitance" vessels. This effect reduces venous return by enlarging the effective blood volume reservoir and therefore reduces end-diastolic, pulmonary, and systemic venous pressures. The clinical consequence of this reduction in preload is to reduce pulmonary and hepatic congestion and, more important, diastolic wall stress. As described in Chapter 21, increased wall stress is a major signaling pathway for hypertrophy and other changes in gene expression that are important in producing the dilated cardiomyopathy phenotype of ventricular dilatation and systolic dysfunction. Because a chronically failing heart is usually operating on a flat portion of the preload-performance relationship (see Fig. 23–2), pharmacological reduction in preload does not ordinarily reduce cardiac output in that setting, but it may do so in acute situations.

Studies of vasodilators in the 1980s demonstrated that they were well tolerated and effective in improving symptoms in patients with HF. These short-term trials eventually led to the first mortality-based clinical trial in chronic HF, the Vasodilator HF Trial (V-HeFT-I).[46] V-HeFT-I was a comparison of the $alpha_1$-adrenergic receptor blocking agent prazosin, the combination of isosorbide dinitrate and hydralazine, and placebo for their effects on total mortality.[47] In this trial, prazosin was not different from placebo, but isosorbide dinitrate–hydralazine reduced mortality at 2 years by 34 percent ($p < 0.03$) but did not reduce mortality over the entire period of follow-up by the log-rank test ($p = 0.09$). On the basis of these statistically marginal results (because of a relatively underpowered sample size as opposed to an inadequate effect size), the Food and Drug Administration (FDA) has not approved the hydralazine–isosorbide dinitrate combination for the treatment of HF.

V-HeFT-I introduced the idea that the natural history of HF could be favorably influenced by medical therapy, and it also provided strong support to the vasodilator approach to treating HF. However, subsequent clinical trials with "pure" vasodilating agents (i.e., those that are not also neurohumoral inhibitors) have not demonstrated a reduction in mortality, and, in fact, the powerful vasodilators flosequinan[48] and epoprostenol[49] markedly (by respective values of 43 and 29 percent) *increased mortality* despite salutary effects on exercise tolerance in earlier, smaller studies. Therefore, vasodilation per se is not a particularly effective method for improving the natural history of chronic HF, but it is an important strategy for dealing with acute, decompensated HF.

Nitrovasodilators

Despite the fact that nitrovasodilators are among the oldest vasodilators in common clinical practice, the cellular mechanisms by which these drugs lead to the relaxation of vascular smooth muscle have only become apparent since 1990. It is now understood that these drugs mimic the activity of nitric oxide and its congeners. These autocrine and paracrine signaling autacoids are formed in endothelial and smooth muscle cells throughout the vasculature as well as in many other cell types, including cardiac muscle cells (see also Chap. 19).[50,51] Nitrogen oxides were originally identified as the bioactive factor (endothelium-derived relaxing factor [EDRF]) responsible for endothelium-dependent relaxation of blood vessels. Their primary mechanism of action in vascular smooth muscle cells is based on their ability to bind to a heme moiety in soluble guanylyl cyclase, with a subsequent increase in intracellular cyclic guanosine monophosphate. The pharmacological activity of each of the nitrovasodilators depends on their biotransformation into nitrogen oxides within the blood and vascular tissue.[50]

Organic Nitrates

The organic nitrates are powerful venodilators and mild arteriolar vasodilators and produce the most extensive epicardial coronary vasodilation of any class of vasodilator. Because of their relatively selective vasodilating effects on the epicardial coronary vasculature, organic nitrates may directly increase systolic and diastolic ventricular function by improving coronary blood flow in patients with ischemic cardiomyopathy, in addition to their activity in reducing ventricular filling pressure, wall stress, and myocardial oxygen consumption.[52] In acute myocardial infarction, however, the effect of the routine use of nitrovasodilators on mortality remains controversial.

Experience with the newer nitrovasodilators, including isosorbide mononitrate, in the treatment of HF, is limited in comparison with their use in the treatment of angina. The spectrum of activity of 5-isosorbide mononitrate would not be expected to differ from that of isosorbide dinitrate in HF. Although isosorbide mononitrate's greater bioavailability and longer elimination half-life may provide a convenient pharmacokinetic profile, only isosorbide dinitrate among the nitrate formulations has been shown to increase exercise tolerance[53] and, in combination with hydralazine, may have prolonged survival in patients with HF.[46]

Although it has never been approved for this purpose by the FDA, intravenous nitroglycerin or glyceryl trinitrate (TNG) is widely used to lower filling pressures and increase cardiac output in decompensated HF. When administered at doses ranging from 10 to 100 μg/min intravenously, TNG is effective in this regard (Fig. 23–5)[54] and in particular should be considered when there is any question of active myocardial ischemia. The main problem with longer term (>24 hours) use of organic nitrates is the development of tolerance (see Chap. 50).

Most of the data on the efficacy of intermittent versus continuous NTG have been obtained in patients with angina rather than chronic congestive HF.[55] Indeed, it is somewhat controversial whether patients with HF should be exposed to a long nitrate-free period. Nevertheless, it seems prudent to recommend nitrate-free intervals in patients receiving chronic doses of isosorbide dinitrate, which can usually be achieved by providing the last dose of isosorbide dinitrate in the early evening. In addition, there is some evidence that the simultaneous administration of hydralazine (see later) can attenuate nitrate tolerance.[56]

Nitroprusside

Intravenous nitroprusside is an effective venous and arterial vasodilator that acts to reduce both ventricular preload and afterload. Because of the fact that it is quickly metabolized to cyanide and nitric oxide, its onset of action is rapid and upward titration can usually be achieved expeditiously to produce an optimal and predictable hemodynamic effect. For these reasons, nitroprusside is commonly used in intensive care settings for the management of acutely decompensated

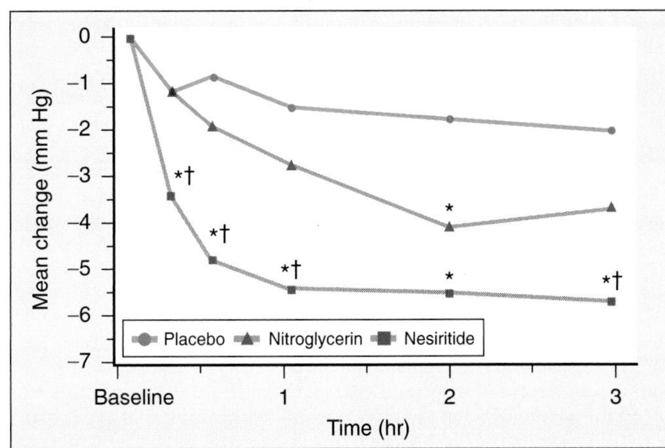

FIGURE 23–5 Changes from baseline in pulmonary capillary wedge pressure in patients in decompensated heart failure treated with placebo, nitroglycerin, or nesiritide. (From Publication Committee for the VMAC Investigators: Intravenous nesiritide vs nitroglycerin for treatment of decompensated congestive heart failure. A randomized controlled trial. JAMA 287:1531, 2002.)

HF when blood pressure is adequate to maintain cerebral, coronary, and renal perfusion. Nitroprusside has balanced effects on afterload and preload, and ventricular filling pressures are rapidly reduced by an increase in venous compliance.[57]

Nitroprusside is among the most effective afterload-reducing agents because of its spectrum of vasodilating activity on different vascular beds. It reduces systemic vascular resistance, increases aortic wall compliance, and, at optimal doses, improves ventricular-vascular coupling. Nitroprusside also decreases pulmonary vascular resistance and improves other components of right ventricular afterload, including the amplitude and timing of reflected pressure waves during ejection.[58]

Nitroprusside should not be used in active ischemia because its powerful intramyocardial afterload-reducing effects may "steal" coronary blood flow from segments of myocardium supplied by epicardial vessels with high-grade lesions. This phenomenon is probably the reason why nitroprusside increased mortality in a study of acute myocardial infarction.[59] In the setting of ischemia, any indicated vasodilator therapy should be delivered by organic nitrates, which are less powerful intramyocardial afterload-reducing agents than nitroprusside and which produce greater epicardial vasodilation.

"Directly Acting" and Other Vasodilators

HYDRALAZINE

Hydralazine, an effective afterload-reducing agent whose cellular mechanism of action remains poorly understood, is best used in chronic HF when combined with isosorbide dinitrate to provide more effective venodilation.[46] This combination produces a more balanced form of vasodilation; in addition, some evidence indicates that hydralazine can attenuate nitrate tolerance by acting as a reducing agent.[56] In HF, hydralazine reduces right and LV afterload by reducing systemic as well as pulmonary artery input impedance and vascular resistance.[60] Unlike the results when hydralazine is used to treat hypertension, the reduction in afterload is usually accompanied by only minor reflex increases in sympathetic nervous system activity, unless symptomatic hypotension occurs. These hemodynamic changes result in an increase in forward stroke volume and reductions in ventricular systolic wall stress and the regurgitant fraction in mitral or aortic regurgitation. Hydralazine's effect on regional blood flow consists of an increase in renal and skeletal muscle blood flow.[61]

One of the problems with the use of hydralazine is its short half-life, which necessitates dosing four times daily. In addition, side effects that may necessitate dose adjustment or withdrawal of hydralazine therapy are common. For example, in V-HeFT-I,[46] 20 percent of patients complained of symptoms that could have been related to hydralazine. The most common complaints—headache and dizziness—could also have been due to the concomitantly administered nitrates. However, with time, the symptoms diminish or respond to a reduction in dose.

Hydralazine metabolism is primarily through hepatic acetylation, although many additional potential metabolic pathways have been described.[62] Therefore, patients with a "slow acetylator" phenotype have a prolonged elimination half-life of the drug. At the usual doses and dosing intervals of hydralazine, these patients are at greater risk for arthritis or other components of a lupus-like syndrome.

Because of the somewhat equivocal results obtained with hydralazine-isosorbide dinitrate in V-HeFT-I[46] and the superiority of the ACEI enalapril to this combination in V-HeFT-II,[63] hydralazine-isosorbide dinitrate is reserved for subjects who cannot tolerate ACEIs or who have need for additional afterload reduction (blood pressure remaining high normal or greater in the presence of full-dose ACE inhibition). Another potential use for hydralazine-isosorbide dinitrate is in American blacks, who in V-HeFT-II had better clinical responses to the combination than to enalapril.[64] A trial evaluating the effects of combination therapy with nitrates and hydralazine in African American patients (A-HeFT) is being conducted.

Natriuretic Peptides

The contribution of the natriuretic peptides ANP, BNP, and related proteins, including urodilatin and fragments of the pro-ANP protein, to the physiological adaptations that accompany HF and their potential role in pharmacotherapy for this syndrome have been the subject of intensive research efforts by cardiovascular and renal pharmacologists for more than a decade.[65] Apart from C-type natriuretic peptide, which is synthesized in endothelial (and other) cells in a number of organs and tissues and has limited natriuretic activity, plasma levels of these peptides are increased in most patients with HF (see Chap. 21) and exhibit both vasodilator effects and a direct natriuretic effect on the kidney.[66]

The natriuretic peptides act at both particulate (i.e., membrane-bound) guanylyl cyclase–linked (GC-A and GC-B or NPR-A [natriuretic peptide receptor A] and NPR-B) receptors and so-called clearance receptors (NPR-C) that are linked through inhibitory GTP-binding proteins to adenylyl cyclase or through stimulatory GTP-binding proteins to phospholipase C. Aside from actions that indirectly affect renal function, such as inhibition of AVP release by the pituitary, inhibition of aldosterone synthesis by adrenal zona glomerulosa cells, sympathoinhibitory effects, and relaxant effects on systemic vascular resistance and venous capacitance, natriuretic peptides directly affect renal solute and water homeostasis. Acting predominantly through guanylyl cyclase (GC-A and GC-B)–linked receptors, natriuretic peptides alter the hemodynamic forces regulating glomerular filtration and tubular Na^+ resorption, particularly in the distal nephron.

Infusions of ANP have been shown to cause afferent arteriolar dilation and efferent arteriolar constriction, which results in an increase in GFR.[5] Even when infused at concentrations that do not affect the GFR, ANP induces natriuresis by inhibiting the resorptive capacity of the proximal tubular epithelium largely by inhibiting the actions of locally acting antinatriuretic agents such as angiotensin II and by augmenting the activity of intrarenal dopamine. In the distal nephron, particularly in the medullary portion of the collecting duct, there is evidence that natriuretic peptides, acting through GC-A receptors, decrease Na^+ influx from the tubular lumen through amiloride-sensitive epithelial Na^+ channels. The result is a natriuresis with minimal effect on urinary potassium excretion. ANP, which is likewise synthesized and released by vascular endothelial cells,[67] may also be important in regulating blood pressure, particularly during physiological stress. For example, the blood pressure of mice that have had their pro-ANP gene disrupted by gene-targeting techniques—and therefore have no detectable circulating ANP—is very sensitive to dietary salt intake.[68] Little evidence has been presented for any clinically significant direct effect of ANP[69] or BNP on ventricular function.

Nesiritide (Human Brain Natriuretic Peptide)

Although ANP has a favorable pharmacological profile in HF, therapeutic trials with ANP have been disappointing because of its short biological half-life, end-organ resistance, the development of pharmacological tolerance, and undesirable hemodynamic effects.[70] Results with BNP have been much more promising.[71-73] When infused continuously into patients with HF, recombinant hBNP (nesiritide) produced vasodilator and cardiac output–increasing effects.[54,71-74] The vasodilation was not accompanied by neurohormonal activation, apparently because of sympathoinhibition.[75] Although BNP was natriuretic and diuretic in one study,[71] in another study, approximately half of the subjects were resistant to the natriuretic effects of BNP.[72] In clinical trials involving patients hospitalized for decompensated HF, nesiritide has been shown to improve hemodynamics and clinical status.[54,73,74] Moreover, nesiritide is less arrhythmogenic than dobutamine.[76] Compared with intravenous nitroglycerin, when administered at a dose of 2 µg/kg as a bolus followed by an infusion of 0.01 µg/kg/min, nesiritide produced faster relief of dyspneic symptoms and quicker reductions in elevated pulmonary capillary wedge pressure (see Fig. 23–5).[54]

Another approach to the use of natriuretic peptides is to deliver them subcutaneously, whereby they could then be used to treat chronic HF. This approach works in animal models of HF,[77] and initial studies in humans are promising.[78]

NEUTRAL ENDOPEPTIDASE INHIBITORS

Because receptor-mediated clearance and metabolism by the zinc metallopeptidase neutral endopeptidase (NEP) are the two predominant mechanisms for natriuretic peptide inactivation and removal, two approaches have been taken to lengthening the biological half-life of endogenous and exogenously infused natriuretic peptides.[79] Analogs of ANP have been developed that bind to ANP-R_2 receptors with high affinity but exhibit little biological activity. Several classes of NEP inhibitors have also been developed that alone or in combination with ANP-R_2 antagonists induce natriuresis and delay the clearance of exogenously infused ANP. NEP antagonists have been shown to increase plasma ANP levels and induce natriuresis with little effect on potassium excretion in patients with HF. However, in limited clinical trials in patients with HF, NEP inhibitors had relatively little efficacy.[80]

NEUTRAL ENDOPEPTIDASE–ANGIOTENSIN-CONVERTING ENZYME (VASOPEPTIDASE) INHIBITION

The combination of an NEP antagonist with an ACEI has been shown to result in more sustained natriuretic effects than an NEP antagonist alone in experimental animal models of HF, in part because of the inhibition of angiotensin II–mediated effects but also because of the fact that both NEP and ACE degrade bradykinin, a vasodilatory and natriuretic peptide.[81]

There is some evidence that ACE inhibition in HF patients may favorably affect the release or clearance, or both, of endogenous ANP, but not BNP, by resetting the relationship between ANP levels and atrial pressure.[82] With these actions in mind, single agents with dual metalloproteinase inhibitor activity (i.e., NEP and ACE inhibition) have been developed that address the mechanisms contributing to both pharmacological tolerance and end-organ resistance to natriuretic peptides in HF.[84] Indeed, both renal (natriuresis) and humoral (decrease in renin) responses to omapatrilat are superior to those to an ACEI in subjects with HF.[83] When omapatrilat was compared with the ACEI lisinopril in two phase II trials, the results were quite promising.[84] Unfortunately, large clinical trials with omapatrilat in HF have failed to demonstrate a clear benefit of NEP-ACE inhibition over ACE inhibition alone.[85] In addition, omapatrilat was associated with a slightly higher incidence of angioedema than enalapril alone.[86]

CALCIUM ANTAGONISTS

Although all three classes of calcium channel antagonists (i.e., phenylalkylamines such as verapamil, benzothiazepines such as diltiazem, and dihydropyridines such as nifedipine, nitrendipine, felodipine, nicardipine, isradipine, or amlodipine) are effective arteriolar vasodilators, none has been shown to produce sustained improvement in symptoms or natural history in patients with HF with predominant systolic ventricular dysfunction. Indeed, some of these agents appear to worsen symptoms and may increase mortality in patients with systolic dysfunction.[86] The reason for these adverse effects or lack of efficacy of calcium channel blockers in HF is unclear. It may be related to the known negative inotropic effects of these drugs, to reflex neurohumoral activation, or a combination of these and other effects.

Second-generation calcium channel antagonists of the dihydropyridine class, such as amlodipine, nicardipine, and felodipine, have fewer negatively inotropic effects than earlier drugs of this class as a result of their higher degrees of vasoselectivity. All three have been evaluated in medium- or large-scale randomized trials,[83–88] where they have not shown efficacy but have had acceptable adverse event profiles. Therefore, highly vasoselective dihydropyridine calcium antagonists can be used in patients with ischemic cardiomyopathy to treat angina that is uncontrolled by beta blockers and nitrates.

Positive Inotropic Agents

Cardiac Glycosides

Cardiac glycosides are used to treat chronic HF in patients in sinus rhythm and to control the response of the ventricular rate to supraventricular arrhythmias, including atrial fibrillation.[89] Digoxin is the most commonly prescribed cardiac glycoside because of its convenient pharmacokinetics, alternative routes of administration, and the widespread availability of serum drug level measurements.

Mechanisms of Action

Digoxin is a complex agent in that its mode of action, inhibition of Na^+,K^+-ATPase, affects multiple cellular processes, including several critical to cardiac myocyte function (see Chap. 19).[89] Digoxin is also extremely toxic, not surprising in view of its apparent role in nature as a toxin evolved by plants to kill mammals. Cardiac glycosides bind to a specific high-affinity site on the extracytoplasmic face of the alpha subunit of Na^+,K^+-ATPase, the enzymatic equivalent of the cellular "sodium pump."[89] The affinity of the subunit for cardiac glycosides varies among species and among the three known mammalian subunit isoforms, each of which is encoded by a separate gene.[89]

Cardiac glycoside binding to and inhibition of the Na^+,K^+-ATPase sodium pump are reversible and entropically driven. Under physiological conditions, these drugs preferentially bind to the enzyme after phosphorylation of a beta-aspartate on the cytoplasmic face of the alpha subunit, thus stabilizing what is known as the E_2P conformation.[89,90] Extracellular K^+ promotes dephosphorylation at this site, resulting in a decrease in the cardiac glycoside binding affinity for the enzyme.[90] This action presumably explains why increased extracellular K^+ tends to reverse some manifestations of digitalis toxicity.

POSITIVE INOTROPIC EFFECT. Cardiac glycosides increase the velocity and extent of shortening of cardiac muscle, thereby resulting in an upward and leftward shift of the ventricular function curve (Frank-Starling) relating cardiac performance to filling volume or pressure (see Fig. 23–2). This process occurs in normal as well as failing myocardium and in atrial as well as ventricular muscle. The effect appears to be sustained for periods of weeks or months without evidence of desensitization or tolerance.[91]

The positive inotropic effect is due to an increase in the availability of cytosolic Ca^{2+} during systole, thus increasing the velocity and extent of sarcomere shortening. The increase in intracellular $[Ca^{2+}]$ is a consequence of cardiac glycoside–induced inhibition of sarcolemmal Na^+,K^+-ATPase.[89,90] Inhibition of Na^+,K^+-ATPase causes an increase in intracellular Na^+, which is then exchanged for extracellular Ca^{2+} through the Na^+/Ca^{2+} exchanger.[92] The net effect of these adjustments is to increase intracellular Ca^{2+} during systole, which increases systolic function.

In part because cardiac glycosides produce an increase in contractile function without increasing the heart rate, the positive inotropic effects are more energetically efficient than the effects of beta-adrenergic agonists and higher doses of PDEIs.[93] This difference may be one of the reasons why low-dose digoxin does not increase mortality in patients with HF.[92]

ANTIADRENERGIC PROPERTIES. Na^+,K^+-ATPase is involved in baroreflex afferent signaling and may be upregulated in the carotid sinus in HF.[94] Decreased baroreflex control is one of the mechanisms responsible for an increase in generalized and cardiac[95] adrenergic activity in HF. Inhibition of Na^+,K^+-ATPase by ouabain modulates baroreflex function toward normal in animal models of HF,[94] which is likely to be the mechanism by which cardiac glycosides inhibit adrenergic activity in HF.

ELECTROPHYSIOLOGICAL ACTIONS. Cardiac glycosides have complex electrophysiological effects that are a combination of indirect, parasympathetic, and direct effects on specialized cardiac pacemaker and conduction tissues.[96] At low to moderate therapeutic serum concentrations (0.5 to 1.9 ng/ml), digoxin usually decreases automaticity and increases maximal diastolic resting membrane potential in atrial and atrioventricular (AV) nodal cells as a result of augmented vagal tone and decreased sympathetic nervous system activity. These effects are accompanied by prolongation of the effective refractory period and decreased AV nodal conduction velocity. At higher, toxic digoxin levels or in the presence of underlying disease, patients are susceptible to sinus bradycardia or arrest, prolongation of AV conduction, or heart block. At toxic levels, cardiac glycosides can also increase sympathetic nervous system activity, potentially contributing to the generation of arrhythmias.

Increased intracellular Ca^{2+} loading and increased sympathetic tone both contribute to an increased rate of spontaneous (phase 4) diastolic depolarization and also to delayed afterdepolarizations that may reach threshold and generate propagated action potentials. The combination of increased automaticity and depressed conduction in the His-Purkinje network predisposes to arrhythmias, including ventricular tachycardia and fibrillation. Data from the Digitalis Investigation Group (DIG) Trial[97] suggest that the increase in ventricular arrhythmia manifested in chronic HF as an increase in sudden death extends down to digoxin serum levels of 1.0 ng/ml, inasmuch as higher concentrations were associated with an increase in mortality.

Clinical Observations

Despite the use of cardiac glycosides for more than 200 years in the treatment of HF, the debate over their use in chronic HF continues. Small and medium-sized trials conducted in the 1970s and 1980s yielded equivocal results. However, in the early 1990s, two relatively large digoxin withdrawal studies, the Randomized Assessment of Digoxin and Inhibitors of Angiotensin-Converting Enzyme (RADIANCE)[98,99] and the Prospective Randomized Study of Ventricular Function and Efficacy of Digoxin (PROVED),[99,100] provided strong support for clinical benefit from digoxin. In these studies,[98-100] worsening HF and HF hospitalizations developed in more patients withdrawn from digoxin to placebo treatment than patients maintained with a therapeutic regimen of digoxin. However, because withdrawal studies are difficult to interpret, a large placebo-controlled mortality trial, the DIG trial, was conducted.[92]

The DIG trial had all-cause mortality as its primary endpoint and had secondary endpoints of hospitalization and worsening HF.[92] This trial enrolled 6800 patients with Classes I to III HF with an average LV ejection fraction of 28 percent, and patients were monitored for an average of 37 months. Remarkably, the DIG trial finished with a relative risk ratio of 1.00 (confidence intervals of 0.91 and 1.07, $p = 0.80$), which indicates that at the doses (0.125 to 0.375 mg/d, with 70 percent receiving 0.25 mg/d) and serum levels of digoxin studied, this positive inotropic agent does *not* increase mortality in chronic HF. The data indicated a strong trend ($p = 0.06$) toward a decrease in deaths assigned to a progressive pump failure etiology, balanced by an increase in sudden and other non–pump failure cardiac deaths ($p = 0.04$).[92] The number of patients hospitalized was statistically significantly reduced (by 4 percent) by digoxin therapy, and the total number of hospitalizations per subject was significantly reduced by 6 percent.[93] Therefore, evidence of efficacy was seen in the DIG trial, but in view of its large size and power, this evidence is modest.

One of the most important findings to emerge from the DIG trial was that mortality was directly related to the digoxin serum level.[97] In addition, data from other studies have demonstrated that the beneficial effects of digoxin on ventricular function[101] and neurohormonal activation[101,102] occur at the "safe" lower serum levels of 0.5 to 1.0 ng/ml. Moreover, in men in the DIG trial, trough levels between 0.6 and 0.8 ng/ml actually reduced mortality.[97] This information means that if digoxin is used in subjects with HF, *trough levels should be kept between 0.5 and 1.0 ng/ml.*

Overall, clinical trial results support the routine use of digoxin in patients in sinus rhythm who have mild to moderate HF, which is why most HF practice guidelines recommend the use of digoxin. Because the DIG trial,[92] as well as RADIANCE[98] and PROVED,[100] were conducted in patients with Class II to III (stage 2) HF, no firm recommendation is possible for patients with more advanced HF in sinus rhythm. In addition, digoxin is indicated in all patients with HF with atrial fibrillation in whom ventricular response slowing is required. However, in both the sinus rhythm and atrial fibrillation settings, digoxin must be used in such a way as to avoid overt toxicity or an increase in sudden death without obvious toxicity. There is some evidence that digoxin is less efficacious in women than men,[103] but this is probably based on higher serum levels and more toxicity in the former when patients in the DIG trial were prescribed doses on the basis of a nomogram rather than trough levels. Although the numbers were too small to derive statistical significance in the DIG trial, women exhibited a trend for higher (>1.0 ng/ml) levels to be associated with increased mortality and lower levels for lower mortality than in placebo-treated patients.[97]

Pharmacokinetics and Dosing

Orally administered digoxin is variably absorbed, depending on the preparation, but Lanoxin is 60 to 80 percent absorbed. Digoxin is approximately 25 percent protein bound in plasma, has a large volume of distribution (4 to 7 liter/kg), and crosses both the blood-brain barrier and the placenta. Digoxin is eliminated primarily by renal mechanisms, both glomerular filtration and tubular secretion. Tubular excretion is through the energy-dependent membrane-bound efflux pump/transport enzyme, P-glycoprotein, which is modulated by many other drugs. Digoxin is largely excreted in the urine unchanged with a clearance rate proportional to the GFR, which results in the excretion of approximately one-third of body stores daily. The half-life for digoxin elimination of 36 to 48 hours in patients with normal or near-normal renal function permits once-daily or every-other-day dosing.[104]

In the presence of an elevated blood urea nitrogen/creatinine ratio (i.e., "prerenal azotemia"), digoxin clearance more closely parallels urea clearance, indicating that under these circumstances some of the drug filtered through the glomerulus undergoes tubular reabsorption.[104] In patients with HF, increased cardiac output and renal blood flow in response to treatment with vasodilators or sympathomimetic agents may increase renal digoxin clearance and necessitate dosage adjustment.

Digoxin can be loaded at a dose of 0.75 to 1.25 mg orally (or intravenously at doses 25 percent lower) over a 24-hour period in three to four divided doses and then given at a maintenance dose, or a daily maintenance dose of 0.0625 to 0.25 mg/d orally can be started, depending on renal function, body size, and the presence or absence of coadministered drugs causing pharmacokinetic interactions. In the absence of loading doses, nearly steady-state blood levels are achieved in four to five half-lives, or about 1 week after initiation of maintenance therapy if normal renal function is present. If given intravenously, administration should be carried out over at least 15 minutes to avoid vasoconstrictor responses to a more rapid injection. Intramuscular digoxin is absorbed unpredictably, causes local pain, and is not recommended.

Patients with HF usually have a reduced volume of distribution and reduced renal function, and both may be influenced by other treatment and by the ebb and flow of the HF. Although nomograms on digoxin dosing have been published, these nomograms should not be used in patients with HF because of the narrow therapeutic index and the unpredictability of the numerous factors that can alter digoxin pharmacokinetics. Instead, patients should be started on a dose as just described and trough levels (see later) measured 1 to 2 weeks later and at frequent intervals (every 1 to 3 months) thereafter.

DRUG INTERACTIONS WITH DIGOXIN. Multiple drugs interact with digoxin at multiple levels, including reduced renal tubular excretion by drugs inhibiting P-glycoprotein renal tubular transport,[105] induction of gut P-glycoprotein,[106] alterations in gut flora by antibiotics causing less gut metabolism of digoxin before absorption, displacement from plasma protein-binding sites, or reduction in renal function. A partial list of these interactions is given in Table 23-4. Among these interactions are drugs that are routinely used in patients with HF, including carvedilol and amiodarone, in whose presence digoxin doses should be lowered.

TABLE 23–4 Partial List of Drugs Interacting with Digoxin		
Drug	Effect on Serum Digoxin Level	Mechanism
Amiodarone	Increases	? ↓ Renal clearance
Verapamil	Increases	↓ Renal clearance
Nifedipine	Increases	↓ Renal clearance
Diltiazem	Increases	↓ Renal clearance
Quinidine	Increases	Displacement of protein binding, ↓ renal clearance
Propafenone	Increases	↓ Renal clearance
Captopril	? Increases	? Renal clearance
Carvedilol	Increases	↑ Oral bioavailability
Spironolactone	Increases	↓ Renal clearance
Amiloride	Increases	↓ Renal clearance
Triamterene	Increases	↓ Renal clearance
Salbutamol	Decreases	Unknown
Macrolide antibiotics (erythromycin, clarithromycin)	Increases	Altered gut flora, ↓ renal clearance
Tetracycline	Increases	Altered gut flora
Indomethacin	Increases	↓ Renal clearance
Alprazolam	Increases	? ↓ Renal clearance
Itraconazole	Increases	↓ Renal clearance
Rifampin	Decreases	Induction of gut P-glycoprotein
Sucralfate	Decreases	Decreased gut absorption
Cholestyramine	Decreases	Decreased gut absorption
Cyclosporine	Increases	↓ Renal clearance
St. John's wort	Increases	↓ Renal clearance

THERAPEUTIC DRUG MONITORING

Digoxin has an extremely low therapeutic index, and its use should be carefully monitored by serum blood levels. The various clinical conditions and drug interactions that can alter digoxin's pharmacokinetics are also reflected in the serum digoxin level. As discussed earlier, on the basis of the dose range of the positive inotropic effects,[101] the neurohormonal inhibition effects,[102] and the DIG trial mortality data,[97] the optimal trough digoxin serum level is 0.5 to 1.0 ng/ml. This concentration range is also the one that should be used to control the ventricular rate response to atrial fibrillation in patients with HF, particularly because digoxin is not a very effective agent in this regard in the setting of high amounts of adrenergic activity.[107] Blood samples for measurement of serum digoxin levels should be taken at least 6 to 8 hours following the last digoxin dose, and patients should be instructed to take their digoxin in the evening so that any level determined during the day is a trough measurement.

DIGITALIS TOXICITY

In patients with HF, overt clinical toxicity tends to emerge at serum concentrations greater than 2.0 ng/ml, but substantial overlap in serum levels exists among patients exhibiting symptoms and signs of toxicity and those with no clinical evidence of intoxication. Disturbances in cardiac impulse formation, conduction, or both are the hallmarks of digitalis toxicity. Among the common electrocardiographic manifestations are ectopic beats of AV junctional or ventricular origin, first-degree AV block, an excessively slow ventricular rate response to atrial fibrillation, or an accelerated AV junctional pacemaker. These manifestations may require only dosage adjustment and monitoring. Sinus bradycardia, sinoatrial arrest or exit block, and second- or third-degree AV conduction delay often respond to atropine, but temporary ventricular pacing is sometimes necessary and should be available.

MANAGEMENT. Oral potassium administration is often useful for atrial, AV junctional, or ventricular ectopic rhythms, even when the serum potassium is in the normal range, unless high-grade AV block is also present. However, $[K^+]$ must be monitored carefully to avoid hyperkalemia, especially in patients with renal failure. Magnesium may be useful in patients with atrial fibrillation in an accessory pathway in whom digoxin administration has facilitated a rapid accessory pathway-mediated ventricular response; again, careful monitoring is required to avoid hypermagnesemia.[108] Neurological or gastrointestinal complaints can also be manifestations of digitalis toxicity. Occasionally, gynecomastia results from digoxin administration, apparently because of the similarity of the glycoside structure to that of estrogens.

ANTIDIGOXIN IMMUNOTHERAPY. Potentially life-threatening digoxin or digitoxin toxicity can be reversed by antidigoxin immunotherapy. Purified Fab fragments from digoxin-specific antisera are available at most poison control centers and larger hospitals in North America and Europe. Clinical experience in adults and children has established the effectiveness and safety of antidigoxin Fab in treating life-threatening digoxin toxicity, including cases of massive ingestion with suicidal intent.[109] Doses of Fab are calculated by using a simple formula based on either the estimated dose of drug ingested or the total-body digoxin burden and are administered intravenously in saline over a period of 30 to 60 minutes.

Adrenergic Agonists

Mechanism of Action

The most powerful way to increase contractility in the human heart is by the use of a beta-adrenergic receptor agonist. Beta-agonists operate through the mechanism that regulates contractility and heart rate on a beat-to-beat basis in the intact heart (see also Chap. 19).[110] As depicted in Figure 23–6, this system is composed of two cell surface membrane receptors (beta$_1$ and beta$_2$); two G proteins (the stimulatory G protein, $G_{\alpha s}$, and the inhibitory G protein, $G_{\alpha i}$); the adenylyl cyclase enzyme (which converts Mg-ATP to cAMP); cAMP-activated protein kinase (protein kinase A); compartmentalized phosphodiesterases, which modulate cAMP levels to produce selective signaling; and target structures whose phosphorylation leads to a positive inotropic effect by changes in Ca^{2+} handling (phospholamban, the ryanodine release channel, and slow inward current calcium channels). An important point in the function of beta-adrenergic pathways is that they are not all cAMP dependent[110]; in Figure 23–6 the beta$_1$ receptor is depicted with direct activation of voltage-sensitive Ca^{2+} channels as well as cAMP-dependent activation. The end result is a powerful positive inotropic as well as positive chronotropic effect.

In the failing human heart, beta-adrenergic pathways undergo *desensitization*, a pharmacological term encompassing the regulatory changes that occur in receptors, G proteins, and adenylyl cyclase.[111,112] In advanced HF, the degree of beta-adrenergic receptor desensitization approaches 50 to 60 percent of the maximum capacity of signal transduction,[113,114] and in severe HF, beta-agonists may no longer be able to support myocardial function.[115] However, the vast majority of patients with advanced HF still exhibit a substantial inotropic response to beta-agonists,[114] which is the basis for their usefulness as inotropic agents in the treatment of decompensated HF.

All beta-agonists are given intravenously for short-term support of decompensated HF. They are all arrhythmogenic to some extent through direct mechanisms as well as through increasing the skeletal muscle deposition of potassium[40] and decreasing serum magnesium. Their administration should be carefully monitored and the lowest possible effective doses used. In addition, all beta-agonists are subject to the development of desensitization phenomena when used continuously, another reason to keep the doses low and use short term or intermittently. Beta-agonists all have short (in minutes) half-lives, which is an advantage for powerful inotropes that may have adverse effects. As shown in Table 23–5,[116,117] from a therapeutic standpoint, it is important to understand how beta-agonists differ from one another with respect to intrinsic activity; affinity for binding to beta$_1$, beta$_2$, and alpha$_1$ receptors; and affinity for the cardiac adrenergic neuronal reuptake system (uptake$_1$). Neuronal reuptake is an important consideration in the heart, which has the most active uptake$_1$ system of any organ and uses neuronal reuptake to terminate the majority of the action of released norepinephrine.

Although beta$_1$- and beta$_2$-adrenergic receptors are coupled to positive inotropic and chronotropic responses through cAMP-dependent and -independent mechanisms, these two receptors have important differences. For one thing, beta$_1$ receptors are positioned inside or near the synaptic cleft area to mediate the effects of released norepinephrine, which also means that catecholamines that have high affinity for neuronal reuptake do not reach myocardial beta$_1$ receptors unless neuronal reuptake is functionally decreased (as it is in myocardial failure) or absent (as it is in a recently [<2 years] transplanted heart). In addition, a growing body of evidence indicates that chronic beta$_1$ receptor agonist occupancy or pathway activation, or both, is more deleterious than beta$_2$ receptor activation.[110,118] However, from an acute support standpoint, both receptors can be used in supporting cardiac function in decompensated patients.

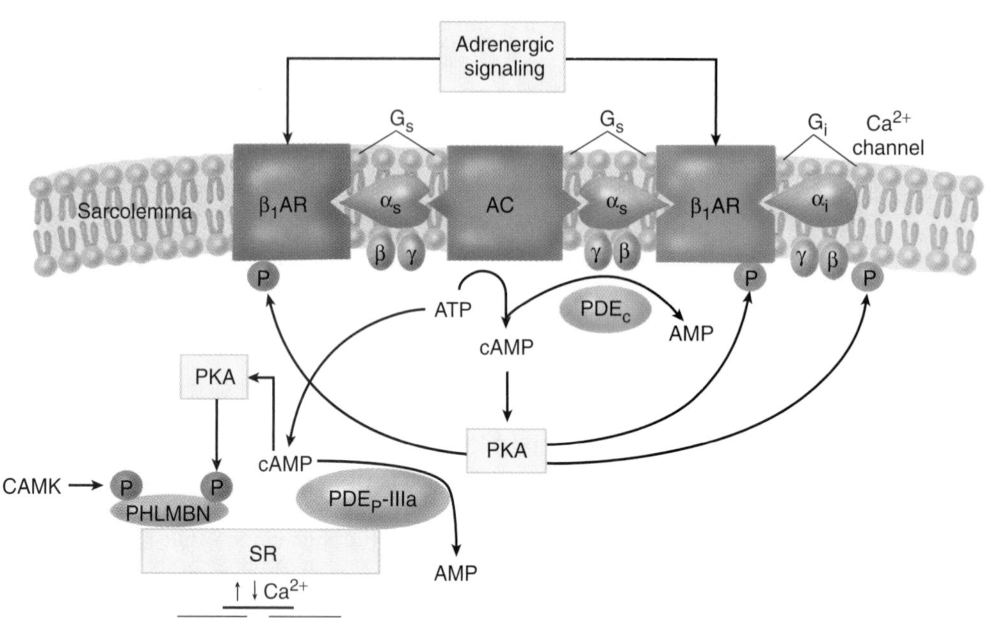

FIGURE 23–6 Schematic representation of selected components of the cardiac myocyte beta$_1$- and beta$_2$-adrenergic receptor pathways. The beta$_1$-adrenergic receptor is illustrated with direct coupling through $G_{\alpha s}$ to voltage-sensitive Ca^{2+} channels as well as to Ca^{2+} channels by cyclic adenosine monophosphate (cAMP)-dependent protein kinase A (PKA) phosphorylation. AC = adenylyl cyclase; AR = adrenergic receptor; ATP = adenosine triphosphate; CAMK = calmodulin-activated kinase; PDE = phosphodiesterase; PHLMBN = phospholamban; SR = sarcoplasmic reticulum.

NEURONAL REUPTAKE AFFINITIES FOR SYMPATHOMIMETIC AMINES. Table 23–5 lists the adrenergic receptor and neuronal reuptake (uptake$_1$) affinities for catecholamines that are used therapeutically to increase cardiac performance or increase systemic vascular resistance or blood pressure. Although the primary action of uptake$_1$ is to terminate the action of norepinephrine, the functional status of uptake$_1$ is also an important determinant of catecholamine therapeutic action when these agents are administered exogenously. For

TABLE 23–5 Pharmacological Characteristics of Various Adrenergic Agonists Used to Treat Decompensated Heart Failure

Agent	Beta$_1$-Receptor Affinity (K_d, nM)	Beta$_2$-Receptor Affinity (K_d, nM)	Alpha$_1$-Receptor Affinity (K_d, nM)	Uptake$_1$ Affinity (nM)	Intrinsic Activity* for Human Beta$_1$ Receptors
Dobutamine	470	570	130	190,330	0.5
Dopamine	25,000	100,000	36,000	130,230	0.2
Epinephrine	20	20	160	1,400	1.0
Isoproterenol	20	20	>10,000	9,000	1.0
Norepinephrine	20	400	200	500,670	1.0
Phenylephrine	>10,000	>10,000	1,000	>10,000	0

Median inhibitory concentration (IC_{50}) data were converted to affinity constants using the Cheng-Prusoff equation.

Some data from Iverson LL (ed): The Uptake and Storage of Noradrenaline in Sympathetic Nerves. Cambridge, UK, Cambridge University Press, 1967.

*Relative to isoproterenol = 1.0 in nonfailing isolated human RV trabeculae. Affinity data are based on radioligand-cold ligand competition curves in (1) human ventricular myocardial membrane preparations (beta$_1$, beta$_2$, alpha$_1$ in nonfailing hearts, norepinephrine, epinephrine, isoproterenol), (2) human recombinant beta$_2$ receptors in COS cell membranes (isoproterenol, norepinephrine, and epinephrine), (3) DTT$_1$ cell membranes (beta$_2$, dobutamine, and dopamine), and rat heart membranes (alpha$_1$, dobutamine). Additional alpha$_1$-agonist affinity data are derived from irreversible dibenamine antagonism in rabbit aorta, with relative affinities corrected for human/rabbit alpha$_1$ receptor–norepinephrine K values (dopamine, phenylephrine, epinephrine). Uptake$_1$ data are from the human recombinant protein cloned from SK-N-SH neuroblastoma cells (norepinephrine, dopamine),[119] rabbit brain synaptosomes (dobutamine, dopamine, isoproterenol),[120] or the original data for rat heart (epinephrine, norepinephrine, phenylephrine).

example, epinephrine, which has an affinity for uptake$_1$ that is slightly lower than that of norepinephrine, is a much more potent therapeutic catecholamine when administered to denervated cardiac transplant hearts than to innervated hearts.[119,120] When the heart is innervated, uptake$_1$ removes much of the systemically administered epinephrine before it can reach myocardial beta$_1$-adrenergic receptors, which are preferentially located within the synaptic cleft area. In contrast, isoproterenol, which has essentially no affinity for uptake$_1$, is equally effective in innervated and denervated hearts.[121,122]

The failing human heart has a functional impairment in uptake$_1$ that essentially creates functional denervation, which in the case of catecholamines with higher affinity for uptake$_1$ can offset some of the postsynaptic desensitization changes. Another way in which uptake$_1$ can influence drug action is to compete with neurotransmitter norepinephrine for neuronal reuptake, which increases the amount of norepinephrine available in the synaptic cleft area. As can be observed in Table 23–5, the substituted synthetic catecholamine, dobutamine, and the endogenous catecholamine, dopamine, have even higher affinity for uptake$_1$ than does norepinephrine, and at least in the case of dopamine, this higher affinity contributes to its predominant inotropic action, which is to potentiate norepinephrine release.

Dobutamine

Dobutamine is a very useful inotropic agent for moderately decompensated HF.[127] As available clinically, dobutamine is a racemic mixture that stimulates both beta$_1$- and beta$_2$-adrenergic receptor subtypes (binding at an approximately 3:1 ratio)[124] and either binds to but does not activate alpha-adrenergic receptors ([+] enantiomer) or stimulates alpha$_1$ and alpha$_2$ receptor subtypes ([−] enantiomer). As discussed earlier, dobutamine also has a relatively high affinity for uptake$_1$. The affinity constants for racemic dobutamine binding to beta$_1$, beta$_2$, and alpha$_{1B}$ receptors are given in Table 23–5, where it can seen that dobutamine is relatively nonselective for binding to beta$_1$ versus beta$_2$ receptors and binds to alpha$_1$ receptors and uptake$_1$ at a slightly higher affinity. When compared with isoproterenol, in human cardiac preparations, dobutamine is a partial beta-agonist with an intrinsic activity of approximately 0.5.[125] The binding to alpha receptors by each isomer of dobutamine results in a mixture of antagonist and agonist action that, when coupled with some peripheral vascular beta$_2$-agonism, usually produces a net mild degree of vasodilation at lower (≤5 μg/kg/min) doses. At these doses, dobutamine reduces aortic impedance and systemic vascular resistance, thus reducing afterload and improving ventricular-vascular coupling by reducing aortic impedance.[126,127] In contrast, dopamine (see later) may either have no effect or increase ventricular afterload by increasing systemic vascular resistance and by causing a more rapid return of reflected aortic pressure waves, depending on the infusion rate. Therefore, dobutamine is preferable to dopamine for most patients with advanced decompensated HF who have not responded adequately to intravenous diuretics.

The neuronal reuptake inhibition of dobutamine means that in subjects with preserved neuronal uptake mechanisms, dobutamine may increase synaptic cleft area norepinephrine concentrations in the heart in addition to its intrinsic receptor-mediated actions. Dobutamine does not stimulate dopaminergic receptors and, unlike dopamine, does not selectively alter renal blood flow.[128] The importance of the vascular effects of dobutamine has been demonstrated by experiments in animals with artificial hearts.[129,130] Even in the presence of a mechanical heart, dobutamine increased cardiac output by 10 to 15 percent and decreased systemic vascular resistance. Interestingly, dobutamine also decreases venous capacitance and increases right atrial pressure, possibly as a result of alpha$_1$-adrenergic agonism of the (−) enantiomer.[130] These experiments also demonstrated that the (+) enantiomer is responsible for the racemic drug's favorable effects on aortic input impedance, wave reflectance, and systemic vascular resistance.[129] The LV afterload–reducing effects are also responsible for the reduction in functional mitral regurgitation often observed concomitantly with dobutamine infusions in patients with large dilated ventricles and high LV end-diastolic pressure.[131] Dobutamine also causes a mild decline in pulmonary vascular resistance that is present regardless of chronic background vasodilator therapy.

At higher doses, the (−) isomer of dobutamine begins to exert alpha$_1$-adrenergic agonist action, thereby preventing progressive vasodilation and usually leading to minimal changes in preload and afterload. The advantage of this alpha-adrenergic effect of dobutamine is that because preload and afterload do not change dramatically, dobutamine can be administered without pulmonary artery catheter monitoring of LV filling pressure. Another advantage of the relative lack of vasodilation coupled to the partial agonist action is that dobutamine does not produce much increase in the heart rate at doses of 10 μg/kg/min or less. Because of its partial agonist activity, desensitization to prolonged infusions of dobutamine is not pronounced.[132] Dobutamine infusions are initiated at 2 to 3 μg/kg/min and are titrated upward according to the patient's hemodynamic response (usually not higher than 20 μg/kg/min).[127,128]

The limitations of dobutamine are that it (1) is a relatively weak beta-agonist,[125] (2) only modestly lowers elevated pulmonary artery pressure, (3) eventually produces desensitization phenomena when used chronically,[132,133] and (4) cannot be effectively used in the presence of high levels of beta-adrenergic receptor blockade.[119,120] The first three of these limitations can be overcome by combining dobutamine with a phosphodiesterase inhibitor (see below), which results in additive effects on myocardial performance,[134] substantial reductions in pulmonary wedge and pulmonary artery pressure,[134] and a protective effect on desensitization[133] related to being able to lower the dobutamine dose. The fourth limitation is best dealt with by avoiding dobutamine and using a PDEI alone in patients receiving carvedilol or high doses of beta$_1$-blocking agents; in the presence of carvedilol, dobutamine produces little or no increase in stroke volume and increases systemic vascular resistance.[119,120] On the other hand, favorable hemodynamic responses to the PDEIs, enoximone or milrinone, are enhanced by either carvedilol[119,120] or metoprolol.[120]

Dopamine

Dopamine is an endogenous catecholamine that is the precursor to norepinephrine in the catecholamine synthetic pathway. When administered therapeutically, dopamine is a complex agent. Dopamine, through its direct effects, is a weak partial beta-agonist. When initially administered, it releases norepinephrine through a tyramine-like effect.[135] It is a potent (relative to its receptor affinities) neuronal uptake inhibitor and by direct action acts as an agonist at dopamine D_1 postsynaptic vasodilator receptors[136] and D_2 presynaptic receptors on blood vessels and in the kidney.[137] The affinities for beta$_1$, beta$_2$, and alpha$_{1B}$ receptors are shown in Table 23–5, where it can be seen that dopamine has extremely low affinity for all three adrenergic receptors.

At lower doses (≤2 μg/kg/min), dopamine causes a relatively selective dilation of splanchnic and renal arterial beds. This effect may be useful in promoting renal blood flow and maintaining GFR in selected patients who become refractory to diuretics, especially when caused by marginal renal perfusion. Dopamine also has direct renal tubular effects that promote natriuresis. At intermediate (2 to 10 μg/kg/min) infusion rates, dopamine, by virtue of its tyramine and neuronal uptake-inhibiting properties, enhances norepinephrine release from vascular and myocardial adrenergic neurons, thereby resulting in increased cardiac beta-adrenergic receptor activation and an increase in peripheral vascular resistance. In patients with advanced HF, who often have depleted intracardiac norepinephrine stores, dopamine is a less effective positive inotropic drug than are other "directly" acting inotropes.[128,129] At higher infusion rates (5 to 20 μg/kg/min), peripheral vasoconstriction occurs as a result of direct alpha-adrenergic receptor stimulation. Increases in systemic vascular resistance are common even at intermediate infusion rates. On initial administration, tachycardia and arrhythmia tend to be more pronounced than with dobutamine[128] and are related to cardiac norepinephrine release.[135,138]

In patients with advanced, decompensated HF, dopamine should not be used as a positive inotropic agent but rather should be used in low doses for renal perfusion and in intermediate to high doses to increase peripheral resistance. The latter property is often necessary for a variety of reasons, including sepsis, iatrogenic overvasodilation, and brain injury.

OTHER ADRENERGIC AGONISTS

EPINEPHRINE. Epinephrine is an endogenous full beta-agonist catecholamine that, like dobutamine, produces relatively balanced effects between vasodilation and vasoconstriction. This balance between vasodilation and vasoconstriction occurs because epinephrine has relatively equal high affinities for $beta_1$, $beta_2$, and $alpha_1$ receptors (see Table 23-5). Epinephrine has a moderately high affinity for neuronal reuptake, which means that the majority of administered drug may not reach $beta_1$-adrenergic receptors in the normal heart. However, neuronal reuptake is markedly reduced in the failing heart,[139,140] which allows epinephrine to reach more $beta_1$-adrenergic receptors in this setting. Epinephrine is an excellent positive inotropic agent in the denervated, transplanted heart[121,122] because neuronal reuptake is no longer a factor. The dose of epinephrine usually ranges from 0.05 to 0.50 μg/kg/min.

When cardiogenic shock is profound, calcium is often added to an epinephrine infusion to produce synergistic increases in contractility[141] and an increase in vascular tone. This combination, made by adding 1 gm of $CaCl_2$ to 250 ml of intravenous solution containing epinephrine and called Epi-Cal, has never been subjected to a clinical trial and should be used in resuscitative settings only.

ISOPROTERENOL. Isoproterenol is a full, nonselective beta-agonist that produces powerful positive chronotropic, inotropic, and vasodilator responses. At therapeutic doses, isoproterenol does not bind to the neuronal uptake system (see Table 23-5). As a therapeutic inotrope, isoproterenol has only one indication—postoperatively, after heart transplantation. Isoproterenol is useful in this setting because an increase in heart rate is not a problem in the presence of normal coronary arteries and the chronotropic stimulation is useful in the newly transplanted heart, which often has a sluggish sinus node mechanism. The pulmonary vasodilator properties of isoproterenol are also useful in this setting, in which pulmonary artery pressure and pulmonary vascular resistance are usually elevated. The dose of isoproterenol ranges from 0.005 to 0.05 μg/kg/min.

NOREPINEPHRINE. As shown in Table 23-5, norepinephrine is a moderately (10- to 30-fold) $beta_1$ versus $beta_2$ receptor-selective agonist with relatively high affinity for $alpha_1$ receptors and for $uptake_1$. This constellation of properties means that norepinephrine is a powerful vasoconstrictor but not a very powerful inotrope in hearts with functioning neuronal uptake. Norepinephrine does not have any recommended uses in subjects with cardiac decompensation; subjects who need peripheral vascular resistance support (such as in sepsis, iatrogenic overvasodilation, or brain injury) are served better by dopamine or dopamine plus phenylephrine administration.

Phosphodiesterase Inhibitors (PDEI)

MECHANISMS OF ACTION. The enzyme phosphodiesterase type IIIa is associated with the sarcoplasmic reticulum (SR) in human cardiac myocytes (see Fig. 23–6),[142,143] platelets, and vascular smooth muscle, where it breaks down cAMP into AMP. Type IIIa phosphodiesterase has an SR-anchoring moiety[143] that accounts for its compartmentalization in cardiac myocytes and vascular smooth muscle. Elevations in cAMP in the vicinity of the SR can then activate locally compartmentalized protein kinase A, which phosphorylates phospholamban and relieves this molecule's inhibition of SR function (see Chap. 19).[144] Thus, specific type III PDEIs, particularly at low doses, may have a relatively selective effect on phospholamban phosphorylation[145] and SR function, which explains why they lower diastolic Ca^{2+} and increase systolic Ca^{2+} in cultured cardiac myocytes. This SR-selective effect is probably the reason why highly type III–specific PDEIs increase contractile function without as much of an increase in heart rate. This is similar to the phenotype of transgenic mice with phospholamban knockout, which exhibit an increase in contractility without an increase in heart rate.[146] However, PDEIs also increase the calcium channel current,[147] and higher doses increase the phosphorylation of phosphoproteins other than phospholamban,[145] similar in effect to beta-agonists.[148]

Type III PDEIs are also potent vasodilators, particularly on venous capacitance and pulmonary vascular beds. The vasodilator properties of PDEIs substantially exceed that of beta-agonists,[119,120,134] including isoproterenol. The reason for this superior vasodilation effect appears to be that, in vascular smooth muscle, PDEI-induced elevations in cAMP activate protein kinase G,[149] which leads to prominent vasodilation that is not unlike a nitrovasodilator effect in its regional distribution. PDEIs are among the best agents for lowering pulmonary artery pressure and pulmonary vascular resistance, which is one of the reasons why they have assumed an important role in postoperative cardiac surgical regimens, including cardiac transplantation.[150-152] The effect of PDEIs on LV function curves is shown in Figure 23–2; PDEIs as inotrope-vasodilators move the LV function curve both upward and leftward.

As with beta-agonists, a PDEI's inotropic response is blunted in failing versus nonfailing hearts (Fig. 23-7).[134,153] In the failing human heart, the reason for blunting of the response to PDEIs is not an alteration in myocardial type III phosphodiesterase[142] but rather upregulation of the inhibitory G protein, $G\alpha$,[154-156] because a decrease in $G_{\alpha i}$[157] leads to augmentation of the PDEI response.[158] However, by comparison with beta-agonists, little or no subsensitivity develops to the inotrope-vasodilator effects of more potent type III PDEIs such as milrinone[159] and enoximone.[119,159,160]

As discussed previously, the substantial preload- and pulmonary artery pressure-reducing properties of PDEIs are both a strength and a weakness of this class of agents, inasmuch as before their acute intravenous administration, it is necessary to be certain of an elevated LV filling pressure. Therefore, in the absence of elevated right-sided venous pressure in a subject with biventricular failure, pulmonary artery catheter-determined documentation of a pulmonary wedge mean pressure greater than 15 mm Hg is desirable before administering a PDEI intravenously. Otherwise, a precipitous drop in blood pressure may accompany drug administration.

PDEIs are absorbed orally, and their attractive hemodynamic profile has led to multiple clinical trials in chronic HF. The increase in cardiac output from PDEIs is preferentially distributed to skeletal muscle,[161] which should theoretically increase maximum exercise responses. Such does appear to be the case.[160,162] In addition, in a dilated, failing heart, PDEIs have a favorable energetic effect,[163] and PDEIs improve diastolic[164,165] as well as systolic[166] function. All these observations suggest that PDEIs would be useful in the long-term treatment of chronic HF.

CLINICAL OBSERVATIONS. In placebo-controlled clinical trials, selective type III PDEIs given in doses that produce large hemodynamic effects are associated with increased mortality.[166-168] Moreover, agents with PDEI activity and K^+ channel antagonism (vesnarinone),[169] as well as PDEI activity and Ca^{2+} sensitization (pimobendan, see later),[170] are also associated with increased mortality. The basis for the increase in mortality is increased sudden death,[168,171] presumably on an arrhythmic basis.

Despite these discouraging results, PDEIs continue in development for the treatment of chronic HF through two new approaches. One is a "low-dose" approach[172] that takes advantage of the fact that doses that are one-sixth to one-third those used in earlier clinical trials are hemodynamically active,[173] increase exercise tolerance,[160] do not increase the heart rate,[160] are not proarrhythmic,[160] and apparently do not increase mortality.[133,160] That a positive inotropic agent can increase mortality at higher doses but be safely given at low doses has been established by the DIG trial,[92,97] but it remains to be seen whether the same is true for PDEIs. The second approach to the safe, long-term use of PDEIs in chronic HF is to combine them with a beta-blocking agent.[175,176] This combination is possible because the site of action of PDEIs is beyond the beta-adrenergic receptor (see Fig. 23–6), and the combination appears to produce additive efficacy and subtractive adverse effects.[174] Treatment with beta-blocking agents actually enhances the hemodynamic effects of PDEIs[119,120,158] because of a beta blocker–related reduction in upregulated $G_{\alpha i}$.[157] As discussed earlier, one practical consequence of these findings and realizations is that subjects receiving beta-blocking agents chronically who decompensate to the point of needing positive inotropic support should be treated with a PDEI rather than dobutamine or some other beta-agonist.[119,120]

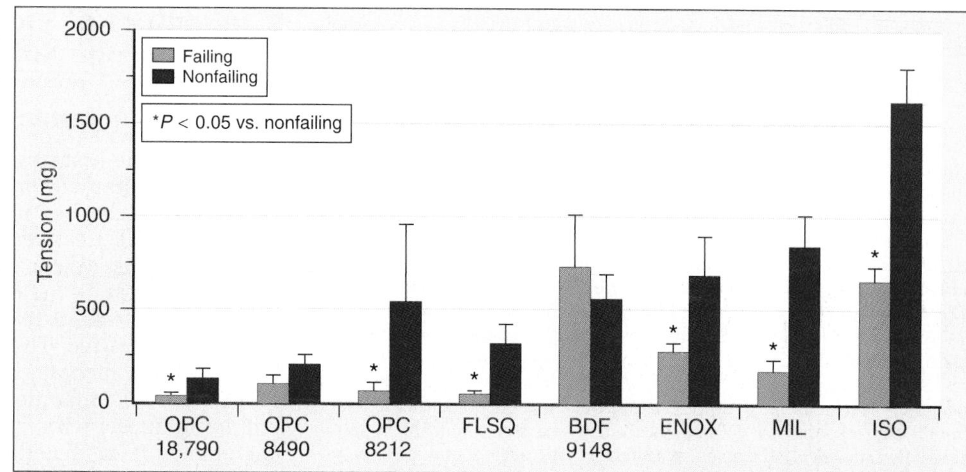

FIGURE 23–7 Effects of various inotropic agents on the systolic tension response in nonfailing and failing human right ventricular trabeculae, mean + standard error of the mean. ENOX = enoximone; FLSQ = flosequinan; ISO = isoproterenol; MIL = milrinone; OPC 8212 = vesnarinone.

Individual Agents

AMRINONE. Amrinone was the first type III PDEI approved for the treatment of decompensated HF.[176] Because amrinone causes thrombocytopenia and may be associated with rapid subsensitivity in subjects with advanced HF,[177] it is no longer widely used to treat decompensated HF.

MILRINONE. Unlike amrinone, milrinone rarely causes thrombocytopenia.[178] Although milrinone is a highly selective type III PDEI, other actions capable of producing an inotropic effect have been described, including stimulation of the Ca^{2+} release channel,[179] Ca^{2+} channel agonism, and effects on sarcolemmal Ca^{2+}-ATPase.[180]

Milrinone produces sustained inotropic and vasodilator effects when administered intravenously.[181] The elimination half-life is 2.3 hours, and milrinone is usually administered as a 25- to 75-μg/kg bolus over a 10- to 20-minute period, followed by a continuous infusion of 0.25 to 0.75 μg/kg/min.[182] Development of oral milrinone has been abandoned because of the increase in mortality in the Prospective Randomized Milrinone Survival Evaluation (PROMISE) trial,[166] which was conducted at doses that are at least four times higher than the minimum effective hemodynamic dose.[182] Milrinone is mostly (80 percent) excreted by the kidney unchanged, and in renal failure the continuous-infusion dose should be decreased by 50 percent.

ENOXIMONE. Enoximone is approved for intravenous use in Europe and is in development in the United States for oral use as low-dose enoximone alone and in combination with $beta_1$-selective blockade. Enoximone is a highly selective type III PDEI with no other known pharmacological actions at therapeutic plasma concentrations. Enoximone rarely causes thrombocytopenia and produces sustained hemodynamic effects with intravenous[183] or oral[160] administration.

Enoximone is about one-tenth as potent as milrinone for inhibiting type III phosphodiesterase, which translates to oral and intravenous doses of enoximone being approximately 10 times those of milrinone. The intravenous loading dose is 0.25 to 0.75 mg/kg, with the continuous infusion rate being 1.25 to 7.5 μg/kg/min. Enoximone is extensively metabolized by the liver to sulfoxide derivatives, including at least one active metabolite.[184] Sulfoxide metabolites (about 75 percent within 24 hours in subjects with HF) are eliminated by the kidney, and dose reductions in renal failure are the same as with milrinone.[185] Enoximone doses should also be reduced in patients with hepatic failure.

PHOSPHODIESTERASE INHIBITORS WITH CALCIUM SENSITIZER ACTIVITY

MECHANISM OF ACTION. These positive inotropic agents act in part by increasing the sensitivity of troponin C or some other part of the myofibrillar Ca^{2+}-binding apparatus to ionized calcium. This property alone would prolong contraction time and decrease diastolic function, which would not be desirable in an inotropic agent. However, all agents that have gone on to clinical development are also PDEIs, and this property "cancels" the increased contraction time and provides favorable effects on diastolic function.[186,187] Under these circumstances, the advantage of Ca^{2+} sensitization is that the pharmacological effect of the drug does not rely on increasing systolic calcium concentrations, although this action occurs if the compound also has PDEI activity. Another advantage would be in not increasing the heart rate, but again, PDEI activity would lead to a chronotropic effect at higher doses. The combination of not increasing intracellular Ca^{2+} or the heart rate would confer an energetic advantage to Ca^{2+} sensitizers.

The mixed-action Ca^{2+} sensitizers levosimendan and pimobendan have undergone the most clinical experience, and their hemodynamic profiles,[186,188] including increasing the heart rate at higher doses, do not differ from those of milrinone and enoximone. This similarity occurs because, as discussed subsequently, the dominant pharmacological action of both compounds is type III phosphodiesterase inhibition.

PIMOBENDAN. This agent is available in oral form for the treatment of HF, but only in Japan. Pimobendan has weak Ca^{2+}-sensitizing properties through facilitating the interaction of Ca^{2+} with troponin C,[189] its major mechanism of action being phosphodiesterase inhibition.[190] In several medium-sized trials, pimobendan increased exercise performance or improved quality of life, or both,[191] but its development in the United States and Europe was put on hold when a strong trend (relative risk 1.8, confidence interval 0.9 to 3.5) toward an increase in mortality was noted in the Pimobendan in Congestive Heart Failure (PICO) trial, which was conducted in subjects with mild to moderate HF.[170]

LEVOSIMENDAN. This drug is available in some European countries in intravenous form. Levosimendan was discovered as part of a screening strategy for identifying compounds that bind to a troponin C affinity column,[192] and levosimendan does bind to free troponin C. However, other data indicate that levosimendan does not bind to the human troponin C-troponin I complex,[193] which is the natural state of the regulatory thin filament proteins.

Levosimendan is in clinical development in the United States in intravenous form. Intravenous levosimendan has been evaluated in two clinical trials. In an acute myocardial infarction study conducted in Russia, patients were randomly assigned to receive levosimendan or a placebo.[194] Not surprisingly, the positive inotropic agent produced better circulatory support, with the secondary endpoints of death, worsening HF, or development of HF being lower in prevalence during the 6-hour infusion period and at 24 hours as well.[194] Only the highest dose (0.4 μg/kg/min) of levosimendan exacerbated myocardial ischemia.[194] In another study in which approximately 40 percent of the subjects were taking beta blockers, levosimendan performed better than dobutamine in terms of hemodynamic response.[195] This result is also expected because by virtue of their respective sites of action, beta blockade would inhibit the response to dobutamine but not to levosimendan. In this study, the statistical advantage of levosimendan over dobutamine was confined to patients receiving beta blockade.[195] These studies do not provide evidence that levosimendan is superior to other PDEI-positive inotropic agents currently available in intravenous form.

In the studies with levosimendan, the hemodynamic and even clinical benefits have extended beyond the duration of the infusion period.[194,195] The explanation for this is a hemodynamically active metabolite with an elimination half-life of 70 to 80 hours.[196] Sustained action beyond the duration of infusion could be an advantage for levosimendan as an intermittently administered agent delivered to outpatients but could be a disadvantage in terms of short-term use when drug action of an inotropic agent is not required or desired beyond a brief period of support.

Neurohormonal Inhibitors

Without question, the greatest advance in the treatment of chronic HF has been the application of agents that inhibit harmful neurohormonal systems that are activated to support the failing heart (see Chaps. 19 and 21). This generally useful paradigm had multiple origins, including work done in the late 1970s and early 1980s that documented the nature and extent of neurohormonal activation in chronic HF,[197] the association of systemic neurohormonal activation with adverse outcomes,[198] observations in the failing human heart that excessive adrenergic activation produces harmful biological effects,[113,199] and astute clinical observations regarding the degree of improvement effected by inhibitors of the adrenergic[200-202] and renin-angiotensin[203,204] systems. By the middle to late 1980s, influential commentaries on the validity of the "neurohormonal hypothesis" were being articulated,[197,205] and all of these developments ultimately culminated in the performance of large-scale clinical trials that demonstrated that inhibition of the renin-angiotensin[206,207] (see Fig. 24–6) and adrenergic[208-212] (see Fig. 24–5) systems improved the natural history of chronic HF caused by primary or secondary cardiomyopathies.

The general mechanisms by which neurohormonal activation worsens and neurohormonal inhibition improves the natural history of myocardial dysfunction and remodeling are discussed in Chapter 21. In essence, multiple neurohormonal signaling pathways, such as beta$_1$-, beta$_2$-, and alpha$_1$-adrenergic receptor,[118] angiotensin II AT$_1$ receptor,[213] endothelin-1 ET$_A$ receptor,[214] and tumor necrosis factor-alpha receptor pathways,[215] are activated in the failing heart and promote maladaptive growth, remodeling, and progressive myocardial dysfunction.[216] Inhibition of these systems may prevent or reverse these adverse biological processes, thereby leading to improvement in the natural history of HF. Therapy targeting individual neurohormonal or cytokine systems is now discussed.

Inhibitors of the Renin-Angiotensin-Aldosterone System (see also Chap. 38)

Angiotensin-Converting Enzyme Inhibitors

ACEIs were the first consistent and substantial success story of medical therapy improving the natural history of chronic HF, and this class of neurohormonal inhibitors remains a mainstay in HF treatment. ACEIs were originally developed within the vasodilator paradigm, but when their clinical results proved to be out of proportion to their relatively weak vasodilator effects, it became apparent that another mechanism was operative. That general mechanism, as elucidated by the Pfeffers' laboratory in elegant studies in animal models of myocardial infarction [217,218] and then in humans[203,204] including those with chronic HF,[219] is the prevention of angiotensin II–mediated remodeling.[216]

RATIONALE AND MECHANISM OF ACTION. Figure 23–8 shows the pathways for angiotensin II formation, which occurs systemically as well as locally in cardiac and vascular tissues. Note that generation of angiotensin II is accomplished by two pathways, one that uses converting enzyme found in high abundance in endothelium and one that uses the protease chymase, which is found in interstitial cells. Transmyocardial studies in the intact human heart have indicated that more than 80 percent of the generation of angiotensin II is by the ACE pathway,[220] but studies in isolated human heart preparations[221] and in model systems[222] have emphasized the contribution of the chymase pathway. If the chymase pathway is important in producing ventricular remodeling in the failing heart, angiotensin receptor-blocking agents (ARBs) would be more effective than ACEIs in decreasing angiotensin II signaling. If, on the other hand, ACEIs are just as effective clinically as ARBs, by inference, the ACE pathway is the dominant mechanism for generating angiotensin II in the failing heart. Finally, if ACEIs are superior to ARBs, additional properties of ACEIs, such as increasing bradykinin,[223] are presumably responsible. From the results of clinical trials with ACEIs and ARBs in chronic HF (see later), it appears that ACEIs are at least as effective as ARBs, supporting the idea that the ACE pathway is dominant in angiotensin II formation in the failing human heart.

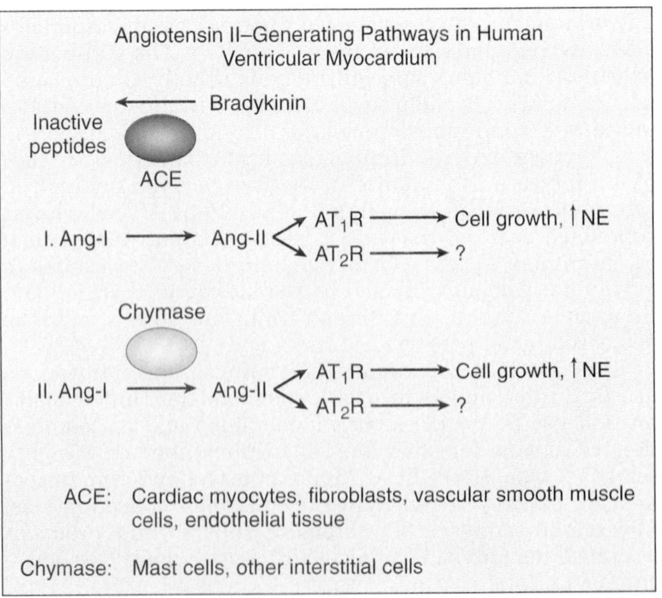

FIGURE 23–8 Pathways of angiotensin II formation. ACE = angiotensin-converting enzyme; Ang-1 = angiotensin I; AT$_1$R = angiotensin II type 1 receptor; AT$_2$R = angiotensin II type 2 receptor; NE = norepinephrine.

As shown in Table 23–6, increased levels of angiotensin II have several adverse effects on the cardiovascular system, including cardiac myocyte hypertrophy, myocyte apoptosis, prejunctional facilitation of norepinephrine release, and mitogenic effects on fibroblasts. Most, if not all, of these effects are mediated by the AT_1 subtype. In addition, most of these biological effects of angiotensin II contribute to the development of hypertrophy and remodeling.

CLINICAL OBSERVATIONS. Two types of studies demonstrate the consistent efficacy of ACEIs in HF: post-myocardial infarction studies and clinical trials in chronic HF. As shown in Table 23–7, more of the former types of studies than the latter types have been conducted. All placebo-controlled chronic HF trials, with the exception of the "asymptomatic" Studies of Left Ventricular Dysfunction (SOLVD) Prevention Study,[224] demonstrated a reduction in mortality. As can be observed in Table 23–7, the Class IV Cooperative North Scandinavian Enalapril Survival Study (CONSENSUS I) had a much larger effect size than the SOLVD Treatment Trial, which in turn had a larger effect size than the SOLVD Prevention Trial. Although only these three placebo-controlled mortality trials have been conducted in patients with chronic HF, it seems obvious that ACEIs reduce mortality in direct relation to the degree of severity of chronic HF. Although not placebo controlled, the V-HeFT-II trial provided evidence that ACEIs improve the natural history of HF through mechanisms other than vasodilation, inasmuch as subjects treated with enalapril had significantly lower mortality than subjects treated with the nonneurohormonal inhibitor-vasodilator combination of hydralazine plus isosorbide dinitrate.[63] Although only one ACEI, enalapril, has been used in placebo-controlled mortality trials in chronic HF, as can be observed in Table 23–7, multiple ACEIs have proven to be more or less equally effective when administered in oral form within the first week of the ischemic event in post-myocardial infarction trials.[225-227] ACEIs also have a proven track record in preventing HF in two settings: enalapril in asymptomatic LV dysfunction (see Table 23–7)[224] and ramipril in cardiovascular at-risk patients without LV dysfunction.[228] These observations support the conclusion that the effects of ACE inhibition on the natural history of chronic HF, post-myocardial infarction LV dysfunction, or

TABLE 23–6 Biological Responses Mediated by Angiotensin II Receptors in the Human Cardiovascular System

Biologic Response	Receptor Mediation
Cardiac myocyte growth	AT_1
Positive inotropic response (minimal)	AT_1
Myocyte apoptosis	AT_1, AT_2
Aldosterone release	AT_1
Norepinephrine release	AT_1
Cardiac myocyte toxicity	Beta-adrenergic via norepinephrine release
Fibroblast proliferation	AT_1
Smooth muscle proliferation	AT_1
Vasoconstriction	AT_1

TABLE 23–7 Crude, Annualized Mortality Rates in Renin-Angiotensin-Aldosterone System Inhibitor Placebo-Controlled Trials Conducted in Chronic Heart Failure (HF) from Systolic Dysfunction, Left Ventricular (LV) Dysfunction after Myocardial Infarction, or in Patients Without LV Dysfunction at Risk for HF*

Trial Name	Agent	NYHA Class	No. of Subjects Enrolled	12-Month Placebo Mortality (%)	12-Month Effect Size (%)	*P* Value 12 Months (Full F/U)
ACEIs						
CHF						
CONSENSUS-I[217]	Enalapril	IV	253	52	↓31	0.01 (0.003)
SOLVD-Rx[218]	Enalapril	I-III	2569	15	↓21	0.02 (0.004)
SOLVD-Asx[235]	Enalapril	I, II	4228	5	0	0.82 (0.30)
Totals		I-IV	7050	11	↓16	0.02
POST-MI						
SAVE[236]	Captopril	—	2231	12	↓18	0.11 (0.02)
AIRE[237]	Ramipril	—	1986	20	↓22	0.01 (0.002)
TRACE[238]	Trandolapril	—	1749	26	↓16	0.046 (0.001)
Totals			5966	19	↓18	0.001
ARBs						
CHF						
Val-HeFT[253]	Valsartan	II-IV	5010	9	0	NS
CHARM-Alternative[254]	Candesartan	II-IV	2028	8	↓14	NS
CHARM-Added[255]	Candesartan	II-IV	2548	8	↓12	NS
Totals		II-IV	9586	9	↓6	NS
Aldosterone Antagonists						
CHF						
RALES[18]	Spironolactone	III, IV	1663	24	↓25	(<0.001)
POST-MI						
EPHESUS[21]	Eplerenone	I	6632	12	↓15	(0.005)

AIRE = Acute Infarction Ramipril Efficacy; CHARM = candesartan in heart failure—assessment of reduction in mortality and morbidity; CHF = congestive heart failure; CONSENSUS = Cooperative North Scandinavian Enalapril Survival Study; EPHESUS = Eplerenone Post-Acute Myocardial Infarction Heart Failure Efficacy and Survival Study; MI = myocardial infarction; RALES = Randomized Aldactone Evaluation Study; SAVE = Survival and Ventricular Enlargement; SOLVD = Studies of Left Ventricular Dysfunction; TRACE = Trandolapril Cardiac Evaluation; Val-HeFT = Valsartan Heart Failure Trail.

*Twelve-month mortality rates are taken from survival curves when data not directly available in published material.

TABLE 23–8 Properties of Widely Used Angiotensin-Converting Enzyme Inhibitors

Agent	Half-Life (hr)	Recommended Starting Dose (mg)	Recommended Target Dose (mg)	Relative Tissue Binding
Captopril	3	6.25	50 t.i.d.	+
Enalapril	11	2.5-5	10 b.i.d.	+
Lisinopril	12	5	20 qd	+
Ramipril	9-18	2.5	5 b.i.d.	++
Quinapril	2 (25)	5	20 b.i.d.	+++
Trandolapril	6	1	1-2 b.i.d.	NA

NA = not available.

HF prevention in cardiovascular at-risk patients are class effects.

In summary, an ACEI is considered mandatory treatment in chronic HF, asymptomatic LV systolic dysfunction, or in the setting of cardiovascular disease with any risk factor for the development of HF. The doses employed should be at least the average dose used to lower mortality in HF or post-myocardial infarction trials (Table 23–8). The only consistent adverse effect noted with ACEIs is a low-level (5 percent greater than placebo) increase in cough. In such patients, an angiotensin II AT_1 receptor–blocking agent can be substituted.

Angiotensin II AT_1 Receptor-Blocking Agents

RATIONALE AND MECHANISM OF ACTION. It has been shown in numerous studies that ACEIs do not completely inhibit tissue-based RAASs[229] and that after several months of treatment, "escape" can occur with an increase in systemic angiotensin II[230] or aldosterone levels (see Fig. 23–8).[231] These observations set the stage for additional RAAS inhibitor strategies, including the use of ARBs and aldosterone antagonists.

Multiple ARBs approved for the treatment of hypertension are now on the market in the United States (Table 23–9). Three of these, losartan, valsartan, and candesartan, have been extensively evaluated in the setting of HF. The rationale for the use of these agents in HF is derived from information presented in Table 23–6, showing that virtually all the adverse biological effects relevant to a failing, remodeled heart are mediated by the AT_1 receptor. Moreover, ARBs antagonize the effects of angiotensin II regardless of its origin (through the ACE or chymase pathway; see Fig. 23–8). All these compounds are selective, high-affinity antagonists of AT_1 receptors.

Hemodynamic studies and studies with ARBs in HF have demonstrated effects that are similar to those of ACEIs; that is, these agents reduce pulmonary wedge and pulmonary artery pressure moderately, are mild preload reducers, and increase cardiac output.[232-234] Heart rate is not affected unless baroreflexes are excessively activated by hypotension. Maximum exercise time is also improved to a similar degree with each type of RAS inhibitor.[235,236] The combination of an ACEI and an ARB produces additive hemodynamic effects[237,238] as well as additive effects on prevention of remodeling.[239]

CLINICAL OBSERVATIONS. Clinical trial data on ARBs have, on balance, demonstrated that (1) in HF populations not treated with ACEIs, they are about as effective as ACEIs in reducing mortality[240-243] or mortality and morbidity, including patients intolerant of ACEIs (see Fig. 24–6)[242,243]; (2) on a background of ACEIs, they reduce HF hospitalizations[242,243]; (3) when given in addition to ACEIs in general cohorts of patients with symptomatic HF, they have a modest beneficial[244] or no[242] effect on mortality (Table 23–7); and (4) in subgroups of patients receiving ACEIs and beta blockers they have been reported either to increase mortality[242] or to decrease HF hospitalizations and mortality.[244] In addition, in diastolic dysfunction the ARB candesartan has reduced hospitalizations for HF.[245] ARBs are well tolerated in HF populations and do not produce the most common side effect associated with ACEIs, cough.[240,241] In a large trial comparing the ACEI captopril and the ARB valsartan (the valsartan in acute myocardial infarction [VALIANT] trial) in patients with impaired LV function following acute myocardial infarction, no difference in mortality was observed.[246] Furthermore, the combination of these drugs produced no further reduction in mortality, although the number of adverse events increased.

As discussed in Chapter 24, the clinical trial data for ARBs in HF from systolic dysfunction currently support their use in ACE-intolerant patients, added to ACEIs in patients not treated with beta-blocking agents, and added to ACEIs and beta blockers in patients with preserved blood pressures. With regard to the last use, there may be a drug- or dose-specific aspect of ARB use,[242,244] and only candesartan has demonstrated benefit.[244]

Aldosterone Receptor Antagonists

RATIONALE AND MECHANISM OF ACTION. As discussed previously, aldosterone levels are not reduced by long-term treatment with ACEIs.[231] There are numerous lines of evidence that aldosterone produces harmful myocardial effects, including the promotion of fibrosis[247] and ventricular arrhythmias.[248] These effects are probably mediated through the mineralocorticoid receptor, which is supported by evidence in transgenic mice overexpressing an enzyme that leads to increased aldosterone receptor occupancy of this receptor.[249] In these experiments, mice developed a cardiomyopathy with increased interstitial fibrosis.[249] These observations provide the rationale for the use of aldosterone receptor antagonists as therapy in addition to ACE inhibition in HF.

CLINICAL OBSERVATIONS. The first evidence that this approach could produce a major clinical benefit was provided by the Randomized Aldactone Evaluation Study (RALES) trial,[18] which evaluated the addition of the competitive aldosterone antagonist spironolactone versus placebo to standard HF therapy in stage 3 (New York Heart Association [NYHA] Class III or IV) patients, the primary endpoint being all-cause mortality. As can be seen in Table 23–7, in RALES,[18] spironolactone produced a 30 percent reduction in total mortality when compared with placebo ($p = 0.001$). The beneficial effect of spironolactone appeared to be on both

TABLE 23–9 Properties of Widely Used Angiotensin Receptor Blockers			
Agent	Half-Life (hr)	Recommended Starting Dose (mg)	Recommended Target Dose (mg)
Losartan	2	25	50-100 qd
Valsartan	6	40	80-160 b.i.d.
Irbesartan	11-15	75	150 qd
Candesartan	9	4	16-32 qd
Telmisartan†	24	20	80 qd
Eprosartan	5-9	200	400 b.i.d.

*Indicates half-life of the active metabolite.
†Decreases digoxin clearance.

TABLE 23–10 Biological Responses Mediated by Adrenergic Receptors in the Human Heart	
Biological Response	Adrenergic Receptor Mediation
Positive inotropic response	β_1, β_2, α_1 (minimal)
Positive chronotropic response	β_1, β_2
Myocyte toxicity	$\beta_1 >> \beta_2$
Myocyte apoptosis	β_1
Cardiac myocyte growth	$\beta_1 >> \beta_2$, α_1
Fetal gene induction	$\beta_1 >> \beta_2$, α_1
Proarrhythmic	β_1, β_2, α_1

sudden and pump failure–related deaths. Although the mechanism behind the benefit of spironolactone has not been fully elucidated, prevention of extracellular matrix remodeling[247] and prevention of increasing potassium levels are leading contenders. In RALES, serum potassium levels were 0.3 mEq/liter higher in the spironolactone group than in the placebo group (p = 0.001),[18] which could have played a major role in reducing sudden or even pump failure–related deaths.

Although spironolactone was well tolerated in RALES,[18] it has antiandrogenic and progesterone-like effects and is associated with a small incidence of gynecomastia, impotence, and menstrual irregularities, which may lead to discontinuation. Newer generation aldosterone antagonists are associated with a much lower incidence of these adverse effects and should be considered for patients intolerant of spironolactone. Eplerenone[19,20] is a selective aldosterone inhibitor that has been evaluated in the Eplerenone Post-Acute Myocardial Infarction Heart Failure Efficacy and Survival Study (EPHESUS) (see Fig. 23–4).[21] Patients with LV ejection fractions less than 40 percent were randomly assigned 3 to 14 days after myocardial infarction to therapy with eplerenone or placebo. During a mean follow-up of 16 months, eplerenone significantly improved mortality (relative risk 0.85, 95 percent confidence interval 0.75 to 0.96, p = 0.008) (see Table 23–7). Gynecomastia, impotence, and breast tenderness were not increased by eplerenone.

Both spironolactone and eplerenone can produce hyperkalemia, particularly in patients with advanced HF with compromised renal function when administered on a background of ACE inhibition or in patients receiving potassium supplementation. For that reason, when initiating aldosterone antagonist therapy in a patient with HF, it is prudent to lower the level of potassium supplementation and check the potassium serum level frequently until a steady state of potassium balance has been achieved. In addition, in HF there is inadequate information regarding the efficacy of aldosterone antagonists when added to background therapy of ACEIs and beta blockers. It is likely that the presence of a beta blocker, because of its antirenin effects, further reduces the tolerability of aldosterone antagonists in patients with advanced HF; for example, in a clinical trial in which spironolactone was mandated background therapy along with ACEIs or ARBs and beta blockers, the proportion of patients who could tolerate spironolactone was only 55 percent.[250]

From the results of RALES[18] and EPHESUS,[21] a case can be made for all patients with HF related to systolic dysfunction being treated with an aldosterone antagonist, with eplerenone being used if endocrine-related side effects of spironolactone are observed.

Antiadrenergic Agents

Rationale and Mechanism of Action

Adrenergic Dysfunction in the Failing Human Heart (see also Chaps. 19 and 21)

The failing human heart is adrenergically activated to maintain cardiac performance over the short term by increasing contractility[251] and heart rate. In contrast, in the resting state, no adrenergic support occurs in normally functioning human left ventricles.[251] Multiple lines of evidence[252-255] indicate that it is increased cardiac adrenergic drive rather than an increase in circulating norepinephrine that is both ini-tially supportive and then ultimately damaging to the failing human heart. Norepinephrine, the adrenergic neurotransmitter, is a beta$_1$-selective agonist[256] with an affinity for beta$_1$ receptors that is approximately 20-fold greater than for beta$_2$ receptors and 10-fold greater than for alpha$_1$ receptors (see Table 23–5).

As shown in Table 23–10, human cardiac myocytes have three adrenergic receptors (beta$_1$, beta$_2$, and alpha$_1$) that are coupled to both beneficial and to harmful biological responses.[111,112,118,257] Beta-adrenergic receptors are coupled through the stimulatory G protein G_s to the effector enzyme adenylyl cyclase (see Fig. 23–6), which converts the substrate Mg-ATP to cAMP. cAMP is a positive inotropic and chronotropic second messenger and is also strongly growth promoting. In younger (<50 years) nonfailing human left or right ventricles, the beta$_1$/beta$_2$ ratio is 70 to 80:30 to 20,[257] but in failing[111,257] or older[258] human ventricles, 35 to 40 percent of the total number of beta receptors are beta$_2$ as a result of selective downregulation in the beta$_1$ subtype. Alpha$_1$ receptors are coupled through a different G protein (G_q) to the effector enzyme phospholipase C, which through the second messenger diacylglycerol activates the growth-promoting protein kinase C family. Because alpha$_1$ receptors are upregulated in the failing heart,[259,260] the cardiac myocyte adrenergic receptor profile changes from predominantly (>70 percent of the total adrenergic receptor population) beta$_1$ to more of a mixed, 2:1:1 (beta$_1$/beta$_2$/alpha$_1$) ratio in end-stage HF.[111,112,118] Beta$_2$ receptors are also present on adrenergic nerve terminals in the heart, where they facilitate norepinephrine release.[261] The beta$_3$ receptor may also be present in the human heart as a counterregulatory receptor coupled to the inhibitory G protein G_i,[262] and some evidence also existed for a beta$_4$ receptor[263]; however, this now appears to be discounted.

Cardiac Damage Induced by Receptor Activation

Norepinephrine is an exceptionally cardiotoxic substance that produces cardiac myocyte injury in concentrations found in the failing human heart. As shown in Table 23–5, norepinephrine is mildly $beta_1$ receptor selective (10- to 30-fold compared with the binding affinity to $beta_2$ receptors, 10-fold compared with $alpha_1$), and its cytotoxicity appears to be mediated through beta- rather than alpha-adrenergic receptors.[264] In transgenic mice, cardiac overexpression of human $beta_1$ receptors,[264-266] $beta_2$ receptors,[267,268] $G_{\alpha s}$,[269] or $G_{\alpha q}$[270] can produce an overtly cardiomyopathic phenotype and, ultimately, chamber dilation and systolic dysfunction. Although direct comparisons have yet to be made, it appears that approximately 10-fold higher levels of expression of human $beta_2$ versus $beta_1$ receptors are required to produce histopathology.[264,265,268] Overexpression of $G_{\alpha s}$ is also associated with increased markers of apoptosis, which can be produced in cardiac myocytes by norepinephrine exposure.[271,272] Norepinephrine-mediated apoptosis is mediated through $beta_1$ receptors,[272] and apoptosis is prominent in cardiac $beta_1$ receptor–overexpressing mice.[265] Finally, cardiac expression of a constitutively activated $alpha_1$ receptor produces concentric hypertrophy,[273] and cardiac overexpression of $alpha_{1C}$ receptors produces a cardiomyopathy.[274] These data from model systems incontrovertibly indicate that chronic adrenergic signaling is a harmful compensatory mechanism in the failing human heart. The data are quite convincing for chronic $beta_1$ receptor signaling and less convincing but likely for chronic $beta_2$ and $alpha_1$ receptor pathway activation. The compensatory as well as adverse effects of adrenergic signaling pathways are summarized in Figure 23–1 and Table 23–10.

Interestingly, when components of the beta-adrenergic–adenylyl cyclase–phospholamban phosphorylation pathway are transgenically manipulated beyond the level of $G_{\alpha s}$, no overt pathology is apparent despite marked and sustained increases in contractility.[146,266,275] This finding may mean that $G_{\alpha s}$-coupled cAMP-independent pathways that include calcium channel activation[276] may mediate the majority of myocardial damage in beta-adrenergic receptor– and $G_{\alpha s}$-overexpressing animals.

In the failing heart, beta-adrenergic signal transduction is reduced secondary to desensitization changes at the level of $beta_1$ and $beta_2$ receptors, the inhibitory G protein ($G_{\alpha i}$), and an enzyme responsible for modulating receptor activity by phosphorylation (beta-adrenergic receptor kinase) as well as by changes in expression of the adenylyl cyclase enzyme itself.[111,118,154-156,258,277,278] In an end-stage failing heart, 50 to 60 percent of the total signal-transducing potential is lost, but substantial signaling capacity remains.[116] These and other data from model systems[279] suggest that the beta-adrenergic receptor pathway desensitization changes present in the failing human heart are adaptive changes and that a potentially effective therapeutic strategy would be to add to this endogenous antiadrenergic strategy by inhibiting receptor signal transduction.[111,118,199,205,280]

Thus, the chronically increased adrenergic drive present in the failing human heart delivers adverse biological signals to the cardiac myocyte through $beta_1$-, $beta_2$-, and possibly $alpha_1$-adrenergic receptors. Elimination of these adverse signals is the fundamental reason for using antiadrenergic agents in the treatment of chronic HF.[118]

Beta-Adrenergic Receptor–Blocking Agents

Because of their clinical availability, beta-adrenergic blocking agents were the first antiadrenergic agents used to treat chronic HF.[200] Although three classes of beta blockers are now available for clinical use, only the "second-generation" $beta_1$ receptor–selective antagonists or the "third-generation" beta blocker-vasodilators are tolerated to an acceptable degree by subjects with chronic HF.[281] Second-generation compounds are tolerated because they do not block cardiac pre- or postjunctional $beta_2$ receptors,[118,261,281,282] and third-generation compounds are tolerated because their afterload-reducing properties mitigate the cardiac output–reducing effects of beta-adrenergic withdrawal.[118,281,283] The receptor-binding profiles of beta-blocking agents that have been used successfully to treat HF are given in Table 23–11.

Regardless of the type of beta-blocking agent used, the treatment approach that must be taken in subjects with chronic HF is to start with extremely low doses (1/8 to 1/16 of the target dose) (Table 23–12) and gradually increase the dose every 1 to 2 weeks until full beta-blocking doses are achieved.[281] When this approach is taken, more than 90 percent of subjects with mild to moderate (stage 2) and more than 70 percent of subjects with advanced (stage 3) HF can tolerate beta blockade. The general mechanism of action of beta blockade in the failing and adversely remodeled heart has been reviewed extensively.[112,118,216,284] Both second- and third-generation beta-blocking agents improve intrinsic systolic function and reverse remodeling in primary or secondary cardiomyopathy in a time-dependent fashion that begins after an initial period of myocardial depression related to withdrawal of beta-adrenergic support.[112,115,216] However, these effects are not uniform across all treated subjects, and

TABLE 23–11 Adrenergic Receptor Blocking Affinities of Beta-Blocking Agents in Human Receptors*

Generation/ Class	Compound	K($beta_1$)† (nM)	K($beta_2$) (nM)	$Beta_1$/$Beta_2$ Selectivity	K($alpha_1$) (nM)	$Beta_1$/$Alpha_1$ Selectivity
First/nonselective	Propranolol‡	4.1	8.5	2.1	—	—
Second/selective $beta_1$	Metoprolol	45	3,345	74	—	—
	Bisoprolol	121	14,390	119	—	—
Third/beta blocker–vasodilator	Carvedilol‡	4.0	29	7.3	9.4	2.4
	Bucindolol‡	3.6	5.0	1.4	238	66 (19)*
	Nebivolol	0.7	225	352	330	471

*Beta receptors are the average of data from radiological binding data in myocardial membranes and recombinant receptors, and inhibition in functional assays; $alpha_1$ receptors are from myocardial membranes. Metoprolol and bisoprolol data are from radiological binding data in myocardial membranes. Nebivolol data are from another laboratory, in guinea pig receptor preparations.[4]

†K($beta_1$) = average of high-affinity dissociation constant determined from ^{125}I-CYP competition curves in human ventricular myocardial membranes, dissociation constant determined from competition curves in transfected cells expressing recombinant human $beta_1$ receptors, and dissociation constant determined from inhibition of isoproterenol-mediated stimulation of muscle contraction in preparations of nonfailing human heart. K($beta_2$) = average of low-affinity dissociation constant determined from ^{125}I-CYP competition curves, dissociation constant determined from simple curve fitting in transfected cells expressing recombinant human $beta_2$ receptors, and dissociation constant determined from inhibition of isoproterenol-mediated stimulation of adenylyl cyclase in membrane preparations of human heart. K($alpha_1$) = dissociation constant determined from ^{125}I-BE2254 competition curves in human ventricular myocardial membranes.

‡Based on an $alpha_1$ K_i of 69 nM in human saphenous vein ring segments (Tackett RL, personal communication, 1999).

TABLE 23–12 Starting and Target Doses for Beta Blockers

Agent	Starting Dose	Target Dose <75-85 kg	Target Dose ≥75-85 kg
Metoprolol CR/XL	12.5 or 25 mg PO qd*	200 mg PO qd	200 mg PO qd
Bisoprolol†	1.25 mg PO qd	5 mg PO qd	10 mg PO qd
Carvedilol	3.125 mg PO b.i.d.	25 mg PO b.i.d.	50 mg PO b.i.d.

*Starting dose should be half of above if disease is Class III or IV or if the patient has severe right-sided heart failure or is tenuous.

†Not approved by the Food and Drug Administration for heart failure in the United States.

some subjects may deteriorate and have an adverse clinical response to beta blockade.[285] The specific mechanism by which beta blockers produce a time-dependent improvement in systolic function and reversal of remodeling has also been investigated.[286,287] In the failing, remodeled human heart, both second- and third-generation beta-blocking agents produce changes in myocardial gene expression that would be expected to increase systolic function and reverse remodeling.[286] These changes in gene expression fall within a family of genes that constitute the so-called fetal gene program, shown several years ago to be associated with the development of pathological hypertrophy and systolic dysfunction in rodent models of cardiomyopathy.[288]

As discussed earlier and shown in Table 23–10, the beta$_1$ receptor pathways have much greater pathological potential than the beta$_2$ or alpha$_1$ pathways, and as shown in Table 23–5, norepinephrine, the adrenergic neurotransmitter, is a beta$_1$-selective agonist. These two realities mean that beta$_1$-selective blocking agents have equal or nearly equal therapeutic potential compared with agents that block beta$_1$, beta$_2$, and alpha$_1$ receptor pathways.[256] Accordingly, a study that compared gene expression changes between equal beta$_1$-blocking doses of the second-generation compound metoprolol and the third-generation beta blocker carvedilol found no difference in their respective abilities to reverse partially fetal gene induction.[286]

Unlike members of the ACEI, ARB, and aldosterone antagonist classes of neurohormonal inhibitors, beta-blocking agents are more diverse in their pharmacological effects and they are therefore discussed individually. However, as shown in Table 23–11, all beta blockers have in common the property of competitive antagonism of beta$_1$-adrenergic receptors.

Metoprolol

Metoprolol is a second-generation beta$_1$ receptor–selective blocking agent with an approximately 75-fold higher affinity for human beta$_1$- than beta$_2$-adrenergic receptors. Metoprolol, in its long-acting, controlled-release form (metoprolol succinate, CR/XL), is approved for the treatment of HF in the United States. Metoprolol is also approved for hypertension and ischemic heart disease indications.

The first placebo-controlled multicenter trial with a beta-blocking agent was the Metoprolol in Dilated Cardiomyopathy (MDC) trial, which used the shorter acting tartrate preparation at a target dose of 50 mg three times a day.[208] The MDC trial compared metoprolol tartrate with placebo in subjects with symptomatic HF caused by idiopathic dilated cardiomyopathy. The sample size estimate was based on an expected 50 percent reduction by metoprolol in the combined endpoint of all-cause mortality and deterioration of the patient to the point of requiring listing for heart transplantation. The MDC trial had in addition numerous prespecified secondary endpoints, including mortality alone, number of hospitalizations, LV function, quality of life, and exercise tolerance.[208] In the MDC trial, metoprolol at an average dose of 108 mg/d reduced the prevalence of the primary endpoint by 34 percent, which was not quite statistically significant ($p = 0.058$).[208] The benefit was due entirely to a reduction by metoprolol in the morbidity component of the primary endpoint (a reduction of 90 percent), with no favorable trends in the mortality component of the primary endpoint. In addition, when compared with placebo, metoprolol improved LV function, quality of life, number of hospitalizations, and exercise tolerance at 12 months.[208]

THE MERIT-HF TRIAL. Despite the salutary clinical effects demonstrated for metoprolol tartrate in MDC,[288] this agent was not selected by at least two trial steering committees (BEST and MERIT-HF) for use in a phase III, placebo-controlled mortality trial, primarily because of its pharmacokinetic properties. Metoprolol tartrate given at a 50-mg dose has relatively short elimination and pharmacological half-lives in non–slow metabolizer subjects (respectively 3 to 4 hours and 6 hours), which ideally necessitates dosing three times a day. Although it is possible to increase the metoprolol tartrate dose to attain twice-daily beta$_1$ receptor blockade,[286] higher (100 mg) doses produce large peak blood levels that may produce adverse effects. At lower doses (≤50 mg twice a day), the short pharmacological half-life and rapid receptor offset kinetics[289] of metoprolol tartrate mean that a "beta blocker withdrawal" syndrome is more likely to occur, especially if doses are missed or delayed, a situation that could predispose patients with HF to sudden death. Thus, a more efficacious formulation of metoprolol was developed, metoprolol CR/XL, which because of its controlled-release profile has operational elimination and pharmacological half-lives of 12 to 15 hours plus very shallow, near-plateau plots of plasma concentration versus time.[290]

The steering committee of the Metoprolol CR/XL Randomized Interventional Trial in Congestive Heart Failure (MERIT-HF) therefore selected the succinate continuous release, coated metoprolol succinate pellet formulation for use in a placebo-controlled mortality trial.[291] MERIT-HF was stopped prematurely because of a 34 percent reduction in mortality in the metoprolol arm (Table 23–13; see Fig. 24–5).[292] MERIT-HF enrolled 3991 subjects with ischemic and nonischemic dilated cardiomyopathy who had Classes II to IV HF.[292] The average dose of metoprolol achieved in MERIT-HF was larger than in the MDC trial, 159[212] versus 108[208] mg. The majority (97 percent) of patients enrolled in MERIT-HF were categorized as having Class II or III HF, and on the basis of the annualized mortality rate of 11 percent in the placebo group and the baseline LV ejection fraction of 28 percent, this landmark clinical trial[212] enrolled subjects with mild to moderate HF and moderate to severe systolic dysfunction. Notably, in MERIT-HF, mortality from sudden death or progressive pump failure was reduced.[212] In addition, mortality was reduced across most demographic groups, including older versus younger subjects, nonischemic versus ischemic etiology, and lower versus higher ejection fractions.[212] However, almost no mortality reduction was noted in the relatively small number of female subjects enrolled (23 percent of the total),[212] which suggests that gender may influence the response to beta blockade in HF populations.

The CR/XL preparation used in MERIT-HF produces a relatively constant blood level of metoprolol for 24 hours, but the bioavailability of the CR preparation is approximately 70 percent that of the conventional formulation. However, when compared with 50 mg twice daily of the conventional formulation, 100 mg/d of the CR preparation produces similar trough levels and average degrees of reduction in exercise heart rate, indicating bioequivalence of the two preparations. The reduced fluctuation in blood levels for the CR versus the conventional formulation provides the potential for improved tolerability of the CR formulation in patients with HF. In addition, as discussed previously, the much more shallow slope of the CR plasma concentration curve at the end of the dosing interval would theoretically reduce the potential of producing a beta blocker withdrawal effect. Although these differences in pharmacokinetics could account for greater efficacy of the CR preparation in reducing mortality, a direct comparison of metoprolol tartrate with the CR succinate preparation in subjects with chronic HF indicated no obvious difference in LV function or clinical improvement between the two preparations.[292]

A mortality trial (Carvedilol or Metoprolol European Trial [COMET]) comparing metoprolol tartrate with carvedilol demonstrated 17 percent greater mortality reduction in favor of carvedilol, with respective mean daily doses of the two beta blockers being 85 and 42 mg.[293] This

TABLE 23–13 Beta Blocker Trials Conducted in Chronic Heart Failure, with 12-Month Mortality Rates Taken from Survival Curves When Data Not Directly Available in Published Material

Trial Name	Agent	NYHA Class	Heart Failure Stage, 1-4*	No. of Subjects Enrolled	12-Month Placebo Mortality (%)	12-Month Effect Size (%)
Stage 2 Populations of Patients						
CIBIS-I	Bisoprolol	"III,IV"	2	641	11	↓20
Carvedilol U.S.	Carvedilol	II,III	2	1,094	10	↓66
CIBIS-II	Bisoprolol	"III,IV"	2	2,647	13	↓33
MERIT-HF	Metoprolol CR	II-IV	2	3,991	11	↓35
Stage 3 Populations of Patients						
BEST	Bucindolol	III,IV	3	2,708	17	↓10[†]
COPERNICUS	Carvedilol	"Severe HF"	3	2,289	18	↓38
Beta blocker totals		II-IV	2-3	13,370	14	↓32
Post-MI Populations of Patients						
CAPRICORN	Carvedilol	I	1	1,959	11	↓23
BEAT	Bucindolol	I	1	343	21	↓12

BEAT = bucindolol evaluation in acute myocardial infarction trial; BEST = Beta Blocker Evaluation of Survival Trial; CAPRICORN = Carvedilol Post-Infarct Survival Control in Left Ventriular Dysfunction; CIBIS = Cardiac Insufficiency Bisoprolol Study; COPERNICUS = Carvedilol Prospective Randomized Cumulative Survival; MERIT-HF = Metoprolol CR/XL Randomized Interventional Trial in Congestive Heart Failure; NYHA = New York Heart Association.

*See Chapter 21.

[†]Effect size at 2 years.

relatively low average dose of metoprolol also produced less heart rate or blood pressure reduction than carvedilol.[293] In view of the fact that in MERIT-HF the degree of mortality reduction produced by metoprolol CR/XL in the entire cohort[212] as well as in a subpopulation with "severe HF"[294] was essentially identical to that produced by carvedilol in the Carvedilol Prospective Randomized Cumulative Survival (COPERNICUS)[295] trial (see Table 23–13 and Fig. 24–9), at least some of the differential efficacy of carvedilol and metoprolol in COMET was probably due to the lower beta$_1$-blocking doses of immediate-release metoprolol tartrate rather than to an absolute difference in efficacy between metoprolol and carvedilol.[256]

Bisoprolol

Bisoprolol is a second-generation beta$_1$ receptor–selective blocking agent with approximately 120-fold higher affinity for human beta$_1$ versus beta$_2$ receptors (see Table 23–12). Bisoprolol has long elimination (9 to 12 hours in healthy subjects, probably longer in patients with HF) and pharmacological (12 to 14 hours) half-lives, making it suitable for once-daily dosing.[296] Bisoprolol is approved for the treatment of hypertension in the United States and for HF or hypertension in Europe.

The first trial performed with bisoprolol was the Cardiac Insufficiency Bisoprolol Study I (CIBIS-I) trial,[297] which was a placebo-controlled trial of the effects of bisoprolol on mortality in subjects with symptomatic ischemic or nonischemic cardiomyopathy treated for an average follow-up of 22.8 months (see Table 23–13). This trial, sample sized on an unrealistically high expected event rate in the control group, ended up with a statistically insignificant, 20 percent mortality reduction.[297] In addition, the benefit in this trial was confined to subjects with nonischemic cardiomyopathy.[297] Despite the lack of overall statistical significance in CIBIS-I, the reduction in mortality was similar to what has been accomplished with ACEIs and was viewed as encouraging. The results prompted a follow-up trial, CIBIS-II,[211] with more conservative effect size estimates and sample size calculations.

The CIBIS-II trial was stopped by the Data and Safety Monitoring Committee 18 months early because of a 32 percent reduction ($p < 0.001$) in all-cause mortality (see Table 23–13) in the bisoprolol-treated group (see Fig. 24–5).[211] CIBIS-II enrolled 2647 patients with Class III or IV HF caused by ischemic and nonischemic cardiomyopathy; the median follow-up was 1.3 years. In addition to the reduction in mortality, bisoprolol reduced the number of hospitalizations (by 20 percent) and cardiovascular deaths (by 29 percent).[211] In CIBIS-II,[211] deaths classified as sudden were statistically reduced (by 44 percent) in the bisoprolol group, whereas pump failure deaths were nonsignificantly reduced by 26 percent.

This trend toward a greater reduction in sudden versus pump failure deaths was opposite to that obtained in CIBIS-I.[211,297] Another difference between CIBIS-I and CIBIS-II was the effect on ischemic versus nonischemic cardiomyopathy, which also demonstrated opposite trends. In CIBIS-I,[297] the reduction in mortality in the nonischemic group was 47 percent (p = 0.01), whereas in patients with a history of myocardial infarction, a trend toward an increase in mortality (by 11 percent) was noted in the bisoprolol group. One possible explanation for the differences between the CIBIS-I and CIBIS-II trials is the average dose of bisoprolol used; in CIBIS-II the target dose was 10 mg/d,[211] whereas in CIBIS-I it was 5 mg/d.[297]

Although CIBIS-II enrolled patients with Class III (>90 percent of the total) or Class IV symptoms, the annualized placebo mortality was only 13.2 percent (see Table 23–13).[211] This mortality rate is similar to that found in the enalapril arm of the SOLVD Treatment Trial[207] (see Table 23–7), which was composed of 68 percent Class I and II patients. In addition, the average blood pressure of patients enrolled in CIBIS-II was 130/80 mm Hg, which is higher than the blood pressures of the SOLVD patients[207] or the patients enrolled in the U.S. carvedilol trials,[209] who were approximately 50:50 Class II and III. A relatively large proportion of CIBIS-II patients were enrolled in Eastern Europe and Russia, where practice patterns, HF etiology, or symptom interpretation may not be comparable to that in Western Europe and the United States. Nevertheless, the results of CIBIS-II were internally consistent through all major demographic groups,[211] and the impressive results constitute a landmark clinical trial in the development of beta blockade as therapy for chronic HF.

Carvedilol

Carvedilol is currently approved for the treatment of chronic HF in the United States; it is also approved in most other countries. As noted in Table 23–11, carvedilol is a minimally $beta_1$ receptor–selective beta-blocking agent that has high affinity for $alpha_1$-adrenergic receptors as well as ancillary antioxidant action.[298] Because carvedilol is a potent vasodilator, its side effect profile on initiation of therapy and during uptitration is different from that of highly $beta_1$-selective second-generation agents, with orthostatic symptoms being more prominent.[281] At low doses (≤6.25 mg twice daily), carvedilol may exhibit some $beta_1$ selectivity in humans with HF.[299] At higher target doses, carvedilol blocks all three adrenergic receptors coupled to hypertrophy and other adverse biological effects ($beta_1$, $beta_2$, and $alpha_1$ receptors; see Table 23–11) that contribute to remodeling and myocardial dysfunction in the failing human heart.

In addition, because it blocks prejunctional $beta_2$ receptors, carvedilol mildly reduces cardiac adrenergic drive.[300] Perhaps because of its comprehensive antiadrenergic action, the beneficial effects of carvedilol on myocardial function and reversal of remodeling are consistent and substantial.[300-306]

PHARMACODYNAMICS. Carvedilol is a highly lipophilic beta blocker that is stereospecifically metabolized by the liver. The preferential metabolism of the *S* isomer means that *R* isomer concentrations are approximately 2.5 times higher in plasma, and this effect may be even greater in slow metabolizers.[118] The *S* isomer of carvedilol has an affinity constant (K_D) for human cardiac $beta_1$ receptors of 0.4 nM, and the *R* isomer has a K_D of 26 nM (unpublished data) and a net (directly measured) K_D of the racemate of 4 nM (see Table 23-11). The *S* and *R* isomers have comparable K_D values for the human cardiac $alpha_1$ receptor of 9.4 nM. This means that at 2.5-fold higher plasma and presumably myocardial levels of the *R* versus the *S* isomer, the degrees of $beta_1$ and $alpha_1$ receptor blockade are approximately equal, which is what is observed clinically. Carvedilol has an elimination half-life of 4 to 6 hours in normal volunteers or hypertensive subjects, which necessitates twice-daily dosing.[307] However, carvedilol has very slow receptor offset kinetics,[289] the likely explanation for a third compartment with a 14.5-hour elimination half-life observed after intravenous administration. As a result, carvedilol is less prone to beta receptor withdrawal phenomena on dose interruption.

DOSE-RESPONSE RESULTS. Unlike the case of other beta-blocking agents approved for the treatment of HF, there is extensive dose-response information on the efficacy and safety of carvedilol. The Multicenter Oral Carvedilol Heart Failure Assessment (MOCHA) trial[210] demonstrated LV functional and clinical superiority of 25 mg of carvedilol twice daily over 6.25 mg twice daily but clearly defined efficacy of 6.25 mg twice daily compared with placebo. In addition, most,[308-310] but not all,[311] studies comparing carvedilol with $beta_1$-selective antagonists have found at least trends in favor of quantitatively greater effects for carvedilol. On the other hand, in these studies the degree of $beta_1$ receptor blockade, as assessed by exercise heart rate inhibition, has generally been greater with carvedilol.[310] Even if carvedilol does produce a slightly greater degree of improvement in myocardial function and reversal of remodeling, as discussed earlier, it is not yet clear whether this superiority translates into better clinical results in view of the excellent results of $beta_1$-selective compounds in the MERIT-HF[212] and CIBIS-II[211] trials. The COMET trial described previously did show a small advantage (by 17 percent) for carvedilol versus immediate-release metoprolol tartrate for mortality reduction, but heart rate data also indicated a greater degree of $beta_1$ blockade by carvedilol,[293] and so this trial cannot be interpreted as demonstrating superior efficacy of carvedilol versus metoprolol. Data from the MOCHA trial[210] and from CIBIS I[297] and CIBIS II[211] strongly suggest that the responses to beta blockade in terms of survival and improvements in LV ejection fraction are dependent on dose and degree of beta blockade, and the COMET results are probably another example of this.[256]

CLINICAL TRIALS. The database of placebo-controlled clinical trials for carvedilol is the most extensive for any beta blocker in chronic HF. To date, 4037 patients have been enrolled in nine randomized, placebo-controlled phase II and III clinical trials in chronic HF,[209,210,295,300-302,312-316] plus one trial involving 1959 patients after myocardial infarction or LV dysfunction (see Table 23–13).[317] The phase III U.S. Carvedilol Trials Program, composed of four individual trials managed by single Steering and Data and Safety Monitoring committees, was stopped prematurely by the Data and Safety Monitoring Committee because of a highly significant ($p < 0.0001$) 65 percent reduction in mortality by carvedilol versus placebo across all four trials.[209] In addition, one individual trial (MOCHA) demonstrated a highly statistically significant, 73 percent reduction in mortality.[210] However, because these trials were relatively short term and the number of events was small, the data from MOCHA or the rest of the U.S. Carvedilol Trials Program were not considered by the FDA to be conclusive for an indication of mortality reduction. Carvedilol was originally approved by the FDA for delaying progression of the myocardial disease process and lowering the combined risk of morbidity plus mortality on the basis of data from the carvedilol U.S. trials[210,312-314] and then later approved for mortality reduction on the basis of the COPERNICUS trial[295] results.

The COPERNICUS trial investigated "severe" HF with no documentation of NYHA functional class.[295] Patients qualifying by symptoms had to be clinically euvolemic and have an LV ejection fraction less than 25 percent. Compared with placebo, carvedilol reduced the mortality risk at 12 months by 38 percent (see Table 23–13)[295] and the risk of death or HF hospitalization by 31 percent (see Fig. 24–5).[317]

Carvedilol has also been evaluated in a post-myocardial infarction trial in which patients had to exhibit LV dysfunction, the CAPRICORN trial.[316] Although carvedilol did not reduce the primary endpoint of mortality plus cardiovascular hospitalization, it did reduce total mortality (by 23 percent, $p = 0.03$), cardiovascular mortality (by 25 percent, $p < 0.05$), and nonfatal myocardial infarction (by 41 percent, $p = 0.014$).[316]

BUCINDOLOL*

PHARMACOLOGICAL PROPERTIES. Bucindolol is a completely nonselective third-generation beta-blocking agent with mild vasodilator activity that is probably due to weak $alpha_1$ receptor–blocking properties.[118] The pharmacokinetic properties of bucindolol are similar to those of carvedilol, except that there is no stereospecific metabolism. The mild vasodilator properties of bucindolol coupled with its low "inverse agonist" profile[118,318,319] make this beta blocker extremely well tolerated in HF patients,[281] including those with advanced HF.[320] Inverse agonism is the ability of a receptor antagonist to inactivate "active-state" receptors that are precoupled to G proteins and capable of transducing signals without agonist occupancy.[112] In the human heart, the percentage of such precoupled beta-adrenergic receptors identified by high-affinity agonist binding is on the order of 10 to 30 percent of the total. Antagonists with high degrees of inverse agonist activity such as metoprolol have a greater ability than bucindolol to inactivate these active-state receptors, which is probably why bucindolol is associated with less intrinsic myocardial depression and lowers 24-hour Holter-monitored heart rates less than metoprolol or carvedilol.[283] The latter property translates into less symptomatic bradycardia with bucindolol, which is why the BEST trial had a much lower heart rate exclusion criterion (50 beats/min)[320] than other beta blocker HF trials (typically 68 beats/min). Thus, a low inverse agonist profile is a property that increases the tolerability of a beta blocker in subjects with HF.

Although bucindolol has intrinsic sympathomimetic activity in some smaller animal species,[321] because of differences in the stoichiometry of receptor–G protein coupling between animal models and humans, bucindolol has no intrinsic sympathomimetic activity in failing[322-326] or nonfailing[326] functioning human myocardial preparations or in the intact failing human heart.[201,283] Finally, because of its potent $beta_2$ receptor–blocking properties coupled with only mild vasodilation, bucindolol is the only beta-blocking agent that has been shown to lower systemic adrenergic activity in subjects with HF.[210,320,327] Thus, the unique pharmacological

*Not approved by the FDA.

profile of bucindolol allows an agent with comprehensive antiadrenergic activity to be given to patients with advanced, stage 3 HF.

CLINICAL OBSERVATIONS. Bucindolol was the first beta-blocking agent shown to improve LV function in a placebo-controlled trial,[201] and it was the first beta-blocking agent shown to improve load-independent, intrinsic systolic function.[202] In those and subsequent phase II trials,[328,329] bucindolol was well tolerated, in marked contrast to previous[330,331] and subsequent[332] experience with the nonselective first-generation agent propranolol. Bucindolol was the second beta-blocking agent to be evaluated in a multicenter trial, in which bucindolol produced a dose-related improvement in LV function and a dose-unrelated prevention of deterioration in LV function in subjects with symptomatic ischemic and nonischemic cardiomyopathy treated for a 12-week period.[329] On the basis of these data, doses of bucindolol with very high degrees of beta blockade[329] (100 mg twice daily for subjects heavier than 75 kg, 50 mg twice daily for subjects less than 75 kg) were chosen for use in phase III trials.

THE BEST TRIAL. The largest of these phase III trials, the Beta Blocker Evaluation of Survival Trial (BEST),[320] randomly assigned 2708 subjects with advanced (Class III or IV) HF to placebo or bucindolol. As can be observed from the 12-month placebo mortality rates in Table 23-13, BEST[320] was conducted in subjects with advanced HF comparable to that investigated in COPERNICUS.[295] In the BEST subject population as a whole, bucindolol produced a statistically nonsignificant (p = 0.10), 10 percent reduction in total mortality that was heterogeneous with respect to race.[320] That is, the 76 percent of subjects in BEST who were not black had a statistically significant (p = 0.01), 19 percent reduction in mortality, whereas the 24 percent who were black had a nonsignificant trend for an increase (by 17 percent) in mortality (interaction p value < 0.05). Because BEST was the first beta blocker mortality trial to enroll a substantial percentage of black patients and is the first reported beta blocker study in advanced HF, it is uncertain whether the demographically heterogeneous findings can be extrapolated to other beta-blocking agents or to less advanced HF.

Of note is that in the U.S. Carvedilol Trials conducted in mild to moderate HF, an agent with a similar pharmacological profile produced a similar degree of improvement in LV function and clinical parameters in blacks and nonblacks.[333] In addition, in a small single-center experience[334] and in the small number of black subjects investigated in MERIT-HF,[335] metoprolol appeared to improve LV function[334] or reduce HF hospitalizations[325] in blacks to a similar degree as in whites. Therefore, the apparent lack of favorable effect of bucindolol in blacks in BEST may be due to the more advanced nature of HF investigated in BEST or the unique characteristics of the population of black patients in this trial. However, there are also potential drug-specific explanations for the bucindolol versus carvedilol or metoprolol data in blacks, including the greater degree of vasodilation with carvedilol being beneficial in an HF population with a high incidence of a history of hypertension, the beta$_1$ selectivity of metoprolol, or the norepinephrine-lowering property of bucindolol producing too much withdrawal of adrenergic support (see later for moxonidine) in the black population of BEST.

Norepinephrine lowering is a beta$_2$ receptor blockade–mediated response, and the black population of BEST had higher baseline systemic norepinephrine levels than nonblacks.[320] In addition, 67 percent of blacks in BEST were homozygous for an alpha$_{2C}$-adrenergic receptor loss-of-function polymorphism that is associated with an increased risk for developing HF, presumably because of increased adrenergic activity (Liggett S, Bristow MR, unpublished observations). This would could have predisposed black patients to being susceptible to the adverse sympatholytic effects of bucindolol.[327] From previous trials it is known that black hypertensives respond less well to beta-blocking agents or ACEIs[336] than nonblacks and that blacks with HF also do not respond well to ACEIs.[337] Thus, the most beneficial therapy for favorably affecting the natural history of HF, ACEIs and beta-blocking agents, may be less effective or even ineffective in a population group that represents 12 percent of the U.S. population.

In the BEST population as a whole, bucindolol produced statistically favorable effects on multiple secondary endpoints, including cardiovascular deaths, HF hospitalizations, the combined endpoint of mortality plus hospitalization, the need for cardiac transplantation, left and right ventricular function, and the incidence of myocardial infarction.[320,337] Bucindolol is the first beta blocker to demonstrate reduction in myocardial infarction in a population with chronic HF or ischemic cardiomyopathy.[337] In addition, in an immediate post-myocardial infarction trial, a study that was ended early by the sponsor, bucindolol did not significantly reduce mortality (reduction by 12 percent, p = not significant) but substantially (by at least 30 percent, $p < 0.05$) reduced all myocardial reinfarction–related endpoints and was well tolerated.[338] These data suggest that the sympatholytic and comprehensive antiadrenergic effects of bucindolol may have had heightened efficacy in certain subpopulations with LV dysfunction, such as those with active ischemia or even adrenergic receptor polymorphisms in which more powerful antiadrenergic action is desired.[339]

NEBIVOLOL*

Nebivolol is another third-generation beta blocker–vasodilator in development, which is approved in Europe for the treatment of hypertension. Nebivolol has limited but favorable experience[340,341] in HF trials. As can be observed in Table 23-12, nebivolol is markedly beta$_1$ selective and, as such, it is unique among third-generation compounds available or in development for HF. Another unique feature of nebivolol is that its vasodilatory action appears to be due to the generation of nitric oxide.[342] Interestingly, in a small study comparing nebivolol and placebo, nebivolol improved intrinsic systolic function and resulted in regression of hypertrophy in South African blacks with mild to moderate HF.[340] Although it is likely that the populations of patients differ substantially (such as more subjects with a history of hypertension in the carvedilol U.S. data), it is worth noting that carvedilol and nebivolol, both of which have substantial vasodilator properties, have shown some success in black populations with mild to moderate HF.

Class Recommendations for the Use of Beta-Blocking Agents in Chronic Heart Failure

Table 23–14 summarizes the class effects of beta-blocking agents, related to competitive antagonism of beta$_1$-adrenergic receptors, that have been observed in large, placebo-controlled HF clinical trials. Doses are shown in Table 23–11. Patients with mild to moderate compensated HF from nonischemic or ischemic dilated cardiomyopathy and NYHA Class II to III symptoms (stage 2 subjects) who are receiving standard treatment, including diuretics and ACEIs, and who do not have a contraindication to beta blockade, are candidates for treatment with a beta-blocking agent.[118,134,343,344] For the present, this group would include black patients, although the data supporting use in such patients are not extensive.

Euvolemic patients with advanced, Class III or IV (stage 3) HF should also be routinely treated with a beta blocker on the basis of data from the COPERNICUS[295] and MERIT-HF trials.[294] For patients with decompensated Class III or IV HF, beta blockers remain contraindicated, but this position could change pending the outcome of current trials such as Enoximone Plus Metoprolol in Subjects With Advanced Chronic Heart Failure (EMPOWER), which combines a type III PDEI with a beta blocker, on the basis of encouraging phase II data.[175]

When patients with HF reach a maintenance dose of a beta blocker, treatment should be maintained indefinitely because of the risk of deterioration after drug withdrawal.[345] As discussed earlier (see Positive Inotropic Agents) if it is necessary to treat a decompensated patient receiving maintenance beta blockade with a positive inotropic agent, a PDEI rather than a beta-agonist should be used because the hemodynamic effects of PDEIs are not antagonized by beta blockade.[119,120,158,174]

Which Beta-Blocker Should Be Used to Treat Chronic Heart Failure?

From the preceding discussions, it is apparent that beta-blocking agents are more pharmacologically diverse in mechanism of action than ACEIs or even ARBs. On the other hand, the predominance of the beta$_1$ receptor over other adrenergic receptor pathways in protein abundance, binding affinity for norepinephrine, and pathological potential leads to a thera-

*Not approved by the FDA.

TABLE 23–14 Class Clinical Effects of Beta-Adrenergic Blocking Agents in Chronic Heart Failure

Effect	Studies	Beta Blockers
Reduction in total mortality	CIBIS-II, MERIT-HF, COPERNICUS	Metoprolol CR/XL, bisoprolol, carvedilol
Reduction in CV mortality	CIBIS-II, MERIT-HF, COPERNICUS, BEST	Metoprolol CR/XL, bisoprolol, carvedilol, bucindolol
Reduction in CV or HF hospitalizations	MDC, MERIT-HF, CIBIS-II, U.S. Carvedilol, BEST	Metoprolol tartrate, metoprolol CR/XL, bisoprolol, carvedilol, bucindolol
Improved HF symptoms	MDC, MERIT-HF, CIBIS-II, U.S. Carvedilol	Metoprolol tartrate, metoprolol CR/XL, bisoprolol, carvedilol
Reduced need for cardiac transplantation	MDC, BEST	Metoprolol tartrate, bucindolol
Reduction in myocardial infarction	BEST	Bucindolol

BEST = Beta Blocker Evaluation of Survival Trial; CIBIS = Cardiac Insufficiency Bisoprolol Study; COPERNICUS = Carvedilol Prospective Randomized Cumulative Survival; CV = cardiovascular; HF = heart failure; MDC = Metoprolol in Dilated Cardiomyopathy; MERIT-HF = Metoprolol CR/XL Randomized Interventional Trial in Congestive Heart Failure.

peutic class effect for any competitive antagonist that binds with high affinity to $beta_1$-adrenergic receptors without possessing intrinsic sympathomimetic activity. Although data indicating that carvedilol is superior to metoprolol have been generated in direct comparison trials,[293,300] these trials were flawed by the use of a lower $beta_1$-blocking dose of the formulation of metoprolol in comparison with carvedilol.[256] However, the COMET trial[293] has demonstrated that lower $beta_1$-blocking doses of immediate-release metoprolol given twice daily are inferior to higher $beta_1$ receptor–blocking doses of carvedilol. Therefore, lower doses of shorter acting $beta_1$-selective blocking agents such as metoprolol tartrate or atenolol (for which there is no controlled experience in HF) *cannot be* recommended as equivalent to therapy with higher doses of carvedilol, controlled-release (CR/XL) metoprolol, or bisoprolol. Of course, there remains the possibility that carvedilol is truly superior to $beta_1$-selective agents delivered to the same degree of $beta_1$ receptor blockade, but no study demonstrating this has been conducted.

Because of the pharmacological heterogeneity among beta-blocking agents, the degree of polymorphic variation in key components of adrenergic mechanisms, and the clinical diversity of HF subpopulations, there remains an excellent possibility that antiadrenergic therapy with beta-blocking agents will evolve to a more tailored and targeted approach involving individual types of agents being more effective for subsets of polymorphic receptor variants or other determinants of antiadrenergic response, or both.[338]

Limitations of Beta Blocker Therapy in Chronic Heart Failure

Despite their proven efficacy in HF in patients with primary or secondary dilated cardiomyopathy, it is important to emphasize that beta blockers have limitations to general application in HF populations. First and foremost is that many patients with HF have contraindications to beta blockade, such as reactive airway disease, sinus node or conduction system disease with bradycardia, and advanced HF with hemodynamic decompensation. Another problem is that even in mild to moderate HF, initiation of therapy and uptitration of beta-blocking agents can be difficult and require both persistence and a knowledge of management maneuvers[281] that allow target doses to be achieved. A third problem is that for reasons that are not yet clear, some patients do not respond to beta blockade in terms of favorable effects on myocardial function, and these individuals may have a worse outcome than patients treated with placebo.[285] Some, but not all, of these problems might be overcome by the development of more efficacious or better tolerated compounds; the use of other, more effective types of antiadrenergic therapy; or the use of a combination of beta blockers with positive inotropic agents.[174,175] The importance of the beta blocker data set is not that it demonstrates a "cure" for chronic HF but rather that it has now been shown that in some patients, the prognosis can be substantially improved by medical therapy. This observation should provide an impetus to develop further types of treatment that improve the biological properties of the failing heart.

OTHER ANTIADRENERGIC AGENTS

The success of beta-blocking agents and the realization that many subjects have contraindications to them have prompted attempts to develop antiadrenergic approaches other than beta receptor blockade. An obvious approach would be to inhibit norepinephrine synthesis or release, but these approaches have not produced much success. In small studies conducted in less advanced HF, clonidine, which inhibits norepinephrine release through $alpha_2$ receptor agonist activity, has been well tolerated and has produced some evidence of clinical benefit.[346,347] In a medium-sized trial, the imidazoline receptor agonist moxonidine powerfully lowered norepinephrine in a dose-related fashion and produced evidence of reverse remodeling at higher doses.[348] However, in this trial, moxonidine also produced dose-related increases in adverse events that were greater than in the placebo group.[348] In addition, a phase III trial of high-dose moxonidine (MOXCON) had to be stopped because of a marked (by >50 percent) increase in mortality.[349] These data indicate that a drug that powerfully lowers adrenergic activity in a potentially insurmountable manner is not a good strategy in the treatment of chronic stable HF.

THE NEXT GENERATION OF HEART FAILURE TREATMENT

As can be observed by the effects of ACEIs, aldosterone antagonists, and beta blocker therapy (see Tables 23-7 and 23-13), medical therapy of HF has improved substantially over the past 15 years. This neurohormonal inhibitor approach to HF has been remarkably successful and has resulted in cumulated reductions in mortality of 30 to 40 percent. Unfortunately, we appear to have reached a limit in further antagonism of neurohormonal-cytokine systems inasmuch as most recent trials attempting to add additional neurohormonal-cytokine inhibition to background therapy of ACE inhibition and beta blockade have been unsuccessful. This list of failures includes certain endothelin antagonists, tumor necrosis factor-alpha inhibitors, and an NEP-ACEI. This experience indicates the limits of neurohormonal inhibition and strongly signals that different drug development approaches are now needed. Fortunately, these approaches are under way, with new small molecules, cell replacement therapy, gene therapy, and new devices all being examined. From the standpoint of small-molecule drug or gene therapy, major developmental programs exist targeting fetal gene induction, metabolism, apoptosis, and SR dysfunction. These are all novel approaches that target correction of maladaptive mechanisms, and it is likely that some of them will be successful in the near term.

Diuretics

1. Rouse D, Suki WN: Effects of neural and humoral agents on the renal tubules in congestive heart failure. Semin Nephrol 14:412, 1994.
2. Abassi Z, Winawer J, Skorecki KL: Control of extracellular fluid volume and the pathophysiology of edema formation. *In* Brenner BM (ed): Brenner and Rector's the Kidney. 7th ed. Philadelphia, WB Saunders, 2004, pp 777-856.
3. Maddox DA, Brenner BM: Glomerular ultrafiltration. *In* Brenner BM (ed): Brenner and Rector's the Kidney. 7th ed. Philadelphia, WB Saunders, 2004, pp 353-412.
4. Schrier RW, Abraham WT: Hormones and hemodynamics in heart failure. N Engl J Med 341:577, 1999.
5. Sladek CD, Kapoor JR: Neurotransmitter/neuropeptide interactions in the regulation of neurohypophyseal hormone release. Exp Neurol 171:200, 2001.
6. Benigni A, Perico N, Remuzzi G: Endothelin antagonists and renal protection. J Cardiovasc Pharmacol 35(4 Suppl 2):S75, 2000.
7. Haas M: The Na-K-Cl cotransporters. Am J Physiol 267:C869, 1994.
8. Raftery EB: Hemodynamic effects of diuretics in heart failure. Br Heart J 72:44, 1994.
9. Dunn CJ, Fitton A, Brogden RN: Torsemide. An update of its pharmacological properties and therapeutic efficacy. Drug Eval 49:121, 1995.
10. Wiemer G, Fink E, Linz W, et al: Furosemide enhances the release of endothelial kinins, nitric oxide and prostacyclin. J Pharmacol Exp Ther 271:1611, 1994.
11. Greenberg S, McGowan C, Xie J, Summer WR: Selective pulmonary and venous smooth muscle relaxation by furosemide: A comparison with morphine. J Pharmacol Exp Ther 270:1077, 1994.
12. Canessa C, Schild L, Buell G, et al: Amiloride-sensitive epithelial Na^+ channel is made of three homologous subunits. Nature 367:463, 1994.
13. Daleau P, Turgeon J: Triamterene inhibits the delayed rectifier potassium current (K_K) in guinea pig ventricular myocytes. Circ Res 74:1114, 1994.
14. Wang L, Sheldon RS, Mitchell B, et al: Amiloride-quinidine interaction: Adverse outcomes. Clin Pharmacol Ther 56:659, 1994.
15. Wingo CS, Cain BD: The renal H-K-ATPase: Physiological significance and role in potassium homeostasis. Annu Rev Physiol 55:323, 1993.
16. Farquharson CA, Struthers AD: Spironolactone increases nitric oxide bioactivity, improves endothelial vasodilator dysfunction, and suppresses vascular angiotensin I/angiotensin II conversion in patients with chronic heart failure. Circulation 101:594, 2000.
17. Funder JW: Aldosterone action. Annu Rev Physiol 55:115, 1993.
18. Pitt B, Zannad F, Remme WJ, et al: The effect of spironolactone on morbidity and mortality in patients with severe heart failure. Randomized Aldactone Evaluation Study Investigators. N Engl J Med 341:709, 1999.
19. Delyani JA: Mineralocorticoid receptor antagonists: The evolution of utility and pharmacology. Kidney Int 57:1408, 2000.
20. Hameedi A, Chadow HL: The promise of selective aldosterone receptor antagonists for the treatment of hypertension and congestive heart failure. Curr Hypertens Rep 2:378, 2000.
21. Pitt B, Remme W, Zannad F, et al, Eplerenone Post-Acute Myocardial Infarction Heart Failure Efficacy and Survival Study Investigators: Eplerenone, a selective aldosterone blocker, in patients with left ventricular dysfunction after myocardial infarction. N Engl J Med 348:1309, 2003.
22. White WB, Duprez D, St Hillaire R, et al: Effects of the selective aldosterone blocker eplerenone versus the calcium antagonist amlodipine in systolic hypertension. Hypertension 41:1021, 2003.
23. Schrier RW, Martin PY: Recent advances in the understanding of water metabolism in heart failure. Adv Exp Med Biol 449:415, 1998.
24. Burrell LM, Phillips PA, Stephenson JM, et al: Vasopressin and a nonpeptide antidiuretic hormone receptor antagonist (OPC-31260). Blood Press 3:137, 1994.
25. Naitoh M, Suzuki H, Murakami M, et al: Effects of oral AVP receptor antagonists OPC-21268 and OPC-31260 on congestive heart failure in conscious dogs. Am J Physiol 267:H2245, 1994.
26. Yamamura Y, Ogawa H, Yamashita H, et al: Characterization of a novel aquaretic agent, OPC-31260, as an orally effective, nonpeptide vasopressin V_2 receptor antagonist. Br J Pharmacol 105:787, 1992.
27. Hirano T, Yamamura Y, Nakamura S, et al: Effects of the V(2)-receptor antagonist OPC-41061 and the loop diuretic furosemide alone and in combination in rats. J Pharmacol Exp Ther 292:288, 2000.
28. Gheorghiade M, Niazi I, Ouyang J, et al, Tolvaptan Investigators: Vasopressin V2-receptor blockade with tolvaptan in patients with chronic heart failure: Results from a double-blind, randomized trial. Circulation 107:2690, 2003.
29. Abraham WT, Oren RM, Crisman TS, et al: Effects of an oral, non-peptide, selective V_2 receptor vasopressin antagonist in patients with chronic heart failure. J Am Coll Cardiol 29:169A, 1997.
30. Tahara A, Tomuira Y, Wada KI, et al: Pharmacological profile of YM087, a novel potent nonpeptide vasopressin V1A and V2 receptor antagonist, in vitro and in vivo. J Pharmacol Exp Ther 282:301, 1997.
31. Udelson JE, Smith WB, Hendrix GH, et al: Acute hemodynamic effects of conivaptan, a dual V(1A) and V(2) vasopressin receptor antagonist, in patients with advanced heart failure. Circulation 104:2417, 2001.
32. Russell SD, Selaru P, Pyne DA, et al: Rationale for use of an exercise end point and design for the ADVANCE (A Dose evaluation of a Vasopressin ANtagonist in CHF patients undergoing Exercise) trial. Am Heart J 145:179, 2003.
33. Van Kerckhoven R, Lankhuizen I, van Veghel R, et al: Chronic vasopressin V(1A) but not V(2) receptor antagonism prevents heart failure in chronically infarcted rats. Eur J Pharmacol 49:135, 2002.
34. Brater DC: Diuretic resistance: Mechanisms and therapeutic strategies. Cardiology 84:57, 1994.
35. Wilcox CS: Diuretics. *In* Brenner BM (ed): Brenner and Rector's the Kidney. 7th ed. Philadelphia, WB Saunders, 2004, pp 2345-2381.
36. Morsing P, Velazquez H, Wright FS, Ellison DH: Adaptation of distal convoluted tubule of rats. II. Effects of chronic thiazide infusion. Am J Physiol 261:F137, 1991.
37. Dzau VJ, Packer M, Lilly LS, et al: Prostaglandins in severe congestive heart failure. Relation to activation of the renin-angiotensin system and hyponatremia. N Engl J Med 310:347, 1984.
38. Good JM, Brady AJB, Noormohamed FH, et al: Effect of intense angiotensin II suppression on the diuretic response to furosemide during chronic ACE inhibition. Circulation 90:220, 1994.
39. Bailey MA, Giebisch G: Control of renal potassium excretion. *In* Brenner BM (ed): Brenner and Rector's the Kidney. 7th ed. Philadelphia, WB Saunders, 2004, pp 453-496.
40. Brown MJ, Brown DC, Murphy MB: Hypokalemia from beta2-receptor stimulation by circulating epinephrine. N Engl J Med 309:1414, 1983.
41. Haffner CA, Kendall MJ: Metabolic effects of beta 2-agonists. J Clin Pharm Ther 17:155, 1992.
42. Siscovick DS, Raghunathan TE, Psaty BM, et al: Diuretic therapy for hypertension and the risk of primary cardiac arrest. N Engl J Med 330:1852, 1994.
43. Ramsay LE, Yeo WW, Jackson PR: Metabolic effects of diuretics. Cardiology 84:48, 1994.

Vasodilators

44. Cohn JN, Franciosa JA: Vasodilator therapy of cardiac failure. N Engl J Med 297:27, 1977.
45. Kass DA, Kelly RP: Ventriculo-arterial coupling: Concepts, assumptions, and applications. Ann Biomed Eng 20:41, 1992.
46. Cohn JN, Archibald DG, Ziesche S, et al: Effect of vasodilator therapy on mortality in chronic congestive heart failure. Results of a Veterans Administration Cooperative Study. N Engl J Med 314:1547, 1986.
47. Cohn JN: Effect of vasodilator therapy on mortality in chronic congestive heart failure. Eur Heart J 9(Suppl A):171, 1988.
48. Packer M, Rouleau J, Swedberg K, et al: Effect of flosequinan on survival in chronic heart failure: Preliminary results of the PROFILE study [abstract]. Circulation 88(Suppl 1):301, 1993.
49. Califf RM, Adams KF, McKenna WJ, et al: A randomized controlled trial of epoprostenol therapy for severe congestive heart failure: The Flolan International Randomized Survival Trial (FIRST). Am Heart J 134:44, 1997.
50. Harrison DG, Bates JN: The nitrovasodilators. New ideas about old drugs. Circulation 87:1461, 1993.
51. Hare JM, Keaney JF Jr, Balligand JL, et al: Role of nitric oxide in parasympathetic modulation of β-adrenergic myocardial contractility in normal dogs. J Clin Invest 95:360, 1995.
52. Fallen EL, Nahmias C, Scheffel A, et al: Redistribution of myocardial blood flow with topical nitroglycerin in patients with coronary artery disease. Circulation 91:1381, 1995.
53. Leier CV, Huss P, Magouin RD, Unverferth DV: Improved exercise capacity and differing arterial and venous tolerance during chronic isosorbide dinitrate therapy for congestive heart failure. Circulation 67:817, 1983.
54. Publication Committee for the VMAC Investigators (Vasodilatation in the Management of Acute CHF): Intravenous nesiritide vs nitroglycerin for treatment of decompensated congestive heart failure: A randomized controlled trial. JAMA 287:1531, 2002.
55. Parker JD, Parker AB, Farrell B, et al: Intermittent transdermal nitroglycerin therapy. Decreased anginal threshold during the nitrate-free interval. Circulation 91:973, 1995.
56. Munzel T, Kurz S, Rajagopalan S, et al: Hydralazine prevents nitroglycerin tolerance by inhibiting activation of a membrane-bound NADH oxidase. A new action for an old drug. J Clin Invest 98:1465, 1996.
57. Risoe C, Simonsen S, Rootwelt K, et al: Nitroprusside and regional vascular capacitance in patients with severe congestive heart failure. Circulation 85:997, 1992.
58. Kussmaul WG, Altschuler JA, Matthai WH, et al: Right ventricular-vascular interaction in congestive heart failure. Importance of low-frequency impedance. Circulation 88:1010, 1993.
59. Cohn JN, Franciosa JA, Francis GS, et al: Effect of short-term infusion of sodium nitroprusside on mortality rate in acute myocardial infarction complicated by left ventricular failure: Results of a Veterans Administration cooperative study. N Engl J Med 306:1129, 1982.
60. Ginks WR, Redwood DR: Hemodynamic effects of hydralazine at rest and during exercise in patients with chronic heart failure. Br Heart J 44:259, 1980.
61. Leier CV: Regional blood flow responses to vasodilators and inotropes in congestive heart failure. Am J Cardiol 62:86E, 1988.
62. Hofstra AH: Metabolism of hydralazine: Relevance to drug-induced lupus. Drug Metab Rev 26:485, 1994.
63. Cohn JN, Johnson G, Ziesche S, et al: A comparison of enalapril with hydralazine-isosorbide dinitrate in the treatment of chronic congestive heart failure. N Engl J Med 325:303, 1991.
64. Carson P, Ziesche S, Johnson G, et al: Racial differences in response to therapy for heart failure: Analysis of the vasodilator-heart failure trials. Vasodilator-Heart Failure Trial Study Group. J Card Fail 5:178, 1999.
65. Vesely DL, Douglass MA, Dietz JR, et al: Three peptides from the atrial natriuretic factor prohormone amino terminus lower blood pressure and produce diuresis, natriuresis, and/or kaliuresis in humans. Circulation 90:1129, 1994.
66. Nakamura M, Arakawa N, Yoshida H, et al: Vasodilatory effects of C-type natriuretic peptide on forearm resistance vessels are distinct from those of atrial natriuretic peptide in chronic heart failure. Circulation 90:1210, 1994.
67. Suga SI, Nakao K, Itoh H, et al: Endothelial production of C-type natriuretic peptide and its marked augmentation by transforming growth factor-β. Possible existence of "vascular natriuretic peptide system." J Clin Invest 90:1145, 1992.

68. John SWM, Krege JH, Oliver PM, et al: Genetic decreases in atrial natriuretic peptide and salt-sensitive hypertension. Science 267:679, 1995.
69. Semigran MJ, Aroney CN, Herrmann HC, et al: Effects of atrial natriuretic peptide on myocardial contractile and diastolic function in patients with heart failure. J Am Coll Cardiol 20:98, 1992.
70. Connelly TP, Francis GS, Williams KJ, et al: Interaction of intravenous atrial natriuretic factor with furosemide in patients with heart failure. Am Heart J 127:392, 1994.
71. Marcus LS, Hart D, Packer M, et al: Hemodynamic and renal excretory effects of human brain natriuretic peptide infusion in patients with congestive heart failure: A double-blind, placebo-controlled, cross-over trial. Circulation 94:3184, 1996.
72. Abraham WT, Lowes BD, Ferguson DA, et al: Systemic hemodynamic, neurohormonal, and renal effects of a steady-state infusion of human brain natriuretic peptide in patients with advanced hemodynamically decompensated heart failure. J Card Fail 4:37, 1998.
73. Colucci WS, Elkayam U, Horton DP, et al: Intravenous nesiritide, a natriuretic peptide, in the treatment of decompensated congestive heart failure. Nesiritide Study Group. N Engl J Med 343:246, 2000.
74. Mills RM, Hobbs RE, Young JB: "BNP" for heart failure: Role of nesiritide in cardiovascular therapeutics. Congest Heart Fail 8:270, 2002.
75. Abramson BL, Ando S, Notarius CF, et al: Effect of atrial natriuretic peptide on muscle sympathetic activity and its reflex control in human heart failure. Circulation 99:1810, 1999.
76. Burger AJ, Horton DP, LeJemtel T, et al, Prospective Randomized Evaluation of Cardiac Ectopy with Dobutamine or Natrecor Therapy: Effect of nesiritide (B-type natriuretic peptide) and dobutamine on ventricular arrhythmias in the treatment of patients with acutely decompensated congestive heart failure: The PRECEDENT study. Am Heart J 44:1102, 2002.
77. Chen HH, Grantham JA, Schirger JA, et al: Subcutaneous administration of brain natriuretic peptide in experimental heart failure. J Am Coll Cardiol 36:1706, 2000.
78. Chen HH, Nordstrom LJ, Redfield MM, et al: Subcutaneous BNP administration in symptomatic human heart failure: A novel therapeutic strategy for congestive heart failure [abstract]. J Am Coll Cardiol 35:240, 2000.
79. Kentsch M, Otter W: Novel neurohormonal modulators in cardiovascular disorders. The therapeutic potential of endopeptidase inhibitors. Drugs R D 1:331, 1999.
80. Margulies KB, Burnett JC Jr: Neutral endopeptidase 24.11: A modulator of natriuretic peptides. Semin Nephrol 13:71, 1993.
81. Trippodo NC, Panchal BC, Fox M: Repression of angiotensin II and potentiation of bradykinin contribute to the synergistic effects of dual metalloprotease inhibition in heart failure. J Pharmacol Exp Ther 272:619, 1995.
82. Vera WG, Fournie-Zaluski MC, Pham I, et al: Hypotensive and natriuretic effects of RB 105, a new dual inhibitor of angiotensin converting enzyme and neutral endopeptidase in hypertensive rats. J Pharmacol Exp Ther 272:343, 1995.
83. Chen HH, Lainchbury JG, Harty G, Burnett JC: The superior renal and humoral actions of acute dual NEP/ACE inhibition by vasopeptidase inhibitor versus ACE inhibition alone in experimental mild heart failure: Properties mediated via potentiation of endogenous cardiac natriuretic peptides [abstract]. J Am Coll Cardiol 35:270, 2000.
84. Kostis JB, Rouleau JL, Pfeffer MA, et al: Beneficial effects of vasopeptidase inhibition on mortality and morbidity in heart failure: Evidence from the omapatrilat heart failure program [abstract]. J Am Coll Cardiol 35:240, 2000.
85. Packer M, Califf RM, Konstam MA, et al: Comparison of omapatrilat and enalapril in patients with chronic heart failure: The Omapatrilat Versus Enalapril Randomized Trial of Utility in Reducing Events (OVERTURE). Circulation 106:920, 2002.
86. Elkayam U: Calcium channel blockers in heart failure. Cardiology 89:38, 1998.
87. Cohn JN, Ziesche S, Smith R, et al: Effect of the calcium antagonist felodipine as supplementary vasodilator therapy in patients with chronic heart failure treated with enalapril: V-HeFT III. Vasodilator-Heart Failure Trial (V-HeFT) Study Group. Circulation 96:856, 1997.
88. Packer M, O'Connor CM, Ghali JK, et al: Effect of amlodipine on morbidity and mortality in severe chronic heart failure. Prospective Randomized Amlodipine Survival Evaluation Study (PRAISE) Group. N Engl J Med 335:1107, 1996.

Positive Inotropic Agents

89. Hauptman PJ, Kelly RA: Digitalis. Circulation 99:1265, 1999.
90. Blaustein MP: Physiological effects of endogenous ouabain: Control of intracellular Ca^{2+} stores and cell responsiveness. Am J Physiol 264:C1367, 1993.
91. Schmidt TA, Allen PD, Colucci WS, et al: No adaptation to digitalization as evaluated by digitalis receptor (Na,K-ATPase) quantification in explanted hearts from donors without heart disease and from digitalized recipients with end-stage heart failure. Am J Cardiol 70:110, 1992.
92. The Digitalis Investigation Group: The effect of digoxin on mortality and morbidity in patients with heart failure. N Engl J Med 336:525, 1997.
93. Holubarsch C, Hasenfuss G, Just H, Alpert NR: Positive inotropism and myocardial energetics: Influence of β receptor agonist stimulation, phosphodiesterase inhibition, and ouabain. Cardiovasc Res 28:994, 1994.
94. Wang W, Chen JS, Zucker IH: Carotid sinus baroreceptor sensitivity in experimental heart failure. Circulation 81:1959, 1990.
95. Esler M, Kaye D, Lambert G, et al: Adrenergic nervous system in heart failure. Am J Cardiol 80(11A):7L, 1997.
96. Kelly RA, Smith TW: Pharmacologic treatment of heart failure. *In* Hardman JG, Limbird LT (eds): Goodman and Gilman's Pharmacological Basis of Therapeutics. 9th ed. New York, McGraw-Hill, 1996, pp 809-838.
97. Rathore SS, Curtis JP, Wang Y, et al: Serum digoxin concentration and the efficacy of digoxin therapy in the treatment of heart failure: An analysis of the Digitalis Investigation Group (DIG) trial. JAMA 289:871, 2003.
98. Packer M, Gheorghiade M, Young JB, et al: Withdrawal of digoxin from patients with chronic heart failure treated with angiotensin-converting-enzyme inhibitors. RADIANCE study. N Engl J Med 329:1, 1993.
99. Young JB, Gheorghiade M, Uretsky BF, et al: Superiority of "triple" drug therapy in heart failure: Insights from the PROVED and RADIANCE trials. Prospective Randomized Study of Ventricular Function and Efficacy of Digoxin. Randomized Assessment of Digoxin and Inhibitors of Angiotensin-Converting Enzyme. J Am Coll Cardiol 32:686, 1998.
100. Uretsky BF, Young JB Shahidi FE, et al: Randomized study assessing the effect of digoxin withdrawal in patients with mild to moderate chronic congestive heart failure: Results of the PROVED trial. PROVED Investigative Group. J Am Coll Cardiol 22:955, 1993.
101. Slatton ML, Irani WN, Hall SA, et al: Does digoxin provide additional hemodynamic and autonomic benefit at higher doses in patients with mild to moderate heart failure and normal sinus rhythm? J Am Coll Cardiol 29:1206, 1997.
102. Gheorghiade M, Hall VB, Jacobsen G, et al: Effects of increasing maintenance dose of digoxin on left ventricular function and neurohormones in patients with chronic heart failure treated with diuretics and angiotensin-converting enzyme inhibitors. Circulation 92:1801, 1995.
103. Rathore SS, Wang Y, Krumholz HM: Sex-based differences in the effect of digoxin for the treatment of heart failure. N Engl J Med 347:1403, 2002.
104. Magnani B, Malini PL: Cardiac glycosides. Drug interactions of clinical significance. Drug Saf 12:97, 1995.
105. Fromm MF, Kim RB, Stein CM, et al: Inhibition of P-glycoprotein-mediated drug transport: A unifying mechanism to explain the interaction between digoxin and quinidine. Circulation 99:552, 1999.
106. Greiner B, Eichelbaum M, Fritz P, et al: The role of intestinal P-glycoprotein in the interaction of digoxin and rifampin. J Clin Invest 104:147, 1999.
107. Goldman S, Probst P, Selzer A, Cohn K: Inefficacy of "therapeutic" serum levels of digoxin in controlling the ventricular rate in atrial fibrillation. Am J Cardiol 35:651, 1975.
108. Merrill JJ, DeWeese G, Wharton JM: Magnesium reversal of digoxin-facilitated ventricular rate during atrial fibrillation in the Wolff-Parkinson-White syndrome Am J Med 97:25, 1994.
109. Bosse GM, Pope TM: Recurrent digoxin overdose and treatment with digoxin-specific Fab antibody fragments. J Emerg Med 12:179, 1994.
110. Port JD, Bristow MR: Altered beta-adrenergic receptor gene regulation and signaling in chronic heart failure. J Mol Cell Cardiol 33:887, 2001.
111. Bristow MR: Changes in myocardial and vascular receptors in heart failure. J Am Coll Cardiol 22(Suppl A):61, 1993.
112. Bristow MR: Mechanism of action of beta-blocking agents in heart failure. Am J Cardiol 80(11A):261, 1997.
113. Bristow MR, Ginsburg R, Minobe WA, et al: Decreased catecholamine sensitivity and β-adrenergic-receptor density in failing human hearts. N Engl J Med 307:205, 1982.
114. Fowler MB, Laser JA, Hopkins GL, et al: Assessment of the β-adrenergic receptor pathway in the intact failing human heart: Progressive receptor down-regulation and subsensitivity to agonist response. Circulation 74:1290, 1986.
115. Ginsburg R, Esserman L, Bristow MR: Myocardial performance and extracellular ionized calcium in a severely failing human heart. Ann Intern Med 98:603, 1983.
116. Pacholczyk T, Blakely RD, Amara SG: Expression cloning of a cocaine- and antidepressant-sensitive human noradrenaline transporter. Nature 350:350, 1991.
117. Mitchell PD, Smith GW, Wells E, West PA: Inhibition of $uptake_1$ by dopexamine hydrochloride in vitro. Br J Pharmacol 92:265, 1987.
118. Bristow MR: β-Adrenergic receptor blockade in chronic heart failure. Circulation 101:558, 2000.
119. Lowes BD, Tsvetkova T, Eichhorn EJ, et al: Milrinone vs. dobutamine in heart failure subjects treated chronically with carvedilol. Int J Cardiol 81:141, 2001.
120. Metra M, Nodari S, D'Aloia A, et al: Beta-blocker therapy influences the hemodynamic response to inotropic agents in patients with heart failure. A randomized comparison of dobutamine and enoximone before and after chronic treatment with metoprolol or carvedilol. J Am Coll Cardiol 40:1248, 2002.
121. Gilbert EM, Eiswirth CC, Mealey PC, et al: β-Adrenergic supersensitivity of the transplanted human heart is presynaptic in origin. Circulation 79:344, 1989.
122. von Scheidt W, Bohm M, Schneider B, et al: Isolated presynaptic inotropic beta-adrenergic supersensitivity of the transplanted denervated human heart in vivo. Circulation 85:1056, 1992.
123. Scrutinio D, Napoli V, Passantino A, et al: Low-dose dobutamine responsiveness in idiopathic dilated cardiomyopathy: Relation to exercise capacity and clinical outcome. Eur Heart J 21:927, 2000.
124. Maccarrone C, Malta E, Raper C: β-Adrenoceptor selectivity of dobutamine: In vivo and in vitro studies. J Cardiovasc Pharmacol 6:132, 1984.
125. Wollmering MM, Wiechmann RJ, Port JD, et al: Dobutamine is a partial agonist with an intrinsic activity of 0.5 in human myocardium [abstract]. J Am Coll Cardiol 17:283, 1991.
126. Binkley PF, VanFossen DV, Nunziata E, et al: Influence of positive inotropic therapy on pulsatile hydraulic load and ventricular-vascular coupling in congestive heart failure. J Am Coll Cardiol 15:1127, 1990.
127. Leier CV: Current status of non-digitalis positive inotropic drugs. Am J Cardiol 69:120G, 1992.
128. Leier CV, Heban PT, Huss P, et al: Comparative systemic and regional hemodynamic effects of dopamine and dobutamine in patients with cardiomyopathic heart failure. Circulation 58:466, 1978.
129. Binkley PF, Murray KD, Watson KM, et al: Dobutamine increases cardiac output of total artificial heart. Implications for vascular contribution of inotropic agents to augmented ventricular function. Circulation 84:1210, 1991.
130. Cork RC, Gallo JA Jr, Copeland JG: Acute effects of dobutamine and isoproterenol after implantation of a total artificial heart. J Heart Lung Transplant 11:253, 1992.
131. Keren G, Laniado S, Sonnenblick EH, LeJemtel LH: Dynamics of functional mitral regurgitation during dobutamine therapy in patients with severe congestive heart failure. A Doppler echocardiographic study. Am Heart J 118:748, 1989.

132. Gilbert EM, Larrabee PA, Volkman AK, et al: Does dobutamine tolerance result from myocardial β-receptor down-regulation [abstract]? J Am Coll Cardiol 19:253, 1992.
133. Lee HR, Hershberger RE, Port JD, et al: Low-dose enoximone in subjects awaiting cardiac transplantation: Clinical results and effects on β-adrenergic receptors. J Thorac Cardiovasc Surg 102:246, 1991.
134. Gilbert EM, Hershberger RE, Wiechmann RJ, et al: Pharmacologic and hemodynamic effects of combined β-agonist stimulation and phosphodiesterase inhibition in the failing human heart. Chest 108:1524, 1995.
135. Port JD, Gilbert EM, Larrabee P, et al: Neurotransmitter depletion compromises the ability of indirect-acting amines to provide inotropic support in the failing human heart. Circulation 81:929, 1990.
136. Nichols AJ, Ruffolo RR Jr, Brooks DP: The pharmacology of fenoldopam. Am J Hypertens 3(Suppl):116, 1990.
137. Lokhandwala MF, Amenta F: Anatomical distribution and function of dopamine receptors in the kidney. FASEB J 5:3023, 1991.
138. Anderson FL, Port JD, Reid BB, et al: Effect of therapeutic dopamine administration on myocardial catecholamine and neuropeptide Y concentrations in the failing ventricles of patients with idiopathic dilated cardiomyopathy. J Cardiovasc Pharmacol 20:800, 1992.
139. Abraham WT, Lowes BD, Roden RL, et al: Mechanism of increased cardiac adrenergic activity in heart failure: Evidence for decreased cardiac neuronal norepinephrine reuptake. Circulation 96(Suppl 1):92, 1997.
140. Rundqvist B, Elam M, Eisenhofer G, Friberg P: Increased cardiac adrenergic drive precedes generalized sympathetic activation human heart failure. Circulation 95:516, 1997.
141. Bristow MR, Daniels JR, Kernoff RS, Harrison DC: Effect of compound D600, practolol and alterations in magnesium on ionized calcium relationships in the intact dog heart. Circ Res 41:574, 1977.
142. Movsesian MA, Smith CJ, Krall J, et al: Sarcoplasmic reticulum-associated cyclic adenosine 5′-monophosphate phosphodiesterase activity in normal and failing human hearts. J Clin Invest 88:15, 1991.
143. Leroy M-J, Degerman E, Taira M, et al: Characterization of two recombinant PDE_3 (cGMP-inhibited cyclic nucleotide phosphodiesterase) isoforms, RcGIP1 and HcGIP2, expressed in NIH 3006 murine fibroblasts and Sf9 cells. Biochemistry 35:10194, 1996.
144. Koss KL, Kranias EG: Phospholamban: A prominent regulator of myocardial contractility. Circ Res 79:1059, 1996.
145. Edes I, Kiss E, Kitada Y, et al: Effects of levosimendan, a cardiotonic agent targeted to troponin C, on cardiac function and on phosphorylation and Ca^{2+} sensitivity of cardiac myofibrils and sarcoplasmic reticulum in guinea pig hearts. Circ Res 77:107, 1995.
146. Luo W, Grupp IL, Ponniah S, et al: Targeted ablation of the phospholamban gene is associated with markedly enhanced myocardial contractility and loss of β-agonist stimulation. Circ Res 75:401, 1994.
147. Kajimoto K, Hagiwara N, Kasanuki H, Hosoda S: Contribution of phosphodiesterase isozymes to the regulation of the L-type calcium current in human cardiac myocytes. Br J Pharmacol 121:1549, 1997.
148. Walaas SI, Czernik AJ, Olstad OK, et al: Protein kinase C and cyclic AMP-dependent protein kinase phosphorylate phospholemman, an insulin and adrenaline-regulated membrane phosphoprotein, at specific sites in the carboxy terminal domain. Biochem J 304:635, 1994.
149. Jiang H, Colbran JL, Francis SH, Corbin JD: Direct evidence for cross-activation of cGMP-dependent protein kinase by cAMP in pig coronary arteries. J Biol Chem 267:1015, 1992.
150. Kikura M, Levy JH, Michelsen LG, et al: The effect of milrinone on hemodynamics and left ventricular function after emergence from cardiopulmonary bypass. Anesth Analg 85:16, 1997.
151. Paulus S, Lehot JJ, Bastien O, et al: Enoximone and acute left ventricular failure during weaning from mechanical ventilation after cardiac surgery. Crit Care Med 22:74, 1994.
152. Chen EP, Bittner HB, Davis RD, Van Tright P: Hemodynamic and inotropic effects of milrinone after heart transplantation in the setting of recipient pulmonary hypertension. J Heart Lung Transplant 17:669, 1998.
153. Feldman MD, Copelas L, Gwathmey JK, et al: Deficient production of cyclic AMP: Pharmacologic evidence of an important cause of contractile dysfunction in patients with end-stage heart failure. Circulation 75:331, 1987.
154. Feldman AM, Cates AE, Veazey WB, et al: Increase of the 40,000-mol wt pertussis toxin substrate (G protein) in the failing human heart. J Clin Invest 82:189, 1988.
155. Neumann J, Schmitz W, Scholz H, et al: Increase in myocardial G_i-proteins in heart failure. Lancet 2:936, 1988.
156. Bristow MR, Anderson FL, Port JD, et al: Differences in β-adrenergic neuroeffector mechanisms in ischemic versus idiopathic dilated cardiomyopathy. Circulation 84:1024, 1991.
157. Sigmund M, Jakob H, Becker H, et al: Effects of metoprolol on myocardial β-adrenoceptors and G_α-proteins in patients with congestive heart failure. Eur J Clin Pharmacol 51:127, 1996.
158. Böhm M, Deutsch HJ, Hartmann D, et al: Improvement of postreceptor events by metoprolol treatment in patients with chronic heart failure. J Am Coll Cardiol 30:992, 1997.
159. Shipley JB, Tolman D, Hastillo A, Hess ML: Milrinone: Basic and clinical pharmacology and acute and chronic management. Am J Med Sci 311:286, 1996.
160. Lowes B, Higginbotham M, Petrovich L, et al: Low dose enoximone improves exercise capacity in chronic heart failure. J Am Coll Cardiol 36:501, 2000.
161. Leier CV, Meiler SEL, Matthews S, Unverferth DV: A preliminary report of the effects of orally administered enoximone on regional hemodynamics in congestive heart failure. Am J Cardiol 60:27C, 1987.
162. Dibianco R, Shabetai R, Kostuk W, et al: A comparison of oral milrinone, digoxin, and their combination in the treatment of patients with chronic heart failure. N Engl J Med 320:677, 1989.
163. Monrad ES, Baim DS, Smith HS, et al: Effects of milrinone on coronary hemodynamics and myocardial energetics in patients with congestive heart failure. Circulation 71:972, 1985.
164. Monrad ES, McKay RG, Baim DS, et al: Improvement in indexes of diastolic performance in patients with congestive heart failure treated with milrinone. Circulation 70:1030, 1984.
165. Ludmer PL, Wright RF, Arnold JM, et al: Separation of the direct myocardial and vasodilator actions of milrinone administered by an intracoronary infusion technique. Circulation 73:130, 1986.
166. Packer M, Carver JR, Chesebro JH, et al: Effect of oral milrinone on mortality in severe chronic heart failure. PROMISE Study Research Group. N Engl J Med 325:1468, 1991.
167. Uretsky BF, Jesup M, Konstam MA, et al: Multicenter trial of oral enoximone in patients with moderate to moderately severe congestive heart failure: Lack of benefit compared to placebo. Enoximone Multicenter Trial Group. Circulation 82:774, 1990.
168. Cowley AJ, Skene AM, on behalf of the Enoximone Investigators: Treatment of severe heart failure: Quantity or quality of life? A trial of enoximone. Br Heart J 72:226, 1994.
169. Cohn JN, Goldstein SO, Greenberg BH, et al: A dose-dependent increase in mortality with vesnarinone among patients with severe heart failure. N Engl J Med 339:1810, 1998.
170. Lubsen J, Just H, Hjalmarsson AC, et al: Effect of pimobendan on exercise capacity in patients with heart failure: Main results from the Pimobendan in Congestive Heart Failure (PICO) trial. Heart 76:223, 1996.
171. Teerlink JR, Jalaluddin M, Anderson S, et al: Ambulatory ventricular arrhythmias in patients with heart failure do not specifically predict an increased risk of sudden death. PROMISE (Prospective Randomized Milrinone Survival Evaluation) Investigators. Circulation 101:40, 2000.
172. Bristow MR, Lowes BD: Low-dose inotropic therapy of ambulatory heart failure. Coron Artery Dis 5:112, 1994.
173. Gilbert EM, Bristow MR, Mason JW: The acute hemodynamic response to low dose enoximone (MDL 17,043): An oral dose-range study. Am J Cardiol 82:57C, 1987.
174. Lowes BD, Simon MA, Tsekova TO, Bristow MR: Inotropes in the β-blocker era. Clin Cardiol 23(Suppl 3):11, 2000.
175. Shakar SF, Abraham WT, Gilbert EM, et al: Combined oral positive inotropic and beta-blocker therapy for the treatment of refractory Class IV heart failure. J Am Coll Cardiol 31:1336, 1998.
176. Benotti JR, Grossman W, Braunwald E, et al: Hemodynamic assessment of amrinone: A new inotropic agent. N Engl J Med 299:1373, 1978.
177. Maisel AS, Wright CM, Carter SM, et al: Tachyphylaxis with amrinone therapy: Association with sequestration and down-regulation of lymphocyte beta-adrenergic receptors. Ann Intern Med 110:195, 1989.
178. Kikura M, Lee MK, Safon RA, et al: The effects of milrinone on platelets in patients undergoing cardiac surgery. Anesth Analg 81:44, 1995.
179. Holmberg SR, Williams AJ: Phosphodiesterase inhibitors and the cardiac sarcoplasmic reticulum calcium release channel: Differential effects of milrinone and enoximone. Cardiovasc Res 25:537, 1991.
180. Cody V, Wojtczak A, Davis FB, et al: Structure-activity relationships of milrinone analogues determined in vitro in a rabbit heart membrane Ca^{2+}-ATPase model. J Med Chem 38:1990, 1995.
181. Siostrzonek P, Koreny M, Delle-Karth G, et al: Milrinone therapy in catecholamine-dependent critically ill patients with heart failure. Acta Anaesth Scand 44:403, 2000.
182. Seino Y, Takano T, Hayakawa H, et al: Hemodynamic effects and pharmacokinetics of oral milrinone for short-term support in acute heart failure. Cardiology 86:34, 1995.
183. Gibeline P, Dadoun-Dybal M, Candito M, et al: Hemodynamic effects of prolonged enoximone infusion (7 days) in patients with severe chronic heart failure. Cardiovasc Drugs Ther 7:333, 1993.
184. Okerholm RA, Chan KY, Lang JF, et al: Biotransformation and pharmacokinetic overview of enoximone and its sulfoxide metabolite. Am J Cardiol 60:21C, 1987.
185. Burns AM, Park GR: Prolonged action of enoximone in renal failure. Anaesthesia 46:864, 1991.
186. Boknik P, Neumann J, Kaspereit G, et al: Mechanisms of the contractile effects of levosimendan in the mammalian heart. J Pharmacol Exp Ther 280:277, 1997.
187. Remme WJ, Kruijssen DA, van Hoogenhuyze DC, et al: Hemodynamic, neurohumoral, and myocardial energetic effects of pimobendan, a novel calcium-sensitizing compound, in patients with mild to moderate heart failure. J Cardiovasc Pharmacol 24:730, 1994.
188. Lilleberg J, Sundberg S, Nieminen MS: Dose-range study of a new calcium sensitizer, levosimendan, in patients with left ventricular dysfunction. J Cardiovasc Pharmacol 26(Suppl):63, 1995.
189. Hagemeijer F: Calcium sensitization with pimobendan: Pharmacology, haemodynamic improvement, and sudden death in patients with chronic congestive heart failure. Eur Heart J 14:551, 1993.
190. Bethke T, Eschenhagen T, Klimkiewicz A, et al: Phosphodiesterase inhibition by enoximone in preparations from nonfailing and failing human hearts. Arzneimittelforschung 42:437, 1992.
191. Kubo SH, Gollub S, Bourge R, et al: Results of a multicenter trial. The Pimobendan Multicenter Research Group. Circulation 85:942, 1992.
192. Haikala H, Kaivola J, Nissinen E, et al: Cardiac troponin C as a target protein for a novel calcium sensitizing drug, levosimendan. J Mol Cell Cardiol 27:1859, 1995.
193. Kleerekoper Q, Putkey JA: Drug binding to cardiac troponin C. J Biol Chem 274:23932, 1999.
194. Moiseyev VS, Poder P, Andrejevs N, et al: Safety and efficacy of a novel calcium sensitizer, levosimendan, in patients with left ventricular failure due to an acute myocardial infarction. A placebo-controlled, double-blind study (RUSSLAN). Eur Heart J 23:1422, 2002.
195. Follath F, Cleland JG, Just H, et al: Efficacy and safety of intravenous levosimendan compared with dobutamine in severe low-output heart failure (the LIDO study): A randomized double-blind trial. Lancet 360:196, 2002.
196. Kivikko M, Lehtonen L, Colucci WS: Sustained hemodynamic effects of intravenous levosimendan. Circulation 107:81, 2003.

Neurohormonal Inhibitors

197. Francis GS, Goldsmith SR, Levine TB, et al: The neurohumoral axis in congestive heart failure. Ann Intern Med 101:370, 1984.
198. Packer M, Lee WH, Kessler PD, et al: Role of neurohormonal mechanisms in determining survival in patients with severe chronic heart failure. Circulation 75(Suppl 4):80, 1987.
199. Bristow MR, Kantrowitz NE, Ginsburg R, Fowler MB: β-Adrenergic function in heart muscle disease and heart failure. J Mol Cell Cardiol 17(Suppl 2):41, 1985.
200. Waagstein F, Hjalmarson A, Varnauskas E, Wallentin I: Effect of chronic beta-adrenergic receptor blockade in congestive cardiomyopathy. Br Heart J 37:1022, 1975.
201. Gilbert EM, Anderson JL, Deitchman D, et al: Long-term β-blocker vasodilator therapy improves cardiac function in idiopathic dilated cardiomyopathy: A double-blind, randomized study of bucindolol versus placebo. Am J Med 88:223, 1990.
202. Eichhorn EJ, Bedotto JB, Malloy CR, et al: Effect of beta-adrenergic blockade on myocardial function and energetics in congestive heart failure: Improvements in hemodynamic, contractile, and diastolic performance with bucindolol. Circulation 82:473, 1990.
203. Pfeffer MA, Lamas GA, Vaughan DE, et al: Effect of captopril on progressive ventricular dilation after anterior myocardial infarction. N Engl J Med 319:80, 1988.
204. Sharpe N, Smith H, Murphy J, Hannan S: Treatment of patients with symptomless left ventricular dysfunction after myocardial infarction. Lancet 365:255, 1988.
205. Fowler MB, Bristow MR: Rationale for beta-adrenergic blocking drugs in cardiomyopathy. Am J Cardiol 55:D120, 1985.
206. The CONSENSUS Trial Study Group: Effects of enalapril on mortality in severe congestive heart failure. Results of the Cooperative North Scandinavian Enalapril Survival Study (CONSENSUS). N Engl J Med 316:429, 1987.
207. The SOLVD Investigators: Effect of enalapril on survival in patients with reduced left ventricular ejection fractions and congestive heart failure. N Engl J Med 325:293, 1991.
208. Waagstein F, Bristow MR, Swedberg K, et al: Beneficial effects of metoprolol in idiopathic dilated cardiomyopathy. Metoprolol in Dilated Cardiomyopathy (MDC) Trial Study Group. Lancet 342:1441, 1993.
209. Packer M, Bristow MR, Cohn JN, et al: Effect of carvedilol on morbidity and mortality in patients with chronic heart failure. U.S. Carvedilol Heart Failure Study Group. N Engl J Med 334:1349, 1996.
210. Bristow MR, Gilbert EM, Abraham WT, et al: Carvedilol produces dose-related improvements in left ventricular function and survival in subjects with chronic heart failure. MOCHA Investigators. Circulation 94:2807-2816, 1996.
211. The Cardiac Insufficiency Bisoprolol Study II (CIBIS-II): A randomised trial. Lancet 353:9, 1999.
212. MERIT-HF Study Group: Effect of metoprolol CR/XL in chronic heart failure: Metoprolol CR/XL Randomized Intervention Trial in Congestive Heart Failure (MERIT-HF). Lancet 353:2001, 1999.
213. Inagami T: Molecular biology and signaling of angiotensin receptors: An overview. J Am Soc Nephrol 10(Suppl 11):2, 1999.
214. Mulder P, Richard V, Bouchart F, et al: Selective ET_A receptor blockade prevents left ventricular remodeling and deterioration of cardiac function in experimental heart failure. Cardiovasc Res 39:600, 1998.
215. Torre-Amione G, Bozkurt B, Deswal A, Mann DL: An overview of tumor necrosis factor alpha and the failing human heart. Curr Opin Cardiol 14:206, 1999.
216. Eichhorn EJ, Bristow MR: Medical therapy can improve the biologic properties of the chronically failing heart: A new era in the treatment of heart failure. Circulation 94:2285, 1996.

Inhibitors of the Renin-Angiotensin-Aldosterone System

217. Pfeffer JM, Pfeffer MA, Braunwald E: Hemodynamic benefits and prolonged survival with long-term captopril therapy in rats with myocardial infarction and heart failure. Circulation 75:1149, 1987.
218. Pfeffer JM, Pfeffer MA, Mirsky I, Braunwald E: Regression of left ventricular hypertrophy and prevention of left ventricular dysfunction by captopril in the spontaneously hypertensive rat. Proc Natl Acad Sci USA 79:3310, 1982.
219. Greenberg B, Quinones MA, Koilpillai C, et al: Effects of long-term therapy on cardiac structure and function in patients with left ventricular dysfunction. Results of the SOLVD echocardiography substudy. Circulation 91:2573, 1995.
220. Zisman LS, Abraham WT, Meixell GE, et al: Angiotensin II formation in the intact human heart: Predominance of the angiotensin-converting enzyme pathway. J Clin Invest 96:1490, 1995.
221. Urata H, Hoffmann S, Ganten D: Tissue angiotensin II system in the human heart. Eur Heart J 15(Suppl):68, 1994.
222. Wei CC, Meng QC, Palmer R, et al: Evidence for angiotensin-converting enzyme and chymase-mediated angiotensin II formation in the interstitial fluid space of the dog heart in vivo. Circulation 99:2583, 1999.
223. Liu YH, Yang XP, Mehta D, et al: Role of kinins in chronic heart failure and in the therapeutic effect of ACE inhibitors in kininogen-deficient rats. Am J Physiol 278:H507, 2000.
224. The SOLVD Investigators: Effect of enalapril on mortality and the development of heart failure in asymptomatic patients with reduced left ventricular ejection fractions. N Engl J Med 327:685, 1992.
225. Pfeffer MA, Braunwald E, Moye LA, et al: Effect of captopril on mortality and morbidity in patients with left ventricular dysfunction after myocardial infarction. Results of the survival and ventricular enlargement trial. The SAVE Investigators. N Engl J Med 327:669, 1992.
226. The Acute Infarction Ramipril Efficacy (AIRE) Study Investigators: Effect of ramipril on mortality and morbidity of survivors of acute myocardial infarction with clinical evidence of heart failure. Lancet 342:821, 1993.
227. Kober L, Torp-Pedersen C, Carlsen JE, et al: A clinical trial of the angiotensin-converting-enzyme inhibitor trandolapril in patients with left ventricular dysfunction after myocardial infarction. Trandolapril Cardiac Evaluation (TRACE) Study Group. N Engl J Med 333:1670, 1995.
228. Arnold JMO, Yusuf S, Young J, et al: Prevention of heart failure in patients without known left ventricular dysfunction: The Heart Outcomes Prevention Study (HOPE). Circulation 107:1284, 2003.
229. Ruzicka M, Leenen FHH: Relevance of blockade of cardiac and circulatory angiotensin-converting enzyme for the prevention of volume overload-induced cardiac hypertrophy. Circulation 91:16, 1995.
230. Borghi C, Boschi S, Ambrosioni E, et al: Evidence of a partial escape of renin-angiotensin-aldosterone blockade in patients with acute myocardial infarction treated with ACE inhibitors. J Clin Pharmacol 33:40, 1993.
231. Pitt B: "Escape" of aldosterone production in patients with left ventricular dysfunction treated with an angiotensin converting enzyme inhibitor: Implications for therapy. Cardiovasc Drugs Ther 9:145, 1995.
232. Gottlieb SS, Kickstein K, Fleck E, et al: Hemodynamic and neurohormonal effects of the angiotensin II antagonist losartan in patients with congestive heart failure. Circulation 88:1602, 1993.
233. Havranek EP, Thomas I, Smith WB, et al: Dose-related beneficial long-term hemodynamic and clinical efficacy of irbesartan in heart failure. J Am Coll Cardiol 33:1174, 1999.
234. Mazayev VP, Fomina IG, Kazkov EN, et al: Valsartan in heart failure patients previously untreated with an ACE inhibitor. Int Cardiol 65:239, 1998.
235. Guazzi M, Palermo P, Pontone G, et al: Synergistic efficacy of enalapril and losartan on exercise performance and oxygen consumption at peak exercise in congestive heart failure. Am J Cardiol 84:1038, 1999.
236. Riegger GA, Bouzo H, Petr P, et al: Improvement in exercise tolerance and symptoms of congestive heart failure during treatment with candesartan cilexetil. Symptom, Tolerability, Response to Exercise Trial of Candesartan Cilexetil in Heart Failure (STRETCH) Investigators. Circulation 100:2224, 1999.
237. Hamroff G, Katz SD, Mancini D, et al: Addition of angiotensin II receptor blockade to maximal angiotensin-converting enzyme inhibition improves exercise capacity in patients with severe congestive heart failure. Circulation 99:990, 1999.
238. Baruch L, Anand I, Cohen IS, et al: Augmented short- and long-term hemodynamic and hormonal effects of an angiotensin receptor blocker added to angiotensin converting enzyme inhibitor therapy in patients with heart failure. Vasodilator Heart Failure Trial (V-HeFT) Study Group. Circulation 99:2658, 1999.
239. McKelvie RS, Yusuf S, Pericak D, et al: Comparison of candesartan, enalapril, and their combination in congestive heart failure: Randomized evaluation of strategies for left ventricular dysfunction (RESOLVD) pilot study. The RESOLVD Pilot Study Investigators. Circulation 100:1056, 1999.
240. Pitt B, Segal R, Martinez FA, et al: Randomized trial of losartan versus captopril in patients over 65 with heart failure (Evaluation of Losartan in the Elderly Study, ELITE). Lancet 349:747, 1997.
241. Pitt B, Poole-Wilson PA, Segal R, et al: Effect of losartan compared with captopril on mortality in patients with symptomatic heart failure: Randomised trial—The Losartan Heart Failure Survival Study ELITE II. Lancet 355:1582, 2000.
242. Cohn JN, Tognoni G, Valsartan Heart Failure Trial Investigators: A randomized trial of the angiotensin-receptor blocker valsartan in chronic heart failure. N Engl J Med 345:1667, 2001.
243. Granger CB, McMurray JJV, Yusuf S, et al, for the CHARM Investigators. Effects of candesartan in patients with chronic heart failure and reduced left ventricular systolic function intolerant to angiotensin-converting-enzyme inhibitors: The CHARM-Alternative Trial. Lancet 362:772, 2003.
244. McMurray JJV, Ostergren J, Swedberg K, et al, for the CHARM Investigators: Effects of candesartan in patients with chronic heart failure and reduced left ventricular systolic function taking angiotensin-converting-enzyme inhibitors: The CHARM-Added Trial. Lancet 362:767, 2003.
245. Yusuf S, Pfeffer MA, Swedberg K, et al, for the CHARM Investigators. Effects of candesartan in patients with chronic heart failure and preserved left-ventricular ejection fraction: The CHARM-Preserved Trial. Lancet 362:777, 2003.
246. Pfeffer MA, McMurray JJV, Velazquez EJ, et al: Valsartan, captopril, or both in myocardial infarction complicated by heart failure, left ventricular dysfunction, or both. N Engl J Med 349:1893, 2003
247. Weber KT, Brilla CG, Campbell SE, et al: Myocardial fibrosis: Role of angiotensin II and aldosterone. Basic Res Cardiol 8:107, 1998.341.
248. Ramires FJ, Mansor A, Coelho O, et al: Effect of spironolactone on ventricular arrhythmias in congestive heart failure secondary to idiopathic dilated or to ischemic cardiomyopathy. Am J Cardiol 85:1207, 2000.
249. Qin W, Rudolph AE, Bond BR, et al: Transgenic model of aldosterone-driven cardiac hypertrophy and heart failure. Circ Res 93:69, 2003.
250. Bristow MR, Saxon LA, Boehmer J, et al: Cardiac resynchronization therapy with or without an implantable defibrillator in advanced chronic heart failure: The COMPANION trial. N Engl J Med 350:2140, 2004.

Antiadrenergic Agents

251. Haber HL, Christopher LS, Gimple LW, et al: Why do patients with congestive heart failure tolerate the initiation of β-blocker therapy? Circulation 88:1610, 1993.
253. Goldsmith SR, Francis GS, Cohn JN: Norepinephrine infusions in congestive heart failure. Am J Cardiol 56:802, 1985.
254. Bristow MR, Minobe W, Rasmussen R, et al: β-Adrenergic neuroeffector abnormalities in the failing human heart are produced by local, rather than systemic mechanisms. J Clin Invest 89:803, 1992.
255. Kaye DM, Lefkovits J, Jennings GL, et al: Adverse consequences of high sympathetic nervous activity in the failing human heart. J Am Coll Cardiol 26:1257, 1995.

256. Bristow MR, Feldman AM, Adams KF, Goldstein S: Selective versus nonselective β-blockade for heart failure therapy—Are there lessons to be learned from the COMET Trial? J Card Fail 9:444, 2003.
257. Bristow MR, Ginsburg R, Fowler M, et al: β_1 and β_2-adrenergic receptor subpopulations in normal and failing human ventricular myocardium: Coupling of both receptor subtypes to muscle contraction and selective β_1 receptor down-regulation in heart failure. Circ Res 59:297, 1986.
258. White M, Roden R, Minobe W, et al: Age-related changes in β-adrenergic neuroeffector systems in the human heart. Circulation 90:1225, 1994.
259. Vago T, Bevilacqua M, Norbiato G, et al: Identification of α_1-adrenergic receptors on sarcolemma from normal subjects and patients with idiopathic dilated cardiomyopathy: Characteristics and linkage to GTP-binding protein. Circ Res 64:474, 1989.
260. Bristow MR, Port JD, Gilbert EM: The role of adrenergic receptor regulation in the treatment of heart failure. Cardiovasc Drugs Ther 3:971, 1989.
261. Newton GE, Parker JD: Acute effects of β_1-selective and nonselective β-adrenergic receptor blockade on cardiac sympathetic activity in congestive heart failure. Circulation 94:353, 1996.
262. Gauthier C, Tavernier G, Charpentier F, et al: Functional β_3-adrenoceptor in the human heart. J Clin Invest 98:556, 1996.
263. Kaumann AJ, Molenaar P: Modulation of human cardiac function through 4 beta-adrenergic populations. Naunyn Schmiedebergs Arch Pharmacol 355:667, 1997.
264. Engelhardt S, Hein L, Wiesman F, Lohse MJ: Progressive hypertrophy and heart failure in β_1-adrenergic receptor transgenic mice. Proc Natl Acad Sci USA 96:7059, 1999.
265. Bisognano JD, Weinberger HD, Bohlmeyer TJ, et al: Myocardial-directed overexpression of the human β_1-adrenergic receptor in transgenic mice. J Mol Cell Cardiol 32:817, 2000.
266. Perez JM, Rathz DA, Petrashevskaya NN, et al: β_1-Adrenergic receptor polymorphisms confer differential function and predisposition to heart failure. Nat Med 10:1300, 2003.
267. Freeman K, Lerman I, Kranias EG, et al: Alterations in cardiac adrenergic signaling and calcium cycling differentially affect the progression of cardiomyopathy. J Clin Invest 107:967, 2001.
268. Liggett SB, Tepe NM, Lorenz JN, et al: Early and delayed consequences of β_2-adrenergic receptor overexpression in mouse hearts: Critical role for expression level. Circulation 101:1707, 2000.
269. Iwase M, Bishop SP, Uechi M, et al: Adverse effects of chronic endogenous sympathetic drive induced by cardiac $G_{s\alpha}$ overexpression. Circ Res 78:517, 1996.
270. D'Angelo DD, Sakatra Y, Lorenz JN, et al: Transgenic Gαq overexpression induces cardiac contractile failure in mice. Proc Natl Acad Sci USA 94:8121, 1997.
271. Communal C, Singh K, Pimental DR, Colucci WS: Norepinephrine stimulates apoptosis in adult rat ventricular myocytes by activation of the β-adrenergic receptor. Circulation 98:1329, 1998.
272. Communal C, Singh K, Sawyer DB, Colluci WS: Opposing effects of β_1- and β_2-adrenergic receptors on cardiac myocyte apoptosis. Role of a pertussis-toxin sensitive G protein. Circulation 100:2210, 1999.
273. Milano CA, Dolber PC, Rockman HA, et al: Myocardial expression of a constitutively active α_{1B}-adrenergic receptor in transgenic mice induces cardiac hypertrophy. Proc Natl Acad Sci USA 91:10109, 1994.
274. Lemire I, Ducharme A, Tardif JC, et al: Cardiac-directed overexpression of wild-type alpha1B-adrenergic receptor induces dilated cardiomyopathy. Am J Physiol 281:H931, 2001.
275. Gao MH, Lai C, Roth DM, et al: Adenylylcyclase increases responsiveness to catecholamine stimulation in transgenic mice. Circulation 99:1618, 1999.
276. Kim SJ, Yatani A, Vatner DE, et al:. Differential regulation of inotropy and lusitropy in overexpressed Gsalpha myocytes through cAMP and Ca^{2+} channel pathways. J Clin Invest 103:1089, 1999.
277. Bristow MR, Hershberger RE, Port JD, et al: β_1- and β_2-adrenergic receptor mediated adenylate cyclase stimulation in nonfailing and failing human ventricular myocardium. Mol Pharmacol 35:295, 1989.
278. Ungerer M, Parruti G, Bohm M, et al: Expression of β-arrestins and β-adrenergic receptor kinases in the failing human heart. Circ Res 74:206, 1994.
279. Tan LB, Benjamin IJ, Clark WA: β-Adrenergic receptor desensitization may serve a cardioprotective role. Cardiovasc Res 26:608, 1992.
280. Bristow MR: Pathophysiologic and pharmacologic rationales for clinical management of chronic heart failure with beta-blocking agents. Am J Cardiol 71:12C, 1993.
281. Eichhorn EJ, Bristow MR: Practical guidelines for initiation of beta-adrenergic blockade in patients with chronic heart failure. Am J Cardiol 79:794, 1997.
282. Newton GE, Azevedo ER, Parker JD: Inotropic and sympathetic responses to the intracoronary infusion of a beta2-receptor agonist: A human in vivo study. Circulation 99:2402, 1999.
283. Bristow MR, Roden RL, Lowes BD, et al: The role of third generation β-blocking agents in chronic heart failure. Clin Cardiol 21(Suppl 1):I3, 1998.
284. Bristow MR, Gilbert EM: Improvement in cardiac myocyte function by biologic effects of medical therapy: A new concept in the treatment of heart failure. Eur Heart J 16(Suppl F):20, 1995.
285. Lechat P, Escolano S, Golmard JL, et al: Prognostic value of bisoprolol-induced hemodynamic effects in heart failure during the Cardiac Insufficiency Bisoprolol Study (CIBIS). Circulation 96:2197, 1997.
286. Lowes BD, Gilbert EM, Abraham WT, et al: Myocardial gene expression in dilated cardiomyopathy treated with beta-blocking agents. N Engl J Med 346:1357, 2002.
287. Abraham WT, Gilbert EM, Lowes BD, et al: Coordinate changes in myosin heavy chain isoform gene expression are selectively associated with alterations in dilated cardiomyopathy phenotype. Mol Med 8:750, 2002.
288. Nadal-Ginard B, Mahdavi V: Molecular basis of cardiac performance. Plasticity of the myocardium generated through protein isoform switches. J Clin Invest 84:1693, 1989.
289. Asano K, Zisman LS, Yoshikawa T, et al: Bucindolol, a nonselective β_1- and β_2-adrenergic receptor antagonist, decreases β-adrenergic receptor density in cultured embryonic chick cardiac myocyte membranes. J Cardiovasc Pharmacol 37:678, 2001.
290. Sandberg A, Abrahamsson B, Regardh C-G, et al: Pharmacokinetic and biopharmaceutic aspects of once daily treatment with metoprolol CR/ZOK: A review article. J Clin Pharm 30:S2, 1990.
291. The International Steering Committee: Rationale, design, and organization of the Metoprolol CR/XL Randomized Intervention Trial in Heart Failure (MERIT-HF). Am J Cardiol 80(9B):54J, 1997.
292. Kukin ML, Mannino MM, Freudenberger RS, et al: Hemodynamic comparison of twice daily metoprolol tartrate with once daily metoprolol succinate in congestive heart failure. J Am Coll Cardiol 35:45, 2000.
293. Poole-Wilson PA, Swedberg K, Cleland JGF, et al, for the COMET Investigators: Comparison of carvedilol and metoprolol on clinical outcomes in patients with chronic heart failure in the Carvedilol Or Metoprolol European Trial (COMET): Randomised controlled trial. Lancet 362:7, 2003.
294. Goldstein S, Fagerberg B, Hjalmarson A, et al, for the MERIT-HF Study Group: Metoprolol controlled release/extended release in patients with severe heart failure. J Am Coll Cardiol 38:932, 2001.
295. Packer M, Fowler MB, Roecker EB, et al, for the Carvedilol Prospective Randomized Cumulative Survival (COPERNICUS) Study Group: Effect of carvedilol on the morbidity of patients with severe chronic heart failure: Results of the Carvedilol Prospective Randomized Cumulative Survival (COPERNICUS) study. Circulation 106:2194, 2002.
296. Le Coz F, Sauleman P, Poirier JM, et al: Oral pharmacokinetics of bisoprolol in resting and exercising healthy volunteers. J Cardiovasc Pharmacol 18:28, 1991.
297. CIBIS Investigators and Committees: A randomized trial of beta-blockade in heart failure: The Cardiac Insufficiency Bisoprolol Study (CIBIS). Circulation 90:1765, 1994.
298. Noguchi N, Nishino K, Niki E: Antioxidant action of the antihypertensive drug, carvedilol, against lipid peroxidation. Biochem Pharmacol 59:1069, 2000.
299. Lindenfeld JA, Lowes BD, Bristow MR: Hypotension with dobutamine. Beta-adrenergic antagonist selectivity at low doses of carvedilol. Ann Pharmacother 33:1266, 1999.
300. Metra M, Nardi M, Giubbini R, Dei Cas L: Effects of short- and long-term carvedilol administration on rest and exercise hemodynamic variables, exercise capacity and clinical conditions in patients with idiopathic dilated cardiomyopathy. J Am Coll Cardiol 24:1678, 1994.
301. Olsen SL, Gilbert EM, Renlund DG, et al: Carvedilol improves left ventricular function and symptoms in heart failure: A double-blind randomized study. J Am Coll Cardiol 25:1225, 1995.
302. Krum H, Sakner-Bernstein JD, Goldsmith RL, et al: Double-blind, placebo-controlled study of the long-term efficacy of carvedilol in patients with severe chronic heart failure. Circulation 92:1499, 1995.
303. Lowes BD, Gill EA, Abraham WT, et al: The effect of carvedilol on left ventricular mass, chamber geometry and mitral regurgitation in chronic heart failure. Am J Cardiol 83:1201, 1999.
304. Doughty RN, Whalley GA, Gamble G, et al: Left ventricular remodeling with carvedilol in patients with congestive heart failure due to ischemic heart disease. J Am Coll Cardiol 29:1060, 1997.
305. Doughty RN, Whalley GA, Gamble G, et al: Effects of carvedilol on left ventricular regional wall motion in patients with heart failure caused by ischemic heart disease. J Card Fail 6:11, 2000.
306. O'Keefe JH Jr, Magalski A, Stevens TL, et al: Predictors of improvement in left ventricular ejection fraction with carvedilol for congestive heart failure. J Nucl Cardiol 7:3, 2000.
307. McTavish D, Campoli-Richards D, Sorkin EM: Carvedilol: A review of its pharmacodynamic and pharmacokinetic properties, and therapeutic efficacy. Drugs 45:232, 1993.
308. Gilbert EM, Abraham WT, Olsen S, et al: Comparative hemodynamic, left ventricular functional, and antiadrenergic effects of chronic treatment with metoprolol versus carvedilol in the failing heart. Circulation 94:2817, 1996.
309. Bristow MR, Abraham WT, Yoshikawa T, et al: Second- and third-generation beta-blocking drugs in chronic heart failure. Cardiovasc Drugs Ther 11:291, 1997.
310. Metra M, Nodari S, Giubbini R, et al: Differential effects of beta-blockers in patients with heart failure. A prospective, randomized, double-blind comparison of the long-term effects of metoprolol versus carvedilol. Circulation 102:546, 2000.
311. Kukin ML, Kalman J, Charney RH, et al: Prospective, randomized comparison of effect of long-term treatment with metoprolol or carvedilol on symptoms, exercise, ejection fraction, and oxidative stress in heart failure. Circulation 99:2645, 1999.
312. Packer M, Colucci WS, Sackner-Bernstein JD, et al: Double-blind, placebo-controlled study of the effects of carvedilol in patients with moderate to severe heart failure: The PRECISE Trial. Circulation 94:2793, 1996.
313. Colucci WS, Packer M, Bristow MR, et al: Carvedilol inhibits clinical progression in patients with mild symptoms of heart failure. Circulation 94:2800, 1996.
314. Cohn JN, Fowler MB, Bristow MR, et al: Effect of carvedilol in severe chronic heart failure J Card Fail 3:173, 1997.
315. Australia-New Zealand Heart Failure Research Collaborative Group: Effects of carvedilol, a vasodilator-β-blocker, in patients with congestive heart failure due to ischemic heart disease. Circulation 92:212, 1995.
316. Australia/New Zealand Heart Failure Research Collaborative Group: Randomised, placebo-controlled trial of carvedilol in patients with congestive heart failure due to ischaemic heart disease. Lancet 349:375, 1997.
317. Packer M, Fowler MB, Roecker EB, et al: Carvedilol Prospective Randomized Cumulative Survival (COPERNICUS) Study Group: Effect of carvedilol on the morbidity of patients with severe chronic heart failure: Results of the carvedilol prospective randomized cumulative survival (COPERNICUS) study. Circulation 106:2194, 2002.
318. Lowes BD, Chidiac P, Olsen S, et al: Clinical relevance of inverse agonism and guanine nucleotide modulatable binding properties of adrenergic receptor blocking agents. Circulation 90(Suppl 1):543, 1994.

319. Yoshikawa T, Port JD, Asano K, et al: Cardiac adrenergic receptor effects of carvedilol. Eur Heart J 17(Suppl B):8, 1996.
320. BEST Trial Investigators: A trial of the beta-adrenergic blocker bucindolol in patients with advanced heart failure. N Engl J Med 344:1659, 2001.
321. Willette RN, Mitchell MP, Ohlstein EH, et al: Evaluation of intrinsic sympathomimetic activity of bucindolol and carvedilol in rat heart. Pharmacology 56:30, 1998.
322. Hershberger RE, Wynn JR, Sundberg L, Bristow MR: Mechanism of action of bucindolol in human ventricular myocardium. J Cardiovasc Pharmacol 15:959, 1990.
323. Maack C, Cremers B, Flesch M, et al: Different intrinsic activities of bucindolol, carvedilol and metoprolol in human failing myocardium. Br J Pharmacol 130:1131, 2000.
324. Brixius K, Bundkirchen A, Bolck B, et al: Nebivolol, bucindolol, metoprolol and carvedilol are devoid of intrinsic sympathomimetic activity in human myocardium. Br J Pharmacol 133:1330, 2001.
325. Bristow MR, Larrabee P, Minobe W, et al: Receptor pharmacology of carvedilol in the human heart. J Cardiovasc Pharmacol 19(Suppl 1):68, 1992.
326. Sederberg J, Wichman WE, Lindenfeld J, et al: Bucindolol has no intrinsic sympathomimetic activity in nonfailing human ventricular preparations [abstract]. J Am Coll Cardiol 35:207, 2000.
327. Bristow MR, Krause-Steinrauf H, Nuzzo R, et al: Effect of baseline changes in adrenergic activity on clinical outcomes in the Beta-blocker Evaluation of Survival Trial (BEST). Circulation (in press).
328. Pollock SG, Lystash J, Tedesco C, et al: Usefulness of bucindolol in congestive heart failure. Am J Cardiol 66:603, 1990.
329. Bristow MR, O'Connell JB, Gilbert EM, et al: Dose-response of chronic β-blocker treatment in heart failure from either idiopathic dilated or ischemic cardiomyopathy. Circulation 89:1632, 1994.
330. Stephen SA: Unwanted effects of propranolol. Am J Cardiol 18:463, 1966.
331. Epstein SE, Braunwald E: The effect of beta adrenergic blockade on patterns of urinary sodium excretion: Studies in normal subjects and in patients with heart disease. Ann Intern Med 65:20, 1968.
332. Talwar KK, Bhargava B, Upasani PT, et al: Hemodynamic predictors of early intolerance and long-term effects of propranolol in dilated cardiomyopathy. J Card Fail 2:273, 1996.
333. Yancy C, Fowler MB, Colucci WS, et al: Race and the response to adrenergic blockade with carvedilol in patients with chronic heart failure. N Engl J Med 344:1358, 2001.
334. Freudenberger R, Kalman J, Mannino M, et al: Effect of race in the response to metoprolol in patients with congestive heart failure secondary to idiopathic dilated or ischemic cardiomyopathy. Am J Cardiol 80:1372, 1997.
335. Goldstein S, Deedwania P, Gottlieb S, Wikstrand J; MERIT-HF Study Group: Metoprolol CR/XL in black patients with heart failure (from the metoprolol CR/XL randomized intervention trial in chronic heart failure). Am J Cardiol 92:478, 2003.
336. Carson P, Ziesche S, Johnson G, Cohn J: Racial differences in response to therapy for heart failure: Analysis of the vasodilator-heart failure trials. J Card Fail 5:178, 1999.
337. Domanski M, Krause-Steinrauf H, Deedwania P, et al: The effect of diabetes on outcome of advanced heart failure patients in the BEST Trial. J Am Coll Cardiol 42:914, 2003.
338. Torp-Pedersen C, Kober L, Ball S, et al: The incomplete bucindolol evaluation in acute myocardial infarction trial (BEAT). Eur J Heart Fail 4:495, 2002.
339. Bristow MR: Anti-adrenergic therapy of chronic heart failure: Surprises and new opportunities. Circulation 107:1100, 2003.
340. Wisenbaugh T, Katz I, Davis J, et al: Long-term (3 month) effects of a new beta-blocker (nebivolol) on cardiac performance in dilated cardiomyopathy. J Am Coll Cardiol 21:1094, 1993.
341. Uhlir O, Dvorak I, Gregor P, et al: Nebivolol in the treatment of cardiac failure: A double-blind controlled clinical trial. J Card Fail 3:271, 1997.
342. Cockcroft JR, Chowienczyk PJ, Brett SE, et al: Nebivolol vasodilates human forearm vasculature: Evidence for an L-arginine/NO-dependent mechanism. J Pharmacol Exp Ther 274:1067, 1995.
343. Abraham WT: Beta blockers; the new standard of therapy for mild heart failure. Arch Intern Med 160:1237, 2000.
344. Metra M, Nodari S, D'Aloia A, et al: A rationale for the use of beta blockers as standard treatment for heart failure. Am Heart J 139:511, 2000.
345. Swedberg K, Hjalmarson A, Waagstein F, Wallentin I: Adverse effects of beta-blockade withdrawal in patients with congestive cardiomyopathy. Br Heart J 44:134, 1980.
346. Manolis AJ, Olympios C, Sifaki M, et al: Chronic sympathetic suppression in the treatment of chronic congestive heart failure. Clin Exp Hypertens 20:717, 1998.
347. Zhang YH, Zhu J, Song YC: Suppressing sympathetic activation with clonidine on ventricular arrhythmias in congestive heart failure. Int J Cardiol 65:233, 1998.
348. Swedberg K, Bristow MR, Cohn JN, et al, for the MOXSE Investigators: The effects of moxonidine SR, an imidazoline agonist, on plasma norepinephrine in patients with congestive heart failure. Circulation 105:1797, 2002.
349. Cohn JN, Pfeffer MA, Rouleau J, et al, for the MOXCON Investigators: Adverse mortality effect of central sympathetic inhibition with sustained-release moxonidine in patients with heart failure (MOXCON). Eur J Heart Fail 5:659, 2003.

CHAPTER 24

Management of Heart Failure

Michael R. Bristow • Brian D. Lowes

Heart failure (HF) is a specific term used to define the clinical syndrome that ensues when the heart is unable to pump enough blood to supply the metabolic needs of the body (see Chaps. 19 and 21). The clinical syndrome of HF is caused by *cardiac failure*, a term used to define the various types of pump dysfunction that may cause HF. Cardiac failure may be produced by processes involving the pericardium, heart valves, coronary circulation, or myocardium (Table 24–1). Of these etiologies, the most common cause of chronic HF is myocardial dysfunction, termed *myocardial failure*. Myocardial failure is usually divided into two general types, *systolic dysfunction* and *diastolic dysfunction*, to reflect the dominant abnormalities of contraction and relaxation, respectively. Subjects with myocardial failure can have symptomatic HF or asymptomatic ventricular dysfunction.

As typically used, HF generally refers to the chronic syndrome, or *chronic HF*. The qualifier "congestive" should not be used in association with HF inasmuch as many HF patients receiving modern medical treatment do not manifest congestive symptoms or signs. Rather, HF symptoms usually relate to impaired exercise tolerance, plus or minus symptoms related to fluid overload. Symptoms of exercise intolerance are typically assessed by the New York Heart Association (NYHA) functional classification (see Chap. 7),[1] where

I = no symptoms
II = symptoms with moderate or marked levels of activity
III = symptoms with mild activity
IV = symptoms at rest

Because of its high prevalence (~2 percent of the adult population,[2,3] lifetime risk for men or women ~20 percent)[4] and frequent hospitalizations, the clinical syndrome of HF is among the most costly medical problems in the United States (see Chap. 22).[5] Despite improvements in the treatment of HF introduced since the early 1980s, including the general availability of cardiac transplantation and better medical treatment, clinical outcome following the onset of symptoms remains characterized by high mortality, morbidity, and progression of symptoms. For example, even in recent clinical trials showing benefit of new agents superimposed on successful older treatment, annualized mortality (percentage) and hospitalization rates (number of hospitalizations per patient per year) in the active treatment groups have been, respectively, 5 to 9 percent and 0.3 to 0.4 in Classes II and III[6-8] and 14 to 18 percent and 0.6 to 0.8 in Classes III and IV HF.[9,10] Furthermore, HF is the only cardiovascular disorder in the United States that is increasing in prevalence,[11] and since the prevalence is directly related to age,[12] the incidence and prevalence of HF will continue to increase on the basis of population demographics (Fig. 24–1). At present, an estimated 4.5 million patients have HF in the United States,[11] plus at least as many additional subjects with asymptomatic left ventricular dysfunction.[13] As can be observed in Figure 24–1, by 2050 the number of subjects with symptomatic HF will increase to more than 7 million on the basis of an increase in the number of persons older than 65 years,[14] in whom the prevalence of HF is 6 percent.[2]

Pathophysiology of Heart Failure due to Primary or Secondary Dilated Cardiomyopathies

The discussion of pathophysiology here is confined to primary and secondary dilated cardiomyopathy (see Chap. 59), the cause of the majority of cases of HF, as it may relate to medical therapy. More detailed discussion of the pathophysiology of myocardial failure is given in Chapter 21. HF caused by pericardial (see Chap. 64), valvular (see Chap. 57), and ischemic (see Chap. 50) heart disease is discussed elsewhere.

As depicted in Figure 24–2, two interrelated processes, chamber remodeling and myocardial systolic dysfunction, are thought to play critical roles in the development and progression of primary and secondary dilated cardiomyopathy.[15,16] Although both are the products of changes that occur at the cardiac myocyte level, changes in the interstitium also contribute.[17] In the remodeling process, cardiac myocytes become longer without a proportional increase in transverse diameter, which explains the increase in chamber diameter without an increase in wall thickness.[18] Factors known to contribute to the cellular and chamber remodeling process are activation of "compensatory mechanisms" that include the renin-angiotensin-aldosterone system (RAAS) and the adrenergic nervous system.[16] Although the remodeling process does increase the number of contractile elements as new sarcomeres are laid down in series, the law of Laplace dictates that diastolic wall stress will be markedly increased (see Chap. 19). Also, the elongated and remodeled cardiac myocyte is poorly contractile,[19] in part due to the activation of a "fetal" gene program that can directly cause contractile dysfunction.[20] The end result of these processes is a poorly contractile, dilated ventricular chamber that at some point can no longer adequately support the circulatory requirements of daily living. These processes are progressive in most patients with established chronic HF,[21] and the pace[22] and degree[23] of this progression are directly related to prognosis. This is why the pharmacological therapy of HF, discussed in detail in Chapter 23, is aimed at inhibiting the mechanistic processes that promote systolic dysfunction and remodeling.[16,20,21]

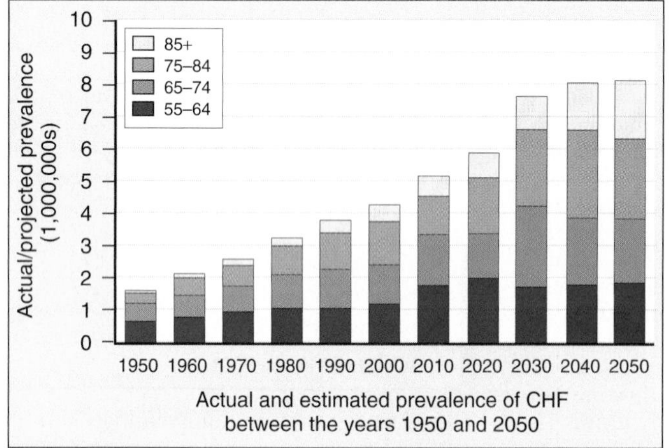

FIGURE 24–1 Effect of the aging population on the prevalence of heart failure, based on data from the National Heart, Lung, and Blood Institute (www.nhlbi.nih.gov/health/public/heart/other/CHF) and the U.S. Bureau of the Census. CHF = congestive heart failure.

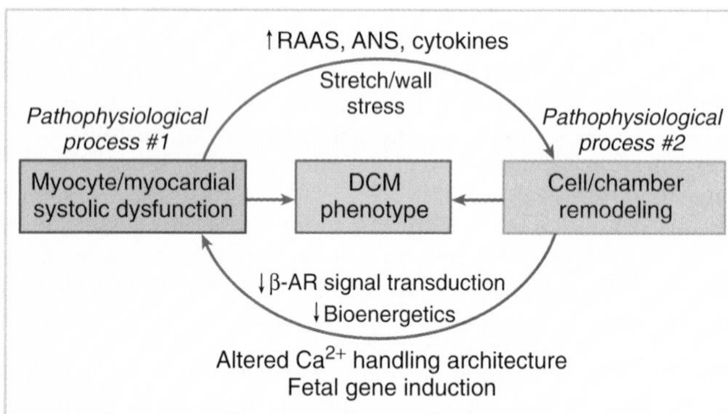

FIGURE 24–2 Relationship between contractile dysfunction and remodeling. RAAS = renin-angiotensin-aldosterone system; ANS = adrenergic nervous system; DCM = dilated cardiomyopathy; β-AR = beta-adrenergic receptor.

TABLE 24–1 General Etiologies of Cardiac Failure

General Cause	Specific Examples
Pericardial	Tamponade, pericardial constriction
Valvular	Aortic or mitral regurgitation
Myocardial	Idiopathic dilated cardiomyopthy, familial dilated cardiomyopathy, ischemic cardiomyopathy, valvular cardiomyopathy
Coronary vascular	Acute ischemic episodes
Rhythm disturbances	Tachycardia-induced heart failure

Diagnosis of Heart Failure: Determination of Etiology and Prognosis

One of the major problems in HF is its initial diagnosis, since the earliest symptoms of HF are often mistaken for other medical problems, including bronchial asthma, chronic obstructive pulmonary disease, pneumonia, and other pulmonary and nonpulmonary problems (see Chap. 22). Numerous studies have documented the lack of sensitivity and specificity of HF signs and symptoms,[24] and the initial diagnosis is often first made by the radiologist from a chest radiograph demonstrating pulmonary edema and cardiomegaly. Because of these realities, alternative means of initially diagnosing HF have and are being developed, such as point-of-care blood tests. Two of these tests, brain natriuretic peptide (BNP)[25] and N-terminal pro-BNP,[26] have been shown to improve the accuracy of HF diagnosis in an urgent care setting. The utility of these tests would appear to markedly improve the sensitivity of the diagnosis of HF, while at the same time reducing costs by limiting the number of unnecessary diagnostic echocardiograms.[27,28]

DETECTION OF SYSTOLIC DYSFUNCTION (see Chap. 20). An algorithm for diagnosing and evaluating HF is given in Figure 24-3. If HF is suspected because of symptoms (dyspnea, dyspnea on exertion, paroxysmal nocturnal dyspnea, orthopnea, peripheral edema, easy fatigability), radiographic or biochemical data, or a high natriuretic peptide concentration, an echocardiogram needs to be obtained. In the limited number of subjects who cannot be imaged by ultrasound for technical reasons, radionuclide ventriculography or magnetic resonance imaging (MRI) can be used to detect ventricular systolic dysfunction. An echocardiogram is the initial test of choice because it evaluates valvular and pericardial causes of HF, as well as being able to detect systolic dysfunction, and it may also be able to detect diastolic dysfunction. An echocardiogram (see Chap. 11) provides immediate information about whether the etiology is a pericardial, valvular, or myocardial process. HF needs to be diagnosed as early as possible so that mortality- and morbidity-lowering treatment can be initiated.

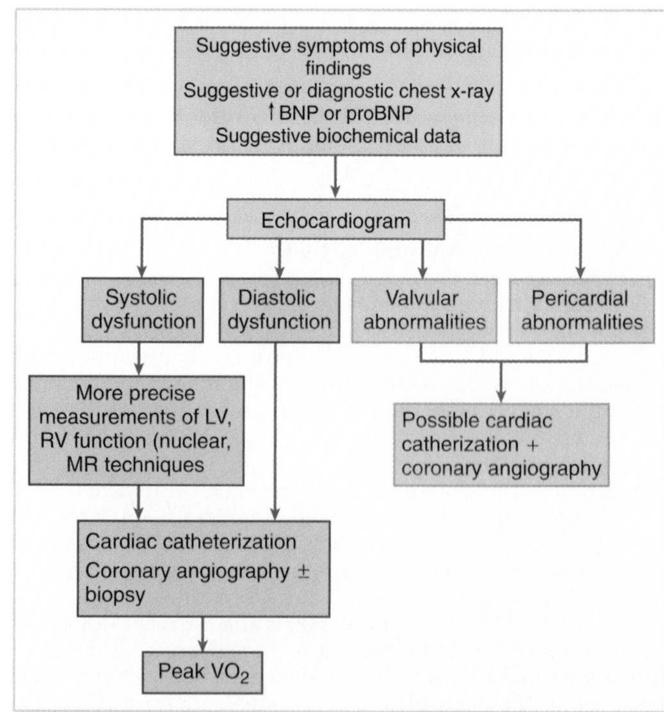

FIGURE 24–3 Algorithm for establishing the diagnosis of heart failure and determining etiology and prognosis. LV = left ventricular; MR = magnetic resonance; RV = right ventricular; BNP = brain natriuretic peptide; VO_2 = oxygen consumption.

If impaired left ventricular systolic function is detected by echocardiography, more precise measurement of the function of both ventricles may be indicated via radionuclide ventriculography (see Chap. 13). This imaging modality is able to measure left ventricular systolic function more precisely, which is important from a prognostic standpoint,[22,23] and for monitoring the response to beta blocker therapy, a treatment that favorably affects systolic function (see later).[16] Radionuclide ventriculography can also measure right ventricular function, which is another prognostic index in chronic HF.[29] When right ventricular structural abnormalities are suspected, cardiac MRI is indicated (see Chap. 14) because this modality is currently the best available imaging method for visualizing right ventricular pathology and function.

DIASTOLIC DYSFUNCTION (see Chap. 20). The diagnosis of diastolic dysfunction is largely one of exclusion. That is, to make the diagnosis of diastolic dysfunction, two pieces of data are required: documentation of normal or near-normal systolic function and unequivocal evidence of HF. The latter may be provided by unambiguous documentation of acute episodes of decompensation (e.g., pulmonary edema on a chest radiograph plus symptoms of breathlessness or right-sided failure) or chronic myocardial dysfunction resulting in high filling pressure, decreased cardiac output, and impaired functional capacity. Although echocardiographic and radionuclide ventriculographic data can contribute to a diagnosis of diastolic dysfunction, neither are considered sufficiently definitive to establish the diagnosis on the basis of isolated measurements. Importantly, diastolic dysfunction as the cause of HF in a relatively young (<60-year-old) patient suggests an infiltrative process, and an endomyocardial biopsy may be indicated.

Once the diagnosis of HF has been established, additional data need to be gathered. In general, the goals of this additional work-up are to determine the etiology and establish a general prognosis. The diagnostic work-up of HF should seek to determine the etiology, as outlined in Figure 24-3, unless the patient is so infirm that no form of intervention would be possible. Cardiac catheterization is often indicated to eliminate the possibility of coronary artery disease and other processes for whom specific management is required. Examples of indications for cardiac catheterization in a patient with newly diagnosed HF and various echocardiographic data are given in Table 24-2.

ENDOMYOCARDIAL BIOPSY. Perhaps the most controversial diagnostic test in the work-up of heart muscle disease is endomyocardial biopsy (see Chap. 17). This procedure in inexperienced hands can be associated with complications, including death in rare cases (<1 percent). On the other hand, in the presence of unexplained heart muscle disease, endomyocardial biopsy yields important diagnostic and prognostic information in 11 percent of patients,[30] a figure high enough to justify biopsy provided that experienced personnel are available to perform it and interpret the results.

In cases of systolic dysfunction caused by a primary or secondary dilated cardiomyopathy, precise determination of the degree of left and right ventricular dysfunction has important prognostic value. Additional clinical characteristics that may have an impact on the prognosis are the degree of pulmonary hypertension, the presence or absence of high-grade ventricular arrhythmia, and the extent of coronary artery disease. Valuable prognostic information can be gained by measuring peak oxygen consumption, which in chronic HF correlates with prognosis independently of left ventricular function.[31]

Management of Acute, New-Onset Heart Failure

TRANSIENT HEART FAILURE. (Management of episodes of acute decompensation in patients with chronic HF is discussed later.) Although chronic HF is the most commonly encountered form of symptomatic myocardial dysfunction, HF may also be acute and not superimposed on chronic pump dysfunction. Such manifestations can occur in the postoperative state following cardiac surgery,[32] in the setting of severe brain injury,[33] secondary to ischemic insults, or after the sudden onset of an inflammatory process or any pathophysiological mechanism that rapidly produces myocardial injury. The general pathophysiological mechanism involved is either some form of "stunning" of functional myocardium (see Chap. 19) or abrupt loss of functioning tissue that occurs before compensatory mechanisms can stabilize function. In both of these situations, myocardial function is adequate to support the circulation once recovery has occurred, and in the case of mechanisms that may produce stunning, such as cardiopulmonary bypass, other ischemic insults, and severe brain injury (where the stunning is probably related to massive release of catecholamines),[31] myocardial function may be completely normal on recovery.

TABLE 24–2 Indications for Cardiac Catheterization after Evaluation for Heart Failure and Performance of an Echocardiogram

Echo, Clinical Findings	Cardiac Catheterization or Other Procedure
Significant pericardial effusion, evidence of tamponade	Right heart catheterization, pericardiocentesis
Thickened pericardium, evidence of cardiac compression	Right and left heart catheterization ± endomyocardial biopsy if restriction suspected
Severe aortic or mitral regurgitation, LVE with decreased systolic function	Right and left heart catheterization, coronary angiography in anticipation of possible surgery
Aortic stenosis	Right heart catheterization, coronary angiography in anticipation of surgery
Mitral stenosis	Right and left heart catheterization, coronary angiography in anticipation of possible surgery or balloon valvuloplasty
LVE, decreased systolic function with valvular abnormalities < severe	Right and left heart catheterization, coronary angiography, possible endomyocardial biopsy if coronary arteries normal
Normal LV size, function	Right and left heart catheterization, coronary angiography, possible endomyocardial biopsy if coronary arteries normal, to rule out an infiltrative process
Hypertrophic cardiomyopathy with ASH, ± mitral regurgitation	Coronary angiography if surgery (myectomy, ± mitral valve replacement) contemplated
Normal LV size, decreased systolic function, no history of anthracyclines	Right and left heart catheterization, coronary angiography, endomyocardial biopsy if coronary arteries normal to rule out inflammatory heart disease
RV dysfunction, arrhythmia	MRI (to rule out ARVC)
RV dysfunction, isolated	Right heart catheterization (to rule out PAH)

ARVC = arrhythmic RV cardiomyopathy; ASH = asymmetrical septal hypertrophy; Echo = echocardiogram; LV = left ventricular; LVE = LV enlargement; PAH = pulmonary arterial hypertension; RV = right ventricular.

Management of episodes of acute HF caused by an evanescent process depressing myocardial function is therapy with diuretics, support of pump function with positive inotropic agents (see Chap. 23) and/or, if extremely severe, with mechanical devices (see Chap. 25) to the extent necessary to provide adequate perfusion of critical organs. Once function has recovered, no further treatment may be necessary. In the case of ischemia caused by coronary artery disease or another mechanism that may persist to cause recurrent problems, treatment of the underlying process is the management goal. Further details of the treatment of transient myocardial failure are given later in the section on the treatment of decompensated chronic HF.

NEW-ONSET, PERSISTENT HEART FAILURE. The most common manifestation of acute, new-onset HF is superimposition on a chronic process that has previously been subclinical and in which myocardial function has been supported by the compensatory mechanisms depicted in Figure 24–2. Therefore, most episodes of new-onset HF are actually the first episode of decompensation, similar to what occurs in established chronic HF.

How much myocardial functional loss can be countered by compensatory mechanisms? The quantitative relationship between degree of myocardial loss and development of myocardial pump dysfunction has been examined in two settings: following myocardial infarction[34] and after individual cardiac myocyte "dropout" from anthracycline cardiotoxicity.[35] The experimental model data from acute myocardial infarction[34] are more relevant to acute-onset HF superimposed on previously normal cardiac function, whereas the anthracycline data generated in patients[35] represent decompensation superimposed on a chronic myocardial process that has previously been stabilized by compensatory mechanisms. The conclusion from the myocardial infarction studies conducted in animal models was that loss of 30 percent or less of the left ventricle in rats[34] and 25 percent or less in dogs is relatively well tolerated, whereas in rats, infarcts in excess of 46 percent were associated with severe hemodynamic compromise.

ANTHRACYCLINE-INDUCED CARDIOMYOPATHY. Investigation of the structure-function relationship in anthracycline-induced cardiomyopathy (see Chap. 83) was conducted in the intact human heart in patients receiving the antitumor agent doxorubicin (Adriamycin).[35-37] Myocardial damage in this unique form of drug-induced heart disease consists of vacuolization and myofibrillar loss in individual cardiac myocytes, which are typically surrounded by myocytes that are unaffected.[35,36] By morphometrically counting the number of affected myocytes relative to the total in a field of endomyocardial biopsy material, it is possible to determine the percentage of cells that are nonfunctional because of the anthracycline process.[36,37] The degree of myocardial damage can then be related to the degree of myocardial dysfunction, as assessed by right-heart catheterization performed at rest and with exercise.[35-37] In anthracycline cardiomyopathy it is not until more than 15 percent of cells are damaged that detectable myocardial dysfunction develops, and moderate dysfunction does not develop until more than 25 percent of cardiac myocytes are involved.[35-37] In other words, as in myocardial infarction, in anthracycline-associated cardiomyopathy a certain amount of myocardial damage can be tolerated with the aid of compensatory mechanisms. In anthracycline cardiomyopathy, these compensatory mechanisms rely heavily on adrenergic stimulation, since hypertrophy is inhibited by the effects of anthracyclines on myocardial protein synthesis.[38,39]

Therefore, data from these model systems suggest that the initial, sudden onset of HF occurs when compensatory mechanisms can no longer sustain normal myocardial function. Consequently, myocardial function and structural measurements usually indicate a chronic remodeling process at the initial evaluation for HF.

Management of Chronic Heart Failure

Pharmacological Therapy for Chronic Heart Failure Caused by Systolic Dysfunction

The pharmacological treatment of chronic HF is best understood by subdividing the patient population into four groups as described in Table 24–3. This "HF stage" classification system reflects the average symptomatic status of the patient inasmuch as patients typically move from one NYHA class to another within the stage groups, and is not the same as the American College of Cardiology/American Heart Association (ACC/AHA) Task Force stage classification that begins with stage A being an at-risk patient without HF or myocardial dysfunction.[40] In general, the average symptomatic status is directly related to hospitalization frequency and is also related to mortality risk as demonstrated in Figure 24–4. Important differences between the HF stage–ordered classification and the NYHA functional class are that the stage classification (1) begins with some level of disability as opposed to asymptomatic status, (2) ends with a more advanced level of disability than is generally reflected by the NYHA Class IV category, and (3) recognizes the reality that patients with HF often move from one level of symptoms to another, for example, typically exhibiting Class III symptoms that transiently increase to Class IV depending on medical management and other factors.

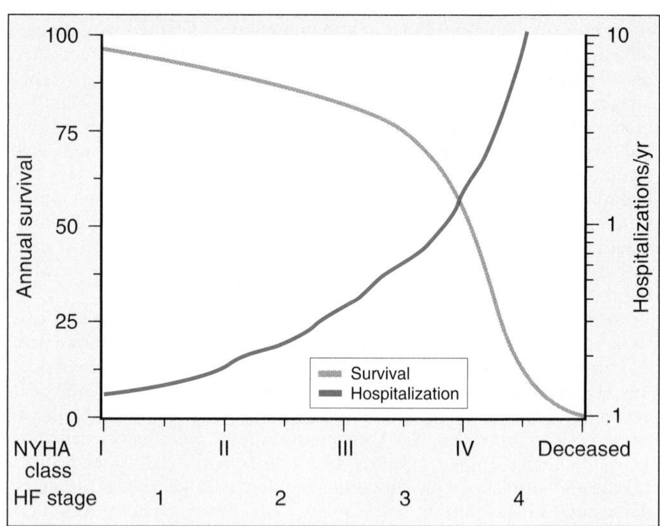

FIGURE 24–4 Plot of the relationship between survival or hospitalization frequency and New York Heart Association (NYHA) class or heart failure (HF) stage in chronic HF.

As outlined in Table 24–3, the goals of treatment for chronic HF are to (1) relieve symptoms and improve functional capacity, (2) reduce disability and hospitalizations, (3) delay progression of or reverse remodeling and myocardial dysfunction, and (4) reduce mortality. Depending on the stage that a particular HF patient is in, one or more of these goals may be more important than the others and dictate the type of agent to be developed or used once efficacy and safety are established.

STAGE 1 (MYOCARDIAL DYSFUNCTION WITH NO OR MILD HEART FAILURE, NYHA CLASS I/II SYMPTOMS). As for any chronic disease process, the most effective way to deal with the HF problem is to treat it early, before irreversible damage has developed. The goals of treatment of stage 1 HF (see Table 24–3) are to prevent progression of the underlying pathophysiological processes of remodeling and dysfunction and thereby prevent disease progression and overt development of the HF syndrome. However, only limited data actually support this generally accepted belief. Clinical trial experience is confined to one study—the Studies of Left Ventricular Dysfunction (SOLVD) Prevention Trial (see Table 23–7).[41] That trial demonstrated that the angiotensin-converting enzyme (ACE) inhibitor enalapril reduced the probability of development of overt HF by 37 percent and reduced the combined endpoint of mortality plus HF hospitalizations by 20 percent.[41]

TABLE 24–3 Goals and Pharmacological Treatment for Various Stages of Heart Failure

Stage	Goals (in order of importance)	Treatment
1 (asymptomatic–mild)	Reverse or prevent progressive remodeling and dysfunction	ACE inhibitors ? Beta-blocking agents ? ARBs
	Prevent overt heart failure or progressive symptoms	ACE inhibitors ? Beta-blocking agents ? ARBs
2 (mild–moderate)	Reverse or prevent progressive remodeling and dysfunction	ACE inhibitors Beta-blocking agents ARBs
	Improve symptoms and functional capacity	Diuretics ACE inhibitors ARBs Digoxin
	Reduce disability and hospitalizations	Diuretics ACE inhibitors Beta-blocking agents ARBs Digoxin
	Reduce mortality	ACE inhibitors Beta-blocking agents
3 (advanced)	Reduce mortality	ACE inhibitors Spironolactone Beta-blocking agents
	Reduce disability and hospitalizations	Diuretics ACE inhibitors Beta-blocking agents Spironolactone ? Positive inotropic agents, including digoxin
	Improve symptoms and functional capacity	Diuretics ACE inhibitors Spironolactone ? Positive inotropic agents, including digoxin
4 (severe)	Reduce disability and hospitalizations	Diuretics ACE inhibitors Positive inotropic agents, for periods of decompensation
	Improve symptoms and functional capacity	Diuretics ACE inhibitors Positive inotropic agents, for periods of decompensation
	Reduce mortality	ACE inhibitors ? Beta-blocking agents + positive inotropes

ACE = angiotensin-converting enzyme; ARB = angiotensin receptor blocker.

Although it is likely that beta-adrenergic blocking agents will reduce mortality in stage 1 HF, because of the sample size and therefore the cost considerations of performing placebo-controlled trials in this patient population, to date no beta blocker clinical trial has examined this patient population. Similarly, trials with other neurohormonal antagonists will probably not be performed until efficacy has been demonstrated in later-stage HF.

STAGE 2 (MILD TO MODERATE HEART FAILURE, NYHA CLASS II/III SYMPTOMS). This is the HF stage in which the majority of clinical trial data are available, because of the prevalence and relative stability of these patients. As a result, recommendations for medical therapy for Class II to III or stage 2 HF can be given with a high degree of certainty, as outlined in Table 24–3. The goals of therapy in this stage are, similar to stage 1, centered around reversal or prevention of progression of remodeling and dysfunction because the potential for reversibility of the dilated cardiomyopathy phenotype still exists. As remodeling/dysfunction is attenuated or reversed, the other treatment goals outlined in Table 24–3 will be realized, and all are important in stage 2 HF.

ACE inhibitors[42-44] (see Table 23–7) and beta-blocking agents[6-8,45] (Fig. 24–5) have been shown to reduce mortality and hospitalizations in patients with stage 2 HF. ACE inhibitors also improve symptoms and tend to improve functional capacity in this stage of HF,[44] whereas beta-blocking agents have produced variable results on symptoms and functional capacity.[45] Angiotensin-receptor blockers (ARBs) can reduce the combined endpoint of cardiovascular mortality and HF hospitalizations when administered on top of an ACE inhibitor in stage 2 patients with preserved blood pressures (average systolic blood pressure >120 mm Hg),[46,47] mostly by reducing HF hospitalizations. However, in one of these trials (Val-Heft)[46] there was an increase in mortality in patients treated with the ARB valsartan on top of ACE inhibition and beta blockade. This adverse effect was not found in the CHARM-Added Trial, which investigated the ARB candesartan.[47] In both trials ARBs were effective in lowering mortality and HF morbidity in patients intolerant of ACE inhibitors (Fig. 24–6).[46,48]

On balance, digoxin has generally improved symptoms and functional capacity in patients in sinus rhythm with mild to moderate HF,[49] slightly reduces hospitalizations but does not reduce mortality.[50] Other, nonapproved positive inotropic agents have also improved functional capacity.[51,52] However, positive inotropic agents other than digoxin have been associated with increased mortality when used chronically in HF, and it is unclear whether newer

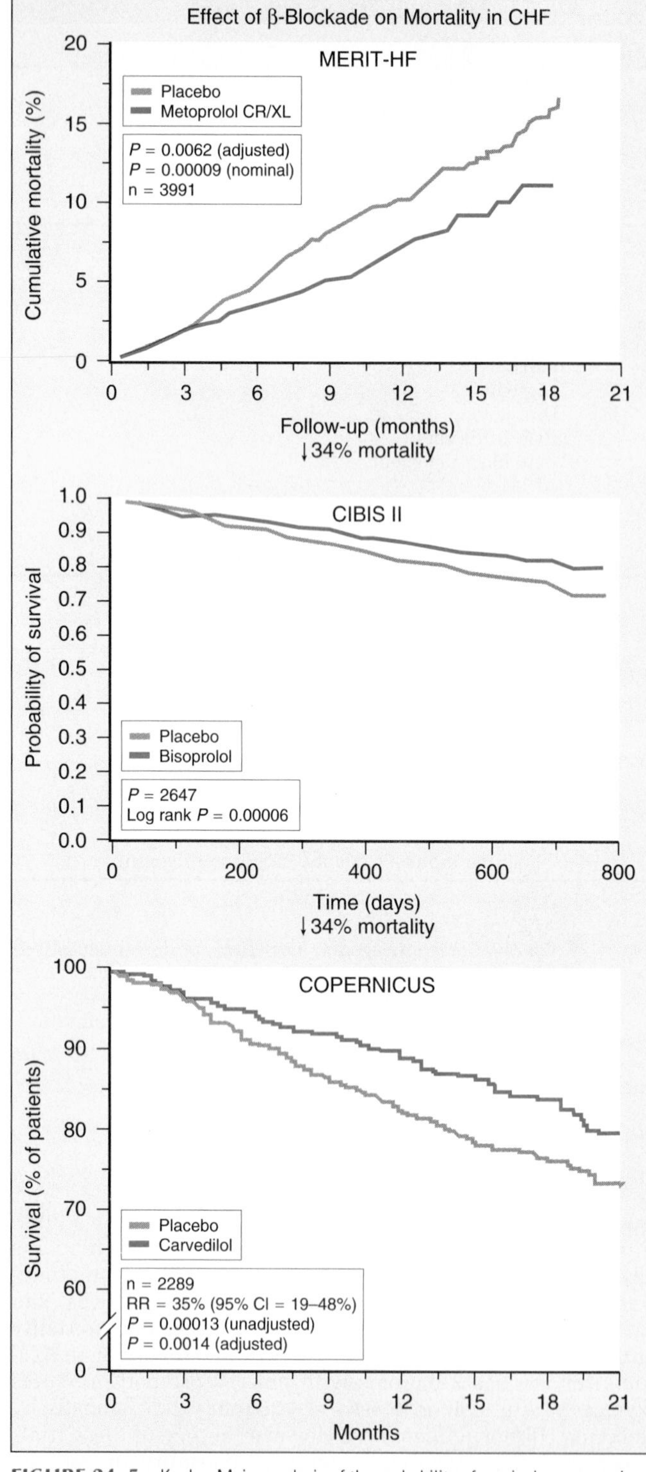

FIGURE 24–5 Kaplan-Meier analysis of the probability of survival among patients in the placebo and beta-blocker groups in the MERIT-HF **(top)**, CIBIS II **(middle)**, and COPERNICUS **(bottom)** trials. CHF = chronic heart failure; CI = confidence interval. (Data from The Cardiac Insufficiency Bisoprolol Study II [CIBIS II]. Lancet 353:9-13, 1999; Metoprolol CR/XL randomized intervention trial in congestive heart failure [MERIT-HF]. Lancet 353:2001-2007, 1999; and Packer M, Coats AJ, Fowler MB, et al, for The Carvedilol Prospective Randomized Cumulative Survival Study Group: Effect of carvedilol on survival in severe chronic heart failure. N Engl J Med. 344:1651-1658, 2001.)

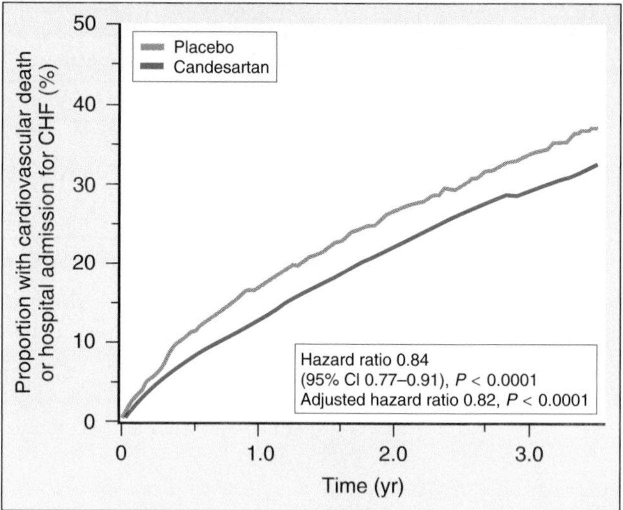

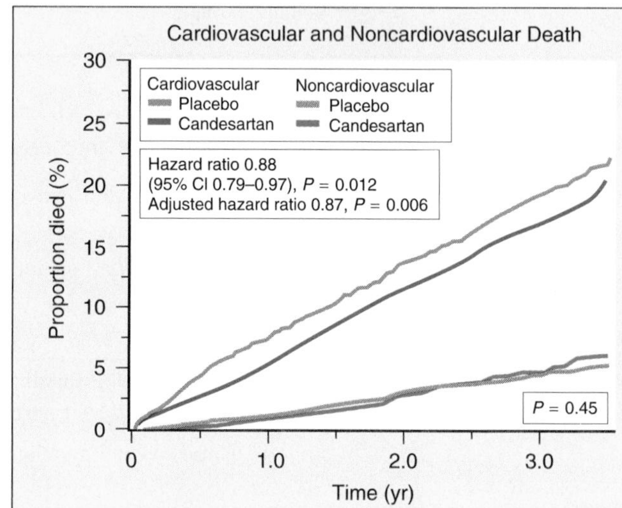

FIGURE 24–6 **A,** Effect of candesartan on cardiovascular mortality or hospital admission for congestive heart failure (CHF) in the CHARM trials. Three groups of patients include (1) patients with left ventricular ejection fraction less than 0.40 who could not tolerate angiotensin-converting enzyme (ACE) inhibitors; (2) patients in whom angiotensin-receptor blocker was given in addition to the ACE inhibition; and (3) patients with HF and preserved ejection fraction. **B,** Kaplan-Meier curves of cardiovascular or noncardiovascular deaths. (From Pfeffer MA, Swedberg K, Granger CB, et al: Effects of candesartan on mortality and morbidity in patients with chronic heart failure. The CHARM-Overall programme. Lancet 362:759-766, 2003.)

strategies such as low-dose administration[52,53] or combination with beta-blocking agents[54] will mitigate theses adverse effects.

If digoxin is used, the trough serum level should be kept at or below 1.0 ng/ml,[55] because levels above that are associated with increased mortality. Keeping digoxin levels low also mitigates adverse effects on women,[55,56] which at least in part are due to higher levels related to smaller volumes of distribution compared to men given the same fixed doses.

Although never subjected to large-scale trials, loop diuretics are a cornerstone of symptomatic HF treatment beginning in stage 2.[57] The goals of diuretic therapy are to reduce congestive symptoms, reduce wall stress, and attenuate the harmful signaling of remodeling/dysfunction mechanisms outlined in Table 24–3. In stage 2, a loop diuretic alone usually suffices, along with potassium replacement to maintain serum levels well into the normal range. Diuretics should be used in conjunction with dietary salt restriction, initially avoiding added salt and then avoiding foods prepared with salt such as canned foods and processed foods.

The aldosterone antagonist, K^+-sparing minimal diuretic spironolactone, has been shown to lower mortality in stage 3 patients (see later), and results with the newer aldosterone antagonist eplerenone in a post-myocardial infarction setting[58] (see Fig. 23–4) suggest that aldosterone inhibition added to an ACE inhibitor would be effective in lowering mortality and morbidity in stage 2 HF.

In summary, patients in stage 2 should be treated with an ACE inhibitor, a beta-adrenergic blocker, a diuretic, and sodium restriction; digoxin is optional. If patients cannot tolerate an ACE inhibitor, typically because of cough, they can be treated with an ARB. If blood pressure is relatively preserved (≥120 mm Hg), an ARB can be added to an ACE inhibitor or an ACE inhibitor and a beta blocker. For lower blood pressures an ARB should be added with caution, particularly on top of a beta blocker and an ACE inhibitor. Another option is the addition of an aldosterone antagonist to an ACE inhibitor and beta blocker, although in stage 2 HF this is not yet supported by clinical trial data.

STAGE 3 (ADVANCED HEART FAILURE, NYHA CLASS III/IV SYMPTOMS). As shown in Figure 24–4, in stage 3 HF the hospitalization rate and mortality begin to increase markedly. Therefore, the main goal of therapy in advanced, stage 3 HF is to lower the probability of HF-related hospitalization and mortality. ACE inhibitors (see Table 23–7) and the aldosterone antagonist spironolactone[9] have been shown to be effective in this regard. Beta-blocking agents, which are quantitatively more effective than ACE inhibitors in stage 2 HF, appear to be less effective in reducing mortality and hospitalizations in more advanced HF.[8] However, if patients with advanced HF and severe left ventricular dysfunction (left ventricular ejection fraction [LVEF] < 0.25) are carefully selected (compensated, no fluid overload) they can benefit substantially from beta blockade, with annualized mortality reductions in the 30 to 40 percent range (see Fig. 24–5).[59,60]

In terms of symptom relief and improvement of functional capacity in stage 3 patients, inhibitors of the RAAS, diuretics, and possibly positive inotropic agents have had some success in controlled trials. For diuretics, in stage 3 HF it is often necessary to add the powerful thiazide-like diuretic metolazone plus a K^+-sparing compound (spironolactone if it is tolerated) to control fluid retention. Dietary salt restriction should be intensified. Trials of inotropic agents in this patient population have not prolonged survival thus far,[61-63] but promising low-dose and combined beta blocker–inotrope approaches are currently being evaluated.[52-54]

STAGE 4 (SEVERE HEART FAILURE, NYHA CLASS III/IV SYMPTOMS WITH FREQUENT OR SUSTAINED DECOMPENSATION). When subjects progress to stage 4, i.e., severe HF despite optimal medical management, as shown in Table 24–3, the goals of therapy change to include palliation of symptoms, reducing rates of hospitalization, and in subjects who are eligible, bridging to cardiac transplantation (see also Chap. 26). In general, reversal of the intrinsic biological processes of remodeling and dysfunction are not possible in this stage. The only treatment shown to be effective in lowering mortality in this stage of HF is ACE inhibition,[64] but despite this treatment, when subjects reach stage 4 HF, the possibility of salvage by medical therapy is indeed remote.

Although for ethical reasons no randomized study has provided convincing proof, in subjects who periodically decompensate to incipient or overt cardiogenic shock, the administration of non–glycoside-positive inotropic agents appear to be life saving. Currently, no orally administered positive inotropic agents are approved for palliation of advanced HF, but investigational agents[52,53,65] have shown enough promise to initiate Phase III clinical trials in this regard. Until an oral agent is available, the standard treatment for palliation of advanced HF will remain intermittent or continuous administration of intravenous inotropic agents such as dobutamine,[66] milrinone,[67] enoximone,[68] or levosimendan (see Chap. 23).[69]

SUMMARY OF PLACEBO CONTROLLED PHASE III CLINICAL TRIALS MEASURING MORTALITY AS A PRIMARY ENDPOINT. Tables 23–7 and 23–13 list the clinical trials discussed earlier, with all data expressed as 12-month event rate rates and event rate reductions. As successful therapy is developed, the next generation of clinical trials is conducted on a background of that therapy, and as a result any efficacy signal must be detected as one that is additive with the background therapy. By adding the risk reductions given in these tables, it is possible to estimate the cumulative degree of reduction in mortality ("combined mortality reduction") referenced back to placebo. Only therapies that have produced a statistically significant reduction in mortality have the cumulative risk reduction calculated. Compared to placebo, 12 months of treatment with ACE inhibitors produces an average reduction in mortality of 17 percent. Beta blockers, whose trials were conducted on a background of ACE inhibitors, lowered mortality further, by an average of 32 percent. This figure yields a cumulative reduction in mortality, referenced back to placebo, of 44 percent. Spironolactone, also evaluated on a background of ACE inhibitors, produces a reduction in mortality of 25 percent and a cumulative reduction of 38 percent.

PHARMACOLOGICAL THERAPY IN SPECIALIZED SUBGROUPS

THE BLACK POPULATION. Some HF demographic groups have exhibited responses to pharmacological treatment that appears to be different from that of other groups or the population as a whole. One of them is American blacks, who in the Beta-Blocker Evaluation of Survival Trial[10] (BEST) exhibited a worse response to beta blockade than did the rest of the population. American blacks treated with bucindolol had a statistically insignificant 17 percent increase in mortality as compared with a statistically significant 19 percent reduction in mortality in the rest of the population.[10]

However, blacks treated with carvedilol in the U.S. Carvedilol Trials fared as well as the remainder of the population,[70] perhaps because they had only stage 2 HF as opposed to the stage 3 subjects in BEST. Another possibility for the difference in response to beta blockade in BEST and the U.S. Carvedilol Trials is that the more powerful vasodilator properties of carvedilol were beneficial in a population enriched in hypertensive heart disease.[10,70] What is certain is that blacks with HF have quite different associated demographics, including a lower prevalence of ischemic cardiomyopathy, more hypertension by history, a higher prevalence of diabetes, and a younger subject population.[10,70,71]

Another likely factor influencing therapeutic response of blacks is gene polymorphisms enriched in the black population compared to nonblacks. An example of this is the alpha$_{2C}$-receptor deletion polymorphism α_{2C}Del322-325, which leads to loss of function[72] in a receptor that ordinarily inhibits norepinephrine release. This polymorphism is present in the homozygous state in more than 50 percent of the American black population but in fewer than 10 percent of American whites.[73] How this relates to an increased adrenergic drive in blacks is not yet clear, but this polymorphism is associated with an approximate fivefold increase in the risk of developing HF.[73] Thus, it is not clear whether genetic modifier mechanisms or race-associated demographic conditions account for the difference in response to beta blockers and ACE inhibitors that has been noted in clinical trials. The scientific basis for these differences needs to be further elucidated, and more effective treatment of blacks with HF needs to be developed. For the present, it is prudent to carefully utilize beta blockers in black patients with stage 3 HF and to consider the alternative of hydralazine/isosorbide dinitrate instead of ACE inhibitor treatment.[74]

WOMEN. Gender may also influence pharmacological treatment.[75-77] Women with HF have a better prognosis than men,[12] greater functional incapacity for the same degree of left ventricular dysfunction,[75] a higher prevalence of diastolic dysfunction,[76,77] and a higher percentage of elderly individuals.[76] Some or all of these factors may contribute to the tendency for lower effect sizes in women versus men in the few clinical trials that have enrolled enough women to report differences in response versus men.[8,10] However, based on currently available data, there is no reason to treat women with HF any different than men. This includes the use of digoxin, as long as trough long serum levels are kept at or below 1.0 ng/ml.[55]

DIABETICS. Another common subgroup in HF populations is patients with diabetes. Diabetes mellitus is a risk factor for developing HF,[4] and most HF cohorts have a prevalence of diabetes that is higher than 20 percent. In addition, the presence of diabetes in patients with systolic dysfunction confers a greater risk of mortality, but only in patients who have coronary artery disease.[78,79] Pharmacological therapy for the diabetic patient with HF should be the same as for nondiabetics, with extra attention paid to tight control of hyperglycemia. Medical therapy of diabetic HF patients should include beta-blocking agents, which have clinical effects that are at least as beneficial as in nondiabetics, with acceptable safety profiles.[79,80]

Pharmacological Therapy for Chronic Heart Failure Caused by Diastolic Dysfunction

As many as 30 to 50 percent of patients with symptomatic HF exhibit diastolic rather than systolic dysfunction (see Chaps. 20 and 21).[3,77,81] Diastolic dysfunction is more common in women[73] and the elderly,[80] and in the latter it may be the dominant form of HF.[82] Additional risk factors for diastolic dysfunction include a history of hypertension[83] and diabetes mellitus.[84] Most studies indicate that patients with diastolic dysfunction as the primary cause of HF have a better prognosis than do control subjects with systolic dysfunction. As discussed earlier, predominantly diastolic dysfunction in a younger (<60-year-old) patient suggests an infiltrative cardiomyopathic process.

Unlike systolic dysfunction, no medical treatment that reduces mortality in diastolic dysfunction is available. The cornerstone of treatment is careful regulation of ventricular filling pressure by diuretics, in a range that prevents excessive dyspnea and liver congestion but allows for adequate cardiac output. ACE inhibitors and/or spironolactone may make diuretic management easier by preventing excessive activation of the RAAS. In addition, some evidence indicates that ACE inhibitors improve ventricular relaxation,[85] but this improvement does not seem to be translated into benefit in subjects with diastolic HF. A large clinical trial (CHARM-Preserved)[86] comparing an angiotensin receptor–blocking agent (candesartan) to placebo demonstrated a small (18 percent) reduction in HF hospitalizations, without a beneficial effect on the primary endpoint (cardiovascular death or HF hospitalizations) or on mortality. In patients with tachycardia (resting heart rates > 90 beats/min) beta blockers may be used to slow the heart rate and prolong filling time, and beta blockers or amiodarone may be required to control and prevent supraventricular arrhythmias. Finally, phosphodiesterase inhibitors (PDEIs) have been shown to improve diastolic function acutely,[87] but there has been no controlled experience with these agents in chronic therapy.

Adjunctive Pharmacological Therapy

ANTIARRHYTHMIC AGENTS (see Chap. 30). In general, antiarrhythmic therapy in HF patients is reserved for symptomatic arrhythmias or for control of ventricular responses to atrial fibrillation. With regard to treatment of ventricular arrhythmias, the Cardiac Arrhythmia Suppression Trial (CAST),[88,89] which was conducted not in a HF population but in subjects with left ventricular dysfunction after myocardial infarction, convincingly demonstrated that type 1 antiarrhythmic agents (i.e., sodium-channel blockers) increase mortality when used to suppress ventricular premature contractions. The Electrophysiological Study Versus Electrocardiographic Monitoring (ESVEM)[90] extended the evidence for adverse effects of type 1 agents in subjects with left ventricular dysfunction and Holter monitor–documented ventricular arrhythmias or inducible sustained ventricular tachycardia. In the ESVEM trial, sotalol, a beta-blocking agent with type III antiarrhythmic properties, was the most effective agent. However, ESVEM had no placebo control, so it was not possible to precisely measure the efficacy and adverse effects of sotalol.

The antiarrhythmic agent that has undergone the most extensive evaluation for efficacy and safety in populations with HF or left ventricular dysfunction is amiodarone. Similar to sotalol, amiodarone is a type III antiarrhythmic with antiadrenergic properties. In controlled clinical trials in HF or asymptomatic left ventricular dysfunction, amiodarone either has been associated with reduced mortality[91] or has been equivalent to placebo.[92] In other words, amiodarone is the one antiarrhythmic agent that appears to be safe in patients with left ventricular dysfunction and HF. However, amiodarone has pulmonary, thyroid, liver, and other toxicities, and its use should be accompanied by careful surveillance for adverse effects. Additionally, as for all antiarrhythmic agents, amiodarone has negative inotropic effects and may be poorly tolerated by patients with advanced HF.

Treatment of arrhythmias has evolved to catheter-based ablation and implantable defibrillators (see Chap. 31). Current indications for device therapy for ventricular arrhythmias are given later.

ANTICOAGULATION (see Chap. 80). The use of anticoagulation in the form of warfarin in patients with normal sinus rhythm and severe left ventricular dysfunction is an area of considerable controversy. In controlled clinical trials, the risk of arterial thromboembolic events, most of which are stroke, ranges from 0.9 to 5.5 per 100 patient-years.[93,94] Since warfarin convincingly lowers thromboembolism and stroke risk in atrial fibrillation,[95] it is logical that this benefit would extend to subjects with severe left ventricular dysfunction. Such benefit may be particularly true in nonischemic cardiomyopathies, which are associated with a relatively high incidence of left ventricular thrombus.[96] A few small studies generally support a benefit of oral anticoagulation. On the basis of these considerations, many, but not all HF centers routinely administer anticoagulants to all patients with moderate or severe left ventricular dysfunction who do not have a contraindication. However, anticoagulation with warfarin is not without risk, and it must be carefully monitored. In chronic HF, a firm indication for anticoagulation can be made in patients with atrial fibrillation, those with a visualized left ventricular thrombus, and those with a history of a thromboembolic event.[97] Anticoagulation in left ventricular dysfunction with normal sinus rhythm should be considered optional, with the issue to be settled by ongoing clinical trials.

Device Therapy

Implantable Cardioverter-Defibrillators

Implantable cardioverter-defibrillators (ICDs) (see Chap. 31) are now the treatment of choice in patients with left ventricular dysfunction who have survived sudden cardiac death,[98] have symptomatic sustained ventricular tachycardia,[99] have asymptomatic nonsustained but inducible ventricular tachycardia,[9,100] or have an ischemic cardiomyopathy with an LVEF less than 30 percent.[101] Data supporting these recommendations are derived from the Antiarrhythmic Versus Implantable Defibrillator (AVID) Trial,[98] the Multicenter Automatic Defibrillator Implantation Trial (MADIT),[99] the Multicenter Unsustained Tachycardia Trial (MUSTT),[100] and the Multicenter Automatic Defibrillator Implantation Trial II (MADIT II) (Fig. 24–7).[101] The benefit of ICD implantation was most striking in patients with a QRS wider than 0.12 seconds (Fig. 24–7B).

At this point, a major question is whether ICDs can reduce mortality in other left ventricular dysfunction or HF populations, such as patients with nonsustained and noninducible ventricular tachycardia, nonischemic cardiomyopathies,

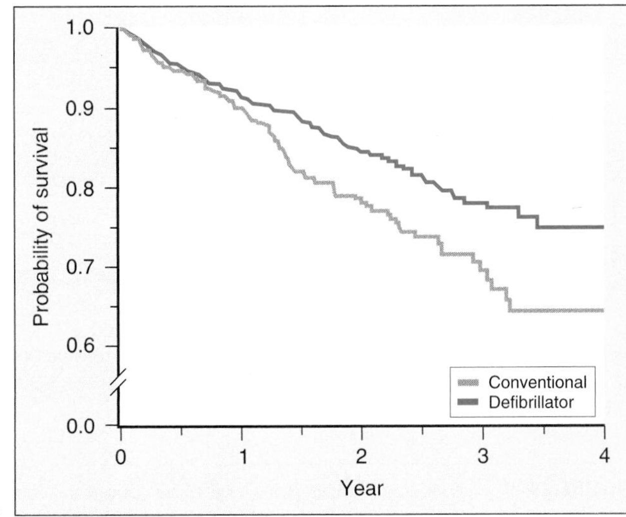

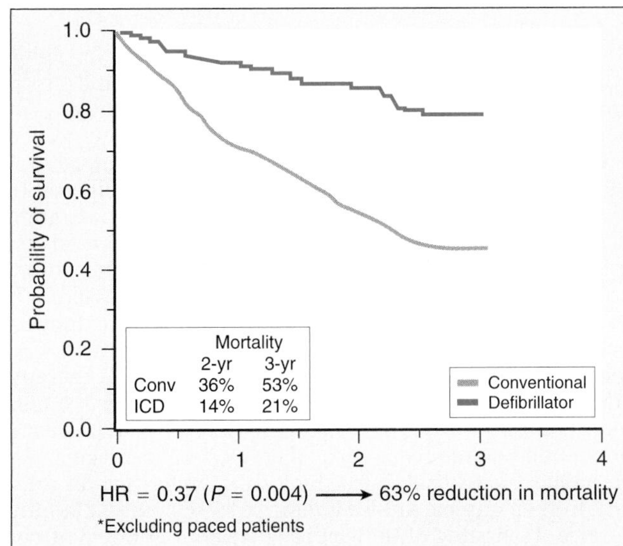

FIGURE 24–7 MADIT II Trial. **A,** Kaplan-Meier estimates of the probability of survival in post-myocardial infarction patients with ejection fraction less than 0.30 assigned to receive an implantable cardioverter-defibrillator (ICD) and the group assigned to receive conventional medical therapy. The difference in survival between the two groups was significant (nominal $p = 0.007$, by the log rank test). **B,** Survival in MADIT II patients with QRS wider than 0.12 seconds. HR = heart rate. (**A,** From Moss AJ, Zareba W, Hall WJ, et al: Prophylactic implantation of a defibrillator in patients with myocardial infarction and reduced ejection fraction. N Engl J Med 346:877, 2002; **B,** Courtesy of Dr. A. J. Moss.)

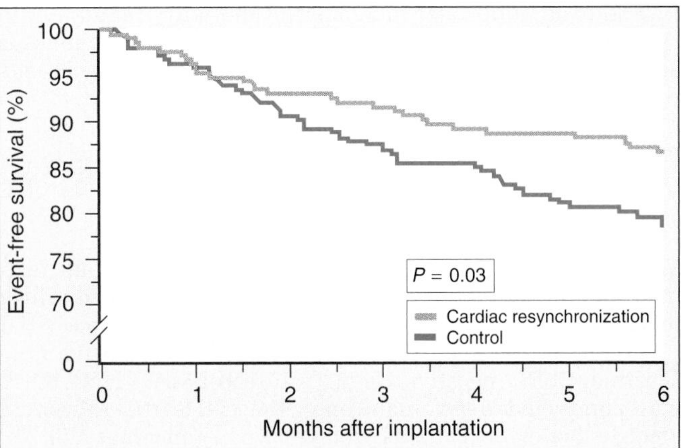

FIGURE 24–8 Kaplan-Meier estimates of the time to death or hospitalization for worsening heart failure in the control and resynchronization groups in the MIRACLE Trial, which enrolled 453 patients with heart failure, an ejection fraction less than 0.35, and a QRS wider than 130 milliseconds. The risk of an event was 40 percent lower in the resynchronization group (95 percent confidence interval, 4 to 63 percent; $p = 0.03$). (Data from Abraham WT, Fisher WG, Smith AL, et al: Cardiac resynchronization in chronic heart failure. N Engl J Med 346:1845-1853, 2002.)

large numbers of premature ventricular contractions, intraventricular conduction delays, and abnormal signal-averaged electrocardiograms, or even in subjects with no evidence of electrophysiological abnormalities. In this regard, the Comparison of Medical Therapy, Pacing and Defibrillation in Chronic Heart Failure (COMPANION) Trial recently evaluated patients with a lengthened QRS (>120 milliseconds), left ventricular dysfunction (LVEF < 0.35), and a HF hospitalization within the past year.[102] In this trial patients were randomized between optimal medical therapy (OPT), OPT + biventricular pacing to provide cardiac resynchronization therapy (CRT), or OPT + CRT and an ICD (CRT-D). The primary endpoint in this trial was time to all-cause death or any hospitalization. In this patient population, the combination of biventricular pacing and an ICD substantially reduced mortality in nonischemic cardiomyopathy patients, by 50 percent ($p < 0.01$) compared to 27 percent in the ischemic cardiomyopathy group.[103] In contrast, in the biventricular pacing without ICD arm, mortality was reduced by only 9 percent (p = NS).[103] These data indicate that the addition of an ICD to biventricular pacing in patients with intraventricular conduction defects and other enrollment criteria used in the COMPANION Trial can reduce mortality in nonischemic cardiomyopathy patients.

Biventricular Pacing

One of the more interesting recent developments in HF is the concept that left ventricular or biventricular pacing (see Chap. 31) may be beneficial in a subset of subjects with intraventricular conduction delay, which may include 15 to 30 percent of subjects with advanced left ventricular dysfunction (Fig. 24–8).[104-106] The biventricular pacing strategy is based on the fact that most subjects with intraventricular conduction delay have dyssynchronous left ventricular contraction, which results in a reduction in ventricular performance and unfavorable myocardial energetics.[107] There is no question that, acutely, biventricular or left ventricular pacing can, by synchronizing left ventricular contraction, improve left ventricular rate of pressure increase (dP/dT)[107,108] and ejection fraction,[109] cardiac index,[108] and myocardial energetics.[107] These favorable myocardial functional effects contribute to a short-term reduction in neurohormonal activation[110] and to an improvement in functional capacity and quality of life over a several-month period.[103,111-113] Moreover, the improvement in systolic function discussed earlier is translated by 6 months into reverse remodeling, with a sustained increase in ejection fraction and a reduction in left ventricular size.[114-116]

The COMPANION Trial, mentioned above, was designed to determine if CRT can improve major clinical outcomes in advanced HF patients with intraventricular conduction defects.[100] CRT or CRT + CRT-D was compared to optimal pharmacological therapy for effects on survival and hospitalizations.[103] In this study both CRT and CRT-D reduced the incidence of the primary endpoint of all-cause mortality or all-cause hospitalization by 19 to 20 percent ($p < 0.02$), secondary to an favorable effects on mortality and HF hospitalizations.[103] CRT alone reduced mortality by 24 percent ($p = 0.06$), whereas, as mentioned earlier, CRT-D reduced mortality by 36 percent ($p < 0.01$).[103] Thus in advanced HF patients with intraventricular conduction defects CRT produces a major reduction (by 35 to 40 percent) in HF hospitalizations and a moderate reduction in mortality; the addition of an

ICD adds an additional increment of mortality reduction, to a degree (by 36 percent) that statistical significance is achieved and the clinical impact is substantial. Thus patients with LVEFs less than 0.35 and QRS durations wider than 120 milliseconds should be considered for CRT or CRD-D therapy, as an adjunct to optimal background pharmacological treatment.

Ventricular Assist Devices (see Chap. 25)

Ventricular assist devices have emerged as a potential treatment of chronic HF, beyond their traditional role as a bridge to transplantation. A randomized, controlled clinical trial (the Randomized Evaluation of Mechanical Assistance for the Treatment of Congestive Heart Failure [REMATCH] Trial)[117] was conducted to evaluate one device (Heartmate vented electric device) in patients who were not transplant eligible. This trial randomized patients with an LVEF less than 0.25, NYHA Class IV symptoms, and the continued need for inotropic therapy to continued medical therapy or an assist device.[117] Patients randomized to an assist device had a 48 percent reduction in death from any cause as well as an improved quality of life (see Fig. 25–12).[118] Unfortunately, long-term survival with this device was still poor (1 year, 52 percent, and 2 years, 25 percent).[118] The frequency of serious adverse events including serious bleeding, infection, and neurological dysfunction was also 2.35 times that noted in the medical therapy group.[118] Despite these limitations, left ventricular assist devices will likely have an expanding role in the treatment of a subset of ultraadvanced HF patients.

OTHER DEVICES. Several other devices in development may have a role in the treatment of HF. For example, external pneumatic counterpulsation, shown to be effective in treating angina,[119] may have a role in treating HF.[120] One of the more interesting approaches to preventing progressive remodeling is a device (the "Acorn" device) that physically prevents ventricular dilation in animal models (see Fig. 20–1).[121] Clearly, devices of various types will increasingly contribute to HF treatment in the future.

Surgical Therapy

CARDIAC TRANSPLANTATION (see Chap. 26). This procedure was the first definitive treatment developed for HF, that is, the first treatment that lowered mortality.[122] The treatment is so successful in advanced or severe stage 3 or 4 HF that to this point no randomized study could have been ethically justified. Survival curves for severe HF (stage 4) subjects from the enalapril arm of the Cooperative New Scandinavian Enalapril Survival (CONSENSUS) Trial,[64] a cohort of stage 3 subjects from 1980 prior to ACE inhibitor treatment, the beta-blocker arms of the Carvedilol Prospective Randomized Cumulative Survival Study (COPERNICUS)[59] and BEST[10] Trials conducted in stage 3 patients, the CRT-D arm of the COMPANION Trial representing the current best available medical and device therapy in stage 3 HF, and cardiac transplantation for stage 3 or 4 patients are shown in Figure 24–9. Survival after transplantation is superior to that with pharmacological or pharmacological + device therapy. However, as can be observed in the COMPANION Trial CRT-D patients,[103] survival with the combination of pharmacological and device therapy is improving and with another incremental improvement it will rival transplantation for outcomes in at least stage 3 patients.

The biggest limitation of cardiac transplantation is not efficacy or safety but rather the limited supply of donors available to apply the treatment. It has been estimated that less than 10 percent of subjects who would benefit from cardiac transplantation can actually receive it on the basis of the upward limit of 2500 usable donors per year in the United

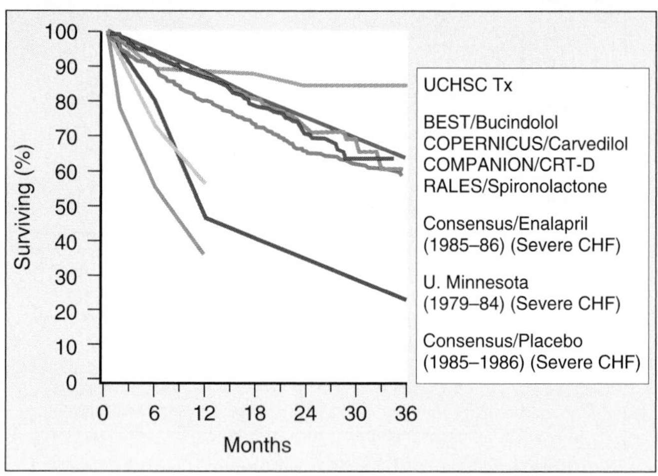

FIGURE 24–9 Survival curves in stage 3 or 4 heart failure, patients treated medically (see text for description of trials) or with cardiac transplantation (UCHSC Tx).

States.[123] Therefore, transplantation is reserved for subjects who have reached stage 4 or late stage 3 HF and are progressing despite application of all medical therapy of proven benefit.

CORONARY ARTERY BYPASS GRAFTING (see Chap. 50). More than 15 years ago, the Coronary Artery Surgery Study (CASS)[124] demonstrated that coronary artery bypass grafting (CABG) is superior to medical therapy from a survival standpoint in subjects with symptomatic triple-vessel coronary artery disease and reduced but not severely depressed LVEFs. In recent years, the benefit of CABG has been extended to patients with LVEFs lower than the 0.35 cutoff in CASS. Many centers have successfully extended CABG therapy to stage 3 HF subjects with LVEFs less than 0.30,[125,126] but no large controlled trials have compared CABG with current recommended standard medical therapy, including beta blockers. One such trial, also including investigation of the addition of surgical anterior ventricular restoration (a form of surgical reshaping of the ventricle without removal of viable myocardium)[127] to CABG (the STICH Trial) is currently being conducted.

MITRAL VALVE RECONSTRUCTION IN LEFT VENTRICULAR DYSFUNCTION (see Chap. 57). Mitral regurgitation occurs to a greater or lesser degree in the remodeled, dilated ventricle. During the past decade surgical approaches to correction of mitral regurgitation without valve replacement have been applied to the failing, remodeled ventricle with low operative mortality and impressive early clinical outcomes.[128] However, no prospective controlled, randomized studies have compared mitral valve reconstruction with the best available medical therapy, which itself can reverse remodeling in patients with mitral regurgitation. Thus, the role of mitral valve reconstruction in the setting of remodeling and mitral regurgitation is somewhat unclear and at the moment should be conservatively confined to cases of severe mitral regurgitation with some preservation of left ventricular function, i.e., with ejection fractions greater than 0.30.

Management of Episodes of Acute Decompensation

As discussed earlier, acute manifestations of HF can either be in the context of new onset or be in subjects with established chronic HF. Treatment of acute episodes of HF are similar in these two scenarios, with the exception that a diagnostic work-up potentially leading to definitive therapy should be done in new cases. Since multiple-treatment modalities may be brought to bear on acute HF episodes, the discussion is

TABLE 24–4 Pharmacological Therapy for Acute, Decompensated Heart Failure

Treatment Modality	Specific Examples
Intravenous diuretics	Furosemide, bumetatide, torsemide
Intravenous positive inotropic agents	Dobutamine, milrinone, enoximone
Intravenous vasodilators	Nitroprusside, nitroglycerine, nesiritide
Blood pressure, renal perfusion support	Intravenous dopamine, intravenous vasopressin

divided into pharmacological and nonpharmacological forms of therapy.

PHARMACOLOGICAL THERAPY (see Chap. 23). Table 24–4 gives the standard treatment modalities typically used to treat acute episodes of HF with advanced, Class IV symptoms. In general, treatment begins with intravenous diuretics, which in subjects with adequate organ perfusion often suffice to produce diuresis accompanied by a prompt drop in preload and relief of symptoms related to pulmonary edema. If peripheral perfusion is compromised or diuresis does not ensue, intravenous dobutamine, an inotropic beta/alpha-adrenergic agonist that produces an increase in cardiac output without substantially dropping preload or blood pressure,[129] or nesiritide (BNP)[130] (see Fig. 23–5), a vasodilator, can be added via a well-secured peripheral line. A PDEI such as milrinone[131,132] or enoximone[133,134] can also be used to treat decompensated HF but should not be administered without pulmonary artery pressure monitoring unless it is certain that left ventricular filling pressure is high (>15 mm Hg). The reason for this precaution is that PDEIs are such potent venodilators that in patients with normal or low filling pressure, they can drop preload to undesirably low levels. Finally, in decompensated subjects who are still receiving beta-blocking agents, a PDEI rather than a beta blocker is the treatment of choice because PDEIs retain full or even have enhanced activity in the presence of beta blockade.[135]

If the situation has not stabilized, additional inotropic support with or without supplemental afterload reduction is indicated and best delivered with the aid of pulmonary artery catheter monitoring. The combination of dobutamine and a PDEI is additive for effects on cardiac output and, via the PDEI, will produce a reduction in pulmonary artery and left ventricular filling pressure.[136,137] The latter may provide welcome unloading of the right ventricle inasmuch as high pulmonary artery pressure can produce limiting right ventricular dysfunction in some patients.

Once optimal inotropic therapy is being delivered, pure vasodilators can be additionally administered to subjects with persistently high systemic or pulmonary vascular resistance. Vasodilators such as nitroprusside or nitroglycerin can also be used in lieu of a positive inotropic agent, particularly in patients with higher systemic vascular resistance. As a vasodilator, nesiritide has the unique property of preferentially increasing renal blood flow[138,139] and theoretically may be of value in patients with compromised renal function; however, nesiritide may also precipitate renal failure and must be used cautiously in this setting.

Finally, in patients with blood pressure so low that renal perfusion is compromised, dopamine may be added to increase perfusion pressure and renal blood flow via this agent's alpha-adrenergic and dopaminergic properties. However, dopamine should not be considered an effective positive inotropic agent because the majority of its weak, partial beta-agonist effect is mediated by norepinephrine release,[140] which results in tachyphylaxis within 12 hours of administration.[135]

TABLE 24–5 Nonpharmacological Therapy for Acute, Decompensated Heart Failure

Treatment Modality	Specific Examples
Oxygenation	Supplemental oxygen, mechanical ventilation
Balloon counterpulsation	Intraaortic balloon pump
VAD	Pulsatile-flow LVAD
Pacing	AV sequential pacemaker; biventricular pacing
Urgent cardiac catheterization	PTCA, mitral valvuloplasty, pericardiocentesis
Urgent cardiac surgery	CABG, AVR, MV repair or replacement, transplantation

AV = atrioventricular; AVR = aortic valve replacement; CABG = coronary artery bypass grafting; LVAD = left ventricular assist device; MV = mitral valve; PTCA = percutaneous transluminal coronary angioplasty; VAD = ventricular assist device.

NONPHARMACOLOGICAL THERAPY. Table 24–5 lists some nonpharmacological therapies that can be used to treat acute episodes of HF. In general, nonpharmacological therapy is used only if drug therapy does not stabilize the patient. Although its effectiveness has never been demonstrated in a controlled clinical trial, use of an intraaortic balloon pump (IABP) can increase cardiac output modestly while increasing effective coronary perfusion pressure. This benefit and the ease of use of this device make it an attractive adjunct in myocardial failure occurring in the context of ischemia. The IABP is also helpful in nonischemic myocardial failure. However, contraindications to IABP use include significant aortic regurgitation and severe peripheral vascular disease. If pharmacological therapy plus IABP does not stabilize the patient, a ventricular assist device should be used in selected individuals, as discussed in Chapter 25.

Because of the success of treating acute myocardial infarction by primary angioplasty[141] with stenting,[142] percutaneous coronary intervention techniques (see Chap. 48) have assumed an important role in treating the most common cause of new-onset acute HF, that arising in the setting of myocardial infarction. In general, the primary goal of treating myocardial failure in the setting of infarction is to establish and maintain patency of the infarct artery in the most expeditious manner possible. The catheterization laboratory is also an ideal setting in which to initiate adjunctive treatment such as an IABP, mechanical ventilation, and optimal pharmacological support guided by hemodynamic monitoring. Other techniques that can be applied in the catheterization laboratory used to treat acute HF treatment include pericardiocentesis for tamponade (see Chap. 64) and relief of severe mitral stenosis by balloon valvuloplasty (see Chap. 57).

Occasionally, urgent cardiac surgery is required for the treatment of acute HF. These procedures include CABG in acute ischemic disorders involving disease of the left main coronary artery or in patients in whom percutaneous coronary intervention is not a technical option, acute aortic or mitral valve surgery, and on rare occasion, transplantation. In general, it is neither desirable nor feasible to perform cardiac transplantation on someone during the initial HF decompensation.

Health Care Delivery Strategies

HEART FAILURE CENTERS. The number of therapeutic options for the care of HF patients is extensive, and access to investigational agents or complex approaches limited to specialized centers, such as transplantation, is often required. Numerous outcomes studies[143-145] have documented the utility of such centers, and there is strong argument[146] for federal support of such a center analogous to what was done in the United States in the early 1970s for cancer. However, it must be appreciated that most patients are cared for by primary care physicians rather than HF specialists or general cardiologists.[147] The sheer number of HF patients dictates that primary care physicians will continue to care for these patients, but it is likely that specialized centers will have an increasing role as treatment becomes even more complex.

HEART FAILURE CLINICS FOR DISEASE MANAGEMENT. It has become evident that a substantial and perhaps a majority of HF patients are not being optimally treated with medications that are clearly indicated, much less given more aggressive treatment options such as some of the surgical and device approaches described earlier. For example, estimates of the percentage of HF patients in the United States being treated with ACE inhibitors are between 50 percent[148] and 71 percent,[149] whereas on the basis of what is achieved in controlled clinical trials, it should be higher than 90 percent.[6,9,10] For beta blockers, the results are even worse, with estimates of 25 percent of the HF population receiving therapy[144,146] as compared with the ideal figure of more than 60 percent.[103] Inadequate medical treatment of HF no doubt extends beyond the appropriate use of ACE inhibitors or beta blockers and probably includes failure to consistently adhere to a low-salt diet, suboptimal use of diuretics, failure to maintain digoxin levels lower than 1.0 ng/ml,[55] inadequate interval follow-up, and numerous other important factors.

The failure to deliver optimal medical care to HF patients is multifactorial. As for other medical conditions, optimal care includes a health care provider with knowledge and the ability to communicate that knowledge, a method of ensuring that the patient has received and understood the knowledge, a system of encouraging adherence to the recommended regimen, and patient compliance. The elderly nature of many HF patients and the incapacitating nature of the HF disease syndrome present special challenges to caregivers. However, many of the challenges to delivering optimal care to HF patients can be met through an integrated specialized clinic approach that uses nurse and physician extenders to deliver and ensure the implementation of care. This disease management approach has been shown to reduce hospitalizations and increase the percentage of patients receiving ideal, guideline-recommended therapy.[150] The end result is lowered cost of HF treatment and likely improved survival.[151]

The biggest challenge to this obvious solution to the delivery of HF care is how to support the additional personnel required in the disease management model. In specialized centers, the costs are usually supported by sponsored research, and in the community, some health care maintenance organizations or hospitals have seen the wisdom of this cost-reducing approach. This model will probably be adopted in direct relation to the availability of financial support for it, which in turn is dependent on the health care system.

Exercise

Until recently, HF patients were instructed to avoid exercise, and at one point, bed rest was offered as a treatment of HF.[152] Bed rest is no longer prescribed, and in fact, exercise now appears to be promising as a treatment of HF. It is not surprising that an exercise regimen can increase functional capacity in subjects with HF, as documented in numerous studies.[153-158] What is surprising is that in small controlled studies, various other aspects of HF thought to be important in prognosis, such as neurohormonal activation,[153-155] symptoms,[157] resting cardiac function,[158] and quality of life,[153] appear to be improved by exercise. What is lacking is a large, well-controlled clinical outcomes trial to test the hypothesis that moderate levels of exercise improve the natural history of HF. Such a trial is currently ongoing (the Anticoagulation Consortium to Improve Outcomes Nationally [ACTION] Trial). Until results are available, it appears prudent to suggest to patients that they maintain at least some level of conditioning with mild to moderate regimens of aerobic exercise in view of the lack of evidence that such exercise is harmful and the potential beneficial effect on symptoms and individual psychology.

Investigational Treatment and Future Directions

In the last 10 years, major progress has been made in the medical treatment of HF. In clinical trials conducted in mild to moderate stage 2 HF, the use of ACE inhibitors and beta-adrenergic blocking agents has reduced mortality by more than 40 percent,[45] and in patients with intraventricular conduction defects the addition of CRT-D to optimal background pharmacological therapy further reduces mortality by more than 60 percent.[103] This progress is beginning to be manifest in improved clinical outcomes in community-based studies.[159] The enormous magnitude of the challenge that remains and the growing number of patients with HF will ensure that efforts to improve pharmacological and device therapy will continue. However, to attain such progress, subjects with HF will need to continue to be enrolled in investigational protocols, typically available at larger, well-organized HF centers. More important, the advances in HF treatment need to be more rapidly translated into application in community practice. This requires a strong cooperative effort among the various components of the health care industry, including pharmaceutical and device companies, academic medical centers, health care delivery organizations, as well as individual physicians.

REFERENCES

1. New York Heart Association: Nomenclature and Criteria for Diagnosis of Diseases of the Heart and Blood Vessels. New York, New York Heart Association, 1963.
2. Schocken DD, Arrieta MI, Leaverton PE, Ross EA: Prevalence and mortality of congestive heart failure in the United States. J Am Coll Cardiol 20:301-306, 1992.
3. Redfield MM, Jacobsen SJ, Burnett JC Jr, et al: Burden of systolic and diastolic ventricular dysfunction in the community: Appreciating the scope of the heart failure epidemic. JAMA 289:194-202, 2003.
4. Lloyd-Jones DM, Larson MG, Leip EP, et al: Lifetime risk for developing congestive heart failure: The Framingham Heart Study. Circulation 106:3068-3072, 2002.
5. O'Connell JB: The economic burden of heart failure. Clin Cardiol 23:II-I6–II-20, 2000.
6. Packer M, Bristow MR, Cohn JN, et al: Effect of carvedilol on morbidity and mortality in patients with chronic heart failure. N Engl J Med 334:1349-1355, 1996.
7. CIBIS-II Investigators and Committees: The Cardiac Insufficiency Bisoprolol Study II (CIBIS-II): A randomised trial. Lancet 353:9-13, 1999.
8. MERIT-HF Study Group: Effect of metoprolol CR/XL in chronic heart failure: Metoprolol CR/XL Randomized Intervention Trial in Congestive Heart Failure (MERIT-HF). Lancet 353:2001-2006, 1999.
9. Pitt B, Zannad F, Remme WJ, et al: The effect of spironolactone on morbidity and mortality in patients with severe heart failure. N Engl J Med 341:709-717, 1999.
10. BEST Trial Investigators: Effect of β-adrenergic blockade on mortality in patients with advanced chronic heart failure: The β-blocker Evaluation of Survival Trial. New Engl J Med 344:1659-1667, 2001.
11. American Heart Association: 2004 Heart and Stroke Statistical Update. Dallas, American Heart Association, 2004.
12. Ho KKL, Anderson KM, Kannel WB, et al: Survival after the onset of congestive heart failure in Framingham Heart Study subjects. Circulation 88:107-115, 1993.
13 Wang TJ, Evans JC, Benjamin EJ, et al: Natural history of asymptomatic left ventricular systolic dysfunction in the community. Circulation 108:977-982, 2003.
14. Hayflick L: How and Why We Age. New York, Ballantine, 1994.

Pathophysiology of Heart Failure due to Primary or Secondary Dilated Cardiomyopathies

15. Bristow MR: Why does the myocardium fail? New insights from basic science. Lancet 352(Suppl 1):8-14, 1998.

16. Eichhorn EJ, Bristow MR: Medical therapy can improve the biologic properties of the chronically failing heart: A new era in the treatment of heart failure. Circulation 94:2285-2296, 1996.
17. Weber KT: Extracellular matrix remodeling in heart failure: A role for de novo angiotensin II generation. Circulation 96:4065-4082, 1997.
18. Gerdes AM, Kellerman SE, Moore JA, et al: Structural remodeling of cardiac myocytes from patients with chronic ischemic heart disease. Circulation 86:426-430, 1992.
19. Davies CH, Davia K, Bennett JG, et al: Reduced contraction and altered frequency response of isolated ventricular myocytes from patients with heart failure. Circulation 92:2540-2549, 1995.
20. Lowes BD, Gilbert EM, Abraham WT, et al: Myocardial gene expression in dilated cardiomyopathy treated with beta-blocking agents. New Engl J Med 346:1357-1365, 2002.
21. Cohn JN: Structural basis for heart failure: Ventricular remodeling and its pharmacological inhibition. Circulation 91:2504-2507, 1995.
22. Cintron C, Johnson G, Francis G, et al: Prognostic significance of serial changes in left ventricular ejection fraction in patients with congestive heart failure. Circulation 87(Suppl 6):17-23, 1993.
23. Cohn JN, Johnson GR, Shabetai R, et al: Ejection fraction, peak exercise oxygen consumption, cardiothoracic ratio, ventricular arrhythmias, and plasma norepinephrine as determinants of prognosis in heart failure. Circulation 87(Suppl 6):5-16, 1993.

Diagnosis of Heart Failure

24. Cleland JGF, Habib F: Assessment and diagnosis of heart failure. J Intern Med 239:317-325, 1996.
25. Maisel AS, Krishnaswamy P, Nowak RM, et al, for The Breathing Not Properly Multinational Study Investigators: Rapid measurement of B-type natriuretic peptide in the emergency diagnosis of heart failure. N Engl J Med. 347:161-167, 2002.
26. Groenning BA, Nilsson JC, Sondergaard L, et al: Detection of left ventricular enlargement and impaired systolic function with plasma *N*-terminal pro brain natriuretic peptide concentration. Am Heart J 143:923-929, 2002.
27. Sim V, Hampton D, Phillips C, et al: The use of brain natriuretic peptide as a screening test for left ventricular systolic dysfunction: Cost-effectiveness in relation to open access echocardiography. Fam Pract 20:570-574, 2003.
28. Lainchbury JG, Campbell E, Frampton CM, et al: Brain natriuretic peptide and *N*-terminal brain natriuretic peptide in the diagnosis of heart failure in patients with acute shortness of breath. J Am Coll Cardiol 42:728-735, 2003.
29. de Groote P, Millaire A, Foucher-Hossein C, et al: Right ventricular ejection fraction is an independent predictor of survival in patients with moderate heart failure. J Am Coll Cardiol 32:948-954, 1998.
30. Felker GM, Hu W, Hare LM, et al: The spectrum of dilated cardiomyopathy: The Johns Hopkins experience with 1278 patients. Medicine (Baltimore) 78:270-283, 1999.
31. Myers J, Gullestad L, Vagelos R, et al: Clinical, hemodynamic, and cardiopulmonary exercise test determinants of survival in patients referred for evaluation of heart failure. Ann Intern Med 129:286-293, 1998.

Management of Acute, New-Onset Heart Failure

32. Hannen EL, Kilburn H, O'Donnell JF, et al: Adult open heart surgery in New York State: An analysis of risk factors and hospital mortality rates. JAMA 264:2768-1774, 1990.
33. White M, Wiechmann RJ, Roden RL, et al: Cardiac β-adrenergic neuroeffector systems in acute myocardial dysfunction related to brain injury: Evidence for catecholamine-mediated myocardial damage. Circulation 92:2183-2189, 1995.
34. Pfeffer MA, Pfeffer JM, Fishbein MC, et al: Myocardial infarct size and ventricular function in rats. Circ Res 44:503-512, 1979.
35. Bristow MR, Mason JW, Billingham ME, Daniels JR: Dose-effect and structure function relationships in doxorubicin cardiomyopathy. Am Heart J 102:709-718, 1981.
36. Billingham ME, Mason JW, Bristow MR, Daniels JR: Anthracycline cardiomyopathy monitored by morphological changes. Cancer Treat Rep 62:865-872, 1978.
37. Bristow MR, Lopez MB, Mason JW, et al: Efficacy and cost of cardiac monitoring in patients receiving doxorubicin. Cancer 50:32-41, 1982.
38. Lewis W, Gonzalez B: Actin isoform synthesis by cultured cardiac myocytes: Effects of doxorubicin. Lab Invest 56:295-301, 1987.
39. Bristow MR: Is too much or too little hypertrophy of individual cardiac myocytes the problem in the failing heart? Heart Fail 10:162-165, 1994.

Management of Chronic Heart Failure

40. Hunt SA, Baker DW, Chin MH, et al: ACC/AHA guidelines for the evaluation and management of chronic heart failure in the adult. Circulation 104:2996-3007, 2001.
41. The SOLVD Investigators: Effect of enalapril on mortality and the development of heart failure in asymptomatic patients with reduced left ventricular ejection fractions. N Engl J Med 327:685-691, 1992.
42. The SOLVD Investigators: Effect of enalapril on survival in patients with reduced left ventricular ejection fractions and congestive heart failure. N Engl J Med 325:293-302, 1991.
43. Packer M, Poole-Wilson PA, Armstrong PW, et al: Comparative effects of low and high doses of the angiotensin-converting enzyme inhibitor, lisinopril, on morbidity and mortality in chronic heart failure. ATLAS Study Group. Circulation 100:2312-2318, 1999.
44. Pfeffer MA: Angiotensin-converting enzyme inhibition in congestive heart failure: Benefit and perspective. Am Heart J 126:789-793, 1993.
45. Bristow MR: β-Adrenergic receptor blockade in chronic heart failure. Circulation 101:558-569, 2000.
46. Cohn JN, Tognoni G, Valsartan Heart Failure Trial Investigators: A randomized trial of the angiotensin-receptor blocker valsartan in chronic heart failure. N Engl J Med 345:1667-1675. 2001.
47. McMurray JJV, Ostergren J, Swedberg K, et al, for The CHARM Investigators: Effects of candesartan in patients with chronic heart failure and reduced left ventricular systolic function taking angiotensin-converting-enzyme inhibitors: The CHARM-Alternative Trial. Lancet 362:772-776, 2003.
48. Granger CB, McMurray JJV, Yusuf S, et al, for The CHARM Investigators: Effects of candesartan in patients with chronic heart failure and reduced left ventricular systolic function taking angiotensin-converting-enzyme inhibitors: The CHARM-Added Trial. Lancet 362:767-761, 2003.
49. Hauptman PJ, Kelly RA: Digitalis. Circulation 99:1265-1270, 1999.
50. Digitalis Investigation Group: The effect of digoxin on mortality and morbidity in patients with heart failure. N Engl J Med 336:525-533, 1997.
51. DiBianco R, Shabetai R, Kostak W, et al: A comparison of oral milrinone, digoxin, and their combination in the treatment of patients with chronic heart failure. N Engl J Med 320:677-683, 1989.
52. Lowes BD, Higginbotham M, Petrovich L, et al: Low-dose enoximone improves exercise capacity in chronic heart failure. J Am Coll Cardiol 36:501-508, 2000.
53. Bristow MR, Lowes BD: Low-dose inotropic therapy of ambulatory heart failure. Coron Artery Dis 5:112-118, 1994.
54. Shakar SF, Abraham WT, Gilbert EM, et al: Combined oral positive inotropic and beta-blocker therapy for the treatment of refractory Class IV heart failure. J Am Coll Cardiol 31:1336-1340, 1998.
55. Rathore SS, Curtis JP, Wang Y, et al: Association of serum digoxin concentration and outcomes in patients with heart failure. JAMA 289:871-878, 2003.
56. Rathore SS, Wang Y, Krumholz HM: Sex-based differences in the effect of digoxin for the treatment of heart failure. N Engl J Med 347:1403-1411, 2002.
57. Taylor HS: Diuretic therapy in congestive heart failure. Cardiol Rev 8:104-114, 2000.
58. Pitt B, Remme W, Zannad F, et al, for The Eplerenone Post-Acute Myocardial Infarction Heart Failure Efficacy and Survival Study Investigators: Eplerenone, a selective aldosterone blocker, in patients with left ventricular dysfunction after myocardial infarction. N Engl J Med 348:1309-1321, 2003.
59. Packer M, Coats AJ, Fowler MB, et al, for The Carvedilol Prospective Randomized Cumulative Survival Study Group: Effect of carvedilol on survival in severe chronic heart failure. N Engl J Med. 344:1651-1658, 2001.
60. Goldstein S, Fagerberg B, Hjalmarson A, et al, for The MERIT-HF Study Group: Metoprolol controlled release/extended release in patients with severe heart failure: Analysis of the experience in the MERIT-HF study. J Am Coll Cardiol. 38:932-938, 2001.
61. Packer M, Carver JR, Chesebro JH, et al: Effect of milrinone on mortality in severe chronic heart failure: The prospective randomized milrinone survival evaluation (PROMISE). N Engl J Med 325:1468-1475, 1991.
62. Cohn JN, Goldstein SO, Greenberg BH, et al: A dose-dependent increase in mortality with vesnarinone among patients with severe heart failure. Vesnarinone Trial Investigators. N Engl J Med 339:1810-1816, 1998.
63. Uretsky BF, Jesup M, Konstam M, et al: Multicenter trial of oral enoximone in patients with moderate to moderately severe congestive heart failure: Lack of benefit compared to placebo. Circulation 82:774-780, 1990.
64. The CONSENSUS Trial Study Group: Effects of enalapril on mortality in severe congestive heart failure. N Engl J Med 316:1429-1435, 1987.
65. Lee HR, Hershberger RE, Port JD, et al: Low-dose enoximone in subjects awaiting cardiac transplantation: Clinical results and effects on beta-adrenergic receptors. J Thorac Cardiovasc Surg 102:246-258, 1991.
66. Sindone AP, Keogh AM, Macdonald PS, et al: Continuous home ambulatory intravenous inotropic therapy in severe heart failure: Safety and cost efficacy. Am Heart J 134:889-900, 1997.
67. Milfred-LaForest SK, Shubert J, Mendoza B, et al: Tolerability of extended-duration intravenous milrinone in patients hospitalized for advanced heart failure and the usefulness of uptitration of oral angiotensin-converting enzyme inhibitors. Am J Cardiol 84:894-899, 1999.
68. Gibelein P, Dadoun-Dybal M, Candito M, et al: Hemodynamic effects of prolonged enoximone infusion (7 days) in patients with severe chronic heart failure. Cardiovasc Drugs Ther 7:333-336, 1993.
69. Follath F, Cleland JG, Just H, et al, for The Steering Committee and Investigators of the Levosimendan Infusion versus Dobutamine (LIDO) Study: Efficacy and safety of intravenous levosimendan compared with dobutamine in severe low-output heart failure (the LIDO study): A randomised double-blind trial. Lancet 360:196-202, 2002.
70. Yancy C, Fowler MB, Colluci WS, et al: Response of black heart failure patients to carvedilol [abstract]. J Am Coll Cardiol 29:84, 1997.
71. Dries DL, Exner DV, Gersh BJ, et al: Racial differences in the outcome of left ventricular dysfunction. N Engl J Med 340:609-616, 1999.
72. Small KM, Forbes SL, Rahman FF, et al: A four-amino acid deletion polymorphism in the third intracellular loop of the human alpha$_{2C}$-adrenergic receptor confers impaired coupling to multiple effectors. J Biol Chem 275:23059-23064, 2000.
73. Small KM, Wagoner LE, Levin AM, et al: Synergistic polymorphisms of beta$_1$- and alpha$_{2C}$-adrenergic receptors and the risk of congestive heart failure. New Engl J Med 347:1135-1142, 2002.
74. Carson P, Ziesche S, Johnson G, Cohn J: Racial differences in response to therapy for heart failure: Analysis of the vasodilator-heart failure trials. Vasodilator-Heart Failure Trial Study Group. J Card Fail 5:178-187, 1999.
75. Daida H, Allison TJ, Johnson BD, et al: Comparison of peak exercise oxygen uptake in men versus women in chronic heart failure secondary to ischemic or idiopathic dilated cardiomyopathy. Am J Cardiol 80:85-88, 1997.
76. Vaccarino V, Chen YT, Wang Y, et al: Sex differences in the clinical care and outcomes of congestive heart failure. Am Heart J 138:835-842, 1999.
77. Bonow RO, Udelson JE: Left ventricular diastolic dysfunction as a cause of congestive heart failure: Mechanisms and management. Ann Intern Med 117:502-510, 1992.
78. Dries D, Sweitzer N, Drazner M, et al: Prognostic impact of diabetes mellitus in patients with heart failure according to the etiology of left ventricular dysfunction. J Am Coll Cardiol 38:421-428, 2001.

79. Domanski M, Krause-Steinrauf H, Deedwania P, et al: The effect of diabetes on outcome of advanced heart failure patients in the BEST Trial. J Am Coll Cardiol 42:914-922, 2003.
80. Bristow MR, Gilbert, EM, Abraham WT, et al: Effect of carvedilol on LV function and mortality in diabetic versus non-diabetic patients with ischemic or nonischemic dilated cardiomyopathy. Circulation 94(Suppl): I-664, 1996.
81. Diller PM, Smucker DR, David B, Graham RJ: Congestive heart failure due to diastolic dysfunction: Frequency and patient characteristics in an ambulatory setting. Arch Fam Med 8:414-420, 1999.
82. Rich MW: Epidemiology, pathophysiology, and etiology of congestive heart failure in older adults. J Am Geriatr Soc 45:968-974, 1997.
83. Iriarte M, Murga N, Sagastagoitia D, et al: Congestive heart failure from left ventricular diastolic dysfunction in systemic hypertension. Am J Cardiol 71:308-312, 1993.
84. Spector KS: Diabetic cardiomyopathy. Clin Cardiol 21:885-887, 1998.
85. Friedrich SP, Lorrell BH, Rousseau MF, et al: Intracardiac angiotensin-converting enzyme inhibition improves diastolic function in patients with left ventricular hypertrophy due to aortic stenosis. Circulation 90:2761-2771, 1994.
86. Yusuf S, Pfeffer MA, Swedberg K, et al, for The CHARM Investigators: Effects of candesartan in patients with chronic heart failure and preserved left-ventricular ejection fraction. The CHARM-Preserved Trial. Lancet 362:767-771, 2003.
87. Mitrovic V, Strasser R, Berwig K, et al: Acute effects of enoximone after intracoronary administration on hemodynamics, myocardial perfusion, and regional wall motion. Z Kardiol 85:856-867, 1996.
88. Echt DS, Liebson PR, Mitchell LB, et al: Mortality and morbidity in patients receiving encainide, flecainide, or placebo. The Cardiac Arrhythmia Suppression Trial. N Engl J Med 324:781-788, 1991.
89. The Cardiac Arrhythmia Suppression Trial Investigators: Effect of the antiarrhythmic agent moricizine on survival after myocardial infarction. N Engl J Med 327:227-233, 1992.
90. Mason JW: A comparison of seven antiarrhythmic drugs in patients with ventricular tachyarrhythmias. Electrophysiologic Study Versus Electrocardiographic Monitoring Investigators. N Engl J Med 329:452-458, 1993.
91. Doval HC, Nul DR, Grancelli HO, et al: Randomised trial of low-dose amiodarone in severe congestive heart failure. Grupo de Estudio de la Sobrevida en la Insufficiencia Cardiaca en Argentina. Lancet 344:493-498, 1994.
92. Singh SN, Fletcher RD, Fisher SG, et al: Amiodarone in patients with congestive heart failure and asymptomatic ventricular arrhythmia. Survival Trial of Antiarrhythmic Therapy in Congestive Heart Failure. N Engl J Med 333:77-82, 1995.
93. Dunkman WB, Johnson GR, Carson PE, et al: Incidence of thromboembolic events in congestive heart failure. The V-HeFT VA Cooperative Studies Group. Circulation 87(Suppl 6):94-101, 1993.
94. Baker DW, Wright RF: Management of heart failure: IV. Anticoagulation for patients with heart failure due to left ventricular dysfunction. JAMA 272:1614-1618, 1994.
95. Hart RG, Haperin JL: Atrial fibrillation and thromboembolism: A decade of progress in stroke prevention. Ann Intern Med 131:688-695, 1999.
96. Falk RH, Foster E, Coats MH: Ventricular thrombi and thromboembolism in dilated cardiomyopathy: A prospective follow-up. Am Heart J 123:136-142, 1992.
97. Garg RK, Gheorghiade M, Jafri SM: Antiplatelet and anticoagulant therapy in the prevention of thromboemboli in chronic heart failure. Prog Cardiovasc Dis 41:225-236, 1998.
98. AVID Investigators: A comparison of antiarrhythmic drug therapy with implantable defibrillators in patients resuscitated from near-fatal ventricular arrhythmias. N Engl J Med 337:1576-1583, 1997.
99. MADIT Investigators: Improved survival with an implanted defibrillator in patients with coronary disease at high risk for ventricular arrhythmia. N Engl J Med 335:1933-1940, 1996.
100. Buxton AE, Lee KL, Fisher JD, et al: A randomized study of the prevention of sudden death in patients with coronary artery disease. N Engl J Med 341:1882-1890, 1999.
101. Moss AJ, Zareba W, Hall WJ, et al, for The Multicenter Automatic Defibrillator Implantation Trial II Investigators: Prophylactic implantation of a defibrillator in patients with myocardial infarction and reduced ejection fraction. N Engl J Med 346:877-883, 2002.
102. Bristow MR, Feldman AM, Saxon L, for the COMPANION Steering Committee: Heart failure management with biventricular pacing: The Comparison of Medical Therapy, Pacing and Defibrillation in Chronic Heart Failure (COMPANION) Trial. J Card Fail 6:276-285, 2000.
103. Bristow MR, Saxon LA, Boehmer J, et al: Cardiac resynchronization therapy with or without an implantable defibrillator in advanced chronic heart failure: The COMPANION Trial. N Engl J Med 350:2140, 2004.
104. Shamim W, Francis DP, Yousufuddin M, et al: Intraventricular conduction delay: A prognostic marker in chronic heart failure. Int J Cardiol 70:171-178, 1999.
105. Baldasseroni S, Opasich C, Gorini M, et al: Left bundle branch block is associated with increased 1-year sudden and total mortality rate in 5517 outpatients with congestive heart failure: A report from the Italian Network on Congestive Heart Failure. Am Heart J 143:398-405, 2002.
106. Werling C, Weisse U, Siemon G, et al. Biventricular pacing in patients with ICD: How many patients are possible candidates? Thorac Cardiovasc Surg 50:67-70, 2002.
107. Kass DA, Chen CH, Curry C, et al: Improved left ventricular mechanics from acute VDD pacing in patients with dilated cardiomyopathy and ventricular conduction delay. Circulation 99:1567-1573, 1999.
108. Leclercq C, Cazeau S, LeBreton H, et al: Acute hemodynamic effects of biventricular DDD pacing in patients with end-stage heart failure. J Am Coll Cardiol 32:1825-1831, 1998.
109. Kerwin WF, Botvinick EH, O'Connell JW, et al: Ventricular contraction abnormalities in dilated cardiomyopathy: Effect of biventricular pacing to correct interventricular dyssynchrony. J Am Coll Cardiol 35:1221-1227, 2000.
110. Saxon L, DeMarco T, Chatterjee K, et al: Chronic biventricular pacing decreases serum norepinephrine in dilated heart failure patients with the greatest sympathetic activation at baseline. Pacing Clin Electrophysiol 22:830, 1999.
111. Cazeau S, Leclercq C, Lavergne T, et al, for The Multisite Stimulation in Cardiomyopathies (MUSTIC) Study Investigators: Effects of multisite biventricular pacing in patients with heart failure and intraventricular conduction delay. N Engl J Med 344:873-880, 2001.
112. Auricchio A, Stellbrink C, Sack S, et al, for The Pacing Therapies in Congestive Heart Failure (PATH-CHF) Study Group: Long-term clinical effect of hemodynamically optimized cardiac resynchronization therapy in patients with heart failure and ventricular conduction delay. J Am Coll Cardiol 39:2026-2033, 2002.
113. Abraham WT, Fisher WG, Smith AL, et al, for The MIRACLE Study Group: Multicenter InSync Randomized Clinical Evaluation: Cardiac resynchronization in chronic heart failure. N Engl J Med 346:1845-1853, 2002.
114. Lau CP, Yu CM, Chau E, et al: Reversal of left ventricular remodeling by synchronous biventricular pacing in heart failure. Pacing Clin Electrophysiol 231722-1725, 000.
115. Saxon LA, De Marco T, Schafer J, et al, for The VIGOR Congestive Heart Failure Investigators: Effects of long-term biventricular stimulation for resynchronization on echocardiographic measures of remodeling. Circulation 105:1304-1310, 2002.
116. St. John Sutton MG, Plappert T, Abraham WT, et al, for The Multicenter InSync Randomized Clinical Evaluation (MIRACLE) Study Group: Effect of cardiac resynchronization therapy on left ventricular size and function in chronic heart failure. Circulation 107:1985-1990, 2003.
117. Rose EA, Moskowitz AJ, Packer M, et al: The REMATCH trial: Rationale, design, and end points. Randomized Evaluation of Mechanical Assistance for the Treatment of Congestive Heart Failure. Ann Thorac Surg 67:723-730, 1999.
118. Rose EA. Gelijns AC. Moskowitz AJ, et al, for The Randomized Evaluation of Mechanical Assistance for the Treatment of Congestive Heart Failure (REMATCH) Study Group: Long-term mechanical left ventricular assistance for end-stage heart failure. N Engl J Med 345:1435-1443, 2001.
119. Arora RR, Chou TM, Jain D, et al: The Multicenter Study of Enhanced External Counterpulsation (MUST-EECP): Effect of EECP on exercise-induced myocardial ischemia and anginal episodes. J Am Coll Cardiol 33:1833-1840, 1999.
120. Soran O, Fleishman B, Demarco T, et al: Enhanced external counterpulsation in patients with heart failure: A multicenter feasibility study. Congest Heart Fail 8:204-208, 227, 2002.
121. Chaudhry PA, Anagnostopouls PV, Mishima T, et al: Acute ventricular reduction with the acorn cardiac support device: Effect on progressive left ventricular dysfunction and dilation in dogs with chronic heart failure. J Card Surg 16:118-126, 2001.
122. Miniati DN, Robbins RC: Heart transplantation: A thirty-year perspective. Annu Rev Med 53:189-205, 2002.
123. Zaroff JG, Rosengard BR, Armstrong WF, et al: Consensus conference report: Maximizing use of organs recovered from the cadaver donor—cardiac recommendations, March 28-29, 2001, Crystal City, Va. Circulation 106:836-841, 2002.
124. Passamani E, Davis KB, Gillespie MJ, Killip T: A randomized trial of coronary artery bypass surgery. Survival of patients with a low ejection fraction. N Engl J Med 312:1665-1671, 1985.
125. Elefteriades JA, Morales DL, Gradel C, et al: Results of coronary artery bypass grafting by a single surgeon in patients with left ventricular ejection fractions ≤ 30 percent. Am J Cardiol 79:1573-1578, 1997.
126. Bax JJ, Poldermans D, Elhendy A, et al: Improvement of left ventricular ejection fraction, heart failure symptoms, and prognosis after revascularization in patients with chronic coronary artery disease and viable myocardium detected by dobutamine stress echocardiography. J Am Coll Cardiol 34:163-169, 1999.
127. Athanasuleas CL, Buckberg GD, Menicanti L, Gharib M, for the RESTORE Group: Optimizing ventricular shape in anterior restoration. Semin Thorac Cardiovasc Surg 13:459-467, 2001.
128. Bolling SF, Pagani FD, Deeb GM, Bach DS: Intermediate-term outcome of mitral reconstruction in cardiomyopathy. J Thorac Cardiovasc Surg 115:381-386, 1998.

Management of Episodes of Acute Decompensation

129. Leier CV, Ebel J, Bush CA: The cardiovascular effects of the continuous infusion of dobutamine in patients with severe cardiac failure. Circulation 56:468-472, 1977.
130. Publication Committee for the VMAC Investigators (Vasodilatation in the Management of Acute CHF): Intravenous nesiritide versus nitroglycerin for treatment of decompensated congestive heart failure: A randomized controlled trial. JAMA 287:1531-1540, 2002.
131. Likoff MJ, Weber KT, Andrews V, et al: Milrinone in the treatment of chronic cardiac failure: A controlled trial. Am Heart J 110:1035-1042, 1985.
132. Biddle TL, Benotti JR, Creager MA, et al: Comparison of intravenous milrinone and dobutamine for congestive heart failure secondary to either ischemic or dilated cardiomyopathy. Am J Cardiol 59:1345-1350, 1987.
133. Gilbert E, for the Enoximone Working Group: Double-blind, placebo-controlled comparison of enoximone and dobutamine infusions in moderate to severe heart failure patients (NYHA III-IV) [abstract]. J Am Coll Cardiol 17:274, 1991.
134. Berti S, Palmieri C, Ravani M, et al: Acute enoximone effect on systemic and renal hemodynamics in patients with heart failure. Cardiovasc Drugs Ther 10:81-87, 1996.
135. Lowes BD, Simon MA, Tsvetkova TO, Bristow MR: Inotropes in the β-blocker era. Clin Cardiol 23(Suppl 3):11-16, 2000.
136. Gage J, Rutman H, Lucido D, LeJemtel TH: Additive effects of dobutamine and amrinone on myocardial contractility and ventricular performance in patients with severe heart failure. Circulation 74:367-373, 1986.
137. Gilbert EM, Hershberger RE, Wiechmann RJ, et al: Pharmacologic and hemodynamic effects of combined β-agonist stimulation and phosphodiesterase inhibition in the failing human heart. Chest 108:1524-1532, 1995.
138. Marcus LS, Hart D, Packer M, et al: Hemodynamic and renal excretory effects of human brain natriuretic peptide infusion in patients with congestive heart failure: A double-blind, placebo-controlled, cross-over trial. Circulation 94:3184-3189, 1996.
139. Abraham WT, Lowes BD, Ferguson DA, et al: Systemic hemodynamic, neurohormonal, and renal effects of a steady-state infusion of human brain natriuretic peptide in

patients with advanced hemodynamically decompensated heart failure. J Card Fail 4:37-44, 1998.
140. Port JD, Gilbert EM, Larrabee P, et al: Neurotransmitter depletion compromises the ability of indirect-acting amines to provide inotropic support in the failing human heart. Circulation 81:929-938, 1990.
141. Grines CI, Browne KF, Marco J, et al: A comparison of immediate angioplasty with thrombolytic therapy for acute myocardial infarction. The Primary Angioplasty in Myocardial Infarction Study Group. N Engl J Med 328:673-679, 1993.
142. Grines CI, Cox DA, Stone GW, et al: Coronary angioplasty with or without stent implantation for acute myocardial infarction. Stent Primary Angioplasty in Myocardial Infarction Study Group. N Engl J Med 341:1949-1956, 1999.

Health Care Delivery Strategies

143. Hanumanthu S, Butler J, Chomsky D, et al: Effect of a heart failure program on hospitalization frequency and exercise tolerance. Circulation 96:2842-2848, 1997.
144. Chapman DB, Torpy J: Development of a heart failure center: A medical center and cardiology practice join forces to improve care and reduce costs. Am J Managed Care 3:431-437, 1997.
145. Nohria A, Chen YT, Morton DJ, et al: Quality of care for patients hospitalized at academic medical centers. Am Heart J 137:1028-1034, 1999.
146. Bristow MR, Abraham WT: Specialized centers for heart failure management. Circulation 96:2755-2757, 1997.
147. Croft JB, Giles WH, Roegner RH, et al: Pharmacologic management of heart failure among older adults by office-based physicians in the United States. J Fam Pract 44:382-390, 1997.
148. Schmedtje JF Jr, Evans GW, Byerly W, et al: Treatment of chronic heart failure in a managed care setting: Baseline results from the Achieving Cardiac Excellence Project. N C Med J 64:4-10, 2003.
149. Roe CM, Motheral BR, Teitelbaum F, Rich MW: Angiotensin-converting enzyme inhibitor compliance and dosing among patients with heart failure. Am Heart J 138:818-825, 1999.
150. Balk AH: The "heart failure nurse" to help us close the gap between what we can and what we do achieve. Eur Heart J 20:632-633, 1999.
151. Stromberg A, Martensson J, Fridlund B, et al: Nurse-led heart failure clinics improve survival and self-care behaviour in patients with heart failure: Results from a prospective, randomised trial. Eur Heart J 24:1014-1023, 2003.

Exercise

152. Burch GE, Giles TD: Prolonged bed rest in the management of patients with cardiomyopathy. Cardiovasc Clin 4:375-387, 1972.
153. Coats AJ, Adamopoulos S, Radaelli A, et al: Controlled trial of physical training in chronic heart failure: Exercise performance, hemodynamics, ventilation, and autonomic function. Circulation 85:2119-2131, 1992.
154. Kiilavuaori K, Naveri H, Leinonen H, Harkonen M: The effect of physical training on hormonal status and exertional response in patients with congestive heart failure. Eur J Cardiol 20:456-464, 1999.
155. Keteyian SJ, Brawner CA, Schairer, et al: Effects of exercise training on chronotropic incompetence in patients with heart failure. Am Heart J 138:233-240, 1999.
156. Braith RW, Welsch MA, Feigenbaum MS, et al: Neuroendocrine activation in heart failure is modified by endurance exercise training. J Am Coll Cardiol 34:1170-1175, 1999.
157. Coats AJ, Adamopoulous S, Meyer TE, et al: Effects of physical training in chronic heart failure. Lancet 335:63-66, 1990.
158. Willenheimer R, Erhardt L, Cline C, et al: Exercise training in heart failure improves quality of life and exercise capacity. Eur Heart J 19:774-781, 1998.
159. Levy D, Kenchaiah S, Larson MG, et al: Long-term trends in the incidence of and survival with heart failure. N Engl J Med 347:1397-1402, 2002.

GUIDELINES *Thomas H. Lee*

Management of Heart Failure

Guidelines for the evaluation and management of heart failure (HF) were published by a joint task force of the American College of Cardiology and the American Heart Association (ACC/AHA) in 2001.[1] These guidelines updated previous sets of recommendations issued by the ACC/AHA in 1995,[2] as well as guidelines from the Agency for Health Care Policy and Research in 1994[3] and the Heart Failure Society of America in 1999.[4]

Reflecting growing appreciation for the importance of prevention of HF, the updated ACC/AHA guidelines classified patients according to four stages, as follows:

Stage A patients are at high risk for developing HF but have no structural disorder of the heart.

Stage B patients have a structural disorder of the heart but have never developed symptoms of HF.

Stage C patients are those with past or current symptoms of HF associated with underlying structural heart disease.

Stage D patients have end-stage disease and require specialized treatment strategies such as mechanical circulatory support, continuous inotropic infusions, cardiac transplantation, or hospice care.

The traditional New York Heart Association (NYHA) functional classification system primarily gauges the severity of symptoms in patients who are in stage C or D. The usefulness of the four-stage system is that it recommends interventions for asymptomatic patients with the goal of preventing signs or symptoms of HF. Figure 24G-1 summarizes the guideline recommendations for therapy by stage.

As with other ACC/AHA guidelines, these recommendations classify interventions into one of three classes as follows, including two levels of the intermediate group:

Class I: conditions for which there is evidence and/or general agreement that a given procedure/therapy is useful and effective

Class II: conditions for which there is conflicting evidence and/or a divergence of opinion about the usefulness/efficacy of performing the procedure/therapy

Class IIa: weight of evidence and opinion in favor of usefulness/efficacy

Class IIb: usefulness/efficacy is less well established by evidence and opinion

Class III: conditions for which there is evidence and/or general agreement that a procedure or therapy is not useful or effective and in some cases may be harmful

The ACC/AHA guidelines also adopted a convention for rating levels of evidence on which recommendations have been based. *Level A* recommendations were derived from data from multiple randomized clinical trials; *level B* recommendations were derived from a single randomized trial or nonrandomized studies; and *level C* recommendations were based on the consensus opinion of experts. The guidelines emphasize that the strength of evidence does not necessarily reflect the strength of a recommendation. A treatment may be controversial despite having been evaluated in controlled clinical trials; conversely, a strong recommendation may be supported only by historical data or by no data at all.

INITIAL EVALUATION OF PATIENT

The ACC/AHA guidelines state that a complete history and physical examination should be the first step in the evaluation of patients with HF (Table 24G-1). This evaluation may provide insight into the cause of the patient's HF and the presence or absence of structural cardiovascular abnormalities. Other issues to be addressed include presence or absence of history of diabetes, rheumatic fever, chest radiation, and exposure to cardiotoxic drugs. The patient's functional and hemodynamic status should also be evaluated to assess prognosis and guide management.

The guidelines recommend that the initial evaluation should include a complete blood count; urinalysis; serum electrolytes, renal and hepatic function, calcium, and magnesium; thyroid function tests; blood lipids; a chest radiograph; and a 12-lead electrocardiogram. Measurement of serum ferritin level and transferrin saturation was considered potentially useful for the detection of hemochromatosis, since this condition is a treatable cause of HF. Only weak support was found for routine screening for human immunodeficiency virus, connective tissue diseases, or pheochromocytoma unless other clinical data suggest that these diagnoses should be suspected.

Echocardiography to assess left ventricular function and detect underlying myocardial, valvular, or pericardial disease was considered

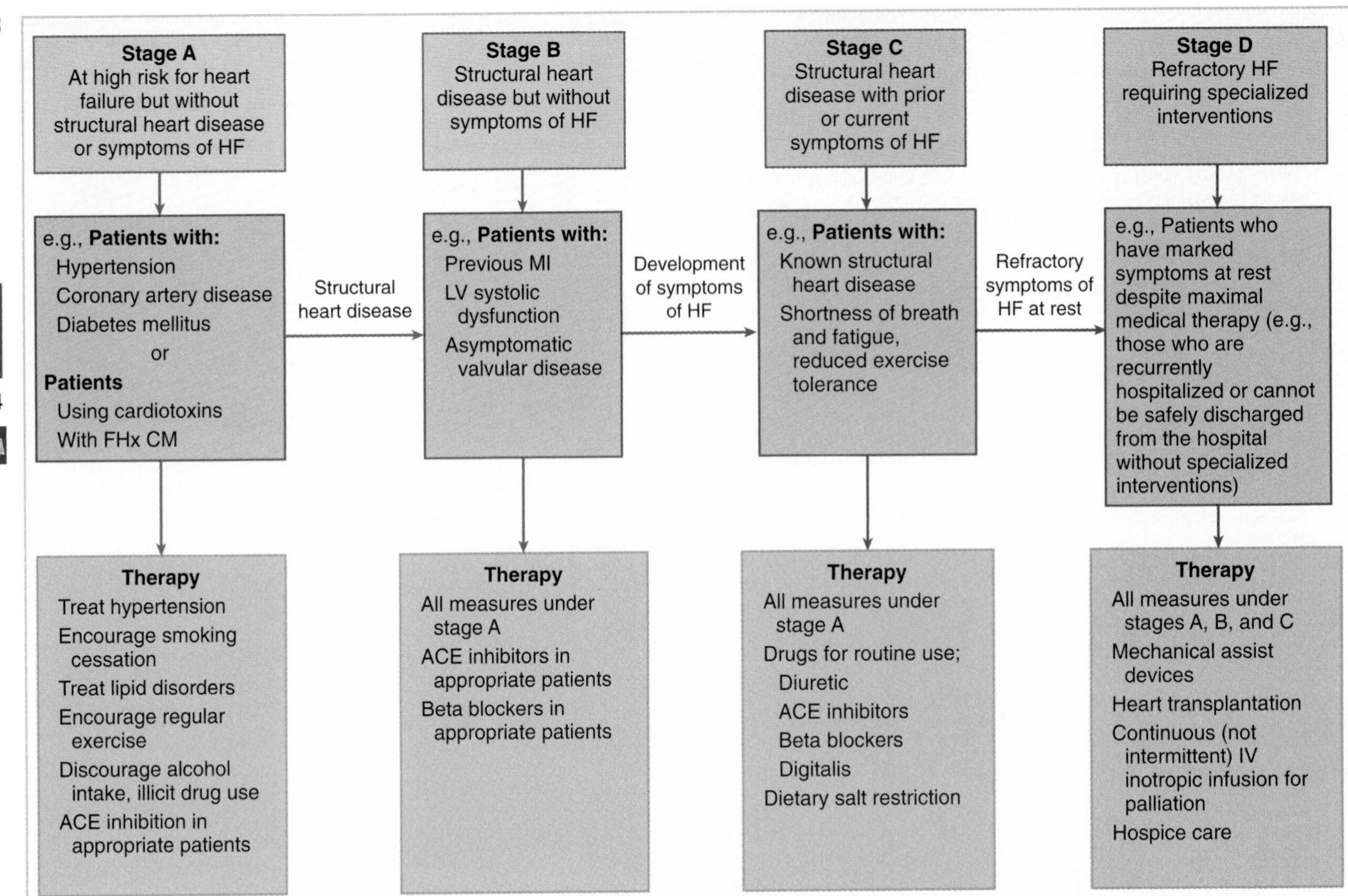

FIGURE 24G–1 Stages in the evolution of heart failure and recommended therapy by stage. FHx CM = family history of cardiomyopathy; HF = heart failure; ACE = angiotensin-converting enzyme; MI = myocardial infarction; LV = left ventricular; IV = intravenous. (From Hunt SA, Baker DW, Chin MH, et al: ACC/AHA guidelines for the evaluation and management of chronic heart failure in the adult: A report of the American College of Cardiology/American Heart Association Task Force on Practice Guidelines [Committee to Revise the 1995 Guidelines for the Evaluation and Management of Heart Failure]. American College of Cardiology, 2001. [http://www.acc.org/ clinical/guidelines/failure/hf_index.htm])

a more valuable initial test than radionuclide ventriculography or magnetic resonance imaging. The guidelines were noncommittal about routine measurement of brain natriuretic peptide; considerable data on this topic have been published since release of these guidelines, and future updates can be expected to offer recommendations on use of this test.

Screening for and assessment of coronary artery disease in patients with HF were given considerable attention in these guidelines, reflecting the frequent coexistence of these conditions and the survival benefit of revascularization of patients with severe coronary disease and left ventricular dysfunction. Coronary angiography was recommended (Class I indication) for patients with angina and HF who would be candidates for revascularization. For patients who have chest pain and HF, the guidelines provide support for bypassing the step of noninvasive testing and proceeding directly to coronary angiography (Class IIa indication). For patients without chest pain, the guidelines consider coronary angiography "reasonable" in younger patients with HF to exclude the diagnosis of coronary disease. However, the guidelines did not support routine coronary angiography in older HF patients without chest pain syndromes and found only weak support (Class IIb) for noninvasive testing for ischemia in such patients.

The guidelines did not recommend routine use of endomyocardial biopsy or ambulatory monitoring to detect arrhythmia.

Ongoing Assessment of Patients with Heart Failure

Although the guidelines support routine assessment of functional and volume status in patients with HF, they recommend restraint in the use of noninvasive testing with the exception of serum electrolytes and renal function. They specifically discourage routine serial measurement of ejection fraction at regular intervals. Instead, they recommend that ejection fraction be reassessed if patients have had a change in clinical status, recovered from a significant clinical event, or received treatment that might affect left ventricular function. Similarly, routine invasive or noninvasive assessment of hemodynamic function is discouraged.

Treatment of Patients at High Risk of Developing Heart Failure (Stage A)

The ACC/AHA guidelines provide strong recommendations (Class I) for control of risk factors for coronary disease and other causes of cardiomyopathy, including hypertension, hyperlipidemia, diabetes, alcohol abuse, cigarette smoking, and hyperthyroidism (Table 24G-2). Patients at risk for HF should also be assessed frequently for evidence that they are developing this condition, and a low threshold for use of angiotensin-converting enzyme (ACE) inhibitors is recommended. The ACC/AHA task force did not find evidence to support life-style interventions for prevention of HF in this population, including exercise, salt restriction, or routine use of nutritional supplements.

Restraint in the use of noninvasive testing was urged in patients without signs or symptoms of HF or structural heart disease. Noninvasive evaluation of left ventricular function was considered probably reasonable (Class IIa) in patients with a strong family history of cardiomyopathy or who were receiving cardiotoxic interventions.

TABLE 24G–1 ACC/AHA Guidelines for Evaluation of Heart Failure

Class	Indication	Level of Evidence*
I (indicated)	1. Thorough history and physical examination to identify cardiac and noncardiac disorders that might lead to the development of heart failure or accelerate the progression of heart failure	C
	2. Initial and ongoing assessment of a patient's ability to perform routine and desired activities of daily living	C
	3. Initial and ongoing assessment of volume status	C
	4. Initial measurement of complete blood count, urinalysis, serum electrolytes (including calcium and magnesium), blood urea nitrogen, serum creatinine, blood glucose, liver function tests, and thyroid-stimulating hormone	C
	5. Serial monitoring of serum electrolytes and renal function	
	6. Initial 12-lead electrocardiogram and chest radiograph	C
	7. Initial two-dimensional echocardiography with Doppler or radionuclide ventriculography to assess left ventricular systolic function	C
	8. Cardiac catheterization with coronary arteriography in patients with angina who are candidates for revascularization	B
IIa (good supportive evidence)	1. Cardiac catheterization with coronary arteriography in patients with chest pain who have not had evaluation of their coronary anatomy and who have no contraindications to coronary revascularization	C
	2. Cardiac catheterization with coronary arteriography in patients with known or suspected coronary artery disease but without angina who are candidates for revascularization	C
	3. Noninvasive imaging to detect ischemia and viability in patients with known coronary artery disease and no angina who are being considered for revascularization	C
	4. Maximal exercise testing with measurement of respiratory gas exchange and/or blood oxygen saturation to help determine whether heart failure is the cause of exercise limitation when the contribution of heart failure is uncertain	C
	5. Maximal exercise testing with measurement of respiratory gas exchange to identify high-risk patients who are candidates for cardiac transplantation or other advanced treatments	B
	6. Echocardiography in asymptomatic first-degree relatives of patients with idiopathic dilated cardiomyopathy	C
	7. Repeat measurement of ejection fraction in patients who have had a change in clinical status or who have experienced or recovered from a clinical event or received treatment that might have had a significant effect on cardiac function	C
	8. Screening for hemochromatosis	C
	9. Measurement of serum antinuclear antibody, rheumatoid factor, urinary vanillylmandelic acid, and metanephrines in selected patients	C
IIb (weak supportive evidence)	1. Noninvasive imaging to define the likelihood of coronary artery disease in patients with left ventricular dysfunction	C
	2. Maximal exercise testing with measurement of respiratory gas exchange to facilitate prescription of an appropriate exercise program	C
	3. Endomyocardial biopsy in patients in whom an inflammatory or infiltrative disorder of the heart is suspected	C
	4. Assessment of HIV status	C
III (not indicated)	1. Endomyocardial biopsy in the routine evaluation of patients with heart failure	C
	2. Routine Holter monitoring or signal-averaged electrocardiography	C
	3. Repeat coronary arteriography or noninvasive testing for ischemia in patients for whom coronary artery disease has previously been excluded as the cause of left ventricular dysfunction	C
	4. Routine measurement of circulating levels of norepinephrine or endothelin	C

ACC = American College of Cardiology; AHA = American Heart Association; HIV = human immunodeficiency virus.
*See guidelines text for definition of level of evidence categories.

Treatment of Patients with Left Ventricular Dysfunction Who Have Not Developed Symptoms (Stage B)

In this population, the goal of therapy is to reduce the risk of further damage to the left ventricle and to minimize the rate of progression of left ventricular dysfunction. The same risk factor modifications supported for stage A patients are also recommended for stage B patients (Table 24G-3). As was true with stage A patients, no evidence was found to support use of exercise and other life-style modifications for this population.

The two major pharmacological interventions that warrant consideration in all stage B patients are ACE inhibitors and beta blockers. In the absence of contraindications, medications in these two classes are recommended for all patients with histories of myocardial infarction, regardless of ejection fraction, and for all patients with diminished ejection fraction, regardless of history of myocardial infarction. In contrast, the guidelines discourage use of digoxin in this population.

Because tachyarrhythmias may hasten the progression of left ventricular dysfunction, the guidelines urge interventions to control ventricular response to supraventricular tachyarrhythmias. They also support surgery to correct valvular disease that causes HF, but note the absence of evidence providing support for the use of vasodilators in patients with aortic insufficiency.

TABLE 24G–2 ACC/AHA Guidelines for Treatment of Patients at High Risk of Developing Heart Failure (Stage A)

Class	Indication	Level of Evidence*
I (indicated)	1. Control of systolic and diastolic hypertension in accordance with recommended guidelines	A
	2. Treatment of lipid disorders, in accordance with recommended guidelines	B
	3. Avoidance of patient behaviors that may increase the risk of heart failure (e.g., smoking, alcohol consumption, and illicit drug use)	C
	4. ACE inhibition in patients with a history of atherosclerotic vascular disease, diabetes mellitus, or hypertension and associated cardiovascular risk factors	B
	5. Control of ventricular rate in patients with supraventricular tachyarrhythmias	B
	6. Treatment of thyroid disorders	C
	7. Periodic evaluation for signs and symptoms of heart failure	C
IIa (good supportive evidence)	Noninvasive evaluation of left ventricular function in patients with a strong family history of cardiomyopathy or in those receiving cardiotoxic interventions	C
IIb (weak supportive evidence)	None	
III (not indicated)	1. Exercise to prevent the development of heart failure	C
	2. Reduction of dietary salt beyond that which is prudent for healthy individuals in patients without hypertension or fluid retention	C
	3. Routine testing to detect left ventricular dysfunction in patients without signs or symptoms of heart failure or evidence of structural heart disease	C
	4. Routine use of nutritional supplements to prevent the development of structural heart disease	C

ACC = American College of Cardiology; AHA = American Heart Association; ACE = angiotensin-converting enzyme.
*See guidelines text for definition of level of evidence categories.

TABLE 24G–3 ACC/AHA Guidelines for Treatment of Asymptomatic Left Ventricular Systolic Dysfunction (Stage B)

Class	Indication	Level of Evidence*
I (indicated)	1. ACE inhibition in patients with a recent or remote history of myocardial infarction regardless of ejection fraction	A
	2. ACE inhibition in patients with a reduced ejection fraction, whether or not they have experienced a myocardial infarction	B
	3. Beta blockade in patients with a recent myocardial infarction regardless of ejection fraction	A
	4. Beta blockade in patients with a reduced ejection fraction, whether or not they have experienced a myocardial infarction	B
	5. Valve replacement or repair for patients with hemodynamically significant valvular stenosis or regurgitation	B
	6. Regular evaluation for signs and symptoms of heart failure	C
	7. Measures listed as Class I recommendations for patients in stage A (see Table 23G–2)	
IIa (good supportive evidence)	None	
IIb (weak supportive evidence)	1. Long-term treatment with systemic vasodilators in patients with severe aortic regurgitation	B
III (not indicated)	1. Treatment with digoxin in patients with left ventricular dysfunction who are in sinus rhythm	C
	2. Reduction of dietary salt beyond that which is prudent for healthy individuals in patients without hypertension or fluid retention	C
	3. Exercise to prevent the development of heart failure	C
	4. Routine use of nutritional supplements to treat structural heart disease or prevent the development of symptoms of heart failure	C

ACC = American College of Cardiology; AHA = American Heart Association; ACE = angiotensin-converting enzyme.
*See guidelines text for definition of level of evidence categories.

Treatment of Patients with Left Ventricular Dysfunction and Current or Prior Symptoms (Stage C)

The measures recommended to prevent or minimize progression of left ventricular dysfunction for stage A and B patients are also supported for stage C patients, who have current or prior symptoms attributable to left ventricular dysfunction (Table 24G–4). However, in contrast with the recommendations for stage B patients, the guidelines support use of moderate sodium restriction as well as daily measurement of weight. Immunization with influenza and pneumococcal vaccines is also encouraged.

Physical activity is also recommended for stage C patients in the 2001 ACC/AHA guidelines, although they also stipulate that most patients should not engage in heavy labor or exhaustive sports. More

TABLE 24G–4 ACC/AHA Guidelines for Treatment of Symptomatic Left Ventricular Systolic Dysfunction (Stage C)

Class	Indication	Level of Evidence*
I (indicated)	1. Diuretics in patients who have evidence of fluid retention	A
	2. ACE inhibition in all patients, unless contraindicated	A
	3. Beta-adrenergic blockade in all stable patients, unless contraindicated. Patients should have no or minimal evidence of fluid retention and should not have required treatment recently with an intravenous positive inotropic agent	A
	4. Digitalis for the treatment of symptoms of heart failure, unless contraindicated	A
	5. Withdrawal of drugs known to adversely affect the clinical status of patients (e.g., nonsteroidal antiinflammatory drugs, most antiarrhythmic drugs, and most calcium-channel blocking drugs)	B
	6. Measures listed as Class I recommendations for patients in stages A and B (see Tables 24G–2 and 24G–3)	
IIa (good supportive evidence)	1. Spironolactone in patients with recent or current Class IV symptoms, preserved renal function, and a normal potassium concentration	B
	2. Exercise training as an adjunctive approach to improve clinical status in ambulatory patients	A
	3. Angiotensin-receptor blockade in patients who are being treated with digitalis, diuretics, and a beta blocker and who cannot be given an ACE inhibitor because of cough or angioedema	A
	4. A combination of hydralazine and a nitrate in patients who are being treated with digitalis, diuretics, and a beta blocker and who cannot be given an ACE inhibitor because of hypotension or renal insufficiency	B
IIb (weak supportive evidence)	1. Addition of an angiotensin-receptor blocker to an ACE inhibitor	B
	2. Addition of a nitrate (alone or in combination with hydralazine) to an ACE inhibitor in patients who are also being given digitalis, diuretics, and a beta blocker	B
III (not indicated)	1. Long-term intermittent use of an infusion of a positive inotropic drug	C
	2. Use of an angiotensin-receptor blocker instead of an ACE inhibitor in patients with heart failure who have not been given or who can tolerate an ACE inhibitor	B
	3. Use of an angiotensin-receptor blocker before a beta blocker in patients with heart failure who are taking an ACE inhibitor	A
	4. Use of a calcium-channel blocking drug as a treatment for heart failure	B
	5. Routine use of nutritional supplements (coenzyme Q10, carnitine, taurine, and antioxidants) or hormonal therapies (growth hormone or thyroid hormone) for the treatment of heart failure	C

ACC = American College of Cardiology; AHA = American Heart Association; ACE = angiotensin-converting enzyme.
*See guidelines text for definition of level of evidence categorises.

detailed recommendations were subsequently provided in an AHA Scientific Statement on Exercise and Heart Failure published in 2003.[5] This Scientific Statement noted the absence of large randomized trials of the impact of exercise on outcome for patients with HF and observed that most available data on this topic preceded the era of treatment of HF with beta blockers. Nevertheless, the authors considered the likely benefit sufficient to support exercise training using an individualized approach. This statement supported use of technologies including gas exchange measurements to provide an objective assessment of functional capacity and direct monitoring (including telemetry monitoring), particularly for initial training sessions. Even fewer data are available on the risks of resistive training in this population, but the Scientific Statement observed that such training seems to offer some physiological benefits and supported the use of small free weights and exercises aimed at strengthening the upper body.

The 2001 ACC/AHA guidelines support use of ACE inhibitors and beta blockers for all stage C patients, in the absence of contraindications, and use of diuretics for patients with fluid overload and digitalis for symptomatic patients (see Table 24G–4). Of note is that these guidelines preceded data published in 2002 indicating worse prognosis for women treated with digoxin[6]; hence, it is possible that support for use of digoxin may be tempered in future revisions. The risks of initiation of beta blockers are considered in detail in these guidelines, but these agents are recommended for "all patients with stable [HF] due to left ventricular systolic dysfunction unless they have a contraindication to their use or have been shown to be unable to tolerate treatment with these drugs."

The guidelines offer qualified support (Class IIa) for use of spironolactone in patients with Class IV HF symptoms based on its effectiveness in one large-scale, long-term trial.[7] They also offer support for use of angiotensin-receptor blockade and hydralazine/nitrate combinations in patients who cannot tolerate an ACE inhibitor, although as a second choice after ACE inhibitors. The recommendations regarding use of angiotensin-receptor blockers will likely be revised to reflect findings from the Valsartan Heart Failure Trial (Val-HeFT).[8]

They recommend withdrawal of drugs from three classes that are known to exacerbate HF or worsen prognosis: nonsteroidal antiinflammatory agents, most antiarrhythmic drugs, and most calcium-channel blocking drugs. Of the latter two classes of drugs, the guidelines observed that only amiodarone and amlodipine had not been shown to adversely affect survival. The guidelines also explicitly discourage use of intermittent infusions of positive inotropic agents and of routine use of nutritional supplements or hormonal therapies.

TREATMENT OF PATIENTS WITH REFRACTORY END-STAGE HEART FAILURE (STAGE D)

Stage D HF patients typically have symptoms at rest, have severely limited functional capacity, and often have frequent hospitalizations for management of symptoms. The ACC/AHA guidelines emphasize the importance of meticulous application of the measures listed as Class I recommendations for patients in stages A, B, and C (see Tables

TABLE 24G–5 ACC/AHA Guidelines for Treatment of Patients with Refractory End-Stage Heart Failure (Stage D)

Class	Indication	Level of Evidence*
I (indicated)	1. Meticulous identification and control of fluid retention 2. Referral for cardiac transplantation in eligible patients 3. Referral to a heart failure program with expertise in the management of refractory heart failure 4. Measures listed as Class I recommendations for patients in stages A, B, and C (see Tables 24G–2 to 24G–4)	B B A
IIa (good supportive evidence)	None	
IIb (weak supportive evidence)	1. Pulmonary artery catheter placement to guide therapy in patients with persistently severe symptoms 2. Mitral valve repair or replacement for severe secondary mitral regurgitation 3. Continuous intravenous infusion of a positive inotropic agent for palliation of symptoms	C C C
III (not indicated)	1. Partial left ventriculectomy 2. Routine intermittent infusions of positive inotropic agents	C B

ACC = American College of Cardiology; AHA = American Heart Association.
*See guidelines text for definition of level of evidence categories.

TABLE 24G–6 ACC/AHA Guidelines: Indications for Cardiac Transplantation

Absolute Indications

- For hemodynamic compromise due to heart failure
  - Refractory cardiogenic shock
  - Documented dependence on IV inotropic support to maintain adequate organ perfusion
  - Peak V_{O_2} < 10 ml/kg/min with achievement of anaerobic metabolism
- Severe symptoms of ischemia that consistently limit routine activity and are not amenable to coronary artery bypass surgery or percutaneous coronary intervention
- Recurrent symptomatic ventricular arrhythmias refractory to all therapeutic modalities

Relative Indications

- Peak V_{O_2} 11–14 ml/kg/min (or 55% predicted) and major limitation of the patient's daily activities
- Recurrent unstable ischemia not amenable to other intervention
- Recurrent instability of fluid balance/renal function not due to patient noncompliance with medical regimen

Insufficient Indications

- Low left ventricular ejection fraction
- History of functional Class III or IV symptoms of heart failure
- Peak V_{O_2} > 15 ml/kg/min (and >55% predicted) without other indications

ACC = American College of Cardiology; AHA = American Heart Association.
From Hunt SA, Baker DW, Chin MH, et al: ACC/AHA guidelines for the evaluation and management of chronic heart failure in the adult: A report of the American College of Cardiology/American Heart Association Task Force on Practice Guidelines (Committee to Revise the 1995 Guidelines for the Evaluation and Management of Heart Failure). American College of Cardiology, 2001. (http://www.acc.org/clinical/guidelines/failure/hf_index.htm)

24G-2 to 24G-4) and consider these patients candidates for specialized treatment strategies, such as mechanical circulatory support, continuous intravenous positive inotropic therapy, referral for cardiac transplantation, or hospice care (Table 24G-5). The guidelines also endorse the use of team management approaches such as HF programs. Detailed specifications of the components of such HF programs were provided in an AHA Scientific Statement published in 2000.[9]

The 2001 ACC/AHA guidelines include explicit cautionary notes about the use of ACE inhibitors and beta blockers for this population. Although consideration of these agents is supported, the guidelines state that "treatment with either agent should not be initiated in patients with systolic blood pressures less than 80 mm Hg or who have signs of peripheral hypoperfusion. In addition, patients should not be started on a beta-blocker if they have significant fluid retention or if they recently required treatment with an intravenous positive inotropic agent." When these medications are used, very low doses should be prescribed at initiation, and patients should be monitored closely for evidence of intolerance. The guidelines note that spironolactone has been shown to be beneficial in patients with advanced HF, but they emphasize that these data are derived from patients with preserved renal function[7] and that spironolactone may induce hyperkalemia in patient with impaired renal function.

The ACC/AHA guidelines recognized the value of continuous intravenous inotropic support for some patients who require a "bridge" strategy while awaiting cardiac transplantation or who cannot otherwise be discharged from hospital. However, the guidelines directly discouraged routine intermittent intravenous infusion of inotropic agents. Similarly, the guidelines did not encourage use of partial left ventriculectomy.

The guidelines also include a summary of indications for cardiac transplantation (Table 24G-6). These indications make explicit that low

TABLE 24G–7 ACC/AHA Guidelines for Management of Concomitant Diseases in Patients with Heart Failure

Class	Indication	Level of Evidence*
I (indicated)	1. Control of systolic and diastolic hypertension in patients with heart failure in accordance with recommended guidelines	A
	2. Nitrates and beta blockers (in conjunction with diuretics) for the treatment of angina in patients with heart failure	B
	3. Coronary revascularization in patients who have both heart failure and angina	A
	4. Anticoagulants in patients with heart failure who have paroxysmal or chronic atrial fibrillation or a previous thromboembolic event	A
	5. Control of the ventricular response in patients with heart failure and atrial fibrillation with a beta blocker (or amiodarone, if the beta blocker is contraindicated or not tolerated)	A
	6. Beta-adrenergic blockade (unless contraindicated) in patients with heart failure to reduce the risk of sudden death. Patients should have no or minimal fluid retention and should not have recently required treatment with an intravenous positive inotropic agent	A
	7. Implantable cardioverter-defibrillator (alone or in combination with amiodarone) in patients with heart failure who have a history of sudden death, ventricular fibrillation, or hemodynamically destabilizing ventricular tachycardia	A
IIa (good supportive evidence)	1. Antiplatelet agents for prevention of myocardial infarction and death in patients with heart failure who have underlying coronary artery disease	B
	2. Digitalis to control the ventricular response in patients with heart failure and atrial fibrillation	A
IIb (weak supportive evidence)	1. Coronary revascularization in patients who have heart failure and coronary artery disease but no angina	B
	2. Restoration of sinus rhythm by electrical cardioversion in patients with heart failure and atrial fibrillation	C
	3. Amiodarone to prevent sudden death in patients with heart failure and asymptomatic ventricular arrhythmias	B
	4. Anticoagulation in patients with heart failure who do not have atrial fibrillation or a previous thromboembolic event	B or C
III (not indicated)	1. Routine use of an implantable cardioverter-defibrillator in patients with heart failure	C
	2. Class I or III antiarrhythmic drugs (except amiodarone) in patients with heart failure for the prevention or treatment of asymptomatic ventricular arrhythmias	A
	3. Ambulatory electrocardiographic monitoring for the detection of asymptomatic ventricular arrhythmias	A

ACC = American College of Cardiology; AHA = American Heart Association.
*See guidelines text for definition of level of evidence categories.

left ventricular ejection fraction and poor functional status are insufficient indications in the absence of demonstrated peak oxygen consumption less than 15 ml/kg/min.

Special Populations and Concomitant Disorders

The ACC/AHA guidelines support consideration of patient-specific needs and coexisting medical conditions. Clinicians are reminded that women, minorities, and the elderly are less likely to receive interventions supported by clinical trials and that differences in the natural history of HF and response to treatment exist among various patient subsets. Specific clinical recommendations (Table 24G-7) emphasize the importance of meticulous management of hypertension, ischemic heart disease, anticoagulation, and supraventricular and ventricular arrhythmias.

The guidelines do not support routine use of implantable cardioverter-defibrillators or use of Class I or III antiarrhythmic drugs except amiodarone. Since these guidelines were issued, additional trials have been published providing insight into the potential beneficial impact of implantable cardioverter-defibrillators for primary prevention of sudden death in patients with dilated cardiomyopathy with or without acute myocardial infarction,[10,11] so future revisions of these guidelines may offer support for these devices in a wider population. Because of the absence of effective therapies other than implantable cardioverter-defibrillators, the guidelines do not support screening for asymptomatic ventricular arrhythmias with ambulatory electrocardiographic monitoring.

Diastolic Dysfunction

Recommendations for management of patients with HF in the absence of left ventricular systolic dysfunction reflect the lack of conclusive data on effective therapies. The major strategies are control of hypertension, control of ventricular rate in patients with atrial fibrillation, and use of diuretics to control pulmonary congestion (Table 24G-8). Because myocardial ischemia can cause diastolic dysfunction, the guidelines offer support for consideration of use of coronary revascularization in patients with coronary disease (Class IIa indication).

TABLE 24G–8 ACC/AHA Guidelines for Management of Heart Failure and Preserved Systolic Function

Class	Indication	Level of Evidence*
I (indicated)	1. Control of systolic and diastolic hypertension, in accordance with published guidelines	A
	2. Control of ventricular rate in patients with atrial fibrillation	C
	3. Diuretics to control pulmonary congestion and peripheral edema	C
IIa (good supportive evidence)	Coronary revascularization in patients with coronary artery disease in whom symptomatic or demonstrable myocardial ischemia is judged to be having an adverse effect on diastolic function	C
IIb (weak supportive evidence)	1. Restoration of sinus rhythm in patients with atrial fibrillation	C
	2. Use of beta-adrenergic blocking agents, ACE inhibitors, angiotensin-receptor blockers, or calcium antagonists in patients with controlled hypertension to minimize symptoms of heart failure	C
	3. Digitalis to minimize symptoms of heart failure	C
III (not indicated)	None	

ACC = American College of Cardiology; AHA = American Heart Association; ACE = angiotensin-converting enzyme.
*See guidelines text for definition of level of evidence categories.

References

1. Hunt SA, Baker DW, Chin MH, et al: ACC/AHA guidelines for the evaluation and management of chronic heart failure in the adult: A report of the American College of Cardiology/American Heart Association Task Force on Practice Guidelines (Committee to Revise the 1995 Guidelines for the Evaluation and Management of Heart Failure). American College of Cardiology, 2001. (http://www.acc.org/clinical/guidelines/failure/ hf_index.htm)
2. Williams JF Jr, Hlatky MA, Bristow MR, et al: Guidelines for the Evaluation and Management of Heart Failure: Report of the American College of Cardiology/American Heart Association Task Force on Practice Guidelines (Committee on Evaluation and Management of Heart Failure). J Am Coll Cardiol 26:1376-1398, 1996.
3. Konstam M, Dracup K, Baker, D, et al: Heart Failure: Evaluation and Care of Patients with Left-Ventricular Systolic Dysfunction. Clinical Practice Guidelines No. 11. AHCPR Publication No. 94-0612. Rockville, MD, Agency for Health Care Policy and Research and the National Heart, Lung, and Blood Institute; Public Health Service, U.S. Department of Health and Human Services, June 1994.
4. Baughman KL, Dec WB, Uklayam U, et al: HFSA guidelines for management of patients with heart failure caused by left ventricular systolic dysfunction–pharmacological approaches. J Card Fail 5:357-382, 1999.
5. Pina IL, Apstein CS, Balady GJ, et al: Exercise and heart failure: A statement from the American Heart Association Committee on Exercise, Rehabilitation, and Prevention. Circulation 107:1210-1225, 2003.
6. Rathore SS, Wang Y, Krumholz HM: Sex-based differences in the effect of digoxin for the treatment of heart failure. N Engl J Med 347:1403-1411, 2002.
7. Pitt B, Zannad F, Remme WJ, et al: The effect of spironolactone on morbidity and mortality in patients with severe heart failure. Randomized Aldactone Evaluation Study Investigators. N Engl J Med 341:709-717, 1999.
8. Cohn JN, Tognoni G: A randomized trial of the angiotensin receptor blocker valsartan in chronic heart failure. N Engl J Med 345:1667-1675, 2001.
9. Grady KL, Dracup K, Kennedy G, et al: Team management of patients with heart failure: A statement for healthcare professionals from the Cardiovascular Nursing Council of the American Heart Association. Circulation 102:2443-2456, 2000.
10. Moss AJ, Zareba W, Hall WJ, et al: Prophylactic implantation of a defibrillator in patients with myocardial infarction and reduced ejection fraction. N Engl J Med 346:877-883, 2002.
11. Bansch D, Antz M, Boczor S, et al: Primary prevention of sudden death in idiopathic dilated cardiomyopathy: The Cardiomyopathy Trial (CAT). Circulation 105:1453-1458, 2002.

CHAPTER 25

Assisted Circulation in the Treatment of Heart Failure

Yoshifumi Naka • Jonathan M. Chen • Eric A. Rose

Although advanced medical therapy benefits increasing numbers of patients with progressive heart failure (see Chap. 24), the overall survival and quality of life for these patients remains limited. Cardiac transplantation has traditionally represented the only treatment to provide substantial individual benefit in this setting. However, with donor availability limited to only 3000 annually worldwide, the overall impact of transplantation on heart failure has been described as "epidemiologically trivial."[1] Improving the survival and quality of life of patients with end-stage heart disease remains the ultimate goal of mechanical circulatory assistance.

Since their inception in the late 1960s, mechanical circulatory assist devices have evolved substantially, with widespread availability today of intraaortic balloon pumps (IABPs) in even small hospitals, to a broad array of sophisticated univentricular, biventricular, short, long-term, and permanent assist devices accessible at designated specialized centers. With this evolution has developed a better understanding of the technological drawbacks limiting current device design as well as a growing comprehension of appropriate indications for insertion and management. The dream of a completely implantable device, a total artificial heart, or a device whose design specifications allow its use for neonates, infants, and children is not only likely to be attainable but also expected to reach clinical trial and application in the near future.

History

The year 2003 marked the 50th anniversary of the first clinical application of the heart-lung machine, introduced by John Gibbon to repair an atrial septal defect in a young woman.[2] Revolutionizing the field of cardiac surgery, the heart-lung machine quickly had broad application in the treatment of pulmonary embolus, cardiogenic shock, and intracardiac defects by Cooley, Stuckey, and DeBakey and their colleagues.[3-5] DeBakey later modified a concept first reported by Dennis in 1962, using left-heart bypass as a means of support for patients who could not be weaned intraoperatively.[6]

Development of the theory of counterpulsation as an adjunct allowing systolic unloading and diastolic augmentation ultimately resulted in the report by Kantrowitz and coworkers in 1968 of clinical application of IABP counterpulsation.[7] Initiatives from the National Heart, Lung, and Blood Institute (NHLBI) helped to develop a family of mechanical assist devices, later versions of which enjoyed refinement in design, materials, and indications through the 1970s and 1980s. Today, ventricular assist devices (VADs) exist for a wide variety of conditions, requiring the clinician to enunciate clearly the needs of the given patient—does the patient need right-sided support, left-sided support, or both? Is recovery of myocardial function anticipated? Can the patient be sent home safely? Is the patient a transplant candidate? As experience with mechanical assistance has grown, the indications for insertion of the devices have become more specific. Only with continued collaboration between industry and clinical investigators, with preliminary application in patients, will incremental progress in this field be made.

Intraaortic Balloon Counterpulsation

Intraaortic balloon counterpulsation (the IABP) represents one of the most commonly used and widely available methods of mechanical circulatory support, employing the concepts of systolic unloading and diastolic augmentation proposed initially by Moulopolous and associates in 1962.[8] Bregman and Casarella[9] modified these concepts for percutaneous use in 1980, and between 1996 and 2001 more than 22,000 IABPs were inserted worldwide.[10]

The IABP, which is an intravascular, catheter-based device with a balloon volume of 30 to 50 ml, is generally positioned within the thoracic aorta distal to the left subclavian artery and proximal to the renal arteries (Fig. 25–1). The balloon itself may be inserted percutaneously or through direct arterial cannulation from the femoral artery, the axillary artery, or, in cases of postcardiotomy shock, directly through a purse-string suture in the thoracic aorta. When used percutaneously, the balloon may be inserted either through the lumen of a larger sheath (between 8 and 9 French) or alone ("sheathless").

With appropriate synchronization, by arterial blood pressure tracing or electrocardiogram, a set volume of gas (usually helium) is injected into the balloon from a bedside console during cardiac diastole and withdrawn during systole. Balloon inflation thus increases diastolic pressure, thereby augmenting coronary blood flow and myocardial oxygen supply; deflation reduces the afterload component of cardiac work during ventricular contraction and thereby decreases myocardial oxygen consumption. The frequency with which the balloon inflates can be timed to each, every other, or every third cardiac cycle, and balloon support may be adjusted by this method.

Whereas IABP assistance affects the myocardial supply/demand ratio considerably, it has only modest effects on cardiac output, limited naturally to the overall contractility and reserve of the ventricular

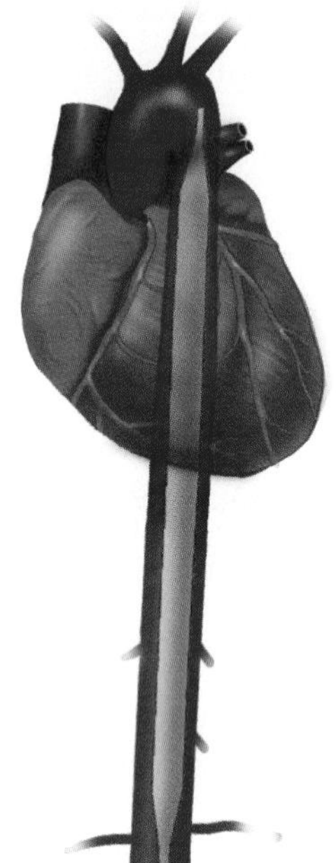

FIGURE 25–1 Schematic representing proper positioning of the intraaortic balloon. (Courtesy of Datascope, Inc.)

TABLE 25–1 Indications for Intraaortic Balloon Counterpulsation

Cardiogenic shock
  Postcardiotomy
  Associated with acute myocardial infarction
  Mechanical complications of myocardial infarction
    Mitral regurgitation
    Ventricular septal defect

In association with coronary artery bypass surgery
  Preoperative insertion
    Patients with severe left ventricular dysfunction
    Patients with intractable ischemic arrhythmias
  Postoperative insertion
    Postcardiotomy cardiogenic shock

In association with nonsurgical revascularization
  Hemodynamically unstable infarct patients
  High-risk coronary angioplasty
    Patients with severe left ventricular dysfunction
    Complex coronary artery disease

Stabilization of cardiac transplant recipient before insertion of ventricular assist device
Postinfarction angina
Ventricular arrhythmias related to ischemia

myocardium. A common misconception is that the institution of IABP counterpulsation should result in an immediate increase in systemic blood pressure; although this event may occur as a net result of the preceding effects, systemic blood pressure is not a parameter by which the efficacy of IABP assistance should be gauged.

Clinical Applications

IABP counterpulsation has traditionally been used in a variety of surgical and nonsurgical patients in the setting of cardiogenic shock and low-output state or unstable angina (Table 25–1). Some have even advocated its use as a bridge to cardiac transplantation, although this strategy has largely been discarded as the waiting time for transplantation has increased substantially. It has been estimated that of the patients who experience cardiogenic shock refractory to medical therapy in the setting of an acute myocardial infarction (AMI), as many as three-quarters may improve with IABP use (see Chap. 47).[11] The goal of IABP application in this setting is to stabilize the patient for either revascularization (catheter based or operative) or insertion of a more durable VAD. For those undergoing insertion intraoperatively as an adjunct to aid in weaning from cardiopulmonary bypass, IABP counterpulsation is used to offset temporary, reversible myocardial dysfunction.

In a cohort of patients undergoing IABP placement for AMI, in-hospital mortality rates varied significantly depending on the indication for insertion. Patients receiving IABP support for refractory angina had 6.4 percent mortality, those receiving IABP support intraoperatively had 7.7 percent mortality, those requiring IABP support to aid in weaning from cardiopulmonary bypass had 25.9 percent mortality, and those receiving IABP support for cardiogenic shock (without percutaneous or operative intervention) had 38.7 percent mortality.[10]

It is estimated that IABP is used in the setting of coronary artery bypass surgery in as many as 5 to 13 percent of cases nationwide, and of the IABP recipients listed in the international registry, 17 percent underwent pump insertion for perioperative indications.[12] Here, preoperative IABP insertion may be especially helpful for those with profound left ventricular dysfunction, and postoperative IABP use may counterbalance the effects of postcardiotomy cardiogenic shock from a variety of causes. Although the efficacy of IABP use in the setting of unstable or postinfarction angina is controversial, generally its use for those with ongoing ischemia, unstable angina, deteriorating hemodynamics, or ischemic ventricular tachyarrhythmias refractory to medical management is well supported.

The use of IABP is absolutely *contraindicated* in the setting of aortic insufficiency and aortic dissection. Relative contraindications for use through a femoral arterial approach are related to the vascular consequences of cannulation: significant aortoiliac or iliofemoral disease and abdominal or descending thoracic aortic aneurysms. In addition, some advocate avoiding the femoral approach in the setting of a recent groin incision at the insertion site or in the setting of morbid obesity, in which transperitoneal cannulation may occur because of anatomical distortion.[13]

INSERTION TECHNIQUE

Before device insertion, accurate examination and documentation of pedal pulses are essential. A balloon should be selected according to the height of the patient. The common femoral artery is then cannulated, a guidewire placed using the Seldinger technique, and a series of dilators placed and withdrawn until either the balloon itself (sheathless) or a larger introducer sheath is finally inserted. In some systems, prior to insertion, the balloon must be purged of any residual air; however, the balloon should not be tested (inflated) before insertion. We have found it easiest to "size" the balloon to the patient by aseptically holding the tip of the balloon above the suprasternal notch and noting the distance to the femoral cannulation site. The balloon is then inserted so that the tip may be seen just below the left subclavian artery (approximately the 2nd or 3rd intercostal space), a location that may be confirmed echocardiographically or on a routine chest radiograph, where the radiopaque tip of the IABP may be seen just at the level of the carina. Counterpulsation should *not* be employed before confirmation of accurate balloon placement.

Alternatively, the balloon may be inserted in the femoral artery or axillary artery using a side-arm graft of polyethylene terephthalate (Dacron) or polytetrafluoroethylene (Gore-Tex) sewn end to side to the artery through which the balloon is passed and secured. At the conclusion of IABP support, the balloon may be withdrawn and the graft closed with a vascular stapler (leaving the artery-graft anastomosis intact). Although more complicated in its approach, this technique maintains the advantage that it reduces impairment to antegrade flow through the artery during and after support and thus minimizes the risk of limb ischemia. The balloon may also be inserted directly through the femoral artery or antegrade through the thoracic aorta through concentric purse-string sutures.

When accurate location has been confirmed, the balloon is connected to the bedside console and synchronized to either the patient's arterial blood pressure tracing or electrocardiogram; in patients with frequent premature contractions, adjusting the timing to arterial blood pressure may be more efficacious. Inflation and deflation must be adjusted assiduously to effect the greatest augmentation. Absolute indications for immediate balloon removal include blood in the gas line leading to the balloon (indicating balloon rupture), inability to adjust the balloon, or ongoing limb ischemia and impending limb threat.

REMOVAL TECHNIQUE

The patient may be weaned slowly from balloon support by adjusting the frequency with which the balloon inflates (e.g., 1 : 1 to 1 : 3). The patient's coagulation profile and platelet count should be normalized with exogenous blood products, if necessary, prior to balloon removal. When hemodynamic stability with minimal support is confirmed, balloon inflation is discontinued and the balloon aspirated of any residual gas. Manual pressure is held on the distal femoral artery, and the balloon and sheath are removed. The proximal femoral artery is allowed to exsanguinate for 2 to 4 seconds to clear any debris, pressure is transferred to the proximal artery, and the distal artery is allowed to purge its debris. Pressure is then applied to the insertion site for at least 30 minutes. Removal under direct vision with potential patch angioplasty is recommended in cases of limb ischemia or in obese patients in whom manual compression may not be adequate.

COMPLICATIONS

The frequency of complications of IABP insertion ranges from 1 to 14 percent (Table 25–2).[10] Over the years, although the overall *rate* of complications has not decreased significantly, the *severity* of complications has diminished. Most of the major morbidities are related to the sequelae of vascular compromise or problems encountered with insertion. The incidence of ischemia has diminished slightly with the advent of smaller introducer sheaths and the development of a sheathless balloon technique. Unfortunately, irreversible limb ischemia resulting from IABP insertion renders most such affected patients poor candidates for later VAD insertion or transplantation and thus represents a condition for which ongoing vigilance in its earlier, potentially reversible, stages is mandatory.

Ventricular Assist Devices

The clinical application of VADs grew from experience with their application in the operating room. Unlike the IABP, VADs function to reduce myocardial work by completely unloading the ventricle while maintaining its output. They may be employed for right ventricular, left ventricular, or biventricular support for short-term (<1 week) or longer term support and for permanent ("destination therapy") use. The device may be completely extracorporeal, paracorporeal, implantable but with percutaneous power support, or totally implantable, and it may provide continuous or pulsatile flow.

BASIC RATIONALE AND TREATMENT GOALS. Hemodynamic eligibility criteria for mechanical cardiac assistance have traditionally been those representative of cardiogenic shock, namely a cardiac index less than 2.0 liter/min/m^2, a systolic blood pressure less than 90 mm Hg, left or right atrial pressures greater than 20 mm Hg, and a systemic vascular resistance greater than 2100 dyne·sec·cm^{-1}.[14] In addition, those with intractable cardiac arrhythmias are considered candidates. The population of patients has expanded from patients in decompensated chronic heart failure to include a large proportion of patients with acute heart failure in cardiogenic shock. Although some reports have demonstrated better outcomes in stable patients awaiting transplantation, favorable results have also been obtained in this emerging population of patients.[15-18]

There are essentially four groups of patients for whom support with different types of VADs is appropriate (Table 25–3). The first group consists of those in whom reversibility of ventricular insult is anticipated, the so-called *bridge-to-recovery* group. Here, patients who may be experiencing postcardiotomy shock despite reasonable preoperative myocardial reserve or who may suffer from a potentially reversible process (e.g., acute myocarditis) benefit from short- to medium-term device support. The management of these patients (even if implantation took place elsewhere) should be continued at a specialized center experienced in weaning. After a short period of myocardial rest with VAD support, the device is weaned at the bedside or in the operating room with guidance from transesophageal echocardiography. Resumption of native myocardial function in this setting may allow device removal (sometimes presaged by myocardial viability as evidenced by positron emission tomography [see Chap. 13]). If hemodynamic decompensation ensues after device removal, a more long-term device or permanent device should be considered.

The second, the *bridge-to-bridge* cohort, consists of patients who experience acute cardiogenic shock, after cardiotomy or without an operation, at a center that does not offer transplantation or long-term assist devices. For these patients, the efficacious institution of short-term assistance and rapid transfer to a center specialized in longer term ventricular assist support are warranted. We have described the success of this strategy, which we call the "hub and spoke" design.[16]

The third group is the traditional *bridge-to-transplantation* cohort, who meet criteria for transplantation and undergo VAD insertion to improve their overall candidacy for transplantation.[17] This decision by necessity limits the cohort to patients younger than 65 years and often involves delineation by blood group; a transplant candidate who is blood type O has a protracted waiting time and thus a lower threshold for device insertion while waiting. Because of concerns regarding infection and the potential need for long-term support, these patients require a more long-term device, preferably implantable, for bridging.

Finally, patients are selected who are *destination therapy* candidates. Several prospective randomized trials including the Randomized Evaluation of Mechanical Assistance for the Treatment of Congestive Heart Failure (REMATCH)[1] and currently the *non*randomized Investigation of Non-Transplant-Eligible Patients who are Inotrope Dependent (INTrEPID) have examined the efficacy of permanent implantable left ventricular assist device (LVAD) insertion for patients who are not transplant candidates (destination therapy).[1] REMATCH demonstrated clear advantages in overall survival and quality of life; INTrEPID is still ongoing. Such long-term expectations, however, challenge the extended durability of

TABLE 25–2 Complications of Intraaortic Balloon Counterpulsation

Minor
Bleeding at the insertion site
Superficial wound infection
Lymphocele
Peritoneal perforation
Major
Limb ischemia requiring thrombectomy, revascularization, or amputation
Aortic dissection
Aortoiliac laceration
Femoral artery pseudoaneurysm
Retroperitoneal hemorrhage
Renal ischemia from malposition
Myocardial ischemia from poor timing of balloon augmentation
Deep wound infection requiring operative débridement

TABLE 25–3 Indications for Ventricular Assist Device Implantation

Intended Use	Therapeutic Goal	Devices	Outcomes		
			Quality of Life	*Short-Term Survival* (days to weeks)	*Long-Term Survival* (months)
Bridge to recovery	Temporary support	IABP	+	++	0
		Centrifugal pump	+	+	0
		ECMO	+	+	0
		Abiomed	+	+	0
		HeartMate	+++	+++	+++
		Novacor	+++	+++	+++
Bridge to bridge	Stabilization to LVAD/BiVAD	Abiomed	+	++	0
		Centrifugal pump	+	+	0
		ECMO	+	+	0
Bridge to transplantation	Support to transplantation	HeartMate	+++	+++	+++
		Novacor	+++	+++	+++
		Thoratec BiVAD	++	++	++
		Abiocor/TAH	++	+	+
		Axial flow pump	+++	++	++
Destination	Permanent support	HeartMate	+++	+++	+++
		Novacor	+++	Undocumented →	
		Abiocor/TAH	+++	Undocumented →	
		LionHeart	+++	Undocumented →	

BiVAD = biventricular assist device; ECMO = extracorporeal membrane oxygenator; IABP = intraaortic balloon pump; LVAD = left ventricular assist device; TAH = total artificial heart.

device design, currently the limiting factor to extended use for this indication. At present, only those who are not transplant candidates are eligible for destination therapy.

Indications for Ventricular Assist Device Support

The indications for VAD insertion are in flux. With further experience, the spectrum of disease for which VADs are implanted continues to expand while our understanding of the timing of implementation and the specific cohorts for which it is appropriate becomes more refined. Broadly speaking, patients in profound shock with end-organ dysfunction and biventricular heart failure need early, efficacious support to avoid permanent end-organ damage and increase their chances of survival. The preferred devices in such a scenario are ones that may provide full ventricular support reestablishing nearly normal hemodynamics and potentially allowing myocardial recovery. If a prolonged support period is expected, a longer term biventricular device may be implanted or, if preferred, a longer term LVAD may be used with concomitant utilization of a short-term right ventricular assist device (RVAD).

POSTCARDIOTOMY SHOCK. Patients undergoing cardiac surgical procedures are at risk for myocardial injury owing to myocardial stunning and ischemia, insufficient myocardial protection, reperfusion injury, and cardiac arrhythmias. These patients may be categorized into two groups: (1) those who had persistent or significant dysfunction prior to surgery (and are unlikely to be weaned from device support) and (2) those who had adequate myocardial reserve prior to surgery (and who may require only a few days of temporary support). In general, for patients who cannot be weaned from cardiopulmonary bypass who maintain otherwise reasonable end-organ function, the best strategy is often the placement of a temporary VAD that may stabilize the patient long enough for transfer to a center with more experience and more choices of long-term devices should the patient be deemed unweanable (*bridge-to-bridge,* see earlier).

Patients undergoing high-risk cardiac surgery may need mechanical ventricular support if the surgical procedure is not successful. Ideally, such patients should be screened for transplant candidacy preoperatively and cardiac surgery scheduled with LVAD back-up in the event that LVAD support and subsequent heart transplantation are needed.

Although postcardiotomy shock represented the indication for which early clinical application of VADs was approved, increasing experience with device support in this population has been discouraging. Conservative estimates at our center support only a 25 percent hospital survival for these patients, refuting the concept of widespread use of VADs for this indication alone.

CARDIOGENIC SHOCK AFTER ACUTE MYOCARDIAL INFARCTION (see also Chap. 47)**.** The survival of patients in cardiogenic shock related to AMI often depends upon the timely institution of circulatory support.[19] Cardiogenic shock is thought to occur when more than 40 percent of ventricular mass is lost to infarction; without some form of cardiac assistance, this condition is associated with 80 percent mortality.[19,20] Even with early revascularization, 1-year survival of these patients remains less than 50 percent.[21] Although it is controversial, it has been our contention that coronary artery bypass grafting (CABG) may be detrimental to those who suffer AMI with cardiogenic shock. Although LVAD support allows myocardial rest, in this setting it is highly unlikely that myocardial recovery sufficient to allow LVAD weaning and explantation would develop. Thus, we advocate early institution of VAD support without CABG for this subset of patients for the reasons described as well as to avoid both another operation involving cardiopulmonary bypass (for the CABG) and additional technical problems of inserting an LVAD with CABG grafts already in place.

DECOMPENSATED CHRONIC HEART FAILURE—TRANSPLANT ELIGIBLE. Because of the increase in waiting times, some patients awaiting cardiac transplantation deteriorate hemodynamically and require increasing doses of intravenous inotropic support. These patients may not have been listed for transplantation at the time of failure, although often they are observed at transplantation centers. Acute decompensation can be triggered by several etiologies, including new ischemic injuries, arrhythmias, and infections. In the absence of an immediately available donor organ, VAD support for this indication allows establishment of hemodynamic stability, improvement in end-organ function, and the opportunity for nutritional support and rehabilitation before transplantation. For these patients, long-term support must be considered.

Some patients are not deemed candidates for transplantation at the time of LVAD implantation for reasons of marginal end-organ function, most commonly renal impairment. For these patients, LVAD support often reverses the injury and allows full recovery of end-organ function, rendering such patients good candidates for transplantation provided that other impaired end-organ function improves as well.

DECOMPENSATED CHRONIC HEART FAILURE—TRANSPLANT INELIGIBLE. Other patients are not candidates for transplantation at the time of LVAD implantation on the basis of age or other absolute criteria. When these patients decompensate, LVAD implantation is performed with the anticipation of permanent use for destination therapy. The precise indications and contraindications for LVAD insertion in this cohort require further study and refinement.

ACUTE MYOCARDITIS AND VENTRICULAR ARRHYTHMIAS. LVAD implantation for acute myocarditis, particularly in young patients, may sometimes be used as a bridge to recovery rather than to transplantation. Unfortunately, it is difficult to determine which patients will benefit from short-term support and which will require long-term devices with subsequent transplantation; thus, we feel that one should prepare for long-term support.[22] We advocate initial insertion of a long-term device to allow expeditious extubation and rehabilitation. After a sufficient degree of rehabilitation has taken place, cardiac function may be evaluated carefully and the device may be explanted if recovery sufficient to sustain reasonable hemodynamics is documented; if no appreciable recovery is demonstrated, the device may be a bridge to transplantation.

Patients with ventricular arrhythmias represent a unique population in that, aside from the arrhythmia, their native cardiac function may not be compromised significantly. If pharmacological therapy and defibrillators have failed, VAD support may be warranted, and it has been successfully implemented in these cases.[23,24] Further, although ventricular decompression often helps to diminish the arrhythmias, if they persist after LVAD insertion, ventricular arrhythmias are generally well tolerated.[25]

Preoperative Risk Assessment

The selection process for VAD implantation must reach a balance between too liberal listing of highest risk patients who have unacceptably high mortality rates and too conservative an approach that overlooks patients who would otherwise have benefited from VAD support. Indeed, judicious use of this resource is essential, as VAD implantation involves a significant social and financial investment.

In 1995 we, in conjunction with investigators from the Cleveland Clinic Foundation, devised a scoring system to predict which patients would have successful outcomes after LVAD implantation.[26,27] This scoring scheme relied upon five clinical factors weighted to determine post-LVAD outcome: urine output, central venous pressure, prothrombin time, the need for mechanical ventilation, and prior median sternotomy. However, as our perioperative management improved, our cohort of potential LVAD patients expanded, and the old score was revised in 2001 to better reflect the current LVAD-eligible population.[28]

The revised score was based on 130 patients receiving vented electric HeartMate devices from 1996 to 2001 (Table 25–4). Interestingly, with the new scoring scale, unlike the old system, preoperative renal insufficiency was not demonstrated to affect survival. After multivariable analysis, the five factors included in the new scoring system are ventilatory support, reoperative surgery, previous LVAD insertion, central venous pressure greater than 16 mm Hg, and prothrombin time greater than 16 seconds. After adding up the scores of these risk factors, a sum greater than five corresponds to 47 percent post-LVAD mortality as opposed to 9 percent mortality for a score less than five.[28]

Perhaps not surprisingly, the urgency of device placement has also been demonstrated to be a factor in survival. In a study by Schmid and colleagues,[15] patients receiving LVADs emergently because of acute heart failure such as AMI, acute myocarditis, and postcardiotomy low-output syndrome had a lower survival to transplantation than those receiving devices for chronic failure or those who did not need devices while awaiting transplantation.[15] In contrast, other data from our institution have suggested that those receiving an LVAD as a bridge to transplantation have a posttransplantation survival comparable to that of patients who did not have an LVAD as a bridge. Clearly, both groups (transplantation with or without prior LVAD) are heterogeneous, and post-transplantation outcome may be in fact best reflective of the relative pretransplantation acuity and comorbidity of the patient (regardless of whether an LVAD bridge was used). Certainly, more data are required to establish the full effect of pretransplantation LVAD support on posttransplantation survival.

CONTRAINDICATIONS. Although the list of contraindications to VAD insertion has diminished substantially in the past decade, several important factors still exist. First, patients with irreversible end-organ failure are poor device candidates. In particular, those with longstanding renal impairment (whose likelihood of improvement with VAD support is small) have prohibitively high morbidity and mortality after VAD insertion because of difficulties in fluid management and the infectious risks of long-term dialysis access. These patients are also unlikely to be candidates for transplantation.

Irreversible neurological injury represents an *absolute* contraindication to VAD insertion. Although this condition may be difficult to assess in the immediate postcardiotomy or acute cardiogenic shock setting, it is important to evaluate prior to VAD insertion (e.g., reduce sedation to help assess even gross neurological function). Because of the very poor outcomes after VAD insertion of patients who experience

TABLE 25–4 Revised Risk Factor Summation Score "LVAD Screening Score"[28]

Variable	Relative Risk	Weight
Mechanical ventilation	5.3	4
Postcardiotomy	3.3	2
Prior LVAD	3.3	2
Central venous pressure >16 mm Hg	2.1	1
Prothrombin time >16 sec	2.1	1
Excluded by multivariable analysis:		
Prior RVAD	3.2	
Coronary artery disease	2.0	
Acute myocardial infarction	1.7	
Urine output <30 ml/hr	1.2	
Reoperative surgery	1.2	

LVAD = left ventricular assist device; RVAD = right ventricular assist device.

severe neurological insults, we aggressively employ a strategy that involves preoperative family consent to discontinue support in the event of catastrophic neurological impairment.[29]

Overwhelming infection and sepsis are also *absolute* contraindications to insertion. Bacteremia may lead to device infection with the potential for device endocarditis, prolonged sepsis, and multiorgan failure and certainly should be treated before LVAD insertion. Once established, however, LVAD infections are often treatable. In a review of our experience with device infection (defined as the presence of a positive culture from the inflow, outflow, diaphragm, pocket, or driveline with leukocytosis or LVAD endocarditis), we demonstrated 15 to 20 percent of patients infected whose survival to transplantation and long-term survival after transplantation were identical to those of noninfected patients.[25,30]

Device Selection

Device selection is invariably influenced by both availability and physicians' experiences. Although much has been published on individual devices, few studies have compared assist devices at a single institution. The Food and Drug Administration (FDA) has approved several assist devices, in addition to the IABP, for these various indications. These devices include (1) the Abiomed biventricular system (BVS) 5000i for postcardiotomy and post-AMI cardiogenic shock; (2) the Thoratec paracorporeal device, the Novacor left ventricular assist system (LVAS), and both the implantable pneumatic (IP) and vented electric (VE) HeartMate LVADs for bridge to transplantation; (3) the HeartMate LVAD for destination therapy; and (4) a variety of investigational implantable devices, including the Arrow LionHeart, the Jarvik, HeartMate II, and MicroMed DeBakey axial flow pumps, and the Cor-Aide centrifugal device for acute cardiogenic shock. In addition to the FDA-approved devices, there are several other VADs in development and clinical use that are discussed later.

Important clinical issues to consider when choosing a device include the expected duration of support, the need for biventricular support, cost, device-related risks (such as the need for anticoagulation and device failure rates), patients' characteristics (especially the size and blood type of the patient), and United Network of Organ Sharing (UNOS) classification rules. Institutional standards of care, ranging from community practice to tertiary heart failure-transplant centers, also influence device selection. With regard to the size of the patient, the implantable HeartMate and Novacor LVADs require the patient's body surface area (BSA) to be greater than 1.5 m^2. Patients whose BSA is less than 1.5 m^2 require support with the Abiomed BVS, a centrifugal pump, the Thoratec paracorporeal device, or other devices in development (see later), depending upon the estimated period of support.

Short-Term Devices

EXTRACORPOREAL CENTRIFUGAL PUMPS. Centrifugal pumps were first introduced as alternatives to roller pumps for cardiopulmonary bypass and have been available since the late 1970s for use as short-term cardiac support. These pumps are widely available, relatively inexpensive, and simple. They may be used for right, left, or biventricular support and require systemic anticoagulation.

One of the most commonly used is the BioMedicus Biopump (Medtronic-BioMedicus, Eden Prairie, MN), which consists of an acrylic pump head with inlet and outlet ports oriented at right angles. An impeller composed of parallel cones is driven by an external motor and, with rotation, creates a vortex that drives blood in proportion to rotational speed. The pump is versatile and may be used as an RVAD (from right atrium or right ventricle to pulmonary artery), as an LVAD (from left atrium or left ventricular apex to aorta), or as part of an extracorporeal membrane oxygenation (ECMO) circuit.

This device has several disadvantages. First, the need for systemic anticoagulation to an activated clotting time of 200 seconds increases the possibility of bleeding complications. Second, there is an appreciable amount of interstitial edema potentially created by increased capillary permeability as part of a systemic inflammatory response. In this setting, fluid management can be extremely difficult, as this device is significantly preload dependent. Finally, the device requires continuous supervision by specially trained personnel, a constraint that can cost as much as $1000 per day.

SHORT-TERM SYSTEMS: EXTRACORPOREAL MEMBRANE OXYGENATION. ECMO provides mechanical cardiac support (univentricular or biventricular) as well as pulmonary support. Although its success has been extensively documented in the neonatal and infant population, the outcomes of its use for adults have been less promising.[31]

The main indications for ECMO are the need for mechanical assistance in the presence of combined pulmonary failure or pure respiratory failure. When it was initially used for postcardiotomy cardiogenic shock, survival was low (25 percent). With experience and improved circuits, survival increased to 40 percent. ECMO's benefits include potential peripheral cannulation and the versatility of small consoles, which together allow potential implementation for both cardiac and pulmonary support in areas outside the operating room. Major limitations, however, include a requirement for sedation or paralysis to effect immobilization and full systemic heparinization. As with the centrifugal pumps (many of which are used in the ECMO circuit), full-time trained personnel are also necessary to manage the ECMO circuit continuously. Complications are common, including leg ischemia, renal failure, bleeding, and oxygenator failure. Overall, the successful use of ECMO in adults has been limited to selected centers.[31]

ABIOMED BVS 5000i. The Abiomed BVS 5000i (Abiomed Cardiovascular, Danvers, MA) is a short-term uni- or biventricular support system composed of external pumps driven by a computer-controlled drive console (Fig. 25–2). Since its initial FDA approval in the setting of postcardiotomy failure, the indications for its use have expanded to include AMI, myocarditis, right ventricular support in conjunction with a long-term left ventricular support device, bridge to recovery, and bridge to transplantation. As a result, the device has become one of the most commonly used means of short-term mechanical cardiac support.[19,32]

The device is an extracorporeal dual-chamber device composed of two 100-ml polyurethane blood sacs, the inlet and outlet portions of which are guarded by polyurethane valves. Although the device fills passively, it ejects blood from a pneumatic drive console that adjusts the duration of systole and diastole to maintain a stroke volume of approximately 80 ml. One advantage of the BVS 5000i system is its weanability; a hand dial on the console allows the device flow to be weaned manually to off. When used in conjunction with transesophageal echocardiography and measures of hemodynamics, this feature allows easy bedside assessment of return of myocardial function.

Other advantages that have made the BVS system popular are ease of insertion and simplicity in operation, obviating the need for a full-time perfusionist at the bedside. The system functions reliably for several days and has even been used as long as 90 days. However, such use commits a patient to systemic anticoagulation for the duration of support. We tend not to use the device for more than 5 to 7 days because if there is no evidence of recovery after this time, we feel its development is unlikely and a more long-term device should be inserted or the support withdrawn. Because of its ease in placement, the 5000i has been particularly helpful in hospitals where there may be a need to transfer the patient to a transplant center for further treatment.[16,32]

Disadvantages of this device include the requirement for continuous anticoagulation, limited mobility compared with implantable devices, and the requirement of intensive care unit (ICU) monitoring and management. Flow rates are also limited compared with those of other devices, with the BVS maximum flow rate of 6 liter/min at times being insufficient to support fully larger or septic patients.

MAJOR CONCERNS FOR LONG-TERM DEVICES. Several key characteristics govern the development of long-term device design and are helpful in considering the advantages and disadvantages of these devices. First, all pulsatile long-term devices require inflow and outflow valves. In some, these are tissue valves; in others, they are mechanical valves and require long-term anticoagulation. The blood contact surface of the device must also be addressed with regard to anticoagulation. To overcome the need for anticoagulation, the HeartMate device employs an innovative textured surface, which ultimately becomes lined with a pseudoneointima less likely to promote thrombus.[33] The disadvantage is that its neointima may also act as an immunologically active entity, which can itself promote a form of autoimmunity and immunological reactivity that limits the ultimate eligibility of its recipients for transplantation.[33-35] Finally, device durability remains a concern for devices expected to function beyond 1 year.[1] The only study to date comparing directly the Novacor and Thoratec HeartMate devices demonstrated these findings; the Novacor patients had a higher rate of neurological disorders despite anticoagulation, and the HeartMate patients demonstrated a higher rate of infectious complications and device malfunction.[36]

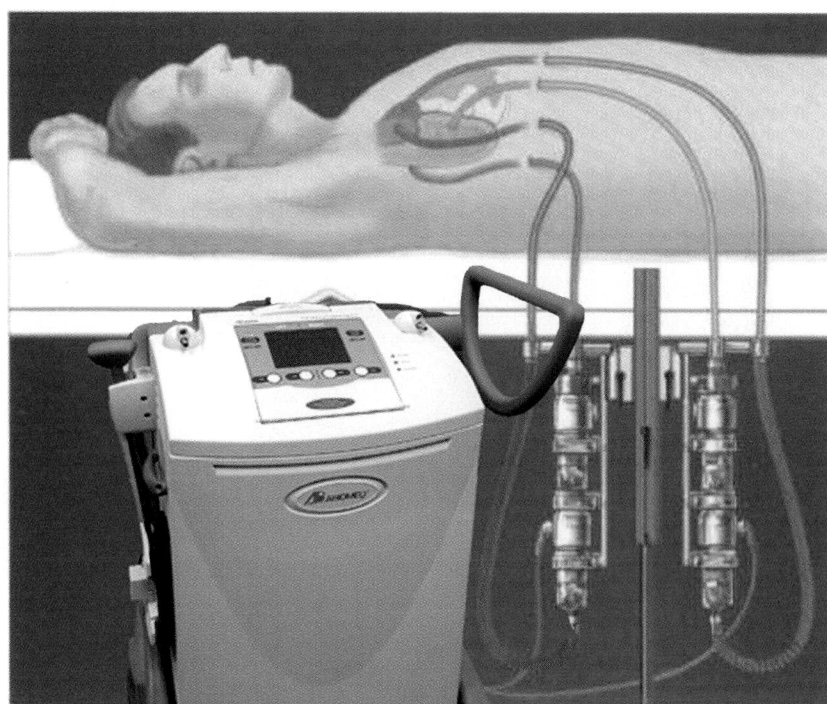

FIGURE 25–2 The Abiomed biventricular system (BVS) 5000i. (Courtesy of Abiomed, Inc.)

Pulsatile Devices

HEARTMATE LEFT VENTRICULAR ASSIST DEVICE (IMPLANTABLE). The HeartMate LVAD (Thoratec Corporation, Pleasanton, CA) was designed in 1975 (Fig. 25–3). The system was originally a pneumatic vented (IP) system requiring a large console that limited patients' mobility outside the hospital. In 1991, a clinical trial of the VE model was begun that allowed greater mobility, with portable battery units worn in a holster.[37] Since then, both models have been associated with a 60 to 70 percent rate of survival to transplantation.[38,39] The worldwide average implant duration is 80 to 100 days, and maximum duration of support has exceeded 2 years. However, of note, in the REMATCH trial, the probability of device failure was demonstrated to be 35 percent at 2 years.[1]

The HeartMate has a titanium alloy external housing, with inflow and outflow conduits that utilize porcine xenograft valves (25 mm). The unique characteristic of the device is its internal blood contact surface, which is made of textured titanium on one side and textured polyurethane on the other (Fig. 25–4). This textured surface results in the deposition of a fibrin-cellular matrix that forms a pseudoneointima. The formation of this surface decreases the need for anticoagulation, as thrombus formation is greatly reduced. Patients with these devices take aspirin (for antiinflammation but not primarily for anticoagulation) with a remarkably low rate of thromboembolic complications and without the need for warfarin (Coumadin).

The device has a pumping capacity in excess of 9 liter/min, a maximal stroke volume of 83 ml, and pulsatile flow is created using a pusher-plate system. The device is operated in either a fixed-rate or automatic mode; in automatic mode, the pump senses when the chamber is full and activates the pusher plate. The pump is inserted into the left upper quadrant of the abdomen either pre- or intraperitoneally. The driveline, consisting of an air vent and power cables, is tunneled subcutaneously and brought out of the skin in the right upper quadrant. Small battery units, worn in a harness, are connected to the cables; battery life is between 4 and 6 hours, depending on the patient's activity level. In case of an

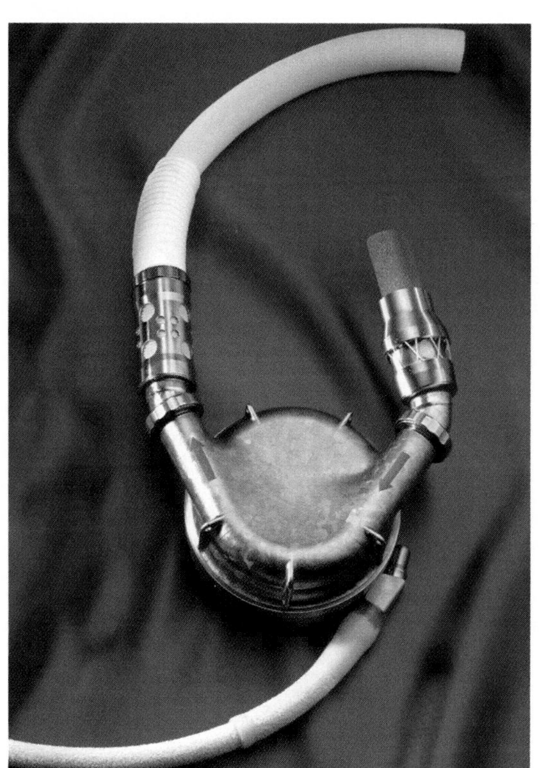

FIGURE 25–3 The HeartMate left ventricular assist device. (Courtesy of Thoratec, Inc.)

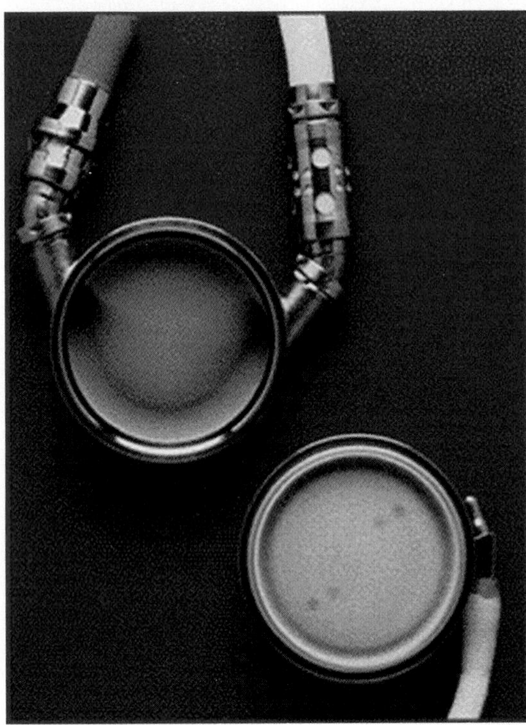

FIGURE 25–4 The inside surface of the HeartMate left ventricular assist device. (Courtesy of Thoratec, Inc.)

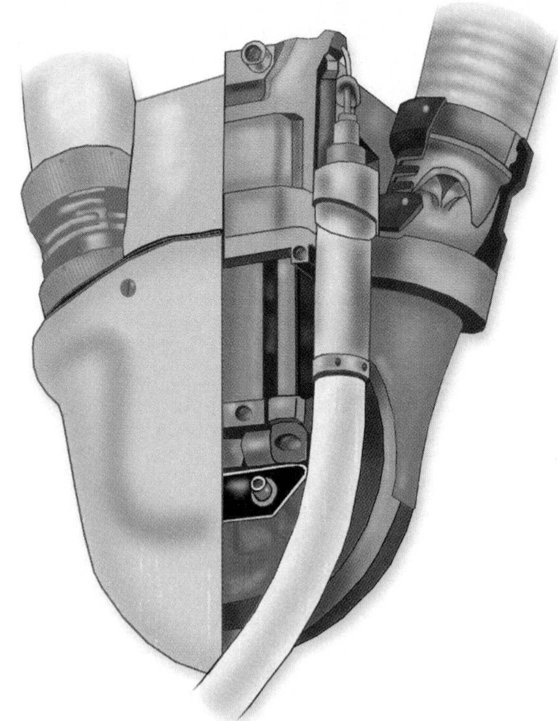

FIGURE 25–5 The Novacor left ventricular assist device. (Courtesy of World Heart Corporation.)

emergency, a portable hand pump can be used to activate the device.

The patient's body size is an important factor in allowing device placement. Because of the size of the device and flow limitations to avoid thromboembolic complications caused by blood stagnation, patients are required to have a BSA greater than 1.5 m^2 for successful implantation.

NOVACOR (IMPLANTABLE). The Novacor (World Heart Corporation, Ottawa, Ontario, Canada) LVAS was first successfully used in 1984 as a bridge to transplantation (Fig. 25–5). Initially, it was designed as a console-based controller system, but since 1993 it has been available with a wearable controller. This system has proved to be reliable, with about 55 to 65 percent of patients surviving to transplantation.[40] The worldwide mean time of LVAS support using this system is 85 days, with the device lasting as long as 962 days.[40]

The device is similar to the overall design of the HeartMate. The pump works using dual pusher plates that compress a polyurethane sac. Twenty-five millimeter bioprosthetic valves are used in both the inflow and outflow tracts. As with the HeartMate device, the pump is placed in the left upper abdominal quadrant, the inflow tract connected to the left ventricular apex and the outflow tract to the ascending aorta. The percutaneous driveline is brought out in the right upper quadrant of the abdomen and connected to a controller worn on a belt system.

However, unlike patients with the HeartMate system, those with the Novacor LVAS require anticoagulation with warfarin to avoid embolic events. The prevalence of embolic cerebrovascular events is estimated as between 27 and 41 percent.[40,41] However, comparison of the HeartMate and Novacor devices in this realm is particularly difficult owing to variation in the definition of "embolism" utilized in the literature.[41] A new inflow cannula made with Gore-Tex was introduced with the hope that it will reduce the rate of cerebrovascular events. Preliminary reports suggest that the Vascutek inflow conduit reduced embolic events to 12 percent.[42]

PARACORPOREAL PULSATILE DEVICES: THORATEC. The Thoratec paracorporeal VAD (Thoratec Corporation, Pleasanton, CA) is a commonly used system for biventricular support (Fig. 25–6). Unlike the Novacor and HeartMate, it is a paracorporeal system that can be applied for univentricular or biventricular support. Because the actual pump chamber is outside the body, this device can be used on patients with body sizes too small to house the HeartMate or Novacor devices (i.e., <1.5 m^2). However, a paracorporeal system also limits mobility and thus presents an obstacle for patients in a long-term setting.

The pump consists of a prosthetic ventricle with a maximum stroke volume of 65 ml and cannulas for ventricular or atrial inflow and arterial outflow. Currently, a large pneumatic drive console is available and a smaller briefcase-sized power driver unit is in trial.[43] Pneumatic drivers provide alternating air pressure to fill and empty the blood pump, and the pump flow rate ranges from 1.3 to 7.2 liter/min. Although inflow cannula placement can occur in either an atrial or ventricular position, ventricular cannula placement is preferred for left-sided support as it allows greater flow rates than does atrial cannulation. Anticoagulation with warfarin is necessary, as in patients with mechanical valves.[43]

This device has been used in more than 1000 patients for uni- and biventricular support for both bridge to transplantation and postcardiotomy recovery. Survival to transplantation has been between 60 and 80 percent, depending upon which ventricle was supported.[43] As with the BVS 5000i, the biggest advantage of this system is its versatility; it is easy to place with less surgical dissection, can be used for patients of various sizes, can be attached to either the atrium or ventricle, and can be used for right- and left-heart support. However, its paracorporeal location potentially limits the patient's activity and thus its use as a permanent device.

THORATEC INTRACORPOREAL VENTRICULAR ASSIST DEVICE. The Thoratec intracorporeal VAD (Thoratec Corporation, Pleasanton, CA) is being designed by the same firm that developed the paracorporeal device and clinical trials are currently anticipated. The intracorporeal

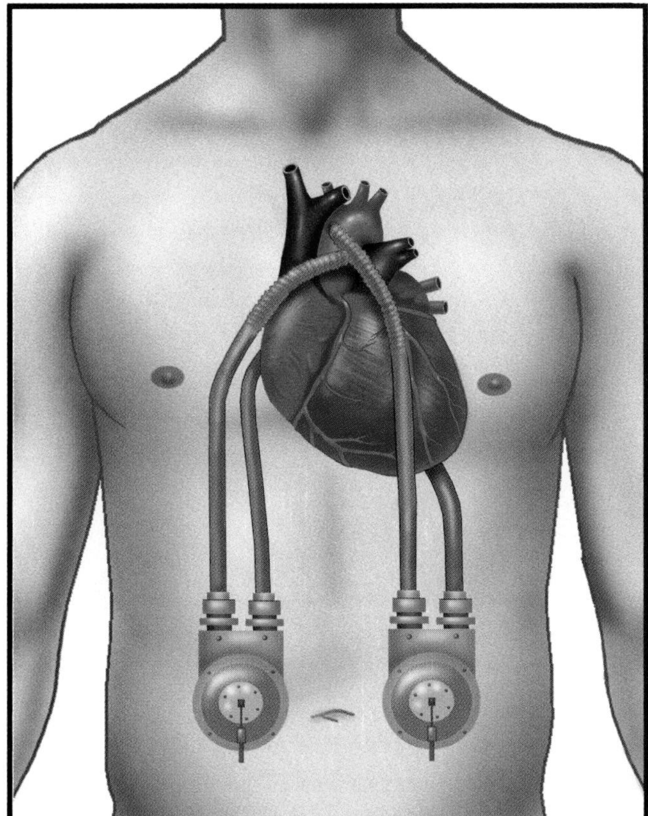

FIGURE 25–6 The Thoratec paracorporeal ventricular assist device. (Courtesy of Thoratec, Inc.)

system is the same size as the external system but is encased in a titanium alloy housing, and its pumps will be placed intracorporeally (not paracorporeally); two drivelines still exit the skin. The advantages of this system are its small size; reliability; implantable right, left, and biventricular support; and technology similar to that of the currently used Thoratec system. It is targeted toward patients who would benefit from long-term support and the benefits of an implanted device.

Total Artificial Heart

CARDIOWEST TOTAL ARTIFICIAL HEART. The CardioWest total artificial heart (TAH) (Syncardia, Tucson, AZ) began as the Jarvik-7 TAH used in the 1980s and is a pneumatic, biventricular, orthotopically implanted TAH with an externalized driveline to its console.[17,44,45] It consists of two spherical polyurethane chambers with polyurethane diaphragms. Inflow and outflow conduits are constructed of Dacron and contain Medtronic Hall (Medtronic, Minneapolis, MN) valves. Despite early obstacles, a new investigational device exemption study began in 1993 and demonstrated support durations of 12 to 186 days with a 93 percent survival to transplantation.[44]

The TAH benefits from the ability to provide complete support and, unlike the other devices, it obviates the presence of the native heart. This is particularly useful in situations in which leaving the native heart in place would be detrimental or impossible (e.g., cardiac tumors).

However, adequate intrathoracic space is required to accommodate the TAH. Fitting criteria include BSA greater than 1.7 m^2, cardiothoracic ratio greater than 0.5, LV diastolic dimension greater than 66 mm, anterior-posterior distance greater than 10 cm, and combined ventricular volume greater than 1500 ml. Careful intraoperative fitting is critical. In addition to size requirements, strict anticoagulation with warfarin, aspirin, and pentoxifylline is needed. As with the Thoratec paracorporeal system, rehabilitation and hospital discharge are unfortunately limited because of the current design of the large console.

ABIOCOR. The AbioCor TAH (Abiomed Cardiovascular, Danvers, MA) consists of an internal thoracic pump, an internal rechargeable battery, internal electronics, and an external battery pack (Fig. 25–7). External power is delivered through a transcutaneous energy transmission coil located under the skin of the chest wall. The AbioCor TAH is an electrohydraulically actuated device implanted in the pericardial space after excision of the native heart. The pump chambers are sutured to atrial tissue and the great vessels by textured Dacron (E.I. du Pont de Nemours, Wilmington, DE) atrial cuffs and grafts. Two polyurethane blood pump chambers with a 60-ml stroke volume produce flow at 8 liter/min. A centrifugal pump moves hydraulic fluid between the ventricles, providing alternate left and right ventricular pulsatile flow. In addition, there is an atrial "balance chamber" that adjusts for left and right atrial pressures. Anticoagulation is maintained with warfarin and clopidogrel.

After extensive animal testing starting in 1998 at the University of Louisville and the Texas Heart Institute, the device received FDA approval for a multicenter limited human testing trial involving patients requiring total heart support who did not qualify for heart transplantation. As of May 2003, 11 patients have been enrolled in the AbioCor clinical trial; 2 patients died in the immediate perioperative period, and 9 survived from 53 to 512 days, with an average support of 5 months. Four patients experienced neurological events significant enough to lead to withdrawal of support. Two patients are currently alive and remain hospitalized.

Axial Flow Pumps

Axial flow pumps represent one of the newest generations of assist devices. They can provide full cardiac support in a much smaller pump with fewer moving parts and a smaller blood contact surface than pusher-plate devices. Their small size allows implantation into smaller patients than most pulsatile pumps and also makes placement and explantation easier. With fewer moving parts, there are fewer points of

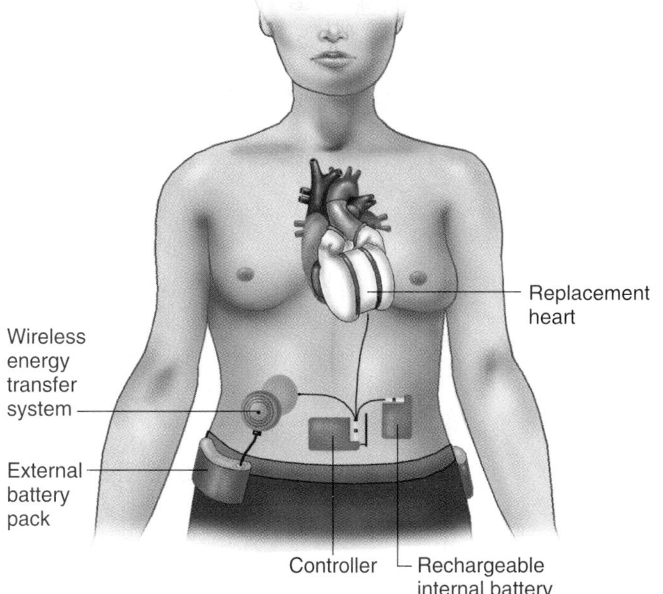

FIGURE 25–7 The AbioCor total artificial heart. (Courtesy of Abiomed, Inc.)

friction; therefore, expected durability is increased. In addition, because of their small size, these pumps represent the most likely candidates for development as pediatric assist devices in the near future. However, the bearings of these devices are lubricated with blood, a characteristic that may ultimately limit durability. In addition, shear rates with resultant hemolysis remain a concern.

In addition to their small size, axial flow pumps are notable for nonpulsatile flow. Metabolic and neurohumoral changes in organ perfusion with nonpulsatile flow have been demonstrated.[46-50] However, both clinical and long-term animal studies have failed to demonstrate significant differences in morbidity and mortality with axial flow pumps (Figs. 25–8 and 25–9).[51,52] Also, many patients maintain some native cardiac function during axial pump support and therefore continue to have pulsatile patterns of blood flow, unlike the situation with many of the pumps previously described (which completely unload the ventricle). Conversely, in the event of a device failure, few options or back-up mechanisms exist for axial flow pumps other than replacement, and because these pumps lack valves, if device malfunction does occur, the patient experiences hemodynamic perturbations equivalent to those seen with severe aortic insufficiency.

Finally, most axial flow pumps generate such negative pressure continuously that there is a potential risk of collapsing the ventricle and causing transient pump cessation (and therefore thrombus formation) and air entrainment (and therefore air emboli). To counteract this, many have device inflow cannulas that have a long tract to stent open the middle of the ventricle and allow more reliable continuous flow throughout the cardiac cycle.[53] Because of this phenomenon, both ventricular preload and cannula placement are of paramount importance with these pumps.

MICROMED DEBAKEY VENTRICULAR ASSIST DEVICE. This pump unit is 1.2 inches in diameter, 3 inches long, and weighs 95 gm (see Fig. 25–8). It is made of titanium casing with an impeller-inducer capable of pumping 10 liter/min. The rest of the pump consists of a titanium inflow cannula, a flowmeter, a Dacron outflow graft (Sulzer, Austin, TX), and a percutaneous cable connecting to a wearable battery-control console.[54] The inflow cannula is inserted into the left ventricular apex, the pump is placed into a small abdominal pocket, and the outflow graft is anastomosed to the ascending or descending aorta. Patients require chronic anticoagulation with warfarin and an antiplatelet agent.[54] A pump index greater than 2.0 to 2.5 liter/min/m^2 is recommended and the pump is started at 7500 rpm and adjusted for an average pump flow of 3.9 to 5.4 liter/min; flow is preload dependent. This pump also has a flow probe on its outflow graft that allows continuous flow monitoring, enabling pump speed adjustment as well as detection of extreme suction (and thus ventricular collapse). The major complication of this device in European clinical trials was late bleeding probably related to the level of anticoagulation (which has since been decreased to a target International Normalized Ratio [INR] of 2.0 to 2.5).[55] Follow-up of patients with the device has demonstrated improved exercise tolerance and the ability to be discharged home with the device while awaiting transplantation.[56]

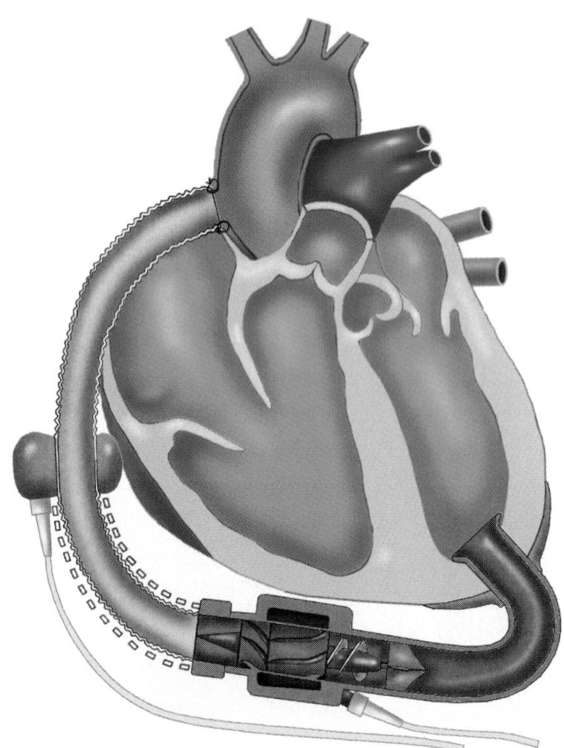

FIGURE 25–8 The MicroMed DeBakey axial flow pump. (Courtesy of Micromed, Inc.)

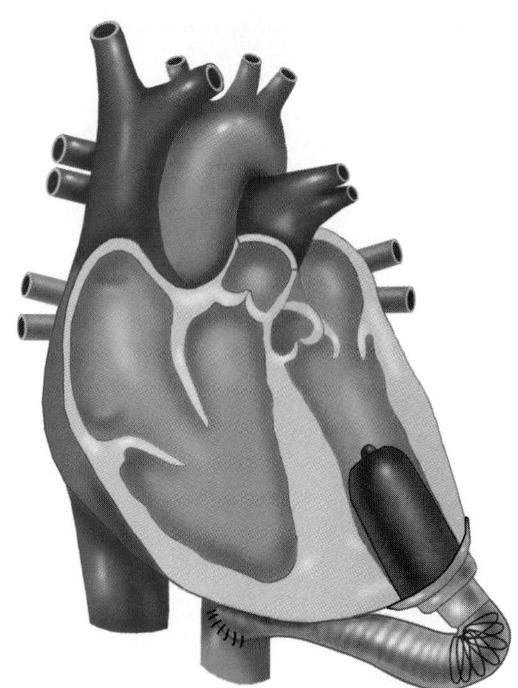

FIGURE 25–9 The Jarvik 2000 axial flow pump. (Courtesy of THI.)

HEARTMATE II. This is an axial flow rotary LVAD made of titanium with a rotor capable of producing flow rates greater than 10 liter/min at speeds greater than 10,000 rpm. As with the DeBakey VAD, the inflow cannula is joined to the apex of the left ventricle with the outflow graft connected to the ascending aorta.[53] Anticoagulation is at present required to keep the INR between 1.5 and 2.5. The pump has a volume of 124 ml and is inserted preperitoneally or within the abdominal musculature. Power and control are supplied by a percutaneous lead that attaches to either a power base unit or portable rechargeable batteries. This system similarly may be operated in either manual or automatic mode.

JARVIK 2000. The titanium Jarvik 2000 pump measures 2.5 cm in diameter, displaces 25 ml, and weighs 90 gm (see Fig. 25–9).[57] The rotor includes titanium impeller blades and is held in place by two ceramic bearings. The impeller rotates at 8000 to 12,000 rpm, producing a flow rate of 7 liter/min. Unlike the DeBakey VAD or the HeartMate II, this pump is positioned inside the ventricle with the outflow graft anastomosed to the descending aorta. The pump can operate in either a fixed-rate or variable mode and has manual rate adjustment capabilities. Two different control and energy systems are currently available: (1) a percutaneous model that, like most other LVAD systems, has a power lead that exits the patient's skin and (2) a modified percutaneous system that uses a titanium pedestal screwed into the skull with a transcutaneous connector that attaches to an external cable (for more permanent use). The fixed skull implantation is thought to provide a low level of repeated trauma and minimize the risk of infection owing to high vascularity of the scalp.

Unlike the other systems, which require a sternotomy, the Jarvik 2000 is implanted through a left thoracotomy incision. The pump is mainly used as a partial decompression device, allowing the aortic valve to open. However, if full decompression is achieved (and the aortic valve remains closed), because the outflow graft is anastomosed to the descending aorta, thrombus can form in areas of stagnation in the ascending aorta more proximally. Similarly to other systems, the pump provides a low pulsatile flow with a narrowing of pulse pressure at higher speeds.[57]

Totally Implantable Pulsatile Devices

ARROW LIONHEART LVD-2000. The Arrow LionHeart LVD-2000 is the first system designed specifically with destination support in mind.[58] It is a completely implantable system with a transcutaneous energy transmission system and a compliance chamber that allows complete implantation with no percutaneous lines or connections (Fig. 25–10). The pump is made of a titanium casing with pumping activated by a pusher plate. Unidirectional blood flow is maintained by two Derlin disc monostrut valves (27-mm inlet; 25-mm outlet). The inflow and outflow tracts are positioned in the ventricular apex and aorta, respectively. Maximum pump flow is 8 liter/min with a stroke volume of 64 ml. The controller is housed in a titanium casing, which also houses rechargeable batteries. The compliance chamber consists of a circular polymer sac (placed in the pleural space) and an attached subcutaneous port infusion system (this chamber loses gas through the polymer and requires replenishment once a month).[58] Recharging of the battery is accomplished through a transcutaneous system with a wand overlying the recharging coil. Patients may be completely disconnected from the external power supply for a short period of time and during that time rely on internal back-up batteries. The internal coil must be positioned under the skin so as to allow no more than 1 cm of tissue thickness between the coil and skin surface.[58]

NOVACOR II. Novacor II (World Heart Corporation, Ottawa, ON, Canada) is a totally implantable pump for the definitive treatment of heart failure. Its unique dual-chamber, four-valve pump requires no volume compensator. The pusher plate is suspended and magnetically driven, thus providing a system with few moving parts (the magnetic drive obviates the need for bearings, cams, or linkages).[59] The two chambers fill alternately, creating pulsatile flow. The system also uses transcutaneous energy transfer technology to supply power. It is currently in preclinical testing.[59]

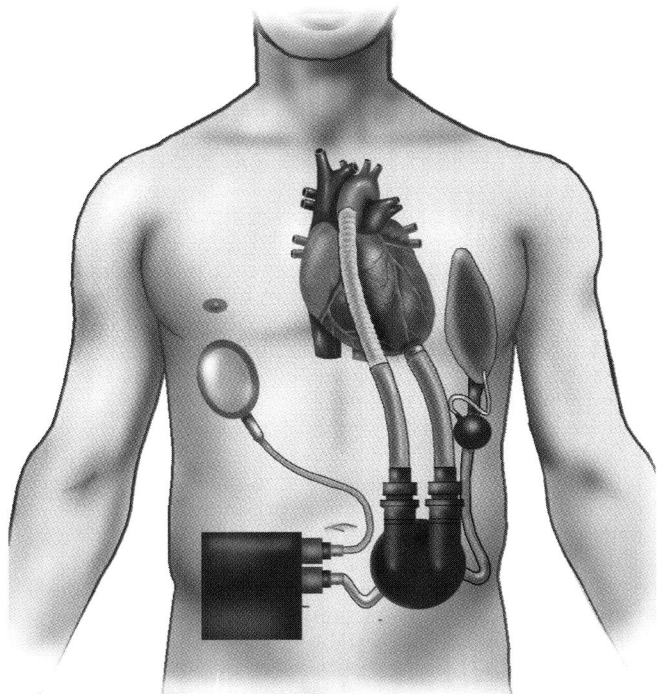

FIGURE 25–10 The Arrow LionHeart implantable left ventricular assist device. (Courtesy of Arrow, Inc.)

Postoperative Management

EARLY POSTOPERATIVE PERIOD. Several factors are important in the postoperative management of patients with mechanical support. Antibiotic prophylaxis is started preoperatively and continues for at least 3 days after implantation. Right-sided heart failure is immediately or prophylactically treated with milrinone and inhaled nitric oxide.[60] In addition, vasodilatory hypotension is treated with intravenous arginine vasopressin.[61] Aprotinin is continued in the postoperative period until bleeding has stopped.[62] Arrhythmias are managed with appropriate pharmacological agents and cardioversion if necessary. Aspirin is used for patients with all devices. Anticoagulation with heparin and, subsequently, warfarin is used in all patients except those receiving the HeartMate device. Physical therapy and nutrition are addressed early.

LATE POSTOPERATIVE PERIOD. Late postoperative care focuses on rehabilitation and monitoring of the immunological changes induced by the LVAD during the wait for heart transplantation.[63] Patients with the vented electric Thoratec LVAD and the Novacor LVAD are eligible for discharge home while awaiting transplantation. General criteria for discharge include physical rehabilitation, echocardiographic evidence of marginal heart function (to keep the patient alive in cases of device failure), and a training course in use and care of the device. Support from the family is very important. When these criteria are met, patients undergo a gradual program with longer trips outside the hospital and final discharge with weekly follow-up visits.[64] Panel-reactive antibody levels are measured in patients with LVADs biweekly to monitor immunological sensitization during device support.

LEFT VENTRICULAR ASSIST DEVICE EXPLANT VERSUS TRANSPLANT. The profound ventricular unloading provided by LVAD support can lead to reverse remodeling evident at genetic, biochemical, and histological levels.[65,66] Long-term LVAD explantation is considered at our institution only if there is significant myocardial recovery as evidenced by improvement of parameters on an exercise testing protocol. LVAD flow is reduced to 2 liter/min as the patient exercises on a treadmill, and right-heart catheterization and echocardiography are performed to determine the adequacy of ventricular function.[67] Although functional recovery allowing LVAD explantation has been reported, our experience has demonstrated that only a minority of patients can be successfully weaned from their devices.[48,68-70] The question of which patients are suitable for bridge to recovery and device explantation requires further clinical evaluation.

COMPLICATIONS AND ADVERSE EVENTS

BLEEDING. Bleeding is a major complication after implantation of LVADs and can occur both in the immediate perioperative period and later postoperatively. Immediate postoperative bleeding occurs in 20 to 40 percent of patients who receive assist devices. Preoperative heart failure leading to hepatic dysfunction, preoperative anticoagulation, coagulopathy caused by blood-device surface interaction, extensive surgical dissection, and prolonged cardiopulmonary bypass time all contribute to higher rates of bleeding after device implantation. In the immediate postoperative period, coagulation parameters as well as complete blood counts must be monitored closely, and deficiencies in platelet count and coagulation factors must be replaced as necessary. Because excessive transfusion of blood products can cause volume overload and subsequently exacerbate right-sided heart failure, care must be taken to avoid unnecessary transfusion. Although meticulous surgical technique is the mainstay of hemostasis, several medications can be used to prevent postoperative bleeding.

It is well established that aprotinin reduces blood loss and blood use in patients receiving assist devices.[62] Desmopressin (DDAVP) may also be used as an adjunct for uremic patients or those taking aspirin. Reexploration for bleeding should be performed in a timely fashion if needed. However, if excessive bleeding is noted at the time of chest closure, the chest may be left open and packed and the patient taken to the ICU, stabilized, and the chest closed when coagulation is normalized.

Bleeding can also occur late postoperatively. All devices except the HeartMate require heparin and subsequently warfarin to achieve an INR of 2.5 to 3.5 postoperatively. Aspirin is added to this regimen as an anti-inflammatory agent in all cases. Care must be taken to maintain adequate levels of anticoagulation. Because LVADs can activate both coagulation and fibrinolytic pathways, there is potential to exacerbate either bleeding or thrombotic complications even late postoperatively.[33] Therefore, clinical signs of late bleeding need to be carefully monitored in those patients.

INFECTION. Infection is one of the most serious complications common after LVAD implantation, affecting short- and long-term survival for patients receiving mechanical circulatory support. Although the definition of device-related infection varies among publications, LVAD infection, in general, can be manifest as driveline, pocket, or bloodstream infections or, ultimately, as device endocarditis.[30] In addition to device-related infections, these patients are susceptible to the common infections seen in critically ill patients such as pneumonia, line sepsis (with multiple catheters and intravenous lines), and urinary tract infections. For these reasons, it is sometimes difficult to identify the source of infection when a patient with LVAD support has positive blood cultures.

The reported infection rates in these patients are from 12 to 55 percent.[30,49] Pocket infection rates have been reported to be 11 to 24 percent for the HeartMate and Novacor systems; the driveline infection rate is even higher and in the range of 18 to 30 percent for the two devices.[30] Again, there is much variability in these data because definitions for these infections have not been standardized. Sepsis accounts for 21 to 25 percent of LVAD deaths and occurs at a rate of 11 to 26 percent.[30]

A variety of microorganisms are responsible for VAD infections. Gram-positive cocci are most commonly seen, but gram-negative bacilli and fungi can be identified. If organisms are identified, timely and appropriate systemic and topical management of infection is necessary. Infection itself is not a contraindication to transplantation in this population, and transplantations have been accomplished successfully in infected patients.[49,50] Topical treatments of driveline infections include immobilization of the exit site, local sterilization, drainage, and, if necessary, surgical débridement. Appropriate drainage of the cavity is needed for an LVAD pocket infection. Device endocarditis can be treated with systemic antibiotics as well as emergent heart transplantation, device explantation, or device replacement.[30]

The interaction between device and human that occurs after VAD implantation is a topic of much interest and is discussed later. LVAD implantation is accompanied by progressive defects in cellular immunity caused by an aberrant state of T-cell activation and apoptosis. These defects together predispose LVAD patients toward susceptibility to infections.[34,35]

THROMBOEMBOLIC EVENTS. Thromboembolism is a major concern in any patient with mechanical circulatory support because of the blood-device interface. The prevalence of embolism varies from 2 to 47 percent, with the majority of events occurring in cerebral distribution in 25 percent, although the definition of embolism varies among publications.[71,72] The HeartMate has the lowest thromboembolic rate of all the devices despite the fact that these patients do not receive warfarin (probably because of the device's promotion of formation of a neointimal surface that reduces thrombus formation).[73] All other devices require heparin in the immediate postoperative period and, subsequently, warfarin as well as antiplatelet agents such as aspirin or clopidogrel.

DEVICE FAILURE. Device failure is also a major concern because the number of heart transplantations is declining and, according to a new UNOS rule, the status of patients awaiting heart transplantation who receive mechanical assist devices changes from 1A to 1B after 30 days of implantation.

Device failure involves a variety of events, although the definition and therefore the reported event rate also vary among publications. Major failures, such as disconnection of the outflow assembly from the pump body or pump diaphragm rupture, require emergent device replacement.[55] Minor failures, such as controller or battery malfunction, usually do not require emergency surgery but do require appropriate treatment such as replacement of controllers.[74]

The HeartMate IP and VE devices are reported to have a failure rate of approximately 10 percent, including major and minor failures.[38,55] Of note, although no system failed within 12 months of implantation, the probability of device failure was 35 percent at 24 months in the REMATCH trial, in which the device was used as destination therapy. However, modifications of the system are aimed at reducing this incidence substantially.[55]

For example, repeated pulsatile flow, especially in the setting of significant afterload (hypertension), can lead to inflow valve damage and regurgitation. Modifications in valve mounting and flow algorithms to reduce intracavitary pressures have been adopted and, it is hoped, will have a significant impact on long-term device durability. In the event of electronic failure, the HeartMate device can be operated by a pneumatic console, and the overall reported survival rate to heart transplantation with the HeartMate is comparable (72 percent) to that of other devices even when back-up components are used.[55]

According to publications in 1999 and 2000, the Novacor LVAS has better durability than the HeartMate, with a failure rate between 0 and 2 percent and devices replaced after 3 to 4 years of support.[36,40] The main failure mode is bearing wear, which can be monitored periodically in vivo. If signs of wear are detected, the patient can be upgraded to UNOS status 1A or device replacement can be scheduled on a nonemergency basis. The Thoratec paracorporeal device is reported to have a lower incidence (3.5 percent) of major failures.[74]

RIGHT-SIDED HEART FAILURE. This complication is reported in 10 to 30 percent of patients who received either HeartMate or Novacor implantable LVADs, and an RVAD was used in 1 to 11 percent of all cases.[55,60,75] In patients with Thoratec paracorporeal devices, the incidence of RVAD use was as high as 38 to 42 percent.[71,74] However, this difference may be related to differences in device selection criteria and device availability among institutions. We reviewed our institutional experience in this area and demonstrated no difference in posttransplantation survival between those who received an RVAD as a bridge and those who did not. Of interest, however, was the fact that there was a significant survival advantage for those who received their RVAD within 24 hours after LVAD insertion compared with those who received it after 24 hours.

In patients with end-stage heart failure, pulmonary vascular resistance is usually elevated because of longstanding left-sided heart failure and is further increased in the early postoperative period by the effects of cardiopulmonary bypass and extensive blood product transfusion.[76] These factors, individually or in combination, can lead to impaired RV contractility, increased RV afterload, and subsequent RV dysfunction.[60] In most cases, unloading and supporting the LV help to reduce pulmonary vascular resistance and improve RV performance. However, it must be noted that complete LV decompression can also reduce the septal contribution to RV function by causing the interventricular septum to bulge toward the left.[77] In this setting, RV contractility may be impaired further by the enhanced preload to the RV from the superlative LVAD output. Interestingly, two independent analyses elucidated low preoperative RV stroke work index and low preoperative mean pulmonary artery pressure as risk factors for either postoperative development of right-sided heart failure or postoperative use of an RVAD, indicating that, in this setting, the failing RV may be unable to generate high pulmonary artery pressures (making the pulmonary artery pressures appear fictitiously low).[60,75]

Because the perioperative use of blood transfusions can contribute to right-sided heart failure, the intraoperative use of aprotinin is strongly recommended.[62] Perioperatively, if there is any indication of right-sided heart failure, such as increased central venous pressure or decreased LVAD flow with appropriate LV decompression and without tamponade, treatment of right-sided heart failure must be initiated immediately with pulmonary vasodilators (inhaled nitric oxide) and inotropic agents to enhance RV contractility.[60] If the RV function does not improve and the LVAD flow still remains suboptimal (<2.4 liter/min/m^2 with central venous pressure >16 mm Hg), RVAD insertion may be required.

MULTISYSTEM ORGAN FAILURE. Multisystem organ failure is another frequent complication in the LVAD population. Because of the significant amount of preoperative end-organ dysfunction and the number of comorbid conditions, some patients with LVADs do not recover fully after device implantation. In many situations, multiple organ failure is the end result of a long cascade of complications including sepsis, bleeding, and other events. At other times, multisystem organ failure may be the result of significant preoperative multiorgan dysfunction that deteriorates after the insult of surgery. In all of these scenarios, multisystem organ failure accounts for 11 to 29 percent of deaths with the device.

IMMUNOLOGICAL PERTURBATION. Itescu and colleagues at out institution have extensively analyzed the immunological interaction of patients with the HeartMate LVAD and demonstrated several important findings.[34,35] First significant T-cell activation was noted, both on the LVAD surface and in the circulation, albeit with defective proliferative responses to stimulation. Second, the circulating T cells demonstrated susceptibility to activation-induced cell death after T-cell receptor engagement. Third, the LVAD recipients demonstrated significant B-cell hyperreactivity. Together, it is thought that these phenomena are responsible for both (1) a progressive defect in cellular immunity (and thus produce an increased risk of infection) and (2) an increased rate of allosensitization.[34]

Few comparable studies have been performed with recipients of other types of devices. Immunological evaluation of the patient-device interaction with the DeBakey axial flow pump (which does not promote a neointimal layer) demonstrated an initial finding of increased markers of apoptosis. However, these markers declined to normal levels after 7 weeks and did not appear to confer an increased risk of infection in this cohort. Clearly, more data are necessary to evaluate these effects fully and to determine whether such findings may be attributable specifically to these devices.

SENSITIZATION. LVAD implantation is thus associated with an increased risk of developing circulating anti-human leukocyte antigen (HLA) class I and II antibodies (sensitization), causing as many as 66 percent of patients with an LVAD to be sensitized prior to transplantation.[34,35] This increased antibody level is associated with a significant risk for early graft failure and poorer survival of patients as a result of complement-mediated humoral rejection.[34] Thus, all efforts are made to reduce the number of necessary blood product (especially platelet) transfusions where possible.[34]

If the patient has become sensitized, donor-specific crossmatching is mandatory prior to transplantation, resulting in an increased waiting time for these patients.[34] Studies have demonstrated that pretransplantation immunomodulatory therapy with intravenously administered cyclophosphamide together with intravenous immunoglobulin successfully diminishes serum alloreactivity and reduces waiting list times and the risk of acute rejection in many LVAD recipients.[35]

Destination Therapy

Because of the constant shortage of available donor organs, the large group of patients who would benefit from circulatory assistance, and the encouraging results from the use of current LVADs as long-term support, a multicenter trial was conducted to evaluate the use of LVADs as permanent devices in the treatment of heart failure. REMATCH was undertaken in 1998 and included 129 patients in 20 centers using the HeartMate VE LVAD (see Figs. 25–3 and 25–4) as the study device. Eligible patients were adults with end-stage heart failure with contraindications to transplantation.[1]

The patients in the study were randomly assigned to receive either an LVAD or maximal medical therapy, with death as the primary endpoint and several secondary endpoints assessing quality of life, complications, and hospitalizations. The study ended in July 2001 and demonstrated a 48 percent reduction in the risk of death in the group treated with LVADs compared with the medically treated group (Fig. 25–11), with superior quality of life measurements demonstrated in the LVAD treatment group. However, patients with devices were more than twice as likely to develop an adverse event and had a higher median number of days spent in and out of the hospital.[1]

The INTrEPID trial is a nonrandomized study currently near completion that assesses destination therapy using the Novacor LVAD. INTrEPID assesses all-cause 6-month mortality as its primary endpoint, and 6-month cardiac mortality and health-related quality of life as its secondary endpoint. To date, enrollment of patients has been completed.

Further analysis of the REMATCH data after study completion has demonstrated improved outcomes across several "eras" of the study (Figs. 25–12 and 25–13).[78] Notably, survival in the LVAD cohort was significantly higher for those

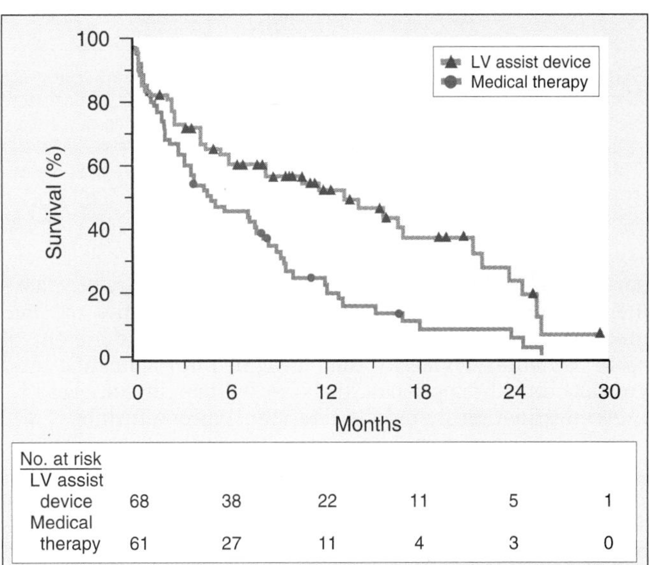

FIGURE 25–11 Comparison of actuarial survival curves from the Randomized Evaluation of Mechanical Assistance for the Treatment of Congestive Heart Failure (REMATCH). LV = left ventricular. (From Rose EA, Gelijns AC, Moskowitz AJ, et al: Long-term mechanical left ventricular assistance for end-stage heart failure. N Engl J Med 345:1435, 2001.)

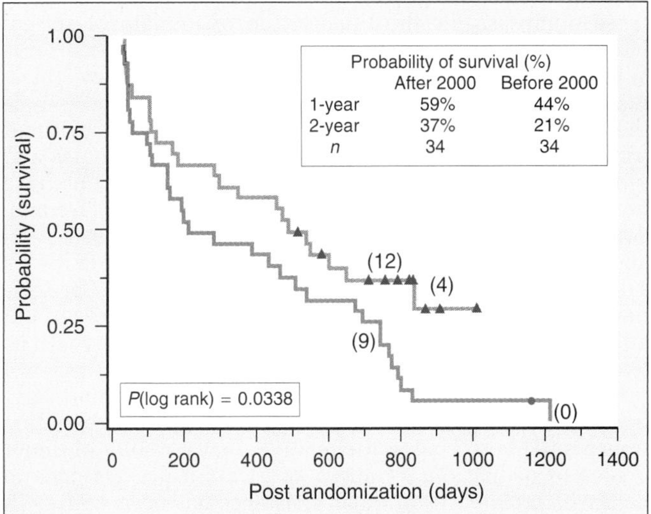

FIGURE 25–12 Randomized Evaluation of Mechanical Assistance for the Treatment of Congestive Heart Failure (REMATCH) left ventricular (LV) assist device "learning curve": comparison of actuarial survival curves of those enrolled in REMATCH before and after 2000. Upper line (blue) denotes those enrolled after 2000, lower line (magenta) denotes those enrolled prior to 2000.[78]

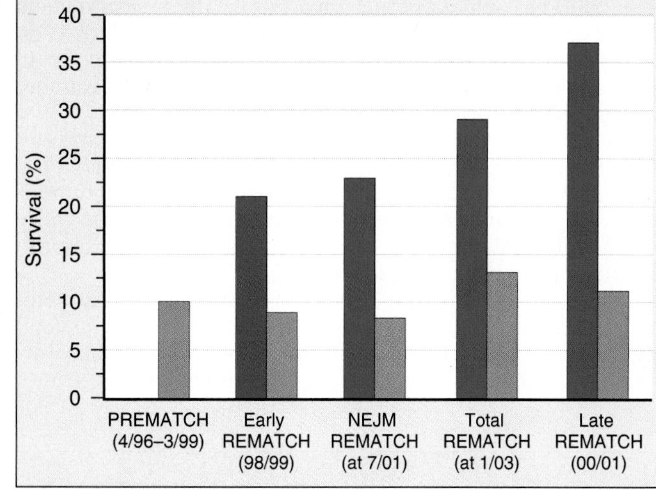

FIGURE 25–13 Comparison of 2-year survival among patients enrolled in the Randomized Evaluation of Mechanical Assistance for the Treatment of Congestive Heart Failure (REMATCH) during different "eras" of study. OMM = optimal medical management cohort; NEJM REMATCH = New England Journal of Medicine reference REMATCH data. *Includes three crossover patients with ventricular assist devices, accounting for 5 percent of OMM patients.[78]

enrolled after 2000, and 2-year survival demonstrated incremental improvement despite little change in the optimal medical management cohort. Certainly, with the advent of more durable devices, other design improvements, and greater clinical experience, the survival benefit conferred by LVAD destination therapy is likely to improve further.

Future Development

Long-term mechanical circulatory support continues to be a source of intense research and development. The obstacles of thrombogenicity (and embolization), device infection, and immunological sensitization remain a target of ongoing research for the currently available VADs. The potential of VADs as destination therapy has further tested the limits of device durability. Finally, the increasing desire to miniaturize pump design to allow complete implantability and pediatric applications continues to drive development.

MINIATURIZED CENTRIFUGAL PUMPS. Years after the invention of centrifugal pumps, researchers are re-evaluating these pumps as the third generation of implantable circulatory assist devices. The Levitronix LVAS (Levitronix, Waltham, MA) is one such pump built on the "maglev" (magnetic levitation) concept, which allows the motor to levitate the rotor magnetically so that rotation is achieved without friction, with less thrombogenicity, with minimal noise and vibration, and with anticipated long-term durability because of lack of metal-to-metal contact. The DuraHeart (Terumo, Ann Arbor, MI) is based on a similar concept and design and may be implemented in patients whose BSA is as low as 1.1 m^2, with flows from 2 to 10 liter/min. It, like the Cor-Aide device (Cor-Aide, Cleveland, OH), has been operated without anticoagulation in animal trials. Whether this strategy will be feasible in clinical applications remains unknown.

PEDIATRIC ASSIST DEVICES. Children with end-stage heart failure are at particular risk for dying while awaiting transplantation owing to the relative unavailability of donor organs in pediatric size ranges. Most clinical experience to date with isolated ventricular assistance has been with children larger than 6 kg; the largest experience in smaller children and neonates has been with ECMO.

Several specific requirements for a pediatric assist device make its development difficult. First, the device must be versatile; children with complex heart disease often require biventricular support or alternatively have only a single functional ventricle. In addition, the ability to include an oxygenator in the support circuit may be required. Second, the cannulas must be small enough to allow ventricular decompression without generating excessive negative pressure (and air entrainment). Third, the device itself must be small enough to be used potentially as an implantable device in larger children and not be cumbersome as a paracorporeal device in smaller infants. Finally, the device must be able to run at flows that are considered low by adult standards but would fully support children (e.g., 0.5 to 1.5 liter/min).

Worldwide, only the Berlin Heart and the Medos pumps have enjoyed significant application in children. Both are essentially miniaturized versions of the Pierce-Donachy paracorporeal biventricular assist device (similar to the Thoratec).[79,80] However, a directive from the NHLBI has been issued to address this need, with expectations of clinical trials in 5 years.

Conclusion

Mechanical circulatory assistance has evolved over the past 20 years from an investigational strategy for the moribund to a standard therapy supporting patients in cardiogenic shock and decompensated heart failure. Although medical therapy has advanced significantly during this time and had a considerable impact on moderate heart failure, its lasting influence on severe heart failure has been less substantial.[81] Today, a wide variety of devices are available for short-, medium-, and long-term and permanent support at a variety of centers worldwide. Indeed, the consistent results with VAD use in this setting have advanced beyond those of pharmacotherapy to the point at which randomly assigning patients between VAD use and medical therapy alone has been questioned as ethically inappropriate.

As experience with device implantation and management has grown, so too has the interest in outcome shifted from mere postoperative survival and safety to more subtle parameters of quality of life.[1] Only with the persistent introduction and trial of new VADs, with sufficient registries to document efficacy, adverse events, and quality of life measures, will innovative therapies continue to develop. The dream of the ideal device—completely implantable, requiring no anticoagulation, available across a wide variety of patients' sizes, and endlessly durable—continues to evade current technology but remains a target of design for the future.

REFERENCES

1. Rose EA, Gelijns AC, Moskowitz AJ, et al: Long term use of a left ventricular assist device for end-stage heart failure. N Eng J Med 345:1435, 2001.
2. Gibbon JH Jr: Application of a mechanical heart and lung apparatus to cardiac surgery. Minn Med 37:171, 1954.
3. Cooley DA, Beall AC Jr, Alexander JK: Acute massive pulmonary embolism: Successful surgical treatment using temporary cardiopulmonary bypass. JAMA 177:283, 1961.
4. Stuckey JH, Newman MM, Dennis C, et al: The use of the heart-lung machine in selected cases of acute myocardial infarction. Surg Forum 8:342, 1957.
5. DeBakey ME: Left ventricular bypass pump for cardiac assistance. Clinical experience. Am J Cardiol 27:3, 1971.
6. Dennis C, Carlens E, Senning A, et al: Clinical use of a cannula for left heart bypass without thoracotomy. Ann Surg 156:623, 1962.
7. Kantrowitz AM, Tjønneland S, Freed PS, et al: Initial clinical experience with intra-aortic balloon pumping in cardiogenic shock. JAMA 203:135, 1968.

Intraaortic Balloon Counterpulsation

8. Moulopoulos SD, Topaz S, Kolff WJ: Diastolic balloon pumping (with carbon dioxide) in the aorta—A mechanical assistance to the failing circulation. Am Heart J 63:669, 1962.
9. Bregman D, Casarella WJ: Percutaneous intraaortic balloon pumping: Initial clinical experience. Ann Thorac Surg 29:153, 1980.
10. Stone GW, Ohman EM, Miller MF, et al: Contemporary utilization and outcomes of intra-aortic balloon counterpulsation in acute myocardial infarction. J Am Coll Cardiol 41:1940, 2003.

11. Pae WE Jr, Pierce WS, Sapirstein JS: Intra-aortic balloon counterpulsation, ventricular assist pumping and the artificial heart. *In* Baue AE, Geha AS, Hammond GL, et al (eds): Glenn's Thoracic and Cardiovascular Surgery. Stamford, Conn, Appleton & Lange, 1996, p 1825.
12. Ghali WA, Ash AS, Hall RE, Moskowitz MA: Variation in hospital rates of intraaortic balloon pump use in coronary artery bypass operations. Ann Thorac Surg 67:441, 1999.
13. Reichenbacher WE, Pierce WS: Treatment of heart failure: Assisted circulation. *In* Braunwald E, Zipes DP, Libby P (eds): Heart Disease: A Textbook of Cardiovascular Medicine. Philadelphia, WB Saunders, 2001, p. 602.
14. Normal JC, Cooley DA, Igo SR, et al: Prognostic indices for survival during postcardiotomy intra-aortic balloon pumping: Methods of scoring and classification, with implications for LVAD utilization. J Thorac Cardiovasc Surg 74:709, 1977.
15. Schmid C, Deng M, Hammel D, et al: Emergency versus elective/urgent left ventricular assist device implantation. J Heart Lung Transplant 17:1024, 1998.
16. Helman DN, Morales DL, Edwards NM, et al: Left ventricular assist device bridge-to-transplant network improves survival after failed cardiotomy. Ann Thorac Surg 68:1187, 1999.
17. Copeland JG, Smith RG, Arabia FA, et al: The CardioWest total artificial heart as a bridge to transplantation. Semin Thorac Cardiovasc Surg 12:238, 2000.
18. Hendry PJ, Masters RG, Mussivand TV, et al: Circulatory support for cardiogenic shock due to acute myocardial infarction: A Canadian experience. Can J Cardiol 15:1090, 1999.
19. Chen JM, DeRose JJ, Slater JP, et al: Improved survival rates support left ventricular assist device implantation early after myocardial infarction. J Am Coll Cardiol 33:1903, 1999.
20. Hands ME, Rutherford JD, Muller JE, et al: The in-hospital development of cardiogenic shock after myocardial infarction: Incidence, predictors of occurrence, outcome and prognostic factors. J Am Coll Cardiol 14:40, 1989.
21. Hochman JS, Sleeper LA, White HD, et al: One-year survival following early revascularization for cardiogenic shock. JAMA 285:190, 2001.
22. Houel R, Vermes E, Tixier DB, et al: Myocardial recovery after mechanical support for acute myocarditis: Is sustained recovery predictable? Ann Thorac Surg 68:2177, 1999.
23. Swartz MT, Lowdermilk GA, McBride LR: Refractory ventricular tachycardia as an indication for ventricular assist device support. J Thorac Cardiovasc Surg 118:1119, 1999.
24. Oz MC, Rose EA, Slater J, et al: Malignant ventricular arrhythmias are well tolerated in patients receiving long-term left ventricular assist devices. J Am Coll Cardiol 24:1688, 1994.
25. Morgan JA, John R, Rao V, et al: Bridging to transplant with the HeartMate left ventricular assist device: The Columbia-Presbyterian experience. J Thorac Cardiovasc Surg 127:1309, 2004.
26. Oz MC, Rose EA, Levin HR: Selection criteria for placement of left ventricular assist devices. Am Heart J 129:173, 1995.
27. Oz MC, Goldstein DJ, Pepino P, et al: Screening scale predicts patients successfully receiving long-term implantable left ventricular assist devices. Circulation 92:II169, 1995.
28. Rao V, Oz MC, Flannery MA, et al: Revised screening scale to predict survival after insertion of a left ventricular assist device. J Thorac Cardiovasc Surg 125:855, 2003.
29. Oz M, Prager KM: Proposed policy for VAD removal. Ann Thorac Surg 73:1688, 2002.
30. Sinha P, Chen JM, Rajasinghe HR, et al: Infections during left-ventricular assist device support do not affect post-transplant outcomes. Circulation 102:III194, 2000.
31. Smedira NG, Moazami N, Golding CM, et al: Clinical experience with 202 adults receiving extracorporeal membrane oxygenation for cardiac failure: Survival at five years. J Thorac Cardiovasc Surg 122:92, 2001.
32. Wassenberg PA: The Abiomed BVS 5000 biventricular support system. Perfusion 15:369, 2000.
33. Spanier T, Oz MC, Levin H, et al: Activation of coagulation and fibrinolytic pathways in patients with left ventricular assist devices. J Thorac Cardiovasc Surg 112:1090, 1996.
34. John R, Lietz K, Schuster M: Immunologic sensitization in recipients of left ventricular assist devices. J Thorac Cardiovasc Surg 125:578, 2003.
35. Itescu S, John R: Interactions between the recipient immune system and the left ventricular assist device surface: Immunological and clinical implications. Ann Thorac Surg 75:S58, 2003.
36. El-Banayosy A, Arusoglu L, Kizner L, et al: Novacor left ventricular assist system versus HeartMate vented electric left ventricular assist system as a long-term mechanical circulatory support device in bridging patients: A prospective study. J Thorac Cardiovasc Surg 119:581, 2000.
37. Frazier OH: First use of an untethered, vented electric left ventricular assist device for long-term support. Circulation 89:2908, 1994.
38. Sun BC, Catanese KA, Spanier TB, et al: 100 long-term implantable left ventricular assist devices: The Columbia Presbyterian interim experience. Ann Thorac Surg 68:688,1999.
39. Poirier VL: Worldwide experience with the TCI HeartMate system: Issues and future perspective. Thorac Cardiovasc Surg 49:316, 1999.
40. Murali S: Mechanical circulatory support with Novacor LVAS: World-wide clinical results. Thorac Cardiovasc Surg 47:321, 1999.
41. Pasque MK, Rogers JG: Adverse events in the use of the HeartMate vented electric and Novacor left ventricular assist devices: Comparing apples and oranges. J Thorac Cardiovasc Surg 124:1063, 2002.
42. Portner PM, Jansen PGM, Oyer PE: Improved outcomes with an implantable left ventricular assist system: A multicenter study. Ann Thorac Surg 71:205, 2001.
43. Farrar DJ: The Thoratec ventricular assist device: A paracorporeal pump for treating acute and chronic heart failure. Semin Thorac Cardiovasc Surg 12:243, 2000.
44. Copeland JG, Arabia FA, Banchy ME, et al: The CardioWest total artificial heart bridge to transplantation: 1993 to 1996 national trial. Ann Thorac Surg 66:1662,1998.
45. Arabia FA, Copeland JG, Smith RG, et al: International experience with the CardioWest total artificial heart as a bridge to heart transplantation. Eur J Cardiothorac Surg 11:S5, 1997.
46. Sezai A, Shiono M, Orime Y, et al: Comparison studies of major organ microcirculations under pulsatile- and nonpulsatile-assisted circulations. Artif Organs 20:139, 1996.
47. Reddy RC, Goldstein AH, Pacella J, et al: End organ function with prolonged nonpulsatile circulatory support. ASAIO J 41:M547, 1995.
48. Yacoub MH: A novel strategy to maximize the efficacy of left ventricular assist devices as a bridge to recovery. Eur Heart J 22:534, 2001.
49. Holman WL, Rayburn BK, McGiffin DC: Infection in ventricular assist devices: Prevention and treatment. Ann Thorac Surg 75:S48, 2003.
50. Nurozler F, Argenziano M, Oz MC, Naka Y: Fungal left ventricular assist device endocarditis. Ann Thorac Surg 71:614, 2001.
51. Macha M, Litwak P, Yamazaki K, et al: Survival for up to six months in calves supported with an implantable axial flow ventricular assist device. ASAIO J 43:311, 1997.
52. Kawahito K, Damm G, Benkowski R, et al: Ex vivo phase 1 evaluation of the DeBakey/NASA axial flow ventricular assist device. Artif Organs 20:47, 1996.
53. Griffith BP, Kormos RL, Borovetz HS, et al: HeartMate II left ventricular assist system: From concept to first clinical use. Ann Thorac Surg 71:S116, 2001.
54. Noon GP, Morley DL, Irwin S, et al: Clinical experience with the MicroMed DeBakey ventricular assist device. Ann Thorac Surg 71:S133, 2001.
55. Frazier OH, Rose EA, Oz MC, et al: HeartMate LVAS Investigators. Left ventricular assist system, multicenter clinical evaluation of the HeartMate vented electric left ventricular assist system in patients awaiting heart transplantation. J Thorac Cardiovasc Surg 122:1186, 2001.
56. Wieselthaler GM, Schima H, Dworschak M, et al: First experience with outpatient care of patients with implanted axial flow pumps. Artif Organs 25:331, 2001.
57. Frazier OH, Myers TJ, Jarvik RK, et al: Research and development of an implantable, axial-flow left ventricular assist device: The Jarvik 2000 Heart. Ann Thorac Surg 71:S125, 2001.
58. Mehta SM, Pae WE, Rosenberg G, et al: The LionHeart LVD-2000: A completely implanted left ventricular assist device for chronic circulatory support. Ann Thorac Surg 71:S156, 2001.
59. Robbins RC, Kown MH, Portner PM, et al: The totally implantable Novacor left ventricular assist system. Ann Thorac Surg 71:S162, 2001.
60. Kavarana MN, Pessin-Minsley MS, Urtecho J, et al: Right ventricular dysfunction and organ failure in left ventricular assist device recipients: A continuing problem. Ann Thorac Surg 73:745, 2002.
61. Argenziano M, Choudhri AF, Oz MC, et al: A prospective randomized trial of arginine vasopressin in the treatment of vasodilatory shock after left ventricular assist device placement. Circulation 96:II-90, 1997.
62. Goldstein DJ, Seldomridge JA, Chen JM, et al: Use of aprotinin in LVAD recipients reduces blood loss, blood use, and perioperative mortality. Ann Thorac Surg 59:1063, 1995.
63. Morrone TM, Buck LA, Catanese KA, et al: Early progressive mobilization of left ventricular assist device patients is safe and optimizes recovery before heart transplantation. J Heart Lung Transplant 15:423, 1996.
64. El-Banayosy A, Fey O, Sarnowski P, et al: Midterm follow-up of patients discharged from hospital under left ventricular assistance. J Heart Lung Transplant 20:53, 2001.
65. Levin HR, Oz MC, Chen JM, et al: Reversal of chronic ventricular dilation in patients with end-stage cardiomyopathy by prolonged mechanical unloading. Circulation 91:2717, 1995.
66. Frazier OH, Benedict CR, Radovancevic B, et al: Improved left ventricular function after chronic left ventricular unloading. Ann Thorac Surg 62:675, 1996.
67. Foray A, Williams D, Reemtsma K, et al: Assessment of submaximal exercise capacity in patients with left ventricular assist devices. Circulation 94:II222, 1996.
68. Mueller J, Wallukat G, Weng Y, et al: Predictive factors for weaning from a cardiac assist device. An analysis of clinical, gene expression, and protein data. J Heart Lung Transplant 20:202, 2001.
69. Helman DN, Maybaum SW, Morales DL, et al: Recurrent remodeling after ventricular assistance: Is long-term myocardial recovery attainable? Ann Thorac Surg 70:1255, 2000.
70. Hetzer R, Muller JH, Weng YG, et al: Midterm follow-up of patients who underwent removal of a left ventricular assist device after cardiac recovery from end-stage dilated cardiomyopathy. J Thorac Cardiovasc Surg 120:843, 2000.
71. McBride LR, Naunheim KS, Fiore AC, et al: Clinical experience with 111 Thoratec ventricular assist devices. Ann Thorac Surg 67:1233, 1999.
72. Thomas CE, Jichici D, Petrucci R, et al: Neurologic complications of the Novacor left ventricular assist device. Ann Thorac Surg 72:1311, 2001.
73. Rafii S, Oz MC, Seldomridge JA, et al: Characterization of hematopoietic cells arising on the textured surface of left ventricular assist devices. Ann Thorac Surg 60:1627, 1995.
74. Korfer R, El-Banayosy A, Arusoglu L, et al: Single-center experience with the Thoratec ventricular assist device. J Thorac Cardiovasc Surg 119:596, 2000.
75. Fukamachi K, McCarthy PM, Smedira NG, et al: Preoperative risk factors for right ventricular failure after implantable left ventricular assist device insertion. Ann Thorac Surg 68:2181, 1999.
76. Cave AC, Manche A, Derias NW, et al: Thromboxane A_2 mediates pulmonary hypertension after cardiopulmonary bypass in the rabbit. J Thorac Cardiovasc Surg 106:959, 1993.
77. Chen JM, Levin HR, Rose EA, et al: Experience with right ventricular assist devices for perioperative right sided circulatory failure. Ann Thorac Surg 61:305, 1996.
78. Park SJ, Frazier OH, Piccioni W, et al: LVAD destination therapy: An extended follow-up of outcomes. J Thorac Cardiovasc Surg (in press).
79. Konertz W, Reul H: Mechanical circulatory support in children. Int J Artif Organs 20:657, 1997.
80. Warnecke H, Berdijs F, Lange P, et al: Mechanical left ventricular support as a bridge to cardiac transplantation in childhood. Eur J Cardiothorac Surg 5:300, 1991.
81. Stevenson LW, Kormos KL: Mechanical cardiac support 2000: Current applications and future trial design. J Am Coll Cardiol 37:341, 2001.

CHAPTER 26

Heart Transplantation

Sharon A. Hunt • Peter C. Kouretas • Leora B. Balsam • Robert C. Robbins

History

Clinical heart transplantation has become a mature clinical science in the last 15 years or so, but its maturation was preceded by several decades of preclinical and preliminary clinical work involving a variety of scientific disciplines. The earliest work defining the optimum surgical methods for excision of the donor heart and implantation of the heart in the orthotopic position happened in the 1950s, and the technique with use of cardiopulmonary bypass and topical hypothermia for donor heart preservation was published as a two-page report by the Shumway group in 1960. The basic surgical technique has changed little since that time and is outlined in this chapter.

The first clinical heart transplant was performed in South Africa in December 1967 and was greeted with much publicity and followed by much surgical enthusiasm for the next year, with just over 100 procedures being performed in 1968. This enthusiasm was soon tempered, however, by the observation of very poor survival rates in these early patients (~15 percent at 1 year) and by 1970 essentially only two centers (Stanford and the Medical College of Virginia) continued to pursue programs in clinical heart transplantation. Working virtually alone in the decade of the 1970s, these programs gradually evolved recipient and donor acceptance criteria, introduced the endomyocardial biopsy as a means to detect the presence of and the adequacy of therapy for rejection, and outlined what have come to be the expected posttransplant complications.

In the 1980s, general advances in the field of immunosuppression, prominently including the clinical introduction of the calcineurin inhibitor cyclosporine, led to a gradual resurgence of interest and clinical activity in the field of heart transplantation. In 1982 an international registry of heart transplantation data was begun by the International Society for Heart and Lung Transplantation (ISHLT) and continues to accrue data today. In 1994, this registry was merged with the overall organ transplant registry in the United States supervised by the United Network for Organ Sharing (UNOS). In the United States reporting of data is mandatory; it is voluntary for the rest of the world, but completeness of reporting is quite good. The data are updated and published annually in the *Journal of Heart and Lung Transplantation* and are available online at the UNOS website (www.UNOS.org).

By the decade of the 1990s, the demand for heart transplantation began to exceed the supply of available donor hearts, and since then the annual numbers of transplants performed has been strictly limited by the numbers of donor hearts available. The annual numbers seem to have plateaued at approximately 4000 procedures worldwide per year.[1]

Heart Transplantation: The Operation

DONOR OPERATIVE TECHNIQUE

Retrieval of the donor heart in the modern era typically occurs as a part of a multiorgan procurement effort. The cardiothoracic team works in conjunction with an abdominal team, which procures the liver and/or kidneys, and communication between the two teams is critical for optimum management of the donor during the retrieval process.

The donor operation is performed via a median sternotomy. The heart and great vessels are carefully inspected for any signs of contusion, infarction, congenital anomalies, and aneurysmal disease and for overall ventricular function. The coronary arteries are palpated to evaluate coronary artery disease. Substantial abnormalities identified in this manner preclude the use of the donor heart for transplantation.

When the abdominal team has completed their dissection, heparin is administered to the donor and the aorta is cannulated for infusion of cardioplegic solution., The left heart is decompressed by incising one of the pulmonary veins; the heart is then allowed to empty and the aortic cross clamp is applied. Cold crystalloid cardioplegia is administered via the aortic root. When the infusion is completed, the heart is rapidly excised by dividing the superior vena cava (SVC), the four pulmonary veins, the aorta, and the pulmonary artery at its bifurcation.

RECIPIENT OPERATIVE TECHNIQUE

The recipient operation for heart transplantation proceeds in two phases. The first step is the excision of the recipient's native organ and the second step is the implantation of the allograft. The recipient is brought to the operating room and appropriate monitoring lines are placed. After induction of general anesthesia and endotracheal intubation, a median sternotomy is performed and the pericardium is opened and reflected laterally. The ascending aorta, SVC, and inferior vena cava (IVC) are dissected free and encircled with tapes. After the recipient is fully heparinized, the high ascending aorta and both venae cavae are cannulated separately, cardiopulmonary bypass (CPB) is instituted, and the patient is cooled to 28°C. Once the donor heart has been delivered to the operating room, the recipient cardiectomy is performed. The aorta is cross-clamped just proximal to the aortic cannulation site. The right and left atrial walls, atrial septum, pulmonary artery, and aorta are divided. Division of the pulmonary artery and aorta is performed just above the semilunar valves (Fig. 26-1).

The donor heart is then brought onto the operative field and prepared for implantation into the recipient. The tissue between the orifices of the four pulmonary veins is excised, leaving a single large opening (Fig. 26-2). The right atrium is opened beginning from the lateral aspect of the IVC and extending into the base of the right atrial appendage (Fig. 26-3). The heart is carefully examined for any valvular or congenital anomalies. The standard or biatrial technique, as originally described by Lower and Shumway, proceeds with anastomoses of the left atrium, right atrium, pulmonary artery, and aorta (Figs. 26-4 and 26-5).

After at least 30 minutes of reperfusion, the patient is gradually weaned from CPB with implementation of the appropriate inotropic support. The cannulas are removed and protamine is administered slowly to reverse the effect of heparin. Temporary atrial and ventricular pacing wires are placed as well as mediastinal and pleural drainage tubes. The sternum is then closed in the standard fashion. Induction immunosuppressive therapy is administered at this time.

In recent years, the bicaval technique for orthotopic heart transplantation has become the preferred approach at most transplant centers.[2,3] Several modifications distinguish the bicaval approach from the standard biatrial technique. First, the recipient SVC is cannulated just below the innominate vein junction and the IVC is cannulated at the diaphragm. Recipient cardiectomy is performed as a two-step procedure. In the first step, the heart is transected at the midatrial level, the aorta and pulmonary artery are divided, and the heart is removed. In the second step, the posterior walls of both atria are removed; on the right side, the SVC and IVC are transected at their junction with the right atrium, and on the left side, the left atrium is trimmed, leaving a cuff of tissue around the pulmonary vein orifices (Fig. 26-6). The donor heart left atrium is trimmed, leaving a single orifice where the pulmonary vein entry sites had been, and the right atrium remains intact. In the bicaval approach, the typical sequence of anastomoses is left atrium, IVC, SVC, pulmonary arteries, and aorta (Figs. 26-7 and 26-8). The left atrial, pulmonary artery, and aortic anastomoses are performed as described in the standard biatrial technique.

The standard biatrial technique is still used in some transplant centers because of the advantage of shorter operative times and avoidance of the potential complications of SVC and IVC thromboses and stenoses. There are several disadvantages of the biatrial technique, however, which has prompted a shift to the bicaval technique in many transplant centers.[3,4] The biatrial technique distorts the atrioventricular geometry, which can result in atrial enlargement, atrioventricular valve insufficiency, impaired atrial function, atrial thromboses, and a propensity toward sinoatrial node dysfunction.[5] Several studies have demonstrated improved atrial function and ventricular function and decreased atrioventricular valvular insufficiency as well as a decreased incidence of arrhythmias and heart block with the bicaval technique.[3,6,7] A reported disadvantage of the bicaval technique is the risk of SVC stenosis, particularly when there is a size mismatch between the donor and recipient. A recent series from Stanford reported a 2.4 percent incidence of this complication.[8]

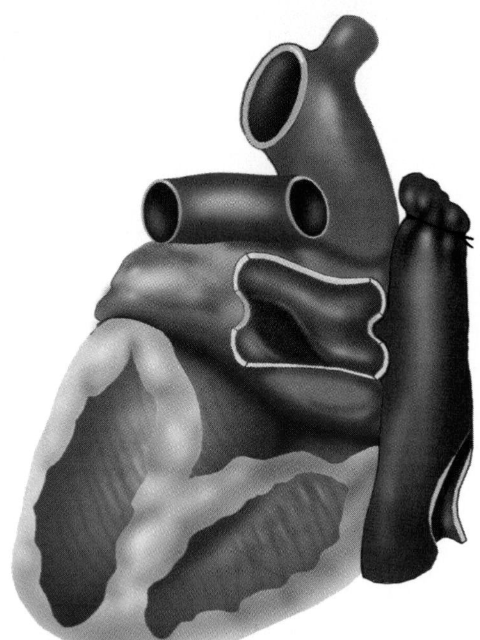

FIGURE 26–2 Creation of donor heart left atrial cuff by incising through the pulmonary vein orifices.

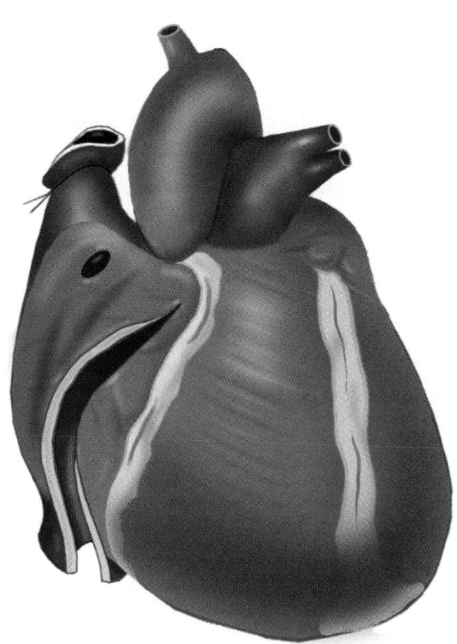

FIGURE 26–3 Creation of the donor heart right atrial cuff.

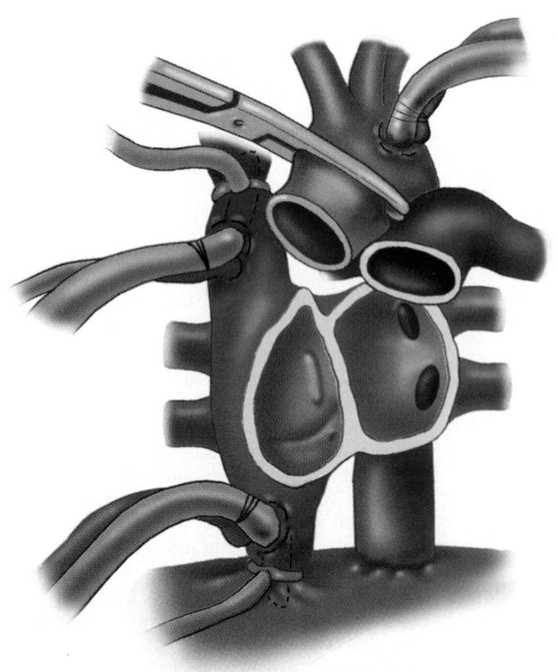

FIGURE 26–1 Completed recipient cardiectomy in preparation for standard orthotopic transplantation.

Recipient Selection

Cardiac recipient selection criteria aim to identify the patients with end-stage heart disease who are most likely to

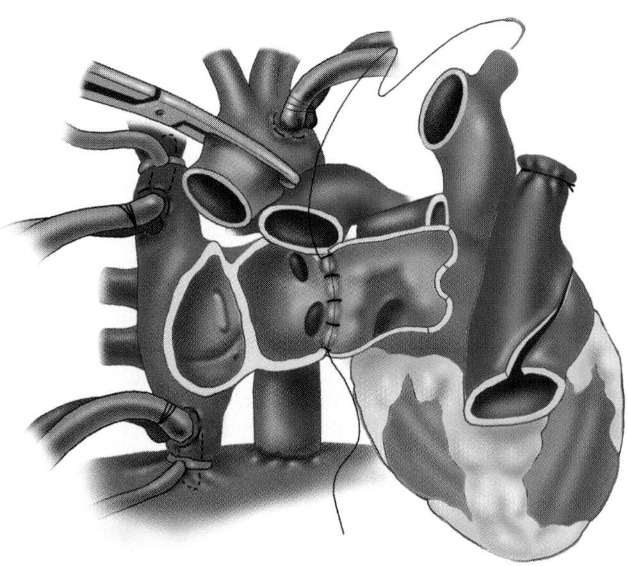

FIGURE 26–4 Commencement of the left atrial anastomosis.

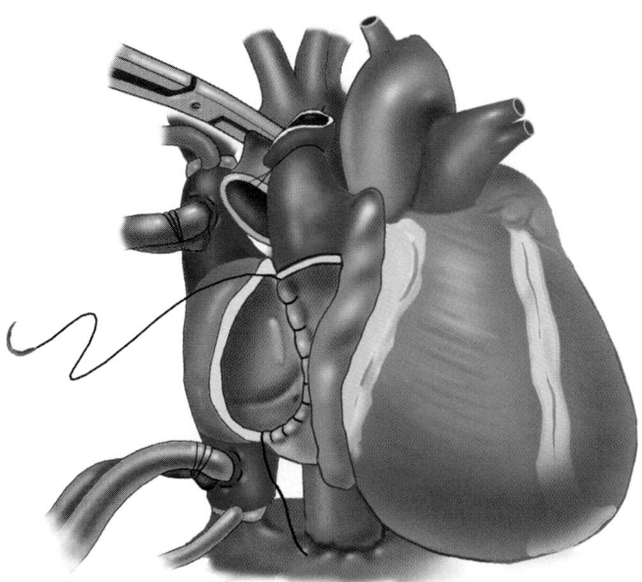

FIGURE 26–5 Commencement of right atrial anastomosis.

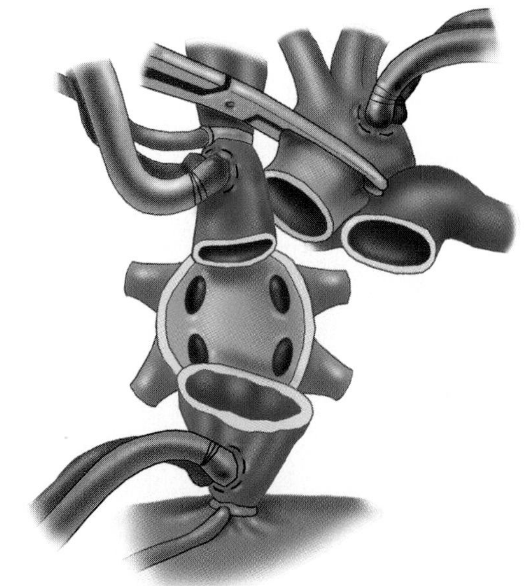

FIGURE 26–6 Creation of superior and inferior vena caval cuffs in preparation for bicaval technique.

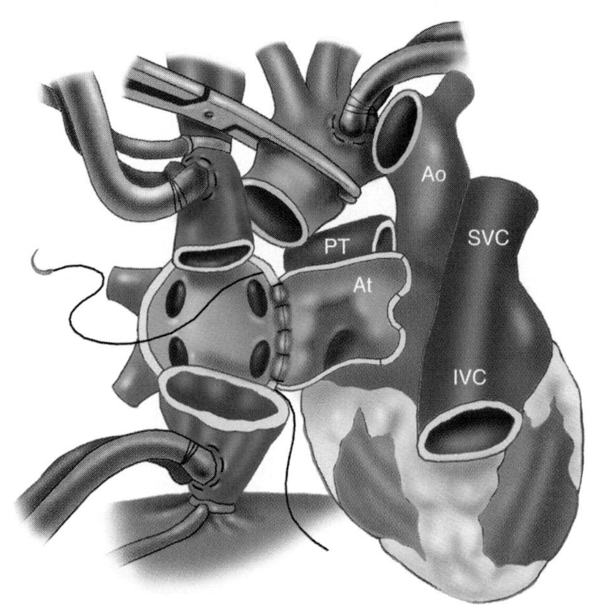

FIGURE 26–7 Commencement of left atrial anastomosis in the bicaval technique.

have the greatest benefit from the scarce societal resource of the donor heart (Table 26–1). The criteria have evolved a great deal over time and continue to do so as experience and expertise at dealing with issues limiting postoperative survival accrue. The most fundamental criterion remains the presence of advanced heart disease that is irremediable by any more conservative forms of therapy. As medical therapy for heart failure has improved over the years, the designation of truly "end-stage" heart disease has become a "moving target" since many patients who are referred for heart transplantation end up improving their clinical status with judicious use of newer therapies.

Most patients eventually accepted for transplantation in the current era have failed aggressive medical management at a heart failure center and usually have required recurrent hospitalizations for heart failure management. Many are hospital-bound with requirement for intravenous inotropic support and/or mechanical support of the circulation. In ambulatory patients the goal is to select those with the very worst prognosis.[9] In this context the measurement of peak oxygen consumption with exercise to anaerobic threshold (VO_2 max) has been shown to be one of the best predictors of prognosis.[10-12] Patients with a VO_2 max less than 15 ml/kg/min have a poor prognosis and a level of 14 ml/kg/min is often considered a basic threshold for transplant eligibility in ambulatory patients.

The other criteria listed in Table 26–1 all are open to interpretation.[13]

Advanced Age

Age criteria for eligibility were initially rigid, but it became apparent that chronological and physiological age could be quite discrepant, and there have been a number of single-

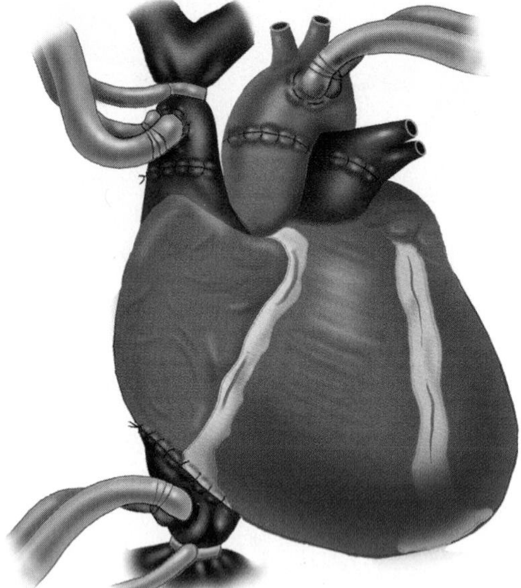

FIGURE 26–8 Completion of bicaval transplant technique, showing the inferior vena caval, superior vena caval, aortic, and pulmonary artery anastomoses.

TABLE 26–1 Cardiac Recipient Selection Criteria
End-stage heart disease not remediable by more conservative measures
Absence of Advanced age Severe peripheral or cerebrovascular disease Irreversible dysfunction of another organ (kidney, liver, lung) unless being considered for multiorgan transplantation History of malignancy with probability of recurrence Inability to comply with complex medical regimen Irreversible pulmonary hypertension (>4 Wood units) Active systemic infection

center reports of excellent post heart transplant survival in carefully selected older recipients. Most programs currently do not have fixed upper age limits, but patients older than 65 years of age are very highly selected for lack of comorbidities.

Severe Peripheral or Cerebrovascular Disease

Since systemic vascular disease contributes to both poor prognosis for survival as well as poor quality of life on a noncardiac basis, and since risk factors contributing to the disease are also major risk factors for development of vascular disease in the allograft, advanced noncardiac vascular disease is a major comorbidity that can preclude eligibility for cardiac transplantation. It would be difficult to design an exact description of the extent of disease that would disqualify a patient, however.

Irreversible Organ Dysfunction

Coexisting disease in other organs that might separately limit a patient's survival has generally been considered a contraindication to heart transplantation, and this has applied primarily to disease of the lungs, kidneys, and liver. With advances in the general area of solid-organ transplantation, some centers have commenced programs in multiorgan transplantation in highly selected patients and referral of patients in need of more than one organ to such a center can be considered.

History of Malignancy

The institution of chronic immunosuppression, a form of therapy known to be associated with a higher-than-usual incidence of malignancy, might favor recurrence of or more aggressive behavior of a prior or current malignancy. There are many reports, however, of long-term successful heart transplantation in patients with a remote history of malignancy that is considered to have essentially no probability of recurrence. Many of these patients have developed their end-stage heart disease as a direct consequence of the chemotherapy and/or radiation therapy that cured their malignancy. In cases in which the malignancy is less remote in history or probability of recurrence less certain, consultation with an oncologist regarding prognosis can be quite helpful.

Inability or Unwillingness to Comply with a Complex Medical Regimen

Psychosocial criteria, including history of compliance with medical regimens and medical follow-up and quality of family or social support structure, have a long history of being considered as factors for transplant eligibility. They are, however, the most difficult ones to quantify or defend. Certainly, the existence of active substance abuse or refusal to take medications should be a major consideration; however, more vague measures of "social worth" (including incarceration status, level of mental retardation, health care coverage status, family support or lack thereof) cannot be considered as major factors.

Irreversible Pulmonary Hypertension

It was discovered in the early days of clinical heart transplantation that a normal donor right ventricle faced with high recipient pulmonary vascular resistance (PVR) and the demand to increase its external workload acutely often failed abruptly, frequently as early as on the operating table. Subsequently, pulmonary hypertension in excess of about 4 Wood units became an exclusion to transplant candidacy. In recent years the concept of reversibility of the pulmonary hypertension seen in some patients with chronic heart failure has been recognized, and it is believed that if reversibility can be demonstrated acutely with pharmacological maneuvers either in the cardiac catheterization laboratory or in the intensive care unit setting with hemodynamic monitoring, a patient can be expected to do well with a transplant since the same reversal could presumably be accomplished in the postoperative setting.[14,15] Thus, the cardiologist often becomes in a sense a patient advocate in the cardiac catheterization laboratory, devising combinations of inotropes and vasodilators to try and demonstrate reversibility of elevated PVR while maintaining adequate systemic pressures.[16,17] Irreversible pulmonary hypertension remains an exclusion from transplant candidacy in most centers unless combined heart and lung transplantation is considered.

Active Systemic Infection

As discussed in the section on malignancy, there is a general and intuitive feeling that the institution of systemic immunosuppression is also contraindicated in the presence of significant active systemic infection since the state of immunosuppression would be expected to be deleterious to defense mechanisms against infection. The existence of a systemic infection is thus considered a (sometimes temporary) contraindication to transplant eligibility. Some infections that are not considered "temporary" include human immunodeficiency virus (HIV) infection and disseminated tuberculosis, although some clinical experience has actually been reported with organ transplantation in HIV-positive patients.

Donor Selection and Management

The selection of donors for heart transplantation is a stepwise process coordinated by the organ procurement organization, the transplant physicians, and the procuring surgeons. A primary screen is performed by a specialist from the organ procurement organization who collects information regarding the medical history, cause of death, body size, ABO blood type, serologies (including HIV, hepatitus B virus [HBV], and hepatitus C virus [HCV]), and clinical course of the potential donor. A secondary screen is performed by a transplant physician who reviews relevant history, physical findings, and test results, including the baseline electrocardiogram, chest radiograph, laboratory data, and echocardiogram. A final screen is performed by the procuring surgeon, who directly inspects the organ, usually at a site distant from the transplant hospital, and works in concert with procurement teams for the donor's other organs.

Guidelines for Donor Selection

Standard guidelines have been established for cardiac donor selection (Table 26–2).[18,19] Potential donors must meet legal requirements for brain death. Donor age younger than 55 years is preferred, although on occasion older donors are considered. Donors with a history of cardiac disease, including prior myocardial infarction or significant valvular or other structural disease or arrhythmia, are usually excluded. In addition, donors with a history of severe chest trauma are excluded because of concern about cardiac contusion. Donors must meet established hemodynamic criteria, including a mean arterial pressure (MAP) higher than 60 mm Hg and a central venous pressure (CVP) of 8 to 12 mm Hg, either on initial evaluation or after appropriate resuscitation maneuvers as described later. Prolonged cardiac arrest, arterial hypoxemia, hypotension, and/or high-dose inotropic support are reasons for exclusion. Donors with a history of active malignancy (excluding basal cell and squamous cell carcinomas of the skin and some isolated brain tumors) are excluded because there is a high probability of transferring malignant cells to the immunosuppressed recipient. Coronary angiography is recommended for most male donors older than 45 years and female donors older than 50 years to evaluate coronary artery stenoses. Serologies for HIV, HBV, and HCV should be negative, although some centers "match" donors who have positive hepatitis serology with seropositive recipients.

TABLE 26–2 Cardiac Donor Selection Criteria
Age < 55 yr
No history of chest trauma or cardiac disease
No prolonged hypotension or hypoxemia
Meets hemodynamic criteria MAP > 60 mm Hg CVP 8-12 mm Hg Inotropic support < 10 μg/kg/min dopamine or dobutamine
Normal ECG
Normal echocardiogram
Normal cardiac angiography*
Negative HBsAg, HCV, and HIV serologies

CVP = central venous pressure; ECG = electrocardiogram; HBsAg = hepatis B surface antigen; HCV = hepatitis C virus; HIV = human immunodeficiency virus; MAP = mean arterial pressure.
*Performed as indicated by donor age and history.

In response to the donor organ shortage, there has been a trend toward liberalizing donor selection criteria. Expansion of the cardiac donor pool has involved accepting hearts of older donors, tolerating longer organ ischemic times, and accepting hearts with some structural abnormalities, including mild left ventricular hypertrophy, mild valvular anomalies, or mild coronary artery disease. Limited information is available regarding the long-term durability of organs derived from this expanded donor pool, though there is some evidence that certain donor factors, such as older age and prolonged ischemic time, may act synergistically to increase recipient mortality risk.[20]

Donor Management

Aggressive hemodynamic and metabolic management of donors has been shown to result in higher organ retrieval rates.[21,22] Brain-injured patients often suffer from hemodynamic instability due to neurogenic shock, excessive fluid loss, and bradycardia. Typical management should include correction of volume deficits, metabolic derangements, and hormonal abnormalities. Fluid should be administered to maintain a CVP between 5 and 10 mm Hg and blood transfusions given sparingly to maintain a hematocrit of 30 percent. When available, cytomegalovirus (CMV)-negative and leukocyte-filtered blood is preferred. Inotropic support should be used as little as possible. Metabolic derangements, including acidosis, hypoxemia, and hypercarbia, should be corrected. Because hormonal abnormalities are common in brain-injured patients, hormonal replacement with arginine vasopressin, triiodothyronine, methylprednisolone, and/or insulin may be necessary.

The Crystal City Guidelines are a consensus statement formulated in 2002 with a goal of improving cardiac donor management and organ utilization.[18] A management strategy for potential organ donors is described in this document. The algorithm begins with conventional management (volume replacement, correction of acidosis, hypoxemia, and anemia, and weaning of inotropes), followed by an initial echocardiogram to identify any structural abnormalities and to evaluate left ventricular function. If the left ventricular ejection fraction (LVEF) is 0.45 or higher, the heart is considered appropriate for transplantation. If the LVEF is less than 0.45, recommendations include hormonal therapy with arginine vasopressin, triiodothyronine, methylprednisolone, and insulin and placement of a pulmonary artery catheter to guide hemodynamic management. The heart should be considered for transplantation only if appropriate hemodynamic criteria are reached (MAP > 60 mm Hg, pulmonary capillary wedge pressure 8 to 12 mm Hg, CVP 4 to 12 mm Hg, SVR 800 to 1200 $dyne \cdot sec^{-1} \cdot cm^{-5}$, cardiac index > 2.4 $liter \cdot min^{-1} \cdot m^{-2}$, and dopamine or dobutamine < 10 $\mu g/kg \cdot min^{-1}$).

Donor and Recipient Matching

Donor/recipient matching parameters for heart transplantation include only ABO compatibility and body size.[19] ABO compatibility is an absolute requirement, because hyperacute rejection may occur within minutes when transplantation is performed across ABO barriers. For reasons involving the limitations on ischemic times as well as laboratory availability, human leukocyte antigen (HLA) matching is not considered to be practical in this field. For cardiac transplantation, height and weight differences up to 20 percent may be tolerated; however, in potential recipients with elevated PVR, a donor whose body size is at least equal to that of the recipient should be chosen to decrease the likelihood of acute right ventricular failure. For potential recipients with an elevated panel reactive antibody (PRA) titer, indicating a high level of presensitization to HLA (often due to prior transfusions or pregnancies), a prospective crossmatch with donor lymphocytes is also necessary. A positive crossmatch occurs if the recipient harbors antibodies against donor HLA. In such an instance, hyperacute rejection is likely, and the donor organ cannot be accepted for that recipient.

Adoption of allocation schemes has facilitated equitable distribution of donor organs. In the United States, the UNOS contracts with the federal government to oversee organ allocation. Under UNOS policy, thoracic organs are distributed based on blood type, medical urgency, and time on the waiting list. Distribution occurs first locally and then regionally. Allocation policies are reviewed and updated on a regular basis with input from transplant physicians as well as organ procurement specialists, patient organizations, and scientists involved in the field of transplantation.

Organ Procurement

Improved techniques in organ preservation have allowed longer safe ischemic times and thus more distant procurement, thereby increasing the donor organ pool.[23] For heart grafts, cold ischemic periods up to 4 to 6 hours are currently considered permissible. As described earlier, donor organ retrieval usually occurs as part of a multiorgan procurement, and often thoracic and abdominal surgical teams will be working simultaneously on the same donor.

Immunosuppression

Postoperative management of the cardiac transplant recipient is similar to that for other postoperative heart surgery, with the important exception of the need to institute immunosuppression. Regimens used to provide suppression of the normal recipient immune response to an allograft vary at different centers and what is considered "state of the art" evolves, seemingly more rapidly over time. All currently used regimens are nonspecific, however, providing general hyporeactivity to foreign antigens rather than donor-specific hyporeactivity. For this reason, current regimens all lead to an unwanted susceptibility to infections and malignant complications in the recipient.

Most cardiac transplantation centers currently introduce immunosuppression with a three-drug regimen commencing immediately at the time of transplant. Most include a calcineurin inhibitor (cyclosporine or tacrolimus), an inhibitor of T-lymphocyte proliferation or differentiation (azathioprine or mycophenolate mofetil or sirolimus), and at least a short course of corticosteroids. Many also include in the perioperative period "induction" therapy with polyclonal (antithymocyte preparations) or monoclonal (mouse CD3 monoclonal antibodies such as Orthoclone OKT3) anti-T cell antibodies to decrease the frequency or severity of early posttransplant rejection. Most recently introduced have been monoclonal antibodies (daclizumab and basiliximab) that block the interleukin-2 receptor and may provide prevention of allograft rejection without additional global immunosuppression.[24] The "tapering" or adjustment of the immunosuppressive regimen after the perioperative period is a process that is highly individualized for each patient and determined by the patient's rejection history and tolerance to and complications from the drugs or modalities used. The following section details the methods for surveillance and therapy for acute allograft rejection.

Physiology of the Transplanted Heart

The cardiac allograft is functionally and anatomically denervated and relies on atypical adaptive mechanisms to meet varying demands for cardiac output. Having no direct neural stimulus to acutely increase heart rate in response to exercise, the allograft responds with the intrinsic Frank-Starling mechanism (the property of cardiac muscle that causes it to increase the force of its contraction in response to increased stretch or tension) to increase cardiac output in response to increased venous return at the onset of exercise. Circulating catecholamine levels later rise and provide a delayed chronotropic response to exercise. Slowing of the heart rate occurs in a likewise delayed fashion as catecholamine levels decline, but cardiac output drops mainly in response to a reduction in venous return and the reverse of the Frank-Starling mechanism.

Despite the theoretical adequacy of these atypical adaptive mechanisms, heart transplant recipients have subnormal capacity for exercise, although they have normal hemodynamic function at rest.[25-27] However, heart transplant recipients have sufficient capacity to perform activities of daily living and at least moderate exercise and generally enjoy an excellent quality of life. A number of lines of evidence suggest that reinnervation may occur in some patients late posttransplant, and a recent study suggested that reinnervation may lead to functional improvement of the transplanted heart.[28]

Since the transplanted heart lacks not only efferent but also afferent innervation, patients are classically unable to experience the sensation of angina pectoris in response to cardiac ischemia or infarction. They may experience symptoms related to the sequelae of ischemia such as dyspnea due to heart failure or arrhythmias or low cardiac output. Clinicians caring for these patients, especially late postoperatively, need to be sensitive to the subtle signs or symptoms that may signal ischemic heart disease.

Expected Postoperative Complications

Rejection

As is the case with any organ graft, the transplanted heart is subject to normal immune responses that, left unchecked, destroy the graft. The immunosuppression described earlier mitigates this reaction to variable extents in individual patients. Detection of cardiac allograft rejection and the attendant need for augmented immunosuppression are generally accomplished in some part on clinical and echocardiographic grounds but usually also with the use of the right ventricular endomyocardial biopsy. Histological grading of biopsy specimens is done with an internationally accepted grading scale[29] and this grade, when integrated with clinical and echocardiographic indices, determines the aggressiveness of augmentation of immunosuppression (Fig. 26–9). Most centers pursue serial biopsies on a surveillance basis during the first year or so after transplant and infrequently thereafter, or as clinically indicated. The endomyocardial biopsy is usually performed under fluoroscopic guidance with the use of a bioptome using a percutaneous approach from the right internal jugular vein (see previous editions of this text for details of this procedure).

Infection

All of the nonspecific immunosuppressive regimens currently used heighten susceptibility of the allograft recipient to infectious complications, particularly with opportunistic organisms. The degree of susceptibility correlates with the intensity of immunosuppression and thus is greatest during the early postoperative period. For this reason, available expertise in the specialty of infectious disease is generally considered an important aspect of institutional qualifications for an excellent transplant program.

Malignancy

The tendency to develop an incidence of malignancy in excess of that seen in the general population is yet another consequence of the current nonspecific forms of immunosuppression, or the "price of immunotherapy" to use the words of the patriarch of the field, Israel Penn. The need to recognize and treat malignancy has become a standard part of the set of clinical skills required for physicians caring for organ transplant recipients. For many years the Cincinnati Transplant Tumor Registry, under the direction of Dr. Penn, maintained a database of de novo malignancies reported in organ transplant recipients.[30] This registry has amply documented that transplant recipients tend to have cancers that are common in the general population with a normal incidence but have a markedly increased incidence of both lymphoproliferative malignancy and carcinomas of the skin.

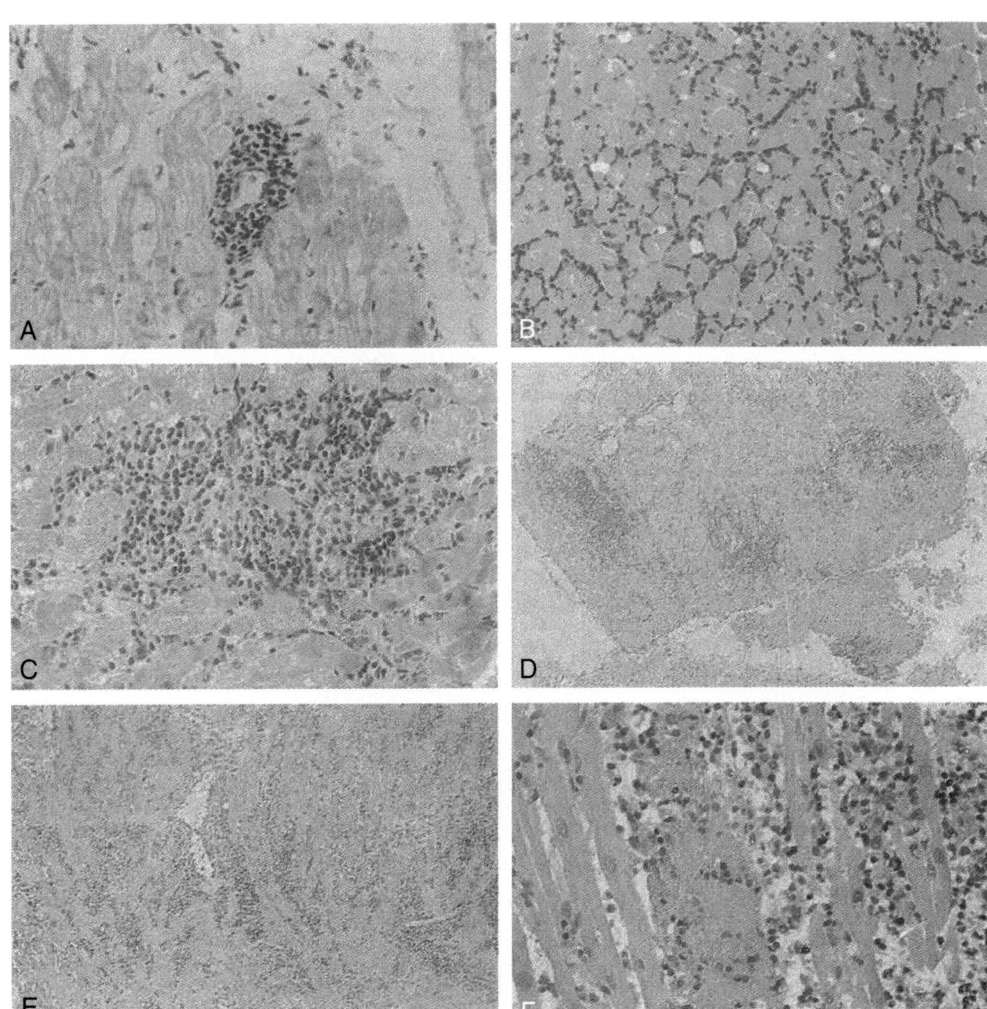

FIGURE 26–9 International Society for Heart and Lung Transplantation (ISHLT) grades of rejection. **A,** Grade 1A: Focal perivascular lymphocytic infiltrate without damage to adjacent myocytes. **B,** Grade 1B: Diffuse interstitial lymphocytic infiltrate without damage to adjacent myocytes. **C,** Grade 2: One focus of dense lymphocytic infiltrate with associated myocyte damage. **D,** Grade 3A: Multiple foci of dense lymphocytic infiltrates with associated myocyte damage. There are intervening areas of uninvolved myocardium. **E,** Grade 3B: Diffuse infiltrate with associated myocyte damage. **F,** Grade 4: Polymorphous infiltrate with extensive myocyte damage, edema, and hemorrhage. (Hematoxylin & eosin.) (From Winters GL, Schoen FJ: Pathology of cardiac transplantation. *In* Silver MD, Gotlieb AI, Schoen FJ [eds]: Cardiovascular Pathology. 3rd ed. Philadelphia, WB Saunders, 2001, pp 725-762.)

The lymphoproliferative malignancies occurring in the context of transplantation (commonly known as *posttransplant lymphoproliferative disorder*) consist mostly of abnormal proliferations of B lymphocytes, and most appear to be driven by the Epstein-Barr virus. The clinical presentations are quite heterogeneous and differ from the well-recognized clinical patterns seen with other lymphomas, with more than 70 percent involving extranodal sites. Reduction of immunosuppression can lead to durable tumor regression in these patients, but this maneuver is truly a "double-edged sword" when used with a life-sustaining allograft such as the heart. Traditional cytotoxic chemotherapy does not have a good response rate with these malignancies, and newer targeted antibody approaches, currently with the anti-CD20 monoclonal antibody rituximab, have been encouraging.[31-33]

Graft Coronary Artery Disease

The development of a chronologically premature and anatomically quite diffuse and often rapidly progressive obliterative pattern of coronary artery disease, a vascular disease that is limited to the allograft, is currently the major complication limiting truly long-term survival in cardiac transplant recipients (see also Chap. 35). Its etiology is likely complex and is thought to involve an interplay of immunologic (HLA and other mismatches), infectious (CMV and others), and more usual (lipid status, diabetes, and other) factors.

Some angiographic evidence of this disease is present by 1 year posttransplant in 10 percent of patients, and 50 percent have some evidence by 5 years (Fig. 26–10). In recent years the use of intravascular ultrasound has provided earlier and more sensitive diagnosis of the intimal thickening that characterizes the disease, and the technique has provided a surrogate endpoint for clinical trials of newer immunosuppressive agents designed to evaluate changes in the incidence of the disease consequent to changed immunosuppression (Fig. 26–11).[34]

As noted earlier, as transplant recipients generally have a high degree of both afferent and efferent denervation, they often do not experience the subjective sensation of angina pectoris. Ischemic sequelae in these patients can include arrhythmias leading to sudden death as well as ischemic left ventricular dysfunction leading to the clinical syndrome of heart failure. The very diffuseness of the disease makes the use of standard revascularization with percutaneous or surgical interventions palliative at best. The prognosis once graft

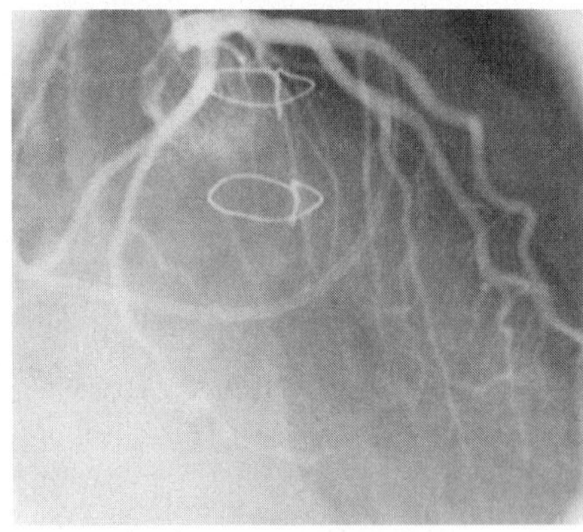

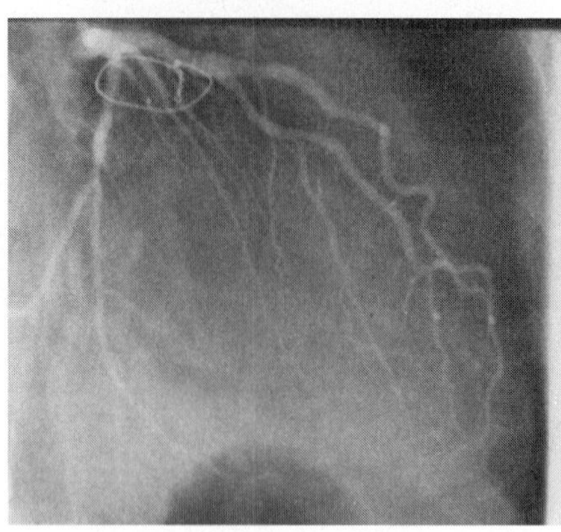

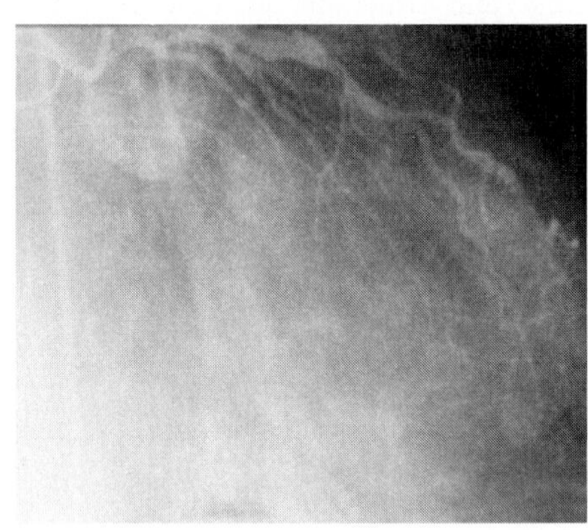

FIGURE 26–10 Graft coronary artery disease—progression by angiography. Serial angiograms obtained at time of transplantation (year 0) and at years 2 and 4 following engraftment show progressive "pruning" of the distal vessels and, by year 4, segmental stenoses of the proximal epicardial coronary arteries. (Courtesy of James C. Fang, Brigham and Women's Hospital, Boston, MA.)

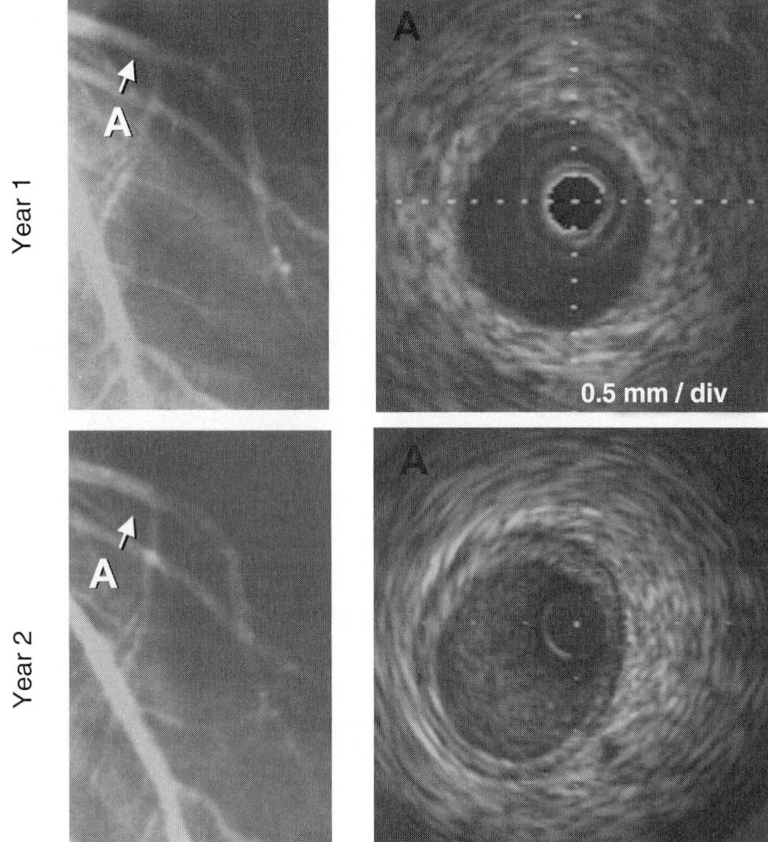

FIGURE 26–11 Graft coronary artery disease—appearance by angiography and intravascular ultrasound. The **left** panels show angiograms obtained on a transplanted heart at years 1 and 2 following engraftment. The **right** panels show intravascular ultrasound images obtained at the same time at the points labeled A in the angiogram. Note the progression of concentric intimal thickening that produces narrowing but not the appearance of a focal stenosis on the angiogram. These paired images show that the angiogram can underestimate the degree of intimal thickening in allograft coronary artery disease owing to the concentric nature of the intimal expansion. (From Lee RT, Braunwald E [eds]: Atlas of Cardiac Imaging. Philadelphia, Churchill Livingstone, 1998.

vasculopathy has led to clinical events is poor, with one study finding only 18 to 20 percent survival in heart transplant recipients 1 year after an ischemic clinical event. No drug or agent has been shown to reverse this disease, and the only definitive therapy available is retransplantation. The overall survival rates reported after retransplantation late after a first transplant are slightly inferior to those after the first transplant, and the use of scarce donor hearts for this purpose is a somewhat contentious issue in the transplant community.

Drug-Related Toxicity

Each of the drugs used in the immunosuppressive regimen comes with its inherent toxicity profile and set of drug interactions. The class of drugs now known as *calcineurin inhibitors* (cyclosporine and tacrolimus) was introduced into clinical heart transplantation in 1980, and the introduction was followed by marked improvement in survival. The class has subsequently provided the cornerstone of otherwise variable immunosuppressive regimens. These drugs have potent inherent nephrotoxicity and have led to the development of end-stage renal disease in many patients despite meticulous monitoring of drug levels. Newer drugs with less nephrotoxicity (but, of course, other toxicities) may eventually replace calcineurin inhibitors.

Overall Results

ISHLT maintains a registry of information regarding nearly 63,000 heart transplants that have been performed worldwide; every year, an annual report is presented containing data regarding survival, risk factors for mortality, and posttransplant functional status.[1] The number of reported heart transplants continues to decline for the past several years (Fig. 26–12). This decline results almost entirely from a decrease in transplants reported by non-U.S. centers. The age distribution of heart transplant recipients has changed in recent years (Fig. 26–13). The proportion of recipients in the 50- to 64-year and greater than 65-year age ranges has increased whereas the proportion in the 35- to 49-year age range has decreased. The age distribution of heart transplant donors, however, has remained relatively stable during the past several years. The major diagnoses in adult heart transplants continue to be idiopathic cardiomyopathy and ischemic cardiomyopathy (Fig. 26–14).

Over the past 20 years, survival after heart transplantation has improved, with 1-year, 5-year, 10-year, and 20-year survival rates of 80, 66, 29, and 16 percent, respectively (Fig. 26–15). Patient half-life (i.e., time to 50 percent survival)

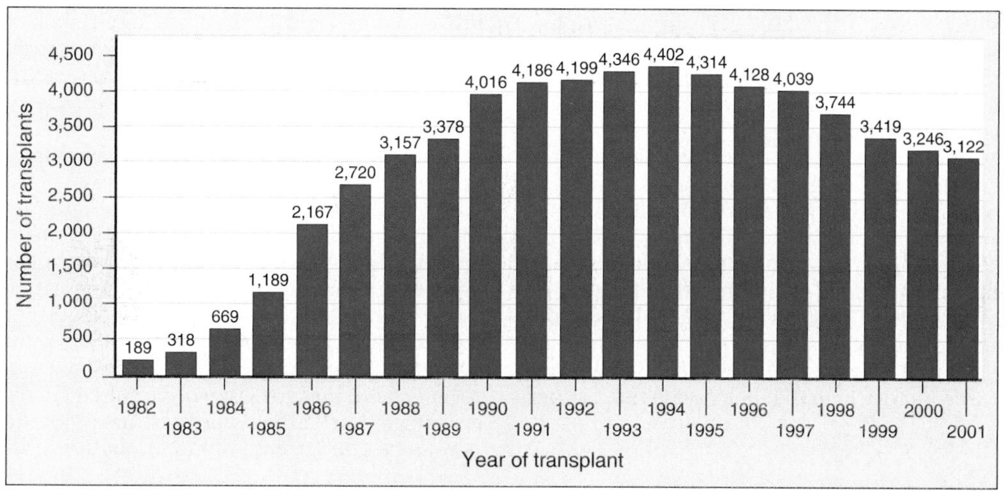

FIGURE 26–12 Number of heart transplants by year. (From Taylor DO, Edwards LB, Mohacsi PJ, et al: The registry of The International Society for Heart and Lung Transplantation: Twentieth official adult heart transplant report—2003. J Heart Lung Transplant 22:616, 2003.)

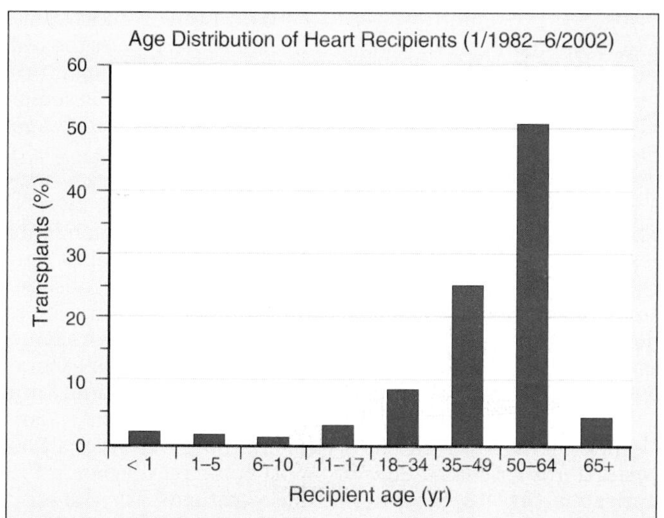

FIGURE 26–13 Age distribution of heart transplant recipients as reported between January 1982 and June 2002. (From Taylor DO, Edwards LB, Mohacsi PJ, et al: The registry of The International Society for Heart and Lung Transplantation: Twentieth official adult heart transplant report—2003. J Heart Lung Transplant 22:616, 2003.)

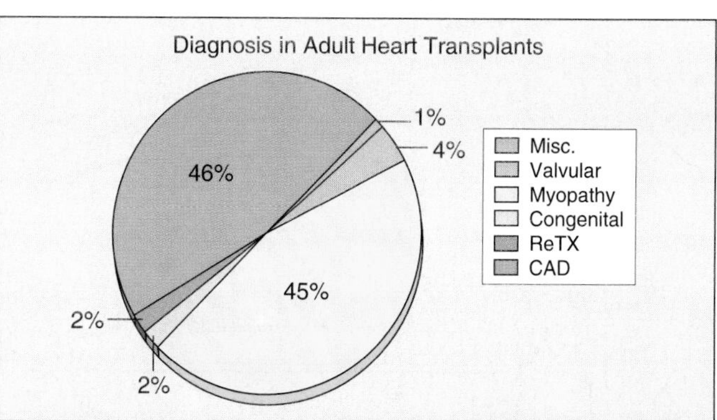

FIGURE 26–14 Diagnoses of adult heart transplant recipients. CAD = coronary artery disease; ReTX = retransplant. (From Taylor DO, Edwards LB, Mohacsi PJ, et al: The registry of The International Society for Heart and Lung Transplantation: Twentieth official adult heart transplant report—2003. J Heart Lung Transplant 22:616, 2003.)

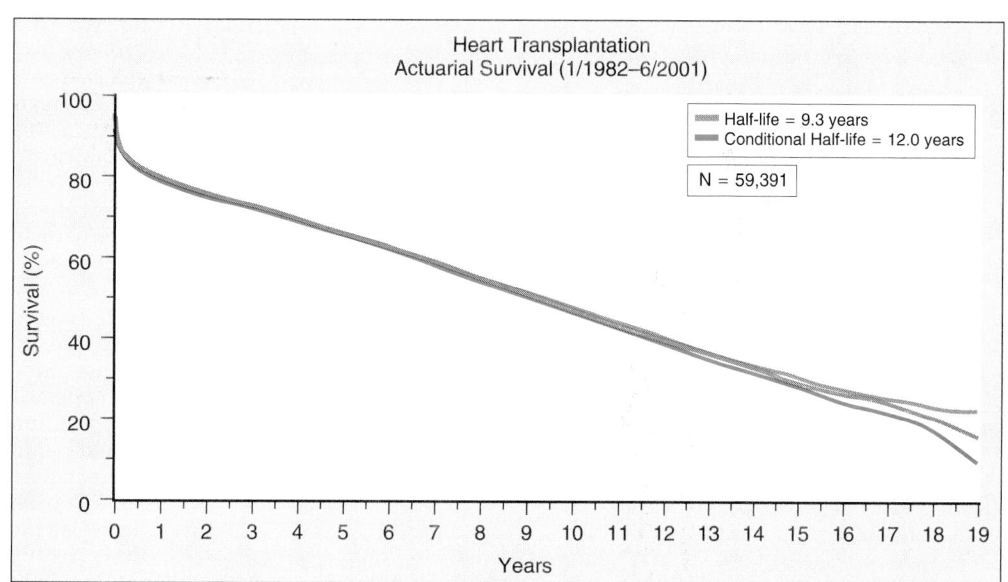

FIGURE 26–15 Actuarial survival for heart transplants performed between January 1982 and June 2001. (From Taylor DO, Edwards LB, Mohacsi PJ, et al: The registry of The International Society for Heart and Lung Transplantation: Twentieth official adult heart transplant report—2003. J Heart Lung Transplant 22:616, 2003.)

is 9.3 years. Survival rates in the first 2 years after transplantation have improved over the last 20 years, but late survival has changed little. When patients transplanted after 1982 are grouped into arbitrary 4- to 5-year eras, survival improves with each successive era (Fig. 26–16).

The ISHLT lists the following as major risk factors for 1-year mortality: underlying diagnosis of congenital heart disease, patient in hospital and/or on ventilator before transplant, PRA >10 percent, and dialysis. Additional risk factors include older donor age, older recipient age, increased donor heart ischemic time, and elevated recipient bilirubin or creatinine. While in the past, an underlying diagnosis of coronary artery disease, retransplantation, the presence of an intra-aortic balloon pump or ventricular assist device at the time of transplant, or a history of malignancy were risk factors for 1-year mortality, they are not risk factors in the most recent cohort of patients. Five-year mortality risk factors include graft coronary artery disease within the first posttransplant year, infection prior to transplant discharge or during the first posttransplant year, cerebrovascular disease at transplant, insulin-dependent diabetes, and underlying diagnosis of coronary artery disease.

Approximately 40 percent of patients are hospitalized in the first posttransplant year, often for treatment of rejection or infection. By the second posttransplant year, only 20 percent are hospitalized. The vast majority report good functional status after transplantation. Nevertheless, less than 40 percent of heart transplant recipients return to work after transplantation. Thus, despite the lack of sufficient donor organs, and the growing importance of device therapy for end-stage heart failure, cardiac transplantation can offer independence and a relatively high quality of life to many.

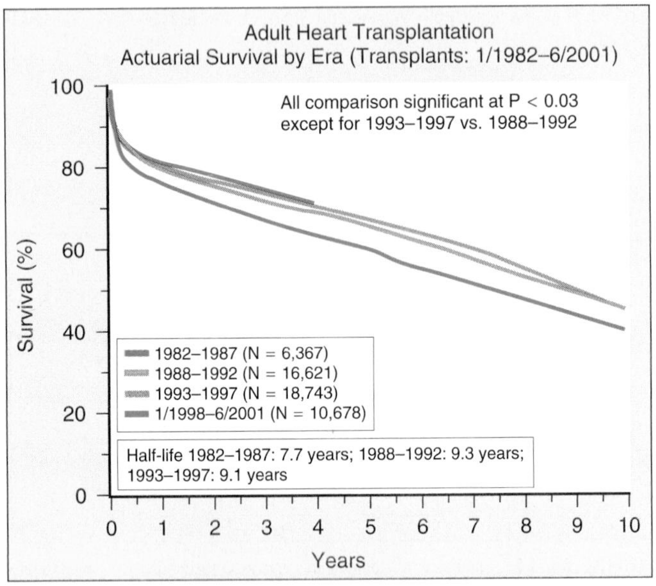

Adult Heart Transplantation
Actuarial Survival by Era (Transplants: 1/1982–6/2001)
All comparison significant at P < 0.03 except for 1993–1997 vs. 1988–1992
Survival (%)
Years
1982–1987 (N = 6,367)
1988–1992 (N = 16,621)
1993–1997 (N = 18,743)
1/1998–6/2001 (N = 10,678)
Half-life 1982–1987: 7.7 years; 1988–1992: 9.3 years; 1993–1997: 9.1 years

FIGURE 26–16 Actuarial survival for heart transplants performed between January 1982 and June 2001 by era of transplantation. (From Taylor DO, Edwards LB, Mohacsi PJ, et al: The registry of The International Society for Heart and Lung Transplantation: Twentieth official adult heart transplant report—2003. J Heart Lung Transplant 22:616, 2003.)

Heart-Lung Transplantation

Since the initial clinical transplants performed by Reitz and associates at Stanford in 1981, the field of heart-lung transplantation has evolved dramatically, particularly over the last several years. Heart-lung transplantation was developed initially for patients suffering from severe pulmonary vascular disease, specifically primary pulmonary hypertension and Eisenmenger syndrome secondary to congenital heart disease. A total of 2190 heart-lung transplants were performed between January 1992 and June 2002 (Fig. 26–17). The diagnostic profile of heart-lung transplant recipients reported to the Registry of the ISHLT through 2002 lists pulmonary hypertension secondary to congenital heart disease as the most frequent diagnosis, accounting for 32 percent of these procedures ($n = 705$). Primary pulmonary hypertension associated with irreversible right heart failure is the second most common indication for heart-lung transplantation, with 24 percent of recipients carrying this diagnosis ($n = 526$). Despite the widespread use of bilateral lung transplantation, cystic fibrosis remains the third most common diagnosis, the indication for 16 percent of these patients ($n = 341$).[35] However, the trend over the past few years has been to reserve combined heart and lung transplantation for patients who are not candidates for double-lung transplantation and cardiac repair because of concomitant end-stage pulmonary and cardiac disease processes.

The technique of heart-lung transplantation has also evolved over the last several years. The standard biatrial technique for the heart transplant has been converted to the bicaval technique (see Figs. 26–6 through 26–8). The physiological advantages of the bicaval technique have already been discussed in the heart transplant section and apply to heart-lung transplantation as well. The second major change in the operative technique is the positioning of the pulmonary hila anterior to the phrenic nerve pedicle.[36] This modification requires less posterior mediastinal dissection, which decreases the rates of phrenic and vagus nerve injury. It also affords

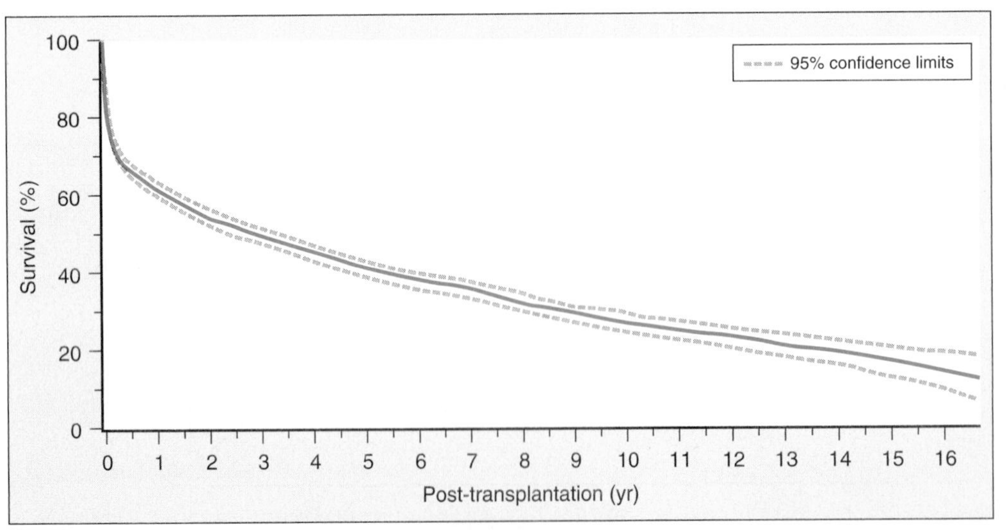

FIGURE 26–17 Actuarial curve showing survival rate after heart-lung transplantation (January 1992 to June 2002).(From Taylor Do, Edwards LB, Mohacsi PJ, et al: The registry of The International Society for Heart and Lung Transplantation: Twentieth official adult heart transplant report—2003. J Heart Lung Transplant 22:616, 2003.)

easier access to the posterior mediastinum for inspection of bleeding while still on CPB.

The actuarial survival for adult heart-lung transplant recipients at 1, 5, and 10 years were 61, 40, and 25 percent, respectively (see Fig. 26–17).[35] Recipients with Eisenmenger syndrome have had significantly better survival rates than those with other congenital anomalies or primary pulmonary hypertension. The cause of early mortality include graft failure, non-CMV infection, and technical complications, together accounting for 80 percent of the deaths. After the first year of transplantation, the most common cause of death is chronic rejection manifested as obliterative bronchiolitis (OB). The overall prevalence of OB in patients surviving heart-lung transplantation longer than 3 months was 64 percent, with an overall mortality greater than 70 percent after 5 years of follow-up.[37] The incidence and severity of transplant coronary artery disease are significantly less when compared with the heart transplantation population but affect approximately 10 percent of patients within 5 years following transplantation.

Heart-lung transplantation continues to be an accepted therapy for selected patients with end-stage cardiopulmonary disease. The goal of restoring the function of heart-lung transplantation without significant long-term morbidity and mortality will require considerable advances in immunosuppression and immunotolerance.

REFERENCES

1. Taylor DO, Edwards LB, Mohacsi PJ, et al: The registry of the International Society for Heart and Lung Transplantation: Twentieth Offiicial Adult Heart Transplant Report 2003. J Heart Lung Transplant 22:616-624, 2003.

Heart Transplantation: The Operation

2. Aziz TM, Burgess MI, El Gamel A, et al: Orthotopic cardiac transplantation technique: A survey of current practice. Ann Thorac Surg 68:1242-1246, 1999.
3. Aziz T, Burgess M, Khafagy R, et al: Bicaval and standard techniques in orthotopic heart transplantation: Medium-term experience in cardiac performance and survival. J Thorac Cardiovasc Surg 118:115-122, 1999.
4. Traversi E, Pozzoli M, Grande A, et al: The bicaval anastomosis technique for orthotopic heart transplantation yields better atrial function than the standard technique: An echocardiographic automatic boundary detection study. J Heart Lung Transplant 17:1065-1074, 1998.
5. Miniati DN, Robbins RC: Techniques in orthotopic cardiac transplantation: A review. Cardiol Rev 9:131-136, 2001.
6. Aziz TM, Saad RA, Burgess MI, et al: Clinical signifiicance of tricuspid valve dysfuntion after orthotopic heart transplantation. J Heart Lung Transplant 21:1101-1108, 2002.
7. Aziz TM, Burgess MI, Rahman AN, et al: Risk factors for tricuspid valve regurgitation after orthotopic heart transplantation. Ann Thorac Surg 68:1247-1251, 1999.
8. Sze DY, Robbins RC, Semba CP, et al: Superior vena cava syndrome after heart transplantation: Percutaneous treatment of a complication of bicaval anastomoses. J Thorac Cardiovasc Surg 116:253-261, 1998.

Recipient Selection

9. Aaronson KD, Schwartz JS, Chen T-M, et al: Development and prospective validation of a clinical index to predict survival in ambulatory patients referred for cardiac transplant evaluation. Circulation 95:2660-2667, 1997.
10. Mancini DM, Eisen H, Kussmaul W, et al: Value of peak exercise consumption for optimal timing of cardiac transplantation in ambulatory patients with heart failure. Circulation 83:778-786, 1991.
11. Osada N, Chaitman BR, Miller LW, et al: Cardiopulmonary exercise testing identifiie low-risk patients with heart failure and severely impaired exercise capacity considered for heart transplantation. J Am Coll Cardiol 31:577-582, 1998.
12. Myers J, Gullestad L, Vagelos R, et al: Clinical, hemodynamic, and cardiopulmonary exercise test determinants of survival in patients referred for evaluation of heart failure. Ann Intern Med 129:286-293, 1998.
13. Cimato TR, Jessup M: Recipient selection in cardiac transplantation: Contraindications and risk factors for mortality. J Heart Lung Transplant 21:1161-1173, 2002.
14. Costard-Jackle, Fowler MB: Inflluence of preoperative pulmonary artery pressure on motality after heart transplantation: Test of potential reversibility of pulmonary hypertension with nitroprusside is useful in defiining a high-risk group. J Am Coll Cardio 19:48-54, 1992.
15. Natale ME, Pina I: Evaluation of pulmonary hypertension in heart transplant candidates. Curr Opin Cardiol 18:136-140, 2003.
16. Haraldsson A, Kieler-Jensen N, Nathorst-Westfelt U, et al: Comparison of inhaled nitric oxide and inhaled aerosolized prostacyclin in the evaluation of heart transplant candidates with elevated pulmonary vascular resistance. Chest 114:780-786, 1998.
17. Sablotzki A, Hentschel T, Gruenig I, et al: Hemodynamic effects of inhaled aerosolized iloprost and inhaled nitric oxide in heart transplant candidates with elevated pulmonary vascular resistance. Eur J Cardiothorac Surg 22:746-752, 2002.
18. Zaroff JG, Rosengard BR, Armstrong WF, et al: Consensus conference report: Maximizing Use of Organs Recovered from the Cadaver Donor—Cardiac Recommendations, March 28-29, 2001, Crystal City, VA. Circulation 106:836-841, 2002.
19. Harringer W, Haverich A: Heart and heart-lung transplantation: Standards and improvements. World J Surg 26:218-225, 2002.
20. Del Rizzo DF, Menkis AH, Pfllugfelder PW, et al: The role of donor age and ischemi time on survival following orthotopic heart transplantation. J Heart Lung Transplant 18:310-319, 1999.
21. Wheeldon DR, Potter CD, Oduro A, et al: Transforming the "unacceptable" donor: Outcomes from the adoption of a standardized donor management technique. J Heart Lung Transplant 14:734-742, 1995.
22. Stoica SC, Satchithananda DK, Charman S, et al: Swan-Ganz catheter assessment of donor hearts: Outcome of organs with borderline hemodynamics. J Heart Lung Transplant 21:615-622, 2002.
23. Jahania MS, Sanchez JA, Narayan P, et al: Heart preservation for transplantation: Principles and strategies. Ann Thorac Surg 68:1983-1987, 1999.
24. Beniaminovitz A, Itescu S, Lietz K, et al: Prevention of rejection in cardiac transplantation by blockade of the interleukin-2 receptor with a monoclonal antibody. N Engl J Med 342:613-619, 2000.

Physiology of the Transplanted Heart

25. Givertz MM, Hartley LH, Colucci W: Long-term sequential changes in exercise capacity and chronotropic responsiveness after cardiac transplantation. Circulation 96:232-237, 1997.
26. Osada N, Chaitman BR, Donohue TJ, et al: Long-term cardiopulmonary exercise performance after heart transplantation. Am J Cardiol 79:451-456, 1997.
27. Mettauer B, Zhao QM, Epailly E, et al: Vo_2 kinetics reveal a central limitation at the onset of subthreshold exercise in heart transplant recipients. J Appl Physiol 88:1228-1238, 2000.
28. Bengel FM, Ueberfuhr P, Schiepel N, et al: Effect of sympathetic reinnervation on cardiac performance after heart transplantation. N Engl J Med 345:731-738, 2001.
29. Billingham ME, Cary NR, Hammond ME, et al: A working formulation for the standardization of nomenclature in the diagnosis of heart and lung rejection: Heart Rejection Study Group. The International Society for Heart Transplantation. J Heart Transplant 9:587-593, 1990.
30. Penn I: Occurrence of cancers in immunosuppressed organ transplant recipients. Clin Transpl 11:147-158, 1998.
31. Cook RC, Connors JM, Gascoyne RD, et al: Treatment of post-transplant lymphoproliferative disease with rituximab monoclonal antibody after lung transplantation. Lancet 354:1698-1699, 1999.
32. Zilz ND, Olson LJ, McGregor CG: Treatment of post-transplant lymphoproliferative disorder with monoclonal CD20 antibody (rituximab) after heart transplantation. J Heart Lung Transplant 20:770-772, 2001.
33. Dotti G, Rambaldi A, Fiocchi R, et al: Anti-CD20 antibody (rituximab) administration in patients with late-occurring lymphomas after solid organ transplant. Haematologica 86:618-623, 2001.
34. Kobashigawa JA: First-year intravascular ultrasound results as a surrogate marker for outcomes after heart transplantation. J Heart Lung Transplant 22:711-714, 2003.

Heart-Lung Transplantation

35. Trulock EP, Edwards LB, Taylor DO, et al: The registry of the International Society for Heart and Lung Transplantation: Twentieth Offiicial Adult Lung and Heart-Lung Transplant Report—2003. J Heart Lung Transplant 22:625-635, 2003.
36. Lick SD, Copeland JG, Rosado LJ, et al: Simplifiied technique of heart-lung transplanttion. Ann Thorac Surg 59:1592-1593, 1995.
37. Reichenspurner H, Girgis RE, Robbins RC, et al: Stanford experience with obliterative bronchiolitis after lung and heart-lung transplantation. Ann Thorac Surg 62:1467-1472, 1996.

PART IV

Arrhythmias, Sudden Death, and Syncope

CHAPTER 27

Genesis of Cardiac Arrhythmias: Electrophysiological Considerations

Michael Rubart • Douglas P. Zipes

Anatomy of the Cardiac Conduction System

Sinus Node

In humans, the sinus node is a spindle-shaped structure composed of a fibrous tissue matrix with closely packed cells. It is 10 to 20 mm long, 2 to 3 mm wide, and thick, tending to narrow caudally toward the inferior vena cava. It lies less than 1 mm from the epicardial surface, laterally in the right atrial sulcus terminalis at the junction of the superior vena cava and right atrium (Figs. 27–1 and 27–2). The artery supplying the sinus node branches from the right (55 to 60 percent of the time) or the left (40 to 45 percent) circumflex coronary artery and approaches the node from a clockwise or counterclockwise direction around the superior vena caval–right atrial junction.

CELLULAR STRUCTURE. Cells from the sinoatrial node region exhibit a wide variety of morphologies, including spindle- and spider-shaped cells, rod-shaped atrial cells with clear striations, and small round cells corresponding to endothelial cells.[1] Only the spindle- and spider-shaped cells exhibit the typical electrophysiological characteristics of pacemaker cells, including the presence of the hyperpolarization-activated current, I_f,[2] and absence of the inwardly rectifying potassium current, I_{K1}, as well as spontaneous beating under physiological conditions.[3,4]

GAP JUNCTIONS AND SINOATRIAL COUPLING. The sinoatrial node requires a delicate balance of intercellular electrical coupling in order to maintain its function as a pacemaker. Excess electrical coupling depresses sinus node automaticity because the sinus node membrane potential is damped by the surrounding atrial myocardium to a more negative potential than the normal maximal diastolic potential, thereby inhibiting spontaneous diastolic depolarization (see Fig. 27–14). Too little coupling may prevent impulse transmission to the adjacent atrial muscle. Restriction of the hyperpolarizing influence of the atrial muscle on the sinus node while maintaining impulse exit into the crista terminalis is achieved by the composition and spatial organization of connexins, proteins that form gap junction channels responsible for intercellular current fluxes (see under Intercalated Discs). Connexin40 and connexin45, but not connexin43, are expressed in the central sinus node (Fig. 27–3). The major part of the crista terminalis–sinus node border exhibits a sharp demarcation boundary of connexin43-expressing atrial myocytes and connexin40/connexin45-expressing myocytes. On the endocardial site a transitional zone between the crista terminalis and the peripheral node exists in which connexin45 and connexin43 are colocalized.[5] This colocalization of different connexin isoforms raises the possibility that individual gap junctional channels in the transitional zone are formed by more than one connexin isoform.[1] These disparate connexin phenotypes may create specific types of hybrid channels with rectifying electrical properties that ensure the maintenance of sinus node pacemaker activity but diminish electrotonic interference from the atrial muscle.[1,6,7]

FUNCTION. Very probably, no single cell in the sinus node serves as *the* pacemaker. Rather, sinus nodal cells function as electrically coupled oscillators that discharge synchronously because of mutual entrainment. Thus, faster discharging cells are slowed by cells firing more slowly, and they themselves are sped so that a "democratically derived" discharge rate occurs.[8] The interaction depends on the degree of coupling and the electrophysiological characteristics of the individual sinoatrial node cell. The resulting rate is not just a simple average of each of the cells. With an individual pacemaker cell coupled to an average of five other cells,[8] each with potentially different electrophysiological properties, the resulting discharge rate is not obvious. In humans, sinus rhythm may result from impulse origin at widely separated sites, with two or three individual

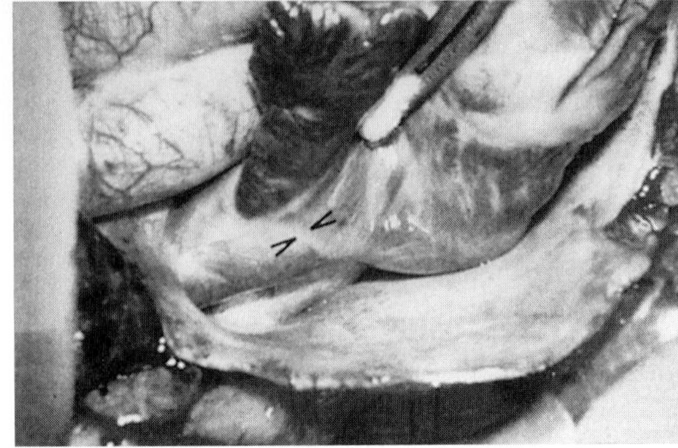

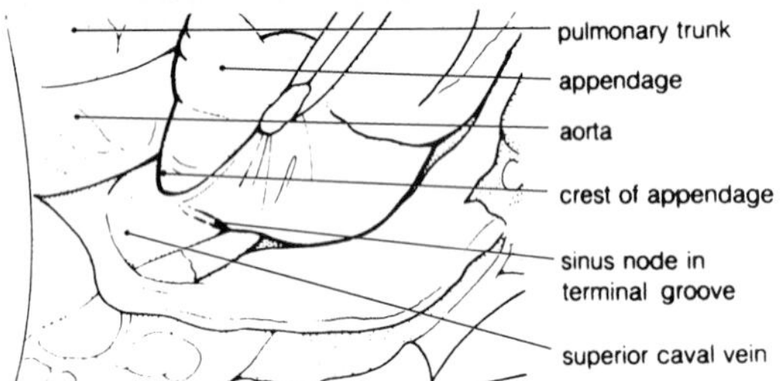

FIGURE 27–1 The human sinus node. This photograph, taken in the operating room, shows the location of the normal cigar-shaped sinus node along the lateral border of the terminal groove at the superior vena cava–atrial junction (arrowheads). (From Anderson RH, Wilcox BR, Becker AE: Anatomy of the normal heart. *In* Hurst JW, Anderson RH, Becker AE, Wilcox BR [eds]: Atlas of the Heart. New York, Gower, 1988, p 1.2.)

wave fronts created that merge to form a single, widely disseminated wave front.[8] Modulated parasystole can occur.

INNERVATION. The sinus node is densely innervated with postganglionic adrenergic and cholinergic nerve terminals.[9] Discrete vagal efferent pathways innervate both the sinus and atrioventricular (AV) regions of the dog and nonhuman primate. Most efferent vagal fibers to the atria appear to converge first at a single fat pad that is located between the medial portion of the superior vena cava and the aortic root, superior to the right pulmonary artery; the fibers then project onto two other fat pads found at the inferior vena cava-left atrial junction and the right pulmonary vein-atrial junction and subsequently project to both atria. Vagal fibers to the sinus and AV nodes also converge at the superior vena cava–aortic root fat pad before projection to the right pulmonary vein and inferior vena cava fat pads.[9] The concentration of norepinephrine is two to four times higher in atrial than in ventricular tissue in canine and guinea pig hearts. Although the sinus nodal region contains amounts of norepinephrine equivalent to those in other parts of the right atrium, acetylcholine, acetylcholinesterase, and choline acetyltransferase (the enzyme necessary for the synthesis of acetylcholine) have all been found in greatest concentration in the sinus node, with the next highest concentration in the right and then the left atrium. The concentration of acetylcholine in the ventricles is only 20 to 50 percent of that in the atria.

Neurotransmitters modulate the sinus node discharge rate by stimulation of beta-adrenergic and muscarinic receptors. Both $beta_1$ and $beta_2$ adrenoceptor subtypes are present in the sinoatrial node. Human sinoatrial nodes contain a more than threefold greater density of beta-adrenergic and muscarinic cholinergic receptors than adjacent atrial tissue.[8] The functional significance of beta adrenoceptor subtype diversity in the sinus node is unclear. Binding of receptor agonists released from sympathetic nerve terminals causes a positive chronotropic response through a $beta_1$ receptor–activated pathway involving the stimulatory guanosine triphosphate (GTP) regulatory protein (G_s), activation of adenylyl cyclase, intracellular accumulation of cyclic adenosine monophosphate (cAMP), stimulation of cAMP-dependent protein kinase A, and phosphorylation of target proteins (including the L-type Ca^{2+} channel, the channels underlying I_f, and the ryanodine-sensitive Ca^{2+} release channel [ryanodine receptor] in the sarcoplasmic reticulum membrane[10]). The second messenger pathway underlying $beta_2$ receptor activation–induced heart rate increase and the key target proteins are currently unknown but most likely involve an inhibitory GTP regulatory protein (G_i).[11] The negative chronotropic response of vagal stimulation is mediated by acetylcholine binding to and ensuing activation of M2 muscarinic receptors. Membrane currents regulated by muscarinic receptor activation include the acetylcholine- and adenosine-sensitive K^+ current ($I_{K(Ach,Ado)}$; see Table 22–3), $I_{Ca,L}$, and I_f. The effect of muscarinic receptor agonist in activating $I_{K(Ach,Ado)}$ is mediated by direct interaction of a G-protein subunit with the $K_{(Ach,Ado)}$ channel and does not require second messengers.[12] Activation of $I_{K(Ach,Ado)}$ causes hyperpolarization of the sinoatrial node cell membrane, resulting in a reduced rate of diastolic depolarization. Muscarinic receptor activation–mediated effects on $I_{Ca,L}$ and I_f are primarily due to a reduction in the intracellular cAMP level, thereby antagonizing the positive chronotropic effects of beta adrenoceptor stimulation.

Besides its negative chronotropic effect, acetylcholine also prolongs intranodal conduction time, at times to the point of sinus nodal exit block. Acetylcholine increases whereas norepinephrine decreases refractoriness in the center of the sinus node. The phase (timing) in the cardiac cycle at which vagal discharge occurs and the background sympathetic tone importantly influence vagal effects on the sinus rate and conduction (see later). After cessation of vagal stimulation, sinus nodal automatically may accelerate transiently (postvagal tachycardia). The neurotransmitters neuropeptide Y (NPY) and vasoactive intestinal peptide (VIP) are localized in sympathetic and parasympathetic nerve terminals, respectively. VIP reversibly increases I_f, whereas NPY reversibly decreases I_f.[13] The role of other peripheral neurotransmitters (such as calcitonin gene-related peptide, substance P) in controlling sinus node electrophysiology is unclear.

Internodal and Intraatrial Conduction

Whether impulses travel from the sinus to the AV node over preferentially conducting pathways has been contested. Anatomical evidence has been interpreted to indicate the presence of three intraatrial pathways. The *anterior internodal pathway* begins at the anterior margin of the sinus node and curves anteriorly around the superior vena cava to enter the anterior interatrial band, called the *Bachmann bundle.* This band continues to the left atrium, with the anterior internodal pathway entering the superior margin of the AV node. The *Bachmann bundle* is a large muscle bundle that appears to conduct the cardiac impulse preferentially from the right to the left atrium. The *middle internodal tract* begins at the superior and posterior margins of the sinus node, travels behind the superior vena cava to the crest of the interatrial septum, and descends in the interatrial septum to the superior margin of the AV node. The *posterior internodal tract* starts at the posterior margin of the sinus node and travels posteriorly around the superior vena cava and along the crista terminalis to the eustachian ridge and then into the interatrial septum above the coronary sinus, where it joins the posterior portion of the AV node. Some fibers from all three tracts bypass the crest of the AV node and enter its more distal segment. These groups of internodal tissue are best referred to as *internodal atrial myocardium,* not tracts, because they do not appear to be histologically discrete specialized tracts, only plain atrial myocardium.

Preferential internodal conduction, that is, higher conduction velocity between the nodes in some parts of the atrium than in other parts, does exist and may be due to fiber orientation, size, geometry, or other factors rather than to specialized tracts located between the nodes. Impulse propagation from the atrium to the AV node occurs through multiple preferential input pathways. On the basis of their conduction velocities, these inputs are divided into fast, slow, and intermediate pathways. Notably, the atrial anterosuperior and posteroinferior inputs or approaches to the AV node are the anatomical substrates constituting the fast and slow pathways of AV nodal reentry.[14,15] The reentrant circuit of the slow/fast type begins counterclockwise with block in the fast pathway located at the apex of the Koch triangle, delay in the slow pathway located near the coronary sinus, then exit from the AV node to the fast pathway and return to the slow pathway through atrial tissue along the base of Koch's triangle. The reentrant circuit of the fast/slow type is clockwise. The term "triangle of Koch," however, has to be used with caution because histological studies of anatomically normal adult hearts demonstrated that the tendon of Todaro, which forms one side of the triangle of Koch, is absent in about two-thirds of hearts.[16]

The Atrioventricular Junctional Area and Intraventricular Conduction System

The normal AV junctional area (Figs. 27–4 and 27–5) can be divided into distinct regions: the transitional cell zone, also called nodal approaches; the compact portion, or the AV node itself; and the penetrating part of the AV bundle (His bundle), which continues as a nonbranching portion.

TRANSITIONAL CELL ZONE. In the rabbit AV node, the transitional cells or nodal approaches are located in posterior, superficial, and deep groups of cells. They differ histologically from atrial myocardium and connect the latter with the compact portion of the AV node. Some fibers may pass from the posterior internodal tract to the distal portion of the AV node or His bundle and provide the anatomical substrate for conduction to bypass AV nodal slowing. However, the importance of this structure is unclear.

The Atrioventricular Node

The compact portion of the AV node is a superficial structure lying just beneath the right atrial endocardium, anterior to the ostium of the coronary sinus, and directly above the insertion of the septal leaflet of the tricuspid valve. It is at the apex of a triangle formed by the tricuspid annulus and the tendon of Todaro, which originates in the central fibrous body and passes posteriorly through the atrial septum to continue with the eustachian valve (see Figs. 27–4 and 27–5; however, see previous comments on the triangle of Koch).[14,15] The compact portion of the AV node is divided from and becomes the penetrating portion of the His bundle at the point where it enters the central fibrous body. In 85 to 90 percent of human hearts, the arterial supply to the AV node is a branch from the right coronary artery that originates at the posterior intersection of the AV and interventricular grooves (crux). A branch of the circumflex coronary artery provides the AV nodal artery in the remaining hearts. Fibers in the lower part of the AV node may exhibit automatic impulse formation. The main function of the AV node is modulation of atrial impulse transmission to the ventricles, thereby coordinating atrial and ventricular contractions (Fig. 27–6).

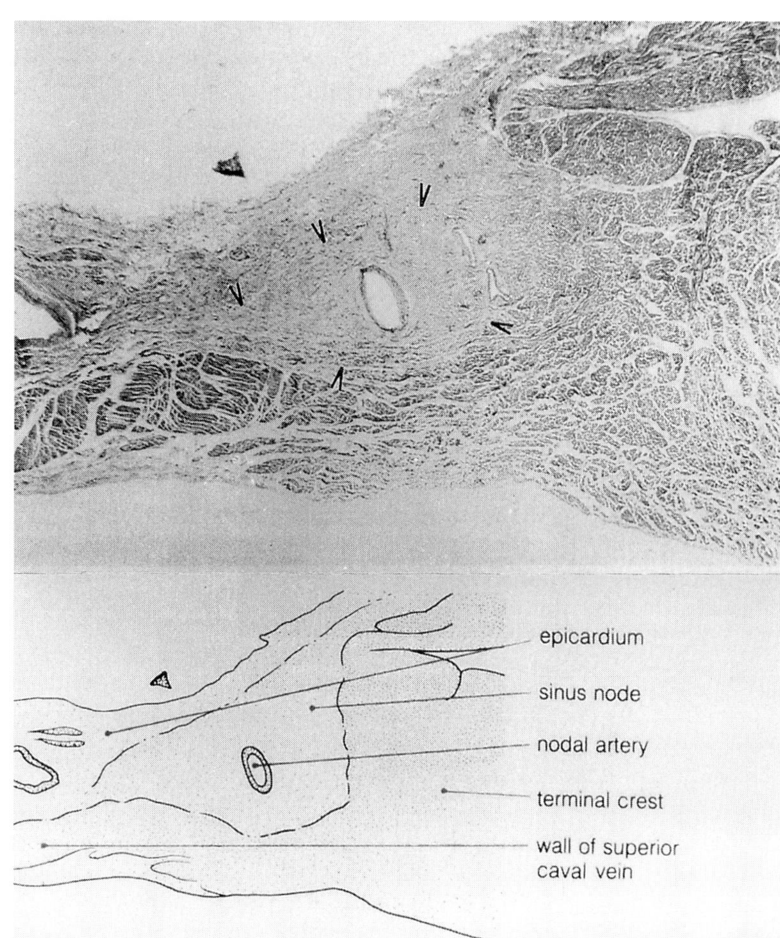

FIGURE 27–2 Histological section taken at right angles to the cigar-shaped sinus node shows that in short axis, the node is a wedge-shaped structure located between the wall of the superior vena cava and the terminal crest. Discrete boundaries between the sinus node and atrial muscle are noted (arrowheads). The node is penetrated by the sinus nodal artery. (From Anderson RH, Wilcox BR, Becker AE: Anatomy of the normal heart. *In* Hurst JW, Anderson RH, Becker AE, Wilcox BR [eds]: Atlas of the Heart. New York, Gower, 1988, p 1.2.)

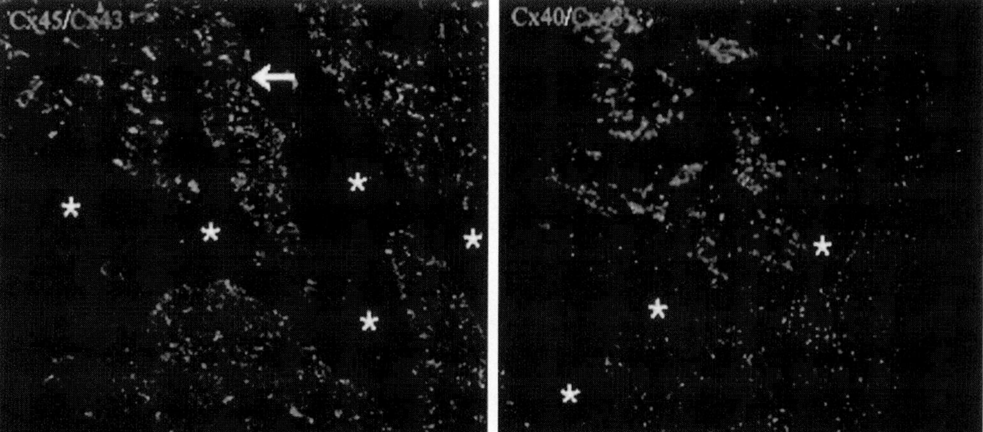

FIGURE 27–3 Sections through the sinoatrial node double labeled with connexin45 (Cx45) and Cx43 **(left)** and Cx43 with Cx40 **(right)**. Regions positive for Cx40/Cx45 (small punctate green signals) showing no detectable Cx43 signal (red) are sharply demarcated from adjacent Cx43-expressing regions of the crista terminalis. A zone of connective tissue (asterisks) contributes to separation between the zones, although elsewhere (arrow) the zones seem to be more closely approximated. (From Coppen SR, Kodama I, Boyett MR, et al: Connexin45, a major connexin of the rabbit sino-atrial node, is co-expressed with connexin43 in a restricted zone at the nodal–crista terminalis border. J Histochem Cytochem 47:907, 1999.)

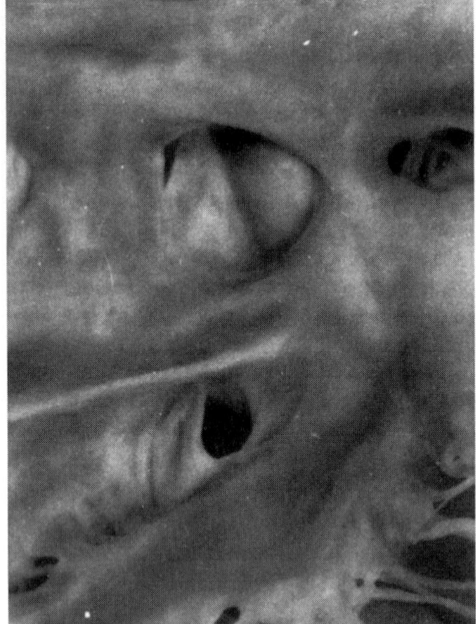

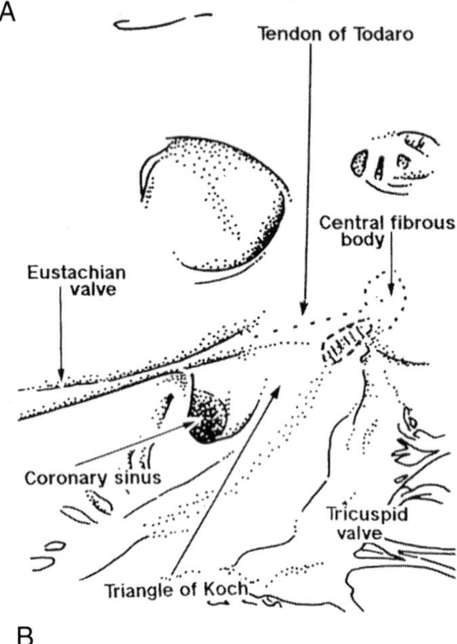

FIGURE 27–4 **A,** hotograph of a normal human heart showing the anatomical landmarks of the triangle of Koch. This triangle is delimited by the tendon of Todaro superiorly, which is the fibrous commissure of the flap guarding the openings of the inferior vena cava and coronary sinus, by the attachment of the septal leaflet of the tricuspid valve inferiorly, and by the mouth of the coronary sinus at the base. **B,** The stippled area adjacent to the central fibrous body is the approximate site of the compact atrioventricular node. (From Janse MJ, Anderson RH, McGuire MA, et al: "AV nodal" reentry: I. "AV nodal" reentry revisited. J Cardiovasc Electrophysiol 4:561, 1993.)

The Bundle of His, or Penetrating Portion of the Atrioventricular Bundle

This structure connects with the distal part of the compact AV node, perforates the central fibrous body, and continues through the annulus fibrosis, where it is called the nonbranching portion as it penetrates the membranous septum (see Fig. 27–5). Proximal cells of the penetrating portion are heterogeneous and resemble those of the compact AV node; distal cells are similar to cells in the proximal bundle branches. Connective tissue of the central fibrous body and membranous septum encloses the penetrating portion of the AV bundle, which may send out extensions into the central fibrous body.[17] However, large well-formed fasciculoventricular connections between the penetrating portion of the AV bundle and the ventricular septal crest are rarely found in adult hearts. Branches from the anterior and posterior descending coronary arteries supply the upper muscular interventricular septum with blood, which makes the conduction system at this site more impervious to ischemic damage unless the ischemia is extensive.

The Bundle Branches, or Branching Portion of the Atrioventricular Bundle

These structures begin at the superior margin of the muscular interventricular septum, immediately beneath the membranous septum, with the cells of the left bundle branch cascading downward as a continuous sheet onto the septum beneath the noncoronary aortic cusp (Fig. 27–7). The AV bundle may then give off other left bundle branches, sometimes constituting a true bifascicular system with an anterosuperior branch, in other hearts giving rise to a group of central fibers, and in still others appearing more as a network without a clear division into a fascicular system. The right bundle branch continues intramyocardially as an unbranched extension of the AV bundle down the right side of the interventricular septum to the apex of the right ventricle and base of the anterior papillary muscle. In some human hearts, the His bundle traverses the right interventricular crest and gives rise to a right-sided narrow stem origin of the left bundle branch. The anatomy of the left bundle branch system may be variable and may not conform to a constant bifascicular division. However, the concept of a trifascicular system remains useful to both the electrocardiographer and the clinician (see Fig. 27–7).

Terminal Purkinje Fibers

These fibers connect with the ends of the bundle branches to form interweaving networks on the endocardial surface of both ventricles that transmit the cardiac impulse almost simultaneously to the entire right and left ventricular endocardium. Purkinje fibers tend to be less concentrated at the base of the ventricle and at the papillary muscle tips. They penetrate the myocardium for varying distances depending on the animal species: In humans, they apparently penetrate only the inner third of the endocardium, whereas in the pig they almost reach the epicardium. Such variations could influence changes produced by myocardial ischemia, for example, because Purkinje fibers appear to be more resistant to ischemia than ordinary myocardial fibers are.

CELLULAR COMPOSITION OF THE ATRIOVENTRICULAR JUNCTIONAL AREA AND THE INTRAVENTRICULAR CONDUCTION SYSTEM. Transitional cells in the rabbit are elongated and smaller than atrial cells, stain more palely, and are separated by numerous strands of connective tissue. They merge at the entrance of the compact portion of the AV node, where the cells are small and spherical, not separated by muscle or connective tissue, and have very few nexuses. They interweave in interconnecting whorls of fasciculi. The AV node is divided on the basis of electrophysiological characteristics into AN, N, and NH regions.[18] In the rabbit, the AN region corresponds to the transitional cell groups of the posterior portion of the node, the NH region to the anterior portion of the bundle of lower nodal cells, and the N region to the small enclosed node where transitional cells merge with midnodal cells. *Dead-end pathways*—groups of cells that form an apparent electrophysiological cul-de-sac that does not contribute to overall conduction in the node—are also found at several sites. Cells in the penetrating bundle remain similar to compact AV nodal cells.

Purkinje cells are found in the His bundle and bundle branches, cover much of the endocardium of both ventricles, and align to form multicellular bundles in longitudinal strands separated by collagen. Although conduction of the cardiac impulse appears to be their major function, free-running Purkinje fibers, sometimes called *false tendons,* which are

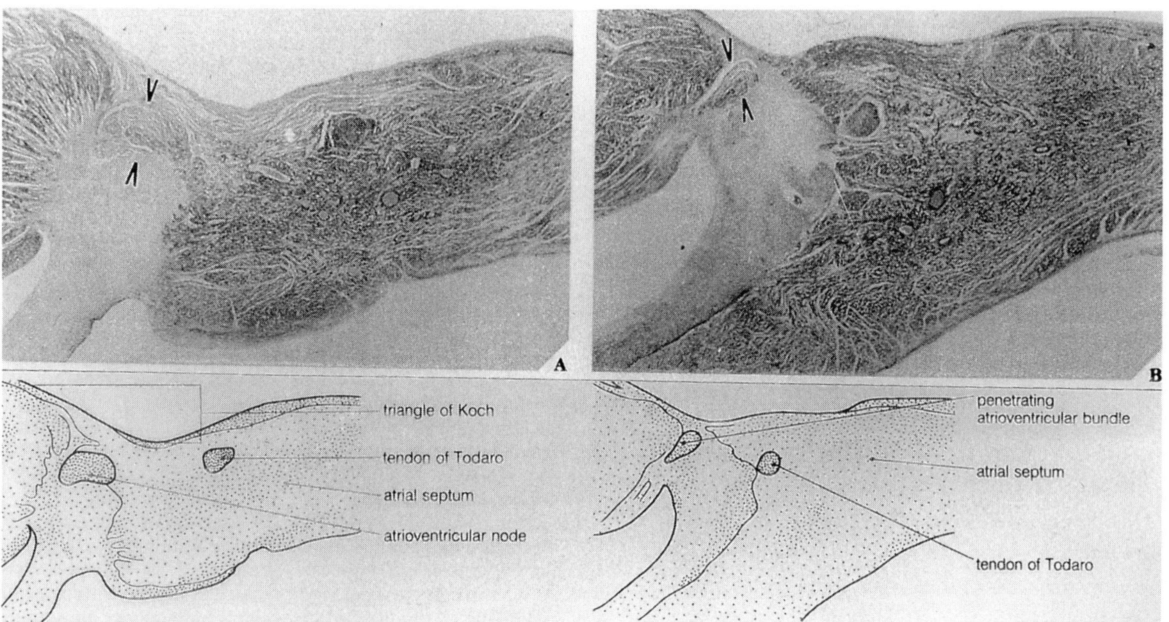

FIGURE 27–5 Sections through the atrioventricular (AV) junction show the position of the AV node (arrowhead) within the triangle of Koch **(A)** and the penetrating AV bundle of His (arrowheads) within the central fibrous body **(B)**. (From Anderson RH, Wilcox BR, Becker AE: Anatomy of the normal heart. *In* Hurst JW, Anderson RH, Becker AE, Wilcox BR [eds]. Atlas of the Heart. New York, Gower, 1988, p 1.2.)

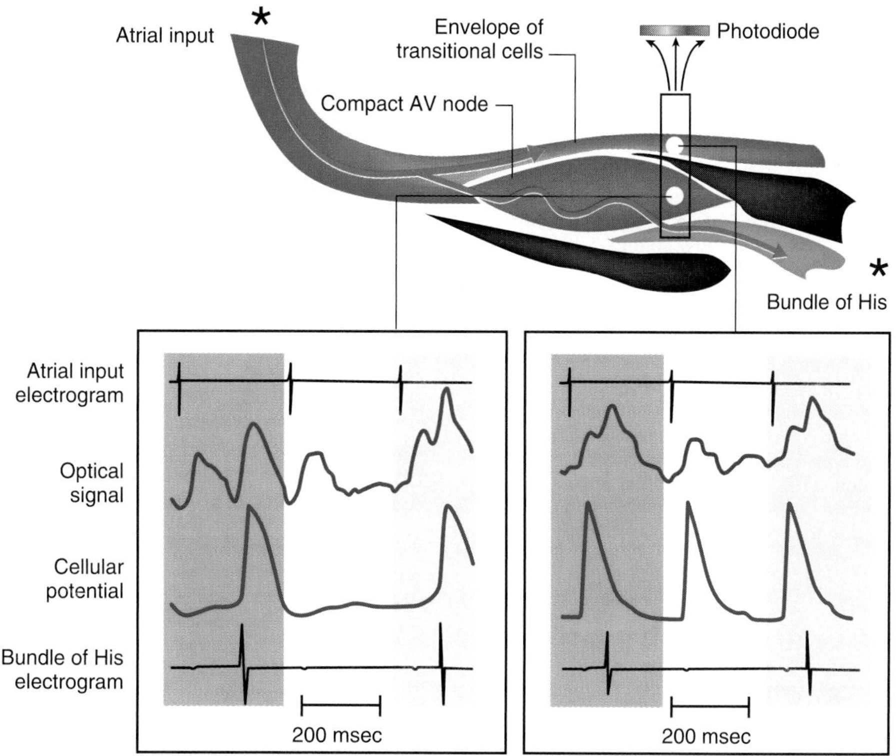

FIGURE 27–6 Multilayer conduction pattern in the atrioventricular (AV) node. Diagram of a cross section through the rabbit AV junction perpendicular to the endocardial atrial surface. The compact node (red) is covered with a superficial layer of transitional cells (blue), providing a connection between the atrial tissue and the compact node. The compact node, in turn, connects to the bundle of His (orange). Connective tissue protrusions are shown in black. Optical recordings of membrane potential changes obtained with a photodiode from the underlying tissue were accompanied by local electrograms from the atrial input to the AV node and from the bundle of His (asterisks). In addition, a microelectrode was used to measure transmembrane potentials at different AV node layers (circles). Each of the **lower panels** illustrates three consecutive heartbeats with simultaneously acquired atrial input and His electrograms, along with optical and microelectrode signals. In the time interval between an atrial input activation and ensuing activation of the bundle of His, two distinct optical action potentials can be identified. The first component corresponds to the depolarization of cells located in the superficial transitional cell layer, whereas the second component reflects the depolarization of cells in the distal portion of the compact AV node. The second beats (white strips) are blocked in the AV node, as indicated by the absence of the signal from the distal portion of the AV node but continued presence of the signal obtained from the transitional cell layer. (From Efimov IR, Mazgalev TN: High resolution three-dimensional fluorescent imaging reveals multiplayer conduction pattern in the atrioventricular node. Circulation 98:54, 1998. By permission of the American Heart Association.)

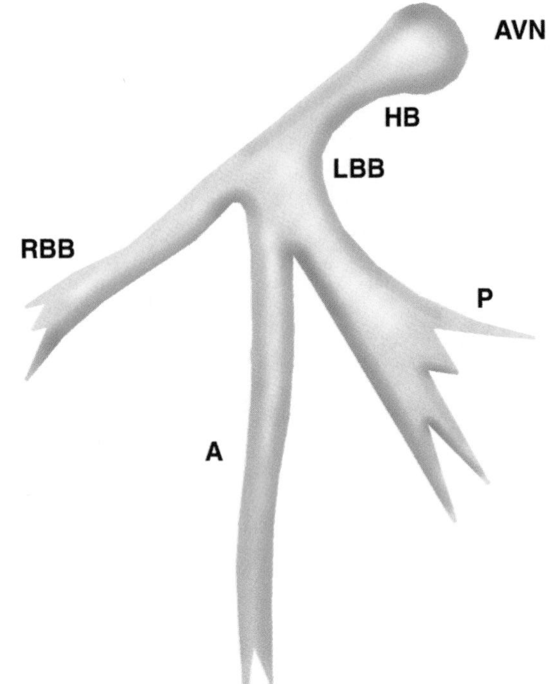

FIGURE 27–7 Schematic representation of the trifascicular bundle branch system. A = anterosuperior fascicle of the left bundle; AVN = atrioventricular node; HB = His bundle; LBB = main left bundle branch; P = posteroinferior fascicle of the left bundle branch; RBB = right bundle branch. (Modified from Rosenbaum MB, Elizari MV, Lazzari JO: The Hemiblocks. Oldsmar, Fla, Tampa Tracings, 1970, cover illustration.)

composed of many Purkinje cells in a series, are capable of contraction. Direct visualization of impulse conduction within the specialized conduction system using high-resolution optical mapping illustrated that action potentials propagate within thin Purkinje fiber bundles from base to apex before activation of the surrounding myocytes occurs.[19] Action potential propagation within the His-Purkinje system and the working myocardium is mediated by connexins. Ventricular myocytes express mainly connexin43 and Purkinje fibers express connexin40 and connexin45.[19,20] The molecular identity of the connexin type that enables impulse transmission at the Purkinje fiber–myocyte junction (PMJ) is unclear. It is also still not clear how the small amount of depolarizing current provided by the thin bundle of Purkinje fibers can activate a much larger mass of ventricular muscle (current-to-load mismatch).[21] It is possible that individual gap junctional channels at the PMJ are formed by more than one connexin isoform.[20] These disparate connexin phenotypes may create specific types of hybrid channels with unique properties that ensure safe conduction at the PMJ. Because Purkinje cells have markedly longer repolarization times than surrounding myocytes (see Fig. 27-15), these connexin hybrids could also decrease entrainment of repolarization at the PMJ and thereby increase repolarization gradients.

Innervation of the Atrioventricular Node, His Bundle, and Ventricular Myocardium

PATHWAYS OF INNERVATION. The AV node and His bundle region are innervated by a rich supply of cholinergic and adrenergic fibers with a density exceeding that found in the ventricular myocardium. Ganglia, nerve fibers, and nerve nets lie close to the AV node. Parasympathetic nerves to the AV node region enter the canine heart at the junction of the inferior vena cava and the inferior aspect of the left atrium, adjacent to the coronary sinus entrance. Nerves in direct contact with AV nodal fibers have been noted, along with agranular and granular vesicular processes, presumably representing cholinergic and adrenergic processes. Acetylcholine release may be concentrated around the N region of the AV node.[9]

In general, autonomic neural input to the heart exhibits some degree of "sidedness," with the right sympathetic and vagal nerves affecting the sinus node more than the AV node and the left sympathetic and vagal nerves affecting the AV node more than the sinus node. The distribution of the neural input to the sinus and AV nodes is complex because of substantial overlapping innervation. Despite the overlap, specific branches of the vagal and sympathetic nerves can be shown to innervate certain regions preferentially, and sympathetic or vagal nerves to the sinus node can be interrupted discretely without affecting AV nodal innervation. Similarly, vagal or sympathetic neural input to the AV node can be interrupted without affecting sinus innervation. Supersensitivity to acetylcholine follows vagal denervation. Stimulation of the right stellate ganglion produces sinus tachycardia with less effect on AV nodal conduction, whereas stimulation of the left stellate ganglion generally produces a shift in the sinus pacemaker to an ectopic site and consistently shortens AV nodal conduction time and refractoriness but inconsistently speeds the sinus nodal discharge rate. Stimulation of the right cervical vagus nerve primarily slows the sinus nodal discharge rate, and stimulation of the left vagus primarily prolongs AV nodal conduction time and refractoriness when sidedness is present. Although neither sympathetic nor vagal stimulation affects normal conduction in the His bundle, either can affect abnormal AV conduction. The negative dromotropic response of the heart to vagal stimulation is mediated by activation of $I_{K(Ach,Ado)}$, which results in hyperpolarization of the AV nodal cells, thereby influencing the conductive properties of the node. The positive dromotropic effect of sympathetic stimulation arises as a consequence of activation of the L-type Ca^{2+} current, $I_{Ca.L}$ (see Table 27-3).

Most efferent sympathetic impulses reach the canine ventricles over the ansae subclaviae, branches from the stellate ganglia. Sympathetic nerves then synapse primarily in the caudal cervical ganglia and form individual cardiac nerves that innervate relatively localized parts of the ventricles. On the right side, the major route to the heart is the recurrent cardiac nerve, and on the left, the ventrolateral cardiac nerve. In general, the right sympathetic chain shortens refractoriness primarily of the anterior portion of the ventricles and the left affects primarily the posterior surface of the ventricles, although overlapping areas of distribution occur.

The intraventricular route of sympathetic nerves generally follows coronary arteries. Functional data suggest that afferent and efferent sympathetic nerves travel in the superficial layers of the epicardium and dive to innervate the endocardium, and anatomical observations support this conclusion. Vagal fibers travel intramurally or subendocardially and rise to the epicardium at the AV groove (Fig. 27-8).[9]

EFFECTS OF VAGAL STIMULATION. The vagus modulates cardiac sympathetic activity at prejunctional and postjunctional sites by regulating the amount of norepinephrine released and by inhibiting cAMP–induced phosphorylation of cardiac proteins such as phospholamban. The latter inhibition occurs at more than one level in the series of reactions constituting the adenylate cyclase-, AMP-dependent protein kinase system. Neuropeptides released from nerve fibers of both autonomic limbs also modulate autonomic responses. For example, NPY released from sympathetic nerve terminals inhibits cardiac vagal effects.[22]

Tonic vagal stimulation produces a greater absolute reduction in sinus rate in the presence of tonic background sympathetic stimulation, a sympathetic-parasympathetic interaction termed *accentuated antagonism*. In contrast, changes in AV conduction during concomitant sympathetic and vagal stimulation are essentially the *algebraic sum* of the individual AV conduction responses to tonic vagal and sympathetic stimulation alone. Cardiac responses to brief vagal bursts begin after a short latency and dissipate quickly; in contrast, cardiac responses to sympathetic stimulation commence and dissipate slowly. The rapid onset and offset of responses to vagal stimulation allow dynamic beat-to-beat vagal modulation of heart rate and AV conduction, whereas the slow temporal response to sympathetic stimulation precludes any beat-to-beat regulation by sympathetic activity. Periodic vagal bursting (as may occur each time a systolic pressure wave arrives at the baroreceptor regions in the aortic and carotid sinuses) induces phasic changes in sinus cycle length and can entrain the sinus node to discharge faster or slower at periods that are identical to those of the vagal burst. In a similar phasic manner, vagal bursts prolong AV nodal conduction time and are influenced by background levels of sympathetic tone. Because the peak vagal effects on sinus rate and AV nodal conduction occur at different times in the

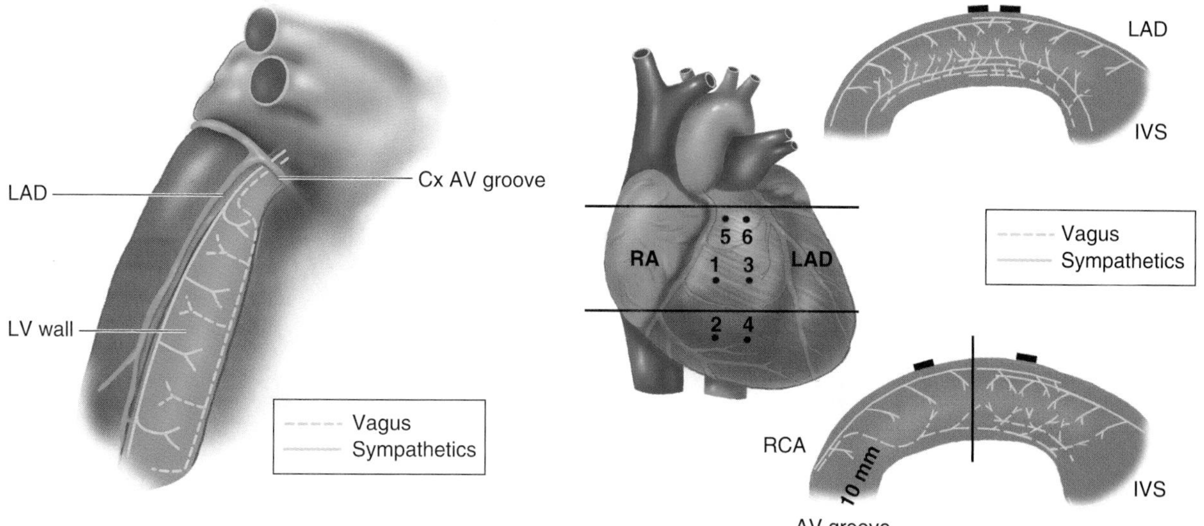

FIGURE 27–8 **Left,** Intraventricular route of sympathetic and vagal nerves to the left ventricle. **Right,** Schematic of the transverse views of the right ventricular (RV) wall showing functional pathways of the efferent sympathetic and vagal nerves. **Top right,** Transverse view of the RV outflow tract at the upper horizontal line on the left. **Bottom right,** Transverse view of the anterolateral wall at the lower horizontal line on the left. The vertical solid line indicates the center of the RV anterolateral wall. Closed circles indicate positions of plunge electrodes labeled 1 to 6. IVS = interventricular septum; LAD = left anterior descending coronary artery; RA = right atrium; RCA = right coronary artery. (From Ito M, Zipes DP: Efferent sympathetic and vagal innervation of the canine right ventricle. Circulation 90:1459, 1994. By permission of the American Heart Association.)

cardiac cycle, a brief vagal burst can slow the sinus rate without affecting AV nodal conduction or can prolong AV nodal conduction time and not slow the sinus rate.[22]

EFFECTS OF SYMPATHETIC STIMULATION. Stimulation of sympathetic ganglia shortens the refractory period equally in the epicardium and underlying endocardium of the left ventricular free wall, although dispersion of recovery properties occurs; that is, different degrees of shortening of refractoriness occur when measured at different epicardial sites. Nonuniform distribution of norepinephrine may, in part, contribute to some of the nonuniform electrophysiological effects because the ventricular content of norepinephrine is greater at the base than at the apex of the heart, with greater distribution to muscle than to Purkinje fibers. Afferent vagal activity appears to be greater in the posterior ventricular myocardium, which may account for the vagomimetic effects of inferior myocardial infarction.[9]

The vagi exert minimal but measurable effects on ventricular tissue: decreasing the strength of myocardial contraction and prolonging refractoriness. Under some circumstances, acetylcholine can cause a positive inotropic effect. It is now clear that the vagus (acetylcholine) can exert direct effects on some types of ventricular fibers as well as exert indirect effects by modulating sympathetic influences.[9]

Arrhythmias and the Autonomic Nervous System

Alterations in vagal and sympathetic innervation can influence the development of arrhythmias and sudden cardiac death from ventricular tachyarrhythmias.[9,23-25] Damage to nerves extrinsic to the heart, such as the stellate ganglia, as well as to intrinsic cardiac nerves from diseases that may affect nerves primarily, such as viral infections, or secondarily, from diseases that cause cardiac damage, may produce cardioneuropathy. Such neural changes may create electrical instability through a variety of electrophysiological mechanisms. For example, myocardial infarction can interrupt afferent and efferent neural transmission and create areas of sympathetic supersensitivity that may be conducive to the development of arrhythmias.[9] Mutations in genes encoding cardiac ion channel subunits also affect channel function in the central autonomic nervous system,[26] resulting in abnormal firing properties of affected neurons.[27] This observation may partially explain the clinical finding that sudden cardiac death in some variants of the long QT syndrome (see Chaps. 28 and 32) is typically preceded by a sympathetic arousal.

Basic Electrophysiological Principles

Physiology of Ion Channels

Electrical signaling in the heart involves the passage of ions through ionic channels. The Na^+, K^+, Ca^{2+}, and Cl^- ions are the major charge carriers, and their movement across the cell membrane creates a flow of current that generates excitation and signals in cardiac myocytes. Ion channels are macromolecular pores that span the lipid bilayer of the cell membrane (Fig. 27–9). Conformational transitions change (gate) a single ion channel from closed to open, which allows selected ions to flow passively down the electrochemical activity gradient at a very high rate (>10^6 ions per second). The high transfer rates and restriction to "downhill" fluxes not stoichiometrically coupled to the hydrolysis of energy-rich phosphates distinguish ionic channel mechanisms from those of other ion-transporting structures such as the sarcolemmal Na^+,K^+-adenosine triphosphatase (ATPase) or the sarcoplasmic reticular Mg^{2+},Ca^{2+}-ATPase. Ion channels may be gated by extracellular and intracellular ligands, changes in transmembrane voltage, or mechanical stress (see Table 27–3). Gating of single ion channels can best be studied by means of the patch-clamp technique (see, e.g., reference 28).

Ion channels are usually named after the strongest permeant ion—Na^+, Ca^{2+}, K^+, Cl^-—but some channels are less or not selective, as in gap junctional channels. Channels have also been named after neurotransmitters, as in acetylcholine-sensitive K^+ channels, $I_{K.Ach}$.

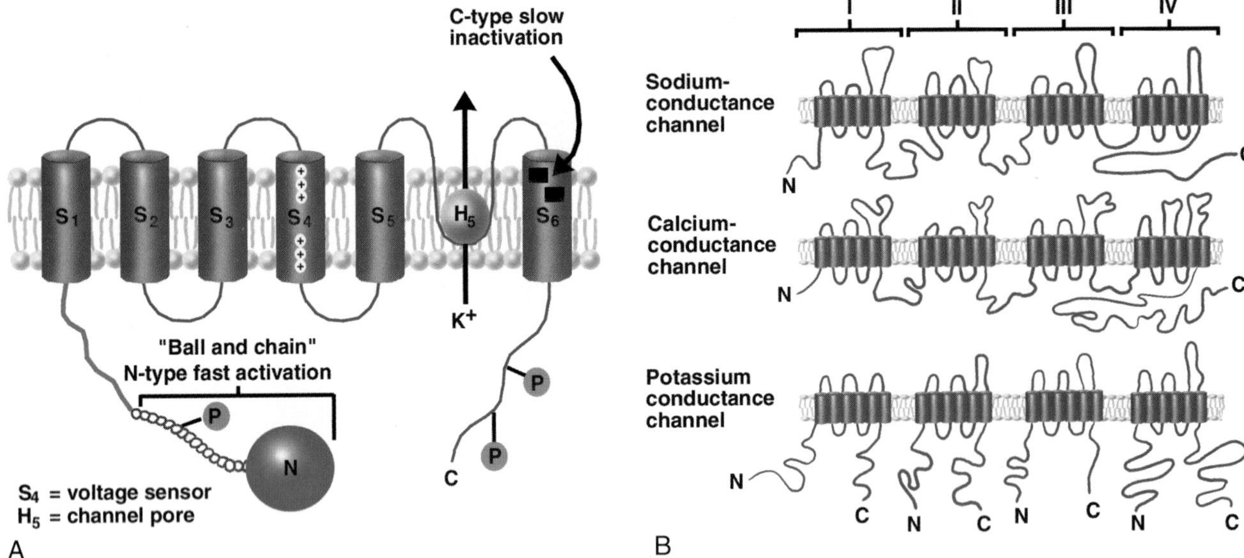

FIGURE 27–9 Structure of ion channels. **A,** Subunit of a voltage-gated potassium channel containing six membrane-spanning domains (S_1 through S_6) linked by intracellular and extracellular sequences of hydrophilic amino acids. One of the subunits (S_4) has positively charged lysine and arginine residues, and this region is thought to form the voltage sensor of the channel. Transmembrane segments S_5 and S_6, along with the intervening peptide chain (H), line the pore through which ions pass into the lipid bilayer. Voltage-dependent "fast" or N-type inactivation is mediated by an N-terminal particle that binds to the activated channel and plugs the permeation pathway. C-type or "slow" inactivation requires conformational changes at the outer side of the channel pore. Both the COOH terminus and the NH_2 terminus have phosphorylation sites (P) that are potential targets for a variety of protein kinases and protein phosphatases. A change in phosphorylation status may then result in altered gating and/or permeation properties of the channel. **B,** Voltage-gated Na^+ and Ca^{2+} channels are composed of a *single* tetramer consisting of four covalently linked repeats of the six-transmembrane-spanning motifs, whereas voltage-gated K^+ channels are composed of four *separate* subunits, each containing a single six-transmembrane-spanning motif. (Modified from Katz AM: Molecular biology in cardiology, a paradigmatic shift. J Mol Cell Cardiol 20:355, 1988.)

The ionic permeability ratio is a commonly used quantitative index of a channel's selectivity. It is defined as the ratio of the permeability of one ion type to that of the main permeant ion type. Permeability ratios of voltage-gated K^+ and Na^+ channels for monovalent and divalent (e.g., Ca^{2+}) cations are usually less than 1:10. Voltage-gated Ca^{2+} channels exhibit a more than thousandfold discrimination against Na^+ and K^+ ions (e.g., P_K/P_{Ca} = 1/3000) and are impermeable to anions.

Because ions are charged, net ionic flux through an open channel is determined by both the concentration and electrical gradient across the membrane (electrodiffusion). The potential at which the passive flux of ions along the chemical driving force is exactly balanced by the electrical driving force is called the reversal or Nernst potential of the channel. In the case of a channel that is perfectly selective for one ion species, the reversal potential equals the thermodynamic equilibrium potential of that ion, E_S, which is given by the Nernst equation in the form

$$E_S = RT/zF\ \ln([S_o]/[S_i])$$

where S_i and S_o are the intracellular and extracellular concentrations of the permeant ion, respectively, z is the valence of the ion, R is the gas constant, F is the Faraday constant, T is the temperature in kelvins, and ln is the logarithm to the base e. At membrane voltages more positive to the reversal potential of the channel, passive ion movement is outward, whereas it is inward at membrane potentials that are more negative to the Nernst potential of that channel. If the current through an open channel is carried by more than one permeant ion, the reversal potential becomes a weighted mean of all Nernst potentials.

As shown in Figures 27–13, 27–14, and 27–15 and Table 27–2, membrane voltages during a cardiac action potential are in the range of −95 to +30 mV. With physiological external K^+ (4 mM; see Table 27–1), E_K is approximately −91 mV, and passive K^+ movement during an action potential is out of the cell. On the other hand, because the calculated reversal potential of a cardiac Ca^{2+} channel is +64 mV (assuming P_K/P_{Ca} = 1/3000, K_i = 150 mM, K_o = 4 mM, Ca_i = 100 nM, Ca_o = 2 mM), passive Ca^{2+} flux is into the cell. With physiological internal and external chloride concentrations (Table 27–1), E_{Cl} is −80 to −35 mV, and passive movement of Cl^- ions through open chloride channels can be both inward and outward at membrane potentials typically occurring during a cardiac action potential. In more general terms, the direction and magnitude of passive ion flux through a single open channel at any given transmembrane voltage are governed by the reversal potential of that ion and its concentration on the two sides of the membrane, with the net flux being larger when ions move from the more concentrated side.

TABLE 27–1 Intracellular and Extracellular Ion Concentrations in Cardiac Muscle

Ion	Extracellular Concentration (mM)	Intracellular Concentration	Ratio of Extracellular to Intracellular Concentration	E_I (mV)
Na	145	15 mM	9.7	+60
K	4	150 mM	0.027	−94
Cl	120	5-30 mM	4-24	−83 to −36
Ca	2	10^{-7} M	2×10^4	+129

Athough intracellular Ca content is about 2 mM, most of this Ca is bound or sequestered in intracellular organelles (mitochondria and sarcoplasmic reticulum).

E_I = equilibrium potential for a particular ion at 37°C.

Modified after Sperelakis N: Origin of the cardiac resting potential. *In* Berne RM, Sperelakis N, Geiger SR (eds): Handbook of Physiology, The Cardiovascular System. Bethesda, Md, American Physiological Society, 1979, p. 193.

ION FLUX THROUGH VOLTAGE-GATED CHANNELS

Changes in transmembrane potential determine ion flux through voltage-gated channels not only through the voltage dependence of the electrochemical driving force on the permeant ion but also through the voltage dependence of channel activation; that is, the fraction of time that a channel permits ions to permeate is determined by the membrane voltage. If the probability of a channel being activated (i.e., the open-state probability of that channel) exhibits voltage dependence, as is the case with the fast Na^+ channel or voltage-dependent K^+ channels in cardiac myocytes, activation increases with membrane depolarization. Note that channels do not have a sharp voltage threshold for opening. The dependence of channel activation on membrane potential is rather a continuous function of voltage and follows a sigmoidal curve (Fig. 27–10). The potential at which activation is half-maximal and the steepness of the activation curve determine the channel's activity during changes in membrane potential. Shifting the activation curve to potentials positive to the midpoint of activation or reducing the steepness of the channel's acti-

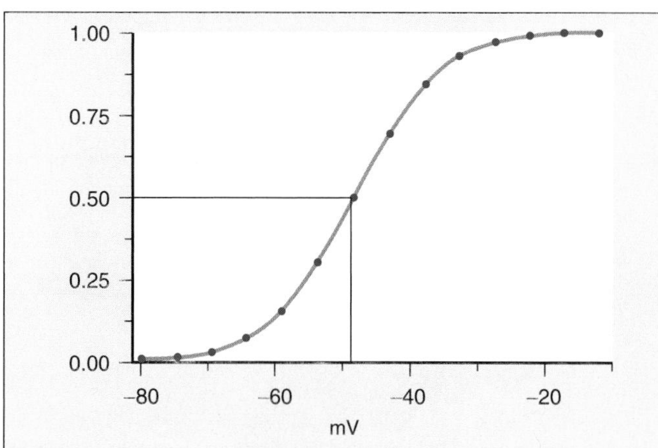

FIGURE 27–10 Voltage dependence of fast Na^+ current activation. Fractional activation (y-axis) is plotted as a function of membrane potential. Voltage at which activation is half-maximal is demarked by a vertical line.

vation curve or both are two possible mechanisms by which ion channel blockers can inhibit ion channel activity.

As indicated in Figure 27–11, open channels enter a nonconducting conformation after a depolarizing change in membrane potential, a process termed *inactivation*.[29] If membrane depolarization persists, the channel remains inactivated and cannot reopen. This steady-state inactivation increases with membrane depolarization in a sigmoidal fashion. Inactivation curves of the various voltage-gated ion channel types in the heart differ in their slopes and midpoints of inactivation. For example, sustained cardiomyocyte membrane depolarization to −50 mV (as may occur in acutely ischemic myocardium) causes almost complete inactivation of the fast, voltage-gated Na^+ channel, whereas the L-type Ca^{2+} channel exhibits only little inactivation at this membrane potential.[30] Activation and inactivation curves can overlap, in which case a steady-state or non-inactivating current flows. The existence of such a "window" current has been verified for both the voltage-gated Na^+ current[31] and the L-type Ca^{2+} current.[32] The L-type window current has been implicated in the genesis of triggered activity arising from early afterdepolarizations (EADs).

Channels recover from inactivation and then enter the closed state from which they can be reactivated (see Fig. 27–11). Rates of recovery from inactivation vary among the different types of voltage-dependent channels and usually follow monoexponential or multiexponential time courses, with the longest time constants ranging from a few milliseconds, as, for example, for the fast sodium channel,[33] to several seconds, as for some subtypes of K^+ channels (see Table 27–3).[34] Together, the activity of voltage-dependent ion channels in cardiomyocytes over the course of an action potential is tightly regulated by the orchestrated interplay of a number of time- and voltage-dependent gating mechanisms, including activation, inactivation, and recovery from inactivation. All of these mechanisms represent potential targets for pharmacological interventions.

PRINCIPLES OF IONIC CURRENT MODULATION

The whole-cell current amplitude, I, is the product of the number of functional channels in the membrane available for opening (N), the probability that a channel will open (P_o), and the single-channel current amplitude (i), or $I = N \cdot P_o \cdot i$. Modulation of current amplitudes in single

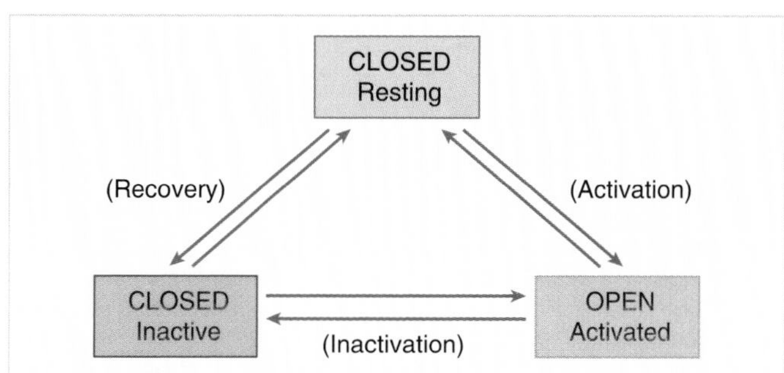

FIGURE 27–11 Simplest scheme for gating of voltage-gated ion channels.

cardiomyocytes therefore results from alterations in N, P_o, i, or any combination of these. Changes in the number of available channels in the cell membrane may result from changes in the expression of ion channel-encoding genes.[35] The magnitude of the single-channel current amplitude is dependent, among other factors, on the ionic concentration gradient across the membrane. For example, an increase in the extracellular Ca^{2+} concentration increases current through a single Ca^{2+} channel. Changes in channel activation can result from phosphorylation/dephosphorylation of the channel protein by second messenger–mediated activation of protein kinases and protein phosphatases, respectively (see also Fig. 27–9).[36] Channel phosphorylation/dephosphorylation causes a shift in the membrane potential dependence of a channel's activation or availability curve, or both, or modification of the sensitivity of channel activation/inactivation to changes in membrane potential. For example, protein kinase A–mediated potentiation of the cardiac sodium current is partially due to a shift of the sodium channel activation curve to more negative potentials.[37]

Molecular Structure of Ion Channels

Voltage-gated potassium channels are composed of four *separate* subunits, each containing six regions of hydrophobic amino acids (S1 through S6) that are thought to form membrane-spanning domains, and these hydrophobic regions are linked by sequences of hydrophilic amino acids that are exposed to the intracellular or extracellular space (see Fig. 27–9A). One of the membrane-spanning subunits (S4) is positively charged, having a cluster of basic amino acids (lysine or arginine), and this region is thought to be part of the voltage sensor. The peptide chain linking S5 and S6 (H5 loop) lines the water-filled pore. Voltage-dependent "fast" inactivation of the channel is mediated by a tethered N-terminal particle ("inactivation ball") that binds to the activated channel and occludes the intracellular mouth of the permeation pathway (see Fig. 27–9A). In contrast to this "tethered ball" mechanism of N-type inactivation, C-type (or "slow") inactivation involves relatively localized changes in conformation of amino acid residues near the external mouth of the channel pore.[29] The rate of C-type inactivation and its recovery strongly determine refractoriness and can be modulated by binding of drugs, for example, dofetilide. Voltage-gated Na^+ and Ca^{2+} channels have a basic structure similar to that of voltage-dependent potassium channels, although, unlike K^+ channels, each Ca^{2+} or Na^+ channel consists of a single (alpha) subunit containing the four repeats of the six transmembrane-spanning domains (see Fig. 27–9B).

A structurally different family of potassium channels is that containing the inwardly rectifying potassium-selective channels (Kir). Kir channels in cardiac myocytes, as in other cells, conduct inward current at membrane potentials negative to E_K and smaller outward currents at membrane potentials positive to E_K. The activity of Kir channels is a function of both the membrane potential and the extracellular K^+ concentration ($[K^+]_o$). As $[K^+]_o$ changes, the channel conducts inward current at potentials negative to the new E_K while a small outward current within a certain potential range positive to the new E_K remains. Structurally, Kir channels resemble voltage-gated K^+ channels, but the subunits lack the S1 to S4 domains, whereas the pore-forming domains and the H5 region are conserved. Kir channel subunits can form heteromultimeric complexes with other proteins, which adds considerable complexity to the behavior of Kir channels. For example, the ATP-sensitive K^+ channel $I_{K.ATP}$ is a heteromeric complex of inwardly rectifying potassium channel subunits and the sulfonylurea receptor. Drugs such as nicorandil, pinacidil, and diazoxide open ATP-sensitive K^+ channels, whereas sulfonylurea compounds (such as glibenclamide) inhibit the activity of $I_{K.ATP}$. Opening of cardiac sarcolemmal K_{ATP} channels underlies electrocardiographic ST segment elevation during acute myocardial ischemia.[38]

The molecular basis of the acetylcholine-activated potassium channel $I_{K.Ach}$ is a heteromultimer of two inwardly rectifying potassium channel subunits. This channel is activated after direct binding of the beta-gamma subunits of G protein. Stimulation of $I_{K.Ach}$ by vagally secreted acetylcholine decreases spontaneous depolarization in the sinus node and slows the velocity of conduction in the AV node.[39] Adenosine, through type 1 purinergic receptor–mediated G protein activation, also increases $I_{K.Ach}$ activity in atrial, sinoatrial node, and AV node cells, thus making this compound a treatment of choice for AV reentry tachycardia.

Intercalated Discs

Another family of ion channel proteins is that containing the gap junctional channels. These dodecameric channels are found in the intercalated discs between adjacent cells. Three types of specialized junctions make up each intercalated disc. The macula adherens or desmosome and fascia adherens form areas of strong adhesion between cells and may provide a linkage for the transfer of mechanical energy from one cell to the next. The *nexus,* also called the *tight* or *gap junction,* is a region in the intercalated disc where cells are in functional contact with each other. Membranes at these junctions are separated by only about 10 to 20 Å and are connected by a series of hexagonally packed subunit bridges. Gap junctions provide low-resistance electrical coupling between adjacent cells by establishing aqueous pores that directly link the cytoplasm of these adjacent cells. Gap junctions allow movement of ions and small molecules between cells, thereby linking the interiors of adjacent cells.

Gap junctions permit a multicellular structure such as the heart to function electrically like an orderly, synchronized, interconnected unit and are probably responsible in part for the fact that conduction in the myocardium is *anisotropic*; that is, its anatomical and biophysical properties vary according to the direction in which they are measured. Usually, conduction velocity is two to three times faster longitudinally, in the direction of the long axis of the fiber, than it is transversely, in the direction perpendicular to this long axis.[40,41] Resistivity is lower longitudinally than transversely. Interestingly, the safety factor for propagation is greater transversely than horizontally. Conduction delay or block occurs more commonly in the longitudinal direction than it does transversely. Cardiac conduction is discontinuous because of resistive discontinuities created by the gap junctions, which have an anisotropic distribution on the cell surface.[42] Because of anisotropy, propagation is discontinuous and can be a cause of reentry.

Gap junctions may also provide "biochemical coupling" that might permit cell-to-cell movement of ATP or other high-energy phosphates. Gap junctions can also change their electrical resistance. When intracellular calcium rises, as in myocardial infarction, the gap junction may close to help "seal off" the effects of injured from noninjured cells. Acidosis increases and alkalosis decreases gap junctional resistance. Increased gap junctional resistance tends to slow the rate of action potential propagation, a condition that could lead to conduction delay or block.[43] Cardiac restricted inactivation of gap junctions decreases transverse conduction velocity to a greater degree than longitudinal conduction, resulting in an increased anisotropic ratio that may play a role in premature sudden death from ventricular arrhythmias.[44]

Connexins are the proteins that form the intercellular channels of gap junctions. An individual channel is created by two hemichannels (connexons), each located in the plasma membrane of adjacent cells and composed of six integral membrane protein subunits (connexins). The hemichannels surround an aqueous pore and thereby create a transmembrane channel (Fig. 27-12). Connexin43, a 43-kDa polypeptide, is the most abundant cardiac connexin, with connexin40 and connexin45 found in smaller amounts. Ventricular muscle expresses connexin43 and connexin45, whereas atrial muscle and components of the specialized conduction system express connexin43, connexin45, and connexin40. Individual cardiac connexins form gap junctional channels with characteristic unitary conductances, voltage sensitivities, and ionic permeabilities.[45] Tissue-specific connexin expression and spatial distribution of gap junctions determine the disparate conduction properties of cardiac tissue. The functional heterogeneity of cardiac gap junctions is further enhanced by the ability of different connexin isoforms to form hybrid gap junctional channels with unique electrophysiological properties. These channel chimeras appear to have a major function in controlling impulse transmission at the sinus node–atrium border, the atrium–AV node transitional zone, and the Purkinje-myocyte border.[7,20]

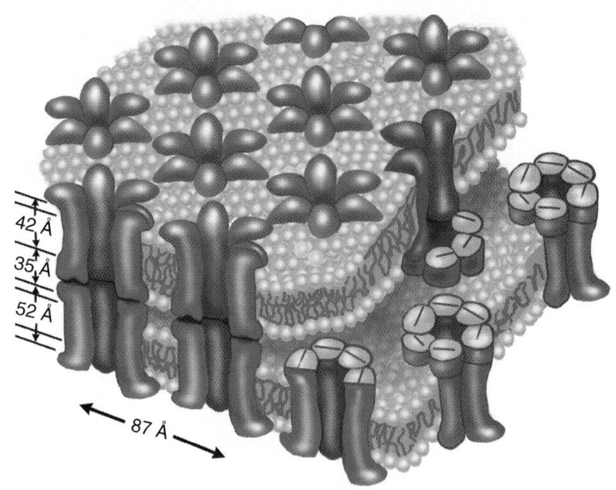

FIGURE 27–12 Model of the structure of a gap junction based on results of x-ray diffraction studies. Individual channels are composed of paired hexamers that travel in the membranes of adjacent cells and adjoin in the extracellular gap to form an aqueous pore that provides continuity of the cytoplasm of the two cells. (From Saffitz JE: Cell-to-cell communication in the heart. Cardiol Rev 3:86, 1995.)

Phases of the Cardiac Action Potential

The cardiac transmembrane potential consists of five phases: phase 0, upstroke or rapid depolarization; phase 1, early rapid repolarization; phase 2, plateau; phase 3, final rapid repolarization; and phase 4, resting membrane potential and diastolic depolarization (see Fig. 27–14). These phases are the result of passive ion fluxes moving down electrochemical gradients established by active ion pumps and exchange mechanisms. Each ion moves primarily through its own ion-specific channel. Impulses spread from one cell to the next without requiring neural input. The transplanted heart dramatically demonstrates this fact. The following discussion explains the electrogenesis of each of these phases. For in-depth coverage, the reader is referred to other reference sources.[46]

General Considerations

Ionic fluxes regulate membrane potential in cardiac myocytes in the following fashion. When only one type of ion channel opens, assuming that this channel is perfectly selective for that ion, the membrane potential of the entire cell would equal the Nernst potential of that ion. Solving the Nernst equation for the four major ions across the plasma membrane, one obtains the following equilibrium potentials: sodium, +60 mV; potassium, −94 mV; calcium, +129 mV; and chloride, −80 to −35 mV. Therefore, if a single K^+-selective channel opens, such as the inwardly rectifying K^+ channel, the membrane potential approaches E_K (−94 mV). If a single Na^+-selective channel opens, the transmembrane potential becomes E_{Na} (+60 mV). A quiescent cardiac myocyte (phase 4) has many more open potassium than sodium channels, and the cell's transmembrane potential is close to E_K (Table 27–2). When two or more types of ion channel open simultaneously, each type tries to make the membrane potential go to the equilibrium potential of that channel. The contribution of each ion type to the overall membrane potential at any given moment is determined by the instantaneous permeability of the plasma membrane to that ion. For example, deviation of the measured resting membrane potential from E_K (see Table 27–1) would predict that other ion types with equilibrium potentials positive to E_K contribute to the resting membrane potential in cardiac myocytes. If it is assumed that Na^+, K^+, and Cl^- are the permeant ions at resting potential, their individual contributions to the resting membrane potential V can be quantified by the GHK *voltage* equation of the form

$$V = RT/F \ln[(P_K\,[K]_o + P_{Na}\,[Na]_o + P_{Cl}[Cl]_i)/(P_K[K]_I + P_{Na}[Na]P_{Cl}[Cl]_o)]$$

where the symbols have the meanings outlined previously. With only one permeant ion, V becomes the Nernst potential for that ion. With several permeant ion types, V is a weighted mean of all the Nernst potentials.

Intracellular electrical activity can be recorded by inserting a glass microelectrode filled with an electrolyte solution and having a tip diameter less than 0.5 µm into a single cell. The electrode produces minimal damage, its entry point apparently being sealed by the cell. The transmembrane potential is recorded by using this electrode in reference to an extracellular ground electrode placed in the tissue bath near the cell membrane and represents the potential difference between intracellular and extracellular voltage (Fig. 27–13). Alternatively, the patch-clamp technique in current clamp mode can be used to measure transmembrane potentials.

TABLE 27–2 Properties of Transmembrane Potentials in Mammalian Hearts

Property	Sinus Nodal Cell	Atrial Muscle Cell	AV Nodal Cell	Purkinje Fiber	Ventricular Muscle Cell
Resting potential (mV)	−50 to −60	−80 to −90	−60 to −70	−90 to −95	−80 to −90
Action potential					
Amplitude (mV)	60-70	110-120	70-80	120	110-120
Overshoot (mV)	0-10	30	5-15	30	30
Duration (msec)	100-300	100-300	100-300	300-500	200-300
V_{max} (V/S)	1-10	100-200	5-15	500-700	100-200
Propagation velocity (m/sec)	<0.05	0.3-0.4	0.1	2-3	0.3-0.4
Fiber diameter (μm)	5-10	10-15	1-10	100	10-16

Modified from Sperelakis N: Origin of the cardiac resting potential. *In* Berne RM, Sperelakis N, Geiger SR (eds): Handbook of Physiology. The Cardiovascular System. Bethesda, Md, American Physiological Society, 1979, p. 190.

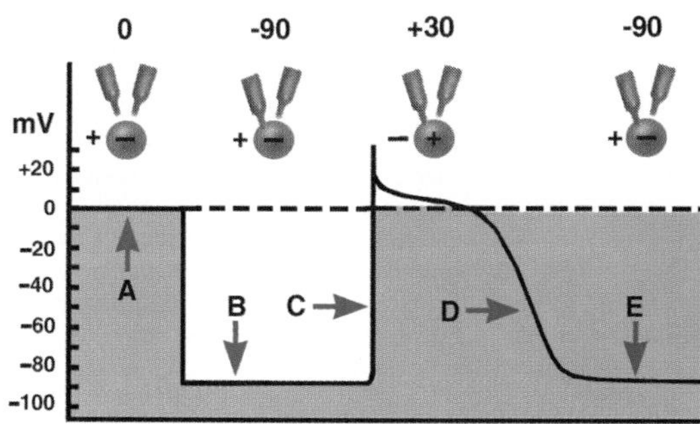

FIGURE 27–13 Demonstration of action potentials recorded during impalement of a cardiac cell. The **upper row** of diagrams shows a cell (circle), two microelectrodes, and stages during impalement of the cell and its activation and recovery. A, Both microelectrodes are extracellular, and no difference in potential exists between them (0 potential). The environment inside the cell is negative and the outside is positive because the cell is polarized. B, One microelectrode has pierced the cell membrane to record the intracellular resting membrane potential, which is −90 mV with respect to the outside of the cell. C, The cell has depolarized and the upstroke of the action potential is recorded. At its peak voltage, the inside of the cell is about +30 mV with respect to the outside of the cell. D, Phase of repolarization, with the membrane returning to its former resting potential (E). (From Cranefield PF: The Conduction of the Cardiac Impulse. Mt Kisco, NY, Futura, 1975.)

Phase 4—The Resting Membrane Potential

The intracellular potential during electrical quiescence in diastole is −50 to −95 mV, depending on the cell type (see Table 27–2). Therefore, the inside of the cell is 50 to 95 mV negative relative to the outside of the cell because of the distribution of ions such as K^+, Na^+, and Cl^-.

Because cardiac myocytes have an abundance of open K^+ channels at rest, the cardiac transmembrane potential (in phase 4) is close to E_K. Potassium outward current through open, inwardly rectifying K^+ channels, I_{K1}, mainly contributes to the resting membrane potential in atrial and ventricular myocytes, as well as in Purkinje cells, under normal conditions. Deviation of the resting membrane potential from E_K is due to movement of monovalent ions with an equilibrium potential greater than the E_K, for example, Cl^- efflux through activated chloride channels, such as $I_{Cl.cAMP}$, $I_{Cl.Ca}$, and $I_{Cl.swell}$.[47] Calcium does not contribute directly to the resting membrane potential, but changes in intracellular free calcium concentration can affect other membrane conductance values. For instance, an increase in sarcoplasmic reticulum Ca^{2+} load can cause spontaneous intracellular Ca^{2+} waves,[48] which in turn activate the Ca^{2+}-dependent chloride conductance $I_{Cl.Ca}$ and thereby lead to spontaneous transient inward currents and concomitant membrane depolarization. Increases in $[Ca^{2+}]_i$ can also stimulate the Na^+/Ca^{2+} exchanger $I_{Na/Ca}$. This protein exchanges three Na^+ ions for one Ca^{2+} ion, the direction being dependent on the sodium and calcium concentrations on the two sides of the membrane and the transmembrane potential difference. At resting membrane potential and during a spontaneous sarcoplasmic reticulum Ca^{2+} release event, this exchanger would generate a net Na^+ influx, possibly causing transient membrane depolarizations (see Fig. 27–23).[49,50] $[Ca^{2+}]_i$ has also been shown to activate I_{K1} in cardiac myocytes, thereby indirectly contributing to cardiac resting membrane potential.[51] Because of the Na-K pump, which pumps Na^+ out of the cell against its electrochemical gradient and simultaneously pumps K^+ into the cell against its chemical gradient, the intracellular K^+ concentration remains high and the intracellular Na^+ concentration remains low. This pump, fueled by an Na^+,K^+-ATPase enzyme that hydrolyzes ATP for energy, is bound to the membrane. It requires both Na^+ and K^+ to function and can transport three Na^+ ions outward for two K^+ ions inward. Therefore, the pump can be electrogenic and generate a net outward movement of positive charges. The rate of Na^+–K^+ pumping to maintain the same ionic gradients must increase as the heart rate increases because the cell gains a slight amount of Na^+ and loses a slight amount of K^+ with each depolarization. Cardiac glycoside–induced block of the Na^+,K^+-ATPase increases contractility through an increase in intracellular Na^+ concentration, which in turn reduces Ca^{2+} extrusion through the Na^+/Ca^{2+} exchanger (see later), ultimately increasing myocyte contractility.[52]

Phase 0—Upstroke or Rapid Depolarization

A stimulus delivered to excitable tissue evokes an action potential characterized by a sudden voltage change caused by transient depolarization followed by repolarization. The action potential is conducted throughout the heart and is responsible for initiating each "heartbeat." Electrical changes in action potential follow a relatively fixed time and voltage relationship that differs according to specific cell types (Figs. 27–14 and 27–15). In nerve, the entire process takes several milliseconds, whereas action potentials in human cardiac fibers last several hundred milliseconds. Normally, the action potential is independent of the size of the depolarizing stimulus if the latter exceeds a certain threshold potential. Small subthreshold depolarizing stimuli depolarize the membrane in proportion to the strength of the stimulus. However, when the stimulus is sufficiently intense to reduce membrane potential to a threshold value in the range of −70 to −65 mV for normal Purkinje fibers, more intense stimuli do not produce larger action potential responses, and an "all-or-none" response results. In contrast, hyperpolarizing pulses, stimuli that render the membrane potential more negative, elicit a response proportional to the strength of the stimulus.

MECHANISM OF PHASE 0. The upstroke of the cardiac action potential in atrial and ventricular muscle and His-Purkinje fibers is due to a sudden increase in membrane

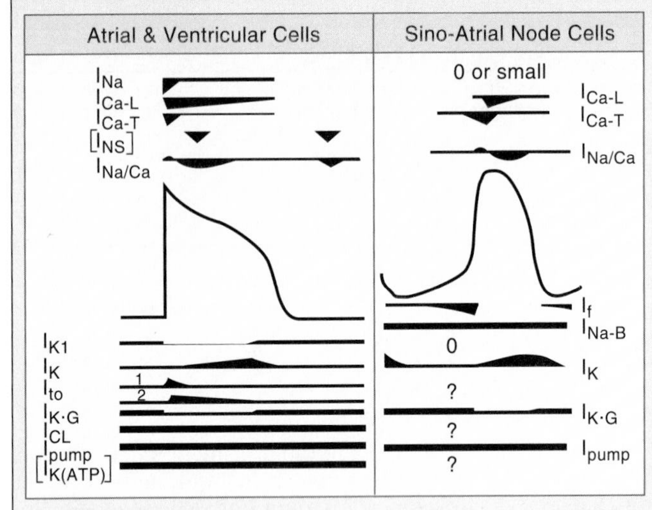

FIGURE 27–14 Currents and channels involved in generating resting and action potentials. The time course of a stylized action potential of atrial and ventricular cells is shown on the left, and that of sinoatrial node cells is on the right. Above and below are the various channels and pumps that contribute the currents underlying the electrical events. See Table 27–3 for identification of the symbols and description of the channels or currents. Where possible, the approximate time courses of the currents associated with the channels or pumps are shown symbolically without an effort to represent their magnitudes relative to each other. I_K incorporates at least two currents, $I_{K\text{-}R}$ and $I_{K\text{-}S}$. There appears to be an ultrarapid component as well, designated $I_{K\text{-}UR}$. The heavy bars for I_{Cl}, I_{pump}, and $I_{K(ATP)}$ indicate only the presence of these channels or pump without implying magnitude of currents because that would vary with physiological and pathophysiological conditions. The channels identified by brackets (I_{NS} and $I_{K(ATP)}$) are active only under pathological conditions. I_{NS} may represent a swelling-activated cation current. For the sinoatrial node cells, I_{NS} and I_{K1} are small or absent. Question marks indicate that experimental evidence is not yet available to determine the presence of these channels in sinoatrial cell membranes. Although it is likely that other ionic current mechanisms exist, they are not shown here because their roles in electrogenesis are not sufficiently well defined. (From Members of the Sicilian Gambit: Antiarrhythmic Therapy: A Pathophysiologic Approach. Mt Kisco, NY, Futura, 1994, p 13.)

conductance to Na^+. An externally applied stimulus or a spontaneously generated local membrane circuit current in advance of a propagating action potential depolarizes a sufficiently large area of membrane at a sufficiently rapid rate to open the Na^+ channels and depolarize the membrane further. When the stimulus activates enough Na^+ channels, Na^+ ions enter the cell, down their electrochemical gradient. The excited membrane no longer behaves like a K^+ electrode, that is, exclusively permeable to K^+, but more closely approximates a Na^+ electrode, and the membrane moves toward the Na^+ equilibrium potential.

The rate at which depolarization occurs during phase 0, that is, the maximum rate of change of voltage over time, is indicated by the expression dV/dt_{max} or $\dot{V}_{max}$ (see Table 27-2), which is a reasonable approximation of the rate and magnitude of Na^+ entry into the cell and a determinant of conduction velocity for the propagated action potential. The transient increase in sodium conductance lasts 1 to 2 milliseconds. The action potential, or more properly the Na^+ current (I_{Na}), is said to be regenerative; that is, intracellular movement of a little Na^+ depolarizes the membrane more, which increases conductance to Na^+ more, which allows more Na^+ to enter, and so on. As this process is occurring, however, $[Na^+]_i$ and positive intracellular charges increase and reduce the driving force for Na^+. When the equilibrium potential for Na^+ (E_{Na}) is reached, Na^+ no longer enters the cell; that is., when the driving force acting on the ion to enter the cell balances the driving force acting on the ion to exit the cell, no current flows. In addition, Na^+ conductance is time dependent, so that when the membrane spends some time at voltages less negative than the resting potential, Na^+ conductance decreases (inactivation; see earlier). Therefore, an intervention that reduces membrane potential for a time (acute myocardial ischemia)—but not to threshold—partially inactivates Na^+ channels, and if threshold is now achieved, the magnitude and rate of Na^+ influx are reduced, causing the conduction velocity to slow.

In cardiac Purkinje fibers and to a lesser extent in ventricular muscle, two different populations of Na^+ channels, or two different modes of operation of the same Na^+ channel, exist. One is responsible for the brief Na^+ current of phase 0, and the other, which is longer lasting, participates in the action potential plateau (steady-state or window current).[31] Tetrodotoxin (TTX) and local anesthetics block both types of channels,

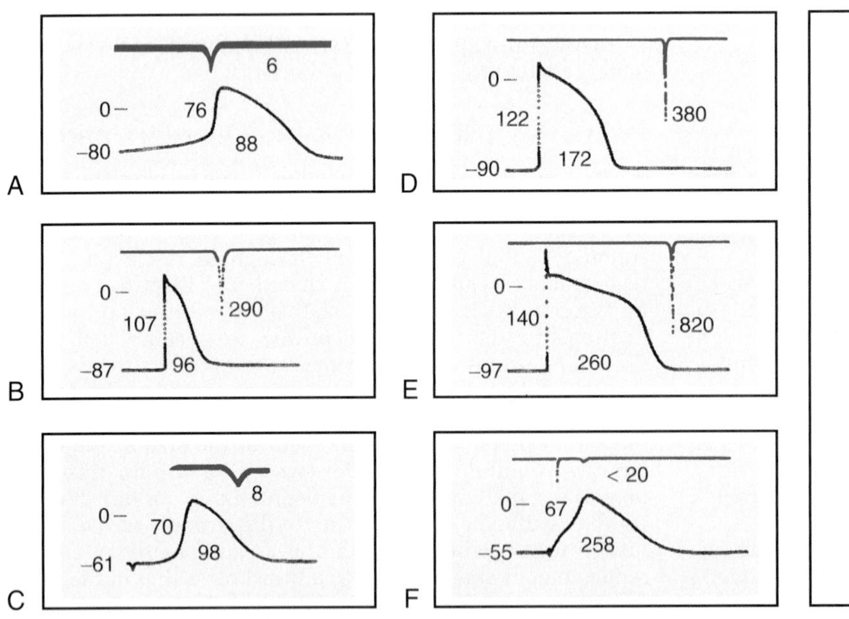

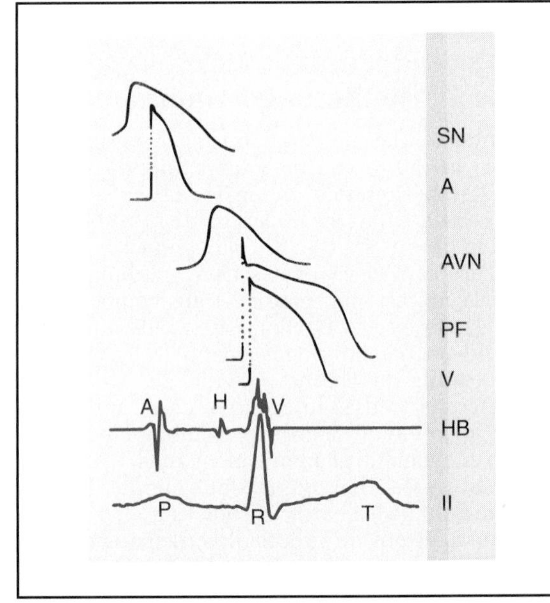

FIGURE 27–15 Action potentials recorded from different tissues in the heart **(left)** remounted along with a His bundle recording and scalar electrocardiogram from a patient **(right)** to illustrate the timing during a single cardiac cycle. In panels **A to F,** the top tracing is dV/dt of phase 0 and the second tracing is the action potential. For each panel the numbers (from left to right) indicate maximum diastolic potential (mV), action potential amplitude (mV), action potential duration at 90 percent of repolarization (milliseconds), and $\dot{V}_{max}$ of phase 0 (V/sec). Zero potential is indicated by the short horizontal line next to the zero on the upper left of each action potential. **A,** Rabbit sinoatrial node. **B,** Canine atrial muscle. **C,** Rabbit atrioventricular node. **D,** Canine ventricular muscle. **E,** Canine Purkinje fiber. **F,** Diseased human ventricle. Note that the action potentials recorded in **A, C,** and **F** have reduced resting membrane potentials, amplitudes, and $\dot{V}_{max}$ when compared with the other action potentials. In the right panel, A = atrial muscle potential; AVN = atrioventricular nodal potential; HB = His bundle recording; II = lead II; PF = Purkinje fiber potential; SN = sinus nodal potential; V = ventricular muscle potential. Horizontal calibration on the left: 50 milliseconds for A and C, 100 milliseconds for B, D, E, and F; 200 milliseconds on the right. Vertical calibration on the left: 50 mV. Horizontal calibration on the right: 200 milliseconds. (Modified from Gilmour RF Jr, Zipes DP: Basic electrophysiology of the slow inward current. *In* Antman E, Stone PH [eds]: Calcium Blocking Agents in the Treatment of Cardiovascular Disorders. Mt Kisco, NY, Futura, 1983, pp 1-37.)

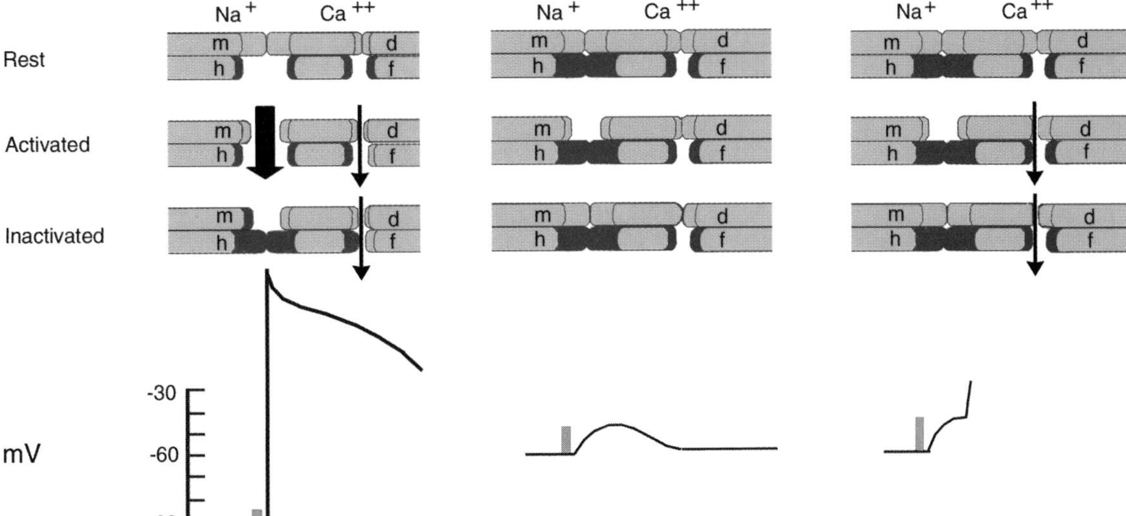

FIGURE 27–16 Schematic representation of membrane channels for rapid and slow inward currents at resting membrane potential **(top row)**, during the activated state **(middle row)**, and during the inactivated state **(bottom row)**. Vertically separated panels depict fibers with a normal resting potential of –90 mV **(left)**, with resting membrane potential reduced to less than –60 mV **(middle)**, and after stimulation of the cell with catecholamines **(right)**. The activation (m) and inactivation (h) gates of the fast channel and the activation (d) and inactivation (f) gates of the slow channel are depicted. During the resting state **(left)**, the activation gates of both channels are closed while the inactivation gates are open. When the cell is stimulated, the m gates of the fast channel open, and for a brief period, the open m gates and h gates allow inward sodium current to flow, depolarize the cell, and produce its upstroke. The action potential is depicted below. The h gates then close the channel and inactivate sodium conductance. Membrane depolarization also activates voltage-gated Ca^{2+} channels (d gates open), allowing influx of Ca^{2+} that contributes to the plateau phase of the action potential. The inactivation gates of the slow Ca^{2+} channel are both voltage and $[Ca^{2+}]_i$ dependent. High and low levels of intracellular free calcium ions, respectively, accelerate and slow inactivation, thereby functioning as a negative feedback mechanism to control intracellular calcium content. When the upstroke of the action potential exceeds the threshold for activation of the slow inward current, the d gates open and allow ingress of the slow inward current that contributes to the plateau phase of the action potential. The f gates of the slow channel close more slowly than the h gates. Although the slow inward channel remains open longer than the fast channel does, less total current flows. When the resting membrane potential is reduced below –60 mV by increasing $[K]_o$ from 4.0 to 14.0 mm **(middle)**, the cell depolarizes to –60 mV and the fast channel becomes inactivated because the h gates remain closed. Even though the m gate may open during activation, the amount of sodium current is too small to elicit an action potential. The inactivation gates of the slow channel (f gates) remain open, and when the cell is excited after the addition of catecholamine **(right)**, the d gates open and permit flow of a slow inward current that causes a slow-response action potential. This action potential resembles those in panels A, C, and F of Figure 27–15. (From Wit AL, Bigger JT Jr: Possible electrophysiological mechanisms for lethal arrhythmias accompanying myocardial ischemia and infarction. Circulation 52[Suppl 3]:96, 1975.)

thereby diminishing the rate of rise of phase 0 and shortening the action potential duration. Furthermore, there may be a background Na^+ current ($I_{Na\text{-}B}$) through a voltage-independent channel in sinus nodal cells that contributes to pacemaker behavior.[8]

GATING OF VOLTAGE-DEPENDENT FAST SODIUM CHANNELS. In this model, three m (activation) gates and one h (inactivation) gate can be considered to be lined up in series in the membrane Na^+ channel (Fig. 27–16), with the m gate on the extracellular side and the h gate on the intracellular side of the membrane. When the membrane is in a resting polarized state, the m gates are almost completely closed, the h gate is open, and no Na^+ can cross the membrane. Although depolarization of the membrane opens the m gates and closes the h gate, the m gates open faster than the h gate closes; that is, activation of the channel proceeds faster than inactivation can occur, and Na^+ flows through the Na^+ channel for about 1 millisecond while both gates are open simultaneously (see Fig. 27–16, left, thick arrow).

When the membrane repolarizes to fairly high negative values, that is, the membrane potential becomes more negative than about –60 mV, the m gates shut rapidly, the h gate opens more slowly (reactivation or recovery from inactivation), and the membrane is once again capable of depolarization. Until that time, the cell is absolutely refractory; that is, no stimulus, regardless of intensity, can activate the cell. If the membrane is activated a second time before reaching a large negative value, all the h gates have not yet reopened and the maximum number of Na^+ channels that can open is reduced. The resulting action potential has reduced $\dot{V}_{max}$, amplitude, duration, and conduction velocity. The state of the gates at any time depends on the membrane potential and the length of time that the potential has been maintained.

A cluster of positively charged arginine and lysine residues in the S4 domain is thought to function as the voltage sensor (m gate), and the peptide loop connecting repeats S3 and S4 binds to the activated channel and occludes the intracellular mouth of the channel pore (h gate; Fig. 27–17). This loop could be regarded as analogous to the N-terminal peptide chain of inactivating voltage-gated potassium channels (see Fig. 27–9A).

The Hodgkin-Huxley theory has been used to describe the voltage dependence of single-channel permeability to sodium, with four hypothetical gating particles making independent transitions between conducting and nonconducting positions to control ion flux. Three m particles control activation and one h particle controls inactivation. The probability that they are all in a position where the channel conducts is m^3h, and for the Na^+ channel,

$$P_{Na} = m^3 \cdot h \cdot P_{Na,max}$$

where P_{Na} is the permeability of the sodium channel at a given voltage, $P_{Na,max}$ is the maximal possible permeability of the channel, m^3 represents the probability that all three activation particles are in a position to make up an open channel (m = 1, gate is permissive; m = 0, gate is nonpermissive), whereas h represents the probability that the Na^+ channel is not inactivated (h = 1, gate is open; h = 0, gate is shut). Because opening and closing of the gates are voltage *and* time dependent, the permeability of the channel (P_{Na}) is some fraction of the maximum possible permeability ($P_{Na,max}$), depending on membrane potential and the period for which the membrane has been at that voltage.

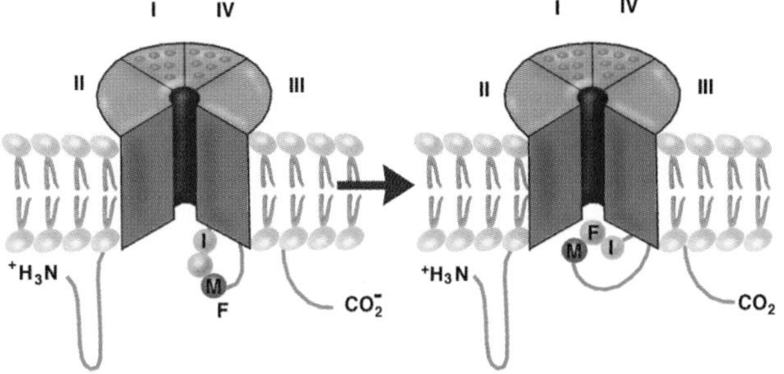

FIGURE 27–17 Mechanism of fast inactivation of sodium channels. The hinged-lid mechanism of sodium channel inactivation is illustrated. The intracellular loop connecting domains III and IV of the sodium channel is depicted as forming a hinged lid. The critical residue (Phe1489F) is shown as occluding the intracellular mouth of the pore. (From Catteral WA: Molecular analysis of voltage gated sodium channels in the heart and other tissues. *In* Zipes DP, Jalife J [eds]: Cardiac Electrophysiology: From Cell to Bedside. 2nd ed. Philadelphia, WB Saunders, 1994, p 1.)

UPSTROKE OF THE ACTION POTENTIAL. In normal atrial and ventricular muscle and in fibers in the His-Purkinje system, action potentials have very rapid upstrokes with a large $\dot{V}_{max}$ and are called *fast responses*. Action potentials in the normal sinus and AV nodes and many types of diseased tissue have very slow upstrokes with a reduced $\dot{V}_{max}$ and are called *slow responses* (Table 27–3; see Fig. 27–15). Upstrokes of slow responses are mediated by a slow inward, predominantly Ca^{2+} current (I_{Ca}) rather than the fast inward I_{Na} (Table 27–4). These potentials received the name *slow response* because the time required for activation and inactivation of the slow inward current ($I_{Ca.L}$) is approximately an order of magnitude slower than that for the fast inward Na^+ current (I_{Na}). Recovery from inactivation also takes longer. Calcium entry and $[Ca^{2+}]_i$ help promote inactivation. Thus, the slow channel opens (activation gates d) and closes (inactivation gates f) more slowly than the fast channel does, remains open for a longer time, and requires more time following a stimulus to be reactivated (see Fig. 27–16). In fact, recovery of excitability outlasts full restoration of maximum diastolic potential, which means that even though the membrane potential has returned to normal, the cell has not recovered excitability completely because the latter depends on elapse of a certain amount of time (i.e., is time dependent) and not just on recovery of a particular membrane potential (i.e., voltage dependence), a phenomenon termed postrepolarization refractoriness.

The threshold for activation of $I_{Ca.L}$, that is, the voltage that the cell must reach to "turn on" the slow inward current, is about −30 to −40 mV. In fibers of the fast response type, $I_{Ca.L}$ is normally activated during phase 0 by the regenerative depolarization caused by the fast sodium current. Current flows through both fast and slow channels during the latter part of the action potential upstroke. However, $I_{Ca.L}$ is much smaller than the peak Na^+ current and therefore contributes little to the action potential until the fast Na^+ current is inactivated, after completion of phase 0. Thus, $I_{Ca.L}$ affects mainly the plateau of action potentials recorded in atrial and ventricular muscle and His-Purkinje fibers. When the fast Na^+ current is inactivated rapidly, such as in frog ventricle, $I_{Ca.L}$ may contribute noticeably to the peak of phase 0. In addition, $I_{Ca.L}$ may play a prominent role in partially depolarized cells in which the fast Na^+ channels have been inactivated, if conditions are appropriate for slow-channel activation.[30,53]

At least two types of calcium current exist in human cardiac myocytes: a slowly inactivating dihydropyridine-sensitive current $I_{Ca.L}$ and a rapidly inactivating dihydropyridine-insensitive current $I_{Ca.T}$. $I_{Ca.L}$ produces depolarization and propagation in sinus and AV nodal cells and contributes to the plateau of atrial and ventricular myocytes. Calcium channel blockers block this channel, which is strongly modulated by neurotransmitters. $I_{Ca.T}$ is activated at membrane potentials intermediate between I_{Na} and $I_{Ca.L}$ and probably contributes inward current to the later stages of phase 4 depolarizations in the sinus node and His-Purkinje cells.[54] A functional role of $I_{Ca.T}$ in normal atrial and ventricular myocytes is less certain. Whether Ca^{2+} influx through open T-type channels provides a sufficient trigger for Ca^{2+} release from the sarcoplasmic reticulum is controversial. The density of T-type Ca^{2+} channels has been found to be increased in myocytes from hearts with experimentally induced hypertrophy,[54] but the role of enhanced T-type channel density under these conditions remains to be determined.

Other significant differences exist between the fast and slow channels (see Table 27-4). Drugs that elevate cAMP levels, such as beta adrenoceptor agonists, phosphodiesterase inhibitors such as theophylline, and the lipid-soluble derivative of cAMP dibutyryl cAMP, increase $I_{Ca.L}$. Binding of the beta adrenoceptor agonist to specific sarcolemmal receptors facilitates the dissociation of two subunits of a regulatory protein (G protein, see Chap. 19), one of which (G_s) activates adenylate cyclase and thus increases intracellular levels of cAMP. The latter binds to a regulatory subunit of a cAMP-dependent protein kinase that promotes phosphorylation of specific phosphorylation sites on the channel protein (see Fig. 27-9A), ultimately resulting in enhanced open-state probability of the channel.

Acetylcholine reduces $I_{Ca.L}$ by decreasing adenylate cyclase activity. However, acetylcholine stimulates cyclic guanosine monophosphate (cGMP) accumulation. cGMP has negligible effects on basal $I_{Ca.L}$ but decreases $I_{Ca.L}$ levels that have been elevated by beta adrenoceptor agonists. This effect is mediated by cAMP hydrolysis through a cGMP-stimulated cyclic nucleotide phosphodiesterase.[55]

DIFFERENCES BETWEEN CHANNELS. Fast and slow channels can be differentiated on the basis of their pharmacological sensitivity. Drugs that block the slow channel with a *fair* degree of specificity include verapamil, nifedipine, diltiazem, and D-600 (a methoxy derivative of verapamil). Antiarrhythmic agents such as lidocaine, quinidine, procainamide, and disopyramide (see Chap. 30) affect the fast channel and not the slow channel. The puffer fish poison TTX, which is too toxic to be used clinically, blocks the fast channel with considerable specificity (see Table 27-4).

Normal action potentials recorded from the sinus node and the N region of the AV node have a reduced resting membrane potential, action potential amplitude, overshoot, upstroke, and conduction velocity compared with action potentials in muscle or Purkinje fibers (see Fig. 27-15).

Slow-channel blockers, but not TTX, suppress sinus and AV nodal action potentials. The prolonged time for reactivation of $I_{Ca.L}$ probably accounts for the fact that sinus and AV nodal cells remain refractory longer than the time that it takes for full voltage repolarization to occur. Thus, premature stimulation immediately after the membrane potential reaches full repolarization leads to action potentials with reduced amplitudes and upstroke velocities. Therefore, slow conduction and prolonged refractoriness are characteristic features of nodal cells. These cells also have a reduced "safety factor for conduction," which means that the stimulating efficacy of the propagating impulse is low and conduction block occurs easily. Membranes of nodal cells probably do have Na channels that are inactivated by the relatively depolarized range of potentials over which activity takes place. Hyperpolarization exposes a fast TTX-sensitive sodium current in nodal cells.

INWARD CURRENTS. Thus, I_{Na} and I_{Ca} represent two important inward currents. Another important inward current is I_f, also called the *pacemaker current*.[2] This current is activated by hyperpolarization and is carried by Na^+ and K^+. It generates phase 4 diastolic depolarization in the sinus node. I_f modulation is one major mechanism by which beta-adrenergic and cholinergic neurotransmitters regulate cardiac rhythm under physiological conditions. Catecholamines increase the probability of channel opening, with no change in single-channel amplitude, and increase the discharge rate, with cholinergic action, in general, having an opposite effect.

A variety of manipulations, including those that block or inactivate I_{Na} (such as administration of TTX or sustained depolarization of the cell membrane with external Ba^{2+} to block K^+ efflux through I_{K1} channels), combined with those that increase $I_{Ca.L}$ (such as administration of catecholamines), can transform a fast channel–dependent fiber (e.g., a Purkinje fiber) to a slow channel–dependent fiber. Whether these artificial in vitro alterations have clinical relevance is not known.

The electrophysiological changes accompanying *acute* myocardial ischemia may represent a depressed form of a fast response in the center of the ischemic zone and a slow response in the border area. Probable slow-response activity has been shown in myocardium resected from patients undergoing surgery for recurrent ventricular tachyarrhythmias (see Fig. 27-15F). Whether and how slow responses play a role in the genesis of ventricular arrhythmias in these patients have not been established.

Phase 1—Early Rapid Repolarization

Following phase 0, the membrane repolarizes rapidly and transiently to nearly 0 mV (early notch), partly because of inactivation of I_{Na} and concomitant activation of several outward currents:

I_{to}. The 4-aminopyridine-sensitive transient outward K^+ current, commonly termed I_{to} (or I_{to1}), is turned on rapidly by depolarization and then rapidly inactivates. Both the density and recovery of I_{to} from inactivation exhibit transmural gradients in the left ventricular free wall, with the density decreasing and reactivation becoming progressively prolonged from epicardium to endocardium.[56] It is currently unknown whether these nonuniformities in I_{to} recovery reflect transmural differences in channel subunit composition or in posttranslational modification of channel proteins that are thought to underlie I_{to} (Kv4.2 and Kv4.3). Gradients in I_{to} channel density and reactivation kinetics give rise to regional differences in action potential shape, with increasingly slower phase 1 restitution kinetics and diminution of the notch along the transmural axis (Fig. 27-18). These regional differences might create transmural voltage gradients, specifically at higher rates, thereby increasing

TABLE 27–3 Synopsis of Ionic Currents in Mammalian Cardiac Myocytes

I_{Na}	Tetrodotoxin-sensitive voltage-gated Na^+ current
$I_{Na\text{-}B}$	Proposed background Na^+ current through a voltage-independent channel in sinus nodal cells
$I_{Ca.L}$	L-type (*l*ong lasting, *l*arge conductance) Ca^{2+} currents through voltage-gated channels blocked by dihydropyridine-type antagonists (e.g., nifedipine), phenylalkylamines (e.g., verapamil), benzothiazepines (e.g., diltiazem), and a variety of divalent ions (e.g., Cd^{2+}), activated by dihydropyridine-type agonists (e.g., Bay K 8644), responsible for phase 0 depolarization and propagation in sinoatrial and AV nodal tissue, and contributing to the plateau of atrial, His-Purkinje, and ventricular cells; main trigger of Ca^{2+} release from the sarcoplasmic reticulum (Ca^{2+}-induced Ca^{2+} release); a noninactivating or "window" component may underlie early afterdepolarizations
$I_{Ca.T}$	T-type (*t*ransient current, *t*iny conductance) Ca^{2+} currents through voltage-gated channels blocked by mibefradil but insensitive to dihydropyridines; may contribute inward current to the later phase of phase 4 depolarization in pacemaker cells
I_f	Hyperpolarization-activated current carried by Na^+ and K^+ in sinoatrial and AV nodal cells and His-Purkinje cells and involved in generating phase 4 depolarization; increases rate of impulse initiation in pacemaker cells
I_{K1}	Inward rectifier K^+ current, voltage-dependent block by Ba^{2+} at micromolar concentrations: responsible for maintaining resting membrane potential in atrial, His-Purkinje, and ventricular cells; channel activity is a function of both membrane potential and $[K^+]_0$; inward rectification appears to result from depolarization-induced internal block by Mg^{2+}
$I_{K.G}$ ($I_{K.Ach}$, $I_{K.Ade}$)	Inwardly rectifying K^+ current activated by muscarinic [M_2] and purinergic (type 1) receptor stimulation via GTP regulatory (G) protein signal transduction; expressed in sinoatrial and AV nodal cells and atrial cells, where it causes hyperpolarization and action potential shortening; activation causes negative chronotropic and dromotropic effects
I_K	K^+ current carried by a voltage-gated K^+ channel (delayed rectifier K^+ channel); composed of the rapid (I_{Kr}) and slow (I_{Ks}) component. I_{Kr} is specifically blocked by dofetilide and sotalol in a reverse-use–dependent manner; inward rectification of I_{Kr} result from depolarization-induced fast inactivation; plays a major role in determining action potential duration
$I_{K.ur}$	K^+ current through a voltage-gated channel with ultrarapid activation, but ultraslow inactivation kinetics; expressed in atrial myocytes; determines action potential duration
I_{to} (I_{to1}, I_A)	Transient outward K^+ current through voltage-gated channels; exhibits fast activation and inactivation kinetics; blocked by 4-aminopyridine in a reverse-use–dependent manner; determines time course of phase 1 repolarization
$I_{Cl.Ca}$ (I_{to2})	4-Aminopyridine–resistant transient outward current carried by Cl^- ions; activated by rises in intracellular calcium; blocked by stilbene derivatives (SITS, DIDS); determines time course of phase 1 repolarization; may underlie spontaneous transient inward currents under conditions of Ca^{2+} overload
$I_{Cl.cAMP}$	Time-independent chloride current regulated by the cAMP/adenylate cyclase pathway; slightly depolarizes resting membrane potential and significantly shortens action potential duration; antagonizes action potential prolongation associated with β-adrenergic stimulation of $I_{Ca.L}$
$I_{Cl.swell}$	Outwardly rectifying, swelling-activated Cl^- current; inhibited by 9-anthracene carboxylic acid; activation causes resting membrane depolarization and action potential shortening
$I_{K.ATP}$	Time-independent K^+ current through channels activated by a fall in intracellular ATP concentration; inhibited by sulfonylurea drugs, such as glibenclamide; activated by pinacidil, nicorandil, cromakalim; causes shortening of action potential duration during myocardial ischemia or hypoxia
$I_{Cir.swell}$	Inwardly rectifying, swelling-activated cation current; permeable to Na^+ and K^+ ($P_{Na}/P_K = 8$); inhibited by Gd^{3+}; depolarizes resting membrane potential and prolongs terminal (phase 3) repolarization
$I_{Na/Ca}$	Current carried by the Na/Ca exchanger; causes a net Na^+ outward current and a Ca^{2+} inward current (reverse mode) or a net Na^+ inward and Ca^{2+} outward current (3 Na^+ for 1 Ca^{2+}), the direction of Na^+ flux being dependent on membrane potential and intracellular and extracellular concentrations of Na^+ and Ca^{2+}; Ca^{2+} influx mediated by $I_{Na/Ca}$ can trigger SR Ca^{2+} release; underlies I_{ti} (transient inward current) under conditions of intracellular Ca^{2+} overload
$I_{Na/K}$	Na^+ outward current generated by Na^+, K^+-ATPase (stoichiometry: 3 Na^+ leave and 2 K^+ enter); inhibited by digitalis
Electroneutral Ion-Exchanging Proteins	
Ca^{2+}-ATPase	Extrudes cytosolic calcium
Na/H	Exchanges intracellular H^+ for extracellular Na^+; cardiac myocytes express isoform NHE 1; specifically inhibited by the benzoylguanidine derivatives HOE 694 and HOE 642; inhibition causes intracellular acidification
Cl^--HCO_3^-	Exchanges intracellular HCO_3^- for external Cl^-; inhibited by SITS
Na^+-K^+-$2Cl^-$	Cotransporter blocked by amiloride

ATP = adenosine triphosphate; AV = atrioventricular; cAMP = cyclic adenosine monophosphate; DIDS = 4,4′-diisothiocyanatostilbene-2,2′-disulfonic acid; GTP = guanosine triphosphate; SITS = 4-acetamido-4′-isothiocyanatostilbene-2,2′-disulfonic acid; SR = sarcoplasmic reticulum.

TABLE 27–4 Characteristics of Fast and Slow Inward Currents in Cardiac Tissue

Characteristic	Fast	Slow
Primary charge carrier	Na	Ca (Na)
Activation threshold* (mV)	−70 to −55	−55 to −30
Magnitude (μA)	1-30	0.1-3.0
Time constant of		
Activation (msec)	<1	<5
Inactivation (msec)	<1	3-80
Inhibitors	Tetrodotoxin, local anesthetics, sustained depolarization at less than −40 mV	Verapamil, D-600, nifedipine, diltiazem, Mn, Co, Ni, La, Ca^{2+}
Resting membrane potential (mV)	−80 to −95	−40 to −70
Conduction velocity (m/sec)	0.3-3.0	0.01-0.10
Rate of rise ($\dot{V}_{max}$) of action potential upstroke (V/sec)	200-1000	1-10
Action potential amplitude (mV)	100-130	35-75
Response to stimulus	All or none	Affected by characteristics of stimulus
Recovery of excitability	Prompt, ends with repolarization	Delayed, outlasts full repolarization
Safety factor for conduction	High	Low
Major current of action potential upstroke in the following:		
SA node	−	+
Atrial myocardium	+	−
AV node (N region)	−	+
His-Purkinje system	+	−
Ventricular myocardium	+	−
Neurotransmitter influence		
Beta-adrenergic	−	↑↑
Alpha-adrenergic	−	↑
Muscarinic, cholinergic	−	↓ In atrium ↓ In ventricle

AV = atrioventricular; SA = sinoatrial.

*Note that the term "threshold" does not stand for a sharp voltage threshold for channel opening but a threshold for reversal of the net membrane current. This situation occurs when the membrane potential reaches a range where just enough Na^+ (or Ca^{2+}) channels open to make an inward current that opposes the sum of outward currents carried by K^+ and other ions.

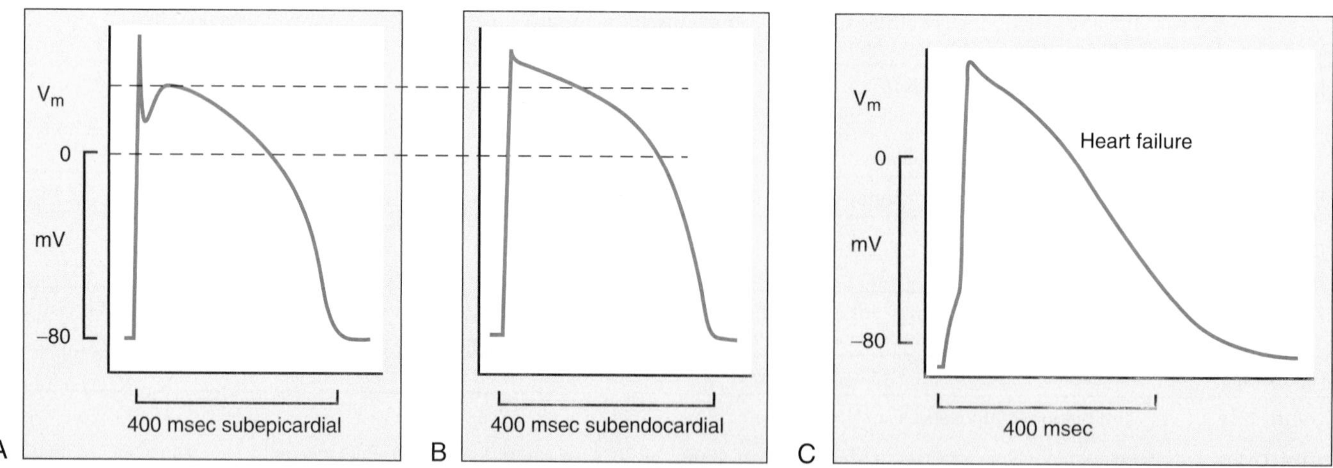

FIGURE 27–18 Action potential plots demonstrating differences in the action potential shape of human ventricular myocytes of subepicardial **(A)** and subendocardial **(B)** origin. Subepicardial myocytes present a prominent notch during phase 1 repolarization of the action potential, most likely caused by a larger I_{to} in these cells. The notch is absent in subendocardial cells. The peak plateau potential is higher in subendocardial than in subepicardial myocytes, and the action potential duration tends to be shorter in subepicardial cells. Recording temperature = 35°C; V_m = membrane potential. **C,** Transmembrane action potential in a human ventricular cardiomyocyte of a failing heart. Note loss of the prominent phase 1 notch and delayed repolarization. (**A** and **B,** From Näbauer M, Beuckelmann DJ, Uberfuhr P, Steinbeck G: Regional differences in current density and rate-dependent properties of the transient outward current in subepicardial and subendocardial myocytes of human left ventricle. Circulation 93:168, 1996. By permission of the American Heart Association. **C,** From Priebe L, Beuckelmann DJ: Simulation studies of cellular electrical properties in heart failure. Circ Res 82:1206-1223, 1998.)

dispersion of repolarization, a putative arrhythmogenic factor (see Brugada syndrome in Chap. 32). Because I_{to} overlaps I_{Na}, changes in I_{to} density or properties can also affect cellular excitability. Downregulation of I_{to} is at least partially responsible for slowing of phase 1 repolarization in failing human myocytes.[57] Studies have demonstrated that these changes in the phase 1 notch of the cardiac action potential cause a reduction in the kinetics and peak amplitude of the action potential–evoked intracellular Ca^{2+} transient because of failed recruitment and synchronization of the sarcoplasmic reticulum Ca^{2+} release through $I_{Ca,L}$. Thus, modulation of I_{to} appears to play a significant physiological role in controlling cardiac excitation-contraction coupling,[58,59] and it remains to be determined whether transmural differences in phase 1 repolarization translate into similar differences in regional contractility.

$I_{Cl.Ca}$. The 4-aminopyridine-resistant, Ca^{2+}-activated chloride current $I_{Cl.Ca}$ (or I_{to2}) also contributes a significant outward current during phase 1 repolarization.[60] This current is activated by the action potential–evoked intracellular Ca^{2+} transient. Therefore, interventions that augment the amplitude of the Ca^{2+} transient associated with the twitch (such as beta-adrenergic receptor stimulation) also enhance outward $I_{Cl.Ca}$. It is not currently known whether human cardiac myocytes express Ca^{2+}-activated chloride channels. Other, time-*in*dependent chloride currents may also play a role in determining the time course of early repolarization, such as the cAMP- or swelling-activated chloride conductances $I_{Cl.cAMP}$ and $I_{Cl.swell}$.[47]

Na/Ca EXCHANGER. A third current contributing to early repolarization is Na^+ outward movement through the Na/Ca exchanger operating in reverse mode (see Fig. 27–14).[61] Overexpression of the exchanger in transgenic mice caused accentuation of the early "notch" in left ventricular myocytes.[62]

Sometimes, a transient depolarization follows phase 1 repolarization. This notch is well defined and separated from phase 2 in Purkinje fibers and left ventricular epicardial and midmyocardial myocytes (see Fig. 27–18).

Phase 2—Plateau

During the plateau phase, which may last several hundred milliseconds, membrane conductance to all ions falls to rather low values. Thus, less change in current is required near plateau levels than near resting potential levels to produce the same changes in transmembrane potential. The plateau is maintained by the competition between outward current carried by K^+ and Cl^- ions and inward current carried by Ca^{2+} moving through open L-type Ca^{2+} channels and Na^+ being exchanged for internal Ca^{2+} by the Na^+/Ca^{2+} exchanger operating in forward mode. After depolarization, potassium conductance falls to plateau levels as a result of inward rectification in spite of the large electrochemical driving force on K^+ ions.

Rectification simply means that membrane conductance changes with voltage. Specifically, inward rectification means that K^+ channels are open at negative potentials but shut at less negative or positive voltages. Membrane depolarization–induced internal block by intracellular ionized magnesium is thought to underlie inward rectification of cardiac I_{K1} channels. The mechanism underlying rectification of the rapid component of the delayed rectifier K^+ current (I_{Kr}) in cardiac cells is the inactivation that channels rapidly undergo during depolarizing pulses. More I_{Kr} channels enter the inactivated state with stronger depolarizations, thereby causing inward rectification. This fast inactivation mechanism is sensitive to changes in extracellular K^+ in the physiological range, with inactivation more accentuated at low extracellular K^+ concentrations.[63] Thus, hypokalemia would decrease outward I_{Kr}, thereby prolonging action potential duration.

Outward K^+ movement carried by the slow component of the delayed rectifier K^+ current (I_{Ks}) also contributes to plateau duration. (1) I_{Ks} density has been shown to be correlated with action potential duration[57] and (2) isolated defects in the KvLQT1 subunit, which in combination with the IsK subunit (minK) reconstitutes the cardiac I_{Ks} current, are associated with abnormally prolonged ventricular repolarization (long QT syndrome type 1; see Chaps. 28 and 32). Although I_{Ks} activates slowly compared with action potential duration, it is only slowly inactivated. Therefore, increases in heart rate can cause this activation to accumulate during successive depolarizations. Thus, cumulative activation can determine the contribution to repolarization of K^+ currents that are active during the plateau of the action potential.[29] In conditions of reduced intracellular ATP concentration (hypoxia, ischemia), K^+ efflux through activated K_{ATP} channels is enhanced, thereby shortening the plateau phase of the action potential. Other ionic mechanisms that control plateau potential and duration include the kinetics of inactivation of the L-type Ca^{2+} current. Reduced efficiency of intracellular free Ca^{2+} to induce Ca^{2+}-dependent inactivation, such as in myocytes from hypertrophic hearts, can result in delayed repolarization. Steady-state components of both I_{Na} and $I_{Ca.L}$ (window currents) can shape the plateau phase.

One type of the long QT syndrome, LQT3, is caused by a defective sodium channel gene, *SCN5A*. One mutation in patients with LQT3 involves a deletion of three amino acids in the S3-S4 cytoplasmic linker loop (see Fig. 27–17 and Chap. 28), which is thought to mediate inactivation. The mutant sodium channel is inactivated only incompletely, which results in prolonged depolarizations. Na^+,K^+-ATPase generates a net outward current by pumping out three Na^+ ions in exchange for two K^+. Noninactivating chloride currents, such as $I_{Cl.swell}$ and $I_{Cl.cAMP}$, may produce significant outward currents during the plateau phase under certain conditions, thereby significantly shortening action potential duration. A nonselective, swelling-induced cation current has been shown to cause action potential prolongation in myocytes from failing ventricles.[64]

Phase 3—Final Rapid Repolarization

In this portion of the action potential, repolarization proceeds rapidly owing at least in part to two currents: time-dependent inactivation of $I_{Ca.L}$, with a decrease in the intracellular movement of positive charges, and activation of repolarizing K^+ currents, including the slow and rapid components of the delayed rectifier K^+ current I_{Ks} and I_{Kr} and the inwardly rectifying K^+ currents I_{K1} and $I_{K.Ach}$, all causing an increase in the movement of positive charges out of the cell. The net membrane current becomes more outward, and the membrane potential shifts to the resting potential. Mutations in the human ether-a-go-go–related gene (*HERG*), which is responsible for I_{Kr}, prolong phase 3 repolarization, thereby predisposing to the development of torsades de pointes. Macrolide antibiotics such as erythromycin, antihistamines such as terfenadine, and antifungal drugs such as ketoconazole all inhibit I_{Kr} and have been implicated in the acquired form of long QT syndrome (see Chaps. 28 and 32). A decrease in I_{K1} activity, as is the case in left ventricular myocytes from failing hearts,[57] causes action potential prolongation by slowing of phase 3 repolarization and resting membrane depolarization (Fig. 27–19). Reduction in the outward

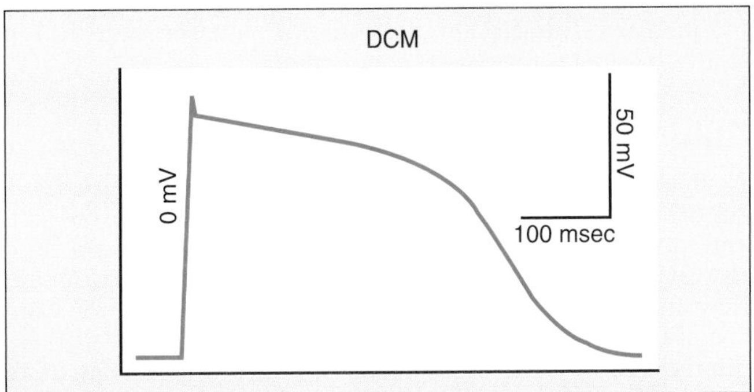

FIGURE 27–19 Transmembrane action potential recording in a ventricular myocyte of a failing human heart caused by idiopathic dilated cardiomyopathy (DCM). Note the marked slowing of phase 3 repolarization compared with an action potential of a nonfailing human ventricular myocyte (see Fig. 27–16). (From Koumi S, Backer CL, Arentzen CE: Molecular and cellular cardiology: Characterization of inwardly rectifying K^+ channel in human cardiac myocytes: Alterations in channel behavior in myocytes isolated from patients with idiopathic dilated cardiomyopathy. Circulation 92:164, 1995.)

potassium current through open inward rectifier K^+ channels renders the failing cardiomyocyte more susceptible to the induction of delayed afterdepolarizations triggered by spontaneous intracellular Ca^{2+} release events and therefore plays a major role in arrhythmogenesis in the failing heart (see Fig. 27–23).

Phase 4—Diastolic Depolarization

Under normal conditions, the membrane potential of atrial and ventricular muscle cells remains steady throughout diastole. I_{K1} is the current responsible for maintaining the resting potential near the K^+ equilibrium potential in atrial, His-Purkinje, and ventricular cells. I_{K1} is the inward rectifier and shuts off during depolarization. It is absent in sinus nodal and AV nodal cells. In other fibers found in certain parts of the atria, in the muscle of the mitral and tricuspid valves, in His-Purkinje fibers, and in the sinus node and distal portion of the AV node, the resting membrane potential does not remain constant in diastole but gradually depolarizes (see Fig. 27–15A). If a propagating impulse does not depolarize the cell or group of cells, it can reach threshold by itself and produce a spontaneous action potential. The property possessed by spontaneously discharging cells is called *phase 4 diastolic depolarization*; when it leads to initiation of action potentials, automaticity results. The discharge rate of the sinus node normally exceeds the discharge rate of other potentially automatic pacemaker sites and thus maintains dominance of the cardiac rhythm. The discharge rate of the sinus node is normally more sensitive to the effects of norepinephrine and acetylcholine than the discharge rate of ventricular muscle cells. Normal or abnormal automaticity at other sites can cause discharge at rates faster than the sinus nodal discharge rate and can usurp control of the cardiac rhythm for one cycle or many (see Chap. 32).

Normal Automaticity

The ionic basis of automaticity is explained by a net gain in intracellular positive charges during diastole. Contributing to this change is a voltage-dependent channel activated by potentials negative to −50 to −60 mV, that is, a hyperpolarization-activated inward pacemaker current. At this potential I_f becomes activated and is carried by a channel relatively nonselective for monovalent cations. Hyperpolarization increases its rate of activation, and at −70 mV the time constant of activation ranges from 2 to 4 seconds. I_f probably underlies the slow diastolic depolarization that occurs between −90 and −60 mV in Purkinje fibers. Although either K^+ or Na^+ ions can serve as ion transporters, I_f carries largely Na^+ at the more negative intracellular voltages. Extracellular K^+ ions activate I_f, but $[Na^+]_o$ does not influence its conductance.

Automaticity in Sinus Nodal Cells

At the reduced membrane potentials of sinus nodal cells, I_f contributes only about 20 percent of the pacemaker current, and automaticity is primarily dependent on I_K and $I_{Ca.L}$. However, sinus nodal cells exhibit significant I_f current if they are hyperpolarized in the range of −50 to −100 mV. Conversely, I_K in normally polarized Purkinje fibers adds little to the pacemaker current. Deactivation of I_K, the presence of an unidentified background inward current, deactivation of $I_{Ca.T}$, and activation of $I_{Ca.L}$ are the essential processes governing the rate of pacemaker depolarization in sinus and AV nodal cells and in Purkinje fibers whose membrane potential has been depolarized to voltages largely positive to the activation range of I_f.

The sinus nodal discharge rate maintains dominance over latent pacemaker sites because it depolarizes more rapidly and because of the mechanism called *overdrive suppression*, a phenomenon characterized by prolonged suppression of normal pacemakers in proportion to the duration and rate of stimulation by a more rapidly discharging pacemaker. The mechanism may be related to active Na extrusion during the more rapid rate that maintains diastolic depolarization of latent pacemakers at a level more negative than the threshold potential for automatic discharge.

The rate of sinus nodal discharge can be varied by several mechanisms in response to autonomic or other influences. The pacemaker locus can shift within or outside the sinus node to cells discharging faster or more slowly. If the pacemaker site remains the same, alterations in the slope of the diastolic depolarization, maximum diastolic potential, or threshold potential can speed or slow the discharge rate. For example, if the slope of diastolic depolarization steepens and if the resting membrane potential becomes less negative or the threshold potential more negative (within limits), discharge rate increases. Opposite changes slow the discharge rate.

Acetylcholine activates K^+ efflux through acetylcholine-sensitive inward rectifier K^+ channels, which are expressed in both sinus nodal and AV nodal cells, thereby shifting the maximum diastolic potential to more negative values. The same mechanism reduces input resistance at diastolic potentials, which means that a greater depolarizing current would be required to achieve "threshold" for firing an action potential.

Studies using fluorescent calcium-sensitive indicators, combined with imaging and simultaneous measurement of transmembrane action potential, suggest that cyclic variations in submembrane Ca^{2+} concentration coupled to activation of the Na^+/Ca^{2+} exchange current modulate sinoatrial node cell beating rate and are a factor in establishing dominance of the sinoatrial node cell pacemaker function (Fig. 27-20).[65]

Passive Membrane Electrical Properties

We have just discussed many of the features of active membrane properties. In addition, it is important to be aware of some features of the passive membrane properties of cardiac myocytes, such as membrane resistance, capacitance, and cable properties.

Although the cardiac cell membrane is resistant to current flow, it also has capacitative properties, which means that it behaves like a battery and can store charges of opposite sign on its two sides: an excess of negative charges inside the membrane balanced by equivalent positive charges outside the membrane. These resistive and capacitative properties cause the membrane to take a certain amount of time to respond to an applied stimulus, rather than responding instantly, because the charges across the capacitative membrane must be altered first. A subthreshold rectangular current pulse applied to the membrane produces a slowly rising and decaying membrane voltage change rather than a rectangular voltage change. A value called the *time constant of the membrane* reflects this property. The time constant tau is equal to the product of membrane resistance R_m and cell capacitance C_m,

$$\text{tau} = R_m \cdot C_m$$

and is the time taken by the membrane voltage to reach 63 percent of its final value after application of a steady current.

When aligned end to end, cardiac cells, particularly the His-Purkinje system, behave like a long cable in which current flows more easily inside the cell and to the adjacent cell across the gap junction than it does across the cell membrane to the outside. When current is injected at a point, most of it flows along inside the cell, but some leaks out. Because of this loss of current, the voltage change of a cell at a site distant from the point of applied current is less than the change in membrane voltage where the stimulus was given. A measure of this property of a cable is called the space or length constant *lambda* (λ), which is the distance along the cable from the point of stimulation at which the voltage at steady state is 1/e (37 percent) of its value at the point of introduction.

Restated, λ describes how far current flows before leaking passively across the surface membrane to a value about one-third of its initial value. This distance is normally about 2 mm for Purkinje fibers, 0.5 mm for the sinus node, and 0.8 mm for ventricular muscle fibers. λ is about 10 times the length of an individual cell. As an example, if e is about 2.7 and a hyperpolarizing current pulse in a Purkinje fiber produces a membrane voltage change of 15 mV at the site of current injection, the membrane potential change one space constant (2 mm) away would be 15/2.7 = 5.5 mV.

Because the current loop in any circuit must be closed, current must flow back to its point of origin. Local circuit currents pass across gap junctions between cells and exit across the sarcolemmal membrane to

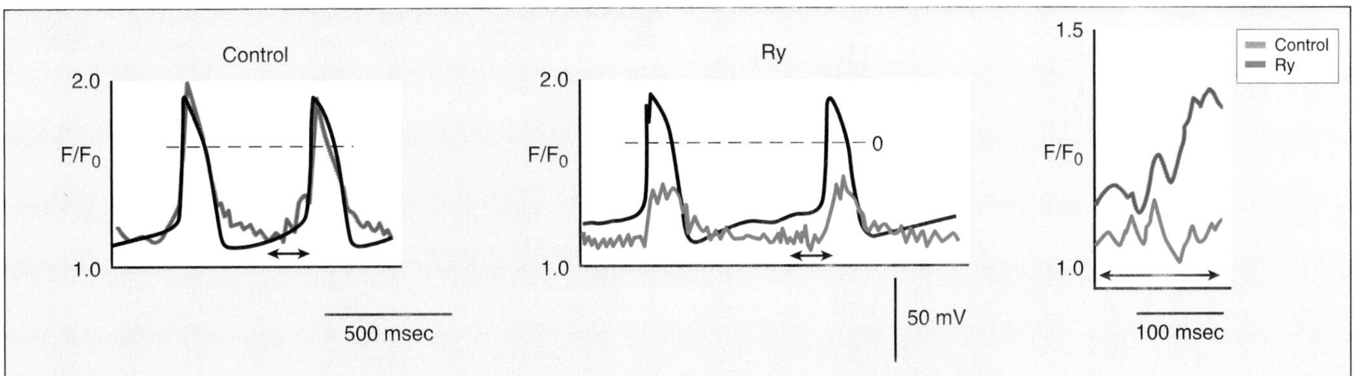

FIGURE 27–20 Ca^{2+} release from the sarcoplasmic reticulum through ryanodine receptors during diastolic depolarization in an isolated rabbit sinoatrial node cell; plot of variations in intracellular calcium concentration (in blue and magenta, respectively) with simultaneously recorded membrane potential. In the control state, the Ca^{2+} waveform exhibits an increase, during the later part of the spontaneous diastolic depolarization, that precedes the rapid upstroke of the action potential (bracketed by arrows and shown at greater resolution in the rightmost panel). This increase is abolished by the specific blocker of the sarcoplasmic reticulum Ca^{2+} release channel, ryanodine (Ry), concurrent with a slowing of the beating rate by this drug. (From Lakatta EG, Maltsev VA, Bogdanov KY, et al: Cyclic variation in intracellular calcium. A critical factor for cardiac pacemaker cell dominance. Circ Res 92:e45, 2003.)

close the loop and complete the circuit. Inward excitation currents in one area (carried by Na^+ in most regions) flow intracellularly along the length of the tissue (carried mostly by K^+), escape across the membrane, and flow extracellularly in a longitudinal direction. The outside local circuit current is the current recorded in an electrocardiogram (ECG; see Chap. 9). Through these local circuit currents the transmembrane potential of each cell influences the transmembrane potential of its neighbor because of the passive flow of current from one segment of the fiber to another across the low-resistance gap junctions.

As discussed earlier, the speed of conduction depends on active membrane properties such as the magnitude of the Na^+ current, a measure of which is $\dot{V}_{max}$. Passive membrane properties also contribute to conduction velocity and include excitability threshold, which influences the capability of cells adjacent to the one that has been discharged to reach threshold; the intracellular resistance of the cell, which is determined by the free ions in the cytoplasm; the resistance of the gap junction; and the cross-sectional area of the cell. Direction of propagation is crucial because of the influence of anisotropy, as mentioned earlier.

Loss of Membrane Potential and Arrhythmia Development

Many acquired abnormalities of cardiac muscle or specialized fibers that result in arrhythmias produce a loss of membrane potential; that is, maximum diastolic potential becomes less negative. This change should be viewed as a symptom of an underlying abnormality, analogous to fever or jaundice, rather than as a diagnostic category in and of itself because both the ionic changes resulting in cellular depolarization and the more fundamental biochemical or metabolic abnormalities responsible for the ionic alterations are probably multicausal. Cellular depolarization can result from elevated $[K^+]_o$ or decreased $[K^+]_i$, an increase in membrane permeability to Na^+ (P_{Na} increases), or a decrease in membrane permeability to K^+ (P_K decreases). Reference to the GHK equation for V (see Phases of the Cardiac Action Potential, General Considerations) illustrates that these changes alone or in combination make membrane diastolic voltage less negative.

Normal cells perfused by an abnormal milieu (e.g., hyperkalemia), abnormal cells perfused by a normal milieu (e.g., healed myocardial infarction), or abnormal cells perfused by an abnormal milieu (e.g., acute myocardial ischemia and infarction) can exist alone or in combination and reduce resting membrane voltage. Each of these changes can have one or more biochemical or metabolic causes. For example, acute myocardial ischemia results in decreased $[K^+]_i$[66] and increased $[K^+]_o$[67], norepinephrine release, and acidosis that may be related to an increase in intracellular Ca^{2+} and Ca^{2+}-induced transient inward currents and accumulation of amphipathic lipid metabolites and oxygen free radicals. All these changes can contribute to the development of an abnormal electrophysiological environment and arrhythmias during ischemia and reperfusion. Knowledge of these changes may provide insight into therapy that actually reverses basic defects and restores membrane potential or other abnormalities to normal.

EFFECTS OF REDUCED RESTING POTENTIAL. The reduced resting membrane potential alters the depolarization and repolarization phases of the cardiac action potential. For example, partial membrane depolarization causes a decrease in the steady-state availability of fast sodium channels, thereby reducing the magnitude of peak I_{Na} during phase 0 of the action potential. The subsequent reduction in $\dot{V}_{max}$ and action potential amplitude prolongs the conduction time of the propagated impulse, at times to the point of block.[30]

Action potentials with reduced upstroke velocity resulting from partial inactivation of I_{Na} are called depressed fast responses (see Fig. 27–15F). Their contours often resemble and can be difficult to distinguish from slow responses, in which upstrokes are due to $I_{Ca.L}$ (see Fig. 27–15F). Membrane depolarization to levels of −60 to −70 mV can inactivate half the Na^+ channels, and depolarization to −50 mV or less can inactivate all the Na^+ channels. At membrane potentials positive to −50 mV, $I_{Ca.L}$ can be activated to generate phase 0 if conditions are appropriate. These action potential changes are likely to be heterogeneous, with unequal degrees of Na^+ inactivation that create areas with minimally reduced velocity, more severely depressed zones, and areas of complete block. These uneven changes are propitious for the development of arrhythmias (Fig. 27–21).

In these cells with reduced membrane potential, refractoriness can outlast voltage recovery of the action potential; that is, the cell can still be refractory or partially refractory after the resting membrane potential returns to its most negative value. Furthermore, if block of the cardiac impulse occurs in a fairly localized area without significant slowing of conduction proximal to the site of block, cells in this proximal zone exhibit short action potentials and refractory periods because unexcited cells distal to the block (still in a polarized state) electrotonically speed recovery in cells proximal to the site of block.

If conduction slows gradually proximal to the site of block, the duration of these action potentials and their refractory periods can be prolonged. Some cells can exhibit abnormal electrophysiological properties even though they have a relatively normal resting membrane potential.

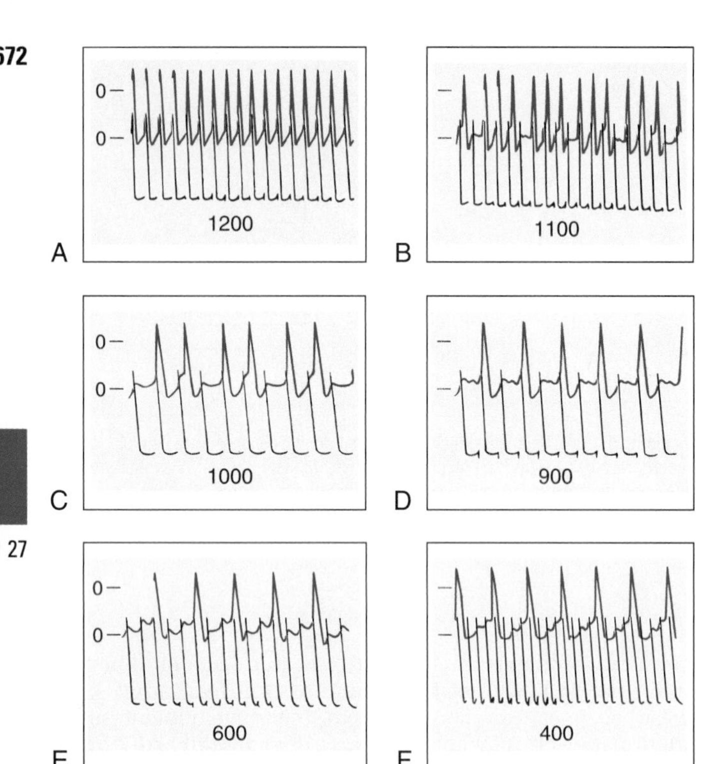

FIGURE 27–21 Rate-dependent conduction from the normal zone into the abnormal zone. When the pacing cycle length in the normal zone was shortened from 1200 to 400 milliseconds (**A** to **F**), increasing degrees of entrance block into the abnormal area occurred and progressed from 1:1 conduction at a cycle length of 1200 milliseconds to 4:3 conduction at 1100 milliseconds, 3:2 conduction at 1000 milliseconds, 2:1 conduction at 900 milliseconds, 3:1 conduction at 600 milliseconds, and 4:1 conduction at 400 milliseconds. Pacing the abnormal zone (not shown) resulted in block to the normal zone (unidirectional propagation). Vertical calibration: 50 mV. Horizontal calibration: 4 seconds in A and B and 2 seconds in C to F. (From Gilmour RF Jr, Heger JJ, Prystowsky EN, et al: Cellular electrophysiologic abnormalities of diseased human ventricular myocardium. Am J Cardiol 51:137, 1983.)

Mechanisms of Arrhythmogenesis

The mechanisms responsible for cardiac arrhythmias (Table 27–5) are generally divided into categories of disorders of impulse formation, disorders of impulse conduction, or combinations of both.[46] It is important to realize, however, that our present diagnostic tools do not permit unequivocal determination of the electrophysiological mechanisms responsible for many clinically occurring arrhythmias or their ionic bases. This is especially true for ventricular arrhythmias. It may be difficult to separate micro-reentry from automaticity clinically, and often one is left with a postulate that a particular arrhythmia is "most consistent with" or "best explained by" one or the other electrophysiological mechanism. Some tachyarrhythmias can be started by one mechanism and perpetuated by another. An episode of tachycardia caused by one mechanism can precipitate another episode caused by a different mechanism. For example, an initiating tachycardia or premature complex caused by abnormal automaticity can precipitate an episode of tachycardia sustained by reentry. However, by using the features of entrainment (see later), arrhythmias caused by macro-reentry circuits can be identified.

Disorders of Impulse Formation

Disorders in this category are characterized by an inappropriate discharge rate of the normal pacemaker, the sinus node (e.g., sinus rates too fast or too slow for the physiological needs of the patient), or discharge of an ectopic pacemaker that controls atrial or ventricular rhythm. Pacemaker discharge from ectopic sites, often called *latent* or *subsidiary pacemakers*, can occur in fibers located in several parts of the atria, the coronary sinus and pulmonary veins, AV valves, portions of the AV junction, and the His-Purkinje system. Ordinarily kept from reaching the level of threshold potential because of overdrive suppression by the more rapidly firing sinus node or electrotonic depression from contiguous fibers, ectopic pacemaker activity at one of these latent sites can become manifest when the sinus nodal discharge rate slows or block occurs at some level between the sinus node and the ectopic pacemaker site and permits *escape* of the latent pacemaker at the latter's normal discharge rate. A clinical example would be sinus bradycardia to a rate of 45 beats/min that permits an AV junctional escape complex to occur at a rate of 50 beats/min.

TABLE 27–5 Mechanisms of Arrhythmogenesis

Disorders of Impulse Formation
Automaticity
  Normal automaticity
    Experimental examples—Normal in vivo or in vitro in sinus node. Purkinje fibers, others
    Clinical examples—Sinus tachycardia or bradycardia inappropriate for the clinical situation, possibly ventricular parasystole
  Abnormal automaticity
    Experimental example—Depolarization-induced automaticity in Purkinje fibers or ventricular muscle
    Clinical example—Possibly accelerated ventricular rhythms after myocardial infarction
Triggered activity
  Early afterdepolarizations
    Experimental examples—EADs produced by barium, hypoxia, high concentrations of catecholamines, drugs such so sotalol, *N*-acetylprocainamide, cesium
    Clinical examples—Possibly idiopathic and acquired long QT syndromes and associated ventricular arrhythmias
  Delayed afterdepolarizations
    Experimental example—DADs produced in Purkinje fibers by digitalis
    Clinical example—Possibly some digitalis-induced arrhythmias

Disorders of Impulse Conduction
Block
  Bidirectional or unidirectional without reentry
    Experimental example—SA, AV, bundle branch, Purkinje-muscle, others
    Clinical examples—SA, AV, bundle branch, others
  Unidirectional block with reentry
    Experimental examples—AV node, Purkinje-muscle junction, infarcted myocardium, others
    Clinical examples—Reciprocating tachycardia in WPW syndrome, AV nodal reentry, VT due to bundle branch reentry, others
  Reflection
    Experimental example—Purkinje fiber with area of inexcitability
    Clinical example—Unknown

Combined Disorders
Interactions between automatic foci
  Experimental examples—Depolarizing or hyperpolarizing subthreshold stimuli speed or slow automatic discharge rate
  Clinical examples—Modulated parasystole
Interactions between automaticity and conduction
  Experimental examples—Deceleration-dependent block, overdrive suppression of conduction, entrance and exit block
  Clinical examples—Similar to experimental

AV = atrioventricular; DAD = delayed afterdepolarization; EAD = early afterdepolarization; SA = sinoatrial; WPW = Wolfe-Parkinson-White.

Alternatively, the discharge rate of the latent pacemaker can speed up inappropriately and usurp control of cardiac rhythm from the sinus node, which has been discharging at a normal rate. A clinical example would be interruption of normal sinus rhythm by a premature ventricular complex or a burst of ventricular tachycardia. It is important to remember that such disorders of impulse formation can be due to speeding or slowing of a *normal* pacemaker mechanism (e.g., phase 4 diastolic depolarization that is ionically normal for the sinus node or for an ectopic site such as a Purkinje fiber but occurs inappropriately fast or slow) or due to an ionically *abnormal* pacemaker mechanism.

A patient with persistent sinus tachycardia at rest or sinus bradycardia during exertion exhibits inappropriate sinus nodal discharge rates, but the ionic mechanisms responsible for sinus nodal discharge may still be normal, although the kinetics or magnitude of the currents may be altered. Conversely, when a patient experiences ventricular tachycardia during an acute myocardial infarction, ionic mechanisms ordinarily not involved in formation of spontaneous impulses for this fiber type may be operative and generate the tachycardia. For example, although pacemaker activity is not generally found in ordinary working myocardium, the effects of myocardial infarction can perhaps depolarize these cells to membrane potentials at which inactivation of I_K and activation of $I_{Ca.L}$ cause automatic discharge. Because the maximum rate that can be achieved by adrenergic stimulation of normal automaticity is generally less than 200 beats/min, it is likely that episodes of faster tachycardia are not due to enhanced normal automaticity.

Abnormal Automaticity

Mechanisms responsible for *normal* automaticity were described earlier. *Abnormal* automaticity can arise from cells that have reduced maximum diastolic potentials, often at membrane potentials positive to −50 mV, when I_K and $I_{Ca.L}$ may be operative.

Automaticity at membrane potentials more negative than −70 mV may be due to I_f. When the membrane potential is between −50 and −70 mV, the cell may be quiescent. Electrotonic effects from surrounding normally polarized or more depolarized myocardium influence the development of automaticity. Abnormal automaticity has been found in Purkinje fibers removed from dogs subjected to myocardial infarction, in rat myocardium damaged by epinephrine, in human atrial samples, and in ventricular myocardial specimens from patients undergoing aneurysmectomy and endocardial resection for recurrent ventricular tachyarrhythmias.

Abnormal automaticity can be produced in normal muscle or Purkinje fibers by appropriate interventions such as current passage that reduces diastolic potential. An automatic discharge rate speeds up with progressive depolarization, and hyperpolarizing pulses slow the spontaneous firing. It is possible that partial depolarization and failure to reach normal maximal diastolic potential can induce automatic discharge in most if not all cardiac fibers. Although this type of spontaneous automatic activity has been found in human atrial and ventricular fibers, its relationship to the genesis of clinical arrhythmias has not been established.

Rhythms resulting from automaticity may be slow atrial, junctional, and ventricular escape rhythms; certain types of atrial tachycardias (such as those produced by digitalis or perhaps those coming from the pulmonary veins); accelerated junctional (nonparoxysmal junctional tachycardia) and idioventricular rhythms; and parasystole (see Chap. 32).

Triggered Activity

Automaticity is the property of a fiber to initiate an impulse *spontaneously,* without need for prior stimulation, so that electrical quiescence does not occur. *Triggered activity* is initiated by afterdepolarizations, which are depolarizing oscillations in membrane voltage induced by one or more preceding action potentials. Thus, triggered activity is pacemaker activity that results *consequent* to a preceding impulse or series of impulses, without which electrical quiescence occurs (Fig. 27–22). This triggering activity is not caused by an automatic self-generating mechanism, and the term *triggered automaticity* is therefore contradictory. These depolarizations can occur before or after full repolarization of the fiber and are best termed *early afterdepolarizations* (EADs) when they arise from a reduced level of membrane potential during phases 2 (type 1) and 3 (type 2) of the cardiac action potential and called *late* or *delayed afterdepolarizations*

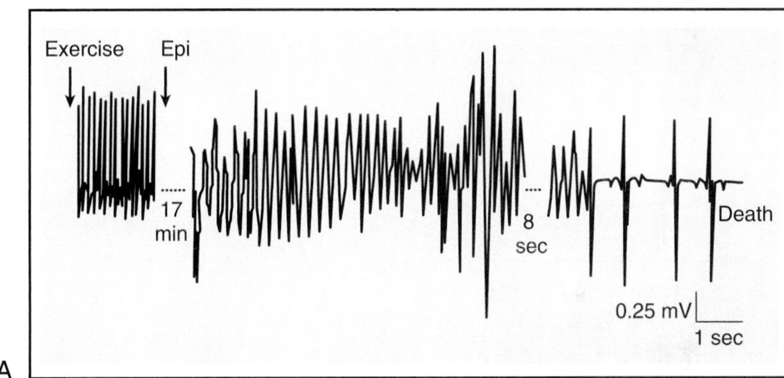

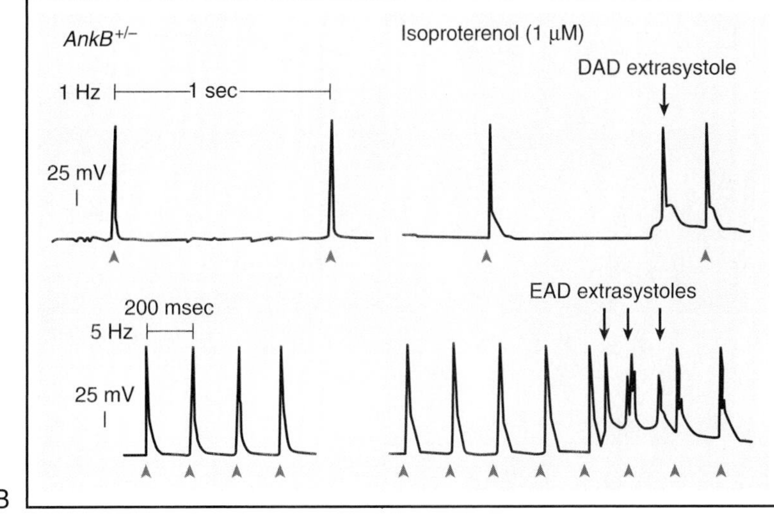

FIGURE 27–22 Polymorphic ventricular tachycardia and sudden death in an animal model of type 4 long QT syndrome. **A,** Electrocardiogram after exercise and administration of epinephrine in a mouse heterozygous for a loss-of-function mutation in the gene encoding ankyrin-B (*AnkB*$^{+/-}$). Polymorphic ventricular tachycardia (torsades de pointes) occurred within about 17 minutes of epinephrine administration, followed by marked bradycardia and death 2 minutes after the arrhythmia. **B,** Transmembrane action potentials in single cardiomyocytes from *AnkB*$^{+/-}$ mice at the frequencies indicated. Acute exposure to isoproterenol induced both delayed and early afterdepolarizations that led to extra beats. (From Mohler PJ, Schott J, Gramolini AO, et al: Ankyrin-B mutation causes type 4 long-QT cardiac arrhythmia and sudden cardiac death. Nature 421:634, 2003.)

TABLE 27–6 Determinants of the Amplitude of Afterdepolarizations

Intervention	Effect on Amplitude of EADs	DADs
Long cycles (basic and premature)	↑	↓
Long action potential duration	↑	↑
Reduced membrane potential	↑	↓
Na channel blockers	No effect	↓
Ca channel blockers	↓	↓
Catecholamines	↑	↑

↑ = increase amplitude; ↓ = decrease amplitude; DADs = delayed afterdepolarizations; EADs = early afterdepolarizations.

(DADs) when they occur after completion of repolarization (phase 4), generally at a more negative membrane potential than that from which EADs arise (Table 27–6). Not all afterdepolarizations may reach threshold potential, but if they do, they can trigger another afterdepolarization and thus self-perpetuate.

EARLY AFTERDEPOLARIZATIONS

A variety of interventions, each of which results in an increase in intracellular positivity, can cause EADs. EADs may be responsible for the lengthened repolarization time and ventricular tachyarrhythmias in several clinical situations, such as the acquired and congenital forms of the long QT syndrome (see Fig. 27–22; see Chap. 32).[68,68a] Left ansa subclavian stimulation increases the amplitude of cesium-induced EADs in dogs and the prevalence of ventricular tachyarrhythmias more than does right ansa subclavian stimulation, possibly because of a greater quantitative effect of the left than the right stellate ganglion on the left ventricle.

Patients with the heritable long QT syndrome have abnormally prolonged cardiac action potential duration and are at increased risk for sudden cardiac death from ventricular tachyarrhythmias. The genesis of long QT syndrome–associated ventricular tachycardia or fibrillation is uncertain. There is mounting evidence that increased intracellular Ca^{2+} concentration related to spontaneous Ca^{2+} release from the sarcoplasmic reticulum in cardiomyocytes coupled with dispersion of repolarization plays a causative role in long QT syndrome–associated cardiac arrhythmia and sudden cardiac death (Fig. 27–23; see Fig. 27–22). Action potential prolongation may increase Ca^{2+} influx through L-type Ca^{2+} channels during a cardiac cycle, causing excessive Ca^{2+} accumulation in the sarcoplasmic reticulum and spontaneous sarcoplasmic reticular Ca^{2+} release. The ensuing elevation of intracellular free calcium may depolarize cardiomyocyte membrane potential by activation of Ca^{2+}-dependent chloride currents or the electrogenic Na^+/Ca^{2+} exchange current, or both, thereby evoking EADs. EADs can trigger a propagated response and thereby elicit an extra beat, potentially launching a tachycardia.

Experimental observations[69] also suggest an important role of transmural or longitudinal heterogeneity of repolarization, or both.[70] Marked transmural dispersion of repolarization can create a vulnerable window for the development of reentry. Multiple studies of isolated ventricular myocytes or tissue preparations have demonstrated spatial dispersion of repolarization along the transmural axes of the left and right ventricular free wall. A prominent spike and dome is apparent in myocytes from epicardium and the M region but not in myocytes from endocardium. Action potential duration-rate relationships are considerably more pronounced in cells isolated from the M region.[69] The ionic basis for electrophysiologi-

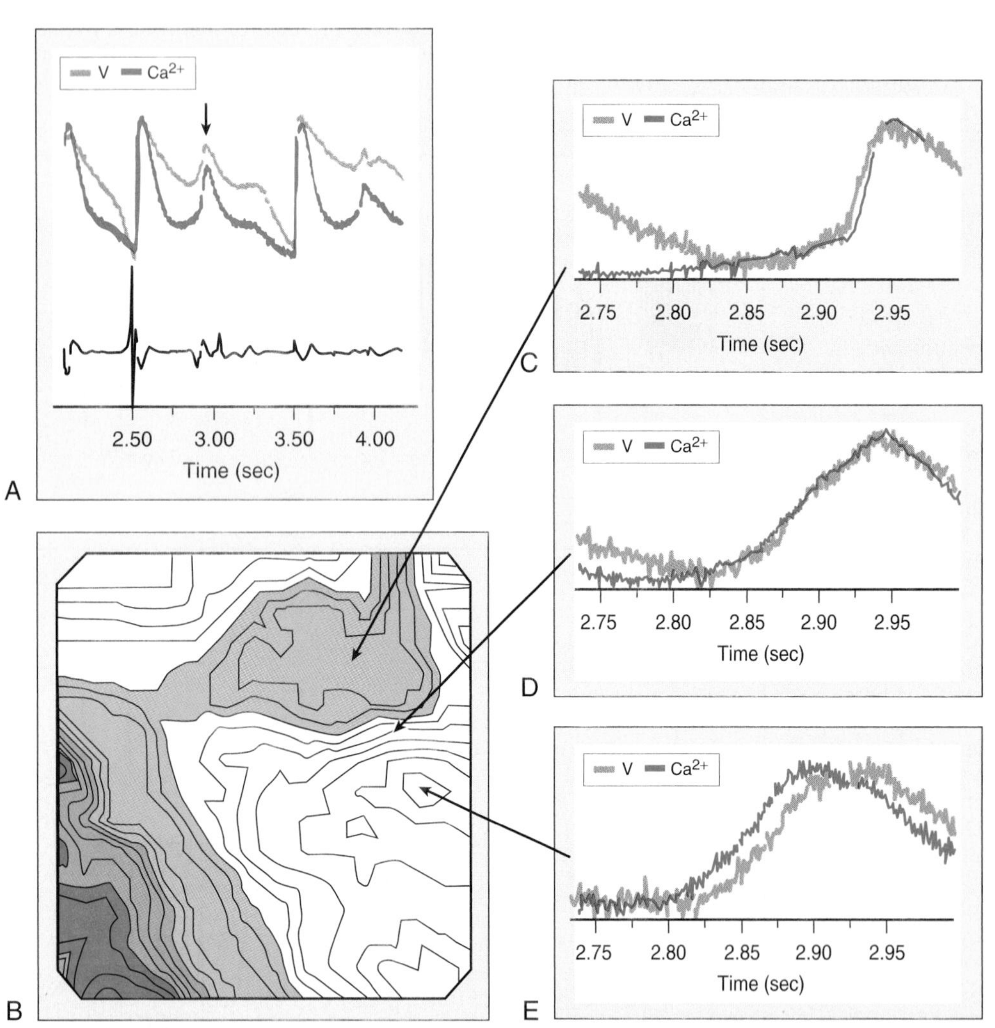

FIGURE 27–23 Primary role of spontaneous increases in intracellular Ca^{2+} $[Ca^{2+}]_i$ in triggering early afterdepolarizations (EADs) in an animal model of type 2 long QT syndrome. Simultaneous mapping of membrane potential (V_m) and intracellular Ca^{2+} concentration using voltage- and Ca^{2+}-sensitive fluorescent dyes, respectively, from the epicardial surface of a Langendorff-perfused isolated rabbit heart exposed to the I_{Kr} inhibitor E4031 and low extracellular concentrations of K^+ and Mg^{2+}. Under these conditions, action potentials are markedly prolonged and spontaneous EADs develop causing polymorphic ventricular tachycardia (torsades de pointes). **A,** Recording of V_m and $[Ca^{2+}]_i$ during an EAD (arrow) and the corresponding depolarizations recorded with bipolar electrogram (bottom trace). **B,** Activation map of the EAD labeled with an arrow in panel A. **C** and **D,** Superimposition of V_m and $[Ca^{2+}]_i$ traces measured at sites remote from the site of origin of the EAD. At those sites, V_m changes precede or are synchronous with those in $[Ca^{2+}]_i$. **E,** Voltage and $[Ca^{2+}]_i$ traces at the first site to fire an EAD. Here, the rise in $[Ca^{2+}]_i$ precedes the rise of V_m. (From Choi B, Burton F, Salama G: Cytosolic Ca^{2+} triggers early afterdepolarizations and torsade de pointes in rabbit hearts with type 2 long QT syndrome. J Physiol (Lond) 543.2:615, 2002.)

cal distinctions among epicardial, midmyocardial, and endocardial myocytes is a large gradient in both the density- and rate-dependent properties of the transient outward K^+ current[56] and a smaller density of the slow component of the delayed rectifier K^+ current I_{Ks} as well as larger late Na^+ currents and inward $I_{Na/Ca}$[71,72] in midmyocardial cells than in myocytes of endocardial and epicardial origin.[56]

Sympathetic stimulation, primarily left, could increase the EAD amplitude to provoke ventricular tachyarrhythmias. Alpha adrenoceptor stimulation also increases the amplitude of cesium-induced EADs and the prevalence of ventricular tachyarrhythmias, both of which are suppressed by magnesium.

In patients with the acquired long QT syndrome and torsades de pointes from drugs such as quinidine, *N*-acetylprocainamide, cisapride, erythromycin, and some class III antiarrhythmic agents, EADs can also be responsible. Such drugs easily elicit EADs experimentally and clinically, whereas magnesium suppresses them. It is possible that multiple drugs can cause summating effects to provoke EADs and torsades de pointes in patients. Activators of ATP-dependent potassium channels, such as pinacidil and nicorandil, can eliminate EADs.[73]

DELAYED AFTERDEPOLARIZATIONS

DADs and triggered activity have been demonstrated in Purkinje fibers, specialized atrial fibers and ventricular muscle fibers exposed to digitalis preparations, pulmonary veins,[74] normal Purkinje fibers exposed to Na-free superfusates from the endocardium of the intact heart, ventricular myocardial cells from failing hearts (Fig. 27-24)[50] and hearts with ankyrin-B mutations (see Fig. 27-22)[68] during beta-adrenergic stimulation, and endocardial preparations 1 day after a myocardial infarction. When fibers in the rabbit, canine, simian, and human mitral valves and in the canine tricuspid valve and coronary sinus are superfused with norepinephrine, they exhibit the capacity for sustained triggered rhythmic activity.

Triggered activity caused by DADs has also been noted in diseased human atrial and ventricular fibers studied in vitro. Left stellate ganglion stimulation can elicit DADs in canine ventricles. In vivo, atrial and ventricular arrhythmias apparently caused by triggered activity have been reported in the dog and possibly in humans. It is tempting to ascribe certain clinical arrhythmias to DADs, such as some arrhythmias precipitated by digitalis or some atrial fibrillations arising from DADs in pulmonary veins. The accelerated idioventricular rhythm 1 day after experimental canine myocardial infarction may be due to DADs, and some evidence suggests that certain ventricular tachycardias, such as those arising in the right ventricular outflow tract, may be due to DADs whereas other data suggest that EADs are responsible.[75]

IONIC BASIS OF DELAYED AFTERDEPOLARIZATIONS. DADs appear to be caused by a transient inward current (I_{ti}) that is small or absent under normal physiological conditions.

When intracellular Ca^{2+} overload occurs, as is the case during adrenergic stimulation, elevated extracellular Ca^{2+} levels, prolonged action potentials, and rapid repetitive stimulation or after large doses of digitalis, spontaneous release of Ca^{2+} from the sarcoplasmic reticulum can activate Cl^- currents[60] or the Na/Ca exchanger[50] and result in transient inward currents and brief membrane depolarizations (see Fig. 27-24). Compounds that reduce the sarcoplasmic Ca^{2+} load (L-type Ca^{2+} channel antagonists, beta-adrenergic receptor blocker) or inhibit sarcoplasmic Ca^{2+} release (thapsigargin, ryanodine, cyclopiazonic acid) suppress DADs. Inhibitors of calmodulin kinase eliminated I_{ti} carried by inward $I_{Na/Ca}$ in isolated rabbit ventricular myocytes,[49] indicating that activation of this enzyme appears to play an important role in cardiac arrhythmogenesis. In addition, drugs that reduce I_{Na} also reduce I_{ti}, relieve Ca^{2+} overload, and

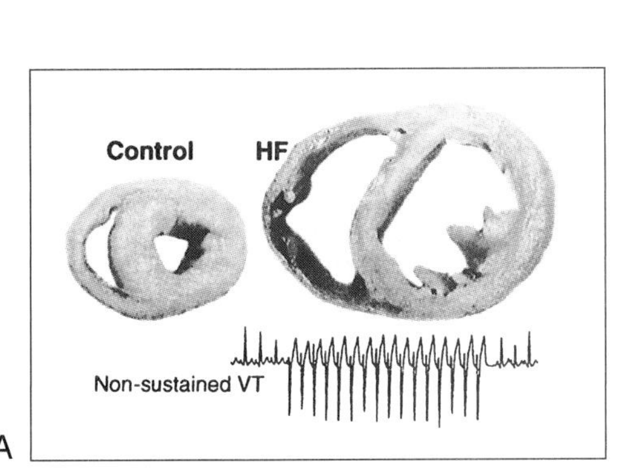

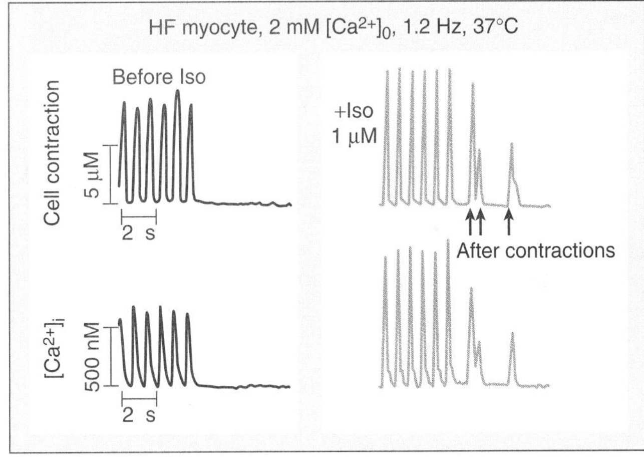

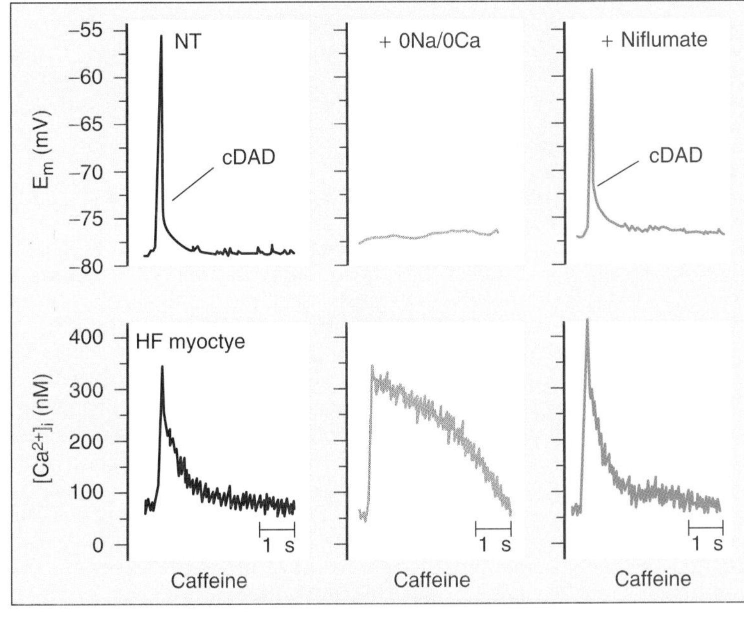

FIGURE 27–24 Ventricular arrhythmia in an animal model of heart failure (aortic constriction-insufficiency in rabbit). **A,** Cross sections of a control and failing heart (HF) and Holter recording of nonsustained ventricular tachycardia (VT) seen in a failing heart. **B,** Spontaneous aftercontractions and increases in $[Ca^{2+}]_i$ in a failing cardiomyocyte after exposure to isoproterenol. **C,** Induction of a delayed afterdepolarization (DAD) by application of caffeine (cDAD) in a cardiomyocyte isolated from a failing rabbit heart. In normal Tyrode's (NT) solution, caffeine causes rapid release of Ca^{2+} from the sarcoplasmic reticulum that leads to increases in intracellular free calcium concentration **(bottom trace),** which in turn causes membrane depolarization. Blocking the Na^+/Ca^{2+} exchange current in Na^+-free and Ca^{2+}-free solution (0Na/0Ca) abolished DADs despite similar increase in $[Ca^{2+}]_i$, whereas blocking the Ca^{2+}-activated Cl^- current with niflumate did not prevent DADs. E_m = membrane voltage. (From Pogwizd SM, Schlotthauer K, Li L, et al: Arrhythmogenesis and contractile dysfunction in heart failure. Circ Res 88:1159, 2001. With permission by the American Heart Association.)

can abolish DADs. DADs most likely play a causative role in arrhythmogenesis in the failing heart. It was found that a given sarcoplasmic reticular Ca^{2+} release produced greater arrhythmogenic inward current in failing cardiomyocytes (because of upregulation of the Na/Ca exchange current), and approximately 50 percent less Ca^{2+} release was required to trigger an action potential in failing myocytes.[50] In addition, downregulation of the inward rectifier K^+ current, I_{K1}, in heart failure allows greater depolarization for a given Na/Ca exchange current. Thus, increased $I_{Na/Ca}$ in concert with reduced I_{K1} (see also Table 27–6) creates a strongly proarrhythmogenic milieu in the failing heart.

Short coupling intervals or pacing at rates more rapid than the triggered activity rate (overdrive pacing) increases the amplitude and shortens the cycle length of the DAD following cessation of pacing (overdrive acceleration) rather than suppressing and delaying the escape rate of the afterdepolarization, as in normal automatic mechanisms. Premature stimulation exerts a similar effect; the shorter the premature interval, the larger the amplitude and shorter the escape interval of the triggered event.

The clinical implication might be that tachyarrhythmias caused by DAD-triggered activity may not be suppressed easily or, indeed, may be precipitated by rapid rates, either spontaneous (such as a sinus tachycardia) or pacing induced. Finally, because a single premature stimulus can both initiate and terminate triggered activity, differentiation from reentry (see later) becomes quite difficult. The response to overdrive pacing may help separate triggered arrhythmias from reentrant ones.

Parasystole

Classically, parasystole has been likened to the function of a fixed-rate asynchronously discharging pacemaker: Its timing is not altered by the dominant rhythm, it produces depolarization when the myocardium is excitable, and the intervals between discharges are multiples of a basic interval (see Chap. 32). Complete *entrance block*, constant or intermittent, insulates and protects the parasystolic focus from surrounding electrical events and accounts for such behavior. Occasionally, the focus can exhibit *exit block*, during which it may fail to depolarize excitable myocardium. In fact, the dominant cardiac rhythm may modulate parasystolic discharge to speed up or slow down its rate. Experimental simulations of parasystole demonstrate that the discharge rate of an isolated, "protected" focus can be modulated by electrotonic interactions with the dominant rhythm across an area of depressed excitability. Brief subthreshold depolarizations induced during the first half of the cardiac cycle of a spontaneously discharging pacemaker delay the subsequent discharge, whereas similar depolarizations induced in the second half of the cardiac cycle accelerate it (Fig. 27–25).

The ionic basis for these rate changes is not totally established, but it is probable that early depolarizing stimuli reactivate outward potassium currents and retard depolarization and late stimuli contribute depolarizing current that enables the cell to reach threshold more quickly. Early hyperpolarizing subthreshold stimuli accelerate and late hyperpolarizing stimuli retard discharge. Similar examples have been noted in human ventricular tissue, and interactions may be predicted according to the general rules of biological oscillators. Numerous clinical examples have been published to support these experimental observations.

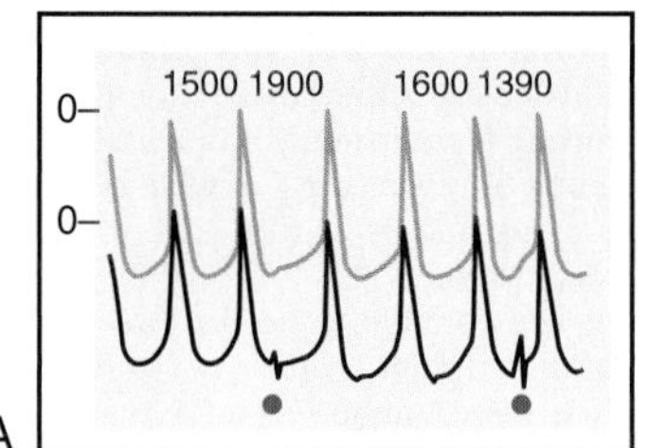

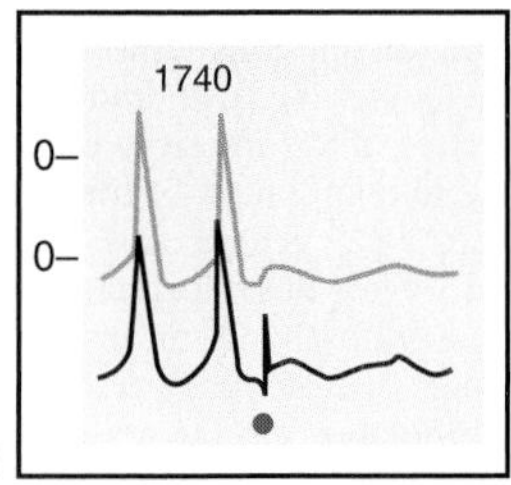

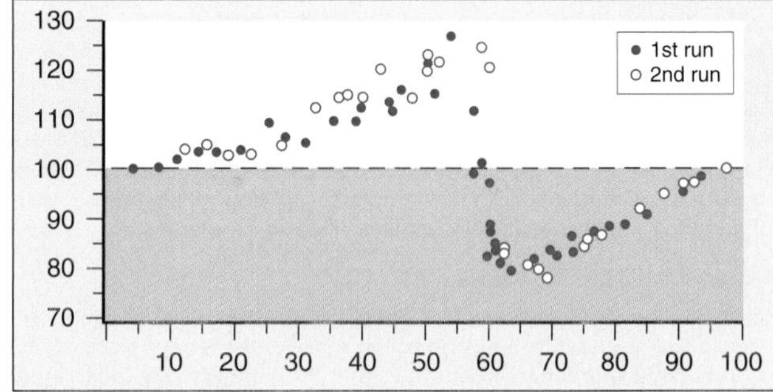

FIGURE 27–25 Modulation of pacemaker activity by subthreshold current pulses in diseased human ventricle. **A,** Two recording sites along the same trabecula in a spontaneously active preparation. Current pulses (indicated by the red dots) 30 milliseconds in duration were injected through the lower microelectrode at various times. The interval between the spontaneous action potentials is given in milliseconds above each cycle. Injection of a subthreshold current pulse through the lower microelectrode relatively early in the spontaneous cycle (about 680 milliseconds after initiation of the rapid portion of the preceding action potential upstroke) produced a subthreshold depolarization in the upper recording and delayed the next spontaneous discharge by 400 to 1900 milliseconds. This response curve would fall in the first half of the curve indicated in C. A current pulse of the same intensity and duration delivered later in the spontaneous cycle (950 milliseconds after the preceding upstroke) accelerated the next discharge by 210 to 1390 milliseconds relative to the previous two action potentials. The response to this current injection falls in the second half of the graph depicted in C. **B,** A stimulus at a precise interval in the cardiac cycle (called the singular point; in this example, 930 milliseconds after the preceding action potential upstroke) abolishes pacemaker activity. **C,** Phase-response curves from experimental data obtained in canine Purkinje fibers in a manner similar to the human experiment shown in A and B. Two different runs are shown. Ordinate = percent increase or decrease in spontaneous cycle length of the "parasystolic focus" (control cycle length equals 100 percent); abscissa = percentage of the "parasystolic focus" spontaneous cycle length during which stimulation was performed. The spontaneous cycle length was maximally prolonged (by 26 percent) or shortened (by 20 percent) by subthreshold depolarizations that entered the parasystolic focus after approximately 50 and 60 percent of the cycle had elapsed, respectively. Very similar curves can be plotted for patients with parasystole (for example, see Figs. 9 and 10 from Zipes DP: Plenary lecture. Cardiac electrophysiology: Promises and contributions. J Am Coll Cardiol 13:1329, 1989). (**A** and **B,** From Gilmour RF Jr, Heger JJ, Prystowsky EN, et al: Cellular electrophysiological abnormalities of diseased human ventricular myocardium. Am J Cardiol 51:137, 1983; **C,** From Jalife J, Moe GK: Effect of electronic potentials on pacemaker activity of canine Purkinje fibers and relation to parasystole. Circ Res 39:801, 1976, By permission of the American Heart Association.)

Disorders of Impulse Conduction

Conduction delay and block[76] can result in bradyarrhythmias or tachyarrhythmias, the former when the propagating impulse is blocked and is followed by asystole or a slow escape rhythm and the latter when the delay and block produce reentrant excitation (see later). Various factors involving both active and passive membrane properties determine the conduction velocity of an impulse and whether conduction is successful. Among these factors are the stimulating efficacy of the propagating impulse, which is related to the amplitude and rate of rise of phase 0, the excitability of the tissue into which the impulse is conducted,[77] and the geometry of the tissue.[30,53]

DECELERATION-DEPENDENT BLOCK. Diastolic depolarization has been suggested as a cause of conduction block at slow rates, so-called bradycardia- or deceleration-dependent block (see Chap. 32). Yet excitability *increases* as the membrane depolarizes until about −70 mV, despite a reduction in action potential amplitude and $\dot{V}_{max}$. Evidently, depolarization-induced inactivation of fast Na^+ channels is offset by other factors such as reduction in the difference between membrane potential and threshold potential and increase in membrane excitability.

PHASE 3 OR TACHYCARDIA-DEPENDENT BLOCK. More commonly, impulses are blocked at rapid rates or short cycle lengths as a result of incomplete recovery of refractoriness caused by incomplete time- or voltage-dependent recovery of excitability (see Chap. 32). For example, such incomplete recovery is the usual mechanism responsible for a nonconducted premature P wave or one that conducts with a functional bundle branch block.

DECREMENTAL CONDUCTION. Decremental conduction is used commonly in the clinical literature but is often misapplied to describe any Wenckebach-like conduction block, that is, responses similar to block in the AV node during which progressive conduction delay precedes the nonconducted impulse. Correctly used, *decremental conduction* refers to a situation in which the properties of the fiber change along its length so that the action potential loses its efficacy as a stimulus to excite the fiber ahead of it. Thus, the stimulating efficacy of the propagating action potential diminishes progressively, possibly as a result of its decreasing amplitude and $\dot{V}_{max}$.

Reentry

Electrical activity during each normal cardiac cycle begins in the sinus node and continues until the entire heart has been activated. Each cell becomes activated in turn, and the cardiac impulse dies out when all fibers have been discharged and are completely refractory. During this absolute refractory period, the cardiac impulse has "no place to go." It must be extinguished and restarted by the next sinus impulse. If, however, a group of fibers not activated during the initial wave of depolarization recover excitability in time to be discharged before the impulse dies out, they may serve as a link to reexcite areas that were just discharged and have now recovered from the initial depolarization. Such a process is given various names, all meaning approximately the same thing: reentry, reentrant excitation, circus movement, reciprocal or echo beat, or reciprocating tachycardia.

ANATOMICAL REENTRY. The earliest studies on reentry were with models that had anatomically defined separate pathways in which it could be shown that they had (1) an area of unidirectional block, (2) recirculation of the impulse to its point of origin, and (3) elimination of the arrhythmia by cutting the pathway. In models with anatomically defined pathways, because the two (or more) pathways have different electrophysiological properties (e.g., a refractory period longer in one pathway than the other), the impulse (1) is blocked in one pathway (site A in Fig. 27-26A) and (2) propagates slowly in the adjacent pathway (serpentine arrow, D to C, Fig. 27-26A). If conduction in this alternative route is sufficiently depressed, the slowly propagating impulse excites tissue beyond the blocked pathway (horizontal lined area in Fig. 27-26A) and returns in a reversed direction along the pathway initially blocked (B to A in Fig. 27-26A) to (3) reexcite tissue proximal to the site of block (A to D in Fig. 27-26A). A clinical arrhythmia caused by anatomical reentry is most likely to have a monomorphic contour.

For reentry of this type to occur, the time for conduction within the depressed but unblocked area and for excitation of the distal segments must exceed the refractory period of the initially blocked pathway (A in Fig. 27-26A) and the tissue proximal to the site of block (D in Fig. 27-26A). Stated another way, continuous reentry requires the anatomical length of the circuit traveled to equal or exceed the reentrant wavelength. The latter is equal to the mean conduction velocity of the impulse multiplied by the longest refractory period of the elements in the circuit. Both values can be different at different points along the reentry pathway, and thus the wavelength value is somewhat contrived.

Conditions for Reentry. The length of the pathway is fixed and determined by the anatomy. Conditions that depress conduction velocity or abbreviate the refractory period promote the development of reentry in this model, whereas prolonging refractoriness and speeding conduction velocity can hinder it. For example, if conduction velocity (0.30 m/sec) and refractoriness (350 milliseconds) for ventricular muscle were normal, a pathway of 105 mm (0.30 m/sec × 0.35 seconds) would be necessary for reentry to occur. However, under certain conditions, conduction velocity in ventricular muscle and Purkinje fibers can be very slow (0.03 m/sec), and if refractoriness is not greatly prolonged (600 milliseconds), a pathway of only 18 mm (0.03 m/sec × 0.60 seconds) may be necessary. Such reentry frequently exhibits an excitable gap, that is, a time interval between the end of refractoriness from one cycle and the beginning of depolarization in the next, when tissue in the circuit is excitable. This condition results because the wavelength of the reentrant circuit is less than the pathway length. Electrical stimulation during this time period can invade the reentrant circuit and reset its timing or terminate the tachycardia.

Rapid pacing can entrain the tachycardia, that is, continuously reset it by entering the circuit and propagating around it in the same way as the reentrant impulse, which increases the tachycardia rate to the pacing rate without terminating the tachycardia (see Fig. 27-28). In reentrant circuits with an excitable gap, conduction velocity determines the revolution time of the impulse around the circuit and, hence, the rate of the tachycardia. Prolongation of refractoriness, unless it is great enough to eliminate the excitable gap and make the impulse propagate in relatively refractory tissue, does not influence the revolution time around the circuit or the rate of the tachycardia. Anatomical reentry occurs in patients with the Wolff-Parkinson-White syndrome, in AV nodal reentry, in some atrial flutters, and in some ventricular tachycardias.

FUNCTIONAL REENTRY. Functional reentry lacks confining anatomical boundaries and can occur in contiguous fibers that exhibit functionally different electrophysiological properties caused by local differences in transmembrane action potential. Dispersion of excitability or refractoriness, or both, as well as anisotropic distributions of intercellular resistance permit initiation and maintenance of reentry.[78] A clinical arrhythmia caused by functional reentry is most likely to be polymorphic because of changing circuits.

Leading Circle Reentry. Leading circle reentry, important in atrial fibrillation (AF), is reentrant excitation during which the reentrant circuit propagates around a functionally refractory core and follows a course along fibers that have a shorter refractory period so that the impulse is blocked in one direction in fibers with a longer refractory period (Fig. 27-27). The maintenance of leading circle reentry is due to repetitive centripetal wavelets that keep the core in a constant state of refractoriness. In addition to refractoriness, the wave front curvature is important in maintaining functional reentry. The curvature of a wave front progressively increases from the periphery to the core. When a critical curvature is reached, propagation fails despite the presence of excitable tissue, forming a central core of reentry.[79]

The pathway length of a functional circuit is determined by the smallest circuit in which the leading wave front is just able to excite tissue ahead that is still relatively refractory. If these parameters change, the size of the circuit can also change and alter the rate of the tachycardia. Shorter wavelengths can predispose to fibrillation. No or a very short excitable gap exists, and the duration of the refractory period of the tissue in the circuit primarily determines the cycle length of the tachycardia because the stimulating efficacy of the head of the next impulse is just sufficient to excite the relatively refractory tissue in the wake of the preceding impulse. Propagating impulses originating outside the circuit cannot easily enter the circuit to reset, entrain, or terminate the reentry.[78]

Theoretically, drugs that prolong refractoriness and do not delay conduction would slow tachycardia as a result of the leading circle mechanism and not affect tachycardia with an excitable gap until the prolongation of refractoriness exceeded the duration of the excitable gap. Drugs that primarily slow conduction would have major effects on tachycardia with an excitable gap and not on tachycardias resulting from the leading circle concept. Mixed circuits with both anatomical and functional pathways obfuscate these differences.

RANDOM REENTRY. Random reentry, also important in AF, occurs when the reentry propagates continuously and randomly and reexcites areas that were excited shortly before by another wavelet.

ANISOTROPIC REENTRY. Anisotropic reentry is due to the structural features responsible for variations in conduction velocity and the time course of repolarization, such as a density of gap junctions at the ends rather than on the side of cells, which can result in block and slowed conduction with subsequent reentry (see Fig. 27-27).[80,81] Even in normal cardiac tissue showing normal transmembrane potentials and uniform refractory periods, conduction can be blocked in the direction parallel to the long axis of fiber orientation, propagate slowly in the direction transverse to the long axis of fiber orientation, and reenter the area of block. Spatial differences in refractoriness may not be necessary for reentry to occur. Such anisotropic reentry has been shown in atrial and ventricular muscle and may be responsible for ventricular tachycardia in epicardial muscle surviving myocardial infarction. An excitable gap may be present.[81]

SPIRAL WAVE REENTRY. Spiral waves of excitation have been demonstrated in cardiac muscle and represent a two-dimensional form of reentry; in three dimensions, spiral waves may be represented by scroll

CH 27

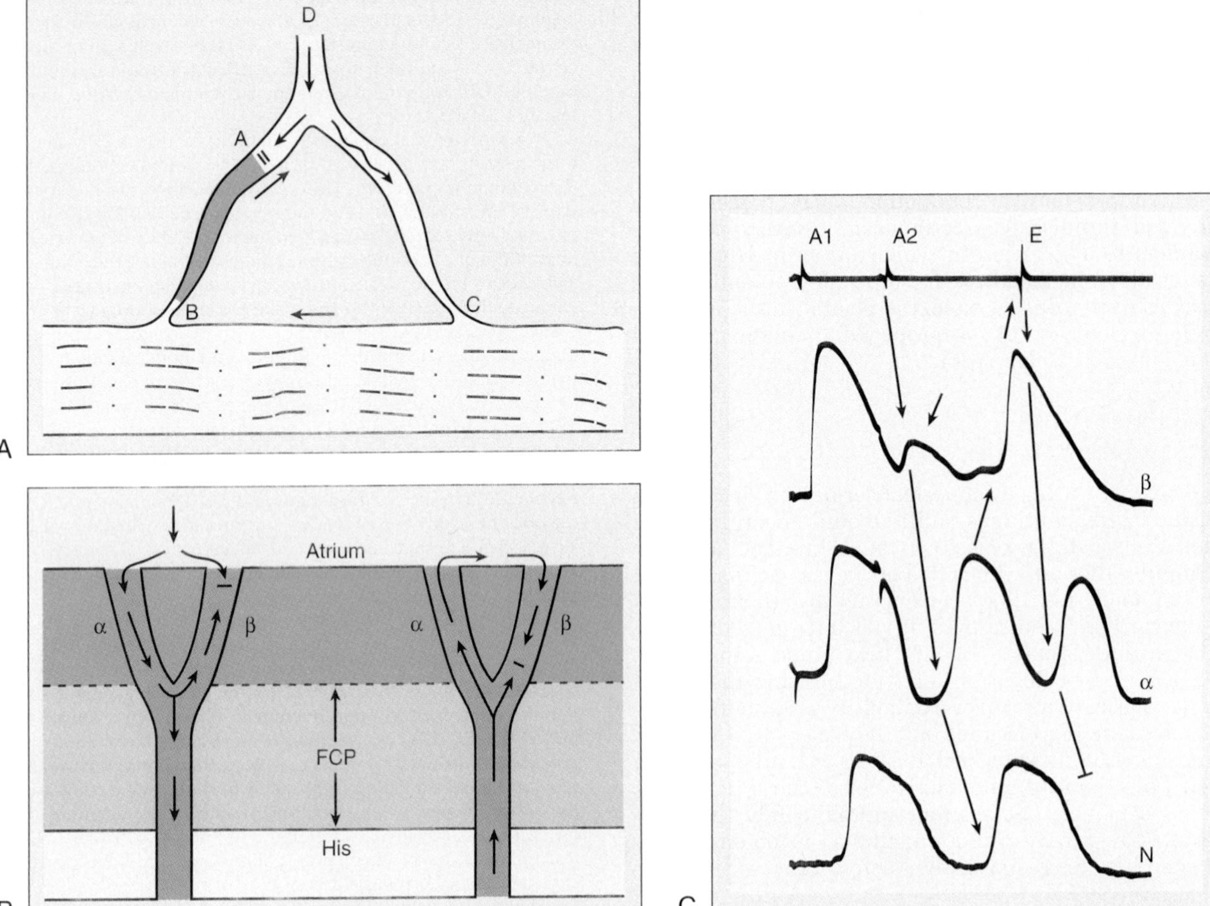

FIGURE 27–26 **A,** Diagram of reentry published by Schmitt and Erlanger in 1928. A Purkinje fiber (D) divides into two pathways (B and C), both of which join ventricular muscle. It is assumed that the original impulse travels down D, is blocked in its anterograde direction at site A (arrow followed by a double bar), but continues slowly down C (serpentine arrow) to excite ventricular muscle. The impulse then reenters the Purkinje twig at B and retrogradely excites A and D. If the impulse continues to propagate through D to the ventricular myocardium and elicits ventricular depolarization, a reentrant ventricular extrasystole results. Continued reentry of this type would produce ventricular tachycardia. **B,** Schematic representation of intranodal dissociation responsible for an atrial echo **(left diagram).** A premature atrial response fails to penetrate the beta (β) pathway, which exhibits a unidirectional block but propagates anterogradely through the alpha (α) pathway. Once the final common pathway (FCP) is engaged, the impulse may return to the atrium through the now-recovered beta pathway to produce an atrial echo. The neighboring **(right)** diagram illustrates the pattern of propagation during generation of a ventricular echo. A premature response in the His bundle traverses the FCP, encounters a refractory beta pathway (unidirectional block), reaches the atrium over the alpha pathway, and returns through a now-recovered beta pathway to produce a ventricular echo. **C,** Actual recordings from the atrium **(top tracing),** with cells impaled in the beta region **(second tracing),** alpha region **(third tracing)**, and N portion of the atrioventricular (AV) node **(bottom tracing)** in an isolated rabbit preparation. The basic response to A1 activated both alpha and beta pathways and the N cell (first tier of action potentials). The premature atrial response A2 caused only a local response in the beta cell (short arrow), was delayed in transmission to the alpha cell, and was further delayed in propagation to the N cell. Following the alpha response, a retrograde spontaneous response occurred in the beta cell and propagated to the atrium (E). This atrial response represents an atrial echo. The echo returned to stimulate the alpha cell but was not propagated to the N cell. It is important that although intranodal reentry has been shown to occur within the rabbit AV node, AV nodal reentry in humans probably occurs over extranodal pathways. (From Mendez C, Moe GK: Demonstrations of a dual AV nodal conduction system in the isolated rabbit heart. Circ Res 19:378, 1966. By permission of the American Heart Association.)

waves. Spiral waves may be stationary when the shape, size, and location of the arc remain unchanged throughout the episode, drifting when the arc migrates away from its site of origin, or anchoring when the drifting core becomes anchored to some small obstacle, such as a blood vessel. One can speculate that a stationary spiral wave could be responsible for a monomorphic tachycardia, a drifting spiral wave responsible for rhythm with changing contours such as torsades de pointes, and an anchoring spiral wave responsible for the transition from a polymorphic to a monomorphic tachycardia (see Fig. 27-27).[82,83] The use of voltage-sensitive probes in combination with high-resolution video imaging to record electrical wave propagation on the surface of the heart has provided experimental evidence for the role of spiral wave reentry in cardiac fibrillation. Experiments in isolated perfused hearts[84] demonstrate that a single rapidly moving rotor or a small number of coexisting but short-lived rotors give rise to ECG patterns of activity indistinguishable from ventricular fibrillation (VF). The rotors can drift and interact with each other and with boundaries in the heart and result in annihilation or formation of new but also short-lived rotors, or both.[84]

REFLECTION. Reflection can be considered a special subclass of reentry. As in reentry, an area of conduction delay is required, and the total time for the impulse to leave and return to its site of origin must exceed the refractory period of the proximal segment. Reflection differs from reentry in that the impulse does not require a circuit but appears to travel along the *same* pathway in both directions.

Tachycardias Caused by Reentry

Reentry is probably the cause of many tachyarrhythmias, including various kinds of supraventricular and ventricular tachycardias, flutter, and fibrillation (see Chap. 32). However, in complex preparations, such as large pieces of tissue in vitro or the intact heart, it becomes much more difficult to prove unequivocally that reentry exists.

Brugada Syndrome

A reentry mechanism has been implicated in the genesis of ventricular tachycardia-fibrillation associated with the inheritable Brugada syndrome, which is characterized by ST segment elevation (unrelated to ischemia, electrolyte abnormalities, or structural heart disease) in the right precordial (V_1 to V_3) ECG leads, often but not always accompanied by an apparent right bundle branch block. The Brugada syndrome appears to be a congenital ion channel disorder because mutations in the cardiac sodium channel gene *SCN5A* have been reported (see Chap. 28).[85] The gene defect causes either acceleration of recovery of the sodium channel from inactivation or a nonfunctional sodium channel. Inhibition of the sodium channel current causes heterogeneous loss of the action potential dome during the plateau phase (phase 2) in the right ventricular epicardium, which leads to a marked dispersion of repolarization and refractoriness and the potential for phase 2 reentry.[86] Whether transmural heterogeneity in Na^+ channel recovery in the right ventricular free wall causes arrhythmia by a similar mechanism remains to be determined.

In addition, many other factors such as stretch, autonomic stimulation, and a host of modulating influences can act on these electrophysiological mechanisms and obscure the cause of many arrhythmias. Initiation or termination of tachycardia by pacing stimuli, the demonstration of electrical activity bridging diastole, fixed coupling, and a variety of other clinically used techniques such as entrainment and resetting curves, although consistent with reentry, do not constitute absolute proof of its existence. The most compelling evidence for reentry is probably provided by entrainment.[87]

Leading circle model

A

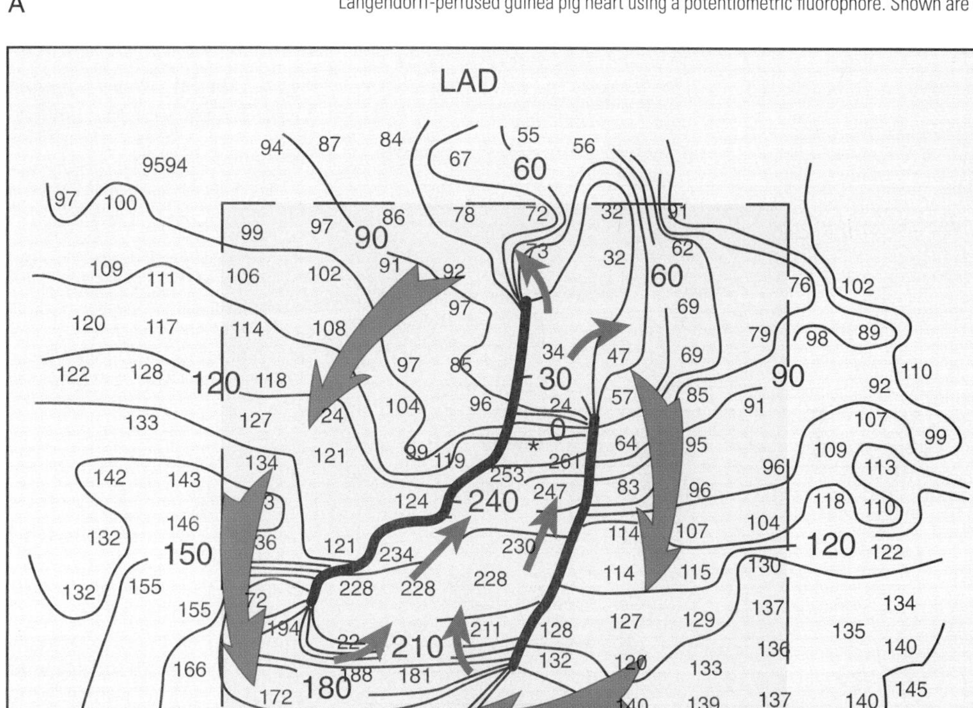

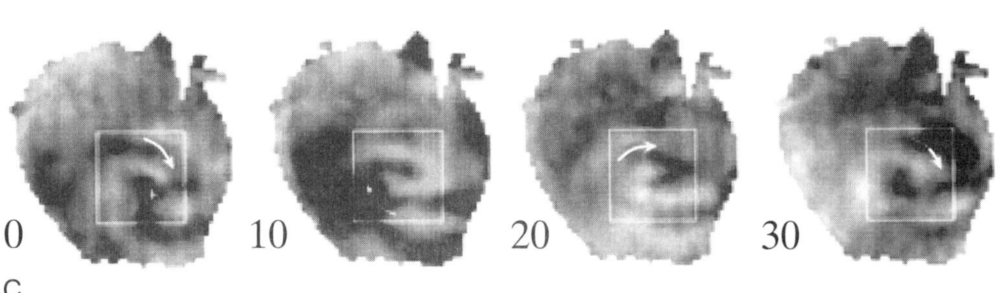

FIGURE 27–27 Functional models of reentry. **A,** *Leading circle model,* a diagrammatic representation of the leading circle model of reentry in isolated left atrium of the rabbit. The central area is activated by converging centripetal wavelets. **B,** *Figure-8-reentry in anisotropic myocardium.* Maps of activation times of a stable reentrant circuit during ventricular tachycardia in the epicardial border zone of a 4-day-old anterior infarct in a dog. The activation times (in milliseconds, small numbers) are shown, as are lines of isochronal activation, at 10-millisecond intervals (larger numbers). The lines of functional block are shown in bold. The circuit consists of clockwise and counterclockwise wave fronts around two functional arcs of block that merge into a central common pathway that usually represents the slow zone of the reentrant circuit. The localization of the functional arcs of block coincides with the spatial disarray of connexin43 gap junctions **C,** *Spiral wave model.* Recording of spiral wave reentry during ventricular fibrillation in a Langendorff-perfused guinea pig heart using a potentiometric fluorophore. Shown are the distributions of membrane potentials at four different times during one rotation on the left ventricular epicardial surface, with white and black being the most positive and most negative membrane potentials, respectively. Numbers are time in milliseconds. Arrows denote direction of wave front propagation. (**A,** From Allessie MA, Bonke FIM, Schopman FJG: Circus movement in rabbit atrial muscle as a mechanism of tachycardia: III. The "leading circle" concept: A new model of circus movement in cardiac tissue without the involvement of an anatomical obstacle. Circ Res 41:9, 1977. By permission of the American Heart Association. **B,** From Peters NS, Coromilas J, Severs NJ, et al: Disturbed connexin43 gap junction distribution correlates with the location of reentrant circuits in the epicardial border zone of healing canine infarcts that cause ventricular tachycardia. Circulation 95:988, 1997. By permission of the American Heart Association. **C,** From Samie FH, Berenfeld O, Anumonwo J, et al: Background potassium current. A determinant of rotor dynamics in ventricular fibrillation. Circ Res 1216, 2001. By permission of the American Heart Association.)

Entrainment

It has been shown that if one could entrain the tachycardia, that is, increase the rate of the tachycardia by pacing, with resumption of the intrinsic rate of the tachycardia when pacing was stopped, the presence of reentry could be established. (Fig. 27–28A). Entrainment represents capture or continuous resetting of the reentrant circuit of the tachycardia by the pacing-induced activation. Each pacing stimulus creates a wave front that travels in an anterograde direction (orthodromic) and resets the tachycardia to the pacing rate. A wave front propagating retrogradely in the opposite direction

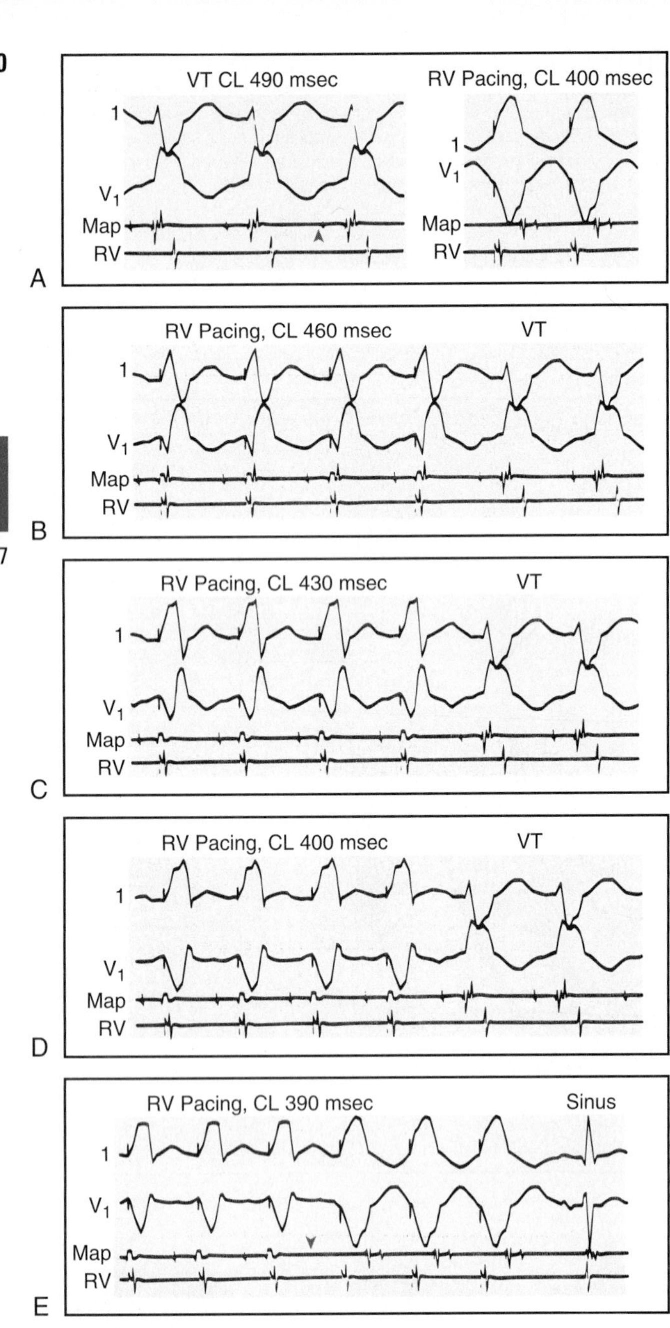

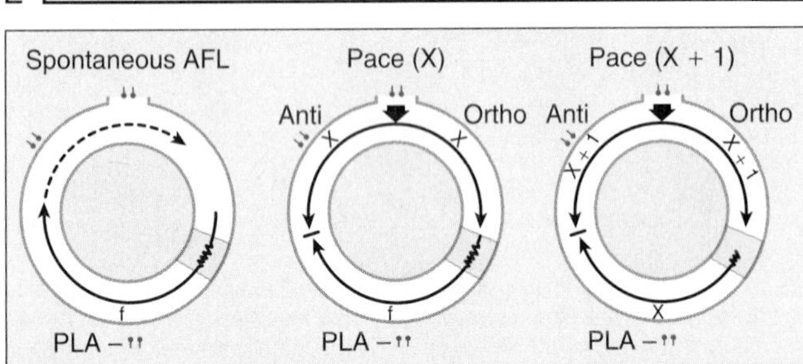

FIGURE 27–28 **Top:** Illustrated criteria for entrainment exemplified in a case of postinfarct ventricular tachycardia (VT). **A, left,** Two electrocardiographic (ECG) leads of a VT and intracardiac recordings from a mapping catheter (Map) at a left ventricular site critical for VT continuation, as well as from the right ventricular apex (RV). Note the diastolic potential (red arrow) during VT. Recordings are similarly arranged in all subsequent panels. **A, right,** RV pacing in the setting of sinus rhythm. **B,** RV pacing at a cycle length (CL) slightly shorter than VT produces a QRS complex that is a blend between fully VT and fully paced ("fusion") complexes. All recordings are accelerated to the paced CL, and after pacing ceases, the same VT resumes. Each fused QRS complex is identical and the last beat is entrained, but surface fusion is absent. **C** and **D,** The same phenomena, but at shorter paced CLs. Note that the fused QRS complex appears more similar to pacing than it does to VT as the pacing CL shortens. B through D thus illustrate a progressive degree of ECG fusion. The Map recording of B through D also shows a progression of fusion, with both the morphology and timing of a portion of the electrogram changing with faster pacing. **E,** Finally, a still shorter paced CL results in a sudden change in both the Map electrogram (block in the small diastolic potential, red arrow) and the surface ECG, which is now fully paced. When pacing ceases, VT has been interrupted. **Bottom:** Diagrammatic representation of the reentrant circuit during spontaneous atrial flutter (AFL) and during transient entrainment of the AFL. **Left,** The reentrant circuit during spontaneous type I AFL. f = circulating wave front of the AFL. **Center,** Introduction of the first pacing impulse (X) during rapid pacing from a high atrial site during AFL. The large arrow indicates entry of the pacing impulse into the reentrant circuit, whereupon it is conducted orthodromically (Ortho) and antidromically (Anti). The antidromic wave front of the pacing impulse (X) collides with the previous beat, in this case the circulating wave front of the spontaneous AFL (f), which results in an atrial fusion beat and, in effect, terminates the AFL. However, the orthodromic wave front from the pacing impulse (X) continues the tachycardia and resets it to the pacing rate. **Right,** Introduction of the next pacing impulse (X + 1) during rapid pacing from the same high atrial site. The large arrow again indicates the entry of the pacing impulse into the reentrant circuit, whereupon it is conducted orthodromically and antidromically. Once again, the antidromic wave front from the pacing impulse (X + 1) collides with the orthodromic wave front of the previous beat. In this case, it is the orthodromic wave front of the previous paced beat (X), and an atrial fusion beat results. The orthodromic wave front from the pacing impulse (X + 1) continues the tachycardia and resets it to the pacing rate. In all three parts, arrows indicate the direction of spread of the impulses; the serpentine line indicates slow conduction through a presumed area of slow conduction (stippled region) in the reentrant circuit, and the red dots with tails indicate bipolar electrodes at the high atrial pacing site, the posteroinferior portion of the left atrium (PLA), and another atrial site. (**Top,** From Zipes DP: A century of cardiac arrhythmia: In search of Jason's golden fleece. J Am Coll Cardiol 34:959, 1999; **Bottom,** from Waldo AL: Atrial flutter. Entrainment characteristics. J Cardiovasc Electrophysiol 8:337, 1997.)

(antidromic) collides with the orthodromic wave front of the previous beat (Fig. 27–28B). These wave front interactions create ECG and electrophysiological features that can be explained only by reentry. Therefore, the criteria of entrainment can be used to prove the reentrant mechanism of a clinical tachycardia and form the basis for localizing the pathway traveled by the tachycardia wave front. Such localization is essential for ablation therapy.[88]

Atrial Flutter (see also Chap. 32)

Reentry is the most likely cause of the usual form of atrial flutter, with the reentrant circuit confined to the right atrium, where it usually travels counterclockwise, in a caudocranial direction in the interatrial septum and in a craniocaudal direction in the right atrial free wall. An area of slow conduction is present in the posterolateral to posteromedial inferior area of the right atrium with a central area of block that can include an anatomical (inferior vena cava) and functional component. It is possible that several different reentrant circuits exist in patients with some types of atrial flutter. However, this area of slow conduction is rather constant and represents the site of successful ablation of atrial flutter. Ablation results are consistent with a macro-reentry circuit.[87-89]

Ventricular Fibrillation (see also Chap. 32)

ELECTRICAL RESTITUTION AND CRITICAL MASS. Substantial experimental support has accumulated in favor of the concept that the onset of VF involves the disintegration of a single spiral wave into many self-perpetuating waves.[84,90] It has been proposed that the breakup of spiral waves is precipitated by oscillations of action potential duration that are of sufficiently large amplitude to cause conduction block along the spiral wave front.

Experimental support for this idea comes from studies demonstrating that if action potential duration restitution (which relates action potential duration to the preceding diastolic interval) contains a region of slope greater than 1, action potential duration alternans is possible and can lead to the formation of reentrant waves.[91,92] Reduction of the slope of the restitution relationship prevented the induction of VF, indicating that the kinetics of electrical restitution appears to be a key determinant of VF. The mass of the tissue appears to be another important factor in the development of fibrillation. In an isolated swine model, it was shown that tissue mass reduction resulted in the termination of VF when a critical mass (19 gm) was reached.[93] In humans, this value appears to be much greater (>111 gm).[92] Similarly, partitioning the atrium into its small segments prevents AF, a concept that has led to a corrective surgical[94] and ablation[95] procedure (see Chap. 30).

LOWER AND UPPER LIMITS OF VULNERABILITY. The cardiac response to electrical stimulation depends on the strength and timing of the stimulus relative to cardiac recovery (coupling interval). A vulnerable zone is present in the T wave during which a stimulus with appropriate strength can induce VF. When the heart is beating spontaneously (e.g., during sinus rhythm), the timing of the vulnerable period corresponds to the T wave on the surface ECG, more precisely, to the latter part of its upslope and its peak.[96] The strength of a stimulus may not be either too low or too high. There is a lower limit of stimulus strength that can induce VF, as well as an upper limit of vulnerability, defined as a current strength at or above which VF cannot be induced.

Propagated graded responses may underlie the mechanisms of ventricular vulnerability to a single premature stimulus. A stimulus delivered during incomplete recovery evokes a gradual response that propagates slowly to neighboring recovered cells and, if its amplitude is large enough, can induce an all-or-none response. This all-or-none response spreads in all directions except into regions near the site of stimulus because of a graded response–induced increase in effective refractory period at the latter site, which results in unidirectional block and reentry (propagated graded-response hypothesis of ventricular vulnerability). When the extrastimulus strength and thus the magnitude of gradual responses increase beyond a critical level, the increase in refractoriness at the site of the stimulus becomes so long that the unidirectional block becomes bidirectional and prevents the formation of reentry (upper limit of vulnerability).[96]

Atrial Fibrillation

SPATIOTEMPORAL ORGANIZATION AND FOCAL DISCHARGE (see also Chap. 32). According to the multiple-wavelet hypothesis, AF is characterized by fragmentation of the wave front into multiple daughter wavelets that wander randomly throughout the atrium and give rise to new wavelets that collide with each other and are mutually annihilated or that give rise to new wavelets in a perpetual activity (for a demonstration of wave front dynamics during fibrillation, see enclosed movie from Samie and colleagues[84]).

The randomness of the irregular electrical activity during AF has been disputed on the basis of both statistical methods and experimental studies. A combination of high-resolution video imaging, ECG recordings, and spectral analysis was used to demonstrate that reentry in anatomically or functionally determined circuits forms the basis of spatiotemporal periodicity during acute AF.[97-99] The cycle length of the source in the left atrium determines the dominant peak in the frequency spectra. The underlying periodicity may stem from a repetitive focal source of activity propagated from an individual pulmonary vein to the remainder of the atrium as fibrillating waves.[100] If a single repetitive focal source of activity that undergoes fractionation underlies maintenance of AF, ablation of this focal source should interrupt AF. Indeed, delivery of radiofrequency energy to discrete sites in the distal pulmonary veins in humans has been shown to eliminate or reduce recurrence of AF.[101]

ELECTRICAL REMODELING OF THE ATRIA. Electrical remodeling of the atria appears to be a key determinant for maintenance of AF.[102] Prolonged rapid atrial pacing in goats and dogs causes electrophysiological alterations of the atria, including shortening and loss of the physiological rate adaptation of refractoriness and decrease in conduction velocity. Because abbreviation of the atrial refractory period is disproportionally larger than reduction of conduction velocity, the wavelength of the reentrant wavelets shortens and thereby promotes reentrant activity (the wavelength is the distance traveled by the depolarization wave front during the duration of its refractory period and equals conduction velocity times refractoriness). The rapid atrial rate also remodels the sinus node.[103]

The ionic basis of shortening of the refractory period and slowing of conduction may be due to a significant reduction in the density of both the L-type Ca^{2+} and the fast Na^{+} currents.[104,105] The electrophysiological changes are paralleled by similar decreases in messenger ribonucleic acid (mRNA) levels of Ca^{2+} and Na^{+} channel genes, which suggests alterations in gene expression as the underlying molecular mechanisms of atrial electrical remodeling.[106] Changes in the density or spatial distribution, or both, of various connexin types may also cause alterations in atrial impulse propagation.[107] Autonomic remodeling also appears to play a key role in both triggering and maintaining AF. Long-term selective vagal denervation of the atria and sinus and AV nodes prevents induction of AF.[108] Heterogeneous sympathetic denervation of the atria favors the development of sustained AF.[109,110]

A variety of interventions attenuate atrial electrical remodeling resulting from short-term rapid atrial pacing, including administration of L-type Ca^{2+} channel blockers,[111] inhibition of reverse mode Na/Ca exchange current[112] and Na/H exchange,[113] and treatment with ascorbate.[114] Digoxin, in contrast, increases tachycardia-induced electrical remodeling of the atria.[115] These findings support the idea that disturbances of the intracellular ionic homeostasis and oxidative stress may electrically remodel the atria by as yet unknown signaling pathways. The signaling pathways underlying long-term tachycardia-fibrillation–induced electrical remodeling, specifically the molecular mechanisms responsible for altered ion channel gene expression, are unknown.

Sinus Reentry (see also Chap. 32)

The sinus node shares with the AV node electrophysiological features such as the potential for *dissociation of conduction*; that is, an impulse can conduct in some nodal fibers but not in others, thereby permitting reentry to occur.[116] The reentrant circuit can be located entirely within the sinus node or involve both the sinus node and atrium. Supraventricular tachycardias caused by sinus node reentry are generally less symptomatic than other supraventricular tachycardias because of slower rates. Ablation of the sinus node may be necessary in an occasional refractory tachycardia.[116]

Atrial Reentry (see also Chap. 32)

Reentry within the atrium, unrelated to the sinus node, can be a cause of supraventricular tachycardia in humans.[117] Atrial reentry appears to be less frequently encountered than other types of supraventricular tachycardia. It has been shown to be due to reentry, automaticity, and afterdepolarizations causing triggered activity. Distinguishing atrial tachycardia caused by automaticity from atrial tachycardia sustained by reentry over quite small areas, that is, microreentry of the leading circle type, is difficult. Multiple foci can be present.

Atrioventricular Nodal Reentry (see also Chap. 32)

Studies employing optical mapping coupled with microelectrode recording have provided detailed insight into the localization and properties of AV nodal conduction and reentrant pathways underlying AV nodal reentrant tachycardia (AVNRT) (Figs. 27–29 and 27–30).[14,15,118] On the basis of conductive properties, multiple, nondiscrete AV nodal input pathways exist, which can be arbitrarily divided into fast, intermediate, and slow pathways (Fig. 27–29). Impulse propagation occurs rapidly over the atrial tissue (red zone in Fig. 27–29D) and slowly toward the AV node through the transi-

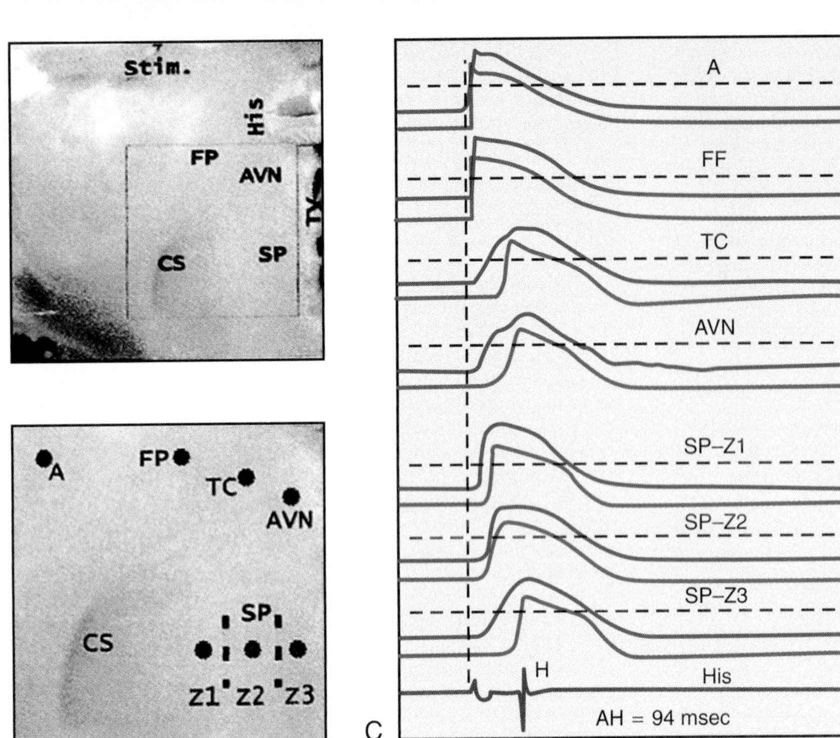

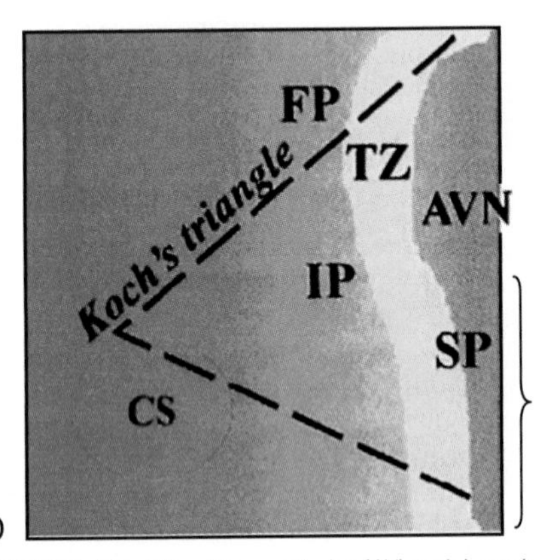

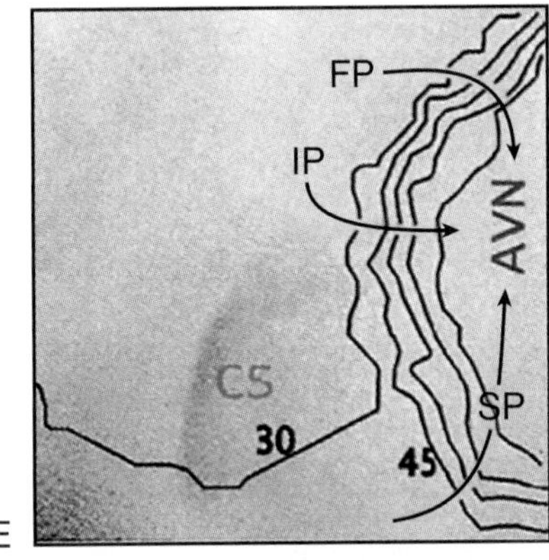

FIGURE 27–29 Atrioventricular (AV) nodal conduction in an isolated, arterially perfused canine preparation. Optical mapping of a potentiometric fluorophore combined with the conventional microelectrode technique were used to delineate the conduction pathways across the AV node. **A,** Endocardial aspect of the preparation. The stimulation electrode (Stim.) and bipolar electrode recording His bundle electrogram (His) are located in the top portion of the picture. The square box next to the tricuspid valve (TV) represents the optical mapping area. AVN = AV node; CS = coronary sinus; FP = fast pathway; SP = slow pathway. **B,** Enlarged picture of optical mapping area to illustrate the sites of microelectrode impalements (dark circles) in atrium (A), fast pathway (FP), transitional cells (TC), AV node (AVN), and three zones (Z1 to Z3) of the slow pathway (SP). **C,** Optical (top, red) and intracellular action potentials (bottom, blue) recorded from different anatomical regions are superimposed and displayed at fast sweep. **D,** Distribution of atrial (red), transitional (yellow), and AV nodal (green) cells in relation to AV nodal inputs (fast [FP], intermediate [IP], and slow [SP] pathways) and posterior extension (AVNPE). **E,** Sketch of the nondiscrete AV nodal input pathways as shown in the optical activation map. (From Wu J, Zipes DP: Mechanisms underlying atrioventricular nodal conduction and the reentrant circuit of atrioventricular nodal reentrant tachycardia using optical mapping. J Cardiovasc Electrophysiol 13:831, 2002.)

tional zone (yellow in Fig. 27–29D) surrounding the AV node. All of the atrial tissue enveloping Koch's triangle (see Fig. 27–29) delivered impulses to the AV node, providing direct evidence to support the concept that slow pathway conduction is present in all normal hearts with or without AVNRT. As seen in Figure 27–29C, conduction delay is associated with a progressive decrease in the upstroke velocity of transmembrane action potentials as well as a progressive lengthening of action potential duration as the impulse approaches the AV node area, suggesting that spatial heterogeneity in the passive (density, cellular distribution, and characteristics of gap junctional channels[118]) or active membrane properties (density or characteristics of ion channels, or both) in the transitional zone underlies AV conduction delay. Optical mapping during echo beats reveals the reentrant pathways underlying the various types of AVNRT (see Fig. 27–30). The reentrant pathway of the slow/fast type starts counterclockwise with block in the fast pathway, delay in conduction across the slow pathway to the compact AV node, then exit from the AV node to the fast pathway and rapid return to the slow pathway through atrial tissue located at the base of Koch's triangle. The reentrant circuit of the fast/slow type is clockwise. In the slow/slow type, anterograde conduction is over the intermediate pathway and retrograde conduction is over the slow pathway. Because slow pathway conduction is involved in each type of AVNRT, this observation explains why ablation of the slow pathway is effective in all types of AVNRT. These results also demonstrate that atrial tissue surrounding Koch's triangle is clearly involved in all three types of AV nodal reentry in these examples (see also Fig. 27–26).

Preexcitation Syndrome

(see also Chap. 32)

In most patients who have reciprocating tachycardias associated with Wolff-Parkinson-White syndrome, the accessory pathway conducts more rapidly than the normal AV node but takes a longer time to recover excitability; that is, the anterograde refractory period of the accessory pathway exceeds that of the AV node at long cycles.[119] Consequently, a premature atrial complex that occurs sufficiently early is blocked anterogradely in the accessory pathway and continues to the ventricle over the normal AV node and His bundle. After the ventricles have been excited, the impulse is able to enter the accessory pathway retrogradely and return to the atrium. A continuous conduction loop of this kind establishes the circuit for the tachycardia. The usual (orthodromic) activation wave during such a reciprocating tachycardia in a patient with an accessory pathway occurs anterogradely over the normal AV node–His-Purkinje system and retrogradely over the accessory pathway, which results in a normal QRS complex (Fig. 27–31).

Because the circuit requires both atria and ventricles, the term *supraventricular tachycardia* is not precisely correct, and the tachycardia is more accurately called *atrioventricular reciprocating tachycardia* (AVRT). The reentrant loop can be interrupted by ablation of the normal AV node–His bundle pathway *or* the accessory pathway.[119,120] Occasionally, the activation wave travels in a reverse (antidromic) direction to the ventricles over the accessory pathway and to the atria retrogradely up the AV node.[119,120] Two accessory pathways can form the circuit in some patients with antidromic AVRT. In

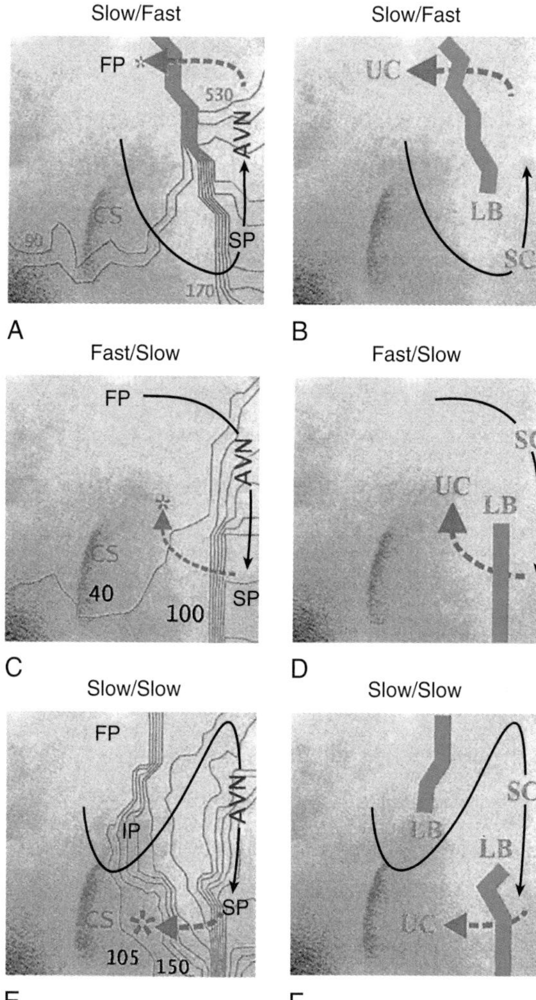

FIGURE 27–30 Reentrant circuits of different types of AV nodal reentrant tachycardia. Pictures of the optical activation maps of A2 obtained from three different experiments at A2 coupling intervals of 190, 220, and 190 milliseconds were merged with the pictures of the mapping area to show the initiation of echo beats in **A** (slow/fast), **C** (fast/slow), and **E** (slow/slow), respectively. The numbers in the maps indicate the activation times in reference to the A2 stimulus. The interrupted black arrow indicates anterograde conduction, and the star and the dashed red arrow represent the site of earliest retrograde atrial activation. The corresponding locations of the lines of block (LB, green), slow anterograde conduction (SC, black arrow), and unidirectional conduction (UC, red) are shown in **B, D,** and **F,** respectively. (From Wu J, Zipes DP: Mechanisms underlying atrioventricular nodal conduction and the reentrant circuit of atrioventricular nodal reentrant tachycardia using optical mapping. J Cardiovasc Electrophysiol 13:831, 2002.)

some patients, the accessory pathway may be capable of only retrograde conduction ("concealed"), but the circuit and mechanism of AVRT remain the same. Less commonly, the accessory pathway can conduct only anterogradely. The pathway can be localized by analysis of the scalar ECG.[121] Patients can have AF as well as AVRT.

Unusual accessory pathways with AV node–like electrophysiological properties, that is, nodofascicular or nodoventricular fibers, can constitute the circuit for reciprocating tachycardias in patients who have some form of the Wolff-Parkinson-White syndrome. Tachycardia in patients with nodoventricular fibers can be due to reentry with these fibers used as the anterograde pathway and the His-Purkinje fibers and a portion of the AV node used retrogradely. In the so-called Lown-Ganong-Levine syndrome (short PR interval and normal QRS complex), conduction over a James fiber that connects the atrium to the distal portion of the AV node and His bundle has been *proposed*, although little functional evidence exists to support the presence of this entity.

Ventricular Tachycardia Caused by Reentry

(see also Chap. 32)

Reentry in the ventricle, both anatomical and functional, as a cause of sustained ventricular tachycardia has been supported by many animal[81] and clinical[122,123] studies (Fig. 27–32). Reentry in ventricular muscle, with or without contribution from specialized tissue, is responsible for many or most ventricular tachycardias in patients with ischemic heart disease. The area of micro-reentry appears to be quite small, and, less uncommonly, a macro-reentry is found around the infarct scar. Surviving myocardial tissue separated by connective tissue provides serpentine routes of activation traversing infarcted areas that can establish reentry pathways. Bundle branch reentry can cause sustained ventricular tachycardia, particularly in patients with dilated cardiomyopathy.[123]

Both figure-of-8 (see Fig. 27–27) and single-circle (see Fig. 27–32) reentrant loops have been described as circulating around an area of functional block in a manner consistent with the leading circle hypothesis or conducting slowly across an apparent area of block created by anisotropy.[81] When intramural myocardium survives, it can form part of the reentrant loop. Structural discontinuities that separate muscle bundles, for example, as a result of naturally occurring myocardial fiber orientation and anisotropic conduction, as well as collagen matrices formed from the fibrosis after a myocardial infarction, establish the basis for slowed conduction, fragmented electrograms, and continuous electrical activity that can lead to reentry. After the infarction, the surviving epicardial border zone undergoes substantial electrical remodeling,[124] including reduced conduction velocity and increased anisotropy associated with the occurrence of reentrant circuits and ventricular tachycardia. Conduction slowing arises from alterations in the spatial distribution[81] and electrophysiological properties of connexin43 gap junctions[125] as well as from reduced sodium current.[126] During acute ischemia, a variety of factors, including elevated $[K]_o$ and reduced pH, combine to create depressed action potentials in ischemic cells that retard conduction and can lead to reentry.[67]

Ventricular Tachycardias Caused by Nonreentrant Mechanisms

In some instances of ventricular tachycardia related to coronary artery disease, but especially in patients without coronary artery disease, nonreentrant mechanisms are important causes of ventricular tachycardias. However, in many patients the mechanism of the ventricular tachycardia remains unknown.

TRIGGERED ACTIVITY. A group of probably nonreentrant ventricular tachycardias occurring in the absence of structural heart disease can be initiated and terminated by programmed stimulation. They are catecholamine dependent and are terminated by the Valsalva maneuver, adenosine, and verapamil. These ventricular tachycardias are generally, but not exclusively, located in the right ventricular outflow tract and may be due to triggered activity, possibly DADs that are cAMP dependent.[75] EADs have been recorded in this tachycardia as well. Left ventricular fascicular tachycardias can be suppressed by verapamil but not generally by adenosine, and some may be due to triggered activity and others to reentry.[75] EADs and triggered activity may be responsible for torsades de pointes.[68,70]

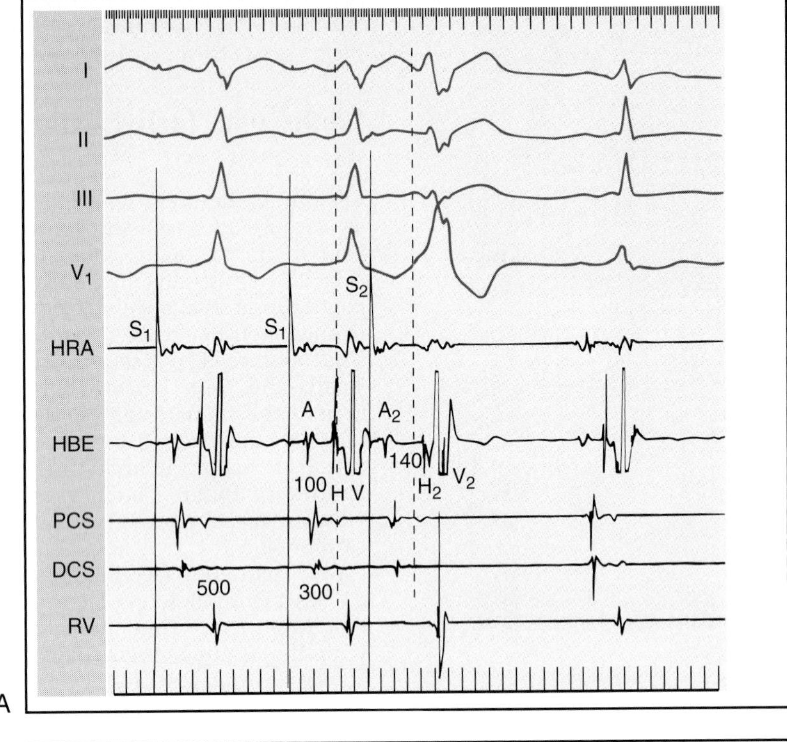

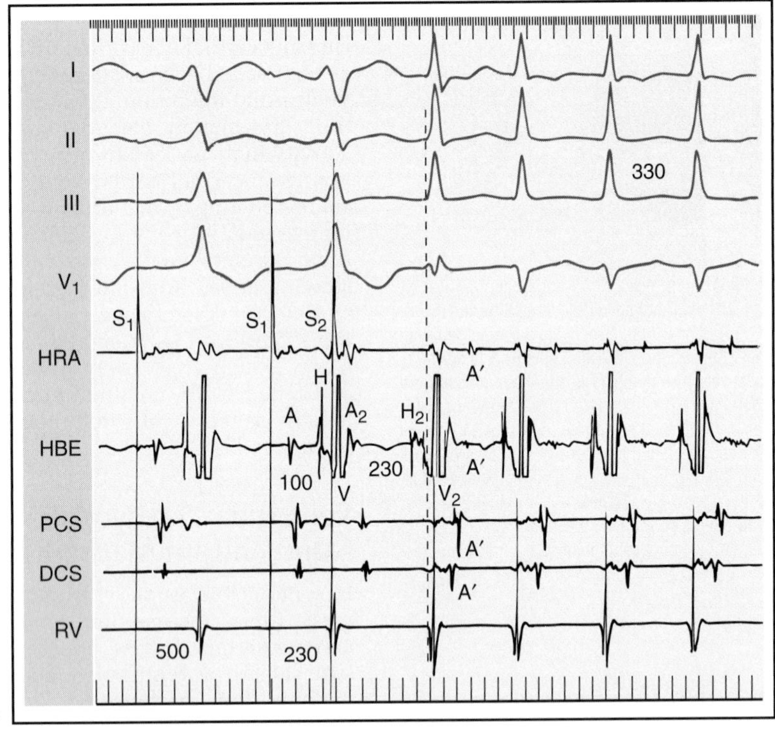

FIGURE 27–31 **A,** Wolff-Parkinson-White syndrome. Following high right atrial pacing at a cycle length of 500 milliseconds (S_1-S_1), premature stimulation at a coupling interval of 300 milliseconds (S_1-S_2) produces physiological delay in atrioventricular (AV) nodal conduction resulting in an increase in the A-H interval from 100 to 140 milliseconds but no delay in the AV interval. Consequently, activation of the His bundle occurs following activation of the QRS complex (second interrupted line), and the QRS complex becomes more anomalous in appearance because of increased ventricular activation over the accessory pathway. I, II, III, and V_1 indicate scalar ECG leads. DCS = distal coronary sinus electrogram; HBE = His bundle electrogram; HRA = high right atrium; PCS = proximal coronary sinus electrogram; RV = right ventricular electrogram. Time lines are in 50- and 10-millisecond intervals. S_1, stimulus of the drive train; S_2, premature stimulus. A, H-V, atrial His bundle, and ventricular activation during the drive train; A_2, H_2, V_2, atrial His bundle, and ventricular activation during the premature stimulus. **B,** Induction of reciprocating atrioventricular tachycardia. Premature stimulation at a coupling interval of 230 milliseconds prolongs the A-H interval to 230 milliseconds and results in anterograde block in the accessory pathway and normalization of the QRS complex (a slight functional aberrancy in the nature of incomplete right bundle branch block occurs). Note that H_2 precedes onset of the QRS complex (interrupted line). Following V_2, the atria are excited retrogradely (A′) beginning in the distal coronary sinus, followed by atrial activation in leads recording from the proximal coronary sinus, His bundle, and high right atrium. A supraventricular tachycardia is initiated at a cycle length of 330 milliseconds. Conventions are as in panel A. (From Zipes DP, Mahomed Y, King RD, et al: Wolff-Parkinson-White syndrome: Cryosurgical treatment. Indiana Med 89:432, 1986.)

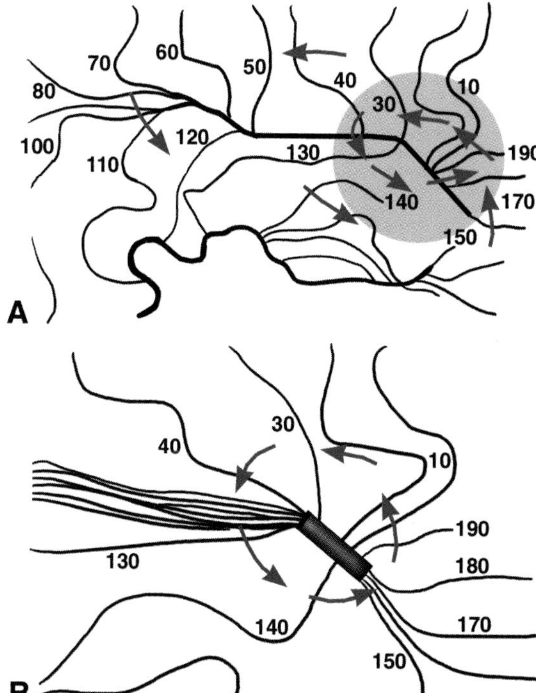

FIGURE 27–32 Model of anisotropic reentry in the epicardial border zone. **A,** The activation map of the single reentrant circuit is shown. The arrows point out the general activation pattern; activation appears to occur around a long line of block. However, parallel isochrones adjacent to the line (isochrones 130 and 140) suggest that activation is also occurring across the line and thereby results in the smaller circuit shown by the arrows in the shaded area. **B,** This circuit is shown enlarged. Rapid activation occurs parallel to the long axis of the fiber orientation (isochrones 10 to 40 and 130 to 150), whereas very slow activation (closely bunched isochrones 50 to 120) occurs transverse to fiber orientation in the circuit. The dark black rectangle is an area of either functional or anatomical block that forms the fulcrum of the circuit. (From Wit AL, Dillon SM: Anisotropic reentry. *In* Zipes DP, Jalife J [eds]: Cardiac Electrophysiology: From Cell to Bedside. Philadelphia, WB Saunders, 1990.)

AUTOMATICITY. Automatic discharge can be responsible for some ventricular tachycardias and does not appear to be suppressed by adenosine. Unless invasive studies are undertaken, mechanisms of ventricular tachycardia can only be conjectured.

REFERENCES

Anatomy of the Cardiac Conduction System

1. Honjo H, Boyett MR, Coppen SR, et al: Heterogeneous expression of connexins in rabbit sinoatrial node cells: Correlation between connexin isotype and cell size. Cardiovasc Res 53:89, 2002.
2. Altomare C, Terragni B, Brioschi C, et al: Heteromeric HCN1-HCN4 channels: A comparison with native pacemaker channels from the rabbit sinoatrial node. J Physiol (Lond) 549:347, 2003.
3. Boyett MR, Honjo H, Kodama I: The sinoatrial node, a heterogeneous pacemaker structure. Cardiovasc Res 47:658, 2000.
4. Lei M, Honjo H, Kodama I, et al: Characterization of the outward K$^+$ current in rabbit sinoatrial node cells. Cardiovasc Res 46:431, 2000.
5. Coppen SR, Kodama I, Boyett MR, et al: Connexin45, a major connexin of the rabbit sino-atrial node, is co-expressed with connexin43 in a restricted zone at the nodal–crista terminalis border. J Histochem Cytochem 47:907, 1999.
6. Martinez AD, Hayrapetyan V, Moreno AP, et al: Connexin43 and connexin45 form heteromeric gap junction channels in which individual components determine permeability and regulation. Circ Res 90:1100, 2002.
7. Bukauskas FF, Bukaukien A, Verselis VH, et al: Coupling asymmetry of heterotypic connexin 45/ connexin 43-EGFP gap junctions: Properties of fast and slow gating mechanisms. Proc Natl Acad Sci USA 99:7113, 2002.
8. Schuessler RB, Boineau JP, Saffitz JE, et al: Cellular mechanisms of sinoatrial activity. *In* Zipes DP, Jalife J (eds): Cardiac Electrophysiology: From Cell to Bedside. 3rd ed. Philadelphia, WB Saunders, 1999, pp 187-195.
9. Schwartz PJ, Zipes DP: Autonomic modulation of cardiac arrhythmias. *In* Zipes DP, Jalife J (eds): Cardiac Electrophysiology: From Cell to Bedside. 3rd ed. Philadelphia, WB Saunders, 1999, pp 300-314.
10. Lakatta EG, Maltsev VA, Bogdanov KY, et al: Cyclic variation of intracellular calcium: A critical factor for cardiac pacemaker cell dominance. Circ Res 92:45, 2003.
11. Steinberg SF: The molecular basis for distinct ß-adrenergic receptor subtype actions in cardiomyocytes. Circ Res 85:1101, 1999.
12. Ackerman MJ, Clapham DE: G proteins and ion channels. *In* Zipes DP, Jalife J (eds): Cardiac Electrophysiology: From Cell to Bedside. 3rd ed. Philadelphia, WB Saunders, 1999, pp 112-118.
13. Chang F, Yu H, Cohen IS: Actions of vasoactive intestinal peptide and neuropeptide Y on the pacemaker current in canine Purkinje fibers. Circ Res 74:157, 1994.
14. Wu J, Wu J, Olgin J, et al: Mechanisms underlying the reentrant circuit of atrioventricular nodal reentry tachycardia in isolated canine nodal preparations using optical mapping. Circ Res 88:1189, 2001.
15. Nikolski V, Efimov IR: Fluorescent imaging of a dual-pathway atrioventricular nodal conduction system. Circ Res 88:e23, 2001.
16. James TN: The tendons of Todaro and the "triangle of Koch": Lessons from eponymous hagiolatry. J Cardiovasc Electrophysiol 10:1478, 1999.
17. Wu J, Zipes DP: Mechanisms underlying atrioventricular nodal conduction and the reentrant circuit of atrioventricular nodal reentrant tachycardia using optical mapping. J Cardiovasc Electrophysiol 13:831, 2002.
18. Mazgalev TN, Van Wagoner DR, Efimov IR: Mechanisms of AV nodal excitability and propagation. *In* Zipes DP, Jalife J (eds): Cardiac Electrophysiology: From Cell to Bedside. 3rd ed. Philadelphia, WB Saunders, 1999, pp 196-205.
19. Tamaddon HS, Vaidya D, Simon AM, et al: High-resolution optical mapping of the right bundle branch in connexin40 knockout mice reveals slow conduction in the specialized conduction system. Circ Res 87:929, 2000.
20. Connen SR, Dupont E, Rothery S, et al: Connexin45 expression is preferentially associated with the ventricular conduction system in mouse and rat heart. Circ Res 82:232, 1998.
21. Rohr S, Kucera JP, Fast VG, et al: Paradoxical improvement of impulse conduction in cardiac tissue by partial uncoupling. Science 275:841, 1997.
22. Levy MN: Time dependency of the autonomic interactions that regulate heart rate and rhythms. *In* Zipes DP, Jalife J (eds): Cardiac Electrophysiology: From Cell to Bedside. 2nd ed. Philadelphia, WB Saunders, 1994, p 454.
23. Olgin JE, Sih HJ, Hanish S, et al: Heterogeneous atrial denervation creates substrate for sustained atrial fibrillation. Circulation 98:2608, 1998.
24. Liu Y, Wu C, Lu L, et al: Sympathetic nerve sprouting, electrical remodeling, and increased vulnerability to ventricular fibrillation in hypercholesterolemic rabbits. Circ Res 92:1145, 2003.
25. Cao J, Chen LS, KenKnight BH, et al: Nerve sprouting and sudden cardiac death. Circ Res 86:816, 2000.
26. Hartmann HA, Colom LV, Sutherland ML, Noebels JL: Selective localization of cardiac SCN5A sodium channels in limbic regions of rat brain. Nat Neurosci 2:593, 1999.
27. Shamsuzzaman ASM, Ackerman MJ, Kara T, et al: Sympathetic nerve activity in the congenital long-QT syndrome. Circulation 107:1844, 2003.

Basic Electrophysiological Principles

28. Inoue M, Bridge JHB: Ca^{2+} sparks in rabbit ventricular myocytes evoked by action potentials. Involvement of clusters of L-type Ca^{2+} channels. Circ Res 92:532, 2003.
29. Rasmusson RL, Morales MJ, Wang S, et al: Inactivation of voltage-gated cardiac K^+ channels. Circ Res 82:739, 1998.
30. Rohr S, Kucera JP, Kléber AG: Slow conduction in cardiac tissue, I. Circ Res 83:781, 1998.
31. Sakmann BFAS, Spindler AJ, Bryant SM, et al: Distribution of a persistent sodium current across the ventricular wall in guinea pigs. Circ Res 87:910, 2000.
32. Kamp TJ, Zhou Z, Zhang S, et al: Pharmacology of L- and T-type calcium channels in the heart. *In* Zipes DP, Jalife J (eds): Cardiac Electrophysiology: From Cell to Bedside. 3rd ed. Philadelphia, WB Saunders, 1999, pp 141-156.
33. Gaspo R, Bosch RF, Bou-Abboud E, et el: Tachycardia-induced changes in Na^+ current in a chronic dog model of atrial fibrillation. Circ Res 81:1045, 1997.
34. Wang Z, Feng J, Shi H, et al: Potential molecular basis of different physiological properties of the transient outward K^+ current in rabbit and human atrial myocytes. Circ Res 84:551, 1999.
35. Yue L, Melnik P, Gaspo R, et al: Molecular mechanisms underlying ionic remodeling in a dog model of atrial fibrillation. Circ Res 87:776, 1999.
36. Antos CL , Frey N, Marx SO, et al: Dilated cardiomyopathy and sudden death resulting from constitutive activation of protein kinase A. Circ Res 89:997, 2001.
37. Zhou J, Shin H, Ji Y, et al: Phosphorylation and ER retention signals are required for protein kinase A–mediated potentiation of cardiac sodium current. Circ Res 91:540, 2002.
38. Li RA, Leppo M, Miki T, et al: Molecular basis of electrocardiographic ST-segment elevation. Circ Res 87:837, 2000.
39. Martynuyk AE, Morey TE, Belardinelli L, et al: Hyperkalemia enhances the effect of adenosine on $I_{K,Ado}$ in rabbit isolated AV nodal myocytes and on AV nodal conduction in guinea pig isolated heart. Circulation 99:312, 1999.
40. Baker LC, London B, Choi B, et al: Enhanced dispersion of repolarization and refractoriness in transgenic mouse hearts promotes ventricular tachycardia. Circ Res 86:396, 2000.
41. Spach MS, Heidlage JF, Dolber PC, et al: Electrophysiological effects of remodeling cardiac gap junctions and cell size. Circ Res 86:302, 2000.
42. Kléber AG, Fast VG, Rohr S: Continuous and discontinuous propagation. *In* Zipes DP, Jalife J (eds): Cardiac Electrophysiology: From Cell to Bedside. 3rd ed. Philadelphia, WB Saunders, 1999, pp 205-213.
43. Morley GE, Vaidya D, Samie FH, et al: Characterization of conduction in the ventricles of normal and heterozygous Cx43 knockout mice using optical mapping. J Cardiovasc Electrophysiol 10:1361, 1999.
44. Gutstein DE, Morley GE, Tamaddon H, et al: Conduction slowing and sudden arrhythmic death in mice with cardiac-restricted inactivation of connexin43. Circ Res 88:333, 2001.

45. Saffitz JE, Yamada KA: Gap junction distribution in the heart. *In* Zipes DP, Jalife J (eds): Cardiac Electrophysiology: From Cell to Bedside. Philadelphia, WB Saunders, 1999, pp 179-187.
46. Zipes DP, Jalife J (eds): Cardiac Electrophysiology: From Cell to Bedside. 3rd ed. Philadelphia, WB Saunders, 2000.
47. Clemo HF, Stambler BS, Baumgarten CM: Swelling-activated chloride current is persistently activated in ventricular myocytes from dogs with tachycardia-induced congestive heart failure. Circ Res 84:157, 1999.
48. Kaneko T, Tanaka H, Oyamada M, et al: Three distinct types of Ca^{2+} waves in Langendorff-perfused rat heart revealed by real-time confocal microscopy. Circ Res 86:1093, 2000.
49. Wu Y, Roden DM, Anderson ME: Calmodulin kinase inhibition prevents development of the arrhythmogenic transient inward current. Circ Res 84:906, 1999.
50. Pogwizd SM, Schlotthauer K, Li L, et al: Arrhythmogenesis and contractile dysfunction in heart failure. Circ Res 88:1159, 2001.
51. Zaza A, Rocchetti M, Brioschi A, et al: Dynamic Ca^{2+}-induced inward rectification of K^+ current during the ventricular action potential. Circ Res 82:947, 1998.
52. Reuter H, Henderson SA, Han T, et al: The Na^+-Ca^{2+} exchanger is essential for the action of cardiac glycosides. Circ Res 90:305, 2002.
53. Kucera JP, Kléber AG, Rohr S: Slow conduction in cardiac tissue, II. Circ Res 83:795, 1998.
54. Balke CW, Marbán E, O'Rourke B: Calcium channels: structure, function, and regulation. *In* Zipes DP, Jalife J (eds): Cardiac Electrophysiology: From Cell to Bedside. Philadelphia, WB Saunders, 1999, pp 8-21.

55. Belardinelli L, Song Y, Shryock JC: Cholinergic control of cardiac electrical activity. *In* Zipes DP, Jalife J (eds): Cardiac Electrophysiology: From Cell to Bedside. Philadelphia, WB Saunders, 1999, pp 294-300.
56. Snyders DJ: Molecular biology of potassium channels. *In* Zipes DP, Jalife J (eds): Cardiac Electrophysiology: From Cell to Bedside. Philadelphia, WB Saunders, 1999, pp 21-31.
57. Priebe L, Beuckelmann DJ: Simulation studies of cellular electrical properties in heart failure. Circ Res 82:1206, 1998.
58. Sah R, Ramirez RJ, Backx PH: Modulation of Ca^{2+} release in cardiac myocytes by changes in repolarization rate. Circ Res 90:165, 2002.
59. Sah R, Ramirez RJ, Oudit GY, et al: Regulation of cardiac excitation-contraction coupling by action potential repolarization: Role of the transient outward potassium current (I_{to}). J. Physiol (Lond) 546:5, 2003.
60. Zygmunt AC, Goodrow RJ, Weigel CM: I_{NaCa} and $I_{Cl(Ca)}$ contribute to isoproterenol-induced delayed afterdepolarizations in midmyocardial cells. Am J Physiol 275:H1979, 1998.
61. Weber CR, Ginsburg KS, Bers DM: Cardiac submembrane $[Na^+]$ transients sensed by Na^+-Ca^{2+} exchange current. Circ Res 92:950, 2003.
62. Yao A, Su Z, Nonaka A, et al: Effects of overexpression of the Na^+-Ca^{2+} exchanger on $[Ca^{2+}]_i$ transients in murine ventricular myocytes. Circ Res 82:657, 1998.
63. Yang T, Snyders DJ, Roden DM: Rapid inactivation determines the rectification and $[K^+]_o$ dependence of the rapid component of the delayed rectifier K^+ current in cardiac cells. Circ Res 80:782, 1997.
64. Clemo HF, Stambler BS, Baumgarten CM: Persistent activation of a swelling-activated cation current in ventricular myocytes from dogs with tachycardia-induced congestive heart failure. Circ Res 83:147, 1998.
65. Lakatta EG, Maltsev VA, Bogdanov KY, et al: Cyclic variation in intracellular calcium. A critical factor for cardiac pacemaker cell dominance. Circ Res 92:e45, 2003.
66. Shivkumar K, Deutsch NA, Lamp ST, et al: Mechanism of hypoxic K loss in rabbit ventricle. J Clin Invest 100:1782, 1997.
67. Kanda A, Watanabe I, Williams ML, et al: Unanticipated lessening of the rise in extracellular potassium during ischemia by pinacidil. Circulation 95:1937,1997.

Mechanisms of Arrhythmogenesis

68. Mohler PJ, Schott J, Gramolini AO, et al: Ankyrin-B mutation causes type 4 long-QT cardiac arrhythmia and sudden cardiac death. Nature 421:634, 2003.
68a. Kass RS, Moss AJ: Long QT syndrome: Novel insights into the mechanisms of cardiac arrhythmias. J Clin Invest 112:810-815, 2003.
69. Antzelevitch C, Shimizu W, Yan G, et al: The M cell: Its contribution to the ECG and to normal and abnormal electrical function of the heart. J Cardiovasc Electrophysiol 10:1124, 1999.
70. Choi B, Burton F, Salama G: Cytosolic Ca^{2+} triggers early afterdepolarizations and torsade de pointes in rabbit hearts with type 2 long QT syndrome. J Physiol (Lond) 543.2:615, 2002.
71. Zygmunt AC, Eddlestone GT, Thomas GP, et al: Larger late sodium conductance in M cells contributes to electrical heterogeneity in canine ventricle. Am J Physiol 281:H689, 2001.
72. Zygmunt AC, Goodrow RJ, Antzelevitch C: I_{NaCa} contributes to electrical heterogeneity within the ventricle. Am J Physiol 278:H2671, 2000.
73. Shimizu W, Kurita T, Matsuo K, et al: Improvement of repolarization abnormalities by a K^+ channel opener in the LQT1 of congenital long-QT syndrome. Circulation 97:1581, 1998.
74. Hwang C, Karagueuzian HS, Chen PS: Idiopathic paroxysmal atrial fibrillation induced by a focal discharge mechanism in the left superior pulmonary vein: Possible roles of the ligament of Marshall. J Cardiovasc Electrophysiol 10:636, 1999.
75. Lerman BB, Stein KM, Markowitz SM, et al: Ventricular tachycardia in patients with structurally normal hearts. *In* Zipes DP, Jalife J (eds): Cardiac Electrophysiology: From Cell to Bedside. Philadelphia, WB Saunders, 1999, pp 640-656.
76. Zipes DP, Jalife J: Atrioventricular block and dissociation. *In* Zipes DP, Jalife J (eds): Cardiac Electrophysiology: From Cell to Bedside. 4th ed. Philadelphia, WB Saunders, 2003, pp 451-458.
77. Hund TJ, Rudy Y: Determinants of excitability in cardiac myocytes: Mechanistic investigation of memory effect. Biophys J 79:3095, 2000.
78. Krinsky V: Qualitative theory of reentry. *In* Zipes DP, Jalife J (eds): Cardiac Electrophysiology: From Cell to Bedside. 3rd ed. Philadelphia, WB Saunders, 1999, pp 320-326.
79. Athill CH, Ikeda T, Kim Y, et al: Transmembrane potential properties at the core of functional reentrant wavefronts in isolated canine atria. Circulation 98:1556, 1998.
80. Uzzaman M, Honjo H, Takagishi Y, et al: Remodeling of gap junctional coupling in hypertrophied right ventricles of rats with monocrotaline-induced pulmonary hypertension. Circ Res 86:871, 2000.
81. Peters NS, Coromilas J, Severs NJ, et al: Disturbed connexin43 gap junction distribution correlates with the location of reentrant circuits in the epicardial border zone of healing canine infarcts that cause ventricular tachycardia. Circulation 95:988, 1997.
82. Beaumont J, Jalife J: Rotors and spiral waves in two dimensions. *In* Zipes DP, Jalife J (eds): Cardiac Electrophysiology: From Cell to Bedside. 3rd ed. Philadelphia, WB Saunders, 1999, pp 327-335.
83. Pertsov AM, Jalife J: Three-dimensional vortex-like reentry. *In* Zipes DP, Jalife J (eds): Cardiac Electrophysiology: From Cell to Bedside. 3rd ed. Philadelphia, WB Saunders, 1999, pp 336-344.
84. Samie FH, Berenfeld O, Anumonwo J, et al: Background potassium current. A determinant of rotor dynamics in ventricular fibrillation. Circ Res 89:1216, 2001.
85. Chen Q, Glenn E, Zhang D, et al: Genetic basis and molecular mechanism for idiopathic ventricular fibrillation. Nature 392:293, 1998.
86. Antzelevitch C, Brugada P, Brugada J, et al: Brugada syndrome. A decade of progress. Circ Res 91:1114, 2002.
87. Waldo AL: Atrial flutter: Mechanisms, clinical features, and management. *In* Zipes DP, Jalife J (eds): Cardiac Electrophysiology: From Cell to Bedside. 3rd ed. Philadelphia, WB Saunders, 1999, pp 468-475.
88. Zipes DP: 50th anniversary historical article. A century of cardiac arrhythmias: In search of Jason's golden fleece. J Am Coll Cardiol 34:959, 1999.
89. Uno K, Kumagai K, Khrestian CM, et al: New insights regarding the atrial flutter reentrant circuit. Circulation 100:1354, 1999.
90. Witkowski FX, Leon LJ, Penkoske PA, et al: Spatiotemporal evolution of ventricular fibrillation. Nature 392:78, 1998.
91. Riccio ML, Koller ML, Gilmour RF: Electrical restitution and spatiotemporal organization during ventricular fibrillation. Circ Res 84:955, 1999.
92. Wu TJ, Yashima M, Doshi R, et al: Relation between cellular repolarization characteristics and critical mass for human ventricular fibrillation. J Cardiovasc Electrophysiol 10:1077, 1999.
93. Kim YH, Garfinkel A, Ikeda T, et al: Spatiotemporal complexity of ventricular fibrillation revealed by tissue mass reduction in isolated swine right ventricle. J Clin Invest 100:2486, 1997.
94. Pagé PL: Surgery for atrial fibrillation and other supraventricular tachyarrhythmias. *In* Zipes DP, Jalife J (eds): Cardiac Electrophysiology: From Cell to Bedside. 3rd ed. Philadelphia, WB Saunders, 1999, pp 1065-1077.
95. Haïssaguerre M, Jaïs P, Shah DC, et al: Catheter ablation for atrial fibrillation: clinical electrophysiology of linear lesions. *In* Zipes DP, Jalife J (eds): Cardiac Electrophysiology: From Cell to Bedside. 3rd ed. Philadelphia, WB Saunders, 1999, pp 994-1008.
96. Chen PS, Swerdlow CD, Hwang C, Karagueuzian HS: Current concepts of ventricular defibrillation. J Cardiovasc Electrophysiol 9:553, 1998.
97. Skanes AC, Manapati R, Berenfeld O, et al: Spatiotemporal periodicity during atrial fibrillation in the isolated sheep heart. Circulation 98:1236, 1998.
98. Manapati R, Skanes AC, Chen J, et al: Stable microreentrant sources as a mechanism of atrial fibrillation in the isolated sheep heart. Circulation 101:194, 2000.
99. Sih HJ, Zipes DP, Berbari EJ, et al: Differences in organization between acute and chronic atrial fibrillation in dogs. J Am Coll Cardiol 36:924, 2000.
100. Jaïs P, Haïssaguerre M, Shah DC, et al: A focal source of atrial fibrillation treated by discrete radiofrequency ablation. Circulation 95:572, 1997.
101. Haissaguerre M, Jais P, Shah DC, et al: Spontaneous initiation of atrial fibrillation by ectopic beats originating in the pulmonary veins. N Engl J Med 339:659, 1998.
102. Olgin JE, Rubart M: Remodeling of the atria and ventricles due to rate. *In* Zipes DP, Jalife J (eds): Cardiac Electrophysiology: From Cell to Bedside. 3rd ed. Philadelphia, WB Saunders, 1999, pp 364-378.
103. Hadian D, Zipes DP, Olgin JE, et al: Short-term rapid atrial pacing produces electrical remodeling of sinus node function in humans. J Cardiovasc Electrophysiol 13:584, 2002.
104. Yue L, Feng J, Gaspo R, et al: Ionic remodeling underlying action potential changes in a canine model of atrial fibrillation. Circ Res 81:512, 1997.
105. Gaspo R, Bosch RF, Bou-Abboud E, Nattel S: Tachycardia-induced changes in Na^+ current in a chronic dog model of atrial fibrillation. Circ Res 81:1045, 1997.
106. Yue L, Melnyk P, Gaspo R, et al: Molecular mechanisms underlying ionic remodeling in a dog model of atrial fibrillation. Circ Res 84:776, 1999.
107. Elvan A, Huang XD, Pressler ML, Zipes DP: Radiofrequency catheter ablation of the atria eliminates pacing-induced sustained atrial fibrillation and reduces connexin 43 in dogs. Circulation 96:1675, 1997.
108. Chio CW, Eble JN, Zipes DP: Efferent vagal innervation of the canine atria and sinus and atrioventricular nodes. The third fat pad. Circulation 9:2573, 1997.
109. Olgin JE, Sih HJ, Hanish S, et al: Heterogeneous atrial denervation creates substrate for sustained atrial fibrillation. Circulation 98:2608, 1998.
110. Jayachandran JV, Sih HJ, Winkle W, et al: Atrial fibrillation produced by prolonged rapid atrial pacing is associated with heterogeneous changes in atrial sympathetic innervation. Circulation 101:1185, 2000.
111. Yu WC, Chen SA, Lee SH, et al. Tachycardia-induced change of atrial refractory period in humans: Rate dependency and effects of antiarrhythmic drugs. Circulation 97:2331, 1998.
112. Miyata A, Hall SD, Zipes DP, et al: KB-R7943 prevents acute, atrial fibrillation-induced shortening of atrial refractoriness in anesthetized dogs. Circulation 106:1410, 2002.

113. Jayachandran JV, Zipes DP, Weksler J, et al: Role of the Na^+/H^+ exchanger in short-term atrial electrophysiological remodeling. Circulation 101:1861, 1999.
114. Carnes CA, Chung MK, Nakayma T, et al: Ascorbate attenuates atrial pacing-induced peroxynitrite formation and electrical remodeling and decreases the incidence of post-operative atrial fibrillation. Circ Res 89:e32, 2001.
115. Sticherling C, Oral H, Horrocks J, et al: Effects of digoxin on acute, atrial fibrillation–induced changes in atrial refractoriness. Circulation 102:2503, 2000.
116. Olgin JE: Sinus tachycardia and sinus node reentry. *In* Zipes DP, Jalife J (eds): Cardiac Electrophysiology: From Cell to Bedside. 3rd ed. Philadelphia, WB Saunders, 1999, pp 459-468.
117. Lesh MD: Catheter ablation of atrial flutter and tachycardia. *In* Zipes DP, Jalife J (eds): Cardiac Electrophysiology: From Cell to Bedside. 3rd ed. Philadelphia, WB Saunders, 1999, pp 1009-1027.
118. Nikolski VP, Jones SA, Lancaster MK, et al: Cx43 and dual-pathway electrophysiology of the atrioventricular node and atrioventricular nodal reentry. Circ Res 92:469, 2003.
119. Miles WM, Zipes DP: Atrioventricular reentry and variants: Mechanisms, clinical features, and management. *In* Zipes DP, Jalife J (eds): Cardiac Electrophysiology: From Cell to Bedside. 3rd ed. Philadelphia, WB Saunders, 1999, pp 488-504.
120. Yee R, Klein GJ, Prystowsky E: The Wolff-Parkinson-White syndrome and related variants. *In* Zipes DP, Jalife J (eds): Cardiac Electrophysiology: From Cell to Bedside. 3rd ed. Philadelphia, WB Saunders, 1999, pp 845-861.
121. Maury P, Metzger J, Zimmermann M: Intermittent anterograde conduction in an accessory pathway during atrial pacing: What is the mechanism? J Cardiovasc Electrophysiol 9:1394, 1998.
122. Callans DJ, Josephson ME: Ventricular tachycardias in the setting of coronary artery disease. *In* Zipes DP, Jalife J (eds): Cardiac Electrophysiology: From Cell to Bedside. 3rd ed. Philadelphia, WB Saunders, 1999, pp 530-536.
123. Galvin JM, Ruskin JN: Ventricular tachycardia in patients with dilated cardiomyopathy. *In* Zipes DP, Jalife J (eds): Cardiac Electrophysiology: From Cell to Bedside. 3rd ed. Philadelphia, WB Saunders, 1999, pp 537-546.
124. Cabo C, Boyden PA: Electrical remodeling of the epicardial border zone in the canine infarcted heart: A computational analysis. Am J Physiol 284:H372, 2002.
125. Yao J, Hussain W, Patel P, et al: Remodeling of gap junctional channel function in epicardial border zone of healing canine infarcts. Circ Res 92:437, 2003.
126. Pu J, Balser JR, Boyden PA: Lidocaine action on Na^+ currents in ventricular myocytes from the epicardial border zone of infarcted hearts. Circ Res 83:431, 1998.

CHAPTER 28

Genetics of Cardiac Arrhythmias

Silvia G. Priori • Carlo Napolitano • Peter J. Schwartz

Cardiac arrhythmias most often occur in the presence of an abnormal substrate that is responsible for a derangement in impulse initiation and conduction. Ischemic heart disease is the primary cause for the development of ventricular fibrillation, and other structural heart diseases (such as hypertrophic and dilated cardiomyopathies) account for most of the remaining cases (see Chaps. 50 and 59). In most postmortem series of cardiac arrest victims, structural abnormalities were absent in approximately 5 to 8 percent[1] of cases, which, for many years, were referred to as cases of idiopathic ventricular fibrillation (IVF).[2] Now, with the help of molecular biology, the substrate of IVF has been partially defined. In little more than a decade, substantial evidence has been collected to demonstrate that genetically determined abnormalities of proteins that control the electrical activity of the heart can cause cardiac arrest in the structurally intact heart. At least nine genes (Table 28–1) have been associated with inherited arrhythmogenic diseases, and it is expected that several more genes will be identified and linked to sudden death in persons with an apparently normal heart (Fig. 28–1).

In this chapter we review the clinical and genetic characteristics of the three most common inherited arrhythmogenic diseases predisposing to arrhythmias and sudden death, the long QT syndrome, Brugada syndrome, and catecholaminergic polymorphic ventricular tachycardia.

Long QT Syndrome

The long QT syndrome (LQTS) is an inherited arrhythmogenic disease characterized by susceptibility to life-threatening ventricular arrhythmias. Two major forms of LQTS have been identified, one transmitted as an autosomal dominant trait (Romano-Ward syndrome) and the second transmitted as an autosomal recessive disease in which the cardiac phenotype is associated with neurosensory deafness (Jervell and Lange-Nielsen syndrome). The electrocardiographic (ECG) marker of LQTS consists of prolonged repolarization (i.e., prolonged QT interval), abnormal morphology of the T wave (Fig. 28–2), and a characteristic polymorphic ventricular tachycardia called torsades de pointes that is most often induced by activation of the sympathetic nervous system.[3]

Clinical Manifestations

Syncope and fainting are the typical manifestations of LQTS, and their occurrence is often precipitated by physical or emotional stress (e.g., fear, anger, loud noises, sudden awakening).[4] Onset of symptoms is typically in the first two decades of life, including the neonatal period, when LQTS can be misdiagnosed as sudden infant death syndrome,[5] but the first symptoms can appear later in life, especially among females.[4] The severity of the clinical manifestations of LQTS is highly variable, ranging from full-blown disease with a markedly prolonged QT interval and recurrent syncope to subclinical forms with borderline QT interval prolongation and no arrhythmias or syncopal events.[6] Thus, risk stratification becomes a crucial step for clinical management.

Clinical Management of Long QT Syndrome (see Chap. 30)

The link between the onset of cardiac events and increased sympathetic activity suggested the use of beta blockers in the treatment of the disease.[3] The efficacy of beta blockade in patients with LQTS has been reassessed in a large collaborative study that showed a significant residual risk for sudden death.[7] Left cardiac sympathetic denervation is also used for patients unresponsive to, or not tolerating, beta-blocking therapy.[3] Because cardiac arrest survivors represent the subset of LQTS patients at higher risk for sudden death despite treatment, prophylactic implantation of an implantable cardioverter defibrillator (ICD) is recommended for them. Permanent pacemaker implantation is indicated in selected LQTS patients who have atrioventricular block or bradycardia- or pause-dependent tachyarrhythmias. The implantation of a pacemaker is not an alternative to beta blocker treatment.

GENETIC BASIS OF LONG QT SYNDROME

The discovery of the genetic basis of LQTS accelerated in the early 1990s with linkage analysis studies performed in large affected kindreds that allowed the mapping of four LQTS loci on chromosomes 11, 3, and 7 (Online Mendelian Inheritance in Man [OMIM] identification numbers 192500, 152427, and 603830). The gene on chromosome 11 (LQT1), *KCNQ1*, was identified in 1996 using positional cloning, and the candidate gene approach allowed the identification of the genes located on chromosomes 7 (LQT2) and 3 (LQT3) as *KCNH2* and *SCN5A*, respectively. Subsequently, the candidate gene approach allowed identification of mutations in two additional genes both located on chromosome 21 and called *KCNE1* (LQT5; OMIM 176261) and *KCNE2* (LQT6; OMIM 603796). All the genes associated with LQT1 to 3 and LQT5 and 6 encode cardiac ion channel subunits.[8] On the basis of this evidence, LQTS was initially considered a "channelopathy." A locus on chromosome 4 was identified in 1995 as responsible for LQT4 (OMIM 600919). The responsible gene was identified as *ANKB*; at variance with the other genes, however,

TABLE 28–1 Genetic Bases of Inherited Arrhythmogenic Diseases

Disease	Inheritance	Locus	Gene	Protein
LQT3	AD	3p21-p23	*SCN5A*	Nav 1.5
LQT4	AD	4q25-q27	*ANKB*	Ankyrin
LQT2	AD	7q35-q36	*KCNE2*	HERG
LQT1	AD	11p15.5	*KCNQ1*	KvLQT1
LQT5	AD	21q22.1-p22.2	*KCNE1*	MinK
LQT6	AD	21q22.1-p22.2	*KCNE2*	MiRP1
JLN1	AR	11p15.5	*KCNQ1*	KvLQT1
JLN2	AR	21q22.1-q22.2	*KCNE1*	MinK
Brugada	AD	3p21-p23	*SCN5A*	Nav1.5
CPVT	AD	1q42-43	*RyR2*	RyR2
CPVT	AR	1p11-13.3	*CASQ2*	CASQ2

AD = autosomal dominant; AR = autosomal recessive; Brugada = Brugada syndrome; CPVT = catecholaminergic polymorphic ventricular tachycardia; JLN = Jervell and Lange-Nielsen type of long QT syndrome; LQT = long QT syndrome.

ANKB encodes not a cardiac ion channel but a structural protein called ankyrin that is most likely implicated in ion channel anchoring to the cellular membrane.[9]

***KCNQ1* (LQT1) AND *KCNE1* (LQT5).** The cardiac delayed rectifier current (I_K) is a major determinant of phase 3 of the cardiac action potential. It comprises two independent components: one rapid (I_{Kr}) and one slow and catecholamine sensitive (I_{Ks}) (see Chap. 27).

The *KCNQ1* gene and the *KCNE1* gene encode, respectively, the alpha (KVLQT1) and beta (MinK) subunits of the potassium channel conducting the I_{Ks} current. *KCNQ1* mutations are found in the LQT1 variant of the disease, which is also the most prevalent genetic form of LQTS. Approximately half of genotyped patients have a mutation on this gene (see Fig. 28–1).

More than 130 different *KCNQ1* mutations (mainly single amino acid substitutions) have been described (see http://pc4.fsm.it:81/cardmoc). Homozygous or compound heterozygous mutations of *KCNQ1* have been associated with the recessive Jervell and Lange-Nielsen form of LQTS (JLN1). LQT5 is a rather uncommon variant of LQTS caused by mutations in the *KCNE1* gene; it accounts for approximately 2 to 3 percent of all genotyped LQTS patients. Mutations in the *KCNE1* gene cause both Romano-Ward (LQT5) and Jervell and Lange-Nielsen (JLN2) syndromes.

Expression studies of mutated proteins suggest multiple mechanisms of functional failure. Defective proteins can coassemble with wild-type protein and exert a dominant negative effect. Other mutations lead to defective proteins that do not assemble with wild-type peptides, resulting in a loss of function that reduces the I_{Ks} current by 50 percent (haploinsufficiency). Finally, defective peptides may not even reach the membrane of the cardiac cell because the mutations interfere with intracellular protein trafficking.[8,10]

***KCNH2* (LQT2) AND *KCNE2* (LQT6).** The *KCNH2* and *KCNE2* genes encode, respectively, the alpha (HERG) and beta (MIRP) subunits of the potassium channel conducting the I_{Kr} current (see Fig. 28–1). Approximately 100 *KCNH2* mutations have been reported (http://pc4.fsm.it:81/cardmoc), suggesting that this is the second most common variant of LQTS, accounting for 35 to 40 percent of mutations in LQTS genotyped patients. Functional expression studies have demonstrated that mutations in the *KCNH2* gene cause a reduction of the I_{Kr} current. *KCNH2* mutants have reduced function compared with the wild-type peptides; therefore, I_{Kr} channels that incorporate mutated subunits carry a reduced I_{Kr} repolarizing current. Defective proteins can have a dominant negative effect on the wild-type subunits or may not interfere with the function of the normal subunits, thus causing haploinsufficiency. Trafficking abnormalities have also been reported as a consequence of *KCNH2* mutations.[11]

Mutations in the *KCNE2* gene are found in the LQT6 variant of LQTS. This gene encodes MiRP1 (MinK-related peptide 1), a small peptide that coassembles with the HERG protein to form the I_{Kr} channel. In the literature worldwide there are only a few examples of *KCNE2* mutations associated with LQTS (http://pc4.fsm.it:81/cardmoc). Accordingly, LQT6 seems the rarest variant of the disease.

***SCN5A* (LQT3).** The *SCN5A* gene encodes the protein of the cardiac sodium channel. This gene was cloned in 1992 and mapped to chromosome 3p21 in 1995. The Na^+ channel protein is a relatively large molecule that folds onto itself to surround the channel pore (see Fig. 28–1).

The first *SCN5A* mutations were clustered in the regions that regulate the inactivation of the channel (delKPQ, R1623Q, N1325S). In vitro expression studies showed that these mutations cause an increased late inward sodium current (I_{Na}). It was concluded that Na^+ channel mutations originate the LQTS phenotype by inducing a gain of function leading to an increase in the Na^+ inward current that prolongs the action potential duration.

Approximately 25 mutations have been reported so far in the literature (http://pc4.fsm.it:81/cardmoc), and the prevalence of LQT3 among LQTS patients is estimated to be 10 to 15 percent.

***ANKB* (LQT4).** Only one family linked to this locus (4q25-q27) has been reported so far. Interestingly, the phenotype of the LQT4 patients differs from the typical LQTS phenotype. In addition to QT interval prolonga-

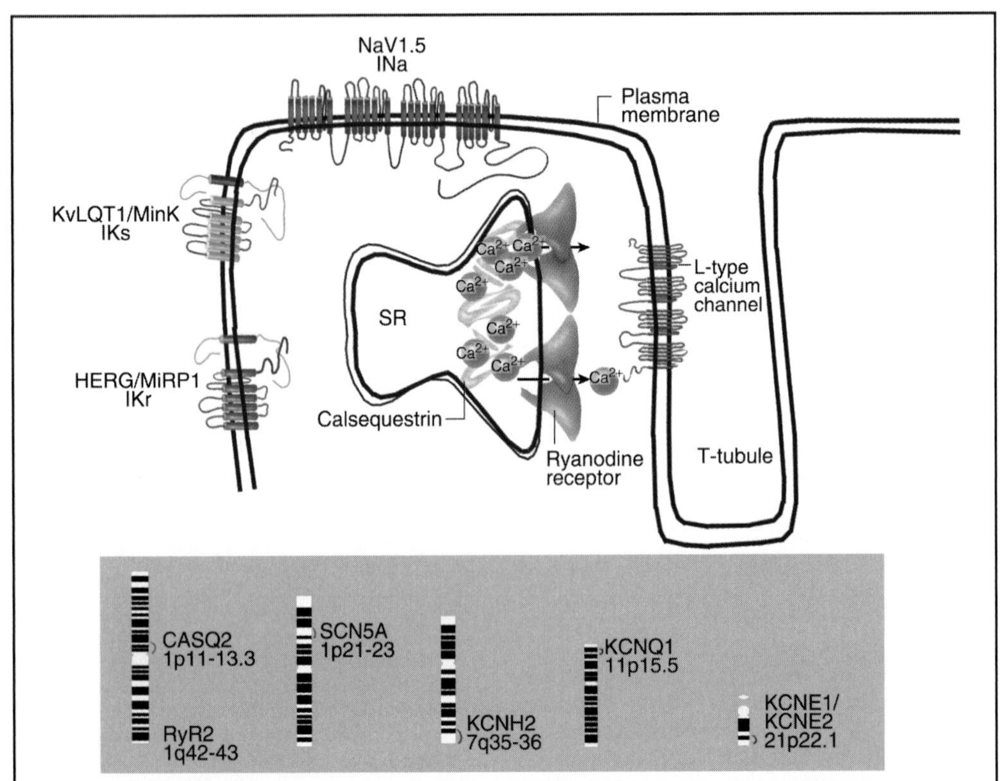

FIGURE 28–1 Genes and proteins in inherited arrhythmogenic diseases: the chromosomal locations of the genes known to cause cardiac inherited disorders. The proteins encoded by each gene are schematically drawn in the figure.

tion, most of the affected individuals present with severe sinus bradycardia, paroxysmal atrial fibrillation (detected in more than 50 percent of the patients), and biphasic T waves. Experimental data for ankyrin knockout mice suggested that this protein, located in the LQT4 critical region, was a plausible candidate gene for LQT4. Subsequently, a missense mutation in the *ANKB* gene was identified in the family linked to the critical region on chromosome 4, confirming that the gene for LQT4 is the *Ankyrin* gene.[9]

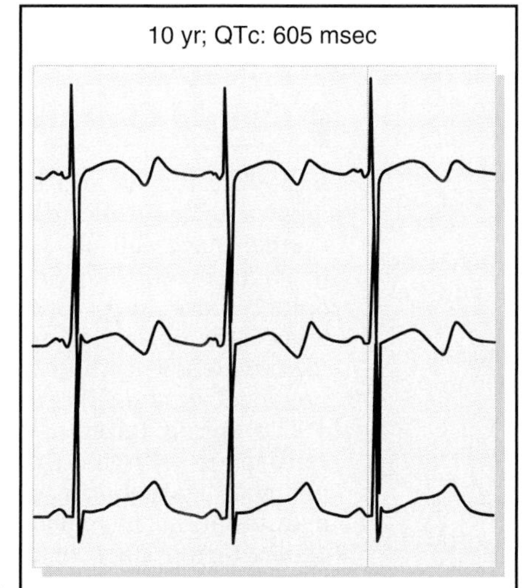

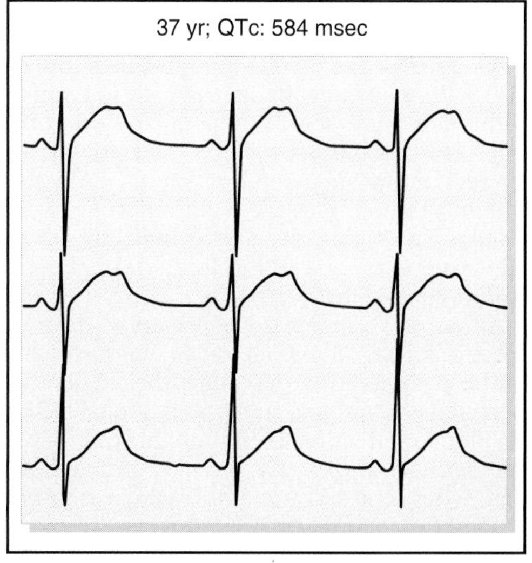

FIGURE 28–2 Electrocardiograms in long QT syndrome (LQTS). Typical electrocardiograms of two LQTS patients, 10 **(A)** and 37 **(B)** years old, showing QT interval prolongation and T wave morphological abnormalities. The genetic defect is LQTS *KCNH2* mutation (HERG) A561V.

GENOTYPE-PHENOTYPE CORRELATION STUDIES. The distinguishing features of the three most common genetic variants of LQTS, namely LQT1, LQT2, and LQT3, have been outlined.[12] Analysis of the ECG patterns revealed a gene-specific morphology of the ST-T wave complex,[13] which may guide genotyping.

Schwartz and coworkers[4] have provided evidence that the triggers for cardiac events differ among the genetic variants of LQTS. This difference is particularly evident for lethal events. LQT1 patients have an increased risk during physical or emotional stress. They experience 90 percent of lethal events in this setting, whereas LQT3 patients experience most of their events (64 percent) at rest or while asleep and only 4 percent do so during exercise. LQT2 patients are at higher risk for lethal events during arousal or emotional states (49 percent) but are also at risk during sleep and at rest (29 percent) and not at all at risk during exercise. There are also triggers that appear highly specific. Indeed, 99 percent of cardiac events that occur while swimming involve LQT1 patients and 80 percent of events related to acoustic stimuli involve LQT2 patients.[4,12]

Natural History and Risk Stratification

The increased availability of data collected for genotyped LQTS patients has allowed the development of risk stratification models based on the genetic substrate. Priori and colleagues have reported information on 647 LQTS patients from 193 genotyped families.[14]

This study showed that a lower cumulative event-free survival was observed among LQT2 versus LQT1 patients, and a similar trend was present among LQT3 versus LQT1 patients. Gender had a different effect across different genotypes. It had no influence in LQT1 patients, whereas a higher risk was present for LQT2 females and LQT3 males. It was also observed that the percentage of genetically affected patients with a normal QT interval ("silent mutation carriers") differed strikingly among genotypes, being much greater ($P < 0.001$) in LQT1 (36 percent) than in LQT2 (19 percent) and especially than in LQT3 (10 percent) patients. Quartiles of QTc distribution were determined within each genetic subgroup and permitted recognition that among LQT1 and LQT2 patients, those with a QTc in the upper quartile had respectively a 5.3- and 8.4-fold risk increase compared with those in the first quartile. In contrast, QTc duration did not differentiate risk among LQT3 patients.

These data were incorporated in a risk quantification model by comparing the event-free survival in 12 categories including, for each genetic locus, the four combinations of gender and QTc below or above 500 milliseconds. This analysis provided the identification of a differential risk within these 12 categories (Fig. 28–3).

In this study, it was assumed that patients with mutations on the same gene share a common risk profile. Risk stratification, however, may be further refined when the location of a mutation is also taken into consideration. In 1997 Donger and colleagues observed in a small subset of patients that mutations located in the carboxyl terminus of the *KCNQ1* gene were associated with a mild clinical phenotype.[14a] In 2002 Moss and associates[15] studied 201 LQT2 patients and showed that individuals with mutations in the pore region were at considerably greater risk for cardiac events than patients with nonpore mutations even though the difference in the incidence of aborted cardiac arrest and sudden death was not statistically significant.

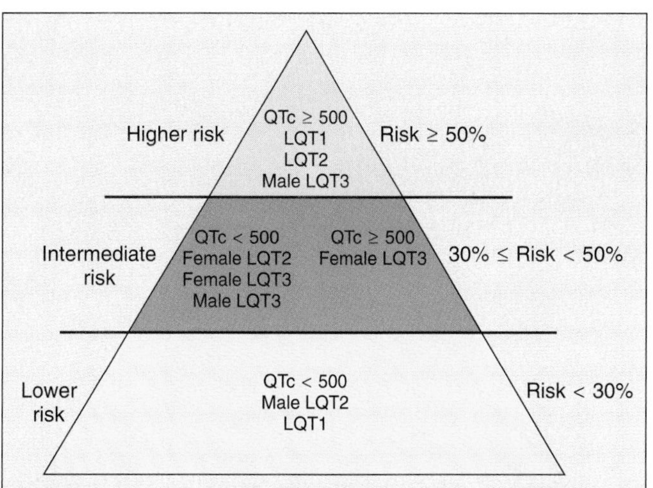

FIGURE 28–3 Risk stratification in the long QT (LQT) syndrome. Shown here is the risk stratification scheme for patients with long QT syndrome according to genotype and gender. The risk groups have been defined on the basis of the probability of experiencing a first cardiac event (syncope, cardiac arrest, or sudden death) by age 40 years. A 50 percent or higher probability of events constitutes the higher risk subgroup, a risk between 30 and 50 percent the intermediate risk group, and a risk less than 30 percent the lower risk group. (Modified from Priori SG, Schwartz PJ, Napolitano C, et al: Risk stratification in the long-QT syndrome. N Engl J Med 348:1866, 2003.)

GENE-SPECIFIC THERAPY. Data collected from small cohorts of LQT3 patients[7,16] have raised concern that beta blockers may not be effective in this subset of patients with LQTS. However, available data are not sufficiently robust to allow definitive conclusions on the role of beta blockers in LQT3. Specifically, it remains unclear whether beta blockers are ineffective and therefore should not be used in LQT3 or whether they at least provide a partial reduction of cardiac events. The main obstacle in reaching conclusive data on this issue is related to the limited number of LQT3 families identified worldwide.

Attempts to devise alternative therapeutic strategies specific for LQT3 patients have emerged. On the basis of the evidence that LQT3 is caused by an increased late I_{Na}, an experimental preparation mimicking LQT3 and LQT2 was developed.[17] In this LQT3 model, the Na^+ channel blocker mexiletine significantly reduced the action potential duration, whereas it did not modify the action potential duration in the LQT2 model. In 1995 the feasibility of this pharmacological intervention was tested in a few genotyped patients, and indeed sodium channel blockade with mexiletine shortened the QT interval among LQT3 patients but not among LQT2 patients.[16] Other authors later confirmed that QT was also shortened in response to another sodium channel blocker, flecainide. However, concerns exist about the use of flecainide in LQT3 patients as Priori and colleagues demonstrated that intravenous flecainide may induce ST segment elevation in the right precordial leads (Brugada-like electrocardiogram).[18]

A gene-specific therapy for LQT2 patients was proposed in 1996 by Compton and associates,[18a] who suggested that one could compensate for the reduced I_{Kr} current by increasing the potassium plasma concentration with exogenous administration of potassium salts and potassium-sparing diuretics.

It is important to remember that, despite the appeal of gene-specific therapy, its place is still in research studies rather than in clinical practice as there is no evidence that it can affect mortality or reduce the number of cardiac events.

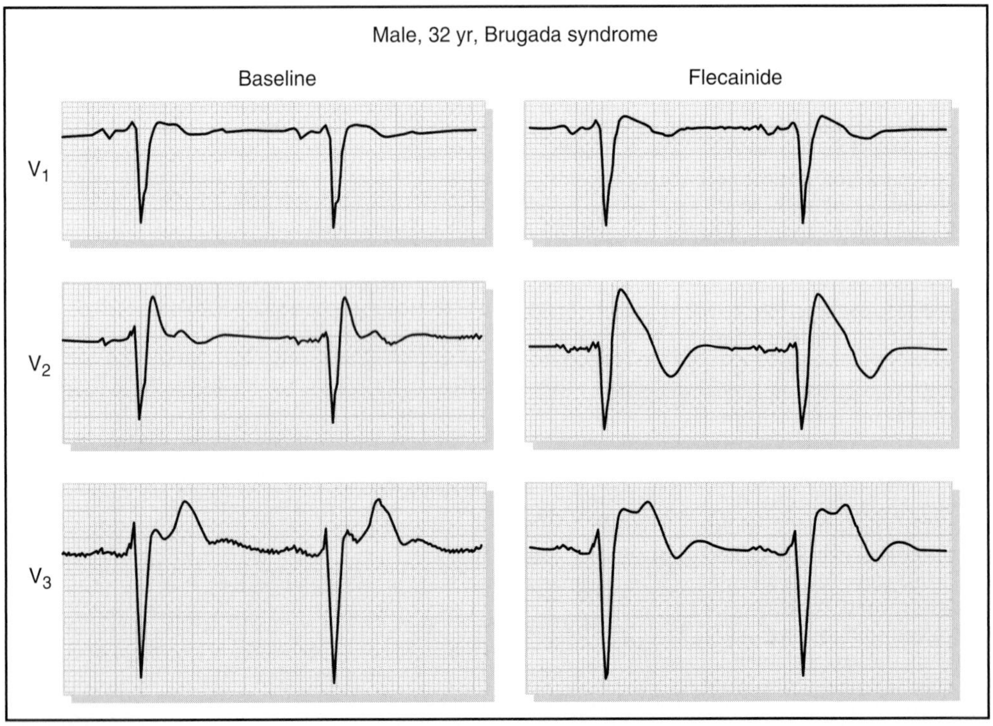

Brugada Syndrome

Clinical Characteristics

In 1992, Brugada and Brugada described a novel autosomal dominant inherited disease occurring in the structurally normal heart and characterized by ST segment elevation in the right precordial leads (V_1 to V_3) (Fig. 28–4), right bundle branch block, and susceptibility to ventricular tachyarrhythmias. This disease is now referred to as Brugada syndrome. Its prevalence is not known, but the disease seems to be more prevalent in countries in the Far East (see Chap. 32).

The age at onset of clinical manifestations (syncope or cardiac arrest) is the third to fourth decade of life, although malignant forms with earlier onset and even with neonatal manifestations have been reported.[19] Cardiac events typically occur during sleep or at rest.[20] Even though the disease is inherited as an autosomal dominant trait, there is a striking male-to-female ratio of 8:1 in clinical manifestations.

Diagnosis

The diagnosis of Brugada syndrome is complicated by the intermittent nature of the ECG pattern. Concealed forms may be unmasked only after performing provocative drug testing with selected Class IC drugs such as ajmaline, flecainide or procainamide.[21] It has been suggested that the autonomic nervous system can modify the ECG phenotype because intravenous administration of isoproterenol attenuates whereas acetylcholine accentuates the ECG abnormalities in affected patients.

Prognostic Indicators and Management

Initial data from Brugada and colleagues published in 1992 and data subsequently published in 1998 provided an alarming estimate of the lethality of the disease when they suggested that the risk of sudden death within 3 years from the time of the clinical diagnosis was close to 30 percent in both asymptomatic and symptomatic patients. Because no drug therapy is effective in preventing arrhythmic events in Brugada syndrome, the only prophylactic treatment to prevent cardiac arrest is the ICD (see Chap. 31). It is therefore reassuring to observe that with the collection of larger groups of patients, the estimated lethality of the disease is much lower than initially feared.[22] In a study by Priori and coworkers,[22] assessment of the natural history of Brugada syndrome showed that 28 percent of patients had a cardiac arrest from birth to age 60. Later, they proposed a novel risk stratification scheme (Fig. 28–5) based on retrospective analysis of the event-free survival in 200 individuals,[23] the

Male, 32 yr, Brugada syndrome

Baseline | Flecainide

V_1 V_2 V_3

FIGURE 28–4 Electrocardiograms in Brugada syndrome. V_1 to V_3 leads show a mild ST segment elevation and an incomplete right bundle branch block, possibly indicating Brugada syndrome. The typical and conclusively diagnostic pattern is unmasked in the same patient by the intravenous administration of flecainide (2 mg/kg). The genetic defect is Brugada *SCN5A* mutation R526H.

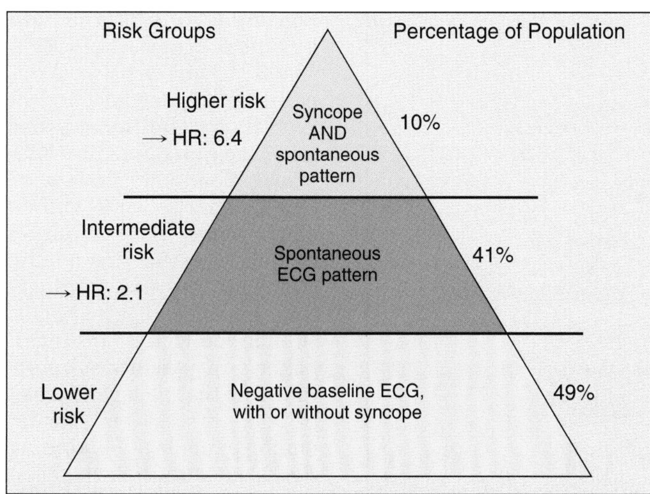

FIGURE 28–5 Risk stratification in Brugada syndrome using the history of syncope and the presence of a spontaneously diagnostic electrocardiographic pattern as the clinical variables for quantification of risk. Hazard ratios are calculated using the lower risk group as a reference. ECG = electrocardiogram; HR = hazard ratio. (From Priori SG, Napolitano C, Gasparini M, et al: Clinical and genetic heterogeneity of right bundle branch block and ST-segment elevation syndrome: A prospective evaluation of 52 families. Circulation 2000; 102:2509, 2000.).

severity of the ECG signs (spontaneously present ST elevation versus ST elevation unmasked only by drug testing), and the occurrence of syncopal events. The latest data from Brugada and colleagues included a larger proportion of asymptomatic individuals and also showed that individuals with the spontaneous ECG pattern are at higher risk for cardiac events.[24]

One area of persistent disagreement in the risk stratification for patients with Brugada syndrome concerns the role of programmed electrical stimulation (PES) to identify individuals at higher risk for cardiac arrest. Brugada and associates[25] showed that PES is highly sensitive in predicting the risk of major cardiac events, whereas Priori,[23] Gasparini,[26] and Eckardt[27] and their coworkers failed to show that it is a good indicator of risk for cardiac events. As a consequence, the use of PES in Brugada syndrome has received a Class IIb recommendation by the Task Force on Sudden Cardiac Death of the European Society of Cardiology.[1]

GENETIC BASIS OF BRUGADA SYNDROME

The understanding of the molecular basis of Brugada syndrome is still limited; so far, only one gene has been identified and it accounts for no more than 20 percent of clinical cases.[10]

In 1998, the gene responsible for some of the cases of Brugada syndrome was identified as the cardiac sodium channel gene (*SCN5A*), the same gene responsible for the LQT3 variant of LQTS.[28] Mutations identified in Brugada syndrome are either missense mutations, in-frame deletions, or mutations (insertions or deletions) leading to frameshifts and early truncation of the protein of the cardiac sodium channel. In vitro functional characterization of *SCN5A* mutations showed that several distinct electrophysiological mechanisms can lead to the clinical phenotype of Brugada syndrome but the overall effect of all the mutations identified leads to a "reduction " in the sodium current (loss of function). This finding is at variance with the effect of *SCN5A* mutations identified in LQT3, in which mutations lead to an excess of sodium inward current (gain of function). Interestingly, overlapping phenotypes of LQT3 and Brugada syndrome have been reported by Bezzina and colleagues,[29] who described the simultaneous presence of QT prolongation and ST segment elevation in a family in which an *SCN5A* mutation (InsD1795) was present. Grant and coworkers[29a] also reported a family with ECG features of both diseases.

Catecholaminergic Polymorphic Ventricular Tachycardia

Catecholaminergic polymorphic ventricular tachycardia (CPVT)[30] was initially described in 1978. It was reported that the disease is characterized by ventricular tachycardia (VT), syncope, and sudden death occurring in familial or in sporadic cases in the absence of structural abnormalities of the heart and in the absence of any ECG abnormality. Three distinguishing features of CPVT were highlighted: (1) a direct relationship between adrenergic activation (physical or emotional stress) and the onset of arrhythmias, (2) a typical pattern of bidirectional VT with an unremarkable resting electrocardiogram (Fig. 28–6), and (3) a structurally normal heart. CPVT (OMIM 604772) has now been recognized as a genetically determined arrhythmogenic disease and its pathophysiological mechanisms are being progressively unveiled (see Chap. 32).

Clinical Features

ELECTROCARDIOGRAPHIC CHARACTERISTICS. The resting electrocardiogram of patients with CPVT is unremarkable with the exception of a sinus bradycardia reported in some patients; atrioventricular conduction is within normal limits and no significant abnormalities are identified by signal-averaging electrocardiography.

Physical activity and acute emotions are the specific triggers for arrhythmias in CPVT patients. The complexity of arrhythmias progressively increases with increase in workload, from isolated premature beats to bigeminy and to runs of nonsustained VT. If the patients continue to exercise, the duration of VT runs progressively increases and the arrhythmia can become sustained. A 180-degree alternating QRS axis on a beat-to-beat basis, the so-called bidirectional VT, is often the distinguishing presentation of CPVT-related arrhythmias. However, later observations have pointed to the fact that CPVT patients can also show irregular polymorphic VT without a "stable" QRS vector alternans. At variance with LQTS, exercise-induced runs of nonsustained supraventricular tachycardia are a relatively common finding among CPVT patients. Triggered activity has been suggested as the most likely arrhythmogenic mechanism in CPVT.

CARDIAC EVENTS AND CLINICAL MANIFESTATIONS. Syncope, triggered by exercise or acute emotion, is often the first manifestation of CPVT even though sudden cardiac death can occur in previously asymptomatic subjects. In approximately 30 percent of cases, the family history reveals one or multiple premature sudden deaths that usually occurred during childhood, even if later onset (after age 20 years) events have been reported. Often, unheralded sudden death occurring in individuals without cardiac structural abnormalities can lead to the postmortem diagnosis of IVF.

GENETIC BASIS

AUTOSOMAL DOMINANT CPVT. Evidence supporting a familial distribution of CPVT has been provided since the initial description of the disease. The distribution of the phenotype in the first reported familial cases was consistent with an autosomal dominant pattern of inheritance.[31] The availability of two large kindreds allowed Swan and coworkers to perform genome-wide linkage analysis and to map the disease locus to chromosome 1q42-43 with a significant logarithm of odds (LOD) score of 4.74.[32]

On the basis of these findings and the evidence that the gene encoding the human cardiac ryanodine receptor (*RyR2*) maps to the CPVT critical region, Priori and colleague performed molecular screening of this gene in families with stress-induced bidirectional VT and successfully identified *RyR2* mutations in four probands, demonstrating that *RyR2* is

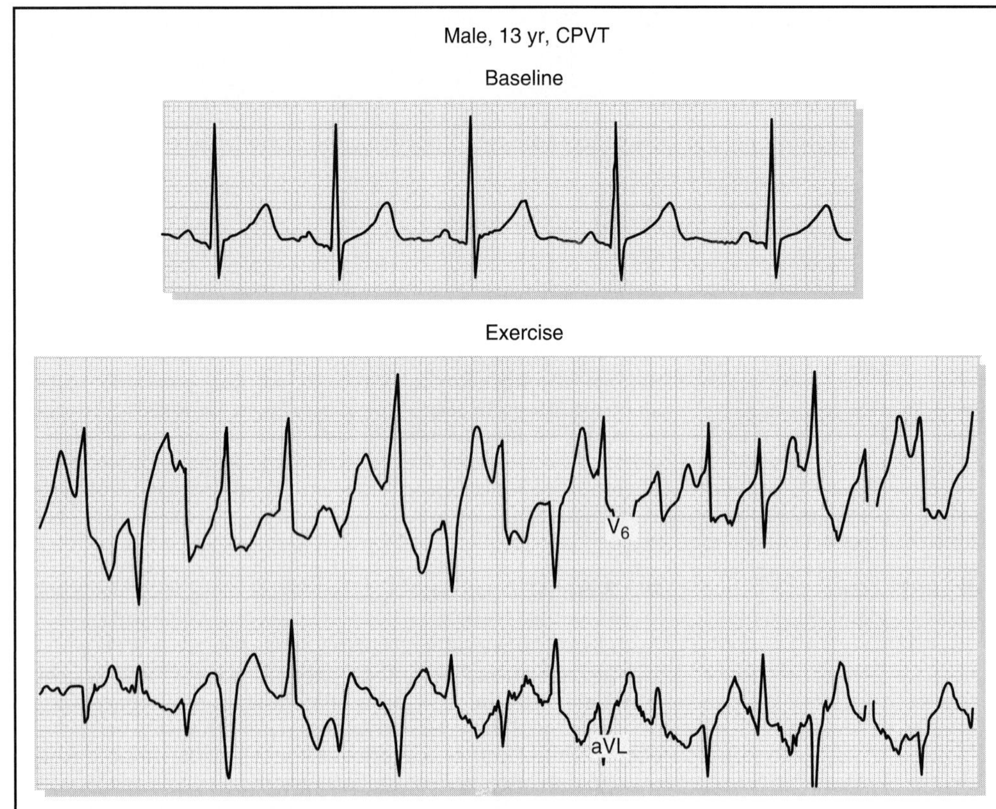

FIGURE 28–6 Electrocardiograms in catecholaminergic polymorphic ventricular tachycardia (CPVT). The findings in a young teenager with CPVT show an unremarkable electrocardiogram at rest **(upper panel)** and the onset of polymorphic or bidirectional ventricular tachycardia during an exercise stress test **(lower panel).** The genetic defect is CPVT *RyR2* mutation 52246L.

the gene for autosomal dominant CPVT.[33] The involvement of the cardiac ryanodine receptor in the genesis of CPVT was shortly afterward confirmed by other groups and by functional characterization of the defective proteins.[34]

RyR2 plays a major role in the regulation of intracellular calcium fluxes and excitation-contraction coupling. This large tetrameric protein is localized across the membrane of the sarcoplasmic reticulum (SR), and it releases Ca^{2+} ions from the SR in response to Ca^{2+} entry through the L-type channels during phase 2 of the action potential. The identification of *RyR2* mutations in CPVT patients constitutes the first demonstration of the involvement of an intracellular ion channel in an inherited arrhythmia and points to the pivotal role of intracellular Ca^{2+} handling in arrhythmogenesis.[35]

An increasing number of *RyR2* mutations is being reported (http://pc4.fsm.it:81/cardmoc), and abnormal variants of this gene have also been linked to an atypical or "concealed" form of arrhythmogenic right ventricular dysplasia (ARVD2) characterized by exercise-induced bidirectional VT.[36]

AUTOSOMAL RECESSIVE CPVT. Lahat and associates in 2001 provided the first evidence for a variant of CPVT inherited as an autosomal dominant trait. They mapped the disease in seven consanguineous Bedouin families in a 16-cM interval on chromosome 1p23-21 with a LOD score of 8.24. Subsequently, they identified *CASQ2* as the gene for this variant of CPVT.[37,38] *CASQ2* encodes calsequestrin, a protein highly expressed in the heart. It serves as a major Ca^{2+} binding protein localized in the terminal cisternae of the SR of cardiac muscle cells, and it binds Ca^{2+} with high capacity and moderate affinity. Thus, calsequestrin is a Ca^{2+} storage protein in the lumen of the SR. CPVT patients of different ethnic backgrounds have been successfully genotyped as carriers of *CASQ2* mutations, suggesting that patients with CPVT should be screened for this gene when an autosomal recessive pattern of inheritance is suspected.

Clinical Management

GENOTYPE-PHENOTYPE CORRELATION IN *RYR2*-CPVT. *RyR2* mutations are found in approximately 50 percent of patients who have a clinical diagnosis of CPVT. Thus, the disease is genetically heterogeneous, and at present no additional genes have been linked to the autosomal dominant variant of CPVT. This lack of knowledge limits the definition of gene-specific therapeutic strategies and risk stratification schemes. The evidence so far collected in small cohorts of patients supports the view that the age of onset of the disease is greater among patients not harboring *RyR2* genetic defects than among RyR2 mutation carriers (20 ± 12 versus 8 ± 2 years) and that among carriers of *RyR2* mutations, males seem to be at higher risk (relative risk = 4.2) of cardiac events at a young age.[39] Furthermore, it has been shown that *RyR2* mutations are not always associated with typical bidirectional VT, because polymorphic VT is present in approximately 40 percent of genotyped probands.[39] The incidence of cardiac events from birth is not different when patients with and without *RyR2* mutations are compared. Both groups present with the majority of cardiac events during childhood, and by age 20, more than 60 percent of the patients experience a first cardiac event (syncope or cardiac arrest).

GENOTYPE-PHENOTYPE CORRELATION IN *CASQ2*-CPVT. Because of the limited number of *CASQ2* genotyped patients, it is not yet possible to compare *CASQ2*- and *RyR2*-related CPVT. Lahat and colleagues reported a mild QT interval prolongation in their initial paper,[37] but it was not confirmed in their subsequent report.

Risk Stratification and Therapy in Catecholaminergic Polymorphic Ventricular Tachycardia

Antiadrenergic treatment with beta blockers is the cornerstone of therapy for CPVT patients.[39] Despite the limited experience available, amiodarone and Class I antiarrhythmic agents appear ineffective (see Chap. 30).

PES is not useful for diagnosis and risk stratification because CPVT patients usually do not have inducible arrhythmias.[39] On the other hand, the highly reproducible pattern of arrhythmia during exercise among CPVT patients allows diagnosis, dose titration, and monitoring. Overall, chronic treatment with full-dose beta-blocking agents can prevent recurrences of syncope in some patients.[39] Nonetheless, Priori and colleagues reported that in approximately 40 percent of their cases, the control of arrhythmias was unsatisfactory despite optimization of therapy with repeated exercise stress testing.[39] They concluded that the use of an ICD may be indicated when exercise stress testing and repeated Holter monitoring suggest that only incomplete protection from arrhythmias is obtained with beta blockers.

REFERENCES

Long QT Syndrome

1. Priori SG, Aliot E, Blomstrom-Lundqvist C, et al: Task Force on Sudden Cardiac Death of the European Society of Cardiology. Eur Heart J 22:1374, 2001.
2. Survivors of out-of-hospital cardiac arrest with apparently normal heart. Need for definition and standardized clinical evaluation. Consensus Statement of the Joint Steering Committees of the Unexplained Cardiac Arrest Registry of Europe and of the Idiopathic Ventricular Fibrillation Registry of the United States. Circulation 95:265, 1997.
3. Schwartz PJ, Priori SG, Napolitano C: The long QT syndrome. *In* Zipes DP, Jalife J (eds): Cardiac Electrophysiology: From Cell to Bedside. Philadelphia, WB Saunders, 2000, pp 597-615.
4. Schwartz PJ, Priori SG, Spazzolini C, et al: Genotype-phenotype correlation in the long-QT syndrome: Gene-specific triggers for life-threatening arrhythmias. Circulation 103:89, 2001.
5. Schwartz PJ, Priori SG, Dumaine R, et al: A molecular link between the sudden infant death syndrome and the long-QT syndrome. N Engl J Med 343:262, 2000.
6. Priori SG, Napolitano C, Schwartz PJ: Low penetrance in the long-QT syndrome: Clinical impact. Circulation 99:529, 1999.
7. Moss AJ, Zareba W, Hall WJ, et al: Effectiveness and limitations of beta-blocker therapy in congenital long-QT syndrome. Circulation 101:616, 2000.
8. Keating MT, Sanguinetti MC: Molecular and cellular mechanisms of cardiac arrhythmias. Cell 104:569, 2001.
9. Mohler PJ, Schott JJ, Gramolini AO, et al: Ankyrin-B mutation causes type 4 long-QT cardiac arrhythmia and sudden cardiac death. Nature 421:634, 2003.
10. Priori SG, Rivolta I, Napolitano C: Genetics of long QT, Brugada and other channellopathies. *In* Zipes DP, Jalife J (eds): Cardiac Electrophysiology. 4th ed. Philadelphia, Elsevier (in press).
11. Zhou Z, Gong Q, Epstein ML, January CT: HERG channel dysfunction in human long QT syndrome. Intracellular transport and functional defects. J Biol Chem 273:21061, 1998.
12. Schwartz PJ, Priori SG: Long QT syndrome—Phenotype genotype considerations. *In* Zipes DP, Jalife J (eds): Cardiac Electrophysiology. 4th ed. Philadelphia, Elsevier (in press).
13. Zhang L, Timothy KW, Vincent GM, et al: Spectrum of ST-T-wave patterns and repolarization parameters in congenital long-QT syndrome: ECG findings identify genotypes. Circulation 102:2849, 2000.
14. Priori SG, Schwartz PJ, Napolitano C, et al: Risk stratification in the long-QT syndrome. N Engl J Med 348:1866, 2003.

14a. Donger C, Denjoy I, Berthet M, et al: KVLQT1 C-terminal missense mutation causes a forme fruste long-QT syndrome. Circulation 96:2778, 1997.

15. Moss AJ, Zareba W, Kaufman ES, et al: Increased risk of arrhythmic events in long-QT syndrome with mutations in the pore region of the human ether-a-go-go-related gene potassium channel. Circulation 105:794, 2002.
16. Schwartz PJ, Priori SG, Locati EH, et al: Long QT syndrome patients with mutations of the *SCN5A* and *HERG* genes have differential responses to Na^+ channel blockade and to increases in heart rate. Implications for gene-specific therapy. Circulation 92:3381, 1995.
17. Priori SG, Napolitano C, Cantu F, et al: Differential response to Na^+ channel blockade, beta-adrenergic stimulation, and rapid pacing in a cellular model mimicking the SCN5A and HERG defects present in the long-QT syndrome. Circ Res 78:1009, 1996.
18. Priori SG, Napolitano C, Schwartz PJ, et al: The elusive link between LQT3 and Brugada syndrome: The role of flecainide challenge. Circulation 102:945, 2000.

18a. Compton SJ, Lux RL, Ramsey MR, et al: Genetically defined therapy of inherited long QT syndrome. Correction of abnormal repolarization by potassium. Circulation 94:1018, 1996.

Brugada Syndrome

19. Priori SG, Napolitano C, Giordano U, et al: Brugada syndrome and sudden cardiac death in children. Lancet 355:808, 2000.
20. Brugada J, Brugada P, Brugada R: The syndrome of right bundle branch block ST segment elevation in V1 to V3 and sudden death—The Brugada syndrome. Europace 1:156, 1999.
21. Brugada R, Brugada J, Antzelevitch C, et al: Sodium channel blockers identify risk for sudden death in patients with ST-segment elevation and right bundle branch block but structurally normal hearts. Circulation 101:510, 2000.
22. Priori SG, Napolitano C, Gasparini M, et al: Clinical and genetic heterogeneity of right bundle branch block and ST-segment elevation syndrome: A prospective evaluation of 52 families. Circulation 102:2509, 2000.
23. Priori SG, Napolitano C, Gasparini M, et al: Natural history of Brugada syndrome. Insights for risk stratification and management. Circulation 105:1342, 2002.
24. Brugada J, Brugada R, Antzelevitch C, et al: Long-term follow-up of individuals with the electrocardiographic pattern of right bundle-branch block and ST-segment elevation in precordial leads V1 to V3. Circulation 105:73, 2002.
25. Brugada P, Geelen P, Brugada R, et al: Prognostic value of electrophysiologic investigations in Brugada syndrome. J Cardiovasc Electrophysiol 12:1004, 2001.
26. Gasparini M, Priori SG, Mantica M, et al: Programmed electrical stimulation in Brugada syndrome: How reproducible are the results? J Cardiovasc Electrophysiol 13:880, 2002.
27. Eckardt L, Kirchhof P, Schulze-Bahr E, et al: Electrophysiologic investigation in Brugada syndrome; yield of programmed ventricular stimulation at two ventricular sites with up to three premature beats. Eur Heart J 23:1394, 2002.
28. Chen Q, Kirsch GE, Zhang D, et al: Genetic basis and molecular mechanism for idiopathic ventricular fibrillation. Nature 392:293, 1998.
29. Bezzina C, Veldkamp MW, van Den Berg MP, et al: A single Na(+) channel mutation causing both long-QT and Brugada syndromes. Circ Res 85:1206, 1999.

29a. Grant AO, Carboni MP, Nipliovera V, et al: Long QT syndrome, Brugada syndrome, and conduction system disease are linked to a single sodium channel mutation. J Clin Invest 110:1201, 2002.

Catecholaminergic Polymorphic Ventricular Tachycardia

30. Napolitano C, Priori SG: Catecholaminergic polymorphic ventricular tachycardia. *In* Zipes DP, Jalife J (eds); Cardiac Electrophysiology. 4th ed. Philadelphia, Elsevier (in press).
31. Fisher JD, Krikler D, Hallidie-Smith KA: Familial polymorphic ventricular arrhythmias: A quarter century of successful medical treatment based on serial exercise-pharmacologic testing. J Am Coll Cardiol 34:2015, 1999.
32. Swan H, Piippo K, Viitasalo M, et al: Arrhythmic disorder mapped to chromosome 1q42-q43 causes malignant polymorphic ventricular tachycardia in structurally normal hearts. J Am Coll Cardiol 34:2035, 1999.
33. Priori SG, Napolitano C, Tiso N, et al: Mutations in the cardiac ryanodine receptor gene (*hRyR2*) underlie catecholaminergic polymorphic ventricular tachycardia. Circulation 103:196, 2001.
34. Wehrens XH, Lehnart SE, Huang F, et al: FKBP12.6 deficiency and defective calcium release channel (ryanodine receptor) function linked to exercise-induced sudden cardiac death. Cell 113:829, 2003.
35. Marks AR, Priori S, Memmi M, et al: Involvement of the cardiac ryanodine receptor/calcium release channel in catecholaminergic polymorphic ventricular tachycardia. J Cell Physiol 190:1, 2002.
36. Tiso N, Stephan D, Nava A: Identification on mutations in the cardiac ryanodine receptor gene in families affected with arrhythmogenic right ventricular cardiomyopathy type 2 (ARVD2). Hum Mol Genet 10:189, 2001.
37. Lahat H, Pras E, Olender T, et al: A missense mutation in a highly conserved region of CASQ2 is associated with autosomal recessive catecholamine-induced polymorphic ventricular tachycardia in Bedouin families from Israel. Am J Hum Genet 69:1378, 2001.
38. Lahat H, Eldar M, Levy-Nissenbaum E, et al: Autosomal recessive catecholamine- or exercise-induced polymorphic ventricular tachycardia. Circulation 103:2822, 2001.
39. Priori SG, Napolitano C, Memmi M, et al: Clinical and molecular characterization of patients with catecholaminergic polymorphic ventricular tachycardia. Circulation 106:69, 2002.

CHAPTER 29

Diagnosis of Cardiac Arrhythmias

John M. Miller • Douglas P. Zipes

Diagnosis of Cardiac Arrhythmias

In the management of clinical arrhythmias, the physician must evaluate and treat the whole patient, not just the rhythm disturbance.[1] Some arrhythmias are hazardous to the patient regardless of the clinical setting (e.g., ventricular fibrillation, VF), whereas others are hazardous because of the clinical setting (e.g., rapidly conducted atrial fibrillation in a patient with severe coronary artery stenoses). Some arrhythmias, such as premature ventricular complexes (PVCs), may be highly symptomatic yet are not associated with any adverse outcome, whereas some patients with atrial fibrillation have no symptoms at all but may still be at significant risk of stroke. Evaluation of the patient begins with a careful history and physical examination and should usually progress from the simplest to the most complex test, from the least invasive and safest to the most invasive and risky, and from the least expensive out-of-hospital evaluations to those that require hospitalization and sophisticated, costly procedures. Occasionally, depending on the clinical circumstances, the physician may wish to proceed directly to a high-risk, expensive procedure, such as an electrophysiological study (EPS), before obtaining a 24-hour electrocardiographic (ECG) recording.

History

Patients with cardiac rhythm disturbances can present with a variety of complaints, but commonly symptoms such as palpitations, syncope, presyncope, or congestive heart failure cause them to seek a physician's help. Their awareness of palpitations and of a regular or irregular cardiac rhythm varies greatly.[2] Some patients perceive slight variations in their heart rhythm with uncommon accuracy, whereas others are oblivious even to sustained episodes of ventricular tachycardia (VT); still others complain of palpitations when they actually have regular sinus rhythm.

In assessing a patient with known or suspected arrhythmia, several key pieces of information should be obtained that can help determine a diagnosis or guide further diagnostic testing. The *mode of onset* of an episode may give clues about the type of arrhythmia or preferred treatment option. For example, palpitations that occur in the setting of exercise, fright, or anger are often caused by catecholamine-sensitive automatic or triggered tachycardias that may respond to adrenergic blocking agents; palpitations that occur at rest or that awaken the patient may be due to vagal initiation, such as atrial fibrillation. Lightheadedness or syncope occurring in the setting of a tightly fitting collar, shaving the neck, or turning the head suggests carotid sinus hypersensitivity. The *mode of termination* of episodes may also be helpful: if palpitations can be reliably terminated by breath-holding, Valsalva, or other vagal maneuvers, it is likely that the atrioventricular (AV) node comprises an integral part of a tachycardia circuit; occasionally, focal atrial tachycardias or VTs terminate with vagal maneuvers. Patients should be asked *how frequently episodes occur, how long they last,* and *how severe their symptoms.* These features can help guide how aggressively and quickly the physician needs to pursue a diagnostic or therapeutic plan (a patient with daily episodes associated with near-syncope or severe dyspnea warrants a more expeditious evaluation than one with infrequent episodes of mild palpitations and no other symptoms). Patients can sometimes report the heart rate during an episode (either rapid or slow, regular or irregular) by counting their pulse directly or using an automatic blood pressure or heart rate monitor. Characteristics of mode of onset and frequency of episodes can guide the choice of diagnostic tests (see later).

A careful drug and dietary history should also be sought; some nasal decongestants can provoke tachycardia episodes, whereas beta-adrenergic blocking eye drops for treatment of glaucoma can drain into tear ducts, be absorbed systemically, and precipitate syncope due to bradycardia. Dietary supplements, particularly those containing ephedrine, can cause arrhythmias. A growing list of drugs can directly or indirectly affect ventricular repolarization and produce long-QT interval–related tachyarrhythmias (see Chaps. 5 and 32). The patient should be questioned about the presence of systemic illnesses that may be associated with arrhythmias such as chronic obstructive pulmonary disease, thyrotoxicosis, pericarditis, or congestive heart failure. A family history of rhythm disturbances is often present in long-QT syndrome, hypertrophic cardiomyopathy, and muscular or myotonic dystrophies.

Physical Examination

Examination of the patient during a symptomatic episode can be revealing. Clearly, heart rate and blood pressure are key measurements to make. Assessment of the jugular venous pressure and waveform can disclose the rapid oscillations of atrial flutter or "cannon" A waves indicative of contraction of the right atrium against a closed tricuspid valve in patients with AV dissociation in disorders such as complete heart block or VT. Variation in the intensity of the first heart sound has the same implications.

Physical maneuvers during a tachycardia can have diagnostic and therapeutic value. The Valsalva maneuver or carotid sinus massage causes a transient increase in vagal tone; tachyarrhythmias that depend on the AV node for continuation can terminate or slow with these maneuvers but may also show no change. Focal atrial tachycardias occasionally terminate in response to vagal stimulation, as do rare VTs. Sinus tachycardia slows slightly following vagal stimulation, returning to its original rate soon thereafter; the ventricular response during atrial flutter and fibrillation and other atrial tachycardias can slow briefly. During wide-QRS tachycardias with a 1:1 relationship between P waves and QRS complexes, vagal influence may terminate or slow a supraventricular tachycardia (SVT) with aberrant interventricular conduction that depends on the AV node for perpetuation; on the other hand, vagal effects on the AV node may transiently block retrograde conduction and thus establish the diagnosis of VT by demonstrating AV dissociation. The effect of either of these physical maneuvers typically lasts only seconds; the physician must be ready to observe or record any changes in rhythm on an ECG when the maneuver is performed or they may not be appreciated.

Carotid massage is performed with the patient supine and comfortable, with the head tipped away from the side being stimulated. Careful auscultation for carotid bruits must always precede any attempt at carotid massage since there have been reports of embolic events associated with massage. The area of the carotid sinus, at the artery's bifurcation, is palpated with two fingers at the angle of the jaw until a good pulse is felt. Even this minimal amount of pressure may induce a hypersensitive response in affected individuals. If there is no initial effect, a side-to-side or rotating motion of the fingers over the site is performed for up to 5 seconds. A negative response is lack of ECG effect after 5 seconds of pressure adequate to cause mild discomfort. Because responses to carotid massage may differ on the two sides, the maneuver can be repeated on the opposite side; both sides should never be stimulated simultaneously.

Physical findings can suggest the presence of structural heart disease (and, thus, generally a clinically more serious situation with worse overall prognosis) even in the absence of an arrhythmia episode. For instance, a laterally displaced or dyskinetic apical impulse, a regurgitant or stenotic murmur, or a third heart sound in an older adult can denote significant myocardial or valvular dysfunction or damage.

Electrocardiogram

The ECG is the primary tool in arrhythmia analysis (see Chap. 9); only an EPS, in which intracardiac catheters are used to record activity from several regions of the heart at one time, is more definitive. Initially, a 12-lead ECG is recorded. In addition, a long continuous recording using the lead that shows distinct P waves is often quite helpful for closer analysis; most commonly, this is one of the inferior leads (2, 3, aVF) and occasionally V_1 or aVR. The ECG obtained during an episode of arrhythmia may be diagnostic by itself, obviating the need for further diagnostic testing. Figure 29–1 depicts an algorithm for diagnosing specific tachyarrhythmias from the 12-lead ECG. A major branch point in the differential diagnosis concerns the QRS duration: Wide-QRS (>0.12-second) tachycardias are often VT, and narrow-QRS (≤0.12-second) tachycardias are almost always SVT, but there is some overlap (Table 29–1).[3] The next most important questions to answer, regardless of QRS width, concern characteristics of P waves. If P waves are not clearly visible, atrial activity can sometimes be recorded by placing the right and left arm leads in various anterior chest positions to discern P waves (so-called Lewis leads) or by applying esophageal electrodes or intracavitary right atrial recordings; the latter methods are not readily available in most clinical situations.

TABLE 29–1 Electrocardiographic Distinctions for Diagnosis of Wide QRS Complex Tachycardia

Favor Supraventricular Tachycardia	Favor Ventricular Tachycardia
Initiation with premature P wave	Initiation with premature QRS complex
"Long-short" sequence preceding initiation	Tachycardia beats identical to PVCs during sinus rhythm
Changes in P-P interval precede changes in R-R interval	Changes in R-R interval precede changes in P-P interval
QRS contours consistent with aberrant conduction (V_1, V_6)	QRS contours inconsistent with aberrant conduction (V_1, V_6)
Slowing or termination with vagal maneuvers	AV dissociation or other non-1:1 AV relationship Fusion beats, capture beats QRS duration >0.14 sec Left axis deviation (especially −90 to 180 degrees) Concordant R wave progression pattern Absence of "rS" complex in any precordial lead

AV = atrioventricular; PVC = premature ventricular complex.

An echocardiogram showing atrial contraction can be helpful. The long rhythm strip may yield important clues by revealing P waves if perturbations occur during the arrhythmia (changes in rate, premature complexes, sudden termination, effect of physical maneuvers, as noted earlier).

Each arrhythmia should be approached in a systematic manner to answer the several key questions; as suggested earlier, many of these relate to P wave characteristics and underscore the importance of assessing the ECG carefully for these. If P waves are visible, are the atrial and ventricular rates identical? Are the P-P and R-R intervals regular or irregular? If irregular, is it a consistent, repeating irregularity? Is there a P wave related to each QRS complex? Does the P wave seem to precede ("long-RP" interval) or follow ("short-RP" interval) the QRS complex (Fig. 29–2)? Are the resultant RP and PR intervals constant? Are all P waves and QRS complexes identical? Is the P wave vector normal or abnormal? Are P, PR, QRS, and QT durations normal? Once these questions are addressed, one needs to assess the significance of the arrhythmia in view of the clinical setting. Should it be treated, and, if so, how? For SVTs with a normal QRS complex, a branching decision tree such as Figure 29–1 may be useful.

THE LADDER DIAGRAM. The ladder diagram, derived from the ECG, is used to depict depolarization and conduction schematically to aid understanding of the rhythm. Straight or slightly slanting lines drawn on a tiered framework beneath an ECG represent electrical events occurring in the various cardiac structures (Fig. 29–3). Since the ECG and therefore the ladder diagram represent electrical activity against a time base, conduction is indicated by the lines of the ladder diagram sloping in a left-to-right direction. A steep line represents rapid conduction, with more slanting lines depicting slower conduction. A short bar drawn perpendicular to a sloping line represents blocked conduction. Activity originating in an ectopic site such as the ventricle is indicated by lines emanating from that tier. Sinus nodal discharge and conduction and, under certain circumstances, AV junctional discharge and conduction can only be inferred; their activity is not directly recorded on a scalar ECG.

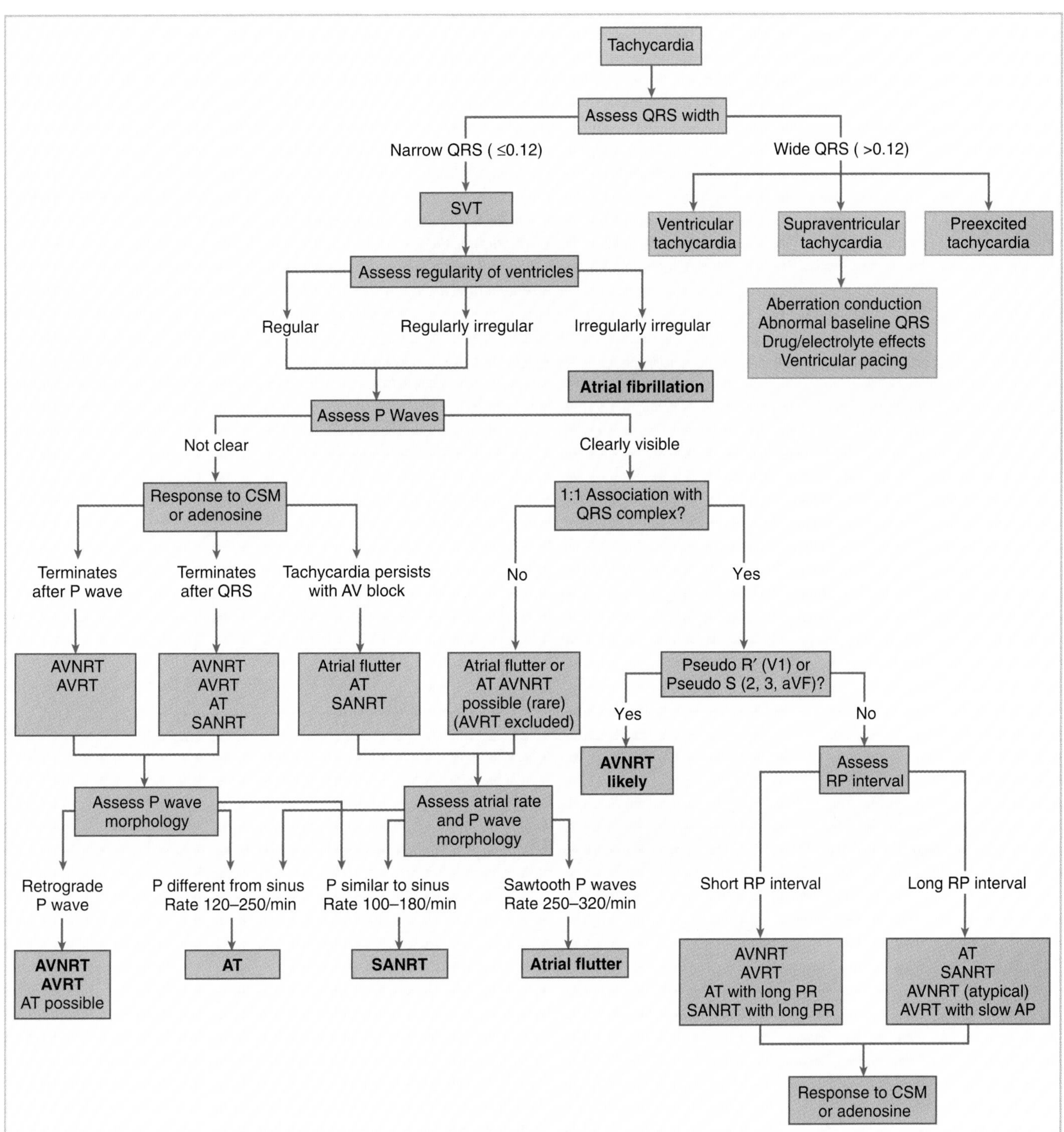

FIGURE 29–1 Stepwise approach to diagnosis of type of tachycardia based on 12-lead electrocardiogram during the episode. The initial step is to determine whether the tachycardia has a wide or narrow QRS complex. For wide-complex tachycardia, see Table 29–1; the remainder of the algorithm is helpful in diagnosing the type of narrow-complex tachycardia. SVT = supraventricular tachycardia; CSM = carotid sinus massage; AV = atrioventricular; AVNRT = AV nodal reentrant tachycardia; AVRT = AV reciprocating tachycardia; AT = atrial tachycardia; SANRT = sinoatrial nodal reentry tachycardia; AP = accessory pathway.

Additional Tests

The following additional tests can be used to evaluate patients who have cardiac arrhythmias. The physician's choice of which test to use depends on the clinical circumstances. For instance, a patient with multiple daily episodes of presyncope is likely to have an event recorded on a 24-hour ambulatory ECG (Holter) monitor, whereas in a patient who complains of infrequent anxiety- or exercise-induced palpitations, exercise stress testing may be more likely to provide a diagnosis.

Exercise Testing (see also Chap. 10)

Exercise can induce various types of supraventricular and ventricular tachyarrhythmias and, uncommonly, bradyarrhythmias.[4] About one third of normal subjects develop ventricular ectopy in response to exercise testing. Ectopy is

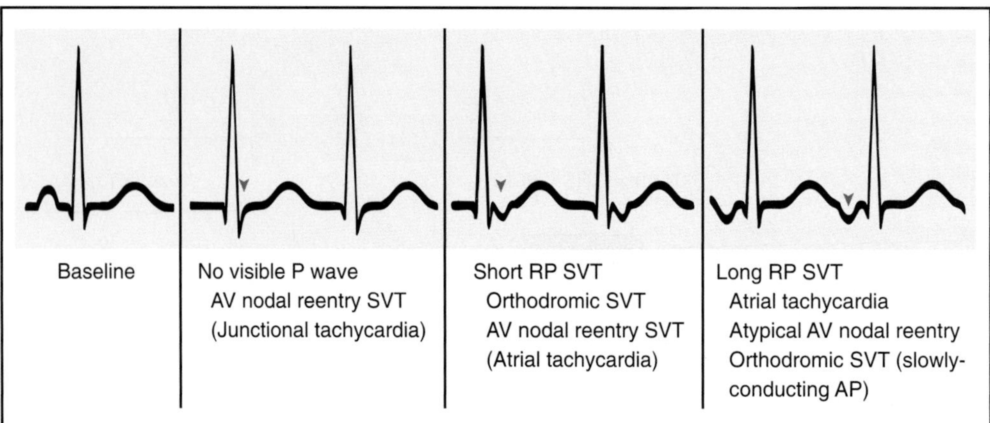

FIGURE 29–2 Differential diagnosis of different types of supraventricular tachycardia (SVT) based on timing of atrial activity (RP and PR intervals). A normal beat is shown at left; different types of tachycardia are listed below the representative electrocardiographic patterns they can produce, categorized by P wave position relative to the QRS complex. Arrow shows the location of the P wave in each example. AV = atrioventricular; AP = accessory pathway.

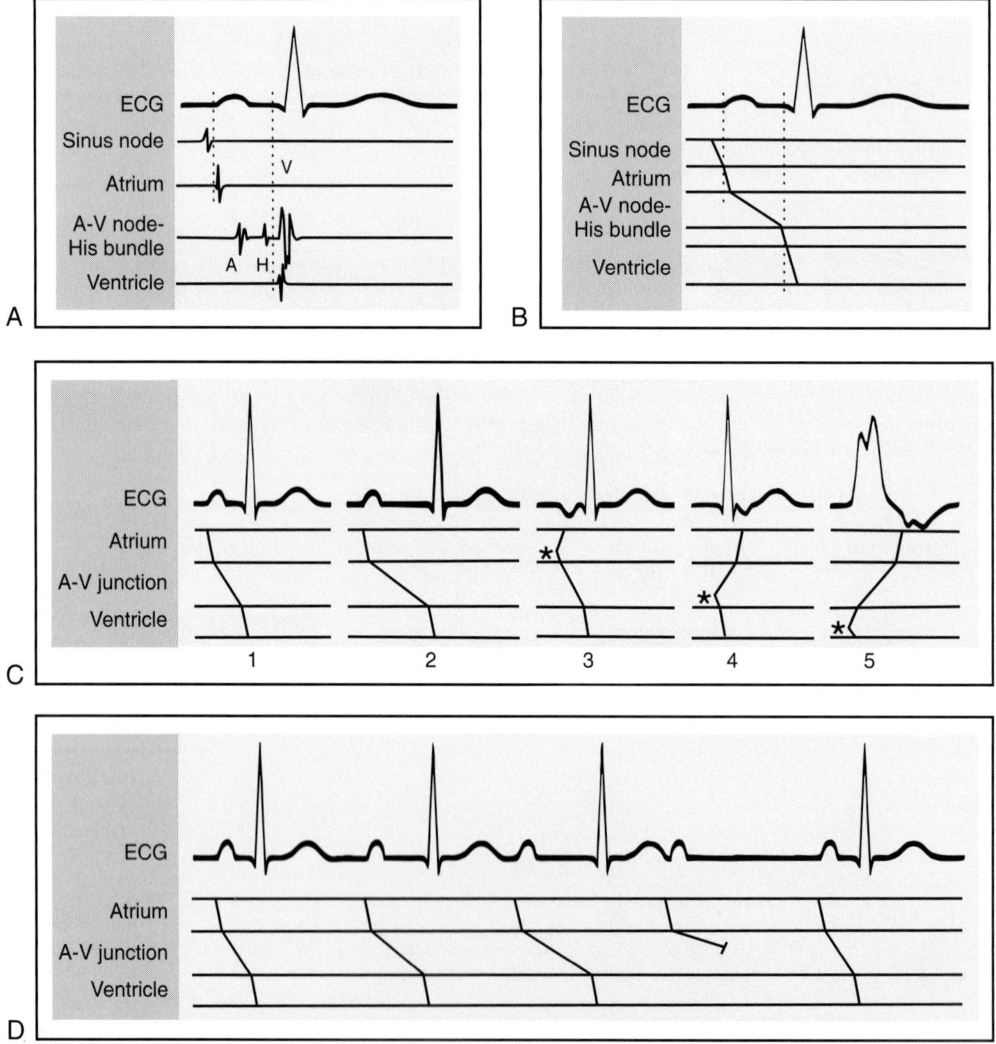

FIGURE 29–3 Intracardiac signals and ladder diagrams. **A,** A single beat is shown with accompanying intracardiac signals from the sinus node, right atrium, atrioventricular (AV) nodal and His bundle regions, and right ventricle. **B,** The same beat is shown with accompanying ladder diagram below. Cardiac regions have been divided into tiers separated by horizontal lines. Vertical dotted lines denote onset of P wave and QRS complexes. Note the relatively steep lines (rapid conduction through atrium, His bundle, and ventricular muscle) and more gently sloping lines as the impulse traverses the sinus and AV nodes (signifying slow conduction). **C,** Several different situations are depicted with accompanying explanatory ladder diagrams. Beat 1 is normal, as in **B**; beat 2 shows first-degree AV delay, with a more gradual slope than normal in the AV nodal tier, signifying very slow conduction in this region. In beat 3, an atrial premature complex is shown (starting in atrial tier as asterisk) producing an inverted P wave on electrocardiogram. In beat 4, an ectopic impulse arises in the His bundle (*) and propagates to the ventricle as well as retrogradely through the AV node to the atrium. In beat 5, a ventricular ectopic complex (*) conducts retrogradely through the His bundle and AV node and eventually to the atrium. **D,** A Wenckebach AV cycle (type 1 second-degree block) is shown. As the PR interval progressively increases from left to right in the figure, the slope of the line in the AV nodal region is progressively less steep until it fails to propagate at all after the fourth P wave (small line perpendicular to sloping AV nodal conduction line), after which the cycle repeats. A = atrial recording; ECG = electrocardiograph; H = His recording; V = ventricular recording.

more likely to occur at faster heart rates, usually in the form of occasional PVCs of constant morphology, or even pairs of PVCs, and is often not reproducible from one stress test to the next. Three to six beats of nonsustained VT can occur in normal patients, especially the elderly, and its occurrence does not establish the existence of ischemic or other forms of heart disease or predict increased cardiovascular morbidity or mortality. Premature supraventricular complexes are often more common during exercise than at rest and increase in frequency with age; their occurrence does not suggest the presence of structural heart disease. A persistent elevation of heart rate after the end of exercise (delay in return to baseline) is associated with a worse cardiovascular prognosis.[5]

Approximately 50 percent of patients who have coronary artery disease develop PVCs in response to exercise testing. Ventricular ectopy appears in these patients at lower heart rates (<130 beats/min) than in the normal population and often occurs in the early recovery period as well. Frequent (>7 PVCs/min) or complex ectopy is associated with a worse prognosis.[6] Exercise reproduced sustained VT or VF in only about 10 percent of patients with spontaneous VT or VF late after myocardial infarction, but those who had it experienced a worse outcome. The relation of exercise to ventricular arrhythmia in patients with structurally normal hearts has no prognostic implications. Stress testing with Holter recording has been used to assess antiarrhythmic drug efficacy.[7]

Patients who have symptoms consistent with an arrhythmia induced by exercise (e.g., syncope, sustained palpitations) should be considered for stress testing. Stress testing may be indicated to uncover more complex grades of ventricular arrhythmia, to provoke supraventricular arrhythmias, to determine the relationship of the arrhythmia to activity, to aid in choosing antiarrhythmic therapy and uncovering proarrhythmic responses, and possibly to provide some insight into the mechanism of the tachycardia. The test can be performed safely and appears more sensitive than a standard 12-lead resting ECG to detect ventricular ectopy. However, prolonged ambulatory recording is more sensitive than exercise testing in detecting ventricular ectopy. Because either technique can uncover serious arrhythmias that the other technique misses, both examinations may be indicated for selected patients.

Long-Term Electrocardiographic Recording

Prolonged ECG recording in patients engaged in normal daily activities is the most useful noninvasive method to document and quantitate the frequency and complexity of an arrhythmia, correlate the arrhythmia with the patient's symptoms, and evaluate the effect of antiarrhythmic therapy on spontaneous arrhythmia.[8] For example, recording normal sinus rhythm during the patient's typical symptomatic episode effectively excludes cardiac arrhythmia as a cause. In addition, some recorders can document alterations in QRS, ST, and T contours (Fig. 29–4).

AMBULATORY ECG (HOLTER) RECORDING. Continuous ECG tape recorders represent the traditional Holter monitor and typically record (on analog tape or digital cards) two or three ECG channels for 24 hours.[9] Interpretative accuracy of long-term recordings varies with the system used, but most computers that scan the recording media are sufficiently accurate to meet clinical needs. All systems can potentially record more information than the physician needs or can assimilate. As long as the system detects important episodes of ectopic activity, VT, or asystolic intervals and semiquantitates these abnormalities, the physician probably receives all the clinical information that is needed. Twenty-five to 50 percent of patients experience a complaint during a 24-hour recording, caused by an arrhythmia in 2 to 15 percent (see Fig. 29–4). The ability to temporally correlate symptoms with ECG abnormalities is one of the strengths of this technique.

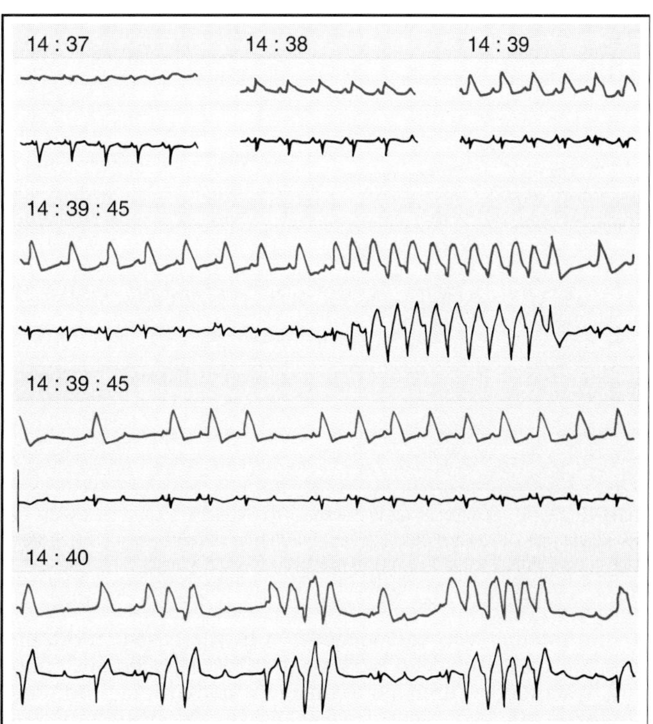

FIGURE 29–4 Long-term electrocardiographic recording in a patient with atypical angina. The top channel reflects an inferior lead, and the bottom channel records an anterior lead. Note progressive ST segment elevation in the inferior lead, eventually resembling a monophasic action potential. Bursts of nonsustained ventricular tachycardia result. Then, sinus slowing and Wenckebach atrioventricular (AV) block occur from a vasodepressor reflex response elicited by ischemia of the inferior myocardial wall or possibly caused by ischemia of the sinus and AV nodes. In the bottom tracing, both AV block and ventricular arrhythmias are apparent. Numbers indicate time (e.g., 2:37 P.M.). (Courtesy of D. A. Chilson, MD.)

Significant rhythm disturbances are fairly uncommon in healthy young persons. However, sinus bradycardia with heart rates of 35 to 40 beats/min, sinus arrhythmia with pauses exceeding 3 seconds, sinoatrial exit block, type 1 (Wenckebach) second-degree AV block (often during sleep), a wandering atrial pacemaker, junctional escape complexes, and premature atrial complexes (PACs) and PVCs are not necessarily abnormal. Frequent and complex atrial and ventricular rhythm disturbances are less commonly observed, however, and type II second-degree AV conduction disturbances (see Chap. 32) are not recorded in normal patients. Elderly patients may have a greater prevalence of arrhythmias, some of which may be responsible for neurological symptoms (Fig. 29–5). The long-term prognosis in asymptomatic healthy subjects with frequent and complex PVCs resembles that of the healthy U.S. population without an increased risk of death.

Most patients who have ischemic heart disease, particularly those after myocardial infarction, exhibit PVCs when monitored for 6 to 24 hours. The frequency of PVCs progressively increases over the first several weeks, decreasing at about 6 months after infarction. Frequent and complex PVCs constitute an independent risk factor and are associated with a twofold to fivefold increased risk of cardiac or sudden death in patients after myocardial infarction. Evidence from the Cardiac Arrhythmia Suppression Trial (CAST) raises the possibility that the ventricular ectopy is a marker identifying the patient at risk rather than being causally related to sudden death, because PVC suppression with flecainide, encainide,

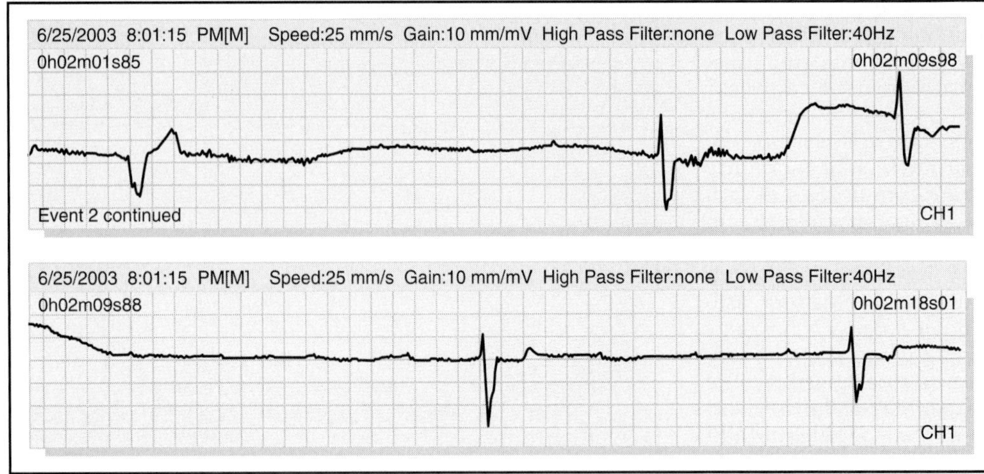

FIGURE 29–5 Continuous electrocardiographic recording from a patient-activated event monitor during an episode of lightheadedness. Sinus rhythm at 75 beats/min with sudden atrioventricular block is present with pauses of longer than 4 seconds and, in the bottom strip, there is an effective heart rate of about 8 beats/min.

or moricizine was associated with increased mortality compared with placebo.[10] Thus, the PVC may be an "innocent bystander," unrelated to the tachyarrhythmia producing sudden death. Although the mechanism responsible for the drug-induced exacerbation of mortality is not clear, it may relate to an increase in ischemia-produced conduction delay due to sodium-channel blocking drugs.

Holter recordings have been used to determine antiarrhythmic drug efficacy. In one study, Holter recordings led to predictions of antiarrhythmic drug efficacy more often than did electrophysiological testing in patients with sustained ventricular tachyarrhythmias, and there was no significant difference in the success of drug therapy as selected by the two methods.[7] The beneficial results of noninvasive compared with invasive assessment of drug efficacy in this study have been challenged.

Long-term ECG recording also has exposed potentially serious arrhythmias and complex ventricular ectopy in patients with left ventricular hypertrophy; in those with mitral valve prolapse; in those who have otherwise unexplained syncope or transient vague cerebrovascular symptoms; in those with conduction disturbances, sinus node dysfunction, bradycardia-tachycardia syndrome, Wolff-Parkinson-White syndrome, increased QT dispersion, and pacemaker malfunction; and after thrombolytic therapy. It has shown that asymptomatic atrial fibrillation occurs far more often than symptomatic atrial fibrillation in patients with that arrhythmia.[11] This has important implications for deciding whether a patient needs chronic anticoagulation based only on recurrent symptoms or a single ECG recording.

Variations of Holter recording have been used for particular applications. Repeated 24-hour recording periods may be needed to obtain enough episodes of PAC triggering atrial fibrillation to warrant proceeding to an EPS and catheter ablation. Some monitoring systems are able to "reconstruct" a full 12-lead ECG from a seven-electrode recording system. This is especially useful when trying to document the ECG morphology of VT before an ablation procedure or a consistent morphology of PACs that may arise from an ablatable focus of atrial fibrillation. Most Holter recording and analysis systems have the ability to place a clearly recognizable deflection on the recording when a pacemaker stimulus is detected. This greatly facilitates diagnosis of potential pacemaker malfunction. Occasionally, ECG artifacts due to alterations in tape recording or playback speed can mimic bradycardias or tachycardias and lead to erroneous therapy. Newer digital Holter systems are less subject to this phenomenon. Finally, most systems can also provide heart rate variability data (see later).

EVENT RECORDING. In many patients, the 24-hour "snapshot" provided by the Holter recording is incapable of documenting the cause of the patient's symptoms. Longer term monitoring is necessary in these cases, which occur frequently, such as with an event recorder.[12] These devices are about the size of a pager and are kept by the patient for 30 days. During that time, digital recordings can be made during symptomatic episodes and transmitted to a receiving station over standard telephone lines at the patient's convenience (see Fig. 29–5). Some of these recorders store more than 30 seconds of ECG before the time when the patient activates the recording. These "loop" recorders record continuously, but only a small window of time is present in memory at any time; when the event button is pressed by the patient, the current window is "frozen" while the device continues recording for another 30 to 60 seconds, depending on how it is configured. Event recorders are highly effective in documenting infrequent events, but the quality of the recordings is more variable than Holter recorders and usually only one channel can be recorded. Using some systems, the patient must be able to press the event button to begin recording; if syncope occurs without warning and the patient is not able to actuate the device, it cannot provide diagnostic information. With other systems, the device automatically begins recording the rhythm when the heart rate falls outside predetermined parameters.

Some pacemakers and implantable defibrillators are capable of providing Holter-like data on occurrence of premature beats or tachycardia episodes and can even store electrograms of these events from the implanted leads. The device can then be interrogated later and the electrograms printed for analysis.

IMPLANTABLE LOOP RECORDER. For patients with infrequent and transient symptoms, neither Holter recorders nor 30-day event recorders may yield diagnostic information. In such patients, implantable loop recorders may be used. This device (about the size of a pack of chewing gum) is inserted under the skin at about the second rib on the left front of the chest and is activated by passing a special magnet over the device.[13] It is capable of recording up to 42 minutes of a single ECG channel that can be partitioned for 1 to 7 episodes, with up to 20 minutes of preactivation ECG saved for subsequent downloading to a programming unit for analysis. Both P waves and QRS complexes can usually be identified. The device can be configured to store patient-activated episodes, automatically activated recordings (heart rate outside preset parameters), or a combination of these (Fig. 29–6). In one report, this device was implanted in 24 patients with recurrent syncope who had undergone extensive evaluation without determining a cause of syncope. Over a mean 5-month period after implant, 21 patients had recurrent syncope; the device was instrumental in establishing the diagnosis in 18 patients.[13]

Heart Rate Variability

Heart rate variability is used to evaluate vagal and sympathetic influences on the sinus node (inferring that the same

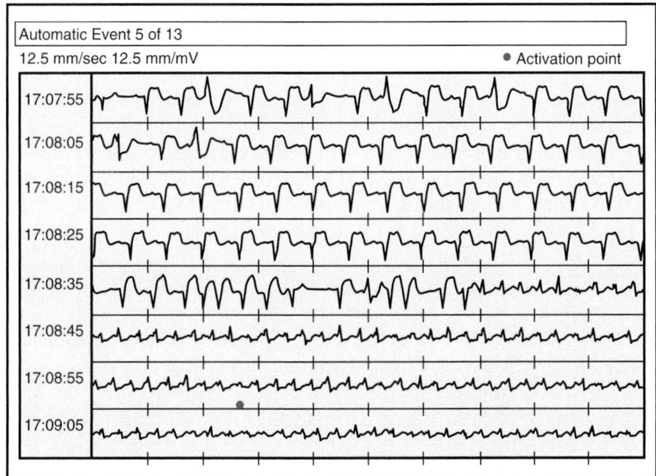

FIGURE 29–6 Recordings from an implantable loop recorder. Each line contains 10 seconds of continuous electrocardiogram from the implanted device. The first four lines show sinus rhythm with premature ventricular complexes; during the fifth line, short runs of atrial tachycardia precede an episode of a faster tachycardia with a different complex (ventricular tachycardia). This episode triggered an automatic activation (red circle) of the device recording (no symptoms associated with the episode).

activity is occurring in the ventricles also) and to identify patients at risk for a cardiovascular event or death.[14] Frequency domain analysis resolves parasympathetic and sympathetic influences better than does time domain analysis, but both types of analysis are useful. R-R variability predicts all-cause mortality as well as does left ventricular ejection fraction or nonsustained VT in patients after myocardial infarction and can be added to other measures of risk to enhance predictive accuracy. Similar results have been obtained in patients with dilated cardiomyopathy.[15] High-frequency components of R-R interval variability reflect vagal activity. Reduced RR interval variability, the marker of increased risk, indicates loss or reduction of the physiological periodic sinus node fluctuations, which can be due to many different influences and may not necessarily represent a particular shift in autonomic modulation. Some investigators have determined that simple heart rate measurement contains as much prognostic information as heart rate variability.[16]

QT Dispersion

Heterogeneity in refractoriness and conduction velocity is a hallmark of reentrant arrhythmias. One index of heterogeneity of ventricular refractoriness can be found in differences in length of the QT interval in surface ECG leads. The most commonly used index to calculate this QT dispersion has been the difference between the longest and shortest QT intervals on the 12-lead ECG, which is often adjusted for heart rate as well as number of leads sampled (when the T wave is flat in some). Other indices have been developed. Abnormally high QT dispersion has been correlated with risk of arrhythmic death in a variety of disorders,[17] although results are not consistent. QT dispersion has been correlated with efficacy and proarrhythmic potential of drug therapy. Different techniques exist for determining dispersion (including automated algorithms), and the results of one study are often difficult to compare with those of another; in addition, seasonal variation in QT dispersion has been shown.[18] It remains to be seen whether QT dispersion measured on a scalar ECG will be a useful clinical tool.[19,20]

Late Potentials

Signal averaging is a method that improves signal-to-noise ratio when signals are recurrent and the noise is random.[21] In conjunction with appropriate filtering and other methods of noise reduction, signal averaging can detect cardiac signals of a few microvolts in amplitude, reducing noise amplitude, such as muscle potentials that are typically 5 to 25 μV, to less than 1 μV. With this method, very low-amplitude electrical potentials generated by the sinus and AV nodes, His bundle, and bundle branches are detectable at the body surface.

One of the constituents of reentrant ventricular arrhythmias in patients with prior myocardial damage is slow conduction. Direct cardiac mapping techniques can record myocardial activation from damaged areas that occurs after the end of the surface ECG QRS complex during sinus rhythm. These delayed signals have very low amplitude that cannot be discerned on routine ECG and correspond to the delayed and fragmented conduction in the ventricles recorded with direct mapping techniques (Fig. 29–7). Signal averaging has been applied clinically most often to detect such late ventricular potentials of 1 to 25 μV. Criteria for late potentials are (1) filtered QRS complex duration greater than 114 to 120 milliseconds, (2) less than 20 μV of root-mean-square signal amplitude in the last 40 milliseconds of the filtered QRS complex, and (3) the terminal filtered QRS complex remains below 40 μV for longer than 39 milli-

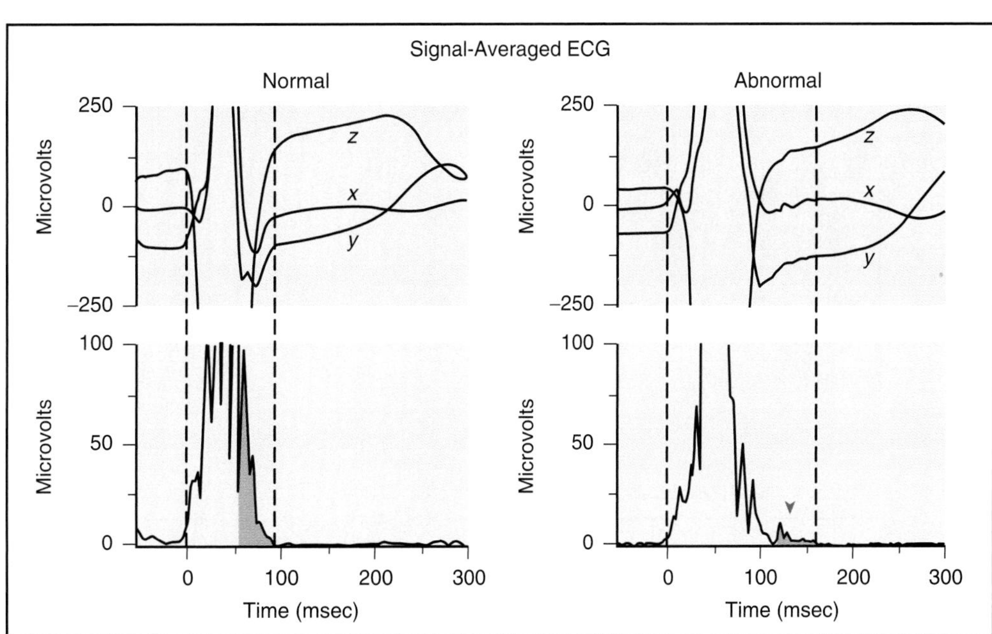

FIGURE 29–7 Signal-averaged electrocardiogram (ECG). Normal **(left)** and abnormal **(right)** results are shown from a patient with prior myocardial infarction and venticular tachycardia. **Bottom panels:** Shaded blue areas at the end of each tracing represent voltage content of last 40 milliseconds of the filtered QRS integral. The small shaded area in the abnormal study denotes prolonged, slow conduction and suggests the potential for reentrant ventricular arrhythmias.

seconds. These late potentials have been recorded in 70 to 90 percent of patients with spontaneous sustained and inducible VT after myocardial infarction, in only 0 to 6 percent of normal volunteers, and in 7 to 15 percent of patients after myocardial infarction who do not have VT. Late potentials can be detected as early as 3 hours after the onset of chest pain, increase in prevalence in the first week after myocardial infarction, and disappear in some patients after 1 year. If not present initially, late potentials usually do not appear later. Early use of thrombolytic agents may reduce the prevalence of late potentials after coronary occlusion. Patients with bundle branch block or paced ventricular rhythms have wide QRS complexes already, rendering the technique less useful in these cases.

Late potentials also have been recorded in patients with VT not related to ischemia, such as dilated cardiomyopathies. Successful surgical resection of the VT can eliminate late potentials but is not necessary to cause tachycardia suppression. The presence of a late potential is a sensitive, but not specific, marker of arrhythmic risk and thus its prognostic use is limited.[22] In specific situations, it can be helpful; for instance, a patient with a prior inferior wall myocardial infarction (normally the last portion of the heart to be activated) who has no late potential has a very low likelihood of having VT episodes.

The high-pass filtering used to record late potentials meeting the criteria just noted is called *time domain analysis* because the filter output corresponds in time to the input signal. Because late potentials are high-frequency signals, Fourier transform can be applied to extract high-frequency content from the signal-averaged ECG, called *frequency domain analysis.* Some data suggest that frequency domain analysis provides useful information not available in the time domain analysis.

Signal averaging has been applied to the P wave to determine risk for developing atrial fibrillation as well as maintenance of sinus rhythm after cardioversion. The overall use of the technique remains limited at present.

T Wave Alternans

Beat-to-beat alternation in the amplitude and/or morphology of the ECG measurement of ventricular repolarization, the ST segment and T wave, has been found in conditions favoring the development of ventricular tachyarrhythmias such as ischemia and long-QT interval syndrome and in patients with ventricular arrhythmias.[23] The electrophysiological basis appears to be the alternation of repolarization of ventricular myocytes.[24] In the presence of a long QT interval, the cellular basis of alternation has been shown to be due to beat-to-beat repolarization changes in midmyocardial cells (M cells).[25] Whether this mechanism applies to different disease states is not known. T wave alternans testing requires exercise or atrial pacing to achieve a heart rate of 100 to 120 beats/min with relatively little atrial or ventricular ectopic activity. The test is less useful in patients with a wide QRS complex (>120 milliseconds). A positive T wave alternans test is associated with a worse arrhythmic prognosis in a variety of disorders, including ischemic heart disease[26] and nonischemic cardiomyopathy.[27] T wave alternans may represent a fundamental marker of an electrically unstable myocardium prone to developing VT or VF, and, as such, ST-T wave analysis for alternans may be useful in the future as a method to risk-stratify patients (Fig. 29–8).

Baroreceptor Reflex Sensitivity Testing

(see Chap. 87)

Acute blood pressure elevation triggers a baroreceptor reflex that augments vagal "tone" to the heart and slows the sinus rate. The increase in sinus cycle length per millimeter of mercury systolic blood pressure increase is a measure of the sensitivity of the baroreceptor reflex and, when reduced, identifies patients susceptible to developing VT and VF.[28,29] The mechanism of the reduction in baroreceptor reflex

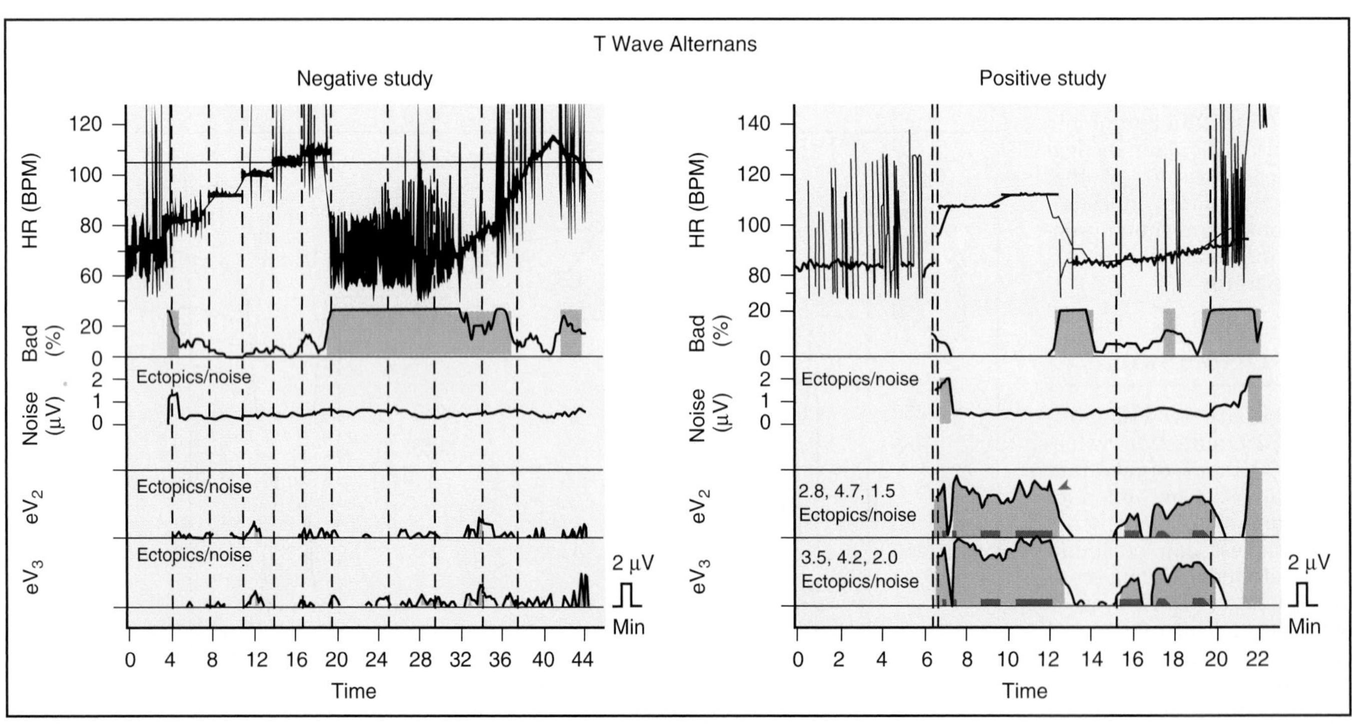

FIGURE 29–8 T wave alternans. Reports of T wave alternans analysis from two patients are shown, displaying heart rate (HR) in beats per minute (BPM), proportion of beats rejected from analysis (% Bad), electrocardiogram noise level (in microvolts), and selected precordial leads (V_2 and V_3) as a function of time. Records in the left panel are from a patient with no structural heart disease; the amplitude of T wave alternans was minimal. The study in the right panel, from a patient hospitalized for sustained ventricular tachycardia after myocardial infarction, shows T wave alternans (blue shaded area, arrow).

sensitivity is not certain. However, this test may be useful to identify patients at risk for developing a serious ventricular arrhythmia after myocardial infarction.

Body Surface Mapping

Isopotential body surface maps are used to provide a complete picture of the effects of the currents from the heart on the body surface. The potential distributions are represented by contour lines of equal potential, and each distribution is displayed instant by instant throughout activation or recovery, or both.[30]

Body surface maps have been used clinically to localize and size areas of myocardial ischemia, localize ectopic foci or accessory pathways, differentiate aberrant supraventricular conduction from ventricular origin, recognize the patient prone to developing arrhythmias, and possibly understand the mechanisms involved. Although these procedures are of interest, their clinical utility has not yet been established. In addition, the technique is cumbersome and the analysis is complex.

Upright Tilt-Table Testing

The tilt-table test is used to identify patients who have a vasodepressor and/or a cardioinhibitory response as a cause of syncope.[31] Patients are positioned on a tilt table in the supine position and are tilted upright to a maximum of 60 to 80 degrees for 20 to 45 minutes, or longer if necessary (Fig. 29–9). Isoproterenol, as a bolus or an infusion, may provoke syncope in patients whose initial upright tilt-table testing shows no abnormalities or after just several minutes of tilt to shorten the time of the test necessary to produce a positive response. An initial intravenous isoproterenol dose of 1 μg/min can be increased in 0.5-μg/min steps until symptoms occur or a maximum of 4 μg/min is given. Isoproterenol induces a vasodepressor response in upright, susceptible patients generally consisting of a decrease in heart rate and blood pressure along with near-syncope or syncope. Intravenous edrophonium chloride, nitroglycerin, and esmolol withdrawal have also been used. Atropine can block the early bradycardia but not the hypotension; beta blockers can inhibit the latter. Tilt-table test results are positive in two thirds to three fourths of patients susceptible to neurally mediated syncope and are reproducible in about 80 percent, but have a 10 to 15 percent false-positive response rate. Repeating an initially negative tilt-table test on a subsequent day rarely yields a positive result. A positive test result is more meaningful when it reproduces symptoms that have occurred spontaneously. Positive responses can be divided into cardioinhibitory, vasodepressor, and mixed categories. Therapy with beta blockers, disopyramide, theophylline, selective serotonin reuptake inhibitors, midodrine, and salt loading or fludrocortisone have each been reported to be successful, as has "tilt training" (in which the patient leans against a wall for prolonged periods to increase tolerance to this body position).

MECHANISM[32]

Vasodepressor reactions, which are thought to be caused by activation of unmyelinated left ventricular vagal C fibers, can be triggered by a variety of events, including increased left ventricular pressure (see Chap. 34). Stimulation of C fibers from vigorous left ventricular contraction on a relatively empty cavity reduces efferent sympathetic tone while increasing efferent vagal tone, possibly producing vasodepression and paradoxical bradycardia. Isoproterenol increases left ventricular contractility while reducing left ventricular volume. A passive upright tilt exaggerates these responses because the tilt also reduces venous return and prevents isoproterenol from increasing cardiac output. Some patients may experience profound bradycardia, whereas others may have a prominent vasodepressor component. Dual-chamber pacing has been shown to benefit some patients with refractory neurocardiogenic syncope.[33] Before pacemaker implantation, some investigators have advocated performing a tilt-table test with temporary pacing catheters in place to simulate how a permanent pacing system would perform; however, correlation between this type of acute testing and long-term pacing results has not been proven.

A variant of the neurocardiogenic response, the postural orthostatic tachycardia syndrome, is characterized by dramatic increases in heart rate during the first 10 minutes of tilt-table testing.[34] This syndrome appears to be distinct from simple orthostatic hypotension as well as standard neurocardiogenic responses and is thought to be due to various forms of autonomic imbalance. Relief of symptoms has been effected with fludrocortisone, beta blockers, or combinations.

ESOPHAGEAL ELECTROCARDIOGRAPHY

Esophageal electrocardiography is a useful noninvasive technique to diagnose arrhythmias. The esophagus is located immediately behind the left atrium, between the left and right pulmonary veins. An electrode in the lumen of the esophagus can record atrial potentials. Bipolar recording is superior to unipolar recording because far-field ventricular events

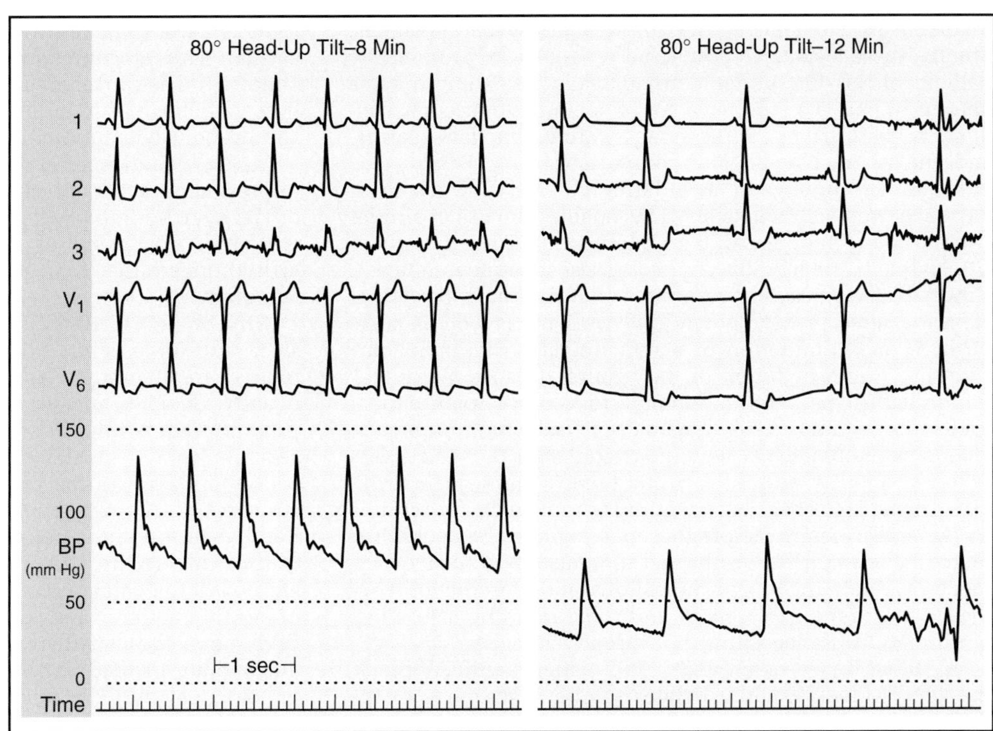

FIGURE 29–9 Head-up tilt-table testing. Surface electrocardiogram (ECG) leads and an arterial blood pressure (BP) tracing are shown. After 8 minutes of head-up tilt at 80 degrees (left), heart rate and BP were normal and the patient was asymptomatic. Four minutes later (right), systolic BP dropped precipitously to 80 mm Hg, the heart rate fell to 50 beats/min, and the patient lost consciousness. ECG artifact at right is seizure activity.

with the former method can lead to possible diagnostic confusion. In addition, atrial and occasionally ventricular pacing can be performed by means of a catheter electrode inserted into the esophagus, and initiation and termination of tachycardias can be accomplished. Optimal electrode position for atrial pacing correlates with patient height and is within about 1 cm of the site at which the maximum amplitude of the atrial electrogram is recorded. When recorded simultaneously with the surface ECG, the esophageal atrial electrogram can be used to differentiate SVT with aberrancy from VT and to define the mechanism of SVTs. For example, if atrial and ventricular depolarizations occur simultaneously during a narrow QRS tachycardia, reentry using an accessory AV pathway (Wolff-Parkinson-White syndrome) can be excluded, and AV nodal reentry is the most likely mechanism for the tachycardia. Complications of transesophageal recording and pacing are uncommon, but the technique is not comfortable for most patients and it is thus not commonly applied.

Invasive Electrophysiological Studies

An invasive EPS involves introducing multipolar catheter electrodes into the venous and/or arterial system and positioning the electrodes at various intracardiac sites to record and/or stimulate cardiac electrical activity. Assessment of AV conduction at rest is made by positioning the catheter along the septal leaflet of the tricuspid valve and measuring the atrial-His interval (an estimate of AV nodal conduction time; normally 60 to 125 milliseconds) and the His-ventricular (HV) interval (a measure of infranodal conduction; normally 40 to 55 milliseconds). The heart is stimulated from portions of the atria or ventricles and from the region of the His bundle, bundle branches, accessory pathways, and other structures. Such studies are performed diagnostically to provide information on the type of clinical rhythm disturbances and insight into its electrophysiological mechanism. They are used therapeutically to terminate a tachycardia by electrical stimulation or electroshock; to evaluate the effects of therapy by determining whether a particular intervention modifies or prevents electrical induction of a tachycardia or whether an electrical device properly senses and terminates an induced tachyarrhythmia; and to ablate myocardium involved in the tachycardia to prevent further episodes. Finally, these tests have been used prognostically to identify patients at risk for sudden cardiac death. The study may be helpful in patients who have AV block, intraventricular conduction disturbance, sinus node dysfunction, tachycardia, and unexplained syncope or palpitations.[35]

The EPS is quite good at initiating VT or SVT when these have occurred spontaneously. This enables the use of similar stimulation techniques after an intervention (drug therapy or surgical or catheter ablation) to assess treatment efficacy. However, false-negative responses (not finding a particular electrical abnormality known to be present) as well as false-positive ones (induction of a nonclinical arrhythmia) may complicate interpretation of the results, because many lack reproducibility. Altered autonomic tone in a supine patient undergoing study, hemodynamic or ischemic influences, changing anatomy (e.g., new infarction) after the study, day-to-day variability, and the fact that the test employs an artificial "trigger" (electrical stimulation) to induce the arrhythmia are several of many factors that may explain the occasional disparity between test results and spontaneous clinical occurrences. Overall, the diagnostic validity and reproducibility of these studies are quite good, and they are quite safe when performed by skilled clinical electrophysiologists.

AV BLOCK (see also Chap. 32). In patients with AV block, the site of block usually dictates the clinical course of the patient and whether a pacemaker is needed. Generally, the site of AV block can be determined from an analysis of the scalar ECG. When the site of block cannot be determined from such an analysis, and when knowing the site of block is imperative for patient management, an invasive EPS is indicated. Candidates include symptomatic patients in whom His-Purkinje block is suspected but not established and patients with AV block treated with a pacemaker who continue to be symptomatic in whom a causal ventricular tachyarrhythmia is sought. Possible candidates are those with second- or third-degree AV block in whom knowledge of the site of block or its mechanism may help direct therapy or assess prognosis and patients suspected of having concealed His bundle extrasystoles. Patients with block in the His-Purkinje system more commonly become symptomatic because of periods of bradycardia or asystole and more commonly require pacemaker implantation than do patients who have AV nodal block.[36] Type I (Wenckebach) AV block in older patients may have clinical implications similar to type II AV block. The results of EPS for evaluating the conduction system must be interpreted with caution, however. In rare cases, the process of recording conduction intervals alters their values. For instance, catheter pressure on the AV node or His bundle can cause a prolongation of the atrial-His or HV interval and lead to erroneous diagnosis and therapy.

INTRAVENTRICULAR CONDUCTION DISTURBANCE. For patients with an intraventricular conduction disturbance, an EPS provides information on the duration of the HV interval, which can be prolonged with a normal PR interval or normal with a prolonged PR interval. A prolonged HV interval (>55 milliseconds) is associated with a greater likelihood of developing trifascicular block (but the rate of progression is slow, 2 to 3 percent annually), having structural disease, and higher mortality. Finding very long HV intervals (>80 to 90 milliseconds) identifies patients at increased risk of developing AV block. The HV interval has a high specificity (~80 percent) but low sensitivity (~66 percent) for predicting the development of complete AV block. During the study, atrial pacing is used to uncover abnormal His-Purkinje conduction. A positive response is provocation of distal His block during 1:1 AV nodal conduction. Once again, sensitivity is low but specificity is high. Functional His-Purkinje block due to normal His-Purkinje refractoriness is not a positive response. Drug infusion, such as that with procainamide or ajmaline, sometimes exposes abnormal His-Purkinje conduction (Fig. 29–10). Ajmaline (not available in the United States) can cause arrhythmias and should be used cautiously.

An EPS is indicated in the patient with symptoms (syncope or presyncope) that appear to be related to a bradyarrhythmia or tachyarrhythmia when no other cause of symptoms is found. For many of these patients, ventricular tachyarrhythmias rather than AV block can be the cause of their symptoms.

SINUS NODE DYSFUNCTION. The demonstration of slow sinus rates, sinus exit block, or sinus pauses temporally related to symptoms suggests a causal relationship and usually obviates further diagnostic studies. Carotid sinus pressure that results in several seconds of complete cardiac asystole or AV block and reproduces the patient's usual symptoms exposes the presence of a hypersensitive carotid sinus reflex. Carotid sinus massage must be done cautiously. Rarely, carotid sinus massage can precipitate a stroke. Neurohumoral agents, adenosine, or stress testing can be employed to evaluate the effects of autonomic tone on sinus node automaticity and sinoatrial conduction time (SACT). EPS should be considered in patients who have symptoms attributable to bradycardia or asystole, such as presyncope or syncope, and for whom noninvasive approaches have provided no explanation for the symptoms.

Sinus Node Recovery Time. Sinus node recovery time (SNRT) is a technique that can be useful to evaluate sinus node function. The interval between the last paced high right atrial response and the first spontaneous (sinus) high right atrial response after termination of pacing is measured to determine the SNRT. Because the spontaneous sinus rate influences the SNRT, the value is corrected by subtracting the spontaneous sinus node cycle length (before pacing) from the SNRT (Fig. 29–11). This value, the CSNRT, is generally less than 525 milliseconds. Prolonged CSNRT has been found in patients suspected of having sinus node dysfunction. Direct recordings of the sinus node electrogram have documented that SNRT is influenced by prolongation of sinoatrial conduction time (the time from the onset of the sinus impulse to the onset of activation of surrounding atrial myocardium), as well as by changes in sinus node automaticity, especially in the first beat after cessation of pacing. After cessation of pacing, the first return sinus cycle can be normal and can be followed by secondary pauses. Secondary pauses appear to be more common in patients whose sinus node dysfunction is caused by sinoatrial exit block (a potential cause of ECG sinus pauses). Finally, it is important to evaluate AV node and His-Purkinje function in patients with sinus node dysfunction, because many also exhibit impaired AV conduction.

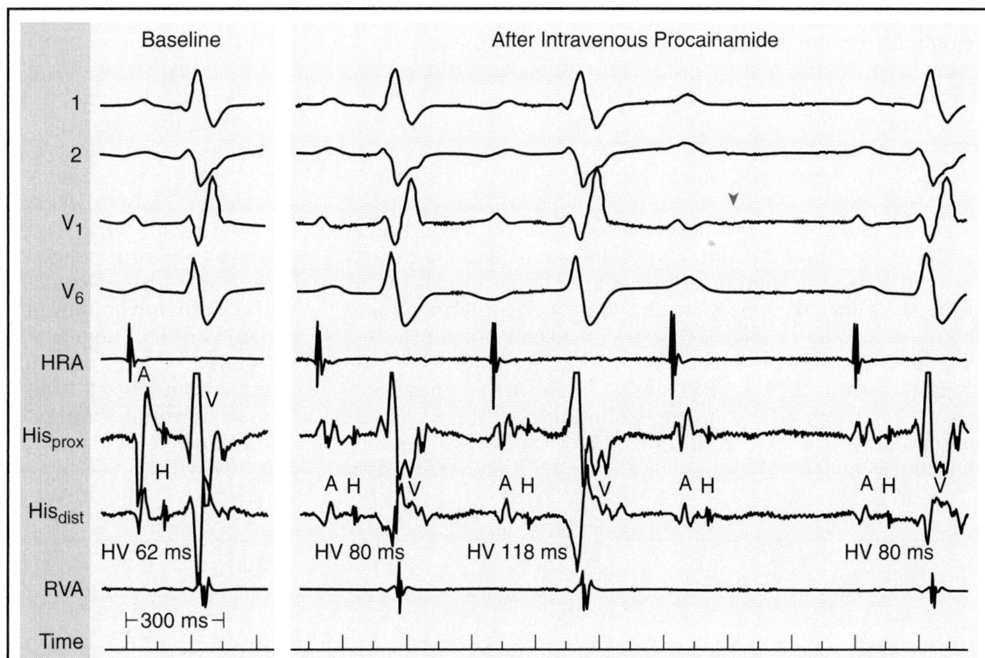

FIGURE 29–10 Testing the His-Purkinje system. A 43-year-old woman with sarcoid underwent electrophysiological study after a syncopal episode. Surface leads 1, 2, V_1, and V_6 are shown with intracardiac recordings from catheters in the high right atrium (HRA), proximal (His_{prox}), and distal (His_{dist}) electrode pairs of a catheter at the atrioventricular junction to record the His potential, and right ventricular apex (RVA). During baseline recording, the HV interval is only slightly prolonged (62 milliseconds). After infusion of intravenous procainamide, the HV interval is longer and infra-His Wenckebach block is present. Arrow denotes "missing" QRS complex due to infra-His block. A = atrial electrogram; H = His potential; V = ventricular electrogram.

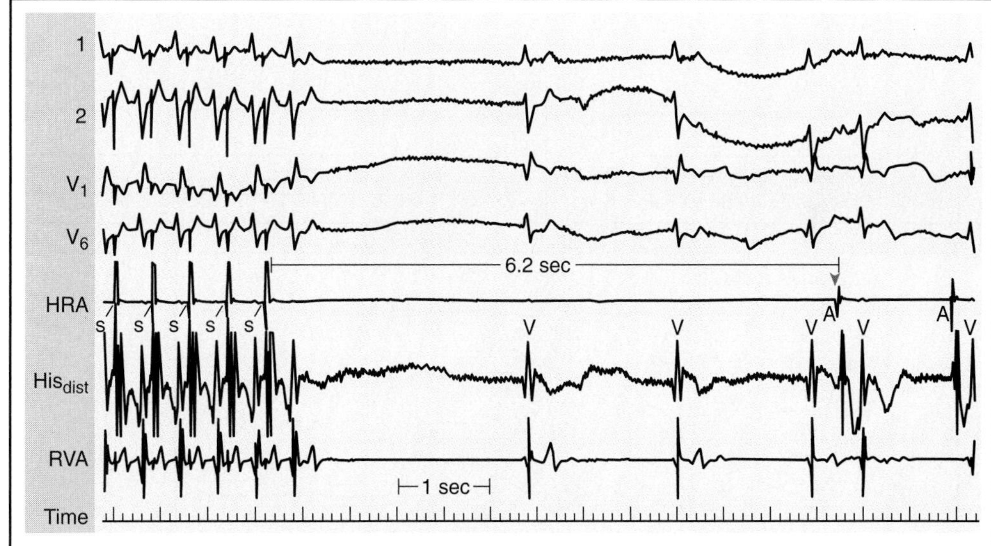

FIGURE 29–11 Abnormal sinus node function. Recordings are similar to those in Figure 23-3. The last five complexes of a 1-minute burst of atrial pacing (S) at a cycle length of 400 milliseconds are shown, after which pacing is stopped. The sinus node does not spontaneously discharge (sinus node recovery time) until 6.2 seconds later (arrow). Three junctional escape beats occurred before this time.

Sinoatrial Conduction Time. SACT can be estimated using simple pacing techniques based on the assumptions that (1) conduction times into and out of the sinus node are equal, (2) no depression of sinus node automaticity occurs, and (3) the pacemaker site does not shift after premature stimulation (see Chap. 32). These assumptions can be erroneous, particularly in patients with sinus node dysfunction. SACT can also be measured directly with extracellular electrodes placed in the region of the sinus node. This direct measurement correlates well with the SACT measured indirectly in patients with normal sinus node function. The sensitivity of the SACT and SNRT tests is only about 50 percent for each test alone and about 65 percent when combined. The specificity, when combined, is about 88 percent, with a low predictive value. Thus, if these tests are abnormal, the likelihood of the patient having sinus node dysfunction is great. However, normal results do not exclude the possibility of sinus node disease. Candidates for invasive EPS to evaluate sinus node function are symptomatic patients in whom sinus node dysfunction has not been established as a cause of the symptoms. Potential candidates are those requiring pacemakers to determine the pacing modality, patients with sinus node dysfunction to determine the mechanism and response to therapy, and patients in whom other causes of symptoms (e.g., tachyarrhythmias) are to be excluded.

TACHYCARDIA. In patients with tachycardias, an EPS can be used to diagnose the arrhythmia, determine and deliver therapy, determine the anatomical site(s) involved in the tachycardia, identify patients at high risk for developing serious arrhythmias, and gain insights into mechanisms responsible for the arrhythmia. The study can differentiate aberrant supraventricular conduction from ventricular tachyarrhythmias when standard ECG criteria fail to make the differentiation.

An SVT is recognized electrophysiologically by the presence of an HV interval equaling or exceeding that recorded during normal sinus rhythm (Fig. 29–12). In contrast, during VT, the HV interval is shorter than normal or the His deflection cannot be recorded clearly owing to superimposition of the larger ventricular electrogram. Only two situations exist when a consistently short HV interval occurs: during retrograde activation of the His bundle from activation originating in the ventricle (i.e., PVC or VT) or during conduction over an accessory pathway (preexcitation syndrome). Atrial pacing at rates exceeding the tachycardia rate can demonstrate the ventricular origin of the wide QRS tachycardia by producing fusion and capture beats and normalization of the HV interval. The only VT that exhibits an HV interval equal to or slightly exceeding the normal sinus HV interval is bundle branch reentry, but His activation will be in the retrograde direction.

An EPS should be considered (1) in patients who have symptomatic, recurrent, or drug-resistant supraventricular or ventricular tachyarrhythmias to help select optimal therapy; (2) in patients with tachyarrhythmias occurring too infrequently to permit adequate diagnostic or therapeutic assessment; (3) to differentiate SVT and aberrant conduction from VT; (4) whenever nonpharmacological therapy such as the use of electrical devices, catheter ablation, or surgery is contemplated; (5) in patients surviving an episode of cardiac arrest (occurring 48 hours after an acute myocardial infarction or without evidence of an acute Q-wave myocardial infarction); and (6) in assessing risk of sustained VT in patients with a prior myocardial infarction, ejection fraction

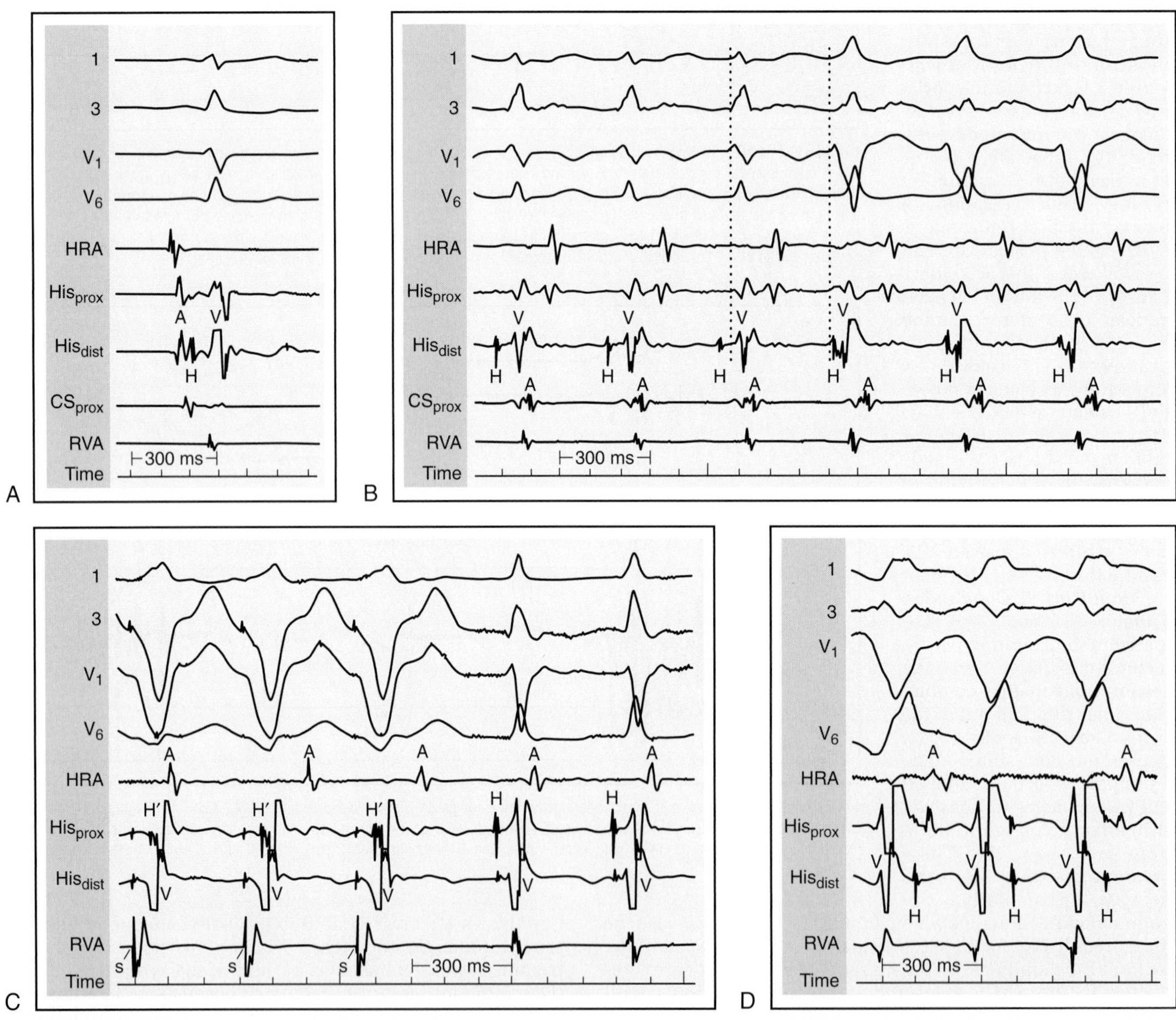

FIGURE 29–12 Bundle of His recordings in different situations similar to those in prior figures (see Figs. 29–10 and 29–11). **A,** Baseline sinus rhythm with normal atrioventricular (AV) conduction. **B,** Orthodromic supraventricular tachycardia with retrograde conduction over a left-sided accessory pathway throughout the tracing. The first three beats have a narrow QRS complex with a normal HV interval; the last three QRS complexes represent a fusion of conduction over the AV node-His and a slowly conducting right-sided accessory pathway. The His potential occurs after the onset of the wide QRS complex (dashed lines). In **C,** three paced ventricular beats are shown with a retrograde His potential (H′), followed by initiation of AV node reentrant supraventricular tachycardia (atrial depolarization near the end of the QRS complex, as seen in HRA tracing). **D,** Ventricular tachycardia with delayed activation of the His potential and complete retrograde AV node block (dissociated atrial complexes). CS_{prox} = proximal coronary sinus; His_{dis} = distal electrode pair; His_{prox} = proximal electrode pair; HRA = high right atrium; RVA = right ventricular apex.

of 0.3 to 0.4, and nonsustained VT on ECG.[37,38] Generally, EPS is not indicated in patients with long-QT syndrome and torsades de pointes.

The process of initiation and termination of SVT or VT with programmed electrical stimulation to test the potential efficacy of pharmacological, electrical, or surgical therapy represents an important application of EPS in patients with tachycardia. The role of drug therapy in clinically significant arrhythmias continues to diminish; although EPS was widely used at one time to predict the efficacy of drug therapy in suppressing spontaneous tachycardia recurrences, the technique is now rarely used for this purpose. Noninvasive stimulation from an implanted pacemaker or defibrillator can be used to test the effects of drug therapy given to try to decrease arrhythmia frequency.

UNEXPLAINED SYNCOPE (see Chap. 34)**.** The three common arrhythmic causes of syncope include sinus node dysfunction, AV block, and tachyarrhythmias. Of the three, tachyarrhythmias are most reliably initiated in the electrophysiology laboratory, followed by sinus node abnormalities and then His-Purkinje block.[39]

The cause of syncope remains uncertain in up to 50 percent of patients, depending in part on the extent of the evaluation. A careful, accurately performed history and physical examination begin the evaluation,[1] followed by noninvasive tests, including a 12-lead ECG, and can lead to a diagnosis in half or more of the patients.[40,41] A small percentage (<5 percent) of patients develops an arrhythmia coincident with syncope or presyncope during a 24-hour ECG recording, whereas a larger percentage (15 percent) have symptoms without an arrhythmia, excluding an arrhythmic cause. Prolonged ECG monitoring with patient-activated transtelephonic event recorders that have memory loops may increase the yield. Signal averaging has a high sensitivity (~75 percent) and specificity (~90 percent) for predicting patients with syncope in whom VT can be induced at EPS.[22] Tilt-table and stress testing can be useful in some patients, as can long-term ECG recordings.

The EPS helps explain the cause of syncope or palpitations when it induces an arrhythmia that replicates the patient's symptoms. Syncopal patients with a nondiagnostic EPS have a low incidence of sudden death and 80 percent remission rate. In those with recurrent syncope, the test is falsely negative in 20 percent, owing to failure to find AV block or sinus node dysfunction. On the other hand, in many patients with structural heart disease, several abnormalities that could account for syncope can be diagnosed at EPS. Deciding which among these abnormalities is responsible for syncope and therefore requires therapy can be difficult. Mortality and incidence of sudden cardiac death are mainly determined by the presence of underlying heart disease.[42]

Syncopal patients considered for EPS are those whose spells remain undiagnosed despite general, neurological, and noninvasive cardiac evaluation, particularly if the patient has structural heart disease. The diagnostic yield is about 70 percent in that group but only about 12 percent in patients without structural heart disease.[43] Therapy for a putative cause found during EPS prevents recurrence of syncope in about 80 percent of patients. Among arrhythmic causes of syncope, intermittent conduction disturbances are the most difficult to diagnose. EPS is poor at establishing this diagnosis despite an array of provocative tests that can be applied. When tachyarrhythmias have been thoroughly sought and excluded and the clinical suspicion of intermittent heart block is high (e.g., bundle branch block or long HV interval), empirical permanent pacing may be justified.

PALPITATIONS. An EPS is indicated in patients with palpitations who have had a pulse documented by medical personnel to be inappropriately rapid without ECG recording or in those suspected of having clinically significant palpitations without ECG documentation.

In patients with syncope or palpitations, the sensitivity of the EPS may be low but may be increased at the expense of specificity. For example, more aggressive pacing techniques (e.g., using three or four premature stimuli), administration of drugs (e.g., isoproterenol), or left ventricular pacing can increase the success rate of ventricular arrhythmia induction, but by precipitating nonclinical ventricular tachyarrhythmias such as nonsustained polymorphic or monomorphic VT or VF. Similarly, aggressive techniques during atrial pacing can induce nonspecific episodes of atrial flutter or atrial fibrillation. A diagnostic dilemma arises when the patient's clinical, symptom-producing arrhythmia is one of these nonspecific arrhythmias that can be produced in the normal patient who has no arrhythmia. In most patients, these arrhythmias are regarded as "nonclinical" (i.e., nonspecific responses to intense stimulation). In other patients, such as those with hypertrophic or dilated nonischemic cardiomyopathy, these may be clinically relevant arrhythmias. However, induction of sustained SVT (e.g., AV nodal reentry, AV reciprocating tachycardia) or monomorphic VT is never an artifact of intense stimulation. Initiation of these arrhythmias in patients who have not had known spontaneous episodes of these tachycardias is uncommon and provides important information that the induced tachyarrhythmia may be clinically significant and responsible for the patient's symptoms. Generally, other abnormalities, such as prolonged sinus pauses after overdrive atrial pacing or His-Purkinje AV block, are not induced in patients who do not or may not experience these abnormalities spontaneously. Induction of these arrhythmias has a high degree of specificity.

COMPLICATIONS OF ELECTROPHYSIOLOGICAL STUDIES. The risks of undergoing only an EPS are small. Because most procedures do not involve left-sided heart access, risk of stroke, systemic embolism, or myocardial infarction is less than that of coronary arteriography. Myocardial perforation with cardiac tamponade, pseudoaneurysms at arterial access sites, and provocation of nonclinical arrhythmias can occur, each with less than 1/500 incidence. Adding therapeutic maneuvers (e.g., ablation) to the procedure increases the incidence of complications. In a European survey[44] based on 4398 patients reported from 68 institutions, procedure-related complications ranged from 3.2 to 8 percent. Five deaths occurred within the perioperative period of the ablation. In a North American Society of Pacing and Electrophysiology (NASPE) survey[45] of 164 hospitals reporting in 1998 on more than 3300 patients who received radiofrequency ablation, complications ranged from 1 to 3 percent, with procedure-related deaths of about 0.2 percent. In a study of 1050 patients undergoing temperature-controlled ablation for supraventricular arrhythmias, 32 (3%) had a major complication. Predictors of major complications were ejection fraction less than 0.35 and multiple ablation targets.[46] The improvement in the complication rate probably reflects the learning curve for radiofrequency ablation. In many centers, diagnostic EPS and even ablation procedures are performed on an outpatient basis. With the increasing use of extensive ablation in the left atrium to treat atrial fibrillation, an increase in systemic thromboembolic complications may be observed.

DIRECT CARDIAC MAPPING: RECORDING POTENTIALS DIRECTLY FROM THE HEART

Cardiac mapping is a method whereby potentials recorded directly from the heart are spatially depicted as a function of time in an integrated manner (Fig. 29-13). The location of recording electrodes (epicardial, intramural, or endocardial) and the recording mode used (unipolar versus bipolar) as well as the method of display (isopotential versus isochronal maps) depend on the problem under consideration. Special electrodes can record monophasic action potentials.

Direct cardiac mapping by means of catheter electrodes (or, less commonly, at the time of cardiac surgery) can be used to identify and localize the areas responsible for rhythm disturbances in patients with

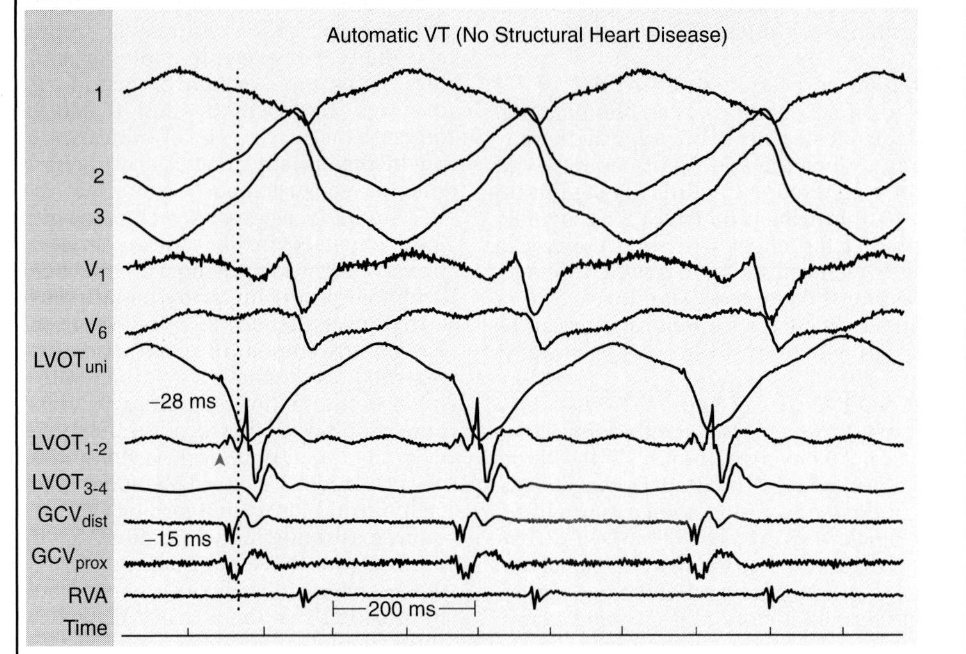

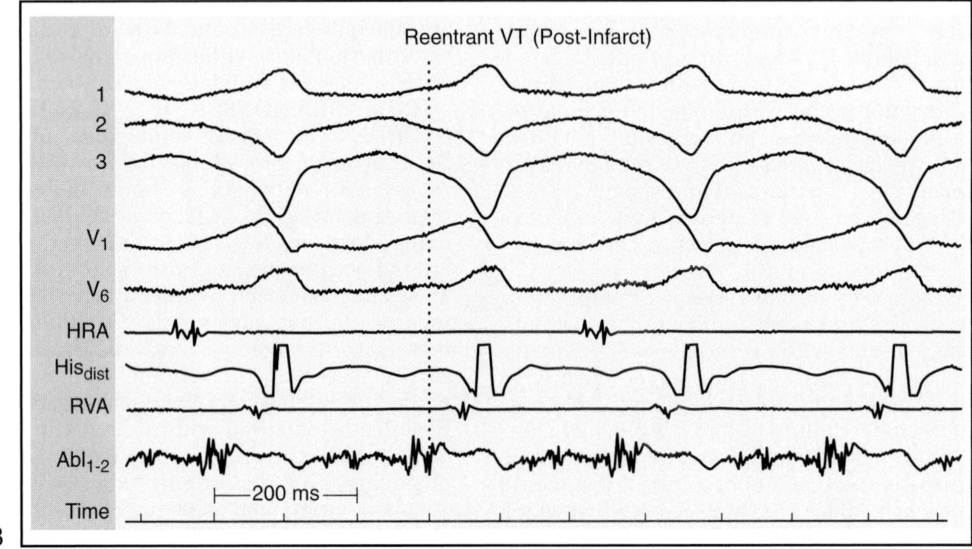

FIGURE 29–13 Endocardial catheter recordings during ventricular tachycardia (VT) in two patients. Dotted lines denote onset of QRS complexes. **A,** A woman without structural heart disease had a sustained VT arising from the left ventricular outflow tract (LVOT). Note unipolar (uni) electrogram with a sharp "QS" complex and the onset (arrow) distal bipolar recording ($LVOT_{1-2}$) preceding right ventricular recordings. They also precede recordings from a multielectrode catheter advanced along the coronary sinus and down the great cardiac vein (GCV_{dist} and GCV_{prox}) on the epicardial surface opposite the endocardial recording. Retrograde 1:1 conduction is present. Ablation at this site (LVOT) terminated the VT. **B,** A patient with reentrant VT due to a prior inferior wall infarction underwent mapping. The ablation catheter on the inferomedial wall shows a very prolonged, fragmented electrogram indicative of slow conduction. The electrogram spans all of the diastolic interval between QRS complexes. Ablation at this site eliminated the VT.

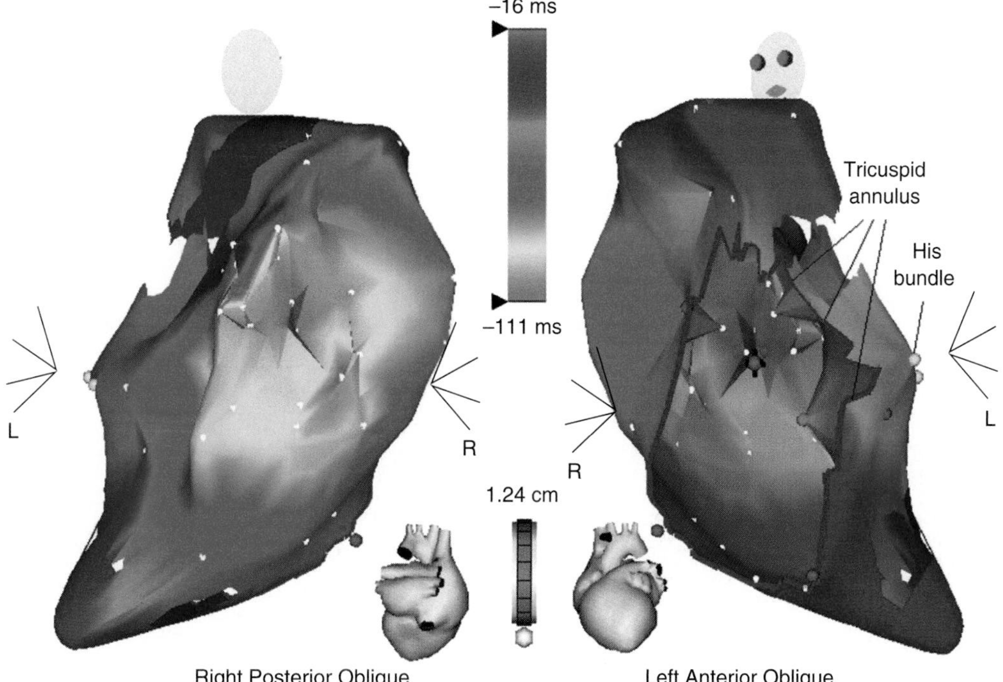

FIGURE 29–14 Electroanatomical map of focal atrial tachycardia. The right atrium is shown in two views (small gray icons at bottom center help with orientation). A color-coded time scale of activation is shown at top center; red indicates earliest activation, purple latest. A distance scale is below. This atrial tachycardia arose in the posterolateral right atrium (red spot) with all other areas activated centrifugally. Ablation at this site eliminated the tachycardia.

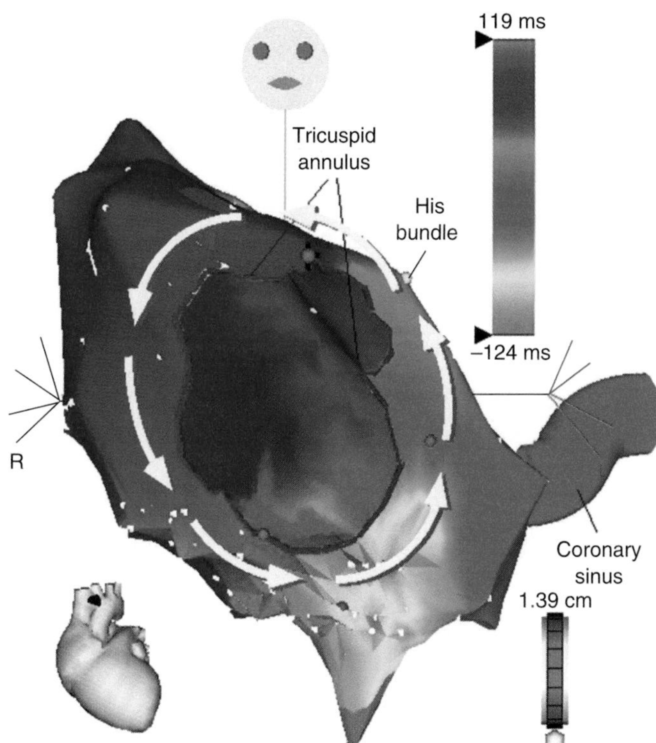

FIGURE 29–15 Electroanatomical map of reentrant atrial flutter. A left anterior oblique view of the right atrium is shown along with a depiction of the coronary sinus. See Figure 29-14 for other details. The electrical wave front propagates around the tricuspid annulus in a counterclockwise direction; in this complete circuit, "early" activation (in red) abuts "late" activation (purple) near the bottom of the tricuspid annulus. The cycle length of the tachycardia was 250 milliseconds, almost completely described by the points shown in the figure (from –124 to +119 milliseconds, a total of 243 milliseconds).

supraventricular and ventricular tachyarrhythmias for catheter or surgical ablation, isolation, or resection. Disorders amenable to this approach include accessory pathways associated with Wolff-Parkinson-White syndrome, the pathway(s) in AV node reentry, AV node/His bundle ablation, sites of origin of atrial tachycardia and VTs, isolated pathways essential for maintenance of reentrant atrial tachycardia or VTs, and various substrates responsible for episodes of atrial fibrillation. Mapping can also be used to delineate the anatomical course of the His bundle to avoid injury during open-heart surgery (usually for congenital heart surgery or septal accessory pathway ablation).

Early efforts at mapping involved moving an electrode from location to location, acquiring data from a single point at a time, and comparing the timing of local activation with some reference recording as well as other mapped sites. Obtaining enough data points to determine where ablation should be performed relied heavily on the memory of the operator. Specialized mapping systems have been developed that use computers to log not only the activation times at various points in the heart but the physical locations from which these were obtained.The mapping information thus acquired can be displayed on a screen showing relative activation times in a color-coded sequence. Using such systems, dozens or even hundreds of sites can be sampled relatively quickly, leading to a clear picture of cardiac activation and potential target sites for ablation (Figs. 29-14 and 29-15). Other mapping systems can acquire data from several thousand points simultaneously using a multipolar electrode array. This is particularly useful in hemodynamically unstable tachycardias or those that terminate spontaneously within just seconds, precluding detailed point-to-point mapping.

REFERENCES

1. Zipes DP, Miles WM: Assessment of the patient with a cardiac arrhythmia. *In* Zipes DP, Jalife J (eds): Cardiac Electrophysiology: From Cell to Bedside. 3rd ed. Philadelphia, WB Saunders, 1999, pp 706-709.
2. Barsky AJ: Palpitations, arrhythmias, and awareness of cardiac activity. Ann Intern Med 134:832-837, 2001.

Electrocardiogram

3. Miller JM, Rothman SA, Hsia HH, Buxton AE: Ventricular tachycardia versus supraventricular tachycardia: ECG recognition. *In* Zipes DP, Jalife J (eds): Cardiac Electrophysiology: From Cell to Bedside. 3rd ed. Philadelphia, WB Saunders, 1999, pp 696-705.

4. Lauer MR, Sung RJ: Exercise-induced cardiac arrhythmias. *In* Zipes DP, Jalife J (eds): Cardiac Electrophysiology: From Cell to Bedside. 3rd ed. Philadelphia, WB Saunders, 1999, pp 710-715.
5. Cole CR, Blackstone EH, Pashkow FJ, et al: Heart-rate recovery immediately after exercise as a predictor of mortality. N Engl J Med 341:1351-1357, 1999.
6. Frolkis JP, Pothier CE, Blackstone EH, Lauer MS: Frequent ventricular ectopy after exercise as a predictor of death. N Engl J Med 348:781-790, 2003.
7. Mason JW: A comparison of electrophysiologic testing with Holter monitoring to predict antiarrhythmic-drug effiicacy for ventricular tachyarrhythmias. Electrophysiologic Stud Versus Electrocardiographic Monitoring Investigators. N Engl J Med 329:445-451, 1993.
8. Crawford MH, Bernstein SJ, Deedwania PC, et al: ACC/AHA Guidelines for Ambulatory Electrocardiography: A report of the American College of Cardiology/American Heart Association Task Force on Practice Guidelines (Committee to Revise the Guidelines for Ambulatory Electrocardiography). Developed in collaboration with the North American Society for Pacing and Electrophysiology. J Am Coll Cardiol 34:912-948, 1999.
9. Kennedy HL: Use of long-term (Holter) electrocardiography recordings. *In* Zipes DP, Jalife J (eds): Cardiac Electrophysiology: From Cell to Bedside. 3rd ed. Philadelphia, WB Saunders, 1999, pp 716-729.
10. Investigators TC: Preliminary report: Effect of encainide and flecainide on mortality i a randomized trial of arrhythmia suppression after myocardial infarction. N Engl J Med 321:406-412, 1989.
11. Page RL, Tilsch TW, Connolly SJ, et al: Asymptomatic or "silent" atrial fiibrillation: Frquency in untreated patients and patients receiving azimilide. Circulation 107:1141-1145, 2003.
12. Zimetbaum PJ, Josephson ME: The evolving role of ambulatory arrhythmia monitoring in general clinical practice. Ann Intern Med 130:848-856, 1999.
13. Krahn AD, Klein GJ, Yee R, Manda V: The high cost of syncope: Cost implications of a new insertable loop recorder in the investigation of recurrent syncope. Am Heart J 137:870-877, 1999.

Heart Rate Variability

14. Stein PK: Assessing heart rate variability from real-world Holter reports. Card Electrophysiol Rev 6:239-244, 2002.
15. Karcz M, Chojnowska L, Zareba W, Ruzyllo W: Prognostic signifiicance of heart rate variability in dilated cardiomyopathy. Int J Cardiol 87:75-81, 2003.
16. Abildstrom SZ, Jensen BT, Agner E, et al: Heart rate versus heart rate variability in risk prediction after myocardial infarction. J Cardiovasc Electrophysiol 14:168-173, 2003.
17. Zabel M, Klingenheben T, Franz MR, Hohnloser SH: Assessment of QT dispersion for prediction of mortality or arrhythmic events after myocardial infarction: Results of a prospective, long-term follow-up study. Circulation 97:2543-2550, 1998.
18. Voon WC, Wu JC, Lai WT, Sheu SH: Seasonal variability of the QT dispersion in healthy subjects. J Electrocardiol 34:285-288, 2001.
19. Zabel M, Malik M: Predictive value of T-wave morphology variables and QT dispersion for postmyocardial infarction risk assessment. J Electrocardiol 34(Suppl):27-35, 2001.
20. Rautaharju PM: Why did QT dispersion die? Card Electrophysiol Rev 6:295-301, 2002.
21. Berbari EJ. High-resolution electrocardiography. *In* Zipes DP, Jalife J (eds): Cardiac Electrophysiology: From Cell to Bedside. 3rd ed. Philadelphia, WB Saunders, 1999, pp 730-736.
22. Kudaiberdieva G, Gorenek B, Goktekin O, et al: Combination of QT variability and signal-averaged electrocardiography in association with ventricular tachycardia in postinfarction patients. J Electrocardiol 36:17-24, 2003.

T Wave Alterans

23. Gold MR, Spencer W: T wave alternans for ventricular arrhythmia risk stratifiication Curr Opin Cardiol 18:1-5, 2003.
24. Rosenbaum DS: T wave alterans: A mechanism of arrhythmogenesis comes of age after 100 years. J Cardiovasc Electrophysiol 12:196-206, 2001.
25. Shimizu W, Antzelevitch C: Cellular and ionic basis for T wave alternans under long-QT conditions. Circulation 99:1499-1507, 1999.
26. Pruvot EJ, Rosenbaum DS: T wave alternans for risk stratifiication and prevention o sudden cardiac death. Curr Cardiol Rep 5:350-357, 2003.
27. Hohnloser SH, Klingenheben T, Bloomfiield D, et al: Usefulness of microvolt T wav alternans for prediction of ventricular tachyarrhythmic events in patients with dilated cardiomyopathy: Results from a prospective observational study. J Am Coll Cardiol 41:2220-2224, 2003.
28. Hoffmann J, Grimm W, Menz V, et al: Heart rate variability and baroreflex sensitivity i idiopathic dilated cardiomyopathy. Heart 83:531-538, 2000.
29. La Rovere MT, Pinna GD, Hohnloser SH, et al: Baroreflex sensitivity and heart rate variability in the identifiication of patients at risk for life-threatening arrhythmias: Implictions for clinical trials. Circulation 103:2072-2077, 2001.
30. Flowers NC, Horan LG: Body surface potential mapping. *In* Zipes DP, Jalife J (eds): Cardiac Electrophysiology: From Cell to Bedside. 3rd ed. Philadelphia, WB Saunders, 1999, pp 737-745.
31. Benditt DG: Head-up tilt-table testing: Rationale, methodology and applications. *In* Zipes DP, Jalife J (eds): Cardiac Electrophysiology: From Cell to Bedside. 3rd ed. Philadelphia, WB Saunders, 1999, pp 746-752.
32. Atiga W, Calkins H: Management of vasovagal syncope. J Cardiovasc Electrophysiol 10:874-886, 1999.
33. Connolly SJ, Sheldon R, Roberts RS, Gent M: The North American Vasovagal Pacemaker Study (VPS): A randomized trial of permanent cardiac pacing for the prevention of vasovagal syncope. J Am Coll Cardiol 33:16-20, 1999.
34. Shen WK, Low PA, Jahangir A, et al: Is sinus node modifiication appropriate for inappropriate sinus tachycardia with features of postural orthostatic tachycardia syndrome? Pacing Clin Electrophysiol 24:217-230, 2001.

Invasive Electrophysiological Studies

35. Zipes DP, DiMarco JP, Gillette PC, et al: Guidelines for clinical intracardiac electrophysiological and catheter ablation procedures: A report of the American College of Cardiology/American Heart Association Task Force on Practice Guidelines (Committee on Clinical Intracardiac Electrophysiologic and Catheter Ablation Procedures), developed in collaboration with the North American Society of Pacing and Electrophysiology. J Am Coll Cardiol 26:555-573, 1995.
36. Rardon DP, Miles WM, Zipes DP: Atrioventricular block and dissociation. *In* Zipes DP, Jalife J (eds): Cardiac Electrophysiology: From Cell to Bedside. 3rd ed. Philadelphia, WB Saunders, 1999, pp 451-458.
37. Moss AJ, Hall WJ, Cannom DS, et al: Improved survival with an implanted defiibrill-tor in patients with coronary disease at high risk for ventricular arrhythmias. N Engl J Med 335:1933-1940, 1996.
38. Buxton AE, Lee KL, Fisher JD, et al: A randomized study of the prevention of sudden death in patients with coronary artery disease. Multicenter Unsustained Tachycardia Trial Investigators. N Engl J Med 341:1882-1890, 1999.
39. Calkins H: Syncope. *In* Zipes DP, Jalife J (eds): Cardiac Electrophysiology: From Cell to Bedside. 3rd ed. Philadelphia, WB Saunders, 1999, pp 873-881.
40. Linzer M, Yang EH, Estes NA III, et al: Diagnosing syncope: I. Value of history, physical examination, and electrocardiography. Clinical Effiicacy Assessment Project of th American College of Physicians. Ann Intern Med 126:989-996, 1997.
41. Linzer M, Yang EH, Estes NA III, et al: Diagnosing syncope: II. Unexplained syncope. Clinical Effiicacy Assessment Project of the merican College of Physicians. Ann Intern Med 127:76-86, 1997.
42. Kapoor WN: Current evaluation and management of syncope. Circulation 106:1606-1609, 2002.
43. Goldschlager N, Epstein AE, Grubb BP, et al: Etiologic considerations in the patient with syncope and an apparently normal heart. Arch Intern Med 163:151-162, 2003.
44. Hindricks G: The Multicentre European Radiofrequency Survey (MERFS): Complications of radiofrequency catheter ablation of arrhythmias. The Multicentre European Radiofrequency Survey (MERFS) Investigators of the Working Group on Arrhythmias of the European Society of Cardiology. Eur Heart J 14:1644-1653, 1993.
45. Scheinman MM, Huang S: The 1998 NASPE Prospective Catheter Ablation Registry. Pacing Clin Electrophysiol 23:1020-1028, 2000.
46. Calkins H, Yong P, Miller JM, et al: Catheter ablation of accessory pathways, atrioventricular nodal reentrant tachycardia, and the atrioventricular junction: Final results of a prospective, multicenter clinical trial. The Atakr Multicenter Investigators Group. Circulation 99:262-270, 1999.

CHAPTER 30

Therapy for Cardiac Arrhythmias

John M. Miller • Douglas P. Zipes

The treatment of patients with cardiac arrhythmias has evolved dramatically in the last 40 years. In the mid-1960s, patients with bradyarrhythmias could be treated with bulky implantable pacemakers with a battery life less than 5 years and fixed-rate pacing; patients with tachyarrhythmias had a limited number of drugs as their only treatment option. In the late 1960s, surgical therapy—and the prospect for cure, not just suppression of tachyarrhythmias—became a reality. It was first applied to Wolff-Parkinson-White syndrome and then extended to other forms of supraventricular tachycardia (SVT) and ventricular tachycardia (VT). Catheter ablation (at first with direct current, delivered from an external defibrillator, and then with radiofrequency current) for cure of tachyarrhythmias was first performed in the 1980s and underwent refinement in subsequent decades. This form of therapy has largely replaced surgical and drug therapy for patients who need treatment for SVT and VT in the absence of structural heart disease and has employed other forms of energy as well. Finally, the implantable cardioverter-defibrillator (ICD) was also developed in the early 1980s and has become standard therapy for patients with serious ventricular arrhythmias in the presence of structural heart disease. Some patients require a combination of these forms of treatment ("hybrid" therapy, such as an ICD and antiarrhythmic drugs or surgery and an ICD).[1] Drug therapy of arrhythmias, at one time the only option, now plays a supporting role in most cases.

Pharmacological Therapy

Principles of clinical pharmacokinetics and pharmacodynamics are covered in Chapter 5.

General Considerations Regarding Antiarrhythmic Drugs

Most of the available antiarrhythmic drugs (Table 30–1) can be classified according to whether they exert blocking actions predominantly on sodium, potassium, or calcium channels and whether they block beta adrenoceptors. The commonly used Vaughan Williams classification is limited because it is based on the electrophysiological effects exerted by an arbitrary concentration of the drug, generally on normal cardiac tissue. Actually, the actions of these drugs are quite complex and depend on tissue type, species, the degree of acute or chronic damage, heart rate, membrane potential, the ionic composition of the extracellular milieu, age (see Chap. 72), and other factors (see Table 30–1). Many drugs exhibit actions that belong in multiple categories or operate indirectly, such as by altering hemodynamics, myocardial metabolism, or autonomic neural transmission. Some drugs have active metabolites that exert effects different from those produced by the parent compound. Not all drugs in the same class have identical effects (e.g., bretylium, sotalol, and amiodarone). Whereas all class III agents are dramatically different, some drugs in different classes have overlapping actions (e.g., classes IA and IC drugs). In vitro studies on healthy fibers usually establish the properties of antiarrhythmic agents rather than their actual antiarrhythmic properties.

Despite these limitations, the Vaughan Williams classification[2] is widely known and provides a useful communication shorthand. It is listed here, but the reader is cautioned that drug actions are more complex than those depicted by the classification. A more realistic view of antiarrhythmic agents is provided by the "Sicilian gambit."[3] This approach to drug classification is an attempt to identify the mechanisms of a particular arrhythmia, determine the vulnerable parameter of the arrhythmia most susceptible to modification, define the target most likely to affect the vulnerable parameter, and then select a drug that will modify the target. This concept provides a framework in which to consider antiarrhythmic drugs (Table 30–2; see Table 30–1).[4]

DRUG CLASSIFICATION (Table 30–3). According to the Vaughan Williams classification, class I drugs predominantly block the fast sodium channel (they can also block potassium channels). They, in turn, are divided into three subgroups:

TABLE 30–1 Actions of Drugs Used in Treatment of Arrhythmias

Drug	Channels: Na* Fast	Med	Slow	Ca	K_r	K_s	Receptors: α	β	M_2	P	Pumps: Na^+, K^+-ATPase	Clinical Effects: LV Function	Sinus Rate	Extracardiac
Quinidine		●A			⊙		○		○			—	↑	⊙
Procainamide		●A			⊙							↓	—	⊙
Disopyramide		●A			⊙				○			↓	—	●
Lidocaine	○											—	—↓	○
Mexiletine	○											—	—	○
Phenytoin	○											—	—	⊙
Flecainide			●A		○							↓	—	○
Propafenone		●A			○			⊙				↓	↓	○
Moricizine	●I											↓	—	○
Propranolol	○							●				↓	↓	○
Nadolol								●				↓	↓	○
Amiodarone	○			⊙	●	⊙	⊙	⊙				—	↓	●
Bretylium					●		⊡	⊡				—	↓	○
Sotalol					●			●				↓	↓	○
Ibutilide					○							—	↓	○
Dofetilide					●							—	—	○
Azimilide					⊙	⊙	○					—	—	○
Verapamil	○			●			⊙					↓	↓	○
Diltiazem				⊙								↓	↓	○
Adenosine										□		—	↓	⊙
Digoxin									○		●	↑	↓	⊙
Atropine									●			—	↑	⊙

Relative potency of blockade or extracardiac side effect: ○ = low; ⊙ = moderate; ● = high. □ = agonist; ⊡ = agonist-antagonist; A = activated state blocker; I = inactivated state blocker; — = minimal effect; ↑ = increase; ↓ = decrease; K_r = rapid component of delayed rectifier K^+ current; K_s = slow component of delayed rectifier K^+ current; M_2 = muscarinic receptor subtype 2; P = A_1 purinergic receptor.
Adapted from Schwartz PJ, Zaza A: Eur Heart J 13:26, 1992. Copyright © 1992, reproduced by permission of Elsevier.
*Fast, med (medium), and slow refer to kinetics of recovery from sodium channel blockade.

Class IA. Drugs that reduce $\dot{V}_{max}$ (rate of rise of action potential upstroke [phase 0]) and prolong action potential duration (see Chap. 77): quinidine, procainamide, disopyramide; kinetics of onset and offset in blocking the Na^+ channel are of intermediate rapidity (<5 seconds).

Class IB. Drugs that do not reduce $\dot{V}_{max}$ and that shorten action potential duration: mexiletine, phenytoin, and lidocaine; fast onset and offset kinetics (<500 milliseconds).

Class IC. Drugs that reduce $\dot{V}_{max}$, primarily slow conduction, and can prolong refractoriness minimally: flecainide, propafenone, and moricizine; slow onset and offset kinetics (10 to 20 seconds).

Class II. Drugs that block beta-adrenergic receptors and include propranolol, timolol, metoprolol, and others.

Class III. Drugs that predominantly block potassium channels (such as I_{Kr}) and prolong repolarization. They include sotalol, amiodarone, and bretylium.

Class IV. Drugs that predominantly block the slow calcium channel ($I_{Ca\text{-}L}$) and include verapamil, diltiazem, nifedipine, and others (felodipine blocks $I_{Ca\text{-}T}$).

A newer model suggests that antiarrhythmic drugs cross the cell membrane and interact with receptors in the membrane channels when the latter are in the rested, activated, or inactivated state (see Table 30–1) and that each of these interactions is characterized by different association and dissociation rate constants. Such interactions are voltage and time dependent. Transitions among rested, activated, and inactivated states are governed by standard Hodgkin-Huxley-type equations. When the drug is bound (associated) to a receptor site at or very close to the ionic channel (the drug probably does not actually "plug" the channel), the latter cannot conduct, even in the activated state.

USE-DEPENDENCE. Some drugs exert greater inhibitory effects on the upstroke of the action potential at more rapid rates of stimulation and after longer periods of stimulation, a characteristic called use-dependence. Use-dependence means that depression of $\dot{V}_{max}$, is greater after the channel has been "used" (i.e., after action potential depolarization rather than after a rest period). It is possible that this use-dependence results from preferential interaction of the antiarrhythmic drug with either the open or the inactive channel, and there is little interaction with the resting channels of the unstimulated cell. Agents in class IB exhibit fast kinetics of onset and offset or use-dependent block of the fast channel; that is, they bind and dissociate quickly from the receptors. Class IC drugs have slow kinetics, and class IA drugs are intermediate. With increased time spent in diastole (slower rate), a greater proportion of receptors become drug free, and the drug exerts less effect. Cells with reduced membrane potentials recover more slowly from drug actions than cells with more negative membrane potentials.

REVERSE USE-DEPENDENCE. Some drugs exert greater effects at slow rates than at fast rates, a property known as reverse use-dependence. This is particularly true for drugs that lengthen repolariza-

TABLE 30–2 Classification of Drug Actions on Arrhythmias Based on Modification of Vulnerable Parameter

Mechanism	Arrhythmia	Vulnerable Parameter (Effect)	Drugs (Effect)
Automaticity			
Enhanced normal	Inappropriate sinus tachycardia Some idiopathic ventricular tachycardias	Phase 4 depolarization (decrease)	Beta-adrenergic blocking agents Na^+ channel blocking agents
Abnormal	Atrial tachycardia	Maximum diastolic potential (hyperpolarization) Phase 4 depolarization (decrease)	M_2 agonist Ca^{2+} or Na^+ channel blocking agents M_2 agonist
	Accelerated idioventricular rhythms	Phase 4 depolarization (decrease)	Ca^{2+} or Na^+ channel blocking agents
Triggered activity			
EAD	Torsades de pointes	Action potential duration (shorten) EAD (suppress)	Beta-adrenergic agonists; vagolytic agents (increase rate) Ca^{2+} channel blocking agents; Mg^{2+}; beta-adrenergic blocking agents
DAD	Digitalis-induced arrhythmias	Calcium overload (unload) DAD (suppress)	Ca^{2+} channel blocking agents Na^+ channel blocking agents
	RV outflow tract ventricular tachycardia	Calcium overload (unload) DAD (suppress)	Beta-adrenergic blocking agents Ca^{2+} channel blocking agents; adenosine
Reentry—Na^+ channel dependent			
Long excitable gap	Typical atrial flutter	Conduction and excitability (depress)	Type IA, IC Na^+ channel blocking agents
	Circus movement tachycardia in WPW	Conduction and excitability (depress)	Type IA, IC Na^+ channel blocking agents
	Sustained uniform ventricular tachycardia	Conduction and excitability (depress)	Na^+ channel blocking agents
Short excitable gap	Atypical atrial flutter	Refractory period (prolong)	K^+ channel blocking agents
	Atrial fibrillation	Refractory period (prolong)	K^+ channel blocking agents
	Circus movement tachycardia in WPW	Refractory period (prolong)	Amiodarone, sotalol
	Polymorphic and uniform ventricular tachycardia	Refractory period (prolong)	Type IA Na^+ channel blocking agents
	Bundle branch reentry	Refractory period (prolong)	Type IA Na^+ channel blocking agents;
	Ventricular fibrillation	Refractory period (prolong)	bretylium
Reentry—Ca^{2+} channel dependent			
	AV nodal reentrant tachycardia	Conduction and excitability (depress)	Ca^{2+} channel blocking agents
	Circus movement tachycardia in WPW	Conduction and excitability (depress)	Ca^{2+} channel blocking agents
	Verapamil-sensitive ventricular tachycardia	Conduction and excitability (depress)	Ca^{2+} channel blocking agents

AV = atrioventricular; DAD = delayed afterdepolarization; EAD = early afterdepolarization; RV = right ventricular; WPW = Wolff-Parkinson-White.

Data from Task Force of the Working Group on Arrhythmias of the European Society of Cardiology: The Sicilian gambit: A new approach to the classification of antiarrhythmic drugs based on their actions on arrhythmogenic mechanisms. Circulation 84:1831, 1991. Copyright 1991, American Heart Association.

tion. The QT interval becomes prolonged more at slow than fast rates. This effect is opposite to what the ideal antiarrhythmic agent would do because prolongation of refractoriness should be increased at fast rates so as to interrupt or prevent a tachycardia and should be minimal at slow rates to avoid precipitating torsades de pointes.

MECHANISMS OF ARRHYTHMIA SUPPRESSION (see Table 30–2). Given the fact that enhanced automaticity, triggered activity, or reentry can cause cardiac arrhythmias (see Chaps. 27 and 32), mechanisms by which antiarrhythmic agents suppress arrhythmias can be postulated. Antiarrhythmic agents can slow the spontaneous discharge frequency of an automatic pacemaker by depressing the slope of diastolic depolarization, shifting the threshold voltage toward zero, or hyperpolarizing the resting membrane potential. Mechanisms by which different drugs suppress normal or abnormal automaticity may not be the same. In general, however, most antiarrhythmic agents in therapeutic doses depress the automatic firing rate of spontaneously discharging ectopic sites while minimally affecting the discharge rate of the normal sinus node. Slow-channel blockers such as verapamil, beta blockers such as propranolol, and some antiarrhythmic agents such as amiodarone also depress spontaneous discharge of the sinus node, whereas drugs that exert vagolytic effects, such as disopyramide or quinidine, can increase the sinus discharge rate. Drugs can also suppress early or delayed afterdepolarizations and eliminate triggered arrhythmias related to these mechanisms.

As mentioned earlier, reentry depends critically on the timing interrelationships between refractoriness and conduction velocity, the presence of unidirectional block in one of the pathways, and other factors that influence refractoriness and conduction, such as excitability. An antiarrhythmic agent can stop reentry that is already present or prevent it from starting if the drug improves or depresses conduction. For example, improved conduction can (1) eliminate the unidirectional block so that reentry cannot begin or (2) facilitate conduction in the reentrant loop so that the returning wave front reenters too quickly, encroaches on fibers that are still refractory, and extinguishes. A drug that depresses conduction can transform the unidirectional block to a bidirectional block and thus terminate reentry or prevent it from

TABLE 30–3 In Vitro Electrophysiological Characteristics of Antiarrhythmic Drugs

Drug	APA	APD	dV/dt	MDP	ERP	CV	PF Phase 4	SN Auto	Memb Res	ET	VFT	Contr	SI Curr	Autonomic Nervous System	Local Anesth.
Quinidine	↓	↑	↓	0	↑	↓	↓	0	↓	↑	↑	0	0	Antivagal; alpha blocker	Yes
Procainamide	↓	↑	↓	0	↑	↓	↓	0	↓	↑	↑	0	0	Slight antivagal	Yes
Disopyramide	↓	↑	↓	0	↑	↓	↓	↓ 0 ↑	↓	↑	↑	↓	0	Central: antivagal, antisympathetic	Yes
Lidocaine	0 ↓	↓	0 ↓	0	↓	0 ↓	↓	0	0 ↓	0 ↑	↑	0	0	0	Yes
Mexiletine	0	↓	0 ↓	0	↓	↓	↓	0	↓	↑	↑	↓	0	0	Yes
Phenytoin	0	↓	↓ 0 ↑	0	↓	0	↓	0	0 ↑	0			0	0	No
Flecainide	↓	0 ↑	↓	0	↑	↓↓	↓	0	↓			↓	0	0	Yes
Propafenone	↓	0 ↑	↓	0	↑	↓↓	↓	0	↓	↑	↑	↓	0 ↓	Antisympathetic	Yes
Moricizine	↓	↓	↓	0	↓	↓	0	0	↓	↑	0		0	0	No
Propranolol	0 ↓	0 ↓	0 ↓	0	↓	0	↓*	↓	↓			↓	0 ↓	Antisympathetic	No
Amiodarone	0	↑	0 ↓	0	↑	↓	↓	↓	0	0	↑	0 ↑	0	Antisympathetic	Yes
Bretylium	0	↑	0	0	↑	0	0 ↓*	0 ↓	0 ↑	0	0 ↑	↓	0	Antisympathetic	Yes
Sotalol	0 ↓	↑	0 ↓	0	↑	0	0 ↓	↓	0 ↓	0	0	↓	0 ↓	Antisympathetic	No
Ibutilide	0	↑	0	0	↑	0	0	↓	0	0		0	0	0	No
Dofetilide	0	↑	0	0	↑	0	0	0	0	0		0	0	0	No
Azimilide	0	↑	0	0	↑	0	0	0	0	0		0	0	0	No
Verapamil	0	↓	0	0	0	0	↓*	↓	0	0	0	↓	↓↓	? Block alpha receptors; enhance vagal	Yes
Adenosine	0	↑	0 ↓	0	↑	0	0 ↓	↓	0	0	0	0	↓	Vagomimetic	No

APA = action potential amplitude; APD = action potential duration; dV/dt = rate of rise of action potential; MDP = maximum diastolic potential; ERP = effective refractory period (longest S_1-S_2 interval at which S_2 fails to produce a response); CV = conduction velocity; PF = Purkinje fiber; SN Auto = sinus nodal automaticity; Memb Res = membrane responsiveness; ET = excitability threshold; VFT = ventricular fibrillation threshold; Contr = contractility; SI Curr = slow inward current; Local Anesth. = local anesthetic effect.

*With a background of sympathetic activity.

occurring by creating an area of complete block in the reentrant pathway. Conversely, a drug that slows conduction without producing block or lengthening refractoriness significantly can promote reentry. Finally, most antiarrhythmic agents share the ability to prolong refractoriness relative to their effects on action potential duration (APD); that is, the ratio of effective refractory period (ERP) to APD exceeds 1.0. If a drug prolongs refractoriness of fibers in the reentrant pathway, the pathway may not recover excitability in time to be depolarized by the reentering impulse and the reentrant propagation ceases. The different types of reentry (see Chap. 27) influence the effects and effectiveness of a drug.

When considering the properties of a drug, it is important that the situation or model, or both, from which conclusions are drawn be defined with care. Electrophysiological, hemodynamic, autonomic, pharmacokinetic, and adverse effects may all differ in normal subjects compared with patients, in normal tissue compared with abnormal tissue, in cardiac muscle compared with specialized conduction fibers, in atrium as opposed to ventricular muscle, and in different species (Table 30–4).

STEREOSELECTIVITY. Drug interactions with a channel, receptor, or enzyme may depend on the three-dimensional geometry of the drug. Many drugs have stereoisomers (molecules with the same atomic composition but different spatial arrangement) that can influence drug effects, metabolism, binding, clearance, and excretion. Most drugs of this type are prescribed as 50:50 mixtures of their two forms (racemates), which may make 50 percent of the dose ineffective for some drugs. Except for timolol, virtually all beta blockers are racemates. *d*-Propranolol exerts antiarrhythmic actions unrelated to beta adrenoceptor blockade, whereas *l*-propranolol blocks the beta receptor. Both enantiomers (mirror images) of sotalol block the potassium channel to prolong APD and suppress arrhythmias equally, but *d*-sotalol does not block the beta adrenoceptor and, alone, can be arrhythmogenic. Racemic propafenone exhibits beta-blocking actions related to the *S* enantiomer. Other drugs with notable stereoselective differences include disopyramide, with one form (*S* [+]) prolonging repolarization and having greater antiarrhythmic effects than *R* (−), which shortens repolarization. The latter form has fewer anticholinergic effects. The (−) enantiomer of verapamil exerts much more negative inotropic and dromotropic effects than the (+) form and may have more potent antiarrhythmic actions. Stereoselectivity affects sodium channel blocking drugs less than it affects beta adrenoceptor, potassium, and calcium blockers.

DRUG METABOLITES. Drug metabolites may add to or alter the effects of the parent compound by exerting similar actions, competing with the parent compound, or mediating drug toxicity. Quinidine has at least four active metabolites but none with a potency exceeding that of the parent drug and none preliminarily implicated in causing torsades de pointes. About 50 percent of procainamide is metabolized to *N*-acetylprocainamide (NAPA). Only the parent drug blocks cardiac sodium channels and slows impulse propagation in the His-Purkinje system. NAPA prolongs repolarization and is a less effective antiarrhythmic drug but competes with procainamide for renotubular secretory sites and can increase the parent drug's elimination half-life. Lidocaine's metabolite can compete with lidocaine for sodium channels and partially reverse block produced by lidocaine.

PHARMACOGENETICS (see Chap. 5). Genetically determined metabolic pathways account for many of the differences in patients' responses to some drugs. The genetically determined activity of hepatic *N*-acetyltransferase regulates the development of antinuclear antibodies and development of the lupus syndrome in response to procainamide. Slow acetylator phenotypes appear more prone to develop lupus than rapid acetylators. About 7 percent of subjects lack debrisoquin 4-hydroxylase. This enzyme (termed $P450_{dbl}$) is needed to metabolize debrisoquin (an antihypertensive drug) and propafenone, to hydroxylate several beta blockers, and to biotransform flecainide. Lack of this enzyme reduces metabolism of the parent compound, leading to increased plasma concentrations of the parent drug and reduced concentrations of metabolites. Propafenone is metabolized by this enzyme to a compound with slightly less antiarrhythmic and beta-adrenergic blocking effects as well as fewer central nervous system side effects. Thus, poor metabolizers may experience more heart rate slowing and neurotoxicity than extensive metabolizers. Quinidine in low doses can inhibit this enzyme and thereby alter concentrations of the drugs and metabolites given in combination that are affected by the $P450_{dbl}$ enzyme, such as propafenone or flecainide.

Understanding stereoselectivity and pharmacogenetics can provide major clues to understanding differences in drug efficacy and toxicity from one patient to the next. Cimetidine and ranitidine also affect drug metabolism, probably by inhibiting hepatic P450-metabolizing enzymes. Other commonly used noncardiovascular medications affect this important metabolic pathway. Drugs such as rifampin, phenobarbital, and phenytoin induce synthesis of larger amounts of cytochrome $P450_{dbl}$, leading to lower concentrations of parent drugs that are extensively metabolized, whereas erythromycin, clarithromycin, fluoxetine, and grapefruit juice inhibit enzyme activity, leading to accumulation of the parent compound. This effect is thought to explain why cisapride, an agent that had been used to increase gastric motility, could cause QT interval prolongation and torsades de pointes in isolated cases. Cisapride blocked the delayed rectifier current I_{Kr} but did not prolong the QT interval significantly in the majority of patients, presumably owing to extensive metabolism. In patients who take an inhibitor of cytochrome P450 (such as erythromycin) along with cisapride, the latter drug can accumulate, leading to QT prolongation and torsades de pointes.

SIDE EFFECTS. Antiarrhythmic drugs produce one group of side effects related to excessive dosage and plasma concentrations, resulting in both noncardiac (e.g., neurological defects) and cardiac (e.g., heart failure, some arrhythmias) toxicity, and another group of side effects unrelated to plasma concentrations, which is termed idiosyncratic. Examples of the latter include procainamide-induced lupus syndrome and some arrhythmias such as quinidine-induced torsades de pointes. The latter phenomenon can occur in individuals with a "forme fruste" of the long QT syndrome (i.e., normal QT interval at rest but markedly prolonged interval in the presence of certain medications).[5] In the future, it is likely that genetic differences will explain many "idiosyncratic" reactions.[6-11]

Proarrhythmia. Drug-induced or drug-exacerbated cardiac arrhythmias (proarrhythmia) constitute a major clinical problem.[12] Proarrhythmia can be manifested as an increase in frequency of a preexisting arrhythmia, sustaining of a previously nonsustained arrhythmia (even making it incessant), or development of arrhythmias the patient has not previously experienced. Electrophysiological mechanisms are probably related to prolongation of repolarization, the development of early afterdepolarizations to cause torsades de pointes, and alterations in reentry pathways to initiate or sustain ventricular tachyarrhythmias. Proarrhythmic events can occur in as many as 5 to 10 percent of patients receiving antiarrhythmic agents. Heart failure increases proarrhythmic risk. Patients with atrial fibrillation treated with antiarrhythmic agents had a relative risk of cardiac death of 4.7 if they had a history of heart failure compared with patients not so treated, who had a relative risk of arrhythmic death of 3.7. Patients without a history of congestive heart failure had no increased risk of cardiac mortality during antiarrhythmic drug treatment.[13] Reduced left ventricular function, treatment with digitalis and diuretics, and longer pretreatment QT interval characterize patients who experience drug-induced ventricular fibrillation (VF). The more commonly known proarrhythmic events occur within several days of beginning drug therapy or changing dosage and are represented by such developments as incessant VT, long QT syndrome, and torsades de pointes. However, in the Cardiac Arrhythmia Suppression Trial (CAST),[14] researchers found that encainide and flecainide reduced spontaneous ventricular arrhythmias but were associated with a total mortality of 7.7 percent, in comparison with 3.0 percent in the group receiving placebo. Deaths were equally distributed throughout the treatment period, raising the important consideration that another kind of proarrhythmic response can occur some time after the beginning of drug therapy. Such late proarrhythmic effects may be related to drug-induced exacerbation of regional myocardial conduction delay caused by ischemia and heterogeneous drug concentrations that can promote reentry. Moricizine also increased mortality, leading to termination of CAST II.

Until the 1970s, when separate surgical treatments were developed to treat Wolff-Parkinson-White syndrome and VT (see later), antiarrhythmic drugs were the only form of treatment for patients with tachyarrhythmias. The availability of catheter ablation (see later) and ICDs (see Chap. 31) to treat a wide variety of arrhythmias has relegated drug therapy to a secondary role. Drugs are still useful to prevent or decrease frequency of recurrences in patients who have relatively infrequent episodes of benign tachycardias, those who have had incomplete success with catheter ablation procedures, and patients with an ICD who have frequent episodes of ventricular arrhythmia resulting in shocks.

Class IA Antiarrhythmic Agents

Quinidine

Quinidine and quinine are isomeric alkaloids isolated from cinchona bark. Although quinidine shares the antimalarial, antipyretic, and vagolytic actions of quinine, the latter lacks the significant electrophysiological and antiarrhythmic effects of quinidine.

ELECTROPHYSIOLOGICAL ACTIONS (Table 30-5; see Tables 30-1, 30-2, and 30-3). Quinidine exerts little effect on automaticity of the isolated or denervated normal sinus node but suppresses automaticity in normal Purkinje fibers, especially in ectopic pacemakers, by decreasing the slope of phase 4 diastolic depolarization and shifting the threshold voltage toward zero. In patients with the sick sinus syndrome, quinidine can depress sinus node automaticity. It does not affect abnormal automaticity in partially depolarized Purkinje fibers. Quinidine produces early afterdepolarizations in experimental preparations and in humans, which may be responsible for torsades de pointes.[15] Because of its significant anticholinergic effect and reflex sympathetic stimulation resulting from alpha-adrenergic blockade that causes peripheral vasodilation, quinidine can increase sinus node discharge rate and can improve atrioventricular (AV) nodal conduction. Direct myocardial effects can prolong AV nodal and His-Purkinje conduction times and refractoriness in an AV accessory pathway. Quinidine slightly prolongs the APD of atrial and ventricular muscle and Purkinje fibers while also prolonging the ERP without significantly changing resting membrane potential. Prolongation of repolarization is more prominent at slow heart rates (reverse use-dependence) owing to block of I_{Kr}. Action potential amplitude, overshoot, and $\dot{V}_{max}$ of phase 0 are reduced, more so during ischemia, hypoxia, and in partially depolarized fibers, especially at fast rates. The open channel has a high affinity for quinidine, resulting in block of a fraction of sodium channels with each action potential upstroke. The time for unblocking by class IA drugs (about 4 seconds) is longer than for class IB drugs but shorter than for class IC drugs. For the duration of the plateau of the action potential (inactivated state) or in depolarized fibers, the rate of unblocking is slow, but it is much faster in polarized fibers. Therefore, faster rates result in more block of sodium channels and less unblocking because of a smaller percentage of time spent in a polarized state (use-dependence). Isoproterenol can modulate the effects of quinidine on reentrant circuits in humans. Quinidine's effect on I_{to} (but not I_K) varies according to the patient's age and may account for its lower efficacy in children than adults.

TABLE 30–4 Clinical Usage Information for Antiarrhythmic Agents*

Drug	Usual Dosage Ranges: Intravenous (mg) Loading	Intravenous (mg) Maintenance	Oral (mg) Loading	Oral (mg) Maintenance
Quinidine	6 to 10 mg/kg at 0.3 to 0.5 mg/kg/min	—	800 to 1000	300 to 600 q6hr
Procainamide	6 to 13 mg/kg at 0.2 to 0.5 mg/kg/min	2 to 6 mg/min	500 to 1000	250 to 1000 q4-6hr
Disopyramide	1 to 2 mg/kg over 15 to 45 min‡	1 mg/kg/hr		100 to 300 q6-8hr
Lidocaine	1 to 3 mg/kg at 20 to 50 mg/min	1 to 4 mg/min	N/A	N/A
Mexiletine	500 mg‡	0.5 to 1.0 gm/24 hr	400 to 600	150 to 300 q8-12hr
Phenytoin	100 mg q5min for ≤1000 mg		1000	100 to 400 q12-24hr
Flecainide	2 mg/kg‡	100 to 200 q12hr		50 to 200 q12hr
Propafenone	1 to 2 mg/kg‡		600 to 900	150 to 300 q8-12hr
Moricizine	N/A	N/A	300	100 to 400 q8hr
Propranolol	0.25 to 0.5 mg q5min to ≤0.20 mg/kg			10 to 200 q6-8hr
Amiodarone	15 mg/min for 10 min, 1 mg/min for 3 hr, 0.5 mg/min thereafter	1 mg/min	800 to 1600 qd for 7-14 days	200 to 600 qd
Bretylium	5 to 10 mg/kg at 1 to 2 mg/kg/min	0.5 to 2 mg/min	N/A	4 mg/kg/d
Sotalol	10 mg over 1 to 2 min‡			80 to 320 q12hr
Ibutilide	1 mg over 10 min	N/A	N/A	N/A
Dofetilide	2 to 5 µg/kg infusion‡	N/A	N/A	0.125 to 0.5 q12hr
Azimilide	N/A	N/A	N/A	100 to 200 qd
Verapamil	5 to 10 mg over 1 to 2 min	0.005 mg/kg/min		80 to 120 q6-8hr
Adenosine	6 to 18 mg (rapidly)	N/A	N/A	N/A
Digoxin	0.5 to 1.0 mg	0.125 to 0.25 qd	0.5 to 1.0	0.125 to 0.25 qd

N/A = not applicable.
*Results presented may vary according to doses, disease state, and intravenous or oral administration.
†Pregnancy class: A, controlled studies show no fetal risk; B, no controlled studies, but no evidence of fetal risk; fetal harm unlikely; C, fetal risk cannot be excluded; drug should be used only if potential benefits outweigh potential risk; D, definite fetal risk; drug should be avoided unless in a life-threatening situation or safer alternatives do not exist; X, contraindicated in pregnancy.
‡Intravenous use investigational.
§Investigational only.

HEMODYNAMIC EFFECTS. Quinidine decreases peripheral vascular resistance and can cause significant hypotension because of its alpha-adrenergic receptor blocking effects. Concomitant administration of vasodilators can exaggerate the potential for hypotension. In some patients, quinidine can increase cardiac output, possibly by reducing afterload and preload. No significant direct myocardial depressant action occurs with orally administered quinidine.

PHARMACOKINETICS (aee Table 30–4). Although orally administered quinidine sulfate and quinidine gluconate exhibit similar degrees of systemic availability, plasma quinidine concentrations peak at about 90 minutes after oral administration of quinidine sulfate and at 3 to 4 hours after oral administration of quinidine gluconate. Intramuscular administration should be avoided because of incomplete absorption and tissue necrosis. Quinidine can be given intravenously if it is infused slowly. Approximately 80 percent of plasma quinidine is protein bound, especially to alpha$_1$-acid glycoprotein, which increases in heart failure. Both the liver and the kidneys remove quinidine, and dose adjustments may be made according to the creatinine clearance. Metabolism is by means of the cytochrome P450 system. Approximately 20 percent is excreted unchanged in the urine. Because congestive heart failure, hepatic disease, or poor renal function can reduce quinidine elimination and increase plasma concentration, the dosage should probably be reduced and the drug given cautiously to patients with these disorders while serum quinidine concentration is monitored. Elimination half-life is 5 to 8 hours after oral administration. Quinidine's effect on repolarization and overall efficacy vary directly with left ventricular function; for the same serum concentration, the QT interval is longer in women and with higher degrees of sympathetic tone.[16,17]

DOSAGE AND ADMINISTRATION (see Table 30–4). The usual oral dose of quinidine sulfate for an adult is 300 to 600 mg four times daily, which results in a steady-state level within about 24 hours. A loading dose of 600 to 1000 mg produces an earlier effective concentration. Similar doses of quinidine gluconate are used intramuscularly, whereas the intravenous (IV) dose of quinidine gluconate is about 10 mg/kg given at a rate of about 0.5 mg/kg/min as blood pressure and electrocardiographic (ECG) parameters are checked frequently. Oral doses of the gluconate are about 30 percent greater than those of sulfate. Important interactions with other drugs occur.

INDICATIONS. Quinidine is a versatile antiarrhythmic agent, useful for treating premature supraventricular and ventricular complexes and sustained tachyarrhythmias. It may prevent spontaneous recurrences of AV nodal reentrant tachycardia (AVNRT) by prolonging atrial and ventricular

Time to Peak Plasma Concentration (Oral) (hr)	Effective Serum or Plasma Concentration (μg/ml)	Half-Life (hr)	Bioavailability (%)	Major Route of Elimination	Pregnancy Class†
1.5 to 3.0	3 to 6	5 to 9	60 to 80	Liver	C
1	4 to 10	3 to 5	70 to 85	Kidneys	C
1 to 2	2 to 5	8 to 9	80 to 90	Kidneys	C
N/A	1 to 5	1 to 2	N/A	Liver	B
2 to 4	0.75 to 2	10 to 17	90	Liver	C
8 to 12	10 to 20	18 to 36	50 to 70	Liver	D
3 to 4	0.2 to 1.0	20	95	Liver	C
1 to 3	0.2 to 3.0	5 to 8	25 to 75	Liver	C
1 to 3	0.1	2	40	Liver	B
4	1 to 2.5	3 to 6	35 to 65	Liver	C
	0.5 to 1.5	56 days	25	Kidneys	D
2 to 4	0.04 to 0.90	8 to 14	20 to 50	Liver	C
2.5 to 4	2.5	12	90 to 100	Kidneys	B
N/A	N/A	6		Kidneys	C
		7 to 13	90	Kidneys	C
	200 to 1000		90 to 100	Kidneys	—
1 to 2	0.10 to 0.15	3 to 8	10 to 35	Liver	C
N/A					C
2 to 6	0.0008 to 0.002	36 to 48	60 to 80	Kidneys	C

refractoriness and depressing conduction in the retrograde fast pathway. In patients with the Wolff-Parkinson-White syndrome, quinidine prolongs the ERP of the accessory pathway and, by so doing, can prevent reciprocating tachycardias and slow the ventricular response from conduction over the accessory pathway during atrial flutter or atrial fibrillation. Quinidine and other antiarrhythmic agents can also prevent recurrences of tachycardia by suppressing the "trigger" (i.e., the premature atrial complex [PAC] or premature ventricular complex [PVC] that initiates a sustained tachycardia).[6]

Quinidine successfully terminates atrial flutter or atrial fibrillation in 20 to 60 percent of patients, with higher success rates if the arrhythmia is of more recent onset and if the atria are not enlarged. Before quinidine is administered to these patients, the ventricular response should be slowed sufficiently with digitalis, propranolol, or verapamil because quinidine-induced slowing of the atrial flutter rate (e.g., from 300 to 230 beats/min) and its vagolytic effect on AV nodal conduction can convert a 2:1 AV response (ventricular rate 150 beats/min) to a 1:1 AV response, with an increase in the ventricular rate (to 230 beats/min).[18] If quinidine is going to be used to try to maintain sinus rhythm after elective cardioversion of patients with atrial fibrillation, it probably should be given for 1 to 2 days before planned cardioversion because this regimen restores sinus rhythm in some patients (thus obviating the need for direct-current cardioversion) and helps maintain sinus rhythm once it is achieved. In addition, early toxicity or patient's intolerance of the drug may be observed and changes made in drug therapy before attempting cardioversion. However, a meta-analysis of six studies testing the effects of quinidine versus control in maintaining sinus rhythm in patients with atrial fibrillation showed that quinidine-treated patients remained in sinus rhythm longer than the control group but had an increased total mortality over the same period.

Quinidine has prevented sudden death in some patients resuscitated after out-of-hospital cardiac arrest and may be combined with other antiarrhythmic agents for increased efficacy in suppressing serious ventricular tachyarrhythmias; however, the majority of these patients have ICDs and drug therapy is strictly adjunctive (i.e., used to decrease the frequency of arrhythmia episodes). It is important to stress that no published data from controlled, randomized studies indicate improved survival in quinidine-treated patients after myocardial infarction and cardiac arrest can occur despite quinidine therapy. Because it crosses the placenta, quinidine can be used to treat arrhythmias in the fetus.

ADVERSE EFFECTS. The most common adverse effects of chronic oral quinidine therapy are gastrointestinal and include nausea, vomiting, diarrhea, abdominal pain, and anorexia. Gastrointestinal side effects may be milder with the gluconate form. Central nervous system toxicity includes tinnitus, hearing loss, visual disturbances, confusion, delirium, and psychosis. Cinchonism is the term usually applied to these side effects. Allergic reactions may be manifested as rash, fever, immune-mediated thrombocytopenia, hemolytic anemia, and, rarely, anaphylaxis. Thrombocytopenia is due to the presence of antibodies to quinidine-platelet complexes, causing platelets to agglutinate and lyse. In patients

TABLE 30–5 In Vivo Electrophysiological Characteristics of Antiarrhythmic Drugs*

	Electrocardiographic Measurements					Electrophysiologic Intervals					
Drug	***Sinus Rate***	***PR***	***QRS***	***QT***	***JT***	***ERP-AVN***	***ERP-HPS***	***ERP-A***	***ERP-V***	***AH***	***HV***
Quinidine	0 ↑	↓ 0 ↑	↑	↑	↑	0 ↑	↑	↑	↑	0 ↓	↑
Procainamide	0	0 ↑	↑	↑	↑	0 ↑	↑	↑	↑	0 ↑	↑
Disopyramide	0 ↑	↓ 0 ↑	↑	↑	↑	↑ 0	↑	↑	↑	↓ 0 ↑	↑
Lidocaine	0	0	0	0 ↓	↓	0 ↓	0 ↑	0	0	0 ↓	0 ↑
Mexiletine	0	0	0	0 ↓	↓	0 ↑	0 ↑	0	0	0 ↑	0 ↑
Phenytoin	0	0	0	0	0	0 ↓	↓	0	0	0 ↑	0
Flecainide	0 ↓	↑	↑	0 ↑	0	↑	↑	↑	↑	↑	↑
Propafenone	0 ↓	↑	↑	0 ↑	0	0 ↑	0 ↑	0 ↑	↑	↑	↑
Moricizine	0 ↓	0 ↑	0 ↑	0	↓	0	0	0 ↑	0 ↑	↑	↑
Propranolol	↓	0 ↑	0	0 ↓	0	↑	0	0	0	0	0
Amiodarone	↓	0 ↑	↑	↑	↑	↑	↑	↑	↑	↑	↑
Bretylium	↓ 0 ↑	0	0	0 ↑	↑	0	↑	↑	↑	↓ 0 ↑	0
Sotalol	↓	0 ↑	0	↑	↑	↑	↑	↑	↑	↑	0
Ibutilide	↓	0 ↓	0	↑	↑	0	0	↑	↑	0	0
Dofetilide	0	0	0	↑	↑	0	0	↑	↑	0	0
Azimilide	0	0	0	↑	↑	0	0	↑	↑	0	0
Verapamil	0 ↓	↑	0	0	0	↑	0	0	0	↑	0
Adenosine	↓ then ↑	↑	0	0	0	↑	0	↓	0	↑	0
Digoxin	↓	↑	0	0	↓	↑	0	↓	0	↑	0

↑ = increase; ↓ = decrease; 0 = no change; 0 ↑ or 0 ↓ = slight or inconsistent increase or decrease; A = atrium; AH = atrio-His interval (an index of atrioventricular nodal conduction); AVN = atrioventricular node; ERP = effective refractory period (longest S_1-S_2 interval at which S_2 fails to produce a response); HPS = His-Purkinje system; HV = His-ventricular interval (an index of His-Purkinje conduction); V = ventricle.

*Results presented may vary according to tissue type, drug concentration, and autonomic tone.

receiving oral anticoagulants, quinidine can cause bleeding. Side effects may preclude long-term administration of quinidine in 30 to 40 percent of patients.

Quinidine can slow cardiac conduction, sometimes to the point of block, manifested as prolongation of the QRS duration or sinoatrial (SA) or AV nodal conduction disturbances. Quinidine-induced cardiac toxicity can be treated with molar sodium lactate. Quinidine can produce syncope in 0.5 to 2.0 percent of patients, most often the result of a self-terminating episode of torsades de pointes. Torsades de pointes may be due to the development of early afterdepolarizations, as noted earlier. Quinidine prolongs the QT interval in most patients, whether or not ventricular arrhythmias occur, but significant QT prolongation (QT interval of 500 to 600 milliseconds) is often a characteristic of patients with quinidine syncope. Many of these patients are also receiving digitalis or diuretics or have hypokalemia; women are more susceptible than men.[17,18] Syncope is unrelated to plasma concentrations of quinidine or duration of therapy, although the majority of episodes occur within the first 2 to 4 days of therapy (often after conversion of atrial fibrillation to sinus rhythm) (see Table 72–3).

Therapy for quinidine syncope requires immediate discontinuation of the drug and avoidance of other drugs that have similar pharmacological effects, such as disopyramide, because cross-sensitivity exists in some patients. Magnesium given intravenously (2 gm over 1 to 2 minutes, followed by an infusion of 3 to 20 mg/min) is the initial drug treatment of choice. Atrial or ventricular pacing can be used to suppress the ventricular tachyarrhythmia and may act by suppressing early afterdepolarizations. For some patients, drugs that do not prolong the QT interval, such as lidocaine or phenytoin, can be tried. When pacing is not available, isoproterenol can be given with caution. The arrhythmia gradually dissipates as quinidine is cleared and the QT interval returns to baseline.

Drugs that induce hepatic enzyme production, such as phenobarbital and phenytoin, can shorten the duration of quinidine's action by increasing its rate of elimination. Quinidine can increase plasma concentrations of flecainide by inhibiting the P450 enzyme system. Quinidine may elevate serum digoxin and digitoxin concentrations by decreasing total-body clearance of digitoxin and by decreasing the clearance, volume of distribution, and affinity of tissue receptors for digoxin.

Procainamide

ELECTROPHYSIOLOGICAL ACTIONS (see Tables 30–1, 30–2, 30–3, and 30–5). The cardiac actions of procainamide on automaticity, conduction, excitability, and membrane responsiveness resemble those of quinidine. Procainamide predominantly blocks the inactivated state of I_{Na}. It also blocks I_{Kr} and I_{KATP}. Like quinidine, procainamide usually prolongs the ERP more than it prolongs the APD and thus may prevent reentry. Compared with disopyramide and quinidine, procainamide exerts the least anticholinergic effects. It does not affect normal sinus node automaticity. In vitro, procainamide decreases abnormal automaticity, with less effect on triggered activity or catecholamine-enhanced normal automaticity.

The electrophysiological effects of NAPA, procainamide's major metabolite, differ from those of the parent compound. NAPA (10 to 40 mg/liter) does not suppress the rate of phase 4 diastolic depolarization of Purkinje fibers and does not alter resting membrane potential, action potential amplitude, or $\dot{V}_{max}$ of phase 0 of the action potential of Purkinje fibers or ventricular muscle. However, NAPA, a K^+ channel blocker (I_{Kr}), exerts a class III action and prolongs the APD of ventricular muscle and Purkinje fibers in a dose-dependent manner. Toxic doses produce early afterdepolarizations, triggered activity, and ventricular tachyarrhythmias, including torsades de pointes. Procainamide appears to exert greater electrophysiological effects than NAPA.

HEMODYNAMIC EFFECTS. Procainamide can depress myocardial contractility in high doses. It does not produce alpha blockade but can result in peripheral vasodilation, possibly through antisympathetic effects on brain or spinal cord that can impair cardiovascular reflexes.

PHARMACOKINETICS (see Table 30–4). Oral administration produces a peak plasma concentration in about 1 hour. Approximately 80 percent of oral procainamide is bioavailable, with 20 percent bound to serum proteins. The overall elimination half-life for procainamide is 3 to 5 hours, with 50 to 60 percent of the drug eliminated by the kidney and 10 to 30 percent eliminated by hepatic metabolism. Prolonged-release forms of procainamide given every 6 hours provide steady-state plasma levels of the drug equivalent to those from an equal total daily dose of short-acting procainamide given every 4 hours.

The drug is acetylated to NAPA, which is excreted almost exclusively by the kidneys. As renal function decreases and in patients with heart failure, procainamide levels—particularly NAPA levels—increase and, because of the risk of serious cardiotoxicity, need to be carefully monitored in such situations. NAPA has an elimination half-life of 7 to 8 hours, but the half-life exceeds 10 hours if high doses of procainamide are used. Small amounts of NAPA are converted back to procainamide by deacetylation. Increased age, congestive heart failure, and reduced creatinine clearance lower the procainamide clearance and necessitate a reduced dosage.

DOSAGE AND ADMINISTRATION (see Table 30–4). Procainamide can be given by the oral, IV, or intramuscular route to achieve plasma concentrations in the range of 4 to 10 mg/ml that produce an antiarrhythmic effect. Occasionally, plasma concentrations exceeding 10 mg/ml have been required, but the probability of adverse effects at these higher plasma concentrations generally precludes long-term administration. Several IV regimens have been used to administer procainamide. Twenty-five to 50 mg can be given over a 1-minute period and then repeated every 5 minutes until the arrhythmia is controlled, hypotension results, or the QRS complex is prolonged more than 50 percent. Doses of 10 to 15 mg/kg at 50 mg/min can also be used. Using this method, plasma concentration falls rapidly during the first 15 minutes after the loading dose, with parallel effects on refractoriness and conduction. A constant-rate IV infusion of procainamide can be given at a dose of 2 to 6 mg/min. The upper limits regarding total IV dose are flexible and range between 1000 and 2000 mg, depending on the patient's response.

Oral administration of procainamide requires a 3- to 4-hour dosing interval at a total daily dose of 2 to 6 gm, with a steady state reached within 1 day. When a loading dose is used, it should be twice the maintenance dose. Frequent dosing is required because of the short elimination half-life in normal subjects. For the prolonged-release forms of procainamide, dosing is at 6- to 12-hour intervals. Although a longer half-life may be seen in some cardiac patients, allowing longer intervals between drug administration, this needs to be documented for the individual patient. Procainamide is well absorbed after intramuscular injection, with virtually 100 percent of the dose bioavailable.

INDICATIONS. Procainamide is used to treat both supraventricular and ventricular arrhythmias in a manner comparable with that of quinidine. Although both drugs have similar electrophysiological actions, either drug can effectively suppress a supraventricular or ventricular arrhythmia that is resistant to the other drug.[7]

Procainamide can be used to convert atrial fibrillation of recent onset to sinus rhythm. As with quinidine, prior treatment with digitalis, propranolol, or verapamil is recommended to prevent acceleration of the ventricular response during atrial fibrillation after procainamide therapy. Procainamide's effect on conduction and refractoriness in the "flutter isthmus" of the right atrial free wall (see later) varies depending on the direction of wave front propagation in the isthmus.[19] Procainamide can block conduction in the accessory pathway of patients with the Wolff-Parkinson-White syndrome and may be used in patients with atrial fibrillation and a rapid ventricular response related to conduction over the accessory pathway. It can produce His-Purkinje block (see Fig. 29–10) and is sometimes administered during electrophysiology study (EPS) to "stress" the His-Purkinje system in evaluating the need for a pacemaker. However, it should be used with caution in patients with evidence of His-Purkinje disease (bundle branch block) in whom a ventricular pacemaker is not readily available.

Procainamide is more effective than lidocaine in acutely terminating sustained VT. Most consistently, procainamide slows the VT rate, a change correlated with the increase in QRS duration.[20] The electrophysiological response to procainamide given intravenously appears to predict the response to the drug given orally. Procainamide appears to affect preferentially the reentrant circuit of the VT compared with other areas of myocardium. The antiarrhythmic response to procainamide does not predict the response to NAPA.

ADVERSE EFFECTS. Multiple adverse noncardiac effects have been reported with procainamide administration and include rashes, myalgias, digital vasculitis, and the Raynaud phenomenon. Fever and agranulocytosis may be due to hypersensitivity reactions, and white blood cell and differential blood cell counts should be performed at regular intervals. Gastrointestinal side effects are less frequent than with quinidine, and adverse central nervous system side effects are less frequent than with lidocaine (although it can cause giddiness, psychosis, hallucinations, and depression). Toxic concentrations of procainamide can diminish myocardial performance and promote hypotension. A variety of conduction disturbances or ventricular tachyarrhythmias can occur that are similar to those produced by quinidine, including prolonged QT syndrome and polymorphic VT. NAPA can also cause QT prolongation and torsades de pointes (see Table 72–3). In the absence of sinus node disease, procainamide does not adversely affect sinus node function. In patients with sinus node dysfunction, procainamide tends to prolong corrected sinus node recovery time and can worsen symptoms in some patients who have the bradycardia-tachycardia syndrome. Procainamide does not increase the serum digoxin concentration.

Arthralgia, fever, pleuropericarditis, hepatomegaly, and hemorrhagic pericardial effusion with tamponade have been described in a systemic lupus erythematosus (SLE)–like syndrome related to procainamide administration. The syndrome occurs more frequently and earlier in patients who are slow acetylators of procainamide and is genetically influenced. Acetylating an aromatic amino group on procainamide to form NAPA appears to block the SLE-inducing effect. Sixty to 70 percent of patients who receive procainamide on a chronic basis develop antinuclear antibodies, with clinical symptoms in 20 to 30 percent, but this is reversible when procainamide is stopped. When symptoms occur, SLE cell preparations are often positive. Positive serological tests are not necessarily a reason to discontinue drug therapy; however, the development of symptoms or a positive anti-

DNA antibody is, unless it is the only effective treatment of a life-threatening arrhythmia (which would be very rare). Corticosteroid administration in these patients may eliminate the symptoms. In this syndrome, in contrast to naturally occurring SLE, the brain and kidney are spared and there is no predilection for females.

Disopyramide

Disopyramide has been approved in the United States for oral but not IV administration to treat patients with ventricular arrhythmias.

ELECTROPHYSIOLOGICAL ACTIONS (see Tables 30–1, 30–2, 30–3, and 30–5). Although structurally different from quinidine and procainamide, disopyramide produces similar electrophysiological effects in vitro. It causes use-dependent block of I_{Na} and non-use-dependent block of I_{Kr}. Along with quinidine, low concentrations tend to prolong APD and induce early afterdepolarizations just as do higher concentrations.[9] Disopyramide also inhibits I_{KATP}. It decreases the slope of phase 4 diastolic depolarization in Purkinje fibers, produces a rate-dependent depression of $\dot{V}_{max}$ of phase 0, prolongs the ERP more than it prolongs the APD, and lengthens conduction time in normal and depolarized Purkinje fibers; it does not affect calcium-dependent action potentials, except possibly at very high concentrations. Disopyramide, like procainamide, reduces the differences in APD between normal and infarcted tissue by lengthening the action potential of normal cells more than that of cells from infarcted regions.

Disopyramide is a muscarinic blocker and can increase the sinus node discharge rate and shorten AV nodal conduction time and refractoriness when the nodes are restrained by cholinergic (vagal) influences. Disopyramide can also slow the sinus node discharge rate by a direct action when given in high concentration and can significantly depress sinus node activity in patients with sinus node dysfunction. Disopyramide exerts greater anticholinergic effects than quinidine and does not appear to affect alpha or beta adrenoceptors.

Disopyramide prolongs atrial and ventricular refractory periods, but its effect on AV nodal conduction and refractoriness is not consistent. Disopyramide prolongs His-Purkinje conduction time, but infra-His block rarely occurs. Disopyramide can be administered safely to patients who have first-degree AV delay and narrow QRS complexes.

HEMODYNAMIC EFFECTS. Disopyramide suppresses ventricular systolic performance and is a mild arterial vasodilator. Patients who have abnormal ventricular function tolerate disopyramide's negative inotropic effects quite poorly. In these patients, the drug should generally be avoided.

PHARMACOKINETICS (see Table 30–4). Disopyramide is 80 to 90 percent absorbed, with a mean elimination half-life of 8 to 9 hours in healthy volunteers but almost 10 hours in patients with heart failure and sometimes longer in some patients with ventricular arrhythmias. Total-body clearance and volume of distribution are lower and mean serum concentration is higher in patients than in normal subjects. Renal insufficiency prolongs the elimination time. Thus, in patients who have renal, hepatic, or cardiac insufficiency, loading and maintenance doses need to be reduced. Peak blood levels after oral administration result in 1 to 2 hours, and bioavailability exceeds 80 percent. The fraction of disopyramide bound to serum protein varies inversely with the total plasma concentration of the drug but may be more stable (30 to 40 percent) at clinically relevant concentrations of 3 μg/ml. It is bound to alpha$_1$-acid glycoprotein and passes through the placenta. About half an oral dose is recovered unchanged in the urine, with about 30 percent as the mono-*N*-dealkylated metabolite. The metabolites appear to exert less effect than the parent compound. Erythromycin inhibits its metabolism.

DOSAGE AND ADMINISTRATION (see Table 30–4). Doses are generally 100 to 200 mg orally every 6 hours, with a range of 400 to 1200 mg/d. A controlled-release preparation can be given as 200 to 300 mg every 12 hours. The IV (investigational) dose is 1 to 2 mg/kg as an initial bolus given over 5 to 10 minutes, which may be followed by an infusion of 1 mg/kg/hr.

INDICATIONS. Disopyramide appears comparable to quinidine and procainamide in reducing the frequency of PVCs and effectively preventing recurrence of VT in selected patients. Disopyramide has been combined with other drugs such as mexiletine to treat patients who do not respond or only partially respond to one drug.

Disopyramide helps prevent recurrence of atrial fibrillation after successful cardioversion as effectively as quinidine and may terminate atrial flutter. In treating patients with atrial fibrillation, particularly atrial flutter, the ventricular rate must be controlled before administering disopyramide, or the combination of a decrease in atrial rate vagolytic effects on the AV node can result in 1:1 AV conduction during atrial flutter. Disopyramide may be useful in preventing episodes of neurally mediated syncope. It has been used in patients with hypertrophic cardiomyopathy (see Chap. 59).

ADVERSE EFFECTS. Three categories of adverse effects follow disopyramide administration. The most common effects are related to the drug's potent parasympatholytic properties and include urinary hesitancy or retention, constipation, blurred vision, closed-angle glaucoma, and dry mouth. Symptoms are less with the sustained-release form. Second, disopyramide can produce ventricular tachyarrhythmias that are commonly associated with QT prolongation and torsades de pointes[8] (see Table 72–3). Some patients can have "cross-sensitivity" to both quinidine and disopyramide and develop torsades de pointes while receiving either drug. When drug-induced torsades de pointes occurs, agents that prolong the QT interval should be used cautiously or not at all. Finally, disopyramide can reduce contractility of the normal ventricle, but the depression of ventricular function is much more pronounced in patients with preexisting ventricular failure. Occasionally, cardiovascular collapse can result.

Class IB Antiarrhythmic Agents

Lidocaine

ELECTROPHYSIOLOGICAL ACTIONS (see Tables 30–1, 30–2, 30–3, and 30–5). Lidocaine blocks I_{Na}, predominantly in the open or possibly inactivated state. It has rapid onset and offset kinetics and does not affect normal sinus node automaticity in usual doses but does depress other normal as well as abnormal forms of automaticity, as well as early and late afterdepolarizations in Purkinje fibers in vitro. Lidocaine has only a modest depressant effect on $\dot{V}_{max}$ and has no effect on maximal diastolic potential of normal muscle and specialized tissue in concentrations of about 1.5 μg/ml. However, faster rates of stimulation, reduced pH,[21] increased extracellular K^+ concentration, and reduced membrane potential—all changes that can result from ischemia—increase the ability of lidocaine to block I_{Na}. Lidocaine reduces the magnitude of the transient inward current responsible for some forms of afterdepolarization. Intracellular calcium activity may be reduced because of the sodium-calcium exchange mechanism. Lidocaine can convert areas of unidirectional block into bidirectional block during ischemia and prevent development of VF by preventing fragmentation of organized large wave fronts into heterogeneous wavelets. Lidocaine may be arrhythmogenic if it depresses conduction but not to the point of bidirectional block, but this does not appear to be an important clinical problem.

Except in very high concentrations, lidocaine does not affect slow channel–dependent action potentials despite its moderate suppression of the slow inward current. In fact, its depressant effect on electrical potentials from ischemic myocardium supports the idea that these ischemic potentials are depressed fast responses rather than slow responses. Lidocaine significantly reduces the APD and the ERP of Purkinje fibers and ventricular muscle because of blockade of sodium channels and decreasing entry of sodium into the cell. It has little effect on atrial fibers and does not affect conduction in accessory pathways. In some in vitro preparations, lidocaine can improve conduction by hyperpolarizing tissues depolarized as a result of stretch or low external potassium concentration.

In vivo, lidocaine has a minimal effect on automaticity or conduction except in unusual circumstances. Patients with preexisting sinus node dysfunction, abnormal His-Purkinje conduction, or junctional or ventricular escape rhythms can develop depressed automaticity or conduction. Part of its effects may be to inhibit cardiac sympathetic nerve activity.

HEMODYNAMIC EFFECTS. Clinically significant adverse hemodynamic effects are rarely noted at usual drug concentrations unless left ventricular function is severely impaired.

PHARMACOKINETICS (see Table 30–4). Lidocaine is used only parenterally because oral administration results in extensive first-pass hepatic metabolism and unpredictable, low plasma levels with excessive metabolites that can produce toxicity. Hepatic metabolism of lidocaine depends greatly on hepatic blood flow, so that clearance of this drug almost equals (and can be approximated by) measurements of this flow. Severe hepatic disease or reduced hepatic blood flow, as in heart failure or shock, can markedly decrease the rate of lidocaine metabolism. Beta adrenoceptor blockers can decrease hepatic blood flow and increase lidocaine serum concentration. Prolonged infusion can reduce lidocaine clearance. Its elimination half-life averages 1 to 2 hours in normal subjects, more than 4 hours in patients after relatively uncomplicated myocardial infarction, more than 10 hours in patients after myocardial infarction complicated by cardiac failure, and even longer in the presence of cardiogenic shock. Maintenance doses should be reduced by one third to one half for patients with low cardiac output. Lidocaine is 50 to 80 percent protein bound and binds to alpha$_1$-acid glycoprotein, which may increase in heart failure and myocardial infarction. A two-compartment model accurately predicts serum concentrations.

DOSAGE AND ADMINISTRATION (see Table 30–4). Although lidocaine can be given intramuscularly, the IV route is most commonly used. Intramuscular lidocaine is given in doses of 4 to 5 mg/kg (250 to 350 mg), resulting in effective serum levels at about 15 minutes and lasting for about 90 minutes. Intravenously, lidocaine is given as an initial bolus of 1 to 2 mg/kg of body weight at a rate of 20 to 50 mg/min, with a second injection of one half of the initial dose 20 to 40 minutes later. Patients treated with an initial bolus followed by a maintenance infusion may experience transient subtherapeutic plasma concentrations at 30 to 120 minutes after initiation of therapy. A second bolus of about 0.5 mg/kg without increasing the maintenance infusion rate reestablishes therapeutic serum concentrations.[9]

If recurrence of arrhythmia appears after a steady state has been achieved (e.g., 6 to 10 hours after starting therapy), a similar bolus should be given and the maintenance infusion rate increased. Increasing the maintenance infusion rate alone without an additional bolus results in a very slow increase in plasma lidocaine concentrations, reaching a new plateau in over 6 hours (four elimination half-lives), and is therefore not recommended. Another recommended IV dosing regimen is 1.5 mg/kg initially and 0.8 mg/kg at 8-minute intervals for three doses. Doses are reduced by about 50 percent for patients with heart failure.

If the initial bolus of lidocaine is ineffective, up to two more boluses of 1 mg/kg may be administered at 5-minute intervals. Patients who require more than one bolus to achieve a therapeutic effect have arrhythmias that respond only to higher lidocaine plasma concentrations, and a greater maintenance dose may be necessary to sustain these higher concentrations. Patients requiring only a single initial bolus of lidocaine should probably receive a maintenance infusion of 30 mg/kg/min, whereas those requiring two or three boluses may need infusions of 40 to 50 mg/kg/min.

Loading doses may also be administered by rapid infusion, and a constant-rate IV infusion may be used to maintain an effective concentration. Maintenance infusion rates in the range of 1 to 4 mg/min produce steady-state plasma levels of 1 to 5 μg/ml in patients with uncomplicated myocardial infarction, but these rates must be reduced during heart failure or shock because of concomitant reduced hepatic blood flow. A loading dose of approximately 75 mg followed by an initial infusion rate of 5.33 mg/min that declines exponentially to 2 mg/min with a half-life of 25 minutes has also been recommended.

INDICATIONS. Lidocaine demonstrates efficacy against ventricular arrhythmias of diverse etiology, the ability to achieve effective plasma concentrations rapidly, and a fairly wide toxic-to-therapeutic ratio with a low incidence of hemodynamic complications and other side effects. However, its first-pass hepatic effect precludes oral use, and it is generally ineffective against supraventricular arrhythmias. In patients with the Wolff-Parkinson-White syndrome, for whom the ERP of the accessory pathway is relatively short, lidocaine generally has no significant effect and may even accelerate the ventricular response during atrial fibrillation.

Lidocaine is used primarily for patients with recurrent ventricular tachyarrhythmias; although once a common usage, lidocaine prophylaxis in patients with acute myocardial infarction is currently not recommended because its ability to reduce the incidence of VF in hospitalized patients with acute myocardial infarction has not been clearly established and it can produce side effects and a possible increase in the risk of developing asystole. It has been effective in patients after coronary revascularization and in patients resuscitated from out-of-hospital VF, although amiodarone has been shown to yield higher rates of survival to hospital admission.[22]

ADVERSE EFFECTS. The most commonly reported adverse effects of lidocaine are dose-related manifestations of central nervous system toxicity: dizziness, paresthesias, confusion, delirium, stupor, coma, and seizures. Occasional sinus node depression and His-Purkinje block have been reported. In patients with atrial tachyarrhythmias, ventricular rate acceleration has been noted. Rarely, lidocaine can cause malignant hyperthermia. Both lidocaine and procainamide can elevate defibrillation thresholds.

Mexiletine

Mexiletine, a local anesthetic congener of lidocaine with anticonvulsant properties, is used for oral treatment of patients with symptomatic ventricular arrhythmias.

ELECTROPHYSIOLOGICAL ACTIONS (see Tables 30–1, 30–2, 30–3, and 30–5). Mexiletine is similar to lidocaine in many of its electrophysiological actions. In vitro, mexiletine shortens the APD and ERP of Purkinje fibers and, to a lesser extent, of ventricular muscle. It depresses $\dot{V}_{max}$ of phase 0 by blocking I_{Na}, especially at faster rates, and depresses automaticity of Purkinje fibers but not of the normal sinus node. Its onset and offset kinetics are rapid. Hypoxia or ischemia can increase its effects on $\dot{V}_{max}$.

Mexiletine can result in severe bradycardia and abnormal sinus node recovery time in patients with sinus node disease but not in patients with a normal sinus node. It does not affect AV nodal conduction and can depress His-Purkinje conduction, but not greatly, unless conduction was abnormal initially. Mexiletine does not appear to affect the ERP of human atrial and ventricular muscle. The duration of the QT interval does not increase. Because of its rate-dependent effects, theoretically, mexiletine might be expected to suppress closely coupled rather than late-coupled ventricular extrasystoles or faster tachycardias.

HEMODYNAMIC EFFECTS. Mexiletine exerts no major hemodynamic effects. It does not depress myocardial performance when given orally, although IV administration can produce hypotension.

PHARMACOKINETICS (see Table 30–4). Mexiletine has been reported to be rapidly and almost completely absorbed after oral ingestion by volunteers, with peak plasma concentrations attained in 2 to 4 hours. Elimination half-life in healthy subjects is approximately 10 hours, and in patients after myocardial infarction it is 17 hours. Therapeutic plasma levels of 0.5 to 2 μg/ml are maintained by oral doses of 200 to 300 mg every 6 to 8 hours. Absorption with less than a 10 percent first-pass hepatic effect occurs in the upper small intestine and is delayed and incomplete in patients who have myocardial infarction and in patients receiving narcotic analgesics, antacids, or atropine-like drugs that retard gastric emptying. Bioavailability of orally administered mexiletine is approximately 90 percent, and about 70 percent of the drug is protein bound. The apparent volume of distribution is large, reflecting extensive tissue uptake. Normally, mexiletine is eliminated metabolically by the liver, with less than 10 percent excreted unchanged in the urine. Doses probably should be reduced in patients with cirrhosis and those with left ventricular failure. Renal clearance of mexiletine decreases as urinary pH increases. Known metabolites exert no electrophysiological effects. Metabolism can be increased by phenytoin, phenobarbital, and rifampin and reduced by cimetidine. It is influenced by the genotype for the *CYP206* gene.

DOSAGE AND ADMINISTRATION (see Table 30–4). The recommended starting dose is 200 mg orally every 8 hours when rapid arrhythmia control is not essential. Doses may be increased or decreased by 50 to 100 mg every 2 to 3 days and are better tolerated when given with food. Total daily dose should not exceed 1200 mg. In some patients, administration every 12 hours can be effective. For rapid loading, 400 mg followed in 8 hours by a 200-mg dose is suggested.

INDICATIONS. Mexiletine is an effective antiarrhythmic agent for treating patients with both acute and chronic ventricular tachyarrhythmias but not with SVTs. Success rates vary from 6 to 60 percent and can be increased in some patients if mexiletine is combined with other drugs such as procainamide, beta blockers, quinidine, disopyramide, or amiodarone. Most studies show no clear superiority of mexiletine over other class I agents. Mexiletine may be very useful in children with congenital heart disease and serious ventricular arrhythmias. In treating patients with a long QT interval, mexiletine may be safer than drugs such as quinidine that increase the QT interval further. Limited experience in treating subsets of patients with long QT syndrome (LQT3, which is related to the *SCN5A* gene for the cardiac sodium channel) suggests a beneficial role (see Chap. 28). It does not appear to alter the prognosis of patients with inducible ventricular tachyarrhythmias after myocardial infarction. It may be effectively combined with propafenone or amiodarone.[23]

ADVERSE EFFECTS. Thirty to 40 percent of patients may require a change in dose or discontinuation of mexiletine therapy as a result of adverse effects, including tremor, dysarthria, dizziness, paresthesia, diplopia, nystagmus, mental confusion, anxiety, nausea, vomiting, and dyspepsia. Cardiovascular side effects are seen most often after IV dosing and include hypotension, bradycardia, and exacerbation of arrhythmia. Adverse effects of mexiletine appear to be dose related, and toxic effects occur at plasma concentrations only slightly higher than therapeutic levels. Therefore, effective use of this antiarrhythmic drug requires careful titration of dose and monitoring of plasma concentration. Lidocaine should be avoided, or the dose reduced, in patients also receiving lidocaine congeners such as mexiletine.

Phenytoin

Phenytoin was employed originally to treat seizure disorders. Its value as an antiarrhythmic agent remains limited.

ELECTROPHYSIOLOGICAL ACTIONS (see Tables 30-1, 30-2, 30-3, and 30-5). Phenytoin effectively abolishes abnormal automaticity caused by digitalis-induced delayed afterdepolarizations in cardiac Purkinje fibers and suppresses certain digitalis-induced arrhythmias in humans. The rate of rise of action potentials initiated early in the relative refractory period is increased, as is membrane responsiveness, possibly reducing the chance for impaired conduction and block. Phenytoin minimally affects sinus discharge rate and AV conduction in humans. As with other class IB agents, phenytoin has little effect on $\dot{V}_{max}$ in normally polarized fibers at slow rates and shows use-dependence and rapid kinetics for onset and termination of effects. Some of phenytoin's antiarrhythmic effects may be neurally mediated because it can modulate both sympathetic and vagal efferent activity. It has no peripheral cholinergic or beta-adrenergic blocking actions. Phenytoin exerts minimal hemodynamic effects.

PHARMACOKINETICS (See Table 30–4). The pharmacokinetics of phenytoin are less than ideal. Absorption after oral administration is incomplete and varies with the brand of drug. Plasma concentrations peak 8 to 12 hours after an oral dose. Ninety percent of the drug is protein bound. Phenytoin has limited solubility at physiological pH, and intramuscular administration is associated with pain, muscle necrosis, sterile abscesses, and variable absorption. Therapeutic serum concentrations of phenytoin (10 to 20 μg/ml) are similar for treating both cardiac arrhythmias and epilepsy. Lower concentrations can suppress certain digitalis-induced arrhythmias or other arrhythmias when decreased plasma protein binding occurs (as in uremia) because a larger fraction of drug is free and pharmacologically active.

METABOLISM. Over 90 percent of a dose is hydroxylated in the liver to presumably inactive compounds; significant genetically determined variation can occur. Elimination half-time is about 24 hours and can be slowed in the presence of liver disease or when phenytoin is administered concomitantly with drugs such as phenylbutazone, warfarin, isoniazid, chloramphenicol, and phenothiazines that compete with phenytoin for hepatic enzymes. Because of the large number of medications that can increase or decrease phenytoin levels during chronic therapy, phenytoin plasma concentration should be determined frequently when changes are made in other medications. Phenytoin has concentration-dependent kinetics for elimination that can cause unexpected toxicity because disproportionately large changes in plasma concentration can follow dose increases.

DOSAGE AND ADMINISTRATION (see Table 30–4). To achieve a therapeutic plasma concentration rapidly, 100 mg of phenytoin should be administered intravenously every 5 minutes until the arrhythmia is controlled, about 1 gm has been given, or adverse side effects result. Generally, 700 to 1000 mg controls the arrhythmia. A large central vein should be used to avoid pain and development of phlebitis produced by the extremely alkalotic (pH 11.0) vehicle in which phenytoin is dissolved. Orally, phenytoin is given as a loading dose of approximately 1000 mg the first day, 500 mg on the second and third days, and 300 to 400 mg daily thereafter. All maintenance doses can be given once or twice daily, depending on the brand, because of the long half-life of elimination.

INDICATIONS. Phenytoin has been used successfully to treat atrial and ventricular arrhythmias caused by digitalis toxicity but is much less effective in treating ventricular arrhythmias in patients with ischemic heart disease or with atrial arrhythmias not due to digitalis toxicity. It may be useful in some patients with the long QT syndrome.

ADVERSE EFFECTS. The most common manifestations of phenytoin toxicity are central nervous system effects of nystagmus, ataxia, drowsiness, stupor, and coma. Progression of such symptoms can be correlated with increases in plasma drug concentration. Nausea, epigastric pain, and anorexia are also relatively common effects of phenytoin. Long-term administration can result in hyperglycemia, hypocalcemia, rashes, megaloblastic anemia, gingival hypertrophy, lymph node hyperplasia (a syndrome resembling malignant lymphoma), peripheral neuropathy, pneumonitis, and drug-induced SLE. Birth defects can also result.[24]

Class IC Antiarrhythmic Agents

Flecainide

Flecainide is approved by the U.S. Food and Drug Administration (FDA) to treat patients with life-threatening ventricular arrhythmias as well as a variety of supraventricular arrhythmias.

ELECTROPHYSIOLOGICAL ACTIONS (see Tables 30-1, 30-2, 30-3, and 30-5). Flecainide exhibits marked use-dependent depressant effects on the rapid sodium channel, decreasing $\dot{V}_{max}$ with slow onset and offset kinetics. Drug dissociation from the sodium channel is very slow, with time constants of 10 to 30 seconds (compared with 4 to 8 seconds for quinidine and less than 1 second for lidocaine).Thus, marked drug effects can occur at physiological heart rates. Flecainide shortens the duration of the Purkinje fiber action potential but prolongs it in ventricular muscle, actions that, depending on the circumstances, could enhance or reduce electrical heterogeneity and create or suppress arrhythmias. Flecainide profoundly slows conduction in all cardiac fibers and, in high concentrations, inhibits the slow Ca^{2+} channel. Conduction time in the atria, ventricles, AV node, and His-Purkinje system is prolonged. It can terminate experimental atrial reentry by causing conduction block in the reentry pathway and eliminate atrial tachycardia (AT) by producing exit block from the focus. Flecainide can also promote reentry. Minimal increases in atrial or ventricular refractoriness or in the QT interval result. Anterograde and retrograde refractoriness in accessory pathways can increase significantly in a use-dependent fashion. Sinus node function remains unchanged in normal subjects but may be depressed in patients with sinus node dysfunction. Pacing and defibrillation thresholds are characteristically slightly increased.

HEMODYNAMIC EFFECTS. Flecainide depresses cardiac performance, particularly in patients with compromised ventricular systolic function. Left ventricular ejection fraction decreases after oral (single dose of 200 to 250 mg) or IV (1 mg) administration. Flecainide should be used cautiously, or not at all, in patients with moderate or severe ventricular systolic dysfunction.

PHARMACOKINETICS (see Table 30–4). Flecainide is at least 90 percent absorbed, with peak plasma concentrations in 3 to 4 hours. Elimination half-life in patients with ventricular arrhythmias is 20 hours, with 85 percent of the drug being excreted unchanged or as an inactive metabolite in urine. Two major metabolites exert fewer effects than the parent drug. Elimination is slower in patients with renal disease and heart failure, and doses should be reduced in these situations. Therapeutic plasma concentrations range from 0.2 to 1.0 μg/ml. About 40 percent of the drug is protein bound. Increases in serum concentrations of digoxin (15 to 25 percent) and propranolol (30 percent) result during coadministration with flecainide. Propranolol, quinidine, and amiodarone may increase flecainide serum concentrations. Five to 7 days of dosing may be required to reach steady state in some patients.

DOSAGE AND ADMINISTRATION (see Table 30–4). The starting dose is 100 mg every 12 hours, increased in increments of 50 mg twice daily, no sooner than every 3 to 4 days, until efficacy is achieved, an adverse effect is noted, or to a maximum of 400 mg/d. Cardiac rhythm and QRS duration should be monitored.

INDICATIONS. Flecainide is indicated for the treatment of life-threatening ventricular tachyarrhythmias, SVTs, and paroxysmal atrial fibrillation. Some experts suggest that therapy should begin in the hospital while the electrocardiogram is being monitored because of the possibility of proarrhythmic events (see later). Serum concentration should not exceed 1.0 μg/ml. Flecainide is particularly effective in almost totally suppressing PVCs and short runs of nonsustained VT, although the importance of such a response to the subsequent outcome of the patient has not been established. As with other class I antiarrhythmic drugs, there are no data from controlled studies to indicate that the drug favorably affects survival or sudden cardiac death, and data from CAST (see later) indicate increased mortality in patients with coronary artery disease. Flecainide produces a use-dependent prolongation of VT cycle length that improves hemodynamic tolerance.

Flecainide is also useful in a variety of SVTs such as atrial flutter and atrial fibrillation,[10] in Wolff-Parkinson-White syndrome, and for AT. Isoproterenol can reverse some of these effects. Flecainide may be more effective than procainamide in the acute termination of atrial fibrillation. It is important to slow the ventricular rate before treating with flecainide to avoid 1:1 AV conduction. Flecainide has been used to treat fetal arrhythmias and arrhythmias in children.[25] It may increase defibrillation thresholds. Flecainide administration may produce ST elevation in lead V_1 characteristic of Brugada syndrome (see Chap. 32) and has been used as a diagnostic tool in patients suspected of having this disorder.

ADVERSE EFFECTS. Proarrhythmic effects are some of the most important adverse effects of flecainide. Its marked slowing of conduction precludes its use in patients with second-degree AV block without a pacemaker and warrants cautious administration in patients with intraventricular conduction disorders. Worsening of existing ventricular arrhythmias or onset of new ventricular arrhythmias can occur in 5 to 30 percent of patients, with the increased percentage in patients with preexisting sustained VT, cardiac decompensation, and higher doses of the drug. Failure of the flecainide-related arrhythmia to respond to therapy, including electrical cardioversion-defibrillation, may result in mortality as high as 10 percent in patients who develop proarrhythmic events. Negative inotropic effects can cause or worsen heart failure. Patients with sinus node dysfunction may experience sinus arrest, and those with pacemakers may develop an increase in pacing threshold. In CAST, patients treated with flecainide had 5.1 percent mortality or nonfatal cardiac arrest compared with 2.3 percent in the placebo group over 10 months.[14] Mortality was highest in those with non-Q-wave infarction, frequent PVCs, and faster heart rates, raising the possibility of drug interaction with ischemia and electrical instability. Exercise can amplify the conduction slowing in the ventricle produced by flecainide and in some cases can precipitate a proarrhythmic response. Therefore, exercise testing has been recommended to screen for proarrhythmia. Central nervous system complaints, including confusion and irritability, represent the most frequent noncardiac adverse effects. The safety of flecainide during pregnancy has not been determined although, as noted previously, it is occasionally used to treat fetal arrhythmias. It is concentrated in breast milk to levels 2.5- to 4-fold higher than in plasma.

Propafenone

Propafenone has been approved by the FDA for treatment of patients with life-threatening ventricular tachyarrhythmias.

ELECTROPHYSIOLOGICAL ACTIONS (see Tables 30-1, 30-2, 30-3, and 30-5). Propafenone blocks the fast sodium current in a use-dependent manner, as well as at rest, in Purkinje fibers and to a lesser degree in ventricular muscle. Use-dependent effects contribute to its ability to terminate experimental atrial fibrillation. The dissociation constant from the receptor is slow, like that of flecainide. Effects are greater in ischemic than normal tissue and at reduced membrane potentials. Propafenone decreases excitability and suppresses spontaneous automaticity and triggered activity. It terminates experimental VT by producing conduction block or by collision of the impulse with an echo wave. Propafenone is a weak blocker of I_{Kr}[26] and beta-adrenergic receptors. Although ventricular refractoriness increases, conduction slowing is the major effect. The active metabolites of propafenone exert important actions, reducing $\dot{V}_{max}$, action potential amplitude and duration in canine Purkinje fibers. Propafenone depresses sinus node automaticity. In patients, the AH, HV, PR, and QRS intervals increase, as do refractory periods of the atria, ventricles, AV node, and accessory pathways. The corrected QT interval increases only as a function of increased QRS duration.

HEMODYNAMIC EFFECTS. Propafenone and 5-hydroxypropafenone exhibit negative inotropic properties at high concentrations in vitro, and large doses depress left ventricular function in vivo. In patients with ejection fractions exceeding 40 percent, the negative inotropic effects are well tolerated, but patients with preexisting left ventricular dysfunction and congestive heart failure may have symptomatic worsening of their hemodynamic status.

PHARMACOKINETICS (see Table 30–4). With more than 95 percent of the drug absorbed, propafenone's maximum plasma concentration occurs in 2 to 3 hours. Systemic bioavailability is dose dependent and ranges from 3 to 40 percent because of variable presystemic clearance. Bioavailability increases as the dose increases, and plasma concentration is therefore nonlinear. A threefold increase in dosage (300 to 900 mg/d) results in a 10-fold increase in plasma concentration, presumably because of saturation of hepatic metabolic mechanisms. Propafenone is 97 percent bound to alpha$_1$-acid glycoprotein, with an elimination half-life of 5 to 8 hours. Maximum therapeutic effects occur at serum concentrations of 0.2 to 1.5 μg/ml. Marked interpatient variability of pharmacokinetics and pharmacodynamics may be due to genetically determined differences in metabolism. About 93 percent of the population are extensive metabolizers and exhibit shorter elimination half-lives (5 to 6 hours), lower plasma concentrations of the parent compound, and higher concentrations of metabolites. Poor metabolizers, because of diminished capacity of the hepatic microsomal cytochrome P450 enzyme system, exhibit an elimination half-life of 15 to 20 hours for the parent compound and virtually no 5-hydroxypropafenone. The (+) enantiomer provides nonspecific beta-adrenergic receptor blockade with 2.5 to 5 percent of the potency of propranolol. Because plasma propafenone concentrations may be 50 times or more higher than propranolol levels, these beta-blocking properties may be relevant. Poor metabolizers have a greater beta-adrenergic receptor blocking effect than extensive metabolizers. Propafenone also blocks the slow calcium channel to a degree about 1 percent that of verapamil.

DOSAGE AND ADMINISTRATION (see Table 30–4). Most patients respond to oral doses of 150 to 300 mg every 8 hours, not exceeding 1200 mg/d. Doses are similar for patients of both metabolizing phenotypes. Concomitant food administration increases bioavailability, as does hepatic dysfunction. No good correlation between plasma propafenone concentration and arrhythmia suppression has been shown. Doses should not be increased more often than every 3 to 4 days. Propafenone increases plasma concentrations of warfarin, digoxin, and metoprolol.

INDICATIONS. Propafenone is indicated for the treatment of SVTs,[11] paroxysmal atrial fibrillation, and life-threatening ventricular tachyarrhythmias and effectively suppresses spontaneous PVCs and nonsustained and sustained VT. Propafenone has also been approved for use in patients with AT, AV node reentry, AV reentry, and atrial flutter or fibrillation. Acute termination of atrial fibrillation episodes was effected with a single 600-mg oral dose of propafenone in 76 percent of patients given the drug (twice the rate of those given placebo).[27] It has been used effectively in the pediatric age group. Propafenone increases the pacing threshold but minimally affects the defibrillation threshold. Sinus rate during exercise is reduced. Propafenone use is associated with higher mortality in cardiac arrest survivors than use of an implantable defibrillator. Sotalol was more effective than propafenone in the Electrophysiology Study Versus Electrocardiographic Monitoring (ESVEM) trial. Propafenone has been combined effectively with mexiletine.

ADVERSE EFFECTS. Minor noncardiac effects occur in about 15 percent of patients, with dizziness, disturbances in taste, and blurred vision the most common and gastrointestinal side effects next. Exacerbation of bronchospastic lung disease can occur because of mild beta-blocking effects. Cardiovascular side effects occur in 10 to 15 percent of patients, including conduction abnormalities such as AV block, sinus node depression, and worsening of heart failure. Proarrhythmic responses, which occur more often in patients with a history of sustained VT and decreased ejection fractions, appear less commonly than with flecainide and may be in the range of 5 percent. The applicability of data from CAST about flecainide to propafenone is not clear, but limiting propafenone's application in a manner similar to that of other class IC drugs seems prudent at present until more information is available. Its beta-blocking actions may make it different, however. The safety of propafenone administration during pregnancy has not been established.

Moricizine (Ethmozine)

Moricizine is a phenothiazine derivative indicated for treatment of patients with ventricular tachyarrhythmias; it has also been used for atrial fibrillation.[28] It was formerly discussed as a class IB antiarrhythmic drug because it shortens Purkinje fiber action potential. However, the intensity of its effect on the Na^+ channel is more like that of a class IA antiarrhythmic drug, whereas the time constants for onset and offset resemble those of class IC agents.

ELECTROPHYSIOLOGICAL ACTIONS. Moricizine decreases I_{Na} predominantly in the inactivated state, with a resultant decrease in $\dot{V}_{max}$ of phase 0 and action potential amplitude (see Tables 30-1, 30-2, 30-3, and 30-5). Maximum diastolic potential is not changed. Moricizine blocks $I_{Ca\text{-}L}$ and I_K and prolongs AV node and His-Purkinje conduction times and QRS duration. The JT interval shortens slightly, whereas the QTc is prolonged 5 percent owing to QRS prolongation. Ventricular refractoriness is prolonged slightly, with no consistent atrial change. No alterations in sinus node automaticity result. Moricizine minimally raises the defibrillation threshold.

HEMODYNAMIC EFFECTS. Moricizine exerts minimal effects on cardiac performance in patients with impaired left ventricular function; an occasional patient with significant left ventricular dysfunction may have worsening of heart failure.

PHARMACOKINETICS (see Table 30–4). After oral ingestion, moricizine undergoes extensive first-pass metabolism, resulting in absolute bioavailability of 35 to 40 percent. Peak plasma concentrations are reached in 0.5 to 2 hours and later if the drug is taken after meals. Protein binding is 95 percent to alpha$_1$-acid glycoprotein and albumin. Antiarrhythmic and electrophysiological actions do not relate to plasma concentrations or to any of its more than 20 metabolites. Plasma elimination half-life is 1.5 to 3.5 hours, with slightly more than half the drug excreted in the feces and slightly less than half excreted in the urine.

DOSAGE AND ADMINISTRATION (see Table 30–4). The usual adult dose is 600 to 900 mg/d, given every 8 hours in divided doses, with increments of 150 mg/d at 3-day intervals. Some patients may be treated every 12 hours. Dosage should be reduced in patients with hepatic or neural disease, AV conduction disturbances, or sinus node dysfunction without a pacemaker and with significant congestive heart failure.

INDICATIONS. Moricizine is indicated for prevention of life-threatening ventricular arrhythmias and has an efficacy about comparable to those of quinidine and disopyramide. Moricizine can have proarrhythmic effects; in CAST, it caused an increase in mortality compared with placebo during initial treatment of patients who had symptomatic or minimally symptomatic ventricular arrhythmias after myocardial infarction.[29] Risk was greater in patients taking diuretics.

ADVERSE EFFECTS. Usually, the drug is well tolerated. Noncardiac adverse effects primarily involve the nervous system and include tremor, mood changes, headache, vertigo, nystagmus, and dizziness. Gastrointestinal side effects include nausea, vomiting, and diarrhea. Worsening of congestive heart failure may rarely occur. Proarrhythmic effects have been reported in 3 to 15 percent of patients, more commonly in patients with severe ventricular arrhythmias. Advancing age increases the susceptibility to adverse effects. Moricizine appears to be relatively safe to use during pregnancy (class B) and is present in small amounts in breast milk.

Class II Antiarrhythmic Agents

Beta Adrenoceptor Blocking Agents

Although many beta adrenoceptor blocking drugs have been approved for use in the United States, acebutolol (PVCs), esmolol (SVT), metoprolol (post-myocardial infarction), atenolol (post-myocardial infarction), propranolol (post-myocardial infarction, SVT, VT), and timolol (post-myocardial infarction) have been approved to treat arrhythmias or to prevent sudden death after myocardial infarction.[30] It is generally considered that no beta blocker offers distinct advantages over others and that, when titrated to the proper dose, all can be used effectively to treat cardiac arrhythmias, hypertension, or other disorders. However, differences in pharmacokinetic or pharmacodynamic properties that confer safety, reduce adverse effects, or affect dosing intervals or drug interactions influence the choice of agent. Also, some beta blockers such as sotalol, pindolol, and carvedilol exert unique actions.

Beta receptors can be separated into those that affect predominantly the heart (beta$_1$) and those that affect predominantly blood vessels and the bronchi (beta$_2$). In low doses, selective beta blockers can block beta$_1$ receptors more than they block beta$_2$ receptors and might be preferable for treating patients with pulmonary or peripheral vascular diseases. In high doses, the "selective" beta$_1$ blockers also block beta$_2$ receptors. Carvedilol also exerts alpha blocking effects and is used primarily in patients with heart failure (see Chap. 23).

Some beta blockers exert intrinsic sympathomimetic activity; that is, they slightly activate the beta receptor. These drugs appear to be as efficacious as beta blockers without intrinsic sympathomimetic actions and may cause less slowing of heart rate at rest and less prolongation of AV nodal conduction time. They have been shown to induce less depression of left ventricular function than beta blockers without intrinsic sympathomimetic activity. Only nonselective beta blockers without intrinsic sympathomimetic activity have been demonstrated to reduce mortality in patients after myocardial infarction (Fig. 30–1).

The following discussion concentrates on the use of propranolol as a prototypical antiarrhythmic agent, generally applicable to other beta blockers.

ELECTROPHYSIOLOGICAL ACTIONS. Beta blockers exert an electrophysiological action by competitively inhibiting catecholamine binding at beta adrenoceptor sites, an effect almost entirely due to the (−)-levorotatory stereoisomer, or by their quinidine-like or direct membrane-stabilizing action (see Tables 30-1, 30-2, 30-3, and 30-5). The latter is a local anesthetic effect that depresses I_{Na} and membrane responsiveness in cardiac Purkinje fibers, occurs at concentrations generally 10 times that necessary to produce beta blockade, and most likely plays an insignificant antiarrhythmic role. Thus, beta blockers exert their major effects in cells most actively stimulated by adrenergic actions. At beta-blocking concentrations, propranolol slows spontaneous automaticity in the sinus node or in Purkinje fibers that are being stimulated by adrenergic tone, producing block of I_f (see Chap. 27). Beta blockers also block $I_{Ca\text{-}L}$ stimulated by beta agonists. In the absence of adrenergic stimulation, only high concentrations of propranolol slow normal automaticity in Purkinje fibers, probably by a direct membrane action.

Concentrations that cause beta receptor blockade but no local anesthetic effects do not alter the normal resting membrane potential, maximum diastolic potential amplitude, $\dot{V}_{max}$, repolarization, or refractoriness of atrial, Purkinje, or ventricular muscle cells in the absence of catecholamine stimulation. However, in the presence of isoproterenol, a pure beta receptor stimulator, beta blockers reverse isoproterenol's accelerating effects on repolarization; in the presence of norepinephrine, beta blockade permits unopposed alpha adrenoceptor stimulation to prolong APD in Purkinje fibers. Propranolol (2×10^{-6} M) reduces the amplitude of digitalis-induced delayed afterdepolarizations and suppresses triggered activity in Purkinje fibers. Propranolol upregulates beta adrenoceptors in part by externalizing receptors from a light vesicle fraction to the sarcolemma.

Concentrations exceeding 3 mg/ml are required to depress $\dot{V}_{max}$ action potential amplitude, membrane responsiveness, and conduction in normal atrial, ventricular, and Purkinje fibers without altering resting membrane potential. These effects probably result from depression of I_{Na}. Propranolol shortens the APD of Purkinje fibers and, to a lesser extent, of atrial and ventricular muscle fibers. Long-term administration of propranolol may lengthen APD. As with the effects of lidocaine, acceler-

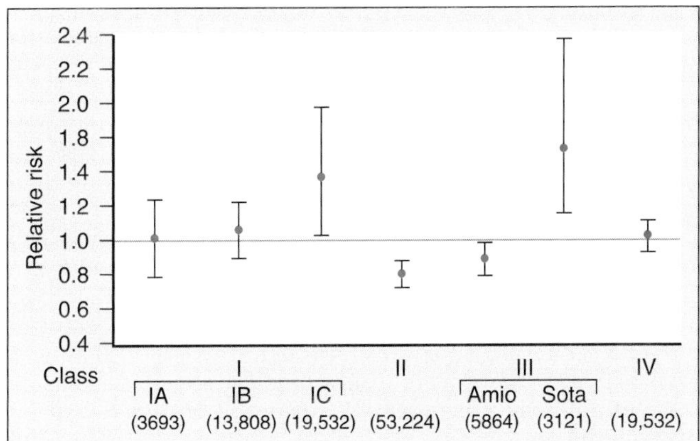

FIGURE 30–1 Meta-analytical data from randomized clinical trials of antiarrhythmic drugs in survivors of acute myocardial infarction. The relative risk is compared with placebo therapy (mean and 95 percent confidence interval) for death during therapy with various electrophysiological classes of compounds. Class I agents, particularly IC, and sotalol increase mortality, whereas beta blockers and amiodarone decrease mortality. Numbers under each drug class refer to number of patients involved in the trials. Amio = amiodarone; Sota = sotalol. (Modified from Teo KK, Yusuf S: *In* Singh BN, Dzau VJ, Vanhoutte PM, Woosley RL [eds]: Cardiovascular Pharmacology and Therapeutics. New York, Churchill Livingstone, 1994, pp 631-643; and Waldo AL, Camm AJ, deRuyter H, et al: Effect of *d*-sotalol on mortality in patients with left ventricular dysfunction after recent and remote myocardial infarction: The SWORD Investigators. Survival With Oral *d*-Sotalol. Lancet 348:7, 1996.)

ation of repolarization of Purkinje fibers is most marked in areas of the ventricular conduction system in which the APD is greatest. At least one beta blocker, sotalol, markedly increases the time course of repolarization in Purkinje fibers and ventricular muscle. Smaller doses of propranolol are required to prevent sympathetically induced shortening of ventricular refractoriness than are required to prevent sympathetically induced sinus acceleration.

Propranolol slows the sinus discharge rate in humans by 10 to 20 percent, although severe bradycardia occasionally results if the heart is particularly dependent on sympathetic tone or if sinus node dysfunction is present. The PR interval lengthens, as do AV nodal conduction time and effective and functional refractory periods (if the heart rate is maintained constant), but refractoriness and conduction in the normal His-Purkinje system remain unchanged even after high doses of propranolol. Therefore, therapeutic doses of propranolol in humans do not exert a direct depressant or "quinidine-like" action but influence cardiac electrophysiology through a beta-blocking action. Beta blockers do not affect conduction in normal ventricular muscle, as evidenced by their lack of effect on the QRS complex, and they insignificantly prolong the uncorrected QT interval.

Because administration of beta blockers that do not have direct membrane action prevents many arrhythmias resulting from activation of the autonomic nervous system, it is thought that the beta-blocking action is responsible for their antiarrhythmic effects. Nevertheless, the possible importance of the direct membrane effect of some of these drugs cannot be discounted totally because beta blockers with direct membrane actions can affect transmembrane potentials of diseased cardiac fibers at much lower concentrations than are needed to affect normal fibers directly. However, indirect actions on arrhythmogenic effects of ischemia are probably most important. Beta blockers reduce myocardial injury during experimental cardiopulmonary resuscitation.

HEMODYNAMIC EFFECTS. Beta blockers exert negative inotropic effects and can precipitate or worsen heart failure. However, beta blockers clearly improve survival in patients with heart failure (see Chap. 23). By blocking beta receptors, these drugs may allow unopposed alpha-adrenergic effects to cause peripheral vasoconstriction and exacerbate coronary artery spasm or pain from peripheral vascular disease in some patients.

PHARMACOKINETICS (see Table 30–4). Although various types of beta blockers exert similar pharmacological effects, their pharmacokinetics differ substantially. Propranolol is almost 100 percent absorbed, but the effects of first-pass hepatic metabolism reduce bioavailability to about 30 percent and produce significant interpatient variability of plasma concentration for a given dose. Reduction in hepatic blood flow, as in patients with heart failure, decreases the hepatic extraction of propranolol; in these patients propranolol may further decrease its own elimination rate by reducing cardiac output and hepatic blood flow. Beta blockers eliminated by the kidney tend to have longer half-lives and exhibit less interpatient variability of drug concentration than beta blockers metabolized by the liver.

DOSAGE AND ADMINISTRATION (see Table 30–4). The appropriate dose of propranolol is best determined by a measure of the patient's physiological response, such as changes in resting heart rate or in the prevention of exercise-induced tachycardia, because wide individual differences exist between the observed physiological effect and plasma concentration. For example, IV dosing is best achieved by titrating the dose to a clinical effect, beginning with doses of 0.25 to 0.50 mg, increasing to 1.0 mg if necessary, and administering doses every 5 minutes until either a desired effect or toxicity is produced or a total of 0.15 to 0.20 mg/kg has been given. In many instances, the short-acting effects of esmolol are preferred. Orally, propranolol is given in four divided doses, usually ranging from 40 to 160 mg/d to more than 1 gm/d. A once-daily long-acting propranolol preparation is available, to which patients may be switched after dosage titration with the short-acting form if needed. Generally, if one agent in adequate doses proves to be ineffective, other beta blockers are also ineffective.

INDICATIONS. Arrhythmias associated with thyrotoxicosis, pheochromocytoma, and anesthesia with cyclopropane or halothane or arrhythmias largely related to excessive cardiac adrenergic stimulation, such as those initiated by exercise, emotion, or cocaine, often respond to beta blocker therapy. Beta-blocking drugs usually do not convert chronic atrial flutter or atrial fibrillation to normal sinus rhythm but may do so if the arrhythmia is of recent onset and in patients who have recently undergone cardiac surgery.[31-34] The atrial rate during atrial flutter or fibrillation is not changed, but the ventricular response decreases because beta blockade prolongs AV nodal conduction time and refractoriness. Esmolol combined with digoxin has been useful. In the absence of heart failure, beta blockers can be more effective than digoxin to control the rate. For reentrant SVTs using the AV node as one of the reentrant pathways, such as AVNRT and orthodromic reciprocating tachycardias in the Wolff-Parkinson-White syndrome or inappropriate sinus tachycardia, or for ATs, beta blockers can slow or terminate the tachycardia and be used prophylactically to prevent a recurrence. Combining beta blockers with digitalis, quinidine, or a variety of other agents may be effective when the beta blocker as a single agent fails. Metoprolol and esmolol may be useful in patients with multifocal AT. These agents must be used with caution in this arrhythmia, however, because a common setting for it is advanced lung disease, often with a bronchospastic component.

Beta blockers may be effective for digitalis-induced arrhythmias such as AT, nonparoxysmal AV junctional tachycardia, PVCs, or VT. If a significant degree of AV block is present during a digitalis-induced arrhythmia, lidocaine or phenytoin may be preferable to propranolol. Beta blockers may also be useful to treat ventricular arrhythmias associated with the prolonged QT interval syndrome and with mitral valve prolapse. For patients with ischemic heart disease, beta blockers generally do not prevent episodes of recurrent monomorphic VT that occur in the absence of acute ischemia but may be effective in some patients, usually at a beta-blocking concentration. It is well accepted that propranolol, timolol, and metoprolol reduce the incidence of overall death and sudden cardiac death after myocardial infarction. The mechanism of this reduction in mortality is not entirely clear and may be related to reduction of the extent of ischemic damage, autonomic effects, a direct antiarrhythmic effect, or combinations of these factors. Beta blockers may have been protective against proarrhythmic responses in CAST and may be more effective in some patients than electrophysiologically guided antiarrhythmic drug therapy for ventricular tachyarrhythmias.

Labetalol, an $alpha_1$- and beta-blocking drug, has been used for ventricular arrhythmias in eclampsia. *Carvedilol,* another alpha- and beta-blocking agent, has been shown to improve survival in moderate to severe heart failure. *Esmolol* is an ultra-short-acting (elimination half-life, 9 minutes), cardioselective beta adrenoceptor blocker that is useful for the rapid control of the ventricular rate in patients with atrial flutter or fibrillation.

ADVERSE EFFECTS. Adverse cardiovascular effects from beta blockers include unacceptable hypotension, bradycardia, and congestive heart failure. The bradycardia may be due to sinus slowing or AV block. Sudden withdrawal of propranolol in patients with angina pectoris can precipitate or worsen angina and cardiac arrhythmias and cause an acute myocardial infarction, possibly owing to heightened sensitivity to beta agonists caused by previous beta blockade (receptor upregulation). Heightened sensitivity may begin several days after cessation of beta blocker therapy and may last 5 or 6 days. Other adverse effects of beta blockers include worsening of asthma or chronic obstructive pulmonary disease, intermittent claudication, Raynaud phenomenon, mental depression, increased risk of hypoglycemia among insulin-dependent diabetic patients, easy fatigability, disturbingly vivid dreams or insomnia, and impaired sexual function. Many of these side effects were noted less frequently when using $beta_1$-selective agents, but even so-called cardioselective beta blockers can exacerbate asthma or diabetic control in individual patients.

Class III Antiarrhythmic Agents

Amiodarone

Amiodarone is a benzofuran derivative approved by the FDA for the treatment of patients with life-threatening ventricular tachyarrhythmias when other drugs are ineffective or are not tolerated. Dronedarone, a noniodinated derivative of amiodarone, is being studied as a potentially less toxic alternative to amiodarone. As of this writing, it has not been approved for use in the United States.[32-34]

ELECTROPHYSIOLOGICAL ACTIONS (see Tables 30-1, 30-2, 30-3, and 30-5). When chronically given orally, amiodarone prolongs APD and refractoriness of all cardiac fibers without affecting resting membrane potential. When acute effects are evaluated, amiodarone and its metabolite, desethylamiodarone, prolong the APD of ventricular muscle but shorten the APD of Purkinje fibers. Injected into the sinus and AV node arteries, amiodarone reduces sinus and junctional discharge rates and prolongs AV nodal conduction time. It decreases the slope of diastolic depolarization of the sinus node and markedly depresses $\dot{V}_{max}$ in guinea pig papillary muscle in a rate- or use-dependent manner. Such depression of $\dot{V}_{max}$ is caused by blocking of inactivated sodium channels, an effect that is accentuated by depolarized and reduced by hyperpolarized membrane potentials. Amiodarone also inhibits depolarization-induced automaticity. Amiodarone depresses conduction at fast rates more than at slow rates (use-dependence), not only by depressing $\dot{V}_{max}$ but also by increasing resistance to passive current flow. It does not prolong repolarization more at slow than fast rates (i.e., does not demonstrate reverse use-dependence) but does exert time-dependent effects on refractoriness, which may in part explain the low incidence of torsades de pointes and high efficacy.

Desethylamiodarone has relatively greater effects on fast-channel tissue and probably contributes notably to antiarrhythmic efficacy. The delay to build up adequate concentrations of this metabolite may explain in part the delay in amiodarone's antiarrhythmic action.

In vivo, amiodarone noncompetitively antagonizes alpha and beta receptors and blocks conversion of thyroxine (T_4) to triiodothyronine (T_3), which may account for some of its electrophysiological effects. Amiodarone exhibits slow-channel blocking effects, and chronic oral therapy slows the spontaneous sinus node discharge rate in anesthetized dogs even after pretreatment with propranolol and atropine. With oral administration it slows the sinus rate by 20 to 30 percent and prolongs the QT interval, at times changing the contour of the T wave and producing U waves.

ERPs of all cardiac tissues are prolonged. His-Purkinje conduction time increases and QRS duration lengthens, especially at fast rates. Amiodarone given intravenously modestly prolongs the refractory period of atrial and ventricular muscle. The PR interval and AV nodal conduction time lengthen. The duration of the QRS complex lengthens at increased rates but less than after oral amiodarone. Thus, far less increase in prolongation of conduction time (except for the AV node), duration of repolarization, and refractoriness occur after IV administration compared with the oral route. Considering these actions, it is clear that amiodarone has class I (blocks I_{Na}), class II (antiadrenergic), and class IV (blocks I_{Ca-L}) actions in addition to class III effects (blocks I_K). Amiodarone's actions approximate those of a theoretically ideal drug that exhibits use-dependent Na^+ channel blockade with fast diastolic recovery from block and use-dependent prolongation of APD. It does not increase and may decrease QT dispersion. Catecholamines can partially reverse some of the effects of amiodarone.

HEMODYNAMIC EFFECTS. Amiodarone is a peripheral and coronary vasodilator. When administered intravenously (150 mg over 10 min, then 1 mg/min infusion) amiodarone decreases heart rate, systemic vascular resistance, left ventricular contractile force, and left ventricular dP/dt. Oral doses of amiodarone sufficient to control cardiac arrhythmias do not depress left ventricular ejection fraction, even in patients with reduced ejection fractions, and ejection fraction and cardiac output may increase slightly. However, because of antiadrenergic actions of amiodarone and because it does exert some negative inotropic action, it should be given cautiously, particularly intravenously, to patients with marginal cardiac compensation.

PHARMACOKINETICS (see Table 30–4). Amiodarone is slowly, variably, and incompletely absorbed, with systemic bioavailability of 35 to 65 percent. Plasma concentrations peak 3 to 7 hours after a single oral dose. There is a minimal first-pass effect, indicating little hepatic extraction. Elimination is by hepatic excretion into bile with some enterohepatic recirculation. Extensive hepatic metabolism occurs with desethylamiodarone as a major metabolite. The plasma concentration ratio of parent to metabolite is 3:2. Both accumulate extensively in the liver, lung, fat, "blue" skin, and other tissues. Myocardium develops a concentration 10 to 50 times that found in the plasma. Plasma clearance of amiodarone is low, and renal excretion is negligible. Doses need not be reduced in patients with renal disease. Amiodarone and desethylamiodarone are not dialyzable. Volume of distribution is large but variable, averaging 60 liter/kg. Amiodarone is highly protein bound (96 percent), crosses the placenta (10 to 50 percent), and is found in breast milk.

The onset of action after IV administration is generally within 1 to 2 hours. After oral administration, the onset of action may require 2 to 3 days, often 1 to 3 weeks, and, on occasion, even longer. Loading doses reduce this time interval. Plasma concentrations relate well to oral doses during chronic treatment, averaging about 0.5 μg/ml for each 100 mg/d at doses between 100 and 600 mg/d. Elimination half-life is multiphasic with an initial 50 percent reduction in plasma concentration 3 to 10 days after cessation of drug ingestion (probably representing elimination from well-perfused tissues) followed by a terminal half-life of 26 to 107 days (mean, 53 days), with most patients in the 40- to 55-day range. To achieve steady state without a loading dose takes about 265 days. Interpatient variability of these pharmacokinetic parameters mandates close monitoring of the patient. Therapeutic serum concentrations range from 1 to 2.5 μg/ml. Greater suppression of arrhythmias may occur up to 3.5 μg/ml, but the risk of side effects increases.

DOSAGE AND ADMINISTRATION (see Table 30–4). An optimal dosing schedule for all patients has not been achieved. One recommended approach is to treat with 800 to 1600 mg/d for 1 to 3 weeks, reduced to 800 mg/d for the next 2 to 4 weeks, then 600 mg/d for 4 to 8 weeks, and finally, after 2 to 3 months of treatment, a maintenance dose of 300 mg or less per day. Maintenance drug can be given once or twice daily and should be titrated to the lowest effective dose to minimize the occurrence of side effects. Doses as low as 100 mg/d can be effective in some patients. Regimens must be individualized for a given patient and clinical situation. Amiodarone may be administered intravenously to achieve more rapid loading and an effect in emergencies at initial doses of 15 mg/min for 10 minutes, followed by 1 mg/min for 6 hours and then 0.5 mg/min for the remaining 18 hours and for the next several days, as necessary. Supplemental infusions of 150 mg over 10 minutes can be used for breakthrough VT or VF. IV infusions can be continued safely for 2 to 3 weeks. IV amiodarone is generally well tolerated even in patients with left ventricular dysfunction. Patients with depressed ejection fractions should receive IV amiodarone with great caution because of hypotension. High-dose oral loading (800 to 2000 mg two or three times a day to maintain trough serum concentrations of 2 to 3 mg/ml) may suppress ventricular arrhythmias in 1 to 2 days.

INDICATIONS. Amiodarone has been used to suppress a wide spectrum of supraventricular and ventricular tachyarrhythmias in utero, in adults, and in children, including AV node and AV entry, junctional tachycardia, atrial flutter and fibrillation, VT and VF associated with coronary artery disease, and hypertrophic cardiomyopathy. Success rates vary widely depending on the population of patients, arrhythmia, underlying heart disease, length of follow-up, definition and determination of success, and other factors. In general, however, amiodarone's efficacy equals or exceeds that of all other antiarrhythmic agents and may be in the range of 60 to 80 percent for most supraventricular tachyarrhythmias and 40 to 60 percent for ventricular tachyarrhythmias. Amiodarone may be useful in improving survival in patients with hypertrophic cardiomyopathy, nonischemic dilated cardiomyopathy,[35] asymptomatic ventricular arrhythmias after myocardial infarction, and ventricular tachyarrhythmia during and after resuscitation from cardiac arrest. Amiodarone given before open-heart surgery,[36] as well as postoperatively, has been shown to decrease the incidence of postoperative atrial fibrillation. Amiodarone is superior to class I antiarrhythmic agents and sotalol in maintaining sinus rhythm in patients with recurrent atrial fibrillation.

Patients who have an ICD receive fewer shocks if they are treated with amiodarone compared with conventional drugs.[37] Amiodarone has little effect on pacing threshold but typically increases the electrical defibrillation threshold slightly.

A number of prospective, randomized, controlled trials have demonstrated improved survival with amiodarone therapy compared with placebo or metoprolol in patients after myocardial infarction. Amiodarone was found to improve survival in patients resuscitated from VF compared with conventional drugs. In patients with congestive heart failure, amiodarone therapy improved survival in one study (in which heart failure was mainly due to nonischemic cardiomyopathy), whereas no benefit was observed in another (primarily ischemic cardiomyopathy patients). The Antiarrhythmics Versus Implantable Defibrillator (AVID) trial was designed to compare mortality between patients treated with antiarrhythmic drugs (empirical amiodarone or EPS- or Holter-guided sotalol) versus an ICD in patients with ejection fraction less than 0.40 who had suffered spontaneous hypotensive VT or cardiac arrest. This study was stopped prematurely when an interim analysis showed that ICD-treated patients survived better after 1 year of treatment.[38]

Some controversy exists regarding the ability to predict the effectiveness of amiodarone in patients with ventricular tachyarrhythmias. Clinical assessment, suppression of spontaneous ventricular arrhythmias as documented by 24-hour ECG recordings, and response to EPS have served as endpoints to judge therapy. In the patient with a history of sustained VT or VF and minimal spontaneous ventricular arrhythmias in between symptomatic episodes, an invasive EPS is indicated to judge drug efficacy. The answer to when, after amiodarone therapy is started, such a study should be done is still not entirely resolved, but the interval should probably be 1 week or longer. In the 10 to 20 percent of patients whose electrically induced, clinical, ventricular tachyarrhythmias become no longer inducible while they are receiving amiodarone, the chances for a spontaneous recurrence of the arrhythmias are low while the patients are taking amiodarone, probably less than 5 to 10 percent at 1 year. For patients whose ventricular tachyarrhythmias are still inducible, the recurrence rate is 40 to 50 percent at 1 year. Patients' hemodynamic responses to the induced arrhythmia may also predict how they tolerate a spontaneous recurrence. Amiodarone slows the VT rate, but it is important to remember that the supine patient in the electrophysiology laboratory may tolerate the same tachycardia better than the patient in an erect position. An ejection fraction greater than 0.4 may predict a good response to amiodarone in patients with VT or VF.

Because of the serious nature of the arrhythmias being treated, the unusual pharmacokinetics of the drug, and its adverse effects, amiodarone therapy should be started with the patient hospitalized and monitored for at least several days. Combining other antiarrhythmic agents with amiodarone may improve efficacy in some patients.

ADVERSE EFFECTS. Adverse effects are reported by about 75 percent of patients treated with amiodarone for 5 years but compel stopping the drug in 18 to 37 percent. The most frequent side effects requiring drug discontinuation involve pulmonary and gastrointestinal complaints. Most adverse effects are reversible with dose reduction or cessation of treatment. Adverse effects are more common when therapy is continued in the long term and at higher doses. Of the noncardiac adverse reactions, pulmonary toxicity is the most serious; in one study it occurred between 6 days and 60 months of treatment in 33 of 573 patients, with 3 deaths. The mechanism is unclear but may involve a hypersensitivity reaction or widespread phospholipidosis, or both. Dyspnea, nonproductive cough, and fever are common symptoms, with crackles on examination, hypoxia, a positive gallium scan, reduced diffusion capacity, and radiographic evidence of pulmonary infiltrates.[39,40] Amiodarone must be discontinued if such pulmonary inflammatory changes occur. Corticosteroids can be tried, but no controlled studies have been done to support their use. A 10 percent mortality results in patients with pulmonary inflammatory changes, often in patients with unrecognized pulmonary involvement that is allowed to progress. Chest radiographs and pulmonary function tests, including carbon monoxide diffusion capacity (DLCO), at 3-month intervals for the first year and then twice a year for several years have been recommended. At maintenance doses less than 300 mg/d, pulmonary toxicity is uncommon. Advanced age, high drug maintenance dose, and reduced predrug diffusion capacity are risk factors for developing pulmonary toxicity. An unchanged DLCO on therapy may be a negative predictor of pulmonary toxicity.

Although asymptomatic elevations of liver enzymes are found in most patients, the drug is not stopped unless values exceed two or three times normal in a patient with initially abnormal values. Cirrhosis occurs uncommonly but may be fatal. Neurological dysfunction, photosensitivity (perhaps minimized by sunscreens), bluish skin discoloration, gastroenterological disturbances, and hyperthyroidism[41] (1 to 2 percent) or hypothyroidism (2 to 4 percent) can occur. Amiodarone appears to inhibit the peripheral conversion of T_4 to T_3 so that chemical changes result, which are characterized by a slight increase in T_4, reverse T_3 and thyroid-stimulating hormone (TSH), and a slight decrease in T_3. Reverse T_3 concentration has been used as an index of drug efficacy. During hypothyroidism, TSH increases greatly, whereas T_3 increases in hyperthyroidism. Thyroid function tests should be obtained approximately every 3 months for the first year while amiodarone is taken and once or twice yearly thereafter, sooner if symptoms develop that are consistent with thyroid dysfunction. Corneal microdeposits occur in almost 100 percent of adults receiving the drug more than 6 months. More serious ocular reactions, including optic neuritis or atrophy with visual loss, or both, have been reported but are rare and causality by amiodarone has not been established.[42]

Cardiac side effects include symptomatic bradycardias in about 2 percent; worsening of ventricular tachyarrhythmias (with occasional development of torsades de pointes)[40] in 1 to 2 percent, possibly higher in women (see Table 72–3); and worsening of congestive heart failure in 2 percent. Possibly because of interactions with anesthetics, complications after open-heart surgery, including pulmonary dysfunction, hypotension, hepatic dysfunction, and low cardiac output, have been noted by some, but not all, investigators.

In general, the lowest possible maintenance dose of amiodarone that is still effective should be used to avoid significant adverse effects. Many supraventricular arrhythmias can be successfully managed with daily doses of 200 mg or less, whereas ventricular arrhythmias generally require higher doses. Adverse effects are uncommon at doses of 200 mg/d or less but still occur. Because of potential toxicity in a variety of organ systems, special multidisciplinary amiodarone clinics have been used by some to attempt to prevent adverse outcomes when using the drug.

Important interactions with other drugs occur, and when they are given concomitantly with amiodarone, the doses of warfarin, digoxin, and other antiarrhythmic drugs should be reduced by one third to one half and the patient observed closely. Drugs with synergistic actions, such as beta blockers or calcium channel blockers, must be given cautiously. Amiodarone's safety during pregnancy has not been established, and it should be used in the pregnant patient only if no alternatives exist.

Bretylium Tosylate

Bretylium is a quaternary ammonium compound that is approved by the FDA for parenteral use only in patients with life-threatening ventricular tachyarrhythmias.

ELECTROPHYSIOLOGICAL ACTIONS (see Tables 30-1, 30-2, 30-3, and 30-5). Bretylium is selectively concentrated in sympathetic ganglia and their postganglionic adrenergic nerve terminals. After initially causing norepinephrine release, bretylium prevents norepinephrine release by depressing sympathetic nerve terminal excitability without depressing preganglionic or postganglionic sympathetic nerve conduction, impairing conduction across sympathetic ganglia, depleting the adrenergic neuron of norepinephrine, or decreasing the responsiveness of adrenergic receptors. It produces a state resembling chemical sympathectomy. During chronic bretylium treatment, the beta-adrenergic responses to circulating catecholamines are increased. The initial release of catecholamines results in several transient electrophysiological responses, such as an increase in the discharge rates of the isolated, perfused sinus node and of in vitro Purkinje fibers, often making quiescent fibers automatic.

Bretylium initially increases conduction velocity and excitability and decreases refractoriness in the rabbit atrium, and partially depolarized fibers may hyperpolarize. Pretreatment with propranolol prevents these early changes. Initial catecholamine release can exacerbate some arrhythmias, such as those caused by digitalis excess or myocardial infarction. Prolonged drug administration lengthens the duration of the action potential and refractoriness of atrial and ventricular muscle and Purkinje fibers, possibly by blocking one or more repolarizing potassium currents. The ratio of ERP to APD does not change, nor do membrane responsiveness and conduction velocity. Bretylium exerts little effect on diastolic excitability. It has little if any effect on sustained VT but can prevent recurrences of VF. It is not clear whether the chemical sympathectomy-like state alone or together with other actions exerts the antifibrillatory effect. Reduced disparity between APD and ERP in regions of normal and infarcted myocardium may account for some of its antifibrillatory effects. Bretylium has no effect on vagal reflexes and does not alter the responsiveness of cholinergic receptors in the heart.

HEMODYNAMIC EFFECTS. Bretylium does not depress myocardial contractility. After an initial increase in blood pressure, the drug can cause significant hypotension by blocking the efferent limb of the baroreceptor reflex. Hypotension results most commonly when patients are sitting or standing but can also occur in the supine position in seriously ill patients. Bretylium reduces the extent of the vasoconstriction and tachycardia reflexes during standing. Orthostatic hypotension can persist for several days after the drug has been discontinued.

PHARMACOKINETICS (see Table 30–4). Bretylium is effective orally as well as parenterally, but it is absorbed poorly and erratically from the gastrointestinal tract and thus is practically useful only intravenously. Bioavailability may be less than 50 percent, and elimination is almost exclusively by renal excretion without significant metabolism or active metabolites being recognized. Elimination half-life is 5 to 10 hours but with fairly wide variability. Doses should be reduced in patients with renal insufficiency. In survivors of VT or VF, bretylium had an elimination half-life of 13.5 hours after single IV dosing, which was similar to previous results in normal subjects. Renal clearance accounted for virtually all elimination. Onset of action after IV administration occurs within several minutes, but full antiarrhythmic effects may not be seen for 30 minutes to 2 hours.

DOSAGE AND ADMINISTRATION (see Table 30–4). Bretylium can be given intravenously in doses of 5 to 10 mg/kg of body weight diluted in 50 to 100 ml of 5 percent dextrose in water and administered over 10 to 20 minutes or more quickly in a life-threatening state. This dose can be repeated in 1 to 2 hours if the arrhythmia persists. The total daily dose probably should not exceed 30 mg/kg. A similar initial dose, but undiluted, can be given intramuscularly. The maintenance IV dose is 0.5 to 2.0 mg/min. Intramuscular injection during cardiopulmonary resuscitation from cardiac arrest and in shock states should be avoided because of unreliable absorption during reduced tissue perfusion. In this situation, bretylium should be given intravenously.

INDICATIONS. Bretylium is used in patients who are in an intensive care setting and who have life-threatening, recurrent ventricular tachyarrhythmias that have not responded to other antiarrhythmic drugs. Bretylium has been effective in treating some patients with drug-resistant tachyarrhythmias and in treating victims of out-of-hospital VF.

ADVERSE EFFECTS. Hypotension, most prominently orthostatic but also supine, appears to be the most significant side effect and can be prevented with tricyclic drugs such as protriptyline. Transient hypertension, increased sinus rate, and worsening of arrhythmias, often those related to digitalis excess or ischemia, may follow initial drug administration and may be due to initial release of catecholamines. Bretylium should be used cautiously or not at all in patients who have a relatively fixed cardiac output, such as those with severe aortic stenosis. Vasodilators or diuretics can enhance these hypotensive effects. Nausea and vomiting can occur after parenteral administration.

Sotalol

Sotalol is a nonspecific beta adrenoceptor blocker without intrinsic sympathomimetic activity that prolongs repolarization.[43] It was approved in 1992 by the FDA to treat patients with life-threatening ventricular tachyarrhythmias and in 1998 for atrial fibrillation.

ELECTROPHYSIOLOGICAL ACTIONS (see Tables 30-1, 30-2, 30-3, and 30-5). Both *d* and *l* isomers have similar effects on prolonging repolarization, whereas the *l* isomer is responsible for virtually all the beta-blocking activity. Sotalol does not block alpha adrenoceptors and does not block the sodium channel (no membrane-stabilizing effects) but does prolong atrial and ventricular repolarization times by reducing I_{Kr}, thus prolonging the plateau of the action potential. Action potential prolongation is greater at slower rates (reverse use-dependence). Resting membrane potential, action potential amplitude, and $\dot{V}_{max}$ are not significantly altered. Sotalol prolongs atrial and ventricular refractoriness, AH and QT intervals, and sinus cycle length. It shortens the excitable gap in reentrant VT.

HEMODYNAMICS. Sotalol exerts a negative inotropic effect only through its beta-blocking action. It can increase the strength of contraction by prolonging repolarization, which occurs maximally at slow heart rates. In patients with reduced cardiac function, sotalol can cause a decrease in cardiac index, an increase in filling pressure, and overt heart failure. Therefore, it must be used cautiously in patients with marginal cardiac compensation but appears to be well tolerated in patients with normal cardiac function.

PHARMACOKINETICS (see Table 30–4). Sotalol is completely absorbed and not metabolized, making it 90 to 100 percent bioavailable. It is not bound to plasma proteins, is excreted unchanged primarily by the kidneys, and has an elimination half-life of 10 to 15 hours. Peak plasma concentrations occur 2.5 to 4.0 hours after oral ingestion, with steady state attained after five or six doses. Effective antiarrhythmic plasma concentration is in the range of 2.5 μg/ml. There is little intersubject variability in plasma levels. Over the dose range of 160 to 640 mg, sotalol displays dose proportionality with plasma concentration. The dose must be reduced in patients with renal disease. The beta-blocking effect is half maximal at 80 mg/d and maximal at 320 mg/d. Significant beta-blocking action occurs at 160 mg/d.

DOSAGE (see Table 30–4). The typical oral dose is 80 to 160 mg every 12 hours, allowing 2 to 3 days between dose adjustments to attain steady state and monitor the electrocardiogram for arrhythmias and QT prolongation. Doses exceeding 320 mg/d can be used in patients when the potential benefits outweigh the risk of proarrhythmia.

INDICATIONS. Approved by the FDA to treat patients with ventricular tachyarrhythmias and atrial fibrillation, sotalol is also useful to prevent recurrence of a wide variety of SVTs, including atrial flutter, AT, AV node reentry, and AV reentry. It also slows the ventricular response to atrial tachyarrhythmias. It appears to be more effective than conventional antiarrhythmic drugs and may be comparable to amiodarone in treating patients with ventricular tachyarrhythmias. Sotalol has been shown to be superior to lidocaine for acute termination of sustained VT and is useful in patients with arrhythmogenic right ventricular dysplasia. Sotalol may be effective in pediatric patients. Unlike most other antiarrhythmic drugs, it may decrease the frequency of ICD discharges[44] and reduce the defibrillation threshold.

ADVERSE EFFECTS. Proarrhythmia is the most serious adverse effect. Overall, new or worsened ventricular tachyarrhythmias occur in about 4 percent, and this response is due to torsades de pointes in about 2.5 percent. The incidence of torsades de pointes increases to 4 percent in patients with a history of sustained VT and is dose related, reportedly only 1.6 percent at 320 mg/d but 4.4 percent at 480 mg/d (see Table 72–3). This proarrhythmic effect was probably the cause of excess mortality in patients given *d*-sotalol (the enantiomer lacking a beta-blocking effect) after an acute myocardial infarction in the Survival With Oral *d*-Sotalol (SWORD) trial. Other adverse effects commonly seen with other beta blockers also apply to sotalol. Sotalol should be used with caution or not at all in combination with other drugs that prolong the QT interval. However, such combinations have been used successfully.

Ibutilide

Ibutilide is an agent released for use in acutely terminating episodes of atrial flutter and fibrillation.

ELECTROPHYSIOLOGICAL ACTIONS (see Tables 30-1, 30-2, 30-3, and 30-5). Like other class III agents, ibutilide prolongs repolarization. Although it is like other class III agents that block outward potassium currents such as I_{Kr}, ibutilide is unique in that it also appears to activate a slow inward sodium current. Administered intravenously, ibutilide causes mild slowing of the sinus rate and has minimal effects on AV conduction or QRS duration, but the QT interval is characteristically prolonged. Ibutilide has no significant effect on hemodynamics.

PHARMACOKINETICS (see Table 30–4). Ibutilide is administered intravenously and has a large volume of distribution. Clearance is predominantly renal, with a drug half-life averaging 6 hours (but with considerable interpatient variability). Protein binding is approximately 40 percent. One of the drug's metabolites has weak class III effects.

DOSAGE AND ADMINISTRATION (see Table 30–4). Ibutilide is given as a rapid IV infusion of 1 mg over 10 minutes. It should not be given in the presence of a QTc interval greater than 440 milliseconds or other drugs that prolong the QT interval or when uncorrected hypokalemia or bradycardia exists. A second 1-mg dose may be given after the first dose is finished if the arrhythmia persists. Patients must have continuous ECG monitoring throughout the dosing period and for 6 to 8 hours thereafter because of the risk of ventricular arrhythmias. Up to 60 percent of patients with atrial fibrillation and 70 percent of those with atrial flutter convert to sinus rhythm after 2 mg of ibutilide.[45]

INDICATIONS. Ibutilide is indicated for termination of an established episode of atrial flutter or fibrillation. It should not be used in patients with frequent, short paroxysms of atrial fibrillation because it merely terminates episodes and is not useful for prevention. Patients whose condition is hemodynamically unstable should proceed to direct-current cardioversion. Ibutilide has been administered at the time of transthoracic electrical cardioversion to increase the likelihood of termination of atrial fibrillation. In one study, all 50 patients given ibutilide before attempted electrical cardioversion achieved sinus rhythm, whereas only 34 of 50 who did not receive the drug converted to sinus rhythm.[46] Of note, all 16 patients who did not respond to electrical cardioversion without ibutilide were successfully electrically cardioverted to sinus rhythm when a second attempt was made after ibutilide pretreatment.

Ibutilide prolongs accessory pathway refractoriness and can temporarily slow the ventricular rate during preexcited atrial fibrillation. The drug can also terminate episodes of sustained uniform morphology VT.

ADVERSE EFFECTS. The most significant adverse effects of ibutilide are QT prolongation and torsades de pointes, which occur in approximately 2 percent of patients given the drug. The adverse effect occurs within the first 4 to 6 hours of dosing, after which the risk is negligible. Thus, patients in whom the drug is used must undergo ECG monitoring for up to 8 hours after dosing. This requirement can make ibutilide's use in emergency departments or private offices problematic. Ibutilide's safety during pregnancy is not well studied. Its use should be restricted to cases in which no safer alternative exists (see Table 72–3).

Dofetilide

Dofetilide is approved for acute conversion of atrial fibrillation to sinus rhythm as well as chronic suppression of recurrent atrial fibrillation.[47]

ELECTROPHYSIOLOGICAL ACTIONS (see Tables 30-1, 30-2, 30-3, and 30-5). The sole electrophysiological effect of dofetilide appears to be block of the rapid component of the delayed rectifier potassium current (I_{Kr}), which is important in repolarization (see Chap. 27). This effect is more prominent in the atria than in the ventricles (30 percent increase in atrial refractory periods versus 20 percent in the ventricles). Dofetilide's effect on I_{Kr} prolongs refractoriness without slowing conduction, which is believed to be largely responsible for its antiarrhythmic effect. It is also responsible for the prolongation of the QT interval on the electrocardiogram, which averages 11 percent but can be much greater. This effect on the QT interval is dose dependent and linear. No other important ECG changes are observed with the drug. It has no significant hemodynamic effects. Dofetilide is more effective than quinidine at converting atrial fibrillation to sinus rhythm.

PHARMACOKINETICS (see Table 30–4). Orally administered dofetilide is absorbed well, with over 90 percent bioavailability. Fifty to 60 percent of the drug is excreted unchanged in urine, with a mean elimination half-life of 7 to 13 hours. The remainder of the drug undergoes hepatic metabolism to inert compounds. Significant drug-drug interactions have been reported in patients using dofetilide; cimetidine, verapamil, ketoconazole, and trimethoprim (alone or in combination with sulfamethoxazole) cause significant elevation in dofetilide serum concentration and should not be used with this drug.

DOSAGE AND ADMINISTRATION (see Table 30–4). Dofetilide is available only as an oral preparation. Dosing is from 0.125 to 0.5 mg twice daily and must be initiated in a hospital setting with continuous ECG monitoring to ensure that inordinate QT prolongation and torsades de pointes do not develop. Physicians must be certified to prescribe the drug. Dosage must be decreased in the presence of impaired renal function or increase in QT interval of more than 50 percent. The drug should not be given to patients with a creatinine clearance less than 20 ml/min or a baseline corrected QT interval greater than 440 milliseconds.

INDICATIONS. IV dofetilide has been used on an investigational basis for termination of an established episode of atrial flutter, fibrillation, or other types of SVT. Oral dofetilide is indicated for prevention of episodes of supraventricular tachyarrhythmias, particularly atrial flutter and fibrillation. Dofetilide's role in therapy for ventricular arrhythmias is less clear. Dofetilide has been shown to have a neutral effect on mortality when given to patients after myocardial infarction.[48]

ADVERSE EFFECTS. The most significant adverse effect of dofetilide is QT interval prolongation with torsades de pointes, occurring in 2 to 4 percent of patients given the drug. Risk is highest in patients with a baseline prolonged QT interval, those who are hypokalemic, those taking some other agent that prolongs repolarization, and after conversion from atrial fibrillation to sinus rhythm (see Table 72–3). The drug is otherwise well tolerated with few side effects. Its use in pregnancy (class C) has not been studied extensively, and it should probably be avoided in this setting if possible.

Azimilide

Azimilide is a new agent (not yet approved by the FDA at the time of this writing) for use in the treatment of atrial flutter and fibrillation.[49]

ELECTROPHYSIOLOGICAL ACTIONS (see Tables 30-1, 30-2, 30-3, and 30-5). Unlike dofetilide, which blocks the rapid component of the delayed rectifier potassium current, azimilide produces a more balanced blockade of both rapid and slow components of I_K. It is presumed that this effect is responsible for the lower rate of proarrhythmia as well as better preservation of drug efficacy at higher heart rates with this agent compared with pure I_{Kr} blockers. Azimilide produces a mild prolongation of the QT interval but no other meaningful ECG changes. Unlike dofetilide and sotalol, which have greater effects on atrial than ventricular refractoriness, azimilide exerts a similar effect on each.[50]

PHARMACOKINETICS (see Table 30–4). Azimilide's pharmacokinetic profile is relatively simple and predictable. It can be taken orally once a day, and its absorption is nearly complete and unaffected by food intake. Few drug interactions have been reported. Azimilide is cleared by the kidney; some metabolism of the drug to inactive compounds occurs. The drug has no significant adverse hemodynamic effects.

DOSAGE AND ADMINISTRATION (see Table 30–4). Azimilide can be taken by mouth once a day at a dose of 100 to 200 mg. The drug is well tolerated, and dosing need not be adjusted in the presence of renal or hepatic disease.

INDICATIONS. Azimilide is indicated for IV administration to terminate an established episode of atrial flutter or fibrillation, as well as orally for long-term prevention of these arrhythmias. Studies are under way to evaluate its efficacy in ventricular arrhythmias.

ADVERSE EFFECTS. The drug is generally well tolerated. As with other class III agents, the most significant adverse effect of azimilide is torsades de pointes, although this arrhythmia appears to be less common with this agent than with other class III medications (occurring in approximately 1 percent of patients given the drug) (see Table 72–3). Azimilide's safety in pregnancy is not known; its use should probably be avoided if possible.

Class IV Antiarrhythmic Agents

Calcium Channel Antagonists: Verapamil and Diltiazem

Verapamil, a synthetic papaverine derivative, is the prototype of a class of drugs that block the slow calcium channel and reduce $I_{Ca\text{-}L}$ in cardiac muscle. Diltiazem has electrophysiological actions similar to those of verapamil. Nifedipine exhibits minimal electrophysiological effects at clinically used doses; felodipine blocks the T-type calcium current (see Chap. 27), and its clinical application has not been established. Neither of these drugs is discussed here.

ELECTROPHYSIOLOGICAL ACTIONS (see Tables 30-1, 30-2, 30-3, and 30-5). By blocking $I_{Ca\text{-}L}$ in all cardiac fibers, verapamil reduces the plateau height of the action potential, slightly shortens muscle action potential, and slightly prolongs total Purkinje fiber action potential. It does not appreciably affect the action potential amplitude, $\dot{V}_{max}$ of phase 0, or resting membrane voltage in cells that have fast-response characteristics related to I_{Na} (atrial and ventricular muscle, the His-Purkinje system). Verapamil suppresses slow responses elicited by a variety of experimental methods as well as triggered sustained rhythmic activity and early and late afterdepolarizations. Verapamil and diltiazem suppress electrical activity in the normal sinus and AV nodes in concentrations that do not suppress action potentials of fast channel-dependent cells. Verapamil depresses the slope of diastolic depolarization in sinus node cells, $\dot{V}_{max}$ of phase 0, maximum diastolic potential, and action potential amplitude in sinus node and AV node cells and prolongs conduction time and the effective and functional refractory periods of the AV node. The AV node blocking effects of verapamil and diltiazem are more apparent at faster rates of stimulation (use-dependence) and in depolarized fibers (voltage dependence). Verapamil slows the activation and delays recovery from inactivation of the slow channel. Unbinding of the drug from its receptor occurs more rapidly in tissue that is hyperpolarized.

Verapamil does exert some local anesthetic activity because the dextrorotatory stereoisomer of the clinically used racemic mixture exerts slight blocking effects on I_{Na}. The levorotatory stereoisomer blocks the slow inward current carried by calcium, as well as other ions, traveling through the slow channel. Verapamil does not modify calcium uptake, binding, or exchange by cardiac microsomes, nor does it affect calcium-activated adenosine triphosphatase. Verapamil does not block beta receptors but may block alpha receptors and potentiate vagal effects on the AV node. Verapamil may also cause other effects that indirectly alter cardiac electrophysiology, such as decreasing platelet adhesiveness or reducing the extent of myocardial ischemia.

In humans, verapamil prolongs conduction time through the AV node (the AH interval) without affecting the P wave or QRS duration or HV interval and lengthens the anterograde and retrograde functional refractory periods and ERPs of the AV node. Spontaneous sinus rate may decrease slightly, an effect only partially reversed by atropine. More commonly, the sinus rate does not change significantly because verapamil causes peripheral vasodilation, transient hypotension, and reflex sympathetic stimulation that mitigates any direct slowing effect verapamil exerts on the sinus node. If verapamil is given to a patient who is also receiving a beta blocker, the sinus node discharge rate may slow because reflex sympathetic stimulation is blocked. Verapamil does not exert a significant direct effect on atrial or ventricular refractoriness or on anterograde or retrograde properties of accessory pathways. However, reflex sympathetic stimulation following IV verapamil administration may increase the ventricular response over the accessory pathway during atrial fibrillation in patients with the Wolff-Parkinson-White syndrome.

HEMODYNAMIC EFFECTS. Because verapamil interferes with excitation-contraction coupling, it inhibits vascular smooth muscle contraction and causes marked vasodilation in coronary and other peripheral vascular beds. Propranolol does not block the vasodilation produced by verapamil. Reflex sympathetic effects may reduce in vivo the marked negative inotropic action of verapamil on isolated cardiac muscle, but the direct myocardial depressant effects of verapamil may predominate when the drug is given in high doses. In patients with well-preserved left ventricular function, combined therapy with propranolol and verapamil appears to be well tolerated, but beta blockade can accentuate the hemodynamic depressant effects produced by oral verapamil. Patients who have reduced left ventricular function may not tolerate the combined blockade of beta receptors and slow channels, and thus in these patients verapamil and propranolol should be used in combination either cautiously or not at all. Verapamil decreases myocardial oxygen demand while decreasing coronary vascular resistance and reduces the extent of ischemic damage in experimental preparations. Such changes may be antiarrhythmic. Diltiazem also reduces ventricular arrhythmias during coronary occlusion in the dog, possibly by preventing calcium overload.

Peak alterations in hemodynamic variables occur 3 to 5 minutes after completion of a verapamil injection, with the major effects dissipating within 10 minutes. Systemic resistance and mean arterial pressure decrease, as does left ventricular dP/dt_{max}, and left ventricular end-diastolic pressure increases. Heart rate, cardiac index, left ventricular minute work, and mean pulmonary artery pressure do not change significantly. Thus, afterload reduction produced by verapamil significantly minimizes its negative inotropic action so that the cardiac index may not be reduced. In addition, when verapamil slows the ventricular rate in a patient with a tachycardia, cardiac slowing may also improve hemodynamics. Nevertheless, caution should be exercised when giving verapamil to patients with severe myocardial depression or those receiving beta blockers or disopyramide because hemodynamic deterioration may progress in some patients.

PHARMACOKINETICS (see Table 30–4). After single oral doses of verapamil, measurable prolongation of AV nodal conduction time occurs in 30 minutes and lasts 4 to 6 hours. After IV administration, AV nodal conduction delay occurs within 1 to 2 minutes and AH interval prolongation is still detectable after 6 hours. Effective plasma concentrations necessary to terminate SVT are in the range of 125 ng/ml after doses of 0.075 to 0.150 mg/kg. After oral administration, absorption is almost complete, but an overall bioavailability of 20 to 35 percent suggests substantial first-pass metabolism in the liver, particularly of the *l*-isomer. The elimination half-life of verapamil is 3 to 7 hours, with up to 70 percent of the drug excreted by the kidneys. Norverapamil is a major metabolite that may contribute to verapamil's electrophysiological actions. Serum protein binding is approximately 90 percent. With diltiazem, the percentage of heart rate reduction in atrial fibrillation is related to plasma concentration.

DOSAGE AND ADMINISTRATION (see Table 30–4). The most commonly used IV dose of verapamil is 10 mg infused over 1 to 2 minutes while cardiac rhythm and blood pressure are monitored. A second injection of equal dose may be given 30 minutes later. The initial effect achieved with the first bolus injection, such as slowing of the ventricular response during atrial fibrillation, may be maintained by a continuous infusion of the drug at a rate of 0.005 mg/kg/min. The oral dose is 240 to 480 mg/d in divided doses. Diltiazem is given intravenously at a dose of 0.25 mg/kg as a bolus over 2 minutes, with a second dose in 15 minutes if necessary; because it is generally better tolerated (less hypotension) for long-term administration, such as for control of ventricular rate during atrial fibrillation, diltiazem is preferred over verapamil in this setting. Orally, doses must be adjusted to the patient's needs, with a 120- to 360-mg range. Various long-acting preparations exist for verapamil and diltiazem.

INDICATIONS. After simple vagal maneuvers have been tried and adenosine given, IV verapamil or diltiazem is the next treatment of choice for terminating sustained sinus node reentry, AV node reentry, or orthodromic AV reciprocating tachycardia associated with an accessory pathway. Verapamil is as effective as adenosine for termination of these arrhythmias. Verapamil should definitely be tried before attempting termination by digitalis administration, pacing, electrical direct-current cardioversion, or acute blood pressure elevation with vasopressors. Verapamil and diltiazem terminate 60 to 90 percent or more episodes of paroxysmal SVTs within several minutes. Verapamil may be of use in some fetal SVTs as well. Although IV verapamil has been given along with IV propranolol, this combination should be used only with great caution.

Verapamil and diltiazem decrease the ventricular response over the AV node during atrial fibrillation or atrial flutter, possibly converting a small number of episodes to sinus rhythm, particularly if the atrial flutter or fibrillation is of recent onset. In addition, verapamil may prevent early recurrence of atrial fibrillation after cardioversion.[51] Some patients who exhibit atrial flutter may develop atrial fibrillation after verapamil administration. As noted earlier, in patients with preexcited ventricular complexes during atrial fibrillation associated with the Wolff-Parkinson-White syndrome, IV verapamil may accelerate the ventricular response; therefore, the IV route is contraindicated in this situation. Verapamil can terminate some ATs. Even though verapamil terminates a left septal VT, hemodynamic collapse can occur if IV verapamil is given to patients with the more common forms of VT because they generally occur in the setting of decreased left ventricular systolic function. A general rule to avoid complications, however, is not to administer IV verapamil to any patient with wide QRS tachycardia unless one is absolutely certain of the nature of the tachycardia and its response to verapamil.

Orally, verapamil or diltiazem can prevent the recurrence of AV node reentrant and orthodromic AV reciprocating tachycardias associated with the Wolff-Parkinson-White syndrome as well as help maintain a decreased ventricular response during atrial flutter or atrial fibrillation in patients without an accessory pathway. In this regard, the effectiveness of verapamil appears to be enhanced when given concomitantly with quinidine, and that of diltiazem is enhanced when given with digoxin. Verapamil generally has not been effective in treating patients who have recurrent ventricular tachyarrhythmias, although it may suppress some forms of VT, such as a left septal VT, as noted earlier. It may also be useful in about two thirds of patients with idiopathic VT that has a left bundle branch block morphology, in patients with hypertrophic cardiomyopathy who have experienced cardiac arrest, in patients with a short-coupled variant of torsades de pointes, in patients with right ventricular dysplasia, and in patients with ventricular arrhythmias related to coronary artery spasm. Whereas data from animal models suggest that verapamil may be useful in reducing or preventing ventricular arrhythmias related to acute myocardial ischemia, calcium antagonists have not been shown to reduce mortality or prevent sudden cardiac death in patients after acute myocardial infarction, except for diltiazem in patients with non-Q-wave infarctions. Verapamil abolishes the wall motion abnormality found in patients with the long QT syndrome.

ADVERSE EFFECTS. Verapamil must be used cautiously in patients with significant hemodynamic impairment or in those receiving beta blockers, as previously noted. Hypotension, bradycardia, AV block, and asystole are more likely to occur when the drug is given to patients who are already receiving beta-blocking agents. Hemodynamic collapse has been noted in infants, and verapamil should be used cautiously in patients younger than 1 year. Verapamil should also be used with caution in patients with sinus node abnormalities because marked depression of sinus node function or asystole can result in some of these patients. Isoproterenol, calcium, glucagon infusion, dopamine, or atropine (which may be only partially effective) or temporary pacing may be necessary to counteract some of the adverse effects of verapamil. Isoproterenol may be more effective for treating bradyarrhythmias and calcium may be used for treating hemodynamic dysfunction secondary to verapamil. AV node depression is common in overdoses. Contraindications to the use of verapamil and diltiazem include the presence of advanced heart failure, second- or third-degree AV block without a pacemaker in place, atrial fibrillation and anterograde conduction over an accessory pathway, significant sinus node dysfunction, most VTs, cardiogenic shock, and other hypotensive states. Although the drugs probably should not be used in patients with overt heart failure, if the latter is due to one of the supraventricular tachyarrhythmias noted earlier, verapamil or diltiazem may restore sinus rhythm or significantly decrease the ventricular rate, leading to hemodynamic improvement. Finally, it is important to note that verapamil can decrease the excretion of digoxin by about 30 percent. Hepatotoxicity may occur on occasion. Verapamil crosses the placental barrier; its use in pregnancy has been associated with impaired uterine contraction, fetal bradycardia, and, possibly, fetal digital defects. It should thus be used only if no good alternatives exist.

Other Antiarrhythmic Agents

Adenosine

Adenosine is an endogenous nucleoside present throughout the body and has been approved by the FDA to treat patients with SVTs.

ELECTROPHYSIOLOGICAL ACTIONS (see Tables 30-1, 30-2, 30-3, and 30-5). Adenosine interacts with A_1 receptors present on the extracellular surface of cardiac cells, activating K^+ channels ($I_{K\,Ach}$, $I_{K\,Ado}$) in a fashion similar to that produced by acetylcholine. The increase in K^+ conductance shortens atrial APD, hyperpolarizes the membrane potential, and decreases atrial contractility. Similar changes occur in the sinus and AV nodes. In contrast to these direct effects mediated through the guanine nucleotide regulatory proteins G_i and G_o, adenosine antagonizes catecholamine-stimulated adenylate cyclase to decrease cyclic adenosine monophosphate accumulation and to decrease $I_{Ca\text{-}L}$ and the pacemaker current I_f in sinus node cells, along with a decrease in $\dot{V}_{max}$. Shifts in pacemaker site within the sinus node and sinus exit block may occur. Adenosine slows the sinus rate in humans, which is followed by a reflex increase in sinus rate. In the N region of the AV node, conduction is depressed, along with decreases in action potential amplitude, duration, and $\dot{V}_{max}$. Transient prolongation of the AH interval results, often with transient first-, second-, or third-degree AV node block. Delay in AV nodal conduction is rate dependent. His-Purkinje conduction is generally not directly affected. Adenosine does not affect conduction in normal accessory pathways. Conduction may be blocked in accessory pathways that have long conduction times or decremental conduction properties. Patients with heart transplants exhibit a supersensitive response to adenosine. Adenosine may mediate the phenomenon of ischemic preconditioning.

PHARMACOKINETICS (see Table 30–4). Adenosine is removed from the extracellular space by washout, enzymatically by degradation to inosine, by phosphorylation to adenosine monophosphate, or by reuptake into cells through a nucleoside transport system. The vascular endothelium and the formed blood elements contain these elimination systems, which result in very rapid clearance of adenosine from the circulation. Elimination half-life is 1 to 6 seconds. Most of adenosine's effects are produced during its first passage through the circulation. Important drug interactions occur: methylxanthines are competitive antagonists, and therapeutic concentrations of theophylline totally block the exogenous adenosine effect. Dipyridamole is a nucleoside transport blocker that blocks reuptake of adenosine, delaying its clearance from the circulation or interstitial space and potentiating its effect. Smaller adenosine doses should be used in patients receiving dipyridamole.

DOSAGE AND ADMINISTRATION (see Table 30–4). To terminate tachycardia, a bolus of adenosine is rapidly injected intravenously at doses of 6 to 12 mg followed by a flush. Pediatric dosing should be 0.1 to 0.3 mg/kg. When given into a central vein and in patients after heart transplantation or in patients receiving dipyridamole, the initial dose should be reduced to 3 mg. Transient sinus slowing or AV node block results, lasting less than 5 seconds.

INDICATIONS. Adenosine has become the drug of first choice to terminate acutely an SVT such as AV node or AV reentry. It is useful in pediatric patients and to judge the effectiveness of ablation of accessory pathways. Adenosine can produce AV block or terminate ATs and sinus node reentry. It results in only transient AV block during atrial flutter or fibrillation and is thus useful only in their diagnosis (not therapy). Adenosine terminates a group of VTs whose maintenance depends on adrenergic drive, which is most often located in the right ventricular outflow tract but found at other sites as well. Adenosine has less potential than verapamil for lowering the blood pressure should tachycardia persist after injection.

Doses as low as 2.5 mg terminate some tachycardias; doses of 12 mg or less terminate 92 percent of SVTs, usually within 30 seconds. Successful termination rates with adenosine are comparable to those achieved with verapamil. Because of its effectiveness and extremely short duration of action, adenosine is preferable to verapamil in most instances, particularly in patients who previously received IV beta adrenoceptor blockers, in those having poorly compensated heart failure or severe hypotension, and in neonates. Verapamil might be chosen first in patients receiving drugs such as theophylline, which is known to interfere with adenosine's actions or metabolism; in patients with active bronchoconstriction; and in those with inadequate venous access.

Adenosine may be useful to help differentiate among causes of wide QRS tachycardias because it terminates many SVTs with aberrancy or reveals the underlying atrial mechanism, and it does not block conduction over an accessory pathway or terminate most VTs. Adenosine in rare cases terminates some VTs (characteristically those of right ventricular outflow tract origin), and therefore tachycardia termination is not completely diagnostic for an SVT. This agent may predispose to the development of atrial fibrillation and possibly can increase the ventricular response in patients with atrial fibrillation conducting over an accessory pathway. Adenosine may also be useful in differentiating conduction over the AV node from that over an accessory pathway during ablative procedures designed to interrupt the accessory pathway. However, this distinction is not absolute because adenosine can block conduction in slowly conducting accessory pathways and does not always effect block in the AV node. Endogenously released adenosine may be important in ischemia and hypoxia-induced AV node block and in post-defibrillation bradyarrhythmias.

ADVERSE EFFECTS. Transient side effects occur in almost 40 percent of patients with SVT given adenosine and are most commonly flushing, dyspnea, and chest pressure. These symptoms are fleeting, lasting less than 1 minute, and are well tolerated. PVCs, transient sinus bradycardia, sinus arrest, and AV block are common when an SVT abruptly terminates. Atrial fibrillation is occasionally observed (12 percent in one study) with adenosine administration,[52] perhaps owing to the drug's effect in shortening atrial refractoriness. Induction of atrial fibrillation can be problematic in patients with the Wolff-Parkinson-White syndrome and rapid AV conduction over the accessory pathway.

Digoxin

Cardiac actions of digitalis glycosides have been recognized for centuries. Digoxin is used for control of supraventricular arrhythmias, mainly control of ventricular rate during atrial fibrillation. The use of digoxin has decreased owing to the availability of agents with greater potency and a wider therapeutic-to-toxic drug concentration range.

ELECTROPHYSIOLOGICAL ACTIONS (see Tables 30-1, 30-2, 30-3, and 30-5). Digoxin acts mainly through the autonomic nervous system, in particular by enhancing both central and peripheral vagal tone. These actions are largely confined to slowing the sinus node discharge rate, shortening atrial refractoriness, and prolonging AV nodal refractoriness. Electrophysiological effects on the His-Purkinje system and ventricular muscle are minimal except in toxic concentrations. In studies of denervated hearts, digoxin has relatively little effect on the AV node and causes a mild increase in atrial refractoriness. Digoxin has a mild antiadrenergic effect in low doses but may enhance central sympathetic tone at higher concentrations, which may be important in the development of digitalis-toxic arrhythmias.

The sinus rate and P wave duration are minimally changed in most patients taking digoxin. The sinus rate may decrease in patients with heart failure whose left ventricular performance is improved by the drug; individuals with significant underlying sinus node disease also have slower sinus rates or even sinus arrest. Similarly, the PR interval is generally unchanged except in patients with underlying AV node disease. QRS and QT intervals are unaffected. The characteristic ST and T wave abnormalities seen with digoxin use do not represent toxicity.

PHARMACOKINETICS (see Table 30–4). Intravenously administered digoxin yields some electrophysiological effect within minutes, with a peak effect occurring after 1.5 to 3 hours. After oral dosing, the peak effect occurs in 4 to 6 hours. The extent of digoxin absorption after oral administration varies depending on the preparation: tablet forms are 60 to 75 percent absorbed, whereas encapsulated gel forms are almost completely absorbed. Ingestion of cholestyramine or an antacid preparation at the same time as digoxin ingestion decreases its absorption. The serum half-life of digoxin is 36 to 48 hours, and the drug is excreted unchanged by the kidneys.

DOSAGE AND ADMINISTRATION (see Table 30–4). In acute loading doses of 0.5 to 1.0 mg, digoxin may be given intravenously or by mouth. Chronic daily oral dosing should be adjusted on the basis of clinical indications and the extent of renal dysfunction. Most patients require from 0.125 to 0.25 mg/d as a single dose; however, as little as 0.125 mg every other day is needed in some patients receiving renal dialysis, whereas young patients may require as much as 0.5 mg/d. Serum digoxin levels may be used to monitor compliance with therapy as well as to determine whether digitalis toxicity is the cause of new symptoms compatible with the diagnosis. However, routine monitoring of digoxin levels is not warranted in patients whose ventricular rate is controlled during atrial fibrillation and who have no symptoms of toxicity.

A large number of pharmacokinetic interactions have been described for digoxin, the most important being with quinidine (which increases serum digoxin concentrations by displacing the drug from tissue binding sites and decreasing renal clearance).

INDICATIONS. Digoxin can be used intravenously to slow the ventricular rate during atrial fibrillation and flutter; it has been used in the past to attempt to convert SVTs to sinus rhythm, but its onset of action is much slower and its success rate less than that of adenosine, verapamil, or beta blockers; thus, it is rarely used in this way at present. Digoxin is more commonly used orally to control the ventricular rate in chronic atrial fibrillation. When the patient with atrial fibrillation is at rest and vagal tone predominates, the ventricular rate can be maintained between 60 and 100 beats/min in 40 to 60 percent of cases. However, when the patient begins to exercise, the decrease in vagal tone and increase in adrenergic tone combine to diminish digoxin's beneficial effects on AV nodal conduction. Patients may experience a marked increase in ventricular rate with even mild exertion. Thus, digoxin is rarely used as a single agent to control the ventricular rate in chronic atrial fibrillation. The drug has little capacity to prevent episodes of paroxysmal atrial fibrillation or to control ventricular rate during episodes. Finally, digoxin is no more effective than placebo at terminating episodes of acute- or recent-onset atrial fibrillation.

ADVERSE EFFECTS. One of the main reasons why digoxin use has decreased is the potential for serious adverse effects and the narrow window between therapeutic and toxic concentrations. Digitalis toxicity produces a variety of symptoms and signs, including headache, nausea and vomiting, altered color perception, halo vision, and generalized malaise. More serious than these are digitalis-related arrhythmias. These include bradycardias related to a markedly enhanced vagal effect (sinus bradycardia or arrest, AV node block) and tachyarrhythmias that may be due to delayed afterdepolarization–mediated triggered activity (atrial, junctional, and fascicular or ventricular tachycardia). Worsening renal function, advanced age, hypokalemia, chronic lung disease, hypothyroidism, and amyloidosis increase the patient's sensitivity to digitalis-related arrhythmias. The diagnosis can be confirmed using serum digoxin levels. Therapy for most bradycardias consists of withdrawal of digoxin; atropine or temporary pacing may be needed in symptomatic patients. Phenytoin can be used for control of atrial tachyarrhythmias, whereas lidocaine has been successful in treating infranodal tachycardias. Life-threatening arrhythmias can be treated with digoxin-specific antibody fragments. Electrical direct-current cardioversion should be performed only when absolutely necessary in the digitalis-toxic patient because life-threatening VT or VF can result, which can be very difficult to control.

Electrotherapy of Cardiac Arrhythmias

Direct-Current Electrical Cardioversion

Electrical cardioversion offers obvious advantages over drug therapy in terminating tachycardia. Under conditions optimal for close supervision and monitoring, a precisely regulated "dose" of electricity can restore sinus rhythm immediately and safely. The distinction between supraventricular and ventricular tachyarrhythmias—crucial to the proper medical management of arrhythmias—becomes less significant, and the time-consuming titration of drugs with potential side effects is obviated.

MECHANISMS. Electrical cardioversion appears to terminate most effectively the tachycardias related to reentry, such as atrial flutter and many cases of atrial fibrillation, AV node reentry, reciprocating tachycardias associated with the Wolff-Parkinson-White syndrome, most forms of VT, ventricular flutter, and VF. The electrical shock, by depolarizing all excitable myocardium and possibly by prolonging refractoriness, interrupts reentrant circuits and establishes electrical homogeneity that terminates reentry. The mechanism by which a shock successfully terminates VF has not been completely explained. If the precipitating factors are no longer present, interrupting the tachyarrhythmia for only the brief time produced by the shock may prevent its return for long periods even though the anatomical and electrophysiological substrates required for the tachycardia are still present.

Tachycardias thought to be due to disorders of impulse formation (automaticity) include parasystole, some forms of AT, ectopic junctional tachycardia (with or without digitalis toxicity), accelerated idioventricular rhythm, and rare forms of VT. An attempt to cardiovert these tachycardias electrically is not indicated in most instances because they typically recur within seconds after the shock. It has not been established whether cardioversion can terminate tachycardias caused by enhanced automaticity or triggered activity.

TECHNIQUE. Before *elective* cardioversion, a careful physical examination, including palpation of all pulses, should be performed. A 12-lead electrocardiogram is obtained before and after cardioversion, as well as a rhythm strip during the electroshock. The patient, who should be informed completely about what to expect, is in a fasting state and "metabolically balanced"; that is, blood gases, pH, and electrolytes should be normal with no evidence of drug toxicity. Withholding digitalis for several days before elective cardioversion in patients without clinical evidence of digitalis toxicity is not necessary, although patients in whom digitalis toxicity is suspected should not be electrically cardioverted until this situation is corrected. Maintenance antiarrhythmic drug administration 1 to 2 days before electrical cardioversion of patients with atrial fibrillation can revert some patients to sinus rhythm, help prevent recurrence of atrial fibrillation once sinus rhythm is restored, and help determine the patient's tolerance for the drug.

Self-adhesive pads applied in the standard apicoanterior or apicoposterior paddle positions have transthoracic impedances similar to those of paddles and are useful in elective cardioversions or other situations in which there is time for their application. Paddles 12 to 13 cm in diameter can be used to deliver maximum current to the heart, but the benefits of these paddles compared with those of paddles 8 to 9 cm in diameter have not been clearly established. Larger paddles may distribute the intracardiac current over a wider area and may reduce shock-induced myocardial necrosis.

A synchronized shock (i.e., one delivered during the QRS complex) is used for all cardioversions except for very rapid ventricular tachyarrhythmias, such as ventricular flutter or VF (Fig. 30–2). Although generally minimal, shock-related myocardial damage increases directly with increases in applied energy, and thus the minimum effective energy should be used. Therefore, shocks are "titrated" when the clinical situation permits. Except for atrial fibrillation, shocks in the range of 25 to 50 joules successfully terminate most SVTs and should be tried initially. If unsuccessful, a second shock of higher energy can be delivered. The starting level to terminate atrial fibrillation with older monophasic machines should be no less than 100 joules, but with newer biphasic systems, energies as little as 25 joules may succeed.[53] Delivered energy can be increased in a stepwise fashion; up to 360 joules can be used safely. Anteroposterior pads may have a

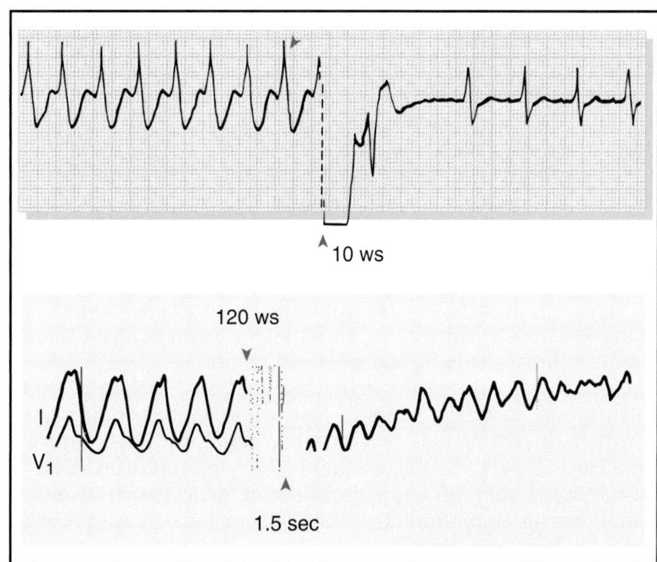

FIGURE 30–2 **Top,** A synchronized shock (note synchronization marks in the apex of the QRS complex [arrow]) during ventricular tachycardia is followed by a single repetitive ventricular response and then normal sinus rhythm. **Bottom,** A shock synchronized to the terminal portion of the QRS complex (arrow) in a patient with atrial fibrillation and conduction to the ventricle over an accessory pathway (Wolff-Parkinson-White syndrome) resulted in ventricular fibrillation that was promptly terminated by a 400-joule shock. Recording was lost for 1.5 seconds (arrow) owing to baseline drift after the shock. ws = watt seconds.

higher efficacy rate by placing more of the atrial mass in the shock vector than is the case for apicoanterior pads. If a shock of 360 joules fails to convert the rhythm, repeated shocks at the same energy may succeed by decreasing chest wall impedance; reversing pad polarity can occasionally help as well. Administration of ibutilide has been shown to facilitate electrical cardioversion of atrial fibrillation to sinus rhythm. Intracardiac defibrillation can be tried if all attempts at external cardioversion fail. For patients with stable VT, starting levels in the range of 25 to 50 joules can be employed. If there is some urgency to terminate the tachyarrhythmia, one can begin with higher energies. To terminate VF, 100 to 200 joules (biphasic; 200 to 360 joules with monophasic machines) is generally used, although much lower energies (<50 joules) terminate VF when the shock is delivered at the onset of the arrhythmia, using adhesive pads in the electrophysiology laboratory, for example.

During elective cardioversion, a short-acting barbiturate such as methohexital, a sedative such as propofol, or an amnesic such as diazepam or midazolam can be used. A physician skilled in airway management should be in attendance, an IV route should be established, and pulse oximetry, the electrocardiogram, and blood pressure should be monitored. All equipment necessary for emergency resuscitation should be immediately accessible. Before cardioversion, 100 percent oxygen may be administered for 5 to 15 minutes by nasal cannula or face mask and is continued throughout the procedure. Manual ventilation of the patient may be necessary to avoid hypoxia during periods of deepest sedation. Adequate sedation of the patient undergoing even urgent cardioversion is essential; some patients who have needlessly been shocked while awake (because of uneasiness of the physician with the arrhythmia) have declined further medical care for their arrhythmias because of concern that they would again undergo cardioversion without appropriate sedation.

In up to 5 percent of patients with atrial fibrillation, sinus rhythm cannot be restored by external countershock despite all the preceding measures including ibutilide pretreatment and biphasic shocks. It is important to distinguish between inability to attain sinus rhythm, indicating inadequate energy delivery to the atria, and inability to maintain sinus rhythm following transient termination of fibrillation; the latter condition (early reinitiation of atrial fibrillation) does not respond to higher energy shocks because fibrillation has already been terminated (but quickly recurs). Pretreatment with an antiarrhythmic drug may help maintain sinus rhythm after subsequent shocks. Patients in whom atrial fibrillation simply cannot be terminated with external shock tend to be very obese or have severe obstructive lung disease. In such cases, internal cardioversion can be performed using specially configured catheters with multiple large electrodes covering several centimeters of the distal portion of the catheter for distributing shock energy. Using standard percutaneous access, these catheters can be situated in the lateral right atrium and coronary sinus to achieve a shock vector across most of the atrial mass. With such configurations, internal shocks of 2 to 15 joules are able to terminate atrial fibrillation in more than 90 percent of patients whose arrhythmia is refractory to transthoracic shock. Esophageal cardioversion has also been reported.

INDICATIONS. As a rule, any tachycardia that produces hypotension, congestive heart failure, or angina and does not respond promptly to medical management should be terminated electrically. Very rapid ventricular rates in patients with atrial fibrillation and Wolff-Parkinson-White syndrome are often best treated by electrical cardioversion. In almost all instances, the patient's hemodynamic status improves after cardioversion. An occasional patient may experience hypotension, reduced cardiac output, or congestive heart failure after the shock. This problem may be related to complications of the cardioversion, such as embolic events, myocardial depression resulting from the anesthetic agent or the shock itself, hypoxia, lack of restoration of left atrial contraction despite return of electrical atrial systole, or postshock arrhythmias. Direct-current countershock of digitalis-induced tachyarrhythmias is contraindicated.

Favorable candidates for electrical cardioversion of atrial fibrillation include patients who (1) have symptomatic atrial fibrillation of less than 12 months' duration and derive significant hemodynamic benefits from sinus rhythm, (2) continue to have atrial fibrillation after the precipitating cause has been removed (e.g., after treatment of thyrotoxicosis), and (3) have a rapid ventricular rate that is difficult to slow. In patients who have indications for chronic warfarin therapy to prevent stroke, the hope of avoiding anticoagulation by restoring sinus rhythm is not a reason to attempt cardioversion because these patients are still at increased risk for thromboembolic events. Several large trials[54] have shown that maintenance of sinus rhythm confers no survival advantage over rate control and anticoagulation; thus, not all patients with newly discovered atrial fibrillation warrant an attempt at restoring sinus rhythm. Treatment must be determined individually.

Unfavorable candidates include patients with (1) digitalis toxicity, (2) no symptoms and a well-controlled ventricular rate without therapy, (3) sinus node dysfunction and various unstable supraventricular tachyarrhythmias or bradyarrhythmias (often the bradycardia-tachycardia syndrome) who finally develop and maintain atrial fibrillation (which in essence represents a "cure" for the sick sinus syndrome), (4) little or no symptomatic improvement with normal sinus rhythm who promptly revert to atrial fibrillation after cardioversion despite drug therapy, (5) a large left atrium and longstanding atrial fibrillation, (6) infrequent episodes of atrial fibrillation that revert spontaneously to sinus rhythm, (7) no mechanical atrial systole after the return of electrical atrial systole, (8) atrial fibrillation and advanced heart block, (9) cardiac surgery planned in the near future, and (10) antiarrhythmic drug intolerance. Atrial fibrillation is likely to recur after cardioversion in patients who have significant chronic obstructive lung disease, congestive heart failure, mitral valve disease (particularly mitral regurgitation), atrial fibrillation longer than 1 year, and an enlarged left atrium (>4.5 cm by echocardiography).

In patients with atrial flutter, slowing the ventricular rate by administering digitalis or terminating the flutter with an antiarrhythmic agent may be difficult, and electrical cardioversion is often the initial treatment of choice. For the patient with other types of SVT, electrical cardioversion may be employed when (1) vagal maneuvers or simple medical management (e.g., IV adenosine and verapamil) has failed to terminate the tachycardia and (2) the clinical setting indicates that fairly prompt restoration of sinus rhythm is desirable because of hemodynamic decompensation or electrophysiological consequences of the tachycardia. Similarly, in patients with VT, the hemodynamic and electrophysiological consequences of the arrhythmias determine the need for and urgency of direct-current cardioversion. Electrical countershock is the initial treatment of choice for ventricular flutter or VF. Speed is essential.

If, after the first shock, reversion of the arrhythmia to sinus rhythm does not occur, a higher energy level should be tried. When transient ventricular arrhythmias result after an unsuccessful shock, a bolus of lidocaine can be given before delivering a shock at the next energy level. If sinus rhythm returns only transiently and is promptly supplanted by the tachycardia, a repeated shock can be tried, depending on the tachyarrhythmia being treated and its consequences. Administration of an antiarrhythmic agent intravenously may be useful before delivering the next cardioversion shock (such as ibutilide in resistant atrial fibrillation). After cardioversion, the patient should be monitored at least until full consciousness has been restored and preferably for several hours thereafter, depending on the duration of recovery from the particular form of sedation or anesthesia used. If ibutilide has been given, the electrocardiogram should be monitored for up to 8 hours because torsades de pointes can develop in the first few hours after administration.

RESULTS. Cardioversion restores sinus rhythm in 70 to 95 percent of patients, depending on the type of tachyarrhythmia. However, sinus rhythm remains after 12 months in less than one third to one half of the patients with chronic atrial fibrillation. Thus, maintenance of sinus rhythm, once established, is the difficult problem, not the immediate termination of the tachycardia. The likelihood of maintaining sinus rhythm depends on the particular arrhythmia, the presence of underlying heart disease, and the response to antiarrhythmic drug therapy. Atrial size decreases after termination of atrial fibrillation and restoration of sinus rhythm, and functional capacity improves.

COMPLICATIONS. Arrhythmias induced by electrical cardioversion are generally caused by inadequate synchronization, with the shock occurring during the ST segment or T wave. Occasionally, a properly synchronized shock can produce VF (see Fig. 30–2). Postshock arrhythmias are usually transient and do not require therapy. Embolic episodes are reported to occur in 1 to 3 percent of the patients converted from atrial fibrillation to sinus rhythm. Prior therapeutic anticoagulation (international normalized ratio, 2.0 to 3.0) consistently for at least 3 weeks should be employed for patients who have no contraindication to such therapy and have had atrial fibrillation present for longer than 2 to 3 days or of indeterminate duration. This approach is particularly true for those who are at high risk for emboli, such as those with mitral stenosis and atrial fibrillation of recent onset, a history of recent or recurrent emboli, a prosthetic mitral valve, an enlarged heart (including left atrial enlargement), or congestive heart failure. (It is important to note that 3 weeks of therapeutic anticoagulation is not the same as simply administering warfarin for 3 weeks.) Anticoagulation with warfarin for at least 4 weeks afterward is recommended because restoration of atrial mechanical function lags behind that of electrical systolic function, and thrombi can still form in largely akinetic atria, although they are electrocardiographically in sinus rhythm. Exclusion of left atrial thrombus by transesophageal echocardiography may not always preclude embolism after cardioversion of atrial fibrillation. Atrial thrombi may be present in patients with nonfibrillation atrial tachyarrhythmias such as atrial flutter and AT in patients with congenital heart disease.[55] The same precardioversion and postcardioversion anticoagulation recommendations apply to these patients as well as to those with atrial fibrillation. Although direct-current shock has been demonstrated in animals to cause myocardial injury, studies in humans indicate that elevations of myocardial enzymes after cardioversion are not common. ST segment elevation (sometimes dramatic) can occur immediately after elective direct-current cardioversion and last for 1 to 2 minutes, although cardiac enzymes and myocardial scintigraphy may be unremarkable. ST elevation lasting longer than 2 minutes usually indicates myocardial injury unrelated to the shock. A decrease in serum K^+ and Mg^{2+} can occur after cardioversion of VT.

Cardioversion of VT can also be achieved by a chest thump. Its mechanism of termination is probably related to a mechanically induced PVC that interrupts a tachycardia and may be related to commotio cordis (see Chap. 75). The thump cannot be timed very well and is probably effective only when delivered during a nonrefractory part of the cardiac cycle. The thump can alter a VT and possibly induce ventricular flutter or VF if it occurs during the vulnerable period of the T wave. Because there may be a slightly greater likelihood of converting a stable VT to VF than of terminating VT to sinus rhythm, the thump version should not be attempted unless a defibrillator is simply unavailable.

Implantable Electrical Devices for Treatment of Cardiac Arrhythmias

Implantable devices that monitor the cardiac rhythm and can deliver competing pacing stimuli and low- and high-energy shocks have been used effectively in selected patients and are discussed fully in Chapter 31.

Ablation Therapy for Cardiac Arrhythmias

The purpose of catheter ablation is to destroy myocardial tissue by delivering electrical energy over electrodes on a catheter placed next to an area of the endocardium integrally related to the onset or maintenance of the arrhythmia, or both. The first catheter ablation procedures were performed using direct-current shocks, but this energy source has been almost wholly supplanted by radiofrequency (RF) energy, which is delivered from an external generator and destroys tissue by controlled heat production.[56] Lasers and microwave energy sources have been used, but not commonly; cryothermal catheter ablation has been approved for use in humans.[57] When a target tissue has been identified at EPS, the tip of the ablation catheter is maneuvered into apposition with this tissue. After stable catheter position and recordings have been ensured, RF energy is delivered between the catheter tip and an indifferent electrode, usually an electrocautery-type grounding pad on the skin of the patient's thigh. Because energies in the RF portion of the electromagnetic spectrum are poorly conducted by cardiac tissue, RF energy instead causes resistive heating in the cells in close proximity to the catheter tip (i.e., these cells transduce the electrical energy into thermal energy). When the tissue temperature exceeds 50°C, irreversible cellular damage and tissue death occur. An expanding front of conducted heat emanates from the region of resistive heating while RF delivery continues, resulting in production of a homogenous hemispheric lesion of coagulative necrosis 3 to 5 mm in radius (Fig. 30–3). RF-induced heating of tissue that has inherent automaticity (His bundle, foci of automatic tachycardias) results in acceleration of a rhythm, whereas RF delivery during a reentrant arrhythmia typically causes slowing and termination of the arrhythmia. In most cases, RF delivery is painless, although ablation of atrial or RV tissue can be uncomfortable for some patients.

COOLED-TIP RADIOFREQUENCY ABLATION. There are situations in which the catheter can be delivered to the correct location but conventional RF energy delivery is unable to eliminate the tachycardia. In some such cases, the amount of damage (either depth or breadth) caused by standard RF is inadequate. Using standard RF, power delivery is usually regulated to maintain a preset catheter tip temperature (typically 55° to 70°C). Tip temperatures greater than 90°C are associated with coagulation of blood elements on the electrode that preclude further energy delivery and could also become detached and embolize. Cooling the catheter tip, by either internal circulation of liquid or continuous fluid infusion through the tip electrode, can prevent excessive heating of the tip and allow greater power delivery, thus effecting a larger lesion size and potentially enhancing efficacy. Cooled-tip ablation has been used to good advantage in cases in which standard (4-mm tip) catheter ablation has failed as well as for primary therapy in atrial flutter and some cases of VT associated with structural heart disease, in which additional damage to already diseased areas is not harmful and may be required to achieve the desired result.[58]

Catheter-delivered cryoablation causes tissue damage by freezing cellular structures. Nitrous oxide is delivered to the catheter tip, where it is allowed to boil, cooling the tip electrode, after which the gas is circulated back to the delivery console. Catheter tip temperature can be regulated, cooling to as low as –70°C. Cooling to 0°C causes reversible loss of function and can be used as a diagnostic test (i.e., termination of a tachycardia when the catheter is in contact with a group of cells critical to its perpetuation). The catheter tip can then be cooled more deeply to effect permanent damage and thus cure of the arrhythmia. Cryoablation appears to cause less endocardial damage and may thus engender less risk of thromboemboli following ablation.[59]

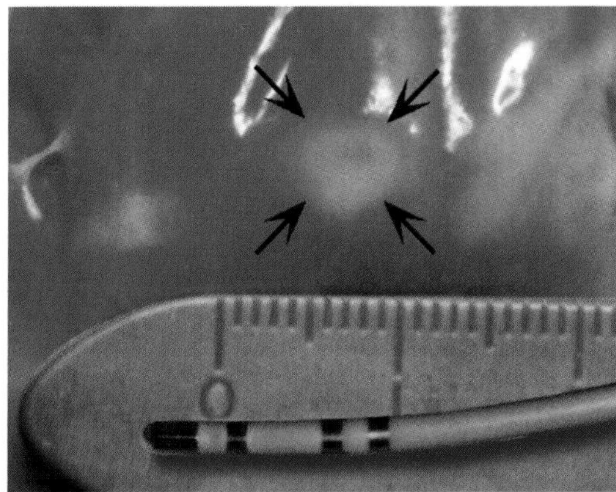

FIGURE 30–3 Radiofrequency lesion in human ventricular myocardium (explanted heart at the time of transplantation). A 30-second application of energy was made at the location denoted by arrows using the tip of the catheter shown. The lesion is 5 mm in diameter and has a clear border. A central depression in the lesion results from partial desiccation of tissue.

RADIOFREQUENCY CATHETER ABLATION OF ACCESSORY PATHWAYS

LOCATION OF PATHWAYS. The safety, efficacy, and cost-effectiveness of RF catheter ablation of an accessory AV pathway have made ablation the treatment of choice in most adult and many pediatric patients who have AV reentrant tachycardia (AVRT) or atrial flutter or fibrillation associated with a rapid ventricular response over the accessory pathway. However, the fact that the lesion size, when RF energy is delivered to an immature heart, can increase as the heart grows makes the long-term outlook for ablation less certain in the very young. RF energy has replaced direct-current shock as the optimal energy source.

An EPS is performed initially to determine that the accessory pathway is part of the tachycardia circuit or capable of rapid AV conduction during atrial fibrillation and to localize the accessory pathway (the optimal site for ablation). Pathways can exist in the right or left free wall or septum of the heart (Fig. 30-4). Septal accessory pathways are further classified as anteroseptal, midseptal, and posteroseptal. Rare parahisian pathways can be distinguished from anteroseptal pathways. Midseptal locations are true septal pathways, whereas those classified as anteroseptal generally have no septal connection but are located anteriorly along the central fibrous body or the right fibrous trigone at the right anterior free wall. Pathways classified as posteroseptal are located posterior to the central fibrous body within the so-called pyramidal space, which is bounded by the posterior superior process of the left ventricle and the inferomedial aspects of both atria. Anteroseptal pathways are found near the His bundle, and accessory pathway activation potential as well as His bundle potential can be recorded simultaneously from a catheter placed at the His bundle region. Midseptal pathways are classified as right midseptal if an accessory pathway potential is recorded through a catheter located in an area bounded anteriorly by the tip electrode of the His bundle catheter and posteriorly by the coronary sinus ostium. Pathways that are located in a similar region but can be ablated only from a left-sided approach are called left midseptal pathways. Right posteroseptal pathways insert along the tricuspid ring in the immediate vicinity of the coronary sinus ostium, whereas left posteroseptal pathways are close to the terminal portion of the coronary sinus and may be located at a subepicardial site around the proximal coronary sinus, within a middle cardiac vein or coronary sinus diverticulum, or subendocardially along the ventricular aspect of the mitral annulus. Pathways at all locations and in all age groups can be ablated successfully. Multiple pathways are present in about 5 percent of patients. Occasional epicardial locations may be more easily approached from within the coronary sinus. Rarely, pathways may connect an atrial appendage with adjacent ventricular epicardium, 2 cm or more from the AV groove (see Chap. 32).

ABLATION SITE. The optimal ablation site can be found by direct recordings of the accessory pathway (Fig. 30-5), although deflections that mimic accessory pathway potentials can be recorded at other sites. The ventricular insertion site can be determined by finding the site of the earliest onset of the ventricular electrogram in relation to the onset of the delta wave. Other helpful guidelines are unfiltered unipolar recordings that register a QS wave and the shortest AV conduction time during maximal preexcitation. A major ventricular potential synchronous with the onset of the delta wave can be a target site in left-sided preexcitation, whereas earlier ventricular excitation in relation to the delta wave can be found for right-sided preexcitation. The atrial insertion site of manifest or concealed pathways (i.e., delta wave present or absent, respectively) can be found by locating the site showing the shortest ventriculoatrial interval during retrograde conduction over the pathway. Reproducible mechanical inhibition of accessory pathway conduction during catheter manipulation and subthreshold stimulation have also been used to determine the optimal site. Accidental catheter trauma should be avoided, however, because it can "hide" the target for prolonged periods. Intracardiac echocardiography can be helpful at times in

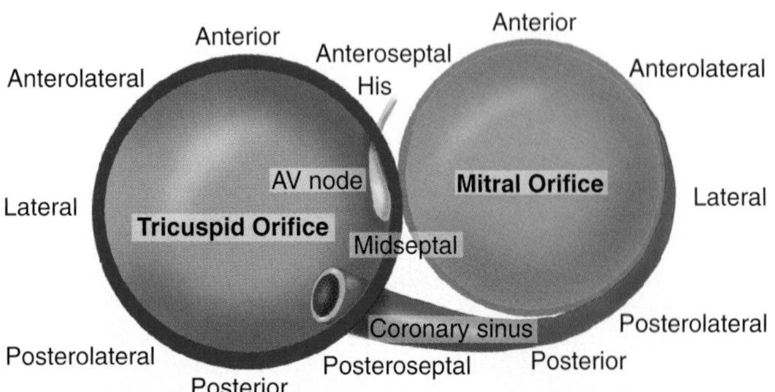

FIGURE 30-4 Locations of accessory pathways by anatomical region. Tricuspid and mitral valve annuli are depicted in a left anterior oblique view. Locations of coronary sinus, atrioventricular node, and bundle of His are shown. Accessory pathways may connect atrial to ventricular myocardium in any of the regions shown. AV = atrioventricular.

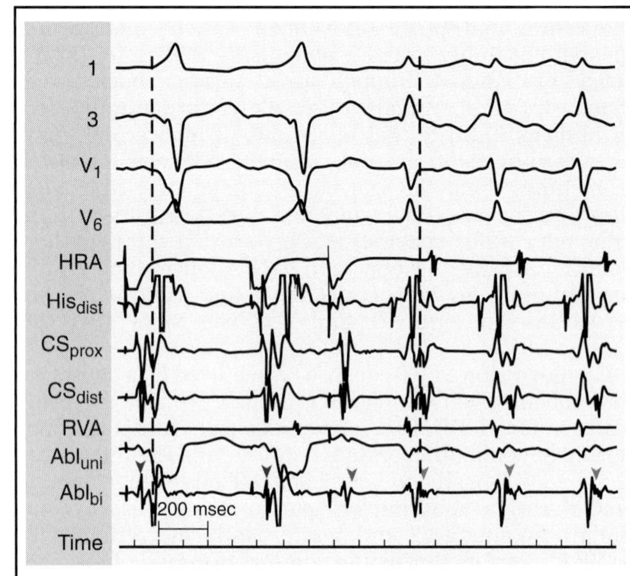

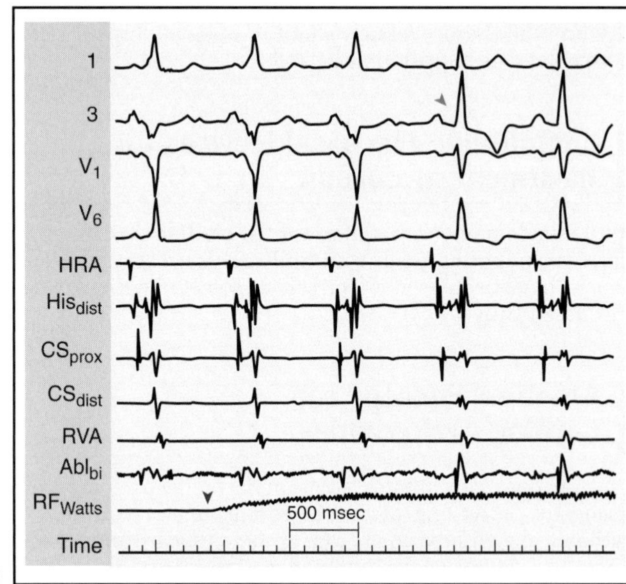

FIGURE 30-5 Wolff-Parkinson-White syndrome. Surface ECG leads 1, 3, V_1, and V_6 are shown with intracardiac recordings from high right atrium (HRA), distal His (His_{dist}) bundle region, proximal (CS_{prox}) and distal (CS_{dist}) coronary sinus, right ventricular apex (RVA), and unipolar (Abl_{uni}) and bipolar (Abl_{bi}) tip electrodes of ablation catheter. Radiofrequency powers in watts (RF_{Watts}) is also shown. **A,** Two beats of atrial pacing are conducted over the accessory pathway (blue arrows in Abl_{bi} recording, from the site of the accessory pathway) resulting in a delta wave on the electrocardiogram; a premature atrial stimulus (center) encounters accessory pathway refractoriness (red arrow) instead conducting over the atrioventricular (AV) node and bundle of His, resulting in a narrow QRS complex and starting an episode of AV reentrant tachycardia. After each narrow QRS complex is an atrial deflection, the earliest portion of which is recorded at the ablation site (green arrows). **B,** Ablation of this pathway is accomplished by delivery of radiofrequency (RF) energy from the ablation catheter tip. Blue arrow denotes onset of radiofrequency energy delivery; two QRS complexes later, the delta wave is abruptly lost (green arrow in lead 3) owing to elimination of conduction over the accessory pathway. T wave inversion in lead 3 is due to "memory" (see Chap. 32).

delineating unusual anatomy, guiding atrial septal puncture for left-sided access, and determining adequacy of catheter contact at ablation sites.

Left-sided accessory pathways often cross the mitral annulus obliquely. Consequently, the earliest site of retrograde atrial activation and the earliest site of anterograde ventricular activation are not directly across the AV groove from each other. Identification of the earliest site of atrial activation is usually performed during orthodromic AVRT or during relatively rapid ventricular pacing, so that retrograde conduction using the AV node does not confuse assessment of the location of the earliest atrial activation.

Successful ablation sites should exhibit stable fluoroscopic and electrical characteristics. During sinus rhythm, the local ventricular activation at the successful ablation site precedes the onset of the ECG delta wave by 10 to 35 milliseconds; during orthodromic AVRT, the interval between the onset of ventricular activation in any lead and local atrial activation is usually 70 to 90 milliseconds (see Fig. 30-5). When thermocouple- or thermistor-tipped ablation catheters are used, a stable rise in catheter tip temperature is a helpful indicator of catheter stability and adequate contact between the catheter and tissue.[60] In such an instance, the tip temperature generally exceeds 50°C. The retrograde transaortic and transseptal approaches have been used with equal success to ablate accessory pathways located along the mitral annulus. Routine EPS performed weeks after the ablation procedure is generally not indicated but should be considered in patients who have recurrent delta wave or symptoms of tachycardia. Catheter-delivered cryoablation may be useful in patients with septal accessory pathways (located near the AV conduction system). Using this system, the catheter tip and adjacent tissue can be reversibly cooled to test a potential site. If the accessory pathway conduction fails while normal AV conduction is preserved, deeper cooling can be performed at the site to complete the ablation. If, however, normal AV conduction is damaged, allowing the catheter to rewarm results in no permanent damage.

Patients with atriofascicular accessory pathways have connections consisting of a proximal portion responsible for conduction delay and decremental conduction properties and a long distal segment located along the endocardial surface of the right ventricular free wall that has electrophysiological properties similar to those of the right bundle branch. The distal end of the right atriofascicular accessory pathway can insert into the apical region of the right ventricular free wall close to the distal right bundle branch or can actually fuse with the latter. Right atriofascicular accessory pathways may actually represent a duplication of the AV conduction system and can be localized for ablation by recording potentials from the rapidly conducting distal component crossing the tricuspid annulus (analogous to the His bundle) and extending to the apical region of the right ventricular free wall. Ablation attempts should be performed more proximally to avoid inadvertently ablating the distal right bundle branch, which could actually be proarrhythmic and create incessant tachycardia by lengthening the reentrant circuit.

Indications. Ablation of accessory pathways is indicated in patients with symptomatic AVRT that is drug resistant or when the patient is drug intolerant or does not desire long-term drug therapy. It is also indicated in patients with atrial fibrillation (or other atrial tachyarrhythmias) and a rapid ventricular response by means of an accessory pathway when the tachycardia is drug resistant or when the patient is drug intolerant or does not desire long-term drug therapy. Other potential candidates include patients with AVRT or atrial fibrillation with rapid ventricular rates identified during EPS of another arrhythmia; asymptomatic patients with ventricular preexcitation whose livelihood, profession, important activities, insurability, mental well-being, or the public safety would be affected by spontaneous tachyarrhythmias or by the presence of the ECG abnormality; patients with atrial fibrillation and a controlled ventricular response by means of the accessory pathway; and patients with a family history of sudden cardiac death. Not all patients with accessory pathways need treatment; however, ablation has such a high success rate and low complication rate that in many centers patients who need any form of therapy are referred for catheter ablation.

Results. From the results of an early survey conducted by the North American Society of Pacing and Electrophysiology (NASPE),[61] successful ablation of left free wall accessory pathways was achieved in 2312 of 2527 (91 percent) patients; of septal accessory pathways, in 1115 of 1279 (87 percent); and of right free wall accessory pathways, in 585 of 715 (82 percent). Significant complications were reported in 94 of 4521 patients (2.1 percent), and there were 13 procedure-related deaths in 4521 studies of patients (0.2 percent). An update of this survey tallied only 651 accessory pathway ablation cases, among which successful ablation was achieved in 94 percent with a 2 percent complication rate and no deaths.[62] In Europe, the complication rate was 4.4 percent, with 3 deaths in 2222 patients.[49] A large study of patients using a temperature-controlled ablation system had similar success rates (overall success, 398 of 465 [93 percent] with an 8 percent recurrence rate).[60]

RADIOFREQUENCY CATHETER MODIFICATION OF THE AV NODE FOR AV NODAL REENTRANT TACHYCARDIAS. AV node reentry is a common cause of SVT episodes. Although controversy still exists about the exact nature of the tachycardia circuit, abundant evidence indicates that two pathways in the region of the AV node participate, one with relatively fast conduction but long refractoriness and the other with shorter refractoriness but slower conduction.[64] PACs can encounter refractoriness in the fast pathway, conduct down the slow pathway, and reenter the fast pathway retrogradely, initiating AV nodal reentrant SVT (Fig. 30–6). Although this is the most common presentation of AV node reentry, some patients have what appears to be propagation in the opposite direction in this circuit (anterograde fast, retrograde slow) as well as a "slow-slow" variant. Two or more of these variants can exist in the same patient (Fig. 30–7).

FAST-PATHWAY ABLATION. Ablation can be performed to eliminate conduction in the fast pathway or the slow pathway. In ablating the fast pathway, the electrode tip is positioned along the AV node–His bundle axis in the anterosuperior portion of the tricuspid annulus. The catheter is gradually withdrawn until the atrial electrogram amplitude equals or exceeds that of the ventricular electrogram and the His bundle recording is either absent or extremely small (0.05 mV). During energy delivery, the electrocardiogram is monitored for PR prolongation or the occurrence of AV block, or both. If accelerated junctional rhythm is noted during delivery of RF energy, the atrium can be paced at a faster rate to ensure integrity of AV conduction. The initial RF pulse is delivered at 15 to 20 watts for 10 to 15 seconds and gradually increased. Endpoints are PR prolongation, elimination of retrograde fast-pathway conduction, and noninducibility of AVNRT. An alternative approach is to apply RF current at the site of earliest retrograde atrial activation during tachycardia. RF current should be discontinued if the PR interval is prolonged by more than 50 percent or if AV block results. At present, fast-pathway ablation is rarely performed because it is associated with a prolonged PR interval, a higher recurrence rate (10 to 15 percent). and a slightly higher risk of complete AV block (2 to 5 percent) compared with slow-pathway ablation. One uncommon situation in which fast-pathway ablation may be preferred is in patients who have a markedly prolonged PR interval at rest and no evidence of anterograde fast-pathway conduction. In such cases, ablation of the anterograde slow pathway may produce complete AV block, whereas retrograde fast-pathway ablation can eliminate SVT without altering AV conduction.

SLOW-PATHWAY ABLATION. The slow pathway can be located by mapping along the posteromedial tricuspid annulus close to the coronary sinus os. Electrogram recordings are obtained with an atrial-to-ventricular electrogram ratio of less than 0.5 and either a multicomponent atrial electrogram or a recording of possible slow-pathway potential.[65] In the anatomical approach, target sites are selected fluoroscopically. A single RF application suffices in many cases, but in others serial RF lesions may be needed, starting at the most posterior site (near the coronary sinus os) and progressing to the more anterior locus (closer to the His bundle recording site). An accelerated junctional rhythm (Fig. 30–8) usually occurs when RF energy is applied at a site that will result in successful elimination of SVT. The success rate with the anatomical or electrogram mapping approach is equivalent, and, most often, combinations of both are used, yielding success rates approaching 100 percent with less than a 1 percent chance of complete heart block. Catheter-delivered cryoablation has been used for treatment of AVNRT with

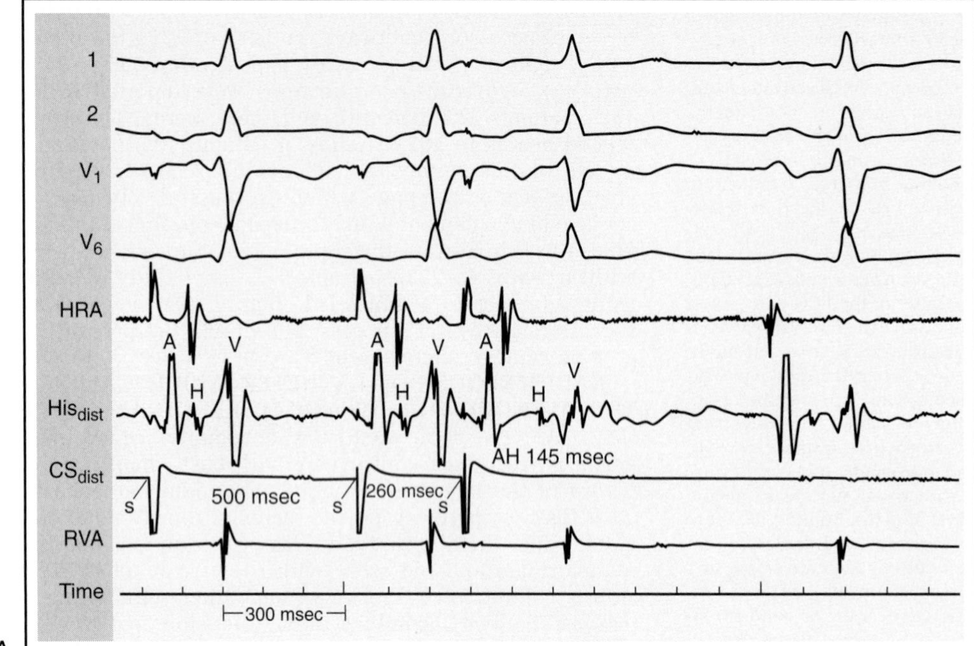

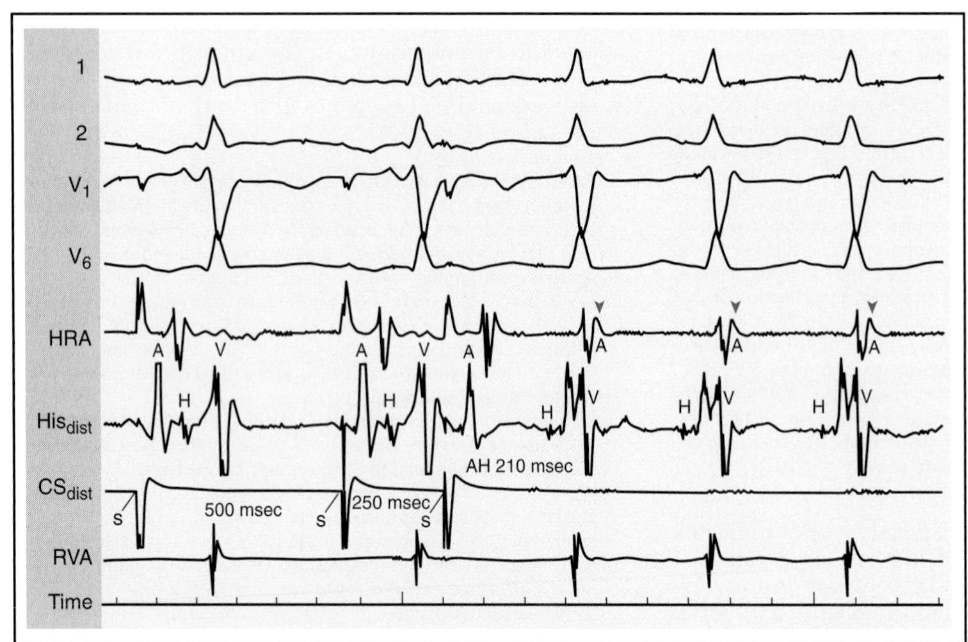

FIGURE 30–6 Atrioventricular (AV) node reentry. **A,** Two atrial paced complexes from the coronary sinus (CS) are followed by an atrial premature stimulus at coupling interval 260 milliseconds, resulting in an AH interval of 145 milliseconds. **B,** The same atrial drive train is followed by an atrial extrastimulus 10 milliseconds earlier than before (250 milliseconds). This results in a marked increase in the AH interval to 210 milliseconds, after which AV nodal reentrant tachycardia ensues because the extrastimulus encounters block in a "fast" AV node pathway, conducts down a "slow" pathway, and then conducts back up the fast pathway in a repeating fashion. Red arrows denote atrial electrograms coincident with QRS complexes, characteristic of the most common type of AV node reentry. Recording as in prior figures.

excellent results.[66] In theory, the ability to "cryomap" (test potential sites for slow-pathway block with moderate, reversible cooling) should almost entirely eliminate the risk of AV block with ablation.

Slow-pathway ablation results in an increase in the anterograde AV block cycle length and AV node ERP without a change in the AH interval or retrograde conduction properties of the AV node. Patients in whom slow-pathway conduction is completely eliminated almost never have recurrent SVT episodes; approximately 40 percent of patients can have evidence of residual slow-pathway function after successful elimination of sustained AVNRT (usually manifested as persistent dual AV node physiology and single AV node echoes during atrial extrastimulation). The surest endpoint for slow-pathway ablation is the elimination of sustained AVNRT both with and without an infusion of isoproterenol.

AVNRT recurs in about 5 percent of patients after slow-pathway ablation. In some patients, the ERP of the fast pathway decreases after slow-pathway ablation, possibly because of electrotonic interaction between the two pathways. Atypical forms of reentry can result after ablation, as can apparent parasympathetic denervation, resulting in inappropriate sinus tachycardia.

At present, the slow-pathway approach is the preferred method for ablation of typical AVNRT. Ablation of the slow pathway is also a safe and effective means for treating atypical AVNRT. In patients with AVNRT undergoing slow-pathway ablation, junctional ectopy during application of RF energy is a sensitive but nonspecific marker of successful ablation, occurring in longer bursts at effective target sites than at ineffective sites. Ventriculoatrial conduction should be expected during the junctional ectopy, and poor ventriculoatrial conduction or actual block may herald subsequent anterograde AV block in patients undergoing RF ablation of the slow pathway. Junctional ectopic rhythm is due to heating of the AV node and does not occur with cryoablation.

Indications. RF catheter ablation for AVNRT can be considered in patients with recurrent, symptomatic, sustained AVNRT that is drug resistant or when the patient is drug intolerant or does not desire long-term drug treatment. The procedure can also be considered in patients with sustained AVNRT identified during EPS or catheter ablation of another arrhythmia or when there is a finding of dual AV node pathway physiology and atrial echoes but without AVNRT during EPS in a patient suspected of having AVNRT clinically.

Results. Results of the NASPE survey indicate that 3052 patients had slow-pathway ablation with a 96 percent reported success rate, whereas 255 had fast-pathway ablation that was successful in 229 (90 percent). Significant complications occurred in 0.96 percent, but no procedure-related deaths were reported.[61] In Europe, the complication rate was 8.0 percent, mostly related to AV block after fast-pathway ablation, and there were no deaths in 815 patients.[61] Most centers currently employ slow-pathway ablation, resulting in a procedural success rate of 98 percent, recurrence rate of less than 2 percent, and incidence of heart block requiring permanent pacing of less than 1 percent.

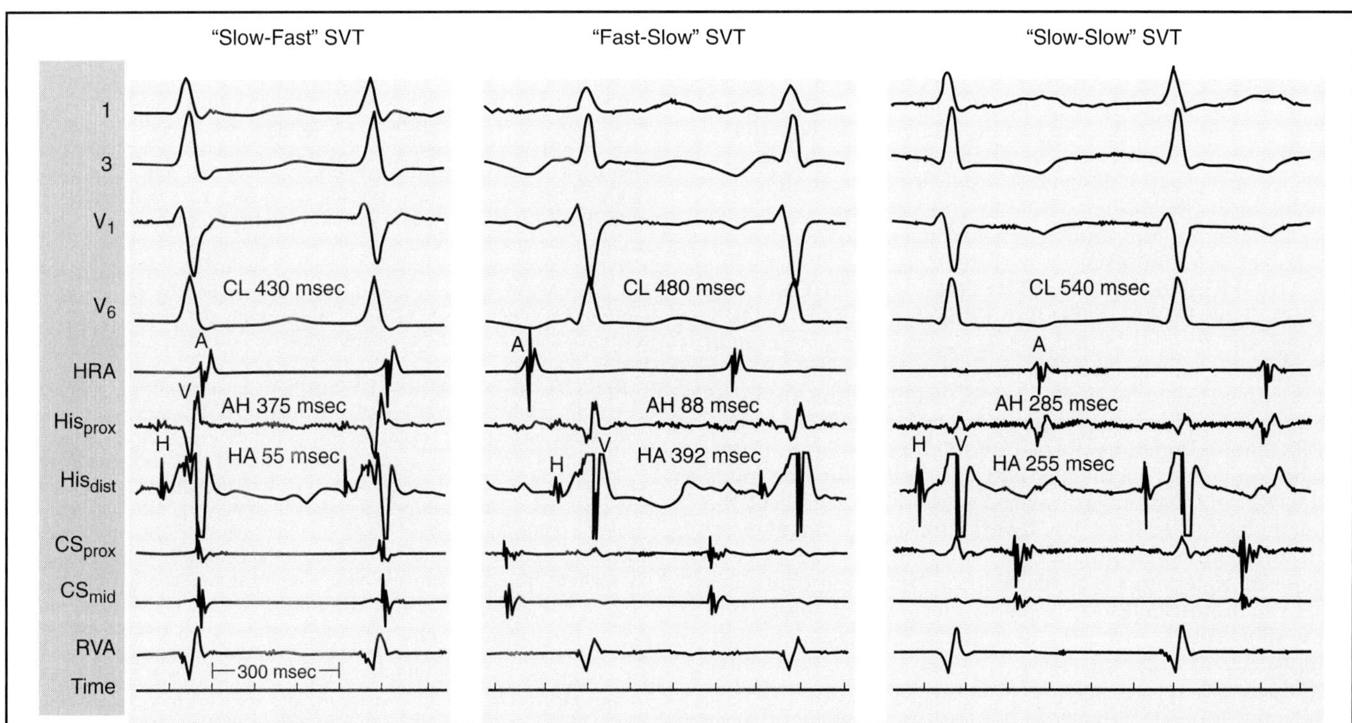

FIGURE 30–7 Three variants of atrioventricular (AV) node reentrant supraventricular tachycardia (SVT) in the same patient. Recordings as in other figures. The left panel shows the most common type of AV node SVT (anterograde slow pathway, retrograde fast); atrial activation is coincident with ventricular activation. The center panel shows "atypical" AV node reentry, with anterograde fast-pathway conduction and retrograde conduction over a slow pathway. A rare variety is shown in the right panel, with anterograde conduction over a slow pathway and retrograde conduction over a second slow pathway. Note the similar atrial activation sequences in the latter two (coronary sinus before right atrium), as distinct from that of slow-fast AV node reentry (coronary sinus and right atrial activation nearly simultaneous). Note also the different P-QRS relationships, from simultaneous activation (left, short RP interval) to P in front of the QRS (middle, long RP interval) and P midway in the cardiac cycle (right). CL = cycle length.

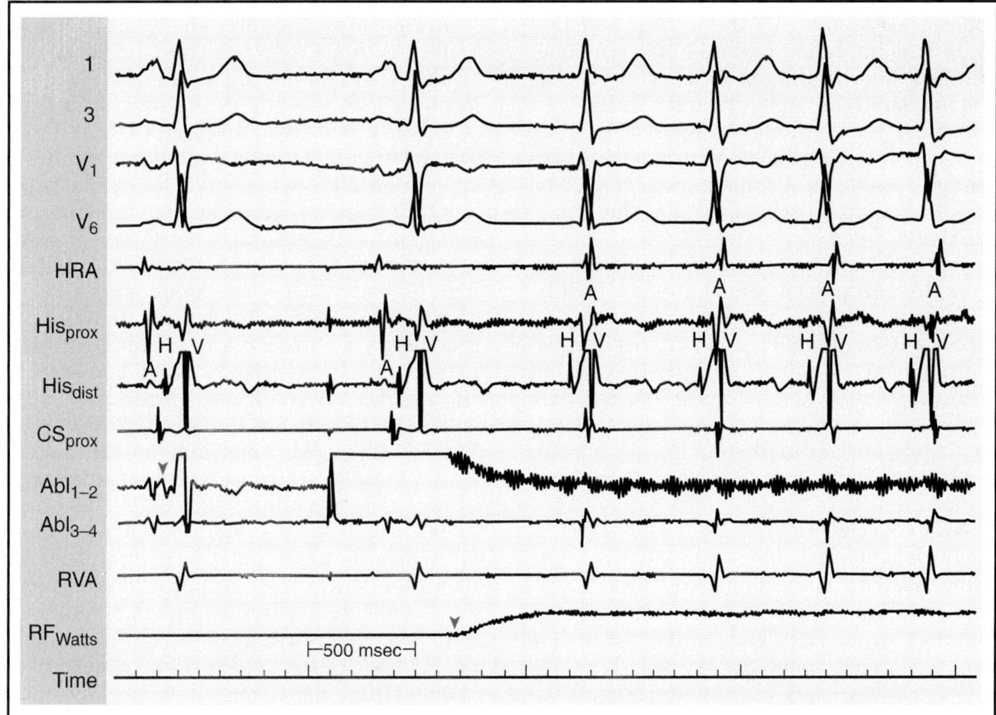

FIGURE 30–8 Atrioventricular (AV) node slow-pathway modification for cure of AV node reentrant supraventricular tachycardia. Recordings as in prior figures. The ablation recording (arrow in Abl_{1-2}) shows a slurred deflection between atrial and ventricular electrogram components; this may represent the AV node slow-pathway deflection (but it is not the bundle of His deflection, which is instead recorded from a separate catheter 15 mm away). Shortly after the onset of radiofrequency delivery (arrow in RF_{Watts}), an accelerated junctional rhythm begins and gradually speeds up further. Retrograde conduction is present during the junctional rhythm. Abl_{3-4} = proximal electrode recording from ablation catheter.

ECTOPIC JUNCTIONAL TACHYCARDIA. Ectopic junctional tachycardia is a rare form of SVT in which the electrocardiogram resembles that in AVNRT but is distinct in that (1) the mechanism is automatic, not reentrant, and (2) the atrium is clearly not involved in the tachycardia. This disorder is most commonly observed in young healthy individuals, women more often than men, and is usually very catecholamine dependent. Ablation must be carried out very near the His bundle, and the risk of heart block requiring pacemaker insertion exceeds 5 percent.[67]

RADIOFREQUENCY CATHETER ABLATION OF ARRHYTHMIAS RELATED TO THE SINOATRIAL NODE. Reentry in or around the sinus node is an uncommon arrhythmia, characterized by episodes of tachycardia with a P wave identical to the sinus P wave, usually with a PR interval longer than in sinus (in physiological sinus tachycardia, the PR interval remains normal or shortens because of catecholamine effects on the AV node as well as on the sinus node). RF applications are placed around the region of the sinus node at sites of early activation (prior to P wave onset) until tachycardia terminates.

Inappropriate sinus tachycardia is a syndrome characterized by high sinus rates with exercise and at rest. Patients complain of palpitations at all times of day that correlate with inappropriately high sinus rates. They may not respond well to beta blocker therapy because of either lack of desired effect or occurrence of side effects. When the sinus node area is to be ablated, it can be identified anatomically as well as electrophysiologically, and ablation lesions are usually placed between the superior vena cava and crista terminalis at sites of early atrial activation. Isoproterenol may be helpful in "forcing" the site of impulse formation to cells with the most rapid discharge rate. Care must be taken to apply RF energy at the most cephalad sites first; initial ablation performed farther down the crista terminalis does not alter the atrial rate at the time but can damage subsidiary pacemaker regions that may be needed after the sinus node is eventually ablated.

Indications. Catheter ablation for sinus node reentrant tachycardia can be performed in patients with recurrent symptomatic episodes of sustained SVT that is drug resistant or when the patient is drug intolerant or does not desire long-term drug treatment. Patients with inappropriate sinus tachycardia should be considered for ablation only after clear failure of medical therapy because ablation results are often less than completely satisfactory. Whenever ablation is performed in the region of the sinus node, the patient should be apprised of the risk of needing a pacemaker after the procedure. Phrenic nerve damage is also a possibility.

Results. Sinus node reentrant tachycardia can be successfully ablated in more than 90 percent of candidates. Results are not as good for inappropriate sinus tachycardia; although a good technical result may be obtained at the time of the procedure, symptoms often persist because of recurrence of rapid sinus rates (at or near preablation rates) or for nonarrhythmic reasons. Multiple ablation sessions are needed in some patients, and about 20 percent eventually undergo pacemaker implantation (not all of whom have relief of palpitations despite a normal heart rate).

RADIOFREQUENCY CATHETER ABLATION OF ATRIAL TACHYCARDIA. ATs are a heterogeneous group of disorders with causes including rapid discharge of a focus (focal tachycardia) and reentry. The former can occur in anyone, irrespective of the presence of structural abnormalities of the atria, whereas reentrant ATs almost always occur in the setting of structurally damaged atria. Symptoms vary from none (in relatively infrequent or slow ATs in patients without heart disease) to syncope (rapid AT with compromised cardiac function) or heart failure (incessant AT over a period of weeks or months). All forms of AT are amenable to catheter ablation.

FOCAL ATRIAL TACHYCARDIA. In focal ATs (automatic or triggered foci or micro-reentry), activation mapping is used to determine the site of the AT by recording the earliest onset of local activation.[68] These tachycardias can behave capriciously and be practically noninducible at EPS despite the patient's complaining of multiple daily episodes for the week prior to EPS. Ten to 15 percent of patients can have multiple atrial foci. Sites tend to cluster near the pulmonary veins in the left atrium and the mouths of the atrial appendages and along the crista terminalis on the right (Fig. 30–9A; see Fig. 29–14). Activation times of these sites typically occur only 15 to 40 milliseconds prior to the onset of the P wave on the electrocardiogram. Care must be taken to avoid inadvertent damage to the phrenic nerve; its location can be determined by pacing at high current at a potential site of ablation, observing for diaphragmatic contraction. Ablation should not be performed at a site at which this is seen, if at all possible.

REENTRANT ATRIAL TACHYCARDIA. As noted, these ATs occur more commonly in the setting of structural heart disease, especially after prior atrial surgery. The region of slow conduction is typically related to an end of an atriotomy scar; this is, however, not in a constant anatomical location but varies from patient to patient depending on the operation performed. Therefore, preprocedure review of operative reports and careful electrophysiological mapping are essential. Because reentry within a complete circuit is occurring, activation can be recorded throughout the entire cardiac cycle. The ablation strategy is to identify regions with mid-diastolic atrial activation during tachycardia that can be proved by pacing techniques to be integral to the tachycardia (see Figs. 29–15 and 30–9B). Such sites are attractive ablation targets because they are composed of relatively few cells (hence electrical silence on the surface electrocardiogram in diastole) and are thus more easily ablated by a typical application of RF energy than other areas. Focal ablation of these sites can then be performed, but in many cases tachycardia can still be initiated (often at a slower rate) or recurs after the procedure. Because these sites are typically located at a relatively narrow zone between the ends of prior scars or surgical incisions and another nonconducting barrier (such as another scar, caval orifice, or valve annulus), another technique is to make a line of ablation lesions from the end of the scar to the nearest electrical barrier. Reentry can thus be prevented. This technique is analogous to that used in curing atrial flutter (see later). Because these patients often have extensive atrial disease with islands of scar that could serve as barriers for additional ATs, specialized mapping techniques may be needed to locate these regions and preemptively connect them with ablation lesions to prevent future AT episodes.

Indications. Catheter ablation for ATs should be considered in patients with recurrent episodes of symptomatic, sustained ATs that are drug resistant, or when the patient is drug intolerant or does not desire long-term drug treatment.

Results. Success rates for ablation of focal AT are from 80 to 95 percent, largely depending on the ability to induce episodes at EPS; when episodes can be initiated with pacing, isoproterenol, or other means, AT can usually be ablated. Reentrant ATs, although more readily induced at EPS, are often harder to eliminate completely; initial success rates are high (90 percent) but recurrences are seen in up to 20 percent of patients, necessitating drug therapy or another ablation procedure. Complications, occurring in 1 to 2 percent of patients, include phrenic nerve damage, cardiac tamponade, and heart block (with rare perinodal ATs).

RADIOFREQUENCY CATHETER ABLATION OF ATRIAL FLUTTER. Atrial flutter may be defined electrocardiographically (most typically, negative sawtooth waves in leads II and III and aVF at a rate of about 300 beats/min) or electrophysiologically (a rapid, organized macro-reentrant AT, the circuit for which is anatomically determined). Understanding the reentrant pathway for all forms of atrial flutter is essential for developing an ablation approach. Reentry in the right atrium, with the left atrium passively activated, constitutes the mechanism of the typical ECG variety of atrial flutter, with caudocranial activation along the right atrial septum and a craniocaudal activation of the right atrial free wall (Fig. 30–10A). In some cases, a zone of slow conduction exists in the low right atrium, which is typically bounded by the tricuspid annulus, the inferior vena cava, and the coronary sinus. In other cases, conduction velocity is more uniform

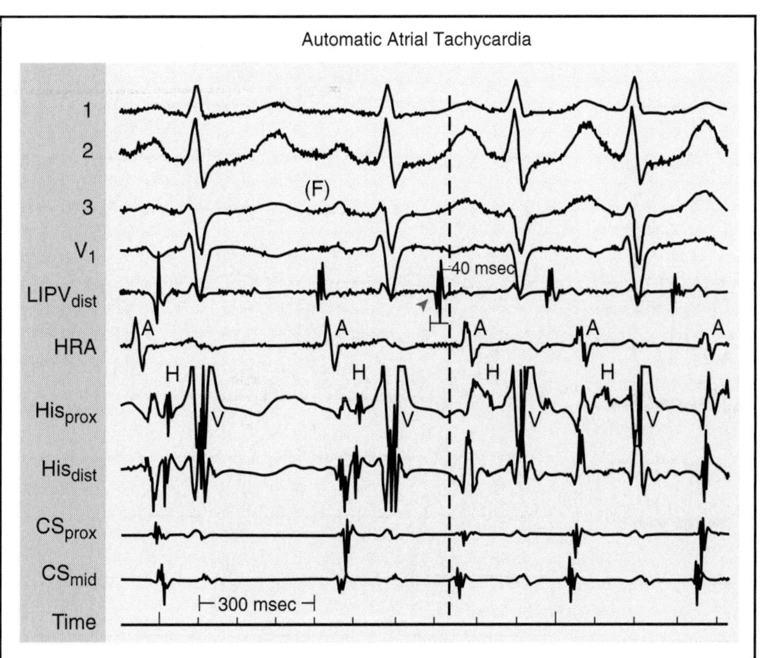

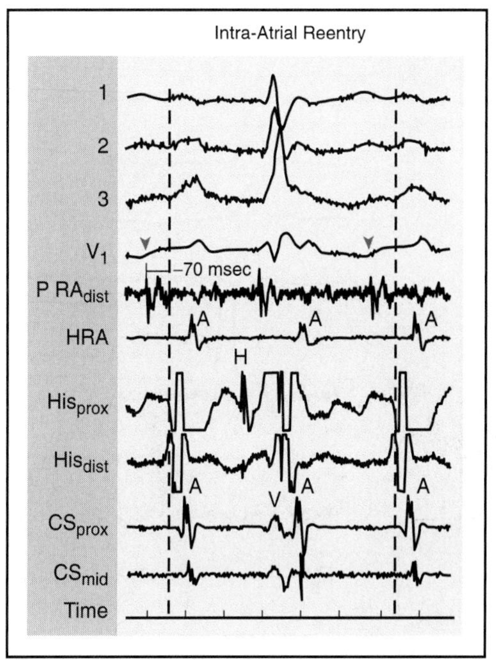

FIGURE 30–9 Atrial tachycardias. **A,** Automatic atrial tachycardia arising in the left inferior pulmonary vein (LIPV). A sinus beat is shown at left, followed by a fusion beat (F) of sinus and tachycardia activation. The last three beats in the panel are atrial tachycardia. The ablation catheter was within the LIPV and recorded a sharp potential (arrow) 40 milliseconds before the P wave onset (dashed line). Ablation at this site terminated the tachycardia. **B,** Intraatrial reentrant tachycardia in a patient who had undergone atrial septal defect repair years earlier. The ablation catheter is in the posterior right atrium (PRA), where a fragmented signal is recorded. A portion of this electrogram (arrows) precedes the P wave onset during tachycardia (dashed line) by 70 milliseconds. Ablation at this site terminated the tachycardia. Recordings as in prior figures.

throughout the large circuit. Placing an ablative lesion between any two anatomical barriers that transects a portion of the circuit necessary for perpetuation of reentry can be curative. Typically, this is across the isthmus of atrial tissue between the inferior vena caval orifice and tricuspid annulus (the cavotricuspid isthmus), a relatively narrow point in the circuit. Successful ablation can be accomplished where the advancing flutter wave front enters this zone in the low inferolateral right atrium, near the exit of this zone at the inferomedial right atrium, or in between these sites. Locations for RF delivery can be guided anatomically or electrophysiologically. Less commonly, the direction of wave front propagation in this large right atrial circuit is reversed ("clockwise" flutter proceeding cephalad up the right atrial free wall and caudad down the septum, with upright flutter waves in the inferior leads [see Fig. 30–10A]). This arrhythmia, which has been called "atypical atrial flutter," may also be ablated using the same techniques as with more typical atrial flutter. These two arrhythmias constitute "cavotricuspid isthmus–dependent" flutter and are distinct from other rapid atrial arrhythmias that may have a similar ECG appearance but utilize different (and often multiple) circuits in other parts of the right or left atrium. Ablation can be more difficult in these cases, which often occur in the setting of advanced lung disease or prior cardiac surgery. A common theme in these complex reentrant arrhythmias is the presence of an anatomically determined zone of inexcitability around which an electrical wave front can circulate. Specialized mapping tools and skills are necessary to effect successful ablation in such cases.

In patients with atrial fibrillation, an antiarrhythmic drug can slow intraatrial conduction to such a degree that atrial flutter results and fibrillation is no longer observed. In some of these, ablation of atrial flutter and having the patient continue to take the antiarrhythmic drug can prevent recurrences of these atrial arrhythmias.

The endpoint of atrial flutter ablation procedures was initially termination of atrial flutter with RF application accompanied by noninducibility of the arrhythmia. However, using these criteria, up to 30 percent of patients had recurrent flutter because of lack of complete and permanent conduction block in the cavotricuspid isthmus. In the last several years, the endpoint of ablation has changed to ensuring a line of bidirectional block in this region by pacing from opposite sides of the isthmus (see Fig. 30–10B) or other techniques.[69] Using these criteria, recurrence rates have fallen to less than 5 percent.

Indications. Candidates for RF catheter ablation include patients with recurrent episodes of atrial flutter that are drug resistant, those who are drug intolerant, or those who do not desire long-term drug therapy.

Results. Regardless of circuit location, atrial flutter can be successfully ablated in more than 90 percent of cases, although patients with complex right or left atrial flutters require more extensive and complex procedures. Recurrence rates are less than 5 percent except in patients with extensive atrial disease, in whom new circuits can develop over time as new areas of conduction delay and block form. Complications are rare, including inadvertent heart block and phrenic nerve paralysis.

ABLATION AND MODIFICATION OF ATRIOVENTRICULAR CONDUCTION FOR ATRIAL TACHYARRHYTHMIAS. In some patients with atrial tachyarrhythmias who have rapid ventricular rates despite optimal drug therapy, RF ablation can be used to eliminate or modify AV conduction to control the ventricular rates. To achieve RF catheter ablation of AV conduction, a catheter is placed across the tricuspid valve and positioned to record the largest His bundle electrogram associated with the largest atrial electrogram. RF energy is applied until complete AV block is achieved and is continued for an additional 30 to 60 seconds. If no change in AV conduction is observed after 15 seconds of RF ablation, the catheter is repositioned and the attempt is repeated. In occasional patients, attempts at RF ablation using this right-sided heart approach fail to achieve heart block. These patients can undergo an attempt from the left ventricle with

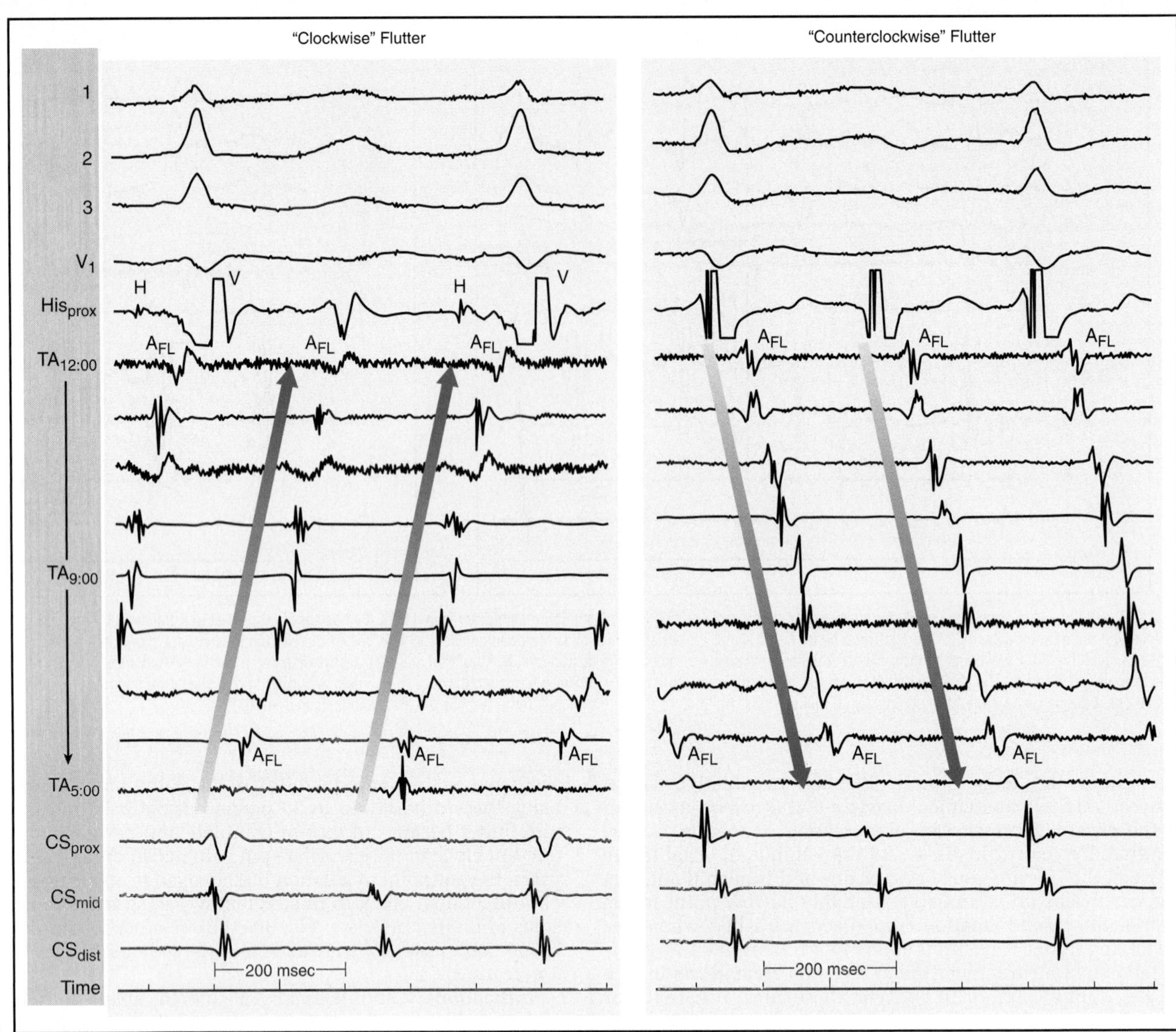

FIGURE 30–10 **A,** Two forms of atrial flutter in the same patient are shown. A "halo" catheter with 10 electrode pairs is situated on the atrial side of the tricuspid annulus (TA), with recording sites displayed from the top of the annulus ("12:00") to the inferomedial aspect ("5:00"), as shown in fluoroscopic views in **B**. On the left, the wave front of atrial activation proceeds in a "clockwise" fashion (arrows) along the annulus, whereas at the right the direction of propagation is the reverse.

a catheter positioned along the posterior interventricular septum just beneath the aortic valve to record a large His bundle electrogram. Energy is applied between the catheter electrode and the skin patch or between catheters in the left and right ventricles. Success rates currently approach 100 percent, with recurrence of AV conduction in less than 5 percent. Improved left ventricular function can result from both control of ventricular rate during atrial fibrillation and withdrawal of rate-controlling medications with negative inotropic action. Permanent ventricular or AV pacing is required after ablation.

In some cases, the AV junction can be modified to slow the ventricular rate without producing complete AV block by ablation in the region of the slow pathway, as described in connection with AV node modification for AV node reentry. Initial success rates for slowing the ventricular response are quite good; however, long-term results are less consistent.[70] Some patients have a gradual increase in ventricular rate to nearly preablation levels, whereas late complete heart block may occur in others. Nonetheless, this procedure can be tried before producing complete AV block.

Indications. Ablation and modification of AV conduction can be considered in (1) patients with symptomatic atrial tachyarrhythmias who have inadequately controlled ventricular rates unless primary ablation of the atrial tachyarrhythmia is possible; (2) similar patients when drugs are not tolerated or the patient does not wish to take them, even though the ventricular rate can be controlled; (3) patients with symptomatic, nonparoxysmal, junctional tachycardia that is drug resistant or in whom drugs are not tolerated or are not desired; (4) patients resuscitated from sudden cardiac death related to atrial flutter or atrial fibrillation with a rapid ventricular response in the absence of an accessory pathway; and (5) patients with a dual-chamber pacemaker and a pacemaker-mediated tachycardia that cannot be treated effectively by drugs or by reprogramming the pacemaker. The last three situations are rarely encountered.

Results. Results from the U.S. survey indicated that the procedure was successful in producing complete AV block in 95 percent of 1600 patients, with significant complications occurring in 21 (1.3 percent) and two procedure-related deaths (0.1 percent).[61] In Europe, the complication rate was

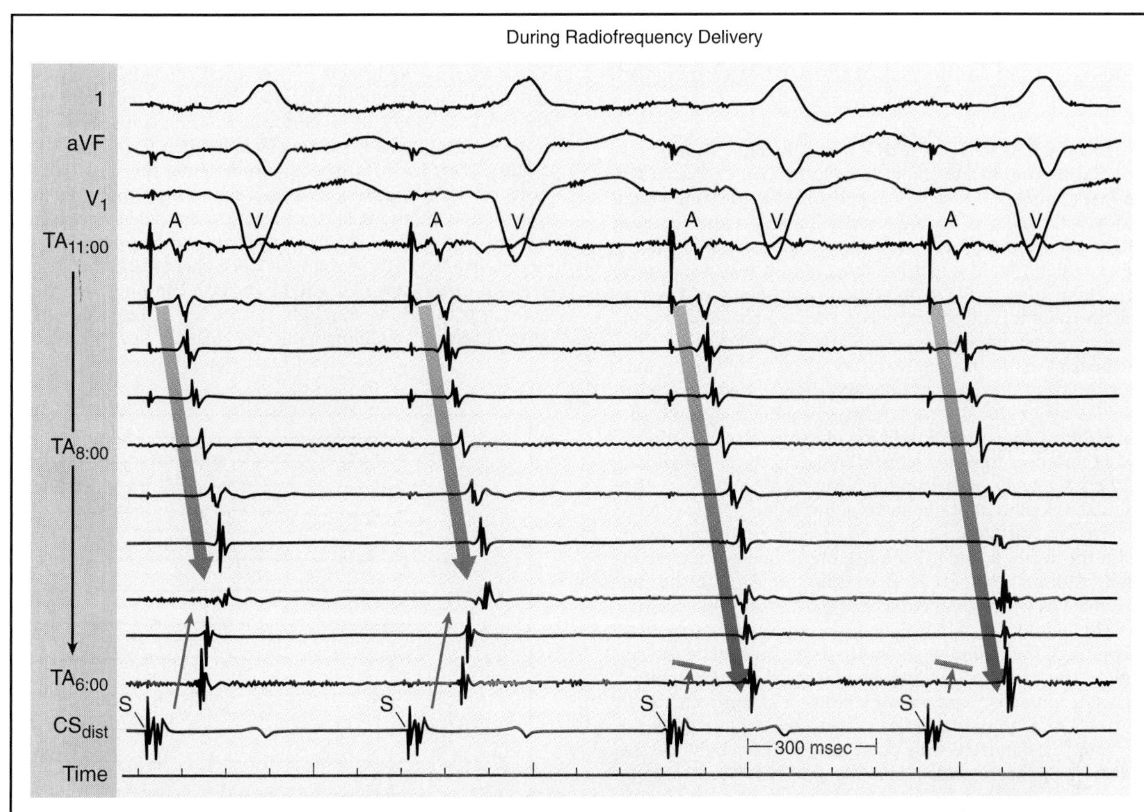

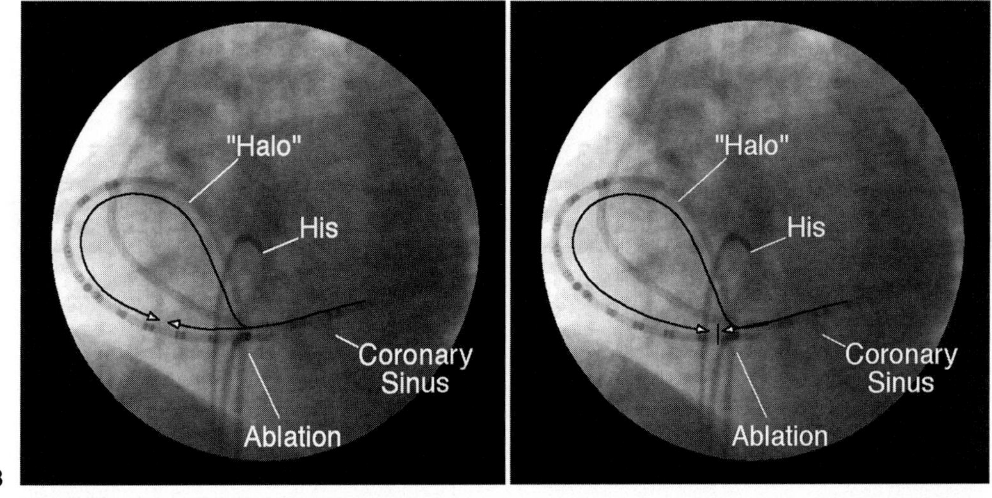

B

FIGURE 30–10, cont'd **B,** Ablation of the isthmus of atrial tissue between the tricuspid annulus and inferior vena caval orifice for cure of atrial flutter. Recordings are displayed from the multipolar catheter around much of the circumference of the tricuspid annulus (see left anterior oblique fluoroscopy images). Ablation of this isthmus is performed during coronary sinus pacing. In the two beats on the left, atrial conduction proceeds in two directions around the tricuspid annulus, as indicated by arrows and recorded along the halo catheter. In the two beats on the right, ablation has interrupted conduction in the floor of the right atrium, eliminating one path for transmission along the tricuspid annulus. The halo catheter now records conduction proceeding all the way around the annulus. This finding demonstrates unidirectional block in the isthmus; block in the other direction may be demonstrated by pacing from one of the halo electrodes and observing a similar lack of isthmus conduction. (The bundle of His recording in the right panel is lost owing to catheter movement.)

3.2 percent, and there was one death in 900 patients.[63] In early studies, up to 4 percent of patients had an episode of sudden death after AV junction ablation despite adequate pacemaker function, presumably because of relative bradycardia after long periods of rapid ventricular rates.[71] In one study, 6 of 100 patients died suddenly when the initial pacing rate was set to 60 beats/min, but none of 135 died suddenly when the rate was set to 90 beats/min for 1 to 3 months after ablation. Improvements in quality of life indices as well as cost-effectiveness have been demonstrated for this procedure.

RADIOFREQUENCY CATHETER ABLATION OF ATRIAL FIBRILLATION. Considerable progress has been made in understanding the pathophysiology of atrial fibrillation. The use of this information has translated directly into therapeutic advances. For example, it is now recognized that a significant proportion of patients with paroxysmal atrial fibrillation in the absence of structural heart disease have a focal origin of the arrhythmia; that is, rapid discharges from a focal source (often in a pulmonary vein) drive the atrium more rapidly than it can uniformly conduct, leading to the ECG appearance of atrial fibrillation. In other cases, a focal source can serve as a "trigger" that initiates episodes of fibrillation (see Chap. 32). In either scenario, if this focus can be located and ablated or its spread to the rest of the atrium eliminated, recurrences of atrial fibrillation are prevented.

LOCATION AND ABLATION OF FOCAL SOURCES. A variety of methods have been used to locate and ablate focal sources of atrial fibrillation. When first applied, PACs were mapped and the site from which they originated was ablated. This technique was limited by the fact that few patients have adequate frequency of PACs or short bursts of fibrillation to serve as either a good target for ablation or a useful indicator of success (i.e.,, elimination of PACs). In addition, the source of PACs or fibrillation in many cases was up to 3 cm deep within a pulmonary vein; ablation at these sites could result in pulmonary vein stenosis. As experience grew, it became clear that the majority of cases of paroxysmal atrial fibrillation originated within pulmonary veins; muscular sleeves extend from the left atrium for several centimeters along the pulmonary vein. Efforts then shifted to electrical isolation of the pulmonary veins to prevent spread of impulses from the sites of initiation to the remainder of the atrium. The advantages of this strategy over focal ablation are that (1) there is a greater likelihood of eliminating fibrillation because multiple veins may be arrhythmogenic, (2) the patient need not have PACs in order to perform the ablation, and (3) the risk of pulmonary vein stenosis may be lower. Although strands of atrial muscle enshroud the pulmonary veins, actual electrical connections may exist at only two or three discrete points. The pulmonary vein isolation strategy can be carried out either with mapping of the pulmonary veins to locate and ablate the discrete points of electrical connection between vein and atrium or with a purely anatomical approach. Mapping uses either a circular electrode catheter (Fig. 30-11) or a multipolar "basket" catheter situated within the ostium of the vein.[72] Pulmonary vein potentials, which might be the origin of fibrillation, appear as either sharp potentials (Fig. 30-12) or complex, fragmented signals following the nearby left atrial recording (Fig. 30-13).

Ablation is performed on the atrial side of the venoatrial junction until the pulmonary vein potentials are eliminated ("entrance block" into the vein). Ablation can be performed during sinus rhythm, atrial pacing, or even during atrial fibrillation (which often terminates during RF application).[73] Some advocate pacing from within the vein to demonstrate the more relevant "exit block" from vein to atrium. Using the anatomical approach, continuous lines of ablation are made that surround venous orifices. This method requires sophisticated mapping tools to be able to record the sites that have already been ablated and the areas that remain. In some cases, gaps in a line of ablation can be proarrhythmic by providing a path for macro-reentry in the left atrium. Some electrophysiologists make an additional line of ablation between the left inferior

FIGURE 30–11 Depiction of catheters for pulmonary vein (PV) isolation. Both left PVs are illustrated with strands of atrial muscle connecting PV to left atrium at discrete points. A circular mapping catheter is shown resting in the ostium of the left lower PV and an ablation catheter with a large-tip electrode is shown adjacent to electrodes of the circular catheter that are recording a PV potential from the nearby strand. A radiofrequency (RF) lesion (between the two venous ostia) is at the site of a previously ablated strand.

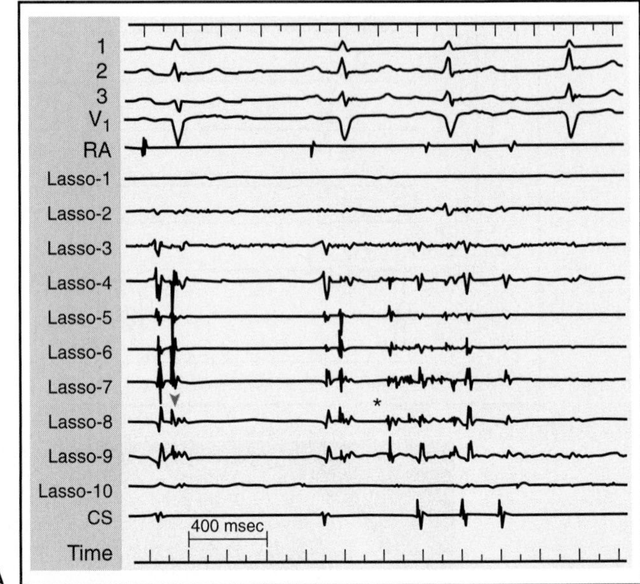

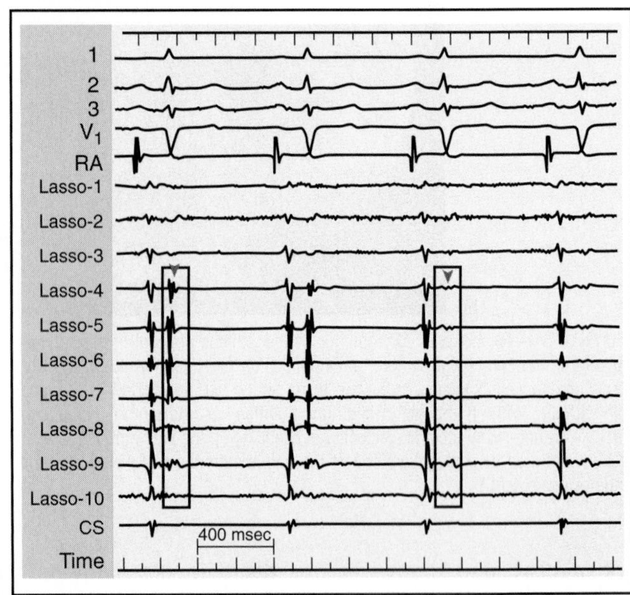

FIGURE 30–12 Sharp pulmonary vein potentials (PVPs). Surface electrocardiographic leads and intracardiac recordings from right atrium (RA), coronary sinus (CS), and a 10-electrode circular catheter (Lasso) situated in the ostium of a pulmonary vein. **A,** Lasso recordings show left atrial electrograms followed by sharp PV potentials in recordings Lasso-4 through Lasso-10 during a sinus beat (arrow points to earliest PVP at Lasso-8 as wave front enters vein); an asterisk marks an ectopic beat from this vein that initiates a very short episode of atrial fibrillation. **B,** Recorded during radiofrequency ablation near Lasso-8 recording site; the same sharp PVPs are seen in the first two beats (left arrow) but are absent during the last two beats (right arrow), leaving only the left atrial recordings. This vein has thus been electrically isolated from the left atrium.

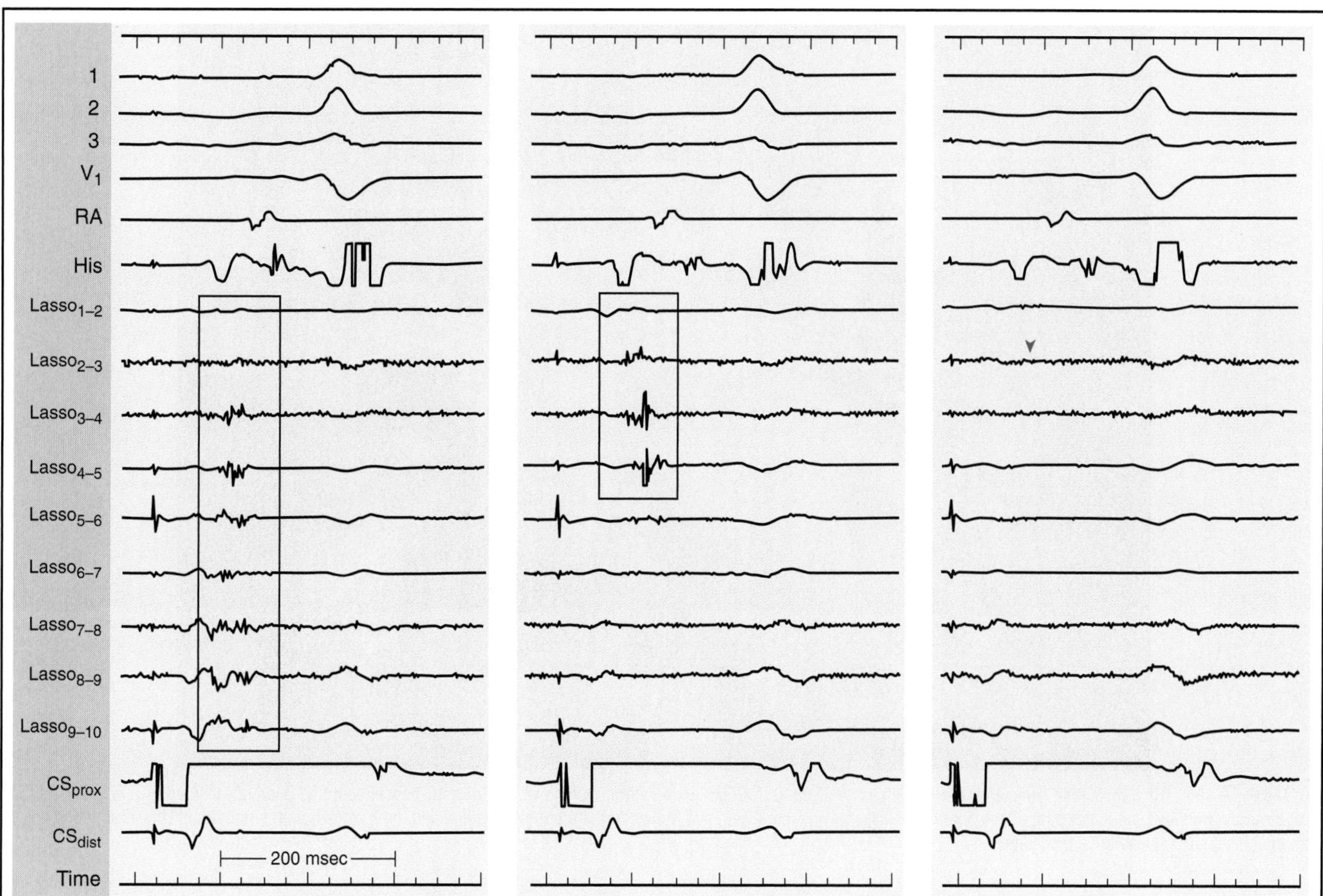

FIGURE 30–13 Low-amplitude, fragmented pulmonary vein potentials (PVPs). Recordings during coronary sinus pacing are similar to those in Figure 30–12. **Left,** Preablation recordings from PV; note fragmented recordings in Lasso-3 through Lasso-9 (within rectangle). **Middle,** Recordings partway through ablation; PVPs are no longer evident in Lasso-5 through Lasso-9. **Right,** Continued ablation eliminates all PVPs (arrow). This vein is now electrically isolated from the left atrium.

pulmonary vein and the mitral annulus to forestall this possibility. In many cases, a "flutter lesion" in the floor of the right atrium is also made because many patients undergoing a purely left atrial procedure have subsequent episodes of flutter. Each method of isolation requires left atrial access using a patent foramen ovale or the septal puncture technique, with full anticoagulation. This approach increases the risk of bleeding complications and still has not entirely prevented thromboemboli related to the procedure. The pulmonary vein isolation approach has been used primarily in younger patients with paroxysmal atrial fibrillation in the absence of structural heart disease; although experience with this technique in patients with chronic atrial fibrillation or those with structural heart disease is limited, preliminary results suggest nearly equivalent success rates. Before the ablation procedure, it is useful to obtain some type of noninvasive study to better define pulmonary venous anatomy, such as a high-resolution computed tomography or magnetic resonance imaging study (Fig. 30-14). This study aids the operator in planning the procedure so that anomalous venous anatomy does not interfere with successful ablation.

As noted earlier, some patients with atrial fibrillation show a transformation to stable atrial flutter when given antiarrhythmic drugs, particularly sodium channel blocking agents. In these patients, performing a flutter ablation and having the patient continue to take the same drug may prevent arrhythmia recurrence.[74]

The maze surgical procedure has become established as a successful technique for permanently restoring sinus rhythm. In 1994, the first reports appeared of replicating the surgically induced lines of block in the atria using catheter ablation in humans. The intent of the procedure is to compartmentalize the atrial muscle into segments too small to support fibrillation wave fronts yet have the segments connected enough to participate in contraction. Several techniques have been used, including creation of long, linear RF lesions limited to either the right or left atrium or both. This technique has been largely supplanted by pulmonary vein isolation, although it has been helpful in some patients who have had recurrent fibrillation after an apparently successful isolation procedure. These may be very long procedures, lasting 5 to 8 hours, and fluoroscopy times over 90 minutes are not uncommon.

Indications. Candidates for focal atrial fibrillation ablation have paroxysmal atrial fibrillation in the absence of structural heart disease and include those whose atrial fibrillation is either refractory to medications or who prefer not to take medications. Patients in whom linear ablation for atrial fibrillation might be considered are those with some degree of structural heart disease and persistent or chronic atrial fibrillation for whom maintenance of sinus rhythm is important and in whom atrial fibrillation recurs despite standard antiarrhythmic drugs or in whom drug therapy is not tolerated or preferred.

Results. Success rates of ablation for atrial fibrillation range from 70 to 85 percent. At present, there does not seem to be a preferred technique (mapping-guided segmental isolation of pulmonary venous ostia versus purely anatomically based ablation). Reasons for failure of ablation include (1) incomplete isolation of an arrhythmogenic vein, (2) restitution of conduction after apparently successful isolation, and (3) nonpulmonary venous sources of fibrillation. The risk of stroke related to extensive left atrial ablation is approximately 2 percent even with rigorous anticoagulation regimens. Pulmonary vein stenosis, more likely if ablation is performed within the vein itself rather than at the ostium, can cause dyspnea and pulmonary arterial hypertension. In some cases, angioplasty and stenting have been necessary.

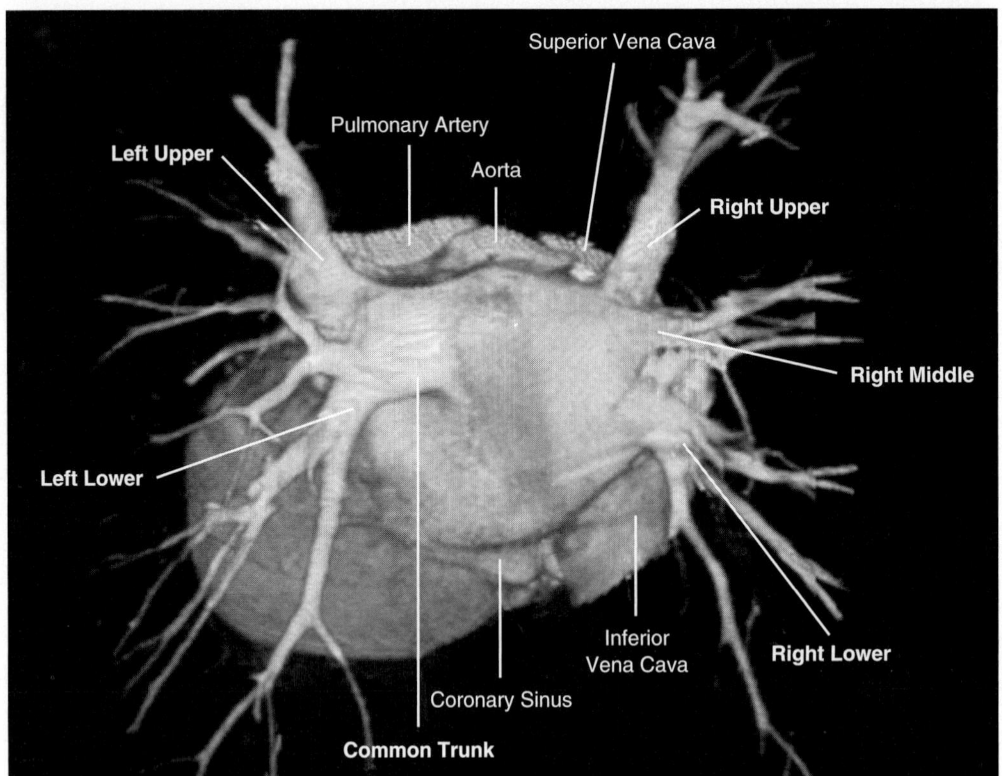

FIGURE 30–14 High-resolution computed tomographic view of the left atrium, viewed from behind to illustrate pulmonary vein (PV) anatomy. Instead of two veins entering the left atrium from each lung, this patient had both left veins emptying into a common trunk before entering the atrium and three veins from the right lung. This information helped plan the pulmonary vein isolation procedure.

Other nonpharmacological modalities for the treatment of atrial fibrillation, such as preventive pacing and implantable atrial defibrillators or atrial rhythm management devices, are discussed in Chapter 31.

RADIOFREQUENCY CATHETER ABLATION OF VENTRICULAR TACHYCARDIA. In general, the success rate for ablation of VTs is lower than that for AV node reentry or AV reentry. This lower success rate may be related to the fact that this procedure is often a last resort in patients with drug-resistant VTs, but it is also related to more difficult mapping in the ventricles. Furthermore, the VT induction must ideally be reproducible, uniform in QRS morphology from beat to beat, sustained, and hemodynamically stable so that the patient can tolerate the VT long enough during the procedure to undergo the extensive mapping necessary to localize optimal ablation target sites. (Patients with several electrocardiographically distinct, uniform morphologies of VT can still be candidates for ablation because in many instances a common reentrant pathway is shared by two or more VT morphologies.) Also, the origin of the VT must be fairly circumscribed and endocardially situated (rare cases of successful ablation only from the epicardial aspect have been reported[75]). Very rapid VT, polymorphic VT, and infrequent, nonsustained episodes are generally not amenable to this form of therapy at this time (see later).

LOCATION AND ABLATION. RF catheter ablation of VT can be divided into idiopathic VT that occurs in patients with essentially normal hearts, VT that occurs in a variety of disease settings but without coronary artery disease, and VT in patients with coronary artery disease and prior myocardial infarction. In the first group, VTs can arise in either ventricle. Right ventricular tachycardias most commonly originate in the outflow tract and have a characteristic left bundle branch block–like, inferior axis morphology; less often, VTs arise in the inflow tract or free wall. Initiation of tachycardia can often be facilitated by catecholamines. The majority of left ventricular VTs are septal in origin and have a characteristic QRS configuration (right bundle branch block, superior axis); other VTs occur less commonly and arise from other areas of the left ventricle, including the left ventricular outflow tract, and are similar in ECG appearance and clinical behavior to those arising in the right ventricular outflow tract (see Fig. 29–13). Abnormal patterns of sympathetic innervation may be present in some. VTs in abnormal hearts without coronary artery disease can be due to bundle branch reentry, most typically observed in patients with dilated cardiomyopathies. In these patients, ablation of the right bundle branch eliminates the tachycardia. VT can occur in right ventricular dysplasia, sarcoidosis, Chagas disease, hypertrophic cardiomyopathy, and a host of other noncoronary disease states (see Chap. 32).

Activation mapping and pace mapping are effective in patients with idiopathic VTs to locate the site of origin of the VT. In activation mapping, the timing of endocardial electrograms sampled by the mapping catheter is compared with the onset of the surface QRS complex. Sites that are activated before the surface QRS onset are near the origin of the VT (Fig. 30–15; see Fig. 29–13). In idiopathic VT, ablation at a site at which the unipolar electrogram shows a "QS" complex may yield greater success than if an "rS" potential is observed (Fig. 30–16). Pace mapping involves stimulation of various ventricular sites to initiate a QRS contour that duplicates the QRS contour of the spontaneous VT, thus establishing the apparent site of origin of the arrhythmia (see Fig. 30–15). This technique is limited by several methodological problems but may be useful when the tachycardia cannot be initiated and when a 12-lead electrocardiogram has been obtained during the spontaneous VT. Presystolic Purkinje potentials as well as very low-amplitude mid-diastolic signals can be recorded during VT from sites at which ablation cures VT in most patients with left ventricular VTs that have a right bundle branch block superior axis. Localization of optimal ablation sites for VT in patients with coronary artery disease and prior infarction is more difficult than in patients with structurally normal hearts because of the altered anatomy and electrophysiology. Pace mapping has lower sensitivity and specificity than it does for idiopathic VT. Furthermore, reentry circuits can sometimes be large and resistant to the relatively small lesions produced by RF catheter ablation in scarred endocardium.

Finding a protected region of diastolic activation used as a critical part of the reentrant circuit is desirable because ablation at this site has a good chance of eliminating the tachycardia (Fig. 30–17). Because of the extensive derangement in electrophysiology caused by the infarction, many areas of the ventricle may have diastolic activation but not be relevant to the perpetuation of the VT. These "bystander sites" make activation mapping more difficult. Pacing techniques such as entrainment can be used to test whether a site is truly part of a circuit or a bystander. Entrainment involves pacing for several seconds during a tachycardia at a rate slightly faster than the VT rate; after pacing ceases and the same tachycardia resumes, the timing of the first complex relative to the last paced beat is an indicator of how close the pacing site is to a part of the VT circuit. During entrainment, part of the ventricle is activated by the paced wave front and part by the VT wave front being forced to exit earlier than it ordinarily would, resulting in a fusion complex on the electrocardiogram. Pacing from within a critical portion of the circuit itself produces an exact QRS match with the VT; fusion occurs only within the circuit and is "concealed" on the surface electrocardiogram. Sites with a low-amplitude, isolated mid-diastolic potential that cannot be dissociated from the tachycardia by pacing perturbations, at which entrainment with concealed fusion can be demonstrated, are highly likely to be successful ablation sites.

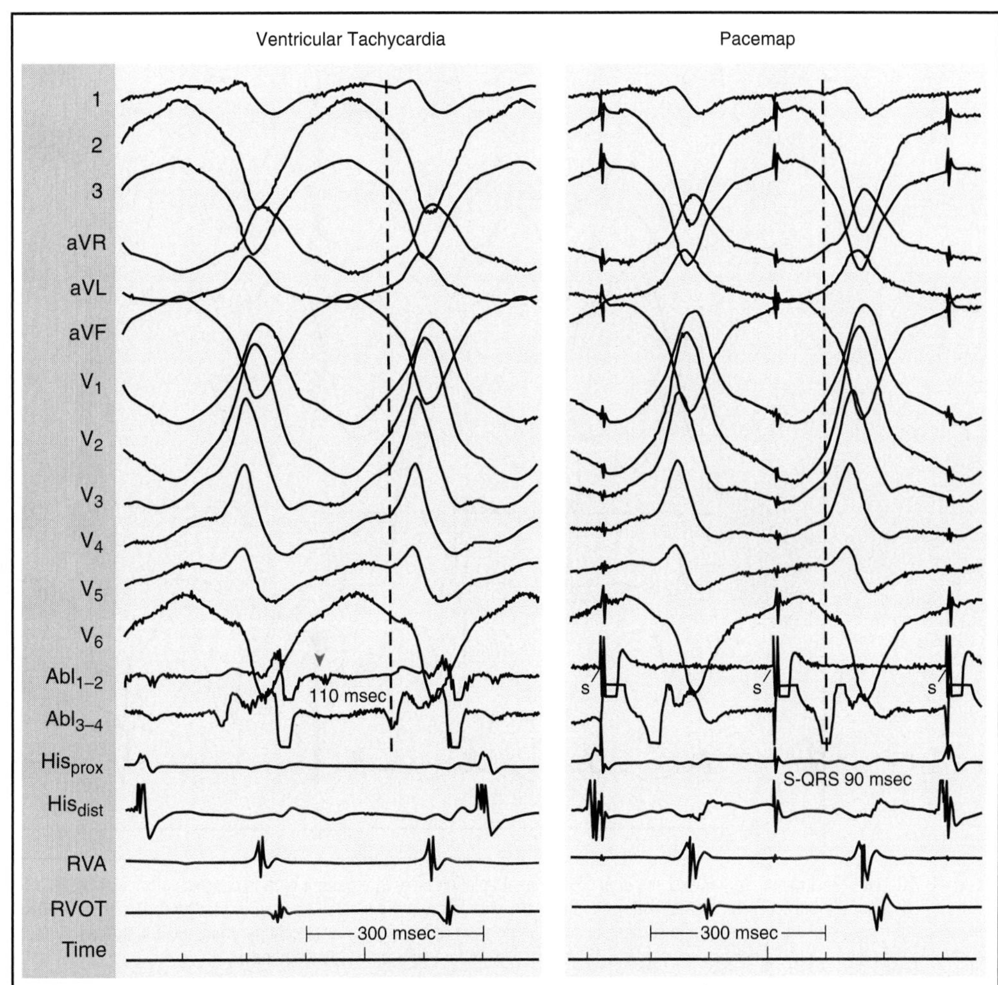

FIGURE 30–15 Ventricular tachycardia and pace mapping. All 12 surface electrocardiographic leads are shown along with intracardiac recordings during ventricular tachycardia (VT). The $Abl_{1\text{-}2}$ recording shows a small deflection occurring early in electrical diastole (arrow) 110 milliseconds before the onset of the QRS (dashed line). In the right panel, pacing is performed from this site. This produces an identical QRS complex in each lead, with a stimulus–QRS onset interval similar to the electrogram–QRS onset interval during VT. Ablation at this site eliminated VT in 2 seconds. RVOT = right ventricular outflow tract.

In a significant proportion of patients with VT in the presence of structural heart disease, activation mapping and entrainment cannot be performed because of poor hemodynamic tolerance of the arrhythmia or inability to initiate sustained tachycardia at EPS. Some investigators have devised techniques to ascertain the location of myocardial regions at which ablation would decrease or eliminate VT recurrences. Such methods generally fall into a category of substrate mapping, in which areas of low electrical voltage or those from which very delayed potentials are recorded during sinus rhythm or at which pacing closely replicates a known VT 12-lead ECG morphology (pace mapping) are targeted for ablation without performing any mapping during VT.[76] Experience with these methods is limited, but results in decreasing the number of VT recurrences are thus far promising.

In patients without structural heart disease, only a single VT is usually present, and catheter ablation of that VT is curative. In patients with extensive structural heart disease, especially those with prior myocardial infarction, multiple VTs are usually present. Catheter ablation of a single VT in such patients may be only palliative and may not eliminate the need for further antiarrhythmic therapy. The genesis of multiple tachycardia morphologies is not clear, although in some cases they are merely different manifestations of one circuit (e.g., different directions of wave front propagation or exit to the ventricle as a whole), and ablation of one may prevent recurrence of others. The presence of multiple VT morphologies contributes to the difficulties in mapping and ablation of VT in these patients because pacing techniques employed to validate recordings at potential sites of ablation may result in a change in morphology to another VT that does not arise in the same region.

After ablation of VT, repeated ventricular stimulation is performed to assess efficacy. In some cases, rapid polymorphic VT or fibrillation is initiated. The clinical significance of these arrhythmias is unclear, but some evidence suggests that they have a low likelihood of spontaneous occurrence during follow-up.

As noted previously, most cases of polymorphic VT and VF are not currently amenable to ablation because of hemodynamic instability and beat-to-beat changes in activation sequence. However, rare reports of successful ablation of these arrhythmias in patients with apparent focal initiation have shown that at least some cases can be managed with ablation. In such cases, repeated episodes of arrhythmia have constant ECG features of the initiating beat or beats suggesting a consistent source, which may be in either ventricle. The electrogram at sites of successful ablation often has very sharp presystolic potentials reminiscent of Purkinje potentials.[77]

Indications. Patients considered for RF catheter ablation of VT in the absence of structural heart disease are those with symptomatic, sustained, monomorphic VT when the tachycardia is drug resistant, when the patient is drug intolerant, or when the patient does not desire long-term drug therapy. Patients with structural heart disease who are candidates for ablation include those with bundle branch reentrant VT and patients with sustained monomorphic VT and an ICD who are receiving multiple shocks not manageable by reprogramming or concomitant drug therapy. Occasionally, nonsustained VT or even severely symptomatic PVCs require RF catheter ablation.

Results. In the U.S. NASPE survey, 429 patients underwent ablation, with an overall success rate of 71 percent. In 224 patients with structurally normal hearts, the success rate

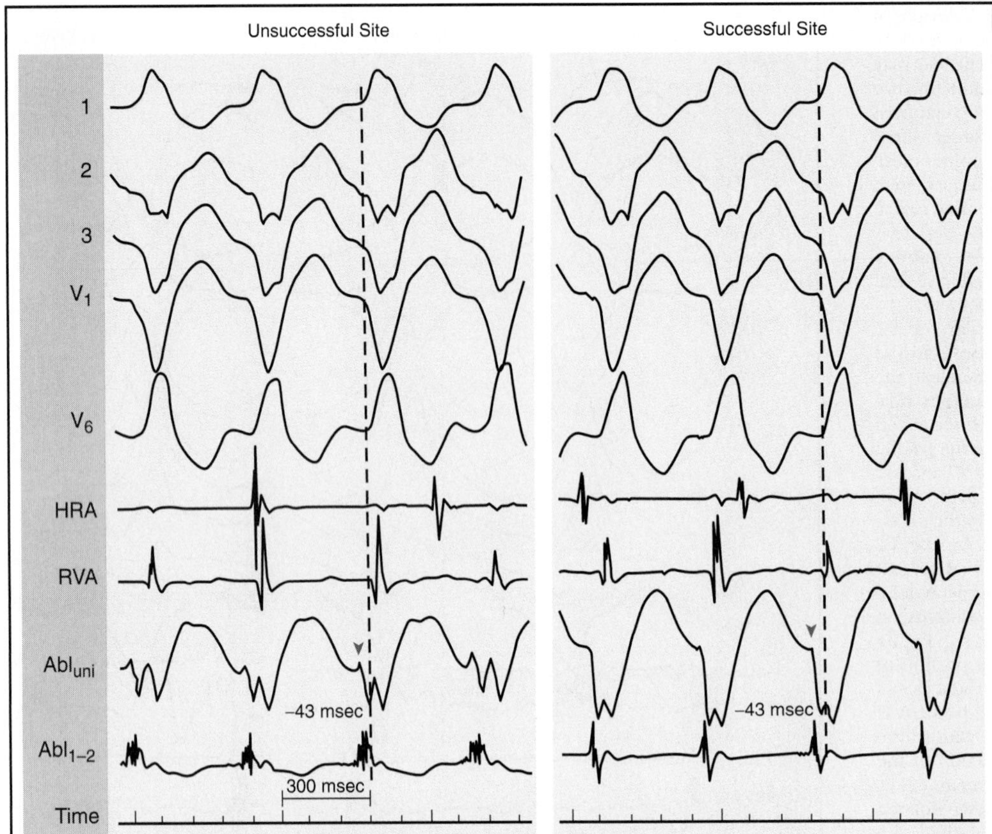

FIGURE 30–16 Recordings from unsuccessful and successful ablation sites in a patient with idiopathic ventricular tachycardia arising in the inferior right ventricular wall. In the recordings from the unsuccessful ablation site, the unipolar signal (arrow) has a small r wave, indicating that a portion of the wave front from the focus of tachycardia was approaching the site from elsewhere. At the successful site, the unipolar recording has a QS configuration, indicating that all depolarization was emanating from this site. In each site, the bipolar recording (Abl_{1-2}) occurs an identical 43 milliseconds before QRS onset (dashed lines).

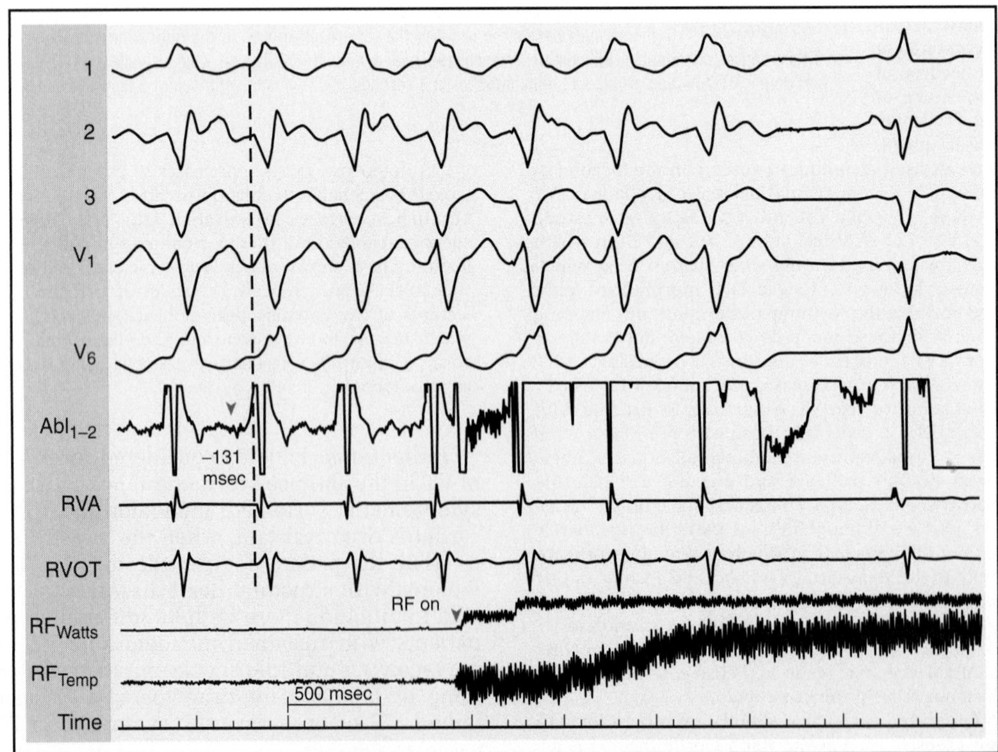

FIGURE 30–17 Radiofrequency (RF) ablation of postinfarct ventricular tachycardia (VT). Recordings are as in previous figures. The electrogram in the ablation recording (Abl_{1-2}, arrow) precedes the QRS onset (dashed line) by 131 milliseconds. Ablation here (RF on) results in slight deceleration of VT before termination in 1.3 seconds. Temperature monitored from the catheter tip had just peaked (approximately 70°C) at the time VT terminated.

was 85 percent. The success rate was 54 percent in 115 patients with VT related to ischemic heart disease and 61 percent in 90 patients with idiopathic cardiomyopathy. There were 13 significant complications (3.0 percent) and, interestingly, considering the nature of the disease, no procedure-related deaths.[61] The complication rate was 7.5 percent in the European survey, and there was one death in 320 patients.[63] Later series suggest a 30 percent "cure" rate for patients (no inducible ventricular arrhythmia of any type, no recurrences), whereas more than 70 percent of patients no longer have recurrences of VT after the procedure, despite inducibility of rapid VT or VF.

NEW MAPPING AND ABLATION TECHNOLOGIES

Multielectrode Mapping Systems. As noted earlier, many of the limitations of ablation are related to inadequate mapping. These problems include only isolated premature complexes during the EPS as opposed to sustained tachycardias (in idiopathic atrial and ventricular tachycardias), nonsustained episodes of VT, poor hemodynamic tolerance of VT, and multiple VT morphologies. Standard mapping techniques sample single sites sequentially and are poorly suited to these situations. New mapping systems are available that enable sampling of many sites simultaneously and incorporate sophisticated computer algorithms for analysis and display of global maps. These mapping systems use a variety of technologies, ranging from multiple electrodes situated on each of several splines of a basket catheter, to the use of low-intensity electrical or magnetic fields to localize the catheter tip in the heart and record and plot activation times on a contour map of the chamber, to the use of complex mathematics to compute "virtual" electrograms recorded from a mesh electrode situated in the middle of a chamber cavity.[78] Some of these systems are capable of generating activation maps of an entire chamber using only one complex, an obvious advantage in patients with only premature complexes, nonsustained arrhythmias, or poor hemodynamic tolerance. Although these mapping systems offer great assistance in selected cases, they are complex and expensive.

EPICARDIAL CATHETER MAPPING. Although the majority of VTs can be ablated from the endocardium, occasional cases are resistant to this therapy. In some of these cases, epicardial ablation may be successful.[75] Much of the work in this area has been performed in patients with VT related to Chagas disease, in whom a majority appear to require epicardial mapping and ablation; it is less frequently necessary in postinfarct or cardiomyopathy patients and those without structural heart disease. The technique for gaining access to the epicardium differs slightly from that for pericardiocentesis. A long spinal anesthesia needle is introduced from a subxiphoid approach under fluoroscopic guidance. As the pericardial surface is approached, a small amount of a radiocontrast agent is injected. If the needle tip is still outside the pericardium, the dye stays where injected; when the pericardial space has been entered, the dye disperses, outlining the heart. A guidewire can then be introduced through the needle and a standard vascular introducer sheath exchanged over the wire. The pericardial space is then accessible for a standard mapping ablation catheter. Standard mapping techniques can then be applied. When a site is selected for possible ablation, coronary arteriography may be warranted to avoid delivery of RF energy near a coronary artery. This is less important in postinfarct VT because the VT substrate is typically in a region of prior transmural infarction. The technique can be applied in patients who have had prior cardiac surgery, although adhesions may obliterate portions of the pericardial space.

CHEMICAL ABLATION. Chemical ablation with alcohol or phenol of an area of myocardium involved in a tachycardia has been used to create AV block in patients not responding to catheter ablation and to eliminate atrial and ventricular tachycardias. Recurrences of tachycardia several days after apparently successful ablation are common. Excessive myocardial necrosis is the major complication, and alcohol ablation should be considered only when other ablative approaches fail or cannot be done.

Surgical Therapy for Tachyarrhythmias

The objectives of a surgical approach to treating a tachycardia are to excise, isolate, or interrupt tissue in the heart critical for the initiation, maintenance, or propagation of the tachycardia while preserving or even improving myocardial function. In addition to a direct surgical approach to the arrhythmia, indirect approaches such as aneurysmectomy, coronary artery bypass grafting, and relief of valvular regurgitation or stenosis can be useful in selected patients by improving cardiac hemodynamics and myocardial blood flow. Cardiac sympathectomy alters adrenergic influences on the heart and has been effective in some patients, particularly those who have recurrent VT with the long QT syndrome.

Supraventricular Tachycardias

Surgical procedures exist for patients (adults and children) with ATs, atrial flutter, AV node reentry, and AV reentry (Fig. 30–18). RF catheter ablation adequately treats the vast majority of these patients and has thus replaced direct surgical intervention except for the occasional patient in whom RF catheter ablation fails or who is having concomitant cardiovascular surgery. In some instances, a prior attempt at RF catheter ablation complicates surgery by obliterating the normal tissue planes that exist in the AV groove of the heart or by rendering tissues too friable. Occasionally, patients with ATs have multiple foci that require surgical intervention.

The maze procedure, developed to treat patients with atrial fibrillation, eliminates the arrhythmia by reducing atrial tissue mass to a size at any instant in time too small to perpetuate the reentrant circuits responsible for atrial fibrillation.[79] It forces atrial activation to proceed along a surgically determined pathway, thus maintaining sinus rhythm with AV nodal conduction. The maze procedure permits organized electrical depolarization of the atria, restores atrial transport function, and in so doing decreases the risk of thromboembolism. Maintenance of sinus rhythm more than 3 months after the procedure approaches 100 percent, although up to 10 percent of patients require pacemakers because of chronotropic incompetence of the sinus node (related to either the surgery or the preexisting atrial pathology). The advent of minimally invasive endoscopic and endovascular techniques may make it possible to perform an equivalent of the maze procedure without thoracotomy in the future. The maze procedure or a variation of it is currently most commonly performed concomitantly with mitral valve surgery rather than as a primary indication. In many centers, intraoperative RF ablation has replaced surgical incisions for performing the maze procedure, although significant complications (such as esophageal erosion) have been reported.[80]

Ventricular Tachycardia

In contrast to patients with supraventricular arrhythmias, candidates for surgical therapy for ventricular arrhythmias often have severe left ventricular dysfunction, which is generally caused by coronary artery disease. The cause of the underlying heart disease influences the type of surgery performed. Candidates are patients with drug-resistant, symptomatic, recurrent ventricular tachyarrhythmias who ideally have a segmental wall motion abnormality (scar or aneurysm) with preserved residual left ventricular function, have not benefited from prior attempts at catheter ablation, or are not candidates for catheter ablation because of hemodynamic

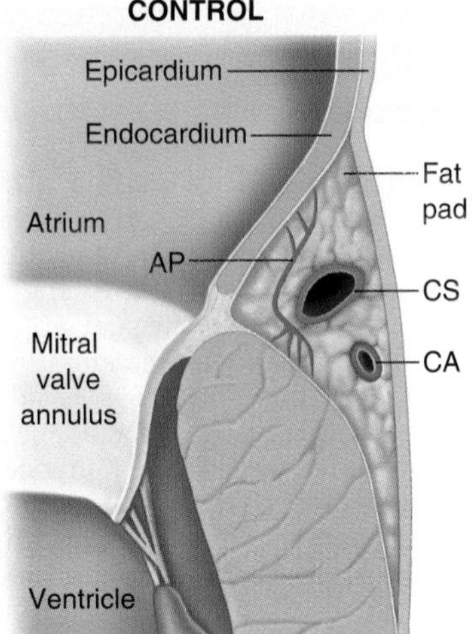

FIGURE 30–18 Schematic diagram showing the two approaches for surgical interruption of an accessory pathway. The left panel depicts the left atrioventricular groove and its vascular contents, the coronary sinus (CS) and circumflex coronary artery (CA). Multiple accessory pathways (APs) course through the fat pad. The middle panel shows the epicardial dissection approach, and the right panel exhibits the endocardial dissection. Both approaches clear out the fat pad and interrupt any accessory pathways. WPW = Wolff-Parkinson-White. (From Zipes DP: Cardiac electrophysiology: Promises and contributions. J Am Coll Cardiol 13:1329, 1989. Reprinted by permission of the American College of Cardiology.)

instability during VT or the presence of left ventricular thrombus. Poorer surgical results are obtained in patients with nonischemic cardiomyopathy.

ISCHEMIC HEART DISEASE. In almost all patients who have VT associated with ischemic heart disease, the arrhythmia, regardless of its configuration on the surface electrocardiogram, arises in the left ventricle or on the left ventricular side of the interventricular septum. The ECG contour of the VT can change from a right bundle branch block to a left bundle branch block pattern without a change in the site of earliest diastolic activation, suggesting that the site of the circuit within the left ventricle remains the same, often near the septum, but its exit pathway is altered.

Indirect surgical approaches, including cardiothoracic sympathectomy, coronary artery bypass grafting, and ventricular aneurysm or infarct resection with or without coronary artery bypass grafting, have been successful in 20 to 30 percent of reported cases. Coronary artery bypass grafting as a primary therapeutic approach has generally been successful only in patients who experience VT during ischemia as well as patients with ischemia-related VF but can sometimes be useful in patients with coronary disease resuscitated from sudden death who have no inducible arrhythmias at EPS. These patients generally have a clear relationship between episodes of ventricular arrhythmia and immediately antecedent severe ischemia and have either no evidence of infarction or minimal wall motion abnormalities with preserved overall left ventricular function. Patients with sustained monomorphic VT or only polymorphic VT rarely have their arrhythmias affected by coronary bypass surgery, although the latter can reduce the frequency of the arrhythmic episodes in some patients and prevent new ischemic events.

Surgical Techniques

Generally, two types of direct surgical procedures are used: resection and ablation (Fig. 30–19).[81] The first direct surgical approach to VT was encircling endocardial ventriculotomy, using a transmural ventriculotomy to isolate areas of endocardial fibrosis that were recognized visually; this procedure is rarely employed now. The rationale for subendocardial resection is based on animal and clinical data indicating that arrhythmias after myocardial infarction arise mostly at the subendocardial borders between normal and infarcted tissues. Subendocardial resection involves peeling off a 1- to 3-mm-thick layer of endocardium, often near the rim of an aneurysm, that has been demonstrated by means of mapping procedures to be the site of earliest activation recorded during the VT. Some VTs can arise from the epicardium. Tachycardias arising from near the base of the papillary muscles are treated using a cryoprobe cooled to –70°C. Cryoablation can also be used to isolate areas of the ventricle that cannot be resected and is often combined with resection. The neodymium:yttrium-aluminum-garnet laser approaches have been used as well with good success, but the equipment is expensive and difficult to work with.

RESULTS. For ventricular tachyarrhythmias, operative mortality ranges from 6 to 23 percent, with success rates defined as absence of recurrence of spontaneous ventricular arrhythmias ranging from 59 to 98 percent. In experienced centers, operative mortality can be as low as 5 percent in stable patients undergoing elective procedures, with 85 to 95 percent of survivors free of inducible or spontaneous ventricular tachyarrhythmias. Long-term recurrence rates range from 2 to 38 percent and correlate with results of the patient's postoperative electrophysiological stimulation study. Operative survival is strongly influenced by the degree of left ventricular dysfunction.

Operative mortality for nonthoracotomy ICD implantation is less than 1 percent, with an annual sudden cardiac death mortality rate of less than 1 percent. Because of the difference in operative survival and shorter hospital stay with ICD therapy compared with direct surgery for VT and the success rates for catheter ablation in patients who have an ICD but experience frequent episodes of VT, few curative surgical procedures are now performed.

Electrophysiological Studies

PREOPERATIVE ELECTROPHYSIOLOGICAL STUDY. In patients for whom direct surgical therapy for VT is planned, a preoperative EPS is usually warranted. This study involves initiation of the VT and electrophysiological mapping to localize the area to be resected, as is done with catheter ablation. A resolution of 4 to 8 cm^2 of ventricular endocardium is thereby achieved, although more accurate anatomical localization of the mapping electrode tip in the ventricle may be possible. Tachycardias that are too rapid, short in duration, or polymorphic cannot be mapped accurately unless multiple catheters or a multielectrode array is used. Administering a drug such as procainamide may slow the VT and transform a nonsustained polymorphic VT into a sustained VT of uniform contour that can be mapped. Preoperative catheter mapping is contraindicated in patients who have known left ventricular thrombus that might be dislodged by the mapping catheter.

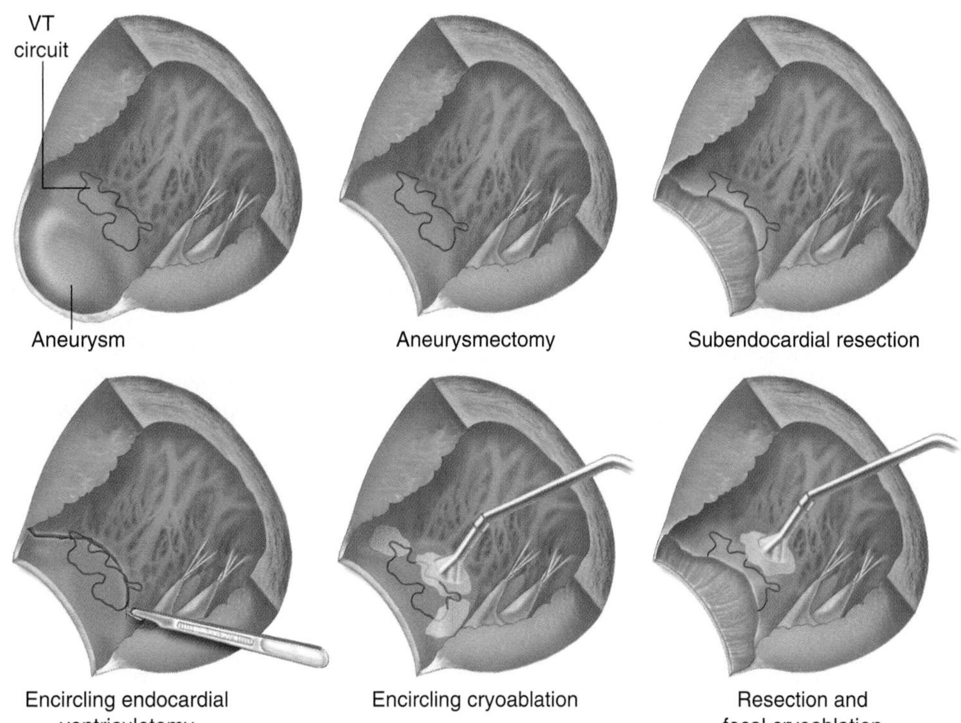

FIGURE 30–19 Schematic diagram showing surgical procedures for treatment of postinfarct ventricular tachycardia (VT) with left ventricular aneurysm. A damaged left ventricle is depicted as opened along the lateral wall and viewing the septum and papillary muscles. The tachycardia circuit (upper left) takes a meandering course near where the aneurysm meets normal myocardium and at times is superficial and at other times coursing deeper (green lines). Simple aneurysmectomy that leaves a portion of the aneurysm for suturing often misses the circuit and thus does not cure the arrhythmia. Using subendocardial resection, a layer of endocardium and subjacent tissue is removed, including at least some of the tachycardia circuit. This resection results in elimination of tachycardia. Encircling endocardial ventriculotomy attempts to isolate the circuit electrically without removing tissue, but it probably actually works by incising portions of the circuit. Cryoablation can be used to encircle the infarct zone or in combination with resection to damaged tissue too deep in the wall to be safely resected.

INTRAOPERATIVE VENTRICULAR MAPPING. Electrophysiological mapping is also performed at the time of surgery, with the surgeon using a handheld probe or an electrode array coupled with computer techniques that instantaneously provide an overall activation map cycle by cycle. The sequence of activation during VT can be plotted and the area of earliest activation determined. Resection or cryoablation of tissue from which these recordings are made usually cures the VT, indicating that they represent a critical portion of the reentrant circuit. However, it is quite clear that such electrical activity can be late following the preceding cycle or early in advance of the next cycle. When the earliest recordable endocardial electrical activity occurs less than 30 milliseconds before the onset of the QRS complex, the critical portions of the circuit may be in the interventricular septum or near the epicardium of the free wall.

The area of earliest recorded electrical activity during VT may not actually represent a critical portion of the tachycardia circuit because the latter may be several centimeters away (e.g., in a small, scarred area). The impulse may then be conducted slowly until it reaches more normally excitable tissue, where it exits and spreads rapidly to the rest of the endocardium to generate a QRS complex. However, this area of early activation is probably closely related to the origin of the tachycardia that, on the basis of the present state of knowledge and results from surgery, warrants surgical intervention at that site. Finding an area from which "continuous electrical activity" is recorded rarely, if ever, indicates that the entire circuit is being recorded. However, it is likely that a critical portion of the tachycardia circuit is close to the area of continuous electrical activity. In some patients, intramural mapping using a plunge needle electrode can be useful, particularly if the origin of the tachycardia is not in the subendocardium. Most centers now employ a strategy of "sequential" subendocardial resection, in which VT is initiated, mapped, and ablated (resected or cryoablated) and stimulation is immediately repeated. If VT can still be initiated, mapping and resection are also repeated until VT can no longer be initiated.

REFERENCES

1. Murgatroyd FD: "Pills and pulses": Hybrid therapy for atrial fiibrillation. J ardiovasc Electrophysiol 13:S40, 2002.

Pharmacological Therapy

2. Vaughan Williams EM: The relevance of cellular to clinical electrophysiology in classifying antiarrhythmic actions. J Cardiovasc Pharmacol 20:S1, 1992.
3. Members of the Sicilian Gambit: Antiarrhythmic Therapy: A Pathophysiologic Approach. Armonk, NY, Futura Publishing Company, 1994.
4. Kowey PR, Marinchak RA, Rials SJ, Bharucha DB: Classifiication and pharmacology o antiarrhythmic drugs. Am Heart J 140:12, 2000.
5. Napolitano C, Schwartz PJ, Brown AM, et al: Evidence for a cardiac ion channel mutation underlying drug-induced QT prolongation and life-threatening arrhythmias. J Cardiovasc Electrophysiol 11:691, 2000.
6. Naccarelli GV, Wolbrette DL, Khan M, et al: Old and new antiarrhythmic drugs for converting and maintaining sinus rhythm in atrial fiibrillation: Comparative effiicacy a results of trials. Am J Cardiol 91:15D, 2003.
7. Sarkozy A, Dorian P: Advances in the acute pharmacologic management of cardiac arrhythmias. Curr Cardiol Rep 5:387, 2003.
8. Choudhury L, Grais IM, Passman RS: Torsades de pointes due to drug interaction between disopyramide and clarithromycin. Heart Dis 1:206, 1999.
9. Somberg JC, Bailin SJ, Haffajee CI, et al: Intravenous lidocaine vs intravenous amiodarone (in a new aqueous formulation) for incessant ventricular tachycardia. Am J Cardiol 90:853, 2002.
10. Aliot E, De Roy L, Capucci A, et al: Safety of a controlled-release fllecainide acetate fomulation in the prevention of paroxysmal atrial fiibrillation in outpatients. Ann Cardio Angeiol (Paris) 52:34, 2003.
11. Kowey PR, Yan GX, Winkel E, et al: Pharmacologic and nonpharmacologic options to maintain sinus rhythm: Guideline-based and new approaches. Am J Cardiol 91:33D, 2003.
12. Naccarelli GV, Wolbrette DL, Luck JC: Proarrhythmia. Med Clin North Am 85:503, 2001.
13. Flaker GC, Blackshear JL, McBride R, et al: Antiarrhythmic drug therapy and cardiac mortality in atrial fiibrillation. The Stroke Prevention in Atrial Fibrillation Investigators J Am Coll Cardiol 20:527, 1992.
14. The Cardiac Arrhythmia Suppression Trial Investigators: Preliminary report: Effect of encainide and fllecainide on mrtality in a randomized trial of arrhythmia suppression after myocardial infarction. N Engl J Med 321:406, 1989.

15. Wyse KR, Ye V, Campbell TJ: Action potential prolongation exhibits simple dose-dependence for sotalol, but reverse dose-dependence for quinidine and disopyramide: Implications for proarrhythmia due to triggered activity. J Cardiovasc Pharmacol 21:316, 1993.
16. Darbar D, Fromm MF, Dellorto S, Roden DM: Sympathetic activation enhances QT prolongation by quinidine. J Cardiovasc Electrophysiol 12:9, 2001.
17. Benton RE, Sale M, Flockhart DA, Woosley RL: Greater quinidine-induced QTc interval prolongation in women. Clin Pharmacol Ther 67:413, 2000.
18. Brembilla-Perrot B, Houriez P, Beurrier D, et al: Predictors of atrial fllutter with 1:1 conduction in patients treated with class I antiarrhythmic drugs for atrial tachyarrhythmias. Int J Cardiol 80:7, 2001.
19. Morita N, Kobayashi Y, Iwasaki YK, et al: Pronounced effect of procainamide on clockwise right atrial isthmus conduction compared with counterclockwise conduction: Possible mechanism of the greater incidence of common atrial fllutter during antiarrhythmi therapy. J Cardiovasc Electrophysiol 13:212, 2002.
20. Rials SJ, Britchkow D, Marinchak RA, Kowey PR: Electropharmacologic effect of a standard dose of intravenous procainamide in patients with sustained ventricular tachycardia. Clin Cardiol 23:171, 2000.

Class IB Antiarrhythmic Agents

CH 30

21. Ye VZ, Wyse KR, Campbell TJ: Lidocaine shows greater selective depression of depolarized and acidotic myocardium than propafenone: Possible implications for proarrhythmia. J Cardiovasc Pharmacol 21:47, 1993.
22. Dorian P, Cass D, Schwartz B, et al: Amiodarone as compared with lidocaine for shock-resistant ventricular fiibrillatio. N Engl J Med 346:884, 2002.
23. Yonezawa E, Matsumoto K, Ueno K, et al: Lack of interaction between amiodarone and mexiletine in cardiac arrhythmia patients. J Clin Pharmacol 42:342, 2002.
24. Azarbayjani F, Danielsson BR: Phenytoin-induced cleft palate: Evidence for embryonic cardiac bradyarrhythmia due to inhibition of delayed rectifiier + channels resulting in hypoxia-reoxygenation damage. Teratology 63:152, 2001.

Class IC Antiarrhythmic Agents

25. Ebenroth ES, Cordes TM, Darragh RK: Second-line treatment of fetal supraventricular tachycardia using flecainide acetate. Pediatr Cardiol 22:483, 2001.
26. Arias C, Gonzalez T, Moreno I, et al: Effects of propafenone and its main metabolite, 5-hydroxypropafenone, on HERG channels. Cardiovasc Res 57:660, 2003.
27. Boriani G, Martignani C, Biffi M, et al: Oral loading with propafenone for conversion o recent-onset atrial fiibrillation: A review on in-hospital treatment. Drugs 62:415, 2002.
28. Geller JC, Geller M, Carlson MD, Waldo AL: Effiicacy and safety of moicizine in the maintenance of sinus rhythm in patients with recurrent atrial fiibrillation. Am J Cardio 87:172, 2001.
29. The Cardiac Arrhythmia Suppression Trial II Investigators: Effect of the antiarrhythmic agent moricizine on survival after myocardial infarction. N Engl J Med 327:227, 1992.

Class II Antiarrhythmic Agents

30. Singh BN, Sarma JSM: Beta-blockers and calcium channel blockers as antiarrhythmic drugs. *In* Zipes DP, Jalife J (eds): Cardiac Electrophysiology: From Cell to Bedside. 3rd ed. Philadelphia, WB Saunders, 1999, pp 903-920.
31. Connolly SJ, Cybulsky I, Lamy A, et al: Double-blind, placebo-controlled, randomized trial of prophylactic metoprolol for reduction of hospital length of stay after heart surgery: The beta-Blocker Length Of Stay (BLOS) study. Am Heart J 145:226, 2003.
32. Sun W, Sarma JS, Singh BN: Chronic and acute effects of dronedarone on the action potential of rabbit atrial muscle preparations: Comparison with amiodarone. J Cardiovasc Pharmacol 39:677, 2002
33. Aimond F, Beck L, Gautier P, et al: Cellular and in vivo electrophysiological effects of dronedarone in normal and postmyocardial infarcted rats. J Pharmacol Exp Ther 292:415, 2000.
34. Camm AJ, Yap YG: What should we expect from the next generation of antiarrhythmic drugs? J Cardiovasc Electrophysiol 10:307, 1999.

Class III Antiarrhythmic Agents

35. Doval HC, Nul DR, Grancelli HO, et al: Randomised trial of low-dose amiodarone in severe congestive heart failure. Grupo de Estudio de la Sobrevida en la Insufiicienci Cardiaca en Argentina (GESICA). Lancet 344:493, 1994.
36. Daoud EG, Strickberger SA, Man KC, et al: Preoperative amiodarone as prophylaxis against atrial fiibrillation after heart surgery. N Engl J Med 337:1785, 1997.
37. Dorian P, Mangat I: Role of amiodarone in the era of the implantable cardioverter defiibrillator. J Cardiovasc Electrophysiol 14(Suppl 9):S78, 2003.
38. The AVID Investigators: Antiarrhythmics Versus Implantable Defiibrillators (AVID) Rationale, design, and methods. Am J Cardiol 75:470, 1995.
39. Ott MC, Khoor A, Leventhal JP, et al: Pulmonary toxicity in patients receiving low-dose amiodarone. Chest 123:646, 2003.
40. van Opstal JM, Schoenmakers M, Verduyn SC, et al: Chronic amiodarone evokes no torsades de pointes arrhythmias despite QT lengthening in an animal model of acquired long-QT syndrome. Circulation 104:2722, 2001.
41. Cardenas GA, Cabral JM, Leslie CA: Amiodarone induced thyrotoxicosis: Diagnostic and therapeutic strategies. Cleve Clin J Med 70:624, 628, 2003.
42. Sreih AG, Schoenfeld MH, Marieb MA: Optic neuropathy following amiodarone therapy. Pacing Clin Electrophysiol 22:1108, 1999.
43. Hohnloser SH, Woosley RL: Sotalol. N Engl J Med 331:31, 1994.
44. Pacifiico A, Hohnloser SH, Williams JH, et al: Prevention of implantable-defiibrillar shocks by treatment with sotalol. *d,l*-Sotalol Implantable Cardioverter-Defiibrillato Study Group. N Engl J Med 340:1855, 1999.
45. Eversole A, Hancock W, Johns T, et al: Ibutilide: Effiicacy and safety in atrial fiibrillati and atrial flutter in a generl cardiology practice. Clin Cardiol 24:521, 2001.
46. Oral H, Souza JJ, Michaud GF, et al: Facilitating transthoracic cardioversion of atrial fiibrillation with ibutilide pretreatment. N Engl J Med 340:1849, 1999.
47. Kalus JS, Mauro VF: Dofetilide: A class III–specifiic antiarrhythmic agent. Ann Pharmcother 34:44, 2000.
48. Pedersen OD, Bagger H, Keller N, et al: Effiicacy of dofetilide in the treatment of atria fiibrillation-fllutter in patients with reduced left ventricular function: A Danish investigations of arrhythmia and mortality on dofetilide (diamond) substudy. Circulation 104:292, 2001.
49. Clemett D, Markham A: Azimilide. Drugs 59:271, discussion, 278, 2000.
50. Abrol R, Page RL: Azimilide dihydrochloride: A new class III anti-arrhythmic agent. Expert Opin Investig Drugs 9:2705, 2000.

Class IV Antiarrhythmic Agents

51. De Simone A, De Pasquale M, De Matteis C, et al: Verapamil plus antiarrhythmic drugs reduce atrial fiibrillation recurrences after an electrical cardioversion (VEPARAF Study) Eur Heart J 24:1425, 2003.

Other Antiarrhythmic Agents

52. Strickberger SA, Man KC, Daoud EG, et al: Adenosine-induced atrial arrhythmia: A prospective analysis. Ann Intern Med 127:417, 1997.

Electrotherapy of Cardiac Arrhythmias

53. Mittal S, Ayati S, Stein KM, et al: Transthoracic cardioversion of atrial fiibrillation: Coparison of rectilinear biphasic versus damped sine wave monophasic shocks. Circulation 101:1282, 2000.
54. Wyse DG, Waldo AL, DiMarco JP, et al: Atrial Fibrillation Follow-up Investigation of Rhythm Management (AFFIRM) Investigators: A comparison of rate control and rhythm control in patients with atrial fiibrillation. N Enl J Med 347:1825, 2002.
55. Klein AL, Grimm RA, Murray RD, et al: Use of transesophageal echocardiography to guide cardioversion in patients with atrial fiibrillation. N Engl J Med 344:1411, 2001.
56. Morady F: Radio-frequency ablation as treatment for cardiac arrhythmias. N Engl J Med 340:534, 1999.
57. Kimman GJ, Szili-Torok T, Theuns DA, Jordaens LJ: Transvenous cryothermal catheter ablation of a right anteroseptal accessory pathway. J Cardiovasc Electrophysiol 12:1415, 2001.
58. Nabar A, Rodriguez LM, Timmermans C, Wellens HJ: Use of a saline-irrigated tip catheter for ablation of ventricular tachycardia resistant to conventional radiofrequency ablation: Early experience. J Cardiovasc Electrophysiol 12:153, 2001.
59. Rodriguez LM, Geller JC, Tse HF, et al: Acute results of transvenous cryoablation of supraventricular tachycardia (atrial fiibrillation, atrial flutter, Wolff-Parkins-White syndrome, atrioventricular nodal reentry tachycardia). J Cardiovasc Electrophysiol 13:1082, 2002.
60. Calkins H, Yong P, Miller JM, et al: Catheter ablation of accessory pathways, atrioventricular nodal reentrant tachycardia, and the atrioventricular junction: Final results of a prospective, multicenter clinical trial. The Atakr Multicenter Investigators Group. Circulation 99:262, 1999.
61. Scheinman MM: Patterns of catheter ablation practice in the United States: Results of the 1992 NASPE survey. North American Society of Pacing and Electrophysiology. Pacing Clin Electrophysiol 17:873, 1994.
62. Scheinman MM, Huang S: The 1998 NASPE prospective catheter ablation registry. Pacing Clin Electrophysiol 23:1020, 2000.
63. Hindricks G: The Multicentre European Radiofrequency Survey (MERFS): Complications of radiofrequency catheter ablation of arrhythmias. The Multicentre European Radiofrequency Survey (MERFS) investigators of the Working Group on Arrhythmias of the European Society of Cardiology. Eur Heart J 14:1644, 1993.
64. Wu J, Wu J, Olgin J, et al: Mechanisms underlying the reentrant circuit of atrioventricular nodal reentrant tachycardia in isolated canine atrioventricular nodal preparation using optical mapping. Circ Res 88:1189, 2001.
65. McGuire MA, de Bakker JM, Vermeulen JT, et al: Origin and signifiicance of doubl potentials near the atrioventricular node. Correlation of extracellular potentials, intracellular potentials, and histology. Circulation 89:2351, 1994.
66. Skanes AC, Dubuc M, Klein GJ, et al: Cryothermal ablation of the slow pathway for the elimination of atrioventricular nodal reentrant tachycardia. Circulation 102:2856, 2000.
67. Scheinman MM, Gonzalez RP, Cooper MW, et al: Clinical and electrophysiologic features and role of catheter ablation techniques in adult patients with automatic atrioventricular junctional tachycardia. Am J Cardiol 74:565, 1994.
68. Chen SA, Tai CT, Chiang CE, et al: Focal atrial tachycardia: Reanalysis of the clinical and electrophysiologic characteristics and prediction of successful radiofrequency ablation. J Cardiovasc Electrophysiol 9:355, 1998.
69. Tada H, Oral H, Sticherling C, et al: Double potentials along the ablation line as a guide to radiofrequency ablation of typical atrial flutter. J Am Coll Cariol 38:750, 2001.
70. Narasimhan C, Blanck Z, Akhtar M: Atrioventricular nodal modifiication and atrioventricular junctional ablation for control of ventricular rate in atrial fibrillation. J Cardivasc Electrophysiol 9:S146, 1998.
71. Ozcan C, Jahangir A, Friedman PA, et al: Long-term survival after ablation of the atrioventricular node and implantation of a permanent pacemaker in patients with atrial fibrillation. N Engl J Med 344:1043, 2001.
72. Marrouche NF, Martin DO, Wazni O, et al: Phased-array intracardiac echocardiography monitoring during pulmonary vein isolation in patients with atrial fiibrillation: Impac on outcome and complications. Circulation 107:2710, 2003.
73. Oral H, Knight BP, Ozaydin M, et al: Segmental ostial ablation to isolate the pulmonary veins during atrial fiibrillation: Feasibility and mechanistic insights. Circulatio 106:1256, 2002.
74. Nabar A, Rodriguez LM, Timmermans C, et al: Effect of right atrial isthmus ablation on the occurrence of atrial fiibrillation: Observations in fou patient groups having type I atrial fllutter with or without associated atrial fiibrillation. Circulation 99:1441, 1999

75. Sosa E, Scanavacca M, d'Avila A: Transthoracic epicardial catheter ablation to treat recurrent ventricular tachycardia. Curr Cardiol Rep 3:451, 2001.
76. Marchlinski FE, Callans DJ, Gottlieb CD, Zado E: Linear ablation lesions for control of unmappable ventricular tachycardia in patients with ischemic and nonischemic cardiomyopathy. Circulation 101:1288, 2000.
77. Haïssaguerre M, Shoda M, Jaïs P, et al: Mapping and ablation of idiopathic ventricular fibrillation. Circulation 106:962, 2002.
78. Strickberger SA, Knight BP, Michaud GF, et al: Mapping and ablation of ventricular tachycardia guided by virtual electrograms using a noncontact, computerized mapping system. J Am Coll Cardiol 35:414, 2000.

79. Gillinov AM, McCarthy PM, Marrouche N, Natale A: Contemporary surgical treatment for atrial fibrillation. Pacing Clin Electrophysiol 26:1641, 2003.
80. Melo J, Adragao PR, Neves J, et al: Electrosurgical treatment of atrial fibrillation with new intraoperative radiofrequency ablation catheter. Thorac Cardiovasc Surg 47(Suppl 3):370, 1999.
81. Miller JM, Rothman SA, Addonizio VP: Surgical techniques for ventricular tachycardia ablation. *In* Singer I (ed): Interventional Electrophysiology. New York, Williams & Wilkins, 1996, pp 641-684.

GUIDELINES *Thomas H. Lee*

Ambulatory Electrocardiography and Electrophysiological Testing

Guidelines for appropriate use of ambulatory electrocardiography (ECG) were first published by the American College of Cardiology/American Heart Association (ACC/AHA) in 1989[1] and updated in 1999.[2] In conjunction with other professional societies, the ACC/AHA issued a statement of requirements for clinical competence in ambulatory ECG in 2001.[3] Guidelines for performance of electrophysiology testing were first published in 1989[4] and updated in 1995[5]; a clinical competence statement was issued by the ACC/AHA for electrophysiology studies and catheter ablation in 2000.[6] The AHA and the North American Society of Pacing and Electrophysiology (NASPE) made recommendations on safety-related issues, such as restrictions on driving, for patients with arrhythmia in 1996.[7] Since then, efforts to update guidelines have focused on appropriateness of use of pacemakers and implantable defibrillators,[8] reflecting rapid advances in knowledge about the ability of implantable defibrillators to improve survival for patients with arrhythmia with or without electrophysiology testing.[9-11] Guidelines on the latter topic are addressed in the appendix to Chapter 31.

Ambulatory Electrocardiography

The evolution of guidelines for use of ambulatory ECG from 1989 to 1999[2] reflected important progress in several areas, including:

- Understanding of the limited usefulness of suppression of ventricular ectopy with drug therapy
- Solid-state digital technology that facilitates transtelephonic transmission of electrocardiographic data
- Technical advances in long-term event recorders
- Improved signal quality and interpretation
- Improved computer arrhythmia interpretation
- Increasingly sophisticated monitoring capacity of pacemakers and implantable defibrillators

As a result of progress in these areas, with increased knowledge about arrhythmias, ambulatory ECG is now considered to be of uncertain appropriateness for many indications for which it was once an accepted strategy.

As with other ACC/AHA guidelines, the indications for use of ambulatory ECG are classified into one of four classes:

- Class I: Conditions for which there is evidence and/or general agreement that the test is useful and effective.
- Class II: Conditions for which there is conflicting evidence and/or a divergence of opinion about the usefulness/efficacy of performing the test.
- Class IIa: Weight of evidence/opinion is in favor of usefulness/efficacy.
- Class IIb: Usefulness/efficacy is less well established by evidence/opinion.
- Class III: Conditions for which there is evidence and/or general agreement that the test is not useful/effective and in some cases may be harmful.

Diagnosis

In the assessment of symptoms that may be due to arrhythmias, ambulatory ECG is quite clearly established for evaluation of syncope (Table 30G–1). When continuous ambulatory ECG is not diagnostic, intermittent recorders may be useful. Ambulatory ECG is also supported for evaluation of recurrent palpitations, particularly if the frequency of these symptoms makes it reasonably likely that they can be correlated with the tracings obtained during a 24-hour monitoring period. The guidelines comment that data on the use of ambulatory ECG for near syncope or dizziness are insufficient to describe the diagnostic performance of this technology for patients with such symptoms.

The ACC/AHA guidelines explicitly discourage ambulatory ECG for patients with syncope or palpitations if other causes have been identified during the clinical evaluation and for patients with cerebrovascular accidents and no other evidence of arrhythmia. The guidelines seek to reduce performance of ambulatory ECG "for completeness" in such cases. Little support is provided for use of ambulatory ECG in cases in which the etiology of the patient's symptoms is unclear but in which the likelihood of detecting an unsuspected arrhythmia is low (class IIb indications).

Assessment of Risk

The ACC/AHA guidelines discouraged the use of ambulatory ECG for either arrhythmia detection or analysis of heart rhythm variability for the purpose of risk assessment among patients without symptoms of arrhythmia, even if they had cardiovascular conditions such as myocardial contusions, left ventricular hypertrophy, or valvular heart disease (see Table 30G–1). Routine use for patients in whom arrhythmia is a common cause of death (left ventricular dysfunction, hypertrophic cardiomyopathy) was considered a class IIb indication. These recommendations preceded data demonstrating the beneficial impact of implantable cardioverter-defibrillators (ICDs) in patients with left ventricular dysfunction after acute myocardial infarction even without symptoms of arrhythmia.[9] These more recent findings may lead to an expanded role for ambulatory ECG in determining which such asymptomatic patients most need these expensive devices.

Efficacy of Antiarrhythmic Therapy

In the absence of data demonstrating that oral antiarrhythmic therapy can improve survival through control of ventricular arrhythmias, ambulatory ECG has a diminished role as a test for evaluation of the efficacy of treatment (see Table 30G–1). Oral antiarrhythmic agents are important for control of supraventricular arrhythmias, but most patients with such arrhythmias do not have episodes every day. Event recorders can be useful for documenting the relationship between symptoms and recurrent arrhythmia and the interval between episodes, which can help guide therapy.

The guidelines provide some support for use of ambulatory ECG for detection of proarrhythmia during initiation of drug therapy, but patients at high risk for such complications tend to have initiation of these medications as inpatients.

TABLE 30G–1 ACC/AHA Guidelines for Ambulatory Electrocardiography for Assessment of Symptoms and Arrhythmias

Indication	Class I (Indicated)	Class IIa (Good Supportive Evidence)	Class IIb (Weak Supportive Evidence)	Class III (Not Indicated)
Assessment of symptoms possibly related to rhythm disturbances	Patients with unexplained syncope, near syncope, or episodic dizziness in whom the cause is not obvious Patients with unexplained recurrent palpitation		Patients with episodic shortness of breath, chest pain, or fatigue that is not otherwise explained Patients with neurological events when transient atrial fibrillation or flutter is suspected Patients with symptoms such as syncope, near syncope, episodic dizziness, or palpitation in whom a probable cause other than an arrhythmia has been identified but in whom symptoms persist despite treatment of this other cause	Patients with symptoms such as syncope, near syncope, episodic dizziness, or palpitation in whom other causes have been identified by history, physical examination, or laboratory tests Patients with cerebrovascular accidents, without other evidence of arrhythmia
Arrhythmia detection to assess risk for future cardiac events in patients without symptoms from arrhythmia			Post-MI patients with LV dysfunction (ejection fraction <40%) Patients with CHF Patients with idiopathic hypertrophic cardiomyopathy	Patients who have sustained myocardial contusion Systemic hypertensive patients with LV hypertrophy Post-MI patients with normal LV function Preoperative arrhythmia evaluation of patients for noncardiac surgery Patients with sleep apnea Patients with valvular heart disease
Measurement of heart rate variability to assess risk for future cardiac events in patients without symptoms from arrhythmia			Post-MI patients with LV dysfunction Patients with CHF Patients with idiopathic hypertrophic cardiomyopathy	Post-MI patients with normal LV function Diabetic subjects to evaluate for diabetic neuropathy Patients with rhythm disturbances that preclude HRV analysis (i.e., atrial fibrillation)
Assessment of antiarrhythmic therapy	To assess antiarrhythmic drug response in individuals in whom baseline frequency of arrhythmia has been characterized as reproducible and of sufficient frequency to permit analysis	To detect proarrhythmic responses to antiarrhythmic therapy in patients at high risk	To assess rate control during atrial fibrillation To document recurrent or asymptomatic nonsustained arrhythmias during therapy in the outpatient setting	

ACC/AHA = American College of Cardiology/American Heart Association; CHF = congestive heart failure; HRV = heart rhythm variability; LV = left ventricular; MI = myocardial infarction.

CH 30

Assessment of Pacemaker and Implantable Cardioverter-Defibrillator Function

Ambulatory ECG was considered to be appropriate for evaluation of function of pacemakers and ICDs, but the role of ambulatory ECG is being eroded by increasing diagnostic and monitoring functions being built into these devices. Ambulatory ECG can provide useful information by correlating symptoms with device activity and by detecting abnormalities in sensing and capture during chronic follow-up (Table 30G–2). However, the ACC/AHA guidelines emphasize that ambulatory ECG should not be used when data available from device interrogation are sufficient to guide clinical management.

Monitoring for Myocardial Ischemia

The 1999 ACC/AHA guidelines do not provide strong support for any indications for routine clinical use of ambulatory ECG monitoring for myocardial ischemia (Table 30G–3). The only indication for which the task force felt there was good supportive evidence was in patients with suspected variant angina. This technology was not considered a first-choice alternative to exercise testing for patients who are unable to exercise.

TABLE 30G–2	ACC/AHA Guidelines for Ambulatory Electrocardiography for Assessment of Pacemaker and Implantable Cardioverter-Defibrillator Function
Class	**Indication**
Class I (indicated)	Evaluation of frequent symptoms of palpitations, syncope, or near syncope to assess device function to exclude myopotential inhibition and pacemaker-mediated tachycardia and to assist in the programming of enhanced features such as rate responsivity and automatic mode switching Evaluation of suspected component failure or malfunction when device interrogation is not definitive in establishing a diagnosis To assess the response to adjunctive pharmacological therapy in patients receiving frequent ICD therapy
Class IIa (good supportive evidence)	
Class IIb (weak supportive evidence)	Evaluation of immediate postoperative pacemaker function after pacemaker or ICD implantation as an alternative or adjunct to continuous telemetric monitoring Evaluation of the rate of supraventricular arrhythmias in patients with implanted defibrillators
Class III (not indicated)	Assessment of ICD or pacemaker malfunction when device interrogation, ECG, or other available data (chest radiograph and so forth) are sufficient to establish an underlying cause or diagnosis Routine follow-up in asymptomatic patients

ACC/AHA = American College of Cardiology/American Heart Association; ECG = electrocardiographic; ICD = implantable cardioverter-defibrillator.

TABLE 30G–3	ACC/AHA Guidelines for Ischemia Monitoring
Class	**Indication**
Class I (indicated)	
Class IIa (good supportive evidence)	Patients with suspected variant angina
Class IIb (weak supportive evidence)	Evaluation of patients with chest pain who cannot exercise Preoperative evaluation for vascular surgery of patients who cannot exercise Patients with known CAD and atypical chest pain syndrome
Class III (not indicated)	Initial evaluation of patients with chest pain who are able to exercise Routine screening of asymptomatic subjects

ACC/AHA = American College of Cardiology/American Heart Association; CAD = coronary artery disease.

Clinical Competence

The ACC/AHA statement on clinical competence recommended that trainees interpret at least 150 ambulatory electrocardiograms under supervision to acquire minimal competence with this technology.[3] A minimum of 25 test interpretations per year was recommended to maintain competence.

Electrophysiological Procedures for Diagnosis

The ACC/AHA guidelines for use of intracardiac electrophysiological procedures from 1989[4] and 1995[6] reflect the emerging role of catheter ablation as a therapeutic strategy but do not fully reflect the reduced importance of antiarrhythmic medications and growing role of ICDs that have occurred. Nevertheless, most of the basic themes of these guidelines remain valid today.

These guidelines, which are older than most of the ACC/AHA guidelines, use a simpler, three-category system for assessment of appropriateness, in which class II indications are not subdivided into indications with more and less support.

Evaluation of Sinus Node Function

Clinical evaluation of sinus node dysfunction is often difficult because of the episodic nature of symptomatic abnormalities and the wide variability in sinus node function among asymptomatic people. Invasive tests of sinus function can test the ability of the sinus node to recover from overdrive suppression and assess sinoatrial conduction by introducing atrial extrastimuli or by atrial pacing.

The ACC/AHA guidelines consider electrophysiological studies of sinus node function most appropriate for patients in whom dysfunction is suspected but not proved after a noninvasive evaluation (Table 30G–4). In contrast, the guidelines consider such studies inappropriate when a documented bradyarrhythmia has been found to be correlated with the patient's symptoms and management is unlikely to be influenced by an electrophysiological study. Studies are also considered inappropriate in asymptomatic patients and those who have sinus pauses only during sleep. When bradyarrhythmias were recognized as the cause of the patient's symptoms, electrophysiological studies were considered to have possible but uncertain appropriateness (class II) if such data might refine treatment choices.

Acquired Atrioventricular Block

The ACC/AHA guidelines emphasized that electrophysiological studies are inappropriate (class III) when ECG findings correlate with symptoms and the findings from electrophysiological studies are unlikely to alter management (e.g., documentation of His bundle conduction rarely improves management for a patient whose other clinical data indicate that placement of a permanent pacemaker is warranted because of symptomatic advanced atrioventricular [AV] block). Similarly, electrophysiological studies are not appropriate for asymptomatic patients with mild degrees of AV block who are not likely to warrant pacemaker implantation. According to these guidelines, electrophysiological studies of AV conduction should be performed when a relationship between symptoms and AV block has not been proved; in such patients, another arrhythmia could be the cause of symptoms.

Chronic Intraventricular Delay

According to ACC/AHA guidelines, the main role of electrophysiological testing in patients with prolonged H-V intervals is not to predict future complications but to determine whether the symptoms of arrhythmia are due to conduction delay or block versus some other arrhythmia. The only class I (clearly appropriate) indication for electrophysiological testing is in symptomatic patients in whom the cause of symptoms is not known. The guidelines specifically discourage such testing of asymptomatic patients and provide only equivocal support for asymptomatic patients with bundle branch block in whom treatment with drugs that might increase conduction delay is being considered.

Narrow and Wide Complex QRS Tachycardia. The ACC/AHA guidelines define different roles for electrophysiological testing in patients with narrow and wide complex tachycardias. In narrow QRS tachycardia, the site of abnormal impulse formation or the reentry circuit can often be determined from information from the 12-lead

TABLE 30G–4 ACC/AHA Guidelines for Clinical Intracardiac Electrophysiological Studies for Evaluation of Specific Electrocardiographic Abnormalities

Indication	Class I (Appropriate)	Class II (Equivocal)	Class III (Inappropriate)
Evaluation of sinus node function	Symptomatic patients in whom sinus node dysfunction is suspected as the cause of symptoms but a causal relation between an arrhythmia and the symptoms has not been established after appropriate evaluation	Patients with documented sinus node dysfunction in whom evaluation of atrioventricular (AV) or ventriculoatrial (VA) conduction or susceptibility to arrhythmias may aid in selection of the most appropriate pacing modality Patients with electrocardiographically documented sinus bradyarrhythmias to determine whether abnormalities are due to intrinsic disease, autonomic nervous system dysfunction, or the effects of drugs so as to help select therapeutic options Symptomatic patients with known sinus bradyarrhythmias to evaluate potential for other arrhythmias as the cause of symptoms	Symptomatic patients in whom an association between symptoms and a documented bradyarrhythmia has been established and choice of therapy would not be affected by results of an electrophysiological study Asymptomatic patients with sinus bradyarrhythmias or sinus pauses observed only during sleep, including sleep apnea
Acquired AV block	Symptomatic patients in whom His-Purkinje block, suspected as a cause of symptoms, has not been established Patients with second- or third-degree AV block treated with a pacemaker who remain symptomatic and in whom another arrhythmia is suspected as a cause of symptoms	Patients with second- or third-degree AV block in whom knowledge of the site of block or its mechanism or response to pharmacological or other temporary intervention may help direct therapy or assess prognosis Patients with premature, concealed junctional depolarizations suspected as a cause of second- or third-degree AV block pattern (i.e., pseudo AV block)	Symptomatic patients in whom the symptoms and presence of AV block are correlated by ECG findings Asymptomatic patients with transient AV block associated with sinus slowing (e.g., nocturnal type I second-degree AV block)
Chronic intraventricular conduction delay	Symptomatic patients in whom the cause of symptoms is not known	Asymptomatic patients with bundle branch block in whom pharmacological therapy that could increase conduction delay or produce heart block is contemplated	Asymptomatic patients with intraventricular conduction delay Symptomatic patients whose symptoms can be correlated with or excluded by ECG events
Narrow QRS tachycardia (QRS complex <0.12 sec)	Patients with frequent or poorly tolerated episodes of tachycardia that do not adequately respond to drug therapy and for whom information about site of origin, mechanism, and electrophysiological properties of the pathways of the tachycardia is essential for choosing appropriate therapy (drugs, catheter ablation, pacing, or surgery) Patients who prefer ablative therapy to pharmacological treatment	Patients with frequent episodes of tachycardia requiring drug treatment for whom there is concern about proarrhythmia or the effects of the antiarrhythmic drug on the sinus node or AV conduction	Patients with tachycardias easily controlled by vagal maneuvers and/or well-tolerated drug therapy who are not candidates for nonpharmacological therapy
Wide complex tachycardias	Patients with wide QRS complex tachycardia in whom correct diagnosis is unclear after analysis of available ECG tracings and for whom knowledge of the correct diagnosis is necessary for care	None	Patients with VT or supraventricular tachycardia with aberrant conduction or preexcitation syndromes diagnosed with certainty by ECG criteria and for whom invasive electrophysiological data would not influence therapy. However, data obtained at baseline electrophysiological study in these patients might be appropriate as a guide for subsequent therapy

TABLE 30G–4 ACC/AHA Guidelines for Clinical Intracardiac Electrophysiological Studies for Evaluation of Specific Electrocardiographic Abnormalities—cont'd			
Indication	**Class I (Appropriate)**	**Class II (Equivocal)**	**Class III (Inappropriate)**
Prolonged QT interval syndrome	None	Identification of a proarrhythmic effect of a drug in patients experiencing sustained VT or cardiac arrest while receiving the drug Patients who have equivocal abnormalities of QT interval duration or TU wave configuration, with syncope or symptomatic arrhythmias, in whom catecholamine effects may unmask a distinct QT abnormality	Patients with clinically manifest congenital QT prolongation, with or without symptomatic arrhythmias Patients with acquired prolonged QT syndrome with symptoms closely related to an identifiable cause or mechanism
Wolff-Parkinson-White syndrome	Patients being evaluated for catheter ablation or surgical ablation of an accessory pathway Patients with ventricular preexcitation who have survived cardiac arrest or who have unexplained syncope Symptomatic patients in whom determination of the mechanism of arrhythmia or knowledge of the electrophysiological properties of the accessory pathway and normal conduction system would help in determining appropriate therapy	Asymptomatic patients with a family history of sudden cardiac death or with ventricular preexcitation but no spontaneous arrhythmia who engage in high-risk occupations or activities and in whom knowledge of the electrophysiological properties of the accessory pathway or inducible tachycardia may help determine recommendations for further activities or therapy Patients with ventricular preexcitation who are undergoing cardiac surgery for other reasons	Asymptomatic patients with ventricular preexcitation, except those in class II
Ventricular premature complexes, couplets, and nonsustained ventricular tachycardia	None	Patients with other risk factors for future arrhythmic events, such as a low ejection fraction, positive signal-averaged ECG, and nonsustained VT on ambulatory ECG recordings in whom electrophysiological studies will be used for further risk assessment and for guiding therapy in patients with inducible VT Patients with highly symptomatic, uniform morphology premature ventricular complexes, couplets, and nonsustained VT who are considered potential candidates for catheter ablation	Asymptomatic or mildly symptomatic patients with premature ventricular complexes, couplets, and nonsustained VT without other risk factors for sustained arrhythmias

ACC/AHA = American College of Cardiology/American Heart Association; ECG = electrocardiographic.

electrocardiogram. Thus, electrophysiological testing was considered more appropriate as a guide to therapy in this setting than as a tool for diagnosis. Class I indications for electrophysiological testing include patients with recurrent tachycardia for whom data from testing may help clinicians choose among drug therapy, catheter ablation, pacing, or surgery. However, testing was not considered useful for patients whose tachycardias were controlled by vagal maneuvers or medications and who are not candidates for nonpharmacological therapy.

In wide complex tachycardias, identification of the site of origin is frequently impossible from ECG tracings alone. However, electrophysiological testing permits accurate diagnosis in virtually all patients. Because knowledge of the mechanism of the arrhythmia is essential for selection of optimal therapy, electrophysiological testing was considered appropriate (class I) for the diagnosis of wide complex tachycardias in these guidelines. However, when the diagnosis is clear from other data and electrophysiological testing is not likely to influence therapy, the guidelines considered it inappropriate.

Prolonged QT Intervals. The ACC/AHA guidelines did not consider electrophysiological testing for any indications for routine use in patients with prolonged QT intervals. Whether catecholamine infusion during testing is useful for revealing patients who are at high risk for complications or whether electrophysiological testing can be used to evaluate proarrhythmic effects in this population was considered uncertain.

Wolff-Parkinson-White Syndrome. Electrophysiological testing is useful for patients with this syndrome for both diagnosis and planning of therapy. The ACC/AHA guidelines considered electrophysiological testing appropriate for patients who were candidates for catheter or surgical ablation, for those who had had cardiac arrests or unexplained syncope, or for patients whose management might be altered by knowledge of the electrophysiological properties of the accessory pathway and normal conduction system. For asymptomatic patients, however, electrophysiological studies were deemed inappropriate except in special situations, such as patients with high-risk occupations or those with a family history of sudden cardiac death.

More recently recognized entities such as Brugada syndrome, catecholaminergic tachycardia, and right ventricular cardiomyopathy were not considered.

Nonsustained Ventricular Tachycardia. For patients with ventricular premature complexes, couplets, and nonsustained ventricular tachycardia, the usefulness of electrophysiological testing is compromised by the lack of therapeutic strategies that have been shown to improve outcomes. There were no clearly appropriate indications for electrophysiological studies in these patients, and the guidelines discouraged testing in patients without other risk factors for sustained arrhythmias. Research published since these guidelines suggests that exceptions would include patients who fit the Multicenter Automatic Defibrillator Implantation Trial (MADIT) or Multicenter Unsustained Tachycardia Trial (MUSTT) criteria. For certain patients with other data suggesting an adverse prognosis, electrophysiological testing was believed to have possible but unproven appropriateness (class II).

Unexplained Syncope

The ACC/AHA guidelines recommend a low threshold for use of electrophysiological testing for patients with unexplained syncope if they also have structural heart disease (Table 30G–5). However, in patients without structural heart disease, the yield of electrophysiological testing is low. Thus, the ACC/AHA guidelines recommend a higher threshold for use of electrophysiological studies in such patients and suggest that head-up tilt testing may be a more useful test.

Survivors of Cardiac Arrest

The ACC/AHA guidelines considered electrophysiological testing appropriate for patients who were survivors of cardiac arrest other than in the earliest phase of acute myocardial infarction (see Table 30G–5). Since publication of these guidelines, acceptance of the usefulness of ICDs has become more widespread, and many of these patients receive such a device without electrophysiological testing or receive limited electrophysiological testing at device implantation. The guidelines considered electrophysiological studies inappropriate when cardiac arrest had occurred within the first 48 hours of myocardial infarction or when the cardiac arrest resulted from clearly definable specific causes.

Unexplained Palpitations

The procedure of choice to determine the cause of palpitations is ambulatory ECG, according to the ACC/AHA guidelines. The guidelines suggest that electrophysiological testing should be reserved for patients with palpitations that are associated with syncope or those in whom electrocardiograms have failed to capture a cause of the palpitations but who have been noted to have a rapid pulse rate by medical personnel (see Table 30G–5). Electrophysiological testing was considered of equivocal value in patients with symptoms so sporadic that they cannot be documented while ambulatory ECGs are performed.

Electrophysiological Studies for Therapeutic Intervention

The 1995 ACC/AHA guidelines for appropriateness of electrophysiological studies for guidance of drug therapy and implantable electrical devices do not fully reflect the decline in role of oral antiarrhythmic therapy and the rise in use of ICDs for treatment of patients who have had cardiac arrests (Table 30G–6). However, the guideline recommendations for the role of catheter ablation are still largely valid. The characteristics that are common among appropriate indications include supraventricular arrhythmias that are symptomatic; that cannot be controlled with medications because of either limited effectiveness, side effects, or inconvenience; or that have caused sudden cardiac death. Catheter ablation is also useful for some patients with ventricular tachycardia, although patients with extensive structural heart disease tend to have multiple sites of origin of their arrhythmia and may therefore be poor candidates for this procedure. Ablation is sometimes useful as an adjunct to ICD implantation to limit the episodes of ventricular tachycardia requiring ICD treatment.

TABLE 30G–5 ACC/AHA Guidelines for Clinical Intracardiac Electrophysiological Studies for Evaluation of Clinical Syndromes

Indication	Class I (Appropriate)	Class II (Equivocal)	Class III (Inappropriate)
Unexplained syncope	Patients with suspected structural heart disease and syncope that remain unexplained after appropriate evaluation	Patients with recurrent unexplained syncope without structural heart disease and a negative head-up tilt test	Patients with a known cause of syncope for whom treatment will not be guided by electrophysiological testing
Survivors of cardiac arrest	Patients surviving cardiac arrest without evidence of an acute Q wave MI Patients surviving cardiac arrest occurring more than 48 hr after the acute phase of MI in the absence of a recurrent ischemic event	Patients surviving cardiac arrest caused by bradyarrhythmia Patients surviving cardiac arrest thought to be associated with a congenital repolarization abnormality (long QT syndrome) in whom the results of noninvasive diagnostic testing are equivocal	Patients surviving a cardiac arrest that occurred during the acute phase (<48 hr) of MI Patients with cardiac arrest resulting from clearly definable specific causes such as reversible ischemia, severe valvular aortic stenosis, or noninvasively defined congenital or acquired long QT syndrome
Unexplained palpitations	Patients with palpitations who have a pulse rate documented by medical personnel as inappropriately rapid and in whom ECG recordings fail to document the cause of the palpitations Patients with palpitations preceding a syncopal episode	Patients with clinically significant palpitations, suspected to be of cardiac origin, in whom symptoms are sporadic and cannot be documented. Studies are performed to determine the mechanisms of arrhythmias, direct or provide therapy, or assess prognosis	Patients with palpitations documented to be due to extracardiac causes (e.g., hyperthyroidism)

ACC/AHA = American College of Cardiology/American Heart Association; ECG = electrocardiographic; MI = myocardial infarction.

TABLE 30G–6 ACC/AHA Guidelines for Clinical Intracardiac Electrophysiological Studies for Therapeutic Intervention

Indication	Class I (Appropriate)	Class II (Equivocal)	Class III (Inappropriate)
Guidance of drug therapy	Patients with sustained VT or cardiac arrest, especially those with prior MI Patients with AVNRT, AV reentrant tachycardia using an accessory pathway, or atrial fibrillation associated with an accessory pathway, for whom chronic drug therapy is planned	Patients with sinus node reentrant tachycardia, atrial tachycardia, atrial fibrillation, or atrial flutter without ventricular preexcitation syndrome, for whom chronic drug therapy is planned Patients with arrhythmias not inducible during control electrophysiological study for whom drug therapy is planned	Patients with isolated atrial or ventricular premature complexes Patients with ventricular fibrillation with a clearly identified reversible cause
Patients who are candidates for or who have implantable electrical devices	Patients with tachyarrhythmias, before and during implantation, and final (predischarge) programming of an electrical device to confirm its ability to perform as anticipated Patients with an implanted electrical antitachyarrhythmia device in whom changes in status or therapy may have influenced the continued safety and efficacy of the device Patients who have a pacemaker to treat a bradyarrhythmia and receive a cardioverter-defibrillator, to test for device interactions	Patients with previously documented indications for pacemaker implantation to test for the most appropriate long-term pacing mode and sites to optimize symptomatic improvement and hemodynamics	Patients who are not candidates for device therapy
Indications for catheter ablation procedures	Patients with symptomatic atrial tachyarrhythmias who have inadequately controlled ventricular rates unless primary ablation of the atrial tachyarrhythmia is possible Patients with symptomatic atrial tachyarrhythmias such as those above but when drugs are not tolerated or the patient does not wish to take them, even though the ventricular rate can be controlled Patients with symptomatic nonparoxysmal junctional tachycardia that is drug resistant or the patient is drug intolerant or does not wish to take it Patients resuscitated from sudden cardiac death caused by atrial flutter or atrial fibrillation with a rapid ventricular response in the absence of an accessory pathway	Patients with a dual-chamber pacemaker and pacemaker-mediated tachycardia that cannot be treated effectively by drugs or by reprogramming the pacemaker	Patients with atrial tachyarrhythmias responsive to drug therapy acceptable to the patient
Radiofrequency catheter ablation for AVNRT	Patients with symptomatic sustained AVNRT that is drug resistant or the patient is drug intolerant or does not desire long-term drug therapy	Patients with sustained AVNRT identified during electrophysiological study or catheter ablation of another arrhythmia The finding of dual AV nodal pathway physiology and atrial echoes but without AVNRT during electrophysiological study in patients suspected of having AVNRT clinically	Patients with AVNRT responsive to drug therapy that is well tolerated and preferred by the patient to ablation The finding of dual AV nodal pathway physiology (with or without echo complexes) during electrophysiological study in patients in whom AVNRT is not suspected clinically

Continued

TABLE 30G–6 ACC/AHA Guidelines for Clinical Intracardiac Electrophysiological Studies for Therapeutic Intervention—cont'd

Indication	Class I (Appropriate)	Class II (Equivocal)	Class III (Inappropriate)
Ablation of atrial tachycardia, flutter, and fibrillation: atrium/atrial sites	Patients with atrial tachycardia that is drug resistant or the patient is drug intolerant or does not desire long-term drug therapy Patients with atrial flutter that is drug resistant or the patient is drug intolerant or does not desire long-term drug therapy	Atrial flutter or atrial tachycardia associated with paroxysmal atrial fibrillation when the tachycardia is drug resistant or the patient is drug intolerant or does not desire long-term drug therapy Patients with atrial fibrillation and evidence of a localized site(s) of origin when the tachycardia is drug resistant or the patient is drug intolerant or does not desire long-term drug therapy	Patients with atrial arrhythmia that is responsive to drug therapy, well tolerated, and preferred by the patient to ablation Patients with multiform atrial tachycardia
Ablation of atrial tachycardia, flutter, and fibrillation: accessory pathways	Patients with symptomatic AV reentrant tachycardia that is drug resistant or the patient is drug intolerant or does not desire long-term drug therapy Patients with atrial fibrillation (or other atrial tachyarrhythmia) and a rapid ventricular response through the accessory pathway when the tachycardia is drug resistant or the patient is drug intolerant or does not desire long-term drug therapy	Patients with AV reentrant tachycardia or atrial fibrillation with rapid ventricular rates identified during electrophysiological study of another arrhythmia Asymptomatic patients with ventricular preexcitation whose livelihood or profession, important activities, insurability, or mental well-being or the public safety would be affected by spontaneous tachyarrhythmias or the presence of the ECG abnormality Patients with atrial fibrillation and a controlled ventricular response through the accessory pathway Patients with a family history of sudden cardiac death	Patients who have accessory pathway–related arrhythmias that are responsive to drug therapy, well tolerated, and preferred by the patient to ablation
Ablation of VT	Patients with symptomatic sustained monomorphic VT when the tachycardia is drug resistant or the patient is drug intolerant or does not desire long-term drug therapy Patients with bundle branch reentrant ventricular tachycardia Patients with sustained monomorphic VT and an ICD who are receiving multiple shocks not manageable by reprogramming or concomitant drug therapy	Nonsustained VT that is symptomatic when the tachycardia is drug resistant or the patient is drug intolerant or does not desire long-term drug therapy	Patients with VT that is responsive to drug, ICD, or surgical therapy and that therapy is well tolerated and preferred by the patient to ablation Unstable, rapid, multiple, or polymorphic VT that cannot be adequately localized by current mapping techniques Asymptomatic and clinically benign nonsustained VT

ACC/AHA = American College of Cardiology/American Heart Association; AV = atrioventricular; AVNRT = AV nodal reentrant tachycardia; ECG = electrocardiographic; ICD = implantable cardioverter-defibrillator; MI = myocardial infarction; VT = ventricular tachycardia.

Clinical Competence

The ACC/AHA statement on clinical competence from 2000[6] recommends that physicians specializing in electrophysiology undergo a minimum of 1 year of specialized training in electrophysiological studies, during which the physician should be the primary operator and analyze 100 to 150 initial diagnostic studies. At least 50 of these studies should involve patients with supraventricular arrhythmias. Because antiarrhythmic devices constitute a major part of current electrophysiology practice, the guidelines suggest that trainees should be the primary operators during at least 25 electrophysiological evaluations of implantable antiarrhythmic devices. For maintenance of competence, a minimum of 100 diagnostic electrophysiological studies per year is recommended. The statement also recommends that specialists in electrophysiology attend at least 30 hours of formal continuing medical education every 2 years to remain abreast of changes in knowledge and technology.

For physicians who perform catheter ablation, the NASPE Ad Hoc Committee on Catheter Ablation recommended that training should include at least 30 ablations, of which at least 15 are accessory pathway ablations.[12] The ACC/AHA statement recommended that physicians who perform ablations maintain a volume of at least 20 to 50 ablations per year.

Personal and Public Safety Issues

The AHA and the NASPE published a medical-scientific statement in 1996 that addressed many of the common issues regarding personal and public safety that arise in the care of patients with arrhythmias.[7] This publication summarized guidelines from other organizations, such as the U.S. Federal Aviation Administration, and the limited data available to estimate the risk of injury to the patient and others related to arrhythmias and provided recommendations about acceptable activities for patients with arrhythmias that may impair consciousness.

The AHA/NASPE guidelines divide patients into three classes. Class A patients should have no restrictions. Class B patients are restricted for a defined time without arrhythmia recurrence, usually after a therapeutic intervention (Table 30G–7). This time period is usually expressed as a subscript indicating the number of months of restriction (e.g., B_3). Patients in class C should have total restriction of potentially hazardous activities. Restrictions were divided into two categories: personal or noncommercial driving and commercial driving or flying. Except where stated otherwise, recommendations for flying were the same as those for commercial drivers. The guidelines noted that recommendations for restriction for commercial drivers might also be relevant to people in other potentially hazardous occupations, such as operators of heavy equipment.

The restrictions imposed by the guidelines vary depending on the severity of the arrhythmia and accompanying symptoms (see Table 30G–7). The duration of the restriction is shorter for patients who did not have impairment of symptoms with their arrhythmias but increases for patients who did have such symptoms and who had ventricular fibrillation or sustained ventricular tachycardia. Patients who had either of these arrhythmias should be totally restricted from commercial driving or flying according to these guidelines.

TABLE 30G–7 AHA/NASPE Guidelines for Safe Resumption of Activities (Classes of Restriction)

Arrhythmia	Private	Commercial
Nonsustained ventricular tachycardia	B_3 if symptoms of impaired consciousness with arrhythmia before treatment A if no impairment of consciousness with arrhythmia	B_6 if symptoms of impaired consciousness with arrhythmia before treatment A if no impairment of consciousness with arrhythmia
Sustained ventricular tachycardia	B_6 B_3 if idiopathic ventricular tachycardia (normal coronary arteries, normal ventricular function) and no impairment of consciousness	C B_6 if idiopathic ventricular tachycardia (normal coronary arteries, normal ventricular function) and no impairment of consciousness
Ventricular fibrillation	B_6	C
Asymptomatic or minimally symptomatic SVT (including WPW syndrome)	A	A
Symptomatic (evidence of hemodynamic compromise) SVT	B until after initiation of therapy that eliminates symptoms	B until after initiation of therapy that eliminates symptoms
Atrial fibrillation treated by catheter ablation of AV node	B	B
SVT with uncontrolled symptoms	C	C
Bradycardia without a pacemaker—no symptoms	A	A
Bradycardia without a pacemaker—syncope or near syncope	C	C
Bradycardia with a pacemaker—not pacemaker dependent*	A	A
Bradycardia with a pacemaker—pacemaker dependent*	B—1 wk	B—4 wk
Vasovagal syncope—mild	A	B_1
Vasovagal syncope—severe		
Treated vasovagal syncope	B_3	B_6
Untreated vasovagal syncope	C	C
Carotid sinus syncope—mild	A	A
Carotid sinus syncope—severe, treated with control	B_1	B_1
Carotid sinus syncope—severe, treated with uncertain control	B_3	B_6
Untreated	C	C

AHA/NASPE = American Heart Association/North American Society of Pacing and Electrophysiology; AV = atrioventricular; SVT = supraventricular tachycardia; WPW = Wolff-Parkinson-White.

Class A = no restriction; class B = restricted for months (in subscript); class C = total restriction.

*Patients who are pacemaker dependent are defined as those who have lost consciousness in the past because of bradyarrhythmias. This group may also include patients immediately after atrioventricular junction ablation or any other patient in whom sudden pacemaker failure would be likely to result in alteration of consciousness.

From Epstein AE, Miles WM, Benditt DG, et al: Personal and public safety issues related to arrhythmias that may affect consciousness: Implications for regulation and physician recommendations. Circulation 94:1147, 1996.

These recommendations were for patients who were treated with either antiarrhythmic drugs or ICDs. The guidelines recommended that noncommercial drivers should be prohibited from all driving for the first 6 months after ICD implantation; after this period, driving can be resumed if ICD discharge has not occurred. The guidelines recommend that all commercial driving be prohibited permanently after ICD implantation.

Special mention was made of patients with long QT syndromes. When the QT prolongation is acquired and due either wholly or in part to reversible factors such as electrolyte abnormalities, most patients can be allowed to drive after correction of these factors. Patients who have symptomatic long QT syndromes should not have driving privileges; those who are asymptomatic with or without treatment can receive driving privileges after a 6-month symptom-free interval.

For patients with supraventricular tachycardias, the guidelines did not impose harsher restrictions on commercial than on private drivers. No restrictions were recommended for patients with minimal or no symptoms with supraventricular tachycardia (see Table 30G–7). For patients who had symptoms suggestive of hemodynamic compromise (e.g., syncope, presyncope, chest pain, or dyspnea), the guidelines recommended restrictions until after initiation of therapy that eliminates symptoms. Patients with supraventricular tachycardia that appears to be successfully ablated can drive after recovery from the procedure. Patients treated with drug therapy should as a minimum have a 1-month symptom-free period before resuming driving, depending on the pretherapy frequency of tachycardia. If symptoms cannot be controlled, permanent full restrictions were recommended.

No restrictions were recommended for patients with bradyarrhythmias who were asymptomatic or who had a pacemaker but were not pacemaker dependent, i.e., patients who lost consciousness in the past because of bradyarrhythmias. "Pacemaker dependent" also included patients immediately after AV junction ablation or any other patient in whom sudden pacemaker failure would be likely to result in alteration of consciousness. Patients who were pacemaker dependent and had received a pacemaker should be restricted for 1 to 4 weeks, depending on whether they were private or commercial drivers. Patients who had had syncope or presyncope related to bradyarrhythmias who had not received a pacemaker should have full permanent restrictions.

No or only mild restrictions were recommended for patients with mild vasovagal syncope or carotid sinus syncope. The guidelines as written (see Table 30G–7) allow the clinician considerable leeway in determining the duration of restriction.

References

1. Knoebel SB, Crawford MH, Dunn MI, et al: Guidelines for ambulatory electrocardiography. A report of the American College of Cardiology/American Heart Association Task Force on Assessment of Diagnostic and Therapeutic Cardiovascular Procedures (Subcommittee on Ambulatory Electrocardiography). J Am Coll Cardiol 12:249, 1989.
2. Crawford MH, Bernstein SJ, Deedwania PC, et al: ACC/AHA guidelines for ambulatory electrocardiography. A report of the American College of Cardiology/American Heart Association Task Force on Practice Guidelines (Committee to Revise the Guidelines for Ambulatory Electrocardiography). J Am Coll Cardiol 34:866, 1999.
3. Kadish AH, Buxton AE, Kennedy HL, et al: ACC/AHA clinical competence statement on electrocardiography and ambulatory electrocardiography. A report of the ACC/AHA/ACP-ASIM Task Force on Clinical Competence (ACC/AHA Committee to Develop a Clinical Competence Statement on Electrocardiography and Ambulatory Electrocardiography). Circulation 104:3169, 2001.
4. Zipes DP, Akhtar M, Denes P, et al: Guidelines for clinical intracardiac electrophysiology studies. A report of the American College of Cardiology/American Heart Association Task Force on Assessment of Diagnostic and Therapeutic Cardiovascular Procedures (Subcommittee to Assess Clinical Intracardiac Electrophysiologic Studies). J Am Coll Cardiol 14:1827, 1989.
5. Zipes DP, DiMarco JP, Gillette PC, et al: Guidelines for clinical intracardiac electrophysiology studies and catheter ablation procedures. A report of the American College of Cardiology/American Heart Association Task Force on Practice Guidelines (Subcommittee on Clinical Intracardiac Electrophysiologic and Catheter Ablation Procedures). J Am Coll Cardiol 26:555, 1995.
6. Tracy CM, Akhtar M, DiMarco JP, et al: American College of Cardiology/American Heart Association Clinical Competence Statement on invasive electrophysiology studies, catheter ablation, and cardioversion. A report of the American College of Cardiology/American Heart Association/American College of Physicians-American Society of Internal Medicine Task Force on Clinical Competence. Circulation 102:2309, 2000.
7. Epstein AE, Miles WM, Benditt DG, et al: Personal and public safety issues related to arrhythmias that may affect consciousness: Implications for regulation and physician recommendations. Circulation 94:1147, 1996.
8. Gregoratos G, Abrams J, Epstein AE, et al: ACC/AHA/NASPE 2002 Guideline Update for Implantation of Cardiac Pacemakers and Antiarrhythmia Devices—summary article: A report of the American College of Cardiology/American Heart Association Task Force on Practice Guidelines (ACC/AHA/NASPE Committee to Update the 1998 Pacemaker Guidelines). J Am Coll Cardiol 40:1703, 2002.
9. Moss AJ, Zareba W, Hall WJ, et al: Prophylactic implantation of a defibrillator in patients with myocardial infarction and reduced ejection fraction. N Engl J Med 346:877, 2002.
10. Bansch D, Antz M, Boczor S, et al: Primary prevention of sudden death in idiopathic dilated cardiomyopathy: The Cardiomyopathy Trial (CAT). Circulation 105:1453, 2002.
11. Ezekowitz JA, Armstrong PW, McAlister FA: Implantable cardioverter defibrillators in primary and secondary prevention: A systematic review of randomized, controlled trials. Ann Intern Med 138:445, 2003.
12. Scheinman MM: Catheter ablation for cardiac arrhythmias, personnel, and facilities. North American Society of Pacing and Electrophysiology Ad Hoc Committee on Catheter Ablation. Pacing Clin Electrophysiol 15:715, 1992.

CHAPTER 31

Cardiac Pacemakers and Cardioverter-Defibrillators

David L. Hayes • Douglas P. Zipes

Implantable devices for the management of cardiac arrhythmias have evolved rapidly since the inception of cardiac pacing in the late 1950s. The collective intelligence of creative biomedical engineers and clinicians, coupled with the advent and increasing sophistication of the microprocessor, has made this possible. What began with asynchronous ventricular pacing as a therapy for patients with Stokes-Adams attacks has made momentous strides every decade. Device therapy is now rapidly expanding with implantable devices for hemodynamic monitoring and heart failure therapy. The rapid technological advancements in cardiac pacemakers have, at least to some degree, served as a catalyst for an even faster evolution in implantable cardioverter-defibrillators (ICDs) and cardiac resynchronization therapy (CRT) devices. The evolution of ICD and CRT technology has been staggering. As the technology for both pacemakers—ICDs and CRT—has evolved, clinical trials have been crucial to prove efficacy. Clinical trials are an integral part of the discipline of implantable device therapy and will remain so as we see further innovative improvements in the years to come.

Pacemaker Nomenclature

Pacemaker nomenclature was established in 1974, and it is necessary to know the nomenclature to understand the discipline of cardiac pacing (Table 31–1).[1] The code was updated in 2002 to include a "generic code" for the expanding field of multisite pacing therapy. The following is a brief description of the elements of the code that are shown in Table 31–1:

- The first position (I) refers to the chamber or chambers in which stimulation occurs: A = atrium; V = ventricle; and D = dual chamber, or both A and V.
- The second position (II) refers to the chamber or chambers in which sensing occurs. The letters are the same as those for the first position. (Manufacturers also use "S" in both the first and the second position to indicate that the device is capable of pacing only a single cardiac chamber.)
- The third position (III) refers to the mode of sensing, or how the pacemaker responds to a sensed event. An "I" indicates that a sensed event inhibits the output pulse and causes the pacemaker to recycle for one or more timing cycles. "T" means that an output pulse is triggered in response to a sensed event. "D" means that both "T" and "I" responses can occur. This designation is restricted to dual-chamber systems. An event sensed in the atrium inhibits the atrial output but triggers a ventricular output. Unlike a single-chamber triggered mode (VVT or AAT), in which an output pulse is triggered immediately on sensing, a dual-chamber mode has a delay between the sensed atrial event and the triggered ventricular output to mimic the normal PR interval. If a native ventricular signal or R wave is sensed, the ventricular output and possibly even the atrial output are inhibited, depending on where sensing occurs.
- The fourth position (IV) of the code indicates both programmability and rate modulation. An "R" in the fourth position indicates that the pacemaker incorporates a sensor to modulate the rate independently of intrinsic cardiac activity, such as with motion or respiration. From a practical standpoint, "R" is the only indicator commonly used in the fourth position.
- The fifth position (V) of the code is now used to indicate whether multisite pacing is present in (0) none of the cardiac chambers, (A) one or both atria, (V) one or both ventricles, or (D) any combination of atria and ventricles. To describe a patient with a DDDR (dual-chamber rate-adaptive) pacemaker with biventricular stimulation, the code would be DDDRV.

Indications for Cardiac Pacing

A joint committee of the American College of Cardiology (ACC), the American Heart

TABLE 31–1 Revised NASPE/BPEG Generic Code for Antibradycardia Pacing

Position	I	II	III	IV	V
Category	**Chamber(s) paced** O = None A = Atrium V = Ventricle D = Dual (A + V)	**Chamber(s) sensed** O = None A = Atrium V = Ventricle D = Dual (A + V)	**Response to sensing** O = None T = Triggered I = Inhibited D = Dual (T + I)	**Rate modulation** O = None R = Rate modulation	**Multisite pacing** O = None A = Atrium V = Ventricle D = Dual (A + V)
Manufacturers' designation only	S = Single (A or V)	S = Single (A or V)			

See text for explanation of use of the code.
BPEG = British Pacing and Electrophysiology Group; NASPE = North American Society of Pacing and Electrophysiology.
From Bernstein AD, Daubert JC, Fletcher RD, et al, and North American Society of Pacing and Electrophysiology/British Pacing and Electrophysiology Group: The revised NASPE/BPEG generic code for antibradycardia, adaptive-rate, and multisite pacing. Pacing Clin Electrophysiol 25:260-264, 2002.

Association (AHA), and the North American Society of Pacing and Electrophysiology (NASPE) has established indications for pacing into categories of "generally indicated," "may be indicated," and "not indicated."[2] Although some indications for permanent pacing are relatively certain or unambiguous, others require considerable expertise and judgment. The clinician prescribing permanent pacing systems should be aware of the published indications and controversies regarding indications.

The clinical need for pacing and appropriate objective data, such as electrocardiographic (ECG) tracings, must be documented clearly in the patient's medical record to ensure reimbursement by Medicare or third-party payers.

Indications are considered in categories of acquired atrioventricular (AV) block, congenital AV block, chronic bifascicular and trifascicular block, sinus node dysfunction, and neurocardiogenic syndromes. Currently, sinus node dysfunction is the most frequent indication for pacing, followed by AV node dysfunction. Pacing for tachyarrhythmias and miscellaneous indications comprises a relatively small percentage. Potential hemodynamic indications for permanent pacing are discussed separately.

Acquired AV Block

AV block is classified traditionally into first-, second-, and third-degree (or complete) heart block (see Chap. 32). Alternatively, it can be defined anatomically as supra-Hisian, intra-Hisian, or infra-Hisian. If the QRS complex is prolonged more than 0.12 second, there is a greater probability that the conduction disturbance is infra-Hisian. Acquired AV block is most commonly idiopathic and related to aging, but it has many potential causes. Indications for permanent pacing in acquired AV block are listed in Table 31–2.

Indications for permanent pacing for AV block that occurs with an acute myocardial infarction (see Chaps. 46 and 47) are more controversial. A pacemaker is generally considered indicated if complete AV block, Mobitz type II block, or bilateral or alternating bundle branch block persists for more than 72 hours after the acute event. Some clinicians consider new and persistent bifascicular block an indication for pacing, and others consider pacing for a new left anterior or left posterior hemiblock alone.

Congenital Complete Heart Block

Although some controversy remains about when to pace patients with congenital complete heart block, there is now a tendency to pace in all these patients and to do so earlier, even if they are asymptomatic. There is a high incidence of unpredictable syncope with significant mortality from initial attacks, a gradual decrease in heart rate, and a high incidence of acquired mitral regurgition.[3] In pediatric patients with congenital complete heart block, pacemaker implantation is recommended for congestive heart failure, average heart rate of less than 50 beats/min in the awake infant, history of

TABLE 31–2 Indications for Permanent Pacing in Atrioventricular Block

Type of AV Block	Pacemaker Necessary	Pacemaker Probably Necessary	Pacemaker not Necessary
Third	Symptomatic congenital CHB Acquired symptomatic AV block Atrial fibrillation with CHB Acquired asymptomatic CHB Neuromuscular diseases with AV block, with or without symptoms	—	AV block of any degree that is expected to resolve and unlikely to recur, e.g., drug toxicity, Lyme disease, sleep apnea, without treatment
Second	Symptomatic second-degree AV block regardless of type Asymptomatic advanced second-degree AV block with asystole ≥ 3.0 sec or escape rate < 40 beats/min in awake patients	Asymptomatic, type I, at intra-His or infra-His level* Hemodynamically symptomatic due to loss of AV synchrony Neuromuscular diseases with AV block, with or without symptoms	Asymptomatic, type I, at supra-His (AV node) level
First		Hemodynamically symptomatic due to loss of AV synchrony with markedly prolonged PR interval, e.g., > 300 msec	Asymptomatic

AV = atrioventricular; CHB = complete heart block.
*Shaw DB, Gowers JI, Kekwick CA, et al: Is Mobitz type I atrioventricular block benign in adults? Heart 90:169, 2004.

syncope or presyncope, significant ventricular ectopy, or exercise intolerance.

Chronic Bifascicular and Trifascicular Block

If bifascicular or trifascicular block is associated with transient complete heart block, whether symptomatic or not, pacing is indicated. Pacing in the patient with bifascicular or trifascicular block and syncope that cannot be attributed to any other cause is a class II ACC/AHA indication. If only fascicular block is noted in the asymptomatic patient, pacing is not indicated.

Sinus Node Dysfunction

Tachycardia-bradycardia syndrome, sick sinus syndrome, symptomatic sinus bradycardia, sinus arrest and sinus pauses, and chronotropic incompetence all are variants of sinus node dysfunction, and often the terms are used synonymously. The degree of bradycardia at which to consider pacing is controversial but is generally accepted to be rates of less than 40 beats/min during waking hours. There is disagreement about the absolute cycle length at which pacing should be considered. Although every patient needs to be considered individually, sinus pauses exceeding 3 seconds during waking hours are often considered abnormal and may warrant pacing if the patient has symptoms consistent with bradycardia. Pauses that occur during sleep are more difficult to categorize. Because of vagal influences, many normal persons display pauses significantly longer than 3 seconds during sleep. Permanent pacing should be considered for any patient who has symptomatic bradyarrhythmias if the cause of the bradyarrhythmia is not reversible or they require a drug, for example, a beta blocker, that produces symptomatic bradycardia. Examples of reversible conditions would include transient AV block secondary to an infectious disease that will respond to appropriate treatment, such as Lyme disease, untreated sleep disorder with secondary conduction abnormalities, and other hypervagal states.

Permanent pacing for patients with sinus node dysfunction after myocardial infarction is reserved for those who have symptoms during bradycardia. If drug therapy results in symptomatic bradycardia, criteria for permanent pacing should follow the guidelines given for sinus node dysfunction in Table 31–3.

Neurocardiogenic Syncope

Permanent pacing may be indicated for some of the several types of neurally mediated syncope.[4] Neurally mediated syncope includes carotid sinus hypersensitivity and vasovagal syncope (see Chap. 34).

The carotid sinus reflex is the physiological response to pressure applied to the carotid sinus. Although this reflex is physiological, some persons have an exaggerated or even pathological response. This reflex has two components: cardioinhibitory and vasodepressor. A cardioinhibitory response results predominantly from increased parasympathetic tone and may be manifested by sinus bradycardia, PR prolongation, or advanced AV block. The vasodepressor response is predominantly due to sympathetic withdrawal and secondary hypotension. Although a pure cardioinhibitory or pure vasodepressor response can occur, a mixed response is most common. Tilt-table testing can provide the physiological environment to reproduce vasovagal syncope. It is important to document whether the predominant cause of symptoms is cardioinhibitory or vasodepressor because therapy differs. Tilt-table testing is often helpful in determining the predominant cause.

Drugs such as beta blockers are commonly used as first-line therapy despite an absence of convincing efficacy data. Although significant controversy persists, vasovagal syncope can be aborted or blunted by dual-chamber pacing, and even if syncope does occur, pacing can prolong consciousness to avoid injury. In the North American Vasovagal Pacemaker Study I (VPS-I),[5] 46 patients with recurrent syncope and a positive tilt test were randomized to dual-chamber pacemaker with a special feature known as "rate drop" or to no pacemaker therapy. (The rate-drop algorithm allows the pacemaker to pace at a faster rate if bradycardia suddenly occurs.) Stopped prematurely because of the benefit observed with pacemaker therapy, the study revealed that only 17 percent of paced patients had recurrent syncope compared with 59 percent of patients without pacing.

The Vasovagal Syncope International Study (VASIS)[6] demonstrated a reduction in syncopal episodes, similar to VPS-I. This group of patients had experienced multiple episodes of vasovagal syncope as part of the inclusion criteria.

In the North American Vasovagal Pacemaker Study II (VPS-II),[7] all patients received a pacemaker implant and were then programmed to no pacing (ODO mode) or DDD with rate-drop response. In contrast to the initial trial,[5] there was no statistically significant improvement in the group of patients programmed to active pacing with rate-drop response.

Syncope and Falls in the Elderly Pacing and Carotid Sinus Evaluation 2 (SAFE PACE-2)[8] study is under way to assess pacing therapy in carotid sinus hypersensitivity (Table 31–4). In the precursor to this study, SAFE PACE-1,[11] there was a strong association between nonaccidental falls and cardioinhibitory carotid sinus hypersensitivity, and these patients should be referred for cardiovascular assessment.

Selection of the Appropriate Pacing Mode

When an indication for pacing has been identified, consideration should be given to selecting the most appropriate

TABLE 31–3 Indications for Permanent Pacing in Sinus Node Dysfunction (SND)

Pacemaker Necessary	Pacemaker Probably Necessary	Pacemaker not Necessary
Symptomatic sinus bradycardia	Symptomatic patients with SND who have documented rates of < 40 beats/min without a clear-cut association between significant symptoms and bradycardia	Asymptomatic SND
Symptomatic sinus bradycardia due to long-term drug therapy of a type and at a dose for which there is no accepted alternative	Syncope of unexplained origin when major abnormalities of sinus node function are discovered or provoked in electrophysiologic studies	

TABLE 31–4 Trials of Pacing Therapy in Neurocardiogenic Syncope

Study	Patient Inclusion Criteria	Endpoint(s)	Treatment Arms	Key Results
VPS-I[5]	≥Six lifetime episodes of syncope *and* Positive HUT test with syncope or presyncope Relative bradycardia	Time to recurrent syncope	Standard drug therapy *vs.* Pacemaker	85% risk reduction for recurrent syncope with pacing
VPS-II[7]	History strongly suggests vasovagal syncope ≥Six lifetime episodes of syncope *or* ≥Three in past 2 yr *or* One episode in past 6 mo *and* Positive HUT test with syncope or presyncope	Time to recurrent syncope Efficacy of RDR	Randomized to DDD or no pacing for 6 mo or until first episode of syncope Rerandomized to DDD pacing with or without RDR	No significant difference between pacing and no pacing
VASIS[6]	≥Three syncopal episodes in prior 2 yr Duration of symptoms > 6 mo	Recurrence of syncope Recurrence of presyncope Need for secondary pacemaker implant or drug therapy	Dual-chamber pacing with hysteresis *vs.* No pacing (no specific therapy)	5% incidence of syncope in paced group vs. 61% without pacing
SAFE PACE-2[8]	Age ≥ 50 yr ≥Two unexplained falls ± one syncopal episode in prior 12 mo >3-sec asystole on CSM No other cause of falls	Recurrent falls Time to first fall Frequency of dizziness or presyncope Health care utilization Quality of life	Pacemaker *vs.* Conventional therapy	In progress
SYDIT[9]	No cardiac disease Age > 35 yr ≥Three syncopal spells in preceding 2 yr Positive HUT test with HR ↓ ≥ 30% and bradycardia ≤ 50 beats/min	Recurrence of syncope	Atenolol vs. DDD pacing with RDR	Significant effect in favor of permanent pacing with recurrent syncope in 4.3% of patients with pacemaker and 25.5% of patients on atenolol
SYNPACE[10]	Symptomatic vasovagal syncope	Recurrence of syncope	Dual-chamber pacemaker with RDR on *vs.* Pacemaker implanted but programmed off	Active pacing not superior in preventing syncopal recurrence

CSM = carotid sinus massage; HR = heart rate; HUT = head-up tilt; RDR = rate drop response; SAFE PACE = Syncope and Falls in the Elderly Pacing and Carotid Sinus Evaluation; SYDIT = Syncope Diagnosis and Treatment Study; SYNPACE = Vasovagal Syncope and Pacing; VASIS = Vasovagal Syncope International Study; VPS = North American Vasovagal Pacemaker Study.

pacing mode for the patient. Factors to consider when choosing the pacing mode include the following:

- Underlying rhythm disturbance
- Overall physical condition
- Associated medical problems
- Exercise capacity
- Chronotropic response to exercise
- Effect of pacing mode on long-term morbidity and mortality

The effect of pacing mode on morbidity and mortality has been the basis of multiple randomized clinical trials.

Many investigators performed retrospective reviews to assess the effect of pacing mode on mortality. Despite the inherent weaknesses of retrospective analyses, it is difficult to dismiss the similar finding among all the studies of a significantly lower mortality with DDD or atrial inhibited (AAI) pacing than with ventricular inhibited (VVI) pacing and significantly lower incidences of atrial fibrillation.

Several prospective trials have been completed (Table 31-5). Andersen and colleagues[12] performed one of the first prospective studies on pacing mode and survival. In patients with sinus node dysfunction randomized to AAI or VVI pacing, the authors demonstrated a higher incidence of atrial fibrillation in the VVI group (14 percent of the AAI group vs. 23 percent of the VVI group; $p = 0.12$) and a higher incidence of thromboembolism in the VVI group than in the AAI group ($p = 0.0083$). Although no difference in mortality could be detected at the initial analysis at 3.3 years, subsequent analysis at 5.5 years showed improved survival and less heart failure in the AAI group.[12] In addition, there was a persistent reduction in the incidences of atrial fibrillation and thromboembolic events.

The Pacemaker Selection in the Elderly (PASE) trial, a prospective, randomized, single-blind trial, compared DDDR and VVIR pacing modes.[13] There was no statistically significant difference in quality of life between DDDR and VVIR pacing modes, but there was a trend toward improved quality of life in patients with sinus node dysfunction randomized to dual-chamber pacing. Perhaps more significant was a crossover of 26 percent of patients from ventricular pacing to dual-chamber pacing because of pacemaker syndrome.

TABLE 31–5 Trials Assessing the Effect of Pacing Mode on Morbidity and Mortality

Study	Patient Inclusion Criteria	Endpoint(s)	Treatment Arms	Key Results
Danish study[12]	Sick sinus syndrome requiring pacing	Mortality Cardiovascular death AF TE events Heart failure AV block	AAI pacing ($n = 110$) *vs.* VVI pacing ($n = 115$)	Cumulative incidence of CV death, PAF, chronic AF, and TE events lower with AAI pacing Less severe heart failure with AAI Multivariate analysis: AAI associated with freedom from TE events, survival from CV death
PASE[13]	Age ≥ 65 yr Need for PPM for prevention or treatment of bradycardia	QOL All-cause mortality First nonfatal CVA or death First hospitalization for CHF AF PM syndrome	Single-blind, randomized, controlled comparison; VVIR pacing *vs.* DDDR pacing	QOL improved significantly, but no difference between pacing modes 26% of patients with VVIR crossover to DDDR due to PM syndrome Trends of borderline statistical significance in endpoints favoring DDDR in patients with SND
CTOPP[14]	Initial PM Life expectancy > 1 yr Not in chronic AF	Cardiovascular mortality or stroke Paroxysmal or chronic AF Hospitalization for CHF QOL 6-min walk	DDDR or AAIR pacing *vs.* VVIR pacing	No difference in QOL, VVI vs. DDD/AAI No statistically significant difference in mortality or stroke No difference in hospitalizations 24% ↓ incidence of chronic or paroxysmal AF with DDD/AAI
MOST[15]	SND requiring PM NSR or atrial standstill at time of implantation	Stroke Health status Cost-effectiveness Total mortality CV mortality AF Heart failure score PM syndrome	DDDR *vs.* VVIR	Lower incidence of AF with DDDR No difference in any other endpoint
UKPACE[16]	AV block requiring PM Age > 70 yr	All-cause mortality Composite endpoint of CV deaths HF hospitalization AF CVA or events Reoperation	DDDR *vs.* VVI or VVIR	No difference in any endpoint
DANPACE[17]	Tachycardia-bradycardia syndrome with normal AV conduction	All-cause mortality CV mortality Incidence of AF and TE events QOL Cost-effectiveness	AAIR *vs.* DDDR	In progress

AF = atrial fibrillation; AV = atrioventricular; CHF = congestive heart failure; CTOPP = Canadian Trial of Physiologic Pacing; CV = cardiovascular; CVA = cardiovascular accident; DANPACE = Danish Pacing Trial; HF = heart failure; MOST = Mode Selection Trial; NSR = normal sinus rhythm; PAF = paroxysmal atrial fibrillation; PASE = Pacemaker Selection in the Elderly; PM = pacemaker; PPM = permanent pacemaker; QOL = quality of life; SND = sinus node dysfunction; TE = thromboembolic; UKPACE = United Kingdom Pacing and Cardiovascular Events.

The Canadian Trial of Physiologic Pacing (CTOPP)[14] compared VVIR with DDDR or AAIR and had primary endpoints of overall mortality and cerebrovascular accidents and secondary endpoints of atrial fibrillation, hospitalizations for congestive heart failure, and death due to a cardiac cause. CTOPP demonstrated that physiological pacing (DDD/AAI) was associated with a reduced incidence of chronic atrial fibrillation but no difference in quality of life or mortality.

The Mode Selection Trial (MOST) also randomized patients with sinus node dysfunction to either VVI or DDD pacing, with primary endpoints of all causes of mortality and cerebrovascular accidents.[15] MOST failed to demonstrate any difference in mortality but did demonstrate a lower incidence of atrial fibrillation with physiological pacing and also reduced the signs and symptoms of heart failure and slightly improved quality of life. The study concluded that, overall, dual-chamber pacing offers significant improvement compared with ventricular pacing.

The United Kingdom Pacing and Cardiovascular Events (UKPACE) trial compared DDD with VVI pacing modes in patients 70 years and older requiring permanent pacing for second- or third-degree AV block.[16] Results of this trial, presented (ACC March 2003) but not yet published, showed no significant difference between pacing modes in the primary endpoint of all-cause mortality or in the composite secondary endpoint of cardiovascular deaths, atrial fibrillation, heart failure hospitalizations, cerebrovascular accidents or thromboembolic events, and reoperation.

With the exception of PASE and UKPACE, the major trials discussed have demonstrated a lower incidence of atrial fibrillation with AAI or dual-chamber pacing.

Only one of the trials discussed demonstrated a lower mortality with physiological pacing. The difference in this trial design that may explain the mortality outcome merits discussion because of the larger implications for cardiac pacing. In the Andersen trial patients, the physiological pacing mode implemented was AAI mode. With AAI pacing, the patient maintains intrinsic AV conduction; perhaps more important, this avoids the abnormal depolarization pattern of right ventricular pacing that would occur with VVI or DDD pacing. There is growing sentiment, and data to support it, that the adverse effects of right ventricular apical pacing can lead to significant left ventricular dysfunction. This knowledge would support an effort to maintain intrinsic ventricular depolarization or pacing from some site that would enable more normal ventricular depolarization.[17]

Modes and Timing Cycles

The advantages and disadvantages of each pacing mode cannot be completely comprehended unless the timing cycle of each is understood.

Single-Chamber Triggered Pacing

Single-chamber triggered pacing (AAT and VVT) releases an output pulse every time a native event is sensed. This feature increases the current drain on the battery, accelerating its rate of depletion, and deforms the inscription of the intrinsic spontaneous complex on the ECG. However, it can serve as an excellent marker for the site of sensing within an intrinsic complex and can prevent inappropriate inhibition from oversensing when the patient does not have a stable escape rhythm. Triggered pacing is used infrequently.

Ventricular-Inhibited Pacing

VVI is a pacing mode that incorporates sensing on the ventricular channel, enabling a sensed ventricular event to inhibit pacemaker output (Fig. 31–1). VVI pacemakers are refractory for an interval after a paced or sensed ventricular event, the ventricular refractory period (VRP). Any ventricular event occurring within the VRP is not sensed and does not reset the ventricular timer.

VVI pacing is the most commonly used pacing mode worldwide. Although VVI pacing protects the patient from lethal bradycardias, it is significantly limited because it does not restore or maintain AV synchrony and does not provide rate responsiveness in the chronotropically incompetent patient, that is, the patient in whom the spontaneous sinus heart rate does not increase in response to a physiological demand. In addition, some patients with VVI pacing experience symptomatic hemodynamic deterioration during ventricular pacing. Adverse hemodynamics associated with a normally functioning pacing system that cause overt symptoms or limit the patient's ability to achieve optimal functional status are referred to as *pacemaker syndrome* (Fig. 31–2). Pacemaker syndrome was initially recognized with VVI pacing but can occur with any pacing mode if there is AV dissociation. The incidence of pacemaker syndrome is difficult to determine and depends on how the syndrome is defined. If the definition is restricted to patients with clinical limitations during any pacing mode that results in AV dissociation, the incidence is probably in the range of 7 to 10 percent of patients with VVI pacing. In a study of patients with DDD pacemakers who were randomized to DDD or VVI pacing mode, some degree of pacemaker syndrome was thought to be present in 83 percent. The most common symptoms reported were shortness of breath, dizziness, fatigue, pulsations in the neck or abdomen, cough, and apprehension. It can be concluded from this study that if patients with VVI pacing have some basis for comparison, they may be more aware of symptoms with VVI pacing.

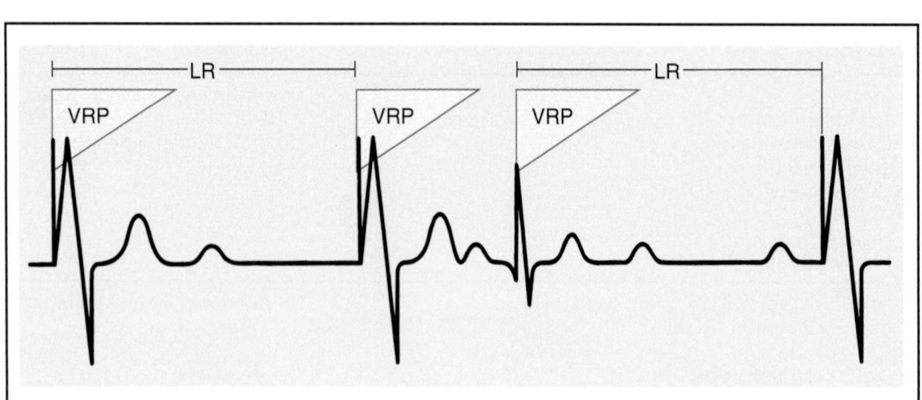

FIGURE 31–1 The VVI timing cycle consists of a defined lower rate limit (LR) and a ventricular refractory period (VRP, represented by triangle). When the LR timer is complete, a pacing artifact is delivered in the absence of a sensed intrinsic ventricular event. If an intrinsic QRS occurs, the LR timer is started from that point. A VRP begins with any sensed or paced ventricular activity.

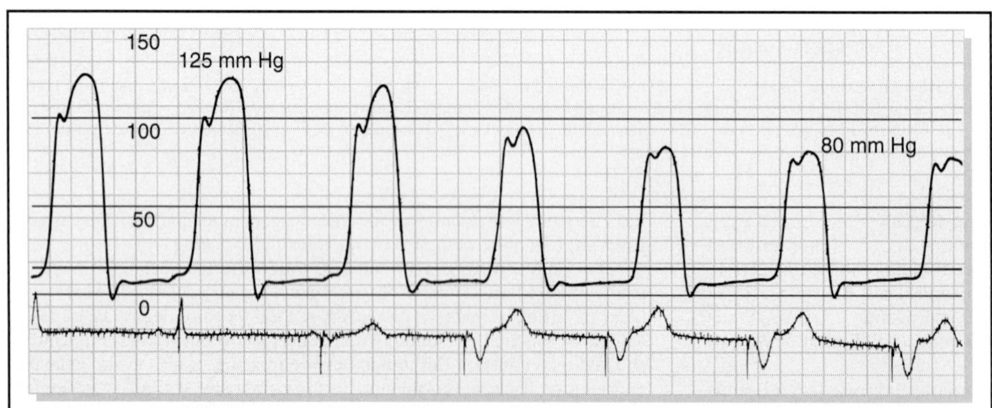

FIGURE 31–2 Hemodynamic tracing from a patient with pacemaker syndrome. In the initial portion of the tracing there is sinus rhythm with intrinsic atrioventricular node conduction with a systolic arterial pressure of approximately 125 mm Hg. This is followed by fusion beats and a progressive decrease in systolic pressure. When the ventricle is completely depolarized by the pacemaker, the systolic pressure decreases to approximately 80 mm Hg. This hemodynamic response is compatible with pacemaker syndrome.

Atrial-Inhibited Pacing

AAI pacing mode incorporates the same timing cycles, with the obvious difference that pacing and sensing occur from the atrium and pacemaker output is inhibited by a sensed atrial event (Fig. 31–3). An atrial paced or sensed event initiates a refractory period during which no spontaneous event is sensed by the pacemaker. When the atrial timing cycle ends, the atrial pacing artifact is delivered regardless of ventricular events because an AAI pacemaker should not sense ventricular events. The single exception to this rule is far-field sensing; that is, the ventricular signal is large enough to be inappropriately sensed by the atrial lead. In this situation, the atrial timing cycle is reset by events sensed in the ventricle. Sometimes this abnormality can be corrected by making the atrial channel less sensitive or by lengthening the refractory period.

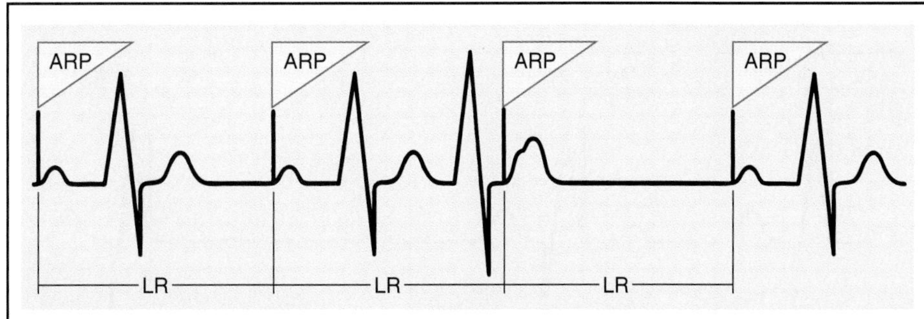

FIGURE 31–3 The AAI timing cycle consists of a defined lower rate (LR) limit and an atrial refractory period (ARP). When the LR cycle is complete, a pacing artifact is delivered in the atrium in the absence of a sensed atrial event. If an intrinsic P wave occurs, the LR timer is started from that point. An ARP begins with any sensed or paced atrial activity. The AAI timing cycle should not be affected by events in the ventricle. In this schematic example, a premature ventricular contraction (PVC) occurs. Appropriately, it is not sensed by the AAI pacemaker, and the atrial pacing artifact occurs in the T wave of the PVC. Even though atrial capture presumably would occur, there is no ventricular event after the paced atrial event because the ventricle is still refractory. However, the timing cycle will be reset by anything that is sensed on the atrial sensing circuit. In this schematic example, a PVC occurs. It is appropriately not sensed, and the pacing artifact is delivered after the PVC. Even though there appears to be atrial depolarization, no intrinsic ventricular depolarization occurs because the ventricle is refractory.

AAI pacing is appropriate for patients with sinus node dysfunction and normal AV conduction. The obvious disadvantage of atrial pacing is lack of ventricular support should AV block occur. If the patient with sinus node dysfunction is assessed carefully for AV node disease at the time of pacemaker implantation, the occurrence of clinically significant AV node disease is very low (<2 percent per year). Assessment before use of an AAI system should include incremental atrial pacing at the time of pacemaker implantation. Although criteria vary among institutions and implanting physicians, the adult patient should be capable of 1:1 AV node conduction to rates of 120 to 140 beats/min.

Dual-Chamber Pacing

AV Sequential, Non-P-Synchronous Pacing

AV sequential, non-P-synchronous pacing (DDI) is a pacing mode with dual-chamber sensing that incorporates atrial sensing as well as ventricular sensing, which prevents competitive atrial pacing (Fig. 31–4). The DDI mode of response is inhibition only; that is, no tracking of P waves can occur. Therefore, the programmed rate, which by definition is the lower rate, because only a single rate exists, is the fastest paced rate that can be seen. DDI is rarely the preimplantation mode of choice but remains a programmable option in most dual-chamber pacemakers. The DDI pacing mode could be considered for patients with intermittent atrial tachyarrhythmias, but DDD or DDDR pacing with mode switching is preferable.

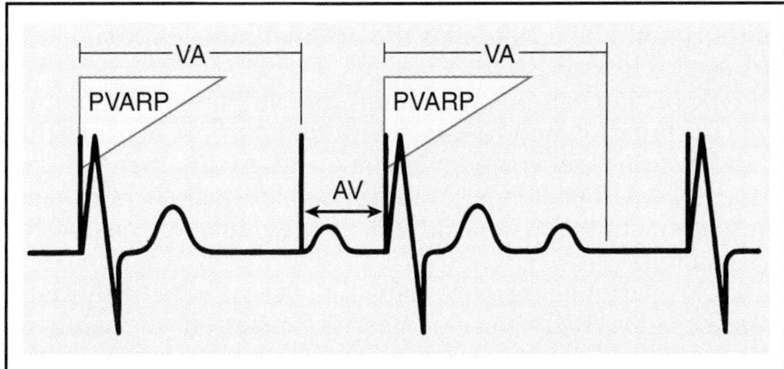

FIGURE 31–4 The timing cycle in DDI pacing consists of a lower rate limit, an atrioventricular (AV) interval, a ventricular refractory period (VRP), and an atrial refractory period (ARP). The VRP is initiated by any sensed or paced ventricular activity, and the ARP is initiated by any sensed or paced atrial activity. The lower rate limit cannot be violated even if the sinus rate is occurring at a faster rate. PVARP = postventricular atrial refractory period; VA = ventriculoatrial.

Atrial Synchronous Pacing

Atrial synchronous (VDD) pacemakers pace only in the ventricle, sense in both chambers, and respond both by inhibition of ventricular output due to intrinsic ventricular activity and by ventricular tracking of P waves. The VDD mode has become increasingly available as a single-lead pacing system. In this system, a single lead is capable of pacing in the ventricle in response to sensing atrial activity by way of a remote electrode situated on the intraatrial portion of the ventricular pacing lead.

In the VDD mode, sensed atrial events initiate the AV interval (AVI). If an intrinsic ventricular event occurs before the termination of the AVI, ventricular output is inhibited and the lower rate timing cycle is reset (Fig. 31–5). If a paced ventricular beat occurs at the end of the AVI, this beat resets the lower rate. If no atrial event occurs, the pacemaker escapes with a paced ventricular event at the lower rate limit; that is, the pacemaker displays VVI activity in the absence of a sensed atrial event. VDD pacing may be appropriate for the patient with normal sinus node function and conduction disease of the AV node.

Dual-Chamber Pacing and Sensing with Inhibition and Tracking

In the dual-chamber pacing and sensing with inhibition and tracking (DDD) mode, the basic timing circuit associated with lower rate pacing is divided into two sections: the ventriculoatrial (VA) interval and the AVI. The AVI may be defined by AV sequential pacing initiated by pacing with subsequent intrinsic ventricular conduction or initiated by a native P wave with subsequent ventricular pacing (Fig. 31–6).

The postventricular atrial refractory period (PVARP) is the period after a sensed or paced ventricular event during which the atrial sensing circuit is refractory. Any atrial event occurring during the PVARP is not sensed by the atrial sensing circuit. If a P wave occurs after the PVARP and is sensed, no atrial pacing artifact is delivered at the end of the VA interval (see Fig. 31–6). Because the maximum tracking rate of the pacemaker is determined by the total atrial refractory period (TARP), the PVARP is a significant determinant

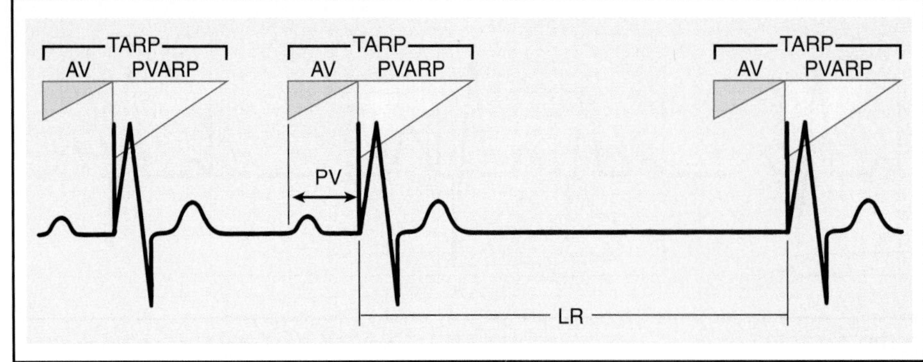

FIGURE 31–5 The timing cycle of VDD consists of a lower rate (LR) limit, an atrioventricular interval (AVI), a ventricular refractory period, a postventricular atrial refractory period (PVARP), and an upper rate limit. A sensed P wave initiates the AVI (during the AVI the atrial sensing channel is refractory). At the end of the AVI a ventricular pacing artifact is delivered if no intrinsic ventricular activity has been sensed; this represents P wave tracking pacing. Ventricular activity, paced or sensed, initiates the PVARP and the ventriculoatrial interval (the LR limit interval minus the AVI). If no P wave activity occurs, the pacemaker escapes with a ventricular pacing artifact at the LR limit. AV = atrioventricular; PV = interval from intrinsic atrial event to paced ventricular event; TARP = total atrial refractory period.

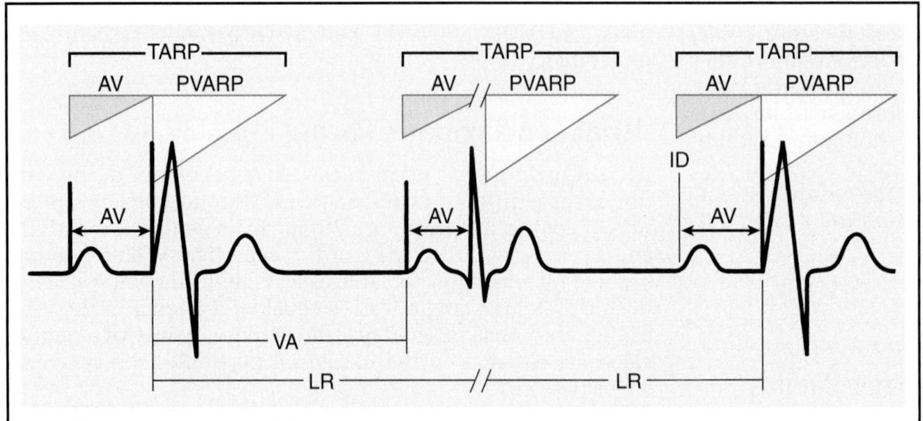

FIGURE 31–6 The timing cycle in DDD consists of a lower rate (LR) limit, an atrioventricular interval (AVI), a postventricular atrial refractory period (PVARP), and an upper rate limit. The AVI and PVARP together comprise the total atrial refractory period (TARP). If intrinsic atrial and ventricular activity occur before the LR times out, both channels are inhibited and no pacing occurs. If no intrinsic atrial or ventricular activity occurs, there is atrioventricular (AV) sequential pacing (first sequence). If no atrial activity is sensed before the ventriculoatrial (VA) interval is completed, an atrial pacing artifact is delivered, which initiates the AVI. If intrinsic ventricular activity occurs before the termination of the AVI, the ventricular output from the pacemaker is inhibited, that is, atrial pacing (second sequence). If a P wave is sensed before the VA interval is completed, output from the atrial channel is inhibited. The AVI is initiated, and if no ventricular activity is sensed before the AVI terminates, a ventricular pacing artifact is delivered, that is, P-synchronous pacing (third sequence). ID = intrinsic deflection.

of the upper rate limit. *The PVARP is especially important for the prevention of endless-loop, or pacemaker-mediated, tachycardia.*

Normal DDD function can appear electrocardiographically as (1) normal sinus rhythm, (2) atrial pacing only, (3) AV sequential pacing, or (4) P-synchronous pacing.

DDD pacing mode is most appropriate for patients with normal sinus node function and AV block. DDD pacing is often considered the mode of choice in neurocardiogenic syndromes with symptomatic cardioinhibition.

DDD pacing has limitations in the patient with sinus node dysfunction, because P-synchronous pacing is not possible in chronic atrial fibrillation or in patients with a paralyzed or nonexcitable atrium. Also, DDD pacing does not restore rate response in the chronotropically incompetent patient.

In any pacemaker capable of P-synchronous pacing, endless-loop tachycardia, also called *pacemaker reentrant tachycardia* or *pacemaker-mediated tachycardia*, can result. If AV synchrony is dissociated by any event, most commonly a premature ventricular complex (PVC), retrograde VA conduction can result in a retrograde P wave (Fig. 31–7). If the retrograde P wave is sensed by the atrial sensing circuit of the pacemaker, the AVI is initiated, resulting in a paced ventricular complex at a cycle length approximately equal to the maximum tracking rate. The paced ventricular event can again result in retrograde VA conduction, perpetuating this rapid reentrant circuit. Endless-loop tachycardia can be prevented by a PVARP that is long enough to prevent sensing of the retrograde P wave. Most pacemakers also have specific algorithms that attempt to recognize and abort endless-loop tachycardia.

Indications for Rate-Adaptive Pacing

Rate-adaptive pacemakers have the ability to increase the pacing rate through sensors that monitor physiological processes such as activity and minute ventilation. Single-chamber rate-adaptive pacing (AAIR, VVIR) has timing cycles that are not significantly different from those of its non–rate-adaptive counterparts. The difference lies in the potential variability of the paced rate. Depending on the sensor incorporated and the level of exertion of the patient, the basic interval shortens from the programmed lower rate limit to an upper rate limit programmed to define the absolute shortest cycle length allowable.

VVIR pacing, like VVI, is generally contraindicated if ventricular pacing results in retrograde (VA) conduction or a decrease in blood pressure. Also, if the sinus node is normal, P-synchronous pacing should be considered the optimal rate-adaptive mode and used when possible.

AAIR pacing can be considered for the patient with sinus node dysfunction and normal AV node function, because this mode restores rate responsiveness and maintains AV synchrony. If AAIR pacing is contemplated, normal AV node conduction must first be determined, as previously discussed for AAI pacing.

DDDR pacemakers are capable of all the variations described for DDD pacemakers. In addition to using P-synchronous pacing as a method for increasing heart rate, the sensor incorporated in the pacemaker can also drive the increase in heart rate. The resulting rhythm can be sinus driven or sensor driven. The ideal patient for DDDR pacing is one with combined sinus node and AV node dysfunction, because this mode allows restoration of rate responsiveness and AV synchrony.

Algorithms for determining the appropriate pacing mode for patients with sinus node disease and AV node disease are shown in Figure 31–8. In Figure 31-8A, a more complex algorithm, most of the available pacing modes are considered. The second algorithm is simpler and assumes that a pacemaker capable of rate adaptation is used (Fig. 31–8B).

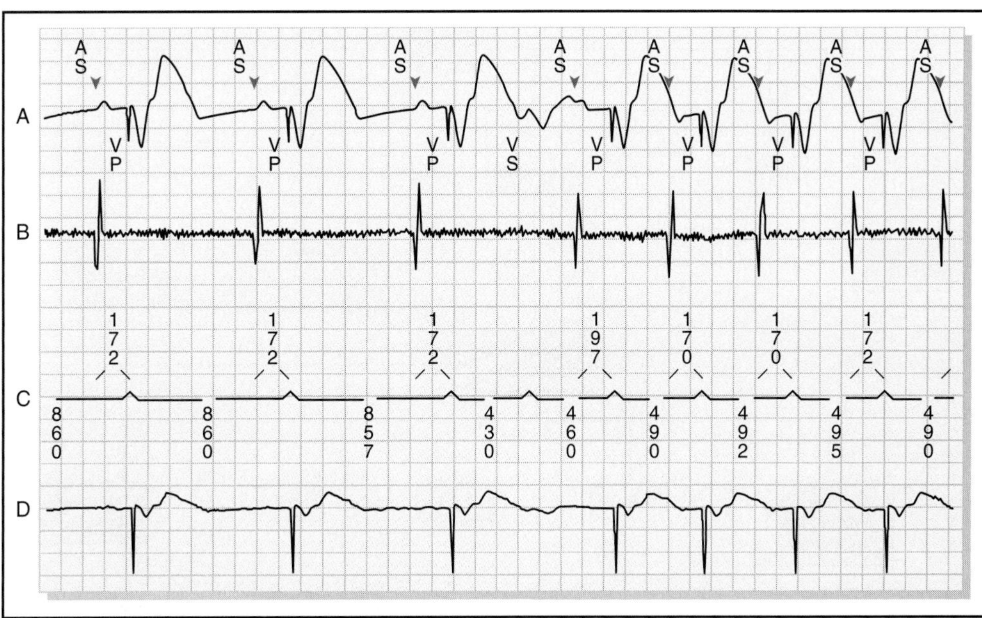

FIGURE 31–7 Electrocardiographic (ECG) example of pacemaker-mediated tachycardia (PMT) in a patient whose device is programmed to the DDD pacing mode. The ECG tracing **(A)** demonstrates P-synchronous pacing. The third paced QRS complex is followed by a ventricular sensed event that is followed by retrograde atrial sensing and subsequent ventricular pacing at a rate of approximately 115 beats/min. This appearance is consistent with PMT, or endless-loop tachycardia. **(B),** Atrial electrogram. **(C),** Marker channel. **(D),** Ventricular electrogram. VP = ventricular paced event; VS = ventricular sensed event; AS = atrial sensed event. Arrows indicate sensed or paced events. Numbers above the line indicate milliseconds between events. Numbers below the line indicate MS between ventricular events.

Selecting the Appropriate Sensor for Rate-Adaptive Pacing

Several varieties of sensors appropriate for rate-adaptive pacing have been developed and are displayed in Figure 31–9 as endpoints of some physiological response.[18] Although a number of sensors have been used clinically (some with clinical potential), only activity sensors, minute-ventilation sensors, and stimulus-T (QT interval) sensors have achieved clinical acceptance.

Activity Sensors

Activity sensing with vibration detection (piezoelectric crystal or accelerometer) has been the most widely used form of rate adaptation because it is simple, easy to apply clinically, and rapid in onset of rate response. The main difference between the piezoelectric crystal sensor and the accelerometer is that the former senses vibration from "up and down" motion and the latter in addition senses anterior and posterior motion. Accelerometers have become the activity sensor of choice, having been shown to have a slightly more physiological response than piezoelectric crystal sensors and, specifically, to have a more appropriate rate response to stair walking.[19]

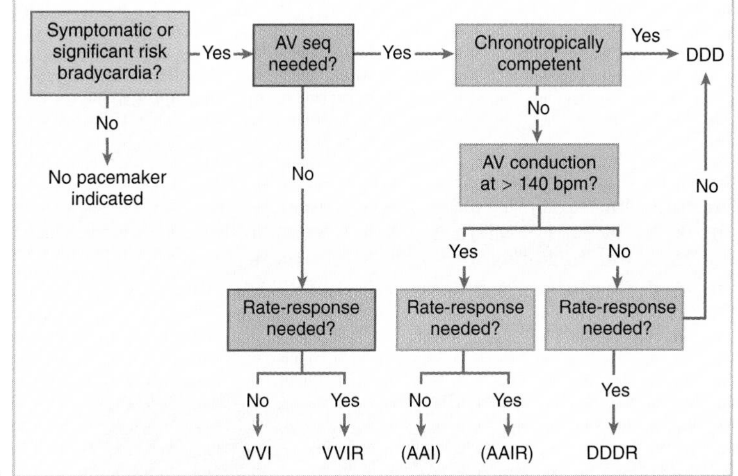

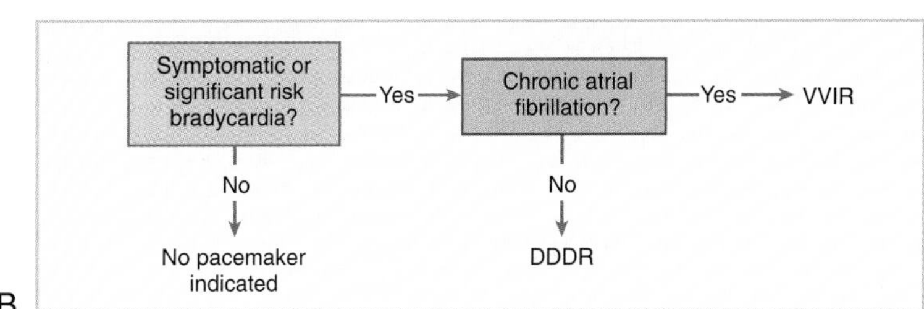

FIGURE 31–8 Algorithms for pacemaker mode selection. **A,** Choice of VVI, VVIR, AAI, AAIR, DDD, or DDDR is allowed. **B,** Only VVIR or DDDR is selected. AV = atrioventricular.

Minute-Ventilation Sensors

The minute-ventilation (respiratory rate × tidal volume) sensor has an excellent correlation with metabolic demand. In a rate-adaptive pacing system, minute volume is determined by emission of a small charge of known current from the pacemaker and measurement of the resulting voltage at the lead tip. When both current and voltage are known, transthoracic impedance can be measured between the ring electrode and the pacemaker. Because transthoracic impedance varies with respiration and its amplitude varies with tidal volume, the impedance measurement can be used to determine respiratory rate and tidal volume. A pacing algorithm uses the minute-volume measurements to alter pacing rate. Long-term reliability of the minute-ventilation sensor has been excellent.

Stimulus-T or QT-Sensing Pacemaker

The interval from the onset of a paced QRS complex to the end of the T wave has been used successfully for rate adaptation for many years. Autonomic activity and heart rate affect the stimulus-T interval, and the relationship allows

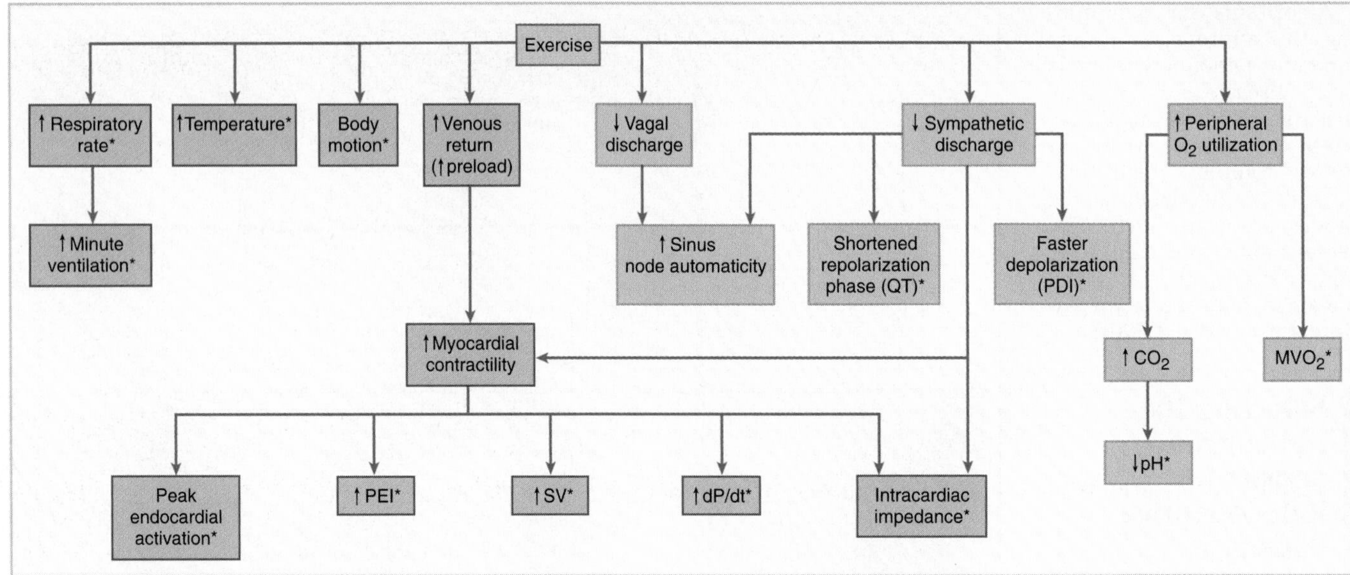

FIGURE 31–9 Physiological responses that have been investigated or clinically used for rate adaptation of permanent pacemakers. *Endpoints used for rate adaptation. PDI = paced depolarization integral; PEI = preejection interval; SV = stroke volume.

measurement of the stimulus-T interval to be used for rate adaptation.

Dual-Sensor Combinations

The overall performance of market-approved single-sensor rate-adaptive systems has been excellent. However, sensors have been combined in an effort to more closely mimic the normal sinus node at all levels of activity and during emotional stress.

The perfect sensor would be resistant to nonphysiological stimuli. A multisensor rate-adaptive pacing system could improve specificity by having one sensor verify or cross-check the other. For example, if one sensor indicated a rate increase and the other did not, a rate increase would not occur. Both sensors would have to indicate a rate increase before it would be allowed.

Pacing for Hemodynamic Improvement

In addition to hemodynamic improvements from pacing when a bradyarrhythmia is corrected, there are also nonbradyarrhythmic indications for permanent pacing for hemodynamic improvement.

Hypertrophic Obstructive Cardiomyopathy

Dual-chamber pacing has been used as a therapeutic modality for some patients with severe, symptomatic, medically refractory hypertrophic obstructive cardiomyopathy (HCM) (see Chap. 59).[20,21] The therapy is based on the concept that the altered septal activation caused by right ventricular apical pacing results in less narrowing of the left ventricular outflow tract and a subsequent decrease in the Venturi effect responsible for systolic anterior motion of the mitral valve.[20]

CLINICAL TRIALS

Pacing in HCM has been the subject of several randomized single-center and multicenter trials (Table 31–6). A single-center randomized crossover trial demonstrated symptomatic improvement in 63 percent of patients with pacing in the DDD mode.[22] However, 42 percent of patients had improvement when the pacemaker was programmed to a low pacing rate in the AAI mode, that is, effectively no pacing, suggesting a significant placebo effect.

In the Pacing in Cardiomyopathy (PIC) study, a multicenter, randomized, crossover study,[23] dual-chamber pacing resulted in a 50 percent reduction of the left ventricular outflow tract gradient, a 21 percent increase in exercise duration, and improvement in New York Heart Association (NYHA) functional class compared with baseline status. When clinical parameters, including chest pain, dyspnea, and subjective health status, were compared between DDD and back-up AAI pacing, there was no significant difference, again suggesting a significant placebo effect.

In the Multicenter Study of Pacing Therapy for Hypertrophic Cardiomyopathy (M-PATHY) trial, no significant differences were evident with randomization between pacing and no pacing, either subjectively or objectively, when exercise capacity, quality of life score, treadmill exercise time, and peak oxygen consumption were compared.[24] The investigators concluded that pacing should not be regarded as a primary treatment for HCM and that subjective benefit without objective evidence of improvement should be interpreted cautiously.

Pacing for the treatment of medically refractory HCM is currently a class IIb indication for pacing by the ACC/AHA guidelines.[2]

When pacing is applied in the patient with HCM, AVI programming is crucial to achieve optimal hemodynamic improvement. Ventricular depolarization must occur as a result of pacing. Therefore, the AVI must be short enough to result in depolarization by the paced event (Fig. 31–10). However, the shortest AVI is not necessarily the best.[22] Some experts have advocated AV node ablation to ensure paced ventricular depolarization if rapid intrinsic AV node conduction prevents total ventricular depolarization by means of the pacing stimulus.

Cardiac Resynchronization Therapy

Cardiac resynchronization therapy is the term applied to reestablishing synchronous contraction between the left ventricular free wall and the ventricular septum in an attempt

TABLE 31–6 Clinical Trials in Pacing for Hypertrophic Obstructive Cardiomyopathy

Study	Patient Inclusion Criteria	Endpoint(s)	Treatment Arms	Key Results
Mayo: Pacing in HCM[22]	Symptomatic HCM despite maximal medical regimen	LVOT gradient Quality of life Exercise duration Oxygen consumption	Blinded crossover of DDD pacing *vs.* No pacing (AAI)	Subjective improvement in ~60% of patients Significant placebo effect from pacing LVOT gradient reduced by mean of 33 ± 29 mm Hg
PIC[23]	Refractory symptoms from HCM despite stable drug regimen NYHA Class II or III Angina or dyspnea LVOT > 30 mm Hg	Exercise tolerance Dyspnea-angina symptom score NYHA Class Quality of life	Blinded crossover of DDD pacing *vs.* No pacing (AAI)	50% ↓ in LVOT gradient 21% ↑ in exercise duration 0.7 ↓ in NYHA Class
M-PATHY[24]	Symptomatic HCM despite maximal medical regimen LVOT ≥ 50 mm Hg	Quality of life Treadmill exercise duration Peak O_2 consumption ΔLVOT gradient ΔLV wall thickness	Blinded crossover of DDD pacing *vs.* No pacing (AAI at 30 beats/min)	No significant subjective or objective improvement with randomization Significant placebo effect

HCM = hypertrophic obstructive cardiomyopathy; LV = left ventricular; LVOT = left ventricular outflow tract; M-PATHY = Multicenter Study of Pacing Therapy for Hypertrophic Cardiomyopathy; NYHA = New York Heart Association; PIC = Pacing in Cardiomyopathy.

Data from Maron BJ, Nishimura RA, McKenna WJ, et al: Assessment of permanent dual-chamber pacing as a treatment for drug-refractory symptomatic patients with obstructive hypertrophic cardiomyopathy: A randomized, double-blind, crossover study (M-PATHY). Circulation 99:2927, 1999.

to improve left ventricular efficiency and, subsequently, to improve functional class. Generally, CRT has been used to describe biventricular or multisite ventricular pacing (Fig. 31–11), but cardiac resynchronization can be achieved by left ventricular pacing only in some patients.

Several randomized clinical trials have now been completed and have demonstrated the safety and efficacy of CRT. These trials are summarized in Table 31–7. In the most recent ACC/AHA/NASPE guidelines[2] for pacing, biventricular pacing in medically refractory, symptomatic NYHA Class III/IV patients with idiopathic dilated or ischemic cardiomyopathy, prolonged QRS interval (≥130 milliseconds), left ventricular end-diastolic diameter of 55 mm or more, and left ventricular ejection fraction of 0.35 or less is included as a class IIa indication. Similarly, the U.S. Food and Drug Administration labeling criteria for CRT are the following:

- NYHA functional Class III or IV
- QRS longer than 130 milliseconds
- Left ventricular ejection fraction of no more than 0.35
- Optimized medical therapy
- Normal sinus rhythm

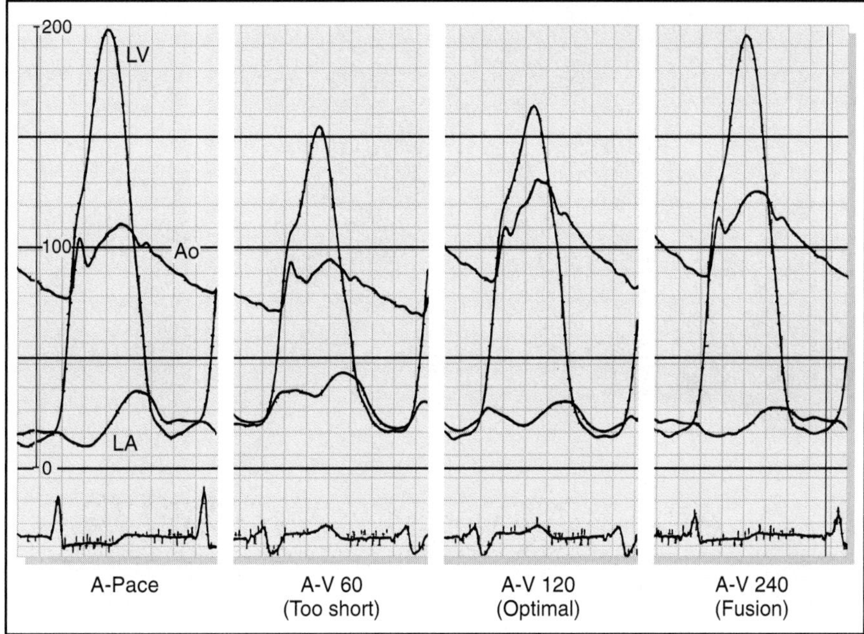

FIGURE 31–10 Pressure tracings at different atrioventricular (AV) intervals in a patient with hypertrophic obstructive cardiomyopathy. In this example, the outflow gradient was minimized at an AV interval of 120 milliseconds. LA = left atrium; LV = left ventricle; Ao = aorta.

CRT is rapidly gaining acceptance. Devices combining CRT and ICD capabilities are also available. The indications for such a device, often designated as *high-voltage CRT*, are discussed in the subsequent ICD section.

Pacing to Prevent Atrial Fibrillation

Multisite and alternate site atrial pacing have been used to prevent recurrent atrial tachyarrhythmias (see Chap. 32), presumably by decreasing the dispersion of refractoriness in the atrium.[25] Various techniques have been used to reduce or prevent atrial tachyarrhythmias (Table 31–8). Biatrial synchronous pacing with leads in the right atrial appendage and coronary sinus allows sensing from the lead in the right atrial appendage to be followed by immediate pacing at the coronary sinus site. The designation of *dual-site atrial pacing* has generally been used to describe one lead in a standard right atrial position and the other lead in the coronary sinus or near the coronary sinus ostium (Fig. 31–12). With both leads connected to the same port, there is simultaneous pacing at both sites. Dual-site pacing has been shown in a randomized clinical trial to decrease the number of episodes of paroxysmal atrial fibrillation and flutter and to increase the interval to

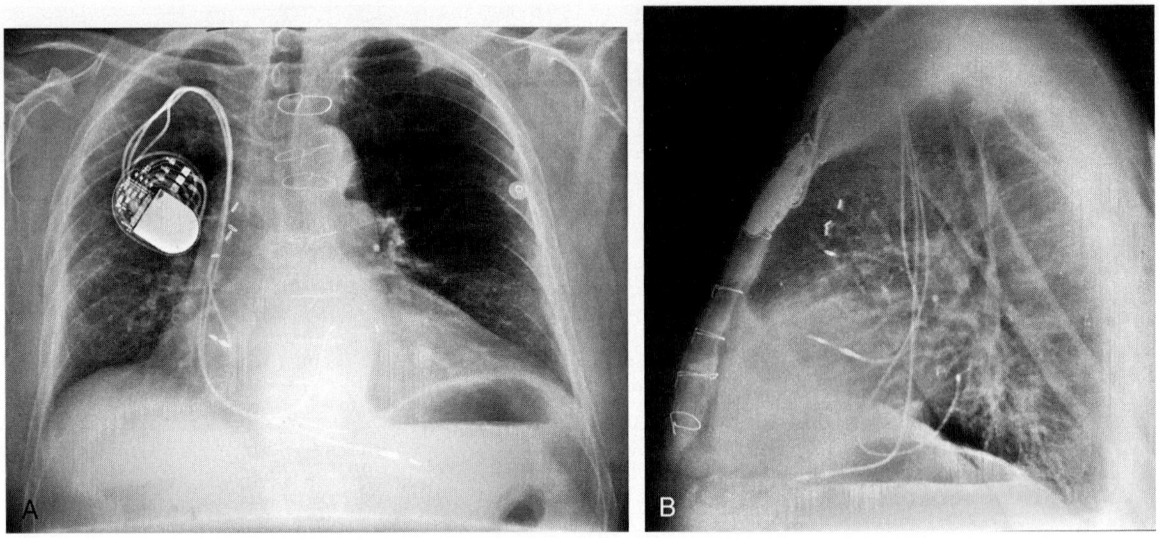

FIGURE 31–11 Posteroanterior **(A)** and lateral **(B)** chest radiographs demonstrating a biventricular pacing system. There are three leads: the first is positioned in the right atrium, a second is positioned in the right ventricular apex, and the third courses posteriorly in the coronary sinus and into the posterolateral cardiac vein.

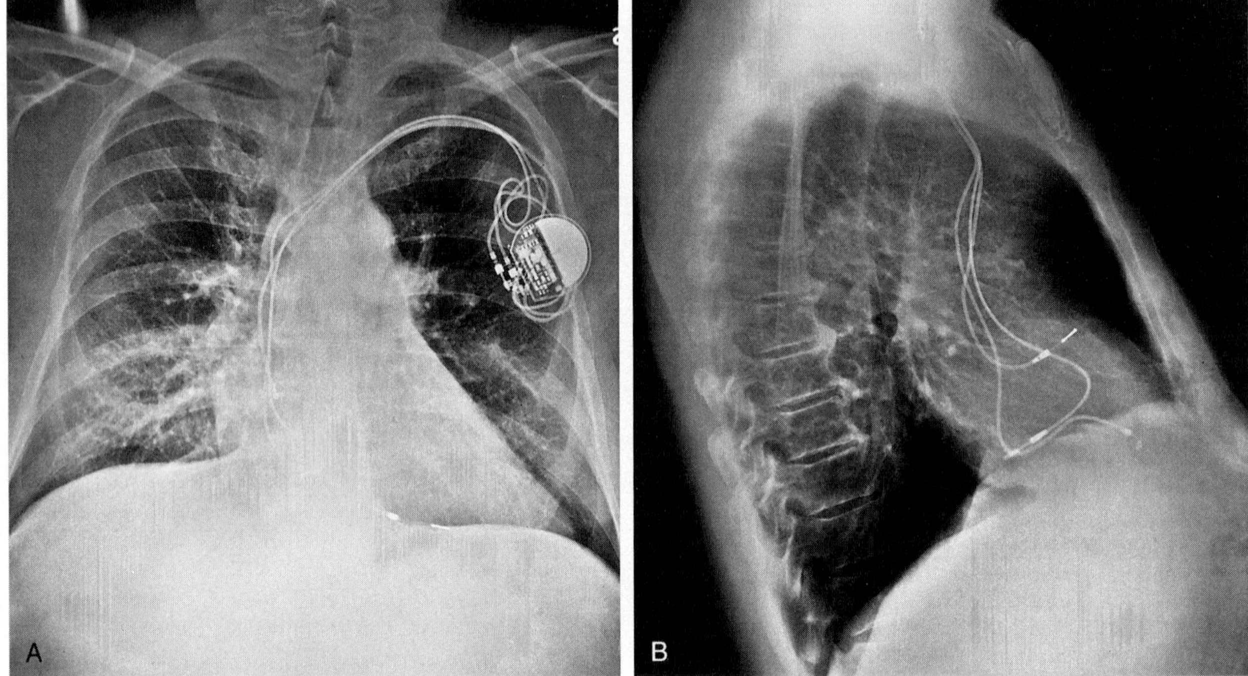

FIGURE 31–12 Posteroanterior **(A)** and lateral **(B)** chest radiographs in a patient with a dual-site atrial pacing system for the prevention of paroxysmal atrial fibrillation. Leads are positioned in the right atrium, near the coronary sinus ostium, and in the right ventricular apex.

recurrent atrial arrhythmias.[30] When "no pacing" was compared with dual-site or single-site atrial pacing, dual-site pacing was better, but single-site atrial pacing also resulted in a significant improvement over no pacing. Single-site atrial septal pacing[31] and Bachmann bundle pacing[32] have also been tested.

In addition to these alternate-pacing techniques, pacing algorithms have been incorporated in contemporary pacemakers in an effort to decrease the number of premature atrial complexes and maintain consistent atrial pacing (see Table 31–8). Multiple algorithms have been developed, and some pacemakers include as many as four different algorithms. A schematic representation of an algorithm that alters atrial pacing rate as a result of an atrial sensed event is shown in Figure 31–13.

Several clinical trials have been completed to assess these atrial pacing algorithms. A reduction in atrial fibrillation burden was demonstrated in two trials: the Atrial Dynamic Overdrive Pacing Trial (ADOPT)[33] (NASPE, 2002) and Atrial Fibrillation Therapy (AFT) trial (results not yet published) (European Society of Cardiology, 2002). Multiple additional trials are under way, but it is likely that atrial pacing algorithms will be included in the majority of future dual-chamber pacemakers.

Pacing in Long-QT Syndrome

The long-QT syndrome is characterized by abnormally prolonged ventricular repolarization and a risk of development

TABLE 31–7 Clinical Trials in Pacing for Congestive Heart Failure				
Study	**Patient Inclusion Criteria**	**Endpoint(s)**	**Treatment Arms**	**Key Results**
InSync	NYHA Class III or IV on stable drug regimen LVEDD > 60 mm, LVEF ≤ 0.35 QRS width ≥ 150 msec	QOL NYHA Class 6-min hall walk	Nonrandomized	Sustained improvement in all three endpoints
MIRACLE	NYHA Class III or IV on stable drug regimen LVEDD ≥ 55 mm, LVEF ≤ 0.35 QRS width ≥ 130 msec	QOL NYHA Class 6-min hall walk	Randomized to pacing or no pacing for 6 mo and then to pacing	Sustained improvement in all three endpoints
PATH-CHF	DCM of any cause NYHA Class III or IV on stable drug regimen QRS ≥ 120 msec PR ≥ 150 msec	Acute maximum LV pressure derivative Aortic pulse pressure Chronic oxygen uptake Anaerobic threshold 6-min walk	Acute hemodynamic and chronic assessment of RV pacing *vs.* LV pacing *vs.* BiV pacing	Acute BiV and LV: ↑ LV pressure derivative and aortic pulse pressure more than RV pacing Sustained chronic improvement in all endpoints
MUSTIC-NSR	NYHA Class III Refractory symptoms on stable drug therapy LVEF < 0.35 LVEDD > 60 mm 6-min walk < 450 m NSR with QRS > 150 msec	Functional capacity QOL Metabolic exercise performance Mortality or need for transplant or LVAD Hospital admission for CHF	BiV pacing *vs.* No pacing with crossover	Sustained improvement in all endpoints Fewer hospital admissions with CRT
MUSTIC-AF	NYHA Class III Refractory symptoms on stable drug therapy LVEF < 0.35 LVEDD > 60 mm 6-min walk < 450 m AF with paced QRS > 200 msec	Functional capacity QOL Metabolic exercise performance Mortality or need for transplant or LVAD Hospital admission for CHF	BiV pacing *vs.* No pacing with crossover	Sustained improvement in all endpoints Fewer hospital admissions with CRT
InSync-III	NYHA Class III or IV on stable drug regimen LVEDD ≥ 60 mm, LVEF ≤ 0.35 QRS width ≥ 130 msec	QOL NYHA Class 6-min hall walk	BiV pacing with optimized AV and VV intervals *vs.* No pacing with crossover	Sustained improvement in all endpoints
CARE-HF	NYHA Class III or IV on stable drug regimen LVEDD ≥ 60 mm, LVEF ≤ 0.35 QRS width ≥ 150 msec or > 120 msec with echo study	Mortality QOL Economic outcomes Echo parameters Neurohormonal measurements	BiV pacing *vs.* No pacing with crossover	Enrollment completed (3/03)
PACMAN	Functional NYHA Class III CHF LVEF < 0.35 DCM of any etiology QRS > 150 msec Optimal medical management Hospitalization at least once in past 12 mo	Functional capacity by 6-min walk Secondary endpoints of QOL, adverse events, ventricular arrhythmias, hospitalizations	Observation over 1 yr with randomization of patients to CRT *vs.* No CRT (1:1 randomization)	Enrollment completed; in follow-up phase
VecToR	NYHA Class III or IV LVEF ≤ 0.35 QRS ≥ 140 msec LVEDD > 54 mm	QOL Mortality Echo parameters	BiV pacing *vs.* No pacing with crossover	In progress
ReLeVent	NYHA Class III or IV LVEF < 0.35 QRS > 140 msec LVEDD > 55 mm	6-min walk LVEDD LVESD Mortality QOL	BiV pacing *vs.* No pacing with crossover	In progress
PAVE	NYHA Class II or III Status post AV nodal ablation Able to complete 6-min hall walk 3 mo stable medical therapy	Exercise tolerance QOL	BiV pacing *vs.* RV pacing	In progress

Continued

TABLE 31–7 Clinical Trials in Pacing for Congestive Heart Failure—cont'd

Study	Patient Inclusion Criteria	Endpoint(s)	Treatment Arms	Key Results
MUSTIC-II	NYHA Class III or IV AF after ablation and paced for > 3 mo LVEDD > 60 mm QRS > 200 msec 6-min walk < 450 m LVEF < 0.35	Exercise tolerance QOL Hospitalization rates Modification of drug therapy	BiV pacing *vs.* No pacing with crossover	In progress

AF = atrial fibrillation; BiV = biventricular; CARE-HF = Cardiac Resynchronization in Heart Failure; CHF = congestive heart failure; CRT = cardiac resynchronization therapy; DCM = dilated cardiomyopathy; echo = echocardiographic; LV = left ventricular; LVAD = left ventricular assist device; LVEDD = left ventricular end-diastolic dimension; LVEF = left ventricular ejection fraction; LVESD = left ventricular end-systolic dimension; MIRACLE = Multicenter InSync Randomized Clinical Evaluation; MUSTIC = Multisite Stimulation in Cardiomyopathy; NSR = normal sinus rhythm; NYHA = New York Heart Association; PACMAN = Pacing for Cardiomyopathy: a European Study; PATH-CHF = Pacing Therapy in Congestive Heart Failure; PAVE = Left Ventricular Post-AV Nodal Ablation Evaluation; QOL = quality of life; ReLeVent = Remodeling of Cardiac Cavities by Long-Term Ventricular-Based Stimulation; RV = right ventricular; VecToR = Ventricular Resynchronization Therapy Randomized.

TABLE 31–8 Clinical Trials in Pacing for Prevention of Atrial Fibrillation

Study	Patient Inclusion Criteria	Endpoint(s)	Treatment Arms	Key Results
SYNBIAPACE	≥1-yr history of recurrent and drug-refractory AA P wave duration ≥ 120 msec and IACT ≥ 100 msec	Time to first AA recurrence	BASP at 70 beats/min *vs.* Single-site HRA at 70 beats/min *or* Single-site HRA at 40 beats/min	Trend to a ↓ in incidence of AA with BASP, but no real benefit of BASP
DAPPAF*	Bradycardia requiring pacing Two documented episodes of AF in prior 3 mo	Time to first recurrence of symptoms of AF Quality of life Safety of DAP	Dual-site right atrial pacing *or* Single-site atrial pacing *vs.* Support pacing mode (control arm)	Dual-site right atrial pacing prolonged or tended to prolong time to recurrent AF in presence of AAD Support pacing poorly tolerated and associated with highest recurrence rates of symptomatic AF
STOP-AF[26]	—	Time to recurrence of PAF	Physiological pacing *vs.* VVI pacing	In progress
PA3[27]	History of PAF with three or more episodes within year before Most recent PAF within 3 mo of entry At least one episode of PAF documented by ECG	Time to recurrence of PAF ≥ 5 min occurring ≥ 2 wk after entry Intervals between successive episodes of PAF Frequency of PAF Proportion of patients who chose to defer ablation	DDDR pacemaker implanted and randomized to atrial pacing or no pacing	Atrial RAP did not prevent PAF over short term in patients with drug-resistant PAF
PIPAF[28,29]	Indication for pacing Documented paroxysmal AAs for at least 1 yr, three episodes Stable drug therapy Fewer than two cardioversions in past year	Time to first recurrence of AA Cumulative arrhythmia duration	Comparison of six different lead and algorithm combinations	In progress

AA = atrial arrhythmia; AAD = antiarrhythmic drug; BASP = biatrial synchronous pacing; DAP = dual-site atrial pacing; DAPPAF = Dual-Site Atrial Pacing to Prevent Atrial Fibrillation; ECG = electrocardiography; HRA = high right atrium; IACT = interatrial conduction time; PA3 = Atrial Pacing Periablation for Prevention of Paroxysmal Atrial Fibrillation; PAF = paroxysmal atrial fibrillation; PIPAF = Pacing in Prevention of Atrial Fibrillation; RAP = rate-adaptive pacing; STOP-AF = Systematic Trial of Pacing for Atrial Fibrillation; SYNBIAPACE = Synchronous Biatrial Pacing.

*Data from Fitts SM, Hill MR, Mehra R, et al: DAPPAF Phase I Investigators: Design and implementation of the Dual Site Atrial Pacing to Prevent Atrial Fibrillation (DAPPAF) clinical trial. J Interv Card Electrophysiol 2:139, 1998.

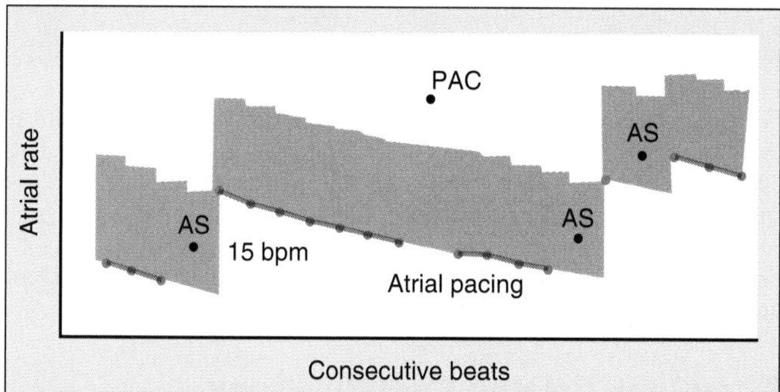

FIGURE 31–13 Schematic representation of an atrial pacing algorithm that increments the atrial pacing rate when a sensed atrial beat (AS) is detected to consistently overdrive the intrinsic atrial rhythm. The pacing rate would decrement after a specified period if no additional ASs were detected. PAC = premature atrial complex.

TABLE 31–9 Measurements During Implantation of Pacemaker or Cardioverter-Defibrillator

Threshold of stimulation Atrium* Ventricle
Measurement of electrogram† Atrium* Ventricle
Measurement of antegrade conduction‡ Wenckebach block point
Defibrillation threshold§

*Necessary only when an atrial lead is being placed.
†Electrogram measurement implies measurement of intrinsic amplitude of P wave (atrium) or QRS (ventricle); actual electrogram can easily be recorded by pacing system analyzer.
‡Necessary only when an AAI or AAIR system is implanted.
§Should be measured during all cardioverter-defibrillator implants.

of life-threatening ventricular tachyarrhythmias (see Chaps. 28 and 32). Therapy must be individualized depending on the clinical situation. Therapeutic options include beta-blocker therapy, permanent pacing, and the ICD (see later).

Pulse Generator Implantation

Only qualified physicians should undertake pacemaker or ICD implantation. The recommended training requirements for pacemaker implantation[34] are as follows: a base of core knowledge for pacemaker follow-up, participation in at least 100 pacemaker follow-up visits, participation in at least 50 initial transvenous pacemaker implantations as the primary operator (recommended that at least one-half of these be dual-chamber), participation in at least 20 revisions of pacing systems, exposure to lead extraction techniques (suggested), and thorough knowledge of recognition and treatment of pacemaker and surgical complications and emergencies. A detailed description of pacemaker and ICD implantation technique can be found in texts devoted to these disciplines.[35] However, certain information related to the implantation technique is important for the referring physician to know.

Almost all pacemakers and defibrillators are now implanted transvenously, with the pulse generator placed in the upper anterior portion of the chest, just anterior to the pectoralis major muscle. Epicardial pacing is usually considered only in persons without reasonable venous access, that is, no access to the right ventricle because of an associated congenital anomaly, a prosthetic tricuspid valve, or an intracardiac right-to-left shunt.

Although multiple venous routes have been used for lead placement, the subclavian and cephalic veins are most commonly used. The subclavian approach involves a subclavian puncture and the use of one or more peel-away introducers. A lateral approach to the subclavian vein, often lateral enough to be the axillary vein, is preferred to minimize the risk of pneumothorax and to avoid subclavian crush injury to the lead, which is more common when a medial approach is used. The cephalic vein is often large enough to accept one or two pacing leads, and this approach avoids the risks associated with blind subclavian puncture. Potential complications of subclavian puncture include pneumothorax, hemopneumothorax, subclavian artery puncture, brachial nerve plexus injury, and thoracic duct injury.

Specific measurements must be obtained at the time of pacemaker or ICD implantation (Table 31–9).

After placement of the pulse generator, posteroanterior and lateral chest radiographs must be obtained to exclude pneumothorax and also to ensure adequate lead positioning. Before hospital dismissal, the pulse generator should be programmed to determine pacing and sensing thresholds for final programming with adequate safety margins. If the pulse generator is being programmed to a rate-adaptive pacing mode, adequate rate response should be assessed by formal or informal stress testing.

Pacemaker Programming

All contemporary pacemakers have many programmable parameters that can be altered to optimize and troubleshoot pacemaker function. A detailed description of pacemaker programming is beyond the scope of this text. A few of the most critical parameters merit mention here, but any caregiver taking responsibility for pacemaker follow-up should have a thorough knowledge of all programming options.

Programming Pulse Width and Voltage Amplitude

Output programming is probably the most important aspect of programming that should be performed routinely. The output must be high enough to allow an adequate pacing margin of safety but should also be programmed with the intent of maximizing pacemaker longevity. A strength-duration curve plots voltage and pulse width thresholds and allows determination of appropriate values to ensure an adequate safety margin. There is no consensus of the best way to program output parameters, but options include doubling the voltage amplitude at threshold, tripling the pulse width at threshold, determining the threshold, or programming output parameters to achieve triple the threshold determined in microjoules. Some pacemakers automatically determine output parameters and others continually do surveillance of the capture threshold and automatically adjust output parameters.

AVI

In dual-chamber pacemakers, the interval corresponding to the intrinsic PR interval, that is, the interval between paced or sensed atrial event and paced ventricular event, must be programmed. Optimization of this interval is critical in some patients to obtain optimal hemodynamic benefit from the pacemaker. As mentioned earlier, there is currently a preference to maintain intrinsic ventricular activation, that is, program a longer AVI, when possible, to avoid the potential adverse effects of right ventricular apical pacing.

Mode Switching

Mode switching is the ability of the pacemaker to automatically change from one mode to another in response to an inappropriately rapid atrial rhythm (Fig. 31–14).[36] Mode switching is particularly useful for patients with paroxysmal supraventricular rhythm disturbances. In the DDD or DDDR pacing modes, if a supraventricular rhythm disturbance occurs and the pacemaker senses the pathological atrial rhythm, rapid ventricular pacing can occur. Any pacing mode that eliminates tracking of the pathological rhythm, that is, DDI, DDIR, DVI, or DVIR, also eliminates the ability to track normal sinus rhythm, which is usually the predominant rhythm. Mode switching avoids this limitation by switching from DDD or DDDR during sinus rhythm to a nontracking mode, such as DDIR, during the pathological atrial rhythm.

Rate-Adaptive Parameters

The goal of programming rate-adaptive pacemakers is to optimize the patient's chronotropic response. Some form of exercise is necessary to optimize rate-adaptive parameters. For patients who are limited to activities of daily living, informal exercise testing, such as walking at casual and brisk paces in the hospital corridor or in the outpatient facility, is often adequate. In determining the appropriate heart rate response, the patient's age and "usual activities" must be taken into consideration. If formal exercise testing is performed, a low-intensity exercise protocol that allows for a gradual increase may be preferable to a standard Bruce protocol. The chronotropic exercise assessment protocol allows for a gradual increase in speed and grade and thus mimics levels of exercise that are likely to occur during activities of daily living.

Pacemaker Complications

Complications can be divided into those related to implantation and those related to failure of a component of the pacing system. There are also problems encountered during follow-up that are actually pseudoabnormalities, that is, a normal response that appears abnormal because of unusual timing or because of idiosyncrasies of the device. Many complications are directly related to the experience of the implanter.

Implant-Related Complications

Most patients undergoing pacemaker implantation have some discomfort at the site of the incision in the early postoperative period. Mild analgesics may be required. Mild ecchymoses around the incision are not uncommon. As previously noted, if subclavian puncture is used for lead placement, several potential complications of this "blind" technique can occur, including the possibility of traumatic pneumothorax and hemopneumothorax, inadvertent arterial puncture, air embolism, arteriovenous fistula, thoracic duct injury, subcutaneous emphysema, and brachial plexus injury.

Hematoma formation at the pulse generator site occurs most commonly when anticoagulant therapy is initiated or reinstituted prematurely. A hematoma must be dealt with on the basis of its secondary consequences. Aspiration is generally not advised, and evacuation of the hematoma should be considered only if there is continued bleeding, potential compromise of the suture line or skin integrity, or pain from the hematoma that cannot be managed with analgesics.

Introduction of the lead or leads into the subclavian artery, the aorta, and the left ventricle usually is readily recognized because of the pulsatile flow of saturated blood. A pacing lead may also be placed in the left ventricle by passing it across an unsuspected atrial or ventricular septal defect (Fig. 31-15). Once the lead is within the subclavian artery, passage into the left ventricle is as easy as passage into the right ventricle via the venous system. Left ventricular lead placement should be recognized if lateral fluoroscopy is used or a lateral chest radiograph is obtained, because the lead is in the posterior aspect of the heart. The ECG during right ventricular pacing usually has a left bundle branch block (LBBB) pattern, and during left ventricular pacing, a right bundle branch block (RBBB) pattern is most common.

Although thresholds may be adequate, lead placement in the arterial circulation is associated with thrombus formation, embolization, and, consequently, stroke. The management of inadvertent left ventricular lead placement is dependent on the time it is discovered after implantation and individual patient needs and associated comorbid conditions.

Patients undergoing device implantation should be made aware of the potential for lead perforation. Although cardiac tamponade is the most dramatic outcome from perforation, lack of symptoms after ventricular perforation by a lead is not uncommon. The only sign may be a rising stimulation threshold. In other patients, the signs can include an RBBB pattern from a lead placed in the right ventricle, intercostal muscle, or diaphragmatic contraction; friction rub after implantation; and pericarditis, pericardial effusion, or cardiac tamponade. (Depending on lead

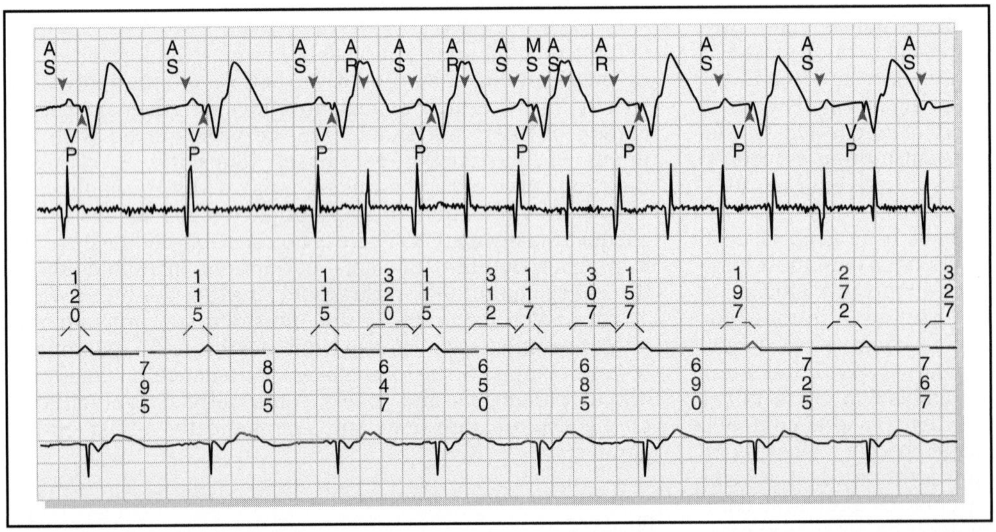

FIGURE 31–14 Electrocardiographic tracing from a patient with a DDD pacemaker. In the initial portion of the tracing, the pacing is in sinus rhythm. This is followed by the onset of an atrial tachyarrhythmia with initial tracking, but mode switching causes reversion to a DDI pacing mode. (The top tracing is the marker channel, the second tracing represents the atrial electrogram, and the third is the timing channel. The lower tracing represents the surface electrocardiogram.) Arrows indicate paced or sensed events or change in operation (mode switch [MS]). AR = atrial event in refractory period; AS = atrial sensed event; VP = ventricular paced event. Numbers above the line indicate milliseconds from one event to another (e.g., AS to VP). Numbers below the line indicate MS between ventricular events.

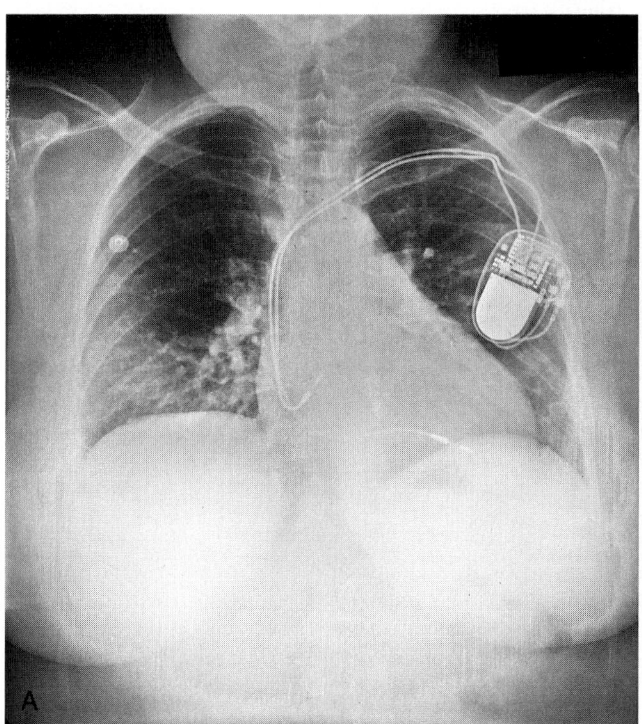

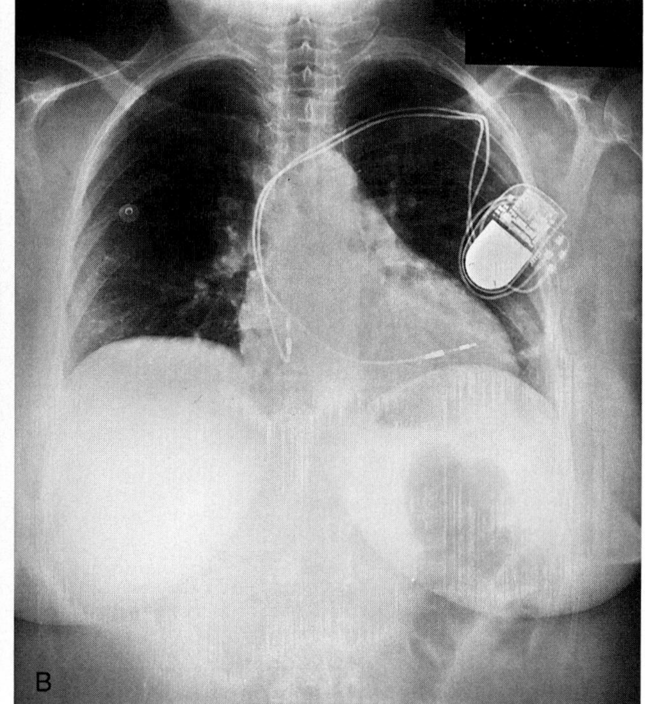

FIGURE 31–15 Posteroanterior chest radiographs of a dual-chamber pacemaker. **A,** Ventricular lead is passing through an atrial septal defect into the left ventricle. **B,** Lead is repositioned in the right ventricular apex.

position, an RBBB pattern is also possible when the lead is within the right ventricular cavity.)

Ventricular perforation may be suggested by radiography, ECG, and echocardiography. Once perforation is identified, lead withdrawal and repositioning are usually uncomplicated, although pericardial bleeding or tamponade results rarely.

Partial or silent inconsequential venous thrombosis of the subclavian vein is not uncommon after transvenous lead placement and is usually clinically insignificant. Such partial or silent thrombosis may limit venous access at the time of pacing system revision. Symptomatic thrombosis of the subclavian vein, with an edematous, painful upper extremity, is a relatively rare but recognized complication. Once again, management must be individualized. Anticoagulation will be necessary in some patients.

Lead-Related Complications

Several lead-related complications deserve attention, including lead dislodgment (Fig. 31–16), loose connector pin (Fig. 31–17), conductor coil (lead) fracture (Fig. 31–18), and insulation break.

Acceptable dislodgment rates should probably be less than 1 percent for ventricular leads and no more than 2 to 3 percent for atrial leads. Dislodgment may be radiographically evident (macrodislodgment) or not radiographically detectable (microdislodgment). Adequate lead position is assessed by posteroanterior and lateral chest radiographs and comparison with any previous chest radiographs.

Intermittent or complete failure of output can occur because of a loose connection at the interface of the lead and connector block (see Fig. 31-17), usually because the lead was inadequately secured at the time of pacemaker implantation. When a connection is loose, manipulating the pulse generator or pocket may reproduce the problem. The poor connection may be evident radiographically.

Loss of integrity of the insulating material is also uncommon and clinically can present as sensing or pacing abnormalities (or both). Both insulation defects and conductor fractures (see Fig. 31-18) can be caused by crush injury, specifically at the costoclavicular space when placement is by the subclavian puncture technique.

Supraventricular and ventricular arrhythmias, often encountered during pacemaker implantation, are usually inconsequential.

Extrasystoles can be seen in the early postimplantation period and are usually morphologically similar to the paced beats because they

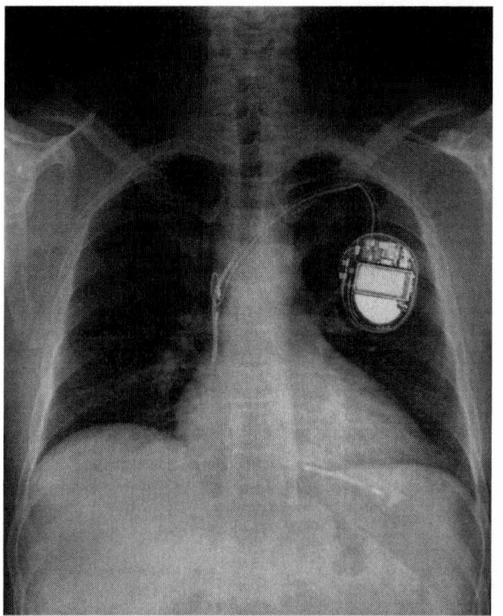

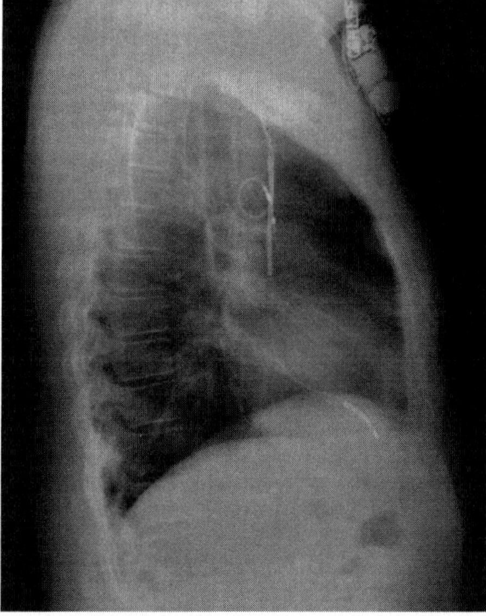

A B

FIGURE 31–16 Posteroanterior chest radiographs of a dual-chamber pacemaker. **A,** The atrial lead, originally positioned in a right atrial appendage position, is clearly no longer apically positioned. **B,** Lateral view also demonstrates definite dislodgment of the ventricular lead.

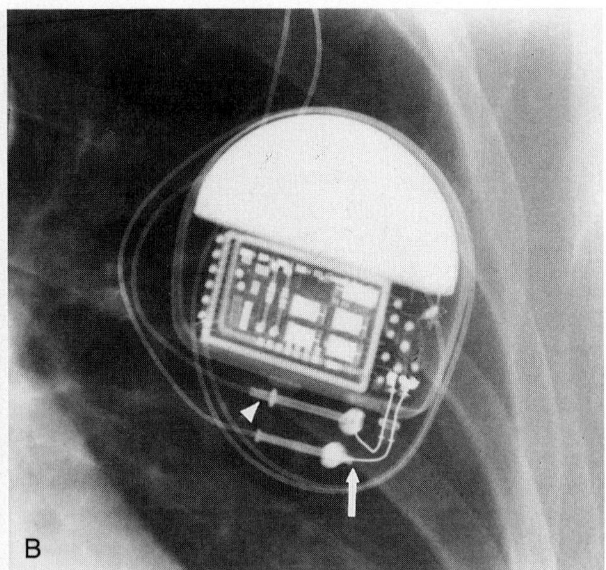

FIGURE 31–17 **A,** Posteroanterior chest radiograph in a patient with a VVI pacemaker and a bifurcated bipolar ventricular lead. The patient presented with recurrent near-syncope and intermittent failure to output. **B,** Close-up of the pacemaker shows that the lower connector pin is not securely in the connector block (arrow). (For comparison, the arrowhead indicates an appropriately engaged connector pin.) (**A** and **B,** From Hayes DL: Pacemaker radiography. *In* Furman S, Hayes DL, Holmes DR Jr [eds]: A Practice of Cardiac Pacing. 3rd ed. Mount Kisco, NY, Futura, 1993, p 361, By permission of Mayo Foundation.)

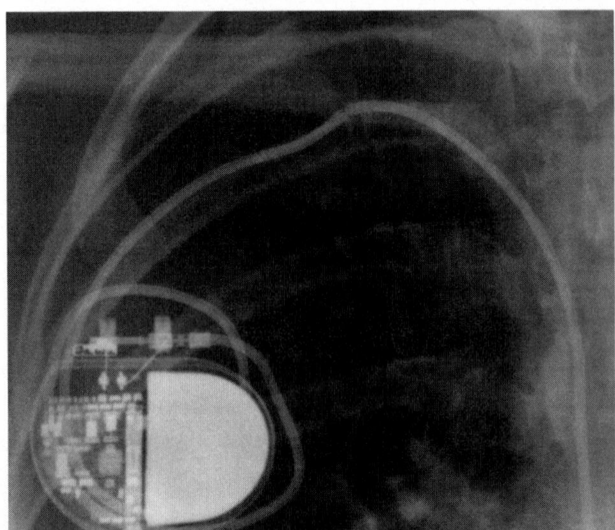

FIGURE 31–18 Close-up view of a portion of the posteroanterior chest radiograph in a patient with a single-chamber pacemaker. The lead has fractured where it passes below the clavicle. The patient presented with intermittent ventricular failure to capture and intermittent failure to output on the ventricular lead. Impedance was intermittently measured at more than 9999 Ω.

originate at the same site as the paced beats but are not preceded by a pacemaker stimulus. Such extrasystoles most often occur during the first 24 to 48 hours after implantation, usually resolve spontaneously, and almost never require pharmacological suppression. Extracardiac stimulation usually involves the diaphragm or pectoral muscle. Diaphragmatic stimulation may be due to direct stimulation of the diaphragm (usually stimulation of the left hemidiaphragm) or stimulation of the phrenic nerve (usually stimulation of the right hemidiaphragm). Diaphragmatic stimulation occurring during the early postimplantation period may be due to either microdislodgment or macrodislodgment of the pacing lead. Stimulation can be minimized or alleviated by decreasing the voltage output or pulse width (or both), but an adequate pacing margin of safety must be maintained after the output parameters are decreased. If the problem cannot be resolved by reprogramming the pacemaker output, lead repositioning will be required.

Pacemaker System Infection

Erosion is an uncommon complication that most commonly occurs because of an indolent infection, although it may also be the result of a pacemaker pocket that is too "tight."

If the patient seeks medical attention before the pacemaker has eroded through the skin, it may be possible to revise the pocket and reimplant the pacemaker. Impending erosion should be dealt with as an emergency because once any portion of the pacemaker has eroded through the skin, the only choice is removal of the pacemaker system and placement of a new system in another site.

Infection may be present even without purulent material; therefore, a specimen for culture should be obtained and proven negative before pocket revision. Adherence of the pacemaker to the skin strongly suggests an infection, and salvage of the site may not be possible.

The incidence of infection after pacemaker implantation should certainly be less than 2 percent and in most series has been less than 1 percent. Careful attention to surgical details and sterile procedures is of paramount importance in avoiding pacemaker site infection. Prophylactic use of antibiotics before implantation and in the immediate postoperative period remains controversial. Most studies do not show any significant difference in the rate of infection between patients who have had prophylactic administration of antibiotics and those who have not. Irrigation of the pacemaker pocket with an antibiotic solution at the time of pacemaker implantation is probably more important in the prevention of infection.

Pacemaker infection may appear as local inflammation or abscess formation in the pacemaker pocket, erosion of part of the pacing system with secondary infection, or sepsis with positive blood culture findings with or without a focus of infection elsewhere.

The most common clinical presentation is localized pocket infection; septicemia is uncommon. Many infectious agents can be responsible, but early infections are most commonly caused by *Staphylococcus aureus*, are aggressive, and are often associated with fever and systemic symptoms. Late infections commonly are caused by *Staphylococcus epidermidis* and are more indolent, usually without fever or systemic manifestation. Treatment for both organisms requires removal of the entire infected pacing system, pacemaker, and leads.

Troubleshooting Electrocardiographic Abnormalities

ECG abnormalities in the paced patient can be broadly grouped into failure to capture, failure to output, sensing abnormalities (undersensing or oversensing), and inappropriate rate change.

FAILURE TO CAPTURE

Failure to capture indicates that a pacing artifact is present without subsequent cardiac depolarization (Fig. 31-19). The possible causes of failure to capture are high thresholds with an inadequately programmed output, partial conductor coil fracture, insulation defect, lead dislodgment or perforation, impending total battery depletion, functional noncapture, poor or incompatible connection at the connector block, circuit failure, air in the pulse generator pocket (unipolar pacemaker), and elevated thresholds due to drugs or metabolic abnormality.

FAILURE TO PACE

Failure to pace, or failure to output, that is, failure to deliver an appropriate pacing stimulus, is often due to oversensing and inhibition of output but could also be due to true failure to output from the pacemaker or circuit interruption that prevents the electrical signal from reaching the heart (Fig. 31-20). The reasons for failure to output are circuit failure, complete or intermittent conductor coil fracture, intermittent or permanently loose set screw, incompatible lead or header, total battery depletion, internal insulation failure (bipolar lead), oversensing of any noncardiac activity, crosstalk (Fig. 31-21), and lack of anodal connector contact (e.g., unipolar lead in bipolar generator, bipolar lead in pacemaker programmed in unipolar mode, air in the pocket of a unipolar device, and unipolar pacemaker not in the pocket).

The differential diagnoses of failure to capture and failure to pace obviously overlap somewhat. For example, ECG manifestations of a conductor coil fracture may include failure to capture because of significant leakage of current at the incomplete fracture site and not enough current remaining to result in stimulation. Nonetheless, the pacemaker stimuli can appear. Alternatively, escaping current can be sensed by the pacemaker and inhibit pacemaker output. If the conductor coil is completely fractured, rendering the circuit incomplete, no pacemaker output will be detected on the ECG. Insulation defects can also be signaled by oversensing and failure to pace or by failure to capture, although the most common consequences of insulation failure are sensing abnormalities.

As the pacemaker battery reaches end stages of depletion, either failure to capture because of decreasing voltage output or failure to pace

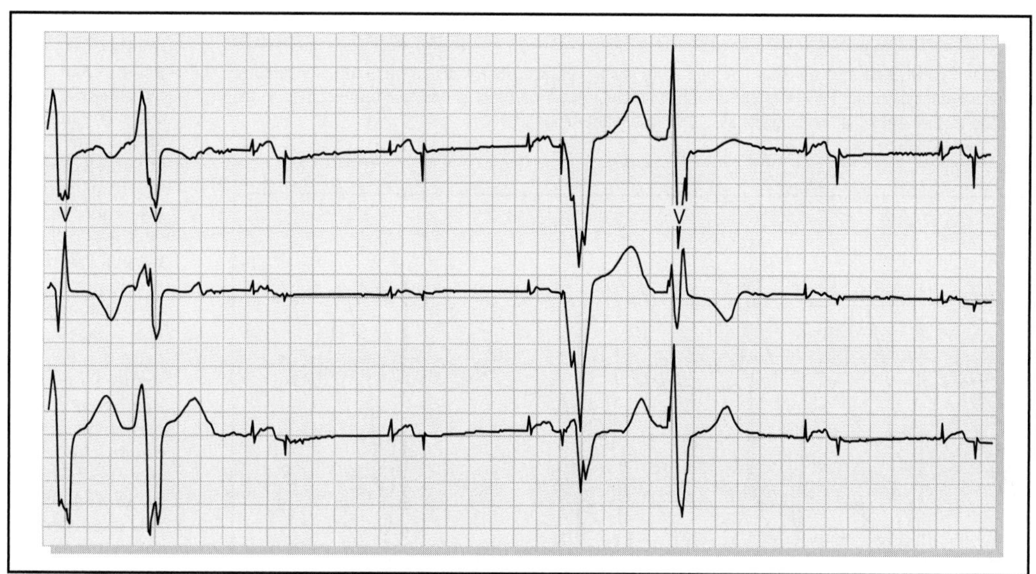

FIGURE 31–19 Electrocardiographic tracing from a patient with a DDDR pacemaker. All but one ventricular pacing artifact fail to result in ventricular depolarization, that is, failure to capture. In this patient, intermittent ventricular failure to capture was due to lead dislodgment.

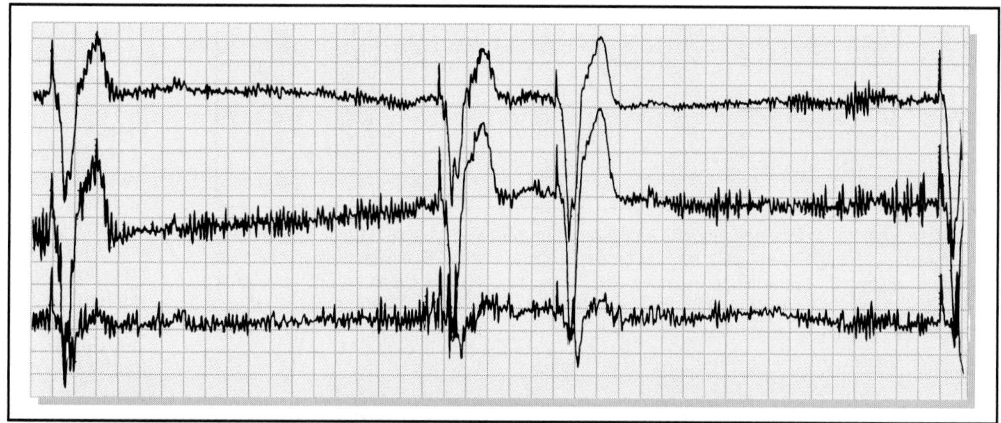

FIGURE 31–20 Electrocardiographic tracings. Patient with a VVIR pacemaker with a lower rate of 70 beats/min. After an initial paced ventricular beat, there is a pause of approximately 2.8 seconds with significant baseline artifact. After two additional paced beats, another pause of approximately 2.8 seconds occurs. This patient had a pacemaker programmed to a unipolar sensing configuration. Sensing of myopotentials led to symptomatic pauses, and reprogramming the pacemaker to a bipolar sensing configuration prevented subsequent myopotential oversensing.

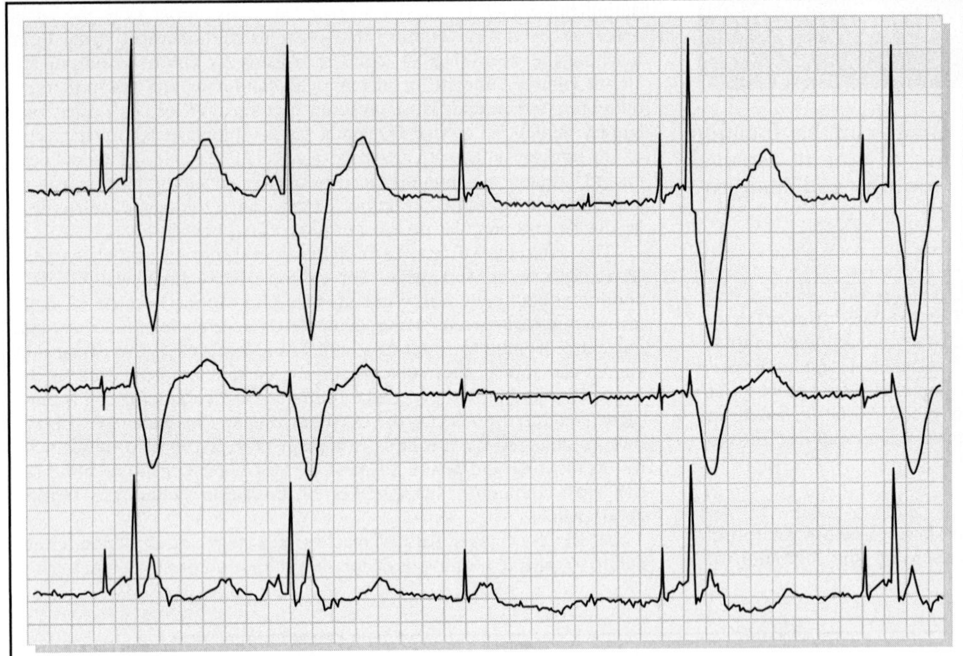

FIGURE 31–21 Patient with a DDD pacemaker. After the third atrial pacing artifact, there is evidence of atrial depolarization, but there is no ventricular pacing output. Failure to deliver the ventricular pacing artifact is due to crosstalk; that is, the atrial pacing output is sensed by the ventricular sensing circuit, with subsequent inhibition.

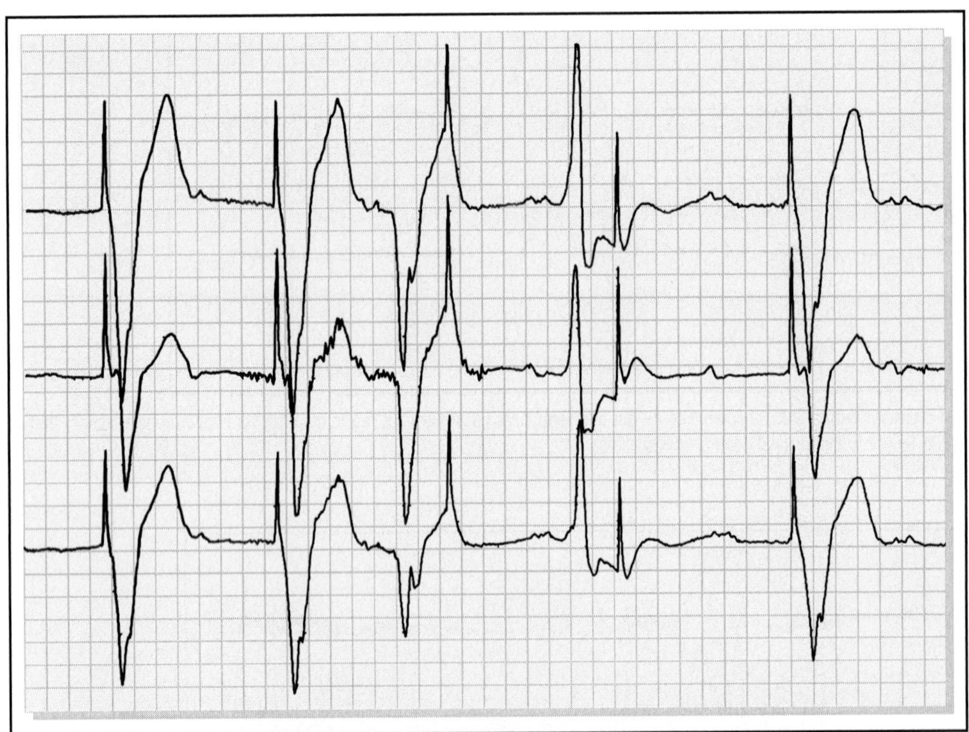

FIGURE 31–22 Electrocardiographic tracing from a patient with a VVI pacemaker with a programmed rate of 70 beats/min. After two paced ventricular complexes, a premature ventricular complex occurs. In approximately 260 milliseconds, a ventricular pacing artifact occurs. This is followed by a P wave with intrinsic atrioventricular nodal conduction and native QRS complex. A pacemaker artifact follows in approximately 220 milliseconds. This represents ventricular undersensing. In this patient, the abnormality occurred because of an insulation failure of the ventricular pacing lead.

because of total battery depletion can occur. This degree of battery depletion should be avoided by appropriate pacemaker follow-up.

Apparent failure to capture is noted if a pacemaker stimulus occurs during the refractory period of a spontaneous beat. This is referred to as *functional noncapture*.

FAILURE TO SENSE

Sensing abnormalities can be divided into *true abnormalities*, including undersensing (a failure to recognize normal intrinsic cardiac activity [Fig. 31–22] and oversensing (unexpected sensing of an intrinsic or extrinsic electrical signal [see Fig. 31–20]), and *functional sensing abnormalities*. The possible causes of sensing abnormalities are lead dislodgment or poor lead positioning, lead insulation failure, circuit failure, magnet application, malfunction of reed switch, electromagnetic interference (EMI), and battery depletion. The morphology of the intrinsic event is different from that measured at implantation.

True undersensing is most commonly due to lead dislodgment or inadequate initial lead placement. Sensing abnormalities can commonly be seen secondary to insulation defects and to intermittent "make-or-break" conductor fracture. A normally functioning pacing system at times fails to detect atrial or ventricular extrasystoles. The intrinsic events measured at the time of implantation generate an electrogram at the electrode tip. If an extrasystole is occurring elsewhere in the heart, the sensing vector is different from that of the normal intrinsic beat, and the resulting voltage generated may not be great enough to be sensed by the pacemaker. This anomaly cannot be anticipated unless extrasystoles of the same morphology occur during implantation and can be measured. It is reasonable to attempt reprogramming the sensitivity to allow the extrasystoles to be sensed, but if this is unsuccessful, it is rarely, if ever, necessary to reposition the lead for this abnormality.

Functional undersensing is present when an intrinsic cardiac event is not sensed because it falls within a programmed refractory period. For example, if an intrinsic atrial event occurs within the PVARP, the event is not, and should not be, sensed. However, without a thorough understanding of the timing cycle, it may appear as though there is true undersensing.

Fusion and pseudofusion beats occur as a result of superimposition of an ineffective pacemaker stimulus on a spontaneously occurring P wave or QRS complex (Fig. 31–23). ("Fusion" is present when the morphology of the cardiac event is a hybrid of the intrinsic morphology and the paced morphology. "Pseudofusion" is present when the pacemaker artifact occurs late enough that the intrinsic morphology is not deformed, but it may appear so because of distortion on the ECG by the superimposed pacing artifact.) Pseudofusion is usually the consequence of pacemaker discharge during the refractory period of intrinsic P or QRS before sufficient intracardiac voltage is generated to activate the sensing circuit. This is most likely to occur when the pacing rate and the intrinsic rate are similar. Also, pseudofusion beats can be the result of a delayed activation due to intraventricular conduction abnormalities.

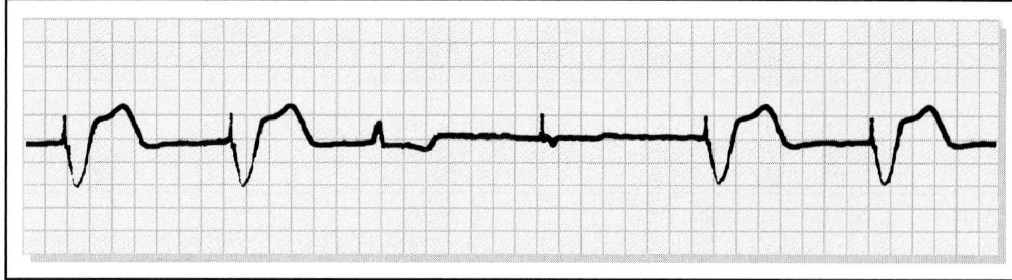

FIGURE 31–23 Electrocardiographic tracing from a patient with a VVI pacemaker. The first two complexes represent fully paced ventricular depolarizations. The third ventricular event is an intrinsic QRS complex, and the fourth event represents a fusion beat. This is followed by two paced ventricular complexes.

Implantable Cardioverter-Defibrillator Therapy

Indications for ICD Therapy

As previously noted, the ACC/AHA/NASPE guidelines for pacemakers and ICDs were updated in 2002.[2] These indications are summarized in Table 31–10, and significant changes from the previous guidelines are discussed in the following sections.

RANDOMIZED CLINICAL TRIALS OF ICD THERAPY

Clinical trials have been designed to determine the effect of ICD therapy (1) in secondary prevention of sudden cardiac death (Table 31-11), that is, in patients who have already experienced a life-threatening ventricular rhythm disturbance, and (2) in primary prevention, that is, in those who have not yet experienced a life-threatening ventricular tachyarrhythmia but are at high risk for sudden cardiac death (Table 31-12). The Antiarrhythmics Versus Implantable Defibrillators (AVID)[45] trial (secondary prevention), Multicenter Automatic Defibrillator Implantation Trial (MADIT)[46] (primary prevention), Cardiac Arrest Study Hamburg (CASH)[37] (secondary prevention), and Multicenter Unsustained Tachycardia Trial (MUSTT)[47] (primary prevention) all have demonstrated significant improvement in overall survival with ICD therapy compared with conventional or pharmacological treatment. No significant difference in overall survival was seen with ICD therapy in the Canadian Implantable Defibrillator Study (CIDS) trial (secondary prevention, probably underpowered) or the Coronary Artery Bypass Graft—Implantable Cardioverter-Defibrillator (CABG-PATCH)[48] study (primary prevention). CABG-PATCH should probably be considered separately because it randomized patients who were to undergo coronary artery bypass grafting to either ICD implantation at the time of bypass surgery or postoperative antiarrhythmic treatment. The study was terminated prematurely when the interim analysis failed to show a survival difference between the two study groups. The deaths in both groups were perioperative and, therefore, could not have been prevented by antiarrhythmic therapy. Analysis of subgroups showed the benefits of the ICD in patients at risk

TABLE 31–10 Implantable Cardioverter-Defibrillator Indications

Class I	Class II	Class III
Cardiac arrest due to VF or VT not due to a transient or reversible cause Spontaneous sustained VT associated with structural heart disease Syncope of undetermined origin with clinically relevant, hemodynamically significant sustained VT or VF induced at EP study when drug therapy is ineffective, not tolerated, or not preferred Nonsustained VT in patients with coronary disease, prior MI, LV dysfunction, and inducible VF or sustained VT at EP study not suppressible by an NYHA Class I antiarrhythmic drug Spontaneous sustained VT in patients without structural heart disease not amenable to other treatments	Patients with LVEF ≤ 30% at least 1 mo post MI and 3 mo post coronary artery revascularization surgery Cardiac arrest presumed due to VF when EP testing is precluded by other medical conditions Severe symptoms (e.g., syncope) attributable to sustained ventricular tachyarrhythmias while awaiting cardiac transplantation Familial or inherited conditions with a high risk for life-threatening ventricular tachyarrhythmias such as long-QT syndrome or hypertrophic cardiomyopathy Nonsustained VT with coronary artery disease, prior MI, and LV dysfunction, and inducible sustained VT or VF at EP study Recurrent syncope of undetermined cause in presence of ventricular dysfunction and inducible ventricular arrhythmias at EP study, when other causes of syncope have been excluded Syncope of unexplained origin or family history of unexplained sudden cardiac death associated with typical or atypical right bundle branch block and ST segment elevation (Brugada syndrome) Syncope in patients with advanced structural heart disease in whom thorough invasive and noninvasive investigations have failed to define a cause	Syncope of undetermined cause in a patient without inducible ventricular tachyarrhythmias and without structural heart disease Incessant VT or VF VF or VT resulting from arrhythmias amenable to surgical or catheter ablation, e.g., atrial arrhythmias associated with WPW, RVOT VT, idiopathic LV tachycardia, or fascicular VT Ventricular tachyarrhythmias due to transient or reversible disorder (e.g., AMI, electrolyte imbalance, drugs, or trauma) when correction of the disorder is considered feasible and likely to substantially reduce the risk of recurrent arrhythmia Significant psychiatric illnesses that may be aggravated by device implantation or may preclude systematic follow-up Terminal illnesses with projected life expectancy < 6 mo Patients with coronary artery disease with LV dysfunction and prolonged QRS duration in absence of spontaneous or inducible sustained or nonsustained VT who are undergoing coronary bypass surgery NYHA Class IV drug-refractory congestive heart failure in patients who are not candidates for cardiac transplantation

AMI = acute myocardial infarction; EP = electrophysiologic; LV = left ventricular; LVEF = left ventricular ejection fraction; MI = myocardial infarction; NYHA = New York Heart Association; RVOT = right ventricular outflow tract; VF = ventricular fibrillation; VT = ventricular tachycardia; WPW = Wolfe-Parkinson-White syndrome.

TABLE 31–11 Secondary Prevention of Sudden Cardiac Death

Study	Patient Inclusion Criteria	Endpoint(s)	Treatment Arms	Key Results
AVID	Survivor of cardiac arrest VT with syncope Symptomatic sustained VT with LVEF ≤ 0.40	Total mortality Mode of death Quality of life Cost benefit	Amiodarone or sotalol	Significant improvement in overall survival with ICD
CASH[37]	Survivor of cardiac arrest	Total mortality Recurrences of arrhythmias requiring CPR Recurrence of unstable VT	ICD Amiodarone, propafenone, or metoprolol	Significant improvement in overall survival with ICD
CIDS	Survivor of cardiac arrest Syncope with symptomatic sustained VT with LVEF ≤ 0.35 or syncope with inducible VT	Total mortality	Amiodarone	No significant improvement in survival with ICD
MAVERIC[38]	Resuscitated VT/VF, SCD Sustained nonsyncopal VT Dilated nonischemic cardiomyopathy with EF ≤ 0.35, syncope, and NSVT or positive SAECG	All-cause mortality Event-free survival Costs Quality of life Cost-effectiveness	Empirical amiodarone EP-guided therapy (drug or nondrug) Immediate ICD implantation	In progress
ASTRID	Patients with Ventak AV 1810 implanted for current indication DFT < 600 V and minimum 1 mV atrial, 5 mV ventricular EGM amplitudes at implantation	Time to first occurrence of inappropriate therapy Health care utilization Quality of life	Standard-features programming Enhanced-features programming	Completed; results not published

ASTRID = Atrial Sensing Trial to Prevent Inappropriate Detections; AVID = Antiarrhythmics Versus Implantable Defibrillators; CASH = Cardiac Arrest Study Hamburg; CIDS = Canadian Implantable Defibrillator Study; CPR = cardiopulmonary resuscitation; DFT = defibrillation threshold; EF = ejection fraction; EGM = electrogram; EP = electrophysiologic; ICD = implantable cardioverter-defibrillator; LVEF = left ventricular ejection fraction; MAVERIC = Midlands Trial of Empirical Amiodarone Versus Electrophysiologically Guided Intervention and Cardioverter Implant in Ventricular Arrhythmias; NSVT = nonsustained ventricular tachycardia; SAECG = signal-averaged electrocardiography; SCD = sudden cardiac death; VF = ventricular fibrillation; VT = ventricular tachycardia.

CH 31

for life-threatening ventricular tachyarrhythmia.[49] The role of ICD therapy for patients with asymptomatic sustained monomorphic ventricular tachycardia and structural heart disease but with an ejection fraction greater than 0.40 is less clear.[50]

Impact of Left Ventricular Function

Patients with coronary artery disease and reduced left ventricular function appear to experience greater benefit with ICD therapy than with drug therapy.[46] In the AVID trial, patients with an ejection fraction greater than 0.35 who received an ICD did not have a significant mortality benefit over those who received amiodarone therapy. Similarly, in post hoc analyses of MADIT-I, patients with a lower left ventricular ejection demonstrated the greatest mortality benefit.[46]

The MADIT-II trial evaluated ICD therapy as primary prevention in 1352 patients with a left ventricular ejection fraction no greater than 0.30 and a previous myocardial infarction.[9] Patients were randomized to ICD or conventional medical therapy. Patients who received an ICD had a 31 percent reduction in mortality (see Fig. 24–7). Based largely on this trial, the most recent ACC/AHA/NASPE guidelines include patients who meet MADIT-II criteria as a class IIa indication for ICD implantation. This significantly expands the patient population eligible for ICD therapy. MADIT-II criteria—previous myocardial infarction and left ventricular ejection fraction of 0.30 or less—have been approved as a reimbursable indication for ICD therapy but with the added criterion of QRS duration longer than 120 milliseconds.

Although MADIT-II addressed patients with reduced left ventricular function secondary to an ischemic event, it did not address patients with symptomatic congestive heart failure or those with an idiopathic dilated cardiomyopathy. In patients with idiopathic dilated cardiomyopathy (see Chap. 59), the combination of poor left ventricular function and nonsustained ventricular tachycardia is associated with an increased risk of sudden death (see Chap. 30).[45] A few trials evaluating ICD therapy as primary prevention in patients with dilated cardiomyopathy have been completed and several are under way (Table 31-13).

Trials evaluating combined CRT and ICD therapy have also been performed, with others in progress. The InSync ICD trial and CONTAK-CD studies included patients who met criteria for CRT and a clinical requirement for ICD therapy, that is, secondary prevention. Both trials demonstrated the safety and efficacy of a combined CRT and ICD device but were not designed as mortality trials.

The Comparison of Medical Therapy, Pacing, and Defibrillation (COMPANION) trial, presented but not published (ACC, 2003), was the first CRT and CRT with cardioverter-defibrillator capability (CRT/ICD) trial designed to assess all-cause mortality. In this trial, 1634 patients with left ventricular dysfunction of either idiopathic or ischemic etiology were randomized to optimized medical therapy, optimized medical therapy and CRT, or optimized medical therapy and CRT with ICD therapy. The study, terminated early by the data safety monitoring board, demonstrated a 43 percent decrease in mortality among patients who received CRT with ICD therapy when compared with the patients receiving only optimized medical therapy ($p = 0.02$). CRT therapy alone insignificantly reduced mortality by approximately 24 percent when compared with medical therapy ($p = 0.12$). Initial reports suggested that there was no difference in response or mortality outcomes between ischemic and nonischemic causes. Both CRT and CRT/ICD therapy decreased hospitalizations by approximately 19 percent over medical therapy alone.

The impact of CRT and CRT/ICD on mortality will be further defined by ongoing studies. The Cardiac Resynchronization in Heart Failure study has completed enrollment and will assess the effect of CRT on all-cause mortality and unplanned cardiovascular hospitalization as the primary endpoints.[51]

TABLE 31–12 Primary Prevention of Sudden Cardiac Death

Study	Patient Inclusion Criteria	Endpoint(s)	Treatment Arms	Key Results
MADIT	Q wave MI ≥ 3 wk Asymptomatic NSVT LVEF ≤ 0.35 Inducible and nonsuppressible VT on EPS with procainamide NYHA Classes I-III	Overall mortality Costs and cost-effectiveness	ICD ($n = 95$) Conventional therapy ($n = 101$)	ICDs reduced overall mortality by 54% ICDs cost $16,900 per life-year saved *vs.* Conventional therapy
CABG-PATCH	Scheduled for elective CABG surgery LVEF < 0.36 Abnormal SAECG	Overall mortality	ICD ($n = 446$) Standard treatment ($n = 454$)	Survival not improved by prophylactic implantation of ICD at time of elective CABG
MUSTT	CAD EF ≤ 0.40 NSVT Inducible VT or VF	Sudden arrhythmic death or spontaneous sustained VT	ICD in nonsuppressible group AAD therapy in suppressible group No therapy	Patients receiving ICD had > 70% risk reduction in arrhythmic death or cardiac arrest and > 50% reduction in total mortality
CAT[39]	Nonischemic DCM LVEF ≤ 0.30 NYHA Class II or III	Total mortality Sudden death Serious arrhythmia	ICD Standard treatment	Cumulative survival was not significantly different between the two groups at 2- and 4-yr follow-up
BEST-ICD[40]	Acute MI EF ≤ 0.40 SDRR < 70 msec or ≥ 109 PVCs/hr or abnormal SAECG	All-cause mortality Cost-effectiveness	Conventional + BB therapy EPS: if inducible, ICD and BB; if noninducible, BB	No significant survival improvement with ICD (concern that too few patients enrolled to draw firm conclusion)
DINAMIT	Acute MI (6-21 d) LVEF ≤ 0.35 HR ≥ 80 beats/min or SDRR < 70 msec	All-cause mortality Quality of life Cost-effectiveness	Conventional therapy ICD	Optimal medical therapy (OMT) *vs.* OMT + ICD Death from any cause NS, $p = 0.66$ Arrhythmic death lower with ICD, $p = 0.009$ Non-arrhythmic death. Risk lower in OMT group, $p = 0.016$
MADIT-II[41]	Prior MI EF ≤ 0.30	All-cause mortality Cost-effectiveness	Conventional therapy ICD	With ICD, 31% reduction in mortality
SCD-HeFT[42]	Ischemic or nonischemic cardiomyopathy EF ≤ 0.35 NYHA Class II or III Appropriate ACE inhibitor No history of sustained VT/VF	All-cause mortality Quality of life Cost-effectiveness Morbidity Incidence of arrhythmias	Placebo and standard therapy *vs.* Amiodarone and standard therapy *vs.* ICD and standard therapy	In progress; enrollment completed Mortality by intention to treat: Amiodarone *vs.* Placebo, NS, $p = 0.529$ ICD *vs.* Placebo, ICD lowers mortality by 23%, $p = 0.007$
DEBUT (SUDS)[43]	Survivor of sudden cardiac arrest from resuscitated VT/VF Probable sudden cardiac arrest with RBBB and ST elevation	All-cause mortality Rhythms via stored EGMs that triggered ICD shocks	ICD *vs.* BB	Study terminated early after no deaths in ICD group vs. four deaths in BB group
PRIDE	VT, VF, or nonischemic cardiomyopathy with EF < 0.35 and NSVT or positive SAECG	All-cause mortality Hospitalization due to CHF	ICD *vs.* EPS and randomization to ICD *vs.* Amiodarone or sotalol Negative EPS: therapy at physician discretion	In progress; follow-up to be completed in 2004

Continued

TABLE 31–12 Primary Prevention of Sudden Cardiac Death—cont'd

Study	Patient Inclusion Criteria	Endpoint(s)	Treatment Arms	Key Results
AMIOVIRT[44]	Patients with nonischemic dilated cardiomyopathy and nonsustained VT and EF ≤ 0.35	Primary Total mortality Secondary Arrhythmia-free survival Quality of life Costs	Amiodarone *vs.* ICD	Mortality and quality of life not significantly different between the two arms
SEDET	Acute MI (1-3 wk) Ineligible for thrombolysis EF ≥ 0.15 to ≤ 0.40 NSVT or ≥ 10 PVCs/hr between 6 and 21 d after MI	All-cause mortality Quality of life Incidence of VT Sudden and nonsudden death Cardiac death Predictive value of BRS and HRV	ICD *vs.* Conventional therapy	In progress
IRIS	Acute MI Fast NSVT > 150 beats/min HR > 100 beats/min at admission	All-cause mortality	ICD *vs.* Conventional therapy	In progress

AAD = antiarrhythmia drug; ACE = angiotensin-converting enzyme; AMIOVIRT = Amiodarone Versus Implantable Cardioverter-Defibrillator Trial; BB = beta blocker; BEST-ICD = Beta-Blocker Strategy Plus Implantable Cardioverter-Defibrillator; BRS = baroreceptor sensitivity; CABG = coronary artery bypass graft; CABG-PATCH = Coronary Artery Bypass Graft Patch Trial; CAD = coronary artery disease; CAT = Cardiomyopathy Trial; CHF = congestive heart failure; DCM = dilated cardiomyopathy; DEBUT (SUDS) = Defibrillator Versus Beta Blockers for Unexplained Death in Thailand (Sudden Unexplained Death Syndrome); DINAMIT = Defibrillator in Acute Myocardial Infarction Trial; EF = ejection fraction; EGM = electrogram; EPS = electrophysiologic study; HR = heart rate; HRV = heart rate variability; ICD = implantable cardioverter-defibrillator; IRIS = Immediate Risk Stratification Improves Survival; LVEF = left ventricular ejection fraction; MADIT = Multicenter Automatic Defibrillator Implantation Trial; MI = myocardial infarction; MUSTT = Multicenter Unsustained Tachycardia Trial; NSVT = nonsustained ventricular tachycardia; NYHA = New York Heart Association; PRIDE = Primary Implantation of Cardioverter-Defibrillator in High-Risk Ventricular Arrhythmias; PVC = premature ventricular contraction; RBBB = right bundle branch block; SAECG = signal-averaged electrocardiography; SCD-HeFT = Sudden Cardiac Death in Heart Failure Trial; SDRR = standard deviation of RR interval; SEDET = South European Defibrillator Trial; VF = ventricular fibrillation; VT = ventricular tachycardia.

There are a number of inherited arrhythmia conditions such as long-QT syndrome,[52] Brugada syndrome, right ventricular arrhythmogenic dysplasia (see Chap. 32), hypertrophic cardiomyopathy (see Chap. 59),[53] and others for which an ICD is often recommended.

The patient with idiopathic ventricular fibrillation should receive an ICD. Some patients with idiopathic ventricular tachycardia and no structural heart disease should probably be considered for catheter ablation before consideration of ICD therapy (see Chap. 32).

ICD Design

The basic components of the ICD are electronic circuitry, power source, and memory, with a microprocessor coordinating the various parts of the system.[54] High-voltage capacitors transform the battery-provided voltage into discharges ranging from less than 1 V for pacing to 750 V for defibrillation. ICDs incorporate a different sensing circuit than most pacemakers. Because of the need to reliably sense low-amplitude signals during ventricular fibrillation and to avoid sensing extracardiac noise and cardiac signals other than ventricular tachycardia or fibrillation, the sensing circuit is designed to automatically adjust either the gain or the sensing threshold.[54]

Virtually all ICD systems are implanted transvenously and include antitachycardia pacing (ATP) and ventricular bradycardia pacing, dual-chamber pacing with rate-adaptive options.[55] In addition, atrial defibrillation capabilities, as well as CRT features, are available in some devices. The longevity of ICDs depends on the frequency of shock delivery, the degree of pacemaker dependency, and other programmable options, but most are expected to last from 5 to 9 years. All currently available ICDs use biphasic shock waveforms, but the specifics of the waveform differ among various manufacturers.

The ICD functions by continuously monitoring the patient's cardiac rate and delivering therapy when the rate exceeds the programmed rate "cutoff." For example, if the ICD is programmed to treat ventricular tachyarrhythmias at a rate cutoff of 175 beats/min, once the ICD detects a rate greater than 175 beats/min it delivers ATP or charges and delivers a shock, depending on the programmed therapy.

ATP has the advantage of terminating a rhythm disturbance without delivery of a shock. ICDs capable of ATP have significant programming flexibility to adjust many aspects of tachycardia detection and therapy, thereby customizing therapy for the individual patient. Different "zones" or "tiers" of therapy can be programmed to detect ventricular tachyarrhythmias to allow slower arrhythmias to be treated with ATP before a shock is delivered but to still allow faster tachycardias to be treated more aggressively. The programming for a hypothetical patient is outlined in Table 31–14. In this patient, slower ventricular tachycardia in the range of 126 to 190 beats/min is treated with ATP therapies in zone 1. If initial ATP therapy (ATP-1) is unsuccessful, a second and different ATP therapy (ATP-2) is automatically delivered. If this is unsuccessful, lower energy shocks are attempted before high-energy shocks are delivered. Shocks are synchronized during ventricular tachycardia (cardioversion) or are asynchronous during ventricular fibrillation (defibrillation). A second zone of therapy is determined for a faster ventricular tachycardia, and still faster ventricular tachycardia or ventricular fibrillation is treated aggressively with a high-energy shock. In addition, current ICDs provide bradycardia support, as single- or dual-chamber devices.

The zones, detection rates of the different zones, specifics of the different therapies, and bradycardia pacing options all are programmable, and programming flexibility varies significantly from device to device.

TABLE 31–13 ICD Trials in Patients with Congestive Heart Failure and ICD/CRT Trials

Study	Patient Inclusion Criteria	Endpoint(s)	Treatment Arms	Key Results
VENTAK-CHF/ CONTAK CD	Indication for ICD Symptomatic CHF on stable drugs, including ACE inhibitors EF ≤ 0.35 QRS > 120 msec	Primary composite endpoint of mortality, HF, hospitalizations, and episodes of ventricular tachycardia or ventricular fibrillation	BiV pacing or no pacing and then crossover (ICD therapy was in both arms)	Composite endpoint insignificant trend favoring CRT Peak V_{O_2}, 6-min hall walk, quality of life, NYHA Class all improved significantly with CRT
DEFINITE	Symptomatic nonischemic cardiomyopathy NSVT Low EF	All-cause mortality	ICD, standard drug therapy, and BB *vs.* Standard drug therapy and BB only	2-year mortality: no ICD, 13.8%; ICD, 8.1%; relative risk reduction (RR), 34%; arrhythmia deaths decrease (RR = 74%); $p = 0.01$).
Defibrillat	Patient with CHF awaiting heart transplant	Total mortality Serious arrhythmias	ICD Standard treatment	In progress
COMPANION	NYHA Classes II-IV EF ≤ 0.35 QRS ≥ 120 msec PR interval > 150 msec No conventional device indications	All-cause mortality and hospitalization Cardiac morbidity Long-term survival Functional capacity in HF patients (substudy)	Optimized medical therapy *vs.* CRT *vs.* CRT/ICD	43% mortality reduction with CRT/ICD 24% mortality reduction with CRT 19% reduction in hospitalization with CRT/ICD and CRT
BELIEVE	NYHA Classes II-IV QRS > 130 msec EF ≤ 0.35 LBBB LVEDD ≥ 55 mm ICD indications	LV-only pacing safe and effective BiV ATP safe and effective	LV CRT + RV ATP vs. BiV CRT + BiV ATP	In progress
MIRACLE-ICD	NYHA Classes II-IV QRS > 130 msec EF < 0.35 LVEDD > 55 mm Indication for ICD	Device safety and efficacy Quality of life 6-min walk		

ACE = angiotensin-converting enzyme; ATP = antitachycardia pacing; BB = beta blocker; BELIEVE = Biventricular Versus Left Ventricular Pacing in Italian Evaluation on Heart Failure Patients with Ventricular Arrhythmias; BiV = biventricular; CHF = congestive heart failure; COMPANION = Comparison of Medical Therapy, Pacing, and Defibrillation in Heart Failure; CRT = cardiac resynchronization therapy; CRT/ICD = CRT with cardioverter-defibrillator capability; Defibrillat = Defibrillator Implantation as a Bridge to Transplantation; DEFINITE = Defibrillators in Nonischemic Cardiomyopathy Treatment Evaluation; EF = ejection fraction; HF, heart failure; ICD = implantable cardioverter-defibrillator; LBBB = left bundle branch block; LV = left ventricular; LVEDD = left ventricular end-diastolic dimension; MIRACLE-ICD = Multicenter InSync Randomized Clinical Evaluation—Implantable Cardioverter-Defibrillator; NSVT = nonsustained ventricular tachycardia; NYHA = New York Heart Association; RV = right ventricular; VENTAK-CHF/CONTAK CD = Ventak-Congestive Heart Failure/Contak Cardioverter-Defibrillator.

TABLE 31–14 Implantable Cardioverter-Defibrillator Therapy

Zone	Tachycardia Rate (beats/min)	Sequence of Therapy Delivered
1	126-160	ATP-1, ATP-2, 1 J, 5 J, 34 J
2	161-200	ATP, 10 J, 34 J
3	>200	34 J

ATP = antitachycardia pacing therapy; ATP-1 = first ATP; ATP-2 = second (and different) ATP.

Device Selection

Considerations about the type of ICD to select for a given patient include whether the patient has bradycardia requiring pacing support, has associated atrial tachyarrhythmias, or would benefit from CRT (or a combination of these). The need for bradycardia support requires a choice between single- and dual-chamber ICD based on the mode selection algorithm already described.

The recent trend in the United States has been to implant more dual-chamber ICDs. However, data from the recent Dual-chamber and VVIT Implantable Defibrillator (DAVID) trial suggest that single-chamber ICD therapy may be advantageous if the patient does not have associated bradyarrhythmias.[56] In 506 patients with a left ventricular ejection fraction of 0.40 or less and no indication for cardiac pacing, dual-chamber pacing offered no clinical advantage over ventricular back-up pacing. Patients whose device was programmed to the DDD pacing at 70 beats/min experienced 1-year survival free of the composite endpoint (time to death or first hospitalization for congestive heart failure) of 73.3 percent compared with 83.9 percent for the VVI (40 beats/min) back-up pacing group (relative hazard, 1.61; 95 percent confidence interval [CI], 1.06 to 2.44). Mortality was also slightly higher (10.1 percent) for the dual-chamber patients than for the patients programmed to VVI at 40 beats/min (6.5 percent; relative hazard, 1.61; 95 percent CI, 0.84 to 3.09). The investigators suggested that the adverse effects of right ventricular apical pacing may account for the differences seen in the study.

If the patient has associated atrial tachyarrhythmias, a dual-chamber ICD capable of detecting and treating atrial tachyarrhythmias should be considered. Some devices also provide the ability to cardiovert atrial tachyarrhythmias.

As previously noted, devices that combine CRT and ICD therapy can be considered for patients who meet CRT criteria.

Issues Unique to ICD Implantation

When the ICD is placed transvenously with the pulse generator in the prepectoral position, the implantation technique and related complications are the same as those for pacemaker implantation, with the exception that complications can arise as a result of determining the defibrillation threshold (DFT). (*DFT* can be defined as the minimal energy that terminates ventricular fibrillation.[54]) Most ICD implantations are performed with conscious sedation and local anesthesia, with mask-supported ventilation. When DFT determination is completed, the patient can be allowed to recover from deeper anesthesia as the pocket is closed.

An acceptable DFT is a value that ensures an adequate safety margin for defibrillation, usually being at least 10 J less than the maximum output of the ICD, which ranges from 30 to 41 J of stored energy. It is difficult to state an "ideal" DFT because ideally it is the lowest achievable DFT with an adequate safety margin.

Generally, the preference is to implant the ICD in the left pectoral region because of a more favorable vector for delivery of the shock. Although successful defibrillation can usually be accomplished with a right-sided implant, the shocking vector is less optimal and may have an effect on achievable DFT.[57] Regardless of whether the ICD is placed on the right or the left side, in a small percentage of patients adequate DFT cannot be achieved with standard lead placement. In this situation, options include repositioning the ventricular lead to an alternative site or adding another lead in a subcutaneous position or within the superior vena cava.

Complications

Frequent ICD discharges may represent a clinical emergency. These discharges may be appropriate or inappropriate (Table 31–15). Appropriate discharges represent frequently occurring ventricular tachycardia or fibrillation or an electrical storm (see Chap. 32). If the device is discharging frequently because the defibrillation is unsuccessful, the device may have been programmed to an inappropriately low shock output or the DFT may have increased, for example, in response to a drug such as amiodarone (see Chap. 30).

Inappropriate discharges are usually the result of detection of a supraventricular tachyarrhythmia, most commonly atrial fibrillation. Inappropriate discharge can also be the result of device failure, for example, lead fracture with generation of make-or-break signals.

TABLE 31–15 Differential Diagnosis and Management of Multiple Implantable Cardioverter-Defibrillator (ICD) Shocks

Clinical Finding	Management
Frequent ventricular tachycardia or ventricular fibrillation (electrical storm)	Reassess antiarrhythmic therapy and programmed ICD therapy
Unsuccessful ICD therapy due to inappropriately low-output shock or elevation of defibrillation threshold	Reprogram ICD Assess potential causes of defibrillation threshold increase (e.g., drugs)
Lead fracture Lead dislodgment	Replace fractured lead Reposition lead
Sensing supraventricular rhythms	Reassess antiarrhythmic therapy Reprogram ICD parameters Ablate supraventricular arrhythmic focus
Oversensing separate pacing system	Reprogram pacemaker or ICD (or both) Reposition pacemaker or ICD leads (or both) Remove pacemaker and replace ICD with another ICD with more sophisticated bradycardia support
Oversensing electromagnetic interference	Avoid source Reprogram ICD
Oversensing intracardiac signals	Reprogram ICD Reposition sensing lead

Modified from Pinsky SL, Fahy GJ: Implantable cardioverter-defibrillators. Am J Med 106:446-458, 1999. Reprinted by permission of Excerpta Medica.

Electromagnetic Interference

EMI is defined as any signal—biological or nonbiological—that is within a frequency spectrum detectable by the sensing circuitry of the pacemaker or ICD. EMI can result in rate alteration, sensing abnormalities, asynchronous pacing, noise reversion, or reprogramming.[58] EMI can also cause failure to deliver antibradycardia pacing, inappropriate delivery of antitachycardia therapy, resetting of programmed parameters, and damage to the pulse generator or myocardial interface.

Other cardiac and extracardiac signals that can be falsely interpreted as a P wave or QRS complex and result in oversensing include T waves (Fig. 31–24), myopotential interference, afterpotential delay, and P waves.

Sources of EMI can be within and outside the hospital. Although multiple sources of EMI in the nonhospital environment can potentially result in single-beat inhibition, few, if any, of these are clinically significant and truly represent a threat to the paced patient.

Several potential sources of EMI require specific mention either because of their real potential for causing significant EMI or because of existing confusion or controversy. Industrial-strength welding equipment, certain degaussing equipment, and induction ovens are identified sources of EMI that can cause significant pacemaker or ICD interference. Most welding equipment used for "hobby" welding should not cause any significant problems. For the pacemaker-dependent patient who does hobby welding or any other activity that raises the clinician's concerns about EMI, the environment should be determined safe for the patient before the activity is condoned.

Currently, there is much interest in the potential EMI that may emanate from cellular telephones[59,60] and antitheft devices.[61] Available information suggests that commercially available cellular phones are safe for the device patient as long as some simple guidelines are followed. The patient should avoid having the "activated" cellular phone directly over the pacemaker or ICD, either from random motion of the phone or by carrying the activated phone in a breast pocket over the device.

Antitheft devices also have potential for pacemaker interference.[61] Practical suggestions are for patients with pacemakers or ICDs to be aware of electronic equipment for surveillance of articles and to avoid leaning on or lingering near such devices. If the patient passes through the equipment at a normal pace, adverse effects are quite unlikely. Any patient who feels unusual in any way when near electronic surveillance equipment should move away.

Hospital sources of potentially significant EMI are electrocautery, cardioversion, defibrillation, magnetic resonance imaging (MRI), lithotripsy,[62] radiofrequency ablation, electroshock therapy, and diathermy. The most important aspect of pacemaker or ICD care after exposure to any of these sources of EMI is to reassess the device to be certain that programmed parameters have not been changed.

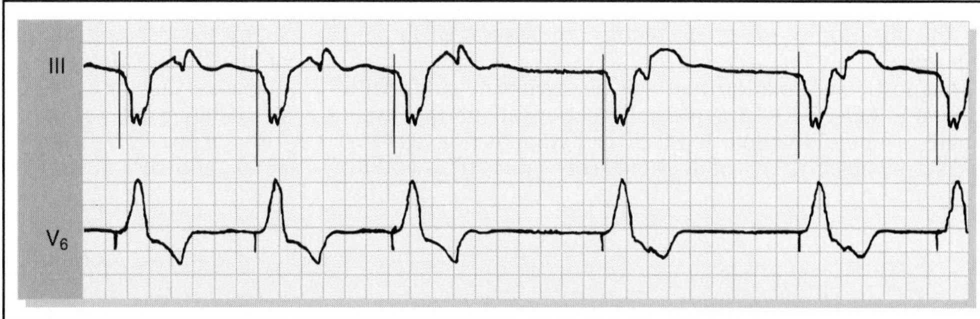

FIGURE 31–24 Electrocardiographic tracing from a patient with a VVI pacemaker programmed to a rate of 70 beats/min (857 milliseconds). The third and fourth VV cycles are longer than the programmed lower rate. Measuring 857 milliseconds backward from the ventricular pacing artifact at the end of the longer cycles locates the point at which there was oversensing. In this case, probably the T wave is sensed. Definite retrograde P waves can be recognized by deformation of the T wave. Although it is possible that the retrograde P wave is being oversensed, the relationship of the P waves does not appear to consistently coincide with the point of oversensing.

One of the most frequent questions asked is how to manage the patient with a pacemaker or ICD during an operative procedure, given the potential effects of electrocautery and guidelines for cardioversion and defibrillation. Routine interrogation of the device and deactivation of ICD therapy should be accomplished before the operation. After the procedure, the device should be reinterrogated and ICD therapy reinitiated. (During the time ICD therapy is "off," the patient must be monitored.) For pacemaker-dependent patients, it is reasonable to program the pacemaker to an asynchronous pacing mode, VOO or DOO, or to achieve the same effect by placing a magnet over the pacemaker throughout the procedure. The potential effects of electrocautery are reprogramming; permanent damage to the pulse generator; pacemaker inhibition; reversion to a fall-back mode, noise reversion mode,[63] or electrical reset; and myocardial thermal damage. The guidelines for cardioversion and defibrillation in the patient with a pacemaker or ICD are as follows: ideally, place paddles in the anteroposterior position, try to keep the paddles at least 4 inches from the pulse generator, have the appropriate pacemaker programmer available, and interrogate the pacemaker after the procedure.

Given the increasing utilization of MRI, potential interference with implantable devices merits mention. MRI is still considered a relative contraindication in patients with a pacemaker or ICD given the potential for induction of rapid hemodynamically unstable ventricular rhythms and the theoretical possibility of heating of the conductor coil and thermal damage at the electrode-myocardial interface. Although there are reports of MRI being performed safely in non–pacemaker-dependent patients, there are also reports of deaths resulting from MRI-induced rhythm disturbances.

Interference from Drugs and Metabolic Abnormalities

Drugs can affect sensing thresholds, pacing thresholds, and DFTs and result in ECG abnormalities.[58,64] Although many drugs have been reported to affect pacing thresholds, class 1C agents are the only drugs that commonly cause a problem. Flecainide and propafenone have the potential to increase pacing thresholds and sensing thresholds. If these drugs are administered to the patient with a pacemaker, especially a pacemaker-dependent patient, thresholds should be monitored for change. Amiodarone does not consistently affect pacing thresholds. Changes in drug therapy must also be monitored closely in the patient with an ICD.[64] In addition to altering pacing thresholds and increasing DFTs, certain drugs have the potential for interaction by altering the detection of ventricular tachycardia and producing proarrhythmic effects. Drug-induced slowing of the rate of ventricular tachycardia can result in inadequate detection of the arrhythmia. The DFT can increase from the administration of amiodarone.[65] Other drugs can theoretically increase the DFT or have been reported to do so in single case reports, but a clinically significant change does not often result.[64]

Electrolyte and metabolic abnormalities can also affect pacing and sensing thresholds. Hyperkalemia is the most common electrolyte abnormality to cause clinically significant problems, but severe acidosis or alkalosis, hypercapnia, severe hyperglycemia, hypoxemia, and hypothyroidism can also alter thresholds.

Device Follow-Up

Patients with pacemakers and ICDs must be followed on a regular schedule. There are different follow-up methods depending on clinician preference. For pacemaker follow-up, some caregivers prefer regular office assessment, others prefer transtelephonic follow-up, and still others prefer a combination of the two techniques. Transtelephonic assessment should include collection of a nonmagnet ECG strip, an ECG strip with magnet applied to the pacemaker, and measurement of magnet rate and pulse duration (pulse duration on both atrial and ventricular channels should be measured for a dual-chamber pacemaker). During an office visit, the same information should be collected. In addition, on some periodic basis, for example, once a year, patients whose device is programmed to a rate-adaptive pacing mode should be assessed to determine whether rate-response is appropriate.

Internet-based device follow-up has been introduced recently and marks the first major change in device follow-up in many years.[66,67]

Follow-up of the patient with an ICD must include periodic visits during which specific information is collected and assessed. In addition, patients may require interim assessment if there are concerns about the appropriateness of delivered therapy or other changes in the patient's medical status or drug regimen that could affect ICD therapy.

The electrophysiologist or an allied professional with ICD expertise and immediate access to the electrophysiologist should perform follow-up procedures. Aspects of follow-up include history with specific emphasis on awareness of delivered therapy and any tachyarrhythmic events, device interrogation, assessment of battery status and charge time, retrieval and assessment of stored diagnostic data, periodic radiographic assessment, and periodic arrhythmic induction in the electrophysiology laboratory to assess DFTs and efficacy.

Diagnostic information that can be retrieved varies with different ICDs. ICDs provide information about the cycle length or rate of the detected tachyarrhythmias (Fig. 31–25), and stored electrograms of detected arrhythmias (Fig. 31–26).

Follow-up protocols for patients with ICDs vary. Many caregivers are comfortable with follow-up every 3 to 6 months for the first 3 to 4 years, after which follow-up frequency increases. Currently, Internet-based retrieval is available but not widely used.

Frequency of DFT testing may depend on the type of ICD system and DFT at implant or change in medications.

COUNTER DATA REPORT -- Page 1 of 2

Date Interrogated: Jun 18, 1999 12:29:28
Counters Last Cleared: Jan 08, 1999 15:49:29

TACHYCARDIA COUNTERS:		BRADYCARDIA PACING COUNTERS:	
VF:	3	Total Brady Pulses:	8653351
FVT:	0	Runs of > 3 Consecutive Pulses:	65535
VT:	0		
ONSET CRITERION MET:	0	PREMATURE EVENT COUNTERS:	
		Isolated Premature Events:	0
		Runs of 2–4 Premature Beats:	0

VF THERAPY	Rx1	Rx2	Rx3	Rx4
INITIATED:	3	0	0	0
SUCCESSFUL:	3	0	0	0
ABORTED:	0	0	0	0
INEFFECTIVE:	0	0	0	0
CONVERTED TO VT:	0	0	0	0
CONVERTED TO FVT:	0	0	0	0
UNDETERMINED:	0	0	0	0

SN PCB200253R Rev 9891A221 Jun 18, 1999 12:29

A

EPISODE DATA REPORT -- Episode 1 of 3

19:53:54 VF detected VF Rx 1 Successful

INTERVAL (ms): VF = 260 VT = 350
STABILITY: OFF
ONSET: OFF

THERAPY SEQUENCE:
VF 1

PRE-DETECTION INTERVALS (ms):

−29.	740 VS	−14.	870 VS
−28.	130 FS	−13.	200 FS
−27.	270 TS	−12.	1200 VP
−26.	120 FS	−11.	330 TS
−25.	240 FS	−10.	150 FS
−24.	1180 VS	−9.	130 FS
−23.	130 FS	−8.	190 FS
−22.	240 FS	−7.	130 FS
−21.	1160 VS	−6.	120 FS
−20.	130 FS	−5.	130 FS
−19.	190 FS	−4.	740 VS
−18.	1010 VS	−3.	160 FS
−17.	210 FS	−2.	120 FS
−16.	190 FS	−1.	140 FS
−15.	120 FS	0.	120 FD

INTERVALS (ms): AFTER LAST Rx START:

1.	440 VS	11.	720 VS
2.	1210 CD	12.	770 VS
3.	530 VS	13.	860 VS
4.	680 VS	14.	1060 VS
5.	710 VS	15.	1080 VS
6.	640 VS	16.	1200 VP
7.	670 VS	17.	1000 VS
8.	670 VS	18.	1040 VS
9.	650 VS	19.	970 VS
10.	710 VS	20.	970 VS

SN PCB200253R Rev 9891A221 Jun 18, 1999 12:29

B

FIGURE 31–25 **A** and **B,** Printouts from an implantable cardioverter-defibrillator (ICD) programmer of a specific episode detected by the ICD. The text includes 29 VV interval lengths before therapy for ventricular fibrillation and 20 VV cycle lengths after therapy, documenting return to a nonpathological ventricular rhythm. FD = fibrillation detected; FS = fibrillation sensed; TS = tachycardia sensed; VS = ventricular sensed event.

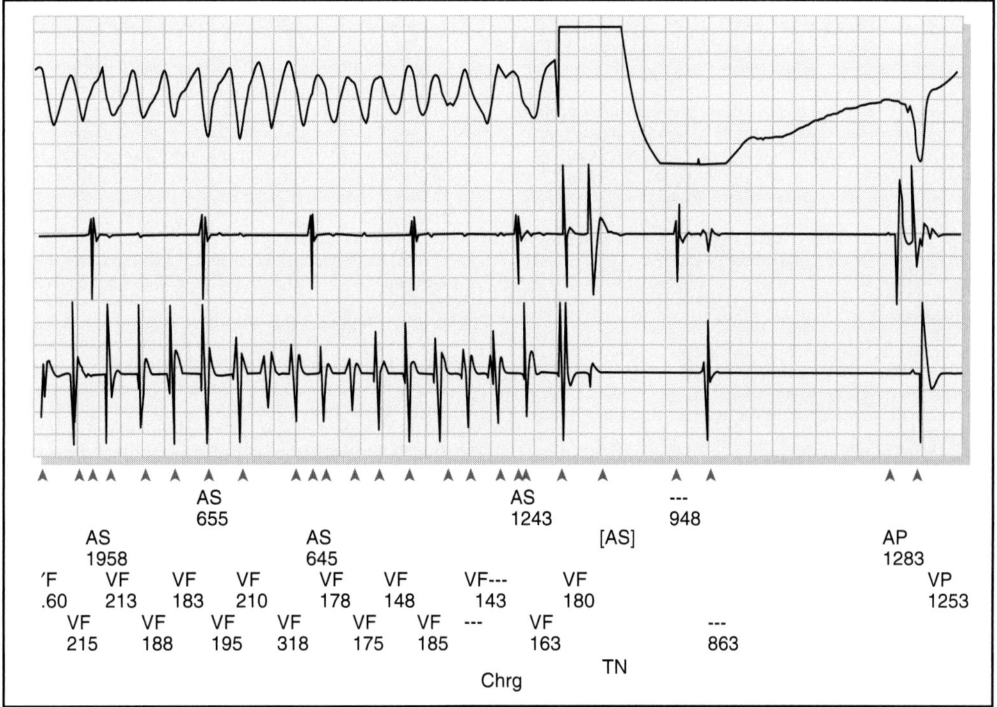

FIGURE 31–26 Stored electrogram from a patient with an episode of ventricular fibrillation and a dual-chamber pacemaker and implantable cardioverter-defibrillator. The **middle** tracing is the atrial electrogram, the **bottom** tracing is the ventricular electrogram, and the **upper** tracing is the surface electrocardiogram. AP = atrial paced event; AS = atrial sensed event; TN = telemetry noise; VF = ventricular fibrillation; VP = ventricular paced event. Chrg = charging. Numbers indicate milliseconds between events.

REFERENCES

Pacing Nomenclature

1. Bernstein AD, Daubert JC, Fletcher RD, et al, North American Society of Pacing and Electrophysiology/British Pacing and Electrophysiology Group: The revised NASPE/BPEG generic code for antibradycardia, adaptive-rate, and multisite pacing. Pacing Clin Electrophysiol 25:260, 2002.

Indications for Cardiac Pacing

2. Gregoratos G, Abrams J, Epstein AE, et al: ACC/AHA/NASPE 2002 guideline update for implantation of cardiac pacemakers and antiarrhythmia devices. Summary article: A report of the American College of Cardiology/American Heart Association Task Force on Practice Guidelines (ACC/AHA/NASPE Committee to Update the 1998 Pacemaker Guidelines). Circulation 106:2145, 2002.
3. Michaelsson M, Jonzon A, Riesenfeld T: Isolated congenital complete atrioventricular block in adult life: A prospective study. Circulation 92:442, 1995.
4. Sheldon R: Pacing to prevent vasovagal syncope. Cardiol Clin 18:81, 2000.
5. Connolly SJ, Sheldon R, Roberts RS, et al: The North American Vasovagal Pacemaker Study (VPS): A randomized trial of permanent cardiac pacing for the prevention of vasovagal syncope. J Am Coll Cardiol 33:16, 1999.
6. Vasovagal Syncope International Study: Is dual-chamber pacing efficacious in treatment of neurally mediated tilt-positive cardioinhibitory syncope? Pacemaker versus no therapy: A multicenter randomised study. Eur J Card Pacing Electrophysiol 3:169, 1993.
7. Connolly SJ, Sheldon R, Thorpe KE, et al, for the VPS-II Investigators: Pacemaker therapy for prevention of syncope in patients with recurrent severe vasovagal syncope. Second Vasovagal Pacemaker Study (VPS-II): A randomized trial. JAMA 289:2224, 2003.
8. Kenny RA, Seifer C: Brief report—SAFE PACE-2 Syncope and Falls in the Elderly Pacing and Carotid Sinus Evaluation: A randomized control trial of cardiac pacing in older patients with falls and carotid sinus hypersensitivity. Am J Geriatr Cardiol 8:87, 1999.
9. Ammirati F, Colivicchi F, Santini M, for the Syncope Diagnosis and Treatment Study Investigators: Permanent cardiac pacing versus medical treatment for the prevention of recurrent vasovagal syncope: A multicenter, randomized, controlled trial. Circulation 104:52, 2001.
10. Raviele A, Giada F, Sutton R, et al: The Vasovagal Syncope and Pacing (SYNPACE) trial: Rationale and study design. Europace 3:336, 2001.
11. Kenny RA, Richardson DA, Steen N, et al: Carotid sinus syndrome: A modifiable risk factor for nonaccidental falls in older adults (SAFE PACE). J Am Coll Cardiol 38:1491, 2001.

Selection of the Appropriate Pacing Mode

12. Andersen HR, Nielsen JC, Thomsen PE, et al: Long-term follow-up of patients from a randomised trial of atrial versus ventricular pacing for sick-sinus syndrome. Lancet 350:1210, 1997.
13. Lamas GA, Orav EJ, Stambler BS, et al, Pacemaker Selection in the Elderly Investigators: Quality of life and clinical outcomes in elderly patients treated with ventricular pacing as compared with dual-chamber pacing. N Engl J Med 338:1097, 1998.
14. Connolly SJ, Kerr CR, Gent M, et al, Canadian Trial of Physiologic Pacing Investigators: Effects of physiologic pacing versus ventricular pacing on the risk of stroke and death due to cardiovascular causes. N Engl J Med 342:1385, 2000.
15. Lamas GA, Lee KL, Sweeney MO, et al: Ventricular pacing or dual-chamber pacing for sinus node dysfunction. N Engl J Med 346:1854, 2002.
16. Toff WD, Skehan JD, De Bono DP, et al: The United Kingdom Pacing and Cardiovascular Events (UKPACE) trial: United Kingdom Pacing and Cardiovascular Events. Heart 78:221, 1997.
17. Andersen HR, Svendsen JH, on behalf of the DANPACE Investigators: The Danish multicenter randomized study on atrial-inhibited versus dual-chamber pacing in sick sinus syndrome (the DANPACE study): Purpose and design of the study. Heart Drug 1:67, 2001.

Indications for Rate-Adaptive Pacing

18. Leung SK, Lau CP: Developments in sensor-driven pacing. Cardiol Clin 18:113, 2000.
19. Alt E, Combs W, Willhaus R, et al: A comparative study of activity and dual sensor: Activity and minute ventilation pacing responses to ascending and descending stairs. Pacing Clin Electrophysiol 21:1862, 1998.

Pacing for Hemodynamic Improvement

20. Sorajja P, Elliott PM, McKenna WJ: Pacing in hypertrophic cardiomyopathy. Cardiol Clin 18:67, 2000.
21. Erwin JP III, Nishimura RA, Lloyd MA, et al: Dual-chamber pacing for patients with hypertrophic obstructive cardiomyopathy: A clinical perspective in 2000. Mayo Clin Proc 75:173, 2000.
22. Nishimura RA, Hayes DL, Ilstrup DM, et al: Effect of dual-chamber pacing on systolic and diastolic function in patients with hypertrophic cardiomyopathy: Acute Doppler echocardiographic and catheterization hemodynamic study. J Am Coll Cardiol 27:421, 1996.
23. Kappenberger L, Linde C, Daubert C, et al, PIC Study Group: Pacing in hypertrophic obstructive cardiomyopathy: A randomized crossover study. Eur Heart J 18:1249, 1997.
24. Maron BJ, Nishimura RA, McKenna WJ, et al: Assessment of permanent dual-chamber pacing as a treatment for drug-refractory symptomatic patients with obstructive hypertrophic cardiomyopathy: A randomized, double-blind, crossover study (M-PATHY). Circulation 99:2927, 1999.
25. Gillis AM: Pacing to prevent atrial fibrillation. Cardiol Clin 18:25, 2000.
26. Charles RG, McComb JM: Systematic Trial of Pacing to Prevent Atrial Fibrillation (STOP-AF). Heart 78:224, 1997
27. Gillis AM, Connolly SJ, Dubuc M, et al, for the PA3 Investigators: Circadian variation of paroxysmal atrial fibrillation. Am J Cardiol 87:794, 2001.
28. Djiane P: The best of cardiac pacing in 2002 [French]. Arch Mal Coeur Vaiss 96(Spec No. 1):35, 2003.

29. Anselme F, Saoudi N, Cribier A: Pacing in Prevention of Atrial Fibrillation—the PIPAF studies. J Interv Card Electrophysiol 4(Suppl 1):177, 2000.
30. Saksena S, Prakash A, Ziegler P, et al: Improved suppression of recurrent atrial fibrillation with dual-site right atrial pacing and antiarrhythmic drug therapy. J Am Coll Cardiol 40:1140, 2002.
31. Padeletti L, Pieragnoli P, Ciapetti C, et al: Randomized crossover comparison of right atrial appendage pacing versus interatrial septum pacing for prevention of paroxysmal atrial fibrillation in patients with sinus bradycardia. Am Heart J 142:1047, 2001.
32. Bailin SJ, Adler S, Giudici M: Prevention of chronic atrial fibrillation by pacing in the region of Bachmann's bundle: Results of a multicenter randomized trial. J Cardiovasc Electrophysiol 12:912, 2001.
33. Carlson MD, Ip J, Messenger J, et al: A new pacemaker algorithm for the treatment of atrial fibrillation: Results of the Atrial Dynamic Overdrive Pacing Trial (ADOPT). J Am Coll Cardiol 42:627, 2003.

Pulse Generator Implantation

34. Hayes DL, Naccarelli GV, Furman S, et al: NASPE policy statement: NASPE training requirements for cardiac implantable electronic devices: Selection, implantation, and follow-up. Pacing Clin Electrophysiol 26:1556-1562. 2003.
35. Ellenbogen KA, Kay GN, Wilkoff BL: Clinical Cardiac Pacing and Defibrillation. 2nd ed. Philadelphia, WB Saunders, 2000.

Pacemaker Programming

36. Fu EY, Ellenbogen KA: Management of atrial tachyarrhythmias in patients with implantable devices. Cardiol Clin 18:37, 2000.

Implantable Cardioverter-Defibrillator Therapy

37. Siebels J, Cappato R, Ruppel R, et al, CASH Investigators: Preliminary results of the Cardiac Arrest Study Hamburg (CASH). Am J Cardiol 72:109F, 1993.
38. Pathmanathan RK, Lau EW, Cooper J, et al: Potential impact of antiarrhythmic drugs versus implantable defibrillators on the management of ventricular arrhythmias: The Midlands trial of empirical amiodarone versus electrophysiologically guided intervention and cardioverter implant registry data. Heart 80:68, 1998.
39. Bansch D, Antz M, Boczor S, et al: Primary prevention of sudden cardiac death in idiopathic dilated cardiomyopathy: The Cardiomyopathy Trial (CAT). Circulation 105:1453, 2002.
40. Raviele A, Bongiorni MG, Brignole M, et al: Which strategy is "best" after myocardial infarction? The Beta-Blocker Strategy plus Implantable Cardioverter Defibrillator Trial: Rationale and study design. Am J Cardiol 83:104D, 1999.
41. Moss AJ, Zareba W, Hall WJ, et al: Prophylactic implantation of a defibrillator in patients with myocardial infarction and reduced ejection fraction. N Engl J Med 346:877, 2002.
42. Bardy GH, Lee KL, Mark DB, et al, and the SCD-HeFT Pilot Investigators: Sudden Cardiac Death in Heart Failure Trial: Pilot study [abstract]. Pacing Clin Electrophysiol 20:1148, 1997.
43. Nademanee K, Veerakul G, Mower M, et al: Defibrillator Versus β-Blockers for Unexplained Death in Thailand (DEBUT): A randomized clinical trial. Circulation 107:E9038, 2003.
44. Strickberger SA, Hummel JD, Bartlett TG, et al: Amiodarone versus implantable cardioverter-defibrillator: Randomized trial in patients with nonischemic dilated cardiomyopathy and asymptomatic nonsustained ventricular tachycardia—AMIOVIRT. J Am Coll Cardiol 41:1707, 2003.
45. The Antiarrhythmics Versus Implantable Defibrillators (AVID) Investigators: A comparison of antiarrhythmic drug therapy with implantable defibrillators in patients resuscitated from near-fatal ventricular arrhythmias. N Engl J Med 337:1576, 1997.
46. Moss AJ, Hall WJ, Cannom DS, et al, Multicenter Automatic Defibrillator Implantation Trial Investigators: Improved survival with an implanted defibrillator in patients with coronary disease at high risk for ventricular arrhythmia. N Engl J Med 335:1933, 1996.
47. Buxton AE, Fisher JD, Josephson ME, et al: Prevention of sudden death in patients with coronary artery disease: The Multicenter Unsustained Tachycardia Trial (MUSTT). Prog Cardiovasc Dis 36:215, 1993.
48. Bigger JT Jr, Coronary Artery Bypass Graft (CABG) Patch Trial Investigators: Prophylactic use of implanted cardiac defibrillators in patients at high risk for ventricular arrhythmias after coronary artery bypass graft surgery. N Engl J Med 337:1569, 1997.
49. Bigger JT Jr, Whang W, Rottman JN, et al: Mechanisms of death in the CABG-PATCH trial: A randomized trial of implantable cardiac defibrillator prophylaxis in patients at high risk of death after coronary artery bypass graft surgery. Circulation 99:1416, 1999.
50. Caruso AC, Marcus FI, Hahn EA, et al: Predictors of arrhythmic death and cardiac arrest in the ESVEM trial: Electrophysiologic Study Versus Electromagnetic Monitoring. Circulation 96:1888, 1997.
51. Cleland JG, Daubert JC, Erdmann E, et al: The CARE-HF study (CArdiac REsynchronisation in Heart Failure study): Rationale, design, and end-points. Eur J Heart Fail 3:481, 2001.
52. Groh WJ, Silka MJ, Oliver RP, et al: Use of implantable cardioverter-defibrillators in the congenital long-QT syndrome. Am J Cardiol 78:703, 1996.
53. Maron BJ, Shen WK, Link MS, et al: Efficacy of implantable cardioverter-defibrillators for the prevention of sudden death in patients with hypertrophic cardiomyopathy. N Engl J Med 342:365, 2000.
54. Pinski SL, Fahy GJ: Implantable cardioverter-defibrillators. Am J Med 106:446, 1999.
55. Higgins SL, Pak JP, Barone J, et al: The first-year experience with the dual-chamber ICD. Pacing Clin Electrophysiol 23:18, 2000.
56. Wilkoff BL, Cook JR, Epstein AE, et al: Dual-chamber pacing or ventricular backup pacing in patients with an implantable defibrillator: The Dual Chamber and VVI Implantable Defibrillator (DAVID) Trial. JAMA 288:3115, 2002.
57. Friedman PA, Rasmussen MJ, Grice S, et al: Defibrillation thresholds are increased by right-sided implantation of totally transvenous implantable cardioverter-defibrillators. Pacing Clin Electrophysiol 22:1186, 1999.

Electromagnetic Interference

58. Pinski SL, Trohman RG: Interference with cardiac pacing. Cardiol Clin 18:219, 2000.
59. Hayes DL, Wang PJ, Reynolds DW, et al: Interference with cardiac pacemakers by cellular telephones. N Engl J Med 336:1473, 1997.
60. Fetter JG, Ivans V, Benditt DG, et al: Digital cellular telephone interaction with implantable cardioverter-defibrillators. J Am Coll Cardiol 31:623, 1998.
61. Groh WJ, Boschee SA, Engelstein ED, et al: Interactions between electronic article surveillance systems and implantable cardioverter-defibrillators. Circulation 100:387, 1999.
62. Chung MK, Streem SB, Ching E, et al: Effects of extracorporeal shock wave lithotripsy on tiered therapy implantable cardioverter-defibrillators. Pacing Clin Electrophysiol 22:738, 1999.
63. Glikson M, Trusty JM, Grice SK, et al: Importance of pacemaker noise reversion as a potential mechanism of pacemaker-ICD interactions. Pacing Clin Electrophysiol 21:1111, 1998.

Interference from Drugs and Metabolic Abnormalities

64. Carnes CA, Mehdirad AA, Nelson SD: Drug and defibrillator interactions. Pharmacotherapy 18:516, 1998.
65. Kopp D, Kall J, Kinder C, et al: Effect of amiodarone and left ventricular mass on defibrillation energy requirements: Monophasic versus biphasic shocks. Pacing Clin Electrophysiol 18:872, 1995.

Device Follow-Up

66. Theuns DAMJ, Res JCJ, Jordaens LJ: Home monitoring in ICD therapy: Future perspectives. Europace 5:139, 2003.
67. Chun SH, Friday KJ, Chan A, et al: Clinical benefit and technical accuracy evaluation of wireless home monitoring pacemaker system: Multicenter clinical trial data. J Am Coll Cardiol 41(Suppl A):139A, 2003.

GUIDELINES *Thomas H. Lee*

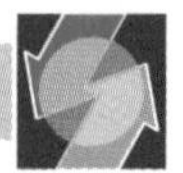

Cardiac Pacemakers and Cardioverter-Defibrillators

Guidelines for implantation of cardiac pacemakers and antiarrhythmia devices were published by the American College of Cardiology/American Heart Association (ACC/AHA) and the North American Society for Pacing and Electrophysiology (NASPE) in 1998[1] and updated in 2002.[2] These guidelines continue to use the ACC/AHA classification system for the indications (class I for generally accepted indications; class IIa when indications are controversial, but the weight of evidence is supportive; class IIb when usefulness or efficacy is less well established; and class III when there is consensus against the usefulness of the intervention). The updated guidelines adopted a convention for rating levels of evidence on which recommendations have been based: *Level A* recommendations were derived from data from multiple randomized clinical trials; *level B* recommendations were derived from a single randomized trial or nonrandomized studies; and *level C* recommendations were based on the consensus opinion of experts.

Indications for Permanent Pacing

(Tables 31G–1 to 31G–10)

Acquired AV Block. For patients with complete or second-degree atrioventricular (AV) block, the ACC/AHA guidelines consider permanent pacing to be appropriate when the abnormality causes complications and is not precipitated by a drug that can be discontinued (see Table 31G–1). Examples of complications include symptomatic bradycardia, congestive heart failure, and confusional states. For asymptomatic patients with complete or advanced second-degree AV block, permanent pacing was considered appropriate for patients with a high risk for development of complications, such as those with periods of asystole of 3 seconds or longer or an escape rate less than 40 beats/min, or patients who have had interventions or neuromuscular diseases that have damaged the AV node.

TABLE 31G–1 ACC/AHA Guidelines for Permanent Pacing in Acquired Atrioventricular Block in Adults

Class	Indication	Level of Evidence (see text)
I (indicated)	1. Third-degree and advanced second-degree AV block at any anatomic level, associated with any one of the following conditions:	
	a. Bradycardia with symptoms (including heart failure) presumed to be due to AV block	C
	b. Arrhythmias and other medical conditions requiring drugs that result in symptomatic bradycardia	C
	c. Documented periods of asystole ≥3.0 sec or any escape rate <40 beats/min in awake, symptom-free patients	B, C
	d. After catheter ablation of the AV junction; there are no trials to assess outcome without pacing, and pacing is virtually always planned in this situation unless the operative procedure is AV junction modification	B, C
	e. Postoperative AV block that is not expected to resolve after cardiac surgery	C
	f. Neuromuscular diseases with AV block, such as myotonic muscular dystrophy, Kearns-Sayre syndrome, Erb dystrophy (limb-girdle), and peroneal muscular atrophy, with or without symptoms, because there may be unpredictable progression of AV conduction disease	B
	2. Second-degree AV block regardless of type or site of block, with associated symptomatic bradycardia	B
IIa (good supportive evidence)	1. Asymptomatic third-degree AV block at any anatomic site with average awake ventricular rates of ≥40 beats/min, especially if cardiomegaly or LV dysfunction is present	B, C
	2. Asymptomatic type II second-degree AV block with a narrow QRS; when type II second-degree AV block occurs with a wide QRS, pacing becomes a class I recommendation	B
	3. Asymptomatic type I second-degree AV block at intra-His or infra-His levels found at electrophysiological study performed for other indications	B
	4. First- or second-degree AV block with symptoms similar to those of pacemaker syndrome	B
IIb (weak supportive evidence)	1. Marked first-degree AV block (>0.30 sec) in patients with LV dysfunction and symptoms of congestive heart failure in whom a shorter AV interval results in hemodynamic improvement, presumably by decreasing left atrial filling pressure	C
	2. Neuromuscular diseases such as myotonic muscular dystrophy, Kearns-Sayre syndrome, Erb dystrophy (limb-girdle), and peroneal muscular atrophy with any degree of AV block (including first-degree AV block), with or without symptoms, because there may be unpredictable progression of AV conduction disease	B
III (not indicated)	1. Asymptomatic first-degree AV block	B
	2. Asymptomatic type I second-degree AV block at the supra-His (AV node) level or not known to be intra-Hisian or infra-Hisian	B, C
	3. AV block expected to resolve and/or unlikely to recur (e.g., drug toxicity, Lyme disease, or during hypoxia in sleep apnea syndrome in absence of symptoms)	B

ACC = American College of Cardiology; AHA = American Heart Association; AV = atrioventricular; LV = left ventricular.

TABLE 31G–2 ACC/AHA Guidelines for Permanent Pacing in Chronic Bifascicular and Trifascicular Block

Class	Indication	Level of Evidence
I (indicated)	1. Intermittent third-degree AV block	B
	2. Type II second-degree AV block	B
	3. Alternating bundle branch block	C
IIa (good supportive evidence)	1. Syncope not demonstrated to be due to AV block when other likely causes have been excluded, specifically VT	B
	2. Incidental finding at electrophysiological study of markedly prolonged HV interval (≥100 msec) in asymptomatic patients	B
	3. Incidental finding at electrophysiological study of pacing-induced infra-His block that is not physiological	B
IIb (weak supportive evidence)	Neuromuscular diseases such as myotonic muscular dystrophy, Kearns-Sayre syndrome, Erb dystrophy (limb-girdle), and peroneal muscular atrophy with any degree of fascicular block, without symptoms, because there may be unpredictable progression of AV conduction disease	C
III (not indicated)	1. Fascicular block without AV block or symptoms	B
	2. Fascicular block with first-degree AV block without symptoms	B

ACC = American College of Cardiology; AHA = American Heart Association; AV = atrioventricular; VT = ventricular tachycardia.

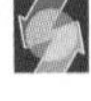

TABLE 31G–3 ACC/AHA Guidelines for Permanent Pacing after the Acute Phase of Myocardial Infarction

Class	Indication	Level of Evidence
I (indicated)	1. Persistent second-degree AV block in the His-Purkinje system with bilateral bundle branch block or third-degree AV block within or below the His-Purkinje system after AMI 2. Transient advanced (second- or third-degree) infranodal AV block and associated bundle branch block; if the site of block is uncertain, an electrophysiological study may be necessary 3. Persistent and symptomatic second- or third-degree AV block	B B C
IIa (good supportive evidence)		
IIb (weak supportive evidence)	Persistent second- or third-degree AV block at the AV node level	B
III (not indicated)	1. Transient AV block in the absence of intraventricular conduction defects 2. Transient AV block in the presence of isolated left anterior fascicular block 3. Acquired left anterior fascicular block in the absence of AV block 4. Persistent first-degree AV block in the presence of bundle branch block that is old or age indeterminate	B B B B

ACC = American College of Cardiology; AHA = American Heart Association; AMI = acute myocardial infarction; AV = atrioventricular.

TABLE 31G–4 ACC/AHA Guidelines for Permanent Pacing in Sinus Node Dysfunction

Class	Indication	Level of Evidence
I (indicated)	1. Sinus node dysfunction with documented symptomatic bradycardia, including frequent sinus pauses that produce symptoms; in some patients, bradycardia is iatrogenic and will occur as a consequence of essential long-term drug therapy of a type and dose for which there are no acceptable alternatives 2. Symptomatic chronotropic incompetence	C C
IIa (good supportive evidence)	1. Sinus node dysfunction occurring spontaneously or as a result of necessary drug therapy, with heart rate <40 beats/min when a clear association between significant symptoms consistent with bradycardia and the actual presence of bradycardia has not been documented 2. Syncope of unexplained origin when major abnormalities of sinus node function are discovered or provoked in electrophysiological studies	C C
IIb (weak supportive evidence)	In minimally symptomatic patients, chronic heart rate <40 beats/min while awake	C
III (not indicated)	1. Sinus node dysfunction in asymptomatic patients, including those in whom substantial sinus bradycardia (heart rate <40 beats/min) is a consequence of long-term drug treatment 2. Sinus node dysfunction in patients with symptoms suggestive of bradycardia that are clearly documented as not associated with a slow heart rate 3. Sinus node dysfunction with symptomatic bradycardia due to nonessential drug therapy	

ACC = American College of Cardiology; AHA = American Heart Association.

TABLE 31G–5 ACC/AHA Guidelines for Permanent Pacemakers that Automatically Detect and Pace to Terminate Tachycardias

Class	Indication	Level of Evidence
I (indicated)	None	
IIa (good supportive evidence)	Symptomatic recurrent supraventricular tachycardia that is reproducibly terminated by pacing in the unlikely event that catheter ablation and/or drugs fail to control the arrhythmia or produce intolerable side effects	C
IIb (weak supportive evidence)	Recurrent supraventricular tachycardia or atrial flutter that is reproducibly terminated by pacing as an alternative to drug therapy or ablation	C
III (not indicated)	1. Tachycardias frequently accelerated or converted to fibrillation by pacing 2. The presence of accessory pathways with the capacity for rapid anterograde conduction whether or not the pathways participate in the mechanism of the tachycardia	

ACC = American College of Cardiology; AHA = American Heart Association.

TABLE 31G–6 ACC/AHA Guidelines for Pacing Recommendations to Prevent Tachycardia

Class	Indication	Level of Evidence
I (indicated)	Sustained pause-dependent VT, with or without prolonged QT, in which the efficacy of pacing is thoroughly documented	C
IIa (good supportive evidence)	High-risk patients with congenital long-QT syndrome	C
IIb (weak supportive evidence)	1. AV reentrant or AV node reentrant supraventricular tachycardia not responsive to medical or ablative therapy 2. Prevention of symptomatic, drug-refractory, recurrent atrial fibrillation in patients with coexisting sinus node dysfunction	C B
III (not indicated)	1. Frequent or complex ventricular ectopic activity without sustained VT in the absence of the long-QT syndrome 2. Torsades de Pointes VT due to reversible causes	

ACC = American College of Cardiology; AHA = American Heart Association; AV = atrioventricular; VT = ventricular tachycardia.

TABLE 31G–7 ACC/AHA Guidelines for Permanent Pacing in Hypersensitive Carotid Sinus Syndrome and Neurocardiogenic Syncope

Class	Indication	Level of Evidence
I (indicated)	Recurrent syncope caused by carotid sinus stimulation; minimal carotid sinus pressure induces ventricular asystole of >3 sec duration in the absence of any medication that depresses the sinus node or AV conduction	C
IIa (good supportive evidence)	1. Recurrent syncope without clear, provocative events and with a hypersensitive cardioinhibitory response 2. Significantly symptomatic and recurrent neurocardiogenic syncope associated with bradycardia documented spontaneously or at the time of tilt-table testing	C B
IIb (weak supportive evidence)		
III (not indicated)	1. A hyperactive cardioinhibitory response to carotid sinus stimulation in the absence of symptoms or in the presence of vague symptoms such as dizziness, lightheadedness, or both 2. Recurrent syncope, lightheadedness, or dizziness in the absence of a hyperactive cardioinhibitory response 3. Situational vasovagal syncope in which avoidance behavior is effective	C C C

ACC = American College of Cardiology; AHA = American Heart Association; AV = atrioventricular.

TABLE 31G–8 ACC/AHA Guidelines for Pacing in Patients with Cardiomyopathy

Indication	Class I (indicated)	Class IIa (good supportive evidence)	Class IIb (weak supportive evidence)	Class III (not indicated)
Hypertrophic cardiomyopathy	Class I indications for sinus node dysfunction or AV block as described previously		Medically refractory, symptomatic hypertrophic cardiomyopathy with significant resting or provoked LV outflow obstruction	1. Patients who are symptomatic or medically controlled 2. Symptomatic patients without evidence of LV outflow obstruction
Dilated cardiomyopathy	Class I indications for sinus node dysfunction or AV block as described previously	Biventricular pacing in medically refractory, symptomatic NYHA Class III or IV patients with idiopathic dilated or ischemic cardiomyopathy, prolonged QRS interval (≥130 msec), LV end-diastolic diameter ≥55 mm, and ejection fraction ≤35%		1. Asymptomatic dilated cardiomyopathy 2. Symptomatic dilated cardiomyopathy when patients are rendered asymptomatic by drug therapy 3. Symptomatic ischemic cardiomyopathy when the ischemia is amenable to intervention
After cardiac transplantation	Symptomatic bradyarrhythmias/ chronotropic incompetence not expected to resolve and other class I indications for permanent pacing		Symptomatic bradyarrhythmias/ chronotropic incompetence that, although transient, may persist for months and require intervention	Asymptomatic bradyarrhythmias after cardiac transplantation

ACC = American College of Cardiology; AHA = American Heart Association; AV = atrioventricular; LV = left ventricular; NYHA = New York Heart Association.

TABLE 31G–9 ACC/AHA Guidelines for Choice of Pacemaker

Type of Pacemaker	Sinus Node Dysfunction	AV Block	Neurally Mediated Syncope or Carotid Sinus Hypersensitivity
Single-chamber atrial	No suspected abnormality of AV conduction and not at increased risk for future AV block Maintenance of AV synchrony during pacing desired Rate response available if desired	Not appropriate	Not appropriate
Single-chamber ventricular	Maintenance of AV synchrony during pacing not necessary Rate response available if desired	Chronic atrial fibrillation or other atrial tachyarrhythmia or maintenance of AV synchrony during pacing not necessary Rate response available if desired	Chronic atrial fibrillation or other atrial tachyarrhythmia Rate response available if desired
Dual-chamber	AV synchrony during pacing desired Suspected abnormality of AV conduction or increased risk for future AV block Rate response available if desired	Rate response available if desired AV synchrony during pacing desired Atrial pacing desired	Sinus mechanism present Rate response available if desired
Single-lead, atrial-sensing ventricular	Not appropriate	Normal sinus node function and no need for atrial pacing Desire to limit the number of pacemaker leads	Not appropriate

ACC = American College of Cardiology; AHA = American Heart Association; AV = atrioventricular.

These recommendations differed from those in the prior ACC/AHA guidelines by supporting a lower threshold for use of pacemakers in patients with asymptomatic advanced second-degree heart block and by emphasizing the prognostic importance of the site of origin of the escape rhythm in cases of advanced AV block. For example, when type II second-degree AV block occurs with a wide QRS, pacing now becomes a class I recommendation, whereas this was a class IIa recommendation in the prior guidelines.

In addition, heart failure is now considered a complication of AV block that justifies a lower threshold for use of permanent pacing. This theme is also apparent in the class IIa recommendations, which consider evidence to be generally supportive for use of pacing in asymptomatic patients with third-degree AV block and ventricular rates or escape rates of 40 beats/min or more, especially if they have cardiomegaly or left ventricular dysfunction.

The guidelines do not support pacing for patients with asymptomatic first-degree or type I second-degree AV block, and they do not support the use of pacing for patients with hypoxia and sleep apnea syndrome in the absence of symptoms. The guidelines were written with awareness of a small study suggesting benefit from atrial pacing for patients with sleep apnea syndrome,[3] but the guideline authors considered support for routine use of pacing in this setting to be premature.

Chronic Bifascicular and Trifascicular Block. Syncope is common among patients with slowing of conduction below the AV node in the fascicles of the right and left bundles, but the risk of sudden death or progression to complete heart block varies among patient subsets. The ACC/AHA guidelines for pacing in these settings (see Table 31G–2) now include alternating bundle branch block as a class I indication for pacing, because this finding is recognized as a reflection of abnormal conduction in all three fascicles. The guidelines also provide some support for pacing in patients with findings of markedly abnormal conduction at electrophysiological studies, even if patients are asymptomatic (class IIa). Pacing is not supported for fascicular block without greater than first-degree AV block or symptoms.

Acute Myocardial Infarction. Symptoms do not play a role in appropriateness for pacing in patients with acute myocardial infarction because of the high risk for sudden death in postinfarction patients with conduction system disturbances (see Table 31G–3). The guidelines emphasize that the requirement for temporary pacing after acute myocardial infarction does not automatically indicate a need for permanent pacing (see Guidelines to Chap. 47). However, permanent pacemakers were supported for use in patients with persistent advanced-degree AV block or transient infranodal AV block and associated bundle branch block. The usefulness of permanent pacemakers for patients with advanced AV block at the AV node level was less clear (class IIb). Permanent pacing was discouraged if the only indication was transient AV conduction disturbances or left anterior hemiblock.

Sinus Node Dysfunction. As noted in the recommendations for pacing for patients with acquired AV block, the ACC/AHA guidelines support pacing for patients with symptoms due to bradycardia that is not due to a drug that can be discontinued. This theme is apparent in the indications for pacing in patients with sinus node dysfunction (see Table 31G–4). Pacing is discouraged in asymptomatic patients, even when resting heart rates are lower than 40 beats/min, and in symptomatic patients when symptoms cannot be proven to be due to bradycardia. A new class IIa recommendation is included in the 2002 guidelines that supports pacing in patients with syncope of unexplained origin when major abnormalities of sinus node function are demonstrated at electrophysiological testing.

Prevention and Termination of Tachyarrhythmias. In some patients with long-QT syndrome, continuous pacing can prevent recurrent tachyarrhythmias. In addition, paroxysmal reentrant tachyarrhythmias can be terminated in some patients through programmed stimulation and short bursts of rapid pacing. However, the ACC/AHA guidelines do not provide support for the routine use of antitachycardia pacemakers without extensive testing before implantation (see Table 31G–5). The 2002 guidelines actually raise the threshold for use of antitachycardia pacemakers by "downgrading" its class I indication for pacing in patients whose recurrent supraventricular tachycardia is unresponsive to antiarrhythmic drugs. This change reflects the Committee consensus that either drugs and/or ablation therapy should be first-line therapies for most patients. The guidelines continue to consider pacing appropriate (class I indication) for patients with sustained pause-dependent ventricular tachycardia, with or without prolonged QT, if the efficacy of pacing has been demonstrated (see Table 31G–6).

Carotid Sinus Syndrome and Neurocardiogenic Syncope. The only class I indication for permanent pacing in the ACC/AHA guidelines in patients with hypersensitive carotid sinus syndrome is

TABLE 31G–10 ACC/AHA Recommendations for ICD Therapy

Class	Indication	Level of Evidence
I (indicated)	1. Cardiac arrest due to VF or VT not due to a transient or reversible cause	A
	2. Spontaneous sustained VT in association with structural heart disease	B
	3. Syncope of undetermined origin with clinically relevant, hemodynamically significant sustained VT or VF induced at electrophysiological study when drug therapy is ineffective, not tolerated, or not preferred	B
	4. Nonsustained VT in patients with coronary disease, prior MI, LV dysfunction, and inducible VF or sustained VT at electrophysiological study not suppressible by a class I antiarrhythmic drug	A
	5. Spontaneous sustained VT in patients without structural heart disease not amenable to other treatments	C
IIa (good supportive evidence)	Patients with ejection fraction ≤30% at least 1 mo post MI and 3 mo post coronary artery revascularization surgery	B
IIb (weak supportive evidence)	1. Cardiac arrest presumed to be due to VF when electrophysiological testing is precluded by other medical conditions	C
	2. Severe symptoms (e.g., syncope) attributable to ventricular tachyarrhythmias in patients awaiting cardiac transplantation	C
	3. Familial or inherited conditions with a high risk for life-threatening ventricular tachyarrhythmias such as long-QT syndrome or hypertrophic cardiomyopathy	B
	4. Nonsustained VT with coronary artery disease, prior MI, LV dysfunction, and inducible sustained VT or VF at electrophysiological study	B
	5. Recurrent syncope of undetermined origin in the presence of ventricular dysfunction and inducible ventricular arrhythmias at electrophysiological study when other causes of syncope have been excluded	C
	6. Syncope of unexplained origin or family history of unexplained sudden cardiac death in association with typical or atypical right bundle branch block and ST segment elevations (Brugada syndrome)	C
	7. Syncope in patients with advanced structural heart disease in whom thorough invasive and noninvasive investigations have failed to define a cause	C
III (not indicated)	1. Syncope of undetermined cause in a patient without inducible ventricular tachyarrhythmias and without structural heart disease	C
	2. Incessant VT or VF	C
	3. VF or VT resulting from arrhythmias amenable to surgical or catheter ablation; e.g., atrial arrhythmias associated with Wolff-Parkinson-White syndrome, RV outflow tract VT, idiopathic LV tachycardia, or fascicular VT	C
	4. Ventricular tachyarrhythmias due to a transient or reversible disorder (e.g., acute MI, electrolyte imbalance, drugs, or trauma) when correction of the disorder is considered feasible and likely to substantially reduce the risk of recurrent arrhythmia	B
	5. Significant psychiatric illnesses that may be aggravated by device implantation or may preclude systematic follow-up	C
	6. Terminal illnesses with projected life expectancy <6 mo	C
	7. Patients with coronary artery disease with LV dysfunction and prolonged QRS duration in the absence of spontaneous or inducible sustained or nonsustained VT who are undergoing coronary bypass surgery	B
	8. NYHA Class IV drug-refractory congestive heart failure in patients who are not candidates for cardiac transplantation	C

ACC = American College of Cardiology; AHA = American Heart Association; ICD = implanted cardioverter-defibrillator; LV = left ventricular; MI = myocardial infarction; NYHA = New York Heart Association; RV = right ventricular; VF = ventricular fibrillation; VT = ventricular tachycardia.

recurrent syncope caused by carotid sinus stimulation in the absence of any drug that depresses the sinus node or AV conduction (see Table 31G–7). However, the guidelines added a new class IIa indication with support for pacing in patients with recurrent neurocardiogenic syncope associated with bradycardia, reflecting recent clinical trials showing the benefit of pacing in this setting. Pacing is discouraged in patients without symptoms or who have syncope without bradycardia.

Cardiomyopathy and after Cardiac Transplantation. For patients with hypertrophic or dilated cardiomyopathy or who have cardiac transplantation, class I indications for permanent pacing are similar to those in other patient populations (see Table 31G–8). The guidelines do not provide much support for the routine use of pacing in patients with hypertrophic cardiomyopathy for the purpose of reducing left ventricular outflow obstruction (class IIb indication). However, the 2002 guidelines add a new class IIa indication of biventricular pacing for patients with dilated cardiomyopathy and prolonged QRS intervals, reflecting multiple trials that have shown clinical and structural benefits from this intervention.

Selection of Pacemakers

The ACC/AHA guidelines provide recommendations (see Table 31G–9) and decision trees to help physicians choose the most appropriate type of pacemaker. These guidelines are aimed at helping physicians match patients' needs to the technology implanted and to anticipate future needs of the patient. Elderly patients should receive devices according to the same indications as younger patients, according to the guidelines.

Follow-Up of Patients with Pacemakers

The ACC/AHA guidelines do not directly address follow-up of patients with pacemakers but instead refer physicians to guidelines from other organizations.[4-8] Examples of reasonable follow-up schedules included twice in the first 6 months after implant of single-chamber pacemakers and then once every 12 months; and, for dual-chamber pacemakers, twice in the first 6 months, then once every 6 months.

Guidelines for transtelephonic monitoring focus on content, not frequency.

Implantable Cardioverter-Defibrillator Therapy

The 2002 ACC/AHA guidelines reflect the continuing expansion of the role of implantable cardioverter-defibrillators (ICDs),[9-11] which are considered clearly appropriate for patients with cardiac arrests not due to transient or reversible causes and for patients with spontaneous sustained ventricular tachycardia associated with structural heart disease (see Table 31G–10). The guidelines note that ICD therapy is most efficacious in patients with sustained ventricular tachycardia and impaired left ventricular performance, whereas VT arising in structurally normal hearts can usually be treated pharmacologically or with catheter ablation.

The guidelines add a new class IIa indication for ICDs for patients with left ventricular ejection fraction less than 0.30 at least 1 month after myocardial infarction and 3 months after coronary artery revascularization surgery, reflecting recent data supporting the use of ICDs for primary prevention of cardiac arrest.[9,11] The Committee agreed that further risk stratification might help define the benefit of an ICD in such patients, and it identified this area as important for future research.

Only limited support (class IIb) was provided for the use of ICDs in patients with syncope of unexplained etiology or family history of unexplained sudden cardiac death in association with electrocardiographic abnormalities typical of Brugada syndrome. ICDs were considered contraindicated in patients in whom a triggering factor for ventricular tachycardia or ventricular fibrillation can be definitely identified, such as ventricular tachyarrhythmias in evolving acute myocardial infarction or electrolyte abnormalities.

See Guidelines in Chapter 30 for recommendations regarding resumption of driving or flying for patients who have received ICDs.

References

1. Gregoratos G, Cheitlin M, Conill A, et al: ACC/AHA guidelines for implantation of cardiac pacemakers and antiarrhythmia devices: A report of the American College of Cardiology/American Heart Association Task Force on Practice Guidelines (Committee on Pacemaker Implantation). J Am Coll Cardiol 31:1175, 1998.
2. Gregoratos G, Abrams J, Epstein AE, et al: ACC/AHA/NASPE 2002 Guideline Update for Implantation of Cardiac Pacemakers and Antiarrhythmia Devices—Summary Article: A Report of the American College of Cardiology/American Heart Association Task Force on Practice Guidelines (ACC/AHA/NASPE Committee to Update the 1998 Pacemaker Guidelines). J Am Coll Cardiol 40:1703-1719, 2002.
3. Garrigue S, Bordier P, Jais P, et al: Benefit of atrial pacing in sleep apnea syndrome. N Engl J Med 346:404-412, 2002.
4. Bernstein AD, Irwin ME, Parsonnet V, et al: Report of the NASPE Policy Conference on Antibradycardia Pacemaker Follow-Up: Effectiveness, needs, and resources. Pacing Clin Electrophysiol 17:1714-1729, 1994.
5. Levine PA, Belott PH, Bilitch M, et al: Recommendations of the NASPE policy conference on pacemaker programmability and follow-up programs. Pacing Clin Electrophysiol 6:1222-1223, 1983.
6. Levine PA: Proceedings of the Policy Conference of the North American Society of Pacing and Electrophysiology on Programmability and Pacemaker Follow-Up Programs. Clin Prog Pacing Electrophysiol 2:145-191, 1984.
7. Medicare Coverage Issues Manual. HCFA Publication No. 6, Thur Rev. 42. Baltimore, U.S. Department of Health and Human Services, Health Care Financing Administration, 1990.
8. Fraser JD, Gillis AM, Irwin ME, et al: Guidelines for pacemaker follow-up in Canada: A consensus statement of the Canadian Working Group on Cardiac Pacing. Can J Cardiol 16:355-376, 2000.
9. Moss AJ, Zareba W, Hall WJ, et al: Prophylactic implantation of a defibrillator in patients with myocardial infarction and reduced ejection fraction. N Engl J Med 346:877-883, 2002.
10. Bansch D, Antz M, Boczor S, et al: Primary prevention of sudden death in idiopathic dilated cardiomyopathy: The Cardiomyopathy Trial (CAT). Circulation 105:1453-1458, 2002.
11. Ezekowitz JA, Armstrong PW, McAlister FA: Implantable cardioverter defibrillators in primary and secondary prevention: A systematic review of randomized, controlled trials. Ann Intern Med 138:445-452, 2003.

CHAPTER 32

Specific Arrhythmias: Diagnosis and Treatment

Jeffrey E. Olgin • Douglas P. Zipes

Sinus Nodal Disturbances

Normal Sinus Rhythm

Normal sinus rhythm is arbitrarily limited to impulse formation beginning in the sinus node at frequencies between 60 and 100 beats/min. A range of 50 to 90 beats/min has been suggested. Infants and children generally have faster heart rates than adults do, both at rest and during exercise. The P wave is upright in electrocardiograph (ECG) leads I, II, and aV_f and negative in lead aV, with a vector in the frontal plane between 0 and +90 degrees. In the horizontal plane, the P vector is directed anteriorly and slightly leftward and can therefore be negative in leads V_1 and V_2 but positive in V_3 to V_6. The PR interval exceeds 120 milliseconds and can vary slightly with the rate. If the pacemaker site shifts, a change in morphology of the P wave can occur. The rate of sinus rhythm varies significantly and depends on many factors, including age, sex, and physical activity (Table 32–1).

The sinus nodal discharge rate responds readily to autonomic stimuli and depends on the effect of the two opposing autonomic influences. Steady vagal stimulation decreases the spontaneous sinus nodal discharge rate and predominates over steady sympathetic stimulation, which increases the spontaneous sinus nodal discharge rate. Single or brief bursts of vagal stimulation can speed, slow, or entrain sinus nodal discharge. A given vagal stimulus produces a greater absolute reduction in heart rate when the basal heart rate has been increased by sympathetic stimulation, a phenomenon known as *accentuated antagonism.*

Sinus Tachycardia

ECG RECOGNITION. *Tachycardia* (Fig. 32–1A) in an adult is defined as a rate faster than 100 beats/min. During sinus tachycardia, the sinus node exhibits a discharge frequency between 100 and 180 beats/min, but it may be higher with extreme exertion. The maximum heart rate achieved during strenuous physical activity decreases with age from near 200 beats/min to less than 140 beats/min. Sinus tachycardia generally has a gradual onset and termination. The P-P interval can vary slightly from cycle to cycle. P waves have a normal contour, but a larger amplitude can develop and the wave can become peaked. They appear before each QRS complex with a stable PR interval unless concomitant atrioventricular (AV) block ensues.

Accelerated phase 4 diastolic depolarization of sinus nodal cells is generally responsible for sinus tachycardia and is usually due to elevated adrenergic tone and/or withdrawal of parasympathetic tone. Carotid sinus massage and the Valsalva or other vagal maneuvers gradually slow sinus tachycardia, which then accelerates to its previous rate on cessation of enhanced vagal tone. More rapid sinus rates can fail to slow in response to a vagal maneuver, particularly those driven by high adrenergic tone.

CLINICAL FEATURES. Sinus tachycardia is common in infancy and early childhood and is the normal reaction to a variety of physiological or pathophysiological stresses such as fever, hypotension, thyrotoxicosis, anemia, anxiety, exertion, hypovolemia, pulmonary emboli, myocardial ischemia, congestive heart failure, or shock. Drugs such as atropine, catecholamines, and thyroid medications, as well as alcohol, nicotine, caffeine, and inflammation, can produce sinus tachycardia. Persistent sinus tachycardia can be a manifestation of heart failure.

In patients with structural heart disease, sinus tachycardia can result in reduced cardiac output or angina or can precipitate another arrhythmia, in part related to the abbreviated ventricular filling time and compromised coronary blood flow. Sinus tachycardia can be a cause of inappropriate defibrillator discharge in patients with an implantable automatic defibrillator. *Chronic inappropriate sinus tachycardia* has been described in otherwise healthy persons, possibly secondary to increased automaticity of the sinus node or an automatic atrial focus located near the sinus node.[1] The abnormality can result from a defect in either sympathetic or vagal nerve control of sinoatrial (SA) automaticity, or an abnormality of the intrinsic heart rate can be present.

MANAGEMENT. Management should focus on the *cause* of the sinus tachycardia. In the hospital inpatient setting, this is

TABLE 32–1 Arrhythmia Characteristics*

Type of Arrhythmia	P Waves: Rate (beats/min)	P Waves: Rhythm	P Waves: Contour	QRS Complexes: Rate (beats/min)	QRS Complexes: Rhythm	QRS Complexes: Contour
Sinus rhythm	60-100	Regular[†]	Normal	60-100	Regular	Normal
Sinus bradycardia	<60	Regular	Normal	<60	Regular	Normal
Sinus tachycardia	100-180	Regular	May be peaked	100-180	Regular	Normal
AV nodal reentry	150-250	Very regular except at onset and termination	Retrograde; difficult to see; lost in QRS complex	150-250	Very regular except at onset and termination	Normal
Atrial flutter	250-350	Regular	Sawtooth	75-175	Generally regular in absence of drugs or disease	Normal
Atrial fibrillation	400-600	Grossly irregular	Baseline undulation, no P waves	100-160	Grossly irregular	Normal
Atrial tachycardia with block	150-250	Regular; may be irregular	Abnormal	75-200	Generally regular in absence of drugs or disease	Normal
AV junctional rhythm	40-100[§]	Regular	Normal	40-60	Fairly regular	Normal
Reciprocating tachycardias using an accessory (WPW) pathway	150-250	Very regular except at onset and termination	Retrograde; difficult to see; monitor the QRS complex	150-250	Very regular except at onset and termination	Normal
Nonparoxysinal AV junctional tachycardia	60-100[¶]	Regular	Normal	70-130	Fairly regular	Normal
Ventricular tachycardia	60-100[¶]	Regular	Normal	110-250	Fairly regular; may be irregular	Abnormal, >0.12 sec
Accelerated idioventricular rhythm	60-100[¶]	Regular	Normal	50-110	Fairly regular; may be irregular	Abnormal, >0.12 sec
Ventricular flutter	60-100[¶]	Regular	Normal; difficult to see	150-300	Regular	Sine wave
Ventricular fibrillation	60-100[¶]	Regular	Normal; difficult to see	400-600	Grossly irregular	Baseline undulations; no QRS complexes
First-degree AV block	60-100**	Regular	Normal	60-100	Regular	Normal
Type I second-degree AV block	60-100**	Regular	Normal	30-100	Irregular[††]	Normal
Type II second-degree AV block	60-100**	Regular	Normal	30-100	Irregular[††]	Abnormal, >0.12 sec
Complete AV block	60-100[¶]	Regular	Normal	<40	Fairly regular	Abnormal, 0.12 sec
Right bundle branch block	60-100	Regular	Normal	60-100	Regular	Abnormal, 0.12 sec
Left bundle branch block	60-100	Regular	Normal	60-100	Regular	Abnormal, >0.12 sec

AV = atrioventricular; WPW = Wolff-Parkinson-White.

Modified from Zipes DP: Arrhythmias. *In* Andreoli K, Zipes DP, Wallace AG, et al (eds): Comprehensive Cardiac Care. 6th ed. St Louis, CV Mosby, 1987.

*In an effort to summarize these arrhythmias in tabular form, generalizations have to be made. For example, the response to carotid sinus massage may be slightly different from what is listed. Acute therapy to terminate a tachycardia may be different from chronic therapy to prevent recurrence. Some of the exceptions are indicated in the footnotes; the reader is referred to the text for a complete discussion.

†P waves initiated by sinus node discharge may not be precisely regular because of sinus arrhythmia.

‡Often, carotid sinus massage fails to slow a sinus tachycardia.

§Any independent atrial arrhythmia may exist or the atria may be captured retrogradely.

	P Waves		QRS Complexes	
	Physical Examination			
Ventricular Response to Carotid Sinus Massage	*Intensity of S_1*	*Splitting of S_2*	*a Waves*	*Treatment*
Gradual slowing and return to former rate	Constant	Normal	Normal	None
Gradual slowing and return to former rate	Constant	Normal	Normal	None, unless symptomatic; atropine
Gradual slowing[‡] and return to former rate	Constant	Normal	Normal	None, unless symptomatic; treat underlying disease
Abrupt slowing caused by termination of tachycardia, or no effect	Constant	Normal	Constant cannon *a* waves	Vagal stimulation, adenosine, verapamil, digitalis, propranolol, DC shock, pacing
Abrupt slowing and return to former rate; flutter remains	Constant; variable if AV block changing	Normal	Flutter waves	DC shock, digitalis, quinidine, propranolol, verapamil, adenosine
Slowing; gross irregularity remains	Variable	Normal	No *a* waves	Digitalis, quinidine, DC shock, verapamil, adenosine
Abrupt slowing and return to normal rate; tachycardia remains	Constant; variable if AV block changing	Normal	More *a* waves than *c-v* waves	Stop digitalis if toxic; digitalis if not toxic; possibly verapamil
None; may be slight slowing	Variables[¶]	Normal	Intermittent cannon waves	None, unless symptomatic; atropine
Abrupt slowing caused by termination of tachycardia, or no effect	Constant but decreased	Normal	Constant cannon waves	See AV nodal reentry above
None, may be slight slowing	Variable[¶]	Normal	Intermittent cannon waves[¶]	None, unless symptomatic: stop digitalis if toxic
None	Variable[¶]	Abnormal	Intermittent cannon waves[¶]	Lidocaine, procainamide, DC shock, quinidine, amiodarone
None	Variable[¶]	Abnormal	Intermittent cannon waves[¶]	None, unless symptomatic: lidocaine, atropine
None	Soft or absent	Soft or absent	Cannon waves	DC shock
None	None	None	Cannon waves	DC shock
Gradual slowing caused by sinus	Constant, diminished	Normal	Normal	None
Slowing caused by sinus slowing and an increase in AV black	Cyclic decrease, then increase after pause	Normal	Normal; increasing *a-c* interval; *a* waves without *c* waves	None, unless symptomatic: atropine
Gradual slowing caused by sinus slowing	Constant	Abnormal	Normal; constant *a-c* interval; *a* waves without *c* waves	Pacemaker
None	Variable**	Abnormal	Intermittent cannon waves**	Pacemaker
Gradual slowing and return to former rate	Constant	Wide	Normal	None
Gradual slowing and return to former rate	Constant	Paradoxical	Normal	None

[¶]Constant if the atria are captured retrogradely.
**Atrial rhythm and rate may vary, depending on whether sinus bradycardia, sinus tachycardia, or another abnormality is the atrial mechanism.
[††]Regular or constant if block is unchanging.

usually obvious (e.g., hemorrhage, sepsis, agitation). In the outpatient setting, the cause may be more elusive. The most common reversible causes include hyperthyroidism, anemia, diabetes, and hypovolemia . Elimination of tobacco, alcohol, coffee, tea, or other stimulants, such as the sympathomimetic agents in nose drops, may be helpful. Drugs such as propranolol or verapamil or fluid replacement in a hypovolemic patient or fever reduction in a febrile patient can be used to help slow the sinus nodal discharge rate. Treatment of inappropriate sinus tachycardia requires beta blockers, calcium-channel blockers, or digitalis, alone or in combination. In severe cases, sinus node radiofrequency or surgical ablation may be indicated.

Sinus Bradycardia

ECG RECOGNITION. Sinus bradycardia (Fig. 32–1B) exists in an adult when the sinus node discharges at a rate slower than 60 beats/min. P waves have a normal contour and occur before each QRS complex, usually with a constant PR interval greater than 120 milliseconds. Sinus arrhythmia often coexists.

CLINICAL FEATURES. Sinus bradycardia can result from excessive vagal and/or decreased sympathetic tone, as an effect of medications, or from anatomical changes in the sinus node. In most cases, symptomatic sinus bradycardia is due to the effects of medication. Asymptomatic sinus bradycardia frequently occurs in healthy young adults, particularly well-trained athletes, and decreases in prevalence with advancing age. During sleep, the normal heart rate can fall to 35 to 40 beats/min, especially in adolescents and young adults, with marked sinus arrhythmia sometimes producing pauses of 2 seconds or longer. Eye surgery, coronary arteriography, meningitis, intracranial tumors, increased intracranial pressure, cervical and mediastinal tumors, and certain disease states such as severe hypoxia, Chagas disease, myxedema, hypothermia, fibrodegenerative changes, convalescence from some infections, gram-negative sepsis, and mental depression can produce sinus bradycardia. Sinus bradycardia also occurs during vomiting or vasovagal syncope (see Chap. 34) and can be produced by carotid sinus stimulation or by the administration of parasympathomimetic drugs, lithium, amiodarone, beta-adrenoceptor blocking drugs, clonidine, propafenone, or calcium antagonists. Conjunctival instillation of beta blockers for glaucoma can produce sinus or AV nodal abnormalities, especially in the elderly.

In most instances, sinus bradycardia is a benign arrhythmia and can actually be beneficial by producing a longer period of diastole and increasing the ventricular filling time. It can be associated with syncope caused by an abnormal autonomic reflex (cardioinhibitory) (see Chap. 34). Sinus bradycardia occurs in 10 to 15 percent of patients with acute myocardial infarction and may be even more prevalent when patients are seen in the early hours of infarction. Unless accompanied by hemodynamic decompensation or arrhythmias, sinus bradycardia is generally associated with a more favorable outcome following myocardial infarction than is the presence of sinus tachycardia. It is usually transient and occurs more commonly during inferior than anterior myocardial infarction; it has also been noted during reperfusion with thrombolytic agents (see Chap. 48). Bradycardia following resuscitation from cardiac arrest is associated with a poor prognosis.

MANAGEMENT. Treatment of sinus bradycardia per se is not usually necessary. For example, if a patient with acute myocardial infarction is asymptomatic, it is probably best to not speed up the sinus rate. If cardiac output is inadequate or if arrhythmias are associated with the slow rate, atropine (0.5 mg intravenously [IV] as an initial dose, repeated if necessary) is usually effective. Lower doses of atropine, particularly when given subcutaneously or intramuscularly, can exert an initial parasympathomimetic effect, possibly via a central action. For symptomatic episodes of sinus bradycardia that are more than momentary or are recurrent (e.g., as during a myocardial infarction) temporary electrical pacing via a transveneous electrode is usually preferable to repeated or prolonged drug therapy. In some patients who experience congestive heart failure or symptoms of low cardiac output as a result of chronic sinus bradycardia, permanent electrical pacing may be needed (see Chap. 31). Atrial pacing is usually preferable to ventricular pacing to preserve sequential AV contraction and is preferable to drug therapy for long-term management of sinus bradycardia. As a general rule, no available drugs increase the heart rate reliably and safely over long periods without important side effects.

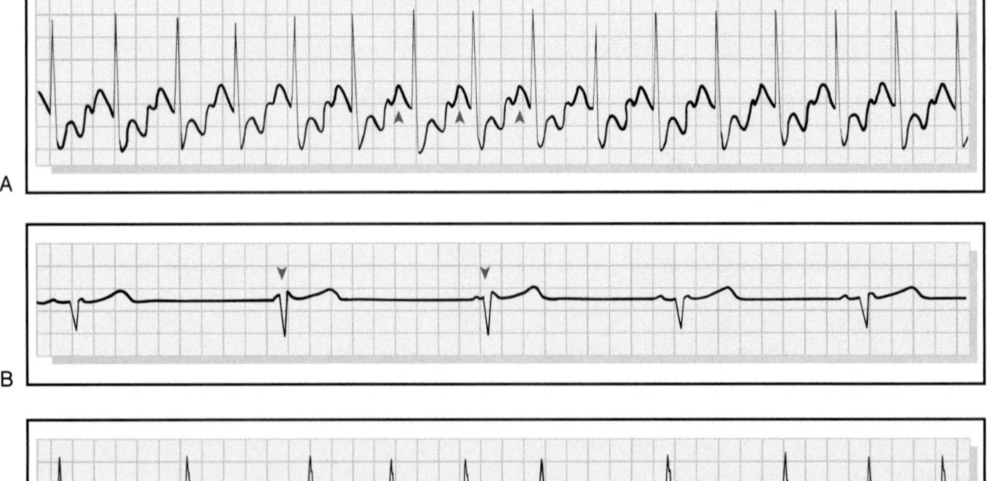

FIGURE 32–1 **A,** Sinus tachycardia (150 beats/min) in a patient during acute myocardial ischemia; note the ST segment depression. P waves are indicated by arrowheads. **B,** Sinus bradycardia at a rate of 40 to 48 beats/min. The second and third QRS complexes (arrowheads) represent junctional escape beats. Note the P waves at the onset of the QRS complex. **C,** Nonrespiratory sinus arrhythmia occurring as a consequence of digitalis toxicity. Monitor leads.

SINUS ARRHYTHMIA

Sinus arrhythmia (Fig. 32-1C) is characterized by a phasic variation in sinus cycle length during which the maximum sinus cycle length minus the minimum sinus cycle length exceeds 120 milliseconds or the maximum sinus cycle length minus the minimum sinus cycle length divided by the minimum sinus cycle length exceeds 10 percent. It is the most frequent form of arrhythmia and is considered to be a normal event. P wave morphology does not usually vary, and the PR interval exceeds 120 milliseconds and remains unchanged since the focus of discharge remains relatively fixed within the sinus node. Occasionally, the pacemaker focus can wander within the sinus node, or its exit to the atrium may change and produce P waves of a slightly different contour (but not retrograde) and a slightly changing PR interval that exceeds 120 milliseconds.

Sinus arrhythmia commonly occurs in the young, especially those with slower heart rates or following enhanced vagal tone, such as after the administration of digitalis or morphine, and decreases with age or with autonomic dysfunction, such as diabetic neuropathy. Sinus arrhythmia appears in two basic forms. In the *respiratory* form, the P-P interval cyclically shortens during inspiration, primarily as a result of reflex inhibition of vagal tone, and slows during expiration; breath-holding eliminates the cycle length variation (see Heart Rate Variability, Chap. 29). Efferent vagal effects alone have been suggested as being responsible for respiratory sinus arrhythmias. *Nonrespiratory* sinus arrhythmia is characterized by a phasic variation in the P-P interval unrelated to the respiratory cycle and may be the result of digitalis intoxication. Loss of sinus rhythm variability is a risk factor for sudden cardiac death (see Chap. 23).

Symptoms produced by sinus arrhythmia are uncommon, but on occasion, if the pauses between beats are excessively long, palpitations or dizziness may result. Marked sinus arrhythmia can produce a sinus pause sufficiently long to produce syncope if not accompanied by an escape rhythm.

Treatment is usually unnecessary. Increasing the heart rate by exercise or drugs generally abolishes sinus arrhythmia. Symptomatic individuals may experience relief from palpitations with sedatives, tranquilizers, atropine, ephedrine, or isoproterenol administration, as in the treatment of sinus bradycardia.

VENTRICULOPHASIC SINUS ARRHYTHMIA. The most common example occurs during complete AV block and a slow ventricular rate, when P-P cycles that contain a QRS complex are shorter than P-P cycles without a QRS complex. Similar lengthening can be present in the P-P cycle that follows a premature ventricular complex (PVC) with a compensatory pause. Alterations in the P-P interval are probably due to the influence of the autonomic nervous system responding to changes in ventricular stroke volume.

SINUS PAUSE OR SINUS ARREST

Sinus pause or sinus arrest (Fig. 32-2) is recognized by a pause in the sinus rhythm. The P-P interval delimiting the pause does not equal a multiple of the basic P-P interval. Differentiation of sinus arrest, which is thought to be due to slowing or cessation of spontaneous sinus nodal automaticity and therefore a disorder of impulse formation from SA exit block (see below) in patients with sinus arrhythmia, can be quite difficult without direct recordings of sinus node discharge.

Failure of sinus nodal discharge results in the absence of atrial depolarization and in periods of ventricular asystole if escape beats initiated by latent pacemakers do not occur (see Fig. 32-2). Involvement of the sinus node by acute myocardial infarction, degenerative fibrotic changes, effects of digitalis toxicity, stroke, or excessive vagal tone all can produce sinus arrest. Transient sinus arrest may have no clinical significance by itself if latent pacemakers promptly escape to prevent ventricular asystole or the genesis of other arrhythmias precipitated by the slow rates. Sinus arrest and AV block have been demonstrated in as many as 30 percent of patients with sleep apnea (see Chap. 68).

Treatment is as outlined earlier for sinus bradycardia. In patients who have a chronic form of sinus node disease characterized by marked sinus bradycardia or sinus arrest, permanent pacing is often necessary. However, as a general rule, chronic pacing for sinus bradycardia is indicated only in symptomatic patients or those with a sinus pause exceeding 3 seconds.[2]

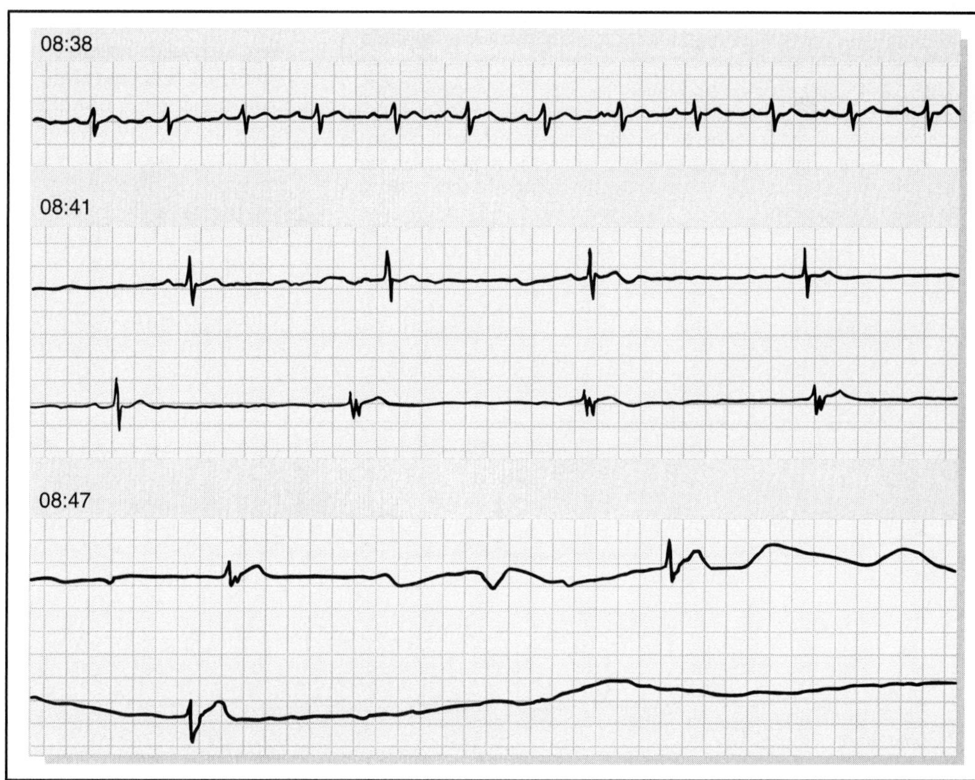

FIGURE 32–2 Sinus arrest. The patient had a long-term electrocardiographic (ECG) recorder connected when he died suddenly of cardiac standstill. The rhythms demonstrate progressive sinus bradycardia and sinus arrest at 8:41 A.M. The rhythm then becomes a ventricular escape rhythm, which progressively slows and finally ceases at 8:47 A.M. Monitor lead. The double ECG strips are continuous recordings.

SINOATRIAL EXIT BLOCK

This arrhythmia is recognized electrocardiographically by a pause resulting from absence of the normally expected P wave (Fig. 32-3). The duration of the pause is a multiple of the basic P-P interval. SA exit block is due to a conduction disturbance during which an impulse formed within the sinus node fails to depolarize the atria or does so with delay (Fig. 32-4). An interval without P waves that equals approximately two, three, or four times the normal P-P cycle characterizes type II second-degree SA exit block. During type I (Wenckebach) second-degree SA exit block, the P-P interval progressively shortens prior to the pause, and the duration of the pause is less than two P-P cycles. (See Chap. 27 for further discussion of Wenckebach intervals.) First-degree SA exit block cannot be recognized by ECG because SA nodal discharge is not recorded. Third-degree SA exit block can be manifested as a complete absence of P waves and is difficult to diagnose with certainty without sinus node electrograms.

Excessive vagal stimulation, acute myocarditis, infarction, or fibrosis involving the atrium, as well as drugs such as quinidine, procainamide, or digitalis, can produce SA exit block. SA exit block is usually transient. It may be of no clinical importance except to prompt a search for the underlying cause. Occasionally, syncope can result if the SA block is prolonged and unaccompanied by an escape rhythm. SA exit block can occur in well-trained athletes.

Therapy for patients who have symptomatic SA exit block is as outlined for sinus bradycardia.

WANDERING PACEMAKER

This variant of sinus arrhythmia involves passive transfer of the dominant pacemaker focus from the sinus node to latent pacemakers that have the next highest degree of automaticity located in other atrial sites (usually lower in the crista terminalis) or in AV junctional tissue. The change occurs in a gradual fashion over the duration of several beats; thus, only one pacemaker at a time controls the rhythm, in sharp contrast with AV dissociation. The ECG (Fig. 32-5) displays a cyclical increase in the R-R interval: a PR interval that gradually shortens and can become less than 120 milliseconds; and a change in the P wave contour, which becomes negative in lead I or II (depending on the site of discharge) or is lost within the QRS complex. Generally, these changes

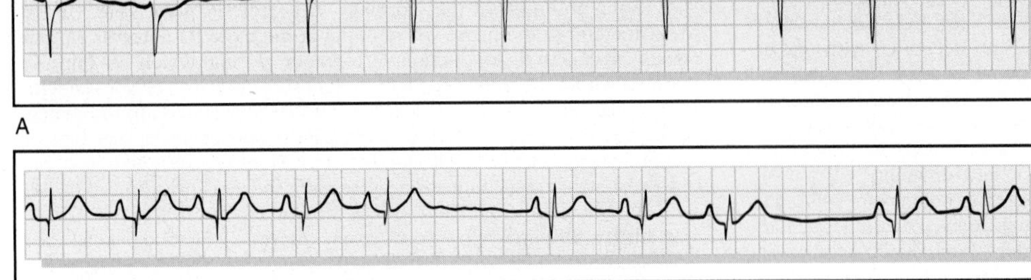

FIGURE 32–3 Sinus nodal exit block. **A,** A type I sinoatrial (SA) nodal exit block has the following features: The P-P interval shortens from the first to the second cycle in each grouping, followed by a pause. The duration of the pause is less than twice the shortest cycle length, and the cycle after the pause exceeds the cycle before the pause. The PR interval is normal and constant. Lead V_1. **B,** The P-P interval varies slightly because of sinus arrhythmia. The two pauses in sinus nodal activity equal twice the basic P-P interval and are consistent with a type II 2:1 SA nodal exit block. The PR interval is normal and constant. Lead III.

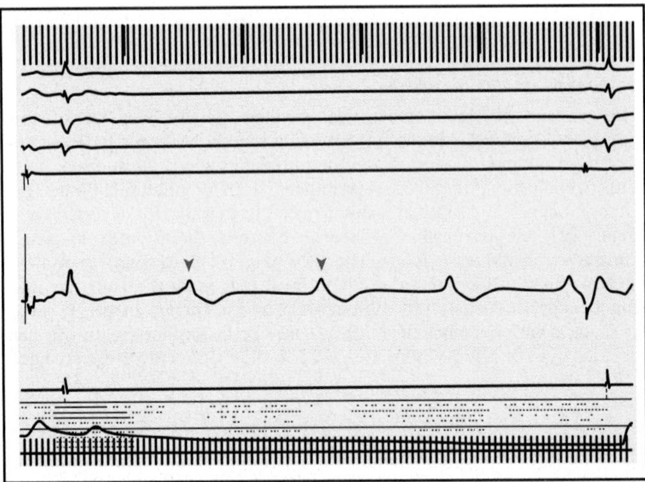

FIGURE 32–4 Sinus node exit block. After a period of atrial pacing (only the last paced cycle is shown), sinus node exit block developed. The tracing demonstrates sinus node potentials (arrowheads), recorded with a catheter electrode, not conducting to the atrium until the last complex. Recordings are leads I, II, III, and V_1, right atrial recording, sinus node recording, and right ventricular apical recording. The bottom tracing is femoral artery blood pressure.

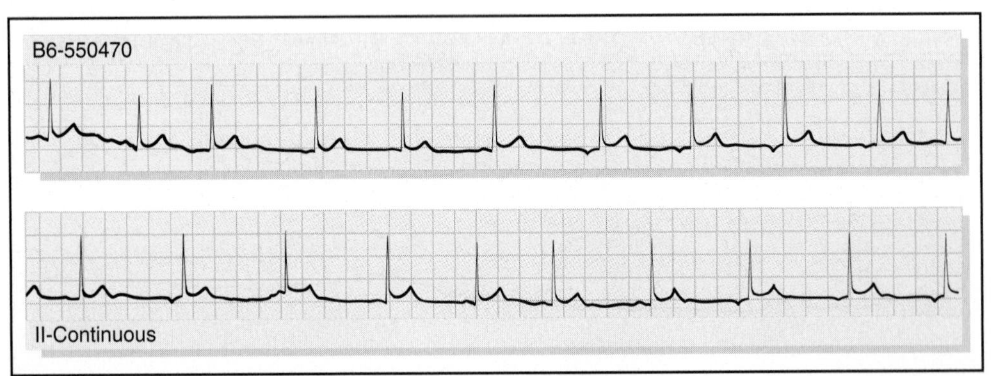

FIGURE 32–5 Wandering atrial pacemaker. As the heart rate slows, the P waves become inverted and then gradually revert toward normal when the heart rate speeds up again. The PR interval shortens to 0.14 second with the inverted P wave and is 0.16 second with the upright P wave. This phasic variation in cycle length with varying P wave contour suggests a shift in pacemaker site and is characteristic of wandering atrial pacemaker.

occur in reverse as the pacemaker shifts back to the sinus node. Wandering pacemaker is a normal phenomenon that often occurs in the very young and particularly in athletes, presumably because of augmented vagal tone. Persistence of an AV junctional rhythm for long periods, however, may indicate underlying heart disease. *Treatment* is not usually indicated but, if necessary, is the same as that for sinus bradycardia (see earlier).

Hypersensitive Carotid Sinus Syndrome

(see also Chap. 34)

ECG RECOGNITION. Hypersensitive carotid sinus syndrome (Fig. 32–6) is characterized most frequently by ventricular asystole caused by cessation of atrial activity from sinus arrest or SA exit block. AV block is observed less frequently, probably in part because the absence of atrial activity from sinus arrest precludes the manifestations of AV block. However, if an atrial pacemaker maintained an atrial rhythm during the episodes, a higher prevalence of AV block would probably be noted. In symptomatic patients, AV junctional or ventricular escapes generally do not occur or are present at very slow rates, thus suggesting that heightened vagal tone and sympathetic withdrawal can suppress subsidiary pacemakers located in the ventricles, as well as supraventricular structures.

CLINICAL FEATURES. Two types of hypersensitive carotid sinus responses are noted. *Cardioinhibitory* carotid sinus hypersensitivity is generally defined as ventricular asystole exceeding 3 seconds during carotid sinus stimulation, although normal limits have not been carefully established. In fact, asystole exceeding 3 seconds during carotid sinus massage is not common but can occur in asymptomatic subjects (see Fig. 32–6). *Vasodepressor* carotid sinus hypersensitivity is generally defined as a decrease in systolic blood pressure of 50 mm Hg or more without associated cardiac slowing or a decrease in systolic blood pressure exceeding 30 mm Hg when the patient's symptoms are reproduced.

Even if a hyperactive carotid sinus reflex is elicited in patients, particularly in older patients who complain of syncope or presyncope, the hyperactive reflex elicited with carotid sinus massage may not necessarily be responsible for these symptoms. Direct pressure or extension on the carotid sinus from head turning, neck tension, and tight collars can also be a source of syncope by reducing blood flow through the cerebral arteries. Hypersensitive carotid sinus reflex is most commonly associated with coronary artery disease. The mechanism responsible for hypersensitive carotid sinus reflex is not known.

MANAGEMENT. Atropine abolishes cardioinhibitory carotid sinus hypersensitivity. However, most symptomatic patients require pacemaker implantation.

Because AV block can occur during periods of hypersensitive carotid reflex, some form of *ventricular* pacing, with or without atrial pacing, is generally required. Atropine and pacing do not prevent the decrease in systemic blood pressure in the vasodepressor form of carotid sinus hypersensitivity, which may result from inhibition of sympathetic vasoconstrictor nerves and possibly from activation of cholinergic sympathetic vasodilator fibers. Combinations of vasodepressor and cardioinhibitory types can occur, and vasodepression can account for continued syncope after pacemaker implantation in some patients. Patients who have a hyperactive carotid sinus reflex that does not cause symptoms require no treatment. Drugs such as digitalis, alpha-methyldopa, clonidine, and propranolol can enhance the response to carotid sinus massage and be responsible for symptoms in some patients. Elastic support hose and sodium-retaining drugs may be helpful in patients with vasodepressor responses.

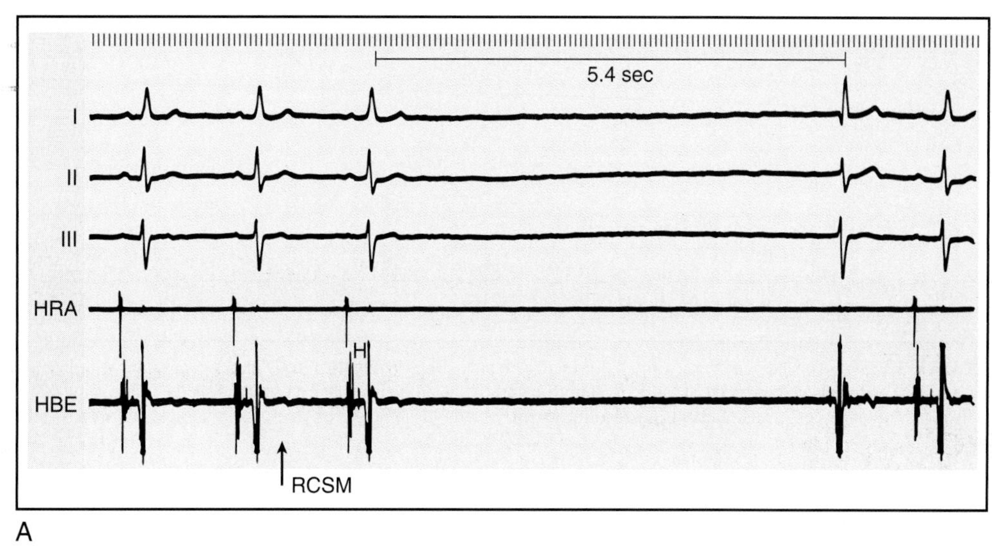

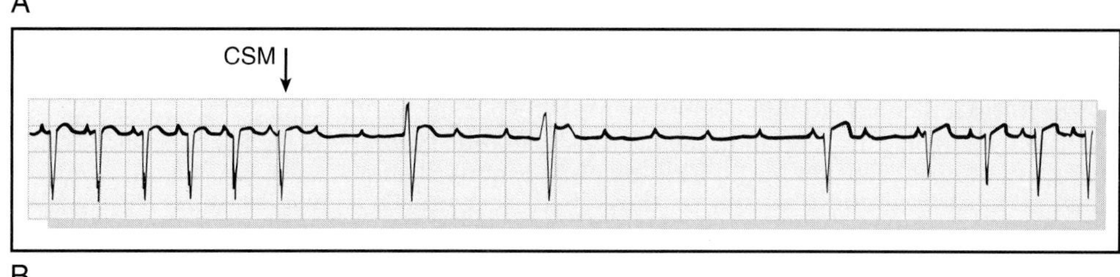

FIGURE 32–6 **A,** Right carotid sinus massage (RCSM) (arrow) results in sinus arrest and a ventricular escape beat (probably fascicular) 5.4 seconds later. Sinus discharge then resumes. **B,** Carotid sinus massage (CSM) (arrow; monitor lead) results in slight sinus slowing but, more important, advanced atrioventricular block. Obviously, an atrial pacemaker without ventricular pacing would be inappropriate for this patient.

Sick Sinus Syndrome

ECG RECOGNITION. *Sick sinus syndrome* is a term that is applied to a syndrome encompassing a number of sinus nodal abnormalities, including (1) persistent spontaneous sinus bradycardia not caused by drugs and inappropriate for the physiological circumstance; (2) sinus arrest or exit block (Fig. 32–7); (3) combinations of SA and AV conduction disturbances; or (4) alternation of paroxysms of rapid regular or irregular atrial tachyarrhythmias and periods of slow atrial and ventricular rates (bradycardia-tachycardia syndrome [Fig. 32–8]). More than one of these conditions can be recorded in the same patient on different occasions, and often their mechanisms can be shown to be causally interrelated and combined with an abnormal state of AV conduction or automaticity. Rapid atrial rates can "remodel" the sinus node and depress its automaticity, so the sinus bradycardia may be functional in part and reversible.[3]

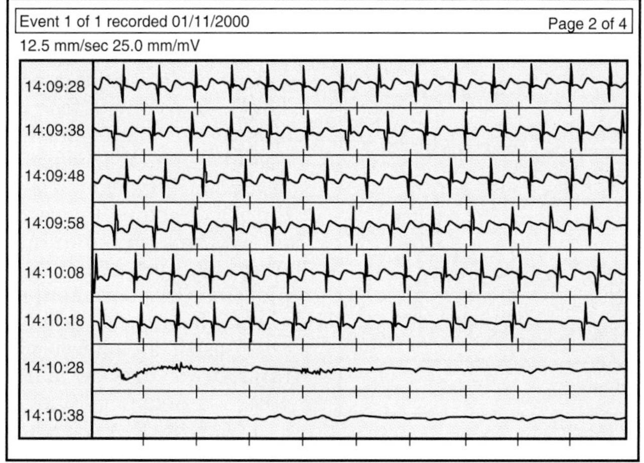

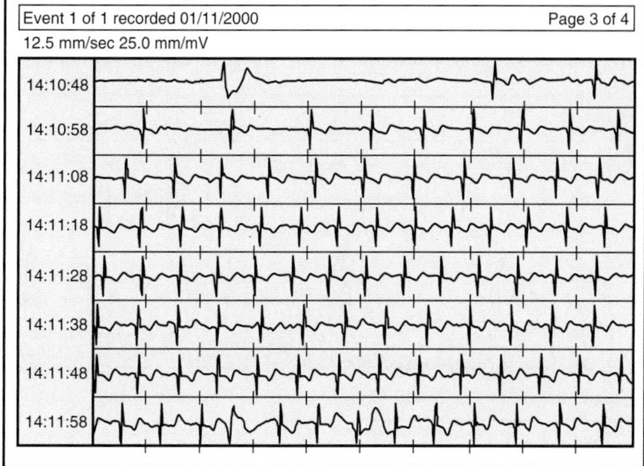

FIGURE 32–7 Continuous recording from an implanted loop recorder in a patient with syncope. The tracing shows paroxysmal sinus node arrest and a sinus pause of nearly 30 seconds. The preceding sinus cycle length appears to lengthen just prior to the pause, suggesting an autonomic component to the pause. There is also a single ventricular escape complex at 14:10:48.

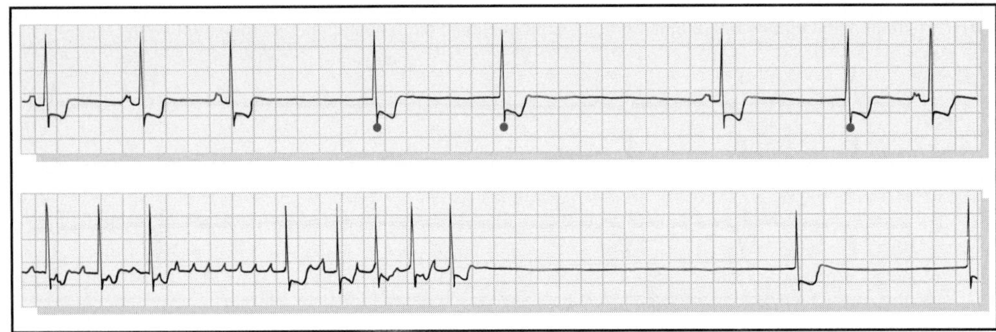

FIGURE 32–8 Sick sinus syndrome with bradycardia-tachycardia. **Top,** Intermittent sinus arrest is apparent with junctional escape beats at irregular intervals (red circles, top). **Bottom,** In this continuous monitor lead recording, a short episode of atrial flutter is followed by almost 5 seconds of asystole before a junctional escape rhythm resumes. The patient became presyncopal at this point.

Patients who have sinus node disease can be categorized as having intrinsic sinus node disease unrelated to autonomic abnormalities or combinations of intrinsic and autonomic abnormalities. Symptomatic patients with sinus pauses and/or SA exit block frequently show abnormal responses on electrophysiological testing and can have a relatively high incidence of atrial fibrillation. In children, sinus node dysfunction most commonly occurs in those with congenital or acquired heart disease, particularly following corrective cardiac surgery. Sick sinus syndrome can occur in the absence of other cardiac abnormalities. The course of the disease is frequently intermittent and unpredictable because it is influenced by the severity of the underlying heart disease. Excessive physical training can heighten vagal tone and produce syncope related to sinus bradycardia or AV conduction abnormalities in otherwise normal individuals.

The anatomical basis of sick sinus syndrome can involve total or subtotal destruction of the sinus node, areas of nodal-atrial discontinuity, inflammatory or degenerative changes in the nerves and ganglia surrounding the node, and pathological changes in the atrial wall. Fibrosis and fatty infiltration occur, and the sclerodegenerative processes generally involve the sinus node and the AV node or the bundle of His and its branches or distal subdivisions.[4] Occlusion of the sinus node artery may be important.

MANAGEMENT. For patients with sick sinus syndrome, treatment depends on the basic rhythm problem but generally involves permanent pacemaker implantation when symptoms are manifested (see Chap. 31). Pacing for the bradycardia, combined with drug therapy to treat the tachycardia, is required in those with bradycardia-tachycardia syndrome.

SINUS NODAL REENTRY TACHYCARDIA

ECG RECOGNITION. The rate of sinus nodal reentrant tachycardia varies from 80 to 200 beats/min but is generally slower than the other forms of supraventricular tachycardia, with an average rate of 130 to 140 beats/min (Fig. 32-9). Electrocardiographically, P waves are identical or very similar to the sinus P wave; the PR interval is related to the tachycardia rate, but generally the RP interval is long, with a shorter PR interval (Fig. 32-10D). AV block can occur without affecting the tachycardia, and vagal maneuvers can slow and then abruptly terminate the tachycardia. Electrophysiologically, the tachycardia can be initiated and terminated by premature atrial and, uncommonly, premature ventricular stimulation (see Fig. 32-9). Initiation of sinus nodal reentry does not depend on a critical degree of intraatrial or AV nodal conduction delay, and the atrial activation sequence is the same as during sinus rhythm. An AV nodal Wenckebach block during the tachycardia is common. The development of a bundle branch block does not affect the cycle length or PR interval during tachycardia.

Sinus nodal reentry may account for 5 to 10 percent of cases of supraventricular tachycardia. It occurs in all age groups without sex predilection. Patients may be slightly older and have a higher incidence of heart disease than do patients with supraventricular tachycardia resulting from other mechanisms. Many may not seek medical attention because the relatively slow rate of the tachycardia does not result in serious symptoms. On the other hand, sinus nodal reentry may be responsible for apparent "anxiety-related sinus tachycardia" in some patients. Drugs such as beta blockers, calcium-channel blockers, and digitalis may be effective in terminating and preventing recurrences of sinus node reentrant tachycardia. Catheter ablation is highly effective in treating this arrhythmia and does not produce sinus node dysfunction.

Disturbances of Atrial Rhythm

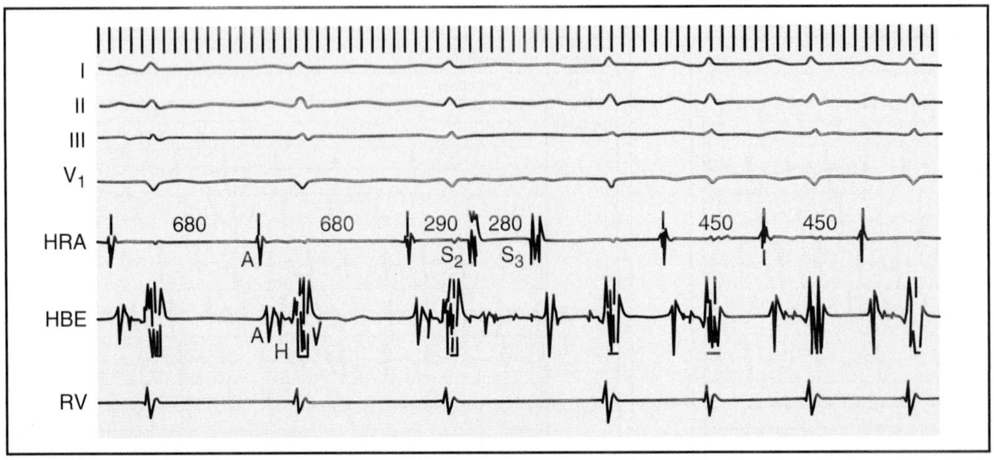

Premature Atrial Complexes

Premature complexes are among the most common causes of an irregular pulse. They can originate from any area in the heart—most frequently from the ventricles, less often from the atria and the AV junctional area, and rarely from the sinus node. Although premature complexes arise commonly in normal hearts, they are more often associated with structural heart disease and increase in frequency with age.

ECG RECOGNITION. The diagnosis of premature atrial complexes (Fig. 32–11) is indicated on the ECG by a premature P wave with a PR

FIGURE 32–9 Sinus node reentry. After three spontaneous sinus-initiated beats, premature stimulation of the high right atrium (S_2, S_3) initiates a sustained tachycardia at a cycle length of 450 milliseconds that has the identical high-low atrial activation sequence characteristic of sinus node discharge. This is sinus node reentry. Leads I, II, III, and V_1 are scalar leads. A = atrial electrogram; H = His electrogram; HBE = His bundle electrogram; HRA = high right atrial electrogram; RV = right ventricular electrogram; V = ventricular electrogram. Numbers are milliseconds.

interval exceeding 120 milliseconds (except in Wolff-Parkinson-White [WPW] syndrome, in which case the PR interval is usually less than 120 milliseconds). Although the contour of a premature P wave can resemble that of a normal sinus P wave, it generally differs. While variations in the basic sinus rate can at times make the diagnosis of prematurity difficult, differences in the contour of the P waves are usually apparent and indicate a different focus of origin. When a premature atrial complex occurs early in diastole, conduction may not be completely normal. The AV junction may still be refractory from the preceding beat and prevent propagation of the impulse (blocked or nonconducted premature atrial complex [Fig. 32–11A]) or cause conduction to be slowed (premature atrial complex with a prolonged PR interval). As a general rule, the RP interval is inversely related to the PR interval; thus, a short RP interval produced by an early premature atrial complex occurring close to the preceding QRS complex is followed by a long PR interval. When premature atrial complexes occur early in the cardiac cycle, the premature P waves can be difficult to discern because they are superimposed on T waves. Careful examination of tracings from several leads may be necessary before the premature atrial complex is recognized as a slight deformity of the T wave. Often, such premature atrial complexes are blocked before reaching the ventricle and can be misinterpreted as a sinus pause or sinus exit block (Fig. 32–11A).

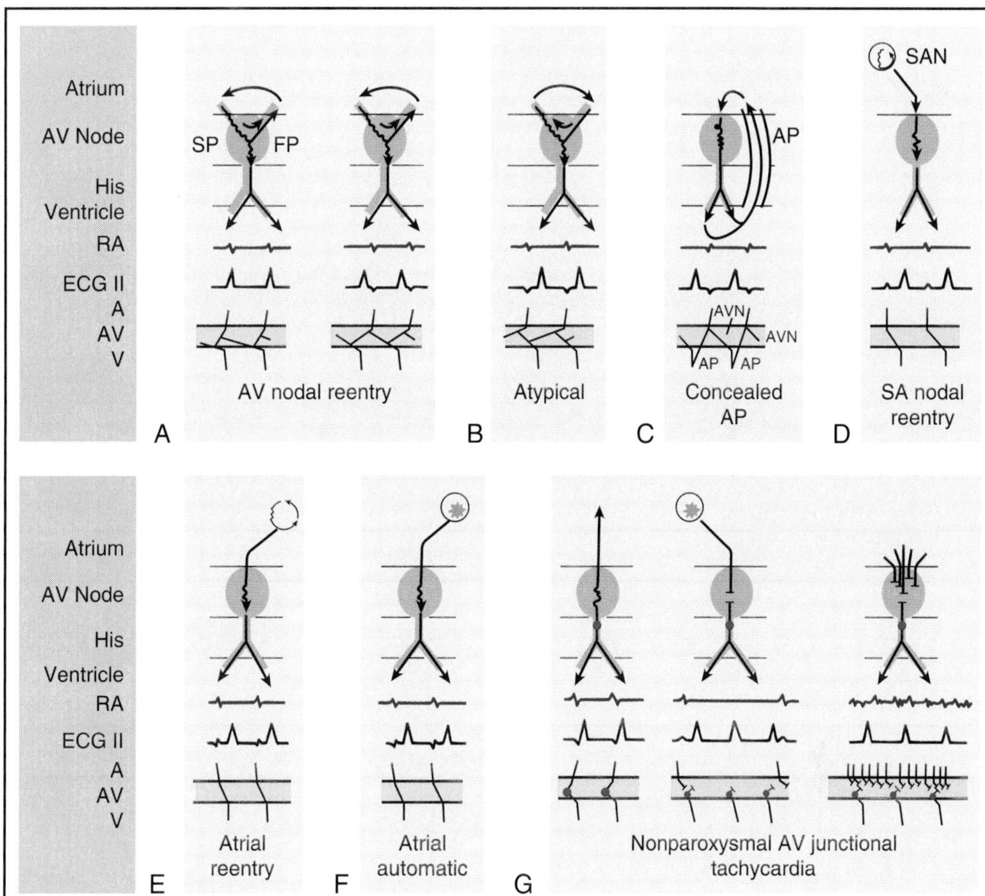

FIGURE 32–10 Diagrammatic representation of various tachycardias. In the upper portion of each example, a schematic of the presumed anatomical pathways is drawn; in the lower half, the electrocardiographic (ECG) appearance and the explanatory ladder diagram are depicted. **A,** Atrioventricular (AV) nodal reentry. In the left example, reentrant excitation is drawn with retrograde atrial activity occurring simultaneously with ventricular activity as a result of anterograde conduction over the slow AV nodal pathway (SP) and retrograde conduction over the fast AV nodal pathway (FP). In the right example, atrial activity occurs slightly later than ventricular activity because of retrograde conduction delay. **B,** Atypical AV nodal reentry caused by anterograde conduction over a fast AV nodal pathway and retrograde conduction over a slow AV nodal pathway. **C,** Concealed accessory pathway (AP). Reciprocating tachycardia is due to anterograde conduction over the AV node (AVN) and retrograde conduction over the accessory pathway. Retrograde P waves occur after the QRS complex. **D,** Sinus nodal reentry. The tachycardia is due to reentry within the sinus node, which then conducts the impulse to the rest of the heart. SA = sinoatrial; SAN = sinoatrial node. **E,** Atrial reentry. Tachycardia is due to reentry within the atrium, which then conducts the impulse to the rest of the heart. **F,** Automatic atrial tachycardia (star indicates origin). Tachycardia is due to automatic discharge in the atrium, which then conducts the impulse to the rest of the heart; it is difficult to distinguish from atrial reentry. **G,** Nonparoxysmal AV junctional tachycardia. Various manifestations of this tachycardia are depicted with retrograde atrial capture, AV dissociation with the sinus node in control of the atria, and AV dissociation with atrial fibrillation. Star indicates sinus node discharge. Red circles indicate site of junctional discharge.

The length of the pause following any premature complex or series of premature complexes is determined by the interaction of several factors. If the premature atrial complex occurs when the sinus node and perinodal tissue are not refractory, the impulse can be conducted into the sinus node, discharge it prematurely, and cause the next sinus cycle to begin from that time. The interval between the two normal P waves flanking a premature atrial complex that has reset the timing of the basic sinus rhythm is less than twice the normal P-P interval, and the pause after the premature atrial complex is said to be "noncompensatory." Referring to Figure 32–11E and F, reset (noncompensatory pause) occurs when the A_1-A_2 interval plus the A_2-A_3 interval is less than two times the A_1-A_1 interval and the A_2-A_3 interval is greater than the A_1-A_1 interval. The interval between the premature atrial complex (A_2) and the following sinus-initiated P wave (A_3) exceeds one sinus cycle but is less than "fully compensatory" (see later) because the A_2-A_3 interval is lengthened by the time that it takes the ectopic atrial impulse to conduct to the sinus node and depolarize it and then for the sinus impulse to return to the atrium. These factors lengthen the return cycle, that is, the interval between the premature atrial complex (A_2) and the following sinus-initiated P wave (A_3) (Fig. 32–11E and F). Premature discharge of the sinus node by an early premature atrial complex can temporarily depress sinus nodal automatic activity and cause the sinus node to beat more slowly initially (Fig. 32–11D). Often when this happens, the interval between the A_3 and the next sinus-initiated P wave exceeds the A_1-A_1 interval.

Less commonly, the premature atrial complex encounters a refractory sinus node or perinodal tissue (Fig. 32–11F), in which case the timing of the basic sinus rhythm is not altered since the sinus node is not reset by the premature atrial complex, and the interval between the two normal, sinus-initiated P waves flanking the premature atrial complex is twice the normal P-P interval. The interval following this premature atrial discharge is said to be a "full compensatory pause," that is, of sufficient duration so that the P-P interval bounding the premature atrial complex is twice the normal P-P interval. However, sinus arrhythmia can lengthen or shorten this pause. Rarely, an *interpolated premature atrial* complex

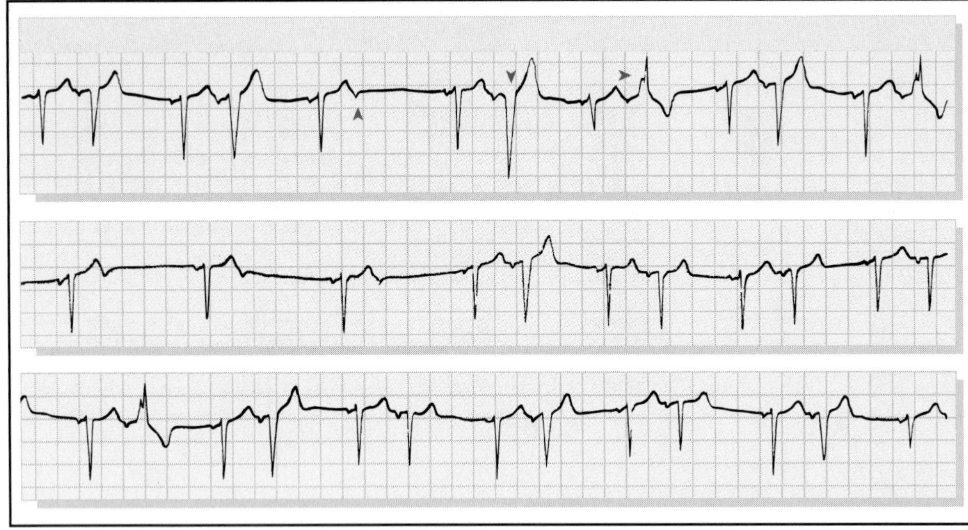
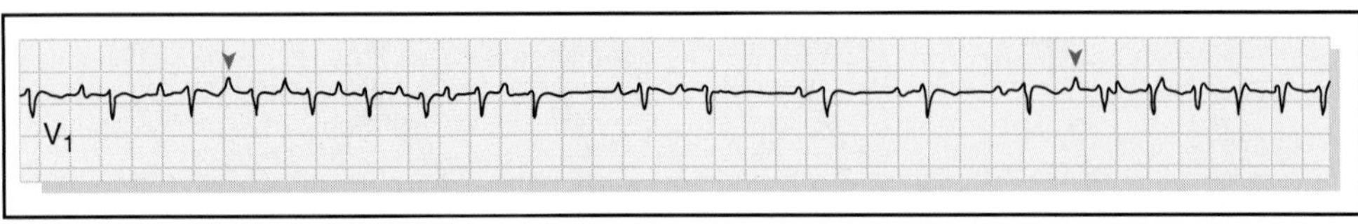

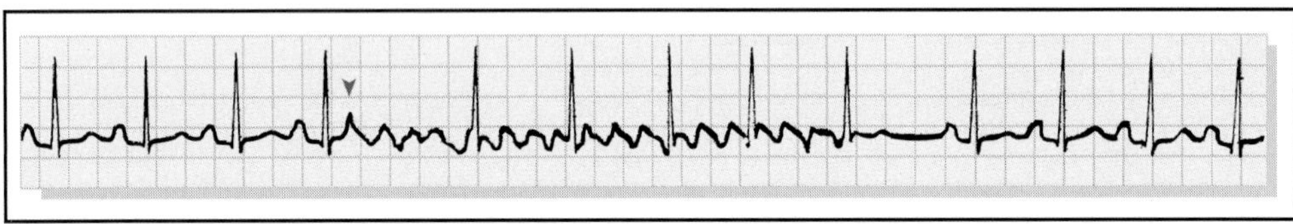
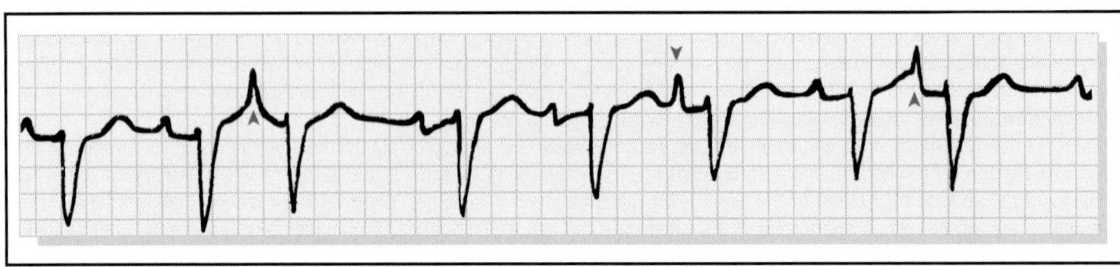

A

B

C

D

FIGURE 32–11 **A,** Premature atrial complexes (PACs) that block conduction entirely or conduct with a functional right or functional left bundle branch block. Depending on the preceding cycle length and coupling interval of the PAC, the latter blocks conduction entirely in the atrioventricular (AV) node (arrowhead ↑) or conducts with a functional left bundle branch block (arrowhead ↓) or functional right bundle branch block (arrowhead →). **B,** A PAC on the left (arrowhead) initiates AV nodal reentry that is due to reentry anterogradely and retrogradely over two slow AV nodal pathways, with a retrograde P wave produced midway in the cardiac cycle. On the right, a PAC (arrowhead) initiates AV nodal reentry as a result of anterograde conduction over the slow pathway and retrograde conduction over the fast pathway (see Fig. 32–10A), which produces a retrograde P wave in the terminal portion of the QRS complex that simulates an r′ wave. **C** and **D,** A PAC (arrowhead ↓) initiating a short run of atrial flutter **(C)** and a PAC (arrowhead ↑) depressing return of the next sinus nodal discharge **(D)**. A slightly later PAC (arrowhead ↓) in **D** does not depress sinus nodal automaticity. **B** to **D,** Monitor leads. *Continued*

may occur. In this case, the pause after the premature atrial complex is very short, and the interval bounded by the normal sinus–initiated P waves on each side of the premature atrial complex is only slightly longer than or equals one normal P-P cycle length. The interpolated premature atrial complex fails to affect the sinus nodal pacemaker, and the sinus impulse following the premature atrial complex is conducted to the ventricles, often with a slightly lengthened PR interval. An interpolated atrial or ventricular premature complex of any type represents the only type of premature systole that does not actually replace the normally conducted beat. Premature atrial complexes can originate in the sinus node and are identified by premature P waves that have a contour identical to that of the normal sinus P wave.

On occasion, when the AV node has had sufficient time to repolarize and conduct without delay, the supraventricular QRS complex initiated by the premature atrial complex can be aberrant in configuration because the His-Purkinje system or ventricular muscle has *not* completely repolarized and conducts with a functional delay or block (Fig. 32–11A). The refractory period of cardiac fibers is directly related to cycle length. (In an adult, the AV nodal effective refractory period is prolonged at shorter cycle lengths.) A slow heart rate (long cycle length) produces a longer His-Purkinje refractory period than does a faster heart rate. As a consequence, a premature atrial complex that follows a long R-R interval (long refractory period) can result in a functional bundle branch block (aberrant ventricular conduction). Since the right bundle branch at long cycles has a longer refractory period than the left bundle branch does, aberration with a right bundle branch block pattern at slow rates occurs more commonly than aberration with a left bundle branch block pattern. At shorter cycles, the refractory period of the left bundle branch exceeds that of the right bundle branch, and a left bundle branch block pattern may be more likely to occur.

CLINICAL FEATURES. Premature atrial complexes can occur in a variety of situations, such as during infection, inflammation, or myocardial ischemia, or they can be provoked by a variety of medications, by tension states, or by tobacco, alcohol, or caffeine. Premature atrial complexes can precipitate or presage the occurrence of sustained supraventricular (Fig. 32–11B and C) and, rarely, ventricular tachyarrhythmias.

MANAGEMENT. Premature atrial complexes generally do not require therapy.[5] In symptomatic patients or when the premature atrial complexes precipitate tachycardias, treatment with digitalis, a beta blocker, or a calcium antagonist can be tried.

Atrial Flutter (see also Chap. 30)

Atrial flutter is now recognized as a macro-reentrant atrial rhythm. Typical atrial flutter (sometimes called *type I*) is a reentrant rhythm in the right atrium constrained anteriorly by the tricuspid annulus[6] and posteriorly by the crista terminalis and eustachian ridge. The flutter can circulate in a counterclockwise direction around the tricuspid annulus in the frontal plane (typical flutter, counterclockwise flutter) or in a clockwise direction (atypical, clockwise, or reverse flutter).[7,8] Since both of these forms of atrial flutter are constrained by anatomical structures, their rates and flutter wave morphology on surface ECG are consistent and predictable (see later).[7] Other forms of atrial flutter are now recognized as distinct types and include atrial macro-reentry caused by incisional scars from prior atrial surgery,[9] idiopathic fibrosis in areas of the atrium, or other anatomical or functional conduction barriers in the atria.[7,8,10] Because the barriers that constrain these atrial flutters are variable, the ECG pattern of these so-called atypical atrial flutters can be varied. Oftentimes, flutter wave morphology changes during the same episode of flutter, which indicates multiple circuits and/or nonfixed conduction barriers.

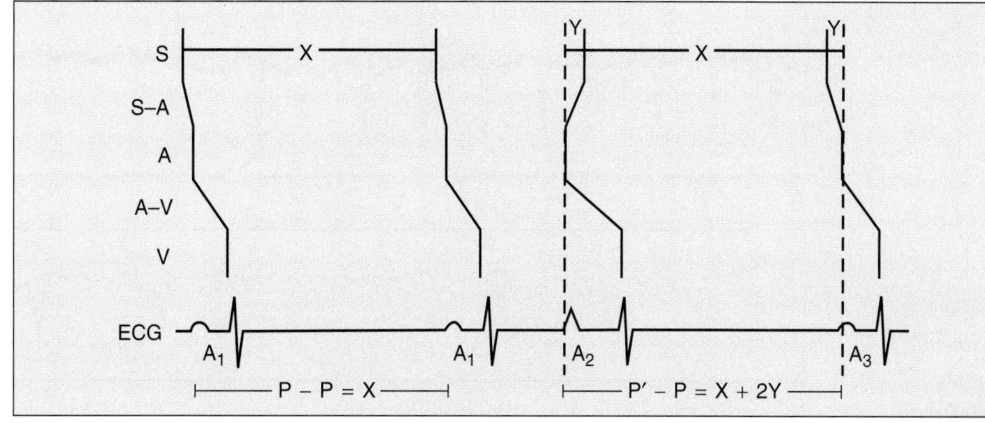

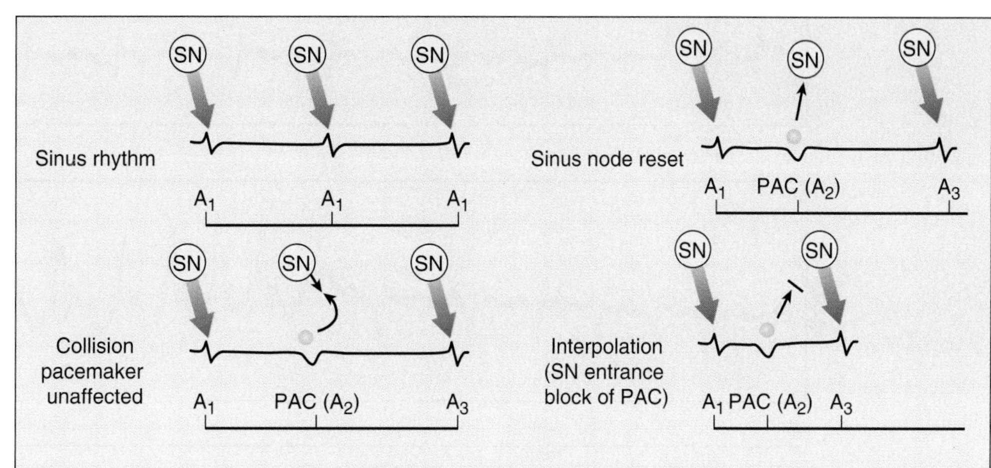

FIGURE 32–11, cont'd **E,** Diagrammatic example of the effects of a PAC. The sinus interval (A_1-A_1) equals X. The third P wave represents a PAC (A_2) that reaches and discharges the sinoatrial (SA) node, which causes the next sinus cycle to begin at that time. Therefore, the P-P (A_2-A_3) interval equals X + 2Y milliseconds, assuming no depression of SA nodal automaticity. **F,** Diagram of interactions of a PAC (yellow circles indicate origin; QRS complexes omitted) with the sinus node (SN) depending on the degree of prematurity. The top represents spontaneous sinus rhythm. The bottom is a late coupled PAC that collides with the exiting sinus impulse and therefore does not affect (or reset) the sinus pacemaker. The next sinus impulse (S_3) occurs at exactly twice the sinus interval. An early coupled PAC in the next diagram is able to penetrate the sinus node and thus resets the pacemaker, thereby resulting in resetting of the sinus node (as depicted in **E**). An even earlier coupled PAC in the lower figure reaches refractory tissue around the sinus node and is thus unable to penetrate the sinus node (SN entrance block); therefore, it does not affect sinus node discharge. The next spontaneous sinus beat (S_3) arrives exactly at the sinus interval. (**E,** Modified from Zipes DP, Fisch C: Premature atrial contraction. Arch Intern Med 128:453, 1971.)

ECG RECOGNITION. The atrial rate during typical atrial flutter is usually 250 to 350 beats/min, although it is occasionally slower, particularly when the patient is treated with antiarrhythmic drugs, which can reduce the rate to the range of 200 beats/min. If such slowing occurs, the ventricles can respond in a 1:1 fashion to the slower atrial rate. Ordinarily, the atrial rate is about 300 beats/min, and in untreated patients the ventricular rate is half the atrial rate, that is, 150 beats/min (Fig. 32–12A and F). A significantly slower ventricular rate (in the absence of drugs) suggests abnormal AV conduction. In children, in patients with the preexcitation syndrome (see Chap. 30), occasionally in patients with hyperthyroidism, and in those whose AV nodes conduct rapidly, atrial flutter can conduct to the ventricle in a 1:1 fashion and produce a ventricular rate of 300 beats/min.

In typical atrial flutter, the ECG reveals identically recurring regular sawtooth flutter waves (see Figs. 32–11C and 32–12B and F) and evidence of continual electrical activity (lack of an isoelectric interval between flutter waves), often best visualized in leads II, III, aV_f, or V_1 (Fig. 32–13). In some instances, transient slowing of the ventricular response, either with carotid sinus massage (see Fig. 32–12B) or with adenosine (see Fig. 32–12F), is necessary to visualize the flutter waves. The flutter waves for (type I) typical atrial flutter are inverted (negative) in these leads because of a counterclockwise reentrant pathway, and sometimes they are upright (positive) when the reentrant loop is clockwise (see Fig. 32–13). When the flutter waves are upright from clockwise rotation, they are often notched. If the AV conduction ratio remains constant, the ventricular rhythm will be regular; if the ratio of conducted beats varies (usually the result of a Wenckebach AV block), the ventricular rhythm will be irregular. Alternation between 2:1 and 4:1 AV conduction often occurs and can be due to two levels of block—2:1 high in the AV node and 3:2 lower down. The irregular ventricular response is frequently due to Wenckebach periodicity. Recurrent alternation of short and long ventricular intervals can be due to concealed conduction. Various degrees of penetration into the AV junction by flutter impulses can also influence AV conduction. The ratio of flutter waves to conducted ventricular complexes is most often an even number (e.g., 2:1, 4:1, and so on).

CLINICAL FEATURES. Atrial flutter is less common than atrial fibrillation. It can occur as a result of atrial dilation from septal defects, pulmonary emboli, mitral or tricuspid valve stenosis or regurgitation, or chronic ventricular failure but can also (rarely) occur without underlying heart disease. Toxic and metabolic conditions that affect the heart, such as thyrotoxicosis, alcoholism, and pericarditis, can cause atrial flutter. Occasionally, it can be congenital, follow surgery for congenital heart disease, or even occur in utero. When it

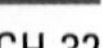

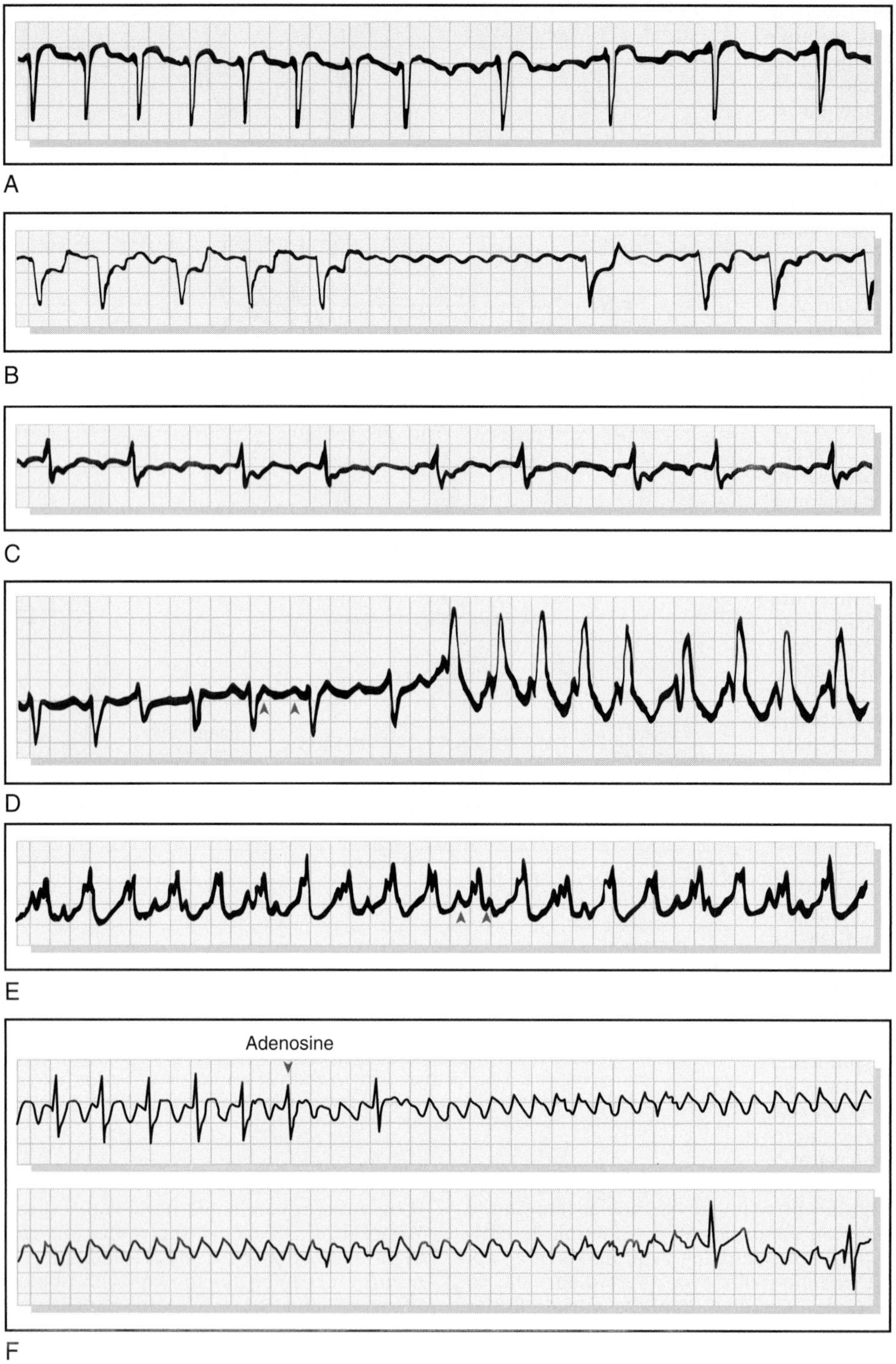

FIGURE 32–12 Various manifestations of atrial flutter. **A,** Atrial flutter at a rate of 300 beats/min conducting impulses to ventricles with a 2:1 block. In the midportion of the tracing, carotid sinus massage converts the block to 4:1, and the ventricular rate slows to 75 beats/min. **B,** Carotid sinus massage produces a transient period of atrioventricular (AV) block clearly revealing the flutter waves. **C,** Quinidine has slowed the atrial flutter rate to approximately 188 beats/min. The block is variable. **D,** Wide QRS complexes with an rSR′ configuration in V_1 begin after a short cycle that follows a long cycle in the midportion of the electrocardiogram strip. This pattern represents a functional right bundle branch block. Arrowheads indicate flutter waves. **E,** The QRS complexes are 0.12 second in duration and have a regular interval at a rate of 200 beats/min. Atrial activity is also regular at a rate of 300 beats/min and independent of ventricular activity (arrows). Thus, atrial flutter is present with a probable ventricular tachycardia, an example of complete AV dissociation. **F,** Adenosine injection given to a patient with a supraventricular tachycardia (SVT) at a rate of 150 beats/min reveals underlying atrial flutter, thus diagnosing the SVT as atrial flutter with 2:1 AV conduction and the flutter waves obscured within the T waves. Monitor leads in **A, B, C, E,** and **F**.

follows reparative surgery of congenital heart disease it usually involves an atriotomy and often occurs years after the surgery. In children, continued episodes of atrial flutter are associated with an increased possibility of sudden death.

Atrial flutter usually responds to carotid sinus massage with a decrease in the ventricular rate in stepwise multiples and returns in reverse manner to the former ventricular rate at the termination of carotid massage (see Fig. 32–12A). *Physical examination* may reveal rapid flutter waves in the jugular venous pulse. If the relationship of flutter waves to conducted QRS complexes remains constant, the first heart sound will have a constant intensity. Occasionally, sounds caused by atrial contraction can be auscultated.

MANAGEMENT. Cardioversion (see Chap. 30) is commonly the initial treatment of choice for atrial flutter since it promptly and effectively restores sinus rhythm. Cardioversion can be accomplished with synchronous direct current (DC), which often requires relatively low energies (<50 J). If the electrical shock results in atrial fibrillation, a second shock at a higher energy level is used to restore sinus rhythm or, depending on clinical circumstances, the atrial fibrillation can be left untreated. The latter can revert to atrial flutter or sinus rhythm. The short-acting antiarrhythmic medication ibutilide can also be given IV to convert atrial flutter. Ibutilide appears to successfully cardiovert about 60 to 90 percent of episodes of atrial flutter.[11,12] However, because this medication prolongs the QT interval, torsades de pointes is a potential complication during and shortly after the infusion. Other medications such as procainamide can be given to chemically convert atrial flutter. *Rapid atrial pacing* with a catheter in the esophagus or the right atrium can effectively terminate type I (counterclockwise and clockwise) and some forms of atypical atrial flutter in most patients and produce sinus rhythm or atrial fibrillation with a slowing of the ventricular rate and concomitant clinical improvement. Although the risk of thromboembolism is lower than that for atrial fibrillation, patients with atrial flutter do appear to have a risk of thromboembolism immediately after conversion to sinus rhythm.[13-15]

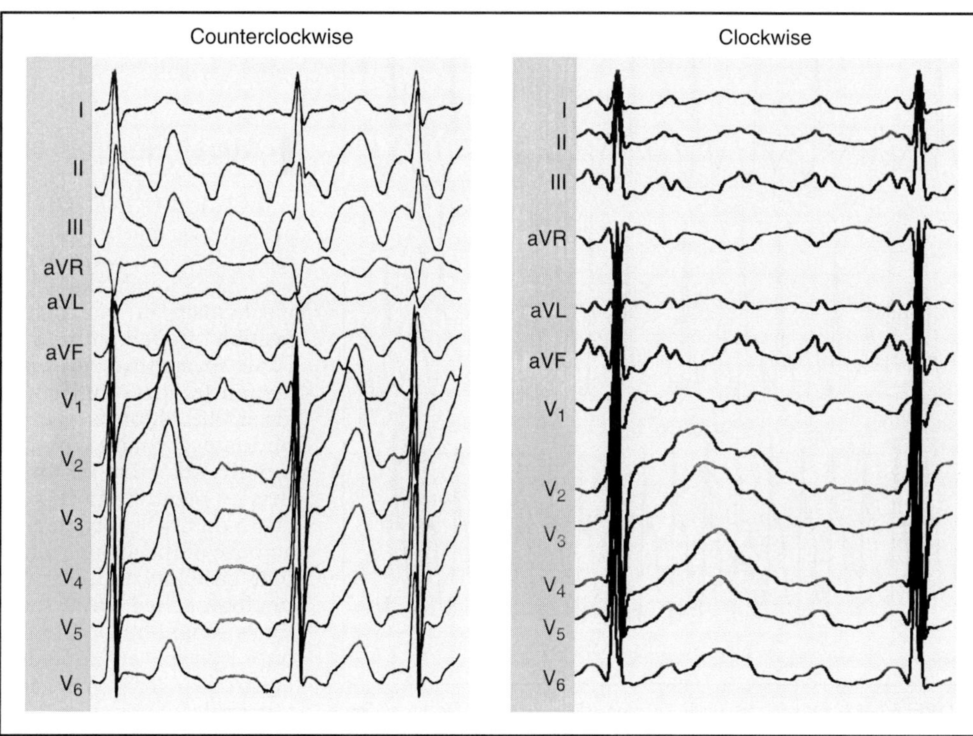

FIGURE 32–13 Twelve-lead electrocardiogram of counterclockwise and clockwise atrial flutter. In counterclockwise atrial flutter, the flutter waves are negative in leads II, III, aVL, and V_6 and upright in V_1. In counterclockwise atrial flutter, the flutter waves are upright in leads II, III, and aVF and often notched.

Verapamil (see Chap. 30) given as an initial bolus of 5 to 10 mg IV, followed by a constant infusion at a rate of 5 mg/kg/min, or *diltiazem* 0.25 mg/kg to slow the ventricular response, can be tried. *Adenosine* produces a transient AV block and can be used to reveal flutter waves if diagnosis of the arrhythmias is in doubt. It will not generally terminate the atrial flutter and can provoke atrial fibrillation. Esmolol, a beta-adrenergic blocker with a 9-minute elimination half-life, can be used to slow the ventricular rate.

If the flutter cannot be electrically cardioverted, terminated by pacing, or slowed by the aforementioned drugs, a *short-acting digitalis preparation* (such as digoxin or deslanoside) can be tried alone or with a calcium antagonist or beta blocker. The dose of digitalis necessary to slow the ventricular response varies and at times can result in toxic levels because it is often difficult to slow the ventricular rate during atrial flutter. Frequently, atrial fibrillation develops after digitalis administration and can revert to normal sinus rhythm on withdrawal of digitalis treatment; occasionally, normal sinus rhythm may occur without intervening atrial fibrillation. IV amiodarone has been shown to slow the ventricular rate as effectively as digoxin.

If the atrial flutter persists, class IA or IC drugs (see Chap. 30) can be tried in an attempt to restore sinus rhythm and prevent recurrence of atrial flutter. Amiodarone, especially in low doses of 200 mg/day, can also prevent recurrences. Side effects of these drugs, especially proarrhythmic responses, must be carefully considered and are dealt with at length in Chapter 30. Sometimes, treatment of the underlying disorder, such as thyrotoxicosis, is necessary to effect conversion to sinus rhythm. In certain instances, atrial flutter can continue, and if the ventricular rate can be controlled with drugs, conversion to sinus rhythm may not be indicated. Therapy with classes I and III drugs should be discontinued if flutter remains.

It is important to reemphasize that class I or III drugs should *not* be used unless the ventricular rate during atrial flutter has been *slowed* with digitalis or with a calcium antagonist or beta-blocking drug. Because of the vagolytic action of quinidine, procainamide, and disopyramide (see Chap. 30), but primarily because of the ability of class I drugs to slow the flutter rate, AV conduction can be *facilitated* sufficiently to result in a 1:1 ventricular response to the atrial flutter (Fig. 32–14).

Prevention of recurrent atrial flutter is often difficult to achieve medically but should be approached as outlined for the prevention of paroxysmal supraventricular tachycardia resulting from AV nodal reentry (see also Chap. 30). If recurrences cannot be prevented, therapy is directed toward controlling the ventricular rate when the flutter does recur with digitalis alone or combined with beta blockers or calcium antagonists. Mounting evidence indicates that the risk of emboli in atrial flutter may be more significant[13-15] than once thought. Because of this and since many patients with atrial flutter also have atrial fibrillation, anticoagulation is usually warranted. However, carefully controlled studies to determine the degree of embolic risk in patients with only atrial flutter are lacking. Long-term anticoagulation, as in atrial fibrillation, should probably be considered until more definitive data are available. Radiofrequency catheter ablation of typical flutter (counterclockwise and clockwise) is highly effective at curing atrial fibrillation and has a long-term success rate of 90 to 100 percent.[16] Because ablation of atrial flutter is highly effective with little risk, it can be offered as an alternative to

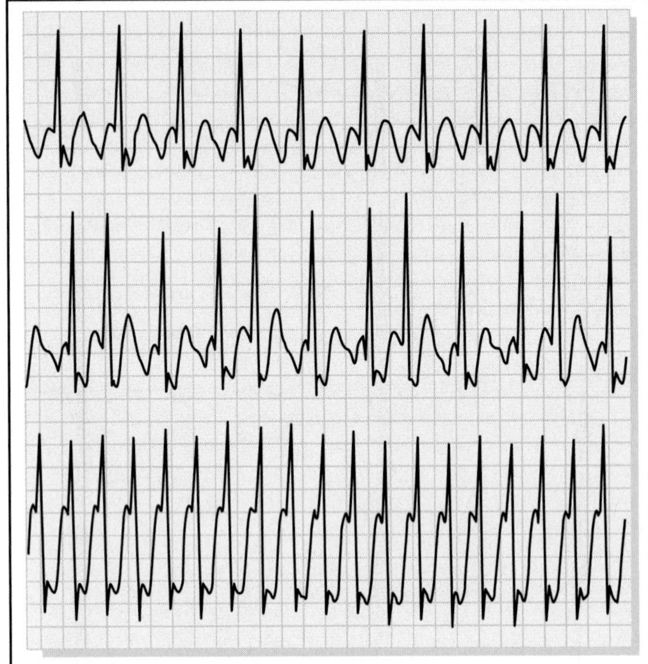

FIGURE 32–14 Atrial flutter with 1:1 conduction caused by flecainide. **Top,** Atrial flutter occurs with 2:1 conduction. **Middle,** 2:1 conduction alternates with 3:2 conduction. **Bottom,** Flecainide administration has been started, and the atrial flutter rate slows, with subsequent 1:1 conduction.

drug therapy. Ablation of other forms of atrial flutter is also effective, although success rates are somewhat lower and more variable.[9,10,17]

Atrial Fibrillation (see also Chap. 30)

ECG RECOGNITION. Atrial fibrillation (Fig. 32–15) is an arrhythmia that is characterized by seemingly disorganized atrial depolarizations without effective atrial contraction. It was once thought that all atrial fibrillation was due to a single mechanism of multiple wavelets propagating in random fashion throughout the atria. It is now apparent that there are likely several mechanisms and that there may be some organization to atrial fibrillation. For example, in many patients atrial fibrillation is due a focal discharge at rapid rates and fibrillatory conduction (heterogeneous conduction due to rapidity of activation) through the atria. Nonetheless, all of these potential mechanisms of atrial fibrillation have a common ECG appearance. During atrial fibrillation, electrical activity of the atrium can be detected on ECG as small, irregular baseline undulations of variable amplitude and morphology, called *f waves*, at a rate of 350 to 600 beats/min. At times, small, fine, rapid f waves can occur and are detectable only by right atrial leads or by intracavitary or esophageal electrodes. The ventricular response is grossly irregular ("irregularly irregular") and, in an untreated patient with normal AV conduction, is usually between 100 and 160 beats/min. In patients with WPW syndrome, the ventricular rate during atrial fibrillation can at times exceed 300 beats/min and lead to ventricular fibrillation. Atrial fibrillation should be suspected when the ECG shows supraventricular complexes at an irregular rhythm and no obvious P waves. The recognizable f waves probably do not represent total atrial activity but depict only the larger vectors generated by the multiple wavelets of depolarization that occur at any given moment.

Each recorded f wave is not conducted through the AV junction, so a rapid ventricular response comparable to the atrial rate does not occur. Many atrial impulses are concealed because of a collision of wavefronts, or they are blocked in the AV junction without reaching the ventricles (i.e., concealed conduction, which accounts for the irregular ventricular rhythm). The refractory period and conductivity of the AV node are determinants of the ventricular rate. When the ventricular rate is very rapid or very slow, it may appear to be more regular. Even though conversion of atrial fibrillation to atrial flutter is accompanied by slowing of the atrial rate, an increase in the ventricular response can result since more atrial impulses are transmitted to the ventricle

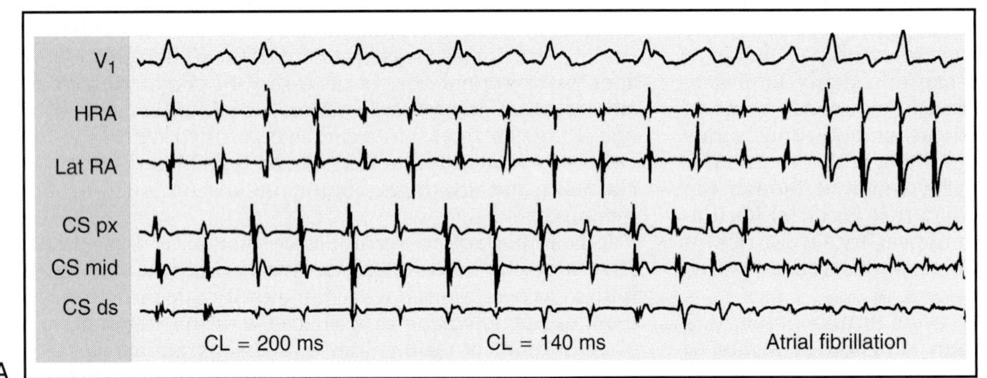

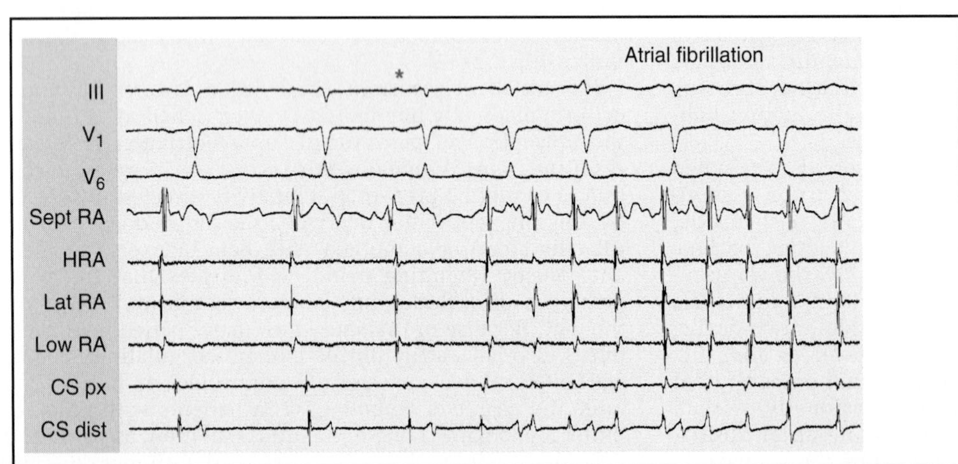

FIGURE 32–15 Atrial fibrillation produced by "focal" mechanisms. **A,** A rapid, regular atrial tachycardia (left side of figure) at a cycle length (CL) of 200 milliseconds degenerates into atrial fibrillation (right side of figure) characterized by rapid, irregular atrial depolarizations. **B,** A premature atrial complex (marked by the asterisk) induces atrial fibrillation (right side of figure). Elimination of these focal triggers for atrial fibrillation can eliminate the atrial fibrillation.

because of less concealed conduction. Also, it is easier to slow the ventricular rate during atrial fibrillation than during atrial flutter with drugs such as digitalis, calcium antagonists, and beta blockers because the increased concealed conduction makes it easier to produce an AV block.

CLINICAL FEATURES. Atrial fibrillation is a common arrhythmia that is found in 1 percent of persons older than 60 years to more than 5 percent of patients older than 69 years. The overall chance of atrial fibrillation developing over a period of two decades in patients older than 30 years, according to Framingham data, is 2 percent. Estimates are that 2.2 million Americans have atrial fibrillation, which occurs more commonly in men than in women.[18] A history of congestive heart failure, valvular heart disease and stroke, left atrial enlargement, abnormal mitral or aortic valve function, treated systemic hypertension, and advanced age are independently associated with the prevalence of atrial fibrillation. Four important aspects of atrial fibrillation are etiology, control of the ventricular rate, prevention of recurrences, and prevention of thromboembolic episodes. Occult or manifested thyrotoxicosis should be considered in patients with recent-onset atrial fibrillation. Atrial fibrillation can be intermittent or chronic and may be influenced by autonomic activity. Atrial fibrillation, whether it is persistent or intermittent, predisposes to stroke. Symptoms as a result of atrial fibrillation are determined by multiple factors, including the underlying cardiac status, the rapid ventricular rate, and loss of atrial contraction.

Physical findings include a slight variation in intensity of the first heart sound, absence of *a* waves in the jugular venous pulse, and an irregularly irregular ventricular rhythm. Often, with fast ventricular rates a significant pulse deficit appears, during which the auscultated or palpated apical rate is faster than the rate palpated at the wrist (pulse deficit) because each contraction is not sufficiently strong to open the aortic valve or transmit an arterial pressure wave through the peripheral artery. If the ventricular rhythm becomes regular in patients with atrial fibrillation, conversion to sinus rhythm, atrial tachycardia, or atrial flutter with a constant ratio of conducted beats or the development of junctional tachycardia or ventricular tachycardia (VT) should be suspected.

EMBOLIZATION AND ANTICOAGULATION. In addition to hemodynamic alterations, the risk of systemic emboli, probably arising in the left atrial cavity or appendage as a result of circulatory stasis, is an important consideration (see Chap. 80). Nonvalvular atrial fibrillation is the most common cardiac disease associated with cerebral embolism. In fact, almost half of cardiogenic emboli in the United States occur in patients with nonvalvular atrial fibrillation. The risk of stroke in patients with nonvalvular atrial fibrillation is five to seven times greater than that in controls without atrial fibrillation. Overall, 20 to 25 percent of ischemic strokes are due to cardiogenic emboli.

Many studies have evaluated the risk of stroke in patients with atrial fibrillation and the benefits of anticoagulation and antiplatelet therapy.[19-25] Patients with mitral stenosis and atrial fibrillation have a 4 to 6 percent incidence of embolism per year. Risk factors that predict stroke in patients with nonvalvular atrial fibrillation include a history of previous stroke or transient ischemic attack (relative risk 2.5), diabetes (relative risk 1.7), history of hypertension (relative risk 1.6), and increasing age (relative risk 1.4 for each decade). Patients with any of these risk factors have an annual stroke risk of at least 4 percent if untreated. Patients whose only stroke risk factor is congestive heart failure or coronary artery disease have stroke rates approximately three times higher than do patients without any risk factors. Left ventricular (LV) dysfunction and a left atrial size greater than 2.5 cm/m^2 on echocardiographic examination are associated with thromboembolism. Patients younger than 60 to 65 years of age who have a normal echocardiogram and no risk factors have an extremely low risk for stroke (1 percent per year). Therefore, the risk of stroke in patients with *lone atrial fibrillation,* that is, idiopathic atrial fibrillation in the absence of any structural heart disease or any of the risk factors discussed previously, is quite low.

The annual rate of stroke for the unanticoagulated control group in five large anticoagulation trials was 4.5 percent but was reduced to 1.4 percent (68 percent risk reduction) for the warfarin-treated group (60 percent risk reduction in men; 84 percent risk reduction in women). Aspirin, 325 mg/d, produced a risk reduction of 44 percent. The annual rate of major hemorrhage was 1 percent for the control group, 1 percent for the aspirin group, and 1.3 percent for the warfarin group. No difference in stroke risk occurs between paroxysmal (intermittent) atrial fibrillation and constant (chronic) atrial fibrillation. Anticoagulation therapy is approximately 50 percent more effective than aspirin therapy for the prevention of ischemic stroke in patients with atrial fibrillation. Risk factors for anticoagulant-associated intracranial hemorrhage include excessive anticoagulation and poorly controlled hypertension. Elderly individuals are at increased risk for anticoagulant-associated brain hemorrhage, especially if overanticoagulated.

From these and other data, it appears that individuals younger than 60 years of age without any clinical risk factors or structural heart disease (lone atrial fibrillation) do not require antithrombotic therapy for stroke prevention because of their low risk. The stroke rate is also low (~2 percent per year) in patients between the ages of 60 and 75 years with lone atrial fibrillation. These patients may be adequately protected from stroke by aspirin therapy. In very elderly (older than 75 years) patients with atrial fibrillation, anticoagulation should be used with caution and carefully monitored because of the potential increased risk of intracranial hemorrhage. Nevertheless, elderly patients with atrial fibrillation are still likely to benefit from anticoagulation because they are at particularly high stroke risk. Food and drugs such as antibiotics and antiarrhythmics (e.g., amiodarone) can influence the effects of warfarin (see Chap. 80).

The following recommendations for antithrombotic therapy can be made: Any patient with atrial fibrillation who has risk factors for stroke (prior stroke or transient ischemic attack, significant valvular heart disease, hypertension, diabetes, age older than 65 years, left atrial enlargement, coronary artery disease, or congestive heart failure) should be treated with warfarin anticoagulation to achieve an international normalized ratio (INR) of 2.0 to 3.0 for stroke prevention if the individual is a good candidate for oral anticoagulation. Patients with contraindications to anticoagulation and unreliable individuals should be considered for aspirin treatment. Patients with atrial fibrillation who do not have any of the preceding risk factors have a low stroke risk (2 percent per year or less) and can be protected from stroke with aspirin. In patients older than 75 years, anticoagulation should be used with caution and monitored carefully to keep the INR less than 3.0 because of the risk of intracranial hemorrhage.

The risk of embolism following cardioversion to sinus rhythm in patients with atrial fibrillation varies from 0 to 7 percent, depending on the underlying risk factors. This risk is independent of the mode of cardioversion, either by chemical (drug) or DC shock. Patients at high risk are those with prior embolism, a mechanical valve prosthesis, or mitral stenosis. Low-risk patients are those younger than 60 years without underlying heart disease. The high-risk group should receive chronic anticoagulation (see later), regardless of whether they will undergo cardioversion. Patients not in the low-risk group who have atrial fibrillation longer than 2 days should receive warfarin to achieve an INR of 2.0 to 3.0 for 3 weeks before elective cardioversion and for 3 to 4 weeks after reversion to sinus rhythm. An alternative strategy is to obtain a transesophageal echocardiogram to exclude the presence of an atrial thrombus. It appears that this technique predicts a group at low risk for the development of thromboembolism following cardioversion, provided that the patients are immediately treated with heparin followed by therapeutic doses of warfarin.[26] Anticoagulation with heparin has been recommended for emergency cardioversion when 3 weeks of anticoagulation or a transesophageal echocardiogram cannot be obtained. No matter which strategy is used, anticoagulation should be continued for at least 4 weeks following cardioversion since atrial contractile function may not fully return until then.[27,28]

These suggestions must be individualized for a given patient. For example, patients at risk of trauma by virtue of occupation, participation in sports, and episodes of dizziness or syncope are at increased risk of bleeding if given anticoagulants and should probably not receive warfarin. Patients should be warned about taking any new drugs, such as nonsteroidal antiinflammatory agents, if they are receiving warfarin.

There are no data to suggest that conversion to sinus rhythm eliminates the risk of thromboembolism and thus that should not be for the sole purpose of doing so. In fact, data from the Atrial Fibrillation Follow-Up Investigation of Rhythm Management (AFFIRM) trial suggest that the strategy of maintaining sinus rhythm is insufficient alone to prevent thromboembolism, and patients who are treated with a strategy of maintaining sinus rhythm should be continued on anticoagulation unless there is a contraindication.[29] Many patients can have asymptomatic recurrences of atrial fibrillation.

Newer strategies for stroke prevention are being developed. Oral thrombin inhibitors (e.g., ximelagatran and Melagatran)[30] have been shown to be effective in preventing postoperative deep vein thrombosis and have just been evaluated in a randomized trial for stroke prevention in atrial fibrillation (Stroke Prevention Using Oral Thrombin Inhibitor in Atrial Fibrillation [SPORTIF V]). Although the results of this study are not currently known, the potential advantage of these agents is their wider therapeutic window, not requiring monitoring like warfarin. Left atrial occlusion, either surgically[31] or with a catheter-based system,[32] is also in the early stages of evaluation as a method for stroke prevention.

MANAGEMENT. The goals of management of the patient with atrial fibrillation are to reduce the risk of thromboembolism (described earlier) and to control symptoms. The latter is accomplished by controlling the ventricular rate during atrial fibrillation and/or restoring and maintaining sinus rhythm. Currently, no clear benefit has been ascribed to one treatment strategy over the other (rate control vs. rhythm control), particularly since antiarrhythmic drugs are only 50 to 70 percent effective and carry risks of proarrhythmia (see later). Data from large clinical studies (e.g., AFFIRM, Pharmacologic Intervention in Atrial Fibrillation [PIAF], and Rate Control versus Electrical Cardioversion [RACE]) all demonstrate that both treatment strategies are reasonable.[29,33,34] In the largest of these studies, AFFIRM, 4060 patients with atrial fibrillation and risk factors for thromboembolism were randomized to either rhythm control or rate control treatment strategy, using standard pharmacological approaches. The study found no differences in mortality or quality of life between the two groups.[29] In both groups, thromboembolic events occurred in those patients in whom anticoagulation was stopped. These studies compared treatment strategies and did not compare sinus rhythm to atrial fibrillation with rate control. In the AFFIRM trial, only 60 percent of the patients in the rhythm control arm were in sinus rhythm at follow-up, and patients were not rigorously monitored for atrial fibrillation recurrences between visits.

The overall treatment strategy (i.e., ventricular rate control or restoration and maintenance of sinus rhythm) should be individualized for each patient and based on whether patients are symptomatic from uncontrolled ventricular rates or from atrial fibrillation itself (i.e., loss of AV synchrony and atrial contraction) and risk for side effects from drugs. It can sometimes be difficult to determine whether a patient's symptoms are due to rapid ventricular rates or the loss of atrial contraction. As a general rule, asymptomatic patients found to be in atrial fibrillation on routine ECG are not likely to require rhythm control, and rate control is usually sufficient. Ambulatory monitoring (see Chap. 30) correlating the patients' ventricular response and rhythm to symptoms and exercise testing can be useful to this end. Trials of aggressive rate control or, conversely, cardioversion and maintenance of sinus rhythm are sometimes necessary to make this determination. Intolerance to medications or excessive risk in one strategy may necessitate switching strategies. Again, a rhythm control strategy should not be an alternative to anticoagulation therapy to reduce stroke risk.

Many elderly patients tolerate atrial fibrillation well without therapy because the ventricular rate is slow as a result of concomitant AV nodal disease. These patients often have associated sick sinus syndrome, and the development of atrial fibrillation represents a cure of sorts. Such patients may demonstrate serious supraventricular and ventricular arrhythmias or asystole after cardioversion, so the likelihood of establishing and maintaining sinus rhythm should be weighed against the risks of cardioversion or other forms of therapy.

Acute Management. A patient with atrial fibrillation discovered for the first time should be evaluated for a precipitating cause, such as thyrotoxicosis, mitral stenosis, pulmonary emboli, or pericarditis. The patient's clinical status determines initial therapy, the objectives being to slow the ventricular rate and restore atrial systole. If sudden onset of atrial fibrillation with a rapid ventricular rate results in acute cardiovascular decompensation, electrical cardioversion is the initial treatment of choice. For other patients, the decision to cardiovert is largely based on the individual clinical situation. The need to restore sinus rhythm must be weighed against the likelihood of successful cardioversion and long-term maintenance of sinus rhythm.

Maintenance of sinus rhythm after cardioversion is influenced by the duration of atrial fibrillation and, in some adults, atrial dilation. Animal studies indicate that atrial fibrillation begets atrial fibrillation: The longer the patient has atrial fibrillation, the greater the likelihood that it will remain because of a process called *electrophysiological remodeling*. Similar electrophysiological abnormalities can be demonstrated in patients following short episodes of atrial fibrillation, but the mechanism(s) and clinical significance are currently unknown.[35-39] Although parameters such as atrial size and duration of atrial fibrillation predict the success of cardioversion in population studies, enlarged atria and atrial fibrillation of long duration are not absolute contraindications to attempted cardioversion. Internal cardioversion via intracavitary catheters can be effective when transthoracic shocks fail, particularly in obese patients or those with significant pulmonary disease.[40,41] However, with the advent of biphasic external defibrillators, the success rates and the energy requirement for cardioversion have improved and the need to perform internal cardioversions has decreased.[43-45] Alternatively, antiarrhythmic drugs that lower defibrillation thresholds such as ibutilide can be used to pretreat the patient and increase the success of DC cardioversion.[42] Atrial contraction may not return immediately after restoration of electrical systole, and clinical improvement may be delayed. DC cardioversion establishes normal sinus rhythm in more than 90 percent of patients, but sinus rhythm remains for 12 months in only 30 to 50 percent. Patients with atrial fibrillation of less than 12 months' duration have a greater chance of maintaining sinus rhythm after cardioversion. For patients who do not require emergent cardioversion, chemical cardioversion with IV antiarrhythmic drugs is effective in 35 to 75 percent of patients, depending on the population studied.[11,46] Although procainamide has been used extensively for years, no well-controlled studies have been performed to determine its efficacy. Outside the United States, IV flecainide has been used with good results.[46] IV amiodarone appears to be less effective, with no difference in conversion rates from placebo. IV ibulitide is also effective in about 35 to 75 percent of patients, depending on the population studied.[11,12,47] In the absence of decompensation, the patient can be treated with drugs such as digitalis, beta blockers, or calcium antagonists to maintain a resting apical rate of 60 to 80 beats/min that does not exceed 100 beats/min after slight exercise. The combined use of digitalis and a beta blocker or calcium antagonist can be helpful in slowing the ventricular rate. Digitalis may be more effective if associated LV dysfunction is present; without such dysfunction, a beta blocker may be preferable to control the ventricular rate.

Long-Term Management. For the *rate control strategy*, digitalis, calcium-channel blockers (diltiazem and verapamil) and beta blockers can be used alone or in combination. For chronic management, digitalis is usually insufficient for adequate rate control during periods of exertion. One should not rely on a resting heart rate during an office visit as the sole evaluation of the adequacy of rate control. Ambulatory monitoring and/or exercise testing can be useful to confirm adequate rate control during activity. In some patients with frequent recurrence and rapid ventricular rates not controlled by drugs or in patients intolerant to drugs, modification or elimination of AV nodal conduction by radiofrequency catheter ablation and implantation of a rate-adaptive VVI (VVIR) pacemaker is acceptable rate control therapy (see Chap. 31). Whenever possible, atrial or dual-chamber pacing is preferable since the incidence of atrial fibrillation and stroke appears to be reduced compared with VVI pacing.

If a decision to *maintain sinus rhythm* has been made, class IA, IC, and III (amiodarone, sotalol) agents can be used to terminate acute-onset atrial fibrillation and prevent recurrences of atrial fibrillation. No one drug, with the possible exception of amiodarone, appears clearly superior, and selection is often based on the side effect profile and risk of proarrhythmia.[46,48] This appears to be true for newer drugs, such as azimilide and dofetilide, as well, although comparative trials have not yet been done.[49,50] Most antiarrhythmic drugs increase the likelihood of maintaining sinus rhythm from about 30 to 50 percent to 50 to 70 percent of patients per year after cardioversion. Before electrical cardioversion, an antiarrhythmic agent is often administered for a few days to help prevent relapse of atrial fibrillation, as well as to convert some patients to sinus rhythm. For those patients who fail drug therapy, new catheter ablation approaches have been applied successfully. Ablation of a focus within the pulmonary vein (Fig. 32–16) or electrical isolation of the pulmonary veins is 70 to 85 percent effective in patients with paroxysmal atrial fibrillation in short-term follow-up studies.[51,52] The surgical Maze procedure has been used to eliminate atrial fibrillation, particularly in combination with valve surgery, with a high success rate (see Chap 30).[53]

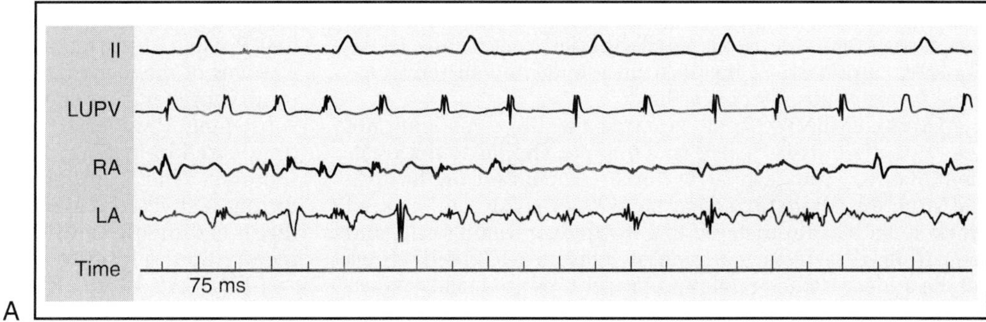

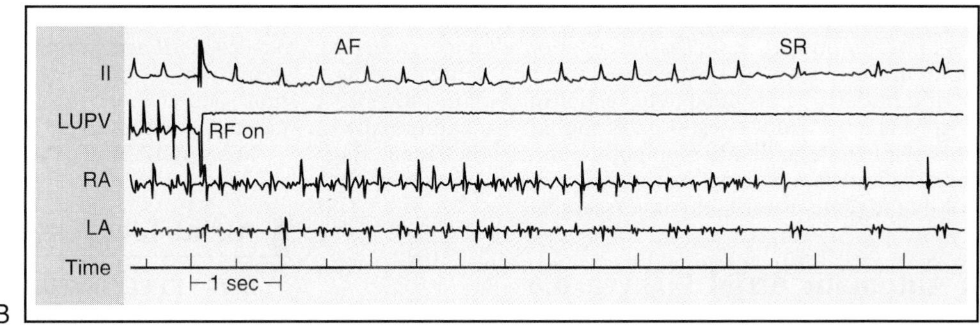

FIGURE 32–16 Focal atrial fibrillation arising from the left upper pulmonary vein (LUPV) **A,** During atrial fibrillation, irregular activity is recorded in the left atrium (LA) and the right atrium (RA). However, with a catheter at the focus in the LUPV, a regular sharp electrogram is recorded. **B,** During radiofrequency (RF) ablation at the site in **A,** the atrial fibrillation terminates within 7 seconds and sinus rhythm ensues.

Atrial Tachycardias

ECG RECOGNITION. Atrial tachycardia (Fig. 32–17) has an atrial rate of generally 150 to 200 beats/min with a P wave contour different from that of the sinus P wave. At onset, there may be some "warming up" of the rate, resulting in a slight increase in heart rate over the initial several complexes. Frequently, atrial tachycardias occur in short, recurrent bursts with spontaneous terminations. P waves are usually found in the second half of the tachycardia cycle (long RP/short PR tachycardia). If the atrial rate is not excessive and AV conduction is not depressed, each P wave can conduct to the ventricles. If the atrial rate increases and AV conduction becomes impaired, a Wenckebach (Mobitz type I) second-degree AV block can ensue. This aberration is sometimes called *atrial tachycardia with block*. When caused by digitalis, other manifestations of digitalis excess are present, such as PVCs. In nearly half the cases of atrial tachycardia with block, the atrial rate is irregular. Characteristic isoelectric intervals between P waves, in contrast to atrial flutter, are usually present in all leads. However, at rapid atrial rates, the distinction between atrial tachycardia with block and atrial flutter can be difficult. Analysis of P wave configuration during tachycardia indicates that a positive or biphasic P wave in V_1 predicts a right atrial focus, whereas a positive P wave in V_1 predicts a left atrial focus.

CLINICAL FEATURES. Although atrial tachycardia occurs commonly in patients with significant structural heart disease such as coronary artery disease, with or without myocardial infarction, cor pulmonale, or digitalis intoxication, it is also seen in patients without structural heart

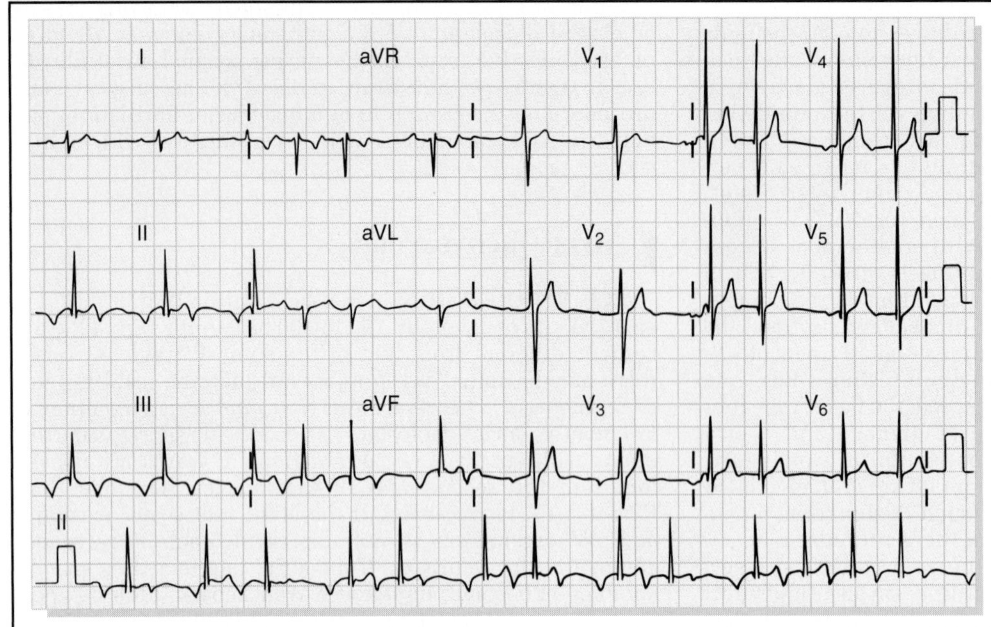

FIGURE 32–17 Atrial tachycardia. This 12-lead electrocardiogram and rhythm strip (bottom) demonstrate an atrial tachycardia at a cycle length of approximately 520 milliseconds. Conduction varies between 3:2 and 2:1. Note the negative P waves in leads II, III, and aVF and, when consecutive P waves are conducted, that the RP interval exceeds the PR interval. Note also that the tachycardia persists despite the development of atrioventricular (AV) block, an important finding that excludes the participation of an AV accessory pathway and sharply differentiates this tachycardia from the one shown in Figure 32–35.

disease. Potassium depletion can precipitate the arrhythmia in patients taking digitalis. The signs, symptoms, and prognosis are usually related to the underlying cardiovascular status and the rate of the tachycardia.

Physical findings during a variable rhythm include variable intensity of the first heart sound as a result of the varying AV block and PR interval. An excessive number of *a* waves can be seen in the jugular venous pulse. Carotid sinus massage or administration of adenosine increases the degree of AV block by slowing the ventricular rate in stepwise fashion without terminating the tachycardia, as in atrial flutter. It should be performed cautiously in patients with digitalis toxicity because serious ventricular arrhythmias can result. Occasionally, carotid sinus massage or adenosine can terminate some forms of atrial tachycardia.

MANAGEMENT. Atrial tachycardia in a patient not receiving digitalis is treated in a manner similar to the treatment of other atrial tachyarrhythmias. Depending on the clinical situation, digitalis, a beta blocker, or a calcium-channel blocker can be administered to slow the ventricular rate, and then if atrial tachycardia remains, class IA, IC, or III drugs can be added. Catheter ablation procedures are usually effective at eliminating the atrial tachycardia, depending on the mechanism and underlying heart disease (see Chap. 30).[9,17] However, atrial tachycardias can occasionally recur at a different site following a successful ablation attempt. If atrial tachycardia appears in a patient receiving digitalis, the drug should initially be assumed to be responsible for the arrhythmia. Therapy includes cessation of digitalis and administration of digitalis antibodies or potassium if low. Often, the ventricular response is not excessively fast, and simply withholding digitalis is all that is necessary.

Automatic Atrial Tachycardia

Three types of atrial tachycardias have been distinguished experimentally: automatic, triggered, and reentrant. The characteristics of automatic and reentrant tachycardias are discussed separately. Entrainment,[63] resetting curve patterns in response to overdrive pacing, the patient's response to adenosine, and recording of monophasic action potentials can be used to help distinguish one mechanism from the other. However, in most cases no clear identification of mechanism can be made clinically.

ECG FEATURES. Automatic atrial tachycardia (see Fig. 32–10F) is characterized electrocardiographically by a supraventricular tachycardia that generally accelerates after its initiation, with heart rates slower than 200 beats/min. The P wave contour differs from the sinus P wave, the PR interval is influenced directly by the tachycardia rate, and AV block can exist without affecting the tachycardia; that is, it continues uninterrupted. Vagal maneuvers do not generally terminate the tachycardia, even though they can produce AV nodal block. Thus, pharmacological or physiological maneuvers that selectively result in AV block do not affect the automatic focus, nor does the development of bundle branch block alter the PR or RP interval unless it is associated with prolongation of the H-V interval.

Initiation of tachycardia with premature atrial stimulation is not generally possible but is independent of intraatrial or AV nodal conduction delay when it occurs. The atrial activation sequence usually differs from a sinus-initiated P wave, and the A-H interval is related to the tachycardia rate. The first P wave of the tachycardia is the same as the subsequent P waves of the tachycardia, in contrast to most forms of reentrant supraventricular tachycardia, in which the initial and subsequent P waves differ. Usually, the tachycardia cannot be terminated by pacing, although it can exhibit overdrive suppression. The introduction of premature atrial complexes during tachycardia merely resets the timing of the tachycardia. It is difficult to differentiate this mechanism from microreentry by the leading-circle concept (see Chap. 27).

CLINICAL FEATURES. Many supraventricular tachycardias associated with AV block are probably due to automatic atrial tachycardia, including atrial tachycardia from digitalis intoxication (see Fig. 32–17). Automatic atrial tachycardia occurs in all age groups and is seen in settings of myocardial infarction, chronic lung disease (especially with acute infection), acute alcohol ingestion, a variety of metabolic derangements, or without any concomitant disease.

MANAGEMENT. Management is as discussed earlier.

Atrial Tachycardia Caused by Reentry

ECG RECOGNITION. Atrial tachycardia caused by reentry (Fig. 32–18; see also Fig. 32–10E). This arrhythmia is electrocardiographically manifest by a P wave that has a contour different from that of the sinus P wave, a PR interval

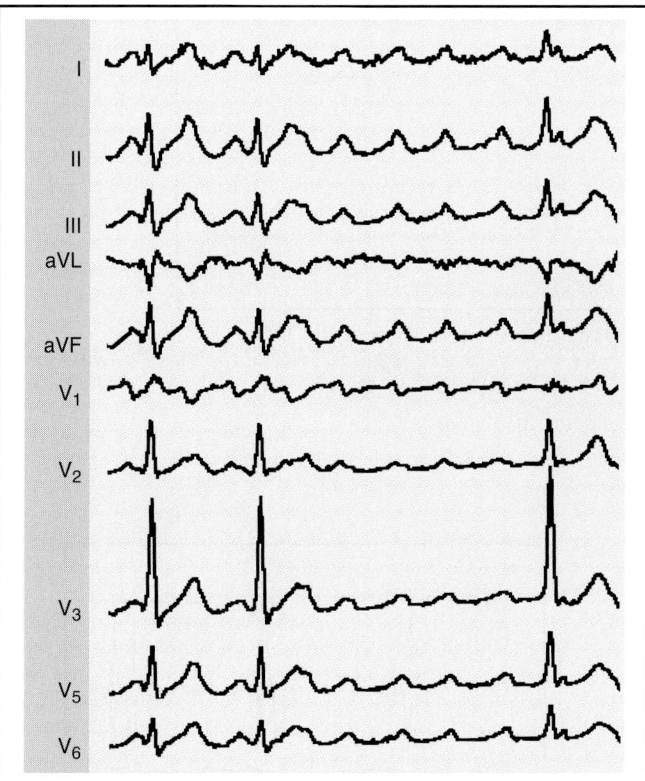

FIGURE 32–18 Macro-reentrant atrial tachycardia in a patient who underwent atrial septal defect repair 10 years earlier. This tachycardia uses a reentrant circuit established by the atriotomy on the lateral atrial wall. Ablation to extend the scar to the tricuspid annulus eliminated this tachycardia.

directly influenced by the tachycardia rate, and the capability to develop an AV block without interrupting the tachycardia. Atrial flutter (described earlier) is the prototypic atrial arrhythmia caused by reentry. Reentry can exist around a surgical scar, anatomical structure, or atriotomy incision.[9] Electrophysiologically, initiation of the tachycardia occurs with premature stimulation during the atrial relative refractory period, which results in a critical degree of intraatrial conduction delay, an atrial activation sequence different from what occurs during sinus rhythm, and an AV nodal conduction time related to the tachycardia rate. Occasionally, more aggressive stimulation is required to initiate some forms of reentrant atrial tachycardias. Vagal maneuvers generally do not terminate the tachycardia and can produce AV block.

CLINICAL FEATURES. Forms of atrial reentry producing atrial tachycardias include those that occur with atrial fibrosis (with pulmonary disease) or surgical atriotomy scars (see Fig. 32–18). The tachycardia can be started and stopped by an atrial extrastimulus. Spontaneous termination can be either sudden, with progressive slowing, or with alternating long-short cycle lengths.

CHAOTIC ATRIAL TACHYCARDIA

Chaotic (sometimes called *multifocal*) atrial tachycardia is characterized by atrial rates between 100 and 130 beats/min, with marked variation in P wave morphology and totally irregular P-P intervals (Fig. 32–19). Generally, at least three P wave contours are noted, with most P waves conducted to the ventricles, although often with variable PR intervals. This tachycardia occurs commonly in older patients with chronic obstructive pulmonary disease and congestive heart failure and may eventually develop into atrial fibrillation. Digitalis appears to be an unusual cause, and theophylline administration has been implicated. Chaotic atrial tachycardia can occur in childhood.

MANAGEMENT. Management is primarily directed toward the underlying disease. Antiarrhythmic agents are often ineffective in slowing either the rate of the atrial tachycardia or the ventricular response. Beta-adrenoreceptor blockers should be avoided in patients with bronchospastic pulmonary disease but can be effective if tolerated. Verapamil and amiodarone have been useful. Potassium and magnesium replacement may suppress the tachycardia.

AV Junctional Rhythm Disturbances

AV JUNCTIONAL ESCAPE COMPLEX

MECHANISM. Automatic fibers that are prevented from initiating depolarization by a pacemaker such as the sinus node, which possesses a more rapid rate of firing, are called *latent pacemakers*. Such latent pacemakers are found in some parts of the atrium, in the AV node–His bundle area, in the right and left bundle branches, in the Purkinje system and in the ventricular outflow tracts. A latent pacemaker can become the dominant pacemaker by default or usurpation, that is, by passive or active mechanisms. A decrease in the number of impulses arriving at a latent pacemaker site, the result of slowing of the sinus node or interruption of propagation of the normal impulse anywhere along its course, allows the latent pacemaker to escape and initiate depolarization passively, by default. An increase in the discharge rate of a latent pacemaker can capture pacemaker control actively, by usurpation. The implication of the two different mechanisms of ectopic impulse formation is important therapeutically.

ECG RECOGNITION. An AV junctional escape beat occurs when the rate of impulse formation of the primary pacemaker, generally the sinus node, becomes less than that of the AV junctional region or when impulses from the primary pacemaker do not penetrate to the region of the escape focus and allow the AV junctional focus to reach threshold and discharge. The interval from the last normally conducted beat to the AV junctional escape beat is a measure of the initial discharge rate of the AV junctional focus and generally corresponds to a rate of 35 to 60

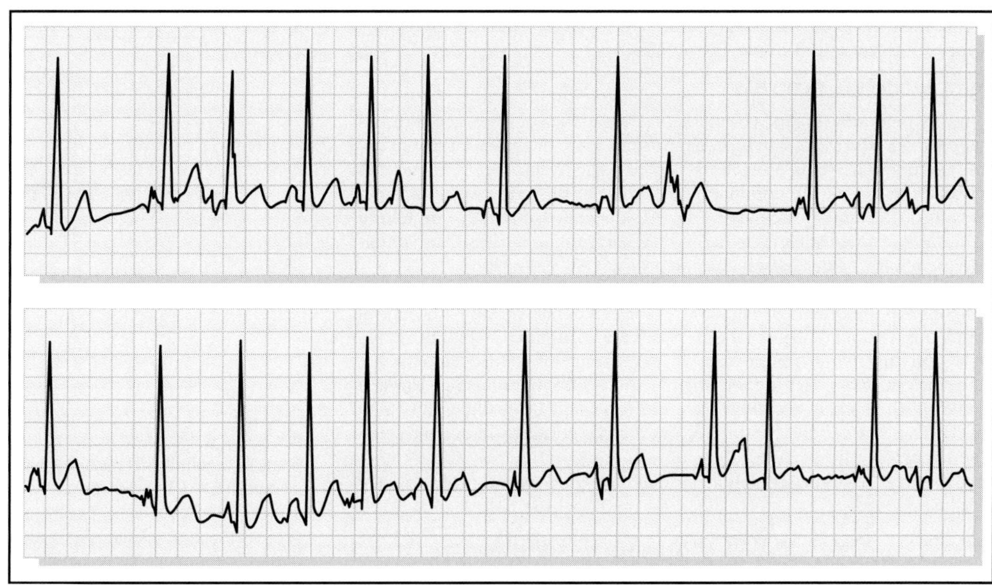

FIGURE 32–19 Chaotic (multifocal) atrial tachycardia. Premature atrial complexes occur at varying cycle lengths and with differing contours.

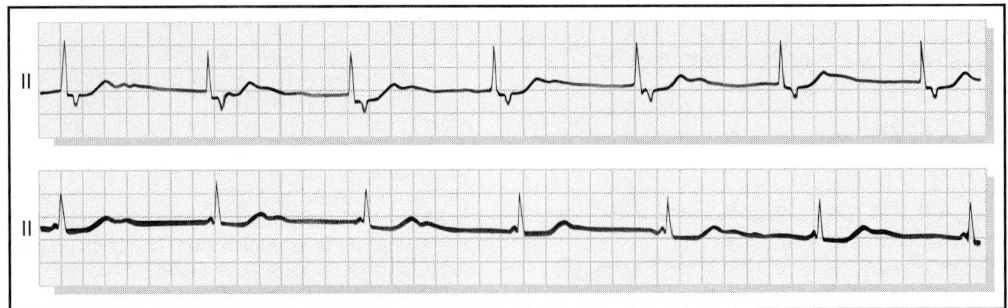

FIGURE 32–20 Atrioventricular (AV) junctional rhythm. **Top,** AV junctional discharge occurs fairly regularly at a rate of approximately 50 beats/min. Retrograde atrial activity follows each junctional discharge. **Bottom,** Recording made on a different day in the same patient. The AV junctional rate is slightly more variable, and retrograde P waves precede onset of the QRS complex. The positive terminal portion of the P wave gives the appearance of AV dissociation, which was not present.

beats/min (see Fig. 32–1B). Although an AV junctional escape rhythm is usually fairly regular, intervals between subsequent escape beats after the initial escape beat can gradually shorten as the rate of discharge of the escape focus increases, the so-called rhythm of development or warm-up phenomenon.

The ECG displays pauses longer than the normal P-P interval, interrupted by a QRS complex of supraventricular configuration with absent, retrograde, fusion, or sinus P waves that do not conduct to the ventricle. If P waves precede the QRS, they have a PR interval generally less than 0.12 second. The exact site of impulse formation (i.e., AN, N, or NH regions; low atrium; or His bundle) is not known and may differ from patient to patient and be influenced by the cause of the arrhythmia.

Treatment, if any, lies in increasing the discharge rate of the higher pacemakers and improving AV conduction and can require pacing. Frequently, no treatment is necessary.

PREMATURE AV JUNCTIONAL COMPLEXES

Premature AV junctional complexes are characterized by an impulse that arises prematurely in the AV junction (the exact site—i.e., AN, N, or NH regions; low atrium; or His bundle—is not known and may vary from patient to patient) and that attempts conduction in anterograde and retrograde directions. If unimpeded in its course, the impulse discharges the atrium to produce a premature retrograde P wave and a premature QRS complex with a supraventricular contour. The retrograde P wave can occur before, during, or after the QRS complex. Alterations in conduction time can influence the PR or RP relationships without a change in the site of origin of the impulse. Premature AV junctional complexes that conduct aberrantly are difficult to distinguish from PVCs observed on scalar ECG.

Treatment of premature AV junctional complexes is not generally necessary. However, since they may arise distal to the AV node, they can occur early in the cardiac cycle and can initiate a ventricular tachyarrhythmia in some instances. Under these circumstances, therapy is approached as for PVCs (see Chap. 30).

AV JUNCTIONAL RHYTHM

If the AV junctional escape complexes continue for a period, the rhythm is called an *AV junctional rhythm* (Fig. 32–20). Since the inherent rate of the AV junctional tissue is 35 to 60 beats/min, the AV junctional tissue can assume the role of the dominant pacemaker at this rate only by passive default of the sinus pacemaker. The ECG displays a normally conducted QRS complex, which can conduct retrogradely to the atrium or can occur independently of atrial discharge and produce AV dissociation.

An AV junctional escape rhythm can be a normal phenomenon in response to the effects of vagal tone, or it can occur during pathological sinus bradycardia or heart block. The escape complex or rhythm serves as a safety mechanism to prevent the occurrence of ventricular asystole. *Physical findings* vary depending on the P-QRS relationship. Large *a* waves in the jugular venous pulse and a loud, soft, or changing intensity of the first heart sound can be present if atrial contraction occurs when the tricuspid valve is shut.

Therapy is discussed under AV junctional escape complexes (see earlier).

NONPAROXYSMAL AV JUNCTIONAL TACHYCARDIA

ECG RECOGNITION. To usurp dominant pacemaker status, AV junctional tissue must exhibit an enhanced discharge rate such as during nonparoxysmal AV junctional tachycardia (Figs. 32–21 and 32–22). The

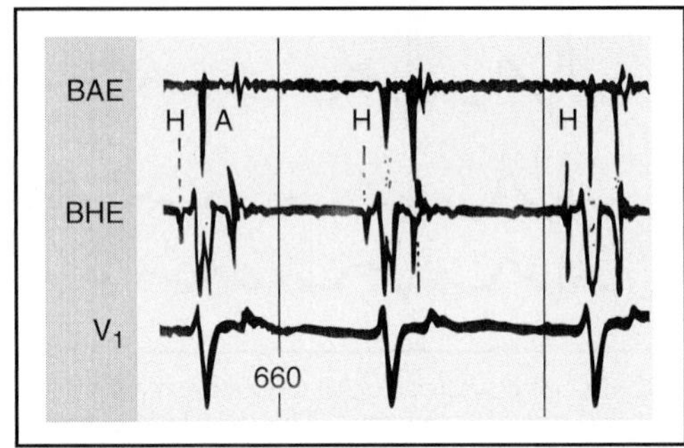

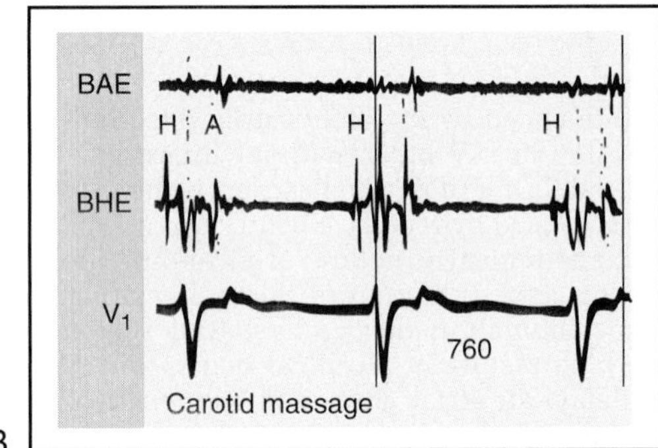

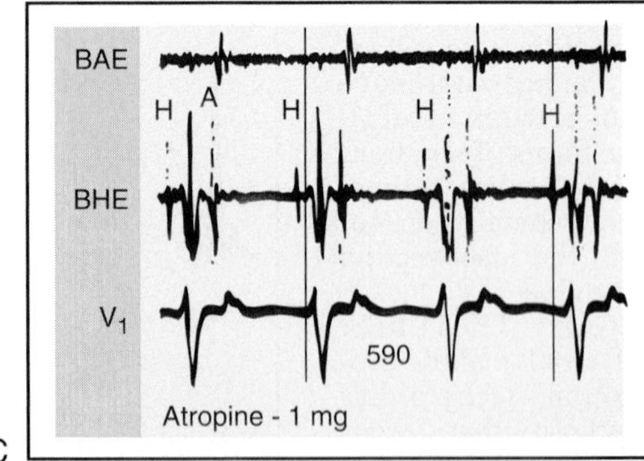

FIGURE 32–21 Nonparoxysmal atrioventricular (AV) junctional tachycardia. **A,** Control. **B,** Response to carotid sinus massage. **C,** Response to atropine 1 mg intravenously. Note that His bundle depolarization is the earliest recordable electrical activity in each cycle. The atria are depolarized retrogradely (low right atrial activity recorded in the BHE precedes high right atrial activity recorded in the BAE). Note also that carotid sinus massage slows the junctional discharge rate while atropine speeds it up. From these tracings alone one could not distinguish the rhythm from some other types of supraventricular tachycardia. However, the onset and termination of this tachycardia were typical of nonparoxysmal AV junctional tachycardia. BAE, bipolar atrial electrogram; BHE, bipolar His electrogram.

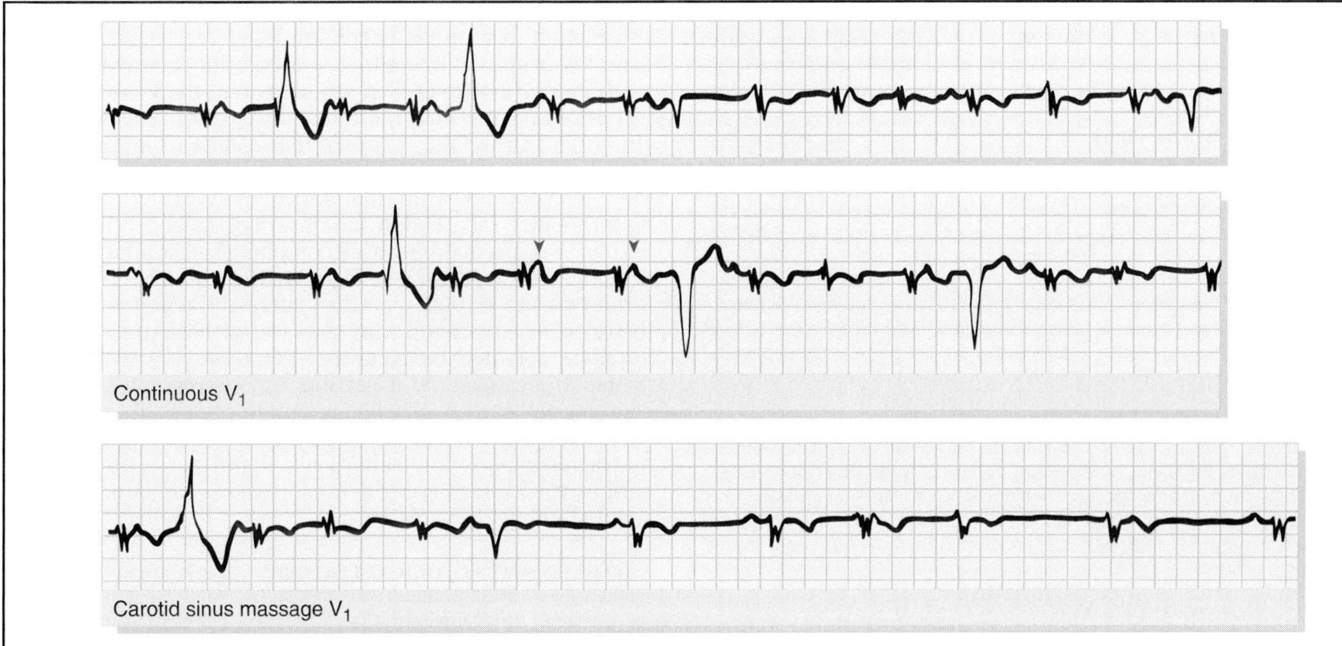

FIGURE 32–22 Nonparoxysmal atrioventricular junctional tachycardia in a healthy young adult. **Top,** This tachycardia occurs at a fairly regular interval ("W-shaped" complexes) and is interrupted intermittently with sinus captures that produce functional right and left bundle branch blocks. **Middle,** Two P waves are indicated by arrowheads. The junctional discharge rate is approximately 120 beats/min (cycle length = 500 milliseconds) and the rhythm irregular, sometimes shortened by sinus captures or delayed by concealed conduction that resets and displaces the junctional focus. **Bottom,** Carotid sinus massage slows the junctional as well as the sinus discharge rates.

tachycardia is usually of gradual onset and termination, hence the modifier *nonparoxysmal.* On occasion, nonparoxysmal AV junctional tachycardia can become manifest abruptly because slowing of the dominant pacemaker may then allow sudden capture and control of the rhythm by the AV junctional focus.

Nonparoxysmal AV junctional tachycardia is recognized by a QRS of supraventricular configuration at a fairly regular rate of 70 to 130 beats/min, but it can be faster. Accepted terminology assigns the label of tachycardia to rates exceeding 100 beats/min. The term *nonparoxysmal AV junctional tachycardia,* although not entirely correct when the rate is 70 to 100 beats/min, has generally been accepted since rates exceeding 60 beats/min in effect represent tachycardia for the AV junctional tissue. Enhanced vagal tone can slow while vagolytic agents can speed up the discharge rate. Although retrograde activation of the atria can occur, the atria are commonly controlled by an independent sinus, atrial, or on occasion, a second AV junctional focus resulting in AV dissociation (see Fig. 32–10G). The ECG diagnosis can be complicated by the presence of entrance and exit blocks at the AV junctional tissue level and incomplete forms of AV dissociation.

The cause of this arrhythmia is probably *accelerated automatic discharge* in or near the His bundle. It is possible that nonparoxysmal AV junctional tachycardia originates in atrial fibers without recognition of the latter's role from analysis of the scalar ECG or on intracardiac electrograms unless a careful search is made. Wenckebach periods can occur, but the presence of exit block has not yet been demonstrated by His bundle recording in humans, and the block can be in the AV node with the origin of the nonparoxysmal AV junctional tachycardia proximal to the site of the His bundle recording.

CLINICAL FEATURES. Nonparoxysmal AV junctional tachycardia occurs most commonly in patients with underlying heart disease, such as inferior infarction or myocarditis (often the result of acute rheumatic fever), or after open-heart surgery. An important cause is excessive digitalis, which can also produce the ECG manifestations of varying degrees of exit block (usually the Wenckebach type) from the accelerated AV junctional focus. Junctional tachycardia occurs commonly during radiofrequency catheter ablation of the slow pathway (see Chap. 30). Nonparoxysmal AV junctional tachycardia can occur in otherwise healthy individuals without symptoms (see Fig. 32–22) or can be a serious and difficult-to-control tachycardia, occasionally chronic, rapid, and long lasting. It can occur congenitally in infants or children and is associated with relatively high mortality.

The clinical features vary depending on the rate of the arrhythmia and the underlying etiology and severity of heart disease. As in most arrhythmias, the physical signs are determined by the relationship of the P wave to the QRS complex and the rate of atrial and ventricular discharge. The first heart sound can therefore be constant or varying, and cannon *a* waves may or may not occur in the jugular venous pulse.

The ventricular rhythm can be regular or irregular, often in a constant fashion. It is especially important to recognize slowing and regularization of the ventricular rhythm in a patient with atrial fibrillation as being caused by nonparoxysmal AV junctional tachycardia and as a possible early sign of *digitalis intoxication* (see Chap. 30). Initially, during atrial fibrillation, the regular ventricular rhythm can result from an AV junctional escape rhythm because the depressed AV conduction caused by digitalis blocks the passage of impulses from the fibrillating atria (see Fig. 32–10G). As digitalis administration is continued, the ventricular rate can then accelerate because of increased discharge of the AV junctional pacemaker but can still be regular. Further digitalis administration can produce a rate that is slow and irregular because of varying degrees of AV junctional exit block. The rhythm can be misdiagnosed as resumption of conduction from the fibrillating atria. The rate can then increase further because of development of VT.

MANAGEMENT. Therapy is directed toward the underlying etiologic factor and functional support of the cardiovascular system. If the rhythm is regular, cardiovascular status is not compromised, and the patient is not taking digitalis, digitalis administration could be considered. If the patient tolerates the arrhythmia well, careful monitoring and attention to the underlying heart disease are usually all that are required in an adult. The arrhythmia generally abates spontaneously. If digitalis toxicity is the cause, treatment with the drug must be stopped and digitalis antibody given or potassium, if it is low. If digitalis is not involved, initial drug therapy with digitalis, calcium-channel blockers, or beta blockers can be tried. Other drug therapy can include agents from classes IA, IC, and III. Catheter ablation of the junctional site can be effective but carries a risk of complete heart block.

Tachycardias Involving the AV Junction

Much confusion exists regarding the nomenclature of tachycardias characterized by a supraventricular QRS complex, a regular R-R interval, and no evidence of ventricular preexcitation. Because it is now apparent that a variety of electrophysiological mechanisms can account for these tachycardias (see Fig. 32–10), the nonspecific term *paroxysmal supraventricular tachycardia* has been proposed to encompass the entire group. This term may be inappropriate because some tachycardias in patients with accessory pathways (see later) are no more supraventricular than they are ventricular in origin in that they may require participation of both the atria and the ventricles in the reentrant pathway and they exhibit a QRS complex of normal contour and duration only because anterograde conduction occurs over the normal AV node–His bundle pathways (see Fig. 32–10C). If conduction over the reentrant pathway reverses direction and travels in an "antidromic" direction (i.e., to the ventricles over the accessory pathway and to the atria over the AV node–His bundle), the QRS complex exhibits a prolonged duration, although the tachycardia is basically the same. The term *reciprocating tachycardia* has been offered as a substitute for paroxysmal supraventricular tachycardia, but use of such a term presumes the mechanism of the tachycardia to be reentrant (which is probably the case for many supraventricular tachycardias). Reciprocating tachycardia is probably the mechanism of many VTs as well. Thus, no universally acceptable nomenclature exists for these tachycardias. In this chapter, descriptive titles, although cumbersome, are used for the sake of clarity. In addition, the mechanism of reentry is assumed to be operative when the weight of evidence supports its presence even though unequivocal proof is not always available.

AV Nodal Reentrant Tachycardia

ECG RECOGNITION. Reentrant tachycardia in the AV node is characterized by a tachycardia with a QRS complex of supraventricular origin, with sudden onset and termination generally at rates between 150 and 250 beats/min (commonly 180 to 200 beats/min in adults) and with a regular rhythm. Uncommonly, the rate may be as low as 110 beats/min and occasionally, especially in children, may exceed 250 beats/min. Unless functional aberrant ventricular conduction or a previous conduction defect exists, the QRS complex is normal in contour and duration. P waves are generally buried in the QRS complex. Often, the P wave is seen just prior to or just after the end of the QRS and causes a subtle alteration in the QRS complex that results in a pseudo-S or pseudo-r′, which may be recognized only on comparison to the QRS complex in normal sinus rhythm (Fig. 32–23). AV nodal reentry recorded at the onset begins abruptly, usually following a premature atrial complex that conducts with a prolonged PR interval (see Figs. 32–10A and 32–11B). The R-R interval can shorten over the course of the first few beats at the onset or lengthen during the last few beats preceding termination of the tachycardia. Variation in cycle length is usually caused by variation in anterograde AV nodal conduction time. Cycle length and/or QRS alternans can occur, usually when the rate is very fast. Carotid sinus massage can slow the tachycardia slightly prior to its termination or, if termination does not occur, can produce only slight slowing of the tachycardia.

ELECTROPHYSIOLOGICAL FEATURES. An atrial complex that conducts with a critical prolongation of AV nodal conduction time generally precipitates AV nodal reentry (Figs. 32–24 to 32–26). Premature ventricular stimulation can also induce AV nodal reentry in about one third of patients. Data from radiofrequency catheter ablation results and mapping support the presence of differential atrial inputs into the AV node, the fast and slow pathways, to explain this tachycardia (see Chaps. 27 and 29). In Figure 32–30, as well as Figure 32–10A and B, the atria are shown as a necessary link between the fast and slow pathways. Whether these pathways are discrete pathways (perhaps due to anisotropy) or functional in nature is not known. In most examples, the retrograde P wave occurs at the onset of the QRS complex, clearly excluding the possibility of an accessory pathway. If an accessory pathway in the ventricle were part of the tachycardia circuit, the ventricles would have to be activated anterogradely before the accessory pathway could be activated retrogradely and depolarize the atria, thus placing the retrograde P wave no earlier than during the ST segment (see Preexcitation Syndrome, Chap. 30).

In approximately 30 percent of instances, atrial activation begins at the end of or just after the QRS complex and gives rise to a discrete P wave on the surface ECG (often appearing as a nubbin of an R in V_1) (see Fig. 32–10A), whereas in most patients, P waves are not seen since they are buried within the inscription of the QRS complex. In the most common variety of AV nodal reentrant tachycardia, the ventriculoatrial (VA) interval (i.e., the interval between the onset of QRS and the onset of atrial activity) is less than 50 percent of the R-R interval, and the ratio of the AV to the VA interval exceeds 1.0. These VA intervals are longer in patients with tachycardia related to accessory pathways, as well as in atypical forms of AV nodal reentry (see Fig. 32–10B).

Slow and Fast Pathways. In most patients, anterograde conduction to the ventricle occurs over the slow (alpha) pathway and retrograde conduction occurs over the fast (beta) pathway (see Chap. 27 and Fig. 32–10A and B). To initiate tachycardia, an atrial complex blocks conduction in the fast pathway anterogradely, travels to the ventricle over the slow

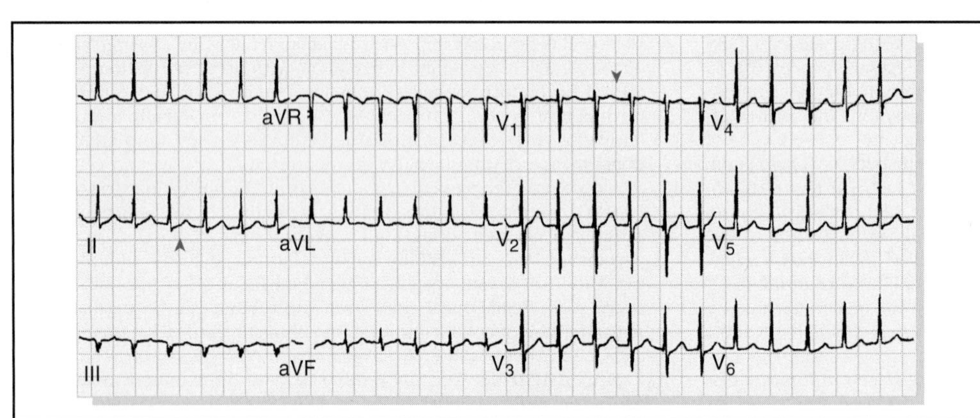

A

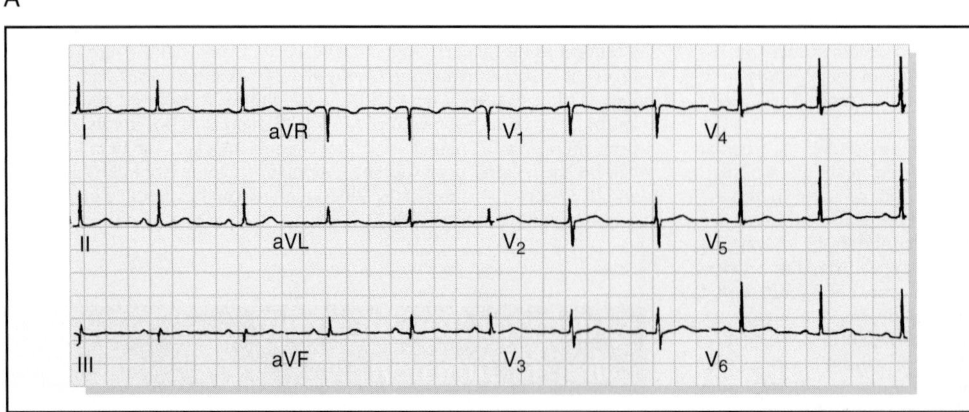

B

FIGURE 32–23 Twelve-lead electrocardiogram of atrioventricular nodal reentrant tachycardia. **A,** During tachycardia a pseudo-r′ is seen in lead V_1 (arrowhead) and pseudo-S waves (arrowhead) are seen in leads II, III, and aVF. **B,** These waves become more obvious when compared with the QRS complexes during sinus rhythm.

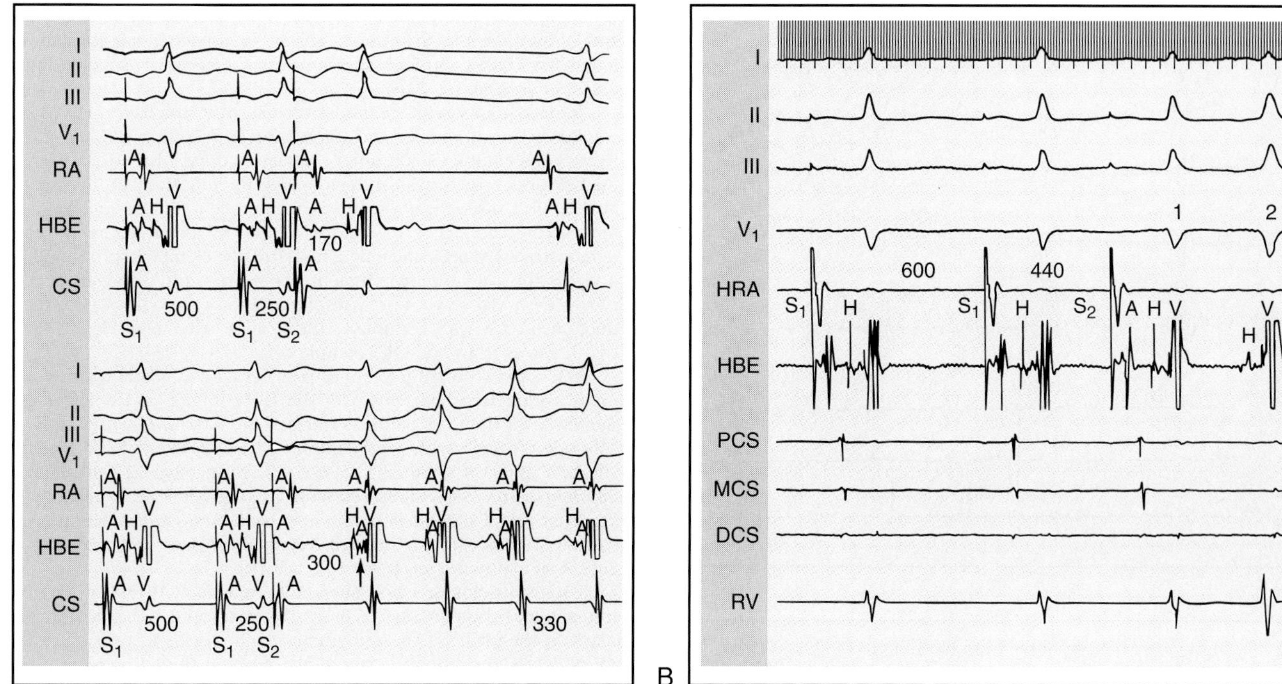

FIGURE 32–24 **A,** Initiation of atrioventricular (AV) nodal reentrant tachycardia in a patient with dual AV nodal pathways. **Upper** and **lower** panels show the last two paced beats of a train of stimuli delivered to the coronary sinus at a pacing cycle length of 500 milliseconds. The results of premature atrial stimulation at an S_1-S_2 interval of 250 milliseconds on two occasions are shown. In the **upper** panel, S_2 was conducted to the ventricle with an A-H interval of 170 milliseconds and was then followed by a sinus beat. In the **lower** panel, S_2 was conducted with an A-H interval of 300 milliseconds and initiated AV nodal reentry. Note that the retrograde atrial activity occurs (arrow) prior to the onset of ventricular septal depolarization and is superimposed on the QRS complex. Retrograde atrial activity begins first in the low right atrium (HBE lead) and then progresses to the high right atrium (RA) and coronary sinus (CS) recordings. **B,** Two QRS complexes in response to a single atrial premature complex. After a basic train of S_1 stimuli at 600 milliseconds, an S_2 at 440 milliseconds is introduced. The first QRS complex in response to S_2 occurs after a short (95 milliseconds) A-H interval caused by anterograde conduction over the fast AV nodal pathway. The first QRS complex is labeled number 1 (in lead V_1). The second QRS complex in response to the S_2 stimulus (labeled number 2) follows a long A-H interval (430 milliseconds) caused by anterograde conduction over the slow AV nodal pathway.

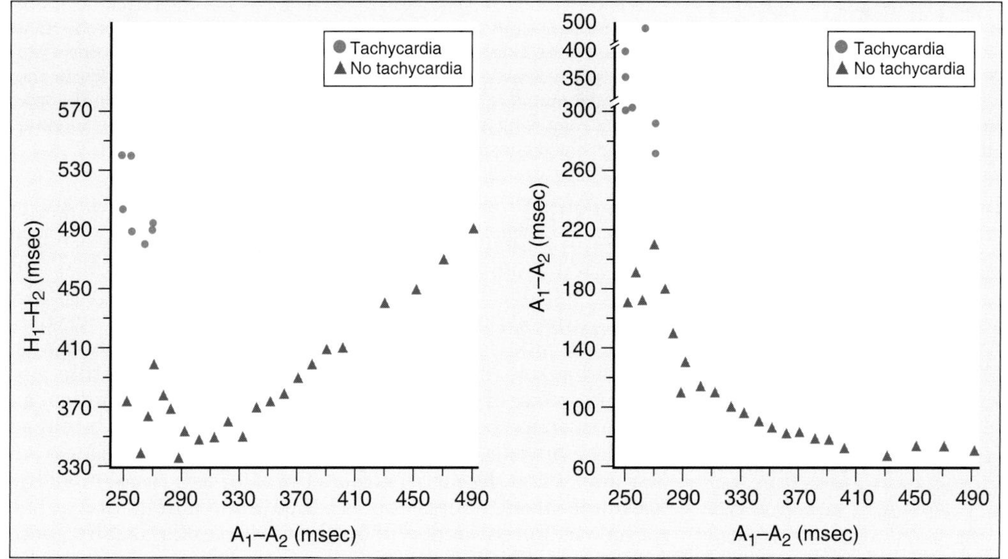

FIGURE 32–25 H_1-H_2 intervals **(left)** and A_2-H_2 intervals **(right)** at various A_1-A_2 intervals with a discontinuous atrioventricular (AV) nodal curve. At a critical A_1-A_2 interval the H_1-H_2 and the A_1-H_2 intervals increase markedly. At the break in the curves, AV nodal reentrant tachycardia is initiated.

pathway, and returns to the atrium over the previously blocked fast pathway ("slow-fast" form). The proximal and distal final pathways for this circus movement appear to be located within the AV node, so as currently conceived, the circus movement occurs over the two atrial approaches and the AV node (see Fig. 32–10A and B). The reentrant loop for typical AV nodal reentry is the anterograde slow AV nodal pathway to the final distal common pathway (probably the distal AV node), to the retrograde fast AV nodal pathway, and then to atrial myocardium. In atypical AV node reentry, the reentry occurs in the opposite direction. In some patients, the His bundle may be incorporated in the reentrant circuit. Less commonly, the reentry pathway can be over two slow pathways, the so-called slow-slow AV node reentry (see Fig. 32-11B). Some data are consistent with intranodal activity.

The cycle length of the tachycardia generally depends on how well the slow pathway conducts because the fast pathway usually exhibits excellent capability for retrograde conduction and has the shorter refractory period in the retrograde direction. Therefore, conduction time in the anterograde slow pathway is a major determinant of the cycle length of the tachycardia.

The Dual-Pathway Concept. Evidence supporting the dual-pathway concept derives from several observations, the most compelling of which is that radiofrequency catheter ablation of *either* the slow pathway or the fast pathway eliminates AV nodal reentry without eliminating AV nodal conduction. Other observations provide supporting proof. For example, in these patients a plot of the A_1-A_2 versus the A_2-H_2 or the A_1-A_2 versus the H_1-H_2 interval shows a discontinuous curve (see Fig. 32–25). The explanation is that at a crucial A_1-A_2 interval the impulse is suddenly blocked in the fast pathway and is conducted with delay over the slow pathway, with sudden prolongation of the A_2-H_2 (or H_1-H_2) interval. Generally, the A-H interval increases at least 50 milliseconds, with only a 10- to 20-millisecond decrease in the coupling interval of the premature atrial complex. Less commonly, dual pathways may be manifest by different PR

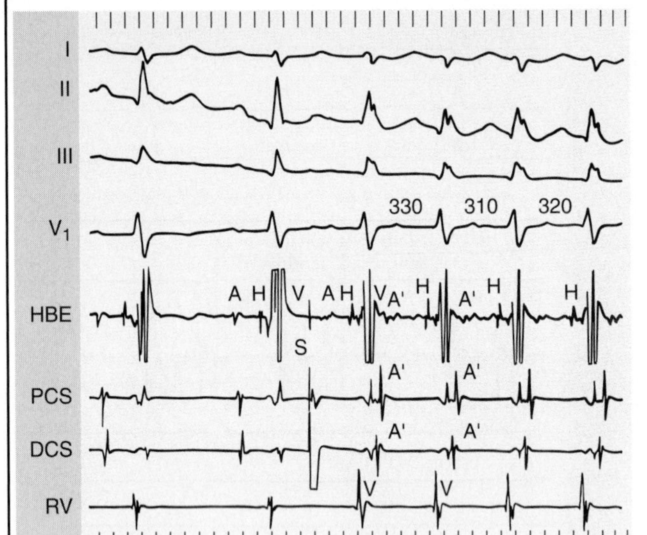

A

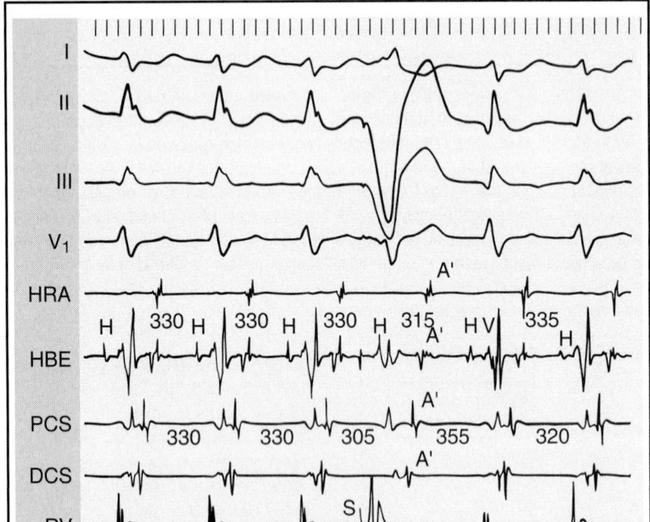

B

FIGURE 32–26 Atrial preexcitation during atrioventricular (AV) reciprocating tachycardia in a patient with a concealed accessory pathway. No evidence of accessory pathway conduction is present in the two sinus-initiated beats shown in **A.** A premature stimulus in the coronary sinus (S) precipitates a supraventricular tachycardia at a cycle length of approximately 330 milliseconds. The retrograde atrial activation sequence begins first in the distal coronary sinus (A′, DCS), followed by activation recorded in the proximal coronary sinus (PCS), low right atrium (HBE), and then the high right atrium (not shown). The QRS complex is normal and identical to the sinus-initiated QRS complex. (The terminal portion is slightly deformed by superimposition of the retrograde atrial recording.) Note that the RP interval is short and the PR interval is long. The shortest VA interval exceeds 65 milliseconds, consistent with conduction over a retrogradely conducting AV pathway. **B,** Premature ventricular stimulation at a time when the His bundle is still refractory from anterograde activation during tachycardia shortens the A-A interval from 330 to 305 milliseconds without a change in the retrograde atrial activation sequence. (Note that no change occurs in the H-H interval when the right ventricular stimulus, S, is delivered. H-H intervals are in milliseconds in the HBE lead.) Thus the ventricular stimulus, despite His bundle refractoriness, still reaches the atrium and produces an identical retrograde atrial activation sequence. The only way that this finding can be explained is via conduction over a retrogradely conducting accessory pathway. Therefore, the patient has a concealed accessory pathway with the Wolff-Parkinson-White syndrome.

or A-H intervals during sinus rhythm or at identical paced rates or by a sudden jump in the A-H interval during atrial pacing at a constant cycle length. Two QRS complexes in response to one P wave provide additional evidence (see Fig. 32–24B).

Some patients with AV nodal reentry may not have discontinuous refractory period curves, and some patients who do not have AV nodal reentry can exhibit discontinuous refractory curves. In the latter patients, dual AV nodal pathways can be a benign finding. Many of these patients also exhibit discontinuous curves retrogradely. Similar mechanisms of tachycardia can occur in children. Triple AV nodal pathways can be demonstrated in occasional patients. Virtually irrefutable proof of dual AV nodal pathways is the simultaneous propagation in opposite directions of two AV nodal wavefronts without collision (see Chap. 27) or the production of two QRS complexes from one P wave (see Fig. 32–24B) or two P waves from one QRS complex.

In less than 5 to 10 percent of patients with AV nodal reentry, anterograde conduction proceeds over the fast pathway and retrograde conduction over the slow pathway (termed the *unusual form* of "fast-slow" AV node reentry), with production of a long VA interval and a relatively short AV interval (generally AV/VA < 0.75; see Fig. 32–10B). The least common form ("slow-slow") exhibits a retrograde P wave midway in the cardiac cycle. Finally, it is possible to have tachycardias that use either the anterograde slow or fast pathways and conduct retrogradely over an accessory pathway (see later).

The ventricles are not needed to maintain AV nodal reentry in humans, and spontaneous AV block has been noted on occasion, particularly at the onset of the arrhythmia. Such block can take place in the AV node distal to the reentry circuit, between the AV node and bundle of His, within the bundle of His, or distal to it (see Chap. 27). Rarely, the block can be located between the reentry circuit in the AV node and the atrium. Most commonly, when block appears, it is below the bundle of His. Termination of the tachycardia generally results from a block in the anterogradely conducting slow pathway ("weak link"), so a retrograde atrial response is not followed by a His or ventricular response. Functional bundle branch block during AV nodal reentrant tachycardia does not modify the tachycardia significantly.

Retrograde Atrial Activation. The sequence of retrograde atrial activation is normal during AV nodal reentrant supraventricular tachycardia, which means that the earliest site of atrial activation during retrograde conduction over the fast pathway is recorded in the His bundle electrogram, followed by electrograms recorded from the os of the coronary sinus and then spreading to depolarize the rest of the right and left atria. During retrograde conduction over the slow pathway in the atypical type of AV nodal reentry, atrial activation recorded in the proximal coronary sinus precedes atrial activation recorded in the low right atrium, which suggests that the slow and fast pathways can enter the atria at slightly different positions.

CLINICAL FEATURES. AV nodal reentry commonly occurs in patients who have no structural heart disease and in the adult population frequently presents in the third and fourth decade of life. Symptoms frequently accompany the tachycardia and range from feelings of palpitations, nervousness, and anxiety to angina, heart failure, syncope, or shock, depending on the duration and rate of the tachycardia and the presence of structural heart disease. Tachycardia can cause syncope because of the rapid ventricular rate, reduced cardiac output, and cerebral circulation or because of asystole when the tachycardia terminates as a result of tachycardia-induced depression of sinus node automaticity. The prognosis for patients without heart disease is usually good.

MANAGEMENT

The Acute Attack. Management of AV nodal reentrant tachycardia depends on the underlying heart disease, how well the tachycardia is tolerated, and the natural history of previous attacks in the individual patient. For some patients, rest, reassurance, and sedation may be all that are required to abort an attack. Vagal maneuvers, including carotid sinus massage, the Valsalva and Mueller maneuvers, gagging, and occasionally exposure of the face to ice water, serve as the first line of therapy. These maneuvers may slightly slow the tachycardia rate, which then can speed up to the original rate following cessation of the attempt, or can terminate it. If vagal maneuvers fail, adenosine is the initial drug of choice. Digitalis, calcium antagonists, beta-adrenoceptor blockers, and adenosine normally depress conduction in the anterogradely conducting slow AV nodal pathway, whereas class IA and IC drugs depress conduction in the retrogradely conducting fast pathway (Table 32–2).

ADENOSINE. Adenosine (see Chap. 30) 6 to 12 mg given rapidly IV is the initial drug of choice and is successful at terminating the tachycardia in about 90 percent of cases.[64] *Verapamil* (see Chap. 30) 5 to 10 mg IV or diltiazem 0.25 to 0.35 mg/kg IV terminates AV nodal reentry successfully in about 2 minutes in approximately 90 percent of instances and is given when simple vagal maneuvers and adenosine fail.

DIGITALIS. Although it may be effective for longer-term management, digitalis has a slower onset of action than the agents described earlier and thus is not as useful in the acute management. If digitalis is used, digoxin can be given, 0.5 to 1 mg IV over a period of 10 to 15 minutes, followed by 0.25 mg every 2 to 4 hours, with a total dose less than 1.5 mg within any 24-hour period. *Oral digitalis* administration to terminate an acute attack is not generally indicated. Vagal maneuvers that were previously ineffective can terminate the tachycardia following digitalis administration and should therefore be repeated.

BETA-ADRENOCEPTOR BLOCKERS. Beta-adrenoceptor blockers must be used cautiously, if at all in patients with heart failure, chronic lung disease, or a history of asthma because their beta-adrenoceptor blocking action depresses myocardial contractility and can produce bronchospasm. Digitalis, calcium antagonists, beta blockers, and adenosine normally depress conduction in the anterogradely conducting slow pathway, whereas classes IA and IC drugs depress conduction in the retrogradely conducting fast pathway.

DC CARDIOVERSION. Before digitalis or a beta blocker is administered, it is advisable to reassess the clinical status of the patient and consider whether DC cardioversion may be advisable. DC shock administered to patients who have received excessive amounts of digitalis can be dangerous and result in serious postshock ventricular arrhythmias (see Chap. 30). Particularly if signs or symptoms of cardiac decompensation occur, DC electrical shock should be considered early. DC shock, synchronized to the QRS complex to avoid precipitating ventricular fibrillation, successfully terminates AV nodal reentry with energies in the range of 10 to 50 J; higher energies may be required in some instances.

PACING. If DC shock is contraindicated or if pacing wires are already in place (either postoperatively or if the patient has a permanent pacemaker), competitive *atrial* or *ventricular pacing* can restore sinus rhythm. In some instances, esophageal pacing can be useful (see Chap. 31).

Classes IA, IC, and III drugs are not usually required to terminate AV nodal reentry. Unless contraindicated, DC cardioversion should generally be attempted before using these agents, which are more often administered to prevent recurrence.

TABLE 32–2 Drugs that Slow Conduction in, and Prolong Refractoriness of, the Accessory Pathway and AV Node

Affected Tissue	Drugs
Accessory pathway AV node	Class IA Class II Class IV Adenosine Digitalis
Both	Class IC Class III (amiodarone)

AV = atrioventricular.

Pressor drugs can terminate AV nodal reentry by inducing reflex vagal stimulation mediated by baroreceptors in the carotid sinus and aorta when systolic blood pressure is acutely elevated to levels of about 180 mm Hg, but they are rarely needed unless the patient is also hypotensive.

Prevention of Recurrences. Initially, one must decide whether the frequency and severity of the attacks warrant long-term therapy. If the attacks of paroxysmal tachycardia are infrequent, well tolerated, and short lasting and either terminate spontaneously or are easily terminated by the patient, no prophylactic therapy may be necessary. If the attacks are sufficiently frequent and/or long lasting to necessitate therapy, the patient can be treated with drugs empirically or on the basis of serial electrophysiological testing. If empirical testing is desirable, digitalis, a long-acting calcium antagonist, or a long-acting beta-adrenoceptor blocker is a reasonable initial choice. The clinical situation and potential contraindications, such as beta blockers in an asthmatic, usually dictate the selection. If digitalis is used, rapid oral digitalization can be accomplished in 24 to 36 hours with digoxin at an initial dose of 1 to 1.5 mg, followed by 0.25 to 0.5 mg every 6 hours for a total dose of 2 to 3 mg. A less rapid oral regimen induces digitalization in 2 to 3 days with an initial dose of 0.75 to 1 mg, followed by 0.25 to 0.5 mg every 12 hours for a total dose of 2 to 3 mg. Alternatively, digoxin administered as a maintenance dose of 0.125 to 0.5 mg achieves digitalization in about 1 week. If any of these drugs are ineffective when taken singly, combinations can be tested.

RADIOFREQUENCY ABLATION. Radiofrequency ablation is more than 95 percent effective at curing patients long term, with a low incidence of complications. Because it is preferable to *cure* the patient of the tachycardia rather than use potentially toxic drugs to suppress it or to implant an antitachycardia device that terminates the tachycardia only after its onset (see Chap. 30), radiofrequency catheter ablation should be considered early in the management of patients with symptomatic recurrent episodes of AV node reentry. The procedure can be offered as an alternative to drug therapy in patients with frequent, symptomatic episodes. For patients who do not wish to take drugs, patients who are drug intolerant, or those in whom drugs are ineffective, radiofrequency catheter ablation is the treatment of choice. It should be considered before long-term therapy with class IA, IC, or III antiarrhythmic drugs. Ablation has replaced surgery in virtually all instances and may be considered the initial treatment of choice in many symptomatic patients.

Reentry over a Concealed (Retrograde-Only) Accessory Pathway

ECG RECOGNITION. The presence of an accessory pathway that conducts unidirectionally from the ventricle to the atrium but not in the reverse direction is not apparent by analysis of the scalar ECG during sinus rhythm because the ventricle is not preexcited (see Fig. 32–26).[65] Therefore, ECG manifestations of WPW syndrome are absent, and the accessory pathway is said to be "concealed." Since the mechanism responsible for most tachycardias in patients who have WPW syndrome is macro-reentry caused by anterograde conduction over the AV node–His bundle pathway and retrograde conduction over an accessory pathway, the latter, even if it only conducts retrogradely, can still participate in the reentrant circuit to cause an *AV reciprocating* tachycardia. Electrocardiographically, a tachycardia resulting from this mechanism can be *suspected* when the QRS complex is normal and the retrograde P wave occurs *after* completion of the QRS complex, in the ST segment, or early in the T wave (see Fig. 32–10C).

MECHANISMS. The cause of unidirectional propagation is not clear and can relate to multiple factors. During sinus rhythm, the atrial impulse probably enters the accessory pathway but is blocked near the ventricular insertion site with both right- and left-sided concealed accessory pathways. During functional block in patients with anterograde conduction over accessory pathways, block occurs near the ventricular insertion site most commonly with left-sided pathways but more often near the atrial insertion site with right-sided accessory pathways.

The P wave follows the QRS complex during tachycardia because the ventricle must be activated before the propagating impulse can enter the accessory pathway and excite the atria retrogradely. Therefore, the retrograde P wave must occur after ventricular excitation, in contrast to AV nodal reentry, in which the atria are usually excited during ventricular activation (see Fig. 32–10A). Also, the contour of the retrograde P wave can differ from that of the usual retrograde P wave since the atria may be activated eccentrically, that is, in a manner other than the normal retrograde activation sequence, which starts at the low right atrial septum as in AV nodal reentry. This eccentric activation occurs because the concealed accessory pathway in most instances is left sided, that is, inserts into the left atrium, which makes the left atrium the first site of retrograde atrial activation and causes the retrograde P wave to be negative in lead I (see Fig. 32–26).

Finally, since the tachycardia circuit involves the ventricles, if a functional bundle branch block occurs in the same ventricle in which the accessory pathway is located, the VA interval and cycle length of the tachycardia can become longer (see Fig. 32–31). This important change ensues because the bundle branch block lengthens the reentrant circuit (see Preexcitation Syndrome). For example, the normal activation sequence for a reciprocating tachycardia circuit with a left-sided accessory pathway but without a functional bundle branch block progresses from the atrium to the AV node–His bundle, to the right and left ventricles, to the accessory pathway, and then to the atrium. However, during a functional left bundle branch block, for example, the tachycardia circuit travels from the atrium to the AV node–His bundle, to the right ventricle, to the septum, to the left ventricle, to the accessory pathway, and then back to the atrium. This increase in the VA interval provides definitive proof that the ventricle and accessory pathway are part of the reentry circuit. The additional time required for the impulse to travel across the septum from the right to the left ventricle before reaching the accessory pathway and atrium lengthens the VA interval, which lengthens the cycle length of the tachycardia by an equal amount, assuming that no other changes in conduction times occur within the circuit. Thus, lengthening of the tachycardia cycle length by more than 35 milliseconds during an ipsilateral functional bundle branch block is diagnostic of a free wall accessory pathway if the lengthening can be shown to be due to VA prolongation only and not to prolongation of the H-V interval (which can develop with the appearance of a bundle branch block). In an occasional patient, the increase in cycle length because of prolongation of VA conduction can be nullified by a simultaneous decrease in the PR (A-H) interval.

The presence of an ipsilateral bundle branch block can facilitate reentry and cause an incessant AV reentrant tachycardia. A functional bundle branch block in the ventricle contralateral to the accessory pathway does not lengthen the tachycardia cycle if the H-V interval does not lengthen.

Septal Accessory Pathway. An exception to these observations occurs in a patient with a concealed septal accessory pathway. First, retrograde atrial activation is normal because it occurs retrogradely up the septum. Second, the VA interval and the cycle length of the tachycardia increase 25 milliseconds or less with the development of an ipsilateral functional bundle branch block.

Vagal maneuvers, by acting predominantly on the AV node, produce a response on AV reentry similar to AV nodal reentry, and the tachycardia can transiently slow and sometimes terminate. Generally, termination occurs in the anterograde direction, so the last retrograde P wave fails to conduct to the ventricle.

ELECTROPHYSIOLOGICAL FEATURES. Electrophysiological criteria supporting the diagnosis of tachycardia involving reentry over a concealed accessory pathway include the fact that initiation of tachycardia depends on a critical degree of AV delay (necessary to allow time for the accessory pathway to recover excitability so that it can conduct retrogradely), but the delay can be in the AV node or His-Purkinje system; that is, a critical degree of A-H delay is not necessary. Occasionally, a tachycardia can start with little or no measurable lengthening of AV nodal or His-Purkinje conduction time. The AV nodal refractory period curve is smooth, in contrast to the discontinuous curve found in many patients with AV nodal reentry. Dual AV nodal pathways can occasionally be noted as a concomitant, but unrelated finding.

Diagnosis of Accessory Pathways. Diagnosis can be accomplished by demonstrating that during ventricular pacing, premature ventricular stimulation activates the atria before retrograde depolarization of the His bundle, thus indicating that the impulse reached the atria before it depolarized the His bundle and must have traveled a different pathway to do so. Also, if the ventricles can be stimulated prematurely during tachycardia at a time when the His bundle is refractory and the impulse still conducts to the atrium, retrograde propagation traveled to the atrium over a pathway other than the bundle of His (see Fig. 32–26B). If the PVC depolarizes the atria without lengthening of the VA interval and with the same retrograde atrial activation sequence, one assumes that the stimulation site (i.e., ventricle) is within the reentrant circuit without intervening His-Purkinje or AV nodal tissue that might increase the VA interval and therefore the A-A interval. In addition, if a PVC delivered at a time when the His bundle is refractory terminates the tachycardia without activating the atria retrogradely, it most likely invaded and blocked conduction in an accessory pathway.

The VA interval (a measurement of conduction over the accessory pathway) is generally constant over a wide range of ventricular paced rates and coupling intervals of PVCs, as well as during the tachycardia in the absence of aberration. Similar short VA intervals can be observed in some patients during AV nodal reentry, but if the VA conduction time or RP interval is the same during tachycardia *and* ventricular pacing at comparable rates, an accessory pathway is almost certainly present. The VA interval is usually less than 50 percent of the R-R interval. The tachycardia can be easily initiated following premature ventricular stimulation that conducts retrogradely in the accessory pathway but blocks conduction in the AV node or His bundle. Atria and ventricles are required components of the macro-reentrant circuit; therefore, continuation of the tachycardia in the presence of AV or VA block excludes an accessory AV pathway as part of the reentrant circuit.

CLINICAL FEATURES. The presence of concealed accessory pathways is estimated to account for about 30 percent of patients with apparent supraventricular tachycardia referred for electrophysiological evaluation. The great majority of these accessory pathways are located between the left ventricle and left atrium and in the posteroseptal area, less commonly between the right ventricle and right atrium. It is important to be aware of a concealed accessory pathway as a possible cause of apparently "routine" supraventricular tachycardia since the therapeutic response may at times not follow the usual guidelines. Tachycardia rates tend to be somewhat faster than those occurring in AV nodal reentry (200 beats/min), but a great deal of overlap exists between the two groups.

Syncope can occur because the rapid ventricular rate fails to provide adequate cerebral circulation or because the tachyarrhythmia depresses the sinus pacemaker and causes a period of asystole when the tachyarrhythmia terminates. Physical examination reveals an unvarying, regular ventricular rhythm with constant intensity of the first heart sound. Jugular venous pressure can be elevated, but the waveform generally remains constant.

MANAGEMENT. The therapeutic approach to terminate this form of tachycardia acutely is as outlined for AV nodal reentry. It is necessary to achieve block of a single impulse from atrium to ventricle or ventricle to atrium. Generally, the most successful method is to produce a transient AV nodal block; therefore, vagal maneuvers, IV adenosine, verapamil or diltiazem, digitalis, and beta blockers are acceptable choices. Radiofrequency catheter ablation and conventional antiarrhythmic agents that prolong the activation time or refractory period in the accessory pathway need to be considered for chronic prophylactic therapy, similar to that discussed for reciprocating tachycardias associated with the preexcitation syndrome. Radiofrequency catheter ablation is curative, has low risk, and should be considered early for symptomatic patients (see Chap. 30).[65] The presence of atrial fibrillation in patients with a *concealed accessory pathway* should not be a greater therapeutic challenge than in patients who do not have such a pathway because anterograde AV conduction occurs only over the AV node and not over an accessory pathway. IV verapamil and digitalis are not contraindicated. However, under some circumstances, such as catecholamine stimulation, anterograde conduction can occur in the apparently concealed accessory pathway.

Preexcitation Syndrome

ECG RECOGNITION. Preexcitation, or the WPW ECG abnormality, occurs when the atrial impulse activates the whole or some part of the ventricle or the ventricular impulse activates the whole or some part of the atrium earlier than would be expected if the impulse traveled by way of the normal specialized conduction system only (Fig. 32–27).[65] This premature activation is caused by muscular connections composed of working myocardial fibers that exist outside the specialized conducting tissue and connect the atrium and ventricle while bypassing AV nodal conduction delay. They are named *accessory AV pathways* or connections and are responsible for the most common variety of preexcitation (incidentally noted in other species such as monkeys, dogs, and cats). The term *syndrome* is attached to this disorder when tachyarrhythmias occur as a result of the accessory pathway. Three basic features typify the ECG abnormalities of patients with the usual form of WPW conduction caused by an AV connection: (1) PR interval less than 120 milliseconds during sinus rhythm; (2) QRS complex duration exceeding 120 milliseconds with a slurred, slowly rising onset of the QRS in some leads (delta wave) and usually a normal terminal QRS portion; and (3) secondary ST-T wave changes that are generally directed in an opposite direction to the major delta and QRS vectors. Analysis of the scalar ECG can be used to localize the accessory pathway (Fig. 32–27D).[66]

In the *WPW syndrome,* the most common tachycardia is characterized by a normal QRS, a regular rhythm, ventricular rates of 150 to 250 beats/min (generally faster than AV nodal reentry), and sudden onset and termination, in most respects behaving like the tachycardia described for conduction over a concealed pathway (see Chap. 27). The major difference between the two is the capacity for anterograde conduction over the accessory pathway during atrial flutter or atrial fibrillation (see later).

Variants

A variety of other anatomical substrates exist and provide the basis for different ECG manifestations of several variations of the preexcitation syndrome (Fig. 32-28).[65] Fibers from the atrium to the His bundle bypassing the physiological delay of the AV node are called *atriohisian tracts* (Fig. 32-28B) and are associated with a short PR interval and a normal QRS complex. Although demonstrated anatomically (see later), the electrophysiological significance of these tracts in the genesis of tachycardias with a short PR interval and a normal QRS complex (Lown-Ganong-Levine [LGL] syndrome) remains to be established. Indeed, evidence does *not* support the presence of a specific LGL syndrome consisting of a short PR interval, normal QRS complex, and tachycardias related to an atriohisian bypass tract.

Another variant of accessory pathway conduction is that due to *atriofascicular* or *nodofascicular* accessory pathways. These fibers result in a unique AV conduction pattern (sometimes referred to as *Mahaim conduction*) characterized by the development of ventricular preexcitation (widened QRS and short H-V interval) with a progressive increase in the AV interval in response to atrial overdrive pacing, as opposed to the behavior of the usual accessory pathway in which preexcitation occurs with short AV intervals (Fig. 32-29). Because the accessory pathways responsible for this conduction pattern usually insert into the right bundle branch, preexcitation generally results in a left bundle branch block pattern. This phenomenon can be due to fibers passing from the AV node to the ventricle, called *nodoventricular fibers* (or nodofascicular if the insertion is into the right bundle branch rather than ventricular muscle) (see Fig. 32-28C). For nodoventricular connections, the PR interval may be normal or short, and the QRS complex is a fusion beat. This pattern of preexcitation can also result from *atriofascicular* accessory pathways. These fibers almost always represent a duplication of the AV node and the distal conducting system and are located in the right ventricular free wall. The apical end lies close to the lateral tricuspid annulus and conducts slowly, with AV node–like properties. After a long course, the distal portion of these fibers, which conducts rapidly, inserts into the distal right bundle branch or the apical region of the right ventricle.[65] No preexcitation is generally apparent during sinus rhythm but can be exposed by premature right atrial stimulation. The absence of retrograde conduction in these pathways produces only an antidromic AV reentry tachycardia ("preexcited" tachycardia) characterized by anterograde conduction over the accessory pathway and retrograde conduction over the right bundle branch–His bundle–AV node, thus making the atrium a necessary part of the circuit. The preexcited tachycardia has a left bundle branch block pattern, long AV interval (because of the long conduction time over the accessory pathway), and short VA interval. A right bundle branch block can be proarrhythmic by increasing the length of the tachycardia circuit (the VA interval is prolonged because of a delay in retrograde activation of the His bundle), and the tachycardia can become incessant.[65]

In patients who have an atriohisian tract, theoretically, the QRS complex would remain normal and the short A-H interval fixed or show very little increase during atrial pacing at more rapid rates. This response is uncommon. Rapid atrial pacing in patients who have nodoventricular or nodofascicular connections shortens the H-V interval and widens the QRS complex, with production of a left bundle branch block contour, but in contrast to the situation in patients who have an AV connection (Fig. 32-30), the AV interval also lengthens. In patients who have fasciculoventricular connections, the H-V interval remains short and the QRS complex unchanged and anomalous during rapid atrial pacing.

ELECTROPHYSIOLOGICAL FEATURES OF PREEXCITATION. If the accessory pathway is capable of anterograde conduction, two parallel routes of AV conduction are possible, one subject to physiological delay over the AV node and the other passing directly without delay from the atrium to the ventricle (Figs. 32-31 to 32-37; see also Figs. 32-28 to 32-30). This direct route of conduction produces the typical QRS complex that is a fusion beat as a result of depolarization of the ventricle in part by the wavefront traveling over the accessory pathway and in part by the wavefront traveling over the normal AV node–His bundle route. The delta wave represents ventricular activation from input over the accessory pathway. The extent of the contribution to ventricular deplorization by the wavefront over each route depends on their relative activation times. If AV nodal conduction delay occurs because of a rapid atrial pacing rate or premature atrial complex, for example, more of the ventricle becomes activated over the accessory pathway and the QRS complex becomes more anomalous in contour. Total activation of the ventricle over the accessory pathway can occur if the AV nodal conduction delay is sufficiently long. In contrast, if the accessory pathway is relatively far from the sinus node, for example, a left lateral accessory pathway, or if the AV nodal conduction time is relatively short, more of the ventricle may be activated by conduction over the normal pathway (see Fig. 32-30). The normal fusion beat during sinus rhythm has a short H-V interval, or His bundle activation actually begins after the onset of ventricular depolarization because part of the atrial impulse bypasses the AV node and activates the ventricle early, at a time when the atrial impulse traveling the normal route just reaches the His bundle. This finding of a short or negative H-V interval occurs *only* during conduction over an accessory pathway or from retrograde His activation during a complex originating in the ventricle, such as a VT.

Pacing the atrium at rapid rates, at premature intervals, or from a site close to the atrial insertion of the accessory pathway accentuates the anomalous activation of the ventricles and shortens the H-V interval even more (His activation may become buried in the ventricular electrogram, as in Fig. 32-30B). The position of the accessory pathway can be determined by careful analysis of the spatial direction of the delta wave in the 12-lead ECG in maximally preexcited beats (see Fig. 32-27).[66] T wave abnormalities can occur after the disappearance of preexcitation with orientation of the T wave according to the site of preexcitation (T wave

Text continued on p. 836

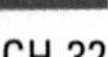

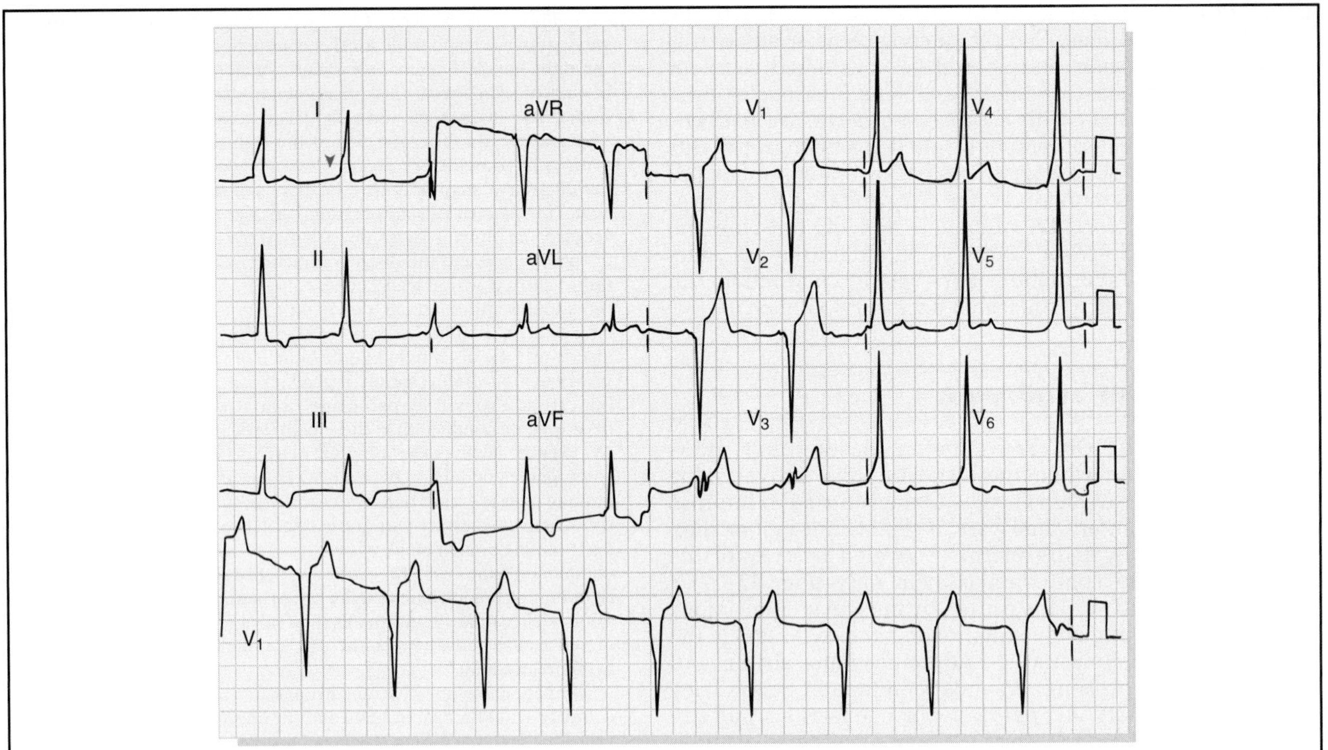

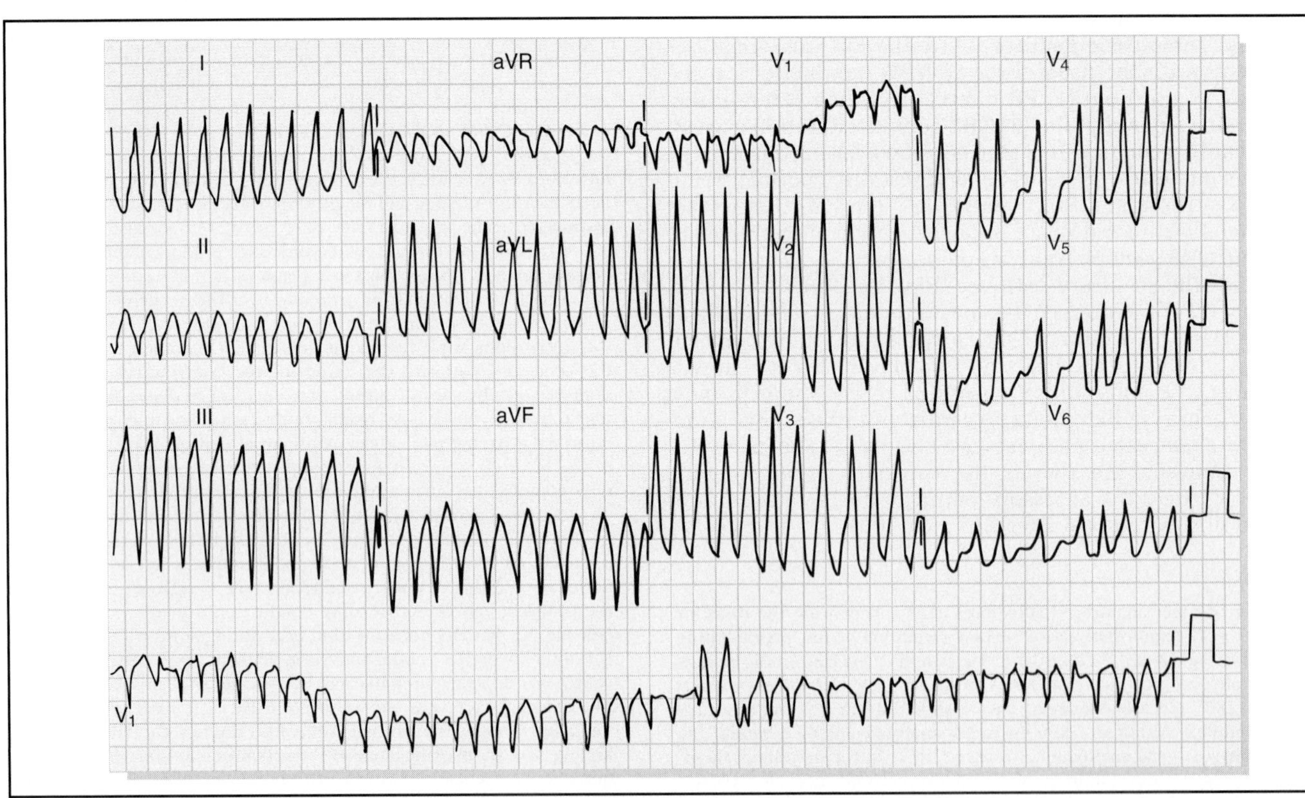

FIGURE 32–27 **A,** Right anteroseptal accessory pathway. The 12-lead electrocardiogram characteristically exhibits a normal to inferior axis. The delta wave is negative in V_1 and V_2, upright in leads I, II, aVL, and aVF, isoelectric in lead III, and negative in aVR. Location was verified at surgery. The arrowhead indicates a delta wave (lead I). **B,** Right posteroseptal accessory pathway. Negative delta waves in leads II, III, and aVF, upright in I and aVL, localize this pathway to the posteroseptal region. The negative delta wave in V_1 with sharp transition to an upright delta wave in V_2 pinpoints it to the right posteroseptal area. Atrial fibrillation is present. Location was verified at surgery. **C,** Left lateral accessory pathway. A positive delta wave in the anterior precordial leads and in leads II, III, and aVF, positive or isoelectric in leads I and aVL, and isoelectric or negative in V_5 and V_6 is typical of a left lateral accessory pathway. Rapid coronary sinus pacing (450-millisecond cycle length) was used to enhance preexcitation (negative P wave in leads I, II, III, aVF, and V_3 through V_6). Location was verified at surgery. **D,** Right free wall accessory pathway. The predominantly negative delta wave in V_1 and the axis more leftward than in **A** indicate the presence of a right free wall accessory pathway. **E,** Logic diagram to determine the location of accessory pathways. Begin with analysis of V_1 to determine whether the delta wave and the QRS complex are negative or positive. That establishes the ventricle in which the accessory pathway is located. Next, determine whether the delta wave and QRS complex are negative in leads II, III, and aVF. If so, the accessory pathway is located in a posteroseptal position. If the accessory pathway is located in the right ventricle, an inferior axis indicates an anteroseptal location, whereas a left axis indicates a right free wall location. If the accessory pathway is located in the left ventricle, an isoelectric or negative delta wave and QRS complex in leads I, aVL, V_5, and V_6 indicate a left lateral (free wall) location.

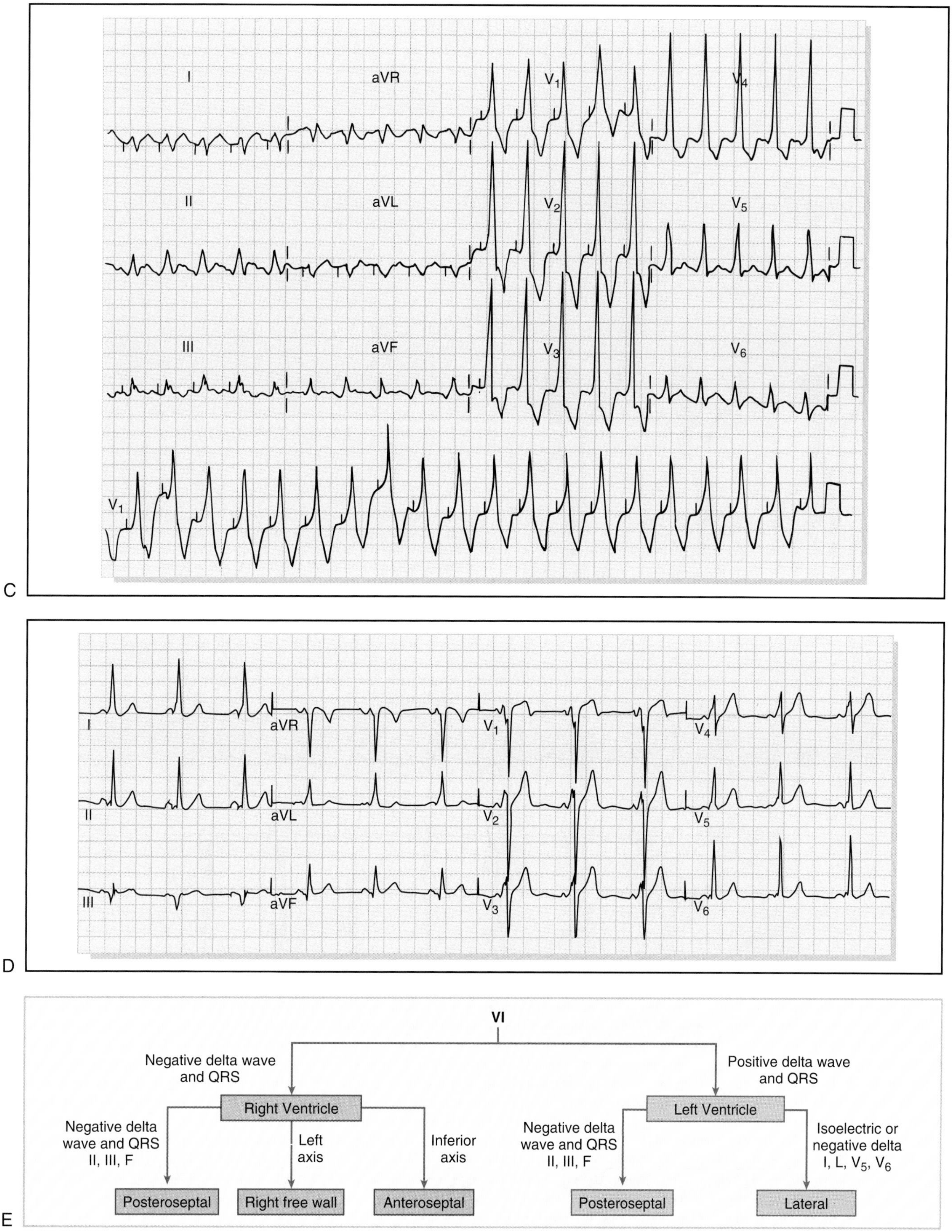

C

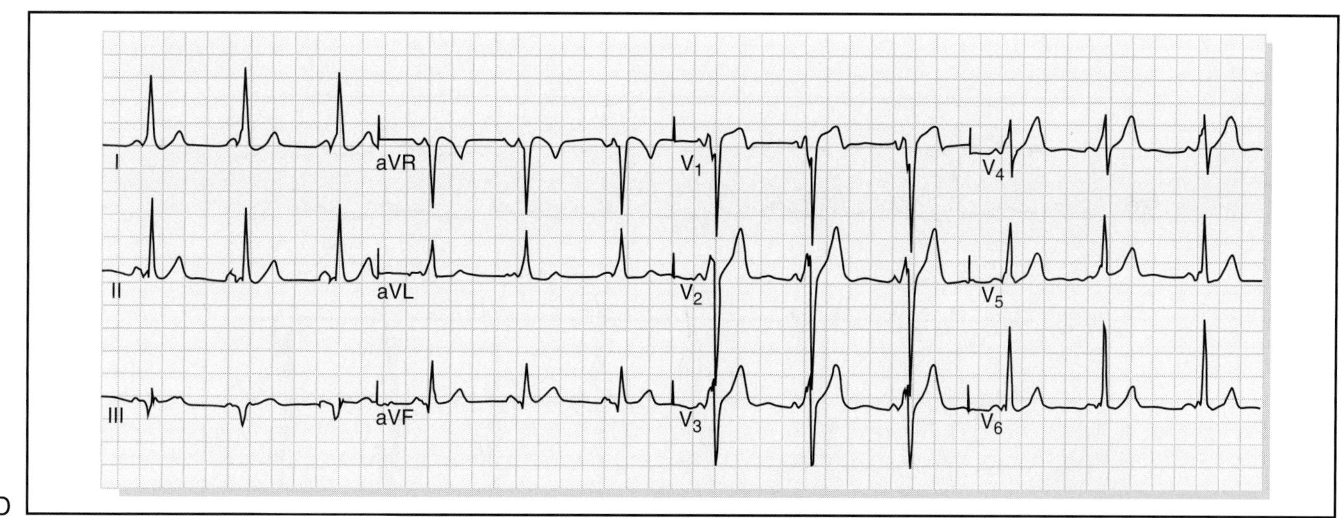

D

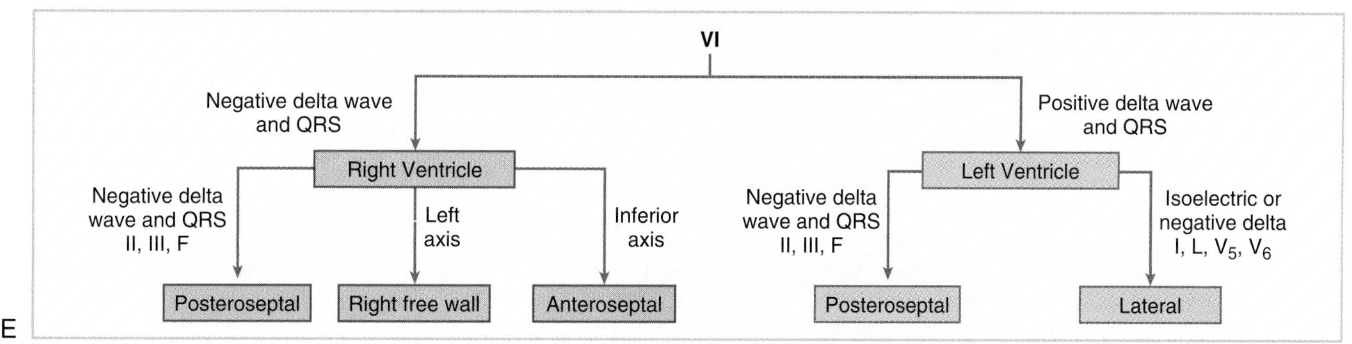

E

FIGURE 32–27 cont'd.

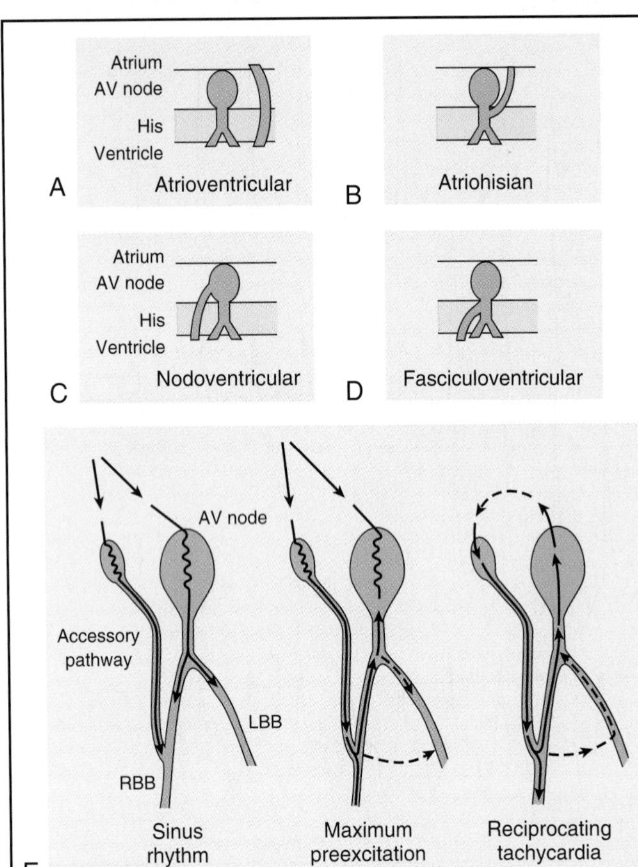

FIGURE 32–28 Schematic representation of accessory pathways. **A,** The "usual" atrioventricular (AV) accessory pathway giving rise to most clinical manifestations of tachycardia associated with Wolff-Parkinson-White (WPW) syndrome. **B,** The very uncommon atriohisian accessory pathway. If Lown-Ganong-Levine syndrome exists, it would have this type of anatomy, which has been demonstrated on occasion histopathologically. **C,** Nodoventricular pathways, original concept, in which anterograde conduction travels down the accessory pathway with retrograde conduction in the bundle branch–His bundle–AV node (see below). **D,** Fasciculoventricular connections, which are not thought to play an important role in the genesis of tachycardias. **E,** The current concept of nodofascicular accessory pathway in which the accessory pathway is an AV communication with AV nodal-like properties. Sinus rhythm results in a fusion QRS complex, as in the usual form of WPW syndrome shown in **A.** Maximum preexcitation results in ventricular activation over the accessory pathway, and the His bundle is activated retrogradely. During reciprocating tachycardia, anterograde conduction occurs over the accessory pathway with retrograde conduction over the normal pathway. LBBB = left bundle branch block; RBBB = right bundle branch block. (**E** from Benditt DG, Milstein S: Nodoventricular accessory connection: A misnomer or a structural/functional spectrum. J Cardiovasc Electrophysiol 1:231, 1990.)

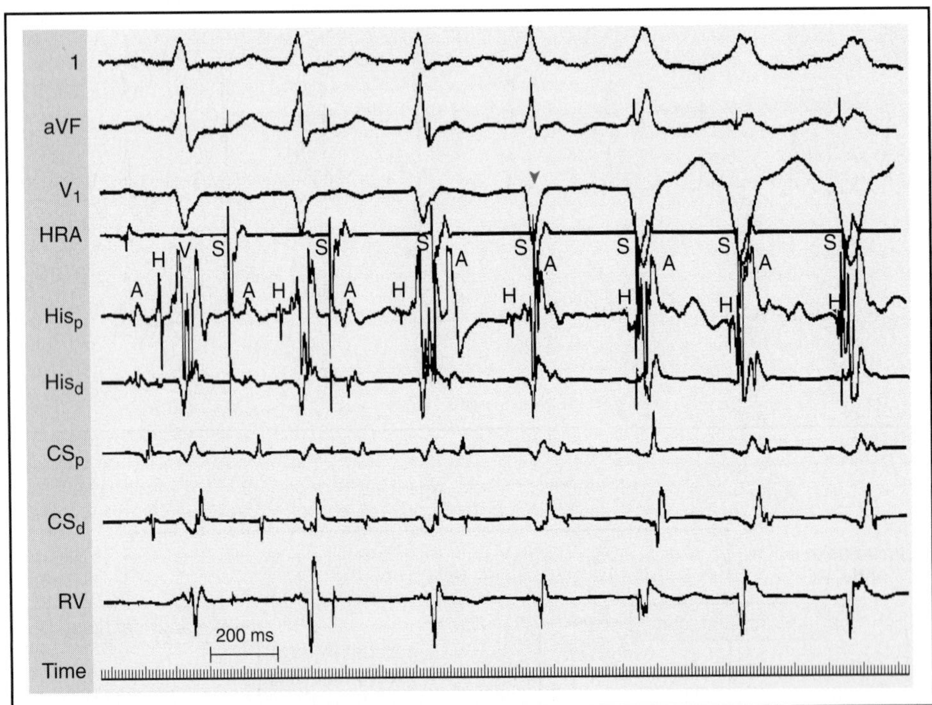

FIGURE 32–29 Development of preexcitation over an atriofascicular accessory pathway. During atrial pacing (S), on the left side of the figure, conduction occurs down the atrioventricular node as evidenced by a normal-appearing QRS complex and a normal H-V interval. The stimulus marked by the arrowhead conducts the impulse down an atriofascicular fiber, which results in a preexcited QRS, as evidenced by a widened QRS and short H-V interval.

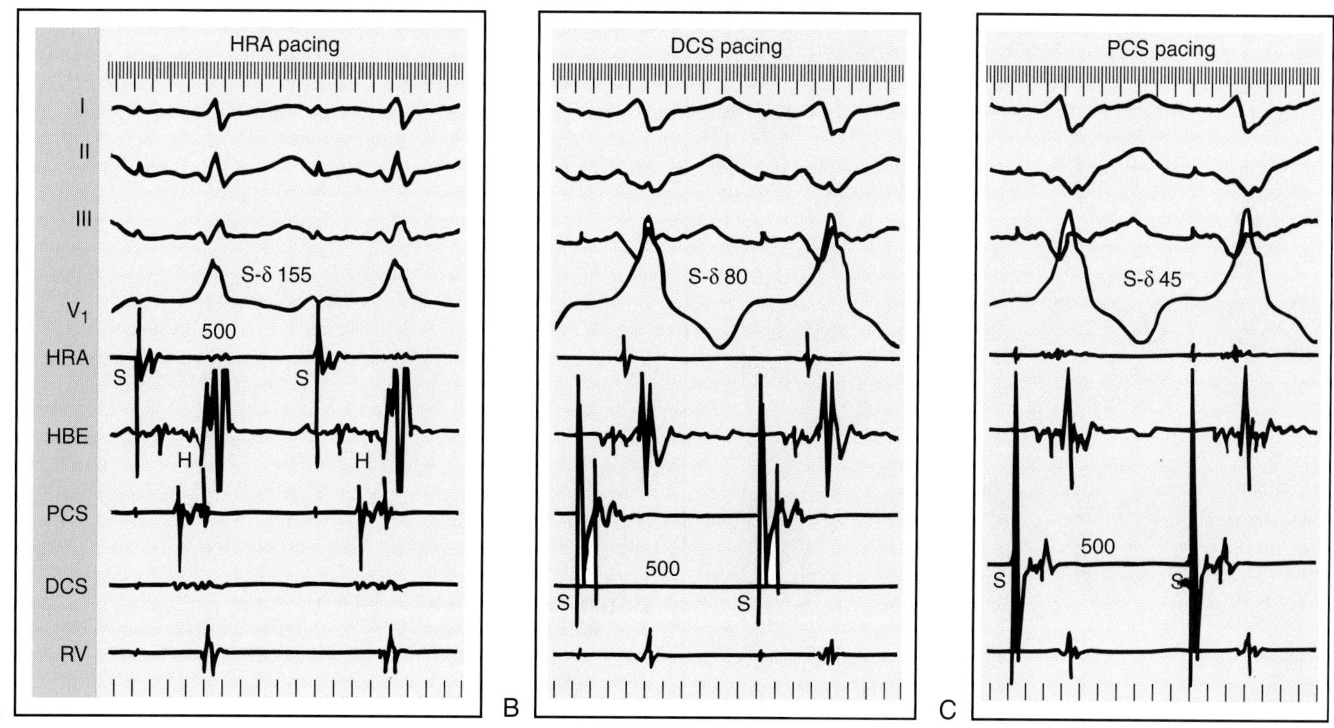

FIGURE 32–30 Atrial pacing at different atrial sites illustrating different conduction over the accessory pathway. **A,** High right atrial pacing at a cycle length of 500 milliseconds produces anomalous activation of the ventricle (note the upright QRS complex in V_1) and a stimulus-delta interval of 155 milliseconds (S-δ 155). This interval indicates that the time from the onset of the stimulus to the beginning of the QRS complex is relatively long because the stimulus is delivered at a fairly large distance from the accessory pathway. Note that His bundle activation (H) occurs at about the onset of the QRS complex. **B,** Atrial pacing occurs through the distal coronary sinus electrode (DCS). At the same pacing cycle length, DCS pacing results in more anomalous ventricular activation and a shorter stimulus-delta interval (80 milliseconds). His bundle activation is now buried within the inscription of the ventricular electrogram in the HBE lead. **C,** Pacing from the proximal coronary sinus electrode (PCS) results in the shortest stimulus-delta interval (45 milliseconds); such an interval indicates that the pacing stimulus is being delivered very close to the atrial insertion of the accessory pathway, which is located in the left posteroseptal region of the atrioventricular groove.

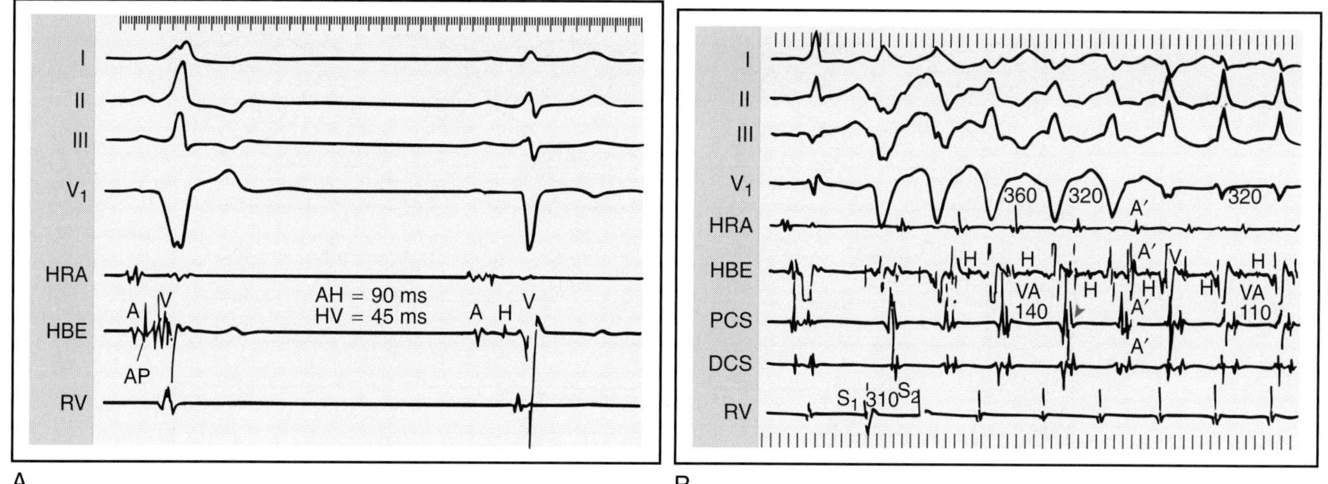

FIGURE 32–31 **A,** Recording of depolarization of an accessory pathway (AP) with a catheter electrode. The first QRS complex illustrates conduction over the AP. In the scalar ECG, a short P-R interval and delta wave (best seen in leads I and V_1) are apparent. His bundle activation is buried within the ventricular complex. In the following complex, conduction has blocked over the AP and a normal QRS complex results. His bundle activation clearly precedes the onset of ventricular depolarization by 45 milliseconds. The A-H interval for this complex is 90 milliseconds. **B,** Influence of functional ipsilateral bundle branch block on the VA interval during an atrioventricular reciprocating tachycardia. Partial preexcitation can be noted in the sinus-initiated complex (first complex). Two premature ventricular stimuli (S_1, S_2) initiate a sustained supraventricular tachycardia that persists with a left bundle branch block for several complexes before finally reverting to normal. The retrograde atrial activation sequence is recorded first in the proximal coronary sinus lead (arrowhead, PCS), then in the distal coronary sinus lead (DCS) and low right atrium (HBE), and then high in the right atrium (HRA). During the functional bundle branch block, the ventriculoatrial interval in the PCS lead is 140 milliseconds, which shortens to 110 milliseconds when the QRS complex reverts to normal. Such behavior is characteristic of a left-sided accessory pathway with prolongation of the reentrant pathway by the functional left bundle branch block. (**A,** From Prystowsky EN, Browne KF, Zipes DP: Intracardiac recording by catheter electrode of accessory pathway depolarization. J Am Coll Cardiol 1:468, 1983.)

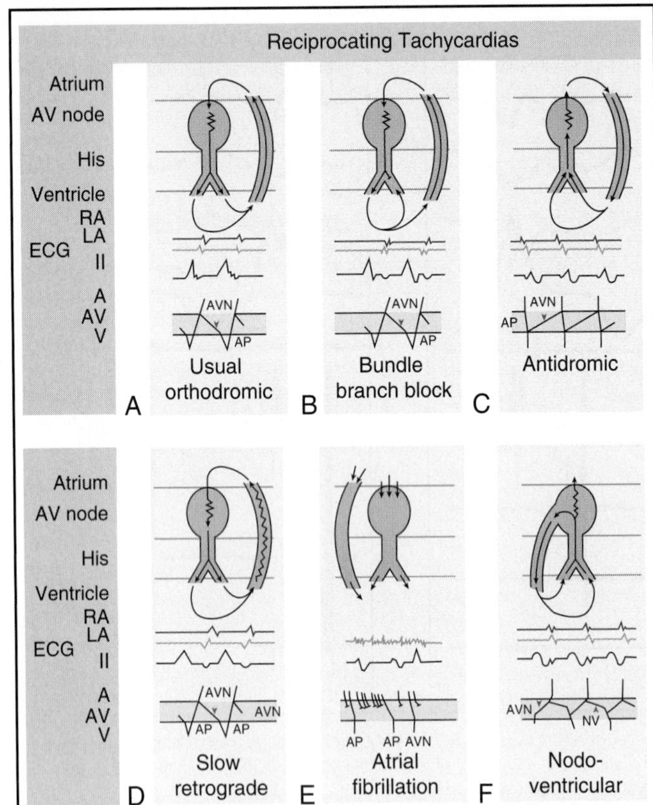

FIGURE 32–32 Schematic diagram of tachycardias associated with accessory pathways. **A,** Orthodromic tachycardia with anterograde conduction (arrow) over the atrioventricular (AV) node–His bundle route and retrograde conduction over the accessory pathway (left sided for this example, as depicted by left atrial activation preceding right atrial activation). **B,** Orthodromic tachycardia and ipsilateral functional bundle branch block. **C,** Antidromic tachycardia with anterograde conduction over the accessory pathway and retrograde conduction (arrow) over the AV node–His bundle. **D,** Orthodromic tachycardia with a slowly conducting accessory pathway (arrow). **E,** Atrial fibrillation with the accessory pathway as a bystander. **F,** Anterograde conduction over a portion of the AV node and a nodoventricular pathway and retrograde conduction over the AV node (arrows).

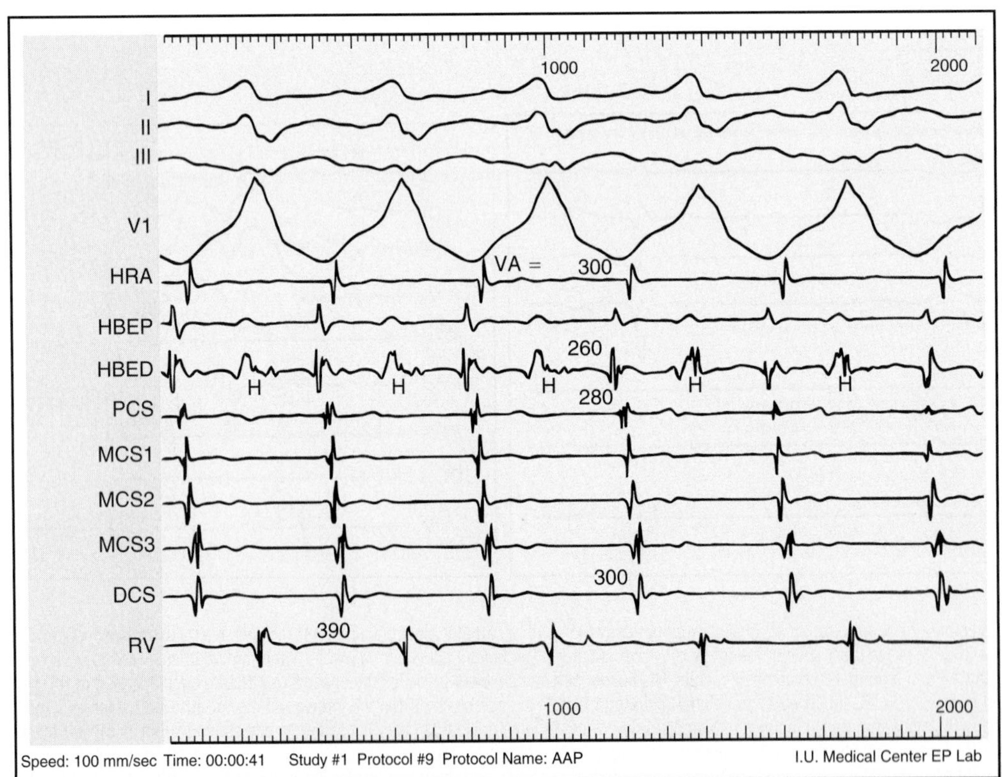

FIGURE 32–33 Antidromic atrioventricular (AV) reciprocating tachycardia. Tachycardia in this example is due to anterograde conduction over the accessory pathway (note the abnormal QRS complex of a left posterior accessory pathway) and a normal retrograde atrial activation sequence (beginning first in the HBED lead), which is due to retrograde conduction over the AV node. Tachycardia cycle length is 390 milliseconds, with a ventriculoatrial (VA) interval of 300 milliseconds measured in the high right atrial lead, 260 milliseconds in the distal His lead, and 280 milliseconds in the proximal coronary sinus lead. I, II, III, and V_1 are scalar leads. DCS = distal coronary sinus lead; HBEP and HBED leads = His bundle electrogram, proximal and distal; HRA = high right atrial electrogram; MCS1-3 = midcoronary sinus leads; PCS = proximal coronary sinus; RV = right ventricular electrogram.

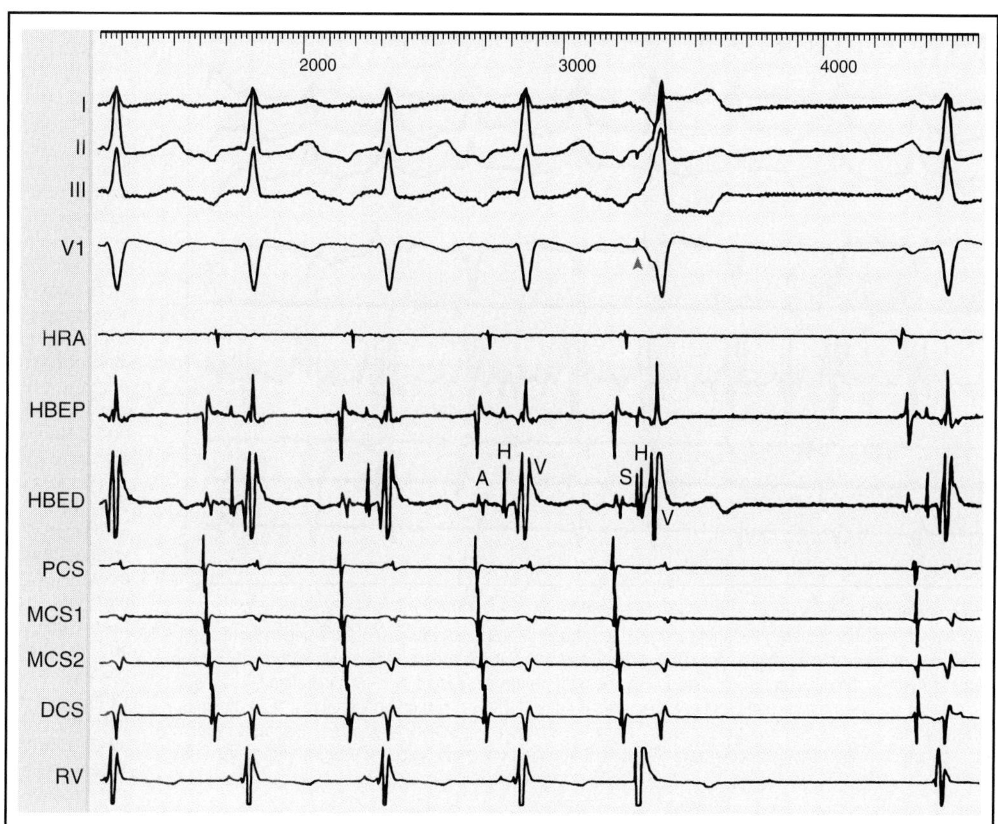

FIGURE 32–34 Termination of the permanent form of atrioventricular (AV) junctional reciprocating tachycardia (PJRT). In the left portion of this example, PJRT is present. The atrial activation sequence is indistinguishable from atypical AV nodal reentry and atrial tachycardia originating in the low right atrium. The response to premature stimulation identifies the tachycardia as PJRT. Premature ventricular stimulation (arrowhead) occurs at a time when the His bundle is refractory from depolarization during the tachycardia (second labeled H). Therefore, premature ventricular stimulation cannot enter the AV node. Furthermore, premature ventricular stimulation does not reach the atrium. Yet premature ventricular stimulation terminates the tachycardia. This detail can be explained only by the PVC invading and blocking in a retrogradely conducting accessory pathway. I, II, III, and V_1 are scalar electrocardiographic leads. DCS = distal coronary sinus electrograms; HBEP, HBED = His bundle electrogram, proximal and distal; HRA = high right atrial electrogram; MCS1, MCS2 = midcoronary sinus electrograms; PCS = proximal coronary sinus electrogram; RV = right ventricular electrogram.

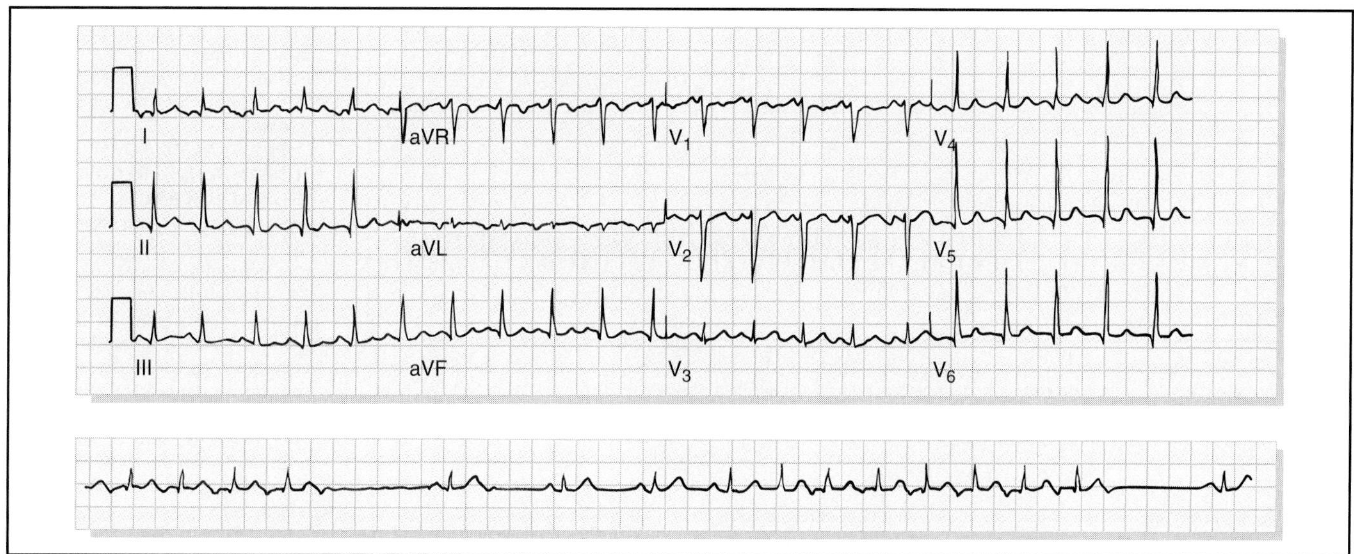

FIGURE 32–35 Permanent form of junctional reciprocating tachycardia (PJRT) in a patient with a left-sided accessory pathway. The 12-lead electrocardiogram demonstrates a long RP interval-short PR interval tachycardia, which in contrast to the usual form of PJRT, exhibits negative P waves in leads I and aVL. The rhythm strips below (lead I) indicate that whenever a nonconducted P wave occurs, the tachycardia always terminates, only to begin again after several sinus beats. This pattern is in marked contrast to that in Figure 32–12, in which the tachycardia continues despite nonconducted P waves.

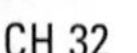

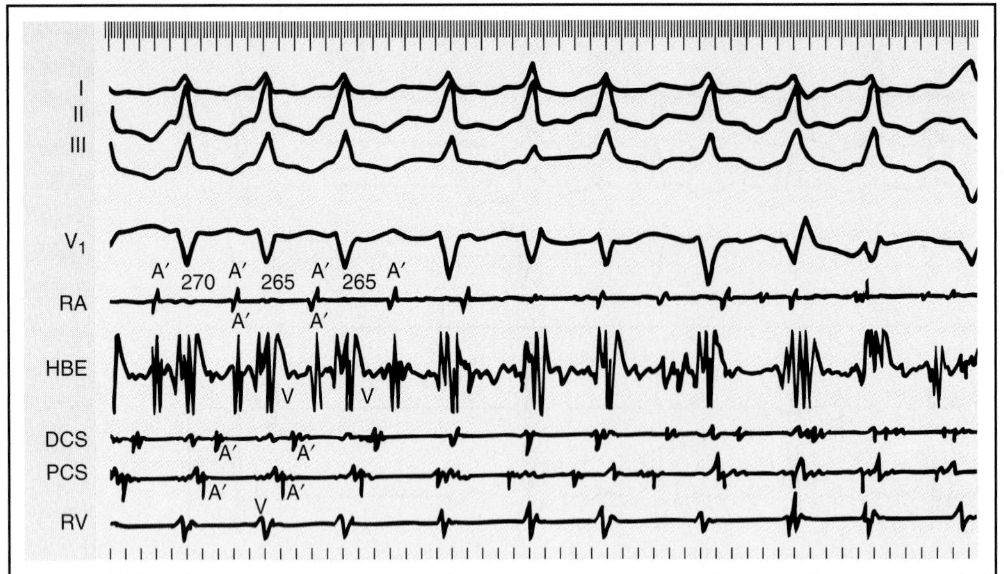

FIGURE 32–36 Atrioventricular (AV) reciprocating tachycardia disorganizing into atrial fibrillation. During sustained AV reciprocating tachycardia at a cycle length of approximately 265 milliseconds, the retrograde atrial activation sequence began first in the right paraseptal region (not shown in this example; location proved at surgery) and was then recorded in the proximal coronary sinus electrogram, followed by atrial activity in the distal coronary sinus, in the low right atrium recorded in the His bundle lead, and then in the high right atrium. Spontaneously, the atrial activation sequence becomes irregular (after the last A′) and atrial fibrillation begins. Note that the last QRS complex reflects conduction over the accessory pathway. Such a transformation occurred repeatedly in this patient and was associated with quickening of the ventricular rate. Atrial fibrillation did not recur following surgical interruption of the accessory pathway.

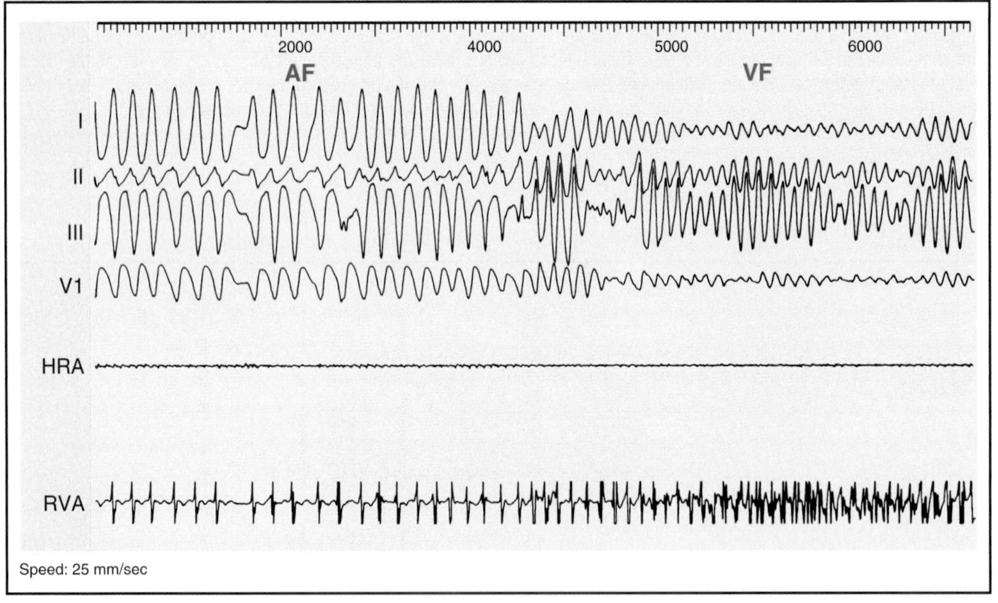

FIGURE 32–37 Atrial fibrillation (AF) becoming ventricular fibrillation (VF). In the left portion of this panel, the electrocardiogram (ECG) demonstrates AF with conduction over an accessory pathway producing a rapid ventricular response, at times in excess of 350 beats/min. In the midportion of the tracing VF can be seen to develop. I, II, III, and V_1 are scalar ECG leads. HRA = high right atrial electrogram; RVA = right ventricular apex electrogram.

memory). A variety of electrical, radionuclide, and echocardiographic techniques can be used to localize the insertion site of the accessory pathway (see Chap. 29).

ACCESSORY PATHWAY CONDUCTION. Even though the accessory pathway conducts more rapidly than the AV node (conduction velocity is faster in the accessory pathway), the accessory pathway usually has a longer refractory period during long cycle lengths (e.g., sinus rhythm); that is, it takes longer for the accessory pathway to recover excitability than it does for the AV node. Consequently, a premature atrial complex can occur sufficiently early to block conduction anterogradely in the accessory pathway and conduct to the ventricle only over the normal AV node–His bundle (see Fig. 32–32A and B). The resultant H-V interval and the QRS complex become normal. Such an event can initiate the most common type of reciprocating tachycardia, one characterized by anterograde conduction over the normal pathway and retrograde conduction over the accessory pathway (*orthodromic AV reciprocating tachycardia*) (see Fig. 32–32). The accessory pathway, which blocks conduction in an anterograde direction, recovers excitability in time to be activated after the QRS complex in a retrograde direction, thereby completing the reentrant loop.

Much less commonly, patients can have tachycardias called *antidromic* tachycardias during which anterograde conduction occurs over the accessory pathway and retrograde conduction over the AV node. The resultant QRS complex is abnormal because of total ventricular activation over the accessory pathway (see Figs. 32–32C and 32–33). In both tachycardias, the accessory pathway is an obligatory part of the reentrant circuit. In patients with bidirectional conduction over the accessory pathway, different fibers can be used anterogradely and retrogradely.

A small percentage of patients have multiple accessory pathways often suggested by various ECG clues, and on occasion, tachycardia can be due to a reentrant loop conducting anterogradely over one accessory pathway and retrogradely over the other. Fifteen to 20 percent of patients may exhibit AV nodal echoes or AV nodal reentry after interruption of the accessory pathway.

PERMANENT FORM OF AV JUNCTIONAL RECIPROCATING TACHYCARDIA. An incessant form of supraventricular tachycardia has been recognized that generally occurs with a long RP interval that exceeds the PR interval (see Figs. 32–34 and 32–35). Usually, a posteroseptal accessory pathway (most often the right ventricular but other locations as well) that conducts very slowly, possibly because of a long and tortuous route, appears responsible. Tachycardia is maintained by anterograde AV nodal conduction and retrograde conduction over the accessory pathway (see Fig. 32–32D). Although anterograde conduction over this pathway has been demonstrated, the long anterograde conduction time over the accessory pathway ordinarily prevents ECG manifestations of accessory pathway conduction during sinus rhythm. Therefore, during sinus rhythm, the QRS duration is prolonged from conduction over this accessory pathway only when conduction times through the AV node–His bundle exceed those in the accessory pathway.[65]

RECOGNITION OF ACCESSORY PATHWAYS. When retrograde atrial activation during tachycardia occurs over an accessory pathway that connects the left atrium to the left ventricle, the earliest retrograde activity is recorded from a left atrial electrode usually positioned in the coronary sinus (see Fig. 32-26). When retrograde atrial activation during tachycardia occurs over an accessory pathway that connects the right ventricle to the right atrium, the earliest retrograde atrial activity is generally recorded from a lateral right atrial electrode. Participation of a septal accessory pathway creates the earliest retrograde atrial activation in the low right portion of the atrium situated near the septum, anterior or posterior, depending on the insertion site. These mapping techniques provide an accurate assessment of the position of the accessory pathway, which can be anywhere in the AV groove except in the intervalvular trigone between the mitral valve and the aortic valve annuli. Recording electrical activity directly from the accessory pathway obviously provides precise localization.

It may be difficult to distinguish AV nodal reentry from participation of a septal accessory connection using the retrograde sequence of atrial activation because activation sequences during both tachycardias are similar. Other approaches to demonstrate retrograde atrial activation over the accessory pathway must be tried and can be accomplished by inducing PVCs during tachycardia to determine whether retrograde atrial excitation can occur from the ventricle at a time when the His bundle is refractory (see Fig. 32-26B). Since VA conduction cannot occur over the normal conduction system because the His bundle is refractory, an accessory pathway must be present for the atria to become excited. No patient with a reciprocating tachycardia from an accessory AV pathway has a VA interval of less than 70 milliseconds measured from the onset of ventricular depolarization to the onset of the earliest atrial activity recorded on an esophageal lead or a VA interval of less than 95 milliseconds when measured to the high right part of the atrium. In contrast, in most patients with reentry in the AV node, intervals from the onset of ventricular activity to the earliest onset of atrial activity recorded in the esophageal lead are less than 70 milliseconds.

Other Forms of Tachycardia in Patients with Wolff-Parkinson-White Syndrome

Patients can have other types of tachycardia during which the accessory pathway is a "bystander," that is, uninvolved in the mechanism responsible for the tachycardia, such as AV nodal reentry or an atrial tachycardia that conducts to the ventricle over the accessory pathway. In patients with atrial flutter or atrial fibrillation, the accessory pathway is not a requisite part of the mechanism responsible for tachycardia, and the flutter or fibrillation occurs in the atrium unrelated to the accessory pathway (see Fig. 32-32E). Propagation to the ventricle during atrial flutter or atrial fibrillation can therefore occur over the normal AV node–His bundle or accessory pathway. Patients with WPW syndrome who have atrial fibrillation almost always have inducible reciprocating tachycardias as well, which can develop into atrial fibrillation (see Fig. 32-36). In fact, interruption of the accessory pathway and elimination of AV reciprocating tachycardia usually prevent recurrence of the atrial fibrillation. Atrial fibrillation presents a potentially serious risk because of the possibility for very rapid conduction over the accessory pathway. At more rapid rates, the refractory period of the accessory pathway can shorten significantly and permit an extremely rapid ventricular response during atrial flutter or atrial fibrillation (see Fig. 32-27B). The rapid ventricular response can exceed the ability of the ventricle to follow in an organized manner; it can result in fragmented, disorganized ventricular activation and hypotension and lead to ventricular fibrillation (see Fig. 32-37). Alternatively, a supraventricular discharge bypassing AV nodal delay can activate the ventricle during the vulnerable period of the antecedent T wave and precipitate ventricular fibrillation. Patients who have had ventricular fibrillation have ventricular cycle lengths during atrial fibrillation in the range of 200 milliseconds or less.

Patients with preexcitation syndrome can have other causes of tachycardia such as AV nodal reentry, sometimes with dual AV nodal curves, sinus nodal reentry, or even VT unrelated to the accessory pathway. Some accessory pathways can conduct anterogradely only; more commonly, pathways conduct retrogradely only. If the pathway conducts only anterogradely, it cannot participate in the usual form of reciprocating tachycardia (see Fig. 32-32A). It can, however, participate in antidromic tachycardia (Fig. 32-32C), as well as conduct to the ventricle during atrial flutter or atrial fibrillation (Fig. 32-32E). Some data suggest that the accessory pathway demonstrates automatic activity, which could conceivably be responsible for some instances of tachycardia.

"WIDE-QRS" TACHYCARDIAS. In patients with preexcitation syndrome, so-called wide-QRS tachycardias can be due to multiple mechanisms, including sinus or atrial tachycardias, AV nodal reentry, and atrial flutter or fibrillation with anterograde conduction over the accessory pathway; orthodromic reciprocating tachycardia with functional or preexisting bundle branch block; antidromic reciprocating tachycardia; reciprocating tachycardia with anterograde conduction over one accessory pathway and retrograde conduction over a second one; tachycardias using nodofascicular or atriofascicular fibers; or VT.

CLINICAL FEATURES. The reported incidence of preexcitation syndrome depends in large measure on the population studied and varies from 0.1 to 3 per 1000 in apparently healthy subjects, with an average of about 1.5 per 1000. The incidence of the ECG pattern of WPW conduction in 22,500 healthy aviation personnel was 0.25 percent with a prevalence of documented tachyarrhythmias of 1.8 percent. Left free wall accessory pathways are most common, followed in frequency by posteroseptal, right free wall, and anteroseptal locations. WPW syndrome is found in all age groups from the fetal and neonatal periods to the elderly, as well as in identical twins. The prevalence is higher in men and decreases with age, apparently because of loss of preexcitation. Most adults with preexcitation syndrome have normal hearts, although a variety of acquired and congenital cardiac defects have been reported, including Ebstein anomaly, mitral valve prolapse, and cardiomyopathies. Patients with Ebstein anomaly (see Chap. 56) often have multiple accessory pathways, right sided either in the posterior septum or in the posterolateral wall, with preexcitation localized to the atrialized ventricle. They often have reciprocating tachycardia with a long VA interval and a right bundle branch block morphology.

The frequency of paroxysmal tachycardia apparently increases with age, from 10 per 100 patients with WPW syndrome in a 20- to 39-year-old age group to 36 per 100 in patients older than 60 years. Approximately 80 percent of patients with tachycardia have a reciprocating tachycardia, 15 to 30 percent have atrial fibrillation, and 5 percent have atrial flutter. VT occurs uncommonly. The anomalous complexes can mask or mimic myocardial infarction (see Chap. 46), bundle branch block, or ventricular hypertrophy, and the presence of the preexcitation syndrome can call attention to an associated cardiac defect. The prognosis is excellent in patients without tachycardia or an associated cardiac anomaly. For most patients with recurrent tachycardia, the prognosis is good, but sudden death occurs rarely, with an estimated frequency of 0.1 percent.

It is highly likely that an accessory pathway is congenital, although its manifestations can be detected in later years and appear to be "acquired." Relatives of patients with preexcitation, particularly those with multiple pathways, have an increased prevalence of preexcitation, thus suggesting a hereditary mode of acquisition. Some children and adults can lose their tendency for the development of tachyarrhythmias as they grow older, possibly as a result of fibrotic or other changes at the site of the accessory pathway insertion. Pathways can lose their ability to conduct anterogradely. Tachycardia beginning in infancy can disappear but frequently recurs. Tachycardia still present after 5 years of age persists in 75 percent of patients regardless of accessory pathway location. Intermittent preexcitation during sinus rhythm and abrupt loss of conduction over the accessory pathway after intravenous ajmaline or procainamide and with exercise suggest that the refractory period of the accessory pathway is long and that the patient is not at risk for a rapid ventricular rate should atrial flutter or fibrillation develop. These approaches are relatively specific, but not very sensitive, with a low positive predictive accuracy. Exceptions to these safeguards can occur.

TREATMENT. Patients with ventricular preexcitation who have only the ECG abnormality, without tachyarrhythmias, do not require electrophysiological evaluation or therapy. However, for patients with frequent episodes of symptomatic tachyarrhythmia, therapy should be initiated.

Three therapeutic options exist: electrical or surgical (see Chap. 30) ablation and pharmacological therapy. Drugs are chosen to prolong conduction time and/or refractoriness in the AV node, the accessory pathway, or both to prevent rapid rates from occurring. If successful, this therapy prevents maintenance of an AV reciprocating tachycardia or a rapid ventricular response to atrial flutter or atrial fibrillation. Some drugs can suppress premature complexes that precipitate the arrhythmias.

Adenosine, verapamil, propranolol, and digitalis all prolong conduction time and refractoriness in the AV node. Verapamil and propranolol do not directly affect conduction in the accessory pathway, and digitalis has had variable effects. Because digitalis has been reported to shorten refractoriness in the accessory pathway and speed the ventricular response in some patients with atrial fibrillation, it is advisable to *not* use digitalis as a single drug in patients with WPW syndrome who have or may have atrial flutter or atrial fibrillation. Since atrial fibrillation can develop *during* the reciprocating tachycardia in many patients (see Fig. 32–36), this caveat probably applies to *all* patients who have tachycardia and WPW syndrome. Rather, drugs that prolong the refractory period in the accessory pathway should be used, such as classes IA and IC drugs (see Chap. 30).

Class IC drugs, amiodarone, and sotalol can affect both the AV node and the accessory pathway. Lidocaine does not generally prolong refractoriness of the accessory pathway. Verapamil and IV lidocaine can *increase* the ventricular rate during atrial fibrillation in patients with WPW syndrome. IV verapamil can precipitate *ventricular fibrillation* when given to a patient with WPW syndrome who has a rapid ventricular rate during atrial fibrillation. This effect does not appear to happen with *oral* verapamil. Catecholamines can expose WPW syndromes, shorten the refractory period of the accessory pathway, and reverse the effects of some antiarrhythmic drugs.

Termination of an Acute Episode. Termination of an acute episode of reciprocating tachycardia, suspected electrocardiographically from a normal QRS complex, regular R-R intervals, a rate of about 200 beats/min, and a retrograde P wave in the ST segment, should be approached similar to AV nodal reentry. After vagal maneuvers, adenosine followed by IV verapamil or diltiazem is the initial treatment of choice. Atrial fibrillation can occur after drug administration, particularly adenosine, with a rapid ventricular response. An external cardioverter-defibrillator should be immediately available if necessary. For atrial flutter or fibrillation, the latter suspected from an anomalous QRS complex and grossly irregular R-R intervals (see Figs. 32–27B and 32–36), drugs must be used that prolong refractoriness in the accessory pathway, often coupled with drugs that prolong AV nodal refractoriness (e.g., procainamide and propranolol). In many patients, particularly those with a very rapid ventricular response and any signs of hemodynamic impairment, electrical cardioversion is the *initial* treatment of choice.

Prevention. For long-term therapy to prevent recurrence, it is not always possible to predict which drugs may be most effective for an individual patient. Some drugs can actually increase the frequency of episodes of reciprocating tachycardia by prolonging the duration of anterograde and not retrograde refractory periods of the accessory pathway, thereby making it easier for a premature atrial complex to block conduction anterogradely in the accessory pathway and initiate tachycardia. Oral administration of two drugs, such as flecainide and propranolol, to decrease conduction capability in both limbs of the reentrant circuit can be beneficial. Class IC drugs, amiodarone, or sotalol, which prolong refractoriness in both the accessory pathway and the AV node, can be effective. Depending on the clinical situation, empirical drug trials or serial electrophysiological drug testing can be used to determine optimal drug therapy for patients with reciprocating tachycardia. For patients who have atrial fibrillation with a rapid ventricular response, induction of atrial fibrillation while the patient is receiving therapy is essential to be certain that the ventricular rate is controlled. Exercise or isoproterenol can be superimposed to be certain that the rate is controlled. Patients who have accessory pathways with very short refractory periods may be poor candidates for drug therapy since the refractory periods may be insignificantly prolonged in response to the standard agents.

Electrical or Surgical Ablation (see Chap. 30). Radiofrequency catheter ablation of the accessory pathway is advisable for patients with frequent symptomatic arrhythmias that are not fully controlled by drugs, in patients who are drug intolerant, or in those who do not wish to take drugs. This option should be considered early in the course of treatment of a symptomatic patient because of its high success rate, low frequency of complications, and potential cost-effectiveness.[68] Rarely, surgical interruption of the accessory pathway may be necessary.

Summary of Electrocardiographic Diagnosis of Supraventricular Tachycardias

ECG clues that permit differentiation among the various supraventricular tachycardias are often present. P waves during tachycardia that are identical to sinus P waves and occur with a long RP interval and a short PR interval are most likely due to sinus nodal reentry, sinus tachycardia, or an atrial tachycardia arising from the right atrium near the sinus node. Retrograde (inverted in leads II, III, and aV_f) P waves generally represent reentry involving the AV junction, either AV nodal reentry or reciprocating tachycardia using a paraseptal accessory pathway. Tachycardia without manifest P waves is probably due to AV nodal reentry (P waves buried in QRS), whereas a tachycardia with an RP interval exceeding 90 milliseconds may be due to an accessory pathway. AV dissociation or AV block during tachycardia excludes the participation of an AV accessory pathway and makes AV nodal reentry less likely. Multiple tachycardias can occur at different times in the same patient. QRS alternans, thought to be a feature of AV reciprocating tachycardia, is more likely a rapid rate–related phenomenon independent of the tachycardia mechanism. RP-PR relationships (Table 32–3) help differentiate supraventricular tachycardias. QRS voltage can increase during supraventricular tachycardia.[69]

TABLE 32–3 Supraventricular Tachycardias

Short RP/Long PR Internal	Long RP/Short PR Internal
AV node reentry	Atrial tachycardia
AV reentry	Sinus node reentry Atypical AV node reentry AVRT with a slowly conducting accessory pathway (e.g., PJRT)

AV = atrioventricular; AVRT = AV reciprocating tachycardia; PJRT = paroxysmal junctional reciprocating tachycardia.

Ventricular Rhythm Disturbances

Premature Ventricular Complexes

ECG RECOGNITION. A PVC is characterized by the premature occurrence of a QRS complex that is abnormal in shape and has a duration usually exceeding the dominant QRS complex, generally greater than 120 milliseconds. The

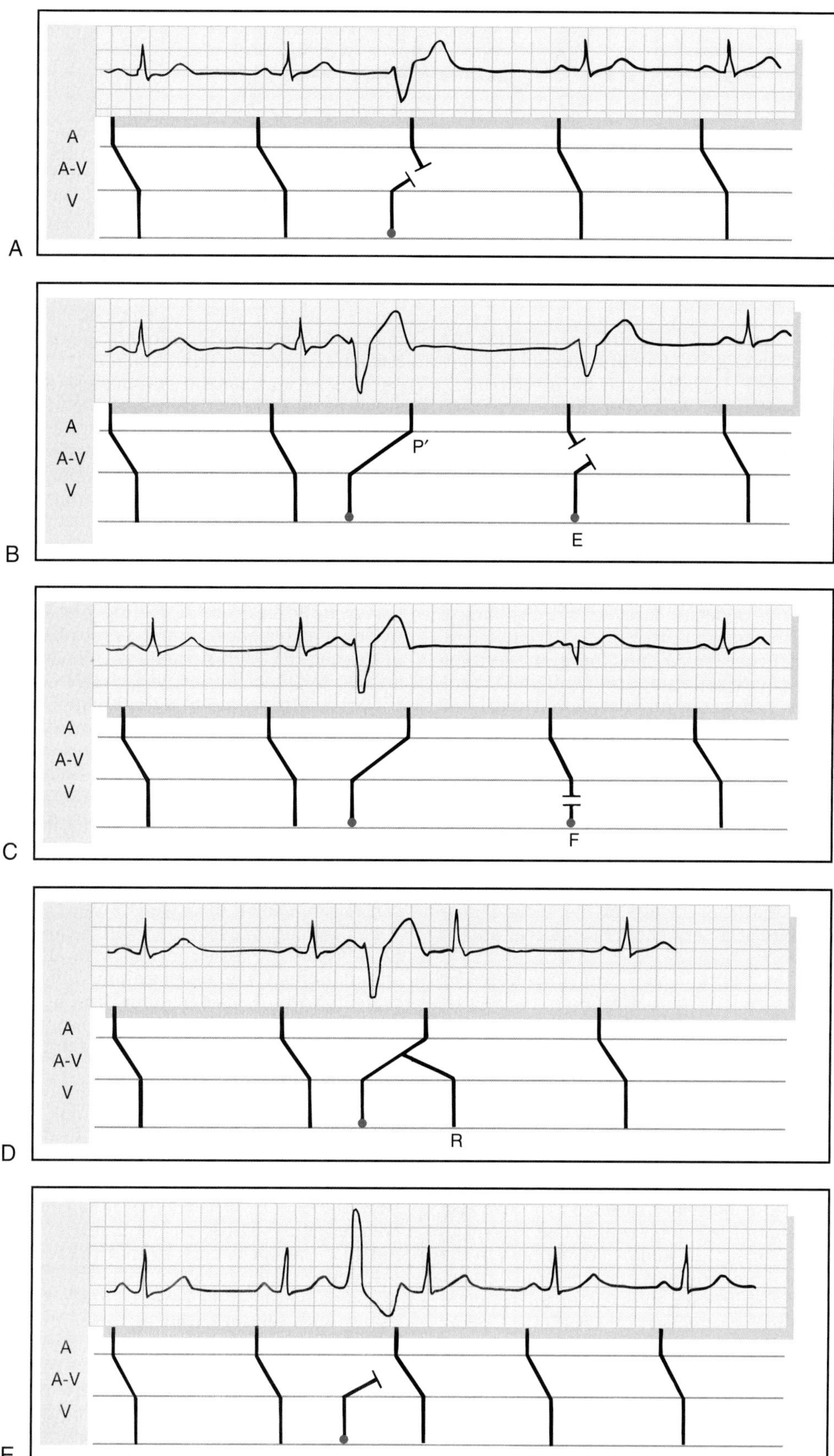

FIGURE 32–38 Premature ventricular complexes (PVCs). **A** to **D** were recorded in the same patient. **A,** A late results in a compensatory pause. **B,** A slower sinus rate and a slightly earlier premature ventricular complex result in retrograde atrial excitation (P). The sinus node is reset, followed by a noncompensatory pause. Before the sinus-initiated P wave that follows the retrograde P wave can conduct the impulse to the ventricle, ventricular escape (E) occurs. **C,** Events are similar to those in **B** except that a ventricular fusion beat (F) results after the PVC because of a slightly faster sinus rate. **D,** The impulse propagating retrogradely to the atrium reverses its direction after a delay and returns to reexcite the ventricles (R) to produce a ventricular echo. **E,** An interpolated PVC is followed by a slightly prolonged PR interval of the sinus-initiated beat. Lead II. Red circles indicate origin of PVCs.

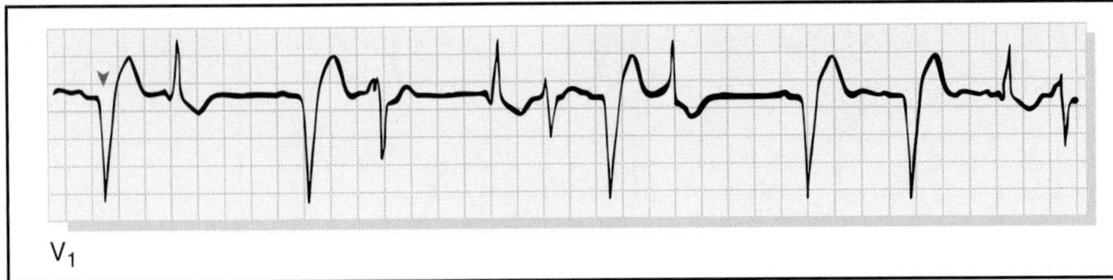

FIGURE 32–39 Multiform premature ventricular complexes (PVCs). The normally conducted QRS complexes exhibit a left bundle branch block contour (arrowhead) and are followed by PVCs with three different morphologies.

T wave is commonly large and opposite in direction to the major deflection of the QRS. The QRS complex is not preceded by a premature P wave but can be preceded by a nonconducted sinus P wave occurring at its expected time. The diagnosis of a PVC can never be made with unequivocal certainty from the scalar ECG since a supraventricular beat or rhythm can mimic the manifestations of ventricular arrhythmia (Fig. 32–38). Retrograde transmission to the atria from the PVC occurs fairly frequently but is often obscured by the distorted QRS complex and T wave. If the retrograde impulse discharges and resets the sinus node prematurely, it produces a pause that is not fully compensatory. More commonly, the sinus node and atria are not discharged prematurely by the retrograde impulse since interference of impulses frequently occurs at the AV junction in the form of collision between the anterograde impulse conducted from the sinus node and the retrograde impulse conducted from the PVC. Therefore, a fully compensatory pause usually follows a PVC: The R-R interval produced by the two sinus-initiated QRS complexes on either side of the premature complex equals twice the normally conducted R-R interval. The PVC may not produce any pause and may therefore be interpolated (Fig. 32–38E), or it may produce a postponed compensatory pause when an interpolated premature complex causes PR prolongation of the first postextrasystolic beat to such a degree that the P wave of the second postextrasystolic beat occurs at a very short RP interval and is therefore blocked.

Interference within the ventricle can result in *ventricular fusion beats* caused by simultaneous activation of the ventricle by two foci—one from the supraventricular impulse and the other from the PVC. On occasion, a fusion beat can be narrower than the dominant sinus beat when a right bundle branch block pattern of a PVC arising in the left ventricle fuses with the sinus-initiated complex conducting through the AV junction (see Fig. 32–32) or when a ventricle with a left bundle branch block pattern is paced artificially and a narrow ventricular fusion beat is produced between the paced and the sinus-conducted beats. Narrow PVCs have also been explained as originating at a point equidistant from each ventricle in the ventricular septum and by arising high in the fascicular system. Whether a compensatory or noncompensatory pause, retrograde atrial excitation, or an interpolated complex, fusion complex, or echo beat occurs (Fig. 32–38D), it is merely a function of how the AV junction conducts and the timing of the events taking place.

The term *bigeminy* refers to pairs of complexes and indicates a normal and premature complex, *trigeminy* indicates a premature complex following two normal beats, a premature complex following three normal beats is called *quadrigeminy,* and so on. Two successive PVCs are termed a *pair* or a *couplet,* whereas three successive PVCs are termed a *triplet.* Arbitrarily, three or more successive PVCs are termed *ventricular tachycardia.* PVCs can have different contours and are often called *multifocal* (Fig. 32–39). More properly they should be called *multiform, polymorphic,* or *pleomorphic* since it is not known whether multiple foci are discharging or whether conduction of the impulse originating from one site is merely changing.

PVCs can exhibit fixed or variable coupling; that is, the interval between the normal QRS complex and the PVC can be relatively stable or variable. Fixed coupling can be due to reentry, triggered activity (see Chap. 27), or other mechanisms. Variable coupling can be due to parasystole, to changing conduction in a reentrant circuit, or to changing discharge rates of triggered activity. Usually, it is difficult to determine the precise mechanism responsible for the PVC based on either constant or variable coupling intervals.

CLINICAL FEATURES. The prevalence of premature complexes increases with age, and they are associated with male sex and a reduced serum potassium concentration. PVCs are more frequent in the morning in patients after myocardial infarction, but this circadian variation is absent in patients with severe LV dysfunction. Symptoms of palpitations or discomfort in the neck or chest can result because of the greater than normal contractile force of the postextrasystolic beat or the feeling that the heart has stopped during the long pause after the premature complex. Long runs of frequent PVCs in patients with heart disease can produce angina, hypotension, or heart failure. Frequent interpolated PVCs actually represent a doubling of the heart rate and can compromise the patient's hemodynamic status. Activity that increases the heart rate can decrease the patient's awareness of the premature systole or reduce their number. Exercise can increase the number of premature complexes in some patients. Premature systoles can be quite uncomfortable in patients who have aortic regurgitation because of the large stroke volume. Sleep is usually associated with a decrease in the frequency of ventricular arrhythmias, but some patients can experience an increase.

PVCs occur in association with a variety of stimuli and can be produced by direct mechanical, electrical, and chemical stimulation of the myocardium. Often they are noted in patients with LV false tendons, during infection, in ischemic or inflamed myocardium, and during hypoxia, anesthesia, or surgery. They can be provoked by a variety of medications, by electrolyte imbalance, by tension states, by myocardial stretch, and by excessive use of tobacco, caffeine, or alcohol. Both central and peripheral autonomic stimulation have profound effects on the heart rate and can produce or suppress premature complexes.

Physical examination reveals the presence of a premature beat followed by a pause that is longer than normal. A fully compensatory pause can be distinguished from one that is not fully compensatory in that the former does not change the timing of the basic rhythm. The premature beat is often accompanied by a decrease in intensity of the heart sounds, often with auscultation of just the first heart sound, which can be sharp and snapping, and a decreased or absent peripheral (e.g., radial) pulse. The relationship of atrial to ventricular systole determines the presence of normal *a* waves or giant *a* waves in the jugular venous pulse, and the length of the PR interval determines the intensity of the first heart sound. The second heart sound can be abnormally split, depending on the origin of the ventricular complex.

The importance of PVCs depends on the clinical setting. In the absence of underlying heart disease, the presence of PVCs usually has no impact on longevity or limitation of activity; antiarrhythmic drugs are not indicated.[71] Patients should be reassured if they are symptomatic (see Chaps. 29 and 30). In men without apparent coronary disease, the incidental detection of ventricular arrhythmias is associated with a twofold increased risk for all-cause mortality and myocardial infarction or death from coronary disease. However, it has not been demonstrated that premature ventricular systoles or complex ventricular arrhythmias play a *precipitating* role in the genesis of sudden death in these patients, and the arrhythmias may simply be a marker of heart disease. Results from electrophysiological testing suggest that patients with PVCs who do not have VT induced at electrophysiological study have a low incidence of subsequent sudden death. Antiarrhythmic therapy given to suppress the premature ventricular systoles or complex ventricular arrhythmias has not been shown to reduce the incidence of sudden death in such apparently healthy men.

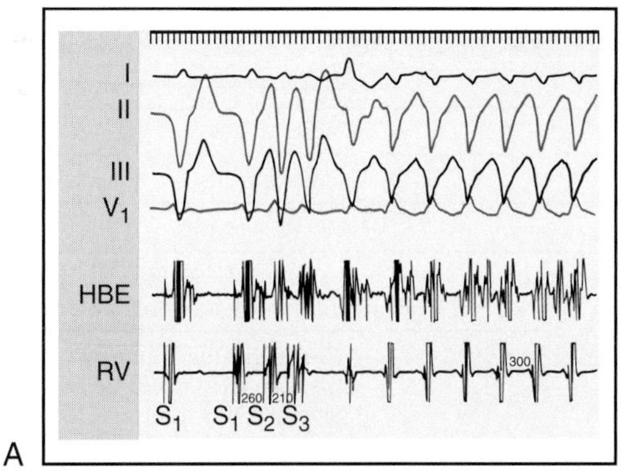

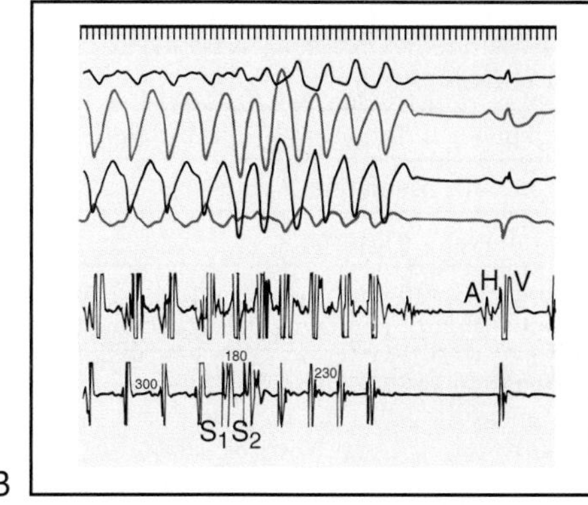

FIGURE 32–40 Initiation and termination of ventricular tachycardia by means of programmed ventricular stimulation. The last two ventricular-paced beats at a cycle length of 600 milliseconds are shown in **A.** A premature stimulus (S_2) at an S_1-S_2 interval of 260 milliseconds and another premature stimulus (S_3) at a cycle length of 210 milliseconds initiate a sustained monomorphic ventricular tachycardia at a cycle length of 300 milliseconds. Two premature ventricular stimuli (S_1-S_2) in **B** create an unstable ventricular tachycardia that persists for several beats at a shorter cycle length (230 milliseconds) and then terminates, followed by sinus rhythm.

In patients suffering from acute myocardial infarction, PVCs once considered to presage the onset of ventricular fibrillation, such as those occurring close to the preceding T wave, more than five or six per minute, bigeminal or multiform complexes, or those occurring in salvoes of two, three, or more, do not occur in about half the patients in whom ventricular fibrillation develops, and ventricular fibrillation does not develop in about half of the patients who have these PVCs. Thus these PVCs are not particularly helpful prognostically. The presence of 1 to more than 10 ventricular extrasystoles per hour can identify patients at increased risk for VT or sudden cardiac death after myocardial infarction but is likewise nonspecific.

MANAGEMENT. In most patients, PVCs (occurring as single PVCs, bigeminy, or trigeminy but excluding nonsustained VT [see later]) do not need to be treated, particularly if the patient does not have an acute coronary syndrome, and treatment is usually dictated by the presence of symptoms attributable to the PVCs. Both fast and slow heart rates can provoke the development of PVCs. PVCs accompanying slow ventricular rates can be abolished by increasing the basic rate with atropine or isoproterenol or by pacing, whereas slowing the heart rate in some patients with sinus tachycardia can eradicate PVCs. In hospitalized patients, IV lidocaine (see Chap. 30) is generally the initial treatment of choice to suppress PVCs. If maximum dosages of lidocaine are unsuccessful, procainamide given IV can be tried. Propranolol can be tried if the other drugs have been unsuccessful. IV magnesium can be useful. For long-term oral maintenance, a variety of classes I,[67] II,[72] and III drugs can be useful to prevent VT. Class IC drugs seem particularly successful in suppressing PVCs, but flecainide and moricizine have been shown to increase mortality in patients treated after myocardial infarction. Amiodarone can be quite effective. Athletes with structural heart disease and ventricular extrasystoles who are in high-risk groups can participate in low-intensity sports only.[5] Thrombolysis therapy does not influence the frequency of ventricular extrasystoles, which are related to residual LV pump performance after myocardial infarction. Low levels of serum potassium and magnesium are associated with higher prevalence rates of ventricular arrhythmias.

Ventricular Tachycardia

ECG RECOGNITION. VT arises distal to the bifurcation of the His bundle in the specialized conduction system, in ventricular muscle, or in combinations of both tissue types. Mechanisms include disorders of impulse formation and conduction considered earlier (see Chap. 27). Autonomic modulation can be important. The ECG diagnosis of VT is suggested by the occurrence of a series of three or more consecutive, abnormally shaped PVCs whose duration exceeds 120 milliseconds, with the ST-T vector pointing opposite the major QRS deflection. The R-R interval can be exceedingly regular or can vary. Patients can have VTs with multiple morphologies originating at the same or closely adjacent sites, probably with different exit paths. Others have multiple sites of origin. Atrial activity can be independent of ventricular activity, or the atria can be depolarized by the ventricles retrogradely (VA association). Depending on the particular type of VT, rates range from 70 to 250 beats/min, and the onset can be paroxysmal (sudden) or nonparoxysmal. QRS contours during the VT can be unchanging (uniform, monomorphic), can vary randomly (multiform, polymorphic, or pleomorphic), can vary in a more or less repetitive manner (torsades de pointes), can vary in alternate complexes (bidirectional VT), or can vary in a stable but changing contour (i.e., right bundle branch contour changing to a left bundle branch contour). VT can be sustained, defined arbitrarily as lasting longer than 30 seconds or requiring termination because of hemodynamic collapse, or nonsustained, when it stops spontaneously in less than 30 seconds. Most commonly, very premature stimulation is required to initiate VT electrically, whereas late coupled ventricular complexes usually initiate its spontaneous onset (Fig. 32–40).

Making the ECG distinction between supraventricular tachycardia with aberration and VT can be difficult at times since features of both arrhythmias overlap and under certain circumstances a supraventricular tachycardia can mimic the criteria established for VT.[73] Ventricular complexes with an abnormal and prolonged configuration indicate only that conduction through the ventricle is abnormal, and such complexes can occur in supraventricular rhythms as a result of preexisting bundle branch block, aberrant conduction during incomplete recovery of repolarization, conduction over accessory pathways, and several other conditions. These complexes do not necessarily indicate the origin of impulse formation or the reason for the abnormal conduction. Conversely, ectopic beats originating in the ventricle can

TABLE 32–4 Major Features in the Differential Diagnosis of Wide QRS Beats Versus Tachycardia

Supports SVT	Supports VT
Slowing or termination by vagal tone	Fusion beats
Onset with premature P wave	Capture beats
RP interval ≤ 100 msec	AV dissociation
P and QRS rate and rhythm linked to suggest that ventricular activation depends on atrial discharge, e.g., 2:1 AV block rSR′ V_1	P and QRS rate and rhythm linked to suggest that atrial activation depends on ventricular discharge, e.g., 2:1 VA block
Long-short cycle sequence	"Compensatory" pause Left axis deviation; QRS duration >140 msec Specific QRS contours (see text)

SVT = supraventricular tachycardia; VT = ventricular tachycardia.

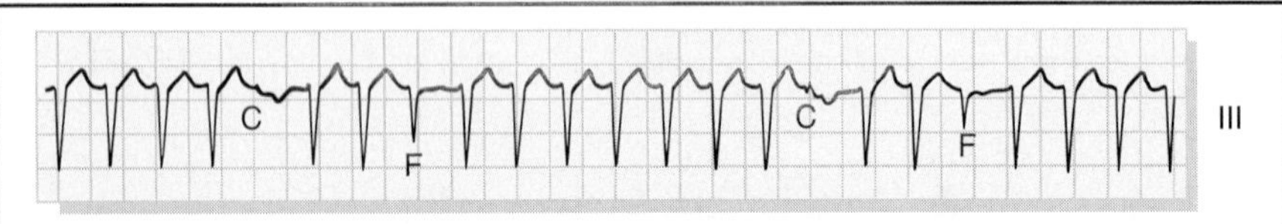

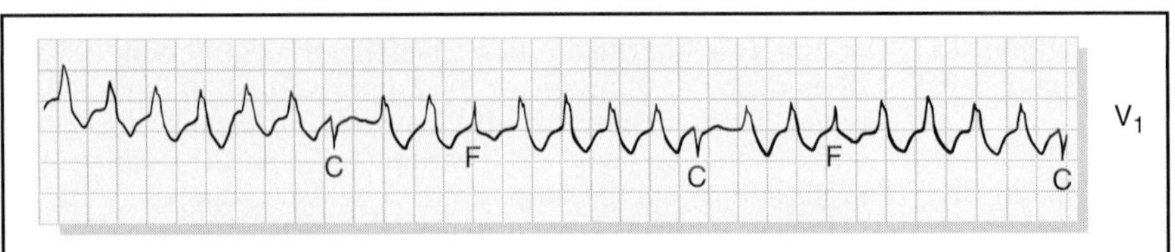

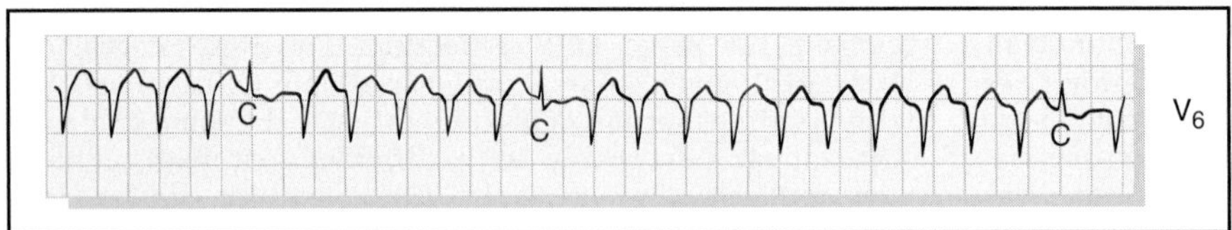

FIGURE 32–41 Fusion and capture beats during ventricular tachycardia. The QRS complex is prolonged, and the R-R interval is regular except for occasional capture beats (C) that have a normal contour and are slightly premature. Complexes intermediate in contour represent fusion beats (F). Thus, even though atrial activity is not clearly apparent, atrioventricular dissociation is present during ventricular tachycardia and produces intermittent capture and fusion beats.

uncommonly have a fairly normal duration and shape. However, VT is the most common cause of tachycardia with a wide QRS complex. A past history of myocardial infarction makes the diagnosis even more likely.

During the course of a tachycardia characterized by wide, abnormal QRS complexes, the presence of fusion beats and capture beats provides maximum support for the diagnosis of VT (Fig. 32–41 and Table 32–4). *Fusion beats* indicate activation of the ventricle from two different foci, with the implication that one of the foci had a ventricular origin. *Capture* of the ventricle by the supraventricular rhythm with a normal configuration of the captured QRS complex at an interval shorter than the tachycardia in question indicates that the impulse has a supraventricular origin. AV dissociation has long been considered a hallmark of VT. However, retrograde VA conduction to the atria from ventricular beats occurs in at least 25 percent of patients, and therefore, VT may not exhibit AV dissociation. AV dissociation can occur uncommonly during supraventricular tachycardias. Even if a P wave appears to be related to each QRS complex, it is at times difficult to determine whether the P wave is conducted anterogradely to the next QRS complex (i.e., supraventricular tachycardia with aberrancy and a long PR interval) or retrogradely from the preceding QRS complex (i.e., a VT). As a general rule, however, AV dissociation during tachycardia with a wide QRS is strong presumptive evidence that the tachycardia is of ventricular origin.

Differentiation Between Ventricular and Supraventricular Tachycardia. While fusion and capture beats and AV dissociation provide the strongest ECG evidence for differentiating VT from supraventricular tachycardia with aberrant conduction, these features are not always present. Therefore, other clues from the ECG may be required to help with this differentiation. Some ECG features characterizing supraventricular arrhythmia with aberrancy are (1) consistent onset of the tachycardia with a premature P wave; (2) a very short RP interval (0.1 second) often requiring an esophageal recording to visualize the P waves; (3) a QRS configuration the same as that occurring from known supraventricular conduction at similar rates; (4) P wave and QRS rate and rhythm linked to suggest that ventricular activation depends on atrial discharge (e.g., an AV Wenckebach block); and (5) slowing or termination of the tachycardia by vagal maneuvers.

Analysis of specific QRS contours can also be helpful in diagnosing VT and localizing its site of origin. For example, QRS contours suggesting VT include left-axis deviation in the frontal plane and a QRS duration exceeding 140 milliseconds with a QRS of normal duration during sinus rhythm. During VT with a right bundle branch block appearance, (1) the QRS complex is monophasic or biphasic in V_1 with an initial deflection different from that of the sinus-initiated QRS complex, (2) the amplitude of the R wave in V_1 exceeds the R′, and (3) a small R and large S wave or a QS pattern in V_6 may be present. With a VT having a left bundle branch block contour, (1) the axis can be rightward with negative deflections deeper in V_1 than in V_6, (2) a broad prolonged (>40 milliseconds) R wave can be noted in V_1, and (3) a small Q–large R wave or QS pattern in V_6 can exist. A QRS complex that is similar in V_1 through V_6, either all negative or all positive, favors a ventricular origin, as does the presence of a 2:1 VA block. (An upright QRS complex in V_1 through V_6 can also occur from conduction over a left-sided accessory pathway.) Supraventricular beats with aberration often have a triphasic pattern in V_1, an initial vector of the abnormal complex similar to that of the normally conducted beats, and a wide QRS complex that terminates a short cycle length following a long cycle (long-short cycle sequence). During atrial fibrillation, fixed coupling, short coupling intervals, a long pause after the abnormal beat, and runs of bigeminy rather than a consecutive series of abnormal complexes all favor a ventricular origin of the premature complex rather than a supraventricular origin with aberration. A grossly irregular, wide QRS tachycardia with ventricular rates exceeding 200 beats/min should raise the question of atrial fibrillation with conduction over an accessory pathway (see Fig. 32–4B). In the presence of a preexisting bundle branch block, a wide QRS tachycardia with a contour different from the contour during sinus rhythm is most likely a VT. Several algorithms, based on these criteria, for distinguishing VT from supraventricular tachycardia with aberrancy have been suggested. Exceptions exist to all the aforementioned criteria, especially in patients who have preexisting conduction disturbances or preexcitation syndrome; when in doubt, one must rely on sound clinical judgment and consider the ECG only one of several helpful ancillary tests.

Termination of a tachycardia by triggering vagal reflexes is considered diagnostic of supraventricular tachycardias. However, VT (especially if originating in the right ventricular outflow tract) can be stopped in a similar manner.

ELECTROPHYSIOLOGICAL FEATURES. Electrophysiologically, VT can be distinguished by a short or negative H-V interval (i.e., H begins after the onset of ventricular depolarization) because of retrograde activation from the ventricles (see Chap. 29). His bundle deflections are not usually apparent during VT because they are obscured by simultaneous ventricular septal depolarization or inadequate catheter position. The latter must be determined during supraventricular rhythm before the onset or after the termination of VT (see Fig. 32–40). His bundle deflections dissociated from ventricular activation are diagnostic, with rare exception. VT can produce QRS complexes of narrow duration and short H-V interval, most likely when the site of origin is close to the His bundle in the fascicles.

Successful electrical induction of VT by premature stimulation of the ventricle (see Fig. 32–40) depends on the characteristics of the VT and the anatomical substrate. Patients with sustained, hemodynamically stable VT and VT secondary to chronic coronary artery disease have monomorphic VT induced (90 percent) more frequently than do patients with nonsustained VT, VT from non–coronary-related causes or acute ischemia, and cardiac arrest (40 to 75 percent).[74] In general, it is more difficult to induce VT with late premature ventricular stimuli than with early premature stimuli, during sinus rhythm than during ventricular pacing, and with one premature stimulus than with two or three. The specificity of VT induction using more than two premature ventricular stimuli begins to decrease (while the sensitivity increases), and nonsustained polymorphic VT or ventricular fibrillation can be induced in patients who have no history of VT. Of patients with stable VT who have inducible sustained monomorphic VT, the latter is induced in about 25 percent with single extrastimuli, in 50 percent with double extrastimuli, and in 25 percent with triple extrastimuli. Occasionally, VT can be initiated only from the left ventricle or from specific sites in the right ventricle. Multiple premature stimuli reduce the need for LV stimulation. Drugs such as isoproterenol, various antiarrhythmic agents, and alcohol can facilitate the induction of VT. Coughing during VT that causes hypotension can help maintain blood pressure.

Termination by pacing depends significantly on the rate of the VT and the site of pacing. Slower VTs are terminated more easily and with fewer stimuli than are more rapid ones. An increasing number of stimuli are required to terminate more rapid VTs, which increases the risks of pacing-induced acceleration of the VT. Subthreshold stimulation and transthoracic stimulation can terminate VT. Atrial pacing, at times, can also induce and terminate VT (see Chap. 29).

CLINICAL FEATURES. Symptoms occurring during VT depend on the ventricular rate, duration of tachycardia, and the presence and extent of the underlying heart disease and peripheral vascular disease. VT can be in the form of short, asymptomatic, nonsustained episodes; sustained, hemodynamically stable events, generally occurring at slower rates or in otherwise normal hearts; or unstable runs, often degenerating into ventricular fibrillation. In some patients who have nonsustained VTs initially, sustained episodes or ventricular fibrillation later develops. The location of impulse formation and therefore the way in which the depolarization wave spreads across the myocardium can also be important. Physical findings depend in part on the P-to-QRS relationship. If atrial activity is dissociated from the ventricular contractions, the findings of AV dissociation are present. If the atria are captured retrogradely, regularly occurring cannon *a* waves appear when atrial and ventricular contractions occur simultaneously and signs of AV dissociation are absent.

More than half the patients treated for symptomatic recurrent VT have ischemic heart disease. The next biggest group has cardiomyopathy (both congestive and hypertrophic), with lesser percentages divided among those with primary electrical disease, mitral valve prolapse, valvular heart disease, congenital heart disease, and miscellaneous causes. LV hypertrophy can lead to ventricular arrhythmias. Coronary artery spasm can cause transient myocardial ischemia with severe ventricular arrhythmias in some patients (during ischemia as well as during the apparent reperfusion period).[74] Complex ventricular arrhythmias can occur *after* coronary artery bypass grafting. In patients resuscitated from sudden cardiac death (see Chap. 33), the majority (75 percent) have severe coronary artery disease, and ventricular tachyarrhythmias can be induced by premature ventricular stimulation in approximately 75 percent. When VT occurs in an ambulatory patient, it is uncommonly induced by R-on-T PVCs. Patients who have sustained VT are more likely to have a reduced ejection fraction (EF), slowed ventricular conduction and electrogram abnormalities, LV aneurysm, and previous myocardial infarction than are patients who have ventricular fibrillation, thus indicating different electrophysiological and anatomical substances. Young patients can also suffer cardiac arrest from VT or ventricular fibrillation, and persistent electrical inducibility of arrhythmias in these patients connotes a poor prognosis. In patients with coronary artery disease, sustained VT displays a circadian variation, with peak frequency in the morning.

Many approaches have been used to assess prognosis in patients with ventricular arrhythmias. Reduced baroreceptor sensitivity and heart period variability apparently caused by reduced vagal activity may indicate an increased risk of VT or sudden cardiac death. The presence of nonsustained VT after myocardial infarction often presages sudden cardiac death. Findings of reduced LV function, spontaneous ventricular arrhythmias, late potentials on signal-averaged ECG, QT interval dispersion, T wave alternans,[75,76] QRS duration, heart rate turbulence, and inducible sustained VTs at electrophysiological study all carry increased risk, further exaggerated when two or more of these features are present in the same patient. However, currently, no noninvasive technique reliably predicts outcome better than does assessment of LV function. LV function and inducibility of VT during electrophysiological study are the two strongest predictors of poor outcome. Early data suggest that T wave alternans may be as good as programmed stimulation.[77] Currently, T wave alternans is being evaluated in a prospective study to determine its value in risk stratification for implantable cardioverter-defibrillator (ICD) implantation. New risk factors such as elevated C-reactive protein, various cytokines, and genotypes may provide useful information in the future. In general, the prognosis for patients with idiopathic VT (see later), in the absence of structural heart disease or a prolonged QT interval, is good and warrants less aggressive treatment than in patients with structural heart disease.

MANAGEMENT. The dramatic changes in the management of VT and aborted sudden death over the past several years have been fueled by several large clinical trials (Table 32–5) and development of the ICD. Management decisions can be stratified into those involved in the acute management (or termination) and those involved in long-term therapy (or prevention of recurrence or sudden death) (see Chap. 33).

Acute Management of Sustained Ventricular Tachycardia. VT that does not cause hemodynamic decompensation can be treated medically to achieve acute termination by administering IV amiodarone, lidocaine, or procainamide, followed by an infusion of the successful drug. Lidocaine is often ineffective; amiodarone,[78] sotalol, and procainamide appear to be superior. In patients in whom procainamide is ineffective or in whom procainamide may be problematic

TABLE 32–5 Clinical Trials in the Treatment of Ventricular Tachycardia and Prevention of Cardiac Arrest

Study	Patient Inclusion	Endpoints	Treatment Arms	Key Results
Primary Prevention Studies				
BHAT[79]	*Post-MI*	Total mortality Sudden cardiac death	Propranolol Placebo	Total mortality and sudden cardiac death reduced in treatment arm
CAST[80]	*Post-MI* ≥6 PVCs/hr LVEF ≤40%	Arrhythmic death	Flecainide Encainide Moricizine Placebo	Arrhythmic death increased with all treatment arms
SWORD[81]	*Post-MI* LVEF <40% or Remote MI NYHA II, III	Total mortality	*d*-Sotalol Placebo	Increased mortality in treatment arm
EMIAT[82]	*Post-MI* LVEF <40%	Total mortality Arrhythmic death	Amiodarone Placebo	Amiodarone reduced arrhythmic death but not total mortality
CAMIAT[83]	*Post-MI* ≥10 PVCs/hr or NSVT	Arrhythmic death Total mortality	Amiodarone Placebo	Amiodarone reduced arrhythmic death but not total mortality
GESICA[84]	*CHF* LVEF ≤35%	Total mortality	Amiodarone Best therapy	Amiodarone reduced mortality. Patients with NSVT had higher mortality
CHF-STAT[85]	*CHF* LVEF ≤40% ≥10% PVCs/hr (asymptomatic)	Total mortality	Amiodarone Placebo	No effect in ischemic cardiomyopathy but trend toward reduced mortality in nonischemic cardiomyopathy
SCD-HeFT[87]	*CHF* LVEF ≤35% NYHA II, III	Total mortality Arrhythmic mortality Cost Quality of life	ICD Amiodarone Placebo	Ongoing
CABG Patch[88]	*CAD undergoing CABG* LVEF <36% Positive SAECG	Total mortality	CABG CABG + ICD	No difference in total mortality
MADIT[89]	*Post-MI* NSVT sustained LVEF ≤35% NYHA I-III Inducible VT not suppressed by procainamide	Total mortality	ICD Antiarrhythmic drug (80% amiodarone)	ICD reduced mortality
MADIT II[100]	*Post-MI* EF ≤30% >10 PVCs/hr or couplets	Total mortality	ICD No ICD	ICD reduced mortality
MUSTT[99]	*Post-MI* LVEF <40% NSVT sustained	Arrhythmic death or cardiac arrest	ICD in nonsuppressible group Antiarrhythmic drug in suppressible group No therapy	ICD reduced mortality
Secondary Prevention Studies				
ESVEM[91,92]	*Cardiac arrest, sustained VT or syncope* ≥10 PVCs/hr Inducible VT	Recurrence of arrhythmia	EP-guided antiarrhythmics (imipramine, mexiletine, procainamide, quinidine, sotalol, pirmenol, propafenone) Holter-guided antiarrhythmics	No difference between Holter- and EP-guided groups. Sotalol group had lowest recurrence rate of VT, arrhythmic death, and total death
CASCADE[93]	*Cardiac arrest* Not associated with acute MI	Cardiac mortality Aborted cardiac arrest	EP- or Holter-guided conventional drug therapy Empirical amiodarone	Amiodarone survival better than conventional drug therapy
CASH[94]	*Cardiac arrest* Not associated with acute MI	Total mortality	Empirical amiodarone Metoprolol Propafenone ICD	Sudden cardiac death mortality lowest in ICD arm. Increased mortality in propafenone arm
AVID[95]	*Cardiac arrest or sustained VT*	Total mortality Cost Quality of life	ICD Drug therapy (empirical amiodarone or EP/Holter-guided sotalol)	Survival better in ICD group, with most of benefit occurring in the first 9 m. Benefit most pronounced in patients with EF <35%
CIDS[96,97]	*Cardiac arrest or sustained VT*	Total mortality	ICD Amiodarone	Survival trended better in ICD group

CABG = coronary artery bypass grafting; CAD = coronary artery disease; CHF = congestive heart failure; EF = ejection fraction; EP = electrophysiology; ICD = implanted cardioverter-defibrillator; LVEF = left ventricular ejection fraction; MI = myocardial infarction; NSVT = nonsustained ventricular tachycardia; NYHA = New York Heart Association; PVC = premature ventricular complex; SAECG = signal-averaged electrocardiogram; VT = ventricular tachycardia.

(severe heart failure, renal failure), IV amiodarone is often effective. In general, an initial amiodarone loading dose of 15 mg/min is given over a 10-minute period. This dose is followed by an infusion of 1 mg/min for 6 hours and then a maintenance dose of 0.5 mg/min for the remaining 18 hours and for the next several days, as necessary. If VT does not terminate or if it recurs, a repeat loading dose can be given. Rarely, sinus bradycardia or AV block can be seen with IV amiodarone. The hypotension associated with IV amiodarone, caused largely by the diluent used in earlier formulations, does not seem to be as frequent a problem and is usually related to the rate of infusion. Bretylium is rarely used in this setting because of the frequently associated hypotension and because amiodarone appears to be more effective.

If the arrhythmia does not respond to medical therapy, electrical DC cardioversion can be used. VT that precipitates hypotension, shock, angina, congestive heart failure, or symptoms of cerebral hypoperfusion should be treated *promptly* with DC cardioversion (see Chaps. 30 and 33). Very low energies can terminate VT, beginning with a synchronized shock of 10 to 50 J. Digitalis-induced VT is best treated pharmacologically. After conversion of the arrhythmia to a normal rhythm, it is essential to institute measures to prevent recurrence.

Striking the patient's chest, sometimes called "thumpversion," can terminate VT by mechanically inducing a PVC that presumably interrupts the reentrant pathway necessary to support it. Chest stimulation at the time of the vulnerable period during the arrhythmia can accelerate the VT or possibly provoke ventricular fibrillation.

In some instances, such as VT associated with a remote myocardial infarction (which is due to reentry), ventricular pacing via a pacing catheter inserted into the right ventricle or transcutaneously at rates faster than the tachycardia can terminate the tachycardia. This procedure incurs the risk of accelerating the VT to ventricular flutter or ventricular fibrillation. In patients with recurrent VT, competitive ventricular pacing can be used to prevent recurrence. Intermittent VT, interrupted by several supraventricular beats, is generally best treated pharmacologically.

A search for reversible conditions contributing to the initiation and maintenance of VT should be made and the conditions corrected if possible. For example, VT related to ischemia, hypotension, or hypokalemia can at times be terminated by antianginal treatment, vasopressors, or potassium, respectively. Correction of heart failure can reduce the frequency of ventricular arrhythmias. Slow ventricular rates that are caused by sinus bradycardia or AV block can permit the occurrence of PVCs and ventricular tachyarrhythmias, which can be corrected by administering atropine, by temporary isoproterenol administration, or by transvenous pacing. Supraventricular tachycardia can initiate ventricular tachyarrhythmias and should be prevented if possible.

Long-Term Therapy for Prevention of Recurrences. The goal of long-term therapy is to prevent sudden cardiac death and recurrence of symptomatic VT. Asymptomatic nonsustained ventricular arrhythmias in low-risk populations (i.e., preserved LV function) often need not be treated. In patients with symptomatic nonsustained tachycardia, beta blockers are frequently effective in preventing recurrences. In patients refractory to beta blockers, class IC agents, sotalol, or amiodarone can be effective. However, class IC agents should be avoided in patients with structural heart disease, especially those with coronary artery disease because of the increased mortality associated with these drugs because of proarrhythmia. Sotalol should be used cautiously because of its potential for prolonging the QT interval and producing torsades des pointes. Patients with nonsustained VT after myocardial infarction and poor LV function are at significant risk for sudden death. The Multicenter Automatic Defibrillator Trial[98] (MADIT) found that patients with prior myocardial infarction and an EF of 0.35 or less who had inducible VT that was not suppressed with drugs[98] had better survival if treated with an ICD, with a hazard ratio of 0.46. In the Multicenter Unsustained Tachycardia Trial (MUSTT),[99] patients with an EF of 0.40 or less with coronary disease and asymptomatic nonsustained VT who had inducible sustained VT at electrophysiological study had a significant reduction in mortality if treated with an ICD. These studies suggest that patients with nonsustained VT and an EF of 0.35 to 0.40 or less should undergo electrophysiological study and, if they have inducible VT (i.e., not suppressed with procainamide), should have an ICD.[89] More recently, the MADIT-II study[100] found that patients with ischemic cardiomyopathy (prior myocardial infarction) with an EF of 0.30 or less and no requirement for ventricular arrhythmia had improved survival if treated with an ICD (hazard ratio of 0.69). This study suggests that patients with prior myocardial infarction and an EF of 0.30 or less ought to have a prophylactic ICD placed, regardless of the results of an electrophysiology study. Each of these trials demonstrated the superiority of the ICD over drugs as primary prevention of sudden cardiac death in patients at risk for a life-threatening ventricular arrhythmia. The Sudden Cardiac Death Heart Failure Trial (SCD-HeFT) is still ongoing and will investigate the role of ICDs in patients with classes II to III heart failure regardless of the presence of nonsustained VT or prior myocardial infarction. Whether additional risk stratifiers (such as T wave alternans) are beneficial is being investigated.

For secondary prevention of sustained VT or cardiac arrest (see Table 32–5 and Chaps. 30 and 33) in patients with structural heart disease, it is now clear from several clinical trials that (1) class I antiarrhythmic drugs produce a worse outcome than do class III antiarrhythmic drugs,[91,92,94] (2) empirical amiodarone results in better survival than does electrophysiology-guided antiarrhythmic drugs,[93] and (3) implantable defibrillators provide better survival than amiodarone does, particularly in patients with a left ventricular ejection fraction (LVEF) less than 0.35.[94-96] Therefore, in patients who have survived a cardiac arrest or who have sustained VT resulting in hemodynamic compromise and poor LV function (EF < 0.35), an ICD is the treatment of choice.[95] For those with higher EFs, amiodarone may produce outcomes similar to those of implanted defibrillators. In patients who refuse a cardioverter-defibrillator, empirical amiodarone is the next best therapy.[93,94] The optimal therapy for patients with coronary disease who have preserved LV function with sustained VT is not currently known. Empirical amiodarone appears to be the safest therapy,[82-84] although Holter-guided sotalol has been advocated.[91,92] Some patients who receive ICDs have frequent shocks because of recurrent VT. In these patients, concomitant therapy with amiodarone may be required to reduce the frequency of VT or slow the rate of the VT to allow it to be pace terminated. Other drugs such as sotalol, procainamide, mexiletine, or flecainide may be required if amiodarone is not effective. Occasionally, a combination of drugs may be effective when a single drug is not. Although radiofrequency ablation (see Chap. 30) of certain types of idiopathic VT (see later) is very effective, ablation for postinfarct VT or that associated with dilated cardiomyopathy is somewhat less effective. In addition, because of the significant mortality associated with these arrhythmias in patients with structural heart disease and depressed LV function, ablation is generally used as an adjunct to ICD placement to reduce the frequency of VT and ICD shocks.[101-103] However, in patients with well-tolerated postinfarct VT and well-preserved LV function or in patients refractory to drugs, it may be used as first-line therapy.[101,103]

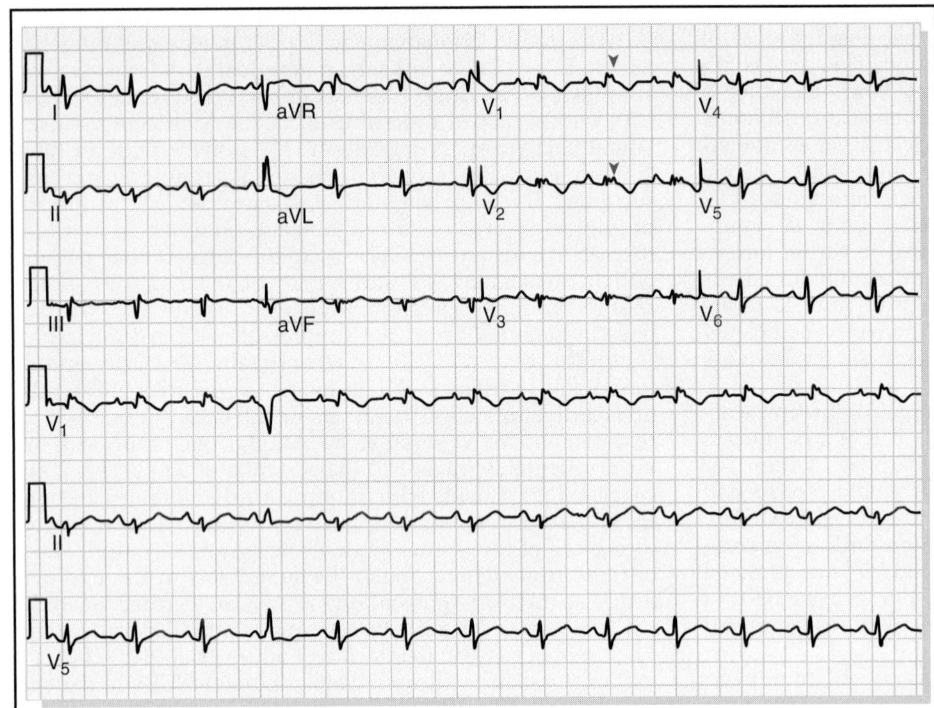

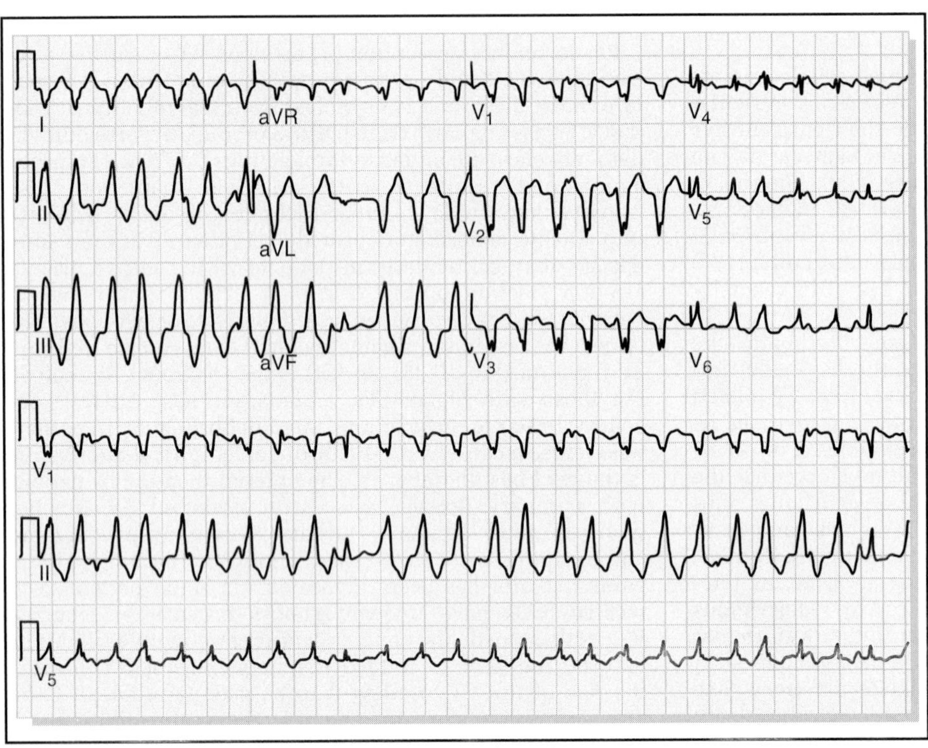

FIGURE 32–42 **A,** Normal sinus rhythm in a patient with arrhythmogenic right ventricular dysplasia. The arrowheads in V_1 and V_2 point to late right ventricular activation called an *epsilon wave.* **B,** Ventricular tachycardia in the same patient with right ventricular dysplasia.

Specific Types of Ventricular Tachycardia

A number of fairly specific types of VT have been identified, and distinction is based on either a constellation of distinctive ECG and electrophysiological features or a specific set of clinical events. Although our understanding of the electrophysiological mechanisms responsible for clinically occurring VTs is still naive, being able to identify different kinds of VTs is the first step toward understanding their mechanisms. These different kinds of VT often carry different prognoses and responses to different therapy. They are distinct from VTs associated with remote myocardial infarction or dilated cardiomyopathies.

Arrhythmogenic Right Ventricular Dysplasia

Patients with arrhythmogenic right ventricular dysplasia have VT that generally has a left bundle branch block contour (since the tachycardia arises in the right ventricle), often with right-axis deviation and T waves inverted over the right precordial leads (Fig. 32–42A). The VT may be due to reentry. Supraventricular arrhythmias can also occur, and exercise can induce the VT in some patients.

Arrhythmogenic right ventricular dysplasia is due to a type of cardiomyopathy, possibly familial in some patients, with hypokinetic areas involving the wall of the right ventricle. In the familial form, the genetic abnormality has been mapped to chromosomes 1 and 14q23-q24[104,105] and, most recently, chromosome 10, which has been implicated in apoptosis.[106,107] Mutations in the gene encoding the ryanodine receptor have also been identified in patients with arrhythmogenic right ventricular dysplasia (see Chap. 28).[108] Arrhythmogenic right ventricular dysplasia can be an important cause of ventricular arrhythmia in children and young adults with apparently normal hearts, as well as in older patients. Initial findings can be subtle and often mimic those of outflow tract VT (see later), that is, manifested only by tachycardia and no symptoms of right-sided heart failure. Right-sided heart failure or asymptomatic right ventricular enlargement can be present with normal pulmonary vasculature. Males predominate, and most patients usually show an abnormal right ventricle by echocardiography, computed tomography, right ventricular angiography, or magnetic resonance imaging, although this abnormality may not be apparent on initial evaluation. Two pathological patterns have been identified: fatty and fibrofatty infiltration. In the latter, myocardial atrophy appears to be the result of injury and myocyte death (perhaps from apoptosis) and culminates in fibrofatty replacement mediated by patchy myocarditis. The fatty degeneration preferentially occurs in the right ventricular inflow and outflow tracts and the apex. The left ventricle can be involved in advanced forms of the disease in up to 60 percent of patients.[104] Sympathetic innervation appears to be abnormal. The ECG during sinus rhythm can exhibit complete or incomplete right bundle branch block and T wave inversions in V_1 to V_3. A terminal notch in the QRS (called an *epsilon wave*) can be present as a result of slowed intraventricular conduction.[104] The signal-averaged ECG can be abnormal. Although there is no clinical trial at this point, ICDs are generally preferable to pharmacological approaches because of the progressive nature of the disease and poor prognosis, particularly if the patients have poorly tolerated VT (resulting in syncope or sudden cardiac death). Radiofrequency catheter ablation can be tried but is often not successful because of the multiple morphologies of VT and the progressive nature of the disease.

Tetralogy of Fallot

Chronic serious ventricular arrhythmias can occur in patients some years after repair of the *tetralogy of Fallot* (see Chap. 56). Sustained VT after repair can be caused by reentry at the site of previous surgery in the right ventricular outflow tract and can be cured by resection or catheter ablation of this area. The signal-averaged ECG can be abnormal. Decreased cardiac output can occur during VT and residual right ventricular outflow obstruction and lead to ventricular fibrillation.

Cardiomyopathies (see also Chap. 59)

Dilated Cardiomyopathy

Both dilated and hypertrophic cardiomyopathies can be associated with VTs and an increased risk of sudden cardiac death. Induction of VT by programmed stimulation does not reliably identify high-risk patients, whereas T wave alternans may be a useful means of risk stratifying patients with dilated cardiomyopathy.[109,110] Because it is difficult to predict patients at risk of sudden death or those who might respond favorably to an antiarrhythmic drug, ICDs have been advocated for patients with life-threatening ventricular arrhythmias and dilated cardiomyopathy. This recommendation has been supported by a large multicenter randomized trial (see Table 32–5) comparing amiodarone with implantable defibrillators in patients with poor ventricular function and symptomatic sustained VT; the study found improved survival in patients who received a defibrillator.[95] Bundle branch reentry may be the basis of some VTs in this population and can be treated by ablating the right bundle branch. Asymptomatic ventricular arrhythmias are common. The role of antiarrhythmic drugs and implantable defibrillators in the primary prevention of sudden cardiac death in patients with dilated cardiomyopathy may be warranted in certain high-risk patients, as discussed earlier. However, ongoing clinical trials will further clarify which patient population will benefit the most and which modality is most effective.

Hypertrophic Cardiomyopathy

The risk of sudden death in patients with hypertrophic cardiomyopathy (see Chap. 59) is increased by the presence of syncope, a family history of sudden death in first-degree relatives, septal thickness greater than 3 cm, or the presence of nonsustained VT on 24-hour ECG recordings. Asymptomatic or mildly symptomatic patients with brief and infrequent episodes of nonsustained VT have a low mortality. The use of electrophysiological testing to identify patients at increased risk of ventricular arrhythmias and sudden death is controversial. Amiodarone has been useful in some patients with mildly symptomatic, nonsustained VT but not in improving survival in patients without arrhythmias. QT dispersion is increased in those with ventricular arrhythmias and sudden death, as is T wave alternans.[111] DDD pacing has been useful in reducing the outflow gradient, but its role in affecting ventricular arrhythmia has not been established. Currently, no totally acceptable way to risk-stratify patients with hypertrophic cardiomyopathy in terms of VT has been identified. In patients believed to be at high risk of sudden death or those with sustained VT or frequent nonsustained VT, an implantable defibrillator may be indicated.[112] Alcohol ablation of the septum via direct injection into the septal branches of the coronary circulation has been used to improve outflow gradients, but its effect on ventricular arrhythmias and sudden cardiac death is not known.

Mitral Valve Prolapse

Patients with mitral valve prolapse (see Chap. 57) frequently have ventricular arrhythmias, although a causal relationship has not been clearly established between the arrhythmia and the mitral valve prolapse. The prognosis for most patients appears good, although sudden death can occur.

Idiopathic Ventricular Fibrillation

Idiopathic ventricular fibrillation can occur in about 1 to 8 percent of cases of out-of-hospital ventricular fibrillation and affects mostly men and those in middle age. Cardiovascular evaluation is normal except for the arrhythmia. Monomorphic VT is rarely induced at electrophysiological study. The natural history is incompletely known, but recurrences are not uncommon. It is important in this entity, as well as in patients with idiopathic VTs (see later), to remember that the arrhythmia may at times be an early manifestation of a developing cardiomyopathy, at least in some patients. Implantable defibrillators are useful therapeutic choices.

Catecholaminergic Polymorphic Ventricular Tachycardia

Catecholaminergic polymorphic ventricular tachycardia is an uncommon form of inherited VT that occurs in children and adolescents without any overt structural heart disease.[113] Patients typically present with syncope or aborted sudden death with highly reproducible, stress-induced VT that is often bidirectional. These patients have no structural heart disease and normal QT intervals. A family history of sudden death or stress-induced syncope is present in about 30 percent of the cases. During exercise, typical responses include initial sinus tachycardia and ventricular extrasystoles followed by salvos of monomorphic or bidirectional VT, which eventually leads to polymorphic VT as exercise continues. Recently, a genetic abnormality resulting in a mutation of the ryanodine receptor gene has been identified in many of these patients; those patients with this mutation appear to have a higher risk and earlier symptom (see Chap. 28).[114] The treatment of choice is beta blockers and ICDs.

Brugada Syndrome

Brugada syndrome is a distinct form of idiopathic ventricular fibrillation in which patients have right bundle branch block and ST segment elevation in the anterior precordial leads without evidence of structural heart disease (Fig. 32–43).[115-118] Mutations in a gene responsible for the sodium channel (*SCN5A*) have been identified in many families with Brugada syndrome.[119-121] Although the mutations are on the same gene as that responsible for one form of long-QT syndrome (long-QT-3) (see later), the site of mutation is different and does not result in a prolonged QT interval.[122] Mutations in the Brugada syndrome result either in acceleration of sodium-channel recovery or in nonfunctional sodium channels. This syndrome, common in apparently healthy young Southeast Asians, probably accounts for approxi-

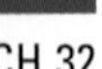

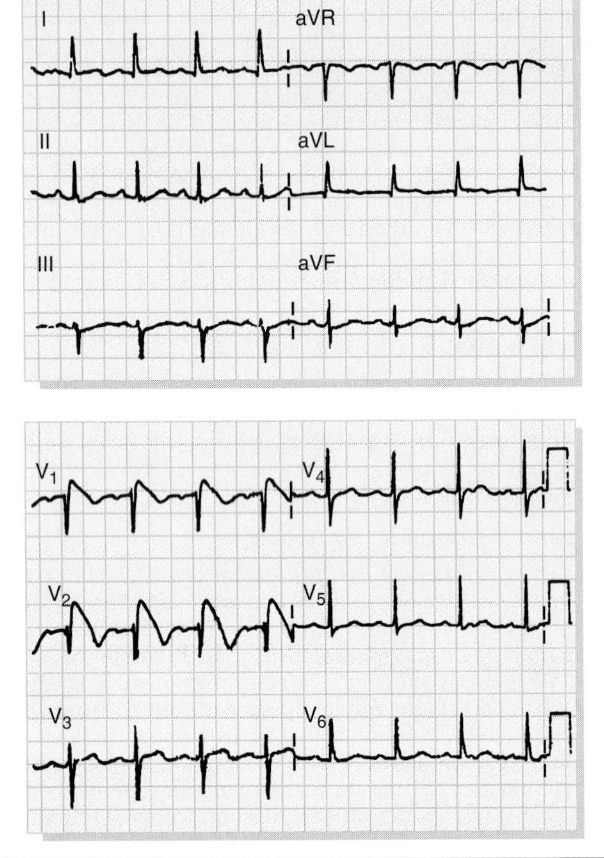

FIGURE 32–43 Twelve-lead electrocardiogram (ECG) of a patient with Brugada syndrome. The ECG is characterized by a right bundle branch block pattern and persistent ST elevation in V_1 through V_3. (From Brugada J, Brugada R, Brugada P: Right bundle branch block and ST segment elevation in leads V_1 through V_3: A marker for sudden death in patients without demonstrable structural heart disease. Circulation 97:457-460, 1998.)

mately 40 to 60 percent of all cases of idiopathic ventricular fibrillation.[119] The precise mechanism of the ECG changes and the development of ventricular fibrillation is not known. It is thought that loss of the action potential dome in the right ventricular epicardium, but not in the endocardium, results in the persistent ST segment elevation.[115] Heterogeneous loss of the action potential dome in the right ventricular epicardium leads to propagation of the dome from sites at which its presence is maintained to sites at which it is lost (phase 2 reentry), resulting in ventricular arrhythmias. Among several agents that can reproduce this ECG phenomenon are sodium-channel blockers. They can expose latent ECG forms of the syndrome and have been proposed as a provocative test. Currently, no pharmacological treatment can reliably prevent ventricular fibrillation in these patients. ICDs are the only effective treatment for preventing sudden death.

Idiopathic Ventricular Tachycardias

Idiopathic VTs with monomorphic contours can be divided into at least three types. Two types, paroxysmal VT and repetitive monomorphic VT, appear to originate from the region of the right ventricular outflow tract (Figs. 32–44 and 32–45). Right ventricular outflow tract VTs have a characteristic ECG appearance of a left bundle branch block contour in V_1 and an inferior axis in the frontal plane. Vagal maneuvers, including adenosine, terminate the VT, whereas exercise, stress, isoproterenol infusion, and rapid or premature stimulation can initiate or perpetuate the tachycardia. Beta blockers and verapamil can suppress this tachycardia as well. The mechanism responsible may be cyclic adenosine monophosphate–triggered activity[123,124] resulting from early or delayed afterdepolarizations. The paroxysmal form is exercise or stress induced, whereas the repetitive monomorphic type occurs at rest with sinus beats interposed between runs of nonsustained VT that may be precipitated by transient increases in sympathetic activity unrelated to exertion. The prognosis for most patients is quite good. Radiofrequency catheter ablation effectively eliminates this focal tachycardia in symptomatic patients. In others, antiarrhythmic drugs can be effective. An anatomical abnormality in the outflow tract of the right ventricle has been recognized in some patients.[123] In a small number of patients, the tachycardia seems to arise in the inflow tract or apex of the right ventricle. A similar tachycardia has been identified in the left ventricle and may mimic that of right ventricular outflow tract tachycardia.[125]

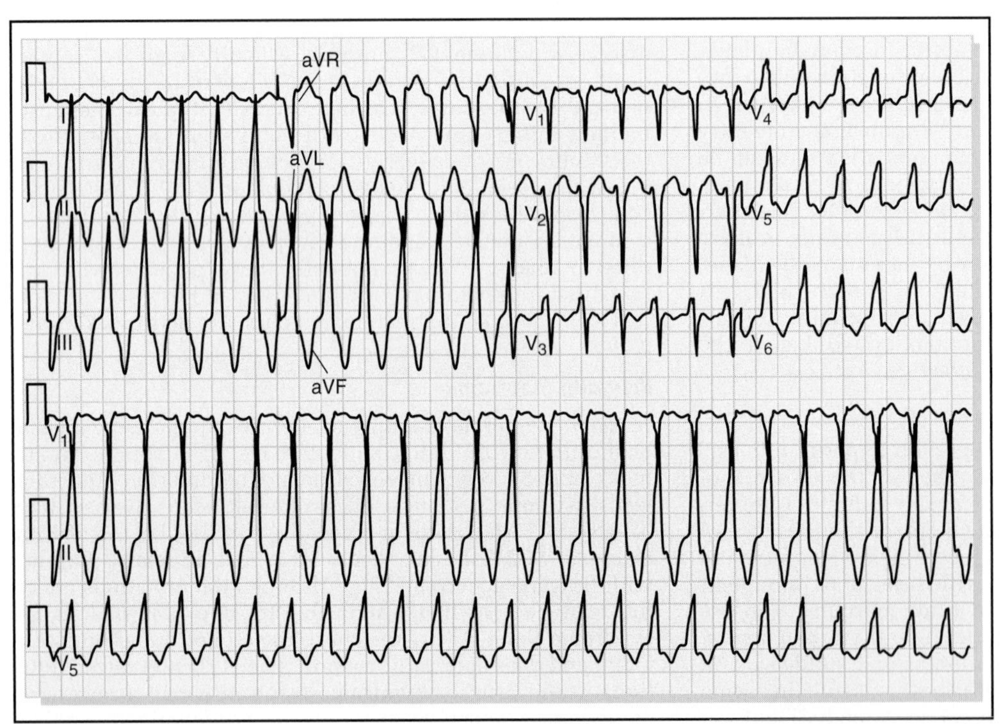

FIGURE 32–44 Ventricular tachycardia originating from the right ventricular outflow tract. This tachycardia is characterized by a left bundle branch block contour in V_1 and an inferior axis.

Left Septal Ventricular Tachycardia

A *left septal VT* has been described as arising in the left posterior septum, often preceded by a fascicular potential, and is sometimes called a *fascicular tachycardia* (Fig. 32–46). Entrainment has been demonstrated, which suggests reentry as a cause of some of the tachycardias. Verapamil or diltiazem suppresses this tachycardia, whereas adenosine does so only rarely. The response to verapamil suggests that the slow inward

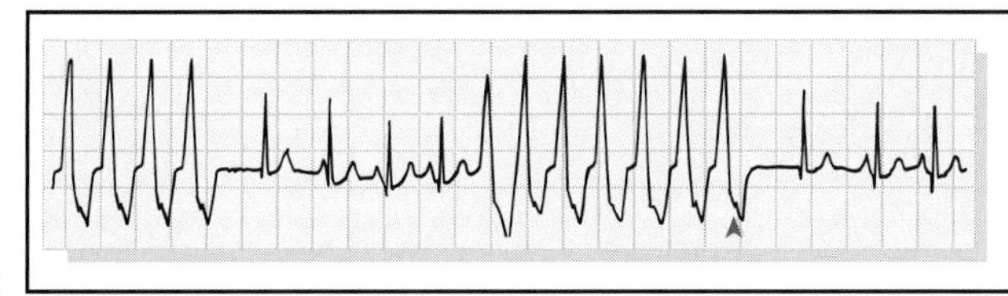

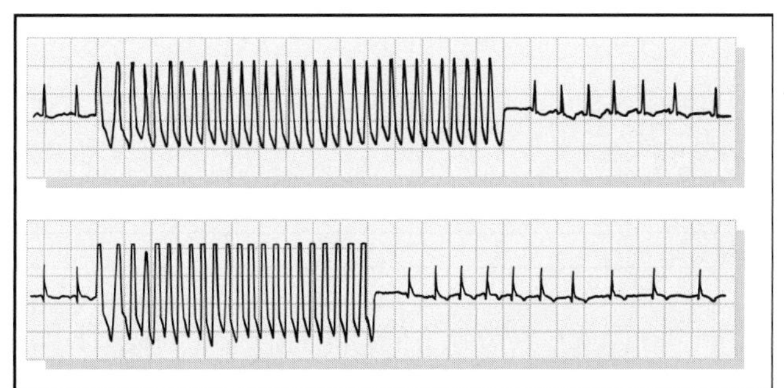

FIGURE 32–45 **A,** Repetitive monomorphic ventricular tachycardia. Short episodes of a monomorphic ventricular tachycardia at a rate of 160 beats/min repeatedly interrupt the normal sinus rhythm. Retrograde atrial capture probably occurs (the arrowhead points to the deflection in the ST segment), and the retrograde P wave of the last complex of the repetitive monomorphic ventricular tachycardia conducts over the normal pathway to produce a QRS complex with a normal contour. **B,** Short runs of a very rapid (260 beats/min) ventricular tachycardia of uniform contour. They probably provoke a compensatory sympathetic response because each is followed by a brief period of sinus tachycardia. The sinus pacemaker appears unstable as changes in P wave morphology result.

current may be important, possibly in a reentrant circuit or via delayed afterdepolarizations. Several mechanisms may be operative, and the group may not be homogeneous. Oral verapamil is not as effective as IV verapamil. Once initiated, the tachycardia is paroxysmal and sustained. It can be started by rapid atrial or ventricular pacing and sometimes by exercise or isoproterenol. Generally, the prognosis is good. Radiofrequency catheter ablation is effective in symptomatic patients. Late potentials have been reported in one-third of patients.

Sudden infant death syndrome is a syndrome of unexplained death that occurs in infancy. The precise cause is not known and is probably due to a variety of etiologies, both cardiac and noncardiac. It is not known what percentage, if any, is due to arrhythmias. Some have suggested that the long-QT (see later) and Brugada syndromes may be responsible in some cases (see Chap. 33).[126,127]

ACCELERATED IDIOVENTRICULAR RHYTHM

ECG RECOGNITION. The ventricular rate, commonly between 60 and 110 beats/min, usually hovers within 10 beats of the sinus rate, so control of the cardiac rhythm shifts between these two competing pacemaker sites. Consequently, fusion beats often occur at the onset and termination of the arrhythmia as the pacemakers vie for control of ventricular depolarization (Fig. 32-47). Because of the slow rate, capture beats are common. The onset of this arrhythmia is generally gradual (nonparoxysmal) and occurs when the rate of the VT exceeds the sinus rate because of sinus slowing or SA or AV block. The ectopic mechanism can also begin after a PVC, or the ectopic ventricular focus can simply accelerate sufficiently to overtake the sinus rhythm. The slow rate and nonparoxysmal onset avoid the problems initiated by excitation during the vulnerable period, and consequently, precipitation of more rapid ventricular arrhythmias is rarely seen. Termination of the rhythm generally occurs gradually as the dominant sinus rhythm accelerates or as the ectopic ventricular rhythm decelerates. The ventricular rhythm can be regular or irregular and can occasionally show sudden doubling, which suggests the presence of exit block. Many characteristics incriminate enhanced automaticity as the responsible mechanism.

The arrhythmia occurs as a rule in patients who have heart disease, such as those with acute myocardial infarction or with digitalis toxicity. It is transient and intermittent, with episodes lasting a few seconds to a minute, and does not appear to seriously affect the patient's clinical course or the prognosis. It commonly occurs at the moment of reperfusion of a previously occluded coronary artery, and it can be found during resuscitation.

MANAGEMENT

Suppressive therapy is rarely necessary because the ventricular rate is generally less than 100 beats/min, but such therapy may be considered when AV dissociation results in loss of sequential AV contraction, when an accelerated idioventricular rhythm occurs together with a more rapid VT, when an accelerated idioventricular rhythm begins with a PVC and causes discharges in the vulnerable period of the preceding T wave, when the ventricular rate is too rapid and produces symptoms, and if ventricular fibrillation develops as a result of the accelerated idioventricular rhythm. This last event appears to be fairly rare. Therapy, when indicated, should be as already noted for VT. Often, simply increasing the sinus rate with atropine or atrial pacing suppresses the accelerated idioventricular rhythm.

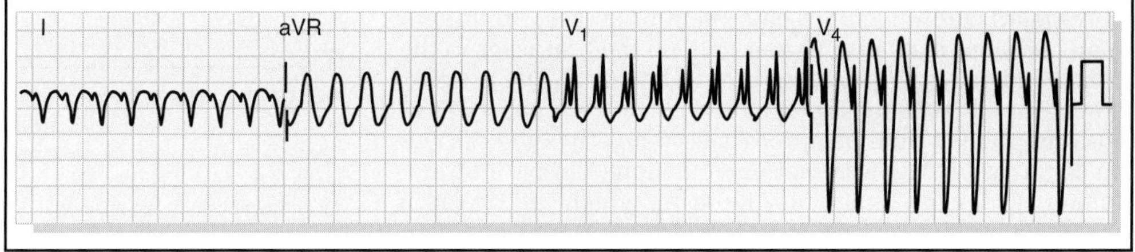

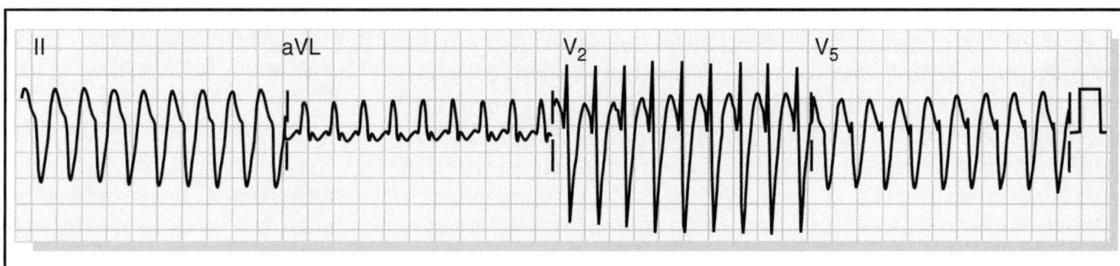

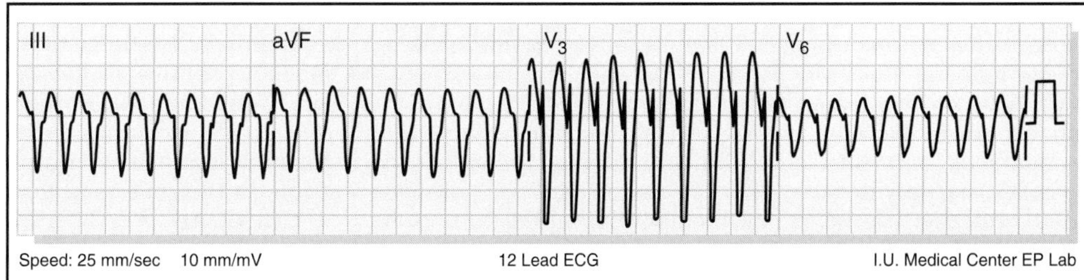

FIGURE 32–46 Left septal ventricular tachycardia. This tachycardia is characterized by a right bundle branch block contour. In this instance, the axis was rightward. The site of the ventricular tachycardia was established to be in the left posterior septum by electrophysiological mapping and ablation.

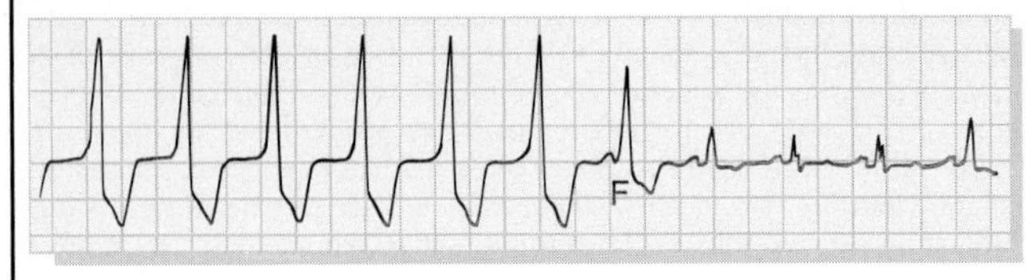

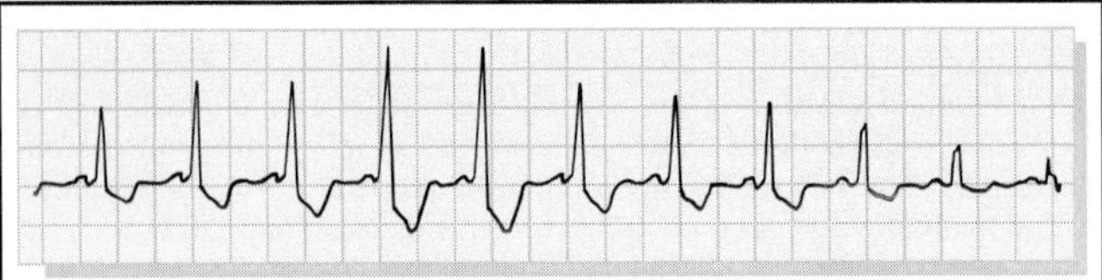

FIGURE 32–47 Accelerated idioventricular rhythm. In this continuous monitor lead recording, an accelerated idioventricular rhythm competes with the sinus rhythm. Wide QRS complexes at a rate of 90 beats/min fuse (F) with the sinus rhythm, which takes control briefly, generates the narrow QRS complexes, and then yields once again to the accelerated idioventricular rhythm as the P waves move "in and out" of the QRS complex. This example of isorhythmic atrioventricular dissociation may be due to hemodynamic modulation of the sinus rate via the autonomic nervous system.

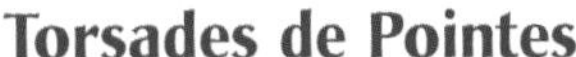

Torsades de Pointes

ECG RECOGNITION. The term *torsades de pointes* refers to a VT characterized by QRS complexes of changing amplitude that appear to twist around the isoelectric line and occur at rates of 200 to 250/min (Fig. 32–48A).[128] Originally described in the setting of bradycardia caused by complete heart block, the term *torsades de pointes* is usually used to connote a *syndrome,* not simply an ECG description of the QRS complex of the tachycardia, characterized by prolonged ventricular repolarization with QT intervals generally exceeding 500 milliseconds. The U wave can also become prominent and merge with the T wave, but its role in this syndrome and in long-QT syndrome is not clear. The abnormal repolarization need not be present or at least prominent on all beats but may be apparent only on the beat prior to the onset of torsades de pointes (i.e., following a PVC). Long-short R-R cycle sequences commonly precede the onset of torsades de pointes from acquired causes. Relatively late PVCs can discharge during termination of the long T wave and precipitate successive bursts of VT during which the peaks of the QRS complexes appear successively on one side and then on the other side of the isoelectric baseline and give the typical twisting appearance with continuous and progressive changes in QRS contour and amplitude. Torsades de pointes can terminate with progressive prolongation in cycle length and larger and more distinctly formed QRS complexes and culminate in a return to the basal rhythm, a period of ventricular standstill, and a new attack of torsades de pointes or ventricular fibrillation.

A less common form, the short-coupled variant of torsades de pointes, is a malignant disease with a high mortality rate and shares several characteristics with idiopathic ventricular fibrillation. The ventricular arrhythmia in this setting is initiated with a close-coupled PVC and usually does not involve preceding pauses or bradycardia.[129]

VT that is similar morphologically to torsades de pointes and occurs in patients *without* QT prolongation, whether spontaneous or electrically induced, should generally be classified as polymorphic VT, not as torsades de pointes. The distinction has important therapeutic implications (see later).

ELECTROPHYSIOLOGICAL FEATURES. The electrophysiological mechanisms responsible for torsades de pointes are not completely understood. Most data suggest that early afterdepolarizations (see Chap. 27) are responsible for

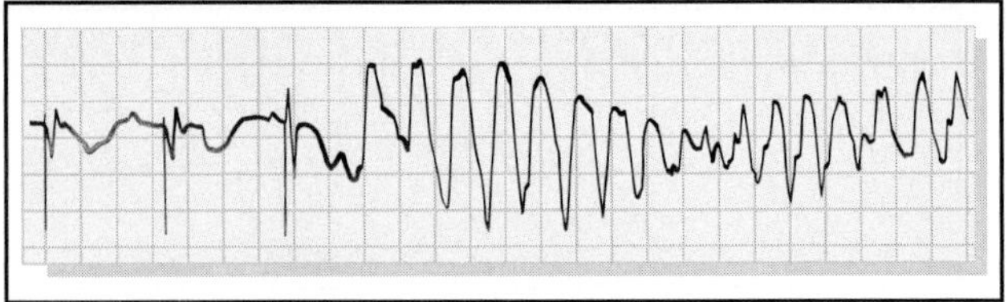

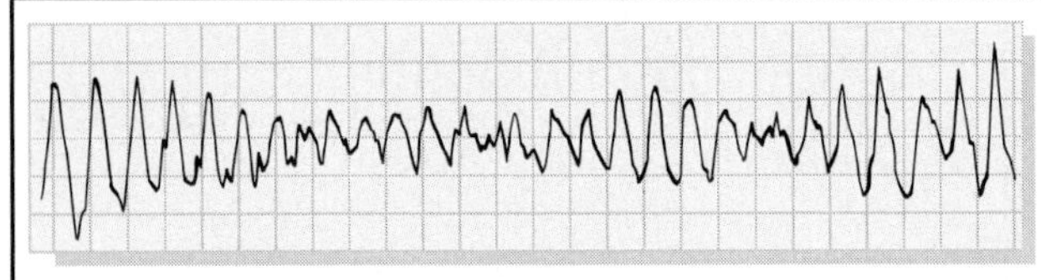

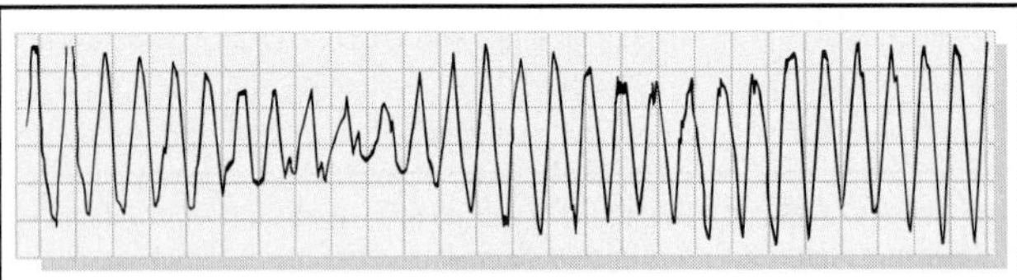

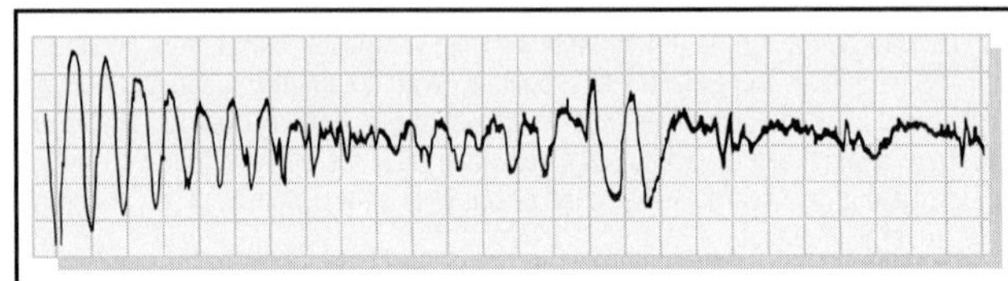

A

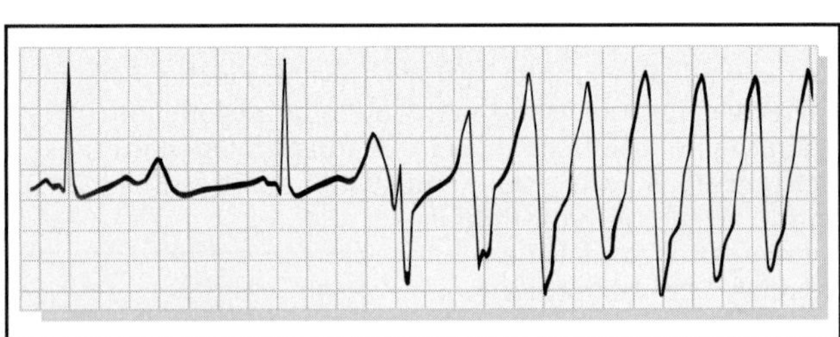

B

FIGURE 32–48 Torsades de pointes. **A** (top four panels), Continuous monitor lead recording. A demand ventricular pacemaker (VVI) had been implanted because of type II second-degree atrioventricular block. After treatment with amiodarone for recurrent ventricular tachycardia, the QT interval became prolonged (about 640 milliseconds during paced beats), and episodes of torsades de pointes developed. In this recording, the tachycardia spontaneously terminates and a paced ventricular rhythm is restored. Motion artifact is noted at the end of the recording as the patient lost consciousness. **B,** Tracing from a young boy with congenital long-QT syndrome. The QTU interval in the sinus beats is at least 600 milliseconds. Note TU wave alternans in the first and second complexes. A late premature complex occurring in the downslope of the TU wave initiates an episode of ventricular tachycardia.

both long-QT syndrome and the torsades de pointes, or at least its initiation. Perpetuation may be due to triggered activity, reentry resulting from dispersion of repolarization produced by the early afterdepolarizations, or abnormal automaticity. Two out-of-phase discharging foci have been experimentally shown to produce a tachycardia similar to torsades de pointes, as have drifting rotors. Dispersion of repolarization from endocardium to epicardium may also play a role. A distinct group of cells, called *M cells,* located in the subepicardium have prolonged repolarization and may play a role in the genesis of torsades de pointes.[130]

CLINICAL FEATURES. Although many predisposing factors have been cited, the most common causes are congenital, severe bradycardia, potassium depletion, and use of medications (such as class IA, IC or III antiarrhythmic drugs). More than 50 drugs have been noted to prolong the QT interval (see Long-QT Syndrome). Clinical features depend on whether the torsades de pointes is due to the acquired or congenital (idiopathic) long-QT syndrome (see later). Symptoms from the tachycardia depend on its rate and duration, as with other VTs, and range from palpitations to syncope and death. Women, perhaps because of a longer QT interval, are at greater risk for torsades de pointes than are men.

MANAGEMENT. The approach to VT with a polymorphic pattern depends on whether it occurs in the setting of a prolonged QT interval. For this practical reason and because the mechanism of the tachycardia can differ depending on whether a long-QT interval is present, it is important to restrict the definition of torsades de pointes to the typical polymorphic VT in the setting of a long QT and/or U wave in the basal complexes. In all patients with torsades de pointes, administration of class IA, possibly some class IC, and class III antiarrhythmic agents (amiodarone and sotalol) can increase the abnormal QT interval and worsen the arrhythmia. IV magnesium is the initial treatment of choice for torsades de pointes from an acquired cause, followed by temporary ventricular or atrial pacing. Isoproterenol, given cautiously because it can exacerbate the arrhythmia, can be used to increase the rate until pacing is instituted. Lidocaine, mexiletine, or phenytoin can be tried. Potassium-channel openers may be useful. The cause of the long QT should be determined and corrected if possible. When the QT interval is normal, polymorphic VT *resembling* torsades de pointes is diagnosed, and standard antiarrhythmic drugs can be given. In borderline cases, the clinical context may help determine whether treatment should be initiated with antiarrhythmic drugs. Torsades de pointes resulting from congenital long-QT syndrome is treated with beta blockade, surgical sympathetic interruption, pacing, and implantable defibrillators (see later). ECGs taken on close relatives can help secure the diagnosis of long-QT syndrome in borderline cases.

Long-QT Syndrome

ECG RECOGNITION. The upper limit for duration of the normal QT interval *corrected* for heart rate (QTc) is often given as 0.44 seconds (Fig. 32–48B). However, the normal corrected QT interval may actually be longer (0.46 seconds for men and 0.47 seconds for women), with a normal range of plus or minus 15 percent of the mean value. Data from Holter recordings are consistent with a normal QTc less than 440 milliseconds.[131] The nature of the U wave abnormality and its relationship to long-QT syndrome is not clear. M cells may be responsible for the U wave (see Chap. 27). The probable risk of life-threatening ventricular arrhythmias developing in patients with idiopathic long-QT syndrome is exponentially related to the length of the QTc interval. T wave "humps" in the ECG suggest the presence of long-QT syndrome and may be caused by early afterdepolarizations. A point score system has been suggested to aid in the diagnosis. Unique T wave contours have been ascribed to specific genotypes causing long-QT syndrome.

CLINICAL FEATURES. Long-QT syndrome can be divided into idiopathic (congenital) and acquired forms.[128] The idiopathic form is a familial disorder that can be associated with sensorineural deafness (Jervell and Lange-Nielsen syndromes, autosomal recessive) or normal hearing (Romano-Ward syndrome, autosomal dominant). A nonfamilial form with normal hearing has been called the *sporadic form*.

The hypothesis that the idiopathic long-QT syndrome results from a preponderance of left sympathetic tone has been replaced by genetic information linking the disorder in different families to sites in several different chromosomes (see Table 28–1). The gene products from several of these mutations have been identified as potassium and sodium channels (see Table 38–1).[133-135] A detailed discussion of the genetics of long-QT syndrome is presented in Chapter 28.

The acquired form has a long-QT interval caused by various drugs (see Table 72–3) such as quinidine, procainamide, *N*-acetylprocainamide, sotalol, amiodarone, disopyramide, phenothiazines, or tricyclic antidepressants; cisapride; nonsedating antihistamines such as astemizole and terfenedine, whose actions can be exacerbated by drugs affecting their metabolism such as ketoconazoles; drugs such as erythromycin, pentamidine, and some antimalarials; electrolyte abnormalities such as hypokalemia and hypomagnesemia; the results of a liquid protein diet and starvation; central nervous system lesions; significant bradyarrhythmias; cardiac ganglionitis; mitral valve prolapse; and probucol. The acquired long-QT syndrome may be a forme fruste of the inherited form.[136,136a]

Patients with congenital long-QT syndrome can initially have syncope, at times misdiagnosed as epilepsy, from VTs that are often caused by torsades de pointes. Sudden death can occur in this group of patients, and it occurs in about 10 percent of pediatric patients without preceding symptoms. It is obvious that in some patients the ventricular arrhythmia becomes sustained and probably results in ventricular fibrillation. Patients with idiopathic long-QT syndrome who are at increased risk for sudden death include those with family members who died suddenly at an early age and those who have experienced syncope. It also appears that the specific mutations carry different risks, with long-QT-1 and long-QT-2 carrying the highest risk for arrhythmias. Although patients with the long-QT-3 mutation tend to have fewer cardiac events, they tend to be more lethal ones. Thus, the cumulative mortality appears to be the same for long-QT-1, long-QT-2, and long-QT-3.[137] Ventricular tachyarrhythmias commonly develop during periods of adrenergic stimulation, such as fright or exertion. However, some phenotypic variation is noted, such that patients with long-QT-1 and long-QT-2 mutations tend be more sympathetically driven, whereas long-QT-3 patients tend to have more events during sleep.[137] Syndactyly has recently been described in some patients with the idiopathic form.

Stress testing can prolong the QT interval and produce T wave alternans, the latter indicative of electrical instability. ECGs should be obtained for all family members when the propositus has symptoms. Patients should undergo prolonged ECG recording with various stresses designed to evoke ventricular arrhythmias, such as auditory stimuli, psychological stress, cold pressor stimulation, and exercise. The Valsalva maneuver can lengthen the QT interval and cause T wave alternans and VT in patients who have prolonged QT syndromes. Catecholamines can be infused in some patients, but this challenge must be performed cautiously, with resuscitative equipment along with alpha and beta antagonists close at hand. Stellate ganglion stimulation and blockade have been useful to provoke or abolish arrhythmias. Premature ventricular stimulation electrically does not generally induce arrhythmias in this syndrome and electrophysiology studies are usually not helpful in the diagnosis. Torsades de pointes commonly develops in patients with the acquired form during periods of bradycardia or after a long pause in the R-R interval, whereas those with the idiopathic form can have a sinus tachycardia preceding the ventricular arrhythmia. Competitive sports are contraindicated for patients with the congenital long-QT syndrome.[5]

MANAGEMENT. For patients who have idiopathic long-QT syndrome but do not have syncope, complex ventricular arrhythmias, or a family history of sudden cardiac death, generally no therapy or treatment with a beta blocker is recommended. In asymptomatic patients with complex ventricular arrhythmias or a family history of early sudden cardiac death, beta-adrenoceptor blockers at maximally tolerated doses are recommended. Implantation of a permanent pacemaker to prevent the bradycardia and/or pauses that may predispose to the development of torsades de pointes may be indicated.[2,138,139] In patients with syncope due to ventricular arrhythmias or aborted sudden death, an ICD is warranted. These patients should also be treated with concomitant beta blockers and perhaps overdrive atrial pacing (via the ICD) to minimize the frequency of ICD discharges. ICD is beneficial in these patient not simply because of the shocking capabilities but because of the ability to continually pace to prevent bradycardia-induced torsades and because of algorithms to prevent post-PVC pauses. The use of ICD in patients without syncope but with a long-QT interval and a strong family history of sudden death is still controversial but may be warranted in these high-risk patients. For patients who continue to have syncope despite maximum drug therapy, left-sided cervicothoracic sympathetic ganglionectomy that interrupts the stellate ganglion and the first three or four thoracic ganglia may be helpful. For patients with the acquired form and torsades de pointes, IV magnesium and atrial or ventricular pacing are initial choices. Class IB antiarrhythmic drugs or isoproterenol (cautiously) to increase the heart rate can be tried. Avoidance of precipitating drugs is mandatory. Potassium-channel–activating drugs such as pinacidil and cromakalim may be useful in both forms of long-QT syndrome.

Bidirectional Ventricular Tachycardia

Bidirectional VT is an uncommon type of VT that is characterized by QRS complexes with a right bundle branch block pattern, alternating polarity in the frontal plane from −60 to −90 degrees to +120 to +130 degrees, and a regular rhythm. The ventricular rate is between 140 and 200 beats/min. Although the mechanism and site of origin of this tachycardia have remained somewhat controversial, most evidence supports a ventricular origin.

Bidirectional VT can be a manifestation of digitalis excess, typically in older patients and in those with severe myocardial disease. When the tachycardia is due to digitalis, the extent of toxicity is often advanced, with a poor prognosis. Catecholaminergic polymorphic VT can present as bidirectional VT.

In addition to digoxin-binding antibodies (Digibind), drugs useful to treat digitalis toxicity such as lidocaine, potassium, phenytoin, and propranolol should be considered if excessive digitalis administration is suspected. Otherwise, the usual therapeutic approach to VT is recommended.

Bundle Branch Reentrant Ventricular Tachycardia

VT secondary to bundle branch reentry is characterized by a QRS morphology determined by the circuit established over the bundle branches or fascicles. Retrograde conduction over the left bundle branch system and anterograde conduction over the right bundle branch create a QRS complex with a left bundle branch block contour and constitute the most common form. The frontal plane axis may be about +30 degrees. Conduction in the opposite direction produces a right bundle branch block contour. Reentry can also occur over the anterior and posterior fascicles. Electrophysiologically, bundle branch reentrant complexes are started after a critical S_2-H_2 or S_3-H_3 delay. The H-V interval of the bundle branch reentrant complex equals or exceeds the H-V interval of the spontaneous normally conducted QRS complex.

Bundle branch reentry is a form of monomorphic sustained VT that is usually seen in patients with structural heart disease such as dilated cardiomyopathy. During follow-up, congestive heart failure is the most common cause of death in this population. Myocardial VTs can also be present. Uncommonly, bundle branch reentry can occur in the absence of myocardial disease.

The therapeutic approach is as for other types of VT. In the acute setting, pace termination is frequently effective. Long-term, catheter ablation effectively eliminates this form of VT.

Ventricular Flutter and Fibrillation (see also Chap. 33)

ECG RECOGNITION. These arrhythmias represent severe derangements of the heartbeat that usually terminate fatally within 3 to 5 minutes unless corrective measures are undertaken promptly. Ventricular flutter is manifested as a sine wave in appearance: regular large oscillations occurring at a rate of 150 to 300/min (usually about 200) (Fig. 32–49A). The distinction between rapid VT and ventricular flutter can be difficult and is usually of academic interest only. Hemodynamic collapse is present with both. Ventricular fibrillation is recognized by the presence of irregular undulations of varying contour and amplitude (Fig. 32–49B). Distinct QRS complexes, ST segments, and T waves are absent. Fine-amplitude fibrillatory waves (0.2 mV) are present with prolonged ventricular fibrillation. These fine waves identify patients with worse survival rates and are sometimes confused with asystole.[140]

MECHANISMS. Ventricular fibrillation occurs in a variety of clinical situations but is most commonly associated with coronary artery disease and as a terminal event (see Chap. 27).[141] Thrombolytic agents reduce the incidence of ventricular arrhythmias and inducible VT after myocardial infarction. Cardiovascular events, including sudden cardiac death from ventricular fibrillation, but not asystole, occur most frequently in the morning and may be related to increased platelet aggregability. Aspirin reduces this mortality. An excess in sudden deaths appears to occur during the winter months.[142] Ventricular fibrillation can occur during antiarrhythmic drug administration, hypoxia, ischemia, atrial fibrillation, and very rapid ventricular rates in the preexcitation syndrome; after electrical shock administered during cardioversion (see Chaps. 30 and 31) or accidentally by improperly grounded equipment; and during competitive ventricular pacing to terminate VT.

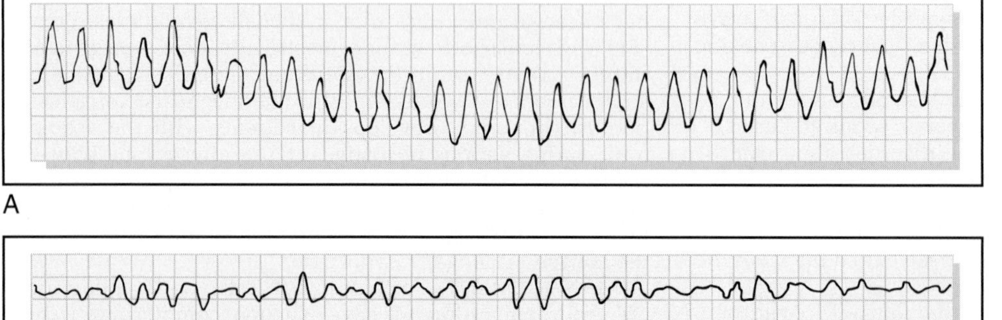

FIGURE 32–49 Ventricular flutter and ventricular fibrillation. **A,** The sine wave appearance of the complexes occurring at a rate of 300 beats/min is characteristic of ventricular flutter. **B,** The irregular undulating baseline typifies ventricular fibrillation.

CLINICAL FEATURES. Ventricular flutter or ventricular fibrillation results in faintness, followed by loss of consciousness, seizures, apnea, and eventually, if the rhythm continues untreated, death. The blood pressure is unobtainable, and heart sounds are usually absent. The atria can continue to beat at an independent rhythm for a time or in response to impulses from the fibrillating ventricles. Eventually, electrical activity of the heart ceases.

In patients resuscitated from out-of-hospital cardiac

arrest, 75 percent have ventricular fibrillation. Bradycardia or asystole, which can occur in 15 to 25 percent of these patients, is associated with a worse prognosis than is ventricular fibrillation and is usually associated with more advanced LV dysfunction. VT commonly precedes the onset of ventricular fibrillation, although frequently no consistent premonitory patterns emerge. Heart rate variability may be decreased.

Although 75 percent of resuscitated patients exhibit significant coronary artery disease, acute transmural myocardial infarction develops in only 20 to 30 percent. In one study, 73 percent had recent coronary artery thrombosis. Those in whom myocardial infarction does *not* develop have an increased recurrence rate for sudden cardiac death or ventricular fibrillation. Patients who have ventricular fibrillation and acute myocardial infarction have a recurrence rate at 1 year of 2 percent. In the past 20 years, there appears to have been an overall decrease in the incidence of sudden cardiac death, parallel to the decrease in death from coronary heart disease.

Predictors of death for resuscitated patients include a reduced EF, abnormal wall motion, history of congestive heart failure, history of myocardial infarction but no acute event, and the presence of ventricular arrhythmias. Patients discharged after an anterior myocardial infarction complicated by ventricular fibrillation appear to represent a subgroup at high risk of sudden death. Ventricular fibrillation can occur in infants, young people, athletes, and persons without known structural heart disease and in unexplained syndromes.

MANAGEMENT. Management should follow basic life support and advanced cardiac life support guidelines (see Chap. 33).[143] *Immediate* nonsynchronized DC electrical shock using 200 to 400 J is mandatory therapy for ventricular fibrillation and for ventricular flutter that has caused loss of consciousness. Automatic external defibrillators have facilitated the ability to defib-rillate early. Cardiopulmonary resuscitation is used only until the defibrillation equipment is readied. Time should not be wasted with cardiopulmonary resuscitation maneuvers if electrical defibrillation can be done promptly. Defibrillation requires fewer joules if done early. If the circulation is markedly inadequate despite return to sinus rhythm, closed-chest massage with artificial ventilation as needed should be instituted. The use of anesthesia during electrical shock is obviously dictated by the patient's condition and is not generally required. After conversion of the arrhythmia to a normal rhythm, it is essential to monitor the rhythm continuously and institute measures to prevent recurrence. Metabolic acidosis quickly follows cardiovascular collapse. If the arrhythmia is terminated within 30 to 60 seconds, significant acidosis does not occur. Judicious use of sodium bicarbonate to reverse the acidosis may be necessary, but its use should not delay administration of epinephrine or defibrillation shocks (see Chap. 33).

If the resuscitation time is short, artificial ventilation by means of a tightly fitting rubber face mask and an AMBU bag is quite satisfactory and eliminates the delay attending intubation by inexperienced personnel. If such a mask and bag are not available, mouth-to-mouth or mouth-to-nose resuscitation is indicated. It is important to reemphasize that there should be *no delay in instituting electrical shock.* If the patient is not monitored and it cannot be established whether asystole or ventricular fibrillation caused the cardiovascular collapse, the electrical shock should be administered *without* wasting precious seconds attempting to obtain an ECG. The DC shock may cause the asystolic heart to begin discharging and also terminate ventricular fibrillation, if the latter is present.

A search for conditions contributing to the initiation of ventricular flutter or fibrillation should be made and the conditions corrected, if possible. Initial medical approaches to prevent recurrence of ventricular fibrillation include IV administration of amiodarone, lidocaine, bretylium, or procainamide. Amiodarone tends to be the most effective and does not produce the ventricular dysfunction and hypotension often seen with bretylium or procainamide. Ventricular fibrillation rarely terminates spontaneously, and death results unless countermeasures are instituted immediately. Subsequent therapy is necessary to prevent recurrence. Implantable defibrillators have become the mainstay of chronic therapy in patients at continued risk for ventricular fibrillation or VT from nonreversible causes (see Chap. 31).

Heart Block

Heart block is a disturbance of impulse conduction that can be permanent or transient depending on the anatomical or functional impairment. It must be distinguished from *interference,* a normal phenomenon that is a disturbance of impulse conduction caused by physiological refractoriness resulting from inexcitability from a preceding impulse. Either interference or block can occur at any site where impulses are conducted, but they are recognized most commonly between the sinus node and atrium (SA block), between the atria and ventricles (AV block), within the atria (intraatrial block), or within the ventricles (intraventricular block). During AV block, the block can occur in the AV node, His bundle, or bundle branches. In some instances of bundle branch block the impulse may only be delayed and not completely blocked in the bundle branch, yet the resulting QRS complex may be indistinguishable from a QRS complex generated by a complete bundle branch block.

The conduction disturbance is classified by severity into three categories. During *first-degree heart block,* conduction time is prolonged but all impulses are conducted. *Second-degree heart block* occurs in two forms: Mobitz types I (Wenckebach) and II. Type I heart block is characterized by a progressive lengthening of the conduction time until an impulse is not conducted. Type II heart block denotes occasional or repetitive sudden block of conduction of an impulse without prior measurable lengthening of conduction time. When no impulses are conducted, *complete* or *third-degree block* is present. The degree of block may depend in part on the direction of impulse propagation. For unknown reasons, normal retrograde conduction can occur in the presence of advanced anterograde AV block. The reverse can also occur. Some electrocardiographers use the term *advanced heart block* to indicate blockage of two or more consecutive impulses.[144]

Certain features of type I second-degree block deserve special emphasis because when actual conduction times are not apparent in the ECG, for example, during SA, junctional, or ventricular exit block (Fig. 32–50), a type I conduction disturbance can be difficult to recognize. During a typical type I block, the increment in conduction time is greatest in the second beat of the Wenckebach group, and the absolute *increase* in conduction time *decreases* progressively over subsequent beats. These two features serve to establish the characteristics of classic Wenckebach group beating: (1) The interval between successive beats progressively decreases, although the conduction time increases (but by a decreasing function); (2) the duration of the pause produced by the nonconducted impulse is less than twice the interval preceding the blocked impulse (which is usually the shortest interval); and (3) the cycle following the nonconducted beat (beginning the Wenckebach group) is longer than the cycle preceding the blocked impulse. Although much emphasis has been placed on this characteristic grouping of cycles, primarily to be able

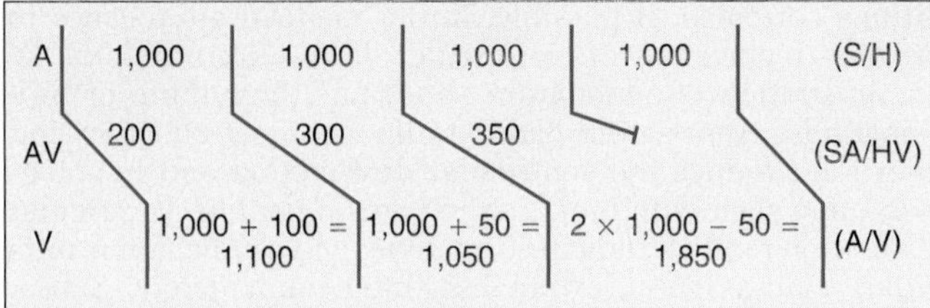

FIGURE 32–50 Typical 4:3 Wenckebach cycle. P waves ("A" tier) occur at a cycle length of 1000 milliseconds. The PR interval ("AV" tier) is 200 milliseconds for the first beat and generates a ventricular response ("V" tier). The PR interval increases by 100 milliseconds in the next complex, which results in an R-R interval of 1100 milliseconds (1000 + 100). The increment in the PR interval is only 50 milliseconds for the third cycle, and the PR interval becomes 350 milliseconds. The R-R interval shortens to 1050 milliseconds (1000 + 50). The next P wave is blocked, and an R-R interval is created that is less than twice the P-P interval by an amount equal to the increments in the PR interval. Thus, the Wenckebach features explained in the text can be found in this diagram. If the increment in the PR interval of the last conducted complex increased rather than decreased (e.g., 150 milliseconds rather than 50 milliseconds), the last R-R interval before the block would increase (1150 milliseconds) rather than decrease and thus become an example of an atypical Wenckebach cycle (see Fig. 32–44). If this were a Wenckebach exit block from the sinus node to the atrium, the sinus node cycle length (S) would be 1000 milliseconds, and the sinoatrial interval would increase from 200 to 300 to 350 milliseconds and culminate in a block. These events would be inapparent in the scalar electrocardiogram (ECG). However, the P-P interval in the ECG would shorten from 1100 to 1050 milliseconds, and finally, there would be a pause of 1850 milliseconds (A). If this rhythm were a junctional rhythm arising from the His bundle and conducting to the ventricle, the junctional rhythm cycle length would be 1000 milliseconds (H), and the H-V interval would progressively lengthen from 200 to 300 to 350 milliseconds, whereas the R-R interval would decrease from 1100 to 1050 milliseconds and then increase to 1850 milliseconds (V). The only clue to the Wenckebach exit block would be the cycle length changes in the ventricular rhythm.

to diagnose a Wenckebach exit block, this typical grouping occurs in fewer than 50 percent of patients who have a type I Wenckebach AV nodal block.

Differences in these cycle length patterns can result from changes in pacemaker rate (e.g., sinus arrhythmia), in neurogenic control of conduction, and in the increment of conduction delay. For example, if the PR increment in the last cycle *increases*, the R-R cycle of the last conducted beat can lengthen rather than shorten. In addition, since the last conducted beat is often at a critical state of conduction, it can become blocked and produce a 5:3 or 3:1 conduction ratio instead of a 5:4 or 3:2 ratio. During a 3:2 Wenckebach structure, the duration of the cycle following the nonconducted beat will be the same as the duration of the cycle preceding the nonconducted beat.

AV Block

An AV block exists when the atrial impulse is conducted with delay or is not conducted at all to the ventricle at a time when the AV junction is not physiologically refractory.

FIRST-DEGREE AV BLOCK. During first-degree AV block, every atrial impulse conducts to the ventricles and a regular ventricular rate is produced, but the PR interval exceeds 0.20 second in adults. PR intervals as long as 1.0 second have been noted and can at times exceed the P-P interval, a phenomenon known as "skipped" P waves. Clinically important PR interval prolongation can result from a conduction delay in the AV node (A-H interval), in the His-Purkinje system (H-V interval), or at both sites. Equally delayed conduction over both bundle branches can uncommonly produce PR prolongation without significant QRS complex aberration. Occasionally, an intraatrial conduction delay can result in PR prolongation. If the QRS complex in the scalar ECG is normal in contour and duration, the AV delay almost always resides in the AV node, rarely within the His bundle itself. If the QRS complex shows a bundle branch block pattern, the conduction delay may be within the AV node and/or His-Purkinje system (Fig. 32–51). In this latter instance, His bundle ECG is necessary to localize the site of conduction delay. Acceleration of the atrial rate or enhancement of vagal tone by carotid massage can cause first-degree AV nodal block to progress to type I second-degree AV block. Conversely, type I second-degree AV nodal block can revert to first-degree block with deceleration of the sinus rate.

SECOND-DEGREE AV BLOCK. Blocking of some atrial impulses conducted to the ventricle at a time when physiological interference is not involved constitutes second-degree AV block (Figs. 32–52 and 32–53; see also Fig. 32–50). The nonconducted P wave can be intermittent or frequent, at regular or irregular intervals, and can be preceded by fixed or lengthening PR intervals. A distinguishing feature is that conducted P waves relate to the QRS complex with recurring PR intervals; that is, the association of P with QRS is not random. Electrocardiographically, typical type I second-degree AV block is characterized by progressive PR prolongation culminating in a nonconducted P wave (see Fig. 32–52), whereas in type II second-degree AV block, the PR interval remains constant prior to the blocked P wave (Fig. 32–54A). In both instances the AV block is intermittent and

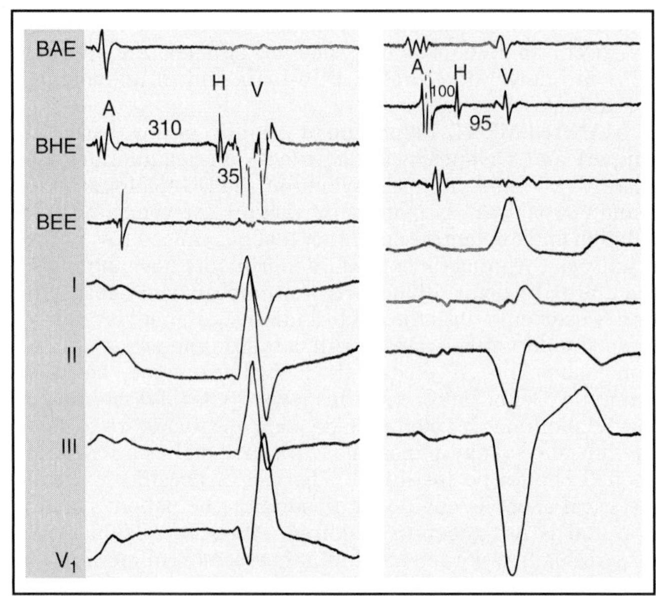

FIGURE 32–51 First-degree atrioventricular (AV) block. One complex during sinus rhythm is shown. **Left panel,** The PR interval measured 370 milliseconds (PA = 25 milliseconds; A-H = 310 milliseconds; H-V = 35 milliseconds) during a right bundle branch block. Conduction delay in the AV node causes the first-degree AV block. **Right panel,** The PR interval is 230 milliseconds (PA = 35 milliseconds; A-H = 100 milliseconds; H-V = 95 milliseconds) during a left bundle branch block. The conduction delay in the His-Purkinje system causes the first-degree AV block.

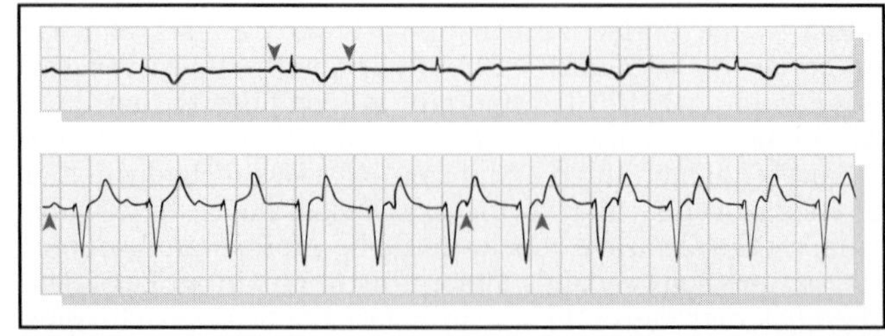

FIGURE 32–52 Unidirectional block. **Top,** During spontaneous sinus rhythm at a rate of 68 beats/min, 2:1 anterograde atrioventricular conduction occurs. In the **bottom** electrocardiogram, 1:1 retrograde conduction is seen during ventricular pacing at a rate of 70 beats/min. P waves are indicated by arrowheads.

generally repetitive and can block several P waves in a row. Often, the eponyms *Mobitz type I* and *Mobitz type II* are applied to the two types of block, whereas the term *Wenckebach block* refers to type I block only. A Wenckebach block in the His-Purkinje system in a patient with a bundle branch block can resemble an AV nodal Wenckebach block very closely (Fig. 32–54B).

Although it has been suggested that type I and type II AV blocks are different manifestations of the same electrophysiological mechanism that differ only quantitatively in the size of the increments, clinically separating second-degree AV block into type I and type II serves a useful function, and in most instances, the differentiation can be made easily and reliably from the surface ECG. Type II AV block often antedates the development of Adams-Stokes syncope and complete AV block, whereas type I AV block with a normal QRS complex is generally more benign and does not progress to more advanced forms of AV conduction disturbance. In older people, type I AV block with or without bundle branch block has been associated with a clinical picture similar to that in type II AV block.

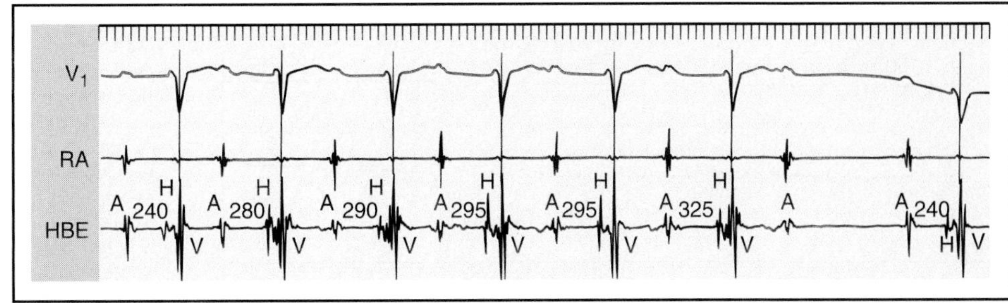

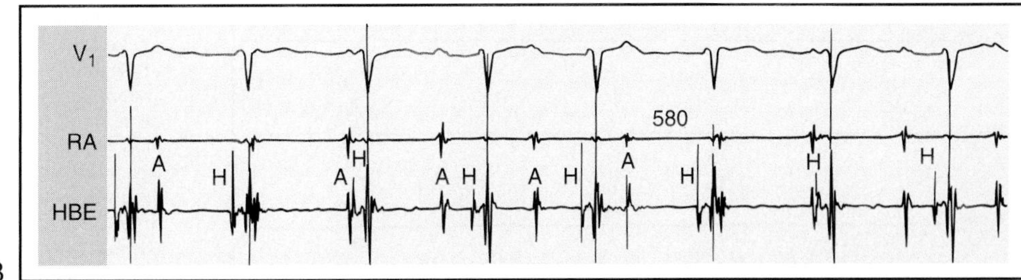

FIGURE 32–53 Type I (Wenckebach) atrioventricular (AV) nodal block **(A)**. During spontaneous sinus rhythm, progressive PR prolongation occurs and culminates in a nonconducted P wave. From the His bundle recording (HBE) it is apparent that the conduction delay and subsequent block occur within the AV node. Since the increment in conduction delay does not consistently decrease, the R-R intervals do not reflect the classic Wenckebach structure. **B** was recorded 5 minutes after the administration of 0.6 mg atropine intravenously. Atropine has had its predominant effect on sinus and junctional automaticity by this time, with little improvement in AV conduction. Consequently, more P waves are blocked and AV dissociation, caused by a combination of AV block and an enhanced junctional discharge rate, is present. At 8 minutes (not shown), when atropine finally improved AV conduction, 1:1 AV conduction occurred.

In a patient with an acute myocardial infarction, type I AV block usually accompanies inferior infarction (perhaps more often if a right ventricular infarction also occurs), is transient, and does not require temporary pacing, whereas type II AV block occurs in the setting of an acute anterior myocardial infarction, can require temporary or permanent pacing, and is associated with a high rate of mortality, generally from pump failure. A high degree of AV block can occur in patients with acute inferior myocardial infarction and is associated with more myocardial damage and a higher mortality rate than in those without AV block.

Although type I conduction disturbance is ubiquitous and can occur in any cardiac tissue in vivo, as well as in vitro, the site of block for the usual forms of second-degree AV block can be judged from the surface ECG with sufficient reliability to permit clinical decisions without requiring invasive electrophysiological studies in most instances. Type I AV block with a normal QRS complex almost always takes place at the level of the AV node, proximal to the His bundle. An exception is the uncommon patient with type I intrahisian block. Type II AV block, particularly in association with a bundle branch block, is localized to the His-Purkinje system. Type I AV block in a patient with a bundle branch block can be due to block in the AV node or in the His-Purkinje system. Type II AV block in a patient with a normal QRS complex can be due to an intrahisian AV block, but the block is likely to be a type I AV nodal block, which exhibits small increments in AV conduction time.

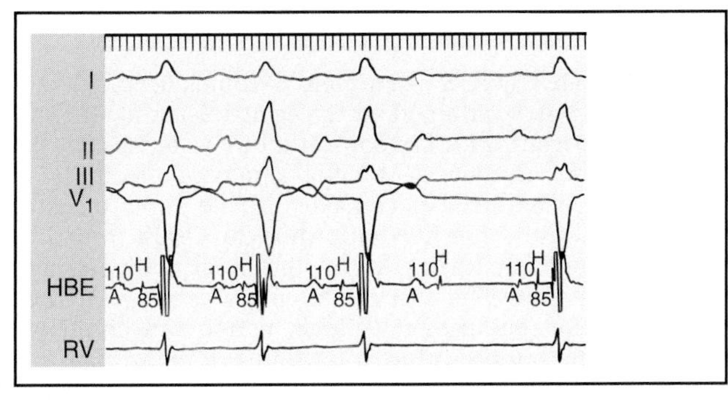

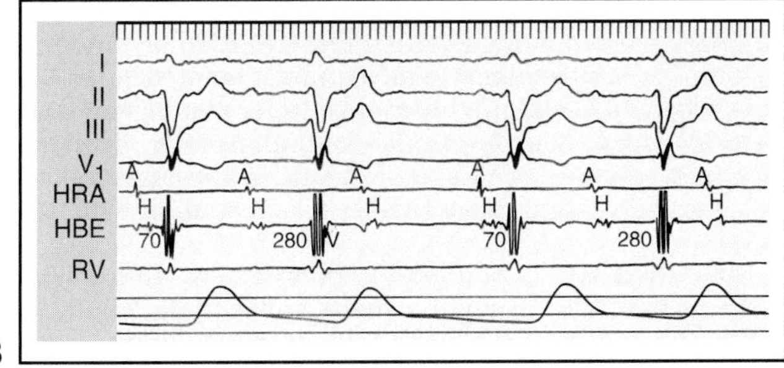

FIGURE 32–54 Type II atrioventricular (AV) block. **A,** The sudden development of a His-Purkinje block is apparent. The A-H and H-V intervals remain constant, as does the PR interval. Left bundle branch block is present. **B,** Wenckebach AV block in the His-Purkinje system. The QRS complex exhibits a right bundle branch block morphology. However, note that the second QRS complex in the 3:2 conduction exhibits a slightly different contour from the first QRS complex, particularly in V_1. This finding is the clue that the Wenckebach AV block might be in the His-Purkinje system. The H-V interval increases from 70 milliseconds to 280 milliseconds, and then block distal to the His bundle results.

DIFFERENTIATING TYPE I FROM TYPE II AV BLOCK. The preceding generalizations encompass the vast majority of patients with second-degree AV block. However, certain caveats must be heeded to avoid misdiagnosis because of subtle ECG changes or exceptions:

1. The 2:1 AV block can be a form of type I or type II AV block (Fig. 32–55). If the QRS complex is normal, the block is more likely to be type I and located in the AV node, and one should search for

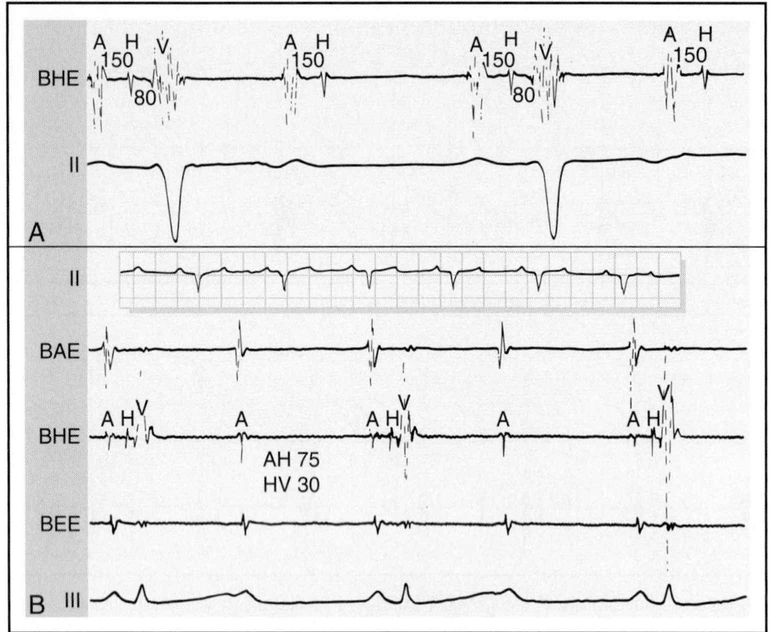

FIGURE 32–55 A 2:1 atrioventricular (AV) block proximal and distal to the His bundle deflection in two different patients. **A,** A 2:1 AV block seen in the scalar electrocardiogram occurs distal to the His bundle recording site in a patient with right bundle branch block and anterior hemiblock. The A-H interval (150 milliseconds) and H-V interval (80 milliseconds) are both prolonged. **B,** A 2:1 AV block proximal to the bundle of His in a patient with a normal QRS complex. The A-H interval (75 milliseconds) and the H-V interval (30 milliseconds) remain constant and normal.

transition of the 2:1 block to a 3:2 block, during which the PR interval lengthens in the second cardiac cycle. If a bundle branch block is present, the block can be located either in the AV node or in the His-Purkinje system.

2. AV block can occur simultaneously at two or more levels and can cause difficulty in distinguishing between types I and II.

3. If the atrial rate varies, it can alter conduction times and cause a type I AV block to stimulate a type II block or change a type II AV block into type I. For example, if the shortest atrial cycle length that just achieved 1:1 AV nodal conduction at a constant PR interval is decreased by as little as 10 or 20 milliseconds, the P wave of the shortened cycle can block conduction at the level of the AV node without an apparent increase in the antecedent PR interval. An apparent type II AV block in the His-Purkinje system can be converted to type I in the His-Purkinje system in some patients by increasing the atrial rate.

4. Concealed premature His depolarizations can create ECG patterns that simulate type I or type II AV block.

5. Abrupt, transient alterations in autonomic tone can cause sudden block of one or more P waves without altering the PR interval of the conducted P wave before or after the block. Thus, an apparent type II AV block would be produced at the AV node. Clinically, a burst of vagal tone usually lengthens the P-P interval, as well as producing an AV block.

6. The response of the AV block to autonomic changes either spontaneous or induced to distinguish type I from type II AV block can be misleading. Although vagal stimulation generally increases and vagolytic agents decrease the extent of type I AV block, such conclusions are based on the assumption that the intervention acts primarily on the AV node and fail to consider rate changes. For example, atropine can minimally improve conduction in the AV node and markedly increase the sinus rate, which results in an *increase* in AV nodal conduction time and the degree of AV block as a result of the faster atrial rate (see Fig. 32-53B). Conversely, if an increase in vagal tone minimally prolongs AV conduction time but greatly slows the heart rate, the net effect on type I AV block may be to improve conduction. In general, however, carotid sinus massage improves and atropine worsens AV conduction in patients with His-Purkinje block, whereas the opposite results are to be expected in patients who have AV nodal block. These two interventions can help differentiate the site of block without invasive study, although damaged His-Purkinje tissue may be influenced by changes in autonomic tone.

7. During type I AV block with high ratios of conducted beats, the increment in PR interval can be quite small and suggest a type II AV block if only the last few PR intervals before the blocked P wave are measured. By comparing the PR interval of the first beat in the long Wenckebach cycle with that of the beats immediately preceding the blocked P wave, the increment in AV conduction becomes readily apparent.

8. The classic AV Wenckebach structure depends on a stable atrial rate and a maximal increment in AV conduction time for the second PR interval of the Wenckebach cycle, with a progressive decrease in subsequent beats. Unstable or unusual alterations in the increment of AV conduction time or in the atrial rate, often seen with long Wenckebach cycles, result in atypical forms of type I AV block in which the last R-R interval can lengthen because the PR increment *increases;* these alterations are common.

9. Finally, it is important to remember that the PR interval in the scalar ECG is made up of conduction through the atrium, the AV node, and the His-Purkinje system. An increment in H-V conduction, for example, can be masked in the scalar ECG by a reduction in the A-H interval, and the resulting PR interval will not reflect the entire increment in His-Purkinje conduction time. Very long PR intervals (200 milliseconds) are more likely to result from AV nodal conduction delay (and block), with or without concomitant His-Purkinje conduction delay, although an H-V interval of 350 milliseconds is quite possible.

First-degree and type I second-degree AV block can occur in normal healthy children, and a Wenckebach AV block can be a normal phenomenon in well-trained athletes, probably related to an increase in resting vagal tone. Occasionally, progressive worsening of the Wenckebach AV conduction disorder can result and the athlete becomes symptomatic and has to decondition. In patients who have chronic second-degree AV nodal block (proximal to the His bundle) without structural heart disease, the course is relatively benign (except in older age groups), whereas in those who have structural heart disease the prognosis is poor and related to the underlying heart disease. *Advanced AV block* indicates a block of two or more consecutive P waves.

Complete AV Block

ECG RECOGNITION. Complete AV block occurs when no atrial activity is conducted to the ventricles and, therefore, the atria and ventricles are controlled by independent pacemakers. Thus, complete AV block is one type of complete AV dissociation. The atrial pacemaker can be sinus or ectopic (tachycardia, flutter, or fibrillation) or can result from an AV junctional focus occurring above the block with retrograde atrial conduction. The ventricular focus is usually located just below the region of the block, which can be above or below the His bundle bifurcation. Sites of ventricular pacemaker activity that are in or closer to the His bundle appear to be more stable and can produce a faster escape rate than can those located more distally in the ventricular conduction system. The ventricular rate in acquired complete heart block is less than 40 beats/min but can be faster in congenital complete AV block. The ventricular rhythm, usually regular, can vary in response to PVCs, a shift in the pacemaker site, an irregularly discharging pacemaker focus, or autonomic influences.

MECHANISMS. Complete AV block can result from block at the level of the AV node (usually congenital) (Fig. 32–56), within the bundle of His, or distal to it in the Purkinje system (usually acquired) (Fig. 32–57). Block proximal to the His bundle generally exhibits normal QRS complexes and rates of 40 to 60 beats/min because the escape focus that controls the ventricle arises in or near the His bundle. In complete AV nodal block, the P wave is not followed by a His deflection, but each ventricular complex is preceded by a His deflection (see Fig. 32–56). His bundle ECG can be useful to differentiate AV nodal from intrahisian block since the latter may carry a more serious prognosis than the former. Intrahisian block is recognized infrequently without invasive studies. In

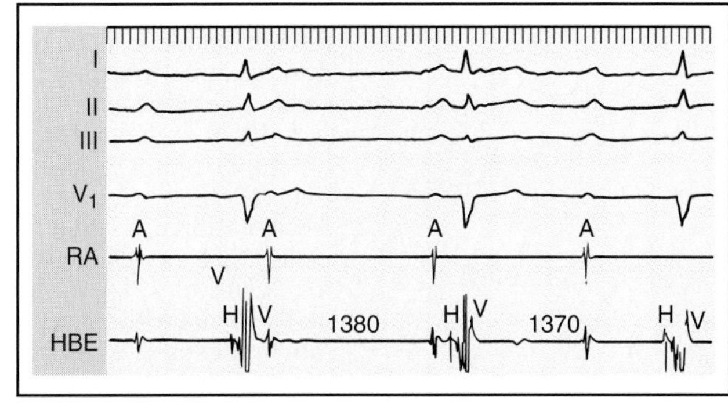

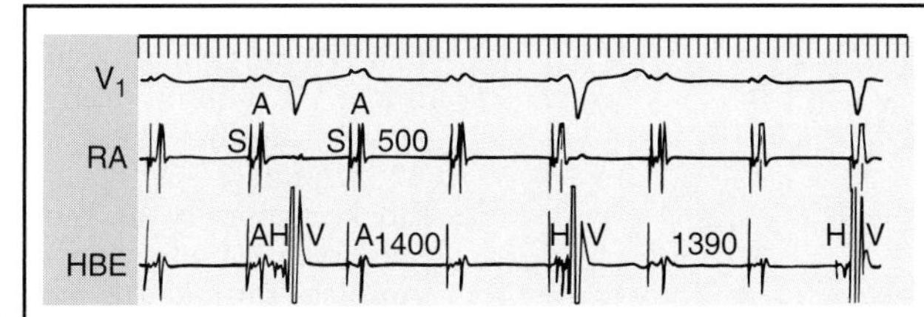

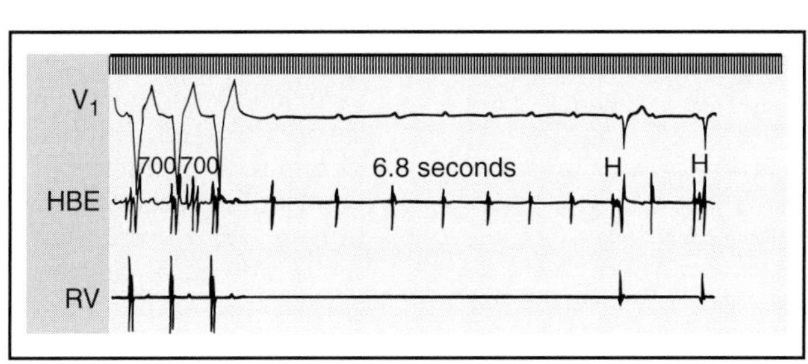

FIGURE 32–56 Congenital third-degree atrioventricular (AV) block. **A,** Complete AV nodal block is apparent. No P wave is followed by a His bundle potential, whereas each ventricular depolarization is preceded by a His bundle potential. **B,** Atrial pacing (cycle length of 500 milliseconds) fails to alter the cycle length of the functional rhythm. Still, no P wave is followed by a His bundle potential. **C,** After 30 seconds of ventricular pacing (cycle length of 700 milliseconds), suppression of the junctional focus results for almost 7 seconds (overdrive suppression of automaticity).

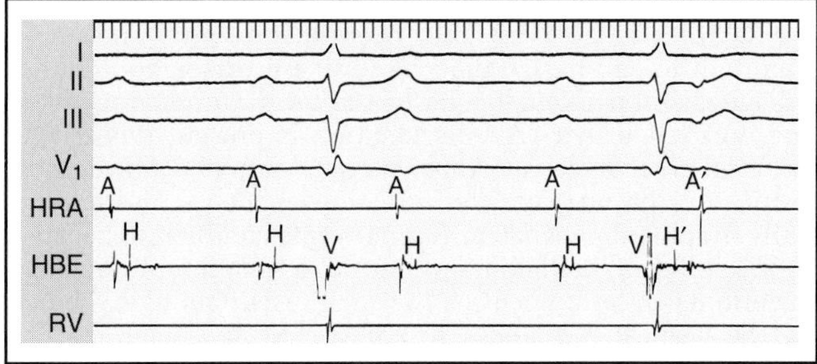

FIGURE 32–57 Complete anterograde atrioventricular (AV) block with retrograde ventriculoatrial conduction. All the sinus P waves are blocked distal to the His bundle, consistent with acquired complete AV block. The ventricles escape at a cycle length of approximately 1800 milliseconds (33 beats/min) and are not preceded by His bundle activation. The ventricular escape rhythm produces a QRS contour with left-axis deviation and right bundle branch block, possibly caused by impulse origin in the posterior fascicle of the left bundle branch. Of interest is the fact that the second ventricular escape beat conducts retrogradely through His (H) and to the atrium (note the low-high atrial activation sequence and the negative P wave in leads II and III). The first ventricular complex does not conduct retrogradely, probably because the His bundle is still refractory from the immediately preceding atrial impulse.

patients with AV nodal block, atropine usually speeds both the atrial and the ventricular rates. Exercise can reduce the extent of AV nodal block. Acquired complete AV block occurs most commonly distal to the bundle of His because of trifascicular conduction disturbance. Each P wave is followed by a His deflection, and the ventricular escape complexes are not preceded by a His deflection (see Fig. 32–57). The QRS complex is abnormal, and the ventricular rate is usually less than 40 beats/min. A hereditary form due to degeneration of the His bundle and bundle branches has been linked to the *SCN5A* gene that is also responsible for long-QT-3.[145]

Paroxysmal AV block in some instances can be due to hyperresponsiveness of the AV node to vagotonic reflexes. Surgery, electrolyte disturbances, myoendocarditis, tumors, Chagas disease, rheumatoid nodules, calcific aortic stenosis, myxedema, polymyositis, infiltrative processes (such as amyloid, sarcoid, or scleroderma), and an almost endless assortment of common and unusual conditions can produce AV block. In adults, rapid rates can sometimes be followed by block, an event known as *overdrive suppression* of conduction. This form of block may be important as a cause of paroxysmal AV block after cessation of a tachycardia.

AV Block in Children. In children, the most common cause of AV block is congenital (see Chap. 56). Under such circumstances, the AV block can be an isolated finding or be associated with other lesions. Connective tissue disease and the presence of anti-Rh_0-negative antibodies in the maternal sera of patients with congenital complete AV block raise the possibility that placentally transmitted antibodies play a role in some instances. Anatomical disruption between the atrial musculature and peripheral parts of the conduction system and nodoventricular discontinuity are two common histological findings. Children are most often asymptomatic; however, in some children symptoms develop that require pacemaker implantation. Mortality from congenital AV block is highest in the neonatal period, is much lower during childhood and adolescence, and increases slowly later in life. Adams-Stokes attacks can occur in patients with congenital heart block at any age. It is difficult to predict the prognosis in an individual patient. A persistent heart rate at rest of 50 beats/min or less correlates with the incidence of syncope, and extreme bradycardia can contribute to the frequency of Adams-Stokes attacks in children with congenital complete AV block. The site of block may not distinguish symptomatic children who have congenital or surgically induced complete heart block from those without symptoms. Prolonged recovery times of escape foci following rapid pacing (see Fig. 32–56C), slow heart rates on 24-hour ECG recordings, and the occurrence of paroxysmal tachycardias may be predisposing factors to the development of symptoms.

CLINICAL FEATURES. Many of the signs of AV block are evidenced at the bedside. First-degree AV block can be recognized by a long *a-c* wave interval in the jugular venous pulse and by diminished intensity of the first heart sound as the PR interval lengthens. In type I second-degree AV block, the heart rate may increase imperceptibly with gradually diminishing intensity of the first heart sound, widening of the *a-c* interval, terminated by a pause, and an *a* wave not followed by a *v* wave. Intermittent ventricular pauses and *a* waves in the neck not followed by *v* waves characterize type II AV block. The first heart sound maintains a constant intensity. In complete AV block, the findings are the same as those in AV dissociation (see later).

Significant clinical manifestations of first- and second-degree AV block usually consist of palpitations or subjective feelings of the heart "missing a beat." Persistent 2:1 AV block can produce symptoms of chronic bradycardia. Complete AV block can be accompanied by signs and symptoms of reduced cardiac output, syncope or presyncope, angina, or palpitations from ventricular tachyarrhythmias. It can occur in twins.

MANAGEMENT. For patients with transient or paroxysmal AV block who present with presyncope or syncope, the diagnosis can be elusive. Ambulatory monitoring (Holter or external loop recorders) can be useful, but on occasion monitoring for longer periods may be necessary and thus an

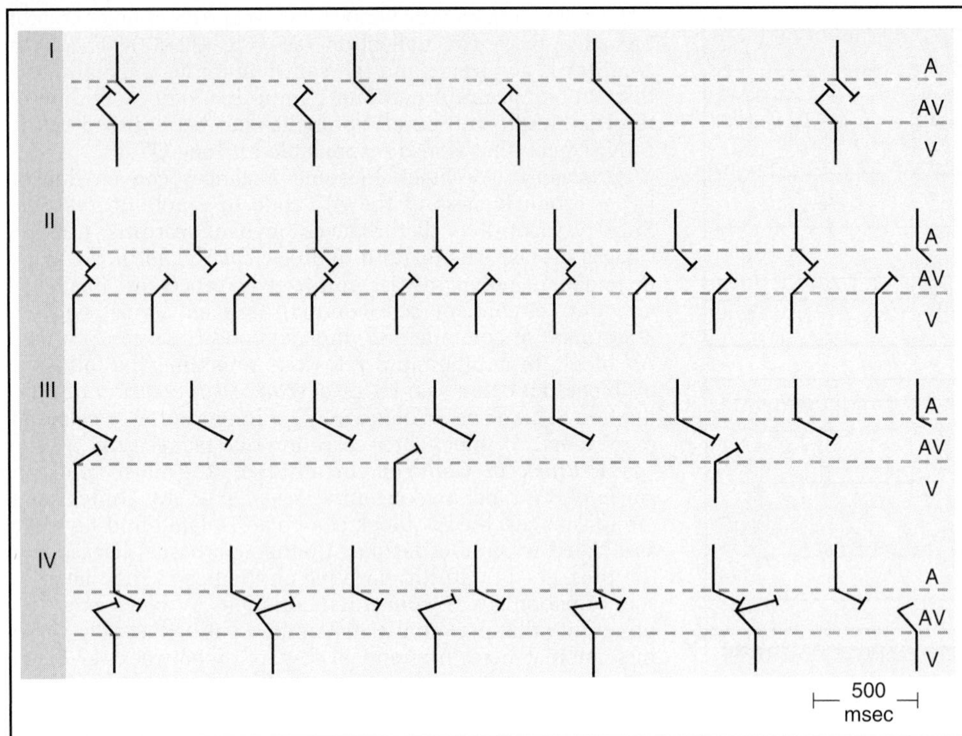

FIGURE 32–58 Diagrammatic illustration of the causes of atrioventricular (AV) dissociation. A sinus bradycardia allowing escape of an AV junctional rhythm that does not capture the atria retrogradely illustrates cause I **(top panel).** Intermittent sinus captures occur (third P wave) and produce incomplete AV dissociation. For cause II, ventricular tachycardia without retrograde atrial capture produces complete AV dissociation (see Figs. 32–22 and 32–41). As the third cause, complete AV block with a ventricular escape rhythm is diagrammed (see Figs. 32–56 and 32–57). The combination of causes II and III is shown in panel IV, which represents a nonparoxysmal AV junctional tachycardia and some degree of AV block.

implantable loop recorder may be needed to establish the diagnosis (see Chap. 29). Drugs cannot be relied on to increase the heart rate for more than several hours to several days in patients with symptomatic heart block without producing significant side effects. Therefore, temporary or permanent pacemaker insertion is indicated in patients with symptomatic bradyarrhythmias. Long-term right ventricular apical pacing can reduce cardiac function. For short-term therapy when the block is likely to be evanescent but still requires treatment or until adequate pacing therapy can be established, vagolytic agents such as atropine are useful for patients who have AV nodal disturbances, whereas catecholamines such as isoproterenol can be used transiently to treat patients who have heart block at any site (see Sinus Bradycardia). Isoproterenol should be used with extreme caution or not at all in patients who have acute myocardial infarction. The use of transcutaneous pacing is preferable.

AV Dissociation

CLASSIFICATION. As the term AV dissociation indicates, dissociated or independent beating of the atria and ventricles defines AV dissociation. AV dissociation is never a *primary* disturbance of rhythm but is a "symptom" of an underlying rhythm disturbance produced by one of three causes or a combination of causes (Fig. 32–58) that prevent the normal transmission of impulses from atrium to ventricle, as follows:

1. Slowing of the dominant pacemaker of the heart (usually the sinus node), which allows escape of a subsidiary or latent pacemaker. AV dissociation by *default* of the primary pacemaker to a subsidiary one in this manner is often a normal phenomenon. It may occur during sinus arrhythmia or sinus bradycardia and permit an independent AV junction rhythm to arise (see Fig. 32–1B).
2. Acceleration of a latent pacemaker that *usurps* control of the ventricles. An abnormally enhanced discharge rate of a usually slower subsidiary pacemaker is pathological and commonly occurs during nonparoxysmal AV junctional tachycardia or VT without retrograde atrial capture (see Figs. 32–22 and 32–41).
3. Block, generally at the AV junction, that prevents impulses formed at a normal rate in a dominant pacemaker from reaching the ventricles and allows the ventricles to beat under the control of a subsidiary pacemaker. Junctional or ventricular escape rhythm during AV block, without retrograde atrial capture, is a common example in which block gives rise to AV dissociation. Complete AV block is *not* synonymous with complete AV dissociation: Patients who have complete AV block have complete AV dissociation, but patients who have complete AV dissociation may or may not have complete AV block (see Figs. 32–56 and 32–57).
4. A combination of causes, for example, when digitalis excess results in the production of nonparoxysmal AV junctional tachycardia associated with SA or AV block.

MECHANISMS. With this classification in mind, it is important to emphasize that the term *AV dissociation* is *not* a diagnosis and is analogous to the term *jaundice* or *fever.* One must state that "AV dissociation is present *due to . . .*" and then give the cause. An accelerated rate of a slower, normally subsidiary pacemaker or a slower rate of a faster, normally dominant pacemaker that prevents conduction because of physiological collision and mutual extinction of opposing wavefronts (interference) or the manifestations of AV block are the basic disturbances producing AV dissociation. The atria in all these cases beat independently from the ventricles, under control of the sinus node or ectopic atrial or AV junctional pacemakers, and can exhibit any type of supraventricular rhythm. If a single pacemaker establishes control of both atria and ventricles for one beat (capture) or a series of beats (sinus rhythm, AV junctional rhythm with retrograde atrial capture, VT with retrograde atrial capture, and so forth), AV dissociation is abolished for that period. Conversely, as stated earlier, whenever the atria and ventricles fail to respond to a single impulse for one beat (PVC without retrograde capture of the atrium) or a series of beats (VT without retrograde atrial capture), AV dissociation exists for that period. The interruption of AV dissociation by one or a series of beats under the control of one pacemaker, either anterogradely or retrogradely, indicates that the AV dissociation is incomplete. Complete or incomplete dissociation can also occur in association with all forms of AV block. Commonly, when AV dissociation occurs as a result of AV block, the atrial rate exceeds the ventricular rate. For example, a subsidiary pacemaker with a rate of 40 beats/min can escape in the presence of a 2:1 AV block when the atrial rate is 78. If the AV block is bidirectional, AV dissociation results.

ECG AND CLINICAL FEATURES. The ECG demonstrates the independence of P waves and QRS complexes. The P wave morphology depends on the rhythm controlling the atria (sinus, atrial tachycardia, junctional, flutter, or fibrillation). During complete AV dissociation, both the QRS complex and the P waves appear regularly spaced without a fixed temporal relationship to each other. When the dissociation is incomplete, a QRS complex of supraventricular contour occurs early and is preceded by a P wave at a PR interval exceeding 0.12 second and within a conductable range. This combination indicates ventricular capture by the supraventricular focus. Similarly, a premature P wave with retrograde morphology and a conductable RP interval may indicate retrograde atrial capture by the subsidiary focus.

Physical findings include a variable intensity of the first heart sound as the PR interval changes, atrial sounds, and *a* waves in the jugular venous pulse lacking a consistent relationship to ventricular contraction. Intermittent large (cannon) *a* waves may be seen in the jugular venous pulse when atrial and ventricular contractions occur simultaneously. The second heart sound can split normally or paradoxically, depending on the manner of ventricular activation. A premature beat representing ventricular capture can interrupt a regular heart rhythm. When the ventricular rate exceeds the atrial rate, a cyclical increase in intensity of the first heart sound is produced as the PR interval shortens, climaxed by a very loud sound (bruit de canon). This intense sound is followed by a sudden reduction in intensity of the first heart sound and the appearance of giant *a* waves as the PR interval shortens and P waves "march through" the cardiac cycle.

MANAGEMENT. Management is directed toward the underlying heart disease and precipitating cause. The individual components *producing the AV dissociation*—not the AV dissociation per se—determine the specific type of antiarrhythmic approach. Therapy ranges from pacemaker insertion in a patient who has AV dissociation resulting from complete AV block to antiarrhythmic drug administration in a patient who has AV dissociation caused by VT.

Other Electrophysiological Abnormalities Leading to Cardiac Arrhythmias

SUPERNORMAL CONDUCTION

Supernormal conduction is the term applied to situations characterized by conduction that is better than expected but generally not as good as normal. The phenomenon almost always occurs when conduction is depressed but can be present in normal cardiac tissues as well. It generally occurs when conduction takes place during the relative refractory period of the preceding complex (Fig. 32-59). The electrophysiological basis can relate, in some examples, to supernormal excitability (see later) but probably to other mechanisms as well. Supernormal conduction has commonly been invoked to explain AV (most probably His-Purkinje rather than AV nodal) conduction that is more rapid than expected or AV conduction that results when AV block is expected.

SUPERNORMAL EXCITATION

Supernormal excitation results when a stimulus, normally subthreshold, occurs during the supernormal period of recovery of the preceding complex and produces a propagated response. Stimuli occurring earlier or later fail to produce a propagated response. Demonstrated in vitro in Purkinje fibers but not ventricular muscle, supernormal excitation occurs during phase 3 of the cardiac action potential, when the membrane potential, closer to threshold at the end of repolarization, requires less current to produce a propagated response. A similar phenomenon occurs during phase 4 diastolic depolarization or during afterdepolarizations that reduce the membrane potential closer to threshold. The phenomenon is most easily recognized when a nonsensing pacemaker, failing because of battery exhaustion and reduced output, produces a propagated response only when discharge falls during a specific period in a cardiac cycle (Fig. 32-60). Similar phenomena probably occur spontaneously with "weak" automatic foci, but recognition of these events clinically is difficult and often speculative.

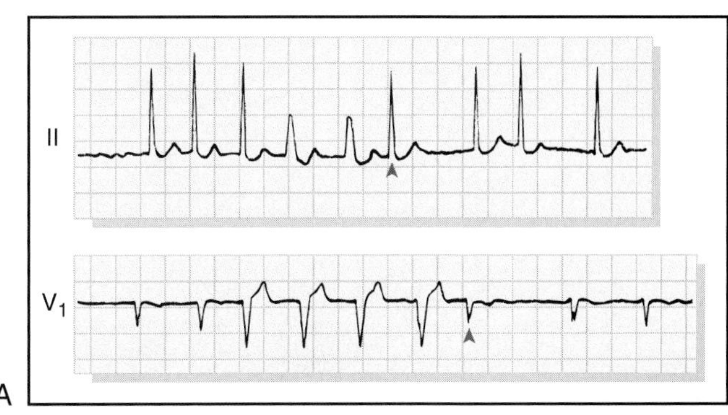

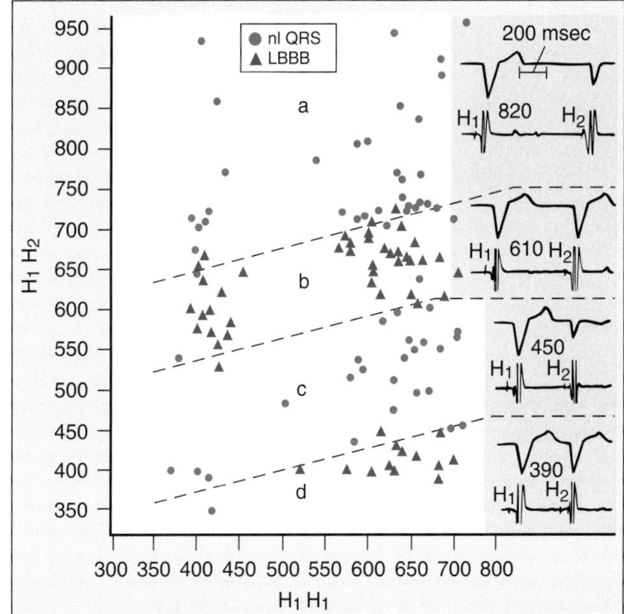

FIGURE 32–59 Supernormal conduction. **A,** Atrial fibrillation with long-short R-R cycle sequences giving rise to QRS complexes conducted with a functional left bundle branch block. In each example, however, a shorter R-R cycle length is terminated by a normal QRS complex (arrowhead), an example of supernormal conduction. **B,** Graph of the intervals and illustrative recordings during an electrophysiological study of the patient whose electrocardiogram is shown in **A**. The H-V interval of the complexes conducted with a left bundle branch block (LBBB) morphology is 45 milliseconds, whereas the H-V interval of those conducted with normal morphology is 35 milliseconds. The graph indicates the premature interval (H_1-H_2, ordinate) plotted against the preceding cycle length (H_1-H_1, abscissa). All H_1-H_1 intervals were taken from complexes with a left bundle branch block morphology. Normal complexes are represented by magenta circles and left bundle branch block contours by blue triangles. Four zones of conduction are identified and illustrated by the four examples to the right. The longest H_1-H_2 intervals are followed by normal intraventricular conduction (zone a), whereas at shorter intervals, left bundle branch block occurs (zone b). When the H_1-H_2 interval shortens further, normal intraventricular conduction returns and the H-V intervals shorten to 35 milliseconds (zone c, supernormal conduction). At the shortest H_1-H_2 interval, left bundle branch block again appears (zone d). (**B,** From Miles WM, Prystowsky EN, Heger JJ, Zipes DP: Evaluation of the patient with wide QRS tachycardia. Med Clin North Am 68:1015, 1984.)

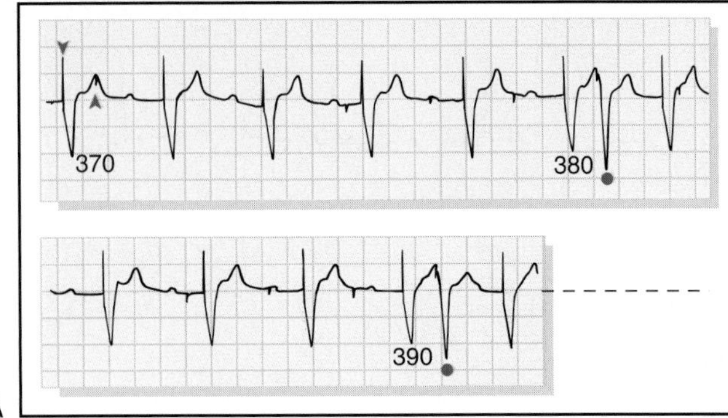

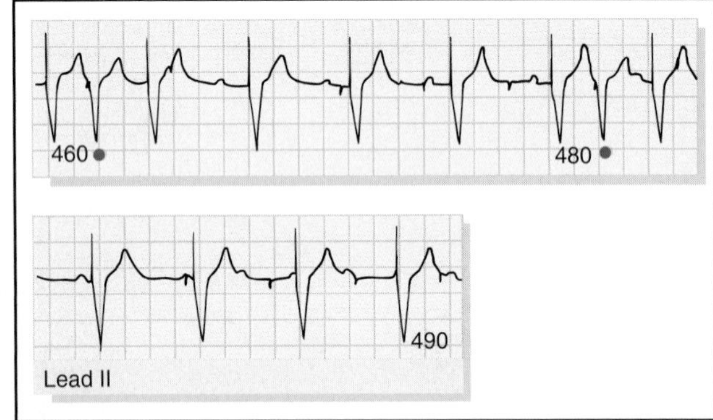

FIGURE 32–60 Supernormal excitation. **A** and **B,** Noncontiguous portions of a continuous electrocardiogram recording with a middle segment removed (dashed line). The patient had a bipolar pacemaker that had exceeded end-of-life status and was no longer consistently producing ventricular depolarization (small negative deflections indicated by the upright arrowhead). A temporary pacemaker was implanted and set at a fixed rate (asynchronous, VOO). These large deflections are indicated by the inverted arrowhead. The numbers in milliseconds indicate the interval between the onset of the QRS complex and the following subthreshold pacemaker stimulus. At intervals of 370 milliseconds (beginning, **A**) and 490 milliseconds (end, **B**), the subthreshold stimulus fails to produce a propagated ventricular response. However, at intervals between 380 and 480 milliseconds, ventricular depolarizations result (red circles). Thus, the period of supernormal excitation is 100 milliseconds in duration, from 380 to 480 milliseconds after the onset of the QRS complex.

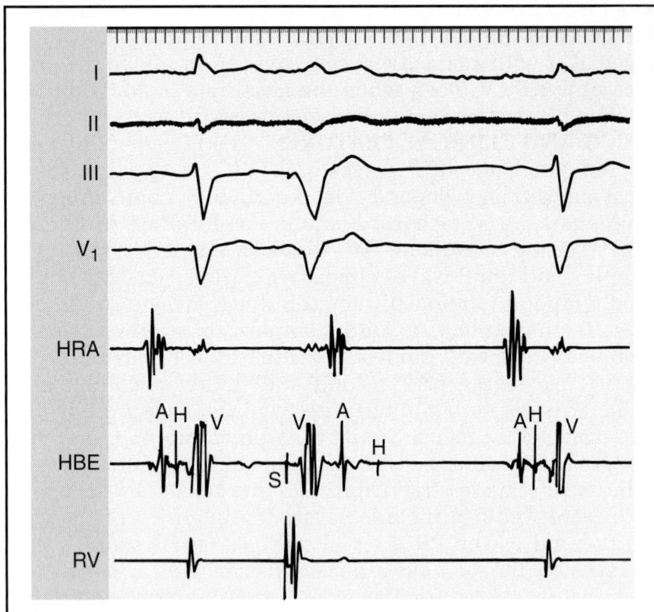

FIGURE 32–61 Concealed conduction. Following the first normally conducted sinus-initiated complex, a premature ventricular complex is stimulated (S). The next spontaneous sinus-initiated P wave is blocked and a fully compensatory pause is produced. The third sinus-initiated P wave is conducted normally. From the His bundle recording it is obvious that the nonconducted sinus beat is blocked distal to the His bundle recording site. Note that the A-H interval of the nonconducted sinus P wave beat is prolonged, which suggests that the retrogradely activated His and invaded the AV node, thereby making it partially refractory to the next sinus beat. Since retrograde conduction into the atrioventricular (AV) node is not recorded and can be surmised only on the basis of the increase in the following A-H interval, it is an example of concealed conduction. Furthermore, since retrograde His and AV node activation by the PVC would not be apparent in the scalar electrocardiogram but is responsible for the compensatory pause, the blocked P wave is an example of concealed conduction.

CONCEALED CONDUCTION

Concealed conduction describes the phenomenon during which impulses penetrate an area of the conduction tissue, the AV node commonly but other areas as well, without emerging. Since transmission of the impulse is concealed, that is, electrically silent in the standard ECG, concealed conduction becomes manifested only by its *effects* on the conduction and/or formation of subsequent impulses.[146] The most common example follows a PVC. Partial retrograde penetration of the AV node by the PVC is *deduced* because the following sinus-initiated P wave blocks conduction to produce a compensatory pause (Fig. 32-61) or conducts with a longer PR interval if the PVC is interpolated. The slower ventricular response when the atrial rate increases from atrial flutter to atrial fibrillation is due to a greater number of atrial impulses being blocked (conducting into, without emerging) in the AV node and is a manifestation of concealed conduction. Concealed conduction occurs in WPW syndrome and can be manifested by unidirectional block anterogradely or retrogradely in an accessory pathway. Concealed junctional extrasystoles can create ECG manifestations of apparent AV block. Strict confirmation of concealed conduction should be the demonstration of conduction, such as in the form of conducted junctional extrasystoles.

PARASYSTOLE

Parasystole (Fig. 32-62) refers to a cardiac arrhythmia characterized electrocardiographically by (1) a varying coupling interval between the ectopic (parasystolic) complex and the dominant (generally, sinus-initiated) complex; (2) a common minimal time interval between interectopic intervals, with the longer interectopic intervals being multiples of this minimal interval; (3) fusion complexes; and (4) presence of the

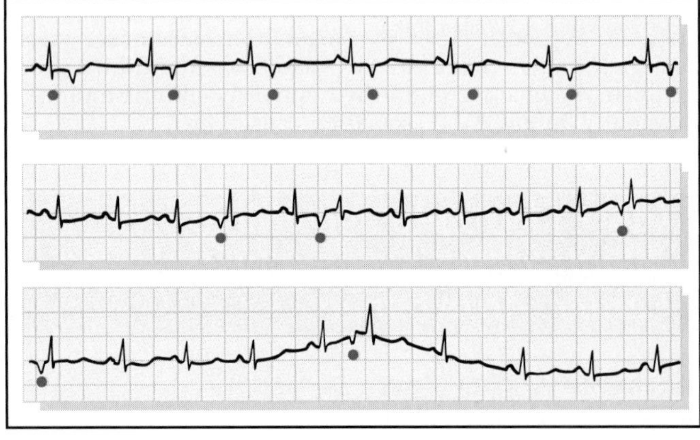

FIGURE 32–62 Atrial parasystole. **Top,** Atrial parasystolic impulses (red circles under the negative P waves) are present at a fixed coupling interval to the dominant sinus rhythm. The reason for the fixed coupling is as follows: Each time that the parasystolic impulse depolarizes the atrium, it also discharges the sinus node. Diastolic depolarization in the sinus node begins at that point (reset) and results in the following sinus P wave (positive P wave). Thus, the constant parasystolic discharge rate (interectopic interval approximately 960 milliseconds), resetting of the sinus node, and constant phase 4 diastolic depolarization in the sinus node combine to result in fixed coupling. **Middle** and **Bottom,** The sinus discharge rate is slightly faster. It is no longer discharged by the parasystolic impulse, which is still occurring at approximately 960 milliseconds (slightly longer interval in the bottom tracing). Variable coupling, the usual manifestation of parasystole, results. Lead II.

parasystolic impulse whenever the cardiac chamber is excitable. Parasystole with exit block is suspected when the parasystolic discharge focus fails to appear even though cardiac tissue is excitable. The analogy commonly invoked to represent parasystole is the behavior of a fixed-rate nonsensing (VOO) pacemaker (see Chap. 31). Parasystole can occur in the sinus and AV nodes, atrium and ventricle, and AV junction. The parasystolic mechanism presumably results from the regular discharge of an automatic focus that is independent of and protected from discharge by the dominant cardiac rhythm. A number of mechanisms have been postulated to explain the apparent protection enjoyed by the parasystolic rhythm.

These classic definitions of parasystole need to be modified because it has been well established that the dominant sinus beats can modulate the discharge rate of the parasystolic rhythm despite entrance block. Thus, wide variations in the modulated parasystolic cycle may occur. The "true," or unmodulated, parasystolic cycle length can be determined by finding two consecutive parasystolic complexes without intervening beats. Phase response curves can be generated. Fixed coupling between the dominant and parasystolic rhythms can occur through a variety of mechanisms, including entrainment. It is possible that modulated parasystole in the presence of supernormal excitability can trigger ventricular fibrillation.

REFERENCES

Individual Cardiac Arrhythmias and Sinus Nodal Disturbances

1. Olgin JE: Inappropriate sinus tachycardia and sinus node reentry. *In* Zipes D, Jalife J (eds): Cardiac Electrophysiology: From Cell to Bedside. 3rd ed. Philadelphia, WB Saunders, 2000, pp 459-468.
2. Gregoratos G, Cheitlin MD, Conill A, et al: ACC/AHA guidelines for implantation of cardiac pacemakers and antiarrhythmia devices: A report of the American College of Cardiology/American Heart Association Task Force on Practice Guidelines (Committee on Pacemaker Implantation). J Am Coll Cardiol 31:1175-1209, 1998.
3. Elvan A, Wylie K, Zipes DP: Pacing-induced chronic atrial fibrillation impairs sinus node function in dogs: Electrophysiological remodeling. Circulation 94:2953-2960, 1996.
4. Bharati S, Lev M: The pathologic changes in the conduction system beyond the age of ninety. Am Heart J 124:486-496, 1992.

Disturbances of Atrial Rhythm

5. Zipes DP, Garson A Jr: 26th Bethesda Conference: Recommendations for determining eligibility for competition in athletes with cardiovascular abnormalities. Task Force 6: Arrhythmias. Med Sci Sports Exerc 26(Suppl):276-283, 1994.
6. Kalman JM, Olgin JE, Saxon LA, et al: Activation and entrainment mapping defines the tricuspid annulus as the anterior barrier in typical atrial flutter. Circulation 94:398-406, 1996.
7. Olgin JE, Kalman JM, Fitzpatrick AP, Lesh MD: Role of right atrial endocardial structures as barriers to conduction during human type I atrial flutter: Activation and entrainment mapping guided by intracardiac echocardiography. Circulation 92:1839-1848, 1995.
8. Kalman JM, Olgin JE, Saxon LA, et al: Electrocardiographic and electrophysiologic characterization of atypical atrial flutter in man: Use of activation and entrainment mapping and implications for catheter ablation. J Cardiovasc Electrophysiol 8:121-144, 1997.
9. Kalman JM, VanHare GF, Olgin JE, et al: Ablation of "incisional" reentrant atrial tachycardia complicating surgery for congenital heart disease: Use of entrainment to define a critical isthmus of conduction. Circulation 93:502-512, 1996.
10. Olgin JE, Jayachandran JV, Engelstein E, et al: Atrial macroreentry involving the myocardium of the coronary sinus—a unique mechanism for atypical flutter. J Cardiovasc Electrophysiol 9:1094-1099, 1998.
11. Stambler BS, Wood MA, Ellenbogen KA, et al: Efficacy and safety of repeated intravenous doses of ibutilide for rapid conversion of atrial flutter or fibrillation. Ibutilide Repeat Dose Study Investigators. Circulation 94:1613-1621, 1996.
12. Abi-Mansour P, Carberry PA, McCowan RJ, et al: Conversion efficacy and safety of repeated doses of ibutilide in patients with atrial flutter and atrial fibrillation. Study Investigators. Am Heart J 136:632–642, 1998.
13. Weiss R, Marcovitz P, Knight BP, et al: Acute changes in spontaneous echo contrast and atrial function after cardioversion of persistent atrial flutter. Am J Cardiol 82:1052-1055, 1998.
14. Kontos MC, Paulsen WH: Impairment of left atrial appendage function after spontaneous conversion of atrial flutter. Clin Cardiol 21:769-771, 1998.
15. Sparks PB, Jayaprakash S, Vohra JK, et al: Left atrial "stunning" following radiofrequency catheter ablation of chronic atrial flutter. J Am Coll Cardiol 32:468-475, 1998.
16. Olgin JE, Lesh MD: The laboratory evaluation and role of catheter ablation for patients with atrial flutter. Cardiol Clin 15:677-688, 1997.
17. Olgin JE, Miles W: Ablation of atrial tachycardias. *In* Singor I, Barold S, Camm A (eds): Nonpharmacological Therapy of Arrhythmias for the 21st Century: The State of the Art. Mount Kisco, NY, Futura, 1998, pp 197-217.
18. Feinberg WM, Cornell ES, Nightingale SD, et al: Relationship between prothrombin activation fragment F1.2 and international normalized ratio in patients with atrial fibrillation. Stroke Prevention in Atrial Fibrillation Investigators. Stroke 28:1101-1106, 1997.
19. Warfarin versus aspirin for prevention of thromboembolism in atrial fibrillation: Stroke Prevention in Atrial Fibrillation II Study. Lancet 343:687-691, 1994.
20. Secondary prevention in non-rheumatic atrial fibrillation after transient ischaemic attack or minor stroke. EAFT (European Atrial Fibrillation Trial) Study Group. Lancet 342:1255-1262, 1993.
21. Ezekowitz MD, Bridgers SL, James KE, et al: Warfarin in the prevention of stroke associated with nonrheumatic atrial fibrillation. Veterans Affairs Stroke Prevention in Nonrheumatic Atrial Fibrillation Investigators. N Engl J Med 327:1406-1412, 1992.
22. Connolly SJ, Laupacis A, Gent M, et al: Canadian Atrial Fibrillation Anticoagulation (CAFA) Study. J Am Coll Cardiol 18:349-355, 1991.
23. The effect of low-dose warfarin on the risk of stroke in patients with nonrheumatic atrial fibrillation. The Boston Area Anticoagulation Trial for Atrial Fibrillation Investigators. N Engl J Med 323:1505-1511, 1990.
24. Petersen P, Boysen G, Godtfredsen J, et al: Placebo-controlled, randomised trial of warfarin and aspirin for prevention of thromboembolic complications in chronic atrial fibrillation. The Copenhagen AFASAK study. Lancet 1:175-179, 1989.
25. Stroke Prevention in Atrial Fibrillation Study. Final results. Circulation 84:527-539, 1991.
26. Klein AL, Grimm RA, Black IW, et al: Cardioversion guided by transesophageal echocardiography: The ACUTE Pilot Study. A randomized, controlled trial. Assessment of Cardioversion Using Transesophageal Echocardiography. Ann Intern Med 126:200-209, 1997.
27. Escudero EM, San Mauro M, Laugle C: Bilateral atrial function after chemical cardioversion of atrial fibrillation with amiodarone: An echo-Doppler study. J Am Soc Echocardiogr 11:365-371, 1998.
28. Omran H, Jung W, Luderitz B: Left atrial appendage function after internal atrial defibrillation. J Cardiovasc Electrophysiol 9(Suppl):97-103, 1998.
29. Wyse DG, Waldo AL, DiMarco JP, et al: A comparison of rate control and rhythm control in patients with atrial fibrillation. N Engl J Med 347:1825-1833, 2002.
30. Hopfner R: Ximelagatran (AstraZeneca). Curr Opin Investig Drugs 3:246-251, 2002.
31. Crystal E, Lamy A, Connolly SJ, et al: Left Atrial Appendage Occlusion Study (LAAOS): A randomized clinical trial of left atrial appendage occlusion during routine coronary artery bypass graft surgery for long-term stroke prevention. Am Heart J 145:174-178, 2003.
32. Sievert H, Lesh MD, Trepels T, et al: Percutaneous left atrial appendage transcatheter occlusion to prevent stroke in high-risk patients with atrial fibrillation: Early clinical experience. Circulation 105:1887-1889, 2002.
33. Hohnloser SH, Kuck KH, Lilienthal J: Rhythm or rate control in atrial fibrillation—Pharmacological Intervention in Atrial Fibrillation (PIAF): A randomised trial. Lancet 356:1789-1794, 2000.
34. Saxonhouse SJ, Curtis AB: Risks and benefits of rate control versus maintenance of sinus rhythm. Am J Cardiol 91:27-32, 2003.
35. Tieleman RG, Van Gelder IC, Crijns HJ, et al: Early recurrences of atrial fibrillation after electrical cardioversion: A result of fibrillation-induced electrical remodeling of the atria? J Am Coll Cardiol 31:167-173, 1998.
36. Franz MR, Karasik PL, Li C, et al: Electrical remodeling of the human atrium: Similar effects in patients with chronic atrial fibrillation and atrial flutter. J Am Coll Cardiol 30:1785-1792, 1997.
37. Daoud EG, Knight BP, Weiss R, et al: Effect of verapamil and procainamide on atrial fibrillation-induced electrical remodeling in humans. Circulation 96:1542-1550, 1997.
38. Olgin JE, Rubart M: Remodeling of the atria and ventricle due to rate. *In* Zipes D, Jalife J (eds): Cardiac Electrophysiology: From Cell to Bedside. 3rd ed. Philadelphia, WB Saunders, 2000, pp 364-378.
39. Sopher SM, Camm AJ: New trials in atrial fibrillation. J Cardiovasc Electrophysiol 9(Suppl):211-215, 1998.
40. Alt E, Ammer R, Schmitt C, et al: A comparison of treatment of atrial fibrillation with low-energy intracardiac cardioversion and conventional external cardioversion. Eur Heart J 18:1796-1804, 1997.
41. Levy S, Ricard P, Lau CP, et al: Multicenter low-energy transvenous atrial defibrillation (XAD) trial results in different subsets of atrial fibrillation. J Am Coll Cardiol 29:750-755, 1997.
42. Oral H, Souza JJ, Michaud GF, et al: Facilitating transthoracic cardioversion of atrial fibrillation with ibutilide pretreatment. N Engl J Med 340:1849-1854, 1999.
43. Mittal S, Ayati S, Stein KM, et al: Transthoracic cardioversion of atrial fibrillation: Comparison of rectilinear biphasic versus damped sine wave monophasic shocks. Circulation. 101:1282-1287, 2000.
44. Page RL, Kerber RE, Russell JK, et al: Biphasic versus monophasic shock waveform for conversion of atrial fibrillation: The results of an international randomized, double-blind multicenter trial. J Am Coll Cardiol 39:1956-1963, 2002.
45. Benditt DG, Samniah N, Iskos D, et al: Biphasic waveform cardioversion as an alternative to internal cardioversion for atrial fibrillation refractory to conventional monophasic waveform transthoracic shock. Am J Cardiol 88:1426-1428, 2001.
46. Viskin S, Barron H, Olgin JE, et al: The treatment of atrial fibrillation: Pharmacologic and non-pharmacological strategies. Curr Probl Cardiol 22:44-108, 1997.
47. Volgman AS, Carberry PA, Stambler B, et al: Conversion efficacy and safety of intravenous ibutilide compared with intravenous procainamide in patients with atrial flutter or fibrillation. J Am Coll Cardiol 31:1414-1419, 1998.
48. Olgin JE, Viskin S: Management of intermittent atrial fibrillation: Drugs to maintain sinus rhythm. J Cardiovasc Electrophysiol 10:433-441, 1999.
49. Lindeboom J, Kingma JH, Crijns HJ, Dunselman PH: Efficacy and safety of intravenous dofetilide for rapid termination of atrial fibrillation and atrial flutter. Am J Cardiol 85:1031-1033, 2000.
50. Sager PT: New advances in class III antiarrhythmic drug therapy. Curr Opin Cardiol 15:41-53, 2000.
51. Pappone C, Oreto G, Rosanio S, et al: Atrial electroanatomic remodeling after circumferential radiofrequency pulmonary vein ablation: Efficacy of an anatomic approach in a large cohort of patients with atrial fibrillation. Circulation 104:2539-2544, 2001.

52. Oral H, Knight BP, Tada H, et al: Pulmonary vein isolation for paroxysmal and persistent atrial fibrillation. Circulation 105:1077-1081, 2002.
53. Jessurun ER, Van Hemel NM, Defauw JJ, et al: A randomized study of combining maze surgery for atrial fibrillation with mitral valve surgery. J Cardiovasc Surg (Torino) 44:9-18, 2003.
54. Jais P, Haissaguerre M, Shah DC, et al: A focal source of atrial fibrillation treated by discrete radiofrequency ablation. Circulation 95:572-576, 1997.
55. Haissaguerre M, Jais P, Shah DC, et al: Spontaneous initiation of atrial fibrillation by ectopic beats originating in the pulmonary veins. N Engl J Med 339:659-666, 1998.
56. Haissaguerre M, Jais P, Shah DC, et al: Catheter ablation of chronic atrial fibrillation targeting the reinitiating triggers. J Cardiovasc Electrophysiol 11:2-10, 2000.
57. Wellens HJ, Lau CP, Luderitz B, et al: Atrioverter: An implantable device for the treatment of atrial fibrillation. Circulation 98:1651-1656, 1998.
58. Bailin SJ, Sulke N, Swerdlow CD: Clinical experience with a dual chamber implantable cardioverter defibrillator in patients with atrial fibrillation and flutter [abstract]. PACE 22:871, 1999.
59. Jung W, Wolpert C, Esmailzadeh B, et al: Clinical experience with implantable atrial and combined atrioventricular defibrillators. J Interv Cardiol Electrophysiol 4(Suppl 1):185-195, 2000.
60. Pollak A, Falk RH: Pacemaker therapy in patients with atrial fibrillation. Am Heart J 125:824-830, 1993.
61. Delfaut P, Saksena S, Prakash A, Krol RB: Long-term outcome of patients with drug-refractory atrial flutter and fibrillation after single- and dual-site right atrial pacing for arrhythmia prevention. J Am Coll Cardiol 32:1900-1908, 1998.
63. Waldo AL: Atrial flutter: Entrainment characteristics. J Cardiovasc Electrophysiol 8:337-352, 1997.

AV Junctional Rhythm Disturbances

64. Glatter KA, Cheng J, Dorostkar P, et al: Electrophysiologic effects of adenosine in patients with supraventricular tachycardia. Circulation 99:1034-1040, 1999.
65. Miles WM, Zipes DP: Atrioventricular reentry and variants: Mechanisms, clinical features, and management. *In* Zipes DP, Jalife J (eds): Cardiac Electrophysiology: From Cell to Bedside. 3rd ed. Philadelphia, WB Saunders, 2000, pp 638-655.
66. Arruda MS, McClelland JH, Wang X, et al: Development and validation of an ECG algorithm for identifying accessory pathway ablation site in Wolff-Parkinson-White syndrome. J Cardiovasc Electrophysiol 9:2-12, 1998.
68. Morady F: Radio-frequency ablation as treatment for cardiac arrhythmias. N Engl J Med 340:534-544, 1999.

Ventricular Rhythm Disturbances

69. Oreto G, Luzza F, Badessa F, et al: QRS complex voltage changes associated with supraventricular tachycardia. J Cardiovasc Electrophysiol 12:1358-1362, 2001.
71. Kennedy HL: Use of long-term (Holter) electrocardiographic recordings. *In* Zipes DP, Jalife J (eds): Cardiac Electrophysiology: From Cell to Bedside. 3rd ed. Philadelphia, WB Saunders, 2000, pp 716-730.
72. Singh BN: Beta-blockers and calcium channel blockers as anti-arrhythmic drugs. *In* Zipes DP, Jalife J (eds): Cardiac Electrophysiology: From Cell to Bedside. 3rd ed. Philadelphia, WB Saunders, 2000, pp 903-921.
73. Miller JM, Hsia HH, Rothman SA, Buxton AE: Ventricular tachycardia versus supraventricular tachycardia with aberration: Electrocardiographic distinctions. *In* Zipes DP, Jalife J (eds): Cardiac Electrophysiology: From Cell to Bedside. 3rd ed. Philadelphia, WB Saunders, 2000, pp 696-705.
74. Myerburg RJ, Kessler KM, Kimura S: Life-threatening ventricular arrhythmias: The link between epidemiology and pathophysiology. *In* Zipes DP, Jalife J (eds): Cardiac Electrophysiology: From Cell to Bedside. 3rd ed. Philadelphia, WB Saunders, 2000, pp 521 530.
75. Armoundas AA, Rosenbaum DS, Ruskin JN, et al: Prognostic significance of electrical alternans versus signal averaged electrocardiography in predicting the outcome of electrophysiological testing and arrhythmia-free survival. Heart 80:251-256, 1998.
76. Hohnloser SH, Klingenheben T, Li YG, et al: T wave alternans as a predictor of recurrent ventricular tachyarrhythmias in ICD recipients: Prospective comparison with conventional risk markers. J Cardiovasc Electrophysiol 9:1258-1268, 1998.
77. Gold MR, Bloomfield DM, Anderson KP, et al: A comparison of T-wave alternans, signal averaged electrocardiography, and programmed ventricular stimulation for arrhythmia risk stratification. J Am Coll Cardiol 36:2247-2253, 2000.
78. Somberg JC, Bailin SJ, Haffajee CI, et al: Intravenous lidocaine versus intravenous amiodarone (in a new aqueous formulation) for incessant ventricular tachycardia. Am J Cardiol 90:853-859, 2002.
79. A randomized trial of propranolol in patients with acute myocardial infarction: I. Mortality results. JAMA 247:1707-1714, 1982.
80. Echt DS, Liebson PR, Mitchell LB, et al: Mortality and morbidity in patients receiving encainide, flecainide, or placebo. The Cardiac Arrhythmia Suppression Trial. N Engl J Med 324:781-788, 1991.
81. Waldo AL, Camm AJ, deRuyter H, et al: Effect of *d*-sotalol on mortality in patients with left ventricular dysfunction after recent and remote myocardial infarction. The SWORD Investigators. Survival with Oral *d*-Sotalol. Lancet 348:7-12, 1996.
82. Julian DG, Camm AJ, Frangin G, et al: Randomised trial of effect of amiodarone on mortality in patients with left-ventricular dysfunction after recent myocardial infarction: EMIAT. European Myocardial Infarct Amiodarone Trial Investigators. Lancet 349:667-674, 1997.
83. Cairns JA, Connolly SJ, Roberts R, Gent M: Randomised trial of outcome after myocardial infarction in patients with frequent or repetitive ventricular premature depolarisations: CAMIAT. Canadian Amiodarone Myocardial Infarction Arrhythmia Trial Investigators. Lancet 349:675-682, 1997.
84. Doval HC, Nul DR, Grancelli HO, et al: Nonsustained ventricular tachycardia in severe heart failure: Independent marker of increased mortality due to sudden death. GESICA-GEMA Investigators. Circulation 94:3198-3203, 1996.
85. Singh SN, Fletcher RD, Fisher SG, et al: Amiodarone in patients with congestive heart failure and asymptomatic ventricular arrhythmia. Survival Trial of Antiarrhythmic Therapy in Congestive Heart Failure. N Engl J Med 333:77-82, 1995.
87. Klein H, Auricchio A, Reek S, Geller C: New primary prevention trials of sudden cardiac death in patients with left ventricular dysfunction: SCD-HEFT and MADIT-II. Am J Cardiol 83:91D-97D, 1999.
88. Bigger JT Jr, Whang W, Rottman JN, et al: Mechanisms of death in the CABG Patch trial: A randomized trial of implantable cardiac defibrillator prophylaxis in patients at high risk of death after coronary artery bypass graft surgery. Circulation 99:1416-1421, 1999.
89. Moss AJ, Hall WJ, Cannom DS, et al: Improved survival with an implanted defibrillator in patients with coronary disease at high risk for ventricular arrhythmia. Multicenter Automatic Defibrillator Implantation Trial Investigators. N Engl J Med 335:1933-1940, 1996.
90. Buxton AE, Lee KL, Fisher JD, et al: A randomized study of the prevention of sudden death in patients with coronary artery disease. Multicenter Unsustained Tachycardia Trial Investigators. N Engl J Med 341:1882-1890, 1999.
91. Mason JW: A comparison of electrophysiologic testing with Holter monitoring to predict antiarrhythmic-drug efficacy for ventricular tachyarrhythmias. Electrophysiologic Study versus Electrocardiographic Monitoring Investigators. N Engl J Med 329:445-451, 1993.
92. Mason JW: A comparison of seven antiarrhythmic drugs in patients with ventricular tachyarrhythmias. Electrophysiologic Study versus Electrocardiographic Monitoring Investigators. N Engl J Med 329:452-458, 1993.
93. Greene HL: The CASCADE Study: Randomized antiarrhythmic drug therapy in survivors of cardiac arrest in Seattle. CASCADE Investigators. Am J Cardiol 72:70F-74F, 1993.
94. Siebels J, Cappato R, Ruppel R, et al: Preliminary results of the Cardiac Arrest Study Hamburg (CASH). CASH Investigators. Am J Cardiol 72:109F-113F, 1993.
95. A comparison of antiarrhythmic-drug therapy with implantable defibrillators in patients resuscitated from near-fatal ventricular arrhythmias. The Antiarrhythmics versus Implantable Defibrillators (AVID) Investigators. N Engl J Med 337:1576-1583, 1997.
96. Cappato R: Secondary prevention of sudden death: The Dutch Study, the Antiarrhythmics Versus Implantable Defibrillator Trial, the Cardiac Arrest Study Hamburg, and the Canadian Implantable Defibrillator Study. Am J Cardiol 83:68D-73D, 1999.
97. Connolly SJ, Gent M, Roberts RS, et al: Canadian Implantable Defibrillator Study (CIDS): Study design and organization. CIDS Co-Investigators. Am J Cardiol 72:103F-108F, 1993.
98. Moss AJ, Hall WJ, Cannom DS, et al: Improved survival with an implanted defibrillator in patients with coronary disease at high risk for ventricular arrhythmia. Multicenter Automatic Defibrillator Implantation Trial Investigators. N Engl J Med 335:1933-1940, 1996.
99. Buxton AE, Lee KL, Fisher JD, et al: A randomized study of the prevention of sudden death in patients with coronary artery disease. Multicenter Unsustained Tachycardia Trial Investigators. N Engl J Med 341:1882-1890, 1999.
100. Moss AJ, Zareba W, Hall WJ, et al: Prophylactic implantation of a defibrillator in patients with myocardial infarction and reduced ejection fraction. N Engl J Med 346:877-883, 2002.
101. Rothman SA, Hsia HH, Cossu SF, et al: Radiofrequency catheter ablation of postinfarction ventricular tachycardia: Long-term success and the significance of inducible nonclinical arrhythmias. Circulation 96:3499-3508, 1997.
102. Strickberger SA, Man KC, Daoud EG, et al: A prospective evaluation of catheter ablation of ventricular tachycardia as adjuvant therapy in patients with coronary artery disease and an implantable cardioverter-defibrillator. Circulation 96:1525-1531, 1997.
103. Miller JM, Engelstein ED, Groh WJ, et al: Radiofrequency catheter ablation for postinfarct ventricular tachycardia. Curr Opin Cardiol 14:30-35, 1999.
104. Corrado D, Basso C, Thiene G, et al: Spectrum of clinicopathologic manifestations of arrhythmogenic right ventricular cardiomyopathy/dysplasia: A multicenter study. J Am Coll Cardiol 30:1512-1520, 1997.
105. Corrado D, Basso C, Schiavon M, Thiene G: Screening for hypertrophic cardiomyopathy in young athletes. N Engl J Med 339:364-369, 1998.
106. Li D, Ahmad F, Gardner MJ, et al: The locus of a novel gene responsible for arrhythmogenic right-ventricular dysplasia characterized by early onset and high penetrance maps to chromosome 10p12-p14. Am J Hum Genet 66:148-156, 2000.
107. Li D, Bachinski LL, Roberts R: Genomic organization and isoform-specific tissue expression of human NAPOR (CUGBP2) as a candidate gene for familial arrhythmogenic right ventricular dysplasia. Genomics 74:396-401, 2001.
108. Tiso N, Stephan DA, Nava A, et al: Identification of mutations in the cardiac ryanodine receptor gene in families affected with arrhythmogenic right ventricular cardiomyopathy type 2 (*ARVD2*). Hum Mol Genet 10:189-194, 2001.
109. Sakabe K, Ikeda T, Sakata T, et al: Comparison of T-wave alternans and QT interval dispersion to predict ventricular tachyarrhythmia in patients with dilated cardiomyopathy and without antiarrhythmic drugs: A prospective study. Jpn Heart J 42:451-457, 2001.
110. Sakabe K, Ikeda T, Sakata T, et al: Predicting the recurrence of ventricular tachyarrhythmias from T-wave alternans assessed on antiarrhythmic pharmacotherapy: A prospective study in patients with dilated cardiomyopathy. Ann Noninvasive Electrocardiol 6:203-208, 2001.
111. Kuroda N, Ohnishi Y, Yoshida A, et al: Clinical significance of T-wave alternans in hypertrophic cardiomyopathy. Circ J 66:457-462, 2002.
112. Primo J, Geelen P, Brugada J, et al: Hypertrophic cardiomyopathy: Role of the implantable cardioverter-defibrillator. J Am Coll Cardiol 31:1081-1085, 1998.
113. Leenhardt A, Lucet V, Denjoy I, et al: Catecholaminergic polymorphic ventricular tachycardia in children: A 7-year follow-up of 21 patients. Circulation 91:1512-1519, 1995.
114. Priori SG, Napolitano C, Memmi M, et al: Clinical and molecular characterization of patients with catecholaminergic polymorphic ventricular tachycardia. Circulation 106:69-74, 2002.

115. Gussak I, Antzelevitch C, Bjerregaard P, et al: The Brugada syndrome: Clinical, electrophysiologic, and genetic aspects. J Am Coll Cardiol 33:5-15, 1999.
116. Alings M, Wilde A: "Brugada" syndrome: Clinical data and suggested pathophysiological mechanism. Circulation 99:666-673, 1999.
117. Brugada P, Geelen P: Some electrocardiographic patterns predicting sudden cardiac death that every doctor should recognize. Acta Cardiol 52:473-484, 1997.
118. Brugada J, Brugada R, Brugada P: Right bundle-branch block and ST-segment elevation in leads V_1 through V_3: A marker for sudden death in patients without demonstrable structural heart disease. Circulation 97:457-460, 1998.
119. Chen Q, Kirsch GE, Zhang D, et al: Genetic basis and molecular mechanism for idiopathic ventricular fibrillation. Nature 392:293-296, 1998.
120. Potet F, Mabo P, Le Coq G, et al: Novel Brugada *SCN5A* mutation leading to ST segment elevation in the inferior or the right precordial leads. J Cardiovasc Electrophysiol 14:200-203, 2003.
121. Viswanathan PC, Benson DW, Balser JR: A common *SCN5A* polymorphism modulates the biophysical effects of an *SCN5A* mutation. J Clin Invest 111:341-346, 2003.
122. Veldkamp MW, Viswanathan PC, Bezzina C, et al: Two distinct congenital arrhythmias evoked by a multidysfunctional Na^+ channel. Circ Res 86:E91-E97, 2000.
123. Lerman BB, Dong B, Stein KM, et al: Right ventricular outflow tract tachycardia due to a somatic cell mutation in G protein subunit alpha 2. J Clin Invest 101:2862-2868, 1998.
124. Markowitz SM, Litvak BL, Ramirez de Arellano EA, et al: Adenosine-sensitive ventricular tachycardia: Right ventricular abnormalities delineated by magnetic resonance imaging. Circulation 96:1192-1200, 1997.
125. Callans DJ, Menz V, Schwartzman D, et al: Repetitive monomorphic tachycardia from the left ventricular outflow tract: Electrocardiographic patterns consistent with a left ventricular site of origin. J Am Coll Cardiol 29:1023-1027, 1997.
126. Schwartz PJ, Stramba-Badiale M, Segantini A, et al: Prolongation of the QT interval and the sudden infant death syndrome. N Engl J Med 338:1709-1714, 1998.
127. Priori SG, Napolitano C, Giordano U, et al: Brugada syndrome and sudden cardiac death in children. Lancet 355:808-809, 2000.
128. Schwartz PJ, Locati EH, Napolitano C: The long QT syndrome. *In* Zipes DP, Jalife J (eds): Cardiac Electrophysiology: From Cell to Bedside. 3rd ed. Philadelphia, WB Saunders, 2000, 788-811.
129. Viskin S, Belhassen B: Polymorphic ventricular tachyarrhythmias in the absence of organic heart disease: Classification, differential diagnosis, and implications for therapy. Prog Cardiovasc Dis 41:17-34, 1998.
130. Shimizu W, Antzelevitch C: Cellular basis for the ECG features of the LQT1 form of the long-QT syndrome: Effects of beta-adrenergic agonists and antagonists and sodium channel blockers on transmural dispersion of repolarization and torsades de pointes. Circulation 98:2314-2322, 1998.
131. Molnar J, Zhang F, Weiss J, et al: Diurnal pattern of QTc interval: how long is prolonged? Possible relation to circadian triggers of cardiovascular events. J Am Coll Cardiol 27:76-83, 1996.
133. Wang Q, Chen Q, Towbin JA: Genetics, molecular mechanisms and management of long QT syndrome. Ann Med 30:58-65, 1998.
134. Priori SG, Barhanin J, Hauer RN, et al: Genetic and molecular basis of cardiac arrhythmias: Impact on clinical management, parts I and II. Circulation 99:518-528, 1999.
135. Wang Q, Chen Q, Li H, Towbin JA: Molecular genetics of long QT syndrome from genes to patients. Curr Opin Cardiol 12:310-320, 1997.
136. Priori SG, Napolitano C, Schwartz PJ: Low penetrance in the long-QT syndrome: Clinical impact. Circulation 99:529-533, 1999.
136a. Roden DM: Drug-induced prolongations of the QT interval. N Engl J Med 350:1013–1022, 2004.
137. Zareba W, Moss AJ, Schwartz PJ, et al: Influence of genotype on the clinical course of the long-QT syndrome. International Long-QT Syndrome Registry Research Group. N Engl J Med 339:960-965, 1998.
138. Viskin S, Fish R, Roth A, Copperman Y: Prevention of torsades de pointes in the congenital long QT syndrome: Use of a pause prevention pacing algorithm. Heart 79:417-419, 1998.
139. Moss AJ: Clinical management of patients with the long QT syndrome: Drugs, devices, and gene-specific therapy. Pacing Clin Electrophysiol 20:2058-2060, 1997.
140. Epstein AE, Ideker RE: Ventricular fibrillation. *In* Zipes DP, Jalife J (eds): Cardiac Electrophysiology: From Cell to Bedside. 3rd ed. Philadelphia, WB Saunders, 2000, pp 927-933.
141. Zipes DP: Warning: The short days of winter may be hazardous to your health. Circulation 100:1590-1592, 1999.
143. Guidelines 2000 for Cardiopulmonary Resuscitation and Emergency Cardiovascular Care. Part 6: Advanced Cardiovascular Life Support: 7C: A Guide to the International ACLS algorithms. The American Heart Association in collaboration with the International Liaison Committee on Resuscitation. Circulation 102:I142-I157, 2000.

Heart Block

144. Rardon DP, Miles WM, Zipes DP: Atrioventricular block and AV dissociation. *In* Zipes DP, Jalife J (eds): Cardiac Electrophysiology: From Cell to Bedside. 3rd ed. Philadelphia, WB Saunders, 2000, pp 935-942.

Other Electyrophysiological Abnormalities Leading to Arrhythmias

145. Probst V, Kyndt F, Potet F, et al: Haploinsufficiency in combination with aging causes *SCN5A*-linked hereditary Lenegre disease. J Am Coll Cardiol 41:643-652, 2003.
146. Fisch C: Electrocardiographic manifestations of exit block, concealed conduction and "supernormal" conduction. *In* Zipes DP, Jalife J (eds): Cardiac Electrophysiology: From Cell to Bedside. 3rd ed. Philadelphia, WB Saunders, 2000, pp 955-976.

CHAPTER 33

Cardiac Arrest and Sudden Cardiac Death

Robert J. Myerburg • Agustin Castellanos

Definitions

Sudden cardiac death (SCD) is natural death from cardiac causes, heralded by abrupt loss of consciousness within 1 hour of the onset of acute symptoms. Preexisting heart disease may or may not have been known to be present, but the time and mode of death are unexpected. This definition incorporates the key elements of "natural," "rapid," and "unexpected." It consolidates previous definitions that have conflicted, largely because the most useful operational definition of SCD in the past differed for the clinician, the cardiovascular epidemiologist, the pathologist, and the scientist attempting to define pathophysiological mechanisms. As causes and mechanisms began to be understood, these differences faded.[1]

Four time elements must be considered in the construction of a definition of SCD to satisfy clinical, scientific, legal, and social considerations: (1) prodromes, (2) onset, (3) cardiac arrest, and (4) biological death (Fig. 33–1). Because the proximate cause of SCD is an abrupt disturbance of cardiovascular function, which is incompatible with maintaining consciousness because of abrupt loss of cerebral blood flow, any definition must recognize the brief time interval between the onset of the mechanism directly responsible for cardiac arrest and the consequent loss of consciousness (Fig. 33–1C). The 1-hour definition, however, refers to the duration of the "terminal event" (Fig. 33–1B), which defines the interval between the onset of symptoms signaling the pathophysiological disturbance leading to cardiac arrest and the onset of the cardiac arrest itself (Fig. 33–1B and C).

Premonitory signs and symptoms are often absent,[2] but nonspecific symptoms can occur during the days or weeks before a cardiac arrest. Prodromes (Fig. 33–1A) are poor predictors of an impending event because of low sensitivity but may be more specific for an imminent cardiac arrest when they begin abruptly. Sudden onset of chest pain, dyspnea, or palpitations and other symptoms of arrhythmias often precede the onset of cardiac arrest. The fourth element, *biological death* (Fig. 33–1D), was an immediate consequence of the clinical cardiac arrest in the past, usually occurring within minutes. However, since the development of community-based interventions and life support systems, patients may now remain biologically alive for a long period of time after the onset of a pathophysiological process that has caused irreversible damage and will ultimately lead to death. In this circumstance, the causative pathophysiological and clinical event is the cardiac arrest itself rather than the factors responsible for the delayed biological death. However, because of legal, forensic, and certain social considerations, biological death must continue to be used as the absolute definition of death. Finally, the forensic pathologist studying *unwitnessed deaths* may use the definition of sudden death for a person known to be alive and functioning normally 24 hours before, and this remains appropriate within obvious limits. The generally accepted clinical-pathophysiological definition of up to 1 hour between onset of the terminal event and biological death requires qualifications for specific circumstances.

The development of community-based intervention systems has also led to inconsistencies in the use of terms considered absolute. *Death* is defined biologically, legally, and literally as an absolute and irreversible event. Thus, SCD can be aborted, or a patient can survive cardiac arrest or cardiovascular collapse; however, survival after (sudden) death is a contradiction in terms. Table 33–1 provides definitions for events and terms related to the concept of SCD—death, cardiac arrest, and cardiovascular collapse.

Epidemiology

Epidemiological Overview

The worldwide incidence of SCD is difficult to estimate because it varies largely as a function of coronary heart disease prevalence in different countries (see Chap. 1).[3] Estimates for the United States, largely based upon retrospective death certificate

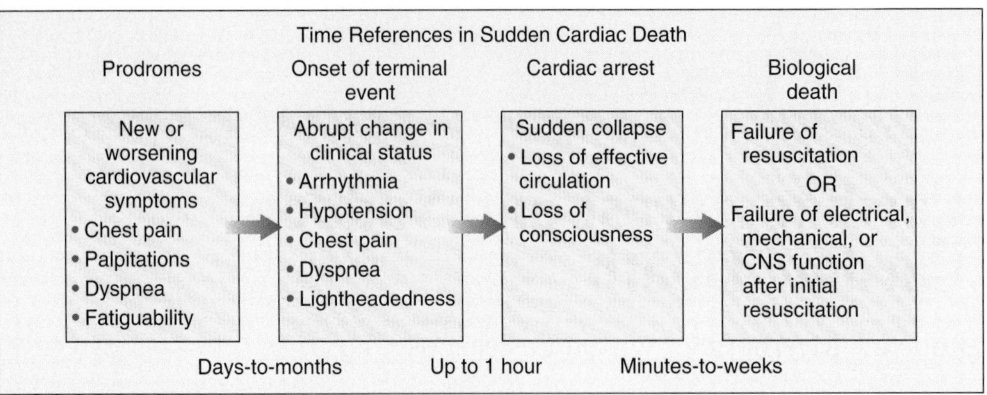

FIGURE 33–1 Sudden cardiac death viewed from four temporal perspectives: (1) prodromes, (2) onset of the terminal event, (3) cardiac arrest, and (4) progression to biological death. Individual variability of the components influences clinical expression. Some victims experience no prodromes, with onset leading almost instantaneously to cardiac arrest; others may have an onset that lasts up to 1 hour before clinical arrest. Some patients may live days to weeks after the cardiac arrest before biological death, often because of irreversible brain damage and dependence upon life support. These factors influence interpretation of the 1-hour definition. The two most relevant clinical factors are onset of the terminal event (2) and the clinical cardiac arrest itself (3); legal and social considerations focus on the time of biological death (4). CNS = central nervous system.

analyses[4-7] and an emergency rescue data base in one study,[8] range from less than 200,000 to more than 450,000 SCDs annually, with the most widely used estimates in the range of 300,000 to 350,000 SCDs annually.[9] The variation is based in part on the definition of sudden death and inclusion criteria used in individual studies, and the correct number can be found only from a carefully designed prospective epidemiological study.

The temporal definition of sudden death strongly influences epidemiological data. Retrospective death certificate studies have demonstrated that a temporal definition of death less than 2 hours after the onset of symptoms results in 12 to 15 percent of all natural deaths being defined as "sudden" and nearly 90 percent of all natural sudden deaths being due to cardiac causes. In contrast, the application of a 24-hour definition of sudden death increases the fraction of all natural deaths falling into the sudden category to more than 30 percent but reduces the proportion of all sudden natural deaths that are due to cardiac causes to 75 percent.

Prospective studies demonstrate that about 50 percent of all coronary heart disease deaths are sudden and unexpected, occurring shortly (instantaneous to 1 hour) after the onset of symptoms. Because coronary heart disease is the dominant cause of both sudden and nonsudden cardiac deaths in the United States, the fraction of total cardiac deaths that are sudden is similar to the fraction of deaths from coronary heart disease that are sudden, although there does appear to be a geographical variation in the fraction of coronary deaths that are sudden.[10] It is also of interest that the age-adjusted decline in coronary heart disease mortality in the United States during the past half-century[11] has not changed the fraction of coronary deaths that are sudden and unexpected,[12] even though there may be a decline in out-of-hospital deaths compared with emergency department deaths.[4] Furthermore, the decreasing age-adjusted mortality does not imply a decrease in absolute numbers of cardiac or sudden deaths because of the growth and aging of the U.S. population and the increasing prevalence of chronic heart disease.[13,14]

TABLE 33–1 Definition of Terms Related to Sudden Cardiac Death

Term	Definition	Qualifiers or Exceptions
Death	Irreversible cessation of all biological functions	None
Cardiac arrest	Abrupt cessation of cardiac pump function, which may be reversible but will lead to death in the absence of prompt intervention	Rare spontaneous reversions, likelihood of successful intervention relates to mechanism of arrest, clinical setting, and time to intervention
Cardiovascular collapse	A (sudden) loss of effective blood flow due to cardiac and/or peripheral vascular factors that may revert spontaneously (e.g., vasodepressor or cardioinhibitory syncope) or only with interventions (e.g., cardiac arrest)	Nonspecific term that includes cardiac arrest and its consequences and also events that characteristically revert spontaneously

FIGURE 33–2 Impact of population subgroups and time from events on the clinical epidemiology of sudden cardiac death (SCD). **A,** Estimates of incidence (percent per year) and the total number of events per year for the general adult population in the United States and for increasingly high risk subgroups. The overall adult population has an estimated sudden death incidence of 0.1 to 0.2 percent per year, accounting for a total of more than 300,000 events per year. With the identification of increasingly powerful risk factors, the incidence *increases* progressively, but it is accomplished by a progressive *decrease* in the total number of events represented by each group. The inverse relationship between incidence and total number of events occurs because of the progressively smaller denominator pool in the highest subgroup categories. Successful interventions among larger population subgroups require identification of specific markers to increase the ability to identify specific patients who are at particularly high risk for a future event. (Note: The horizontal axis for the incidence figures is not linear and should be interpreted accordingly. **B,** The distribution of clinical status of victims at the time of SCD. Nearly two-thirds of cardiac arrests occur as the first clinically manifest event or in the clinical setting of known disease in the absence of strong risk predictors. Less than 25 percent of the victims have high-risk markers based on arrhythmic or hemodynamic parameters. **C,** Idealized curves of SCD risk for a population of patients with known cardiovascular disease but at low risk because of freedom from major cardiovascular events (top curve) and for populations of patients who have survived a major cardiovascular event (bottom curve). Attrition over time is accelerated in both absolute and relative terms for the initial 6 to 18 months after the major cardiovascular event. After the initial attrition, the slopes of the curves for the high-risk and low-risk populations parallel each other, highlighting both the early attrition and the attenuation of risk after 18 to 24 months. These relations have been observed in diverse high-risk subgroups (cardiac arrest survivors, post-myocardial infarction patients with high-risk markers, recent onset of heart failure). AP = angina pectoris; EF = ejection fraction; M.I. = myocardial infarction. (**A,** From Myerburg et al, reference 14; reproduced with permission of the American Heart Association; **B,** modified from Myerburg RJ: Sudden cardiac death: Exploring the limits of our knowledge. J Cardiovasc Electrophysiol 12:369, 2001; **C,** modified from Myerburg RJ, Kessler KM, Castellanos A: Sudden cardiac death: Structure, function, and time-dependence of risk. Circulation 85[Suppl I]:I-2, 1992. Copyright 1992 American Heart Association.)

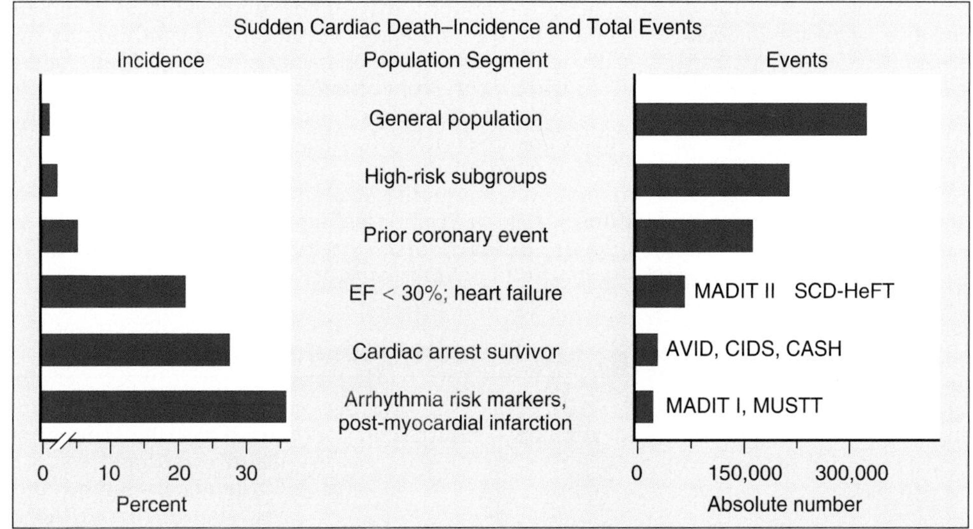

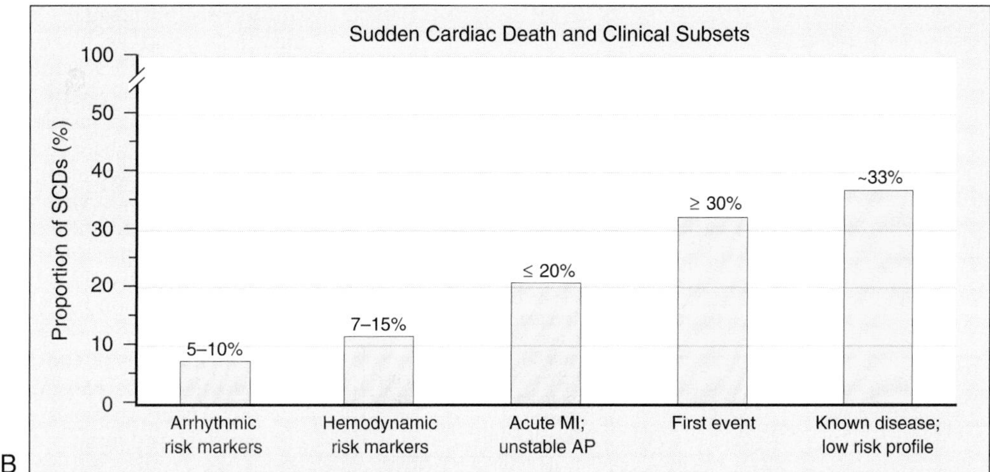

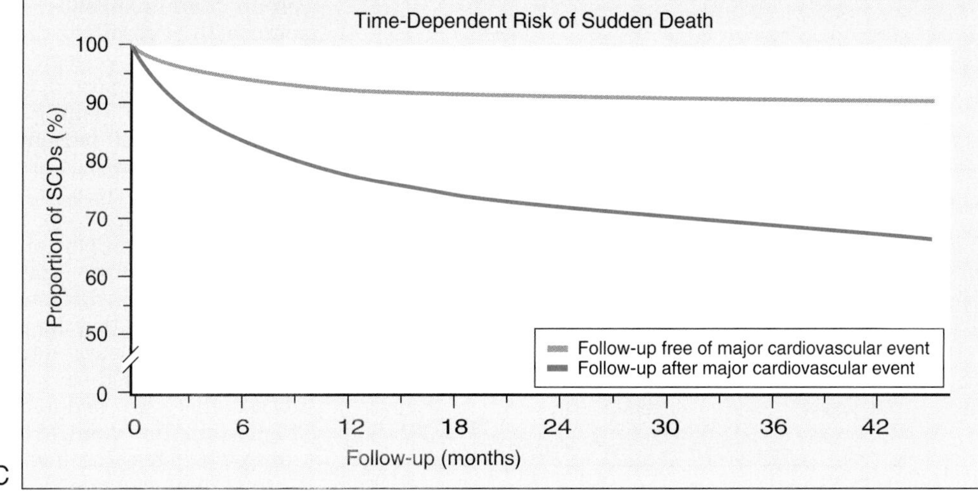

Population Pools and Time Dependence of Risk

Three factors are of primary importance for identifying populations at risk and consideration of strategies for prevention of SCD: (1) the absolute numbers and event rates (incidence) among population subgroups (Fig. 33–2A), (2) the clinical subgroups in which SCDs occur (Fig. 33–2B), and (3) the time dependence of risk (Fig. 33–2C).

POPULATION SUBGROUPS AND SUDDEN CARDIAC DEATH. When the more than 300,000 adult SCDs that occur annually in the United States are viewed as a global incidence in an unselected adult population, the overall incidence is 1 to 2 per 1000 population (0.1 to 0.2 percent) per year (see Fig. 33–2A). This large population base includes victims whose SCDs occur as a first cardiac event as well as those whose SCDs can be predicted with greater accuracy because they are included in higher risk subgroups (see Fig. 33–2B). Any intervention designed for the general population must, therefore, be applied to the 999 per 1000 who do not have an event in order to reach and possibly influence the 1 per 1000 who does. The cost and risk-to-benefit uncertainties limit the nature of such broad-based interventions and demand a higher resolution of risk identification. Figure 33–2A highlights this problem by expressing the incidence (percent per year) of SCD among various subgroups and comparing the incidence figures with the total number of events that occur annually in each subgroup. On moving from the total adult population to a subgroup at higher risk because of the presence of selected coronary risk factors, there may be a 10-fold or greater increase in the incidence of events annually, with the magnitude of increase dependent on the number of risk factors operating in the subgroup. The size of the denominator pool, however, remains very large, and implementation of interventions remains problematic, even at this heightened level of risk. Higher resolution is desirable and can be achieved by identification of more specific subgroups. However, the corresponding absolute number of deaths becomes progressively smaller as the subgroups become more focused (see Fig. 33–2A), limiting the potential benefit of interventions to a much smaller fraction of the total number of patients at risk. Various estimates suggest that at least one-third of all SCDs related to coronary heart disease occur as a first clinical event.

In addition, another one-third occur among subgroups of patients with known coronary heart disease profiled at relatively low risk for SCD (see Fig. 33–2B).[11]

BIOLOGICAL AND CLINICAL TIME-DEPENDENT RISK. Temporal elements in risk of SCD have been analyzed in the context of both biological and clinical chronology. In the former, epidemiological analyses of SCD risk among populations have identified three patterns: diurnal, weekly, and seasonal. General patterns of heightened risk during the morning hours, on Mondays, and during the winter months have been described.[15] In the clinical paradigm, risk of SCD is not linear as a function of time after changes in cardiovascular status.[9,14,16] Survival curves after major cardiovascular events, which identify risk for both sudden and total cardiac death, usually demonstrate that the most rapid rate of attrition occurs during the first 6 to 18 months after the index event (see Fig. 33–2C). Thus, there is a time dependence of risk that focuses the opportunity for maximum efficacy of an intervention during the early period after a conditioning event. Curves that have these characteristics have been generated from among survivors of out-of-hospital cardiac arrest, new onset of heart failure, and unstable angina and from high-risk subgroups of patients having recent myocardial infarction. Even though attrition rates decrease over time, an effective intervention can still cause late diversion of treated versus control risk curves, indicating continuing benefit. *The addition of time as a dimension for measuring risk may increase the resolution within subgroups.*

Age, Heredity, Gender, and Race

AGE. There are two ages of peak incidence of sudden death: between birth and 6 months of age (the sudden infant death syndrome) (see Chap. 56) and between 45 and 75 years of age. Among the adult population, the *incidence* of sudden death caused by coronary heart disease increases as a function of advancing age,[17] in parallel with the age-related increase in incidence of total coronary heart disease deaths. The incidence is 100-fold less in adolescents and adults younger than 30 years (1 in 100,000 per year)[18-20] than it is in adults older than 35 years (1 in 1000 per year) (Fig. 33–3A).[11] In contrast to incidence, however, the *proportion* of deaths caused by coronary heart diseases that are sudden and unexpected decreases with advancing age. In the 20- to 39-year age group, approximately 75 percent of coronary heart disease deaths in men are sudden and unexpected, with the proportion falling to approximately 60 percent in the 45- to 54-year age group and hovering close to 50 percent thereafter. Age also influences the proportion of all cardiovascular causes among all causes of natural sudden death in that the proportion of coronary deaths and of all cardiac causes of death that are sudden is highest in the younger age groups, whereas the fraction of total sudden natural deaths that are due to any cardiovascular cause is higher in the older age groups. At the other end of the age range, only 19 percent of sudden natural deaths among children between 1 and 13 years of age are due to cardiac causes; the proportion increases to 30 percent in the 14- to 21-year-old age group.[21]

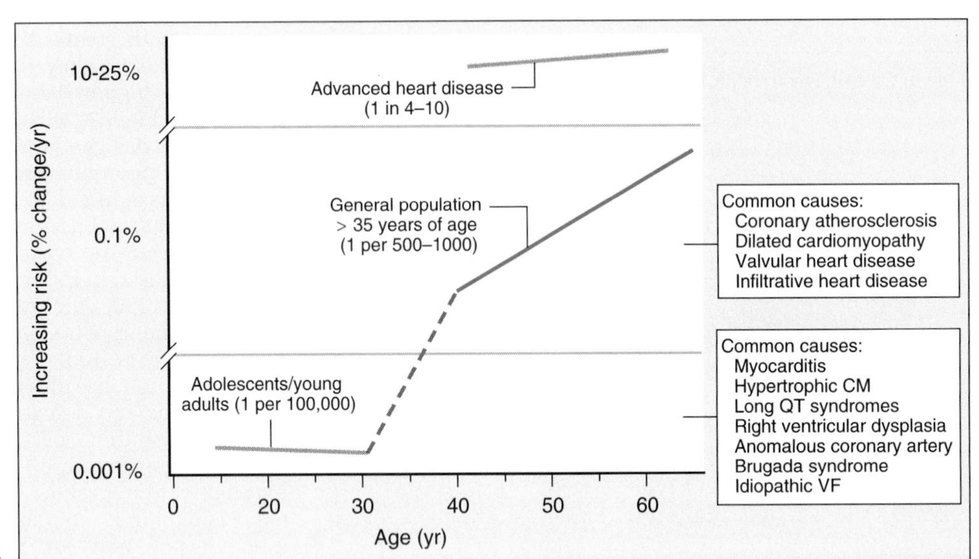

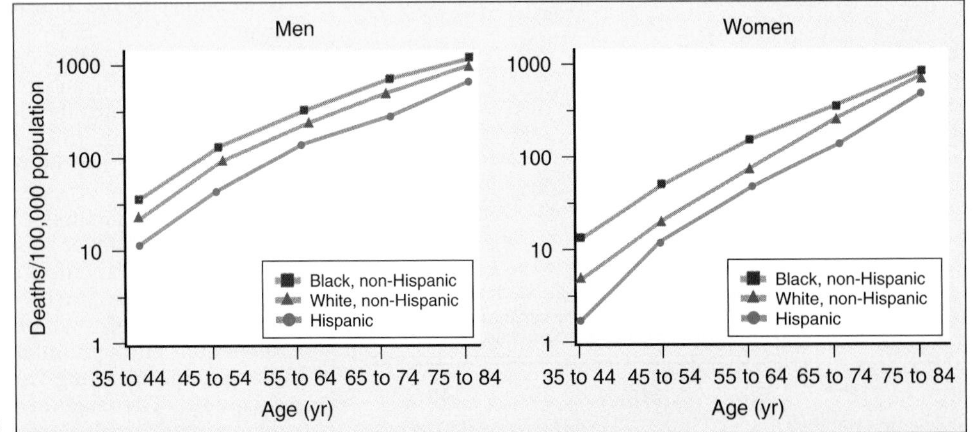

FIGURE 33–3 Age-, gender-, and race-specific risks of sudden cardiac death (SCD). **A,** Age-related and disease-specific risk for SCD. For the general population 35 years of age and older, SCD risk is 0.1 to 0.2 percent per year (1 per 500 to 1000 population). Among the general population of adolescents and adults younger than 30 years, the overall risk of SCD is 1 per 100,000 population or 0.001 percent per year. The risk of SCD increases dramatically beyond the age of 35 years and continues to increase past the age of 70 years. The greatest rate of increase is between 40 and 65 years (vertical axis is discontinuous). Among patients older than 30 years, with advanced structural heart disease and markers of high risk for cardiac arrest, the event rate may exceed 25 percent per year, and age-related risk attenuates. Among adolescents and young adults at risk for SCD because of specific identified causes, it is difficult to ascertain risk for individual patients because of variable expression of the disease state. The major risk is electrical, and the competing risk of mechanical heart dysfunction, as in advanced ischemic heart disease or dilated cardiomyopathy, does not contribute significantly to risk in many of these disorders. Therefore, effective electrical interventions are expected to have a better total mortality benefit (see text for details). **B,** SCD risk as a function of age, gender, and race or culture (white, black, and Hispanic). CM = cardiomyopathy; VF = ventricular fibrillation. (**B,** Modified from Gillum RF: Sudden cardiac death in Hispanic Americans and African Americans. Am J Public Health 87:1461, 1997.)

HEREDITY. Among the less common causes of SCD, hereditary patterns have been reported for specific syndromes[22] such as the congenital long QT interval syndromes,[23] hypertrophic cardiomyopathy,[24] right ventricular dysplasia,[25] the Brugada syndrome,[26] "idiopathic" ventricular tachycardia or fibrillation,[27,28] and yet-to-be-defined patterns of familial SCD in children and young adults (see Chap. 32). Mutations and functioning polymorphisms are being mapped to genes located on many chromosomes as the molecular bases for the entities are being defined. Although patients with stable congenital conducting system abnormalities have a good prognosis, progressive familial conducting system disease, which appears to have a hereditary pattern, carries an increased risk of SCD.[29] Familial sudden death associated with cardiac ganglionitis has been reported, but an inheritance pattern has not been demonstrated in the reports to date.

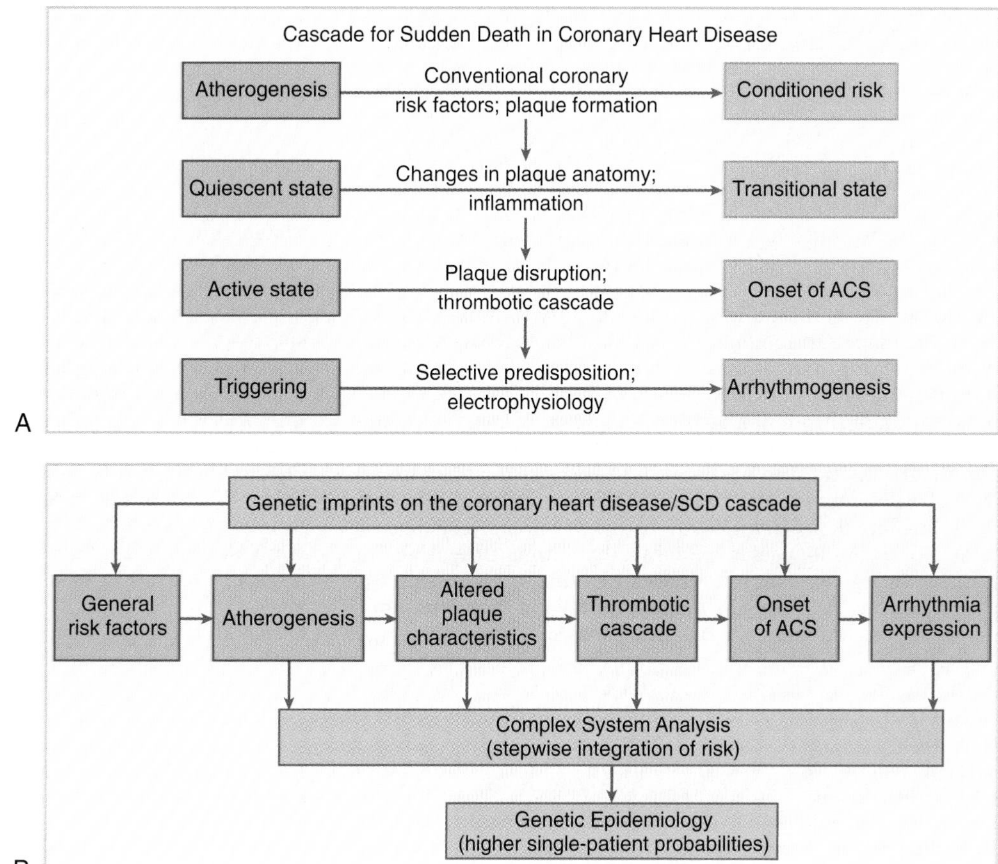

FIGURE 33–4 The coronary atherosclerosis heart disease cascade and genetic imprints on the progression to sudden cardiac death (SCD). **A,** The cascade from conventional risk factors for coronary atherosclerosis to arrhythmogenesis in SCD related to coronary heart disease. The cascade identifies four levels of risk, beginning with lesion initiation and development, progressing to the transition to an active state, then to acute coronary syndromes (ACS), and finally to the specific expression of life-threatening arrhythmias. Multiple factors enter at each level, including specific risk based upon genetic profiles of individual patients. **B,** Positions along multiple sites in the cascade from general risk factors for atherosclerosis to arrhythmic expression leading to SCD. Individual risk based on genetic profiles has been identified for atherogenesis, plaque evolution, the thrombotic cascade, and arrhythmia expression. Stepwise integration of these characteristics for individuals through complex analytical methods offers the hope of a field of genetic epidemiology that may lead to higher single-patient probabilities for SCD risk prediction. By integrating the risk associated with each step in the cascade, profiles become more highly specific for individual risk (see text for details). (Modified from Myerburg RJ: Scientific gaps in the prediction and prevention of sudden cardiac death. J Cardiovasc Electrophysiol 13:709, 2002.)

The multiple specific mutations at gene loci encoding ion channel proteins associated with the various inherited arrhythmia syndromes (see Chap. 28) provide a major advance in the understanding of a genetic and pathophysiological basis for these causes of sudden death. In addition, these observations may provide screening tools for individuals at risk as well as the potential for devising specific therapeutic strategies. These gene loci also serve as candidates for investigation of the role of low-penetrance mutations or polymorphisms in SCD related to more common causes, such as coronary heart disease. An example is a genetic variant in the cardiac sodium channel gene (*SCN5A*) observed among the African-American population (carrier rate = 13.2 percent) that appears to predispose to arrhythmias, even though it is not expressed as a prototypic long QT syndrome under control conditions.[30] Its role in predicting risk of SCD awaits clarification.

To the extent that SCD is an expression of underlying coronary heart disease, hereditary factors that contribute to coronary heart disease risk have been thought to operate nonspecifically for the SCD syndrome. However, studies have identified mutations and relevant polymorphisms along multiple steps of the cascade from atherogenesis to plaque destabilization, thrombosis, and arrhythmogenesis, each of which is associated with increased risk of a coronary event (Fig. 33–4).[31-34] Integration of these individual markers may provide more powerful individual risk prediction in the future. In addition, two population studies suggest that SCD, as an expression of coronary heart disease, clusters in specific families.[35,36] Whether this familial pattern is genetically or environmentally determined, or both, awaits further clarification.

GENDER. The SCD syndrome has a large preponderance in males compared with females during the young adult and early middle-age years because of the protection females enjoy from coronary atherosclerosis before menopause (see Fig. 33–3B).[37-39] Various population studies have demonstrated four- to sevenfold excesses of SCD among males compared with females prior to the 65-year-old and beyond age groups, in which the differences decrease to 2:1 or less. As coronary event risk increases in postmenopausal women, SCD risk increases proportionately.[37-39] Even though the overall risk is much lower in younger women, the classic coronary risk factors are still predictive of events among women,[37,40] including cigarette smoking, diabetes, use of oral contraceptives, and hyperlipidemia.

RACE. A number of studies comparing racial differences in relative risk of SCD in whites and blacks with coronary heart disease in the United States had yielded conflicting and inconclusive data. However, later studies have demonstrated excess risk of cardiac arrest and SCD among blacks compared with whites (see Fig. 33–3D).[39,41] SCD rates among Hispanic populations were smaller.[39] The differences were observed across all age groups.

CH 33

Risk Factors for Sudden Cardiac Death

General Profile of Sudden Cardiac Death Risk

Risk profiling for coronary artery disease, by means of the conventional risk factors for coronary *atherogenesis*, is useful for identifying levels of population risk and individual risk[42] but cannot be used to distinguish individual patients at risk for SCD from those at risk for other manifestations of coronary heart disease. Multivariate analyses of selected risk factors (i.e., age, systolic blood pressure, heart rate, electrocardiographic abnormalities, vital capacity, relative weight, cigarette consumption, and serum cholesterol) have determined that approximately one-half of all SCDs occur among the 10 percent of the population in the highest risk decile, based upon multiple risk factors (Fig. 33–5). Thus, the cumulative risk derived from multiple risk factors exceeds the simple arithmetic sum of the individual risks.[42] The comparison of risk factors in the victims of SCD with those in people who developed any manifestations of coronary artery disease does not provide useful patterns, by either univariate or multivariate analysis, to distinguish victims of SCD from the overall pool. In addition, angiographic and hemodynamic patterns discriminate SCD risk from non-SCD risk only under limited conditions.[43] In contrast, familial clustering of SCD as a specific manifestation of the disease may lead to identification of specific genetic abnormalities that predispose to SCD.[35,36]

Hypertension is a clearly established risk factor for coronary heart disease and also emerges as a highly significant risk factor for incidence of SCD.[44,45] However, there is no influence of increasing systolic blood pressure levels on the ratio of sudden deaths to total coronary heart disease deaths. No relationship has been observed between cholesterol concentration and the proportion of coronary deaths that were sudden. Neither the electrocardiographic pattern of left ventricular hypertrophy nor nonspecific ST-T wave abnormalities influence the proportion of total coronary deaths that are sudden and unexpected; *only intraventricular conduction abnormalities are suggestive of a disproportionate number of SCDs*.[31] The latter is an old observation that is reinforced by data from device trials that suggests the importance of QRS duration as a risk marker.[46] A low vital capacity also suggests a disproportionate risk for sudden versus total coronary deaths. This is of interest because such a relationship was particularly striking in the Framingham Study in the analysis of data on women who had died suddenly.[37,38]

The conventional risk factors used in early studies of SCD are the risk factors for evolution of coronary artery disease. The rationale is based on two facts: (1) coronary disease is the structural basis for 80 percent of SCDs in the United States, and (2) the coronary risk factors are easy to identify because they tend to be present continuously over time (see Fig. 33–4A). However, risk factors specific for fatal arrhythmias are dynamic pathophysiological events and occur transiently.[47,48] Transient pathophysiological events are being modeled epidemiologically[49] in an attempt to express and use them as clinical risk factors for both profiling and intervention.[50]

FUNCTIONAL CAPACITY AND SUDDEN DEATH. The Framingham Study demonstrated a striking relationship between functional classification and death during a 2-year follow-up period. However, the proportion of deaths that were sudden did not vary with functional classification, ranging from 50 to 57 percent in all groups and from those free of clinical heart disease to those in functional class IV.[51] Other studies also suggest that patients with heart failure with better functional capacity are at lower risk of dying, as expected, but a higher proportion of those deaths are sudden.[12]

Life Style and Psychosocial Factors

LIFE STYLE. There is a strong association between *cigarette smoking* and all manifestations of coronary heart disease. The Framingham Study demonstrated that cigarette smokers have a twofold to threefold increase in sudden death risk in each decade of life at entry between 30 and 59 years and that this is one of the few risk factors in which the proportion of coronary heart disease deaths that are sudden increases in association with the risk factor.[51] In addition, in a study of 310 survivors of out-of-hospital cardiac arrest, the recurrent cardiac arrest rate was 27 percent at 3 years of follow-up among those who continued to smoke after their index event compared with 19 percent in those who stopped ($p < 0.04$).[52] Obesity is a second factor that appears to influence the proportion of coronary deaths that occur suddenly.[38,51] With increasing relative weight, the percentage of coronary heart disease deaths that were sudden in the Framingham Study increased linearly from a low of 39 percent to a high of 70 percent. Total coronary heart disease deaths increased with increasing relative weight as well.

Associations between levels of physical activity and SCD have been studied with variable results. Epidemiological observations have suggested a relationship between *low levels of physical activity* and increased coronary heart disease death risk. The Framingham Study, however, showed an *insignif-*

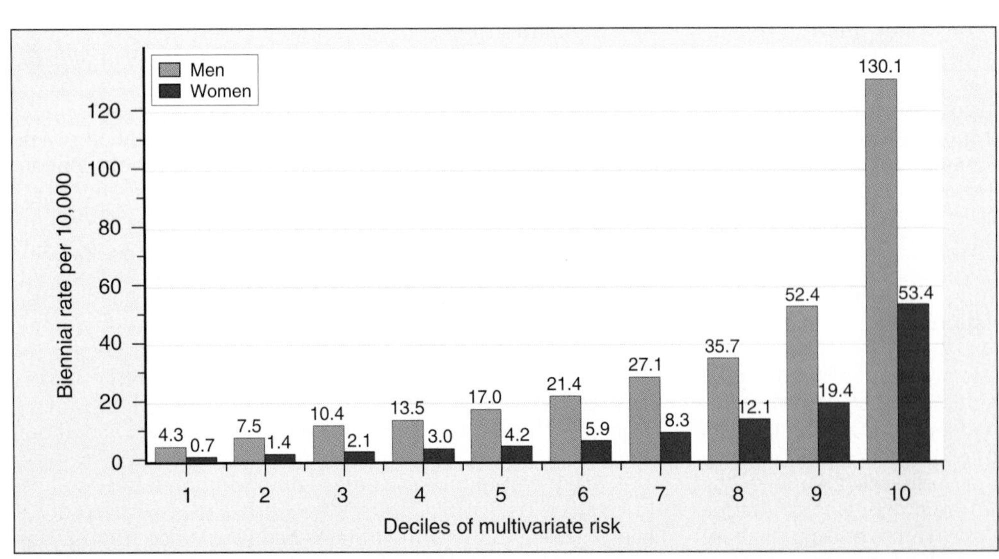

FIGURE 33–5 Risk of sudden death by decile of multivariant risk: 26-year follow-up, the Framingham Study. The variables included are age, systolic blood pressure, left ventricular hypertrophy, intraventricular block on the electrocardiogram, nonspecific electrocardiographic abnormalities, serum cholesterol, heart rate, vital capacity, cigarettes consumed per day, and relative weight. (Modified from Kannel WB, Shatzkin A: Sudden death: Lessons from subsets in population studies. Reprinted by permission of the American College of Cardiology. J Am Coll Cardiol 5[Suppl 6]:141B, 1985.)

icant relationship between low levels of physical activity and incidence of sudden death but a high proportion of sudden to total cardiac deaths at higher levels of physical activity.[51] An association between acute physical exertion and the onset of myocardial infarction has been suggested, particularly among individuals who are habitually physically inactive.[50] A subsequent case-crossover cohort study confirmed this observation for SCD, demonstrating a 17-fold relative increase in SCD associated with vigorous exercise compared with lower level activity or inactive states.[53] However, the absolute risk for events was very low (1 event per 1.5 million exercise sessions). Habitual vigorous exercise markedly attenuated risk. In contrast, SCD among young athletes has a higher incidence than among young nonathletic individuals in the same age range (see Chap. 75).[54] Information about physical activity relationships in various clinical settings, such as overt and silent disease states, is still lacking.

PSYCHOSOCIAL FACTORS. The magnitude of recent life changes in the realms of health, work, home and family, and personal and social factors has been related to myocardial infarction and SCD.[55-59] There is an association with significant elevations of life-change scores during the 6 months before a coronary event, and the association is particularly striking in victims of SCD. Among women, those who die suddenly are less often married, had fewer children, and had greater educational discrepancies with their spouses than did age-related control subjects living in the same neighborhood as the victims of sudden death. A history of psychiatric treatment, cigarette smoking, and greater quantities of alcohol consumption than the control subjects also characterized the sudden death group. Controlling for other major prognostic factors, risk of sudden and total deaths, and other coronary events is affected by social and economic stresses.[60] Alteration of modifiable life-style factors has been proposed as a strategy for reducing risk of SCD in patients with coronary heart disease,[61] although a study of treatment of depression following myocardial infarction failed to demonstrate an effect on event rates.[62] Acute psychosocial stressors have been associated with risk of cardiovascular events, including SCD.[63,64] The risk appears to cluster around the time of the stress and appears to occur among victims at preexisting risk, with the stressor simply advancing the time of an impending event.[63] In contrast, the possibility of physical stress–induced coronary plaque disruption has been suggested.[65]

Sudden Death and Previous Coronary Heart Disease

Although SCD is the first clinical manifestation of coronary heart disease in 20 to 25 percent or more of all coronary heart disease patients[1,9,11] and is the first clinical manifestation in more than 30 percent of coronary heart disease–related SCDs (see Fig. 33–2),[11,66] a previous myocardial infarction can be identified in as many as 75 percent of patients who die suddenly. The high incidence of both recognized and unrecognized prior myocardial infarction in victims of SCD has led to a search for predictors of SCD in survivors of myocardial infarction as well as in patients with other clinical manifestations of coronary heart disease and those with clinically silent disease.

LEFT VENTRICULAR EJECTION FRACTION IN CHRONIC ISCHEMIC HEART DISEASE. A marked reduction of the left ventricular ejection fraction is the most powerful predictor of SCD in patients with chronic ischemic heart disease as well as those at risk for SCD from other causes (see later). Increased risk, independent of other risk factors, is measurable at ejection fractions greater than 40 percent, but the greatest rate of change of risk is between 30 and 40 percent.[67] An ejection fraction equal to or less than 30 percent is the single most powerful independent predictor for SCD, but it has low specificity.

VENTRICULAR ARRHYTHMIAS IN CHRONIC ISCHEMIC HEART DISEASE. Most forms of ambient ventricular ectopic activity (premature ventricular complexes [PVCs] and short runs of nonsustained ventricular tachycardia [VT]) have a benign prognosis in the absence of structural heart disease.[68] An exception is polymorphic forms of nonsustained VT that occur in patients without structural heart disease but can have molecular, functional or drug- or electrolyte-related bases for high-risk arrhythmias.[69] When present in subjects in the coronary-prone age groups, however, PVCs select a subgroup with a higher probability of coronary artery disease and of SCD. Exercise-induced PVCs and short runs of nonsustained VT indicate some level of SCD risk,[70] even in the absence of recognizable structural heart disease. However, the data available to support this hypothesis are conflicting, with the possible exception of polymorphic runs of nonsustained VT.[69] Additional data suggest that PVCs and nonsustained VT during both the exercise and recovery phases of a stress test are predictive of increased risk.[71] Arrhythmias in the recovery phase, previously thought to be benign, appear to predict higher risk than arrhythmias in the exercise phase, and there is a gradient of risk with increasing severity of arrhythmias.

The occurrence of PVCs in survivors of myocardial infarction, particularly if frequent and of complex forms such as repetitive PVCs,[67] predicts an increased risk of SCD and total mortality during long-term follow-up. There are conflicting data on the role of measures of *frequency* and *forms* of ventricular ectopic activity as discriminators of risk, but most studies cite a frequency cutoff of 10 PVCs per hour as a threshold level for increased risk. Several investigators have emphasized that the most powerful predictors among the various forms of PVCs are runs of nonsustained VT, although this relationship is now questioned. Many of the reported studies have been based on a single ambulatory monitor sample recorded 1 week to several months after the onset of acute myocardial infarction, and the duration of the samples has ranged from 1 to 48 hours. Other studies have suggested that ambulatory ventricular arrhythmias in patients with heart failure do not specifically predict an increased risk of death.[72]

The results of the Cardiac Arrhythmia Suppression Trial (CAST) (see Chap. 30), designed to test the hypothesis that PVC suppression by antiarrhythmic drugs alters the risk of SCD after myocardial infarction, were surprising for two reasons.[73] First, the death rate in the randomized placebo group was lower than expected, and second, the death rate among patients in the encainide and flecainide arms exceeded control rates by more than three times. Subgroup analysis demonstrated increased risk in the placebo group for patients with nonsustained VT and with an ejection fraction of 30 percent or less, but excess risk in the treated group was still observed. The excess death rates may be accounted for by the occurrence of ischemic events in the presence of drug. No adverse effect (other than short-term proarrhythmic risk at initiation of therapy) was observed with the other drug in the study (moricizine), but no long-term benefit emerged either.[73] The Survival with Oral *d*-Sotalol (SWORD) study, a comparison of *d*-sotalol with placebo in a post-myocardial infarction population with a low death rate, also demonstrated excess risk in the drug-treated group.[74] Whether the conclusions from CAST, CAST II, and SWORD extend beyond the drugs studied, or to other diseases, remains to be learned.

Left ventricular dysfunction is the major modulator of risk implied by chronic PVCs after myocardial infarction.[67] The risk of death predicted by post-myocardial infarction PVCs is enhanced by the presence of left ventricular dysfunction

(Fig. 33–6); the latter appears to exert its influence most strongly in the first 6 months after infarction. Finally, there are data suggesting that the risk associated with postinfarction ventricular arrhythmias is higher in patients who have non-Q-wave infarctions than in those with transmural infarctions.[75]

Causes of Sudden Cardiac Death

Coronary heart disease and its consequences account for at least 80 percent of SCDs in Western cultures, and the cardiomyopathies cause another 10 to 15 percent (Table 33–2). Coronary heart disease is also the most common cause in many areas of the world in which its prevalence is lower. Despite the established relation between coronary heart disease and SCD, a complete understanding of SCD requires recognition of other causes that, although less common and often quite rare (see Table 33–2), may be recognizable before death, have therapeutic implications, and provide broad insight into the sudden death problem.[76,77] Many of these entities emerge as common causes of SCD in adolescents and young adults, among whom the prevalence of coronary atherosclerosis is much lower (see Fig. 33–3A).

Coronary Artery Abnormalities

Although structural abnormalities of coronary arteries other than coronary atherosclerosis are infrequent causes of SCD, the relative risk of SCD may be quite high for specific abnormalities. Nonatherosclerotic coronary artery abnormalities include congenital lesions, coronary artery embolism, coronary arteritis, and mechanical abnormalities of the coronary arteries. Among the congenital lesions, *anomalous origin of a left coronary artery from the pulmonary artery* (see Chaps. 56 and 75) is relatively common and associated with a high death rate in infancy and early childhood without surgical treatment. The early risk for SCD is not excessively high, but patients who survive to adulthood without surgical intervention are at risk for SCD. Other forms of coronary arterial-venous fistulas are much less frequent and associated with a low incidence of SCD.

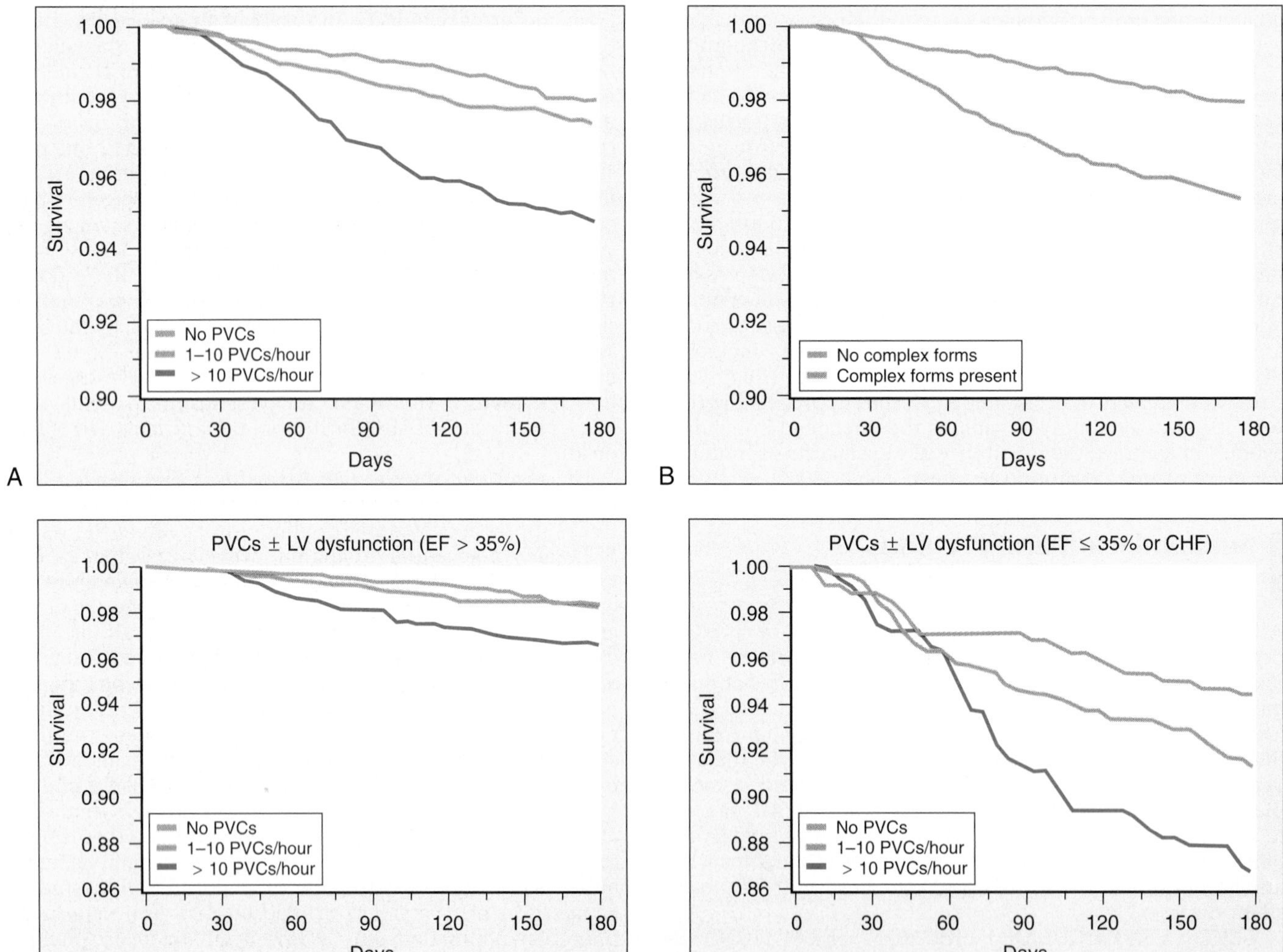

FIGURE 33–6 Prognostic significance of ventricular arrhythmias after myocardial infarction. The Gruppo Italiano per lo Studio della Sopravvivenza nell'Infarto Miocardico (GISSI)-2 data demonstrate that, in the thrombolytic era, frequent premature ventricular complexes (PVCs) carry prognostic information for mortality in the 6 months after an acute myocardial infarction, as previously reported in earlier studies. PVCs occurring at a frequency of greater than 10 per hour **(A)** and the presence of complex forms **(B)** both have an adverse effect on survival, although the latter did not hold up as an independent predictor on multivariate analysis. **C,** When PVCs occurred in the absence of left ventricular (LV) dysfunction (defined as ejection fraction [EF] less than 35 percent or the occurrence of congestive heart failure [CHF] during the event), the predictive power of frequent PVCs was reduced, and in the presence of LV dysfunction **(D)** it was enhanced. (From Maggioni AP, Zuanetti G, Franzosi MG, et al: Prevalence and prognostic significance of ventricular arrhythmias after acute myocardial infarction in the fibrinolytic era: GISSI-2 results. Circulation 87:312, 1993.)

TABLE 33–2 Causes and Contributing Factors in Sudden Cardiac Death

I. Coronary artery abnormalities
  A. Coronary atherosclerosis
    1. Chronic ischemic heart disease with transient supply-demand imbalance—thrombosis, spasm, physical stress
    2. Acute myocardial infarction
    3. Chronic atherosclerosis with change in myocardial substrate
  B. Congenital abnormalities of coronary arteries
    1. Anomalous origin from pulmonary artery
    2. Other coronary arteriovenous fistula
    3. Origin of a left coronary branch from right or noncoronary sinus of Valsalva
    4. Origin of right coronary artery from left sinus of Valsalva
    5. Hypoplastic or aplastic coronary arteries
    6. Coronary-intracardiac shunt
  C. Coronary artery embolism
    1. Aortic or mitral endocarditis
    2. Prosthetic aortic or mitral valves
    3. Abnormal native valves or left ventricular mural thrombus
    4. Platelet embolism
  D. Coronary arteritis
    1. Polyarteritis nodosa, progressive systemic sclerosis, giant cell arteritis
    2. Mucocutaneous lymph node syndrome (Kawasaki disease)
    3. Syphilitic coronary ostial stenosis
  E. Miscellaneous mechanical obstruction of coronary arteries
    1. Coronary artery dissection in Marfan syndrome
    2. Coronary artery dissection in pregnancy
    3. Prolapse of aortic valve myxomatous polyps into coronary ostia
    4. Dissection or rupture of sinus of Valsalva
  F. Functional obstruction of coronary arteries
    1. Coronary artery spasm with or without atherosclerosis
    2. Myocardial bridges

II. Hypertrophy of ventricular myocardium
  A. Left ventricular hypertrophy associated with coronary heart disease
  B. Hypertensive heart disease without significant coronary atherosclerosis
  C. Hypertrophic myocardium secondary to valvular heart disease
  D. Hypertrophic cardiomyopathy
    1. Obstructive
    2. Nonobstructive
  E. Primary or secondary pulmonary hypertension
    1. Advanced chronic right ventricular overload
    2. Pulmonary hypertension in pregnancy (highest risk peripartum)

III. Myocardial diseases and heart failure
  A. Chronic congestive heart failure
    1. Ischemic cardiomyopathy
    2. Idiopathic dilated cardiomyopathy
      (a) Acquired
      (b) Hereditary
    3. Alcoholic cardiomyopathy
    4. Hypertensive cardiomyopathy
    5. Postmyocarditis cardiomyopathy
    6. Peripartum cardiomyopathy
  B. Acute cardiac failure
    1. Massive acute myocardial infarction
    2. Acute myocarditis
    3. Acute alcoholic cardiac dysfunction
    4. Ball-valve embolism in aortic stenosis or prosthesis
    5. Mechanical disruptions of cardiac structures
      (a) Rupture of ventricular free wall
      (b) Disruption of mitral apparatus
        (1) Papillary muscle
        (2) Chordae tendineae
        (3) Leaflet
      (c) Rupture of interventricular septum
    6. Acute pulmonary edema in noncompliant ventricles

IV. Inflammatory, infiltrative, neoplastic, and degenerative processes
  A. Viral myocarditis, with or without ventricular dysfunction
    1. Acute phase
    2. Postmyocarditis interstitial fibrosis
  B. Myocarditis associated with the vasculitides
  C. Sarcoidosis
  D. Progressive systemic sclerosis
  E. Amyloidosis
  F. Hemochromatosis
  G. Idiopathic giant cell myocarditis
  H. Chagas disease

TABLE 33–2 Causes and Contributing Factors in Sudden Cardiac Death—cont'd

I. Cardiac ganglionitis
J. Arrhythmogenic right ventricular dysplasia; right ventricular cardiomyopathy
K. Neuromuscular diseases (e.g., muscular dystrophy, Friedreich ataxia, myotonic dystrophy)
L. Intramural tumors
  1. Primary
  2. Metastatic
M. Obstructive intracavitary tumors
  1. Neoplastic
  2. Thrombotic

V. Diseases of the cardiac valves
  A. Valvular aortic stenosis/insufficiency
  B. Mitral valve disruption
  C. Mitral valve prolapse
  D. Endocarditis
  E. Prosthetic valve dysfunction

VI. Congenital heart disease
  A. Congenital aortic or pulmonic valve stenosis
  B. Right-to-left shunts with Eisenmenger physiology
    1. Advanced disease
    2. During labor and delivery
  C. Late after surgical repair of congenital lesions (e.g., tetralogy of Fallot)

VII. Electrophysiological abnormalities
  A. Abnormalities of the conducting system
    1. Fibrosis of the His-Purkinje system
      (a) Primary degeneration (Lenegre disease)
      (b) Secondary to fibrosis and calcification of the "cardiac skeleton" (Lev disease)
      (c) Postviral conducting system fibrosis
      (d) Hereditary conducting system disease
    2. Anomalous pathways of conduction (Wolff-Parkinson-White syndrome, short refractory period bypass)
  B. Abnormalities of repolarization
    1. Congenital long QT interval syndromes
      (a) Romano-Ward syndrome (without deafness)
      (b) Jervell and Lange-Nielsen syndrome (with deafness)
    2. Acquired (or provoked) long QT interval syndromes
      (a) Drug effect (with genetic predisposition?)
        (1) Cardiac, antiarrhythmic
        (2) Noncardiac
        (3) Drug interactions
      (b) Electrolyte abnormality (response modified by genetic predisposition?)
      (c) Toxic substances
      (d) Hypothermia
      (e) Central nervous system injury
    3. Brugada syndrome—right bundle branch block and ST segment elevations in the absence of ischemia
  C. Ventricular fibrillation of unknown or uncertain cause
    1. Absence of identifiable structural or functional causes
      (a) "Idiopathic" ventricular fibrillation
      (b) Short-coupled torsades de pointes, polymorphic ventricular tachycardia
      (c) Nonspecific fibrofatty infiltration in previously healthy victim (variation of right ventricular dysplasia?)
    2. Sleep-death in Southeast Asians (see VII.B.3, Brugada syndrome)
      (a) Bangungut
      (b) Pokkuri
      (c) Lai-tai

VIII. Electrical instability related to neurohumoral and central nervous system influences
  A. Catecholamine-dependent lethal arrhythmias
  B. Central nervous system related
    1. Psychic stress, emotional extremes
    2. Auditory related
    3. "Voodoo" death in primitive cultures
    4. Diseases of the cardiac nerves
    5. Congenital QT interval prolongation

IX. Sudden infant death syndrome and sudden death in children
  A. Sudden infant death syndrome
    1. Immature respiratory control functions
    2. Susceptibility to lethal arrhythmias (e.g., long QT syndrome)
    3. Congenital heart disease
    4. Myocarditis
  B. Sudden death in children
    1. Eisenmenger syndrome, aortic stenosis, hypertrophic cardiomyopathy, pulmonary atresia
    2. After corrective surgery for congenital heart disease
    3. Myocarditis
    4. Genetic disorders of electrical function (e.g., long QT syndrome)
    5. No identified structural or functional cause

TABLE 33–2 Causes and Contributing Factors in Sudden Cardiac Death—cont'd

X. Miscellaneous
  A. Sudden death during extreme physical activity (seek predisposing causes)
  B. Commotio cordis—blunt chest trauma
  C. Mechanical interference with venous return
    1. Acute cardiac tamponade
    2. Massive pulmonary embolism
    3. Acute intracardiac thrombosis
  D. Dissecting aneurysm of the aorta
  E. Toxic/metabolic disturbances
    1. Electrolyte disturbances
    2. Metabolic disturbances
    3. Proarrhythmic effects of antiarrhythmic drugs
    4. Proarrhythmic effects of noncardiac drugs
  F. Mimics sudden cardiac death
    1. "Cafe coronary"
    2. Acute alcoholic states ("holiday heart")
    3. Acute asthmatic attacks
    4. Air or amniotic fluid embolism

ANOMALOUS ORIGIN OF CORONARY ARTERIES FROM THE INAPPROPRIATE SINUS OF VALSALVA (see Chap. 75). These anatomical variants are associated with increased risk of SCD,[78] particularly during exercise. When the anomalous artery passes between the aortic and the pulmonary artery root, the takeoff angle of the anomalous ostium creates a slit-like opening of the vessel, reducing the effective cross-sectional area for blood flow. Congenitally hypoplastic, stenotic, or atretic left coronary arteries are uncommon abnormalities associated with a high risk of myocardial infarction but not of SCD.

EMBOLISM TO THE CORONARY ARTERIES. Coronary artery emboli occur most commonly in aortic valve endocarditis and from thrombotic material on diseased or prosthetic aortic or mitral valves. Emboli can also originate from left ventricular mural thrombi or as a consequence of surgery or cardiac catheterization. Symptoms and signs of myocardial ischemia or infarction are the most common manifestations. In each of these categories, SCD is a risk resulting from the electrophysiological consequences of the embolic ischemic event.

MUCOCUTANEOUS LYMPH NODE SYNDROME (KAWASAKI DISEASE) (see Chap. 82). This syndrome carries a risk of SCD in association with coronary arteritis. Polyarteritis nodosa and related vesiculitis syndromes can cause SCD presumably because of coronary arteritis, as can coronary ostial stenosis in syphilitic aortitis. The latter has become a rare manifestation of syphilis.

MECHANICAL OBSTRUCTION TO CORONARY ARTERIES. Several types of mechanical abnormalities are listed among causes of SCD. Coronary dissection, with or without dissection of the aorta, occurs in Marfan syndrome (see Chap. 56) and has also been reported after trauma and in the peripartum period of pregnancy. Among the rare mechanical causes of SCD is prolapse of myxomatous polyps from the aortic valve into coronary ostia, as well as dissection or rupture of a sinus of Valsalva aneurysm, with involvement of the coronary ostia and proximal coronary arteries. Finally, deep myocardial bridges over coronary arteries (see Chap. 75) have been reported in association with SCD occurring during strenuous exercise, possibly caused by dynamic mechanical obstruction. However, most myocardial bridges are inconsequential and SCD associated with this anatomy is uncommon.

CORONARY ARTERY SPASM (see Chap. 46). Coronary vasospasm may cause serious arrhythmias and SCD.[79] It is usually associated with some degree of concomitant coronary atherosclerotic disease. Painless myocardial ischemia, associated with either spasm or fixed lesions, is now recognized as a mechanism of previously unexplained sudden death.[79] Different patterns of silent ischemia (e.g., totally asymptomatic, post-myocardial infarction, and mixed silent-anginal pattern) may have different prognostic implications.[80]

VENTRICULAR HYPERTROPHY AND HYPERTROPHIC CARDIOMYOPATHY (see Chaps. 59 and 75). Left ventricular hypertrophy is an independent risk factor for SCD, accompanies many causes of SCD, and may be a physiological contributor to mechanisms of potentially lethal arrhythmias.[44,45] The underlying states resulting in hypertrophy include hypertensive heart disease with or without atherosclerosis, valvular heart disease, obstructive and nonobstructive hypertrophic cardiomyopathy, primary pulmonary hypertension with right ventricular hypertrophy, and advanced right ventricular overload secondary to congenital heart disease. Each of these conditions is associated with risk of SCD, and it has been suggested that patients with severely hypertrophic ventricles are particularly susceptible to arrhythmic death.[81]

Risk of SCD in obstructive and nonobstructive hypertrophic cardiomyopathy was identified in the early clinical and hemodynamic descriptions of this entity.[82] Among patients who have the obstructive form, up to 70 percent of all deaths are sudden. However, survivors of cardiac arrest in this group may have a better long-term outcome than survivors with other causes, and reports have suggested that the risk of *primary* cardiac arrest and SCD in hypertrophic cardiomyopathy is lower than previously thought.[83,84]

A substantial proportion of patients with obstructive and nonobstructive cardiomyopathy have a family history of affected relatives or premature SCDs of unknown cause. Genetic studies have confirmed autosomal dominant inheritance patterns, with a great deal of allele and phenotypic heterogeneity. Most of the mutations are at loci that encode elements in the contractile protein complex, the most common being beta-myosin heavy chain and cardiac troponin T, which together account for more than half of identified abnormalities.[24] In the beta-myosin heavy chain form, there is a relationship between severity of left ventricular hypertrophy and risk of SCD; in the troponin T form, left ventricular hypertrophy is less severe despite SCD risk. Thus, the specific defect, rather than the locus, is more relevant and may be independent of the severity of structural hypertrophy among different loci.[24]

Specific clinical markers have not been especially predictive of SCD in individual patients, although young age at onset, strong family history, magnitude of left ventricular mass, ventricular arrhythmias, and worsening symptoms (especially syncope) appear to indicate higher risk.[82-87] Early studies suggested that a low resting outflow gradient, with a substantial provocable gradient, identified high risk of SCD.[82] A more recent study supports the predictive power of a high resting gradient.[87] The mechanism of SCD in patients with hypertrophic obstructive cardiomyopathy was initially thought to involve outflow tract obstruction, possibly as a consequence of catecholamine stimulation, but later data have focused on lethal arrhythmias as the common mechanism of sudden death in this disease. Risk is also thought to be suggested by PVCs and nonsustained VT on ambulatory recording or the inducibility of potentially lethal arrhythmias during programmed electrical stimulation. However, stable and asymptomatic nonsustained VT has limited predictive power for SCD in these patients. Rapid or polymorphic symptomatic nonsustained tachycardias, or both, have better predictive power.

The question of whether the pathogenesis of the arrhythmias represents an interaction between electrophysiological and hemodynamic abnormalities or is a consequence of electrophysiological derangement of hypertrophied muscle[81] is unanswered. The observation that patients with nonobstructive hypertrophic cardiomyopathy have high-risk arrhythmias and are at increased risk for SCD suggests that an electrophysiological mechanism secondary to the hypertrophied muscle itself plays some role. In athletes younger than 35 years, hypertrophic cardiomyopathy is the most common cause of SCD, in contrast to athletes over the age of 35, among whom ischemic heart disease is the most common cause.[88]

DILATED CARDIOMYOPATHY AND HEART FAILURE. The advent of therapeutic interventions that provide better long-term control of congestive heart failure has improved long-term survival of such patients (see Chaps. 22 and 23). However, the proportion of patients with heart failure who die suddenly is substantial, especially among those who appear clinically stable (i.e., functional class I or II).[89] The mechanism of SCD (VT or ventricular fibrillation [VF] versus bradyarrhythmia or asystole) appears to be related to cause (i.e., ischemic versus nonischemic).[90] The absolute risk of SCD increases with deteriorating left ventricular function, but the ratio of sudden to nonsudden deaths is related inversely to the extent of functional impairment.[89] Among patients with cardiomyopathy who have good functional capacity (class I and II), total mortality risk is considerably lower than it is for those with poor functional capacity (class III and IV)(Fig. 33–7). Unexplained syncope has been observed to be a powerful predictor of SCD in patients who have functional class III or IV disease related to any cause of cardiomyopathy, although ambulatory ventricular arrhythmias do not appear to indicate specific SCD risk in such patients.[72,91,92]

The interaction between post-myocardial infarction ventricular arrhythmia and depressed ejection fraction in determining risk for SCD has been described.[67] The majority of studies addressing the relation between chronic congestive heart failure and SCD focused on patients with ischemic, idiopathic, alcoholic, and postmyocarditis congestive cardiomyopathy. Peripartum cardiomyopathy (see Chap. 74) may also cause SCD.

ACUTE HEART FAILURE. All causes of acute cardiac failure (see Chap. 21), in the absence of prompt interventions, can result in SCD caused by either the circulatory failure itself or secondary arrhythmias. The electrophysiological mechanisms involved have been proposed to be caused by acute stretching of myocardial fibers or the His-Purkinje system, on the basis of its experimentally demonstrated arrhythmogenic effects. However, the roles of neurohumoral mechanisms and acute electrolyte shifts have not been fully evaluated. Among the causes of acute cardiac failure that are associated with SCD are massive acute myocardial infarction, acute myocarditis, acute alcoholic cardiac dysfunction, acute pulmonary edema in any form of advanced heart disease, and a number of mechanical causes of heart failure, such as massive pulmonary embolism, mechanical disruption of intracardiac structures secondary to infarction or infection, and ball-valve embolism in aortic or mitral stenosis (see Table 33–2).

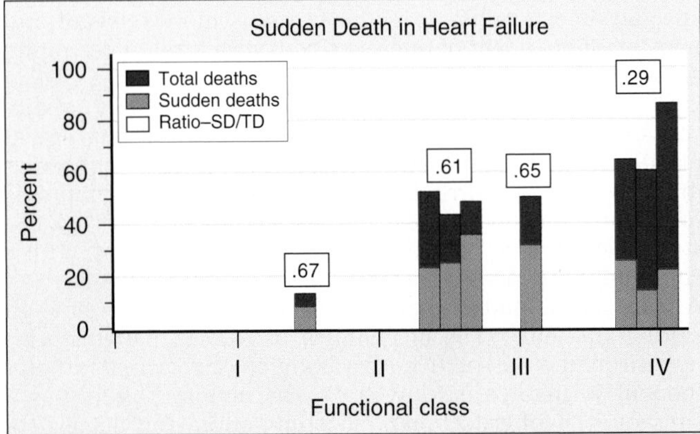

FIGURE 33–7 Risk of sudden cardiac death related to functional classification in heart failure. The relative probability of death being sudden is higher in the patients with better functional capacity who are at lower total mortality risk. SD = sudden death; TD = total death. (Modified from Kjekshus J: Arrhythmia and mortality in congestive heart failure. Am J Cardiol 65:42, 1990.)

INFLAMMATORY, INFILTRATIVE, NEOPLASTIC, AND DEGENERATIVE DISEASES OF THE HEART. Almost all diseases in this category have been associated with SCD, with or without concomitant cardiac failure. Acute viral myocarditis with left ventricular dysfunction (see Chap. 60) is commonly associated with cardiac arrhythmias, including potentially lethal arrhythmias. It is now recognized that serious ventricular arrhythmias or SCD can occur in myocarditis in the absence of clinical evidence of left ventricular dysfunction.[93,94] In a report of 19 SCDs among 1,606,167 previously screened U.S. Air Force recruits, 8 of the 19 (42 percent) had evidence of myocarditis (5 nonrheumatic, 3 rheumatic) at postmortem examination, and 15 (79 percent) suffered their cardiac arrests during strenuous exertion.[95] Viral carditis can also cause damage isolated to the specialized conducting system and result in a propensity to arrhythmias; the rare association of this process with SCD has been reported. Varicella in adults is a rare cause of striking conduction system disorders, but left ventricular function is usually preserved; its relationship to SCD is unclear.

Myocardial involvement in collagen-vascular disorders, tumors, chronic granulomatous diseases, infiltrative disorders, and protozoan infestations varies widely, but in all instances SCD can be the initial or terminal manifestation of the disease process. Among the granulomatous diseases, *sarcoidosis* (see Chap. 59) stands out because of the frequency of SCD associated with it. Roberts and coworkers[96] reported that SCD was the terminal event in 67 percent of sarcoid heart disease deaths; the occurrence of SCD has been related to the extent of cardiac involvement. In a report on the pathological findings in nine patients who died of *progressive systemic sclerosis* (see Chap. 59), eight who died suddenly had evidence of transient ischemia and reperfusion histologically, suggesting that this might represent Raynaud-like involvement of coronary vessels. *Amyloidosis* of the heart (see Chap. 59) may also cause sudden death. An incidence of 30 percent has been reported, and diffuse involvement of ventricular muscle or of the specialized conducting system may be associated with SCD.

ARRHYTHMOGENIC RIGHT VENTRICULAR DYSPLASIA OR RIGHT VENTRICULAR CARDIOMYOPATHY (see Chap. 32). This condition is associated with a high incidence of ventricular arrhythmias, including polymorphic nonsustained VT and VF as well as recurrent sustained monomorphic VT.[97] Although symptomatic monomorphic VT has been well recognized in the syndrome for many years, the risk of SCD was unclear and thought to be relatively low. However, the features of the disease and risks associated with it have now been clarified by a number of studies.[98-100] In a high proportion of victims, perhaps as many as 80 percent, the first manifestation of the disease is "unexplained" syncope or SCD.[98] SCD is often exercise related, and in some areas of the world where screening for hypertrophic cardiomyopathy has excluded the affected athletes from competition, right ventricular dysplasia has emerged as the most common cause of sport-related SCD.[101]

A genetic basis for right ventricular dysplasia is also being explored. A large proportion of the cases (up to an estimated 30 to 50 percent currently) appear to have a familial distribution.[22,99,100] The inheritance pattern is autosomal dominant except in one geographically isolated cluster in which it is autosomal recessive (Naxos disease—plakoglobin locus on chromosome 17).[22] To date, autosomal dominant mutations in two gene loci have been characterized (the ryanodine receptor locus on chromosome 1 [1q42][102] and the desmoplakin domain locus on chromosome 6 [6p24][103]), even though linkage analyses have implicated a heterogeneous distribution of multiple potential loci that may contribute to inheritance patterns (see Chap. 28).[22,25]

VALVULAR HEART DISEASE (see Chap. 57). Before the advent of surgery for valvular heart disease, severe *aortic stenosis* was associated with a high mortality risk. Approximately 70 percent of deaths were sudden, accounting for an absolute SCD mortality rate of 15 to 20 percent among all affected patients.[104] The advent of safe and effective procedures for aortic valve replacement has reduced the incidence of this cause of sudden death, but patients with prosthetic or heterograft aortic valve replacements remain at some risk for SCD caused by arrhythmias, prosthetic valve dysfunction, or coexistent coronary heart disease.[105] The incidence peaks 3 weeks after operation and then levels off after 8 months. Nonetheless, the risk is still appreciably lower than the historical risk among patients before the advent of valve surgery. A high incidence of ventricular arrhythmia has been observed during follow-up of patients with valve replacement, especially those who had aortic stenosis, multiple valve surgery, or cardiomegaly.[106] Sudden death during follow-up was associated with ventricular arrhythmias and thromboembolism. Hemodynamic variables were less predictive. Stenotic lesions of other valves imply a much lower risk of SCD. Regurgitant lesions, particularly chronic aortic regurgitation and acute mitral regurgitation, may cause SCD, but the risk is also lower than with aortic stenosis.

MITRAL VALVE PROLAPSE (see Chap. 57). This entity is prevalent, but probably less than previously thought,[107] and associated with a high incidence of annoying cardiac arrhythmias. However, a risk of SCD, although apparent, is quite low.[108] This uncommon complication appears to correlate with nonspecific ST-T wave changes in the inferior leads on the electrocardiogram (ECG). An association with redundancy of mitral leaflets on the echocardiogram has also been suggested. Reported associations between QT interval prolongation or preexcitation and SCD in mitral prolapse syndrome are less consistent.

ENDOCARDITIS OF THE AORTIC AND MITRAL VALVES (see Chap. 58). This may be associated with rapid death resulting from acute disruption of the valvular apparatus, coronary embolism, or abscesses of valvular rings or the septum; however, such deaths are rarely true sudden deaths as conventionally defined and tachyarrhythmic mechanisms are uncommon. Coronary embolism from valvular vegetations can trigger fatal ischemic arrhythmia on rare occasions.

CONGENITAL HEART DISEASE. The congenital lesions most commonly associated with SCD are aortic stenosis (see Chap. 56) and communications between the left and right sides of the heart with the Eisenmenger physiology. In the latter, the risk of SCD is a function of the severity of pulmonary vascular disease; also, there is an extraordinarily high risk of maternal mortality during labor and delivery in the pregnant patient with Eisenmenger syndrome (see Chap. 74).[109] Potentially lethal arrhythmias and SCD have been described as late complications after surgical repair of complex congenital lesions, particularly tetralogy of Fallot, transposition of the great arteries, and atrioventricular (AV) canal.[110] These patients should be observed closely and treated aggressively when cardiac arrhythmias are identified, although the late risk of SCD may not be as high as previously thought.

ELECTROPHYSIOLOGICAL ABNORMALITIES. Acquired disease of the AV node and His-Purkinje system and the presence of accessory pathways of conduction (see Chap. 32) are two groups of structural abnormalities of specialized conduction that may be associated with SCD. Epidemiological studies have suggested that intraventricular conduction disturbances in coronary heart disease are one of the few factors that can increase the proportion of SCD in coronary heart disease.[51] Several studies from the late 1970s and 1980s had demonstrated increased total mortality and SCD risk during the late in-hospital course and first few months after hospital discharge among patients with anterior myocardial infarctions and right bundle branch block or bifascicular block. In one study, 47 percent of patients who had late hospital VF had had the combination of anteroseptal infarction and bundle branch block. This finding corresponded to a VF incidence of 35 percent among a subgroup that represented only 4.1 percent of a total of 966 myocardial infarctions. In a later study, evaluating the impact of thrombolytic therapy on the prethrombolytic data, the incidence of pure right bundle branch block was actually higher but that of bifascicular block was lower, as were late complications and mortality.[111] These observations suggest a benefit of thrombolytic therapy, but the principle of increased risk among those who develop advanced conduction abnormalities (probably related to infarct size) is not attenuated by the therapy and the condition still requires aggressive management.

Primary fibrosis (Lenegre disease) or secondary mechanical injury (Lev disease) of the His-Purkinje system is commonly associated with intraventricular conduction abnormalities and symptomatic AV block and less commonly with SCD. The identification of people at risk and the efficacy of pacemakers for preventing SCD, rather than only ameliorating symptoms, have been subjects of debate. However, survival appears to depend more on the nature and extent of the underlying disease than on the conduction disturbance itself.

Patients with congenital AV block (see Chap. 32) or nonprogressive congenital intraventricular block, in the absence of structural cardiac abnormalities and with stable heart rate and rhythm, have been characterized as being at low risk for SCD in the past. In contrast, progressive congenital intraventricular blocks and the coexistence of structural congenital defects predicted a high risk and were considered pacemaker indications. Later data suggest that patients with the patterns of congenital AV block previously thought to be benign are at risk for a dilated cardiomyopathy,[112] and routine pacemaker implantation in patients older than 15 years, if not indicated sooner, has been suggested by at least one group.[113] Whether there is mortality benefit from pacemakers or a reduction in the incidence of dilated cardiomyopathy is not yet clear. A hereditary form of AV heart block has also been reported in association with a familial propensity to SCD.[29]

The anomalous pathways of conduction, bundles of Kent in the Wolff-Parkinson-White syndrome and Mahaim fibers, are commonly associated with nonlethal arrhythmias. However, when the anomalous pathways of conduction have short refractory periods, the occurrence of atrial fibrillation may allow the induction of VF during very rapid conduction across the bypass tract (see Chap. 32). The incidence of SCD in patients with short refractory period bypass tracts is unknown because an accurate estimate of its incidence among the population is not available. Patients who have multiple pathways appear to be at higher risk for SCD, as do patients with a familial pattern of anomalous pathways and premature SCD.[114] Family history is relevant because a genetic predisposition to Wolff-Parkinson-White syndrome has been suggested.[115]

THE LONG QT INTERVAL SYNDROMES (see also Chaps. 27 and 32). The *congenital* long QT interval syndrome is a functional abnormality caused by hereditary defects of molecular structure in ion channel proteins and is apparently associated with environmental or neurogenic triggers that can initiate lethal arrhythmias.[116-118] Two hereditary patterns have been described: the much more common autosomal dominant pattern known as the Romano-Ward syndrome and the rare autosomal recessive inheritance pattern, which is associated with deafness, the Jervell and Lange-Nielsen syndrome. There is a broad range of phenotypical expression. Some patients have prolonged QT intervals throughout life without any manifest arrhythmias, whereas others are highly susceptible to symptomatic and potentially fatal ventricular arrhythmias, particularly the torsades de pointes form of VT.[117,119] Moreover, genetic studies have demonstrated that penetrance may be low or variable in some families,[22] making electrocardiographic identification of affected members difficult. The relationship between low penetrance and risk of SCD remains undefined, but such patients are likely to be susceptible to QT-lengthening effects of drugs or serum electrolyte variations, expressed clinically as acquired long QT syndrome (see later).

Higher levels of risk are associated with female gender, greater degrees of QT prolongation or QT alternans, unexplained syncope, family history of premature SCD, and documented torsades de pointes or prior VF. Patients with the syndrome require avoidance of drugs that are associated with QT lengthening and careful medical management, which may include implantable defibrillators.[118,120] Moreover, efforts to identify and manage medically relatives who carry the mutation is an important preventive measure, given the familial pattern of expression of the entity (see Chaps. 27 and 32 for details). Mutations associated with the Romano-Ward inheritance pattern have been identified at loci on chromosomes 3, 4, 7, 11, and 21.[11] The Jervell and Lange-Nielsen form, in which the cardiac manifestations are associated with congenital deafness, has an autosomal recessive inheritance pattern. It is caused by inherited abnormalities of *KvLQT1* (chromosome 11) and *minK* (chromosome 21) or homozygous *KvLQT1* mutations.[22] It is likely that most of the mutations are not true recessives but rather variants with limited penetrance when heterozygous (see Chap. 27).

The *acquired form* of prolonged QT interval syndrome refers to excessive lengthening of the QT interval and the potential for developing torsades de pointes in response to environmental influences. As with congenital long QT, it is more common in women. The syndrome may be due to drug effects or individual patients' idiosyncrasies (particularly related to class IA or class III antiarrhythmic drugs and psychotropic drugs [see Chap. 72]), electrolyte abnormalities, hypothermia, toxic substances, bradyarrhythmia-induced QT adjustments, and central nervous system injury.[121] It has also been reported in intensive weight reduction programs that involve the use of liquid protein diets and in anorexia nervosa. Lithium carbonate can prolong the QT interval and has been reported to be associated with an increased incidence of SCD in cancer patients with preexisting heart disease. Drug interactions have been recognized as a mechanism of prolongation of the QT interval and torsades de pointes.[122] A growing body of evidence is suggesting that inherited polymorphisms or mutations with low penetrance, involving the same gene loci associated with phenotypically expressed long QT syndrome, underlie the susceptibility to the acquired form in many (if not most) instances.[30,123-125] In acquired prolonged QT syndrome, as in the congenital form, torsades de pointes is commonly the specific arrhythmia that triggers or degenerates into VF.

THE BRUGADA SYNDROME (see Chaps. 27 and 32). This disorder is characterized by right bundle branch block and an unusual form of nonischemic ST-T wave elevations in the anterior precordial leads (Fig. 33–8), associated with risk of SCD.[126] It is a familial disorder and occurs most commonly in young and middle-aged males. A mutation involving the cardiac Na^+ channel gene (*SCN5A*) has been observed in a minority of cases,[26] and there are compelling data suggesting that other ion channel defects may be a cause.[127] The right bundle branch block and ST-T wave changes may be intermittent and evoked or exaggerated by Na^+ channel blockers (e.g., flecainide). Risk of SCD is high and appears to be best predicted by the combination of persistent baseline ECG changes, syncope, life-threatening arrhythmias, a strong family history of SCD, and inducibility of ventricular tachyarrhythmias during electrophysiological testing.[128,129]

ELECTRICAL INSTABILITY RESULTING FROM NEUROHUMORAL AND CENTRAL NERVOUS SYSTEM INFLUENCES. Catecholamine-dependent lethal arrhythmias in the absence of QT interval prolongation, with control by beta adrenoceptor blocking agents, have been described.[130] In younger patients, more commonly males, bidirectional or polymorphic VT associated with SCD risk is related to a genetic disorder involving the ryanodine receptor locus, whereas the syndrome not associated with that genotype appears more likely to be in older patients, more commonly women.[131] Several central nervous system–related interactions with cardiac electrical stability have been suggested (see Chap. 85).[132] Epidemiological data also suggest an association between behavioral abnormalities and the risk of SCD. Psychic stress and emotional extremes have been suggested as triggering mechanisms for advanced arrhythmias and SCD for many years,[133,134] but there are only limited, largely observational, data supporting such associations. Stress-induced arrhythmias are better supported than stress-induced mortality risk, the latter requiring more study. Data from the 1994 Los Angeles earthquake identified an increased rate of fatal cardiac events on that day, but the event rate was reduced over the ensuing 2 weeks, suggesting a triggering of events about to happen rather than independent causation.[135] Associations between auditory stimulation and auditory auras and SCD have been reported. The auditory abnormalities in some forms of congenital QT prolongation have also been observed.

A variant of torsades de pointes, characterized by short coupling intervals between a normal impulse and the initiating impulse, has been described (Fig. 33–9).[136] It appears to have familial trends and to be related to alterations in autonomic nervous system activity. The 12-lead ECG demonstrates normal QT intervals, but VF and sudden death are common (see Chaps. 28 and 32).

The phenomenon of "voodoo death" has been studied in developing countries.[137] There appears to be an association between isolation from the tribe, a sense of hopelessness, severe bradyarrhythmias, and sudden death. With cultural changes in many of these areas, the syndrome has become less amenable to observation and study; however, there remain pockets of cultural isolation in which the syndrome may still exist.

SUDDEN INFANT DEATH SYNDROME AND SUDDEN CARDIAC DEATH IN CHILDREN. The sudden infant death syndrome (SIDS) occurs between birth and 6 months of age, is more common in males, and had an incidence of 0.1 to 0.3 percent of live births prior to widespread publication of appropriate sleep positions in at-risk infants.[138] Because of its abrupt nature, a cardiac mechanism has been suspected for many years, but a variety of causes, with central respiratory dysfunction playing a major role, are considered likely. Many cases of SIDS are believed to represent a form of "sleep apnea" that, if prolonged, can lead to hypoxia, cyanosis, and cardiac arrhythmias. Experience with "near misses" and the results of respiratory monitoring, in conjunction with the propensity of the syndrome to occur in premature infants, all suggest impaired central nervous system respiratory control reflexes, possibly owing to immaturity. There has been interest, however, in the possibility of obstructive apnea as another mechanism. Identification of individual infants at risk is difficult, but the risk does not persist beyond the first 6 months of life. Having infants sleep on their backs was anticipated to reduce the incidence of SIDS and appears to have achieved this goal in some studies,[139] but not all studies have demonstrated this improvement.

Primary cardiac causes have been considered the basis of this syndrome in some victims, and a large study of ECGs of infants suggested an association of risk of SIDS with prolonged QT interval as a potential cause.[140] Subsequently, a near-miss survivor was shown to have a de novo mutation of the Na^+ channel gene (*SCN5A*; chromosome 3), validating the concept that long QT may be one of the mechanisms of SIDS.[141] The combination of the relative incidence of SIDS among victims with the longer QT intervals and documentation of long QT–related arrhythmias in near misses supports the notion that a significant fraction of SIDS deaths occur by this mechanism. It does not, however, exclude the respiratory hypothesis as the mechanism for the majority of cases. Other cardiac causes have also been reported. Accessory pathways (two cases) and dispersed or immature AV nodal or bundle branch cells in the annulus fibrosus (four cases) were described among a group of seven SIDS victims studied by detailed histopathology.[142]

Sudden death in children beyond the age group at risk for SIDS is often associated with identifiable heart disease.[20,143] Although one earlier study identified cardiac causes in only 25 percent of victims of sudden natural death between the ages of 1 and 21 years,[21] a later report identified cardiac causes in 65 percent, with cardiac causes attributed in 80 percent of older children and adolescents.[20] About 25 percent of SCDs in children occur in those who have undergone previous surgery for congenital cardiac disease. Of the remaining 75 percent, more than one-half occur in children who have one of four lesions: congenital aortic stenosis, Eisenmenger syndrome, pulmonary stenosis or atresia, or obstructive hypertrophic cardiomyopathy. Neuspiel and Kuller[21] observed 14 cases of myocarditis among 51 SCDs in children (27 percent).

OTHER CAUSES AND CIRCUMSTANCES ASSOCIATED WITH SUDDEN DEATH. SCD can occur during or after extreme physical activity in competing athletes or under special circumstances within the general population, examples of the latter being intense exercise and basic military training. Among adolescent and young adult competitive athletes, the incidence estimate is in the range of 1 per 75,000 annually in Italy,[144] compared with less than 1 per 125,000 for the general nonathlete population in the same age group.[54] However, Maron (see Chap. 75) reported the frequency of sudden unexpected death related to cardiovascular disease during competitive sports to be 1 in 200,000 individual student-athletes per academic year and in 1 in 70,000 over a 3-year high school career. Exercise-related incidence figures are more difficult to ascertain among other populations, but one study reported an incidence of one SCD per 1.5 million exercise sessions in health clubs.[53] The majority of both athletes and nonathletes have a previously known or unrecognized cardiac abnormality. In middle-aged and older adults, in whom coronary disease dominates as the cause of SCD, exercise-related deaths appear to be associated with acute plaque disruptions.[65] Whether exercise contributed to the initiation of plaque disruption or preexisting disruption simply set the stage for the fatal response during exercise remains unclear. Among athletes, hypertrophic cardiomyopathy with or without obstruction, occult congenital or acquired coronary artery disease, and valvular aortic stenosis are the

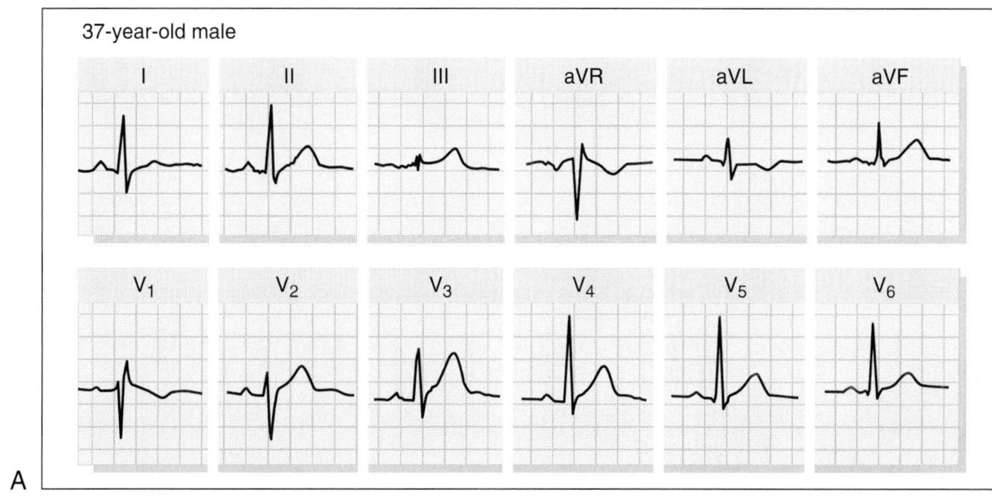

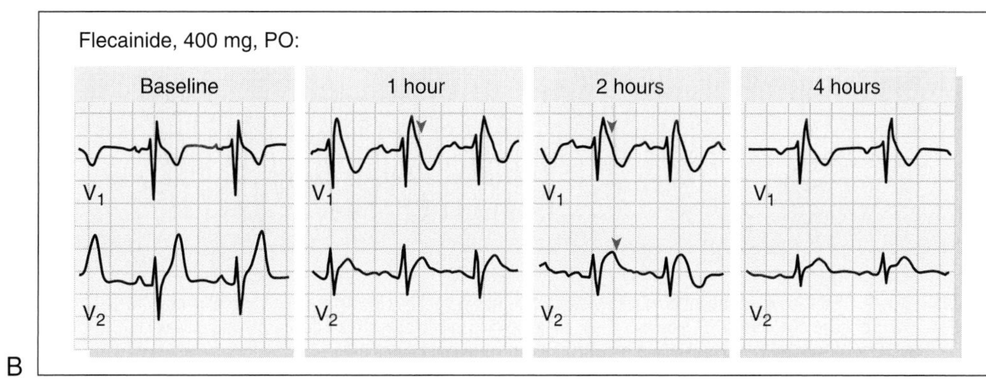

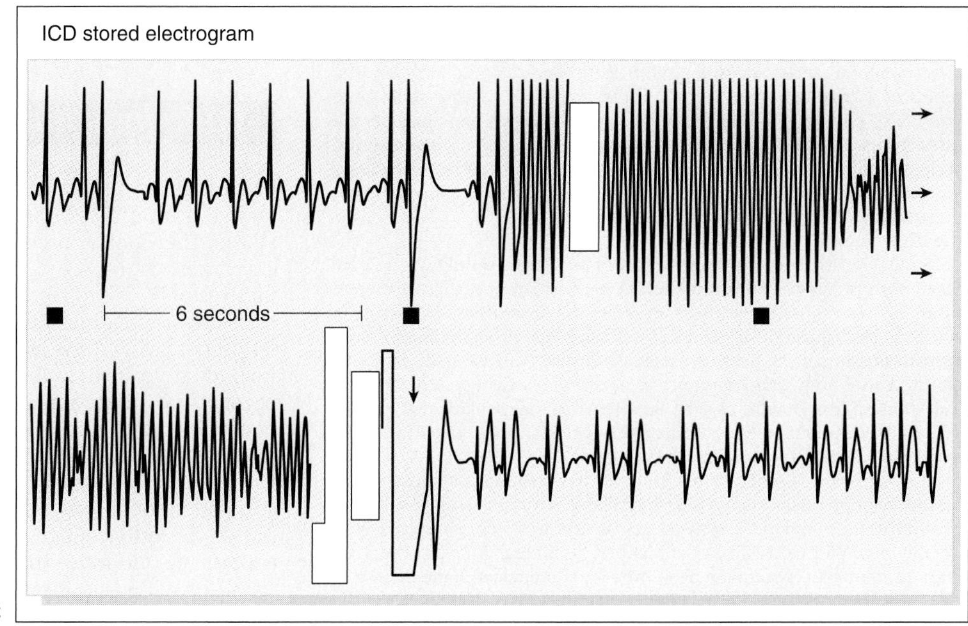

FIGURE 33–8 Electrocardiographic and clinical findings in a 37-year-old man with Brugada syndrome. The patient was resuscitated after out-of-hospital ventricular fibrillation. No structural disease was identified. **A,** The 12-lead electrocardiogram shows an incomplete right bundle branch block pattern, which is not typical for Brugada syndrome. **B,** Typical repolarization changes of Brugada syndrome (arrows) were elicited by a single oral dose of flecainide, 400 mg. The patient received an implantable cardioverter-defibrillator (ICD) and 6 months later had an appropriate shock (arrow) **(C)** as shown on the accompanying electrogram stored in the device.

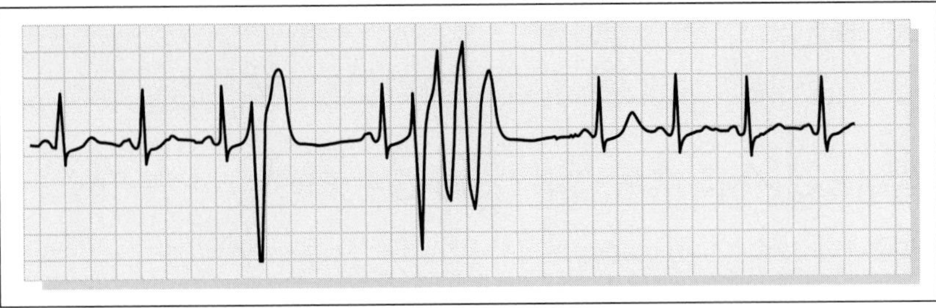
A

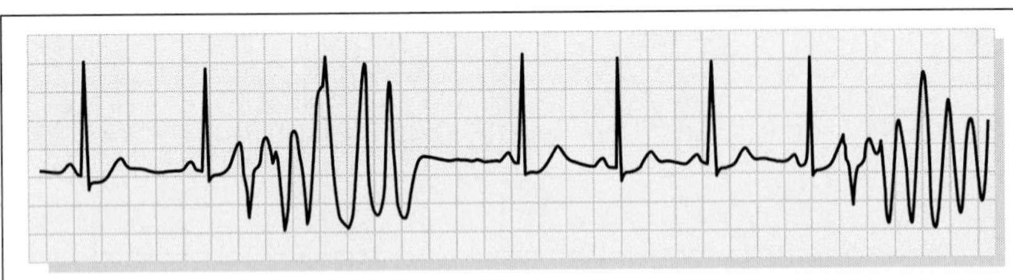
B

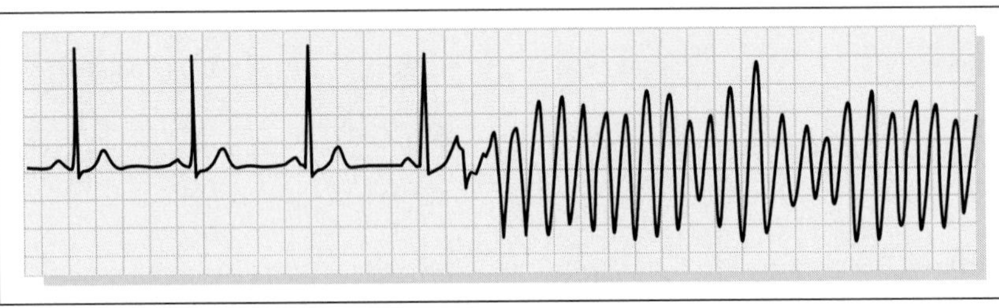
C

FIGURE 33–9 Short-coupled variant of torsades de pointes. This variant has been observed in people without structural heart disease and normal QT intervals. They are subject to spontaneous episodes of polymorphic ventricular tachycardia (torsades de pointes), which may degenerate into ventricular fibrillation. There is a high risk of sudden death in this uncommon syndrome.

most common causes identified after death (see Chap. 75).[88,144-149] In a report of a large cohort of U.S. Air Force recruits,[95] a surprisingly large fraction of people who died suddenly during exertion had unsuspected myocarditis. Diseases attributed to molecular structural abnormalities, such as long QT syndrome and right ventricular dysplasia, are being increasingly recognized as causes of SCD among athletes and exercising nonathletes.[88,146,147] Cardiac trauma (commotio cordis [see Chap. 59]) is the cause in some.[149]

Sudden death from true cardiac causes in athletes should not be confused with precipitous death related to heat stroke or malignant hyperthermia.[150] In the latter, excessive exercise in hot weather, sometimes in association with use of substances that cause heat production, and vasoconstriction impairing heat exchange can cause collapse with markedly elevated core body temperatures and irreversible organ system damage. Ingestion of exogenous dietary supplements, particularly ephedrine-related preparations in excess quantities, is being investigated for a role in precipitating SCD related to arrhythmia.

A small group of such victims, however, have neither previously determined functional abnormality nor identifiable structural abnormalities at postmortem examination. Such events or deaths, when associated with documented VF, are classified as idiopathic.[151] Although long-term survival after an idiopathic potentially fatal event is still unclear, some degree of risk appears to remain.[152] The idiopathic category is decreasing as the subtle molecular causes become better defined, including recognition by postmortem genetic studies. One pattern of so-called idiopathic VT has been associated with an inherited abnormality in calcium handling related to a ryanodine receptor mutation.[27] Limited data suggest that higher risk persists primarily in patients with subtle cardiac structural abnormalities, in contrast to patients who are truly normal. In addition, these events tend to occur in young, otherwise healthy people.

Long before Brugada's description of right bundle branch block, anterior nonischemic ST segment alterations, and sudden death predominantly in young males,[126] a specific pattern of SCD in young males had been observed in Southeast Asia. Syndromes referred to as *bangungut* in the Philippines, *pokkuri* in Japan, and *lai-tai* in Laos were reported. In each there was a tendency for death to occur unexpectedly during sleep, and at one time a toxic cause was suspected. Documented cases were reported in Laotians who came to the United States after the Vietnam War. The mechanism was identified as VF in some of these cases. The fact that these cases continue to occur in a new cultural setting suggested that there might be a hereditary predisposition. It is now accepted that many, if not all, of the subjects have Brugada syndrome.[153]

There also are a number of noncardiac conditions that *mimic* SCD. These include the so-called *cafe coronary* in which food, usually an unchewed piece of meat, lodges in the oropharynx and causes an abrupt obstruction at the glottis. The classic description of a cafe coronary is sudden cyanosis and collapse in a restaurant during a meal accompanied by lively conversation. The *holiday heart syndrome* is characterized by cardiac arrhythmias, most commonly atrial, and other cardiac abnormalities associated with acute alcoholic states. It has not been determined whether potentially lethal arrhythmias occurring in such settings account for reported sudden deaths associated with acute alcoholic states. *Massive pulmonary embolism* (see Chap. 66) can cause acute cardiovascular collapse and sudden death; sudden death in severe acute asthmatic attacks, without prolonged deterioration of the patient's condition, is well recognized. Air or amniotic fluid embolism at the time of labor and delivery may cause sudden death on rare occasions, with the clinical picture mimicking SCD. Peripartum air embolism caused by unusual sexual practices has been reported as a cause of such sudden deaths.

Finally, a number of abnormalities that do not directly involve the heart may cause SCD or mimic it. These include aortic dissection (see Chap. 53), acute cardiac tamponade (see Chap. 64), and rapid exsanguination.

Pathology and Pathophysiology

Pathological studies in SCD victims[154] reflect the epidemiological and clinical observations that coronary atherosclerosis is the major predisposing etiology.[76] Liberthson and coworkers[155] reported that 81 percent of 220 autopsied victims of SCD had significant coronary heart disease. At least one vessel with more than 75 percent stenosis was found in 94 percent of victims, acute coronary occlusion in 58 percent, healed myocardial infarction in 44 percent, and acute myocardial infarction in 27 percent. These observations are consistent with subsequent studies of the frequency of coronary disease in SCD victims, but the focus had evolved from the simple anatomical presence of coronary lesions to the specific associations with unstable plaques (see later).[65,156,157] All of the other causes of SCD (see Table 33–2) collectively account for no more than 15 to 20 percent of cases, but they have provided a large base of enlightening pathological data.[154]

The Pathology of Sudden Death Caused by Coronary Heart Disease

CORONARY ARTERIES. Extensive atherosclerosis has long been recognized as the most common pathological finding in the coronary arteries of victims of SCD. The combined results of a number of studies suggest a general pattern of at least two coronary arteries with 75 percent or greater narrowing among more than 75 percent of the victims. Several studies have demonstrated no specific pattern of distribution of coronary artery lesions that preselect for SCD. In a quantitative analysis comparing coronary artery narrowing at postmortem examination in SCD victims and control subjects, 36 percent of the 5-mm segments of the coronary arteries from the SCD group had 76 to 100 percent cross-sectional area reductions compared with 3 percent in the control group.[158] An additional 34 percent of the sections from the SCD group had 51 to 75 percent reductions in cross-sectional areas. Only 7 percent of the sections from the SCD patients had 0 to 25 percent reductions in cross-sectional areas.

The role of *active coronary artery* lesions, characterized by plaque fissuring, platelet aggregation, and thrombosis, as a major pathophysiological mechanism of the onset of cardiac arrest leading to SCD has become clarified.[65,156,157,159] Among 100 consecutive victims of sudden coronary death, 44 percent had major (more than 50 percent luminal occlusion) recent coronary thrombi, 30 percent had minor occlusive thrombi, and 21 percent had plaque fissuring. Only 5 percent had no acute coronary artery changes; 65 percent of the thrombi occurred at sites of preexisting high-grade stenoses, and an additional 19 percent were found at sites of more than 50 percent stenosis. In a subsequent study by the same investigators, 50 of 168 victims (30 percent) had occlusive intraluminal coronary thrombi, and 73 (44 percent) had mural intraluminal thrombi. Single-vessel disease, acute infarction at postmortem examination, and prodromal symptoms were associated with the presence of thrombi. In a later study, plaque rupture or erosion was observed in 66 percent of culprit vessel lesions among victims of SCD related to coronary heart disease.[48] Disruption, platelet aggregation, and thrombosis associate with markers of inflammation and various conventional risk factors for coronary atherosclerosis, such as cigarette smoking and hyperlipidemia.[160] *Coronary artery spasm,* an established cause of acute ischemia, can also cause SCD[79] and is recognizable in rare instances at postmortem examination.

MYOCARDIUM. Myocardial pathology in SCD caused by coronary heart disease reflects the extensive atherosclerosis usually present. Studies of victims of out-of-hospital SCD and from epidemiological sources indicate that healed myocardial infarction is a common finding in SCD victims, with most investigators reporting frequencies ranging from 40 to more than 70 percent.[155] In one study, 72 percent of men in the 25- to 44-year age group who died suddenly (24 or fewer hours) with no previous clinical history of coronary heart disease had scars of large (63 percent) or small (less than 1 cm cross-sectional area, 9 percent) areas of healed myocardial necrosis. The incidence of acute myocardial infarction is considerably less, with cytopathological evidence of recent myocardial infarction averaging about 20 percent. This estimate corresponds well with results of studies of out-of-hospital cardiac arrest survivors, who have an incidence of new myocardial infarction in the range of 20 to 30 percent. These pathological observations do not provide insight into the likely possibility that many SCDs occur by acute coronary syndrome mechanisms and progress from ischemia to fatal arrhythmias without time for structural markers to become visible. Even though there is an association of troponin elevations during chest pain syndromes with risk of cardiac death subsequently,[161] and troponin elevations occur in a substantial proportion of cardiac arrest survivors,[162] the question of whether the myocardial injury preceded or followed the cardiac arrest is difficult to resolve.

VENTRICULAR HYPERTROPHY. Myocardial hypertrophy can coexist and interact with acute or chronic ischemia but appears to confer an independent mortality risk.[44,45] There is not a close correlation between increased heart weight and severity of coronary heart disease in SCD victims; heart weights are higher in SCD victims than in those whose death is not sudden despite similar prevalences of history of hypertension before death. Hypertrophy-associated mortality risk is also independent of left ventricular function and extent of coronary artery disease.[163] Anderson[81] suggested that left ventricular hypertrophy itself may predispose to SCD. Experimental data also suggest increased susceptibility to potentially lethal ventricular arrhythmias in left ventricular hypertrophy with ischemia and reperfusion.[164] A study of massively enlarged hearts (i.e., weighing more than 1000 gm), however, did not indicate an excess incidence of SCD, but the underlying pathology in that study was dominated by lesions that produce volume overload.

SPECIALIZED CONDUCTING SYSTEM IN SUDDEN CARDIAC DEATH

Fibrosis of the specialized conducting system is a common but nonspecific endpoint of multiple causes. Although this process is associated with AV block or intraventricular conduction abnormalities, its role in SCD is uncertain. Lev and Lenegre diseases, ischemic injury caused by small-vessel disease, and numerous infiltrative or inflammatory processes all can result in such changes. In addition, active inflammatory processes such as myocarditis and infiltrative processes such as amyloidosis, scleroderma, hemochromatosis, and morbid obesity all may damage or destroy the AV node or bundle of His, or both, and result in AV block.[165]

Focal diseases such as sarcoidosis, Whipple disease, and rheumatoid arthritis and fibrotic or fatty infiltration of the AV node or His-Purkinje system with apparent discontinuities[93] can also involve the conducting system (see Chap. 32). These various categories of conducting system disease have been considered as possible pathological substrates for SCD that may be overlooked because of the difficulty in doing careful postmortem examinations of the conducting system routinely. Focal involvement of conducting tissue by tumors (especially mesothelioma of the AV node but also lymphoma, carcinoma, rhabdomyoma, and fibroma) has also been reported, and rare cases of SCD have been associated with these lesions. It has been suggested that abnormal postnatal morphogenesis of the specialized conducting system may be a significant factor in some SCDs in infants and children.

CARDIAC NERVES AND SUDDEN CARDIAC DEATH

Diseases of cardiac nerves have been postulated to have a role in SCD. Neural involvement may be the result of random damage to neural elements within the myocardium (i.e., "secondary" cardioneuropathy) or may be "primary," as in a selective cardiac viral neuropathy. Secondary involvement can be a consequence of ischemic neural injury in coronary heart disease and has been postulated to result in autonomic destabilization, enhancing the propensity to arrhythmias. Nerve sprouting may be important.[166] Some experimental data support this hypothesis, and a clinical technique for imaging cardiac neural fibers suggests a changing pattern over time after myocardial infarction. Viral, neurotoxic, and hereditary causes (e.g., progressive muscular dystrophy and Friedreich ataxia) have been emphasized.

Mechanisms and Pathophysiology

Electrical mechanisms of cardiac arrest are divided into tachyarrhythmic and bradyarrhythmia-asystolic events. The tachyarrhythmias include VF and sustained VT in which adequate blood flow cannot be maintained and perfusion is inadequate to meet the body's needs. Bradyarrhythmia-asystolic events include severe bradyarrhythmias—heart rates slow enough to impede adequate tissue perfusion and inability to generate a mechanical event because of either complete absence of electrical activity (asystole) or dissociation between abnormal spontaneous electrical activity and mechanical function (pulseless electrical activity). It is likely that VF, or VT deteriorating to VF, is the initiating event in the majority of cardiac arrests. After a variable period of time fibrillation may cease, and asystole or pulseless electrical activity emerges. In a significant minority of cases, however, the documented initial recording is asystole or pulseless electrical activity, which can continue as such or transform into VF.[167] More commonly, asystolic events or pulseless electrical activity follows an initial tachyarrhythmic event.

The occurrence of potentially lethal tachyarrhythmias, or of severe bradyarrhythmia or asystole, is the end of a cascade of pathophysiological abnormalities that result from complex interactions between coronary vascular events, myocardial injury, variations in autonomic tone, or the metabolic and electrolyte state of the myocardium (see Fig. 33–4).[12,168,169] There is no uniform hypothesis regarding mechanisms by which these elements interact to lead to the final pathway of lethal arrhythmias. However, Figure 33–10 shows a model of the pathophysiology of SCD in which the central event is the initiation of a potentially fatal arrhythmia. The risk of this event is conditioned by the presence of *structural abnormalities* and modulated by *functional variations*.[170]

Pathophysiological Mechanisms of Lethal Tachyarrhythmias

CORONARY ARTERY STRUCTURE AND FUNCTION. Among the 80 percent of SCDs associated with coronary atherosclerosis, the extent and distribution of chronic arterial narrowing have been well defined by pathological studies. However, the specific mechanisms by which these lesions lead to potentially lethal disturbances of electrical stability are no longer viewed as simply the consequence of steady-state reductions in regional myocardial blood flow in association with variable demands (see Chap. 35).[11,12,168] A simple increase in myocardial oxygen demand, in the presence of a fixed supply, may be a mechanism of exercise-induced arrhythmias and sudden death during intense physical activity or in others whose heart disease had not previously become clinically manifest. However, the dynamic nature of the pathophysiology of coronary events has led to the recognition that superimposed acute lesions create a setting in which alterations in the metabolic or electrolyte state of the myocardium are the common circumstance leading to disturbed electrical stability. Active vascular events, leading to acute or transient reduction in regional myocardial blood flow in the presence of a normal or previously compromised circulation, constitute a common mechanism of ischemia, angina pectoris, arrhythmias, and SCD.[11,79,168,169] Coronary artery spasm or modulation of coronary collateral flow, predisposed to by local endothelial dysfunction, exposes the myocardium to the double hazard of transient ischemia and reperfusion (Fig. 33–11).[151,168] Neurogenic influences may play a role but do not appear to be a sine qua non for the production of spasm. Vessel susceptibility and humoral factors, particularly those related to platelet activation and aggregation, also appear to be important mechanisms.

Transition of stable atherosclerotic plaques to an "active" state because of endothelial damage, with plaque fissuring leading to platelet activation and aggregation followed by thrombosis, is a mechanism that appears to be present in the majority of SCDs related to coronary heart disease (see Chap. 46).[156] Inflammatory responses in atherosclerotic plaques are now viewed as the condition leading to lesion progression, including erosion, disruption, platelet activation, and thrombosis. In addition to causing subacute or acute critical reduction in regional blood flow, these mechanisms produce a series of biochemical alterations that may enhance or retard susceptibility to VF by means of vasomotor modulation.

The final step in the role of coronary artery pathophysiology leading to ischemia-induced arrhythmias is platelet aggregation and thrombosis (see Fig. 33–4; see Chap. 35). Davies and Thomas[159] pointed out that 95 of 100 subjects who died suddenly (less than 6 hours after the onset of symptoms) had acute coronary thrombi, plaque fissuring, or both. This incidence was considerably higher than in many previous reports, but it is noteworthy that only 44 percent of the patients had the largest thrombus occluding 51 percent or more of the cross-sectional area of the involved vessel and only 18 percent of the patients had more than 75 percent occlusion. These findings raise questions about whether mechanical obstruction to flow was dominant or whether the high incidence of nonoccluding thrombi simply reflected the state of activation of the platelets. The discrepancy between the relatively high incidence of acute thrombi in postmortem studies and the low incidence of evolution of new myocardial infarction among survivors of out-of-hospital VF[155,171] highlights this question. Spontaneous thrombolysis, a dominant role of spasm induced by platelet products, or a combination may explain this discrepancy.

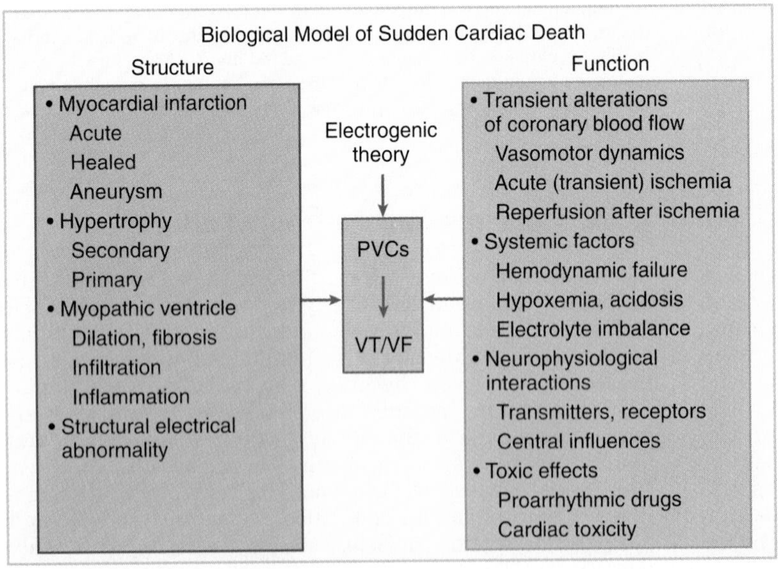

Biological Model of Sudden Cardiac Death

Structure		Function
• Myocardial infarction Acute Healed Aneurysm • Hypertrophy Secondary Primary • Myopathic ventricle Dilation, fibrosis Infiltration Inflammation • Structural electrical abnormality	Electrogenic theory ↓ PVCs → ↓ ← VT/VF	• Transient alterations of coronary blood flow Vasomotor dynamics Acute (transient) ischemia Reperfusion after ischemia • Systemic factors Hemodynamic failure Hypoxemia, acidosis Electrolyte imbalance • Neurophysiological interactions Transmitters, receptors Central influences • Toxic effects Proarrhythmic drugs Cardiac toxicity

FIGURE 33–10 Biological model of sudden cardiac death (SCD). Structural cardiac abnormalities are commonly defined as the causative basis for SCD. However, functional alterations of the abnormal anatomical substrate are usually required to alter stability of the myocardium, permitting a potentially fatal arrhythmia to be initiated. In this conceptual model, short- or long-term structural abnormalities interact with functional modulations to influence the probability that premature ventricular contractions (PVCs) initiate ventricular tachycardia or fibrillation (VT/VF). (From Myerburg RJ, Kessler KM, Bassett AL, Castellanos A: A biological approach to sudden cardiac death: Structure, function, and cause. Am J Cardiol 63:1512, 1989.)

ACUTE ISCHEMIA AND INITIATION OF LETHAL ARRHYTHMIAS. The onset of acute ischemia produces immediate electrical, mechanical, and biochemical dysfunction of cardiac muscle (see Figs. 33-10 and 33-11). The specialized conducting tissue is more resistant to acute ischemia than working myocardium, and therefore the electrophysiological consequences are less intense and delayed in onset in specialized conduction tissue. Experimental studies have also provided data on the long-term consequences of left ventricular hypertrophy and healed experimental myocardial infarction. Tissue exposed to chronic stress produced by long-term left ventricular pressure overload and tissue that has healed after ischemic injury both show lasting cellular electrophysiological abnormalities, including regional changes in transmembrane action potentials and refractory periods.[169] Moreover, acute ischemic injury or acute myocardial infarction in the presence of healed myocardial infarction is more arrhythmogenic than the same extent of acute ischemia in previously normal tissue.[172] In addition to the direct effect of ischemia on normal or previously abnormal tissue, reperfusion after transient ischemia can cause lethal arrhythmias (see Fig. 33-11).[79,169] Reperfusion of ischemic areas can occur by three mechanisms: (1) spontaneous thrombolysis, (2) collateral flow from other coronary vascular beds to the ischemic bed, and (3) reversal of vasospasm. Some mechanisms of reperfusion-induced arrhythmogenesis appear to be related to the duration of ischemia before reperfusion. Experimentally, there is a window of vulnerability beginning 5 to 10 minutes after the onset of ischemia and lasting up to 20 to 30 minutes.

ELECTROPHYSIOLOGICAL EFFECTS OF ACUTE ISCHEMIA. Within the first minutes after experimental coronary ligation there is a propensity to ventricular arrhythmias that abates after 30 minutes and reappears after several hours. The initial 30 minutes of arrhythmias is divided into two periods, the first of which lasts for about 10 minutes and is presumably directly related to the initial ischemic injury. The second period (20 to 30 minutes) may be related either to reperfusion of ischemic areas or to the evolution of different injury patterns in the epicardial and endocardial muscle. Multiple mechanisms of reperfusion arrhythmias have been observed experimentally, including slow conduction and reentry[173] and afterdepolarizations and triggered activity.[164]

At the level of the myocyte, the immediate consequences of ischemia, which include alteration of cell membrane physiology with efflux of K^+, influx of Ca^{2+}, acidosis, reduction of transmembrane resting potentials,[174] and enhanced automaticity in some tissues, are followed by a separate series of changes during reperfusion. Those of particular interest are the possible continued influx of Ca^{2+}, which may produce electrical instability; responses to alpha or beta adrenoceptor stimulation, or both; and afterdepolarizations as triggering responses for Ca^{2+}-dependent arrhythmias. Other possible mechanisms studied experimentally include formation of superoxide radicals in reperfusion arrhythmias and differential responses of endocardial and epicardial muscle activation times and refractory periods during ischemia or reperfusion. The adenosine triphosphate-dependent K^+ current ($I_{K\text{-}ATP}$), which is inactive during normal conditions, is activated during ischemia.[175] Its activation results in a strong efflux of K^+ ions from myocytes, markedly shortening the time course of repolarization and leading to slow conduction and ultimately to inexcitability.[176] The fact that this response is more marked in epicardium than in endocardium leads to a prominent dispersion of repolarization across the myocardium during transmural ischemia. At an intercellular level, ischemia alters the distribution of connexin43, the primary gap junction protein between myocytes.[177] This alteration results in uncoupling of myocytes, a factor that is arrhythmogenic because of altered patterns of excitation and regional changes in conduction velocity.[178]

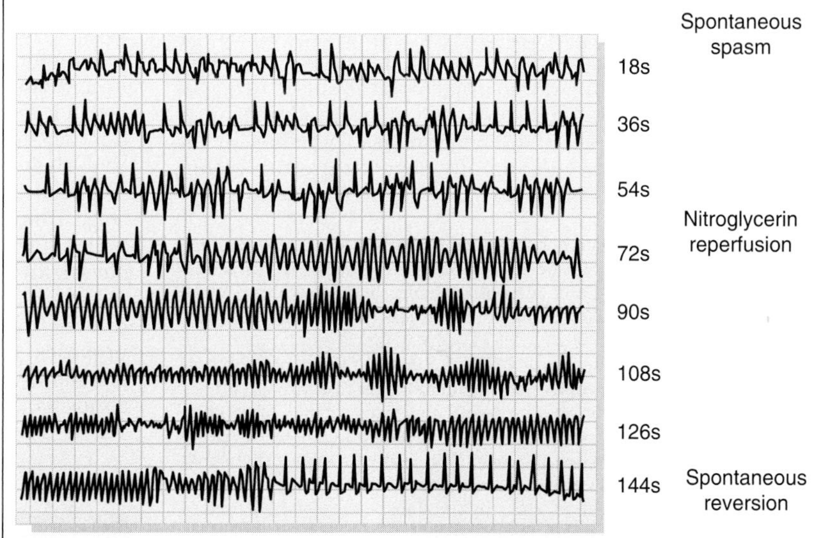

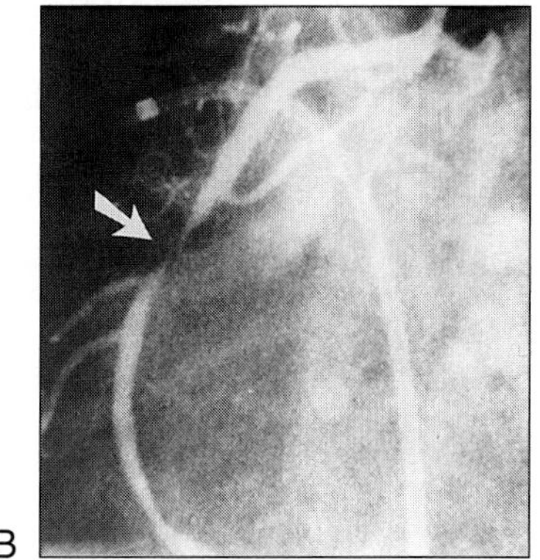

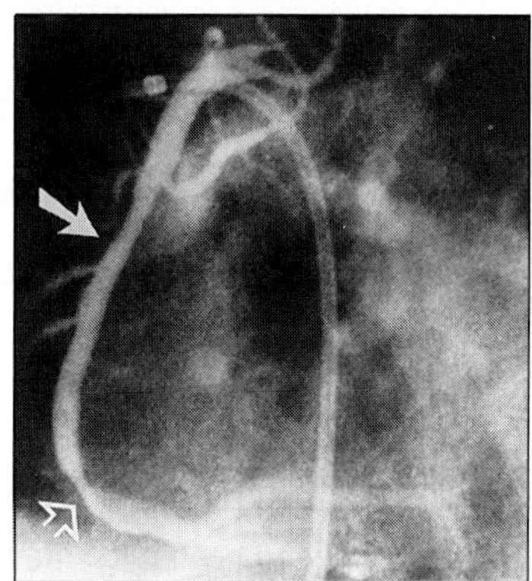

FIGURE 33–11 Life-threatening ventricular arrhythmias associated with acute myocardial ischemia related to coronary artery spasm and with reperfusion. **A,** Continuous lead II electrocardiographic monitor recording during ischemia (time 0 to 55 seconds) caused by spasm of the right coronary artery **(B)**. There is an abrupt transition (time 56 to 72 seconds) from repetitive ventricular ectopy to a rapid polymorphic, prefibrillatory tachyarrhythmia (time 80 to 130 seconds) associated with nitroglycerin-induced reversal of the spasm **(C)**. Closed arrows, site of spasm before and after nitroglycerin; open arrow, lower grade distal lesion.

The importance of the myocardial response to the onset of ischemia has been emphasized on the basis of the demonstration of dramatic cellular electrophysiological changes during the early period after coronary occlusion. However, the state of the myocardium at the time of onset of ischemia is a critical additional factor. Tissue healed after previous injury appears to be more susceptible to the electrical destabilizing effects of acute ischemia, as is chronically hypertrophied muscle. There are data suggesting that remodeling-induced local stretch, regional hypertrophy, or intrinsic cellular alteration may contribute to this vulnerability. Of more direct clinical relevance is the suggestion that K^+ depletion by diuretics and clinical hypokalemia may make ventricular myocardium more susceptible to potentially lethal arrhythmias.

The association of metabolic and electrolyte abnormalities, and neurophysiological and neurohumoral changes,[179] with lethal arrhythmias emphasizes the importance of integrating changes in the myocardial substrate with systemic influences. Most direct among myocardial metabolic changes in response to ischemia are local acute increase in interstitial K^+ levels to values exceeding 15 mM, a fall in tissue pH to below 6.0, changes in adrenoceptor activity, and alterations in autonomic nerve traffic, all of which tend to create and maintain electrical instability, especially if regional in distribution. Other metabolic changes such as cyclic adenosine monophosphate elevation, accumulation of free fatty acids and their metabolites, formation of lysophosphoglycerides, and impaired myocardial glycolysis have also been suggested as myocardial destabilizing influences.[180] These local myocardial changes integrate with systemic patterns of autonomic fluctuation that can be observed as patterns of altered heart rate variability and fractal dynamics,[181] potentially identifying subsets of patients predetermined to be at higher risk for SCD during an ischemic event.

TRANSITION FROM MYOCARDIAL INSTABILITY TO LETHAL ARRHYTHMIAS. Tshe combination of a triggering event and a susceptible myocardium is a fundamental electrophysiological concept for the mechanism of initiation of potentially lethal arrhythmias (see Figs. 33–4 and 33–10). The triggering event may be electrophysiological, ischemic, metabolic, or hemodynamic.[170] The endpoint of their interaction is disorganization of patterns of myocardial activation into multiple uncoordinated reentrant pathways (i.e., VF). Clinical, experimental, and pharmacological data all suggest that triggering events in the absence of myocardial instability are unlikely to initiate lethal arrhythmias. Therefore, in the absence of myocardial vulnerability, many triggering events, such as frequent and complex PVCs, may be innocuous.[170]

The onset of ischemia is accompanied by abrupt reductions in transmembrane resting potential and amplitude and in duration of the action potentials in the affected area with little change in remote areas. When ischemic cells depolarize to resting potentials less than −60 mV, they may become inexcitable and of little electrophysiological importance (see Chap. 27). As they are depolarizing to that range, however, or repolarizing as a consequence of reperfusion, the membranes pass through ranges of reduced excitability, upstroke velocity, and time courses of repolarization. These characteristics result in slow conduction and electrophysiological heterogeneity. When this occurs in ischemic myocardium that is adjacent to nonischemic tissue, it creates a setting for the key elements of reentry—slow conduction and unidirectional block—which makes the myocardium vulnerable to reentrant arrhythmias. When premature impulses are generated in this environment, regardless of their electrical mechanism (i.e., reentrant, triggered activity, automaticity), they may further alter the dispersion of recovery between ischemic tissue, chronically abnormal tissue, and normal cells, ultimately leading to complete disorganization and VF.

The dispersion of refractory periods produced by acute ischemia, which provides the substrate for reentrant tachycardias and VF, may be further enhanced by a healed ischemic injury. The time course of repolarization is lengthened after healing of ischemic injury and shortened by acute ischemia. The coexistence of the two appears to make the ventricle more susceptible to sustained arrhythmias in some experimental models.[172]

Bradyarrhythmias and Asystolic Arrest

The basic electrophysiological mechanism in this form of arrest is failure of normal subordinate automatic activity to assume the pacemaking function of the heart in the absence of normal function of the sinus node or AV junction, or both. Bradyarrhythmic and asystolic arrests are more common in severely diseased hearts and with cardiac arrest in patients with a number of end-stage disorders, both cardiac and noncardiac. These mechanisms may result, in part, from diffuse involvement of subendocardial Purkinje fibers in advanced heart disease. Systemic influences that increase extracellular K^+ concentration, such as anoxia, acidosis, shock, renal failure, trauma, and hypothermia, can result in partial depolarization of normal or already diseased pacemaker cells in the His-Purkinje system, with a decrease in the slope of spontaneous phase 4 depolarization and ultimate loss of automaticity. These processes can produce global dysfunction of automatic cell activity, in contrast to the regional dysfunction more common in acute ischemia. Functionally depressed automatic cells (e.g., owing to increased extracellular K^+ concentration) are more susceptible to overdrive suppression. Under these conditions, brief bursts of tachycardia may be followed by prolonged asystolic periods, with further depression of automaticity by the consequent acidosis and increased local K^+ concentration or by changes in adrenergic tone. The ultimate consequence may be degeneration into VF or persistent asystole.

Pulseless Electrical Activity

Pulseless electrical activity, formerly called electromechanical dissociation, is separated into *primary* and *secondary forms*. The common denominator in both is continued electrical rhythmicity of the heart in the absence of effective mechanical function. The secondary form includes the causes that result from an abrupt cessation of cardiac venous return, such as massive pulmonary embolism, acute malfunction of prosthetic valves, exsanguination, and cardiac tamponade from hemopericardium. The primary form is the more familiar; in it, none of these obvious mechanical factors are present but ventricular muscle fails to produce an effective contraction despite continued electrical activity (i.e., *failure of electromechanical coupling*). It usually occurs as an end-stage event in advanced heart disease, but it can occur in patients with acute ischemic events or, more commonly, after electrical resuscitation from a prolonged cardiac arrest. Although it is not thoroughly understood, it appears that diffuse disease, metabolic abnormalities, or global ischemia provides the pathophysiological substrate. The proximate mechanism for failure of electromechanical coupling may be abnormal intracellular Ca^{2+} metabolism, intracellular acidosis, or perhaps adenosine triphosphate depletion.

Clinical Characteristics of the Patient with Cardiac Arrest

Although the pathological anatomy associated with SCD related to coronary artery disease reflects the presence of the changes associated with acute coronary syndromes in the majority of cases, only a minority of survivors of out-of-hospital VF have clinical evidence of a new transmural myocardial infarction.[171,182,183] In the Seattle study, only one of five survivors had new transmural infarctions.[182] Nonetheless, many have enzyme elevations, with nonspecific ECG changes suggesting myocardial damage, which may be due to transient ischemia as a triggering event or a consequence of the loss of myocardial perfusion during the cardiac arrest.[162] The former supports the concept of transient pathophysiological changes associated with acute coronary syndromes as the trigger for cardiac arrest. The recurrence rate in survivors of out-of-hospital cardiac arrest was low in the subgroup of patients who had documentation of a new transmural myocardial infarction. In contrast, it was found to be 30 percent at 1 year and 45 percent at 2 years in the survivors who did not have a new transmural myocardial infarction.[182,183] Recurrence rates decreased subsequently,[171] possibly owing in part to long-term interventions. However, it is not known whether the decrease resulted from a change in the natural history, changes in preventive strategies for underlying disease, or long-term interventions for controlling arrhythmic risk.

Clinical cardiac arrest and SCD can be described in the framework of the same four phases of the event used to establish temporal definitions (see Fig. 33–1): prodromes, onset of the terminal event, the cardiac arrest, and progression to biological death or survival.

Prodromal Symptoms

Patients at risk for SCD can have prodromes such as chest pain, dyspnea, weakness or fatigue, palpitations, syncope, and a number of nonspecific complaints. Several epidemiological and clinical studies demonstrated that such symptoms can presage coronary events, particularly myocardial infarction and SCD, and result in contact with the medical system weeks to months before SCD. Among a group of patients successfully resuscitated after out-of-hospital cardiac arrest, 28 percent reported retrospectively that they had had new or changing angina pectoris or dyspnea in the 4 weeks before arrest and 31 percent had seen a physician during this time, but only 12 percent because of these symptoms.[182]

Attempts to identify early prodromal symptoms that are specific for the patient at risk for SCD have not been successful. Although several studies reported that 12 to 46 percent of fatalities occurred in patients who had seen a physician 1 to 6 months before death, such visits were more likely to presage myocardial infarction or nonsudden deaths, and the majority of complaints responsible for those visits were not heart related. However, patients who have chest pain as a prodrome to SCD appear to have a higher probability of intraluminal coronary thrombosis at postmortem examination.[184] Fatigue has been a particularly common symptom in the days or weeks before SCD in a number of studies, but this symptom is nonspecific. The symptoms that occur within the last hours or minutes before cardiac arrest are more specific for heart disease and may include symptoms of arrhythmias, ischemia, or heart failure. Liberthson and associates[155] reported specific cardiac symptoms at a mean interval of about 3.8 hours before collapse in 24 percent of victims of SCD. However, most studies have reported such symptoms even less commonly, particularly when victims whose deaths were instantaneous were included.

Onset of the Terminal Event

The period of 1 hour or less between acute changes in cardiovascular status and the cardiac arrest itself is defined as the "onset of the terminal event." A report on ambulatory recordings fortuitously obtained during the onset of an unexpected cardiac arrest indicated dynamic changes in cardiac electrical activity during the minutes or hours before the event.[185] This report suggested that increasing heart rate and advancing grades of ventricular ectopy are common antecedents of VF. Alterations in autonomic nervous system activity may also contribute to the onset of the event. Studies of short-term variations of heart rate variability, or related measures, have identified changes that correlate with the occurrence of ventricular arrhythmias.[186] Although these recordings suggest transient electrophysiological destabilization of the myocardium, the extent to which these objective observations are paralleled by clinical symptoms or events is less well documented.[187] SCDs caused by either arrhythmias or acute circulatory failure mechanisms correlate with a high incidence of acute myocardial disorders at the onset of the terminal event; such disorders are more likely to be ischemic when the death is due to arrhythmias and to be associated with low-output states or myocardial anoxia when the deaths are due to circulatory failure.

Abrupt, unexpected loss of effective circulation can be caused by cardiac arrhythmias or mechanical disturbances, but the majority of such events that terminate in SCD are arrhythmic. Hinkle and Thaler[188] classified cardiac deaths among 142 subjects who died during a follow-up of 5 to 10 years. Class I was labeled arrhythmic death and class II was death caused by circulatory failure. The distinction between the two classes was based on whether circulatory failure preceded (class II) or followed (class I) the disappearance of the pulse. Among deaths that occurred less than 1 hour after the onset of the terminal illness, 93 percent were due to arrhythmias; in addition, 90 percent of deaths caused by heart disease were initiated by arrhythmic events rather than circulatory failure. Deaths caused by circulatory failure occurred predominantly among patients who could be identified as having terminal illnesses (95 percent were comatose), were associated more frequently with bradyarrhythmias than with VF as the terminal arrhythmias, and were dominated by noncardiac events as the terminal illness. In contrast, 98 percent of the arrhythmic deaths were associated primarily with cardiac disorders.

Clinical Features of Cardiac Arrest

The cardiac arrest itself is characterized by abrupt loss of consciousness caused by lack of adequate cerebral blood flow. It is an event that uniformly leads to death in the absence of an active intervention, although spontaneous reversions occur rarely. The most common cardiac mechanism is VF, followed by asystole–pulseless electrical activity or severe bradyarrhythmias and sustained VT. Other mechanisms include rupture of the ventricle, cardiac tamponade, acute mechanical obstruction to flow, and acute disruption of a major blood vessel.

The potential for successful resuscitation is a function of the setting in which cardiac arrest occurs, the mechanism of the arrest, and the underlying clinical status of the victim. Closely related to the potential for successful resuscitation is the decision of whether to attempt to resuscitate.[189]

At present, there are fewer low-risk patients with otherwise uncomplicated myocardial infarctions weighting in-hospital cardiac arrest statistics than previously. Bedell and coworkers[190] reported that only 14 percent of patients receiving in-hospital cardiopulmonary resuscitation (CPR) were discharged from the hospital alive and that 20 percent of these patients died within the ensuing 6 months. Although 41 percent of the patients had suffered an acute myocardial infarction, 73 percent had a history of congestive heart failure and 20 percent had had prior cardiac arrests. The mean age of 70 years may have influenced the outcome statistics, but patients with high-risk complicated myocardial infarction and those with other high-risk markers heavily influenced the population of patients at risk for in-hospital cardiac arrest. Noncardiac clinical diagnoses were dominated by renal failure, pneumonia, sepsis, diabetes, and a history of cancer. The strong male preponderance consistently reported in out-of-hospital cardiac arrest studies is not present in in-hospital patients, but the better prognosis of VT or VF mechanisms, compared with bradyarrhythmic or asystolic mechanisms, persists (27 percent survival versus 8 percent survival). However, the proportion of arrests that are due to in-hospital VT or VF is considerably less (33 percent), with the combination of respiratory arrest, asystole, and electromechanical dissociation dominating the statistics (61 percent). In a more recent report, de Vos and colleagues[191] observed 22 percent survival to hospital discharge. Adverse risks were age older than 70 years, prior stroke or renal failure, or heart failure on admission. Better outcomes were predicted by prior angina pectoris or admission because of ventricular arrhythmias.

The important risk factors for death after CPR are listed in Table 33–3. The facts that the fraction of out-of-hospital cardiac arrest survivors who are discharged from the hospital alive may now equal or exceed the fraction of in-hospital cardiac arrest victims who are discharged alive and that the postdischarge mortality rate for in-hospital cardiac arrest survivors is higher than that for out-of-hospital cardiac arrest survivors[190] are telling clinical statistics. Not only do they emphasize the success of preventive measures for cardiac arrest in low-risk in-hospital patients, causing those statistics to be dominated by higher risk patients, but also they suggest the need for newer strategies for rapid in-hospital responses[192] in addition to emphasizing the need for improvement in prehospital and in-hospital care of out-of-hospital cardiac arrest victims.

Among elderly persons, the outcomes after community-based responses to out-of-hospital cardiac arrest are not as good as for younger victims. In one study comparing persons younger than 80 years (mean age = 64 years) with those in their 80s and 90s, survival to hospital discharge among the younger group was 19.4 percent compared with 9.4 percent for octogenarians and 4.4 percent for nonagenerians.[193]

TABLE 33–3 Predictors of Mortality after In-Hospital Cardiopulmonary Resuscitation

Before Arrest
Hypotension (systolic BP <100 mm Hg)
Pneumonia
Renal failure (BUN >50 mg/dl)
Cancer
Homebound life style
During Arrest
Arrest duration >15 min
Intubation
Hypotension (systolic BP <100 mm Hg)
Pneumonia
Homebound life style
After Resuscitation
Coma
Need for pressors
Arrest duration >15 min

BP = blood pressure; BUN = blood urea nitrogen.
Modified from Bedell SE, Delbanco TL, Cook EF, Epstein FH: Survival after cardiopulmonary resuscitation in the hospital. N Engl J Med 309:569, 1983. Copyright Massachusetts Medical Society.

However, when the groups were analyzed according to markers favoring survival (e.g., VF, pulseless VT), the incremental benefit was even better for the elderly than the younger patients (36, 24, and 17 percent, respectively). This finding suggests that age is only a weak predictor of an adverse outcome and should not be used in isolation as a reason not to resuscitate. Unfortunately, the frequency of ventricular tachyarrhythmias compared to nonshockable rhythms is lower among elderly persons.[193,194] Long-term neurological status and length of hospitalization were similar among older and younger surviving patients.

Progression to Biological Death

The time course for progression from cardiac arrest to biological death is related to the mechanism of the cardiac arrest, the nature of the underlying disease process, and the delay between onset and resuscitative efforts. The onset of irreversible brain damage usually begins within 4 to 6 minutes after loss of cerebral circulation related to unattended cardiac arrest, and biological death follows quickly. In large series, however, it has been demonstrated that a limited number of victims can remain biologically alive for longer periods and may be resuscitated after delays in excess of 8 minutes before beginning basic life support and in excess of 16 minutes before advanced life support. Despite these exceptions, it is clear that the probability of a favorable outcome deteriorates rapidly as a function of time after unattended cardiac arrest. Younger patients with less severe cardiac disease and the absence of coexistent multisystem disease appear to have a higher probability of a favorable outcome after such delays.

Irreversible injury of the central nervous system usually occurs before biological death, and the interval may extend to a period of weeks in patients who are resuscitated during the temporal gap between brain damage and biological death. In-hospital cardiac arrest caused by VF is less likely to have a protracted course between the arrest and biological death, with patients either surviving after a prompt intervention or succumbing rapidly because of inability to stabilize cardiac rhythm or hemodynamics.

The patients whose cardiac arrest is due to sustained VT with cardiac output inadequate to maintain consciousness can remain in VT for considerably longer periods, with blood flow that is marginally sufficient to maintain viability. Thus, there is a longer interval between the onset of cardiac arrest and the end of the period that allows successful resuscitation. The lives of such patients usually end in VF or an asystolic arrest if the VT is not actively or spontaneously reverted. Once the transition from VT to VF or to a bradyarrhythmia occurs, the subsequent course to biological death is similar to that in patients in whom VF or bradyarrhythmias are the initiating event.

The progression in patients with asystole or bradyarrhythmias as the initiating event is more rapid. Such patients, whether in an in-hospital or out-of-hospital environment, have a poor prognosis because of advanced heart disease or coexistent multisystem disease. They tend to respond poorly to interventions, even if the heart is successfully paced. Although a small subgroup of patients with bradyarrhythmias associated with electrolyte or pharmacological abnormalities may respond well to interventions, the majority progress rapidly to biological death. The infrequent cardiac arrests caused by mechanical factors such as tamponade, structural disruption, and impedance to flow by major thromboembolic obstructions to right or left ventricular outflow are reversible only in the instances in which the mechanism is recognized and an intervention is feasible. The vast majority of these events lead to rapid biological death, although prompt relief of tamponade may save some lives.

Hospital Course of Survivors of Cardiac Arrest

The conditions of patients who are resuscitated immediately from *primary* VF associated with acute myocardial infarction usually stabilize promptly, and they require no special management after the early phase of the infarction (see Chap. 47). The management after *secondary cardiac arrest in myocardial infarction* is dominated by the hemodynamic status of the patient. Among survivors of *out-of-hospital cardiac arrest,* the initial 24 to 48 hours of hospitalization are characterized by a tendency to ventricular arrhythmias, which usually respond well to antiarrhythmic therapy. The overall rate of recurrent cardiac arrest is low, 10 to 20 percent, but the mortality rate in patients who have recurrent cardiac arrests is about 50 percent. Only 5 to 10 percent of in-hospital deaths after out-of-hospital resuscitation are due to recurrent cardiac arrhythmias.[182,183] Patients who have recurrent cardiac arrest have a high incidence of either new or preexisting AV or intraventricular conduction abnormalities.[171]

The most common causes of death in hospitalized survivors of out-of-hospital cardiac arrest are noncardiac events related to central nervous system injury.[171,195] These include anoxic encephalopathy and sepsis related to prolonged intubation and hemodynamic monitoring lines. Fifty-nine percent of deaths during index hospitalization after prehospital resuscitation have been reported to be due to such causes. Approximately 40 percent of those who arrive in hospital in coma never awaken after admission to the hospital and die after a median survival of 3.5 days. Two-thirds of those who regain consciousness have no gross deficits, and an additional 20 percent have persisting cognitive deficits only. Of the patients who do awaken, 25 percent do so by admission, 71 percent by the first hospital day, and 92 percent by the third day. A small number of patients awakened after prolonged hospitalization. Among those who die in hospital, 80 percent do not awaken before death. Two studies suggest a potential benefit of therapeutic hypothermia for patients with post-cardiac arrest coma (see Post-Cardiac Arrest Care in Survivors of Out-of-Hospital Cardiac Arrest).[196,197]

Cardiac causes of delayed death during hospitalization after out-of-hospital cardiac arrest are most commonly related to hemodynamic deterioration, which accounts for about one-third of deaths in hospitals. Among all deaths, those that occurred within the first 48 hours of hospitalization were usually due to hemodynamic deterioration or arrhythmias regardless of the neurological status; later deaths were related to neurological complications. Admission characteristics most predictive of subsequent awakening included motor response, pupillary light response, spontaneous eye movement, and blood glucose level below 300 mg/dl.

Clinical Profile of Survivors of Out-of-Hospital Cardiac Arrest

The clinical features of survivors of out-of-hospital cardiac arrest are heavily influenced by the type and extent of the underlying disease associated with the event. Causation is dominated by coronary heart disease, which accounts for approximately 80 percent of out-of-hospital cardiac arrest in the United States[9] and is commonly extensive. The cardiomyopathies collectively account for another 10 to 15 percent, with all other structural heart diseases plus functional abnormalities and toxic or environmental causes accounting for the remainder (see Table 33–2).[76,198]

Ambient ventricular arrhythmias have been reported in the majority of survivors of prehospital cardiac arrest who had serial ambulatory monitor recordings. These arrhythmias show trends to higher grades of ventricular ectopy in victims of recurrent cardiac arrest compared with long-term survivors. Repetitive PVCs were strongly associated with a history of congestive heart failure or previous myocardial infarction.

LEFT VENTRICULAR FUNCTION. Left ventricular function is abnormal in the majority of survivors of out-of-hospital cardiac arrest, often severely so, but there is a wide variation, ranging from severe dysfunction to normal or near-normal measurements (Fig. 33–12).[199] The severity of myocardial dysfunction estimated shortly after cardiac arrest commonly improves within the first 24 hours of hospitalization.[200] Failure to begin improvement within that time frame is an adverse short-term prognostic sign. In a study of resuscitated out-of-hospital cardiac arrest victims admitted to hospital and subsequently discharged alive and neurologically intact, 47 percent had acute coronary syndromes identified during work-up and had a mean ejection fraction of 42 percent, compared with 32 percent among nonsurvivors.[201] Among survivors to hospital discharge, a reduced ejection fraction is an adverse long-term prognostic sign.

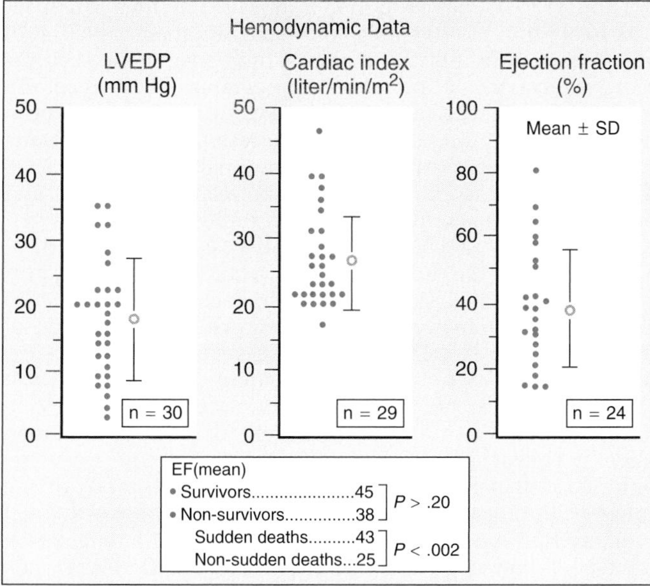

FIGURE 33–12 Hemodynamic data from victims of prehospital cardiac arrest studied during initial postarrest hospitalization. These data indicate a broad range of cardiac function and a statistically insignificant difference between ejection fraction at entry in long-term survivors and in victims of recurrent cardiac arrest. However, patients who died suddenly had significantly higher ejection fraction than those who died of nonsudden cardiac causes. LVEDP = left ventricular end-diastolic pressure. (From Myerburg RJ, Conde CA, Sung RJ, et al: Clinical, electrophysiologic and hemodynamic profile of patients resuscitated from prehospital cardiac arrest. Am J Med 68:568, 1980.)

CORONARY ANGIOGRAPHY. Studies of survivors of out-of-hospital cardiac arrest have shown that as a group this population tends to have extensive disease but no specific pattern of abnormalities. Acute coronary lesions, usually multifocal, are present in a majority of survivors.[168] Significant lesions in two or more vessels are present in at least 70 percent of patients who have any coronary lesion. Among patients who have recurrent cardiac arrests, the incidence of triple-vessel disease is higher than among those who do not. However, the frequency of moderate to severe stenosis of the left main coronary artery does not differ between cardiac arrest survivors and the overall population of patients with symptomatic coronary heart disease.

EXERCISE TESTING. Exercise testing is no longer commonly used to evaluate the need for, and response to, antiischemic therapy in survivors of out-of-hospital cardiac arrest, except when there is a question of transient ischemia as a mechanism for onset. The probability of a positive test related to ischemia is relatively low, although termination of testing because of fatigue is common.[171] Mortality during follow-up is greater in patients who have angina or failure of a normal rise in systolic blood pressure occurring during exercise.

ELECTROCARDIOGRAPHIC OBSERVATIONS. Among survivors of out-of-hospital cardiac arrest, the 12-lead ECG (see Chap. 9) has proved of value only for discriminating risk of recurrence among those whose cardiac arrest was associated with new transmural myocardial infarction. Patients who develop documented new Q waves in association with a clinical picture suggesting that an acute myocardial infarction began before the cardiac arrest itself are at lower risk for recurrence.[171] In contrast, nonspecific ECG markers of ischemia, associated with elevations of troponin or creatine kinase MB, indicate higher risk of recurrence.[162] A higher incidence of repolarization abnormalities (ST segment depression, flat T waves, prolonged QT) occurs in out-of-hospital cardiac arrest survivors than in post-myocardial infarction patients, and these might be markers for increased risk. Prolonged QRS duration is associated with increased mortality risk in patients with heart failure,[202] although it is not clear that this observation applies to sudden death specifically or to post-cardiac arrest victims in particular.

BLOOD CHEMISTRY. Lower serum K^+ levels are observed in survivors of cardiac arrest than in patients with acute myocardial infarction or stable coronary heart disease. This finding is probably a consequence of resuscitation interventions rather than a preexisting hypokalemic state owing to chronic diuretic use or other causes. Low ionized Ca^{2+} levels, with normal total calcium levels, were also observed during resuscitation from out-of-hospital cardiac arrest. Higher resting lactate levels have been reported in out-of-hospital cardiac arrest survivors than in normal subjects. Lactate levels correlated inversely with ejection fractions and directly with PVC frequency and complexity.

LONG-TERM PROGNOSIS. Studies from the early 1970s in both Miami[182] and Seattle[183] indicated that the risk of recurrent cardiac arrest in the first year after surviving an initial VT-VF event was about 30 percent and at 2 years was 45 percent. Total mortality at 2 years was about 60 percent in both studies. More recent total mortality data from the control groups of the secondary prevention implantable cardioverter-defibrillator (ICD) trials demonstrated a 2-year mortality rate between 20 and 25 percent.[203-205] The apparent improved outcomes, independent of the benefit provided by ICD therapy, are probably attributable to the current interventions used among survivors, such as beta adrenoceptor blockers, antiischemic procedures, amiodarone, and other therapies that were not available or in general use at the earlier time. Risk of recurrent cardiac arrest and all-cause mortality is higher during the first 12 to 24 months after the index event and relates best to ejection fraction during the first 6 months (Fig. 33–13).

Management of Cardiac Arrest

Community-Based Interventions

The initial systems responding to out-of-hospital cardiac arrests as developed in the United States were integrated into fire departments as primary emergency rescue systems. They employed paramedical personnel trained in CPR and the use of CPR monitoring equipment, defibrillators, and specific intravenous drug therapy. Although the initial out-of-hospital intervention experience in Miami and Seattle[182,183] reported in the mid-1970s yielded only 14 and 11 percent survivals to discharge, respectively, later improvements in the systems saved more lives (Fig. 33–14A).[206] By the early 1980s both had increased survival rates to about 25 percent[171,206] and by the late 1980s to 30 percent or more. Improvements correlated with the addition of emergency medical technicians as another tier of responders to provide CPR and earlier defibrillation. Survival rates have decreased since then, presumably because of the extension of rescue systems into less densely populated regions,[207] in addition to increased traffic congestion and verticalization of buildings in urban areas (see Fig. 33–14A). Generally, rural areas have lower success rates,[208,209] and the national success rate for the United States is probably 5 percent or less.

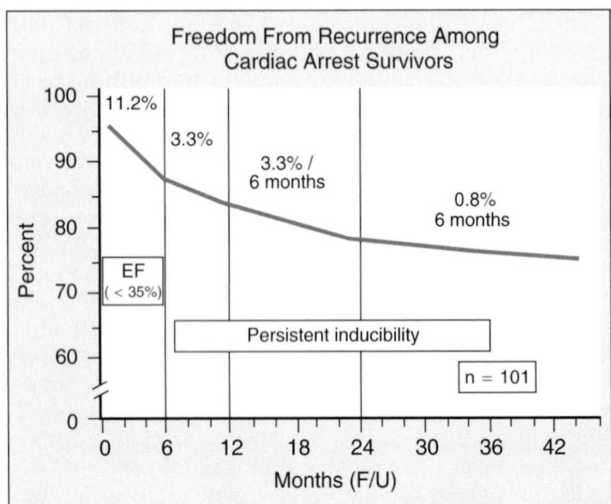

FIGURE 33–13 Time dependence of recurrences among survivors of cardiac arrest. Actuarial analysis of occurrences among a population of 101 cardiac arrest survivors with coronary artery disease is demonstrated. The risk was highest in the first 6 months (11.2 percent) and then fell to 3.3 percent per 6 months for the next three 6-month blocks. After 24 months, the rate fell to 0.8 percent per 6 months. A low ejection fraction (EF) was the most powerful predictor of death during the first 6 months; subsequently, persistent inducibility during programmed stimulation, despite drug therapy or surgery, was the most powerful predictor. F/U = follow-up. (Modified from Furukawa T, Rozanski JJ, Nogami A, et al: Time-dependent risk of and predictors for cardiac arrest recurrence in survivors of out-of-hospital cardiac arrest with chronic coronary artery disease. Circulation 80:599, 1989. The figure is reproduced from Myerburg RJ, Kessler KM, Castellanos A: Sudden cardiac death: Structure, function, and time-dependence of risk. Circulation 85[Suppl I]:I-2, 1992. Copyright 1992 American Heart Association.)

Reports from very densely populated areas (i.e., Chicago and New York City) have also provided disturbing outcome data. The Chicago study reported that only 9 percent of out-of-hospital cardiac arrest victims survived to be hospitalized and that only 2 percent were discharged alive.[41] Moreover, outcomes in blacks were far worse than in whites (0.8 percent versus 2.6 percent). The fact that a large majority had bradyarrhythmias, asystole, or pulseless electrical activity on initial contact with emergency medical services suggests prolonged times between collapse and emergency medical service arrival or absent or ineffective bystander interventions, or both. The New York City report indicated a survival-to-hospital discharge rate of only 1.4 percent.[210] Among those who had bystander CPR, the rate increased to 2.9 percent, and bystander CPR plus VF as the initial rhythm yielded a further increase to 5.3 percent. Finally, for those whose arrests occurred after the arrival of emergency medical services, the success rate increased further to 8.5 percent. These trends suggest that delays and breaks in the "chain of survival"[211] have a major negative impact on results of emergency medical services in densely populated areas.

IMPORTANCE OF ELECTRICAL MECHANISMS. Several sources have identified a disturbing trend in initial rhythms recorded by emergency rescue personnel.[7,212,213] Compared with data from the 1970s and 1980s, there has been a decrease in the number of events in which ventricular tachyarrhythmias are the initial rhythm recorded, with a consequent reduction in the proportion of victims who have rhythms amenable to cardioversion-defibrillation (Fig. 33–15). Some studies now suggest that less than one-half of victims are in shockable rhythms at initial contact. This fact is associated with a reduction in cumulative survival probabilities from community-based interventions,[7] even though data from studies employing nonconventional automated external defibrillator (AED) strategies suggest improvement for outcomes in VT or VF victims.[212,213] Because this finding does not appear to be related to time from 911 summons to arrival, it is likely that pre-911 delays in recognition and reaction to an event may be playing a role, which suggests a need for more extensive public education programs. Thus "response times" may not be as close to true "down times" as one would hope, impairing the potential for success. The 4- to 6-minute time for a desirable response is not optimal. By 4 minutes significant circulatory and ischemic changes have occurred, and beyond that time conditions worsen rapidly.[214]

The electrical mechanism of out-of-hospital cardiac arrest, as defined by the initial rhythm recorded by emergency rescue personnel, has a powerful impact on outcome. The subgroup of patients who are in sustained VT at the time of first contact, although small, has the best outcome (Fig. 33–16). Eighty-eight percent of patients in cardiac arrest related to VT were successfully resuscitated and admitted to the hospital alive, and 67 percent were ultimately discharged alive.[171] However, this relatively low-risk group represents only 7 to 10 percent of all cardiac arrests. Because of the inherent time lag between collapse and initial recordings, it is likely that many more cardiac arrests begin as rapid sustained VT and degenerate into VF before arrival of rescue personnel.

Patients who have a bradyarrhythmia or asystole at initial contact have the worst prognosis; only 9 percent of such patients in the Miami study were admitted to the hospital alive and none was discharged.[171] In a later experience there was some improvement in outcome, although the improvement was limited to patients in whom the initial bradyarrhythmia recorded was an idioventricular rhythm that responded promptly to chronotropic agents in the field. Bradyarrhythmias also have adverse prognostic implications after defibrillation from VF in the field. Patients who developed a heart rate less than 60 beats/min after defibrillation regardless of the specific bradyarrhythmic mechanism had a poor prognosis, with 95 percent of such patients dying either before hospitalization or in the hospital.[182]

The outcome in the group of patients in whom VF is the initial rhythm recorded is intermediate between the outcomes associated with sustained VT and bradyarrhythmia and asystole. Figure 33–16 demonstrates that 40 percent of such patients were successfully resuscitated and admitted to the hospital alive and 23 percent were ultimately discharged alive.[171] Later data indicate improvement in outcome. The proportion of each of the electrophysiological mechanisms responsible for cardiac arrest varied among the earlier reports, with VF ranging from 65 to more than 90 percent of the study populations and bradyarrhythmia and asystole ranging from 10 to 30 percent. However, in reports from densely populated metropolitan areas, the ratios of tachyarrhythmic to bradyarrhythmic or pulseless activity events were reversed, and outcomes were far worse.[41,210]

A

History of Community-Based EMS Systems		
1971–1974	Initial Miami/Seattle outcomes	14%, 11%
1978–1985	Peak Miami/Seattle outcomes	25–35%
1984	Rural outcomes: Standard basic life support Ambulance-based expanded access	 3% 19%
1991	Estimated cumulative U.S. survival	1–3%
1992–1994	Major metropolitan population centers	≤ 2%
1996	Dade County, Florida, outcomes	9%
1996–1998	Current U.S. EMS outcomes, cumulative	< 5%
1999	"Optimized" systems (OPALS)	5%

B

AED Deployment Strategies				
Deployment	**Examples**	**Rescuers**	**Advantages**	**Limitations**
Emergency vehicles	Police cars Fire engines Ambulances	Trained emergency personnel	Experienced users Broad deployment Objectivity	Deployment time Arrival delays Community variations
Public access sites	Public buildings Stadiums, malls Airports Airliners	Security personnel Designated rescuers Random lay persons	Population density Shorter delays Lay and emergency personnel access	Low event rates Inexperienced users Panic and confusion
Multi-family dwellings	Apartments Condominiums Hotels	Security personnel Designated rescuers Family members	Familiar locations Defined personnel Shorter delays	Infrequent use Low event rates Geographic factors
Single-family dwellings	Private homes Apartments Neighborhood "Heart Watch"	Family members Security personnel Designated rescuers	Immediate access Familiar setting	Acceptance Victim may be alone One-time user; panic

FIGURE 33–14 Out-of-hospital cardiac arrest survival and deployment strategies for automated external defibrillators (AEDs). **A,** The history of out-of-hospital cardiac arrest survival statistics demonstrates that standard emergency rescue systems are not sufficient to have a meaningful impact on sudden cardiac death in the community. **B,** Various deployment strategies for nonconventional responders with access to AEDs. For each example, the type of rescuer and the advantages and limitations of each strategy are provided. It is unlikely that any single strategy will dominate; rather, there will be a cumulative benefit from the additive effect of multiple approaches. EMS = emergency medical service; OPALS = Ontario Prehospital Advanced Life Support. (From Myerburg RJ: Sudden cardiac death: Exploring the limits of our knowledge. J Cardiovasc Electrophysiol 12:369, 2001.)

Both improved prehospital care and improvements in in-hospital technology and practices can contribute to better outcomes, as described in the chain of survival concept.[211] Of these two general factors, the influence of prehospital care has been studied in more detail. The importance of early defibrillation for improving outcome is supported by a number of studies (Fig. 33–17).[214-218] In rural communities, earlier defibrillation by ambulance technicians yielded a 19 percent survival compared with only 3 percent for standard CPR. In another report, an analysis of the relationship between response delay and survival to hospital discharge revealed a 48 percent survival for response times of 2 minutes or less compared with less than 10 percent survival when responses were longer than 10 minutes (Fig. 33–18A).[215] Mean response time was approximately 13 minutes, and overall survival was 5 percent. It was 9.5 percent for those in VT or VF on first contact. These observations have motivated the search for strategies that shorten response times, such as deploying automatic external defibrillators in public places[218] and for use by nonconventional responders.[212,216,217] Preliminary data suggest that this strategy may improve outcome by substantial increments based upon the rationale of shortening response times (see later and Fig. 33–18B).

A second element in prehospital care that appears to contribute to outcome is the role of bystander CPR by laypeople awaiting the arrival of emergency rescue personnel.[219,220] It has been reported that although there was no significant difference in the percentage of patients successfully resuscitated and admitted to the hospital alive with (67 percent) or without (61 percent) bystander intervention, almost twice as many prehospital cardiac arrest victims were ultimately discharged alive when they had had bystander CPR (43 percent) than when such support was not provided (22 percent). Central nervous system protection, expressed as early regaining of consciousness, is the major protective element of bystander CPR. The rationale for bystander intervention is further highlighted by the relation between time to defibrillation and survival when analyzed as a function of time to initiation of basic CPR. It has been reported that more than 40 percent of victims whose defibrillation and other advanced life support activities were instituted more than 8

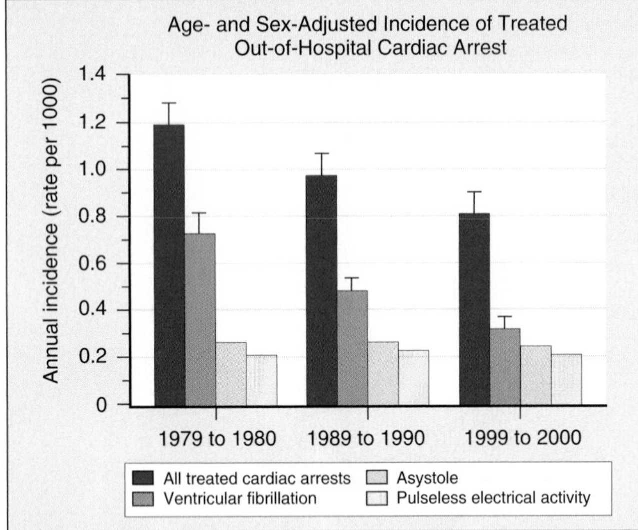

FIGURE 33–15 Changing incidence of ventricular fibrillation in the community. Between 1980 and 2000, there was a progressive decrease in the ventricular fibrillation event rate in the Seattle, Washington, community for unexplained reasons. Of note is the fact that there was not a concomitant increase in nonshockable rhythms. The proportion of events with ventricular fibrillation at initial contact is decreasing, as observed in several other studies. (Modified from Cobb LA, Fahrenbruch CE, Olsufka M, Copass MK: Changing incidence of out-of-hospital ventricular fibrillation, 1980-2000. JAMA 288:3008, 2002.)

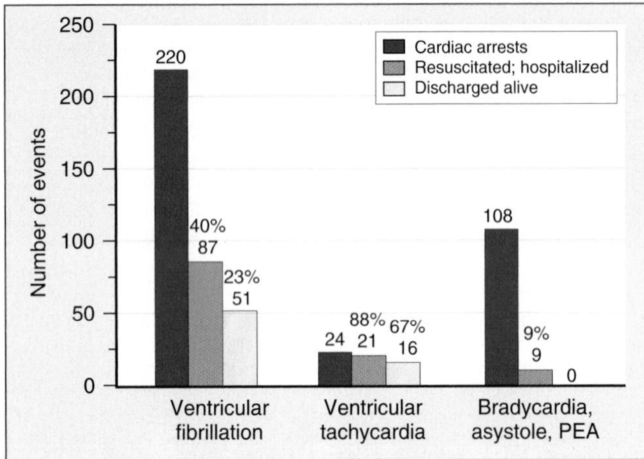

FIGURE 33–16 Survival after out-of-hospital cardiac arrest as function of the initial electrophysiological mechanism recorded by emergency rescue personnel. The mechanisms among 352 out-of-hospital cardiac arrest victims are separated into three categories: ventricular fibrillation (n = 220; 62 percent); ventricular tachycardia (n = 24; 7 percent); and bradycardia, asystole, and pulseless electrical activity (PEA) (n = 108; 31 percent). The purple bars illustrate the total number of events in each category. The blue bars illustrate the number and percentage of patients who were initially resuscitated in the field and reached the hospital alive in each category, and the yellow illustrate the percentage of total events in which patients were discharged from the hospital alive for each category. The data are derived from the Miami, Florida, experience.[211]

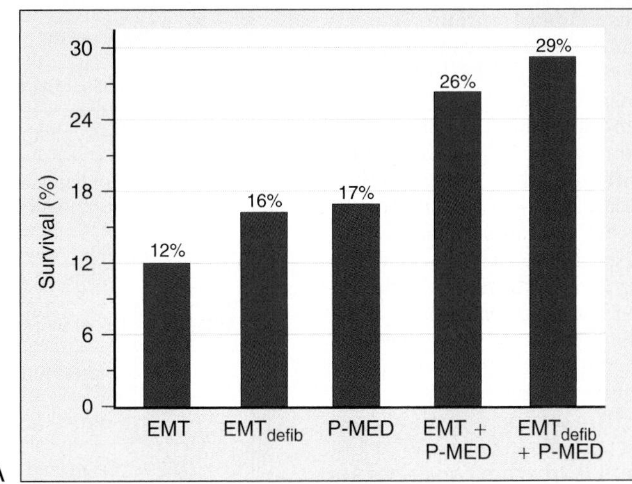

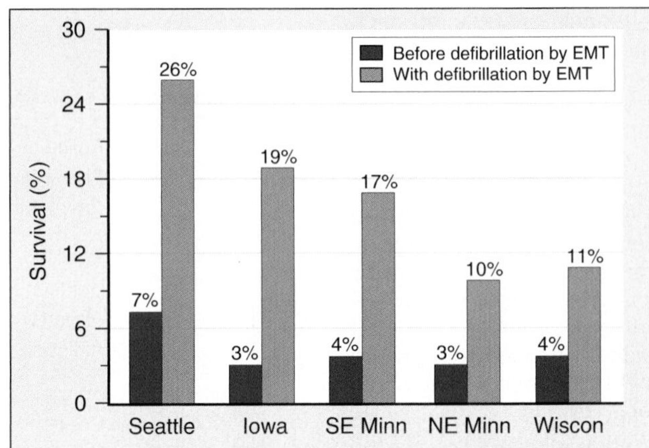

FIGURE 33–17 Impact of emergency rescue system design and immediate defibrillation on out-of-hospital cardiac arrest survival. **A,** Percent survival to hospital discharge with rescue activities by standard emergency medical technician (EMT) trained in cardiopulmonary resuscitation (CPR), EMTs allowed to defibrillate immediately (EMT_{defib}), initial response by paramedics (P-MED), two-tiered system with EMT and P-MED, and two-tiered system with EMTs allowed to defibrillate if they are the first responders plus P-MED. Training of first-responders (EMT_{defib}) and a two-tiered system have the best outcome. **B,** Comparison of outcomes observed in five geographic areas with EMTs providing only CPR (purple) versus EMTs trained to defibrillate as first responders (blue). In each group, there was a marked improvement in outcome when EMT personnel were trained and permitted to defibrillate. (Modified from Ornato JP, Om A: Community experience in treating out-of-hospital cardiac arrest. *In* Akhtar M, Myerburg RJ, Ruskin JN [eds]: Sudden Cardiac Death: Prevalence, Mechanisms and Approach to Diagnosis and Management. Baltimore, Williams & Wilkins, 1994, p 450.)

minutes after collapse survived if basic CPR had been initiated less than 2 minutes after onset of the arrest.[206] A period of CPR before defibrillation may also be helpful,[219] particularly if the time to defibrillation exceeds 4 minutes from onset of arrest.[214,221]

The time from onset of cardiac arrest to advanced life support influences outcome statistics. Improvement in both early neurological status and survival occurs in patients defibrillated by first responders, even if they are minimally trained emergency technicians allowed to carry out defibrillation as part of basic life support, compared with outcomes associated with awaiting more highly trained paramedics. Thus, the time to defibrillation plays a central role in determining outcome in cardiac arrest caused by VF. The development and deployment of AEDs (see Chap. 31) in the community hold promise for progress in the future.[218] This technology is potentially applicable with a number of different strategic models, each with its own benefits and limitations (see Fig. 33–14B).

Among the strategies that have yielded identifiable benefit to date are deployment in police vehicles,[212,213,217] airliners and airports,[224,225] casinos,[226] and more general community-based sites.[213,218] Police AED deployment data have been inconsistent among various studies,[209,212,213,217] possibly because of appropriateness for various types of communities and specific deployment strategies used, but data suggest that in large metropolitan areas there is benefit (Fig. 33–19).[212] Initial airline data were similarly uncertain, but a report on data from a large airline with a well-organized system sug-

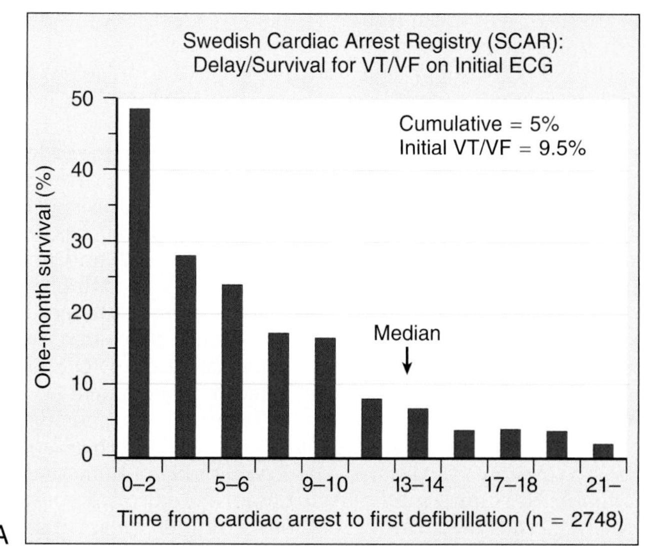

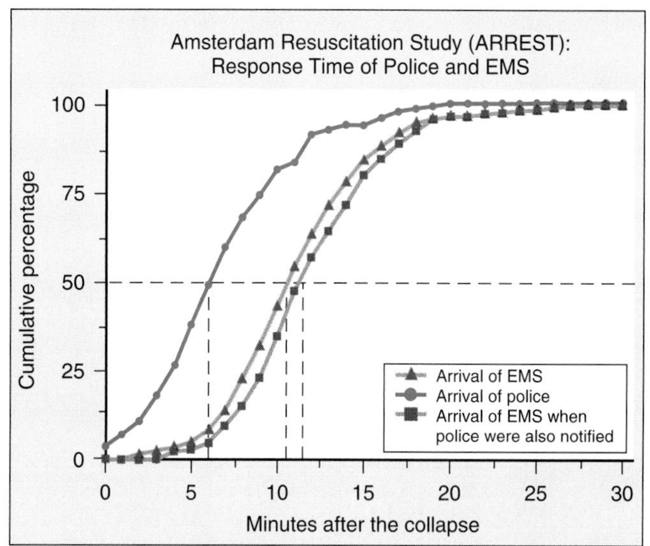

FIGURE 33–18 Influence of response time on survival from out-of-hospital cardiac arrest. **A,** The time from onset of cardiac arrest to initial defibrillation attempt is related to 1-month survival on the basis of data from the Swedish Cardiac Arrest Registry.[214] The cumulative survival rate was 5 percent, and the survival rate for victims whose initial rhythm was ventricular tachycardia (VT) or ventricular fibrillation (VF) was 9.5 percent. The median response time was nearly 13 minutes. Thirty-day survival ranged from a maximum of 48 percent with responses of less than 2 minutes to less than 5 percent with response time greater than 15 minutes. **B,** The potential for faster response systems, based on the Amsterdam Resuscitation Study, is demonstrated, comparing response times of police vehicles with those of conventional emergency medical systems (EMS). At the 50th percentile of response times, police vehicles provided a nearly 5-minute improvement in arrival time (approximately 6 minutes).[215]

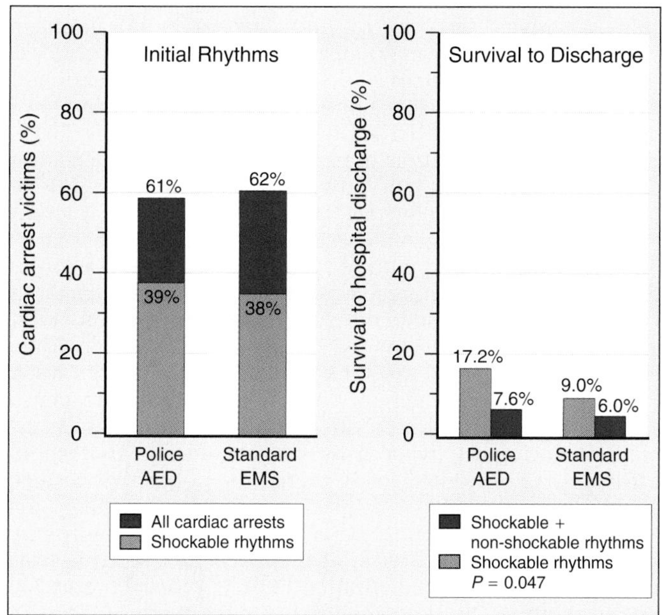

FIGURE 33–19 Rhythms at initial contact and survival statistics from the Miami–Dade County, Florida, police automated external defibrillator (AED) project. Shockable rhythms were observed in just under 40 percent in both the police AED program and the standard emergency medical system (EMS) historical control data. Those with shockable rhythms had improved survival to hospital discharge, with only a small improvement when both shockable and nonshockable rhythms were included in the analyzed data. (Modified from Myerburg RJ, Fenster J, Velez M, et al: Impact of community-wide police car deployment of automated external defibrillators on out-of-hospital cardiac arrest. Circulation 106:1058, 2002. Reproduced with permission of the American Heart Association).

gested benefit (Fig. 33–20A).[222] Similar encouraging results have been reported from deployment of AEDs in the Chicago airport system.[223] Finally, the special circumstance of casinos, in which continuous television monitoring alerts security officers to medical problems immediately, yielded impressive survival rates (Fig. 33–20B).[224] For more general community sites, defined as true public access including single-family dwellings, data are not yet available to determine benefit. However, there appears to be a great deal of variability of efficiency on the basis of expected event rates at different types of community sites.[218]

Management of Cardiac Arrest and Post-Cardiac Arrest Care

Management of the cardiac arrest victim is divided into five elements: (1) initial assessment, (2) basic life support, (3) advanced life support and definitive resuscitative efforts, (4) post-cardiac arrest care, and (5) long-term management. The first of these can be applied by a broad population base, which includes physicians and nurses as well as paramedical personnel, emergency rescue technicians, and laypeople educated in bystander intervention. The requirements for specialized knowledge and skills become progressively more focused as the patient moves through post-cardiac arrest management and into long-term follow-up care.[189]

Initial Assessment and Basic Life Support

This activity includes both diagnostic maneuvers and elementary interventions. The first action of the persons or persons in attendance when an individual collapses unexpectedly must be *confirmation that collapse is due to (or suspected to be due to) a cardiac arrest.* A few seconds of evaluation for response to voice, observation for respiratory movements and skin color, and simultaneous palpation of major arteries for the presence or absence of a pulse yield sufficient information to determine whether a life-threatening incident is in progress. Once a life-threatening incident is suspected or confirmed, contact with an available emergency medical rescue system (911) should be an immediate priority.[189]

The absence of a carotid or femoral pulse, particularly if confirmed by the absence of an audible heartbeat, is a primary diagnostic criterion. For lay responders, the pulse check is no longer recommended.[189] Skin color may be pale or intensely cyanotic. Absence of respiratory efforts or the presence of

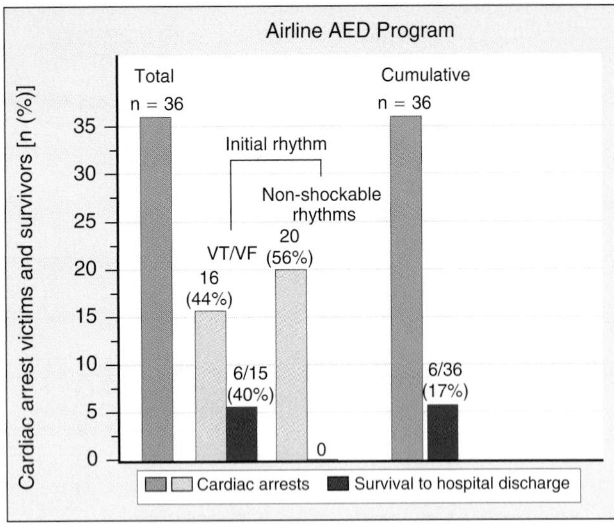

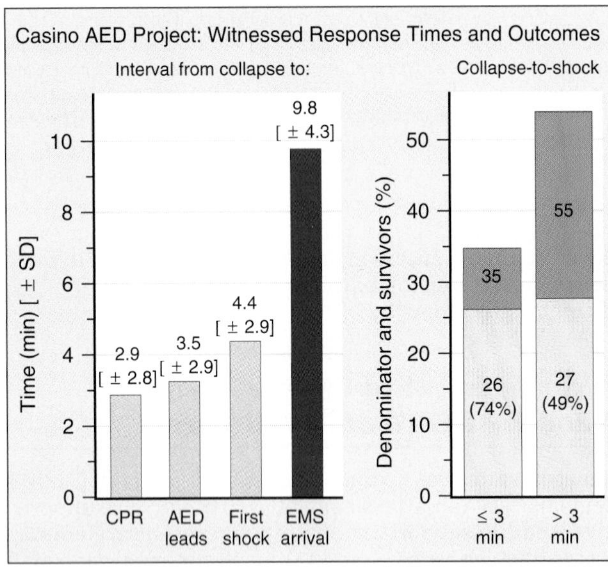

FIGURE 33–20 Outcomes of automated external defibrillator (AED) deployment programs at specific public sites. **A,** The data on outcomes after deployment of AEDs on a major airline demonstrated that approximately 44 percent of the cardiac arrests were associated with a documented ventricular tachycardia or fibrillation (VT/VF) mechanism and 40 percent of those victims survived. There were no survivors among the 56 percent of the victims who had nonshockable rhythms. Cumulative survival for the program was 17 percent. **B,** The results of AED deployment in the controlled environment of casinos. Because the onset of cardiac arrest can frequently be witnessed, short intervals from onset of collapse to cardiopulmonary resuscitation (CPR) and AED shocks were achieved. Response times were reduced by more than 50 percent compared with the standard emergency medical system (EMS). For those found in VT/VF, survival was better than expected from other community-based systems and approached 60 percent for VT/VF with a witnessed onset. When response time was less than 3 minutes, survival for VT/VF was more than 70 percent. (**A,** Modified from Page RL, Joglar JA, Kowal RC, et al. Use of automated external defibrillators by a U.S. airline. N Engl J Med 343:1210, 2000; **B,** modified from Valenzuela TD, Roe DJ, Nichol G, et al. Outcomes of rapid defibrillation by security officers after cardiac arrest in casinos. N Engl J Med 343:1206, 2000.)

only agonal respiratory efforts, in conjunction with an absent pulse, is diagnostic of cardiac arrest; however, respiratory efforts can persist for a minute or more after the onset of the arrest. In contrast, absence of respiratory efforts or severe stridor with persistence of a pulse suggests a primary respiratory arrest that will lead to a cardiac arrest in a short time. In the latter circumstance, initial efforts should include exploration of the oropharynx in search of a foreign body and the Heimlich maneuver, particularly if the incident occurs in a setting in which aspiration is likely (e.g., restaurant death or cafe coronary).

CHEST THUMP. When the diagnosis of a pulseless collapse (presumed cardiac arrest) is established, a blow to the chest (precordial thump, "thump-version") may be attempted by a properly trained rescuer. It has been recommended to be reserved as an advanced life support activity.[189] Caldwell and coworkers[225] supported its use on the basis of a prospective study in 5000 patients. Precordial thumps successfully reverted VF in 5 events, VT in 11, asystole in 2, and undefined cardiovascular collapse in 2 others in which the electrical mechanism was unknown. In no instance was conversion of VT to VF observed. Because the latter is the only major concern about the precordial thump technique and electrical activity can be initiated by mechanical stimulation in the asystolic heart, the technique is considered optional for responding to a *pulseless* cardiac arrest in the absence of monitoring when a defibrillator is not immediately available. It should not be used unmonitored for the patient with a rapid tachycardia without complete loss of consciousness. For attempted thump-version in cardiac arrest, one or two blows should be delivered firmly to the junction of the middle and lower thirds of the sternum from a height of 8 to 10 inches, but the effort should be abandoned if the patient does not immediately develop a spontaneous pulse and begin breathing. Another mechanical method, which requires that the patient is still conscious, is so-called cough-induced cardiac compression or cough-version. It is a conscious act of forceful coughing by the patient that may support forward flow by cyclic increases in intrathoracic pressure during VF or may cause conversion of sustained VT. Data supporting its successful use exist but are limited, and it is not considered an alternative to conventional techniques.

THE ABCS OF CARDIOPULMONARY RESUSCITATION. The goal of this activity is to maintain viability of the central nervous system, heart, and other vital organs until definitive intervention can be achieved. The activities included within basic life support encompass both the initial responses outlined earlier and their natural flow into establishing ventilation and perfusion. This range of activities can be carried out not only by professional and paraprofessional personnel but also by trained emergency technicians and laypeople. Time is the key issue, and there should be minimal delay between the diagnosis and preparatory efforts in the initial response and the institution of basic life support. This principle has measurable impact for both out-of-hospital and in-hospital cardiac arrest. Survival to discharge for in-hospital cardiac arrests, considering all etiologies and mechanisms, was reported to be 33 percent when CPR was initiated within the first minute compared with 14 percent when the time was more than 1 minute (odds ratio, 3.06).[192] When VF was the initial rhythm, the corresponding figures were 50 and 32 percent. In the out-of-hospital setting if only one witness is present, notification of emergency personnel (telephone 911) is the only activity that should precede basic life support.

AIRWAY. Clearing the airway is a critical step in preparing for successful resuscitation. This process includes tilting the head backward and lifting the chin in addition to exploring the airway for foreign bodies—including dentures—and removing them. The Heimlich maneuver should be performed if there is reason to suspect a foreign body lodged in the oropharynx. This maneuver entails wrapping the arms around the victim from the back and delivering a sharp thrust to the upper abdomen with a closed fist. If it is not possible for the person in attendance to carry out the maneuver because of insufficient physical strength, mechanical dislodgment of the foreign body can sometimes be achieved by abdominal thrusts with the unconscious patient in a supine position. The Heimlich maneuver is not entirely benign; ruptured abdominal viscera in the victim have been reported, as has an instance in which the rescuer disrupted his own aortic root and died. If there is strong suspicion that respiratory arrest precipitated cardiac arrest, particularly in the presence of a mechanical airway obstruction, a second precordial thump should be delivered after the airway is cleared.

BREATHING. With the head properly placed and the oropharynx clear, mouth-to-mouth respiration can be initiated if no specific rescue equipment is available. To a large extent, the procedure used for establishing ventilation depends on the site at which the cardiac arrest occurs. A variety of devices are available, including plastic oropharyngeal airways, esophageal obturators, the masked Ambu bag, and endotracheal tubes. Intubation is the preferred procedure, but time should not be sacrificed even in the in-hospital setting while awaiting an endotracheal tube or a person trained to insert it quickly and properly. Thus, in the in-hospital setting, temporary support with Ambu bag ventilation is the usual method until endotracheal intubation can be carried out, and in the out-of-hospital setting mouth-to-mouth resuscitation is used while awaiting emergency rescue personnel. The effect of the acquired immunodeficiency syndrome and hepatitis B transmission on attitudes toward mouth-to-mouth resuscitation by bystanders and even professional personnel in hospitals is an area of concern, but currently available data assessing risk of infection suggest that it is minimal.[189] The impact of this concern on attitudes toward, and outcomes of, resuscitative efforts has not been assessed.

Conventional CPR ventilatory techniques require that the lungs be inflated twice in succession after every 15 chest compressions.[189] Techniques of CPR based on the hypothesis that increased intrathoracic pressure is the prime mover of blood, rather than cardiac compression itself, have been evaluated; the cyclic ventilatory techniques are altered in these procedures (see later). However, clinical applicability is still not clarified.[226]

CIRCULATION (Fig. 33–21). This element of basic life support is intended to maintain blood flow (i.e., circulation) until definitive steps can be taken. The rationale is based on the hypothesis that chest compression allows the heart to maintain an externally driven pump function by sequential emptying and filling of its chambers, with competent valves favoring the forward direction of flow. In fact, the application of this technique has proved successful when used as recommended.[189] The palm of one hand is placed over the lower sternum and the heel of the other rests on the dorsum of the lower hand. The sternum is then depressed with the resuscitator's arms straight at the elbows to provide a less tiring and more forceful fulcrum at the junction of the shoulders and back (see Fig. 33–21). By using this technique, sufficient force is applied to depress the sternum about 4 to 5 cm, with abrupt relaxation, and the cycle is carried out at a rate of about 100 compressions per minute. Despite the fact that this conventional technique produces measurable carotid artery flow and a record of successful resuscitations, the absence of a pressure gradient across the heart in the presence of an extrathoracic arterial-venous pressure gradient has led to a concept that it is not cardiac compression per se but rather a pumping action produced by pressure changes in the entire thoracic cavity that optimizes systemic blood flow during resuscitation. Experimental work in which the chest is compressed during ventilations rather than between them (simultaneous compression-ventilation) had demonstrated better extrathoracic arterial flow. However, increased carotid artery flow does not necessarily equate with improved cerebral perfusion, and the reduction in coronary blood flow caused by elevated intrathoracic pressures by certain techniques may be too high a price for the improved peripheral flow. In addition, a high thoracoabdominal gradient has been demonstrated during experimental simultaneous compression-ventilation, which could divert flow from the brain in the absence of concomitant abdominal binding. On the basis of these observations, new mechanically assisted techniques, including an active decompression phase (i.e., active compression-decompression), have been evaluated for improved circulation during CPR.[226,227] More clinical studies are needed before establishing their general clinical applications.

Advanced Life Support and Definitive Resuscitation

This next step in the resuscitative sequence is designed to achieve definitive stabilization of the patient.[189] The implementation of advanced life support is not intended to suggest an abrupt cessation of basic life support activities but rather a merging and transition from one level of activity to the next. In the past, advanced life support required judgments and technical skills that removed it from the realm of activity of lay bystanders and even emergency medical technicians, limiting these activities to specifically trained paramedical

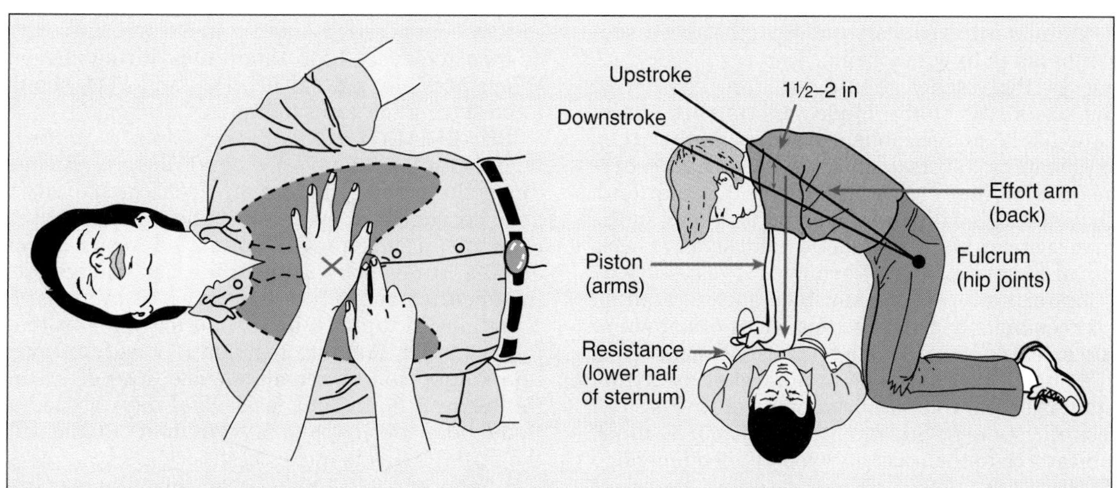

FIGURE 33–21 External chest compression. **Left,** Locating the correct hand position on the lower half of the sternum. **Right,** Proper position of the rescuer, with shoulders directly over the victim's sternum and elbows locked. (From Standards and guidelines for Cardiopulmonary Resuscitation [CPR] and Emergency Cardiac care [ECC]. National Academy of Sciences-National Research Council. JAMA 255:2906, 1986. Copyright 1986, the American Medical Association.)

personnel, nurses, and physicians. With further education of emergency technicians, most community-based CPR programs now permit them to carry out advanced life support activities. In addition, the development and testing of automatic external defibrillators that have the ability to sense and analyze cardiac electrical activity and prompt the user to deliver definitive electrical intervention[228] provides a role for less highly trained rescue personnel (i.e., police, ambulance drivers) and even untrained lay bystanders[218,223] for rapid defibrillation.

The general goals of advanced life support are to revert the cardiac rhythm to one that is hemodynamically effective, optimize ventilation, and maintain and support the restored circulation. Thus, during advanced life support, the patient's cardiac rhythm is promptly cardioverted or defibrillated as the first priority if appropriate equipment is immediately available. There is increasing evidence that a short period of closed-chest cardiac compression immediately before defibrillation enhances the probability of survival.[214,219,221] After the initial attempt to restore a hemodynamically effective rhythm, the patient is intubated and oxygenated, if needed, and the heart is paced if a bradyarrhythmia or asystole occurs. An intravenous line is established to deliver medications. After intubation, the goal of ventilation is to reverse hypoxemia and not merely achieve a high alveolar oxygen pressure (PO_2). Thus, oxygen rather than room air should be used to ventilate the patient; if possible, the arterial PO_2 should be monitored. Respirator support in hospital and an Ambu bag by means of an endotracheal tube, or facemasks in the out-of-hospital setting, are usually used.

DEFIBRILLATION-CARDIOVERSION (Fig. 33–22). Rapid conversion to an effective cardiac electrical mechanism is a key step for successful resuscitation. Delay should be minimal, even when conditions for CPR are optimal. When VF or a rapid VT is recognized on a monitor or by telemetry, defibrillation should be carried out immediately with a shock of 200 joules. From data based on monophasic waveforms, up to 90 percent of VF victims weighing up to 90 kg can be successfully resuscitated with a 200-joule shock, and a 300- or 360-joule shock may be used if this is not successful.[189] Failure of the initial shocks to cardiovert to an effective rhythm is a poor prognostic sign. After failure of three shocks up to a maximum of 360 joules of energy, CPR should be continued while the patient is intubated and intravenous access achieved. Epinephrine, 1 mg intravenously (IV), is administered and followed by repeated defibrillation attempts at 360 joules. Epinephrine may be repeated at 3- to 5-minute intervals with defibrillator shocks in between,[189] but high-dose epinephrine does not appear to provide added benefit.[229] Vasopressin, 40 units intravenously one time, has been suggested as an alternative to epinephrine.[230]

Simultaneously, the rescuer should focus on ventilation to correct the chemistry of the blood, efforts that render the heart more likely to reestablish a stable rhythm (i.e., improved oxygenation, reversal of acidosis, and improvement of the underlying electrophysiological condition). Although adequate oxygenation of the blood is crucial in the immediate management of the metabolic acidosis of cardiac arrest, additional correction can be achieved if necessary by intravenous administration of sodium bicarbonate. Sodium bicarbonate is recommended for circumstances of known or suspected preexisting bicarbonate-responsive causes of acidosis, certain drug overdoses, and prolonged resuscitation runs.[189] The more general role for bicarbonate during cardiac arrest has been questioned, but in any circumstance, much less sodium bicarbonate than was previously recommended is adequate for treatment of acidosis in this setting. Excessive quantities can be deleterious. Although some investigators have questioned the use of sodium bicarbonate at all because risks of alkalosis, hypernatremia, and hyperosmolality may

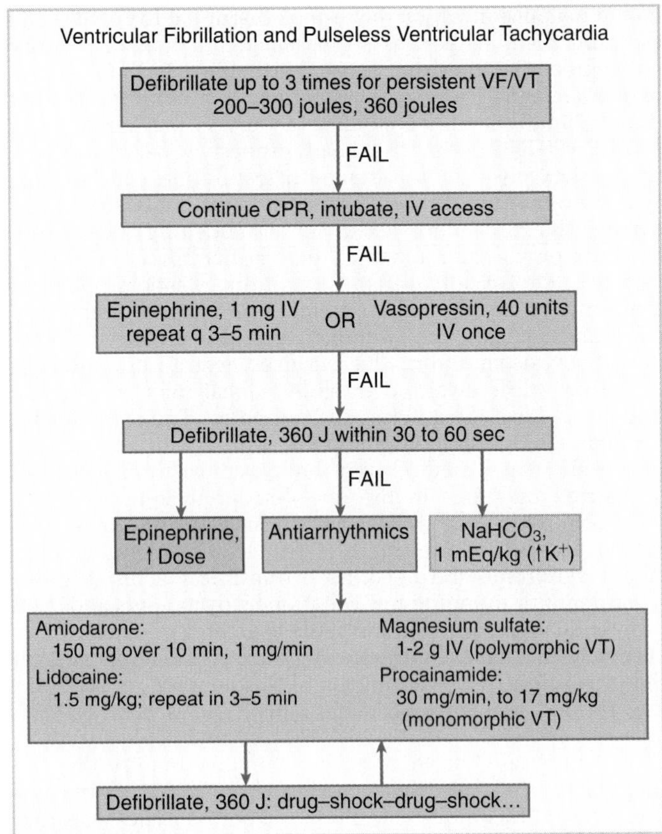

FIGURE 33–22 Advanced life support for ventricular fibrillation (VF) and pulseless ventricular tachycardia (VT). If initial defibrillation fails, the patient should be intubated and intravenous (I.V.) access immediately established while cardiopulmonary resuscitation (CPR) is continued. Epinephrine, 1 mg intravenously, should be administered and may be repeated several times with additional attempts to defibrillate with 360-joule shocks. If the conversion is still unsuccessful, epinephrine may be administered again, although it is unlikely that higher doses would provide any further benefit. Sodium bicarbonate should be administered at this time only if the patient is known to be hyperkalemic, but intravenous antiarrhythmic drugs should be tried (see text). Additional attempts to defibrillate should follow the administration of each drug attempted. (Modified from Emergency Cardiac Care Committee and Subcommittees, American Heart Association: Guidelines for cardiopulmonary resuscitation and emergency cardiac care. JAMA 268:2172, 1992. American Medical Association. See original reference for further details.)

outweigh its benefits, the circumstances cited may benefit from administration of 1 mEq/kg sodium bicarbonate while CPR is being carried out. Up to 50 percent of this dose may be repeated every 10 to 15 minutes during the course of CPR. When possible, arterial pH, PO_2, and PCO_2 should be monitored during the resuscitation.

PHARMACOTHERAPY (see Chap. 30). For the patient who continues to have VT or VF despite direct-current cardioversion after epinephrine, electrical stability of the heart may be achieved by intravenous administration of antiarrhythmic agents during continued resuscitation (see Fig. 33–22). Intravenous amiodarone has emerged as the initial treatment of choice (150 mg over 10 minutes, followed by 1 mg/min for up to 6 hours and 0.5 mg/min thereafter) (see Fig. 33–22).[167] Another regimen is 1 mg/min over the next 3 hours, followed by a maintenance dose of 0.5 mg/min over the next 18 hours and for several days as necessary. Additional bolus dosing, to a maximum of 500 mg, can be tried if the initial bolus is unsuccessful.

A bolus of 1.0 to 1.5 mg/kg of lidocaine may be given intravenously and the dose repeated in 2 minutes for patients in whom amiodarone is unsuccessful and possibly for those who have an acute transmural myocardial infarction as the triggering mechanism for the cardiac arrest. Intravenous procainamide (loading infusion of 100 mg per 5 minutes to a total dose of 500 to 800 mg, followed by continuous infusion at 2 to 5 mg/min) is rarely used in this setting any longer, but may be tried for persisting, hemodynamically stable arrhythmias.

For patients in whom acute hyperkalemia is the triggering event for resistant VF or who have hypocalcemia or are toxic from Ca^{2+} entry blocking drugs, 10 percent calcium gluconate, 5 to 20 ml infused at a rate of 2 to 4 ml/min, may be helpful.[189] Calcium should not be used routinely during resuscitation, even though ionized Ca^{2+} levels may be low during resuscitation from cardiac arrest. Some resistant forms of polymorphic VT or torsades de pointes, rapid monomorphic VT or ventricular flutter (rate ≥ 260/min), or resistant VF may respond to intravenous beta blocker therapy (propranolol, 1 mg IV boluses to a total dose of up to 15 to 20 mg; metoprolol, 5 mg IV, up to 20 mg) or intravenous $MgSO_4$ (1 to 2 gm IV given over 1 to 2 minutes).

BRADYARRHYTHMIC AND ASYSTOLIC ARREST; PULSELESS ELECTRICAL ACTIVITY (Fig. 33–23). The approach to the patient with bradyarrhythmic or asystolic arrest or pulseless electrical activity differs from the approach to patients with tachyarrhythmic events (VT or VF).[189] When this form of cardiac arrest is recognized, efforts should focus first on establishing control of the cardiorespiratory status (i.e., continue CPR, intubate, and establish intravenous access), then reconfirming the rhythm (in two leads if possible), and finally taking actions that favor the emergence of a stable spontaneous rhythm or attempt to pace the heart. Possible reversible causes, particularly for bradyarrhythmia and asystole, should be considered and excluded (or treated) promptly. These include hypovolemia, hypoxia, cardiac tamponade, tension pneumothorax, preexisting acidosis, drug overdose, hypothermia, and hyperkalemia. Epinephrine (1.0 mg IV every 3 to 5 minutes) and atropine (1.0 to 2.0 mg intravenously) are commonly used in an attempt to elicit spontaneous electrical activity or increase the rate of a bradycardia. These have had only limited success, as have intravenous isoproterenol infusions in doses up to 15 to 20 μg/min. In the absence of an intravenous line, epinephrine (1 mg [i.e., 10 ml of a 1:10,000 solution]) may be given by the intracardiac route, but there is danger of coronary or myocardial laceration. Sodium bicarbonate, 1 mEq/kg, may be tried for known or strongly suspected preexisting hyperkalemia or bicarbonate-responsive acidosis.

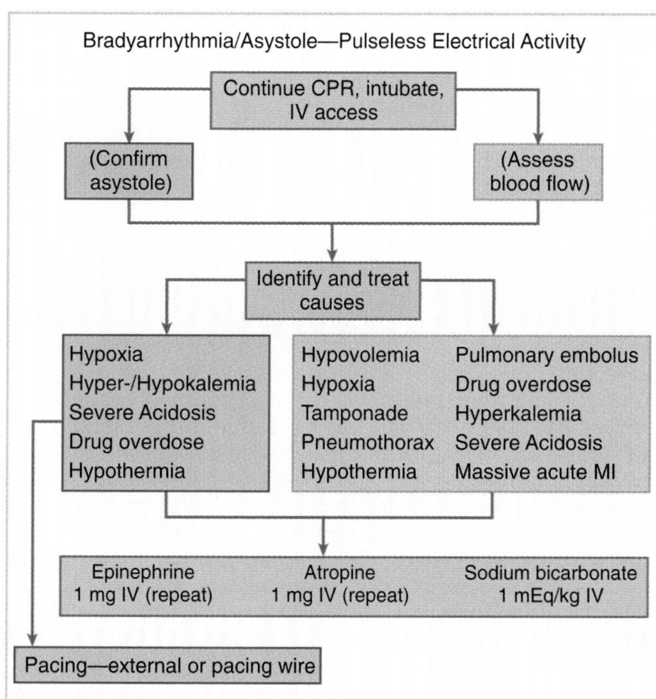

FIGURE 33–23 Advanced cardiac life support for patients with severe bradyarrhythmia, asystole, and pulseless electrical activity. The patient in any of these states should have continued cardiopulmonary resuscitation (CPR) and be intubated, with intravenous (I.V.) access established, before pharmacological treatment. The initial activity is to confirm persisting asystole or attempt to assess blood flow in patients thought to have pulseless electrical activity. An immediate attempt should be made to identify and treat reversible or treatable causes of these forms of cardiac arrest. Epinephrine is generally administered first, and atropine or bicarbonate, or both, may be administered subsequently. An attempt to pace the heart with an external device or an intracardiac pacing catheter is advisable, although usually not successful, except for certain reversible bradyarrhythmias. M.I. = myocardial infarction. (Modified from Emergency Cardiac Care Committee and Subcommittees, American Heart Association: Guidelines for cardiopulmonary resuscitation and emergency cardiac care. JAMA 268:2172, 1992. Copyright 1992, American Medical Association. See original reference for further details.)

Pacing of the bradyarrhythmic or asystolic heart has been limited in the past by the unavailability of personnel capable of carrying out such procedures at the scene of cardiac arrests. With the development of more effective external pacing systems, the role of pacing and its influence on outcome must now be reevaluated. Unfortunately, all data to date suggest that the *asystolic* patient continues to have a very poor prognosis despite new techniques.[231]

The published standards for CPR and emergency cardiac care[189] include a series of teaching algorithms to be used as guides to appropriate care. Figures 33–22 and 33–23 provide the algorithms for VF and pulseless VT, asystole (or cardiac standstill), and pulseless electrical activity. These general guides are not to be interpreted as inclusive of all possible approaches or contingencies. The special circumstance of CPR in pregnant women requires additional attention to effects of drugs on the gravid uterus and the fetus, mechanical and physiological influences of pregnancy on the efficacy of CPR, and risk of complications such as ruptured uterus and lacerated liver.

STABILIZATION. As soon as electrical resuscitation from VT, VF, bradycardia, asystole, or pulseless electrical activity is achieved, the focus of attention shifts to maintaining a stable electrical, hemodynamic, and central nervous system status. For electrical stability, a continuous infusion of an effective drug, based on observation during the cardiac arrest run, is commonly used. This drug may be lidocaine, 1 to 4 mg/min depending on size and clinical factors; intravenous amiodarone, 10 mg/kg/d (if this drug was required in the initial resuscitation); or procainamide, 2 to 4 mg/min. Occasionally, a continuous infusion of propranolol or esmolol is used. Catecholamines are used in cardiac arrest not only in an attempt to achieve better electrical stability (e.g., conversion from fine to coarse VF, or increasing the rate of spontaneous contraction during bradyarrhythmias) but also for their inotropic and peripheral vascular effects. Epinephrine is the first choice among the catecholamines for use in cardiac arrest because it increases myocardial contractility, elevates perfusion pressure, may convert electromechanical dissociation to electromechanical coupling, and improves chances for defibrillation. Because of its adverse effects on renal and mesenteric flow, norepinephrine is a less desirable agent despite its inotropic effects. When the chronotropic effect of epinephrine is undesirable, dopamine or dobutamine is preferable to norepinephrine for inotropic effect. Isoproterenol may be used for the treatment of primary or postdefibrillation bradycardia when heart rate control is the primary goal of therapy intended to improve cardiac output. Calcium chloride, 2 to 4 mg/kg, is sometimes used in patients with pulseless electrical activity that persists after administration of catecholamines. The efficacy of this intervention is uncertain. Stimulation of alpha adrenoceptors may be important during definitive resuscitative efforts. For instance, the alpha adrenoceptor–stimulating effects of epinephrine and higher dosages of dopamine, producing elevation of aortic diastolic pressures by peripheral vasoconstriction with increased cerebral and myocardial flow, have been reemphasized.

Post-Cardiac Arrest Care

For successfully resuscitated cardiac arrest victims, whether the event occurred in or out of hospital, post-cardiac arrest care includes admission to an intensive care unit and continuous monitoring for a minimum of 48 to 72 hours. Some elements of postarrest management are common to all resuscitated patients, but prognosis and certain details of management are specific for the clinical setting in which the cardiac arrest occurred. The major management categories include (1) primary cardiac arrest in acute myocardial infarction, (2) secondary cardiac arrest in acute myocardial infarction, (3) cardiac arrest associated with noncardiac disorders, and (4) survival after out-of-hospital cardiac arrest.

Primary Cardiac Arrest in Acute Myocardial Infarction

VF in patients with acute myocardial infarction free of concomitant hemodynamic complications (i.e., primary VF) (see also Chap. 47) is now less common in hospitalized patients than the 15 to 20 percent incidence before the availability of cardiac care units. The events that do occur are almost always successfully reverted by prompt interventions in properly equipped emergency departments or cardiac care units. After successful resuscitation, patients are often maintained with a lidocaine infusion at 2 to 4 mg/min. Antiarrhythmic support is usually discontinued after 24 hours if arrhythmias do not recur (see Chap. 30). The occurrence of VF during the early phase of acute myocardial infarction (i.e., first 24 to 48 hours) is not an indication for subsequent electrophysiological testing or long-term antiarrhythmic or device therapy. Rapid sustained VT producing the clinical picture of cardiac arrest in acute myocardial infarction is treated similarly; its intermediate- and long-term implications are the same as those of VF. Cardiac arrest caused by bradyarrhythmias or asystole in acute inferior wall myocardial infarction, in the absence of primary hemodynamic consequences, is uncommon and may respond to either atropine or pacing. The prognosis is good, with no special long-term care required in most instances. Rarely, symptomatic bradyarrhythmias that require permanent pacemakers persist in survivors. In contrast to inferior myocardial infarction, bradyarrhythmic cardiac arrest associated with large anterior wall infarctions (and AV or intraventricular block) has a poor prognosis.

Secondary Cardiac Arrest in Acute Myocardial Infarction

This condition is defined as cardiac arrest occurring in association with, or as a result of, hemodynamic or mechanical dysfunction. The immediate mortality among patients in this setting ranges from 59 to 89 percent, depending on the severity of the hemodynamic abnormalities and size of the myocardial infarction. Resuscitative efforts commonly fail in such patients, and when they are successful, the post-cardiac arrest management is often difficult. When secondary cardiac arrest occurs by the mechanisms of VT or VF, aggressive hemodynamic or antiischemic measures may help achieve rhythm stability. If recurrences of the arrhythmia continue, intravenous amiodarone has emerged as the antiarrhythmic therapy of choice.[167] Lidocaine may also be tried if the mechanism appears to be ischemic but is less likely to be successful in this setting than in primary VF. The success of interventions and prevention of recurrent cardiac arrest are related closely to the outcome of managing the hemodynamic status. The incidence of cardiac arrest caused by bradyarrhythmias or asystole, or by electromechanical dissociation, is higher in the secondary form of cardiac arrest in acute myocardial infarction. Such patients usually have large myocardial infarctions and major hemodynamic abnormalities and may be acidotic and hypoxemic. Even with aggressive therapy, the prognosis after a bradyarrhythmic or asystolic arrest in such patients is poor, and patients are resuscitated only rarely from electromechanical dissociation. All patients in circulatory failure at the onset of arrest are in a high-risk category, with only a 2 percent survival rate among hypotensive patients in one study.[190]

CARDIAC ARREST AMONG IN-HOSPITAL PATIENTS WITH NONCARDIAC ABNORMALITIES. These patients fall into two major categories: (1) those with life-limiting diseases such as malignancies, sepsis, organ failure, end-stage pulmonary disease, and advanced central nervous system disease and (2) those with acute toxic or proarrhythmic states that are potentially reversible. In the former category, the ratio of tachyarrhythmic to bradyarrhythmic cardiac arrest is low[190] and the prognosis for surviving cardiac arrest is poor. Although the data may be somewhat skewed by the practice of assigning "do not resuscitate" orders to patients with end-stage disease, available data for attempted resuscitations show a poor outcome. Only 7 percent of cancer patients, 3 percent of renal failure patients, and no patients with sepsis or acute central nervous system disease were successfully resuscitated and discharged from the hospital. For the few successfully resuscitated patients in these categories, postarrest management is dictated by the underlying precipitating factors.

Most antiarrhythmic drugs (see Chap. 30), a number of drugs used for noncardiac purposes, and electrolyte disturbances can precipitate potentially lethal arrhythmias and cardiac arrest. The class IA and class III antiarrhythmic drugs can cause proarrhythmic responses by lengthening the QT interval and generating torsades de pointes. The class IC drugs rarely cause torsades de pointes but cause excess SCD risk in patients with recent myocardial infarction, possibly by interacting with ischemia or other transient risk factors. Among other categories of drugs, the phenothiazines, tricyclic antidepressants, lithium, terfenadine interacting with ketoconazole (or other blockers of enzymes in the hepatic P450 system), pentamidine, cocaine, erythromycin, and cardiovascular drugs that are not antiarrhythmics—such as lidoflazine—are recognized causes. Beyond these, a broad array of pharmacological and pathophysiological-metabolic causes have been reported. Hypokalemia, hypomagnesemia, and perhaps hypocalcemia are the electrolyte disturbances most closely associated with cardiac arrest. Acidosis and hypoxia can potentiate the vulnerability associated with electrolyte disturbances. Proarrhythmic effects are often prewarned by prolongation of the QT interval, although this electrocardiographic change is not always present.[121]

Cardiac arrest caused by torsades de pointes is managed by intravenous administration of magnesium, pacing, or treatment with isoproterenol and removal of the offending agent. Class IC drugs may cause a rapid, sinusoidal VT pattern, especially among patients with poor left ventricular function. This VT has a tendency to recur repetitively after cardioversion until the drug has begun to clear and has been controlled by propranolol in some patients. When the patient's condition can be stabilized until the offending factor is removed (e.g., proarrhythmic drugs) or corrected (e.g., electrolyte imbalances, hypothermia), the prognosis is excellent. The recognition of torsades de pointes (see Chap. 32) and the identification of its risk by prolongation of the QT interval in association with the offending agent are helpful in managing these patients.

POST–CARDIAC ARREST CARE IN SURVIVORS OF OUT-OF-HOSPITAL CARDIAC ARREST. The initial management of survivors of out-of-hospital cardiac arrest centers on stabilizing the cardiac electrical status, supporting hemodynamics, and providing supportive care for reversal of organ damage that has occurred as a consequence of the cardiac arrest. The in-hospital risk of recurrent cardiac arrest is relatively low, and arrhythmias account for only 10 percent of in-hospital deaths after successful prehospital resuscitation.[232] However, the mortality rate during the index hospitalization is 50 percent, indicating that nonarrhythmic mortality dominates the mechanisms of early postresuscitation deaths (30 percent hemodynamic, 60 percent central nervous system related). Antiarrhythmic therapy, usually intravenous amiodarone, is used in an attempt to prevent recurrent cardiac arrest among patients who demonstrate residual electrophysiological instability and recurrent arrhythmia during the first 48 hours of postarrest hospitalization. Patients who have either preexisting or new AV or intraventricular conduction disturbances are at particularly high risk for recurrent cardiac arrest.[232] The routine use of temporary pacemakers has been evaluated in such patients but was not found to be helpful for preventing early recurrent cardiac arrest. Invasive techniques for hemodynamic monitoring are used in a patient whose condition is unstable but not routinely for those whose condition is stable on admission.

Anoxic encephalopathy is a strong predictor of in-hospital death. A suggested addition to the management of this condition is the use of induced mild hypothermia to reduce metabolic demands and cerebral edema.[196,197] When this strategy is applied promptly to the postarrest survivor who remains unconscious upon hospital admission, there is a modest but measurable survival benefit. During the later convalescent period, continued attention to central nervous system status, including physical rehabilitation, is of primary importance for an optimal outcome. Respiratory support by conventional methods is used as necessary. Management of other organ system injury (e.g., renal, hepatic), as well as early recognition and treatment of infectious complications, also contributes to ultimate survival.

Long-Term Management of Survivors of Out-of-Hospital Cardiac Arrest

When the survivor of an out-of-hospital cardiac arrest has awakened and achieved electrical and hemodynamic stability, usually between 1 and 7 days after the event, decisions must be made regarding the nature and extent of the work-up required to establish a long-term management strategy. The goals of the work-up are to identify the specific etiological and triggering cause of the cardiac arrest, clarify the functional status of the patient's cardiovascular system, and establish long-term therapeutic strategies. The extent of the work-up is largely dictated by the degree of central nervous system recovery and the factors already known to have contributed to the cardiac arrest. For instance, patients who have limited return of central nervous system function usually do not undergo extensive work-ups, and patients whose cardiac arrests were triggered by an acute transmural myocardial infarction have work-ups similar to those for other patients with acute myocardial infarction (see Chap. 47).

Survivors of out-of-hospital cardiac arrest not associated with acute myocardial infarction who have good return of neurological function appear to have a long-term survival probability commensurate with their age, gender, and extent of disease when treated according to existing guidelines.[201] These patients should undergo diagnostic work-ups to define the cause of cardiac arrest and tailor long-term therapy, the latter targeted to both the underlying disease and strategies for prevention of recurrent cardiac arrests or SCD. The work-up includes cardiac catheterization with coronary angiography if coronary atherosclerosis is known or considered to be the possible cause of the event,[233] an evaluation of the functional significance of coronary lesions by stress-imaging techniques if indicated, determination of functional and hemodynamic status, and estimation of baseline susceptibility to recurrent life-threatening arrhythmias and of the expected response to long-term therapy.

GENERAL CARE. The general management of survivors of cardiac arrest is determined by the specific cause and the pathophysiology of the underlying process. For patients with ischemic heart disease (see Chaps. 49 and 50), who constitute approximately 80 percent of cardiac arrest victims, interventions to prevent myocardial ischemia, optimization of therapy for left ventricular dysfunction, and attention to general medical status are all addressed. Although there are limited data suggesting that revascularization procedures may improve the recurrence rate and total mortality rates after survival from out-of-hospital cardiac arrest,[234] no properly controlled prospective studies have validated this impression for either bypass surgery or percutaneous interventions. Moreover, a randomized trial of prophylactic implantable defibrillators versus usual therapy in patients with low ejection fractions undergoing coronary bypass surgery in the absence of a history of cardiac arrest or other life-threatening arrhythmia or arrhythmia markers (the Coronary Artery Bypass Graft Patch Trial [CABG-Patch]) revealed no mortality benefit of implantable defibrillators after revascularization.[235] The indications for revascularization after a cardiac arrest are limited to those who have a generally accepted indication for angioplasty or surgery,[171] including (but not limited to) a documented ischemic mechanism for the cardiac arrest.

Although no data from placebo-controlled trials are available to define a benefit of various antiischemic strategies (including beta blockers or other medical antiischemic therapy) for long-term management after out-of-hospital cardiac arrest, medical, catheter interventional, or surgical antiischemic therapy, rather than antiarrhythmic drug therapy, is generally considered the primary approach to long-term management of the subgroup of prehospital cardiac arrest survivors in whom transient myocardial ischemia was the inciting factor. Moreover, in an uncontrolled observation comparing cardiac arrest survivors who had ever received beta blockers after the index event with those who had not received the drug, a significant improvement in long-term outcome was observed among those who had received beta blockers.[236] Further evaluation of the specific role of revascularization procedures and antiischemic medical therapy after out-of-hospital cardiac arrest is needed.

The long-term management of the consequences of left ventricular dysfunction by conventional means such as digitalis preparations and chronic diuretic use has been evaluated in several studies. Data from the Multiple Risk Factor Intervention Trial (MRFIT) suggested a higher mortality rate in the special intervention group, presumably related to diuretic use and K^+ depletion, and other data regarding the relation between K^+ depletion and arrhythmias have focused attention on routine use of such drugs. Although the facts are currently far from conclusive, it is advisable that diuretic use should be accompanied by careful monitoring of electrolytes. The use of digoxin in survivors of out-of-hospital cardiac arrest should be tailored to specific indications for left ventricular dysfunction.

The various pharmacological strategies (such as angiotensin-converting enzyme inhibitors, carvedilol and other beta-adrenergic blocking agents, and spironolactone) that have been shown to provide a clinical and mortality benefit in patients with left ventricular dysfunction, with or without heart failure, provide an SCD benefit in conjunction with total mortality benefit. The extent to which there is a specific SCD benefit for cardiac arrest survivors is uncertain, although some primary prevention trials suggest that such benefit occurs.

Prevention of Cardiac Arrest and Sudden Cardiac Death

Therapeutic strategies to prevent SCD can be classified into five categories: (1) prevention of recurrent events in survivors of cardiac arrest or hemodynamically compromising VT (secondary prevention); (2) prevention of an initial event among patients at high risk because of advanced heart disease with ejection fractions less than or equal to 35 percent (primary prevention); (3) primary prevention in patients with less advanced common or uncommon structural heart diseases and ejection fractions greater than 35 percent; (4) primary prevention in patients with structurally normal hearts, subtle or minor structural abnormalities, or molecular disorders associated with electrophysiological properties that establish risk for ventricular arrhythmias; and (5) primary prevention among the general population (Table 33–4). The last category includes the substantial proportion of SCDs that occur as a first cardiac event among victims previously free of known disease (see earlier).[169]

Four modes of antiarrhythmic therapy, which are not mutually exclusive, may be considered for patients at risk for cardiac arrest: antiarrhythmic drug therapy, surgery, catheter ablation, and implantable defibrillator therapy. The choice of therapy is based on estimation of the potential benefit determined by evaluation of the individual patient and available efficacy and safety data.

Antiarrhythmic Drug Strategies

The earliest approach, historically, to the management of risk of out-of-hospital cardiac arrest and VT with hemodynamic compromise was the use of pharmacological agents. This approach was based initially on the assumption that the high frequency of ambient ventricular arrhythmias constituted a triggering mechanism for potentially lethal arrhythmias and that the electrophysiological pathophysiology or instability of the myocardium that predisposed to potentially lethal arrhythmias could be modified by antiarrhythmic drugs. The therapeutic strategy for the former was the suppression of ambient ventricular arrhythmias by antiarrhythmic drugs, and the strategy for the latter was the suppression of inducibility of VT or VF during programmed electrical stimulation studies. Observational data suggested that suppression of ambient arrhythmias, identified on ambulatory recorders, could be achieved by the empirical use of amiodarone, beta-adrenergic blocking agents, or membrane-active antiarrhythmic drugs. On the basis of historical expectations, it was suggested, but not proved, that such suppressive techniques would improve mortality risk. For the membrane-active drugs, the observations that post-cardiac arrest survivors who had been treated with class I antiarrhythmic drugs had a worse outcome than those who were not treated challenged the concept of benefit,[236] and that skepticism was definitively reinforced by the results of CAST,[73] which demonstrated that certain class I antiarrhythmic drugs were neutral or did harm. In contrast, beta blocker therapy might have some benefit in such patients,[236,237] and amiodarone might also be effective for some patients.[238]

Another study, the Electrophysiologic Study Versus Electrocardiographic Monitoring (ESVEM) trial, designed to compare the value of ambulatory monitoring with programmed electrical stimulation techniques for predicting therapeutic outcome,[239] suggested that the class III antiarrhythmic drug sotalol was superior to class I membrane-active antiarrhythmic agents for patients with life-threatening ventricular tachyarrhythmias but provided no comparison with amiodarone or beta blockers. In summary, ambient arrhythmia suppression as a technique for reduction of risk enjoyed a short period of popularity for VT-VF survivors but in time yielded to the apparent greater benefits of amiodarone, and perhaps beta blockers,[240] prescribed empirically. The combination of amiodarone and beta blocker therapy in the post-myocardial infarction patient has been suggested as a strategy that provides greater benefit than either drug alone from subgroup analysis of the European Myocardial Infarct Amiodarone Trial (EMIAT) and Canadian Amiodarone Myocardial Infarction Trial (CAMIAT),[241] and another study reinforced the benefit of beta blockers for specific prevention of SCD in unselected post-myocardial infarction patients.[242]

TABLE 33–4 Categories of Therapeutic Strategies for Prevention of Recurrent Cardiac Arrest and Sudden Cardiac Death (SCD)

Prevention Targets	Clinical Examples	Estimate of Risk	Data Sources
Secondary*	Survivors of cardiac arrest; VF/VT	High	Observational; RCT: (+) control
Primary			
Advanced structural cardiac disease	CAD/DCM, EF < 35%	High	Observational; RCT: (+) control RCT: (–) control
Lower grade structural disease	CAD/DCM, EF > 35% RVD, sarcoidosis, HCM	Variable	Observational; RCT: Subgroup analyses
Functional cardiac disorders†	Long QT syndrome, Brugada syndrome	Variable	Observational
SCD as primary event in CAD†	Family history of SCD, risk factors for CAD	Low	Epidemiological; genetic (?)

Much of the data for secondary prevention, identified as a high-risk population because of the occurrence of a prior cardiac arrest, has derived from observational data and, more recently, from randomized controlled trials (RCTs), all of which have employed an active-therapy control group [(+) control], comparing outcomes between groups treated with implantable cardioverter-defibrillators (ICDs) and antiarrhythmic drugs (see Table 33–5).

RCTs are not feasible for primary prevention in patients with these lower risk conditions. However, some information can be acquired from subgroup analysis of larger studies: Decisions for ICD implantation in these patients must be judgment based rather than evidence based. Suggestions of familial clustering of sudden death, as a specific expression of coronary artery disease (CAD), raise the question of primary prevention in patients at risk for SCD using epidemiological and perhaps genetic markers in the future.

DCM = dilated cardiomyopathy; EF = ejection fraction; HCM = hypertrophic cardiomyopathy; RVD = right ventricular dysplasia; VF = ventricular fibrillation; VT = ventricular tachycardia.

Ambulatory Electrocardiographic Recording and Empirical Therapy

The development of reliable methods of analysis of ambulatory recordings led some investigators to study the usefulness of such recordings for profiling risk of sustained tachyarrhythmic events and to measure suppressibility of ambient arrhythmias as a specific and individualized means of evaluating drug therapy for prevention of SCD. This strategy is now obsolete as a primary approach in the cardiac arrest survivor, but ambulatory monitoring is still used for profiling the risk of developing life-threatening sustained arrhythmias in individuals with certain forms of structural or electrophysiological disease who are considered at high risk. For example, the strategies used in the Multicenter Automatic Defibrillator Implantation Trial (MADIT)[243] and the Multicenter Unsustained Tachycardia Trial (MUSTT)[244] employed identification of nonsustained VT in post-myocardial infarction patients with other risk markers for early mortality. Although the ambient arrhythmias were not a target for therapy in the design of the studies, they have established the usefulness of this technique for identifying risk. Similarly, ambulatory recordings, particularly among patients with symptoms, are used as an aid to risk profiling in disorders such as hypertrophic cardiomyopathy, long QT interval syndrome, and right ventricular dysplasia and in patients with dilated cardiomyopathy or heart failure.

Other investigators provided data suggesting the possibility that ambient arrhythmia suppression might be equivalent to suppression of inducible arrhythmias by programmed electrical stimulation for predicting outcome.[239] Moreover, analysis of the CAST data base also suggested an association between the ease of suppression of ambient ventricular arrhythmias and survival,[245] supporting the concept of a meaningful relationship between *suppressibility* of ambient arrhythmias and survival. Under circumstances in which amiodarone or beta-adrenergic blocking agents, or both, are used for primary prevention of cardiac arrest (and secondary prevention if ICDs are not available), baseline and follow-up ambulatory monitors are still used as a possible indicator of drug efficacy. This approach appears to have a rational basis for evaluating ambient arrhythmia responses, but there is still a level of uncertainty regarding its translation to actual cardiac arrest events.

Finally, empirical antiarrhythmic therapy, predominantly amiodarone, for prevention of recurrent cardiac arrest or other life-threatening arrhythmias has been observed to have a relative benefit in several studies. Whether it has an absolute mortality benefit can be determined only with data from placebo-controlled trials, which are not available. Moreover, several controlled trials have now suggested that empirical amiodarone is less effective than implantable defibrillators in reducing risk of death among survivors of life-threatening arrhythmic events (Antiarrhythmics Versus Implantable Defibrillators [AVID], Canadian Implantable Defibrillator Study [CIDS], and the Cardiac Arrest Study Hamburg [CASH]), particularly when the ejection fraction is less than 35 percent (see Chap. 31).[203-205]

PROGRAMMED ELECTRICAL STIMULATION

The second major antiarrhythmic strategy was based on suppression of inducibility of sustained ventricular arrhythmias, considered to be a marker of risk during electrophysiological testing. The use of programmed electrical stimulation to identify benefit on the basis of suppression of inducibility by an antiarrhythmic drug gained popularity for evaluating long-term therapy among survivors of out-of-hospital cardiac arrest. It evolved as the preferred method of management despite concerns about the sensitivity and specificity of the various pacing protocols and the extent to which the myocardial status at the time of the programmed electrical stimulation study reflected that present at the time of the clinical cardiac arrest. Nonetheless, most studies demonstrated limitations based on observations that a relatively small fraction of cardiac arrest survivors (an average of less than 50 percent on the basis of multiple studies) had inducible arrhythmias.

Drug suppression of inducibility during electrophysiological testing as an endpoint for either secondary prevention of SCD or primary prevention in high-risk post-myocardial infarction patients has yielded to the benefits of ICD therapy in most subgroups, with a few exceptions among primary prevention categories. It still has use, however, for risk profiling in a number of clinical circumstances.[243,244,246,247] Despite a large, albeit somewhat conflicting, data base on the role of electrophysiological testing for risk profiling, results of the secondary prevention trials among cardiac arrest survivors suggest that routine electrophysiological testing among such individuals is no longer necessary, particularly if ICD therapy is available to the patient. All of the secondary prevention trials demonstrated a benefit of the ICD over antiarrhythmic therapy, usually using amiodarone, without a determination that risk profiling by electrophysiological testing offered any benefit.[203-205] Under conditions in which a potentially reversible trigger for cardiac arrest can be identified, and perhaps among some cardiac arrest survivors in whom transient ischemia was the initiating mechanism and the ejection fraction is greater than 40 percent, there might be a persistent limited role for such testing as a guide to therapy. In contrast, several primary prevention trials such as MADIT[243] and MUSTT[244] used electrophysiological testing to profile risk and demonstrated large benefits. MADIT II,[248] which enrolled patients with lower ejection fractions than MADIT or MUSTT and did not employ arrhythmia markers, also demonstrated a survival benefit of ICD therapy. The extent to which MADIT II differs from MADIT and MUSTT and the question of whether the electrophysiological testing criteria in the latter are necessary have yet to be resolved. Until then, electrophysiological testing is used as the indicator leading to ICD use among candidates defined by MADIT and MUSTT criteria.

The implications of induced nonsustained forms of VT are more controversial. Although it has been suggested that induction of nonsustained ventricular rhythms may indicate risk, it is generally considered nonspecific in the absence of structural heart disease or when an aggressive protocol is used. The use of the suppression of nonsustained arrhythmias as an endpoint of therapy is not considered valid.

The significance of *non*inducibility at baseline electrophysiological stimulation testing in relation to risk and long-term management is also controversial. In the past, opinions ranged from the conclusion that potentially high-risk patients free of inducible ventricular arrhythmias were electrophysiologically stable and required no long-term antiarrhythmic therapy to the other extreme that such patients remained at risk but did not have an objective endpoint of therapy by this method and therefore must be treated by other techniques. Despite these conflicting opinions, it is generally accepted now that survivors of cardiac arrest without clearly identifiable transient and treatable causes remain at high risk regardless of inducibility status. Some out-of-hospital cardiac arrests can be clearly demonstrated to result from transient ischemia, and this subgroup appears to achieve benefit from antiischemic therapy.[201]

SURGICAL INTERVENTION STRATEGIES

The previously popular antiarrhythmic surgical techniques now have limited applications. Intraoperative map-guided cryoablation techniques may be used for patients who have inducible, hemodynamically stable sustained monomorphic VT during electrophysiological testing and have suitable ventricular and coronary artery anatomy, amenable to catheter ablation. However, they have little applicability to survivors of out-of-hospital cardiac arrest because the type of arrhythmia favoring this surgical approach is infrequently observed among cardiac arrest survivors. It can be used for patients whose arrhythmia frequency requires frequent ICD shocks as adjustive therapy to the device. In contrast, coronary revascularization procedures have a clearly defined role for cardiac arrest survivors in whom an ischemic mechanism was responsible for the event and suitable surgical anatomy is present.[234]

CATHETER ABLATION THERAPY

The use of catheter ablation techniques to treat ventricular tachyarrhythmias has been most successful for the benign focal tachycardias that originate in the right ventricle or left side of the interventricular septum (see Chap. 30) and for some reentrant VTs. With rare exceptions, catheter ablation techniques are not used for the treatment of higher risk ventricular tachyarrhythmias or for definitive therapy in patients at risk for progression of the arrhythmic substrate. For VT caused by bundle branch reentrant mechanisms, which occur in cardiomyopathies as well as other structural cardiac disorders, ablation of the right bundle branch to interrupt the reentrant cycle has been successful.[249] However, this has limited applicability to the large number of patients with structural heart disease at risk for SCD or those who have survived a cardiac arrest. On the other hand, the use of catheter ablation techniques for patients with ICDs who are having multiple tachyarrhythmic events is an appropriate and helpful adjunctive treatment strategy[250] rather than a preferred primary therapy for prevention of SCD.

Implantable Defibrillators

The development of the ICD added a new dimension to the management of patients at high risk for cardiac arrest (see Chap. 31). After the early reports by Mirowski and coworkers[251] and Echt and colleagues,[252] multiple observational studies confirmed that ICDs could achieve rates of sudden death consistently less than 5 percent at 1 year and total death rates in the 10 to 20 percent range among populations who have high mortality risks, as predicted by mortality surrogates such as historical controls or time to first appropriate shock.[253-256] Yet, determination of the mortality benefit of ICDs remained uncertain and they were debated for many years.[257] More than 16 years elapsed between the first clinical use of an implanted defibrillator[258] and publication of the first major randomized clinical trial comparing implantable defibrillator therapy with antiarrhythmic drug therapy.[243] Through that period of time, reports had documented the ability of implantable devices to revert potentially fatal arrhythmias but could not identify a valid relative or absolute mortality benefit because of confounding factors such as competing risks for sudden and nonsudden death and determination of whether appropriate shocks represented the interruption of an event that would have been fatal. Despite these limitations, ICD therapy continued to increase its relative position among other forms of therapy for survivors of out-of-hospital cardiac arrest and, to a lesser extent, for those considered to be at high risk for a primary cardiac arrest on the basis of specific clinical markers.

With publication of the results of MADIT,[243] information on the relative benefit of defibrillators over antiarrhythmic drug therapy (largely amiodarone) for primary prevention of SCD in a very high-risk population became available (Table 33–5; see also Fig. 33–24). The outcome demonstrated a 59 percent reduction in relative risk of total mortality at 2 years of follow-up (54 percent cumulative) and a 19 percent reduction in absolute risk of dying at 2 years of follow-up. One year later, the first adequately powered secondary prevention trial of ICDs versus antiarrhythmic drugs was published. This study, the AVID trial, demonstrated a 27 percent reduction in relative risk of total mortality at 2 years of follow-up with an absolute risk reduction of 7 percent.[203] The AVID trial was followed shortly by reports of two other studies—CIDS[204] and CASH[205]—both limited by the power of the enrollment numbers but suggesting trends toward similar benefits (see Table 33–5). As a consequence of the secondary prevention trials, ICDs have emerged as the preferred therapy for survivors of out-of-hospital cardiac arrest or hemodynamically important VT. A subgroup analysis of AVID suggested that the benefit is limited to patients with ejection fractions less than 35 percent; above that value, the outcome with either amiodarone or an ICD might be equivalent.[238]

Whereas the studies cited documented the ability of implantable devices to revert potentially fatal arrhythmias and subsequently showed a relative benefit over amiodarone in some groups of patients, the absence of placebo-controlled trials still prevents quantitation of the true magnitude of any mortality benefit because of the inability of positive-

TABLE 33–5 Summary of Major Implantable Cardioverter-Defibrillator Trials for Prevention of Sudden Cardiac Deaths

		2-Year Outcomes (%)			
Trial	**Study Group**	***Control***	***ICDs***	***Rel RR***	***Abs RR***
Secondary prevention*					
AVID[202] (n = 1061)	VF, VT-syncope, VT: EF ≤ 40%	25	18	−27	−7
CIDS[203] (n = 659)	VF, VT-syncope, VT: EF ≤ 35% and CL < 400 ms	21	15	−30	−6
CASH[204] (n = 346)	Cardiac arrest survivors (VF, VT)	20 (combined)	12	−37	−8
		2-Year (MADIT, CABG-Patch, MADIT-2) and 5-Year (MUSTT, SCD-HeFT) Outcomes (%)			
		Control	***ICDs***	***Rel RR***	***Abs RR***
Primary prevention†					
MADIT[242] (n = 196)	Prior MI, EF ≤ 35%, NS VT, inducible VT, failed IV PA	32	13	−59	−19
MUSTT[243] (n = 704)	Prior MI, EF ≤ 40%, NS VT, inducible VT	55	24	−58	−31
CABG-Patch[234] (n = 900)	Coronary bypass surgery, EF < 36%, SAECG (+)	18	18	0	0
MADIT-2[248] (n = 1232)	Prior MI (>1 month), EF ≤ 30%	22	16	−28	−6
SCD-HeFT (n = 2521)‡	Class II-III CHF, EF ≤ 35%	36	29	−23	−7

Abs RR = absolute risk reduction; CHF = congestive heart failure; CL = cycle length; EF = ejection fraction; EP = electrophysiological; ICD = implantable cardioverter-defibrillator; IV PA = intravenous procainamide; MI = myocardial infarction; NS = nonsustained; Rel RR = relative risk reduction; SAECG = signal-averaged electrocardiogram; VF = ventricular fibrillation.

*Three major randomized trials for secondary prevention among survivors of out-of-hospital cardiac arrest, or high-risk ventricular tachycardia (VT), have been completed: the Antiarrhythmics Versus Implantable Defibrillators (AVID) trial, the Canadian Implantable Defibrillator Study (CIDS), and the Cardiac Arrest Study of Hamburg (CASH). Each used an active control, randomized design, comparing ICDs with antiarrhythmic drug (AAD) therapy, primarily amiodarone. The cumulative data, as well as the individual data from the larger studies, support the idea that the ICD is preferable to drug therapy for this high-risk population. However, the large relative benefits translated to more modest absolute benefits, with a large residual risk among the ICD-treated groups in each study.

†Four primary prevention trials among patients presumed to be at high risk but who have not had spontaneous life-threatening ventricular arrhythmias have been completed: the Multicenter Automatic Defibrillator Implantation Trial (MADIT), the Multicenter Unsustained Tachycardia Trial (MUSTT), the coronary artery bypass surgery/implantable defibrillator trial (CABG-Patch), and the Multicenter Automatic Defibrillator Implantation Trial-2 (MADIT-2). MADIT showed an advantage of ICD therapy over AAD therapy, MUSTT showed superiority of electrophysiologically (EP) guided evaluation leading to ICD therapy compared with that leading to drug therapy, and CABG-Patch showed no benefit to ICDs for patients undergoing routine coronary bypass surgery. MADIT-2 showed a benefit of ICD therapy compared with usual therapy for post-myocardial infarction patients with an EF ≤ 30%. The other large primary prevention trial, the Sudden Cardiac Death in Heart Failure Trail (SCD-HeFT), was in progress (along with a number of smaller trials) at time of writing.

‡Presented as a late-breaking trial at the Annual Scientific Sessions of the American College of Cardiology, March 8, 2004. No difference shown between amidiarone and control.

controlled trials to identify the absolute benefit of an intervention.[259] Despite these limitations, implantable defibrillator therapy is now the preferred therapy for survivors of cardiac arrest at risk for recurrences and for primary prevention in patients in a number of high-risk categories. Major questions still unanswered include the relative benefit of amiodarone versus defibrillators among lower risk subgroups of survivors of out-of-hospital cardiac arrest, the role of beta blockers, and the role of antiischemic surgical and medical therapy as definitive approaches.

A much larger issue, and one that has not yet been defined, is the use of implantable defibrillators among patients thought to be at intermediate levels of risk for cardiac arrest but who have not yet had an event. Several trials are in progress to determine whether preventive defibrillator therapy is an effective means of preventing the first cardiac arrest. Many of the trials are studying cost efficacy in addition to medical efficacy. One of the more important strategies being tested involves a comparison of defibrillator therapy and empirical amiodarone therapy with placebo in patients with heart failure without symptomatic arrhythmias or a history of cardiac arrest (see Chaps. 30 and 31).

Application of Therapeutic Strategies to Specific Groups of Patients

SECONDARY PREVENTION AFTER SURVIVING CARDIAC ARREST. As populations of cardiac arrest survivors began to accumulate from community-based emergency rescue activities, long-term therapeutic strategies intended to reduce recurrent cardiac arrest rates and total mortality risks emerged as a mandate for clinical investigators. The problem that affects all long-term strategies for cardiac arrest survivors, however, is the lack of a reliable concurrent natural history denominator against which to compare the results of interventions. This lack is a consequence of ethical concerns about withholding therapy in a placebo-controlled study model for patients at such high risk for dying[259] in conjunction with the likelihood that general therapies used in such patients may also improve total mortality risk. Earlier approaches to long-term therapy centered on the use of antiarrhythmic drug therapy, largely guided by the results of electrophysiological testing or the empirical use of antiarrhythmic drugs, particularly amiodarone. During the evolution of therapeutic strategies, various observational and positive-controlled studies suggested first that suppression of inducible ventricular arrhythmias yielded a better outcome than failure of suppression, then that amiodarone was better than class I antiarrhythmic drugs, and finally that ICDs were better than amiodarone. Therefore, ICD therapy has emerged as preferred therapy, absent absolute benefit data. Electrophysiological testing for secondary prevention—once routine—is now considered of questionable necessity and is commonly not performed.

Anatomically based antiarrhythmic surgery enjoyed a short period of popularity for secondary prevention, limited by the observation that surgical antiarrhythmic procedures appeared to provide benefit to only a small subset of such patients.[260] As the implantable defibrillator came into wider use, it also began to supplant pharmacological antiarrhythmic approaches, with the possible exception of amiodarone, even before the randomized clinical trials demonstrated relative ICD benefit. In the late 1990s, information from randomized clinical trials—AVID, CIDS, and CASH—provided compelling support for the use of ICDs as preferred therapy for secondary prevention of cardiac arrest related to ventricular tachyarrhythmias (Fig. 33–24).

PRIMARY PREVENTION OF OUT-OF-HOSPITAL CARDIAC ARREST WITH ADVANCED HEART DISEASE.

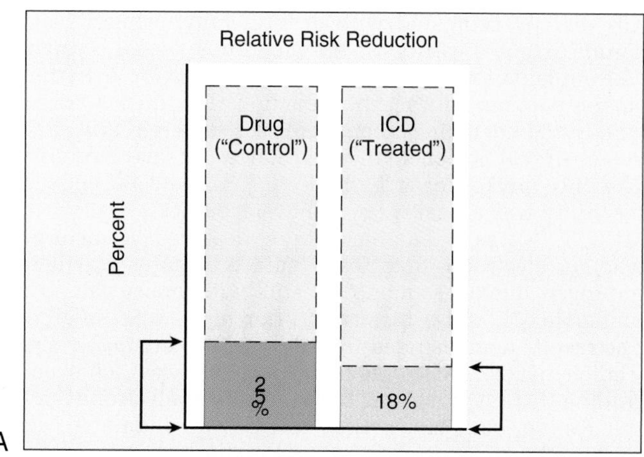

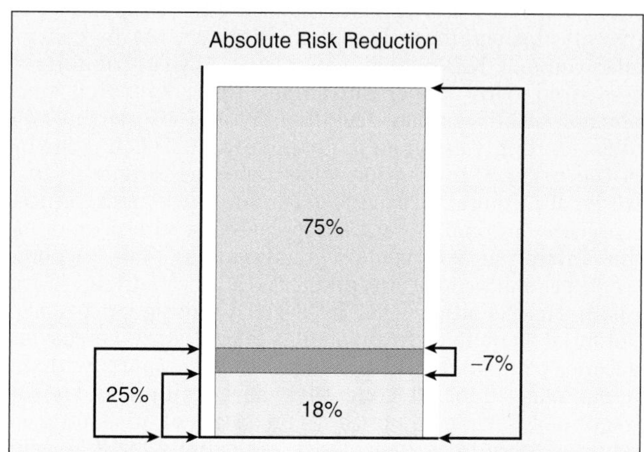

FIGURE 33–24 Relative and absolute benefit of implantable cardioverter-defibrillators (ICDs) in the Antiarrhythmics Versus Implantable Defibrillators (AVID) study. **A,** The ICD-treated subgroup had 18 percent mortality at 2 years versus 25 percent in the drug-treated group, a 27 percent *relative* reduction in the population having events. **B,** When relative reduction is extrapolated to the total target population, the *absolute* reduction of fatal events in the total population is 7 percent. (From Myerburg RJ, Mitrani R, Interian A Jr, Castellanos A: Interpretation of outcomes of antiarrhythmic clinical trials: Design features and population impact. Circulation 97:1514, 1998. Copyright 1998, American Heart Association.)

Because SCD is frequently the initial clinical expression of underlying structural heart disease or occurs in identified patients profiled to be at low risk (see Fig. 33–2), there has been a longstanding interest in therapeutic strategies targeted to primary prevention. After the disappointing outcome of CAST[73] and the disturbing suggestions of lack of efficacy or adverse effects of the class I antiarrhythmic drugs generally when used for primary or secondary prevention of SCD,[73,236] interest shifted to the use of amiodarone and implantable defibrillators. Two major trials of amiodarone in post-myocardial infarction patients,[261,262] one of which required ejection fractions less than 40 percent, demonstrated no total mortality benefit even though both trials demonstrated antiarrhythmic benefit, expressed as a reduction in arrhythmic deaths or resuscitated VF. Subgroup analyses suggested that the concomitant use of beta blockers did confer a mortality benefit.[241]

In parallel with the amiodarone trials, the randomized controlled trial comparing antiarrhythmic therapy (primarily amiodarone) with ICD therapy (MADIT) was carried out (see Table 33–5).[243] This trial randomly assigned patients with ejection fractions less than 35 percent, nonsustained VT during ambulatory recording, and inducible VT that was not suppressible by procainamide. This very high-risk group demonstrated a 54 percent reduction in total mortality with

ICD therapy compared with drug therapy, primarily amiodarone as noted earlier. At the same time, a trial comparing ICD implantation with no specific therapies for arrhythmias among patients with ejection fractions less than 36 percent who were undergoing coronary bypass surgery (CABG-Patch) demonstrated no benefit of defibrillators for total mortality.[235] The only marker for arrhythmic risk required for entry into the study was a positive signal-averaged ECG. A third trial, MUSTT,[244] was a complex study designed to determine whether electrophysiologically guided therapy provides an improved outcome among patients with nonsustained VT, inducible VT, and a history of prior myocardial infarction. The results demonstrated that although a statistically significant beneficial effect on total mortality was achieved by guiding therapy according to the results of electrophysiological testing, compared with patients with inducible tachycardia who did not receive therapy, the subgroup patients who received ICDs because they failed to respond to drug therapy did significantly better. There was 24 percent mortality among ICD-treated patients at 5 years of follow-up compared with 55 percent among those receiving electrophysiologically guided drug therapy and 48 percent among those randomly assigned to no therapy. MADIT II is the latest of the primary prevention trials reported to date.[248] In this study, ICD therapy provided a mortality benefit compared with conventional therapy among patients with prior myocardial infarction and ejection fractions less than 30 percent. Another study, still in progress, is the Sudden Cardiac Death–Heart Failure Trial (SCD-HeFT), designed to test the potential benefit of implantable defibrillators versus amiodarone, compared with placebo, among patients with functional class II or III congestive heart failure and ejection fractions less than 35 percent. The results of this study, when reported, should further clarify indications for ICD therapy for primary prevention in high-risk subgroups.

PRIMARY PREVENTION IN PATIENTS WITH LESS ADVANCED COMMON HEART DISEASES OR UNCOMMON DISEASES. Primary prevention trials have been designed to enroll populations of patients with advanced heart disease that were estimated to be at very high risk for SCD and total mortality as a consequence of the severity of the underlying disease. Most of the clinical trials testing the question of relative efficacy of antiarrhythmic versus ICD therapy have used the ejection fraction as the marker for advanced disease, with the qualifying criteria in the range of 30 to 40 percent or less. Moreover, in the secondary prevention trial AVID, a subgroup analysis suggested that there was no relative benefit of ICD therapy over amiodarone for patients with ejection fractions between 36 and 40 percent; all of the benefits accrued to those with ejection fractions of 35 percent or less.[238] This observation is important because it raises a question about therapeutic options—for both primary and secondary prevention strategies—when ejection fractions are greater than 35 percent. However, as a retrospective analysis, the observation calls for confirmation in a controlled trial.

Whereas the risk for SCD and total mortality is highest among patients with advanced structural heart disease and low ejection fractions or limited functional capacity, or both, a substantial portion of the total SCD burden occurs among patients with coronary heart disease or the various nonischemic cardiomyopathies with ejection fractions between 35 and 40 percent and higher. In addition, among patients with heart failure related to various forms of cardiomyopathy, whereas the total mortality risk is considerably lower among patients in functional class I or early class II than among those with late class III or class IV status, the probability of a death being sudden is higher in the former group.[263] Despite this observation, there are no data available to guide therapy for primary prevention of cardiac arrest in such patients.[12,169,264] This limitation is confounded by the fact that the patients in these categories generally have low event rates but cumulatively account for large numbers of SCDs (see Fig. 33–2A). In addition, certain other structural entities that are associated with some elevation of risk of sudden death in the absence of a severely reduced ejection fraction, such as some patterns of viral myocarditis, hypertrophic cardiomyopathy, right ventricular dysplasia, and sarcoidosis, are managed without the benefit of clinical trials to guide therapeutic decisions (see Table 33–4). Patients with symptomatic ventricular arrhythmias related to structural disorders such as right ventricular dysplasia, in which most of the mortality risk is arrhythmic, are often advised to have ICDs even in the absence of a prior cardiac arrest or hemodynamically significant VT. Whether antiarrhythmic therapy would be just as effective remains unknown, but the judgment of using defibrillators in patients with a disorder whose fatal expression is primarily arrhythmic carries the strength of logic, often supported by risk profiling based on observational data on clinical markers. Among the entities in which family history is helpful for defining risk, clinical judgment is made easier when there is a strong family history of SCD. Specific support for this approach derives from genetic studies in hypertrophic cardiomyopathy, in which a limited number of the known mutations appear to be associated with specific risk of SCD.[24] In addition, clinical observational data support the use of ICDs in high-risk subsets of patients with hypertrophic cardiomyopathy.[265]

PRIMARY PREVENTION IN PATIENTS WITH STRUCTURALLY NORMAL HEARTS OR MOLECULAR DISORDERS OF CARDIAC ELECTRICAL ACTIVITY. A new category of interest in primary preventive therapy has emerged. Clinically subtle or inapparent structural disorders or entities with pure electrophysiological expression, such as the congenital long QT interval syndromes, the Brugada syndrome, and idiopathic VF, have received increasing attention. The decision-making process for secondary prevention strategies for patients with the long QT interval syndrome is relatively easy. Individuals who have survived a cardiac arrest or potentially fatal arrhythmic event, especially when there is a family history of SCD, are generally treated with ICDs. Beta blockers are still considered useful for affected family members who have not had an event and perhaps for some subgroups with patients with syncope of undocumented mechanism.[119,120] In contrast, individuals who express the electrocardiographic phenotype of long QT interval syndrome without a family history of SCD or the absence of symptomatic arrhythmias, or both, are generally treated with beta blocker therapy at this time. Between these extremes are the asymptomatic affected family members of patients with symptomatic long QT syndrome. Given the complexity of the pathophysiology of potentially fatal arrhythmias among such patients, the threshold for considering ICD therapy is decreasing.[119] Genetic screening may ultimately prove useful for identifying specific risk, particularly if individual arrhythmic risk is demonstrated to be determined by one or more modifier genes interacting with the defect responsible for an ion channel pore defect (Fig. 33–25).[77] For the present, many such clinical therapeutic decisions remain judgment based rather than data driven. In this context, a family history of premature SCD in affected relatives appears to be useful for the decision-making process for preventive therapy in this general category of patients (see Chap. 28).

Among the other molecular arrhythmia syndromes, the Brugada syndrome is one in which management strategies remain problematic and debated.[266,267] The ICD is accepted as the preferred secondary prevention strategy among cardiac arrest survivors and symptomatic affected individuals even though it is based solely on observational data. However, primary prevention approaches for affected relatives, especially if asymptomatic, are unclear. Studies suggest that syncope associated with ECG changes suggestive of the disorder at baseline is a marker of risk sufficient to warrant ICD

Interactions Between Gene Products	
Direct ion channel modifiers:	
α-subunits	β-subunits
KvLQT1	minK
HERG	MiRP1
SCN5A	SCN1B
Related modifiers:	
Ion channel constructs	Ca^{2+}-handling
KvLQT1 + minK	RyR2
HERG + MiRP1	
SCN5A + SCN1B	
Integrated physiological functions:	
Arrhythmogenic constructs	Autonomic function
I_{K^+}, I_{Na^+}, $I_{Ca^{2+}}$ variants	β_1-AR functional polymorphisms
Gene/Non-Gene Interactions	
Molecular structure	Functional triggers
Inherited ion channel variants	β-adrenergic function (non-gene)
Reactive polymorphisms	Transient pathophysiological states;
Acquired (induced) DNA alterations	Pharmacological/metabolic factors

FIGURE 33–25 Gene-gene and gene-nongene interactions and risk profiling for sudden cardiac death. Genetic characteristics contribute to risk prediction at multiple points in the clinical-epidemiological cascade from the onset of atherogenesis to sudden cardiac death. Genetically determined influences on electrophysiology appear to play a complex role in the final step of the cascade—the onset of a fatal arrhythmia during an acute coronary syndrome. Multiple genes influencing inherent characteristics of ion channel structure and function, their integration with calcium handling and arrhythmogenesis, and individual variations in beta-adrenergic responses to stimulation all appear to play a role in this limited part of the overall cascade. Analysis of the interactions between direct modification of ion channel structure and function, other factors in arrhythmogenesis, and other activities that can be predicted by genetic profiling may provide greater power of prediction for individual risk of arrhythmias in the acutely ischemic setting. Genetically controlled variations, including polymorphisms that are expressed only in pathophysiological states ("reactive" polymorphisms) and acquired DNA alterations, may also play a role. Genetic factors then integrate with nongenetic factors as indicated. The chromosomes containing gene loci currently known to participate in control of several molecular characteristics are indicated. β_1-AR = beta$_1$-adrenergic receptor. (From Myerburg RJ: Scientific gaps in the prediction and prevention of sudden cardiac death. J Cardiovasc Electrophysiol 13:709, 2002.)

therapy[267] and that baseline ECG changes associated with inducibility of ventricular tachyarrhythmias during electrophysiological testing are also a marker of risk.[266] Conversely, the absence of right bundle branch block and ST-T wave changes without provocation suggested lower risk. However, a family history of SCD remains an important factor in judgment-based decisions. Similar arguments, but supported by even less data, apply to affected family members of patients with right ventricular dysplasia.

PRIMARY PREVENTION AMONG THE GENERAL POPULATION, INCLUDING ADOLESCENTS AND YOUNG ADULTS. To have a major impact on the problem of SCD among the general population, we need to move beyond the identification of high-risk patients who have specific clinical entities, advanced or subtle, that predict a high risk of SCD. Rather, it is necessary to find among the general population small subgroups of patients at specific risk for SCD as a manifestation of underlying heart disease, if and when that disease becomes manifest. As an example, the studies that have demonstrated familial clustering of SCD as the first expression of underlying coronary artery disease, suggesting genetic or behavioral predisposition, may provide some help for the future.[35,36] The report of a common genetic "variant" in the cardiac Na^+ channel gene (*SCN5A* on chromosome 3) among blacks with apparent susceptibility to arrhythmias and proarrhythmic responses to antiarrhythmic drugs[30] supports this concept. With a population frequency of affected individuals in the range of 13 percent, a valuable marker of risk may be offered if additional genetic epidemiological studies support the possibility that this is a marker of specific SCD risk during pathophysiological events. If highly specific markers can be found, either related to electrophysiological properties or along multiple points in the cascade of coronary events (see Fig. 33–4), preventive therapy before the first expression of an underlying disease may lead to a major impact on the population problem of SCD. Short of that, successes will be limited to community-based intervention and to the subgroups that are easier to identify and in whom it is more justifiable to use prophylactic interventional therapy on the basis of population size and magnitude of risk.[9,12,169,268]

Adolescents and young adults, including athletes (see Chap. 75), constitute a group for special consideration. The SCD risk among these groups is an order of magnitude of 1 percent of that of the general adult population older than 35 years (see Fig. 33–3A).[88,147,198,269] However, most of the causes of SCD among these populations are not characterized by advanced life-limiting structural heart disease, and therefore surviving cardiac arrest victims can, with appropriate long-term therapy, be expected to have significant extensions of life. Because the majority of deaths are arrhythmic, the ability to identify individuals at risk in advance of a life-threatening arrhythmic event offers more long-term impact than in the case of older populations. Among both the general young population and athletes, identification of individuals at risk may lead to prevention of events that are triggered by physical activity.[270,271] Strategies for screening adolescents, young adults, and athletes to identify the entities that create a risk have met with limited acceptance despite some data indicating both feasibility[146,272] and suggestions of cost-effectiveness.[271] ECG screening of the general adolescent population, including athletes, can identify many of those at potential risk because of congenital long QT syndrome, hypertrophic cardiomyopathy, right ventricular dysplasia, and Brugada syndrome. Although ECG screening in the adolescent and athletic subgroups is imperfect and commonly accompanied by depolarization and repolarization patterns that may be difficult to interpret, this strategy can lead to further testing in appropriate individuals. Echocardiography has also been suggested as a screening method, but it is more expensive and less cost efficient and does not recognize conditions such as long QT syndrome and Brugada syndrome. One study has demonstrated a reduction in SCDs among athletes with the use of widespread screening.[144]

Sudden Death and Public Safety

The unexpectedness of SCD has raised questions concerning secondary risk to the public created by people in the throes of a cardiac arrest. There are no data from controlled studies available to guide public policy regarding people at high risk for potentially lethal arrhythmias and for abrupt incapacitation. In a report of observations on 1348 sudden deaths caused by coronary heart disease in people 65 years of age or younger during a 7-year period in Dade County, Florida, 101 (7.5 percent) of the deaths occurred in people who were engaged in activities at the time of death that were potentially hazardous to the public (e.g., driving motor vehicles, working at altitude, piloting aircraft), and 122 (9.1 percent) of the victims had occupations that could create potential hazards to others if an abrupt loss of consciousness had occurred while they were at work.[273] There were no catastrophic events as a result of these cardiac arrests, only minor property damage in 19 and minor injuries in 5.

Other studies have also led to the conclusion that risk to the public is small. In specific reference to private automobile drivers, most of the data show that sudden death at the wheel usually involves enough of a prodrome to allow the driver to get to the roadside before losing consciousness.[274,275] An analysis of recurrent VT-VF events among cardiac arrest survivors suggested limitation of driving privileges for the first 8 months after the index event on the basis of the clustering of recurrent event rates early after the index event.[16,276] Therefore, although there are likely to be isolated instances in which cardiac arrest causes public hazards in the future, the risk appears to be small; and because it is difficult to identify specific individuals at risk, sweeping restrictions to avoid such risks appear unwarranted. The exceptions are people with multisystem disease, particularly senility, and individual circumstances that require specific consideration, such as high-risk patients who have special responsibilities—school bus drivers, aircraft pilots, train operators, and truck drivers.[16,273,276]

REFERENCES

Definitions

1. Torp-Pedersen C, Kober L, Elming H, Burchart H: Classification of sudden and arrhythmic death. Pacing Clin Electrophysiol 20:245, 1997.
2. Deedwania P: Global risk assessment in the presymptomatic patient. Am J Cardiol 88:17J, 2001.

Epidemiology

3. Priori SG, Aliot E, Blomstrom-Lundqvist C, et al: Task Force on Sudden Cardiac Death of the European Society of Cardiology. Eur Heart J 22:1374, 2001.
4. Gillum RF: Sudden coronary death in the United States: 1980-1985. Circulation 79:756, 1989.
5. Escobedo LG, Zack MM: Comparison of sudden and nonsudden coronary deaths in the United States. Circulation 93:2033, 1996.
6. American Heart Association. 2001 Heart and Stroke Statistical Update. Dallas, American Heart Association, 2000.
7. Zheng ZJ, Croft JB, Giles WH, Mensah GA: Sudden cardiac death in the United States, 1989 to 1998. Circulation 104:2158, 2001.
8. Cobb LA, Fahrenbruch CE, Olsufka M, Copass MK: Changing incidence of out-of-hospital ventricular fibrillation, 1980-2000. JAMA 288:3008, 2002.
9. Myerburg RJ, Kessler KM, Castellanos A: Sudden cardiac death: Epidemiology, transient risk, and intervention assessment. Ann Intern Med 119:1187, 1993.
10. Gillum RF: Geographic variations in sudden coronary death. Am Heart J 119:380, 1990.
11. Myerburg RJ: Sudden cardiac death: Exploring the limits of our knowledge. J Cardiovasc Electrophysiol 12:369, 2001.
12. Huikuri H, Castellanos A, Myerburg RJ: Sudden death due to cardiac arrhythmias. N Engl J Med 345:1473, 2001.
13. Braunwald E: Cardiovascular medicine at the turn of the millennium: Triumphs, concerns, and opportunities. N Engl J Med 337:1360, 1997.
14. Myerburg RJ, Kessler KM, Castellanos A: Sudden cardiac death: Structure, function, and time-dependence of risk. Circulation 85(Suppl I):I-2, 1992.
15. Arntz HR, Willich SN, Schreiber C, et al: Diurnal, weekly and seasonal variation of sudden death. Population-based analysis of 24,061 consecutive cases. Eur Heart J 21:315, 2000.
16. Larsen GC, Stupey MR, Wallace CG, et al: Recurrent cardiac events in survivors of ventricular fibrillation or tachycardia: Implications for driving restrictions. JAMA 271:1335, 1994.
17. Holmberg M, Holmberg S, Herlitz J: Incidence, duration and survival of ventricular fibrillation in out-of-hospital cardiac arrest patients in Sweden. Resuscitation 44:7, 2000.
18. Wren C, O'Sullivan JJ, Wright C: Sudden death in children and adolescents. Heart 83:410, 2000.
19. Kuisma M, Souminen P, Korpela R: Paediatric out-of-hospital cardiac arrests: Epidemiology and outcome. Resuscitation 30:141, 1995.
20. Steinberger J, Lucas RV Jr, Edwards JE, Titus JL: Causes of sudden, unexpected cardiac death in the first two decades of life. Am J Cardiol 77:992, 1996.
21. Neuspiel DR, Kuller LH: Sudden and unexpected natural death in childhood and adolescence. JAMA 254:1321, 1985.
22. Priori SG, Barhanin J, Hauer RNW, et al: Genetic and molecular basis of cardiac arrhythmias: Impact on clinical management. Circulation 99:518, 1999.
23. Schwartz PJ, Priori SG, Spazzolini C, et al: Genotype-phenotype correlation in the long-QT syndrome: Gene-specific triggers for life-threatening arrhythmias. Circulation 103:89, 2001.
24. Marian AJ, Roberts R: Molecular genetic basis of hypertrophic cardiomyopathy: Genetic markers for sudden cardiac death. J Cardiovasc Electrophysiol 9:88, 1998.
25. Danieli GA, Rampazzo A: Genetics of arrhythmogenic right ventricular cardiomyopathy. Curr Opin Cardiol 17:218, 2002.
26. Chen Q, Kirsch GE, Zhang D, et al: Genetic basis and molecular mechanism for idiopathic ventricular fibrillation. Nature 392:293, 1998.
27. Priori SG, Napolitano C, Memmi M, et al: Clinical and molecular characterization of patients with catecholaminergic polymorphic ventricular tachycardia. Circulation 106:69, 2002.
28. Lahat H, Pras E, Olender T, et al: A missense mutation in a highly conserved region of *CASQ2* is associated with autosomal recessive catecholamine-induced polymorphic ventricular tachycardia in Bedouin families from Israel. Am J Hum Genet 69:1378, 2001.
29. Brookfield L, Bharati S, Denes P, et al: Familial sudden death: Report of a case and review of the literature. Chest 94:989, 1988.
30. Splawski I, Timothy KW, Tateyama M, et al: Variant of SCN5A sodium channel implicated in risk of cardiac arrhythmia. Science 297:1333, 2002.
31. Boerwinkle E, Ellsworth DL, Hallman DM, Biddinger A: Genetic analysis of atherosclerosis: A research paradigm for the common chronic diseases. Hum Mol Genet 5:1405, 1996.
32. Faber BC, Cleutjens KB, Niessen RL, et al: Identification of genes potentially involved in rupture of human atherosclerotic plaques. Circ Res 89:547, 2001.
33. Topol EJ, McCarthy J, Gabriel S, et al: Single nucleotide polymorphisms in multiple novel thrombospondin genes may be associated with familial premature myocardial infarction. Circulation 104:2641, 2001.
34. Spooner PM, Albert C, Benjamin EJ, et al: Sudden cardiac death, genes, and arrhythmogenesis: Consideration of new population and mechanistic approaches from a National Heart, Lung, and Blood Institute Workshop. Part I: Circulation 103:2361; Part II: Circulation 103:2447, 2001.
35. Friedlander Y, Siscovick DS, Weinmann S, et al: Family history as a risk factor for primary cardiac arrest. Circulation 97:155, 1998.
36. Jouven X, Desnos M, Guerot C, Ducimetiere P: Predicting sudden death in the population: The Paris Prospective Study I. Circulation 99:1978, 1999.
37. Schatzkin A, Cupples LA, Heeren T, et al: The epidemiology of sudden unexpected death: Risk factors for men and women in the Framingham Heart Study. Am Heart J 107:1300, 1984.
38. Schatzkin A, Cupples LA, Heeren T, et al: Sudden death in the Framingham Heart Study: Differences in incidence and risk factors by sex and coronary disease status. Am J Epidemiol 120:888, 1984.
39. Gillum RF: Sudden cardiac death in Hispanic Americans and African Americans. Am J Public Health 87:1461, 1997.
40. Albert CM, Chae CU, Grodstein F, et al: Prospective study of sudden cardiac death among women in the United States. Circulation 107:2096, 2003.
41. Becker LB, Han BH, Mayer PM, et al: Racial differences in the inci-dence of cardiac arrest and subsequent survival. N Engl J Med 329:600, 1993.
42. Grundy SM, Balady GJ, Criqui MH, et al: Primary prevention of coronary heart disease: Guidance from Framingham: A statement for healthcare professionals from the AHA Task Force on Risk Reduction. Circulation 97:1876, 1998.
43. Holmes DR, Davis K, Gersh BJ, et al: Risk factor profiles of patients with sudden cardiac death and death from other cardiac causes: A report from the Coronary Artery Surgery Study (CASS). J Am Coll Cardiol 13:524, 1989.
44. Verdecchia P, Schillaci G, Borgioni C, et al: Prognostic significance of serial changes in left ventricular mass in essential hypertension. Circulation 97:48, 1998.
45. Haider AW, Larson MG, Benjamin EJ, Levy D: Increased left ventricular mass and hypertrophy are associated with increased risk for sudden death. J Am Coll Cardiol 32:1454, 1998.
46. Essebag V, Eisenberg MJ: Expanding indications for defibrillators after myocardial infarction: Risk stratification and cost effectiveness. Card Electrophysiol Rev 7:43, 2003.
47. Myerburg RJ, Kessler KM, Kimura S, et al: Life-threatening ventricular arrhythmias: The link between epidemiology and pathophysiology. *In* Zipes DP, Jalife J (eds): Cardiac Electrophysiology. 2nd ed. Philadelphia, WB Saunders, 1995, p 723.
48. Taylor AJ, Burke AP, O'Malley PG, et al: A comparison of the Framingham risk index, coronary artery calcification, and culprit plaque morphology in sudden cardiac death. Circulation 101:1243, 2000.
49. Maclure M: The case-crossover design: A method for studying transient effects on the risk of acute events. Am J Epidemiol 33:144, 1991.
50. Mittleman MA, Maclure M, Tofler GH, et al: Triggering of acute myocardial infarction by heavy physical exertion: Protection against triggering by regular exertion. N Engl J Med 329:1677, 1993.
51. Kannel WB, Thomas HE: Sudden coronary death: The Framingham study. Ann NY Acad Sci 382:3, 1982.
52. Hallstrom AP, Cobb LA, Ray R: Smoking as a risk factor for recurrence of sudden cardiac arrest. N Engl J Med 314:271, 1986.
53. Albert CM, Mittleman MA, Chae CU, et al: Triggering of sudden death from cardiac causes by vigorous exertion. N Engl J Med 343:1355, 2000.
54. Thiene G, Basso C, Corrado D: Is prevention of sudden death in young athletes feasible? Cardiologia 44:497, 1999.
55. Rozanski A, Blumenthal JA, Kaplan J: Impact of psychological factors on the pathogenesis of cardiovascular disease and implications for therapy. Circulation 99:2192, 1999.
56. Krantz DS, Sheps DS, Carney RM, Natelson BH: Effects of mental stress in patients with coronary artery disease: Evidence and clinical implications. JAMA 283:1800, 2000.
57. Hemingway H, Malik M, Marmot M: Social and psychosocial influences on sudden cardiac death, ventricular arrhythmia and cardiac autonomic function. Eur Heart J 22:1082, 2001.
58. Thomas SA, Friedmann E, Wimbush F, Schron E: Psychological factors and survival in the cardiac arrhythmia suppression trial (CAST): A reexamination. Am J Crit Care 6:116, 1997.

59. Irvine J, Basinski A, Baker B, et al: Depression and risk of sudden cardiac death after acute myocardial infarction: Testing for the confounding effects of fatigue. Psychosom Med 61:729, 1999.
60. Williams RB, Barefoot JC, Califf RM, et al: Prognostic importance of social and economic resources among medically treated patients with angiographically documented coronary artery disease. JAMA 267:520, 1992.
61. de Vreede-Swagemakers JJ, Gorgels AP, Weijenberg MP, et al: Risk indicators for out-of-hospital cardiac arrest in patients with coronary artery disease. J Clin Epidemiol 52:601, 1999.
62. The Enhancing Recovery in Coronary Heart Disease Patients (ENRICHD) Randomized Trial Writing Committee: Effects of treating depression and low perceived social support on clinical events after myocardial infarction. JAMA 289:3106, 2003.
63. Leor J, Poole WK, Kloner RA: Sudden cardiac death triggered by an earthquake. N Engl J Med 334:413, 1996.
64. Lampert R, Joska T, Burg MM, et al: Emotional and physical precipitants of ventricular arrhythmia. Circulation 106:1800, 2002.
65. Burke AP, Farb A, Malcom GT, et al: Plaque rupture and sudden death related to exertion in men with coronary artery disease. JAMA 281:921, 1999.
66. de Vreede-Swagemakers JJ, Gorgels AP, Dubois-Arbouw WI, et al: Out-of-hospital cardiac arrest in the 1990's: A population-based study in the Maastricht area on incidence, characteristics and survival. J Am Coll Cardiol 30:1500, 1997.
67. Bigger JT, Fleiss JL, Kleiger R, et al: The relationships among ventricular arrhythmias, left ventricular dysfunction, and mortality in the 2 years after myocardial infarction. Circulation 69:250, 1984.
68. Kennedy HL, Whitlock JA, Sprague MK, et al: Long-term follow-up of asymptomatic healthy subjects with frequent and complex ventricular ectopy. N Engl J Med 312:193, 1985.
69. Viskin S, Belhassen B: Polymorphic ventricular tachyarrhythmias in the absence of organic heart disease: Classification, differential diagnosis, and implications for therapy. Prog Cardiovasc Dis 41:17, 1998.
70. Jouven X, Zureik M, Desnos M, et al: Long-term outcome in asymptomatic men with exercise-induced premature ventricular depolarizations. N Engl J Med 343:826, 2000.
71. Frolkis JP, Pothier CE, Blackstone EH, Lauer MS: Frequent ventricular ectopy after exercise as a predictor of death. N Engl J Med 348:781, 2003.
72. Teerlink JR, Jalaluddin M, Anderson S, et al: Ambulatory ventricular arrhythmias in patients with heart failure do not specifically predict an increased risk of sudden death. PROMISE (Prospective Randomized Milrinone Survival Evaluation) Investigators. Circulation 101:40, 2000.
73. Echt DS, Liebson PR, Mitchell LB, et al: Mortality and morbidity in patients receiving encainide, flecainide, or placebo: The Cardiac Arrhythmia Suppression Trial. N Engl J Med 324:781, 1991.
74. Waldo AL, Camm AJ, deRuyter H, et al, for the SWORD Investigators: Effect of d-sotalol on mortality in patients with left ventricular dysfunction after recent and remote myocardial infarction. Lancet 348:7, 1996.
75. Maisel AS, Scott N, Gilpin E, et al: Complex ventricular arrhythmias in patients with Q wave versus non-Q wave myocardial infarction. Circulation 72:963, 1985.

Causes of Sudden Cardiac Death

76. Myerburg RJ, Interian A Jr, Mitrani RM, et al: Frequency of sudden cardiac death and profiles of risk. Am J Cardiol 80:10F, 1997.
77. Myerburg RJ: Scientific gaps in the prediction and prevention of sudden cardiac death. J Cardiovasc Electrophysiol 13:709, 2002.
78. Frescura C, Basso C, Thiene G, et al: Anomalous origin of coronary arteries and risk of sudden death: A study based on an autopsy population of congenital heart disease. Hum Pathol 29:689, 1998.
79. Myerburg RJ, Kessler KM, Mallon SM, et al: Life-threatening ventricular arrhythmias in patients with silent myocardial ischemia due to coronary artery spasm. N Engl J Med 326:1451, 1992.
80. Sheps DS, Heiss G: Sudden death and silent myocardial ischemia. Am Heart J 117:177, 1989.
81. Anderson KP: Sudden death, hypertension, and hypertrophy. J Cardiovasc Pharmacol 6(Suppl 3):S498, 1984.
82. Braunwald E, Morrow AG, Cornell WP, et al: Idiopathic hypertrophic subaortic stenosis: Clinical, hemodynamic, and angiography manifestations. Am J Med 29:924, 1960.
83. Maron BJ, Spirito P: Impact of patient selection biases on the perception of hypertrophic cardiomyopathy and its natural history. Am J Cardiol 72:970, 1993.
84. Maron BJ, Casey SA, Poliac LC, et al: Clinical course of hypertrophic cardiomyopathy in a regional United States cohort. JAMA 281:650, 1999.
85. McKenna WJ, Behr ER: Hypertrophic cardiomyopathy: Management, risk stratification, and prevention of sudden death. Heart 87:169, 2002.
86. Elliott PM, Gimeno Blanes JR, Mahon NG, et al: Relation between severity of left-ventricular hypertrophy and prognosis in patients with hypertrophic cardiomyopathy. Lancet 357:420, 2001.
87. Maron MS, Olivotto I, Betocchi S, et al: Effect of left ventricular outflow tract obstruction on clinical outcome in hypertrophic cardiomyopathy. N Engl J Med 348:295, 2003.
88. Maron BJ, Shirani J, Poliac LC, et al: Sudden death in young competitive athletes. Clinical, demographic, and pathological profiles. JAMA 276:199, 1996.
89. Cleland JG, Chattopadhyay S, Khand A, et al: Prevalence and incidence of arrhythmias and sudden death in heart failure. Heart Fail Rev 7:229, 2002.
90. Stevenson WE, Stevenson LW, Middlekauff HR, et al: Sudden death prevention in patients with advanced ventricular dysfunction. Circulation 88:2953, 1993.
91. Middlekauff HR, Stevenson WG, Stevenson LW, et al: Syncope in advanced heart failure: High sudden death risk regardless of syncope etiology. J Am Coll Cardiol 21:110, 1993.
92. Knight BP, Goyal R, Pelosi F, et al: Outcome of patients with nonischemic dilated cardiomyopathy and unexplained syncope treated with an implantable defibrillator. J Am Coll Cardiol 33:1964, 1999.
93. Corrado D, Basso C, Thiene G: Sudden cardiac death in young people with apparently normal heart. Cardiovasc Res 50:399, 2001.
94. Theleman KP, Kuiper JJ, Roberts WC: Acute myocarditis (predominately lymphocytic) causing sudden death without heart failure. Am J Cardiol 88:1078, 2001.
95. Phillips M, Rabinowitz M, Higgins JR, et al: Sudden cardiac death in Air Force recruits. JAMA 256:2696, 1986.
96. Roberts WC, McAllister HA, Ferrans VJ: Sarcoidosis of the heart: A clinicopathologic study of 35 necropsy patients (group 1) and review of 78 previously described necropsy patients (group 11). Am J Med 63:86, 1977.
97. Corrado D, Basso C, Nava A, Thiene G: Arrhythmogenic right ventricular cardiomyopathy: Current diagnostic and management strategies. Cardiol Rev 9:259, 2001.
98. Thiene G, Nava A, Corrado D, et al: Right ventricular cardiomyopathy and sudden death in young people. N Engl J Med 318:129, 1988.
99. Fontaine G, Fontaliran F, Hebert JL, et al: Arrhythmogenic right ventricular dysplasia. Annu Rev Med 50:17, 1999.
100. Corrado D, Basso C, Thiene G, et al: Spectrum of clinicopathologic manifestations of arrhythmogenic right ventricular cardiomyopathy/dysplasia: A multicenter study. J Am Coll Cardiol 30:1512, 1997.
101. Furlanello F, Bertoldi A, Dallago M, et al: Cardiac arrest and sudden death in competitive athletes with arrhythmogenic right ventricular dysplasia. Pacing Clin Electrophysiol 21:331, 1998.
102. Tiso N, Stephan DA, Nava A, et al: Identification of mutations in the cardiac ryanodine receptor gene in families affected with arrhythmogenic right ventricular cardiomyopathy type 2 (ARVD2). Hum Mol Genet 10:189, 2001.
103. Rampazzo A, Nava A, Malacrida S, et al: Mutation in human desmoplakin domain binding to plakoglobin causes a dominant form of arrhythmogenic right ventricular cardiomyopathy. Am J Hum Genet 71:1200, 2002.
104. Sorgato A, Faggiano P, Aurigemma GP, et al: Ventricular arrhythmias in adult aortic stenosis: Prevalence, mechanisms, and clinical relevance. Chest 113:482, 1998.
105. McGiffin DC, O'Brien MF, Galbraith AJ, et al: An analysis of risk factors for death and mode-specific death after aortic valve replacement with allograft, xenograft, and mechanical valves. J Thorac Cardiovasc Surg 106:895, 1993.
106. Konishi Y, Matsuda K, Nishiwaki N, et al: Ventricular arrhythmias late after aortic and/or mitral valve replacement. Jpn Circ J 49:576, 1985.
107. Freed LA, Levy D, Levine RA, et al: Prevalence and clinical outcome of mitral valve prolapse. N Engl J Med 341:1, 1999.
108. Chugh SS, Kelly KL, Titus JL: Sudden cardiac death with apparently normal heart. Circulation 102:649, 2000.
109. Weiss BM, Hess OM: Pulmonary vascular disease and pregnancy: Current controversies, management strategies, and perspectives. Eur Heart J 21:104, 2000.
110. Gatzoulis MA, Balaji S, Webber SA, et al: Risk factors for arrhythmia and sudden cardiac death late after repair of tetralogy of Fallot: A multicentre study. Lancet 356:975, 2000.
111. Melgarejo-Moreno A, Galcera-Tomas J, Garcia-Alberola A, et al: Incidence, clinical characteristics, and prognostic significance of right bundle-branch block in acute myocardial infarction: A study in the thrombolytic era. Circulation 96:1139, 1997.
112. Udink ten Cate FE, Breur JM, Cohen MI, et al: Dilated cardiomyopathy in isolated congenital complete atrioventricular block: Early and long-term risk in children. J Am Coll Cardiol 37:1129, 2001.
113. Balmer C, Fasnacht M, Rahn M, et al: Long-term follow up of children with congenital complete atrioventricular block and the impact of pacemaker therapy. Europace 4:345, 2002.
114. Vidaillet HJ, Pressley JC, Henke E, et al: Familial occurrence of accessory atrioventricular pathways (preexcitation syndrome). N Engl J Med 317:65, 1987.
115. Gollob MH, Green MS, Tang AS, et al: Identification of a gene responsible for familial Wolff-Parkinson-White syndrome. N Engl J Med 344:1823, 2001.
116. Priori SG, Bloise R, Crotti L: The long QT syndrome. Europace 3:16, 2001.
117. Priori SG, Schwartz PJ, Napolitano C, et al: Risk stratification in the long-QT syndrome. N Engl J Med 348:1866, 2003.
118. Locati EH, Zareba W, Moss AJ, et al: Age- and sex-related differences in clinical manifestations in patients with congenital long-QT syndrome: Findings from the International LQTS Registry. Circulation 97:2237, 1998.
119. Moss AJ, Zareba W, Hall WJ, et al: Effectiveness and limitations of beta-blocker therapy in congenital long-QT syndrome. Circulation 101:616, 2000.
120. Zareba W, Moss AJ, Schwartz PJ, et al: Influence of genotype on the clinical course of the long-QT syndrome. N Engl J Med 339:960, 1998.
121. Fu EY, Clemo HF, Ellenbogen KA: Acquired QT prolongation: Mechanisms and implications. Cardiol Rev 6:319, 1998.
122. Woosley RL, Chen Y, Freiman JP, Gillis RA: Mechanism of cardiotoxic actions of terfenadine. JAMA 269:1532, 1993.
123. Sesti F, Abbott GW, Wei J, et al: A common polymorphism associated with antibiotic-induced cardiac arrhythmia. Proc Natl Acad Sci USA 97:10613, 2000.
124. Napolitano C, Schwartz PJ, Brown AM, et al: Evidence for a cardiac ion channel mutation underlying drug-induced QT prolongation and life-threatening arrhythmias. J Cardiovasc Electrophysiol 11:691, 2000.
125. Makita N, Horie M, Nakamura T, et al: Drug-induced long-QT syndrome associated with a subclinical SCN5A mutation. Circulation 106:1269, 2002.
126. Brugada J, Brugada R, Brugada P: Right bundle-branch block and ST-segment elevation in leads V1 through V3: A marker for sudden death in patients without demonstrable structural heart disease. Circulation 97:457, 1998.
127. Alings M, Wilde A: "Brugada" syndrome: Clinical data and suggested pathophysiological mechanism. Circulation 99:666, 1999.
128. Priori SG, Napolitano C, Gasparini M, et al: Natural history of Brugada syndrome: Insights for risk stratification and management. Circulation 105:1342, 2002.
129. Brugada J, Brugada R, Antzelevitch C, et al: Long-term follow-up of individuals with the electrocardiographic pattern of right bundle-branch block and ST-segment elevation in precordial leads V1 to V3. Circulation 105:73, 2002.

130. Coumel P, Rosengarten MD, Leclercq JF, Attuel P: Role of sympathetic nervous system in non-ischaemic ventricular arrhythmias. Br Heart J 47:137, 1982.
131. Priori SG, Napolitano C, Memmi M, et al: Clinical and molecular characterization of patients with catecholaminergic polymorphic ventricular tachycardia. Circulation 106:69, 2002.
132. Skinner JE: Neurocardiology. Brain mechanisms underlying fatal cardiac arrhythmias. Neurol Clin 11:325, 1993.
133. Krantz DS, Sheps DS, Carney RM, Natelson BH: Effects of mental stress in patients with coronary artery disease: Evidence and clinical implications. JAMA 283:1800, 2000.
134. Lampert R, Joska T, Burg MM, et al: Emotional and physical precipitants of ventricular arrhythmia. Circulation 106:1800, 2002.
135. Leor J, Poole WK, Kloner RA: Sudden cardiac death triggered by an earthquake. N Engl J Med 334:413, 1996.
136. Leenardt A, Glaser E, Burguera M, et al: Short-coupled variant of torsades de pointes: A new electrocardiographic entity in the spectrum of idiopathic ventricular tachyarrhythmias. Circulation 89:206, 1994.
137. Burrell RJW: The possible bearing of curse death and other factors in Bantu culture in the etiology of myocardial infarction. *In* James TN, Keyes JW (eds): The Etiology of Myocardial Infarction. Boston, Little, Brown, 1963, pp 95-100.
138. Hauck FR, Hunt CE: Sudden infant death syndrome in 2000. Curr Probl Pediatr 30:237, 2000.
139. Gibson E, Fleming N, Fleming D, et al: Sudden infant death syndrome rates subsequent to the American Academy of Pediatrics supine sleep position. Med Care 36:938, 1998.

140. Schwartz PJ, Stramba-Badiale M, Segantini A, et al: Prolongation of the QT interval and the sudden infant death syndrome. N Engl J Med 338:1709, 1998.
141. Schwartz P, Priori S, Dumaine R, et al: A molecular link between the sudden infant death syndrome and the long-QT syndrome. N Engl J Med 343:262, 2000.
142. Marino TA, Kane BM: Cardiac atrioventricular junctional tissues in hearts from infants who died suddenly. J Am Coll Cardiol 5:1178, 1985.
143. Topaz O, Edwards JE: Pathologic features of sudden death in children, adolescents, and young adults. Chest 87:476, 1985.
144. Corrado D, Basso C, Schiavon M, Thiene G: Screening for hypertrophic cardiomyopathy in young athletes. N Engl J Med 339:364, 1998.
145. Virmani R, Burke AP, Farb A, Kark JA: Causes of sudden death in young and middle-aged competitive athletes. Cardiol Clin 15:439, 1997.
146. Maron BJ, Thompson PD, Puffer JC, et al: Cardiovascular preparticipation screening of competitive athletes. A statement for health professionals from the Sudden Death Committee (clinical cardiology) and Congenital Cardiac Defects Committee (cardiovascular disease in the young), American Heart Association. Circulation 94:850, 1996.
147. Myerburg RJ, Mitrani R, Interian A Jr, Castellanos A: Identification of risk of cardiac arrest and sudden cardiac death in athletes. *In* Estes NAM, Salem DN, Wang PJ (eds): Sudden Cardiac Death in the Athlete. Armonk, NY, Futura, 1998, p 25.
148. Basso C, Maron BJ, Corrado D, Thiene G: Clinical profile of congenital coronary artery anomalies with origin from the wrong aortic sinus leading to sudden death in young competitive athletes. J Am Coll Cardiol 35:1493, 2000.
149. Maron BJ, Link MS, Wang PJ, Estes NA 3rd: Clinical profile of commotio cordis: An under appreciated cause of sudden death in the young during sports and other activities. J Cardiovasc Electrophysiol 10:114, 1999.
150. Armstrong LE, Maresh CM: Effects of training, environment, and host factors on the sweating response to exercise. Int J Sports Med 19(Suppl 2):S103, 1998.
151. Joint Steering Committees of the Unexplained Cardiac Arrest Registry of Europe and of the Idiopathic Ventricular Fibrillation Registry of the United States: Survivors of out-of-hospital cardiac arrest with apparently normal heart: Need for definition and standardized clinical evaluation. Circulation 95:265, 1997.
152. Meissner MD, Lehmann MH, Steinman RT: Ventricular fibrillation in patients without significant structural heart disease: A multicenter experience with implantable cardioverter-defibrillator therapy. J Am Coll Cardiol 21:1406, 1993.
153. Nademanee K, Veerakul G, Nimmannit S, et al: Arrhythmogenic marker for the sudden unexplained death syndrome in Thai men. Circulation 96:2595, 1997.

Pathology and Pathophysiology

154. Virmani R, Burke AP, Farb A: Sudden cardiac death. Cardiovasc Pathol 10:211, 2001.
155. Liberthson RR, Nagel EL, Hirschman JC, et al: Pathophysiologic observations in prehospital ventricular fibrillation and sudden cardiac death. Circulation 49:790, 1974.
156. Farb A, Tang AL, Burke AP, et al: Sudden coronary death: Frequency of active coronary lesions, inactive coronary lesions, and myocardial infarction. Circulation 92:1701, 1995.
157. Farb A, Burke AP, Tang AL, et al: Coronary plaque erosion without rupture into a lipid core: A frequent cause of coronary thrombosis in sudden coronary death. Circulation 93:1354, 1996.
158. Warnes CA, Roberts WC: Sudden coronary death: Relation of amount and distribution of coronary narrowing at necropsy to previous symptoms of myocardial ischemia, left ventricular scarring, and heart weight. Am J Cardiol 54:65, 1984.
159. Davies MJ, Thomas A: Thrombosis and acute coronary artery lesions in sudden cardiac ischemic death. N Engl J Med 310:1137, 1984.
160. Burke AP, Farb A, Malcom GT, et al: Coronary risk factors and plaque morphology in men with coronary disease who died suddenly. N Engl J Med 336:1276, 1997.
161. Antman EM, Tanasijevic MJ, Thompson B, et al: Cardiac-specific troponin I levels to predict the risk of mortality in patients with acute coronary syndromes. N Engl J Med 335:1342, 1996.
162. Mullner M, Hirschl MM, Herkner H, et al: Creatine kinase-MB fraction and cardiac troponin T to diagnose acute myocardial infarction after cardiopulmonary resuscitation. J Am Coll Cardiol 28:1220, 1996.
163. Cooper RS, Simmons BE, Castaner A, et al: Left ventricular hypertrophy is associated with worse survival independent of ventricular function and number of coronary arteries severely narrowed. Am J Cardiol 65:441, 1990.
164. Furukawa T, Bassett AL, Furukawa N, et al: The ionic mechanism of reperfusion-induced early afterdepolarizations in the feline left ventricular hypertrophy. J Clin Invest 91:1521, 1993.
165. Cohle SD, Suarez-Mier MP, Aguilera B: Sudden death resulting from lesions of the cardiac conduction system. Am J Forensic Med Pathol 23:83, 2002.
166. Liu YB, Wu CC, Lu LS, et al: Sympathetic nerve sprouting, electrical remodeling, and increased vulnerability to ventricular fibrillation in hypercholesterolemic rabbits. Circ Res 92:1145, 2003.
167. Dorian P, Cass D, Schwartz B, et al: Amiodarone as compared with lidocaine for shock-resistant ventricular fibrillation. N Engl J Med 347:368, 2002.
168. Mehta D, Curwin J, Gomes JA, Fuster V: Sudden death in coronary artery disease: Acute ischemia versus myocardial substrate. Circulation 96:3215, 1997.
169. Myerburg RJ, Kessler KM, Kimura S, Castellanos A: Sudden cardiac death: Future approaches based on identification and control of transient risk factors. J Cardiovasc Electrophysiol 3:626, 1992.
170. Myerburg RJ, Kessler KM, Bassett AL, Castellanos A: A biological approach to sudden cardiac death: Structure, function, and cause. Am J Cardiol 63:1512, 1989.
171. Myerburg RJ, Kessler KM, Zaman L, et al: Survivors of prehospital cardiac arrest. JAMA 247:1485, 1982.
172. Furukawa T, Moroe K, Mayrovitz HN, et al: Arrhythmogenic effects of graded coronary blood flow reductions superimposed on prior myocardial infarction in dogs. Circulation 84:368, 1991.
173. Coronel R, Wilms-Schopman FJG, Opthof T, et al: Reperfusion arrhythmias in isolated perfused pig hearts: Inhomogeneities in extra-cellular potassium, ST and QT potentials, and transmembrane action potentials. Circ Res 71:1131, 1992.
174. Vermeulen JT, Tan HL, Rademaker H, et al: Electrophysiologic and extracellular ionic changes during acute ischemia in failing and normal rabbit myocardium. J Mol Cell Cardiol 28:123, 1996.
175. Remme CA, Schumacher CA, de Jong JW, et al: K(ATP) channel opening during ischemia: Effects on myocardial noradrenaline release and ventricular arrhythmias. Cardiovasc Pharmacol 38:406, 2001.
176. Furukawa T, Kimura S, Furukawa N, et al: Role of cardiac ATP-regulated potassium channels in differential responses of endocardial and epicardial cells to ischemia. Circ Res 68:1693, 1991.
177. Beardslee MA, Lerner DL, Tadros PN, et al: Dephosphorylation and intracellular redistribution of ventricular connexin43 during electrical uncoupling induced by ischemia. Circ Res 87:656, 2000.
178. Yao JA, Hussain W, Patel P, et al: Remodeling of gap junctional channel function in epicardial border zone of healing canine infarcts. Circ Res 92:437, 2003.
179. Schwartz PJ: The autonomic nervous system and sudden death. Eur Heart J 19(Suppl F):F-72, 1998.
180. McLennan PL: Myocardial membrane fatty acids and the antiarrhythmic actions of dietary fish oil in animal models. Lipids 36(Suppl):S-111, 2001.
181. Makikallio TH, Koistinen J, Jordaens L, et al: Heart rate dynamics before spontaneous onset of ventricular fibrillation in patients with healed myocardial infarcts. Am J Cardiol 83:880, 1999.

Clinical Characteristics of the Patient with Cardiac Arrest

182. Liberthson RR, Nagel EL, Hirschman JC, Nussenfeld SR: Prehospital ventricular fibrillation: Prognosis and follow-up course. N Engl J Med 291:317, 1974.
183. Baum RS, Alvarez H, Cobb LA: Survival after resuscitation from out-of-hospital ventricular fibrillation. Circulation 50:1231, 1974.
184. Davies MJ, Bland JM, Hangartner JRW, et al: Factors influencing the presence or absence of acute coronary artery thrombi in sudden ischaemic death. Eur Heart J 10:203, 1989.
185. Bayes de Luna A, Coumel P, Leclercq JF: Ambulatory sudden death: Mechanisms of production of fatal arrhythmia on the basis of data from 157 cases. Am Heart J 117:151, 1989.
186. Huikuri HV, Seppanen T, Koistinen MJ, et al: Abnormalities in beat-to-beat dynamics of heart rate before the spontaneous onset of life-threatening ventricular tachyarrhythmias in patients with prior myocardial infarction. Circulation 93:1836, 1996.
187. Huikuri HV, Makikallio TH, Raatikainen MJ, et al: Prediction of sudden cardiac death: Appraisal of the studies and methods assessing the risk of sudden arrhythmic death. Circulation 108:110, 2003
188. Hinkle LE, Thaler HT: Clinical classification of cardiac deaths. Circulation 65:457, 1982.
189. American Heart Association: International Guidelines 2000 for CPR and ECC. Circulation 102(Suppl I):I-1, 2000.
190. Bedell SE, Delbanco TL, Cook EF, Epstein FH: Survival after cardiopulmonary resuscitation in the hospital. N Engl J Med 309:569, 1983.
191. de Vos R, Koster RW, De Haan RJ, et al: In-hospital cardiopulmonary resuscitation: Pre-arrest morbidity and outcome. Arch Intern Med 159:845, 1999.
192. Herlitz J, Bang A, Alsen B, Aune S: Characteristics and outcome among patients suffering from in hospital cardiac arrest in relation to the interval between collapse and start of CPR. Resuscitation 53:21, 2002.
193. Kim C, Becker L, Eisenberg MS: Out-of-hospital cardiac arrest in octogenarians and nonagenarians. Arch Intern Med 160:3439, 2000.
194. Tresch DD, Thakur RK, Hoffmann RG, et al: Should the elderly be resuscitated following out-of-hospital cardiac arrest? Am J Med 86:145, 1989.
195. Kette F, Sbrojavacca R, Rellini G, et al: Epidemiology and survival rate of out-of-hospital cardiac arrest in northeast Italy: The F.A.C.S. study. Friuli Venezia Giulia Cardiac Arrest Cooperative Study. Resuscitation 36:153, 1998.
196. The Hypothermia after Cardiac Arrest Study Group: Mild therapeutic hypothermia to improve the neurologic outcome after cardiac arrest. N Engl J Med 346:549, 2002.
197. Bernard SA, Gray TW, Buist MD, et al: Treatment of comatose survivors of out-of-hospital cardiac arrest with induced hypothermia. N Engl J Med 346:557, 2002.

198. Myerburg RJ: Sudden cardiac death in persons with normal (or near normal) hearts. Am J Cardiol 79(Suppl 6A):3, 1997.
199. Gorgels AP, Gijsbers C, de Vreede-Swagemakers J, et al: Out-of-hospital cardiac arrest—The relevance of heart failure. The Maastricht Circulatory Arrest Registry. Eur Heart J 24:1204, 2003.
200. Laurent I, Monchi M, Chiche JD, et al: Reversible myocardial dysfunction in survivors of out-of-hospital cardiac arrest. J Am Coll Cardiol 40:2110, 2002.
201. Bunch TJ, White RD, Gersh BJ, et al: Long-term outcomes of out-of-hospital cardiac arrest after successful early defibrillation. N Engl J Med 348:2626, 2003.
202. Iuliano S, Fisher SG, Karasik PE, et al: QRS duration and mortality in patients with congestive heart failure. Am Heart J 143:1085, 2002.
203. The Antiarrhythmics versus Implantable Defibrillators (AVID) Investigators: A comparison of antiarrhythmic-drug therapy with implantable defibrillators in patients resuscitated from near-fatal ventricular arrhythmias. N Engl J Med 337:1576, 1997.
204. Connolly SJ, Gent M, Roberts RS, et al, on behalf of the CIDS Investigators: Canadian Implantable Defibrillator Study (CIDS): A randomized trial of the implantable cardioverter defibrillator against amiodarone. Circulation 101:1297, 2000.
205. Kuck KH, Cappato R, Siebels J, Ruppel R: Randomized comparison of antiarrhythmic drug therapy with implantable defibrillators in patients resuscitated from cardiac arrest: The Cardiac Arrest Study Hamburg (CASH). Circulation 102:748, 2000.

Management of Cardiac Arrest

206. Cobb LA, Weaver WD, Fahrenbrush CE: Community-based interventions for sudden cardiac death: Impact, limitations, and charges. Circulation 85(Suppl I): I-98, 1992.
207. Stults KR, Brown DD, Schug VL, Bean JA: Prehospital defibrillation performed by emergency medical technicians in rural communities. N Engl J Med 310:219, 1984.
208. Stapczynski JS, Svenson JE, Stone CK: Population density, automated external defibrillator use, and survival in rural cardiac arrest. Acad Emerg Med 4:552, 1997.
209. Groh WJ, Newman MM, Beal PE, et al: Limited response to cardiac arrest by police equipped with automated external defibrillators: Lack of survival benefit in suburban and rural Indiana—The police as responder automated defibrillation evaluation (PARADE). Acad Emerg Med 8:324, 2001.
210. Lombardi G, Gallagher J, Gennis P: Outcome of out-of-hospital cardiac arrest in New York City: The Pre-Hospital Arrest Survival Evaluation (PHASE) Study. JAMA 271:678, 1994.
211. Cummins RO, Ornato JP, Thies WH, Pepe PE: Improving survival from sudden cardiac arrest: The "chain of survival" concept: A statement for heart professionals from the Advanced Cardiac Life Support Subcommittee and the Emergency Cardiac Care Committee, American Heart Association. Circulation 83:1832, 1991.
212. Myerburg RJ, Fenster J, Velez M, et al: Impact of community-wide police car deployment of automated external defibrillators on out-of-hospital cardiac arrest. Circulation 106:1058, 2002.
213. Capucci A, Aschieri D, Piepoli MF, et al: Tripling survival from sudden cardiac arrest via early defibrillation without traditional education in cardiopulmonary resuscitation. Circulation 106:1065, 2002.
214. Weisfeldt ML, Becker LB: Resuscitation after cardiac arrest: A 3-phase time-sensitive model. JAMA 288:3035, 2002.
215. Holmberg M, Holmberg S, Herlitz J: The problem of out-of-hospital cardiac arrest: Prevalence of sudden death in Europe today. Am J Cardiol 83:88D, 1999.
216. Waalewijn RA, de Vos R, Koster RW: Out-of-hospital cardiac arrests in Amsterdam and its surrounding areas: Results from the Amsterdam resuscitation study (ARREST) in "Utstein" style. Resuscitation 38:157, 1998.
217. White RD, Hankins DG, Bugliosi TF: Seven years' experience with early defibrillation by police and paramedics in an emergency medical services system. Resuscitation 39:145, 1998.
218. Becker L, Eisenberg M, Fahrenbruch C, Cobb L: Public locations of cardiac arrest: Implications for public access defibrillation. Circulation 97:2106, 1998.
219. Cobb LA, Fahrenbruch CE, Walsh TR, et al: Influence of cardiopulmonary resuscitation prior to defibrillation in patients with out-of-hospital ventricular fibrillation. JAMA 281:1182, 1999.
220. Dowie R, Campbell H, Donohoe R, Clarke P: "Event tree" analysis of out-of-hospital cardiac arrest data: Confirming the importance of bystander CPR. Resuscitation 56:173, 2003.
221. Wik L, Hansen TB, Fylling F, et al: Delaying defibrillation to give basic cardiopulmonary resuscitation to patients with out-of-hospital ventricular fibrillation: A randomized trial. JAMA 289:1389, 2003.
222. Page RL, Joglar JA, Kowal RC, et al. Use of automated external defibrillators by a U.S. airline. N Engl J Med 343:1210, 2000.
223. Caffrey SL, Willoughby PJ, Pepe PE, Becker LB: Public use of automated external defibrillators. N Engl J Med 347:1242, 2002.
224. Valenzuela TD, Roe DJ, Nichol G, et al. Outcomes of rapid defibrillation by security officers after cardiac arrest in casinos. N Engl J Med 343:1206, 2000.
225. Caldwell G, Miller G, Quinn E, et al: Simple mechanical methods for cardioversion: Defense of the precordial thump and cough version. Br Med J (Clin Res Ed) 291:627, 1985.
226. Plaisance P, Lurie KG, Payen D: Inspiratory impedance during active compression-decompression cardiopulmonary resuscitation: A randomized evaluation in patients in cardiac arrest. Circulation 101:989, 2000.
227. Mauer D, Wolcke B, Dick W: Alternative methods of mechanical cardiopulmonary resuscitation. Resuscitation 44:81, 2000.
228. Kerber RE, Becker LB, Bourland JD, et al: Automatic external defibrillators for public access defibrillation: Recommendations for specifying and reporting arrhythmia analysis algorithm performance, incorporating new waveforms, and enhancing safety: A statement for health professionals from the American Heart Association Task Force on Automatic External Defibrillation, Subcommittee on AED Safety and Efficacy. Circulation 95:1677, 1997.
229. Gueugniaud PY, Mols P, Goldstein P, et al: A comparison of repeated high doses and repeated standard doses of epinephrine for cardiac arrest outside the hospital: European Epinephrine Study Group. N Engl J Med 339:1595, 1998.
230. Wenzel V, Lindner KH: Arginine vasopressin during cardiopulmonary resuscitation: Laboratory evidence, clinical experience and recommendations, and a view to the future. Crit Care Med 30(4 Suppl):S157, 2002.
231. Cummins RO, Graves JR, Larsen MP, et al: Out-of-hospital transcutaneous pacing by emergency medical technicians in patients with asystolic cardiac arrest. N Engl J Med 328:1377, 1993.
232. Myerburg RJ, Conde CA, Sung RJ, et al: Clinical, electrophysiologic and hemodynamic profile of patients resuscitated from prehospital cardiac arrest. Am J Med 68:568, 1980.
233. Spaulding CM, Joly LM, Rosenberg A, et al: Immediate coronary angiography in survivors of out-of-hospital cardiac arrest. N Engl J Med 336:1629, 1997.
234. Kelly P, Ruskin JN, Vlahakes GJ, et al: Surgical coronary revascularization in survivors of prehospital cardiac arrest. J Am Coll Cardiol 15:267, 1990.
235. Bigger JT Jr, for the Coronary Artery Bypass Graft (CABG) Patch Trial Investigators: Prophylactic use of implanted cardiac defibrillators in patients at high risk for ventricular arrhythmias after coronary-artery bypass graft surgery. N Engl J Med 337:1569, 1997.
236. Hallstrom AP, Cobb LA, Yu BH, et al: An antiarrhythmic drug experience in 941 patients resuscitated from an initial cardiac arrest between 1970 and 1985. Am J Cardiol 68:1025, 1991.

Prevention of Cardiac Arrest and Sudden Cardiac Death

237. Steinbeck G, Andresen S, Bach P, et al: A comparison of electrophysiologically guided antiarrhythmic drug therapy with beta-blocker therapy in patients with symptomatic sustained ventricular tachyarrhythmias. N Engl J Med 327:987, 1992.
238. Domanski MJ, Sakseena S, Epstein AE, et al, for the AVID Investigators: Relative effectiveness of the implantable cardioverter-defibrillator and antiarrhythmic drugs in patients with varying degrees of left ventricular dysfunction who have survived malignant ventricular arrhythmias. J Am Coll Cardiol 34:1090, 1999.
239. Mason JW, for The Electrophysiologic Study versus Electrocardiographic Monitoring Investigators: A comparison of electrophysiologic testing with Holter monitoring to predict antiarrhythmic-drug efficacy for ventricular tachyarrhythmias. N Engl J Med 329:445, 1993.
240. Reiter MJ, Reiffel JA: Importance of beta blockade in the therapy of serious ventricular arrhythmias. Am J Cardiol 82:9-I, 1998.
241. Boutitie F, Boissel JP, Connolly SJ, et al, for the EMIAT and CAMIAT Investigators: Amiodarone interaction with beta-blockers: Analysis of the merged EMIAT (European Myocardial Infarct Amiodarone Trial) and CAMIAT (Canadian Amiodarone Myocardial Infarction Trial) databases. The EMIAT and CAMIAT Investigators. Circulation 99:2268, 1999.
242. Huikuri HV, Tapanainen JM, Lindgran K, et al: Prediction of sudden cardiac death after myocardial infarction in the beta-blocking era. J Am Coll Cardiol 42:652, 2003.
243. Moss AJ, Hall WJ, Cannom DS, et al, for the Multicenter Automatic Defibrillator Implantation Trial Investigators: Improved survival with an implanted defibrillator in patients with coronary disease at high risk for ventricular arrhythmia. N Engl J Med 335:1933, 1996.
244. Buxton AE, Lee KL, Fisher JD, et al: A randomized study of the prevention of sudden death in patients with coronary artery disease. Multicenter Unsustained Tachycardia Trial Investigators. N Engl J Med 341:1882, 1999.
245. Goldstein S, Brooks MM, Ledingham R, et al: The association between ease of suppression of ventricular arrhythmias and survival. Circulation 91:79, 1995.
246. Priori SG, Aliot E, Blomstrom-Lundqvist C, et al: Task force report: Task Force on Sudden Cardiac Death of the European Society of Cardiology. Eur Heart J 22:1374, 2001.
247. Priori SG, Aliot E, Blomstrom-Lundqvist C, et al: Update of the guidelines on sudden cardiac death of the European Society of Cardiology. Eur Heart J 24:13, 2003.
248. Moss AJ, Zareba W, Hall WJ, et al: Prophylactic implantation of a defibrillator in patients with myocardial infarction and reduced ejection fraction. N Engl J Med 346:877, 2002.
249. Blanck Z, Dhala A, Deshpande S, et al: Bundle branch reentrant ventricular tachycardia. J Cardiovasc Electrophysiol 4:253, 1993.
250. Strickberger SA, Man KC, Daoud EG: A prospective evaluation of catheter ablation of ventricular tachycardia as adjuvant therapy in patients with coronary artery disease and an implantable cardioverter-defibrillator. Circulation 96:1525, 1997.
251. Mirowski M, Reid PR, Winkle RA, et al: Mortality in patients with implanted automatic defibrillators. Ann Intern Med 98:585, 1983.
252. Echt DS, Armstrong K, Schmidt P, et al: Clinical experience, complications, and survival in 70 patients with the automatic implantable cardioverter/defibrillator. Circulation 71:289, 1985.
253. Kelly PA, Cannom DS, Garan H, et al: The automatic implantable defibrillator (AICD): Efficacy, complications and survival in patients with malignant ventricular arrhythmias. J Am Coll Cardiol 11:1278, 1988.
254. Tchou PJ, Kadri N, Anderson J, et al: Automatic implantable cardioverter-defibrillators and survival of patients with left ventricular dysfunction and malignant ventricular arrhythmias. Ann Intern Med 109:529, 1988.
255. Myerburg RJ, Luceri RM, Thurer R, et al: Time to first shock and clinical outcome in patients receiving automatic implantable cardioverter-defibrillators. J Am Coll Cardiol 14:508, 1989.
256. Newman D, Sauve MJ, Herre J, et al: Survival after implantation of the cardioverter defibrillator. Am J Cardiol 69:699, 1992.
257. Myerburg RJ, Castellanos A: Clinical trials of implantable defibrillators. N Engl J Med 337:1621, 1997.
258. Mirowski M, Reid PR, Mower MM, et al: Termination of malignant ventricular arrhythmias with an implanted automatic defibrillator in human beings. N Engl J Med 303:322, 1980.

259. Myerburg RJ, Mitrani R, Interian A Jr, Castellanos A: Interpretation of outcomes of antiarrhythmic clinical trials: Design features and population impact. Circulation 97:1514, 1998.
260. Morris JJ, Rastogi A, Stanton MS, et al: Operation for ventricular tachyarrhythmias: Refining current treatment strategies. Ann Thorac Surg 58:1490, 1994.
261. Julian DG, Camm AJ, Frangin G, et al, for the European Myocardial Infarct Amiodarone Trial Investigators: Randomised trial of effect of amiodarone on mortality in patients with left-ventricular dysfunction after recent myocardial infarction: EMIAT. Lancet 349:667, 1997.
262. Cairns JA, Connolly SJ, Roberts R, Gent M, for the Canadian Amiodarone Myocardial Infarction Arrhythmia Trial Investigators: Randomised trial of outcome after myocardial infarction in patients with frequent or repetitive ventricular premature depolarisations: CAMIAT. Lancet 349:675, 1997.
263. MERIT-HF Study Group: Effect of metoprolol CR/XL in chronic heart failure: Metoprolol CR/XL Randomised Intervention Trial in Congestive Heart Failure (MERIT-HF). Lancet 353:2001, 1999.
264. Zipes DP, Wellens HJ: Sudden cardiac death. Circulation 98:2334, 1998.
265. Maron BJ, Shen WK, Link MS, et al: Efficacy of implantable cardioverter-defibrillators for the prevention of sudden death in patients with hypertrophic cardiomyopathy. N Engl J Med 342:365, 2000.
266. Brugada J, Brugada R, Antzelevitch C, et al: Long-term follow-up of individuals with the electrocardiographic pattern of right bundle-branch block and ST-segment elevation in precordial leads V_1 to V_3. Circulation 105:73, 2002.
267. Priori SG, Napolitano C, Gasparini M, et al: Natural history of Brugada syndrome: Insights for risk stratification and management. Circulation 105:1342, 2002.
268. Yusuf S, Sleight P, Pogue J, et al: Effects of an angiotensin-converting enzyme inhibitor, ramipril, on cardiovascular events in high-risk patients. The Heart Outcomes Prevention Evaluation Study Investigators. N Engl J Med 342:748, 2000.
269. Van Camp SP, Bloor CM, Mueller FO, et al: Nontraumatic sports death in high school and college athletes. Med Sci Sports Exerc 27:641, 1995.
270. Basilico FC: Cardiovascular disease in athletes. Am J Sports Med 27:108, 1999.
271. Fuller CM: Cost effectiveness analysis of screening of high school athletes for risk of sudden cardiac death. Med Sci Sports Exerc 32:887, 2000.
272. Maron BJ, Thompson PD, Puffer JC, et al: Cardiovascular preparticipation screening of competitive athletes: Addendum: An addendum to a statement for health professionals from the Sudden Death Committee (Council on Clinical Cardiology) and the Congenital Cardiac Defects Committee (Council on Cardiovascular Disease in the Young), American Heart Association. Circulation 97:2294, 1998.

Sudden Death and Public Safety

273. Myerburg RJ, Davis JH: The medical ecology of public safety: I. Sudden death due to coronary heart disease. Am Heart J 68:586, 1964.
274. Christian MS: Incidence and implications of natural deaths of road users. BMJ 297:1021, 1988.
275. Halinen MO, Jaussi A: Fatal road accidents caused by sudden death of the driver in Finland and Vaud, Switzerland. Eur Heart J 15:888, 1994.
276. Epstein AE, Miles WM, Benditt DG, et al: Personal and public safety issues related to arrhythmias that may affect consciousness: Implications for regulation and physician recommendations. A medical/scientific statement from the American Heart Association and the North American Society of Pacing and Electrophysiology. Circulation 94:1147, 1996.

CHAPTER 34

Hypotension and Syncope

Hugh Calkins • Douglas P. Zipes

Definition

Syncope is a sudden transient loss of consciousness and postural tone with spontaneous recovery. Loss of consciousness results from a reduction of blood flow to the reticular activating system located in the brain stem and does not require electrical or chemical therapy for reversal. The metabolism of the brain, in contrast to that of many other organs, is exquisitely dependent on perfusion. Consequently, cessation of cerebral blood flow leads to loss of consciousness within approximately 10 seconds. Restoration of appropriate behavior and orientation after a syncopal episode is usually immediate. Retrograde amnesia is uncommon. Syncope is an important clinical problem because it is common, is costly, is often disabling, may cause injury, and may be the only warning sign before sudden cardiac death.[1] Patients with syncope account for 1 percent of hospital admissions and 3 percent of emergency department visits. Elderly persons have a 6 percent annual incidence of syncope. Surveys of young adults have revealed that up to 50 percent report a prior episode of loss of consciousness; most of these episodes are isolated events that never come to medical attention. The Framingham Study, in which biennial examinations were performed on 7814 individuals, reported the incidence of a first report of syncope to be 6.2 per 1000 person-years follow-up.[2] The annual cost of evaluating and treating patients with syncope has been estimated to be $800 million.[3] Patients who experience syncope also report a markedly reduced quality of life.[4] The prognosis of patients with syncope varies greatly with the diagnosis. In the Framingham Study, for example, participants with syncope, including those with syncope of unknown origin, had increased mortality compared with participants without syncope. The highest mortality was observed among those with a cardiac cause of syncope. In contrast, the subgroup of participants with neurally mediated syncope (including orthostatic hypotension and medication-related syncope) did not experience increased mortality.[2]

Classification

The causes of syncope can be classified into six primary groups: vascular, cardiac, neurologic-cerebrovascular, psychogenic, metabolic-miscellaneous, and syncope of unknown origin (Table 34–1). A similar subclassification of the causes of syncope can be applied to the other diagnostic groups. Table 34–1 shows the types and relative frequencies with which various etiologies of syncope were established in three prospective clinical trials.[5-7] Vascular causes of syncope are most common, followed by cardiac causes of syncope. Psychogenic causes of syncope are now being recognized with increased frequency.[5-9] Some of the causes of syncope shown in Table 34–1 are not causes of "true syncope," which results from sudden transient global cerebral hypoperfusion. These "nonsyncopal" conditions (shown by an asterisk) include conditions in which consciousness is lost as a result of metabolic disorders, epilepsy, or alcohol as well as conditions in which consciousness is only apparently lost (i.e., conversion reaction).

Although knowledge of the common conditions that can cause syncope is essential and allows the clinician to arrive at a probable cause of syncope in the majority of patients, it is equally important for the clinician to be aware of several of the less common but potentially lethal causes of syncope, such as the long QT syndrome, arrhythmogenic right ventricular dysplasia, Brugada syndrome, hypertrophic cardiomyopathy, and pulmonary emboli.[10-12] It is also important to recognize that the distribution of the causes of syncope varies with age. In young individuals, neurally mediated syncope is by far most common, but neurally mediated syncope is an unusual type of syncope in elderly persons. Common causes of syncope in elderly persons include orthostatic hypotension, postprandial hypotension, medication, aortic stenosis, carotid sinus hypersensitivity, and bradyarrhythmias (i.e., sick sinus syndrome, heart block).

Vascular Causes of Syncope

Vascular causes of syncope, particularly reflex-mediated syncope and orthostatic hypotension, are by far the most common causes, accounting for at least one-third of all syncopal episodes.[13] In contrast, subclavian steal syndrome is an exceedingly uncommon cause of syncope, accounting for less than 0.1 percent of syncopal episodes.

ORTHOSTATIC HYPOTENSION. When a person stands, 500 to 800 ml of blood is displaced to the abdomen and lower extremities, resulting in an abrupt drop in venous return to the heart. This drop leads to a decrease in cardiac output and stimulation of aortic, carotid, and cardiopulmonary baroreceptors that trigger a reflex increase in sympathetic outflow. As a result, heart rate, cardiac contractility, and vascular resistance increase to maintain a stable systemic blood pressure on standing. Orthostatic hypotension, which is defined as a 20 mm Hg drop in systolic blood pressure or a 10 mm Hg drop in diastolic blood pressure within 3 minutes of standing, results from a defect in any portion of this blood pressure control system. Orthostatic hypotension can be asymptomatic or

TABLE 34–1 Causes of Syncope

Causes	Relative Frequency (%)		
	Sarasin et al[7] *(n = 611)*	*Ammirati et al*[5] *(n = 195)*	*Alboni et al*[6] *(n = 356)*
Vascular	**62**	**42**	**58**
Anatomic			
Subclavian steal			
Orthostatic	24	6	2
Autonomic insufficiency			
Idiopathic			
Hypovolemia			
Drug-induced			
Reflex mediated			
Carotid sinus hypersensitivity	1	2	14
Neurally mediated syncope	37	30	33
Glossopharyngeal syncope			
Situational (cough, swallow, micturition)		4	7
Adenosine sensitive			2
Cardiac	**10**	**21**	**23**
Anatomic	4	3	3
Aortic stenosis			
Aortic dissection			
Atrial myxoma			
Cardiac tamponade			
Hypertrophic obstructive cardiomyopathy			
Mitral stenosis			
Myocardial ischemia/infarction			
Pulmonary embolus			
Pulmonary hypertension			
Arrhythmias			
Bradyarrhythmias	5	11	15
Sinus node dysfunction/bradycardia			
Atrioventricular block			
Tachycarrhythmias	2	7	5
Supraventricular arrhythmias			
Ventricular arrhythmias (including long QT syndrome)			
Neurologic / Cerebrovascular*	**5**	**14**	**0.70**
Arnold-Chiari malformation			
Migraine			
Seizure (partial complex, temporal lobe)		3	0.20
Vertebral-basilar insufficiency/transient ischemic attack		11	0.50
Metabolic / Miscellaneous	**2**	**1**	**0**
Metabolic*			
Drugs/alcohol			
Hyperventilation (hypocapnea)			
Hypoglycemia			
Hypoxemia			
Miscellaneous			
Cerebral syncope			
Hemorrhage			
Psychogenic syncope*	**1.50**	**6**	**0.20**
Hysterical			
Anxiety/panic disorder			
Somatization disorders			
Syncope of unknown origin	**14**	**18**	**18**

*Disorders resembling syncope.

associated with symptoms such as lightheadedness, dizziness, blurred vision, weakness, palpitations, tremulousness, and syncope. These symptoms are often worse immediately on arising in the morning or after meals or exercise. Syncope that occurs after meals, particularly in elderly people, can result from a redistribution of blood to the gut. A decline in systolic blood pressure of about 20 mm Hg approximately 1 hour after eating has been reported in up to one third of elderly nursing home residents. Although usually asymptomatic, it can result in lightheadedness or syncope.

Drugs that either cause volume depletion or result in vasodilation are the most common cause of orthostatic hypotension (Table 34–2). Elderly patients are particularly susceptible to the hypotensive effects of drugs because of reduced baroreceptor sensitivity, decreased cerebral blood flow, renal sodium wasting, and an impaired thirst mechanism that develops with aging. Orthostatic hypotension can also result from neurogenic causes, which can be subclassified into primary and secondary autonomic failure.[13,14] Primary causes are generally idiopathic, whereas secondary causes are associated with a known biochemical or structural anomaly or are seen as part of a particular disease or syndrome. There are three types of primary autonomic failure. Pure autonomic failure (Bradbury-Eggleston syn-

TABLE 34–2 Causes of Orthostatic Hypotension

Drugs
Diuretics
Alpha-adrenergic blocking drugs
  Terazosin (Hytrin), labetalol
Adrenergic neuron blocking drugs
  Guanethidine
Angiotensin-converting enzyme inhibitors
Antidepressants
  Monoamine oxidase inhibitors
Alcohol
Diuretics
Ganglion-blocking drugs
  Hexamethonium, mecamylamine
Tranquilizers
  Phenothiazines, barbiturates
Vasodilators
  Prazosin, hydralazine, calcium channel blockers
Centrally acting hypotensive drugs
  Methyldopa, clonidine

Primary Disorders of Autonomic Failures
Pure autonomic failure (Bradbury-Eggleston syndrome)
Multiple system atrophy (Shy-Drager syndrome)
Parkinson disease with autonomic failure

Secondary Neurogenic
Aging
Autoimmune disease
  Guillain-Barré syndrome, mixed connective tissue disease, rheumatoid arthritis
  Eaton-Lambert syndrome, systemic lupus erythematosus
Carcinomatosis autonomic neuropathy
Central brain lesions
  Multiple sclerosis, Wernicke encephalopathy
  Vascular lesions or tumors involving the hypothalamus and midbrain
Dopamine beta-hydroxylase deficiency
Familial hyperbradykinism
General medical disorders
  Diabetes, amyloid, alcoholism, renal failure
Hereditary sensory neuropathies, dominant or recessive
Infections of the nervous system
  Human immunodeficiency virus infection, Chagas disease, botulism, syphilis
Metabolic disease
  Vitamin B_{12} deficiency, porphyria, Fabry disease. Tangier disease
Spinal cord lesions

Adapted from Bannister SR (ed): Autonomic Failure, 2nd ed. Oxford, Oxford University Press, 1988, p 8.

drome) is an idiopathic sporadic disorder characterized by orthostatic hypotension, usually in conjunction with evidence of more widespread autonomic failure such as disturbances in bowel, bladder, thermoregulatory, and sexual function. Patients with pure autonomic failure have reduced supine plasma norepinephrine levels. Multiple system atrophy (Shy-Drager syndrome) is a sporadic, progressive, adult-onset disorder characterized by autonomic dysfunction, parkinsonism, and ataxia in any combination. The third type of primary autonomic failure is Parkinson disease with autonomic failure. A small subset of patients with Parkinson disease may also experience autonomic failure, including orthostatic hypotension. In addition to these forms of chronic autonomic failure is a rare acute panautonomic neuropathy. This neuropathy generally occurs in young people and results in widespread severe sympathetic and parasympathetic failure with orthostatic hypotension, loss of sweating, disruption of bladder and bowel function, fixed heart rate, and fixed dilated pupils.

Postural orthostatic tachycardia syndrome (POTS) is a milder form of chronic autonomic failure and orthostatic intolerance characterized by the presence of symptoms of orthostatic intolerance, an increase of 28 beats/min or more in heart rate, and absence of a significant change in blood pressure within 5 minutes of standing or upright tilt.[13] POTS appears to result from a failure of the peripheral vasculature to vasoconstrict appropriately under orthostatic stress. POTS can also be associated with syncope related to neurally mediated hypotension (see later).

REFLEX-MEDIATED SYNCOPE. There are many reflex-mediated syncopal syndromes (see Table 34–1). In each case, the reflex is composed of a trigger (the afferent limb) and a response (the efferent limb). This group of reflex-mediated syncopal syndromes has in common the response limb of the reflex, which consists of increased vagal tone and a withdrawal of peripheral sympathetic tone and leads to bradycardia, vasodilation, and, ultimately, hypotension, presyncope, or syncope. What distinguishes these causes of syncope are the specific triggers. For example, micturition syncope results from activation of mechanoreceptors in the bladder; defecation syncope results from neural inputs from gut wall tension receptors; and swallowing syncope results from afferent neural impulses arising from the upper gastrointestinal tract. The two most common types of reflex-mediated syncope, carotid sinus hypersensitivity and neurally mediated hypotension, are discussed later.

Neurally Mediated Hypotension or Syncope. The term *neurally mediated hypotension* or *syncope* (also known as neurocardiogenic, vasodepressor, and vasovagal syncope and as "fainting") has been used to describe a common abnormality of blood pressure regulation characterized by the abrupt onset of hypotension with or without bradycardia. Triggers associated with the development of neurally mediated syncope are those that either reduce ventricular filling or increase catecholamine secretion.[13-15] They include the sight of blood, pain, prolonged standing, a warm environment or hot shower, and stressful situations. In these types of situations, patients with this condition experience severe lightheadedness or syncope, or both. It has been proposed that these clinical phenomena result from a paradoxical reflex that is initiated when ventricular preload is reduced by venous pooling. This reduction leads to a reduction in cardiac output and blood pressure, which is sensed by arterial baroreceptors. The resultant increased catecholamine levels, combined with reduced venous filling, lead to a vigorously contracting volume-depleted ventricle. The heart itself is involved in this reflex by virtue of the presence of mechanoreceptors, or C-fibers, consisting of nonmyelinated fibers found in the atria, ventricles, and pulmonary artery. It has been proposed that vigorous contraction of a volume-depleted ventricle leads to activation of these receptors in susceptible individuals. These afferent C-fibers project centrally to the dorsal vagal nucleus of the medulla, leading to a "paradoxical" withdrawal of peripheral sympathetic tone and an increase in vagal tone, which, in turn, causes vasodilation and bradycardia. The ultimate clinical consequence is syncope or presyncope. Not all neurally mediated syncope results from activation of mechanoreceptors. In humans, it is well known that the sight of blood or extreme emotion can trigger syncope. These observations suggest that higher neural centers can also participate in the pathophysiology of vasovagal syncope. In addition, central mechanisms can contribute to the production of neurally mediated syncope.

Carotid Sinus Hypersensitivity. Syncope caused by *carotid sinus hypersensitivity* results from stimulation of carotid sinus baroreceptors, which are located in the internal carotid artery above the bifurcation of the common carotid artery. Carotid sinus hypersensitivity is diagnosed by applying gentle pressure over the carotid pulsation just below the angle of the jaw, where the carotid bifurcation is located. Pressure should be applied for 5 to 10 seconds. Studies have highlighted the importance of performing carotid sinus massage in both the supine and upright positions.[16,17] The main complications associated with performing carotid sinus massage are neurological. One study reported that persistent neurological complications are uncommon, occurring in 1 per 1000 patients.[18] Because of this complication, carotid sinus massage should be avoided in patients with prior transient ischemic attacks, strokes within the past 3 months, and carotid bruits.

A normal response to carotid sinus massage is a transient decrease in the sinus rate or slowing of atrioventricular (AV) conduction, or both. Carotid sinus hypersensitivity is defined as a sinus pause of more than 3 seconds duration and a fall in systolic blood pressure of 50 mm Hg or more. The response to carotid sinus massage can be classified as cardioinhibitory (asystole), vasodepressive (fall in systolic blood pressure), or mixed. Carotid sinus hypersensitivity is detected in approximately one third of elderly patients with syncope. Carotid sinus hypersensitivity is also commonly detected in elderly patients presenting after falls, with one study reporting the presence of carotid sinus hypersensitivity in approximately one fourth of patients presenting to an emergency room after falls.[19] It is important to recognize, however, that carotid sinus hypersensitivity is also commonly observed in asymptomatic elderly patients. Thus, the diagnosis of carotid sinus hypersensitivity should be approached cautiously after excluding alternative causes of syncope. Carotid sinus hypersensitivity is suggested in patients older than 40 years with syncope of unexplained cause following the initial history, physical examination, and electrocardiogram (ECG).[1] Once it is diagnosed, dual-chamber pacemaker implantation is recommended for patients with recurrent syncope resulting from carotid sinus hypersensitivity.[20]

Cardiac Causes of Syncope

Cardiac causes of syncope, particularly tachyarrhythmias and bradyarrhythmias (see Chap. 32), are the second most common causes, accounting for 10 to 20 percent of syncopal episodes. Ventricular tachycardia (VT) is the most common tachyarrhythmia that can cause syncope. Supraventricular tachycardia can also cause syncope, although the great majority of patients with supraventricular arrhythmias present with less severe symptoms such as palpitations, dyspnea, and lightheadedness. Bradyarrhythmias that can result in syncope include sick sinus syndrome as well as AV block. Anatomical causes of syncope include obstruction to blood flow, such as a massive pulmonary embolus, an atrial myxoma, or aortic stenosis.

Neurological Causes of Syncope

Neurological causes of syncope, including migraines, seizures, Arnold-Chiari malformations, and transient ischemic attacks, are surprisingly uncommon, accounting for less than 10 percent of all cases of syncope. The majority of patients in whom a "neurological" cause of syncope is established are found in fact to have had a seizure rather than true syncope.

Metabolic-Miscellaneous Causes of Syncope

Metabolic causes of syncope are rare, accounting for less than 5 percent of syncopal episodes. The most common metabolic causes of syncope are hypoglycemia, hypoxia, and hyperventilation. Establishing hypoglycemia as the cause of syncope requires demonstration of hypoglycemia during the syncopal episode. Although hyperventilation-induced syncope has been generally considered to be due to a reduction in cerebral blood flow, one study demonstrated that hyperventilation alone was not sufficient to cause syncope. This observation suggests that hyperventilation-induced syncope may also have a psychological component. Psychiatric disorders may also cause syncope. It has been reported that up to 25 percent of patients with syncope of unknown origin may have psychiatric disorders for which syncope is one of the presenting symptoms.[8,9] Cerebral syncope is a rare type of syncope resulting from cerebral vasoconstriction induced by orthostatic stress.[21]

RELATIONSHIP BETWEEN PROGNOSES AND THE CAUSE OF SYNCOPE. The prognosis for patients with syncope varies greatly with the diagnosis. Syncope of unknown origin or syncope with a noncardiac etiology (including reflex-mediated syncope) is generally associated with a benign prognosis. In contrast, syncope with a cardiac cause is associated with up to 30 percent mortality at 1 year.[1]

Diagnostic Tests

Identification of the precise cause of syncope is often challenging. Because syncope usually occurs sporadically and infrequently, it is extremely difficult to either examine a patient or obtain an ECG during an episode of syncope. For this reason, the primary goal in the evaluation of a patient with syncope is to arrive at a presumptive determination of the cause of syncope.

History and Physical Examination

The history and physical examination are by far the most important components of the evaluation of a patient with syncope (see Chap. 7). Several studies have reported that the probable cause of syncope can be identified on the basis of the history and physical examination alone in more than 25 percent of patients.[5-7] Maximal information can be obtained from the clinical history when it is approached in a systematic and detailed fashion. Initial evaluation should begin by determining whether the patient did, in fact, experience a syncopal episode. Every effort should be made to differentiate true syncope from alterations in consciousness resulting from nonsyncopal conditions such as metabolic and psychiatric disorders. Although falls can be differentiated from syncope by the absence of loss of consciousness, an overlap between symptoms of falls and syncope has been reported.[16,22] This overlap may reflect the fact that elderly individuals may experience amnesia for the episode of loss of consciousness. When evaluating a patient with syncope, particular attention should then be focused on (1) determining whether the patient has a history of cardiac disease or a family history of cardiac disease, syncope, or sudden death; (2) identifying medications that may have played a role in syncope; (3) quantifying the number and chronicity of prior syncopal and presyncopal episodes; (4) identifying precipitating factors including body position; and (5) quantifying the type and duration of prodromal and recovery symptoms. It is also useful to obtain careful accounts from witnesses who may have been present. The features of the clinical history most helpful in determining whether syncope resulted from neurally mediated hypotension, an arrhythmia, or a seizure are summarized in Table 34–3.

The clinical histories obtained from patients with syncope related to AV block and VT are similar. In each case, syncope

TABLE 34–3 Differentiating Syncope Caused by Neurally Mediated Hypotension, Arrhythmias, and Seizures

	Neurally Mediated Hypotension	Arrhythmias	Seizure
Demographics/clinical setting	Female > male gender Younger age (<55 yr) More episodes (>2) Standing, warm room, emotional upset	Male > female gender Older age (>54 yr) Fewer episodes (<3) Any setting	Younger age (<45 yr) Any setting
Premonitory symptoms	Longer duration (>5 sec) Palpitations Blurred vision Nausea Warmth Diaphoresis Lightheadedness	Shorter duration (<6 sec) Palpitations less common	Sudden onset or brief aura (déjà vu, olfactory, gustatory, visual)
Observations during the event	Pallor Diaphoretic Dilated pupils Slow pulse, low blood pressure Incontinence may occur. Brief clonic movements may occur.	Blue, not pale Incontinence can occur. Brief clonic movements can occur.	Blue face, no pallor Frothing at the mouth Prolonged syncope (duration >5 minutes) Tongue biting Horizontal eye deviation Elevated pulse and blood pressure Incontinence more likely* Tonic clonic movements if grand mal
Residual symptoms	Residual symptoms common Prolonged fatigue common (>90%) Oriented	Residual symptoms uncommon (unless prolonged unconsciousness) Oriented	Residual symptoms common Aching muscles Disoriented Fatigue Headache Slow recovery

*May be observed with any of these causes of syncope but more common with seizures.

typically occurs with less than 5 seconds of warning and few if any prodromal and recovery symptoms. Demographic features suggesting that syncope results from an arrhythmia such as VT or AV block include male gender, less than three prior episodes of syncope, and increased age. Features of the clinical history that point toward a vasovagal cause of syncope include palpitations, blurred vision, nausea, warmth, diaphoresis, or lightheadedness before syncope and the presence of nausea, warmth, diaphoresis, or fatigue after syncope.

The historical features of syncope were evaluated in 341 consecutive patients who were interviewed with a standard questionnaire.[6] A vascular cause of syncope was identified in 58 percent, a cardiac cause in 23 percent, a neurological or psychiatric cause in 1 percent, and syncope of unknown origin was diagnosed in 18 percent. This study initially evaluated the predictive ability of variables that are not part of the presentation of syncope: age, gender, and the presence of suspected cardiac disease (based on the initial evaluation that comprised the clinical history and ECG). Multivariate analysis revealed that the presence of suspected cardiac disease was the only independent predictor of a cardiac cause of syncope (odds ratio 16). The historical variables of syncope were then examined separately among the 191 patients with suspected cardiac disease and the 146 patients without suspected cardiac disease . The absence of suspected cardiac disease on the basis of the initial evaluation allowed a cardiac cause of syncope to be excluded in 142 of the 146 patients without suspected cardiac disease (97 percent). Among patients with suspected cardiac disease, variables that were predictive of a cardiac cause of syncope on multivariate analysis included duration of symptoms less than 4 years, history of presyncope, and blurred vision prior to syncope. Variables predictive of vascular syncope included duration of symptoms greater than 4 years, history of presyncope, and nausea. Among patients without suspected cardiac disease, the only variable predictive of a cardiac cause of syncope was palpitations before loss of consciousness. The only variable predictive of vascular syncope among patients without suspected cardiac disease was a duration of prodromal symptoms greater than 10 seconds. The authors concluded that the absence of suspected cardiac disease on initial evaluation together with the absence of palpitations prior to syncope allows exclusion of a cardiac cause of syncope. Although the presence of suspected cardiac disease is a strong predictor of a cardiac cause of syncope, its specificity is low.

The clinical history is also valuable in distinguishing seizures from syncope. Features of the clinical history that are useful in distinguishing seizures from syncope include orientation following an event, a blue face or not becoming pale during the event, frothing at the mouth, aching muscles, feeling sleepy after the event, and a duration of unconsciousness of more than 5 minutes. Tongue biting strongly points toward a seizure rather than syncope as the cause of loss of consciousness. Other findings suggestive of a seizure as a cause of the syncopal episode include (1) an aura before the episode, (2) horizontal eye deviation during the episode, (3) an elevated blood pressure and pulse during the episode, and (4) a headache following the event. Urinary or fecal incontinence can be observed in association with either a seizure or a syncopal episode but occurs more commonly in association with a seizure. Grand mal seizures are usually associated with tonic-clonic movements. It is important to note that syncope caused by cerebral ischemia can result in decorticate rigidity with clonic movements of the arms. Akinetic or petit mal seizures can be recognized by the patient's lack of responsiveness in the absence of a loss of postural tone. Temporal lobe seizures can also be confused with syncope. These seizures last several minutes and are characterized by confusion, changes in the level of consciousness, and autonomic signs such as flushing. Vertebral basilar insufficiency should be considered as the cause of syncope if syncope occurs in association with other symptoms of brain stem ischemia (i.e., diplopia, tinnitus, focal weakness or sensory loss, vertigo, or dysarthria). Migraine-mediated syncope is often associated with a throbbing unilateral headache, scintillating scotomata, and nausea.

In one study, a standardized questionnaire was administered to 102 patients with seizure and 569 patients with syncope.[23] The clinical symptoms reported by patients with syncope were compared with those reported by patients with seizure. Patients with seizure were more likely to have had a cut tongue, bedwetting, prodromal déjà vu, preoccupation, mood changes, hallucinations or trembling before loss of consciousness, postictal confusion, muscle pain, headaches, observed convulsive movements, head turning, unresponsiveness during loss of consciousness, and blue skin observed by a bystander. Patients with syncope were more likely to experience presyncope, have syncope associated with prolonged sitting or standing, or have presyncope with prolonged sitting or standing, warm environments, and exercise. Patients with syncope were also more likely to experience diaphoresis, dyspnea, chest pain, palpitations, warmth, nausea, and vertigo. The authors then developed a simple point score of diagnostic criteria that distinguishes seizures from syncope with 85 percent accuracy.

PHYSICAL EXAMINATION. After obtaining a careful history, evaluation should continue with a physical examination. In addition to a complete cardiac examination, particular attention should be focused on determining whether structural heart disease is present, defining the patient's level of hydration, and detecting the presence of significant neurological abnormalities suggestive of a dysautonomia or a cerebrovascular accident. Orthostatic vital signs are a critical component of the evaluation. The patient's blood pressure and heart rate should be obtained while he or she is supine and should then be obtained each minute for approximately 3 minutes. The three abnormalities that should be searched for are (1) early orthostatic hypotension, defined as a 20 mm Hg drop in systolic blood pressure or a 10 mm Hg drop in diastolic blood pressure within 3 minutes of standing; (2) POTS, which is defined as an increase of 28 beats/min or more within 5 minutes of standing with symptoms of orthostatic intolerance. The significance of POTS lies in its close overlap with neurally mediated syncope.[13]

Laboratory Tests

BLOOD TESTS. The routine use of blood tests, such as serum electrolytes, cardiac enzymes, glucose, and hematocrit levels, is of low diagnostic value.[24-26] As a result, the routine use of laboratory tests is not recommended for patients with syncope. Under rare circumstances, aspects of the patient's clinical presentation may suggest the diagnostic value of this type of testing.

CAROTID SINUS MASSAGE. Carotid sinus hypersensitivity is diagnosed by carotid massage, as outlined earlier.

TILT-TABLE TESTING. The tilt-table test (see Chap. 29) is a standard and widely accepted diagnostic test for evaluating patients with syncope.[1,27] To the extent that upright tilt testing provides diagnostic evidence indicating susceptibility to neurally mediated syncope, it is considered the "gold standard" for establishing this diagnosis. The American College of Cardiology published an expert consensus document that contains specific recommendations for performing and interpreting the results of this test.[27] Upright tilt testing is generally performed for 30 to 45 minutes at an angle between 60 and 80 degrees (with 70 degrees the most common). The sensitivity of the test can be increased, with an associated fall in specificity, by the use of longer tilt durations, steeper tilt angles, and provocative agents such as isoproterenol or nitroglycerin.[28-30] When isoproterenol is employed as a provocative agent, it is recommended that the infusion rate be increased incrementally from 1 to 3 μg/min in order to increase the heart rate to 25 percent greater than baseline. When nitroglycerin is employed, a fixed does of 400 μg nitroglycerine spray should be administered sublingually with the patient in the upright position. These two provocative approaches are equivalent in diagnostic accuracy. In the absence of pharmacological provocation, the specificity of the test has been estimated to be 90 percent.

There is general agreement that upright tilt testing is indicated in patients with recurrent syncope, in high-risk patients with a single syncopal episode for whom there is no evidence of structural heart disease or other causes of syncope have been excluded, and in the evaluation of patients for whom the cause of syncope has been determined (i.e., asystole) but the presence of neurally mediated syncope on upright tilt would influence treatment.[27] There is also general agreement that upright tilt-table testing is not necessary for patients who have experienced only a single syncopal episode that was highly typical for neurally mediated syncope and during which no injury occurred. Tilt-table testing is not useful in establishing a diagnosis of situation syncope (i.e., postmicturition syncope).[31]

ECHOCARDIOGRAPHY. Although echocardiograms are commonly used in the evaluation of patients with syncope, little objective evidence exists to support their use in patients with a normal physical examination and a normal ECG. The rationale for obtaining an echocardiogram in patients with syncope is to stratify the patient's risk by excluding the possibility of occult cardiac disease not apparent after the history, physical examination, and electrocardiography. The only situations in which an echocardiogram would be considered diagnostic of the cause of syncope are severe left ventricular outflow obstruction (see Chaps. 57 and 59) and atrial myxoma (see Chap. 11). Current guidelines recommend that an echocardiogram should not be obtained routinely for all patients with syncope but should be obtained when cardiac disease is suspected.[1]

STRESS TESTS, CARDIAC CATHETERIZATIONS. Myocardial ischemia is an unlikely cause of syncope and, when present, is usually accompanied by angina (see Chap. 49). Exercise stress testing and cardiac catheterization are unlikely to establish a diagnosis in patients presenting with syncope unless the clinical suspicion of ischemia is high.[32] The use of stress tests in the evaluation of patients with syncope is best reserved for those in whom syncope or presyncope occurred during or immediately after exertion or in association with chest pain. It should be noted that even among patients with syncope during exertion, exercise stress testing is highly unlikely to trigger another event. Patients suspected of having severe aortic stenosis or obstructive hypertrophic cardiomyopathy should not undergo exercise stress testing because it may precipitate a cardiac arrest. Current guidelines suggest that exercise stress testing be performed in patients who experience syncope during or shortly after exercise.[1] Exercise stress testing is not recommended for patients with non-exercise-related syncope.[32] Coronary angiography is recommended in patients with syncope suspected to be due, directly or indirectly, to myocardial ischemia.

ELECTROCARDIOGRAPHY. The 12-lead ECG is another important component in the work-up of a patient with syncope. The initial ECG results in establishment of a diagnosis in approximately 5 percent of patients and suggests a diagnosis in another 5 percent of patients.[24] Specific findings that can identify the probable cause of syncope include QT prolongation (long QT syndrome), the presence of a short PR interval and a delta wave (Wolff-Parkinson-White syndrome), the presence of a right bundle branch block pattern with ST segment elevation (Brugada syndrome), evidence of an acute myocardial infarction, high-grade AV block, or T wave inversion in the right precordial leads (arrhythmogenic right ventricular dysplasia) (see Chap. 32). Any abnormality of the baseline ECG is an independent predictor of cardiac syncope or increased mortality and suggests the need to pursue an evaluation of cardiac causes of syncope.[1] Most patients with syncope have a normal ECG. This finding is useful as it suggests a low likelihood of a cardiac cause of syncope and is associated with an excellent prognosis, particularly when observed in a young patient with syncope. Despite the low diagnostic yield of electrocardiography, the test is inexpensive and risk free. For these reasons, an ECG is considered a standard part of the evaluation of virtually all patients with syncope.[1,24]

SIGNAL-AVERAGED ELECTROCARDIOGRAPHY. Signal-averaged electrocardiography (SAECG) is a noninvasive technique used for the detection of low-amplitude signals in the terminal portion of the QRS complex (late potentials), which are a substrate for ventricular arrhythmias (see Chap. 29). In contrast to a standard ECG, the role of SAECG in the evaluation of patients with syncope is not well established. Studies in selected populations of patients have reported that SAECG has a sensitivity of 73 to 89 percent and a specificity of 89 to 100 percent for the prediction of inducible VT in patients with syncope.[24] Despite these encouraging results, no studies have evaluated the role of SAECG in unselected populations of patients. Furthermore, it is unknown whether SAECG can replace an electrophysiology (EP) study in the evaluation of patients with syncope in the setting of significant structural heart disease. These facts, combined with the inability of SAECG to provide the additional information routinely obtained during EP testing regarding sinus node function, AV conduction, and the presence of inducible supraventricular arrhythmias, limit the role of SAECG as a diagnostic tool in syncope. Another limitation of this technique is that criteria for the use of SAECG as a diagnostic tool in patients with a bundle branch block or nonspecific intraventricular conduction delay have not been developed. At present, SAECG testing is not recommended as a standard part of the evaluation of patients with syncope.[1,24] Perhaps one of the best uses of SAECG testing at present is to evaluate patients with possible arrhythmogenic right ventricular dysplasia.[10,33]

HOLTER RECORDING. Continuous ECG monitoring using telemetry or Holter monitoring, or both, is commonly performed in patients with syncope but is unlikely to identify the cause of syncope (see Chap. 29). The information provided by ECG monitoring at the time of syncope is extremely valuable because it allows an arrhythmic cause of syncope to be established or excluded. However, because of the infrequent and sporadic nature of syncope, the diagnostic yield of Holter monitoring in the evaluation of patients with syncope and presyncope is approximately 4 percent.[24] Another clinically useful finding is the detection of symptoms in the absence of an arrhythmia. This finding is observed in up to 15 percent of patients undergoing continuous ECG monitoring.[24] It is important to emphasize that the absence of an arrhythmia and symptoms during continuous ECG monitoring may not exclude an arrhythmia as the cause of syncope. In patients suspected of having an arrhythmia as the cause of syncope, additional evaluation such as EP testing or event monitoring should be considered. Holter or inpatient telemetric monitoring is indicated in patients with syncope suspected to result from an arrhythmia on the basis of features of the clinical history, an abnormal ECG, or the presence of structural heart disease.[1,24] Holter monitoring is most likely to be diagnostic when it is used in the occasional patient with frequent (i.e., daily) episodes of syncope or presyncope.

EVENT RECORDERS. Transtelephonic event monitors are small, portable ECG recording devices that are carried or worn continuously by the patient and can be activated by the patient to record a rhythm strip (see Chap. 29). The tracings can be stored and transmitted over telephone lines at a later time. Some event monitors, referred to as continuous-loop event monitors, are worn continuously and allow capture of both retrospective and prospective ECG recordings, whereas other types of event monitors record only when they are activated by the patient. Continuous-loop event monitors are preferred when used in the evaluation of a patient with syncope. These devices are often programmed with 4 minutes of retrospective memory and 1 minute of prospective memory on activation. Event monitors are indicated in the evaluation of patients with infrequent but recurrent episodes of presyncope or syncope, particularly when potentially malignant causes of syncope have been excluded.[1,24,34,35] When they are used in selected populations of patients, a diagnostic yield as high has 25 percent may be observed. However, a much lower diagnostic yield can be expected in less selected populations. One study, for example, reported that among 172 patients with syncope, no patient experienced frank syncope during the monitoring period.[35] A significant arrhythmia was detected in 6 percent of patients in association with less severe symptoms.

IMPLANTABLE EVENT RECORDERS. In some patients, episodes of syncope are extremely infrequent, occurring once or twice a year. In this population of patients, a traditional event monitor is unlikely to be diagnostic because of the prolonged length of recording that would be needed to record an event successfully. To address this problem, an implantable event monitor has been developed (Medtronic Reveal, Minneapolis, MN) (see Chap. 29). This lightweight and small device (61 × 19 × 8 mm), with a projected longevity of 18 to 24 months, incorporates two electrodes within its can and is implanted in the subcutaneous tissue of the chest. If necessary, the incision can be extended later to allow insertion of a pacemaker or implantable cardioverter-defibrillator. The ECG signal is stored in a circular buffer capable of recording up to 42 minutes of rhythm. The device can be configured to trigger automatically on the basis of programmed detection criteria as well as with a handheld activator.

In one series, a symptom-ECG correlation was reported in 50 of 85 patients (59 percent) during 10 ± 4 months of follow-up.[36] An arrhythmia was detected in 21 of the patients and sinus rhythm was detected in 29. Complications included two infections, one erosion, and one painful pocket requiring device reinsertion. The authors of the study subsequently performed a randomized trial to evaluate the diagnostic utility of the Reveal device compared with conventional testing.[37] Sixty patients with unexplained syncope after an initial evaluation consisting of a history, physical examination, and echocardiogram were enrolled. Patients with an ejection fraction less than 35 percent were excluded. Patients were randomly assigned to initial implantation of the Reveal monitor versus a standard evaluation consisting of an external event monitor, a tilt test, and an EP study. A diagnosis was established in 14 of 27 patients assigned to prolonged monitoring compared with 6 of 30 patients undergoing conventional testing. Although this implantable monitor provides a new tool for use in evaluating patients with syncope, a limitation of this diagnostic strategy is that it is expensive and requires that the patient experience another episode of syncope to establish a diagnosis. Current guidelines suggest that implantable event monitors be used in selected patients with recurrent and infrequent episodes of syncope when it is thought that there is a high probability of an arrhythmic cause of syncope.[1]

ELECTROPHYSIOLOGY TESTING. EP testing can provide important diagnostic and prognostic information in patients presenting with syncope (see Chaps. 29 and 30). The results of EP testing can be useful in establishing a diagnosis of sick sinus syndrome, carotid sinus hypersensitivity, heart block, supraventricular tachycardia, or VT. The indications for EP testing in the evaluation of patients with syncope have been established on the basis of an American College of Cardiology/American Heart Association Task Force Report.[20] There is general agreement that EP testing should be performed in patients with suspected structural heart disease and unexplained syncope (class 1 indication) and that EP testing should not be performed in patients with a known cause of syncope for whom treatment would not be influenced by the findings of the test (class 3 indication). The role of EP testing in evaluating patients with recurrent unexplained syncope who do not have structural heart disease and have had a negative tilt-table test remains controversial.

Sinus node function is evaluated during EP testing primarily by determining the sinus node recovery time (SNRT). The SNRT is determined by pacing the right atrium at cycle lengths between 600 and 350 milliseconds for 30 to 60 seconds. The SNRT is defined as the interval between the last paced atrial depolarization and the first spontaneous atrial depolarization resulting from activation of the sinus node. The SNRT is corrected for the underlying sinus cycle length (SCL) and expressed as the corrected SNRT (CSNRT = SNRT − SCL). A corrected SNRT greater than 525 milliseconds is generally considered abnormal. A secondary pause is defined as an inappropriately long pause among the beats that follow the first sinus recovery beat after atrial overdrive pacing. Evaluation of secondary pauses increases the sensitivity of the SNRT in the detection of sinus node dysfunction. Other, less widely used assays for evaluating sinus node function include the sinoatrial conduction time and the sinus node refractory period. Although the sinoatrial conduction time is a sensitive indicator of sinus node dysfunction, it lacks a high degree of specificity and has been of limited value in evaluating the need for a permanent pacemaker. Determination of sinus node refractoriness is another technique that has been reported to be useful in identifying patients with sinus node dysfunction. However, the usefulness of this parameter in selecting patients with syncope for pacemaker implantation has not been determined. Identification of sinus node dysfunction as the cause of syncope is uncommon during EP tests (<5 percent). It is also important to note that the absence of evidence of sinus node dysfunction during EP testing does not exclude a bradyarrhythmia as the cause of syncope.

During EP testing, AV conduction is assessed by measuring the AV nodal to His bundle conduction time (A-H interval) and the His bundle to ventricular conduction time (H-V interval) and also by determining the response of AV conduction to incremental atrial pacing and atrial premature stimuli. The findings obtained during EP testing that allow AV block to be established as the probable cause of syncope include an H-V interval of 100 milliseconds or more or infra-His block. Among studies that have reported the results of EP testing in evaluating patients with syncope, AV block was identified as the probable cause of syncope in approximately 10 to 15 percent of patients. Donateo and colleagues reported the results of a systematic evaluation of patients with syncope in the setting of a bundle branch block on their baseline ECG.[38] Of 347 patients referred for evaluation of syncope, 55 had a baseline bundle branch block pattern. Systematic evaluation of these patients, including EP testing, resulted in a diagnosis of cardiac syncope in 25 patients (45 percent): AV block in 20, sick sinus syndrome in 2, VT in 1, and aortic stenosis in 2. Neurally mediated syncope was diagnosed in 22 patients (40 percent) and syncope remained unexplained in 8 (15 percent).

It is uncommon for a supraventricular tachycardia to cause syncope unless the patient has underlying heart disease, the rate is extremely rapid, or the patient has a propensity for the development of neurally mediated syncope. The typical pattern that is observed is the development of syncope or near syncope at the onset of the supraventricular arrhythmia because of an initial drop in blood pressure. The patient often regains consciousness despite the continuation of the arrhythmia owing to the activation of a compensatory mechanism. Completion of a standard EP test allows accurate identification of most types of supraventricular arrhythmias that may have caused syncope. The study should be repeated during an isoproterenol infusion to increase the sensitivity of the study, particularly for detecting idiopathic VT or AV nodal reentrant tachycardia (see Chap. 32). A supraventricular arrhythmia is diagnosed as the probable cause of syncope in less than 5 percent of patients who undergo EP testing for evaluation of syncope of unknown origin.

VT is the most common abnormality that is uncovered during EP testing in patients with syncope. Among studies that have reported the results of EP testing in evaluating patients with syncope, VT was identified as the probable cause of syncope in approximately 20 percent of patients. An approximately 50 percent incidence of appropriate implantable defibrillator discharges has been reported in both patients with syncope who have inducible VT on EP testing and patients who present with a sustained ventricular arrhythmia and undergo cardiac defibrillator implantation.[39] In the past, an EP test was interpreted as positive for VT when sustained monomorphic VT was induced. The induction of polymorphic VT and ventricular fibrillation were considered to represent nonspecific responses to EP testing. More recent data suggest that the induction of polymorphic VT and ventricular fibrillation should also be considered abnormal findings during EP testing performed in a patient with syncope.[40,41] An analysis of data obtained as part of the Antiarrhythmics Versus Implantable Defibrillators (AVID) registry and an AVID syncope substudy showed no difference in the incidence of arrhythmic events among patients with syncope with inducible VT (<200 beats/min), inducible rapid VT (>200 beats/min), and inducible polymorphic VT or ventricular fibrillation.[40] In contrast, ejection fraction was highly predictive of arrhythmic events. At 1 year of follow-up, 15 percent of patients with an ejection fraction greater than 30 percent had an arrhythmic event compared with 38 percent of patients with syncope with an ejection fraction less than 30 percent.

Approximately 30 percent of patients with syncope referred for EP testing to evaluate syncope of unknown origin have a presumptive diagnosis established. Clinical factors identified as predictors of a positive response to EP testing include impaired ventricular function, male sex, prior myocardial infarction, bundle branch block, injury, and nonsustained VT.

Approximately 70 percent of patients referred for evaluation of syncope demonstrate a normal response to EP testing. A negative EP test has generally been considered predictive of a low risk of sudden death. However, studies have suggested that EP testing may have less predictive value in patients with markedly impaired ventricular function. One study reported that 7 of 14 patients with an idiopathic dilated cardiomyopathy who presented with syncope, had a negative EP test, and underwent placement of an implantable defibrillator received appropriate shocks for ventricular arrhythmias during 24 months of follow-up.[42] A similar study involving 46 patients with a nonischemic cardiomyopathy and a negative EP test reported that 33 percent of these patients received appropriate defibrillator therapy during follow-up.[43] Fonarow and colleagues reported the outcome of 147 patients referred for cardiac transplantation who had a nonischemic cardiomyopathy and syncope.[44] Management of patients, including whether to use an implantable defibrillator, was determined by their cardiologist. EP testing was not performed. The outcomes of the 25 patients who received an implantable defibrillator were compared with those of the 122 patients managed with conventional therapy alone. During a mean follow-up of 22 months, there were 31 deaths,

18 sudden, in patients treated with conventional therapy, whereas there were 2 deaths, neither sudden, in patients treated with an implantable defibrillator. An appropriate shock was received by 40 percent of defibrillator patients. The findings of these studies suggest that more sensitive diagnostic tests to evaluate patients' risk for sudden death or greater use of implantable cardioverter-defibrillators, or both, may be needed in this group of patients.

TEST TO SCREEN FOR NEUROLOGICAL CAUSES OF SYNCOPE. Syncope as an isolated symptom rarely has a neurological cause. Neurological causes of syncope are established in less than 5 percent of patients with syncope.[5-7] As a result, widespread use of tests to screen for neurological conditions is rarely diagnostic. In many institutions, computed tomography (CT) scans (see Chap. 15), electroencephalograms (EEGs), and carotid duplex scans are overused, being obtained for more than 50 percent of patients with syncope. A diagnosis is almost never uncovered that was not first suspected on the basis of a careful history and neurological examination. Transient ischemic attacks that result from carotid disease are not accompanied by loss of consciousness. No studies have suggested that carotid Doppler ultrasonography is beneficial in patients with syncope. Current guidelines for the evaluation of syncope suggest that EEGs be obtained only when there is a relatively high likelihood of epilepsy.[1] CT and magnetic resonance imaging should be avoided in patients with uncomplicated syncope.

Approach to the Evaluation of Patients with Syncope

Figure 34–1 outlines the approach to the diagnostic evaluation of a patient presenting with syncope proposed by the European Society of Cardiology Task Force on Syncope.[1] The initial evaluation begins with a careful history, physical examination, and 12-lead ECG. Various clinical features can help suggest a specific cause of the syncope (Table 34–4). On the basis of this initial evaluation performed in either an emergency department or outpatient setting, the probable cause of syncope can be identified in approximately 25 percent of patients. Common causes or types of syncope that can be identified at this initial stage include orthostatic hypotension, situational syncope, and neurally mediated syncope. This initial evaluation should also allow identification of patients who probably had a seizure rather than syncope. In another large group of patients the probable cause of syncope can be suspected and later confirmed with directed diagnostic testing. Causes or types of syncope that fall into this category include left ventricular outflow tract obstruction, neurally mediated syncope with a suggestive but not diagnostic clinical presentation, arrhythmias related to the long QT syndrome, Wolff-Parkinson-White syndrome, the Brugada syndrome, or arrhythmogenic right ventricular dysplasia as well as neurological causes of syncope. Among the remaining patients, the next step in the evaluation depends on the presence of structural heart disease as well as the physician's clinical suspicion that an arrhythmia may have been the cause of syncope. An echocardiogram is often obtained at this point to help determine whether structural heart disease is present. If the patient has significant structural heart disease or a clinical history suggestive of an arrhythmia, an EP test would be an appropriate next step. On the other hand, if structural heart disease is absent and the clinical history is not suggestive of an arrhythmia, the evaluation can be continued with a tilt test, event monitor, or clinical follow-up, depending on the severity and chronicity of the patient's symptoms. With this approach, a probable cause of syncope can be determined in 75 percent of patients.[5]

Management of Patients

The approach to treatment of a patient with syncope depends largely on the diagnosis that is established. For example, the appropriate treatment of a patient with syncope related to AV

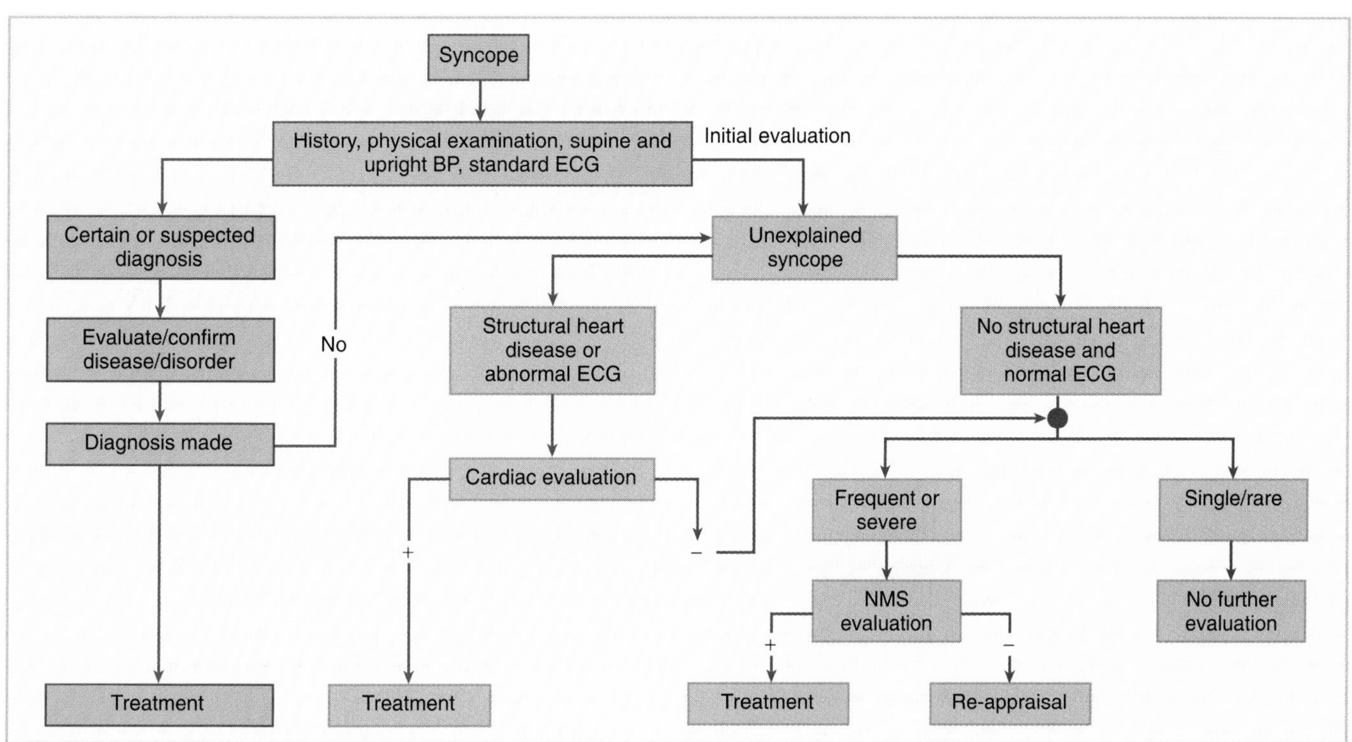

FIGURE 34–1 Diagnostic evaluation of syncope. BP = blood pressure; ECG = electrocardiogram; NMS = neurally mediated syncope.

TABLE 34–4 Clinical Features Suggestive of Specific Causes

Symptom or Finding	Diagnostic Consideration
After sudden unexpected pain, unpleasant sight, sound, or smell	Vasovagal syncope
During or immediately after micturition, cough, swallow, or defecation	Situational syncope
With neuralgia (glossopharyngeal or trigeminal)	Bradycardia or vasodepressor reaction
On standing	Orthostatic hypotension
Prolonged standing at attention	Vasovagal syncope
Well-trained athlete after exertion	Neurally mediated
Changing position (from sitting to lying, bending, turning over in bed)	Atrial myxoma, thrombus
Syncope with exertion	Aortic stenosis, pulmonary hypertension, pulmonary embolus, mitral stenosis, idiopathic hypertrophic subaortic stenosis, coronary artery disease, neurally mediated
With head rotation, pressure on carotid sinus (as in tumors, shaving, tight collars)	Carotid sinus syncope
Associated with vertigo, dysarthria, diplopia, and other motor and sensory symptoms of brain stem ischemia	Transient ischemic attack, subclavian steal, basilar artery migraine
With arm exercise	Subclavian steal
Confusion after episode	Seizure

block or sick sinus syndrome would probably involve placement of a permanent pacemaker (see Chap. 31), treatment of a patient with syncope related to the Wolff-Parkinson White syndrome would probably involve catheter ablation (see Chap. 30), and treatment of a patient with syncope related to VT would probably involve placement of an implantable defibrillator (see Chap. 31). For other types of syncope, optimal management may involve discontinuation of an offending pharmacological agent, an increase in salt intake, or education of the patient.

Other issues that need to be considered include the indication for hospitalization of a patient with syncope and duration of driving restrictions. Generally, hospital admission is indicated when there is concern regarding a potentially life-threatening cause of syncope or when significant injury has occurred. It would therefore be prudent to hospitalize a 65-year-old man with a prior history of a myocardial infarction and heart failure who presents with an initial episode of syncope that occurs without warning or residual symptoms. In this type of patient, the probability of VT as the cause of syncope is high. On the other hand, the evaluation of a young patient who presents with a clinical history suggestive of neurally mediated syncope and no clinical evidence of cardiac disease could be performed on an outpatient basis.

Physicians who care for patients with syncope are often asked to address the issue of driving risk. Patients who experience syncope while driving pose a risk both to themselves and to others. Although some would argue that all patients with syncope should never drive again because of the theoretical possibility of a recurrence, this is an impractical solution that would be ignored by many patients. Factors that should be considered when making a recommendation for a particular patient include (1) the potential for recurrent syncope, (2) the presence and duration of warning symptoms, (3) whether syncope occurs while seated or only when standing, (4) how often and in what capacity the patient drives, and (5) whether any state laws may be applicable. When considering these issues, physicians should note that acute illnesses, including syncope, are unlikely to cause a motor vehicle accident. The American Heart Association and the Canadian Cardiovascular Society have published guidelines concerning this issue. For noncommercial drivers, it is generally recommended that driving be restricted for several months. If the patient remains asymptomatic for several months, driving can then be resumed.

Neurally Mediated Syncope

Because neurally mediated syncope is so common, therapy is outlined in detail. Treatment begins with a careful history with particular attention focused on identifying precipitating factors, quantifying the degree of salt intake and current medication use, and determining whether the patient has a prior history of peripheral edema, hypertension, asthma, or other conditions that may alter the approach used to treat neurally mediated syncope. For many patients, particularly those with infrequent episodes associated with an identifiable precipitant, education about avoidance of predisposing factors and a moderate increase in salt intake are effective treatment. Patients can also be instructed to lie down at the beginning of symptoms or to cross their legs (if sitting) and squeeze them together. For others, treatment involves removal or avoidance of drugs that predispose to orthostatic hypotension or volume depletion, such as vasodilators and diuretics. One study reported that the actuarial probabilities of remaining syncope free 1 and 2 years after a positive tilt test were 72 and 60 percent, respectively.[45] The most powerful predictor of recurrence of syncope was the logarithm of the number of preceding syncopal spells.

Treatment with pharmacological agents is usually targeted at patients in whom syncope is recurrent or has been associated with physical injury. The medications that are generally relied on to treat neurally mediated syncope include beta blockers, fludrocortisone, serotonin reuptake inhibitors, and midodrine.[46] Despite the widespread use of these agents, none of these pharmacological agents have been demonstrated to be effective by the results of multiple large prospective randomized clinical trials. Perhaps the most carefully studied pharmacological agents are serotonin reuptake inhibitors such as paroxetine.[47] Several very small studies have reported that midodrine is effective.[48,49] Although beta blockers are considered by many as first-line therapy, a prospective randomized clinical trial reported that atenolol was ineffective.[50] Another study reported that a placebo was as effective as propranolol and nadolol in the treatment of neurally mediated syncope.[51]

Although pacemakers have also been found to be valuable in the treatment of some patients with neurally mediated syncope in several clinical trials, the Second Vasovagal Pacemaker Study, in which all subjects received pacemakers but pacing was activated in 50 percent of patients, showed no benefit of pacing.[52,53] Because of the variable results of these clinical trials and the profound implications of pacemaker implantation, considerable restraint should be exercised when considering the implantation of a pacemaker for treatment of neurally mediated syncope. The development of asystole during tilt-table testing is not considered to be an absolute indication for pacemaker implantation. Over the past several years, a number of studies have reported the efficacy of "orthostatic training" in the treatment of neurally mediated syncope.[54] This simple, inexpensive, and widely available approach deserves further study.

REFERENCES

Definition

1. Brignole M, Alboni P, Benditt D, et al, Task Force on Syncope, European Society of Cardiology: Guidelines on management (diagnosis and treatment) of syncope. Eur Heart J 22:1256, 2001.
2. Soteriades ES, Evand JC, Larson MG, et al: Incidence and prognosis of syncope. N Engl J Med 347:878, 2002.
3. Nyman JA, Krahn AD, Bland PC, et al: The costs of recurrent syncope of unknown origin in elderly patients. Pacing Clin Electrophysiol 22:1386, 1999.
4. Rose MS, Koshman ML, Spreng S, Sheldon R: The relationship between health-related quality of life and frequency of spells in patients with syncope. J Clin Epidemiol 53:1209, 2000.

Classification

5. Ammirati F, Colivicchi F, Santini M: Diagnosing syncope in clinical practice. Implementation of a simplified diagnostic algorithm in a multicentre prospective trial—The OESIL 2 study (Osservatorio Epidemiologico della Sincope nel Lazio). Eur Heart J 21:935, 2000.
6. Alboni P, Brignole M, Menozzi C, et al: Diagnostic value of history in patients with syncope with or without heart disease. J Am Coll Cardiol 37:1921, 2001.
7. Sarasin FP, Louis-Simonet M, Carballo D, et al: Prospective evaluation of patients with syncope: A population-based study. Am J Med 111:177, 2001.
8. Kapoor WN, Fortunato M, Hanusa BH, Schulberg HC: Psychiatric illnesses in patients with syncope. Am J Med 99:505, 1995.
9. Ventura R, Maas R, Rüppel R, et al: Psychiatric conditions in patients with recurrent unexplained syncope. Europace 3:311, 2001.
10. Nava A, Bauce B, Basso C, et al: Clinical profile and long-term follow-up of 37 families with arrhythmogenic right ventricular cardiomyopathy. J Am Coll Cardiol 36:226, 2000.
11. Elliott PM, Poloniecki J, Dickie S, et al: Sudden death in hypertrophic cardiomyopathy: Identification of high risk patients. J Am Coll Cardiol 36:2212, 2000.
12. Wilde A, Antzelevitch C, Borggrefe M, et al: Proposed diagnostic criteria for Brugada syndrome: Consensus report. Circulation 106:2514, 2002.
13. Grubb BP, Karas B: Clinical disorders of the autonomic nervous system associated with orthostatic intolerance: An overview of classification, clinical evaluation, and management. Pacing Clin Electrophysiol 22:798, 1999.
14. The Consensus Committee of the American Autonomic Society and the American Academy of Neurology: Consensus statement on the definition of orthostatic hypotension, pure autonomic failure, and multiple system atrophy. Neurology 46:1470, 1996.
15. Goldstein DS, Holmes C, Frank SM, et al: Sympathoadrenal imbalance before neurocardiogenic syncope. Am J Cardiol 91:53, 2003.
16. Kenny RAM, Richardson DA, Steen N, et al: Carotid sinus syndrome: A modifiable risk factor for nonaccidental falls in older adults (SAFE PACE). J Am Coll Cardiol 38:1491, 2001.
17. Morillo CA, Camacho ME, Wood MA, et al: Diagnostic utility of mechanical, pharmacological and orthostatic stimulation of the carotid sinus in patients with unexplained syncope. J Am Coll Cardiol 34:1587, 1999.
18. Richardson DA, Bexton R, Shaw RE, et al: Complications of carotid sinus massage—A prospective series of older patients. Age Ageing 29:413, 2000.
19. Richardson DA, Bexton RS, Shaw FE, Kenny RA: Prevalence of cardioinhibitory carotid sinus hypersensitivity in patients 50 years or over presenting to the accident and emergency department with "unexplained" or "recurrent" falls. Pacing Clin Electrophysiol 20:820, 1997.
20. Gregoratos G, Abrams J, Epstein A, et al: ACC/AHA/NASPE 2002 guideline update for implantation of cardiac pacemakers and antiarrhythmia devices: Summary article. A report of the American College of Cardiology/American Heart Association Task Force on practice guidelines (ACC/AHA/NASPE Committee to Update the 1998 Pacemaker Guidelines). Circulation 106:2145, 2002.
21. Grubb, BP, Samoil D, Kosinski D, et al: Cerebral syncope: Loss of consciousness associated with cerebral vasoconstriction in the absence of systemic hypotension. Pacing Clin Electrophysiol 21:652, 1998.

Diagnostic Tests

22. Close J, Ellis M, Hooper R, et al: Prevention of falls in the elderly trial (PROFET), a randomized controlled trial. Lancet 353:93, 1999.
23. Sheldon R, Rose S, Ritchie D, et al: Historical criteria that distinguish syncope from seizures. J Am Coll Cardiol 40:142, 2002.
24. Linzer M, Yang EH, Estes M, et al, for the Clinical Efficacy Assessment Project of the American College of Physicians: Clinical guideline. Diagnosing syncope. Part 1: Value of history, physical examination, and electrocardiography. Ann Intern Med 126:989, 1997.

25. Linzer M, Yang EH, Estes M III, et al, for the Clinical Efficacy Assessment Project of the American College of Physicians: Clinical guideline. Diagnosing syncope. Part 2: Unexplained syncope. Ann Intern Med 127:76, 1997.
26. Link MS, Lauer EP, Homoud MK, et al: Low yield of rule-out myocardial infarction protocol in patients presenting with syncope. Am J Cardiol 88:706, 2001.
27. Benditt DG, Ferguson DW, Grubb BP, et al: Tilt table testing for assessing syncope. J Am Coll Cardiol 28:263, 1996.
28. Takase B, Uehata A, Nishioka TI, et al: Different mechanisms of isoproterenol-induced and nitroglycerin-induced syncope during head-up tilt in patients with unexplained syncope: Important role of epinephrine in nitroglycerin-induced syncope. J Cardiovasc Electrophysiol 12:791, 2001.
29. Calkins H. Isoproterenol-provoked versus nitroglycerin-provoked tilt tests: Do they differ? J Cardiovasc Electrophysiol 12:797, 2001.
30. Raviele A, Giada F, Brignole M, et al: Comparison of diagnostic accuracy of sublingual nitroglycerin test and low-dose isoproterenol test in patients with unexplained syncope. Am J Cardiol 85:1194, 2000.
31. Sumiyoshi M, Nakata Y, Mineda Y, et al: Response to head-up tilt testing in patients with situational syncope. Am J Cardiol 82:1117, 1998.
32. Doi A, Tsuchihashi K, Kyuma M, et al: Diagnostic implications of modified treadmill and head-up tilt tests in exercise-related syncope: Comparative studies with situational and/or vasovagal syncope. Can J Cardiol 18:960, 2002.
33. Nasir K, Rutgerg J, Tandri H, et al: Utility of SAECG in arrhythmogenic right ventricle dysplasia. Ann Noninvasive Electrocardiol 8:112, 2003.
34. Fogel RI, Evans JJ, Prystowsky EN: Utility and cost of event recorders in the diagnosis of palpitations, presyncope, and syncope. Am J Cardiol 79:207, 1997.
35. Zimetbaum P, Kim KY, Ho KKL, et al: Utility of patient-activated cardiac event recorders in general clinical practice. Am J Cardiol 79:371, 1997.
36. Krahn AD, Klein GJ, Yee R, et al: Use of an extended monitoring strategy in patients with problematic syncope. Reveal Investigators. Circulation 99:406, 1999.
37. Krahn AD, Klein GJ, Yee R, Skanes AC: Randomized assessment of syncope trial. Conventional diagnostic testing versus a prolonged monitoring strategy. Circulation 104:46, 2001.
38. Donateo P, Brignole M, Alboni P, et al: A standardized conventional evaluation of the mechanism of syncope in patients with bundle branch block. Europace 4:357, 2002.
39. Andrews NP, Fogel RI, Pelargonio G, et al: Implantable defibrillator event rates in patients with unexplained syncope and inducible sustained ventricular tachyarrhythmias. J Am Coll Cardiol 34:2023, 1999.
40. Steinberg JS, Beckman K, Greene HL, et al: Follow-up of patients with unexplained syncope and inducible ventricular tachyarrhythmias: Analysis of the AVID registry and an AVID substudy. J Cardiovasc Electrophysiol 12:996, 2001.
41. Link MS, Costeas XF, Griffith JL, et al: High incidence of appropriate implantable cardioverter-defibrillator therapy in patients with syncope of unknown etiology and inducible ventricular arrhythmias. J Am Coll Cardiol 29:370, 1997.
42. Knight BP, Goyal R, Pelosi F, et al: Outcome of patients with nonischemic dilated cardiomyopathy and unexplained syncope treated with an implantable defibrillator. J Am Coll Cardiol 33:1964, 1999.
43. Russo AM, Verdino R, Schorr C, et al: Occurrence of implantable defibrillator events in patients with syncope and nonischemic dilated cardiomyopathy. Am J Cardiol 88:1444, 2001.
44. Fonarow GC, Feliciano Z, Boyle NG, et al: Improved survival in patients with nonischemic advanced heart failure and syncope treated with an implantable cardioverter-defibrillator. Am J Cardiol 85:981, 2000.

Approach to the Evaluation of Patients with Syncope and Management of Patients

45. Sheldon R, Rose S, Flanagan P, et al: Risk factors for syncope recurrence after a positive tilt table test in patients with syncope. Circulation 93:973, 1996.
46. Atiga W, Rowe P, Calkins H: Management of vasovagal syncope. J Cardiovasc Electrophysiol 10:874, 1999.
47. Girolamo ED, Iorio CD, Sabatini P, et al: Effects of paroxetine hydrochloride, a selective serotonin reuptake inhibitor, on refractory vasovagal syncope: A randomized, double-blind, placebo-controlled study. J Am Coll Cardiol 33:1227, 1999.
48. Ward CR, Gray JC, Gilroy JJ, et al: Midodrine: A role in the management of neurocardiogenic syncope. Heart 79:45, 1998.
49. Kaufmann H, Saadia D, Voustianiouk A: Midodrine in neurally mediated syncope: A double-blind, randomized, crossover study. Ann Neurol 52:342, 2002.
50. Madrid AH, Ortega J, Rebollo JG, et al: Lack of efficacy of atenolol for the prevention of neurally mediated syncope. J Am Coll Cardiol 37:554, 2001.
51. Flevari P, Livanis EG, Theodorakis GN, et al: Vasovagal syncope: A prospective, randomized, crossover evaluation of the effect of propranolol, nadolol and placebo on syncope recurrence and patients' well-being. J Am Coll Cardiol 40:499, 2002.
52. Connolly SJ, Sheldon R, Roberts RS, Gent M: The North American Vasovagal Pacemaker Study: A randomized trial of permanent cardiac pacing for the prevention of vasovagal syncope. J Am Coll Cardiol 33:16, 1999.
53. Connolly SJ, Sheldon R, Thorpe K, et al, for the VPS II Investigators: Pacemaker therapy for prevention of syncope in patients with recurrent severe vasovagal syncope. Second Vasovagal Pacemaker Study (VPS II): A randomized trial. JAMA 289:2224, 2003.
54. Girolamo ED, Iorio CD, Leonzio L, et al: Usefulness of a tilt training program for the prevention of refractory neurocardiogenic syncope in adolescents: A controlled study. Circulation 100:1798, 1999.

PART V

Preventive Cardiology

CHAPTER 35

The Vascular Biology of Atherosclerosis

Peter Libby

The 20th century witnessed a remarkable evolution in concepts concerning the pathogenesis of atherosclerosis. This disease has a venerable history, having left traces in the arteries of Egyptian mummies. Apparently uncommon in antiquity, atherosclerosis became epidemic as populations increasingly survived early mortality caused by infectious diseases. Also, many societies adopted dietary habits that may promote atherosclerosis, such as a surfeit of saturated fats, and curtailed physical activity (see Chaps. 1, 36, and 39).

Until very recently, most physicians viewed arteries as inanimate tubes rather than living, dynamic tissue. More than 100 years ago, Virchow recognized the participation of cells in atherogenesis. A controversy raged between Virchow, who viewed atherosclerosis as a proliferative disease, and Rokitansky, who believed that atheromata derived from healing and resorption of thrombi.[1] Experiments performed in the early part of the 20th century used dietary modulation to produce fatty lesions in the arteries of rabbits and ultimately identified cholesterol as the culprit. These observations, followed by the characterization of human lipoprotein particles at mid-century, promoted the concept of insudation of lipids as a cause for atherosclerosis.[1] We now recognize that elements of all these pathogenic theories participate in atherogenesis. This chapter summarizes evidence from human studies, animal experimentation, and in vitro work and highlights a synoptic view of atherogenesis, taking into account advances in vascular biology that have deepened our understanding of the process.

Acquaintance with the vascular biology of atherosclerosis should prove useful to the practitioner. Our daily contact with this common disease lulls us into a complacent belief that we understand it better than we actually do. For example, we are just beginning to learn why atherosclerosis affects certain regions of the arterial tree preferentially, and why its clinical manifestations occur only at certain times. Atherosclerosis can involve both large and mid-size arteries diffusely. Postmortem and intravascular ultrasonography studies have revealed widespread intimal thickening in patients with atherosclerosis. Many asymptomatic individuals have intimal lesions in their coronary or carotid arteries even in the early decades of life. At the same time, atherosclerosis is a focal disease that constricts areas of affected vessels much more than others. Understanding of the biological basis of the predilection of certain sites to develop atheroma is just beginning to emerge.[2]

Atherosclerosis also displays heterogeneity in time, being a disease with both chronic and acute manifestations. Few human diseases have a longer "incubation" period than atherosclerosis, which begins to affect arteries of many North Americans in the second and third decades of life (Fig. 35–1).[3] Indeed, one in six American teenagers have abnormal thickening of the coronary arteries.[4] Yet typically, symptoms of atherosclerosis do not occur until several decades later, characteristically occurring even later in women. Despite this indolent time course and prolonged period of clinical inactivity, the dreaded complications of atheroma such as myocardial infarction, unstable angina, or stroke typically occur suddenly.

Another poorly understood issue regarding atherogenesis is its role in causing narrowing, or stenosis, of some vessels and ectasia of others. Typically, we fear stenoses

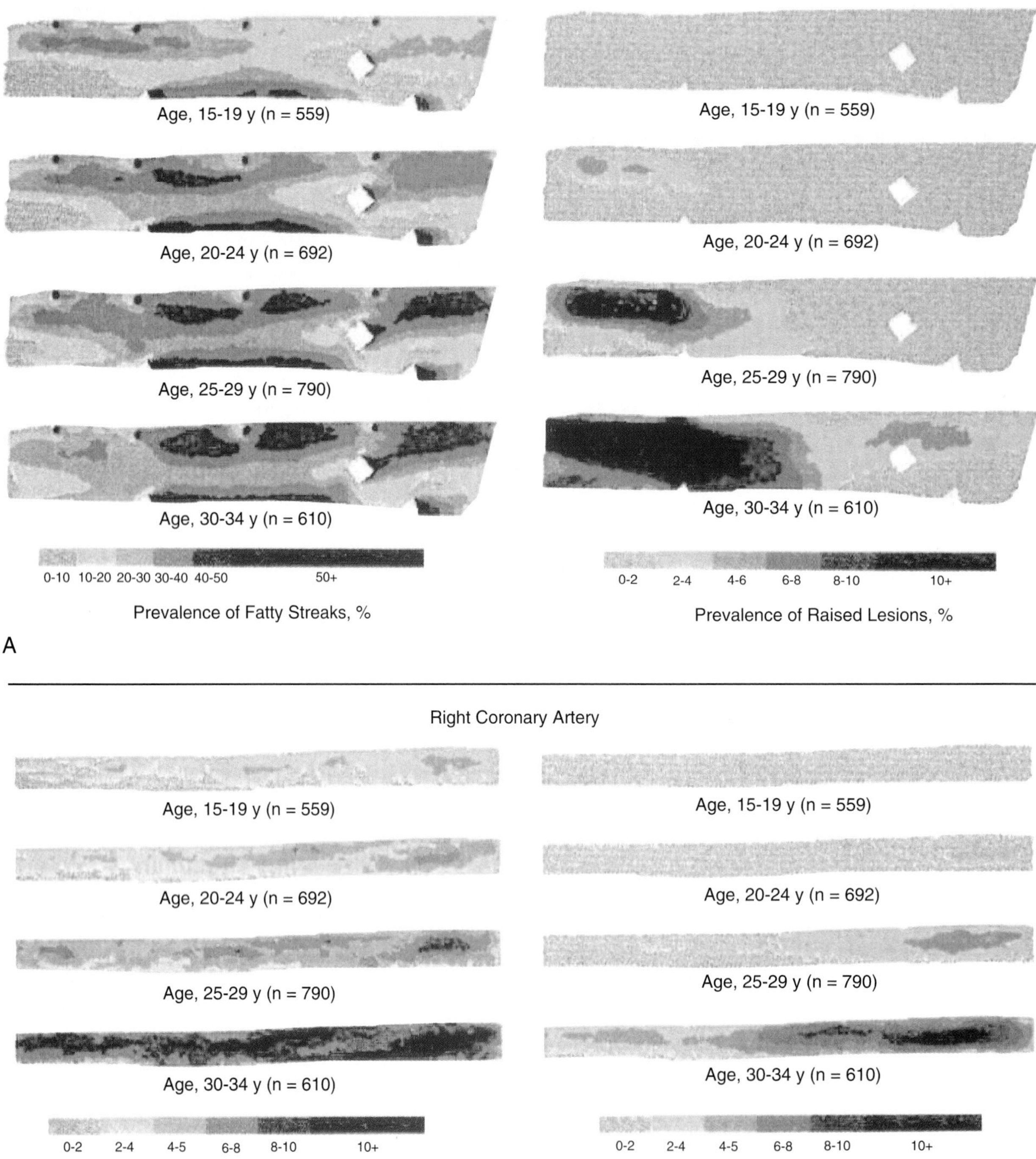

FIGURE 35–1 Prevalence maps of fatty streaks and raised lesions in the abdominal aorta. Composite data from the Pathobiological Determinants of Atherosclerosis In Youth (PDAY) Study show pseudocolored representation of morphometric analysis of more than 2800 aortas from Americans younger than 35 years of age who succumbed for noncardiac reasons. **A,** Note the early involvement of the dorsal surface of the infrarenal abdominal aorta by fatty streaks followed by raised lesions. **B,** A similar but slightly slower progression of lesions affects the right coronary artery. The scales at the bottoms of the panels show the coding of the pseudocoloring. (From Strong JP, Malcolm GT, McMahan CA, et al: Prevalence and extent of atherosclerosis in adolescents and young adults. JAMA 281:727, 1999.)

in coronary atherosclerosis. However, aneurysm is a common manifestation of this disease in other vessels, including the aorta. Even in the life history of a single atherosclerotic lesion, a phase of ectasia known as positive remodeling, or compensatory enlargement, precedes the formation of stenotic lesions.[5] Contemporary vascular biology is beginning to shed light on some of these apparent contradictions, or paradoxes, in understanding atherosclerosis.

Structure of the Normal Artery

Intima

Understanding the pathogenesis of atherosclerosis first requires knowledge of the structure and biology of the normal artery and its indigenous cell types. Normal arteries have a well-developed trilaminar structure (Fig. 35–2). The innermost layer, the tunica intima, is thin at birth in humans and many nonhuman species. Although often depicted as a monolayer of endothelial cells abutting directly on a basal lamina, the structure of the adult human intima is actually much more complex and heterogeneous. The endothelial cell of the arterial intima constitutes the crucial contact surface with blood. Arterial endothelial cells possess many highly regulated mechanisms of capital importance in vascular homeostasis that often go awry during the pathogenesis of arterial diseases.

For example, the endothelial cell provides one of the only surfaces, either natural or synthetic, that can maintain blood in a liquid state during protracted contact (Fig. 35–3). This remarkable blood compatibility derives in part from the expression of heparan sulfate proteoglycan molecules on the surface of the endothelial cell. These molecules, like heparin, serve as a cofactor for antithrombin III, causing a conformational change that allows this inhibitor to bind to and inactivate thrombin. The surface of the endothelial cell also contains thrombomodulin, which binds thrombin molecules and can exert antithrombotic properties by activating proteins S and C. Should a thrombus begin to form, the normal endothelial cell possesses potent fibrinolytic mechanisms associated with its surface. In this regard, the endothelial cell can produce both tissue- and urokinase-type plasminogen activators. These enzymes catalyze the activation of plasminogens to form plasmin, a fibrinolytic enzyme. (For a complete discussion of the role of endothelium in hemostasis and fibrinolysis, see Chapter 80.)

The endothelial monolayer rests on a basement membrane containing nonfibrillar collagen types, such as type IV collagen, laminin, fibronectin, and other extracellular matrix molecules. With aging, human arteries develop a more complex intima containing arterial smooth muscle cells and fibrillar forms of interstitial collagen (types I and III). The smooth muscle cell produces these extracellular matrix constituents of the arterial intima. The presence of a more complex intima, known by pathologists as *diffuse intimal thickening*, characterizes most adult human arteries. Some locales in the arterial tree tend to develop thicker intimas than other regions, even in the absence of atherosclerosis. For example, the proximal left anterior descending coronary artery often contains an intimal cushion of smooth muscle

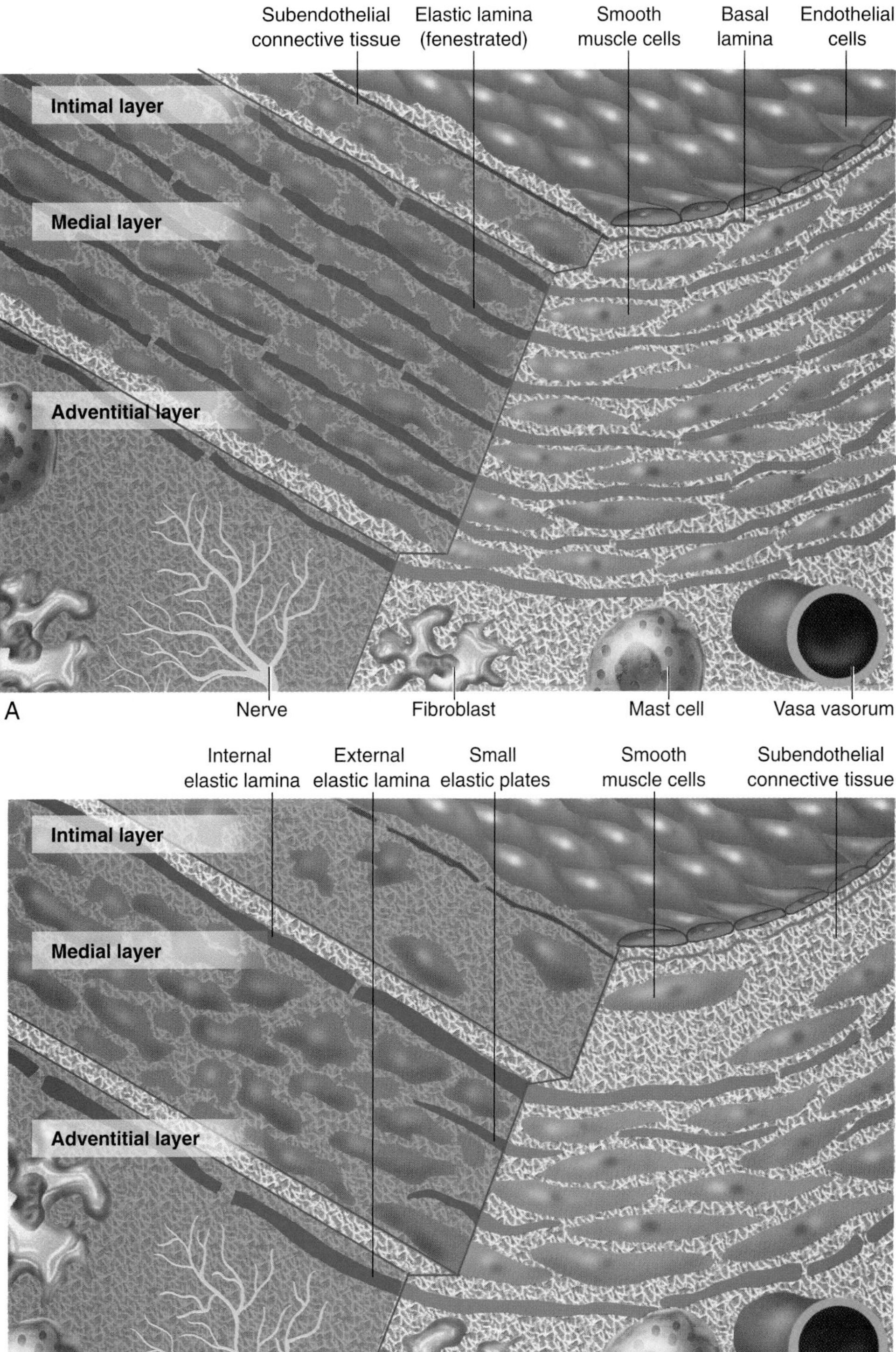

FIGURE 35–2 The structure of normal arteries. **A,** Elastic artery. Note the concentric laminae of elastic tissue that form "sandwiches" with successive layers of smooth muscle cells. Each level of the elastic arterial tree has a characteristic number of elastic laminae. **B,** Muscular artery. The smooth muscle cells are surrounded by a collagenous matrix but lack the concentric rings of well organized elastic tissue characteristic of the larger arteries.

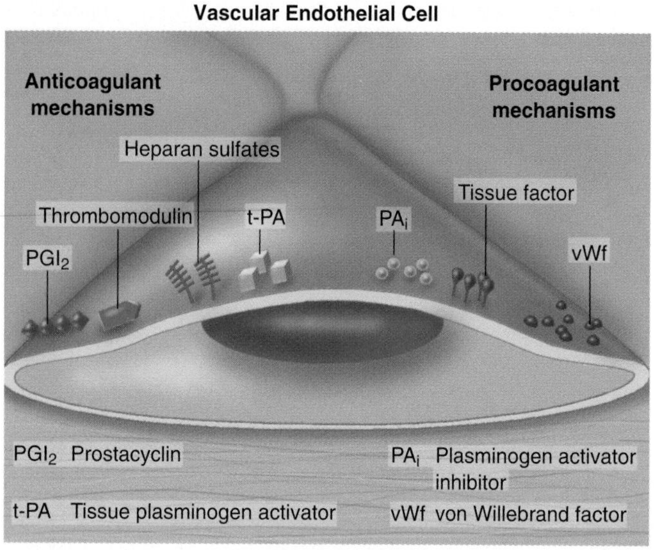

Vascular Endothelial Cell

FIGURE 35–3 The endothelial thrombotic balance. This diagram depicts the anticoagulant profibrinolytic functions of the endothelial cell **(left)** and certain procoagulant and antifibrinolytic functions **(right)**. PA_i = plasminogen activator inhibitor; PGI_2 = prostacyclin; t-PA = tissue type plasminogen activator; vWf = von Willebrand factor.

cells more fully developed than that in typical arteries (see Chap. 54). The diffuse intimal thickening process does not necessarily go hand in hand with lipid accumulation and may occur in individuals without substantial burdens of atheroma. The internal elastic membrane bounds the tunica intima abluminally and serves as the border between the intimal layer and the underlying tunica media.

Tunica Media

The tunica media lies under the media and internal elastic lamina. The media of elastic arteries such as the aorta have well developed concentric layers of smooth muscle cells, interleaved with layers of elastin-rich extracellular matrix (see Fig. 35–2A). This structure appears well adapted to the storage of the kinetic energy of left ventricle systole by the walls of great arteries. The lamellar structure also doubtless contributes to the structural integrity of the arterial trunks. The media of smaller muscular arteries usually have a less stereotyped organization (see Fig. 35–2B). Smooth muscle cells in these smaller arteries generally embed in the surrounding matrix in a more continuous than lamellar array. The smooth muscle cells in normal arteries seldom proliferate. Indeed, rates of both cell division and cell death are quite low under usual circumstances. In the normal artery, a state of homeostasis of extracellular matrix also typically prevails. Because extracellular matrix neither accumulates nor atrophies, rates of arterial matrix synthesis and dissolution usually balance each other. The external elastic lamina bounds the tunica media abluminally, forming the border with the adventitial layer.

Adventitia

The adventitia of arteries has typically received little attention, although appreciation of its potential roles in arterial homeostasis and pathology has recently increased. The adventitia contains collagen fibrils in a looser array than usually encountered in the intima. Vasa vasorum and nerve endings localize in this outermost layer of the arterial wall. The adventitia has a sparser cellular population than do other arterial layers. Cells encountered in this layer include fibroblasts and mast cells (see Fig. 35–2).

Atherosclerosis Initiation

Extracellular Lipid Accumulation

The first steps in atherogenesis in humans remain largely conjectural. However, integration of observations of tissues obtained from young humans with the results of experimental studies of atherogenesis in animals provides hints in this regard. Upon initiation of an atherogenic diet, one typically rich in cholesterol and saturated fat, small lipoprotein particles accumulate in the intima (Fig. 35–4, 1&2).[6] These lipoprotein particles appear to decorate the proteoglycan of the arterial intima and tend to coalesce into aggregates (Fig. 35–5).[7] Detailed kinetic studies of labeled lipoprotein particles indicate that a prolonged residence time characterizes sites of early lesion formation in rabbits. The binding of lipoproteins to proteoglycan in the intima captures and retains these particles, accounting for their prolonged residence time.[7,8] Lipoprotein particles bound to proteoglycan have increased susceptibility to oxidative or other chemical modifications, considered by many investigators to be an important component of the pathogenesis of early atherosclerosis (see Fig. 35–4, 2).[7,9-11] Other studies suggest that permeability of the endothelial monolayer increases at sites of lesion predilection to low-density lipoprotein (LDL). Contributors to oxidative stress in the nascent atheroma could include NADH/NADPH oxidases expressed by vascular cells,[12] lipoxygenases expressed by infiltrating leukocytes,[13] or the enzyme myeloperoxidase.[14]

Leukocyte Recruitment

Another hallmark of atherogenesis, leukocyte recruitment and accumulation, also occurs early in lesion generation (Fig. 35–6; see also Fig. 35–4, 3). The normal endothelial cell generally resists adhesive interactions with leukocytes. Even in inflamed tissues, most recruitment and trafficking of leukocytes occurs in postcapillary venules, not in arteries. However, very early after initiation of hypercholesterolemia, leukocytes adhere to the endothelium and diapedese between endothelial cell junctions to enter the intima, where they begin to accumulate lipids and become foam cells (see Fig. 35–4, 5&6). In addition to the monocyte, T lymphocytes also tend to accumulate in early human and animal atherosclerotic lesions. The expression of certain leukocyte adhesion molecules on the surface of the endothelial cell regulates the adherence of monocytes and T cells to the endothelium. Two broad categories of leukocyte adhesion molecules exist. Members of the immunoglobulin superfamily include structures such as vascular cell adhesion molecule-1 (VCAM-1).[15,16] This adhesion molecule holds particular interest in the context of early atherogenesis because it interacts with an integrin (very late antigen-4 [VLA-4]) characteristically expressed by only those classes of leukocytes that accumulate in nascent atheroma, monocytes, and T cells. Moreover, studies in rabbits and mice have shown expression of VCAM-1 on endothelial cells overlying very early atheromatous lesions. Other members of the immunoglobulin superfamily of leukocyte adhesion molecules include intercellular adhesion molecule-1 (ICAM-1). This molecule is more promiscuous, both in the types of leukocytes it binds and because of its wide and constitutive expression at low levels by endothelial cells in many parts of the circulation.

Selectins constitute the other broad category of leukocyte adhesion molecules. The prototypical selectin, E-selectin (E for "endothelial," the cell type that selectively expresses this particular family member), probably has little to do with early atherogenesis. E-selectin preferentially recruits polymorphonuclear leukocytes, a cell type seldom if ever found in early atheroma (but an essential protagonist in acute

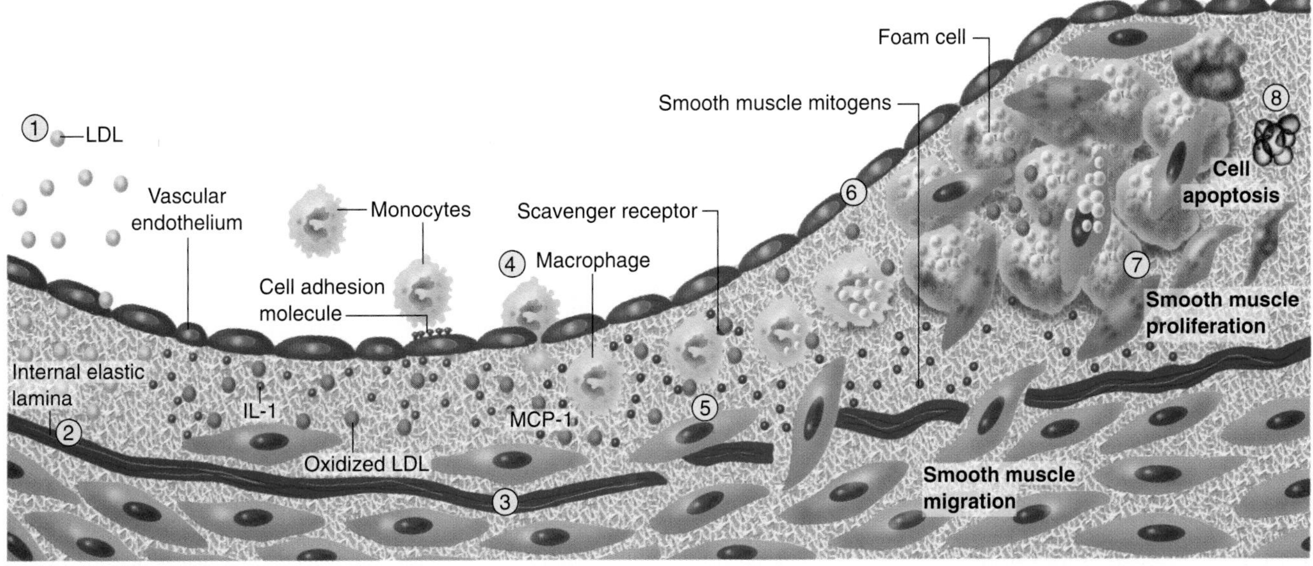

FIGURE 35–4 Schematic of the evolution of the atherosclerotic plaque. **1:** Accumulation of lipoprotein particles in the intima. The modification of these lipoproteins is depicted by the darker color. Modifications include oxidation and glycation. **2:** Oxidative stress, including products found in modified lipoproteins, can induce local cytokine elaboration. **3:** The cytokines thus induced increase expression of adhesion molecules for leukocytes that cause their attachment and chemoattractant molecules that direct their migration into the intima. **4:** Blood monocytes, upon entering the artery wall in response to chemoattractant cytokines such as monocyte chemoattractant protein 1 (MCP-1), encounter stimuli such as macrophage colony stimulating factor (M-CSF) that can augment their expression of scavenger receptors. **5:** Scavenger receptors mediate the uptake of modified lipoprotein particles and promote the development of foam cells. Macrophage foam cells are a source of mediators such as further cytokines and effector molecules such as hypochlorous acid, superoxide anion (O_2^-), and matrix metalloproteinases. **6:** Smooth muscle cells in the intima divide other smooth muscle cells that migrate into the intima from the media. **7:** Smooth muscle cells can then divide and elaborate extracellular matrix, promoting extracellular matrix accumulation in the growing atherosclerotic plaque. In this manner, the fatty streak can evolve into a fibrofatty lesion. **8:** In later stages, calcification can occur (not depicted) and fibrosis continues, sometimes accompanied by smooth muscle cell death (including programmed cell death, or apoptosis) yielding a relatively acellular fibrous capsule surrounding a lipid-rich core that may also contain dying or dead cells and their detritus. IL-1 = interleukin-1; LDL = low-density lipoprotein.

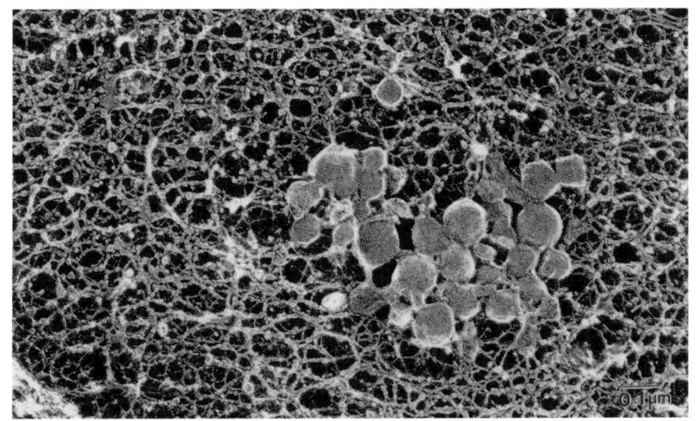

FIGURE 35–5 Scanning electron micrograph of a freeze etch preparation of rabbit aorta following an intravenous injection of human low-density lipoprotein (LDL). Round LDL particles decorate the strands of proteoglycan found in the subendothelial region of the intima. By binding LDL particles, proteoglycan molecules can retard their traversal of the intima and promote their accumulation. Proteoglycan-associated LDL appears particularly susceptible to oxidative modification. Accumulation of extracellular lipoprotein particles is one of the first morphological changes noted after initiation of an atherogenic diet in experimental animals. (From Nievelstein PF, Fogelman AM, Mottino G, Frank JS: Lipid accumulation in rabbit aortic intima 2 hours after bolus infusion of low density lipoprotein: A deep-etch and immunolocalization study of ultrarapidly frozen tissue. Arterioscler Thromb 11:1795, 1991.)

inflammation and host defenses against bacterial pathogens).[17] Moreover, endothelial cells overlying atheroma do not express high levels of this adhesion molecule. Other members of this family, including P-selectin (P for "platelet," the original source of this adhesion molecule), may play a greater role in leukocyte recruitment in atheroma, because endothelial cells overlying human atheroma do express this adhesion molecule.[18,19] Selectins tend to promote saltatory or rolling locomotion of leukocytes over the endothelium. Adhesion molecules belonging to the immunoglobulin superfamily tend to promote tighter adhesive interactions and immobilization of leukocytes. Studies in genetically altered mice have proven roles for VCAM-1 and P-selectin (including both platelet- and endothelial-derived P-selectin) in experimental atherosclerosis.[20-22]

Once adherent to the endothelium, leukocytes must receive a signal to penetrate the endothelial and enter the arterial wall (see Fig. 35–4, 4). The current concept of directed migration of leukocytes involves the action of protein molecules known as chemoattractant cytokines, or chemokines.[23] Two groups of chemokines have particular interest in recruiting the mononuclear cells characteristic of the early atheroma. One such molecule, known as monocyte chemoattractant protein-1 (MCP-1), is produced by the endothelium in response to oxidized lipoprotein and other stimuli. Cells intrinsic to the normal artery, including endothelium and smooth muscle, can produce this chemokine when stimulated by inflammatory mediators, as do many other cell types. MCP-1 selectively promotes the directed migration, or chemotaxis, of monocytes. Studies conducted with genetically modified mice lacking MCP-1 or its receptor CCR-2 have delayed and attenuated atheroma formation when placed on an atherosclerosis-prone hyperlipidemic genetic background.[24,25] Human atherosclerotic lesions express increased levels of MCP-1 compared with uninvolved vessels. Thus, several chemokines appear causally to contribute to monocyte recruitment during atherogenesis in vivo. Interleukin-8, a chemokine that binds to CXCR2 on leukocytes, also participates in experimental atherosclerosis.[26] Another unique cell-surface-bound chemokine, fractalkine, also appears to contribute to atherogenesis.[27] Another group of chemoattractant cytokines may heighten lymphocyte accumulation in

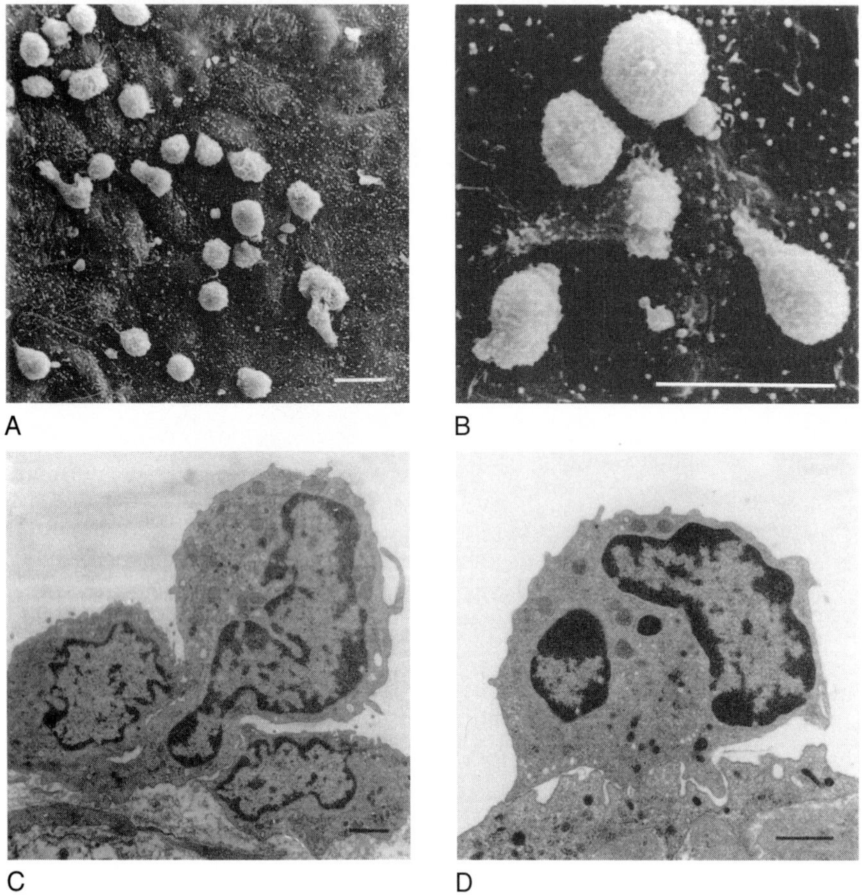

FIGURE 35–6 Electron microscopic examination of leukocyte interactions with the artery wall in hypercholesterolemic nonhuman primates. **A** and **B,** Scanning electron micrographs that demonstrate the adhesion of mononuclear phagocytes to the intact endothelium 12 days after initiating a hypercholesterolemic diet. **C** and **D,** Transmission electron micrographs. Note the abundant interdigitations and intimate association of the monocyte with the endothelium in part C. In part D, a monocyte appears to diapedese between two endothelial cells to enter the intima. (From Faggiotto A, Ross R, Harker L: Studies of hypercholesterolemia in the nonhuman primate. I. Changes that lead to fatty streak formation. Arteriosclerosis 4:323, 1984.)

plaques as well. Atheroma express a trio of lymphocyte-selective chemokines (IP-10, I-TAC, and MIG).[28] Gamma interferon, a cytokine known to be present in atheromatous plaques, induces the genes encoding this family of T-cell chemoattractants.

Focality of Lesion Formation

The spatial heterogeneity of atherosclerosis has proved challenging to explain in mechanistic terms. Equal concentrations of blood-borne risk factors such as lipoproteins bathe the endothelium throughout the vasculature. It is difficult to envisage how injury due to inhaling cigarette smoke could produce any local rather than global effect on arteries. Yet, atheromata typically form focally, as revealed by studies of morphology, lipid accumulation, and adhesion molecule expression. Some have invoked a multicentric origin hypothesis of atherogenesis, positing that atheroma arise as benign leiomyomata of the artery wall. The monotypia of various molecular markers such as glucose-6-phosphate dehydrogenase isoforms in individual atheroma supports this "monoclonal hypothesis" of atherogenesis.[29] However, the location of sites of lesion predilection at proximal portions of arteries after branch points or bifurcations at flow dividers suggests a hydrodynamic basis for early lesion development. Arteries without many branches (e.g., the internal mammary or radial arteries) tend not to develop atherosclerosis.

Two concepts can help one understand how local flow disturbances might render certain foci sites of lesion predilection. Locally disturbed flow could induce alterations that promote the steps of early atherogenesis. Alternatively, the laminar flow that usually prevails at sites that do *not* tend to develop early lesions may elicit antiatherogenic homeostatic mechanisms (atheroprotective functions).[30] The endothelial cell experiences the laminar shear stress of normal flow and the disturbed flow (usually yielding decreased shear stress) at predilected sites. In vitro data suggest that laminar shear stress can augment the expression of genes that may protect against atherosclerosis, including forms of the enzymes superoxide dismutase, or nitric oxide synthase. Superoxide dismutase can reduce oxidative stress by catabolizing the reactive and injurious superoxide anion. Endothelial nitric oxide synthase produces the well known endogenous vasodilator nitric oxide (•NO). However, beyond its vasodilating actions, •NO can resist inflammatory activation of endothelial functions such as expression of the adhesion molecule VCAM-1. Nitric oxide appears to exert this antiinflammatory action at the level of gene expression by interfering with the transcriptional regulator nuclear factor kappa B (NFκB). Nitric oxide actually increases the production of an intracellular inhibitor (IκBα) of this important transcription factor. The NFκB system regulates numerous genes involved in inflammatory responses in general and in atherogenesis in particular.[31] These examples show how basic vascular biology has yielded insights into previously obscure yet important aspects of atherogenesis. Future study of the molecular regulation of vascular cell function by mechanical stimuli should clarify the mechanisms of lesion formation at particular sites in the circulation.

Likewise, study of vascular developmental biology may aid understanding of the tendency of certain arteries to develop atherosclerosis at different rates and in different ways (see Chap. 54). Smooth muscle cells vary in embryological origin in different regions.[32] For example, upper body arteries can recruit smooth muscle from neurectoderm, whereas in the lower body smooth muscle cells derive principally from mesoderm. Coronary artery smooth muscle cells arise from an anlage known as the pro-epicardial organ.[33] After injury or transplantation, arteries can repopulate with smooth muscle cells derived from bone marrow.[34,35] How this heterogeneity in the origin of smooth muscle cells might affect human atherosclerosis and help explain some of the poorly understood issues regarding dispersion of atheroma in time and space remains intriguing yet speculative. (See Chapter 54 for further discussion of the cellular and molecular heterogeneity of blood vessels.)

Intracellular Lipid Accumulation: Foam Cell Formation

The monocyte, once recruited to the arterial intima, can there imbibe lipid and become a foam cell, or lipid-laden macrophage (see Fig. 35–4, 5). Most cells can express the classic cell surface receptor for LDL, but that receptor does not mediate foam cell accumulation (see Chap. 39). This is evident clinically, as patients lacking functional LDL receptors (familial hypercholesterolemia homozygotes) still develop tendinous xanthomata filled with foamy macrophages. The LDL receptor does not mediate foam cell formation because of its exquisite regulation by cholesterol. As soon as a cell collects enough cholesterol from low-density lipoprotein capture for its metabolic needs, an elegant transcriptional control mechanism quenches expression of the receptor (see Chap. 39).

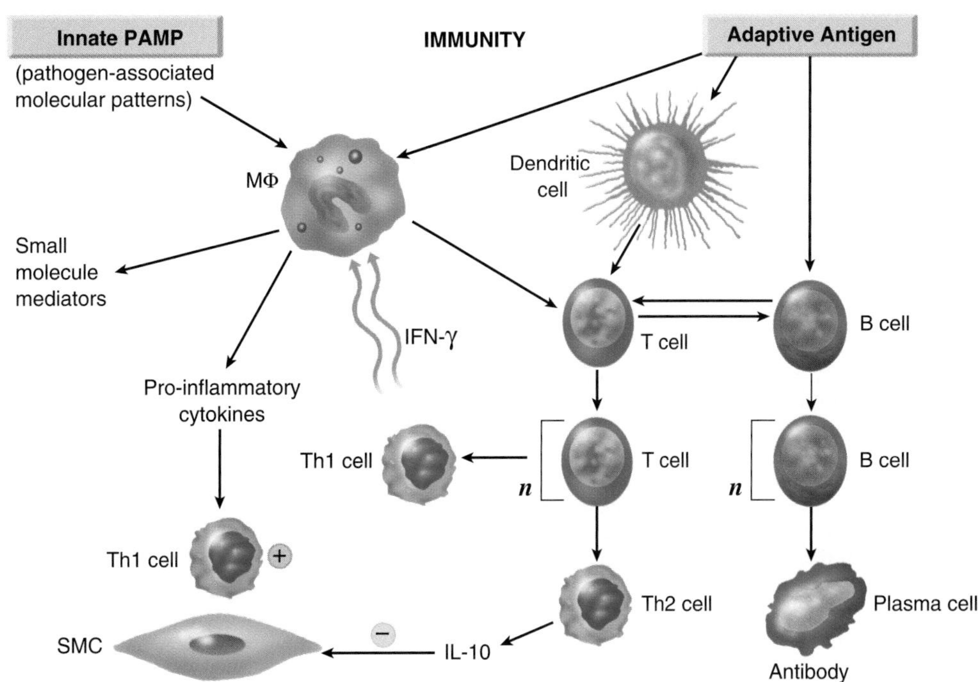

FIGURE 35–7 Innate and adaptive immunity in atherosclerosis. A diagram of the pathways of innate **(left)** and adaptive **(right)** immunity operating during atherogenesis. IFN-γ = interferon gamma; IL = interleukin; MΦ = macrophage; SMC = smooth muscle cell; Th = T helper cell. (Adapted from Hansson G, Libby P, Schoenbeck U, Yan Z-Q: Innate and adaptive immunity in the pathogenesis of atherosclerosis. Circ Res 91:281, 2002.)

Instead of the classic LDL receptor, various molecules known as *scavenger receptors* appear to mediate the excessive lipid uptake characteristic of foam cell formation.[36] The longest studied of these receptors belong to the scavenger receptor-A family. These surface molecules bind modified rather than native lipoproteins and apparently participate in their internalization. Atherosclerosis-prone mice with mutations that delete functional scavenger receptor-A have less exuberant fatty lesion formation than those with functional scavenger receptor-A molecules.[37] Other receptors that bind modified lipoprotein and that may participate in foam cell formation include CD36 and macrosialin, the latter exhibiting preferential binding specificity for oxidized forms of LDL. (See Chap. 39 for a table of scavenger receptors.)

Once macrophages have taken up residence in the intima and become foam cells, they not infrequently replicate. The factors that trigger macrophage cell division in the atherosclerotic plaque likely include macrophage-colony stimulating factor. This co-mitogen and survival factor for mononuclear phagocytes exists in human and experimental atheromatous lesions. Again, atherosclerosis-prone mice lacking functional macrophage-colony stimulating factor have retarded fatty lesion development as well.[38] Other candidates for macrophage mitogens or co-mitogens include interleukin-3 and granulocyte-macrophage colony stimulatory factor.

Up to this point in the development of the nascent atheroma, the lesion consists primarily of lipid-engorged macrophages. Complex features such as fibrosis, thrombosis, and calcification do not characterize the fatty streak, the precursor lesion of the complex atheroma (see Fig. 35–1). Several lines of evidence suggest that such fatty streaks may be reversible, at least to some extent.

Evolution of Atheroma

Innate and Adaptive Immunity: Mechanisms of Inflammation in Atherogenesis

Over the last decade, basic and clinical evidence have converged to demonstrate a fundamental role for inflammation in atherogenesis (see Chap. 36).[39,40] The macrophage foam cells recruited to the artery wall early in this process serve not only as a reservoir for excess lipid. In the established atherosclerotic lesion, these cells also provide a rich source of proinflammatory mediators, both proteins such as cytokines and chemokines and various eicosanoids and lipids such as platelet-activating factor. These phagocytic cells also can elaborate large quantities of oxidant species such as superoxide anion in the milieu of the atherosclerotic plaque.[41] This ensemble of inflammatory mediators can promote inflammation in the plaque and thus contribute to the progression of lesions. The term *innate immunity* describes this type of amplification of the inflammatory response that does not depend on antigenic stimulation (Fig. 35–7).

In addition to innate immunity, mounting evidence supports a prominent role for antigen-specific or adaptive immunity in plaque progression.[39,40] In addition to the mononuclear phagocytes, dendritic cells in atherosclerotic lesion can present antigens to the T cells that constitute an important minority of the leukocytes in the atherosclerotic lesion. Candidate antigens for stimulating this adaptive immune response include modified lipoproteins, heat shock proteins, beta-2 glycoprotein 1b, and infectious agents. The antigen-presenting cells (macrophages, dendritic cells, or endothelial cells) allow the antigen to interact with T cells in a manner that triggers their activation. The activated T cells then can secrete copious quantities of cytokines that can modulate atherogenesis.

The helper T cells (bearing CD4) fall into two general categories. The T helper 1 subtype elaborates proinflammatory cytokines such as interferon gamma, lymphotoxin, CD40 ligand, and tumor necrosis factor-alpha. This panel of Th1 cytokines can in turn activate vascular wall cells and orchestrate alterations in plaque biology that can lead to plaque destabilization and heightened thrombogenicity. On the other hand, helper T cells slanted toward the production of Th2 cytokines such as interleukin-10 may serve as inhibitors of inflammation in the context of atherogenesis.[42] Cytolytic T cells (bearing CD8) can express fas ligand and other cytotoxic factors that can promote cytolysis and apoptosis of target cells, including smooth muscle and endothelial cells, and macrophages.[43,44] The death of all three of these cell types can occur in the atherosclerotic lesion and may contribute to plaque progression and complications (see Fig. 35–4, 8). The role of B cells and antibody in atherosclerosis remains incompletely explored. Humoral immunity may have either atheroprotective or atherogenic properties, depending on the circumstances.

Smooth Muscle Cell Migration and Proliferation

While the early events in atheroma initiation involve primarily altered endothelial function and recruitment and accumulation of leukocytes, the subsequent evolution of atheroma into more complex plaques involves smooth muscle cells as well (see Fig. 35–4, 6&7). Smooth muscle cells in the normal arterial tunica media differ considerably from those in the intima of an evolving atheroma.[45,46] Whereas some smooth muscle cells likely arrive in the arterial intima early in life, others that accumulate in advancing atheroma likely arise from cells that have migrated from the underlying media into the intima. The chemoattractants for smooth muscle cells likely include molecules such as platelet-derived growth factor (PDGF), a potent smooth muscle cell chemoattractant secreted by activated macrophages and overexpressed in human atherosclerosis. These smooth muscle cells in the atherosclerotic intima can also multiply by cell division. Estimated rates of division of smooth muscle cells in the human atherosclerotic lesion are on the order of less than 1 percent. However, even such indolent replication might yield considerable smooth muscle cell accumulation over the decades of lesion evolution.

Smooth muscle cells in the atherosclerotic intima appear to exhibit a less mature phenotype than the quiescent smooth muscle cells in the normal arterial medial layer. Instead of expressing primarily isoforms of smooth muscle myosin characteristic of adult smooth muscle cells, those in the intima have higher levels of the embryonic isoform of smooth muscle myosin.[46] Thus, smooth muscle cells in the intima appear to recapitulate an embryonic phenotype. These intimal smooth muscle cells in atheroma appear morphologically distinct as well. They contain more rough endoplasmic reticulum and fewer contractile fibers than do normal medial smooth muscle cells.

Although replication of smooth muscle cells in the steady state appears infrequent in mature human atheroma, bursts of smooth muscle cell replication may occur during the life history of a given atheromatous lesion. For example, and as will be discussed in considerable detail later, episodes of plaque disruption with thrombosis may expose smooth muscle cells to potent mitogens, including the coagulation factor thrombin itself. Thus, accumulation of smooth muscle cells during atherosclerosis and growth of the intima may not occur in a continuous and linear fashion. Rather, "crises" may punctuate the history of an atheroma, during which bursts of smooth muscle replication and/or migration may occur (Fig. 35–8).

Smooth Muscle Cell Death During Atherogenesis

In addition to smooth muscle cell replication, death of these cells can also participate in the complication of the atherosclerotic plaque (see Fig. 35–4, 8). At least some smooth muscle cells in advanced human atheroma exhibit fragmentation of their nuclear DNA characteristic of programmed cell death, or apoptosis.[43,44] Apoptosis can occur in response to inflammatory cytokines known to be present in the evolving atheroma. In addition to soluble cytokines that can trigger programmed cell death, the T cells in atheroma can participate in eliminating some smooth muscle cells. In particular, certain T cell populations known to accumulate in plaques can express *fas* ligand on their surface. *Fas* ligand can engage *fas* on the surface of smooth muscle cells and, in conjunction with soluble proinflammatory cytokines, lead to death of the smooth muscle cell.[43,47]

Thus, smooth muscle cell accumulation in the growing atherosclerotic plaque probably results from a tug-of-war between cell replication and cell death.[43] Contemporary cell and molecular biological research has identified candidates for mediating both the replication and the attrition of smooth muscle cells, a concept that originated from the careful morphological observations of Virchow almost a century and a half ago. Referring to the smooth muscle cells in the intima, Virchow noted that early atherogenesis involves a "multiplication of their nuclei." However, he recognized that cells in lesions can "hurry on to their own destruction" because of death of smooth muscle cells.

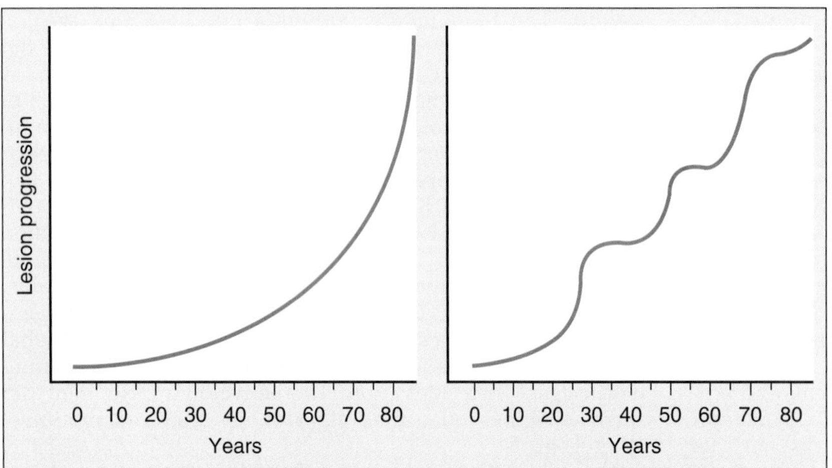

FIGURE 35–8 The time course of atherosclerosis. Traditional teaching held that atheroma formation followed an inexorably progressive course with age, depicted in the left-hand curve. Current thinking suggests an alternative model, a step function rather than a monotonically upward course of lesion evolution in time (right-hand curve). According to this latter model, "crises" can punctuate periods of relative quiescence during the life history of a lesion. Such crises might follow an episode of plaque disruption, with mural thrombosis, and healing, yielding a spurt in smooth muscle proliferation and matrix deposition. Intraplaque hemorrhage due to rupture of a friable microvessel might produce a similar scenario. Such episodes might usually be clinically inapparent. Extravascular events such as an intercurrent infection with systemic cytokinemia or endotoxemia could elicit an "echo" at the level of the artery wall, evoking a round of local cytokine gene expression by "professional" inflammatory leukocytes resident in the lesion. The episodic model of plaque progression shown on the right fits human angiographic data better than the continuous function, depicted on the left.

Arterial Extracellular Matrix

Extracellular matrix rather than cells themselves makes up much of the volume of an advanced atherosclerotic plaque. Thus, extracellular constituents of plaque also require consideration. The major extracellular matrix macromolecules that accumulate in atheroma include interstitial collagens (types I and III) and proteoglycans such as versican, biglycan, aggrecan, and decorin.[48,49] Elastin fibers can also accumulate in atherosclerotic plaques. The vascular smooth muscle cell produces these matrix molecules in disease, just as it does during development and maintenance of the normal artery (see Fig. 35–4, 7). Stimuli for excessive collagen production by smooth muscle cells include PDGF and transforming growth factor-beta (TGF-β), a constituent of platelet granules and a product of many cell types found in lesions.

Much like the accumulation of smooth muscle cells, extracellular matrix secretion also depends on a balance. In this case, the biosynthesis of the extracellular matrix molecules is balanced by breakdown catalyzed in part by catabolic enzymes known as matrix metalloproteinases (MMPs). Dissolution of extracellular matrix macromolecules undoubtedly plays a role in the migration of smooth muscle cells as they penetrate into the intima from the media through a dense extracellular matrix, traversing the elastin-rich internal elastic lamina. In injured arteries, overexpression of such proteinase inhibitors (known as tissue inhibitors of metalloproteinases) can delay smooth muscle accumulation in the intima of injured arteries.[50]

Extracellular matrix dissolution also likely plays a role in the arterial remodeling that accompanies lesion growth. During the first part of the life history of an atheromatous lesion, growth of the plaque is outward, in an abluminal direction, rather than inward in a way that would lead to luminal stenosis. This outward growth of the intima leads to an increase in the caliber of the entire artery. This so-called "positive" remodeling or "compensatory enlargement" must involve turnover of extracellular matrix molecules to accommodate the circumferential growth of the artery. Luminal stenosis tends to occur only after the plaque burden exceeds some 40 percent of the cross-sectional area of the artery.[5]

Angiogenesis in Plaques

The smooth muscle cell is not alone in its proliferation and migration within the evolving atherosclerotic plaque. Endothelial migration and replication also occur as plaques develop in microcirculation, characterized by plexi of newly formed vessels. Such plaque neovessels usually require special stains for visualization. However, histological examination with appropriate markers for endothelial cells reveals a rich neovascularization in evolving plaques. These microvessels likely form in response to angiogenic peptides overexpressed in atheroma. These angiogenesis factors include acidic and basic fibroblast growth factors, vascular endothelial growth factor,[51,52] placental growth factor,[53] and oncostatin M.[54]

These microvessels within plaques probably have considerable functional significance.[55] For example, the abundant microvessels in plaques provide a relatively large surface area for the trafficking of leukocytes, which could include both entry and exit of leukocytes. Indeed, in the advanced human atherosclerotic plaque, microvascular endothelium displays the mononuclear-selective adhesion molecules such as VCAM-1 much more prominently than does the macrovascular endothelium overlying the plaque. The microvascularization of plaques may also allow growth of the plaque overcoming diffusion limitations on oxygen and nutrient supply, analogous with the concept of tumor angiogenic factors and growth of malignant lesions. Consistent with this view, administration of inhibitors of angiogenesis to mice with experimentally induced atherosclerosis limits lesion expansion.[56] Finally, the plaque microvessels may be friable and prone to rupture like the neovessels in the diabetic retina.[57] Hemorrhage and thrombosis in situ could promote a local round of smooth muscle cell proliferation and matrix accumulation in the area immediately adjacent to the microvascular disruption (Fig. 35–9). This scenario illustrates a special case of one of the "crises" described earlier in the evolution of the atheromatous plaque (see Fig. 35–8). Attempts to augment myocardial perfusion by enhancing new vessel growth by transfer of angiogenic proteins or their genes might have adverse effects on lesion growth or clinical complications of atheroma by these mechanisms.

Plaque Mineralization

Plaques often develop areas of calcification as they evolve. Indeed, both Virchow and Rokitansky recognized morphological features of bone formation in atherosclerotic plaques in early microscopic descriptions of atherosclerosis. In recent years, understanding of the mechanism of mineralization during evolution of atherosclerotic plaques has advanced. Some subpopulations of smooth muscle cells may foster calcification by enhanced secretion of cytokines such as bone morphogenetic proteins, homologues of transforming growth factor-beta.[58] Atheromatous plaques can also contain proteins with gamma carboxylated glutamic acid residues specialized in sequestering calcium and thus promoting mineralization.[59]

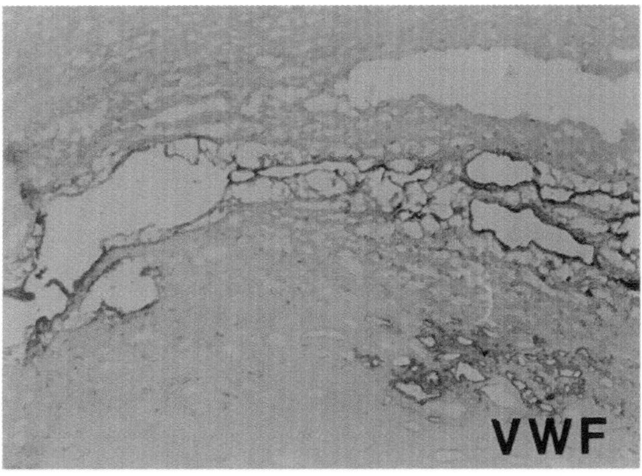

A

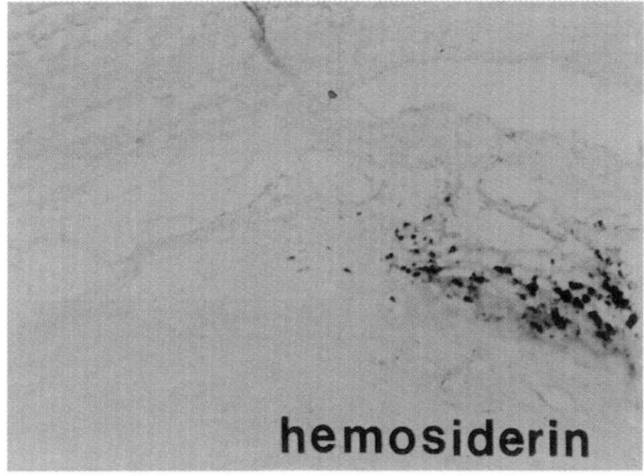

B

FIGURE 35–9 Intraplaque hemorrhage. A typical human atherosclerotic plaque stained for von Willebrand factor **(A)** and iron by Prussian blue **(B)**. The von Willebrand factor stains the endothelial cells that line the microvascular channels and lakes. Note the extravasated von Willebrand factor, which colocalizes with iron deposition, indicating hemosiderin deposition consistent with an intraplaque hemorrhage. (After Brogi E, Winkles JA, Underwood R, et al: Distinct patterns of expression of fibroblast growth factors and their receptors in human atheroma and non-atherosclerotic arteries: Association of acidic FGF with plaque microvessels and macrophages. J Clin Invest 92:2408, 1993.)

Arterial Stenoses and Their Clinical Implications

The previous sections have discussed the initiation and evolution of the atherosclerotic plaque. These phases of the atherosclerotic process generally last many years, during which time the affected individual often has no symptoms. After the plaque burden exceeds the capacity of the artery to remodel outward, encroachment on the arterial lumen begins. During the chronic asymptomatic or stable phase of lesion evolution, growth probably occurs discontinuously, with periods of relative quiescence punctuated by episodes of rapid progression (see Fig. 35–8). Human angiographic studies support this discontinuous growth of coronary artery stenoses.[60] Eventually, the stenoses can progress to a degree that impedes blood flow through the artery. Lesions that produce stenoses of greater than 60 percent can cause flow limitations under conditions of increased demand. This type of athero-occlusive disease commonly produces chronic stable angina pectoris or intermittent claudication upon increased demand. Thus, the symptomatic phase of atherosclerosis usually occurs many decades after lesion initiation.

In many cases of myocardial infarction, however, no history of prior stable angina heralds the acute event. Several kinds of clinical observation suggest that many myocardial infarctions result not from high-grade stenoses but from lesions that do not limit flow.[61,62] For example, in individuals who have undergone coronary arteriography in the months preceding myocardial infarction, the culprit lesion most often shows less than 50 percent stenosis. In a compilation of four such serial angiographic studies, only approximately 15 percent of acute myocardial infarctions arise from lesions with degrees of stenosis greater than 60 percent on an antecedent angiogram.

Instead of progressive growth of the intimal lesion to a critical stenosis, we now recognize that thrombosis, complicating a not necessarily occlusive plaque, most often causes episodes of unstable angina or acute myocardial infarction. Angiographic studies performed in individuals undergoing thrombolysis support this view. In one such study, almost half of patients undergoing thrombolysis for a first myocardial infarction had an underlying stenosis of less than 50 percent once the acute thrombus was lysed.

These findings do not imply that small atheromata cause most myocardial infarctions. Indeed, culprit lesions of acute myocardial infarction may actually be sizeable.[63] However, they may not produce a critical luminal narrowing because of the phenomenon of compensatory enlargement.[5,64,65] Of course, critical stenoses do cause myocardial infarctions. In fact, the high-grade stenoses are more likely to cause acute myocardial infarction than nonocclusive lesions. However, because the noncritical stenoses by far outnumber the tight focal lesions in a given coronary tree, the lesser stenoses cause more infarctions even though high-grade stenoses have a greater individual probability of causing myocardial infarction.

Thrombosis and Atheroma Complication

This evolution in our view of the pathogenesis of the acute coronary syndromes places new emphasis on thrombosis as the critical mechanism of transition from chronic to acute atherosclerosis. Understanding of the mechanisms of coronary thrombosis has advanced considerably. We now appreciate that a physical disruption of the atherosclerotic plaque commonly causes acute thrombosis. Several major modes of plaque disruption provoke most coronary thrombi. The first mechanism, accounting for some two thirds of acute myocardial infarctions, involves a fracture of the plaque's fibrous cap (Fig. 35–10). Another mode involves a superficial erosion of the intima (Fig. 35–11), accounting for up to one-quarter of acute myocardial infarctions in highly selected referral cases from medical examiners on individuals who have succumbed to sudden cardiac death. Superficial erosion appears more frequently in women than in men as a mechanism of coronary sudden death.[66]

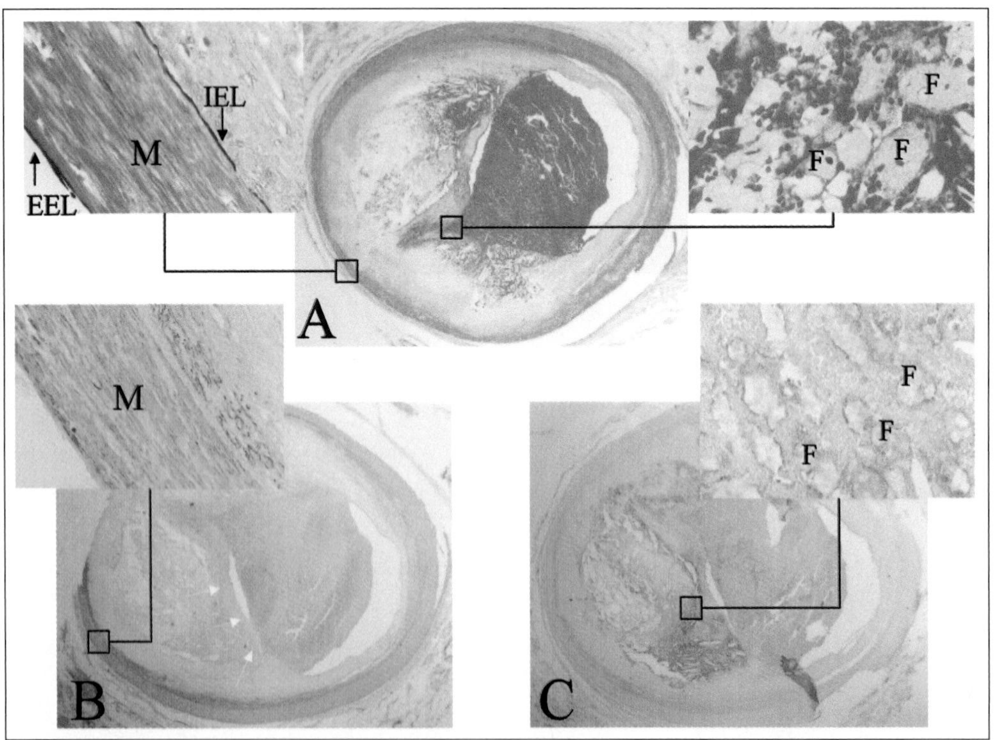

FIGURE 35–10 An example of a ruptured plaque that caused a fatal thrombosis. **A,** Movat stain. **B,** Immunostaining with HHF-35 discloses smooth muscle cells. Note the paucity of smooth muscle cells in the fibrous cap (white arrowheads), in contrast with the abundant smooth muscle cells in the medial layer (inset, M denotes the tunica media). **C,** Macrophage staining (CD-68) shows accumulation of the inflammatory cells near the fibrous cap (inset, F denotes foam cell). EEL = external elastic lamina; IEL = internal elastic lamina. (From Bezerra HG, Higuchi ML, Gutierrez PS, et al: Atheromas that cause fatal thrombosis are usually large and frequently accompanied by vessel enlargement. Cardiovasc Pathol 10:189, 2001.)

Plaque Rupture and Thrombosis

The rupture of the plaque's fibrous cap probably reflects an imbalance between the forces that impinge on the plaque's cap and the mechanical strength of the fibrous cap.[67] Interstitial forms of collagen provide most of the biomechanical resistance to disruption to the fibrous cap. Hence, the

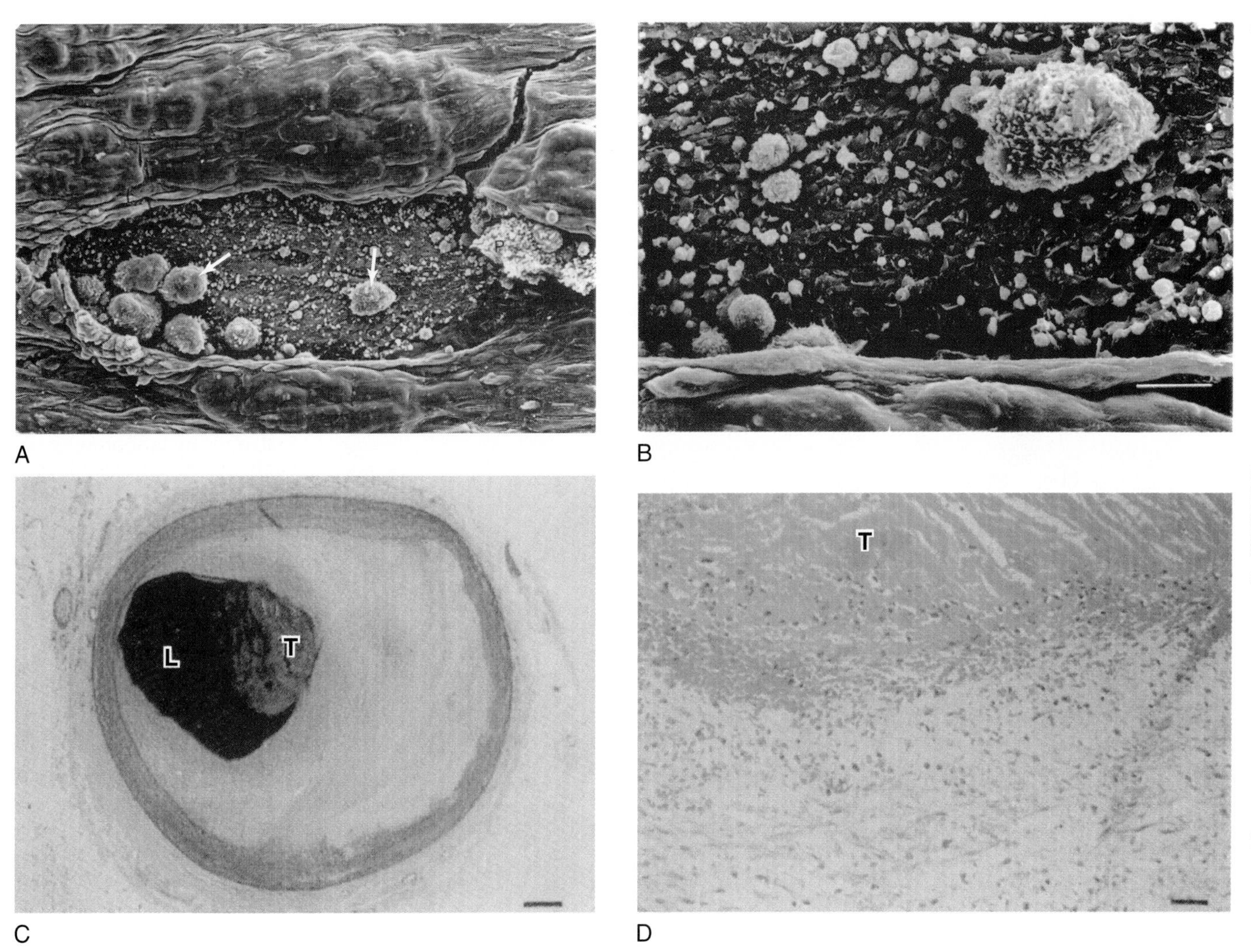

FIGURE 35–11 Superficial erosion of experimental atherosclerotic lesions shown by scanning electron microscopy. Advanced atherosclerotic plaques can promote thrombosis by superficial erosion of the endothelial layer, exposing the blood and platelets to the subendothelial basement membrane containing collagen platelet activation and thrombosis. **A,** In the low-power view, the rent in the endothelium is evident. Leukocytes have adhered to the subendothelium, which is beginning to be covered with a carpet of platelets (arrows). **B,** The high-power view shows a field selected from the center of part A that shows the leukocytes and platelets adherent to the subendothelium. **C,** A low-power histological section through a coronary artery thrombosed due to superficial erosion. **D,** A higher power histological section through a coronary artery thrombosed due to superficial erosion. L = lumen; T = thrombus. (**A** & **B,** from Faggiotto A, Ross R: Studies of hypercholesterolemia in the nonhuman primate. II. Fatty streak conversion to fibrous plaque. Arteriosclerosis 4: 341, 1984. **C** & **D,** from Farb A, Burke AP, Tang AL, et al: Coronary plaque erosion without rupture into a lipid core: A frequent cause of coronary thrombosis in sudden coronary death. Circulation 93:1354, 1996.)

metabolism of collagen probably participates in regulating the propensity of a plaque to rupture (Fig. 35–12). Factors that decrease collagen synthesis by smooth muscle cells can impair their ability to repair and maintain the plaque's fibrous cap. For example, the T-cell–derived cytokine interferon gamma potently inhibits smooth muscle cell collagen synthesis. On the other hand, as already noted, certain mediators released from platelet granules during activation can increase smooth muscle cell collagen synthesis, tending to reinforce the plaque's fibrous structure. Such mediators include TGF-β and PDGF.

In addition to reduced de novo collagen synthesis by smooth muscle cells, increased catabolism of the extracellular matrix macromolecules that comprise the fibrous cap can also contribute to weakening of this structure and rendering it susceptible to rupture and hence thrombosis. The same matrix-degrading enzymes thought to contribute to smooth muscle migration and arterial remodeling can also contribute to weakening of the fibrous cap (see Fig. 35–12). Macrophages in cases of advanced human atheroma overexpress matrix metalloproteinases and elastolytic cathepsins that can break down the collagen and elastin of the arterial extracellular matrix.[68,69] Thus, the strength of the plaque's fibrous cap is under dynamic regulation, linking the inflammatory response in the intima with the molecular determinants of plaque stability and hence thrombotic complications of atheroma. The thinning of the plaque's fibrous cap, a result of reduced collagen synthesis and increased degradation, probably explains why pathological studies have shown that thin fibrous cap characterizes atherosclerotic plaques that have ruptured and caused fatal myocardial infarction.[70]

Another feature of the so-called "vulnerable" atherosclerotic plaque defined by pathological analysis is a relative lack of smooth muscle cells (see Fig. 35–10B). As explained earlier, inflammatory mediators both soluble and associated with the surface of T-lymphocytes can provoke programmed cell death of smooth muscle cells. "Dropout" of smooth muscle cells from regions of local inflammation within plaques probably contributes to the relative lack of smooth muscle cells at places where plaques rupture. Since these cells are the source of the newly synthesized collagen needed to repair and maintain the matrix of the fibrous cap, the lack

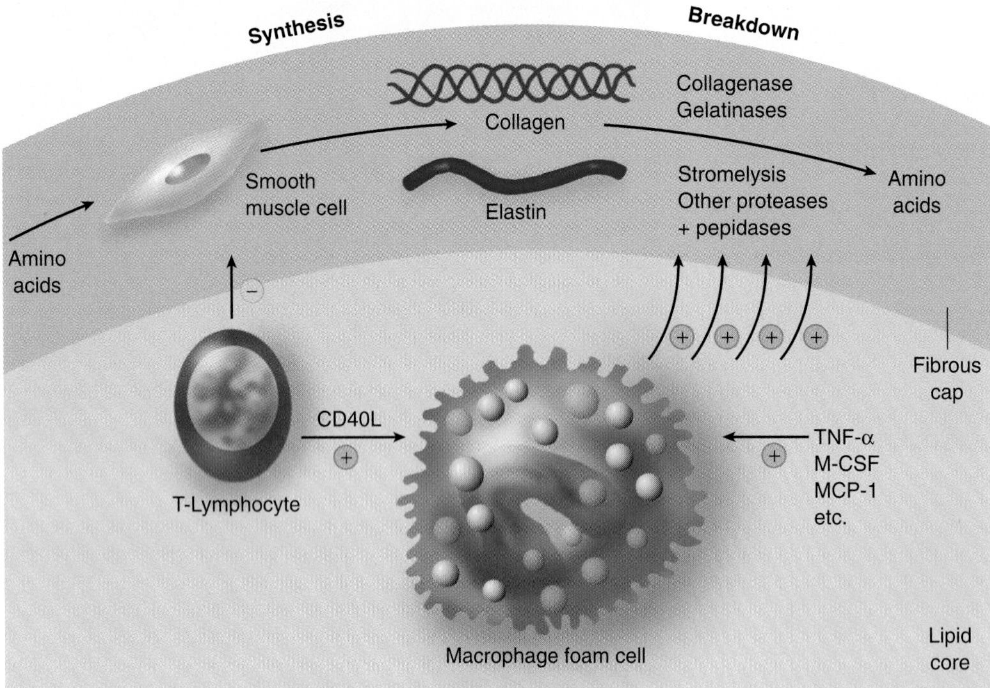

FIGURE 35–12 A schematic relating extracellular matrix metabolism to intimal inflammation during atherogenesis. The lymphocyte can elaborate gamma interferon (γ-IFN) that inhibits smooth muscle cell collagen production. The lymphocyte can also signal either by elaboration of soluble mediators or by contact activation of macrophages. Other cytokines produced in response to products of oxidized lipoproteins, among other stimuli, can further activate the macrophage. The activated phagocyte can release collagen degrading matrix metalloproteinases, and elastolytic enzymes including certain nonmetalloenzymes, such as cathepsins S and K. These enzymes promote matrix catabolism. Thus, in states characterized by heightened intimal inflammation, the extracellular matrix that confers biomechanical strength to the plaque's fibrous cap is under double attack: decreased synthesis and increased degradation. This results in a weakening and thinning of the fibrous cap, features associated in pathological studies with fatal atheromatous plaque disruptions and thrombosis. (From Libby P: The molecular bases of the acute coronary syndromes. Circulation 91:2844, 1995.)

of smooth muscle cells may contribute to weakening of the fibrous cap and hence the propensity of that plaque to rupture.[63]

A prominent accumulation of macrophages and a large lipid pool is a third microanatomical feature of the so-called "vulnerable" atherosclerotic plaque. From a strictly biomechanical viewpoint, a large lipid pool can serve to concentrate biomechanical forces on the shoulder regions of plaques, common sites of rupture of the fibrous cap. From a metabolic standpoint, the activated macrophage characteristic of the plaque's core region produces the cytokines and the matrix-degrading enzymes thought to regulate aspects of matrix catabolism and smooth muscle cell apoptosis in turn. Apoptotic macrophages as well as smooth muscle cells can generate particulate tissue factor, a potential instigator of microvascular thrombosis after spontaneous or iatrogenic plaque disruption. The success of lipid-lowering therapy in reducing the incidence of acute myocardial infarction or unstable angina in patients at risk may result from a reduced accumulation of lipid and decrease in inflammation and plaque thrombogenicity. Recent animal studies and monitoring of peripheral markers of inflammation in humans support this concept.[71-76]

Thrombosis due to Superficial Erosion of Plaques

The foregoing section discusses the pathophysiology of rupture of the plaque's fibrous cap. The pathobiology of superficial erosion is much less well understood. In experimental atherosclerosis in the nonhuman primate, areas of endothelial loss and platelet deposition occur in the more advanced plaques (see Fig. 35–11). In humans, superficial erosion appears more likely to cause fatal acute myocardial infarction in women and in individuals with hypertriglyceridemia and diabetes mellitus.[77,78] However, the underlying molecular mechanisms remain obscure. Apoptosis of endothelial cells could contribute to desquamation of endothelial cells in areas of superficial erosion. Likewise, matrix metalloproteinases such as certain gelatinases specialized in degrading the nonfibrillar collagen found in the basement membrane, such as collagen type IV, might also sever the tetherings of the endothelial cell to the subjacent basal lamina and promote their desquamation.[79]

Most plaque disruptions do not give rise to clinically apparent coronary events. Careful pathoanatomical examination of hearts obtained from individuals who have succumbed to noncardiac death have shown a surprisingly high incidence of focal plaque disruptions with limited mural thrombi. Moreover, hearts fixed immediately after explantation from individuals with severe but chronic stable coronary atherosclerosis and who had undergone transplantation for ischemic cardiomyopathy show similar evidence for ongoing but asymptomatic plaque disruption. Experimentally, in atherosclerotic nonhuman primates, mural platelet thrombi can complicate plaque erosions without causing arterial occlusion. Therefore, repetitive cycles of plaque disruption, thrombosis in situ, and healing probably contribute to lesion evolution and plaque growth. Such episodes of thrombosis and healing constitute one type of "crisis" in the history of a plaque that may cause a burst of smooth muscle cell proliferation, migration, and matrix synthesis. The TGF-β and PDGF released from platelet granules stimulate collagen synthesis by smooth muscle cells, as noted earlier. Thrombin, generated at sites of mural thrombosis, potently stimulates smooth muscle cell proliferation. The late-stage or "burned out" fibrous and calcific atheroma may represent a late stage of a plaque previously lipid-rich and vulnerable but now rendered fibrous and hypocellular due to a wound healing response mediated by the products of thrombosis.

Diffuse and Systemic Nature of Plaque Vulnerability and Inflammation in Atherogenesis

Studies at autopsy of atherosclerotic plaques that caused fatal thrombosis brought the notion of the vulnerability of high-risk plaque to the fore. This stimulated many investigators to seek ways of identifying and treating such high-risk atherosclerotic lesions.[80-84] However, current evidence suggests that such high-risk plaques are indeed numerous in a given coronary tree. Moreover, the inflammation thought to characterize the so-called vulnerable plaque appears widespread. Studies using various imaging modalities have underscored the multiplicity of such high-risk plaques. Careful analysis of angiograms of individuals with acute coronary syndromes has demonstrated evidence for plaque ulceration or thrombosis in more than one lesion in many cases.[85] Individuals with multiple unstable lesions by angiographic criteria tend to have worse outcomes during follow-up. Angioscopic studies have also shown multiple sites of intracoronary thrombosis in patients with acute coronary syndromes.[86] Systematic studies by intravascular ultrasonography of the coronary arterial system in individuals with acute coronary syndromes have revealed that more than 80 percent of such individuals have more than one disrupted atherosclerotic plaque.[87]

Several concordant lines of evidence support the systemic and diffuse nature of inflammation in individuals with acute coronary syndromes. Maseri's group demonstrated a transmyocardial gradient in the inflammatory marker myeloperoxidase when sampling from the great cardiac vein (draining the left coronary territory) in individuals with both left and right coronary artery culprit lesions.[88] Moreover, several studies have shown that various systemic markers of inflammation such as C-reactive protein increase in patients at risk for acute coronary syndromes. This is so even in the absence of biochemical evidence of myocardial injury (e.g., elevated troponin levels) that might elicit a secondary acute phase response.[89] Thus, a combination of imaging studies and investigations using inflammatory markers support the diffuse and systemic nature of instability of atheromata in individuals with or at risk for acute coronary syndromes. This recognition has important therapeutic implications. In addition to revascularization strategies, such individuals should have systemic therapy aimed at stabilizing the usually multiple high-risk lesions that may cause recurrent events.

Special Cases of Arteriosclerosis

Restenosis after Arterial Intervention

(see Chap. 52)

The problem of restenosis after percutaneous arterial intervention represents a special case of arteriosclerosis. After balloon angioplasty, luminal narrowing recurs in approximately one-third of cases within 6 months (see Chap. 52). Initially, work on the pathophysiology of restenosis after angioplasty focused on smooth muscle proliferation. A good deal of the thinking regarding the pathobiology of restenosis depended on extension to the human situation of the results of withdrawal of an overinflated balloon in a previously normal rat carotid artery. Study of this very well standardized preparation promoted precise understanding of the kinetics of intimal thickening after this type of injury. However, the attempts to transfer this information to cases of human restenosis met with considerable frustration. This disparity between the balloon withdrawal injury of animal arteries and human restenosis is not surprising. The substrate of animal studies was usually a normal rather than an atherosclerotic artery, with all the attendant cellular and molecular differences highlighted earlier. Moreover, a high-pressure inflation of an angioplasty balloon only vaguely resembles the overinflated balloon withdrawal injury commonly practiced in rats.

Although smooth muscle cell proliferation appears prominent in the simple experimental models of intimal thickening, observations on human specimens showed relatively low rates of smooth muscle cell proliferation and called into question therapeutic targeting of this process. Moreover, intravascular ultrasonographic studies in humans and considerable evidence from animal experimentation suggested that a substantial proportion of the loss of luminal caliber after balloon angioplasty resulted from a constriction of the vessel from the adventitial side ("negative remodeling").[5,90] These observations renewed interest in adventitial inflammation with scar formation and wound contraction as a mechanism of arterial constriction following balloon angioplasty.[91]

The widespread introduction of stents has changed the face of the restenosis problem. The process of in-stent stenosis, in contrast with restenosis after balloon angioplasty, depends uniquely on intimal thickening, as opposed to "negative remodeling." The stent provides a firm scaffold that prevents constriction from the adventitia. Histological analyses reveal that a great deal of the volume of the in-stent restenotic lesion is made up of "myxomatous" tissue, comprising occasional stellate smooth muscle cells embedded in a loose and highly hydrated extracellular matrix.[92]

The introduction of stents has reduced the clinical impact of restenosis because of the very effective increase in luminal diameter achieved by this technique. Even if a considerable degree of lumen loss occurs due to intimal thickening, the luminal caliber remains sufficient to alleviate the patient's symptoms because of the excellent dilation achieved. Radiation treatment, presumably targeting smooth muscle proliferation and matrix synthesis, proved useful as a therapeutic approach to limiting in-stent restenosis. Currently, stents that elaborate antiproliferative and antiinflammatory substances have shown great benefit in terms of preventing in-stent stenosis (see Chap. 52).[93-95]

Accelerated Arteriosclerosis after Transplantation

Since the advent of effective immunosuppressive therapy such as cyclosporin, the major limitation to long-term survival of cardiac allografts is the development of an accelerated form of arterial hyperplastic disease (see Chap. 26). We favor the term *arteriosclerosis* ("hardening of the arteries") rather than *atherosclerosis* ("gruel-hardening") to describe this process because of the inconstant association with lipids (the "gruel" in atherosclerosis).[96] This form of arterial disease often presents a diagnostic challenge. The patient may not experience typical anginal symptoms because of the interruption of cardiac denervation after transplantation. In addition, graft coronary disease is concentric and diffuse, not only affecting the proximal epicardial coronary vessels but also penetrating smaller intramyocardial branches (Fig. 35–13). For this reason, the angiogram, well suited to visualizing focal and eccentric stenoses, consistently underestimates the degree of transplantation arteriosclerosis.

In most centers, a majority of patients undergoing transplantation have atherosclerotic disease and ischemic cardiomyopathy. However, a sizeable minority of patients undergo heart transplantation for idiopathic dilated cardiomyopathy and may have few if any risk factors for atherosclerosis. Even in the absence of traditional risk factors, this latter group of individuals shares the risk of developing accelerated arteriosclerosis. This observation suggests that the pathophysiology of this form of accelerated arteriosclerosis differs from that of usual atherosclerosis.

The selective involvement of the engrafted vessels with sparing of the host's native arteries suggests that accelerated arteriopathy does not merely result from the immunosuppressive therapy or other systemic factors in the transplantation recipient. Rather, these observations suggest that the immunological differences between the host and the recipient vessels might contribute to the pathogenesis of this

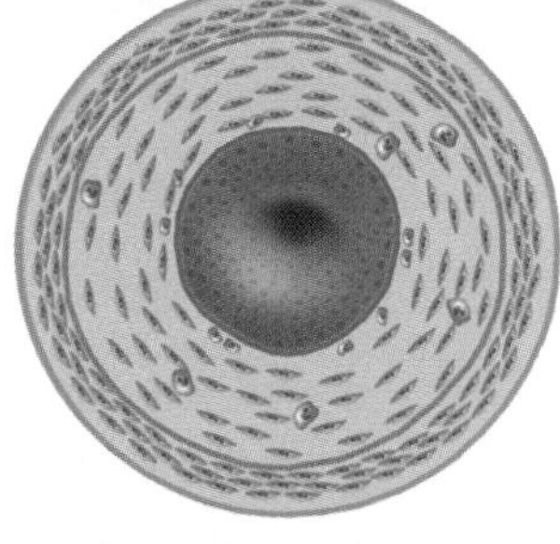

FIGURE 35–13 Comparison of usual atherosclerosis and transplantation arteriosclerosis. Usual atherosclerosis **(left panel)** characteristically forms an eccentric lesion with a lipid core and fibrous capsule. In contrast, the lesion of transplantation-associated accelerated arteriosclerosis **(right panel)** characteristically has a concentric intimal expansion without a clear central lipid core.

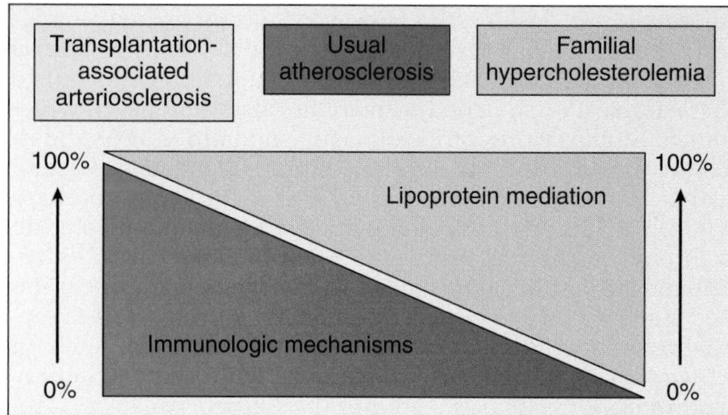

FIGURE 35–14 A multifactorial view of the pathogenesis of atherosclerosis. This diagram depicts two extreme cases of atherosclerosis. One **(far left)** represents accelerated arteriosclerosis that can occur in the transplanted heart in the absence of traditional coronary risk factors. This disease likely represents primarily immune-mediated arterial intimal disease. The other extreme **(far right)** depicts the case of a child who may succumb to rampant atherosclerosis in the first decade of life due solely to an elevated low-density lipoprotein (LDL) level caused by a mutation in the LDL receptor (homozygous familial hypercholesterolemia). Between these two extremes lie the vast majority of patients with atherosclerosis, probably involving various mixtures of immune and inflammatory and/or lipoprotein-mediated disease. One can further consider that this diagram extends to a third dimension that would involve other candidate risk factors such as homocysteine, lipoprotein (a), infection, tobacco abuse, and so on.

disease. Considerable evidence from both human and experimental studies currently supports this viewpoint. Endothelial cells in the transplanted coronary arteries express histocompatibility antigens that can engender an allogeneic immune response from host T cells. The activated T cells can secrete cytokines (e.g., interferon-gamma) that can augment histocompatibility gene expression, recruit leukocytes by induction of adhesion molecules, and activate macrophages to produce smooth muscle cell chemoattractants and growth factors. Interruption of interferon-gamma signaling can prevent experimental graft coronary disease in mice.[97] This disease appears to occur despite cyclosporin therapy, because this immunosuppressant is relatively ineffective as a suppressor of the endothelial allogeneic response. Indeed, immunosuppressive agents that more effectively suppress the endothelial allogeneic response appear effective in retarding graft arteriosclerosis.

The data summarized suggest that graft arteriosclerosis represents an extreme case of the immunologically driven arterial hyperplasia (Fig. 35–14) that can occur in the absence of other risk factors. On the other extreme, patients with homozygous familial hypercholesterolemia can develop fatal atherosclerosis in the first decade of life due solely to an elevation in LDL cholesterol. The vast majority of patients with atherosclerosis fall somewhere between these two extremes. Analysis of usual atherosclerotic lesions shows evidence for a chronic immune response and lipid accumulation. Therefore, by studying the extreme cases, such as transplantation arteriopathy and familial hypercholesterolemia, one can gain insight into elements of the pathophysiology that contribute to the multifactorial form of atherosclerosis that affects the majority of patients.

Aneurysmal Disease

Atherosclerosis produces not only stenoses but also aneurysmal disease (see Chap. 53). Why does a single disease process manifest itself in directionally opposite manner, for example, most commonly producing stenoses in the coronary arteries but causing ectasia of the abdominal aorta? In particular, aneurysmal disease characteristically affects the infrarenal abdominal aorta. This region is highly prone to the development of atherosclerosis. Data from the Pathobiological Determinants of Atherosclerosis In Youth Study (PDAY) show that the dorsal surface of the infrarenal abdominal aorta has a particular predilection for development of fatty streaks and raised lesions in Americans younger than 35 years of age who succumbed for noncardiac reasons (see Fig. 35–1).[3] Due to the absence of vasa vasorum, the relative lack of blood supply to the tunica media in this portion of the abdominal aorta might explain the regional susceptibility of this portion of the arterial tree to aneurysm formation. In addition, the lumbar lordosis of the biped human may alter the hydrodynamics of blood flow in the distal aorta, yielding flow disturbances that may promote lesion formation.

Histological examination shows considerable distinction between occlusive atherosclerotic disease and aneurysmal disease. In typical cases of coronary artery atherosclerosis, expansion of the intimal lesion produces stenotic lesions. The tunica media underlying the expanded intima is often thinned, but its general structure remains relatively well preserved. In contrast, transmural destruction of the arterial architecture occurs in patients with aneurysmal disease. In particular, the usually well defined laminar structure of the normal tunica media disappears with obliteration of the elastic laminae. The medial smooth muscle cells, usually well preserved in typical stenotic lesions, are notable for their paucity in the media of advanced aortic aneurysms.

Study of the pathophysiology that underlies these anatomical pathological findings has proved frustrating. Informative animal models are not available. The human specimens obtainable for analysis generally represent the late stages of this disease. Nonetheless, recent work has identified several mechanisms that may underlie the peculiar pathological features of aneurysmal disease. Widespread destruction of the elastic laminae suggests a role for degradation of elastin, collagen, and other constituents of the arterial extracellular matrix.[98] Many studies have documented overexpression of matrix-degrading proteinases, including matrix metalloproteinases in human aortic aneurysm specimens. Indeed, current clinical trials are testing the hypothesis that matrix metalloproteinase inhibitors can reduce the expansion of aneurysms.[99] Recent experimental work has implicated angiotensin II as a potentiator of aneurysm formation in atherosclerotic mice.[100]

Thus, heightened elastolysis may explain the breakdown of the usually ordered structure of the tunica media in cases of this disease. A slant toward T helper cell Th2 populations in cases of aneurysmal as opposed to occlusive disease may contribute to the overexpression of certain elastolytic enzymes.[101] In addition, aortic aneurysms show evidence for considerable inflammation, particularly in the adventitia.[102] The lymphocytes that characteristically abound on the adventitial side of aneurysmal tissue suggest that apoptosis of smooth muscle cells triggered by inflammatory mediators including soluble cytokines and *fas* ligand, elaborated by these inflammatory cells, may contribute to smooth muscle cell destruction and promote aneurysm formation.[103] Although extracellular matrix degradation and smooth muscle cell death also occur in sites where atherosclerosis causes stenosis, they appear to predominate in regions of aneurysm formation and to affect the tunica media much more extensively, for reasons that remain obscure.

Infection and Atherosclerosis

Recently, interest has increased in the possibility that infections may cause atherosclerosis. A considerable body of seroepidemiological evidence supports a role for certain bacteria, notably *Chlamydia pneumoniae*, and certain viruses, notably cytomegalovirus, in the origin of atherosclerosis.[104–106] The seroepidemiological studies have spurred a number of in vivo and in vitro experiments that lend varying degrees of support to this concept. In evaluation of the seroepidemiological evidence, several caveats apply. First, confounding factors should be carefully considered.[107] For example, smokers may have a higher incidence of bronchitis due to *C. pneumoniae*. Therefore, evidence of infection with *C. pneumoniae* may merely serve as a marker for tobacco use, a known risk factor for atherosclerotic events. Additionally, a strong bias favors publication of studies with positive findings over studies with negative findings. Thus, meta-analyses of seroepidemiological studies may be slanted toward the positive merely because of underreporting of negative findings. Finally, atherosclerosis is a common and virtually ubiquitous disease in developed countries. In most societies, many adults have serological evidence of prior infections with Herpes viridae such as cytomegalovirus and respiratory pathogens such as *C. pneumoniae*. It is difficult to sort out coincidence from causality when the majority of the population studied has evidence of both infection and atherosclerosis.

Although proof that bacteria or viruses can cause atherosclerosis remains elusive, it is quite plausible that infections can potentiate the action of traditional risk factors, such as hypercholesterolemia. Based on the vascular biology of atherosclerosis discussed in this chapter, a number of scenarios might apply. First, cells within the atheroma itself can be a site for infection. For example, macrophages existing in an established atherosclerotic lesion might become infected with *C. pneumoniae*, which could spur their activation and accelerate the inflammatory pathways that we currently believe operate within the atherosclerotic intima. Specific microbial products, such as lipopolysaccharides, heat shock proteins, or other virulence factors might act locally at the level of the artery wall to potentiate atherosclerosis in infected lesions.[108-114]

Extravascular infection might also influence the development of atheromatous lesions and provoke their complication. For example, circulating endotoxin or cytokines produced in response to a remote infection can act locally at the level of the artery wall to promote the activation of vascular cells and of leukocytes in preexisting lesions, producing an "echo" at the level of the artery wall of a remote infection.[105] Also, the acute phase response to an infection in a nonvascular site might affect the incidence of thrombotic complications of atherosclerosis by increasing fibrinogen or plasminogen activator inhibitor or otherwise altering the balance between coagulation and fibrinolysis. Such disturbance in the prevailing prothrombotic, fibrinolytic balance could critically influence whether a given plaque disruption will produce a clinically inapparent transient or nonocclusive thrombus, or sustained and occlusive thrombi that could cause an acute coronary event.

Acute infections might also produce hemodynamic alterations that could trigger coronary events. For example, the tachycardia and increased metabolic demands of fever could augment the oxygen requirements of the heart, precipitating ischemia in an otherwise compensated individual. These various scenarios illustrate how infectious processes, either local in the atheroma or extravascular, might aggravate atherogenesis, particularly in preexisting lesions or in concert with traditional risk factors. However, recent clinical trials have not shown that treatment with azithromycin for 12 weeks can reduce recurrent coronary events in survivors of myocardial infarction.[115] Even if the findings of ongoing studies with more prolonged antibiotic treatment were positive, they would not establish a role for a particular infectious agent, nor could they prove that the antibiotic effect of the agents tested, rather than some other action not related to their antimicrobial effect, produces benefit.[116,117]

REFERENCES

1. Libby P, Aikawa M, Schonbeck U: Cholesterol and atherosclerosis. Biochim Biophys Acta 1529:299, 2000.
2. Gimbrone MA Jr, Nagel T, Topper JN: Biomechanical activation: An emerging paradigm in endothelial adhesion biology. J Clin Invest 100:S61, 1997.
3. Strong JP, Malcom GT, McMahan CA, et al: Prevalence and extent of atherosclerosis in adolescents and young adults: Implications for prevention from the Pathobiological Determinants of Atherosclerosis in Youth Study. JAMA 281:727, 1999.
4. Tuzcu EM, Kapadia SR, Tutar E, et al: High prevalence of coronary atherosclerosis in asymptomatic teenagers and young adults: Evidence from intravascular ultrasound. Circulation 103:2705, 2001.
5. Pasterkamp G, de Kleijn DP, Borst C: Arterial remodeling in atherosclerosis, restenosis and after alteration of blood flow: Potential mechanisms and clinical implications. Cardiovasc Res 45:843, 2000.
6. Kruth HS: The fate of lipoprotein cholesterol entering the arterial wall. Curr Opin Lipidol 8:246, 1997.
7. Camejo G, Hurt-Camejo E, Wiklund O, et al: Association of apo B lipoproteins with arterial proteoglycans: Pathological significance and molecular basis. Atherosclerosis 139:205, 1998.
8. Williams KJ, Tabas I: The response-to-retention hypothesis of atherogenesis reinforced. Curr Opin Lipidol 9:471, 1998.
9. Witztum JL, Berliner JA: Oxidized phospholipids and isoprostanes in atherosclerosis. Curr Opin Lipidol 9:441, 1998.
10. Rong JX, Rangaswamy S, Shen L, et al: Arterial injury by cholesterol oxidation products causes endothelial dysfunction and arterial wall cholesterol accumulation. Arterioscler Thromb Vasc Biol 18:1885, 1998.
11. Tabas I: Nonoxidative modifications of lipoproteins in atherogenesis. Ann Rev Nutr 19:123, 1999.
12. Ushio-Fukai M, Alexander RW, Akers M, et al: p38 Mitogen-activated protein kinase is a critical component of the redox-sensitive signaling pathways activated by angiotensin II: Role in vascular smooth muscle cell hypertrophy. J Biol Chem 273:15022, 1998.
13. Cyrus T, Witztum JL, Rader DJ, et al: Disruption of the 12/15-lipoxygenase gene diminishes atherosclerosis in apo E-deficient mice. J Clin Invest 103:1597, 1999.
14. Sugiyama S, Okada Y, Sukhova GK, et al: Macrophage myeloperoxidase regulation by granulocyte macrophage colony-stimulating factor in human atherosclerosis and implications in acute coronary syndromes. Am J Pathol 158:879, 2001.
15. Nakashima Y, Raines EW, Plump AS, et al: Upregulation of VCAM-1 and ICAM-1 at atherosclerosis-prone sites on the endothelium in the apoE-deficient mouse. Arterioscler Thromb Vasc Biol 18:842, 1998.
16. Iiyama K, Hajra L, Iiyama M, et al: Patterns of vascular cell adhesion molecule-1 and intercellular adhesion molecule-1 expression in rabbit and mouse atherosclerotic lesions and at sites predisposed to lesion formation. Circ Res 85:199, 1999.
17. Ley K: The role of selectins in inflammation and disease. Trends Mol Med 9:263, 2003.
18. Vora DK, Fang ZT, Liva SM, et al: Induction of P-selectin by oxidized lipoproteins: Separate effects on synthesis and surface expression. Circ Res 80:810, 1997.
19. Dong ZM, Brown AA, Wagner DD: Prominent role of P-selectin in the development of advanced atherosclerosis in ApoE-deficient mice. Circulation 101:2290, 2000.
20. Ley K, Huo Y: VCAM-1 is critical in atherosclerosis. J Clin Invest 107:1209, 2001.
21. Cybulsky MI, Iiyama K, Li H, et al: A major role for VCAM-1, but not ICAM-1, in early atherosclerosis. J Clin Invest 107:1255, 2001.
22. Dong ZM, Chapman SM, Brown AA, et al: The combined role of P- and E-selectins in atherosclerosis. J Clin Invest 102:145, 1998.
23. Luster AD: Chemokines: Chemotactic cytokines that mediate inflammation. N Engl J Med 338:436, 1998.

24. Gu L, Okada Y, Clinton S, et al: Absence of monocyte chemoattractant protein-1 reduces atherosclerosis in low-density lipoprotein-deficient mice. Mol Cell 2:275, 1998.
25. Boring L, Gosling J, Cleary M, et al: Decreased lesion formation in CCR2-/- mice reveals a role for chemokines in the initiation of atherosclerosis. Nature 394:894, 1998.
26. Boisvert WA, Curtiss LK, Terkeltaub RA: Interleukin-8 and its receptor CXCR2 in atherosclerosis. Immunol Res 21:129, 2000.
27. Lesnik P, Haskell CA, Charo IF: Decreased atherosclerosis in CX3CR1-/- mice reveals a role for fractalkine in atherogenesis. J Clin Invest 111:333, 2003.
28. Mach F, Sauty A, Iarossi AS, et al: Differential expression of three T lymphocyte-activating CXC chemokines by human atheroma-associated cells. J Clin Invest 104:1041, 1999.
29. Murry CE, Gipaya CT, Bartosek T, et al: Monoclonality of smooth muscle cells in human atherosclerosis. Am J Pathol 151:697, 1997.
30. Gimbrone MA Jr, Resnick N, Nagel T, et al: Hemodynamics, endothelial gene expression, and atherogenesis. Ann N Y Acad Sci 811:1, 1997.
31. Collins T, Cybulsky MI: NF-kappaB: Pivotal mediator or innocent bystander in atherogenesis? J Clin Invest 107:255, 2001.
32. Majesky MW: Vascular smooth muscle diversity: Insights from developmental biology. Curr Atheroscler Rep 5:208, 2003.
33. Landerholm TE, Dong XR, Lu J, et al: A role for serum response factor in coronary smooth muscle differentiation from proepicardial cells. Development 126:2053, 1999.
34. Shimizu K, Mitchell RN: Stem cell origins of intimal cells in graft arterial disease. Curr Atheroscler Rep 5:230, 2003.
35. Saiura A, Sata M, Hirata Y, et al: Circulating smooth muscle progenitor cells contribute to atherosclerosis. Nat Med 7:382, 2001.
36. Miller YI, Chang MK, Binder CJ, et al: Oxidized low density lipoprotein and innate immune receptors. Curr Opin Lipidol 14:437, 2003.

37. Sakaguchi H, Takeya M, Suzuki H, et al: Role of macrophage scavenger receptors in diet-induced atherosclerosis in mice. Lab Invest 78:423, 1998.
38. Rajavashisth T, Qiao JH, Tripathi S, et al: Heterozygous osteopetrotic (op) mutation reduces atherosclerosis in LDL receptor-deficient mice. J Clin Invest 101:2702, 1998.
39. Hansson GK, Libby P, Schonbeck U, et al: Innate and adaptive immunity in the pathogenesis of atherosclerosis. Circ Res 91:281, 2002.
40. Binder CJ, Chang MK, Shaw PX, et al: Innate and acquired immunity in atherogenesis. Nat Med 8:1218, 2002.
41. Griendling KK, Harrison DG: Out, damned dot: Studies of the NADPH oxidase in atherosclerosis. J Clin Invest 108:1423, 2001.
42. Pinderski LJ, Fischbein MP, Subbanagounder G, et al: Overexpression of interleukin-10 by activated T lymphocytes inhibits atherosclerosis in LDL receptor-deficient mice by altering lymphocyte and macrophage phenotypes. Circ Res 90:1064, 2002.
43. Geng YJ, Libby P: Progression of atheroma: A struggle between death and procreation. Arterioscler Thromb Vasc Biol 22:1370, 2002.
44. Littlewood TD, Bennett MR: Apoptotic cell death in atherosclerosis. Curr Opin Lipidol 14:469, 2003.
45. Nagai R, Suzuki T, Aizawa K, et al: Phenotypic modulation of vascular smooth muscle cells: Dissection of transcriptional regulatory mechanisms. Ann N Y Acad Sci 947:56, 2001.
46. Manabe I, Nagai R: Regulation of smooth muscle phenotype. Curr Atheroscler Rep 5:214, 2003.
47. Boyle JJ, Weissberg PL, Bennett MR: Tumor necrosis factor-{alpha} promotes macrophage-induced vascular smooth muscle cell apoptosis by direct and autocrine mechanisms. Arterioscler Thromb Vasc Biol 23:1553, 2003.
48. Wight TN: Versican: A versatile extracellular matrix proteoglycan in cell biology. Curr Opin Cell Biol 14:617, 2002.
49. Williams KJ: Arterial wall chondroitin sulfate proteoglycans: Diverse molecules with distinct roles in lipoprotein retention and atherogenesis. Curr Opin Lipidol 12:477, 2001.
50. Dollery CM, Humphries SE, McClelland A, et al: In vivo adenoviral gene transfer of TIMP-1 after vascular injury reduces neointimal formation. Ann N Y Acad Sci 878:742, 1999.
51. Couffinhal T, Kearney M, Witzenbichler B, et al: Vascular endothelial growth factor/vascular permeability factor (VEGF/VPF) in normal and atherosclerotic human arteries. Am J Pathol 150:1673, 1997.
52. Ramos MA, Kuzuya M, Esaki T, et al: Induction of macrophage VEGF in response to oxidized LDL and VEGF accumulation in human atherosclerotic lesions. Arterioscler Thromb Vasc Biol 18:1188, 1998.
53. Pipp F, Heil M, Issbrucker K, et al: VEGFR-1-selective VEGF homologue P1GF is arteriogenic: Evidence for a monocyte-mediated mechanism. Circ Res 92:378, 2003.
54. Vasse M, Pourtau J, Trochon V, et al: Oncostatin M induces angiogenesis in vitro and in vivo. Arterioscler Thromb Vasc Biol 19:1835, 1999.
55. Libby P: Current concepts of the pathogenesis of the acute coronary syndromes. Circulation 104:365, 2001.
56. Moulton KS, Heller E, Konerding MA, et al: Angiogenesis inhibitors endostatin or TNP-470 reduce intimal neovascularization and plaque growth in apolipoprotein E-deficient mice. Circulation 99:1726, 1999.
57. Kolodgie FD, Gold HK, Burke AP, et al: Intraplaque hemorrhage and progression of coronary atheroma. N Engl J Med 349:2316, 2003.
58. Doherty TM, Asotra K, Fitzpatrick LA, et al: Calcification in atherosclerosis: Bone biology and chronic inflammation at the arterial crossroads. Proc Natl Acad Sci U S A 100:11201, 2003.
59. Bini A, Mann KG, Kudryk BJ, et al: Noncollagenous bone matrix proteins, calcification, and thrombosis in carotid artery atherosclerosis. Arterioscler Thromb Vasc Biol 19:1852, 1999.
60. Yokoya K, Takatsu H, Suzuki T, et al: Process of progression of coronary artery lesions from mild or moderate stenosis to moderate or severe stenosis: A study based on four serial coronary arteriograms per year. Circulation 100:903, 1999.
61. Naghavi M, Libby P, Falk E, et al: From vulnerable plaque to vulnerable patient: A call for new definitions and risk assessment strategies: Part I. Circulation 108:1664, 2003.
62. Naghavi M, Libby P, Falk E, et al: From vulnerable plaque to vulnerable patient: A call for new definitions and risk assessment strategies: Part II. Circulation 108:1772, 2003.
63. Bezerra HG, Higuchi ML, Gutierrez PS, et al: Atheromas that cause fatal thrombosis are usually large and frequently accompanied by vessel enlargement. Cardiovasc Pathol 10:189, 2001.
64. Schoenhagen P, Ziada KM, Kapadia SR, et al: Extent and direction of arterial remodeling in stable versus unstable coronary syndromes: An intravascular ultrasound study. Circulation 101:598, 2000.
65. Schoenhagen P, Stone GW, Nissen SE, et al: Coronary plaque morphology and frequency of ulceration distant from culprit lesions in patients with unstable and stable presentation. Arterioscler Thromb Vasc Biol 23:1895, 2003.
66. Virmani R, Burke AP, Farb A, et al: Pathology of the unstable plaque. Prog Cardiovasc Dis 44:349, 2002.
67. Lee R, Libby P: The unstable atheroma. Arterioscler Thromb Vasc Biol 17:1859, 1997.
68. Sukhova GK, Shi GP, Simon DI, et al: Expression of the elastolytic cathepsins S and K in human atheroma and regulation of their production in smooth muscle cells. J Clin Invest 102:576, 1998.
69. Sukhova GK, Schonbeck U, Rabkin E, et al: Evidence for increased collagenolysis by interstitial collagenases-1 and -3 in vulnerable human atheromatous plaques. Circulation 99:2503, 1999.
70. Kolodgie FD, Burke AP, Farb A, et al: The thin-cap fibroatheroma: A type of vulnerable plaque: The major precursor lesion to acute coronary syndromes. Curr Opin Cardiol 16:285, 2001.
71. Aikawa M, Rabkin E, Okada Y, et al: Lipid lowering by diet reduces matrix metalloproteinase activity and increases collagen content of rabbit atheroma: A potential mechanism of lesion stabilization. Circulation 97:2433, 1998.
72. Aikawa M, Sugiyama S, Hill C, et al: Lipid lowering reduces oxidative stress and endothelial cell activation in rabbit atheroma. Circulation 106:1390, 2002.
73. Aikawa M, Voglic SJ, Sugiyama S, et al: Dietary lipid lowering reduces tissue factor expression in rabbit atheroma. Circulation 100:1215, 1999.
74. Fukumoto Y, Libby P, Rabkin E, et al: Statins alter smooth muscle cell accumulation and collagen content in established atheroma of Watanabe heritable hyperlipidemic rabbits. Circulation 103:993, 2001.
75. Ridker PM, Rifai N, Pfeffer MA, et al: Long-term effects of pravastatin on plasma concentration of C-reactive protein. The Cholesterol and Recurrent Events (CARE) Investigators. Circulation 100:230, 1999.
76. Libby P, Aikawa M: Stabilization of atherosclerotic plaques: New mechanisms and clinical targets. Nat Med 8:1257, 2002.
77. Burke A, Farb A, Malcom G, et al: Coronary risk factors and plaque morphology in men with coronary disease who died suddenly. N Engl J Med 336:1276, 1997.
78. Burke AP, Farb A, Malcom GT, et al: Effect of risk factors on the mechanism of acute thrombosis and sudden coronary death in women. Circulation 97:2110, 1998.
79. Rajavashisth TB, Liao JK, Galis ZS, et al: Inflammatory cytokines and oxidized low density lipoproteins increase endothelial cell expression of membrane type 1-matrix metalloproteinase. J Biol Chem 274:11924, 1999.
80. Madjid M, Naghavi M, Malik BA, et al: Thermal detection of vulnerable plaque. Am J Cardiol 90:36L, 2002.
81. Stefanadis C, Vavuranakis M, Toutouzas P: Vulnerable plaque: The challenge to identify and treat it. J Interv Cardiol 16:273, 2003.
82. Schaar JA, De Korte CL, Mastik F, et al: Characterizing vulnerable plaque features with intravascular elastography. Circulation 108:2636, 2003.
83. Tearney GJ, Yabushita H, Houser SL, et al: Quantification of macrophage content in atherosclerotic plaques by optical coherence tomography. Circulation 107:113, 2003.
84. MacNeill BD, Lowe HC, Takano M, et al: Intravascular modalities for detection of vulnerable plaque: Current status. Arterioscler Thromb Vasc Biol 23:1333, 2003.
85. Goldstein JA, Demetriou D, Grines CL, et al: Multiple complex coronary plaques in patients with acute myocardial infarction. N Engl J Med 343:915, 2000.
86. Asakura M, Ueda Y, Yamaguchi O, et al: Extensive development of vulnerable plaques as a pan-coronary process in patients with myocardial infarction: An angioscopic study. J Am Coll Cardiol 37:1284, 2001.
87. Rioufol G, Finet G, Ginon I, et al: Multiple atherosclerotic plaque rupture in acute coronary syndrome: A three-vessel intravascular ultrasound study. Circulation 106:804, 2002.
88. Buffon A, Biasucci LM, Liuzzo G, et al: Widespread coronary inflammation in unstable angina. N Engl J Med 347:5, 2002.
89. Libby P, Ridker PM, Maseri A: Inflammation and atherosclerosis. Circulation 105:1135, 2002.
90. Mintz GS, Kent KM, Pichard AD, et al: Contribution of inadequate arterial remodeling to the development of focal coronary artery stenoses: An intravascular ultrasound study. Circulation 95:1791, 1997.
91. Libby P, Simon DI, Rogers C: Inflammation and arterial injury. *In* Topol EJ (ed): Textbook of Interventional Cardiology. 4th ed. Philadelphia, Elsevier Science, 2003, p 381.
92. Orford JL, Selwyn AP, Ganz P, et al: The comparative pathobiology of atherosclerosis and restenosis. Am J Cardiol 86:6H, 2000.
93. Moses JW, Leon MB, Popma JJ, et al: Sirolimus-eluting stents versus standard stents in patients with stenosis in a native coronary artery. N Engl J Med 349:1315, 2003.
94. Marks AR: Sirolimus for the prevention of in-stent restenosis in a coronary artery. N Engl J Med 349:1307, 2003.
95. Bennett MR: In-stent stenosis: Pathology and implications for the development of drug eluting stents. Heart 89:218, 2003.
96. Libby P, Zhao DX: Allograft arteriosclerosis and immune-driven angiogenesis. Circulation 107:1237, 2003.
97. Nagano H, Mitchell RN, Taylor MK, et al: Interferon-gamma deficiency prevents coronary arteriosclerosis but not myocardial rejection in transplanted mouse hearts. J Clin Invest 100:550, 1997.

98. Thompson RW: Reflections on the pathogenesis of abdominal aortic aneurysms. Cardiovasc Surg 10:389, 2002.
99. Thompson RW, Baxter BT: MMP inhibition in abdominal aortic aneurysms: Rationale for a prospective randomized clinical trial. Ann N Y Acad Sci 878:159, 1999.
100. Manning MW, Cassi LA, Huang J, et al: Abdominal aortic aneurysms: Fresh insights from a novel animal model of the disease. Vasc Med 7:45, 2002.
101. Schonbeck U, Sukhova GK, Gerdes N, et al: T(H)2 predominant immune responses prevail in human abdominal aortic aneurysm. Am J Pathol 161:499, 2002.
102. McMillan WD, Pearce WH: Inflammation and cytokine signaling in aneurysms. Ann Vasc Surg 11:540, 1997.
103. Henderson EL, Geng YJ, Sukhova GK, et al: Death of smooth muscle cells and expression of mediators of apoptosis by T lymphocytes in human abdominal aortic aneurysms. Circulation 99:96, 1999.
104. Danesh J: Coronary heart disease, *Helicobacter pylori*, dental disease, *Chlamydia pneumoniae*, and cytomegalovirus: Meta-analyses of prospective studies. Am Heart J 138:S434, 1999.
105. Libby P, Egan D, Skarlatos S: Roles of infectious agents in atherosclerosis and restenosis: An assessment of the evidence and need for future research [review]. Circulation 96:4095, 1997.
106. O'Connor S, Taylor C, Campbell LA, et al: Potential infectious etiologies of atherosclerosis: A multifactorial perspective. Emerg Infect Dis 7:780, 2001.
107. Ridker PM: Are associations between infection and coronary disease causal or due to confounding? [editorial; comment]. Am J Med 106:376, 1999.
108. Kol A, Sukhova GK, Lichtman AH, et al: Chlamydial heat shock protein 60 localizes in human atheroma and regulates macrophage TNF-alpha and matrix metalloproteinase expression. Circulation 98:300, 1998.
109. Kol A, Bourcier T, Lichtman AH, et al: Chlamydial and human heat shock protein 60s activate human vascular endothelium, smooth muscle cells, and macrophages. J Clin Invest 103:571, 1999.
110. Kalayoglu MV, Byrne GI: Induction of macrophage foam cell formation by *Chlamydia pneumoniae*. J Infect Dis 177:725, 1998.
111. Kalayoglu MV, Byrne GI: A *Chlamydia pneumoniae* component that induces macrophage foam cell formation is chlamydial lipopolysaccharide. Infect Immun 66:5067, 1998.
112. Kalayoglu MV, Hoerneman B, LaVerda D, et al: Cellular oxidation of low-density lipoprotein by *Chlamydia pneumoniae*. J Infect Dis 180:780, 1999.
113. Kol A, Lichtman AH, Finberg RW, et al: Heat shock protein (HSP) 60 activates the innate immune response: CD14 is an essential receptor for HSP60 activation of mononuclear cells. J Immunol 164:13, 2000.
114. Kalayoglu MV, Libby P, Byrne GI: *Chlamydia pneumoniae* as an emerging risk factor in cardiovascular disease. JAMA 288:2724, 2002.
115. O'Connor CM, Dunne MW, Pfeffer MA, et al: Azithromycin for the secondary prevention of coronary heart disease events: The WIZARD study: A randomized controlled trial. JAMA 290:1459, 2003.
116. Cannon CP, McCabe CH, Belder R, et al: Design of the Pravastatin or Atorvastatin Evaluation and Infection Therapy (PROVE IT)-TIMI 22 trial. Am J Cardiol 89:860, 2002.
117. Grayston JT: Secondary prevention antibiotic treatment trials for coronary artery disease. Circulation 102:1742, 2000.

CHAPTER 36

Risk Factors for Atherothrombotic Disease

Paul M. Ridker • Peter Libby

Cardiovascular disease is the single most common cause of death in the developed world and accounts for almost 1 million fatalities each year in the United States alone. Of these cardiovascular deaths, nearly half result directly from coronary artery disease and another 20 percent from stroke. Given our current understanding of atherothrombosis, it is historically surprising that the conceptual basis for considering specific "cardiovascular risk factors" did not formally exist until the initial findings of the Framingham Heart Study began to appear in the early 1960s.

From an epidemiological perspective, a "risk factor" is a characteristic or feature of an individual or population that is present early in life and is associated with an increased risk of developing future disease. The risk factor of interest may be an acquired behavior (such as smoking), an inherited trait (such as familial hyperlipidemia), or a laboratory measure (such as cholesterol or C-reactive protein). For a risk factor to be causal, the marker of interest must predate the onset of disease and must have biological plausibility. Most risk factors used in daily practice have demonstrated a consistent graded-response effect and are substantiated by a large series of consistent prospective epidemiological studies in broad populations. Several risk factors, such as hyperlipidemia and hypertension, are modifiable, and trials have demonstrated that lowering these factors reduces vascular risk.

This chapter reviews in two parts the epidemiological evidence underlying risk factors for atherothrombosis. The first section describes the conventional risk factors of smoking, hypertension, hyperlipidemia, insulin resistance and diabetes, physical activity, and obesity as well as general strategies for reducing risk related to these disorders. This section also briefly reviews evidence relating mental stress, depression, and vascular risk.

Not all coronary events occur in individuals with multiple traditional risk factors, however, and in some individuals isolated abnormalities of inflammation, hemostasis, and/or thrombosis appear to play critical roles. In particular, nearly half of all myocardial infarctions and strokes occur among individuals without hyperlipidemia. Thus, the second section of the chapter reviews in detail a series of novel atherothrombotic risk factors, including high sensitivity C-reactive protein (hsCRP) and other markers of inflammation, homocysteine, and lipoprotein(a). This chapter also reviews data regarding hemostatic and thrombotic markers of risk, including fibrinogen, D-dimer, and abnormalities of intrinsic fibrinolysis. In each case, we present the evidence that describes whether these novel risk indicators add to risk prediction over and above conventional factors.

Conventional Risk Factors

Smoking

Cigarette consumption remains the single most important modifiable risk factor for coronary artery disease and the leading preventable cause of death in the United States, where it accounts for more than 400,000 deaths annually.[1] Of these, ischemic heart disease causes 35 to 40 percent of all smoking-related deaths, with an additional 8 percent attributable to second-hand smoke exposure. Despite the relative stability (25 percent) in prevalence of current smokers in the United States, rates of tobacco use are increasing among adolescents, young adults, and women.[2,3] Close to 1 million young Americans begin smoking each year.[4] Although increased recognition of the hazards of smoking might be hoped to slow these trends, nearly 1 billion individuals now smoke worldwide. Smoking has a particularly large impact in the Third World. Almost one-half billion individuals worldwide will eventually die of smoking-related complications.[5] Even among nonsmokers, we now recognize that inhaled smoke, whether from passive exposure or from cigar and pipe consumption, also increases coronary risk.[6,7] Passive smoking exposure can cause endothelial dysfunction in the coronary circulation even among otherwise healthy young nonsmokers.[8] The impact of passive smoking is complex, as this exposure also results in increased bronchial responsiveness and concomitant pulmonary dysfunction.[9]

Landmark studies in the early 1950s first reported strong positive associations between cigarette smoke exposure and coronary heart disease. Over the next 50 years, an exceptionally consistent series of prospective studies have documented clearly the effects of smoking on coronary risk. These studies suggest that, compared with nonsmokers, persons who consume 20 or more cigarettes daily have a two- to threefold increase in total coronary heart disease. Moreover, these effects depend on dose; consumption of as few as one to four cigarettes daily increases coronary artery disease risk. Such "light" levels of smoking have a major impact on myocardial infarction and all-cause mortality even among smokers who do not report inhalation.[10] Smoking acts synergistically with oral contraceptive agents, placing younger women taking oral contraceptives at even higher relative risk. In addition to myocardial infarction, cigarette consumption directly relates to increased rates of sudden death, aortic aneurysm formation, symptomatic peripheral vascular disease, and ischemic stroke. As for coronary disease, the risk of ischemic stroke directly increases with the number of cigarettes consumed. Recent prospective evidence also has linked cigarette consumption to elevated risk of hemorrhagic stroke, including both intracranial hemorrhage and subarachnoid hemorrhage, again in a dose-response manner.[11] Not surprisingly, continued smoking is also a major risk factor for recurrent myocardial infarction.[12]

Historically, cigarette consumption was prevalent among men before women and, at least in the United States, smoking prevalence remains lower among women than men. However, this gender gap has markedly narrowed, with overall consumption rates among women now in excess of 20 percent. Native Americans and those with less education have higher rates, whereas black and Hispanic women appear to consume less than white women (Fig. 36–1). Due to adverse synergy with oral contraceptives, young female smokers who take oral contraceptives have particularly elevated risks of premature coronary disease and stroke. Smoking is especially hazardous among women with diabetes.[13]

Beyond acute unfavorable effects on blood pressure, sympathetic tone, and a reduction in myocardial oxygen supply, smoking affects atherothrombosis by several other mechanisms. In addition to accelerating atherosclerotic progression,[14] long-term smoking may enhance oxidation of low-density lipoprotein (LDL) cholesterol and impairs endothelium-dependent coronary artery vasodilation. This latter effect has now been linked directly to dysfunctional endothelial nitric oxide biosynthesis following chronic as well as acute cigarette consumption.[15-17] In addition, smoking has adverse hemostatic and inflammatory effects, including increased levels of hsCRP, soluble intercellular adhesion molecule-1 (ICAM-1), fibrinogen, and homocysteine.[18-20] Additionally, smoking is associated with spontaneous platelet aggregation,[21] increased monocyte adhesion to endothelial cells,[22] and adverse alterations in endothelial derived fibrinolytic and antithrombotic factors, including tissue-type plasminogen activator and tissue pathway factor inhibitor.[23-25] Compared with nonsmokers, smokers have an increased prevalence of coronary spasm and may have reduced thresholds for ventricular arrhythmia. Accruing evidence suggests that insulin resistance represents an additional mechanistic link between smoking and premature atherosclerosis.[26]

Cessation of cigarette consumption constitutes the single most important intervention in preventive cardiology. In a recent major overview, smoking cessation reduced coronary heart disease mortality by 36 percent as compared with mortality in subjects who continued smoking, an effect that did not vary by age, gender, or country of origin.[27] In this analysis, the reduction in nonfatal myocardial reinfarction among those who stopped smoking (relative risk, 0.68; 95 percent confidence interval, 0.57-0.82) was almost identical to the overall reduction in total cardiovascular mortality (RR, 0.64; 95 percent CI, 0.58-0.71). These 35 to 40 percent risk reductions are at least as great as other secondary prevention interventions that have received far more attention from physicians, including the use of aspirin, statins, beta-blockade, and angiotensin-converting enzyme inhibitors. Similar benefits are present among persons with severe as well as mild systemic atherosclerosis.[28] Consistent data show that smoking cessation has immediate economic benefit across the health care system.[29]

In broad-based population studies, reductions in smoking from any mechanism improve health outcomes, particularly when linked to life-style changes, including exercise and dietary control.[30] Trials of nicotine replacement therapy using either transdermal nicotine or nicotine chewing gum have proven to greatly increase abstention rates after cessation. Such pharmacological programs, as well as physician-guided counseling, are cost-effective and should be provided as a standard prevention service.[31] Patients need to recognize that "low yield" cigarettes do not appear to reduce risks of myocardial infarction. Unfortunately, although the elevated cardiovascular risks associated with smoking decrease significantly after cessation, the risks of cancer of the lungs, pancreas, and stomach persist for more than a decade, as do the risks of developing chronic obstructive pulmonary disease. While smoking cessation has clear benefit, smoking reduction alone appears to have only marginal effect.[32]

Poor patient and physician understanding of the importance of smoking cessation continue. The observation that smoking predicts better outcome following various reperfusion strategies (the so-called "smoker's paradox") is not due to any benefit of smoking but simply to the fact that smokers are likely to undergo such procedures at a much younger age and hence have on average lower comorbidity. Despite public health legislation, the tobacco industry continues its aggressive targeting of young adults, who are most susceptible to new addiction.[33,34] Thus, primary prevention remains the most important population-based component of any smoking reduction strategy.

Hypertension (see Chaps. 37 and 38)

In contrast to cigarette consumption, hypertension is often a silent cardiovascular risk factor, and its prevalence is steadily increasing. Of the estimated 50 million Americans with high blood pressure, almost one-third evade diagnosis and only one-fourth receive effective treatment.[35] In the most recent National Health and Nutrition Examination Survey, 28.7 percent of subjects evaluated had a measured blood pressure greater than 140/90 mm Hg or reported use of antihypertensive medications, an increase of almost 4 percent from similar survey data a decade earlier.[36] Hypertension prevalence was highest in non-Hispanic blacks (33.5 percent), increased with age (reaching more than 65 percent after the age of 60 years), and tended to be more prevalent in women than men. Although 68 percent of

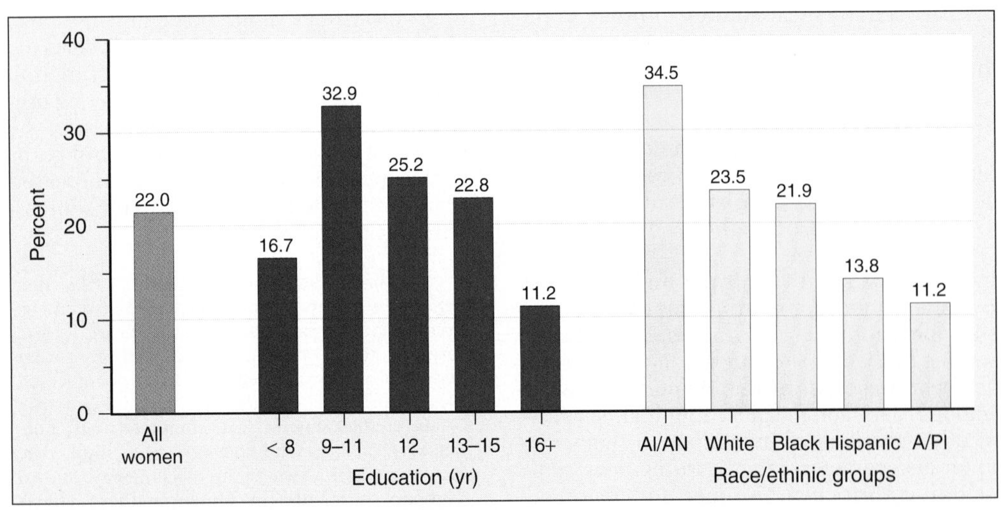

FIGURE 36–1 Prevalence of current smoking among American women aged 18 and older by education and by race/ethnicity. (From the National Health Interview Survey, US Department of Health and Human Services, Centers for Disease Control and Prevention.) AI/AN = American Indian/Alaska Native; A/PI = Asian/Pacific Islander.

the study participants were aware of their hypertension, only 58 percent were under therapy and 31 percent had their hypertension controlled (Fig. 36–2). Thus, in contrast to hyperlipidemia, hypertension prevalence is increasing and treatment rates remain poor, highlighting the need for programs targeting prevention. These trends are even more worrisome in Europe, where the prevalence of hypertension is 60 percent higher than in the United States and Canada. In sample surveys from nine nations, an average blood pressure observed in the European centers was 136/83 mm Hg, compared with an average blood pressure of 122/77 mm Hg in U.S. and Canadian centers.[37]

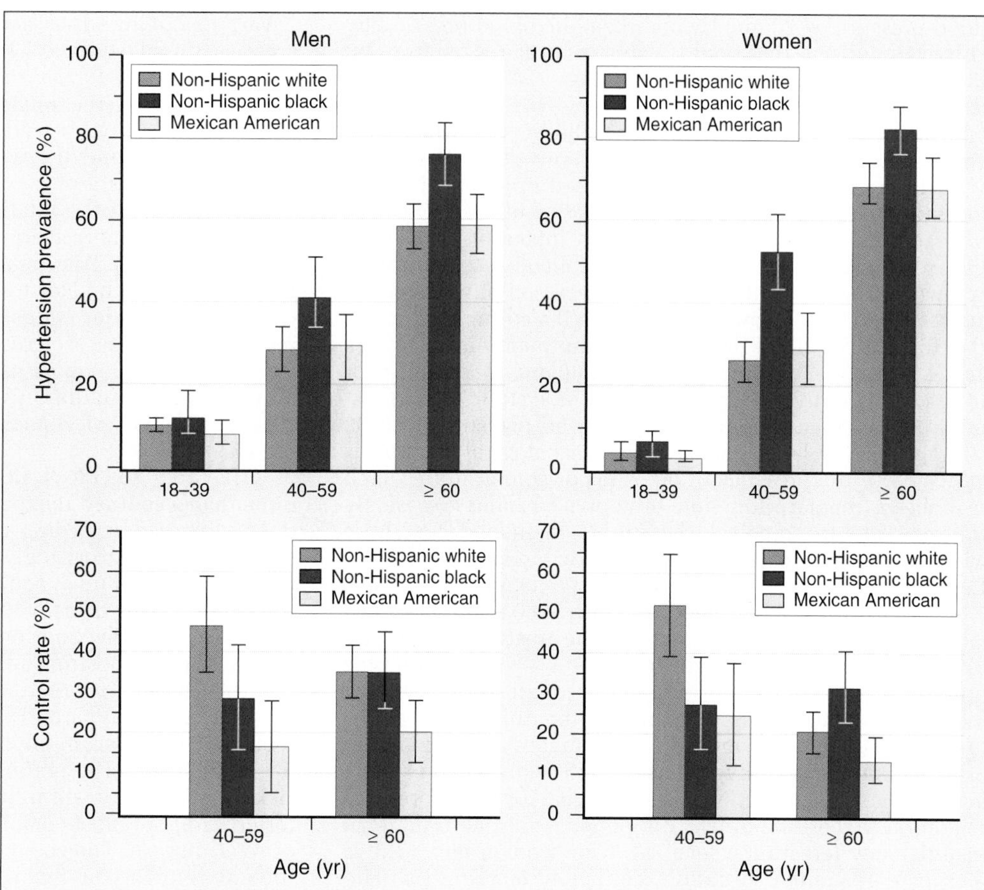

FIGURE 36–2 Hypertension prevalence **(top)** and hypertension control rates **(bottom)** by age and ethnicity among American men and women. (From Hajjar I, Kotchen TA: Trends in prevalence, awareness, treatment, and control of hypertension in the United States, 1988-2000. JAMA 290:199, 2003.)

Part of the complexity of hypertension as a risk factor relates to changing definitions of risk and an understanding that systolic blood pressure and pulse pressure may be of greater importance than diastolic blood pressure, contrary to decades of clinical teaching. Most epidemiological studies now recognize the joint contributions of systolic *and* diastolic blood pressure to the development of cardiovascular risk, an issue that has markedly changed strategies for risk detection.[38,39] Isolated systolic hypertension, in particular, is at least as important as diastolic blood pressure for the outcomes of total cardiovascular mortality and stroke.[40,41] These effects are greatest among older individuals and among those with known cardiovascular disease. Isolated systolic hypertension thus appears to represent a distinct pathophysiological state in which elevated blood pressure reflects reduced arterial elasticity not necessarily associated with increased peripheral resistance or an elevation in mean arterial pressure. In the Framingham Heart Study, even high-normal blood pressure (systolic blood pressure 130 to 139 mm Hg, diastolic blood pressure 85 to 89 mm Hg, or both) augments risk of cardiovascular disease twofold compared with lower levels.[42]

Pulse pressure, a potential surrogate for vascular wall stiffness, also potently predicts both first and recurrent myocardial infarction.[43] Defined as the difference between systolic and diastolic blood pressure, pulse pressure appears to predict independently cardiovascular events, particularly heart failure.[44-46] These data also stress the importance of arterial compliance and stiffness in atherogenesis as well as in the development of left ventricular hypertrophy. Several studies suggest that 24-hour ambulatory monitoring of blood pressure may provide a stronger predictor of cardiovascular morbidity and mortality when compared to office-based measures.[47] While ambulatory blood pressure monitoring has the advantage of correctly classifying as normal patients with "white-coat hypertension," recent data indicate that isolated ambulatory hypertension (in the setting of normal office blood pressure) also strongly correlates with cardiovascular morbidity.[48]

The importance of these changing definitions of hypertension is reflected by intervention trials that specifically target isolated systolic hypertension, all of which have shown benefit.[49-51] At the same time, major overviews continue to demonstrate that blood pressure reductions as small as 4 to 5 mm Hg result in large and clinically significant reductions in risk for stroke, vascular mortality, congestive heart failure, and total coronary heart disease in middle age, among the elderly, and in high-risk groups such as those with diabetes and peripheral arterial disease.[52] Among compliant patients, sodium reduction and weight loss can be effective.[53] However, not all patients respond to such measures, and the long-term success of nonpharmacological approaches to hypertension control has often proven disappointing. By contrast, relatively simple therapies such as low-dose diuretics can have major public health benefit. In an overview of 42 clinical trials that included 192,000 patients, low-dose diuretics compared to placebo yielded reductions of 21 percent in total coronary heart disease, 49 percent in congestive heat failure, 29 percent in stroke, and 19 percent in cardiovascular mortality.[54] Although combined therapy was often superior, none of the other first-line therapies for hypertension, including beta blockers, angiotensin-converting enzyme inhibitors, angiotensin receptor blockers, or calcium channel blockers, were significantly better than low-dose diuretics. Combined low-dose therapies, however, have considerable efficacy in terms of both blood pressure reduction and event prevention. In a comprehensive analysis of 354 randomized trials, regimens of multiple drugs given at low doses were estimated capable of reducing systolic blood pressure by 20 mm Hg and diastolic blood pressure by 11 mm Hg, effects that could result in stroke reductions of 63 percent and coronary heart disease risk reductions of 46 percent.[55]

In response to these observations, the most recent report from the Joint National Committee on Prevention, Detection, Evaluation, and Treatment of High Blood Pressure (JNC VII) continues to stress weight control, adoption of the DASH diet with sodium restriction and increased intake of potassium- and calcium-rich foods, moderation of alcohol consumption to fewer than two drinks daily, and increased physical activity (see Chap. 41).[35] However, the JNC VII also suggests a new classification of blood pressure, with normal defined as less than 120 mm Hg systolic and less than 80 mm Hg diastolic for adults and "pre-hypertension" defined as systolic blood pressure 120 to 139 mm Hg or diastolic blood pressure 80 to 89 mm Hg. In this latter category, pharmacological therapy is indicated in the presence of other major comorbidities such as diabetes, renal dysfunction, or known vascular disease. By contrast, pharmacological therapy is mandated for those with either stage 1 hypertension (systolic blood pressure 140-159 mm Hg or diastolic blood pressure 90-99 mm Hg) or stage 2 hypertension (systolic blood pressure >160 mm Hg or diastolic blood pressure >100 mm Hg). The treatment of hypertension is discussed at length in Chapter 38; a thiazide-type diuretic should be the first drug in almost all patients except those with hyponatremia or gout, and the diuretic should be the cornerstone of any multidrug combination. The majority of patients with overt hypertension will require two or more medications to achieve JNC VII target goal for blood pressure reduction. According to JNC VII, patients with chronic renal insufficiency (creatinine level >1.3 for women and >1.5 in men or a glomerular filtration rate below 60 ml/m^2) should also be targeted for blood pressure reduction, both for the prevention of cardiovascular disease and to slow progression to end-stage renal disease. Finally, as described later, patients with obesity, the metabolic syndrome, and frank diabetes represent high-risk groups. For all of these patients, target blood pressure should be in the "optimal" range of lower than 120/80 mm Hg.

Hyperlipidemia (see Chap. 39)

THE CHOLESTEROL HYPOTHESIS. The relationship between cholesterol and atherosclerosis currently enjoys wide acceptance.[56] In the 1850s, the German pathologist Virchow recognized in human atheromata "numerous plates of cholesterine . . . which display themselves even to the naked eye as glistening lamellae . . . which lie together in large numbers . . . and altogether produce a glittering reflection." In 1913, the Russian experimentalists Anitchkow and Chalatow observed that rabbits fed an egg-rich diet developed lipid-laden arterial lesions reminiscent of human atheromata. Later experiments identified cholesterol as the constituent of eggs that produced arterial lesions.

The biochemistry of cholesterol metabolism advanced throughout the 20th century. The advent of the ultracentrifuge enabled the characterization of the lipoprotein fractions in blood and furnished the foundation for detailed study of lipid metabolism. Armed with the ability to assay lipoproteins and cholesterol, translational investigators began to make clinical correlations. Cross-sectional studies of geographically dispersed populations revealed a relationship between serum cholesterol levels and coronary heart disease (CHD) death. Comparative study of ethnic Japanese living in Japan, the Hawaiian Islands, and the continental United States showed that in this relatively genetically homogeneous population, CHD death rates tracked with the environmentally induced augmentation in total serum cholesterol levels.

Various confounding factors can limit the validity of such cross-sectional studies. Thus, the emergence of data from cohort studies, such as that begun in Framingham in the 1950s, bolstered the relationship between cholesterol and CHD.[56] This study, as well as others performed in different populations around the world, established more firmly the concept of cholesterol as a culprit in coronary heart disease. Substantiation of the relationship between total cholesterol and CHD risk emerged from the Multiple Risk Factor Intervention (MRFIT) Trial, studies in the United Kingdom and Europe such as the Northwick Park Study and the Prospective Cardiovascular Munster (PROCAM) Cohort, and more recently the Atherosclerosis Risk in Communities (ARIC) study. The ARIC cohort has particular relevance to current clinical practice in the United States because it included substantial numbers of women and members of racial minority groups.

THE CHOLESTEROL CONTROVERSY. Although built on more than a century of experimental and clinical observation, doubt lingered regarding the role of cholesterol in atherosclerosis until surprisingly recently. Through the beginning of the 1990s, a cloud of controversy enveloped the role of cholesterol-lowering therapy in CHD risk reduction.[56] Despite the evidence that high cholesterol levels correlated with coronary death, the proposition that cholesterol-lowering therapy could reduce CHD morbidity remained unproven. Critics pointed to the apparently "J-shaped curve" describing the relationship of serum cholesterol with mortality. Advocates of the cholesterol hypothesis countered that the heightened risk for all-cause death in individuals with low levels of cholesterol might reflect comorbidities such as cancer, inanition, or liver disease. The goal of reducing CHD mortality by drug therapy eluded convincing proof for decades. Indeed, some cholesterol-lowering medications appeared to cause an increase in the incidence of some events, including noncoronary death. In the pioneering coronary drug project, estrogen treatment led to excess mortality in the cohort of men studied. The World Health Organization study of clofibrate showed increased noncoronary death. Dietary interventions to lower cholesterol often proved ineffective. Such results challenged the validity of cholesterol as a therapeutic target.

CLINICAL TRIALS SUBSTANTIATE THE CHOLESTEROL HYPOTHESIS (see Chap. 39). In the 1980s, clinical trial evidence first established a protective effect of pharmacological cholesterol reduction on coronary morbidity. The Lipid Research Clinic study showed that bile acid–binding resins could lower cholesterol levels in individuals with high baseline levels. A decrease in coronary morbidity accompanied the drop in serum cholesterol. However, total mortality did not change significantly. This finding fueled the fire of the skeptics.

Vindication of the cholesterol hypothesis awaited clinical trials of cholesterol lowering using the hydroxymethylglutaryl coenzyme A (HMG-CoA) reductase inhibitors. These drugs lowered LDL cholesterol more effectively than previously available agents. We now possess unassailable clinical trial evidence that lowering of LDL cholesterol can reduce coronary events in broad swaths of the population (see Chap. 39). First shown in survivors of myocardial infarction with relatively high cholesterol levels, recent clinical trials have extended the benefits of HMG-CoA reductase inhibitors to individuals without known atherosclerotic disease and with average levels of cholesterol. The ensemble of large clinical trials of HMG-CoA reductase inhibitors have substantiated a decrease in total mortality in the study populations. The HMG-CoA reductase inhibitors lowered LDL cholesterol levels 20 to 60 percent and reduced coronary events by up to one-third over a 5-year period. This result has vitiated previous concerns regarding increased noncardiac mortality due to cholesterol lowering. In addition, two very recent studies, the REVERSAL trial, which monitored intravascular coronary ultrasound, and the PROVE-IT trial of clinical endpoints, both demonstrate the benefit of aggressive as compared to moderate LDL cholesterol reduction.[56a,56b]

LOW-DENSITY LIPOPROTEIN CHOLESTEROL FULFILLS KOCH'S POSTULATES. The case for LDL cholesterol as a coronary heart disease risk factor meets most of the criteria established by Koch in the 19th century to inculpate an etiological agent in a disease. Although Koch's postulates deal with an infectious organism, the degree of rigor required to prove causality can apply to other agents of disease. High cholesterol levels consistently predict risk of future cardiovascular events in human populations. Animal studies in multiple species show a causal relationship between hypercholesterolemia and atherosclerosis. Knowledge of the LDL receptor pathway (see Chap. 39) plus emerging understanding of the vascular biology of atherosclerosis (see Chap. 35) provide biological plausibility for the involvement of LDL in atherogenesis. The human mutations in the LDL receptor produce hypercholesterolemia on a monogenic basis that causes rampant atherosclerosis as early as the first decade of life in individuals with homozygous familial hypercholesterolemia. Finally, intervention in large clinical trials to lower LDL cholesterol by a variety of pathways (bile acid–binding resins, intestinal bypass surgery, HMG-CoA reductase inhibitors) shows a reduction in cardiovascular events. Thus, LDL cholesterol fulfills these modified Koch's postulates as one etiological agent in atherosclerosis.

"AVERAGE" IS NOT NECESSARILY "NORMAL." The clinical chemistry laboratory establishes normal values based on the distribution of the variable in question in the general population. Several independent lines of evidence suggest that what we regard as "normal" cholesterol levels in Western society by these criteria exceed levels that good health requires, or that our species might normally have under different societal circumstances. The first line of evidence comes from comparing levels of cholesterol across different populations. Certain rural, agrarian societies have total cholesterol levels well below those accepted as normal in Western societies. Another line of evidence derives from phylogeny. Contemporary human beings have much higher total cholesterol levels than those of many other species of higher organisms that thrive nonetheless. While the current Adult Treatment Panel III defines "optimal" LDL cholesterol as below 100, the true optimum for our species may be considerably lower based on transcultural and phylogenetic considerations. Current clinical trials may inform further revisions of the guidelines and our concepts of "normal" in this regard.

THE RISK OF HYPERCHOLESTEROLEMIA BEGINS EARLY. Our current national guidelines use the Framingham Risk Equation. This instrument weights age heavily. However, for many patients and doctors, the relevant horizon of cardiovascular risk extends over a lifetime rather than 10 years, as predicated by the National Cholesterol Education Program Adult Treatment Panel III (NCEP ATP III) guidelines. For this reason, it is practically important to know whether cholesterol levels measured early in life influence long-term cardiovascular risk. Several data sets speak to this question. First, in the Bogalusa Heart Study, the burden of risk factors for atherosclerosis including hypercholesterolemia correlate with autopsy-proven fatty streak and raised lesion formation in the arterial tree. Studies performed on Johns Hopkins medical students upon matriculation with long-term follow-up suggested that cholesterol levels in the third decade correlate with long-term risk of myocardial infarction. A recent compilation of three major observational studies underscored the importance of cholesterol levels in young adulthood to long-term cardiovascular risk.[57] Thus, substantial evidence suggests that the burden of risk for cardiovascular disease begins in young adulthood. Well-known autopsy studies from the Korean and Vietnam conflicts, and recent explorations of coronary anatomy by intravascular ultrasonography, in conjunction with the Bogalusa Heart Study mentioned earlier, suggest that atherosclerosis can affect adolescents in our society. Because drug therapy will almost certainly prove neither cost-effective nor medically appropriate in primary prevention in younger populations, intensive life-style modification to reduce coronary risk due to lipid disorders should become a societal priority.

HIGH-DENSITY LIPOPROTEIN CHOLESTEROL. Several studies have found that CHD risk correlates inversely with high-density lipoprotein (HDL) cholesterol levels. Indeed, patients with angiographically proven coronary artery disease more often have low levels of HDL than high levels of LDL, as defined by current criteria. The process of reverse cholesterol transport may explain in part the apparent protective role of HDL against coronary death. According to this concept, HDL could ferry cholesterol from the vessel wall, augmenting peripheral catabolism of cholesterol. HDL can also carry antioxidant enzymes that may reduce the levels of oxidized phospholipids in atheromatous lesions that may enhance atherogenesis (see Chaps. 35 and 39). We lack a consistent body of clinical trial data on intervention to raise HDL cholesterol, in contrast to the case of LDL discussed previously. Yet, the consistency of the observational data, both cross-sectional and prospective, strongly support the HDL level as a "negative" risk factor, as incorporated in the ATP III guidelines.

TRIGLYCERIDE-RICH LIPOPROTEINS IN CARDIOVASCULAR RISK. In contrast to the compelling evidence favoring a causal role for LDL in atherogenesis, the role of triglycerides still engenders controversy. A number of issues foster this confusion. First, as triglyceride levels tend to vary inversely with HDL levels, demonstration of an unequivocal effect of triglycerides on cardiovascular events and mortality independent of HDL levels has proven elusive. Secondly, the level of triglycerides in the blood depends exquisitely on diet. Sampling serum for triglyceride levels in the fasting state avoids some of the variability in this measurement. However, most humans are in the postprandial state much of the day. The actual exposure of the artery wall to triglyceride-rich lipoprotein particles such as very-low-density lipoproteins (see Chap. 39) may indeed constitute a factor that promotes atherosclerosis that would be missed by the fasting lipid profile. For these reasons among others, current guidelines do not establish a target value of triglycerides. In view of the tight link of triglyceride levels with known risk factors for atherosclerosis (low HDL cholesterol level, uncontrolled diabetes, hypothyroidism), however, elevated triglyceride levels should enter into the overall risk assessment for an individual and stimulate consideration of the reason for triglyceride elevation (see Chap. 39).

Metabolic Syndrome, Insulin Resistance, and Diabetes (see Chap. 40)

Almost 35 million Americans have some degree of abnormal glucose tolerance, a condition along with obesity that markedly increases risk for type 2 diabetes and premature atherothrombosis.[58] Patients with diabetes have two- to eightfold higher rates of future cardiovascular events as compared with age- and ethnically matched nondiabetic individuals,[59] and three-fourths of all deaths among diabetic patients result from coronary heart disease.[60] Compared to unaffected individuals, diabetic patients have a greater atherosclerotic burden both in the major arteries and in the microvascular circulation. Not surprisingly, diabetic patients have substantially increased rates of atherosclerotic complications both in

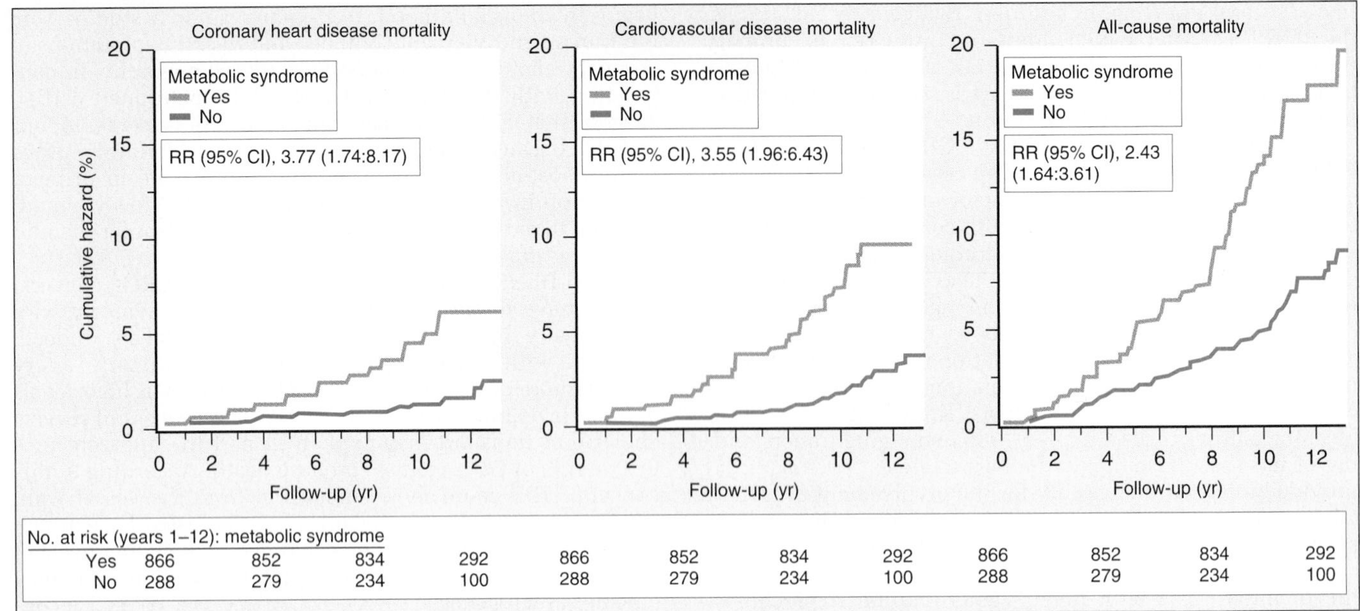

FIGURE 36–3 Cumulative hazard (unadjusted Kaplan-Meier hazard curves) for coronary heart disease, cardiovascular disease, and all-cause mortality among individuals with and without metabolic syndrome. (From Lakka H, Laaksonen DE, Lakka TA, et al: The metabolic syndrome and total and cardiovascular disease mortality in middle-aged men. JAMA 288:2709, 2002.)

the settings of primary prevention and after coronary interventional procedures. Moreover, the risk of cardiovascular disease starts to increase long before the onset of clinical diabetes, suggesting a "ticking clock" phenomenon. In an analysis of data from the Nurses Health Study of women who eventually developed type 2 diabetes, the relative risk of myocardial infarction was elevated threefold *before* the diagnosis of diabetes, a cardiovascular event rate almost as high as the rate in patients with frank diabetes at study entry.[61] These effects are amplified in ethnic minority populations[62] and in patients with other concomitant risk factors[63,64] and reflect subclinical disease in both the diabetic and the nondiabetic patient.[65] Thus, insulin resistance and diabetes rank among the major cardiovascular risk factors.

Although hyperglycemia is associated with microvascular disease, insulin resistance itself promotes atherosclerosis even before it produces frank diabetes, and available data corroborate the role of insulin resistance as an independent risk factor for atherothrombosis. This finding has prompted recommendations for increased surveillance for the metabolic syndrome, a cluster of glucose intolerance and hyperinsulinemia accompanied by hypertriglyceridemia, low HDL levels, hypofibrinolysis, hypertension, microalbuminuria, a predominance of small, dense LDL particles, and central obesity. Although several formal definitions of the metabolic syndrome have been proposed, the definition adopted by the National Cholesterol Education Program Adult Treatment Panel[66] requires at least three of the following five criteria: waist circumference greater than 102 cm in men and 88 cm in women; serum triglyceride levels of at least 150 mg/dl, HDL cholesterol less than 40 mg/dl in men and less than 50 mg/dl in women; blood pressure of at least 130/85 mm Hg; and serum glucose concentration of at least 110 mg/dl. Using these criteria, the prevalence of metabolic syndrome in the United States is almost 25 percent, or nearly 50 million (see Table 40–2).[67]

Several studies document that individuals with the metabolic syndrome have elevated vascular event rates. In the Kuopio Ischaemic Heart Disease Risk Factor Study, patients with metabolic syndrome showed markedly increased rates of coronary, cardiovascular, and all-cause mortality (Fig. 36–3).[68] However, not all individuals with metabolic syndrome have similar risk and, indeed, other markers may help to stratify clinical risk.[69] In particular, data from the Women's Health Study indicate that an hsCRP level greater than 3 mg/liter adds important prognostic information on cardiovascular risk at all levels of the metabolic syndrome (Fig. 36–4).[70] This observation is important, because levels of C-reactive protein measured with a high-sensitivity assay (hsCRP) also predict incident type 2 diabetes.[71-74a] Almost identical data regarding the additive value of hsCRP to the metabolic syndrome in terms of future vascular risk prediction derives from the West of Scotland Coronary Prevention Study.[75] As hsCRP levels correlate with systemic hypofibrinolysis and with basal insulin levels,[76] hsCRP evaluation may well become a routine part of the definition of metabolic syndrome.[77] As reviewed later in this chapter in sections

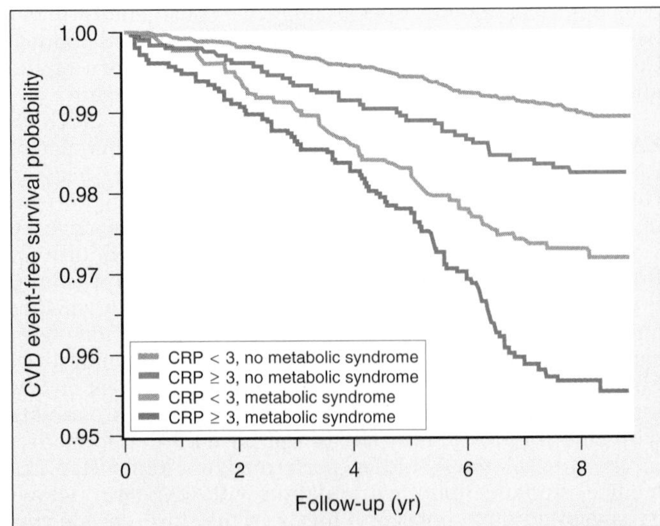

FIGURE 36–4 High-sensitivity C-reactive protein (CRP) adds prognostic information on risk among individuals with and without the metabolic syndrome. CVD = cardiovascular disease. (From Ridker PM, Buring JE, Cook NR, Rifai N: C-reactive protein, the metabolic syndrome, and risk of incident cardiovascular events: An 8-year follow-up of 14,719 initially healthy American women. Circulation 107:391, 2003.)

describing inflammatory markers, this conclusion is emerging in part from observations that atherosclerosis and type 2 diabetes share a common inflammatory basis.[78]

In addition to systemic metabolic abnormalities, hyperglycemia causes accumulation of advanced glycation end products associated with vascular damage.[79,80] Diabetic patients have markedly impaired endothelial and smooth muscle function and appear to have increased leukocyte adhesion to vascular endothelium, a critical early step in atherogenesis.[81] Diabetic nephropathy, detected by microalbuminuria, accelerates these adverse processes. Among individuals with non-insulin-dependent diabetes, microalbuminuria predicts both cardiovascular and all-cause mortality.[82] Abnormalities of endogenous fibrinolysis are also prevalent among diabetic and prediabetic patients, and therapies targeting plasminogen activator inhibitor have been proposed as a novel pathway for disease prevention in this setting.[83] The proinflammatory atherogenic mediator soluble CD40 ligand is elevated among diabetic patients and declines during thiazolidinedione therapy.[84] These effects, in concert with the impaired endothelium-dependent (nitric oxide–mediated) vasodilation common among diabetic patients, contribute to endothelial cell dysfunction and accelerated atherogenesis.[85] Chapters 40, 42, and 51 review the data about therapeutic interventions in patients with diabetes or the metabolic syndrome.

Exercise, Weight Loss, and Obesity

Regular physical exercise reduces myocardial oxygen demand and increases exercise capacity, both of which correlate with lower levels of coronary risk. The cardioprotective effects of exercise include adiposity, diabetes incidence, lowered blood pressure, and improvement of dyslipidemia, plasma rheology, and vascular inflammation. Exercise also enhances endothelial dysfunction, insulin sensitivity, and endogenous fibrinolysis.[86] It is thus not surprising that prospective epidemiological studies almost universally demonstrate strong graded associations between levels of physical activity and reduced rates of cardiovascular morbidity and all-cause mortality.

Recent observational studies cast doubt on the long-held belief that exercise must be vigorous to be beneficial. Exercise levels achieved with as little as 30 minutes of walking daily provide major coronary benefits. In the Women's Health Initiative, walking briskly for 30 minutes five times per week was associated with a 30 percent reduction in vascular events over a 3.5-year follow-up, an effect that persisted after adjustment for body mass index, age, and ethnicity (Fig. 36–5).[87] The Nurses Health Study yielded similar data: 3 hours of brisk walking per week conferred as much protection as did 1.5 hours of vigorous exercise per week.[88] In men participating in the Health Professional Follow-Up Study, 30 minutes of daily walking was associated with an 18 percent reduction in coronary risk. In that study, contrary to commonly given medical advice, resistance exercise and weight training were also found to have cardiovascular benefit.[89] Accumulated episodes of exercise, even if brief, have further demonstrated benefit, suggesting that prolonged vigorous work is not needed for risk reduction.[90] Smaller but consistent benefits of modest exercise have been observed for incident stroke, independent of hypertension.[91] Thus, a "no pain, no gain" approach to the prescription of physical activity to reduce vascular risk now appears passé.[92]

On the basis of these data, a joint statement from the Centers for Disease Control and the American College of Sports Medicine recommends that every American should accumulate at least 30 minutes of moderate-intensity physical activity daily.[93] Unfortunately, 7 of 10 American adults fail to meet this very modest level of activity, and one in three reports no leisure time activity at all.[94] Even though a

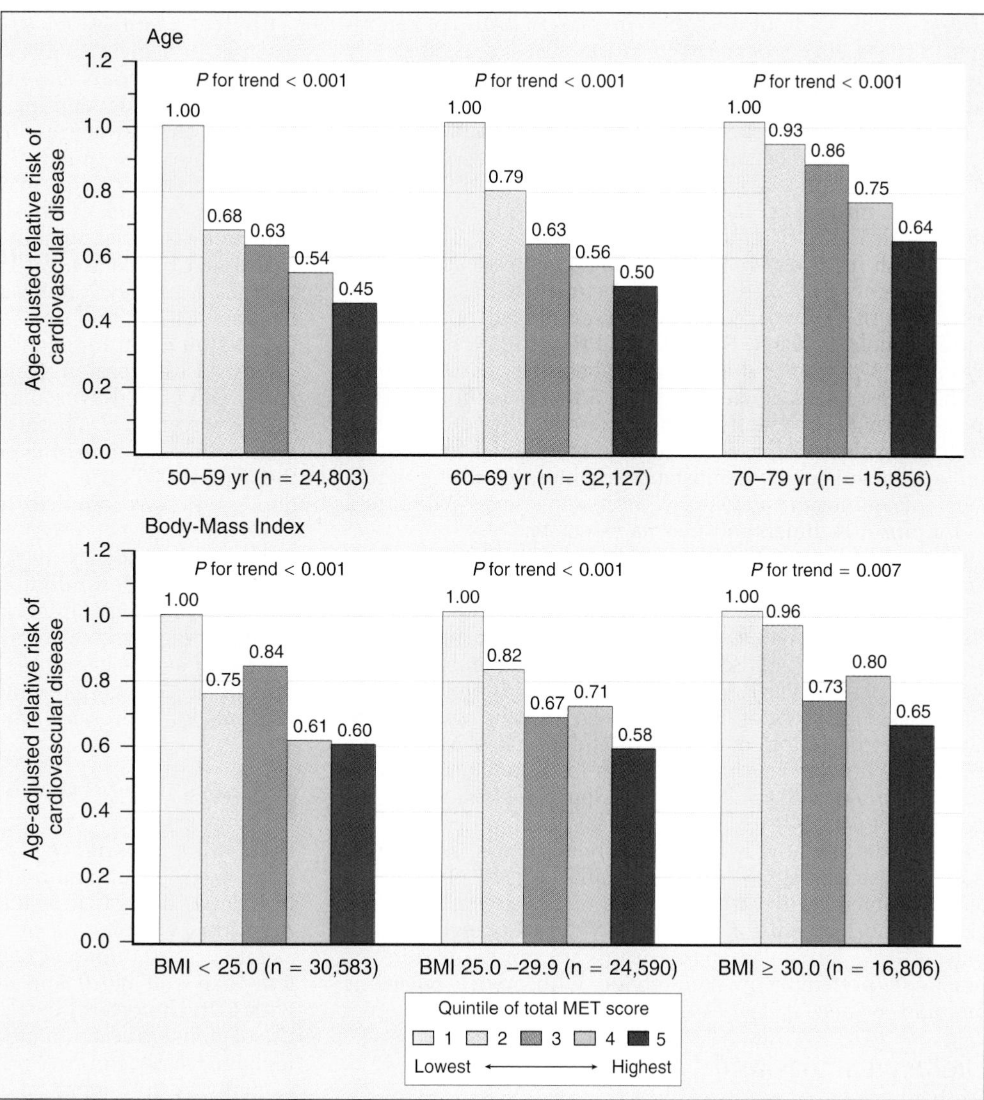

FIGURE 36–5 Relative risks of cardiovascular disease according to quintile of energy expenditure (MET Score) from recreational activities stratified by age **(top)** and body mass index **(bottom)**. (From Manson JE, Greenland P, LaCroix AZ, et al: Walking compared with vigorous exercise for the prevention of cardiovascular events in women. N Engl J Med 347:716, 2002.)

dose-response relationship is widely recognized between level of exercise and coronary risk, many experts worry that motivation to exercise might be undercut by even the slightly more aggressive recommendations from the Institute of Medicine to increase leisure time activity from 30 to 60 minutes daily.[95]

A recognized problem with the "30 minutes of walking per day" approach to vascular risk reduction is that this modest amount of exercise may not be adequate to reduce weight or maintain a healthy body mass index. In descriptive studies, long-term weight reduction requires more aggressive approaches among formerly obese patients, although one randomized trial showed short-term benefits of a less aggressive approach.[96]

Regular exercise affects multiple risk factors for atherosclerosis. In a recent meta-analysis of intervention trials, aerobic exercise was associated with a mean reduction of systolic blood pressure of 5 mm Hg among hypertensive participants, a level comparable to many drug interventions.[97] The degree of blood pressure reduction did not vary by frequency or intensity of exercise, and other studies show that walking alone has comparable effects.[98] Although exercise has been seen traditionally as having only modest effects on total and LDL cholesterol levels, improvements in HDL cholesterol level and reductions in triglycerides occur consistently, and more recent data indicate an increase in the average size of LDL particles without a change in plasma LDL concentration.[99] These effects occur even in the absence of clinically significant weight loss and were related more strongly with amount than intensity of exercise.

Exercise further improves insulin sensitivity and glycemic control with major benefits for diabetic patients. An analysis of 14 intervention trials of at least 8 weeks' duration showed clinically important reductions in glycated hemoglobin, along with reduced requirements for therapy.[100] These data agree with prospective epidemiological observations that moderate-intensity activity is associated with a reduced incidence of diabetes[101] and with randomized intervention studies such as the U.S. Diabetes Prevention Program, in which a 58 percent reduction in diabetes risk was observed with modest levels of exercise and a 5 to 7 percent reduction in body weight.[102] Finally, regular exercise lowers C-reactive protein levels,[103] improves coronary endothelial function,[104] and appears to benefit hemostatic variables, including tissue-type plasminogen activator, fibrinogen, von Willebrand factor, fibrin D-dimer, and plasma viscosity.[105]

Controversy remains as to whether obesity itself is a true risk factor for cardiovascular disease or whether its impact on vascular risk is mediated solely through interrelations with glucose intolerance, insulin resistance, hypertension, physical inactivity, and dyslipidemia. From an epidemiological perspective, obesity alone associates with elevated vascular risk regardless of activity levels, and the waist-to-hip ratio, a surrogate for centripetal or abdominal obesity, independently predicts vascular risk both in women and in older men.[106] Among U.S. adults, the prevalence of obesity (defined as a body mass index of 30 or greater) has doubled over the past decade and now reaches 30 percent across the population.[107] Even among children, particularly girls, obesity is a major problem, with rates in excess of 10 percent for white girls and 20 percent for black girls.[108] Thus, weight control must play a fundamental role in all preventive cardiology practices, preferably in conjunction with advice regarding diet and exercise.

Dietary Factors and Cardiovascular Risk (see Chaps. 41 and 42)

The fundamental role of diet, nutrition, and obesity in cardiovascular risk is discussed in detail in Chapter 41.

Mental Stress, Depression, and Cardiovascular Risk

Mental stress and depression both predispose to increased vascular risk and from a clinician's perspective should be considered as modifiable risk factors. The adrenergic stimulation of mental stress can augment myocardial oxygen requirements and aggravate myocardial ischemia. Mental stress can cause coronary vasoconstriction, particularly in atherosclerotic coronary arteries, and hence can influence myocardial oxygen supply as well. Recent studies have further linked mental stress to platelet and endothelial dysfunction,[109] the metabolic syndrome,[110,111] and the induction of ventricular arrhythmias.[112,113]

Acute stress such as that associated with natural disasters has long been recognized as a risk factor for coronary events.[114,115] More recently, work-related stress has gained recognition as a source of vascular risk. Work stress has two components: job strain (which combines high work demands and low job control) and effort-reward imbalance (which more closely reflects economic factors in the workplace). Both components are associated with an approximate doubling of risk for myocardial infarction and stroke in European[116] and Japanese populations.[117] Other psychological metrics, including anger and hostility scales, have also been associated with elevated vascular risk.

Clinical depression strongly predicts coronary heart disease. In a meta-analysis of 11 studies involving initially healthy individuals, those with depression had a significantly higher risk of developing coronary disease during follow-up, with clinical depression (RR, 2.7) being more important than depressive mood (RR, 1.5).[118] While depression is also associated with an increased prevalence of hypertension, smoking, and lack of physical activity, the effects of depression on overall risk remain after adjusting for these and other traditional risk factors.[119] Thus, findings that depressed individuals also have increased platelet activation, elevated levels of hsCRP, and decreased heart rate variability support depression as an independent predictor of events.

Onset of depression after myocardial infarction is common and predicts cardiovascular mortality independent of cardiac disease severity.[120] Whether therapy for postinfarction depression reduces recurrent event rates remains controversial. In the SADHART trial, a substantial proportion of cardiac depression was found to remit spontaneously, emphasizing the need for placebo-controlled studies.[121] By contrast, in the Enhancing Recovery in Coronary Heart Disease Patients (ENRICHD) trial, random allocation between usual care and formal psychosocial intervention resulted in modest improvements in measures of clinical depression but no significant improvement in event-free survival.[122] Ongoing studies will thus be critical to determine whether more aggressive interventions for depression can improve vascular outcomes.[123]

Novel Atherosclerotic Risk Factors

Despite the importance of blood lipids, half of all myocardial infarctions occur among individuals without overt hyperlipidemia. In fact, in a major prospective study of healthy American women, 77 percent of all future cardiovascular events occurred among patients with LDL cholesterol levels less than 160 mg/dl and 46 percent occurred among those with LDL cholesterol levels less than 130 mg/dl.[124] While the use of global prediction models like those developed in Framingham greatly improves the detection of heart disease risk, as many as 20 percent of all events occur in the absence of any of the major classic vascular risk factors.

This fact challenges several basic issues related to national screening programs for risk detection and disease prevention.

However, clinical data continue to accrue demonstrating the hazard of relying solely on classic risk factors. In one recent analysis of more than 120,000 patients with coronary heart disease, 15 percent of the men and 19 percent of the women had no evidence of hyperlipidemia, hypertension, diabetes, or smoking and more than half had only one of these general risk factors.[125] In another large analysis, between 85 and 95 percent of participants with coronary disease had at least one conventional risk factor, but so too did those participants without coronary disease despite follow-up for as long as 30 years.[126] Thus, because of the considerable need to improve vascular risk detection, much research over the past decade has focused on the identification and evaluation of novel atherosclerotic risk factors.[127,128]

When evaluating any novel risk factor as a potential new screening tool, clinicians need to consider (1) whether there is a standardized and reproducible assay for the marker of interest; (2) whether there is a consistent series of prospective studies demonstrating that a given parameter predicts future risk; (3) whether the novel marker adds to the predictive value of lipid screening; and (4) whether there is evidence that the novel marker adds to global risk prediction scores such as that in the Framingham Heart Study. The following section applies these basic epidemiological requirements to a series of novel risk factors, including hsCRP and other markers of inflammation, lipoprotein(a), homocysteine, and markers of fibrinolytic and hemostatic function such as fibrinogen, D-dimer, tissue plasminogen activator (t-PA), and plasminogen activator inhibitor (PAI-1) antigens (Table 36–1). Physicians should also consider the relative magnitude of novel markers in terms of risk prediction, particularly in comparison to lipid screening. Figure 36–6 shows data describing the relative efficacy of several variables measured at baseline in two large cohorts of initially healthy middle-aged men and women.

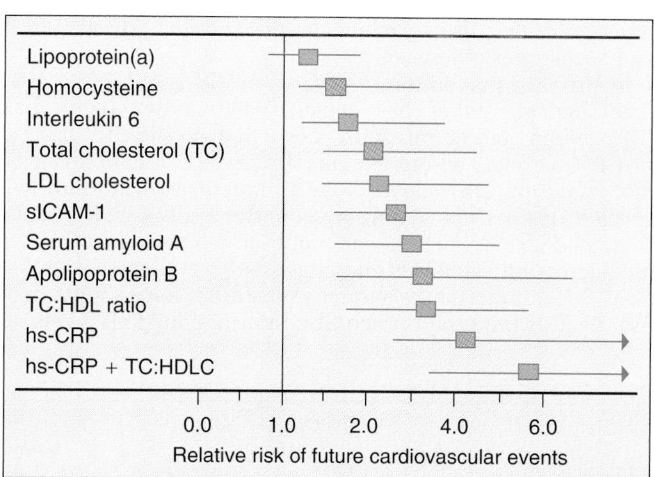

FIGURE 36–6 Relative risks of future myocardial infarction among apparently healthy women according to baseline levels of lipoprotein(a), homocysteine, interleukin-6, total cholesterol, low-density lipoprotein (LDL) cholesterol, soluble intercellular adhesion molecule-1 (sICAM-1), serum amyloid A, apolipoprotein B, the ratio of total cholesterol to high-density lipoprotein cholesterol (TC:HDLC), high-sensitivity C-reactive protein (hsCRP), and the combination of hsCRP with the TC:HDLC. (From Ridker PM: Clinical application of C-reactive protein for cardiovascular disease detection and prevention. Circulation 107:363, 2003.)

C-Reactive Protein (CRP)

Inflammation characterizes all phases of atherothrombosis and provides a critical pathophysiological link between plaque formation and acute rupture, leading to occlusion and infarction.[129] Formation of the fatty streak, the earliest phase of atherogenesis, involves recruitment of leukocytes due to the expression of adhesion molecules on endothelial cells in turn triggered by inflammatory cytokines such as interleukin-1 and tumor necrosis factor-alpha. Subsequent migration of inflammatory cells into the subendothelial space requires chemotaxis controlled by chemokines induced by the primary cytokines. Mononuclear cells within this initial infiltrate as well as intrinsic vascular cells subsequently release growth factors that stimulate proliferation of the smooth muscle cells and lead to plaque progression. The thrombotic complications of plaques often involve physical disruption, usually associated with signs of both local and systemic inflammation.[130] Other proinflammatory cytokines such as CD40 ligand can in turn induce tissue factor expression and promote thrombus formation. Moreover, the primary proinflammatory cytokines result in the expression of messenger cytokines such as interleukin-6, which can travel from local sites of inflammation to the liver, where it triggers a change in the program of protein synthesis characteristic of the acute phase response. The acute phase reactant, CRP, a simple downstream marker of inflammation, has now emerged as a major cardiovascular risk factor.[131]

Composed of five 23 kD subunits, CRP is a circulating member of the pentraxin family that plays a major role in the human innate immune response. Although it is primarily derived from the liver, recent data indicate that cells within human coronary arteries, particularly in the atherosclerotic intima, can elaborate CRP.[132,133] More than simply a marker of inflammation, CRP may influence directly vascular vulnerability through several mechanisms, including enhanced expression of local adhesion molecules, increased expression of endothelial PAI-1, reduced endothelial nitric oxide bioactivity, altered LDL uptake by macrophages, and colocalization with complement within atherosclerotic lesions.[134-137] Moreover, the expression of human CRP in CRP-

TABLE 36–1 Assessment of the Clinical Utility of Novel Markers of Cardiovascular Risk

Marker	Assay Conditions Standardized?	Prospective Studies Consistent?	Additive to Total Cholesterol and High-Density Lipoprotein Cholesterol?	Additive to Framingham Risk?
Lipoprotein(a)	–	+/–	+/–	–
Homocysteine	+	+	+/–	–
Tissue plasminogen activator and plasminogen activator inhibitor-1	+/–	+	+/–	–
Lipoprotein density	–	+/–	–	–
Fibrinogen	–	+	+	–
High-sensitivity C-reactive protein	+	+	+	+

transgenic mice directly enhances intravascular thrombosis[138] and accelerates atherogenesis.[138a]

In primary prevention, a large series of prospective epidemiological studies has demonstrated convincingly that CRP, when measured with new high-sensitivity assays (hsCRP), strongly and independently predicts risk of myocardial infarction, stroke, peripheral arterial disease, and sudden cardiac death even among apparently healthy individuals (Fig. 36–7).[124,139-143] These data apply to women as well as to men across all age levels and consistently to diverse populations. Most importantly, a number of studies have shown that hsCRP adds important prognostic information at all levels of LDL cholesterol and at all levels of risk as determined by the Framingham Risk Score (Fig. 36–8).[124,144] In the largest study to date, hsCRP levels predicted subsequent risk better than LDL cholesterol level. However, because hsCRP levels reflect a component of vascular risk quite different from that of cholesterol, the addition of hsCRP to lipid evaluation provides a major opportunity to improve global risk prediction. In clinical terms, absolute vascular risk is higher among individuals with elevated hsCRP and low levels of LDL cholesterol than among individuals with elevated levels of LDL cholesterol but low levels of hsCRP, yet current guidelines consider only the latter group at high risk (Fig. 36–9).

Additional data corroborating the ability of hsCRP to predict vascular risk after adjustment for traditional risk factors have been provided by several large cohorts in both the United States and Europe.[144a,b,c] These confirmatory studies include data from the Reykjavik Heart Study in which a 50 percent increase in risk associated with hsCRP was observed not only after control for Framingham covariates but also after additional control for diabetes, triglycerides, body mass index, and indices of pulmonary function.[144c] In that study, the odds ratio for hsCRP was identical to that of hypertension and statistically similar to that of smoking—data that demonstrate the clinical importance of inflammation in a population with much higher baseline cholesterol levels than those observed in contemporary U.S. cohorts.

Largely on the basis of these data, the American

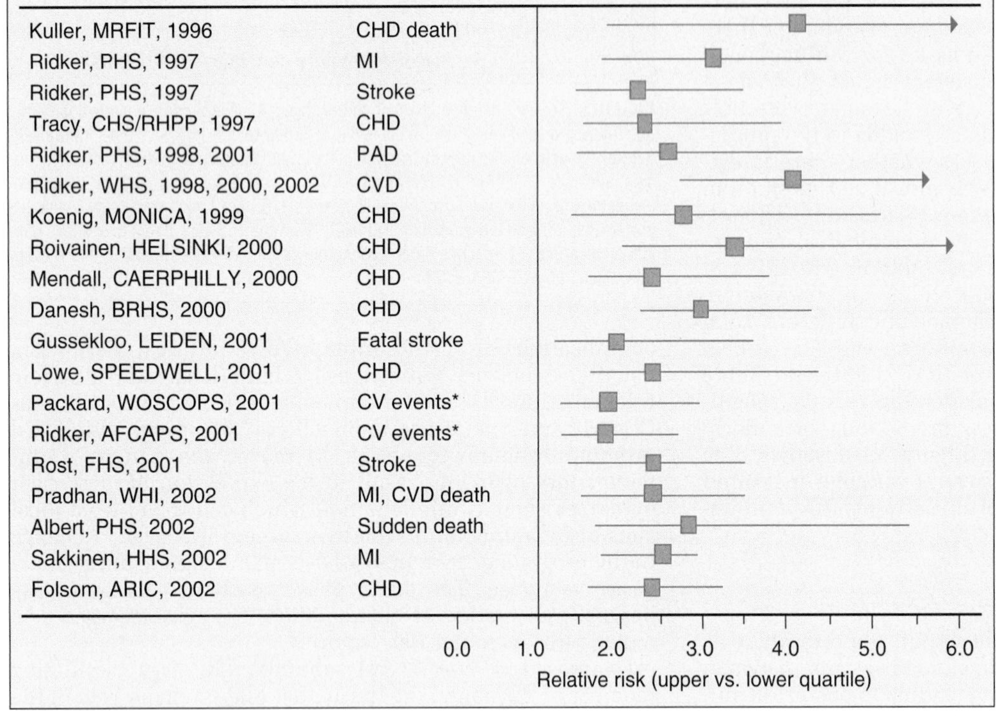

FIGURE 36–7 Prospective studies relating baseline high-sensitivity C-reactive protein levels to the risk of first cardiovascular events. CHD = coronary heart disease; CV = cardiovascular; CVD = cardiovascular disease; MI = myocardial infarction; PAD = pulmonary artery disease. (From Ridker PM: Clinical application of C-reactive protein for cardiovascular disease detection and prevention. Circulation 107:363, 2003.)

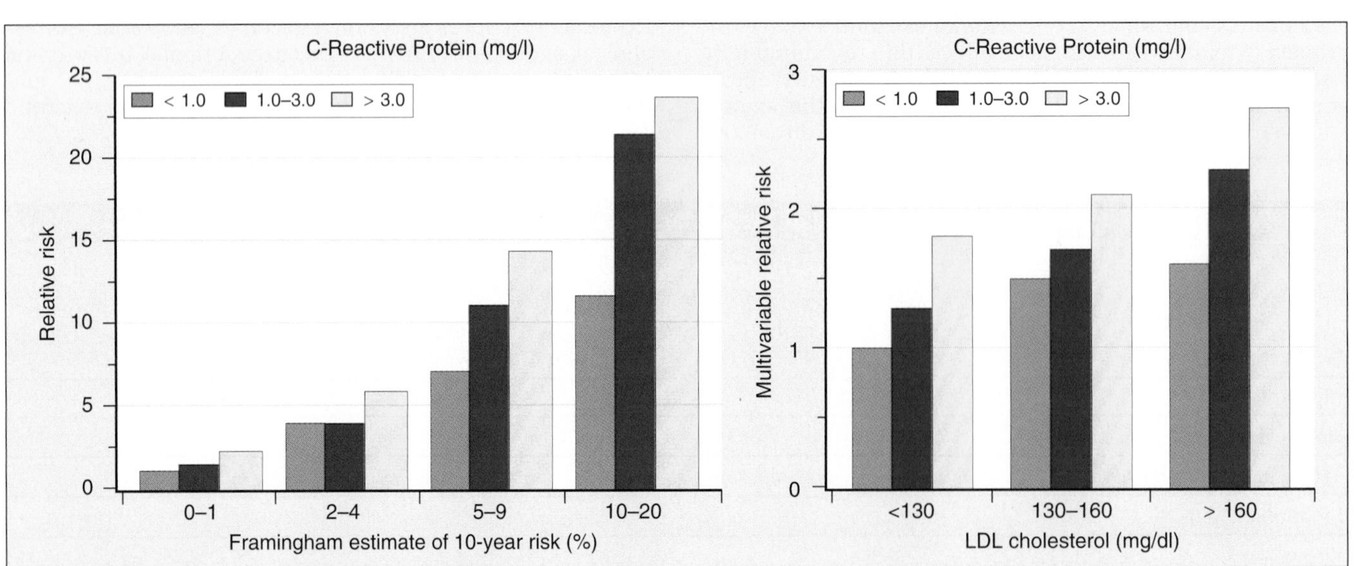

FIGURE 36–8 High-sensitivity C-reactive protein adds prognostic information at all levels of low-density lipoprotein (LDL) cholesterol after multivariate adjustment for traditional risk factors **(right)** and at all levels of the Framingham risk score **(left)**. (From Ridker PM, Rifai N, Rose L, et al: Comparison of C-reactive protein and low-density lipoprotein cholesterol levels in the prediction of first cardiovascular events. N Engl J Med 347:1557, 2002.)

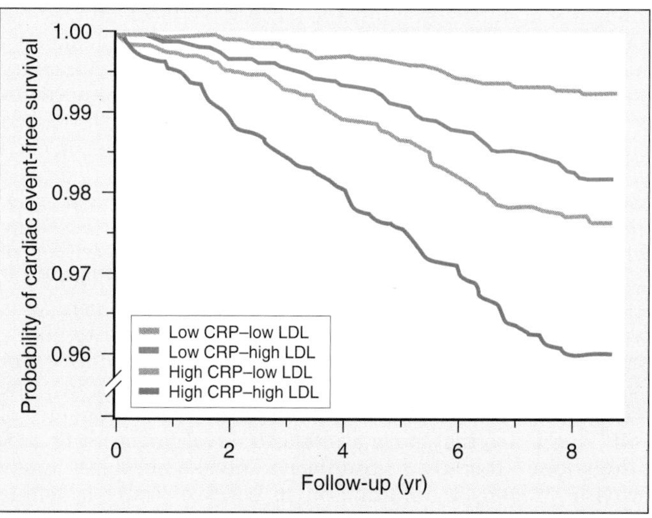

FIGURE 36–9 Cardiovascular event-free survival among apparently healthy individuals according to baseline levels of high-sensitivity C-reactive protein (CRP) and low-density lipoprotein (LDL) cholesterol. (From Ridker PM, Rifai N, Rose L, et al: Comparison of C-reactive protein and low-density lipoprotein cholesterol levels in the prediction of first cardiovascular events. N Engl J Med 347:1557, 2002.)

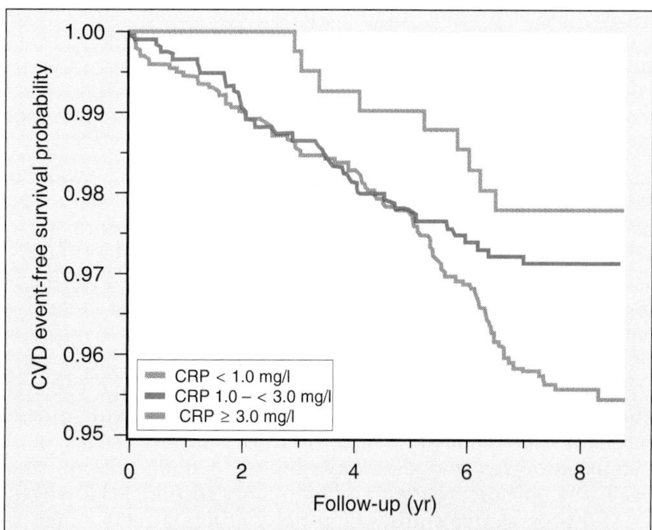

FIGURE 36–10 Cardiovascular disease (CVD) event-free survival among individuals with the metabolic syndrome, stratified by high-sensitivity C-reactive protein (CRP) levels at baseline. (From Ridker PM: Clinical application of C-reactive protein for cardiovascular disease detection and prevention. Circulation 107:363, 2003.)

Heart Association and the Centers for Disease Control and Prevention recently issued the first guidelines for the use of hsCRP in clinical practice.[145] In brief, hsCRP levels of less than 1, 1 to 3, and greater than 3 mg/liter should be interpreted as low, moderate, and high vascular risk, respectively. Screening for hsCRP should be done at the discretion of the physician as a part of global risk evaluation, not as a replacement for LDL and HDL testing. Although hsCRP predicts risk across the full population spectrum, its greatest utility is likely to be among those at "intermediate risk"; that is, individuals with anticipated 10-year event rates between 5 and 20 percent. Values of hsCRP in excess of 10 mg/liter may represent an acute-phase response due to an underlying inflammatory disease or intercurrent infection and should lead to repeat testing in approximately 2 to 3 weeks; consistently high values, however, represent very high risk of future cardiovascular disease because risk appears linear across the full range of hsCRP.[145a] Because hsCRP levels are stable over long periods of time, have no circadian variation, and are not affected by food intake, screening can easily be done on an outpatient basis at the time of cholesterol evaluation.

Levels of hsCRP greater than 3 mg/liter also appear to predict recurrent coronary events, thrombotic complications after angioplasty, poor outcome in the setting of unstable angina, and vascular complications after bypass surgery.[146-150] All of these data support the concept that inflammation plays a critical role throughout the atherothrombotic process. Additionally, hsCRP has prognostic utility in cases of acute ischemia even without troponin elevation, data suggesting that an enhanced inflammatory response at the time of hospital admission can determine subsequent plaque rupture.[151] These findings help explain why individuals with elevated hsCRP levels are also more likely to benefit from aggressive interventions compared to those with low levels.[152,153]

Elevated levels of hsCRP predict not only cardiovascular events but also the onset of type 2 diabetes mellitus,[71,72] perhaps because hsCRP levels correlate with several components of the metabolic syndrome, including those not easily measured in clinical practice such as insulin sensitivity, endothelial dysfunction, and hypofibrinolysis. Thus, hsCRP assessment also adds prognostic information at all levels of the metabolic syndrome.[70,75] Even among individuals with the ATP-III definition of metabolic syndrome, knowledge of hsCRP levels less than 1, 1 to 3, and greater than 3 mg/liter further defines low-, moderate-, and high-risk groups for future vascular events (Fig. 36–10).

Of commercially available novel risk factors, hsCRP has the greatest magnitude of predictive value. Further, unlike homocysteine, fibrinogen, and lipoprotein(a), hsCRP adds important prognostic information to global risk prediction. It is important to recognize, however, that no direct evidence to date shows that lowering hsCRP per se will reduce vascular risk. Nonetheless, smoking cessation, weight loss, diet, and exercise all reduce hsCRP levels and all lower cardiac risk. Thus the primary use of hsCRP at this time should be for improved targeting of primary prevention efforts directed at these modifiable risk factors.

Statins lower hsCRP levels in a manner largely unrelated to the magnitude of LDL cholesterol reduction.[154,155] Data in both primary and secondary prevention indicate that the relative benefit of statin therapy in terms of event reduction may be greater in the presence of elevated hsCRP levels. In the AFCAPS/TexCAPS trial, for example, lovastatin appeared to lower cardiovascular event rates even for those with below-median levels of LDL cholesterol but above-median levels of hsCRP.[156] By contrast, lovastatin did not reduce events among those with neither hyperlipidemia nor inflammation. These observations have led to the hypothesis that statin therapy prevents first vascular events not only among patients with elevated LDL cholesterol levels, but also among those with elevated levels of hsCRP. This critical hypothesis is now under direct investigation.[157]

In addition to statins, treatment with fibrates and niacin may also lower hsCRP levels, as does the use of thiazolidinediones. By contrast, oral preparations of hormone replacement therapy tend to increase hsCRP levels. While aspirin does not directly lower hsCRP levels, the utility of aspirin in preventing first vascular events appears to be greatest among patients with elevated hsCRP levels.

The hsCRP levels correlate only modestly with underlying atherosclerotic disease as measured by carotid intimal medial thickness or by coronary calcification. This observation suggests that hsCRP does not simply reflect the presence of subclinical disease but rather indicates an increased propensity for plaque disruption and/or thrombosis. Autopsy data support this hypothesis: elevated hsCRP levels occur more often among patients with frankly ruptured plaques than among those with erosive disease or among those who died of nonvascular causes.[158] Two recent studies showed that hsCRP levels predict incident hypertension and add prognostic information on vascular risk at all levels of blood pressure.[159,160] In patients with other conditions such as allograft atherosclerosis[161] and chronic renal failure and dialysis,[162] hsCRP levels have proven to predict strongly poor short- and long-term cardiovascular outcome.

Although inflammation clearly participates in vascular injury and hsCRP provides an inexpensive and clinically useful measure of this process, it remains uncertain as to what stimulus initiates the underlying proinflammatory response (see also Chap. 35). Patients with chronic inflammatory diseases such as rheumatoid arthritis tend to have elevated hsCRP levels and on average somewhat higher vascular risk, but a causal relationship in this setting has been difficult to establish. Patients with low-grade infections such as gingivitis or those who chronically carry *Chlamydia pneumoniae, Helicobacter pylori*, herpes simplex virus, and cytomegalovirus may also have higher vascular risk on the basis of a chronic systemic inflammatory response. However, careful prospective studies of antibody titers directed against these agents have not consistently found evidence of association, and a large antibiotic trial did not show reduced recurrent events in myocardial infarction survivors.[163] Whether novel targeted antiinflammatory therapies, including specific cytokine inhibitors, can improve coronary outcomes is an active area of research.

Given the robustness of laboratory and epidemiological data and the low cost of testing, we believe hsCRP evaluation will likely become a routine part of coronary risk prediction. In outpatient settings, hsCRP should be evaluated at the time of cholesterol screening if the practitioner wishes to use it as an adjunct to global risk prediction. For individuals with an LDL cholesterol level greater than 160 mg/dl, a finding of elevated hsCRP should provide an additional impetus for the physician to institute aggressive primary prevention and may help motivate some patients to comply with life-style modifications and, when indicated, pharmacotherapy.

For individuals with LDL cholesterol levels between 130 and 160 mg/dl, the finding of an elevated hsCRP level indicates substantial risk and should again lead to better adherence to preventive efforts and perhaps to earlier use of pharmacological approaches to risk reduction. For individuals with LDL cholesterol levels below 130 mg/dl, it is also clear that an elevated hsCRP value confers elevated risk. However, while post hoc analyses suggest that such patients may benefit from statin therapy, clinical trials testing this issue have only recently begun. Such individuals should thus aggressively undergo exercise, weight loss, and smoking cessation programs. In this setting, an elevated hsCRP level should provide considerable motivation to improve life-style, particularly for those previously told they were not at risk because of an absence of hyperlipidemia. Simple clinical algorithms for the use of hsCRP in primary care have recently become available.[164]

Approaches to hsCRP evaluation in secondary prevention and in acute coronary ischemia are evolving. A major area of concern is in the emergency room evaluation of patients with troponin-negative acute coronary ischemia. Because elevations in several inflammatory markers including hsCRP and myeloperoxidase occur in this setting and predict poor short-term outcomes, some form of inflammatory biomarker may aid the evaluation of chest pain (see also Chap. 45).

Other Markers of Inflammation

While hsCRP is by far the best-characterized inflammatory biomarker for clinical use, several other markers of inflammation have shown promise in terms of predicting vascular risk. These include cytokines such as interleukin-6,[152,165] soluble forms of certain cell adhesion molecules such as intercellular adhesion molecule (sICAM-1), P-selectin, or the mediator CD40 ligand,[166-170] as well as markers of leukocyte activation such as myeloperoxidase.[171] Other inflammatory markers associated with lipid oxidation such as lipoprotein-associated phospholipase A2[172,173] and pregnancy-associated plasma protein A have also shown promise.[174] However, each of these emerging biomarkers has analytical issues that need careful evaluation before routine clinical use. For example, the half-life of some is too short for clinical diagnostic testing, whereas the ability of others to predict risk in settings of broad populations has proved marginal thus far.[175] Nonetheless, several of these inflammatory biomarkers can shed critical pathophysiological light on the atherothrombotic process, particularly at the time of plaque rupture. For example, soluble CD40 ligand may provide insight into the efficacy of specific antithrombotic agents independent of CRP[176] and also may have a role as a novel target for thiazolidinedione therapy.[84] Similarly, myeloperoxidase may provide prognostic information in cases of acute ischemia over and above that associated with troponin or CRP.[130,177,178] Thus, continued evaluation of other inflammatory biomarkers may well provide novel targets for or monitors of therapy, particularly in the setting of acute coronary ischemia.

Homocysteine

Homocysteine is a sulfhydryl-containing amino acid derived from the demethylation of dietary methionine. Patients with rare inherited defects of methionine metabolism can develop severe hyperhomocysteinemia (plasma levels >100 μmol/liter) and have markedly elevated risk of premature atherothrombosis as well as venous thromboembolism. The mechanisms that account for these effects remain uncertain but include endothelial dysfunction, accelerated oxidation of LDL cholesterol, impairment of flow-mediated endothelial-derived relaxing factor with subsequent reduction in arterial vasodilation, platelet activation, increased expression of monocyte chemoattractant protein (MCP-1), and interleukin-8 leading to a proinflammatory response, and oxidative stress.[179-183]

In contrast to severe hyperhomocysteinemia, mild to moderate elevations of homocysteine (plasma levels >15 μmol/liter) are more common in the general population, primarily due to insufficient dietary intake of folic acid.[184] Other patient groups who tend to have elevated levels of homocysteine include those receiving folate antagonists such as methotrexate and carbamazepine, and those with impaired homocysteine metabolism due to hypothyroidism or to renal insufficiency.

A common polymorphism in the methylene tetrahydrofolate reductase (*MTHFR*) gene that encodes a thermolabile protein has also been linked to elevated homocysteine levels and to increased vascular risk, at least among individuals homozygous for the variant. Familial association studies report higher homocysteine levels among offspring of parents with premature coronary artery disease.[185] However, the clinical importance of the *MTHFR* polymorphism appears modest, and heterozygous individuals display little evidence of elevated homocysteine levels even among those with low folate intake. In a recent meta-analysis of 40 observational studies, individuals homozygous for the *MTHFR* 677 TT variant had only a 16 percent increase in relative risk (OR, 1.16; 95 percent CI, 1.05-1.28), and this observation was evident only in studies originating in Europe.[186] Thus, in populations in whom folate fortification exists, such as those in North America, no compelling evidence supports genetic evaluation of *MTHFR* to predict vascular risk.[187,188]

Until recently, total plasma homocysteine (the combination of free homocysteine, bound homocysteine, and mixed disulfides) was measured predominantly by high-performance liquid chromatography, which is accurate but requires a sophisticated analytic setting. Reliable and less expensive immunoassays have become available, however, that have made wider screening of homocysteine possible. Although a nonfasting evaluation of total plasma homocysteine suffices for most clinical purposes, measurement of homocysteine levels 2 to 6 hours after ingestion of an oral methionine load (0.1 gm/kg body mass) can identify individuals with impaired homocysteine metabolism despite normal fasting levels.

Despite availability of newer assays, measurement of homocysteine remains controversial and recent guidelines do not advocate their use. Several reasons suggest that this conservative approach is warranted for most patients. First, although early cross-sectional and retrospective studies reported strong positive associations between plasma homocysteine levels and risk, such study designs are subject to epidemiological bias and cannot establish a causal relationship, as homocysteine levels increase after myocardial infarction and stroke. This overestimation of effect appears to have been borne out now that a large series of prospective studies are available. In several recent meta-analyses, the magnitude and strength of association between baseline homocysteine levels and risk of subsequent disease has proven substantially smaller than previously reported.[189-192] Although there is some heterogeneity between the prospective studies, on average these meta-analyses report a 25 percent lower homocysteine level being associated with an approximate 11 percent lower risk of coronary heart disease, an estimate far smaller than hypothesized. Some of this reduction may reflect the introduction of folate fortification in 1998 to reduce the incidence of neural tube defects (see Chap. 41). However, many of the prospective studies began well before fortification and others have shown predictive value even among individuals taking and those not taking multivitamin supplements.[193] Fortification of the food supply has greatly reduced the frequency of low folate and elevated homocysteine levels, particularly for persons initially in the moderately elevated range.[194] Thus, the number of individuals potentially identifiable by general screening for homocysteine has decreased considerably.

Enthusiasm for population-based homocysteine evaluation has also been limited by a lack of evidence demonstrating that screening adds to standard lipid evaluation or to the Framingham risk score. Unlike inflammatory markers such as hsCRP, there is no evidence that homocysteine evaluation can identify high-risk populations who might benefit differentially from non-vitamin interventions such as statin therapy.[195] The cost of screening compared to the cost of folate supplementation has also been an issue. Folic acid, given in doses of up to 400 μg/day, can reduce homocysteine levels approximately 25 percent, and the addition of vitamin B12 will likely reduce levels another 7 percent.[196,197] Because this therapy is inexpensive and has low toxicity in the absence of vitamin B12 deficiency, vitamin supplementation may be a more cost-effective approach for high-risk groups than screening.[198] Finally, although several randomized trials are underway to evaluate the efficacy of folate and vitamin B supplementation to reduce vascular risk in general populations and in the setting of renal failure,[199-201] few have been reported to date, and concern has been raised that fortification may reduce the power of these trials to detect true differences.[202,203] For example, in the recent Vitamin Intervention for Stroke Prevention trial, moderate reduction in homocysteine with folic acid had no effect on vascular outcomes during two years follow-up.[203a]

There remain specific patient populations for whom homocysteine evaluation may prove appropriate, including those lacking traditional risk factors, in the setting of renal failure, or among those with premature atherosclerosis or a family history of myocardial infarction and stroke at a young age. In secondary prevention, persuasive data show that elevated homocysteine levels predict worse mortality, although no specific intervention has yet proven effective in this regard.[204,205] In the Swiss Heart Study, participants undergoing angioplasty appeared to have lower rates of restenosis, target lesion revascularization, and coronary events when given folate, vitamin B6, and vitamin B12,[206,207] although these data have not been reproduced elsewhere and predate widespread use of coronary stenting.

Current investigations are testing the potential input of homocysteine on nonthrombotic disease. Following observations in hyperhomocysteinemic hypertensive rats[208] and upon associations between homocysteine levels and extent of ventricular hypertrophy in renal failure patients,[209] investigators in the Framingham Study recently found plasma homocysteine levels to be associated with an increase in risk for congestive heart failure among adults without prior myocardial infarction.[210]

Fibrinogen and Fibrin D-Dimer

Plasma fibrinogen influences platelet aggregation and blood viscosity, interacts with plasminogen binding, and, in combination with thrombin, mediates the final step in clot formation and the response to vascular injury. In addition, fibrinogen associates positively with age, obesity, smoking, diabetes, and LDL cholesterol level, and inversely with HDL cholesterol level, alcohol use, physical activity, and exercise level.[211] Fibrinogen, like CRP, an acute phase reactant, increases during inflammatory responses.

Given these relationships, it is not surprising that fibrinogen was among the first "novel" risk factors evaluated. Early reports from the Gothenburg,[212] Northwick Park, and Framingham heart studies all found significant positive associations between fibrinogen levels and future risk of cardiovascular events. Since then, multiple other prospective studies have confirmed these findings[213,214] and in two recent meta-analyses, individuals with levels in the upper third had significantly elevated relative risks compared to those with the lowest levels (RR, 1.8; 95 percent CI, 1.6 to 2.0).[215,216] Fibrinogen levels also indicate increased risk of stroke and peripheral arterial disease.[217] In most studies, these effects were independent of other traditional risk factors, although in other settings fibrinogen was predictive only among those with concomitant elevation of lipoprotein(a)[218] or homocysteine.[219]

Despite the consistency of these data, fibrinogen evaluation has found limited use in clinical practice for several reasons. First, assay standardization for fibrinogen has been inadequate, and analytic consistency across reference laboratories remains poor. Second, at least in comparison to CRP, the predictive value of fibrinogen is modest. This likely results from a wider variation within individuals for fibrinogen levels than CRP and poorer assay characteristics for fibrinogen. Moreover, in several studies that evaluated both CRP and fibrinogen, only CRP independently predicted future vascular events.[143] Third, fibrinogen levels are elevated in certain groups, including women, persons taking estrogen, and smokers, thus complicating the interpretation of study results. Last, despite two decades of evaluation, we still lack data demonstrating additive value in risk assessment in primary prevention over Framingham scoring.

Fibrates and niacin lower fibrinogen levels but statin therapy does not, an effect different than that observed for CRP. To date, three clinical trials have evaluated the potential benefits of fibrinogen reduction, and all have found disappointing results. In the Bezafibrate Infarction Prevention Trial,[220] there was no reduction in event rates with active therapy despite a significant reduction in fibrinogen levels and despite evidence that within the study population baseline fibrinogen levels predicted vascular risk.[221] In a second trial of more than 1500 patients with peripheral vascular disease, bezafibrate reduced fibrinogen levels 13 percent but again had no significant effect on clinical outcomes.[222]

Finally, in the HERS trial and within the Women's Health Initiative, hormone replacement therapy lowered fibrinogen levels but had no benefit on outcome.[223]

Fibrin D-dimer reflects the extent of fibrin turnover in the circulation, and epidemiological evidence has found D-dimer levels to have modest predictive value for future vascular events.[224-226] As with fibrinogen, these studies, when taken together, suggest an approximate relative risk of 1.7 to 1.8 comparing those in the top to bottom thirds of the D-dimer distribution.[227] Following myocardial infarction, D-dimer levels also predict recurrent events[228] and like CRP, D-dimer predicts poor outcome in troponin-negative ischemia.[229] These studies have pathophysiological interest, and evidence has accumulated that genetic determinants of fibrinogen and D-dimer may lead to altered fibrin clot structure in susceptible individuals.[230] As with fibrinogen, however, the utility of D-dimer assessment for arterial thrombosis prediction appears limited in clinical settings. This finding contrasts markedly with the strong clinical utility of D-dimer evaluation in the setting of suspected venous thromboembolism.[231]

Markers of Fibrinolytic Function (Plasminogen Activator Inhibitor-1, Tissue Plasminogen Activator, Clot Lysis)

Impaired fibrinolysis can result from an imbalance between the clot-dissolving enzymes t-PA or urokinase-type plasminogen activator and their endogenous inhibitors, primarily PAI-1. Plasma levels of PAI-1 peak in the morning, whereas concentrations of t-PA demonstrate a less prominent circadian variation. On this basis, a relative hypofibrinolytic state may prevail in the morning that, along with increased platelet reactivity, may contribute to the increased risk of myocardial infarction seen in this time period. Visceral obesity yields enhanced PAI-1 production from adipocytes, and thus impaired fibrinolysis may help explain how weight gain and obesity influence atherothrombosis. Individuals with the insulin resistance syndrome commonly have impaired fibrinolysis, and, in the setting of metabolic syndrome, PAI-1 levels as well as CRP predict adverse vascular outcomes in addition to the onset of type 2 diabetes.[232]

Clinically, patients with isolated PAI-1 deficiencies have excess rates of hemorrhage, whereas genetically mediated PAI-1 excess may lead to spontaneous thrombosis. A consistent series of prospective studies has linked abnormalities of fibrinolysis to increased risk of arterial thrombosis. For example, prospective associations exist between PAI-1 antigen and activity levels and the risk of first and recurrent myocardial infarction. Perhaps paradoxically, individuals at risk for future coronary as well as cerebral thrombosis consistently also have elevated levels of circulating t-PA antigen.[233] These latter effects may represent evidence of underlying endothelial dysfunction among individuals at risk or a direct relationship between t-PA and PAI-1, or they may represent a biological response to impaired fibrinolysis. In this regard, reduced clot lysis time, an overall indicator of net fibrinolytic function, also predicts coronary risk. As reviewed earlier, several studies indicate that levels of D-dimer, a peptide released by plasmin's action on fibrin, also predicts myocardial infarction, peripheral atherosclerosis, and recurrent coronary events. These observations have recently been confirmed in women both taking and not taking hormone replacement therapy, an important issue because conjugated estrogens decrease PAI-1 antigen concentrations.[234,235]

Despite these data, the clinical use of fibrinolytic markers to determine coronary risk may offer marginal value, and no data available suggest that measures of fibrinolysis adds to traditional risk scores. Direct measurement of PAI-1 activity is difficult in clinical settings and requires special anticoagulants and precise phlebotomy techniques to avoid degranulation of platelets, a rich source of PAI-1. In addition, markers of fibrinolytic function such as PAI-1 have a wide circadian variation limiting use in outpatient settings as a risk determinant. Nonetheless, the recognition that fibrinolytic function contributes to atherothrombosis has yielded several practical applications. For example, PAI-1-resistant thrombolytic agents may provide a means to increase the efficacy of thrombolytic therapy for acute myocardial infarction. Further, the renin-angiotensin system plays an important role in the regulation of fibrinolysis, and angiotensin-converting enzyme inhibitors may favorably affect fibrinolytic balance.[236-238] Finally, well-described polymorphisms in the PAI-1 promoter and other components of the fibrinolytic system may contribute to interindividual differences in fibrinolytic function.[239,240]

Lipoprotein(a) (see Chap. 39)

Lipoprotein(a) consists of an LDL particle with its apo B-100 component linked by a disulfide bridge to apo(a), a variable-length protein that has sequence homology to plasminogen. The apo(a) component of lipoprotein(a) is a complex molecule composed in part of varying numbers of cysteine-rich kringle IV repeats that result in great heterogeneity. As such, plasma lipoprotein(a) concentrations vary inversely with apo(a) isoform size but also may vary even within isoform size based on differential levels of production. Underlying its molecular complexity, more than 25 heritable forms of lipoprotein(a) exist, demonstrating the importance of the genome in determining plasma levels, an important issue for risk prediction across different population groups.[241]

Although the biological function of lipoprotein(a) remains uncertain, the close homology between lipoprotein(a) and plasminogen has raised the possibility that this lipoprotein may inhibit endogenous fibrinolysis by competing with plasminogen binding on the endothelium. More recent data suggest that lipoprotein(a) binds and inactivates tissue factor pathway inhibitor and may upregulate the expression of plasminogen activator inhibitor, further linking lipoproteins and thrombosis.[242,243] Lipoprotein(a) also colocalizes within atherosclerotic lesions and may have local actions. Thus, several mechanisms may contribute to a role of lipoprotein(a) in atherothrombosis.

Although many retrospective and cross-sectional studies suggest a positive association between lipoprotein(a) and vascular risk, lipoprotein(a) levels rise after ischemia and with the acute phase response, and thus these studies cannot determine a causal relationship. A series of prospective studies that avoid this bias generally support this association, however. A recent meta-analysis of 27 prospective studies with a mean follow-up period of 10 years found that individuals with lipoprotein(a) levels in the top third of the distribution had a risk 1.6 times higher than those with lipoprotein(a) levels in the bottom third.[244] Adjustment for classic cardiovascular risk factors only modestly attenuated these effects, in part because there is little correlation between lipoprotein(a) and other markers of risk.

Whether the assessment of lipoprotein(a) truly adds prognostic information to overall risk in primary prevention remains uncertain, because in most studies lipoprotein(a) has been predictive only among those already known to be at high risk. For example, recent data from the Italian Longitudinal Study on Aging, the Prospective Cardiovascular Munster study, the Bruneck Heart Study, and the PRIME study suggest that high serum lipoprotein(a) level is an important risk factor primarily among individuals with type 2 diabetes[245,246] or overt hyperlipidemia.[247-249] Other investigators have found that lipoprotein(a) signifies elevated risk in limited situations such as the presence of hyperfibrinogenemia or elevated homocysteine level.[250,251] Several prospective evaluations have shown that lipoprotein(a) predicts risk in a nonlinear manner such that risk increases are very small until lipoprotein(a) levels within the top 5 to 10 percent are reached.[252,253] Large-scale prospective studies confirm these relationships but also find that lipoprotein(a) has modest predictive value in comparison with other novel risk factors.[142,154] Finally, some investigators have advocated lipoprotein(a) assessment in certain patient groups, such as those with established coronary disease[254] or renal failure, although data remain controversial.[255,256] Thus, in terms of general population screening, lipoprotein(a) evaluation appears to have limited utility.

Beyond these epidemiological considerations, several practical issues hamper lipoprotein(a) evaluation in clinical settings. Most importantly, standardization of commercial lipoprotein(a) assays remains problematic. A recent working group of the International Federation of Clinical Chemistry has reported that much of the inaccuracy of commercial lipoprotein(a) determination results from the use of techniques sensitive to apo(a) size.[257] Recognition of this issue, wider use of assays unaffected by apo(a) heterogeneity, and the establishment of reference standards should improve these limitations. We also have only limited data on risk prediction in non-white groups, although lipoprotein(a) levels vary widely on an ethnic basis. Finally, except for high-dose niacin, few interventions lower lipoprotein(a) level. This limitation, as well as the observation that LDL cholesterol reduction markedly reduces any hazard associated with lipoprotein(a), has also dampened enthusiasm for screening. Ongoing genetic investigation is yielding important insights into lipoprotein(a) regulation,[258] and the development of peptides that inhibit lipoprotein(a) assembly raise novel pathways for risk reduction that will require direct testing in clinical trials.[259] Evidence that children with recurrent ischemic stroke have elevated lipoprotein(a) levels also supports the potential use of this biomarker in unusual high-risk settings.[260]

Lipoprotein Subclasses, Particle Size, and Particle Concentration (see Chap. 39)

Although standard chemical measures for total and LDL cholesterol form the basis for current lipid screening and reduction guidelines, the amount of cholesterol carried by individual lipoprotein particles may influence their function and vary widely between individuals. Therefore, measures of core lipid composition and lipoprotein particle size and concentration might provide a better measure of risk prediction.[261] Several lines of evidence indicate that small LDL particles may be more atherogenic than large LDL particles and contribute to the dyslipidemia of diabetes.[262] Currently, a number of technologies are available for evaluation of LDL subclasses and particle size. Studies using density gradient ultracentrifugation and gradient gel electrophoresis have generally found that lipoprotein subclass identifies individuals at higher risk for coronary disease[263] and have successfully shown a preferential benefit of lipid-lowering therapy among patients with small, dense LDL particles as compared to large LDL particles.[264]

Recent studies have also found LDL particle concentration as measured by nuclear magnetic resonance to correlate well with coronary arterial lumen diameter after statin therapy[265] and to have predictive value for future vascular events. For example, in both the Women's Health Study[266] and the Cardiovascular Health Study,[267] LDL particle concentration measured by nuclear magnetic resonance predicted incident vascular events better than standard measurement of LDL cholesterol. These relationships remain complex, however, and have not always been consistent.[268] In addition, standardization across technologies available for lipoprotein subclassification has remained problematic. Thus, although intriguing pathophysiological information regarding lipid reduction with statins has come from studies of nuclear magnetic resonance spectroscopy as well as density gradient studies,[269] it remains unclear whether these novel methods of lipid evaluation greatly add to standard lipid screening. To date, no studies have tested whether such methods add to traditional scoring systems such as the Framingham Heart Study.

Future Directions in Cardiovascular Risk Assessment

Some 40 percent of the U.S. adult population is at "intermediate risk" but do not currently qualify for intensive risk factor intervention despite the presence of one or more traditional risk factors.[270] In the immediate future, the most important novel tool to improve risk stratification among these individuals will be the inflammatory biomarker hsCRP as an adjunct to global risk prediction. As reviewed earlier, strong evidence shows that hsCRP adds prognostic information at all levels of LDL cholesterol, at all levels of the Framingham risk score, and at all levels of the metabolic syndrome. Thus, hsCRP evaluation, along with standard lipid screening, will likely become common practice in the near future. Ongoing trials based on hsCRP evaluation will also probably have an impact on clinical practice guidelines.[157] The pathophysiological implications that follow from the inflammatory hypothesis of atherothrombosis should lead to novel interventions for primary prevention as well as the treatment of acute ischemia.

Direct Plaque Imaging

Aside from the use of inflammatory markers such as hsCRP, future strategies to detect vascular disease will likely take several forms. Most prominent may be the noninvasive detection of atherosclerotic plaque. At this time, a number of studies indicate that coronary calcification as detected by computed tomography can detect high-risk individuals and perhaps permit monitoring of lipid-lowering therapy.[271,272] It remains highly controversial, however, as to whether this approach is cost-effective or has an acceptable false-negative rate.[273] Enrollment in many such studies may be biased by referral patterns or self-selection by patients. Part of the difficulty with coronary calcification as a clinical surrogate is that CT imaging probably detects the very plaques least likely to rupture and does not detect the noncalcified, thin-walled lesions that appear to cause most clinical events. Thus, while coronary calcium provides a noninvasive measure of atherosclerotic burden, patients with low calcium scores cannot be dismissed as being at low risk. Further, the clinical determinants of calcification are largely unknown and may not reflect propensity to plaque rupture. Recent data demonstrating that hsCRP elevation corresponds to an approximate doubling of risk of plaque rupture at all levels of coronary calcium demonstrates the complexity of this approach.[274] Considerable public health concern has also been raised regarding the consequences of false-positive findings from imaging techniques such as coronary calcium scores. For example, in one recent study of currently asymptomatic individuals, 41 percent of all future vascular events occurred among those with coronary artery calcium scores (CACS) less than 100 and 17 percent occurred among those with CACS of zero.[274a] Thus, absence of CACS does not preclude risk of coronary events. Current guidelines do not support the routine use of coronary computed tomographic imaging.

A recent study showed that provision of calcium scores did not effectively motivate patients' adherence to risk reduction regimens.[275] Several other modalities for the noninvasive assessment of atherosclerosis are also available, ranging from those that are well documented and inexpensive (such as the ankle-brachial index) to those that are exploratory (such as thermography and magnetic resonance scanning). Perhaps the best studied noninvasive approach is the ultrasonic measurement of carotid intimal medial thickness. While somewhat operator dependent, this technique has proved to have strong predictive value in general population studies,[276,277] and no additional expense is required because most centers already have the required sonographic tools in place. Although carotid intimal medial thickness undoubtedly provides a valid research tool, its practical applicability in practice remains unproven. Whether any imaging technique will prove cost-effective as a screening tool is currently under study in the Multiethnic Study of Atherosclerosis (MESA) being funded by the National Heart, Lung, and Blood Institute.[278]

The availability of a wide array of genetic data should also change coronary risk prediction in the future, and many large-scale evaluations of polymorphism and haplotype patterns designed to understand better the atherothrombotic process are well underway. For venous thrombosis, genetic detection of factor V Leiden and of a common promoter polymorphism in the prothrombin gene have already entered wide clinical practice. Proteomic studies that go a step further and evaluate all the products of these genes (and their posttranscriptional changes) have also already had an impact in our understanding of venous thromboembolism. By contrast, although family history contributes importantly to determining risk of myocardial infarction or stroke, studies of single nucleotide polymorphisms in arterial thrombosis have largely been disappointing to date. Continued methodological concerns about the reproducibility of published results and generalizability to usual populations suggest that the use of genetic data to predict arterial risk will take several more years of research to come to fruition. However, there is little doubt that major gene-environment and gene-gene interactions exist that, when carefully uncovered, will lead to novel methods of detection and prevention.

REFERENCES

1. Annual smoking-attributable mortality, years of potential life lost, and economic costs—United States, 1995-1999. MMWR Morb Mortal Wkly Rep 51:300, 2002.
2. U.S. Department of Health and Human Services: Women and Smoking. A Report of the Surgeon General. Rockville, Md, U.S. Department of Health and Human Services, Public Health Service, Office of the Surgeon General, 2001.
3. Cigarette smoking among adults—United States, 2000. MMWR Morb Mortal Wkly Rep 51:642, 2002.
4. Incidence of initiation of cigarette smoking—United States, 1965-1996. MMWR Morb Mortal Wkly Rep 47:837, 1998.
5. Peto R, Lopez AD, Boreham J, et al: Mortality from smoking worldwide. Br Med Bull 52:12, 1996.
6. Kawachi I, Colditz GA, Speizer FE, et al: A prospective study of passive smoking and coronary heart disease. Circulation 95:2374, 1997.
7. He J, Vupputuri S, Allen K, et al: Passive smoking and the risk of coronary heart disease: A meta-analysis of epidemiologic studies. N Engl J Med 340:920, 1999.
8. Otsuka R, Watanabe H, Hirata K, et al: Acute effects of passive smoking on the coronary circulation in healthy young adults. JAMA 286:436, 2001.
9. Janson C, Chinn S, Jarvis D, et al: Effect of passive smoking on respiratory symptoms, bronchial responsiveness, lung function, and total serum IgE in the European Community Respiratory Health Survey: A cross-sectional study. Lancet 358:2103, 2001.
10. Prescott E, Scharling H, Osler M, Schnohr P: Importance of light smoking and inhalation habits on risk of myocardial infarction and all cause mortality: A 22 year follow up of 12,149 men and women in The Copenhagen City Heart Study. J Epidemiol Community Health 56:702, 2002.
11. Kurth T, Kase CS, Berger K, et al: Smoking and the risk of hemorrhagic stroke in men. Stroke 34:1151, 2003.
12. Rea TD, Heckbert SR, Kaplan RC, et al: Smoking status and risk for recurrent coronary events after myocardial infarction. Ann Intern Med 137:494, 2002.
13. Al-Delaimy WK, Manson JE, Solomon CG, et al: Smoking and risk of coronary heart disease among women with type 2 diabetes mellitus. Arch Intern Med 162:273, 2002.
14. Howard G, Wagenknecht LE, Burke GL, et al: Cigarette smoking and progression of atherosclerosis: The Atherosclerosis Risk in Communities (ARIC) Study. JAMA 279:119, 1998.
15. Barua RS, Ambrose JA, Srivastava S, et al: Reactive oxygen species are involved in smoking-induced dysfunction of nitric oxide biosynthesis and upregulation of endothelial nitric oxide synthase: An in vitro demonstration in human coronary artery endothelial cells. Circulation 107:2342, 2003.
16. Barua RS, Ambrose JA, Eales-Reynolds LJ, et al: Dysfunctional endothelial nitric oxide biosynthesis in healthy smokers with impaired endothelium-dependent vasodilatation. Circulation 104:1905, 2001.
17. Tsuchiya M, Asada A, Kasahara E, et al: Smoking a single cigarette rapidly reduces combined concentrations of nitrate and nitrite and concentrations of antioxidants in plasma. Circulation 105:1155, 2002.
18. Tracy RP, Psaty BM, Macy E, et al: Lifetime smoking exposure affects the association of C-reactive protein with cardiovascular disease risk factors and subclinical disease in healthy elderly subjects. Arterioscler Thromb Vasc Biol 17:2167, 1997.
19. Blann AD, Steele C, McCollum CN: The influence of smoking on soluble adhesion molecules and endothelial cell markers. Thromb Res 85:433, 1997.
20. Bazzano LA, He J, Muntner P, et al: Relationship between cigarette smoking and novel risk factors for cardiovascular disease in the United States. Ann Intern Med 138:891, 2003.
21. Fusegawa Y, Goto S, Handa S, et al: Platelet spontaneous aggregation in platelet-rich plasma is increased in habitual smokers. Thromb Res 93:271, 1999.
22. Adams MR, Jessup W, Celermajer DS: Cigarette smoking is associated with increased human monocyte adhesion to endothelial cells: Reversibility with oral L-arginine but not vitamin C. J Am Coll Cardiol 29:491, 1997.
23. Newby DE, McLeod AL, Uren NG, et al: Impaired coronary tissue plasminogen activator release is associated with coronary atherosclerosis and cigarette smoking: Direct link between endothelial dysfunction and atherothrombosis. Circulation 103:1936, 2001.
24. Matetzky S, Tani S, Kangavari S, et al: Smoking increases tissue factor expression in atherosclerotic plaques: Implications for plaque thrombogenicity. Circulation 102:602, 2000.
25. Barua RS, Ambrose JA, Saha DC, Eales-Reynolds LJ: Smoking is associated with altered endothelial-derived fibrinolytic and antithrombotic factors: An in vitro demonstration. Circulation 106:905, 2002.
26. Reaven G, Tsao PS: Insulin resistance and compensatory hyperinsulinemia: The key player between cigarette smoking and cardiovascular disease? J Am Coll Cardiol 41:1044, 2003.
27. Critchley JA, Capewell S: Mortality risk reduction associated with smoking cessation in patients with coronary heart disease: A systematic review. JAMA 290:86, 2003.
28. van Domburg RT, Meeter K, van Berkel DF, et al: Smoking cessation reduces mortality after coronary artery bypass surgery: A 20-year follow-up study. J Am Coll Cardiol 36:878, 2000.
29. Lightwood JM, Glantz SA: Short-term economic and health benefits of smoking cessation: Myocardial infarction and stroke. Circulation 96:1089, 1997.
30. Hu FB, Stampfer MJ, Manson JE, et al: Trends in the incidence of coronary heart disease and changes in diet and lifestyle in women. N Engl J Med 343:530, 2000.
31. The Tobacco Use and Dependence Clinical Practice Guideline Panel, Staff, and Consortium Representatives: A clinical practice guideline for treating tobacco use and dependence: A U.S. Public Health Service report. JAMA 283:3244, 2000.
32. Godtfredsen NS, Holst C, Prescott E, et al: Smoking reduction, smoking cessation, and mortality: A 16-year follow-up of 19,732 men and women from The Copenhagen Centre for Prospective Population Studies. Am J Epidemiol 156:994, 2002.
33. Landman A, Ling PM, Glantz SA: Tobacco industry youth smoking prevention programs: Protecting the industry and hurting tobacco control. Am J Public Health 92:917, 2002.
34. Neuman M, Bitton A, Glantz S: Tobacco industry strategies for influencing European Community tobacco advertising legislation. Lancet 359:1323, 2002.
35. Chobanian AV, Bakris GL, Black HR, et al: The Seventh Report of the Joint National Committee on Prevention, Detection, Evaluation, and Treatment of High Blood Pressure: The JNC 7 report. JAMA 289:2560, 2003.
36. Hajjar I, Kotchen TA: Trends in prevalence, awareness, treatment, and control of hypertension in the United States, 1988-2000. JAMA 290:199, 2003.
37. Wolf-Maier K, Cooper RS, Banegas JR, et al: Hypertension prevalence and blood pressure levels in 6 European countries, Canada, and the United States. JAMA 289:2363, 2003.
38. Glynn RJ, L'Italien GJ, Sesso HD, et al: Development of predictive models for long-term cardiovascular risk associated with systolic and diastolic blood pressure. Hypertension 39:105, 2002.
39. Domanski M, Mitchell G, Pfeffer M, et al: Pulse pressure and cardiovascular disease-related mortality: Follow-up study of the Multiple Risk Factor Intervention Trial (MRFIT). JAMA 287:2677, 2002.
40. Staessen JA, Gasowski J, Wang JG, et al: Risks of untreated and treated isolated systolic hypertension in the elderly: Meta-analysis of outcome trials. Lancet 355:865, 2000.
41. O'Donnell CJ, Ridker PM, Glynn RJ, et al: Hypertension and borderline isolated systolic hypertension increase risks of cardiovascular disease and mortality in male physicians. Circulation 95:1132, 1997.
42. Vasan RS, Larson MG, Leip EP, et al: Impact of high-normal blood pressure on the risk of cardiovascular disease. N Engl J Med 345:1291, 2001.
43. Mitchell GF, Moye LA, Braunwald E, et al: Sphygmomanometrically determined pulse pressure is a powerful independent predictor of recurrent events after myocardial infarction in patients with impaired left ventricular function. SAVE investigators. Survival and Ventricular Enlargement. Circulation 96:4254, 1997.
44. Chae CU, Pfeffer MA, Glynn RJ, et al: Increased pulse pressure and risk of heart failure in the elderly. JAMA 281:634, 1999.
45. Vaccarino V, Holford TR, Krumholz HM: Pulse pressure and risk for myocardial infarction and heart failure in the elderly. J Am Coll Cardiol 36:130, 2000.
46. Haider AW, Larson MG, Franklin SS, Levy D: Systolic blood pressure, diastolic blood pressure, and pulse pressure as predictors of risk for congestive heart failure in the Framingham Heart Study. Ann Intern Med 138:10, 2003.
47. Staessen JA, Thijs L, Fagard R, et al: Predicting cardiovascular risk using conventional vs ambulatory blood pressure in older patients with systolic hypertension. Systolic Hypertension in Europe Trial Investigators. JAMA 282:539, 1999.
48. Bjorklund K, Lind L, Zethelius B, et al: Isolated ambulatory hypertension predicts cardiovascular morbidity in elderly men. Circulation 107:1297, 2003.
49. Liu L, Wang JG, Gong L, et al: Comparison of active treatment and placebo in older Chinese patients with isolated systolic hypertension. Systolic Hypertension in China (Syst-China) Collaborative Group. J Hypertens 16:1823, 1998.
50. SHEP Cooperative Research Group: Prevention of stroke by antihypertensive drug treatment in older persons with isolated systolic hypertension: Final results of the Systolic Hypertension in the Elderly Program (SHEP). JAMA 265:3255, 1991.
51. Staessen JA, Fagard R, Thijs L, et al: Randomised double-blind comparison of placebo and active treatment for older patients with isolated systolic hypertension. The Systolic Hypertension in Europe (Syst-Eur) Trial Investigators. Lancet 350:757, 1997.
52. Mehler PS, Coll JR, Estacio R, et al: Intensive blood pressure control reduces the risk of cardiovascular events in patients with peripheral arterial disease and type 2 diabetes. Circulation 107:753, 2003.

53. Whelton PK, Appel LJ, Espeland MA, et al: Sodium reduction and weight loss in the treatment of hypertension in older persons: A randomized controlled trial of nonpharmacologic interventions in the elderly (TONE). TONE Collaborative Research Group. JAMA 279:839, 1998.
54. Psaty BM, Lumley T, Furberg CD, et al: Health outcomes associated with various antihypertensive therapies used as first-line agents: A network meta-analysis. JAMA 289:2534, 2003.
55. Law MR, Wald NJ, Morris JK, Jordan RE: Value of low dose combination treatment with blood pressure lowering drugs: Analysis of 354 randomised trials. BMJ 326:1427, 2003.
56. Libby P, Aikawa M, Schonbeck U: Cholesterol and atherosclerosis. Biochim Biophys Acta 1529:299, 2000.
56a. Nissen SE, Tuzcu EM, Schoenhagen P, et al: Effect of intensive compared with moderate lipid-lowering therapy on progression of coronary atherosclerosis. JAMA 291:1071, 2004.
56b. Cannon CP, Braunwald E, McCabe CH, et al: Intensive versus moderate lipid lowering with statins after acute coronary syndromes. N Engl J Med 350:1495, 2004.
57. Stamler J, Daviglus ML, Garside DB, et al: Relationship of baseline serum cholesterol levels in 3 large cohorts of younger men to long-term coronary, cardiovascular, and all-cause mortality and to longevity. JAMA 284:311, 2000.
58. Grundy SM, Howard B, Smith S Jr, et al: Prevention Conference VI: Diabetes and Cardiovascular Disease: Executive summary: Conference proceeding for healthcare professionals from a special writing group of the American Heart Association. Circulation 105:2231, 2002.
59. Howard BV, Rodriguez BL, Bennett PH, et al: Prevention Conference VI: Diabetes and Cardiovascular disease: Writing Group I: Epidemiology. Circulation 105:e132, 2002.
60. Gu K, Cowie CC, Harris MI: Mortality in adults with and without diabetes in a national cohort of the U.S. population, 1971-1993. Diabetes Care 21:1138, 1998.
61. Hu FB, Stampfer MJ, Haffner SM, et al: Elevated risk of cardiovascular disease prior to clinical diagnosis of type 2 diabetes. Diabetes Care 25:1129, 2002.
62. Gillum RF, Mussolino ME, Madans JH: Diabetes mellitus, coronary heart disease incidence, and death from all causes in African American and European American women: The NHANES I epidemiologic follow-up study. J Clin Epidemiol 53:511, 2000.
63. Garber AJ: Attenuating CV risk factors in patients with diabetes: Clinical evidence to clinical practice. Diabetes Obes Metab 4(Suppl 1):S5, 2002.
64. Henry P, Thomas F, Benetos A, Guize L: Impaired fasting glucose, blood pressure and cardiovascular disease mortality. Hypertension 40:458, 2002.
65. Kuller LH, Velentgas P, Barzilay J, et al: Diabetes mellitus: Subclinical cardiovascular disease and risk of incident cardiovascular disease and all-cause mortality. Arterioscler Thromb Vasc Biol 20:823, 2000.
66. Executive Summary of the Third Report of the National Cholesterol Education Program (NCEP) Expert Panel on Detection, Evaluation, and Treatment of High Blood Cholesterol in Adults (Adult Treatment Panel III). JAMA 285:2486, 2001.
67. Ford ES, Giles WH, Dietz WH: Prevalence of the metabolic syndrome among U.S. adults: Findings from the third National Health and Nutrition Examination Survey. JAMA 287:356, 2002.
68. Lakka HM, Laaksonen DE, Lakka TA, et al: The metabolic syndrome and total and cardiovascular disease mortality in middle-aged men. JAMA 288:2709, 2002.
69. Isomaa B, Almgren P, Tuomi T, et al: Cardiovascular morbidity and mortality associated with the metabolic syndrome. Diabetes Care 24:683, 2001.
70. Ridker PM, Buring JE, Cook NR, Rifai N: C-reactive protein, the metabolic syndrome, and risk of incident cardiovascular events: An 8-year follow-up of 14,719 initially healthy American women. Circulation 107:391, 2003.
71. Pradhan AD, Manson JE, Rifai N, et al: C-reactive protein, interleukin 6, and risk of developing type 2 diabetes mellitus. JAMA 286:327, 2001.
72. Freeman DJ, Norrie J, Caslake MJ, et al: C-reactive protein is an independent predictor of risk for the development of diabetes in the West of Scotland Coronary Prevention Study. Diabetes 51:1596, 2002.
73. Albert CM, Campos H, Stampfer MJ, et al: Blood levels of long-chain n-3 fatty acids and the risk of sudden death. N Engl J Med 346:1113, 2002.
74. Barzilay JI, Abraham L, Heckbert SR, et al: The relation of markers of inflammation to the development of glucose disorders in the elderly: The Cardiovascular Health Study. Diabetes 50:2384, 2001.
74a. Hu FB, Meiss JB, Li TY, et al: Inflammatory markers and risk of developing type 2 diabetes in women. Diabetes 53:693, 2004.
75. Sattar N, Gaw A, Scherbakova O, et al: Metabolic syndrome with and without C-reactive protein as a predictor of coronary heart disease and diabetes in the West of Scotland Coronary Prevention Study. Circulation 108:414, 2003.
76. Pradhan AD, Cook NR, Buring JE, et al: C-reactive protein is independently associated with fasting insulin in nondiabetic women. Arterioscler Thromb Vasc Biol 23:650, 2003.
77. Festa A, D'Agostino R Jr, Howard G, et al: Chronic subclinical inflammation as part of the insulin resistance syndrome: The Insulin Resistance Atherosclerosis Study (IRAS). Circulation 102:42, 2000.
78. Pradhan AD, Ridker PM: Do atherosclerosis and type 2 diabetes share a common inflammatory basis? Eur Heart J 23:831, 2002.
79. Bierhaus A, Hofmann MA, Ziegler R, Nawroth PP: AGEs and their interaction with AGE-receptors in vascular disease and diabetes mellitus. I. The AGE concept. Cardiovasc Res 37:586, 1998.
80. Wautier JL, Guillausseau PJ: Diabetes, advanced glycation endproducts and vascular disease. Vasc Med 3:131, 1998.
81. Eckel RH, Wassef M, Chait A, et al: Prevention Conference VI: Diabetes and Cardiovascular Disease: Writing Group II: Pathogenesis of atherosclerosis in diabetes. Circulation 105:e138, 2002.
82. Valmadrid CT, Klein R, Moss SE, Klein BE: The risk of cardiovascular disease mortality associated with microalbuminuria and gross proteinuria in persons with older-onset diabetes mellitus. Arch Intern Med 160:1093, 2000.
83. Sobel BE: Effects of glycemic control and other determinants on vascular disease in type 2 diabetes. Am J Med 113(Suppl 6A):12S, 2002.
84. Varo N, Vicent D, Libby P, et al: Elevated plasma levels of the atherogenic mediator soluble CD40 ligand in diabetic patients: A novel target of thiazolidinediones. Circulation 107:2664, 2003.
85. Beckman JA, Creager MA, Libby P: Diabetes and atherosclerosis: Epidemiology, pathophysiology, and management. JAMA 287:2570, 2002.
86. Thompson PD, Buchner D, Pina IL, et al: Exercise and physical activity in the prevention and treatment of atherosclerotic cardiovascular disease: A statement from the Council on Clinical Cardiology (Subcommittee on Exercise, Rehabilitation, and Prevention) and the Council on Nutrition, Physical Activity, and Metabolism (Subcommittee on Physical Activity). Circulation 107:3109, 2003.
87. Manson JE, Greenland P, LaCroix AZ, et al: Walking compared with vigorous exercise for the prevention of cardiovascular events in women. N Engl J Med 347:716, 2002.
88. Manson JE, Hu FB, Rich-Edwards JW, et al: A prospective study of walking as compared with vigorous exercise in the prevention of coronary heart disease in women. N Engl J Med 341:650, 1999.
89. Tanasescu M, Leitzmann MF, Rimm EB, et al: Exercise type and intensity in relation to coronary heart disease in men. JAMA 288:1994, 2002.
90. Lee IM, Sesso HD, Paffenbarger RS Jr: Physical activity and coronary heart disease risk in men: Does the duration of exercise episodes predict risk? Circulation 102:981, 2000.
91. Hu FB, Stampfer MJ, Colditz GA, et al: Physical activity and risk of stroke in women. JAMA 283:2961, 2000.
92. Lee IM, Rexrode KM, Cook NR, et al: Physical activity and coronary heart disease in women: Is "no pain, no gain" passe? JAMA 285:1447, 2001.
93. Pate RR, Pratt M, Blair SN, et al: Physical activity and public health: A recommendation from the Centers for Disease Control and Prevention and the American College of Sports Medicine. JAMA 273:402, 1995.
94. Schoenborn CA, Barnes PM: Leisure-time physical activity among adults: United States, 1997-98. Advanced data from vital and health statistics; no.325. Hyattsville, Md, National Center for Health Statistics, 2002.
95. Institute of Medicine: Dietary reference intakes for energy, carbohydrates, fiber, fat, protein, and amino acids. Washington, DC, The National Academies Press, 2002.
96. Irwin ML, Yasui Y, Ulrich CM, et al: Effect of exercise on total and intra-abdominal body fat in postmenopausal women: A randomized controlled trial. JAMA 289:323, 2003.
97. Whelton SP, Chin A, Xin X, He J: Effect of aerobic exercise on blood pressure: A meta-analysis of randomized, controlled trials. Ann Intern Med 136:493, 2002.
98. Kelley GA, Kelley KS, Tran ZV: Walking and resting blood pressure in adults: A meta-analysis. Prev Med 33:120, 2001.
99. Kraus WE, Houmard JA, Duscha BD, et al: Effects of the amount and intensity of exercise on plasma lipoproteins. N Engl J Med 347:1483, 2002.
100. Boule NG, Haddad E, Kenny GP, et al: Effects of exercise on glycemic control and body mass in type 2 diabetes mellitus: A meta-analysis of controlled clinical trials. JAMA 286:1218, 2001.
101. Hu FB, Sigal RJ, Rich-Edwards JW, et al: Walking compared with vigorous physical activity and risk of type 2 diabetes in women: A prospective study. JAMA 282:1433, 1999.
102. Knowler WC, Barrett-Connor E, Fowler SE, et al: Reduction in the incidence of type 2 diabetes with lifestyle intervention or metformin. N Engl J Med 346:393, 2002.
103. Ford ES: Does exercise reduce inflammation? Physical activity and C-reactive protein among U.S. adults. Epidemiology 13:561, 2002.
104. Hambrecht R, Wolf A, Gielen S, et al: Effect of exercise on coronary endothelial function in patients with coronary artery disease. N Engl J Med 342:454, 2000.
105. Wannamethee SG, Lowe GD, Whincup PH, et al: Physical activity and hemostatic and inflammatory variables in elderly men. Circulation 105:1785, 2002.
106. Rexrode KM, Carey VJ, Hennekens CH, et al: Abdominal adiposity and coronary heart disease in women. JAMA 280:1843, 1998.
107. Flegal KM, Carroll MD, Ogden CL, Johnson CL: Prevalence and trends in obesity among U.S. adults, 1999-2000. JAMA 288:1723, 2002.
108. Ogden CL, Flegal KM, Carroll MD, Johnson CL: Prevalence and trends in overweight among U.S. children and adolescents, 1999-2000. JAMA 288:1728, 2002.
109. Ghiadoni L, Donald AE, Cropley M, et al: Mental stress induces transient endothelial dysfunction in humans. Circulation 102:2473, 2000.
110. Brunner EJ, Hemingway H, Walker BR, et al: Adrenocortical, autonomic, and inflammatory causes of the metabolic syndrome: Nested case-control study. Circulation 106:2659, 2002.
111. Hjemdahl P: Stress and the metabolic syndrome: An interesting but enigmatic association. Circulation 106:2634, 2002.
112. Lampert R, Jain D, Burg MM, et al: Destabilizing effects of mental stress on ventricular arrhythmias in patients with implantable cardioverter-defibrillators. Circulation 101:158, 2000.
113. Lampert R, Joska T, Burg MM, et al: Emotional and physical precipitants of ventricular arrhythmia. Circulation 106:1800, 2002.
114. Krantz DS, Santiago HT, Kop WJ, et al: Prognostic value of mental stress testing in coronary artery disease. Am J Cardiol 84:1292, 1999.
115. Krantz DS, Sheps DS, Carney RM, Natelson BH: Effects of mental stress in patients with coronary artery disease: Evidence and clinical implications. JAMA 283:1800, 2000.
116. Kivimaki M, Leino-Arjas P, Luukkonen R, et al: Work stress and risk of cardiovascular mortality: Prospective cohort study of industrial employees. BMJ 325:857, 2002.
117. Iso H, Date C, Yamamoto A, et al: Perceived mental stress and mortality from cardiovascular disease among Japanese men and women: The Japan Collaborative Cohort Study for Evaluation of Cancer Risk Sponsored by Monbusho (JACC Study). Circulation 106:1229, 2002.
118. Rugulies R: Depression as a predictor for coronary heart disease: A review and meta-analysis. Am J Prev Med 23:51, 2002.
119. Wulsin LR, Singal BM: Do depressive symptoms increase the risk for the onset of coronary disease? A systematic quantitative review. Psychosom Med 65:201, 2003.

120. Bush DE, Ziegelstein RC, Tayback M, et al: Even minimal symptoms of depression increase mortality risk after acute myocardial infarction. Am J Cardiol 88:337, 2001.
121. Glassman AH, O'Connor CM, Califf RM, et al: Sertraline treatment of major depression in patients with acute MI or unstable angina. JAMA 288:701, 2002.
122. Berkman LF, Blumenthal J, Burg M, et al: Effects of treating depression and low perceived social support on clinical events after myocardial infarction: The Enhancing Recovery in Coronary Heart Disease Patients (ENRICHD) Randomized Trial. JAMA 289:3106, 2003.
123. Frasure-Smith N, Lesperance F: Depression: A cardiac risk factor in search of a treatment. JAMA 289:3171, 2003.
124. Ridker PM, Rifai N, Rose L, et al: Comparison of C-reactive protein and low-density lipoprotein cholesterol levels in the prediction of first cardiovascular events. N Engl J Med 347:1557, 2002.
125. Khot UN, Khot MB, Bajzer CT, et al: Prevalence of conventional risk factors in patients with coronary heart disease. JAMA 290:898, 2003.
126. Greenland P, Knoll MD, Stamler J, et al: Major risk factors as antecedents of fatal and nonfatal coronary heart disease events. JAMA 290:891, 2003.
127. Ridker PM: Evaluating novel cardiovascular risk factors: Can we better predict heart attacks? Ann Intern Med 130:933, 1999.
128. Hackam DG, Anand SS: Emerging risk factors for atherosclerotic vascular disease: A critical review of the evidence. JAMA 290:932, 2003.
129. Libby P, Ridker PM, Maseri A: Inflammation and atherosclerosis. Circulation 105:1135, 2002.
130. Buffon A, Biasucci LM, Liuzzo G, et al: Widespread coronary inflammation in unstable angina. N Engl J Med 347:5, 2002.
131. Ridker PM: Clinical application of C-reactive protein for cardiovascular disease detection and prevention. Circulation 107:363, 2003.
132. Calabro P, Willerson JT, Yeh ET: Inflammatory cytokines stimulated C-reactive protein production by human coronary artery smooth muscle cells. Circulation 108:1930, 2003.

133. Jabs WJ, Theissing E, Nitschke M, et al: Local generation of C-reactive protein in diseased coronary artery venous bypass grafts and normal vascular tissue. Circulation 108:1428, 2003.
134. Pasceri V, Willerson JT, Yeh ET: Direct proinflammatory effect of C-reactive protein on human endothelial cells. Circulation 102:2165, 2000.
135. Zwaka TP, Hombach V, Torzewski J: C-reactive protein-mediated low density lipoprotein uptake by macrophages: Implications for atherosclerosis. Circulation 103:1194, 2001.
136. Venugopal SK, Devaraj S, Yuhanna I, et al: Demonstration that C-reactive protein decreases eNOS expression and bioactivity in human aortic endothelial cells. Circulation 106:1439, 2002.
137. Devaraj S, Xu DY, Jialal I: C-reactive protein increases plasminogen activator inhibitor-1 expression and activity in human aortic endothelial cells: Implications for the metabolic syndrome and atherothrombosis. Circulation 107:398, 2003.
138. Danenberg HD, Szalai AJ, Swaminathan RV, et al: Increased thrombosis after arterial injury in human C-reactive protein-transgenic mice. Circulation 108:512, 2003.
138a. Paul A, Ko KW, Yechoor V, et al: C-reactive protein accelerates the progression of atherosclerosis in apolipoprotein E-deficient mice. Circulation 109:647, 2004.
139. Pradhan AD, Manson JE, Rossouw JE, et al: Inflammatory biomarkers, hormone replacement therapy, and incident coronary heart disease: Prospective analysis from the Women's Health Initiative observational study. JAMA 288:980, 2002.
140. Albert CM, Ma J, Rifai N, et al: Prospective study of C-reactive protein, homocysteine, and plasma lipid levels as predictors of sudden cardiac death. Circulation 105:2595, 2002.
141. Ridker PM, Cushman M, Stampfer MJ, et al: Inflammation, aspirin, and the risk of cardiovascular disease in apparently healthy men. N Engl J Med 336:973, 1997.
142. Ridker PM, Hennekens CH, Buring JE, Rifai N: C-reactive protein and other markers of inflammation in the prediction of cardiovascular disease in women. N Engl J Med 342:836, 2000.
143. Ridker PM, Stampfer MJ, Rifai N: Novel risk factors for systemic atherosclerosis: A comparison of C-reactive protein, fibrinogen, homocysteine, lipoprotein(a), and standard cholesterol screening as predictors of peripheral arterial disease. JAMA 285:2481, 2001.
144. Albert MA, Glynn RJ, Ridker PM: Plasma concentration of C-reactive protein and the calculated Framingham Coronary Heart Disease Risk Score. Circulation 108:161, 2003.
144a. Ballantyne CM, Hoogeveen RC, Bang H, et al: Lipoprotein-associated phospholipase A2, high-sensitivity C-reactive protein, and risk for incident coronary heart disease in middle-aged men and women in the Atherosclerosis Risk In Communities (ARIC) Study. Circulation 109:837, 2004.
144b. Koenig W, Löwel H, Baumert J, Meisinger C: C-reactive protein modulates risk prediction based on the Framingham Score: Implications for future risk assessment. Circulation 109:1349, 2004.
144c. Danesh J, Wheeler JG, Hirschfield GM, et al: C-reactive protein and other circulating markers of inflammation in the prediction of coronary heart disease. N Engl J Med 350:1387, 2004.
145. Pearson TA, Mensah GA, Alexander RW, et al: Markers of inflammation and cardiovascular disease: Application to clinical and public health practice: A statement for healthcare professionals from the Centers for Disease Control and Prevention and the American Heart Association. Circulation 107:499, 2003.
145a. Ridker PM, Cook N. Clinical usefulness of very high and very low levels of C-reactive protein across the full range of Framingham risk scores. Circulation 109:1955, 2004.
146. Ridker PM, Rifai N, Pfeffer MA, et al: Inflammation, pravastatin, and the risk of coronary events after myocardial infarction in patients with average cholesterol levels. Cholesterol and Recurrent Events (CARE) Investigators. Circulation 98:839, 1998.
147. Liuzzo G, Biasucci LM, Gallimore JR, et al: The prognostic value of C-reactive protein and serum amyloid a protein in severe unstable angina. N Engl J Med 331:417, 1994.
148. Mueller C, Buettner HJ, Hodgson JM, et al: Inflammation and long-term mortality after non-ST elevation acute coronary syndrome treated with a very early invasive strategy in 1042 consecutive patients. Circulation 105:1412, 2002.
149. Milazzo D, Biasucci LM, Luciani N, et al: Elevated levels of C-reactive protein before coronary artery bypass grafting predict recurrence of ischemic events. Am J Cardiol 84:459, A9, 1999.
150. Chew DP, Bhatt DL, Robbins MA, et al: Incremental prognostic value of elevated baseline C-reactive protein among established markers of risk in percutaneous coronary intervention. Circulation 104:992, 2001.
151. Lindahl B, Toss H, Siegbahn A, et al: Markers of myocardial damage and inflammation in relation to long-term mortality in unstable coronary artery disease. FRISC Study Group. Fragmin during Instability in Coronary Artery Disease. N Engl J Med 343:1139, 2000.
152. Lindmark E, Diderholm E, Wallentin L, Siegbahn A: Relationship between interleukin 6 and mortality in patients with unstable coronary artery disease: Effects of an early invasive or noninvasive strategy. JAMA 286:2107, 2001.
153. Dibra A, Mehilli J, Braun S, et al: Association between C-reactive protein levels and subsequent cardiac events among patients with stable angina treated with coronary artery stenting. Am J Med 114:715, 2003.
154. Albert MA, Danielson E, Rifai N, Ridker PM: Effect of statin therapy on C-reactive protein levels: The pravastatin inflammation/CRP evaluation (PRINCE): A randomized trial and cohort study. JAMA 286:64, 2001.
155. Ridker PM, Rifai N, Pfeffer MA, et al: Long-term effects of pravastatin on plasma concentration of C-reactive protein. The Cholesterol and Recurrent Events (CARE) Investigators. Circulation 100:230, 1999.
156. Ridker PM, Rifai N, Clearfield M, et al: Measurement of C-reactive protein for the targeting of statin therapy in the primary prevention of acute coronary events. N Engl J Med 344:1959, 2001.
157. Ridker PM: Rosuvastatin in the primary prevention of cardiovascular disease among patients with low LDL cholesterol and elevated high sensitivity C-reactive protein (hsCRP): Rationale and design of the JUPITER trial. Circulation 108:2292, 2003.
158. Burke AP, Tracy RP, Kolodgie F, et al: Elevated C-reactive protein values and atherosclerosis in sudden coronary death: Association with different pathologies. Circulation 105:2019, 2002.
159. Sesso HD, Buring JE, Rifai N, et al: C-reactive protein and the risk of developing hypertension: Is hypertension an inflammatory disease? JAMA 290:2945, 2003.
160. Blake GJ, Rifai N, Buring JE, Ridker PM: Blood pressure, C-reactive protein, and risk of future cardiovascular events. Circulation 108:2993, 2003.
161. Labarrere CA, Lee JB, Nelson DR, et al: C-reactive protein, arterial endothelial activation, and development of transplant coronary artery disease: A prospective study. Lancet 360:1462, 2002.
162. Wanner C, Zimmermann J, Schwedler S, Metzger T: Inflammation and cardiovascular risk in dialysis patients. Kidney Int Suppl 80:99, May 2002.
163. O'Connor CM, Dunne MW, Pfeffer MA, et al: Azithromycin for the secondary prevention of coronary heart disease events: The WIZARD study: A randomized controlled trial. JAMA 290:1459, 2003.
164. Ridker PM: Cardiology Patient Page. C-reactive protein: A simple test to help predict risk of heart attack and stroke. Circulation 108:e81, 2003.
165. Ridker PM, Rifai N, Stampfer MJ, Hennekens CH: Plasma concentration of interleukin-6 and the risk of future myocardial infarction among apparently healthy men. Circulation 101:1767, 2000.
166. Ridker PM, Hennekens CH, Roitman-Johnson B, et al: Plasma concentration of soluble intercellular adhesion molecule 1 and risks of future myocardial infarction in apparently healthy men. Lancet 351:88, 1998.
167. Ridker PM, Buring JE, Rifai N: Soluble P-selectin and the risk of future cardiovascular events. Circulation 103:491, 2001.
168. Malik I, Danesh J, Whincup P, et al: Soluble adhesion molecules and prediction of coronary heart disease: A prospective study and meta-analysis. Lancet 358:971, 2001.
169. Pradhan AD, Rifai N, Ridker PM: Soluble intercellular adhesion molecule-1, soluble vascular adhesion molecule-1, and the development of symptomatic peripheral arterial disease in men. Circulation 106:820, 2002.
170. Schonbeck U, Varo N, Libby P, et al: Soluble CD40L and cardiovascular risk in women. Circulation 104:2266, 2001.
171. Zhang R, Brennan ML, Fu X, et al: Association between myeloperoxidase levels and risk of coronary artery disease. JAMA 286:2136, 2001.
172. Packard CJ, O'Reilly DS, Caslake MJ, et al: Lipoprotein-associated phospholipase A2 as an independent predictor of coronary heart disease. West of Scotland Coronary Prevention Study Group. N Engl J Med 343:1148, 2000.
173. Ballantyne CM, Houri J, Notarbartolo A, et al: Effect of ezetimibe coadministered with atorvastatin in 628 patients with primary hypercholesterolemia: A prospective, randomized, double-blind trial. Circulation 107:2409, 2003.
174. Bayes-Genis A, Conover CA, Overgaard MT, et al: Pregnancy-associated plasma protein A as a marker of acute coronary syndromes. N Engl J Med 345:1022, 2001.
175. Blake GJ, Dada N, Fox JC, et al: A prospective evaluation of lipoprotein-associated phospholipase A(2) levels and the risk of future cardiovascular events in women. J Am Coll Cardiol 38:1302, 2001.
176. Heeschen C, Dimmeler S, Hamm CW, et al: Soluble CD40 ligand in acute coronary syndromes. N Engl J Med 348:1104, 2003.
177. Baldus S, Heeschen C, Meinertz T, et al: Myeloperoxidase serum levels predict risk in patients with acute coronary syndromes. Circulation 108:1440, 2003.
178. Brennan ML, Penn MS, Van Lente F, et al: Prognostic value of myeloperoxidase in patients with chest pain. N Engl J Med 349:1595, 2003.
179. Welch GN, Loscalzo J: Homocysteine and atherothrombosis. N Engl J Med 338:1042, 1998.
180. Chambers JC, Ueland PM, Obeid OA, et al: Improved vascular endothelial function after oral B vitamins: An effect mediated through reduced concentrations of free plasma homocysteine. Circulation 102:2479, 2000.

181. Bellamy MF, McDowell IF, Ramsey MW, et al: Hyperhomocysteinemia after an oral methionine load acutely impairs endothelial function in healthy adults. Circulation 98:1848, 1998.
182. Poddar R, Sivasubramanian N, DiBello PM, et al: Homocysteine induces expression and secretion of monocyte chemoattractant protein-1 and interleukin-8 in human aortic endothelial cells: Implications for vascular disease. Circulation 103:2717, 2001.
183. Werstuck GH, Lentz SR, Dayal S, et al: Homocysteine-induced endoplasmic reticulum stress causes dysregulation of the cholesterol and triglyceride biosynthetic pathways. J Clin Invest 107:1263, 2001.
184. Jacques PF, Bostom AG, Wilson PW, et al: Determinants of plasma total homocysteine concentration in the Framingham Offspring cohort. Am J Clin Nutr 73:613, 2001.
185. Kark JD, Sinnreich R, Rosenberg IH, et al: Plasma homocysteine and parental myocardial infarction in young adults in Jerusalem. Circulation 105:2725, 2002.
186. Klerk M, Verhoef P, Clarke R, et al: MTHFR 677C→T polymorphism and risk of coronary heart disease: A meta-analysis. JAMA 288:2023, 2002.
187. Wilson PW: Homocysteine and coronary heart disease: How great is the hazard? JAMA 288:2042, 2002.
188. Malinow MR, Bostom AG, Krauss RM: Homocyst(e)ine, diet, and cardiovascular diseases: A statement for healthcare professionals from the Nutrition Committee, American Heart Association. Circulation 99:178, 1999.
189. Wald DS, Law M, Morris JK: Homocysteine and cardiovascular disease: Evidence on causality from a meta-analysis. BMJ 325:1202, 2002.
190. Homocysteine and risk of ischemic heart disease and stroke: A meta-analysis. JAMA 288:2015, 2002.
191. Kelly PJ, Rosand J, Kistler JP, et al: Homocysteine, MTHFR 677C→T polymorphism, and risk of ischemic stroke: Results of a meta-analysis. Neurology 59:529, 2002.
192. Ford ES, Smith SJ, Stroup DF, et al: Homocyst(e)ine and cardiovascular disease: A systematic review of the evidence with special emphasis on case-control studies and nested case-control studies. Int J Epidemiol 31:59, 2002.
193. Ridker PM, Manson JE, Buring JE, et al: Homocysteine and risk of cardiovascular disease among postmenopausal women. JAMA 281:1817, 1999.
194. Jacques PF, Selhub J, Bostom AG, et al: The effect of folic acid fortification on plasma folate and total homocysteine concentrations. N Engl J Med 340:1449, 1999.
195. Ridker PM, Shih J, Cook TJ, et al: Plasma homocysteine concentration, statin therapy, and the risk of first acute coronary events. Circulation 105:1776, 2002.
196. Lowering blood homocysteine with folic acid based supplements: Meta-analysis of randomised trials. Homocysteine Lowering Trialists' Collaboration. BMJ 316:894, 1998.
197. Wald DS, Bishop L, Wald NJ, et al: Randomized trial of folic acid supplementation and serum homocysteine levels. Arch Intern Med 161:695, 2001.
198. Tice JA, Ross E, Coxson PG, et al: Cost-effectiveness of vitamin therapy to lower plasma homocysteine levels for the prevention of coronary heart disease: Effect of grain fortification and beyond. JAMA 286:936, 2001.
199. Spence JD, Howard VJ, Chambless LE, et al: Vitamin Intervention for Stroke Prevention (VISP) trial: Rationale and design. Neuroepidemiology 20:16, 2001.
200. The VITATOPS (Vitamins to Prevent Stroke) Trial: Rationale and design of an international, large, simple, randomised trial of homocysteine-lowering multivitamin therapy in patients with recent transient ischaemic attack or stroke. Cerebrovasc Dis 13:120, 2002.
201. MacMahon M, Kirkpatrick C, Cummings CE, et al: A pilot study with simvastatin and folic acid/vitamin B12 in preparation for the Study of the Effectiveness of Additional Reductions in Cholesterol and Homocysteine (SEARCH). Nutr Metab Cardiovasc Dis 10:195, 2000.
202. Bostom AG, Selhub J, Jacques PF, Rosenberg IH: Power Shortage: Clinical trials testing the "homocysteine hypothesis" against a background of folic acid-fortified cereal grain flour. Ann Intern Med 135:133, 2001
203. Shemin D, Bostom AG, Selhub J: Treatment of hyperhomocysteinemia in end-stage renal disease. Am J Kidney Dis 38:S91, 2001.
203a. Toole JF, Malinow MR, Chambless LE, et al: Lowering homocysteine in patients with ischemic stroke to prevent recurrent stroke, myocardial infarction, and death. JAMA 291:565, 2004.
204. Nygard O, Nordrehaug JE, Refsum H, et al: Plasma homocysteine levels and mortality in patients with coronary artery disease. N Engl J Med 337:230, 1997.
205. Al-Obaidi MK, Stubbs PJ, Collinson P, et al: Elevated homocysteine levels are associated with increased ischemic myocardial injury in acute coronary syndromes. J Am Coll Cardiol 36:1217, 2000.
206. Schnyder G, Roffi M, Pin R, et al: Decreased rate of coronary restenosis after lowering of plasma homocysteine levels. N Engl J Med 345:1593, 2001.
207. Schnyder G, Roffi M, Flammer Y, et al: Effect of homocysteine-lowering therapy with folic acid, vitamin B12, and vitamin B6 on clinical outcome after percutaneous coronary intervention: The Swiss Heart study: A randomized controlled trial. JAMA 288:973, 2002.
208. Miller A, Mujumdar V, Palmer L, et al: Reversal of endocardial endothelial dysfunction by folic acid in homocysteinemic hypertensive rats. Am J Hypertens 15:157, 2002.
209. Blacher J, Demuth K, Guerin AP, et al: Association between plasma homocysteine concentrations and cardiac hypertrophy in end-stage renal disease. J Nephrol 12:248, 1999.
210. Vasan RS, Beiser A, D'Agostino RB, et al: Plasma homocysteine and risk for congestive heart failure in adults without prior myocardial infarction. JAMA 289:1251, 2003.
211. Margaglione M, Cappucci G, Colaizzo D, et al: Fibrinogen plasma levels in an apparently healthy general population: Relation to environmental and genetic determinants. Thromb Haemost 80:805, 1998.
212. Wilhelmsen L, Svardsudd K, Korsan-Bengtsen K, et al: Fibrinogen as a risk factor for stroke and myocardial infarction. N Engl J Med 311:501, 1984.
213. Folsom AR, Rosamond WD, Shahar E, et al: Prospective study of markers of hemostatic function with risk of ischemic stroke. The Atherosclerosis Risk in Communities (ARIC) Study Investigators. Circulation 100:736, 1999.
214. Ma J, Hennekens CH, Ridker PM, Stampfer MJ: A prospective study of fibrinogen and risk of myocardial infarction in the Physicians' Health Study. J Am Coll Cardiol 33:1347, 1999.
215. Danesh J, Collins R, Appleby P, Peto R: Association of fibrinogen, C-reactive protein, albumin, or leukocyte count with coronary heart disease: Meta-analyses of prospective studies. JAMA 279:1477, 1998.
216. Maresca G, Di Blasio A, Marchioli R, Di Minno G: Measuring plasma fibrinogen to predict stroke and myocardial infarction: An update. Arterioscler Thromb Vasc Biol 19:1368, 1999.
217. Lee AJ, Fowkes FG, Lowe GD, et al: Fibrinogen, factor VII and PAI-1 genotypes and the risk of coronary and peripheral atherosclerosis: Edinburgh Artery Study. Thromb Haemost 81:553, 1999.
218. Cantin B, Gagnon F, Moorjani S, et al: Is lipoprotein(a) an independent risk factor for ischemic heart disease in men? The Quebec Cardiovascular Study. J Am Coll Cardiol 31:519, 1998.
219. Acevedo M, Pearce GL, Kottke-Marchant K, Sprecher DL: Elevated fibrinogen and homocysteine levels enhance the risk of mortality in patients from a high-risk preventive cardiology clinic. Arterioscler Thromb Vasc Biol 22:1042, 2002.
220. Secondary prevention by raising HDL cholesterol and reducing triglycerides in patients with coronary artery disease: The Bezafibrate Infarction Prevention (BIP) study. Circulation 102:21, 2000.
221. Tanne D, Benderly M, Goldbourt U, et al: A prospective study of plasma fibrinogen levels and the risk of stroke among participants in the bezafibrate infarction prevention study. Am J Med 111:457, 2001.
222. Meade T, Zuhrie R, Cook C, Cooper J: Bezafibrate in men with lower extremity arterial disease: Randomised controlled trial. BMJ 325:1139, 2002.
223. Hulley S, Grady D, Bush T, et al: Randomized trial of estrogen plus progestin for secondary prevention of coronary heart disease in postmenopausal women. Heart and Estrogen/progestin Replacement Study (HERS) Research Group. JAMA 280:605, 1998.
224. Cushman M, Lemaitre RN, Kuller LH, et al: Fibrinolytic activation markers predict myocardial infarction in the elderly. The Cardiovascular Health Study. Arterioscler Thromb Vasc Biol 19:493, 1999.
225. Smith FB, Lee AJ, Fowkes FG, et al: Hemostatic factors as predictors of ischemic heart disease and stroke in the Edinburgh Artery Study. Arterioscler Thromb Vasc Biol 17:3321, 1997.
226. Lowe GD, Yarnell JW, Sweetnam PM, et al: Fibrin D-dimer, tissue plasminogen activator, plasminogen activator inhibitor, and the risk of major ischaemic heart disease in the Caerphilly Study. Thromb Haemost 79:129, 1998.
227. Danesh J, Whincup P, Walker M, et al: Fibrin D-dimer and coronary heart disease: Prospective study and meta-analysis. Circulation 103:2323, 1998.
228. Moss AJ, Goldstein RE, Marder VJ, et al: Thrombogenic factors and recurrent coronary events. Circulation 99:2517, 1999.
229. Menown IB, Mathew TP, Gracey HM, et al: Prediction of Recurrent Events by D-Dimer and Inflammatory Markers in Patients with Normal Cardiac Troponin I (PREDICT) Study. Am Heart J 145:986, 2003.
230. Mills JD, Ariens RA, Mansfield MW, Grant PJ: Altered fibrin clot structure in the healthy relatives of patients with premature coronary artery disease. Circulation 106:1938, 2002.
231. Wells PS, Anderson DR, Rodger M, et al: Evaluation of D-dimer in the diagnosis of suspected deep-vein thrombosis. N Engl J Med 349:1227, 2003.
232. Festa A, D'Agostino R Jr, Tracy RP, Haffner SM: Elevated levels of acute-phase proteins and plasminogen activator inhibitor-1 predict the development of type 2 diabetes: The insulin resistance atherosclerosis study. Diabetes 51:1131, 2002.
233. Thogersen AM, Jansson JH, Boman K, et al: High plasminogen activator inhibitor and tissue plasminogen activator levels in plasma precede a first acute myocardial infarction in both men and women: Evidence for the fibrinolytic system as an independent primary risk factor. Circulation 98:2241, 1998.
234. Brown NJ, Abbas A, Byrne D, et al: Comparative effects of estrogen and angiotensin-converting enzyme inhibition on plasminogen activator inhibitor-1 in healthy postmenopausal women. Circulation 105:304, 2002.
235. Pradhan AD, LaCroix AZ, Trevisan M, et al: Tissue plasminogen activator antigen and D-dimer as markers for atherothrombotic risk among healthy post-menopausal women: A report from the women's health initiative observational study. Circulation 2004, in press.
236. Vaughan DE, Rouleau JL, Ridker PM, et al: Effects of ramipril on plasma fibrinolytic balance in patients with acute anterior myocardial infarction. HEART Study Investigators. Circulation 96:442, 1997.
237. Brown NJ, Agirbasli MA, Williams GH, et al: Effect of activation and inhibition of the renin-angiotensin system on plasma PAI-1. Hypertension 32:965, 1998.
238. Pretorius M, Rosenbaum D, Vaughan DE, Brown NJ: Angiotensin-converting enzyme inhibition increases human vascular tissue-type plasminogen activator release through endogenous bradykinin. Circulation 107:579, 2003.
239. Festa A, D'Agostino R Jr, Rich SS, et al: Promoter (4G/5G) plasminogen activator inhibitor-1 genotype and plasminogen activator inhibitor-1 levels in blacks, Hispanics, and non-Hispanic whites: The Insulin Resistance Atherosclerosis Study. Circulation 107:2422, 2003.
240. Boekholdt SM, Bijsterveld NR, Moons AH, et al: Genetic variation in coagulation and fibrinolytic proteins and their relation with acute myocardial infarction: A systematic review. Circulation 104:3063, 2001.
241. Hobbs HH, White AL: Lipoprotein(a): Intrigues and insights. Curr Opin Lipidol 10:225, 1999.
242. Caplice NM, Panetta C, Peterson TE, et al: Lipoprotein(a) binds and inactivates tissue factor pathway inhibitor: A novel link between lipoproteins and thrombosis. Blood 98:2980, 2001.
243. Buechler C, Ullrich H, Ritter M, et al: Lipoprotein(a) up-regulates the expression of the plasminogen activator inhibitor 2 in human blood monocytes. Blood 97:981, 2001.

244. Danesh J, Collins R, Peto R: Lipoprotein(a) and coronary heart disease: Meta-analysis of prospective studies. Circulation 102:1082, 2000.
245. Solfrizzi V, Panza F, Colacicco AM, et al: Relation of lipoprotein(a) as coronary risk factor to type 2 diabetes mellitus and low-density lipoprotein cholesterol in patients > or = 65 years of age (The Italian Longitudinal Study on Aging). Am J Cardiol 89:825, 2002.
246. Koschinsky ML, Marcovina SM: The relationship between lipoprotein(a) and the complications of diabetes mellitus. Acta Diabetol 40:65, 2003.
247. von Eckardstein A, Schulte H, Cullen P, Assmann G: Lipoprotein(a) further increases the risk of coronary events in men with high global cardiovascular risk. J Am Coll Cardiol 37:434, 2001.
248. Kronenberg F, Kronenberg MF, Kiechl S, et al: Role of lipoprotein(a) and apolipoprotein(a) phenotype in atherogenesis: Prospective results from the Bruneck study. Circulation 100:1154, 1999.
249. Luc G, Bard JM, Arveiler D, et al: Lipoprotein(a) as a predictor of coronary heart disease: The PRIME Study. Atherosclerosis 163:377, 2002.
250. Foody JM, Milberg JA, Robinson K, et al: Homocysteine and lipoprotein(a) interact to increase CAD risk in young men and women. Arterioscler Thromb Vasc Biol 20:493, 2000.
251. Cantin B, Despres JP, Lamarche B, et al: Association of fibrinogen and lipoprotein(a) as a coronary heart disease risk factor in men (The Quebec Cardiovascular Study). Am J Cardiol 89:662, 2002.
252. Sweetnam PM, Bolton CH, Downs LG, et al: Apolipoproteins A-I, A-II and B, lipoprotein(a) and the risk of ischaemic heart disease: The Caerphilly study. Eur J Clin Invest 30:947, 2000.
253. Sharrett AR, Ballantyne CM, Coady SA, et al: Coronary heart disease prediction from lipoprotein cholesterol levels, triglycerides, lipoprotein(a), apolipoproteins A-I and B, and HDL density subfractions: The Atherosclerosis Risk in Communities (ARIC) Study. Circulation 104:1108, 2001.

254. Glader CA, Birgander LS, Stenlund H, Dahlen GH: Is lipoprotein(a) a predictor for survival in patients with established coronary artery disease? Results from a prospective patient cohort study in northern Sweden. J Intern Med 252:27, 2002.
255. Longenecker JC, Klag MJ, Marcovina SM, et al: Small apolipoprotein(a) size predicts mortality in end-stage renal disease: The CHOICE study. Circulation 106:2812, 2002.
256. Longenecker JC, Coresh J, Marcovina SM, et al: Lipoprotein(a) and prevalent cardiovascular disease in a dialysis population: The choices for healthy outcomes in caring for ESRD (CHOICE) study. Am J Kidney Dis 42:108, 2003.
257. Marcovina SM, Albers JJ, Scanu AM, et al: Use of a reference material proposed by the International Federation of Clinical Chemistry and Laboratory Medicine to evaluate analytical methods for the determination of plasma lipoprotein(a). Clin Chem 46:1956, 2000.
258. Holmer SR, Hengstenberg C, Kraft HG, et al: Association of polymorphisms of the apolipoprotein(a) gene with lipoprotein(a) levels and myocardial infarction. Circulation 107:696, 2003.
259. Sharp RJ, Perugini MA, Marcovina SM, McCormick SP: A synthetic peptide that inhibits lipoprotein(a) assembly. Arterioscler Thromb Vasc Biol 23:502, 2003.
260. Strater R, Becker S, von Eckardstein A, et al: Prospective assessment of risk factors for recurrent stroke during childhood: A 5-year follow-up study. Lancet 360:1540, 2002.
261. Otvos JD, Jeyarajah EJ, Cromwell WC: Measurement issues related to lipoprotein heterogeneity. Am J Cardiol 90:22i, 2002.
262. Sniderman AD, Scantlebury T, Cianflone K: Hypertriglyceridemic hyperapoB: The unappreciated atherogenic dyslipoproteinemia in type 2 diabetes mellitus. Ann Intern Med 135:447, 2001.
263. Lamarche B, Tchernof A, Moorjani S, et al: Small, dense low-density lipoprotein particles as a predictor of the risk of ischemic heart disease in men. Prospective results from the Quebec Cardiovascular Study. Circulation 95:69, 1997.
264. Zambon A, Hokanson JE, Brown BG, Brunzell JD: Evidence for a new pathophysiological mechanism for coronary artery disease regression: Hepatic lipase-mediated changes in LDL density. Circulation 99:1959, 1999.
265. Rosenson RS, Otvos JD, Freedman DS: Relations of lipoprotein subclass levels and low-density lipoprotein size to progression of coronary artery disease in the Pravastatin Limitation of Atherosclerosis in the Coronary Arteries (PLAC-I) trial. Am J Cardiol 90:89, 2002.
266. Blake GJ, Otvos JD, Rifai N, Ridker PM: Low-density lipoprotein particle concentration and size as determined by nuclear magnetic resonance spectroscopy as predictors of cardiovascular disease in women. Circulation 106:1930, 2002.
267. Kuller L, Arnold A, Tracy R, et al: Nuclear magnetic resonance spectroscopy of lipoproteins and risk of coronary heart disease in the cardiovascular health study. Arterioscler Thromb Vasc Biol 22:1175, 2002.
268. Campos H, Moye LA, Glasser SP, et al: Low-density lipoprotein size, pravastatin treatment, and coronary events. JAMA 286:1468, 2001.
269. Otvos JD, Shalaurova I, Freedman DS, Rosenson RS: Effects of pravastatin treatment on lipoprotein subclass profiles and particle size in the PLAC-I trial. Atherosclerosis 160:41, 2002.
270. Greenland P, Smith SC Jr, Grundy SM: Improving coronary heart disease risk assessment in asymptomatic people: Role of traditional risk factors and noninvasive cardiovascular tests. Circulation 104:1863, 2001.
271. Keelan PC, Bielak LF, Ashai K, et al: Long-term prognostic value of coronary calcification detected by electron-beam computed tomography in patients undergoing coronary angiography. Circulation 104:412, 2001.
272. Achenbach S, Ropers D, Pohle K, et al: Influence of lipid-lowering therapy on the progression of coronary artery calcification: A prospective evaluation. Circulation 106:1077, 2002.
273. Detrano RC, Wong ND, Doherty TM, et al: Coronary calcium does not accurately predict near-term future coronary events in high-risk adults. Circulation 99:2633, 1999.
274. Park R, Detrano R, Xiang M, et al: Combined use of computed tomography coronary calcium scores and C-reactive protein levels in predicting cardiovascular events in nondiabetic individuals. Circulation 106:2073, 2002.
274a. Greenland P, LaBree L, Azen SP, et al: Coronary artery calcium score combined with Framingham score for risk prediction in asymptomatic individuals. JAMA 291:210, 2004.
275. O'Malley PG, Feuerstein IM, Taylor AJ: Impact of electron beam tomography, with or without case management, on motivation, behavioral change, and cardiovascular risk profile: A randomized controlled trial. JAMA 289:2215, 2003.
276. Hodis HN, Mack WJ, LaBree L, et al: The role of carotid arterial intima-media thickness in predicting clinical coronary events. Ann Intern Med 128:262, 1998.
277. O'Leary DH, Polak JF, Kronmal RA, et al: Carotid-artery intima and media thickness as a risk factor for myocardial infarction and stroke in older adults. Cardiovascular Health Study Collaborative Research Group. N Engl J Med 340:14, 1999.
278. Bild DE, Bluemke DA, Burke GL, et al: Multi-ethnic study of atherosclerosis: Objectives and design. Am J Epidemiol 156:871, 2002.

CHAPTER 37

Systemic Hypertension: Mechanisms and Diagnosis

Norman M. Kaplan

Recognition, Definitions, Prevalence, and Consequences of Hypertension

As the population grows older and more obese, the incidence of hypertension continues to increase, not only in the United States but in all developed and developing societies (Fig. 37–1).[1] At the same time, despite the widely recognized dangers of uncontrolled hypertension, the disease remains inadequately treated in the majority of patients.[2] Such inadequate management has been noted not only in closely observed communities[2] but also in carefully monitored antihypertensive drug trials.[3] As a consequence, cardiovascular risk remains high among the majority of hypertensive persons, whether treated or not.

Despite these disturbing figures, management of hypertension is now the leading indication for both visits to physicians and the use of prescription drugs in the United States.[4] Clearly, more attention is being directed toward hypertension, but adequate hypertension control remains elusive, in large part because of the asymptomatic nature of the disease for the first 15 to 20 years, even as it progressively damages the cardiovascular system. Asymptomatic patients are often unwilling to alter life style or take medication to forestall some far-off, poorly perceived danger, particularly when they are made uncomfortable in the process.

In view of these built-in barriers to effective control of the individual patient, population-wide application of preventive measures becomes inherently more attractive. Although the specific mechanisms for most hypertension remain unknown, it is highly likely that the process could be slowed, if not prevented, by the prevention of obesity, moderate reduction in sodium intake, higher levels of physical activity, and avoidance of excessive alcohol consumption.[5] Since hypertension will eventually develop in most people during their lifetime (Table 37–1),[6] the need for more widespread adoption of potentially effective and totally safe preventive measures is obvious. In the meantime, better management of those already afflicted must be practiced, starting with careful documentation of the diagnosis.

Measurement of Blood Pressure

Blood pressure typically changes considerably through the day and night. Such variability is seldom recognized by the relatively few office readings taken by most practitioners but can easily be identified by automatically recorded measurements taken throughout the day and night (Fig. 37–2). This variability can often be attributed to physical activity or emotional stress but is frequently without obvious cause. In a few patients, markedly elevated levels clearly indicate serious disease requiring immediate treatment. In most cases, however, initial readings are not high enough to indicate immediate danger, and the diagnosis of hypertension should be substantiated by repeated readings. The reason for such caution is obvious: The diagnosis of hypertension imposes psychological and socioeconomic burdens on an individual and usually implies the need for commitment to lifelong therapy.

Both transient and persistent elevations in blood pressure are common when the reading is taken in the physician's office or hospital. To identify the patient's usual range of blood pressure, more widespread use of out-of-the-office readings, either with semiautomatic inexpensive devices or with automatic ambulatory recorders, is encouraged both to establish the diagnosis and to monitor the patient's response to therapy.[7,8] A large body of data provides normal ranges for both home self-recorded and automatic ambulatory measurements.[9] Both average about 10/5 mm Hg lower than the average of multiple office readings. A closer correlation between the presence of various types of target organ damage, specifically, left ventricular hypertrophy (LVH), carotid wall thickness, proteinuria, and retinopathy, has been noted with ambulatory levels than with office levels. More importantly, increasing evidence supports a closer relation to future cardiovascular events with readings from ambulatory monitoring than with office readings (Fig. 37–3).[10] However, in the absence of adequate long-term follow-up, evidence of the risks associated with home monitoring, and the limited availability of ambulatory monitoring, office readings will continue to be the basis for the diagnosis and management of hypertension for most patients.

OUT-OF-THE-OFFICE MEASUREMENTS. A "white-coat effect," that is, a higher blood pressure on readings taken in the office than out of the office, is present in most patients. Therefore, whenever possible, office readings should be supplemented by out-of-the-office measurements, particularly when there is an apparent discrepancy between the level of blood pressure and the degree of target organ damage, in which case white coat hypertension should be suspected. In as many as one third of patients with office readings that remain elevated despite the use of three or more drugs, hypertension is found to be well controlled by out-of-the-office readings.[11] Purely white coat hypertension, that is, persistently elevated office readings at or above 140/90 mm Hg but persistently normal out-of-the-office

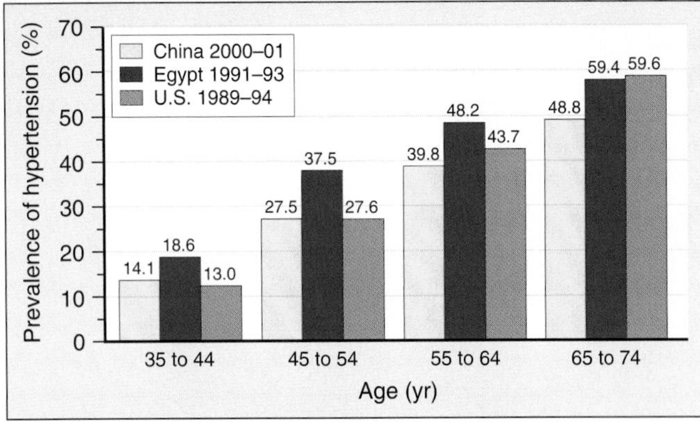

FIGURE 37–1 International Society of Hypertension prevalence of hypertension among three populations, ages 35 to 74 years: InterASIA (2000-2001), the Egyptian National Hypertension Project (1991-1993), and the Third National Health and Nutrition Examination Survey (1989-1994). (From Gu D, Reynolds K, Wu X, et al: Prevalence, awareness, treatment, and control of hypertension in China. Hypertension 40:925, 2002.)

TABLE 37–1 Residual Lifetime Risk of Hypertension According to Baseline Age*

	Women (%)		Men (%)	
Time, yrs	*55 yrs old* (*n* = 709)	*65 yrs old* (*n* = 549)	*55 yrs old* (*n* = 589)	*65 yrs old* (*n* = 438)
10	52	64	56	72
15	72	81	78	85
20	83	89	88	90
25	91	N/A	93	N/A

N/A = not applicable.
Modified from Vasan RS et al: JAMA 2002;287:1003-1010.
*For 55-year-old subjects, the risk for developing hypertension over 25 years represents their lifetime risk. For 65-year-old subjects, the risk for developing hypertension over 20 years indicates their lifetime risk.

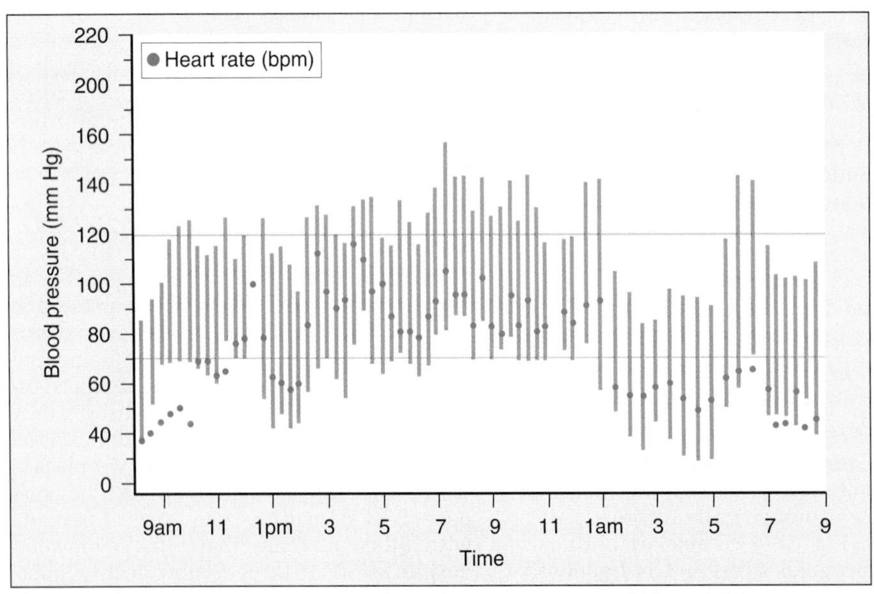

FIGURE 37–2 Computer printout of blood pressure readings obtained by ambulatory blood pressure monitoring over a 24-hour period beginning at 9 AM in a 50-year-old man with hypertension receiving no therapy. The patient slept from midnight until 6 AM. Solid circles indicate heart rate. (From Zachariah PK, Sheps SG, Smith RL: Defining the roles of home and ambulatory monitoring. Diagnosis 10:39, 1988. Copyright 1988, Medical Economics Publishing Company, Pradell, NJ. All rights reserved.)

readings at or below 135/85, is found in 20 to 30 percent of patients. The possibility of white-coat hypertension is increased in patients with these characteristics: (1) office blood pressure between 140 and 159 systolic or 90 and 99 diastolic; (2) female gender; (3) nonsmoking; (4) recent onset of hypertension; and (5) small left ventricular mass by echocardiography.[12] Obviously, the likelihood is also greater if only a few office readings have been taken.

Most such patients are free of the target organ damage and metabolic abnormalities (dyslipidemia, hyperinsulinemia) that are often found in patients with sustained hypertension, and follow-up for up to 10 years has found no increase in cardiovascular events.[12] Therefore, close observation and lifestyle modifications but not antihypertensive drug therapy seem appropriate management for such patients. On the other hand, a smaller portion of patients, particularly elderly subjects on treatment, may have "reverse white-coat" or "masked" hypertension, that is, normal office but elevated ambulatory readings.[13]

In addition to their role in the recognition of white coat and masked hypertension, out-of-the-office readings are essential for the recognition of persistently elevated pressures soon after arising, when the largest proportion of sudden deaths, myocardial infarctions, and strokes occur. The morning surge is dependent on physical activity after awakening and is related to increased sympathetic nervous activity.[14] The best way to blunt the early morning surge in pressure is to use antihypertensive drug formulations that provide full 24-hour coverage and to take them as early in the morning as possible. In view of the usual nocturnal fall in pressure (see Fig. 37–2), addition of the maximal antihypertensive effect of medication taken before bedtime could incite myocardial and cerebral ischemia during sleep.

Although a nocturnal fall or dipping in pressure is usual, little or no fall has been more frequently noted in various groups of hypertensive patients who have a more serious degree of target organ damage or subsequent major cardiovascular events. These groups include patients with LVH, diabetes, or renal damage and black patients. A smaller proportion of patients, mostly elderly, have excessive dipping, beyond 20 percent of the average daytime systolic level, and that too is associated with increased risk of cardiovascular morbidity.[15] Recognition of such abnormal nocturnal patterns of blood pressure then is another indication for more widespread use of automatic recordings.

BLOOD PRESSURE RESPONSE TO EXERCISE. Another source of potentially useful prognostic information is the blood pressure response to exercise, usually ascertained by treadmill testing. An exaggerated response in normotensive adults has been associated with a threefold greater likelihood of hypertension developing over the next 5 to 15 years[16] and a twofold greater cardiovascular mortality over a 21-year follow-up[17] compared to those without an exaggerated response during exercise. Since most normotensive subjects with an exaggerated response do not develop hypertension, exercise tests should not be done for predictive purposes. If, however, a supernormal response is noted, the subject should be advised to start a slowly progressive aerobic exercise program to moderate the response and, perhaps, delay the onset of hypertension.

DOCUMENTATION OF HYPERTENSION. For most patients who are in no immediate danger from markedly elevated pressure, that is, below approximately 170/110 mm Hg, the following guidelines are offered:

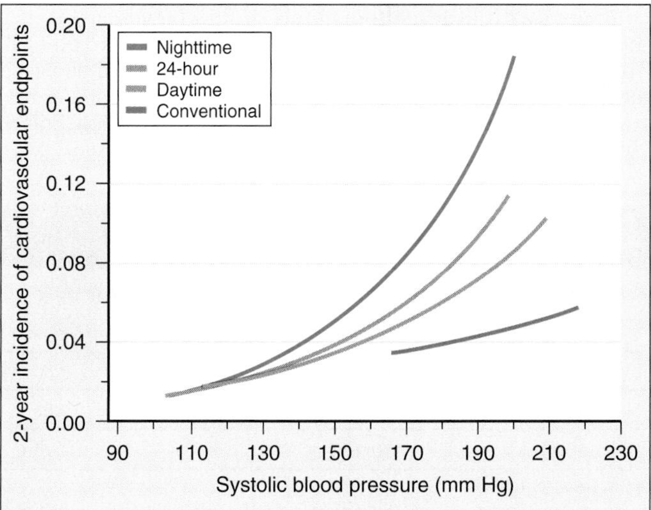

FIGURE 37–3 The relation of systolic blood pressure by conventional (office) or 24-hour daytime and nighttime ambulatory measurements at entry as predictors of the 2-year incidence of cardiovascular endpoints in the placebo-treated older patients with systolic hypertension. Incidence is given as a fraction (i.e., 0.02 is an incidence of 2 events per 100 people). Using multiple Cox regression, the event rate was standardized to female gender, mean age of 69.6 years, no previous cardiovascular complications, nonsmoking status, and residence in western Europe. (Modified from Staessen JA, Thijs L, Fagard R, et al: Predicting cardiovascular risk using conventional vs. ambulatory blood pressure in older patients with systolic hypertension. JAMA 282:539, 1999.)

1. Multiple readings should be obtained with appropriate technique (Table 37–2). If possible, the readings should be taken under varying conditions and at various times for at least 4 to 6 weeks with a semiautomatic home device. If the diagnosis must be established more rapidly, a set of readings obtained by an automatic monitor over a single 24-hour period will be adequate.
2. Although the logical approach would be to calculate the average values from multiple readings when deciding whether hypertension is present, even a single high measurement should not be disregarded. In large populations, antecedent office measurements have been found to predict a greater likelihood of subsequent cardiovascular disease above and beyond current blood pressure levels.[18]
3. Elderly patients may have markedly sclerotic brachial arteries that are not occluded until very high pressures are exerted by the balloon; therefore, cuff levels may be considerably higher than those measured intraarterially. In patients with high cuff readings but little or no hypertensive retinopathy, cardiac hypertrophy, or other evidence of longstanding hypertension, "pseudohypertension" should be suspected and ruled out before treatment is begun.
4. Elderly persons with elevated systolic pressure should be monitored carefully for significant falls in pressure either with sudden upright posture or after meals. These changes reflect a progressive loss of autonomic responsiveness with age.

Definition of Hypertension

Blood pressure is distributed in a typical bell-shaped curve within the overall population. As seen in the 22-year follow-

TABLE 37–2 Guidelines in Measuring Blood Pressure

Conditions for the patient	*Posture:* For patients who are older than 65 years, diabetic, or receiving antihypertensive therapy, check for postural changes by taking readings after 5 min supine and immediately and 2 min after patient stands. Sitting pressures are usually adequate for routine follow-up. Patient should sit quietly with back supported for 5 min and arm supported at level of heart. *Circumstances:* No caffeine for preceding hour. No smoking for preceding 30 min. No exogenous adrenergic stimulants, e.g., phenylephrine in nasal decongestants. Quiet, warm setting. Home readings should be taken under varying circumstances throughout the day; for monitoring of therapy, an occasional reading taken soon after arising is usually adequate.
Equipment	Cuff size: The bladder should encircle and cover two-thirds of the length of the arm; if not, place the bladder over the brachial artery; if bladder is too small, spuriously high readings may result. Manometer: Aneroid gauges and electronic devices should be calibrated every 6 mo against a mercury manometer. For infants, use Doppler ultrasound equipment.
Technique	*Number of readings:* On each occasion, take at least two readings separated by as much time as practical. If readings vary by more than 5 mm Hg, take additional readings until two are close. For diagnosis, obtain at least three sets of readings at least 1 week apart; with home measurements, obtain multiple readings over 3-4 weeks. Initially, take pressure in both arms; if pressure differs, use arm with higher pressure. If arm pressure is elevated, take pressure in one leg, particularly in patients younger than 30 yr. *Performance:* Inflate the bladder quickly to a pressure 20 mm Hg above the systolic, as recognized by disappearance of the radial pulse. Deflate the bladder 3 mm Hg every second. Record the Korotkoff phase V (disappearance) except in children (<10 yrs), in whom use of phase IV (muffling) may be preferable. If Korotkoff sounds are weak, have the patient raise the arm and open and close the hand five to 10 times, after which the bladder should be inflated quickly. *Recordings:* Note the pressure, patient position, which arm, and cuff size (e.g., 140/90, seated, right arm, large adult cuff).

up of the almost 350,000 men screened for the Multiple Risk Factor Intervention Trial (MRFIT), the long-term risks for cardiovascular mortality associated with various levels of pressure rise progressively over the entire range of blood pressure, with no threshold that clearly identifies potential danger (Fig. 37–4).[19] Therefore, the definition of hypertension is somewhat arbitrary and usually taken as that level of pressure associated with a doubling of long-term risk. Perhaps the best operational definition is "the level at which the benefits (minus the risks and costs) of action exceed the risks and costs (minus the benefits) of inaction."

For the individual patient, hypertension should be diagnosed when most readings are at a level known to be associated with a significantly higher cardiovascular risk without treatment. The recommendations of the Sixth Joint National Committee (JNC-6) are shown in Table 37–3.[7] Note that systolic levels of 130 to 139 mm Hg and diastolic levels of 85 to 89 mm Hg are classified as high normal blood pressure, a classification associated with a significant increase in the risk of cardiovascular events over time (Fig. 37–5).[20] In view of this heightened risk, the JNC-7 report[8] defines levels above 120/80 to as high as 140/90 as "prehypertension." Therefore, persons with above-normal systolic or diastolic pressures should be advised that they may be at increased risk and counseled to follow better health habits in the hope of slowing the progression toward definite hypertension.

The criteria shown in Table 37–3 are based on at least three sets of measurements taken over at least a 3-month interval. Even more readings may be needed to establish a patient's usual level. Even though they are diagnosed as hypertensive, not all persons with usual levels above 140/90 mm Hg need be treated with drugs, although all should be advised to use the various life-style modifications described in Chapter 38. The threshold for institution of drug therapy should be based on the overall cardiovascular risk profile.

HYPERTENSION IN CHILDREN AND ADOLESCENTS. Upper limits of normal in children of various ages were

TABLE 37–3 JNC-6 Classification of Blood Pressure for Adults Aged 18 Years and Older*

Category	Blood Pressure (mm Hg)		
	Systolic		*Diastolic*
Optimal†	<120	*and*	<80
Normal	<130	*and*	<85
High-normal	130-139	*or*	85-89
Hypertension‡			
Stage 1	140-159	*or*	90-99
Stage 2	160-179	*or*	100-109
Stage 3	≥180	*or*	N ≥ 110

Adapted from The Sixth Report of the Joint National Committee on Prevention, Detection, Evaluation and Treatment of High Blood Pressure. Arch Intern Med 157:2413, 1997. Copyright 1997, American Medical Association.

*Not taking antihypertensive drugs and not acutely ill. When systolic and diastolic blood pressure levels fall into different categories, the higher category should be selected to classify the individual's blood pressure status. For example, 160/92 mm Hg should be classified as stage 2 hypertension, and 174/120 mm Hg should be classified as stage 3 hypertension. Isolated systolic hypertension is defined as systolic blood pressure 140 mm Hg or greater and diastolic blood pressure less than 90 mm Hg and staged approximately (e.g., 170/82 mm Hg is defined as stage 2 isolated systolic hypertension). In addition to classifying stages of hypertension on the basis of average blood pressure levels, clinicians should specify the presence or absence of target organ disease and additional risk factors. This specificity is important for risk classification and treatment (see Table 37–5).

†Optimal blood pressure with respect to cardiovascular risk is less than 120/80 mm Hg. However, unusually low readings should be evaluated for clinical significance.

‡Based on the average of two or more readings taken at each of two or more visits after an initial screening.

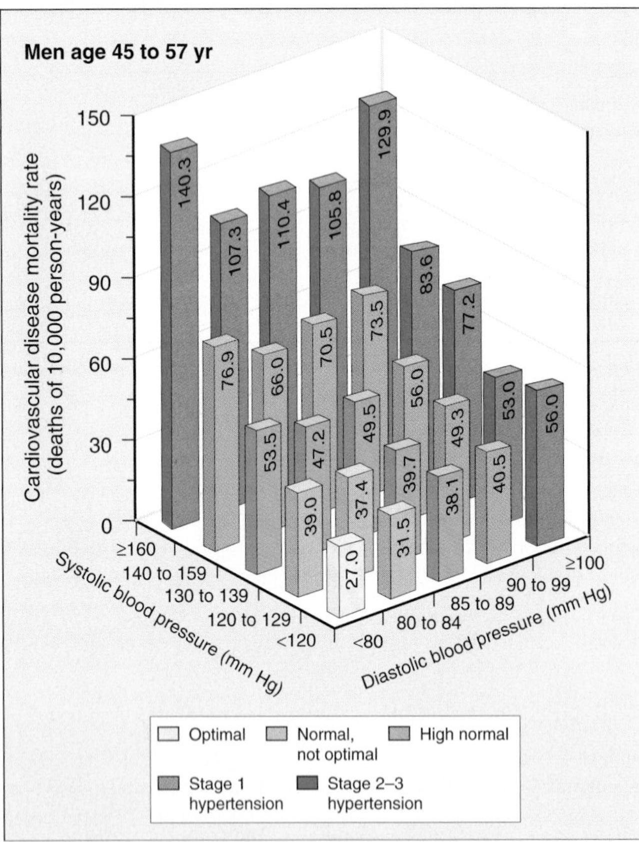

FIGURE 37–4 Age-adjusted cardiovascular disease mortality rate by systolic and diastolic blood pressure level used to define each JNC-VI stratum among the men aged 45 to 57 years enrolled in the Multiple Risk Factor Intervention Trial from 1973 to 1975 and followed through 1996. (Modified from Domanski M, Mitchell G, Pfeffer M, et al: Pulse pressure and cardiovascular disease-related mortality. JAMA 287:268, 2002.)

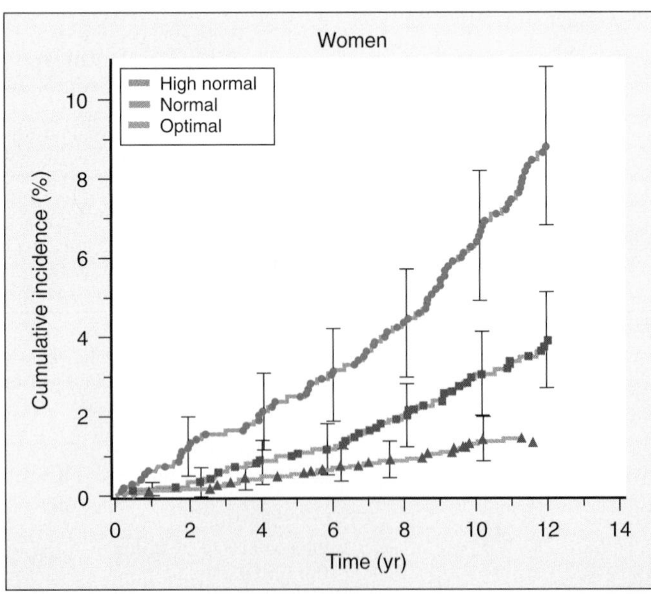

FIGURE 37–5 Cumulative incidence of cardiovascular events in women without hypertension, according to blood-pressure category at the baseline examination. Vertical bars indicate 95 percent confidence intervals. Optimal blood pressure is a systolic pressure of less than 120 mm Hg and a diastolic pressure of less than 80 mm Hg. High-normal blood pressure is a systolic pressure of 130 to 139 mm Hg or a diastolic pressure of 85 to 89. If the systolic and diastolic pressure readings for a subject were in different categories, the higher of the two categories was used. (Modified from Vasan RS, Larson MG, Leip EP, et al: Impact of high-normal blood pressure on the risk of cardiovascular disease. N Engl J Med 345:1295, 2001.)

proposed in the JNC-6 report (Table 37–4).[7] Increasing evidence documents a tracking of blood pressure during childhood with an association between levels at 6 months through adolescence.[21] Appropriate management for asymptomatic post-pubertal children with sustained elevations in blood pressure remains uncertain. Such patients should be monitored carefully, with particular emphasis placed on regular exercise and weight reduction for those who are overweight in the hope of preventing progression of the disease. If lifestyle modifications are not successful, antihypertensive agents should probably be prescribed for patients with sustained levels of blood pressure above the 95th percentile for age and height.

Prevalence of Hypertension

The prevalence of hypertension in the United States rises progressively with age in both men and women (Fig. 37–6).[22] The prevalence of hypertension among blacks is greater at every age beyond adolescence, and hypertension acts as an even stronger risk factor for coronary artery disease among blacks than among whites.[23] The prevalence of hypertension in Mexican Americans is lower than in non-Hispanic whites despite their greater obesity.[24]

After age 50, isolated systolic hypertension increasingly becomes the more common pattern. In the NHANES III survey of a representative sample of the U.S. population, among those not being adequately treated, isolated systolic hypertension was present in 54 percent of hypertensive subjects between the ages of 50 and 59 years and in 87 percent of hypertensive subjects older than 60 years of age.[25] As a consequence of arterial stiffness, systolic levels continue to rise with age, whereas diastolic levels tend to plateau during the fifth decade and to fall thereafter.[26]

SECONDARY HYPERTENSION. Once hypertension has been recognized, it is helpful to know whether some identifiable or secondary process—perhaps curable by surgery or more easily controlled by a specific drug—may be present (Table 37–5).

Most surveys to determine the relative proportion of various identifiable forms of hypertension are biased as a result of the selection process, with only the increasingly suspect population "funneled" to an investigator interested in a particular disease. Thus, estimates as high as 20 percent for certain secondary forms of hypertension have been reported, particularly among those resistant to usual therapy. However, these figures do not reflect the incidence in the population at large. Estimates more likely to be indicative of the situation in usual clinical practice almost all find about 90 percent of hypertensive patients to have primary (essential or idiopathic) disease, with renal parenchymal disease the most common secondary cause, followed by renovascular disease and various adrenal disorders.

SCREENING FOR SECONDARY HYPERTENSION. Because of the relatively low frequency of the various secondary diseases, the clinician should be selective in carrying out various screening and diagnostic tests. The presence of features inappropriate for the usual case of uncomplicated primary hypertension is an indication for additional tests (Table 37–6). However, for the 9 in 10 hypertensive patients without these features, a hematocrit, urine analysis, automated blood biochemical profile (including plasma glucose, potassium, creatinine, and total and high-density lipoprotein cholesterol), and an electrocardiogram are all

TABLE 37–4 Ninety-Fifth Percentile of Blood Pressure by Selected Ages in Girls and Boys in the 50th and 75th Height Percentiles

	Girls' SBP/DBP		Boys' SBP/DBP	
Age (yr)	*50th Percentile for Height*	*75th Percentile for Height*	*50th Percentile for Height*	*75th Percentile for Height*
1	104/58	105/59	102/57	104/58
6	111/73	112/73	114/74	115/75
12	123/80	124/81	123/81	125/82
17	129/84	130/85	136/87	138/88

DBP = diastolic blood pressure; SBP = systolic blood pressure.

Adapted from The Sixth Report of the Joint National Committee on Prevention, Detection, Evaluation and Treatment of High Blood Pressure. Arch Intern Med 157:2413, 1997. Copyright 1997, American Medical Association.

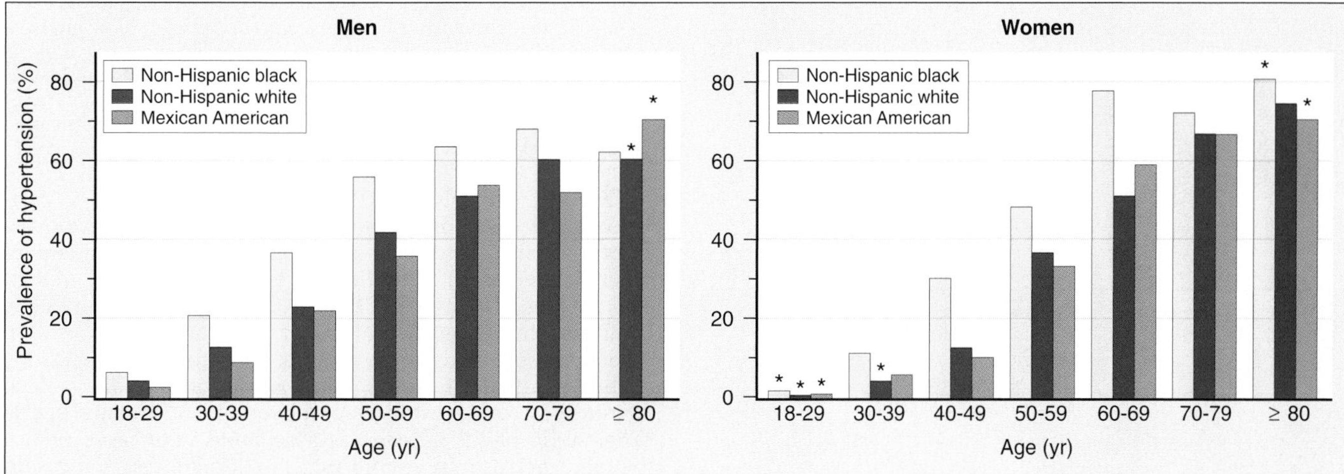

FIGURE 37–6 Prevalence of high blood pressure by age and race or ethnicity for men and women 18 years and older in the U.S. population. Data bars marked with an asterisk are based on a sample size that did not meet the minimum requirements of the National Health and Nutrition Examination Survey (NHANES) III design or relative SEM greater than 30 percent. (Data from Burt VL, Whelton P, Roccella EJ, et al: Prevalence of hypertension in the US adult population: Results from the Third National Health and Nutrition Examination Survey 1988-91. Hypertension 25:305, 1995.)

TABLE 37–5 Types of Hypertension

Systolic and Diastolic Hypertension	Primary, essential or idiopathic Identifiable (secondary) Renal Renal parenchymal disease Acute glomerulonephritis Chronic nephritis Polycystic disease Diabetic nephropathy Hydronephrosis Renovascular Renal artery stenosis Intrarenal vasculitis Renin-producing tumors Renoprival Primary sodium retention (Liddle syndrome, Gordon syndrome) Endocrine Acromegaly Hypothyroidism Hyperthyroidism Hypercalcemia (hyperparathyroidism) Adrenal Cortical Cushing syndrome Primary aldosteronism Congenital adrenal hyperplasia Medullary: pheochromocytoma Extraadrenal chromaffin tumors Apparent mineralocorticoid excess (licorice) Carcinoid Exogenous hormones Estrogen Glucocorticoids Mineralocorticoids Sympathomimetics Erythropoietin Tyramine-containing foods and monoamine oxidase inhibitors Coarctation of the aorta Pregnancy-induced hypertension Neurological disorders Increased intracranial pressure Sleep apnea (usually obstructive) Quadriplegia Acute porphyria Familial dysautonomia Guillain-Barré syndrome Acute stress, including surgery Psychogenic hyperventilation Hypoglycemia Burns Alcohol withdrawal Sickle cell crisis Postresuscitation Perioperative Increased intravascular volume Exogenous causes Alcohol abuse Nicotine Immunosuppressive drugs Heavy metal toxicity
Systolic Hypertension	Increased cardiac output Aortic valvular insufficiency Arteriovenous fistula, patent ductus Thyrotoxicosis Paget disease of bone Beriberi Rigidity of the aorta

TABLE 37–6 Features of "Inappropriate" Hypertension

Onset before 20 or after 50 years of age
Level of blood pressure >180/110 mm Hg
Organ damage Funduscopic findings of grade 2 or higher Serum creatinine >1.5 mg/100 ml Cardiomegaly or left ventricular hypertrophy
Features indicative of secondary causes Unprovoked hypokalemia Abdominal bruit Variable pressures with tachycardia, sweating, tremor Family history of renal disease
Poor response to therapy that is usually effective

that is required. Although some practitioners would include other tests, an inordinate number of screening tests for relatively rare diseases will increase the likelihood of a false-positive result. For example, according to Bayes' theorem, at a prevalence rate of 2 percent for renovascular hypertension, which is probably higher than seen in the overall hypertensive population, the predictive value of an abnormal renogram suggestive of this diagnosis is only 10 percent, and an abnormal renogram is more likely to be a false-positive finding than be true-positive.

If a secondary cause for hypertension is suspected from the initial evaluation, additional diagnostic studies should be obtained in a sequential manner (Table 37-7). More about these and other identifiable causes will be provided at the end of this chapter.

Natural History of Untreated Hypertension

The changing pattern of blood pressure with age—rising systolic and falling diastolic levels—primarily reflects atherosclerotic rigidity of large capacitance arteries and a faster reflection of the pulse wave from arteriosclerotic stiffness of smaller peripheral arteries.[26] Both the rising systolic and falling diastolic levels logically are associated with an increased risk for atherosclerotic vascular diseases. The resultant widening pulse pressure has been widely reported to be the best prognostic indicator of cardiovascular risk. However, an analysis of data from almost one million adults in 61 prospective studies found that, for predicting mortality from both stroke and coronary disease, the systolic blood pressure is slightly more informative than the diastolic blood pressure and that pulse pressure is much less informative.[27]

SYMPTOMS AND SIGNS. Uncomplicated hypertension is almost always asymptomatic, so that patients may be unaware of the consequent progressive cardiovascular damage for as long as 10 to 20 years. Only if blood pressure is measured frequently and people are made aware that hypertension may be harmful even if asymptomatic will the majority of people with unrecognized or inadequately treated hypertension be managed effectively. Symptoms often attributed to hypertension—headache, tinnitus, dizziness, and fainting—may be observed just as commonly in the normotensive population. Moreover, many symptoms attributed to the elevated blood pressure are psychogenic in origin, often reflecting hyperventilation induced by anxiety over the diagnosis of a lifelong, insidious disease that threatens well-being and survival.[28] Even headache, long considered a frequent symptom of hypertension, is poorly related to the level of blood pressure.

COURSE OF UNTREATED HYPERTENSION. The relationship between increasing blood pressure and cardiovascular mortality is direct, continuous, and independent of other risk factors. The findings in the long follow-up of subjects screened for the MRFIT study (see Fig. 37–4)[19] have been confirmed by the meta-analysis of the relationship between blood pressure and cardiovascular mortality in almost one million adults in 61 prospective observational studies.[27] Each 20 mm Hg rise in systolic blood pressure or 10 mm Hg rise in diastolic blood pressure is associated with more than a twofold increase in mortality from stroke and a twofold increase in mortality from coronary disease.

As noted in Figure 37–5, even minimal hypertension is accompanied by significant increases in cardiovascular mortality. These figures may be misleading, however, since they

TABLE 37–7 Overall Guide to Work-up for Identifiable Causes of Hypertension

	Diagnostic Procedure	
Diagnosis	***Initial***	***Additional***
Chronic renal disease	Urinalysis, serum creatinine, renal sonography	Isotopic renogram, renal biopsy
Renovascular disease	Captopril-enhanced isotopic renogram, duplex sonography	Magnetic resonance or CT angiogram, aortogram
Coarctation	Blood pressure in legs	Echocardiogram, aortogram
Primary aldosteronism	Plasma and urinary potassium, plasma renin and aldosterone	Plasma or urinary aldosterone after saline load, adrenal CT and venous sampling
Cushing syndrome	Morning plasma cortisol after 1 mg dexamethasone at bedtime	Urinary cortisol after variable doses of dexamethasone, adrenal CT, and scintiscans
Pheochromocytoma	Plasma metanephrine Spot urine for metanephrine	Urinary catechols; plasma catechols (basal and after 0.3 mg clonidine) Adrenal CT and scintiscans

CT = computed tomography.

seem to imply that most hypertensive subjects, including those with minimally elevated pressure, will experience adverse consequences of hypertension, and rather quickly. In fact, the usual presentation of data as *relative* risk suggests a much greater danger than is shown when data are presented as *absolute* risk. The issue is well identified in the data from the Pooling Project,[29] which includes many prospective follow-up studies, including the Framingham cohort. These data indicate that white men with diastolic pressures of 80 to 87 mm Hg had a 52 percent greater relative risk of having a major coronary event over an 8.6-year period than did those with diastolic pressures below 80. However, this large increased relative risk translates to an absolute excess risk of only 3.5 men per 100 over the 8.6-year interval. Obviously, the majority of those with even higher diastolic pressures did not suffer a major coronary event.

Nonetheless, because so many persons have hypertension, the fact that even a minority of them will suffer a premature cardiovascular event in the course of their disease makes hypertension a major societal problem. In fact, when the cardiovascular death rates for various levels of systolic or diastolic blood pressure are multiplied by the proportion of people in the population who have these various levels, the majority of excess deaths attributable to hypertension are found to occur among those with minimally elevated pressure (Fig. 37–7).

As the public and the medical profession have become aware of the overall societal consequences of even mild hypertension, enthusiasm for early recognition and aggressive treatment of hypertension has continued to mount. A closer look at the issue of deciding on the need for therapy is provided in Chapter 38. However, further consideration of the natural course of hypertension, as it applies to the individual patient, is needed to answer a basic question: Are the blood pressure and the consequent risk high enough to justify medical intervention? Unless the risk is high enough to mandate some form of intervention, there seems to be no need to identify and label the person as hypertensive, since psychological and socioeconomic burdens accompany this label; unless risks clearly outweigh these burdens, caution is obviously advised.

We are thus left with a dilemma: For hypertensive subjects as a group, even among those with the least elevated pressures, risk is increased; for the individual hypertensive subject, the risk may not justify the labeling or treatment of the condition.

Assessment of Individual Risk

Guidelines are available to help practitioners resolve this dilemma in dealing with the individual patient. These guidelines are based on the overall assessment of cardiovascular

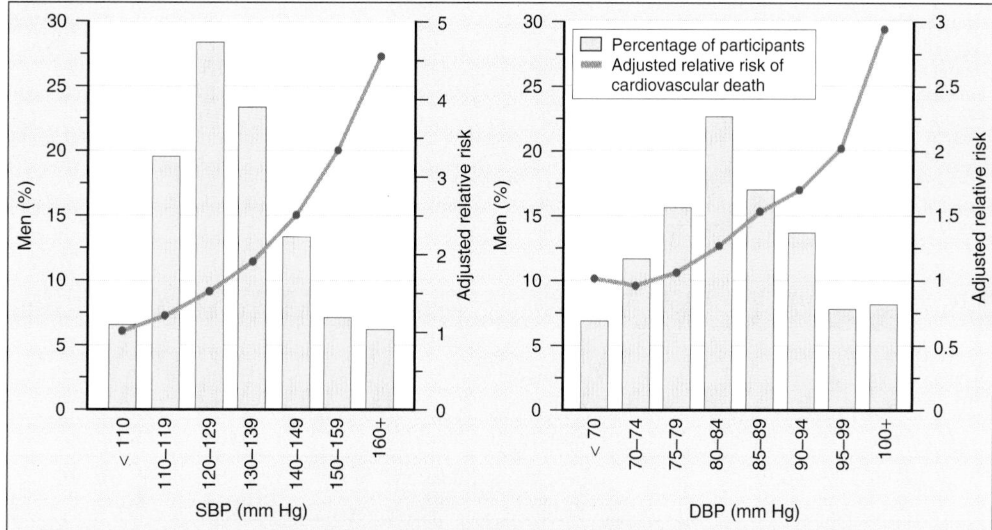

FIGURE 37–7 **Left,** Percentage distribution of systolic blood pressure (SBP) for men screened for the Multiple Risk Factor Intervention Trial who were 35 to 57 years old and had no history of myocardial infarction ($n = 347,978$) (shaded bars) and corresponding 12-year rates of cardiovascular mortality by SBP level adjusted for age, race, total serum cholesterol level, cigarettes smoked per day, reported use of medications for diabetes mellitus, and estimated household income (using census tract of residence). **Right,** Percentage distribution of diastolic blood pressure (DBP) in the same group ($n = 356,222$). (From National High Blood Pressure Education Program Working Group: National High Blood Pressure Education Program Working Group report on primary prevention of hypertension. Arch Intern Med 153:186, 1993. Copyright 1993, American Medical Association.)

risk and the biological aggressiveness of the hypertension. They are intended to apply only to those with stage 1 (formerly referred to as mild) hypertension, that is, systolic pressure between 140 and 159 mm Hg or diastolic pressure between 90 and 99 mm Hg; those with higher levels have been shown to be at high enough risk from the hypertension per se to justify immediate intervention. Recall, however, that most hypertensive persons are in the range between 140 and 159 mm Hg systolic or 90 and 99 mm Hg diastolic (Fig. 37–7). On the other hand, patients at high overall cardiovascular risk, even with high normal blood pressure, are deemed to be in need of active drug therapy.[7]

OVERALL CARDIOVASCULAR RISK. The Framingham Study and other epidemiological surveys have clearly defined certain risk factors for premature cardiovascular disease in addition to hypertension (see Chap. 36). For varying levels of blood pressure, the Framingham data show the increasing likelihood of a vascular event over the next 10 years for both men and women at various ages as more and more risk factors are added (Fig. 37–8). For example, a 55-year-old man with a systolic blood pressure of 160 mm Hg who is otherwise at low risk would have a 13.7 percent chance of a vascular event in the next 10 years. A man of the same age with the same pressure but with all the additional risk factors (elevated serum total cholesterol, low high-density lipoprotein cholesterol, cigarette smoking, glucose intolerance, and LVH on the electrocardiogram) has a 59.5 percent chance. Obviously, the higher the overall risk, the more intensive the interventions should be.

Several approaches have been taken to apply the Framingham risk data to individual patients. As perhaps first and best articulated by a group of New Zealand physicians,[30] the degree of risk from hypertension can be categorized with reasonable accuracy by taking into account (1) the level of blood pressure, (2) the biological nature of the hypertension based on the degree of target organ damage, and (3) the coexistence of other risks. The JNC-6 report provides a stratification of risk into three groups based on known components of risk (Table 37–8) and levels of blood pressure, which are, in turn, used as the basis for deciding upon initial treatment (Table 37–9). According to this stratification, active drug

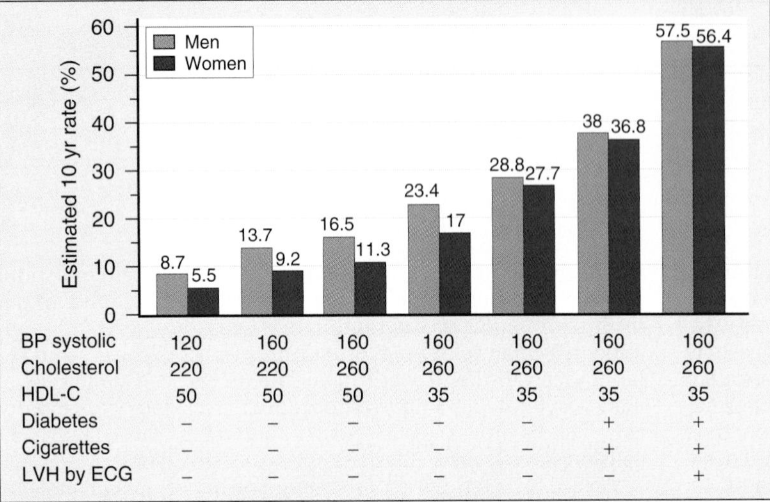

FIGURE 37–8 Estimated 10-year risk of coronary artery disease in hypothetical 55-year-old men and women according to levels of various risk factors. Lipid units are milligrams per deciliter. BP = blood pressure; ECG = electrocardiogram; HDL-C = high-density lipoprotein cholesterol; LVH = left ventricular hypertrophy. (From O'Donnell CJ, Kannel WB: Cardiovascular risks of hypertension: Lessons from observational studies. J Hypertens 16(Suppl 6):3, 1998.)

TABLE 37–8 Components of Cardiovascular Risk Stratification in Patients with Hypertension

Major Risk Factors	Target Organ Damage/Clinical Cardiovascular Disease
Smoking	Heart diseases
Dyslipidemia	Left ventricular hypertrophy
Diabetes mellitus	Angina or prior myocardial infarction
Age >60 yr	Prior coronary revascularization
Sex (men and postmenopausal women)	Heart failure
Family history of cardiovascular disease	Stroke or transient ischemic attack
Women >65 yr or men >55 yr	Nephropathy
	Peripheral arterial disease
	Retinopathy

From The Sixth Report of the Joint National Committee on Prevention, Detection, Evaluation and Treatment of High Blood Pressure. Arch Intern Med 157:2413. 1997. Copyright 1997, American Medical Association.

TABLE 37–9 Risk Stratification and Treatment*

Blood Pressure Stages (mm Hg)	Risk Group A (No risk factors: no TOD/CCD)	Risk Group B (At least 1 risk factor, not including diabetes: no TOD/CCD)	Risk Group C (TOD/CCD and/or diabetes, with or without other risk factors)
High-normal (130-139/85-89)	Life-style modification	Life-style modification	Drug therapy
Stage 1 (140-159/90-99)	Life-style modification (up to 12 months)	Life-style modification (up to 6 months)	Drug therapy
Stages 2 and 3 (>160/>100)	Drug therapy	Drug therapy	Drug therapy

CCD = clinical cardiovascular disease; TOD = target organ disease.

From The Sixth Report of the Joint National Committee on Prevention, Detection, Evaluation and Treatment of High Blood Pressure. Arch Intern Med 157:2413, 1997. Copyright 1997, American Medical Association.

*Note: For example, a patient with diabetes and a blood pressure of 142/94 mm Hg plus left ventricular hypertrophy should be classified as having stage 1 hypertension with target organ disease (left ventricular hypertrophy) and with another major risk factor (diabetes). This patient would be categorized as "stage 1, risk group C," and recommended for immediate initiation of pharmacological treatment. Life-style modification should be adjunctive therapy for all patients recommended for pharmacological therapy.

therapy is recommended for high-risk patients even if blood pressure is only high normal, whereas life-style modifications are recommended for low-risk patients even if blood pressure is as high as 159/99 mm Hg. In the 2003 JNC-7 report, drug therapy is recommended for the majority of patients with blood pressure above 140/90 mm Hg.[8]

Both the 1997 JNC-6 and the 1999 WHO-ISH[31] guidelines identify a large number of patients in whom risk is considered high enough to warrant drug therapy who would not be so identified by other risk estimates.[32] Although there is an increasing acceptance of using an overall coronary risk of 15 percent or higher over 10 years as an appropriate criterion for antihypertensive drug therapy, risk evaluation remains an inexact science. The addition of echocardiography and carotid ultrasonography markedly elevates the estimate of risk in patients who are considered low-risk by JNC-6 or WHO-ISH criteria.[33] Those procedures have not been advocated, however, largely on the basis of cost-benefit analysis.

It is obvious that since the course of the blood pressure cannot be predicted with certainty, even hypertensive subjects who are not treated should be monitored, and recognition of their hypertension should motivate them to follow good health habits. In this way, no harm should be done, and the potential benefit may be considerable if progression of the disease can be slowed by life-style modifications.

Complications of Hypertension

The purpose of risk assessment is to assist clinicians in determining the appropriate treatment of individual patients to best protect against the various complications associated with hypertension. The higher the degree of risk, the more likely that various cardiovascular diseases will develop prematurely through acceleration of atherosclerosis, the pathological hallmark of uncontrolled hypertension. If untreated, about 50 percent of hypertensive patients die of coronary heart disease or congestive failure, about 33 percent of stroke, and 10 to 15 percent of renal failure. Those with rapidly accelerating hypertension die more frequently of renal failure, as do those who are diabetic once proteinuria or other evidence of nephropathy develops. It is easy to underestimate the role of hypertension in producing the underlying vascular damage that leads to these cardiovascular catastrophes. Death is usually attributed to stroke or myocardial infarction instead of to the hypertension that was largely responsible. Moreover, hypertension may not persist after a myocardial infarction or stroke.

The biological aggressiveness of a given level of hypertension varies among individuals. This inherent propensity to induce vascular damage can best be ascertained by examination of the eyes, heart, and kidney.

FUNDUSCOPIC EXAMINATION (see also Chap. 8). Vascular changes in the fundus reflect both hypertensive retinopathy and arteriosclerotic retinopathy. The two processes first induce narrowing of the arteriolar lumen (grade 1) and then sclerosis of the adventitia and/or thickening of the arteriolar wall, visible as arteriovenous nicking (grade 2). Progressive hypertension induces rupture of small vessels, seen as hemorrhage and exudate (grade 3) and eventually papilledema (grade 4). The grade 3 and 4 changes are clearly indicative of an accelerated-malignant form of hypertension, whereas the lesser changes have been correlated with the risk of coronary disease.[34]

CARDIAC INVOLVEMENT. Hypertension places increased tension on the left ventricular myocardium that is manifested as stiffness and hypertrophy, which accelerates the development of atherosclerosis within the coronary vessels. The combination of increased demand and lessened supply increases the likelihood of myocardial ischemia and thereby leads to a higher incidence of myocardial infarction, arrhythmias, and congestive failure in hypertensive patients.

Abnormalities in Left Ventricular Function. Even before LVH develops, changes in both systolic and diastolic function can be seen. Those patients with minimally increased left ventricular muscle mass may have supernormal contractility as reflected by an increased inotropic state with a high percentage of fractional shortening and increased wall stress.[35] The earliest functional cardiac changes in hypertension are in left ventricular diastolic function, with lower E/A ratio and longer isovolemic relaxation time (see Chap. 11).[36]

With increasing hemodynamic load, either systolic or diastolic dysfunction may evolve and progress to different forms of congestive heart failure (Fig. 37–9).[37] In addition, impaired coronary flow reserve and thallium perfusion defects may be observed in hypertensive patients without obstructive coronary disease.[38] Hypertensive black patients are at a higher risk for progression to heart failure and death from left ventricular dysfunction than are similarly treated white patients.[39]

Left Ventricular Hypertrophy. Hypertrophy as a response to the increased afterload associated with elevated systemic vascular resistance can be viewed as necessary and protective up to a certain point. Beyond that point, a variety of dysfunctions accompany LVH, including lower coronary vasodilatory capacity, depressed left ventricular wall mechanics, and abnormal left ventricular diastolic filling pattern.[40]

Whereas LVH is identified by electrocardiography in only 5 to 10 percent of hypertensive patients, LVH is found by echocardiography in nearly 30 percent of unselected hypertensive adults and up to 90 percent of persons with severe hypertension.[41] The patterns of LVH differ by the type of hemodynamic load: volume overload leads to eccentric hypertrophy, whereas pure blood pressure overload leads to an increase in LV wall thickness without concomitant increase in cavity volume (i.e., concentric hypertrophy). The pattern of LVH can also be modified by increased arterial stiffness, increased pulse wave velocity, and blood viscosity.

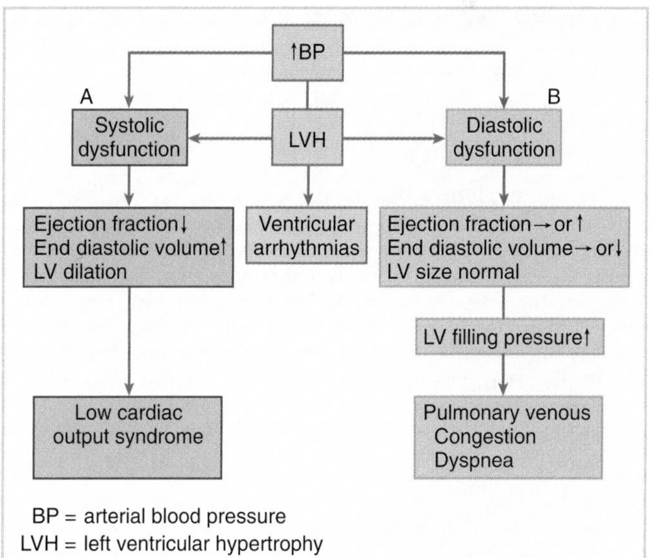

FIGURE 37–9 Consequences of systolic and diastolic dysfunction related to hypertension. **A,** Systolic dysfunction and congestive heart failure caused by impaired ventricular contraction may occur late in the evolution of hypertensive heart disease. **B,** Diastolic dysfunction is the most common manifestation of the effect of hypertension on cardiac function and can also lead to congestive heart failure from increased filling pressures. BP = blood pressure; LV = left ventricular; LVH = left ventricular hypertrophy. (From Shepherd RFJ, Zachariah PK, Shub C: Hypertension and left ventricular diastolic function. Mayo Clin Proc 64:1521, 1989. By permission of the Mayo Foundation.)

In one series of 913 patients with varying stages of hypertension, these percentages of various patterns were found by echocardiography: normal geometry, 19 percent; concentric remodeling, 11 percent; eccentric hypertrophy, 47 percent; and concentric hypertrophy, 23 percent.[42] The presence of LVH is consistently and strongly related to subsequent cardiovascular morbidity and mortality.

Since the presence of LVH may connote a number of deleterious effects of hypertension on cardiac function, a great deal of effort has been expended in showing that treatment of hypertension will cause LVH to regress. Treatment with all antihypertensive drugs except those that further activate sympathetic nervous system activity, for example, direct vasodilators such as hydralazine when used alone, has been shown to cause LVH regression. With regression, left ventricular function usually improves and cardiovascular morbidity decreases.[43]

Congestive Heart Failure (see Chap. 22). The various alterations of systolic and diastolic function seen with LVH obviously can progress into congestive heart failure (CHF). A 20 mm Hg increment in systolic blood pressure conferred a 56 percent increased risk for CHF in the Framingham cohort.[44] Hypertension remains the major preventable factor in the disease that is now the leading cause of hospitalization in the United States for adults older than 65 years of age. It is likely that antihypertensive treatment does not completely prevent CHF but postpones its development by several decades.

Most episodes of CHF in hypertensive patients are associated with systolic dysfunction as reflected in a reduced ejection fraction. However, about 40 percent of episodes of CHF are associated with diastolic dysfunction and preserved left ventricular systolic function. For example, in a series of patients with acute pulmonary edema and systolic blood pressure above 160 mm Hg, an exacerbation of diastolic dysfunction was responsible rather than systolic dysfunction in almost half the cases.[37] Vasan and Benjamin[45] explain the susceptibility of hypertensive patients, particularly those with LVH, to diastolic heart failure:

> When hemodynamically challenged by stress (such as exercise, tachycardia, increased afterload, or excessive preload), persons with hypertension are unable to increase their end-diastolic volume (i.e., they have limited preload reserve), because of decreased left ventricular relaxation and compliance. Consequently, a cascade begins, in which the left ventricular end-diastolic blood pressure rises, left atrial pressure increases, and pulmonary edema develops.

Coronary Heart Disease. As detailed elsewhere (see Chap. 36), hypertension is a major risk factor for myocardial infarction (MI), and ischemia. Moreover, the prevalence of silent MI is significantly increased in hypertensive subjects,[46] and they have a greater risk for mortality after an initial MI.[47] Hypertension may play an even greater role in the pathogenesis of coronary heart disease than is commonly realized, since preexisting hypertension may go unrecognized in patients first seen after an MI. Although acute rises in blood pressure may follow the onset of ischemic pain, the blood pressure often falls immediately after the infarct if pump function is impaired.

Once an MI occurs, the prognosis is affected by both the preexisting and the subsequent blood pressure. The 28-day case fatality rate among 635 men who had an acute MI was 24.5 percent in those with prior systolic blood pressure below 140 mm Hg, 35.6 percent with prior systolic blood pressure of 140 to 159 mm Hg, and 48.2 percent with prior systolic blood pressure of 160 mm Hg or higher.[48] On the other hand, an increase in post-MI mortality has been noted among those whose blood pressure fell significantly, presumably a reflection of poor pump function.[49] If the blood pressure of these subjects remained elevated, the prognosis was even worse, likely representing a severe load on a damaged myocardium, so that care must be taken with patients who have either lower or higher blood pressure after an infarction.

RENAL FUNCTION. Renal dysfunction too subtle to be recognized may be responsible for the development of most cases of primary (essential) hypertension. As discussed later (see Renal Retention of Sodium), increased renal retention of salt and water may be a mechanism initiating primary hypertension, but the retention is so small that it escapes detection. With detailed study, both structural damage and functional derangements reflecting intraglomerular hypertension often reflected by microalbuminuria can be found in most hypertensive persons. Microalbuminuria in hypertensive patients has been correlated with left ventricular hypertrophy and carotid artery thickness.[50] As hypertension-induced nephrosclerosis proceeds, the plasma creatinine level begins to rise, and eventually, renal insufficiency may develop. However, despite the epidemiological evidence for an association between hypertension and renal disease, some investigators question the relationship, postulating that the renal damage seen in hypertensive patients is usually secondary to underlying renal diseases that may, in turn, be aggravated by the presence of hypertension.

CEREBRAL INVOLVEMENT. Hypertension may accelerate cognitive decline with age.[51] Hypertension, particularly systolic, is a major risk factor for both ischemic stroke and intracerebral hemorrhage. Cerebral white matter lesions are a common finding by brain magnetic resonance imaging (MRI), seen in 41 percent of asymptomatic, middle-aged hypertensive patients[52] and brain atrophy is more common past the age 67 years in hypertensive than in normotensive subjects.[53] Blood pressure usually rises further during the acute phases of a stroke, and caution is advised in lowering blood pressure during this crucial period.

Mechanisms of Primary (Essential) Hypertension

No single or specific cause is known for most cases of hypertension, and the condition is referred to as *primary* in preference to *essential*. Since persistent hypertension can develop only in response to an increase in cardiac output or a rise in peripheral resistance, defects may be present in one or more of the multiple factors that affect these two forces (Fig. 37–10). The interplay of various derangements in factors affecting cardiac output and peripheral resistance may precipitate the disease, and these abnormalities may differ in both type and degree in different patients.

Hemodynamic Patterns

Before describing specific abnormalities in the various factors shown in Figure 37–10 to affect the following basic equation

$$\text{blood pressure} = \text{cardiac output} \times \text{peripheral resistance}$$
$$(BP = CO \times PR)$$

the hemodynamic patterns that have been measured in patients with hypertension will be considered. One cautionary factor should be kept in mind: Development of the disease is slow and gradual. By the time that blood pressure becomes elevated, the initiating factors may no longer be apparent because they may have been "normalized" by multiple compensatory interactions. Nonetheless, when a group of untreated young hypertensive patients was studied initially, cardiac output was normal or slightly increased and peripheral resistance was normal.[54] Over the next 20 years, cardiac output fell progressively while peripheral resistance rose. In

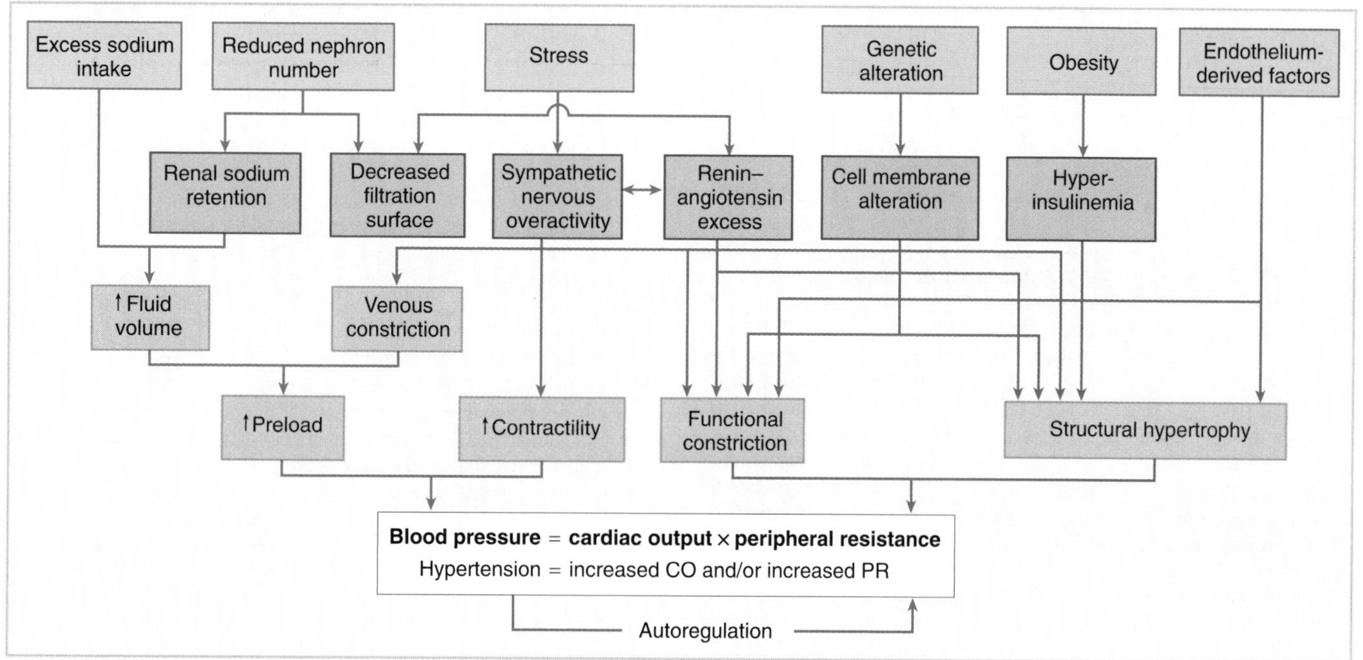

FIGURE 37–10 Some of the factors involved in the control of blood pressure that affect the basic equation blood pressure = cardiac output (CO) × peripheral resistance (PR). (From Kaplan NM: Clinical Hypertension. 8th ed. Baltimore, Lippincott Williams & Wilkins, 2002, p 63.)

a much larger study involving more than 2600 subjects in Framingham who were monitored for 4 years by echocardiography, an increased cardiac index and end-systolic wall stress were related to the development of hypertension,[55] and in a 10-year follow-up of 4700 young people, an increased heart rate, presumably associated with a reflection of increased cardiac output, has been found to be a predictor of future hypertension.[56]

Regardless of how hypertension begins, eventually increased peripheral resistance becomes the primary hemodynamic fault of sustained hypertension.

Genetic Predisposition

As discussed in Chapter 70 and shown in Figure 37–10, genetic alterations may initiate the cascade to permanent hypertension. In studies of twins and family members in which the degree of familial aggregation of blood pressure levels is compared with the closeness of genetic sharing, the genetic contributions have been estimated to range from 30 to 60 percent.[57] Unquestionably, multiple environmental factors play a role, interacting with multiple genes to skew the distribution of blood pressure to higher levels (Fig. 37–11).[58] Essential hypertension is almost certainly a polygenic disorder, involving multiple genes, each having small effects on blood pressure.[59] Linkage genome scans on more than 6000 relatives of hypertensive patients have failed to find regions with large effects.[60]

A number of rare forms of hypertension have been found to be caused by a monogenic abnormality, including glucocorticoid-remediable aldosteronism, Liddle syndrome, and apparent mineralocorticoid excess.[61] Virtually all of these involve renal sodium transport in some manner. A monogenic form should be suspected with a strong family history of early onset of hypertension.

In addition to the search for specific causes of hypertension, genetic profiling may make it possible to direct antihypertensive therapy more precisely. For now, children and siblings of hypertensive patients should be more carefully screened. They should be vigorously advised to avoid environmental factors known to aggravate hypertension and increase cardiovascular risk (e.g., smoking, inactivity, and excess sodium).

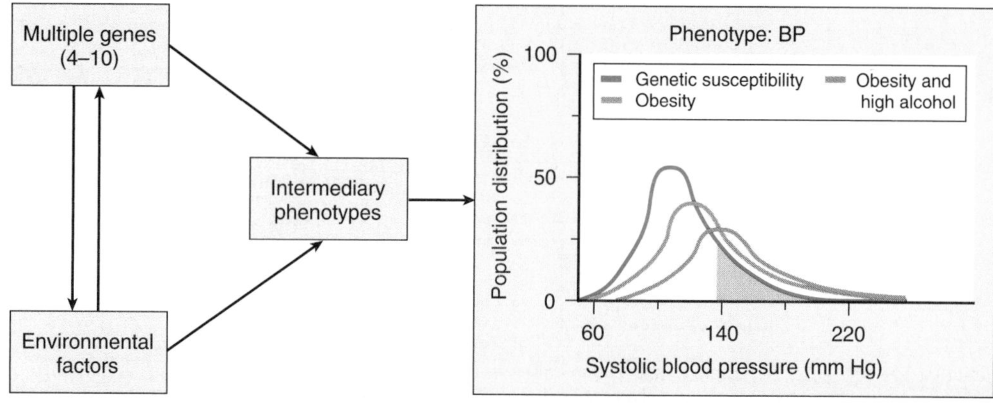

FIGURE 37–11 Interaction among genetic and environmental factors in the development of hypertension. Left side of the figure shows how environmental factors and multiple genes responsible for high blood pressure (BP) interact and affect intermediary phenotypes. The result of these intermediary phenotypes is blood pressure with a normal distribution skewed to the right. The magenta line indicates the theoretical blood pressure of the population that is not affected by hypertensinogenic factors; the shaded area indicates systolic blood pressure in the hypertensive range and the brown lines and blue lines indicate populations in which one (obesity) or two (obesity plus high alcohol intake) hypertensinogenic factors have been added. (From Carretero OA, Oparil S: Essential hypertension. Circulation 101:329, 2000.)

The Fetal Environment

Environmental factors may come into play very early. Low birth weight as a consequence of fetal undernutrition has been repeatedly found to be followed by an increased incidence of high blood pressure later in life with an overall estimate that a 1 kg lower birth weight is associated with a 2 to 4 mm Hg higher systolic blood pressure in adulthood.[62] However, an analysis of 55 studies that reported regression coefficients of systolic blood pressure on birth weight found progressively weaker associations with increased numbers of participants in the studies and a common inappropriate adjustment for current weight and other confounding factors, leading to the conclusion that "birth weight is of little relevance to blood pressure levels in later life."[63] Moreover, increasing weight gain during childhood has been found to have an even greater impact on adult blood pressure.[62]

Despite these objections to the role of the "low birth weight" hypothesis originally proposed by Professor David Barker, increasing evidence for an effect of intrauterine growth retardation on nephrogenesis provides support for the hypothesis of Brenner and colleagues that a reduced number of nephrons eventuates in hypertension (Fig. 37–12).[64] In

addition to experimental evidence,[65] even stronger support comes from a postmortem study of patients with primary hypertension who were found to have half the total number of glomeruli per kidney than matched normotensive control subjects.[66] This lower nephron number presumably was congenital and not acquired after development of hypertension, since there were very few obsolescent glomeruli in the hypertensive subjects' kidneys.

These data fit nicely with Brenner's explanation for the inexorable progression of renal damage once it begins and the concept that hypertension may begin by renal sodium retention induced by the decreased filtration surface area. Other subtle acquired renal injuries induced by vasoconstriction may also contribute to the development of sodium-sensitive hypertension.[67]

Renal Retention of Sodium

A considerable amount of circumstantial evidence supports a role for sodium in the genesis of hypertension (Table 37–10). To induce hypertension, some of that excess sodium must be retained by the kidneys. Such retention could arise in a number of ways, including the following:

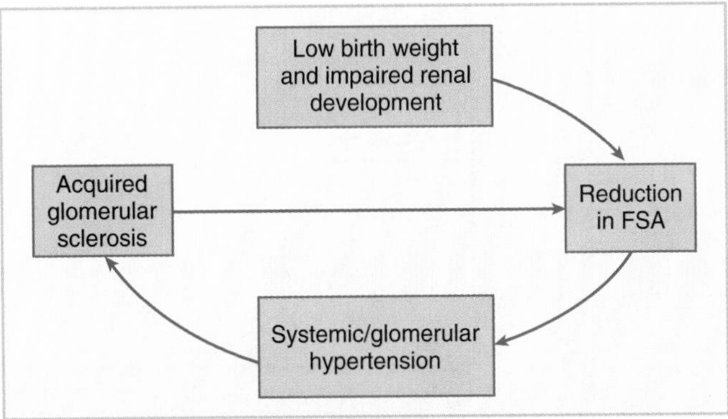

FIGURE 37–12 The risk of essential hypertension and progressive renal injury developing in adult life is increased as a result of congenital oligonephropathy, an inborn deficit of filtration surface area (FSA) caused by impaired renal development. Low birth weight resulting from intrauterine growth retardation or prematurity contributes to this oligonephropathy. Systemic and glomerular hypertension in later life results in progressive glomerular sclerosis, further reducing FSA and thereby perpetuating a vicious cycle that leads, in the extreme, to end-stage renal failure. (From Brenner BM, Chertow GM: Congenital oligonephropathy: An inborn cause of adult hypertension and progressive renal injury? Curr Opin Nephrol Hypertens 2:691, 1993.)

- A decrease in filtration surface by a congenital or acquired deficiency in nephron number or function.
- A resetting of the normal pressure-natriuresis relationship wherein a rise in pressure invokes an immediate increase in renal sodium excretion, thereby shrinking fluid volume and returning the pressure to normal—the Guyton hypothesis.
- Nephron heterogeneity, described as the presence of "a subpopulation of nephrons that is ischemic either from afferent arteriolar vasoconstriction or from an intrinsic narrowing of the lumen. Renin secretion from this subgroup of nephrons is tonically elevated. This increased renin secretion then interferes with the compensatory capacity of intermingled normal nephrons to adaptively excrete sodium and, consequently, perturbs overall blood pressure homeostasis."[68]
- An acquired inhibitor of the sodium pump or other abnormalities in sodium transport.[69]

Thus, more than enough ways are available to incite renal retention of even a very small bit of the excess sodium typically ingested that could eventually expand body fluid volume. Individuals who are more sodium sensitive have been found to have more markers of endothelial damage, nondipping of nocturnal blood pressure, and increased mortality[70] than do those who are less sodium sensitive.

Vascular Hypertrophy

Both excess sodium intake and renal sodium retention would presumably work primarily on increasing fluid volume and cardiac output. A number of other factors may work primarily on the second part of the equation BP = CO × PR (see Fig. 37–10). Most of these factors can cause both functional contraction and structural remodeling and hypertrophy. These pressor-growth promoters may result in both vascular contraction and hypertrophy simultaneously, but perpetuation of hypertension involves hypertrophy. Various hormonal mediators, such as angiotensin II and endothelin, may serve as the initiator of what eventuates as increased peripheral resistance. To explain this process, Lever and Harrap[71] have postulated that

> Most forms of secondary hypertension have two pressor mechanisms: a primary cause, e.g., renal clip, and a second process, which is slow to develop, capable of maintaining hypertension after removal of the primary cause, and probably self-perpetuating in nature. We suggest that essential hypertension also has two mechanisms, both based upon cardiovascular hypertrophy: (1) a growth-promoting process in children (equivalent to the primary cause in secondary hypertension) and (2) a self-perpetuating mechanism in adults.

TABLE 37–10 Evidence for Role of Sodium in Primary (Essential) Hypertension
In multiple populations, the rise in blood pressure with age is directly correlated with increasing levels of sodium intake.
Multiple, scattered groups who consume little sodium (<50 mmol/d) have little or no hypertension. When they consume more sodium, hypertension appears.
Hypertension develops in animals given sodium loads, if genetically predisposed.
In some people, large sodium loads given over short periods cause an increase in vascular resistance and blood pressure.
An increased concentration of sodium is present in the vascular tissue and blood cells of most hypertensives.
Sodium restriction to a level below 100 mmol/d will lower blood pressure in most people. The antihypertensive action of diuretics requires an initial natriuresis.

These investigators have built on the original proposal of Folkow[72] of a "positive feedback interaction" wherein even mild functional pressor influences, if repeatedly exerted, may lead to structural hypertrophy, which in turn reinforces and perpetuates the elevated pressure (Fig. 37–13).

This scheme to explain an immediate pressor action and a slow hypertrophic effect is thought to be common to the action of pressor-growth promoters. When present in high concentrations over long periods, as with angiotensin II in renal artery stenosis, each of these pressor-growth promoters causes hypertension. No marked excess of any known pressor hormone is identifiable in the majority of hypertensive patients. Nonetheless, a lesser excess of one or more may have been responsible for initiation of the process sustained by positive feedback. If this double process is fundamental to the pathogenesis of primary hypertension, the difficulty in recognizing the initiating causal factor is easily explained. As formulated by Lever,[73]

> The primary cause of hypertension will be most apparent in the early stages; in the later stages, the cause will be concealed by an increasing contribution from hypertrophy . . . A particular form of hypertension may wrongly be judged to have 'no known cause' because each mechanism considered is insufficiently abnormal by itself to have produced the hypertension. The cause of essential hypertension may have been considered already but rejected for this reason.

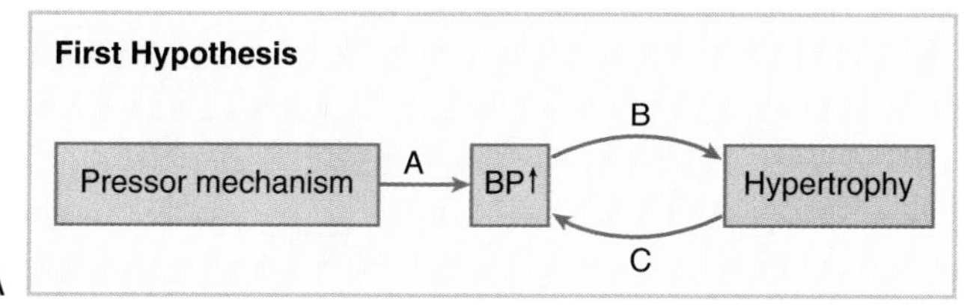

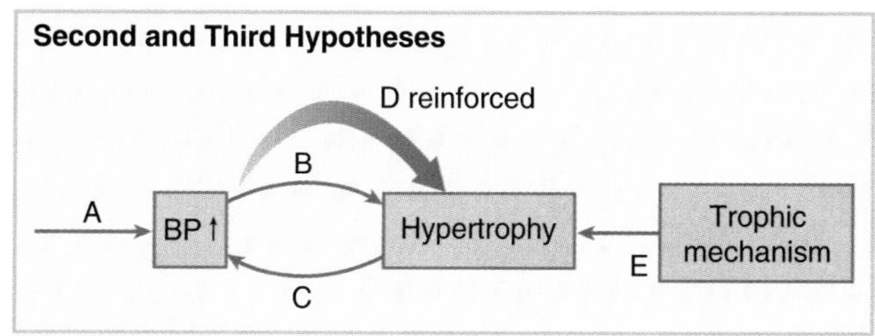

FIGURE 37–13 Hypotheses for the initiation and maintenance of hypertension. **A,** Folkow's first proposal that minor overactivity of a pressor mechanism (A) raises blood pressure (BP) slightly, which initiates positive feedback (B-C-B) and a progressive rise in blood pressure. **B,** As in part **A,** with two additional signals: D, an abnormal or "reinforced" hypertrophic response to pressure; and E, increase in a humoral agent causing hypertrophy directly. (From Lever AF, Harrap SB: Essential hypertension: A disorder of growth with origins in childhood? J Hypertens 10:101, 1992.)

Endothelial Cell Dysfunction

These pressor-growth promoters have traditionally been assumed to be circulating and passing through an inert endothelium. Over the past decade, the endothelial cell has been recognized to be an active participant, the source of multiple relaxing and constricting substances, most having a local, paracrine influence on underlying smooth muscle cells (Fig. 37–14).[74]

NITRIC OXIDE (see Chap. 44). Hypertensive patients have been shown to have a reduced vasodilatory response to various stimuli of nitric oxide release that appears to be independent of the origin of the hypertension and the degree of gross vascular structural alteration. Impaired nitric oxide–mediated vasodilation may promote abnormal vascular remodeling and serves as a marker of future cardiovascular events. Nitric oxide–mediated forearm responsiveness has been restored by normalization of blood pressure by antihypertensive drugs with different modes of action.

ENDOTHELIN. A number of endothelium-derived constricting factors are shown in Figure 37–14. Of these,

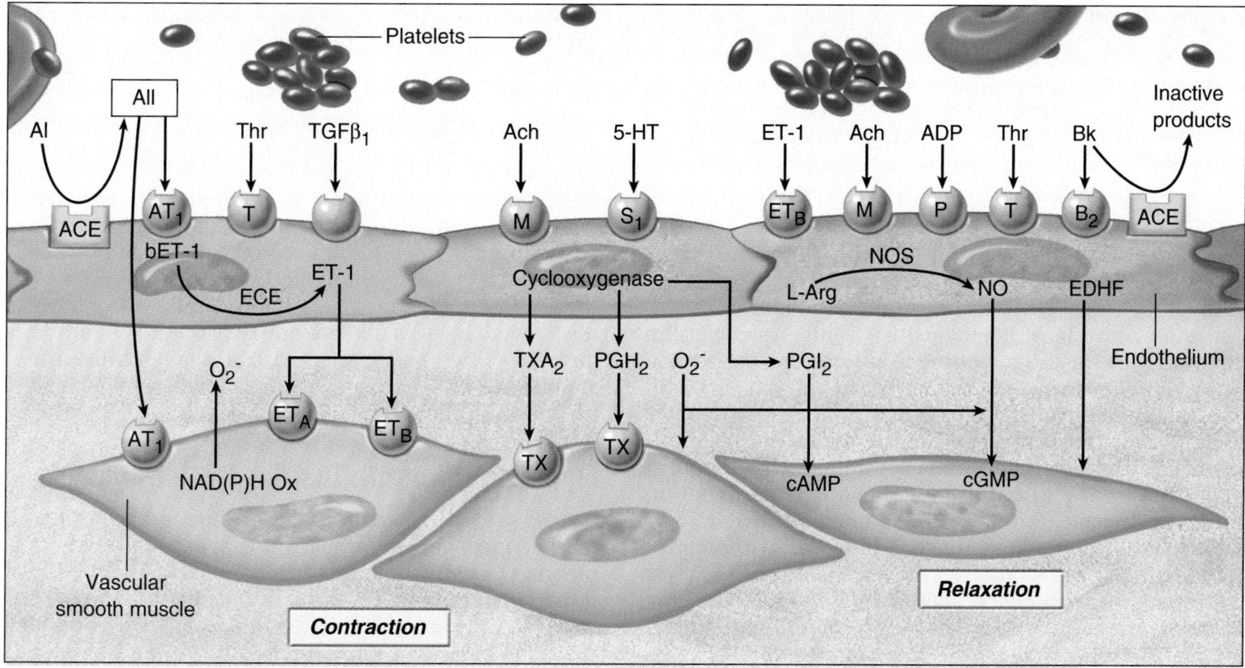

FIGURE 37–14 Endothelium-derived vasoactive substances. Various blood- and platelet-derived substances can activate specific receptors (orange circles) on the endothelial membrane to release relaxing factors such as nitric oxide (NO), prostacyclin (PGI_2), and an endothelium-derived hyperpolarizing factor (EDHF). Other contracting factors are released, such as endothelin-1 (ET-1), angiotensin (A), and thromboxane A_2 (TXA_2), as well as prostaglandin H_2 (PGH_2). ACE = angiotensin-converting enzyme; Ach = acetylcholine; 5-HT = 5-hydroxytryptamine, or serotonin; BK = bradykinin; ECE = endothelin-converting enzyme; L-Arg = L-arginine; NOS = nitric oxide synthase; O_2^- = superoxide; TGF-β_1 = transforming growth factor-beta$_1$; Thr = thrombin. (From Ruschitzka F, Corti R, Noll G, Lüscher TF, et al: A rationale for treatment of endothelial dysfunction in hypertension. J Hyperten 17(Suppl 1):25, 1999.)

endothelin-1 appears to be of particular importance because it causes pronounced and prolonged vasoconstriction and because blockade of its receptors improves endothelium-dependent vasodilation in hypertensive patients.[75] Its role in human hypertension, however, remains uncertain.

A large number of circulating hormones and locally acting substances may be involved in the development of hypertension. Support exists for each of those shown as potential instigators in Figure 37–10.

Sympathetic Nervous Hyperactivity

Young hypertensive patients tend to have increased levels of circulating catecholamines, augmented sympathetic nerve traffic in muscles, faster heart rate, and heightened vascular reactivity to alpha-adrenergic agonists.[76] These changes could raise blood pressure in a number of ways—either alone or in concert with stimulation of renin release by catecholamines—by causing arteriolar and venous constriction, by increasing cardiac output, or by altering the normal renal pressure-volume relationship.

Repetitive stress or an accentuated, exaggerated response to stress is the logical means by which sympathetic activation would arise. Among middle-aged men in Framingham, the development of hypertension over an 18- to 20-year period was associated with heightened anxiety and anger intensity and suppressed expression of anger at baseline.[77] Similarly, among middle-aged men, the systolic pressure reaction to mental stress was positively correlated with higher systolic blood pressures 10 years later.[78] Moreover, the association between progressively lower socioeconomic status and the incidence of hypertension could obviously involve increased levels of stress.

Sympathetic nervous activity could be activated from the brain without the mediation of stress or emotional distress. Hypertension has been induced in animals by various neurogenic defects. An intriguing association has been reported but not well documented between hypertension, increased central sympathetic outflow, and compression of the ventrolateral medulla by loops of the posterior inferior cerebellar artery seen by magnetic resonance tomography.[79]

Whatever the specific role of sympathetic activity in the pathogenesis of hypertension, it appears to be involved in the increased cardiovascular morbidity and mortality that affect hypertensive patients during the early morning hours as noted earlier in this chapter.[14] Increased alpha-sympathetic activity occurs in the early morning in association with the assumption of upright posture after overnight recumbency, raising blood pressure abruptly and markedly. This rise must be at least partly responsible for the increase in cardiovascular catastrophes in the early morning hours.

Renin-Angiotensin System

Both as a direct pressor and as a growth promoter, the renin-angiotensin mechanism is likely involved in the pathogenesis of hypertension. All functions of renin are mediated through the synthesis of angiotensin II. This system is the primary stimulus for the secretion of aldosterone and hence mediates mineralocorticoid responses to varying sodium intake and volume load. When sodium intake is reduced or effective plasma volume shrinks, the increase in renin-angiotensin II stimulates aldosterone secretion, which in turn is responsible for a portion of the enhanced renal retention of sodium and water (Fig. 37–15). As noted elsewhere (see Chap. 79), aldosterone may have additional pathological roles, including a contribution to myocardial fibrosis.

According to the feedback shown in Figure 37–15, any rise in blood pressure inhibits release of renin from the renal juxtaglomerular cells. Therefore, primary (essential) hypertension would be expected to be accompanied by low, suppressed levels of plasma renin activity (PRA). However, when large populations of hypertensive subjects are surveyed, only about 30 percent have low PRA levels, whereas 50 percent have normal levels and the remaining 20 percent have high levels.

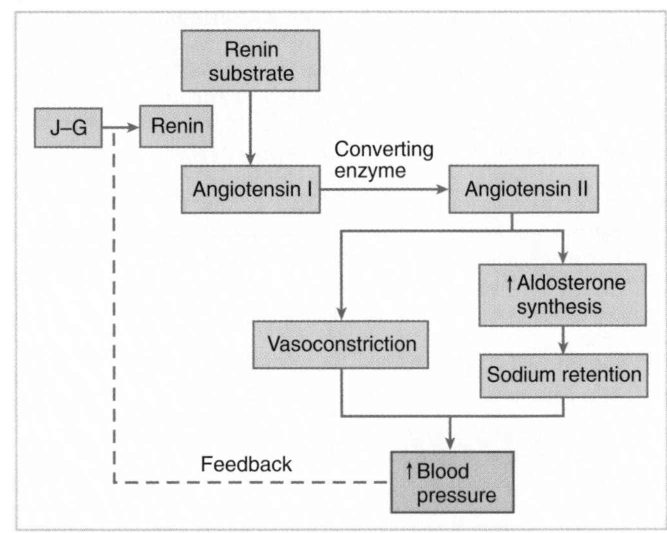

FIGURE 37–15 Overall scheme of the renin-angiotensin mechanism. J-G = juxtaglomerular.

NORMAL- AND HIGH-RENIN HYPERTENSION. A number of explanations have been offered for these "inappropriately normal" or high levels, beyond the proportion expected in a normal gaussian distribution curve. One of the more attractive explanations is the concept of "nephron heterogeneity,"[68] which assumes a mixture of normal and ischemic nephrons caused by afferent arteriolar narrowing. Excess renin from the ischemic nephrons could raise the total blood renin level to varying degrees and cause normal or high renin levels in patients with primary hypertension.

Williams and coworkers[80] have found that about half of normal-renin hypertensive subjects are nonmodulators; that is, they do not normally increase aldosterone secretion in response to sodium restriction and do not normally increase renal blood flow in response to sodium loading. Such nonmodulation in the presence of usual high sodium intake would help explain the pathogenesis of both sodium-sensitive hypertension and the continued secretion of renin due to a defective feedback mechanism.

The renin-angiotensin system is active in multiple organs, either from in situ synthesis of various components or by transport from renal juxtaglomerular cells through the circulation. Most of the important pathophysiological effects are mediated through the angiotensin II type I receptor, but some effects may involve the type II receptor. The presence of the complete system in endothelial cells, the brain, the heart, and the adrenal cortex broadens the potential role of this mechanism even beyond its previously accepted boundaries. As described in Chapter 38, drugs that inhibit the renin-angiotensin mechanism have assumed a major role in the treatment of hypertension.

Hyperinsulinemia/Insulin Resistance

An association between hypertension and hyperinsulinemia has been recognized for many years, particularly with accompanying obesity but also in about 20 percent of nonobese hypertensive patients. Virtually all obese people are hyperinsulinemic secondary to insulin resistance and even more so if the obesity is predominantly visceral—abdominal or upper body—wherein decreased hepatic uptake of insulin contributes to the hyperinsulinemia. The hyperinsulinemia of hypertension also arises as a consequence of resistance to the effects of insulin on peripheral glucose utilization.

The cause of the insulin resistance in nonobese hypertensive persons is unknown. It could reflect a simple reduced ability of insulin to reach skeletal muscle cells, wherein its major peripheral actions on glucose metabolism occur. This impairment may in turn result from a defect in the usual vasodilatory effect of insulin mediated through increased synthesis of nitric oxide, which normally counters the multiple pressor effects of insulin. These pressor effects include activation of sympathetic activity, a trophic action on vascular hypertrophy, and increased renal sodium reabsorption (Fig. 37–16).

The failure of vasodilation to antagonize the multiple pressor effects of insulin presumably eventuates in a rise in blood pressure that may be either a primary cause of hypertension or, at least, a secondary potentiator. In addition, the underlying insulin resistance is often associated with the metabolic syndrome, including dyslipidemia and diabetes along with hypertension, which combine to be a major risk factor for premature coronary disease.

Other Possible Mechanisms

The preceding description of the possible roles of the various mechanisms portrayed in Figure 37–10 does not exhaust the list of putative contributors to the pathogenesis of primary hypertension. Defects in ion transport across cell membranes and deficiencies of various vasodepressor hormones may also be involved. Moreover, a number of associations between hypertension and other conditions have been noted and may offer additional insight into the potential causes and possible prevention of the disease.

ASSOCIATION OF HYPERTENSION WITH OTHER CONDITIONS

Obesity

Hypertension is more common among obese individuals and adds to their increased risk for ischemic heart disease, particularly if it is abdominal or visceral in location as part of the metabolic syndrome. In the Framingham study, the incidence of hypertension was increased 46 percent in men and 75 percent in women who were overweight, defined as a body mass index of 25.0 to 29.9, compared to normal-weight persons.[81] Even small amounts of weight gain are associated with a marked increase in the incidence of hypertension and coronary events. Unfortunately, there is a worldwide epidemic of obesity, perhaps most widespread in the United States, where the prevalence of obesity, defined as a body mass index above 30, increased by 50 percent from 1980 to 1995.[82] Obesity is rapidly increasing among U.S. children, and children seem particularly vulnerable to the hypertensive effects of weight gain.[83] Therefore, avoidance of childhood obesity in the hope of avoiding subsequent hypertension is important. The evidence that weight reduction will lower established hypertension is discussed later.

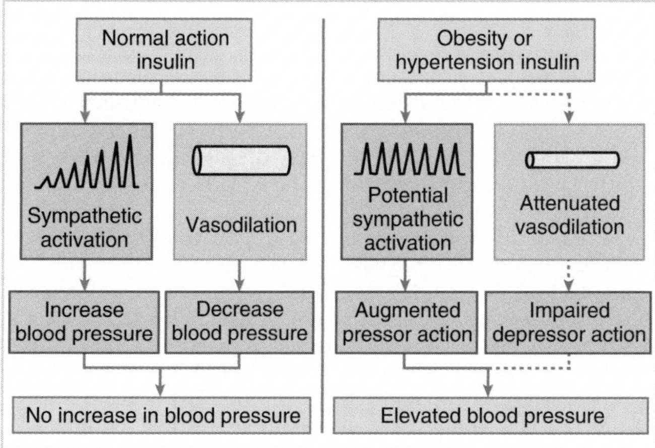

FIGURE 37–16 **Left,** Insulin's actions in normal humans. Although insulin causes a marked increase in sympathetic neural outflow, which would be expected to increase blood pressure, it also causes vasodilation, which would decrease blood pressure. The net effect of these two opposing influences is no change or a slight decrease in blood pressure. There may be an imbalance between the sympathetic and vascular actions of insulin in conditions such as obesity or hypertension. **Right,** Insulin may cause potentiated sympathetic activation or attenuated vasodilation. An imbalance between these pressor and depressor actions of insulin may result in elevated blood pressure. (From Anderson EA, Mark AL: Cardiovascular and sympathetic actions of insulin: The insulin hypothesis of hypertension revisited. Cardiovasc Risk Factors 3:159, 1993.)

Sleep Apnea

One of the contributors to hypertension in obese persons is obstructive sleep apnea. Snoring and sleep apnea are often associated with hypertension, which may in turn be induced by increased sympathetic activity and endothelin release in response to hypoxemia during apnea.[84] Relief of sleep apnea may alleviate hypertension.

Physical Inactivity

Physical fitness can help prevent hypertension, and persons who are already hypertensive can lower their blood pressure by means of regular aerobic exercise. The relationship may involve a restoration of age-related declines in endothelium-dependent vasodilation.[85]

Alcohol Intake

Alcohol in small amounts (less than one or two usual portions a day) provides protection from coronary disease, congestive heart failure, stroke, and dementia[86] and, at least in women, reduces the incidence of hypertension.[87] In larger amounts (more than two portions a day and even more so when drunk in binges), alcohol increases blood pressure and arterial stiffness. The reduction in coronary disease in persons who ingest small amounts of alcohol may reflect an improvement in lipid profile, a reduction in factors that encourage thrombosis, and an improvement in insulin sensitivity.

The pressor effect of larger amounts of alcohol primarily reflects an increase in cardiac output and heart rate, possibly a consequence of increased sympathetic nerve activity. Alcohol also alters cell membranes and allows more calcium to enter, perhaps by inhibition of sodium transport.

Smoking (see Chap. 36)

Cigarette smoking raises blood pressure, probably through the nicotine-induced release of norepinephrine from adrenergic nerve endings. In addition, smoking causes an acute and marked reduction in radial artery compliance independent of the increase in blood pressure. When smokers quit, a rise in blood pressure may occur, probably reflecting a gain in weight.

Hematological Findings

Higher hematocrits are found in hypertensive persons and are associated with abnormal left ventricular filling on echocardiography.[88] Whole-blood viscosity is increased by about 10 percent in persons with untreated mild hypertension, comparable to the increase in their peripheral resistance.[89]

Hyperuricemia

Hyperuricemia is present in 25 to 50 percent of individuals with untreated primary hypertension, about five times the frequency found in normotensive persons. Hyperuricemia probably reflects decreased renal blood flow, presumably a reflection of nephrosclerosis.

Hypercholesterolemia

Hypercholesterolemia frequently coexists with hypertension, at least in part because it impairs endothelium-dependent vasodilation. Lipid-lowering therapy restores the bioavailability of nitric oxide, reduces arterial stiffness, and lowers blood pressure.[90] In addition to these conditions often associated with hypertension, distinctive features of hypertension may be important in various special groups of people.

Hypertension in Special Groups

Blacks

Although, on average, blood pressure in black persons is not higher than in white persons during adolescence, adult blacks have hypertension more frequently, with higher rates of morbidity and mortality. These higher rates may reflect a higher incidence of low birth weight from intrauterine growth retardation, a lesser tendency for the pressure to fall during sleep, hyperresponsivity to stress, and impaired nitric oxide–induced vasodilation,[91] but the lower socioeconomic status and lesser access to adequate health care of black persons as a group are probably more important. In particular, blacks suffer more renal damage, even with apparently effective blood pressure control, which leads to a significantly greater prevalence of end-stage disease.[92] When given a high-sodium diet, most blacks but not whites tend to have renal vasoconstriction and an increase in the glomerular filtration rate, thus providing a possible mechanism for increased glomerular sclerosis. Hypertension in blacks has been characterized as having a relatively greater component of fluid volume excess, including a higher prevalence of low PRA and greater responsiveness to diuretic therapy.

Perhaps black persons as a group evolved the physiological machinery that would offer protection in their ancestral habitat, hot, arid climates in which avid sodium conservation was necessary for survival because the diet was relatively low in sodium. When they migrate to areas where sodium intake is excessive, they are then more susceptible to "sodium overload." In addition, blacks may also be more susceptible to hypertension because as a group they tend to ingest less potassium.[93]

TABLE 37–11 Most Common Causes for Chronic Hypertension in Childhood

Newborn
Renal artery stenosis or thrombosis
Congenital renal structural abnormalities
Coarctation of the aorta
Bronchopulmonary dysplasia
Infancy to 6 yr
Renal structural and inflammatory diseases
Coarctation of the aorta
Renal artery stenosis
Wilms tumor
6-10 yr
Renal structural and inflammatory diseases
Renal artery stenosis
Essential (primary) hypertension
Renal parenchymal diseases
Adolescence
Primary hypertension
Renal parenchymal diseases

From Loggie JMH: Hypertension in children. Heart Dis Stroke 3:147, 1994.

Women

In general, women suffer less cardiovascular morbidity and mortality than men do for any degree of hypertension.[94] Moreover, before menopause, hypertension is less common in women than in men, perhaps reflecting the lower blood volume afforded women by menses. Eventually, however, more women than men have a hypertension-related cardiovascular complication because there are more elderly women than elderly men and hypertension is both more common and more dangerous in the elderly.

Children and Adolescents

As in adults, care is needed in establishing the presence of persistently elevated blood pressure in children when using the upper limits of normal shown in Table 37–4. Surveillance of blood pressure as children grow older shows an overall tracking of systolic levels,[21] but the positive predictive value of a blood pressure reading above the 95th percentile in a 10-year-old boy being at a hypertensive level at age 20 is only 0.44.[95] Nonetheless, most authorities[96] agree that children with "significant" hypertension (levels above the 95th percentile) should be given a limited work-up for target organ damage and secondary causes (perhaps including an echocardiogram and probably including a renal isotopic scan); if results of these tests are negative, the children should be carefully monitored and given nonpharmacological therapy. Those with "severe" hypertension (levels above the 99th percentile) should be more rapidly and completely evaluated and given appropriate pharmacological therapy.

EPIDEMIOLOGY. The older the child is, the more likely it is that the hypertension is of unknown cause, that is, primary or essential. In prepubertal children, chronic hypertension is more likely caused by congenital or acquired renal parenchymal or vascular disease (Table 37–11). In adolescents, primary hypertension is the most likely diagnosis. Factors that increase the likelihood for early onset of hypertension include a positive family history of hypertension, obesity, poor physical fitness, and an increase in thickness of the interventricular septum during systole on echocardiography.

MANAGEMENT. Once persistently elevated blood pressure is identified in children and adolescents and an appropriate work-up has been performed, weight reduction if the patient is overweight, regular dynamic exercise, and moderate restriction of dietary sodium should be encouraged. Those children deemed to be in need of drug therapy are usually treated in the way adults are managed, as described in Chapter 38.

The Elderly

As more people live longer, more hypertension, particularly systolic, will be seen. By the usual criteria of the average of three blood pressure measurements on one occasion at or above 140 mm Hg systolic and/or 90 mm Hg diastolic or the taking of antihypertensive medication, 54 percent of men and women aged 65 to 74 years have hypertension; among blacks, the prevalence is 72 percent.[22] Most of this hypertension is isolated systolic hypertension (>140/<90 mm Hg). Partly because systolic levels are more resistant to therapy and partly because practitioners are often hesitant to treat older patients, the rate of control among the elderly is much lower than among persons younger than 65 years of age.[97] The risks of both pure systolic and combined systolic and diastolic hypertension at every level are greater in the elderly, at least to age 80, than in younger patients as a result of the adverse effects of age-related atherosclerosis and concomitant conditions. It comes as no surprise that elderly subjects achieved even greater reductions in coronary disease and heart failure by effective therapy than did younger hypertensive subjects in multiple clinical trials.[98]

There is evidence, however, that hypertension is no longer a risk factor for cardiovascular disease in those older than 80 years of age.[99] The limited data from seven placebo-controlled trials involving 1670 hypertensive subjects 80 years of age or older reveal significant reductions in major cardiovascular events—strokes by 34 percent, heart failure by 39 percent—in those given antihypertensive drug therapy, but no benefit for mortality.[100] Obviously, more evidence is needed and will be provided by ongoing trials in very old subjects.

As noted before, elderly patients may display three features that reflect age-related cardiovascular changes. The first is pseudohypertension from markedly sclerotic arteries that do not collapse under the blood pressure cuff and therefore cause much higher cuff pressures than present within the vessels. The second feature, seen in 20 to 30 percent of the elderly population, is postural and postprandial hypotension, which usually reflects a progressive loss of baroreceptor responsiveness with age. A standing blood pressure reading should always be taken in patients older than 65 years, particularly if seated or supine hypertension is noted; if postural hypotension is present, maneuvers to overcome the precipitous falls in pressure should be attempted before the seated and supine hypertension is cautiously treated. More about the special therapeutic challenges often found in the elderly is provided in Chapter 38.

The third, increasing arterial stiffness, is largely responsible for the progressively higher levels of systolic pressure (and lower levels of diastolic pressure) with age. Current measures of arterial stiffness have many limitations, but considerable effort is being expended to make them clinically useful.[101] They may prove to be valuable in managing the elderly hypertensive patient.

Patients with Diabetes Mellitus (see Chap. 51)

Hypertension and diabetes coexist more commonly than predicted by chance. They act in a synergistic manner to markedly accelerate cardiovascular damage, which is in turn largely responsible for the premature disabilities and higher rates of mortality that afflict diabetic patients.[102] Among some 1500 diabetic subjects included in the NHANES III survey, 71 percent were hypertensive but only 12 percent had good control—that is, blood pressure below 130/80 mm Hg—whereas 55 percent had blood pressure above 140/90 mm Hg.[103] Not only is hypertension more common in diabetic patients, but it also tends to be more persistent, with less of the usual nocturnal fall in pressure. The absence of a nocturnal fall in pressure may reflect autonomic neuropathy or incipient diabetic nephropathy. Since ambulatory monitoring is not generally available, home measurements of early morning blood pressure should be used. Patients with readings above 130/85 mm Hg are more likely to develop nephropathy and other complications.[104]

When hypertensive, patients with diabetes mellitus may confront some unusual problems. With progressive renal insufficiency, they may have few functional juxtaglomerular cells, and as a result, the syndrome of hyporeninemic hypoaldosteronism may appear, usually manifested by hyperkalemia. If hypoglycemia develops because of too much insulin or other drugs, severe hypertension may occur as a result of stimulated sympathetic nervous activity. Diabetic neuropathy may add to the postural hypotension that is commonly seen in elderly hypertensive individuals. As will be noted in Chapter 38, diabetic patients are also susceptible to special problems associated with antihypertensive therapy. On the other hand, successful control of blood pressure has clearly been shown to protect such patients from the otherwise inexorable progress of diabetic nephropathy. Even more encouraging are the results of large trials documenting the ability of life-style modifications to prevent the onset of diabetes.

Identifiable (Secondary) Forms of Hypertension (see Tables 37–5 and 37–7)

Oral Contraceptive and Postmenopausal Estrogen Use

The use of estrogen-containing oral contraceptive pills is probably the most common cause of secondary hypertension in young women. Most women who take them experience a slight rise in blood pressure. In a prospective cohort study of almost 70,000 nurses, over the 4 years between 1989 and 1993, those who were current users of oral contraceptives had an overall risk for hypertension 50 percent higher than never-users and 10 percent higher than former users.[105] The 50 percent increase in relative risk translated to 41 cases per 10,000 person-years of oral contraceptive use. The incidence of hypertension is likely even less with present-day lower dose formulations.

The dangers of oral contraceptives should be kept in proper perspective. While it is true that use of these drugs is associated with increased morbidity and mortality, the absolute numbers are quite small, as noted in the nurses study.[105] Most adverse effects, including hypertension, occur in women older than 35 years of age who smoke and have other cardiovascular risk factors.[106]

CLINICAL FEATURES. In most women, the hypertension is mild; however, in some, it may accelerate rapidly and cause severe renal damage. When use of the pill is discontinued, blood pressure falls to normal within 3 to 6 months in about half the patients. Whether the pill caused permanent hypertension in the other half or just uncovered primary hypertension at an earlier time is not clear.

MECHANISMS OF HYPERTENSION. Oral contraceptive use probably causes hypertension by volume expansion, since both estrogens and the synthetic progestogens used in oral contraceptive pills cause sodium retention. Although plasma renin levels rise in response to increased levels of angiotensinogen, angiotensin-converting enzyme (ACE) inhibition did not alter blood pressure any more in women with oral contraceptive–induced hypertension than in women with essential hypertension.[107]

MANAGEMENT. The use of estrogen-containing oral contraceptives should be restricted in women older than 35 years, particularly if they also smoke or are hypertensive or obese. Women given the pill should be properly monitored as follows: (1) The initial supply should be limited; (2) they should be asked to return for a blood pressure check before an additional supply is provided; and (3) if blood pressure has risen, an alternative contraceptive method should be offered. If the pill remains the only acceptable contraceptive method, the elevated blood pressure can be reduced with appropriate therapy. In view of the possible role of aldosterone, use of a diuretic-spironolactone combination seems appropriate. In women who stop taking oral contraceptives, evaluation for secondary hypertensive diseases should be postponed for at least 3 months to allow changes in the renin-angiotensin-aldosterone system to remit. If the hypertension does not recede, additional work-up and therapy may be needed.

POSTMENOPAUSAL ESTROGEN USE. Millions of women take estrogen replacement therapy after menopause. Estrogen replacement therapy does not appear to induce hypertension, even though it does induce the various changes in the renin-angiotensin-aldosterone system seen with oral contraceptive use. In fact, most controlled trials find a decrease in daytime ambulatory blood pressure and a greater dipping of nocturnal blood pressure in estrogen replacement therapy users[108] and most hypertensive women have a fall in blood pressure with transdermal estradiol.[109] Such lower blood pressures may reflect a number of effects, including improved endothelium-dependent vasodilation and reduced muscle sympathetic nerve activity.

Renal Parenchymal Disease (see Chap. 86)

Subtle renal dysfunction has been previously described as a likely initiator of primary hypertension, and renal parenchymal disease is the most common cause of secondary hypertension, responsible for 2 to 5 percent of cases. As chronic glomerulonephritis has become less common, hypertensive nephrosclerosis and, to an even greater degree, diabetic nephropathy have become the most common causes of chronic renal disease.[110] The prevalence of chronic renal disease, defined by a reduction in glomerular filtration rate to less than 60 ml/min/1.73 m^2 or persistent albuminuria of more than 300 mg/day, is estimated to be 11 percent (19.2 million) of the adult U.S. population.[111] The higher prevalence of hypertension among U.S. blacks is probably responsible for their significantly higher rate of end-stage renal disease with hypertension as the underlying cause in as many as half of these patients.

As previously noted, even microalbuminuria, 30 to 300 mg/day, is closely related to target organ damage in hypertensive persons,[50] and it likely should be looked for routinely in the evaluation of every new hypertensive patient in a "spot" urine collection. Measurement of serum creatinine is routine but by itself is an inadequate screening test for significant renal damage, particularly in elderly patients.[112] Therefore, a creatinine clearance should be calculated with either the Cockcroft-Gault formula or the Modification of Diet in Renal Disease (MDRD) equation, taking age, gender, and body weight into account.

Once it begins, renal disease is usually progressive, following the concept that a loss of filtration surface leads to both glomerular and systemic hypertension, which engenders more glomerular sclerosis, setting up a cycle of progressive disease (see Fig. 37–12). Therefore, it is critical to identify renal damage early, since removal of causal or aggravating factors can prevent the otherwise inexorable progress of renal damage. These factors include obstruction of the urinary tract, depletion of effective circulating volume, nephrotoxic agents, and, most importantly, uncontrolled hypertension.

In addition to these and other factors involved in chronic renal disease, a number of acute conditions may be responsible for renal damage and hypertension.

ACUTE RENAL DISEASES. Hypertension may appear with any sudden, severe insult to the kidneys that either markedly impairs excretion of salt and water, which leads to volume expansion, or reduces renal blood flow, which sets off the renin-angiotension-aldosterone mechanism. Bilateral ureteral obstruction is an example of the former; sudden bilateral renal artery occlusion, as by cholesterol emboli, is an example of the latter. Relief of either may dramatically reverse severe hypertension. Such reversal of hypertension has been particularly striking in men with high-pressure chronic retention of urine, who may manifest both renal failure and severe hypertension, both of which may be ameliorated by relief of the obstruction.[113] Some collagen diseases may also produce rapidly progressive vasculitis and renal damage.

Two commonly used classes of drugs—nonsteroidal antiinflammatory drugs and inhibitors of the renin-angiotensin system—may suddenly worsen renal function in patients with preexisting renal diseases. Nonsteroidal antiinflammatory drugs, by blocking synthesis of prostaglandins, which act as vasodilators within the kidney, may cause an abrupt loss of renal function. Renin-angiotensin inhibitors, both ACE inhibitors and angiotensin II receptor blockers (ARBs), may precipitate acute renal failure in patients with bilateral renovascular disease whose renal profusion is dependent on high levels of renin-angiotensin.[114]

CHRONIC RENAL DISEASES. All chronic renal diseases are associated with a higher prevalence of hypertension, and the presence of hypertension accelerates the progression of renal damage. Although it is uncertain that hypertension by itself can lead to renal failure in persons who are not black, there is no doubt that hypertension can accelerate the progress of all underlying renal diseases.

The control of hypertension can slow or stop the progression of renal diseases and of cardiovascular sequelae (Fig. 37-17).[115] As noted in the Heart Outcomes Prevention Evaluation (HOPE) trial,[116] the presence of microalbuminuria was associated with an increase in cardiovascular morbidity and mortality in subjects with microalbuminuria (26.4 percent) compared with those without microalbuminuria (15.4 percent). With the further lowering of blood pressure by the addition of the ACE inhibitor ramipril, individuals with microalbuminuria had even greater reduction in their risk. This protection may reflect special advantages of ACE inhibition, but the lowering of blood pressure must also be a factor.

Uncertainty remains as to the goal of antihypertensive therapy in patients with chronic renal disease. In two large trials of nondiabetic patients with chronic renal disease, more intensive therapy to reach a goal of 125/75 mm Hg did not slow the rate of fall of glomerular filtration rate more than did less intensive therapy to a level of 140/85 mm Hg, except in patients with more than 1 g of proteinuria per day.[117,118]

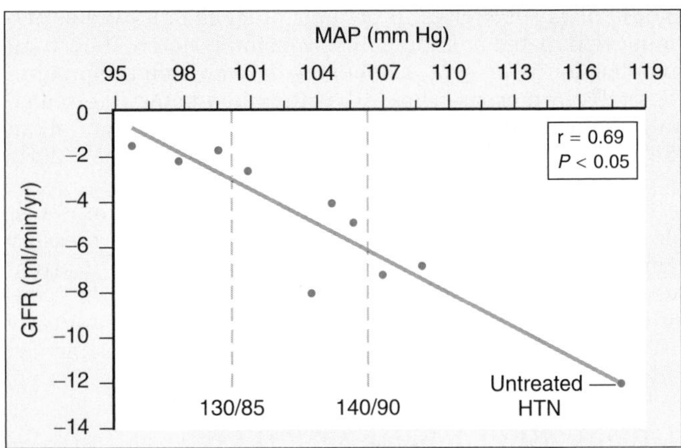

FIGURE 37–17 Relationship between achieved blood pressure control and declines in glomerular filtration rate (GFR) in six clinical trials of patients with diabetic renal disease and three trials of patients with nondiabetic renal disease. HTN = hypertension; MAP = mean arterial pressure. (From Bakris GL, Williams M, Dworkin L, et al: Preserving renal function in adults with hypertension and diabetes: A consensus approach. Am J Kidney Dis 36:646, 2000.)

Issues as to the preferred choices of antihypertensive agents in patients with chronic renal disease are addressed in Chapter 38. Suffice it to note that an ACE inhibitor or an ARB is always indicated as the initial choice, almost always in combination with a diuretic. With whatever drugs chosen, but particularly with ACE inhibitors and ARBs, caution is needed in lowering blood pressure in the presence of previously unrecognized bilateral renovascular disease, which has been found in as many as 20 percent of patients with progressive renal damage.[114] However, a modest increase in serum creatinine, averaging 30 percent above baseline, has been found to predict a better preservation of renal function, presumably reflecting a successful reduction in intraglomerular pressure.[119]

DIABETIC NEPHROPATHY (see Chaps. 51 and 86). The most impressive protection against progressive renal damage by reduction of elevated blood pressure has been seen in patients with diabetic nephropathy.[110] Such protection has been observed to extend to diabetic retinopathy and neuropathy, both in normotensive[120] and hypertensive[121] type 2 diabetic patients with proteinuria. The consensus advice is to start antihypertensive therapy in diabetic patients with or without nephropathy at a blood pressure of 140/90 mm Hg or higher and to reach a level of 130/80 mm Hg or lower.[115] Such intensive control of hypertension has been shown to be much more cost-effective than either intensive glycemic control or reduction in hypercholesterolemia.[122]

Hypertension During Chronic Dialysis and after Renal Transplantation

In patients with end-stage renal disease who are on dialysis, hypertension is a significant risk factor for mortality. Beyond the primary influence of excess fluid volume, hypertension can be accentuated by the accumulation of endogenous inhibitors of nitric oxide synthase. With neither the vasoconstrictor effects of renal renin nor the vasodepressor actions of various renal hormones, blood pressure may be particularly labile and sensitive to changes in fluid volume. Among patients receiving maintenance hemodialysis every 48 hours, elevated blood pressures tend to fall progressively after dialysis is completed, remain depressed during the remainder of the first 24 hours, and rise again during the second day as a consequence of excessive fluid retention. By increasing the time of dialysis treatment and thereby reducing dry weight, blood pressure can be better controlled.[123] As with other forms of renal disease, ACE inhibitors may provide special benefits to hemodialysis patients.[124]

Although successful renal transplantation may cure primary hypertension, various problems can result, with about half of the recipients becoming hypertensive within 1 year. These problems include stenosis of the renal artery at the site of anastomosis, rejection reactions, high doses of adrenal steroids and cyclosporine or tacrolimus, and excess renin derived from the retained diseased kidneys. ACE inhibitor therapy may obviate the need to remove the native diseased kidneys to relieve hypertension caused by their persistent secretion of renin. The source of the donor kidney may also play a role in the subsequent development of hypertension in the recipient. More hypertension has been observed when donors had a family history of hypertension or when the donors had died of subarachnoid hemorrhage and had probably been hypertensive.

Renovascular Hypertension

Renovascular hypertension is among the most common secondary forms of hypertension and is not easily recognizable. The prevalence of proven renovascular hypertension in the overall hypertensive population is unknown, but significant renal artery disease (defined as a 60 percent or greater reduction of diameter on duplex sonography) has been found in 6.8 percent of 824 elderly people in North Carolina[125] and in 7 percent of hypertensive patients undergoing coronary angiography (defined as a 70 percent or greater stenosis on renal angiography).[126]

It has long been known that the presence of renovascular disease does not, in itself, prove that the renovascular lesion is responsible for renovascular hypertension. Therefore, screening should focus on those hypertensive patients who have multiple features known to be associated with renovascular hypertension. The greater the number of clues, the more extensive the search (Table 37–12). The search likely should start with renal arteriography in those who are at high likelihood, since no other screening study can rule out the presence of the disease.

Classification

In adults, the two major types of renovascular disease tend to appear at different times and affect the sexes differently (Table 37–13). Atherosclerotic disease affecting mainly the proximal third of the main renal artery is seen mostly in older men. Fibroplastic disease involving mainly the distal two-thirds and branches of the renal arteries appears most commonly in younger women. As the population grows older, 80 percent of cases are caused by atherosclerotic disease and fewer than 20 percent by fibroplastic disease. Although the nonatherosclerotic stenoses may involve all layers of the renal artery, the most common is medial fibroplasia.

A number of other intrinsic and extrinsic causes of renovascular hypertension are known, including cholesterol emboli within the renal artery or compression of this vessel by nearby tumors. Most renovascular hypertension develops from partial obstruction of one main renal artery, but only a branch need be involved; segmental disease has been found in about 10 percent of cases. On the other hand, if apparent complete occlusion of the renal artery is slow in developing, enough collateral flow will become available to preserve the viability of the kidney. In this way, the seemingly nonfunctioning kidney may be responsible for continued renin secretion and hypertension. If recognized, such totally occluded vessels can sometimes be repaired, with return of renal function and relief of hypertension.[127]

Renovascular stenosis is often bilateral, although usually one side is clearly predominant. The possibility of bilateral disease should be suspected in those with renal insufficiency, particularly if rapidly progressive oliguric renal failure develops without evidence of obstructive uropathy and even more so if it develops after the start of ACE inhibitor or ARB therapy.[114]

Mechanisms

The sequence of changes in patients with renovascular hypertension starts with the release of increased amounts of renin when sufficient ischemia is induced to diminish pulse pressure against the juxtaglomerular cells in the renal afferent arterioles. A reduction in renal perfusion pressure by 50 percent leads to an immediate and persistent increase in renin secretion from the ischemic kidney, along with

TABLE 37–12 Clinical Clues for Renovascular Hypertension

History
- Onset of hypertension before 30 or after 50 years of age
- Abrupt onset of hypertension
- Severe or resistant hypertension
- Symptoms of atherosclerotic disease elsewhere
- Negative family history of hypertension
- Smoker
- Worsening renal function with angiotensin-converting enzyme inhibition
- Recurrent flash pulmonary edema

Examination
- Abdominal bruits
- Other bruits
- Advanced fundal changes

Laboratory
- Secondary aldosteronism
  - Higher plasma renin
  - Low serum potassium
  - Low serum sodium
- Proteinuria, usually moderate
- Elevated serum creatinine
- >1.5 cm difference in kidney size on sonography

Adapted from McLaughlin K, Jardine AG, Moss JG. Renal artery stenosis. Br Med J 320:1124, 2000.

TABLE 37–13 Features of the Two Major Forms of Renal Artery Disease

Cause	Incidence (%)	Age (yr)	Location of Lesion in Renal Artery	Natural History
Atherosclerosis	80-90	>50	Proximal 2 cm; branch disease rare	Progression in 50%, often to total occlusion
Fibromuscular dysplasias				
Intimal	1-2	Birth-25	Midportion of main renal artery and/or branches	Progression in most cases; dissection and/or thrombosis common
Medial	10-20	25-50	Distal segment of main renal artery and/or branches	Progression in 33%; dissection and/or thrombosis rare
Periarterial	1-2	15-30	Middle to distal segments of main renal artery or branches	Progression in most cases; dissection and/or thrombosis common

From Kaplan NM: Kaplan's Clinical Hypertension. 8th ed. Baltimore, Lippincott Williams & Wilkins, 2002, p 385.

suppression of secretion from the contralateral one. With time, renin levels fall (but not to the low level expected from the elevated blood pressure), accompanied by an expanded body fluid volume and increased cardiac output.

Diagnosis

The presence of the clinical features listed in Table 37–12, found in perhaps 5 to 10 percent of all hypertensive persons, indicates the need for a screening test for renovascular hypertension. A positive screening test result, or very strong clinical features, calls for more definitive confirmatory tests. Recurrent flash pulmonary edema has been associated with renovascular hypertension, so this clinical manifestation has been added to the indication for diagnostic work-up.[128] The initial diagnostic study in most patients should be noninvasive and, if abnormal, followed by a study of renal perfusion to ensure that any renovascular lesion is pathogenic, to decide whether revascularization is indicated (Fig. 37–18).[129]

There are problems with all screening studies. Considerable asymmetry of renal blood flow, 25 percent or more, was found in 148 hypertensive patients with patent renal arteries on prior angiography.[130] Such normal asymmetry likely is responsible for the low sensitivity and specificity of captopril-enhanced renal scans. On the other hand, the sensitivity of renal duplex sonography for the detection of hemodynamically significant renovascular disease has been reported to be only 50 percent.[131] The accuracy of ultrasonography is very much operator-dependent, often requiring scanning times of 1 hour or longer, so its use has been limited. However, a strong association with the outcome of revascularization has been reported with the use of a resistance index to assess flow in segmental arteries.[132] Patients with high resistance-index values above 80, reflecting marked intrarenal vascular disease, had generally poor outcomes. Those with lower values had generally good outcomes.

Over the past few years, both contrast-enhanced computed tomography and magnetic resonance angiography have been increasingly used to screen for renovascular hypertension. Magnetic resonance angiography will likely be more widely used, since it avoids the possibility of dye-induced nephrotoxicity and ionizing radiation as well as its greater potential for an assessment of renal function.

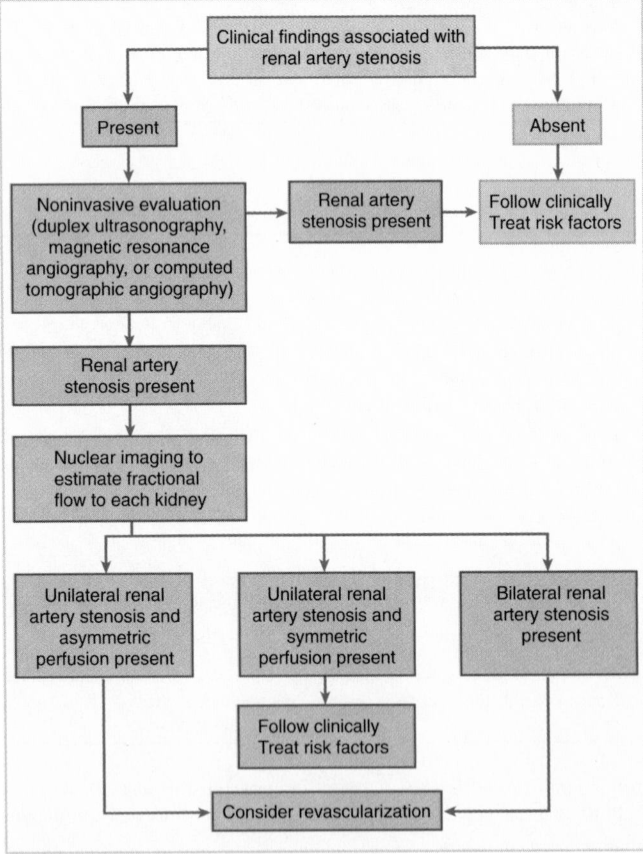

FIGURE 37–18 Algorithm for evaluating patients in whom renal artery stenosis is suspected. Clinical follow-up includes periodic reassessment with duplex ultrasonography, magnetic resonance angiography, and nuclear imaging to estimate fractional blood flow to each kidney. The treatment of risk factors includes smoking cessation and the use of aspirin, lipid-lowering agents, and antihypertensive therapy. (Modified from Safian RD, Textor SC: Renal-artery stenosis. N Engl J Med 344:431, 2001.)

Management

MEDICAL. The availability of ACE inhibitors can be considered a two-edged sword; one edge provides better control of renovascular hypertension than may be possible with other antihypertensive medications, while the other edge exposes the already ischemic kidney to further loss of blood flow by removing the high level of angiotensin II that was supporting its circulation. Other antihypertensive drugs may be almost as effective as ACE inhibitors and perhaps safer, but there are no comparative data.

ANGIOPLASTY (see Chap. 55). Angioplasty has been shown to improve blood pressure (at least transiently) in 60 to 70 percent of patients, more with fibromuscular disease than with atherosclerosis, as is also the case for surgery. In three small but controlled trials, balloon angioplasty was shown to provide a modest but significantly greater reduction in blood pressure than medical therapy.[133] Placement of an arterial stent reduced the likelihood of restenosis and is increasingly performed as the initial procedure to preserve renal function.[134]

SURGERY. Revascularization by surgery is indicated in patients whose hypertension is not well controlled or whose renal function deteriorates with medical therapy and in those with only a transient response to angioplasty or in whom lesions are not amenable to that procedure. Surgery is recommended more to preserve renal function than to relieve hypertension and should be undertaken before serum creatinine level rises above 3 mg/dl.[129]

Renin-Secreting Tumors

Made up of juxtaglomerular cells or hemangiopericytomas, renin-secreting tumors have been found mostly in young patients with severe hypertension, very high renin levels in both peripheral blood and the kidney harboring the tumor, and secondary aldosteronism manifested by hypokalemia.[135] The tumor can generally be recognized by selective renal angiography, usually performed for suspected renovascular hypertension, although a few are extrarenal. More commonly, children with Wilms tumors (nephroblastoma) may have hypertension and high plasma renin and prorenin levels that revert to normal after nephrectomy.[136]

Adrenal Causes of Hypertension

Adrenal causes of hypertension include primary excesses of aldosterone, cortisol, and catecholamines; more rarely, excess deoxycorticosterone is present along with congenital adrenal hyperplasia. Together, these conditions cause less than 1 percent of all hypertensive diseases, although, as will be noted, primary aldosteronism may be more common than previously thought. Each can usually be recognized with relative ease, and patients suspected of having these disorders can be screened by readily available tests.

More of a problem than the diagnosis of these adrenal disorders is the need to exclude their presence because of the increasing identification of incidental adrenal masses when abdominal computed tomography (CT) is done to diagnose intraabdominal pathological conditions. Unsuspected adrenal tumors have been found on about 1 percent of abdominal CT scans obtained for reasons unrelated to the adrenal gland. As delineated in Table 37–7, screening for hormonal excess should be performed if an adrenal tumor is found. Most of these "incidentalomas" appear to be nonfunctional on the basis of normal basal adrenal hormone levels. When more detailed studies are done, however, a significant number show incomplete suppression of cortisol by dexamethasone, that is, subclinical Cushing disease that does not appear to progress to overt hypercortisolism but may be associated with insulin resistance and osteopenia.[137]

The benign nature of smaller tumors can usually be assured by appropriate imaging studies. The threat of malignancy can probably be best excluded by adrenal scintigraphy with NP-59, a radioiodinated derivative of cholesterol. Benign lesions almost always take up the isotope, whereas malignant ones almost always do not. Most tumors larger than 4 cm are resected, since a significant number of them are malignant.

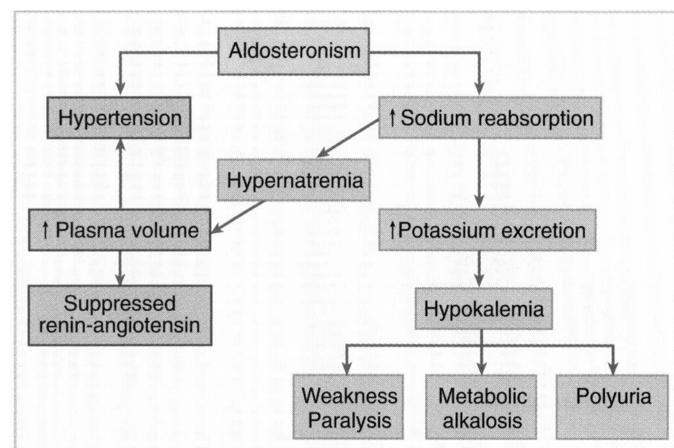

FIGURE 37–19 Pathophysiology of primary aldosteronism.

Primary Aldosteronism

This disease has been considered to be relatively rare in unselected populations, but it has been recognized in considerably more patients screened by a plasma aldosterone/renin activity ratio.[138]

PATHOPHYSIOLOGY OF MINERALOCORTICOID EXCESS. A number of syndromes with mineralocorticoid excess have been recognized (Table 37–14), with primary aldosteronism being by far the most common. Until recently, the most frequently found source of hyperaldosteronism was a solitary aldosterone-producing adenoma. Recently, as milder forms of hyperaldosteronism have been recognized by measurements of plasma renin and aldosterone, bilateral adrenal hyperplasia (BAH) has become far more common.

Aldosterone excess from any source causes hypertension and renal potassium wastage, which should induce hypokalemia (Fig. 37–19). However, the majority of patients with aldosteronism caused by BAH are normokalemic.[138] The lack of overt hypokalemia could be explained in numerous ways: (1) potassium wastage has lowered the serum potassium level, but not yet to hypokalemic levels; (2) with milder degrees of aldosteronism, as are typical with BAH, the excess of aldosterone induces hypertension without causing potassium wastage, a scenario that has never been experimentally or clinically recognized; or (3) the BAH is related to the typical progressive increase in adrenal nodular hyperplasia with age that has no relationship to hypertension.[139] The third explanation would fit with the long-held belief that BAH is simply a form of low-renin hypertension, that is, primary (essential) hypertension with plasma renin levels that are known to fall progressively with age while plasma aldosterone levels remain stable.[140]

This third explanation could account for the common finding of an increased aldosterone/renin ratio, due not to increased aldosterone but to decreased renin as well as the presence of BAH in the majority of normokalemic hypertensive patients reported in recent series.[138] In an analysis of the aldosterone/renin ratio in 505 patients with essential hypertension, an elevated ratio was found to be a measure of low renin alone without increased aldosterone in 36 percent and the positive predictive value of the ratio to identify patients with increased aldosterone and low renin was only 34 percent.[141]

This examination of the pathophysiology of hyperaldosteronism does not deny the existence of autonomous hypersecretive from hyperplastic glands. However, most patients with an elevated aldosterone/renin ratio and BAH do not have autonomous hyperaldosteronism.[142]

DIAGNOSIS. Despite the enthusiasm to screen virtually all hypertensive patients with an aldosterone/renin ratio measurement,[138] there are good reasons to limit use of the test and, rather than using a ratio that could be high entirely because of a low renin level, to simply confirm an elevated plasma aldosterone level, above 15 ng/dl, and a low renin level. This more conservative view is based on the strong likelihood that only a very few normokalemic patients harbor an adenoma that should be resected and that there is no need to identify the presence of bilateral hyperplasia in normokalemic patients, mainly because identification of BAH usually requires an expensive, difficult, and occasionally harmful study, bilateral adrenal venous sampling.[143]

Therefore, screening is recommended only for hypertensive subjects who have a higher likelihood of primary aldosteronism, including those with (1) unprovoked, unexplainable hypokalemia; (2) hypokalemia induced by diuretics but resistant to correction; (3) family history of aldosteronism; or (4) hypertension resistant to appropriate therapy wherein the resistance cannot be explained. Hyperaldosteronism has been found in as many as 20 percent of resistant hypertensive patients, but BAH is the usual finding and therapy with the aldosterone blocker spironolactone significantly reduced blood pressure,[144] alleviating the need for extensive evaluation for aldosteronism in most such patients.

If the screening plasma aldosterone and renin levels are suggestive, a saline suppression study, either oral or intravenous, should be done to document autonomy of hyperaldosteronism (Fig. 37–20). If the aldosteronism persists, either a CT or an MRI scan should look for adrenal pathological lesions. If a solitary adenoma larger than 1 cm is present, the diagnosis of an aldosterone-producing adenoma can be reasonably ensured and consideration given to adrenalectomy. Because some nodularity is common even with a single hypersecreting adenoma, however, most experts suggest adrenal venous sampling before surgery is recommended.[145]

OTHER FORMS OF MINERALOCORTICOID EXCESS. Table 37–14 lists a number of other causes for real or apparent mineralocorticoid excess. One, familial glucocorticoid-remediable aldosteronism, is caused by a mutation in the genes involved in coding for the aldosterone synthase enzyme normally found only in the outer zona glomerulosa and the 11-beta-hydroxylase enzyme in the zona fasciculata. The chimeric

TABLE 37–14 Syndromes of Mineralocorticoid Excess

Adrenal origin
Aldosterone excess (primary)
Aldosterone-producing adenoma
Bilateral hyperplasia
Primary unilateral adrenal hyperplasia
Glucocorticoid-remediable aldosteronism (familial hyperaldosteronism, type I)
Adrenal carcinoma
Extraadrenal tumors
Deoxycorticosterone excess
Deoxycorticosterone-secreting tumors
Congenital adrenal hyperplasia
11β-hydroxylase deficiency
17α-hydroxylase deficiency
Cortisol excess
Cushing syndrome from ACTH-producing tumor
Glucocorticoid receptor resistance
Renal origin
Activating mutation of mineralocorticoid receptor
Pseudohypoaldosteronism, type II (Gordon)
11β-hydroxysteroid dehydrogenase deficiency
Congenital: apparent mineralocorticoid excess
Acquired: licorice, carbenoxolone

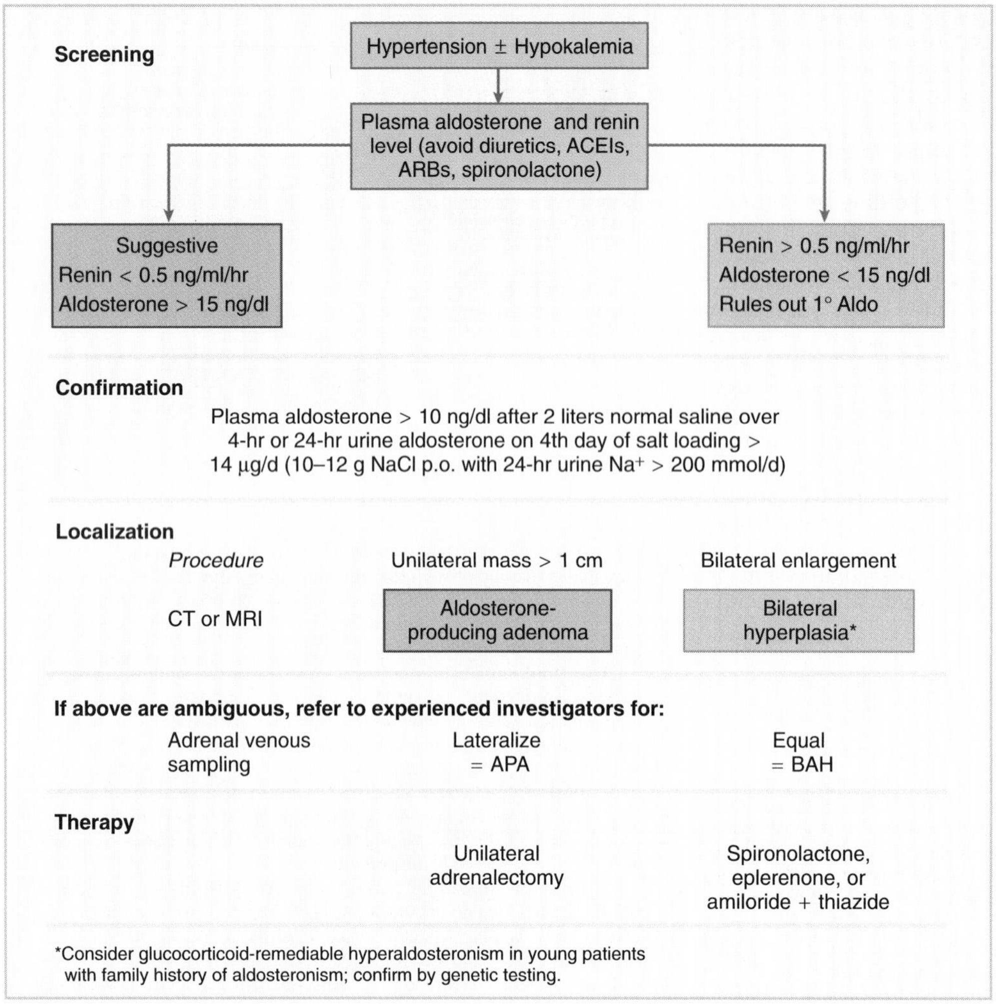

Screening

Hypertension ± Hypokalemia

↓

Plasma aldosterone and renin level (avoid diuretics, ACEIs, ARBs, spironolactone)

Suggestive	
Renin < 0.5 ng/ml/hr Aldosterone > 15 ng/dl	Renin > 0.5 ng/ml/hr Aldosterone < 15 ng/dl Rules out 1° Aldo

Confirmation

Plasma aldosterone > 10 ng/dl after 2 liters normal saline over 4-hr or 24-hr urine aldosterone on 4th day of salt loading > 14 μg/d (10–12 g NaCl p.o. with 24-hr urine Na^+ > 200 mmol/d)

Localization

Procedure	Unilateral mass > 1 cm	Bilateral enlargement
CT or MRI	Aldosterone-producing adenoma	Bilateral hyperplasia*

If above are ambiguous, refer to experienced investigators for:

Adrenal venous sampling	Lateralize = APA	Equal = BAH

Therapy

Unilateral adrenalectomy	Spironolactone, eplerenone, or amiloride + thiazide

*Consider glucocorticoid-remediable hyperaldosteronism in young patients with family history of aldosteronism; confirm by genetic testing.

FIGURE 37–20 A diagnostic flow chart for evaluating and treating patients with primary aldosteronism. 1º Aldo = primary aldosteronism; ACEI = angiotensin-converting enzyme inhibitor; APA = aldosterone-producing adenoma; ARB = angiotensin II receptor blocker; BAH = bilateral adrenal hyperplasia; CT = computed tomography; MRI = magnetic resonance imaging; 18-OH-B, 18-hydroxycorticosterone. (Modified from Kaplan NM: Kaplan's Clinical Hypertension. 8th ed. Baltimore, Lippincott Williams & Wilkins, 2002, p 464.)

gene induces an enzyme that catalyzes the synthesis of 18-hydroxylated cortisol in the zona fasciculata. Since this zone is under the control of adrenocorticotropic hormone (ACTH), the glucocorticoid suppressibility of the syndrome is explained. The diagnosis should be made by genetic testing for the chimeric gene and treatment provided with glucocorticoid suppression.[146]

Another rare form is apparent mineralocorticoid excess caused by deficiency of the enzyme 11-beta-hydroxysteroid dehydrogenase type 2 (11β-OHSD2) in the renal tubule, where it normally converts cortisol (which has the ability to act on the mineralocorticoid receptor) to cortisone (which does not). Persistence of high levels of cortisol induces all the features of mineralocorticoid excess. The 11β-OHSD enzyme may be congenitally absent (the syndrome of apparent mineralocorticoid excess) or inhibited by the glycyrrhetenic acid contained in licorice.[147] Another unusual syndrome with hypertension and hypokalemia but suppressed mineralocorticoid secretion is Liddle syndrome, wherein the kidney reabsorbs excess sodium and wastes potassium because of a mutation in the beta or gamma subunits of the epithelial sodium channel.[148]

THERAPY. Once the diagnosis of primary aldosteronism is made and the type of adrenal disorder has been established, the choice of therapy is easy: Patients with a solitary adenoma should have the tumor resected, now more and more frequently done by laparoscopic surgery, and those with bilateral hyperplasia should be treated with an aldosterone blocker, either spironolactone or eplerenone and, if necessary, a thiazide diuretic or other antihypertensive drugs.[149] When an adenoma is resected, about half the patients will become normotensive, whereas the others, although improved, remain hypertensive, either from preexisting primary hypertension or from renal damage caused by prolonged secondary hypertension.

Cushing Syndrome

(see Chap. 79)

Hypertension occurs in about 80 percent of patients with Cushing syndrome. If left untreated, it can cause marked LVH and CHF. As with hypertension of other endocrine causes, the longer it is present, the less likely it is to disappear when the underlying cause is relieved.

MECHANISM OF HYPERTENSION. Blood pressure can increase for a number of reasons.[150] Secretion of mineralocorticoids can also be increased along with cortisol. The excess cortisol can overwhelm the ability of renal 11β-OHSD2 to convert it to the inactive cortisone, and renal mineralocorticoid receptors are activated by the excess cortisol to retain sodium and expand fluid volume. Cortisol stimulates the synthesis of renin substrate and the expression of angiotensin II receptors, which may be responsible for enhanced pressor effects.

DIAGNOSIS. The syndrome should be suspected in patients with truncal obesity, thin skin, muscle weakness, and osteoporosis. If clinical features are suggestive, the diagnosis can be either ruled out or virtually ensured by the measurement of free cortisol in a 24-hour urine sample or the simple overnight dexamethasone suppression test.[151] In normal subjects, the level of plasma cortisol in a sample drawn at 8 AM after a bedtime dose of 1 mg of dexamethasone should be lower than 2 μg/100 ml. If the level is higher, additional work-up is in order to establish both the diagnosis of cortisol excess and the pathological type. A lack of suppression may be noted in patients who are depressed or are alcohol abusers.

When an abnormal screening test result is present, most authorities continue to recommend an additional high-dose dexamethasone suppression test at 2.0 mg every 6 hours for 2 days, with measurement of urinary free cortisol excretion and plasma cortisol levels. If Cushing syndrome is caused by excess pituitary ACTH drive with bilateral adrenal hyperplasia, urinary free cortisol will be suppressed to below 40 percent of the control value with the 2.0 mg dose. Plasma ACTH assays provide an additional means of differentiating pituitary and ectopic ACTH excess from adrenal tumors with ACTH suppression. The response to corticotropin-releasing hormone and inferior petrosal sinus sampling may be needed to identify a pituitary cause of the syndrome.

THERAPY. In about two-thirds of patients with Cushing syndrome, the process begins with overproduction of ACTH by the pituitary, which leads to bilateral adrenal hyperplasia. Although pituitary hyperfunction may reflect a hypothalamic disorder, the majority of patients have discrete pituitary adenomas that can usually be resected by selective transsphenoidal microsurgery.

If an adrenal tumor is present, it should be removed surgically. With earlier diagnosis and more selective surgical therapy, it is hoped that more patients with Cushing syndrome will be cured without a need for lifelong glucocorticoid replacement therapy and with permanent relief of their hypertension. Temporarily, and rarely permanently, therapy may require one of a number of drugs.[152]

Congenital Adrenal Hyperplasia

Enzymatic defects may induce hypertension by interfering with cortisol biosynthesis. Low levels of cortisol lead to increased ACTH, which increases the accumulation of precursors proximal to the enzymatic block, specifically deoxycorticosterone, which induces mineralocorticoid hypertension. The more common of these is 11-hydroxylase deficiency, which has been attributed to various mutations in the gene[153] and leads to virilization (from excessive androgens) and hypertension with hypokalemia (from excessive deoxycorticosterone). The other is 17-hydroxylase deficiency, which also causes hypertension from excess deoxycorticosterone but, in addition, causes failure of secondary sexual development because sex hormones are also deficient.[154] Affected children are hypertensive, but the defect in sex hormone synthesis may not become obvious until after puberty. Thereafter, affected males display ambiguity of sexual development and fail to mature.

Pheochromocytoma (see Chap. 79)

The wild fluctuations in blood pressure and dramatic symptoms of pheochromocytoma usually alert both the patient and the physician to the possibility of this diagnosis. However, such fluctuations may be missed, or, as occurs in half the patients, the hypertension may be persistent, with headache, sweating, and palpitations. On one hand, the spells that are typical of a pheochromocytoma may be incorrectly attributed to migraine, menopause, or panic attacks. On the other, some patients with severe paroxysmal hypertension do not have a pheochromocytoma but rather marked anxiety.[155] Unfortunately, if the diagnosis of pheochromocytoma is missed, severe complications can arise from exceedingly high blood pressure and damage to the heart by catecholamines. Stroke and hypertensive crises with encephalopathy and retinal hemorrhage may occur, probably because blood pressure levels soar in vessels unprepared by a chronic hypertensive condition. Fortunately, a single blood test will detect the disease with virtual certainty,[156] so diagnostic indecision should be minimized.

PATHOPHYSIOLOGY. Tumors arising from chromaffin cells, that is, pheochromocytomas, occur at all ages anywhere along the sympathetic chain and rarely in aberrant sites. About 15 percent of pheochromocytomas are extraadrenal, that is, paragangliomas. Paragangliomas below the head and neck are often functional; those in the head and neck usually present with a mass effect.

Of the 85 percent of pheochromocytomas that arise in the adrenal medulla, 10 percent are bilateral and another 10 percent are malignant. Familial pheochromocytomas are inherited as an autosomal dominant trait alone or in one of four syndromes with recognized genetic mutations: in about half of patients with multiple endocrine neoplasia types 2A or 2B, in 25 percent of those with von Hippel-Lindau disease, and rarely in those with neurofibromatosis type 1. Such germline mutations have been found in 25 percent of 271 patients with sporadic, nonsyndromic, nonfamilial pheochromocytoma, a much higher prevalence than the generally reported 10 percent of pheochromocytomas.[157] Therefore, a higher index of suspicion for familial syndromes is needed, particularly in young patients or those with multiple extraadrenal tumors, prompting a thorough family history and a careful search for other components of a hereditary syndrome. Genetic testing should become more readily available.

Secretion from nonfamilial pheochromocytomas varies considerably, with small tumors tending to secrete larger proportions of active catecholamines. If the predominant secretion is epinephrine, which is formed primarily in the adrenal medulla, the symptoms reflect its effects, mainly systolic hypertension caused by increased cardiac output, tachycardia, sweating, flushing, and apprehension. If norepinephrine is predominantly secreted, as from some of the adrenal tumors and from almost all extraadrenal tumors, the symptoms include both systolic and diastolic hypertension from peripheral vasoconstriction but less tachycardia, palpitations, and anxiety.

DIAGNOSIS. Many more hypertensive patients have variable blood pressure and "spells" than the 0.1 percent or so who harbor a pheochromocytoma. Spells with paroxysmal hypertension may occur with a number of stresses, and a large number of conditions may involve transient catecholamine release. A pheochromocytoma should be suspected in patients with hypertension that is either paroxysmal or persistent and accompanied by the symptoms and signs listed in Table 37-15. In addition, children and patients with rapidly accelerating hypertension should be screened. Those whose tumors secrete predominantly epinephrine are prone to postural hypotension from a contracted blood volume and blunted sympathetic reflex tone. Suspicion should be heightened if activities such as bending over, exercise, palpation of the abdomen, smoking, or dipping snuff cause repetitive spells that begin abruptly, advance rapidly, and subside within minutes.

High levels of catecholamines can induce myocarditis (see Chap. 60), which can progress to cardiomyopathy and left ventricular failure. Electrocardiographic changes of ischemia can also be seen. Beta blockers given to such patients can raise the pressure and induce coronary spasm through blockade of beta-mediated vasodilation.

LABORATORY CONFIRMATION. The easiest and best procedure is a plasma free metanephrine assay,[156] which provides better sensitivity and specificity than other blood or urine catecholamine assays. The test has been found to be equally sensitive for detection of pheochromocytomas in children as part of one of the autosomal dominant familial disorders.[158]

At the Mayo Clinic, measures of urinary metanephrine and catecholamine excretion provided equal sensitivity and better specificity than plasma free metanephrine assays, so the urinary assays are recommended for testing low-risk patients to avoid false-positive results.[159]

If basal levels are equivocal, a clonidine suppression test can be performed, using the plasma free metanephrine assay.[160]

LOCALIZATION OF THE TUMOR. Once the diagnosis has been made, medical therapy should be started and the tumor localized by CT or MRI, which usually demonstrates these typically large tumors with ease. In the few patients in whom localization is not possible by CT or MRI, radioisotopes that localize in chromaffin tissue are available for imaging.

THERAPY. Once diagnosed and localized, pheochromocytomas should be resected. Although preoperative alpha-adrenergic blockade has been recommended, fewer operative and postoperative problems were encountered in one series of patients who had been treated with a calcium channel blocker.[161] If the tumor is unresectable, chronic medical therapy with the alpha blocker phenoxybenzamine (Dibenzyline) or the inhibitor of catechol synthesis alpha-methyltyrosine (Demser) can be used.

Other Causes of Hypertension

A host of other causes of hypertension are known (see Table 37–5). One that is probably becoming more common is ingestion of various drugs, prescribed (e.g., cyclosporine,

TABLE 37–15 Features Suggestive of Pheochromocytoma

Hypertension: Persistent or Paroxysmal
- Markedly variable blood pressures (± orthostatic hypotension)
- Sudden paroxysms (± subsequent hypertension) in relation to
  - Stress: anesthesia, angiography, parturition
  - Pharmacological provocation: histamine, nicotine, caffeine, beta blockers, glucocorticoids, tricyclic antidepressants
  - Manipulation of tumors: abdominal palpation, urination
- Rare patients persistently normotensive
- Unusual settings
  - Childhood, pregnancy, familial
  - Multiple endocrine adenomas: medullary carcinoma of the thyroid (MEN-2), mucosal neuromas (MEN-2B)
  - von Hippel-Lindau syndrome
  - Neurocutaneous lesions: neurofibromatosis

Associated Symptoms
- Sudden spells with headache, sweating, palpitations, nervousness, nausea, and vomiting
- Pain in chest or abdomen

Associated Signs
- Sweating, tachycardia, arrhythmia, pallor, weight loss

MEN = multiple endocrine neoplasia.

tacrolimus, and erythropoietin), over-the-counter (e.g., ephedra), and illicit (e.g., cocaine). As previously noted, obstructive sleep apnea has been well characterized as a cause of significant, and reversible, hypertension.

Coarctation of the Aorta (see Chap. 56)

Congenital narrowing of the aorta can occur at any level of the thoracic or abdominal aorta. It is usually found just beyond the origin of the left subclavian artery or distal to the insertion of the ligamentum arteriosum. With less severe postductal lesions, symptoms may not appear until the teenage years or later, particularly during pregnancy.

Hypertension in the arms, weak or absent femoral pulses, and a loud murmur heard over the back are the classic features of coarctation. The pathogenesis of the hypertension can be more complicated than simple mechanical obstruction; a generalized vasoconstrictor mechanism is likely involved. The lesion can be detected by two-dimensional echocardiography, and aortography proves the diagnosis. Once repaired, patients may continue to have hypertension that should be carefully monitored[162] and treated.

Hormonal Disturbances

Hypertension is seen in as many as half of patients with a variety of hormonal disturbances, including acromegaly,[163] hypothyroidism,[164] and hyperparathyroidism.[165] Diagnosis of the latter two conditions has been made easier by readily available blood tests, and affected hypertensive patients can be relieved of their high blood pressure by correction of the hormonal disturbance. Such relief happens more frequently in patients with hypothyroidism than in those with hyperparathyroidism.

Perioperative Hypertension

If at all possible, preexisting hypertension should be well controlled before elective surgery, with particular attention to correction of diuretic-induced hypokalemia. Caution is advised in abruptly discontinuing antihypertensive agents preoperatively, in particular beta-blockers or clonidine. Fortunately, intravenous formulations of most classes are available if oral intake is not possible. A skin patch of clonidine can treat the patient through surgery.

Hypertension may appear or worsen in the perioperative period, perhaps more commonly with cardiac than noncardiac surgery (Table 37–16).[166] Patients at high risk for cardiac events have been found to be protected by the use of beta-blockers prior to either cardiac or noncardiac surgery.[167]

Hypertension is of particular concern after heart transplantation, appearing for a number of reasons but in particular because the denervation of cardiac volume receptors prevents the normal suppression of the renin-angiotensin mechanism with volume expansion.[168] Reduction of dietary sodium intake and ACE inhibitor or ARB therapy should be especially beneficial.

TABLE 37–16 Hypertension Associated with Cardiac Surgery

Preoperative
- Anxiety, angina, etc.
- Discontinuation of antihypertensive therapy
- Rebound from beta blockers in patients with coronary artery disease

Intraoperative
- Induction of anesthesia: tracheal intubation; nasopharyngeal, urethral, or rectal manipulation
- Precardiopulmonary bypass (during sternotomy and chest retraction)
- Cardiopulmonary bypass
- Postcardiopulmonary bypass (during surgery)

Postoperative
- Early (within 2 h)
  - Obvious cause: hypoxia, hypercarbia, ventilatory difficulties, hypothermia, shivering, arousal from anesthesia
  - With no obvious cause: after myocardial revascularization; less frequently after valve replacement; after resection of aortic coarctation
- Late (weeks to months)
  - After aortic valve replacement by homografts

Data from Estafanous FG, Tarazi RC: Systemic arterial hypertension associated with cardiac surgery. Am J Cardiol 46:685, 1980.

Hypertension During Pregnancy (see Chap. 74)

In about 12 percent of first pregnancies in previously normotensive women, hypertension appears after 20 weeks (gestational hypertension) and in about half this hypertension will progress to preeclampsia when complicated by proteinuria, edema, or hematological or hepatic abnormalities, which, in turn, increase the risk of progress to eclampsia, defined by the occurrence of convulsions. Women with hypertension predating pregnancy have an even higher incidence of preeclampsia and a greater likelihood of early delivery of small-for-gestational-age babies.

Preeclampsia is of unknown cause but occurs more frequently in primigravid women and in pregnancies involving either men or women who were the product of a pregnancy complicated by preeclampsia,[169] supporting a genetic role. Additional predisposing factors include increased age, black race, multiple gestations, concomitant heart or renal disease, and chronic hypertension.

The diagnosis is usually based on a rise in pressure of 30/15 mm Hg or more to a level above 140/90 mm Hg. As with other forms of hypertension, the diagnosis is most precisely made by ambulatory blood pressure monitoring.[170]

Clinical Features

The features shown in Table 37–17 should help distinguish gestational hypertension and preeclampsia from chronic,

TABLE 37–17 Differences Between Preeclampsia and Chronic Hypertension

Feature	Preeclampsia	Chronic Hypertension
Age (yr)	Young (<20)	Older (>30)
Parity	Primigravida	Multigravida
Onset	After 20 wk of pregnancy	Before 20 wk of pregnancy
Weight gain and edema	Sudden	Gradual
Systolic blood pressure	<160 mm Hg	>160 mm Hg
Funduscopic findings	Spasm, edema	Arteriovenous nicking, exudates
Left ventricular hypertrophy	Rare	More common
Proteinuria	Present	Absent
Plasma uric acid	Increased	Normal
Blood pressure after delivery	Normal	Elevated

primary hypertension. The distinction should be made because management and prognosis are different: Gestational hypertension is self-limited and less commonly recurs in subsequent pregnancies, whereas chronic hypertension progresses and usually complicates subsequent pregnancies. Separation may be difficult because of a lack of knowledge of prepregnancy blood pressure and because of the usual tendency for high pressure to fall considerably during the middle trimester so that hypertension present before pregnancy may not be recognized.

Mechanisms

The hemodynamic features of gestational hypertension are a further rise in cardiac output than usually seen in normal pregnancy, accompanied by profound vasoconstriction that reduces intravascular capacity even more than blood volume that may reflect increased central and peripheral sympathetic activity.[171] The mother may be particularly vulnerable to encephalopathy because of her previously normal blood pressure. As is described in more detail under Hypertensive Crisis, cerebral blood flow is normally maintained constant over a fairly narrow range of mean arterial pressure, roughly between 60 and 100 mm Hg in normotensive individuals. In a previously normotensive young woman, an acute rise in blood pressure to 150/100 mm Hg can exceed the upper limit of autoregulation and result in a "breakthrough" of cerebral blood flow (acute dilation) that leads to cerebral edema and convulsions.

Increasingly strong evidence indicates that preeclampsia starts from deficient trophoblast invasion that, in some manner, sets off a systemic maternal inflammatory response. A variety of triggers have been proposed,[172] but the specific mechanisms remain unknown.

Prevention

Beyond delay of pregnancy until after the teens and better prenatal care, the only other maneuver that has been shown to prevent preeclampsia is the use of low doses of aspirin.[173]

Treatment

The only cure for preeclampsia is delivery, which removes the diseased placenta. To achieve this apparently simple end, the clinician must detect the symptomless prodromal condition by screening all pregnant women, admit to hospital those with advanced preeclampsia so as to keep track of an unpredictable situation, and time preemptive delivery to maximize the safety of mother and baby.

Caution is advised in the use of drugs for gestational hypertension, traditionally limited to methyldopa. Drug treatment of maternal blood pressure does not improve perinatal outcome and may be associated with fetal growth retardation. Most authorities recommend antihypertensive drugs only if diastolic pressures remain above 100 mm Hg.[174] The only drugs that are contraindicated are ACE inhibitors and ARB because of their propensity to induce neonatal renal failure.

Chronic Hypertension

If pregnancy begins while a woman is receiving antihypertensive drug therapy, the medications, including diuretics but excluding ACE inhibitors and ARBs, are usually continued in the belief that the mother should be protected and that the fetus will not suffer from any sudden hemodynamic shifts such as occur when therapy is first begun. However, despite modern treatment, the incidence of perinatal mortality and fetal growth retardation remains higher in patients with chronic hypertension.

Management of Eclampsia

With appropriate care of gestational hypertension, eclampsia hardly ever supervenes; when it does, however, maternal and fetal mortality increase markedly. Excellent results have been reported with the use of magnesium sulfate to prevent and treat convulsions.[175] Caution is needed to avoid volume overload, since pulmonary edema is the most common cause of maternal mortality. When compared with women who were normotensive, the overall prognosis for women who had hypertension during pregnancy is not as good, probably because of causes other than preeclampsia, including unrecognized chronic primary hypertension.

After delivery, transient or persistent hypertension can develop in the mother. In many, early primary hypertension may have been masked by the hemodynamic changes of pregnancy. Peripartum cardiomyopathy is a rare form of left ventricular systolic dysfunction appearing during the last month of pregnancy or within a few months after delivery in the absence of known causes.[176]

Hypertensive Crisis

Definitions

A number of clinical circumstances require rapid reduction of blood pressure (Table 37–18). These circumstances can be separated into *emergencies,* which require immediate reduction of blood pressure (within 1 hour), and *urgencies,* which can be treated more slowly. A persistent diastolic pressure exceeding 130 mm Hg is often associated with acute vascular damage; some patients may suffer vascular damage from lower levels of pressure, whereas others are able to withstand even higher levels without apparent harm. As discussed subsequently, the rapidity of the rise may be more important than the absolute level in producing acute vascular damage. Therefore, in practice, all patients with diastolic blood pressure above 130 mm Hg should be treated, some more rapidly with parenteral drugs and others more slowly with oral agents.

When the rise in pressure causes retinal hemorrhages, exudates, or papilledema, the term *accelerated-malignant hypertension* is used. *Hypertensive encephalopathy* is characterized by headache, irritability, alterations in consciousness, and other manifestations of central nervous dysfunction with sudden and marked elevations in blood pressure.

Incidence

Fewer than 1 percent of patients with primary hypertension progress to an accelerated-malignant phase. The incidence is probably falling as a consequence of more widespread

TABLE 37–18 Circumstances Requiring Rapid Treatment of Hypertension

Accelerated-malignant hypertension with papilledema
Cerebrovascular Hypertensive encephalopathy Atherothrombotic brain infarction with severe hypertension Intracerebral hemorrhage Subarachnoid hemorrhage
Cardiac Acute aortic dissection Acute left ventricular failure Acute or impending myocardial infarction After coronary bypass surgery
Renal Acute glomerulonephritis Renal crises from collagen-vascular diseases Severe hypertension after kidney transplantation
Excessive circulating catecholamines Pheochromocytoma crisis Food or drug interactions with monoamine oxidase inhibitors Sympathomimetic drug use (cocaine) Rebound hypertension after sudden cessation of antihypertensive drugs
Eclampsia
Surgical Severe hypertension in patients requiring immediate surgery Postoperative hypertension Postoperative bleeding from vascular suture lines
Severe body burns
Severe epistaxis
Thrombotic thrombocytopenic purpura

From Kaplan NM: Kaplan's Clinical Hypertension. 8th ed. Baltimore, Lippincott Williams & Wilkins, 2002, p 340.

treatment of hypertension. Any hypertensive disease can initiate a crisis. Some, including pheochromocytoma and renovascular hypertension, do so at a higher rate than seen with primary hypertension. However, since hypertension is of unknown cause in more than 90 percent of all patients, most hypertensive crises appear in the setting of preexisting primary hypertension.

PATHOPHYSIOLOGY. Whenever blood pressure rises and remains above a critical level, various processes set off a series of local and systemic effects that cause further rises in pressure and vascular damage eventuating in accelerated-malignant hypertension.

Studies in animals and humans by Strandgaard and Paulson have elucidated the mechanism of hypertensive encephalopathy.[177] First, they directly measured the caliber of pial arterioles over the cerebral cortex in cats whose blood pressure was varied over a wide range of infusion by vasodilators or angiotensin II. As the pressure fell, the arterioles became dilated; as the pressure rose, they become constricted. Thus, constant cerebral blood flow was maintained by means of autoregulation, which is dependent on the cerebral sympathetic nerves. However, when mean arterial pressure rose above 180 mm Hg, the tightly constricted vessels could no longer withstand the pressure and suddenly dilated. This dilation began in an irregular manner, first in areas with less muscle tone and then diffusely with production of generalized vasodilation. This "breakthrough" of cerebral blood flow hyperperfuses the brain under high pressure and thereby causes leakage of fluid into the perivascular tissue and results in cerebral edema and the syndrome of hypertensive encephalopathy.

In human subjects, cerebral blood flow was measured repetitively by an isotopic technique while blood pressure was lowered or raised with vasodilators or vasoconstrictors in a manner similar to that used in the animal studies.[177] Curves depicting cerebral blood flow as a function of arterial pressure demonstrated autoregulation with a constancy of flow over mean pressures in normotensive persons from about 60 to 120 mm Hg and in hypertensive patients from about 110 to 180 mm Hg (Fig. 37-21). This "shift to the right" in hypertensive patients is the result of structural thickening of the arterioles as an adaptation to the chronically elevated pressure. When pressure was raised beyond the upper limit of autoregulation, the same "breakthrough" with hyperperfusion occurred as was seen in the animal studies. In previously normotensive persons whose vessels have not been altered by prior exposure to high pressure, breakthrough occurred at a mean arterial pressure of about 120 mm Hg; in hypertensive patients, the breakthrough occurred at about 180 mm Hg.

These studies confirm clinical observations. In previously normotensive persons, severe encephalopathy occurs with relatively little hypertension. In children with acute glomerulonephritis and in women with eclampsia, convulsions can occur as a result of hypertensive encephalopathy, with blood pressure readings as low as 150/100 mm Hg. Obviously, chronically hypertensive patients withstand such pressures without difficulty; however, when pressure increases significantly, encephalopathy can develop even in these patients.

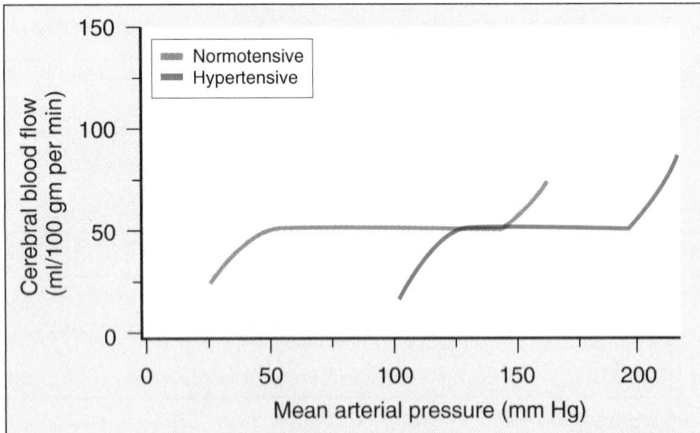

FIGURE 37–21 Idealized curves of cerebral blood flow at varying levels of systemic blood pressure in normotensive and hypertensive subjects. Rightward shift in autoregulation is shown with chronic hypertension. (Adapted from Strandgaard S, Olesen J, Skinhtoi E, Lassen NA: Autoregulation of brain circulation in severe arterial hypertension. Br Med J 1:507, 1973.)

Manifestations and Course

The symptoms and signs of hypertensive crises are usually dramatic (Table 37–19), likely reflecting acute damage to endothelium and platelet activation.[178] However, some patients may be relatively asymptomatic despite markedly elevated pressure and extensive organ damage. Young black men are particularly prone to hypertensive crisis with severe renal insufficiency but little obvious prior distress. Even in elderly persons, however, hypertension can initially present in an accelerated-malignant phase.

If left untreated, patients die quickly of brain damage or more gradually of renal damage. Before effective therapy was available, fewer than 25 percent of patients with malignant hypertension survived 1 year and only 1 percent survived 5 years. With therapy, including renal dialysis, more than 90 percent survive 1 year and about 80 percent survive 5 years.

Differential Diagnosis

The presence of hypertensive encephalopathy or accelerated-malignant hypertension demands immediate, aggressive therapy to lower blood pressure effectively, often before the specific cause is known. However, certain serious diseases, as well as psychogenic problems, can mimic a hypertensive crisis (Table 37–20) and management of these conditions usually requires different diagnostic and therapeutic approaches. In particular, blood pressure should not be lowered too abruptly in a patient with a stroke.[179] Specific therapy for hypertensive crises is described in Chapter 38.

TABLE 37–19 Clinical Characteristics of Hypertensive Crisis
Blood pressure: usually >140 mm Hg diastolic
Funduscopic findings: hemorrhages, exudates, papilledema
Neurological status: headache, confusion, somnolence, stupor, visual loss, focal deficits, seizures, coma
Cardiac findings: prominent apical impulse, cardiac enlargement, congestive failure
Renal: oliguria, azotemia
Gastrointestinal: nausea, vomiting

From Kaplan NM: Kaplan's Clinical Hypertension. 8th ed. Baltimore, Lippincott Williams & Wilkins, 2002, p 341.

TABLE 37–20 Conditions That Can Mimic a Hypertensive Crisis
Acute left ventricular failure
Uremia from any cause, particularly with volume overload
Cerebrovascular accident
Subarachnoid hemorrhage
Brain tumor
Head injury
Epilepsy (postictal)
Collagen diseases, particularly lupus, with cerebral vasculitis
Encephalitis
Sympathomimetics: cocaine, amphetamines, etc.
Hypercalcemia
Acute anxiety with hyperventilation syndrome

REFERENCES

Recognition, Definitions, and Prevalence

1. Gu D, Reynolds K, Wu X, et al: Prevalence, awareness, treatment, and control of hypertension in China. Hypertension 40:920, 2002.
2. Lloyd-Jones DM, Evans JC, Larson MG, Levy D: Treatment and control of hypertension in the community: A prospective analysis. Hypertension 40:640, 2002.
3. Mancia G, Grassi G: Systolic and diastolic blood pressure control in antihypertensive drug trials. J Hypertens 20:1461, 2002.
4. Cherry DK, Woodwell DA: National Ambulatory Medical Care Survey: 2002 summary. Advance data from vital and health statistics; No. 328. Hyattsville, MD, National Center for Health Statistics, 2002.
5. Whelton PK, He J, Appel LJ, et al: Primary prevention of hypertension: Clinical and public health advisory from the National Blood Pressure Education Program. JAMA 288:1882, 2002.
6. Vasan RS, Beiser A, Seshadri S, et al: Residual lifetime risk for developing hypertension in middle-aged women and men. The Framingham Heart Study. JAMA 287:1003, 2002.
7. Joint National Committee: The sixth report of the Joint National Committee on detection, evaluation, and treatment of high blood pressure (JNC VI). Arch Intern Med 157:2413, 1997.
8. Joint National Committee: The seventh report of the Joint Committee on Prevention, Detection, Evaluation, and Treatment of High Blood Pressure (JNC-7 Express). JAMA 289:2560, 2003.
9. Appel L, Robinson K, Guallar E: Utility of blood pressure monitoring outside of the clinic setting. Evidence Report/Technology Assessment No. 63. AHRQ Publication No. 03-E004. Rockville, MD: Agency for Healthcare Research and Quality, 2002.
10. Staessen JA, Thijs L, Fagard R, et al: Predicting cardiovascular risk using conventional vs ambulatory blood pressure in older patients with systolic hypertension. JAMA 282:539, 1999.
11. Brown MA, Buddle ML, Martin A: Is resistant hypertension really resistant? Am J Hypertens 14:1263, 2001.
12. Verdecchia P, O'Brien E, Pickering T, et al: When can the practicing physician suspect white coat hypertension? Statement from the Working Group on Blood Pressure Monitoring of the European Society of Hypertension. Am J Hypertens 16:87, 2003.
13. Wing LMH, Brown MA, Beilin LJ, et al: 'Reverse white-coat hypertension' in older hypertensives. J Hypertens 20:639, 2002.
14. Marfella R, Gualdiero P, Siniscalchi M, et al: Morning blood pressure peak, QT intervals, and sympathetic activity in hypertensive patients. Hypertension 41:237, 2003.
15. Kario K, Pickering TG, Matsuo T, et al: Stroke prognosis and abnormal nocturnal blood pressure falls in older hypertensives. Hypertension 38:852, 2001.
16. Matthews CE, Pate RP, Jackson KL, et al: Exaggerated blood pressure response to dynamic exercise and risk of future hypertension. J Clin Epidemiol 51:29, 1998.
17. Kjeldsen SE, Mundal R, Sandvik L, et al: Supine and exercise systolic blood pressure predict cardiovascular death in middle-aged men. J Hypertens 19:1343, 2001.
18. Vasan RS, Massaro JM, Wilson PWF, et al: Antecedent blood pressure and risk of cardiovascular disease. The Framingham Heart Study. Circulation 105:48, 2002.
19. Domanski M, Mitchell G, Pfeffer M, et al: Pulse pressure and cardiovascular disease-related mortality: Follow-up study of the Multiple Risk Factor Intervention Trial (MRFIT). JAMA 287:2677, 2002.
20. Vasan RS, Larson MG, Leip EP, et al: Impact of high-normal blood pressure on the risk of cardiovascular disease. N Engl J Med 345:18:1291, 2001.
21. Fuentes RM, Notkola I-L, Shemeikka S, et al: Tracking of systolic blood pressure during childhood: A 15-year follow-up population-based family study in eastern Finland. J Hypertens 20:195, 2002.
22. Burt VL, Whelton P, Roccella EJ, et al: Prevalence of hypertension in the US adult population. Results from the Third National Health and Nutrition Examination Survey, 1988-1991. Hypertension 25:3050, 1995.
23. Jones DW, Chambless LE, Folsom AR, et al: Risk factors for coronary heart disease in African Americans. Arch Intern Med 162:2565, 2002.
24. Lorenzo C, Serrano-Rios M, Martinez-Larrad MT, et al: Prevalence of hypertension in Hispanic and non-Hispanic white populations. Hypertension 39:203, 2002.
25. Franklin SS, Jacobs MJ, Wong ND, et al: Predominance of isolated systolic hypertension among middle-aged and elderly US hypertensives. Analysis based on National Health and Nutrition Examination Survey (NHANES) III. Hypertension 37:869, 2001.
26. Lakatta EG, Levy D: Arterial and cardiac aging: Major shareholders in cardiovascular disease enterprises. Part I: Aging arteries: A "set up" for vascular disease. Circulation 103:139, 2003.
27. Prospective Studies Collaboration: Age-specific relevance of usual blood pressure to vascular mortality: A meta-analysis of individual data for one million adults in 61 prospective studies. Lancet 360:1903, 2002.
28. Kaplan NM: Anxiety-induced hyperventilation: A common cause of symptoms in patients with hypertension. Arch Intern Med 157:945, 1997.
29. The Pooling Project Research Group: Relationship of blood pressure, serum cholesterol, smoking habit, relative weight and ECG abnormalities to incidence of major coronary events. Final report of the pooling project. J Chronic Dis 31:201, 1978.
30. Baker S, Priest P, Jackson R: Using thresholds based on risk of cardiovascular disease to target treatment for hypertension: Modelling events averted and number treated. Br Med J 320:680, 2000.
31. Guidelines Subcommittee 1999 World Health Organization: International Society of Hypertension guidelines for the management of hypertension. J Hypertens 17:151, 1999.
32. Yikona JI, Wallis EJ, Ramsay LE, Jackson PR: Coronary and cardiovascular risk estimation in uncomplicated mild hypertension: A comparison of risk assessment methods. J Hypertens 20:2173, 2002.
33. Cuspidi C, Ambrosioni E, Mancia G, et al: Role of echocardiography and carotid ultrasonography in stratifying risk in patients with essential hypertension: The Assessment of Prognostic Risk Observational Survey. J Hypertens 20:1307, 2002.
34. Wong TY, Klein R, Sharrett AR, et al: Retinal arteriolar narrowing and risk of coronary heart disease in men and women: The Atherosclerosis Risk in Communities Study. JAMA 287:1153, 2002.
35. Schussheim AE, Devereux RB, de Simone G: Usefulness of subnormal midwall fractional shortening in predicting left ventricular exercise dysfunction in asymptomatic patients with systemic hypertension. Am J Cardiol 79:1070, 1997.
36. Aeschbacher BC, Hutter D, Fuhrer J, et al: Diastolic dysfunction precedes myocardial hypertrophy in the development of hypertension. Am J Hypertens 14:106, 2001.
37. Gandhi SK, Powers JC, Nomeir A-M, et al: The pathogenesis of acute pulmonary edema associated with hypertension. N Engl J Med 344:17, 2001.
38. Gimelli A, Schneider-Eicke J, Neglia D, et al: Homogeneously reduced versus regionally impaired myocardial blood flow in hypertensive patients: Two different patterns of myocardial perfusion associated with degree of hypertrophy. J Am Coll Cardiol 31:366, 1998.
39. Dries DL, Exner DV, Gersh BJ, et al: Racial differences in the outcome of left ventricular dysfunction. N Engl J Med 340:609, 1999.
40. Kozàkovà M, de Simone G, Morizzo C, Palombo C: Coronary vasodilator capacity and hypertension-induced increase in left ventricular mass. Hypertension 41:224, 2003.
41. Schmieder RE, Messerli FH: Hypertension and the heart. J Hum Hypertens 14:597, 2000.
42. Wachtell K, Rokkedal J, Bella JN, et al: Effect of electrocardiographic left ventricular hypertrophy on left ventricular systolic function in systemic hypertension. Am J Cardiol 87:54, 2001.
43. Verdecchia P, Schillaci G, Borgioni C, et al: Prognostic significance of serial changes in left ventricular mass in essential hypertension. Circulation 97:48, 1998.
44. Haider AW, Larson MG, Franklin SS, Levy D: Systolic blood pressure, diastolic blood pressure, and pulse pressure as predictors of risk for congestive heart failure in the Framingham Heart Study. Ann Intern Med 138:10, 2003.
45. Vasan RS, Benjamin EJ: Diastolic heart failure. N Engl J Med 344:56, 2001.
46. Boon D, Piek JJ, van Montfrans GA: Silent ischaemia and hypertension. J Hypertens 18:1355, 2000.
47. Haider AW, Chen L, Larson MG, et al: Antecedent hypertension confers increased risk for adverse outcomes after initial myocardial infarction. Hypertension 30:1020, 1997.
48. Njølstad I, Arnesen E: Preinfarction blood pressure and smoking are determinants for a fatal outcome of myocardial infarction. Arch Intern Med 158:1326, 1998.
49. Flack JM, Neaton J, Grimm R Jr, et al: Blood pressure and mortality among men with prior myocardial infarction. Circulation 92:2437, 1995.
50. Leoncini G, Sacchi G, Ravera M, et al: Microalbuminuria is an integrated marker of subclinical organ damage in primary hypertension. J Hum Hypertens 16:399, 2002.
51. Reinprecht F, Elmståhl S, Janzon L, André-Petersson L: Hypertension and changes of cognitive function in 81-year-old men: A 13-year follow-up of the population study 'Men Born in 1914', Sweden. J Hypertens 21:57, 2003.
52. Sierra C, de la Sierra A, Mercader J, et al: Silent cerebral white matter lesions in middle-aged essential hypertensive patients. J Hypertens 20:519, 2002.
53. Goldstein IB, Bartzokis G, Guthrie D, Shapiro D: Ambulatory blood pressure and brain atrophy in the healthy elderly. Neurology 59:713, 2002.

Mechanisms of Primary (Essential) Hypertension

54. Lund-Johnson P: Central haemodynamics in essential hypertension at rest and during exercise: A 20-year follow-up study. J Hypertens 7(Suppl):52, 1989.
55. Post WS, Larson MG, Levy D: Hemodynamic predictors of incident hypertension. Hypertension 24:585, 1994.
56. Kim J-R, Kiefe CI, Liu K, et al: Heart rate and subsequent blood pressure in young adults: The CARDIA study. Hypertension 33:640, 1999.
57. Iliadou A, Lichtenstein P, Morgenstern R, et al: Repeated blood pressure measurements in a sample of Swedish twins: Heritabilities and associations with polymorphisms in the renin-angiotensin-aldosterone system. J Hypertens 20:1543, 2002.
58. Carretero OA, Oparil S: Essential hypertension. Circulation 101:329, 2000.
59. Luft FC: Hypertension as a complex genetic trait. Semin Nephrol 22:115, 2002.
60. Province MA, Kardia SLR, Ranade K, et al: A meta-analysis of genome-wide linkage scans for hypertension: The National Heart, Lung and Blood Institute Family Blood Pressure Program. Am J Hypertens 16:144, 2003.
61. Lifton RP, Gharavi AG, Geller DS: Molecular mechanisms of human hypertension [review]. Cell 104:545, 2001.
62. Law CM, Shiell AW, Newsome CA, et al: Fetal, infant, and childhood growth and adult blood pressure: A longitudinal study from birth to 22 years of age. Circulation 105:1088, 2002.
63. Huxley R, Neil A, Collins R: Unravelling the fetal origins hypothesis: Is there really an inverse association between birthweight and subsequent blood pressure? Lancet 360:659, 2002.
64. Brenner BM, Chertow GM: Congenital oligonephropathy: An inborn cause of adult hypertension and progressive renal injury? Curr Opin Nephrol Hypertens 2:691, 1993.
65. Moritz KM, Wintour EM, Dodic M: Fetal uninephrectomy leads to postnatal hypertension and compromised renal function. Hypertension 39:1071, 2002.
66. Keller G, Zimmer G, Mall G, et al: Nephron number in patients with primary hypertension. N Engl J Med 348:101, 2003.
67. Johnson RJ, Herrera-Acosta J, Schreiner GF, Rodríguez-Iturbe B: Subtle acquired renal injury as a mechanism of salt-sensitive hypertension. N Engl J Med 346:913, 2002.
68. Sealey JE, Blumenfeld JD, Bell GM, et al: On the renal basis for essential hypertension: Nephron heterogeneity with discordant renin secretion and sodium excretion causing a hypertensive vasoconstriction-volume relationship. J Hypertens 6:763, 1988.
69. Aperia A: Regulation of sodium/potassium ATPase activity. Curr Hypertens Rep 3:165, 2001.

70. Weinberger MH, Fineberg NS, Fineberg SE, Weinberger M: Salt sensitivity, pulse pressure and death in normal and hypertensive humans. Hypertension 37:429, 2001.
71. Lever AF, Harrap SB: Essential hypertension: A disorder of growth with origins in childhood? J Hypertens 10:101, 1992.
72. Folkow B: "Structural factor" in primary and secondary hypertension. Hypertension 16:89, 1990.
73. Lever AF: Slow pressor mechanisms in hypertension: A role for hypertrophy of resistance vessels? J Hypertens 4:515, 1986.
74. Cosentino F, Lüscher TF: Effects of blood pressure and glucose on endothelial function. Curr Hypertens Rep 3:79, 2001.
75. Cardillo C, Campia U, Kilcoyne CM, et al: Improved endothelium-dependent vasodilation after blockade of endothelin receptors in patients with essential hypertension. Circulation 105:452, 2002.
76. Esler M, Rumantir M, Lambert G, Kaye D: The sympathetic neurobiology of essential hypertension. Am J Hypertens 14(Suppl):139S, S2001.
77. Markovitz JH, Matthews KA, Kannel WB, et al: Psychological predictors of hypertension in the Framingham Study: Is there tension in hypertension? JAMA 270:2439, 1993.
78. Carroll D, Smith GD, Shipley MJ, et al: Blood pressure reactions to acute psychological stress and future blood pressure status: A 10-year follow-up of men in the Whitehall II study. Psychosomatic Med;63:737, 2001.
79. Schobel HP, Frank H, Naraghi R, et al: Hypertension in patients with neurovascular compression is associated with increased central sympathetic outflow. J Am Soc Nephrol 13:35, 2002.
80. Williams GH, Fisher NDL, Hunt SC, et al: Effects of gender and genotype on the phenotypic expression of nonmodulating essential hypertension. Kidney Int 57:1404, 2000.
81. Wilson PWF, D'Agostino R, Sullivan L, et al: Overweight and obesity as determinants of cardiovascular risk. The Framingham experience. Arch Intern Med 162:1867, 2002.
82. Flegal KM, Carroll MD, Ogden CL, Johnson CL: Prevalence and trends in obesity among US adults, 1999-2000. JAMA 288:1723, 2002.
83. Ogden CL, Flegal KM, Carroll MD, Johnson CL: Prevalence and trends in overweight among US children and adolescents, 1999-2000. JAMA 288:1728, 2002.
84. Malhotra A, White DP: Obstructive sleep apnea. Lancet 360:237, 2002.
85. DeSouza CA, Shapiro LF, Clevenger CM, et al: Regular aerobic exercise prevents and restores age-related declines in endothelium-dependent vasodilation in healthy men. Circulation 102:1351, 2000.
86. Mukamal KJ, Kuller LH, Fitzpatrick AL, et al: Prospective study of alcohol consumption and risk of dementia in older adults. JAMA 289:1405, 2003.
87. Thadhani R, Camargo CA Jr, Stampfer MJ, et al: Prospective study of moderate alcohol consumption and risk of hypertension in young women. Arch Intern Med 162:569, 2002.
88. Schunkert H, Koenig W, Bröckel U, et al: Haematocrit profoundly affects left ventricular diastolic filling as assessed by Doppler echocardiography. J Hypertens 18:1483, 2000.
89. Devereux RB, Case DB, Alderman MH, et al: Possible role of increased blood viscosity in the hemodynamics of systemic hypertension. Am J Cardiol 85:1265, 2000.
90. Ferrier KE, Muhlmann MH, Baguet J-P, et al: Intensive cholesterol reduction lowers blood pressure and large artery stiffness in isolated systolic hypertension. J Am Coll Cardiol 39:1020, 2002.

Hypertension in Special Groups

91. Kahn DF, Duffy SJ, Tomasian D, et al: Effects of black race on forearm resistance vessel function. Hypertension 40:195, 2002.
92. Marcantoni C, Ma L-J, Federspiel C, Fogo AB: Hypertensive nephrosclerosis in African Americans versus Caucasians. Kidney Int 62:172, 2002.
93. Morris RC Jr, Sebastian A, Forman A, et al: Normotensive salt sensitivity. Hypertension 33:18, 1999.
94. O'Donnell CJ, Kannel WB: Cardiovascular risks of hypertension: Lessons from observational studies. J Hypertens 16(Suppl 6):S3, 1998.
95. Gillman MW, Cook N, Rosner B, et al: Identifying children at high risk for the development of essential hypertension. J Pediatr 122:837, 1993.
96. Lieberman E: Hypertension in childhood and adolescence. *In* Kaplan N (ed): Kaplan's Clinical Hypertension, 8th ed. Philadelphia, Lippincott Williams & Wilkins, 2002.
97. Hyman DJ, Pavlik VN: Characteristics of patients with uncontrolled hypertension in the United States. N Engl J Med 345:479, 2001.
98. Staessen JA, Gasowski J, Wang JG, et al: Risks of untreated and treated isolated systolic hypertension in the elderly. Lancet 355:865, 2000.
99. Arima H, Tanizaki Y, Kiyohara Y, et al: Validity of the JNC VI recommendations for the management of hypertension in a general population of Japanese elderly. The Hisayama study. Arch Intern Med 163:361, 2003.
100. Gueyffier F, Bulpitt C, Boissel J-P, et al: Antihypertensive drugs in very old people. Lancet 353:793, 1999.
101. O'Rourke MF, Staessen JA, Vlachopoulos C, et al: Clinical applications of arterial stiffness: Definitions and reference values. Am J Hypertens 15:426, 2002.
102. Mooradian AD: Cardiovascular disease in type 2 diabetes mellitus: Current management guidelines. Arch Intern Med 163:33, 2003.
103. Geiss LS, Rolka DB, Engelgau MM: Elevated blood pressure among U.S. adults with diabetes, 1988-1994. Am J Prev Med 22:42, 2002.
104. Kamoi K, Mihakoshi M, Soda S, et al: Usefulness of home blood pressure measurement in the morning in type 2 diabetic patients. Diabetes Care 25:2218, 2002.

Identifiable (Secondary) Forms of Hypertension

105. Chasan-Taber L, Willett WC, Manson JE, et al: Prospective study of oral contraceptives and hypertension among women in the United States. Circulation 94:483, 1996.
106. Seibert C, Barbouche E, Fagan J, et al: Prescribing oral contraceptives for women older than 35 years of age. Ann Intern Med 138:54, 2000.
107. Ribstein J, Halimi J-M, du Cailar G, Mimran A: Renal characteristics and effect of angiotensin suppression in oral contraceptive users. Hypertension 33:90, 1999.
108. Butkevich A, Abraham C, Phillips RA: Hormone replacement therapy and 24-hour blood pressure profile on postmenopausal women. Am J Hypertens 13:1039, 2000.
109. Modena MG, Molinari R, Muia N Jr, et al: Double-blind randomized placebo-controlled study of transdermal estrogen replacement therapy on hypertensive postmenopausal women. Am J Hypertens 12:1000, 1999.
110. Remuzzi G, Schieppati A, Ruggenenti P: Nephropathy in patients with type 2 diabetes. N Engl J Med 346:1145, 2002.
111. Coresh J, Astor BC, Greene T, et al: Prevalence of chronic kidney disease and decreased kidney function in the adult US population: Third National Health and Nutrition Examination Survey. Am J Kidney Dis 41:1, 2003.
112. Swedko PJ, Clark HD, Paramsothy K, Akbari A: Serum creatinine is an inadequate screening test for renal failure in elderly patients. Arch Intern Med 163:356, 2003.
113. Ghose RR, Harinda V: Unrecognized high pressure chronic retention of urine presenting with systemic arterial hypertension. Br Med J 298:1626, 1989.
114. Textor SC, Wilcox CS: Ischemic nephropathy/azotemic renovascular disease. Semin Nephrol 20:489, 2000.
115. Bakris GL, Williams M, Dworkin L, et al: Preserving renal function in adults with hypertension and diabetes: A consensus approach. Am J Kidney Dis 36:646, 2000.
116. The Heart Outcomes Prevention Evaluation Study Investigators: Effects of an angiotensin-converting-enzyme inhibitor, ramipril, on cardiovascular events in high-risk patients. N Engl J Med 342:145, 2000.
117. Lazarus JM, Bourgoignie JJ, Buckalew VM, et al: Achievement and safety of a low blood pressure goal in chronic renal disease: The modification of diet in renal disease study group. Hypertension 29:641, 1997.
118. Wright JT Jr, Bakris G, Greene T, et al: Effect of blood pressure lowering and antihypertensive drug class on progression of hypertensive kidney disease: Results from the AASK trial. JAMA 288:2421, 2002.
119. Palmer BF: Renal dysfunction complicating the treatment of hypertension. N Engl J Med 347:1256, 2002.
120. Schrier RW, Estacio RO, Esler A, Mehler P: Effects of aggressive blood pressure control in normotensive type 2 diabetic patients on albuminuria, retinopathy and strokes. Kidney Int 61:1086, 2002.
121. Gæde P, Vedel P, Larsen N, et al: Multifactorial intervention and cardiovascular disease in patients with type 2 diabetes. N Engl J Med 348:383, 2003.
122. The CDC Diabetes Cost-effectiveness Group: Cost-effectiveness of intensive glycemic control, intensified hypertension control, and serum cholesterol level reduction for type 2 diabetes. JAMA 287:2542, 2002.
123. Rahman M, Dixit A, Donley V, et al: Factors associated with inadequate blood pressure control in hypertensive hemodialysis patients. Am J Kidney Dis 33:498, 1999.
124. Efrati S, Zaidenstein R, Dishy V, et al: ACE inhibitors and survival of hemodialysis patients. Am J Kidney Dis 40:1023, 2002.
125. Hansen KJ, Edwards MS, Craven TE, et al: Prevalence of renovascular disease in the elderly: A population-based study. J Vasc Surg 36:443, 2002.
126. Rihal CS, Textor SC, Breen JF, et al: Incidental renal artery stenosis among a prospective cohort of hypertensive patients undergoing coronary angiography. Mayo Clin Proc 77:309, 2002.
127. Oskin TC, Hansen KJ, Deitch JS, et al: Chronic renal artery occlusion: Nephrectomy versus revascularization. J Vasc Surg 29:140, 1999.
128. Block MJ, Trost DW, Pickering TG, et al: Prevention of recurrent pulmonary edema in patients with bilateral renovascular disease through renal artery stent placement. Am J Hypertens 12:1, 1999.
129. Safian RD, Textor SC: Renal-artery stenosis. N Engl J Med 344:431, 2001.
130. van Onna M, Houben AJHM, Kroon AA, et al: Asymmetry of renal blood flow in patients with moderate to severe hypertension. Hypertension 41:108, 2003.
131. de Haan MW, Kroon AA, Flobbe K, et al: Renovascular disease in patients with hypertension: Detection with duplex ultrasound. J Human Hypertens 16:501, 2002.
132. Radermacher J, Chavan A, Bleck J, et al: Use of Doppler ultrasonography to predict the outcome of therapy for renal-artery stenosis. N Engl J Med 344:410, 2001.
133. Nordmann AJ, Woo K, Parkes R, Logan AG: Balloon angioplasty or medical therapy for hypertensive patients with atherosclerotic renal artery stenosis? A meta-analysis of randomized controlled trials. Am J Med 114:44, 2003.
134. Leertouwer TC, Derkx FHM, Pattynama PMT, et al: Functional effects of renal artery stent placement on treated and contralateral kidneys. Kidney Int 62:574, 2002.
135. Haab F, Duclos JM, Guyenne T, et al: Renin secreting tumors: Diagnosis, conservative surgical approach and long term results. J Urol 153:1781, 1995.
136. Leckie BJ, Birnie G, Carachi R: Renin in Wilms' tumor: Prorenin as an indicator. J Clin Endocrinol Metab 79:1742, 1994.
137. Hadjidakis D, Tsagarakis S, Roboti C, et al: Does subclinical hypercortisolism adversely affect the bone mineral density in patients with adrenal incidentalomas? Clin Endocrinol 58:72, 2003.
138. Gordon RD, Stowasser M, Rutherford JC: Primary aldosteronism: Are we diagnosing and operating on too few patients? World J Surg 25:941, 2001.
139. Tracy RE, White S: A method for qualifying adrenocortical nodular hyperplasia at autopsy: Some use of the methods in illuminating hypertension and atherosclerosis. Ann Diagn Pathol 6:20, 2002.
140. Padfield PL: Primary aldosteronism, a common entity? The myth persists. J Hum Hypertens 16:159, 2002.
141. Schwartz GL, Chapman AB, Boerwinkle E, et al: Screening for primary aldosteronism: Implications of an increased plasma aldosterone/renin ratio. Clin Chem 48:1919, 2002.
142. Rossi E, Regolisti G, Negro A, et al: High prevalence of primary aldosteronism using postcaptopril plasma aldosterone to renin ratio as a screening test among Italian hypertensives. Am J Hypertens 15:896, 2002.
143. Magill SB, Raff H, Shaker JL, et al: Comparison of adrenal vein sampling and computed tomography in the differentiation of primary aldosteronism. J Clin Endocrinol Metab 86:1066, 2001.

144. Lim PO, Jung RT, MacDonald TM: Is aldosterone the missing link in refractory hypertension? Aldosterone-to-renin ratio as a marker of inappropriate aldosterone activity. J Human Hypertens 16:153, 2002.
145. Rossi GP, Sacchetto A, Chiesura-Corona M, et al: Identification of the etiology of primary aldosteronism with adrenal vein sampling in patients with equivocal computed tomography and magnetic resonance findings: Results in 104 consecutive cases. J Clin Endocrinol Metab 86:1083, 2001.
146. Dluhy RG, Lifton RP: Glucocorticoid-remediable aldosteronism. J Clin Endocrinol Metab 84:4341, 1999.
147. Cooper M, Stewart PM: The syndrome of apparent mineralocorticoid excess. Q J Med 91:453, 1998.
148. Yamashita Y, Koga M, Takeda Y, et al: Two sporadic cases of Liddle's syndrome caused by de novo ENaC mutations. Am J Kidney Dis 37:499, 2001.
149. Lim PO, Young WF, MacDonald TM: A review of the medical treatment of primary aldosteronism. J Hypertens 19:353, 2001.
150. Whitworth JA, Mangos GJ, Kelly JJ: Cushing, cortisol, and cardiovascular disease. Hypertension 36:912, 2000.
151. Boscaro M, Barzon L, Fallo F, Sonino N: Cushing's syndrome. Lancet 357:783, 2001.
152. Chu JW, Matthias DF, Belanoff J, et al: Successful long-term treatment of refractory Cushing's disease with high-dose mifepristone (RU 486). J Clin Endocrinol Metab 86:3568, 2001.
153. Chabre O, Portrat-Doyen S, Chaffanjon P, et al: Bilateral laparoscopic adrenalectomy for congenital adrenal hyperplasia with severe hypertension, resulting from two novel mutations in splice donor sites of CYP11B1. J Clin Endocrinol Metab 85:4060, 2000.
154. Hermans C, de Plaen J-F, de Nayer P, Maiter D: Case report: 17 α-Hydroxylase/17,20-lase deficiency: A rare cause of endocrine hypertension. Am J Med 312:126, 1996.
155. Mann SJ: Severe paroxysmal hypertension (pseudopheochromocytoma). Arch Intern Med 159:670, 1999.
156. Lenders JWM, Pacak K, Walther MM, et al: Biochemical diagnosis of pheochromocytoma: Which test is best? JAMA 287:1427, 2002.
157. Neumann HPH, Bausch B, McWhinney SR, et al: Germ-line mutations in nonsyndromic pheochromocytoma. N Engl J Med 346:1459, 2002.
158. Weise M, Merke DP, Pacak K, et al: Utility of plasma free metanephrines for detecting childhood pheochromocytoma. J Clin Endocrinol Metab 87:1955, 2002.
159. Sawka AM, Jaeschke R, Singh RJ, Young WF Jr: A comparison of biochemical tests for pheochromocytoma: Measurement of fractionated plasma metanephrines compared with the combination of 24-hour urinary metanephrines and catecholamines. J Clin Endocrinol Metab 88:553, 2003.
160. Eisenhofer G: Biochemical diagnosis of pheochromocytoma. Ann Intern Med 134:317, 2001.
161. Ulchaker JC, Goldfarb DA, Bravo EL, Novick AC: Successful outcomes in pheochromocytoma surgery in the modern era. J Urol 161:764, 1999.
162. Swan L, Goyal S, Hsia C, et al: Exercise systolic blood pressures are of questionable value in the assessment of the adult with a previous coarctation repair. Heart 89:189, 2003.
163. Colao A, Baldelli R, Marzullo P, et al: Systemic hypertension and impaired glucose tolerance are independently correlated to the severity of the acromegalic cardiomyopathy. J Clin Endocrinol Metab 85:193, 2000.
164. Fommei E, Iervasi G: The role of thyroid hormone in blood pressure homeostasis: Evidence from short-term hypothyroidism in humans. J Clin Endocrinol Metab 87:1996, 2002.
165. Silverberg SJ: Cardiovascular disease in primary hyperparathyroidism. J Clin Endocrinol Metab 85:3513, 2000.
166. Vuylsteke A, Feneck RO, Jolin-Mellgård Å, et al: Perioperative blood pressure control: A prospective study of patient management in cardiac surgery. J Cardiothor Vasc Anesth 14:269, 2000.
167. Auerbach AD, Goldman L: β-blockers and reduction of cardiac events in noncardiac surgery: Scientific review. JAMA 287:1435, 2002.
168. Eisen HJ: Hypertension in heart transplant recipients: More than just cyclosporine. J Am Coll Cardiol 41:433, 2003.
169. Esplin MS, Fausett MB, Fraser A, et al: Paternal and maternal components of the predisposition to preeclampsia. N Engl J Med 344:867, 2001.
170. Hermida RC, Ayala DE, Mojón A, et al: Differences in circadian blood pressure variability during gestation between healthy and complicated pregnancies. Am J Hypertens 16:200, 2003.
171. Greenwood JP, Scott EM, Walker JJ, et al: The magnitude of sympathetic hyperactivity in pregnancy-induced hypertension and preeclampsia. Am J Hypertens 16:194, 2003.
172. Leach RE, Romero R, Kim YM, et al: Pre-eclampsia and expression of heparin-binding EGF-like growth factor. Lancet 360:1215, 2002.
173. Duley L, Henderson-Smart D, Knight M, King J: Antiplatelet drugs for prevention of pre-eclampsia and its consequences: Systematic review. Br Med J 322:329, 2001.
174. National High Blood Pressure Education Program Working Group on High Blood Pressure in Pregnancy: Report of the National High Blood Pressure Education Program Working Group on High Blood Pressure in Pregnancy. Am J Obstet Gynecol 183:S1, 2000.
175. The Magpie Trial Collaborative Group: Do women with pre-eclampsia, and their babies, benefit from magnesium sulphate? The Magpie Trial: A randomized placebo-controlled trial. Lancet 359:1877, 2002.
176. Pearson GD, Veille J-C, Rahimtoola, et al: Peripartum cardiomyopathy. JAMA 283:1183, 2000.
177. Strandgaard S, Paulson OB: Cerebral blood flow and its pathophysiology in hypertension. Am J Hypertens 2:486, 1989.
178. Preston RA, Jy W, Jinenez JJ, et al: Effects of severe hypertension on endothelial and platelet microparticles. Hypertension 41:211, 2003.
179. Chalmers J, Beilin L, Mancia G, et al: International Society of Hypertension (ISH): Statements on blood pressure and stroke. J Hypertens 21:649, 2003.

CHAPTER 38

Systemic Hypertension: Therapy

Norman M. Kaplan

As noted at the beginning of Chapter 37, the number of patients being treated for hypertension has expanded markedly during the past 30 years so that hypertension is now the leading reason for visits by nonpregnant adults to physicians' offices. Nonetheless, in various developed countries—from the United Kingdom and Canada, which have national health schemes that cover everyone, to the United States, with its sporadic coverage—only a third or less of hypertensive patients have their disease under good control.[1] This apparent paradox of expanded coverage but continued poor control is the consequence of multiple factors, including (1) worsening life-style habits, particularly weight gain and physical inactivity, which engender hypertension; (2) poor adherence to long-term prescribed medications; (3) lack of appreciation of the risks associated with even small degrees of elevated blood pressure; and (4) physicians' unwillingness to prescribe the therapy needed to lower the often recalcitrant systolic hypertension so common in elderly patients. Nonetheless, when therapy is pushed to reach appropriate goals, at least two thirds of patients can achieve control.[2] Relatively few patients are truly resistant to therapy.

Fundamental to the difficulty of controlling hypertension is the inherent nature of the disease: induced by common but unhealthy life styles, asymptomatic, and persistent, with overt consequences delayed by 10 to 30 years so that the costs of therapy, both in money and in adverse effects, seem on the surface to outweigh benefits to be derived from adherence to the regimen. Furthermore, behind the inherent nature of the disease lurks yet another disquieting feature of the therapy of most hypertension: it may not benefit the majority of patients who adhere faithfully to their treatment. Even among such elderly patients as enrolled in the Systolic Hypertension in the Elderly Program (SHEP) trial, 111 would need to be treated for 5 years to prevent one cardiovascular death and 19 treated to prevent one cardiovascular event.[3] Because of the costs and side effects of therapy, the use of medication as a preventive measure has not been deemed appropriate.

Yet another element, the issue of cost-effectiveness, has been introduced into the debate about the value of treating all patients with any degree of hypertension. As the escalating costs of health care consume a greater share of society's resources, two opposing forces have risen: one, the need for less expensive illness care, and the other, the relatively large cost of prevention when indiscriminately applied to low-risk subjects. Therefore, it is likely that antihypertensive therapy will be more selective and targeted in the future.

Benefits of Therapy

The treatment of hypertension is aimed not at simple reduction of blood pressure but at prevention of the cardiovascular complications that are known to accompany the high pressure. During the past 35 years, many randomized controlled trials (RCTs) have tested the ability of antihypertensive drugs to prevent strokes and heart attacks.[4] Few other aspects of clinical practice have as strong an evidence base as does the treatment of hypertension.

A meta-analysis of 27 large RCTs wherein systolic blood pressures were provided portrays the effects of therapy in 136,124 patients (Fig. 38–1).[4] Beyond the progressive reduction in cardiovascular mortality that is directly correlated with the degree of systolic blood pressure lowering, reduction in morbidity from stroke and, to a larger degree, from myocardial infarction has also been clearly documented. Over the 35 years encompassed by these trials, benefits of treatment were first documented for patients with severe hypertension, then for those with moderate disease, and only later for those with lesser degrees of hypertension.[3]

The protection against stroke has been shown to apply even to a limited number of patients older than 80 years.[5] In the six trials that included 1670 patients older than 80 years, the half who were treated with either diuretics or dihydropyridine (DHP) calcium antagonists had a 36 percent reduction in stroke, a 39 percent reduction in heart failure, and a statistically significant 22 percent reduction in major coronary events.[5] Moreover, in the one RCT in which dementia was carefully ascertained, treatment of elderly patients with isolated systolic hypertension based on a DHP–calcium channel blocker (CCB) reduced the incidence of dementia by 55 percent over an 8-year follow-up.[6]

The difficulty in showing clear benefits of treatment in the larger part of the hypertensive population, those with stage 1 or blood pressures from 140/90 to 160/100 mm Hg, must be reconciled with the fact that even though their individual risk is relatively low, their sheer number causes them to make the major contribution to the overall population risk from hypertension, as shown in Figure 37–7. This fact has given rise to two important guidelines for clinical practice: first, the critical need for prevention of hypertension by population-wide life-style modifications[7]; and second, the rationale for considering blood pressure in the larger context of overall cardiovascular risk.[8]

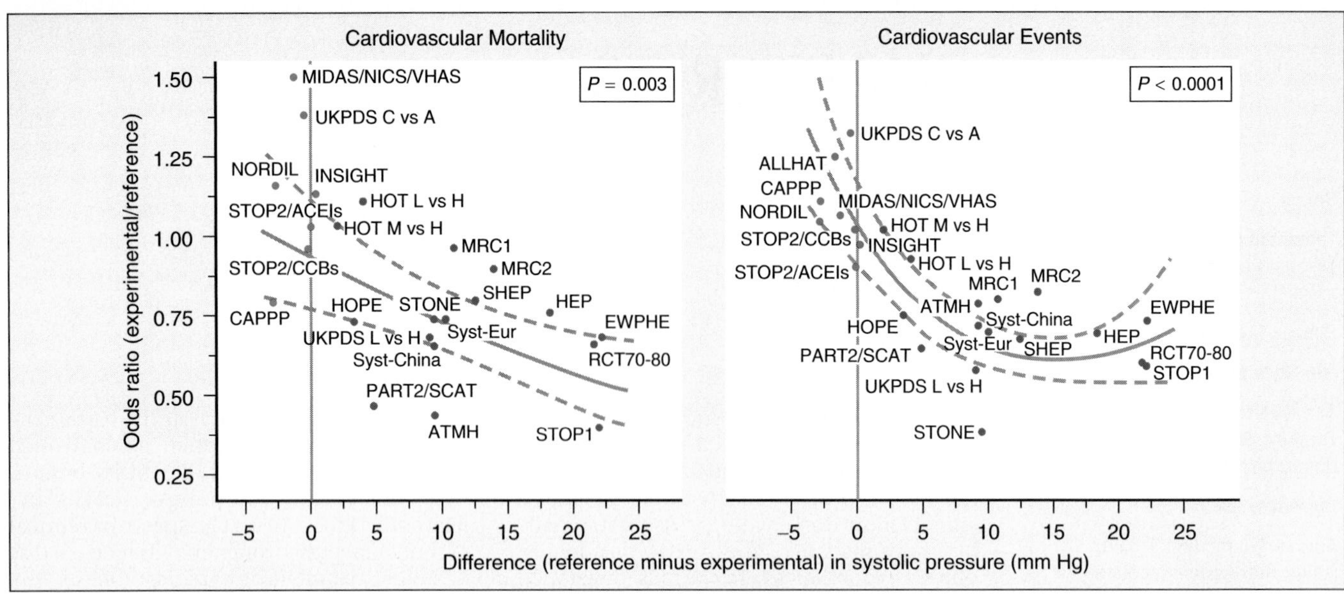

FIGURE 38–1 Relation between the odds ratio for cardiovascular mortality and all cardiovascular events and corresponding differences in systolic blood pressure minus the effect of placebo in 27 published randomized controlled trials of the treatment of hypertension. Magenta dots denote trials that compared new with old drugs. (Modified from Staessen JA, Wang J-G, Thijs L: Cardiovascular protection and blood pressure reduction. Lancet 358:1309, 2001.)

Threshold for Therapy

The value of life-style modifications is documented in the next section of this chapter. The rationale for a broader look at risk beyond blood pressure that was first formalized by a group of investigators from New Zealand[8] has now been incorporated into virtually all guidelines from expert committees.[9,10] The threshold for institution of active drug therapy has generally been taken as an absolute risk of cardiovascular disease of 15 percent or higher in 10 years. The World Health Organization–International Society of Hypertension report provides additional data on the absolute effects of treatment on patients at various levels of cardiovascular risk (Table 38–1).[10] As shown, relatively small benefits have been seen in RCTs of about 5 years' duration in low-risk patients, although with more intensive therapy to lower blood pressure by 20/10 mm Hg, they too can achieve more impressive protection.

As noted in the previous chapter, these relatively crude risk estimates may mark many more patients for antihypertensive

TABLE 38–1 Absolute Effects of Treatment on Cardiovascular Risk

- From the results of randomized, controlled trials, it appears that each reduction of 10 to 14 mm Hg in systolic blood pressure and 5 to 6 mm Hg in diastolic blood pressure confers about two fifths less stroke, one sixth less coronary heart disease, and, in Western populations, one third fewer major cardiovascular events overall.
- In patients with grade I hypertension, monotherapy with most agents produces reductions in blood pressure of about 10/5 mm Hg. In patients with higher grades of hypertension, it is possible to achieve sustained blood pressure reductions of 20/10 mm Hg or more, particularly if combination drug therapy is used.
- The estimated absolute effects of such blood pressure reductions on cardiovascular disease (CVD) risk (fatal plus nonfatal stroke or myocardial infarction) are as follows:

Group of Patients	Absolute Risk (CVD Events over 10 Years) (%)	Absolute Treatment Effects (CVD Events Prevented per 1000 Patient-Years)	
		10/5 mm Hg	*20/10 mm Hg*
Low risk	<15	<5	<8
Medium risk	15-20	5-7	8-11
High risk	20-30	7-10	11-17
Very high risk	>30	>10	>17

- Between these strata, the estimated absolute treatment benefits range from less than 5 events prevented per thousand patient-years of treatment (low risk) to more than 17 events prevented per thousand patient-years of treatment (very high risk).
- The absolute benefits for stroke and coronary artery disease will be augmented by smaller absolute benefits for congestive heart failure and renal disease.
- These estimates of benefit are based on relative risk reductions observed in trials of about 5 years' duration. Longer term treatment over decades could produce larger risk reductions.

From Guidelines Subcommittee: 1999 World Health Organization–International Society of Hypertension guidelines for the management of hypertension. J Hypertens 17:151, 1999.

drug therapy than provided by more careful assessments. On the other hand, the argument has been made that drug therapy should be considered in more presumably low-risk patients even in the absence of evidence that they benefit, largely because there have been no adequate outcome trials in low-risk patients with blood pressure below 140/90 mm Hg. Recall the evidence from the Framingham Study showing that presumably low-risk subjects with high-normal blood pressure—that is, 130 to 139 systolic and 85 to 89 diastolice—had three to four times more cardiovascular events over a 12-year follow-up than occurred among those with lower blood pressure (see Fig. 37–5).[11] On the basis of such evidence, a more liberal approach has been advocated in the 2003 Joint National Committee (JNC)-7 Express report[1]: all patients with sustained blood pressure greater than140/90 are recommended for antihypertensive drug therapy along with appropriate life-style modifications.

These recommendations have placed the decision to treat individual patients with different levels of blood pressure and degrees of overall cardiovascular risk into a much more rational framework. If drug therapy is *not* given, close surveillance must still be provided because from 10 to 17 percent of the placebo-treated patients in various RCTs had progression of their blood pressure to a level above that considered an indication for active treatment. Moreover, all patients should be strongly advised to use the appropriate life-style modifications (see Life-Style Modifications).

Systolic Pressure in Elderly Patients

Current guidelines recommend that therapy be given to elderly patients with isolated systolic hypertension (ISH) because they generally have a higher absolute risk of cardiovascular disease and therefore derive greater benefit from treatment. As previously noted, in the data from eight RCTs involving elderly patients with ISH, those given drugs achieved impressive reductions in cardiovascular morbidity compared with those given placebo,[12] and in the one trial in which cognitive function was specifically monitored, those given drug therapy had a 55 percent reduction in onset of dementia over an 8-year follow-up.[6]

It should be noted that the diagnosis of ISH in these trials was based on a systolic level of 160 mm Hg or higher. A large percentage of elderly persons have systolic pressures above 140 but below 160 with diastolic pressures below 90. As yet there are no data to document benefit in this population, but because many of them are inherently at high risk, the JNC-7 report recommends active drug therapy for those with systolic levels above 140 mm Hg.[1]

USE OF SURROGATE ENDPOINTS. All of the preceding discussion of the benefits of therapy and the threshold for treatment has involved "hard" endpoints: morbidity and mortality. Some argue that softer endpoints should also be taken into account, using as surrogates one or another sign of cardiovascular damage that may be easier to assess and quicker to appear. These include regression of left ventricular hypertrophy (LVH) or carotid artery stenosis and reduction of proteinuria. Most, however, hold to the need for the hard endpoints for large outcome trials.

Goal of Therapy

When the decision has been made to treat, the clinician must consider the goal of therapy. In the past, most physicians assumed that the effects of reduction of blood pressure on cardiovascular risk would fit a straight line downward (line A in Fig. 38–2), justifying the opinion "the lower, the better." However, data from multiple large trials indicated a more

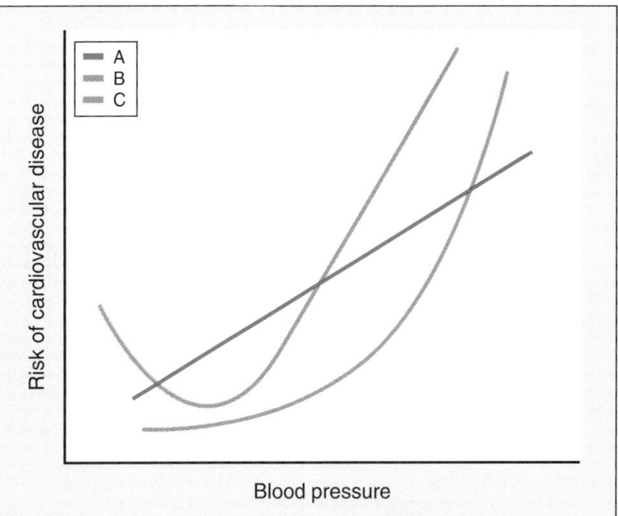

FIGURE 38–2 Three models representing hypothetical relationships between levels of blood pressure and risk of cardiovascular disease. (See text.)

gradual decline in risk when pressures were reduced to moderate levels (line B in Fig. 38–2). Subsequently, evidence has been presented suggesting a J curve, i.e., a fall in risk until some critical level of pressure below which the risk goes back up (line C in Fig. 38–2).[13] The J curve has been claimed for coronary events with falls in diastolic pressure below 85 in patients with diastolic hypertension and for strokes with falls below 65 mm Hg in patients with ISH.

In an attempt to ascertain the presence of a J curve, the Hypertension Optimal Treatment (HOT) trial was performed.[14] Almost 19,000 patients with an initial mean blood pressure of 170/105 mm Hg were randomly allocated to one of three target diastolic pressures: 90, 85, or 80 mm Hg. Diastolic pressures were significantly reduced in all three groups, but at the end, only 4 mm Hg separated them, and it was not possible to prove or disprove a J curve. The least cardiovascular mortality was seen at a blood pressure of 139/86 mm Hg; the least morbidity at 138/83 mm Hg. In the absence of a placebo group, the absolute degree of protection could not be ascertained, but most of the benefit was noted in the 1500 diabetic patients who had a 51 percent reduction in major cardiovascular events in those in the below 80 mm Hg target group compared with the below 90 mm Hg target group.

Another analysis of evidence for a J curve was based on data for individual patients from seven RCTs involving over 40,000 patients given either placebo or drug therapy.[15] A J curve between both systolic and diastolic pressures and cardiovascular mortality was seen, but it occurred in both the treated and the nontreated groups, with the nadir being 5 mm Hg lower in the treated patients (Fig. 38–3). The authors concluded that "The increased risk of events observed with low blood pressure was not related to antihypertensive treatment. . . . Poor health conditions leading to low blood pressure and an increased risk for death probably explain the J-shaped curve."[15]

Certainly, poor general health may cause low blood pressure and increase the risk for death. Nonetheless, excessive antihypertensive treatment may increase cardiovascular morbidity and mortality. The problem may be even more ominous in elderly patients with ISH, whose diastolic pressures are often low before therapy is started. In the SHEP trial, an increased risk for death and stroke was seen with a fall in diastolic pressure below 65 mm Hg.[16]

Nevertheless, the major clinical problem is not overtreatment but undertreatment. Even in carefully conducted clinical trials in which good control should be at a maximum, systolic blood pressures usually remain above 140 mm Hg even though diastolic levels can usually be brought down to below 90 mm Hg. Moreover, even with presumably adequate control, target organ damage may not be reversed. Hypertensives who were treated down to an average level of 128/80 mm Hg maintained a greater left ventricular mass than that seen in normotensive persons, although less than that seen in untreated patients.[17]

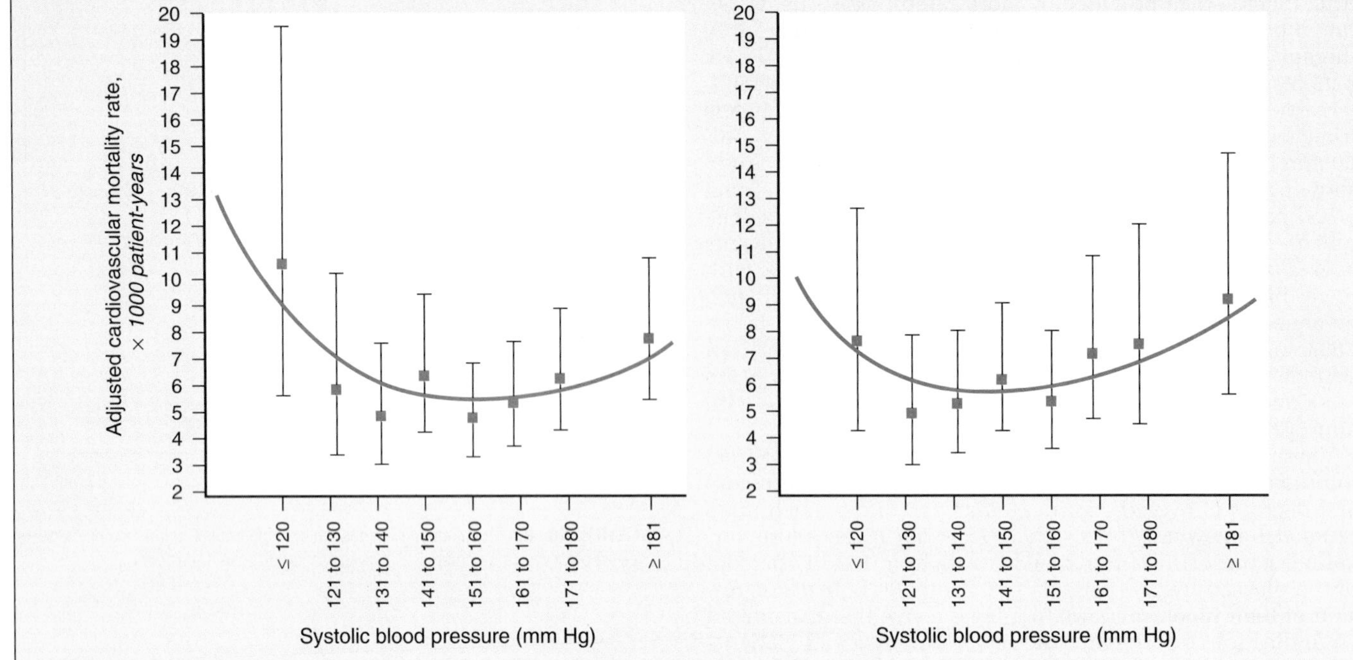

FIGURE 38–3 Age- and sex-adjusted rates of events in eight categories of achieved systolic blood pressure and predicted continuous relationship in active control **(left)** and treatment **(right)** groups from seven randomized controlled trials. (Modified from Boutitie F, Gueyffier F, Pocock S, et al: J-shaped relationship between blood pressure and mortality in hypertensive patients: New insights from a meta-analysis of individual-patient data. Ann Intern Med 136:443, 2002.)

In conclusion, the optimal goal of antihypertensive therapy in most patients with combined systolic and diastolic hypertension who were not at high risk is a blood pressure of less than 140/90 mm Hg. The greatest benefit is probably derived from lowering the diastolic pressure to 80 to 85 mm Hg. Not only is there no proven benefit with more intensive control, but also added cost and probable increased side effects are associated with more aggressive antihypertensive therapy.

In elderly patients with ISH, the goal should be a systolic blood pressure of 140 to 145 mm Hg, as that was the level reached in the RCTs wherein benefit was shown. Caution is advised if, inadvertently, diastolic pressures fall below 65 mm Hg. In such an event, less than ideal reductions in systolic levels need to be balanced against the potential for harm if diastolic levels fall below that level.[13]

More intensive therapy to attain a diastolic pressure of 80 mm Hg or lower may be desirable in some groups, including the following:

- Black patients, who are at greater risk for hypertensive complications and who may continue to have progressive renal damage despite a diastolic pressure of 85 to 90 mm Hg.
- Patients with diabetes mellitus, in whom a blood pressure of less than 130/85 mm Hg reduces the incidence of cardiovascular events.[14] In the United Kingdom Prospective Diabetes Study population of 3642 type 2 diabetic hypertensives, no threshold of risk for systolic pressure was noted: the lower the systolic blood pressure down to 110 mm Hg, the lower was the risk of both micro- and macrovascular complications related to diabetes.[18] (No data on diastolic pressures were provided.)
- Patients with slowly progressive chronic renal disease excreting more than 1 to 2 gm of protein per day, in whom reducing the blood pressure to 125/75 mm Hg may slow the rate of loss of renal function.[19] However, in the African American Study of Kidney Disease (AASK) trial involving 1094 blacks with nondiabetic hypertensive renal disease, those given more therapy to reach a level of 128/78 mm Hg had no better preservation of renal function than those treated to a higher level of 141/85 mm Hg.[19]

Despite the difficulties in achieving the appropriate goal of therapy, good control can be achieved in most patients if they are given enough antihypertensive medication in a progressive manner. Control is enhanced when access to health care is readily available and frequent contact with the same physician is maintained. In addition, the use of life-style modifications markedly improves the chances of adequate control.[1]

Life-Style Modifications

Life-style modifications are indicated for virtually all hypertensives (Table 38–2). Adverse life-style habits are ubiquitous in those with hypertension and may play a major role in the development of the disease. Multiple modifications of life style can lower blood pressure, and their use has been highly correlated with the control of hypertension in the Third National Health and Nutrition Examination Survey (NHANES III) population.[1] Life-style changes are the only maneuvers that have been found to delay, if not stop, the development of hypertension.[7]

Observational and trial data support the importance of multiple simultaneous modifications of life style to accomplish the greatest benefit. Although success in modifying life style may be as difficult or even more difficult to achieve than having patients continue long-term antihypertensive drug therapy, even a small persistent reduction in blood pressure can have a major protective effect on cardiovascular diseases. Moreover, even modest improvements in life style have been shown to reduce the incidence of type 2 diabetes, a common contributor to hypertension.[20]

AVOIDANCE OF TOBACCO. Even though smoking cigarettes has long been known to be a major risk factor for cardiovascular disease, almost 25 percent of U.S. adults now smoke. Part of their risk comes from the major pressor effect of tobacco, which is easily missed because patients are not

TABLE 38–2 Life-Style Modifications to Manage Hypertension

Modification	Recommendation	Approximate Systolic Blood Pressure Reduction (range)
Weight reduction	Maintain normal body weight (body mass index 18.5-24.9 kg/m^2)	50-20 mm Hg/10 kg
Adopt DASH eating plan	Consume a diet rich in fruits, vegetables, and low-fat dairy products with a reduced content of saturated and total fat	8-14 mm Hg
Dietary sodium reduction	Reduce dietary sodium intake to no more than 100 mmol/d (2.4 gm sodium or 6 gm sodium chloride)	2-8 mm Hg
Physical activity	Engage in regular aerobic physical activity such as brisk walking (at least 30 min/d, most days of the week)	4-9 mm Hg
Moderation of alcohol consumption	Limit consumption to no more than two drinks (1 oz or 30 ml ethanol; 24 oz beer, 10 oz wine, or 3 oz 80-proof whiskey) per day in most men and to no more than one drink per day in women and lighter weight persons	2.5-4 mm Hg

DASH = Dietary Approaches to Stop Hypertension.
From Joint National Committee: The seventh report of the Joint National Committee on Prevention, Detection, Evaluation, and Treatment of High Blood Pressure (JNC-7 Express). JAMA 289:2560, 2003.

allowed to smoke in places where blood pressures are recorded. With automatic monitoring, the effect is easy to demonstrate, and blood pressure usually falls immediately when smokers quit.

Tolerance does not develop to the pressor effect of nicotine and sympathetic outflow increases with each cigarette, leading to an increase in arterial stiffness. The noxious effects of smoking include an increase in insulin resistance, visceral obesity, and a particularly detrimental effect on progression of nephropathy. Those who smoke must be told to stop on every contact with a health practitioner. Nicotine replacement therapies are effective and have minimal pressor effects, probably because they provide a lesser and slower rise in plasma nicotine.

WEIGHT REDUCTION. Obesity is growing rapidly in the United States and in all developed and developing societies. The consequences of even small amounts of increased weight are impressive. Over 18 years, women with an initial body mass index (BMI) of 24 were five times more likely to have diabetes and twice as likely to have hypertension as women with a BMI of 21 or lower.[21] In many people, most of this increased weight is deposited in the upper body, constituting a major component of the metabolic syndrome (see Chap. 40), which is now present in almost half of U.S. men and women older than 60. Such upper body obesity is a risk factor for hypertension independent of BMI. Upper body obesity is also more commonly associated with obstructive sleep apnea (see Chap. 68), which is much more common than now recognized, found in more than 10 percent of hypertensives.[22] Obstructive sleep apnea can lead to sustained hypertension, and relief of apnea can lower blood pressure.

In virtually every study of weight reduction, systolic blood pressure is reduced, even if the degree of weight loss is small; each 1.0-kg decrease in body weight is associated with an average blood pressure reduction of 1.6/1.3 mm Hg.

PHYSICAL ACTIVITY. An increase in physical activity is almost always essential for weight reduction. Even without weight loss, however, physical activity can lower the incidence of hypertension and diabetes and protect against cardiovascular disease.[20] The blood pressure falls during aerobic exercise and remains lower for the remainder of the day. The overall antihypertensive effect is greater with longer duration but not with more intensive aerobic exercise.[23]

DIETARY CHANGES

Dietary Sodium Restriction. Evidence incriminating the typically high sodium content of the diet of persons living in developed, industrialized societies was presented earlier as a cause of hypertension. When hypertension is present, modest salt restriction may help lower the blood pressure. In an analysis by He and MacGregor of 28 well-controlled intervention studies that lasted at least 4 weeks in which daily intake (based on urinary sodium excretion) was reduced by a median of 78 mmol per 24 hours, blood pressures fell an average of 5.0/2.7 mm Hg in 734 hypertensive subjects and 2.0/1.0 mm Hg in 2220 normotensive subjects (Fig. 38–4).[24] There was a dose-response relationship—the more sodium reduction, the greater the blood pressure decline. However, the maintenance of dietary sodium restriction over 6 months or longer in 11 controlled trials averaged only 33 mmol per 24 hours and was associated with only a 1.1/0.6 mm Hg reduction in blood pressure.[25]

Not all hypertensive persons respond to a moderate degree of sodium restriction to the recommended level of 100 mmol

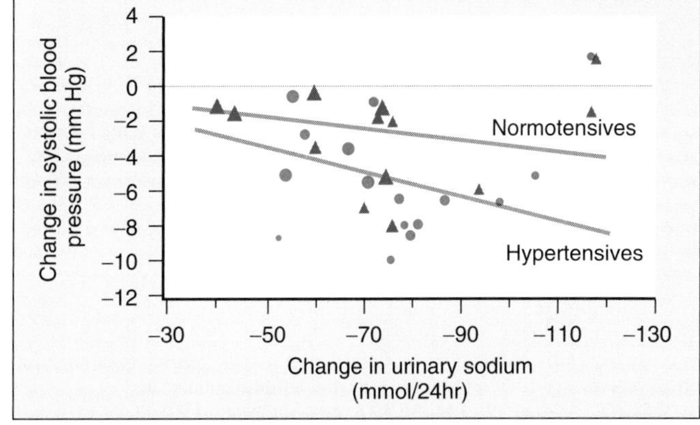

FIGURE 38–4 Relationship between the net change in urinary sodium excretion and systolic blood pressure. The blue triangles represent normotensive and the magenta circles represent hypertensive subjects. The slope is weighted by the inverse of the variance of the net change in systolic blood pressure. The size of the circle is in proportion to the weight of the trial. (Modified from He FJ, MacGregor GA: Effect of modest salt reduction on blood pressure: A meta-analysis of randomized trials. Implications for public health. J Hum Hypertens 16:766, 2002.)

sodium or 2.4 gm/d. Blacks and elderly patients may be more responsive to sodium restriction, perhaps because of their lower renin responsiveness. Nevertheless, even if the blood pressure does not fall with moderate degrees of sodium restriction, patients may still benefit. Multiple cardiovascular and noncardiovascular ill effects have been noted with high sodium intake. In a prospective follow-up of 2400 Finnish men and women, a 100 mmol per 24 hours higher sodium excretion was accompanied by a 45 percent increase in the hazard ratio for cardiovascular disease and a 26 percent increase in all-cause mortality.[26]

However, rigid degrees of sodium restriction not only are difficult for patients to achieve but also may be counterproductive. The marked stimulation of renin-aldosterone and sympathetic nervous activity that accompanies rigid sodium restriction may prevent the blood pressure from falling and increase the amount of potassium wastage if diuretics are used concomitantly.

Therefore, I consider sodium restriction to be useful for all persons, as a preventive measure in those who are normotensive and, more certainly, as partial therapy in those who are hypertensive. The easiest way to accomplish moderate sodium restriction is to substitute natural foods for processed foods because natural foods are low in sodium and high in potassium whereas most processed foods have had sodium added and potassium removed. It is hoped that food processors will gradually reduce the large amounts of salt they often add to processed foods, but in the meantime, patients should be asked to avoid foods whose label indicates more than 300 mg of sodium per portion. Additional guidelines include the following:

- Add no sodium chloride to food during cooking or at the table.
- If a salty taste is desired, use a half sodium and half potassium chloride preparation (such as Lite-Salt) or a pure potassium chloride substitute.
- Avoid or minimize the use of "fast foods," many of which have high sodium content.
- Recognize the sodium content of some antacids and proprietary medications. (For example, Alka-Seltzer contains more than 500 mg of sodium; Rolaids are virtually sodium free.)

POTASSIUM SUPPLEMENTATION. Some of the advantages of a lower sodium intake may be related to its tendency to increase body potassium content, both by a coincidental increase in dietary potassium intake and by a decrease in potassium wastage if diuretics are being used. Low dietary potassium intake is associated with an increased risk of stroke that may be independent of an effect on blood pressure.[27]

Potassium supplements have been shown to reduce the blood pressure an average of 3.1/2.0 mm Hg in 33 RCTs, with the effect being greater in blacks and in the presence of higher dietary sodium intake.[28] Nonetheless, potassium supplements are too costly and potentially hazardous for routine use in normokalemic hypertensive persons. Patients should be protected from potassium depletion and encouraged to increase dietary potassium intake, which may be enough to lower blood pressure.

CALCIUM SUPPLEMENTS. In 42 mostly short-term studies of either calcium supplements (in 33) or dietary intervention (in 9) in 4560 nonpregnant adults, the blood pressure fell 1.44/0.84 mm Hg.[29] Because calcium supplements sometimes raise blood pressure and increase the risk of kidney stones, the best course is to ensure that calcium intake is not inadvertently reduced by reduction of milk and cheese consumption in an attempt to reduce saturated fat and sodium intake.

MAGNESIUM SUPPLEMENTS. A meta-analysis of 20 RCTs of magnesium supplements, averaging 15.4 mmol per 24 hours, found a statistically insignificant fall in blood pressure of 0.6/0.8 mm Hg.[30]

OTHER DIETARY CONSTITUENTS. Significant reductions in blood pressure were observed in a controlled trial of 690 normotensive persons, half of whom ate a diet rich in fruits and vegetables.[31] This fall in blood pressure could reflect increases in fiber, potassium, or other ingredients. Some lowering of the blood pressure has been noted in studies of high fiber intake and high doses of omega-3 fatty acids from fish oil. Supplements of vitamin C have had various effects on blood pressure.

In 11 carefully controlled trials involving 522 subjects who consumed an average of five cups of caffeine-containing coffee, the mean blood pressure rose 2.4/1.2 mm Hg.[32] A pressor response has been noted with decaffeinated coffee as well. Even though consumption of tea has been found to be associated with a lower risk of myocardial infarction, it too may raise blood pressure.

MODERATION OF ALCOHOL. Alcohol is a two-edged sword. Too much, particularly in a binge, raises blood pressure and can have lethal effects; too little can deny multiple cardiovascular benefits (see Chap. 36). The "safe" level of regular alcohol consumption with regard to hypertension in men is less than two portions per 24 hours, although even less was found to increase the incidence in black men.[33] A portion is defined as about 12 ml of alcohol—the equivalent of 12 oz of beer, 4 oz of wine, or 1.5 oz of liquor. Among women, the incidence of hypertension was reduced by 14 percent in those who consumed an average of one half-portion per 24 hours and was increased by 31 percent in those who drank more than two portions per 24 hours.[34] On the other hand, regular consumption of moderate amounts of alcohol reduces the risk of coronary disease, heart failure, ischemic stroke, diabetes, and dementia, perhaps at least in part through an antiinflammatory mechanism.[35]

RELAXATION TECHNIQUES. Most studies of various cognitive-behavioral therapies have shown transient but not sustained lowering of blood pressure. However, more impressive effects were found in 45 hypertensives who received 10 hours of individualized stress management; after 6 months, ambulatory blood pressure levels were reduced by 6.1/4.3 mm Hg.[36] Perhaps acting in ways beyond relaxation, slow breathing guided by a device has also been found to lower blood pressure.[37]

COMBINED THERAPIES. When several life-style modifications are combined, additional antihypertensive effects may accrue. Perhaps the best study is the placebo arm of the Treatment of Mild Hypertension Study (TOMHS),[38] in which 234 mildly hypertensive persons followed a 48-month regimen of moderate sodium restriction, weight loss, regular exercise, and moderation of alcohol use. Despite relatively small changes in weight (average loss of 6.6 pounds), sodium intake (reduction of 10 percent), exercise level, and alcohol consumption, these patients had an 8.6/8.6 mm Hg decline in blood pressure at the end of the 4-year program. Moreover, they experienced improvements in lipid profile and reduction in left ventricular mass.

Nonetheless, despite the need to rely on life-style modifications in the hope of preventing hypertension and in managing the disease once it has developed, the limited success of achieving significant life-style changes in clinical practice must be recognized. Therefore, although life-style changes should be pursued, patients must not be denied the proven benefits of antihypertensive drug therapy.

Antihypertensive Drug Therapy

If the life-style modifications just described are not adequate to bring the blood pressure to goal (<140/90 mm Hg for most, <130/80 mm Hg for those with diabetes or renal insufficiency) or if the level of hypertension at the onset is so high that immediate drug therapy is deemed necessary (>160/100 mm Hg), the JNC-7 report provides an overall algorithm for treatment (Fig. 38–5).[1]

General Guidelines

When drug therapy is decided upon, the guidelines listed in Table 38–3 should be followed in order to provide effective 24-hour control of hypertension in a manner that encourages adherence to the regimen. The approach is based on known pharmacological principles and proven ways to improve adherence.[39]

For the majority of patients who do not require more intensive immediate therapy, once the selection of the most appropriate agent for initial therapy has been made (by a process that is discussed further in the next section), a relatively low dose of a single drug should be started, aiming for a reduction of 5 to 10 mm Hg in blood pressure at each step. Many physicians, by nature and training, wish to control a patient's

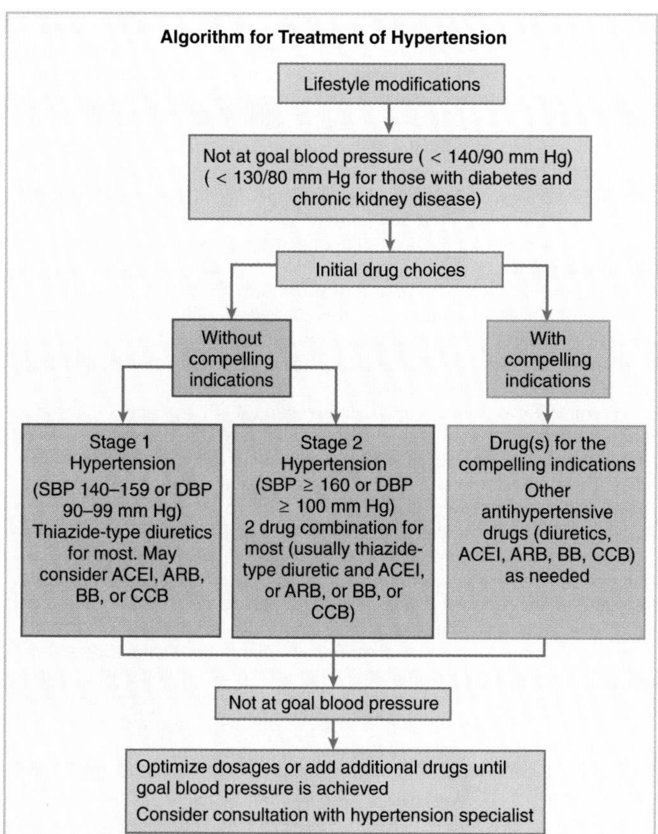

FIGURE 38–5 Treatment of hypertension according to the level of blood pressure and cardiovascular risk as recommended by Joint National Committee (JNC)-7. ACEI = angiotensin-converting enzyme inhibitor; ARB = angiotensin II receptor blocker; BB = beta blocker; CCB = calcium channel blocker; DBP = diastolic blood pressure; SBP = systolic blood pressure. (Modified from Joint National Committee: The seventh report of the Joint Committee on Prevention, Detection, Evaluation, and Treatment of High Blood Pressure (JNC-7 Express). JAMA 289:2560, 2003.)

hypertension rapidly and completely. Regardless of which drugs are used, this approach often leads to undue fatigue, weakness, and postural dizziness, which many patients find intolerable, particularly when they felt well before therapy was begun. Although hypokalemia and other electrolyte abnormalities may be responsible for some of these symptoms, a more likely explanation has been provided by the studies of Strandgaard and Haunsø.[40] As shown in Figure 38–6, they demonstrated the constancy of cerebral blood flow by autoregulation over a range of mean arterial pressures from about 60 to 120 mm Hg in normal subjects and from 110 to 180 mm Hg in patients with hypertension. This shift to the right protects hypertensive patients from a surge of blood flow, which could cause cerebral edema. However, the shift also predisposes hypertensive patients to cerebral ischemia when blood pressure is lowered.

The lower limit of autoregulation necessary to preserve a constant cerebral blood flow in hypertensive patients is a mean of about 110 mm Hg. Thus, acutely lowering the pressure from 160/110 mm Hg (mean = 127) to 140/85 mm Hg (mean = 102) may induce cerebral hypoperfusion, although hypotension in the accepted sense has not been produced. This observation provides a probable explanation for what many patients experience at the start of antihypertensive therapy (i.e., fatigue, lethargy, and dizziness), even though blood pressure levels do not seem inordinately low.

Thus, the approach to antihypertensive therapy should be gradual in order to avoid symptoms related to overly intensive blood pressure reduction. Fortunately, as shown in the middle of Figure 38–6, if therapy is continued for a period, the curve of cerebral autoregulation shifts back toward normal, allowing patients to tolerate greater reductions in blood pressure without experiencing symptoms.

TABLE 38–3 Guidelines to Improve Maintenance of Antihypertensive Therapy
Be aware of the problem and be alert to signs of inadequate intake of medications Recognize and manage depression
Articulate the goal of therapy: to reduce blood pressure to near normotension with few or no side effects
Educate the patient about the disease and its treatment Provide individual assessments of current risks and potential benefits of control Involve the patient in decision-making Provide written instructions Encourage family support
Maintain contact with the patient Encourage visits and calls to allied health personnel Allow the pharmacist to monitor therapy Give feedback to the patient through home blood pressure readings Make contact with patients who do not return
Keep care inexpensive and simple Do the least work-up needed to rule out secondary causes Obtain follow-up laboratory data only yearly unless indicated more often Use home blood pressure readings Use nondrug, low-cost therapies Use once-daily doses of long-acting drugs Use generic drugs and break larger doses of tablets in half If appropriate, use combination tablets Use calendar blister packs (if and when they are marketed) Tailor medication to daily routines Use detailed clinical protocols monitored by nurses and assistants
Prescribe according to pharmacological principles Add one drug at a time Start with small doses, aiming for reductions of 5 to 10 mm Hg at each step Have medication taken immediately on awakening in the morning or after 4 AM if patient awakens to void
Be willing to stop unsuccessful therapy and try a different approach
Anticipate and address side effects Adjust therapy to ameliorate side effects that do not disappear spontaneously
Continue to add effective and tolerated drugs, stepwise, in sufficient doses to achieve the goal of therapy
Provide feedback and validation of success

STARTING DOSAGES. The need to start with a fairly small dose also reflects a greater responsiveness of some patients to doses of medication that may be appropriate for the majority. All drugs exert increasing effect with increasing doses, portrayed by a log-linear dose-response curve (Fig. 38–7).[41] However, different patients require different absolute amounts of drug for their own dose response.

As a hypothetical example, for the majority of patients, 50 mg of the beta blocker atenolol would provide a moderate response, shown as point A on the therapeutic effect curve, whereas a dose of 25 mg would provide only a minimal response. At dose A, providing the significant albeit partial response, the side effects would be minimal, as shown by point A′ on the curve of toxic effect. If a starting dose of 100 mg were used, the therapeutic effect would be near maximal (point B) but the side effects would be much greater as well (point B′). Therefore, a lower starting dose is preferable for most patients.

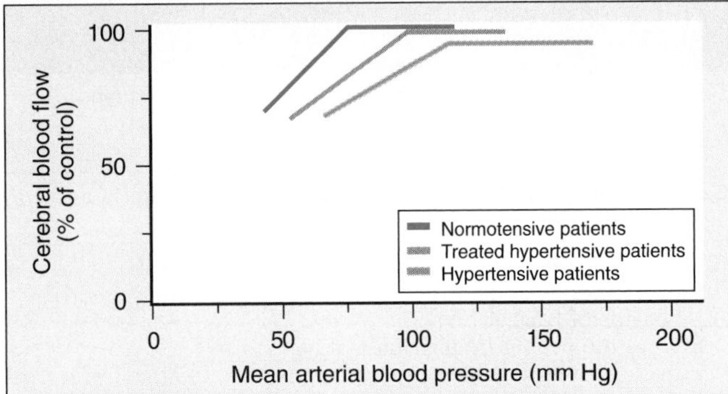

FIGURE 38–6 Mean cerebral blood flow autoregulation curves from normotensive, severely hypertensive, and effectively treated hypertensive patients are shown. (Modified from Strandgaard S: Autoregulation of cerebral blood flow in hypertensive patients. The modifying influence of prolonged antihypertensive treatment on the tolerance to acute, drug-induced hypotension. Circulation 53:720, 1976; and Strandgaard S, Haunsø S: Why does antihypertensive treatment prevent stroke but not myocardial infarction? Lancet 2:658, 1987.)

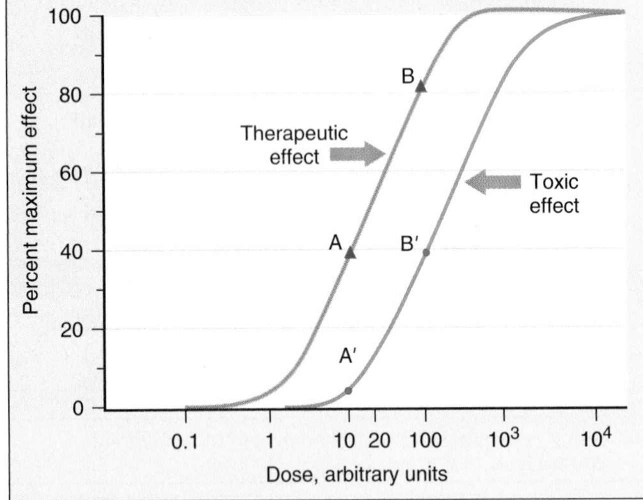

FIGURE 38–7 Theoretical therapeutic and toxic logarithmic-linear dose-response curves. The horizontal axis is the logarithmic scale with arbitrary dose units. The vertical axis is a linear scale showing percentage of maximum possible response. (Modified from Fagan TC: Remembering the lessons of basic pharmacology. Arch Intern Med 154:1430, 1994. Copyright 1994 American Medical Association.)

However, the response to a given dose is not the same for all patients but rather assumes a bell-shaped curve; some patients are very sensitive to that dose and some very resistant, with the majority having a moderate response. Therefore, a significant minority of patients—the very sensitive ones—would have a near-maximal response to the 25-mg dose and would better be started on 12.5 mg in order to achieve a moderate therapeutic effect (point A) with minimal side effects (point A′). Without knowing how individual patients will respond, the safest and easiest approach is to start at a dose that probably is not enough for most patients.

To allow autoregulation of blood flow to maintain perfusion to vital organs when perfusion pressure is lowered, the decline in pressure should be relatively small and gradual. More precipitous reductions in pressure, as frequently occur with larger starting doses, may induce considerable hypoperfusion that results in symptoms that are at least bothersome (fatigue, impotence) and that may be potentially hazardous (postural hypotension, coronary ischemia). It is far better to start low and go slow.

CHOICE OF INITIAL DRUG. In the past, the choice of initial drug was largely based on perceived differences in the efficacy of lowering blood pressure and the likelihood of side effects. Although comparative trials did show some differences, largely determined by age and race,[42] most found that moderate doses of all classes of drugs provided similar efficacy.[3] This conclusion is hardly surprising because the formulations of virtually all antihypertensive drugs are designed to do the same thing: lower the blood pressure at least 10 percent in the majority of hypertensive patients. More than that would probably be unacceptable to patients; less than that would be unacceptable to practitioners.

Recommendations for the choice of initial therapy have been increasingly based on the "compelling" indications of other conditions that frequently coexist with hypertension (Table 38–4).[9,10] In the last 10 years, large trials have examined the ability of different classes to reduce morbidity and mortality, and the results of these outcome trials should now direct the choice of therapy.

The first clear documentation of superiority of one class was a meta-analysis of 19 RCTs comparing outcomes with high and low doses of diuretics and beta blockers, all against placebo (Table 38–5).[43] Low doses of diuretic were seen to protect better against coronary disease than high doses of diuretic or beta blockers.

From 1995 to 2000, eight trials involving 37,872 patients compared different regimens against one other (Table 38–6).[44] The relative risk for stroke was lower for CCB-based therapy than for therapy based on diuretics with or without beta blockers, but the risks for coronary disease and heart failure were lower for therapy based on angiotensin-converting enzyme inhibitors (ACEIs) than for CCB-based therapy. Two points need to be considered in interpreting the data in Table 38–6: (1) in all trials, the primary drug was often admixed with other drugs in order to reach the goal of therapy, and (2) the data comparing ACEI versus CCB came from one large trial that found no significant differences between the two[45] and a much smaller trial that found a highly significant difference.[46] The authors of the meta-analysis concluded that "the evidence suggestive of greater benefits of stroke and lesser benefits for coronary heart disease with calcium-antagonist-based regimens is not sufficiently reliable to allow precise assessments."[45]

THREE RANDOMIZED CLINICAL TRIALS. Since 2000, the results of two larger RCTs comparing different agents in predominantly[2] or exclusively[47] elderly patients have been published. In addition, another large RCT compared an angiotensin II (AII) receptor blocker (ARB) against a beta blocker in the ability to protect hypertensives with LVH.[48]

In brief, the Antihypertensive and Lipid-Lowering Treatment to Prevent Heart Attack Trial (ALLHAT), the largest RCT now available, compared regimens based on a diuretic (chlorthalidone) against either an ACEI (lisinopril) or a CCB (amlodipine) in high-risk hypertensive patients older than 55 years (mean age of 67).[2] Diuretic-based therapy was as effective as ACEI- or CCB-based therapy in preventing the primary endpoint, major coronary events; superior to both in preventing heart failure; and superior to the ACEI in preventing stroke. A large part of the differences in the secondary outcomes may reflect the greater reduction in blood pressure achieved with the diuretic. Moreover, only 35 percent of the patients were treated with their primary drug alone. As with virtually all trials, most patients required more than one drug to achieve the goal of therapy.

A second large outcome trial compared a diuretic-based regimen (hydrochlorothiazide) against an ACEI-based regimen (enalapril) in 6083 hypertensive patients aged 65 to 84.[47] Despite similar reductions in blood pressure, averaging 26/12 mm Hg, those in the ACEI group had an 11 percent greater reduction than the diuretic group in the primary endpoints of cardiovascular events or death. This difference was almost entirely related to a decrease in myocardial infarction in the men, whereas women showed no differences in outcomes, and there was no difference in stroke in either men or women.

In the Losartan Intervention For Endpoint reduction (LIFE) trial, 9193 hypertensive subjects with LVH ascertained by electrocardiography were assigned to either a beta blocker (atenolol) or an ARB (losartan).[48] With equal degrees of blood pressure reduction, those receiving the ARB had a 13 percent lower relative risk of the primary endpoints (death, myocardial infarction, or stroke). This difference was entirely composed of a 25 percent lower risk of stroke; myocardial infarctions were slightly *more* common in those given the ARB, even though more regression of LVH was seen with the ARB. In the LIFE trial, only 11 percent of the patients took only their primary drug and more than 80 percent of both groups also received hydrochlorothiazide.

AN OVERALL ALGORITHM. On the basis of these data and more and in agreement with the JNC-7 algorithm (see Fig. 38–5), the algorithm shown in Figure 38–8 seems to be an appropriate approach to the treatment of stage 1 hypertension. A low-dose thiazide diuretic should be the foundation but is likely to be adequate by itself in only about 30

TABLE 38–4 Indications and Contraindications for the Use of Antihypertensive Drugs

Class of Drug	Indications	Contraindications
Diuretics	Heart failure Advanced age Systolic hypertension	Gout
Beta blockers	Angina or previous myocardial infarction Heart failure Tachyarrhythmias Migraine	Asthma or chronic obstructive pulmonary disease Heart block
Alpha blockers	Prostatic hypertrophy	Incipient heart failure
Calcium channel blockers	Advanced age Systolic hypertension Cyclosporine-induced hypertension	Heart block (verapamil, diltiazem)
ACE inhibitors	Heart failure or left ventricular dysfunction Previous myocardial infarction Diabetic or other nephropathy or proteinuria	Pregnancy Bilateral renal artery stenosis Hyperkalemia
Angiotensin receptor blockers	ACE inhibitor–associated cough Diabetic or other nephropathy Congestive heart failure	Pregnancy Bilateral renal artery stenosis Hyperkalemia

ACE = angiotensin-converting enzyme.

TABLE 38–5 Randomized Controlled Trials in Hypertension: First Drug Therapy

	Relative Risk Versus Placebo			
Agent	***Stroke***	***Coronary Heart Disease***	***Congestive Heart Failure***	***Cardiovascular Mortality***
High-dose thiazide diuretic (50-100 mg)*	0.49	0.99	0.17	0.78
Low-dose thiazide diuretic (12.5-25 mg)*	0.66	0.72	0.58	0.76
Beta blocker	0.71	0.93	0.58	0.89

*Doses are for hydrochlorothiazide or its equivalent.

Modified from Psaty BM, Smith NL, Siscovick DS, et al: Health outcomes associated with antihypertensive therapies used as first-line agents, JAMA 277:739, 1997.

TABLE 38–6 Prospective Overview of Randomized Trials for Hypertension

	Relative Risks (Confidence Interval)					
Therapy	***Stroke***	***CHD***	***CHF***	***Major CV Events***	***CV Death***	***Total Mortality***
ACEI versus placebo (4 trials; 12,124 patients)	0.70 (0.57-0.85)	0.80 (0.72-0.89)	0.84 (0.68-1.04)	0.79 (0.73-0.86)	0.74 (0.64-0.85)	0.84 (0.76-0.94)
CCB versus placebo (2 trials; 5220 patients)	0.61 (0.44-0.85)	0.79 (0.59-1.06)	0.72 (0.48-1.07)	0.72 (0.59-0.87)	0.72 (0.52-0.98)	0.87 (0.70-1.09)
ACEI versus D/βB (3 trials; 16,161 patients)	1.05 (0.92-1.19)	1.00 (0.88-1.14)	0.92 (0.77-1.09)	1.00 (0.93-1.08)	1.00 (0.87-1.15)	1.03 (0.93-1.14)
CCB versus D/βB (5 trials; 23,454 patients)	0.87 (0.77-0.98)	1.12 (1.0-1.26)	1.12 (0.95-1.33)	1.02 (0.95-1.10)	1.05 (0.92-1.2)	1.01 (0.92-1.11)
ACEI versus CCB (2 trials; 4871 patients)	1.02 (0.85-1.21)	0.81 (0.68-0.97)	0.82 (0.67-1.0)	0.92 (0.83-1.01)	1.04 (0.87-1.24)	1.03 (0.91-1.18)

ACEI = angiotensin-converting enzyme inhibitor; CCB = calcium channel blocker; D/βB = diuretic/beta-blacker; CHD = coronary heart disease; CHF = congestive heart failure; CV = cardiovascular.

From Neal B, MacMahon S, Chapman N—Blood Pressure Lowering Treatment Trialists' Collaboration: Effects of ACE inhibitors, calcium antagonists, and other blood-pressure-lowering drugs: Results of prospectively designed overviews of randomised trials. Blood Pressure Lowering Treatment Trialists' Collaboration. Lancet 356:1955, 2000.

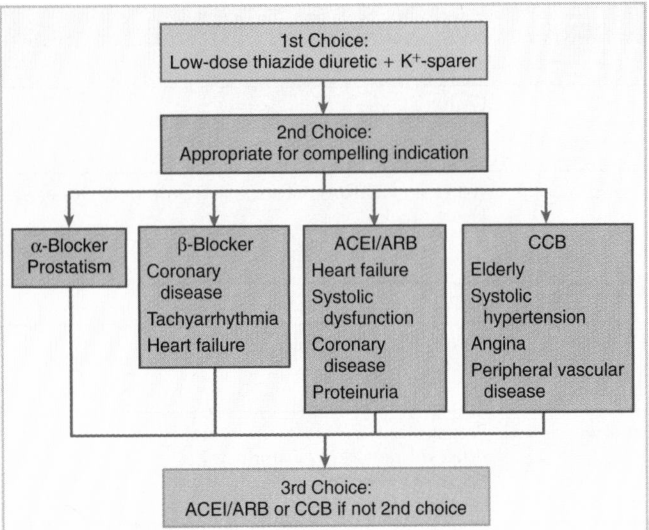

FIGURE 38–8 An algorithm for therapy of hypertension. ACEI = angiotensin-converting enzyme inhibitor; ARB = angiotensin II receptor blocker; CCB = calcium channel blocker.

percent of patients. The remainder should then be given whatever choice seems appropriate for their coexisting conditions (see Table 38–4). On the basis of these short-term efficacy trials, those with only hypertension could logically be given an ACEI if they are younger or nonblack or a CCB if they are older or black. In fact, because the differential responses in blood pressure reduction are largely removed when a diuretic is also given, there seems little reason to favor any drug class in the absence of a specific indication or contraindication.

COMBINATION THERAPY. Because a low dose of a thiazide diuretic potentiates the effect of all other drug classes and because most patients, particularly those with diabetes, renal disease, or levels of blood pressure above 160/100, require two or more drugs for adequate control, a combination of a low-dose diuretic and the appropriate second choice may logically be used at the onset of therapy as recommended by JNC-7. Other combinations are also available and may improve control of hypertension by lowering the cost and improving adherence to therapy.

COMPLETE COVERAGE WITH ONCE-DAILY DOSING. A number of choices within each of the six major classes of antihypertensive drugs now available provide full 24-hour efficacy. Therefore, single daily dosing should be feasible for virtually all patients, resulting in improved adherence to therapy. The use of longer acting agents avoids the potential for inducing too great a peak effect in order to provide an adequate effect at the end of the dosing interval (the trough). Moreover, because many patients occasionally skip a dose of their drugs, there is an additional value in using agents with an inherently long duration of action that covers the skipped dose as well.

Long-acting choices are available within each class. However, because patients differ not only in terms of degree of response but also in terms of the duration of effect, the prudent course is to document the patient's response at the end of the dosing interval by home or ambulatory monitoring. With this approach, the abrupt surge in blood pressure that occurs on awakening is blunted, and, it is hoped, patients can be better protected from the increased incidence of cardiovascular catastrophes at this critical time.

If short-acting medications are taken at bedtime to ensure coverage in the early morning, ischemia to vital organs might be induced by the combination of the maximal effect of the drug within the first 3 to 6 hours after intake and the usual nocturnal decline in pressure. Therefore, the safest course is to take medications with a 24-hour duration of action as early in the morning as possible.

With the general principles of therapy in mind, particulars about the various classes of drugs available are now covered.

Diuretics (see also Chap. 23)

Diuretics may be divided into four major groups by their primary site of action within the tubule, starting in the proximal portion and moving to the collecting duct: (1) agents acting on the proximal tubule, such as carbonic anhydrase inhibitors, which have limited antihypertensive efficacy; (2) loop diuretics; (3) thiazides and related sulfonamide compounds; and (4) potassium-sparing agents (Table 38–7). A thiazide is the usual choice, often in combination with a potassium-sparing agent. Loop diuretics should be reserved for patients with renal insufficiency or resistant hypertension. The availability of a more specific aldosterone blocker, eplerenone, may considerably broaden the use of this class of drug beyond that of spironolactone.

MECHANISM OF ACTION. All diuretics initially lower the blood pressure by increasing urinary sodium excretion and by reducing plasma volume, extracellular fluid volume, and cardiac output. Within 6 to 8 weeks, the lowered plasma, extracellular fluid volume, and cardiac output return toward normal. At this point and beyond, the lower blood pressure is related to a decline in peripheral resistance, thereby improving the underlying hemodynamic defect of hypertension. The mechanism responsible for the lowered peripheral resistance may involve a vasorelaxant effect, but initial diuresis is needed because diuretics fail to lower the blood pressure when the excreted sodium is returned or when given to patients who have nonfunctioning kidneys and are undergoing long-term dialysis. With the shrinkage in blood volume and lower blood pressure, increased secretion of renin and

TABLE 38–7 Representative Diuretics and Potassium-Sparing Agents

Agent	Daily Dose (mg)	Duration of Action (hr)
Thiazides		
Bendroflumethiazide (Naturetin)	1.25-5.0	>18
Cyclothiazide (Anhydron)	0.125-1	18-24
Hydrochlorothiazide (Esidrix, HydroDIURIL, Oretic)	6.25-50	12-18
Methyclothiazide (Enduron)	2.5-5.0	>24
Trichlormethiazide (Metahydrin, Naqua)	1-4	>34
Related Sulfonamide Compounds		
Chlorthalidone (Hygroton)	12.5-50	24-72
Indapamide (Lozol)	1.25-2.5	24
Metolazone (Mykrox, Zaroxolyn)	0.5-10	24
Loop Diuretics		
Bumetanide (Bumex)	0.5-5	4-6
Ethacrynic acid (Edecrin)*	25-100*	12*
Furosemide (Lasix)	40-480	4-6
Torsemide (Demadex)	5-40	12
Potassium-Sparing Agents		
Amiloride (Midamor)	5-10	24
Eplerenone (Inspra)	50-200	24
Spironolactone (Aldactone)	25-100	8-12
Triamterene (Dyrenium)	50-100	12

*No longer available in the United States.

aldosterone retards the continued sodium diuresis. Both renin-induced vasoconstriction and aldosterone-induced sodium retention prevent continued diminution of body fluids and progressive reduction in blood pressure while diuretic therapy is continued.

CLINICAL EFFECTS. With daily diuretic therapy, systolic pressure usually falls about 10 mm Hg, although the degree depends on various factors, including the initial height of the pressure, the quantity of sodium ingested, the adequacy of renal function, and the intensity of the counterregulatory renin-aldosterone response. Those with initially lower renin or aldosterone levels, including many elderly or black hypertensives, tend to have a greater antihypertensive effect.[49] The antihypertensive effect of the diuretic persists indefinitely, although it may be overwhelmed by excessive dietary sodium intake.

If other antihypertensive drugs are used, a diuretic may also be needed. Without a concomitant diuretic, antihypertensive drugs that do not block the renin-aldosterone mechanism may cause sodium retention. This mechanism probably reflects the success of the drugs in lowering the blood pressure and may involve the abnormal renal pressure-natriuresis relationship that is presumably present in primary hypertension. Just as more pressure is needed to excrete a given load of sodium in a hypertensive individual, so does a lowering of pressure toward normal lead to sodium retention.

The critical need for adequate diuretic therapy to keep intravascular volume slightly diminished has been repeatedly documented. Drugs that inhibit the renin-aldosterone mechanism, such as ACEIs, or drugs that induce some natriuresis themselves, such as calcium antagonists, may continue to work without the need for concomitant diuretics. However, a diuretic enhances the effectiveness of all other types of drugs, including calcium antagonists. Moreover, the results of multiple comparative trials including ALLHAT[2] and those shown in Tables 38–5 and 38–6 reconfirm the cardiovascular protective effects of diuretic-based therapy.

The benefits of diuretics may be even greater in patients who are more sodium sensitive, perhaps as a consequence of genetic variants. In a case-controlled study, the hypertensives who carried the alpha-adducin gene variant were found to have an even lower risk for coronary and stroke events when given a diuretic than with other agents.[50]

DOSAGE AND CHOICE OF AGENT. Most patients with mild to moderate hypertension and serum creatinine concentrations less than 1.5 mg/dl respond to the lower doses of the various diuretics (thiazides and related compounds) listed in Table 38–7. An amount equivalent to 12.5 mg of hydrochlorothiazide is usually adequate. For uncomplicated hypertension, a single morning dose of hydrochlorothiazide provides a 24-hour antihypertensive effect. The nonthiazide agent indapamide has special properties that make it an attractive choice. With renal damage, manifested by a serum creatinine level exceeding 1.5 mg/dl or creatinine clearance less than 30 ml/min, thiazides are usually not effective, and repeated daily doses of furosemide, one or two doses of torsemide, or a single dose of metolazone is usually needed. The combination of a thiazide with a loop diuretic may provide even better efficacy by countering the distal nephron hypertrophy seen with loop diuretics alone.

SIDE EFFECTS. A number of biochemical changes often accompany successful diuresis, including a decrease in plasma potassium level and increases in glucose, insulin, and cholesterol levels (Fig. 38–9). Most of these are minimized or absent with low doses of diuretic.

HYPOKALEMIA. The degree of potassium wastage and hypokalemia is directly related to the dose of diuretic; serum potassium level falls an average of 0.7 mmol/liter with 50 mg of hydrochlorothiazide, 0.4 with 25, and little if any with 12.5.[3] Hypokalemia related to high doses of diuretic may precipitate potentially hazardous ventricular ectopic activity and increase the risk of primary cardiac arrest, even in patients not known to be susceptible because of concomitant digitalis therapy or myocardial irritability.

The following maneuvers should help prevent diuretic-induced hypokalemia:

- Use the smallest dose of diuretic needed.
- Use a moderately long-acting (12- to 18-hour) diuretic, such as hydrochlorothiazide, because longer acting drugs (e.g., chlorthalidone) may increase potassium loss.
- Restrict sodium intake to less than 100 mmol/d.
- Increase dietary potassium intake.
- Use a combination of a thiazide with a potassium-sparing agent except in patients with renal insufficiency or in association with an ACEI or ARB.
- Use a concomitant beta blocker, an ACEI, or an ARB, which diminishes potassium loss by blunting the diuretic-induced rise in renin and aldosterone.

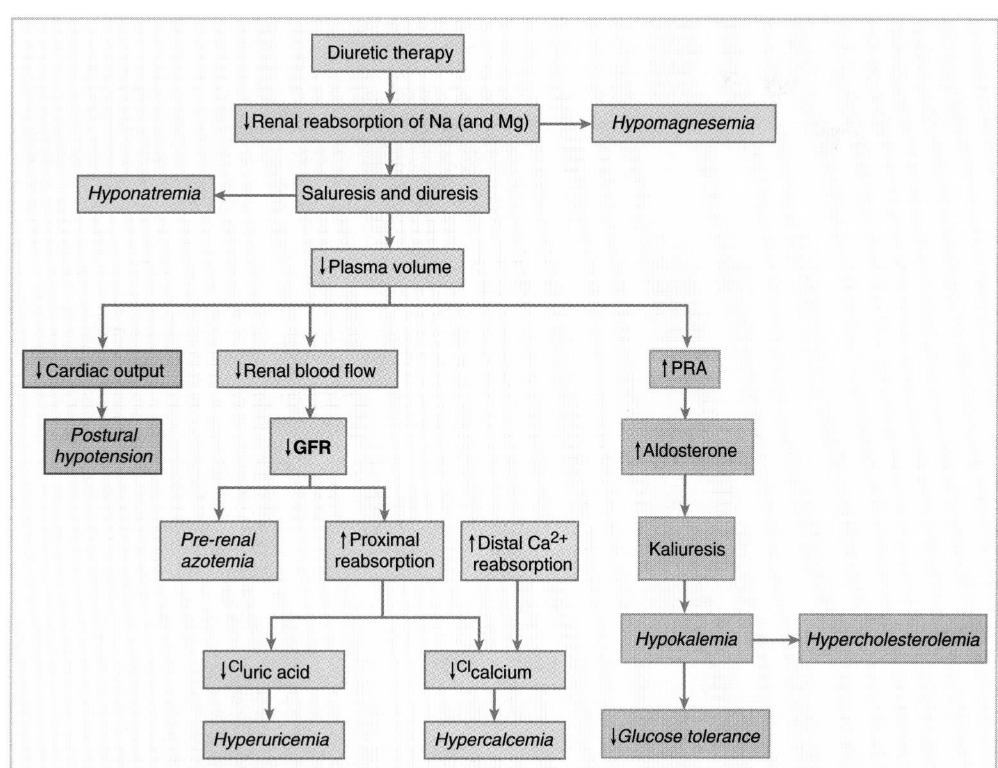

FIGURE 38–9 The mechanisms by which chronic diuretic therapy may lead to various complications. The mechanism for hypercholesterolemia remains in question, although it is shown as arising through hypokalemia. Cl = clearance; GFR = glomerular filtration rate; PRA = plasma renin activity. (Modified from Kaplan NM: Kaplan's Clinical Hypertension. 8th ed. Baltimore, Lippincott Williams & Wilkins, 2002, p 246.)

HYPOMAGNESEMIA. In some patients, concomitant diuretic-induced magnesium deficiency prevents restoration of intracellular deficits of potassium, so that hypomagnesemia should be corrected. Magnesium deficiency may also be responsible for some of the arrhythmias ascribed to hypokalemia.

HYPERURICEMIA. The serum uric acid level is elevated in as many as one third of untreated hypertensive patients. With long-term high-dose diuretic therapy, hyperuricemia appears in another third of patients as a consequence of increased proximal tubule reabsorption accompanying volume contraction and may precipitate acute gout. Because asymptomatic hyperuricemia does not cause urate deposition, most investigators agree that it need not be treated.

HYPERGLYCEMIA AND INSULIN RESISTANCE. High doses of diuretics may impair glucose tolerance and precipitate diabetes mellitus, probably because they increase insulin resistance and hyperinsulinemia.

HYPERCALCEMIA. A slight rise in serum calcium levels, less than 0.5 mg/dl, is frequently seen with thiazide diuretic therapy and is accompanied by a 40 to 50 percent decrease in urinary calcium excretion. Thiazide therapy thereby protects against renal stones and osteoporosis.

HYPONATREMIA. Thiazides may cause insidious hyponatremia, usually in elderly women.

ERECTILE DYSFUNCTION. An increase in the incidence of impotence was noted among men who took 15 mg of chlorthalidone, with the diuretic being the only one of five classes of agents attended by this effect.[51]

RENAL CELL CARCINOMA. A significant but numerically small increase in renal cell carcinoma among diuretic users has been documented.[52]

SULFA SENSITIVITY. Ethacrynic acid, the only diuretic that does not have a sulfonamide structure, is no longer available. A slow rechallenge with a sulfonamide diuretic may be successful in overcoming sulfa sensitivity.

LOOP DIURETICS. Loop diuretics are usually needed in the treatment of hypertensive patients with renal insufficiency, defined here as a serum creatinine level exceeding 1.5 mg/dl. Furosemide has been most widely used, although metolazone may be as effective and requires only a single daily dose. Many physicians use furosemide in the management of uncomplicated hypertension, but this drug provides less antihypertensive action when given once or twice a day than do longer acting diuretics, which maintain the slight volume contraction that is needed for the antihypertensive effect of diuretics.

POTASSIUM-SPARING AGENTS. These drugs are normally used in combination with a thiazide diuretic. Of the four currently available, two (eplerenone and spironolactone) are aldosterone antagonists; the other two (triamterene and amiloride) are direct inhibitors of potassium secretion. In combination with a thiazide diuretic, they diminish the amount of potassium wasting. Although they are more expensive than thiazides alone, they may decrease the total cost of therapy by reducing the need to monitor and treat potassium depletion. Moreover, low doses of spironolactone have been found to prevent myocardial fibrosis and reduce mortality in patients with heart failure.[53]

Eplerenone is a more selective aldosterone antagonist than spironolactone and exerts an impressive antihypertensive effect without the gynecomastia and menstrual irregularities sometimes seen with spironolactone.[54] In view of the increasing evidence that even normal levels of aldosterone induce fibrosis in various tissues,[55] such a selective aldosterone blocker may find much wider use as a potassium sparer.

An Overview of Diuretics in Hypertension

A low dose of a thiazide diuretic should almost always be the initial choice of drug therapy for most hypertensives. If not the first choice, a diuretic should certainly be the second drug used. In those with more severe hypertension or renal damage, larger doses of a thiazide or a loop-acting agent are needed. The potential for multiple adverse effects that can be associated with diuretics requires appropriate surveillance but, overall, they remain the least expensive choice and one that may provide other benefits, e.g., protection against osteoporosis, as well.

Adrenergic Inhibitors

A number of drugs that inhibit the adrenergic nervous system are available, including some that act centrally on vasomotor center activity, peripherally on neuronal catecholamine discharge, or by blocking alpha- or beta-adrenergic receptors, or both (Table 38–8); some act at numerous sites. Figure 38–10, a schematic view of the ending of an adrenergic nerve and the effector cell with its receptors, depicts how some of these drugs act.

An important aspect of sympathetic activity involves the feedback of norepinephrine to alpha- and beta-adrenergic receptors located on the neuronal surface, i.e., presynaptic receptors. Presynaptic alpha-adrenergic receptor activation inhibits release, whereas presynaptic beta activation stimulates further norepinephrine release. The presynaptic receptors have a role in the action of some of the drugs to be discussed.

Drugs That Act Within the Neuron

Reserpine, guanethidine, and related compounds act differently to inhibit the release of norepinephrine from peripheral adrenergic neurons.

RESERPINE. Reserpine, the most active and widely used of the derivatives of the rauwolfia alkaloids, depletes the postganglionic adrenergic neurons of norepinephrine by inhibiting its uptake into storage vesicles, exposing it to degradation by cytoplasmic monoamine oxidase. The peripheral effect is predominant, although the drug enters the brain and depletes central catecholamine stores as well. This effect probably accounts for the sedation and depression accompanying reserpine use. The drug has certain advantages: only one dose a day is needed; in combination with a diuretic, the antihypertensive effect is significant; little postural hypotension is noted; and many patients experience no side effects. The drug has a relatively flat dose-response curve, so that a dose of only 0.05 mg/d gives almost as much antihypertensive effect as 0.125

TABLE 38–8 Adrenergic Inhibitors Used in Treatment of Hypertension

Peripheral Neuronal Inhibitors
Reserpine
Guanethidine (Ismelin)
Guanadrel (Hylorel)
Bethanidine (Tenathan)
Central Adrenergic Inhibitors
Methyldopa (Aldomet)
Clonidine (Catapres)
Guanabenz (Wytensin)
Guanfacine (Tenex)
Alpha Receptor Blockers
Alpha$_1$ and alpha$_2$ receptor
Phenoxybenzamine (Dibenzyline)
Phentolamine (Regitine)
Alpha$_1$ receptor
Doxazosin (Cardura)
Prazosin (Minipress)
Terazosin (Hytrin)
Beta Receptor Blockers
Acebutolol (Sectral)
Atenolol (Tenormin)
Betaxolol (Kerlone)
Bisoprolol (Zebeta)
Carteolol (Cartrol)
Metoprolol (Lopressor, Toprol)
Nadolol (Corgard)
Penbutolol (Levatol)
Pindolol (Visken)
Propranolol (Inderal)
Timolol (Blocadren)
Alpha and Beta Receptor Blockers
Labetalol (Normodyne, Trandate)
Carvedilol (Coreg)

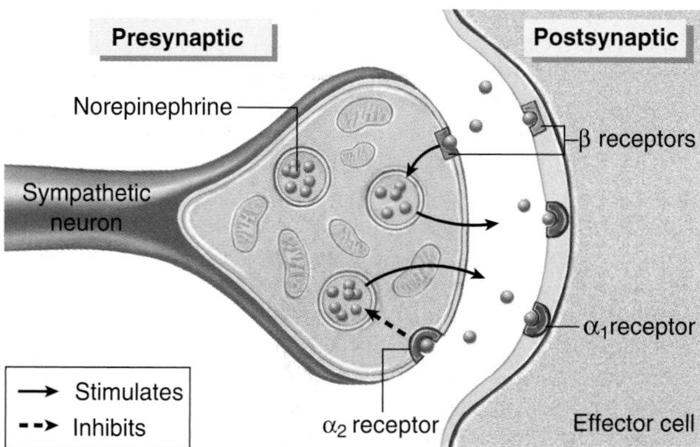

FIGURE 38–10 Simplified schematic view of the adrenergic nerve ending showing that norepinephrine (NE) is released from its storage granules when the nerve is stimulated and enters the synaptic cleft to bind to alpha$_1$ and beta receptors on the effector cell (postsynaptic). In addition, a short feedback loop exists in which NE binds to alpha$_2$ and beta receptors on the neuron (presynaptic) to inhibit or to stimulate further release, respectively.

or 0.25 mg/d but with fewer side effects. Although it remains popular in some places and is recommended as an inexpensive choice where resources are limited, use of reserpine has progressively declined because it has no commercial sponsor.

GUANETHIDINE. This agent and a series of related guanidine compounds, including guanadrel, bethanidine, and debrisoquine, act by inhibiting the release of norepinephrine from the adrenergic neurons. Blood pressure is reduced mainly when the patient is upright, owing to gravitational pooling of blood in the legs, because compensatory sympathetic nervous system–mediated vasoconstriction is blocked. This effect results in the most common side effect, postural hypotension. Unlike reserpine, guanethidine has a steep dose-response curve, so that it can be successfully used in treating hypertension of any degree in daily doses of 10 to 300 mg. As other drugs have become available, guanethidine and related compounds have been relegated mainly to the treatment of severe hypertension unresponsive to all other agents.

Drugs That Act on Receptors

Predominantly Central Alpha-Agonists

Of these, only clonidine has much current use, although methyldopa remains one of the few drugs approved for treatment of pregnancy-induced hypertension (see also Chap. 74).

METHYLDOPA. The primary site of action of methyldopa is within the central nervous system, where alpha-methylnorepinephrine, derived from methyldopa, is released from adrenergic neurons and stimulates central alpha-adrenergic receptors, reducing the sympathetic outflow from the central nervous system. The blood pressure falls mainly as a result of a decrease in peripheral resistance with little effect on cardiac output. Renal blood flow is well maintained, and significant postural hypotension is unusual.

Methyldopa need be given no more than twice daily, in doses ranging from 250 to 3000 mg/d.

Side effects include some that are common to centrally acting drugs that reduce sympathetic outflow: sedation, dry mouth, impotence, and galactorrhea. However, methyldopa causes some unique side effects that are probably of an autoimmune nature because a positive antinuclear antibody test result is obtained in about 10 percent of patients who take the drug, and red cell autoantibodies occur in about 20 percent. Inflammatory disorders in various organs have been reported, most commonly involving the liver (with diffuse parenchymal injury similar to that in viral hepatitis).

CLONIDINE. Although of different structure, clonidine shares many features with methyldopa. It acts at the same central sites, has similar antihypertensive efficacy, and causes many of the same bothersome but less

serious side effects (e.g., sedation, dry mouth). It does not, however, induce the autoimmune and inflammatory side effects.

The drug has a fairly short biological half-life, so that when it is discontinued, the inhibition of norepinephrine release disappears within about 12 to 18 hours and plasma catecholamine levels rise. This effect is responsible for the rapid rebound of the blood pressure to pretreatment levels and the occasional appearance of withdrawal symptoms, including tachycardia, restlessness, and sweating. If the rebound requires treatment, clonidine may be reintroduced or alpha-adrenergic receptor antagonists given.

Clonidine is available in a *transdermal* preparation, which may provide smoother blood pressure control for as long as 7 days with fewer side effects. Bothersome skin rashes preclude its use in perhaps one fourth of patients, however.

GUANABENZ. This drug differs in structure from but shares many characteristics with both methyldopa and clonidine, acting primarily as a central alpha-agonist.

GUANFACINE. This drug is also similar to clonidine but is longer acting, which enables once-daily dosing and minimizes rebound hypertension. This agent, although used less than clonidine, is the preferred choice of a central alpha-agonist.

Alpha-Adrenergic Receptor Antagonists

These agents may have many attractive features but their use has been limited, initially because of the potential for postural hypotension, more recently because of a greater likelihood of fluid retention that may provoke congestive heart failure.[56] The first of this class was prazosin but the two now used, doxazosin and terazosin, have slower onset and longer duration of action so that they may be given once daily with less propensity for first-dose hypotension.

Selective alpha blockers are as effective as other antihypertensives.[38] When given to patients whose condition is poorly controlled by two or more agents, they may reduce blood pressure even more than anticipated. The favorable hemodynamic changes—a fall in peripheral resistance with maintenance of cardiac output—make them an attractive choice for patients who wish to remain physically active. In addition, blood lipids and insulin sensitivity are not adversely altered and may actually improve with alpha blockers, unlike the adverse effects observed with diuretics and beta blockers.[57]

Despite these attractive features, alpha blockers have not been widely used for hypertension. Their use is likely to diminish further because of the ALLHAT trial data.[56] In this large, double-blind, randomized trial involving older patients with hypertension, the alpha-adrenergic blocker doxazosin, when compared with the diuretic chlorthalidone, was associated with significantly higher risks for stroke and congestive heart failure but no increase in mortality.

The higher risk of stroke could be due to the lesser reduction of blood pressure with the alpha blocker than the diuretic. The design of the study may be largely responsible for the increased risk of congestive heart failure. Many of the enrollees were at high risk for heart failure and had to stop abruptly whatever drugs they had been taking, including diuretics or ACEIs, that were effectively keeping them out of failure, and switched to 1 mg of doxazosin. The resultant fluid retention may have precipitated congestive heart failure.

Nonetheless, the ALLHAT data clearly indicate the need to use a diuretic with the alpha blocker, particularly in those with LVH or other risk factors for congestive heart failure. Meanwhile, alpha blockers are now being used primarily for relief of prostatism. By decreasing the tone of the smooth muscle at the bladder neck and prostate, they relieve the obstructive symptoms of prostatic hypertrophy.

Beta-Adrenergic Receptor Antagonists (see also Chaps. 23 and 50)

In the 1980s, beta-adrenergic receptor blockers became the most popular form of antihypertensive therapy after diuretics, reflecting their relative effectiveness and freedom from many bothersome side effects. Because beta blockers have been found to reduce mortality if taken either before or after acute myocardial infarction (i.e., secondary prevention), it was assumed that they might offer special protection against initial coronary events (i.e., primary prevention). However, in large clinical trials, a beta blocker provided less protection than did a low-dose diuretic (see Table 38–5).[43] Nevertheless, their efficacy in treatment of congestive heart failure has stimulated their use.

THE VARIOUS BETA BLOCKERS. Beta blockers now available in the United States are shown in Figure 38–11. Pharmacologically, those now available differ considerably from one another with respect to degree of absorption, protein binding, and bioavailability. However, the three most important differences affecting their clinical use are cardioselectivity, intrinsic sympathomimetic activity, and lipid solubility. Despite these differences, they all seem to be about equally effective as antihypertensives.

Cardioselectivity. Cardioselectivity refers to the relative blocking effect on the $beta_1$-adrenergic receptors in the heart compared with that on the $beta_2$ receptors in the bronchi, peripheral blood vessels, and elsewhere. Such cardioselectivity can easily be shown using small doses in acute studies; with the rather high doses used to treat hypertension, much of this selectivity is lost. However, more cardioprotective drugs may be better tolerated in patients with reactive airway disease or peripheral vascular disease.[58]

Intrinsic Sympathomimetic Activity. Some of these drugs have intrinsic sympathomimetic activity, interacting with beta receptors to cause a measurable agonist response but at the same time blocking the greater agonist effects of endogenous catecholamines. As a result, although in usual doses they lower the blood pressure about the same degree as do other beta blockers, they cause a smaller decline in heart rate, cardiac output, and renin levels.

Lipid Solubility. Atenolol and nadolol are among the least lipid soluble of the beta blockers so that they escape hepatic metabolism and are excreted unchanged. Lipid-soluble agents, e.g., metoprolol and propranolol, are taken up and metabolized in the liver and so are more bioavailable after intravenous than oral administration.

Mechanism of Action. Despite these and other differences, the various beta blockers now available are approximately equipotent as antihypertensive agents. A number of possible mechanisms are likely to be involved in their antihypertensive action. For those without intrinsic sympathomimetic activity, cardiac output falls 15 to 20 percent and renin release is reduced about 60 percent. Central nervous system beta-adrenergic receptor blockade may reduce sympathetic discharge.

At the same time that beta blockers lower blood pressure through various means, their blockade of peripheral beta-adrenergic receptors inhibits vasodilation, leaving alpha receptors open to catecholamine-mediated vasoconstriction. Over time, however, vascular resistance tends to return to normal, which presumably preserves the antihypertensive effect of a reduced cardiac output.

Clinical Effects. Even in small doses, beta blockers begin to lower the blood pressure within a few hours. Although progressively higher doses have usually been given, careful study has shown a near-maximal effect from smaller doses. Beta blockers are particularly well suited for younger and middle-aged hypertensive patients, especially nonblacks, and for patients with tachyarrhythmias, myocardial ischemia, and high levels of stress. Because the hemodynamic responses to physical stress are reduced, however, they may interfere with the ability to exercise.

SPECIAL USES FOR BETA BLOCKERS

COEXISTING ISCHEMIC HEART DISEASE. Even without evidence that beta blockers protect patients from initial coronary events, the antiarrhythmic and antianginal effects of these drugs make them especially valuable in hypertensive patients with coexisting coronary disease.

COEXISTING HEART FAILURE. As described elsewhere (see Chap. 23), beta blockers have been found to reduce mortality in patients with congestive heart failure.

HYPERKINETIC HYPERTENSION. Some hypertensive patients have increased cardiac output that may persist for many years. Beta blockers should be particularly effective in such patients but may reduce their ability to exercise.

MARKED ANXIETY. The somatic manifestations of anxiety—tremor, sweating, and tachycardia—can be helped without the undesirable effects of methods commonly used to control anxiety, such as alcohol and tranquilizers.

PERIOPERATIVE STRESS. Beta blockers have been found to reduce cardiovascular events in high-risk patients who have noncardiac surgery.[59]

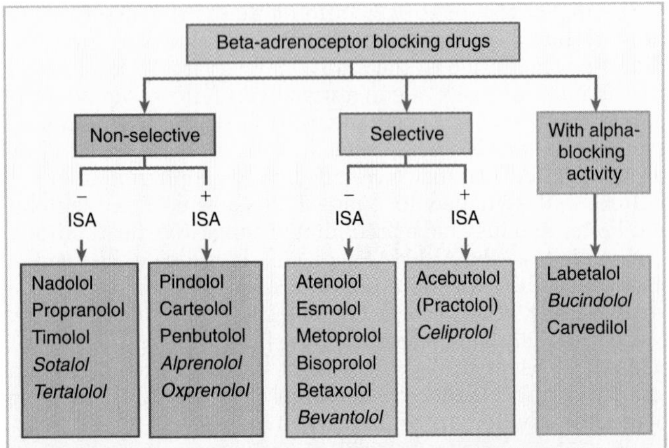

FIGURE 38–11 Classification of beta-adrenoreceptor blockers on the basis of cardioselectivity and intrinsic sympathomimetic activity. Drugs not approved for use in the United States for treatment of hypertension are in italics. ISA = intrinsic sympathomimetic activity. (Modified from Kaplan NM: Kaplan's Clinical Hypertension. 8th ed. Baltimore, Lippincott Williams & Wilkins, 2002, p 262.)

SIDE EFFECTS. Most of the side effects of beta blockers are related to their major pharmacological action, the blockade of beta-adrenergic receptors. Certain concomitant problems may worsen when beta-adrenergic receptors are blocked, including peripheral vascular disease and bronchospasm. However, in a meta-analysis of 29 studies, cardioselective beta blockers did not have clinically significant adverse respiratory effects in patients with mild to moderate reactive airway disease or chronic obstructive pulmonary disease, leading the authors to conclude that these drugs should not be withheld from such patients who have an indication for their use.[58]

The most common side effect is fatigue, probably a consequence of decreased cardiac output and peripheral and cerebral blood flow. Sexual dysfunction was also increased by use of beta blockers in RCTs involving patients with myocardial infarction, congestive heart failure, or hypertension, but depression was not.[60] However, the effect on depression remains uncertain and others have reported an increase in suicide among users of beta blockers compared with ACEIs or CCBs.[61]

The use of beta blockers increases the incidence of diabetes,[62] presumably through a decrease in insulin sensitivity. Diabetic patients may have additional problems with beta blockers, more so with nonselective ones. The responses to hypoglycemia, both the symptoms (except sweating) and the counterregulatory hormonal changes that raise blood glucose levels, are partially dependent on sympathetic nervous activity. Diabetic patients who are susceptible to hypoglycemia may not be aware of the usual warning signals and may not rebound as quickly.

Perturbations of lipoprotein metabolism accompany the use of beta blockers. Nonselective agents cause greater rises in triglycerides and reductions in cardioprotective high-density lipoprotein cholesterol levels. When a beta blocker is suddenly discontinued, angina pectoris and myocardial infarction may occur. Because patients with hypertension are more susceptible to coronary disease, they should be weaned gradually and given appropriate coronary vasodilator therapy.

Caution is advised in the use of beta blockers in patients suspected of harboring a pheochromocytoma (see Chaps. 37 and 79) because unopposed alpha-adrenergic agonist action may precipitate a serious hypertensive crisis if this disease is present. The use of beta blockers during pregnancy has been clouded by scattered case reports of various fetal problems.

AN OVERVIEW OF BETA BLOCKERS IN HYPERTENSION. Beta blockers are specifically recommended for hypertensive patients with concomitant coronary disease, particularly after a myocardial infarction, congestive heart failure, or tachyarrhythmias (see Table 38–4). If a beta blocker is chosen, the agents that are more cardioselective offer the likelihood of fewer perturbations of lipid and carbohydrate metabolism and greater adherence of patients to therapy; only one dose a day is needed, and side effects are probably minimized.

Alpha- and Beta-Adrenergic Receptor Antagonists

The combination of an alpha and a beta blocker in a single molecule is available in the forms of labetalol and carvedilol, with the latter agent approved for treatment of heart failure as well. The fall in pressure results mainly from a decrease in peripheral resistance, with little or no decline in cardiac output. The most bothersome side effects are related to postural hypotension; the most serious side effect is hepatoxicity. Intravenous labetalol is used to treat hypertensive emergencies.

Vasodilators

In the past, direct-acting arteriolar vasodilators were used mainly as third drugs, when combinations of a diuretic and adrenergic blocker failed to control blood pressure. However, with the availability of vasodilators of different types, i.e., ACEIs, ARBs, and CCBs, which can be easily tolerated when used as first or second drugs, wider and earlier application of vasodilators in therapy of hypertension has evolved.

Direct Vasodilators

Hydralazine is the most widely used agent of this type. Minoxidil is more potent but is usually reserved for patients with severe, refractory hypertension associated with renal failure. Nitroprusside and nitroglycerin are given intravenously for hypertensive crises and are discussed later (see Therapy for Hypertensive Crises).

HYDRALAZINE. Hydralazine, in combination with a diuretic and a beta blocker, has been used frequently to treat severe hypertension. The drug acts directly to relax the smooth muscle in precapillary resistance vessels, with little or no effect on postcapillary venous capacitance vessels. As a result, blood pressure falls by a reduction in peripheral resistance, but in the process a number of compensatory processes, which are activated by the arterial baroreceptor arc, blunt the decrease in pressure and cause side effects. With concomitant use of a diuretic to overcome the tendency for fluid retention and an adrenergic inhibitor to prevent the reflex increase in sympathetic activity and rise in renin, the vasodilator is more effective and causes few, if any, side effects.

The drug need be given only twice a day. Its daily dose should be kept below 400 mg to prevent the lupus-like syndrome that appears in 10 to 20 percent of patients who receive more. This reaction, although uncomfortable to the patient, is almost always reversible. The reaction is uncommon with daily doses of 200 mg or less and is more common in slow acetylators of the drug.

MINOXIDIL. This drug vasodilates by opening potassium channels in vascular smooth muscle. Its hemodynamic effects are similar to those of hydralazine, but minoxidil is even more effective and may be used once a day. It is particularly useful in patients with severe hypertension and renal failure. Even more than with hydralazine, diuretics and adrenergic receptor blockers must be used with minoxidil to prevent the reflex increase in cardiac output and fluid retention. Pericardial effusions have appeared in about 3 percent of those given minoxidil, in some without renal or cardiac failure. The drug also causes hair to grow profusely, and the facial hirsutism precludes use of the drug in most women.

Calcium Channel Blockers (see also Chap. 50)

These drugs are among the most popular classes of agents used in the treatment of hypertension. Claims of multiple serious side effects of their use, mostly based on biased observational studies, have been repudiated by data from multiple RCTs including ALLHAT, wherein coronary events were the same for the CCB as for the diuretic or ACEI and mortality from noncardiovascular causes was significantly lower in the CCB group than the diuretic or ACEI group.[2]

MECHANISMS OF ACTION. All currently available CCBs interact with the same L-type voltage-gated plasma membrane channel but at different sites and with different consequences. DHPs have the greatest peripheral vasodilatory action with little effect on cardiac automaticity, conduction, or contractility. However, comparative trials have shown that verapamil and diltiazem, which do affect these properties, are also effective antihypertensives, and they may cause fewer side effects related to vasodilation, such as flushing and ankle edema.

CLINICAL USE. CCBs are effective in hypertensive patients of all ages and races.[42] Against placebo in RCTs, DHP-CCBs reduced cardiovascular events and deaths (see Table 38–6).[44] Compared with other classes of drugs, they may protect better against stroke but less well against heart failure.[2,44]

CCBs have been found to be particularly effective in prevention of stroke in elderly hypertensives, perhaps because they tend to have a greater antihypertensive effect than seen in younger patients.[63] They also appear to lower blood pressure in blacks better than other classes,[64] but with equal degrees of blood pressure reduction as among the blacks in the ALLHAT trial,[2] they are no better in cardioprotection than a diuretic or an ACEI.

Calcium antagonists may cause at least an initial natriuresis, probably by producing renal vasodilation, which may lessen the need for concurrent diuretic therapy. In fact, unlike all other antihypertensive agents, they may have their effectiveness reduced rather than enhanced by concomitant dietary sodium restriction, whereas most careful studies show an enhancement of their effect by concomitant diuretic therapy.[65]

The use of CCBs has been contentious in two important groups of hypertensives: those with diabetes and those with nephropathy. Concerning the use of CCBs in patients with type 2 diabetes, a DHP-CCB, nitrendipine, provided excellent protection in those enrolled in the Systolic Hypertension in Europe (Syst-Eur) trial, even better than that provided by a diuretic in the SHEP trial.[66] Therapy based on the DHP-CCB felodipine provided a 51 percent reduction in major cardiovascular events in the 1501 patients with diabetes enrolled in the HOT trial.[14] Among the almost 12,000 diabetics in the ALLHAT trial, the CCB amlodipine was as protective as the ACEI or diuretic.[2]

Concerning the use of CCBs in patients with nephropathy, experts agree that an ACEI or ARB should be the first drug used.[67] However, in order to provide the degree of blood pressure reduction required to protect such patients maximally, additional drugs are almost always required. A CCB is an appropriate choice as the third drug, with a diuretic as the second. Clearly, a CCB is not as renoprotective as an ACEI[19] or an ARB[68] when used as the initial drug, but, if needed to achieve the goal of therapy, a CCB is just as clearly an appropriate addition.[69]

On the basis of a greater reduction in proteinuria seen with non–DHP-CCBs than with DHP-CCBs, some believe a non–DHP-CCB should be used.[67] However, the addition of a DHP-CCB does not interfere with the renoprotective effect of ACEIs or ARBs.[70] Moreover, renal function, assessed by estimated glomerular filtration rate, was better preserved by the DHP-CCB than by either the diuretic or the ACEI in ALLHAT.[2]

SIDE EFFECTS. Side effects preclude the use of these drugs in perhaps 10 percent of patients. Most side effects—headaches, flushing, local ankle edema—are related to the vasodilation for which the drugs are given. With slow-release and longer acting formulations, vasodilative side effects are reduced. It should be no surprise that, in a few patients, the antihypertensive effect of the short-acting agents, particularly liquid nifedipine, may be so marked as to reduce blood flow and induce ischemia of vital organs, calling for a moratorium on their use.[71]

A potentially serious adverse effect of the use of calcium antagonists to treat hypertension was described in a case-control study in which more hypertensive patients who had a myocardial infarction were taking short-acting calcium antagonists than hypertensive patients who had not had an infarct.[72] The most likely explanation for the finding is exclusion bias, which is an inherent problem with case-control studies in which the cases are at greater risk for the complication than the controls; i.e., higher risk patients are excluded from the control group but not from the case group.[73] The decrease in coronary events in large RCTs with *long-acting* DHPs is the best proof of the safety of these agents. Similar claims based on case-control studies that calcium antagonists increase cancer and gastrointestinal bleeding have also been refuted.[2]

Calcium antagonists may be unique in not having their antihypertensive efficacy blunted by nonsteroidal anti-inflammatory drugs (NSAIDs).[74]

AN OVERVIEW OF CALCIUM CHANNEL BLOCKERS. CCBs have been found to reduce stroke more but heart attacks less than other therapies while having similar effects on overall mortality.[44] They work well and are usually well tolerated across the entire spectrum of hypertensives. They have some particular niches: coexisting angina and cyclosporine or NSAID use. If chosen, an inherently long-acting, second-generation DHP seems the best choice because it maintains better blood pressure control in the critical early morning hours and on throughout the next day if the patient misses a dose.[75] Rate-slowing CCBs, e.g., verapamil or diltiazem, may be preferable in certain circumstances.

Angiotensin-Converting Enzyme Inhibitors

Activity of the renin-angiotensin system may be inhibited in four ways, three of which can be applied clinically. The first, use of beta-adrenergic receptor blockers to inhibit the release of renin, was discussed earlier. The second, direct inhibition of renin activity by specific renin inhibitors, is being investigated.[76] The third, inhibition of the enzyme that converts the inactive decapeptide angiotensin I to the active octapeptide AII, is being widely used with orally effective ACEIs. The fourth, blockade of angiotensin's actions by a competitive receptor blocker, is the basis for the fastest growing class of antihypertensive agents—the ARBs. ARBs may offer additional benefits, but their immediate advantage is the absence of cough that often accompanies ACEIs as well as less angioedema. The ARBs are considered after the ACEIs.

MECHANISM OF ACTION. The first of the ACEIs, captopril, was synthesized as a specific inhibitor of the converting enzyme that, in the classic pathway shown in Figure 86–1, breaks the peptidyl dipeptide bond in angiotensin I, preventing the enzyme from attaching to and splitting the angiotensin I structure. Because AII cannot be formed and angiotensin I is inactive, the ACEI paralyzes the classic renin-angiotensin system, thereby removing the effects of most endogenous AII as both a vasoconstrictor and a stimulant to aldosterone synthesis.

Interestingly, with long-term use of ACEIs, the plasma AII levels actually return to previous values while the blood pressure remains lowered,[77] which suggests that the antihypertensive effect may involve other mechanisms. Because the same enzyme that converts angiotensin I to AII is also responsible for inactivation of the vasodilating hormone bradykinin by inhibiting the breakdown of bradykinin, ACEIs increase the concentration of a vasodilating hormone while they decrease the concentration of a vasoconstrictor hormone. The increased plasma kinin levels may contribute to the vasodilation and other beneficial effects of ACEIs,[78] but they are also probably responsible for the most common and bothersome side effects of their use, a dry, hacking cough and, less frequently, angioedema.[79]

Regardless of their mechanism of action, ACEIs lower blood pressure mainly by reducing peripheral resistance with little, if any, effect on heart rate, cardiac output, or body fluid volumes, probably reflecting preservation of baroreceptor reflexes.[80] As they restore endothelium-dependent relaxation, resistance arteries become less thickened and more responsive.[81]

CLINICAL USE. In patients with uncomplicated primary hypertension, ACEIs as monotherapy provide antihypertensive effects that are equal to those with other classes, but they are somewhat less effective in blacks and elderly people because of their lower renin levels.[42] Addition of a diuretic, even as little as 6.25 mg of hydrochlorothiazide, enhances the efficacy of an ACEI.[82] More important, ACEI-based therapy has provided significant protection against cardiovascular disease and death when compared against placebo and comparable if not better protection than other classes of drugs (see Table 38–6).[44] In the ALLHAT trial involving predominantly elderly, high-risk hypertensives, ACEI-based therapy was equal to diuretic- or CCB-based therapies in most regards except against strokes in the black enrollees,[2] probably because of less antihypertensive efficacy. In the Australian National Blood Pressure Study, involving elderly but lower risk hypertensives, ACEI-based therapy provided better protection against cardiovascular events than diuretic-based therapy for the men but not for the women.[47]

ACEIs have been impressively effective in treatment of hypertensives (and nonhypertensives) with coronary disease or congestive heart failure as detailed in Chapters 23 and 50. Another area in which they have become the drug of choice is chronic renal disease, whether diabetic[67] or nondiabetic[83] in origin. The high levels of renin, arising in the JG cells within the renal afferent arterioles, flood the glomeruli and renal efferent arterioles, providing ACEIs (and ARBs) the opportunity to dilate these vessels selectively and lower intraglomerular pressure more effectively than other classes of drugs. These hemodynamic effects may lower renal perfusion and glomerular filtration. However, because acute increases of serum creatinine of up to 30 percent that stabilize within the first 2 months of ACEI therapy are associated with *better* long-term renoprotection,[84] such rises should not prompt withdrawal of the drug.

Whether ACEIs (and ARBs) provide renal (and cardiac) protection beyond their antihypertensive effects remains in question. The issue has been most intensively studied in patients with proteinuria because it is so easy to measure. Controlled trials suggest that the antiproteinuric effect of an ACEI is directly related to its antihypertensive effect,[85] but there are inadequate data to be sure. As noted later (see Angiotensin II Receptor Blockers, Clinical Use), the potential for an additional antihypertensive effect of an ARB added to an ACEI also remains uncertain.

These drugs have been a mixed blessing for patients with renovascular hypertension. On the one hand, they usually control the blood pressure effectively.[86] On the other hand, the removal of the high levels of AII that they produce may deprive the stenotic kidney of the hormonal drive to its blood flow, thereby causing a marked decline in renal perfusion so that patients with solitary kidneys or bilateral disease may develop acute and sometimes persistent renal failure.

Another potential special indication for ACEI therapy may be in protection against recurrent stroke. In a study of 6105 patients who had a history of prior stroke or transient ischemic attack, the ACEI perindopril plus a diuretic provided a 43 percent relative reduction in recurrent stroke.[87] By itself, the ACEI had an inconsequential effect.

SIDE EFFECTS. Most patients who take an ACEI experience neither the side effects nor the biochemical changes often accompanying other drugs that may be of even more concern even though they are not as obvious; neither rises in lipids, glucose, or uric acid nor reductions in potassium levels are noted. To be sure, ACEIs may have both specific and nonspecific adverse effects. Among the specific ones are rare rashes, loss of taste, and leukopenia. In addition, they may cause a hypersensitivity reaction with angioneurotic edema[79] or a cough that, although often persistent, is infrequently associated with pulmonary dysfunction.[88] The cough, affecting more than 10 percent of women and about half as many men, may not disappear for 3 weeks after the ACEI is discontinued. If a cough appears in a patient who needs an ACEI, an ARB should be substituted.

The antihypertensive efficacy of ACEIs may be blunted by large (300 mg) doses of aspirin and most NSAIDs, with the apparent exception of celecoxib.[89] Finally, patients with renal insufficiency or those taking potassium supplements or potassium-sparing agents may not be able to excrete potassium loads and therefore may develop hyperkalemia.[90]

AN OVERVIEW OF ANGIOTENSIN-CONVERTING ENZYME INHIBITORS. The rationale for the use of ACEIs in the treatment of hypertension has steadily expanded beyond their proven efficacy as antihypertensive agents. In particular, they have been shown to provide special advantages in three large groups of patients: those with heart failure, coronary ischemia, or nephropathy. As seen in Table 38–4, they are clearly the drugs of choice for such patients. Moreover, the evidence from the Heart Outcomes Prevention Evaluation (HOPE) trial[91] has led to the recommendation that an ACEI be given to all patients at high risk for coronary disease, whether hypertensive or not. Although an ACEI-based therapy did not outperform a diuretic or a CCB in the ALLHAT trial,[2] their proven special benefits ensure their continued growth.

Even as ACEIs have become increasingly popular, their position has been threatened by the introduction of ARBs, agents acting at a more distal site of the renin-angiotensin system.

Angiotensin II Receptor Blockers

MECHANISMS OF ACTION. ARBs displace AII from its specific AT_1 receptor, antagonizing all of its known effects and resulting in a dose-dependent fall in peripheral resistance and little change in heart rate or cardiac output.[92] As a consequence of the competitive displacement, circulating levels of AII increase and at the same time the blockade of the renin-angiotensin mechanism is more complete, including any AII that is generated through pathways that do not involve ACEI. No obvious good or bad effects of the increased AII levels have been noted (along with the higher renin levels, as seen with ACEIs).

The major obvious difference between ARBs and ACEIs is the absence of an increase in kinin levels that may be responsible for some of the beneficial effects of ACEIs and probably even more of their side effects. Direct comparisons between the two types of drugs show little difference in antihypertensive efficacy, but cough is not provoked by the ARB[93] although angioedema has been reported.[94] Losartan has a uricosuric effect that is not seen with other ARBs.[95] As seen with ACEIs, ARBs have been found to improve endothelial dysfunction[96] and correct the altered structure of resistance arteries in patients with hypertension.[97]

CLINICAL USE. In the recommended doses, all six currently available ARBs have comparable antihypertensive efficacy and all are potentiated by addition of a diuretic. The dose-response curve is fairly flat for all, although increasing doses of candesartan have an increasing effect.[98] Moreover, in this study, the effect of candesartan persisted for 36 hours after a purposely missed dose whereas the effect of losartan was largely dissipated after 12 hours.

The addition of ARB to a presumed maximal dose of an ACEI was not shown to increase the antihypertensive effect[99] but did reduce the progression of nondiabetic nephropathy.[100] ARB-based therapy has been shown to reduce the progress of renal damage in patients with type 2 diabetes with nephropathy.[68,70,101] Their use in heart failure is described in Chapter 23. Therapy based on the ARB losartan caused LVH to regress and reduced the number of cardiovascular events more than therapy based on the beta blocker atenolol in the LIFE trial of hypertensives with LVH.[48]

SIDE EFFECTS. Whether or not they are more effective than ACEIs, ARBs are easier to take. In various clinical trials, side effects were generally no greater than with placebo, and the agent was better tolerated than other antihypertensive agents. Fetal toxicity, hyperkalemia, hypotension, and renal impairment are almost certain to be noted occasionally because they are expected consequences of blockade of the renin-angiotensin mechanism, but, as yet, no major surprises have surfaced.

OVERVIEW OF ANGIOTENSIN II RECEPTOR BLOCKERS. As reflected in the fast growth of the use of ARBs, they are surely being prescribed for many more patients than the 10 percent or so who are intolerant of an ACEI. With the intensely competitive market for the six (or more) of these agents now being heavily promoted, their use will surely continue to grow. However, caution is advised; additional outcome data are needed to know whether they are as good as the proven ACEIs. All current expert guidelines recommend ARBs only for those who should receive an ACEI but are intolerant, usually because of cough. Many outcome trials now in progress should provide proof of their value beyond that found in type II diabetic nephropathy.[102]

Other Agents

The first of the most promising new class of drugs, neutral endopeptidase inhibitors, was waylaid by a high incidence of angioedema. An old vasodilator now used extensively for coronary ischemia, the nitrate isosorbide, has been shown to be an attractive agent[103] but is not likely to be tested properly because of the lack of a commercial sponsor. Meanwhile, glitazones, which are now used for the treatment of diabetes, have been shown to lower blood pressure in nondiabetic hypertensives, logically as a consequence of improved insulin sensitivity.[104]

Special Considerations in Therapy

WITHDRAWAL OF DRUGS. As many as 20 percent of treated patients with well-controlled hypertension are able to maintain normotension for as long as 1 year after withdrawal of their drugs.[105] Considering how difficult it may be to achieve adequate control, withdrawal seems inappropriate if the therapy is causing no adverse effects.

RESISTANT HYPERTENSION. There are numerous causes of resistance to therapy, usually defined as the failure of diastolic blood pressure to fall below 90 mm Hg despite the use of three or more drugs (Table 38–9). Patients often do not respond well because they do not take their medications. On the other hand, what appears to be a poor response on the basis of office readings of blood pressure may be disclosed to be an adequate response when ambulatory or home readings are obtained.[106] A number of factors may be responsible for a poor response even if the appropriate medication is taken regularly. Most common is volume overload owing either to inadequate diuretic or to excessive dietary sodium intake. Larger doses or more potent diuretics often bring resistant hypertension under control.

ANESTHESIA IN HYPERTENSIVE PATIENTS. In the absence of significant cardiac dysfunction, hypertension adds little to the cardiovascular risks of surgery. If possible, however, hypertension should be well controlled by means of medications before anesthesia and surgery to reduce the risk of myocardial ischemia. Therefore, patients taking antihypertensive medications should continue these drugs, if necessary using dermal or intravenous formulations, as long as the anesthesiologist is aware of their use and takes reasonable precautions to prevent wide swings in pressure. The very short-acting beta blocker esmolol has been successful in preventing surges in blood pressure during intubation, and the use of the beta blocker bisoprolol reduced cardiac events in high-risk patients undergoing vascular surgery.[107]

Hypertension is often observed during and immediately after coronary bypass surgery (see Chap. 50). Various intravenous agents have been used successfully to lower the pressure. Nitroprusside has been the usual choice during the postoperative period, but esmolol, labetalol, or nicardipine may be better choices.

HYPERTENSIVE CHILDREN. Almost nothing is known about the effects of various antihypertensive medications given to children over long periods. In the absence of adequate data, an approach similar to that advocated for adults is advised.[108] Emphasis should be placed on weight reduction in hypertensive children who are obese in the hope of attempting to control hypertension without the need for drug therapy.

HYPERTENSION DURING PREGNANCY. This topic is discussed in Chapters 37 and 74.

HYPERTENSION IN ELDERLY PERSONS. Some elderly persons may have high blood pressure as measured by the sphygmomanometer but may have less or no hypertension when direct intraarterial readings are made, i.e., pseudohypertension related to rigid arteries that do not collapse under the cuff.

If either the systolic pressure alone or both systolic and diastolic levels are elevated, careful lowering of blood pressure with either diuretics or DHP calcium antagonists has been unequivocally documented to reduce cardiovascular morbidity in older hypertensive patients,[12] extending to those older than 80 years.[5] Care is needed because they may have a number of problems with the medications (Table 38–10). In view of the reduced effectiveness of the baroceptor reflex and the failure of peripheral resistance to rise appropriately with

TABLE 38–9 Causes of Inadequate Responsiveness to Therapy

Pseudoresistance	
"White coat" or office elevations	
Pseudohypertension in the elderly	
Nonadherence to Therapy	
Side effects of medication	
Cost of medication	
Lack of consistent and continuous primary care	
Inconvenient and chaotic dosing schedules	
Instructions not understood	
Inadequate education of patients	
Organic brain syndrome (e.g., memory deficit)	
Drug-Related Causes	
Doses too low	
Inappropriate combinations (e.g., two centrally acting adrenergic inhibitors)	
Rapid inactivation (e.g., hydralazine)	
Drug interactions	
Nonsteroidal antiinflammatory drugs	Oral contraceptives
Sympathomimetics	Adrenal steroids
Nasal decongestants	Licorice (chewing tobacco)
Appetite suppressants	Cyclosporine
Cocaine	Erythropoietin
Caffeine	Cholestyramine
Antidepressants (monoamine oxidase inhibitors, tricyclics)	
Excessive volume contraction with stimulation of renin and aldosterone	
Hypokalemia (usually diuretic induced)	
Rebound after clonidine withdrawal	
Associated Conditions	
Smoking	
Increasing obesity	
Sleep apnea	
Insulin resistance or hyperinsulinemia	
Ethanol intake more than 1 oz/d (>three portions)	
Anxiety-induced hyperventilation or panic attacks	
Chronic pain	
Intense vasoconstriction (Raynaud, arteritis)	
Secondary Hypertension	
Renal insufficiency	
Renovascular hypertension	
Pheochromocytoma	
Primary aldosteronism	
Volume Overload	
Excess sodium intake	
Progressive renal damage (nephrosclerosis)	
Fluid retention related to reduction of blood pressure	
Indequate diuretic therapy	

Modified from The sixth report of the Joint National Committee on Prevention, Detection, Evaluation and Treatment of High Blood Pressure. Arch Intern Med 157:2413, 1997. Copyright 1997, American Medical Association.

TABLE 38–10 Factors That Might Contribute to Increased Risk of Pharmacological Treatment of Hypertension in Elderly Persons	
Factors	**Potential Complications**
Diminished baroreceptor activity	Orthostatic hypotension
Decreased intravascular volume	Orthostatic hypotension, dehydration
Sensitivity to hypokalemia	Arrhythmia, muscle weakness
Decreased renal and hepatic function	Drug accumulation
Polypharmacy	Drug interaction
Central nervous system changes	Depression, confusion

standing, postural hypotension should be carefully looked for and, if present, addressed before starting antihypertensive therapy. All drugs should be given in slowly increasing doses to prevent excessive lowering of the pressure.

For those who start with systolic pressures exceeding 160 mm Hg, the goal of therapy should be a level around 140 mm Hg with caution about further reductions in already low diastolic levels.[16]

PATIENTS WITH HYPERTENSION AND DIABETES. Special attention should be given to diabetic patients with hypertension. The two commonly coexist and multiply the cardiovascular risks of each alone. Fortunately, evidence from several trials now documents the protection provided by *intensive* control of hypertension, in concert with management of the diabetes and the dyslipidemia that commonly accompanies the two. Most diabetic hypertensive patients need two or more antihypertensive drugs to bring their pressure to below 130/80 mm Hg, which is probably the highest level that should be tolerated. The benefits of such intensive management were clearly documented in a 7.8-year follow-up of 160 patients with type 2 diabetes and hypertension with microalbuminuria.[109] In the half given more intensive management, the risks of having a cardiovascular event, nephropathy, retinopathy, or autonomic neuropathy were all reduced by 50 percent or more.

An ACEI or ARB should be included if proteinuria is present. A diuretic and a beta blocker are appropriate, and a long-acting DHP is likely to be required.

HYPERTENSIVE PATIENTS WITH IMPOTENCE. Erectile dysfunction is common in hypertensive patients, even more so in those who are also diabetic. The problem may be exacerbated by diuretic therapy, even in appropriately low doses.[51] Fortunately, sildenafil usually returns erectile ability even in the presence of various antihypertensive drugs with no greater likelihood of adverse events than in those not receiving antihypertensive therapy.[110]

HYPERTENSION WITH CONGESTIVE HEART FAILURE. Cardiac output may fall so markedly in hypertensive patients who are in heart failure with systolic dysfunction that their blood pressure is reduced, obscuring the degree of hypertension; often, however, the diastolic blood pressure is raised by intense vasoconstriction while the systolic pressure falls as a result of the reduced stroke volume. Lowering the blood pressure may, by itself, relieve the heart failure. Chronic unloading has been most efficiently accomplished with ACEIs, and beta blockers have been shown to reduce morbidity and mortality further in ACEI-treated patients in heart failure.

As noted in Chapter 37, LVH is frequently found by echocardiography, even in patients with mild hypertension. All antihypertensive drugs except direct vasodilators have been shown to cause LVH to regress, and regression may continue for as long as 5 years of treatment.

HYPERTENSION WITH ISCHEMIC HEART DISEASE. The coexistence of ischemic heart disease makes antihypertensive therapy even more essential because relief of the hypertension may ameliorate the coronary disease. Beta blockers and calcium antagonists are particularly useful if angina or arrhythmias are present. Caution is needed to avoid decreased coronary perfusion that may be responsible for the J curve seen in several trials (see Goal of Therapy).[14]

The often markedly high levels of blood pressure during the early phase of an acute myocardial infarction may reflect sympathetic nervous hyperreactivity to pain. Antihypertensive drugs that do not decrease cardiac output may be utilized cautiously in the immediate postinfarction period, whereas beta blockers and ACEIs have been shown to provide long-term benefit.

Therapy for Hypertensive Crises

When diastolic blood pressure exceeds 140 mm Hg, rapidly progressive damage to the arterial vasculature is demonstrable experimentally, and a surge of cerebral blood flow may rapidly lead to encephalopathy (see Chap. 37). If such high pressures persist or if there are any signs of encephalopathy, the pressures should be lowered using parenteral agents in patients considered to be in immediate danger or oral agents in those who are alert and in no other acute distress.[111]

A number of drugs for this purpose are currently available (Table 38–11). If diastolic pressure exceeds 140 mm Hg and the patient has any complications, such as an aortic dissection, a constant infusion of nitroprusside is most effective and almost always lowers the pressure to the desired level. Constant monitoring with an intraarterial line is mandatory because a slightly excessive dose may lower the pressure abruptly to levels that induce shock. The potency and rapidity of action of nitroprusside have made it the treatment of choice for life-threatening hypertension. However, because nitroprusside acts as a venous and arteriolar dilator, venous return and cardiac output are lowered and intracranial pressures may increase. Therefore, other parenteral agents are being more widely used. These include labetalol and the calcium antagonist nicardipine.

With any of these agents, intravenous furosemide is often needed to lower the blood pressure further and prevent retention of salt and water. Diuretics should not be given if volume depletion is initially present. For patients in less immediate danger, oral therapy may be used. Almost every drug has been used and most, with repeated doses, reduce high pressures. The prior preference for liquid nifedipine by mouth or sublingually has been diminished because of occasional ischemic complications resulting from too rapid reduction in blood pressure.[71] Oral doses of other short-acting formulations may be used, including furosemide, propranolol, captopril, or felodipine. A safer course for any patients, particularly if their current high pressures are simply a reflection of stopping previously effective oral medication and they are asymptomatic, is simply to restart the previous medication and monitor their response closely. If their nonadherence to therapy was caused by side effects, appropriate changes should be made.

Most centers are seeing fewer patients in hypertensive crisis, presumably because more patients are diagnosed and treated before the disease enters this malignant course. The continued successful treatment of many more hypertensive persons will prevent the more frequent long-range cardiovascular complications of hypertension.

TABLE 38–11 Parenteral Drugs for Treatment of Hypertensive Emergency

Drug*	Dose	Onset of Action	Adverse Effects†
Diuretics			
Furosemide	20-40 mg in 1-2 min, repeated and higher doses with renal insufficiency	5-15 min	Volume depletion, hypokalemia
Vasodilators			
Nitroprusside (Nipride, Nitropress)	0.25-10 μg/kg/min as IV infusion	Immediate	Nausea, vomiting, muscle twitching, sweating, thiocyanate and cyanide intoxication
Nitroglycerin (Nitro-Bid IV)	5-100 μg/min as IV infusion	2-5 min	Headache, vomiting, methemoglobinemia, tolerance with prolonged use
Fenoldopam (Corlopam)	0.1-0.6 μg/kg/min as IV infusion	4-5 min	Reflex tachycardia, increased intraocular pressure, headache
Nicardipine‡ (Cardene I.V.)	5-15 mg/h IV	5-10 min	Headache, nausea, flushing, tachycardia, local phlebitis
Hydralazine (Apresoline)	10-20 mg IV 10-50 mg IM	10-20 min 20-30 min	Tachycardia, flushing, headache, vomiting, worsening of angina
Enalaprilat (Vasotec I.V.)	1.25-5 mg every 6 hr	15 min	Precipitous fall in pressure in high-renin states; response variable
Adrenergic Inhibitors			
Phentolamine	5-15 mg IV	1-2 min	Tachycardia, flushing, headache
Esmolol (Brevibloc)	200-500 μg/kg/min for 4 min, then 50-300 μg/kg/min IV	1-2 min	Hypotension, nausea
Labetalol (Normodyne, Trandate)	20-80 mg IV bolus every 10 min 2 mg/min IV infusion	5-10 min	Vomiting, scalp tingling, burning in throat, dizziness, nausea, heart block, orthostatic hypotension

From Kaplan NM: Kaplan's Clinical Hypertension. 8th ed. Baltimore, Lippincott Williams & Wilkins, 2002, p 348.
*In order of rapidity of action.
†Hypotension may occur with any.
‡Intravenous formulations of other calcium channel blockers are also available.

CH 38

REFERENCES

1. Joint National Committee: The seventh report of the Joint Committee on Prevention, Detection, Evaluation, and Treatment of High Blood Pressure (JNC-7 Express). JAMA 289:2560, 2003.
2. ALLHAT Officers and Coordinators for the ALLHAT Collaborative Research Group: Major outcomes in high-risk hypertensive patients randomized to angiotensin-converting enzyme inhibitor or calcium channel blocker vs diuretic. JAMA 288:2981, 2002.
3. Kaplan NM: Treatment of hypertension: Drug therapy. *In* Kaplan NM: Kaplan's Clinical Hypertension. 8th ed. Philadelphia, Lippincott Williams & Wilkins, 2002, pp 237-338.
4. Staessen JA, Wang J-G, Thijs L: Cardiovascular protection and blood pressure reduction. Lancet 358:1305, 2001.
5. Gueyffier F, Bulpitt C, Boissel J-P, et al: Antihypertensive drugs in very old people: A subgroup meta-analysis of randomised controlled trials. Lancet 353:793, 1999.
6. Forette F, Seux M-L, Staessen JA, et al: The prevention of dementia with antihypertensive treatment: New evidence from the Systolic Hypertension in Europe (Syst-Eur) study. Arch Intern Med 162:2046, 2002.
7. Whelton PK, He J, Appel LJ, et al: Primary prevention of hypertension: Clinical and public health advisory from the National High Blood Pressure Education Program. JAMA 288:1882, 2002.
8. Jackson R: Updated New Zealand cardiovascular disease risk-benefit prediction guide. BMJ 320:709. 2000.

Threshold for and Goal of Therapy

9. European Society of Hypertension-European Society of Cardiology Guidelines Committee: 2003 European Society of Hypertension-European Society of Cardiology guidelines for the management of arterial hypertension. J Hypertens 21:1011, 2003.
10. Guidelines Subcommittee: 1999 World Health Organization–International Society of Hypertension guidelines for the management of hypertension. J Hypertens 17:151, 1999.
11. Vasan RS, Larson MG, Leip EP, et al: Impact of high-normal blood pressure on the risk of cardiovascular disease. N Engl J Med 345: 1291, 2001.
12. Staessen JA, Gasowski J, Wang JG, et al: Risks of untreated and treated isolated systolic hypertension in the elderly. Lancet 355:865, 2000.
13. Kaplan NM: What is goal blood pressure for the treatment of hypertension? Arch Intern Med 161:1480, 2001.
14. Hansson L, Zanchetti A, Carruthers SG, et al: Effects of intensive blood-pressure lowering and low-dose aspirin in patients with hypertension: Principal results of the Hypertension Optimal Treatment (HOT) randomised trial. Lancet 351:1755, 1998.
15. Boutitie F, Gueyffier F, Pocock S, et al: J-shaped relationship between blood pressure and mortality in hypertensive patients: New insights from a meta-analysis of individual-patient data. Ann Intern Med 136:438, 2002.
16. Somes GW, Pahor M, Shorr RI, et al: The role of diastolic blood pressure when treating isolated systolic hypertension. Arch Intern Med 159:2004, 1999.
17. Mancia G, Carugo S, Grassi G, et al: Prevalence of left ventricular hypertrophy in hypertensive patients without and with blood pressure control: Data from the PAMELA population. Hypertension 39:744, 2002.
18. Adler AI, Stratton IM, Neil HAW, et al: Association of systolic blood pressure with macrovascular and microvascular complications of type 2 diabetes (UKPDS 36). BMJ 321:412, 2000.
19. Wright JT Jr, Bakris G, Greene T, et al: Effect of blood pressure lowering and antihypertensive drug class on progression of hypertensive kidney disease. Results from the AASK trial. JAMA 288:2421, 2002.

Life-Style Modifications

20. Diabetes Prevention Program Research Group: Reduction in the incidence of type 2 diabetes with lifestyle intervention or metformin. N Engl J Med 346:393, 2002.
21. Willett WC, Dietz WH, Colditz GA: Guidelines for healthy weight. N Engl J Med 341:427, 1999.
22. Sjöström C, Lindberg E, Elmasry A, et al: Prevalence of sleep apnoea and snoring in hypertensive men: A population based study. Thorax 57:602, 2002.
23. Whelton SP, Chin A, Xin X, He J: Effect of aerobic exercise on blood pressure: A meta-analysis of randomized, controlled trials. Ann Intern Med 136:493, 2002.
24. He FJ, MacGregor GA: Effect of modest salt reduction on blood pressure: A meta-analysis of randomized trials. Implications for public health. J Hum Hypertens 16:761, 2002.
25. Hooper L, Bartlett C, Smith GD, Ebrahim S: Systematic review of long term effects of advice to reduce dietary salt in adults. BMJ 325:628, 2002.
26. Tuomilehto J, Jousilahti P, Rastenyte D, et al: Urinary sodium excretion and cardiovascular mortality in Finland: A prospective study. Lancet 357:848, 2001.
27. Bazzano LA, He J, Ogden LG, et al: Dietary potassium intake and risk of stroke in US men and women: National Health Nutrition Examination Survey I Epidemiologic Follow-up Study. Stroke 32:1473, 2001.
28. He J, Whelton PK: What is the role of dietary sodium and potassium in hypertension and target organ injury? Am J Med Sci 317:152, 1999.
29. Griffith LE, Guyatt GH, Cook RJ, et al: The influence of dietary and nondietary calcium supplementation on blood pressure. Am J Hypertens 12:84, 1999.
30. Jee SH, Miller ER, Guallar E, et al: The effect of magnesium supplementation on blood pressure: A meta-analysis of randomized clinical trials. Am J Hypertens 15:691, 2002.
31. John JH, Ziebland S, Yudkin P, et al: Effects of fruit and vegetable consumption on plasma antioxidant concentrations and blood pressure: A randomised controlled trial. Lancet 359:1969, 2002.
32. Jee SH, He J, Whelton PK, et al: The effect of chronic coffee drinking on blood pressure. Hypertension 33:647, 1999.
33. Fuchs FD, Chambless LE, Whelton PK, et al: Alcohol consumption and the incidence of hypertension: The Atherosclerosis Risk in Communities Study. Hypertension 37:1242, 2001.

34. Thadhani R, Camargo CA Jr, Stampfer MJ, et al: Prospective study of moderate alcohol consumption and risk of hypertension in young women. Arch Intern Med 162:569, 2002.
35. Albert MA, Glynn RJ, Ridker PM: Alcohol consumption and plasma concentration of C-reactive protein. Circulation 107:443, 2003.
36. Linden W, Lenz JW, Con AH: Individualized stress management for primary hypertension: A randomized trial. Arch Intern Med 161:1071, 2001.
37. Rosenthal T, Alter A, Peleg E, Gavish B: Device-guided breathing exercises reduce blood pressure: Ambulatory and home measurements. Am J Hypertens 14:74, 2001.
38. Neaton JD, Grimm RH Jr, Prineas RJ, et al: Treatment of mild hypertension study (TOMHS). JAMA 270:713, 1993.

Antihypertensive Drug Therapy

39. Haynes RB, McDonald HP, Garg AX: Helping patients follow prescribed treatment: Clinical applications. JAMA 288:2880, 2002.
40. Strandgaard S, Haunsø S: Why does antihypertensive treatment prevent stroke but not myocardial infarction? Lancet 2:658, 2987.
41. Fagan TC: Remembering the lessons of basic pharmacology. Arch Intern Med 154:1430, 1994.
42. Materson BJ, Reda DJ, Cushman WC, et al: Single-drug therapy for hypertension in men. N Engl J Med 328:914, 1993.
43. Psaty BM, Smith NL, Siscovick DS, et al: Health outcomes associated with antihypertensive therapies used as first-line agents. JAMA 277:739, 1997.
44. Blood Pressure Lowering Treatment Trialists' Collaboration: Effects of ACE inhibitors, calcium antagonists, and other blood-pressure-lowering drugs. Lancet 355:1955, 2000.
45. Hansson L, Lindholm LH, Ekbom T, et al: Randomised trial of old and new antihypertensive drugs in elderly patients. Lancet 354:1751, 1999.
46. Schrier RW, Estacio RO: Additional follow-up from the ABCD trial in patients with type 2 diabetes and hypertension. N Engl J Med 343:1969, 2000.
47. Wing LMH, Reid CM, Ryan P, et al: A comparison of outcomes with angiotensin-converting-enzyme inhibitors and diuretics for hypertension in the elderly. N Engl J Med 348:583, 2003.
48. Dalhöf B, Devereux RB, Kjeldsen SE, et al: Cardiovascular morbidity and mortality in the Losartan Intervention For Endpoint reduction in hypertension study (LIFE): A randomized trial against atenolol. Lancet 359:995, 2002.

Diuretics

49. Chapman AB, Schwartz GL, Boerwinkle E, Turner ST: Predictors of antihypertensive response to a standard doze of hydrochlorothiazide for essential hypertension. Kidney Int 61:1047, 2002.
50. Psaty BM, Smith NL, Heckbert SR, et al: Diuretic therapy, the α-adducin gene variant, and the risk of myocardial infarction or stroke in persons with treated hypertension. JAMA 287:1680, 2002.
51. Grimm RH Jr, Grandits GA, Prineas RJ, et al: Long-term effects on sexual function of five antihypertensive drugs and nutritional hygienic treatment of hypertensive men and women. Hypertension 29:8, 1997.
52. Grossman E, Messerli FH, Goldbourt U: Antihypertensive therapy and the risk of malignancies. Eur Heart J 22:1343, 2001.
53. Pitt B, Zannad F, Remme WJ, et al: The effect of spironolactone of morbidity and mortality in patients with severe heart failure. N Engl J Med 341:709, 1999.
54. Weinberger MH, Roniker B, Krause SL, Weiss RJ: Eplerenone, a selective aldosterone blocker, in mild-to-moderate hypertension. Am J Hypertens 15:709, 2002.
55. Young MJ, Funder JW: Mineralocorticoid receptors and pathophysiological roles for aldosterone in the cardiovascular system. J Hypertens 20:1465, 2002.

Adrenergic Inhibitors

56. ALLHAT Officers and Coordinators for the ALLHAT Collaborative Research Group: Major cardiovascular events in hypertensive patients randomized to doxazosin vs chlorthalidone. JAMA 283:1967, 2000.
57. Levy D, Walmsley P, Levenstein M: Principal results of the hypertension and lipid trial (HALT): A multicenter study of doxazosin in patients with hypertension. Am Heart J 131:966, 1996.
58. Salpeter SR, Ormiston TM, Salpeter EE: Cardioselective β-blockers in patients with reactive airway disease: A meta-analysis. Ann Intern Med 137:715, 2002.
59. Auerbach AD, Goldman L: β-Blockers and reduction of cardiac events in noncardiac surgery. Scientific review. JAMA 287:1435, 2002.
60. Ko DT, Hebert PR, Coffey CS, et al: β-Blocker therapy and symptoms of depression, fatigue, and sexual dysfunction. JAMA 288:351, 2002.
61. Sørensen HT, Mellemkjaer L, Olsen JH: Risk of suicide in users of β-adrenoceptor blockers, calcium channel blockers and angiotensin converting enzyme inhibitors. Br J Clin Pharmacol 52:313, 2001.
62. Gress TW, Nieto FJ, Shahar E, et al: Hypertension and antihypertensive therapy as risk factors for type 2 diabetes mellitus. N Engl J Med 342:905, 2000.

Vasodilators

63. Lernfelt B, Landahl S, Johansson P, et al: Haemodynamic and renal effects of felodipine in young and elderly patients. Eur J Clin Pharmacol 54:595, 1998.
64. Sareli P, Radevski IV, Valtchanova ZP, et al: Efficacy of different drug classes used to initiate antihypertensive treatment in black subjects: Results of a randomized trial in Johannesburg, South Africa. Arch Intern Med 161:965, 2001.
65. Stergiou GS, Malakos JS, Achimastos AD, Mountokalakis TD: Additive hypotensive effect of a dihydropyridine calcium antagonist to that produced by a thiazide diuretic. J Cardiovasc Pharmacol 29:412, 1997.
66. Tuomilehto J, Rastenyte D, Birkenhäger WH, et al: Effects of calcium-channel blockade in older patients with diabetes and systolic hypertension. N Engl J Med 340:677, 1999.
67. Remuzzi G, Schieppati A, Ruggenenti P: Nephropathy in patients with type 2 diabetes. N Engl J Med 346:1145, 2002.
68. Lewis EJ, Hunsicker LG, Clarke WR, et al: Renoprotective effect of the angiotensin-receptor antagonist irbesartan in patients with nephropathy due to type 2 diabetes. N Engl J Med 345:851, 2001.
69. Zanchetti A, Ruilope LM: Antihypertensive treatment in patients with type-2 diabetes mellitus: What guidance from recent controlled randomized trials? J Hypertens 20:2099, 2002.
70. Brenner BM, Cooper ME, de Zeeuw D, et al: Effects of losartan on renal and cardiovascular outcomes in patients with type 2 diabetes and nephropathy. N Engl J Med 345:861, 2001.
71. Grossman E, Messerli FH, Grodzicki T, Kowey P: Should a moratorium be placed on sublingual nifedipine capsules given for hypertensive emergencies and pseudoemergencies? JAMA 276:1328, 1996.
72. Psaty BM, Heckbert SR, Koepsell TD, et al: The risk of myocardial infarction associated with antihypertensive drug therapies. JAMA 274:620, 1995.
73. Leader S, Mallick R, Roht L: Using medication history to measure confounding by indication in assessing calcium channel blockers and other antihypertensive therapy. J Hum Hypertens 15:153, 2001.
74. Celis H, Thijs L, Staessen JA, et al: Interaction between nonsteroidal anti-inflammatory drug intake and calcium-channel blocker-based antihypertensive treatment in the Syst-Eur trial. J Hum Hypertens 15:613, 2001.
75. Elliott HL, Elawad M, Wilkinson R, Singh SP: Persistence of antihypertensive efficacy after missed doses: Comparison of amlodipine and nifedipine gastrointestinal therapeutic system. J Hypertens 20:333, 2002.
76. van Paassen P, de Zeeuw D, Navis G, de Jong PE: Renal and systemic effects of continued treatment with renin inhibitor remikiren in hypertensive patients with normal and impaired renal function. Nephrol Dial Transplant 15:637, 2000.
77. Forclaz A, Maillard M, Nussberger J, et al: Angiotensin II receptor blockade: Is there truly a benefit of adding an ACE inhibitor? Hypertension 41:31, 2003.
78. Pretorius M, Rosenbaum D, Vaughan DE, Brown NJ: Angiotensin-converting enzyme inhibition increases human vascular tissue-type plasminogen activator release through endogenous bradykinin. Circulation 103:579, 2003.
79. Nussberger J, Cugno M, Cicardi M: Bradykinin-mediated angioedema. N Engl J Med 347:621, 2002.
80. Grassi G, Turri C, Dell'Oro R, et al: Effect of chronic angiotensin converting enzyme inhibition on sympathetic nerve traffic and baroreflex control of the circulation in essential hypertension. J Hypertens 16:1789, 1998.
81. Taddei S, Virdis A, Ghiadoni L, et al: Restoration of nitric oxide availability after calcium antagonist treatment in essential hypertension. Hypertension 37:943, 2001.
82. Cheng A, Frishman WH: Use of angiotensin-converting enzyme inhibitors as monotherapy and in combination with diuretics and calcium channel blockers. J Clin Pharmacol 38:477, 1998.
83. Levey AS: Nondiabetic kidney disease. N Engl J Med 347:1505, 2002.
84. Bakris GL, Weir MR: Angiotensin-converting enzyme inhibitor-associated elevations in serum creatinine. Arch Intern Med 160:685, 2000.
85. Haas M, Leko-Mohr Z, Erler C, Mayer G: Antiproteinuric versus antihypertensive effects of high-dose ACE inhibitor therapy. Am J Kidney Dis 40:458, 2002.
86. Losito A, Gaburri M, Errico R, et al: Survival in patients with renovascular disease and ACE inhibition. Clin Nephrol 52:339, 1999.
87. PROGRESS Collaborative Group: Randomised trial of a perindopril-based blood-pressure-lowering regimen among 6105 individuals with previous stroke or transient ischaemic attack. Lancet 358:1033, 2001.
88. Wood R: Bronchospasm and cough as adverse reactions to the ACE inhibitors captopril, enalapril, lisinopril. Br J Clin Pharmacol 39:265, 1995.
89. White WB, Kent J, Taylor A, et al: Effects of celecoxib on ambulatory blood pressure in hypertensive patients on ACE inhibitors. Hypertension 39:929, 2002.
90. Schepkens H, Vanholder R, Billiouw J-M, Lameire N: Life-threatening hyperkalemia during combined therapy with angiotensin-converting enzyme inhibitors and spironolactone: An analysis of 25 cases. Am J Med 110:438, 2001.
91. Heart Outcomes Prevention Evaluation (HOPE) Study Investigators: Effects of an angiotensin-converting-enzyme inhibitor, ramipril, on cardiovascular events in high-risk patients. N Engl J Med 342:145, 2000.
92. Burnier M, Brunner HR: Angiotensin II receptor antagonists. Lancet 355:637, 2000.
93. Tanser PH, Campbell LM, Carranza J, et al: Candesartan cilexetil is not associated with cough in hypertensive patients with enalapril-induced cough. Am J Hypertens 13:214, 2000.
94. Warner KK, Visconti JA, Tschampel MM: Angiotensin II receptor blockers in patients with ACE inhibitor–induced angioedema. Ann Pharmacother 34:526, 2000.
95. Würzner G, Gerster J-C, Chiolero A, et al: Comparative effects of losartan and irbesartan on serum uric acid in hypertensive patients with hyperuricaemia and gout. J Hypertens 19:1855, 2001.
96. Klingbeil AU, John S, Schneider MP, et al: Effect of AT_1 receptor blockade on endothelial function in essential hypertension. Am J Hypertens 16:123, 2003.
97. Schiffrin EL, Park JB, Intengan HD, Touyz RM: Correction of arterial structure and endothelial dysfunction in human essential hypertension by the angiotensin receptor antagonist losartan. Circulation 101:1653, 2000.
98. Lacourcière Y, Asmar R: A comparison of the efficacy and duration of action of candesartan cilexetil and losartan as assessed by clinic and ambulatory blood pressure after a missed dose, in truly hypertensive patients. Am J Hypertens 12:1181, 1999.
99. Agarwal R: Add-on angiotensin receptor blockade with maximized ACE inhibition. Kidney Int 59:2282, 2001.
100. Nakao N, Yoshimura A, Morita H, et al: Combination treatment of angiotensin-II receptor blocker and angiotensin-converting-enzyme inhibitor in non-diabetic renal disease (COOPERATE): A randomized controlled trial. Lancet 361:117, 2003.

101. Parving H-H, Lehnert H, Bröchner-Mortensen J, et al: The effect of irbesartan on the development of diabetic nephropathy in patients with type 2 diabetes. N Engl J Med 345:870, 2001.
102. Brunner HR, Gavras H: Angiotensin blockade for hypertension: A promise fulfilled. Lancet 359:990, 2002.
103. Stokes GS, Barin ES, Gilfillan KL: Effects of isosorbide mononitrate and AII inhibition on pulse wave reflection in hypertension. Hypertension 41:297, 2003.
104. Raji A, Seely EW, Bekins SA, et al: Rosiglitazone improves insulin sensitivity and lowers blood pressure in hypertensive patients. Diabetes Care 26:172, 2003.

Special Considerations in Therapy

105. Nelson MR, Reid CM, Krum H, et al: Short-term predictors of maintenance of normotension after withdrawal of antihypertensive drugs in the Second Australian National Blood Pressure Study (ANBP2). Am J Hypertens 16:39, 2003.
106. Redon J, Campos C, Narciso ML, et al: Prognostic value of ambulatory blood pressure monitoring in refractory hypertension. Hypertension 31:712, 1998.
107. Poldermans D, Boersma E, Bax JJ, et al: The effect of bisoprolol on perioperative mortality and myocardial infarction in high-risk patients undergoing vascular surgery. N Engl J Med 341:1789, 1999.
108. Flynn JT: Pharmacologic management of childhood hypertension: Current status, future challenges. Am J Hypertens 15(Suppl):30S, 2002.
109. Gæde P, Vedel P, Larsen N, et al: Multifactorial intervention and cardiovascular disease in patients with type 2 diabetes. N Engl J Med 348:383, 2003.
110. Kloner RA, Brown M, Prisant LM, Collins M, for the Sildenafil Study Group: Effect of sildenafil in patients with erectile dysfunction taking antihypertensive therapy. Am J Hypertens 14:70, 2001.
111. Mansoor GA, Frishman WH: Comprehensive management of hypertensive emergencies and urgencies. Heart Dis 4:358, 2002.

GUIDELINES *Thomas H. Lee*

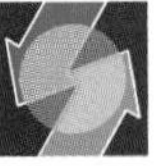

Treatment of Hypertension

The major U.S. guidelines for management of hypertension are issued by the Joint National Committee on Prevention, Detection, Evaluation, and Treatment of High Blood Pressure, a group coordinated by the National Heart Lung and Blood Institute (NHLBI). Their seventh and most recent guidelines were published in 2003, and are known as JNC-7.[1] Other recent recommendations have been published in other countries, such as guidelines from the British Hypertension Society.[2] In 2003, recommendations regarding blood pressure control in patients with diabetes were issued by the American College of Physicians,[3] and for African Americans by the International Society on Hypertension in Blacks.[4]

Initial Evaluation

JNC-7 updated NHLBI recommendations from prior guidelines issued in 1997[5] in several important ways. First, JNC-7 introduced the concept of "prehypertension," which is systolic blood pressures of 120 to 139 mm Hg or a diastolic blood pressure of 80 to 89 mm Hg. JNC-7 recommended a more aggressive approach to patients with blood pressures in this range, with an emphasis on lifestyle modifications to prevent cardiovascular disease. JNC-7 describes "normal" blood pressure as systolic pressures below 120 mm Hg and diastolic blood pressures below 80 mm Hg. Stage 1 hypertension is systolic blood pressure 140 to 159 mm Hg or diastolic blood pressure 90 to 99 mm Hg. Patients with higher blood pressures have Stage 2 hypertension.

JNC-6 gives recommendations for follow-up of patients after initial measurement of blood pressure (Table 38G–1). These recommendations should be guided by the blood pressure and other clinical data, including past blood pressure measurements, other cardiovascular risk factors, or target organ disease. JNC-7 recommends routine laboratory tests before initiation of therapy that include 12-lead electrocardiogram; urinalysis; blood glucose and hematocrit; serum potassium, creatinine, and calcium; and lipid profile. More extensive testing for identifiable causes of hypertension is not indicated routinely.

Initial Management Strategy

The goal of treatment according to JNC-7 is to reduce blood pressure to below 140 mm Hg systolic and 90 mm Hg diastolic; in patients with concomitant diabetes or renal disease, the goal is blood pressure below 130/80 mm Hg.

These guidelines recommend that initial management be based upon the patient's blood pressure stage and other medical issues (Table 38G–2). Life-style modifications should be encouraged for all patients, including those with normal blood pressures, and should be used as the sole therapy for patients with prehypertension unless they have clinical evidence of "compelling indications." These indications include heart failure, postmyocardial infarction, high coronary artery disease risk, diabetes, chronic kidney disease, and need for recurrent stroke prevention.

Recommended life-style modifications include:

- Weight reduction to maintain normal body weight (body mass index 18.5 to 24.9 kg/m^2)
- Adoption of the Dietary Approaches to Stop Hypertension (DASH) eating plan[6]
- Dietary sodium reduction to no more than 100 mmol per day (2.4 g sodium or 6 g sodium chloride)
- Physical activity—at least 30 minutes per day, most days of the week
- Limit alcohol intake to no more than 2 drinks (1 oz or 30 ml ethanol; e.g., 24 oz beer, 10 oz wine, or 3 oz 80-proof whiskey) per day in most men and to no more than 1 drink per day in women and lighter weight persons.

Drug Therapy

JNC-7 guidelines recommend thiazide-type diuretics as the initial therapy for most patients with hypertension, either alone or in combination with one of the other classes. Table 38G–3 describes JNC-7's list of "compelling indications" and recommended therapies. The guidelines note that most patients who are hypertensive will require two or more antihypertensive agents to achieve their blood pressure goals. When blood pressure is more than 20/10 mm Hg above goal, the guidelines recommend that clinicians consider initiating therapy with two drugs.

Guidelines from other organizations vary slightly in thresholds for initiating therapy. For example, the British Hypertension Society's guidelines support initiation of drug therapy for all patients with systolic blood pressure ≥ 160 mm Hg or sustained diastolic blood pressure ≥ 100 mm Hg despite nonpharmacological measures. Drug treatment is also indicated in patients with sustained systolic blood pressures of 140 to 159 mm Hg or diastolic blood pressures of 90 to 99 mm Hg if target organ damage is present, or there is evidence of established cardiovascular disease, or diabetes, or the 10-year coronary heart disease risk is greater than 15%. For most patients, these guidelines recommend a target of reducing systolic pressure below 140 mm Hg and diastolic pressure below 85 mm Hg. For patients with diabetes a lower target is recommended. These guidelines recommend initiation of therapy with a diuretic unless there is a contraindication or a compelling indication for another drug class.

For patients with hypertension and diabetes, the 2003 recommendations from the American College of Physicians include a target blood pressure of no more than 135/80 mm Hg.[3] These guidelines recommend thiazide diuretics or ACE inhibitors as first-line agents for blood pressure control in most patients.

TABLE 38G–1 Joint National Committee (JNC)-6 Guidelines for Follow-Up Based on Initial Blood Pressure Measurements for Adults

Initial Blood Pressure* (mm Hg)		
Systolic	*Diastolic*	*Follow-Up Recommended*
<130	<85	Recheck in 2 yr
130-139	85-89	Recheck in 1 yr (provide information about life-style modifications)
140-159	90-99	Confirm within 2 mo (provide information about life-style modifications)
160-179	100-109	Evaluate or refer to source of care within 1 mo
≧180	≧110	Evaluate or refer to source of care immediately or within 1 wk depending on clinical situation

*If systolic and diastolic categories are different, follow recommendations for shorter time follow-up.

TABLE 38G–2 Joint National Committee (JNC)-7 Guidelines for Classification and Management of Hypertension in Adults

				Initial Drug Therapy	
Blood Pressure Classification	**Systolic Blood Pressure (mm Hg)**	**Diastolic Blood Pressure (mm Hg)**	**Life-style Modification**	***Without Compelling Indications***	***With Compelling Indications****
Normal	<120	And <80	Encourage	No antihypertensive drug indicated	Drug(s) for compelling indications†
Prehypertension	120-139	Or 80-89	Yes		
Stage 1 hypertension	140-159	Or 90-99	Yes	Thiazide-type diuretics for most	Drug(s) for compelling indications.† Other antihypertensive drugs (diuretics, ACEI, ARB, BB, CCB) as needed
Stage 2 hypertension	≧160	Or ≧100	Yes	Two-drug combination for most (usually thiazide-type diuretic and ACEI or ARB or BB or CCB)	

ACEI, angiotensin-converting enzyme inhibitor; ARB, angiotensin receptor blocker; BB, beta blocker; CCB, calcium channel blocker.
*Heart failure, postmyocardial infarction, high coronary artery disease risk, diabetes, chronic kidney disease, recurrent stroke prevention.
†Treat patients with chronic kidney disease or diabetes to blood pressure goal of <130/80 mm Hg.

TABLE 38G–3 Joint National Committee (JNC)-7 Guidelines for Recommended Drugs for Patients with Compelling Indications

	Recommended Drugs					
Compelling Indication	***Diuretic***	***Beta Blocker***	***ACE Inhibitor***	***Angiotensin Receptor Blocker***	***Calcium Channel Blocker***	***Aldosterone Antagonist***
Heart failure	+	+	+	+		+
Postmyocardial infarction		+	+			+
High coronary disease risk	+	+	+		+	
Diabetes	+	+	+	+	+	
Chronic kidney disease			+	+		
Recurrent stroke prevention	+		+			

ACE = angiotensin-converting enzyme.

Guidelines developed for treatment of African Americans recommend lower thresholds for drug therapy and more aggressive treatment strategies.[4] These guidelines recommend a lower blood pressure target (130/80 mm Hg) for African Americans with hypertension who also have conditions such as heart disease, kidney disease, or diabetes. This statement notes that physicians should have a low threshold for using more than one drug for treatment of hypertension in blacks.

FOLLOW-UP AND REFERRAL TO SPECIALISTS

In follow-up, the JNC-7 guidelines recommend that most patients should be seen at approximately monthly intervals until the blood pressure goal is reached. More frequent visits are recommended for patients with Stage 2 hypertension or with complicating comorbid conditions. Serum potassium and creatinine should be monitored at least 1 to 2 times per year. After blood pressure is at goal and stable, follow-up visits can be scheduled at 3- to 6-month intervals. Low-dose aspirin therapy should be considered only after blood pressure is controlled due to risk of hemorrhagic stroke in patients with uncontrolled hypertension.

References

1. Chobanian AV, et al: The Seventh Report of the Joint National Committee on Prevention, Detection, Evaluation, and Treatment of High Blood Pressure. NIH Publication No. 03-5233, 2003.
2. Ramsay LE, Williams B, Johnston GD, et al: Guidelines for management of hypertension: Report of the third working party of the British Hypertension Society. J Hum Hypertens 13:569, 1999.
3. Snow V, Weiss KB, Mottur-Pilson C, for the Clinical Efficacy Assessment Subcommittee of the American College of Physicians: The evidence base for tight blood pressure control in the management of type 2 diabetes mellitus. Ann Intern Med 138:587, 2003.
4. Douglas JG, Bakris GL, Epstein M, et al: Management of high blood pressure in African Americans: Consensus Statement of the Hypertension in African Americans Working Group of the International Society of Hypertension in Blacks. Arch Intern Med 163:525, 2003.
5. Sheps SG, et al: The Sixth Report of the Joint National Committee on Prevention, Detection, Evaluation, and Treatment of High Blood Pressure. NIH Publication No. 98-4080, 1997.
6. Sacks FM, Svetkey LP, Vollmer WM, et al: Effects on blood pressure of reduced dietary sodium and the Dietary Approaches to Stop Hypertension (DASH) diet. DASH-Sodium Collaborative Research Group. N Engl J Med 344:3, 2001.

CHAPTER 39

Lipoprotein Disorders and Cardiovascular Disease

Jacques Genest • Peter Libby • Antonio M. Gotto, Jr.

The lipid fractions of blood have proved to be among the most potent and best substantiated risk factors for atherosclerosis in general and coronary heart disease (CHD) in particular. Chapter 35 discusses the biological basis of atherosclerosis. Chapter 36 presents the observational data on lipids as a key component of the palette of cardiovascular risk factors. This chapter deals with the fundamentals of lipid metabolism, the therapeutic approaches to treatment of lipid disorders, and the evidence base regarding their clinical use.

Although the term *hyperlipidemia* has long been used in clinical practice, the term *dyslipoproteinemia* more appropriately reflects the disorders of the lipid and lipoprotein transport pathways associated with arterial diseases. *Dyslipidemia* encompasses disorders often encountered in clinical practice such as low high-density lipoprotein (HDL) cholesterol level and elevated triglyceride level but an average total plasma cholesterol level. Certain rare lipoprotein disorders can cause overt clinical manifestations, but most common dyslipoproteinemias themselves only rarely cause symptoms or produce clinical signs that are evident on physical examination. Rather, they require laboratory tests for detection. Dyslipoproteinemias constitute a major risk factor for atherosclerosis and coronary artery disease, and their proper recognition and management can reduce cardiovascular and total mortality rates. Thus the fundamentals of lipidology presented here have importance for the daily practice of cardiovascular medicine.

Lipoprotein Transport System

Biochemistry of Lipids

The lipid transport system has evolved to carry hydrophobic molecules (fat) from sites of origin to sites of utilization through the aqueous environment of plasma. The proteins (apolipoproteins) that mediate this process are conserved throughout evolution in organisms with a circulatory system. Most apolipoproteins derive from an ancestral gene and contain both hydrophilic and hydrophobic domains. This amphipathic structure enables these proteins to bridge the interface between the aqueous environment of plasma and the phospholipid constituents of the lipoprotein.[1] The major types of lipids that circulate in plasma include cholesterol and cholesteryl esters, phospholipids, and triglycerides (Fig. 39–1).

Cholesterol is an essential component of mammalian cell membranes and furnishes the substrate for steroid hormones and bile acids. Many cell functions depend critically upon membrane cholesterol, and cells tightly regulate cholesterol content. Most of the cholesterol in plasma circulates in the form of cholesteryl esters, in the core of lipoprotein particles. The enzyme lecithin:cholesterol acyltransferase (LCAT) forms cholesteryl esters by transferring a fatty acyl chain from phosphatidyl choline to cholesterol.

Triglycerides consist of a three-carbon glycerol backbone covalently linked to three fatty acids. The fatty acid composition varies in terms of chain length and presence of double bonds (degree of saturation). Triglyceride molecules are nonpolar and hydrophobic. Hydrolysis of triglycerides by lipases generates free fatty acids used for storage or energy utilization.

Phospholipids are constituents of all cellular membranes and consist of a glycerol molecule linked to two fatty acids. The fatty acids differ in length and in the presence of a single (monounsaturated) or multiple (polyunsaturated) double bonds. The third carbon of the glycerol moiety carries a phosphate group to which one of four molecules is linked: choline (forming phosphatidyl choline—or lecithin), ethanolamine (forming phosphatidylethanolamine), serine (forming phosphatidyl serine), or inositol (forming phosphatidylinositol). A related phospholipid, sphingomyelin, has special functions in the plasma membrane in the formation of membrane microdomains, such as rafts and caveolae. The structure of sphingomyelin resembles that of phosphatidylcholine. The backbone of sphingolipids uses serine rather than glycerol. Phospholipids are polar molecules, more soluble than triglycerides or cholesterol or its esters. Phospholipids participate in signal transduction pathways: hydrolysis by membrane-associated phospholipases generates second messengers such as diacyl

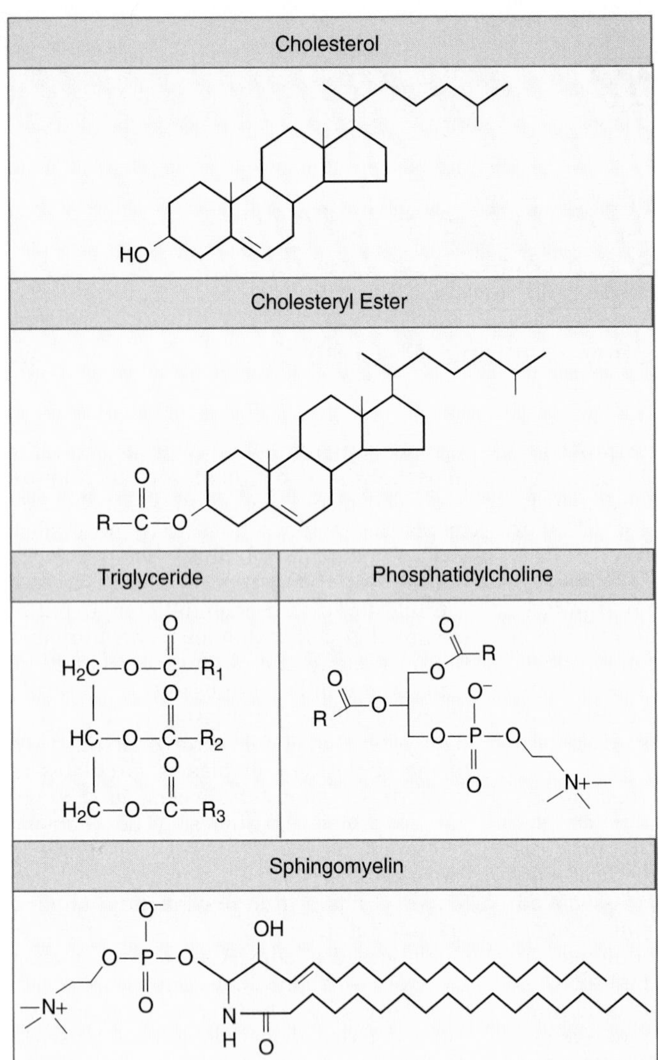

FIGURE 39–1 Biochemical structure of the major lipid molecules: cholesterol, cholesteryl esters, triglycerides, and phospholipids (phosphatidylcholine and sphingomyelin).

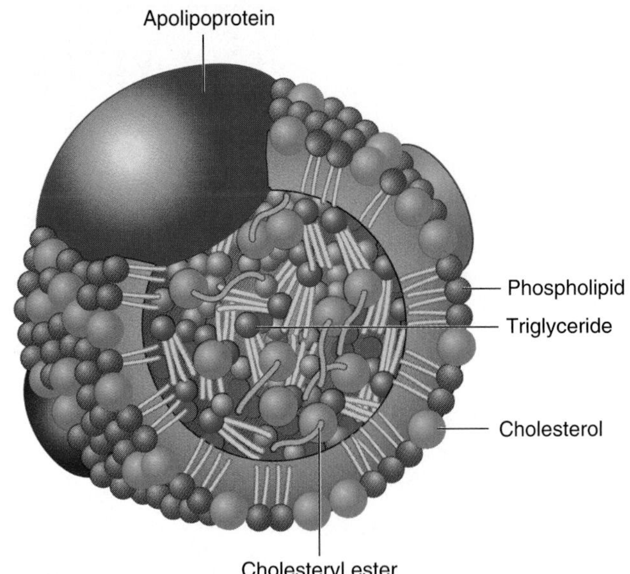

FIGURE 39–2 Structure of lipoproteins. Phospholipids are oriented with their polar head toward the aqueous environment of plasma. Free cholesterol is inserted within the phospholipid layer. The core of the lipoprotein is made up of cholesteryl esters and triglycerides. Apolipoproteins are involved in the secretion of the lipoprotein, provide structural integrity, and act as cofactors for enzymes or as ligands for various receptors.

glycerols, lysophospholipids, phosphatidic acids, and free fatty acids such as arachidonate that can regulate many cell functions.

Lipoproteins, Apolipoproteins, Receptors, and Processing Enzymes

The apolipoprotein coating packages the hydrophobic cholesteryl esters and triglycerides in the core of spherical lipoprotein particles, enabling their transport in blood (Fig. 39–2). Lipoproteins vary in size, density in the aqueous environment of plasma, and lipid and apolipoprotein content (Fig. 39–3, Table 39–1). The classification of lipoproteins reflects their density in plasma (1.006 gm/ml) as gauged by flotation in the ultracentrifuge. The triglyceride-rich lipoproteins consisting of chylomicrons and very-low-density lipoprotein (VLDL) have a density less than 1.006 gm/ml. The rest of the ultracentrifuged plasma consists of low-density lipoprotein (LDL), HDL, and lipoprotein(a).

APOLIPOPROTEINS, RECEPTORS, AND PROCESSING PROTEINS. Apolipoproteins have four major roles: (1) assembly and secretion of the lipoprotein (apo B_{100} and B_{48}); (2) structural integrity of the lipoprotein (apo B, apo E, apo AI, apo AII); (3) coactivators or inhibitors of enzymes (apo AI, CI, CII, CIII); and (4) binding or docking to specific receptors and proteins for cellular uptake of the entire particle or selective uptake of a lipid component (apo AI, B_{100}, E) (Table 39–2). The role of several apolipoproteins (AIV, AV, D, and J) remain incompletely understood.

Many proteins regulate the synthesis, secretion, and metabolic fate of lipoproteins; their characterization has provided insight in molecular cellular physiology and provided targets for drug development (Table 39–3). The discovery of the LDL receptor furnished a landmark in understanding cholesterol metabolism and receptor-mediated endocytosis. The LDL receptor regulates the entry of cholesterol into cells, as tight control mechanisms alter its expression on the cell surface, depending on need. Other receptors for lipoproteins include several that bind VLDL but not LDL. The LDL receptor-related peptide, which mediates the uptake of chylomicron remnants and VLDL, preferentially recognizes apolipoprotein E (apo E).[2] The LDL receptor-related peptide interacts with hepatic lipase. A specific VLDL receptor has also been isolated.[3] The interaction between hepatocytes and the various lipoproteins containing apo E is complex and involves cell surface proteoglycans that provide a scaffolding for lipolytic enzymes (lipoprotein lipase and hepatic lipase) involved in remnant lipoprotein recognition.[4-6] Macrophages express receptors that bind modified (especially oxidized) lipoproteins. These scavenger lipoprotein receptors mediate the uptake of oxidized LDL into macrophages. In contrast to the exquisitely regulated LDL receptor, high cellular cholesterol content does not suppress scavenger receptors, enabling the intimal macrophages to accumulate abundant cholesterol, become foam cells, and form fatty streaks. Endothelial cells can also take up modified lipoproteins through a specific receptor, such as Lox-1.[7]

At least two physiologically relevant receptors bind HDL particles: the scavenger receptor class B (SR-B1; also named CLA-1 in humans)[8] and the adenosine triphosphate-binding cassette transporter A1 (ABCA1). SR-B1 is a ligand for HDL (also for LDL and VLDL, but with less affinity). SR-B1 mediates the selective uptake of HDL cholesteryl esters in steroidogenic tissues, hepatocytes, and endothelium. The ABCA1 mediates cellular phospholipid (and possibly cholesterol) efflux and contributes importantly to the formation of HDL particles.

Lipoprotein Metabolism and Transport

The lipoprotein transport system has two major roles: the efficient transport of triglycerides from the intestine and the liver to sites of utilization (fat tissue or muscle) and the transport of cholesterol to peripheral tissues, for membrane synthesis and for steroid hormone production or to the liver for bile acid synthesis.

TABLE 39–1 Plasma Lipoprotein Composition

	Origin	Density (gm/ml)	Size (nm)	% Protein	[Cholesterol] in plasma†	[Triglyceride] in fasting plasma‡	Major apo	Other apo
Chylomicrons	Intestine	<0.95	100-1000	1-2	0.0	0	B48	AI, C's
VLDL	Liver	<1.006	40-50	10	0.1-0.4	0.2-1.2	B100	AI, C's
IDL	VLDL	1.006-1.019	25-30	18	0.1-0.3	0.1-0.3	B100, E	
LDL	IDL	1.019-1.063	20-25	25	1.5-3.5	0.2-0.4	B100	
HDL	Tissues	1.063-1.210	6-10	40-55	0.9-1.6	0.1-0.2	AI	AII, AIV
Lipoprotein (a)	Liver	1.051-1.082	25	30-50			B100, (a)	

apo = apolipoproteins; HDL = high-density lipoprotein; IDL = intermediate-density lipoprotein; LDL = low-density lipoprotein; VLDL = very-low-density lipoprotein.
†In mmol/L; for mg/dl, multiply by 38.67.
‡In mmol/L; for mg/dl, multiply by 88.5.

INTESTINAL PATHWAY (CHYLOMICRONS TO CHYLOMICRON REMNANTS). Life requires fats. The human body derives essential fatty acids that it cannot make from the diet. Fat typically furnishes 20 to 40 percent of daily calories. The major portion of fats ingested is in the form of triglycerides. For an individual consuming 2000 kcal/day, with 30 percent in the form of fat, this represents approximately 66 gm of triglycerides per day and approximately 250 mg (0.250 gm) of cholesterol.

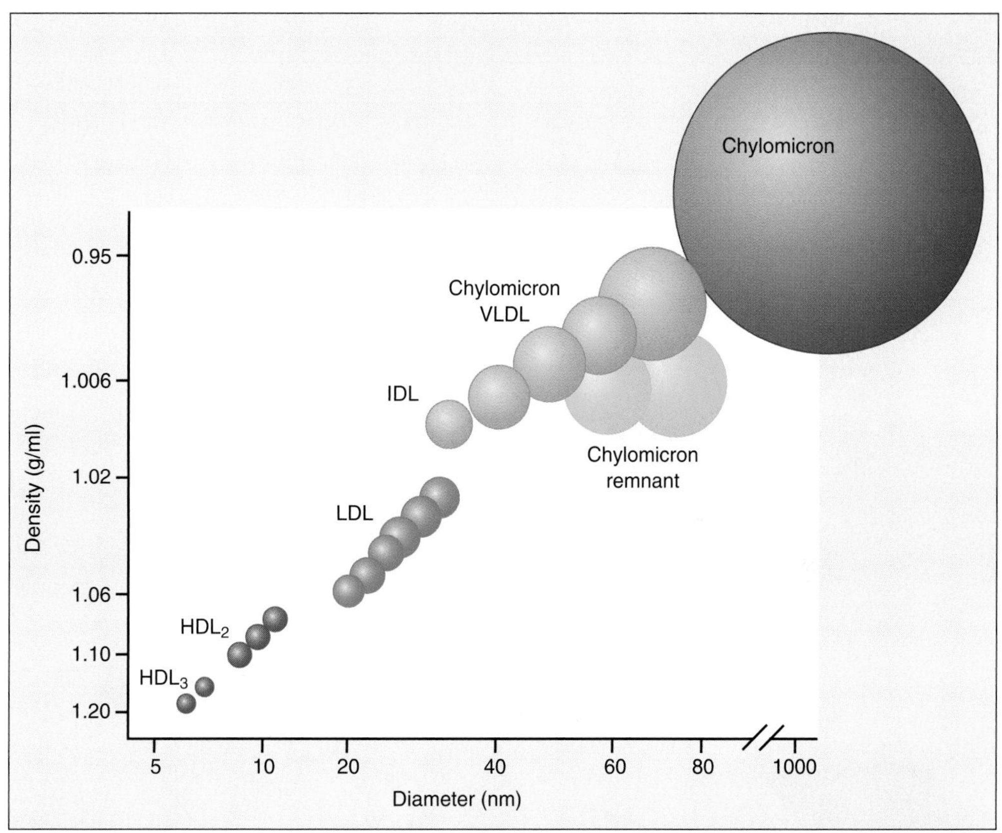

FIGURE 39–3 Relative size of plasma lipoproteins according to their hydrated density. HDL = high-density lipoprotein; IDL = intermediate-density lipoprotein; LDL = low-density lipoprotein.

Upon ingestion, pancreatic lipases hydrolyze triglycerides into free fatty acids and mono- or diglycerides. Emulsification by bile salts leads to the formation of intestinal micelles. Micelles resemble lipoproteins in that they consist of phospholipids, free cholesterol, bile acids, di- and monoglycerides, free fatty acids, and glycerol. The mechanism of micelle uptake by the intestinal brush border cells still engenders debate. Recent work has identified Niemann-Pick C1-like 1 protein as an intestinal cholesterol transporter, and potential target for the cholesterol absorption inhibitor ezetimibe[8a] (see below). The advent of selective inhibitors of cholesterol uptake (ezetimibe; see later) has rekindled interest in the mechanisms of intestinal fat absorption. After uptake into intestinal cells, fatty acids re-esterified to form triglycerides and packaged into chylomicrons inside the intestinal cell enter the portal circulation (Fig. 39–4, part 1). Chylomicrons contain apo B48, the amino-terminal component of apo B100. In the intestine, the apo B gene is modified during transcription into mRNA with a substitution of a uracil for a cytosine by an apo B48 editing enzyme complex (ApoBec). This mechanism involves a cytosine deaminase and leads to a termination codon at residue 2153 and a truncated form of apo B. Only intestinal cells express ApoBec.

Chylomicrons rapidly enter the plasma compartment after meals. In capillaries of adipose tissue or muscle cells in the peripheral circulation, chylomicrons encounter lipoprotein lipase (LPL), an enzyme attached to heparin sulfate and present on the luminal side of endothelial cells (Fig. 39–4, part 2). LPL activity is modulated by apo CII (an activator) and by apo CIII (an inhibitor).[9] Lipoprotein lipase has broad specificity for triglycerides; it cleaves all fatty acyl residues attached to glycerol, generating three molecules of free fatty acid for each molecule of glycerol. Muscle cells rapidly take up fatty acids. Adipose cells can store triglycerides made from fatty acids for energy utilization, a process that requires insulin. Fatty acids can also bind to fatty acid–binding proteins and travel to the liver, where they are repackaged in VLDL. Peripheral resistance to insulin can thus increase the delivery of free fatty acids to the liver with a consequent increase in VLDL secretion and increased apo B particles in plasma. As discussed later, this is one of the consequences of the metabolic syndrome (see Chap. 40). The remnant particles, derived from chylomicron following LPL action, contain apo E and enter the liver for degradation and reutilization of its core constituents (Fig. 39–4, part 3).

TABLE 39–2 Apolipoproteins

	Predominant Lipoprotein	Molecular Weight (kDa)	Plasma Concentration (mg/dl)	Chromosome	Role	Human Disease
Apo AI	HDL	28.3	90-160	11q23	ACAT activation, structural	HDL deficiency
Apo AII	HDL	17	25-45	1q21-23	Structural	
Apo AIV	HDL	45	10-20	11q23	Structural, absorption	
Apo AV	VLDL, HDL			11q23	TRL metabolism[72]	
Apo B100	LDL, VLDL	512	50-150	2q23-24	Structural, LDL-R binding	Hypobetalipoproteinemia
Apo B48	Chylomicrons	241	0-100	2q23-24	Structural	
Apo CI	Chylomicrons	6.63	5-6	19q13.2	TRL metabolism	
Apo CII	Chylomicrons, VLDL	8.84	3-5	19q13.2	LPL activation	Hyperchylomicronemia
Apo CIII	Chylomicrons, VLDL	8.76	10-14	11q23	LPL inhibition	Hypertriglyceridemia
Apo D	HDL	33	4-7	3q26.2	LCAT	
Apo E	Chylomicrons remnant, IDL	34	2-8	19q13.2	LDL-R, ApoE-R binding	Type III
Apo J	HDL	70	10	18p21	Complement system	
Apo(a)	Lipoprotein(a)	250-800	0-200	6q27	Tissue injury?	

Apo = apolipoprotein; ApoE-R = Apo E receptor; HDL = high-density lipoprotein; IDL = intermediate-density lipoprotein; LCAT = lecithin:cholesterol acyltransferase; LDL = low-density lipoprotein; LDL-R = LDL receptor; TRL = triglyceride-rich lipoprotein; VLDL = very-low-density lipoprotein.

CH 39

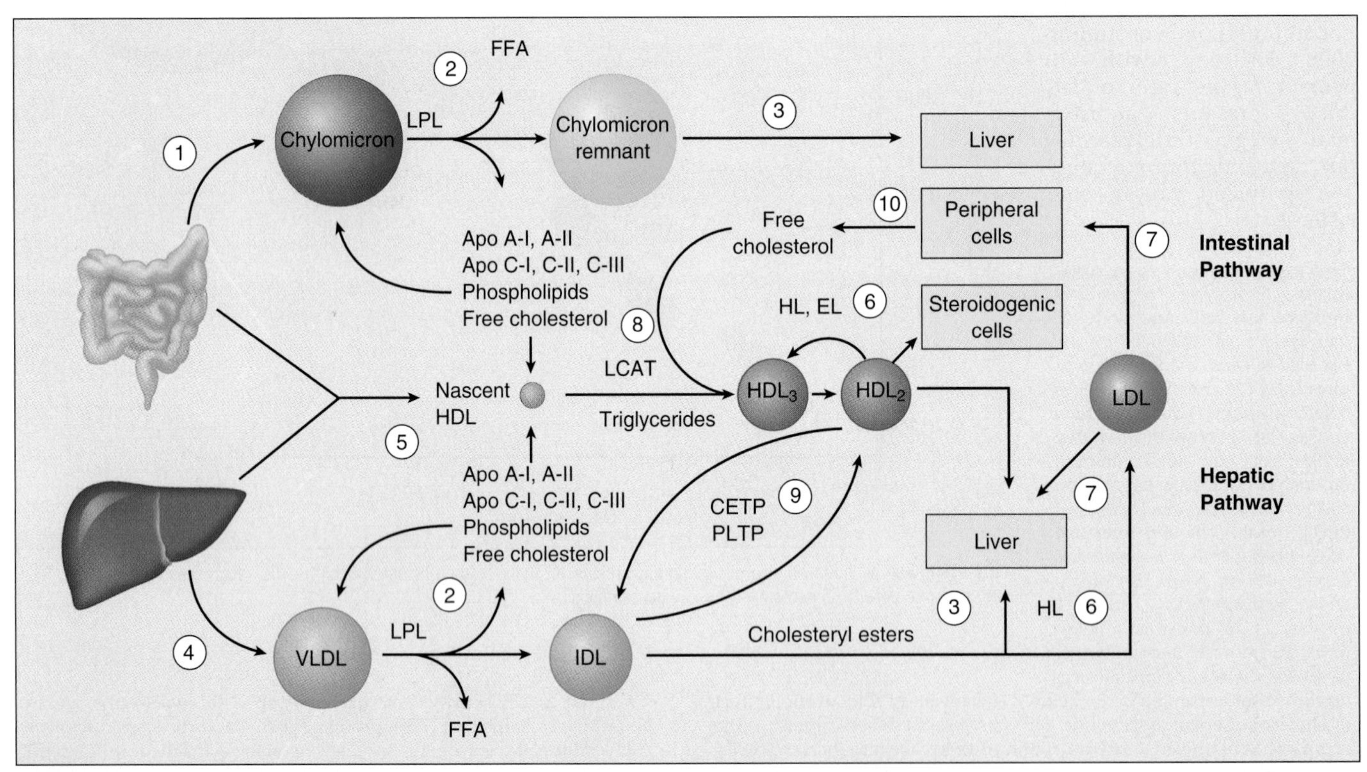

FIGURE 39–4 Schematic diagram of the lipid transport system. Numbers in circles refer to explanation in text. Apo = apolipoprotein; CETP = cholesteryl ester transfer protein; EL = endothelial lipase; FFA = free fatty acids; HL = hepatic lipase; HDL = high-density lipoprotein; IDL = intermediate-density lipoprotein; LCAT = lecithin cholesterol acyltransferase; LDL = low-density lipoprotein; LPL = lipoprotein lipase; PLTP = phospholipid transfer protein; VLDL = very-low-density lipoprotein.

TABLE 39–3 Lipoprotein Processing Enzymes, Receptors, Modulating Proteins

Abreviation	Name	Role	Chromosome	Human Disease
ABCA1	ATP binding cassette AI	Cellular phospholipid efflux	9q31	Tangier disease
ABCG5/G8	ATP binding cassette G5 and G8	Intestinal sitosterol transporter	21	Sitosterolemia
ACAT1	Acyl:CoA cholesterol acyl-transferase 1	Cholesterol esterification	1q22.3	Cellular cholesterol esterification
ACAT2	Acyl:CoA cholesterol acyl-transferase 2	Cholesterol esterification	6q25.3	Cellular cholesterol esterification
ApoE-R	ApoE containing lipoprotein	TRL uptake	1p34	
CD36	Fatty acid translocase	Fatty acid transport	7q11.2	See ref. 73
CETP	Cholesteryl ester transfer protein	Lipid exchange in plasma	16q21	Elevated HDL cholesterol
EL	Endothelial lipase	Tg hydrolysis	18q21.1	See ref. 79
HL	Hepatic lipase	Tg hydrolysis	15q21	Remnant accumulation[75,76]
HSL (LIPE)	Hormone-sensitive lipase	Fatty acid release from adipocytes	19q13.2	
LCAT	Lecithin:cholesterol acyltransferase	Cholesterol esterification	16q22.1	LCAT deficiency, low HDL
LDL-R	Low-density lipoprotein receptor	LDL uptake	19p13	Familial hypercholesterolemia
Lox1	Scavenger receptor	OxLDL uptake, endothelium	12p12-13	Oxidized lipoprotein uptake
LPL	Lipoprotein lipase	Tg hydrolysis	8p22	Hyperchylomicronemia
LRP1	LDL-R–related protein	Protease uptake, many ligands	19q12	
LRP2	LDL-R–related protein 2 (megalin)	Protease uptake, apo J	2q24-31	See ref. 74
MTP	Microsomal triglyceride transfer	Apo B assembly	4q22-24	Abetalipoproteinemia
NPC1	Niemann-Pick C gene product	Cellular cholesterol transport	18q11-12	Niemann-Pick type C
NPC1L1	Niemann-Pick C1-like 1 protein	Intestinal cholesterol absorption	7p13	See ref. 8a
PLTP	Phospholipid transfer protein	Lipid exchange in plasma	20q12	See ref. 77
PCSK9	Proprotein convertase, subtilisin/kexin type 9	Protein cleavage	1p34.1	Hypercholesterolemia
SRA	Scavenger receptor A	OxLDL uptake, macrophages	8p21	
SR-B1	Scavenger receptor B1	HDL CE uptake	12	See ref. 78
VLDL-R	Very-low-density lipoprotein receptor	VLDL uptake	9q24	

CE = cholesterol esters; HDL = high-density lipoprotein; LDL = low-density lipoprotein; OxLDL = oxidized low-density lipoprotein; Tg = triglyceride; TRL = triglyceride-rich lipoprotein; VLDL = very-low-density lipoprotein.

HEPATIC PATHWAY (VERY-LOW-DENSITY LIPOPROTEIN TO INTERMEDIATE-DENSITY LIPOPROTEIN). Food is not always available, and dietary fat content is not always constant. The body must ensure readily available triglyceride molecules for energy demands. Hepatic secretion of VLDL particles serves this function (Fig. 39–4, part 4). VLDLs are triglyceride-rich lipoproteins smaller than chylomicrons (see Table 39–1 and Fig. 39–3). They contain apo B100 as their main lipoprotein. As opposed to apo B48, apo B100 contains a domain recognized by the LDL receptor (the apo B/E receptor). VLDL particles follow the same catabolic pathway through lipoprotein lipase as chylomicrons (Fig. 39–4, part 2). During hydrolysis of triglyceride-rich lipoproteins by LPL, an exchange of proteins and lipids takes place: VLDL particles (and chylomicrons) acquire apo Cs and apo E, in part from HDL particles. VLDLs also exchange triglycerides for cholesteryl esters from HDL (mediated by cholesteryl ester transfer protein [CETP]) (Fig. 39–4, parts 5 and 9). Such bidirectional transfer of constituents between lipoproteins serves several purposes, allowing lipoproteins to acquire specific apolipoproteins that will dictate their metabolic fate; transfer of phospholipids onto nascent HDL particles mediated by phospholipid transfer protein (PLTP)[10] (during the loss of core triglycerides, the phospholipid envelope becomes redundant and is shed off to apo AI to form new HDL particles); and transfer of cholesterol from HDL to VLDL remnants so it can be metabolized in the liver. This exchange constitutes a major part of the reverse cholesterol transport pathway.

After hydrolysis of triglycerides partly depletes VLDL of triglycerides, VLDL particles have relatively more cholesterol, shed several apolipoproteins (especially the C apolipoproteins), and acquire apo E. The VLDL remnant lipoprotein, called *intermediate-density lipoprotein*, is taken up by the liver via its apo E moiety (Fig. 39–4, part 3) or further delipidated by hepatic lipase to form an LDL particle (Fig. 39–4, part 6). There are at least four receptors for triglyceride-rich lipoprotein (TRL), TRL remnants, and apo B–containing lipoproteins: the VLDL receptor, the remnant receptor, the LDL receptor (also called the apo B/E receptor), and the LDL receptor–related peptide. A common feature of most hepatic receptors is their recognition of apo E, which mediates uptake of several classes of lipoproteins, including VLDL and intermediate-density lipoprotein. The interaction between apo E and its ligand is complex and involves the "docking" of TRL on heparan sulfate proteoglycans before presentation of the ligand to its receptor.

LOW-DENSITY LIPOPROTEINS. LDL particles contain predominantly cholesteryl esters packaged with the protein moiety apo B100. Normally, triglycerides constitute only 4 to 8 percent of the LDL mass. In the presence of elevated plasma triglyceride levels, LDL particles can become enriched in triglycerides and depleted in core cholesteryl esters. LDL particle size variation results from changes in core constituents, with an increase in triglycerides and a relative decrease in cholesteryl esters leading to smaller, denser LDL particles.

The LDL particles in most higher mammals, including humans and nonhuman primates, serve as the main carriers of cholesterol. In other mammals, such as rodents or rabbits, VLDL and HDL particles transport most of the cholesterol. The cholesterol molecule is required for membrane biosynthesis, steroid hormone production, or bile acid synthesis in the liver. Cells can either make cholesterol from acetate through enzymatic reactions requiring at least 33 steps or obtain it as cholesteryl esters from LDL particles. Cells internalize LDL via the LDL receptor (LDL-R) (Fig. 39–5A). LDL particles contain one molecule of apo B. While several domains of apo B are highly lipophilic and associate with phospholipids, a region surrounding residue 3500 binds with high affinity and saturability to the LDL-R. The LDL-R localizes in a region of the plasma membrane rich in the protein clathrin (Figs. 39–4, part 7 and 39–5A). Once bound to the receptor, clathrin polymerizes and forms an endosome that contains LDL bound to its receptor, a portion of the plasma membrane, and clathrin. This internalized particle then fuses with a lysosome that will release its catalytic enzymes (cholesteryl ester hydrolase, cathepsins), which in turn will release free cholesterol and degrade apo B. The LDL-R will detach itself from its ligand and recycle to the plasma membrane.

Cells tightly regulate cholesterol content by (1) cholesterol synthesis in the smooth endoplasmic reticulum (via the rate-limiting step hydroxymethylglutaryl coenzyme A [HMG-CoA] reductase); (2) receptor-mediated endocytosis of LDL (two mechanisms under the control of the steroid-responsive element binding protein [SREBP]); (3) cholesterol efflux from plasma membrane to cholesterol acceptor particles (predominantly HDL); and (4) intracellular cholesterol esterification via the enzyme acyl-CoA: cholesteryl acyltransferase (ACAT) (see Fig. 39–5A, B). The SREBP coordinately regulates the first two pathways at the level of gene transcription. Cellular cholesterol binds to a protein called SCAP (SREPB cholesterol-activated protein), which is located on the endoplasmic reticulum. Cholesterol inhibits the interaction of SCAP with SREPB. In the absence of cholesterol, SCAP will mediate the cleavage of SREBP at two sites by specific proteases and release an amino (NH_2) fragment of SREBP. The SREBP NH_2 fragment will migrate to the nucleus and increase the transcriptional activity of genes involved in cellular cholesterol and fatty acid homeostasis. Cleavage of SREBP depends on a proprotein convertase related to the subtilisin/kexin family of convertases.[11] The ACAT pathway is regulated at the level of protein regulation by cholesterol content in membranes.[12] Humans express two separate forms of ACAT. ACAT1 and ACAT2 derive from different genes and mediate cholesterol esterification in cytoplasm and in the endoplasmic reticulum lumen for lipoprotein assembly and secretion.[13]

Regulation of cholesterol efflux depends in part on the ABCA1 pathway, controlled in turn by hydroxysterols (especially 22-OH cholesterol, which acts as a ligand for the liver-specific receptor [LXR] family of transcriptional regulatory factors). In conditions of cellular cholesterol excess, the cell can decrease its input of cholesterol by decreasing the de novo synthesis of cholesterol. The cell can also decrease the amount of cholesterol that enters the cell via the LDL-R, increase the amount stored as cholesteryl esters, and promote the removal of cholesterol by increasing its movement to the plasma membrane for efflux.

HIGH-DENSITY LIPOPROTEIN AND REVERSE CHOLESTEROL TRANSPORT. Epidemiological studies consistently have shown an inverse relationship between plasma levels of HDL cholesterol and the presence of coronary artery disease. HDL promotes reverse cholesterol transport and can prevent lipoprotein oxidation and exert antiinflammatory actions in vitro. In a process called *selective uptake of cholesterol*, HDL also provides cholesterol to steroid hormone–producing tissues and the liver through the scavenger SR-B1 receptor (see Fig. 39–5C).[14,15]

The metabolism of HDL is complex and only partly understood. The complexity arises from the consideration that HDL particles acquire their components from several sources while these components also are metabolized at different sites. Apolipoprotein AI, the main protein of HDL, is synthesized in the intestine and the

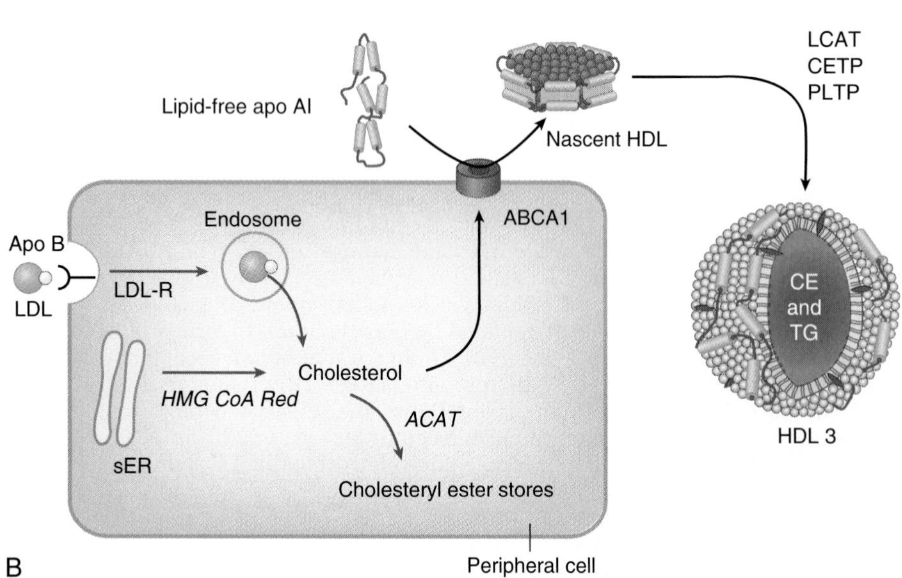

FIGURE 39–5 Cellular cholesterol homeostasis in various tissues. **A,** Cholesterol homeostasis (hepatocytes). **B,** Cellular cholesterol efflux (peripheral cells). *See opposite page for definitions and parts C and D.*

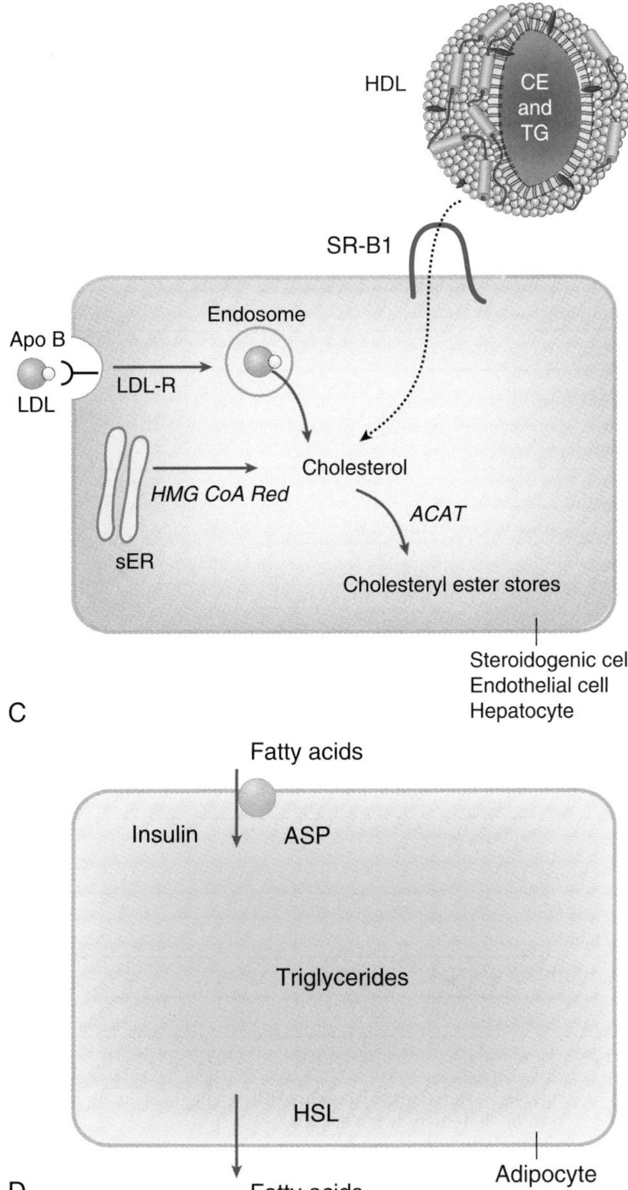

FIGURE 39–5—cont'd **C,** Selective uptake of cholesterol (adrenal cells, hepatocytes, endothelial cells). **D,** Adipocytes. ABCA1 = ATP-binding cassette transporter A1; ACAT = acyl–coenzyme A:cholesterol acyltransferase; Apo = apolipoprotein; ASP = acylation-stimulating protein; CE = cholesterol esters; CETP = cholesteryl ester transfer protein; HDL = high-density lipoprotein; HMG CoA Red = hydroxymethylglutaryl coenzyme A reductase; HSL = hormone-sensitive lipase; IDL = intermediate-density lipoprotein; LCAT = lecithin cholesterol acyltransferase; LDL = low-density lipoprotein; LDL-R = low-density lipoprotein receptor; LRP = low-density lipoprotein receptor–related peptide; PLTP = phospholipid transfer protein; sER = smooth endoplasmic reticulum; SR-B1 = scavenger receptor B1; TG = triglycerides; VLDL = very-low-density lipoprotein; VLDL-R = very-low-density lipoprotein receptor.

liver. Lipid-free apo AI acquires phospholipids from cell membranes and from redundant phospholipids shed during hydrolysis of triglyceride-rich lipoproteins. Lipid-free apo AI binds to ABCA1 and promotes its phosphorylation via cyclic adenosine monophosphate, which increases the net efflux of phospholipids and cholesterol onto apo AI to form a nascent HDL particle (Fig. 39–4, part 10).[16,17] This particle, containing apo AI and phospholipids (and little cholesterol) resembles a flattened disk in which the phospholipids form a bilayer surrounded by two molecules of apo AI arranged in a circular fashion at the periphery of the disk (see Fig. 39–5B). These nascent HDL particles will mediate further cellular cholesterol efflux. Currently, standard laboratory tests do not measure these HDL precursors because they contain little or no cholesterol. Upon reaching a cell membrane, the nascent HDL particles will capture membrane-associated cholesterol and promote the efflux of free cholesterol onto other HDL particles (see Fig. 39–4, part 10). Conceptually, the formation of HDL particles appears to be a two-step phenomenon, the first step being ABCA1-mediated and the second probably not dependent on ABCA1.[18] The plasma enzyme LCAT, an enzyme activated by apo AI, then esterifies the free cholesterol (see Figs. 39–4, part 8, and 39–5B). LCAT transfers an acyl chain (a fatty acid) from the R2 position of a phospholipid to the 3′OH residue of cholesterol, resulting in the formation of a cholesteryl ester (see Fig. 39–1).

Because cholesteryl esters are hydrophobic, they move to the core of the lipoprotein and the HDL particle now assumes a spherical configuration (a particle denoted HDL_3). With further cholesterol esterification, the HDL particle increases in size to become the more buoyant HDL_2. Cholesterol within HDL particles can exchange with triglyceride-rich lipoproteins via cholesteryl ester transfer protein (CETP), which mediates an equimolar exchange of cholesterol from HDL to triglyceride-rich lipoprotein and triglyceride movement from triglyceride-rich lipoprotein onto HDL (Fig. 39–4, part 9). Phospholipid transfer protein (PLTP) mediates the transfer of phospholipids between triglyceride-rich lipoprotein and HDL particles. Triglyceride-enriched HDL are denoted HDL_{2b}. Hepatic lipase can hydrolyze triglycerides within these particles, converting them back to HDL_3 particles.

One mechanism of reverse cholesterol transport includes the uptake of cellular cholesterol and its esterification by LCAT, transport by large HDL particles, and exchange for one triglyceride molecule by CETP. Originally on an HDL particle, the cholesterol molecule can now be taken up by hepatic receptors on a triglyceride-rich lipoprotein or LDL particle. HDL particles, therefore, act as shuttles between tissue cholesterol, triglyceride-rich lipoprotein, and the liver.

The catabolism of HDL particles has been a matter of debate among lipoprotein researchers. The protein component of HDL particles is exchangeable with lipoproteins of other classes. The kidneys appear to be a route of elimination of apolipoprotein AI and other HDL apolipoproteins.[19] The lipid component of HDL particles also follow a different metabolic route (see Fig. 39–5A, B, and C).

Lipoprotein Disorders

Definitions

Time and new knowledge have brought necessary changes to the classification of lipoprotein disorders. The original classification of lipoprotein disorders by Fredrickson, Lees, and Levy was based on the measurement of total plasma cholesterol and triglycerides and analyzed lipoproteins patterns after separation by electrophoresis. This classification recognized elevations of chylomicrons (type I), VLDL or pre-beta lipoproteins (type IV), "broad beta" disease (or type III hyperlipoproteinemia), beta lipoproteins (LDL) (type II), and elevations of both chylomicrons and VLDL (type V). In addition, the combined elevations of pre-beta (VLDL) and beta (LDL) lipoproteins was recognized as type IIb hyperlipoproteinemia. Though providing a useful conceptual framework, this classification has some drawbacks: it does not include HDL cholesterol, and it does not differentiate severe monogenic lipoprotein disorders from the more common polygenic disorders. Subsequently, the World Health Organization, the European Atherosclerosis Society and, more recently, the National Cholesterol Education Program have classified lipoprotein disorders on the basis of arbitrary cut-points.

A practical approach describes the lipoprotein disorder by the absolute plasma levels of lipids (cholesterol and triglycerides) and lipoprotein cholesterol levels (LDL and HDL cholesterol) and considers clinical manifestations of hyperlipoproteinemia in the context of biochemical characterization. For example, a young patient presenting with eruptive xanthomas and a plasma triglyceride level of 11.3 mmol/liter (1000 mg/dl) is likely to have familial hyperchylomicronemia. An obese, hypertensive middle-aged man with a cholesterol level of 6.4 mmol/liter (247 mg/dl), a triglyceride level of 3.1 mmol/liter (274 mg/dl), a HDL cholesterol level of 0.8 mmol/liter (31 mg/ml), and a calculated LDL cholesterol level of 4.2 mmol/liter (162 mg/dl) likely has the metabolic syndrome, the concomitant conditions of which, such as hypertension, hyperglycemia, and hyperuricemia, should be sought.

The clinical usefulness of apolipoprotein levels has stirred debate. Although a useful research tool in general, the measurement of apolipoproteins AI and B practically may add little substantial information to that provided by the conventional lipid profile. Taken as a single measurement, the apo B level provides information on the number of potentially atherogenic particles and can be used as a goal of lipid-lowering therapy.[20] Similarly, LDL particle size correlates highly with plasma HDL cholesterol and triglyceride levels, and most studies do not show it to be an independent cardiovascular risk factor. The presence of small, dense LDL particles can be related to features of the metabolic syndrome, which is characterized by the presence of abdominal obesity, peripheral insulin resistance, high blood pressure, and dyslipoproteinemia with elevated plasma triglycerides and reduced HDL cholesterol levels. In some studies, improvement in LDL particle size correlated with angiographic improvement of coronary artery disease. Other studies showed that large LDL particles correlate with recurrent coronary events in survivors of myocardial infarction.[21] It remains uncertain whether in addition to LDL particle number reduction, a change in LDL particle size will bring further clinical benefit.[22]

Genetic Lipoprotein Disorders

Understanding of the genetics of lipoprotein metabolism has expanded rapidly. Classification of genetic lipoprotein disorders usually requires a biochemical phenotype in addition to a clinical phenotype. With the exception of familial hypercholesterolemia, monogenic disorders tend to be infrequent or very rare. Disorders considered heritable on careful family study may be difficult to characterize unambiguously because of age, gender, penetrance, and gene-gene and environmental interactions. Most common lipoprotein disorders encountered clinically result from the interaction of increasing age, lack of physical exercise, weight gain, and a suboptimal diet with individual genetic make-up.

Genetic lipoprotein disorders can affect LDL, lipoprotein(a), remnant lipoproteins, triglyceride-rich lipoproteins (chylomicrons and VLDL), or HDL (Table 39–4). Within each of these, genetic disorders can cause an excess or a deficiency of a specific class of lipoprotein.

TABLE 39–4 Genetic Lipoprotein Disorders

Disorder	Gene	Figure 4
LDL Particles		
Familial hypercholesterolemia	LDL-R	7
Familial defective apo B-100	Apo B	7
Autosomal dominant hypercholesterolemia	PCSK9	
Abetalipoproteinemia	MTP	
Hypobetalipoproteinemia	Apo B	
Familial sitosterolemia	ABCG5/ABCG8	
Lipoprotein(a)		
Familial lipoprotein(a) hyperlipoproteinemia	Apo (a)	
Remnant Lipoproteins		
Dysbetalipoproteinemia type III	Apo E	3
Hepatic lipase deficiency	HL	6
Triglyceride-rich Lipoproteins		
Lipoprotein lipase deficiency	LPL	2
Apo CII deficiency	Apo CII	2
Familial hypertriglyceridemia	Polygenic	
Chylomicron retention disease	?	
Familial combined hyperlipidemia	Polygenic	
HDL Particles		
Apo AI deficiency	Apo AI	
Familial HDL deficiency/Tangier disease	ABCA1	10
Familial LCAT deficiency syndromes	LCAT	8
CETP deficiency	CETP	9
Niemann-Pick disease types A and B	SMPD1	

CETP = cholesteryl ester transfer protein; HDL = high-density lipoprotein; LCAT = lecithin cholesterol acyltransferase.

Low-Density Lipoproteins (Type II Hyperlipidemia)

FAMILIAL HYPERCHOLESTEROLEMIA. Familial hypercholesterolemia is the most thoroughly studied lipoprotein disorder. The elucidation of the pathway by which complex molecules enter the cell by receptor-mediated endocytosis and the discovery of the LDL receptor represent landmarks in cell biology and clinical medicine. Affected subjects have an elevated LDL cholesterol level greater than the 95th percentile for age and gender. In adulthood, clinical manifestations include corneal arcus, tendinous xanthomas over the extensor tendons (metacarpophalangeal joints, Achilles tendons), and xanthelasmas. Transmission is autosomal codominant. The prevalence of familial hypercholesterolemia is estimated at approximately 1:500, although this prevalence is higher in populations with founder effects. Patients with familial hypercholesterolemia are at high risk of developing coronary artery disease (CAD) by the third to fourth decade in men and approximately 8 to 10 years later in women. Diagnosis is based on elevated plasma LDL cholesterol level, family history of premature CAD, and the presence of xanthomas. A molecular diagnosis is sometimes required. Defects of the *LDL-R* gene cause an accumulation of LDL particles in plasma and thus alter the function of the LDL-R protein and cause familial hypercholesterolemia (Fig. 39–4, part 7). To date, there are well over 600 identified mutations of the *LDL-R* gene (see http://www.umd.necker.fr).[23]

FAMILIAL DEFECTIVE APO B. Mutations within the apo B gene that lead to an abnormal ligand-receptor interaction can cause a form of familial hypercholesterolemia clinically indistinguishable from the primary form. This disorder, familial defective apo B 100, is caused by several mutations at the postulated binding site to the LDL-R (Fig. 39–4, part 7). These consist of apo $B_{Arg3500Gln}$, apo $B_{Arg3500Trp}$, and apo $B_{Arg3531Cys}$.[24] The apo $B_{Arg3500Gln}$ results from a G→A substitution at nucleotide 3500 within exon

26 of the apo B gene. The defective apo B has a reduced affinity (20 to 30 percent of control) for the LDL-R. LDL particles with defective apo B have a plasma half-life three- to fourfold greater than the half-life of normal LDL. Because of their increased half-life, these LDL particles can more readily undergo oxidative modifications that can enhance their atherogenicity. Affected subjects usually have elevated LDL cholesterol levels up to 400 mg/dl (10.4 mmol/liter) but may also have normal levels. Familial defective apo B 100 has a prevalence similar to that of familial hypercholesterolemia (1/500). In subjects with the classic presentation of familial hypercholesterolemia, the prevalence of familial defective apo B 100 is reported to be 1 in 50 to 1 in 20. The reasons for the variability of plasma LDL cholesterol levels remain unexplained.

Mutations within the apo B gene can lead to truncations of the mature apo B_{100} peptide. Many such mutations cause a syndrome characterized by reduced LDL and VLDL cholesterol but little or no clinical manifestations and no known risk of cardiovascular disease. Apo B truncated close to its amino terminus loses the ability to bind lipids, producing a syndrome similar to abetalipoproteinemia, a rare recessive lipoprotein disorder of infancy that causes mental retardation and growth abnormalities. Abetalipoproteinemia is caused by a mutation in gene coding for the microsomal triglyceride transfer protein (MTP) required for assembly of apo B–containing lipoproteins in the liver and the intestine.[25] The resulting lack of apo B–containing lipoproteins in plasma causes a marked deficiency of fat-soluble vitamins (A, D, E, and K) that circulate in lipoproteins.

An autosomal dominant form of hypercholesterolemia has been mapped to chromosome 1p34.1. The genetic basis for this condition is mutation within the proprotein convertase, subtilisin/kexin type 9 gene (*PCSK9*). *PCSK9* codes for a protein identified as neural apoptosis-regulated convertase 1 (NARC1), a novel proprotein convertase belonging to the subtilase family of convertases. It is related to subtilisin/kexin isoenzyme-1 (site-1 protease) required for cleavage of SREBP.[11]

SITOSTEROLEMIA. A rare condition of increased intestinal absorption and decreased excretion of plant sterols (sitosterol and campesterol) can mimic severe familial hypercholesterolemia, with extensive xanthoma formation. Premature atherosclerosis, often apparent clinically before adulthood, occurs frequently in patients with sitosterolemia. Diagnosis requires specialized analysis of plasma sterols demonstrating an elevation in sitosterol, campesterol, cholestanol, sitostanol, and campestanol. Interestingly, plasma cholesterol is normal or reduced, and triglycerides are normal. Positional cloning techniques have localized the defect to chromosome 2p21. Mutations in the adenosine triphosphate binding cassette G5 and G8 genes (*ABCG5* and *ABCG8*) have been found in patients with sitosterolemia. The gene products of *ABCG5* and *ABCG8* are half ABC transporters and are thought to form a heterodimer characteristic of the full ABC transporters. The complex is located in the villous border of intestinal cells and actively pumps plant sterols back into the intestinal lumen. A defect in either of the genes renders the complex inactive, and absorption of plant sterols (rather than their elimination) ensues. *ABCG5* and *ABCG8* mutations leading to sitosterolemia are very rare.[26]

LIPOPROTEIN(A) (see Chap. 36)**.** Lipoprotein(a) consists of an LDL particle linked covalently with one molecule of apo (a). The apo (a) moiety consists of a protein with a high degree of homology with plasminogen. The apo (a) gene appears to have arisen from the plasminogen gene by nonhomologous recombination. The apo (a) gene has multiple repeats of one of the kringle motifs (kringle IV), varying in number from 12 to more than 40 in each individual. Plasma lipoprotein(a) levels depend almost entirely on genetics and correlate inversely with the number of kringle repeats and, therefore, with the molecular weight of apo (a).[27] Few environmental factors or medications modulate plasma lipoprotein(a) levels. The pathogenesis of lipoprotein(a) may result from an antifibrinolytic potential and/or ability to bind oxidized lipoproteins. Some prospective epidemiological studies have shown a positive (albeit weak) association between lipoprotein(a) and coronary artery disease (see Chap. 36).[28]

Triglyceride-Rich Lipoproteins

In subjects with the metabolic syndrome and in diabetic patients, elevation of plasma triglyceride level occurs most often in the presence of visceral (abdominal) obesity and a diet rich in calories, carbohydrates, and saturated fats. Severe elevation of plasma triglycerides can result from genetic disorders of the processing enzymes or apolipoproteins and poorly controlled diabetes.

FAMILIAL HYPERTRIGLYCERIDEMIA (TYPE IV HYPERLIPOPROTEINEMIA). Familial hypertriglyceridemia is not associated with clinical signs such as corneal arcus, xanthoma, and xanthelasmas. Plasma triglycerides, VLDL cholesterol, and VLDL triglycerides are moderately to markedly elevated; LDL cholesterol level is usually low, and HDL cholesterol level is also reduced. Total cholesterol is normal or elevated, depending on VLDL cholesterol levels. Fasting plasma concentrations of triglycerides are in the range of 2.3 to 5.7 mmol/liter (200 to 500 mg/dl). After a meal, plasma triglycerides may exceed 11.3 mmol/liter (1000 mg/dl). The disorder is found in first-degree relatives, but phenotypic variability is related to gender, age, hormone use (especially estrogens), and diet. Alcohol intake potently stimulates hypertriglyceridemia in these subjects, as does caloric or carbohydrate intake. The relationship with coronary artery disease is not as strong as with familial combined hyperlipidemia and has not been found consistently. Depending on criteria used, the prevalence of familial hypertriglyceridemia ranges from 1 in 100 to 1 in 50. The disorder is highly heterogeneous and likely results from several genes, with a strong environmental influence. An unrelated disorder, familial glycerolemia, a chromosome X-linked genetic disorder, may mimic familial hypertriglyceridemia because most measurement techniques for triglycerides use the measurement of glycerol after enzymatic hydrolysis of triglycerides.[29] The diagnosis of familial hyperglycerolemia requires ultracentrifugation of plasma and analysis of glycerol.

The metabolic defect in familial hypertriglyceridemia is hepatic overproduction of VLDL (Fig. 39–4, part 4); the catabolism (uptake) of VLDL particles can be normal or reduced. Lipolysis by LPL appears not to be a limiting factor, although the triglyceride load, especially in the postprandial state, may limit processing of VLDL particles. The genetic basis of familial hypertriglyceridemia is unknown, and the candidate approach to find the gene or genes involved (apo B, LDL, apo CIII) has not yielded fruit thus far. Treatment is based first on lifestyle modifications, including withdrawal of hormones (estrogens and progesterone), limiting alcohol intake, reducing caloric intake, and increasing exercise. The decision to treat this disorder with medications depends on global cardiovascular risk.

An infrequent disorder characterized by severe elevation in plasma triglyceride levels (both VLDL and chylomicrons) is associated with a fat-rich diet, obesity, and poorly controlled diabetes. Recognized as type V hyperlipidemia, the pathogenesis is multifactorial and results from overproduction of both VLDL and chylomicrons and decreased catabolism of these particles.

FAMILIAL HYPERCHYLOMICRONEMIA (TYPE I HYPERLIPIDEMIA). This is a rare disorder of severe hypertriglyceridemia associated with elevations in fasting plasma triglycerides greater than 11.3 mmol/liter (>1000 mg/dl). These patients have recurrent bouts of pancreatitis and eruptive xanthomas. Interestingly, severe hypertriglyceridemia can also be associated with xerostomia, xerophthalmia, and behavioral abnormalities. The hypertriglyceridemia results from a markedly reduced or absent LPL activity or, more rarely, the absence of its activator, apo CII (Fig. 39–4, part 2).[30] These defects lead to a lack of hydrolysis of chylomicrons and VLDL and their accumulation in plasma, especially after meals. Extreme elevations of plasma triglycerides (>113 mmol/liter; >10 000 mg/dl) can result.

Plasma from a patient with very high triglycerides is milky white, and a clear band of chylomicrons can be seen on top of the plasma after it stands overnight in a refrigerator. Populations with a founder effect can have high prevalence of LPL mutations. At least 60 LPL mutations can cause LPL deficiency. LPL_{188}, $LPL_{asn291ser}$, and LPL_{207} are frequently associated hyperchylomicronemia. Heterozygotes for the disorder tend to have an increase in fasting plasma triglycerides and smaller, denser LDL particles. Many patients with complete LPL deficiency present in childhood fail to thrive and have recurrent bouts of pancreatitis. To underscore the importance of LPL's role, the LPL knockout mouse leads to a perinatal lethal phenotype.[31] The treatment of acute pancreatitis includes intravenous hydration and avoidance of fat in the diet (including in parenteral nutrition). Plasma filtration is required only rarely. Chronic treatment includes avoidance of alcohol and dietary fats. To make the diet more palatable, short-chain fatty acids (which are not incorporated in chylomicrons) can be used to supplement the diet.

TYPE III HYPERLIPOPROTEINEMIA. Type III hyperlipoproteinemia, also referred to as *dysbetalipoproteinemia* or *broad beta disease*, is a rare genetic lipoprotein disorder characterized by an accumulation in plasma of remnant lipoprotein particles. On lipoprotein agarose gel electrophoresis, a typical pattern of a broad band between the pre-beta (VLDL) and beta (LDL) lipoproteins is observed, hence the name "broad beta disease." Patients with this disease clearly have increased cardiovascular risk. The clinical presentation consists of pathognomonic tuberous xanthomas and palmar striated xanthomas. The lipoprotein profile shows increased cholesterol and triglyceride levels and reduced HDL cholesterol. Remnant lipoproteins (partly catabolized chylomicrons and VLDL) accumulate in plasma and accumulate cholesterol esters. The defect is due to abnormal apo E, which does not bind to hepatic receptors using

apo E as a ligand (Fig. 39-4, part 3).[32] The ratio of VLDL cholesterol to triglycerides, normally less than 0.7 mmol/liter (<0.30 mg/dl), is elevated in patients with type III hyperlipoproteinemia, owing to cholesteryl ester enrichment of remnant particles. The diagnosis includes plasma ultracentrifugation for lipoprotein separation, lipoprotein electrophoresis, and apo E phenotyping or genotyping. Patients with type III hyperlipoproteinemia have the apo E2/2 phenotype or genotype. There are three common alleles for apo E: apo E2, E3, and E4. The apo E2 allele has markedly decreased binding to the apo B/E receptor.

In a normal population, the prevalence of the apo E2/2 phenotype is approximately 0.7 to 1.0 percent. Type III hyperlipoproteinemia occurs in approximately 1 percent of subjects bearing the apo E2/2 phenotype. The reasons for the relative rarity of type III dyslipoproteinemia are not fully understood. As discussed previously, a second "hit" is thought to impart the full expression of the disorder. Other rare mutations of the apo E gene can cause type III hyperlipoproteinemia.[32] Apo E–deficient mice currently serve as a model for the study of atherosclerosis.[13] In general, type III dyslipoproteinemia responds well to dietary therapy, correction of other metabolic abnormalities (diabetes, obesity), and, in cases requiring drug therapy, fibric acid derivatives or statins.

FAMILIAL COMBINED HYPERLIPIDEMIA. One of the most common familial lipoprotein disorders is familial combined hyperlipoproteinemia. Described initially in survivors of myocardial infarction, the definition of familial combined hyperlipoproteinemia has undergone several refinements. It is characterized by the presence of elevated total cholesterol and/or triglyceride levels based on arbitrary cut-points in several members of the same family. Advances in analytical techniques have added the measurement of LDL cholesterol and, in some cases, apo B levels. Because of the lack of a clear-cut clinical or biochemical marker, considerable overlap exists between familial combined hyperlipoproteinemia, familial dyslipidemic hypertension, the metabolic syndrome, and hyperapobetalipoproteinemia. Genetic heterogeneity probably underlies familial combined hyperlipoproteinemia, which has a prevalence of approximately 1 in 50 and accounts for 10 to 20 percent of patients with premature CAD.[33] The condition has few clinical signs; corneal arcus, xanthomas, and xanthelasmas occur infrequently. The biochemical abnormalities include elevation of plasma total and LDL cholesterol levels (>90th to 95th percentile) and/or an elevation of plasma triglycerides (>90th to 95th percentile)—a type IIb lipoprotein phenotype, often in correlation with low HDL cholesterol and elevated apo B levels; small, dense LDL particles are seen frequently. For a diagnosis of familial combined hyperlipoproteinemia, the disorder must be identified in at least one first-degree relative. The underlying metabolic disorder appears to be hepatic overproduction of apo B–containing lipoproteins, delayed postprandial triglyceride-rich lipoprotein clearance, and increased flux of free fatty acids (FFA) to the liver.

Experimental data have shown that hepatic apo B secretion is substrate driven, the most important substrates being FFA and cholesteryl esters. Increased delivery of FFA to the liver, as occurs in states of insulin resistance, leads to increased hepatic apo B secretion (see Chap. 40). Familial combined hyperlipoproteinemia has complex genetics. It was initially considered an autosomal codominant trait; modifying factors include gender, age of onset, and comorbid states such as obesity, lack of exercise, and diet. Initial reports of linkage with the apo AI-CIII-AIV and LPL genes remain unsubstantiated. A novel locus on chromosome 1 in Finnish families currently appears to be a promising candidate gene related to familial combined hyperlipoproteinemia.[34]

Recent reports of the acylation-stimulating protein (ASP), also known as complement C3desARG pathway, suggests that abnormal peripheral uptake of FFA may underlie some cases of familial combined hyperlipoproteinemia and the insulin-resistance metabolic syndrome.[35] A putative receptor for ASP has been identified recently as the orphan receptor C2L5, the complement C5 receptor that also binds complement C3desARG.[36] Abnormal binding of ASP to peripheral cells has been reported in subjects with familial combined hyperlipoproteinemia. Abnormal ASP binding causes decreased uptake of FFAs into adipocytes and subsequent increased flux of FFAs to the liver (see Fig. 39-5D). FFAs are a major substrate for hepatic apo B-containing lipoprotein assembly and secretion.

High-Density Lipoproteins

Reduced plasma levels of HDL cholesterol consistently correlate with the development or presence of CAD (see Chap. 36). Most cases of reduced HDL cholesterol are secondary to elevated plasma triglycerides or apo B levels and often keep company with other features of the metabolic syndrome. Primary forms of reduced HDL cholesterol have been identified in cases of premature CAD and helped shed light on the complex metabolism of HDL particles. Genetic disorders of HDL can result from decreased production or abnormal maturation and increased catabolism. Genetic lipoprotein disorders leading to moderate to severe elevations in plasma triglycerides cause a reduction in HDL cholesterol levels. Familial hyperchylomicronemia, familial hypertriglyceridemia, and familial combined hyperlipoproteinemia are all associated with reduced HDL cholesterol levels. In complex disorders of lipoprotein metabolism such as familial combined hyperlipidemia, the metabolic syndrome, and common forms of hypertriglyceridemia, several factors most likely correlate to low HDL cholesterol level. Plasma triglycerides and HDL cholesterol levels vary inversely. For several reasons, patients with elevated apo B levels also have reduced HDL cholesterol levels. First, decreased lipolysis of triglyceride-rich lipoproteins (each VLDL contains one molecule of apo B) decrease the substrate (phospholipids) available for HDL maturation. Second, triglyceride enrichment of HDL increases their catabolic rate and hence reduces their plasma concentration. Third, exchange of lipids between HDL and triglyceride-rich lipoprotein is reduced, leading to a more rapid disappearance of HDL from plasma.[37] The inverse relationship between HDL cholesterol levels and plasma triglycerides reflects the interdependency of the metabolism of triglyceride-rich lipoproteins and HDL particles.

APO AI GENE DEFECTS. Primary defects affecting production of HDL particles consist predominantly of apo AI-CIII-AIV gene defects. More than 46 mutations affect the structure of apo AI,[38] leading to a marked reduction in HDL cholesterol levels. Not all of these defects are associated with premature cardiovascular disease. Clinical presentations can vary from extensive atypical xanthomatosis and corneal infiltration of lipids to no manifestations at all. Treatment of these apo AI gene defects generally fails to raise HDL cholesterol levels. Other mutations of apo AI lead to increased catabolic rate of apo AI and may not be associated with cardiovascular disease. One such mutation, apo AI_{Milano} (apo $AI_{Arg173Cys}$), may be associated with longevity despite very low HDL levels.[38]

LCAT, CETP DEFICIENCY. Genetic defects in the HDL-processing enzymes give rise to interesting phenotypes. Deficiencies of LCAT, the enzyme that catalyzes the formation of cholesteryl esters in plasma, cause corneal infiltration of neutral lipids and hematological abnormalities due to abnormal constitution of red blood cell membranes. LCAT deficiency can lead to an entity called "fish eye disease" because of the characteristic pattern of corneal infiltration observed in affected individuals.[39]

Patients without CETP have very elevated HDL cholesterol levels, enriched in cholesteryl esters. Because CETP facilitates the transfer of HDL cholesteryl esters into triglyceride-rich lipoproteins, a deficiency of this enzyme causes accumulation of cholesteryl esters within HDL particles. CETP deficiency is not associated with premature CAD but may not afford protection against CAD.[40,41]

TANGIER DISEASE AND FAMILIAL HIGH-DENSITY LIPOPROTEIN DEFICIENCY. A rare disorder of HDL deficiency was identified in a proband from the Chesapeake Bay island of Tangier in the United States. The proband, whose sister was also affected, had markedly enlarged yellow tonsils and nearly absent HDL cholesterol levels, an entity now called *Tangier disease.* The cellular defect in Tangier disease consists of a reduced cellular cholesterol efflux in skin fibroblasts and macrophages from affected subjects.[42] A more common entity, familial HDL deficiency, was also found to result from decreased cellular cholesterol. The genetic defect in Tangier disease and in familial HDL deficiency results from mutations at the ATP binding cassette A1 gene (*ABCA1*) that encodes the ABCA1 transporter (see Fig. 39–5B).[43-45] At least 50 mutations have been reported within ABCA1, causing Tangier disease (homozygous or compound heterozygous mutations) or familial HDL deficiency (heterozygous mutations). Although subjects with Tangier disease and familial HDL deficiency are at increased risk for CAD, their very low levels of LDL cholesterol appear to have a protective effect. ABCA1 appears to shuttle from the late endosomal compartment to the plasma membrane and act as a membrane-bound transporter of phospholipids (and possibly cholesterol) onto acceptor proteins such as apo AI and apo E. Hydroxysterols regulate ABCA1 via the LXR/RXR nuclear receptor pathway. ABCA1 undergoes phosphorylation via protein kinase A and acts as a receptor for apo AI.

OTHER CHOLESTEROL TRANSPORT DEFECTS. Niemann-Pick type C disease is a disorder of lysosomal cholesterol transport. In patients with Niemann-Pick type C disease, mental retardation and neurological manifestations occur frequently. The cellular phenotype involves markedly decreased cholesterol esterification and cellular cholesterol transport defect to the Golgi apparatus. Unlike Tangier disease/familial HDL deficiency, the cellular defect in Niemann-Pick type C disease appears proximal to the transport of cholesterol to the plasma membrane. The gene for Niemann-Pick type C disease (*NPC1*) has been mapped to 18q21 and the gene codes for a 1278-amino acid protein, the role of which appears to be involved in cholesterol shuttling between the late endosomal pathway and the plasma membrane. The NPC1 gene product shares homology with the morphogen receptor *patched* and the SREBP cleavage activating protein (SCAP).[46] Niemann-Pick type I disease (subtypes A and B), caused by mutations at the sphingomyelin phosphodiesterase-1 (*SMPD-1*) gene, is associated with a low HDL cholesterol level. The *SMPD-1* gene codes for a lysosomal (acidic) and secretory sphingomyelinase. The cause of the low HDL cholesterol level in Niemann-Pick A and B patients appears to be due to a decrease in LCAT reaction because of abnormal HDL constituents.[47]

Secondary Causes of Hyperlipidemia and the Metabolic Syndrome

Several clinical disorders lead to alterations in lipoprotein status (Table 39–5).

HORMONAL CAUSES. Hypothyroidism, a not infrequent cause of secondary lipoprotein disorders, often manifests with elevated LDL cholesterol, triglycerides, or both. An elevated level of thyroid-stimulating hormone is key to the diagnosis, and the lipoprotein abnormalities often revert to normal after correction of thyroid status. Rarely, hypothyroidism may uncover a genetic lipoprotein disorder such as type III hyperlipidemia. Estrogens can elevate plasma triglycerides and HDL cholesterol levels, probably because of increases in both hepatic VLDL and apo AI production. In postmenopausal women, estrogens may reduce LDL cholesterol by 0 to 15 percent. The use of estrogens for the treatment of lipoprotein disorders is no longer recommended because of the slight increase in cardiovascular risk with prolonged use of estrogens in the postmenopausal period (see Chaps. 42 and 73).[48a] Rarely, pregnancy is associated with severe increases in plasma triglycerides, on a background of lipoprotein lipase deficiency. Such cases present a serious threat to mother and child and must be referred to specialized centers. Male sex hormones and anabolic steroids can increase hepatic lipase activity and have been used in the treatment of hypertriglyceridemia in men. Growth hormone can reduce LDL cholesterol and augment HDL cholesterol but is not recommended in the treatment of lipoprotein disorders.

TABLE 39–5 Secondary Causes of Dyslipoproteinemias

Metabolic	Diabetes Lipodystrophy Glycogen storage disorders
Renal	Chronic renal failure Glomerulonephritis
Hepatic	Obstructive liver disease Cirrhosis
Hormonal	Estrogens Progesterones Growth hormone Thyroid disorders (hypothyroidism) Corticosteroids
Lifestyle	Physical inactivity Obesity Diet rich in fats, saturated fats Alcohol intake
Medications	Retinoic acid derivatives Glucocorticoids Exogenous estrogens Thiazide diuretics Beta-adrenergic blockers (selective) Testosterone Immunosuppresive medications (cyclosporine) Antiviral medications (human immunodeficiency virus protease inhibitors)

METABOLIC CAUSES. The most frequent secondary cause of dyslipoproteinemia is probably the constellation of metabolic abnormalities seen in patients with the metabolic syndrome (see Chaps. 40 and 42). The finding of increased visceral fat (abdominal obesity), elevated blood pressure, and peripheral insulin resistance often clusters with increased plasma triglycerides and a reduced HDL cholesterol level. Overt diabetes, especially type 2 diabetes, frequently elevates plasma triglycerides and reduces HDL cholesterol. These abnormalities have prognostic implications in patients with type 2 diabetes. Poor control of diabetes, obesity, and moderate to severe hyperglycemia can yield severe hypertriglyceridemia with chylomicronemia and increased VLDL cholesterol levels. Subjects with juvenile diabetes can also have severe hypertriglyceridemia when the diabetes is poorly controlled. Familial lipodystrophy (complete or partial) may be associated with increased VLDL secretion. Dunnigan lipodystrophy, a genetic disorder with features of the metabolic syndrome, is caused by mutations within the Lamin A/C gene and is associated with limb-girdle fat atrophy. Excess plasma triglycerides often accompany glycogen storage disorders.

RENAL DISORDERS. In subjects with glomerulonephritis and protein-losing nephropathies, a marked increase in secretion of hepatic lipoproteins can raise LDL cholesterol levels, which may approach the levels seen in subjects with familial hypercholesterolemia. By contrast, patients with chronic renal failure have a pattern of hypertriglyceridemia with reduced HDL cholesterol. Patients with end-stage renal disease, including those on hemodialysis or chronic ambulatory peritoneal dialysis, have a poor prognosis and accelerated atherosclerosis and should undergo aggressive treatment of lipoprotein disorders. After organ transplantation, the immunosuppressive regimen (glucocorticoids and cyclosporine) typically elevates triglycerides and reduces HDL cholesterol levels. Because transplant patients generally have an increase in cardiovascular risk, a secondary hyperlipidemia may warrant treatment. Patients receiving the combination of statin plus cyclosporine merit careful dose titrations and monitoring for myopathy.

LIVER DISEASE. Obstructive liver disease, especially primary biliary cirrhosis may lead to the formation of an abnormal lipoprotein termed *lipoprotein-x*. This type of lipoprotein is found in cases of LCAT deficiency and consists of an LDL-like particle but with a marked reduction in cholesteryl esters. Extensive xanthoma formation on the face and palmar areas can result from accumulation of lipoprotein-x.

LIFESTYLE. Factors contributing to obesity, such as an imbalance between caloric intake and energy expenditure, lack of physical activity, and a diet rich in saturated fats and refined sugars, contribute in large part to the lipid and lipoprotein lipid levels within a population (see Chaps. 36 and 41).

MEDICATION. Several medications can alter lipoproteins. Thiazide diuretics can increase plasma triglyceride levels. Beta blockers, especially non-beta-1 selective, increase triglycerides and lower HDL cholesterol levels. Retinoic acid and estrogens can increase triglyceride levels, sometimes dramatically. Corticosteroids and immunosuppressive agents can increase plasma triglyceride levels and lower HDL cholesterol levels. Estrogens can increase plasma HDL cholesterol significantly and may also increase triglyceride concentrations.

In clinical practice, many dyslipoproteinemias, other than the genetic forms mentioned earlier, share an important environmental cause. Lifestyle changes (diet, exercise, reduction of abdominal obesity) should be the cornerstone of the treatment of most dyslipidemias. The effects of marked alterations in lifestyle, reduction in dietary fats, especially saturated fats, and exercise can lead to an improved cardiovascular prognosis. Translating these findings into practice, however, has been more difficult. For example, dietary manipulations as performed in a physician's office lead to relatively small reductions in plasma lipid and lipoprotein cholesterol levels (see Chaps. 36, 41, and 42).

Drugs that Affect Lipid Metabolism (Table 39–6)

Resins

The bile acid–binding resins interrupt the enterohepatic circulation of bile acids by inhibiting their reabsorption in the intestine (bile acids, which contain cholesterol, are more than 90 percent reabsorbed via this pathway). Currently, their main use is adjunctive therapy in patients with severe hypercholesterolemia due to increased LDL cholesterol. Since bile acid–binding resins are not absorbed systemically (they remain in the intestine and are eliminated in the stool), they are considered safe in children. Cholestyramine (Questran) is used in 4-gm unit doses as powder, and colestipol (Colestid) is used in 5-gm unit doses; a 1-gm tablet of colestipol is available. Effective doses range from 2 to 6 unit doses/day, always taken with meals. The most important side effects are predominantly gastrointestinal, with constipation, a sensation of fullness, and gastrointestinal discomfort. Hypertriglyceridemia can result from the use of these drugs. Decreased drug absorption dictates careful scheduling of medications 1 hour before or 3 hours after the patient takes bile acid–binding resins. Bile acid–binding resins can be used in combination with statins and/or cholesterol absorption inhibitors in cases of severe hypercholesterolemia.

TABLE 39–6 Current Lipid-Lowering Medications

Generic Name	Trade Name	Recommended Dose Range
Statins		
Atorvastatin	Lipitor	10-80 mg
Fluvastatin	Lescol	20-80 mg
Lovastatin	Mevacor	20-80 mg
Pravastatin	Pravachol	10-40 mg
Rosuvastatin	Crestor	10-40 mg
Simvastatin	Zocor	10-80 mg
Bile Acid Absorption Inhibitors		
Cholestyramine	Questran	2-24 gm
Colestipol	Colestid	5-30 gm
Colesevelam	WelChol	3.8-4.5 gm
Cholesterol Absorption Inhibitors		
Ezetimibe	Zetia (Ezetrol)	10 mg
Fibrates*		
Bezafibrate	Bezalip	400 mg
Fenofibrate	Tricor (Lipidil Micro)	67-200 mg
Gemfibrozil†	Lopid	600-1200 mg
Niacin‡		
Nicotinic acid		1-3 gm

*Avoid in patients with renal insufficiency.
†Not recommended in combination with statins.
‡Use with caution in patients with diabetes or glucose intolerance.

Hydroxymethylglutaryl–Coenzyme A Reductase Inhibitors (Statins)

Statins inhibit HMG-CoA reductase and prevent the formation of mevalonate, the rate-limiting step of sterol synthesis. To maintain cellular cholesterol homeostasis, expression of the LDL-R increases and the rate of cholesteryl ester formation declines. These homeostatic adjustments to HMG-CoA reductase inhibition increase LDL cholesterol clearance from plasma and decrease hepatic production of VLDL and LDL. In addition to blocking the synthesis of cholesterol, statins also interfere with the synthesis of lipid intermediates with important biological effects. In the cholesterol synthetic pathway, intermediate molecules of dimethylallyl pyrophosphate are metabolized by prenyl transferase into geranyl pyrophosphate and subsequently into farnesyl pyrophosphate. This step occurs before the formation of squalenes.[49] These intermediates, geranylgeranyl and farnesyl, are used for protein prenylation, a mechanism by which a lipid moiety attaches covalently to a protein, allowing anchoring into cell membranes and enhancing its biological activity. This is the case for the GTP-binding proteins Rho A, Rac, and Ras. Indeed, statins may increase HDL cholesterol in part by preventing the geranylgeranylation of Rho A and phosphorylation of perisome proliferator–activated receptor alpha (PPARα), a factor that regulates apo AI transcription.[49] Altered protein prenylation may also mediate some of the putative effects of statins not related to a reduction in LDL cholesterol levels.

Atherosclerosis is an inflammatory disease.[50] Statins decrease C-reactive protein, induce apoptosis in smooth muscle cells, alter collagen content of atherosclerotic plaques, alter endothelial function, and decrease the inflammatory component of plaques.[51,52] Some investigators argue that statins possess effects independent of their inhibition of HMG CoA reductase. In clinical practice, the role of these possible LDL-independent actions is difficult to assess. It remains speculative that clinically important differences exist in efficacy between statins for a given percentage reduction in LDL cholesterol.

Statins are generally well tolerated; side effects include reversible elevation in transaminases and myositis, which causes discontinuation of the drug in less than 1 percent of patients. The currently available drugs are fluvastatin (Lescol), 20 to 80 mg/day; lovastatin (Mevacor), 20 to 80 mg/day; pravastatin (Pravachol), 20 to 40 mg/day; simvastatin (Zocor), 10 to 80 mg/day; atorvastatin (Lipitor), 10 to 80 mg/day; and rosuvastatin (Crestor), 10 to 40 mg/day. Concomitant drugs that interfere with the metabolism of statins by inhibiting the cytochrome P450 3A4 and 2C9 systems can increase plasma concentrations of statins. These include antibiotics, antifungal medications, certain antiviral drugs, grapefruit juice, cyclosporine, amiodarone, and several others.

Cholesterol Absorption Inhibitors

The development of selective inhibitors of intestinal sterol absorption has significantly advanced the treatment of lipoprotein disorders. Ezetimibe is the first such compound. Ezetimibe appears to limit selective uptake of cholesterol and other sterols by intestinal epithelial cells, perhaps by interfering with the Niemann-Pick C1-like 1 protein 1.[8a] It is particularly indicated for patients with LDL cholesterol levels above target on maximally tolerated statin dose. Ezetimibe lowers LDL cholesterol by about 18 percent and is additive to the effect of statins.[53] Because ezetimibe also prevents the intestinal absorption of sitosterol, it might be the drug of choice in cases of sitosterolemia. The current dose of ezitimibe is 10 mg/day.

Fibric Acid Derivatives (Fibrates)

Three derivatives of fibric acid are currently available in the United States and two more are available in Canada and Europe. Gemfibrozil (Lopid) is used at a dose of 600 mg twice a day and is indicated in cases of hypertriglyceridemia and in the secondary prevention of cardiovascular diseases in patients with a low HDL cholesterol levels. These latter recommendations are based on the Veterans Administration HDL Intervention Trial (VA-HIT). Fenofibrate (Tricor, Lipidil Micro) is used to treat hypertriglyceridemia and combined hyperlipoproteinemia. The dose is 200 mg/day and a new formulation is available to vary the dose from 67 mg (especially in cases of renal failure) to 267 mg/day. Clofibrate (Atromid) is still available in some centers, although its use has declined since the introduction of newer molecules. Ciprofibrate (Lypanthyl, Lipanor) and bezafibrate (Bezalip) are more widely used in Europe. The main indications for the use of fibrates is hypertriglyceridemia when diet and lifestyle changes are not sufficient. Another indication is in the prevention of cardiovascular diseases in patients with elevated plasma triglycerides and low HDL cholesterol. The mechanism of action of fibrates involves interaction with the nuclear transcription factor PPARα that regulates the transcription of the LPL, apo CII, and apo AI genes. The side effects of fibrates include cutaneous manifestations, gastrointestinal effects (abdominal discomfort, increased bile lithogenicity), erectile dysfunction, elevated transaminases, interaction with oral anticoagulants, and elevated plasma homocysteine, especially with fenofibrate and, to a lesser extent, with bezafibrate.[54] Because fibrates augment LPL activity, LDL cholesterol levels may rise in patients with hypertriglyceridemia treated with this class of medications. Fibrates, especially gemfibrozil, can inhibit the glucuronidation of statins, and thus retard their elimination. For this reason, combination of gemfibrozil with statins may increase the risk of myotoxicity.

Nicotinic Acid (Niacin)

Niacin has been used for decades for the treatment of dyslipidemias and is particularly effective in increasing HDL cholesterol and lowering triglyceride levels. The effect of niacin on LDL cholesterol is more modest. Effective doses of niacin are in the range of 3000 mg/day, in three separate doses. It is preferable to use an escalating dose schedule to reach the full dose in 2 to 3 weeks rather than starting with the full dose. Slow-release forms of niacin decrease the side effect profile of the drug. Skin flushing can be attenuated by taking a daily aspirin. Niacin decreases the hepatic secretion of VLDL from the liver and decreased FFA mobilization for the periphery. Although niacin has been shown in the long-term follow-up of the Coronary Drug Project to decrease mortality at 15 years, its use has been hampered by significant and sometimes common minor side effects and much less frequent serious adverse actions, and by the development of statins. Side effects of niacin include flushing, hyperuricemia, hyperglycemia, hepatotoxicity, acanthosis nigricans, and gastritis. Close laboratory monitoring of side effects is warranted. Long-acting niacin has the advantage of a once- or twice-daily dosing schedule, but older preparations of slow-release niacin were potentially more hepatotoxic. Niacin effectively raises HDL cholesterol levels and, in combination with low-dose statin, can retard the angiographic progression of CAD and decrease adverse cardiac events.[55] Recent work has identified cell surface receptors for nicotinic acid that belong to the G-protein–coupled heptahelical superfamily. This discovery may speed the elucidation of the molecular mechanism of nicotinic acid's effects on lipid metabolism.[56,57]

Fish Oils

Fish oils are rich in polyunsaturated fatty acids such as eicosapentaenoic acid or docosahexaenoic acid, with the first double in the omega-3 position. These fatty acids lower plasma triglyceride levels and have antithrombotic properties. Although employed in the treatment of hypertriglyceridemia, their use is reserved in cases of severe hypertriglyceridemia refractory to conventional therapy. Fish oils decrease VLDL synthesis and decrease VLDL apo B. The response to fish oils depends on dose, requiring a daily intake of 10 to 15 gm of eicosapentaenoic acid or docosahexaenoic acid for a significant benefit on plasma triglyceride levels.

Phytosterols

Phytosterols are derivatives of cholesterol from plants and trees. They interfere with the formation of micelles in the intestine and prevent intestinal cholesterol absorption. They can be obtained as "neutraceuticals" or can be incorporated in soft margarines. The sterols may prove useful for the adjunctive management of lipoprotein disorders and are part of the therapeutic lifestyle change regimen in the current guidelines (see later).

Other Medications

Probucol was used as an antioxidant and had modest effects on plasma lipoprotein levels. The lack of conclusive evidence that probucol has beneficial effects and profound reduction in HDL levels and prolongation of QT interval led to its withdrawal. A recent study indicates that it may have a role in the prevention of restenosis after coronary angioplasty if used before the procedure.[58] Thyroxine is no longer used as a lipid modulator unless hypothyroidism has been documented.

Monitoring of Lipid Therapy

After initiation of medical therapy, the response should be checked within the first 3 months, along with transaminases and creatinine kinase. Thereafter, clinical judgment should dictate the interval between follow-up visits. Although frequent visits are probably not useful in the detection of serious side effects, they serve to encourage compliance and adherence to diet and lifestyle changes.

Clinical Trials of Drugs Affecting Lipid Metabolism

Numerous pathological, epidemiological, genetic, and interventional trials have validated the central tenet of the "lipid hypothesis," which proposes a causal relationship between dyslipidemia and atherogenesis and identifies lipid modification as a risk-reducing strategy for CHD (see Chap. 36). A number of small trials using dietary or drug therapies have demonstrated the angiographic benefit of managing elevated total cholesterol and LDL cholesterol. Early clinical trials using bile-acid sequestrants, fibrates, or nicotinic acid reported modest reductions in coronary risk with modest reductions in LDL cholesterol. We refer readers interested in these earlier trials to previous editions of this textbook.

The advent of the HMG-CoA reductase inhibitors, or statins, in the mid-1980s made possible more aggressive reduction of LDL cholesterol. By the late 1990s, several large-scale, prospective randomized trials with these drugs had reported robust reductions in relative cardiovascular risks, compared with placebo (Tables 39–7 and 39–8, Fig. 39–6).[59-63] This section discusses the more recently representative or in-progress trials in this area, in the context of some of the unanswered questions about the effects of cholesterol treatment. The focus on statin trials reflects the widespread contemporary interest and clinical success of this category of drugs. Ample reviews have considered the results of the older trials.

Treating High-Risk Patients

As the interaction of multiple coronary risk factors has received greater clinical importance, recommendations for clinical practice have increasingly embraced the concept of global risk management. In the 2001 U.S. Adult Treatment Panel (ATP III) guidelines, the patient's overall risk for developing CHD in the next 10 years determines the intensity of lipid intervention.[64] This global risk is calculated using an algorithm that considers not only total cholesterol but also HDL cholesterol, smoking, age, hypertension, and gender (see Chap. 36).

Because global risk assessment shifts emphasis away from abnormal lipids alone to the patient's overall risk profile, it raises an important issue for the future of lipid management. That is, should the decision to initiate lipid modification for cardiovascular risk reduction be based on high risk or high cholesterol? Recent trials have evaluated this question (Table 39–9).

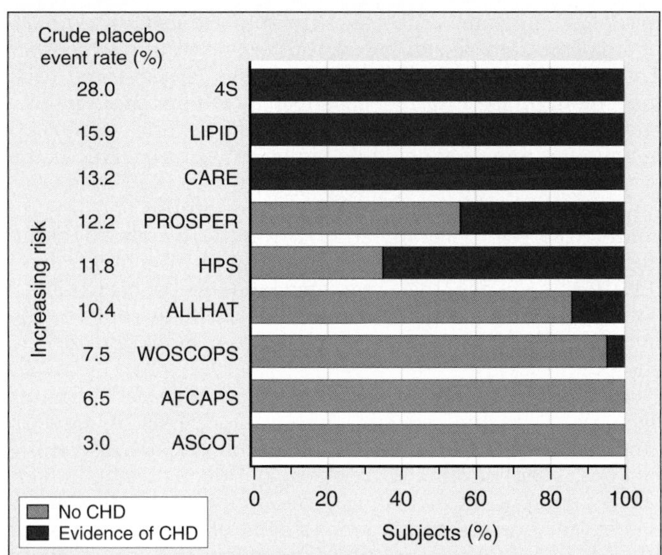

FIGURE 39–6 Clinical trials of statin therapy have demonstrated benefits in patients across the spectrum of coronary disease.

TABLE 39–7 Primary Prevention Trials of Statin Therapy

	WOSCOPS	AFCAPS/ TexCAPS
N (% women)	6596 (0)	6605 (15)
Duration (yrs)	4.9	5.2
Intervention	Pravastatin, 40 mg/day	Lovastatin, 20-40 mg/day
Baseline lipids (mg/dl)		
Total cholesterol	272	221
LDL cholesterol	192	150
HDL cholesterol	44	36 men; 40 women
Triglycerides	164	158
% Lipid changes, treatment vs. placebo		
Total cholesterol	−20	−19
LDL cholesterol	−26	−26
HDL cholesterol	+5	+5
Triglycerides	−12	−13
Endpoints (% changes in risk), treatment vs. placebo		
Nonfatal MI/CHD death	**−31**	−25
Fatal/nonfatal MI	—	−40
Acute major coronary events	—	**−37**
Total mortality	−22	+3 (NS)
CHD mortality	−28	too few
Revascularizations	−37	−33
Stroke	−11 (NS)	—

AFCAPS/TexCAPS = Air Force/Texas Coronary Atherosclerosis Prevention Study; CHD = coronary heart disease; HDL = high-density lipoprotein; LDL = low-density lipoprotein; MI = myocardial infarction; NS = nonsignificant; WOSCOPS = West of Scotland Coronary Prevention Study; **bold** = study's primary endpoint; — = not reported.

TABLE 39–8 Secondary Prevention Trials of Statin Therapy

	4S	CARE	LIPID
N (% women)	4444 (19)	4159 (14)	9014 (17)
Duration (yrs)	5.4	5	6.1
Intervention	Simvastatin, 10-40 mg/day	Pravastatin, 40 mg/day	Pravastatin, 40 mg/day
Baseline lipids (mg/dl)			
Total cholesterol	261	209	218
LDL cholesterol	188	139	150
HDL cholesterol	46	39	36
Triglycerides	135	155	138
% Lipid changes, treatment vs. placebo			
Total cholesterol	−26	−20	−18
LDL cholesterol	−36	−28	−25
HDL cholesterol	+7	+5	+5
Triglycerides	−17	−14	−11
Endpoints (% changes in risk), treatment vs. placebo			
Nonfatal MI/CHD death	−34	**−24**	−24
Fatal/nonfatal MI	−42	−25	−24
Acute major coronary events	—	—	−29
Total mortality	**−30**	−9 (NS)	−22
CHD mortality	−42	−20	**−24**
Revascularizations	−37	−27	−20
Stroke	−30	−31	−19

CARE = Cholesterol and Recurrent Events; CHD = coronary heart disease; HDL = high-density lipoprotein; LDL = low-density lipoprotein; LIPID = Long-term Intervention with Pravastatin in Ischemic Disease; MI = myocardial infarction; NS = nonsignificant; 4S = Scandinavian Simvastatin Survival Study; **bold** = study's primary endpoint; — = not reported.

THE HEART PROTECTION STUDY. The Medical Research Council/British Heart Foundation Heart Protection Study (HPS) evaluated the role of statin therapy in at-risk patients for whom guidelines at the time would not have recommended drug intervention.[65] Participants in the HPS had increased risk for vascular disease, but many did not meet existing criteria for hypolipidemic therapy. The two-by-two factorial design of the HPS intended to analyze the effect of simvastatin, 40 mg/day, versus placebo with or without a combination of antioxidant vitamins (600 mg alpha tocopherol, 250 mg ascorbic acid, 20 mg beta carotene) on the risk of major vascular events.

Patients were selected on the basis of being at increased risk for CHD because of either the presence of documented coronary atherosclerosis or having risk factors considered to confer a level of risk equivalent to having CHD. The trial thus enrolled not only individuals with prior myocardial infarction, unstable or stable angina, coronary artery bypass grafting, or angioplasty eligible for randomization, but also patients with occlusive disease of noncoronary arteries, diabetes, or treated hypertension. The study included patients from 40 to 80 years of age and with total serum cholesterol concentrations of at least 135 mg/dl (3.5 mmol/liter).

The combination of antioxidant vitamins did not affect morbidity or mortality. Simvastatin treatment, on the other hand, reduced the risk for any major vascular event by 24 percent ($p < 0.0001$), with an absolute risk reduction of 5.4 percent (25.2 percent in the placebo group minus 19.8 percent in the simvastatin group). The all-cause mortality rate fell by 13 percent ($p = 0.0003$), with a significant 17 percent reduction ($p < 0.0001$) in deaths attributed to any vascular cause. There was no increase in noncardiac causes of mortality, such as neoplasia, respiratory disease, or other nonvascular deaths.

The HPS population included individuals who would qualify as traditional candidates for primary prevention because of their history of no previous coronary event. A substantial number of individuals without known CHD (n = 7150) had a CHD-equivalent risk profile: diabetes (n = 3982), peripheral vascular disease (n = 2701), or cerebrovascular disease

TABLE 39–9 Trials of Statin Therapy in High-Risk Patients

	HPS	ALL-HAT LLT	ASCOT LLA	PROSPER
N (% women)	20536 (24.7)	10355 (48.8)	10305 (18.8)	5804 (51.7)
Duration (yrs)	5	4.8	3.3	3.2
Percent with Hx of CVD or CHD	65%	14%	14%	44%
Statin crossover rate	17%	26.1%	9%	10%
Intervention	Simvastatin, 40 mg/day vs. placebo	Pravastatin, 20-40 mg/day vs. usual care	Atorvastatin, 10 mg/day vs. placebo	Pravastatin, 40 mg/day vs. placebo
Baseline lipids, mg/dL (mmol/liter)				
Total cholesterol	228 (5.9)	224 (5.8)	213 (5.5)	221 (5.7)
LDL cholesterol	132 (3.4)	146 (3.8)	132 (3.4)	147 (3.8)
HDL cholesterol	41 (1.06)	48 (1.2)	50 (1.3)	50 (1.3)
Triglycerides	124 (1.4)	152 (1.7)	152 (1.7)	58 (1.5)
% Lipid changes, treatment vs. placebo				
Total cholesterol	−20	−10	−24	NR
LDL cholesterol	−29	−17	−35	−34
HDL cholesterol	+3	+1	0	+5
Triglycerides	−21	—	−17	−13
Endpoints (% changes in risk), treatment vs. placebo				
Major cardiovascular events	**−24**	—	—	**+15**
Nonfatal MI/CHD death	−27	NS	**+36**	−19
Fatal/nonfatal MI	—	—	—	—
Total mortality	−13	**NS**	NS	NS
CHD mortality	−17	NS	NS	−24
Revascularizations	−24	—	—	NS
Stroke	−25	NS	−27	NS

HPS = Heart Protection Study; ALL-HAT LLT = Antihypertensive and Lipid-Lowering Treatment to Prevent Heart Attack Trial; ASCOT LLA = Anglo-Scandinavian Cardiac Outcomes Trial Lipid Lowering Arm; PROSPER = Prospective Study of Pravastatin in the Elderly at Risk; LDL = low-density lipoprotein; HDL = high-density lipoprotein; MI = myocardial infarction; CHD = coronary heart disease; NS = nonsignificant; **bold** = study's primary endpoint; — = not reported.

(n = 1820). Statin treatment exhibited clinical benefit regardless of the presence of known vascular disease, baseline LDL cholesterol level, age, or sex.

PROSPER. Coronary and cerebrovascular atherosclerosis in the elderly is a growing clinical problem because of the population's increasing longevity. Older chronological age in and of itself should not exclude patients from receiving therapy, especially if an otherwise healthy older patient's remaining years of life could benefit from prevention of the morbidity associated with a coronary event. Indeed, age is one of the most potent cardiovascular risk factors.

The Prospective Evaluation of Pravastatin in the Elderly (PROSPER) assessed the impact of treatment with pravastatin 40 mg/day versus placebo in 5804 men and women aged 70 to 82 years of age with a history of vascular disease (coronary, cerebrovascular, or peripheral vascular) or a risk factor profile consistent with high risk (smoking, hypertension, or diabetes).[66] Participants in this study had plasma total cholesterol levels between 155 and 350 mg/dl (4.0 to 9.0 mmol/liter) and triglyceride concentrations less than 530 mg/dl (6.0 mmol/liter). Women accounted for more than half of the individuals in PROSPER.

The mean follow-up was 3.2 years and the composite primary endpoint included coronary death, nonfatal myocardial infarction, and fatal or nonfatal stroke. Pravastatin treatment reduced the relative risk for this endpoint significantly by 15 percent ($p = 0.014$) and for CHD death by 24 percent ($p = 0.043$). The treatment showed similar benefit across many subgroups: those with versus those without prior vascular disease; men versus women; tertiles of baseline LDL cholesterol; current smokers versus nonsmokers; and those with and those without a history of hypertension. Participants in the lowest tertile of baseline HDL cholesterol (<1.11 mmol/liter) experienced greater benefit than those in the higher tertiles.

Lipid-modifying treatment had no effect on the risk for stroke or on cognitive function, both of which are important endpoints in an older population. There were no safety differences between pravastatin and placebo, except for a greater number of new cancer diagnoses in pravastatin patients that is inconsistent with the overall clinical experience with this drug and may have arisen from recruitment of patients with occult disease. Despite these concerns, as a whole, the results of PROSPER favor treatment of the elderly to reduce CHD risk and affirm the findings of subgroup analyses from earlier statin trials.

ALLHAT (LIPID-LOWERING ARM). The large Antihypertensive and Lipid-Lowering Treatment to Prevent Heart Attack Trial (ALLHAT) sought to determine whether cholesterol lowering with open-label pravastatin 20 to 40 mg/day (plus resin, if needed) would reduce total mortality in 10,355 moderately hypercholesterolemic, hypertensive men and women, aged 55 years or older, with at least one other CHD risk factor, as compared with usual care.[67] The ALLHAT patients met lipid criteria of a LDL cholesterol level of 120 to 189 mg/dl (3.1 to 5 mmol/liter) (or 100 to 129 mg/dl [2.6 to 3.3 mmol/liter] in those with CHD) and triglycerides less than 350 mg/dl (<3.9 mmol/liter).

In contrast with other studies in this section, ALLHAT reported no benefit and no harm of treatment compared with usual care on any study endpoint. Several aspects of this trial may help explain this null finding.[68] The study may have been underpowered because of difficulties related to patient recruitment. The trial was open-labeled, and there was declining adherence in the pravastatin group and a high crossover rate to statin therapy in the usual-care group (by 6 years, more than 25 percent of these patients were receiving a statin). Indeed, the absolute difference in total cholesterol between the pravastatin and the usual-care group by the end of the trial was only 9.6 percent, which was approximately half of the reduction achieved in other statin trials.

ASCOT. The lipid-lowering arm of the Anglo-Scandinavian Cardiac Outcomes Trial (ASCOT) assessed the clinical effect of atorvastatin, 10 mg/day, versus placebo in 10,305 hypertensive patients with a total cholesterol level of less than 250 mg/dl (6.5 mmol/liter) and a high-risk profile.[69] Although the trial excluded individuals with previous myocardial infarction, current angina, or cerebrovascular disease within 3 months before randomization, the randomized patients had evidence of other vascular disease or CHD risk equivalents (left ventricular hypertrophy, other electrocardiographic abnormalities, peripheral arterial disease, previous cerebrovascular disease, diabetes), or several other CHD risk factors.

Originally planned to have a follow-up period of 5 years, the ASCOT ended early after a median follow-up of 3.3 years, after 100 primary endpoint events had occurred in the atorvastatin group compared with 154 in the placebo group. The relative risk reduction was 36 percent ($p = 0.0005$), and the benefit became apparent within a year of the study's initiation. Benefit was similar across prespecified subgroups. Atorvastatin reduced the relative risk for stroke by 27 percent ($p = 0.024$) and for total cardiovascular events by 21 percent ($p = 0.0005$). Total mortality and adverse events did not differ between the treatment groups.

The ASCOT and ALLHAT are the only two published lipid-lowering clinical trials performed in hypertensive patients. The statin crossover rate in the placebo group was only 9 percent in ASCOT compared with approximately 26 percent in the usual-care group of ALLHAT. Adherence to the study drug was also better in ASCOT than in ALLHAT.

CARDS. Because of their high risk for developing CHD, diabetic patients warrant aggressive lipid modification, according to U.S. guidelines (see Chap. 40). However, few trials have evaluated the effects of lipid modification on clinical endpoints in this population, and the evidence of benefit derives largely from subgroup analyses. The Collaborative Atorvastatin Diabetes Study (CARDS) is a multicenter, randomized, placebo-controlled, primary-prevention study in patients with type 2 diabetes.[70] Entry criteria included not only diabetes but also at least one other CHD risk factor: current smoking, hypertension, retinopathy, or micro- or macroalbuminuria. The trial enrolled individuals with LDL cholesterol levels less than 160 mg/dl (4.14 mmol/liter) and triglycerides less than 600 mg/dl (6.78 mmol/liter). The study included 2838 men and women, 40 to 75 years of age. The trial utilized a fixed dosage of atorvastatin of 10 mg/day compared with placebo. The primary efficacy parameter is the time from randomization to the occurrence of a first primary endpoint event, which may include major coronary events, revascularizations, stroke, unstable angina, or resuscitated cardiac arrest. The study was stopped prematurely for benefit.[71]

Does Lipid Lowering Benefit Patients with Acute Coronary Syndromes?

Earlier secondary prevention statin studies generally selected patients who were at least 3 to 6 months postcoronary event and stabilized. Substantial interest has turned to the question of statin treatment in the period immediately following an acute coronary syndrome. Conflicting observational data, however, have reported either a beneficial or a null effect of early statin treatment on subsequent coronary risk.[72,73]

The Myocardial Ischemia Reduction and Aggressive Cholesterol Lowering (MIRACL) trial examined the premise that early and intensive treatment with high-dose atorvastatin therapy begun immediately after the onset of an acute coronary event might produce beneficial clinical effects in a much larger cohort (n = 3086).[74] The composite primary endpoint of MIRACL included nonfatal acute myocardial infarction, cardiac arrest, or symptomatic myocardial ischemia. Atorvastatin resulted in a modest albeit statistically significant 16 percent improvement in relative risk for the primary endpoint ($p = 0.048$). The major effect of early atorvastatin was a reduction in recurrent myocardial ischemia, which was decreased by 26 percent ($p = 0.02$). While statistically significant, the clinical benefits observed in MIRACL were not as robust as those seen in the larger and longer 4S and LIPID trials. However, MIRACL does provide reassurance regarding the safety of aggressive lipid lowering with a statin in the immediate aftermath of an acute coronary event.

Several other trials in this emerging area have been completed or are in progress. The Aggrastat-to-Zocor (A-2-Z) study will first randomize postacute coronary event patients to treatment with tirofiban and unfractionated versus low-molecular-weight heparin, then re-randomize them to receive either simvastatin, 40 to 80 mg/day, versus diet plus simvastatin, 20 mg/day.[75] Its results are expected in 2004. The Pravastatin or Atorvastatin Evaluation and Infection Therapy (PROVE-IT) trial compared pravastatin, 40 mg/day, with atorvastatin, 80 mg/day, in 4162 postacute coronary event patients.[76] This study also has an antibiotic treatment arm. The lipid-lowering arm of PROVE-IT showed that in patients who have recently survived an acute coronary syndrome, an intensive statin regimen that yielded a median LDL cholesterol of 62 mg/dl (1.60 mmol/liter) provided greater protection against death or major cardiovascular events than less aggressive therapy that lowered LDL cholesterol to a median of 95 mg/dl (2.46 mmol/liter), a level below the upper limit recommended by ATP-III as a target for this category of patients. Thus, PROVE-IT suggests that ACS survivors benefit from early statin treatment to levels of LDL cholesterol considerably below current target levels.[76a]

Medical Therapy Versus Revascularization

The Atorvastatin versus Revascularization Treatment (AVERT) trial evaluated the potential benefits of aggressive lipid lowering with open-label atorvastatin, 80 mg/day, versus usual care on ischemic events in a cohort of 341 patients with stable atherosclerosis who were scheduled to undergo an elective percutaneous revascularization procedure.[77] Follow-up was 18 months. Qualification requirements included at least one native coronary vessel with 50 percent or greater stenosis and an LDL cholesterol level in excess of 115 mg/dl. Exclusion criteria included triglycerides in excess of 500 mg/dl, ejection fraction less than 40 percent, inability to complete 4 minutes of exercise on a standard Bruce protocol, left main or triple vessel coronary atherosclerosis, or recent unstable angina or myocardial infarction (<14 days).

The composite primary endpoint in the AVERT trial encompassed the incidence of ischemic events, defined as cardiac death, resuscitation after cardiac arrest, nonfatal myocardial infarction, stroke, worsening angina, or revascularization (coronary artery bypass graft or repeat angioplasty). The patients randomized to usual care received percutaneous coronary interventions, and approximately one-third of the patients with treated lesions underwent placement of a coronary stent. The patients treated with angioplasty could receive hypolipidemic therapy as part of usual care. Lipid-lowering drugs were administered in 73 percent of patients in this group at some time during the follow-up (71 percent of the total group received statins). Despite this crossover, the atorvastatin group had lower total cholesterol, LDL cholesterol, and triglycerides relative to usual care.

A total of 22 ischemic events occurred in the group randomized to receive aggressive lipid-lowering therapy, compared with 37 events in the usual-care group (36 percent reduction; $p = 0.048$). The difference in the treatment arms tended toward statistical significance, since the significance level was adjusted to 0.045 because of the performance of two interim analyses. Atorvastatin treatment significantly delayed the time to the first event ($p = 0.027$) compared with usual care, but 54 percent of angioplasty patients compared with 41 percent of atorvastatin patients had improvement of Canadian Cardiovascular Society (CCS) classification of angina symptoms ($p = 0.009$). Seventeen serious adverse events were reported in the atorvastatin group, although none were attributed to atorvastatin. Twenty-eight of the patients in the angioplasty group had serious adverse events; six of these patients had events attributable to the angioplasty.

These results support a strategy of aggressive lipid-lowering therapy to complement revascularization in patients with stable angina. The multicenter, randomized Clinical Outcomes Utilizing Revascularization and Aggressive Drug Evaluation (COURAGE) trial may elucidate the issue further through its investigation of whether combining percutaneous coronary intervention with maximal statin intervention will provide greater benefits than statin intervention alone in more than 3000 patients.[78] The COURAGE protocol targets global risk reduction, emphasizing (1) lifestyle modification; (2) maximal use of drugs to lower blood pressure to Joint National Committee on Prevention, Detection, Evaluation, and Treatment of High Blood Pressure (JNC) VI goals; (3) maximal use of simvastatin, 80 mg/day, to lower cholesterol to below current US goals for secondary prevention; and (4) maximal use of drug to alleviate anginal symptoms with or without the best interventional devices to conduct percutaneous coronary intervention. Patients will be treated to a target LDL cholesterol level of 60 to 85 mg/dl and will be followed for a minimum of 3 years. The main outcome will be all-cause mortality or nonfatal myocardial infarction.

What Are the Optimal Limits of Therapy?

No statin clinical trial has rigorously identified a threshold below which LDL cholesterol reduction was not beneficial. Therefore, the optimal LDL cholesterol goal for therapy remains unclear. The Reversal of Atherosclerosis with Lipitor (REVERSAL) trial used intravascular ultrasonography to examine the effect of differing degrees of lipid-lowering on plaque volume. Over 18 months, patients treated with pravastatin (40 mg/day) had a 25 percent drop in LDL cholesterol, and those randomized to atorvastatin (80 mg/day) had a 46 percent decrease, to an average LDL cholesterol level of 79 mg/dl. The more aggressive lipid-lowering regimen reduced lesion volume.[78a] Trials that are tracking clinical events in patients treated to different levels of LDL cholesterol are currently underway. The Study of the Effectiveness of Additional Reductions in Cholesterol and Homocysteine (SEARCH) will examine the effect of high-dosage (80 mg/day) versus low-dosage simvastatin (20 mg/day), with or without folic acid, on clinical endpoints in approximately 12,000 CHD patients. Participants had total cholesterol greater than 135 mg/dl, or greater than 174 mg/dl if no previous statin use, and the high-dosage group will have an LDL cholesterol goal of 70 mg/dl compared with a goal of 100 mg/dl in the low-dosage patients. Will a greater reduction in LDL cholesterol using high-dose therapy translate into greater clinical benefit? The primary efficacy endpoint will be the effect of such treatment on the incidence of CHD death and nonfatal myocardial infarction. The secondary objective will be to assess the effect of high-dose compared with low-dose therapy on stroke, other mortality, and conditions requiring hospitalization. The use of folic acid supplementation will test the hypothesis that reducing homocysteine will reduce CHD risk.[79]

Similarly, the Treating to New Targets (TNT) trial will assess whether lowering LDL cholesterol levels beyond current recommendations with high-dosage versus low-dosage atorvastatin in patients with clinically evident CHD will lower clinical coronary event rates.[80] Patients aged 35 to 75 years with prior myocardial infarction, prior or present angina with objective evidence of atherosclerotic CHD, or prior coronary revascularization procedures and LDL cholesterol and triglyceride levels of 130 to 250 mg/dl (3.36 to 6.46 mmol/liter) and less than 600 mg/dl (6.77 mmol/liter), respectively, will undergo an 8-week open-label treatment phase with atorvastatin. Those patients attaining LDL cholesterol levels less than 130 mg/dl (3.36 mmol/liter) will be randomized to double-blind treatment with atorvastatin 10 mg/d or 80 mg/d; the anticipated LDL cholesterol goals at these dosages are 100 mg/dl (2.58 mmol/liter) and 75 mg/dl (1.93 mmol/liter), respectively. A projected total of 8600 patients will receive randomized treatment for an average of 5 years or until the number of primary coronary events reaches 750. The main efficacy measure is the occurrence of CHD death or nonfatal myocardial infarction. Secondary outcome measures include the incidence of any coronary event (primary event, coronary artery bypass grafting or other coronary revascularization, documented angina), cerebrovascular events, peripheral vascular disease, hospitalization with a primary diagnosis of CHD, any cardiovascular event, and all-cause mortality.

Fibrate Trials

VA-HIT. Of recent fibrate trials, perhaps the most necessary to mention is the Veteran's Affairs Cooperative Studies Program High Density Lipoprotein Cholesterol Intervention Trial (VA-HIT), a multicenter, randomized study that assessed the effects of gemfibrozil at a dose of 1200 mg/day versus dietary therapy on the incidence of cardiovascular events in 2531 men with known CHD and low baseline HDL cholesterol levels.[81] Enrollment criteria for VA-HIT required a HDL cholesterol level of 40 mg/dl (1.03 mmol/liter) or less or LDL cholesterol level of less than 140 mg/dl (3.6 mmol/liter) and triglycerides at 300 mg/dl (3.39 mmol/liter) or less.

The mean age of subjects in the VA-HIT was 64 years, with more than 75 percent of the patients older than 60 years of age. The participants in the VA-HIT had a mean body mass index of 29, a waist-hip ratio of 0.96, and a 25 percent prevalence of diabetes mellitus. Approximately 57 percent of the population was hypertensive and 20 percent were smokers. Baseline lipids in the VA-HIT revealed a total cholesterol level of 175 mg/dl, HDL cholesterol of 32 mg/dl, LDL cholesterol of 111 mg/dl, and triglycerides of 161 mg/dl. Gemfibrozil therapy resulted in essentially minimal alterations in total cholesterol and LDL levels. Total cholesterol was decreased by 4 percent as compared with placebo, and no significant change was demonstrable with LDL cholesterol concentrations. Triglycerides, on the other hand, fell by 31 percent and HDL cholesterol increased by 6 percent. The primary endpoint of the VA HIT was the combination of CHD death and nonfatal myocardial infarction. Patients randomized to receive placebo accounted for 275 events, compared with 219 events in the gemfibrozil group. The decline in coronary events represented a 22 percent risk reduction that was statistically significant ($p = 0.006$). The event curves began to diverge at approximately 2 years after the beginning of the trial.

A number of safety analyses were performed and found no differences in death from malignancies or violent deaths, and the only adverse event observed more frequently in the gemfibrozil group was dyspepsia. The VA-HIT reinforces the importance of targeting low HDL cholesterol as a major coronary risk factor.

BIP. The Bezafibrate Infarction Prevention (BIP) study reported no reduction in fatal and nonfatal myocardial infarction and CHD death in a cohort of 3090 men and women with CHD, total cholesterol of 180 to 250 mg/dl, HDL cholesterol less than 45 mg/dl (1.2 mmol/liter), triglycerides less than 300 mg/dl (3.4 mmol/liter), and LDL cholesterol less than 180 mg/dl (4.7 mmol/liter), who were treated with either bezafibrate, 400 mg/day, or placebo.[19] Despite producing an increase in HDL cholesterol of 14 percent and reduction in triglycerides of 25 percent compared with placebo, fibrate treatment did not reduce CHD risk. After 6.2 years, the reduction in the cumulative probability of the primary endpoint was 7.3 percent ($p = 0.24$). However, a substantial risk reduction with bezafibrate (39.5 percent; $p = 0.02$) was observed post hoc in the small subgroup of patients with elevated triglycerides at baseline (>200 mg/dl [2.3 mmol/liter]).

The lack of effect in BIP can be in part explained by the use of adjuvant open-label lipid-modifying drugs in the placebo group: 15 percent of patients in the placebo group were receiving this additional treatment before the end of the study, compared with 11 percent in the bezafibrate group. Also, compared with the VA-HIT, the BIP cohort had a lower placebo event rate, fewer diabetic participants, higher baseline HDL and LDL cholesterol levels, and lower baseline triglycerides.

ACCORD. The Action to Control Cardiovascular Risk in Diabetes (ACCORD) study, sponsored by the US National Heart, Lung, and Blood Institute, anticipates enrolling 10,000 patients with type 2 diabetes mellitus (from www.accordtrial.org, accessed April 14, 2004). The trial will compare effects on cardiovascular disease events of three strategies: intensive glycemic control; increasing HDL cholesterol and lowering triglycerides (with good LDL cholesterol and glycemic control); and intensive blood pressure control (in the context of good glycemic control). The lipid-modification arm of ACCORD will evaluate a fibrate intended to lower triglycerides and increase HDL cholesterol, combined with a statin to lower the LDL cholesterol level. The ACCORD study, therefore, will assess the effect of multiple risk factor intervention in diabetic patients and will also provide valuable information about the use of the statin-fibrate combination in preventing clinical events. In January 2003, the ACCORD main trial began a 30-month recruiting period. Follow-up will continue until 2009.[82]

In recent years, our understanding of cardiovascular risk management has grown increasingly sophisticated, largely because of the growing dominance of global risk assessment as the conceptual basis of treatment decisions. The clinical trial database has undergone a parallel evolution, in which early clinical trials of lipid modification using strategies capable of only modest lipid changes yielded important, but less than robust, results. The arrival of statin therapy made possible substantially greater LDL cholesterol reductions, and the trials using these drugs in the middle to late 1990s provided the most compelling evidence of benefit seen to date (see Fig. 39–6). With the database thus expanded, the questions being asked in trials have by necessity become increasingly specific. We no longer wonder whether reducing cholesterol will yield coronary benefit—it does—and therefore clinical trialists must turn toward the next direction: identifying the optimal conditions for achieving benefit. What kinds of patients will most likely benefit? What are the optimal goals of therapy? What clinical presentations of atherosclerotic disease will treatment affect most? The answers to these questions will shape the future of cardiovascular guidelines.

Overall Approach to the Treatment of Lipoprotein Disorders

Patients with lipoprotein disorders should undergo comprehensive evaluation and management in the context of a global risk reduction program (see Chap. 42). Most patients with dyslipoproteinemias lack symptoms, except for those with severe hypertriglyceridemia who can present with acute pancreatitis and those with familial lipoprotein disorders who have cutaneous manifestations (xanthomas, xanthelasmas). In the evaluation of patients with dyslipidemia, secondary causes should be sought and treated. The clinical evaluation should include a thorough history, including a complete family history that may reveal clues as to the genetic cause but also to the genetic susceptibility to cardiovascular disease. The physician should seek and address other risk factors (cigarette smoking, diabetes) and institute a management plan to improve lifestyle, such as diet, physical activity, and alcohol intake. Such interventions should make use of nonphysician health professionals (e.g., those with training in diet and nutrition or smoking cessation). The ATP III Therapeutic Lifestyle Change program offers one such approach. Concomitant medication use in addition to lifestyle change will often be needed to achieve current guideline goals.

The physical examination should include a search for xanthomas (in extensor tendons, including hands, elbows, knees, Achilles tendons, and palmar xanthomas); the presence of xanthelasmas, corneal arcus, and corneal opacifications. The blood pressure, waist circumference, weight, and height should be recorded and signs of vascular compromise must be carefully examined. A complete cardiovascular examination must be performed. The evaluation of peripheral pulses

TABLE 39–10 Laboratory Tests for the Diagnosis of Lipoprotein Disorders			
Lipid Profile	**May Help in Diagnosis**	**Specialized Centers**	**Research Tools**
Cholesterol Triglycerides HDL cholesterol LDL cholesterol*	Lipoprotein separation by UTC† Apo B Apo AI Apo E genotype/ phenotype Lipoprotein(a)	LDL particle size LPL assay LCAT assay Apo E levels Apolipoprotein separation by PAGE LDL-R assay Apo CII, CIII	Molecular diagnosis

Apo = apolipoprotein; HDL = high-density lipoprotein; LCAT = lecithin cholesterol acyltransferase; LDL = low-density lipoprotein; LDL-R = LDL receptor; LPL = lipoprotein lipase.
*Calculated as LDL cholesterol = cholesterol (triglycerides/2.2 + HDL cholesterol) in mmol/liter (or triglycerides divided by 5 in mg/dl); valid for triglycerides <4.5 mmol/liter (<400 mg/dl). LDL cholesterol can also be directly measured in plasma.
†Ultracentrifugation.

and the determination of the ankle-brachial index may reveal important clues for the presence of peripheral vascular disease (see Chap. 54).

The diagnosis of lipoprotein disorders depends on laboratory measurements (Table 39–10). The lipid profile generally suffices for most lipoprotein disorders, and specialized laboratories can refine the diagnosis and provide expertise for extreme cases. Additional tests often involve considerable expense and may not increase the predictive value beyond that of the lipid profile, although they can help in refining the diagnosis. To assess baseline risk in individuals on lipid-lowering therapy, the medication should be stopped for 1 month before a lipid profile is measured. Many tests are available in specialized centers (see Table 39–10) but should not be requested unless results of the test will alter clinical judgment and influence treatment.

After diagnosis of a lipid disorder (based on at least two lipid profiles), secondary causes should be evaluated by measurement of thyroid stimulating hormone and glucose. Patients who will receive medications should have measurement of baseline liver function (alanine aminotransferase [ALT]) and creatinine kinase. A decision to treat high-risk subjects (for example, patients with an acute coronary syndrome or post-myocardial infarction or coronary revascularization) should be implemented immediately and should commence concomitantly with lifestyle changes.[51]

Target Levels (see Chap. 42)

The National Cholesterol Education Program Adult Treatment Panel III (NCEP ATP III)[64] has made recommendations for the treatment of hypercholesterolemia. Target levels depend on overall risk of cardiovascular death or nonfatal myocardial infarction. Patients with CAD or atherosclerosis of other vascular beds (carotids or peripheral vascular disease), adults with diabetes, and those patients with an estimated 10-year risk of developing CAD of greater than 20 percent fall into a high-risk category and merit aggressive treatment, including medications along with lifestyle modifications, exercise, and diet to achieve a primary target of an LDL cholesterol level less than 2.6 mmol/liter (100 mg/dl). In subjects with triglycerides greater than 200 mg/dl, ATP III presents a secondary target of a non-HDL cholesterol level less than 3.4 mmol/liter (130 mg/dl). Many of these individuals have the metabolic syndrome.

Lifestyle Changes

TREATMENT. The therapeutic options consist of lifestyle modifications, treatment of secondary causes, and, if possible, diet and medications.

DIET (see Chap. 41). Individuals with dyslipoproteinemias should always adopt dietary therapy. High-risk subjects should have medications started concomitantly with a diet because in many cases, diet may not suffice to reach target levels. The diet should have three objectives. First, it should allow the patient to reach and maintain ideal body weight. Second, it should provide a well-balanced diet with fruits, vegetables, and whole grains and it should be restricted in saturated fats and refined carbohydrates. Dietary counseling should involve a professional dietitian. Often, the help of dietitians, weight loss programs, or diabetic outpatient centers can aid sustained weight loss. Currently, the ATP III and the American Heart Association[16] recommend a diet in which protein intake represents 15 to 20 percent of calories, fats represent less than 35 percent, with only 7 percent from saturated fats, and the remaining calories derive from carbohydrates. Cholesterol intake should be less than 300 mg/day.

Treatment of Combined Lipoprotein Disorders

Combined lipoprotein disorders, characterized by an increase in plasma total cholesterol and triglycerides, frequently occur in clinical practice and represent difficult challenges. Patients with combined lipoprotein disorders have an increase in LDL cholesterol and LDL particle number (as reflected by an increase in total or LDL apo B), small, dense LDL particles, increased VLDL cholesterol and VLDL triglycerides, and a reduced HDL cholesterol level. Patients with this pattern of combined dyslipidemia often have obesity and the metabolic syndrome. Treatment should begin with lifestyle modifications, with a diet reduced in total calories and saturated fats, weight reduction, and increased exercise. Drug treatment, when warranted, aims to correct the predominant lipoprotein abnormality. Statins can reduce plasma triglyceride levels, particularly in individuals with high baseline triglyceride levels. Fibrates reduce triglycerides and may change the composition of LDL particles to a larger and less dense phenotype. Although fibric acid derivatives have a role in the secondary prevention of cardiovascular diseases in subjects with low HDL cholesterol levels, they can paradoxically increase LDL cholesterol levels (because of increased lipoprotein lipase activity). Plasma total homocysteine levels may increase with fenofibrate and to a lesser extent with bezafibrate. In view of gemfibrozil's effects on glucuronidation of statins, we advise against its use in combination therapy. The combination of a statin with a fibrate has proven highly effective in correcting the combined dyslipoproteinemias. Patients taking a fibrate plus a statin merit close medical follow-up for evidence of hepatotoxicity or myositis within the first 6 weeks of therapy and every 6 months thereafter. Other combinations, including fibric acid derivatives with bile acid–binding resins and niacin with bile acid–binding resins, have also proved to be useful in specific cases. The combination of fibrates or statins with niacin requires experience and care because of the risk of hepatotoxicity and myositis. The search for correctable causes (e.g., uncontrolled diabetes, obesity, hypothyroidism, and alcohol use) of combined dyslipidemia and the benefit of lifestyle modifications require reemphasis. Often, the help of dietitians, weight loss programs, or diabetic outpatient centers is highly beneficial.

EXTRACORPOREAL LOW-DENSITY LIPOPROTEIN FILTRATION. Patients with severe hypercholesterolemia, especially those with homozygous familial hypercholesterolemia or severe heterozygous familial hypercholesterolemia may warrant treatment by extracorporeal LDL elimination. These techniques use selective filtration, adsorption, or precipitation of LDL (or apo B–containing particles) after plasma separation. Specialized centers have LDL-pheresis available. This approach can dramatically reduce the risk of developing cardiovascular disease and improve survival.[83]

Novel Approaches

The development of novel pharmaceutical agents for the treatment of lipoprotein disorders will likely continue because cardiovascular disease due to atherosclerosis represents the largest burden of disease for the near future. Better targeting of high-risk individuals will allow optimization of expensive therapies. The finding that subjects who were previously identified as being at relatively low risk of CAD on the basis of their LDL cholesterol levels but who have an elevated C-reactive protein level derive benefit from a statin in the primary prevention of CAD may radically alter the concept of cardiovascular risk stratification.[84,85] If cardiovascular risk can be better identified using markers of inflammation, in addition to conventional risk factors, physicians' attitudes should embrace these findings. This hypothesis is undergoing rigorous testing in a clinical trial.[85]

The burgeoning field of pharmacogenetics might, in the near future, allow treatment of patients on the basis of their genetic make-up. Genetic screening may become a useful clinical tool, as technology improves and rapid genotyping for diagnostic and prognostic purposes becomes available for clinicians. Other than cost issues, the ethics of screening for genetic predisposition to disease and access to information represent daunting challenges. The discovery that the apo E4 allele carries the risk of early-onset Alzheimer disease, one of the familial forms of the disorder, illustrates the ethical complexities of genetic testing in the realm of lipoprotein disorders.

Drug Development and Future Directions

Novel proteins that regulate the synthesis of lipids have become therapeutic targets for drug development. The development of competitive inhibitors of HMG-CoA reductase leading to statin drugs provides a good example. These drugs have an important impact on cardiovascular morbidity and mortality reduction in high-risk individuals. Inhibitors of pancreatic lipases are being used to treat obesity.[86] Future potential drug targets might include inhibition of apo B secretion by inhibiting the microsomal triglyceride transfer protein, which is crucial in the assembly of apo B–containing lipoproteins.[87] Hepatic steatosis may limit this therapeutic option in humans. Selective inhibition of ACAT may also provide a therapeutic target to inhibit cholesterol absorption through the intestinal wall, inhibit secretion from the liver of apo B–containing lipoproteins, and interfere with foam cell formation.[12] Drugs that increase cellular cholesterol efflux to increase HDL cholesterol levels may also prove useful in the treatment of dyslipoproteinemias.

Other therapeutic modalities in the treatment of atherosclerosis by modulating lipoprotein metabolism include the development of inhibitors of CETP to increase HDL cholesterol levels[87a] or modulation of LCAT, and inhibitors of bile acid transport to decrease intestinal cholesterol uptake. Clinical studies currently in progress are testing the effect of CETP inhibitors on human atherosclerosis. Pharmacological modulation of HDL cholesterol levels, other than by niacin, has not led to results proportional to those achieved for LDL cholesterol. Potential modulators of HDL cholesterol levels include SR-B1, ABCA1 pathways, apo A1, and its homologues and mimetics.[88]

Gene Therapy

Severe, homozygous, monogenic disorders may eventually be treated by gene therapy. The initial trials of gene therapy in cases of homozygous familial hypercholesterolemia have not led to a major improvement and have largely been abandoned. However, the lifelong burden of these rare disorders and the potential for cure makes this approach very appealing. Other diseases, such as abetalipoproteinemia, LPL deficiency, Niemann-Pick type C disease, sitosterolemia, and Tangier disease may become therapeutic targets for gene therapy. If the approach to correct these disorders is successful, the more widespread applications of gene-based therapies for the purpose of reducing potential cardiovascular risk will become a daunting medical, social, and ethical problem.

REFERENCES

1. Sorci-Thomas MG, Curtiss L, Parks JS, et al: The hydrophobic face orientation of apolipoprotein A-I amphipathic helix domain 143-164 regulates lecithin:cholesterol acyltransferase activation. J Biol Chem 273:11776, 1998.
2. Hiltunen TP, Luoma JS, Nikkari T, Yla-Herttuala S: Expression of LDL receptor, VLDL receptor, LDL receptor-related protein, and scavenger receptor in rabbit atherosclerotic lesions: Marked induction of scavenger receptor and VLDL receptor expression during lesion development. Circulation 97:1079, 1998.
3. Nimpf J, Schneider WJ: The VLDL receptor: An LDL receptor relative with eight ligand binding repeats, LR8. Atherosclerosis 141:191, 1998.
4. Mahley RW, Ji ZS: Remnant lipoprotein metabolism: Key pathways involving cell-surface heparan sulfate proteoglycans and apolipoprotein E. J Lipid Res 40:1, 1999.
5. Brown ML, Ramprasad MP, Umeda PK, et al: A macrophage receptor for apolipoprotein B48: Cloning, expression, and atherosclerosis. Proc Natl Acad Sci U S A 97:7488, 2000.
6. de Man FH, de Beer F, van der Laarse A, et al: Lipolysis of very low density lipoproteins by heparan sulfate proteoglycan-bound lipoprotein lipase. J Lipid Res 38:2465, 1997.
7. Sawamura T, Kume N, Aoyama T, et al: An endothelial receptor for oxidized low-density lipoprotein. Nature 386:73, 1997.
8. Acton S, Rigotti A, Landschulz KT, et al: Identification of scavenger receptor SR-BI as a high density lipoprotein receptor. Science 271:518, 1996.
8a. Altmann SW, Davis HR Jr, Zhu LJ, et al: Niemann-Pick C1 like 1 protein is critical for intestinal cholesterol absorption. Science 303:1201, 2004.
9. Mann CJ, Troussard AA, Yen FT, et al: Inhibitory effects of specific apolipoprotein C-III isoforms on the binding of triglyceride-rich lipoproteins to the lipolysis-stimulated receptor. J Biol Chem 272:31348, 1997.
10. van Tol A: Phospholipid transfer protein. Curr Opin Lipidol 13:135, 2002.
11. Abifadel M, Varret M, Rabes JP, et al: Mutations in PCSK9 cause autosomal dominant hypercholesterolemia. Nat Genet 34:154, 2003.
12. Willner EL, Tow B, Buhman KK, et al: Deficiency of acyl CoA:cholesterol acyltransferase 2 prevents atherosclerosis in apolipoprotein E-deficient mice. Proc Natl Acad Sci U S A 100:1262, 2003.
13. Zhang SH, Reddick RL, Piedrahita JA, Maeda N: Spontaneous hypercholesterolemia and arterial lesions in mice lacking apolipoprotein E. Science 258:468, 1992.
14. O'Connell BJ, Genest J Jr: High-density lipoproteins and endothelial function. Circulation 104:1978, 2001.
15. Li XA, Titlow WB, Jackson BA, et al: High density lipoprotein binding to scavenger receptor, class B, type I activates endothelial nitric-oxide synthase in a ceramide-dependent manner. J Biol Chem 277:11058, 2002.
16. Oram JF: HDL apolipoproteins and ABCA1: Partners in the removal of excess cellular cholesterol. Arterioscler Thromb Vasc Biol 23:720, 2003.
17. Haidar B, Denis M, Krimbou L, et al: cAMP induces ABCA1 phosphorylation activity and promotes cholesterol efflux from fibroblasts. J Lipid Res 43:2087, 2002.
18. Fielding PE, Nagao K, Hakamata H, et al: A two-step mechanism for free cholesterol and phospholipid efflux from human vascular cells to apolipoprotein A-1. Biochemistry 39:14113, 2000.
19. Hammad SM, Stefansson S, Twal WO, et al: Cubilin, the endocytic receptor for intrinsic factor-vitamin B(12) complex, mediates high-density lipoprotein holoparticle endocytosis. Proc Natl Acad Sci U S A 96:10158, 1999.
20. Grundy SM: Low-density lipoprotein, non-high-density lipoprotein, and apolipoprotein B as targets of lipid-lowering therapy. Circulation 106:2526, 2002.
21. Campos H, Moye LA, Glasser SP, et al: Low-density lipoprotein size, pravastatin treatment, and coronary events. JAMA 286:1468, 2001.
22. Sacks FM, Campos H: Clinical review 163: Cardiovascular endocrinology: Low-density lipoprotein size and cardiovascular disease: A reappraisal. J Clin Endocrinol Metab 88:4525, 2003.
23. Wilson DJ, Gahan M, Haddad L, et al: A World Wide Web site for low-density lipoprotein receptor gene mutations in familial hypercholesterolemia: Sequence-based, tabular, and direct submission data handling. Am J Cardiol 81:1509, 1998.
24. Hansen PS, Defesche JC, Kastelein JJ, et al: Phenotypic variation in patients heterozygous for familial defective apolipoprotein B (FDB) in three European countries. Arterioscler Thromb Vasc Biol 17:741, 1997.
25. Wetterau JR, Aggerbeck LP, Bouma ME, et al: Absence of microsomal triglyceride transfer protein in individuals with abetalipoproteinemia. Science 258:999, 1992.

26. Berge KE, Tian H, Graf GA, et al: Accumulation of dietary cholesterol in sitosterolemia caused by mutations in adjacent ABC transporters. Science 290:1771, 2000.
27. Mooser V, Mancini FP, Bopp S, et al: Sequence polymorphisms in the apo(a) gene associated with specific levels of Lp(a) in plasma. Hum Mol Genet 4:173, 1995.
28. Danesh J, Collins R, Peto R: Lipoprotein(a) and coronary heart disease: Meta-analysis of prospective studies. Circulation 102:1082, 2000.
29. Sjarif DR, Sinke RJ, Duran M, et al: Clinical heterogeneity and novel mutations in the glycerol kinase gene in three families with isolated glycerol kinase deficiency. J Med Genet 35:650, 1998.
30. Santamarina-Fojo S: The familial chylomicronemia syndrome. Endocrinol Metab Clin North Am 27:551, viii, 1998.
31. Weinstock PH, Bisgaier CL, Aalto-Setala K, et al: Severe hypertriglyceridemia, reduced high density lipoprotein, and neonatal death in lipoprotein lipase knockout mice: Mild hypertriglyceridemia with impaired very low density lipoprotein clearance in heterozygotes. J Clin Invest 96:2555, 1995.
32. Mahley RW, Huang Y, Rall SC Jr: Pathogenesis of type III hyperlipoproteinemia (dysbetalipoproteinemia): Questions, quandaries, and paradoxes. J Lipid Res 40:1933, 1999.
33. Genest JJ Jr, Martin-Munley SS, McNamara JR, et al: Familial lipoprotein disorders in patients with premature coronary artery disease. Circulation 85:2025, 1992.
34. Pajukanta P, Nuotio I, Terwilliger JD, et al: Linkage of familial combined hyperlipidaemia to chromosome 1q21-q23. Nat Genet 18:369, 1998.
35. Murray I, Kohl J, Cianflone K: Acylation-stimulating protein (ASP): Structure-function determinants of cell surface binding and triacylglycerol synthetic activity. Biochem J 342:41, 1999.
36. Kalant D, Cain SA, Maslowska M, et al: The chemoattractant receptor-like protein C5L2 binds the C3a des-Arg77/acylation-stimulating protein. J Biol Chem 278:11123, 2003.
37. Lamarche B, Uffelman KD, Carpentier A, et al: Triglyceride enrichment of HDL enhances in vivo metabolic clearance of HDL apo A-I in healthy men. J Clin Invest 103:1191, 1999.
38. Sorci-Thomas MG, Thomas MJ: The effects of altered apolipoprotein A-I structure on plasma HDL concentration. Trends Cardiovasc Med 12:121, 2002.
39. Kuivenhoven JA, Jukema JW, Zwinderman AH, et al: The role of a common variant of the cholesteryl ester transfer protein gene in the progression of coronary atherosclerosis. The Regression Growth Evaluation Statin Study Group. N Engl J Med 338:86, 1998.
40. Kuivenhoven JA, Pritchard H, Hill J, et al: The molecular pathology of lecithin:cholesterol acyltransferase (LCAT) deficiency syndromes. J Lipid Res 38:191, 1997.
41. Zhong S, Sharp DS, Grove JS, et al: Increased coronary heart disease in Japanese-American men with mutation in the cholesteryl ester transfer protein gene despite increased HDL levels. J Clin Invest 97:2917, 1996.
42. Ma K, Cilingiroglu M, Otvos JD, et al: Endothelial lipase is a major genetic determinant for high-density lipoprotein concentration, structure, and metabolism. Proc Natl Acad Sci U S A 100:2748, 2003.
43. Marcil M, Brooks-Wilson A, Clee SM, et al: Mutations in the ABC1 gene in familial HDL deficiency with defective cholesterol efflux. Lancet 354:1341, 1999.
44. Rust S, Rosier M, Funke H, et al: Tangier disease is caused by mutations in the gene encoding ATP-binding cassette transporter 1. Nat Genet 22:352, 1999.
45. Bodzioch M, Orso E, Klucken J, et al: The gene encoding ATP-binding cassette transporter 1 is mutated in Tangier disease. Nat Genet 22:347, 1999.
46. Carstea ED, Morris JA, Coleman KG, et al: Niemann-Pick C1 disease gene: Homology to mediators of cholesterol homeostasis. Science 277:228, 1997.
47. Lee CY, Krimbou L, Vincent J, et al: Compound heterozygosity at the sphingomyelin phosphodiesterase-1 (SMPD1) gene is associated with low HDL cholesterol. Hum Genet 112:552, 2003.
48. Herrington DM, Vittinghoff E, Lin F, et al: Statin therapy, cardiovascular events, and total mortality in the Heart and Estrogen/Progestin Replacement Study (HERS). Circulation 105:2962, 2002.
48a. Anderson GL, Limacher M, Assaf AR: Effects of conjugated equine estrogen in postmenopausal women with hysterectomy: The Women's Health Initiative randomized controlled trial. JAMA 291:1701, 2004.
49. Martin G, Duez H, Blanquart C, et al: Statin-induced inhibition of the Rho-signaling pathway activates PPARalpha and induces HDL apoA-I. J Clin Invest 107:1423, 2001.
50. Libby P, Ridker PM, Maseri A: Inflammation and atherosclerosis. Circulation 105:1135, 2002.
51. Genest J, Pedersen TR: Prevention of cardiovascular ischemic events: High-risk and secondary prevention. Circulation 107:2059, 2003.
52. Libby P, Aikawa M: Stabilization of atherosclerotic plaques: New mechanisms and clinical targets. Nat Med 8:1257, 2002.
53. Gagne C, Bays HE, Weiss SR, et al: Efficacy and safety of ezetimibe added to ongoing statin therapy for treatment of patients with primary hypercholesterolemia. Am J Cardiol 90:1084, 2002.
54. Bissonnette R, Treacy E, Rozen R, et al: Fenofibrate raises plasma homocysteine levels in the fasted and fed states. Atherosclerosis 155:455, 2001.
55. Brown BG, Zhao XQ, Chait A, et al: Simvastatin and niacin, antioxidant vitamins, or the combination for the prevention of coronary disease. N Engl J Med 345:1583, 2001.
56. Wise A, Foord SM, Fraser NJ, et al: Molecular identification of high and low affinity receptors for nicotinic acid. J Biol Chem 278:9869, 2003.
57. Soga T, Kamohara M, Takasaki J, et al: Molecular identification of nicotinic acid receptor. Biochem Biophys Res Commun 303:364, 2003.
58. Cote G, Tardif JC, Lesperance J, et al: Effects of probucol on vascular remodeling after coronary angioplasty. Multivitamins and Protocol Study Group. Circulation 99:30, 1999.
59. Downs JR, Clearfield M, Weis S, et al: Primary prevention of acute coronary events with lovastatin in men and women with average cholesterol levels: Results of AFCAPS/TexCAPS. Air Force/Texas Coronary Atherosclerosis Prevention Study. JAMA 279:1615, 1998.
60. Shepherd J, Cobbe SM, Ford I, et al: Prevention of coronary heart disease with pravastatin in men with hypercholesterolemia. West of Scotland Coronary Prevention Study Group. N Engl J Med 333:1301, 1995.
61. Sacks FM, Pfeffer MA, Moye LA, et al: The effect of pravastatin on coronary events after myocardial infarction in patients with average cholesterol levels. Cholesterol and Recurrent Events Trial investigators. N Engl J Med 335:1001, 1996.
62. Prevention of cardiovascular events and death with pravastatin in patients with coronary heart disease and a broad range of initial cholesterol levels. The Long-Term Intervention with Pravastatin in Ischaemic Disease (LIPID) Study Group. N Engl J Med 339:1349, 1998.
63. Randomised trial of cholesterol lowering in 4444 patients with coronary heart disease: The Scandinavian Simvastatin Survival Study (4S). Lancet 344:1383, 1994.
64. Executive Summary of the Third Report of the National Cholesterol Education Program (NCEP) Expert Panel on Detection, Evaluation, And Treatment of High Blood Cholesterol In Adults (Adult Treatment Panel III). JAMA 285:2486, 2001.
65. MRC/BHF Heart Protection Study of cholesterol lowering with simvastatin in 20,536 high-risk individuals: A randomised placebo-controlled trial. Lancet 360:7, 2002.
66. Shepherd J, Blauw GJ, Murphy MB, et al: Pravastatin in elderly individuals at risk of vascular disease (PROSPER): A randomised controlled trial. Lancet 360:1623, 2002.
67. Major outcomes in moderately hypercholesterolemic, hypertensive patients randomized to pravastatin vs usual care: The Antihypertensive and Lipid-Lowering Treatment to Prevent Heart Attack Trial (ALLHAT-LLT). JAMA 288:2998, 2002.
68. Pasternak RC: The ALLHAT lipid lowering trial—less is less. JAMA 288:3042, 2002.
69. Sever PS, Dahlof B, Poulter NR, et al: Prevention of coronary and stroke events with atorvastatin in hypertensive patients who have average or lower-than-average cholesterol concentrations, in the Anglo-Scandinavian Cardiac Outcomes Trial—Lipid Lowering Arm (ASCOT-LLA): A multicentre randomised controlled trial. Lancet 361:1149, 2003.
70. Colhoun HM, Thomason MJ, Mackness MI, et al: Design of the Collaborative AtoRvastatin Diabetes Study (CARDS) in patients with type 2 diabetes. Diabet Med 19:201, 2002.
71. Colhoun HM, Thomason MJ, Mackness MI, et al: Design of the collaborative Ato Rvastatin Diabetes Study (CARDS) in patients with type 2 diabetes. Diabet Med 19:201, 2002.
72. Stenestrand U, Wallentin L: Early statin treatment following acute myocardial infarction and 1-year survival. JAMA 285:430, 2001.
73. Newby LK, Kristinsson A, Bhapkar MV, et al: Early statin initiation and outcomes in patients with acute coronary syndromes. JAMA 287:3087, 2002.
74. Schwartz GG, Olsson AG, Ezekowitz MD, et al: Effects of atorvastatin on early recurrent ischemic events in acute coronary syndromes: The MIRACL study: A randomized controlled trial. JAMA 285:1711, 2001.
75. Blazing MA, De Lemos JA, Dyke CK, et al: The A-to-Z Trial: Methods and rationale for a single trial investigating combined use of low-molecular-weight heparin with the glycoprotein IIb/IIIa inhibitor tirofiban and defining the efficacy of early aggressive simvastatin therapy. Am Heart J 142:211, 2001.
76. Cannon CP, McCabe CH, Belder R, et al: Design of the Pravastatin or Atorvastatin Evaluation and Infection Therapy (PROVE IT)-TIMI 22 trial. Am J Cardiol 89:860, 2002.
76a. Cannon CP, Braunwald E, McCabe CH, et al: Intensive versus moderate lipid lowering with statins after acute coronary syndromes. N Engl J Med 350:1495, 2004.
77. Pitt B, Waters D, Brown WV, et al: Aggressive lipid-lowering therapy compared with angioplasty in stable coronary artery disease. Atorvastatin versus Revascularization Treatment Investigators. N Engl J Med 341:70, 1999.
78. Chiquette E, Chilton R: Aggressive medical management of coronary artery disease versus mechanical revascularization. Curr Atheroscler Rep 5:118, 2003.
78a. Nissen SE, Tuzcu EM, Schoenhagen P, et al: Effect of intensive compared with moderate lipid-lowering therapy on progression of coronary atherosclerosis: A randomized controlled trial. JAMA 291:1071, 2004.
79. McMahon M, Kirkpatrick C, Cummings CE, et al: A pilot study with simvastatin and folic acid/vitamin B_{12} in preparation for the Study of the Effectiveness of Additional Reductions in Cholesterol and Homocysteine (SEARCH). Nutr Metab Cardiovasc Dis 10:195, 2000.
80. Waters DD, Guyton JR, Herrington DM, et al: Treating to New Targets (TNT): Does lowering low-density lipoprotein in cholesterol levels below currently recommended guidelines yield incremental clinical benefits. Am J Cardiol 193:154, 2004.
81. Rubins HB, Robins SJ, Collins D, et al: Gemfibrozil for the secondary prevention of coronary heart disease in men with low levels of high-density lipoprotein cholesterol. Veterans Affairs High-Density Lipoprotein Cholesterol Intervention Trial Study Group. N Engl J Med 341:410, 1999.
82. Secondary prevention by raising HDL cholesterol and reducing triglycerides in patients with coronary artery disease: The Bezafibrate Infarction Prevention (BIP) study. Circulation 102:21, 2000.
83. Nishimura S, Sekiguchi M, Kano T, et al: Effects of intensive lipid lowering by low-density lipoprotein apheresis on regression of coronary atherosclerosis in patients with familial hypercholesterolemia: Japan Low-density Lipoprotein Apheresis Coronary Atherosclerosis Prospective Study (L-CAPS). Atherosclerosis 144:409, 1999.
84. Ridker PM, Rifai N, Rose L, et al: Comparison of C-reactive protein and low-density lipoprotein cholesterol levels in the prediction of first cardiovascular events. N Engl J Med 347:1557, 2002.
85. Ridker PM: Rosuvastatin in the primary prevention of cardiovascular disease among patients with low levels of low-density lipoprotein cholesterol and elevated high-sensitivity C-reactive protein: Rationale and design of the JUPITER trial. Circulation 108:2292, 2003.
86. Hvizdos KM, Markham A: Orlistat: A review of its use in the management of obesity. Drugs 58:743, 1999.
87. Narcisi TM, Shoulders CC, Chester SA, et al: Mutations of the microsomal triglyceride-transfer-protein gene in abetalipoproteinemia. Am J Hum Genet 57:1298, 1995.
87a. Brousseau ME, Schaefer EJ, Wolfe ML, et al: Effects of an inhibitor of cholesteryl ester transfer protein on HDL cholesterol. N Engl J Med 350:1505, 2004.
88. Nissen SE, Tsunoda T, Tuzcu EM, et al: Effect of recombinant ApoA-I Milano on coronary atherosclerosis in patients with acute coronary syndromes: A randomized controlled trial. JAMA 290:2292, 2003.

CHAPTER 40

Diabetes Mellitus, the Metabolic Syndrome, and Atherosclerotic Vascular Disease

Joshua A. Beckman • Peter Libby • Mark A. Creager

Vascular diseases account for most morbidity and mortality in patients with diabetes mellitus.[1-3] Diabetes causes microvascular diseases, such as nephropathy, neuropathy, and retinopathy, and macrovascular disease, that is, atherosclerosis. Atherosclerosis of the coronary, cerebral, and peripheral arteries accounts for approximately 80 percent of mortality and 75 percent of hospitalizations in persons with diabetes.

Approximately 8 percent of the U.S. population has diabetes, undiagnosed in half the cases.[4] The prevalence of diabetes follows that of obesity, which affected approximately 18 percent of the U.S. population in 1998.[5,6] Hispanics, blacks, Native Americans, and Asian Indians bear a disproportionate burden of diabetic cardiovascular disease.[7] The predilection for these ethnic groups to develop obesity and glucose intolerance on a western diet may have a genetic basis, because the ability to store fat may have conferred a survival advantage in populations subject to famine. This selective pressure could enrich the population in genes that facilitate fat storage, the so-called "thrifty gene" hypothesis.[8,9]

The prevalence of diabetes is increasing within the U.S. population (Fig. 40–1) and has grown from approximately 2 million cases in the early 1960s to 15 million in 2000. Americans born in 2000 will have an estimated 36 percent chance of developing diabetes in their lifetime.[10] Current estimates project 22 million cases by 2025.[11] When viewed in the light of the rapidly expanding diabetic population, these data raise the specter of a reversal in the improvement in cardiovascular outcomes over the last two decades. The general population in the United States has enjoyed an impressive decline in the mortality associated with heart disease in the last decades. However, the drop in cardiovascular mortality in diabetic men and women has lagged well behind that of the general population.[12]

Cardiovascular disease in diabetes also impacts the economic resources of the health care system. Data from a managed care organization on the 1-year costs of treating more than 85,000 patients with diabetes compared with age- and sex-matched nondiabetic counterparts attributes the largest proportion (17 percent) of the excess costs associated with diabetes to coronary artery disease (CAD).[13] In comparison, end-stage renal disease accounted for only 11 percent of the excess costs of treatment.

Better implementation of therapies that reduce cardiovascular risk in diabetic patients will require moving beyond the traditional primary focus on glycemic control.[14] A working knowledge of the effects of diabetes mellitus on the heart and blood vessels will aid physicians caring for these patients.

Diagnostic Criteria for Diabetes Mellitus

In 1997, the American Diabetes Association (ADA) promulgated new criteria for the diagnosis of diabetes mellitus.[15] These criteria use a single blood glucose determination after an 8-hour fast (fasting plasma glucose [FPG]) as the major diagnostic criterion (Table 40–1). An FPG of less than 110 mg/dl is considered normal. A new diagnostic category known as impaired fasting glucose (IFG) encompasses FPGs higher than 110 but lower than 126 mg/dl. An FPG of higher than 126 mg/dl establishes the diagnosis of diabetes mellitus. Type 2 diabetes mellitus, previously known as non-insulin-dependent or adult-onset diabetes, represents 90 percent of the diabetic population. Type 1 diabetes, known previously as insulin-dependent or juvenile-onset diabetes, accounts for the remaining 10 percent. Both forms of diabetes confer independent risk for cardiovascular events, although patients with type 1 diabetes generally develop cardiovascular disease at a much younger age than those with type 2 diabetes.

Epidemiology of Cardiovascular Disease in Diabetes Mellitus

The clinical manifestations of diabetes-related atherosclerosis occur in every major vascular territory, notably the coronary, cerebral, and peripheral (limb) arteries.

Coronary Artery Disease

Patients with diabetes have a twofold to fourfold increase in the risk of CAD.[16] In the Multiple Risk Factor Intervention (MRFIT) study, more than 5000 men (of ~350,000 screened) who reported taking medications for diabetes were followed for an average of 12 years.[17] For every age stratum, ethnic background, and risk factor level, men with diabetes had an absolute risk of CAD death more than 3 times higher than that in the nondiabetic cohort, even after adjustment for established risk factors.[18] Another large cohort of 11,554 white men and 666 black men between 35 and 64 years of age, screened from 1967 to 1973 and followed prospectively for 22 years, showed similar findings.[18]

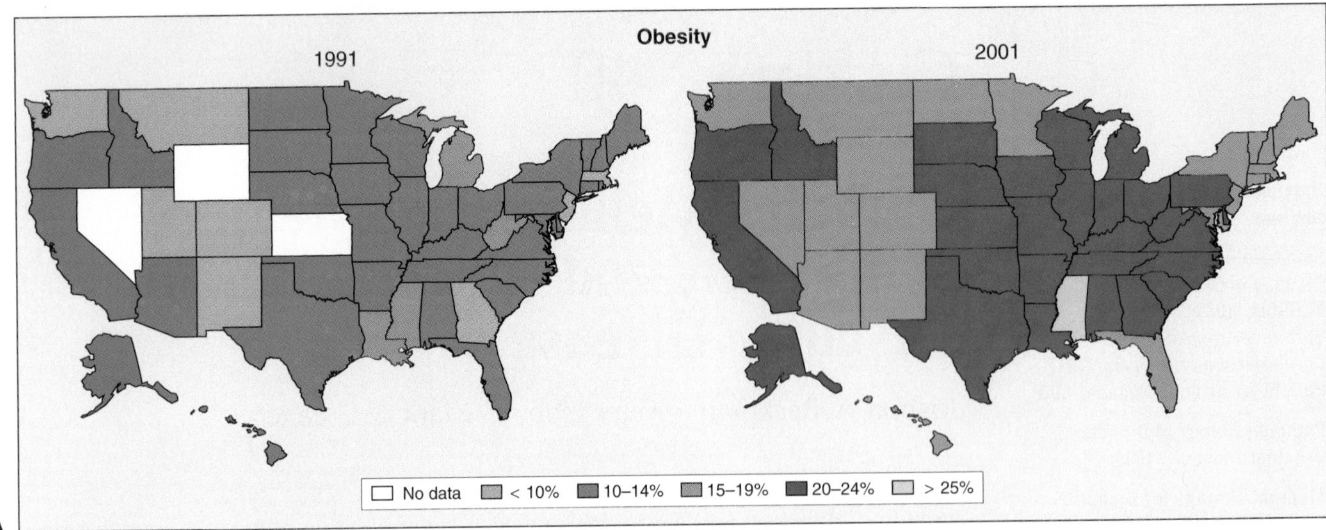

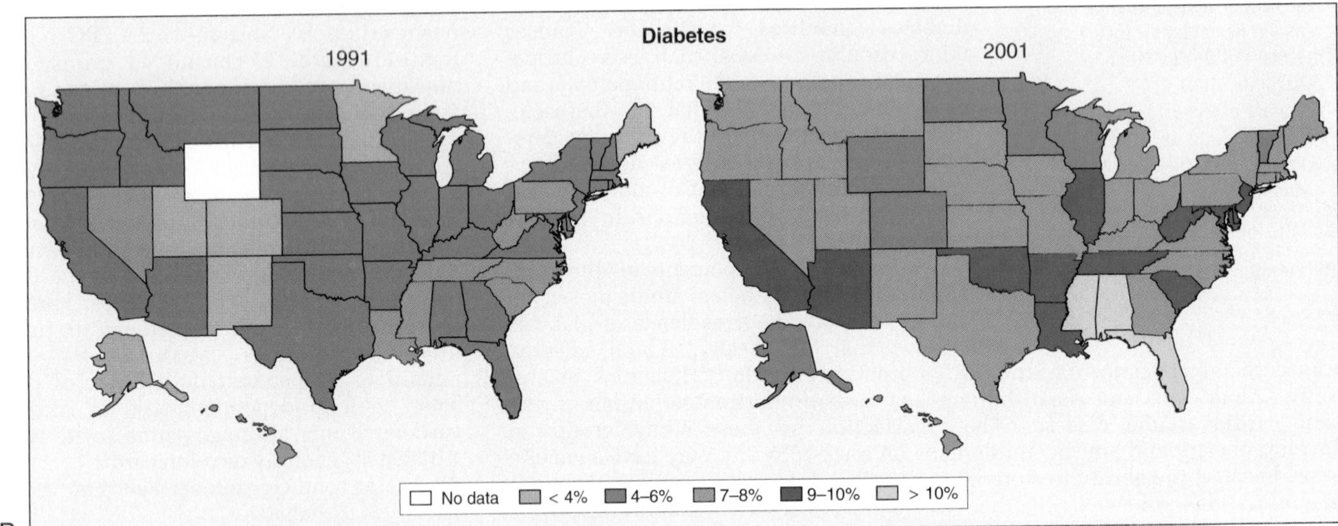

FIGURE 40–1 Obesity and diabetes mellitus in U.S. adults. Over the 10-year period of 1991 to 2001, the prevalence of obesity and diabetes among U.S. adults increased in every region of the nation. Obesity is associated with the development of type 2 diabetes mellitus and may serve as the root cause underlying the increased prevalence of type 2 diabetes. (From Mokdad AH, Ford ES, Bowman BA, et al: Prevalence of obesity, diabetes, and obesity-related health risk factors, 2001. JAMA 289:76-79, 2003.) (See also Chap. 41.)

TABLE 40–1 Criteria for the Diagnosis of Diabetes Mellitus*

Normal	Impaired Fasting Glucose	Diabetes Mellitus
FPG < 110 mg/dl	FPG ≥ 110 mg/dl and <126 mg/dl (IFG)	FPG ≥ 126 mg/dl
2-hr PG < 140 mg/dl	2-hr PG ≥ 140 mg/dl and <200 mg/dl (IGT)	2-hr PG ≥ 200 mg/dl Symptoms of diabetes mellitus and random plasma glucose concentration ≥200 mg/dl

FPG = fasting postload glucose; IFG = impaired fasting glucose; IGT = impaired glucose tolerance; PG = postload glucose.
Data from American Diabetes Association: Clinical practice recommendations. Diabetes Care 22(Suppl 1): S5-S19, 1999.
*Rather than employing the classic glucose tolerance curve with multiple time points sampled, the new criteria employ, in parallel to the FPG measurements, a 2-hr PG set of criteria. The plasma sample is obtained 2 hr following an oral administration of 75 gm of anhydrous glucose in aqueous solution.

In the general population, women experience relative protection from myocardial infarction and usually develop CAD approximately 10 years later than men. However, diabetes blunts the cardiovascular benefit of female gender.[19] Diabetic U.S. women of either European or African ancestry have this heightened risk.[20] Diabetes increases the risk of death after myocardial infarction in women more than men (see Chap. 51).[21] In the First National Health and Nutrition Examination Survey (NHANES) and the NHANES Epidemiologic Follow-Up Survey conducted 10 years apart, age-adjusted mortality decreased in nondiabetic men and women, less so in diabetic men, but increased by 23 percent in diabetic women.[12]

Multiple studies support the notion that acute and long-term adverse cardiovascular events have substantially increased in patients with diabetes. A Finnish epidemiological survey compared the rates of myocardial infarction in nondiabetic and diabetic populations (Fig. 40–2).[22] In this study, patients with diabetes but without prior myocardial infarction had the same level of risk for subsequent acute coronary

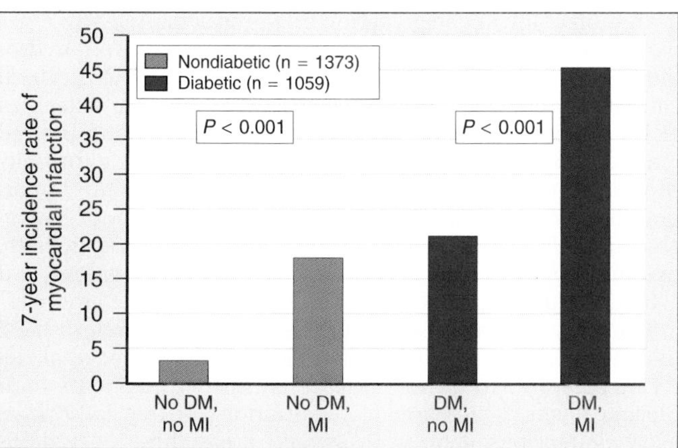

FIGURE 40–2 Marked increase in risk of coronary artery disease in patients with type 2 diabetes mellitus (DM). These data show a striking increase in the risk of first or recurrent myocardial infarction (MI) in diabetic patients compared with nondiabetic subjects in a population-based study in Finland over a 7-year follow-up period. These data also show that the diabetic patient without history of previous myocardial infarction has an approximately equal risk for first myocardial infarction as a nondiabetic subject who has already sustained myocardial infarction. These data support recent recommendations from the American Diabetes Association to treat diabetic subjects as if they already have established coronary artery disease. (From Haffner SM, Lehto S, Ronnemaa T, et al: Mortality from coronary heart disease in subjects with type 2 diabetes and in nondiabetic subjects with and without prior myocardial infraction. N Engl J Med 339:229-234, 1998.)

events as did nondiabetic persons with a history of previous myocardial infarction.

In the six-nation OASIS study, diabetic patients presenting with unstable angina or non-Q wave myocardial infarction had increased rates of stroke, congestive heart failure, and death during the index hospitalization compared with nondiabetic patients.[23] In the Gruppo Italiano per lo Studio della Sopravvivenza nell'Infarto Miocardico-2 (GISSI-2) study of thrombolytic therapy in patients with myocardial infarction, diabetes increased the rate of death in men by 40 percent and women by 90 percent.[24] In the Should We Emergently Revascularize Occluded Coronaries for Cardiogenic Shock (SHOCK) trial, which evaluated a strategy of early revascularization in patients with myocardial infarction complicated by cardiogenic shock, 31.1 percent of the patients had diabetes—a much greater percentage than in the population in general.[25] Moreover, the patients with diabetes experienced a 36 percent excess in mortality compared to patients without diabetes.[26] In the Finnish contribution to the WHO MONICA Project (World Health Organization Multinational Monitoring of Trends and Determinants of Cardiovascular Disease), 1-year mortality was 38 percent higher for diabetic men and 86 percent higher for diabetic women.[21] In a follow-up study of more than 5000 patients who presented to an emergency department with symptoms suggestive of myocardial infarction, diabetic patients had a 53.5 percent 5-year mortality rate compared with 23.3 percent among nondiabetic patients.[27] These trends toward an increasing risk of death among diabetic subjects are even greater in younger patients. In a statewide analysis of myocardial infarction, the risk of death in diabetic subjects was 87 percent greater than in nondiabetics aged 30 to 49 years but only 17 percent greater in the 70- to 89-year age group.[28]

Cerebrovascular Disease

Diabetes mellitus increases the frequency of cerebral atherosclerosis and the risk of stroke. Among patients presenting with a stroke, the prevalence of diabetes is thrice that of matched controls, and diabetes increases the risk of stroke up to fourfold.[29-31] In the MRFIT study, diabetic subjects who required medication for glucose control were threefold as likely to develop a stroke as nondiabetic subjects.[17] Similarly, in more than 12,000 male and female subjects followed for 6 to 8 years in the Atherosclerosis Risk in Communities Study, the relative risk of an ischemic stroke was increased nearly fourfold by the presence of diabetes.[32] Moreover, insulin resistance varies inversely with the risk of stroke.[29] Diabetic subjects have more severe carotid atherosclerosis as assessed by ultrasonography and a fivefold excess prevalence of calcified carotid atheroma as observed on dental panoramic radiographs.[33]

Diabetes puts younger patients at particular risk for stroke. Diabetes decreases the age at presentation for stroke compared to persons who do not have diabetes. One in 10 stroke victims is younger than 55 years of age, and diabetes increases the stroke risk more than 10-fold in this age group.[34] In the Baltimore-Washington Cooperative Young Stroke Study of 296 cases of incident ischemic stroke subjects aged 18 to 44 years, diabetes markedly increased the risk of stroke.[35] The age-adjusted odds ratio for stroke was 3.3 for black women, 4.2 for black men, 6.2 for white women, and 23.1 for white men (Fig. 40–3).

Most studies have shown that diabetes increases the risk of stroke more in women than men.[36,37] In the Renfrew/Paisley Study, a 20-year follow-up study in Scotland of 7052 men and 8354 women aged 45 to 64 years, diabetic women had a nearly threefold excess in stroke.[38] The 52 percent increase in diabetic men did not achieve statistical significance.[38] Further, diabetic women also had a higher risk of death from stroke. In another study of 16,600 patients, diabetes accounted for 16 percent of stroke-related mortality in men and 33 percent in women.[39] Diabetes augments the risk of stroke more among blacks and Caribbean Hispanics than whites. In the Northern Manhattan Stroke Study, the odds ratio for stroke risk was 1.8 for blacks and 2.1 for Caribbean Hispanics compared to whites.[40] Diabetes also increased the risk of stroke-related dementia more in blacks and Hispanics than in whites.[41]

Diabetes worsens stroke outcome as well. Diabetes doubles the risk of recurrent stroke,[42] more than trebles the risk of stroke-related dementia,[41] and markedly increases mortality, both total and stroke related.[37,39,43] In the Renfrew-Paisley

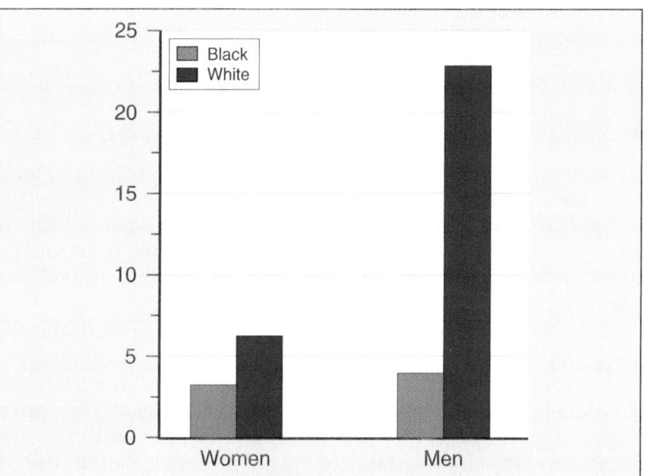

FIGURE 40–3 Odds ratio for stroke in diabetic patients aged 18 to 44 years. These data show a marked increase in the risk of stroke in diabetic persons compared to nondiabetic persons, highlighting a marked increase in risk among young adults. These data support recommendations to treat hypertension aggressively in patients with diabetes to reduce the risk of stroke and death. (From Rohr J, Kittner S, Feeser B, et al: Traditional risk factors and ischemic stroke in young adults: The Baltimore-Washington Cooperative Young Stroke Study. Arch Neurol 53:603-607, 1996.)

study, diabetes raised the relative risk of death after stroke by 290 percent in men and 400 percent in women over 20 years of follow-up.[44]

Peripheral Arterial Disease

Diabetes increases the incidence of peripheral arterial disease (PAD) twofold to fourfold.[2] Diabetic patients more often have femoral bruits and absent pedal pulses.[45] The prevalence of PAD in unselected persons with diabetes, based on decreased ankle-brachial indices (see Chap. 54) ranges from 12 to 16 percent.[46] In whites of European ancestry, the prevalence of PAD ranges from 7 percent in those with normal glucose tolerance to 20.9 percent in patients with diabetes requiring multiple medications.[47]

The duration of diabetes and the severity of hyperglycemia correlate with the prevalence and severity of PAD.[48,49] In addition to increasing the frequency of PAD, diabetes affects the distribution of atherosclerosis in the lower extremity. PAD in diabetic patients typically affects tibial and peroneal arteries, as well as femoral and popliteal arteries. Moreover, the atherosclerotic lesions in diabetic patients are more likely to manifest vascular calcification than those in nondiabetic cohorts.[49,50]

In addition to an increased frequency of lower extremity atherosclerosis, diabetes mellitus augments the likelihood of developing the symptomatic forms of PAD. In the Framingham study, diabetes mellitus increased the risk of claudication by 350 percent in men and 860 percent in women.[51] The duration of diabetes also increases the risk of developing claudication in most but not all studies.[48,52] Diabetes also increases the risk of developing critical limb ischemia and tissue loss and more than doubles the risk of critical limb ischemia in men with intermittent claudication and toe pressures of less than 40 mm Hg.[45] Diabetes is the most common cause of amputation in the United States.[53] The relative risk for amputation is increased 12.7-fold in diabetic compared with nondiabetic persons in the Medicare population in Minnesota. In the highest-risk age group, diabetic persons aged 65 to 74 years, the relative risk of amputation increases 23.5-fold. These trends extend beyond the United States. The Global Lower Extremity Amputation Study Group reports that the percentage of patients with diabetes may reach as high as 90 percent in patients undergoing their first ever amputations in populations studied in North America, Europe, and east Asia.[54]

Pathophysiology of Diabetic Vascular Disease

Diabetes involves metabolic abnormalities, including hyperglycemia, dyslipidemia, and insulin resistance, that disrupt normal arterial function and render arteries susceptible to atherosclerosis. Diabetes specifically alters the function of vascular endothelium and smooth muscle cells, as well as platelets, in ways that promote atherogenesis.

Diabetes impairs the vasodilator function of endothelial cells and decreases the bioavailability of nitric oxide (NO).[55] Moreover, each of the fundamental metabolic disturbances in diabetes, including hyperglycemia, increased free fatty acid concentrations, and insulin resistance, can individually decrease NO bioavailability and attenuate endothelial function.[56-58]

Hyperglycemia decreases NO production from endothelial NO synthase (eNOS) and increases its degradation via generation of reactive oxygen species. Hyperglycemia triggers the production of reactive oxygen species in vascular cells through enzymatic (protein kinase C [PKC] and NADPH oxidases) and nonenzymatic sources of oxidant stress (e.g., the formation of advanced glycation end products [AGEs]).[59,60] As oxidative stress increases, the eNOS cofactor tetrahydrobiopterin becomes oxidized and uncouples eNOS, which causes this enzyme to produce superoxide anion instead of NO.[61] Superoxide anion quenches NO in a diffusion-limited reaction to produce peroxynitrite.[62] Peroxynitrite inhibits prostacyclin synthase and endothelium-dependent hyperpolarizing factor activity.[63,64] Similar to the effects of hyperglycemia, free fatty acids activate intracellular enzymatic oxidant sources, including PKC, NADPH oxidases, and eNOS, yielding analogous increases in superoxide anion.[65]

The excess adipose tissue that usually accompanies type 2 diabetes mellitus releases excess fatty acids. Reduced skeletal muscle uptake of free fatty acids further augments their plasma levels.[66] Increased concentrations of free fatty acids exert deleterious actions in several areas. Free fatty acids independently activate intracellular enzymatic oxidant sources, including PKC, NADPH oxidases, and eNOS, yielding analogous increases in superoxide anion to hyperglycemia.[65] Indeed, free fatty acids likely represent an independent source of pathogenic oxygen-derived free radicals in insulin-resistant states prior to hyperglycemia—a state associated with impaired vascular function.[67] In healthy humans, free fatty acid infusion impairs endothelial function, and the coinfusion of an antioxidant restores it.[68] Moreover, free fatty acids interfere with intracellular signaling pathways to cause not only muscle and visceral insulin resistance but vascular insulin resistance as well.[69]

In diabetes, hyperglycemia and increased free fatty acids increase the concentration in the cell of the metabolite diacylglycerol.[70] Diacylglycerol, in turn, is a classic activator of a family of enzymes, known as PKC, that perform key regulatory functions by phosphorylating proteins important in metabolic control. Recent work has implicated activation of the PKC family in cardiovascular complications of diabetes.[71] Activation of PKC can inhibit the expression of eNOS, augment cytokine-induced tissue factor gene expression and procoagulant activity in human endothelial cells, and increase the production of proinflammatory cytokines, the proliferation of vascular wall cells, and the production of extracellular matrix macromolecules that accumulate during atherosclerotic lesion formation.[71,72] In vivo evidence supports a role of PKC activation in the pathogenesis of various aspects of vascular dysfunction in vivo. Administration of a selective inhibitor of PKC-β to diabetic rats improves retinal blood flow and prevents impaired endothelial function in healthy humans exposed to hyperglycemia (Fig. 40–4).[73,74]

Although typically associated with impairments in skeletal glucose muscle uptake, many tissues in the diabetic patient demonstrate insulin resistance, including adipose, liver, and endothelial cells.[75] Normal vascular function requires intact endothelial insulin signaling. For example, in genetically engineered mice that lack the endothelial cell insulin receptor, vascular eNOS concentration decreases 60 percent.[76] Endothelial insulin resistance alters the pattern of activation of intracellular signaling pathways, favoring stimulation of mitogen-activated protein (MAP) kinases over phosphatidylinositol kinase. Preferential activation of the MAP kinase pathway decreases NO production, increases endothelin production, stimulates the transcription of pro-inflammatory genes, and increases the tendency to coagulation.[77]

Recent work has identified a novel potential mechanism for mediating impaired endothelial-dependent vasodilator function. An endogenous competitive inhibitor of NO synthase, known as asymmetrical dimethylarginine (ADMA), increases directly with insulin resistance in nondiabetic subjects and glycemic control in diabetes[78,79] and improves with glycemic control.[80] The accumulation of ADMA may result from inhibition of its catabolism due to reduction in activity of the enzyme dimethylarginine dimethylaminohydrolase.[81] Recent evidence suggests that dysregulation of this enzyme may raise levels of ADMA in diabetics.[82] These new findings provide yet another potential molecular pathway of impaired vascular function in diabetes.

Diabetes also disturbs vascular function through nonenzymatic glycation of macromolecules. In states of hyperglycemia and increased oxidative stress, many proteins and even lipids undergo nonenzymatic glycation. For example, hemoglobin A1c, the glycated form of hemoglobin, provides the clinician with an integrated gauge of hyperglycemia. Glycated proteins can form structures known as AGEs that actually cause the macromolecule to take on a brown hue, similar to burnt sugar. Numerous chemical studies have characterized the structure of AGEs, which appear to contribute to the pathobiology of complications of diabetes, notably the accelerated vascular disease characteristic of this condition.[83-87] Recent studies have shown accumulation of AGE-modified proteins in diabetic subjects. The presence of glycated forms of low-density lipoprotein (LDL) can engender an immune response and contribute to macrovascular disease.[88] Phospholipids and apolipoproteins can form AGEs.[83] AGE-modified LDL apoprotein and LDL lipid increase in diabetic subjects compared to nondiabetics.[85]

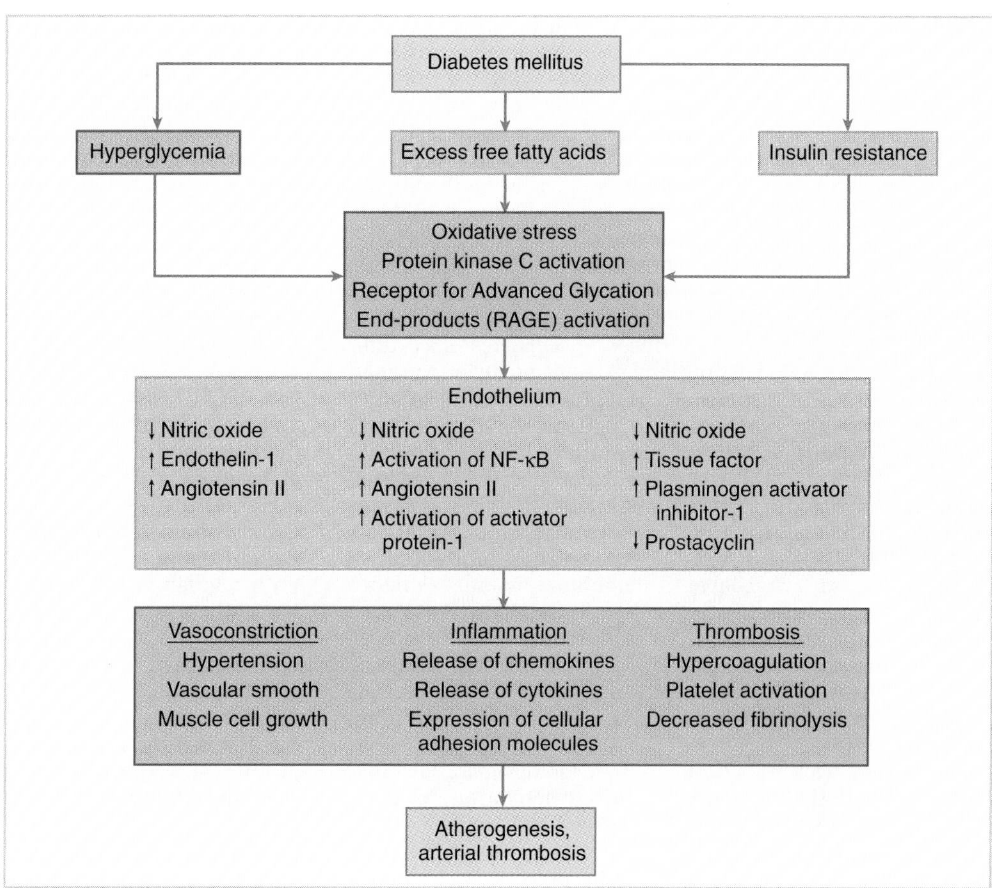

FIGURE 40–4 Endothelial dysfunction in diabetes. Normally, the endothelium maintains vascular homeostasis by promoting vasodilation, minimizing inflammation, and preventing thrombosis. In diabetes, hyperglycemia, excess free fatty acid release, dyslipidemia, and insulin resistance increase reactive oxygen species production, formation of advanced glycation end-products (AGE), and activation of protein kinase C, diminishing the bioavailability of nitric oxide and decreasing its potent vasodilatory, antiinflammatory, and antithrombotic effects. Diabetes impairs endothelial function and promotes vasoconstriction, inflammation, and thrombosis. Decreasing nitric oxide and increasing endothelin 1 and angiotensin II concentrations increases vascular tone and vascular smooth muscle cell growth and migration. Activation of inflammatory transcription factors nuclear factor-kappa B (NF-κB) and activator protein 1 induces liberation of leukocyte-attracting chemokines, production of inflammatory cytokines, and expression of cell adhesion molecules. Attenuated nitric oxide and prostacyclin activate platelets, whereas increases in plasmin activator inhibitor-1 and tissue factor create a prothrombotic milieu.

Cells have several surface receptors for AGEs that mediate their biological effects. Exposure to AGE-modified proteins can elicit the production of inflammatory cytokines from vascular cells, cause impaired endothelial-dependent vasodilator function, and augment endothelial expression of various leukocyte adhesion molecules implicated in atherogenesis in vivo.[85] One extensively characterized receptor for AGE is known as RAGE. Recent experiments support a functional role for RAGE in development of experimental atherosclerosis. Mice lacking the apolipoprotein E gene are susceptible to atherosclerosis. Administration of an antibody fragment that neutralizes RAGE attenuates atherosclerosis in these mutant mice. This beneficial effect on atherosclerotic lesion development does not depend on a change in blood sugar or lipoprotein profile,[90] supporting a role for AGE in atherogenesis.

Through decreases in NO, increases in oxidative stress, AGE production and activation of its receptor, and insulin resistance, diabetes increases vascular inflammation via the activation and nuclear translocation of intracellular transcription factors, nuclear factor (NF)-κB and activator protein 1 (AP-1).[91-93] These factors cause the expression of genes responsible for producing chemokines, cytokines, leukocyte adhesion molecules, and proinflammatory mediators, such as tumor necrosis factor-alpha.[94,95] Diabetes further aggravates plaque progression by causing endothelial cells to produce cytokines that decrease collagen production by vascular smooth muscle cells and to enhance endothelial cell production of matrix metalloproteinases and tissue factor.[96] These changes may decrease the stability of the atherosclerotic plaque's fibrous cap, increasing the likelihood and severity of plaque rupture and thrombosis (see also Chap. 35).

Numerous basic science and clinical studies indicate an increased level of oxidative stress in diabetes.[84] The reactive oxygen species in turn can augment the formation of reactive carbonyl species. Nonoxidative reactions can also increase the concentrations of reactive carbonyl compounds under hyperglycemic conditions. The reactive carbonyl species can derivatize proteins and lipids. Among the products of reactions of proteins with reactive oxygen and carbonyl species are the AGEs, discussed earlier. There is little doubt that products of glycoxidation accumulate in diabetic patients. However, they accumulate in nondiabetic elderly individuals as well.[84] Recent evidence suggests that overwhelming detoxifying mechanisms of the reactive carbonyl groups may account for the increase in oxidant and carbonyl stress in diabetics.

Diabetes impairs vascular smooth muscle function and augments the production of vasoconstrictor mediators including endothelin 1,[97] which causes vascular smooth muscle growth and inflammation.[98] Levels of other atherogenic mediators, including angiotensin II and vasoconstrictor prostanoids, increase in diabetes as well.[2] Patients with type 2 diabetes have impaired vasodilation, possibly reflecting an abnormality in NO signal transduction.[55] Moreover, diabetic patients have attenuated vasoconstriction to endothelin 1 and angiotensin.[99,100] The relative contribution of the sympathetic nervous system to vascular smooth muscle function remains unclear. Experimentally, norepinephrine re-uptake by sympathetic nerve neurons is reduced.[101] Diabetes may alter subcellular calcium distribution,[102] resulting in augmented vasoconstriction in response to norepinephrine and phenylephrine. However, most diabetic patients have peripheral autonomic impairment at the time of diagnosis, and vascular beds regulated by these nerves have decreased arterial resistance.[103,104] Akin to endothelial cells, diabetes activates atherogenic mechanisms within vascular smooth muscle cells, including PKC, RAGE, NF-κB, and the production of oxidative stress.[65,105] Diabetes heightens vascular smooth muscle cell migration in atherosclerotic lesions.[106] Advanced atherosclerotic lesions have fewer vascular smooth muscle cells in diabetic patients than in nondiabetic patients, possibly resulting in decreased resiliency of the fibrous cap and thereby increasing the risk of rupture and luminal thrombosis.[107]

Platelet abnormalities occur in diabetes that parallel those found in endothelial cells, including activation of PKC, decreased production of platelet-derived NO, and increased oxidative stress.[108-110] Diabetes impairs platelet calcium homeostasis,[111] which may contribute importantly to abnormal platelet activity since calcium regulates platelet shape change, secretion, aggregation, and thromboxane formation. Moreover, platelets from patients with diabetes have increased expression of the adhesive glycoproteins Ib and IIb/IIIa.[2] Type 2 diabetes and its associated metabolic abnormalities favor an imbalance in the coagulation/fibrinolytic systems that support clot formation and stability. Type 2 diabetes increases plasminogen activator inhibitor type 1 levels, impairing fibrinolytic capacity in atherosclerotic lesions.[112] Moreover, diabetes increases the expression of tissue factor and the levels of plasma coagulation factors, and it decreases levels of endogenous anticoagulants.[113,114] These various abnormalities may contribute to heightened susceptibility to the thrombotic complications of atherosclerosis.

Medical Therapy for Diabetic Vascular Disease

Over the last decade, treatment of diabetes has evolved from a focus on hyperglycemia to a broader view encompassing all of the metabolic disturbances associated with diabetes: insulin resistance, dyslipidemia, hypertension, and thrombosis (see Fig. 40–3). Each of these abnormalities plays an important role in cardiovascular disease development and progression.

Treatment of Hyperglycemia and Insulin Resistance

Hyperglycemia, a fundamental component of diabetes, adversely affects vascular function and directly correlates with cardiovascular events. In the United Kingdom Prospective Diabetes Study (UKPDS), hemoglobin A1c levels above 6.2 percent were associated with an increased risk of macrovascular disease.[115] For each 1 percent elevation in hemoglobin A1c, coronary heart disease (CHD) risk increased by 11 percent. A meta-analysis of nearly 100,000 diabetic patients found that increases in plasma glucose concentrations correlated with augmented cardiovascular risk, beginning with glucose concentrations below the diabetic threshold.[116] Data concerning the role of glucose intolerance are inconsistent. Large trials such as the Honolulu Heart Program demonstrated an increasing risk of CHD with greater glycemia, whereas the Paris Prospective Study did not.[117,118] However, in UKPDS, it appeared that the relative risk of CHD did not increase in association with hemoglobin A1c levels above 7 percent, suggesting a threshold.

Several clinical trials have sought to determine whether intensive treatment of blood glucose levels can reduce the risk of CHD associated with diabetes. In the Diabetes Control and Complications Trial (DCCT), 1441 patients with type 1 diabetes (mean age 27 years) without significant retinopathy at baseline were randomized to intensive glycemic control (external insulin pump or ≥3 insulin injections per day) or conventional therapy (1 or 2 insulin injections per day).[119] Patients were followed prospectively for a mean of 6.5 years, with regular assessments of microvascular and macrovascular outcomes. After 5 years, the cumulative incidence of retinopathy was approximately 50 percent less in the intensive-treatment group than in the conventional-treatment group ($p < 0.001$). Intensive therapy also reduced the risk of macrovascular disease (cardiovascular and peripheral vascular disease) by 41 percent, although the difference between groups lacked statistical significance. A second, smaller Veterans Affairs (VA) study that tested the feasibility of intensive blood glucose control in type 2 diabetics also showed no significant differences in cardiovascular endpoints between treatment arms.[120] These two trials had a number of important limitations. Both lacked adequate power to detect a difference in macrovascular events between treatment groups, given the small number of events in each group. In the DCCT, the low event rate probably resulted from the relative youth of the study population and, in the VA study, likely resulted from a small patient population and a short follow-up period.

Larger, adequately powered studies, such as UKPDS, showed a nonsignificant trend in favor of intensive blood glucose control in terms of reduction of myocardial infarction.[121] This trial randomized 3867 patients with newly diagnosed type 2 diabetes to intensive therapy (diet plus oral therapy or insulin) or to conventional therapy. Patients entered into the study had a low background prevalence of CHD and a low rate of CHD risk factors, and were followed for approximately 10 years. As in the DCCT, microvascular endpoints were improved in the intensive-therapy arm. There was also a trend for a reduced rate of myocardial infarction in the group receiving intensive blood glucose control ($p = 0.052$).[121]

More recent data support the notion that tight glycemic control may decrease the rate of cardiovascular morbidity and mortality. In the Epidemiology of Diabetes Interventions and Complications study, the long-term follow-up study of patients in the DCCT trial, type 1 subjects underwent carotid ultrasound 1 to 2 years after the end of DCCT and again 4 years later.[122] The subjects in the intensive glycemic control arm had significantly less progression of their carotid intima-media thickness (IMT) than the patients in the usual control arm. Recently, in the STOP-Noninsulin-Dependent Diabetes Mellitus (NIDDM) trial, patients with impaired glucose tolerance were randomized to acarbose, an alpha-glucosidase inhibitor, or matching placebo and followed for an average of 3.3 years.[123] Patients taking acarbose had significantly fewer cardiovascular events (including myocardial infarction, new angina, revascularization, cardiovascular death, congestive heart failure, cerebrovascular events, and PAD) than subjects taking placebo. Ongoing clinical trials with more aggressive glycemic control may enable a better evaluation of the hypothesis that glycemic control serves an important role in the prevention of cardiovascular disease.

Insulin resistance may provide the crucial link between hyperglycemia and cardiovascular disease (Table 40–2). This collective occurrence of multiple metabolic abnormalities in an individual patient has been termed variously, *syndrome X*, the *insulin resistance syndrome*, and *cardiovascular dysmetabolic syndrome*, or simply *metabolic syndrome*. Data from a number of studies indicate that insulin resistance independently predicts cardiovascular disease risk. In a large triethnic population comprising equal numbers of subjects with diabetes, hyperglycemia, and normal glucose tolerance, insulin resistance correlated positively with atherosclerosis as assessed by carotid intima-media thickness.[124] Since insulin resistance typically precedes the development of hyperglycemia, these findings may explain, in part, the elevated risk of CHD in individuals with newly diagnosed type 2 diabetes. Indeed, the severity of insulin resistance directly correlates with rates of myocardial infarction,[125] stroke,[29,32] and PAD.[126] In UKPDS, improving insulin resistance with metformin decreased macrovascular events. This result has engendered some controversy because the addition of metformin to sulfonylurea therapy seemed to increase cardiovascular risk.[53,127] The recent availability of the thiazolidinediones (TZDs) provides a second approach to improve insulin sensitivity and glycemic control.[128] TZDs bind and activate peroxisome proliferator-activated receptor-γ (PPAR-γ), a nuclear receptor that regulates functions of adipose, inflammatory, and vascular cells.[129] In addition to improving insulin sensitivity, PPAR-γ agonists may have antiinflammatory activity and directly retard atherogenesis.[130] TZDs also may decrease the concentration of small, dense LDL[131] and augment LDL resistance to oxidation.[132] However, total, LDL, and HDL cholesterol concentrations increase,[133,134] making the net effect on the lipid profile unclear. TZDs have complex effects as activation of PPAR-γ may theoretically promote foam cell formation.[135,136] Ongoing clinical trials will determine whether improvements in insulin resistance with TZDs or other drugs will decrease cardiovascular morbidity and mortality in patients with diabetes.

Treatment of Dyslipidemia in Diabetes

(see also Chap. 39)

Even though patients with diabetes typically have LDL cholesterol levels in the average range, these patients often have elevated triglycerides, decreased high-density lipoprotein (HDL) cholesterol, and more small, dense LDL. Increased delivery of free fatty acids to the liver due to excess adipose efflux and impaired skeletal muscle uptake increases hepatic production of very low density lipoprotein (VLDL) and cholesteryl ester synthesis (Fig. 40–5).[137] Overproduction of triglyceride-rich lipoproteins and impaired clearance by lipoprotein lipase lead to hypertriglyceridemia in diabetes.[138,139]

TABLE 40–2 Components of the Metabolic Syndrome

Variable	Parameter
Hyperglycemia	>110 mg/dl
Dyslipidemia	HDL cholesterol Men < 40 mg/dl Women < 50 mg/dl Triglycerides > 150 mg/dl
Obesity	Waist circumference Men > 40 in Women > 35 in
Hypertension	Blood pressure >130/85 mm Hg
Age	Men > 45 yr Women > 55 yr

HDL = high-density lipoprotein.

Adapted from Executive Summary of the Third Report of the National Cholesterol Education Program (NCEP) Expert Panel on Detection, Evaluation, and Treatment of High Blood Cholesterol in Adults (Adult Treatment Panel III). JAMA 285:2486, 2001.

Triglyceride levels tend to vary inversely with HDL levels as cholesteryl ester transfer protein mediates exchanges of cholesterol from HDL to VLDL.[137] The combination of elevated triglycerides and low HDL is more common than elevated total and LDL cholesterol in diabetic patients with CAD.[140] In addition to abnormalities of concentration, functional defects in the HDL of diabetic subjects and a diminished capacity to prevent LDL oxidation also may promote atherogenesis.[141] Increased concentrations of small, dense LDL in diabetic person results from abnormal cholesterol and triglyceride transfer between VLDL and LDL and depends on increased levels of VLDL, particularly when triglyceride concentrations are higher than 130 mg/dl.[137] Small, dense LDL particles are proatherogenic. They bind readily to intimal proteoglycans, which enhances their retention in the intima, promoting their oxidative modification and hence take-up by macrophages and smooth muscle cells.[142]

Life-style modification should be the first prescription to improve the lipid profile. Indeed, each component of diabetic dysmetabolism improves with weight loss, exercise, and dietary modification. Strict glycemic control may lessen hepatic VLDL production.[138] Large clinical trials have demonstrated the benefits of pharmacological interventions. Lipid-lowering therapy, particularly with 3-hydroxy-3-methylglutaryl coenzyme A reductase inhibitors, or statins, results in a proportionally greater cardiovascular risk reduction in diabetic than in nondiabetic subjects (Table 40–3).[143,144] In the Scandinavian Simvastatin Survival Study

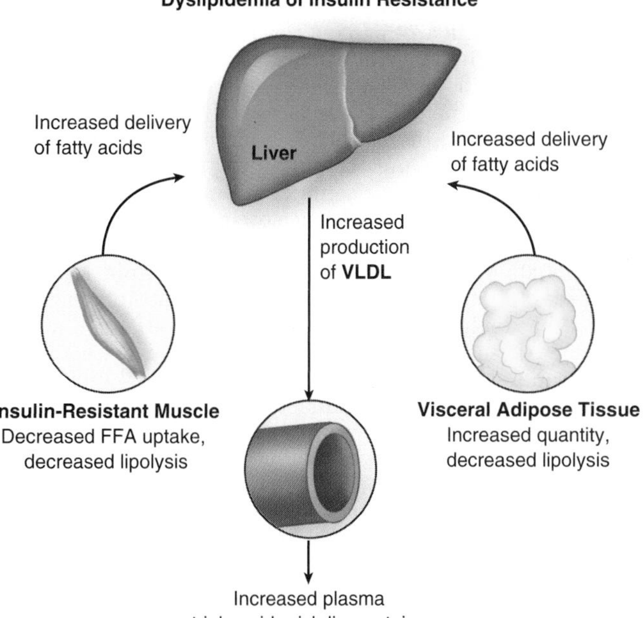

FIGURE 40–5 Pathogenesis of diabetic dyslipidemia. Increased production of very low density lipoprotein (VLDL) from the liver results from increased delivery of fatty acids because of decreased utilization by muscle and increased delivery of fatty acids from visceral abdominal fat to the liver via the portal circulation. Decreased catabolism of postprandial triglyceride-rich lipoprotein particles due to reduced lipoprotein lipase activity (lipolysis) accentuates diabetic dyslipidemia. FFA = free fatty acid.

TABLE 40–3 Statin Therapy in Diabetes

Trial*	No. of Patients	Indication	Drug	Duration (yr)	CV Outcome	Risk Reduction (%)
AFCAPS/ TexCAPS	155	PP, average TC Low HDL	Lovastatin	5.2	FMI, NFMI, SD	43
4S	202	Stable CAD Elevated TC	Simvastatin	5.3	Fatal CHD + NFMI	51
CARE	602	Stable CAD Average TC	Pravastatin	5	Fatal CHD + NFMI + CR	22
LIPID	782	Stable CAD Average TC	Pravastatin	6.1	Fatal CHD + NFMI	17
HPS	5983	Diabetes	Simvastatin	4.8	MI + CVA + CR + NCR	33

*The trials are identified as follows: AFCAPS = Air Force Coronary Artery Prevention Study; 4S = Scandinavian Simvastatin Survival Study; CARE = Cholesterol and Recurrent Events; CAD = coronary artery disease; CHD = coronary heart disease; CR = coronary revascularization; CV = cardiovascular; CVA = cerebrovascular accident; FMI = fatal myocardial infarction; HDL = high-density lipoprotein; HPS = heart protection study; LIPID = Long-term Intervention with Pravastatin in Ischemic Disease; MI = myocardial infarction; NCR = noncoronary revascularization; NFMI = nonfatal myocardial infarction; PP = Primary prevention; SD = sudden death; TC = total cholesterol.

(4S) trial, simvastatin reduced total mortality by 43 percent in diabetics compared with 29 percent in nondiabetics.[144] Similarly, myocardial infarction was reduced by 55 percent versus 32 percent in diabetic and nondiabetic cohorts, respectively.[144] In the Cholesterol and Recurrent Events (CARE) trial, which included subjects with average LDL levels and CAD, pravastatin reduced the absolute risk of coronary events for diabetic and nondiabetic patients by 8.1 percent and 5.2 percent, respectively.[143] In the Heart Protection Study (HPS), which included 5963 subjects with diabetes, simvastatin decreased the risk of coronary death, nonfatal myocardial infarction, stroke, or revascularization by 25 percent in the diabetic subgroup.[145] The reduction risk even extended to patients with pretreatment LDL cholesterol levels below 100 mg/dL.

Fibric acid derivatives address particularly the increased triglyceride and decreased HDL concentrations characteristic of diabetic dyslipidemia. In the VA High-Density Lipoprotein Cholesterol Intervention Trial (VA-HIT), treatment with gemfibrozil resulted in a 24 percent risk reduction for myocardial infarction in the diabetic subjects, who represented one fourth of enrolled subjects, an outcome similar to that observed in nondiabetic subjects.[146]

In the Diabetes Atherosclerosis Intervention Study (DAIS), fenofibrate limited angiographic progression of coronary artery lesions in a diabetic cohort, but the event reduction did not achieve statistical significance owing to the small sample size in this angiographic trial.[147] Akin to TZDs, fibrates may have antiatherogenic effects independent of lipid lowering. Fibrates bind to PPAR-α, which exerts anti-inflammatory effects that include the reduction of endothelial cell activation by pro-inflammatory cytokines and decreased tissue factor production by human macrophages.[148-150] Fibric acid derivatives may prove of value, typically as a second lipid agent in diabetic patients with persistently elevated triglycerides and low HDL. Combinations of statins and fibrates warrant careful monitoring for muscle injury. Despite concern over worsening glycemic control, nicotinic acid may be useful in diabetic persons to increase HDL.

Treatment of Hypertension in Diabetic Patients

Hypertension and insulin resistance frequently occur together as part of the metabolic syndrome.[151,152] The addition of hypertension to the clinical picture of diabetes amplifies the already high cardiovascular disease risk in these patients. Aggressive blood pressure control prevents further cardiovascular events more in diabetics than nondiabetics.[153] Indeed, the Appropriate Blood Pressure Control in Diabetes (ABCD) trial investigated the effect of aggressive blood pressure control in type 2 diabetic patients with PAD. The intensively treated group (128/75 mm Hg) had no increased risk of cardiovascular events over 4 years of follow-up.[154,155]

The role of specific classes of antihypertensive drugs in reducing cardiovascular morbidity and mortality in patients with diabetes has engendered controversy. Two trials compared the effects of calcium-channel blockers and angiotensin-converting enzyme (ACE) inhibitors in patients with type 2 diabetes.[156,157] In these trials, the ACE inhibitor reduced cardiovascular endpoints more effectively than the dihydropyridine calcium-channel blockers. The results of these two studies suggest that calcium-channel blockers do not benefit and might even harm diabetic patients at high risk for cardiovascular events. Neither the UKPDS nor the Systolic Hypertension in Europe Trial (Sys-Eur) has supported the findings of the two smaller trials noted earlier and, indeed, have shown beneficial effects for both ACE inhibitors and calcium-channel blockers in patients with diabetes (Table 40–4). Also, in UKPDS,[158] 1148 hypertensive patients with type 2 diabetes responded equally well to captopril or atenolol in terms of achieving blood pressure control and had similar reductions in the risk of macrovascular disease. Aggressive blood pressure reduction with either agent significantly reduced stroke and deaths due to diabetes. Myocardial infarction declined 21 percent in the group randomized to tight blood pressure control (p = NS). Although blood pressure in the UKPDS subgroup assigned to tight blood pressure control was good (averaging 144/82 mm Hg), data from the Syst-Eur trial[153,159] and the HOT trial[160] indicate that achieving even lower blood pressure with calcium-channel blockers further lowers the rate of cardiovascular complications compared with moderate blood pressure control. Achieving ADA target blood pressure (130/80 mm Hg) almost always requires more than one agent.[53,160,161]

Modulation of the renin-angiotensin system has particular importance in diabetic patients. ACE inhibitors reduce nephropathy and end-stage renal disease in patients with type 1 diabetes, and angiotensin receptor blockers reduce risk of these microvascualar disorders in patients with type 2 diabetes.[162-164] In the recent Heart Outcomes and Prevention Evaluation (HOPE) study, ramipril significantly decreased the rates of myocardial infarction, stroke, and death in patients with diabetes and a mean blood pressure of 140/80 mm Hg.[165] In the Losartan Intervention For Endpoint (LIFE) study,[166] 1195 diabetic subjects were enrolled as part of the cohort. All

TABLE 40–4 Treatment of Hypertension in Diabetes

Trial*	No. of Patients	Population	Drug	Duration (yr)	BP Control: Tight (mm Hg)	BP Control: Less Tight	CV Outcome	Risk Reduction (%)
Placebo Controlled Trials								
SHEP	583	Elderly T2	Chlorthalidone	5	143/68	155/72	CHD	56
							CV mortality	34
HOT	1501	T2, 50-80 yr	Felodipine	3	140/81	144/85	CV events	51
							MI	50
Syst-Eur	492	T2	Nitrendipine	2	153/76	182/81	CVA	69
							CV mortality	70
UKPDS	1148	T2	Captopril or atenolol	8.4	144/82	154/87	CVA	44
							Death	37
HOPE	3547	T2 + 1 RF	Ramipril	4.5	140/77	143/77	MI	22
							CVA	33
							Mortality	24
Drug Comparison Trials			**Initial Therapy**		**Drug 1**	**Drug 2**		
CAPP	572	DM	Captopril vs. diuretic or beta blocker	7	155/89	153/88	FMI/NFMI + CVA/CVD	41
LIFE	1195	DM + LVH	Losartan vs. atenolol	4.8	146/79	148/79	CV events	22
							Mortality	39

DM = diabetes mellitus; LVH = left ventricular hypertrophy; RF = Risk factor; T2 = Type 2 diabetic patients; for other abbreviations see Table 40–3.
*The trials are identified as follows: SHEP = Systolic Hypertension in the Elderly; HOT = Hypertension Optimal Treatment; Syst-Eur = Systolic Hypertension in Europe; UKPDS = United Kingdom Prospective Diabetes Study; HOPE = Heart Outcomes and Prevention Evaluation; CAPP = Captopril Prevention Project; LIFE = Losartan Intervention for Endpoint.

subjects were hypertensive and had evidence of left ventricular hypertrophy. Subjects were randomized to losartan or atenolol. Despite equivalent blood pressure lowering, the subjects randomized to losartan experienced a 39 percent reduction in all-cause mortality, a 37 percent reduction in cardiovascular mortality, and a 21 percent reduction in stroke.[166]

Comprehensive Risk Factor Modification

Aggressive modification of every risk factor may produce results with greater than additive benefit than expected from treatment of each individual risk factor. The Steno-2 trial randomized 160 subjects to intensive multifactorial risk factor modification including dietary modification (fat intake <30 percent of total consumption), light to moderate exercise three to five times per week, smoking cessation courses, ACE inhibitors, multivitamins, aspirin, intensive glucose control, and lipid modification or to conventional therapy.[167] This combination of interventions significantly and markedly reduced the rate of cardiovascular events from 85 events among 35 patients in the conventional arm to 33 events among 19 patients in the intensive risk factor modification group. Aggressive therapies to modify the risks of cardiovascular disease will diminish the clinical manifestations of vascular disease and should be implemented (Fig. 40–6).

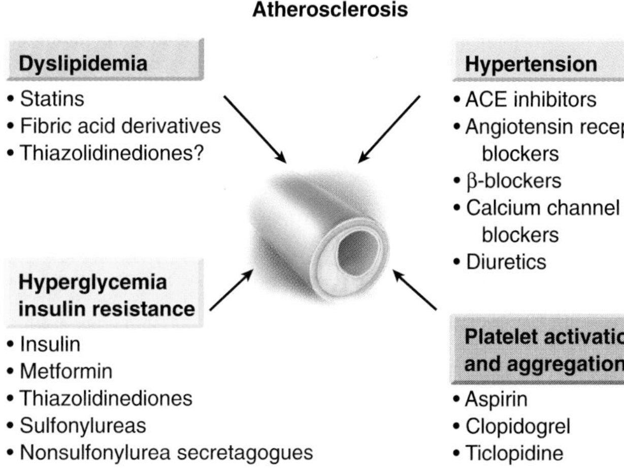

FIGURE 40–6 Antiatherosclerosis therapy in diabetes. To stem the onset and progression of atherosclerosis, patients with diabetes require therapy for each metabolic abnormality. Statins and fibric acid derivatives improve the lipid profile and decrease the risk of myocardial infarction and death. The clinical benefit of thiazolidinediones for cardiovascular outcomes therapy is under investigation. Treatment of hypertension decreases the rate of myocardial infarction and stroke in diabetes. Therapy should include angiotensin-converting enzyme (ACE) inhibitors for their proven microvascular and atherosclerotic benefits. The heightened thrombotic potential of the diabetic state supports the use of platelet antagonists such as aspirin and clopidogrel. Although strict treatment of hyperglycemia does not significantly reduce the incidence of myocardial infarction or death, the improvement in microvascular outcomes itself warrants vigorous pursuit of rigorous glycemic control in diabetes.

Conclusion

Atherosclerosis and its complications cause most deaths and much of the disability in patients with diabetes mellitus. Intensive treatment of the entire scope of metabolic abnormalities beyond hyperglycemia alone significantly reduces the rates of adverse cardiovascular events. As the prevalence of patients with diabetes increases, strategies to ensure the appropriate and aggressive use of medical therapy will help stem the tide of death and disability in this high-risk population.

REFERENCES

1. Resnick HE, Shorr RI, Kuller L, et al: Prevalence and clinical implications of American Diabetes Association–defined diabetes and other categories of glucose

dysregulation in older adults: The health, aging and body composition study. J Clin Epidemiol 54:869-876, 2001.

2. Beckman JA, Creager MA, Libby P: Diabetes and atherosclerosis: epidemiology, pathophysiology, and management. JAMA 287:2570-2581, 2002.
3. Grundy SM, Benjamin IJ, Burke GL, et al: Diabetes and cardiovascular disease: A statement for healthcare professionals from the American Heart Association. Circulation 100:1134-1146, 1999.
4. Mokdad AH, Ford ES, Bowman BA, et al: Prevalence of obesity, diabetes, and obesity-related health risk factors, 2001. JAMA 289:76-79, 2003.
5. Mokdad AH, Bowman BA, Engelgau MM, Vinicor F: Diabetes trends among American Indians and Alaska natives—1990–1998. Diabetes Care 24:1508-1509, 2001.
6. Wilson PW, Kannel WB, Silbershatz H, D'Agostino RB: Clustering of metabolic factors and coronary heart disease. Arch Intern Med 159:1104-1109, 1999.
7. Brancati FL, Kao WH, Folsom AR, et al: Incident type 2 diabetes mellitus in African American and white adults: The Atherosclerosis Risk in Communities Study. JAMA 283:2253-2259, 2000.
8. Carter JS, Pugh JA, Monterrosa A: Non-insulin-dependent diabetes mellitus in minorities in the United States. Ann Intern Med 125:221-232, 1996.
9. Lindeman RD, Romero LJ, Hundley R, et al: Prevalences of type 2 diabetes, the insulin resistance syndrome, and coronary heart disease in an elderly, biethnic population. Diabetes Care 21:959-966, 1998.
10. Narayan KMV, Boyle JP, Thompson TJ, et al: Lifetime risk for diabetes mellitus in the United States. JAMA 290:1884-1890, 2003.
11. Fujimoto WY: The importance of insulin resistance in the pathogenesis of type 2 diabetes mellitus. Am J Med 108(Suppl 6a):9S-14S, 2000.
12. Gu K, Cowie CC, Harris MI: Diabetes and decline in heart disease mortality in U.S. adults. JAMA 281:1291-1297, 1999.
13. Selby JV, Ray GT, Zhang D, Colby CJ: Excess costs of medical care for patients with diabetes in a managed care population. Diabetes Care 20:1396-1402, 1997.
14. Libby P, Plutzky J: Diabetic macrovascular disease: The glucose paradox? Circulation 106:2760-2763, 2002.
15. Report of the Expert Committee on the Diagnosis and Classification of Diabetes Mellitus. Diabetes Care 20:1183-1197, 1997.
16. Kris-Etherton PM: AHA Science Advisory. Monounsaturated fatty acids and risk of cardiovascular disease. American Heart Association. Nutrition Committee. Circulation 100:1253-1258, 1999.
17. Stamler J, Vaccaro O, Neaton JD, Wentworth D: Diabetes, other risk factors, and 12-year cardiovascular mortality for men screened in the Multiple Risk Factor Intervention Trial. Diabetes Care 16:434-444, 1993.
18. Lowe LP, Liu K, Greenland P, et al: Diabetes, asymptomatic hyperglycemia, and 22-year mortality in black and white men. The Chicago Heart Association Detection Project in Industry Study. Diabetes Care 20:163-169, 1997.
19. Hu FB, Stampfer MJ, Solomon CG, et al: The impact of diabetes mellitus on mortality from all causes and coronary heart disease in women: 20 years of follow-up. Arch Intern Med 161:1717-1723, 2001.
20. Gillum RF, Mussolino ME, Madans JH: Diabetes mellitus, coronary heart disease incidence, and death from all causes in African American and European American women: The NHANES I epidemiologic follow-up study. J Clin Epidemiol 53:511-518, 2000.
21. Miettinen H, Lehto S, Salomaa V, et al: Impact of diabetes on mortality after the first myocardial infarction. The FINMONICA Myocardial Infarction Register Study Group. Diabetes Care 21:69-75, 1998.
22. Haffner SM, Lehto S, Ronnemaa T, et al: Mortality from coronary heart disease in subjects with type 2 diabetes and in nondiabetic subjects with and without prior myocardial infarction. N Engl J Med 339:229-234, 1998.
23. Malmberg K, Yusuf S, Gerstein HC, et al: Impact of diabetes on long-term prognosis in patients with unstable angina and non-Q-wave myocardial infarction: Results of the OASIS (Organization to Assess Strategies for Ischemic Syndromes) Registry. Circulation 102:1014-1019, 2000.
24. Zuanetti G, Latini R, Maggioni AP, et al: Influence of diabetes on mortality in acute myocardial infarction: Data from the GISSI-2 study. J Am Coll Cardiol 22:1788-1794, 1993.
25. Hochman JS, Sleeper LA, Webb JG, et al: Early revascularization in acute myocardial infarction complicated by cardiogenic shock. SHOCK Investigators: Should We Emergently Revascularize Occluded Coronaries for Cardiogenic Shock. N Engl J Med 341:625-634, 1999.
26. Shindler DM, Palmeri ST, Antonelli TA, et al: Diabetes mellitus in cardiogenic shock complicating acute myocardial infarction: A report from the SHOCK Trial Registry. SHould we emergently revascularize Occluded Coronaries for cardiogenic shocK? J Am Coll Cardiol 36(3 Suppl A):1097-1103, 2000.
27. Herlitz J, Karlson BW, Lindqvist J, Sjolin M: Rate and mode of death during five years of follow-up among patients with acute chest pain with and without a history of diabetes mellitus. Diabet Med 15:308-314, 1998.
28. Abbud ZA, Shindler DM, Wilson AC, Kostis JB: Effect of diabetes mellitus on short- and long-term mortality rates of patients with acute myocardial infarction: A statewide study. Myocardial Infarction Data Acquisition System Study Group. Am Heart J 130:51-58, 1995.
29. Adachi H, Hirai Y, Tsuruta M, et al: Is insulin resistance or diabetes mellitus associated with stroke? An 18-year follow-up study. Diabetes Res Clin Pract 51:215-223, 2001.
30. Jamrozik K, Broadhurst RJ, Forbes S, et al: Predictors of death and vascular events in the elderly: The Perth Community Stroke Study. Stroke 31:863-868, 2000.
31. Wannamethee SG, Perry IJ, Shaper AG: Nonfasting serum glucose and insulin concentrations and the risk of stroke. Stroke 30:1780-1786, 1999.
32. Folsom AR, Rasmussen ML, Chambless LE, et al: Prospective associations of fasting insulin, body fat distribution, and diabetes with risk of ischemic stroke. The Atherosclerosis Risk in Communities (ARIC) Study Investigators. Diabetes Care 22:1077-1083, 1999.
33. Friedlander AH, Maeder LA: The prevalence of calcified carotid artery atheromas on the panoramic radiographs of patients with type 2 diabetes mellitus. Oral Surg Oral Med Oral Pathol Oral Radiol Endod 89:420-424, 2000.
34. You RX, McNeil JJ, O'Malley HM, et al: Risk factors for stroke due to cerebral infarction in young adults. Stroke 28:1913-1918, 1997.
35. Rohr J, Kittner S, Feeser B, et al: Traditional risk factors and ischemic stroke in young adults: The Baltimore-Washington Cooperative Young Stroke Study. Arch Neurol 53:603-607, 1996.
36. Kuusisto J, Mykkanen L, Pyorala K, Laakso M: Non-insulin-dependent diabetes and its metabolic control are important predictors of stroke in elderly subjects. Stroke 25:1157-1164, 1994.
37. Stegmayr B, Asplund K: Diabetes as a risk factor for stroke: A population perspective. Diabetologia 38:1061-1068, 1995.
38. Hart CL, Hole DJ, Smith GD: Risk factors and 20-year stroke mortality in men and women in the Renfrew/Paisley study in Scotland. Stroke 30:1999-2007, 1999.
39. Tuomilehto J, Rastenyte D, Jousilahti P, et al: Diabetes mellitus as a risk factor for death from stroke: Prospective study of the middle-aged Finnish population. Stroke 27:210-215, 1996.
40. Sacco RL, Boden-Albala B, Abel G, et al: Race-ethnic disparities in the impact of stroke risk factors: The Northern Manhattan Stroke Study. Stroke 32:1725-1731, 2001.
41. Luchsinger JA, Tang MX, Stern Y, et al: Diabetes mellitus and risk of Alzheimer's disease and dementia with stroke in a multiethnic cohort. Am J Epidemiol 154:635-641, 2001.
42. Hankey GJ, Jamrozik K, Broadhurst RJ, et al: Long-term risk of first recurrent stroke in the Perth Community Stroke Study. Stroke 29:2491-2500, 1998.
43. Jorgensen H, Nakayama H, Raaschou HO, Olsen TS: Stroke in patients with diabetes. The Copenhagen Stroke Study. Stroke 25:1977-1984, 1994.
44. Hart CL, Hole DJ, Smith GD: Comparison of risk factors for stroke incidence and stroke mortality in 20 years of follow-up in men and women in the Renfrew/Paisley Study in Scotland. Stroke 31:1893-1896, 2000.
45. Abbott RD, Brand FN, Kannel WB: Epidemiology of some peripheral arterial findings in diabetic men and women: Experiences from the Framingham Study. Am J Med 88:376-381, 1990.
46. Meijer WT, Hoes AW, Rutgers D, et al: Peripheral arterial disease in the elderly: The Rotterdam Study. Arterioscler Thromb Vasc Biol 18:185-192, 1998.
47. Beks PJ, Mackaay AJ, de Neeling JN, et al: Peripheral arterial disease in relation to glycaemic level in an elderly Caucasian population: The Hoorn study. Diabetologia 38:86-96, 1995.
48. Katsilambros NL, Tsapogas PC, Arvanitis MP, et al: Risk factors for lower extremity arterial disease in non-insulin-dependent diabetic persons. Diabet Med 13:243-246, 1996.
49. Jude EB, Oyibo SO, Chalmers N, Boulton AJ: Peripheral arterial disease in diabetic and nondiabetic patients: A comparison of severity and outcome. Diabetes Care 24:1433-1437, 2001.
50. Mozes G, Keresztury G, Kadar A, et al: Atherosclerosis in amputated legs of patients with and without diabetes mellitus. Int Angiol 17:282-286, 1998.
51. Kannel WB, McGee DL: Update on some epidemiologic features of intermittent claudication: The Framingham Study. J Am Geriatr Soc 33:13-18, 1985.
52. Fowkes FG, Housley E, Riemersma RA, et al: Smoking, lipids, glucose intolerance, and blood pressure as risk factors for peripheral atherosclerosis compared with ischemic heart disease in the Edinburgh Artery Study. Am J Epidemiol 135:331-340, 1992.
53. Diabetes-related amputations of lower extremities in the Medicare population—Minnesota, 1993-1995. MMWR Morb Mortal Wkly Rep 47:649-652, 1998.
54. Group TG: Epidemiology of lower extremity amputation in centres in Europe, North America, and East Asia: The Global Lower Extremity Amputation Study Group. Br J Surg 87:328-337, 2000.
55. Beckman JA, Goldfine AB, Gordon MB, et al: Oral antioxidant therapy improves endothelial function in type 1 but not type 2 diabetes mellitus. Am J Physiol Heart Circ Physiol 285:H2392-H2398, 2003.
56. Williams SB, Goldfine AB, Timimi FK, et al: Acute hyperglycemia attenuates endothelium-dependent vasodilation in humans in vivo. Circulation 97:1695-1701, 1998.
57. Steinberg HO, Tarshoby M, Monestel R, et al: Elevated circulating free fatty acid levels impair endothelium- dependent vasodilation. J Clin Invest 100:1230-1239, 1997.
58. Steinberg HO, Chaker H, Leaming R, et al: Obesity/insulin resistance is associated with endothelial dysfunction: Implications for the syndrome of insulin resistance. J Clin Invest 97:2601-2610, 1996.
59. Nishikawa T, Edelstein D, Du XL, et al: Normalizing mitochondrial superoxide production blocks three pathways of hyperglycaemic damage. Nature 404:787-790, 2000.
60. Brownlee M: Biochemistry and molecular cell biology of diabetic complications. Nature 414:813-820, 2001.
61. Shinozaki K, Kashiwagi A, Nishio Y, et al: Abnormal biopterin metabolism is a major cause of impaired endothelium-dependent relaxation through nitric oxide/O_2^- imbalance in insulin-resistant rat aorta. Diabetes 48:2437-2445, 1999.
62. Beckman JS, Koppenol WH: Nitric oxide, superoxide, and peroxynitrite: The good, the bad, and ugly. Am J Physiol 272:C1424-C1437, 1996.
63. Zou M, Yesilkaya A, Ullrich V: Peroxynitrite inactivates prostacyclin synthase by heme-thiolate-catalyzed tyrosine nitration. Drug Metab Rev 31:343-349, 1999.
64. Liu Y, Terata K, Chai Q, et al: Peroxynitrite inhibits Ca^{2+}-activated K^+ channel activity in smooth muscle of human coronary arterioles. Circ Res 91:1070-1076, 2002.
65. Inoguchi T, Li P, Umeda F, et al: High glucose level and free fatty acid stimulate reactive oxygen species production through protein kinase C–dependent activation of NAD(P)H oxidase in cultured vascular cells. Diabetes 49:1939-1945, 2000.
66. Goldstein BJ: Insulin resistance as the core defect in type 2 diabetes mellitus. Am J Cardiol 90:3G-10G, 2002.
67. Steinberg HO, Baron AD: Vascular function, insulin resistance, and fatty acids. Diabetologia 45:623-634, 2002.
68. Pleiner J, Schaller G, Mittermayer F, et al: FFA-induced endothelial dysfunction can be corrected by vitamin C. J Clin Endocrinol Metab 87:2913-2917, 2002.

69. Griffin ME, Marcucci MJ, Cline GW, et al: Free fatty acid–induced insulin resistance is associated with activation of protein kinase C theta and alterations in the insulin signaling cascade. Diabetes 48:1270-1274, 1999.
70. Itani SI, Ruderman NB, Schmieder F, Boden G: Lipid-induced insulin resistance in human muscle is associated with changes in diacylglycerol, protein kinase C, and I kappa B-alpha. Diabetes 2002;51(7):2005-11.
71. Koya D, King GL: Protein kinase C activation and the development of diabetic complications. Diabetes 47:859-866, 1998.
72. Terry CM, Callahan KS: Protein kinase C regulates cytokine-induced tissue factor transcription and procoagulant activity in human endothelial cells. J Lab Clin Med 127:81-93, 1996.
73. Ishii H, Jirousek MR, Koya D, et al: Amelioration of vascular dysfunctions in diabetic rats by an oral PKC beta inhibitor. Science 272:728-731, 1996.
74. Beckman JA, Goldfine AB, Gordon MB, et al: Inhibition of protein kinase C beta prevents impaired endothelium-dependent vasodilation caused by hyperglycemia in humans. Circ Res 90:107-111, 2002.
75. Kaburagi Y, Yamauchi T, Yamamoto-Honda R, et al: The mechanism of insulin-induced signal transduction mediated by the insulin receptor substrate family. Endocr J 46(Suppl):S25-S34, 1999.
76. Vicent D, Ilany J, Kondo T, et al: The role of endothelial insulin signaling in the regulation of vascular tone and insulin resistance. J Clin Invest 111:1373-1380, 2003.
77. Montagnani M, Golovchenko I, Kim I, et al: Inhibition of phosphatidylinositol 3-kinase enhances mitogenic actions of insulin in endothelial cells. J Biol Chem 277:1794-1799, 2002.
78. Stuhlinger MC, Abbasi F, Chu JW, et al: Relationship between insulin resistance and an endogenous nitric oxide synthase inhibitor. JAMA 287:1420-1426, 2002.
79. Paiva H, Lehtimaki T, Laakso J, et al: Plasma concentrations of asymmetric-dimethyl-arginine in type 2 diabetes associate with glycemic control and glomerular filtration rate but not with risk factors of vasculopathy. Metabolism 52:303-307, 2003.
80. Asagami T, Abbasi F, Stuelinger M, et al: Metformin treatment lowers asymmetric dimethylarginine concentrations in patients with type 2 diabetes. Metabolism 51:843-846, 2002.
81. Ito A, Tsao PS, Adimoolam S, et al: Novel mechanism for endothelial dysfunction: Dysregulation of dimethylarginine dimethylaminohydrolase. Circulation 99:3092-3095, 1999.
82. Lin KY, Ito A, Asagami T, et al: Impaired nitric oxide synthase pathway in diabetes mellitus: Role of asymmetric dimethylarginine and dimethylarginine dimethylaminohydrolase. Circulation 106:987-992, 2002.
83. Wendt T, Bucciarelli L, Qu W, et al: Receptor for advanced glycation endproducts (RAGE) and vascular inflammation: Insights into the pathogenesis of macrovascular complications in diabetes. Curr Atheroscler Rep 4:228-237, 2002.
84. Baynes JW, Thorpe SR: Role of oxidative stress in diabetic complications: A new perspective on an old paradigm. Diabetes 48:1-9, 1999.
85. Brownlee M: Negative consequences of glycation. Metabolism 49(2 Suppl 1):9-13, 2000.
86. Stitt AW, Bucala R, Vlassara H: Atherogenesis and advanced glycation: Promotion, progression, and prevention. Ann N Y Acad Sci 811:115-127, 1997; discussion, 127-129.
87. Wautier JL, Guillausseau PJ: Diabetes, advanced glycation end products, and vascular disease. Vasc Med 3:131-137, 1998.
88. Witztum JL: Role of modified lipoproteins in diabetic macroangiopathy. Diabetes 46(Suppl 2):S112-S114, 1997.
89. Schmidt AM, Yan SD, Wautier JL, Stern D: Activation of receptor for advanced glycation end products: A mechanism for chronic vascular dysfunction in diabetic vasculopathy and atherosclerosis. Circ Res 84:489-497, 1999.
90. Park L, Raman KG, Lee KJ, et al: Suppression of accelerated diabetic atherosclerosis by the soluble receptor for advanced glycation end products. Nat Med 4:1025-1031, 1998.
91. Morigi M, Angioletti S, Imberti B, et al: Leukocyte-endothelial interaction is augmented by high glucose concentrations and hyperglycemia in a NF-κB–dependent fashion. J Clin Invest 101:1905-1915, 1998.
92. El Bekay R, Alvarez M, Monteseirin J, et al: Oxidative stress is a critical mediator of the angiotensin II signal in human neutrophils: Involvement of mitogen-activated protein kinase, calcineurin, and the transcription factor NF-kappaB. Blood 102:662-671, 2003.
93. Pieper GM, Riaz ul-Haq: Activation of nuclear factor-kappaB in cultured endothelial cells by increased glucose concentration: Prevention by calphostin C. J Cardiovasc Pharmacol 30:528-532, 1997.
94. Rosen P, Nawroth PP, King G, et al: The role of oxidative stress in the onset and progression of diabetes and its complications: A summary of a Congress Series sponsored by UNESCO-MCBN, the American Diabetes Association, and the German Diabetes Society. Diabetes Metab Res Rev 17:189-212, 2001.
95. Schmidt AM, Stern D: Atherosclerosis and diabetes: The RAGE connection. Curr Atheroscler Rep 2:430-436, 2000.
96. Uemura S, Matsushita H, Li W, et al: Diabetes mellitus enhances vascular matrix metalloproteinase activity: Role of oxidative stress. Circ Res 88:1291-1298, 2001.
97. Park JY, Takahara N, Gabriele A, et al: Induction of endothelin-1 expression by glucose: An effect of protein kinase C activation. Diabetes 49:1239-1248, 2000.
98. Browatzki M, Schmidt J, Kubler W, Kranzhofer R: Endothelin-1 induces interleukin-6 release via activation of the transcription factor NF-kappaB in human vascular smooth muscle cells. Basic Res Cardiol 95:98-105, 2000.
99. Ang C, Hillier C, Cameron AD, et al: The effect of type 1 diabetes mellitus on vascular responses to endothelin-1 in pregnant women. J Clin Endocrinol Metab 86:4939-4942, 2001.
100. McAuley DF, McGurk C, Nugent AG, et al: Vasoconstriction to endothelin-1 is blunted in non-insulin-dependent diabetes: A dose-response study. J Cardiovasc Pharmacol 36:203-208, 2000.
101. Tesfamariam B, Cohen RA: Enhanced adrenergic neurotransmission in diabetic rabbit carotid artery. Cardiovasc Res 29:549-554, 1995.
102. Fleischhacker E, Esenabhalu VE, Spitaler M, et al: Human diabetes is associated with hyperreactivity of vascular smooth muscle cells due to altered subcellular Ca^{2+} distribution. Diabetes 48:1323-1330, 1999.
103. Stansberry KB, Hill MA, Shapiro SA, et al: Impairment of peripheral blood flow responses in diabetes resembles an enhanced aging effect. Diabetes Care 20:1711-1716, 1997.
104. Takahashi T, Nishizawa Y, Emoto M, et al: Sympathetic function test of vasoconstrictor changes in foot arteries in diabetic patients. Diabetes Care 21:1495-1501, 1998.
105. Hattori Y, Hattori S, Sato N, Kasai K: High-glucose-induced nuclear factor kappaB activation in vascular smooth muscle cells. Cardiovasc Res 46:188-197, 2000.
106. Suzuki LA, Poot M, Gerrity RG, Bornfeldt KE: Diabetes accelerates smooth muscle accumulation in lesions of atherosclerosis: Lack of direct growth-promoting effects of high glucose levels. Diabetes 50:851-860, 2001.
107. Fukumoto H, Naito Z, Asano G, Aramaki T: Immunohistochemical and morphometric evaluations of coronary atherosclerotic plaques associated with myocardial infarction and diabetes mellitus. J Atheroscler Thromb 5:29-35, 1998.
108. Assert R, Scherk G, Bumbure A, et al: Regulation of protein kinase C by short-term hyperglycaemia in human platelets in vivo and in vitro. Diabetologia 44:188-195, 2001.
109. Martina V, Bruno GA, Zumpano E, et al: Administration of glutathione in patients with type 2 diabetes mellitus increases the platelet constitutive nitric oxide synthase activity and reduces PAI-1. J Endocrinol Invest 24:37-41, 2001.
110. Schaeffer G, Wascher TC, Kostner GM, Graier WF: Alterations in platelet Ca^{2+} signalling in diabetic patients is due to increased formation of superoxide anions and reduced nitric oxide production. Diabetologia 42:167-176, 1999.
111. Li Y, Woo V, Bose R: Platelet hyperactivity and abnormal Ca^{2+} homeostasis in diabetes mellitus. Am J Physiol Heart Circ Physiol 280:H1480-H1489, 2001.
112. Pandolfi A, Cetrullo D, Polishuck R, et al: Plasminogen activator inhibitor type 1 is increased in the arterial wall of type 2 diabetic subjects. Arterioscler Thromb Vasc Biol 21:1378-1382, 2001.
113. Bruno G, Cavallo-Perin P, Bargero G, et al: Hyperfibrinogenemia and metabolic syndrome in type 2 diabetes: A population-based study. Diabetes Metab Res Rev 17:124-130, 2001.
114. Carr ME: Diabetes mellitus: A hypercoagulable state. J Diabetes Complications 15:44-54, 2001.
115. Turner RC: The U.K. Prospective Diabetes Study: A review. Diabetes Care 21(Suppl 3):C35-C38, 1998.
116. Coutinho M, Gerstein HC, Wang Y, Yusuf S: The relationship between glucose and incident cardiovascular events: A metaregression analysis of published data from 20 studies of 95,783 individuals followed for 12.4 years. Diabetes Care 22:233-240, 1999.
117. Rodriguez BL, Lau N, Burchfiel CM, et al: Glucose intolerance and 23-year risk of coronary heart disease and total mortality: The Honolulu Heart Program. Diabetes Care 22:1262-1265, 1999.
118. Fontbonne A, Charles MA, Thibult N, et al: Hyperinsulinaemia as a predictor of coronary heart disease mortality in a healthy population: The Paris Prospective Study, 15-year follow-up. Diabetologia 34:356-361, 1991.
119. The effect of intensive treatment of diabetes on the development and progression of long-term complications in insulin-dependent diabetes mellitus. The Diabetes Control and Complications Trial Research Group. N Engl J Med 329:977-986, 1993.
120. Abraira C, Colwell J, Nuttall F, et al: Cardiovascular events and correlates in the Veterans Affairs Diabetes Feasibility Trial. Veterans Affairs Cooperative Study on Glycemic Control and Complications in Type 2 Diabetes. Arch Intern Med 157:181-188, 1997.
121. Intensive blood-glucose control with sulphonylureas or insulin compared with conventional treatment and risk of complications in patients with type 2 diabetes (UKPDS 33). UK Prospective Diabetes Study (UKPDS) Group. Lancet 352:837-853, 1998.
122. Nathan DM, Lachin J, Cleary P, et al: Intensive diabetes therapy and carotid intima-media thickness in type 1 diabetes mellitus. N Engl J Med 348:2294-2303, 2003.
123. Chiasson JL, Josse RG, Gomis R, et al: Acarbose treatment and the risk of cardiovascular disease and hypertension in patients with impaired glucose tolerance: The STOP-NIDDM trial. JAMA 290:486-494, 2003.
124. Howard G, O'Leary DH, Zaccaro D, et al: Insulin sensitivity and atherosclerosis. The Insulin Resistance Atherosclerosis Study (IRAS) Investigators. Circulation 93:1809-1817, 1996.
125. Lempiainen P, Mykkanen L, Pyorala K, et al: Insulin resistance syndrome predicts coronary heart disease events in elderly nondiabetic men. Circulation 100:123-128, 1999.
126. Schaper NC, Nabuurs-Franssen MH, Huijberts MS: Peripheral vascular disease and type 2 diabetes mellitus. Diabetes Metab Res Rev 16(Suppl 1):S11-S15, 2000.
127. Effect of intensive blood-glucose control with metformin on complications in overweight patients with type 2 diabetes (UKPDS 34). UK Prospective Diabetes Study (UKPDS) Group. Lancet 352:854-865, 1998.
128. Aronoff S, Rosenblatt S, Braithwaite S, et al: Pioglitazone hydrochloride monotherapy improves glycemic control in the treatment of patients with type 2 diabetes: A 6-month randomized placebo-controlled dose-response study. The Pioglitazone 001 Study Group. Diabetes Care 23:1605-1611, 2000.
129. Plutzky J: Peroxisome proliferator-activated receptors in vascular biology and atherosclerosis: Emerging insights for evolving paradigms. Curr Atheroscler Rep 2:327-335, 2000.
130. Marx N, Sukhova G, Murphy C, et al: Macrophages in human atheroma contain PPARgamma: Differentiation-dependent peroxisomal proliferator-activated receptor gamma (PPARgamma) expression and reduction of MMP-9 activity through PPARgamma activation in mononuclear phagocytes in vitro. Am J Pathol 153:17-23, 1998.
131. Tack CJ, Smits P, Demacker PN, Stalenhoef AF: Troglitazone decreases the proportion of small, dense LDL and increases the resistance of LDL to oxidation in obese subjects. Diabetes Care 21:796-799, 1998.
132. Cominacini L, Young MM, Capriati A, et al: Troglitazone increases the resistance of low-density lipoprotein to oxidation in healthy volunteers. Diabetologia 40:1211-1218, 1997.

133. Parulkar AA, Pendergrass ML, Granda-Ayala R, et al: Nonhypoglycemic effects of thiazolidinediones. Ann Intern Med 134:61-71, 2001.
134. Ghazzi MN, Perez JE, Antonucci TK, et al: Cardiac and glycemic benefits of troglitazone treatment in NIDDM. The Troglitazone Study Group. Diabetes 46:433-439, 1997.
135. Nagy L, Tontonoz P, Alvarez JG, et al: Oxidized LDL regulates macrophage gene expression through ligand activation of PPARgamma. Cell 93:229-240, 1998.
136. Tontonoz P, Nagy L, Alvarez JG, et al: PPARgamma promotes monocyte/macrophage differentiation and uptake of oxidized LDL. Cell 93:241-252, 1998.
137. Sniderman AD, Scantlebury T, Cianflone K: Hypertriglyceridemic hyperapob: The unappreciated atherogenic dyslipoproteinemia in type 2 diabetes mellitus. Ann Intern Med 135:447-459, 2001.
138. Malmstrom R, Packard CJ, Caslake M, et al: Defective regulation of triglyceride metabolism by insulin in the liver in NIDDM. Diabetologia 40:454-462, 1997.
139. Nesto RW, Libby P: Diabetes mellitus and the cardiovascular system. *In* Braunwald E, Zipes DP, Libby P (eds): Heart Disease. 6th ed. Philadelphia, WB Saunders, 2001, pp 2133-2150.
140. Rubins HB, Robins SJ, Collins D, et al: Distribution of lipids in 8,500 men with coronary artery disease. Department of Veterans Affairs HDL Intervention Trial Study Group. Am J Cardiol 75:1196-1201, 1995.
141. Gowri MS, Van der Westhuyzen DR, Bridges SR, Anderson JW: Decreased protection by HDL from poorly controlled type 2 diabetic subjects against LDL oxidation may be due to the abnormal composition of HDL. Arterioscler Thromb Vasc Biol 19:2226-2233, 1999.
142. Williams KJ, Tabas I: The response-to-retention hypothesis of atherogenesis reinforced. Curr Opin Lipidol 9:471-474, 1998.
143. Goldberg RB, Mellies MJ, Sacks FM, et al: Cardiovascular events and their reduction with pravastatin in diabetic and glucose-intolerant myocardial infarction survivors with average cholesterol levels: Subgroup analyses in the cholesterol and recurrent events (CARE) trial. The Care Investigators. Circulation 98:2513-2519, 1998.
144. Pyörala K, Pedersen TR, Kjekshus J, et al: Cholesterol lowering with simvastatin improves prognosis of diabetic patients with coronary heart disease: A subgroup analysis of the Scandinavian Simvastatin Survival Study (4S). Diabetes Care 20:614-620, 1997.
145. Collins R, Armitage J, Parish S, et al: MRC/BHF Heart Protection Study of cholesterol-lowering with simvastatin in 5963 people with diabetes: A randomised placebo-controlled trial. Lancet 361:2005-2016, 2003.
146. Rubins HB, Robins SJ, Collins D, et al: Gemfibrozil for the secondary prevention of coronary heart disease in men with low levels of high-density lipoprotein cholesterol. Veterans Affairs High-Density Lipoprotein Cholesterol Intervention Trial Study Group. N Engl J Med 341:410-418, 1999.
147. Effect of fenofibrate on progression of coronary-artery disease in type 2 diabetes: The Diabetes Atherosclerosis Intervention Study, a randomised study. Lancet 357:905-910, 2001.
148. Marx N, Sukhova GK, Collins T, et al: PPARalpha activators inhibit cytokine-induced vascular cell adhesion molecule-1 expression in human endothelial cells. Circulation 99:3125-3131, 1999.
149. Marx N, Mackman N, Schonbeck U, et al: PPARalpha activators inhibit tissue factor expression and activity in human monocytes. Circulation 103:213-219, 2001.
150. Neve BP, Corseaux D, Chinetti G, et al: PPARalpha agonists inhibit tissue factor expression in human monocytes and macrophages. Circulation 103:207-212, 2001.
151. Sowers JR, Epstein M: Diabetes mellitus and associated hypertension, vascular disease, and nephropathy: An update. Hypertension 26:869-879, 1995.
152. Gress TW, Nieto FJ, Shahar E, et al: Hypertension and antihypertensive therapy as risk factors for type 2 diabetes mellitus. Atherosclerosis Risk in Communities Study. N Engl J Med 342:905-912, 2000.
153. Tuomilehto J, Rastenyte D, Birkenhager WH, et al: Effects of calcium-channel blockade in older patients with diabetes and systolic hypertension. Systolic Hypertension in Europe Trial Investigators. N Engl J Med 340:677-684, 1999.
154. Mehler PS, Jeffers BW, Estacio R, Schrier RW: Associations of hypertension and complications in non-insulin-dependent diabetes mellitus. Am J Hypertens 10:152-161, 1997.
155. Mehler PS, Coll JR, Estacio R, et al: Intensive blood pressure control reduces the risk of cardiovascular events in patients with peripheral arterial disease and type 2 diabetes. Circulation 107:753-756, 2003.
156. Tatti P, Pahor M, Byington RP, et al: Outcome results of the Fosinopril versus Amlodipine Cardiovascular Events Randomized Trial (FACET) in patients with hypertension and NIDDM. Diabetes Care 21:597-603, 1998.
157. Estacio RO, Schrier RW: Antihypertensive therapy in type 2 diabetes: Implications of the appropriate blood pressure control in diabetes (ABCD) trial. Am J Cardiol 82:9R-14R, 1998.
158. Efficacy of atenolol and captopril in reducing risk of macrovascular and microvascular complications in type 2 diabetes: UKPDS 39. UK Prospective Diabetes Study Group. BMJ 317:713-720, 1998.
159. Staessen JA, Fagard R, Thijs L, et al: Randomised double-blind comparison of placebo and active treatment for older patients with isolated systolic hypertension. The Systolic Hypertension in Europe (Syst-Eur) Trial Investigators. Lancet 350:757-764, 1997.
160. Hansson L, Zanchetti A, Carruthers SG, et al: Effects of intensive blood-pressure lowering and low-dose aspirin in patients with hypertension: Principal results of the Hypertension Optimal Treatment (HOT) randomised trial. HOT Study Group. Lancet 351:1755-1762, 1998.
161. Sowers JR, Epstein M, Frohlich ED: Diabetes, hypertension, and cardiovascular disease: An update. Hypertension 37:1053-1059, 2001.
162. Parving HH, Hommel E, Jensen BR, Hansen HP: Long-term beneficial effect of ACE inhibition on diabetic nephropathy in normotensive type 1 diabetic patients. Kidney Int 60:228-234, 2001.
163. Kvetny J, Gregersen G, Pedersen RS: Randomized placebo-controlled trial of perindopril in normotensive, normoalbuminuric patients with type 1 diabetes mellitus. QJM 94:89-94, 2001.
164. Lewis EJ, Hunsicker LG, Clarke WR, et al: Renoprotective effect of the angiotensin-receptor antagonist irbesartan in patients with nephropathy due to type 2 diabetes. N Engl J Med 345:851-860, 2001.
165. Effects of ramipril on cardiovascular and microvascular outcomes in people with diabetes mellitus: Results of the HOPE study and MICRO-HOPE substudy. Heart Outcomes Prevention Evaluation Study Investigators. Lancet 355:253-259, 2000.
166. Lindholm LH, Ibsen H, Dahlof B, et al: Cardiovascular morbidity and mortality in patients with diabetes in the Losartan Intervention For Endpoint reduction in hypertension study (LIFE): A randomised trial against atenolol. Lancet 359:1004-1010, 2002.
167. Gaede P, Vedel P, Larsen N, et al: Multifactorial intervention and cardiovascular disease in patients with type 2 diabetes. N Engl J Med 348:383-393, 2003.

CHAPTER 41

Nutrition and Cardiovascular Disease

Ronald M. Krauss

Appropriate nutritional practices are of central importance in managing risk for atherosclerotic cardiovascular disease. Indeed, many of the current dietary guidelines for the health of the general population aim to prevent cardiovascular disease. These recommendations are based on considerable evidence for nutritional influences on cardiovascular disease risk and a smaller but compelling number of studies indicating that certain dietary modifications can reduce that risk. Additional dietary interventions can benefit patients at higher risk because of specific conditions such as dyslipidemia, hypertension, and obesity. Because of the complexities of testing specific nutrient effects and the inherent difficulties of conducting randomized, controlled clinical endpoint trials for nutritional interventions, they generally cannot be subjected to the same evidence-based criteria that are used to assess drug treatments. Nevertheless, a body of information supports a number of dietary interventions for reducing cardiovascular disease risk and calls into question others that are promoted without an adequate scientific basis.

For dietary recommendations to be effective, they must be provided to patients in a manner that promotes implementation and long-term adherence. The involvement of dietitians and other trained members of a health care team can greatly aid this goal. Of critical importance is the commitment of the health care provider to nutritional guidance and the ability to convey this in terms that patients can accept and readily integrate into their daily lives. Ensuring the patient's understanding of the principles and the goals of the dietary recommendations is an essential element of this process.

The information in this chapter is consistent with dietary guidelines prepared in recent years by the American Heart Association (AHA),[1] the Adult Treatment Panel III of the National Cholesterol Education Program,[2] the National Heart, Lung, and Blood Institute (NHLBI) Joint National Committee on Prevention, Detection, Evaluation and Treatment of High Blood Pressure,[3] and the NHLBI Clinical Guidelines on the Identification, Evaluation, and Treatment of Overweight and Obesity in Adults.[4]

Effects of Overall Dietary Pattern and Specific Food Categories on Cardiovascular Disease

Observational Evidence

Numerous epidemiological studies have identified dietary patterns and food categories associated with reduced risk of cardiovascular disease.[5] Although the interpretation of these studies is limited by their observational nature, the imprecision of the dietary information collected, and the difficulty of correcting for confounding effects of other health behaviors, nevertheless they represent the only feasible approach for drawing conclusions regarding the overall impact of dietary pattern and intake of specific food categories on health outcomes. These analyses permit the general conclusion that lower risk for cardiovascular disease is promoted by emphasis on intake of fruits and vegetables, whole grains, nuts and legumes, fish (preferably fatty), poultry and lean meats, low fat and fat-free dairy products, and liquid vegetable oils. Major nutrient characteristics of these diets include high density of micronutrients and fiber, moderate amounts of unsaturated fats, including omega-3 fatty acids, and lower content of saturated and *trans* fatty acids, sugars, and starches with a high glycemic effect. The relation of these nutrients to cardiovascular disease risk are described further later in the chapter. Epidemiological studies have reported that adherence to such patterns is associated with reductions in cardiovascular disease risk of 30 percent or more.[6-9] However, it is important to recognize that the nutrient composition of these dietary patterns agrees with current recommended dietary intakes for overall health.

A large number of epidemiological studies have reported relationships of specific food categories within these dietary patterns to cardiovascular disease risk, and these studies have formed the basis for recommended intakes of these foods in current dietary guidelines.[1]

FRUITS AND VEGETABLES. Consumption of fruits and vegetables of three or more servings per day versus less than once per day was associated with a 27 percent reduction in cardiovascular disease risk,[10] consistent with results from other studies in which there was a graded risk reduction associated with higher intakes.[11-13] Data suggest that intake of green leafy vegetables and foods rich in carotenoids and vitamin C contribute particularly strongly to this relationship. Based on these data, together with evidence from the Dietary Approaches to Stop Hypertension (DASH) trial, described further later,[14,15] consumption of at least five portions per day of a variety of fruits and vegetables is generally recommended for maintaining cardiovascular health.[1]

WHOLE GRAINS AND FIBER. Consumption of whole grains has been associated with reduced cardiovascular disease risk in a number of studies.[16,17] While this effect may be related to fiber intake,[18,19] not all studies have indicated that the relationship with fiber intake is independent of other variables.[20] There is indeed reason to implicate effects of other nutrients in whole grains that are shared by other plant foods, particularly, vitamins, phytoestrogens, phenols, omega-3 fatty acids, resistant starch, and minerals.

Another issue surrounding intake of whole grains is the potential inverse relationship with consumption of sugars and starches with a high glycemic effect, which may have adverse effects on cardiovascular risk.[21] The magnitude of glycemia, namely the blood glucose elevation following consumption of a dietary carbohydrate, primarily reflects the rate of starch digestion and absorption from the intestine, and this in turn can lead to undesirable metabolic consequences, such as a greater rate of increase in postprandial insulin and an increase in plasma triglycerides.[22] A value ("glycemic index") can be assigned to a food based on the magnitude of blood glucose elevation following consumption of this food in relation to that following a standard food (white bread).[22] However, the reliability of this index as a measure of metabolic effects of meals, and the relation of glycemic load (the quantity of foods with high glycemic index) to disease risk has been challenged.[23]

This food category therefore illustrates the general difficulty of statistically dissociating the effects of a single food category from others that are part of an overall dietary pattern. Nevertheless, a recent meta-analysis indicated an average 27 percent reduction in coronary heart disease independently associated with whole grain consumption and suggested an intake of at least three servings per day for cardiovascular health.[24]

LEGUMES. Increased intake of legumes (e.g., peas, beans, soybeans, lentils) has been associated with reduced cardiovascular disease risk in some,[25,26] but not all[11] analyses. In the case of soy, beneficial effects may derive from cholesterol-lowering effects of soy protein as well as vascular effects of soy isoflavones,[27] but there is little direct evidence for reduced cardiovascular risk.

NUTS. Several large studies have indicated an association of nut consumption with reduced cardiovascular disease risk.[28-30] Women who consumed 5 oz. of nuts per week had a 35 percent lower risk of nonfatal myocardial infarction compared with those eating less than 1 oz. per month,[29] while men who consumed nuts twice per week or more had a 47 percent reduction in risk for sudden cardiac death and a 30 percent reduction in total coronary heart disease mortality compared with those who rarely or never consume nuts.[30] As with other complex plant foods, it is difficult to determine which components of nuts may be responsible for these beneficial associations. Nuts are good sources of monounsaturated fatty acids, fiber, minerals, and flavonoids. Walnuts are particularly rich in polyunsaturated fatty acids such as linoleic and alpha-linolenic acid. Recent studies of almond intake have indicated beneficial effects on plasma lipoproteins,[31] but comparisons with the effects of other nuts have not been reported.

FISH AND FISH OIL. There is strong evidence that consumption of fish, especially those species with high content of omega-3 fatty acids, confers protection from ischemic heart disease[32,33] and that this relationship is particularly strong for coronary heart disease mortality and sudden cardiac death, which has been reported to be on average 52 percent lower in men consuming fish at least once weekly versus men consuming less.[34] Although fish have a number of important nutritive qualities, it is likely that their major cardiovascular benefit is due to their content of the omega-3 fatty acids, eicosapentanoic acid (EPA) and docosahexanoic acid (DHA). Increased plasma levels of these fatty acids predicted a considerable reduction in sudden cardiac death,[35] a result consistent with that of a report indicating that intake of 5.5 gm per/mo of EPA plus DHA (equivalent to one portion of fatty fish per week) was associated with a 50 percent lower incidence of primary cardiac arrest compared with individuals consuming no fish.[36] This effect appears to be related to enrichment of membrane phospholipids with omega-3 fatty acids and a resulting reduction in risk for abnormal cardiac electrical conductivity.[36] Other properties of these fatty acids that may benefit risk for coronary heart disease include antiplatelet and antiinflammatory effects, as well as reduction in plasma triglycerides at higher doses.[33]

Based on these studies, as well as results of intervention trials with omega-3 fatty acids described later, the AHA has recommended consumption of two portions of fish per week,[1] particularly those fish rich in omega-3 fatty acids (e.g., salmon, mackerel, albacore tuna, swordfish, herring, sardines, lake trout). Because these fish (particularly predatory fish such as swordfish and some types of tuna) can contain significant quantities of contaminants including methylmercury, polychlorinated biphenyls, and dioxin, the U.S. Environmental Protection Agency and the U.S. Food and Drug Administration (FDA) have provided guidelines for maximal intakes, an issue of particular concern for children and women of childbearing age. In most cases, however, the recommendation of two portions per week falls within these guidelines.

Clinical trials have supported evidence from epidemiological studies[32] that higher intakes of fish may particularly benefit patients with coronary heart disease (Table 41–1).[33] In the Gruppo Italiano per lo Studio della Sopravvivenza nell'Infarto Miocardio (GISSI) secondary prevention trial,[37,38] a supplement containing a total of 0.85 gm/d of EPA and DHA resulted in reductions of 45 percent and 30 percent in sudden and cardiovascular death. Total mortality and sudden death were reduced after 3 and 4 months of treatment, respectively, consistent with reduction of arrhythmia by the treatment. Based on the overall evidence to date, the AHA has recommended that supplemental EPA plus DHA at doses of up to 1 gm/d may be considered for risk reduction in patients with coronary heart disease in consultation with their physician.[33] Supplements also could be a component of the medical management of hypertriglyceridemia, a setting in which even larger doses (2 to 4 gm/d) are required. The availability of high-quality omega-3 fatty acid supplements, free of contaminants, is an important prerequisite to their use.

ALCOHOL. Moderate alcohol consumption (one to three alcoholic beverages per day) is strongly and consistently associated with lower risk for coronary heart disease than either abstention or higher intakes.[39] Some data have suggested that wine, particularly red varieties, is of particular benefit, possibly due to its content of polyphenols such as resveratrol that may have direct benefits on vascular reactivity, thrombosis, and oxidative stress.[40] However, most studies have not documented such a differential benefit of red versus white wine, and it appears likely that the major benefit of alcohol consumption is related to an increase in high-density lipoprotein (HDL) cholesterol and perhaps to other effects such as reduced fibrinogen, platelet aggregation, and inflammation.[39,41,42] In a recent study, men who consumed alcohol three or four times per week had a 37 percent reduction in risk for myocardial infarction compared to men who drank less than once per week, and the risk reduction was no greater with more frequent consumption.[43] Current recommendations from the AHA[1] and the U.S. Dietary Guidelines Advisory Committee are that men who drink alcohol may consume up to two alcoholic beverages per day, and women no more than one per day, in part because of alcohol-related breast cancer risk. Because of the potential hazards associated with habituation to alcohol, the potential for adverse effects such as hepatoxicity and aggravation of hypertriglyceridemia, and the favorable benefit/risk ratio of other dietary practices and therapeutic interventions, individuals should not begin to consume alcohol as a means of reducing coronary disease risk.[44]

Clinical Trials (see Table 41–1)

Relatively few clinical trials have examined the effects of overall dietary patterns or specific food categories on

TABLE 41–1 Trials of Dietary Interventions and Coronary Events

Trial	Patients in Intervention Group	Dietary Intervention	Dietary Fat (Energy) in Treatment Group, %	Energy From P and S Fat in Treatment Group, %	Overall Trial Duration, y	Change in Serum Cholesterol Level, %†	Change in CHD, %‡
Low-Fat Approach							
MRC (low fat)	123 male MI patients	Reduce total fat	22	NR	3	−5	+5
DART	1015 male MI patients	Reduce total fat	32	NR	2	−4	−9
High-Polyunsaturated-Fat Approach							
Finnish Mental Hospital Study	676 men without CHD	Reduce saturated fat, increase polyunsaturated fat	35	P = 13; S = 9	6	−15	−44§
Los Angeles Veteran Study	424 men; most had no evidence of existing CHD	Reduce saturated fat, increase polyunsaturated fat	40	P = 16; S = 9	8	−13§	−20 in CHD, −31§ in cardiovascular events
Oslo Diet-Heart Study	206 male MI patients	Reduce saturated fat, increase polyunsaturated fat	39	P = 21; S = 9	5	−14§	−25§
MRC (soy oil)	199 male MI patients	Reduce saturated fat, increase polyunsaturated fat	46	P:S ratio = 2	4	−15§	−12
Minnesota Coronary Survey	4393 men and 4664 women	Reduce saturated fat, increase polyunsaturated fat	38	P = 15; S = 9	1‖	−14§	0
Increase Omega-3 Fatty Acid							
DART	1015 male MI patients	Fish twice per week or fish oil (1.5 gm/d)	NR	NR	2	NR	−16 on CHD events, −29§ in total mortality
GISSI-Prevenzione	5666 MI patients, primarily men	Fish oil (EPA + DHA, 1 gm/d)	NR	NR	3.5	0	−30§ in cardiovascular death, −45§ in sudden death
Indian Experiment of Infarct Survival 4	242 MI patients, primarily men	Fish oil (EPA, 1.08 gm/d) or mustard oil (ALA, 2.9 gm/d)	NR	NR	1	0	−30‡ in fish oil group, −19 in mustard oil group
Whole-Diet Approach							
Lyon Diet Heart Study	302 MI patients, primarily men	High ALA intake and Mediterranean diet	31	P:S ratio = 0.7	3.8	0	−72§
Indian Experiment of Infarct Survival	204 MI patients, primarily men	High intake of fruits, vegetables, nuts, fish, and pulses	24	P:S ratio = 1.2	1	−9§	−40§

ALA = α-linolenic acid; CHD = coronary heart disease; DART = Diet and Reinfarction Trial; DHA = docosahexaenoic acid; EPA = eicosapentaenoic acid; GISSI = Gruppo Italiano per lo Studio della Sopravvivenza nell'Infarto Miocardico; MI = myocardial infarction; NR = not reported; MRC = Medical Research Council; P = polyunsaturated fat; S, saturated fat.

*From Hu FB, Willett WC: Optimal diets for prevention of coronary artery disease: JAMA 288:2569, 2002.

†Change in cholesterol level refers to the percentage change in serum cholesterol level in the treatment group compared with the change in the control group.

‡Change in CHD refers to the percentage difference in coronary event rates in the treatment group compared with the control group.

§$P < .05$

‖The total duration of the study was 4.5 years, but the mean duration of the intervention was only 1 year.

cardiovascular disease endpoints. Early randomized trials (Wadsworth Veterans Affairs Hospital, Oslo Diet-Heart, Finnish Mental Hospital Study) tested the effectiveness of cholesterol-lowering diets enriched in polyunsaturated fatty acids.[45] These trials showed a 25 to 50 percent reduction in cardiovascular disease endpoints over 5 to 12 years in conjunction with a 13 to 15 percent reduction in blood cholesterol levels. Notably, these diets were not low in total fat (30 to 40 percent of calories).

More recently, the Lyon Diet Heart Study tested the effects of a Mediterranean-style diet in 423 patients with documented coronary artery disease who were followed for a mean of 3.8 years.[46] Compared with the control diet, the experimental diet had increased amounts of fruits, vegetables, legumes, and fiber and reductions of meats, butter, and cream (but not cheese). In addition, the diet contained a margarine enriched in alpha-linolenic acid, an omega-3 fatty acid precursor of the longer chain EPA plus DHA found in fatty fish. Total fat was approximately 31 percent in both diets. Despite lower content of dietary saturated fat, there were no differences in plasma lipids, lipoproteins, or other major risk factors between the two diets. There were, however, significant reductions in all outcome measures, including all-cause mortality (56 percent), cardiac mortality (65 percent), and nonfatal myocardial infarction (70 percent) (Fig. 41–1).[45,46] Although many components of the dietary program may have contributed to these results, the authors suggested a particularly important role for increased omega-3 fatty acid intake.

The effects of a very low fat diet in the context of an intensive life-style intervention have been evaluated in the Life-Style Heart Trial[47] and a more recent multicenter extension of this program.[48] The regimen includes a vegetarian diet with 10 percent total fat, as well as aerobic exercise training, stress management, smoking cessation, and psychosocial support. In the Life-Style Heart Trial, 48 men with coronary artery disease were allocated to intervention and control groups, and 35 completed a 5-year follow-up. In the experimental group, the average percent diameter stenosis at baseline decreased 1.75 absolute percentage points after 1 year (a 4.5

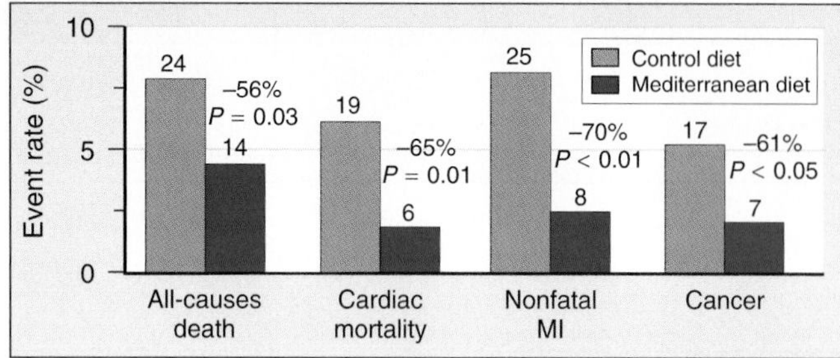

FIGURE 41–1 The effect of a Mediterranean diet on total mortality, coronary disease events, and cancer in men after acute myocardial infarction (MI): the Lyon Heart Study. (From Sacks FM, Katan M: Randomized clinical trials on the effects of dietary fat and carbohydrate on plasma lipoproteins and cardiovascular disease. Am J Med 113:13S, 2002.)

percent relative improvement) and by 3.1 absolute percentage points after 5 years (a 7.9 percent relative improvement). In contrast, the average percent diameter stenosis in the control group increased by 2.3 percentage points after 1 year (a 5.4 percent relative worsening) and by 11.8 percentage points after 5 years (a 27.7 percent relative worsening) (p = .001 between groups). Twenty-five cardiac events occurred in 28 experimental group patients versus 45 events in 20 control group patients during the 5-year follow-up (risk ratio for any event for the control group, 2.47 [95 percent confidence interval, 1.48 to 4.20]). Among major cardiovascular risk factors, the intervention program versus control resulted in a significant 40 percent versus 1 percent reduction of low-density lipoprotein (LDL) cholesterol and a 17 percent versus 4 percent reduction in body weight, with no significant changes in HDL, cholesterol, triglyceride, or blood pressure. Thus, this approach offers an effective means of coronary disease risk reduction, although the magnitude of the contribution of the very low fat diet per se, in the context of the overall program and in comparison with more moderate dietary regimens, has not been established.

Effects of Specific Dietary Components on Risk Factors for Cardiovascular Disease

The effects of dietary patterns and specific food categories on cardiovascular disease risk may operate in part through their effects on risk factors. The major diet-related risk factors are obesity, plasma lipids and lipoproteins, and blood pressure. Other factors for which dietary benefits are less well established include homocysteine, inflammation, and oxidative stress. Other than antiplatelet effects of omega-3 fatty acids, there is little indication of dietary effects on thrombosis.

Overweight and Obesity

Overweight and obesity, defined respectively as body mass index higher than 25 and more than 30 kg/m^2, respectively,[4] are progressively increasing in prevalence in the United States and globally.[49] These conditions are associated with numerous comorbidities affecting cardiovascular disease risk, notably dyslipidemia, hypertension, diabetes, and metabolic syndrome.[49,50] The underlying guidelines for prevention and treatment of excess body weight as articulated in the AHA Dietary Guidelines target both diet and physical activity[1]:

1. Match intake of energy (calories) to overall energy needs; limit consumption of foods with a high-caloric density and/or low nutritional quality, including those with a high content of sugars.
2. Maintain a level of physical activity that achieves fitness and balances energy expenditure with energy intake; for weight reduction, expenditure should exceed intake.

These principles, which agree with those of the NHLBI,[4] recognize that weight reduction requires achieving a negative energy balance. In this regard, carefully controlled metabolic studies have established that at a given level of physical activity, reduced energy intake will result in weight loss irrespective of the macronutrient (carbohydrate, fat, protein) composition of the diet over a rather wide range.[51,52] Nonetheless, considerable controversy persists as to whether diets with differing macronutrient composition differ in their effectiveness in achieving short-term or long-term weight loss. A detailed discussion of this controversy exceeds the scope of this chapter, but arguments based on observational data, or on intervention programs that incorporate dietary change with increases in physical activity and other behavioral changes, do not adequately address the question of diet composition per se as a factor that affects the efficacy of weight loss. In fact, studies of individuals who have achieved long-term weight loss indicate that these individuals employ a number of behavioral changes to control dietary fat intake, have higher levels of physical activity (especially strenuous activity), and maintain a greater frequency of self-weighing.[53]

However, even this information does not help to establish whether alternate dietary strategies, such as very-low-carbohydrate and/or high-protein diets may prove even more effective, based on either their metabolic effects or their influence on eating behavior. Only recently have studies specifically tested the efficacy of such dietary approaches.[54-56] Results to date suggest that at least over periods up to 6 months, average weight loss is higher for diets with very low carbohydrate content (e.g., <35 g/day) than with diets containing more conventional amounts of carbohydrate that are restricted in total fat (Table 41–2).[57] Possible explanations for this finding include the restricted food choices, and the possibility that higher dietary content of protein and/or lower content of carbohydrates, especially simple sugars and rapidly digested starches with lower glycemic effects, increase satiety. Differing effects of these diets on body fat or body composition have not been demonstrated. However, questions remain regarding the long-term safety and overall health effects of such diets, particularly since they lack many of the foods associated with maintaining cardiovascular and overall health, including fruits, vegetables, and whole grains. Additionally, they are high in saturated and *trans* fats and cholesterol, although as described later, the expected effects of these fats on LDL cholesterol levels appear to be attenuated. Another major concern is whether diets with extreme deviations from conventional food choices, i.e., very low in either carbohydrate or fat, can be effectively sustained over the long term (e.g., years). In the case of low-fat diets, this appears possible at least for highly motivated individuals,[48,53] and for population groups such as East Asians, but it remains undetermined for very-low-carbohydrate/high-protein/high-fat diets, regimens for which little long-term population experience exists. There are also specific concerns regarding long-term consequences of high protein intake, particularly in the setting of renal or hepatic impairment.[58]

Plasma Lipids

TOTAL AND LDL CHOLESTEROL. Dietary management of LDL cholesterol remains a major goal of coronary artery disease risk management.[2] Although diet-induced lowering of LDL cholesterol has not been firmly proved to reduce coronary disease risk, this conclusion is reasonable based both on the results of dietary trials designed to lower LDL described

TABLE 41–2 Comparison of Low-Carbohydrate and Reduced-Fat Diets

Variable	Low-Carbohydrate Diet*	Reduced-Fat Diet†
Caloric restriction	Not necessary; ketosis may help reduce intake	Necessary
Food choices	Highly restricted	Moderately restricted
Initial rate of weight loss	Rapid, with increased diuresis	Gradual, with some diuresis
Weight loss	Dependent on duration	Dependent on duration
Weight maintenance	Unproven over the long term	Unproven over the long term
Cholesterol		
LDL	No change	Decrease
HDL	Greater increase	Increase
Triglycerides	Greater decrease	Decrease
Potential long-term concerns	Calciuria (renal stones and decreased bone mass) Relatively high-protein content (patients with renal or hepatic disease) Atherogenicity (high saturated fat, trans fat, and cholesterol levels and relative absence of fruits, vegetables, and whole grains	None

*A low-carbohydrate diet is defined as one that provides <35 gm of carbohydrate per day. The Atkins diet begins with a stricter limitation (20 gm/day) for at least the first 2 weeks, with a gradual increase of 5 gm/week to achieve a rate of weight loss of approximately 2 lb (0.9 kg) per week until a weight within 5 to 10 lb (2.3 to 4.5 kg) of the goal is achieved. Carbohydrate intake is then further increased by 10 gm/week until weight loss ceases.

†A reduced-fat diet is defined as one in which fat constitutes <30% of the total caloric intake; under certain circumstances (e.g., in some patients with the metabolic syndrome), fat intake of ≤35% of the total caloric intake is recommended.

LDL = low-density lipoprotein; HLD = high-density lipoprotein.

From Bonow RO, Eckel RH: Diet, obesity, and cardiovascular risk. N Engl J Med 348:2057, 2003.

earlier and the relation of drug-induced reductions in LDL cholesterol to decreases in coronary disease morbidity and mortality. Nutritional factors known to increase LDL cholesterol levels include saturated and *trans* fatty acids, dietary cholesterol, and excess body weight. While total fat intake tends to correlate with that of saturated fat, there is no evidence that LDL levels rise due to increased dietary total fat intake per se. In fact, as mentioned earlier, trials employing high total and unsaturated fat consumption resulted in lower LDL cholesterol and reduced heart disease risk. Moreover, recent studies have indicated that at least over the short term, very low carbohydrate diets with high levels of total fat and protein blunt the expected increases in LDL cholesterol expected from high saturated fat intake.[54-56]

Substitution of carbohydrate and/or unsaturated fatty acids for saturated and *trans* fatty acids results in reduction of LDL cholesterol. Many studies have assessed the quantitative effects of these dietary changes on LDL and other lipids and lipoproteins, as recently summarized and reviewed (Fig. 41–2).[59,60] When substituted for carbohydrate, the greatest increases in LDL cholesterol result from C12 : 0 (lauric), C14 : 0 (myristic), and C16 : 0 (palmitic) fatty acids found in dairy fat, meat, and tropical oils, with equivalent changes induced by *trans* monounsaturated fatty acids found in baked goods, stick margarine, and in fried "fast foods" such as french fries. In contrast, 18 : 0 fatty acid (stearic), which is found in many of the same foods, generally does not raise LDL cholesterol levels. No increases in LDL cholesterol follow intake of monounsaturated fatty acids, principally 18 : 1 (oleic), a major component of olive and canola oils, and polyunsaturated fatty acids of the omega-6 series, principally 18 : 2 (linoleic), found in vegetable and seed oils such as corn, safflower, and sunflower oils. Current guidelines recommend consumption of less than 10 percent of calories as saturated fat for the general population and further limitation to 7 percent or less for those with a level of LDL cholesterol higher than that recommended for their overall risk status.[1,2] For *trans* fatty acids, it is recommended that intake be reduced to a minimum, a goal that will be easier to achieve once *trans* fatty acid content is indicated on food labels.

With the exception of egg yolk and shellfish, dietary cholesterol is found in foods of animal origin that are also high

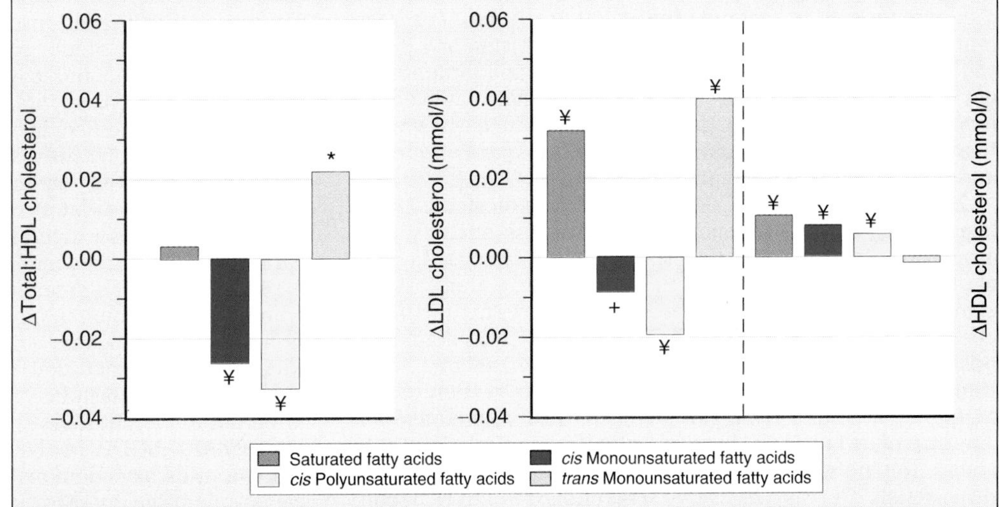

FIGURE 41–2 Predicted changes (Δ) in the ratio of serum total to HDL cholesterol and in LDL- and HDL-cholesterol concentrations when carbohydrates constituting 1 percent of energy are replaced isoenergetically with saturated, *cis* monosaturated, *cis* polyunsaturated, or *trans* monounsaturated fatty acids. *$p < 0.05$; +$p < 0.01$; ¥$p < 0.001$. (From Mensink RP, Zock PL, Kester AD, Katan MB: Effects of dietary fatty acids and carbohydrates on the ratio of serum total to HDL cholesterol and on serum lipids and apolipoproteins: A meta-analysis of 60 controlled trials. Am J Clin Nutr 77:1146, 2003.)

in saturated fat. On average, an increase of 100 mg/d of dietary cholesterol increases total serum cholesterol about 2 to 3 mg/dl, of which approximately 70 percent is in the LDL fraction. This effect of added cholesterol varies considerably among individuals and is attenuated at higher cholesterol intakes. The LDL cholesterol increase would predict approximately a 1 to 2 percent increase in coronary heart disease risk, with possibly offsetting effects of concomitantly increased HDL cholesterol. An effect of this magnitude is difficult to detect in epidemiological data and may contribute to the reported lack of association of egg yolk intake with coronary disease risk for amounts up to 1 or more eggs (~215 mg cholesterol) per day, except in patients with diabetes.[61] Based on available data, as well as the infeasibility of consuming diets with markedly restricted cholesterol content, current guidelines[1,2] recommend limiting intake to less than 300 mg/d for the general population and less than 200 mg/d for individuals at increased risk for heart disease by National Cholesterol Education Program criteria.

Although there is wide interindividual variation in response to these changes,[62,63] the reductions in LDL cholesterol that may be expected with adoption of diets low in saturated fat and cholesterol are generally in the range of 5 to 10 percent. Near-maximal response of LDL cholesterol to dietary change occurs as early as 3 to 4 weeks, and thereafter it can be determined whether additional therapeutic measures will be required to achieve the desired LDL cholesterol target.

Some epidemiological analyses have shown positive independent associations of saturated fat intake with coronary heart disease risk, but the relationships have been relatively weak and inconsistent.[64] This likely reflects several factors including the relatively small average effects of saturated fat on LDL cholesterol and the possible offsetting increases in HDL cholesterol as described later. On the other hand, *trans* fatty acid intake appears to have a stronger relationship with coronary heart disease risk,[64] perhaps reflecting the finding that HDL cholesterol levels are not increased by *trans* fat or perhaps the existence of other adverse effects of these fatty acids on disease mechanisms.

Other nutritional measures that can reduce LDL cholesterol include weight loss, which may be particularly effective in some cases, and addition of plant sterol and stanol esters,[65] viscous fiber (in particular, beta-glucan, a component of oat fiber),[66] soy protein,[27] and nuts.[31] LDL cholesterol has been found to fall by a mean of 28 percent on a diet that combines diet components in amounts (per 1000 kcal) that have been reported to be beneficial individually: plant sterols 1.0 gm, soy protein 21.4 gm, viscous fibers 9.8 gm, and almonds 14 gm.[67] This reduction was comparable to that achieved by lovastatin 10 mg/d (30.9 percent) and significantly greater than with a diet low in saturated fat (4.5 percent of energy) and cholesterol (8.0 percent).

HDL CHOLESTEROL. Although HDL cholesterol correlates inversely and independently with risk for coronary artery disease, it remains uncertain whether changes in HDL cholesterol, and in particular those induced by diet, predict changes in risk. There are two general categories of nutritional effect on HDL: those due to changes in dietary fatty acid composition and those due to factors that also affect plasma triglyceride levels, as described in the next section. Since dietary fatty acids have major effects on LDL as well as HDL cholesterol, it is necessary to examine these effects jointly to assess the potential impact of HDL change on coronary disease risk. The ratio of LDL or total cholesterol to HDL cholesterol permits assessment of these joint effects. A review of 60 dietary trials has indicated that the plasma cholesterol to HDL cholesterol ratio did not change if saturated fatty acids replaced an isocaloric amount of dietary carbohydrates. However, this ratio decreased if *cis* unsaturated fatty acids replaced saturated fatty acids (see Fig. 41–2).[59] The effect on total:HDL cholesterol of replacing *trans* fatty acids with a mix of carbohydrates and *cis* unsaturated fatty acids was almost twice as large as that of replacing saturated fatty acids. Lauric acid greatly increased total cholesterol, but much of its effect was on HDL cholesterol, resulting in a lower ratio of total:HDL cholesterol for oils rich in lauric acid, such as coconut oil. As discussed earlier, the tandem effects of dietary saturated fatty acids as well as dietary cholesterol on total and HDL cholesterol may contribute to the relatively weak relationship of these nutrients to coronary heart disease risk.

TRIGLYCERIDE AND THE ATHEROGENIC DYSLIPIDEMIA OF OBESITY, DIABETES, AND THE METABOLIC SYNDROME. Elevated plasma triglyceride independently but rather weakly predicts coronary heart disease risk. Its principal cardiovascular significance is as a component of, and a marker for, the atherogenic dyslipidemia commonly found in patients with excess adiposity, the metabolic syndrome, and type 2 diabetes mellitus (see Chaps. 39 and 40).[68] The triad of lipid abnormalities in these conditions consists of elevated plasma triglyceride (≥150 mg/dl), reduced HDL cholesterol, and a relative excess of small, dense LDL particles with total LDL cholesterol levels that are generally average.[69] Adiposity itself is the principal nutritionally related influence on atherogenic dyslipidemia. Among nutrients, the major determinant of this dyslipidemic triad is carbohydrate.[70] In general, simple sugars and rapidly hydrolyzed starches have a greater glyceridemic effect than more complex carbohydrates and those consumed in conjunction with higher intake of fiber. The glyceridemic effects of carbohydrates tend to correlate with their glycemic effects.[22] Dietary carbohydrate-induced increases in plasma triglyceride are often accompanied by decreases in HDL cholesterol and increases in levels of small, dense LDL particles.[71] Although there is no direct evidence that these diet-induced changes contribute to increased coronary heart disease risk, it has been reported that dietary glycemic load, a measure of the quantity of high glycemic foods related to high plasma triglyceride and low HDL cholesterol, strongly and independently predicts coronary heart disease risk.[21] Hence, limitation of sugars and high glycemic/glyceridemic carbohydrates is advisable in patients with this form of dyslipidemia.

Blood Pressure

Current recommendations for nonpharmacological management of elevated blood pressure include weight reduction, moderation in alcohol consumption, limitation of sodium intake, and increased intake of certain other minerals (see Chap. 38).[1,3] Another important therapeutic modality for reducing blood pressure is the DASH combination diet.[14,15] Taken together, the evidence supporting these recommendations described later reinforces the roles of multiple components of an overall dietary pattern in promoting cardiovascular and general health.

BODY WEIGHT. Numerous clinical trials reviewed elsewhere[1,3] have documented a substantial and significant relation between change in weight and change in blood pressure. It has been estimated that a reduction of more than 1 mm Hg in systolic and diastolic blood pressure may occur for each kilogram of weight loss.

DIETARY SODIUM. Numerous observational studies and clinical trials have demonstrated that a high intake of sodium can result in an increase in blood pressure.[72] Meta-analyses of randomized trials have shown that on average, reducing sodium intake by about 80 mmol (1.8 gm)/d yields systolic and diastolic blood pressure reductions of about 4 and 2 mm Hg in hypertensive patients and smaller reductions in normotensive subjects.[73] Although the blood pressure response to change in salt intake varies among individuals, in part because of genetic factors and other variables such as age, classification of individuals as "responders" or "nonresponders" can be difficult.[74]

The Trials of Hypertension Prevention documented that sodium reduction, alone or combined with weight loss, can lower incidence of hypertension by about 20 percent (Fig. 41–3).[75] In the Trials of Nonpharmacologic Interventions in the Elderly, a reduced salt intake with or without weight loss significantly reduced blood pressure and the need for antihypertensive medication in older persons.[76] In both trials, the dietary interventions reduced total sodium intake to about 100 mmol/d. Although the DASH-sodium trial has shown that further blood pressure reduction can be achieved by lowering sodium intake to 50 mmol/d (see later), such a limitation is extremely difficult to implement because of the high sodium content of many prepared foods. Overall, the available data support the current AHA population guideline of limiting salt intake to 6 gm/d, the equivalent of 100 mmol of sodium (2400 mg) per day.[1] Careful selection of foods and limitation of added salt can substantially lower sodium intake, and these measures can be particularly beneficial in hypertensive patients.

ALCOHOL. Observational data have consistently demonstrated a relationship between heavy drinking (three or more standard drinks per day) and higher blood pressure.[77] Clinical trials of reducing alcohol consumption have yielded less conclusive findings.[78] As stated previously, the totality of the evidence supports a recommendation to limit alcohol intake to no more than two drinks per day for men and one drink per day for women.

POTASSIUM, MAGNESIUM, AND CALCIUM INTAKE. As reviewed elsewhere,[72,79] observational data have provided evidence that increased intakes of these minerals are associated with lower blood pressure. Clinical trials have also documented a beneficial impact of potassium supplements on blood pressure, but the evidence for calcium and magnesium is less consistent.[72,79] A meta-analysis of randomized trials of the effects of potassium supplementation[80] found that, on average, supplementation of diets with 60 to 120 mmol/d reduced systolic and diastolic blood pressure by 4.4 and 2.5 mm Hg in hypertensive patients and by 1.8 and 1.0 mm Hg in normotensive subjects. Because a high dietary intake of potassium, magnesium, and calcium can be achieved from food sources and because diets rich in these minerals provide a variety of other nutrients, the preferred strategy for increasing mineral intake is through foods rather than supplements.

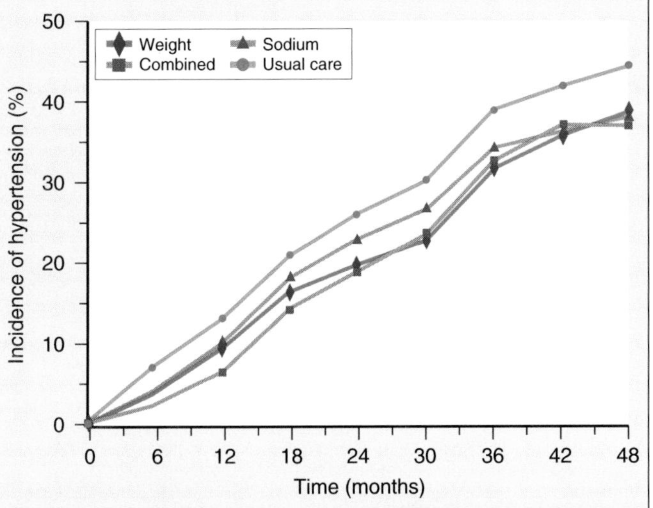

FIGURE 41–3 Plot of the incidence of hypertension for the respective randomized groups through 48 months of follow-up, from life-table analysis in the Trials of Hypertension Prevention, Phase II. (From The Trials of Hypertension Prevention Collaborative Research Group: Effects of weight loss and sodium reduction intervention on blood pressure and hypertension incidence in overweight people with high-normal blood pressure. The Trials of Hypertension Prevention, Phase II. Arch Intern Med 157:657, 1997.)

DIETARY PATTERN. The DASH study[14,81] found that a diet rich in fruits and vegetables (five to nine servings per day) and low-fat dairy products (two to four servings a day), and with reduced saturated and total fat content, reduced systolic and diastolic blood pressure by 5.5 and 3.0 mm Hg more than did a control diet of equal sodium content that produced no differences in sodium or body weight. As with other interventions, reductions were substantially greater in hypertensive than normotensive subjects, and reductions were larger in black than nonblack subjects. In a second trial, the DASH-sodium study, progressive sodium restriction in the DASH diet (from a daily intake of 150 to 100 mmol and 50 mmol) further reduced blood pressure, such that the DASH diet with the lowest sodium intake led to a mean systolic blood pressure that was 7.1 mm Hg lower in participants without hypertension and 11.5 mm Hg lower in participants with hypertension.[15,82] However, particularly among normotensive and nonblack subjects, most of the blood pressure reduction could be accounted for by the DASH diet rather than additional sodium restriction.

Due to the multifactorial dietary intervention of DASH, its mechanisms of effectiveness cannot be determined. However, the diet was rich in potassium, calcium, and magnesium, and hence the findings are consistent with the possibility that these elements contributed to the observed reductions in blood pressure. A similar conclusion may be drawn from the Vanguard study, a trial that used a dietary regimen based on prepackaged foods.[83]

OTHER DIETARY EFFECTS ON BLOOD PRESSURE. Limited data support the possible beneficial effects of additional dietary measures on blood pressure. These include fish,[84] whole grains (in particular, oats),[85] and protein (in particular, soy).[86-88] The suggestion that soy isoflavone content may contribute to this benefit is consistent with a recent report that polyphenols in dark chocolate can also promote blood pressure reduction.[89]

Other Cardiovascular Risk Factors Related to Diet (see also Chap. 36)

HOMOCYSTEINE. Recent meta-analyses have concluded that elevated plasma homocysteine levels modestly increase the risk for ischemic heart disease and stroke.[90,91] Folic acid, as well as pyridoxine and cyanocobalamin (vitamins B_6 and B_{12}), are the major dietary components influencing plasma homocysteine levels.[92] There is as yet little information regarding the potential benefit of plasma homocysteine reduction on cardiovascular disease risk. A placebo-controlled, randomized trial of a daily regimen of folic acid 1 mg, cyanocobalamin 400 μg, and pyridoxine 10 mg significantly reduced a composite endpoint for adverse cardiovascular outcomes in patients undergoing coronary angioplasty.[93] Although, as expected, plasma homocysteine levels were substantially reduced by treatment, it cannot be determined to what extent this contributed to the outcome. Nevertheless, if this finding is confirmed by other ongoing studies, this could provide a basis for future recommendations of supplemental vitamin therapy for high-risk patients. However, such studies may be difficult to carry out, since population levels of plasma homocysteine in the United States have decreased since fortification of cereal grain flour mandated by the FDA in 1998, and it has been shown that folic acid supplementation causes only modest further reductions in homocysteine in coronary artery disease patients who are exposed to cereal products.[94] Administration of folic acid supplements in the absence of adequate cyanocobalamin may lead to masking of pernicious anemia.[92]

DIETARY INFLUENCES ON C-REACTIVE PROTEIN. A number of nutritional factors influence C-reactive protein, a well-established coronary artery disease risk factor (see Chap. 36).[95] Chief among these is adiposity, which in turn appears to exert its effect by increasing insulin resistance.[96] Weight loss reduces C-reactive protein levels.[97] Glycemic load is positively associated with plasma C-reactive protein levels[98] and inversely with alcohol intake,[42] but prospective clinical studies of these effects have not been reported. Higher glycemic loads associate with elevated levels of C-reactive protein in both normal and overweight women (Fig. 41–4). The "portfolio" diet containing multiple supplements that lowered plasma LDL cholesterol also lowered C-reactive protein to a level similar to that obtained with low-dose statin therapy.[67]

ANTIOXIDANT VITAMINS. Despite the evidence supporting the role of oxidative stress in atherogenesis and observational data relating antioxidant intake to reduced risk of cardiovascular disease, there is insufficient evidence from clinical trials to support the use of antioxidant vitamins for the prevention of ischemic heart disease.[99,100] Notably, no benefit was observed with a supplement of 600 mg of vitamin E, 250 mg of vitamin C, and 20 mg of beta carotene daily in the randomized, placebo-controlled Heart Protection Study trial of 20,536 high-risk individuals. In a smaller study, the cardiovascular protective effects of statin plus niacin therapy in patients with coronary artery disease were attenuated by coadministration of a mixture of antioxidants that also resulted in reductions of large HDL particles.[101] It is possible that the observational studies reflect confounding effects of other dietary or lifestyle practices that correlate with antioxidant consumption either in foods or supplements or that longer-term consumption is necessary to achieve benefits.

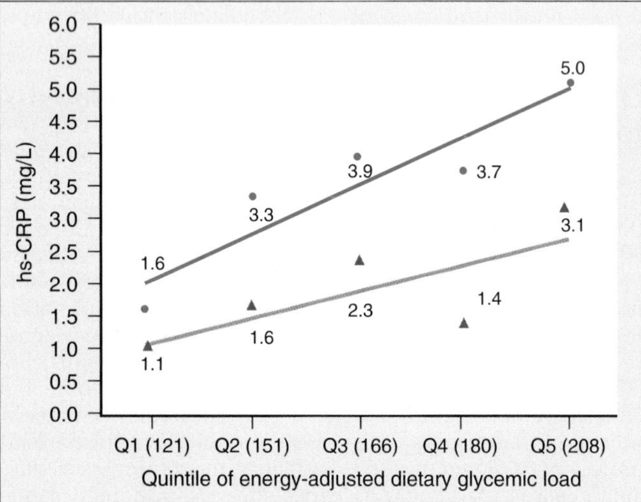

FIGURE 41–4 Adjusted geometric mean plasma concentrations of high-sensitivity C-reactive protein (hs-CRP) by quintiles (Q1 to Q5) of energy-adjusted dietary glycemic load in 244 women in two body mass index categories: BMI < 25 (▲ and blue regression line) and BMI ≥ 25 (● and magenta regression line). Multiple linear regression models were used to adjust for potential confounding factors, including age; randomized treatment status; smoking status; BMI; physical activity levels; alcohol intake; parental history of myocardial infarction before the age of 60 years; history of diabetes mellitus; history of hypertension; history of high cholesterol; postmenopausal hormone use; and intakes of dietary fiber, folate, protein, cholesterol, and total energy. $p = 0.01$ for the interaction between BMI and dietary glycemic load. Mean dietary glycemic load for each quintile is shown in parentheses. (From Liu S, Manson JE, Buring JE, et al: Relation between a diet with a high glycemic load and plasma concentrations of high-sensitivity C-reactive protein in middle-aged women. Am J Clin Nutr 75:492, 2002.)

However, given the available data, no recommendation can be made at this time for the use of antioxidant supplements to reduced cardiovascular disease risk.

Lp(a). This risk factor for cardiovascular disease and stroke is under strong genetic regulation, and dietary influences on plasma Lp(a) levels are modest and variable. Increased *trans* fatty acid intake can lead to variable but generally small increases in Lp(a) levels,[102] in contrast to the effects of saturated fatty acids, which reduce Lp(a).[103]

Conclusion

In conclusion, physicians caring for individuals with or at risk of cardiovascular diseases should emphasize the need for implementing "heart healthy" nutritional measures such as those outlined here. Often, nutritional counseling should use allied health professionals such as dietitians for therapeutic nutritional intervention. The epidemic of obesity and its attendant cardiovascular risks warrant heightened attention to nutrition by practitioners and public alike.

REFERENCES

General Dietary Guidelines

1. Krauss RM, Eckel RH, Howard B, et al: AHA Dietary Guidelines—revision 2000: A statement for healthcare professionals from the Nutrition Committee of the American Heart Association. Circulation 102:2284, 2000.
2. Expert Panel on Detection, Evaluation, and Treatment of High Blood Cholesterol in Adults. Executive Summary of the Third Report of The National Cholesterol Education Program (NCEP) Expert Panel on Detection, Evaluation, and Treatment of High Blood Cholesterol in Adults (Adult Treatment Panel III). JAMA 285:2486, 2001.
3. Chobanian AV, Bakris GL, Black HR, et al: The Seventh Report of the Joint National Committee on Prevention, Detection, Evaluation, and Treatment of High Blood Pressure: The JNC 7 report. JAMA 289:2560, 2003.
4. National Heart, Lung, and Blood Institute. Clinical Guidelines on the Identification, Evaluation, and Treatment of Overweight and Obesity in Adults: The Evidence Report. Rockville, MD, National Heart, Lung, and Blood Institute, 1998.

Diets and Nutrients to Prevent Cardiovascular Disease

5. Hu FB, Willett WC: Optimal diets for prevention of coronary heart disease. JAMA 288:2569, 2002.
6. Stampfer MJ, Hu FB, Manson JE, et al: Primary prevention of coronary heart disease in women through diet and lifestyle. N Engl J Med 343:16, 2000.
7. Hu FB, Rimm EB, Stampfer MJ, et al: Prospective study of major dietary patterns and risk of coronary heart disease in men. Am J Clin Nutr 72:912, 2000.
8. Trichopoulou A, Costacou T, Bamia C, Trichopoulos D: Adherence to a Mediterranean diet and survival in a Greek population. N Engl J Med 348:2599, 2003.
9. Barzi F, Woodward M, Marfisi RM, et al: Mediterranean diet and all-causes mortality after myocardial infarction: Results from the GISSI-Prevenzione trial. Eur J Clin Nutr 57:604, 2003.
10. Bazzano LA, He J, Ogden LG, et al: Fruit and vegetable intake and risk of cardiovascular disease in U.S. adults: The First National Health and Nutrition Examination Survey Epidemiologic Follow-up Study. Am J Clin Nutr 76:93, 2002.
11. Joshipura KJ, Hu FB, Manson JE, et al: The effect of fruit and vegetable intake on risk for coronary heart disease. Ann Intern Med 134:1106, 2001.
12. Liu S, Lee IM, Ajani U, et al: Intake of vegetables rich in carotenoids and risk of coronary heart disease in men: The Physicians' Health Study. Int J Epidemiol 30:130, 2001.
13. Liu S, Manson JE, Lee IM, et al: Fruit and vegetable intake and risk of cardiovascular disease: The Women's Health Study. Am J Clin Nutr 72:922, 2000.
14. Appel LJ, Moore TJ, Obarzanek E, et al: A clinical trial of the effects of dietary patterns on blood pressure. DASH Collaborative Research Group. N Engl J Med 336:1117, 1997.
15. Sacks FM, Svetkey LP, Vollmer WM, et al: Effects on blood pressure of reduced dietary sodium and the Dietary Approaches to Stop Hypertension (DASH) diet. DASH-Sodium Collaborative Research Group. N Engl J Med 344:3, 2001.
16. Liu S, Stampfer MJ, Hu FB, et al: Whole-grain consumption and risk of coronary heart disease: Results from the Nurses' Health Study. Am J Clin Nutr 70:412, 1999.
17. Jacobs DR Jr, Meyer KA, Kushi LH, Folsom AR: Whole-grain intake may reduce the risk of ischemic heart disease death in postmenopausal women: The Iowa Women's Health Study. Am J Clin Nutr 68:248, 1998.
18. Wolk A, Manson JE, Stampfer MJ, et al: Long-term intake of dietary fiber and decreased risk of coronary heart disease among women. JAMA 281:1998, 1999.
19. Bazzano LA, He J, Ogden LG, et al: Dietary fiber intake and reduced risk of coronary heart disease in U.S. men and women: The National Health and Nutrition Examination Survey I Epidemiologic Follow-up Study. Arch Intern Med 163:1897, 2003.
20. Liu S, Buring JE, Sesso HD, et al: A prospective study of dietary fiber intake and risk of cardiovascular disease among women. J Am Coll Cardiol 39:49, 2002.
21. Liu S, Willett WC, Stampfer MJ, et al: A prospective study of dietary glycemic load, carbohydrate intake, and risk of coronary heart disease in U.S. women. Am J Clin Nutr 71:1455, 2000.

22. Jenkins DJ, Kendall CW, Augustin LS, et al: Glycemic index: Overview of implications in health and disease. Am J Clin Nutr 76:266S, 2002.
23. Pi-Sunyer FX: Glycemic index and disease. Am J Clin Nutr 76:290S, 2002.
24. Anderson JW, Hanna TJ, Peng X, Kryscio RJ: Whole-grain foods and heart disease risk. J Am Coll Nutr 19:291S, 2000.
25. Bazzano LA, He J, Ogden LG, et al: Legume consumption and risk of coronary heart disease in U.S. men and women: NHANES I Epidemiologic Follow-up Study. Arch Intern Med 161:2573, 2001.
26. Kushi LH, Meyer KA, Jacobs DR Jr: Cereals, legumes, and chronic disease risk reduction: Evidence from epidemiologic studies. Am J Clin Nutr 70:451S, 1999.
27. Erdman JW Jr: AHA Science Advisory: Soy protein and cardiovascular disease: A statement for healthcare professionals from the Nutrition Committee of the AHA. Circulation 102:2555, 2000.
28. Sabate J: Nut consumption, vegetarian diets, ischemic heart disease risk, and all-cause mortality: Evidence from epidemiologic studies. Am J Clin Nutr 70:500S, 1999.
29. Hu FB, Stampfer MJ, Manson JE, et al: Frequent nut consumption and risk of coronary heart disease in women: Prospective cohort study. BMJ 317:1341, 1998.
30. Albert CM, Gaziano JM, Willett WC, Manson JE: Nut consumption and decreased risk of sudden cardiac death in the Physicians' Health Study. Arch Intern Med 162:1382, 2002.
31. Jenkins DJ, Kendall CW, Marchie A, et al: Dose response of almonds on coronary heart disease risk factors: Blood lipids, oxidized low-density lipoproteins, lipoprotein(a), homocysteine, and pulmonary nitric oxide: A randomized, controlled, crossover trial. Circulation 106:1327, 2002.
32. Marckmann P, Gronbaek M: Fish consumption and coronary heart disease mortality: A systematic review of prospective cohort studies. Eur J Clin Nutr 53:585, 1999.
33. Kris-Etherton PM, Harris WS, Appel LJ: Fish consumption, fish oil, omega-3 fatty acids, and cardiovascular disease. Circulation 106:2747, 2002.
34. Albert CM, Hennekens CH, O'Donnell CJ, et al: Fish consumption and risk of sudden cardiac death. JAMA 279:23, 1998.
35. Albert CM, Campos H, Stampfer MJ, et al: Blood levels of long-chain n-3 fatty acids and the risk of sudden death. N Engl J Med 346:1113, 2002.
36. Siscovick DS, Raghunathan T, King I, et al: Dietary intake of long-chain n-3 polyunsaturated fatty acids and the risk of primary cardiac arrest. Am J Clin Nutr 71:208S, 2000.
37. Gruppo Italiano per lo Studio della Sopravvivenza nell'Infarto Miocardico: Dietary supplementation with n-3 polyunsaturated fatty acids and vitamin E after myocardial infarction: results of the GISSI-Prevenzione trial. Lancet 354:447, 1999
38. Marchioli R, Barzi F, Bomba E, et al: Early protection against sudden death by n-3 polyunsaturated fatty acids after myocardial infarction: Time-course analysis of the results of the Gruppo Italiano per lo Studio della Sopravvivenza nell'Infarto Miocardico (GISSI)-Prevenzione. Circulation 105:1897, 2002.

Alcohol Consumption and Cardiovascular Disease

39. Vogel RA: Alcohol, heart disease, and mortality: A review. Rev Cardiovasc Med 3:7, 2002.
40. Goldberg IJ, Mosca L, Piano MR, Fisher EA: AHA Science Advisory: Wine and your heart: A science advisory for healthcare professionals from the Nutrition Committee, Council on Epidemiology and Prevention, and Council on Cardiovascular Nursing of the American Heart Association. Stroke 32:591, 2001.
41. Sierksma A, van der Gaag MS, Kluft C, Hendriks HF: Moderate alcohol consumption reduces plasma C-reactive protein and fibrinogen levels: A randomized, diet-controlled intervention study. Eur J Clin Nutr 56:1130, 2002.
42. Albert MA, Glynn RJ, Ridker PM: Alcohol consumption and plasma concentration of C-reactive protein. Circulation 107:443, 2003.
43. Mukamal KJ, Conigrave KM, Mittleman MA, et al: Roles of drinking pattern and type of alcohol consumed in coronary heart disease in men. N Engl J Med 348:109, 2003.
44. Pearson TA: AHA Science Advisory: Alcohol and heart disease. Nutrition Committee of the American Heart Association. Am J Clin Nutr 65:1567, 1997.

Diet, Lifestyle Modification, Obesity, and Cardiovascular Disease

45. Sacks FM, Katan M: Randomized clinical trials on the effects of dietary fat and carbohydrate on plasma lipoproteins and cardiovascular disease. Am J Med 113(Suppl 9B):13S, 2002.
46. de Lorgeril M, Salen P, Martin JL, et al: Mediterranean diet, traditional risk factors, and the rate of cardiovascular complications after myocardial infarction: Final report of the Lyon Diet Heart Study. Circulation 99:779, 1999.
47. Ornish D, Scherwitz LW, Billings JH, et al: Intensive lifestyle changes for reversal of coronary heart disease. JAMA 280:2001, 1998.
48. Koertge J, Weidner G, Elliott-Eller M, et al: Improvement in medical risk factors and quality of life in women and men with coronary artery disease in the Multicenter Lifestyle Demonstration Project. Am J Cardiol 91:1316, 2003.
49. Mokdad AH, Ford ES, Bowman BA, et al: Prevalence of obesity, diabetes, and obesity-related health risk factors. JAMA 289:76, 2001
50. Eckel RH: Obesity and heart disease: A statement for healthcare professionals from the Nutrition Committee, American Heart Association. Circulation 96:3248, 1997.
51. Lean ME, Han TS, Prvan T, et al: Weight loss with high and low carbohydrate 1200 kcal diets in free living women. Eur J Clin Nutr 51:243, 1997.
52. Hirsch J, Hudgins LC, Leibel RL, Rosenbaum M: Diet composition and energy balance in humans. Am J Clin Nutr 67:551S, 1998.
53. McGuire MT, Wing RR, Klem ML, Hill JO: Behavioral strategies of individuals who have maintained long-term weight losses. Obes Res 7:334, 1999.
54. Samaha FF, Iqbal N, Seshadri P, et al: A low-carbohydrate as compared with a low-fat diet in severe obesity. N Engl J Med 348:2074, 2003.
55. Foster GD, Wyatt HR, Hill JO, et al: A randomized trial of a low-carbohydrate diet for obesity. N Engl J Med 348:2082, 2003.
56. Westman EC, Yancy WS, Edman JS, et al: Effect of 6-month adherence to a very low carbohydrate diet program. Am J Med 113:30, 2002.
57. Bonow RO, Eckel RH: Diet, obesity, and cardiovascular risk. N Engl J Med 348:2057, 2003.
58. St Jeor ST, Howard BV, Prewitt TE, et al: Dietary protein and weight reduction: A statement for healthcare professionals from the Nutrition Committee of the Council on Nutrition, Physical Activity, and Metabolism of the American Heart Association. Circulation 104:1869, 2001.
59. Mensink RP, Zock PL, Kester AD, Katan MB: Effects of dietary fatty acids and carbohydrates on the ratio of serum total to HDL cholesterol and on serum lipids and apolipoproteins: A meta-analysis of 60 controlled trials. Am J Clin Nutr 77:1146, 2003.
60. National Academy of Sciences and Institute of Medicine: Dietary Reference Intakes: Energy, carbohydrate, fiber, fat, fatty acids, cholesterol, protein, and amino acids. Washington, DC, National Academies Press, 2002.
61. Hu FB, Stampfer MJ, Rimm EB, et al: A prospective study of egg consumption and risk of cardiovascular disease in men and women. JAMA 281:1387, 1999.
62. Dreon DM, Krauss RM: Diet-gene interactions in human lipoprotein metabolism. J Am Coll Nutr 16:313, 1997.
63. Schaefer EJ, Lamon-Fava S, Ausman LM, et al: Individual variability in lipoprotein cholesterol response to National Cholesterol Education Program Step 2 diets. Am J Clin Nutr 65:823, 1997.
64. Hu FB, Manson JE, Willett WC: Types of dietary fat and risk of coronary heart disease: A critical review. J Am Coll Nutr 20:5, 2001.
65. Lichtenstein AH, Deckelbaum RJ: AHA Science Advisory. Stanol/sterol ester-containing foods and blood cholesterol levels: A statement for healthcare professionals from the Nutrition Committee of the Council on Nutrition, Physical Activity, and Metabolism of the American Heart Association. Circulation 103:1177, 2001.
66. Van Horn L: Fiber, lipids, and coronary heart disease: A statement for healthcare professionals from the Nutrition Committee, American Heart Association. Circulation 95:2701, 1997.
67. Jenkins DJ, Kendall CW, Marchie A, et al: Effects of a dietary portfolio of cholesterol-lowering foods versus lovastatin on serum lipids and C-reactive protein. JAMA 290:502, 2003.
68. Grundy SM: Hypertriglyceridemia, atherogenic dyslipidemia, and the metabolic syndrome. Am J Cardiol 81:18B, 1998.
69. Berneis KK, Krauss RM: Metabolic origins and clinical significance of LDL heterogeneity. J Lipid Res 43:1363, 2002.
70. Parks EJ, Hellerstein MK: Carbohydrate-induced hypertriacylglycerolemia: Historical perspective and review of biological mechanisms. Am J Clin Nutr 71:412, 2000.
71. Krauss RM: Dietary and genetic effects on low-density lipoprotein heterogeneity. Annu Rev Nutr 21:283, 2001.

Dietary Factors and Blood Pressure Control

72. Kotchen TA, McCarron DA: Dietary electrolytes and blood pressure: A statement for healthcare professionals from the American Heart Association Nutrition Committee. Circulation 98:613, 1998.
73. Graudal NA, Galloe AM, Garred P: Effects of sodium restriction on blood pressure, renin, aldosterone, catecholamines, cholesterols, and triglyceride: A meta-analysis. JAMA 279:1383, 1998.
74. Obarzanek E, Proschan MA, Vollmer WM, et al: Individual blood pressure responses to changes in salt intake: Results from the DASH-Sodium Trial. Hypertension 42:459, 2003.
75. Trials of Hypertension Prevention Collaborative Research Group. Effects of weight loss and sodium reduction intervention on blood pressure and hypertension incidence in overweight people with high-normal blood pressure: The Trials of Hypertension Prevention, Phase II. Arch Intern Med 157:657, 1997.
76. Whelton PK, Appel LJ, Espeland MA, et al: Sodium reduction and weight loss in the treatment of hypertension in older persons: A randomized controlled trial of nonpharmacologic interventions in the elderly (TONE). TONE Collaborative Research Group. JAMA 279:839, 1998.
77. Klatsky AL: Alcohol and cardiovascular disease—more than one paradox to consider. Alcohol and hypertension: does it matter? Yes. J Cardiovasc Risk 10:21, 2003.
78. Cushman WC, Cutler JA, Hanna E, et al: Prevention and Treatment of Hypertension Study (PATHS): Effects of an alcohol treatment program on blood pressure. Arch Intern Med 158:1197, 1998.
79. Vaskonen T: Dietary minerals and modification of cardiovascular risk factors. J Nutr Biochem 14:492, 2003.
80. Whelton PK, He J, Cutler JA, et al: Effects of oral potassium on blood pressure: Meta-analysis of randomized controlled clinical trials. JAMA 277:1624, 1997.
81. Svetkey LP Simons-Morton D, Vollmer WM, et al: Effects of dietary patterns on blood pressure: Subgroup analysis of the Dietary Approaches to Stop Hypertension (DASH) randomized clinical trial. Arch Intern Med 159:285, 1999.
82. Vollmer WM, Sacks FM, Ard J, et al: Effects of diet and sodium intake on blood pressure: Subgroup analysis of the DASH-Sodium trial. Ann Intern Med 135:1019, 2001.
83. Resnick LM, Oparil S, Chait A, et al: Factors affecting blood pressure responses to diet: The Vanguard study. Am J Hypertens 13:956, 2000.
84. Bao DQ, Mori TA, Burke V, et al: Effects of dietary fish and weight reduction on ambulatory blood pressure in overweight hypertensives. Hypertension 32:710, 1998.
85. Saltzman E, Das SK, Lichtenstein AH, et al: An oat-containing hypocaloric diet reduces systolic blood pressure and improves lipid profile beyond effects of weight loss in men and women. J Nutr 131:1465, 2001.
86. Burke V, Hodgson JM, Beilin LJ, et al: Dietary protein and soluble fiber reduce ambulatory blood pressure in treated hypertensives. Hypertension 38:821, 2001.
87. Teede HJ, Dalais FS, Kotsopoulos D, et al: Dietary soy has both beneficial and potentially adverse cardiovascular effects: A placebo-controlled study in men and postmenopausal women. J Clin Endocrinol Metab 86:3053, 2001.
88. Rivas M, Garay RP, Escanero JF, et al: Soy milk lowers blood pressure in men and women with mild to moderate essential hypertension. J Nutr 132:1900, 2002.

89. Taubert D, Berkels R, Roesen R, Klaus W: Chocolate and blood pressure in elderly individuals with isolated systolic hypertension. JAMA 290:1029, 2003.
90. Bautista LE, Arenas IA, Penuela A, Martinez LX: Total plasma homocysteine level and risk of cardiovascular disease: A meta-analysis of prospective cohort studies. J Clin Epidemiol 55:882, 2002.
91. Homocysteine Cooperative Research Group. Homocysteine and risk of ischemic heart disease and stroke: A meta-analysis. JAMA 288:2015, 2002.
92. Malinow MR, Bostom AG, Krauss RM: Homocyst(e)ine, diet, and cardiovascular diseases: A statement for healthcare professionals from the Nutrition Committee, American Heart Association. Circulation 99:178, 1999.
93. Schnyder G, Roffi M, Flammer Y, et al: Effect of homocysteine-lowering therapy with folic acid, vitamin B_{12}, and vitamin B_6 on clinical outcome after percutaneous coronary intervention: The Swiss Heart study: A randomized controlled trial. JAMA 288:973, 2002.
94. Bostom AG, Jacques PF, Liaugaudas G, et al: Total homocysteine-lowering treatment among coronary artery disease patients in the era of folic acid–fortified cereal grain flour. Arterioscler Thromb Vasc Biol 22:488, 2002.

Other Dietary Factors and Cardiovascular Risk

95. Pearson TA, Mensah GA, Alexander RW, et al: Markers of inflammation and cardiovascular disease—application to clinical and public health practice: A statement for healthcare professionals from the Centers for Disease Control and Prevention and the American Heart Association. Circulation 107:499, 2003.
96. McLaughlin T, Abbasi F, Lamendola C, et al: Differentiation between obesity and insulin resistance in the association with C-reactive protein. Circulation 106:2908, 2002.
97. Esposito K, Pontillo A, Di Palo C, et al: Effect of weight loss and lifestyle changes on vascular inflammatory markers in obese women: A randomized trial. JAMA 289:1799, 2003.
98. Liu S, Manson JE, Buring JE, et al: Relation between a diet with a high glycemic load and plasma concentrations of high-sensitivity C-reactive protein in middle-aged women. Am J Clin Nutr 75:492, 2002.
99. Tribble DL: AHA Science Advisory. Antioxidant consumption and risk of coronary heart disease: Emphasis on vitamin C, vitamin E, and beta-carotene: A statement for healthcare professionals from the American Heart Association. Circulation 99:591, 1999.
100. Morris CD, Carson S: Routine vitamin supplementation to prevent cardiovascular disease: A summary of the evidence for the U.S. Preventive Services Task Force. Ann Intern Med 139:56, 2003.
101. Brown BG, Zhao XQ, Chait A, et al: Simvastatin and niacin, antioxidant vitamins, or the combination for the prevention of coronary disease. N Engl J Med 345:1583, 2001.
102. Lichtenstein AH: Dietary *trans* fatty acid. J Cardiopulm Rehabil 20:143, 2000.
103. Ginsberg HN, Kris-Etherton P, Dennis B, et al: Effects of reducing dietary saturated fatty acids on plasma lipids and lipoproteins in healthy subjects: The DELTA Study, protocol 1. Arterioscler Thromb Vasc Biol 18:441, 1998.

CHAPTER 42

Primary and Secondary Prevention of Coronary Heart Disease

J. Michael Gaziano • JoAnn E. Manson • Paul M. Ridker

Both primary and secondary prevention of coronary heart disease (CHD) have indisputable public health importance. Given the prevalence of CHD, preventing even a small proportion of cases would save thousands of lives, avoid inestimable suffering, and save billions of health care dollars. In addition, measures that prevent CHD may also mitigate other manifestations of atherosclerosis, such as stroke and peripheral artery disease, and may have an impact on hypertension, diabetes, cancer, cognitive function, depression, and other chronic conditions as well. Because cardiovascular diseases (CVDs) will soon become the number one killer worldwide,[1] widespread deployment of affordable preventive strategies should have high priority in both developed and developing countries.[2]

The great strides made over the last 50 years toward understanding the pathophysiology of atherosclerosis and identifying a large number of life-style, biochemical, and genetic factors potentially associated with CHD have contributed to significant declines in age-adjusted cardiovascular mortality (Fig. 42–1). The first step toward prevention entails using these factors to predict who is likely to experience atherosclerotic events. Several scores have been developed that use different risk factors to estimate an individual's risk of future cardiovascular events. Yet the process of disease prevention must push beyond using factors to predict future events and move toward establishing interventions that definitively reduce risk. Weighing the benefits of given interventions against their risks and costs has led to the establishment of guidelines for health providers and the general public. Implementing these guidelines, however, remains a difficult task. Lack of time is certainly one hurdle. Delivering only those cardiovascular-related preventive services recommended by the U.S. Preventive Services Task Force would take the representative clinician a minimum of 1.5 hours per day.[3] Lack of reimbursement also limits the delivery of preventive interventions.

This chapter defines risk factors in a novel way. First, we discuss the various types of risk factors and their utility in predicting risk. Then we present a scheme for prioritizing preventive interventions that divides these interventions into the following three categories:

- Class 1 interventions are those for risk factors with a clear causal relationship with heart disease where the benefits of intervention have been established.
- Class 2 interventions are those for risk factors that appear to have a causal relationship with heart disease and for which the data suggest that intervention will probably reduce coronary events, but for which there are limited data regarding the benefits, risks, and costs of the intervention.
- Class 3 interventions are those for which an independent causal relationship with heart disease is suspected but as yet unproved.

The chapter then examines 13 potentially modifiable risk factor domains and interventions, with information on prevalence, associated risk, benefit of treatment, cost efficacy, and recommendations/guidelines for each. It concludes with a discussion of multiple risk factor interventions.

About Risk Factors

In addition to detailed descriptions of the natural history and epidemiology of atherosclerosis and coronary disease, the Framingham Heart Study gave modern medicine the term *risk factor.* In a 1961 report, Kannel and colleagues described "factors of risk" associated with the development of CHD.[4] Since then, the term has become an integral part of the language of epidemiology, cardiology, and a host of other disciplines.

"Risk factor" generally applies to a parameter that can predict a future cardiovascular event. For the purposes of risk prediction, what matters is the predictive value of the risk factor, the feasibility of assessing it, and the cost of assessment. Age, for example, is a useful predictor, because it is strongly associated with cardiovascular risk and can be assessed easily and at no cost. However, when trying to identify potential targets for intervention, it is worth considering which factors can be modified to lower risk, such as smoking. Risk factors can be divided into four basic categories (Table 42–1): predisposing factors, risk-modifying behaviors, metabolic risk factors, and disease markers.

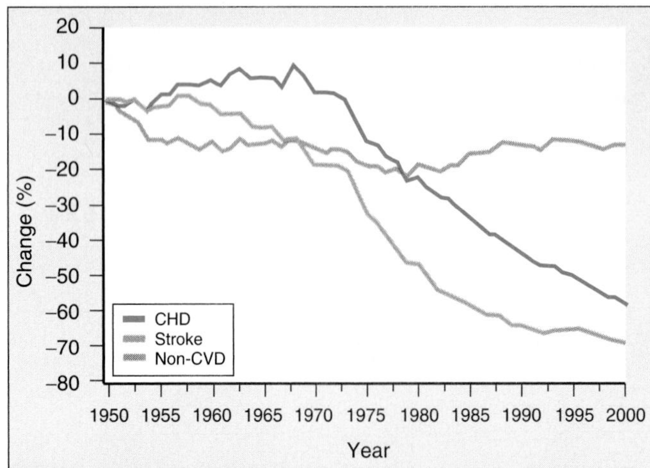

FIGURE 42–1 Change in age-adjusted mortality from coronary heart disease (CHD), stroke, and non-CVD in the United States, 1950 to 2000. CVD = cardiovascular disease. (From Morbidity and Mortality: 2002 Chart Book on Cardiovascular, Lung, and Blood Diseases. Bethesda, MD, National Heart, Lung, and Blood Institute, 2002, p 23.) (See also Chap. 36.)

TABLE 42–1 Four Basic Categories of Risk Factors

Category	Risk Factors
Predisposing factors	Age, sex, family history, genes
Risk-modifying behaviors	Smoking, atherogenic diet, alcohol intake, physical activity
Metabolic risk factors	Dyslipidemias, hypertension, obesity, diabetes, metabolic syndrome
Disease markers	Calcium score, catheterization results, stress test results, left ventricular hypertrophy on echocardiogram, personal history of vascular disease (prior myocardial infarction or stroke, angina, peripheral vascular disease), inflammatory state

These distinctions may be useful but are somewhat arbitrary. At times it may be difficult to classify a factor in a distinct category. For example, family history could represent an individual's genes *or* behaviors that are passed from one generation to the next. Is hypertension a metabolic risk factor that results in part from the influence of risk-modifying behaviors such as an atherosclerotic diet or physical inactivity, or is it a marker of endothelial dysfunction and atherosclerosis? Similarly, an inflammatory state as measured by high-sensitivity C-reactive protein (hs-CRP) could be considered as a metabolic intermediate, such as high cholesterol, or may be a marker of ongoing atherosclerosis. The four categories of risk factors described earlier are useful in considering potential targets for intervention but require evaluation in clinical trials to confirm any suspected modifiability.

In this framework, predisposing factors such as genes interact with behavioral factors and lead to metabolic abnormalities that may eventually lead to cardiovascular disease. For example, an atherogenic diet and lack of exercise in a genetically susceptible individual increase low-density lipoprotein (LDL) cholesterol, which leads to endothelial dysfunction, fatty streaks, atherosclerotic plaques, and eventually to cardiovascular events. Metabolic factors can interact in similar ways to accelerate this process.

For a factor to be useful in prediction, it must be easy and inexpensive to measure—a major potential limitation for expensive techniques such as screening with electron-beam computed tomography (CT). Further, the false-positive rate associated with screening must be low to avoid unnecessary and potentially hazardous consequences. Although predictive value is *necessary* to infer that modification of a risk factor will lead to reduced risk, it is not *sufficient*. The benefit of intervention must clearly exceed any risks and be worth the cost. Then it must be implemented in appropriate populations.

Figure 42–2 describes a way of classifying risk factors by their ability to predict disease and their proven utility for modifying the chance of future events. Although some risk factors that correctly predict disease may be targets for future interventions, we consider only those factors for which there is strong evidence that modification reduces cardiovascular risk. Several preventive medications, such as aspirin, and cardiovascular interventions have been added to the list of interventions that modify risk because of their ability to lower the risk of future events, and therefore they must be considered when addressing prevention for a patient. This chapter considers only those factors that modify intermediate or long-term risk. Interventions used acutely to modify short-term risk, such as aspirin in the setting of an acute myocardial infarction, are considered elsewhere in this text (see Chap. 47).

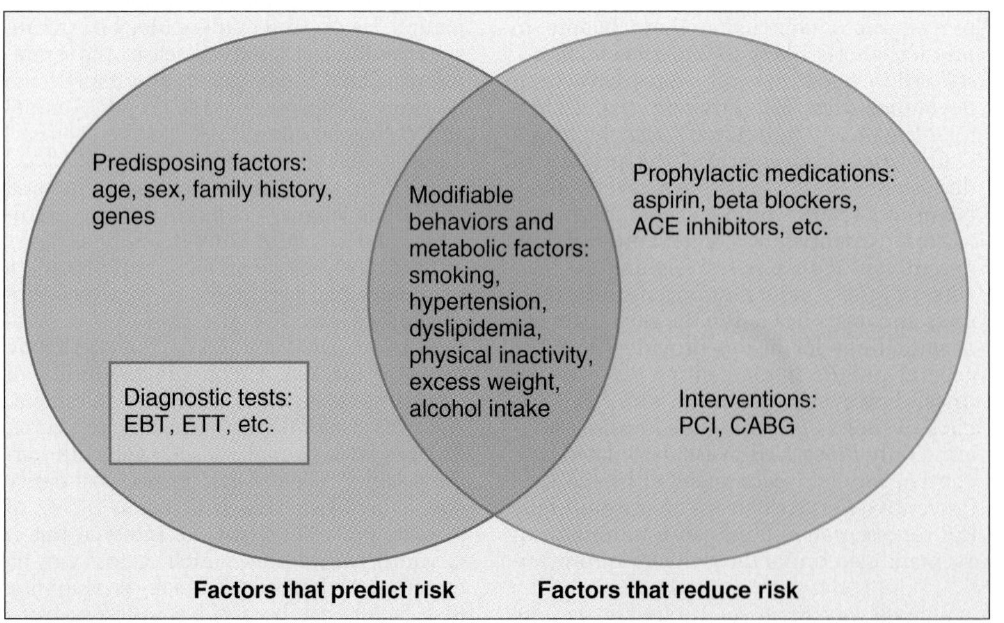

FIGURE 42–2 Classification of risk factors by their ability to predict disease and their proven utility for modifying the chance of future events. EBT = electron-beam tomography; ETT = exercise tolerance test; ACE = angiotensin-converting enzyme; PCI = percutaneous coronary intervention; CABG = coronary artery bypass graft. (See also Chap. 36.)

Predicting Risk

A fundamental step in establishing individual or population-wide preventive strategies involves assessing the risk of development of clinically relevant outcomes because the cost efficacy of any intervention varies according to global risk in a given individual or population. Since absolute risk among those with known disease is higher than among those at lower risk, fewer high-risk individuals require treatment to save one life or prevent one event in comparison to those at lower risk, even if relative risk reductions are identical in both groups. To illustrate this concept, assume that an intervention reduces mortality by 25 percent in both primary and secondary prevention. Furthermore, assume that a high-risk individual with CHD has a 20 percent chance of death from cardiovascular disease over the next 10 years while a low-risk individual has a 1 percent chance of death over the same period. To save a life among those at high risk, one would have to treat only 20 patients (4 of whom are destined to die) for 10 years so that a 25 percent relative risk reduction would result in 1 life saved (3 deaths instead of 4). On the other hand, one would have to treat 400 low-risk patients (4 of whom are also destined to die) so that the same 25 percent relative risk reduction would yield 3 deaths instead of 4. Thus, the total cost per lives saved is considerably lower ($\frac{1}{20}$ the cost) among individuals at higher absolute risk. Assessing an individual's absolute risk enables cost-effective targeting of interventions. Accordingly, the National Cholesterol Education Program (NCEP) Adult Treatment Panel (ATP) III[5] and the Seventh Joint National Committee on Prevention, Detection, Evaluation, and Treatment of High Blood Pressure (JNC-7)[6] now use absolute risk to gauge the intensity of intervention. The American Diabetes Association also recommends a tiered approach to management based on absolute risk.[7]

Assessing Individual Risk

A crude way to categorize individuals as being at higher or lower risk is by the presence or absence of cardiovascular disease. Those with known cardiovascular disease, including coronary, cerebrovascular, or peripheral artery disease, are on average at much higher risk than those without known disease. Approximately 80% of those with known cardiovascular disease will die of some form of cardiovascular disease, whereas those without known cardiovascular disease have approximately half that cardiovascular disease mortality rate. As discussed later in this chapter, those with cardiovascular disease generally warrant aggressive preventive interventions. Risk reduction in those with known cardiovascular disease is referred to as *secondary prevention*, as opposed to primary prevention among those without overt cardiovascular disease. Individuals with diabetes comprise a second high-risk group. Rates of cardiovascular disease events and mortality among diabetic patients considerably exceed those in the general population; thus, patients with diabetes warrant aggressive preventive interventions. Another group of patients that is at exceedingly high risk for cardiovascular disease events and death are those with chronic renal failure, many of whom have diabetes.

For those without overt cardiovascular disease or diabetes, other predictive risk factors should be used to assess overall risk. Several risk prediction strategies have been developed using some of the predictive risk factors outlined in Figure 42–2. Framingham Heart Study investigators have developed a useful tool to assess risk of a first cardiovascular event based on age, gender, total or LDL cholesterol, high-density lipoprotein (HDL) cholesterol, systolic and diastolic blood pressure, and history of diabetes and cigarette smoking (Fig. 42–3).[8] Point-based weights are assigned to the presence and/or level of each risk factor. Once the points have been assigned and summed, the total score can be translated to an estimated absolute risk of a CHD event occurring within the next 10 years. The National Heart, Lung, and Blood Institute has made available an online version of the 10-year risk calculator (hin.nhlbi.nih.gov/atpiii/calculator.asp), as well as versions that can be downloaded to a clinician's desktop computer (hin.nhlbi.nih.gov/atpiii/riskcalc.htm) or handheld device (hin.nhlbi.nih.gov/atpiii/atp3palm.htm).

Risk assessment scales are also available from the Framingham investigators for the secondary prevention of myocardial infarction and stroke. However, since all patients with prior evidence of cardiovascular disease have high risk for recurrent events and require aggressive preventive efforts, the utility of these tools is unclear.

The European Society of Cardiology (ESC) has also assembled recommendations for the prevention of heart disease that stratify preventive interventions according to whether a patient is at high, intermediate, or low risk.[9] Those with known CHD constitute the highest-risk category because most of these individuals have a greater than 20 percent chance of subsequent events over the next 10 years. Individuals without known CHD are assessed for risk with a modified Framingham assessment tool. This tool, presented in a series of easy-to-use charts, allows clinicians to assess risk over the next 10 years based on age, gender, smoking status, diabetes, level of cholesterol, and blood pressure (Fig. 42–4). Those for whom the risk of a primary event exceeds 20 percent over the next 10 years are recommended for aggressive management. Those for whom risk is lower are prescribed a less intense and less costly approach.

A third method of assessing absolute risk in men has emerged from the Prospective Cardiovascular Munster (PROCAM) Study, a long-term follow-up study of more than 5000 men aged 35 to 65 years recruited between 1979 and 1985. Risk factors included in the PROCAM algorithm include cigarette smoking, systolic blood pressure, LDL cholesterol, HDL cholesterol, fasting triglycerides, diabetes, family history of myocardial infarction, and age. Answers to questions regarding these factors is tallied into a point score, just as with the Framingham algorithm, and this point score is converted into a 10-year absolute risk of fatal or nonfatal myocardial infarction or sudden cardiac death.[10] Scores for women are not yet available.

These scores provide a good initial method for assessing risk at low cost. A number of diagnostic tests and novel biochemical markers have emerged as potential ways to augment these simple scores. Calcium scores determined by electron-beam CT and exercise tolerance tests represent two such diagnostic tests for which substantial data are available. Another is hs-CRP, a marker of inflammation that holds promise in providing incremental predictive value. As reviewed in Chapter 36, hs-CRP adds prognostic information at all levels of LDL cholesterol, at all levels of the metabolic syndrome, and at all levels of the Framingham Risk Score. However, these tests entail costs and potential consequences, and their utility in prevention remains controversial.

Although the various risk prediction scores tend to categorize individuals similarly, there are differences. Compared to the ESC score, the Framingham Heart Study score tends to predict slightly higher overall risk.[11] However, for the purposes of broad categorization of individuals, there is generally good agreement between the two scores.

Assessing Risk at a Population Level: Incidence, Prevalence, and Population-Attributable Risk

Sound public policy also requires evaluation of the impact of different factors on the *population*. Population risk depends not only on the strength of the risk factor–disease association and the benefit of intervention but also on how common the factor is in the general population. These concepts are captured in incidence, prevalence, and population-attributable risk. Although incidence rates reflect the frequency of new cases of disease or a risk factor over a given period, prevalence reflects the proportion of individuals with a given condition or factor at a single point. Population-attributable risk, or how much of the population's risk of disease is attributable to a

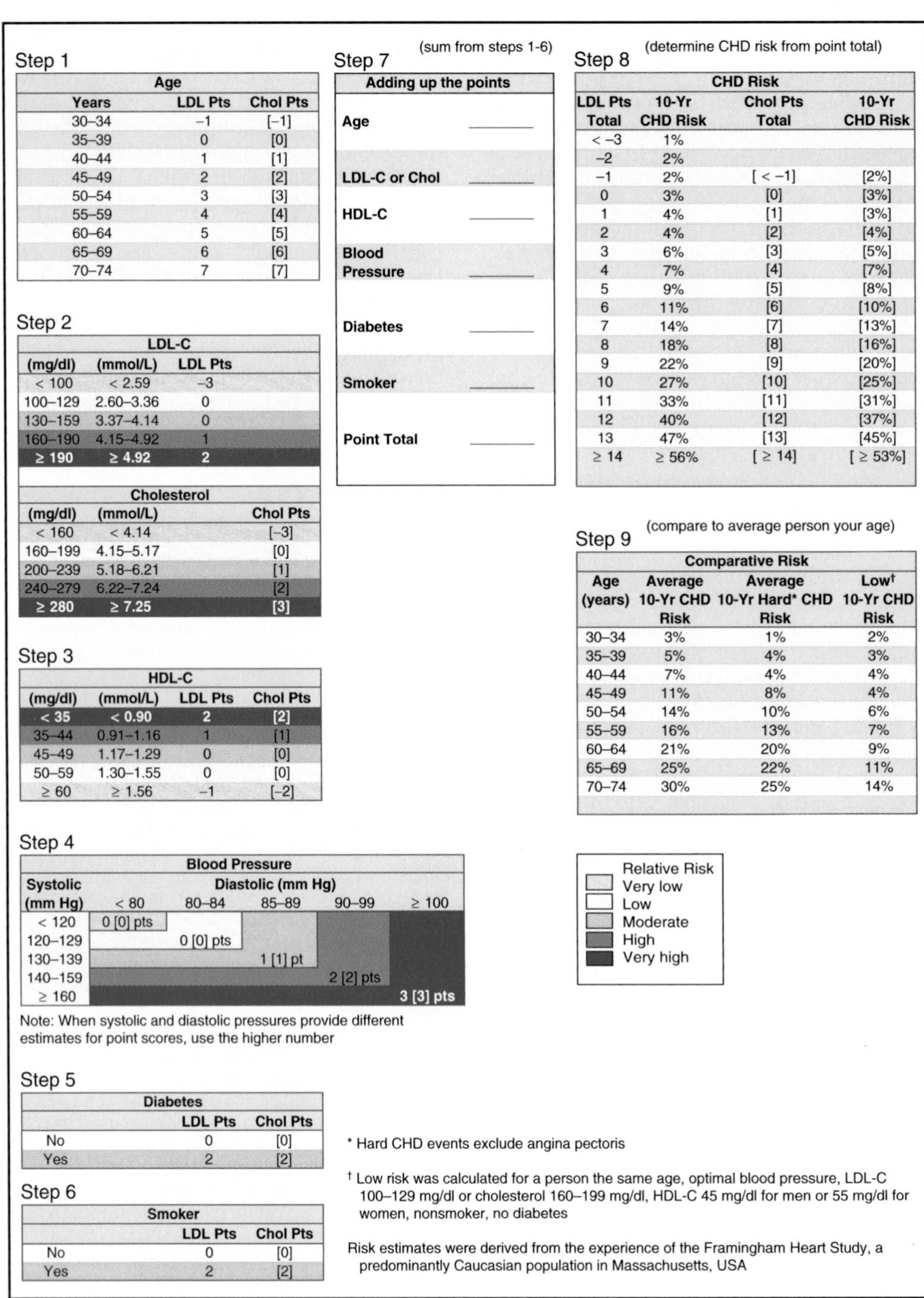

Step 1

Age		
Years	LDL Pts	Chol Pts
30–34	−1	[−1]
35–39	0	[0]
40–44	1	[1]
45–49	2	[2]
50–54	3	[3]
55–59	4	[4]
60–64	5	[5]
65–69	6	[6]
70–74	7	[7]

Step 2

LDL-C		
(mg/dl)	(mmol/L)	LDL Pts
< 100	< 2.59	−3
100–129	2.60–3.36	0
130–159	3.37–4.14	0
160–190	4.15–4.92	1
≥ 190	≥ 4.92	2

Cholesterol		
(mg/dl)	(mmol/L)	Chol Pts
< 160	< 4.14	[−3]
160–199	4.15–5.17	[0]
200–239	5.18–6.21	[1]
240–279	6.22–7.24	[2]
≥ 280	≥ 7.25	[3]

Step 3

HDL-C			
(mg/dl)	(mmol/L)	LDL Pts	Chol Pts
< 35	< 0.90	2	[2]
35–44	0.91–1.16	1	[1]
45–49	1.17–1.29	0	[0]
50–59	1.30–1.55	0	[0]
≥ 60	≥ 1.56	−1	[−2]

Step 4

Blood Pressure					
Systolic	Diastolic (mm Hg)				
(mm Hg)	< 80	80–84	85–89	90–99	≥ 100
< 120	0 [0] pts				
120–129		0 [0] pts			
130–139			1 [1] pt		
140–159				2 [2] pts	
≥ 160					3 [3] pts

Note: When systolic and diastolic pressures provide different estimates for point scores, use the higher number

Step 5

Diabetes		
	LDL Pts	Chol Pts
No	0	[0]
Yes	2	[2]

Step 6

Smoker		
	LDL Pts	Chol Pts
No	0	[0]
Yes	2	[2]

Step 7 (sum from steps 1-6)

Adding up the points	
Age	_____
LDL-C or Chol	_____
HDL-C	_____
Blood Pressure	_____
Diabetes	_____
Smoker	_____
Point Total	_____

Step 8 (determine CHD risk from point total)

CHD Risk			
LDL Pts Total	10-Yr CHD Risk	Chol Pts Total	10-Yr CHD Risk
< −3	1%		
−2	2%		
−1	2%	[< −1]	[2%]
0	3%	[0]	[3%]
1	4%	[1]	[3%]
2	4%	[2]	[4%]
3	6%	[3]	[5%]
4	7%	[4]	[7%]
5	9%	[5]	[8%]
6	11%	[6]	[10%]
7	14%	[7]	[13%]
8	18%	[8]	[16%]
9	22%	[9]	[20%]
10	27%	[10]	[25%]
11	33%	[11]	[31%]
12	40%	[12]	[37%]
13	47%	[13]	[45%]
≥ 14	≥ 56%	[≥ 14]	[≥ 53%]

Step 9 (compare to average person your age)

Comparative Risk			
Age (years)	Average 10-Yr CHD Risk	Average 10-Yr Hard* CHD Risk	Low† 10-Yr CHD Risk
30–34	3%	1%	2%
35–39	5%	4%	3%
40–44	7%	4%	4%
45–49	11%	8%	4%
50–54	14%	10%	6%
55–59	16%	13%	7%
60–64	21%	20%	9%
65–69	25%	22%	11%
70–74	30%	25%	14%

Relative Risk
Very low
Low
Moderate
High
Very high

* Hard CHD events exclude angina pectoris

† Low risk was calculated for a person the same age, optimal blood pressure, LDL-C 100–129 mg/dl or cholesterol 160–199 mg/dl, HDL-C 45 mg/dl for men or 55 mg/dl for women, nonsmoker, no diabetes

Risk estimates were derived from the experience of the Framingham Heart Study, a predominantly Caucasian population in Massachusetts, USA

A

FIGURE 42–3 Coronary heart disease (CHD) score sheets for calculating 10-year CHD risk according to age, total cholesterol (TC) (or low-density lipoprotein cholesterol [LDL-C]), high-density lipoprotein cholesterol (HDL-C), blood pressure, diabetes, and smoking. **A,** Score sheet for men based on the Framingham experience in men 30 to 74 years of age at baseline. Average risk estimates are based on typical Framingham subjects, and estimates of idealized risk are based on optimal blood pressure, TC of 160 to 199 mg/dl (or LDL of 100 to 129 mg/dl), HDL-C of 45 mg/dl, no diabetes, and no smoking.

given factor, is driven by the proportion of the public with a given risk factor and the magnitude of the associated risk.

Population-attributable risk also reflects the shape of the relationship between the exposure and the disease. Many factors increase risk in a linear fashion, so population-attributable risk can be computed against an ideal standard or a low-risk individual. For example, the relationship between hypertension and heart disease and stroke is linear. Thus, lowering blood pressure at any level in the pathological range reduces risk. In contrast, the shape of the risk curve for obesity appears nonlinear, with risk increasing logarithmically (Fig. 42–5). Thus, each incremental pound gained is associated with much more risk in those who are already overweight. Population-attributable risk is an important concept for determining resource allocation between various preventive interventions.

Preventive Intervention Strategies for Modifiable Risk Factors

Some predictive risk factors are potential targets for intervention. A crucial step in developing preventive intervention

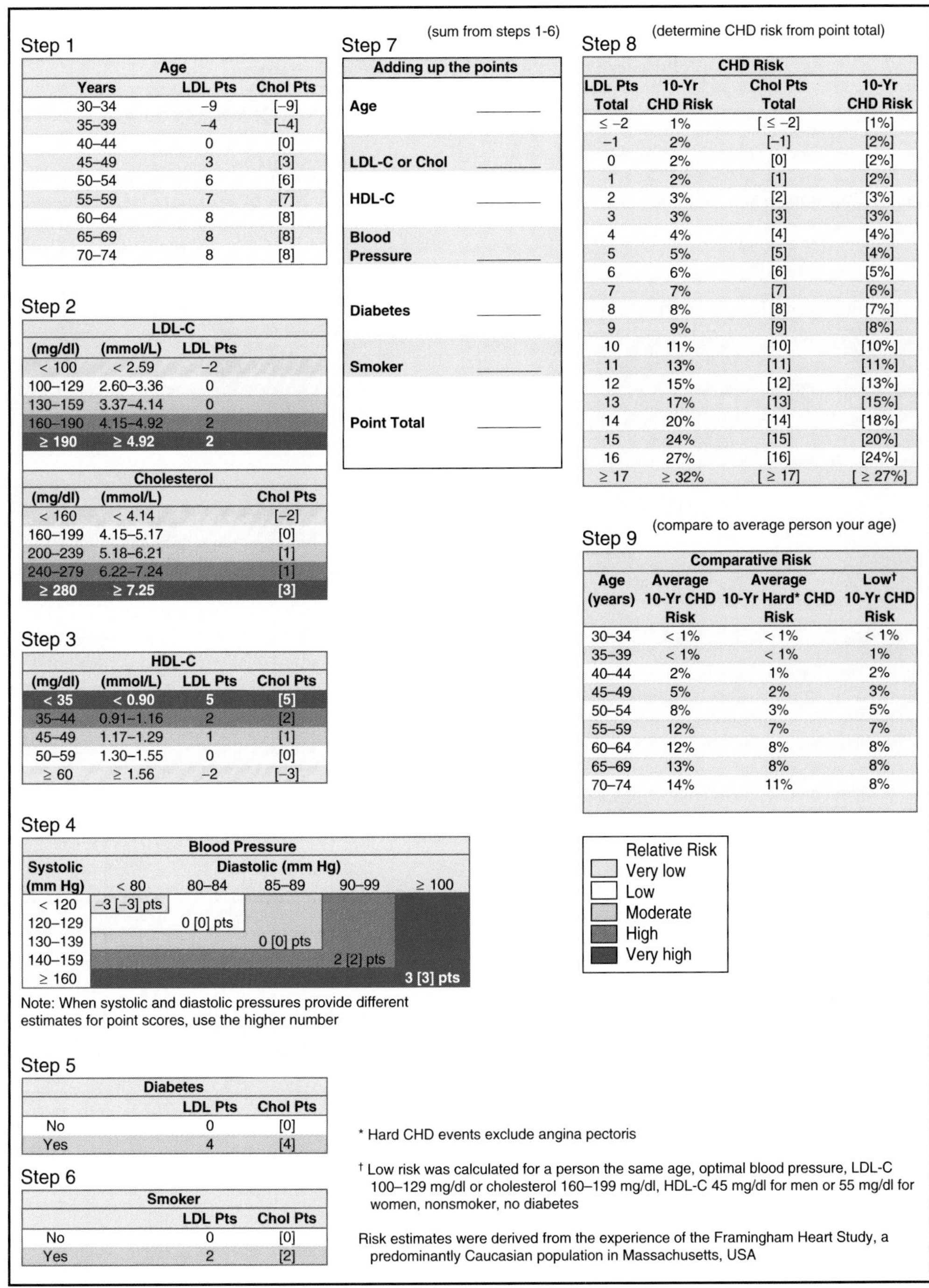

Step 1

Age		
Years	LDL Pts	Chol Pts
30–34	−9	[−9]
35–39	−4	[−4]
40–44	0	[0]
45–49	3	[3]
50–54	6	[6]
55–59	7	[7]
60–64	8	[8]
65–69	8	[8]
70–74	8	[8]

Step 2

LDL-C		
(mg/dl)	(mmol/L)	LDL Pts
< 100	< 2.59	−2
100–129	2.60–3.36	0
130–159	3.37–4.14	0
160–190	4.15–4.92	2
≥ 190	≥ 4.92	2

Cholesterol		
(mg/dl)	(mmol/L)	Chol Pts
< 160	< 4.14	[−2]
160–199	4.15–5.17	[0]
200–239	5.18–6.21	[1]
240–279	6.22–7.24	[1]
≥ 280	≥ 7.25	[3]

Step 3

HDL-C			
(mg/dl)	(mmol/L)	LDL Pts	Chol Pts
< 35	< 0.90	5	[5]
35–44	0.91–1.16	2	[2]
45–49	1.17–1.29	1	[1]
50–59	1.30–1.55	0	[0]
≥ 60	≥ 1.56	−2	[−3]

Step 4

Blood Pressure					
Systolic (mm Hg)	Diastolic (mm Hg)				
	< 80	80–84	85–89	90–99	≥ 100
< 120	−3 [−3] pts				
120–129		0 [0] pts			
130–139			0 [0] pts		
140–159				2 [2] pts	
≥ 160					3 [3] pts

Note: When systolic and diastolic pressures provide different estimates for point scores, use the higher number

Step 5

Diabetes		
	LDL Pts	Chol Pts
No	0	[0]
Yes	4	[4]

Step 6

Smoker		
	LDL Pts	Chol Pts
No	0	[0]
Yes	2	[2]

Step 7 (sum from steps 1-6)

Adding up the points	
Age	_______
LDL-C or Chol	_______
HDL-C	_______
Blood Pressure	_______
Diabetes	_______
Smoker	_______
Point Total	_______

Step 8 (determine CHD risk from point total)

CHD Risk			
LDL Pts Total	10-Yr CHD Risk	Chol Pts Total	10-Yr CHD Risk
≤ −2	1%	[≤ −2]	[1%]
−1	2%	[−1]	[2%]
0	2%	[0]	[2%]
1	2%	[1]	[2%]
2	3%	[2]	[3%]
3	3%	[3]	[3%]
4	4%	[4]	[4%]
5	5%	[5]	[4%]
6	6%	[6]	[5%]
7	7%	[7]	[6%]
8	8%	[8]	[7%]
9	9%	[9]	[8%]
10	11%	[10]	[10%]
11	13%	[11]	[11%]
12	15%	[12]	[13%]
13	17%	[13]	[15%]
14	20%	[14]	[18%]
15	24%	[15]	[20%]
16	27%	[16]	[24%]
≥ 17	≥ 32%	[≥ 17]	[≥ 27%]

Step 9 (compare to average person your age)

Comparative Risk			
Age (years)	Average 10-Yr CHD Risk	Average 10-Yr Hard* CHD Risk	Low† 10-Yr CHD Risk
30–34	< 1%	< 1%	< 1%
35–39	< 1%	< 1%	1%
40–44	2%	1%	2%
45–49	5%	2%	3%
50–54	8%	3%	5%
55–59	12%	7%	7%
60–64	12%	8%	8%
65–69	13%	8%	8%
70–74	14%	11%	8%

Relative Risk
Very low
Low
Moderate
High
Very high

* Hard CHD events exclude angina pectoris

† Low risk was calculated for a person the same age, optimal blood pressure, LDL-C 100–129 mg/dl or cholesterol 160–199 mg/dl, HDL-C 45 mg/dl for men or 55 mg/dl for women, nonsmoker, no diabetes

Risk estimates were derived from the experience of the Framingham Heart Study, a predominantly Caucasian population in Massachusetts, USA

B

FIGURE 42–3, cont'd B, Score sheet for women based on Framingham experience in women 30 to 74 years of age at baseline. Average risk estimates are based on typical Framingham subjects, and estimates of idealized risk are based on optimal blood pressure, TC of 160 to 199 mg/dl (or LDL of 100 to 129 mg/dl), HDL-C of 55 mg/dl, no diabetes, and no smoking. Use of the LDL-C categories is appropriate when fasting LDL-C measurements are available. Pts = points. (From Wilson PW, D'Agostino RB, Levy D, et al: Prediction of coronary heart disease using risk factor categories. Circulation 97:1837-1847, 1998.)

is the establishment of cause and effect. Data from several types of research are needed to establish a causal relationship between exposure and disease (Table 42–2). Basic research provides insight into the mechanisms underlying atherogenesis and helps elucidate the biological plausibility of potential interventions to modify these effects. Basic research has proven particularly successful in drug discovery. The development of preventive strategies also depends heavily on a number of complementary methods of population research, including descriptive studies (cross-sectional surveys and cross-cultural analyses), analytical studies (case-control and prospective cohort studies), and intervention studies (randomized trials).

Each of these strategies has strengths and weaknesses. Descriptive studies (case reports, case series, cross-sectional surveys, cross-cultural studies, and studies of population-based temporal trends) have considerable value for their ability to generate hypotheses. However, their design prevents adequate control for potential factors that may confound apparent associations. Observational studies (case-

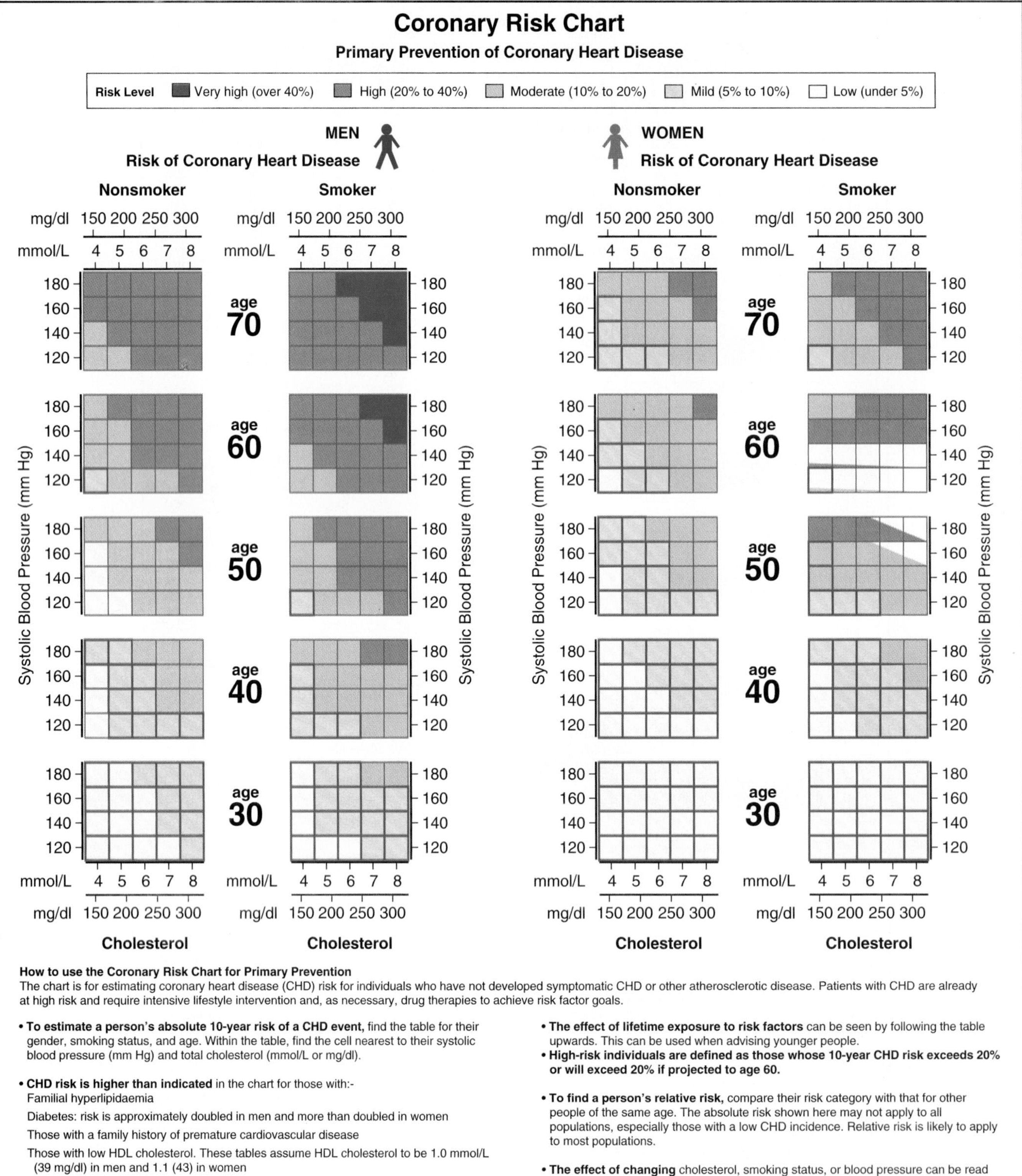

FIGURE 42–4 Risk assessment tool using cholesterol levels, blood pressure, and smoking status devised by a European task force on coronary prevention. (From Wood D, DeBacker G, Faergeman O, et al: Prevention of coronary heart disease in clinical practice: Recommendations of the Second Joint Task Force of European and other Societies on Coronary Prevention. Eur Heart J 19:1434-1503, 1998.)

control and prospective cohort studies) give researchers greater control over potential confounders. They are extremely useful in establishing risk attributable to a single factor, particularly when the effect of a given factor is large, as is the case for smoking and lung cancer. Yet when searching for small-to-moderate effects, the amount of uncontrolled confounding in observational studies may be as large as the probable risk reduction itself. In such cases, randomized trials are essential for confirming causation. Even when causality is not in question, trials help quantify the magni-

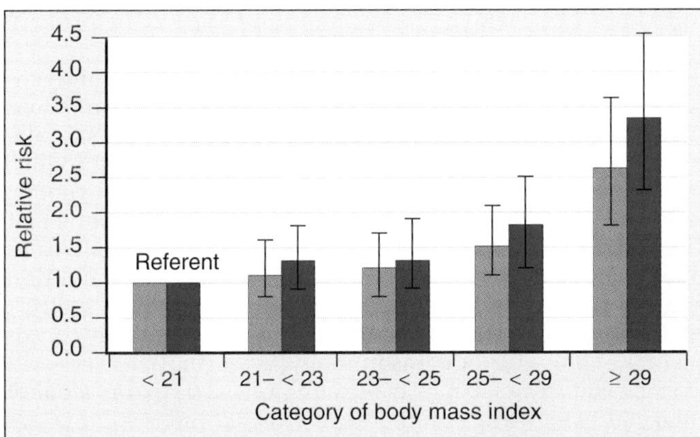

FIGURE 42–5 Association between body mass index and relative risk of nonfatal myocardial infarction and fatal coronary heart disease among women. Light bars show the relative risks for age and smoking. The vertical lines represent 95 percent confidence intervals.

TABLE 42–2 Types of Studies Used in Establishing Preventive Strategies

Basic research
  In vitro studies
  Animal studies

Clinical investigation

Epidemiological studies
  Descriptive studies
    Case reports
    Cross-sectional surveys
    Cross-cultural comparison studies
    Temporal trend studies
  Analytical studies
    Observational
      Case-control studies
      Cohort studies
    Intervention (randomized trials)

Cost-efficacy studies
Meta-analyses

tude of an intervention's effect. In addition, when the intervention is associated with competing risks and benefits, randomized trials are needed to determine the net clinical effect of the intervention.

Once a factor has been established as causally related to disease, interventions to modify the factor must be developed and tested. This is of critical importance because the magnitude of associated risk is not necessarily related to the magnitude of benefit derived from the intervention. Such lack of correlation may be due to the inability of the intervention to achieve the necessary change, or a change in the parameter may not result in the necessary change in risk in a proportional manner. An example is the difference between the observed risk associated with a 1-mm Hg rise in blood pressure and the lower-than-anticipated benefit on CHD derived from reducing blood pressure by this amount.[8,12] Similarly, even though elevated levels of homocysteine have been implicated as a risk factor for CHD and folic acid reduces homocysteine levels, evidence is not yet available from randomized trials indicating that reducing homocysteine levels with folic acid reduces vascular risk. In a similar manner, although hs-CRP is a strong independent predictor of vascular risk, data are not yet available demonstrating that reduction of hs-CRP per se will result in reduced risk.

In addition to providing information on the causal nature of an association, randomized trials generally provide the best data on the magnitude of benefit and risk from a given intervention. This information is essential for assessing cost efficacy and developing preventive strategies.

Cost Efficacy of Preventive Interventions

(see also Chap. 2)

Once reasonable estimates of benefit and risk have been established for a given factor, cost-effectiveness analyses can help establish guidelines for intervention. The common currency used to compare interventions is the quality-adjusted life-year (QALY) or disability-adjusted life-year (DALY). Estimates derived from cost- and risk-benefit analyses are dependent on the underlying assumptions made in a given analysis. In particular, because prevention measures have a long time horizon (decades or more), the consequences of initial assumptions can be much more significant than those of interventions with a short time horizon. Nonetheless, the cost-effectiveness of interventions to prevent heart disease is important because of the prevalence of CHD and the high cost of treatment.

Cost-effectiveness estimates are calculated as the ratio of net cost to gain in life expectancy. Interventions with an incremental cost-effectiveness ratio less than $40,000 per QALY are comparable to other chronic interventions such as hypertension management and hemodialysis. Those with a cost-effectiveness ratio under $20,000 per QALY are very favorable, whereas those exceeding $40,000 per QALY tend to be higher than generally accepted by most insurers.

Interventions at an Individual and Population Level

Three complementary approaches may be used to reduce the population burden of cardiovascular disease: (1) therapeutic interventions for secondary prevention in patients with known cardiovascular disease, (2) identification and targeting of high-risk individuals for primary prevention through mass screening or case finding, and (3) general recommendations disseminated throughout the population. Each of these approaches has merit in different situations. For example, targeted interventions such as specialized cardiac rehabilitation and life-style programs show the greatest efficacy among motivated individuals who hope to avoid a recurrent myocardial infarction, whereas mass screening programs for high blood pressure and hyperlipidemia are cost-effective. Population-wide campaigns against cigarette smoking offer an example of an effective public health approach. Implementation of the first two strategies requires risk assessment at the individual level, while the latter one requires knowledge of risk at the population level.

Classification of Interventions for Modifiable Risk Factors

Implementation of preventive strategies requires a practical, systematic approach to prioritizing interventions and allocating resources. The American College of Cardiology's Bethesda conferences placed risk factors into four categories according to the likelihood that modification of the factor will result in lower risk.[13] These categories include (1) factors for which interventions have been proved to reduce risk; (2) factors for which interventions are likely to lower the incidence of events; (3) factors clearly associated with CHD risk that, if modified, might lower the incidence of coronary events; and (4) factors associated with CHD risk that cannot be modified or, if modified, are not likely to decrease risk

(Table 42–3). Adapting this useful classification scheme to clinical practice requires consideration of cost efficacy. We present a modified classification scheme of interventions for major modifiable risk factors based not only on the strength of the association and evidence of benefit of intervention but also on cost efficacy (Table 42–4).

CLASS 1 INTERVENTIONS. Class 1 interventions have a clear causal relationship with heart disease (Table 42–5). Solid data, generally from randomized clinical trials, demonstrate the magnitude of the intervention's benefit, as well as its risks and cost. Cigarette smoking, hypertension, and dyslipidemias are causally related to CHD, and the corresponding interventions—smoking cessation, blood pressure management, and lipid profile management—all are cost-effective in both primary and secondary prevention. For management of hypertension and dyslipidemia, extensive trial and cost efficacy data enable a tiered approach based on absolute risk at baseline. Other pharmacological approaches proven to be beneficial and cost-effective include aspirin, beta blockers, and angiotensin-converting enzyme (ACE) inhibitors in secondary prevention and aspirin in primary prevention.

CLASS 2 INTERVENTIONS. Class 2 includes interventions for which the available data (largely basic research and human observational studies) strongly indicate a causal relationship and suggest that intervention will probably reduce the incidence of events but for which data on the benefits, risks, and costs of intervention are limited. Class 2 factors that clearly increase the risk of CHD include diabetes, obesity, and physical inactivity. Light-to-moderate alcohol consumption and the use of oral anticoagulants appear to reduce the risk of CHD. Trial data on interventions are forthcoming for several of these factors. It is unlikely, however, that there will ever be data from large-scale randomized trials on alcohol intake. Despite their limitations, class 2 interventions are useful in assessing global risk and have the potential to lower the risk of initial or recurrent CHD. Although it makes sense to invest more resources to modify these factors in individuals at highest risk, guidelines for class 2 factors do not generally distinguish between high- and low-risk individuals.

TABLE 42–3 Evidence Supporting the Association of Risk Factors with Cardiovascular Disease, the Usefulness of Measuring Them, and Their Responsiveness to Intervention

	Evidence for Association with CVD		Clinical	Response to	
Risk Factor	*Epidemiological*	*Clinical Trials*	Measurement Useful?	*Nonpharmacological Therapy*	*Pharmacological Therapy*
Category I (Risk Factors for which Interventions Have Been Proved to Lower CVD Risk)					
Cigarette smoking	+++	++	+++	+++	++
LDL cholesterol	+++	+++	+++	+++	+++
High-fat/high-cholesterol diet	+++	++	++	++	–
Hypertension	+++	+++ (Stroke)	+++	+	+++
Left ventricular hypertrophy	+++	+	++	–	++
Category II (Risk Factors for which Interventions Are Likely to Lower CVD Risk)					
Diabetes mellitus	+++	+	+++	++	+++
Physical inactivity	+++	++	++	++	–
HDL cholesterol	+++	+	+++	++	+
Triglycerides; small, dense LDL	++	++	+++	++	+++
Obesity	+++	–	+++	++	+
Postmenopausal status (women)	+++	–	+++	–	+++
Category III (Factors Associated with Increased CVD Risk that, if Modified, Might Lower Risk)					
Psychosocial factors	++	+	+++	+	–
Lipoprotein (a)	+	–	+	–	+
Homocysteine	++	–	+	++	++
Oxidative stress	+	–	–	+	++
No alcohol consumption	+++	–	++	++	–
Category IV (Factors Associated with Increased CVD Risk but Cannot be Modified)					
Age	+++	–	+++	–	–
Male gender	+++	–	+++	–	–
Low socioeconomic status	+++	–	++	–	–
Family history of early-onset CVD	+++	–	+++	–	–

+ = weak, somewhat consistent evidence; ++ = moderately strong, rather consistent evidence; +++ = very strong, consistent evidence; – = poor or nonexistent evidence. CVD = cardiovascular disease; HDL = high-density lipoprotein; LDL = low-density lipoprotein.

Modified from Pearson TA. McBride PE, Miller NH, Smith SC: 27th Bethesda Conference: Matching the intensity of risk factor management with the hazard for coronary disease events. Task Force 8. Organization or preventive cardiology service. J Am Coll Cardiol 27:1039-1047, 1996.

TABLE 42–4	Classification Scheme for Modifiable Risk Factors
Class	Definition
1	Basic research and human observational studies indicate a clear causal relationship Intervention data (typically from randomized trials) demonstrate the magnitude of the benefit and risk Interventions are cost-effective
2	Basic research and human observational studies indicate a causal relationship Intervention data from large-scale trials are limited Lack of adequate intervention data precludes determination of cost-effectiveness
3	Basic research and human observational studies demonstrate associations, but the independent nature of a causal relationship is not yet clear Interventions are not yet available or have not been adequately tested

TABLE 42–5 Cardiovascular Disease Risk Factors and Interventions

Risk Factor	Intervention	Secondary Prevention	Primary Prevention
Cigarette smoking	Smoking cessation	Class 1	Class 1
High blood pressure	Blood pressure management	Class 1	Class 1
High cholesterol	Cholesterol lowering	Class 1	Class 1
Low HDL	Increase HDL	Class 1, 2	Class 2
High triglycerides	Triglyceride lowering	Class 2	Class 2
Pharmacotherapy	Aspirin therapy Beta blockers ACE inhibitors Oral anticoagulants	Class 1 Class 1 Class 1 Class 1, 2	Class 2 — — —
Diabetes	Diabetes control	Class 2	Class 2
Obesity	Weight reduction	Class 2	Class 2
Physical inactivity	Increase activity	Class 2	Class 2
Dietary factors	Improved diet Moderate alcohol consumption	Class 3 Class 2, 3	Class 3 Class 2, 3
Menopause	Hormone replacement therapy	Class 2	Class 2

ACE = angiotensin-converting enzyme; HDL = high-density lipoprotein.

CLASS 3 INTERVENTIONS. Class 3 interventions are currently under active investigation. For many factors in this class, data are incomplete and an independent causal relationship with CHD cannot be inferred. For others where data are promising, such as homocysteine and C-reactive protein, interventions are not yet available or widely tested even though causal relationships are apparent. Thus, although these factors may have utility for risk assessment, their role in preventing CHD is uncertain. For these reasons, dietary practices such as the consumption of nutritional supplements, psychological factors, the use of hormone replacement therapy after menopause, and novel biochemical and genetic markers are currently considered class 3 factors. It is possible that the identification of high risk may in and of itself provide motivation for better compliance with life-style modifications. For example, individuals with elevated levels of hs-CRP may be more likely to comply with dietary advice and smoking cessation if they understand that they are, in fact, at elevated vascular risk. In several instances, an intervention has proven efficacy in secondary prevention but data are not yet available to support that intervention in primary prevention. For this reason, a factor may be a class 1 intervention for secondary prevention but a class 2 intervention with respect to primary prevention.

Class 1 Interventions

Cigarette Smoking/Cessation (see Chap. 36)

PREVALENCE. In the United States, per capita cigarette consumption rose dramatically in the first half of the 20th century. More than 65 percent of men born between 1911 and 1920 were smoking by 1945.[14] Annual per capita consumption of cigarettes hit an astonishing 4286 (more than 200 packs per year) in 1963, but has since declined to 1875.[15] The prevalence of smoking among men peaked at 55 percent in 1955 and, among women, 10 years later at 34 percent.[16] Since then, smoking rates have declined substantially, although the rate of decline differs by gender. Among men, smoking rates have declined by approximately half, whereas among women, rates have dropped by only one-third, primarily because of increasing smoking rates among women younger than 30 years. Currently, approximately 25 percent of men aged 18 and older are smokers, as compared with 21 percent of women.[17] Smoking rates among high school seniors rose from 30 percent in the mid-1980s to approximately 36.5 percent by 1997[18] but now appear to be on a gradual downward trend.[19] Smoking rates tend to be higher among blacks, those with lower socioeconomic status, and those with a high school education or less.[20]

ASSOCIATED RISK. Smoking increases the risk of CHD (see Chap. 36). By the middle of the 20th century, seminal studies linking smoking and heart disease had been published. The Surgeon General's report in 1964 reaffirmed the epidemiological relationship between the two, and by 1983 the Surgeon General firmly established cigarette smoking as the leading avoidable cause of cardiovascular disease. The Surgeon General's 1989 report presented definitive data from observational case-control and cohort studies, largely among men, that demonstrated that smoking doubles the incidence of CHD and increases CHD mortality by 50 percent, and that these risks increase with age and the number of cigarettes smoked. Similar increases in the relative risk for CHD have been observed among women.

In the United States, cigarette smoking is the leading preventable cause of death and accounts for an estimated 440,000 deaths each year—more than 40 percent of which result from cardiovascular disease—and almost 6 million years of potential life lost.[21] Worldwide, smoking rates continue to rise, with the greatest increases in the developing world[22]; 1 million more deaths were attributable to tobacco in 2000 than in 1990.[23]

BENEFIT OF INTERVENTION. Although data from large-scale, randomized trials concerning the risk reduction associated with smoking cessation are limited, observational studies demonstrate clear benefits of smoking cessation. Smokers who quit reduce their excess risk of a coronary event by 50 percent in the first year or two after cessation, with much of this gain in the first few months. This period is followed by a more gradual decline, with the risk of former smokers approaching that of never smokers after 5 to 15 years.

COST EFFICACY. Smoking cessation is highly cost-effective in both primary and secondary prevention. The intervention is usually short term and thus low cost. In fact, smoking cessation programs generally cost less than continued smoking. The gains in life expectancy are large, and the earlier in life an individual stops smoking, the larger the potential gain—a 35-year-old male smoker may add 3 years to his life expectancy on cessation. Costs vary, depending on the intensity of intervention and the use of pharmacological agents, from $1100 to $4500 (in 1995 dollars) for every QALY saved.[24]

GUIDELINES/RECOMMENDATIONS. Clinical practice guidelines from the U.S. Public Health Service recognize that tobacco dependence is a chronic condition that generally requires repeated intervention.[25] They recommend asking patients about tobacco use at every visit, a strategy supported by the U.S. Preventive Services Task Force.[26] The Public Health Service guidelines support a combination of counseling and pharmacological therapy, when necessary. Three types of counseling and behavioral therapies appear to be particularly effective: (1) provision of problem solving and skills training, (2) provision of social support in treatment, and (3) help securing social support outside of treatment. Six first-line pharmacotherapies that reliably increase long-term smoking abstinence were also identified. These are sustained-release bupropion hydrochloride, nicotine gum, nicotine patch, nicotine inhaler, nicotine nasal spray, and nicotine lozenge.

In view of the addictive nature of smoking and the tendency to increase smoking over time, smoking reduction—as opposed to smoking cessation—is not an acceptable strategy. The efficacy of smoking intervention programs ranges from a 6 percent 1-year success rate for physician counseling to 18 percent for self-help programs and 20 to 40 percent for cessation programs with pharmacological interventions with nicotine gum or patches.[27]

Although it is important to counsel patients at all stages about the hazards of smoking and the benefits of quitting, the period soon after a cardiac event is an opportune time to encourage a patient to make an effort to stop smoking.

FUTURE CHALLENGES. In the United States, the prevalence of smoking is increasing among young women, particularly minority women. Worldwide, intense public health efforts are needed to reverse the alarming rise in smoking rates occurring in many developing countries. The low rates of success in cessation efforts offer a challenge to clinicians, and greater emphasis must be placed on preventing smoking in the first place.

Hypertension/Blood Pressure Control

(see also Chap. 38)

PREVALENCE. As defined by JNC-7,[6] an estimated 50 million Americans are hypertensive and another 45 million fall into a new category called *prehypertension* (Table 42–6). High blood pressure is more common among blacks than whites and among men than women. The prevalence of hypertension clearly increases with age, from 9 percent of those aged 19 to 24 years to 75 percent of those older than 75 years.[28] Data from the Framingham Heart Study suggest that normotensive individuals at age 55 have a 90 percent lifetime risk for developing hypertension.[29] In the United States, hypertension prevalence appears to be increasing, and control rates remain low (~30 percent).[30]

ASSOCIATED RISK. Elevated systolic or diastolic blood pressure is clearly associated with an increased risk of CHD (see Chaps. 36 and 37). The best estimate for the magnitude of associated risk derives from a meta-analysis of nine large prospective, observational studies with 420,000 participants who accrued more than 4850 CHD events during follow-up.[12] A 7-mm Hg increase in diastolic blood pressure over any baseline reading was associated with a 27 percent increase in CHD risk and a 42 percent increase in stroke risk. Hypertension is also associated with increased risk of heart failure, stroke, and kidney disease. The shape of the cardiovascular disease risk curve is linear. For individuals aged 40 to 70 years, each increment of 20 mm Hg in systolic blood pressure or 10 mm Hg in diastolic blood pressure doubles the risk of cardiovascular disease across a blood pressure range from 115/75 to 185/115 mm Hg.[31]

BENEFIT OF INTERVENTION. Beginning in the late 1960s, a number of randomized trials confirmed the protective effect of treating mild to moderate hypertension. These early trial data led to the establishment of treatment guidelines in the 1970s. The most precise estimates of risk reduction have come from meta-analyses reporting that lowering diastolic blood pressure by 5 to 6 mm Hg results in a 42 percent reduction in the risk of stroke and a 15 percent reduc-

TABLE 42–6 Classification and Management of Blood Pressure (BP) for Adults

			Management		
				Initial Drug Therapy	
BP classification	Systolic BP (mm Hg)	Diastolic BP (mm Hg)	Lifestyle Modification	*Without Compelling Indication*	*With Compelling Indication*
Normal	<120	*and* <80	Encourage		
Prehypertension	120-139	*or* 80-89	Yes	None indicated	Drugs for compelling indications* (treat to BP target <130/80)
Stage 1 hypertension	140-159	*or* 90-99	Yes	Thiazide-type diuretics for most. May consider ACEI, ARB, BB, CCB, or combination	Drug(s) for compelling indications* Other antihypertensive drugs (diuretics, ACEI, ARB, BB, CCB) as needed
Stage 2 hypertension	≥160	*or* ≥100	Yes	Two-drug combination for most (usually thiazide-type diuretic and ACEI or ARB or BB or CCB)	

ACEI = angiotensin-converting enzyme inhibitor; ARB = angiotensin-receptor blocker; BB = beta blocker; CCB = calcium channel blocker.
From Chobanian AV, Bakris GL, Black HR, et al: The Seventh Report of the Joint National Committee on Prevention, Detection, Evaluation, and Treatment of High Blood Pressure: The JNC 7 Report. JAMA 289:2560-2572, 2003.
*Patients with chronic kidney disease or diabetes.

tion in the risk of CHD events.[32] Ogden and colleagues applied the risk stratification system of JNC-6 to data from the National Health and Nutrition Examination Survey Epidemiologic Follow-up Study and found that the absolute benefits of antihypertensive therapy depended on baseline blood pressure as well as the presence or absence of additional cardiovascular disease risk factors, preexisting clinical cardiovascular disease, or target organ damage. Among individuals with stage 1 hypertension and additional cardiovascular risk factors, sustaining a 12-mm Hg decrease in systolic blood pressure for 10 years would prevent 1 death for every 11 patients treated. In the presence of cardiovascular disease or target-organ damage, such a reduction would prevent 1 death for every 9 patients treated.[33]

The Antihypertensive and Lipid-Lowering Treatment to Prevent Heart Attack Trial (ALLHAT) demonstrated the efficacy of thiazide diuretics compared with other antihypertensive agents.[34]

COST EFFICACY. Detection and management of hypertension are highly cost-effective in both primary and secondary prevention (see Chap. 2). However, more aggressive management in those at high risk based on the existence of cardiovascular disease or diabetes is warranted based on greater cost efficacy. In secondary prevention, for agents such as diuretics and beta blockers, the cost is below $10,000 per QALY for patients with established CHD, even when blood pressure is only mildly elevated.[35] In primary prevention, cost ranges between $10,000 and $20,000 per QALY among individuals with moderate to severe elevations in blood pressure. However, the cost approaches an unacceptable range of $100,000 per QALY for higher-priced medications. In contrast to some estimates for lipid lowering, cost efficacy decreases with increasing age. Given these issues, careful cost-efficacy evaluation is needed for newer recommendations from JNC-7 since this guideline suggests the use of multiple agents and favors intervention for a wider group of individuals, including those with minor elevations of blood pressure.

GUIDELINES/TREATMENT. The U.S. Preventive Services Task Force recommends routine blood pressure testing of all adults.[36] The JNC-7[6] defines four levels of blood pressure according to the risk imparted (see Table 42–6).

Recommendations for intervention from the JNC-7 are based on the level of blood pressure and the level of absolute risk. The absolute risk strata are defined according to the presence or absence of target-organ disease, clinical cardiovascular disease, diabetes, and cardiovascular risk factors such as smoking, hyperlipidemia, age older than 60 years, gender, and family history of early-onset cardiovascular disease. The JNC-7 sets a blood pressure goal of 140/90 mm Hg for lower-risk patients and 130/80 mm Hg for those with cardiovascular disease, diabetes, or chronic kidney disease. Since the relationship of blood pressure to risk of cardiovascular disease is linear, a significant portion of the population-attributable risk occurs among those with blood pressure in the JNC-7 category of prehypertension—a systolic blood pressure of 120 to 139 mm Hg or a diastolic pressure of 80 to 89 mm Hg.

For all individuals with blood pressure of 120/80 mm Hg or greater, JNC-7 recommends life-style modifications, including smoking cessation, weight reduction if needed, increased physical activity, limited alcohol intake, limited sodium intake, maintenance of adequate potassium and calcium intake, and adoption of the Dietary Approaches to Stop Hypertension (DASH) eating plan—a diet with a reduced content of saturated and total fat that is also rich in fruits, vegetables, and low-fat dairy products (see Chap. 41).[37,38]

Initiation of drug therapy depends on blood pressure and the absolute level of risk. For example, among individuals with stage 1 hypertension but no evidence of end-organ damage, vascular disease, or diabetes and one cardiovascular disease risk factor, life-style modification and drug therapy is recommended. Data from ALLHAT indicate that a thiazide-type diuretic should be the preferred agent for first-step antihypertensive therapy.[34] For individuals with stage 2 hypertension, combination therapy that usually includes a thiazide-type diuretic is the starting point for therapy. The guidelines also recommend initiating therapy with two drugs, one of which is a diuretic, when blood pressure is more than 20/10 mm Hg above the target level. The specific therapeutic agents recommended by JNC-7 are provided in Table 42–7 and discussed at length in Chapter 38. Most patients require more than one agent to achieve their blood pressure goal.

Guidelines from the ESC stratify initial therapy somewhat differently.[9] Drug therapy is recommended for individuals with less than 20 percent absolute risk and blood pressure in excess of 160/95 mm Hg only after at least 6 months of life-style modification; for individuals with greater than 20 percent absolute risk if their blood pressure exceeds 140/90 mm Hg after 3 months of life-style modification; and immediately for individuals whose blood pressure exceeds 180/100 mm Hg, regardless of absolute risk. As with the JNC-7 recommendations, life-style modifications should always be used as an adjunct to drug therapy.

FUTURE CHALLENGES. In the developed world, the prevalence of hypertension is increasing as populations age. In the United States, the proportion of patients with hypertension managed appropriately has decreased, thus reversing a two-decade trend.[39] Approximately 40 percent of those with hypertension do not know they have this condition and are not being treated for it, and only one-third of patients treated for hypertension have their blood pressure under control.[6] In

TABLE 42–7 Compelling Indications for Individual Antihypertensive Drug Classes

High-Risk Indications with Compelling Indication	Recommended Drugs					
	Diuretic	*Beta Blocker*	*ACE Inhibitor*	*ARB*	*CCB*	*Aldosterone Antagonist*
Heart failure	×	×	×	×	×	×
Prior myocardial infarction		×	×			×
High CHD risk	×	×	×		×	
Diabetes	×	×	×	×	×	
Chronic kidney disease				×	×	
Prior stroke	×		×			

ACE = angiotensin-converting enzyme; ARB = angiotensin-receptor blocker; CCB = calcium-channel blocker; CHD = coronary heart disease.
From Chobanian AV, Bakris GL, Black HR, et al: The Seventh Report of the Joint National Committee on Prevention, Detection, Evaluation, and Treatment of High Blood Pressure: The JNC 7 Report. JAMA 289:2560-2572, 2003.

developing countries, hypertension rates are rising rapidly with urbanization and changes in life-style habits. The attributable risk for hypertension tends to be greater in the developing world because the low rates of detection and treatment in such countries result in a proportionately higher rate of hypertensive heart disease and stroke.[40]

Hypercholesterolemia/Lipid Control

(see also Chap. 39)

PREVALENCE. Mean age-adjusted cholesterol levels have declined modestly in the United States since the early 1960s.[28] Even with this decline, half of all American adults have cholesterol levels greater than 200 mg/dl, and 18 percent have cholesterol levels higher than 240 mg.[28]

ASSOCIATED RISK. Elevated serum cholesterol is causally associated with increased risk of CHD. Specifically, a 10 percent increase in serum cholesterol is associated with a 20 to 30 percent increase in risk for CHD, and elevations earlier in life may be associated with higher increases in risk.[41,42]

BENEFIT OF INTERVENTION. Clear benefits have been demonstrated for dietary and pharmacological treatments that lower serum cholesterol (see Chap. 39).[43] A number of completed large-scale primary and secondary prevention trials using 3-hydroxy-3-methylglutaryl coenzyme A reductase inhibitors (statins), beginning with the Scandinavian Simvastatin Survival Study, have demonstrated significant reductions in fatal and nonfatal CHD in a variety of populations. These include patients with established CHD; those with coronary disease, other occlusive arterial disease, or diabetes but usual cholesterol levels; those without clinically evident atherosclerotic cardiovascular disease and average total and LDL cholesterol levels; elderly individuals at risk of vascular disease; and hypertensive patients with average or lower-than-average cholesterol levels. Some,[44] but not all,[45] trial data support the early initiation of statin therapy following myocardial infarction or coronary artery bypass grafting.

A meta-analysis of five primary and secondary trials (30,817 participants and >166,000 person-years of follow-up) demonstrated that statin therapy for an average duration of 5.4 years was associated with average reductions of 20 percent in total cholesterol, 28 percent in LDL, and 13 percent in triglycerides and a 5 percent increase in HDL. Compared with placebo, statin therapy in these trials reduced the risk of major coronary events by 31 percent and all-cause mortality by 21 percent, with similar reductions in men and women, as well as in those younger and older than 65 years.[46] Cholesterol-lowering trials also demonstrate reductions in stroke.[47] These data indicate that long-term compliance is important for successful intervention. Indeed, long-term daily compliance is far more important in determining outcome efficacy than any demonstrated differences between statins in terms of potency.

Several early trials raised concerns that cholesterol lowering might increase the risk of nonvascular mortality. However, data from the large statin trials provide reassuring data that cholesterol reduction does not increase the risk of nonvascular mortality.

COST EFFICACY. The cost efficacy of nonpharmacological interventions to lower LDL cholesterol is unclear (see Chap. 2). Pharmacological intervention, however, is clearly cost-effective under certain conditions, and available data permit tailoring recommendations to the level of baseline CHD risk. Early analyses of cholesterol reduction for secondary prevention (which used data from cholestyramine trials) resulted in very costly interventions, largely because the available drugs were relatively ineffective. In contrast, data for statin therapy are remarkably consistent.

For example, in the Scandinavian Simvastatin Survival Study, the direct cost per life-year saved was $5400 for men and $10,500 for women. As expected, cost decreased as the baseline cholesterol level increased. For example, the direct cost per life saved was $11,400 for a man with a baseline total cholesterol of 213 mg/dl (5.5 mmol/liter) and $6700 for a man with a cholesterol level of 309 mg/dl (8.0 mmol/liter). Furthermore, the direct cost tended to be lower with increasing age, a finding in stark contrast to early estimates based on the Coronary Heart Disease Policy Model.

To determine a more modern cost-effectiveness of statin therapy, Prosser and colleagues[48] applied data from several large-scale, long-term, randomized, controlled trials of statins to the Coronary Heart Disease Policy. They divided men and women aged 35 to 85 years with LDL levels higher than 160 mg/dl into 240 risk subgroups according to age, sex, and the presence of four major CHD risk factors (smoking status, blood pressure, LDL level, and HDL level).[48] In primary prevention, statins failed to reach a cost-effectiveness ratio of $50,000 per QALY in any of the risk subgroups and ranged as high as $1.4 million per QALY. In contrast, primary prevention with a Step I diet ranged from $1900 per QALY to $500,000. In secondary prevention, statin therapy was clearly cost-effective, ranging from $1800 per QALY for a man aged 45 to 54 years to $40,000 for a woman aged 35 to 44 years. Statin therapy is also effective and cost-effective for secondary prevention in patients 75 to 84 years of age.[48,49] All of these QALY evaluations are highly sensitive to drug cost and can be expected to decline substantially as statin agents transition into generic drugs.

GUIDELINES/TREATMENT. All patients with cardiovascular disease should be screened for serum cholesterol levels. In primary prevention, some controversy remains regarding screening. The NCEP recommends routine screening of all adults older than 20 years,[5] the American College of Physicians (ACP) recommends screening only men ages 35 to 65 and women ages 45 to 65,[50] and the U.S. Preventive Services Task Force recommends screening all men aged 35 and older and all women aged 45 and older.[26]

To reduce the prevalence of hyperlipidemia in the United States, the NCEP issued its first *Adult Treatment Panel* (ATP) report in 1988. The latest one was published in 2002.[5] Under the latest NCEP guidelines, the number of U.S. adults eligible for lipid modification has increased from 52 million to 65 million for therapeutic life-style changes, and from approximately 13 million to 36 million for drug therapy. The goals of intervention are based on the level of CHD risk for an individual (Fig. 42–6).

The ATP III guidelines recommend different therapeutic targets depending on a patients' overall risk, which includes calculation of his or her Framingham risk score (see Fig. 42–3). Patients with existing CHD (or a CHD risk equivalent such as diabetes or peripheral arterial disease) are at the highest risk for a cardiovascular event and thus have the lowest LDL target (<100 mg/dl) and receive the most intensive treatment (Table 42–8). Patients without CHD are treated depending on their overall risk. Those with two or more risk factors, or zero or one risk factor and a 10-year overall risk less than 20 percent, should be treated to an LDL target less than 130 mg/dl. Patients with lower risk should be treated to a target LDL less than 160 mg/dl.

As part of its first-line Therapeutic Life-style Changes, the NCEP recommends a diet that includes 25 to 35 percent of calories from fat, with saturated fat accounting for less than 7 percent of fat intake and cholesterol intake limited to less than 200 mg/d. Carbohydrates, predominantly from whole grains and other foods rich in complex carbohydrates, should account for 50 to 60 percent of calories, and protein for 15 percent. These guidelines also recommend including 20 to 30 gm/d of dietary fiber (especially soluble fiber), as well

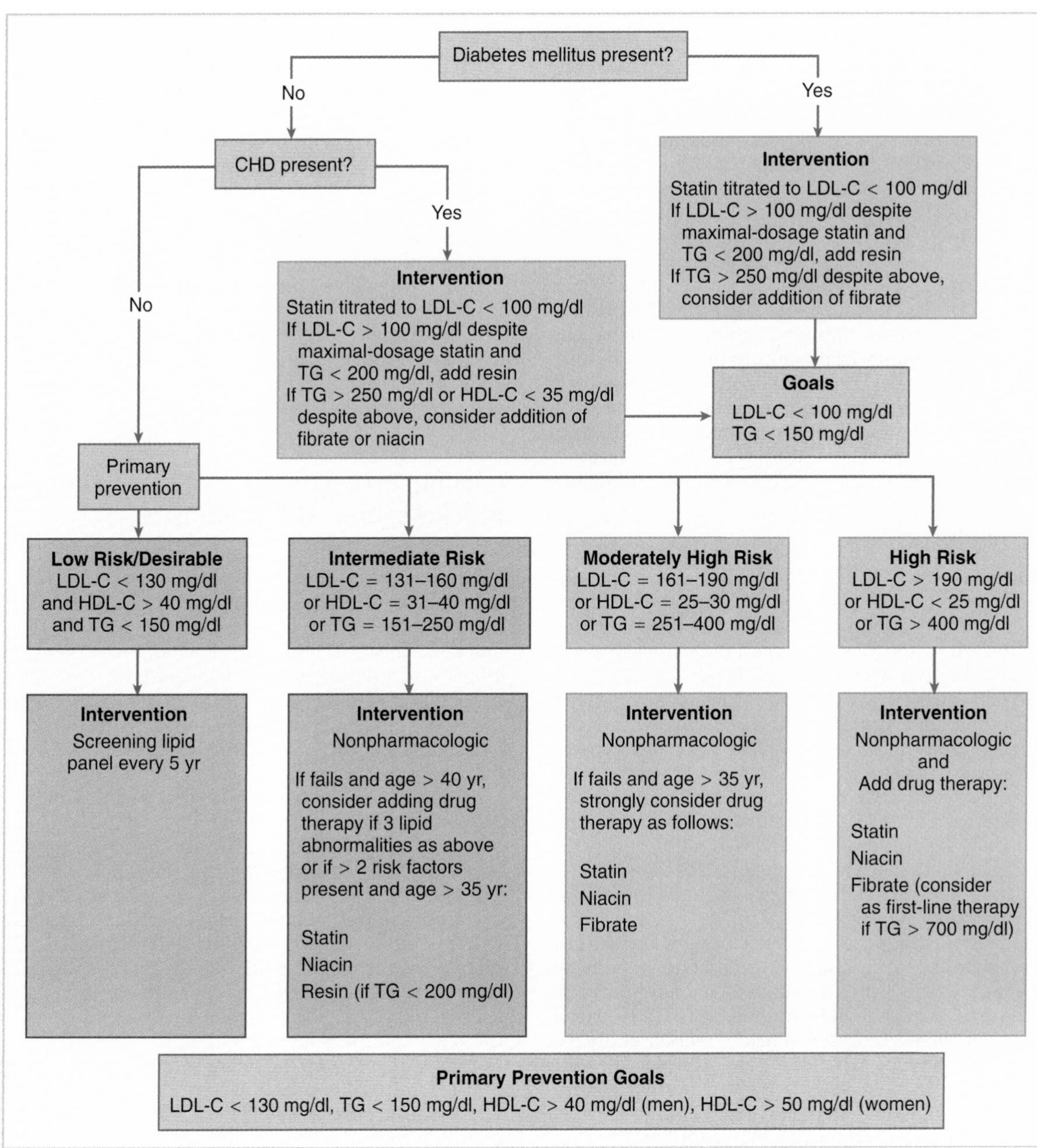

FIGURE 42–6 Algorithm for lipid-lowering therapy based on findings from intervention trials. CHD = coronary heart disease; HDL-C = high-density lipoprotein cholesterol; LDL-C = low-density lipoprotein cholesterol; TG = triglycerides. (From Third Report of the National Cholesterol Education Program [NCEP] Expert Panel on Detection, Evaluation, and Treatment of High Blood Cholesterol in Adults [Adult Treatment Panel III]: Final report. Circulation 106:3143-3421, 2002.) (See also Chap. 39.)

TABLE 42–8 Low-Density Lipoprotein (LDL) Goals for Three Risk Levels

Risk Level	LDL Goal (mg/dl)
CHD and CHD risk equivalent*	<100
Multiple (2+) risk factors	<130†
0-1 risk factor	<160

CHD = coronary heart disease.
From Third Report of the National Cholesterol Education Program (NCEP) Expert Panel on Detection, Evaluation, and Treatment of High Blood Cholesterol in Adults (Adult Treatment Panel III) final report. Circulation 106:3143-3421, 2002.
*Diabetes, chronic kidney disease.
†LDL goal for individuals with multiple risk factors and a 10-yr overall risk >20% is <100 mg/dl.

as 2 gm of plant stanols/sterols. Weight management and increased physical activity are also stressed.

Since patients may find it difficult to understand percent calories, translating these guidelines into grams of fat, protein, and other dietary constituents may be helpful. Such reporting is now mandated on labels of all food sold in the United States. Professional counseling with a dietitian may also be helpful. If dietary therapy does not achieve the target LDL level, drug therapy should be started (see Chap. 39). In all cases, drug therapy should be an adjunct to dietary therapy and increased physical activity.

A variety of drugs are available for lowering total and LDL cholesterol (see Chap. 39). The most commonly used are the statins. Others include niacin, fibrates, bile acid sequestrants, and cholesterol absorption inhibitors.

Guidelines from the ESC also have three tiers.[9] Although the target is identical for all patients (total cholesterol of

≤190 mg/dl [5 mmol/liter] and LDL cholesterol of ≤115 mg/dl [3 mmol/liter]) the timing and intensity of drug therapy are different. For individuals with CHD, diet and drug therapy are initiated simultaneously. In primary prevention, if either the absolute 10-year risk of a CHD event or the projected risk at age 60 is greater than 20 percent, life-style modifications are recommended and lipids are checked in 3 months. If at 3 months the total or LDL cholesterol level is above target, drug therapy may be instituted. For those with a current or projected risk less than 20 percent, life-style advice but not drug therapy is recommended.

FUTURE CHALLENGES. Additional randomized trial data are needed to clarify the role of cholesterol screening and the association between reducing serum cholesterol and stroke prevention. Ongoing trials comparing intensive LDL reduction to moderate LDL reduction will be important for determining appropriate targets for intervention across different risk levels. Although cholesterol levels are falling or stable in industrialized countries, they are rising in developing countries as "Western" diets are increasingly adopted.

HDL and Triglycerides (see also Chap. 39)

PREVALENCE. Low HDL and high triglyceride levels tend to coincide and often result from metabolic phenomena that are distinct from those leading to high levels of LDL cholesterol. Thus, low HDL and high triglyceride levels can occur alone or in combination with high LDL levels.

ASSOCIATED RISK. HDL cholesterol has emerged as an important independent predictor of CHD—every 1 mg/dl decrease in HDL cholesterol causes a 3 to 4 percent increase in coronary artery disease.[5] Furthermore, an emerging body of evidence indicates that the ratio of total or LDL cholesterol to HDL cholesterol may be a better predictor of CHD risk than LDL alone. Data from the Physicians' Health Study, for example, suggest that a 1-unit decrease in this ratio (which is easily achievable with statin drugs) reduces the risk of myocardial infarction by 53 percent.

Imprecision in triglyceride measurements, within-individual variability, and complex interactions between triglycerides and other lipid parameters may obscure the impact of triglycerides in the development of CHD. However, fasting triglyceride levels represent a useful marker of the risk for CHD, particularly when HDL levels are considered.[51] This independence suggests that some triglyceride-rich lipoproteins are atherogenic. Meta-analyses suggest that elevated triglycerides are an independent risk factor for CHD.[52,53]

BENEFIT OF INTERVENTION. Gemfibrozil, an agent that increases HDL and lowers triglyceride levels, reduces risk among those with high total and LDL cholesterol. In the Veterans Affairs High-Density Lipoprotein Cholesterol Intervention Trial (VA-HIT), a 22 percent reduction in cardiovascular events was observed with gemfibrozil treatment in a population with low HDL (<40 mg/dl [1 mmol/liter]).[54] This risk reduction occurred in the absence of any substantial change in LDL cholesterol, data that support the potential for agents targeted at HDL and triglyceride levels. It remains unclear, however, whether therapy targeted at increasing HDL will necessarily reduce vascular risk since diverse metabolic pathways lead to changes in HDL and may be differentially affected by different pharmacological strategies.

RECOMMENDATIONS. Screening of patients with cardiovascular disease should include a full fasting lipid profile, including total cholesterol, HDL, and triglycerides. For patients without cardiovascular disease, screening for HDL remains controversial, with the NCEP recommending for screening and the ACP recommending against it. Because HDL and the ratio of total cholesterol to HDL cholesterol powerfully predict risk and aid in the detection of individuals who have elevated LDL despite moderate levels of total cholesterol, it seems prudent to check HDL along with total cholesterol.

All patients with low HDL and/or high triglycerides should receive recommendations for life-style modifications that include a diet low in saturated fat and increased physical activity.[5] In secondary prevention, individuals with high LDL who also have low HDL or high triglycerides should be treated aggressively and consideration given to combination therapy (see Chap. 39). Further, for those with known disease who have low HDL and normal LDL, consideration can be given to pharmacological intervention based on the results of VA-HIT. In primary prevention, nonpharmacological interventions are warranted for individuals who have a normal LDL level but a low HDL and/or high triglycerides because trial data regarding drug therapy in such cases are insufficient. Intervention data regarding patients with isolated elevated triglyceride levels are needed.

Cardiac Protection with Aspirin, Beta Blockers, and ACE Inhibitors

Several pharmacological interventions have proved highly effective in the prevention of cardiovascular disease. Pharmacological reduction of risk during or immediately after the development of CHD has been demonstrated for aspirin, beta blockers, and ACE inhibitors. Each of these agents has proven efficacy in intermediate and longer-term secondary prevention among various subgroups of patients. Aspirin is also an effective primary prevention agent for some groups.

ASPIRIN IN SECONDARY PREVENTION. Aspirin therapy in patients with existing cardiovascular disease (see Chaps. 36 and 50) reduces the risk of subsequent events by 25 percent. Meta-analyses demonstrate clear reductions in mortality and nonfatal cardiovascular disease events among those with prior myocardial infarction, stroke, bypass surgery, angioplasty, peripheral vascular surgery, or angina.[55]

Unless contraindicated, aspirin should be used by most patients with known cardiovascular disease. Other antiplatelet agents with demonstrated efficacy such as ticlopidine and clopidogrel should be considered for patients with aspirin allergy or intolerance. However, the cost efficacy of these agents is less favorable than the cost efficacy of aspirin. Data from the Coronary Heart Disease Policy Model suggest that extending the use of aspirin therapy for secondary prevention from current levels to all eligible patients for 25 years would have an estimated cost-effectiveness ratio of about $11,000 per QALY gained. Clopidogrel alone in all patients or in routine combination with aspirin had an incremental cost of more than $130,000 per QALY gained.[56]

ASPIRIN IN PRIMARY PREVENTION. Five large-scale trials, performed primarily in men, have assessed the benefits of low-dose aspirin in the prevention of cardiovascular disease. Taken together, these studies suggest a benefit of prophylactic aspirin in primary prevention among men.[57] However, concerns over increased risk of hemorrhagic stroke have not been fully assessed, and data in women remain limited.

In 1997, the American Heart Association recommended against the use of aspirin for primary prevention, largely on the basis of the unknown benefit-risk ratio. Five years later, the U.S. Preventive Services Task Force concluded that there was sufficient evidence that aspirin decreases the incidence of CHD in adults at increased risk for heart disease.[58] Among individuals with a 10-year risk of CHD of 6 percent or greater, the Task Force determined that the benefits of taking aspirin outweighed the increased risk of gastrointestinal bleeding or hemorrhagic stroke. The ESC recommends low-dose aspirin (75 mg) in primary prevention only for men at particularly high risk of CHD.[9]

For women, the Women's Health Study, which is scheduled to end in 2005, is addressing the benefit-risk ratio of aspirin therapy for primary prevention of cardiovascular disease.

BETA BLOCKERS. A number of trials have demonstrated the long-term efficacy of beta blockade after myocardial infarction in reducing mortality, and meta-analyses suggest a 23 percent mortality reduction with long-term use.[59] Long-term use of beta blockers also lowers the risk of recurrent cardiovascular events. Cross-trial comparisons suggest that the higher the level of beta blockade, as measured by heart rate reduction relative to the control group, the greater the benefit. Beta blockade after myocardial infarction and in the setting of congestive heart failure is also extremely cost-effective. Data from the Coronary Heart Disease Policy Model suggest that implementing beta-blocker therapy in all first-myocardial infarction survivors annually over 20 years would prevent 62,000 myocardial infarctions and result in 72,000 fewer CHD deaths; the cost-effectiveness of beta-blocker therapy would be less than $11,000 per QALY gained, even under unfavorable assumptions.[60]

ACE INHIBITORS. The benefit of ACE inhibitors among individuals at high risk for CHD events is substantial. Following myocardial infarction, the use of an ACE inhibitor is associated with a 7 percent reduction in mortality at 30 days.[61,62] Among individuals with a low ejection fraction after myocardial infarction, total mortality is reduced by 26 percent (see Chap. 50). A meta-analysis of six randomized, controlled trials suggests that long-term ACE inhibitor therapy reduces the risk of major clinical outcomes by 22 percent.[63] Findings from the Heart Outcomes Prevention Evaluation (HOPE) Study suggest that the benefits of ACE inhibitors extend to those with clinical CHD (see Chap. 50) and diabetes, even in the absence of left ventricular dysfunction.[64] Results from the Candesartan in Heart Failure Assessment of Reduction in Mortality and Morbidity (CHARM) trials indicate that the use of an angiotensin-receptor blocker such as candesartan among patients with heart failure can prevent 1 death for every 63 patients treated, prevent 1 first hospitalization with heart failure for 23 patients treated, and prevent 1 new case of diabetes for every 71 patients treated.[65]

RECOMMENDATIONS. For secondary prevention, aspirin, beta blockers, and ACE inhibitors are cost-effective and should be considered standard therapy in appropriate patients—aspirin for any patient with cardiovascular disease, beta blockers after myocardial infarction, and ACE inhibitors in patients with a low ejection fraction, as well as in others with cardiovascular disease and diabetes. All three agents are recommended for secondary prevention by the American Heart Association, the American College of Cardiology, and the ESC. The U.S. Preventive Services Task Force recommends aspirin in primary prevention for those with 5-year cardiovascular disease risk of 3 percent or higher.

Class 2 Interventions

Class 2 interventions relate to risk factors that appear to have strong causal associations with CHD risk and for which intervention has the potential to reduce risk but for which intervention data are limited (see Table 42–4). Factors in this category include diabetes, obesity, physical inactivity, and alcohol intake. In general, cost efficacy data are not available because of a lack of adequate intervention data.

Diabetes/Diabetes Control, Prediabetes, and Metabolic Syndrome (see also Chap. 40)

PREVALENCE. In the United States, nearly 17 million people—6.2 percent of the U.S. population—have diabetes mellitus; approximately 90 percent of cases are type 2 diabetes.[66] Fully one-third of people with diabetes are not aware they have this disease. The prevalence of diabetes appears to have increased over the last decade, which may be a reflection of increasing body mass index (BMI).[67] Another alarming trend is the recent increase in type 2 diabetes (formerly called *adult-onset diabetes*) among children, who account for more than 30 percent of new cases in some parts of the U.S.[68,69]

ASSOCIATED RISK. Diabetes is a powerful risk factor for atherosclerotic disease, its complications, and cardiovascular-related mortality. By age 40 years, CHD is the leading cause of death in both diabetic men and women, with surveys showing CHD listed on 69 percent of death certificates in a representative national cohort of adults with diabetes.[70] Age-adjusted rates for CHD are two to three times higher among diabetic men and three to seven times higher among diabetic women than among their counterparts without diabetes.[71] During 10 years of follow-up in the Health Professionals Follow-Up Study, the multivariate relative risks for fatal CHD were 3.84 (95 percent confidence interval [CI], 3.12 to 4.71) for those with diabetes only, 7.88 (95 percent CI, 6.86 to 9.05) for those with myocardial infarction only, and 13.41 (95 percent CI, 10.49 to 17.16) for those with both diabetes and myocardial infarction compared with men without diabetes or prior myocardial infarction at baseline.[72] Similar, though not quite as pronounced, associations were observed among women in the Nurses' Health Study over a 20-year period.[73] Thus, individuals with diabetes must be considered at high risk for CHD, regardless of the presence or absence of other risk factors.

BENEFIT OF TREATMENT. Maintaining normoglycemia may reduce the risk of microvascular (renal and eye) disease. However, data demonstrating reduced risk of CHD with tight glycemic control are scant. In the Diabetes Complications and Control Trial (DCCT), an apparent reduction in CHD events among patients with type 1 diabetes assigned to intensive therapy did not achieve statistical significance, possibly because of the small number of events in this relatively young cohort. Although oral hypoglycemic agents and insulin can improve glycemic control, their role in the reduction of risk from macrovascular complications of type 2 diabetes mellitus remains unclear.[74,75] The recent HOPE trial showed that ACE inhibitor therapy reduced the onset of diabetes.[64,76]

Aggressive multifactorial intervention among diabetics does appear effective in reducing CHD events. In a recent trial of 160 patients with type 2 diabetes and microalbuminuria who were allocated to conventional care or intensive therapy (life-style and pharmacological interventions intended to maintain glycosylated hemoglobin below 6.5 percent, total cholesterol below 175 mg/dl, triglycerides below 150 mg/dl, and blood pressure below 130/80 mm Hg), rates of incident cardiovascular events were more than halved over an 8-year follow-up period (hazard ratio 0.47; 95 percent CI, 0.24 to 0.73).[77] Given beneficial results among diabetic patients enrolled in cardiovascular event reduction trials of statins, aspirin, and ACE inhibitors, these data regarding the continued importance of life-style management are important. Improved screening must also be undertaken if the diabetic population is to benefit from these advances; in a recent study of Medicare beneficiaries with diabetes, half had not undergone lipid evaluation.[78] Most important with regard to cardiovascular disease, subgroup analyses of large placebo-controlled trials of cholesterol- and triglyceride-lowering therapy indicate that individuals with diabetes benefit as much from these therapies as do nondiabetics.[5]

GUIDELINES/RECOMMENDATIONS. Diet and exercise are integral components of the treatment strategy for patients with diabetes. In many patients with type 2 diabetes, glycemic control can be achieved by modest weight loss through diet and exercise.[79]

In contrast with patients with type 1 diabetes, those with type 2 diabetes are much more likely to have multiple coronary risk factors than is the case in the general population. Thus, aggressive modification of associated risk factors—including treatment of hypertension, aggressive reduction of serum cholesterol, reduction of weight, and increased physical activity—is of paramount importance in reducing the risk of CHD among people with diabetes.

Guidelines from the American Diabetes Association call for treating patients with diabetes and hypertension to a target blood pressure lower than 130/80 mm Hg. Although initial drug therapy with any drug class may be indicated for hypertension, some drug classes (ACE inhibitors, beta blockers, and diuretics) have shown particular benefits in reducing cardiovascular disease events among diabetic patients.[80] Current guidelines from the NCEP consider diabetes to be a CHD equivalent.[5] Thus, even for diabetic patients without previous CHD, the LDL cholesterol goal is lower than 100 mg/dl.[7] Life-style changes should be attempted first and supplemented with a statin when necessary or if starting

LDL levels are higher than 130 mg/dl. If the HDL level is less than 40 mg/dl, a fibrate may also be used. Initial therapy for hypertriglyceridemia is improved glycemic control. Additional triglyceride lowering can be achieved with high-dose statins (for subjects with both high LDL and triglyceride levels), a fibrate, or niacin. Administration of a drug that inhibits intestinal absorption of cholesterol, such as ezetimibe, also appears to raise HDL.[81] The American Diabetes Association also recommends daily low-dose aspirin therapy among diabetics with evidence of large-vessel disease (those with a history of myocardial infarction, vascular bypass procedure, stroke or transient ischemic attack, peripheral vascular disease, claudication, and/or angina), as well as among those without evidence of cardiovascular disease but who are at high risk for it based on cardiovascular risk factors such as smoking, hypercholesterolemia, hypertension, or obesity.[82]

Prediabetes and Metabolic Syndrome. The *metabolic syndrome* is a cluster of metabolic abnormalities that includes insulin resistance, dyslipidemia, hypertension, and excess weight, particularly around the waist (see Chaps. 36 and 40). The syndrome is quite common. In age-adjusted estimates from the National Health and Nutrition Examination Survey (NHANES) III, approximately 24 percent of U.S. adults met the criteria for metabolic syndrome.[83] Individuals with this syndrome are at increased risk for diabetes and cardiovascular disease and at increased risk of mortality from cardiovascular disease.[84]

Benefits of Treatment. Two recent randomized clinical trials demonstrate that patients with metabolic syndrome or impaired glucose tolerance benefit markedly from life-style interventions. In the Finnish Diabetes Prevention Study, 522 overweight individuals with impaired glucose tolerance received no intervention or individualized counseling with regard to reducing weight, total fat intake, and physical activity. Over a 3.2-year follow-up period, weight loss was significantly greater in the active intervention group, and the incidence of type 2 diabetes was reduced from 23 percent to 11 percent, a risk reduction of almost 60 percent ($p < 0.001$).[85] Using this simple intervention, 5 subjects with impaired glucose tolerance treated for 5 years would prevent one case of incident type 2 diabetes. In a critical test of this hypothesis, the Diabetes Prevention Program randomly assigned 3234 nondiabetic American patients with abnormal glucose metabolism to either placebo, metformin, or a life-style reduction program targeting weight loss and exercise.[86] In this trial, the life-style intervention reduced the incidence of type 2 diabetes by 58 percent as compared to placebo, whereas metformin reduced risk by 31 percent. Most important, the life-style-induced reduction was significantly greater than that achieved with pharmacological therapy.

Taken together, these two pivotal trials demonstrate that type 2 diabetes can be prevented or delayed, an effect that in turn will likely reduce atherosclerotic complications in this high-risk group. However, precise estimates for reduction in risk of cardiovascular disease events are unknown, and therefore cost efficacy data are not available.

The population impact of life-style intervention is likely to be large. In a prospective study of women, more than 90 percent of all incident cases of diabetes occurred among those who failed to exercise, had a BMI greater than 25, smoked, or had poor dietary habits.[87] The impact of exercise cannot be underestimated, because nearly one-third of all diabetic patients report a life-long pattern of minimal physical exertion.[88] Although a 2-hour postchallenge glucose measure provides improved sensitivity for risk detection in nondiabetic patients compared to fasting glucose levels, the clinical utility of this approach appears modest.[89]

Recommendations. Both the ATP III[5] and JNC-7[6] guidelines address the metabolic syndrome. Patients are classified as having it if they have three or more of the following: waist size > 40 inches for men or > 35 inches women; blood pressure > 135/85 mm Hg; HDL < 40 mg/dl for men or 50 mg/dl for women; triglycerides > 150 mg/dl; and fasting blood sugar > 100 mg/dl.

The main target of therapy is the underlying insulin-resistant state. The safest and most effective strategies for reducing insulin resistance include weight reduction in overweight and obese patients and increased physical activity. Although drugs that can improve insulin resistance are available, there is no clear evidence that they reduce CHD risk in patients with metabolic syndrome. There is evidence that drug therapy to improve the lipid profile, lower blood pressure, and treat the prothrombotic state reduces cardiac risk in this population.[5]

Obesity/Weight Loss (see also Chap. 41)

PREVALENCE. Over the past four decades, the proportion of the U.S. population considered to be overweight (BMI ≥ 25.0) and obese (BMI ≥ 30.0) has risen steadily (Fig. 42–7). In the National Health Examination Survey (1960 to 1962), an estimated 31.6 percent of men and women met the definition for overweight (BMI of 25.0 to 29.9 kg/m^2), of whom 13.4

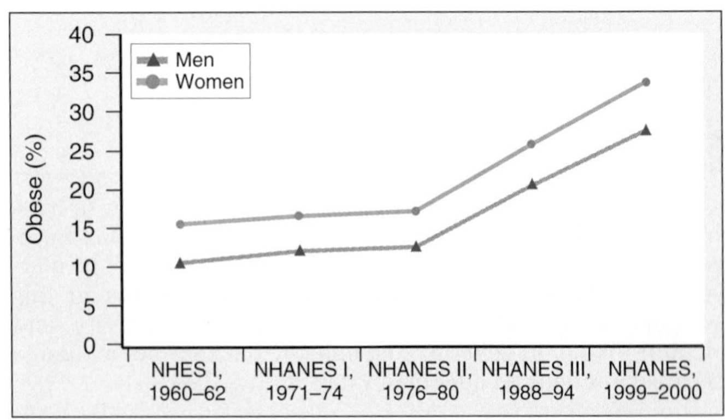

FIGURE 42-7 Percentage of U.S. adults classified as obese (body mass index > 30 kg/m^2) in health surveys from 1960 to 2000. NHES = National Health Examination Survey; NHANES = National Health and Nutrition Examination Survey. (Data from Flegal KM, Carroll MD, Ogden CL, Johnson CL: Prevalence and trends in obesity among U.S. adults, 1999-2000. JAMA 288:1723-1727, 2002.)

percent were obese (BMI > 30 kg/m^2).[90] Today, people who are overweight or obese make up a majority of the U.S. population, with the 1999 to 2000 NHANES showing 64.5 percent of men and women classified as overweight, of whom 30.5 percent were obese.[91]

The prevalence of overweight and obesity in children and adolescents is rising in parallel with that in adults. An estimated 15 percent of those aged 6 to 19 years and 10.4 percent of those aged 2 to 5 years are considered overweight or obese,[92] an alarming trend in view of the fact that early obesity is a strong predictor of later cardiovascular disease. Of considerable concern, excess weight may explain the surprising and dramatic increases in type 2 diabetes among children. In some parts of the United States, more than 30 percent of new cases of type 2 diabetes are in children, and most of these are attributable to obesity.[68,69]

ASSOCIATED RISK. Because various measures have been used to define overweight and obesity, reports on the magnitude of their association with CHD are not entirely consistent. Whether excess weight is an independent risk factor for CHD is disputed because its impact on CHD risk may be mediated, at least in part, by other coronary risk factors such as hypertension, dyslipidemia, glucose intolerance, and possibly hemostatic and inflammatory factors. However, obesity clearly associates with CHD and is thus an important and easily assessed marker of risk.

Data from numerous cohort and metabolic studies provide consistent evidence linking excess weight and inactivity with impaired health. Excess weight increases the risks of metabolic disorders such as hypertension, dyslipidemia, insulin resistance, and glucose intolerance. For example, in the Marks and Spencer Cardiovascular Risk Factor Study of 14,077 middle-aged women, highly significant age-adjusted differences were observed across seven categories of BMI (<20 to >30 kg/m^2) for systolic and diastolic blood pressure, serum total cholesterol, LDL cholesterol, HDL cholesterol, triglycerides, apolipoprotein A1, apolipoprotein B, and fasting blood glucose.[93] Excess weight is associated with increases in inflammatory markers such as C-reactive protein and fibrinogen in adults and children, increases that have been associated with elevated risks of cardiovascular disease.[94-96] Excess weight is also strongly linked to increased risk of CHD, ischemic stroke, type 2 diabetes mellitus, and a host of other chronic conditions.[97-101]

The distribution of body fat may also play a role in the development of CHD, with abdominal adiposity posing a substantially greater risk in both women[102] and men.[103] A waist circumference greater than 35 inches in women and greater than 40 inches in men is an easily measured marker of increased CHD risk.

The personal and economic burdens of excess weight are enormous. Recent estimates from six large prospective cohorts suggest that excess weight accounts for an estimated 280,000 to 320,000 deaths a year in the United States, more than 80 percent of which occur among individuals with BMI greater than 30 kg/m^2.[104] Data from a national survey of almost 10,000 U.S. adults suggest that obesity is associated with more chronic disorders and poorer health-related quality of life than smoking or problem drinking.[105] Medical spending for weight-related conditions accounted for an estimated 9 percent of the total annual U.S. medical expenses in 1998, or $78 billion,[106,107] an amount that rivals expenditures on smoking-related conditions.

BENEFIT OF INTERVENTION. No large-scale randomized trials of weight reduction as an isolated intervention are available on which to estimate the benefits of weight loss in lowering risk of CHD. However, sufficient information is available from numerous observational studies and small or short-term randomized clinical trials[97,108] to conclude that weight loss offers substantial health benefits (Table 42–9).

TABLE 42–9 Benefits of Weight Loss and Physical Activity among Overweight/obese Individuals or Those with Insufficient Daily Activity

Disease/Risk Factor	Weight Loss	Physical Activity
Hypertension	↓↓↓[97]	↓↓↓[109]
Type 2 diabetes mellitus	↓↓↓[85,86,110]	↓↓[85,86,110]
Lipid profile	Definite improvement[97]	Definite improvement[111]
Coronary heart disease	↓↓[108]	↓↓↓[108]
Stroke	↓[112]	↓↓[113]
Colorectal cancer	↓[114]	↓↓[114]
Breast cancer	↓[115]	↓[115]
Osteoarthritis	↓↓[116]	↓[117]
Osteoporosis	↔	↓↓↓[118,119]
Gallbladder disease	↓[120]	↓[121]
Sleep apnea	↓↓[122]	Unknown
Mental health	Probable improvement[123]	Probable improvement[123]

From Manson JE, Skerrett PJ, Greenland P, VanItallie TB: The escalating pandemics of obesity and sedentary lifestyle: A call to action for clinicians. Arch Intern Med 164:249-258, 2004.
↓↓↓: strong decrease in risk; ↓↓: moderate decrease in risk; ↓: slight decrease in risk; ↔: no benefit.

Modest weight loss, on the order of 5 percent to 10 percent, is associated with a significant improvement in blood pressure among individuals with and without hypertension.[97] Modest weight loss is also associated with improvements in the lipoprotein profile—lower levels of serum triglycerides, higher levels of HDL cholesterol, and small reductions in total and LDL cholesterol—as well as improvements in glucose tolerance and/or insulin resistance.[97] It is also associated with improvements in sleep apnea.[124]

There is little consensus, however, on the ideal approach to weight reduction.[125] Promoting life-style changes to encourage weight reduction has been universally disappointing. Although 25 percent of American men and 43 percent of American women may attempt to lose weight in any given year,[126] failure rates are exceedingly high. One reason may be that most individuals who are trying to lose weight are not following recommendations to reduce calorie intake and engage in at least 150 minutes of leisure time activity per week.[126] Effective treatment strategies generally involve a multifaceted approach, including dietary counseling, behavioral modification, increased physical activity, and psychosocial support. For some obese patients, pharmacotherapy or bariatric surgery may be necessary.[127]

COST EFFICACY. Without precise estimates of the benefit and with substantial variability in the intervention strategy, it is currently impossible to estimate the cost-benefit ratio of weight loss programs or interventions.

RECOMMENDATIONS/GUIDELINES. Numerous options are available for helping patients lose weight. Guidelines produced by the National Heart, Lung, and Blood Institute and the North American Association for the Study of Obesity[97] emphasize a three-part strategy for weight loss that includes caloric restriction, structured physical activity, and behavior therapy for all patients with a BMI greater than 30 kg/m^2 and those with a BMI of 25.0 to 29.9 kg/m^2 and a history of CHD or two or more disease risk factors.

Physical Inactivity/Exercise

(see also Chaps. 36 and 43)

PREVALENCE. Physical activity is an exceptionally common modifiable risk factor for CHD. Data from the Behavioral Risk Factor Surveillance System (BRFSS) suggest that 75 percent of adult Americans do not meet the current recommendation of 30 minutes of leisure-time physical activity on most, if not all, days of the week.[128] Nearly one-third do not engage in any leisure-time physical activity.[129] Lack of sufficient physical activity is also endemic among children. Only a minority of schoolchildren have daily physical education classes,[130,131] while walking and bicycling by children has declined.[132] In contrast, the time spent in sedentary activities such as watching television, playing video games, or using a computer has dramatically increased.[133] Older individuals, who are most at risk for cardiovascular disease, are less likely to be physically active than younger individuals, and women tend to be less active than men.

ASSOCIATED RISK. Data from more than 40 observational studies demonstrate clear evidence of an inverse linear dose-response relation between volume of physical activity and all-cause mortality rates in younger and older men and women. Minimal adherence to current physical activity guidelines, which yield an energy expenditure of about 1000 kcal/wk, is associated with a significant 20 to 30 percent reduction in risk of all-cause mortality.[134]

Data available in the mid-1950s showed that CHD rates were lower among bus conductors and mail carriers than sedentary bus drivers and postal supervisors. By incorporating estimates of leisure-time activity in their analyses, these investigators found that civil servants with sedentary jobs who engaged in vigorous sports were half as likely to suffer myocardial infarction as those who did not engage in leisure-time physical activity. Since then, a number of observational studies have reported similar inverse associations between activity level from work or play and CHD. In a 1990 meta-analysis of 27 observational cohort studies, Berlin and Colditz demonstrated that the risk of CHD in sedentary individuals was almost twice that of active individuals after controlling for other coronary risk factors. Long-term prospective studies of men and women consistently demonstrate that regular physical activity protects against death from CHD.[135-137] These benefits apply to activities as simple as brisk walking, which has been shown to reduce the risk of CHD in women[138] and men,[139,140] as well as the risk of type 2 diabetes.[110] Shifting even late in life from a sedentary life style to a more active one confers a reduction in mortality from CHD.[141,142] Physical activity is also associated with a decreased risk of stroke in men[143,144] and women,[145] primarily because of its beneficial effects on body weight, blood pressure, serum cholesterol, and glucose tolerance.

Although no large-scale, randomized trials of physical activity are available, numerous trials of moderate size and duration have been conducted among healthy individuals, those at high risk for cardiovascular disease, and those with existing cardiovascular disease. Despite differences in design, these trials generally demonstrate a benefit.[108] The ideal intensity, frequency, and duration of physical activity, however, have still not been determined.

BENEFIT OF INTERVENTION. While cessation of activity appears to result in increased risk of CHD, the lack of large-scale, randomized, primary prevention trials on the benefits of physical activity makes it difficult to determine the precise benefit of exercise in terms of CHD reduction. Physical activity does, however, have clearly demonstrated benefits on cardiovascular risk factors. Exercise increases HDL, reduces LDL[146] and triglycerides, increases insulin sensitivity,[147,148] and reduces blood pressure in both hypertensive and normotensive individuals.[149] Exercise also improves endothelial function.[150]

In secondary prevention, cardiac rehabilitation programs with an exercise component tend to report benefit in reducing subsequent events. Pooled data from many of these trials suggest reductions in total and cardiovascular mortality of about 25 percent.[151]

GUIDELINES/TREATMENT. For secondary prevention, guidelines from the American Heart Association/American College of Cardiology recommend encouraging patients to be physically active. An "exercise prescription" might include walking, jogging, cycling, swimming, or other aerobic activity for 30 to 60 minutes on at least most days of the week, supplemented with an increase in daily life-style activities such as walking up stairs when possible.[152] Strength training may offer additional cardiovascular and other benefits.[153] Structured exercise programs may enhance long-term compliance. For primary prevention, the U.S. Surgeon General's recommendation is an excellent starting point—every adult should accumulate 30 minutes of moderately intense physical activity on most, if not all, days of the week.[154]

Moderate Alcohol Consumption

Alcohol consumption has complex effects on cardiovascular disease. Observational studies demonstrate that heavy alcohol intake increases total mortality and cardiovascular disease mortality. In contrast, more than 100 prospective studies show an inverse association between moderate drinking and risk of heart attack, ischemic stroke, peripheral vascular disease, sudden cardiac death, and death from all cardiovascular causes.[155] The effect is relatively consistent, corresponding to a 20 to 45 percent reduction in risk. An association between moderate alcohol consumption and decreased cardiovascular risk has been observed in both primary and secondary prevention and among men and women. Mechanisms underlying the effect of moderate alcohol consumption, defined as one or two drinks daily, include raising HDL levels, improving fibrinolytic capacity, and reducing platelet aggregation and hs-CRP.[156]

RECOMMENDATIONS. While the association of alcohol and CHD is likely to be causal, any individual or public health recommendation must consider the complexity of alcohol's metabolic, physiological, and psychological effects. With alcohol, the difference between daily intake of small-to-moderate quantities and large quantities may be the difference between preventing and causing disease. For appropriate patients, a discussion of alcohol intake can be a part of routine preventive counseling. In general, one or two drinks per day may be safe for men. For women, because of their generally smaller BMIs and potential differences in liver metabolism, lower levels may be more prudent. However, counseling must be individualized—other medical problems, including other coronary risk factors (particularly hypertension and diabetes), liver disease, tendency toward excess use, family history of alcoholism, and possibly a family history of breast and colon cancer, should be taken into account when discussing alcohol consumption.

Oral Anticoagulants (see also Chaps. 50 and 80)

Oral anticoagulants prevent embolic events in patients with prosthetic heart valves and atrial fibrillation. Less certain is their role, either alone or in combination with aspirin, in the secondary prevention of events in those with CHD. The results of randomized, controlled trials are inconsistent, a troubling issue because oral anticoagulants have significant bleeding as a side effect.

A meta-analysis provided a comprehensive summary of data on high-, moderate-, and low-intensity oral anticoagulants alone or in combination with aspirin versus placebo or aspirin alone among those with cardiovascular disease.[157] In this analysis, high- and moderate-intensity oral anticoagulation reduced myocardial infarction and stroke rates when compared with placebo but increased the risk of hemorrhage. The combination of low-intensity oral anticoagulation plus aspirin did not appear to confer any benefit over aspirin alone, whereas the combination of moderate- or high-intensity oral anticoagulation plus aspirin did appear to offer promising benefits. These findings require confirmation from ongoing clinical trials.

Class 3 Interventions

Class 3 interventions relate to risk factors that are currently under investigation (see Table 42–3). For some of them, a causal relationship with CHD cannot be determined because of limited data. For others, where causal relationships are apparent, interventions are not yet available or tested.

Postmenopausal Estrogen Therapy

(see also Chap. 73)

RISK ASSOCIATED WITH MENOPAUSE. Before age 45, cardiovascular disease afflicts relatively few women in the United States and other developed countries. By age 60, however, it is the leading cause of death among women.[158] Although men exhibit a higher incidence of CHD at every age, as well as higher mortality rates from it, the gap narrows substantially after both natural menopause and bilateral oophorectomy.

A wide range of factors may explain the increased risk of CHD after menopause. These include adverse changes in lipid and glucose metabolism that result in an increase in LDL cholesterol and a decrease in HDL cholesterol, an increase in glucose intolerance, and changes in hemostatic factors and vascular function. These changes have long been attributed to the decline in endogenous estrogen that accompanies menopause. Physiological effects of exogenous estrogen are consistent with a cardioprotective effect. Estrogen reduces LDL and increases HDL levels; reduces Lp(a) lipoprotein, plasminogen-activator inhibitor type 1, and insulin levels; inhibits oxidation of LDL; and improves endothelial vascular function.[159] The effects of estrogen on inflammation are complex, as levels of fibrinogen decrease while levels of hs-CRP increase. Many of these effects are minimal when estrogen is given transdermally, suggesting a first-pass effect. Estrogen may also play one or more roles in maintaining normal hemostasis and improving glucose tolerance.

Considerable evidence from observational studies had suggested that the use of postmenopausal hormone therapy reduced the risk of CHD. A meta-analysis of 40 cohort and case-control studies suggested a 50 percent reduction in the risk of CHD associated with current estrogen use.[160] In an early study from the Nurses' Health Study, the largest prospective cohort study to address this question, current users of estrogen had about half the risk of CHD (relative risk, 0.51; 95 percent CI, 0.37 to 0.70) as nonusers did. The association appeared even stronger among women with known CHD. Such data provided the foundation for widespread use of postmenopausal hormone therapy to prevent cardiovascular disease.

EFFECTS OF INTERVENTION. Data from seven recent randomized trials (five on secondary prevention and two on primary prevention) not only failed to support the possible benefit of hormone therapy on CHD but indicated that combined estrogen and progestin may actually *increase* CHD risk.[161] This abrupt about-face with regard to the possible benefits of hormone therapy illustrates the problem of confounding and the importance of randomized, controlled trials.

The first secondary prevention trial, the Heart and Estrogen/progestin Replacement Study (HERS), found no cardiovascular benefit of estrogen-progestin supplementation even with extended follow-up.[162] Subsequent trials found no beneficial effect of hormone therapy or an increased risk of CHD events.[163-166]

One arm of the large, ongoing Women's Health Initiative was designed to evaluate the relative benefits and risks of estrogen plus progestin among 16,608 postmenopausal women aged 50 to 79 years with an intact uterus at baseline over a planned 8.5-year period. However, after a mean of 5.2 years of follow-up, the trial's data and safety monitoring board recommended stopping the trial because the test statistic for invasive breast cancer exceeded the stopping boundary for this adverse effect, and the global index statistic supported risks exceeding benefits. At this time, the estimated hazard ratios were 1.29 (95 percent CI, 1.02 to 1.63) for CHD; 1.41 (95 percent CI, 1.07 to 1.85) for stroke; and 2.13 (95 percent CI, 1.39 to 3.25) for pulmonary embolism. The hazard ratio for total cardiovascular disease was 1.22 (95 percent CI, 1.09 to 1.36).[161] The absolute excess cardiovascular risks per 10,000 person-years attributable to estrogen plus progestin were seven more CHD events, eight more strokes, and eight more pulmonary emboli.

The use of unopposed estrogen, other forms of estrogen, selective estrogen receptor modulators, and phytoestrogens in cardiovascular risk prevention remains unproven (see Chap. 73).[167]

RECOMMENDATIONS. Hormone therapy is no longer recommended as an approach to the prevention of cardiovascular disease. The U.S. Preventive Services Task Force recommends against the routine use of estrogen and progestin for the prevention of chronic conditions, including cardiovascular disease, in postmenopausal women.[168] Guidelines from the North American Menopause Society state that estrogen/progestin therapy should not be used for primary or secondary prevention of CHD.[169] Furthermore, in 2003 the U.S. Food and Drug Administration revised the labeling for all postmenopausal hormone therapies containing estrogen alone or estrogen plus a progestogen to include a boxed warning that highlights the increased risk for heart disease, myocardial infarction, stroke, and breast cancer.[170]

Dietary Factors (see also Chap. 41)

Diet clearly has an impact on CHD risk. Cross-cultural studies suggest that diet plays a role in CHD as well as other chronic diseases. For example, the Ni-Hon-San study demonstrated that Japanese immigrants who moved to Hawaii and California developed CHD and ischemic stroke at rates comparable to lifetime residents of the United States. However, understanding the specific components of the Western diet that impart this risk has been challenging. Dietary research is hampered by the complexity and difficulty of measuring dietary components.

Observational Studies

Observational studies have suggested a number of dietary factors that may increase the risk of CHD. One of the key features of the Western life style is an excess of caloric intake relative to caloric expenditure. One of the most consistent findings in observational dietary research is that individuals who consume higher amounts of fresh fruits and vegetables have lower rates of heart disease[171] and stroke.[172] Other components of the Western diet that have been implicated in increasing the risk of CHD include saturated and *trans* fats, simple carbohydrates that represent a glycemic load, and lack of fiber.

Metabolic trials suggest that diet is an important component of any prevention program for several reasons. It can have a potentially profound effect on weight reduction, which can improve dyslipidemia, hypertension, and diabetes. Even without weight loss, a healthy diet can improve the lipid profile and deliver nutrients that have salutary effects on the cardiovascular system. In the DASH Trial, 459 adults with systolic blood pressure lower than 160 mm Hg and diastolic pressure lower than 80 to 95 mm Hg were randomized to (1) a control diet low in fruits, vegetables, and dairy products and with a fat content of 37 percent; (2) a diet rich in fruits and vegetables; or (3) a combination diet rich in fruits, vegetables, and low-fat dairy products. Both of the intervention diets substantially reduced systolic and diastolic blood pressure in individuals with and without hypertension.[37]

A review of data from 147 metabolic studies, prospective cohort studies, and clinical trials suggests that at least three dietary strategies are effective in preventing CHD. These include substituting nonhydrogenated unsaturated fats for saturated and *trans* fats; increasing consumption of omega-3 fatty acids from fish, fish oil supplements, or plant sources; and adhering to a diet high in fruits, vegetables, nuts, and whole grains and low in refined grain products.[173]

Diet Trials with CHD Endpoints

Trial data exploring the impact of dietary changes alone on CHD events are limited. The Lyon Diet Heart Study randomized 605 survivors of a first myocardial infarction to a Mediterranean-type diet or a "prudent Western-type diet." After a mean follow-up of 46 months, the risk of cardiac death or acute myocardial infarction was 65 percent lower for those consuming the Mediterranean diet.[174] In the Gruppo Italiano per lo Studio della Sopravvivenza nell'Infarto Miocardico (GISSI), 11,324 survivors of a recent myocardial infarction were randomized to daily supplements containing 1 gm of n-3 polyunsaturated fatty acids, 300 mg of vitamin E, both, or neither for 3.5 years. Treatment with the n-3 polyunsaturated fatty acids, but not vitamin E, lowered the relative risk of the primary endpoint, which included death, nonfatal myocardial infarction, and stroke, by 10 percent (95 percent CI, 1 to 18).[175] This benefit was primarily attributable to a decrease in the risk of death rather than nonfatal myocardial infarction or stroke.

Specific Foods and Nutrients

A host of foods and micronutrients are under investigation as agents for reducing the risk of cardiovascular disease (see Chap. 41). These include whole grains, fiber, fish and fish oils, soy protein, folate, vitamin B_6, and antioxidants such as vitamin E and ubiquinone (coenzyme Q_{10}). Observational studies tend to report lower rates of CHD events among those who take antioxidant vitamins and folate supplements; however, studies are inconsistent and the effects are modest.

The importance of randomized clinical trials with regard to "heart healthy" foods and nutrients is best illustrated by briefly describing the ups and downs of vitamin E. Basic research strongly suggests that oxidative stress plays an important role in the development of atherosclerotic disease and that vitamin E may delay or prevent various steps in atherosclerosis. By the mid-1990s, observational data strongly suggested that high doses of vitamin E reduced the risk of CHD, particularly with regard to secondary prevention.[176] Completed secondary prevention trials, however, have demonstrated that vitamin E supplementation has little impact on CHD risk.[175,177,178] Several large, ongoing trials will determine whether vitamin E supplementation is effective for the primary prevention of cardiovascular disease.

RECOMMENDATIONS. Given the limited trial data, it is difficult to answer the patient question, "What should I eat to prevent heart disease?" Elements of that answer should include the following:

- Total caloric intake must be balanced with energy expenditure.
- Minimize intake of saturated and *trans* fat as well as rapidly digested carbohydrates. Instead, select monounsaturated and polyunsaturated fats and whole grains.
- Maximize fruit and vegetable intake. The U.S. Department of Agriculture recommends at least two servings of fresh fruit and at least three servings of fresh vegetables per day.
- Adequate intake of omega-3 fatty acids also appears to reduce the incidence of cardiovascular disease and especially sudden cardiac death.[179] Inclusion of two or three servings of fish per week (particularly fatty fish) may help prevent cardiovascular events.

Psychosocial Factors/Counseling

(see also Chaps. 36 and 84)

Like diet, the study of psychosocial factors as potential risk factors for CHD is hampered by imprecision in definitions and widely accepted metrics. Psychosocial factors such as depression, chronic hostility, social isolation, and perceived lack of social support have been consistently linked with risk of CHD.[180] Further data are needed, however, to confirm these relationships and establish the efficacy of interventional strategies. Data are inconsistent regarding associations between vascular risk and other psychological factors such as work-related stress, type A behavior, and anxiety.

Studies of therapeutic interventions, although not blinded, suggest a role for improving psychosocial factors as part of prevention programs, particularly in secondary prevention. The strongest evidence comes from post–myocardial infarction patients.[181] Although abundant data suggest that stress and depression are prevalent and predict events after myocardial infarction, data on interventions are limited. A meta-analysis of 37 small studies of health education and stress-management programs for CHD patients suggested that such efforts might reduce cardiac mortality by 34 percent and recurrent myocardial infarction by 29 percent, quite possibly through favorable effects on blood pressure, cholesterol, body weight, smoking behavior, physical activity, and dietary habits.[181]

The Enhancing Recovery in Coronary Heart Disease Patients (ENRICHD) randomized trial recruited 2481 patients (26 percent with perceived low social support, 39 percent with clinical depression, and 34 percent with both low social support and depression) within 4 weeks of myocardial infarction.[182] Half were randomized to cognitive behavioral therapy and drug therapy, if needed, and half to usual medical care. The intervention did not increase event-free survival. It did improve depression and social isolation, although the relative improvement in the intervention group compared with the usual care group was less than expected due to substantial improvement in usual care patients.

Preliminary evidence suggests that pharmacotherapy for depression following myocardial infarction, revascularization, or the diagnosis of coronary disease may improve morbidity and mortality. The Sertraline Antidepressant Heart Attack Randomized Trial (SADHART) demonstrated the safety of this selective serotonin re-uptake inhibitor as a treatment for recurrent depression in cardiovascular patients. Sertraline had no more impact on left ventricular ejection fraction, treatment-emergent ventricular premature complex runs, or other cardiac measures than placebo.[183] Scores on depression and mood scales were better in the sertraline group, particularly among those who had been depressed before their heart attacks, a group in which postattack depression is especially likely. Of note, rates of second heart attacks, heart failure, episodes of chest pain, or heart-related deaths were lower in the sertraline group than the placebo group. In the ENRICHD trial, antidepressant use was also associated with significantly lower risks of nonfatal myocardial infarction or death.[182]

Novel Biochemical and Genetic Markers

(see also Chap. 36)

Hemostatic and inflammatory markers, novel lipid parameters, cellular adhesion molecules, indicators of prior infection, and markers of oxidative stress all have been linked to steps in atherogenesis, thrombosis, or cardiovascular disease events (reviewed in detail in Chap. 36). Of these novel risk factors, only hs-CRP has been shown to add prognostic information over and above that provided by global risk prediction models such as the Framingham Risk Score. Recent guidelines from the Centers for Disease Control and Prevention and the American Heart Association encourage the use of hs-CRP as an adjunct to risk prediction, particularly among those at "intermediate risk."[184] In part, this endorsement of hs-CRP reflects the low cost of evaluation, particularly in comparison to other screening approaches based on imaging techniques such as CT scans for coronary calcium.

Other novel risk factors such as Lp(a) lipoprotein and homocysteine have more limited use in general screening but are likely to be helpful in settings of premature disease and in families affected by atherosclerosis who lack clusters of traditional risk factors. Novel markers such as the cytokine interleukin-6, the adhesion molecule known as intercellular adhesion molecule 1, CD40 ligand, myeloperoxidase, and lipoprotein-associated phospholipase A_2 have shown efficacy in several settings but currently lack standardized commercial assays for evaluation. A common limitation to all these novel markers is that no data yet exist that lowering levels leads to reduced vascular risk, and thus their use is largely limited to risk identification and motivation for life-style change. For example, although statin therapy lowers hs-CRP levels and post hoc analyses of completed statin trials suggest survival benefits for those with elevated hs-CRP levels, prospective trials directly testing the use of hs-CRP to target statin therapy are only now being initiated. Similarly, although folate lowers homocysteine levels, evidence that this approach lowers vascular risk is lacking. The potential clinical utility of these markers[185] and current evidence regarding their modification are covered in Chapter 36.

A number of common genetic polymorphisms have been associated with coronary risk factors. For example, carriers of a common mutation in the *MTHFR* gene have elevated levels of homocysteine, and there are multiple inherited abnormalities of lipid metabolism linked both to hyperlipidemia and elevated vascular risk. Similarly, almost half of the variance in hs-CRP is heritable. However, as discussed in Chapter 36, there is no evidence that screening for any of these polymorphisms substantially adds to information more easily obtained from direct plasma measures of homocysteine, lipids, or hs-CRP. This finding for arterial thrombosis is in marked contrast to findings for venous thromboembolism, where evaluation for factor V Leiden and the prothrombin mutation has proven clinically useful. Thus, although genetic screening holds great promise for identifying individuals at risk for subsequent events, its role in primary or secondary prevention remains unproven for atherothrombotic disease at this time. However, one can envision a time when genetic assays will play a role in identifying at-risk individuals and targeting therapies to reduce their risk of subsequent events.[186]

Multiple Risk Factor Intervention Programs

Although most prevention studies focus on changing a single factor, several have attempted to measure the impact of simultaneously changing multiple risk factors. In theory, the potential for synergistic effects between risk factors could lead to substantial reductions in risk that are multiplicative and offer the possibility of meaningful reductions in the risk of cardiovascular disease.[187]

Although these multiple risk factor intervention trials (Table 42–10) have made major contributions to our understanding of cardiovascular risk, as well as our knowledge of what makes for effective—and ineffective—intervention strategies, their results have been mixed. It is clear that intervention on multiple levels can reduce risk factors and that this reduction can be sustained over time. In a Belgian study that was part of the World Health Organization (WHO) European Collaborative Trial in the Multifactorial Prevention of Coronary Heart Disease, an intervention program composed of face-to-face counseling about eating habits, smoking, and physical activity substantially reduced predictors of coronary risk when compared with a control program that offered no such advice. The effect was sustained for 5 years.

A common result from multiple risk factor intervention trials is a change in risk factor levels or composite scores among those receiving intervention. However, this change has not always translated into lower event rates. Explanations for this inconsistency include the possibility that the magnitude of intervention was too small or that control patients may also have improved their health habits over time. What is clear from these trials, however, is that multiple simultaneous interventions can reduce cardiovascular risk when the planned interventions are large enough and are adequately implemented.

In an analysis of seven multiple intervention trials, Kornitzer plotted change in the multiple logistic function of risk against the reduction in risk of CHD. The strong linear relationship (Fig. 42–8) suggests that as long as risk factors are truly modified, event rates will also be reduced.

Summary of Recommendations

In this section we outline a general approach to a patient. The appropriate strategy for any given patient begins with an assessment of the overall risk of a first or subsequent cardiovascular event. Patients can be classified into two broad groups: (1) those with overt cardiovascular disease, including previous myocardial infarction, stroke, peripheral vascular disease, angina, or prior vascular procedure and (2) those without overt cardiovascular disease. Those without cardiovascular disease can be further subdivided into three risk strata: diabetics, high-risk nondiabetics, and low-risk nondiabetics. Those with cardiovascular disease and diabetes are generally straightforward to identify. Stratifying the remaining group requires the use of an algorithm such as those developed by the Framingham Heart Study (see Fig. 42–3) or the ESC.

Table 42–11 summarizes the interventional approach for all three classes. Many of these activities can be undertaken by allied health professionals in a prevention program. Case management models of prevention have been demonstrated as useful among higher-risk groups following myocardial infarction or bypass surgery.[188]

Current data strongly support a role for risk factors in the prediction of future risk and in the modification of that risk in both primary and secondary prevention of CHD. For several risk factors—cigarette smoking, dyslipidemias, and hypertension—the strength and consistency of association with atherosclerotic disease indicate a causal relationship, and the benefits of intervention are well documented in both primary and secondary prevention. There is little doubt that diabetes, physical inactivity, and obesity increase the risk of CHD and that light-to-moderate alcohol consumption reduces the risk, but the precise magnitude of the effect attributable to intervention for these factors has been difficult to docu-

TABLE 42–10 Multiple Intervention Trials

Trial	Population	Intervention
Multiple Risk Factor Intervention Trial[189]	12,866 men aged 35-57 yr at high risk for CHD; average 7-yr follow-up	Stepped-care therapy for high BP, counseling for smoking cessation, and dietary advice for high cholesterol; *or* usual care
Oslo Trial[190]	1232 men aged 40-49 yr with coronary risk in upper quartile; 5-yr follow-up	Diet similar to AHA step 1, counseling to stop smoking; *or* usual care
WHO Multifactorial Trial[191]	60,881 men aged 40-59 yr from 80 factories in Belgium, Italy, Poland, and United Kingdom; average 6 yr of intervention and follow-up	Educational materials or individual counseling regarding diet, smoking cessation, physical activity, and BP; drug therapy as needed for BP control; *or* no intervention
North Karelia Project[192]	11,992 men and women aged 25-59 yr; 10-yr follow-up	Population-based prevention program with outreach for smoking cessation and for reducing BP, serum cholesterol and other CVD risk factors
Goteborg Primary Prevention Trial[193]	Random sample of 20,000 men aged 47–55 yr; average 10 yr of intervention and follow-up	Antihypertensive treatment in subjects with SBP > 175 mm Hg or DBP > 115 mm Hg, dietary advice for subjects with serum cholesterol levels > 260 mg/dl, and smoking cessation advice; *or* usual care
Minnesota Heart Health Program[194]	400,000 residents aged 30-74 yr from 6 (3 paired) Midwestern communities; 5- to 6-yr intervention program	Individual counseling and community outreach on decreasing BP and serum cholesterol, smoking cessation, and increasing physical activity; *or* no intervention
Pawtucket Heart Health Program[195]	140,000 residents aged 18-64 yr of Pawtucket, RI, and a reference community; 7-yr intervention program	Community-wide educational programs designed to help individuals lower cholesterol and BP, stop smoking, maintain healthy weight, and increase physical activity
Stanford Five-City Project[196]	320,300 residents of 5 California cities (2 intervention, 3 comparison); 5-yr intervention program	Individual counseling and community outreach regarding decreasing BP and serum cholesterol, smoking cessation, and increasing physical activity
Lifestyle Heart Trial[187]	48 men and women aged 35-75 yr with ischemic heart disease; 4-yr intervention and follow-up	Low-fat vegetarian diet, moderate aerobic exercise, stress management training, smoking cessation, and group support; *or* usual care
Heidelberg Trial[197]	113 men and women recruited after coronary angiography for stable angina pectoris; 6-yr intervention and follow-up	Intervention group: AHA step 3 diet, 30 min of exercise daily, and two 60-min group counseling sessions per week; *or* advice about the AHA step 1 diet and encouragement of moderate aerobic exercise
Stanford Coronary Risk Intervention Project[198]	300 men and women < age 75 yr without severe congestive heart failure, pulmonary disease, intermittent claudication, or noncardiac life-threatening illness	Low-fat diet (<20% of calories from fat and <75 mg of cholesterol/d), physical activity, and counseling for smoking cessation, with cholesterol-lowering medication as needed; *or* usual care with personal physician

AHA = American Heart Association; BMI = body mass index; BP = blood pressure; CAD = coronary artery disease; CHD = coronary heart disease; CVD = cardiovascular disease; DBP = diastolic BP; HDL-C = high-density lipoprotein cholesterol; LDL-C = low-density lipoprotein cholesterol; MI = myocardial infarction; SBP = systolic BP; WHO = World Health Organization.

ment. For these factors low-cost behavioral interventions appear warranted.

Future Challenges

Primary and secondary prevention have contributed substantially to the reduction in CHD mortality rates. Yet challenges remain. First, as the population ages, the number of individuals with factors that put them at risk for cardiovascular disease will increase even if age-adjusted risk factor rates decline. Similarly, the number of people living with cardiovascular disease will increase, thus necessitating greater secondary preventive efforts.

Second, trends of several modifiable risk factors are troubling. Obesity and physical inactivity are epidemic among all

Change in Risk Factor(s)	Impact on Endpoint(s)
Coronary risk factors declined in both groups, though to a greater degree in intervention group	Nonsignificant change in CHD death: 17.9/1000 in intervention group, 19.3/1000 in usual care group
LDL-C (13%), triglycerides (20%), tobacco consumption (45%), and weight were lower in intervention group than usual care group; in both groups, physical activity and BP unchanged vs. baseline	Significant reduction in fatal MI, nonfatal MI, sudden death, and cerebrovascular accidents in intervention vs. control; 55% decrease in CHD death and 32% decrease in total mortality
Coronary risk predictors were significantly lower in intervention group during first 5 yr of trial; by trial's end, differences were statistically significant only for high-risk subjects who received face-to-face counseling	Nonsignificant differences in all-cause mortality (–5.3%), total CHD (–10.2%; $p = 0.07$), fatal CHD (6.9%), and nonfatal MI (–14.8%; $p = 0.06$) for intervention group vs. nonintervention group
In intervention group, 28% decrease in smoking, 3% decrease in serum cholesterol, and 3% decrease in BP vs. reference group	Age-adjusted CHD mortality decreased 22% in intervention group, 12% in reference group, and 11% in all of Finland ($p < 0.05$)
BP, serum cholesterol, and smoking all decreased markedly in both intervention and control groups	No significant differences in total mortality, stroke, and CHD incidence
Generally favorable, though not statistically significant changes in intervention group vs. reference group	No significant difference in CAD death rate
Small, not statistically significant decreases in serum cholesterol and BP in Pawtucket; slightly less smoking in the reference community	Projected CVD rates significantly (16%) less in Pawtucket during education program, but dropped to 8% after education program
Statistically significant reductions in community averages of plasma cholesterol level (2%), BP (4%), resting pulse rate (3%), and smoking rate (13%) in intervention communities vs. reference communities	Decreased composite total mortality risk scores (15%) and CHD risk scores (16%) in intervention communities vs. reference communities
After 4 yr, participants in intervention group were exercising more, practicing more stress management, and consuming less cholesterol and fewer fat calories than those in usual care group	In intervention group after 4 yr, significant reductions in frequency, duration, and severity of angina; fewer revascularizations (21% vs. 60%); and regression of atherosclerotic lesions (vs. continued worsening in usual care group)
Nonsignificant reductions in total cholesterol and triglycerides, maintenance of BMI, and significant increase in physical work capacity among those in intervention group	As assessed by coronary arteriography, significantly slower progression of coronary artery stenosis in intervention group, combined with significant improvements in myocardial perfusion
Significant improvements in percent body fat, weight, BP, LDL-C, triglycerides, HDL-C, and exercise capacity in treatment group vs. controls	Although progression of coronary artery disease occurred in both groups, intervention group had a 47% lower rate of progression per individual and a 58% lower rate of progression in diseased vessel segments than reference group

sectors of the population, including children. These factors will tend to increase rates of diabetes and hypertension and slow the favorable trends in mean lipid levels.

Third, in addition to developing a better understanding of the mechanistic and epidemiological determinants of atherosclerotic disease, we must pay more attention to finding effective strategies for prioritizing factors in prevention programs, implementing existing guidelines for risk factor modification, and developing low-cost interventions for factors for which guidelines are not yet available. Many life-style changes are difficult to achieve and even harder to maintain over the long term. Such interventions need to involve not only the affected individuals but also families, workplaces, schools, and even whole communities.

Finally, for clinicians, identifying a successful strategy for each patient is of critical importance. Further research on cost-benefit and risk-benefit ratios will enable better targeting of interventions for maximal individual and societal benefit. More widespread use of multifaceted self-help and health professional–directed prevention programs should help sustain the decline in cardiovascular disease mortality rates in the United States.

TABLE 42–11 Modifiable Risk Factors for the Prevention of Cardiovascular Disease

Factor	Effect	Intervention	Comment
Class 1 Risk Factors and Interventions in the Prevention of Cardiovascular Disease			
Smoking	2-3-fold increased risk	Smoking cessation with behavior and pharmacological intervention	Smoking cessation results in a 60% reduction in CHD risk by 3 yr; about half of that benefit occurs in first 3-6 mo after quitting. Interventions are cost-effective in both primary and secondary prevention
Hypertension	7 mm Hg increase in BP over baseline increases risk of CVD by 27%	Life-style modifications, weight loss, limited alcohol intake, aerobic exercise, and medications	A 5- to 6-mm Hg reduction in BP results in 42% reduction in risk of stroke and 16% reduction in risk of CVD. Extensive trial and cost-efficacy data support a tiered approach based on underlying risk
Dyslipidemias			
Hypercholesterolemia	10% increase in serum cholesterol increases risk of CVD by 20-30%	Dietary changes, lipid-lowering medications	Reduction in serum cholesterol by 10% reduces CVD death by 10% and CVD events by 18%. Treatment for >5 yr reduces CVD events by 25%. Extensive trial and cost-efficacy data support a tiered approach based on underlying risk
Elevated fasting triglyceride levels and low HDL levels	Increases risk	Diet, exercise, and lipid-lowering therapy	HDL and triglyceride measures are useful markers of CHD risk, and limited trial data suggest that intervention reduces risk
Pharmacological Therapies			
Aspirin in secondary prevention	Reduces CVD events by 25%	Daily low-dose aspirin	Reduces risk among those with any form of CVD
Beta blockers following MI	Reduces CVD events by 18%	Daily beta blocker use	Trial data suggest that the benefit may increase with increasing dose
ACE inhibitors for patients with low EF and following MI	Reduces CVD events by 22% in those with low EF and by 7% following MI	Daily ACE inhibitor use	Trial data suggest that the benefit may increase with increasing dose
Class 2 Risk Factors and Interventions in the Prevention of Cardiovascular Disease			
Insulin-dependent diabetes	Increases risk 2-4-fold in men and 3-7-fold in women	Maintaining normoglycemia with diet, exercise, weight management, and insulin	Trial data strongly suggest that tight control with insulin reduces risk of microvascular disease and may reduce the risk of CVD events
NIDDM	Increases risk 2-4-fold in men and 3-7-fold in women	Maintaining normoglycemia with diet, exercise, weight management, oral agents, and insulin as needed	Tight control appears to reduce microvascular disease, but data on the risk of CHD are not available. Those with NIDDM are likely to have multiple coronary risk factors that should be aggressively modified
Obesity and physical inactivity	Increases risk	Diet, exercise, and weight management programs	In addition to improving other CVD risk factors, maintaining ideal body weight and a physically active life style may reduce risk of MI as much as 50%, but trial data are limited
Moderate alcohol intake (one drink per day)	Decreases risk of MI by 30-50%	Discussion of alcohol intake with all patients	Risk/benefit ratio for moderate alcohol consumption may vary widely by gender and is based on underlying risk of CHD; recommendations must be made individually with careful regard for conditions such as hypertension, diabetes, liver disease, history of alcohol abuse, risk of breast cancer
Pharmacological Therapies			
Aspirin in primary prevention	Pooled trial data in men suggest a 33% reduction in risk of first MI	Daily or alternate-day low-dose aspirin	Prophylactic aspirin use in older men, particularly with risk factors, may reduce risk of MI. Data among women are limited but forthcoming

TABLE 42–11 Modifiable Risk Factors for the Prevention of Cardiovascular Disease—cont'd

Category	Specific Factors	Comment
Class 3 Factors and Interventions in the Prevention of Cardiovascular Disease		
Menopause	Increases CVD risk. Evidence from large RCTs suggests that hormone replacement therapy may increase, not decrease, this risk, and long-term use is associated with increased risk of endometrial and breast cancer	The combination of estrogen and progestin is not recommended as a strategy for decreasing the risk of heart disease in postmenopausal women
Dietary factors	Fruit and vegetable intake, type and amount of fat, type and amount of carbohydrate, fiber, *trans*-fatty acids, dietary antioxidants, dietary bioflavonoids, dietary folate, fish and fish oils, garlic, etc.	USDA recommends 5 servings of fruit and vegetables per day. Reduction in saturated and *trans*-fatty acid intake appears to be warranted
Dietary supplements	Multivitamins, antioxidant supplements, folate, vitamins B_{12} and B_6, fish oils, etc.	Randomized trials of antioxidant supplements have been disappointing. Randomized trial data on antioxidants and folate are forthcoming
Psychological factors	Depression, lack of social support, stress, type A personality, etc.	Trials of antidepressants in secondary prevention are forthcoming
Novel biochemical markers	Fibrinogen, homocysteine, Lp(a), t-PA, von Willebrand factor, factor VII, C-reactive protein, soluble adhesion molecules (sICAM, sVCAM), antibodies to various infectious agents, measures of oxidative stress, etc.	Additional observational data are needed to clarify the role of these factors in clinical practice
Novel genetic markers	LDL receptor, factor V Leiden, ACE, etc.	Potential genetic markers and therapies are emerging at a rapid rate

ACE = angiotensin-converting enzyme; BP = blood pressure; CHD = coronary heart disease; CVD = cardiovascular disease; EF = ejection fraction; HDL = high-density lipoprotein; LDL = low-density lipoprotein; Lp(a) = lipoprotein little A antigen; MI = myocardial infarction; NIDDM = non-insulin-dependent diabetes mellitus; RCTs = randomized controlled trials; sICAM = soluble intercellular adhesion molecule; sVCAM = soluble vascular cell adhesion molecule; t-PA = tissue-type plasminogen activator; USDA = U.S. Department of Agriculture.

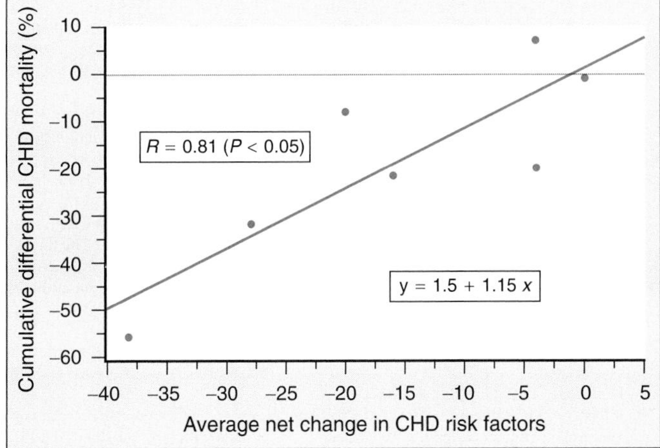

FIGURE 42–8 For seven trials, four of which made up the World Health Organization European Collaborative Trial in Multifactorial Prevention of Coronary Heart Disease, Kornitzer plotted the difference in a composite risk factor score between treated and untreated groups and showed a statistically significant correlation between the magnitude of risk factor improvement and coronary heart disease (CHD) mortality. (From Kornitzer M: Changing individual behavior. *In* Marmot M, Elliott P [eds]: Coronary Heart Disease Epidemiology: From Aetiology to Public Health. Oxford, Oxford University Press, 1992, p 492.)

REFERENCES

1. Murray CJL, Lopez AD: The Global Burden of Disease. Cambridge, MA, Harvard School of Public Health, 1996.
2. Howson CP, Reddy SK, Ryan TJ, Bale JR: Control of Cardiovascular Diseases in Developing Countries. Washington, DC, National Academy Press, 1998.
3. Yarnall KS, Pollak KI, Ostbye T, et al: Primary care: Is there enough time for prevention? Am J Public Health 93:635-641, 2003.
4. Kannel WB, Dawber TR, Kagan A, et al: Factors of risk in the development of coronary heart disease—six year follow-up experience: The Framingham Study. Ann Intern Med 55:33-50, 1961.
5. Third Report of the National Cholesterol Education Program (NCEP) Expert Panel on Detection, Evaluation, and Treatment of High Blood Cholesterol in Adults (Adult Treatment Panel III) final report. Circulation 106:3143-3421, 2002.
6. Chobanian AV, Bakris GL, Black HR, et al: The Seventh Report of the Joint National Committee on Prevention, Detection, Evaluation, and Treatment of High Blood Pressure: The JNC-7 Report. JAMA 289:2560-2572, 2003.
7. Haffner SM: Management of dyslipidemia in adults with diabetes. Diabetes Care 26(Suppl 1):S83-S86, 2003.
8. Wilson PW, D'Agostino RB, Levy D, et al: Prediction of coronary heart disease using risk factor categories. Circulation 97:1837-1847, 1998.
9. Wood D, De Backer G, Faergeman O, et al: Prevention of coronary heart disease in clinical practice: Recommendations of the Second Joint Task Force of European and other Societies on Coronary Prevention. Eur Heart J 19:1434-1503, 1998.
10. Assmann G, Cullen P, Schulte H: Simple scoring scheme for calculating the risk of acute coronary events based on the 10-year follow-up of the prospective cardiovascular Munster (PROCAM) study. Circulation 105:310-315, 2002.
11. Orford JL, Sesso HD, Stedman M, et al: A comparison of the Framingham and European Society of Cardiology coronary heart disease risk prediction models in the normative aging study. Am Heart J 144:95-100, 2002.
12. MacMahon S, Peto R, Cutler J, et al: Blood pressure, stroke, and coronary heart disease: I. Prolonged differences in blood pressure: Prospective observational studies corrected for the regression dilution bias. Lancet 335:765-774, 1990.
13. Pearson TA, McBride PE, Miller NH, Smith SC: 27th Bethesda Conference: Matching the intensity of risk factor management with the hazard for coronary disease events. Task Force 8. Organization of preventive cardiology service. J Am Coll Cardiol 27:1039-1047, 1996.

Cigarette Smoking

14. Strategies to control tobacco use in the United States: A blueprint for public health action in the 1990s. NIH Publication No. 92-3316. Bethesda, MD, U.S. Department of Health and Human Services, Public Health Service, National Institutes of Health, National Cancer Institute, 1991.
15. Cigarette report for 2001. Federal Trade Commission, 2003. (http://www.ftc.gov/os/2003/06/2001cigreport.pdf)
16. Office on Smoking and Health: Percentage of smoking prevalence among U.S. adults, 18 years of age and older, 1955-1994. National Center for Chronic Disease and Prevention, Centers for Disease Control and Prevention, 1996. (http://www.cdc.gov/tobacco/prevali.htm)
17. Cigarette smoking among adults—United States, 2000. MMWR Morb Mortal Wkly Rep 51:642-645, 2002.
18. Johnston LD, O'Malley PM, Bachman JG: National survey results on drug use from the Monitoring the Future study, 1975-1998. Vol I: secondary school students. NIH Publication No. 99-4660. Rockville, MD, National Institutes of Health, National Institute on Drug Abuse, 1999.
19. Trends in cigarette smoking among high school students—United States, 1991–2001. MMWR Morb Mortal Wkly Rep 51:409-412, 2002.

20. Cigarette smoking among adults—United States, 1997. MMWR Morb Mortal Wkly Rep 48:993-996, 1999.
21. Annual smoking—attributable mortality, years of potential life lost, and economic costs: United States, 1995-1999. MMWR Morb Mortal Wkly Rep 51:300-303, 2002.
22. Jha P, Chaloupka FJ: Curbing the epidemic: Governments and the economics of tobacco control. Washington, DC, World Bank, 1999.
23. Reducing risks, promoting healthy life: World Health Report 2002. Geneva, World Health Organization, 2002.
24. Cromwell J, Bartosch WJ, Fiore MC, et al: Cost-effectiveness of the clinical practice recommendations in the AHCPR guideline for smoking cessation. Agency for Health Care Policy and Research. JAMA 278:1759-1766, 1997.
25. A clinical practice guideline for treating tobacco use and dependence: A U.S. Public Health Service report. The Tobacco Use and Dependence Clinical Practice Guideline Panel, Staff, and Consortium Representatives. JAMA 283:3244-3254, 2000.
26. U.S. Preventive Services Task Force: Guide to Clinical Preventive Services. 3rd ed. Rockville, MD, Agency for Healthcare Research and Quality, 2000-2003.
27. Thomson CC, Rigotti NA: Hospital- and clinic-based smoking cessation interventions for smokers with cardiovascular disease. Prog Cardiovasc Dis 45:459-479, 2003.

Hypertension

28. National Center for Health Statistics: Health, United States, 2002. Hyattsville, MD, U.S. Department of Health and Human Services, Centers for Disease Control and Prevention, 2002.
29. Vasan RS, Beiser A, Seshadri S, et al: Residual lifetime risk for developing hypertension in middle-aged women and men: The Framingham Heart Study. JAMA 287:1003-1010, 2002.
30. Hajjar I, Kotchen TA: Trends in prevalence, awareness, treatment, and control of hypertension in the United States, 1988-2000. JAMA 290:199-206, 2003.
31. Lewington S, Clarke R, Qizilbash N, et al: Age-specific relevance of usual blood pressure to vascular mortality: A meta-analysis of individual data for one million adults in 61 prospective studies. Lancet 360:1903-1913, 2002.
32. Collins R, Peto R, MacMahon S, et al: Blood pressure, stroke, and coronary heart disease: II. Short-term reductions in blood pressure: Overview of randomised drug trials in their epidemiological context. Lancet 335:827-838, 1990.
33. Ogden LG, He J, Lydick E, Whelton PK: Long-term absolute benefit of lowering blood pressure in hypertensive patients according to the JNC-VI risk stratification. Hypertension 35:539-543, 2000.
34. Major outcomes in high-risk hypertensive patients randomized to angiotensin-converting enzyme inhibitor or calcium channel blocker versus diuretic: The Antihypertensive and Lipid-Lowering Treatment to Prevent Heart Attack Trial (ALLHAT). JAMA 288:2981-2997, 2002.
35. Pearce KA, Furberg CD, Psaty BM, Kirk J: Cost-minimization and the number needed to treat in uncomplicated hypertension. Am J Hypertens 11:618-629, 1998.
36. Guide to Clinical Preventive Services. 2nd ed. Baltimore, MD, Williams & Wilkins, 1996.
37. Appel LJ, Moore TJ, Obarzanek E, et al: A clinical trial of the effects of dietary patterns on blood pressure. DASH Collaborative Research Group. N Engl J Med 336:1117-1124, 1997.
38. Sacks FM, Svetkey LP, Vollmer WM, et al: Effects on blood pressure of reduced dietary sodium and the Dietary Approaches to Stop Hypertension (DASH) diet. DASH-Sodium Collaborative Research Group. N Engl J Med 344:3-10, 2001.
39. The sixth report of the Joint National Committee on Prevention, Detection, Evaluation, and Treatment of High Blood Pressure. Arch Intern Med 157:2413-2446, 1997.
40. Bertrand E: Cardiovascular disease in developing countries. *In* Dalla Volta S (ed): Cardiology. New York, McGraw-Hill, 1999, pp 825-834.

Dyslipidemia

41. Law MR, Wald NJ, Thompson SG: By how much and how quickly does reduction in serum cholesterol concentration lower risk of ischaemic heart disease? BMJ 308:367-372, 1994.
42. Law MR, Wald NJ, Wu T, et al: Systematic underestimation of association between serum cholesterol concentration and ischaemic heart disease in observational studies: Data from the BUPA study. BMJ 308:363-366, 1994.
43. Maron DJ, Fazio S, Linton MF: Current perspectives on statins. Circulation 101:207-213, 2000.
44. Schwartz GG, Olsson AG, Ezekowitz MD, et al: Effects of atorvastatin on early recurrent ischemic events in acute coronary syndromes. The MIRACL Study: A randomized controlled trial. JAMA 285:1711-1718, 2001.
45. Newby LK, Kristinsson A, Bhapkar MV, et al: Early statin initiation and outcomes in patients with acute coronary syndromes. JAMA 287:3087-3095, 2002.
46. LaRosa JC, He J, Vupputuri S: Effect of statins on risk of coronary disease: A meta-analysis of randomized controlled trials. JAMA 282:2340-2346, 1999.
47. Warshafsky S, Packard D, Marks SJ, et al: Efficacy of 3-hydroxy-3-methylglutaryl coenzyme A reductase inhibitors for prevention of stroke. J Gen Intern Med 14:763-774, 1999.
48. Prosser LA, Stinnett AA, Goldman PA, et al: Cost-effectiveness of cholesterol-lowering therapies according to selected patient characteristics. Ann Intern Med 132:769-779, 2000.
49. Ganz DA, Kuntz KM, Jacobson GA, Avorn J: Cost-effectiveness of 3-hydroxy-3-methylglutaryl coenzyme A reductase inhibitor therapy in older patients with myocardial infarction. Ann Intern Med 132:780-787, 2000.
50. Guidelines for using serum cholesterol, high-density lipoprotein cholesterol, and triglyceride levels as screening tests for preventing coronary heart disease in adults. American College of Physicians. Ann Intern Med 124:515-517, 1996.
51. Gaziano JM, Hennekens CH, O'Donnell CJ, et al: Fasting triglycerides, high-density lipoprotein, and risk of myocardial infarction. Circulation 96:2520-2525, 1997.
52. Austin MA, Hokanson JE, Edwards KL: Hypertriglyceridemia as a cardiovascular risk factor. Am J Cardiol 81:7B-12B, 1998.
53. Assmann G, Schulte H, Funke H, von Eckardstein A: The emergence of triglycerides as a significant independent risk factor in coronary artery disease. Eur Heart J 19(Suppl M):M8-M14, 1998.
54. Rubins HB, Robins SJ, Collins D, et al: Gemfibrozil for the secondary prevention of coronary heart disease in men with low levels of high-density lipoprotein cholesterol. Veterans Affairs High-Density Lipoprotein Cholesterol Intervention Trial Study Group. N Engl J Med 341:410-418, 1999.

Secondary Prevention

55. Collaborative meta-analysis of randomised trials of antiplatelet therapy for prevention of death, myocardial infarction, and stroke in high risk patients. BMJ 324:71-86, 2002.
56. Gaspoz JM, Coxson PG, Goldman PA, et al: Cost-effectiveness of aspirin, clopidogrel, or both for secondary prevention of coronary heart disease. N Engl J Med 346:1800-1806, 2002.
57. Eidelman RS, Hebert PR, Weisman SM, Hennekens CH: An update on aspirin in the primary prevention of cardiovascular disease. Arch Intern Med 163:2006-2010, 2003.
58. Aspirin for the primary prevention of cardiovascular events: Recommendation and rationale. Ann Intern Med 136:157-160, 2002.
59. Freemantle N, Cleland J, Young P, et al: Beta blockade after myocardial infarction: Systematic review and meta regression analysis. BMJ 318:1730-1737, 1999.
60. Phillips KA, Shlipak MG, Coxson P, et al: Health and economic benefits of increased beta-blocker use following myocardial infarction. JAMA 284:2748-2754, 2000.
61. Indications for ACE inhibitors in the early treatment of acute myocardial infarction: Systematic overview of individual data from 100,000 patients in randomized trials. ACE Inhibitor Myocardial Infarction Collaborative Group. Circulation 97:2202-2212, 1998.
62. Domanski MJ, Exner DV, Borkowf CB, et al: Effect of angiotensin-converting enzyme inhibition on sudden cardiac death in patients following acute myocardial infarction: A meta-analysis of randomized clinical trials. J Am Coll Cardiol 33:598-604, 1999.
63. Teo KK, Yusuf S, Pfeffer M, et al: Effects of long-term treatment with angiotensin-converting-enzyme inhibitors in the presence or absence of aspirin: A systematic review. Lancet 360:1037-1043, 2002.
64. Yusuf S, Sleight P, Pogue J, et al: Effects of an angiotensin-converting enzyme inhibitor, ramipril, on cardiovascular events in high-risk patients. The Heart Outcomes Prevention Evaluation Study Investigators. N Engl J Med 342:145-153, 2000.
65. Pfeffer MA, Swedberg K, Granger CB, et al: Effects of candesartan on mortality and morbidity in patients with chronic heart failure: The CHARM-Overall programme. Lancet 362:759-766, 2003.

Diabetes, Metabolic Syndrome, and Obesity

66. National Diabetes Fact Sheet: General Information and National Estimates on Diabetes in the United States, 2000. Atlanta, Centers for Disease Control and Prevention, 2002.
67. Harris MI, Flegal KM, Cowie CC, et al: Prevalence of diabetes, impaired fasting glucose, and impaired glucose tolerance in U.S. adults. The Third National Health and Nutrition Examination Survey, 1988–1994. Diabetes Care 21:518-524, 1998.
68. Type 2 diabetes in children and adolescents. American Diabetes Association. Diabetes Care 23:381-389, 2000.
69. Fagot-Campagna A, Pettitt DJ, Engelgau MM, et al: Type 2 diabetes among North American children and adolescents: An epidemiologic review and a public health perspective. J Pediatr 136:664-672, 2000.
70. Gu K, Cowie CC, Harris MI: Mortality in adults with and without diabetes in a national cohort of the U.S. population, 1971-1993. Diabetes Care 21:1138-1145, 1998.
71. Barrett-Connor EL, Cohn BA, Wingard DL, Edelstein SL: Why is diabetes mellitus a stronger risk factor for fatal ischemic heart disease in women than in men? The Rancho Bernardo Study. JAMA 265:627-631, 1991.
72. Hu FB, Stampfer MJ, Solomon CG, et al: The impact of diabetes mellitus on mortality from all causes and coronary heart disease in women: 20 years of follow-up. Arch Intern Med 161:1717-1723, 2001.
73. Cho E, Rimm EB, Stampfer MJ, et al: The impact of diabetes mellitus and prior myocardial infarction on mortality from all causes and from coronary heart disease in men. J Am Coll Cardiol 40:954-960, 2002.
74. Intensive blood glucose control with sulphonylureas or insulin compared with conventional treatment and risk of complications in patients with type 2 diabetes (UKPDS 33). UK Prospective Diabetes Study (UKPDS) Group. Lancet 352:837-853, 1998.
75. Abraira C, Colwell J, Nuttall F, et al: Cardiovascular events and correlates in the Veterans Affairs Diabetes Feasibility Trial. Veterans Affairs Cooperative Study on Glycemic Control and Complications in Type II Diabetes. Arch Intern Med 157:181-188, 1997.
76. Gerstein HC, Mann JF, Pogue J, et al: Prevalence and determinants of microalbuminuria in high-risk diabetic and nondiabetic patients in the Heart Outcomes Prevention Evaluation Study. The HOPE Study Investigators. Diabetes Care 23(Suppl 2):B35-B39, 2000.
77. Gaede P, Vedel P, Larsen N, et al: Multifactorial intervention and cardiovascular disease in patients with type 2 diabetes. N Engl J Med 348:383-393, 2003.
78. Arday DR, Fleming BB, Keller DK, et al: Variation in diabetes care among states: Do patient characteristics matter? Diabetes Care 25:2230-2237, 2002.
79. Markovic TP, Jenkins AB, Campbell LV, et al: The determinants of glycemic responses to diet restriction and weight loss in obesity and NIDDM. Diabetes Care 21:687-694, 1998.
80. Arauz-Pacheco C, Parrott MA, Raskin P: Treatment of hypertension in adults with diabetes. Diabetes Care 26(Suppl 1):S80-S82, 2003.
81. Ballantyne CM, Houri J, Notarbartolo A, et al: Effect of ezetimibe coadministered with atorvastatin in 628 patients with primary hypercholesterolemia: A prospective, randomized, double-blind trial. Circulation 107:2409-2415, 2003.
82. Colwell JA: Aspirin therapy in diabetes. Diabetes Care 26(Suppl 1):S87-S88, 2003.
83. Ford ES, Giles WH, Dietz WH: Prevalence of the metabolic syndrome among U.S. adults: Findings from the Third National Health and Nutrition Examination Survey. JAMA 287:356-359, 2002.

84. Wilson PW, Grundy SM: The metabolic syndrome: practical guide to origins and treatment: Parts I and II. Circulation 108:1422-1424 and 1537-1540, 2003.
85. Tuomilehto J, Lindstrom J, Eriksson JG, et al: Prevention of type 2 diabetes mellitus by changes in lifestyle among subjects with impaired glucose tolerance. N Engl J Med 344:1343-1350, 2001.
86. Knowler WC, Barrett-Connor E, Fowler SE, et al: Reduction in the incidence of type 2 diabetes with lifestyle intervention or metformin. N Engl J Med 346:393-403, 2002.
87. Hu FB, Manson JE, Stampfer MJ, et al: Diet, lifestyle, and the risk of type 2 diabetes mellitus in women. N Engl J Med 345:790-797, 2001.
88. Nelson KM, Reiber G, Boyko EJ: Diet and exercise among adults with type 2 diabetes: Findings from the Third National Health and Nutrition Examination Survey (NHANES III). Diabetes Care 25:1722-1728, 2002.
89. Smith NL, Barzilay JI, Shaffer D, et al: Fasting and 2-hour postchallenge serum glucose measures and risk of incident cardiovascular events in the elderly: The Cardiovascular Health Study. Arch Intern Med 162:209-216, 2002.
90. Flegal KM, Carroll MD, Kuczmarski RJ, Johnson CL: Overweight and obesity in the United States: Prevalence and trends, 1960-1994. Int J Obes Relat Metab Disord 22:39-47, 1998.
91. Flegal KM, Carroll MD, Ogden CL, Johnson CL: Prevalence and trends in obesity among U.S. adults, 1999-2000. JAMA 288:1723-1727, 2002.
92. Ogden CL, Flegal KM, Carroll MD, Johnson CL: Prevalence and trends in overweight among U.S. children and adolescents, 1999-2000. JAMA 288:1728-1732, 2002.
93. Ashton WD, Nanchahal K, Wood DA: Body mass index and metabolic risk factors for coronary heart disease in women. Eur Heart J 22:46-55, 2001.
94. Ford ES, Galuska DA, Gillespie C, et al: C-reactive protein and body mass index in children: Findings from the Third National Health and Nutrition Examination Survey, 1988-1994. J Pediatr 138:486-492, 2001.
95. Duncan BB, Schmidt MI, Chambless LE, et al: Fibrinogen, other putative markers of inflammation, and weight gain in middle-aged adults—the ARIC study. Atherosclerosis Risk in Communities. Obes Res 8:279-286, 2000.
96. Visser M, Bouter LM, McQuillan GM, et al: Elevated C-reactive protein levels in overweight and obese adults. JAMA 282:2131-2135, 1999.
97. Clinical Guidelines on the Identification, Evaluation, and Treatment of Overweight and Obesity in Adults. National Institutes of Health, National Heart, Lung, and Blood Institute, Obesity Education Initiative, 1998. (http://www.nhlbi.nih.gov/guidelines/obesity/ob_gdlns.htm)
98. Overweight, Obesity, and Health Risk: National Task Force on the Prevention and Treatment of Obesity. Arch Intern Med 160:898-904, 2000.
99. Thompson D, Edelsberg J, Colditz GA, et al: Lifetime health and economic consequences of obesity. Arch Intern Med 159:2177-2183, 1999.
100. Oster G, Thompson D, Edelsberg J, et al: Lifetime health and economic benefits of weight loss among obese persons. Am J Public Health 89:1536-1542, 1999.
101. Must A, Spadano J, Coakley EH, et al: The disease burden associated with overweight and obesity. JAMA 282:1523-1529, 1999.
102. Rexrode KM, Carey VJ, Hennekens CH, et al: Abdominal adiposity and coronary heart disease in women. JAMA 280:1843-1848, 1998.
103. Rexrode KM, Buring JE, Manson JE: Abdominal and total adiposity and risk of coronary heart disease in men. Int J Obes Relat Metab Disord 25:1047-1056, 2001.
104. Allison DB, Fontaine KR, Manson JE, et al: Annual deaths attributable to obesity in the United States. JAMA 282:1530-1538, 1999.
105. Sturm R, Wells KB: Does obesity contribute as much to morbidity as poverty or smoking? Public Health 115:229-235, 2001.
106. Finkelstein EA, Fiebelkorn IC, Wang G: National medical spending attributable to overweight and obesity: How much, and who's paying? Health Aff (Millwood) 22:Web supplement, 2003.
107. Finkelstein EA, Fiebelkorn IC, Wang G: National medical spending attributable to overweight and obesity. Health Affairs, 2003. (http://www.healthaffairs.org/WebExclusives/Finkelstein_Web_Excl_051403.htm)
108. Stefanick ML. Exercise and weight loss. *In* Hennekens CH (ed): Clinical Trials in Cardiovascular Disease: A Companion Guide to Braunwald's Heart Disease. Philadelphia, WB Saunders, 1999, pp 375-391.
109. Halbert JA, Silagy CA, Finucane P, et al: The effectiveness of exercise training in lowering blood pressure: A meta-analysis of randomised controlled trials of 4 weeks or longer. J Hum Hypertens 11:641-649, 1997.
110. Hu FB, Sigal RJ, Rich-Edwards JW, et al: Walking compared with vigorous physical activity and risk of type 2 diabetes in women: A prospective study. JAMA 282:1433-1439, 1999.
111. Hardman AE: Interaction of physical activity and diet: Implications for lipoprotein metabolism. Public Health Nutr 2:369-276, 1999.
112. Rexrode KM, Hennekens CH, Willett WC, et al: A prospective study of body mass index, weight change, and risk of stroke in women. JAMA 277:1539-1545, 1997.

Physical Activity

113. Fletcher GF: Exercise in the prevention of stroke. Health Rep 6:106-110, 1994.
114. Shike M: Diet and lifestyle in the prevention of colorectal cancer: An overview. Am J Med 106:11S-15S; discussion 50S-51S, 1999.
115. McTiernan A: Associations between energy balance and body mass index and risk of breast carcinoma in women from diverse racial and ethnic backgrounds in the U.S. Cancer 88:1248-1255, 2000.
116. Ettinger WH Jr, Burns R, Messier SP, et al: A randomized trial comparing aerobic exercise and resistance exercise with a health education program in older adults with knee osteoarthritis. The Fitness Arthritis and Seniors Trial (FAST). JAMA 277:25-31, 1997.
117. Messier SP, Loeser RF, Mitchell MN, et al: Exercise and weight loss in obese older adults with knee osteoarthritis: A preliminary study. J Am Geriatr Soc 48:1062-1072, 2000.
118. Berard A, Bravo G, Gauthier P: Meta-analysis of the effectiveness of physical activity for the prevention of bone loss in postmenopausal women. Osteoporos Int 7:331-337, 1997.
119. Bonaiuti D, Shea B, Iovine R, et al: Exercise for preventing and treating osteoporosis in postmenopausal women. Cochrane Database Syst Rev CD000333, 2002.
120. The Surgeon General's Call to Action to Prevent and Decrease Overweight and Obesity. Rockville, MD, U.S. Department of Health and Human Services, Public Health Service, Office of the Surgeon General, 2001.
121. Leitzmann MF, Rimm EB, Willett WC, et al: Recreational physical activity and the risk of cholecystectomy in women. N Engl J Med 341:777-784, 1999.
122. Peppard PE, Young T, Palta M, et al: Longitudinal study of moderate weight change and sleep-disordered breathing. JAMA 284:3015-3021, 2000.
123. Physical Activity and Health: A report of the Surgeon General. U.S. Department of Health and Human Services, Centers for Disease Control and Prevention, 1996. (http://www.cdc.gov/nccdphp/sgr/sgr.htm)
124. Peppard PE, Young T, Palta M: Longitudinal study of moderate weight change and sleep-disordered breathing. JAMA 284:3015-3021, 2000.
125. Schmitz MK, Jeffery RW: Public health interventions for the prevention and treatment of obesity. Med Clin North Am 84:491-512, viii, 2000.
126. Serdula MK, Mokdad AH, Williamson DF, et al: Prevalence of attempting weight loss and strategies for controlling weight. JAMA 282:1353-1358, 1999.
127. The Practical Guide: Identification, Evaluation, and Treatment of Overweight and Obesity in Adults. NIH Publication No. 00-4084. Washington DC, National Heart, Lung, and Blood Institute, North American Association for the Study of Obesity, 2000. (available online at<http://www.nhlbi.nih.gov/guidelines/obesity/practgde.htm>)
128. Physical activity trends—United States, 1990–1998. MMWR Morb Mortal Wkly Rep 50:166-169, 2001.
129. Healthy People 2010: Understanding and Improving Health. U.S. Department of Health and Human Services, 2000. (http://www.healthypeople.gov/Document/pdf/uih/2010uih.pdf)
130. Lowry R, Wechsler H, Kann L, Collins JL: Recent trends in participation in physical education among U.S. high school students. J Sch Health 71:145-152, 2001.
131. National Institute of Child Health and Human Development Study of Early Child Care and Youth Development Network: Frequency and intensity of physical activity of third grade children in physical education. Arch Pediatr Adolesc Med 157:185-190, 2003.
132. U.S. Department of Transportation: Nationwide Personal Transportation Survey. Washington DC, Federal Highway Administration, 1997.
133. Rideout VJ, Foehr UG, Roberts DF, Brodie M: Kids and media at the new millennium: A comprehensive national analysis of children's media use. Menlo Park, CA, Kaiser Family Foundation, 1999.
134. Lee IM, Skerrett PJ: Physical activity and all-cause mortality: What is the dose-response relation? Med Sci Sports Exerc 33:S459-S471; discussion S493-S494, 2001.
135. Folsom AR, Arnett DK, Hutchinson RG, et al: Physical activity and incidence of coronary heart disease in middle-aged women and men. Med Sci Sports Exerc 29:901-909, 1997.
136. Leon AS, Myers MJ, Connett J: Leisure time physical activity and the 16-year risks of mortality from coronary heart disease and all-causes in the Multiple Risk Factor Intervention Trial (MRFIT). Int J Sports Med 18(Suppl 3):S208-S215, 1997.
137. Rosengren A, Wilhelmsen L: Physical activity protects against coronary death and deaths from all causes in middle-aged men: Evidence from a 20-year follow-up of the primary prevention study in Goteborg. Ann Epidemiol 7:69-75, 1997.
138. Manson JE, Greenland P, LaCroix AZ, et al: Walking compared with vigorous exercise for the prevention of cardiovascular events in women. N Engl J Med 347:716-725, 2002.
139. Hakim AA, Curb JD, Petrovitch H, et al: Effects of walking on coronary heart disease in elderly men: The Honolulu Heart Program. Circulation 100:9-13, 1999.
140. Tanasescu M, Leitzmann MF, Rimm EB, et al: Exercise type and intensity in relation to coronary heart disease in men. JAMA 288:1994-2000, 2002.
141. Gregg EW, Cauley JA, Stone K, et al: Relationship of changes in physical activity and mortality among older women. JAMA 289:2379-2386, 2003.
142. Wannamethee SG, Shaper AG, Walker M: Changes in physical activity, mortality, and incidence of coronary heart disease in older men. Lancet 351:1603-1608, 1998.
143. Lee IM, Hennekens CH, Berger K, et al: Exercise and risk of stroke in male physicians. Stroke 30:1-6, 1999.
144. Lee IM, Paffenbarger RS Jr: Physical activity and stroke incidence: The Harvard Alumni Health Study. Stroke 29:2049-2054, 1998.
145. Hu FB, Stampfer MJ, Colditz GA, et al: Physical activity and risk of stroke in women. JAMA 283:2961-2967, 2000.
146. Stefanick ML, Mackey S, Sheehan M, et al: Effects of diet and exercise in men and postmenopausal women with low levels of HDL cholesterol and high levels of LDL cholesterol. N Engl J Med 339:12-20, 1998.
147. Henriksen EJ: Effects of acute exercise and exercise training on insulin resistance. J Appl Physiol 93:788-796, 2002.
148. Schmitz KH, Jacobs DR Jr, Hong CP, et al: Association of physical activity with insulin sensitivity in children. Int J Obes Relat Metab Disord 26:1310-1316, 2002.
149. Whelton SP, Chin A, Xin X, He J: Effect of aerobic exercise on blood pressure: A meta-analysis of randomized, controlled trials. Ann Intern Med 136:493-503, 2002.
150. Stewart KJ: Exercise training and the cardiovascular consequences of type 2 diabetes and hypertension: Plausible mechanisms for improving cardiovascular health. JAMA 288:1622-1631, 2002.
151. Jolliffe JA, Rees K, Taylor RS, et al: Exercise-based rehabilitation for coronary heart disease. Cochrane Database Syst Rev 3, 2003.
152. Smith SC Jr, Blair SN, Bonow RO, et al: AHA/ACC Guidelines for Preventing Heart Attack and Death in Patients with Atherosclerotic Cardiovascular Disease: 2001 Update. A statement for healthcare professionals from the American Heart Association and the American College of Cardiology. J Am Coll Cardiol 38:1581-1583, 2001.
153. Pollock ML, Franklin BA, Balady GJ, et al: Resistance exercise in individuals with and without cardiovascular disease: Benefits, rationale, safety, and prescription: An advisory from the Committee on Exercise, Rehabilitation, and Prevention, Council on Clinical Cardiology, American Heart Association. Position paper endorsed by the American College of Sports Medicine. Circulation 101:828-833, 2000.

154. Physical Activity and Health: A Report of the Surgeon General. Washington, DC, U.S. Department of Health and Human Services, Centers for Disease Control and Prevention, 1996.

Alcohol Intake

155. Goldberg IJ, Mosca L, Piano MR, Fisher EA: AHA Science Advisory: Wine and your heart: A science advisory for healthcare professionals from the Nutrition Committee, Council on Epidemiology and Prevention, and Council on Cardiovascular Nursing of the American Heart Association. Circulation 103:472-475, 2001.
156. Rimm EB, Williams P, Fosher K, et al: Moderate alcohol intake and lower risk of coronary heart disease: Meta-analysis of effects on lipids and haemostatic factors. BMJ 319:1523-1528, 1999.
157. Anand SS, Yusuf S: Oral anticoagulant therapy in patients with coronary artery disease: A meta-analysis. JAMA 282:2058-2067, 1999.

Hormone Therapy

158. Anderson R: Deaths: Leading Causes for 2000. National Vital Statistics Reports. Vol 50, No. 16. Hyattsville, MD, National Center for Health Statistics, 2002.
159. Manson JE, Martin KA: Clinical practice: Postmenopausal hormone-replacement therapy. N Engl J Med 345:34-40, 2001.
160. Grodstein F, Stampfer MJ: The epidemiology of postmenopausal hormone therapy and cardiovascular disease. *In* Goldhaber SZ, Ridker PM (eds): Thrombosis and Thromboembolism. New York, Marcel Dekker, 2002, pp 67-78.
161. Rossouw JE, Anderson GL, Prentice RL, et al: Risks and benefits of estrogen plus progestin in healthy postmenopausal women: Principal results From the Women's Health Initiative randomized controlled trial. JAMA 288:321-333, 2002.
162. Grady D, Herrington D, Bittner V, et al: Cardiovascular disease outcomes during 6.8 years of hormone therapy: Heart and Estrogen/progestin Replacement Study follow-up (HERS II). JAMA 288:49-57, 2002.

163. Herrington DM, Reboussin DM, Brosnihan KB, et al: Effects of estrogen replacement on the progression of coronary artery atherosclerosis. N Engl J Med 343:522-529, 2000.
164. Clarke SC, Kelleher J, Lloyd-Jones H, et al: A study of hormone replacement therapy in postmenopausal women with ischaemic heart disease: The Papworth HRT atherosclerosis study. Br J Obstet Gynaecol 109:1056-1062, 2002.
165. Waters DD, Alderman EL, Hsia J, et al: Effects of hormone replacement therapy and antioxidant vitamin supplements on coronary atherosclerosis in postmenopausal women: A randomized controlled trial. JAMA 288:2432-2440, 2002.
166. Cherry N, Gilmour K, Hannaford P, et al: Oestrogen therapy for prevention of reinfarction in postmenopausal women: A randomised placebo controlled trial. Lancet 360:2001-2008, 2002.
167. Lissin LW, Cooke JP: Phytoestrogens and cardiovascular health. J Am Coll Cardiol 35:1403-1410, 2000.
168. Postmenopausal hormone replacement therapy for the primary prevention of chronic condition: Recommendations and rationale. U.S. Preventive Services Task Force. Am Fam Physician 67:358-364, 2003.
169. Amended report from the NAMS Advisory Panel on Postmenopausal Hormone Therapy. Menopause 10:6-12, 2003.
170. FDA approves new labels for estrogen and estrogen with progestin therapies for postmenopausal women following review of Women's Health Initiative data. Washington, DC, U.S. Food and Drug Administration, 2003. (http://www.fda.gov/bbs/topics/NEWS/2003/NEW00863.html)

Diet

171. Ness AR, Powles JW: Fruit and vegetables, and cardiovascular disease: A review. Int J Epidemiol 26:1-13, 1997.
172. Joshipura KJ, Ascherio A, Manson JE, et al: Fruit and vegetable intake in relation to risk of ischemic stroke. JAMA 282:1233-1239, 1999.
173. Hu FB, Willett WC: Optimal diets for prevention of coronary heart disease. JAMA 288:2569-2578, 2002.
174. de Lorgeril M, Salen P, Martin JL, et al: Mediterranean diet, traditional risk factors, and the rate of cardiovascular complications after myocardial infarction: Final report of the Lyon Diet Heart Study. Circulation 99:779-785, 1999.
175. Dietary supplementation with n-3 polyunsaturated fatty acids and vitamin E after myocardial infarction: Results of the GISSI-Prevenzione trial. Gruppo Italiano per lo Studio della Sopravvivenza nell'Infarto miocardico. Lancet 354:447-455, 1999.
176. Tribble DL: AHA Science Advisory. Antioxidant consumption and risk of coronary heart disease: Emphasis on vitamin C, vitamin E, and beta-carotene: A statement for healthcare professionals from the American Heart Association. Circulation 99:591-595, 1999.
177. MRC/BHF Heart Protection Study of antioxidant vitamin supplementation in 20,536 high-risk individuals: A randomised placebo-controlled trial. Lancet 360:23-33, 2002.
178. Yusuf S, Dagenais G, Pogue J, et al: Vitamin E supplementation and cardiovascular events in high-risk patients. The Heart Outcomes Prevention Evaluation Study Investigators. N Engl J Med 342:154-160, 2000.
179. Kris-Etherton PM, Harris WS, Appel LJ: Fish consumption, fish oil, omega-3 fatty acids, and cardiovascular disease. Circulation 106:2747-2757, 2002.

Psychosocial Factors

180. Allan R, Scheidt S. Psychosocial factors. *In* Hennekens CH (ed): Clinical Trials in Cardiovascular Disease: A Companion Guide to Braunwald's Heart Disease. Philadelphia, WB Saunders, 1999, pp 315-323.
181. Dusseldorp E, van Elderen T, Maes S, et al: A meta-analysis of psychoeduational programs for coronary heart disease patients. Health Psychol 18:506-519, 1999.
182. Effects of treating depression and low perceived social support on clinical events after myocardial infarction: The Enhancing Recovery in Coronary Heart Disease Patients (ENRICHD) Randomized Trial. JAMA 289:3106-3116, 2003.
183. Glassman AH, O'Connor CM, Califf RM, et al: Sertraline treatment of major depression in patients with acute MI or unstable angina. JAMA 288:701-709, 2002.

Novel Risk Markers

184. Pearson TA, Mensah GA, Alexander RW, et al: Markers of inflammation and cardiovascular disease: Application to clinical and public health practice: A statement for healthcare professionals from the Centers for Disease Control and Prevention and the American Heart Association. Circulation 107:499-511, 2003.
185. Ridker PM: Evaluating novel cardiovascular risk factors: Can we better predict heart attacks? Ann Intern Med 130:933-937, 1999.
186. Libby P, Ridker PM: Novel inflammatory markers of coronary risk: Theory versus practice. Circulation 100:1148-1150, 1999.

Global Risk Modification

187. Ornish D, Hart JA: Multiple risk factor intervention trials. *In* Hennekens CH (ed): Clinical Trials in Cardiovascular Disease: A Companion Guide to Braunwald's Heart Disease. Philadelphia, WB Saunders, 1999, pp 432-446.
188. DeBusk RF, West JA, Miller NH, Taylor CB: Chronic disease management: Treating the patient with disease(s) versus treating disease(s) in the patient. Arch Intern Med 159:2739-2742, 1999.
189. Multiple Risk Factor Intervention Trial. Risk factor changes and mortality results. Multiple Risk Factor Intervention Trial Research Group. JAMA 248:1465-1477, 1982.
190. Hejermann I: A randomized primary preventive trial in coronary heart disease: The Oslo study. Prev Med 12:181-184, 1983.
191. European Collaborative Trial of Multifactorial Prevention of Coronary Heart Disease: Final report on the 6-year results. World Health Organization European Collaborative Group. Lancet 1:869-872,1986.
192. Puska P, Tuomilehto J, Nissinen A, Salonen J: Ten years of the North Karelia project. Acta Med Scand Suppl 701:66-71, 1985.
193. Wilhelmsen L, Berglund G, Elmfeldt D, et al: The Multifactor Primary Prevention Trial in Goteborg, Sweden. Eur Heart J 7:279-288, 1986.
194. Luepker RV, Rastam L, Hannan PJ, et al: Community education for cardiovascular disease prevention. Morbidity and mortality results from the Minnesota Heart Health Program. Am J Epidemiol 144:351-362, 1996.
195. Carelton RA, Lasater TM, Assaf AR et al: The Pawtucket Heart Health Program: Community changes in cardiovascular risk factors and projected disease risk. Am J Public Health 85:777-785, 1995.
196. Farquhar JW, Fortmann SP, Flora JA, et al: Effects of communitywide education on cardiovascular disease risk factors. The Stanford Five-City Project. JAMA 264:359-365, 1990.
197. Niebauer J, Hambrecht R, Velich T, et al: Attenuated progression of coronary artery disease after 6 years of multifactorial risk intervention: Role of physical exercise. Circulation 96:2534-2541, 1997.
198. Haskell WL, Alderman EL, Fair JM, et al: Effects of intensive multiple risk factor reduction on coronary atherosclerosis and clinical cardiac events in men and women with coronary artery disease. The Stanford Coronary Risk Intervention Project (SCRIP). Circulation 89:975-990, 1994.

CHAPTER 43

Comprehensive Rehabilitation of Patients with Cardiovascular Disease

Richard C. Pasternak

Fifty years ago, patients who survived a myocardial infarction were confined to bed for 2 months or longer and then urged to limit their activity indefinitely. Avoidance of physical activity was likewise advocated for those with angina. The realization that bed rest hindered recovery and contributed to complications radically altered the rehabilitation of cardiac patients. Early efforts aimed at progressive activity gradually coalesced into formal cardiac rehabilitation programs. Although such programs initially emphasized exercise training before and after hospital discharge, contemporary programs have evolved into comprehensive multidisciplinary efforts that, in addition to exercise training, include modification of other risk factors as well as personal and vocational adjustment and education.

In the United States alone, well more than 1 million individuals per year become candidates for cardiac rehabilitation.[1] Unfortunately, up to 90 percent of patients who could benefit from cardiac rehabilitation do not get it; of those who do, 25 to 50 percent drop out within weeks to months.[2] Women and older patients are less likely to participate in a program than are men and younger patients.[3]

Numerous factors contribute to this dismal participation rate, including transportation issues, motivation, comorbidities, misunderstanding of the value of these programs, reimbursement issues, and suboptimal referral rates. Of 100 consecutive patients undergoing coronary artery bypass grafting (CABG) at a major teaching hospital, 78 percent of those who did not participate in a cardiac rehabilitation program cited lack of physician referral.[4]

HISTORY OF CARDIAC REHABILITATION

Until fairly recently, the treatment of patients with heart disease generally followed this Hippocratic suggestion: "In every movement of the body, whenever one begins to endure pain, it will be relieved by rest."[5] By the time Herrick clinically described the link between coronary thrombosis and myocardial infarction in 1912,[6] absolute bed rest for 6 to 8 weeks was the standard first step in recovery and rehabilitation. Lewis, for example, recommended that during this period, "the patient is to be guarded by day and night nursing and helped in every way to avoid voluntary movement or effort."[7] The rationale for immobility was that exertion could lead to ventricular aneurysm formation and ventricular rupture, and the hypoxia associated with exertion could lead to arrhythmia, recurrent myocardial infarction, or sudden death. Following discharge from the hospital, even moderately stressful activity such as climbing stairs was discouraged for a year or more, and return to work or normal activity was the exception rather than the rule.[8]

Dramatic successes in medical rehabilitation achieved during the course of World War II[8] helped clinicians question the benefits of extended immobility. Vilifying extended bed rest as something that "saps morale, provokes desperation, unleashes anxiety, and ushers in hopelessness of the capacity of resuming a normal life,"[9] Levine advocated limited early activity after myocardial infarction. Early mobilization first took the form of "chair therapy," described by Levine and Lown in 1951. It encouraged patients to sit in a chair for 1 to 2 hours a day as soon as the first day following myocardial infarction.[10] Other attempts at early mobilization coupled with results from the Dallas Bed Rest Study[11] demonstrating that deconditioning was associated with greater immobility gradually began to convince clinicians that early mobilization was beneficial rather than harmful. By the early 1970s, clinical practice in the United States varied considerably—the duration of enforced bed rest varied from 1 day to 4 weeks after myocardial infarction and the duration of hospitalization varied from 2 to 6 weeks.[12]

Early mobilization came to be called phase I or inpatient cardiac rehabilitation.[13] Its goal was to condition the patient to carry out safely activities of daily living following discharge. Such programs entailed prescribing activity in rigid steps with successively higher metabolic equivalents (METs). Early phase I programs included up to 14 separate steps.[12] Comprehensive rehabilitation programs eventually grew to include four phases (Table 43-1).

Early rehabilitation programs focused almost exclusively on exercise. Over time they have evolved to encompass what the World Health Organization called the "sum of activity required to ensure cardiac patients the best possible physical, mental, and social conditions so that [patients] may, by their own efforts, regain as normal as possible a place in the community and lead an active life."[14]

Contemporary Cardiac Rehabilitation

Although exercise remains a central part of modern cardiac rehabilitation, it has broadened to include all relevant aspects of secondary prevention (Table 43–2). In addition to risk factor management, the goals of such a secondary prevention program include reduction in both symptoms and risk of premature death and improvement in quality of life. Strategies to improve adherence to all medical therapies and life-style changes are employed. An additional goal is to provide information to patients' family members and others.

TABLE 43–1 Traditional Terminology for the Phases of Cardiac Rehabilitation

Phase I
Inpatient rehabilitation, usually lasting for the duration of hospitalization. It emphasizes a gradual, progressive approach to exercise and an education program that helps the patient understand the disease process, the rehabilitation process, and initial preventive efforts to slow the progression of disease.

Phase II
Multifaceted outpatient rehabilitation, lasting 2 to 3 mo. Emphasizes safe physical activity to improve conditioning with continued behavior modification aimed at smoking cessation, weight loss, healthy eating, and other factors to reduce disease risk. Initiate an exercise prescription.

Phase III
Supervised rehabilitation, lasting 6 to 12 mo. Establishes a prescription for safe exercise that can be performed at home or in a community service facility, such as a senior center or YMCA, and continues to emphasize risk factor reduction.

Phase IV
Maintenance, indefinite

Modern rehabilitation programs generally include three stages: inpatient rehabilitation, outpatient rehabilitation, and maintenance (Fig. 43–1). Responsibilities may lie with different or overlapping groups, e.g., a physical therapy department for an inpatient program and a nurse-managed cardiac rehabilitation specialist for an outpatient program. Because hospital stays after uncomplicated acute myocardial infarction or cardiac procedures have decreased in the United States, comprehensive inpatient rehabilitation is not possible. It is still routine, however, in many other countries. Outpatient programs are traditionally conducted in hospital-based cardiac rehabilitation centers. Community-based centers or home-based programs can also provide a beneficial experience for selected and motivated patients.[15,16]

Inpatient Cardiac Rehabilitation

As soon as it is safe to do so when a patient has been stabilized after initial treatment of an acute coronary syndrome or CABG, he or she should be encouraged to sit in a chair and begin to take a few steps, even in intensive care units. Limited range-of-motion exercises are also advisable, except in unstable patients. When the patient has been transferred out of intensive care, assisted walking should be encouraged unless the patient remains symptomatic. Activity levels are gradually increased during hospitalization with encouragement to perform activities of daily living. Pharmacological therapies to improve the patient's risk factor profile and improve long-term event-free survival should be initiated in the hospital or at discharge.

Short stays make it difficult to do more than introduce patients to the disease process, the factors that maintain it, and strategies for reducing risk. Patients should, however, become familiar with the symptoms of recurrent ischemia, heart failure, and hypertension and should be instructed in the proper response to symptoms if they arise. They should also be provided with key telephone numbers of the responsible physician as well as other important contacts, including hospitals and cardiac rehabilitation programs.

Patients are often overwhelmed during the hospital stay by the volume of new information they must assimilate. Thus, an appropriate trend in inpatient programs is an emphasis on evaluation of risks and a focus on referral to and participation in an appropriate outpatient cardiac rehabilitation program.

Outpatient Cardiac Rehabilitation

The traditional outpatient cardiac rehabilitation model is a formal, institution-based program conducted by a team of rehabilitation professionals. Current programs include efforts that were once accomplished as part of phase II and phase III programs (see Fig. 43–1). Programs now offer the structure, support, and feedback that many individuals need in order to make important behavioral changes (see Table 43–2).

Alternatives to Hospital-Based Cardiac Rehabilitation

Because enrollment in traditional hospital-based cardiac rehabilitation programs is suboptimal, relatively costly, and, under some circumstances, not reimbursed by insurance, a number of alternative models have been devised and tested. These include modified protocols with early transition to community-based or independent programs; physician-supervised, nurse-managed programs; community-based programs supervised by exercise physiologists guided by a computerized management system based on national guidelines; and home-based programs. Small, randomized trials suggest that such alternatives may be as effective as a hospital-based rehabilitation program for some patients.[15-17]

Maintenance

Following more structured outpatient programs are long-term "maintenance" programs, often conducted in the same facilities as structured programs but with fewer staff. In the absence of formal guidelines or reimbursement for these programs, there is less consistency to what they offer. The model for many programs is a supervised health club, for which patients pay a monthly fee.

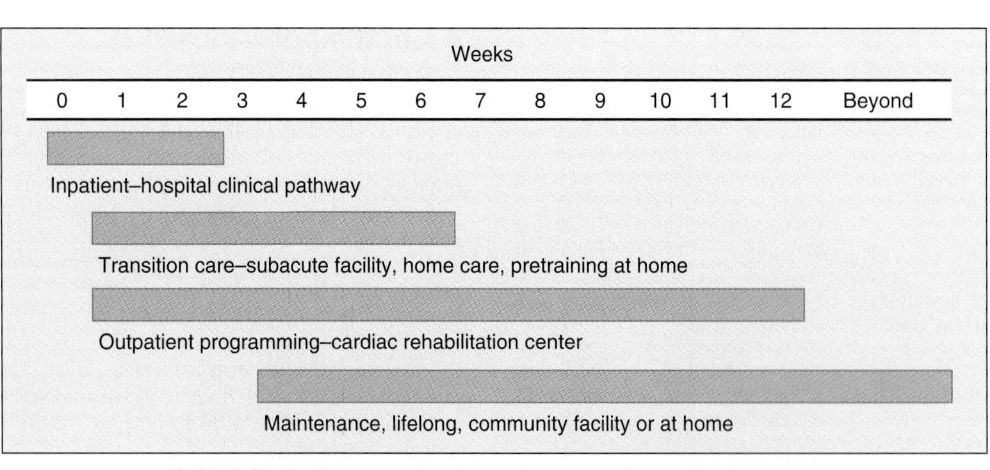

FIGURE 43–1 Recommended continuum of care for cardiac rehabilitative services.

Evidence Base for Cardiac Rehabilitation

Considerably less clinical research has been focused on cardiac rehabilitation than

TABLE 43–2 Components of Cardiac Rehabilitation and Associated Goals

Initial Evaluation
Take medical history and perform physical examination
Measure risk factors
Obtain electrocardiograms at rest and during exercise
Provide vocational counseling
Determine level of risk
Goal: formulation of preventive plan in collaboration with primary care physician

Management of Lipid Levels
Assess and modify diet, physical activity, and drug therapy
Primary goal: LDL cholesterol level < 100 mg/dl
Secondary goals: non-HDL cholesterol level < 130 mg/dl, HDL cholesterol level > 45 mg/dl, triglyceride level < 200 mg/dl

Management of Hypertension
Measure blood pressure frequently at rest and during exercise
If resting systolic pressure is 130 to 139 mm Hg or diastolic pressure is 85 to 89 mm Hg, recommend life-style modifications, including exercise, weight management, sodium restriction, and moderation of alcohol intake; if patient has diabetes or chronic renal or heart failure, consider drug therapy
If resting systolic pressure is ≥140 mm Hg or diastolic pressure is ≥90 mm Hg, recommend drug therapy
Monitor effects of intervention in collaboration with primary care physician
Goal: blood pressure < 140/90 mm Hg (or < 130/85 mm Hg if patient has diabetes or chronic heart or renal failure); optimal < 120/80 mm Hg

Cessation of Smoking
Document smoking status (never smoked, stopped smoking in remote past, stopped smoking recently, or currently smokes)
Determine patient's readiness to quit; if ready, pick a date for quitting
Offer nicotine replacement therapy, bupropion, or both
Offer behavioral advice and group or individual counseling
Goal: long-term abstinence

Weight Reduction
Consider for patients with BMI > 25 or waist circumference > 102 cm (in men) or > 88 cm (in women), particularly if associated with hypertension, hyperlipidemia, or insulin resistance or diabetes
Provide behavioral and nutritional counseling with follow-up to monitor progress in achieving goals
Goals: loss of 5 to 10% of body weight and modification of associated risk factors

Management of Diabetes
Identify candidates on the basis of the medical history and baseline glucose test
Develop a regimen of dietary modification, weight control, and exercise combined with oral hypoglycemic agents and insulin therapy
Monitor glucose control before and after exercise sessions and communicate results to primary care physician
For newly detected diabetes, refer patient to primary care physician for evaluation and treatment
Goals: normalization of fasting plasma glucose level (80 to 110 mg/dl) or glycosylated hemoglobin level (<7.0%) and control of associated obesity, hypertension, and hyperlipidemia

Psychosocial Management
Identify psychosocial problems such as depression, anxiety, social isolation, anger, and hostility by means of an interview, standardized questionnaires, or both
Provide individual or group counseling, or both, for patients with clinically significant psychosocial problems
Provide stress reduction classes for patients
Goal: absence of clinically significant psychosocial problems and acquisition of stress management skills

Physical Activity Counseling and Exercise Training
Assess current physical activity and exercise tolerance with monitored exercise stress test
Identify barriers to increased physical activity
Provide advice regarding increasing physical activity
Develop an individualized regimen of aerobic and resistance training, specifying frequency, intensity, duration, and types of exercise
Goals: increases in regular physical activity, strength, and physical functioning, expenditure of at least 1000 kcal/wk in physical activity

BMI = body mass index; HDL = high-density lipoprotein; LDL = low-density lipoprotein.
Adapted from Balady GJ, Ades PA, Comoss P, et al: Core components of cardiac rehabilitation/secondary prevention programs: A statement for healthcare professionals from the American Heart Association and the American Association of Cardiovascular and Pulmonary Rehabilitation Writing Group. Circulation 102:1069, 2000.

on many other areas of cardiology. Yet, we possess sufficient evidence upon which to base recommendations for rehabilitation following acute myocardial infarction, CABG, or percutaneous coronary intervention. In 1995, the federal Agency for Health Care Policy Research issued a clinical practice guideline with the Public Health Service and the National Heart, Lung, and Blood Institute.[2] Standards for exercise training relevant to cardiac rehabilitation have been issued and updated by the American Heart Association.[18]

Numerous randomized clinical trials of exercise-based cardiac rehabilitation have been conducted in North America and Europe. Although they have generally demonstrated a trend toward reduced mortality, virtually all of these trials had insufficient statistical power to demonstrate the efficacy of cardiac rehabilitation.

Two early meta-analyses that each included approximately 4500 patients concluded that exercise-based cardiac rehabilitation reduced both total and cardiac mortality by 20 to 25 percent but had little effect on nonfatal myocardial infarction or sudden death.[19,20] In a 19-year follow-up of one of the trials included in these meta-analyses, the U.S. National Exercise and Heart Disease Project, all-cause mortality risk estimates were nonsignificantly lower in the intervention group after 3 years (relative risk, 0.69; 95 percent confidence interval [CI], 0.39 to 1.25) but rose gradually with increased follow-up—0.84 after 5 years, 0.95 after 10 years, 1.02 after 15 years, and 1.09 after 19 years.[21] These results suggest either that protective mechanisms associated with cardiac rehabilitation operate in the short term or that patients stop performing the protective activities they engaged in as part of the program.

The latest meta-analysis of exercise-based cardiac rehabilitation, conducted for the Cochrane Collaboration (Fig. 43–2),[22] adds approximately 4000 patients to the prior meta-analyses. Using data from 36 trials and almost 8500 patients, the investigators were able to analyze separately exercise-only and comprehensive programs. The pooled effect estimate for total mortality demonstrated a 27 percent reduction in total mortality for the exercise-only programs (odds ratio [OR], 0.73; 95 percent CI, 0.54 to 0.98) and a 13 percent reduction for comprehensive interventions (OR, 0.87; 95 percent CI, 0.71 to 1.05). The exercise-only interventions appeared to reduce total cardiac mortality slightly more than comprehensive interventions (OR, 0.69; 95 percent CI, 0.51 to 0.94 for exercise only and OR, 0.74; 95 percent CI, 0.57 to 0.96 for comprehensive programs). Neither had an effect on nonfatal myocardial infarction. In addition to confirming the results of the prior meta-analyses that exercise-based cardiac rehabilitation reduces cardiac mortality without reducing the risk of recurrent infarction, the work by Jolliffe and colleagues supports the role of exercise as a critical component of rehabilitation.[22]

Most of the studies in the three meta-analyses preceded widespread use of acute thrombolytic therapy, primary angioplasty, and early revascularization as well as standard secondary prevention therapies including statins and angiotensin-converting enzyme (ACE) inhibitors. Thus, trials that include contemporary rehabilitation programs and emphasize adherence to comprehensive secondary prevention efforts might show greater effects on total and cardiovascular mortality and also affect recurrent myocardial infarction.

Exercise training can affect cardiovascular and overall health in numerous ways. Smoking cessation has an almost immediate effect on cardiovascular health. Even modest reductions in blood pressure result in a 15 percent reduction in the risk of coronary heart disease (CHD) events and a 42 percent reduction in risk of stroke.[23] Reducing serum cholesterol by 10 percent reduces the risk of a CHD event by 15 percent.[24] Among overweight individuals, modest weight loss corresponding to 5 to 10 percent of starting body weight is associated with significant improvements in blood pressure, serum lipids, and glucose tolerance or insulin resistance, or both.[25] (See Chaps. 41 and 42 for details of risk reduction for specific factors.)

A prospective, 1-year controlled study demonstrated the beneficial effects of early short-term intensive cardiac rehabilitation on traditional cardiac risk factors. Within 1 to 4 weeks of hospital discharge for acute myocardial infarction or CABG, 109 patients began a multidisciplinary ambulatory cardiac rehabilitation program. At the study's end, 9 to 10 months later, there was a high rate of aspirin intake, a low rate of smoking (14 percent of the patients), a 15 percent increase in physical capacity, a decrease in resting heart rate of 7 beats/min, and a 4 mg/dl increase in high-density lipoprotein (HDL) cholesterol.[26]

In summary, the aggregate evidence from randomized controlled trials demonstrates that exercise-based cardiac rehabilitation can prevent premature morbidity and mortality. Although there is insufficient evidence to determine whether interventions that include exercise and comprehensive risk factor reduction are the equivalent of exercise-only interventions, most studies were conducted before the current era of aggressive management of coronary disease and newer secondary prevention strategies. Given that the age of large prospective randomized trials for cardiac rehabilitation is probably over, cost, local access to available services, and national consensus guidelines are likely to drive clinicians' choices.

Components of a Cardiac Rehabilitation Program

It is now widely recognized that cardiac rehabilitation and comprehensive secondary rehabilitation programs are integral to the complete management of patients with cardiovascular disease. The most comprehensive statement addressing the core requirements came from the American Association of Cardiovascular and Pulmonary Rehabilitation[27] and has been reviewed and endorsed by the American College of Cardiology and the American Heart Association (see Table 43–2).

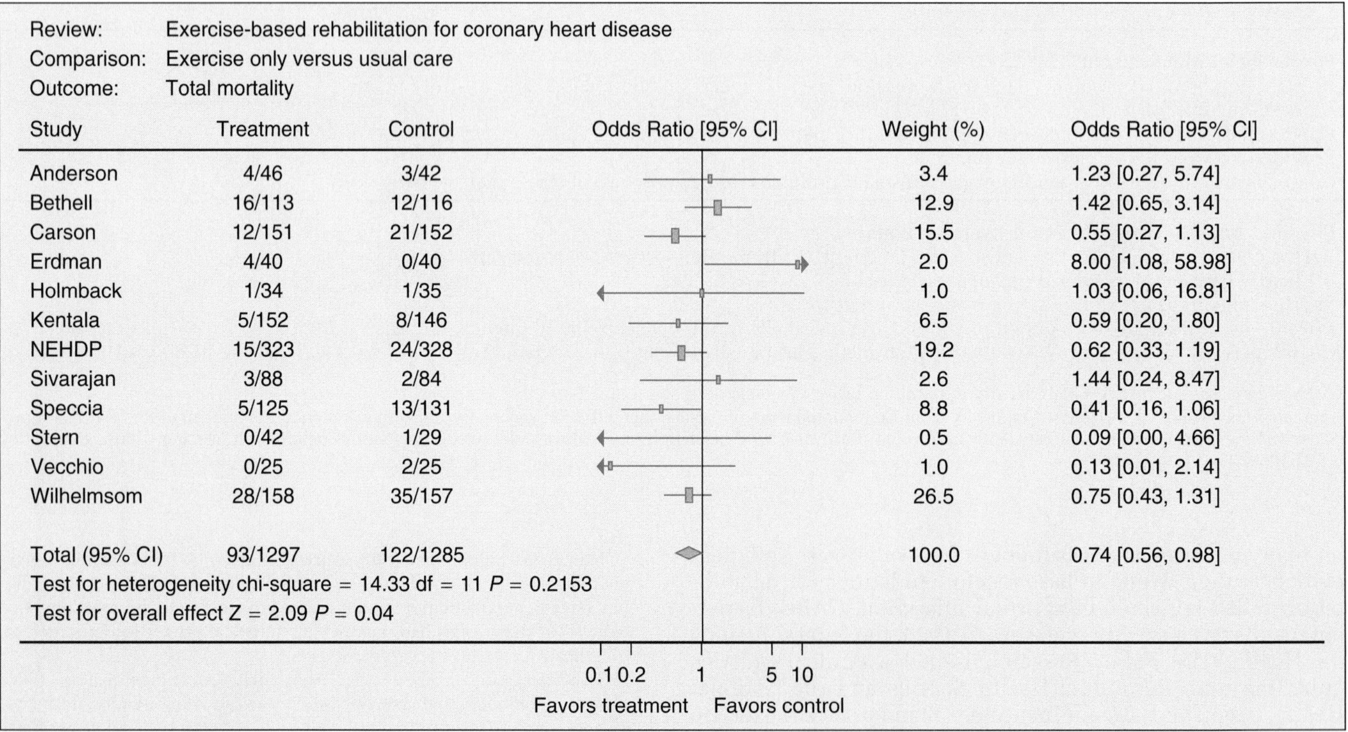

FIGURE 43–2 Meta-analysis of the effect of exercise-based rehabilitation for coronary heart disease on mortality. For information on individual studies listed (left-hand column), see references. (From Jolliffe JA, Rees K, Taylor RS, et al: Exercise-based rehabilitation for coronary heart disease. Cochrane Database Syst Rev [1]:CD001800, 2001 [jajollif@exeter.ac.uk].)

Exercise

Definition of Terms

A variety of terms are used to describe exercise-related activity, often with overlapping definitions. The following are used in this chapter:

- *Physical activity.* Any body movement produced by skeletal muscles that results in energy expenditure beyond resting expenditure.
- *Exercise.* Physical activity that is planned, structured, repetitive, and purposeful, usually aimed at improving or maintaining physical fitness.
- *Physical fitness.* Attributes that people have or achieve related to the ability to perform physical activity, including cardiorespiratory fitness, muscle strength, body composition, and flexibility.
- *Dose.* The total amount of energy expended in physical activity.
- *Intensity.* The absolute or relative rate of energy expenditure during activity. Absolute intensity reflects the rate of energy expenditure during exercise and is usually expressed in metabolic equivalents (METs). Relative intensity refers to the percentage of aerobic power utilized during exercise and is usually expressed as percentage of maximal heart rate or percentage of maximum oxygen consumption (VO_{2max}) (Table 43–3).
- *Metabolic equivalents.* One MET equals the resting metabolic rate of 3.5 ml O_2/kg/min (Table 43–4).
- *Moderate-intensity activity.* Activity performed at a relative intensity of 40 to 60 percent of $\bar{V}O_{2max}$ or an absolute intensity of 4 to 6 METs.
- *Vigorous-intensity activity.* Activity performed at a relative intensity of greater than 60 percent of $\bar{V}O_{2max}$ or an absolute intensity greater than 6 METs.

Exercise Physiology

Exercise induces a large increase in cardiac output that provides for the metabolic needs of exercising muscles, prevents hyperthermia, and ensures adequate blood flow to essential organs. This increase results from changes in both heart rate and stroke volume.

HEART RATE. Within seconds of increased physical activity, the heart rate begins to increase. During strenuous activity, heart rate can attain values of 160 to 180 beats/min. Rates as high as 240 beats/min have been observed during short periods of maximal exercise. Vagal withdrawal rather than an increase in sympathetic tone is the likely cause of the almost instantaneous acceleration in heart rate with exercise, whereas later increases stem from reflex activation of pulmonary stretch receptors and increased levels of circulating adrenal catecholamines. The increase in heart rate during exercise accounts for more of the increase in cardiac output than does the increase in stroke volume. Stroke volume normally reaches its maximum when cardiac output has increased by only half its maximum, and further increases in cardiac output occur by increasing the heart rate alone.

STROKE VOLUME. Exercise affects both physiological mechanisms that influence stroke volume—increased venous return (increased preload) and more forceful contractions (increased inotropy). In the upright position at rest, the diminished venous return to the heart (compared with the supine position) results in smaller stroke volume and cardiac output. During upright exercise, however, stroke volume can approach the maximum stroke volume observed in the recumbent position, achieved in part by increased venous tone and skeletal muscle compression. Exercise also increases inotropy because of catecholamine release.

DISTRIBUTION OF CARDIAC OUTPUT. Sympathetic activity dominates during exercise. Increases in plasma norepinephrine and epinephrine levels constrict the majority of vascular beds, except those in the exercising muscles and the coronary and cerebral circulations. During light and moderate exercise, cutaneous blood flow increases to facilitate body cooling, whereas more vigorous exercise causes a progressive decrease in skin flow. The kidneys and splanchnic tissue can tolerate considerable reductions in blood flow through increased extraction of oxygen from the available blood supply. The heart's limited reserve—it extracts approximately 75 percent of the oxygen in the coronary blood flow at rest—requires that it meet increased oxygen demands during exercise by an increase in coronary blood flow. Cerebral blood flow also increases during exercise.

The cessation of exercise rapidly decreases heart rate and cardiac output because of a decrease in sympathetic drive and the reactivation of vagal activity, while systemic vascular resistance remains lower for some time. As a result, arterial pressure often falls to below preexercise levels for several hours after exercise and then returns to normal levels.

CARDIOVASCULAR RESPONSE TO DIFFERENT TYPES OF EXERCISE. Contraction of large muscle groups that results in movement (*isotonic exercise*) places a volume load on the heart reflected by significant increases in both cardiac output and oxygen consumption and a fall in systemic vascular resistance. Constant muscular contraction of smaller

TABLE 43–3 Classification of Physical Activity Intensity

	Relative Intensity			Endurance-Type Activity, Absolute Intensity in Healthy Adults (age), METS					Strength-Type Exercise/Relative Intensity*
Intensity	*VO_{2max}*[†] *(%)*	*Maximum Heart Rate*[‡] *(%)*	*RPE*[§]	*Young (20-39)*	*Middle-Aged (40-64)*	*Old (65-79)*	*Very Old (80+)*	*RPE*[§]	*Maximum Voluntary Contraction*
Very light	<20	<35	<10	<2.4	<2.0	<1.6	<1.0	<10	<30
Light	20-39	35-54	10-11	2.4-4.7	2.0-3.9	1.6-3.1	1.1-1.9	10-11	30-49
Moderate	40-59	55-69	12-13	4.8-7.1	4.0-5.9	3.2-4.7	2.0-2.9	12-13	50-69
Hard	60-84	70-89	14-16	7.2-10.1	6.0-8.4	4.8-6.7	3.0-4.25	14-16	70-84
Very hard	≥85	≥90	17-19	≥10.2	≥8.5	≥6.8	≥4.25	17-19	≥85
Maximum[‖]	100	100	20	12.0	10.0	8.0	5.0	20	100

MET = metabolic equivalent.

From Fletcher GF, Balady GJ, Amsterdam EA, et al: Exercise standards for testing and training: A statement for healthcare professionals from the American Heart Association. Circulation 104:1694, 2001.

*Based on 8 to 12 repetitions for persons younger than 50 to 60 years and 10 to 15 repetitions for persons older than 50 to 60 years.

[†]VO_2, measured oxygen intake.

[‡]Maximum heart rate indicates 220 minus age or peak heart rate on exercise test.

[§]Borg rating of relative perceived exertion (RPE), scale of 6 to 20.

[‖]Maximum values are mean values achieved during maximum exercise by healthy adults. Absolute intensity values are approximate mean values for men. Mean values for women are approximately 1 to 2 METs lower than those for men.

TABLE 43–4 Energy Requirements of Common Daily Activities*

Activities	METs
Leisure activities	
Mild	
Playing the piano	2.3
Canoeing (leisurely)	2.5
Golf (with cart)	2.5
Walking (2 mph)	2.5
Dancing (ballroom)	2.9
Moderate	
Walking (3 mph)	3.3
Cycling (leisurely)	3.5
Calisthenics (no weight)	4.0
Golf (without cart)	4.4
Swimming (slow)	4.5
Walking (4 mph)	4.5
Vigorous	
Chopping wood	4.9
Tennis (doubles)	5.0
Ballroom (fast) or square dancing	5.5
Cycling (moderately)	5.7
Skiing (water or downhill)	6.8
Climbing hills (no load)	6.9
Swimming	7.0
Walking (5 mph)	8.0
Jogging (10-min mile)	10.2
Rope skipping	12.0
Squash	12.1
Activities of daily living	
Lying quietly	1.0
Sitting; light activity	1.5
Walking from house to car or bus	2.5
Watering plants	2.5
Loading and unloading car	3.0
Taking out trash	3.0
Walking the dog	3.0
Household tasks, moderate effort	3.5
Vacuuming	3.5
Lifting items continuously	4.0
Raking lawn	4.0
Gardening (no lifting)	4.4
Mowing lawn (power mower)	4.5

MET = metabolic equivalent or a unit of sitting, resting oxygen uptake.
*These activities can often be done at variable intensities, assuming that the intensity is not excessive and that the courses are flat (no hills) unless so specified. Categories are based on experience or tolerance; if an activity is perceived to be more than indicated, it should be judged accordingly.

TABLE 43–5 Possible Mechanisms for Exercise-Induced Reductions in Morbidity and Mortality

Cardiovascular influences
Reduction of resting and exercise heart rates
Reduction of resting and exercise blood pressures
Reduction of myocardial oxygen demand at submaximal levels of physical activity
Expansion of plasma volume
Increase in myocardial contractility
Increase in peripheral venous tone
Favorable changes in fibrinolytic system
Increased endothelium-dependent vasodilation
Increased gene expression for nitric oxide synthase
Enhanced parasympathetic tone
Possible increases in coronary blood flow, coronary collateral vessels, and myocardial capillary density
Metabolic influences
Reduction of obesity
Enhanced glucose tolerance
Improved lipid profile
Life-style influences
Decreased likelihood of smoking
Possible reduction of stress, depression
Short-term reduction of appetite

From Shephard RJ, Balady GJ: Exercise as cardiovascular therapy. Circulation 99:963, 1999.

CH 43

muscle groups without movement (*isometric exercise*) tends to exert a pressure load rather than a volume load on the heart that is characterized by increases in systemic vascular resistance and blood pressure with minimal changes in cardiac output and oxygen consumption. *Resistance exercises* such as weight lifting produce muscular contraction with movement and thus, depending on intensity, can produce both volume and pressure loads. Most activities usually combine all three types of exercise.

CHRONIC ADAPTATIONS TO EXERCISE. Over time, regular exercise increases the ability of the cardiovascular system to deliver oxygen to the tissues while at the same time improving the ability of muscles to use oxygen. The combination of increased cardiac output and peripheral adaptations that improve oxygen extraction associated with regular exercise can increase maximum oxygen consumption twofold to threefold. Regular exercise also reduces resting heart rate and blood pressure. By improving functional work capacity, it also reduces the metabolic and circulatory demands of activities of daily living.

Possible Biological Mechanisms for the Benefits of Exercise (Table 43–5)

Physical activity appears to lower cardiovascular disease risk by effects on traditional coronary risk factors, as discussed subsequently. Regular exercise may also improve fibrinolytic and endothelial vasodilator function.

WEIGHT. Exercise by itself yields modest weight loss, with exercise randomized clinical trials showing losses of 2 to 3 kg in the exercise group. However, exercise appears to complement dietary approaches to weight loss—the combination achieves an average weight loss of 8.5 kg.[28] Exercise may play an even more important role in maintenance of weight loss. A meta-analysis of studies of long-term weight loss maintenance found that groups who exercised more had significantly greater weight loss maintenance than those who exercised less.[29] Exercise also improves body composition and fat distribution, both of which are linked to cardiovascular mortality.[30]

BLOOD PRESSURE. Cohort and clinical studies indicate that exercise reduces blood pressure independent of weight loss. A meta-analysis of 54 randomized, controlled trials that included 2419 participants whose intervention and control groups differed only in aerobic exercise demonstrated a clear association between exercise and blood pressure. Aerobic exercise was associated with a 3.84 mm Hg (95 percent CI, 4.97 to 2.72 mm Hg) reduction in mean systolic blood pressure and a 2.58 mm Hg (95 percent CI, 3.35 to 1.81 mm Hg) reduction in diastolic blood pressure. Reductions occurred in men and women, hypertensive and normotensive participants, and overweight and normal-weight participants.[31] The reduction in blood pressure related to aerobic exercise did not differ significantly according to frequency or intensity of aerobic exercise.

DIABETES MELLITUS. Physical activity has beneficial effects on both glucose metabolism and insulin sensitivity.[32] Even moderate-intensity activities such as walking are associated with both prevention of diabetes[33] and reductions in cardiovascular disease and mortality among individuals with diabetes.[34,35] The Diabetes Prevention Program demonstrated the powerful effect that physical activity and weight loss can exert in preventing the onset of type 2 diabetes in individuals at high risk for this disease. Compared with usual care, there was a 58 percent reduction in the onset of type 2 diabetes over 2.8 years among individuals randomly assigned to a life-style intervention that produced an average

4-kg decrease in body weight and an 8-MET-hr/wk increase in physical activity.[36]

LIPIDS. Despite the extensive research focused on the effects of exercise on lipid levels, the benefits of exercise are not precisely known owing to the heterogeneity of study methods, populations, and exercise interventions. A meta-analysis of 52 exercise training trials lasting more than 12 weeks that included 4700 subjects demonstrated an average 4.6 percent increase in HDL levels and reductions in triglyceride and low-density lipoprotein (LDL) concentrations of 3.7 and 5.0 percent, respectively.[37] In the largest and most carefully controlled of these trials, the *HE*alth, *RI*sk factors, Exercise *T*raining, *A*nd *GE*netics (HERITAGE) study, 5 months of exercise training among 675 normolipidemic subjects induced a 1.1-mg/dl increase in HDL among men along with a 5.9-mg/dl decrease in triglycerides and a 0.9-mg/dl decrease in LDL. Among women, HDL increased 1.4 mg/dl, triglycerides decreased 0.6 mg/dl, and LDL decreased 4.4 mg/dl.[38] It is possible that larger exercise-related increases in HDL may occur in individuals with baseline hypertriglyceridemia or in studies of longer duration, but few studies have addressed the effect of exercise in subjects with lipid disorders.

Exercise may also alter the distribution of lipid fractions. Among 111 sedentary, overweight men and women with mild to moderate dyslipidemia randomly assigned to 8 months of exercise or a nonexercise control group, exercising at a caloric equivalent of 17 to 18 miles per week at an intensity equivalent to that of jogging at a moderate pace significantly decreased the concentrations of both small LDL and total LDL particles and increased the average size of LDL particles without changing the plasma LDL cholesterol concentration. The total HDL concentration, concentration of large HDL particles, and average size of HDL particles were also increased, whereas the concentrations of triglycerides and total very low-density lipoprotein triglycerides decreased.[39] The dose of exercise appeared to contribute more to plasma lipoprotein concentrations than the intensity of exercise.

A patient's genotype may influence the impact of exercise duration or intensity on cardiovascular risk factors. Exerting a larger fraction of the total energy expenditure in high-intensity activities, for example, may lead to greater improvements in HDL and triglycerides among individuals with the ApoE4 allele.[40]

THROMBOSIS. Exercise training favorably affects the fibrinolytic system by reducing plasma fibrinogen and plasminogen activator inhibitor-1 levels and increasing tissue plasminogen activator (t-PA) levels. Among 3810 British men observed for 20 years after an initial screening, physical activity showed an inverse dose-response relationship with fibrinogen, plasma and blood viscosity, platelet count, coagulation factors VIII and IX, von Willebrand factor, fibrin D-dimer, tissue plasminogen activator antigen, C-reactive protein, and white cell count.[41] Among sedentary older men, 3 months of aerobic exercise increased endothelial capacity to release t-PA by 55 percent to levels similar to those of young adults and older endurance-trained men.[42] Acute exercise may increase platelet activation and reactivity, especially in sedentary individuals, and thus increase the risk of myocardial infarction or unstable angina. Regular exercise, in comparison, appears to reduce platelet aggregability.

ENDOTHELIAL FUNCTION. Arterial tone and platelet aggregation depend in part on release of nitric oxide from the vascular endothelium. Patients with atherosclerosis or coronary risk factors have impaired endothelium-dependent dilation. Exercise can limit or reverse this dysfunction among patients with coronary disease,[43,44] peripheral arterial disease,[45] heart failure,[46] and diabetes.[47]

AUTONOMIC FUNCTION. Heart rate is modulated by the interplay between sympathetic and parasympathetic activity. Chronic activation of the sympathetic nervous system or neutralization of parasympathetic (vagal) tone, or both, increases the risk of adverse cardiovascular events as well as mortality, especially among patients with heart disease.[48] One measure of autonomic function is heart rate variability. Low heart rate variability has been associated with increased risk of CHD and mortality.[49] Among healthy older adults[50] and those with coronary disease, exercise training significantly improves heart rate variability.[51]

Benefits of Exercise

Data from more than 40 observational studies demonstrate clear evidence of an inverse linear dose-response relation between volume of physical activity and all-cause mortality rates in younger and older men and women. Minimal adherence to current physical activity guidelines, which yield an energy expenditure of about 1000 kcal/wk, is associated with a significant 20 to 30 percent reduction in risk of all-cause mortality.[52]

Exercise capacity is an important prognostic factor in patients with cardiovascular disease. It also predicts mortality among individuals with symptoms that suggested CHD. Among 6213 consecutive men referred for treadmill exercise testing for clinical reasons and observed for a mean of 6.2 years, peak exercise capacity measured in METs was the strongest predictor of the risk of death among both normal subjects and those with cardiovascular disease. Each 1-MET increase in exercise capacity conferred a 12 percent improvement in survival.[53]

Exercise training is useful for patients with angina pectoris who are not candidates for revascularization or who choose not to have it. The symptomatic improvement in exercise tolerance after exercise training results primarily from a reduction in the heart rate and systolic blood pressure or rate-pressure product at submaximal workloads. It is also possible that exercise training improves myocardial oxygen delivery by altering the coronary vasomotor response to exercise.[43]

Although no large studies have directly addressed the benefits of exercise training following coronary revascularization, it is likely to be beneficial in this population as well. The Exercise Training Intervention after Coronary Angioplasty (ETICA) trial randomly assigned 118 consecutive patients to 6 months of exercise training or a control group. Trained patients demonstrated a significant 26 percent increase in peak O_2 and improvement in quality of life.[54] Over almost 3 years of follow-up, the exercise-trained patients had fewer cardiac events (11.9 versus 32.2 percent) and hospital readmissions (18.6 versus 46 percent) than subjects assigned to usual care. In the trained subjects, residual coronary stenosis was reduced by 30 percent and recurrent cardiac events by 29 percent.

Exercise Testing

Exercise testing (see Chap. 10) offers important information regarding a patient's cardiovascular status. Determination of functional capacity in patients referred for cardiac rehabilitation is essential for developing an appropriate exercise prescription (Table 43–6). Thus, exercise testing may be performed as part of cardiac rehabilitation to provide necessary information for the development of the exercise prescription, to assess the impact of exercise training occurring as part of the cardiac rehabilitation program, and to provide feedback to the patient.[55]

Principles of Exercise Prescription

Exercise therapy must be individualized on the basis of the patient's specific characteristics, abilities, and comorbidities. In fact, much like pharmacological therapy, it requires a prescription with a careful consideration of both appropriate dosage and possible side effects (see Table 43–6).

TABLE 43–6 Exercise Prescription for Endurance and Resistance Training

Endurance Training	
Frequency	3-5 d/wk
Intensity	See Table 43–3 and text
Duration	20-60 min
Modality	
Lower extremity	Walking Jogging/running Stairclimber Cycling
Upper extremity	Arm ergometry
Combined	Rowing Cross-country ski machine Combined arm-leg cycle Swimming Aerobics
Resistance Training	
Frequency	2-3 d/wk
Intensity	1-3 sets of 8-15 RM for each muscle group
Modality	
Lower extremity	Legs extensions, curls, presses Adductors-abductors
Upper extremity	Biceps curls Triceps extensions Bench-overhead presses Lateral pulldowns-raises Benchovers–seated rowing

RM = maximum number of times a load can lifted before fatigue.
From Shephard RJ, Balady GJ: Exercise as cardiovascular therapy. Circulation 99:963, 1999.

AEROBIC EXERCISE PRESCRIPTION FOR PATIENTS WITH CARDIOVASCULAR DISEASE

Adequate exercise training is a function of variables that include type of exercise, intensity, frequency, duration, and total energy expenditure.

TYPE OF EXERCISE. Walking is the preferred initial mode of exercise because it requires no special training or equipment and can be performed at any time of day. Because the energy cost of walking varies little from person to person, it is relatively simple to specify the dose of exercise in terms of a distance to be covered within a specified time. However, depending on patients' preferences, other activities such as stationary cycling or rowing may be substituted.

INTENSITY (see also Table 43-3). It was once thought that aerobic training response required exercise at an intensity sufficient to achieve 60 to 80 percent of an individual's maximal Vo_2. For many individuals, however, the largest reduction in overall mortality over time occurs with moving from the lowest to the next lowest quintile of fitness.[56] Thus, for sedentary older adults—the most likely beneficiaries of cardiac rehabilitation programs—aerobic fitness can be enhanced by exercise intensities as low as 40 percent of Vo_{2max}.[57] For some individuals, effort insufficient to augment aerobic power may nevertheless confer some health benefits.

For most patients, exercise intensity should be prescribed at 50 to 80 percent of Vo_{2max} as determined by an exercise test or by the estimated numbers of METs achieved. A training heart rate is generally designated as 65 to 85 percent of the maximal measured heart rate from the exercise test.[58] If an exercise test is not initially performed, a target of 20 beats/min above the resting heart rate is adequate until test results are available. For patients who develop symptoms, ST depression, or arrhythmias, a target of approximately 10 beats/min below the rate at which these occurred should be used.

FREQUENCY. At the beginning of cardiac rehabilitation, as many as three sessions per week may be undertaken under medical supervision. These supervised sessions can be tapered off as home exercise becomes increasingly important. Eventually, aerobic exercise should be performed on most days of the week.[27,58,59]

DURATION. With increasing fitness, patients should be encouraged to achieve a minimum of 30 minutes of aerobic exercise per day.[27,59] This is best accomplished in a single bout of exercise but may be divided into two or three parts. However, divided exercise produce less cardiovascular fitness.

TOTAL ENERGY EXPENDITURE. Because many of the benefits of exercise depend upon the total dose of exercise, patients should be encouraged to engage in as many activities as is practical. They can, at least partially, make up for a "deficit" on one day with a greater dose on the next. In addition to duration, the exercise prescription should specify the pace of activities such as walking or jogging.

ADVANCING THE PRESCRIPTION. As patients become more conditioned, the exercise prescription should be advanced. The scale developed by Borg (see Table 43–3) is useful for this. In general, exercise should be performed at a rate of perceived exertion (RPE) of 13 to 15 on the Borg scale. For some individuals an RPE of 14 to 15 represents exercise too strenuous to sustain, as evidenced by heart rates over target. When this is the case, less aggressive targets should be used. As the RPE falls with improving fitness, the intensity of exercise may be increased, usually in increments of 5 to 10 percent of the maximal heart rate. Most asymptomatic patients should have as a goal the ability to exercise at 85 percent of their peak heart rate for the full exercise session. For symptomatic or high-risk patients or those who experience ischemia or arrhythmias with exercise, repeated exercise testing may be required before safely advancing the prescription.

RESISTANCE TRAINING PRESCRIPTION FOR PATIENTS WITH CARDIOVASCULAR DISEASE

Range-of-motion and resistance exercises are necessary to counter the muscle atrophy induced by aging, surgery, or bed rest. Following CABG, range-of-motion exercises are needed to prevent the development of adhesions and help avoid muscle weakness or loss. Although stretching or flexibility activities can begin as early as 24 hours after CABG or 2 days after myocardial infarction, low-level resistance training should not begin until 2 to 3 weeks after myocardial infarction.[60] In general, surgical patients should avoid strength-training exercises that pull on the sternum for 3 months after CABG surgery.

Otherwise, selected patients should begin the same type of strength-training program recommended for healthy older adults. Patients should start with a weight low enough to allow one set of 10 to 15 repetitions and increase weight slowly (2 to 5 pounds/wk for arms and 5 to 10 pounds/wk for legs). Given the slow course of muscle hypertrophy, current recommendations call for at least two sessions of resistance exercise per week. The prescription for resistance training may differ depending on comorbid conditions and other limitations. Pure isometric exercise is not recommended for cardiac rehabilitation.

Electrocardiographic Monitoring

Practice varies considerably regarding the number of electrocardiographically monitored exercise sessions. Guidelines recommend using as few monitored sessions as possible.[18] The decision should be based on the patient's risk (Table 43–7), available staff, and the exercise setting. Electrocardiographic (ECG) monitoring is generally performed with either hardwired or telemetric systems and should be continuous. Telephonic home ECG monitoring has been used and appears to be effective in selected circumstances.[61]

Safety of Exercise Training and Cardiac Rehabilitation

Among patients with coronary artery disease, the risk of an adverse event during exercise testing is up to 100-fold higher than during usual activity. Even so, exercise training as part of a cardiac rehabilitation program is quite safe, with exceedingly low rates of coronary events reported in the rehabilitation setting. In a survey of 167 supervised programs, the

TABLE 43–7 Criteria for Electrocardiographic Monitoring During Exercise
Severely depressed left ventricular function (ejection fraction < 30%)
Resting complex ventricular arrhythmia
Ventricular arrhythmias appearing or increasing with exercise
Decrease in systolic blood pressure with exercise
Survivors of sudden cardiac death
Survivors of myocardial infarction complicated by congestive heart failure, cardiogenic shock, serious ventricular arrhythmias, or some combination of the three
Severe coronary artery disease and marked exercise-induced ischemia (ST segment depression greater than or equal to 2 mm)
Inability to self-monitor heart rate because of physical or intellectual impairment

From Cardiac Rehabilitation: Clinical Practice Guideline No. 17. Bethesda, Md, Agency for Health Care Policy and Research, National Heart, Lung, and Blood Institute, 1995; and Fletcher GF, Balady GJ, Amsterdam EA, et al: Exercise standards for testing and training: A statement for healthcare professionals from the American Heart Association. Circulation 104:1694, 2001.

incidence rate of cardiac events was quite low: 8.9 per million patient-hours of exercise for cardiac arrest, 3.4 per million patient-hours for myocardial infarction, and 1.3 per million patient-hours for fatalities.[58] In a 16-year follow-up of medically supervised exercise in a single cardiac rehabilitation center, five major cardiovascular complications (three nonfatal myocardial infarctions and two cardiac arrests) were recorded during 292,254 patient exercise hours, yielding an incidence rate of 17.1 per million patient-hours of exercise.[62]

The rate of sudden cardiac arrests among exercising individuals with known cardiovascular disease appears to be considerably higher, approximately 1 per 60,000 person-hours,[18] supporting the concept that supervised exercise, even among higher risk individuals, is far safer in the setting of cardiac rehabilitation.

Strength training is also a safe mode of exercise for cardiac rehabilitation, even among deconditioned patients. A review of 12 studies of resistance training in cardiac rehabilitation in men demonstrated improvements in muscular strength and endurance as well as absence of anginal symptoms, ischemic ST segment depression, abnormal hemodynamics, complex ventricular dysrhythmias, and cardiovascular complications.[2] Unfortunately, similar data for women are lacking. Table 43–8 lists the clinical circumstances in which exercise as part of cardiac rehabilitation is potentially dangerous and thus contraindicated.

Nutrition (see also Chap. 41)

Nutrition has direct effects on weight, serum lipids, blood pressure, blood sugar and insulin sensitivity, cardiac rhythm, endothelial function, and oxidative stress, all factors associated with cardiovascular health and disease.[63] Poor nutrition can thus increase the risk of coronary events, and healthy eating can decrease the risk.

At least five randomized trials with clinical endpoints have demonstrated that different approaches to diet can provide significant reductions in cardiac events such as myocardial infarction and sudden cardiac death.[64-68] Although not all diet studies have demonstrated benefits, more recent ones have been strikingly positive, with reductions in coronary events from 40 to 72 percent and mortality reductions as high as 30 percent.[63] The choice of diet to be recommended as part of

TABLE 43–8 Clinical Contraindications for Inpatient and Outpatient Cardiac Rehabilitation Exercise
Unstable angina
Resting SBP ≥ 180 mm Hg or resting DBP ≥ 100 mm Hg (evaluate on case-by-case basis)
Orthostatic blood pressure drop > 20 mm Hg with symptoms
Critical aortic stenosis
Acute systemic illness or fever
Uncontrolled atrial or ventricular arrhythmia
Uncontrolled sinus tachycardia (>120 beats/min)
Uncompensated CHF
Third-degree AV block (without pacemaker)
Active pericarditis or myocarditis
Recent embolism
Thrombophlebitis
Resting ST displacement (≥2 mm); ≥3 mm if patient is taking digitalis)
Uncontrolled diabetes
Severe orthopedic problems that would prohibit exercise
Other metabolic problems such as acute thyroiditis, hypo- or hyperkalemia, hypovolemia

AV = atrioventricular; CHF = congestive heart failure; DBP = diastolic blood pressure; SBP = systolic blood pressure.

Adapted from American College of Sports Medicine: Guidelines for Graded Exercise Testing and Prescription. 5th ed. Baltimore, Williams & Wilkins, 1995, p 179.

comprehensive cardiac rehabilitation should be based on both existing evidence of a beneficial effect and the social and cultural needs of the patient.

Intervention

Nutritional evaluation, counseling, and tracking must occur as part of a comprehensive cardiac rehabilitation program. Assessment of dietary patterns must begin before active participation with specific goals determined and communicated to the patient. For patients who are overweight (body mass index > 25 kg/m^2), a healthy eating strategy must include a specific weight management component. Interventions to promote weight loss should focus on adjusting caloric intake and increasing caloric expenditure with increased daily physical activity and regular exercise. Referral for medical intervention in the form of pharmacotherapy or bariatric surgery may be considered for patients whose obesity is seriously detrimental to their health. A rate of weight loss of 1 to 2 pounds per week or 1 percent of body weight per week is considered safe.[25]

In spite of intense public debate regarding the relative merits of low-fat versus low-carbohydrate diets, the optimal eating strategy for losing weight is not likely to be resolved soon.[69] It is possible that the specific components of a diet are not as important as achieving continued caloric restriction. Data from the National Weight Control Registry, which has enrolled approximately 3000 women and men who lost more than 30 pounds and kept them off for at least a year, suggest three important strategies for successful weight loss: exercise (an average of 400 calories per day, or the equivalent of 1 hour of brisk walking), consumption of fewer calories (registry members consumed, on average, 1400 calories a day), and a lower fat diet rich in fruits and vegetables and low in sugars and sweets.[70]

Two useful basic plans have been developed. Each one can be easily adapted into cardiac rehabilitation programs.

- The dietary component of the National Cholesterol Education Program's *Therapeutic Lifestyle Changes*[71]: 25 to 35 percent of calories from fat, saturated fat less than 7 percent of caloric intake, and cholesterol intake less than 200 mg/d. Carbohydrates (from whole grains and other foods rich in complex carbohydrates) constitute 50 to 60 percent of calories, protein 15 percent, and 20 to 30 gm of dietary fiber (especially soluble fiber) per day.
- The *Dietary Approaches to Stop Hypertension* (DASH) eating plan[72]: this diet, which emerged from the randomized DASH trial, is low in saturated fat, cholesterol, and total fat, and emphasizes fruits, vegetables, low-fat dairy foods, whole-grain products, fish, poultry, and nuts.

Increased intake of omega-3 fatty acids from fish, fish oil supplements, or plant sources should also be encouraged. Omega-3 fatty acids may reduce the risk of cardiac events, in particular sudden cardiac death.[73]

Regardless of specific nutrition issues, long-term dietary adherence remains problematic. A successful cardiac rehabilitation program provides patients with not only specific dietary information but also critically important strategies to improve adherence based on sound principles from behavioral medicine (see Chap. 84).

Smoking

Cigarette smoking is the leading cause of preventable death,[74] more than 40 percent of which results from smoking-related cardiovascular disease. Tobacco smoke contains a multitude of cardiotoxic substances, of which nicotine is probably the most important.[75] The smoke of as little as one cigarette elevates blood pressure and heart rate, probably related to nicotine-induced release of catecholamines. Cigarette smoking increases platelet activation and impairs fibrinolysis,[76] adversely affects the lipoprotein profile by raising triglycerides and lowering HDL,[77] lowers the threshold for arrhythmia,[78] impairs endothelial function,[79,80] and promotes the progression of atherosclerosis.[81]

Cessation of smoking yields a 50 percent reduction in the risk of a coronary event in the first year or two after quitting, with the risk of former smokers approaching that of nonsmokers after 5 to 15 years. Patients who quit smoking have a 36 percent reduction in crude relative risk of mortality compared with those who continue smoking.[82] A 20-year follow-up of patients after CABG showed that those who continued smoking had a 1.75 relative risk of cardiac death compared with those who stopped smoking for at least 1 year after surgery.[83]

Smoking cessation efforts conducted during the course of a comprehensive cardiac rehabilitation program can have a significant impact on smoking rates. In a study of a combined educational and behavioral intervention, 17 to 26 percent of patients stopped smoking.[84] In a later example, among 109 patients referred to a 2- to 3-month multidisciplinary ambulatory cardiac rehabilitation program within 1 to 4 weeks after hospital discharge for acute myocardial infarction or CABG, smoking rates dropped to 14 percent at 12 months.[26]

Smoking Cessation Intervention

The period following an acute coronary event, revascularization procedure, or diagnosis of cardiovascular disease is an ideal time to encourage patients to stop smoking. Providing information about the link between smoking and cardiovascular disease at this vulnerable time may supply the motivation to stop smoking. This motivation must be carefully nurtured and supported with effective interventions. Guidelines from the U.S. Public Health Service[85] recommend a combination of behavioral counseling and pharmacological therapy for nicotine withdrawal. Social support and training in problem solving appear to be effective behavioral interventions. First-line pharmacotherapies include sustained-release bupropion hydrochloride and nicotine replacement (Table 43–9). These therapies have been demonstrated to be safe, even among patients with CHD.[86] However, current clinical guidelines recommend that these first-line therapies not be used in patients with unstable angina or a myocardial infarction in the previous 2 weeks because there are few data to support their use in this period.[87]

Exposure to passive smoke may explain why counseling the patient alone may not be sufficient for smoking cessation. In a survey of 103 consecutive patients attending a hospital-based 10-week multidisciplinary cardiac rehabilitation program, 40 percent reported living with someone else who smoked, most often a spouse.[88] Thus, interventions to modify the smoking behavior of other members of the cardiac patient's household may be needed to achieve optimum secondary prevention. Smokers who are depressed are more likely to relapse after hospitalization or during cardiac rehabilitation; thus, assessment and treatment of depression should proceed in concert with, or prior to, smoking cessation efforts.

Psychosocial Factors

A wide variety of psychosocial factors influence outcomes in CHD patients. Detection of and intervention for many of these can and should occur in connection with cardiac rehabilitation. Depression and perceived lack of social support are common among patients with CHD, affecting one third or more of this population.[89] Both are associated with increases in cardiac morbidity and mortality up to eightfold among patients with CHD.[90,91] Following myocardial infarction, depression is a risk factor for mortality independent of the severity of cardiac disease,[92] and there is some evidence that depression during admission for myocardial infarction is more closely linked to long-term survival than depression after the event.[93] Although major depression is clearly detrimental, even minimal symptoms of depression increase the risk of mortality after myocardial infarction.[94]

Depression and low social support may predispose a patient to be nonadherent to medications, exercise programs, and other secondary prevention efforts.[95] Depression and stress may also affect biological factors that increase risk of cardiac events, such as ventricular irritability, low heart rate variability, and increased platelet activation.[96,97] Other factors including anxiety, life stress, vital exhaustion (defined as a combination of fatigue, lack of energy, feelings of hopelessness, and loss of libido), and hostility[98] have been shown to influence CHD outcomes. Hostility has attracted attention as the possible "toxic" element of a type A personality. Studies have linked its presence to increased risk.

Two meta-analyses have assessed the impact of psychosocial interventions in cardiac rehabilitation. Linden and colleagues demonstrated that psychosocially treated patients showed greater reductions in psychological distress, systolic blood pressure, heart rate, and cholesterol level, whereas patients who did not receive psychosocial treatment showed significantly greater mortality and cardiac recurrence rates during the first 2 years of follow-up.[99] A meta-analysis by Dusseldorp and colleagues that included 37 studies suggested that psychosocial interventions were associated with a 34 percent reduction in cardiac mortality, a 29 percent reduction in recurrence of myocardial infarction, and significant beneficial effects on blood pressure, cholesterol, body weight, smoking, physical activity, and eating habits.[100]

TABLE 43–9 First-Line Medications to Treat Nicotine Addiction

Medication	Advantages	Side Effects	Considerations
Nicotine patch	Easy to use, steady-state blood levels	Skin reactions, disturbed sleep	Available over the counter, low liability for long-term use
Nicotine gum	Can be used ad libitum	Sore mouth, hiccups, dyspepsia, sore jaw	Compliance can be increased with careful instructions: chew slowly and intermittently, avoid acidic beverages. Available over the counter
Nicotine inhaler	Can be used ad libitum	Mouth-throat irritation, coughing,	Acidic beverages reduce nicotine absorption
Nicotine nasal spray	Can be used ad libitum; causes rapid rise in blood nicotine levels	Nasal irritation or congestion, rhinitis	More likely to be abused than other therapies
Nicotine lozenge	Can be used ad libitum; oral substitute for cigarettes	Sore mouth, dyspepsia, hiccups	Available over the counter
Sustained-release bupropion	Nonnicotine treatment; easy to use and well tolerated	Insomnia, dry mouth	Can be safely used with nicotine replacement therapy; avoid in patients with seizure disorder, history of alcoholism, or severe uncontrolled hypertension

Adapted from Thomson CC, Rigotti NA: Hospital- and clinic-based smoking cessation interventions for smokers with cardiovascular disease. Prog Cardiovasc Dis 45:459, 2003.

In the Enhancing Recovery in Coronary Heart Disease Patients (ENRICHD) trial, 2481 patients with recent myocardial infarction were randomly assigned to 6 months of cognitive behavioral therapy or usual care. In the treatment arm, an antidepressant was prescribed for patients who did not respond within 5 weeks to this therapy or with high scores on the Hamilton Rating Scale for Depression. Psychosocial outcomes were significantly better in the treatment group.[89] There were no significant differences, however, in survival or recurrent myocardial infarction. This null result may be attributed to frequent interventions in the control group—among patients with depression, 28 percent of those in the treatment arm and 20.6 percent of those in the control arm were taking an antidepressant. The interventions employed in the ENRICHD trial can be adjusted and adapted into cardiac rehabilitation programs.

Easing the stress and distress that follow myocardial infarction, revascularization, or a diagnosis of CHD may be one avenue by which comprehensive cardiac rehabilitation programs improve survival. A 3-month nonrandomized trial evaluated 150 men who received either standard medical care (n = 72) or an accelerated comprehensive rehabilitation program that included counseling sessions aimed at coping with stress. At the program's end, rehabilitation patients reported more improvement and less deterioration in mood than control patients. After 9 years of follow-up, the most significant predictors of mortality were left ventricular ejection fraction less than 50 percent (odds ratio, 3.2; 95 percent CI, 1.1 to 9.8) and rehabilitation (odds ratio, 0.2; 95 percent CI, 0.1 to 0.7).[101]

Pharmacotherapy may be an important adjunct to behavioral therapy in treating depression. In the Sertraline Antidepressant Heart Attack Randomized Trial (SADHART), sertraline therapy was judged to be safe following an acute coronary syndrome.[102] The incidence of severe adverse cardiovascular events was 14.5 percent in the sertraline group and 22.4 percent in the placebo group. In the ENRICHD trial, subgroup analysis of patients taking a selective serotonin reuptake inhibitor antidepressant showed significant improvements in cardiac outcomes. Use of a serotonin reuptake inhibitor was associated with a 43 percent lower risk of myocardial infarction and a 42 percent lower risk of death.[89]

Intervention

A rehabilitation program provides an excellent setting in which to identify patients who are significantly depressed, isolated, excessively stressed, or easily angered and to begin appropriate interventions that may act synergistically with other component of the program. Exercise, for example, may help improve depression, and the dynamics of a group setting may provide the seeds of a potentially helpful social support network.[103]

Some cardiac rehabilitation programs offer psychological interventions as a component of the program itself. These include group psychotherapy, individual psychotherapy, behavior counseling, and relaxation or stress management classes. All programs should include an assessment or screening for the presence of psychosocial problems and should provide an opportunity for referral to other experts if conditions merit.

Other Therapy (Aspirin, Statins, Angiotensin-Converting Enzyme Inhibitors, Beta Blockers)

Pharmacotherapy for secondary prevention is covered in detail in Chapters 39 and 42. Participation in cardiac rehabilitation should enhance adherence to recommended pharmacological interventions.[59]

Education

Education of patients is such an integral part of any cardiac rehabilitation program that it was included as a critical component of cardiac rehabilitation in the 1995 Agency for Health Care Policy and Research guideline[2] and is required for certification by the American Association of Cardiovascular and Pulmonary Rehabilitation. Structural aspects of the cardiac rehabilitation program, training expertise, and interests of the staff as well as the needs, abilities, and cultural differences among the patients all influence the important process of information delivery and behavior change that constitute education of patients. Timing of education is of critical importance, because the initial period in outpatient cardiac rehabilitation often represents a time when motivation is likely to be high, but also when there are major deficits in knowledge and important misconceptions. The experience of group cardiac rehabilitation is optimal for improving this situation in a supportive environment in which both experienced professionals and other patients experiencing similar conditions combine their communication efforts to build knowledge and assist with behavior change.

Several principles of behavior change are helpful in improving the participant's motivation as well as an individual's ability to comprehend and digest a broad array of information. None of these principles are mutually exclusive, and many are often combined in programs, depending on staff organization and patients' needs.[104]

LEARNING NEEDS. In many cases, learning depends on what the individual perceives as his or her need to learn. Thus, after a recent cardiovascular event or procedure, learning can be enhanced by structuring information around patient-specific events and findings (the use of anatomical models and diagrams), and such information can be blended with advice on behavior change and awareness of warning signs.

OUTCOME MODEL. Many individuals find it easier to change behavior when specific goals or targets are placed on the horizon. Such a process involves knowing not only what ideal goals should be from the professional standpoint, but also the optimal achievable goals from the patient's perspective. It is also essential to know what resources are available and what experience the individual has had with respect to specific goals. Specific and reasonable outcome goals can be elucidated. Some have found it useful to document these goals explicitly in the form of "contracts."

SELF-EFFICACY. A concept based on Bandura's social learning theory[105] has become important in understanding both barriers to behavior change and strategies to improve healthy behaviors. Self-efficacy concepts tested in the cardiac rehabilitation setting have been shown to improve learning and behavior change. There are two critical components of the self-efficacy concept. The first is an "outcome expectancy," which is an individual's belief that a particular behavior will lead to a specific outcome. The second is an "efficacy expectation" that he or she can be successful in modifying the behavior necessary to produce the outcome. Self-esteem appears to be a critical component of this concept; thus, individuals with low self-esteem are often both less motivated and less able to make behavior change. Strategies that improve self-esteem or self-efficacy, or both, have been shown to improve life-style risk factor change.

STAGES OF CHANGE. The stages of change model, also called the transtheoretical model, developed by Prochaska and DiClemente[106] has been widely applied to smoking cessation and is also being used to understand and improve behavior change efforts for other risk factors. This model generally defines four stages in the process of behavior change: precontemplation, contemplation, action, and maintenance. When an individual's current stage has been identified, educational interventions are targeted to that specific stage. Thus, for an individual who is not yet thinking of stopping smoking (precontemplation), efforts need to be directed at understanding why that patient smokes and what it might take for him or her to consider smoking cessation. Strategies for someone already in the process of planning to stop smoking are quite different—that patient not only needs specific information about why smoking is bad but also needs help with strategies to aid in smoking cessation, including preparation for withdrawal symptoms. Similar strategies could be applied to individuals beginning exercise.

PERFORMED LEARNING STYLE. People understand and remember new information in a variety of different ways. This model emphasizes assessment of which mode of learning suits an individual best (e.g., oral, pictorial, graphic).

Although it would be impractical to tailor all educational efforts to highly specific individual needs, clearly the option of independent learning modalities within a cardiac rehabilitation setting is optimal. Most successful programs include classes (some of which are optional), the opportunities for one-on-one learning, written materials, video materials, and now Internet-based materials.

In addition to imparting knowledge and assisting with behavior change, education of patients in the context of cardiac rehabilitation should optimally be responsive to other learning needs:

- Inclusion of family members and significant others in teaching
- Maintenance of change and prevention of relapse
- Provision of learning resources in different forms—written, video, computer (Internet based)
- Access to other community resources (e.g., local American Heart Association)

Sexual Activity after Myocardial Infarction

Issues of sexual activity must also be addressed. Because patients are often reluctant to discuss sexuality or sexual dysfunction, members of the cardiac rehabilitation team should address these issues, including the possible effect of medications on sexual function. The most common sexual problems encountered by cardiac patients are reduced or extinguished libido and avoidance of sexual activity. Men also commonly experience impotence or premature or delayed ejaculation. Factors contributing to sexual dysfunction include depression, fear of precipitating a cardiovascular event on the part of the individual or his or her partner, and medications, particularly beta blockers and diuretics.

The hemodynamic response to usual sexual activity approximates the maximal heart rate attained with other customary activities, such as walking up one or two flights of stairs.[107] The response may be significantly higher with an unfamiliar partner, in unfamiliar circumstances, or after excessive eating or alcohol consumption. Low-risk patients (those with mild, stable angina, successful coronary revascularization, uncomplicated myocardial infarction, or mild valvular disease) can be safely encouraged to initiate or resume sexual activity or to receive treatment for sexual dysfunction. It is important to stress that sildenafil or other phosphodiesterase-5 inhibitors must not be used by patients taking nitrates in any form. Higher risk patients should receive further cardiological evaluation before recommendations are made regarding sexual activity.[108] Patients should be encouraged to report symptoms lasting more than 10 minutes after sexual activity.

Successful education of the patient in cardiac rehabilitation depends upon the educator's ability to communicate and knowledge of appropriate learning and behavior strategies. Opportunities to obtain competence in these areas are important, and ongoing assessment of abilities allows individual participants to benefit greatly from the cardiac rehabilitation experience and to continue to benefit when the formal program has been completed.

Adherence

To state the obvious, interventions proved to improve outcomes require implementation and adherence to have their desired effect. Patients often have difficulty adhering to even a single intervention such as taking a statin for high cholesterol.[109] Comprehensive cardiac rehabilitation entails more than a dozen separate interventions, making adherence quite complex. Indeed, up to half of individuals who begin a cardiac rehabilitation program fail to complete it.

A review of studies examining participation in and adherence to cardiac rehabilitation reveals several factors consistently associated with participation. These include referral by physicians, specific cardiac diagnoses, reimbursement issues, self-efficacy, perceived benefits of cardiac rehabilitation, distance and transportation, self-motivation, family composition, social support, self-esteem, and occupation. Factors associated with nonadherence include being older, being female, having fewer years of formal education, depression, and difficulty in perceiving the benefits of cardiac rehabilitation.[110]

Successful cardiac rehabilitation depends upon implementation and integration at the levels of the patient, provider, and system. Because these programs are multidisciplinary, often hospital based, and interact at all three levels when optimally designed and utilized, they represent an ideal opportunity to enhance adherence to all secondary prevention interventions. A number of interventions are available to improve adherence at all levels (Table 43–10). The most effective interventions—those with multiple components and a continued maintenance intervention—can be delivered through a model in which physicians provide advice and other members of the health care team provide more in-depth behavioral counseling and follow-up.

Adherence to smoking cessation, dietary change, and psychosocial interventions presents challenges specific to the problems themselves. For example, counseling designed to identify and deal with "triggers" to unhealthy behaviors improves adherence to both smoking cessation and caloric restriction. Uniquely, successful smoking cessation requires specific counseling regarding withdrawal symptoms. Group sessions help some patients with stress reduction and anger management techniques, but depression generally requires individual attention. Indeed, inadequate attention to depression often leads to poor adherence with other behavior changes and medical interventions as well.[95]

A case management system can provide an important framework for the delivery of care by integrating the patient, family, environment, life style, and community.[111] In this model, a single individual, usually a nurse or exercise physiologist, coordinates all aspects of care, engaging physicians and other specialists when necessary.

Rehabilitation for Other Populations

Cardiac rehabilitation is also beneficial for patients with a variety of other cardiovascular diseases. Medicare provides payments for cardiac rehabilitation only for the diagnoses of myocardial infarction, coronary artery bypass surgery, and stable angina. Unfortunately, reimbursement is not available for patients who have undergone percutaneous revascularization, heart transplantation, and heart valve surgery or for patients with heart failure. Insurance coverage by other third-party payers varies considerably throughout the United States.

TABLE 43–10 Interventions to Improve Adherence with Cardiac Rehabilitation

Focus on the Patient
- Simplify medication regimens
- Provide explicit instructions and teach the patient how to follow the prescribed treatment
- Encourage the use of prompts to help patients remember treatment regimens
- Use systems to reinforce adherence and maintain contact
- Encourage the support of family and friends
- Reinforce and reward adherence
- Increase patients' visits for persons unable to achieve treatment goal
- Increase the convenience and access to care
- Involve patients in their care through self-monitoring

Focus on Provider and Medical Office
- Implement prevention guidelines
- Use reminders to prompt physicians to attend to prevention
- Identify a patient advocate in the office
- Develop a standardized treatment plan to structure care
- Use feedback from past performance to foster change in future care
- Remind patients of appointments and follow up missed appointments

Focus on the Health Delivery System
- Use case management by nurses
- Use telemedicine when possible
- Collaborate with pharmacists
- Develop and use critical care pathways

Adapted from National Cholesterol Education Program (NCEP) Expert Panel on Detection, Evaluation, and Treatment of High Blood Cholesterol in Adults (Adult Treatment Panel III): Third Report of the National Cholesterol Education Program (NCEP) Expert Panel on Detection, Evaluation, and Treatment of High Blood Cholesterol in Adults (Adult Treatment Panel III) final report. Circulation 106:3143, 2002.

HEART FAILURE (see also Chap. 24)

Exercise intolerance is a cardinal symptom of heart failure. In addition to myocardial dysfunction, other contributors to this syndrome include abnormalities in peripheral blood flow, skeletal muscle morphology, and metabolism. For many years, bed rest was a primary treatment for congestive heart failure. However, pioneering work from Duke in the late 1980s showed significant improvements in exercise capacity and associated physiological changes with progressive exercise. Since then, a profusion of mostly small, short-term trials has generally demonstrated benefits of exercise in a variety of aspects of heart failure domains. These include increased peak oxygen consumption, improvement in autonomic regulation of cardiovascular activity, improved endothelial function and skeletal muscle function, and favorable effects on ventilatory function as well as improvements in the ability to perform activities of daily living, anxiety, depression, and general well-being.[112] There is, however, no clear evidence yet that exercise therapy improves survival in patients with heart failure.

EXERCISE PRESCRIPTION FOR PATIENTS WITH HEART FAILURE. Guidelines from the Agency for Health Care Policy and Research[2] and from the American Heart Association[112] recommend exercise training for patients with stable heart failure. Because an exercise prescription specifically tailored for patients with heart failure has not yet been devised, it is prudent to use the American Heart Association's exercise standards for exercise testing and training for patients with cardiovascular disease[18] as a template for an individual prescription.

Among patients with advanced disease, exercise prescriptions based on heart rate may not be accurate, given their limited chronotropic reserve. Widespread use of beta blockers in this population also makes it impractical to use heart rate alone to measure exercise intensity. Instead, a peak Vo_2 of 70 to 80 percent may provide a better target for the intensity of exercise. For debilitated patients or those unused to aerobic activity, lower intensity activities (peak Vo_2 of 60 to 65 percent) with programmed periods of rest may be adequate. The duration of exercise should include an adequate warm-up period that may be longer (10 to 15 minutes) than for other cardiac rehabilitation patients. The warm-up period is followed by an exercise period of 20 to 30 minutes at the desired intensity and a cool-down period. Three to five times per week is the usual frequency for training. Resistance training can strengthen individual muscle groups. Guidelines from the American Association of Cardiovascular and Pulmonary Rehabilitation[27] call for direct monitoring and supervision at first, possibly followed by home training.

SAFETY OF REHABILITATION FOR PATIENTS WITH HEART FAILURE. No large-scale trials have focused specifically on the safety of exercise training for patients with heart failure. There is, however, little evidence that exercise worsens left ventricular function or increases the size of heart chambers. Data from the European Heart Failure Training Group confirm the beneficial effects of exercise rehabilitation on functional capacity.[113] In the randomized Exercise Rehabilitation Trial, 12 months of exercise training improved peak oxygen uptake and strength with no significant differences in total mortality, hospitalization for heart failure, or worsening of heart failure.[114] Contraindications for exercise among patients with heart failure are similar to those for patients with coronary artery disease (see Table 43–7).

REHABILITATION FOR CARDIAC TRANSPLANTATION PATIENTS

Candidates for heart transplantation are generally quite debilitated and deconditioned. Following transplantation, persistent heart failure, diminished aerobic capacity, muscle atrophy, and premature coronary atherosclerosis are common. Functional capacity during exercise testing is reduced to 50 percent in heart transplant recipients compared with age-matched healthy control subjects.[115] Case series and several small clinical studies[116-118] have demonstrated that exercise training has the potential for reversing or diminishing physiological abnormalities in heart transplant patients. Thus, training that includes both aerobic and resistance exercise is recommended before and after transplantation.[2,112,118]

Most studies of rehabilitation before or after heart transplantation have followed a standard cardiac rehabilitation model, with exercise sessions conducted three or four times per week from 8 to 12 weeks at moderate intensity. Improvements in aerobic capacity range from 20 to 50 percent. Resistance training offers an opportunity to increase lean muscle mass and bone density.[116]

Published studies to date do not address the progressive, diffuse atherosclerosis that tends to occur after heart transplantation, which is a common cause of late cardiac graft failure and patients' death (see Chaps. 26 and 35). Cardiac rehabilitation and secondary prevention interventions could delay or prevent progression of coronary artery disease in the transplanted heart. Coping with the ongoing medical consequences of heart transplantation presents a substantial challenge to patients. A multidisciplinary cardiac rehabilitation program that includes exercise, education, nutrition, and behavioral interventions is ideally suited to these patients.

REHABILITATION FOR PATIENTS WITH ARRHYTHMIAS

Patients with a variety of arrhythmias can benefit from cardiac rehabilitation. Indeed, exercise can potentially suppress some arrhythmias at rest, possibly because of exercise-induced vagal withdrawal and increased sympathetic stimulation.[18,119] However, exercise programs for these patients vary widely. At one end of the spectrum, those with nonsustained ventricular arrhythmias and normal myocardial function generally require only a few sessions of electrocardiogram-monitored exercise before graduating to a nonmonitored or home exercise program. At the other end, patients with an implantable cardioverter-defibrillator (ICD) related to prior ventricular fibrillation require a much longer period of electrocardiogram-monitored exercise. Unfortunately, exercise training for patients with arrhythmias has received little attention in the literature.

ATRIAL FIBRILLATION. Exercise improves exercise performance in patients with atrial fibrillation to the same extent that it does in those without it.[120] For patients with controlled ventricular rates during atrial fibrillation, the use of a target heart range during exercise is preferred to a specific heart rate. Uncontrolled ventricular rate during atrial fibrillation is a contraindication to exercise training because it can lead to hemodynamic instability.

PREMATURE VENTRICULAR COMPLEXES. Frequent premature ventricular complexes may decrease coronary perfusion, cardiac output, and blood pressure. These, in turn, can lead to ventricular arrhythmias. Thus, patients with frequent premature ventricular complexes should be closely monitored during exercise, and the appearance of exercise-induced arrhythmias should mandate reducing the intensity of exercise or stopping altogether.

PACEMAKER. For patients with pacemakers enrolled in a cardiac rehabilitation program, it is essential to identify the rhythm and conduction history for which the pacemaker has been implanted. Both the exercise prescription and its monitoring must be tailored to the characteristics of the device.

IMPLANTABLE CARDIOVERTER-DEFIBRILLATOR. Patients with an ICD are often physically or psychologically disabled by their disease or the possibility of a sudden ICD discharge, or both. Thus, an important part of cardiac rehabilitation involves allaying fears that activity or exercise will cause a discharge. Baseline exercise testing can help determine whether exercise provokes ventricular arrhythmias as well as establishes the upper limit of exercise (10 to 15 beats/min below the device trigger point). A slow progression from low to moderate exercise intensity may be necessary because of prior deconditioning and to avoid overshooting the target heart rate. Perceived exertion (the Borg scale; see Table 43-3) offers a good guide for increasing exercise intensity. Given these caveats, exercise-based cardiac rehabilitation can offer substantial benefits to patients with ICDs. In a 12-week study of comprehensive cardiac rehabilitation among 16 patients who had undergone implantation of an ICD, no ventricular arrhythmias or device discharges occurred during the exercise components of the program, exercise times increased by 16 percent, and anxiety and depression decreased significantly.[121]

Cardiac Rehabilitation for Elderly Patients (see also Chap. 72)

Given the high prevalence of CHD among those older than 65 years,[1] elderly persons represent a large proportion of potential candidates for cardiac rehabilitation. In addition to improving cardiovascular health and reducing risk factors for cardiovascular and other chronic diseases,[122] rehabilitation programs can enhance functional independence and overall well-being.[123] The benefits of cardiac rehabilitation do not appear to be age limited and are beneficial[124] and cost-effective[125] even in the ninth decade of life. As at other ages, a cardiac rehabilitation program under the direction of trained personnel is often the ideal setting for the provision of education, counseling, and behavioral and exercise interventions for elderly individuals.

In general, the exercise prescription described earlier is appropriate for older patients. However, because the exercise capacity of elderly people is usually lower than that of younger individuals (Table 43–11), activities that require lower levels of energy expenditure (40 to 50 percent of $\dot{V}O_{2max}$) are generally necessary, especially during the first weeks of a rehabilitation program. For individuals who require lower intensity activity, lengthening the duration of activity per session can increase caloric expenditure. Individuals for whom physical or psychosocial problems limit exercise duration may require more frequent episodes of exercise. Guidelines for other comprehensive secondary prevention efforts in elderly persons have been elaborated by the American Heart Association.[126]

Cardiac Rehabilitation for Patients with Diabetes (see also Chaps. 40 and 51)

Of the rapidly growing population of patients with diabetes, more than half exhibit hypertension, an atherogenic lipid profile, abdominal obesity, and endothelial dysfunction. Diabetes increases the risk of cardiovascular disease two- to fourfold,[127] and cardiovascular disease contributes to approximately 70 percent of deaths among individuals with diabetes.[128] The well-established beneficial effects of weight loss and exercise on insulin resistance and the other metabolic disorders associated with diabetes make this population particularly well suited for a comprehensive cardiac rehabilitation program.

Data from cohort studies involving diabetic men[35] and women[129] have demonstrated 35 to 45 percent reductions in risk of cardiovascular disease and mortality with walking and other forms of physical activity. In the Steno-2 study, conducted among 160 patients with type 2 diabetes and microalbuminuria, random assignment to a targeted, multifactorial, risk factor reduction intervention reduced the risk of cardiovascular disease by 53 percent and the risk of microvascular complications such as nephropathy, retinopathy, and autonomic neuropathy by approximately 60 percent after 8 years compared with standard care.[130]

Exercise Prescription and Precautions

Although the balance of benefits and risks of exercise-based cardiac rehabilitation is quite favorable for most patients with diabetes, some precautions are warranted. Given the potential complications of poor glycemic control, peripheral and autonomic neuropathy, and diabetic retinopathy, exercise prescriptions must be individualized. Detailed guidelines for exercise testing and training are available from the American College of Sports Medicine[131] and the American Diabetes Association.[132] In general, the exercise prescription for individuals with uncomplicated diabetes calls for 30 to 45

TABLE 43–11 Age-Associated Changes in Physiological Response to Aerobic Exercise

Reduced aerobic capacity—a decline in maximum oxygen consumption of 8-10%/yr in nontrained populations
Reduced maximum heart rate of 1 beat/min/yr
More rapid increase in systolic blood pressure with exercise
Attenuated elevation in left ventricular ejection fraction

minutes of aerobic exercise three or four times per week and resistance training one or two times per week, with appropriate warm-up and cool-down periods. The intensity of aerobic exercise is generally set at 55 to 80 percent of maximum heart rate for patients with multiple risk factors, autonomic neuropathy, or no exercise testing and at 50 to 60 percent of maximum heart rate for patients with a low initial level of fitness.

Contraindications to exercise based on glycemic control exist for type 1 diabetes,[132] but guidelines for type 2 diabetes are less definitive. Among more than 550 individuals with type 2 diabetes not requiring insulin and with baseline glucose levels ranging from 60 to 400 mg/dl (3.3 to 22.2 mmol/liter) monitored for 24 hours after exercise, no episodes of ketosis or hypoglycemia were observed and the occurrence of hypoglycemia was 2 percent.[133] Thus, patients with type 2 diabetes who do not require insulin may not need routine blood glucose testing while exercising. Supplementary food is generally not necessary unless exercise is exceptionally vigorous or long. Recurrent episodes of hypoglycemia should lead to downward adjustment of preexercise medications or ingestion of carbohydrate before exercise. Evening exercise sessions can occasionally induce early morning hypoglycemia and thus necessitate a bedtime snack or a change in the timing of exercise sessions. Emergency equipment, including glucose tablets or gels and glucagon injection kits, should be readily available to treat hypoglycemic episodes.

Screening for sensory deficits, cutaneous lesions, ingrown toenails, or foot deformities is an important part of intake evaluation for exercise rehabilitation programs. Such patients should be encouraged to examine their feet before and after exercise and to wear proper footwear, with orthotics when necessary. Many patients with autonomic neuropathy have decreased maximum heart rates and resting tachycardia; thus, targets for exercise should be based on perceived exertion rather than heart rate. Swimming, bicycling, rowing, and arm or chair calisthenics may be appropriate for patients with severe neuropathy.[131,132]

Patients with active proliferative diabetic retinopathy, as well as those with moderate or severe nonproliferative diabetic retinopathy, should avoid exercise that involves straining because of concern about vitreous hemorrhage or traction retinal detachment retinopathy.[134] Patients with nonproliferative retinopathy can engage in most forms of exercise with minimal risk of progressive disease.[131,132,135]

Cardiac Rehabilitation for Obese Patients

Mirroring trends in the general population, the majority of candidates for cardiac rehabilitation are overweight or obese. In one survey of 449 consecutive cardiac rehabilitation patients, 88 percent were overweight or obese.[136]

Most controlled exercise training studies among overweight or obese patients show modest improvements in weight (2 to 3 kg), body mass index, and percentage of body fat.[137] Adding a behavioral intervention and increasing the caloric expenditure can significantly increase weight loss.[138,139]

The exercise prescription for most overweight or obese patients should be much like that for other cardiac rehabilitation patients (see Table 43–6). Low-impact exercises, such as brisk walking or cycle ergometry, may be performed with greater duration and frequency and less intensity.

Cardiac Rehabilitation for Patients with Chronic Obstructive Pulmonary Disease

Patients with chronic obstructive pulmonary disease who have suffered a cardiac event or have been diagnosed with cardiovascular disease can generally take part in and benefit from a standard cardiac rehabilitation program. Patients with resting or exercise-induced hypoxia (oxygen saturation < 88 percent) should receive continuous supplemental oxygen during exercise training. Close monitoring generally precludes the use of a home-based program.

CARDIAC REHABILITATION FOR PATIENTS WITH END-STAGE RENAL DISEASE (see also Chap. 86)

Cardiovascular disease is the leading cause of morbidity and mortality in patients with end-stage renal disease, accounting for more than half of deaths.[140] The benefits of exercise training among renal disease patients with cardiovascular disease should be similar to those derived by the cardiac rehabilitation population at large, but such programs are underused in this high-risk cohort. Because of possible limitations in exercise capacity, careful selection of rehabilitation candidates and appropriate medical supervision are important.

As a result of age, poor nutrition, deconditioning, and advanced cardiovascular disease, many patients with end-stage renal disease have reduced exercise capacity. Exercising to target heart rates 50 to 70 percent of those achieved on exercise tests may lead to improvements in exercise capacity and symptoms similar to those attained by individuals able to exercise at higher intensities.[2] Given that ventricular arrhythmias are common among patients with end-stage renal disease undergoing hemodialysis and last for several hours afterward,[141] it is prudent to schedule exercise training sessions and hemodialysis on alternate days.

Cost-Effectiveness of Cardiac Rehabilitation

In the current era of cost containment, cost-effectiveness has become an important element in determining which primary and secondary prevention therapies to pursue. Interventions are generally compared using the quality-adjusted life-year (QALY) or disability-adjusted life-year (DALY). Interventions with an incremental cost-effectiveness ratio under $20,000 per QALY are generally considered to be quite favorable (see Chap. 2).

A cost-effectiveness analysis suggests that cardiac rehabilitation improves life expectancy by 0.2 years at a cost below $5000 per life-year saved.[142] It is more cost effective than many other post-myocardial infarction treatment interventions (Table 43–12).

Modified protocols may be even more cost-effective. Carlson and colleagues randomly assigned 80 low- to moderate-risk cardiac patients to a traditional cardiac rehabilitation program or a modified program for 6 months. The traditional program included three supervised exercise sessions per week with an ECG monitor for the first 3 months as well as one-on-one education about risk factors. The modified program discontinued ECG monitoring after the first month and gradually moved patients to an off-site exercise regimen supplemented with educational support and telephone follow-up. Patients in the modified program had

TABLE 43–12 Comparative Cost-Effectiveness of Treatments for Coronary Heart Disease

Intervention	Cost-Effectiveness ($/LYS)
Cardiac rehabilitation versus usual care	$2130-4950
Smoking cessation	$220-728
Statin therapy	
Secondary prevention	$9630
Primary prevention	$17,000-38,000
Coronary artery bypass grafting versus medical care	$8500-114,000

LYS = life-year saved.
From Ades PA, Pashkow FJ, Nestor JR: Cost-effectiveness of cardiac rehabilitation after myocardial infarction. J Cardiopulm Rehabil 17:222, 1997.

higher rates of off-site exercise over 6 months and total exercise during the final 3 months; other measures, such as lipid levels and maximal oxygen uptake, were the same in both groups. The modified protocol cost $830 less per patient ($1519 versus $2349) and required 30 percent less staff (full-time equivalents) than the traditional protocol.[17]

The number needed to treat (NNT) is an estimate of the number of patients who must be treated to achieve an additional favorable outcome or prevent an additional adverse outcome. Oldridge and colleagues determined the NNT for mortality in three meta-analyses of cardiac rehabilitation trials as 32, 46, and 72.[143] The result compares favorably with the NNT for other common secondary prevention interventions such as aspirin (67)[144] and beta blockers (42).[145] Among patients with stable chronic heart failure, Georgiou and colleagues determined that long-term exercise therapy increased life expectancy by 1.82 years over a 15.5-year period at a cost of $1773 per life-year saved.[146]

Disease Management

As cardiac rehabilitation has evolved from specifically phased programs (I to IV) to more complex multidisciplinary programs that respond to patients' needs after a cardiac event or procedure (in hospital) or after the onset of angina, newer models for the delivery of comprehensive secondary prevention services have appeared.

Case management models for cardiac rehabilitation have been successfully utilized and have demonstrated improved risk factor[16,84] and clinical[147] outcomes. In these models, a case manager (usually a cardiac nurse or exercise physiologist) develops an individualized program that optimizes preventive management across the individual's spectrum of risk factors and behaviors. For those at lower risk, such programs can be carried out remotely, facilitated by telephone or computer-based systems. These programs also allow continued surveillance of prevention issues beyond the duration of customary cardiac rehabilitation programs, often at relatively low cost. Alternatively, many traditional cardiac rehabilitation programs have added a "maintenance" phase to allow patients to continue cardiac rehabilitation at a lower level of supervision following completion of a formal program. Unfortunately, reimbursement is not generally available for such programs.

Case management and newer cardiac rehabilitation models overlap with health care delivery strategies, commonly referred to as "disease management." Disease management programs have arisen from both academia and the largely for-profit disease management industry. Because the latter has often focused on programs that provide a clear and early return on investment, they tend to enroll higher risk individuals (e.g., patients with heart failure). Nevertheless, secondary prevention disease management programs are being tested and utilized. As the health care information technology infrastructure improves, such programs are likely to be integrated into the delivery of comprehensive cardiac rehabilitation. Unfortunately, reimbursement for cardiac rehabilitation remains one of the key barriers to more complete delivery of this crucial service.

Acknowledgment

The author gratefully acknowledges the superb and expert editorial collaboration by Patrick J. Skerrett.

REFERENCES

1. American Heart Association: Heart Disease and Stroke Statistics—2003 Update. Dallas, American Heart Association, 2003.
2. Agency for Health Care Policy and Research: Cardiac Rehabilitation: Clinical Practice Guideline No. 17 (AHCPR Publication No. 96-0672). Bethesda, Md, National Heart, Lung, and Blood Institute, 1995.
3. Evenson KR, Rosamond WD, Luepker RV: Predictors of outpatient cardiac rehabilitation utilization: The Minnesota Heart Surgery Registry. J Cardiopulm Rehabil 18:192, 1998.
4. Pasquali SK, Alexander KP, Lytle BL, et al: Testing an intervention to increase cardiac rehabilitation enrollment after coronary artery bypass grafting. Am J Cardiol 88:1415, A6, 2001.

History of Cardiac Rehabilitation

5. Hippocrates: The Genuine Works of Hippocrates. Huntington, NY, RE Krieger, 1972.
6. Herrick JB: Clinical features of sudden obstruction of the coronary arteries. JAMA 59:2015, 1912.
7. Lewis T: Diseases of the Heart. New York, Macmillan, 1933.
8. White PD, Rusk HA, Lee PR, Williams B: Rehabilitation of the Cardiovascular Patient. New York, McGraw-Hill, 1958.
9. Levine SA: Some harmful effects of recumbency in the treatment of heart disease. JAMA 126:80, 1944.
10. Levine SA, Lown B: The "chair" treatment of acute coronary thrombosis. Trans Assoc Am Physicians 64:316, 1951.
11. Saltin B, Blomqvist G, Mitchell JH, et al: Response to exercise after bed rest and after training. Circulation 38:VII1-78, 1968.
12. Wenger NK, Hellerstein HK, Blackburn H, Castranova SJ: Uncomplicated myocardial infarction. Current physician practice in patient management. JAMA 224:511, 1973.
13. Wenger NK, Gilbert C, Skoropa M: Cardiac conditioning after myocardial infarction. An early intervention program. J Card Rehabil 2:17, 1971.
14. World Health Organization: Rehabilitation of Patients with Cardiovascular Disease (Technical Report Series No. 270). Geneva, World Health Organization, 1964.

Contemporary Cardiac Rehabilitation

15. Arthur HM, Smith KM, Kodis J, McKelvie R: A controlled trial of hospital versus home-based exercise in cardiac patients. Med Sci Sports Exerc 34:1544, 2002.
16. Gordon NF, English CD, Contractor AS, et al: Effectiveness of three models for comprehensive cardiovascular disease risk reduction. Am J Cardiol 89:1263, 2002.
17. Carlson JJ, Johnson JA, Franklin BA, VanderLaan RL: Program participation, exercise adherence, cardiovascular outcomes, and program cost of traditional versus modified cardiac rehabilitation. Am J Cardiol 86:17, 2000.

Evidence Base for Cardiac Rehabilitation

18. Fletcher GF, Balady GJ, Amsterdam EA, et al: Exercise standards for testing and training: A statement for healthcare professionals from the American Heart Association. Circulation 104:1694, 2001.
19. Oldridge NB, Guyatt GH, Fischer ME, Rimm AA: Cardiac rehabilitation after myocardial infarction. Combined experience of randomized clinical trials. JAMA 260:945, 1988.
20. O'Connor GT, Buring JE, Yusuf S, et al: An overview of randomized trials of rehabilitation with exercise after myocardial infarction. Circulation 80:234, 1989.
21. Dorn J, Naughton J, Imamura D, Trevisan M: Results of a multicenter randomized clinical trial of exercise and long-term survival in myocardial infarction patients: The National Exercise and Heart Disease Project (NEHDP). Circulation 100:1764, 1999.
22. Jolliffe JA, Rees K, Taylor RS, et al: Exercise-based rehabilitation for coronary heart disease. Cochrane Database Syst Rev, 2003.
23. Chobanian AV, Bakris GL, Black HR, et al: The Seventh Report of the Joint National Committee on Prevention, Detection, Evaluation, and Treatment of High Blood Pressure: The JNC 7 report. JAMA 289:2560, 2003.
24. Gould AL, Rossouw JE, Santanello NC, et al: Cholesterol reduction yields clinical benefit: Impact of statin trials. Circulation 97:946, 1998.
25. Obesity Education Initiative: Clinical guidelines on the identification, evaluation, and treatment of overweight and obesity in adults. National Institutes of Health, National Heart, Lung, and Blood Institute, 1998. (http://www.nhlbi.nih.gov/guidelines/obesity/ob_gdlns.htm)
26. Detry JR, Vierendeel IA, Vanbutsele RJ, Robert AR: Early short-term intensive cardiac rehabilitation induces positive results as long as one year after the acute coronary event: A prospective one-year controlled study. J Cardiovasc Risk 8:355, 2001.

Components of a Cardiac Rehabilitation Program

27. American Association of Cardiovascular and Pulmonary Rehabilitation: Guidelines for Cardiac Rehabilitation and Secondary Prevention Programs. 3rd ed. Champaign, Ill, Human Kinetics, 1999.
28. Blair SN: Evidence for success of exercise in weight loss and control. Ann Intern Med 119:702, 1993.
29. Anderson JW, Konz EC, Frederich RC, Wood CL: Long-term weight-loss maintenance: A meta-analysis of US studies. Am J Clin Nutr 74:579, 2001.
30. Brochu M, Poehlman ET, Ades PA: Obesity, body fat distribution, and coronary artery disease. J Cardiopulm Rehabil 20:96, 2000.
31. Whelton SP, Chin A, Xin X, He J: Effect of aerobic exercise on blood pressure: A meta-analysis of randomized, controlled trials. Ann Intern Med 136:493, 2002.
32. Henriksen EJ: Effects of acute exercise and exercise training on insulin resistance. J Appl Physiol 93:788, 2002.
33. Hu FB, Sigal RJ, Rich-Edwards JW, et al: Walking compared with vigorous physical activity and risk of type 2 diabetes in women: A prospective study. JAMA 282:1433, 1999.
34. Gregg EW, Gerzoff RB, Caspersen CJ, et al: Relationship of walking to mortality among US adults with diabetes. Arch Intern Med 163:1440, 2003.
35. Tanasescu M, Leitzmann MF, Rimm EB, Hu FB: Physical activity in relation to cardiovascular disease and total mortality among men with type 2 diabetes. Circulation 107:2435, 2003.
36. Knowler WC, Barrett-Connor E, Fowler SE, et al: Reduction in the incidence of type 2 diabetes with lifestyle intervention or metformin. N Engl J Med 346:393, 2002.
37. Leon AS, Sanchez OA: Response of blood lipids to exercise training alone or combined with dietary intervention. Med Sci Sports Exerc 33:S502; discussion S528, 2001.

38. Couillard C, Despres JP, Lamarche B, et al: Effects of endurance exercise training on plasma HDL cholesterol levels depend on levels of triglycerides: Evidence from men of the Health, Risk Factors, Exercise Training and Genetics (HERITAGE) Family Study. Arterioscler Thromb Vasc Biol 21:1226, 2001.
39. Kraus WE, Houmard JA, Duscha BD, et al: Effects of the amount and intensity of exercise on plasma lipoproteins. N Engl J Med 347:1483, 2002.
40. Bernstein MS, Costanza MC, James RW, et al: Physical activity may modulate effects of ApoE genotype on lipid profile. Arterioscler Thromb Vasc Biol 22:133, 2002.
41. Wannamethee SG, Lowe GD, Whincup PH, et al: Physical activity and hemostatic and inflammatory variables in elderly men. Circulation 105:1785, 2002.
42. Smith DT, Hoetzer GL, Greiner JJ, et al: Effects of ageing and regular aerobic exercise on endothelial fibrinolytic capacity in humans. J Physiol (Lond) 546:289, 2003.
43. Hambrecht R, Wolf A, Gielen S, et al: Effect of exercise on coronary endothelial function in patients with coronary artery disease. N Engl J Med 342:454, 2000.
44. Gokce N, Vita JA, Bader DS, et al: Effect of exercise on upper and lower extremity endothelial function in patients with coronary artery disease. Am J Cardiol 90:124, 2002.
45. Brendle DC, Joseph LJ, Corretti MC, et al: Effects of exercise rehabilitation on endothelial reactivity in older patients with peripheral arterial disease. Am J Cardiol 87:324, 2001.
46. Linke A, Schoene N, Gielen S, et al: Endothelial dysfunction in patients with chronic heart failure: Systemic effects of lower-limb exercise training. J Am Coll Cardiol 37:392, 2001.
47. Maiorana A, O'Driscoll G, Cheetham C, et al: The effect of combined aerobic and resistance exercise training on vascular function in type 2 diabetes. J Am Coll Cardiol 38:860, 2001.
48. Curtis BM, O'Keefe JH Jr: Autonomic tone as a cardiovascular risk factor: The dangers of chronic fight or flight. Mayo Clin Proc 77:45, 2002.
49. Dekker JM, Crow RS, Folsom AR, et al: Low heart rate variability in a 2-minute rhythm strip predicts risk of coronary heart disease and mortality from several causes: The ARIC Study. Atherosclerosis Risk In Communities. Circulation 102:1239, 2000.
50. Stein PK, Ehsani AA, Domitrovich PP, et al: Effect of exercise training on heart rate variability in healthy older adults. Am Heart J 138:567, 1999.
51. Iellamo F, Legramante JM, Massaro M, et al: Effects of a residential exercise training on baroreflex sensitivity and heart rate variability in patients with coronary artery disease: A randomized, controlled study. Circulation 102:2588, 2000.
52. Lee I-M, Skerrett PJ: Physical activity and all-cause mortality—What is the dose-response relation? Med Sci Sports Exerc 33(6 Suppl):S459, 2001.
53. Myers J, Prakash M, Froelicher V, et al: Exercise capacity and mortality among men referred for exercise testing. N Engl J Med 346:793, 2002.
54. Belardinelli R, Paolini I, Cianci G, et al: Exercise training intervention after coronary angioplasty: The ETICA trial. J Am Coll Cardiol 37:1891, 2001.
55. Rodgers GP, Ayanian JZ, Balady G, et al: American College of Cardiology/American Heart Association Clinical Competence Statement on Stress Testing. A Report of the American College of Cardiology/American Heart Association/American College of Physicians–American Society of Internal Medicine Task Force on Clinical Competence. Circulation 102:1726, 2000.
56. Blair SN, Kampert JB, Kohl HW 3rd, et al: Influences of cardiorespiratory fitness and other precursors on cardiovascular disease and all-cause mortality in men and women. JAMA 276:205, 1996.
57. American College of Sports Medicine Position Stand. The recommended quantity and quality of exercise for developing and maintaining cardiorespiratory and muscular fitness, and flexibility in healthy adults. Med Sci Sports Exerc 30:975, 1998.
58. Ades PA: Cardiac rehabilitation and secondary prevention of coronary heart disease. N Engl J Med 345:892, 2001.
59. Smith SC J., Blair SN, Bonow RO, et al: AHA/ACC guidelines for preventing heart attack and death in patients with atherosclerotic cardiovascular disease: 2001 update. J Am Coll Cardiol 38:1581, 2001.
60. Pollock ML, Franklin BA, Balady GJ, et al: AHA Science Advisory. Resistance exercise in individuals with and without cardiovascular disease: Benefits, rationale, safety, and prescription: An advisory from the Committee on Exercise, Rehabilitation, and Prevention, Council on Clinical Cardiology, American Heart Association; Position paper endorsed by the American College of Sports Medicine. Circulation 101:828, 2000.
61. Shaw DK, Sparks KE, Jennings HS 3rd: Transtelephonic exercise monitoring: A review. J Cardiopulm Rehabil 18:263, 1998.
62. Franklin BA, Bonzheim K, Gordon S, Timmis GC: Safety of medically supervised outpatient cardiac rehabilitation exercise therapy: A 16-year follow-up. Chest 114:902, 1998.
63. Hu FB, Willett WC: Optimal diets for prevention of coronary heart disease. JAMA 288:2569, 2002.
64. Burr ML, Fehily AM, Gilbert JF, et al: Effects of changes in fat, fish, and fibre intakes on death and myocardial reinfarction: Diet and reinfarction trial (DART). Lancet 2:757, 1989.
65. Singh RB, Rastogi SS, Verma R, et al: Randomised controlled trial of cardioprotective diet in patients with recent acute myocardial infarction: Results of one year follow up. BMJ 304:1015, 1992.
66. Singh RB, Dubnov G, Niaz MA, et al: Effect of an Indo-Mediterranean diet on progression of coronary artery disease in high risk patients (Indo-Mediterranean Diet Heart Study): A randomised single-blind trial. Lancet 360:1455, 2002.
67. Ornish D, Scherwitz LW, Billings JH, et al: Intensive lifestyle changes for reversal of coronary heart disease. JAMA 280:2001, 1998.
68. de Lorgeril M, Salen P, Martin JL, et al: Mediterranean diet, traditional risk factors, and the rate of cardiovascular complications after myocardial infarction: Final report of the Lyon Diet Heart Study. Circulation 99:779, 1999.
69. Ware JH: Interpreting incomplete data in studies of diet and weight loss. N Engl J Med 348:2136, 2003.
70. Wing RR, Hill JO: Successful weight loss maintenance. Annu Rev Nutr 21:323, 2001.
71. National Cholesterol Education Program (NCEP) Expert Panel on Detection, Evaluation, and Treatment of High Blood Cholesterol in Adults (Adult Treatment Panel III): Third Report of the National Cholesterol Education Program (NCEP) Expert Panel on Detection, Evaluation, and Treatment of High Blood Cholesterol in Adults (Adult Treatment Panel III) final report. Circulation 106:3143, 2002.
72. Sacks FM, Svetkey LP, Vollmer WM, et al: Effects on blood pressure of reduced dietary sodium and the Dietary Approaches to Stop Hypertension (DASH) diet. DASH-Sodium Collaborative Research Group. N Engl J Med 344:3, 2001.
73. Leaf A, Kang JX, Xiao YF, Billman GE: Clinical prevention of sudden cardiac death by n-3 polyunsaturated fatty acids and mechanism of prevention of arrhythmias by n-3 fish oils. Circulation 107:2646, 2003.
74. Annual smoking-attributable mortality, years of potential life lost, and economic costs—United States, 1995-1999. MMWR Morb Mortal Wkly Rep 51:300, 2002.
75. Benowitz NL, Gourlay SG: Cardiovascular toxicity of nicotine: Implications for nicotine replacement therapy. J Am Coll Cardiol 29:1422, 1997.
76. Fisher SD, Zareba W, Moss AJ, et al: Effect of smoking on lipid and thrombogenic factors two months after acute myocardial infarction. Am J Cardiol 86:813, 2000.
77. Craig WY, Palomaki GE, Haddow JE: Cigarette smoking and serum lipid and lipoprotein concentrations: An analysis of published data. BMJ 298:784, 1989.
78. Sheps DS, Herbst MC, Hinderliter AL, et al.: Production of arrhythmias by elevated carboxyhemoglobin in patients with coronary artery disease. Ann Intern Med 113:343, 1990.
79. Neunteufl T, Heher S, Kostner K, et al: Contribution of nicotine to acute endothelial dysfunction in long-term smokers. J Am Coll Cardiol 39:251, 2002.
80. Winkelmann BR, Boehm BO, Nauck M, et al: Cigarette smoking is independently associated with markers of endothelial dysfunction and hyperinsulinaemia in nondiabetic individuals with coronary artery disease. Curr Med Res Opin 17:132, 2001.
81. Howard G, Wagenknecht LE, Burke GL, et al: Cigarette smoking and progression of atherosclerosis: The Atherosclerosis Risk in Communities (ARIC) Study. JAMA 279:119, 1998.
82. Critchley JA, Capewell S: Mortality risk reduction associated with smoking cessation in patients with coronary heart disease: A systematic review. JAMA 290:86, 2003.
83. van Domburg RT, Meeter K, van Berkel DF, et al: Smoking cessation reduces mortality after coronary artery bypass surgery: A 20-year follow-up study. J Am Coll Cardiol 36:878, 2000.
84. DeBusk RF, Miller NH, Superko HR, et al.: A case-management system for coronary risk factor modification after acute myocardial infarction. Ann Intern Med 120:721, 1994.
85. A clinical practice guideline for treating tobacco use and dependence: A US Public Health Service report. The Tobacco Use and Dependence Clinical Practice Guideline Panel, Staff, and Consortium Representatives. JAMA 283:3244, 2000.
86. Joseph AM, Fu SS: Safety issues in pharmacotherapy for smoking in patients with cardiovascular disease. Prog Cardiovasc Dis 45:429, 2003.
87. Fiore MC, Bailey WC, Cohen SJ, et al: Treating tobacco use and dependence: Clinical practice guideline. Rockville, Md, U.S. Department of Health and Human Services, Public Health Service, 2000.
88. Hevey D, Slack K, Cahill A, et al: Rates of smoking in the households of cardiac patients. J Cardiovasc Risk 9:271, 2002.
89. Berkman LF, Blumenthal J, Burg M, et al, Enhancing Recovery in Coronary Heart Disease Patients Investigators (ENRICHD): Effects of treating depression and low perceived social support on clinical events after myocardial infarction: The Enhancing Recovery in Coronary Heart Disease Patients (ENRICHD) Randomized Trial. JAMA 289:3106, 2003.
90. Berkman LF, Leo-Summers L, Horwitz RI: Emotional support and survival after myocardial infarction. A prospective, population-based study of the elderly. Ann Intern Med 117:1003, 1992.
91. Frasure-Smith N, Lesperance F, Gravel G, et al: Social support, depression, and mortality during the first year after myocardial infarction. Circulation 101:1919, 2000.
92. Frasure-Smith N, Lesperance F: Depression and other psychological risks following myocardial infarction. Arch Gen Psychiatry 60:627, 2003.
93. Lesperance F, Frasure-Smith N, Talajic M, Bourassa MG: Five-year risk of cardiac mortality in relation to initial severity and one-year changes in depression symptoms after myocardial infarction. Circulation 105:1049, 2002.
94. Bush DE, Ziegelstein RC, Tayback M, et al: Even minimal symptoms of depression increase mortality risk after acute myocardial infarction. Am J Cardiol 88:337, 2001.
95. DiMatteo MR, Lepper HS, Croghan TW: Depression is a risk factor for noncompliance with medical treatment: Meta-analysis of the effects of anxiety and depression on patient adherence. Arch Intern Med 160:2101, 2000.
96. Stein PK, Carney RM, Freedland KE, et al: Severe depression is associated with markedly reduced heart rate variability in patients with stable coronary heart disease. J Psychosom Res 48:493, 2000.
97. Markovitz JH, Shuster JL, Chitwood WS, et al: Platelet activation in depression and effects of sertraline treatment: An open-label study. Am J Psychiatry 157:1006, 2000.
98. Rozanski A, Blumenthal JA, Kaplan J: Impact of psychological factors on the pathogenesis of cardiovascular disease and implications for therapy. Circulation 99:2192, 1999.
99. Linden W, Stossel C, Maurice J: Psychosocial interventions for patients with coronary artery disease: A meta-analysis. Arch Intern Med 156:745, 1996.
100. Dusseldorp E, van Elderen T, Maes S, et al: A meta-analysis of psychoeducational programs for coronary heart disease patients. Health Psychol 18:506, 1999.
101. Denollet J, Brutsaert DL: Reducing emotional distress improves prognosis in coronary heart disease: 9-year mortality in a clinical trial of rehabilitation. Circulation 104:2018, 2001.
102. Glassman AH, O'Connor CM, Califf RM, et al: Sertraline treatment of major depression in patients with acute MI or unstable angina. JAMA 288:701, 2002.
103. Burnett RE, Blumenthal JA: Biobehavioral aspects of coronary artery disease: Considerations for prognosis and treatment. *In* Pollock ML, Schmidt DH (eds): Heart Disease and Rehabilitation. 3rd ed. Champaign, Ill, Human Kinetics, 1995, pp 41-55.

104. Hansen M, Streff MM: Patient education: Practical guidelines. *In* Pollock ML, Schmidt DH (eds): Heart Disease and Rehabilitation. 3rd ed. Champaign, Ill, Human Kinetics, 1995, pp 277-286.
105. Bandura A: Social Learning Theory. Englewood Cliffs, NJ, Prentice Hall, 1977.
106. Prochaska JO, DiClemente CC: Stages of change in the modification of problem behaviors. Prog Behav Modif 28:183, 1992.
107. Falk RH: The cardiovascular response to sexual activity: Do we know enough? Clin Cardiol 24:271, 2001.
108. DeBusk R, Drory Y, Goldstein I, et al: Management of sexual dysfunction in patients with cardiovascular disease: Recommendations of The Princeton Consensus Panel. Am J Cardiol 86:175, 2000.
109. Jackevicius CA, Mamdani M, Tu JV: Adherence with statin therapy in elderly patients with and without acute coronary syndromes. JAMA 288:462, 2002.
110. Daly J, Sindone AP, Thompson DR, et al: Barriers to participation in and adherence to cardiac rehabilitation programs: A critical literature review. Prog Cardiovasc Nurs 17:8, 2002.
111. Ades PA, Balady GJ, Berra K: Transforming exercise-based cardiac rehabilitation programs into secondary prevention centers: A national imperative. J Cardiopulm Rehabil 21:263, 2001.

Rehabilitation for Other Populations

112. Pina IL, Apstein CS, Balady GJ, et al: Exercise and heart failure: A statement from the American Heart Association Committee on exercise, rehabilitation, and prevention. Circulation 107:1210, 2003.
113. Experience from controlled trials of physical training in chronic heart failure. Protocol and patient factors in effectiveness in the improvement in exercise tolerance. European Heart Failure Training Group. Eur Heart J 19:466, 1998.
114. McKelvie RS, Teo KK, Roberts R, et al: Effects of exercise training in patients with heart failure: The Exercise Rehabilitation Trial (EXERT). Am Heart J 144:23, 2002.
115. Keteyian S, Shepard R, Ehrman J, et al: Cardiovascular responses of heart transplant patients to exercise training. J Appl Physiol 70:2627, 1991.
116. Braith RW, Welsch MA, Mills RM Jr, et al: Resistance exercise prevents glucocorticoid-induced myopathy in heart transplant recipients. Med Sci Sports Exerc 30:483, 1998.
117. Kavanagh T, Mertens DJ, Shephard RJ, et al: Long-term cardiorespiratory results of exercise training following cardiac transplantation. Am J Cardiol 91:190, 2003.
118. Kobashigawa JA, Leaf DA, Lee N, et al: A controlled trial of exercise rehabilitation after heart transplantation. N Engl J Med 340:272, 1999.
119. Billman GE: Aerobic exercise conditioning: A nonpharmacological antiarrhythmic intervention. J Appl Physiol 92:446, 2002.
120. Vanhees L, Schepers D, Defoor J, et al: Exercise performance and training in cardiac patients with atrial fibrillation. J Cardiopulm Rehabil 20:346, 2000.
121. Fitchet A, Doherty PJ, Bundy C, et al: Comprehensive cardiac rehabilitation programme for implantable cardioverter-defibrillator patients: A randomised controlled trial. Heart 89:155, 2003.
122. Marchionni N, Fattirolli F, Fumagalli S, et al: Improved exercise tolerance and quality of life with cardiac rehabilitation of older patients after myocardial infarction: Results of a randomized, controlled trial. Circulation 107:2201, 2003.
123. Richardson LA, Buckenmeyer PJ, Bauman BD, et al: Contemporary cardiac rehabilitation: Patient characteristics and temporal trends over the past decade. J Cardiopulm Rehabil 20:57, 2000.
124. Vonder Muhll I, Daub B, Black B, et al: Benefits of cardiac rehabilitation in the ninth decade of life in patients with coronary heart disease. Am J Cardiol 90:645, 2002.
125. Paniagua D, Lopez-Jimenez F, Londono JC, et al: Outcome and cost-effectiveness of cardiopulmonary resuscitation after in-hospital cardiac arrest in octogenarians. Cardiology 97:6, 2002.
126. Williams MA, Fleg JL, Ades PA, et al: Secondary prevention of coronary heart disease in the elderly (with emphasis on patients > or = 75 years of age): An American Heart Association scientific statement from the Council on Clinical Cardiology Subcommittee on Exercise, Cardiac Rehabilitation, and Prevention. Circulation 105:1735, 2002.
127. Marks JB, Raskin P: Cardiovascular risk in diabetes: A brief review. J Diabetes Complications 14:108, 2000.
128. 1102Gu K, Cowie CC, Harris MI: Mortality in adults with and without diabetes in a national cohort of the U.S. population, 1971-1993. Diabetes Care 21:1138, 1998.
129. Hu FB, Stampfer MJ, Solomon C, et al: Physical activity and risk for cardiovascular events in diabetic women. Ann Intern Med 134:96, 2001.
130. Gaede P, Vedel P, Larsen N, et al: Multifactorial intervention and cardiovascular disease in patients with type 2 diabetes. N Engl J Med 348:383, 2003.
131. Albright A, Franz M, Hornsby G, et al: American College of Sports Medicine position stand. Exercise and type 2 diabetes. Med Sci Sports Exerc 32:1345, 2000.
132. Ruderman N, Devlin JT, Schneider S, Kriska A: Handbook of Exercise in Diabetes. 2nd ed. Alexandria, Va, American Diabetes Association, 2002.
133. Badenhop DT, Dunn CB, Eldridge S: Monitoring and management of cardiac rehabilitation patients with type 2 diabetes. Clin Exerc Physiol 3:71, 2001.
134. Aiello LP, Wong J, Cavallerano JD, et al: Retinopathy. *In* Ruderman N, Devlin JT, Schneider S, Kriska A (eds): Handbook of Exercise in Diabetes. 2nd ed. Alexandria, Va, American Diabetes Association, 2002, pp 401-413.
135. Rauramaa R, Salonen JT, Seppanen K, et al: Inhibition of platelet aggregability by moderate-intensity physical exercise: A randomized clinical trial in overweight men. Circulation 74:939, 1986.
136. Bader DS, Maguire TE, Spahn CM, et al: Clinical profile and outcomes of obese patients in cardiac rehabilitation stratified according to National Heart, Lung, and Blood Institute criteria. J Cardiopulm Rehabil 21:210, 2001.
137. Lavie CJ, Milani RV: Benefits of cardiac rehabilitation and exercise training. Chest 117:5, 2000.
138. Savage PD, Brochu M, Poehlman ET, Ades PA: Reduction in obesity and coronary risk factors after high caloric exercise training in overweight coronary patients. Am Heart J 146:317, 2003.
139. Savage PD, Lee M, Harvey-Berino J, et al: Weight reduction in the cardiac rehabilitation setting. J Cardiopulm Rehabil 22:154, 2002.
140. Collins AJ: Cardiovascular mortality in end-stage renal disease. Am J Med Sci 325:163, 2003.
141. Meier P, Vogt P, Blanc E: Ventricular arrhythmias and sudden cardiac death in end-stage renal disease patients on chronic hemodialysis. Nephron 87:199, 2001.

Cost Effectiveness of Cardiac Rehabilitation

142. Ades PA, Pashkow FJ, Nestor JR: Cost-effectiveness of cardiac rehabilitation after myocardial infarction. J Cardiopulm Rehabil 17:222, 1997.
143. Oldridge N, Perkins A, Marchionni N, et al: Number needed to treat in cardiac rehabilitation. J Cardiopulm Rehabil 22:22, 2002.
144. Weisman SM, Graham DY: Evaluation of the benefits and risks of low-dose aspirin in the secondary prevention of cardiovascular and cerebrovascular events. Arch Intern Med 162:2197, 2002.
145. Freemantle N, Cleland J, Young P, et al: Beta blockade after myocardial infarction: Systematic review and meta regression analysis. BMJ 318:1730, 1999.
146. Georgiou D, Chen Y, Appadoo S, et al: Cost-effectiveness analysis of long-term moderate exercise training in chronic heart failure. Am J Cardiol 87:984, 2001.

Disease Management

147. Haskell WL, Alderman EL, Fair JM, et al.: Effects of intensive multiple risk factor reduction on coronary atherosclerosis and clinical cardiac events in men and women with coronary artery disease. The Stanford Coronary Risk Intervention Project (SCRIP). Circulation 89:975, 1994.

DISCLOSURE INDEX

The following contributors have indicated that they have a relationship that, in the context of their participation in the writing of a chapter for the seventh edition of *Braunwald's Heart Disease,* could be perceived by some people as a real or apparent conflict of interest, but do not consider that it has influenced the writing of their chapter. Codes for the disclosure information (institution[s] and nature of relationship[s]) are provided below.

Relationship Codes

A—Stock options or bond holdings in a for-profit corporation or self-directed pension plan
B—Research grants
C—Employment (full or part-time)
D—Ownership or partnership
E—Consulting fees or other remuneration received by the contributor or immediate family
F—Nonremunerative positions, such as board member, trustee, or public spokesperson
G—Receipt of royalties
H—"Speaker's bureau"

Institution and Company Codes

001—ARCA Discovery, Inc.
002—Abbott Labs
003—Adelphi, Inc.
004—Aderis Pharmaceuticals, Inc.
005—Actelion
006—Ajinomoto Pharmaceuticals
007—Alexion Pharmaceuticals
008—Alliance Medical
009—Alza
010—American Association for Cancer Research
011—American Cancer Society
012—American College of Cardiology
013—American Heart Association
014—American Society of Echocardiography
015—Amersham Health
016—Amersham, Inc.
017—Arrow
018—Asahi Chemical Company
019—Astra Zeneca, Inc.
020—Avant Immunotherapeutics
021—Aventis
022—Avon Foundation
023—BASF
024—Baxter Pharmaceuticals
025—Bayer
026—Bayer Diagnostics
027—Berkeley Heart Lab
028—Berlex
029—Best Med
030—Beth Israel Deaconess Medical Center
031—Bioheart Scientific
032—Biomarin Pharmaceuticals
033—Biosite, Inc.
034—Blue Cross Blue Shield of Michigan
035—Boeringer Ingelheim
036—Boston Scientific Corporation
037—Bracco
038—Bristol Meyers Squibb, Co.
039—British Biotech
040—Burrill and Company
041—C2R
042—Cardiac Dimensions
043—Cardiofocus
044—Cardiovascular Biosciences
045—Cardiovascular Imaging Solutions
046—Cell Therapeutics
047—Centocor
048—Chiron
049—Churchill Livingstone
050—Columbia University
051—Cordis Corporation
052—Corvas BMS
053—Covalent
054—Cryocor
055—CTI, Inc.
056—Cubist Pharmaceuticals
057—Current Medicine LLC
058—Current Science
059—CV Therapeutics, Inc.
060—CVRx
061—Dade Behring
062—Denver Health Medical Center
063—Discovery East
064—Discovery, Inc.
065—Doris Duke Foundation
066—EBR systems
067—Eli Lilly and Company
068—Encysive
069—Esperion Therapeutics
070—Excerpta Medica
071—Exhale Therapeutics
072—eV3
073—Fondation Leducq (Paris)
074—Fujisawa
075—Genentech
076—Genvec
077—Genzyme
078—Glaxo Smith Kline
079—GMP Companies, Inc.
080—Goldant
081—GSK
082—GTC Therapeutics
083—Guerbet
084—Guidant Corporation
085—Interleukin Genetics
086—Intraluminal
087—Johnson and Johnson
088—Johnson and Johnson—Merck Consumer Pharmaceuticals
089—K-23 National Institute of Health
090—King Pharmaceuticals
091—KOS
092—Lancet International
093—Life Sentry
094—Lippincott
095—MC Communications
096—McGraw Hill
097—McNeil
098—Medical Decision Point
099—Medicines Company
100—Medreviews
101—Medtronic, Inc.
102—Merck & Co., Inc.
103—Merck Frosst/Schering Plough
104—Merck-Schering Plough Corp.
105—Michael Marcus and Associates Science Partners, LLC
106—Micromed
107—Millennium Pharmaceuticals
108—Mitsubishi
109—Molecular Insight Pharmaceuticals
110—Momenta Pharmaceuticals
111—Mylan
112—Myogen, Inc.
113—National Cancer Institute
114—National Heart, Lung and Blood Institute
115—NCME
116—New York University School of Medicine
117—NIH/NCRR Research Resource for Complex Physiologic Signals
118—Nitromed
119—Novartis, Inc.
120—Novonordisk Pharmaceuticals
121—Nuvelo
122—Octagon Corporation
123—Omnisonics
124—Ortho Biotech, Inc.
125—Ortho-Clinical Diagnostics
126—Ortho-McNeil
127—Otsuka
128—Pacific Mountain Affiliate
129—Paion
130—Pfizer, Inc.

131—Pharmacia Diagnostics
132—Pharmacia-Upjohn, Inc.
133—Philips
134—Philips Canada
135—Pierre Fabre
136—Point Biomedical
137—Procter and Gamble
138—Radiant Medical
139—Reliant Pharmaceuticals
140—Restore Medical
141—Rey Institute for Nonlinear Dynamics in Medicine
142—Roche Diagnostics
143—Sankyo
144—Sanofi-Synthelabo, Inc.
145—Sanyo
146—Scientific American Medicine Editorial Board
147—Scios, Inc.
148—Servier
149—Schering Plough Corp.
150—Siemens
151—SmithKline Beecham
152—St. Jude Medical
153—Stanford University
154—Sunol Molecular
155—Takeda
156—Terumo Cardiovascular Systems Corporation
157—Terumo Heart, Inc.
158—Thoratec
159—TJ Martel Foundation
160—Transneuronix
161—TYCO
162—United Therapeutics, Inc.
163—University of Colorado Health Sciences Center
164—University of Wisconsin, Medical School
165—Vasogen
166—Vasogenix
167—Vertex
168—Vicaron
169—Volcano Therapeutics
170—Women's Health Initiative
171—Wyeth
172—ZLB Behring

Contributors

Antman, Elliot, B-033, B-038, B-039, B-047, B-052, B-061, B-067, B-075, B-102, B107, B-142, B-154
Antman, Karen, A-055; B-011, B-022, B-113, B-159; E-019, E-065, E-110, E-146; F-010, F-011, F-092; G-094
Armstrong, William F., E-019, E-152; H-038
Baim, Donald S., E-036
Barsky, Arthur, B-130
Beckman, Joshua A., B-067, B-130; E-038; H-067, H-102, H-119
Beller, George A., B-038
Bonow, Robert O., B-114; E-038, E-090, E-130, E-155
Braunwald, Eugene, B-021, B-038, B-059, B-067, B-107, B-121; E-045, E-073, E-084, E-095, E-110, E-147; F-012, F-116, F-170; G-057, G-096
Bristow, Michael, A-001, A-064, A-112; E-019, E-041, E-042, E-053, E-060, E-077, E-081, E-084, E-102, E-108, E-111, E-119, E-147
Calkins, Hugh, B-080, B-101, B-152; E-080
Cannon, Christopher, B-038, B-102, B-144; F-018, F-019, F-025, F-078, F-099, F-125, F-130, F-167; H-021, H-038, H-047, H-067, H-075, H-102, H-107, H-144
Creager, Mark A., B-028, B-038, B-067, B-130, B-144, B-171; E-003, E-007, E-028, E-038, E-076, E-077, E-091, E-100, E-127, E-130, E-144, E-165; G-058; H-038, H-127, H-144
Dilsizian, Vasken, B-037, B-112, B-133; E-109; H-038, H-074
Douglas, Pamela S., E-012, E-014, E-102, E-119; F-012, F-014
Eagle, Kim A., C-021, C-034, C-130; E-012; F-114
Eisenhauer, Andrew C., B-84, B-101; E-101
Fleisher, Lee A., B-024; E-024
Gaziano, J. Michael, B-023, B-097, B-142, B-171; E-097; H-130
Genest, Jacques, E-019, E-103, E-130; H-019
Goldhaber, Sam, B-019, B-021; E-021, E-025, E-129, E-130, E-137
Gotto, Antonio M., E-019, E-025, E-038, E-102, E-119 E-130, E-139; F-069
Groh, William, B-067, B-084, B-101
Hayes, David, A-084, A-101; B-084, B-101, B-141; H-084, H-101, H-152
Hoffman, Gary, B-047; E-047; H-130, H-171
Isselbacher, Eric M., H-101, H-130
Kabbani, Samer, E-102, E-144; F-102, F-144
Kaplan, Norman, H-002, H-019, H-119, H-130, H-145, H-148
Karchmer, A. W., A-130; B-025, B-074, B-102, B-126, B-168; E-056, E-130, E-168
Klein, Irwin L., B-090, B-142; E-038
Konkle, Barbara A, B-006, B-025, B-046, B-120, B-122, B-171, B-172; E-025, E-078, E-082, E-120, E-171
Krauss, Ronald M., B-102, B-130; E-002, E-019, E-091, E-102, E-130; H-002, H-104
Libby, Peter, B-019, B-025, B-038, B-102, B-107, B-119, B-130, B-143, B-151; E-019, E-020, E-25, E-038, E-085, E-102, E-107, E-119, E-130, E-135, E-143, E-144, E-149, E-151; H-019, H-025, H-038, H-102, H-119, H-130
Linas, Stuart, E-019, E-062; E-102, E-130; H-019, H-102, H-130
Lipshultz, Steve, B-130, B-132, B-142; E-035
Lowes, Brian D, B-089; C-163; E-112; H-081, H-130
Mark, Daniel, B-008, B-101, B-130, B-137
McCullough, Peter A., E-002, E-015, E-033, E-119, E-124, E-147
McLaughlin, Vallerie, B-068, B-112, B-130; E-005, E-071, E-162; H-005, H-162
Miller, John, B-084, B-101; E-084, E-101
Morrow, David, B-021, B-026, B-061, B-107, B-142, B-154
Myerburg, Robert, E-137, E-144; H-028, H-084, H-137
Nabel, Elizabeth, E-036
Naka, Yoshifumi, E-157
Nesto, Richard W., H-081, H-102, H-130
Olgin, Jeffrey, A-101, A-102; E-036, E-101, E-171
Opie, Lionel, F-102
Pasternak, Richard C., E-019, E-038, E-088, E-091, E-102, E-130, E-144; H-038, H-091, H-102, H-104, H-130, H-144
Pennell, Dudley J., B-083, B-150, B-161; D-045; E-008, E-015, E-038, E-108; G-049
Popma, Jeffrey J., B-002, B-036, B-051, B-072, B-084, B-086, B-101, B-138; H-036, H-051, H-101, H-107, H-149
Port, J. David, A-001, A-112; F-013, F-128; G-112; H-019
Priori, Silvia, B-059, B-101, B-130
Pyeritz, Reed E., E-032, E-077, E-102, E-104; H-102, H-104
Rich, Stuart, A-162; C-162
Ridker, Paul M, B-019, B-038, B-119, B-131; E-002
Robertson, David, No information supplied.
Robertson, Rose Marie, No information supplied.
Roden, Dan, B-038; E-009, E-019, E-059, E-077, E-078, E-087; F-066
Rose, Eric, B-017, B-106, B-158
Rosenfield, Kenneth, A-123; B-002, B-036, B-051; E-002, E-036, E-051; H-067
Schwartz, Janice, A-136; E-054, E-140, E-160; G-096
Smallhorn, Jeffrey F., B-134
Sweitzer, Nancy K., B-147; H-078, H-147
Udelson, James E., B-038, B-090, B-127; E-038, E-076, E-090, E-109, E-127; H-038, H-081
Yancy, Clyde W. Jr., B-078, B-118, B-147; E-101; H-078, H-101, H-147
Zipes, Douglas P., A-043; B-101; D-105; E-004, E-040, E-043, E-059, E-077, E-079, E-093, E-101, E-156; F-012

INDEX

Note: Page numbers followed by f and t indicate figures and tables, respectively.